MW01056967

# 2018

# Current Procedural Coding Expert

CPT® codes with Medicare essentials enhanced for accuracy

**POWER UP YOUR CODING** with Optum360, your trusted
coding partner for 32 years. **Visit optum360coding.com.**

## Notice

The *2018 Current Procedural Coding Expert* is designed to be an accurate and authoritative source of information about the CPT® coding system. Every effort has been made to verify the accuracy of the listings, and all information is believed reliable at the time of publication. Absolute accuracy cannot be guaranteed, however. This publication is made available with the understanding that the publisher is not engaged in rendering legal or other services that require a professional license.

## American Medical Association Notice

CPT © 2017 American Medical Association. All rights reserved.

Fee schedules, relative value units, conversion factors and/or related components are not assigned by the AMA, are not part of CPT, and the AMA is not recommending their use. The AMA does not directly or indirectly practice medicine or dispense medical services. The AMA assumes no liability for data contained or not contained herein.

CPT is a registered trademark of the American Medical Association.

## Our Commitment to Accuracy

Optum360 is committed to producing accurate and reliable materials.

To report corrections, please visit www.optumcoding.com/accuracy or email accuracy@optum360.com. You can also reach customer service by calling 1.800.464.3649, option 1.

## Copyright

Property of Optum360, LLC. Optum360 and the Optum360 logo are trademarks of Optum360, LLC. All other brand or product names are trademarks or registered trademarks of their respective owner.

Copyright © 2017 Optum360, LLC

All rights reserved. No part of this publication may be reproduced or transmitted in any form or by any means electronic or mechanical, including photocopy, recording or storage in a database or retrieval system, without the prior written permission of the publisher.

Made in the USA

ISBN 978-1-62254-330-4

## Acknowledgments

Marianne Randall, CPC, *Product Manager*
Karen Schmidt, BSN, *Technical Director*
Stacy Perry, *Manager, Desktop Publishing*
Lisa Singley, *Project Manager*
Karen H. Kachur, RN, CPC, *Clinical/Technical Editor*
Elizabeth Leibold, RHIT, *Clinical/Technical Editor*
Tracy Betzler, *Senior Desktop Publishing Specialist*
Hope M. Dunn, *Senior Desktop Publishing Specialist*
Katie Russell, *Desktop Publishing Specialist*
Kate Holden, *Editor*

## About the Contributors

### Karen H. Kachur, RN, CPC

Ms. Kachur has expertise in CPT/HCPCS and ICD-9-CM coding, in addition to physician billing, compliance, and fraud and abuse. Prior to joining Optum360, she worked for many years as a staff RN in a variety of clinical settings, including medicine, surgery, intensive care, and psychiatry. In addition to her clinical background, Ms. Kachur served as assistant director of a hospital utilization management and quality assurance department and has extensive experience as a nurse reviewer for Blue Cross/Blue Shield. She is an active member of the American Academy of Professional Coders (AAPC).

### Elizabeth Leibold, RHIT

Ms. Leibold has more than 25 years of experience in the health care profession. She has served in a variety of roles, ranging from patient registration to billing and collections, and has an extensive background in both physician and hospital outpatient coding and compliance. She has worked for large health care systems and health information management services companies, and has wide-ranging experience in facility and professional component coding, along with CPT expertise in interventional procedures, infusion services, emergency department, observation, and ambulatory surgery coding. Her areas of expertise include chart-to-claim coding audits and providing staff education to both tenured and new coding staff. She is an active member of the American Health Information Management Association (AHIMA).

OPTUM360°®

# CODING TOOLS THIS
# EFFICIEN
## ARE BUILT FOR **CODING PROFESSIONALS**

**MedicalReferenceEngine.com** is the precision coding solution for **searching regulatory content.**

## POWERFUL

**Robust Medicare content.** Search this essential repository of up-to-date national and local regulations and policy from CMS. Also included are dozens of Optum360® reference books.

**Powerful lookup tools.** CodeLogic™ search engine technology allows you to search across all three code sets simultaneously. View LCD/NCD, lay descriptions, illustrations and Internet Only Manual references for each code.

## EFFICIENT

**Flexible customization options.** Set bookmarks to easily locate previously viewed documents. Save frequently performed searches. Create multiple search preferences to easily toggle between criteria when working on numerous projects.

**Access forms and fee schedules.** Easily find Medicare fee schedules and frequently used forms.

## ACCURATE

**Continuously adding pertinent content.** Search with confidence for the most up-to-date regulatory information needed to achieve compliance.

**Customized email alerts**. Maintain compliance with alerts to newly updated rules and regulations.

Includes
## 20+
essential
Optum360
references,
plus regulatory
content.

# SCHEDULE A DEMO TODAY

 CLICK
**optum360coding.com/mre**

 CALL
**1-800-464-3649, option 1**

© 2017 Optum360, LLC. All rights reserved. WF342211 4/17

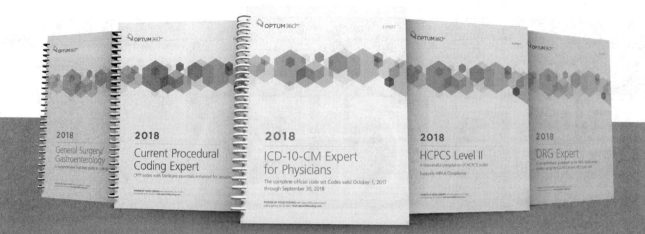

# Keep your go-to coding resources up to date.

Stay current and compliant with our 2018 edition code books.
With more than 30 years in the coding industry, Optum360® is proud to
be your trusted resource for coding, billing and reimbursement resources.
Our 2018 editions include tools for ICD-10-CM/PCS, CPT®, HCPCS, DRG,
specialty-specific coding and much more.

## SAVE UP TO 25% ON ADDITIONAL CODING RESOURCES

**Visit us at optum360coding.com**
and enter promo code **FOBA18ED**
to save 25%.

**Call 1-800-464-3649, option 1,**
and be sure to mention promo
code **FOBA18ED** to save 20%.

CPT is a registered trademark of the American Medical Association.

Excludes custom fee and bookstore items, data files, online coding tools and educational courses. Cannot be combined with any other offer. Offer not valid for
Partner or Medallion accounts. © 2017 Optum360, LLC. All rights reserved.  WF345835  SPRJ3632

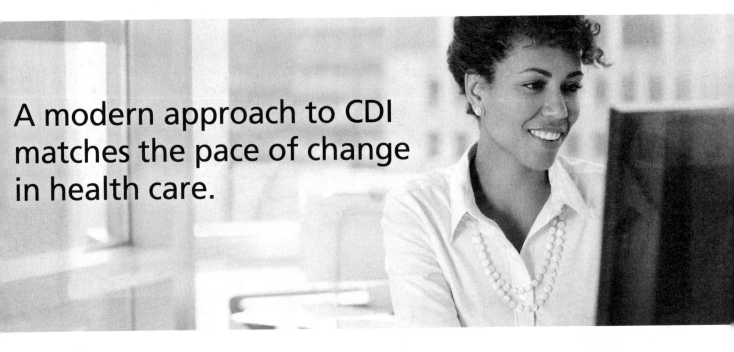

## A modern approach to CDI matches the pace of change in health care.

**The move to value-based care increases the need for accuracy in clinical documentation—across every patient and payer.**

A modern CDI approach makes the work of CDI specialists more efficient by automatically reviewing every patient record and prioritizing those that require intervention.

Using case-finding logic and state-of-the-art natural language processing, Optum CDI 3D connects clinical indicators to identify records with gaps or deficiencies and enables timely documentation improvement, cleaner claims, faster reimbursement and accurate reporting.

Optum CDI 3D, together with Optum's market-leading Enterprise CAC, provides unmatched capabilities in a single, fully integrated CDI and coding solution.

**Modernizing your CDI program starts here.**
Visit optum360.com/CDI3D to learn more.

### OPTUM CDI 3D

- Automates 100-percent record review and identifies clinical documentation improvement opportunities

- Identifies co-morbidities, HACs and patient safety indicators

- Streamlines the query loop between CDIS and physicians

- Enhances code assignment efficiency, compliance and quality reporting

Visit: optum360.com/CDI3D
Email: optum360@optum.com

© 2017 Optum360, LLC. All rights reserved. 2/17
U.S. Patent Nos. 6,915,254; 7,908,552; 8,682,823; 8,731,954; and other patents pending

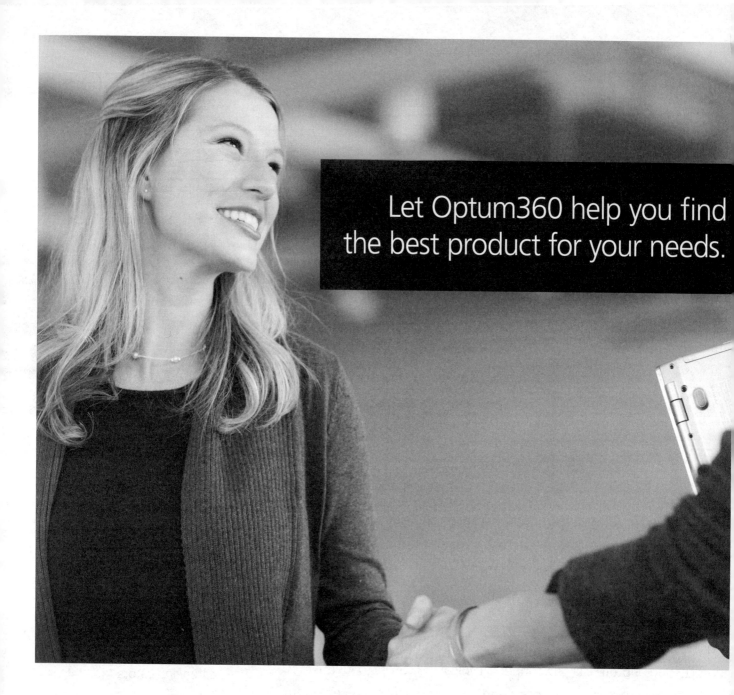

Let Optum360 help you find the best product for your needs.

Together with you, Optum360® can help drive financial results across your organization with industry-leading resources that cut through the complexity of medical coding challenges.

**Let us help you find the best coding solution, at the best price.**

Contact your Medallion representative directly or call Customer Service at 1-800-464-3649, option 1.

© 2017 Optum360, LLC. All rights reserved. WF351448 SPRJ3539 4/17

# OPTUM360°®

## Optum360 **Learning**

### Earn your CEUs with US

You've worked hard for your coding credentials, and now you need an easy way to maintain your certification.

Optum360® offers the most complete training in the marketplace, designed to address exactly what you and your organization need. We offer eLearning courses you can take online at your desk; you can invite a specialist to your office for on-the-job preparation; or ask our consulting professionals to create a tailor-made program specific for your organization.

Our strategy is simple — education must be concise, relevant and accurate. Choose the delivery method that works best for you:

- **eLearning:** Web-based courses offered at the most convenient times for your learners. eLearning courses are interactive, task-focused and developed around practical scenarios. These self-paced courses include "try-it" functionality, knowledge checks and downloadable resources.

- **Instructor-led training (ILT):** On-site or remote courses, built specifically for your organization.

- **Webinars:** Online courses, geared toward a broad market of learners, delivered in a live or recorded setting.

- **Podcasts and videos:** Physician-focused online courses available when and where convenient.

## NO MATTER HOW YOU CHOOSE TO EARN YOUR CEUs, OPTUM360 IS HERE TO HELP YOU.

 VISIT
**optum360coding.com/learning**

 CALL
**1-800-464-3649, option 1**

# RE NEW

## It's time to renew your Optum360 coding tools.

## SAVE UP TO 25%*

when you renew your 2018 coding essentials.

| ITEM # | TITLE<br>INDICATE THE ITEMS YOU WISH TO PURCHASE | QUANTITY | PRICE<br>PER PRODUCT | TOTAL |
|---|---|---|---|---|
| | | | | |
| | | | | |
| | | | | |
| | | | | |
| | | | | |

| | | |
|---|---|---|
| | Subtotal | |
| (AK, DE, HI, MT, NH & OR are exempt) | Sales Tax | |
| 1 item $10.95 • 2–4 items $12.95 • 5+ CALL | Shipping & Handling | |
| | **TOTAL AMOUNT ENCLOSED** | |

## Save up to 25% when you renew.

**PROMO CODE: RENEW18B**

Visit **optum360coding.com** and enter the promo code above.

Call **1-800-464-3649, option 1,** and mention the promo code above.

Fax this order form with purchase order to **1-801-982-4033.** *Optum360 no longer accepts credit cards by fax.*

Mail this order form with payment and/or purchase order to:
**Optum360, PO Box 88050, Chicago, IL 60680-9920.**
*Optum360 no longer accepts credit cards by mail.*

Name

Address

Customer Number      Contact Number

○ CHECK ENCLOSED (PAYABLE TO OPTUM360)

○ BILL ME ○ P.O.#

( )
Telephone
( )
Fax
@
E-mail

Optum360 respects your right to privacy. We will not sell or rent your email address or fax number to anyone outside Optum360 and its business partners. If you would like to remove your name from Optum360 promotions, please call 1-800-464-3649, option 1.

*Save 20% when you order by phone, fax or mail; save 25% when you order online. Save 15% on AMA and custom fee products. Offer excludes digital coding tools, workers' comp and bookstore products.

© 2017 Optum360, LLC. All rights reserved. WF337935  SPRJ3517

# Contents

CPT © 2017 American Medical Association. All Rights Reserved.                              © 2017 Optum360, LLC

# Introduction

Welcome to Optum360's *Current Procedural Coding Expert*, an exciting Medicare coding and reimbursement tool and definitive procedure coding source that combines the work of the Centers for Medicare and Medicaid Services, American Medical Association, and Optum360 experts with the technical components you need for proper reimbursement and coding accuracy. Handy snap in tabs are included to indicate those sections used most often for easy reference.

This approach to CPT® Medicare coding utilizes innovative and intuitive ways of communicating the information you need to code claims accurately and efficiently. *Includes* and *Excludes* notes, similar to those found in the ICD-10-CM manual, help determine what services are related to the codes you are reporting. Icons help you crosswalk the code you are reporting to laboratory and radiology procedures necessary for proper reimbursement. CMS-mandated icons and relative value units (RVUs) help you determine which codes are most appropriate for the service you are reporting. Add to that additional information identifying age and sex edits, ambulatory surgery center (ASC) and ambulatory payment classification (APC) indicators, and Medicare coverage and payment rule citations, and *Current Procedural Coding Expert* provides the best in Medicare procedure reporting.

*Current Procedural Coding Expert* includes the information needed to submit claims to federal contractors and most commercial payers, and is correct at the time of printing. However, CMS, federal contractors, and commercial payers may change payment rules at any time throughout the year. *Current Procedural Coding Expert* includes effective codes that will not be published in the AMA's Physicians' Current Procedural Terminology (CPT) book until the following year. Commercial payers will announce changes through monthly news or information posted on their websites. CMS will post changes in policy on its website at http://www.cms.gov/transmittals. National and local coverage determinations (NCDs and LCDs) provide universal and individual contractor guidelines for specific services. The existence of a procedure code does not imply coverage under any given insurance plan.

*Current Procedural Coding Expert* is based on the AMA's Physicians' Current Procedural Terminology coding system, which is copyrighted and owned by the physician organization. The CPT codes are the nation's official, Health Information Portability and Accountability Act (HIPAA) compliant code set for procedures and services provided by physicians, ambulatory surgery centers (ASCs), and hospital outpatient services, as well as laboratories, imaging centers, physical therapy clinics, urgent care centers, and others.

## Getting Started with *Current Procedural Coding Expert*

*Current Procedural Coding Expert* is an exciting tool combining the most current material at the time of our publication from the AMA' CPT 2018, CMS's online manual system, the Correct Coding initiative, CMS fee schedules, official Medicare guidelines for reimbursement and coverage, the Integrated outpatient coding Editor (I/OCE), and Optum360's own coding expertise.

These coding rules and guidelines are incorporated into more specific section notes and code notes. Section notes are listed under a range of codes and apply to all codes in that range. Code notes are found under individual codes and apply to the single code.

Material is presented in a logical fashion for those billing Medicare, Medicaid, and many private payers. The format, based on customer comments, better addresses what customers tell us they need in a comprehensive Medicare procedure coding guide.

Designed to be easy to use and full of information, this product is an excellent companion to your AMA CPT manual, and other Optum360 and Medicare resources.

For mid-year code updates, official errata changes, correction notices, and any other changes pertinent to the information in *Current Procedural Coding Expert*, see our product update page at https://www.optum360coding.com/ProductUpdates/. The password for 2018 is PROCEDURE2018.

**Note:** The AMA releases code changes quarterly as well as errata or corrections to CPT codes and guidelines and posts them on their web site. Some of these changes may not appear in the AMA's CPT book until the following year. *Current Procedural Coding Expert* incorporates the most recent errata or release notes found on the AMA's web site at our publication time, including new, revised and deleted codes. *Current Procedural Coding Expert* identifies these new or revised codes from the AMA website errata or release notes with an icon similar to the AMA's current new ● and revised ▲ icons. For purposes of this publication, new CPT codes and revisions that won't be in the AMA book until the next edition are indicated with a ● and a ▲ icon. For the next year's edition of *Current Procedural Coding Expert*, these codes will appear with standard black new or revised icons, as appropriate, to correspond with those changes as indicated in the AMA CPT book. CPT codes that were new for 2017 and appeared in the 2017 *Current Procedural Coding Expert* but did not appear in the CPT code book until 2018 are identified in appendix B as "Web Release New and Changed Codes."

## General Conventions

Many of the sources of information in this book can be determined by color.

- All CPT codes and descriptions and the Evaluation and Management guidelines from the American Medical Association are in **black text**.

- Includes, Excludes, and other notes appear in blue text. The resources used for this information are a variety of Medicare policy manuals, the *National Correct Coding Initiative Policy Manual* (NCCI), AMA resources and guidelines, and specialty association resources and our Optum360 clinical experts.

## Resequencing of CPT Codes

The American Medical Association (AMA) uses a numbering methodology of resequencing, which is the practice of displaying codes outside of their numerical order according to the description relationship. According to the AMA, there are instances in which a new code is needed within an existing grouping of codes but an unused code number is not available. In these situations, the AMA will resequence the codes. In other words, it will assign a code that is not in numeric sequence with the related codes. However, the code and description will appear in the CPT manual with the other related codes.

An example of resequencing from *Current Procedural Coding Expert* follows:

|   | 21555 | Excision, tumor, soft tissue of neck or anterior thorax, subcutaneous; less than 3 cm |
|---|-------|------|
| # | 21552 | 3 cm or greater |
|   | 21556 | Excision, tumor, soft tissue of neck or anterior thorax, subfascial (eg, intramuscular); less than 5 cm |
| # | 21554 | 5 cm or greater |

Note that codes 21552 and 21554 are out of numeric sequence. However, as they are indented codes, they are in the correct place.

In *Current Procedural Coding Expert* the resequenced codes are listed twice. They appear in their resequenced position as shown above as well as in their original numeric position with a note indicating that the code is out of numerical sequence and where it can be found. (See example below.)

| *51797* | **Resequenced code. See code following 51729.** |
|---------|------|

© 2017 Optum360, LLC

This differs from the AMA CPT book, in which the coder is directed to a code range that contains the resequenced code and description, rather than to a specific location.

Resequenced codes will appear in brackets in the headers, section notes, and code ranges. For example:

> 27327-27329 [27337, 27339] Excision Soft Tissue Tumors Femur/Knee. Codes [27337, 27339] are included in section 27327-27329 in their resequenced positions.

> Code also toxoid/vaccine (90476-90749 [90620, 90621, 90625, 90630, 90644, 90672, 90673, 90674, 90750, 90756])

> This shows codes 90620, 90621, 90625, 90630, 90644, 90672, 90673, 90674, 90750, and 90756 are resequenced in this range of codes.

## Code Ranges for Medicare Billing

Appendix E identifies all resequenced CPT codes. Optum360 will display the resequenced coding as assigned by the AMA in its CPT products so that the user may understand the code description relationships.

Each particular group of CPT codes in *Current Procedural Coding Expert* is organized in a more intuitive fashion for Medicare billing, being grouped by the Medicare rules and regulations as found in the official CMS online manuals, that govern payment of these particular procedures and services, as in this example:

### 99221-99233 Inpatient Hospital Visits: Initial and Subsequent
**CMS:** 100-4,11,40.1.3 Independent Attending Physician Services; 100-4,12,100.1.1 Teaching Physicians E/M Services; 100-4,12,30.6.10 Consultation Services; 100-4,12,30.6.15.1 Prolonged Services With Direct Face-to-Face Patient Contact; 100-4,12,30.6.4 Services Furnished Incident to Physician's Service; 100-4,12,30.6.9 Hospital Visit and Critical Care on Same Day

## Icons

● **New Codes**
Codes that have been added since the last edition of the AMA CPT book was printed.

▲ **Revised Codes**
Codes that have been revised since the last edition of the AMA CPT book was printed.

● **New Web Release**
Codes that are new for the current year but will not be in the AMA CPT book until 2019.

▲ **Revised Web Release**
Codes that have been revised for the current year, but will not be in the AMA CPT book until 2019.

\# **Resequenced Codes**
Codes that are out of numeric order but apply to the appropriate category.

★ **Telemedicine Services**
Codes that may be reported for telemedicine services. Modifier 95 must be appended to code.

○ **Reinstated Code**
Codes that have been reinstated since the last edition of the book was printed.

**Pink Color Bar—Not Covered by Medicare**
Services and procedures identified by this color bar are never covered benefits under Medicare. Services and procedures that are not covered may be billed directly to the patient at the time of the service.

**Yellow Color Bar—Unlisted Procedure**
Unlisted CPT codes report procedures that have not been assigned a specific code number. An unlisted code delays payment due to the extra time necessary for review.

**Green Color Bar—Resequenced Codes**
Resequenced codes are codes that are out of numeric sequence—they are indicated with a green color bar. They are listed twice, in their resequenced position as well as in their original numeric position with a note that the code is out of numerical sequence and where the resequenced code and description can be found.

INCLUDES **Includes notes**
Includes notes identify procedures and services that would be bundled in the procedure code. These are derived from AMA, CMS, NCCI, and Optum360 coding guidelines. This is not meant to be an all-inclusive list.

EXCLUDES **Excludes notes**
Excludes notes may lead the user to other codes. They may identify services that are not bundled and may be separately reported, OR may lead the user to another more appropriate code. These are derived from AMA, CMS, NCCI, and Optum360 coding guidelines. This is not meant to be an all-inclusive list.

**Code Also**   This note identifies an additional code that should be reported with the service and may relate to another CPT code or an appropriate HCPCS code(s) that should be reported along with the CPT code when appropriate.

**Code First**   Found under add-on codes, this note identifies codes for primary procedures that should be reported first, with the add-on code reported as a secondary code.

◤ **Laboratory/Pathology Crosswalk**
This icon denotes CPT codes in the laboratory and pathology section of CPT that may be reported separately with the primary CPT code.

⁂ **Radiology Crosswalk**
This icon denotes codes in the radiology section that may be used with the primary CPT code being reported.

TC **Technical Component Only**
Codes with this icon represent only the technical component (staff and equipment costs) of a procedure or service. Do not use either modifier 26 (physician component) or TC (technical component) with these codes.

26 **Professional Component**
Only codes with this icon represent the physician's work or professional component of a procedure or service. Do not use either modifier 26 (physician component) or TC (technical component) with these codes.

50 **Bilateral Procedure**
This icon identifies codes that can be reported bilaterally when the same surgeon provides the service for the same patient on the same date. Medicare allows payment for both procedures at 150 percent of the usual amount for one procedure. The modifier does not apply to bilateral procedures inclusive to one code.

80 **Assist-at-Surgery Allowed**
Services noted by this icon are allowed an assistant at surgery with a Medicare payment equal to 16 percent of the allowed amount for the global surgery for that procedure. No documentation is required.

80 **Assist-at-Surgery Allowed with Documentation**
Services noted by this icon are allowed an assistant at surgery with a Medicare payment equal to 16 percent of the allowed amount for the global surgery for that procedure. Documentation is required.

+ **Add-on Codes**
This icon identifies procedures reported in addition to the primary procedure. The icon "**+**" denotes add-on codes. An add-on code is neither a stand-alone code nor subject to multiple procedure rules since it describes work in addition to the primary procedure.

According to Medicare guidelines, add-on codes may be identified in the following ways:

- The code is found on Change Request (CR) 7501 or successive CRs as a Type I, Type II, or Type III add-on code.

- The add-on code most often has a global period of "ZZZ" in the Medicare Physician Fee Schedule Database.

- The code is found in the CPT book with the icon "**+**" appended. Add-on code descriptors typically include the phrases "each additional" or "(List separately in addition to primary procedure)."

⊘ **Modifier 51 Exempt**
Codes identified by this icon indicate that the procedure should not be reported with modifier 51 (Multiple procedures).

⑤⑦ **Optum360 Modifier 51 Exempt**
Codes identified by this Optum360 icon indicate that the procedure should not be reported with modifier 51 (Multiple procedures). Any code with this icon is backed by official AMA guidelines but was not identified by the AMA with their modifier 51 exempt icon.

▱ **Correct Coding Initiative (CCI)**
*Current Procedural Coding Expert* identifies those codes with corresponding CCI edits. The CCI edits define correct coding practices that serve as the basis of the national Medicare policy for paying claims. The code noted is the major service/procedure. The code may represent a column 1 code within the column 1/column 2 correct coding edits table or a code pair that is mutually exclusive of each other.

✖ **CLIA Waived Test**
This symbol is used to distinguish those laboratory tests that can be performed using test systems that are waived from regulatory oversight established by the Clinical Laboratory Improvement Amendments of 1988 (CLIA). The applicable CPT code for a CLIA waived test may be reported by providers who perform the testing but do not hold a CLIA license.

⑥③ **Modifier 63 Exempt**
This icon identifies procedures performed on infants that weigh less than 4 kg. Due to the complexity of performing procedures on infants less than 4 kg, modifier 63 may be added to the surgery codes to inform the payers of the special circumstances involved.

**A2** – **Z3** **ASC Payment Indicators**
This icon identifies ASC status payment indicators. They indicate how the ASC payment rate was derived and/or how the procedure, item, or service is treated under the revised ASC payment system. For more information about these indicators and how they affect billing, consult Optum360's *Outpatient Billing Editor*.

**A2**    Surgical procedure on ASC list in 2007; payment based on OPPS relative payment weight.

**B5**    Alternative code may be available; no payment made.

     Active HCPCS code in current year and next calendar year, status indicator and/or APC assignment has changed; or active HCPCS code that will be discontinued at the end of the current calendar year.

**D5**    Deleted/discontinued code; no payment made.

**F4**    Corneal tissue acquisition; hepatitis B vaccine; paid at reasonable cost.

**G2**    Non-office-based surgical procedure added in CY 2008 or later; payment based on OPPS relative payment weight.

**H2**    Brachytherapy source paid separately when provided integral to a surgical procedure on ASC list; payment based on OPPS rate.

**J7**    OPPS pass-through device paid separately when provided integral to a surgical procedure on ASC list; payment contractor-priced.

**J8**    Device-intensive procedure; paid at adjusted rate.

**K2**    Drugs and biologicals paid separately when provided integral to a surgical procedure on ASC list; payment based on OPPS rate.

**K7**    Unclassified drugs and biologicals; payment contractor-priced.

**L1**    Influenza vaccine; pneumococcal vaccine. Packaged item/service; no separate payment made.

**L6**    New technology intraocular lens (NTIOL); special payment.

**N1**    Packaged service/item; no separate payment made.

     New code for the next calendar year or existing code with substantial revision to its code descriptor in the next calendar year as compared to current calendar year for which we requested comments in the proposed rule, final APC assignment; comments will not be accepted on the final APC assignment for the new code.

     New code for the next calendar year or existing code with substantial revision to its code descriptor in the next calendar year as compared to current calendar year, interim APC assignment; comments will be accepted on the interim APC assignment for the new code.

     New code for the next calendar year or existing code with substantial revision to its code descriptor in the next calendar year as compared to current calendar year, proposed APC assignment; comments will be accepted on the proposed APC assignment for the new code.

**P2**    Office-based surgical procedure added to ASC list in CY 2008 or later with MPFS nonfacility practice expense (PE) RVUs; payment based on OPPS relative payment weight.

**P3**    Office-based surgical procedure added to ASC list in CY 2008 or later with MPFS nonfacility PE RVUs; payment based on MPFS nonfacility PE RVUs.

**R2**    Office-based surgical procedure added to ASC list in CY 2008 or later without MPFS nonfacility PE RVUs; payment based on OPPS relative payment weight.

**Z2**    Radiology or diagnostic service paid separately when provided integral to a surgical procedure on ASC list; payment based on OPPS relative payment weight.

**Z3**    Radiology or diagnostic service paid separately when provided integral to a surgical procedure on ASC list; payment based on MPFS nonfacility PE RVUs.

**A**   **Age Edit**
This icon denotes codes intended for use with a specific age group, such as neonate, newborn, pediatric, and adult. This edit is based on CMS I/OCE designations or age specifications in the CPT code descriptors. Carefully review the code description to ensure the code you report most appropriately reflects the patient's age.

**M**   **Maternity**
This icon identifies procedures that by definition should be used only for maternity patients generally between 12 and 55 years of age based on CMS I/OCE designations.

♀   **Female Only**
This icon identifies procedures designated by CMS for females only based on CMS I/OCE designations.

♂   **Male Only**
This icon identifies procedures designated by CMS for males only based on CMS I/OCE designations.

🚑   **Facility RVU**
This icon precedes the facility RVU from CMS's 2017 physician fee schedule (PFS). It can be found under the code description.

New codes include no RVU information.

〜     **Nonfacility RVU**

This icon precedes the nonfacility RVU from CMS's 2017 PFS. It can be found under the code description.

New codes include no RVU information.

**FUD:**   Global days are sometimes referred to as "follow-up days" or FUDs. The global period is the time following surgery during which routine care by the physician is considered postoperative and included in the surgical fee. Office visits or other routine care related to the original surgery cannot be separately reported if provided during the global period. The statuses are:

000   No follow-up care included in this procedure

010   Normal postoperative care is included in this procedure for ten days

090   Normal postoperative care is included in the procedure for 90 days

MMM   Maternity codes; usual global period does not apply

XXX   The global concept does not apply to the code

YYY   The carrier is to determine whether the global concept applies and establishes postoperative period, if appropriate, at time of pricing

ZZZ   The code is related to another service and is always included in the global period of the other service

**CMS:**   This notation indicates that there is a specific CMS guideline pertaining to this code in the CMS Online Manual System which includes the internet-only manual (IOM) *National Coverage Determinations Manual* (NCD). These CMS sources present the rules for submitting these services to the federal government or its contractors and are included in appendix G of this book.

**AMA:**   This indicates discussion of the code in the American Medical Association's *CPT Assistant* newsletter. Use the citation to find the correct issue. This includes citations for the current year and the preceding six years. In the event no citations can be found during this time period, the most recent citations that can be found are used.

⚡     **Drug Not Approved by FDA**

The AMA CPT Editorial Panel is publishing new vaccine product codes prior to Food and Drug Administration approval. This symbol indicates which of these codes are pending FDA approval at press time.

Ⓐ–Ⓨ   **OPPS Status Indicators (OPSI)**

Status indicators identify how individual CPT codes are paid or not paid under the latest available hospital outpatient prospective payment system (OPPS). The same status indicator is assigned to all the codes within an ambulatory payment classification (APC). Consult your payer or other resource to learn which CPT codes fall within various APCs.

Ⓐ   Services furnished to a hospital outpatient that are paid under a fee schedule or payment system other than OPPS

- Ambulance Services
- Separately payable clinical diagnostic laboratory services
- Separately payable non-implantable prosthetics and orthotics
- Physical, occupational, and speech therapy
- Diagnostic mammography
- Screening mammography

Ⓑ   Codes that are not recognized by OPPS when submitted on an outpatient hospital Part B bill type (12x and 13x).

Ⓒ   Inpatient procedures

Ⓓ   Discontinued codes

Ⓔ1   Items, codes, and services:

- Not covered by any Medicare outpatient benefit category
- Statutorily excluded by Medicare
- Not reasonable and necessary

Ⓔ2   Items and services for which pricing information and claims data are not available

Ⓕ   Corneal tissue acquisition; certain CRNA services and hepatitis B vaccines

Ⓖ   Pass-through drugs and biologicals

Ⓗ   Pass-through device categories

Ⓙ1   Hospital Part B services paid through a comprehensive APC

Ⓙ2   Hospital Part B services that may be paid through a comprehensive APC

Ⓚ   Nonpass-through drugs and nonimplantable biologicals, including therapeutic radiopharmaceuticals

Ⓛ   Influenza vaccine; pneumococcal pneumonia vaccine

Ⓜ   Items and services not billable to the MAC

Ⓝ   Items and services packaged into APC rates

Ⓟ   Partial hospitalization

Ⓠ1   STV-packaged codes

Ⓠ2   T-packaged codes

Ⓠ3   Codes that may be paid through a composite APC

Ⓠ4   Conditionally packaged laboratory tests

Ⓡ   Blood and blood products

Ⓢ   Procedure or service, not discounted when multiple

Ⓣ   Procedure or service, multiple procedure reduction applies

Ⓤ   Brachytherapy sources

Ⓥ   Clinic or emergency department visit

Ⓨ   Nonimplantable durable medical equipment

# Appendixes

**Appendix A: Modifiers**—This appendix identifies modifiers. A modifier is a two-position alpha or numeric code that is appended to a CPT or HCPCS code to clarify the services being billed. Modifiers provide a means by which a service can be altered without changing the procedure code. They add more information, such as anatomical site, to the code. In addition, they help eliminate the appearance of duplicate billing and unbundling. Modifiers are used to increase the accuracy in reimbursement and coding consistency, ease editing, and capture payment data.

**Appendix B: New, Changed, and Deleted Codes**—This is a list of new, changed, and deleted CPT codes for the current year. This appendix also includes a list of web release new and changed codes, which indicate official code changes in *Current Procedural Coding Expert* that will not be in the CPT code book until the following year.

**Appendix C: Evaluation and Management Extended Guidelines**—This appendix presents an overview of evaluation and management (E/M) services that augment the official AMA CPT E/M services. It includes tables that distinguish documentation components of each E/M code and the federal documentation guidelines (1995 and 1997) currently in use by the Centers for Medicare and Medicaid Services (CMS).

**Appendix D: Crosswalk of Deleted Codes**—This appendix is a cross-reference from a deleted CPT code to an active code when one is available. The deleted code cross-reference will also appear under the deleted code description in the tabular section of the book.

Introduction

**Appendix E: Resequenced Codes**—This appendix contains a list of codes that are not in numeric order in the book. AMA resequenced some of the code numbers to relocate codes in the same category but not in numeric sequence.

**Appendix F: Add-on, Modifier 51 Exempt, Optum360 Modifier 51 Exempt, Modifier 63 Exempt, and Modifier 95 Telemedicine Services codes**—This list includes add-on codes that cannot be reported alone, codes that are exempt from modifier 51, codes that should not be reported with modifier 63, and codes identified by the ★ icon to which modifier 95 may be appended when the service is provided as a synchronous telemedicine service.

**Appendix G: Medicare Internet-only Manual – IOM References (Pub 100)**—This appendix contains a verbatim printout of the Medicare Internet Only Manual references that pertain to specific codes. The reference, when available, is listed after the header in the CPT section. For example:

### 93784-93790 Ambulatory Blood Pressure Monitoring
**CMS:** 100-3,20.19 Ambulatory Blood Pressure Monitoring (20.19); 100-4,32,10.1 Ambulatory Blood Pressure Monitoring Billing Requirements

Since appendix G contains these references from the *Medicare National Coverage Determinations (NCD) Manual*, Pub 100-3, chapter 20, section 20.19, and the *Medicare Claims Processing Manual*, Pub 100-4, chapter 32, section 10.1, there is no need to search the Medicare website for the applicable reference.

**Appendix H: Quality Payment Program (QPP)**—Previously, this appendix contained lists of the numerators and denominators applicable to the Medicare PQRS. However, with the implementation of the Quality Payment Program (QPP) mandated by passage of the Medicare Access and Chip Reauthorization Act (MACRA) of 2015, the PQRS system will be obsolete. This appendix now contains information pertinent to that legislation as well as a comprehensive overview of the QPP.

**Appendix I: Medically Unlikely Edits**—This appendix contains the published medically unlikely edits (MUEs). These edits establish maximum daily allowable units of service. The edits will be applied to the services provided to the same patient, for the same CPT code, on the same date of service when billed by the same provider. Included are the physician and facility edits.

**Appendix J: Inpatient-Only Procedures**—This appendix identifies services with the status indicator "C." Medicare will not pay an OPPS hospital or ASC when these procedures are performed on a Medicare patient as an outpatient. Physicians should refer to this list when scheduling Medicare patients for surgical procedures. CMS updates this list quarterly.

**Appendix K: Place of Service and Type of Service**—This appendix contains lists of place-of-service codes that should be used on professional claims and type-of-service codes used by the Medicare Common Working File.

**Appendix L: Multianalyte Assays with Algorithmic Analyses**—This appendix lists the administrative codes for multianalyte assays with algorithmic analyses. The AMA updates this list three times a year.

**Appendix M: Glossary**—This appendix contains general terms and definitions as well as those that would apply to or be helpful for billing and reimbursement.

**Appendix N: Listing of Sensory, Motor, and Mixed Nerves**—This appendix lists a summary of each sensory, motor, and mixed nerve with its appropriate nerve conduction study code.

**Appendix O: Vascular Families**—Appendix O contains a table of vascular families starting with the aorta. Additional information can be found in the interventional radiology illustrations located behind the index.

**Appendix P: Interventional Radiology Illustrations**—This appendix contains illustrations specific to interventional radiology procedures.

**Note:** All data current as of November 8, 2017.

# Anatomical Illustrations

## Body Planes and Movements

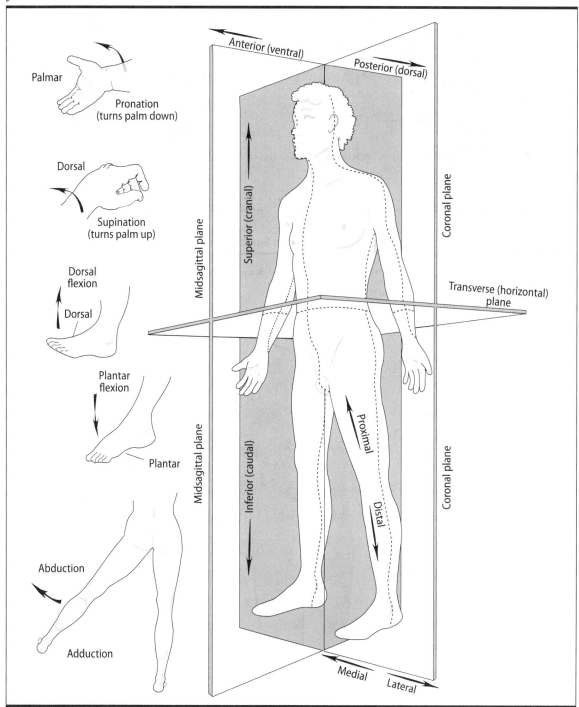

# Integumentary System

## Skin and Subcutaneous Tissue

## Nail Anatomy

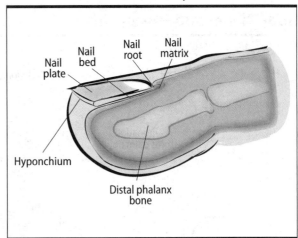

## Assessment of Burn Surface Area

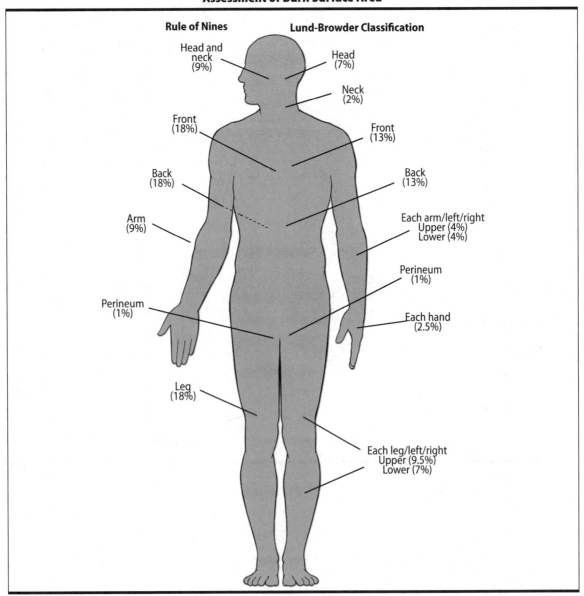

CPT © 2017 American Medical Association. All Rights Reserved.

© 2017 Optum360, LLC

# Musculoskeletal System

## Bones and Joints

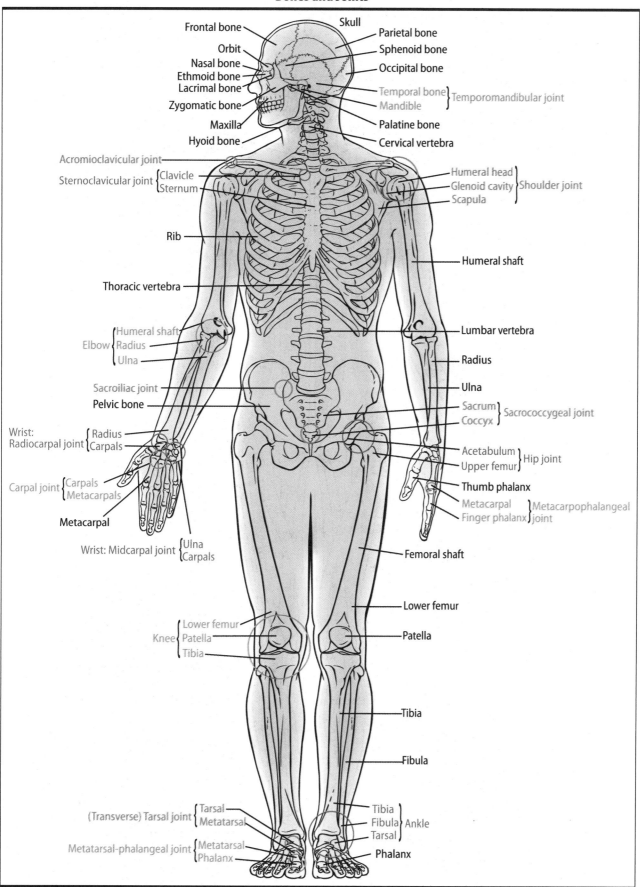

© 2017 Optum360, LLC      CPT © 2017 American Medical Association. All Rights Reserved.

## Muscles

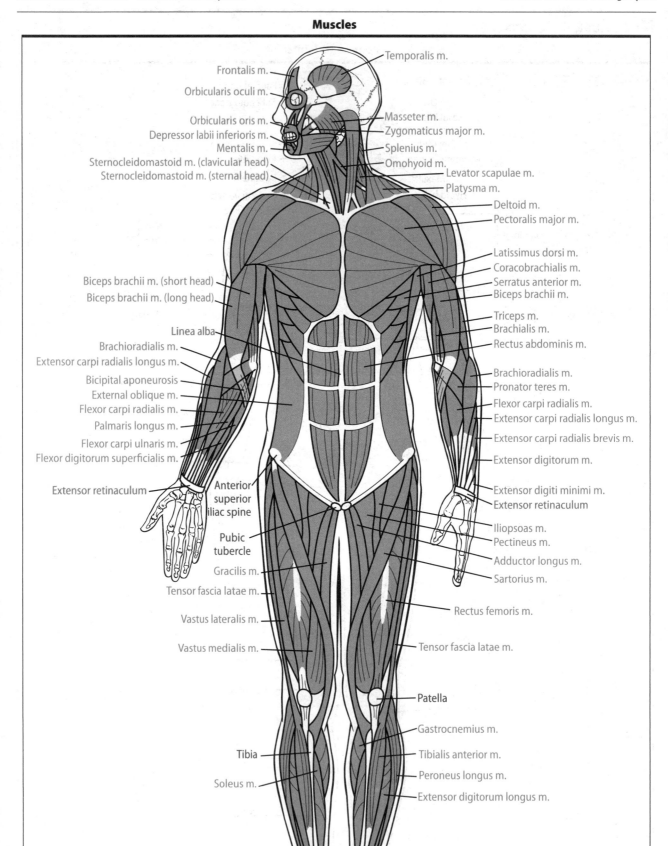

Temporalis m.

Frontalis m.

Orbicularis oculi m.

Orbicularis oris m.

Depressor labii inferioris m.

Mentalis m.

Sternocleidomastoid m. (clavicular head)

Sternocleidomastoid m. (sternal head)

Masseter m.

Zygomaticus major m.

Splenius m.

Omohyoid m.

Levator scapulae m.

Platysma m.

Deltoid m.

Pectoralis major m.

Latissimus dorsi m.

Coracobrachialis m.

Serratus anterior m.

Biceps brachii m.

Triceps m.

Brachialis m.

Rectus abdominis m.

Biceps brachii m. (short head)

Biceps brachii m. (long head)

Linea alba

Brachioradialis m.

Extensor carpi radialis longus m.

Bicipital aponeurosis

External oblique m.

Flexor carpi radialis m.

Palmaris longus m.

Flexor carpi ulnaris m.

Flexor digitorum superficialis m.

Extensor retinaculum

Brachioradialis m.

Pronator teres m.

Flexor carpi radialis m.

Extensor carpi radialis longus m.

Extensor carpi radialis brevis m.

Extensor digitorum m.

Extensor digiti minimi m.

Extensor retinaculum

Anterior superior iliac spine

Pubic tubercle

Gracilis m.

Tensor fascia latae m.

Vastus lateralis m.

Vastus medialis m.

Iliopsoas m.

Pectineus m.

Adductor longus m.

Sartorius m.

Rectus femoris m.

Tensor fascia latae m.

Patella

Gastrocnemius m.

Tibialis anterior m.

Peroneus longus m.

Extensor digitorum longus m.

Tibia

Soleus m.

Superior extensor retinaculum

Lateral maleolus

Medial maleolus

CPT © 2017 American Medical Association. All Rights Reserved.

© 2017 Optum360, LLC

## Head and Facial Bones

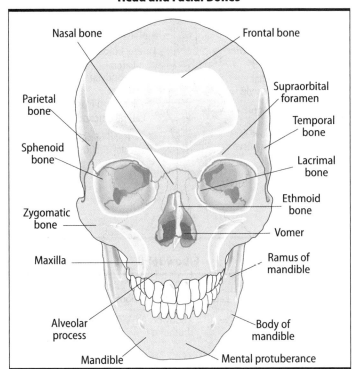

- Nasal bone
- Frontal bone
- Parietal bone
- Supraorbital foramen
- Temporal bone
- Sphenoid bone
- Lacrimal bone
- Zygomatic bone
- Ethmoid bone
- Vomer
- Maxilla
- Ramus of mandible
- Alveolar process
- Body of mandible
- Mandible
- Mental protuberance

## Nose

- Nasal bones
- Lateral nasal cartilages
- Septal cartilage
- Greater alar cartilage
- Lateral crus
- Septal cartilage
- Medial crus

## Shoulder (Anterior View)

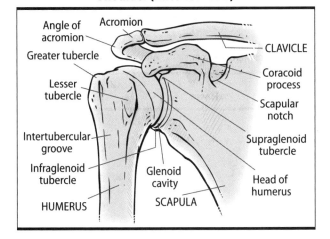

- Angle of acromion
- Acromion
- Greater tubercle
- CLAVICLE
- Lesser tubercle
- Coracoid process
- Intertubercular groove
- Scapular notch
- Infraglenoid tubercle
- Supraglenoid tubercle
- HUMERUS
- Glenoid cavity
- Head of humerus
- SCAPULA

## Shoulder (Posterior View)

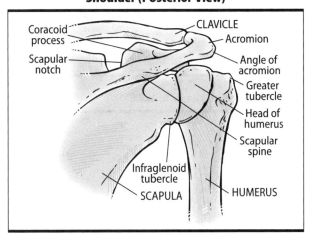

- Coracoid process
- CLAVICLE
- Scapular notch
- Acromion
- Angle of acromion
- Greater tubercle
- Head of humerus
- Scapular spine
- Infraglenoid tubercle
- SCAPULA
- HUMERUS

## Shoulder Muscles

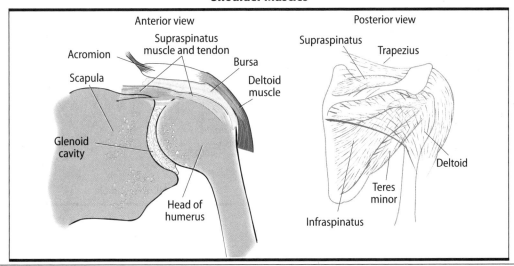

Anterior view
- Acromion
- Supraspinatus muscle and tendon
- Bursa
- Scapula
- Deltoid muscle
- Glenoid cavity
- Head of humerus

Posterior view
- Supraspinatus
- Trapezius
- Deltoid
- Teres minor
- Infraspinatus

© 2017 Optum360, LLC

### Elbow (Anterior View)

### Elbow (Posterior View)

### Elbow Muscles

### Elbow Joint

### Lower Arm

### Hand

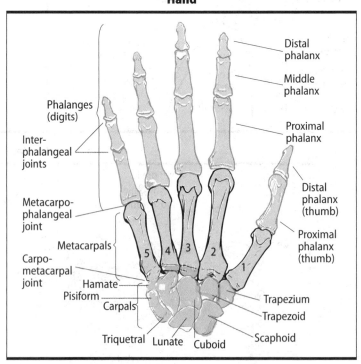

CPT © 2017 American Medical Association. All Rights Reserved.
© 2017 Optum360, LLC

## Hip (Anterior View)

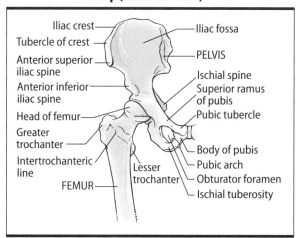

Iliac crest
Tubercle of crest
Anterior superior iliac spine
Anterior inferior iliac spine
Head of femur
Greater trochanter
Intertrochanteric line
FEMUR
Iliac fossa
PELVIS
Ischial spine
Superior ramus of pubis
Pubic tubercle
Lesser trochanter
Body of pubis
Pubic arch
Obturator foramen
Ischial tuberosity

## Hip (Posterior View)

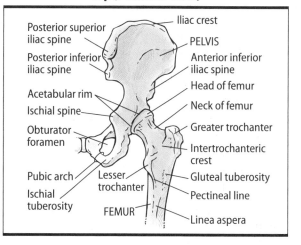

Posterior superior iliac spine
Posterior inferior iliac spine
Acetabular rim
Ischial spine
Obturator foramen
Pubic arch
Ischial tuberosity
FEMUR
Lesser trochanter
Iliac crest
PELVIS
Anterior inferior iliac spine
Head of femur
Neck of femur
Greater trochanter
Intertrochanteric crest
Gluteal tuberosity
Pectineal line
Linea aspera

## Knee (Anterior View)

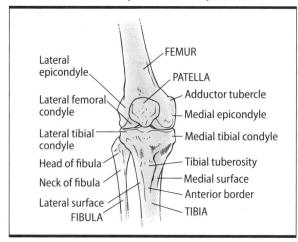

Lateral epicondyle
Lateral femoral condyle
Lateral tibial condyle
Head of fibula
Neck of fibula
Lateral surface
FIBULA
FEMUR
PATELLA
Adductor tubercle
Medial epicondyle
Medial tibial condyle
Tibial tuberosity
Medial surface
Anterior border
TIBIA

## Knee (Posterior View)

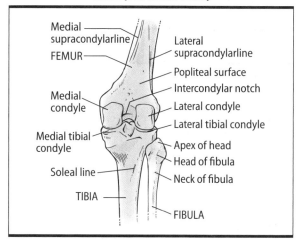

Medial supracondylarline
FEMUR
Medial condyle
Medial tibial condyle
Soleal line
TIBIA
Lateral supracondylarline
Popliteal surface
Intercondylar notch
Lateral condyle
Lateral tibial condyle
Apex of head
Head of fibula
Neck of fibula
FIBULA

## Knee Joint (Anterior View)

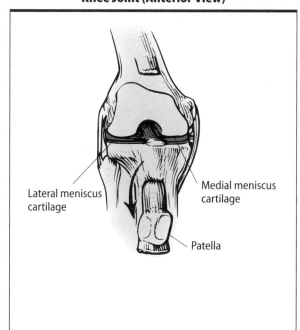

Lateral meniscus cartilage
Medial meniscus cartilage
Patella

## Knee Joint (Lateral View)

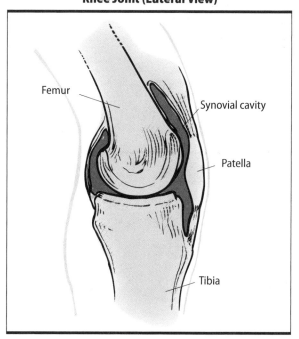

Femur
Synovial cavity
Patella
Tibia

© 2017 Optum360, LLC    CPT © 2017 American Medical Association. All Rights Reserved.    **xiii**

**Anatomical Illustrations—Musculoskeletal System**

Anatomical Illustrations—Musculoskeletal System

## Lower Leg

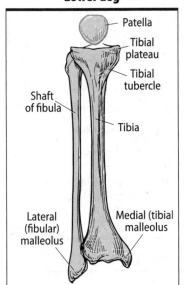

Patella

Tibial plateau

Tibial tubercle

Shaft of fibula

Tibia

Lateral (fibular) malleolus

Medial (tibial) malleolus

## Ankle Ligament (Lateral View)

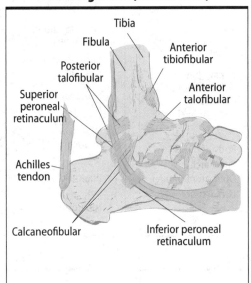

Tibia

Fibula

Anterior tibiofibular

Posterior talofibular

Anterior talofibular

Superior peroneal retinaculum

Achilles tendon

Calcaneofibular

Inferior peroneal retinaculum

## Ankle Ligament (Posterior View)

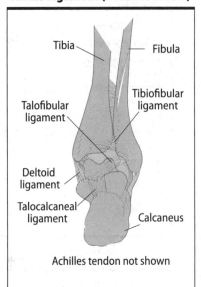

Tibia

Fibula

Talofibular ligament

Tibiofibular ligament

Deltoid ligament

Talocalcaneal ligament

Calcaneus

Achilles tendon not shown

## Foot Tendons

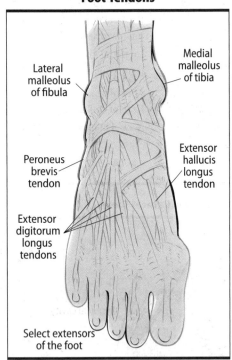

Lateral malleolus of fibula

Medial malleolus of tibia

Peroneus brevis tendon

Extensor hallucis longus tendon

Extensor digitorum longus tendons

Select extensors of the foot

## Foot Bones

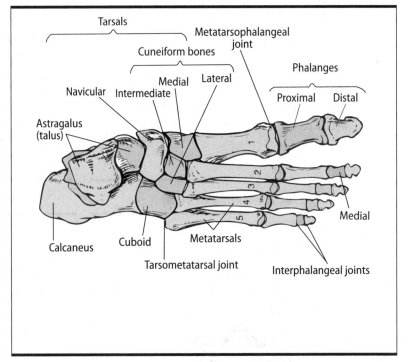

Tarsals

Metatarsophalangeal joint

Cuneiform bones

Phalanges

Medial

Lateral

Navicular

Intermediate

Proximal

Distal

Astragalus (talus)

Medial

Calcaneus

Cuboid

Metatarsals

Tarsometatarsal joint

Interphalangeal joints

CPT © 2017 American Medical Association. All Rights Reserved.

© 2017 Optum360, LLC

## Respiratory System

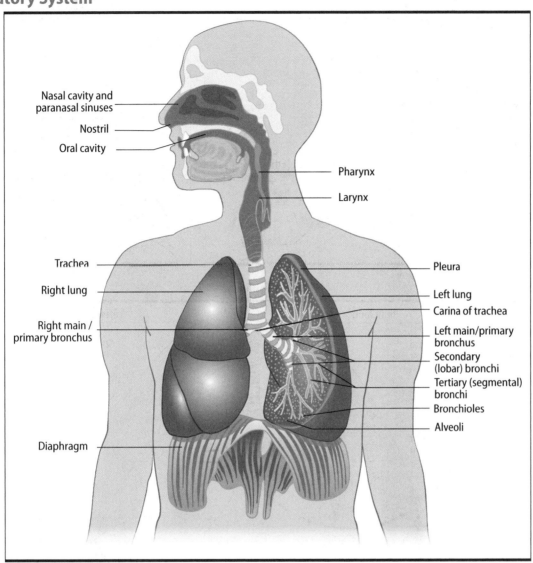

Nasal cavity and paranasal sinuses

Nostril

Oral cavity

Pharynx

Larynx

Trachea

Right lung

Right main / primary bronchus

Diaphragm

Pleura

Left lung

Carina of trachea

Left main/primary bronchus

Secondary (lobar) bronchi

Tertiary (segmental) bronchi

Bronchioles

Alveoli

### Upper Respiratory System

Paranasal sinuses drain into nose via ducts under nasal conchae

Frontal sinus

Olfactory bulb and nerves

Sphenoid sinus

Window in nasal septum reveals lateral nasal wall

Orifice of auditory tube

Naris

Soft palate

**Nasal cavity from front**

Epiglottis

Nasal conchae

Larynx

Vocal cords

Meati

Cricoid cartilage

Trachea

Septum

### Nasal Turbinates

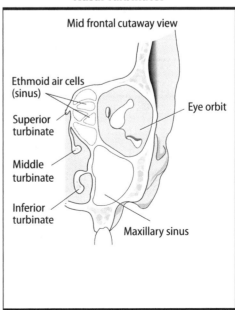

Mid frontal cutaway view

Ethmoid air cells (sinus)

Eye orbit

Superior turbinate

Middle turbinate

Inferior turbinate

Maxillary sinus

**Anatomical Illustrations—Respiratory System**

### Paranasal Sinuses

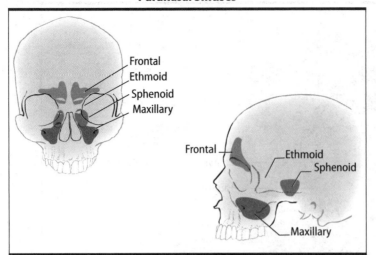

Frontal
Ethmoid
Sphenoid
Maxillary

Frontal
Ethmoid
Sphenoid
Maxillary

### Lower Respiratory System

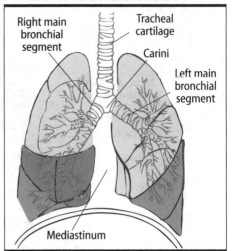

Right main bronchial segment
Tracheal cartilage
Carini
Left main bronchial segment
Mediastinum

### Lung Segments

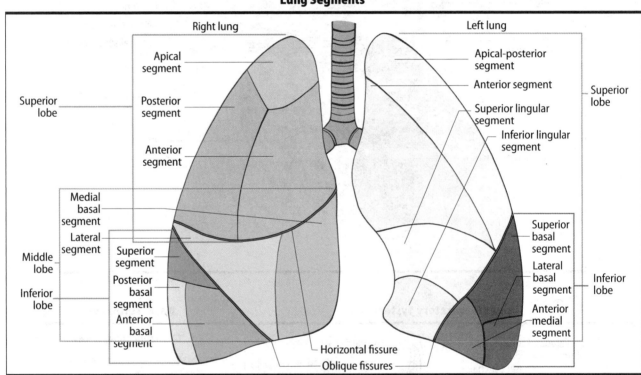

Right lung
Left lung

Superior lobe

Apical segment
Posterior segment
Anterior segment

Medial basal segment
Lateral segment
Superior segment
Posterior basal segment
Anterior basal segment

Middle lobe
Inferior lobe

Apical-posterior segment
Anterior segment
Superior lingular segment
Inferior lingular segment

Superior lobe

Superior basal segment
Lateral basal segment
Anterior medial segment

Inferior lobe

Horizontal fissure
Oblique fissures

### Alveoli

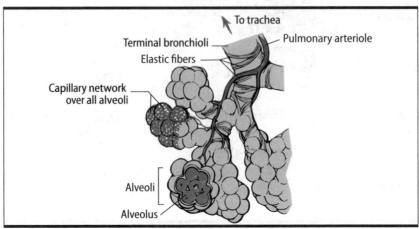

To trachea
Terminal bronchioli
Elastic fibers
Pulmonary arteriole
Capillary network over all alveoli
Alveoli
Alveolus

CPT © 2017 American Medical Association. All Rights Reserved.
© 2017 Optum360, LLC

# Arterial System

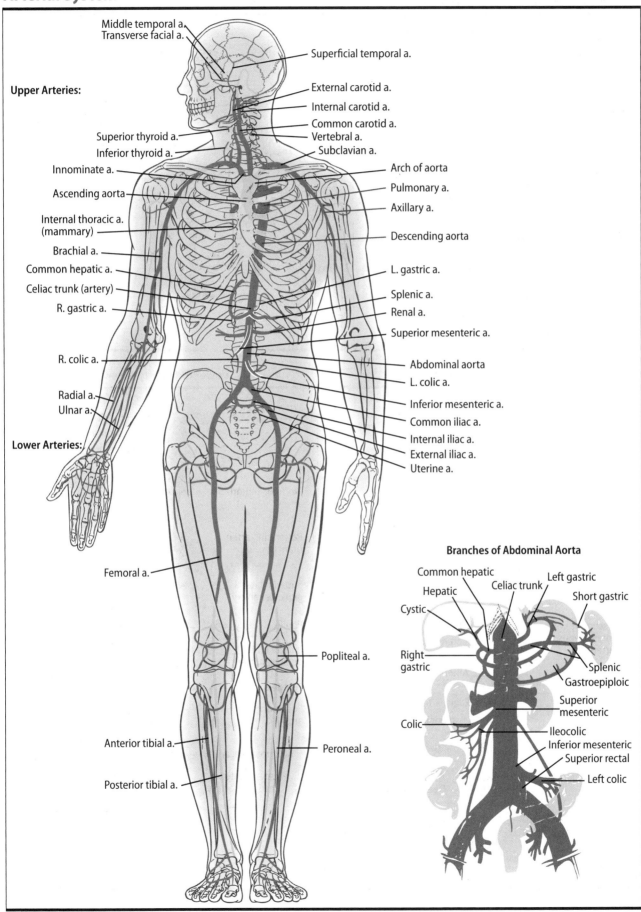

Upper Arteries:

Middle temporal a.
Transverse facial a.
Superficial temporal a.
External carotid a.
Internal carotid a.
Common carotid a.
Vertebral a.
Subclavian a.
Superior thyroid a.
Inferior thyroid a.
Innominate a.
Arch of aorta
Ascending aorta
Pulmonary a.
Axillary a.
Internal thoracic a. (mammary)
Descending aorta
Brachial a.
Common hepatic a.
L. gastric a.
Celiac trunk (artery)
Splenic a.
R. gastric a.
Renal a.
Superior mesenteric a.
R. colic a.
Abdominal aorta
L. colic a.
Radial a.
Inferior mesenteric a.
Ulnar a.
Common iliac a.
Internal iliac a.
External iliac a.
Uterine a.

Lower Arteries:

Femoral a.
Popliteal a.
Anterior tibial a.
Peroneal a.
Posterior tibial a.

## Branches of Abdominal Aorta

Common hepatic
Hepatic
Cystic
Left gastric
Celiac trunk
Short gastric
Right gastric
Splenic
Gastroepiploic
Superior mesenteric
Colic
Ileocolic
Inferior mesenteric
Superior rectal
Left colic

© 2017 Optum360, LLC

CPT © 2017 American Medical Association. All Rights Reserved.

### Internal Carotid and Arteries and Branches

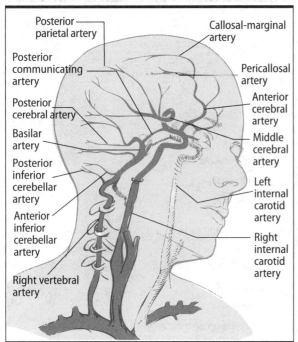

Posterior parietal artery
Posterior communicating artery
Posterior cerebral artery
Basilar artery
Posterior inferior cerebellar artery
Anterior inferior cerebellar artery
Right vertebral artery
Callosal-marginal artery
Pericallosal artery
Anterior cerebral artery
Middle cerebral artery
Left internal carotid artery
Right internal carotid artery

### External Carotid Arteries and Branches

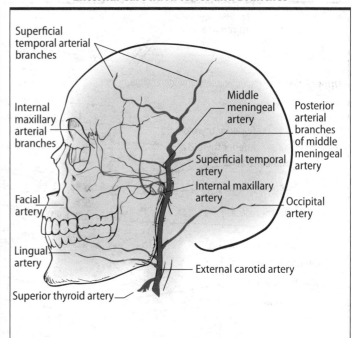

Superficial temporal arterial branches
Internal maxillary arterial branches
Facial artery
Lingual artery
Superior thyroid artery
Middle meningeal artery
Posterior arterial branches of middle meningeal artery
Superficial temporal artery
Internal maxillary artery
Occipital artery
External carotid artery

### Upper Extremity Arteries

Subclavian artery
Axillary Artery
Posterior circumflex humeral artery
Inferior ulnar collateral artery
Recurrent interosseous artery
Ulnar artery
Thoracoacromial artery
Anterior humeral circumflex artery
Deep brachial artery
Brachial artery
Superior ulnar collateral artery
Radial collateral artery
Radial recurrent artery
Common interosseous artery
Anterior interosseous artery
Radial artery
Posterior interosseous artery
Superficial palmar branch of radial artery
Deep palmar arch
Digital arteries

### Lower Extremity Arteries

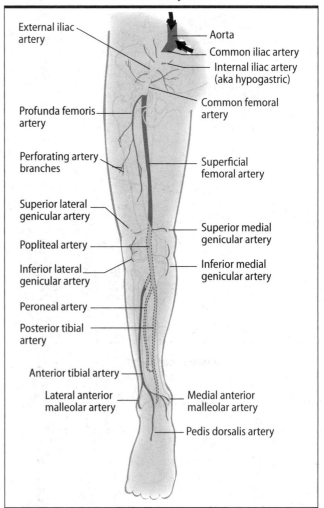

External iliac artery
Profunda femoris artery
Perforating artery branches
Superior lateral genicular artery
Popliteal artery
Inferior lateral genicular artery
Peroneal artery
Posterior tibial artery
Anterior tibial artery
Lateral anterior malleolar artery
Aorta
Common iliac artery
Internal iliac artery (aka hypogastric)
Common femoral artery
Superficial femoral artery
Superior medial genicular artery
Inferior medial genicular artery
Medial anterior malleolar artery
Pedis dorsalis artery

CPT © 2017 American Medical Association. All Rights Reserved.

© 2017 Optum360, LLC

## Venous System

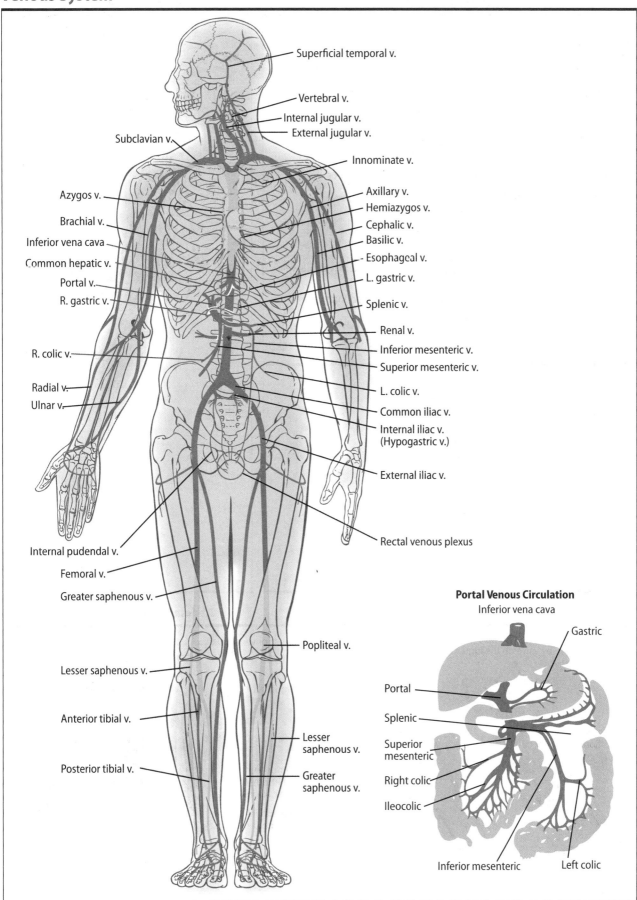

Superficial temporal v.

Vertebral v.

Internal jugular v.

External jugular v.

Subclavian v.

Innominate v.

Azygos v.

Axillary v.

Hemiazygos v.

Brachial v.

Cephalic v.

Inferior vena cava

Basilic v.

Common hepatic v.

Esophageal v.

Portal v.

L. gastric v.

R. gastric v.

Splenic v.

Renal v.

R. colic v.

Inferior mesenteric v.

Superior mesenteric v.

Radial v.

L. colic v.

Ulnar v.

Common iliac v.

Internal iliac v.
(Hypogastric v.)

External iliac v.

Rectal venous plexus

Internal pudendal v.

Femoral v.

Greater saphenous v.

**Portal Venous Circulation**
Inferior vena cava

Gastric

Popliteal v.

Portal

Lesser saphenous v.

Splenic

Superior
mesenteric

Anterior tibial v.

Lesser
saphenous v.

Right colic

Posterior tibial v.

Greater
saphenous v.

Ileocolic

Inferior mesenteric

Left colic

CPT © 2017 American Medical Association. All Rights Reserved.

## Head and Neck Veins

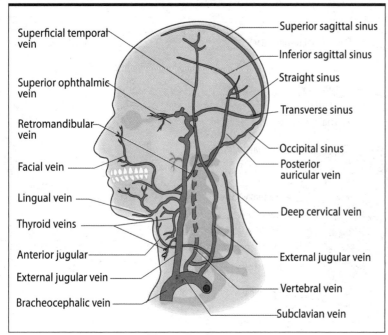

- Superficial temporal vein
- Superior ophthalmic vein
- Retromandibular vein
- Facial vein
- Lingual vein
- Thyroid veins
- Anterior jugular
- External jugular vein
- Bracheocephalic vein
- Superior sagittal sinus
- Inferior sagittal sinus
- Straight sinus
- Transverse sinus
- Occipital sinus
- Posterior auricular vein
- Deep cervical vein
- External jugular vein
- Vertebral vein
- Subclavian vein

## Upper Extremity Veins

- Axillary
- Cephalic
- Brachial
- Basilic
- Median cubital
- Median forearm

## Venae Comitantes

- Artery
- Venae comitantes

## Venous Blood Flow

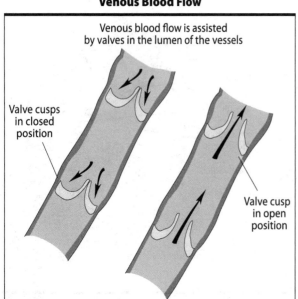

Venous blood flow is assisted by valves in the lumen of the vessels

- Valve cusps in closed position
- Valve cusp in open position

## Abdominal Veins

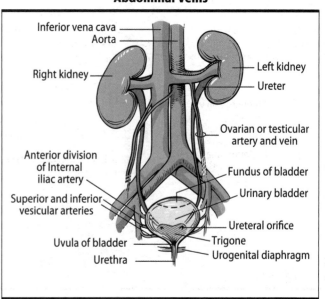

- Inferior vena cava
- Aorta
- Right kidney
- Left kidney
- Ureter
- Ovarian or testicular artery and vein
- Anterior division of Internal iliac artery
- Superior and inferior vesicular arteries
- Fundus of bladder
- Urinary bladder
- Ureteral orifice
- Trigone
- Uvula of bladder
- Urogenital diaphragm
- Urethra

CPT © 2017 American Medical Association. All Rights Reserved.

© 2017 Optum360, LLC

# Cardiovascular System

## Coronary Veins

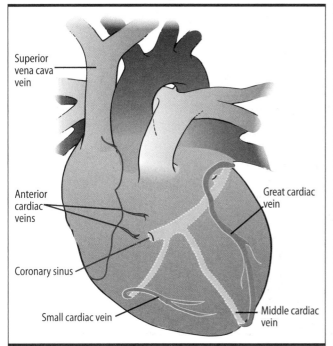

- Superior vena cava vein
- Anterior cardiac veins
- Coronary sinus
- Small cardiac vein
- Great cardiac vein
- Middle cardiac vein

## Anatomy of the Heart

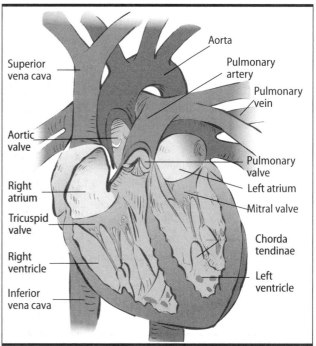

- Superior vena cava
- Aortic valve
- Right atrium
- Tricuspid valve
- Right ventricle
- Inferior vena cava
- Aorta
- Pulmonary artery
- Pulmonary vein
- Pulmonary valve
- Left atrium
- Mitral valve
- Chorda tendinae
- Left ventricle

## Heart Cross Section

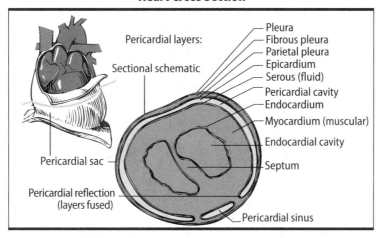

- Pericardial layers:
- Sectional schematic
- Pericardial sac
- Pericardial reflection (layers fused)
- Pleura
- Fibrous pleura
- Parietal pleura
- Epicardium
- Serous (fluid)
- Pericardial cavity
- Endocardium
- Myocardium (muscular)
- Endocardial cavity
- Septum
- Pericardial sinus

## Heart Valves

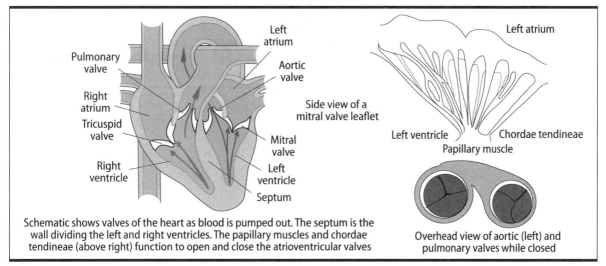

- Pulmonary valve
- Right atrium
- Tricuspid valve
- Right ventricle
- Left atrium
- Aortic valve
- Mitral valve
- Left ventricle
- Septum

Side view of a mitral valve leaflet

- Left atrium
- Left ventricle
- Papillary muscle
- Chordae tendineae

Schematic shows valves of the heart as blood is pumped out. The septum is the wall dividing the left and right ventricles. The papillary muscles and chordae tendineae (above right) function to open and close the atrioventricular valves

Overhead view of aortic (left) and pulmonary valves while closed

© 2017 Optum360, LLC　　　　　CPT © 2017 American Medical Association. All Rights Reserved.

## Heart Conduction System

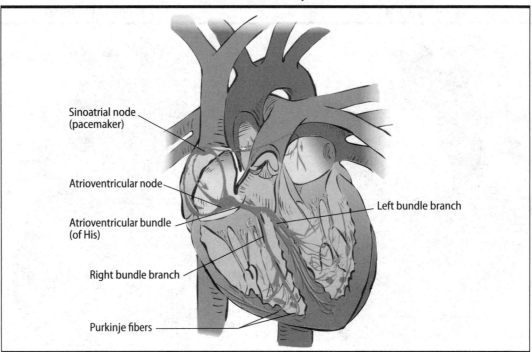

Sinoatrial node (pacemaker)

Atrioventricular node

Atrioventricular bundle (of His)

Right bundle branch

Purkinje fibers

Left bundle branch

## Coronary Arteries

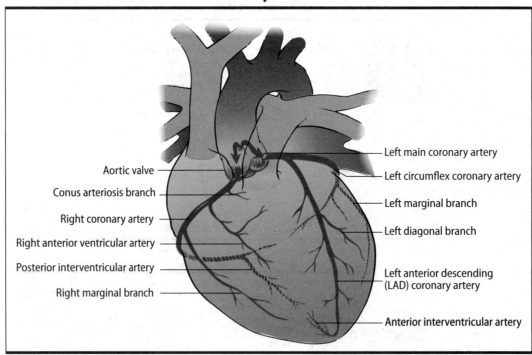

Aortic valve

Conus arteriosis branch

Right coronary artery

Right anterior ventricular artery

Posterior interventricular artery

Right marginal branch

Left main coronary artery

Left circumflex coronary artery

Left marginal branch

Left diagonal branch

Left anterior descending (LAD) coronary artery

Anterior interventricular artery

CPT © 2017 American Medical Association. All Rights Reserved.
© 2017 Optum360, LLC

# Lymphatic System

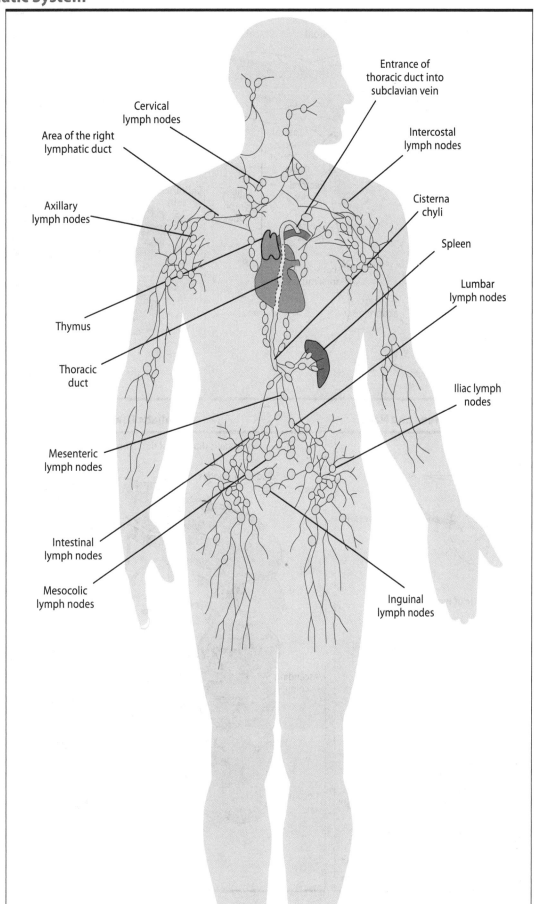

Cervical lymph nodes

Area of the right lymphatic duct

Axillary lymph nodes

Thymus

Thoracic duct

Mesenteric lymph nodes

Intestinal lymph nodes

Mesocolic lymph nodes

Entrance of thoracic duct into subclavian vein

Intercostal lymph nodes

Cisterna chyli

Spleen

Lumbar lymph nodes

Iliac lymph nodes

Inguinal lymph nodes

CPT © 2017 American Medical Association. All Rights Reserved.

Anatomical Illustrations—Lymphatic System

### Axillary Lymph Nodes

### Lymphatic Capillaries

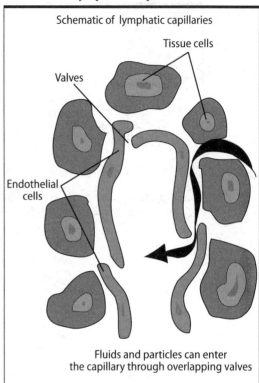

Schematic of lymphatic capillaries

Fluids and particles can enter
the capillary through overlapping valves

### Lymphatic System of Head and Neck

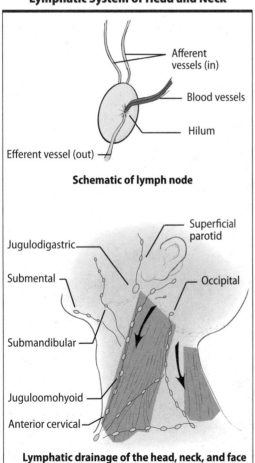

**Schematic of lymph node**

**Lymphatic drainage of the head, neck, and face**

### Lymphatic Drainage

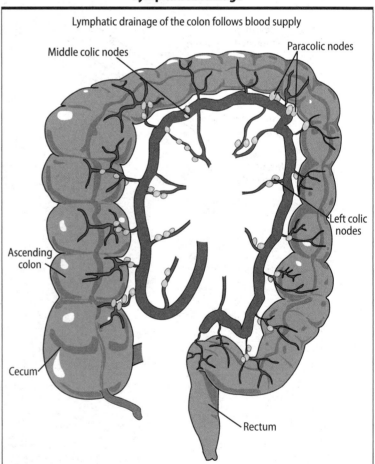

Lymphatic drainage of the colon follows blood supply

CPT © 2017 American Medical Association. All Rights Reserved.

© 2017 Optum360, LLC

## Spleen Internal Structures

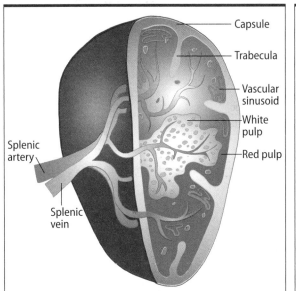

Capsule

Trabecula

Vascular sinusoid

White pulp

Red pulp

Splenic artery

Splenic vein

## Spleen External Structures

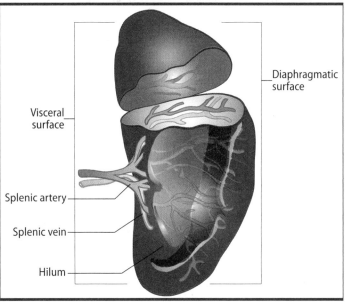

Diaphragmatic surface

Visceral surface

Splenic artery

Splenic vein

Hilum

## Digestive System

### Gallbladder

### Stomach

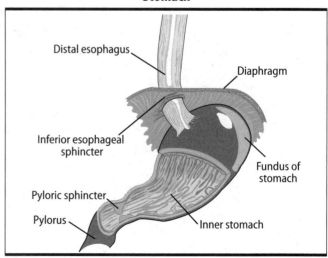

    CPT © 2017 American Medical Association. All Rights Reserved.    © 2017 Optum360, LLC

## Mouth (Upper)

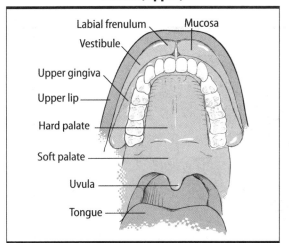

Labial frenulum
Mucosa
Vestibule
Upper gingiva
Upper lip
Hard palate
Soft palate
Uvula
Tongue

## Mouth (Lower)

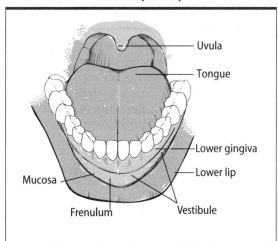

Uvula
Tongue
Lower gingiva
Lower lip
Vestibule
Mucosa
Frenulum

## Pancreas

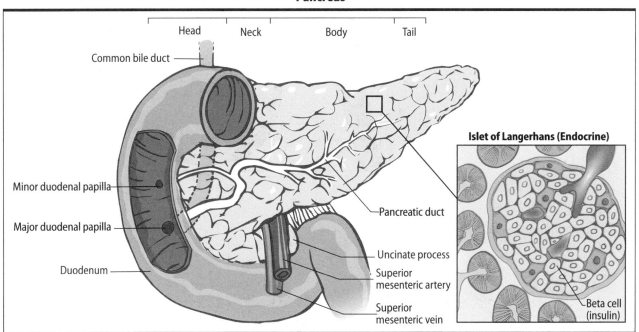

Head    Neck    Body    Tail

Common bile duct

Minor duodenal papilla

Major duodenal papilla

Duodenum

Pancreatic duct

Uncinate process

Superior mesenteric artery

Superior mesenteric vein

### Islet of Langerhans (Endocrine)

Beta cell (insulin)

## Liver

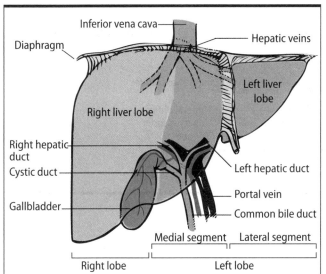

Inferior vena cava
Hepatic veins
Diaphragm
Left liver lobe
Right liver lobe
Right hepatic duct
Cystic duct
Gallbladder
Left hepatic duct
Portal vein
Common bile duct
Medial segment    Lateral segment
Right lobe    Left lobe

## Anus

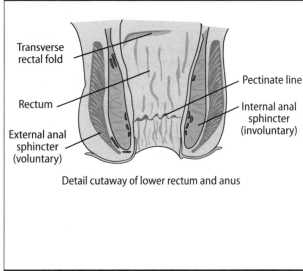

Transverse rectal fold
Rectum
External anal sphincter (voluntary)
Pectinate line
Internal anal sphincter (involuntary)

Detail cutaway of lower rectum and anus

© 2017 Optum360, LLC    CPT © 2017 American Medical Association. All Rights Reserved.

# Genitourinary System

**Urinary System**

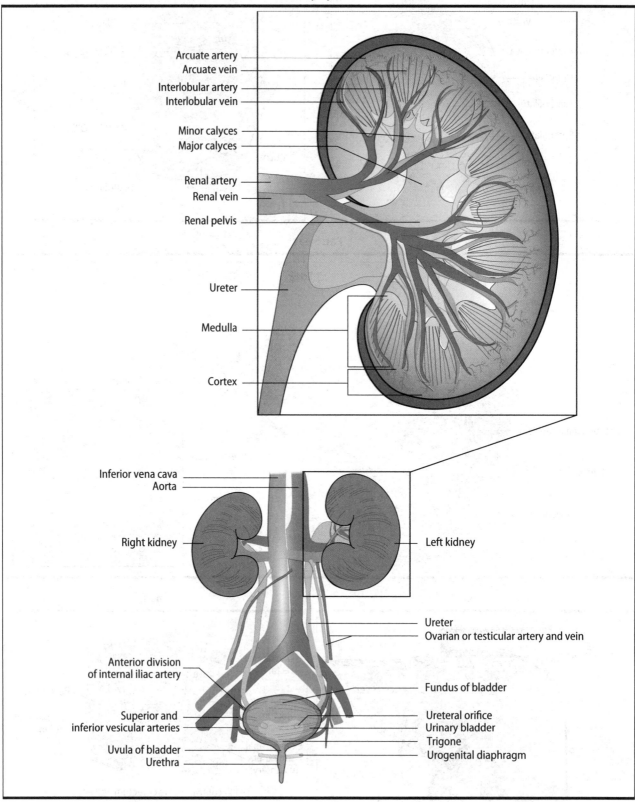

CPT © 2017 American Medical Association. All Rights Reserved.

## Nephron

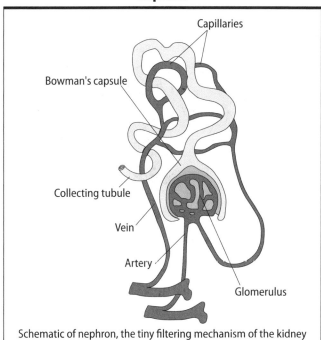

Schematic of nephron, the tiny filtering mechanism of the kidney

## Male Genitourinary

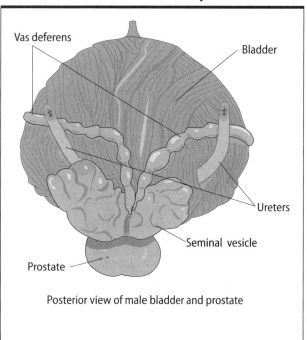

Posterior view of male bladder and prostate

## Testis and Associate Structures

## Male Genitourinary System

### Female Genitourinary

### Female Reproductive System

### Female Bladder

### Female Breast

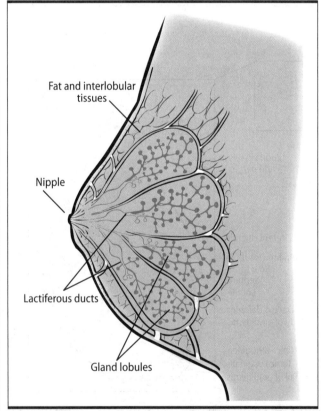

CPT © 2017 American Medical Association. All Rights Reserved.
© 2017 Optum360, LLC

## Endocrine System

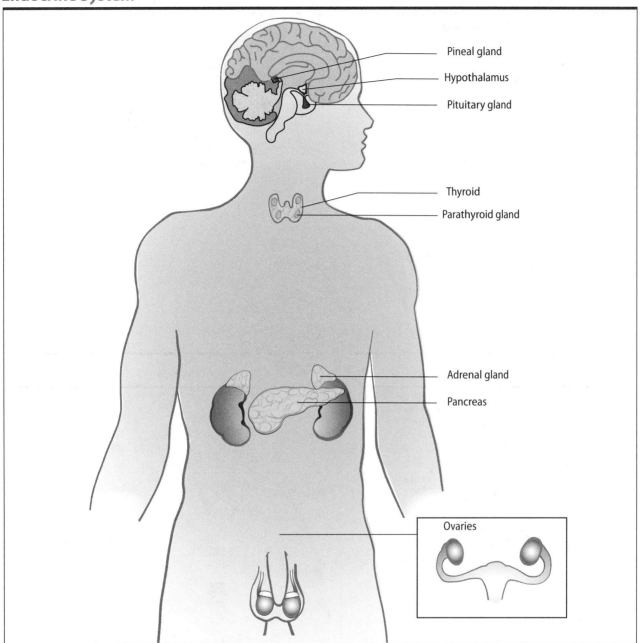

Pineal gland

Hypothalamus

Pituitary gland

Thyroid

Parathyroid gland

Adrenal gland

Pancreas

Ovaries

## Structure of an Ovary

Primary follicles

Primordial follicles

Oocyte

Secondary follicle

Blood vessels

Vesicular (graafian) follicle

Degenerating corpus luteum (corpus albicans)

Corpus luteum

Corona radiata

Ovulated ovum

Developing corpus luteum

## Thyroid and Parathyroid Glands

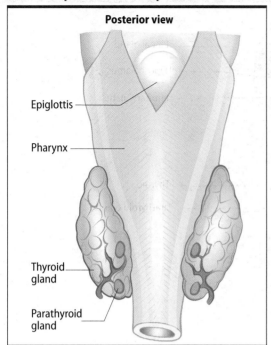

### Posterior view

Epiglottis

Pharynx

Thyroid gland

Parathyroid gland

## Adrenal Gland

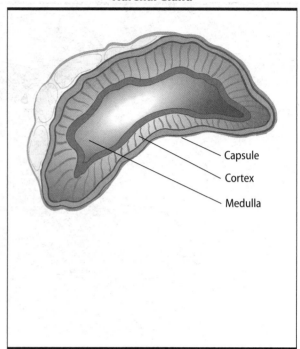

Capsule

Cortex

Medulla

## Thyroid

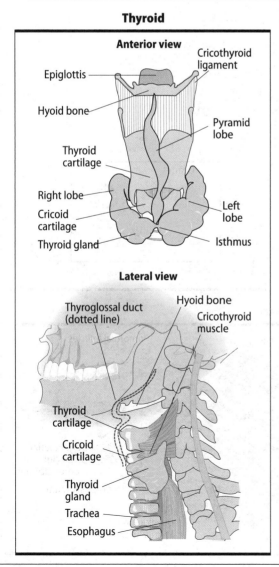

### Anterior view

Epiglottis

Cricothyroid ligament

Hyoid bone

Pyramid lobe

Thyroid cartilage

Right lobe

Cricoid cartilage

Left lobe

Thyroid gland

Isthmus

### Lateral view

Thyroglossal duct (dotted line)

Hyoid bone

Cricothyroid muscle

Thyroid cartilage

Cricoid cartilage

Thyroid gland

Trachea

Esophagus

## Thymus

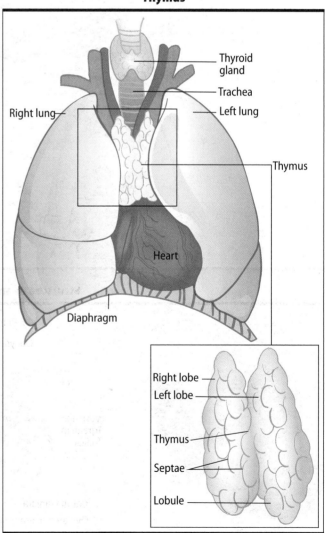

Thyroid gland

Trachea

Left lung

Right lung

Thymus

Heart

Diaphragm

Right lobe

Left lobe

Thymus

Septae

Lobule

CPT © 2017 American Medical Association. All Rights Reserved.
© 2017 Optum360, LLC

# Nervous System

## Brain

## Cranial Nerves

CPT © 2017 American Medical Association. All Rights Reserved.

© 2017 Optum360, LLC

## Spinal Cord and Spinal Nerves

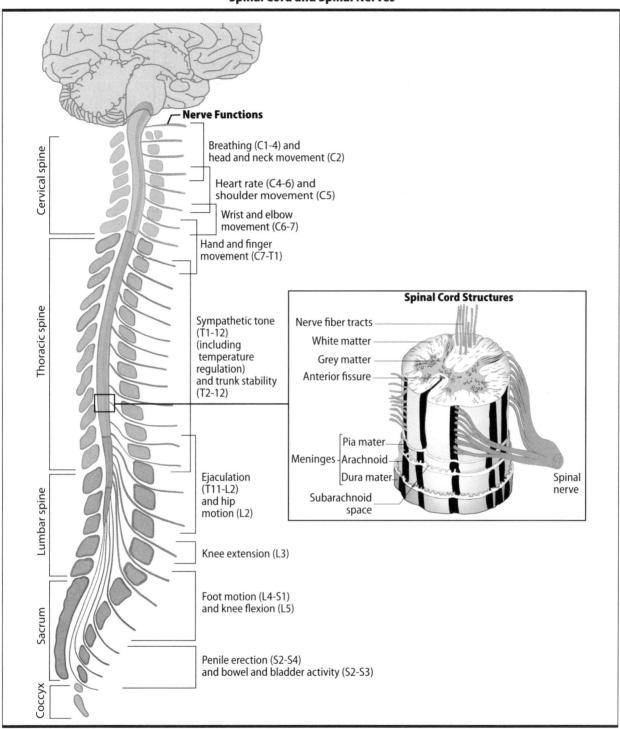

**Nerve Functions**

Breathing (C1-4) and head and neck movement (C2)

Heart rate (C4-6) and shoulder movement (C5)

Wrist and elbow movement (C6-7)

Hand and finger movement (C7-T1)

Sympathetic tone (T1-12) (including temperature regulation) and trunk stability (T2-12)

Ejaculation (T11-L2) and hip motion (L2)

Knee extension (L3)

Foot motion (L4-S1) and knee flexion (L5)

Penile erection (S2-S4) and bowel and bladder activity (S2-S3)

Cervical spine

Thoracic spine

Lumbar spine

Sacrum

Coccyx

**Spinal Cord Structures**

Nerve fiber tracts

White matter

Grey matter

Anterior fissure

Meninges — Pia mater / Arachnoid / Dura mater

Subarachnoid space

Spinal nerve

CPT © 2017 American Medical Association. All Rights Reserved.

**Nerve Cell**

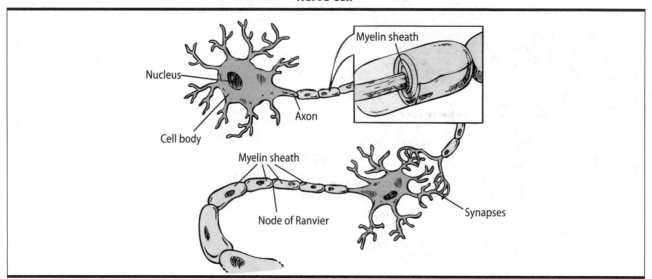

CPT © 2017 American Medical Association. All Rights Reserved.　　　　© 2017 Optum360, LLC

# Eye

## Eye Structure

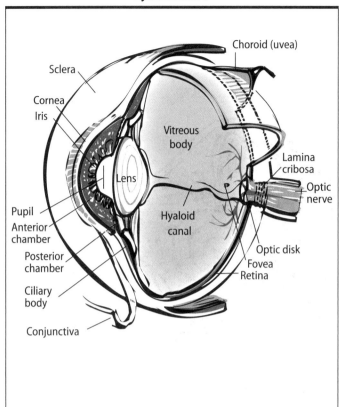

Sclera
Cornea
Iris
Pupil
Anterior chamber
Posterior chamber
Ciliary body
Conjunctiva
Choroid (uvea)
Vitreous body
Lens
Hyaloid canal
Lamina cribosa
Optic nerve
Optic disk
Fovea
Retina

## Posterior Pole of Globe/Flow of Aqueous Humor

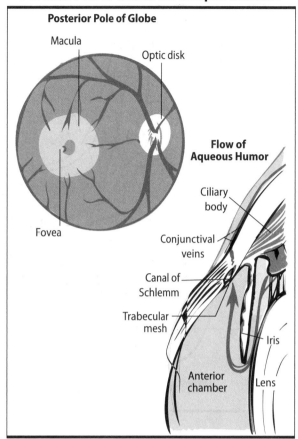

**Posterior Pole of Globe**

Macula
Optic disk
Fovea

**Flow of Aqueous Humor**

Ciliary body
Conjunctival veins
Canal of Schlemm
Trabecular mesh
Iris
Anterior chamber
Lens

## Eye Musculature

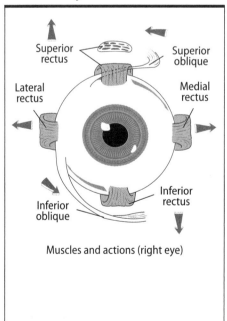

Superior rectus
Superior oblique
Lateral rectus
Medial rectus
Inferior oblique
Inferior rectus

Muscles and actions (right eye)

## Eyelid Structures

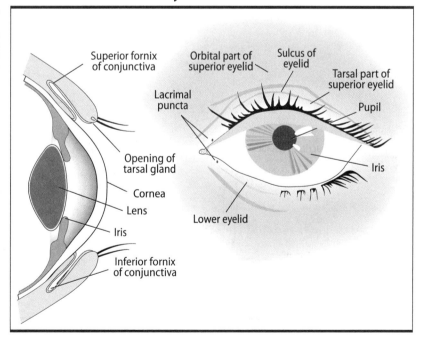

Superior fornix of conjunctiva
Orbital part of superior eyelid
Sulcus of eyelid
Tarsal part of superior eyelid
Lacrimal puncta
Pupil
Opening of tarsal gland
Cornea
Lens
Iris
Lower eyelid
Iris
Inferior fornix of conjunctiva

# Ear and Lacrimal System

## Ear Anatomy

## Lacrimal System

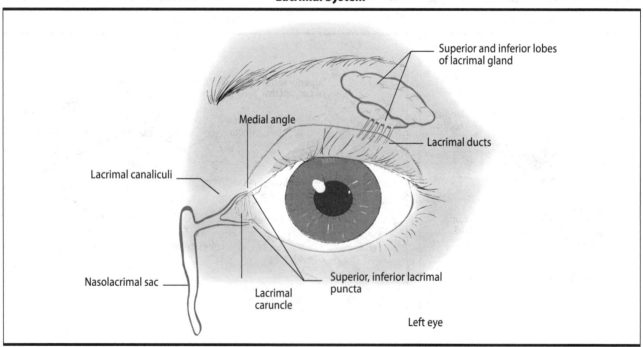

CPT © 2017 American Medical Association. All Rights Reserved.

© 2017 Optum360, LLC

## 0-Numeric

**3-Beta-Hydroxysteroid Dehydrogenase Type II Deficiency**, 81404
**3-Methylcrotonyl-CoA Carboxylase 1**, 81406
**5,10-Methylenetetrahydrofolate Reductase**, 81291

## A

**A Vitamin**, 84590
**Abbe–Estlander Procedure**, 40527, 40761
**ABBI Biopsy**, 19081-19086
**ABCA4**, 81408
**ABCC8**, 81401, 81407
**ABCD1**, 81405
**Abdomen, Abdominal**
  Abscess, 49020, 49040
    Incision and Drainage
      Skin and Subcutaneous Tissue,
        10060-10061
      Open, 49040
        Peritoneal, 49020
        Peritonitis, Localized, 49020
        Retroperitoneal, 49060
        Subdiaphragmatic, 49040
        Subphrenic, 49040
  Angiography, 74175, 75635
  Aorta
    Aneurysm, 0254T, 34701-34712, 34813,
      34830-34832, 34841-34848,
      35081-35103
    Angiography, 75635
    Aortography, 75625, 75630
    Thromboendarterectomy, 35331
  Aortic Aneurysm, 0254T, 34701-34712, 34813,
    34830-34832, 34841-34848, 35081-
    35103
  Artery
    Ligation, 37617
  Biopsy
    Open, 49000
    Percutaneous, 49180
    Skin and Subcutaneous Tissue, 11100,
      11101
  Bypass Graft, 35907
  Cannula/catheter
    Insertion, 49419, 49421
    Removal, 49422
  Catheter
    Removal, 49422
  Celiotomy
    for Staging, 49220
  CT Scan, 74150-74178, 75635
  Cyst
    Destruction/Excision, 49203-49205
    Sclerotherapy, 49185
  Delivery
    with Hysterectomy, 59525
    After Attempted Vaginal Delivery
      Delivery Only, 59620
      Postpartum Care, 59622
      Routine Care, 59618
    Delivery Only, 59514
    Peritoneal Abscess
      Open, 49020
      Peritonitis, localized, 49020
    Postpartum Care, 59515
    Routine Care, 59510
    Tubal Ligation at Time of, 58611
  Drainage, 49020, 49040
    Fluid, 49082-49083
    Retroperitoneal
      Open, 49060
    Skin and Subcutaneous Tissue, 10060-
      10061
    Subdiaphragmatic
      Open, 49040
    Subphrenic
      Open, 49040
  Ectopic Pregnancy, 59130
  Endometrioma, 49203-49205
    Destruction/Excision, 49203-49205
  Excision
    Excess Skin, 15830
    Tumor, Abdominal Wall, 22900
  Exploration, 49000-49084

**Abdomen, Abdominal** — continued
  Exploration — continued
    Blood Vessel, 35840
    Staging, 58960
  Hernia Repair, 49491-49590, 49650-49659
  Incision and Drainage
    Pancreatitis, 48000
  Incision, 49000-49084
    Staging, 58960
  Infraumbilical Panniculectomy, 15830
  Injection
    Air, 49400
    Contrast Material, 49400
  Insertion
    Catheter, 49324, 49418-49421
    Venous Shunt, 49425
  Intraperitoneal
    Catheter Exit Site, 49436
    Catheter Insertion, 49324, 49418-49421,
      49425, 49435
    Catheter Removal, 49422
    Catheter Revision, 49325
    Shunt
      Insertion, 49425
      Ligation, 49428
      Removal, 49429
      Revision, 49426
  Laparoscopy, 49320-49329
  Laparotomy
    with Biopsy, 49000
    Exploration, 47015, 49000-49002, 58960
    Hemorrhage Control, 49002
    Reopening, 49002
    Second Look, 58960
    Staging, 49220, 58960
  Lymphangiogram, 75805, 75807
  Magnetic Resonance Imaging (MRI), 74181-
    74183
    Fetal, 74712-74713
  Needle Biopsy
    Mass, 49180
  Pancreatitis, 48000
  Paracentesis, 49082-49083
  Peritoneal Abscess, 49020
  Peritoneal Lavage, 49084
  Placement Guidance Devices, 49411-49412
  Radical Resection, 51597
  Removal Node(s), 49220
  Repair
    Blood Vessel, 35221
      with
        Other Graft, 35281
        Vein Graft, 35251
    Hernia, 49491-49590, 49650-49659
    Suture, 49900
  Revision
    Venous Shunt, 49426
  Suture, 49900
  Tumor Staging, 58960
  Tumor
    Destruction/Excision, 49203-49205
  Ultrasound, 76700, 76705, 76706
  Unlisted Services and Procedures, 49999
  Wall
    See Abdomen, X–Ray
    Debridement
      Infected, 11005-11006
    Implant
      Fascial Reinforcement, 0437T
    Reconstruction, 49905
    Removal
      Mesh, 11008
      Prosthesis, 11008
    Repair
      Hernia, 49491-49590
        by Laparoscopy, 49650-49651
    Surgery, 22999
    Tumor
      Excision, 22900-22905
  Wound Exploration
    Penetrating, 20102
  X-ray, 74018-74022
**Abdominal Plane Block**
  Bilateral, 64488-64489
  Unilateral, 64486-64487

**Abdominohysterectomy**
  Radical, 58210
  Resection of Ovarian Malignancy, 58951,
    58953-58954, 58956
  Supracervical, 58180
  Total, 58150, 58200
    with Colpo-Urethrocystopexy, 58152
    with Omentectomy, 58956
    with Partial Vaginectomy, 58200
**Abdominoplasty**, 15830, 15847, 17999
**ABG**, 82803, 82805
**ABL1**, 81401
**Ablation**
  Anal
    Polyp, 46615
    Tumor, 46615
  Atria, 33257-33259
  Bone Tumor, 20982-20983
  Colon
    Polyp(s), [45346]
    Tumor, [45346]
  Cryosurgical
    Fibroadenoma, 19105
    Liver Tumor(s), 47381
    Nerve, 0440T-0442T
    Renal mass, 50250
    Renal Tumor
      Percutaneous, 50593
  CT Scan Guidance, 77013
  Endometrial, 58353, 58356, 58563
  Endometrium
    Ultrasound Guidance, 58356
  Endoscopic
    Duodenum/Jejunum, [43270]
    Esophagus, 43229, [43270]
    Hepatobiliary System, [43278]
    Stomach, [43270]
  Endovenous, 36473-36479 [36482, 36483]
  Fractional Laser Fenestration
    Infants and Children, 0479T-0480T
  Heart
    Arrhythmogenic Focus, 93650-93657
      Intracardiac Catheter, 93650-93657
      Open, 33250-33261
    Intracardiac Pacing and Mapping, 93631
      Follow-up Study, 93624
      Stimulation and Pacing, 93623
  Liver
    Tumor, 47380-47383
      Ablation
        Cryoablation, 47381, 47383
        Radiofrequency, 47380, 47382
      Laparoscopic, 47370-47371
        Cryosurgical, 47371
      Open, 47380-47381
  Lung
    Tumor
      Cryoablation, [32994]
      Radiofrequency, 32998
  Magnetic Resonance Guidance, 77022
  Nerve
    Cryoablation, 0440T-0442T
  Open Wound, 0491T-0492T
  Parenchymal Tissue
    CT Scan Guidance, 77013
    Magnetic Resonance Guidance, 77022
    Ultrasound Guidance, 76940
  Prostate, 55873
    Transurethral Waterjet, 0421T
  Pulmonary Tumor
    Cryoablation, [32994]
    Radiofrequency, 32998
  Radiofrequency
    Liver Tumor(s), 47382
    Lung Tumor(s), 32998
    Renal Tumor(s), 50592
    Tongue Base, 41530
  Renal
    Cyst, 50541
    Mass, 50542
      Radiofrequency, 50592
    Tumor, 50593
      Cryotherapy
        Percutaneous, 50593
  Supraventricular Arrhythmogenic Focus,
    33250-33251

**Ablation** — continued
  Tongue Base
    Radiofrequency, 41530
  Turbinate Mucosa, 30801, 30802
  Ultrasound
    Guidance, 76940
    Ultrasound Focused, 0071T-0072T
    Uterine Tumor, 0071T-0072T
  Uterus
    Fibroids, 0404T, 58674
    Leiomyomata, 0071T-0072T
    Tumor
      Ultrasound, Focused, 0071T-0072T
  Vein
    Endovenous, 36473-36479 [36482,
      36483]
  Ventricular Arrhythmogenic Focus, 33261
**ABLB Test**, 92562
**ABO**, 86900
**Abortion**
  See Obstetrical Care
  Incomplete, 59812
  Induced by
    with Hysterotomy, 59100, 59852, 59857
    Amniocentesis Injection, 59850-59852
    Dilation and Curettage, 59840
    Dilation and Evacuation, 59841
    Saline, 59850, 59851
    Vaginal Suppositories, 59855, 59856
  Missed
    First Trimester, 59820
    Second Trimester, 59821
  Septic, 59830
  Spontaneous, 59812
  Therapeutic, 59840-59852
    by Saline, 59850
      with Dilatation and Curettage,
        59851
      with Hysterotomy, 59852
**ABR**, 92585-92586
**Abrasion, Skin**
  Chemical Peel, 15788-15793
  Dermabrasion, 15780-15783
  Lesion, 15786, 15787
**ABS**, 86255, 86403, 86850
**Abscess**
  Abdomen, 49040
    Drainage, 49020, 49040
      Peritoneal
        Open, 49020
        Peritonitis, Localized, 49020
      Retroperitoneal
        Open, 49060
      Skin and Subcutaneous Tissue
        Complicated, 10061
        Multiple, 10061
        Simple, 10060
        Single, 10060
      Subdiaphragmatic
        Open, 49040
      Subphrenic, 49040
    Incision and Drainage
      Open, 49040
  Anal
    Incision and Drainage, 46045, 46050
  Ankle
    Incision and Drainage
      Bone Abscess, 27607
      Deep Abscess, 27603
      Hematoma, 27603
  Appendix
    Incision and Drainage, 44900
  Arm, Lower, 25028
    Bone Abscess, 25035
    Excision, 25145
    Incision and Drainage, 25035
    Sequestrectomy, 25145
  Arm, Upper
    Incision and Drainage, 23930-23935
  Auditory Canal, External, 69020
  Bartholin's Gland
    Incision and Drainage, 56420
  Bladder
    Incision and Drainage, 51080

© 2017 Optum360, LLC                    CPT © 2017 American Medical Association. All Rights Reserved.          [Resequenced]          Index — 1

**Abscess** — continued
Brain
Drainage by
Burr Hole, 61150, 61151
Craniotomy/Craniectomy, 61320, 61321
Excision, 61514, 61522
Incision and Drainage, 61320-61321
Breast
Incision and Drainage, 19020
Carpals
Incision, Deep, 25035
Clavicle
Sequestrectomy, 23170
Drainage
with X–ray, 75989, 76080
Contrast Injection, 49424
Ear, External
Complicated, 69005
Simple, 69000
Elbow
Incision and Drainage, 23930-23935
Sequestrectomy, 24136-24138
Epididymis
Incision and Drainage, 54700
Excision
Olecranon Process, 24138
Radius, 24136
Ulna, 24138
Eyelid
Incision and Drainage, 67700
Facial Bone(s)
Excision, 21026
Femur
with Opening Bone Cortex, 27303
Bursa, 27301
Deep Abscess, 27301
Hematoma, 27301
Finger, 26010-26011
Incision and Drainage, 26010, 26011, 26034
Foot
Incision, 28005
Gums
Incision and Drainage, 41800
Hand
Incision and Drainage, 26034
Hematoma
Incision and Drainage, 27603
Hip
Incision and Drainage, 26990-26992
Humeral Head, 23174
Humerus
Excision, 24134
Incision and Drainage, 23935
Kidney
Incision and Drainage
Open, 50020
Leg, Lower
Incision and Drainage, 27603
Bone Abscess, 27607
Liver
Incision and Drainage, 47010
Open, 47010
Injection, 47015
Marsupialization, 47300
Localization
Nuclear Medicine, 78806, 78807
Lung
Open Drainage, 32200
Lymph Node, 38300, 38305
Incision and Drainage, 38300-38305
Lymphocele
Drainage, 49062
Sclerotherapy, 49185
Mandible
Excision, 21025
Mouth
Dentoalveolar, 41800
Floor of Mouth
Extraoral, 41015-41018
Intraoral, 41000-41009
Incision and Drainage, 40800, 40801, 41005-41009, 41015-41018
Vestibule, 40800-40801

**Abscess** — continued
Nasal Septum
Incision and Drainage, 30020
Nasal
Incision and Drainage, 30000, 30020
Neck
Incision and Drainage, 21501, 21502
Nose
Incision and Drainage, 30000, 30020
Olecranon Process
Incision and Drainage, 23930-23935
Sequestrectomy, 24138
Ovarian
Incision and Drainage, 58820-58822
Abdominal Approach, 58822
Vaginal Approach, 58820
Ovary
Incision and Drainage
Abdominal Approach, 58822
Vaginal Approach, 58820
Palate
Incision and Drainage, 42000
Paraurethral Gland
Incision and Drainage, 53060
Parotid Gland
Drainage, 42300, 42305
Pelvis
Incision and Drainage, 26990-26992
Transrectal, 45000
Perineum
Incision and Drainage, 56405
Perirenal or Renal
Drainage, 50020
Peritoneum
Incision and Drainage
Open, 49020
Pharynx, 42700-42725
Posterior Spine, 22010, 22015
Prostate
Incision and Drainage, 55720-55725
Prostatotomy, 55720, 55725
Transurethral, 52700
Radius
Bone Abscess, 25035
Incision and Drainage, 25028
Incision, Deep, 25035
Sequestrectomy, 24136
Rectum
Incision and Drainage, 45005, 45020, 46040, 46060
Retroperitoneal, 49060
Drainage
Open, 49060
Salivary Gland
Drainage, 42300-42320
Scapula
Sequestrectomy, 23172
Scrotum
Incision and Drainage, 54700, 55100
Shoulder
Bone Cortex, 23035
Incision and Drainage, 23030
Skene's Gland
Incision and Drainage, 53060
Skin
Incision and Drainage, 10060-10061
Complicated, 10061
Multiple, 10061
Simple, 10060
Single, 10060
Puncture Aspiration, 10160
Soft Tissue
Catheter Drainage, 10030
Incision, 20005
Spine
Incision and Drainage, 22010-22015
Subdiaphragmatic
Incision and Drainage
Open, 49040
Sublingual Gland
Drainage, 42310, 42320
Submaxillary Gland
Drainage, 42310, 42320
Subphrenic, 49040
Testis
Incision and Drainage, 54700

**Abscess** — continued
Thigh
Incision and Drainage, 27301
Bone Abscess, 27303
Thoracostomy, 32551
Thorax
Bone Cortex, 21510
Incision and Drainage, 21501, 21502
Throat
Incision and Drainage, 42700-42725
Tongue
Incision and Drainage, 41000-41006
Tonsil
Incision and Drainage, 42700
Ulna
Incision, Deep, 25035
Urethra
Incision and Drainage, 53040
Uvula
Incision and Drainage, 42000
Vagina
Incision and Drainage, 57010
Visceral, 49405
Vulva
Incision and Drainage, 56405
Wrist
Excision, 25145
Incision and Drainage, 25028, 25035
X–ray, 76080
**Absolute Neutrophil Count (ANC)**, 85048
**Absorptiometry**
Dual Energy, 77080
Bone
Appendicular Skeleton, 77081
Axial Skeleton, 77078, 77080
Vertebral, 77080, [77086]
Ordered and Documented (PQRS), 3095F-3096F
Dual Photon
Bone, 78351
Single Photon
Bone, 78350
**Absorption Spectrophotometry**, 82190
Atomic, 82190
**ACADM**, 81400-81401
**ACADS**, 81404-81405
**ACADVL**, 81406
**ACB**, 82045
**ACBE**, 74280
**Accelerometer Data Recording, 3-Axis**, 0381T-0386T
**Access**
Small Bowel via Biliary Tree, Percutaneous, 47541
**Accessory Nerve**
Incision, 63191
Section, 63191
**Accessory, Toes**, 28344
**ACD**, 63075, 63076
**ACE (Angiotensin Converting Enzyme)**
See Angiotensin
**Acellular Immunization**, 90700
**Acetabuloplasty**, 27120, 27122, [29915]
**Acetabulum**
Fracture
with Manipulation, 27222
without Manipulation, 27220
Closed Treatment, 27220, 27222
Open Treatment, 27226-27228
Reconstruction, 27120
with Resection, Femoral Head, 27122
Tumor
Excision, 27076
**Acetaminophen**, [80329, 80330, 80331]
**Acetic Anhydrides**, 84600
**Acetone Body**, 82009, 82010
**Acetone**
Blood or Urine, 82009, 82010
**Acetylcholinesterase**
Blood or Urine, 82013
**AcG**, 85220
**Achilles Tendon**
Incision, 27605, 27606
Lengthening, 27612
Repair, 27650-27654
**Achillotomy**, 27605-27606

**ACI**, 27412, 29870
**Acid**
Adenylic, 82030
Amino
Blood or Urine, 82127-82139
Aminolevulinic
Urine or Blood, 82135
Ascorbic
Blood, 82180
Bile, 82239
Blood, 82240
Deoxyribonucleic
Antibody, 86225-86226
Diethylamide, Lysergic, 80299
Fast Bacilli (AFB)
Culture, 87116
Fast Stain, 88312
Fatty
Blood, 82725
Very Long Chain, 82726
Folic, 82746
RBC, 82747
Gastric, 82930
Glycocholic, 82240
Lactic, 83605
N-Acetylneuraminic, 84275
Perfusion Test
Esophagus, 91013, 91030
Phenylethylbarbituric
Assay, 80184
Phosphatase, 84060-84066
Probes, Nucleic
See Nucleic Acid Probe
Reflux Test, 91034-91038
Salic, 84275
Uric
Blood, 84550
Other Source, 84560
Urine, 84560
**Acidity/Alkalinity**
Blood Gasses, 82800-82805
Body Fluid, Not Otherwise Specified, 83986
Exhaled Breath Condensate, 83987
**ACL Repair**
Arthroscopy aided, 29888
Open, 27407, 27409
**Acne Surgery**
Incision and Drainage
Abscess, 10060, 10061
Puncture Aspiration, 10160
Bulla
Puncture Aspiration, 10160
Comedones, 10040
Cyst, 10040
Puncture Aspiration, 10160
Milia, Multiple, 10040
Pustules, 10040
**Acne Treatment**
Abrasion, 15786, 15787
Chemical Peel, 15788-15793
Cryotherapy, 17340
Dermabrasion, 15780-15783
Exfoliation
Chemical, 17360
**Acoustic**
Evoked Brain Stem Potential, 92585, 92586
Heart Sounds
with Computer Analysis, 93799
Immittance Testing, 92570
Neuroma
Brain Tumor Excision, 61510, 61518, 61520, 61521, 61526, 61530, 61545
Brainstem
Biopsy, 61575, 61576
Decompression, 61575, 61576
Evoked Potentials, 92585
Lesion Excision, 61575, 61576
Mesencephalon
Tractotomy, 61480
Skull Base Surgery
Anterior Cranial Fossa
Bicoronal Approach, 61586
Craniofacial Approach, 61580-61583
Extradural, 61600, 61601

CPT © 2017 American Medical Association. All Rights Reserved. | © 2017 Optum360, LLC

CPT © 2017 American Medical Association. All Rights Reserved.

© 2017 Optum360, LLC

Analysis — *continued*
  Gene — *continued*
    KCNQ2, 81406
    KDM5C, 81407
    Kennedy Disease, 81401
    KIAA0196, 81407
    Killer Cell Immunoglobulin-like Receptor (KIR), 81403
    KIT (v-kit Hardy-Zuckerman 4 feline sarcoma viral oncogene homolog), 81272
      D816 Variant, 81273
    Known Familial Variant Tier 1 or 2, NOS, 81403
    Krabbe Disease, 81401, 81406
    KRAS, 81275-81276, 81405
    L1CAM, 81407
    Lactic Acidosis, 81405-81406
    LAMA2, 81408
    LAMB2, 81407
    LAMP2, 81405
    Langer Mesomelic Dysplasia, 81405
    Laron Syndrome, 81405
    LCT (Lactose Intolerance), 81400
    LDB3, 81406
    LDLR, 81405-81406
    Leber Congenital Amaurosis, 81404, 81406
    Leber Hereditary Optic Neuropathy, 81401
    Legius Syndrome, 81405
    Leigh Syndrome, 81401, 81404-81406
    LEOPARD Syndrome, 81404, 81406, 81442
    LEPR, 81406
    Lethal Congenital Glycogen Storage Disease Heart, 81406
    Leukemia
      Acute Lymphoblastic, 81401
      Acute Lymphocytic, 81401
      Acute Myeloid, 81272, 81310, 81401, 81403
    Leukemias and Lymphomas, 81402
      B-cell, 81261-81264
      T-cell, 81340-81342
    Leukoencephalopathy, 81405-81406
    LHCGR, 81406
    Liddle Syndrome, 81406
    Li-Fraumeni Syndrome, 81405
    LINC00518, 81401
    Lissencephaly, 81405-81406
    LITAF, 81404
    LMNA, 81406
    Loeys Dietz Syndrome, 81410
    Long QT Syndrome, 81413-81414
    LRP5, 81406
    LRRK2, 81401, 81408
    Lujan Syndrome, 81401
    Lynch Syndrome, 81292-81301 *[81288]*, 81317-81319, 81403, 81435-81436
    Machado-Joseph Disease, 81401
    Macular Degeneration/Dystrophy, 81401, 81405-81406
    Male Infertility, 81403
    Malignant Hyperthermia, 81406, 81408
    Mantle Cell Lymphoma, 81401
    MAP2K1, 81406
    MAP2K2, 81406
    Maple Syrup Urine Disease, 81205, 81400, 81405-81406
    MAPT, 81406
    Marfan Syndrome, 81405, 81408, 81410
    Mastocytosis, 81273
    Maturity-Onset Diabetes of the Young (MODY), 81403-81406
    MAX, 81437
    MC4R, 81403
    McArdle Disease, 81401, 81406
    MCCC1, 81406
    MCCC2, 81406
    MCOLN1, 81290, 81412
    MECP2, 81302-81304
    MED12, 81401
    MEFV, 81402, 81404
    MEG3/DLK1, 81401

Analysis — *continued*
  Gene — *continued*
    Melanoma, 81272
      Uveal, 81403
    MEN1, 81404-81405
    Methylglutaconic Aciduria, 81406
    Methylmalonic Acidemia and Homo-cystinuria, 81404-81406
    MFN2, 81406, *[81448]*
    MGMT, *[81287]*
    MHY11, 81408, 81410-81411
    MICA, 81403
    Microsatellite Instability Analysis, 81301
    Miller-Dieker Syndrome, 81405-81406
    Mineralocorticoid Excess Syndrome, 81404
    Mitochondrial Complex Deficiency, 81404-81406
    Mitochondrial DNA Depletion Syndrome, 81404-81405
    Mitochondrial Encephalopathy (MELAS), 81401
    Mitochondrial Respiratory Chain Complex IV Deficiency, 81404-81406
    MLH1, 81292-81294 *[81288]*, 81432-81433, 81435-81436
    MLL/AFF1 (t(4,11)), 81401
    MLL/MLLT3 (t(9;11)), 81401
    MMAA, 81405
    MMAB, 81405
    MMACHC, 81404
    Mowat-Wilson Syndrome, 81404-81405
    MPI, 81405
    MPL, 81402-81403
    MPV17, 81404-81405
    MPZ, 81405, *[81448]*
    MSH2, 81295-81297, 81432-81433, 81435-81436
    MSH6, 81298-81300, 81432-81433, 81435
    MT-ATP6, 81401
    MTHFR, 81291
    MTM1, 81405-81406
    MT-ND4, 81401
    MT-ND5, 81401
    MT-ND6, 81401
    MT-RNR1, 81401, 81430
    MT-TL1, 81401
    MT-TS1, 81401, 81403
    Mucolipidosis, 81290
    Mucolipin 1, 81290
    Mucopolysaccharidosis, 81405-81406
    Muenke Syndrome, 81400
    Multiple Endocrine Neoplasia, 81404-81405
    Muscle-Eye-Brain Disease, 81405-81406
    Muscular Dystrophy
      Amyotrophic Lateral Sclerosis, 81404-81406
      Congenital, 81404, 81408
      Duchenne/Becker Muscular Dystrophy, 81408, *[81161]*
      Emery-Dreifuss, 81404-81406
      Facioscapulohumeral, 81404
      Fukuyama, 81400
      Limb-Girdle, 81404-81406, 81408
      Oculopharyngeal, 81401
      Spinal, 81400, 81403, 81405
    MUT, 81406
    MUTYH, 81401, 81406, 81435
    MYBPC3, 81407, 81439
    Myeloproliferative Disorders, 81219, 81270, 81402-81403
    MYH6, 81407
    MYH7, 81407, 81439
    MYH-associated Polyposis, 81401, 81406
    MYL2, 81405
    MYL3, 81405
    MYLK, 81410
    MYO7A, 81407, 81430
    MYO15A, 81430
    Myoclonic Dystonia, 81406
    Myoclonic Epilepsy (MERRF), 81401
    Myofibrillar Myopathy, 81405
    MYOT, 81405
    Myotonia Congenita, 81406

Analysis — *continued*
  Gene — *continued*
    Myotonic Dystrophy, 81401, 81404
    Myxoid Liposarcoma, 81401
    NDP, 81403-81404
    NDUFA1, 81404
    NDUFAF2, 81404
    NDUFS1, 81406
    NDUFS4, 81404
    NDUFS7, 81405
    NDUFS8, 81405
    NDUFV1, 81405
    NEB, 81400, 81408
    NEFL, 81405
    Nemaline Myopathy, 81408
    Neonatal Alloimmune Thrombocytopenia [NAIT], *[81105, 81106, 81107, 81108, 81109, 81110, 81111, 81112]*
    Nephrogenic Diabetes Insipidus, 81404
    Nephrotic Syndrome, 81407
      Steroid Resistant, 81405
    Neurofibromatosis, 81405-81406
    Neuropathy, *[81448]*
    NF1, 81408
    NF2, 81405-81406
    NHLRC1, 81403
    Niemann-Pick Disease, 81330, 81404, 81406
    NIPA1, 81404
    NLGN3, 81405
    NLGN4X, 81404-81405
    Nocturnal Frontal Lobe Epilepsy, 81405
    NOD2, 81401
    Nonaka Myopathy, 81400, 81406
    Non-small Cell Lung Cancer, 81401
    Nonsyndromic Hearing Loss, 81401, 81403, 81430-81431
    Noonan Spectrum Disorders, 81400, 81405-81406, 81442
    Norrie Disease, 81403-81404
    NOTCH1, 81407
    NOTCH3, 81406
    NPC1, 81404
    NPC2, 81406
    NPHP1, 81405-81406
    NPHS1, 81407
    NPHS2, 81405
    NPM1, 81310
    NPM1/ALK (t(2;5)), 81401
    NRAS, 81311
    NROB1, 81404
    NSD1, 81405-81406
    Nuclear Encoded Mitochondrial Genes, 81440
    Obesity, 81403, 81406
    Oculocutaneous Albinism (IA), 81404
    Oculomotor Apraxia, 81405
    Oncology
      Breast mRNA 81519-81521
      Cardiology (Heart Transplant), 81595
      Colon mRNA Screening, 81525
      Colorectal Screening, 81528
      Gynecologic
        Each Additional Single Drug or Drug Combination, 81536
        First Single Drug or Drug Combination, 81535
      Lung, 81538
      Ovary, 81500-81503
      Prostatic, 81539, 81541, 81551
      Thyroid, 81545
      Tissue of Origin, 81504
      Tumor, Unknown Origin, 81540
    OPA1, 81406-81407
    Optic Atrophy, 81406-81407
    OPTN, 81406
    Ornithine Transcarbamylase Deficiency, 81405
    Osteogenesis Imperfecta, 81408
    Osteoporosis, 81406
    OTC, 81405
    OTOF, 81430
    PABPN1, 81401

Analysis — *continued*
  Gene — *continued*
    PAFAH1B1, 81405-81406
    PAH, 81406
    PALB2, 81406, 81432
    Pancreatic Cancer, 81406
    PARK2, 81405-81406
    Parkinson Disease, 81401, 81405-81406, 81408
    Paroxysmal Nonkinesigenic Dyskinesia, 81406
    PAX2, 81406
    PAX8, 81401
    PC, 81406
    PCA3/KLK3, 81313
    PCCA, 81405-81406
    PCCB, 81406
    PCDH15, 81400, 81406-81407, 81430
    PCDH19, 81405
    PCSK9, 81406
    PDE6A, 81434
    PDE6B, 81434
    PDGFRA, 81314
    PDHA1, 81405-81406
    PDHB, 81405
    PDHX, 81405
    PDX1, 81404
    Pelizaeus-Merzbacher Disease, 81404-81405
    Pendred Syndrome, 81406, 81430-81431
    Peripheral Neuroectodermal Tumor, 81401
    Peripheral Neuropathy, Hereditary, *[81448]*
    Peutz-Jeghers Syndrome, 81405
    Pfeiffer Syndrome, Type 1, 81400
    Phenylketonuria, 81406
    PHEX, 81406
    PHOX2B, 81403-81404
    Pierson Syndrome, 81407
    PIK3CA, 81404
    PINK1, 81405
    Pitt-Hopkins Syndrome, 81405-81406
    PKD1, 81407
    PKD2, 81406
    PKHD1, 81408
    PKLR, 81405
    PKP2, 81406, 81439
    PLCE1, 81407
    PLN, 81403
    PLP1, 81404-81405
    PML/RARalpha, (t(15;17)), 81315-81316
    PMP22, 81324-81326
    PMS2, 81317-81319
    PNKD, 81406
    POLG, 81406
    Polycystic Kidney Disease, 81406-81408
    POMGNT1, 81406
    POMT1, 81406
    POMT2, 81406
    POU1F1, 81405
    PPARG (t(2;3)(q13;p25)), 81401
    PPOX, 81406
    PPP2R2B, 81401
    PQBP1, 81404-81405
    Prader-Willi Syndrome, 81331, 81402
    Precocious Male Puberty, 81406
    Primary Autosomal Recessive Microcephaly, 81407
    Primary Congenital Glaucoma, 81404
    Primary Microcephaly, 81407
    PRKAG2, 81406
    PRKCG, 81406
    PRNP, 81404
    Progressive External Ophthalmoplegia, 81404
    Progressive Myoclonus Epilepsy, 81403-81404
    Promyelocytic Leukemia, 81315-81316
    PROP1, 81404
    Propionic Acidemia, 81405-81406
    Prostate Cancer, 81313
    Prothrombin, Coagulation Factor II (F2), 81240
    PRPF31, 81434
    PRPH2, 81404, 81434

CPT © 2017 American Medical Association. All Rights Reserved.

© 2017 Optum360, LLC

[Resequenced] CPT © 2017 American Medical Association. All Rights Reserved. © 2017 Optum360, LLC

CPT © 2017 American Medical Association. All Rights Reserved.      © 2017 Optum360, LLC

**Antihemophilic Globulin (AHG)**, 85240
**Anti–Human Globulin Consumption Test**
  *See* Coombs Test
**Antihuman Globulin**, 86880-86886
**Anti–inflammatory/Analgesic Agent Prescribed**,
  4016F
**Antimony**, 83015
**Antinuclear Antibodies (ANA)**, 86038, 86039
  Fluorescent Technique, 86255, 86256
**Anti–Phosphatidylserine (Phospholipid) Anti-**
  **body**, 86148
**Anti–Phospholipid Antibody**, 86147
**Antiplasmin, Alpha–2**, 85410
**Antiprotease, Alpha 1**
  *See* Alpha–1 Antitrypsin
**Antistreptococcal Antibody**, 86215
**Antistreptokinase Titer**, 86590
**Antistreptolysin 0**, 86060, 86063
**Antithrombin III**, 85300, 85301
**Antithrombin VI**, 85362-85380
**Antitoxin Assay**, 87230
**Antiviral Antibody**
  *See* Viral Antibodies
**Antrostomy**
  Sinus/Maxillary, 31256-31267
**Antrotomy**
  Sinus
    Maxillary, 31020-31032
    Transmastoid, 69501
**Antrum of Highmore**
  *See* Sinus, Maxillary
**Antrum Puncture**
  Sinus
    Maxillary, 31000
    Sphenoid, 31002
**Anus**
  Ablation, 46615
  Abscess
    Incision and Drainage, 46045, 46050
  Biofeedback, 90911
  Biopsy
    Endoscopic, 46606-46607
  Crypt
    Excision, 46999
  Dilation
    Endoscopy, 46604
  Endoscopy
    Biopsy, 46606-46607
    Dilation, 46604
    Exploration, 46600
    Hemorrhage, 46614
    High Resolution Anoscopy (HRA), 46601,
      46607
    Removal
      Foreign Body, 46608
      Polyp, 46610, 46612
      Tumor, 46610, 46612
  Excision
    Tag, 46230, *[46220]*
  Exploration
    Endoscopic, 46600
    Surgical, 45990
  Fissure
    Destruction, 46940, 46942
    Excision, 46200
  Fistula
    Closure, 46288
    Excision, 46270-46285
    Repair, 46706-46707
  Hemorrhage
    Endoscopic Control, 46614
  Hemorrhoids
    Clot Excision, *[46320]*
    Destruction, 46930
    Excision, 46250-46262
    Injection, 46500
    Ligation, 0249T, 45350, 46221, *[45398]*,
      *[46945]*, *[46946]*
    Stapling, *[46947]*
    Suture, *[46945]*, *[46946]*
  High Resolution Anoscopy, 46601, 46607
  Imperforated
    Repair, 46715-46742
  Incision
    Septum, 46070
    Sphincterotomy, 46200

**Anus** — *continued*
  Lesion
    Destruction, 46900-46917, 46924
    Excision, 45108, 46922
  Manometry, 91122
  Placement
    Seton, 46020
  Polyp, 46615
  Reconstruction, 46742
    with Graft, 46753
    with Implant, 46762
    Congenital Absence, 46730-46740
    Sphincter, 46750, 46751, 46760-46762
  Removal
    Foreign Body, 46608
    Polyp(s), 46610, 46612
      Ablation, 46615
    Seton, 46030
    Suture, 46754
    Tumor(s), 46610, 46612
    Wire, 46754
  Repair
    Anovaginal Fistula, 46715, 46716
    Cloacal Anomaly, 46744-46748
    Fistula, 46706-46707
    Stricture, 46700, 46705
  Sphincter
    Chemodenervation, 46505
    Electromyography, 51784, 51785
    Needle, 51785
  Sphincterotomy, with Fissurectomy, 46200
  Thermal Energy Delivery, 46999
  Tumor, 46615
  Unlisted Procedure, 46999
**Aorta**
  Abdominal
    Aneurysm, 0254T, 34701-34712, 34830-
      34832, 34841-34848, 35081-
      35103
    Screening, 76706
    Thromboendarterectomy, 35331
  Anastomosis
    to Pulmonary Artery, 33606
  Angiogram
    Injection, 93567
  Angioplasty, *[37246, 37247, 37248, 37249]*
  Aortography, 75600-75630
  Ascending
    Graft, 33864
  Balloon
    Insertion, 33967, 33970, 33973
    Removal, 33968, 33971, 33974
  Catheterization
    Catheter, 36200
    Intracatheter, 36160
    Needle, 36160
  Circulation Assist
    Insertion, 33967, 33970, 33973
    Removal, 33968, 33971, 33974
  Conduit to Heart, 33404
  Excision
    Coarctation, 33840-33851
  Graft, 33860-33864, 33875
  Infrarenal
    Endovascular Repair, 34701-34706,
      34709-34712, 34845-34848
  Insertion
    Balloon Device, 33967, 33970, 33973
    Catheter, 36200
    Graft, 33330-33335, 33864
    Intracatheter, 36160
    Needle, 36160
  Removal
    Balloon Assist Device, 33968, 33971,
      33974
  Repair, 33320-33322, 33802, 33803
    Aneurysm
      Abdominal, 0254T, 34701-34712,
        34832, 35081-35103
      Ascending, 33860, 33863-33864
      Sinus of Valsalva, 33720
      Thoracic, 33875, 33877
        Endovascular, 33880-33891
          Radiological S&I, 75956-
            75959
      Thoracoabdominal, 33877

**Aorta** — *continued*
  Repair — *continued*
    Aneurysm — *continued*
      Transverse Arch, 33870
      Aortic Anomalies, 33800-33803
      Aortic Arch, 33852-33853
      Coarctation, 33840-33851
      Graft, 33860-33877
        Ascending, 33864
      Hypoplastic or Interrupted Aortic Arch
        with Cardiopulmonary Bypass,
          33853
        without Cardiopulmonary Bypass,
          33852
      Sinus of Valsalva, 33702-33720
      Thoracic Aneurysm with Graft, 33860-
        33877
        Endovascular, 33880-33891,
          75956-75959
      Translocation Aortic Root, 33782-33783
      Transposition of the Great Vessels,
        33770-33781
  Suspension, 33800
  Suture, 33320-33322
  Thoracic
    Aneurysm, 33880-33889, 75956-75959
    Repair, 75956-75959
    Endovascular, 33880-33891
  Thromboendarterectomy, 35331
  Ultrasound, 76706, 76770, 76775
  Valve
    Implantation, 33361-33369
    Incision, 33415
    Repair, 33390-33391
      Gusset Aortoplasty, 33417
      Left Ventricle, 33414
      Stenosis
        Idiopathic Hypertrophic,
          33416
        Subvalvular, 33415
        Supravalvular, 33417
      Valvuloplasty
        Open
          with Cardiopulmonary
            Bypass, 33390
          Complex, 33391
    Replacement
      with Allograft Valve, 33406
      with Aortic Annulus Enlargement,
        33411-33412
      with Cardiopulmonary Bypass,
        33367-33369, 33405-
        33406, 33410
      with Prosthesis, 33361-33369,
        33405
      with Stentless Tissue Valve, 33410
      with Translocation Pulmonary
        Valve, 33413
      Open, 33405-33413
      Transcatheter, 33361-33369
    Visceral
      Endovascular Repair, 34841-34848
  X-ray with Contrast, 75600-75630
**Aorta–Pulmonary ART Transposition**
  *See* Transposition, Great Arteries
**Aortic Sinus**
  *See* Sinus of Valsalva
**Aortic Stenosis**
  Repair, 33415
    Nikaidoh Procedure, 33782-33783
    Supravalvular, 33417
**Aortic Valve Replacement**
  *See* Replacement, Aortic Valve
**Aortic Valve**
  *See* Heart, Aortic Valve
**Aortocoronary Bypass for Heart Revasculariza-**
  **tion**
  *See* Artery, Coronary, Bypass
**Aortocoronary Bypass**
  *See* Coronary Artery Bypass Graft (CABG)
**Aortography**, 75600, 75605, 75630, 93567
  with Iliofemoral Artery, 75630, 75635
  *See* Angiography
  Serial, 75625
**Aortoiliac**
  Embolectomy, 34151, 34201

**Aortoiliac** — *continued*
  Thrombectomy, 34151, 34201
**Aortopexy**, 33800
**Aortoplasty**
  Supravalvular Stenosis, 33417
**AP**, *[51797]*
**APBI (Accelerated Partial Breast Irradiation)**,
  19296-19298
**APC**, 81201-81203, 81435
**Apert–Gallais Syndrome**
  *See* Adrenogenital Syndrome
**Apexcardiogram**, 93799
**Aphasia Testing**, 96105
**Apheresis**
  Therapeutic, 36511-36516
    with Selective HDL Delipidation and
      Plasma Reinfusion, 0342T
**Apical–Aortic Conduit**, 33404
**Apicectomy**
  with Mastoidectomy, 69530, 69605
  Petrous, 69530
**Apicoectomy**, 41899
**Apnea**
  Central
    Neurostimulator System, 0424T-0436T
**Apoaminotransferase, Aspartate**, 84550
**APOB**, 81401
**APOE**, 81401
**Apolipoprotein**
  Blood or Urine, 82172
**APP**, 81406
**Appendectomy**, 44950-44960
  Laparoscopic, 44970
**Appendiceal Abscess**
  *See* Abscess, Appendix
**Appendico–Stomy**, 44799
**Appendico–Vesicostomy**
**Appendico-Vesicostomy**, 50845
  Cutaneous, 50845
**Appendix**
  Abscess
    Incision and Drainage, 44900
  Excision, 44950-44960
  Incision and Drainage
    Open, 44900
  Laparoscopic, 44970
**Application of External Fixation Device**
  *See* Fixation (Device), Application, External
**Application**
  Allergy Tests, 95044
  Bone Fixation Device
    Multiplane, 20692
    Stereo Computer Assisted, 20696-20697
    Uniplane, 20690
  Caliper, 20660
  Casts, 29000-29086, 29305-29450
  Compression System, 29581-29584
  Cranial Tongs, 20660
  Fixation Device
    Shoulder, 23700
  Halo
    Cranial, 20661
      Thin Skull Osteology, 20664
    Femoral, 20663
    Maxillofacial Fixation, 21100
    Pelvic, 20662
  Injector
    Subcutaneous, On-body, 96377
  Interbody Biomechanical Device, 22853
  Interdental Fixation Device, 21110
  Interlaminar/Interspinous Stabilization/Distrac-
    tion Device, 22867-22870
  Intervertebral Biomechanical Device, 22854,
    22859
  Multi-layer Compression System, 29581-29584
  Neurostimulation, 64550, 64566
    On-body Injector, 96377
  Pulmonary Artery Bands, 33620
  Radioelement
    with Ultrasound, 76965
    Interstitial or Intracavitary, 77761-77763,
      77770-77772
    Surface, 77767-77768, 77789
  Skin Substitute, 15271-15278
  Splint, 29105-29131, 29505-29515
  Stereotactic Frame, 20660, 61800

Index

Audiometry — Benign Neoplasm of Cranial Nerves

[Resequenced]
CPT © 2017 American Medical Association. All Rights Reserved.
© 2017 Optum360, LLC

**Blood Letting**
See Phlebotomy
**Blood Lipoprotein**
See Lipoprotein
**Blood, Occult**
See Occult Blood
**Blood Pressure**
Baroactivation Device, 0266T-0273T
Central Arterial Analysis, Non-Invasive, 93050
Diastolic, 3078F-3080F
Monitoring, 24 hour, 93784-93990
Systolic, 3074F-3075F
Venous, 93770
**Blood Serum**
See Serum
**Blood Transfusion, Autologous**
See Autotransfusion
**Blood Vessel(s)**
See Artery; Vein
Angioscopy
Noncoronary, 35400
Endoscopy
Surgical, 37500-37501
Endothelial Function Assessment, 0337T
Excision
Arteriovenous
Malformation, 63250-63252
Exploration
Abdomen, 35840
Carotid Artery, 35701
Chest, 35820
Extremity, 35860
Femoral Artery, 35721
Neck, 35800
Other Vessel, 35761
Popliteal Artery, 35741
Great
Suture, 33320-33322
Harvest
Endoscopic, 33508
Lower Extremity Vein, 35572
Upper Extremity Artery, 35600
Upper Extremity Vein, 35500
Kidney
Repair, 50100
Repair
Abdomen, 35221, 35251, 35281
with Composite Graft, 35681-
35683
with Other Graft, 35281
with Vein Graft, 35251
See Aneurysm Repair; Fistula, Re-
pair
Aneurysm, 61705-61710
Aorta, 33320-33322
Arteriovenous Malformation, 61680-
61692, 61705-61710, 63250-
63252
Chest, 35211, 35216
with Composite Graft, 35681-
35683
with Other Graft, 35271, 35276
with Vein Graft, 35241, 35246
Direct, 35201-35226
Finger, 35207
Graft Defect, 35870
Great Vessels, 33320-33322
Hand, 35207
Intraabdominal, 35221, 35251, 35281
Intrathoracic, 35211, 35216, 35241,
35246, 35271, 35276
Kidney, 50100
Lower Extremity, 35226, 35256, 35286
with Composite Graft, 35681-
35683
with Other Graft, 35281
with Vein Graft, 35256
Neck, 35201
with Composite Graft, 35681-
35683
with Other Graft, 35261
with Vein Graft, 35231
Upper Extremity, 35206, 35236, 35266
with Composite Graft, 35681-
35683
with Other Graft, 35266

**Blood Vessel(s)** — continued
Repair — continued
Upper Extremity — continued
with Vein Graft, 35236
Shunt Creation
with Bypass Graft, 35686
with Graft, 36825, 36830
with Transposition, 36818-36820
Direct, 36821
Thomas Shunt, 36835
Shunt Revision
with Graft, 36832
Suture Repair, Great Vessels, 33320-33322
**Blood**
Banking
Frozen Blood Preparation, 86930-86932,
88240
Frozen Plasma Preparation, 86927
Physician Services, 86077-86079
Bleeding Time, 85002
Blood Clot
Assay, 85396
Clotting
Factor Test, 85210
Factor, 85250-85293
Inhibitors, 85300-85301
Coagulation Time, 85345-85348
Lysis Time, 85175
Retraction, 85170
Thrombolytic Agents
Tissue Plasminogen Activator (tPA),
4077F
Cell Count
Automated, 85049
B-Cells, 86355
Blood Smear, 85007, 85008
Complete Blood Count (CBC), 85025,
85027
Differential WBC Count, 85004-85007,
85009
Hematocrit, 85014
Hemoglobin, 85018
Hemogram
Added Indices, 85025-85027
Automated, 85025-85027
Manual, 85032
Microhematocrit, 85013
Natural Killer (NK) Cells, 86357
Red Blood Cells, 85032-85041
Red
See Red Blood Cell (RBC), Count
Reticulocyte, 85044-85046
Stem Cells, 86367
T Cell, 86359-86361
White Blood Cell, 85032, 85048, 89055
White
See White Blood Cell, Count
Cell
CD4 and CD8
Including Ratio, 86360
Enzyme Activity, 82657
Exchange, 36511-36513
Sedimentation Rate
Automated, 85652
Manual, 85651
Clot
Assay, 85396
Activity, 85397
ADAMTS-13, 85397
Clot Lysis Time, 85175
Clot Retraction, 85170
Clotting Factor Test, 85210-85244
Clotting Factor, 85250-85293
Clotting Inhibitors, 85300-85303, 85305-
85307, 85335, 85337
Coagulation Time, 85345-85348
Factor Inhibitor Test, 85335
Coagulation
Factor I, 85384, 85385
Factor II, 85210
Factor III, 85730, 85732
Factor IV, 82310
Factor IX, 85250
Factor V, 85220
Factor VII, 85230
Factor VIII, 85244, 85247

**Blood** — continued
Coagulation — continued
Factor X, 85260
Factor XI, 85270
Factor XIII, 85290, 85291
Collection, for Autotransfusion
Intraoperative, 86891
Preoperative, 86890
Feces, 82270, 82272
by Hemoglobin Immunoassay, 82274
Flow Check
Graft, 15860, 90940
Gases
by Pulse Oximetry, 94760
CO2, 82803
HCO3, 82803
Hemoglobin–Oxygen Affinity, 82820
O2 Saturation, 82805, 82810
O2, 82803-82810
pCO2, 82803
pH, 82800, 82803
pO2, 82803, 82820
Gastric Contents, 82271
Harvesting of Stem Cells, 38205-38206
Hemoglobin A1c (HbA1c) Level, 3044F-3046F
Hemoglobin
Concentration, 85046
Quantitative, 88740
Transcutaneous
Carboxyhemoglobin, 88740
Methemoglobin, 88741
Injection
Plasma, 0232T
Nuclear Medicine
Flow Imaging, 78445
Red Cell Survival, 78130, 78135
Red Cell, 78140
Occult, 82270
Osmolality, 83930
Other Sources, 82271
Patch, 62273
Plasma
Exchange, 36514-36516
Frozen Preparation, 86927
Injection, 0232T
Volume, 78110-78111
Platelet
Aggregation, 85576
Automated Count, 85049
Count, 85008
Manual Count, 85032
Phospholipid Neutralization, 85597-
85598
Pool Imaging, 78472, 78473, 78481, 78483,
78494, 78496
Products
Irradiation, 86945
Pooling, 86965
Splitting, 86985
Volume Reduction, 86960
Reticulocyte, 85046
Sample
Fetal, 59030
Smear, 85060
Microorganism Identification, 87205-
87207
Microscopic Examination, 85007-85008
Peripheral, 85060
Sex Chromatin, 88140
Surgical Pathology, 88312-88313, 88319
Stem Cell
Count, 86367
Donor Search, 38204
Erythropoietin Therapy, 3160F, 4090F-
4095F
Harvesting, 38205-38206
Preparation, 38207-38209
Transplantation, 38240-38242
Cell Concentration, 38215
Cryopreservation, 38207, 88240
Plasma Depletion, 38214
Platelet Depletion, 38213
Red Blood Cell Depletion, 38212
T-cell Depletion, 38210
Thawing, 38208-38209, 38241
Tumor Cell Depletion, 38211

**Blood** — continued
Stem Cell — continued
Transplantation — continued
Washing, 38209
Test(s)
Iron Stores, 3160F
Kt/V, 3082F-3084F
Nuclear Medicine
Plasma Volume, 78110, 78111
Platelet Survival, 78191
Red Cell Survival, 78130, 78135
Red Cell Volume, 78120, 78121
Whole Blood Volume, 78122
Panels
Electrolyte, 80051
General Health Panel, 80050
Hepatic Function, 80076
Hepatitis, Acute, 80074
Lipid Panel, 80061
Metabolic Panel, Basic
Basic, 80047-80048
Comprehensive, 80053
Ionized Calcium, 80047
Total Calcium, 80048
Obstetric Panel, 80055, [80081]
Renal Function, 80069
Volume Determination, 78122
Transcutaneous
Carboxyhemoglobin, 88740
Methemoglobin, 88741
Transfusion, 36430, 36440
Exchange, 36455
Newborn, 36450
Partial, 36456
Fetal, 36460
Push
Infant, 36440
Typing
ABO Only, 86900
Antigen Testing, 86902, 86904
Crossmatch, 86920-86923
Other RBC Antigens, 86905
Paternity Testing, 86910, 86911
Rh Phenotype, 86906
Rh(D), 86901
Unlisted Services and Procedures, 85999
Urea Nitrogen, 84520, 84525
Urine, 83491
Viscosity, 85810
Volume
Plasma, 78110-78111
Red Blood Cells, 78120-78121
Whole Blood, 78122
**Bloom Syndrome**
Chromosome Analysis, 88245
Gene Analysis, 81209
Genomic Sequencing Analysis, 81412
**Blot Test, Ink**
See Inkblot Test
**Blotting, Western**
See Western Blot
**Blount Osteotomy**, 27455, 27475-27485
**Blow–Out Fracture**
Orbital Floor, 21385-21395
**Blue, Dome Cyst**
See Breast, Cyst
**BMAC (Breath Methylated Alkane Contour)**, 0085T
**BMPR1A**, 81435
**BMPR2**, 81405-81406
**BMT**, 38240, 38241, 38242
**Boarding Home Care**, 99324-99337
**Bodies, Acetone**
See Acetone Body
**Bodies, Barr**
See Barr Bodies
**Bodies, Carotid**
See Carotid Body
**Bodies, Ciliary**
See Ciliary Body
**Bodies, Heinz**
See Heinz Bodies
**Bodies, Inclusion**
See Inclusion Bodies
**Bodies, Ketone**
See Ketone Bodies

CPT © 2017 American Medical Association. All Rights Reserved.

© 2017 Optum360, LLC

**Brain** — *continued*
  Coverings
    Tumor
      Excision, 61512, 61519
  Craniopharyngioma, 61545
    Excision, 61545
  CT Scan, 0042T, 70450-70470, 70496
  Cyst
    Drainage, 61150, 61151, 62161, 62162
    Excision, 61516, 61524, 62162
  Death Determination, 95824
  Debridement, 62010
  Doppler Transcranial, 93886-93893
  Electrocorticography, 61536, 61538, 61539
  Electroencephalography
    Cerebral Death Evaluation, 95824
    Monitored, 95812-95813
    Recorded, 95816, 95819, 95822, 95827
  Epileptogenic Focus
    Excision, 61534, 61536
    Monitoring, 61531, 61533, 61535, 61760
  Excision
    Amygdala, 61566
    Choroid Plexus, 61544
    Craniopharyngioma, 61545
    Hemisphere, 61543
    Hemispherectomy, 61543
    Hippocampus, 61566
    Meningioma, 61512, 61519
    Other Lobe, 61323, 61539, 61540
    Temporal Lobe, 61537, 61538
  Exploration
    Infratentorial, 61305
    Supratentorial, 61304
  Hematoma
    Drainage, 61154
    Incision and Drainage, 61312-61315
  Implantation
    Chemotherapeutic Agent, 61517
    Electrode, 61210, 61850-61870
    Pulse Generator, 61885, 61886
    Receiver, 61885, 61886
    Reservoir, 61210, 61215
    Thermal Perfusion Probe, 61107, 61210
  Incision
    Corpus Callosum, 61541
    Mesencephalic Tract, 61480
    Subpial, 61567
  Infusion, 64999, 95990-95991
  Insertion
    Catheter, 61210
    Electrode, 61531, 61533, 61850-61870
    Pulse Generator, 61885, 61886
    Receiver, 61885, 61886
    Reservoir, 61210, 61215
  Lesion
    Aspiration, Stereotactic, 61750, 61751
    Excision, 61534, 61536, 61600-61608, 61615, 61616
  Lobectomy, 61537-61540
  Magnetic Resonance Imaging (MRI), 70551-70555
    Intraoperative, 0398T
  Magnetic Stimulation
    Transcranial, 90867-90869
  Magnetoencephalography, 95965-95967
  Mapping, 90867-90869, 95961-95962, 96020
    Motor Function, 64999
  Meningioma
    Excision, 61512, 61519
  Myelography, 70010
  Neurostimulation
    Analysis, 95970-95982
    Electrode
      Implantation, 61210, 61850, 61860, 61863-61864, 61870
      Removal, 61880
      Revision, 61880
    Pulse Generator
      Insertion, 61885-61886
      Removal, 61880
      Revision, 61880
  Nuclear Medicine
    Blood Flow, 78610
    Cerebrospinal Fluid, 78630-78650
    Imaging, 78600-78607

**Brain** — *continued*
  Nuclear Medicine — *continued*
    Imaging — *continued*
      Vascular Flow, 78610
      Shunt Evaluation, 78645
  Perfusion Analysis, 0042T
  Positron Emission Tomography (PET), 78608, 78609
  Radiosurgery
    for Lesion, 61796-61800
    Radiation Treatment Delivery, 77371-77373
  Removal
    Electrode, 61535, 61880
    Foreign Body, 61570, 62163
    Pulse Generator, 61888
    Receiver, 61888
    Shunt, 62256, 62258
  Repair
    Dura, 61618
    Wound, 61571
  Shunt
    Creation, 62180-62192, 62200-62223
    Removal, 62256, 62258
    Replacement, 62160, 62194, 62225-62258
    Reprogramming, 62252
  Skull Base
    Craniofacial Approach, 61580-61585
    Infratemporal Approach, 61590, 61591
    Orbitocranial Zygomatic Approach, 61592
  Skull
    Transcochlear Approach, 61596
    Transcondylar Approach, 61597
    Transpetrosal Approach, 61598
    Transtemporal Approach, 61595
  Stem Auditory Evoked Potential, 92585-92586
  Stereotactic
    Aspiration, 61750, 61751
    Biopsy, 61750, 61751
    Catheter Placement, 64999
    Computer Assisted Navigation, 61781-61782
    Create Lesion, 61720, 61735, 61790, 61791
    Localization for Placement Therapy Fields, 61770
    Navigation, 61781-61782
    Procedure, 61781-61782
    Radiation Treatment, 77432
    Radiosurgery, 61796-61800, 63620-63621, 77371-77373, 77435
    Trigeminal Tract, 61791
  Surface Electrode
    Stimulation, 95961-95962
  Transcranial Magnetic Stimulation (TMS), 90867-90869
  Transection
    Subpial, 61541, 61567
  Tumor
    Excision, 61510, 61518, 61520, 61521, 61526, 61530, 61545, 62164
  Ventriculocisternostomy, 62200-62201
    Torkildsen Type, 62180
  X-ray with Contrast, 70010, 70015

**Brainstem (Brain Stem)**
  *See* Brain
  Auditory Implant, 92640
  Biopsy, 61575, 61576
  Decompression, 61575, 61576
  Evoked Potentials, 92585, 92586
  Lesion
    Excision, 61575, 61576

**Branched-Chain Keto Acid Dehydrogenase E1, Beta Polypeptide Gene Analysis**, 81205
**Branchial Cleft**
  Cyst
    Excision, 42810, 42815
**Branchioma**
  *See* Branchial Cleft, Cyst
**Braun Procedure**, 23405-23406
**BRCA1, BRCA 2**, 81211-81213, 81432-81433, *[81162]*
**BRCA1**, 81214-81215
**BRCA2**, 81216-81217

**Breast**
  Ablation
    Cryosurgery, 19105
    Fibroadenoma, 19105
  Abscess
    Incision and Drainage, 19020
  Augmentation, 19324, 19325
  Biopsy, 19100-19101
    with Localization Device Placement, 19081-19086
      MRI Guided, 19085-19086
      Stereotactic Guided, 19081-19082
      Ultrasound Guided, 19083-19084
    with Specimen Imaging, 19085-19086
    ABBI, 19081-19086
  Cancer Gene Analysis, 81211-81217, 81402, 81406, 81432-81433, *[81162]*
  Catheter Placement for Application Interstitial Radioelement, 19296-19298
  Catheter Placement
    for Interstitial Radioelement Application, 19296-19298, 20555, 41019
  Cryosurgical Ablation, 19105
  Cyst
    Excision, 19120
    Puncture Aspiration, 19000, 19001
  Excision
    Biopsy, 19100-19101
    Capsules, 19371
    Chest Wall Tumor, 19260-19272
    Cyst, 19120
    Lactiferous Duct Fistula, 19112
    Lesion, 19120-19126
      Needle Localization, 19125-19126
    Mastectomy, 19300-19307
    Nipple Exploration, 19110
    Tumors, 19120, 19260, 19271-19272
  Exploration
    Abscess, 19020
    Nipple, 19110
  Implants
    Insertion, 19325, 19340, 19342
    Preparation of Moulage, 19396
    Removal, 19328, 19330
    Soft Tissue Reinforcement, 15777
    Supply, 19396
  Incision
    Capsules, 19370
  Injection
    Radiologic, 19030
  Magnetic Resonance Imaging (MRI), 77058-77059
    with Computer-aided Detection, 0159T
  Mammography, 77065-77067
    Bilateral, 77066-77067
    Computer-Aided Detection, 77065-77067
    Ductogram, 77053-77054
    Galactogram, 77053-77054
      Injection, 19030
    Results Documented and Reviewed, 3014F
    Screening, 3014F, 77067
    Tactile Imaging, 0422T
    Unilateral, 77065
  Mammoplasty
    Augmentation, 19324, 19325
    Reduction, 19318
  Mastectomy
    Complete, 19303
    Gynecomastia, 19300
    Modified Radical, 19307
    Partial, 19301-19302
    Radical, 19303-19306
    Subcutaneous, 19304
      with Axillary Lymphadenectomy, 19302
  Mastopexy, 19316
  Metallic Localization Clip Placement, 19281-19288
  Needle Biopsy, 19100
  Needle Wire Placement, 19281-19288
  Periprosthetic Capsulectomy, 19371
  Periprosthetic Capsulotomy, 19370
  Reconstruction, 19357-19369
    with Free Flap, 19364

**Breast** — *continued*
  Reconstruction — *continued*
    with Latissimus Dorsi Flap, 19361
    with Other Techniques, 19366
    with Tissue Expander, 19357
    with Transverse Rectus Abdominis Myocutaneous (TRAM) Flap, 19367-19369
    Augmentation, 19324, 19325
    Mammoplasty, 19318-19325
    Myocutaneous Flap, 19367-19369
    Nipple and Areola, 19350
      Correction Inverted Nipples, 19355
    Nipple, 19350-19355
    Areola, 19350
    Revision, 19380
  Reduction, 19318
  Removal
    Capsules, 19371
    Modified Radical, 19307
    Partial, 19300-19302
    Radical, 19305-19306
    Simple, Complete, 19303
    Subcutaneous, 19304
  Repair
    Suspension, 19316
  Stereotactic Localization, 19081, 19283
  Tactile Imaging, 0422T
  Tomosynthesis, 77061-77063
  TRAM, 19367-19369
  Tumor
    Excision
      with Ribs, 19260, 19271-19272
      Benign, 19120
      Chest Wall, 19260, 19271-19272
      Malignant, 19120
  Microwave Thermotherapy, 19499
  Ultrasound, 76641-76642
  Unlisted Services and Procedures, 19499
  X-ray
    with Computer-aided Detection, 77065-77067
    Mammography
      Bilateral, Diagnostic, 77065
      Screening, 77067
      Unilateral, Diagnostic, 77066
    Placement Localization Device, 19281-19288
**Breath Methylated Alkane Contour**, 0085T
**Breath Odor Alcohol**
  *See* Alcohol, Breath
**Breath Test**
  Alcohol, Ethyl, 82075
  Heart Transplant Rejection, 0085T
  Helicobacter Pylori, 78267, 78268, 83013, 83014
  Hydrogen, 91065
  Methane, 91065
  Urea, 78267-78268
**Breathing, Inspiratory Positive-Pressure**
  *See* Intermittent Positive Pressure Breathing (IPPB)
**Bricker Operation**
  Intestines Anastomosis, 50820
**Brisement Injection**, 20550-20551
**Bristow Procedure**, 23450-23462
  Capsulorrhaphy, Anterior, 23450-23462
**Brock Operation**, 33470-33475
  Valvotomy, Pulmonary Valve, 33470-33474
**Broken, Nose**
  *See* Fracture, Nasal Bone
**Bronchi**
  Allograft, 32855-32856
  Aspiration
    Catheter, 31720-31725
    Endoscopic, 31629, 31633, 31645-31646
  Biopsy
    Endoscopic, 31625-31629, 31632, 31633
  Bronchial Valve
    Insertion, 31647, *[31651]*
    Removal, 31648-31649
  Bronchodilator
    Home Care, 99503
    Spirometry, 94012, 94060
  Brushing
    Protected Brushing, 31623

**Bronchi** — continued
  Catheterization
    with Bronchial Brush Biopsy, 31717
    Insertion
      with Intracavitary Radioelement,
        31643
  Endoscopy
    Ablation
      Photodynamic Therapy, 96570-
        96571
    Aspiration, 31645, 31646
    Biopsy, 31625, 31628, 31629, 31632,
      31633
    Bronchial Valve Insertion, 31647, [31651]
    Destruction
      Tumor, 31641
    Dilation, 31630-31631, 31636-31638
    Excision
      Lesion, 31640
    Exploration, 31622
      with Balloon Occlusion, 31634,
        31647, [31651]
    Foreign Body Removal, 31635
    Fracture, 31630
    Lesion, 31640, 31641
    Stenosis, 31641
    Tumor, 31640, 31641
  Exploration
    Endoscopic, 31622
  Fracture
    Endoscopy, 31630
  Needle Biopsy, 31629, 31633
  Reconstruction
    Anastomosis, 31775, 32486
    Graft Repair, 31770
    Stenosis, 31775
  Removal
    Foreign Body, 31635
  Repair
    Fistula, 32815, 32906
    Stenosis, 31641, 96570-96571
  Stenosis
    Endoscopic Treatment, 31641
  Stent
    Placement, 31636-31637
    Revision, 31638
  Testing
    Airway Sizing, 31647, [31651]
    Assessment Air Leak, 31647, [31651]
    Bronchospasm Evaluation, 94070, 94617
    Pulmonary Stress Test, 94618
  Tests
    with Antigens, Gases, 95070
    with Chemicals, 95071
  Tumor
    Excision, 31640
  Unlisted Services and Procedures, 31899
**Bronchial Allergen Challenge**
  *See* Bronchial Challenge Test
**Bronchial Alveolar Lavage**, 31624
**Bronchial Brush Biopsy**
  with Catheterization, 31717
**Bronchial Brushings**
  Protected Brushing, 31623
**Bronchial Challenge Test**
  with Antigens or Gases, 95070
  with Chemicals, 95071
  *See also* Allergy Tests
**Bronchial Provocation Test**
  *See* Allergy Tests, Challenge Test, Bronchial
**Bronchoalveolar Lavage**, 31624
**Broncho–Bronchial Anastomosis**, 32486
**Bronchoplasty**, 32501
  Excision Stenosis and Anastomosis, 31775
  Graft Repair, 31770
  Reconstruction, Bronchi, 32501
    Graft Repair, 31770
    Stenosis, 31775
**Bronchopneumonia, Hiberno–Vernal**
  *See* Q Fever
**Bronchopulmonary Lavage**, 31624
**Bronchoscopy**
  Ablation
    Photodynamic Therapy, 96570-96571
  Airway Resizing, 31647, [31651]
  Alveolar Lavage, 31624

**Bronchoscopy** — continued
  Aspiration, 31629, 31633, 31645-31646, 31725
  Assessment Airway Leak, 31647, [31651]
  Balloon Occlusion, 31634, 31647, [31651]
  Biopsy, 31625-31629, 31632, 31633
  Brushing, Protected Brushing, 31623
  Catheter Placement
    Intracavity Radioelement, 31643
  Computer-assisted Image-Guided Navigation,
    31627
  Diagnostic, 31622-31624, 31643
  Dilation, 31630-31631, 31636-31638
  Exploration, 31622
    with Balloon Occlusion, 31634, 31647,
      [31651]
  Fiducial Marker Placement, 31626
  Foreign Body Removal, 31635
  Fracture, 31630
  Insertion Bronchial Valve(s), 31647, 31651
  Needle Biopsy, 31629, 31633
  Removal
    Bronchial Valve(s), 31648-31649
    Foreign Body, 31635
    Tumor, 31640, 31641
  Stenosis, 31641
  Stent Placement, 31631, 31636-31637
  Stent Revision, 31638
  Thermoplasty, 31660-31661
  Tumor
    Destruction, 31641
    Excision, 31640
  via Existing Tracheostomy, 31615
**Bronchospasm Evaluation**, 94060, 94070
  Exercise Test, 94617
  Pulmonology, Diagnostic, Spirometry, 94010-
    94070
**Bronkodyl**
  *See* Theophylline
**Brow Ptosis**
  Repair, 67900
    Reduction of Overcorrection, 67909
**Browne's Operation**, 54324
**Brucella**, 86000
  Antibody, 86622
**Bruise**
  *See* Hematoma
**Brunschwig Operation**, 58240
  Pelvis, Exenteration, 58240
**Brush Biopsy**
  Bronchi, 31717
**Brush Border ab**
  *See* Antibody, Heterophile
**BSCL2**, 81406, [81448]
**BSO**, 58720
**BTD**, 81404
**BTK**, 81406
**Bucca**
  *See* Cheek
**Buccal Mucosa**
  *See* Mouth, Mucosa
**Bulbourethral Gland**
  Excision, 53250
**Bulla**
  Incision and Drainage
    Puncture Aspiration, 10160
  Lung
    Excision–Plication, 32141
    Endoscopic, 32655
**BUN**, 84520-84545
**Bunion Repair**
  with First Metatarsal Medial Cuneiform
    Arthrodesis, 28297
  with Implant, 28291
  with Metatarsal Osteotomy, 28295, 28296
  with Tendon Transplants, 28899
  Bunionectomy, 28299
  Phalanx Osteotomy, 28298-28299
  Simple Ostectomy, 28292
**Bunionectomy**
  with First Metatarsal Medial Cuneiform
    Arthrodesis, 28297
  with Implant, 28291
  with Metatarsal Osteotomy, 28295, 28296
  with Tendon Transplants, 28899
  Phalanx Osteotomy, 28298-28299
  Simple Exostectomy, 28292

**Bunnell Procedure**, 24301
**Burch Operation**, 51840-51841
  Laparoscopic, 58152
**Burgess Amputation**
  Disarticulation, Ankle, 27889
**Burhenne Procedure**, 43500
  Bile Duct, Removal of Calculus, 43264, 47420,
    47425, 47554
**Burkitt Herpes Virus**
  *See* Epstein–Barr Virus
**Burns**
  Anesthesia, 01951-01953
  Debridement, 01951-01953, 15002-15003,
    15004-15005, 16020-16030
  Dressing, 16020-16030
  Escharotomy, 15002-15005, 16035-16036
  Excision, 01951-01953, 15002, 15004-15005
  First Degree Burn, Initial Treatment, 16000
  Initial Treatment, 16000
  Tissue Culture Skin Grafts, 15100-15157
**Burr Hole**
  Anesthesia, 00214
  Skull
    with Injection, 61120
    Aspiration
      Cyst, 61156
      Hematoma, 61156
    Biopsy, Brain, 61140
      Stereotactic, 61750-61751
    Catheterization, 61210
    Drainage
      Abscess, 61150, 61151
      Cyst, 61150, 61151
      Hematoma, 61154, 61156
    Exploration
      Infratentorial, 61253
      Supratentorial, 61250
    Implant
      Catheter, 61210
      Cerebral Monitoring Device, 61210
      Cerebral Thermal Perfusion Probe,
        61107, 61210
      Device for Pressure Recording,
        61210
      EEG Electrode, 61210
      Neurostimulator Array, 61850,
        61863-61868
      Strip Electrodes, 61531
    Injection, Contrast Media, 61120
    Insertion
      Catheter, 61210
      Pump, 61210
      Reservoir, 61210
    Lesion Creation, 61720
    Stereotactic Localization, 61770
    Ventricular Puncture, 61020
      Contrast Media Injection, 61120
      Diagnostic or Therapeutic Injection,
        61026
**Burrow's Operation**, 14000-14350
**Bursa**
  Ankle
    Aspiration, 20605-20606
    Incision and Drainage, 27604
    Injection, 20605-20606
  Arm, Lower
    Aspiration, 20605-20606
    Incision and Drainage, 25031
    Injection, 20605-20606
  Elbow
    Aspiration, 20605-20606
    Excision, 24105
    Incision and Drainage, 23931
    Injection, 20605-20606
  Femur
    Excision, 27062
  Finger
    Aspiration, 20600-20604
    Injection, 20600-20604
  Foot
    Incision and Drainage, 28001
  Hand
    Incision and Drainage, 26025-26030
  Hip
    Aspiration, 20610-20611
    Incision and Drainage, 26991

**Bursa** — continued
  Hip — continued
    Injection, 20610-20611
  Injection, 20600-20611
  Ischial
    Excision, 27060
  Joint
    Aspiration, 20600-20611
    Drainage, 20600-20610
    Injection, 20600-20611
  Knee
    Aspiration, 20610-20611
    Excision, 27340
    Incision and Drainage, 27301
    Injection, 20610-20611
  Leg
    Lower, 27604
    Upper, 27301
  Palm
    Incision and Drainage, 26025, 26030
  Pelvis
    Incision and Drainage, 26991
  Shoulder
    Aspiration, 20610-20611
    Drainage, 23031
    Injection, 20610-20611
  Toe
    Aspiration, 20600-20604
    Injection, 20600-20604
  Wrist
    Aspiration, 20605-20606
    Excision, 25115, 25116
    Incision and Drainage, 25031
    Injection, 20605-20606
**Bursectomy**
  of Hand, 26989
**Bursitis, Radiohumeral**
  *See* Tennis Elbow
**Bursocentesis**
  *See* Aspiration, Bursa
**Buttock**
  Excision
    Excess Skin, 15835
**Button**
  Bone Graft, 20900
  Nasal Septal Prosthesis, 30220
  Voice Prosthesis, 31611
**Butyrylcholine Esterase**
  *See* Cholinesterase
**Bypass Graft**
  with Composite Graft, 35681-35683
  Autogenous
    Three or More Segments
      Two Locations, 35683
    Two Segments
      Two Locations, 35682
  Aortobifemoral, 35540, 35646
  Aortobi-iliac, 35538, 35638
  Aortocarotid, 35526, 35626
  Aortoceliac, 35531, 35631
  Aortofemoral, 35539, 35647
  Aortoiliac, 35537, 35637
  Aortoinnominate, 35526, 35626
  Aortomesenteric, 35531, 35631
  Aortorenal, 35560, 35631
  Aortosubclavian, 35526, 35626
  Axillary Artery, 35516-35522, 35533, 35616-
    35623, 35650, 35654
  Brachial Artery, 35510, 35512, 35522-35525
  Brachial-Ulnar or -Radial, 35523
  Carotid Artery, 33891, 35501-35510, 35601,
    35606, 35642
  Celiac Artery, 35341, 35631-35632
  Coronary Artery
    Arterial, 33533-33536
    Arterial-Venous, 33517-33519, 33521-
      33523, 33530
    Venous Graft, 33510-33516
  Excision
    Abdomen, 35907
    Extremity, 35903
    Neck, 35901
    Thorax, 35905
  Femoral Artery, 35521, 35533, 35539, 35540,
    35556, 35558, 35566, 35621, 35646,
    35647, 35654-35661, 35666, 35700

CPT © 2017 American Medical Association. All Rights Reserved.

© 2017 Optum360, LLC

**Cervix** — *continued*
  Repair
    Cerclage, 57700
      Abdominal, 59325
      Vaginal, 59320
    Suture, 57720
    Stump, 57558
    Suture, 57720
    Unlisted Services and Procedures, 58999
**Cesarean Delivery**
  with Hysterectomy, 59525
  Antepartum Care, 59610, 59618
  Delivery Only, 59514
  Delivery
    After Attempted Vaginal Delivery, 59618
      Delivery Only, 59620
      Postpartum Care, 59622
      Routine Care, 59618
    Routine Care, 59610
  Postpartum Care, 59515
  Routine Care, 59510
  Tubal Ligation at Time of, 58611
  Vaginal after Prior Cesarean
    Delivery and Postpartum Care, 59614
    Delivery Only, 59612
    Routine Care, 59610
**CFH/ARMS2**, 81401
**CFTR**, 81220-81224, 81412
**CGM (Continuous Glucose Monitoring System)**, 95250-95251 *[95249]*
**Chalazion**
  Excision, 67800-67808
    Multiple
      Different Lids, 67805
      Same Lids, 67801
    Single, 67800
    Under Anesthesia, 67808
**Challenge Tests**
  Bronchial Inhalation, 95070-95071
  Cholinesterase Inhibitor, 95857
  Ingestion, 95076, 95079
**Chambers Procedure**, 28300
**Change, Gastrostomy Tube**
  *See* Gastrostomy Tube, Change of
**Change of, Dressing**
  *See* Dressings, Change
**Change**
  Catheter
    Percutaneous with Contrast, 75984
  Fetal Position
    by Manipulation, 59412
  Stent
    (Endoscopic), Bile or Pancreatic Duct,
      *[43275, 43276]*
    Ureteral, 50688
  Tube
    Gastrostomy, 43760
    Percutaneous, with Contrast Monitoring,
      75984
    Tracheotomy, 31502
    Ureterostomy, 50688
**CHCT (Caffeine Halothane Contracture Test)**,
  89049
**CHD7**, 81407
**Cheek**
  Bone
    Excision, 21030, 21034
    Fracture
      Closed Treatment with Manipula-
        tion, 21355
      Open Treatment, 21360-21366
      Reconstruction, 21270
  Fascia Graft, 15840
  Muscle Graft, 15841-15845
  Muscle Transfer, 15845
  Rhytidectomy, 15828
  Skin Graft
    Delay of Flap, 15620
    Full Thickness, 15240, 15241
    Pedicle Flap, 15574
    Split, 15120-15121
  Tissue Transfer, Adjacent, 14040, 14041
  Wound Repair, 13131-13133
**Cheekbone**
  Fracture
    Closed Treatment Manipulation, 21355

**Cheekbone** — *continued*
  Fracture — *continued*
    Open Treatment, 21360-21366
    Reconstruction, 21270
**Cheilectomy**
  Metatarsophalangeal Joint Release, 28289,
    28291
**Cheiloplasty**
  *See* Lip, Repair
**Cheiloschisis**
  *See* Cleft, Lip
**Cheilotomy**
  *See* Incision, Lip
**Chemical**
  Cauterization
    Corneal Epithelium, 65435-65436
    Granulation Tissue, 17250
  Exfoliation, 15788-15793, 17360
  Peel, 15788-15793, 17360
**Chemiluminescent Assay**, 82397
**Chemistry Tests**
  Organ or Disease Oriented Panel
    Electrolyte, 80051
    General Health Panel, 80050
    Hepatic Function Panel, 80076
    Hepatitis Panel, Acute, 80074
    Lipid Panel, 80061
    Metabolic
      Basic, 80047-80048
        Calcium
          Ionized, 80047
          Total, 80048
      Comprehensive, 80053
    Obstetric Panel, 80055, *[80081]*
  Unlisted Services and Procedures, 84999
**Chemocauterization**
  Corneal Epithelium, 65435
    with Chelating Agent, 65436
**Chemodenervation**
  Anal Sphincter, 46505
  Bladder, 52287
  Eccrine Glands, 64650, 64653
  Electrical Stimulation for Guidance, 64617,
    95873
  Extraocular Muscle, 67345
  Extremity Muscle, 64642-64645
  Facial Muscle, 64612, 64615
  Gland
    Eccrine, 64650, 64653
    Parotid, 64611
    Salivary, 64611
    Submandibular, 64611
  Internal Anal Sphincter, 46505
  Larynx, 64617
  Muscle
    Extraocular, 67345
    Extremity, 64642-64645
    Facial, 64612
    Larynx, 64617
    Neck, 64616
    Trunk, 64646-64647
  Neck Muscle, 64615-64616
  Needle Electromyography Guidance, 95874
  Salivary Glands, 64611
  Trunk Muscle, 64646-64647
**Chemonucleolysis**, 62292
**Chemosurgery**
  Destruction
    Benign Lesion, 17110-17111
    Malignant Lesion, 17260-17266, 17270-
      17286
    Premalignant Lesion, 17000-17004
  Mohs Technique, 17311-17315
**Chemotaxis Assay**, 86155
**Chemotherapy**
  Arterial Catheterization, 36640
  Bladder Instillation, 51720
  Brain, 61517
  Cannulation, 36823
  Central Nervous System, 61517, 96450
  Extracorporeal Circulation Membrane Oxygena-
    tion
    Isolated with Chemotherapy Perfusion,
      36823
  Home Infusion Procedures, 99601, 99602

**Chemotherapy** — *continued*
  Intra–Arterial
    Cannulation, 36823
    Catheterization, 36640
    Infusion Pump Insertion, 36260
    Infusion, 96422-96423, 96425
    Push Technique, 96420
  Intralesional, 96405, 96406
  Intramuscular, 96401-96402
  Intravenous, 96409-96417
  Kidney Instillation, 50391
  Peritoneal Cavity, 96446
    Catheterization, 49418
  Pleural Cavity, 96440
  Pump Services
    Implantable, 96522
    Initiation, 96416
    Maintenance, 95990-95991, 96521-
      96522
    Portable, 96521
  Reservoir Filling, 96542
  Subcutaneous, 96401-96402
  Unlisted Services and Procedures, 96549
  Ureteral Instillation, 50391
**Chest Wall**
  Debridement, 11044, 11047
  Manipulation, 94667-94669
  Mechanical Oscillation, 94669
  Reconstruction, 49904
    Lung Tumor Resection, 32504
    Trauma, 32820
  Repair, 32905
    Closure, 32810
    Fistula, 32906
    Lung Hernia, 32800
  Resection, 32503
  Tumor
    Ablation, 32998, *[32994]*
    Excision, 19260-19272
  Unlisted Services and Procedures, 32999
**Chest**
  *See* Mediastinum; Thorax
  Angiography, 71275
  Artery
    Ligation, 37616
  Cavity
    Bypass Graft, 35905
    Thoracoscopy
      Exploration, 32601-32606
      Surgical, 32650-32665
      Therapeutic, 32654-32665
  CT Scan, 71250-71275
  Diagnostic Imaging
    Angiography, 71275
    CT Angiography, 71275
    CT, 71250, 71260, 71270
    Magnetic Resonance Angiography,
      71555
    Magnetic Resonance Imaging (MRI),
      71550-71552
    PET, 78811, 78814
    Ultrasound, 76604
  Exploration
    Blood Vessel, 35820
    Penetrating Wound, 20101
    Postoperative
      Hemorrhage, 35820
      Infection, 35820
      Thrombosis, 35820
  Flail, 21899
  Funnel
    Anesthesia, 00474
    Reconstructive Repair, 21740-21742
    with Thoracoscopy, 21743
  Magnetic Resonance Imaging (MRI), 71550-
    71552
  Repair
    Blood Vessel, 35211, 35216
      with Other Graft, 35271, 35276
      with Vein Graft, 35241, 35246
  Tube, 32551
  Ultrasound, 76604
  Wound Exploration
    Penetrating, 20101
  X–ray, 71045-71048

**Chest** — *continued*
  X–ray — *continued*
    with Computer-aided Detection, 0174T-
      0175T
    Complete (four views) with Fluoroscopy,
      71048, 76000-76001
    Partial (two views) with Fluoroscopy,
      71046, 76000-76001
    Stereo, 71045
**Chiari Osteotomy of the Pelvis**
  *See* Osteotomy, Pelvis
**Chicken Pox (Varicella)**
  Immunization, 90716
**Child Procedure**, 48146
  *See also* Excision, Pancreas, Partial
**Chimerism (Engraftment) Analysis**, 81267-81268
**Chin**
  Cartilage Graft, 21230
  Repair
    Augmentation, 21120
    Osteotomy, 21121-21123
  Rhytidectomy, 15828
  Skin Graft
    Delay of Flap, 15620
    Full Thickness, 15240, 15241
    Pedicle Flap, 15574
    Split, 15120-15121
  Tissue Transfer, Adjacent, 14040, 14041
  Wound Repair, 13131-13133
**Chinidin**, 80194
**Chiropractic Manipulation**
  *See* Manipulation, Chiropractic
**Chiropractic Treatment**
  Spinal
    Extraspinal, 98940-98943
**Chlamydia**
  Antibody, 86631, 86632
  Antigen Detection
    Direct Fluorescent, 87270
    Direct
      Optical Observation, 87810
    Enzyme Immunoassay, 87320
    Immunofluorescence, 87270
    Nucleic Acid, 87485-87492
  Culture, 87110
**Chloramphenicol**, 82415
**Chloride, Methylene**
  *See* Dichloromethane
**Chloride**
  Blood, 82435
  Other Source, 82438
  Panels
    Basic Metabolic, 80047-80048
    Comprehensive Metabolic, 80053
    Electrolyte, 80051
    Renal Function, 80069
  Spinal Fluid, 82438
  Urine, 82436
**Chlorinated Hydrocarbons**, 82441
**Chlorohydrocarbon**, 82441
**Chlorpromazine**, *[80342, 80343, 80344]*
**Choanal Atresia**
  Repair, 30540, 30545
**CHOL**, 82465, 83718-83721
**Cholangiogram**
  Intravenous, 76499
**Cholangiography**
  with Cholecystectomy, 47563, 47605
  Injection, 47531-47533
  Intraoperative, 74300, 74301
  Repair
    with Bile Duct Exploration, 47700
    with Cholecystectomy, 47620
**Cholangiopancreatography**
  with Ablation, *[43278]*
  with Biopsy, 43261
  with Optical Endomicroscopy, 0397T
  with Surgery, 43262-43265 *[43274, 43275,
    43276]*
  *See* Bile Duct, Pancreatic Duct
  Destruction of Calculus, 43264-43265
  Diagnostic, 43260
  Exchange Stent, *[43276]*
  Intraoperative, 74300-74301
  Papillotomy, 43262

CPT © 2017 American Medical Association. All Rights Reserved.        © 2017 Optum360, LLC

**Colonoscopy**
- Ablation Lesions/Polyps/Tumors, [45388]
- Band Ligation, [45398]
- Biopsy, 45380, 45392
- Collection of Specimen, 45378
  - via Colotomy, [45399]
- Decompression, 45393
- Destruction
  - Lesion, [45388]
  - Tumor, [45388]
- Diagnostic, 45378
- Dilation, 45386
- Hemorrhage Control, 45382
- Injection, Submucosal, 45381
- Mucosal Resection, [45390]
- Placement
  - Stent, 45389
- Removal
  - Foreign Body, 45379
  - Polyp, 45384-45385
  - Tumor, 45384-45385
- Surveillance Intervals, 0528F-0529F
- Transabdominal, [45399]
- Ultrasound, 45391-45392
- via Stoma
  - Biopsy, 44389, 44407
  - Decompression, 44408
  - Destruction
    - Polyp, [44401]
    - Tumor, [44401]
  - Dilation, 44405
  - Exploration, 44388
  - Hemorrhage, 44391
  - Injection, Submucosal, 44404
  - Mucosal Resection, 44403
  - Placement
    - Stent, 44402
  - Removal
    - Foreign Body, 44390
    - Polyp, 44392, 44394
    - Tumor, 44392, 44394
  - Ultrasound, 44406-44407
- Virtual, 74261-74263

**Colon–Sigmoid**
- Biopsy
  - Endoscopy, 45331
- Decompression, 45378
  - Volvulus, 45337
- Dilation, 45340
- Endoscopy
  - Ablation
    - Polyp, [45346]
    - Tumor, [45346]
  - Biopsy, 45331
  - Dilation, 45340
  - Exploration, 45330, 45335
  - Hemorrhage, 45334
  - Needle Biopsy, 45342
  - Placement
    - Stent, 45327, 45347
  - Removal
    - Foreign Body, 45332
    - Polyp, 45333, 45338
    - Tumor, 45333, 45338
  - Ultrasound, 45341, 45342
  - Volvulus, 45337
- Exploration
  - Endoscopy, 45330, 45335
- Hemorrhage
  - Endoscopy, 45334
- Needle Biopsy
  - Endoscopy, 45342
- Reconstruction Bladder Using Sigmoid, 50810
- Removal
  - Foreign Body, 45332
- Repair
  - Volvulus
    - Endoscopy, 45337
- Ultrasound
  - Endoscopy, 45341, 45342

**Color Vision Examination**, 92283
**Colorrhaphy**, 44604
**Colostomy**
- with Colorrhaphy, 44605
- with Partial Colectomy, 44141, 44143-44144, 44146

**Colostomy** — continued
- with Partial Colectomy — continued
  - Hartmann Type, 44143
  - Laparoscopic, 44206, 44208
- with Pelvic Exenteration, 45126, 51597, 58240
- with Proctectomy, 45110
  - Laparoscopic, 45395
- with Rectal Repair, 45563, 45805, 45825
- Abdominal
  - with Closure Rectovaginal Fistula, 57307
  - with Creation Sigmoid Bladder, 50810
- Abdominoperineal, 51597, 58240
- Delayed Opening, 44799
- External Fistulization, 44320
  - Paracolostomy Hernia, 44346
  - Revision, 44340
- Home Visit, 99505
- Ileocolostomy, 44160, 44205
- Intestine, Large
  - with Suture, 44605
- Laparoscopic, 44188, 44206, 44208
- Perineal, 50810
- Revision, 44340
  - Paracolostomy Hernia, 44345, 44346

**Colotomy**, 44025
**Colpectomy**
- with Hysterectomy, 58275
  - with Repair of Enterocele, 58280
- Partial, 57106
- Total, 57110

**Colpoceliocentesis**
- See Colpocentesis

**Colpocentesis**, 57020
**Colpocleisis Complete**
- See Vagina, Closure

**Colpocleisis**, 57120
**Colpohysterectomies**
- See Excision, Uterus, Vaginal

**Colpoperineorrhaphy**, 57210
**Colpopexy**, 57280
- Laparoscopic, 57425
- Open, 57280
- Vaginal, 57282-57283

**Colpoplasty**
- See Repair, Vagina

**Colporrhaphy**
- Anterior, 57240, 57289
  - with Insertion of Mesh, 57267
  - with Insertion of Prosthesis, 57267
- Anteroposterior, 57260, 57265
  - with Enterocele Repair, 57265
  - with Insertion of Mesh, 57267
  - with Insertion of Prosthesis, 57267
- Manchester, 58400
- Nonobstetrical, 57200
- Posterior, 57250
  - with Insertion of Mesh, 57267
  - with Insertion of Prosthesis, 57267

**Colposcopy**
- Biopsy, 56821, 57421, 57454-57455, 57460
  - Endometrial, 58110
- Cervix, 57420-57421, 57452-57461
- Endometrium, 58110
- Exploration, 57452
- Loop Electrode Biopsy, 57460
- Loop Electrode Conization, 57461
- Perineum, 99170
- Vagina, 57420-57421, 57452
- Vulva, 56820
  - Biopsy, 56821

**Colpotomy**
- Drainage
  - Abscess, 57010
- Exploration, 57000

**Colpo–Urethrocystopexy**, 58152, 58267, 58293
- Marshall–Marchetti–Krantz procedure, 58152, 58267, 58293
- Pereyra Procedure, 58267, 58293

**Colprosterone**
- See Progesterone

**Column Chromatography/Mass Spectrometry**, 82542
**Columna Vertebralis**
- See Spine

**Combined Heart–Lung Transplantation**
- See Transplantation, Heart–Lung

**Combined Right and Left Heart Cardiac Catheterization**
- See Cardiac Catheterization, Combined Left and Right Heart

**Combined Vaccine**, 90710
**Comedones**
- Opening or Removal of (Incision and Drainage)
  - Acne Surgery, 10040

**Commando–Type Procedure**, 41155
**Commissurotomy**
- Right Ventricular, 33476, 33478

**Common Sensory Nerve**
- Repair, Suture, 64834

**Common Truncus**
- See Truncus, Arteriosus

**Communication Device**
- Non–speech–generating, 92605-92606 [92618]
- Speech–generating, 92607-92609

**Community/Work Reintegration**
- See Physical Medicine/Therapy/ Occupational Therapy
- Training, 97537

**Comparative Analysis Using STR Markers**, 81265-81266
**Compatibility Test**
- Blood, 86920
- Electronic, 86923
- Specimen Pretreatment, 86970-86972

**Complement**
- Antigen, 86160
- Fixation Test, 86171
- Functional Activity, 86161
- Hemolytic
  - Total, 86162
- Total, 86162

**Complete Blood Count**, 85025-85027
**Complete Colectomy**
- See Colectomy, Total

**Complete Pneumonectomy**
- See Pneumonectomy, Completion

**Complete Transposition of Great Vessels**
- See Transposition, Great Arteries

**Complex Chronic Care Management Services**, 99487, 99489, [99490]
**Complex, Factor IX**
- See Christmas Factor

**Complex, Vitamin B**
- See B Complex Vitamins

**Component Removal, Blood**
- See Apheresis

**Composite Graft**, 15760, 15770
- Vein, 35681-35683
  - Autogenous
    - Three or More Segments
      - Two Locations, 35683
    - Two Segments
      - Two Locations, 35682

**Compound B**
- See Corticosterone

**Compound F**
- See Cortisol

**Compression, Nerve, Median**
- See Carpal Tunnel Syndrome

**Compression System Application**, 29581-29584
**Computed Tomographic Angiography**
- Abdomen, 74174-74175
- Abdominal Aorta, 75635
- Arm, 73206
- Chest, 71275
- Head, 70496
- Heart, 75574
- Leg, 73706
- Neck, 70498
- Pelvis, 72191, 74174

**Computed Tomographic Scintigraphy**
- See Emission Computerized Tomography

**Computed Tomography (CT Scan)**
- with Contrast
  - Abdomen, 74160, 74175
  - Arm, 73201, 73206
  - Brain, 70460
  - Cardiac Structure and Morphology, 75572-75573
  - Chest, 71275
  - Ear, 70481
  - Face, 70487

**Computed Tomography (CT Scan)** — continued
- with Contrast — continued
  - Head, 70460, 70496
  - Heart, 75572-75574
  - Leg, 73701, 73706
  - Maxilla, 70487
  - Neck, 70491, 70498
  - Orbit, 70481
  - Pelvis, 72191, 72193
  - Sella Turcica, 70481
  - Spine
    - Cervical, 72126
    - Lumbar, 72132
    - Thoracic, 72129
  - Thorax, 71260
- without Contrast, followed by Contrast
  - Abdomen, 74170
  - Arm, 73202
  - Brain, 70470
  - Ear, 70482
  - Face, 70488
  - Leg, 73702
  - Maxilla, 70488
  - Neck, 70492
  - Orbit, 70482
  - Pelvis, 72194
  - Sella Turcica, 70482
  - Spine
    - Cervical, 72127
    - Lumbar, 72133
    - Thoracic, 72130
  - Thorax, 71270
- without Contrast
  - Abdomen, 74150
  - Arm, 73200
  - Brain, 70450
  - Ear, 70480
  - Face, 70486
  - Head, 70450
  - Heart, 75571
  - Leg, 73700
  - Maxilla, 70486
  - Neck, 70490
  - Orbit, 70480
  - Pelvis, 72192
  - Sella Turcica, 70480
  - Spine, Cervical, 72125
  - Spine, Lumbar, 72131
  - Spine, Thoracic, 72128
  - Thorax, 71250
- Bone
  - Density Study, 77078
- Colon
  - Colonography, 74261-74263
    - Diagnostic, 74261-74262
    - Screening, 74263
  - Virtual Colonoscopy, 74261-74263
- Drainage, 75898
- Follow–up Study, 76380
- Guidance
  - 3D Rendering, 76376-76377
  - Cyst Aspiration, 77012
  - Localization, 77011
  - Needle Biopsy, 77012
  - Radiation Therapy, 77014
- Heart, 75571-75574

**Computer**
- Aided Animation and Analysis Retinal Images, 0380T
- Aided Detection
  - Chest Radiograph, 0174T-0175T
  - Mammography
    - Diagnostic, 77065-77066
    - Magnetic Resonance Imaging (MRI), 0159T
    - Screening, 77067
- Analysis
  - Cardiac Electrical Data, 0206T
  - Electrocardiographic Data, 93228
  - Heart Sounds, Acoustic Recording, 93799
  - Motion Analysis, 96000-96004
  - Pediatric Home Apnea Monitor, 94776
  - Probability Assessment
    - Patient Specific Findings, 99199
  - Stored Data, 99090

CPT © 2017 American Medical Association. All Rights Reserved.

*[Resequenced]*   CPT © 2017 American Medical Association. All Rights Reserved.   © 2017 Optum360, LLC

**Cornea** — *continued*
- Insertion
  - Intrastromal Corneal Ring Segment, 65785
- Lesion
  - Destruction, 65450
  - Excision, 65400
    - with Graft, 65426
    - without Graft, 65420
- Pachymetry, 76514
- Prosthesis, 65770
- Pterygium
  - with Graft, 65426
  - Excision, 65420
- Puncture, 65600
- Relaxing Incisions, 65772, 65775
- Removal
  - Foreign Body, 65220, 65222
  - Lesion, 66600
- Repair
  - with Amniotic Membrane, 65778-65780
  - with Glue, 65286
  - Astigmatism, 65772, 65775
  - Incision, 65772
  - Wedge Resection, 65775
  - Wound
    - Nonperforating, 65275
    - Perforating, 65280, 65285
    - Tissue Glue, 65286
- Reshape
  - Epikeratoplasty, 65767
  - Keratomileusis, 65760
  - Keratophakia, 65765
  - Keratoprosthesis, 65767
- Scraping
  - Smear, 65430
- Tattoo, 65600
- Tear Film Imaging, 0330T
- Tear Osmolarity, 83861
- Thickness Measurement, 76514
- Topography, 92025
- Transplantation
  - Amniotic Membrane, 65780
  - Autograft or Homograft
    - Allograft Preparation, 0290T, 65757
    - Endothelial, 65756
    - Lamellar, 65710
    - Penetrating, 65730-65755
  - Corneal Incisions by Laser
    - Recipient Cornea, 0290T
  - for Aphakia, 65750
- Unlisted Procedure, 66999
**Coronary Angioplasty, Transluminal Balloon**
  - *See* Percutaneous Transluminal Angioplasty
**Coronary Arteriography**
- Anesthesia, 01920
**Coronary Artery**
- Angiography, 93454-93461
- Angioplasty
  - with Atherectomy, *[92933, 92934]*, *[92937, 92938], [92941], [92943, 92944]*
  - with Placement Stent, *[92928, 92929], [92933, 92934], [92937, 92938], [92941], [92943, 92944]*
- Atherectomy, *[92924, 92925]*
- Bypass Graft (CABG), 33503-33505, 33510-33516
  - Arterial Graft
    - Spectroscopy, Catheter Based, 0205T
  - Arterial, 33533-33536
  - Arterial–Venous, 33517-33523
  - Beta Blocker Administered, 4115F
  - Harvest
    - Upper Extremity Artery, 35600
    - Upper Extremity Vein, 35500
  - Reoperation, 33530
  - Venous, 33510-33516
- Ligation, 33502
- Obstruction Severity Assessment, 0206T
- Placement
  - Radiation Delivery Device, *[92974]*
- Reconstruction, 33863-33864
- Repair, 33500-33507

**Coronary Artery** — *continued*
- Revascularization, *[92937, 92938], [92941], [92943, 92944]*
- Thrombectomy, *[92973]*
- Thrombolysis, *[92975], [92977]*
- Translocation, 33506-33507
- Unroofing, 33507
- Ventricular Restoration, 33548
**Coronary Endarterectomy**, 33572
**Coronary Fractional Flow Reserve**, 0501T-0504T
**Coronary**
- Thrombectomy
  - Percutaneous, *[92973]*
**Coroner's Exam**, 88045
**Coronoidectomy**
- Temporomandibular Joint, 21070
**Corpectomy**, 63101-63103
**Corpora Cavernosa, Plastic Induration**
- *See* Peyronie Disease
**Corpora Cavernosa**
- Corpora Cavernosography, 74445
  - Injection, 54230
- Corpus Spongiosum Shunt, 54430
- Dynamic Cavernosometry, 54231
- Glans Penis Fistulization, 54435
- Injection
  - Peyronie Disease, 54200-54205
  - Pharmacologic Agent, 54235
- Irrigation
  - Priapism, 54220
- Peyronie Disease, 54200-54205
- Priapism, 54220, 54430
- Repair
  - Corporeal Tear, 54437
  - Saphenous Vein Shunt, 54420
  - X–ray with Contrast, 74445
**Corpora Cavernosography**, 74445
- Injection, 54230
**Corpus Callosum**
- Transection, 61541
**Corpus Uteri**, 58100-58285
**Corpus Vertebrae (Vertebrale)**
- *See* Vertebral Body
**Correction of Cleft Palate**
- *See* Cleft Palate, Repair
**Correction of Lid Retraction**
- *See* Repair, Eyelid, Retraction
**Correction of Malrotation of Duodenum**
- *See* Ladd Procedure
**Correction of Syndactyly**, 26560-26562
**Correction of Ureteropelvic Junction**
- *See* Pyeloplasty
**Cortex Decortication, Cerebral**
- *See* Decortication
**Cortical Mapping**
- Functional Mapping, 95961-95962
- Noninvasive, 96020
- TMS Treatment
  - Initial, 90867
  - Subsequent, 90868-90869
**Corticoids**
- *See* Corticosteroids
**Corticoliberin**
- *See* Corticotropic Releasing Hormone (CRH)
**Corticosteroid Binding Globulin**, 84449
**Corticosteroid Binding Protein**, 84449
**Corticosteroids**
- Blood, 83491
- Urine, 83491
**Corticosterone**
- Blood or Urine, 82528
**Corticotropic Releasing Hormone (CRH)**, 80412
**Cortisol Binding Globulin**, 84449
**Cortisol**, 80400-80406, 80418, 80420, 80436, 82530
- Stimulation Panel, 80412
- Total, 82533
**Costectomy**
- *See* Resection, Ribs
**Costello Syndrome**, 81442
**Costen Syndrome**
- *See* Temporomandibular
**Costotransversectomy**, 21610
**COTD (Cardiac Output Thermodilution)**, 93561-93562
**Cothromboplastin**
- *See* Proconvertin

**Cotte Operation**, 58400, 58410
- Repair, Uterus, Suspension, 58400, 58410
**Cotting Operation**
- Excision, Nail Fold, 11765
**Cotton (Bohler) Procedure**, 28405
**Cotton Scoop Procedure**, 28118
**Counseling and /or Risk Factor Reduction Intervention – Preventive Medicine, Individual Counseling**
- Behavior Change Interventions, 0403T, 99406-99409
- Caregiver-focused, 96161
- Patient-focused, 96160
- Preventive Medicine, 99411-99412
  - Diabetes, *[0488T]*
**Counseling, Preventive**
- Group, 99411, 99412
- Individual, 99401-99404
- Other, 99429
**Counseling**
- *See* Preventive Medicine
- Smoking and Tobacco Use Cessation, 99406-99407
**Count, Blood Cell**
- *See* Blood Cell Count
**Count, Blood Platelet**
- *See* Blood, Platelet, Count
**Count, Cell**
- *See* Cell Count
**Count, Complete Blood**
- *See* Complete Blood Count (CBC)
**Count, Erythrocyte**
- *See* Red Blood Cell (RBC), Count
**Count, Leukocyte**
- *See* White Blood Cell, Count
**Count, Reticulocyte**
- *See* Reticulocyte, Count
**Counters, Cell**
- *See* Cell Count
**Countershock, Electric**
- *See* Cardioversion
**Coventry Tibial Wedge Osteotomy**
- *See* Osteotomy, Tibia
**Cowper's Gland**
- Excision, 53250
**COX10**, 81405
**COX15**, 81405
**COX6B1**, 81404
**Coxa**
- *See* Hip
**Coxiella Brunetii**
- Antibody, 86638
**Coxsackie**
- Antibody, 86658
**CPAP (Continuous Positive Airway Pressure)**, 94660
**CPB**, 32852, 32854, 33496, 33503-33505, 33510-33523, 33533-33536
**C–Peptide**, 80432, 84681
**CPK**
- Isoenzymes, 82252, 82554
- Isoforms, 82554
- MB Fraction Only, 82553
- Total, 82550
**CPOX**, 81405
**CPR (Cardiopulmonary Resuscitation)**, 92950
**CPT1A**, 81406
**CPT2**, 81404
**CR**, 82565-82575
**Cranial Bone**
- Frontal Bone Flap, 61556-61557
- Halo
  - for Thin Skull Osteology, 20664
- Parietal Bone Flap, 61556
- Reconstruction
  - Extracranial, 21181-21184
  - Temporal Bone
    - Hearing Device, 69710 69711
    - Implantation Cochlear Device, 69930
    - Osseointegrated Implant, 69714-69715
    - Removal Tumor, 69970
    - Resection, 69535
    - Unlisted Procedure, 69979
  - Tumor
    - Excision, 61563-61564
**Cranial Halo**, 20661

**Cranial Nerve II**
- *See* Optic Nerve
**Cranial Nerve V**
- *See* Trigeminal Nerve
**Cranial Nerve VII**
- *See* Facial Nerve
**Cranial Nerve X**
- *See* Vagus Nerve
**Cranial Nerve XI**
- *See* Accessory Nerve
**Cranial Nerve XII**
- *See* Hypoglossal Nerve
**Cranial Nerve**
- Avulsion, 64732-64760, 64771
- Decompression, 61458, 61460, 64716
- Implantation
  - Electrode, 64553, 64568-64569
- Incision, 64732-64746, 64760
- Injection
  - Anesthetic, 64400-64408
  - Neurolytic, 64600-64610
- Insertion
  - Electrode, 64553, 64568-64569
- Neuroplasty, 64716
- Release, 64716
- Repair
  - Suture, with or without Graft, 64864, 64865
- Section, 61460
- Transection, 64732-64760, 64771
- Transposition, 64716
**Cranial Tongs**
- Application
  - Removal, 20660
- Removal, 20665
**Craniectomy**
- with Craniotomy, 61530
- *See* Craniotomy
- Anesthesia, 00211
- Compression
  - Sensory Root Gasserian Ganglion, 61450
- Craniosynostosis, 61558, 61559
  - Multiple Sutures, 61552, 61558-61559
  - Single Suture, 61550
- Decompression, 61322-61323, 61340-61343
  - Cranial Nerves, 61458
  - Sensory Root Gasserian Ganglion, 61450
- Drainage of Abscess, 61320-61321
- Electrode Placement
  - Cortical, 61860, 61870
  - Subcortical, 61863-61864, 61867-61868
- Excision
  - for Osteomyelitis, 61501
  - of Lesion or Tumor, 61500
- Exploratory, 61304-61305, 61458
- Section, 61450, 61460
- Stenosis Release, 61550-61552
- Surgical, 61312-61315, 61320-61323, 61450-61480, 61500-61522
- Tractotomy, 61480
- Wound Treatment, 61571
**Craniofacial and Maxillofacial**
- Unlisted Services and Procedures, 21299
**Craniofacial Procedures**
- Unlisted Services and Procedures, 21299
**Craniofacial Separation**
- Bone Graft, 21436
- Closed Treatment, 21431
- External Fixation, 21435
- Open Treatment, 21432-21436
- Wire Fixation, 21431-21432
**Craniomegalic Skull**
- Reduction, 62115-62117
**Craniopharyngioma**
- Excision, 61545
**Cranioplasty**, 62120
- with Autograft, 62146, 62147
- with Bone Graft, 61316, 62146, 62147
- Bone Graft Retrieval, 62148
- Encephalocele Repair, 62120
- for Defect, 62140, 62141, 62145
**Craniostenosis**
- *See* Craniosynostosis
**Craniosynostosis**
- Bifrontal Craniotomy, 61557
- Extensive Craniectomy, 61558, 61559

**CT Scan** — *continued*
 without Contrast, followed by Contrast — *continued*
   Maxilla, 70488
   Neck, 70492
   Orbit, 70482
   Pelvis, 72194
     and Abdomen, 74178
   Sella Turcica, 70482
   Spine
     Cervical, 72127
     Lumbar, 72133
     Thoracic, 72130
   Thorax, 71270
 without Contrast
   Abdomen, 74150
     and Pelvis, 74176
   Arm, 73200
   Brain, 70450
   Colon, 74261-74263
   Ear, 70480
   Face, 70486
   Head, 70450
   Leg, 73700
   Maxilla, 70486
   Neck, 70490
   Orbit, 70480
   Pelvis, 72192
     and Abdomen, 74176
   Sella Turcica, 70480
   Spine
     Cervical, 72125
     Lumbar, 72131
     Thoracic, 72128
   Thorax, 71250
 3D Rendering, 76376-76377
 Angiography
   Abdomen and Pelvis, 74174
   Abdomen, 74175
   Aorta, 75635
   Heart, 75574
   Leg, 73706, 75635
 Bone
   Density Study, 77078
 Brain, 70450-70470
   Stroke Diagnosis, 3110F-3112F
 Colon
   Diagnostic, 74261-74262
   Screening, 74263
 Drainage, 75989
 Follow–up Study, 76380
 Guidance
   Localization, 77011
   Needle Biopsy, 77012
   Parenchymal Tissue Ablation, 77013
   Radiation Therapy, 77014
   Tissue Ablation, 77013
   Visceral Tissue Ablation, 77013
 Heart
   Evaluation
     Angiography, 75574
     Coronary Calcium, 75571
     Structure and Morphology, 75572-75573
   Hemorrhage Documented, 3110F
   Infarction Documented, 3110F
   Lesion Documented, 3110F
 Optical Coherence Tomography, [92978, 92979]
 Parathyroid Gland, 78072
 Unlisted Procedure, 76497
**CTNNB1**, 81403
**CTRC**, 81405
**CTS**, 29848, 64721
**Cuff, Rotator**
 *See* Rotator Cuff
**Culdocentesis**, 57020
**Culdoplasty**
 McCall, 57283
**Culdoscopy**, 57452
**Culdotomy**, 57000
**Culture**
 Acid Fast Bacilli, 87116
 Amniotic Fluid
   Chromosome Analysis, 88235
 Bacteria
   Aerobic, 87040-87071

**Culture** — *continued*
 Bacteria — *continued*
   Aerobic — *continued*
     Additional Methods, 87077
   Anaerobic, 87073-87076
   Blood, 87040
   Feces, 87045-87046
   Other, 87070-87073
   Screening, 87081
   Urine, 87086, 87088
 Bone Marrow
   Chromosome Analysis, 88237
   Neoplastic Disorders, 88237
 Chlamydia, 87110
 Chorionic Villus
   Chromosome Analysis, 88235
 Fertilized Oocyte
   for In Vitro Fertilization, 89250
     with Co–Culture of Embryo, 89251
     Assisted Microtechnique, 89280, 89281
 Fungus
   Blood, 87103
   Hair, 87101
   Identification, 87106
   Nail, 87101
   Other, 87102
   Skin, 87101
   Source Other Than Blood, 87102
 Lymphocyte, 86821
   Chromosome Analysis, 88230
 Mold, 87107
 Mycobacteria, 87116-87118
 Mycoplasma, 87109
 Oocyte/Embryo
   Extended Culture, 89272
   for In Vitro Fertilization, 89250
     with Co–Culture of Embryo, 89251
 Pathogen
   by Kit, 87084
   Screening Only, 87081
 Skin
   Chromosome Analysis, 88233
 Stool, 87045-87046
 Tissue
   Drug Resistance, 87903-87904
   Homogenization, 87176
   Toxin Virus, 87252, 87253
   Toxin
     Antitoxin, 87230
 Tubercle Bacilli, 87116
 Tumor Tissue
   Chromosome Analysis, 88239
 Typing, 87140-87158
   Culture, 87140-87158
 Unlisted Services and Procedures, 87999
 Yeast, 87106
**Curettage and Dilatation**
 *See* Dilation and Curettage
**Curettage, Uterus**
 *See* Uterus, Curettage
**Curettage**
 *See* Dilation and Curettage
 Anal Fissure, 46940
 Cervix
   Endocervical, 57454, 57456, 57505
   Cornea, 65435, 65436
     Chelating Agent, 65436
   Dentoalveolar, 41830
   Hydatidiform Mole, 59870
   Postpartum, 59160
 Uterus
   Endometrial, 58356
   Postpartum, 59160
**Curettement**
 Skin Lesion, 11055-11057, 17004, 17110, 17270, 17280
   Benign Hyperkeratotic Lesion, 11055-11057
   Malignant, 17260-17264, 17266, 17270-17274, 17280-17284, 17286
   Premalignant, 17000, 17003-17004, 17110-17111
**Curietherapy**
 *See* Brachytherapy

**Custodial Care**
 *See* Domiciliary Services; Nursing Facility Services
**Cutaneolipectomy**
 *See* Lipectomy
**Cutaneous Electrostimulation, Analgesic**
 *See* Application, Neurostimulation
**Cutaneous Tag**
 *See* Skin, Tags
**Cutaneous Tissue**
 *See* Integumentary System
**Cutaneous–Vesicostomy**
 *See* Vesicostomy, Cutaneous
**CVAD (Central Venous Access Device)**
 Insertion
   Central, 36555-36558
   Peripheral, 36568-36569
 Removal, 36589
 Repair, 36575
 Replacement, 36580-36585
 Repositioning, 36597
**CVS**, 59015
**CXL, Collagen Cross-Linking, Cornea**, 0402T
**CXR**, 71045-71048
**Cyanide**
 Blood, 82600
 Tissue, 82600
**Cyanocobalamin**, 82607, 82608
**Cyclic AMP**, 82030
**Cyclic Citrullinated Peptide (CCP), Antibody**, 86200
**Cyclic Somatostatin**
 *See* Somatostatin
**Cyclocryotherapy**
 *See* Cryotherapy, Destruction, Ciliary Body
**Cyclodialysis**
 Destruction
   Ciliary Body, 66740
**Cyclophotocoagulation**
 Destruction
   Ciliary Body, 66710, 66711
**Cyclosporine**
 Assay, 80158
**CYP11B1**, 81405
**CYP17A1**, 81405
**CYP1B1**, 81404
**CYP21A2**, 81402, 81405
**CYP2C19**, 81225
**CYP2C9**, 81227
**CYP2D6**, 81226
**CYP3A4**, [81230]
**CYP3A5**, [81231]
**Cyst**
 Abdomen
   Destruction, 49203-49205
   Excision, 49203-49205
   Laparoscopy with Aspiration, 49322
 Ankle
   Capsule, 27630
   Tendon Sheath, 27630
 Bartholin's Gland
   Excision, 56740
   Marsupialization, 56440
   Repair, 56440
 Bile Duct
   Excision, 47715
 Bladder
   Excision, 51500
 Bone
   Drainage, 20615
   Injection, 20615
 Brain
   Drainage, 61150, 61151, 61156, 62161, 62162
   Excision, 61516, 61524, 62162
 Branchial Cleft
   Excision, 42810, 42815
 Breast
   Excision, 19020
   Puncture Aspiration, 19000, 19001
 Calcaneus, 28100-28103
 Carpal, 25130-25136
 Choledochal
   Excision, 47715
 Ciliary Body
   Destruction, 66770

**Cyst** — *continued*
 Clavicle
   Excision, 23140-23146
 Conjunctiva, 68020
 Dermoid
   Nose
     Excision, 30124, 30125
 Drainage
   Contrast Injection, 49424
     with X–ray, 76080
   Image-guided by catheter, 10030
 Enucleation
   Mandible, 21040
   Maxilla, 21030
   Zygoma, 21030
 Excision
   Cheekbone, 21030
   Clavicle, 23140
     with Allograft, 23146
     with Autograft, 23145
   Femur, 27065-27067, 27355-27358
   Foot, 28090
   Ganglion
     *See* Ganglion
   Hand
     Capsule, 26160
     Tendon Sheath, 26160
   Humerus, 24120-24126
     Proximal, 23150-23156
 Hydatid
   *See* Echinococcosis
 Lymphatic
   *See* Lymphocele
 Maxilla, 21030
 Mediastinum, 32662
 Mouth
   Dentoalveolar, 41800
   Lingual, 41000
   Masticator Space, 41009, 41018
   Sublingual, 41005-41006, 41015
   Submandibular, 41008, 41017
   Submental, 41007, 41016
   Vestibular, 40800-40801
 Olecranon Process, 24120
   with Allograft, 24126
   with Autograft, 24125
 Ovarian, 58925
 Pancreas
   Anastomosis, 48520, 48540
   Excision, 48120
   Marsupialization, 48500
 Pericardial, 32661
   Resection, 33050
 Pilonidal, 11770-11772
 Radius, 24120
   with Allograft, 24126
   with Autograft, 24125
 Scapula, 23140
   with Allograft, 23146
   with Autograft, 23145
 Symphysis Pubis, 27065-27067
 Ulna, 24120, 25120
   with Allograft, 24126, 25125
   with Autograft, 24125, 25126
 Wrist, 25111-25112, 25130, 25135-25136
 Zygoma, 21030
 Facial Bones
   Excision, 21030
 Femur
   Excision, 27065-27067, 27355-27358
 Fibula, 27635-27638
 Finger, 26210, 26215
 Ganglion
   Aspiration/Injection, 20612
 Gums
   Incision and Drainage, 41800
 Hand
   Capsule, 26160
   Tendon Sheath, 26160
 Hip, 27065-27067
 Humerus
   Excision, 23150-23156, 24110
     with Allograft, 24116
     with Autograft, 24115
 Ileum, 27065-27067
 Incision and Drainage, 10060, 10061

© 2017 Optum360, LLC                                        CPT © 2017 American Medical Association. All Rights Reserved.

**Delivery**
  *See* Cesarean Delivery, Vaginal Delivery
  Pharmacologic Agent
    Suprachoroidal, 67299
**Delorme Operation**, 33030
**Denervation, Sympathetic**
  *See* Excision, Nerve, Sympathetic
**Denervation**
  Hip
    Femoral Nerve, 27035
    Obturator Nerve, 27035
    Sciatic Nerve, 27035
  Sympathetic
    Chemodenervation, 64650, 64653
    Neurolytic Agent, 64680-64681
    Transcatheter Percutaneous, 0338T-0339T
**Dengue Vaccine**, 90587
**Dens Axis**
  *See* Odontoid Process
**Denver Developmental Screening Test**, 96101-96103
**Denver Krupin Procedure**, 66180
**Denver Shunt**
  Patency Test, 78291
**Deoxycorticosterone**, 82633
**Deoxycortisol**, 80436, 82634
**Deoxyephedrine**
  *See* Methamphetamine
**Deoxyribonuclease I**
  *See* DNAse
**Deoxyribonuclease**
  Antibody, 86215
**Deoxyribonucleic Acid**
  Antibody, 86225, 86226
**Depilation**
  *See* Removal, Hair
**Depletion**
  Plasma, 38214
  Platelet, 38213
  T–Cell, 38210
  Tumor Cell, 38211
**Deposit Calcium**
  *See* Calcium, Deposits
**Depression Inventory**, 96127
**Depth Electrode**
  Insertion, 61760
**DeQuervain's Disease Treatment**, 25000
**Dermabrasion**, 15780-15783
**Derma–Fat–Fascia Graft**, 15770
**Dermatology**
  Actinotherapy, 96900
  Examination of Hair
    Microscopic, 96902
  Laser Treatment for Psoriasis, 96920-96922
  Photochemotherapy
    Ultraviolet A Treatment, 96912-96913
    Ultraviolet B Treatment, 96910, 96913
  Ultraviolet A Treatment, 96912
  Ultraviolet B Treatment, 96910-96913
  Ultraviolet Light Treatment, 96900-96913
  Unlisted Services and Procedures, 96999
  Whole Body Photography, 96904
**Dermatoplasty**
  Septal, 30620
**Dermoid**
  *See* Cyst, Dermoid
**Derrick–Burnet Disease**
  *See* Q Fever
**DES**, 81405
**Descending Abdominal Aorta**
  *See* Aorta, Abdominal
**Design**
  Collimator, 77338
  IMRT Devices, 77332-77334
**Desipramine**
  Assay, *[80335, 80336, 80337]*
**Desmotomy**
  *See* Ligament, Release
**Desoxycorticosterone**, 82633
**Desoxycortone**
  *See* Desoxycorticosterone
**Desoxyephedrine**
  *See* Methamphetamine
**Desoxynorephedrin**
  *See* Amphetamine

**Desoxyphenobarbital**
  *See* Primidone
**Desquamation**
  *See* Exfoliation
**Destruction**
  with Cystourethroscopy, 52354
  Acne, 17340, 17360
    Cryotherapy, 17340
  Arrhythmogenic Focus
    Heart, 33250, 33251, 33261
  Bladder, 51020, 52214, 52224, 52354
    Endoscopic, 52214
      Large Tumors, 52240
      Medium Tumors, 52235
      Minor Lesions, 52224
      Small Tumors, 52234
  Calculus
    Bile Duct, 43265
    Kidney, 50590
    Pancreatic Duct, 43265
  Chemical Cauterization
    Granulation Tissue, 17250
  Chemosurgery, 17110-17111
  Ciliary Body
    Cryotherapy, 66720
    Cyclodialysis, 66740
    Cyclophotocoagulation, 66710, 66711
    Diathermy, 66700
    Endoscopic, 66711
  Condyloma
    Anal, 46900-46924
    Penis, 54050-54065
    Vagina, 57061-57065
    Vulva, 56501-56515
  Cryosurgery, 17110-17111
  Curettement, 17110-17111
  Cyst
    Abdomen, 49203-49205
    Ciliary Body, 66740, 66770
    Iris, 66770
    Retroperitoneal, 49203-49205
  Electrosurgery, 17110-17111
  Endometrial Ablation, 58356
  Endometriomas
    Abdomen, 49203-49205
    Retroperitoneal, 49203-49205
  Fissure
    Anal, 46940, 46942
  Hemorrhoids
    Thermal, 46930
  Kidney, 52354
    Endoscopic, 50557, 50576
  Laser Surgery, 17110-17111
  Lesion
    Anus, 46900-46917, 46924
    Bladder, 51030
    Choroid, 67220-67225
    Ciliary Body, 66770
    Colon, *[44401]*, *[45388]*
    Conjunctiva, 68135
    Cornea, 65450
    Eyelid, 67850
    Facial, 17000-17108, 17280-17286
    Gastrointestinal, Upper, *[43270]*
    Gums, 41850
    Intestines
      Large, *[44401]*, *[45388]*
      Small, 44369
    Iris, 66770
    Mouth, 40820
    Nerve
      Celiac Plexus, 64680
      Inferior Alveolar, 64600
      Infraorbital, 64600
      Intercostal, 64620
      Mental, 64600
      Neurofibroma, 0419T-0420T
      Other Peripheral, 64640
      Paravertebral Facet Joint, *[64633, 64634, 64635, 64636]*
      Plantar, 64632
      Pudendal, 64630
      Superior Hypogastric Plexus, 64681
      Supraorbital, 64600
      Trigeminal, 64600, 64605, 64610

**Destruction** — *continued*
  Lesion — *continued*
    Nose
      Intranasal, 30117, 30118
    Palate, 42160
    Penis
      Cryosurgery, 54056
      Electrodesiccation, 54055
      Extensive, 54065
      Laser Surgery, 54057
      Simple, 54050-54060
      Surgical Excision, 54060
    Pharynx, 42808
    Prostate, 45320
      Thermotherapy, 53850-53852
        Microwave, 53850
        Radio Frequency, 53852
    Rectum, 45320
    Retina
      Cryotherapy, Diathermy, 67208, 67227
      Photocoagulation, 67210, 67228-67229
      Radiation by Implantation of Source, 67218
    Skin
      Benign, 17110-17111
      Cutaneous Vascular, 17106-17108
      Malignant, 17260-17286
      Photodynamic Therapy, 96567
      Premalignant, 17000-17004
        by Photodynamic Therapy, 96567, 96573-96574
    Spinal Cord, 62280-62282
    Ureter, 52341, 52342, 52344, 52345
    Urethra, 52400, 53265
    Uvula, 42160
    Vagina
      Extensive, 57065
      Simple, 57061
      Vascular, Cutaneous, 17106-17108
    Vulva
      Extensive, 56515
      Simple, 56501
  Molluscum Contagiosum, 17110, 17111
  Muscle Endplate
    Extraocular, 67345
    Extremity, 64642-64645
    Facial, 64612
    Neck Muscle, 64616
    Trunk, 64646-64647
  Nerve, 64600-64681 *[64633, 64634, 64635, 64636]*
    Laryngeal, Recurrent, 31595
    Paravertebral Facet, *[64633, 64634, 64635, 64636]*
  Neurofibroma, 0419T-0420T
  Plantar Common Digital Nerve, 64632
  Polyp
    Aural, 69540
    Nasal, 30110, 30115
    Rectum, 45320
    Urethra, 53260
  Prostate Tissue
    Transurethral
      Thermotherapy, 53850-53852
    Prostate, 55873
  Sinus
    Frontal, 31080-31085
  Skene's Gland, 53270
  Skin Lesion
    Benign
      Fifteen Lesions or More, 17111
      Fourteen Lesions or Less, 17110
    Malignant, 17260-17286
    Premalignant, 17000-17004
      by Photodynamic Therapy, 96567, 96573-96574
      Fifteen or More Lesions, 17004
      First Lesion, 17000
      Two to Fourteen Lesions, 17003
  Skin Tags, 11200, 11201
  Tonsil
    Lingual, 42870
  Tumor or Polyp
    Rectum, 45320

**Destruction** — *continued*
  Tumor
    Abdomen, 49203-49205
    Bile Duct, *[43278]*
    Breast, 19499
    Chemosurgery, 17311-17315
    Colon, *[44401]*, *[45388]*
    Intestines
      Large, *[44401]*, *[45388]*
      Small, 44369
    Mesentery, 49203-49205
    Pancreatic Duct, *[43278]*
    Peritoneum, 49203-49205
    Rectum, 45190, 45320
    Retroperitoneal, 49203-49205
    Urethra, 53220
    Turbinate Mucosa, 30801, 30802
  Unlisted Services and Procedures, 17999
  Ureter
    Endoscopic, 50957, 50976
  Urethra, 52214, 52224, 52354
    Prolapse, 53275
  Warts
    Flat, 17110, 17111
**Determination, Blood Pressure**
  *See* Blood Pressure
**Determination**
  Lung Volume, 94727-94728
**Developmental**
  Screening, 96110
  Testing, 96111
**Device, Orthotic**
  *See* Orthotics
**Device**
  Adjustable Gastric Restrictive Device, 43770-43774
  Aortic Counterpulsation Ventricular Assist, 0451T-0463T
  Contraceptive, Intrauterine
    Insertion, 58300
    Removal, 58301
  Handling, 99002
  Iliac Artery Occlusion Device
    Insertion, 34808
  Intrauterine
    Insertion, 58300
    Removal, 58301
  Multi-leaf Collimator Design and Construction, 77338
  Programming, 93644, *[93260]*, *[93261]*
  Subcutaneous Port
    for Gastric Restrictive Device, 43770, 43774, 43886-43888
  Venous Access
    Collection of Blood Specimen, 36591-36592
    Implanted, 36591
      Venous Catheter, 36592
    Fluoroscopic Guidance, 77001
    Insertion
      Catheter, 36578
      Central, 36560-36566
      Imaging, 75901, 75902
      Obstruction Clearance, 36595, 36596
      Peripheral, 36570, 36571
      Removal, 36590
      Repair, 36576
      Replacement, 36582, 36583, 36585
    Irrigation, 96523
    Obstruction Clearance, 36595-36596
      Imaging, 75901-75902
    Removal, 36590
    Repair, 36576
    Replacement, 36582-36583, 36585
      Catheter, 36578
  Ventricular Assist, 0451T-0463T, 33975-33983, 33990-33993
**Dexamethasone**
  Suppression Test, 80420
**DFNB59**, 81405
**DGUOK**, 81405
**DHA Sulfate**
  *See* Dehydroepiandrosterone Sulfate
**DHCR7**, 81405
**DHEA (Dehydroepiandrosterone)**, 82626

   *[Resequenced]*     CPT © 2017 American Medical Association. All Rights Reserved.     © 2017 Optum360, LLC

**Endoscopy** — continued
Ureter — continued
Destruction — continued
Uterocele, 52300-52301
Diagnostic, 52351
Dilation, 50572, 50575, 50953
Stricture, 52341-52342, 52344-52345
Excision
Tumor, 52355
Exploration, 52351
Incision, 52290
Injection of Implant Material, 52327
Insertion Guide Wire, 52334
Lithotripsy, 52325, 52353
Manipulation of Ureteral Calculus, 52330
Placement
Stent, 50947, 52332
Removal
Calculus, 50961, 50980, 52310-52315, 52320, 52352
Foreign Body, 50961, 50980
Resection, 52305, 52355
via Incision, 50970-50976, 50980
via Stoma, 50951-50957, 50961
via Ureterotomy, 50970-50980
Urethra, 52000, 52010
Biopsy, 52204, 52354
Catheterization, 52005, 52010
Destruction, 52214, 52354
Congenital Posterior Valves, 52400
Lesion, 52214, 52224, 52234-52235, 52240
Polyps, 52285
Evacuation
Clot, 52001
Excision
Tumor, 52355
Exploration, 52351
Incision, 52285
Congenital Posterior Valves, 52400
Ejaculatory Duct, 52402
Internal, 52270, 52275-52276
Meatotomy, 52281, 52285
Injection
for Cystography, 52281
Implant Material, 51715
Steroid, 52283
Insertion
Radioactive Substance, 52250
Stent, 52282
Lithotripsy, 52353
Lysis Fibrosis, 52285
Removal
Stent, 52310
Resection
Congenital Posterior Valves, 52400
Ejaculatory Duct, 52402
Sphincter, 52277
Vasectomy, 52402
Vasotomy, 52402
Uterus
Anesthesia, 00952
Hysteroscopy
with Division
Resection Intrauterine Septum, 58560
with Lysis of Intrauterine Adhesions, 58559
Diagnostic, 58555
Placement
Fallopian Tube, 58565
Removal
Endometrial, 58563
Impacted Foreign Body, 58562
Leiomyomata, 58561
Surgical with Biopsy, 58558
Vagina, 57421
Anesthesia, 00950
Biopsy, 57421, 57454
Exploration, 57452
Vascular
Surgical, 33508, 37500, 37501
Virtual
Colon, 74261-74263
Vulva, 56820

**Endoscopy** — continued
Vulva — continued
With Biopsy, 56821
**Endosteal Implant**
Reconstruction
Mandible, 21248, 21249
Maxilla, 21248, 21249
**Endothelial Function Assessment**, 0337T
**Endothelioma, Dural**
See Meningioma
**Endotoxin**
Bacteria, 87176
**Endotracheal Tube**
Intubation, 31500
**Endovascular**
Repair
Angiography, 0254T, 34701-34711, 75956-75959
Aorta
Abdominal Aneurysm
with Open Exposure, 34714-34813 [34812, 34820, 34833, 34834]
Endograft Placement, 34701-34713
Descending Thoracic, 33880-33891
Open After Failed Endovascular Repair, 34830-34832
Visceral
Fenestrated Endograft, 34841-34848
Modular Endograft, 34845-34848
Unibody Endograft, 34845-34848
Endograft
Aorta, 34701-34706
Iliac Artery, 34707-34711
Infrarenal Artery, 34701-34706
Femoral Artery, 34713
Iliac Artery Bifurcation, 0254T
Iliac Artery, 34702-34708
Imaging Neck, 75956-75959
Infrarenal Abdominal Aorta
with Endograft, 34701-34706, 34709-34711, 34845-34848
Lower Extremity, 37220-37235
Physician Planning 90 Minutes, 34839
Vena Cava, 37191-37193
Visceral Aorta
with Endograft, 34841-34848
Therapy
Ablation
Administration, Pharmacologic Agent, Other Than Thrombolysis, 61650-61651
Vein, 36473-36479
Neurosurgery
Balloon Angioplasty, 61630
Intracranial Balloon Dilatation, 61640-61642
Occlusion
Balloon, Arterial, 61623
Transcatheter, 61624, 61626
Vascular Catheterization, 61630, 61635
**Enema**
Air Contrast, 74280
Contrast, 74270
Diagnostic, 74280
Home Visit for Fecal Impaction, 99511
Intussusception, 74283
Therapeutic
for Intussusception, 74283
**Energies, Electromagnetic**
See Irradiation
**ENERGIX-B**, 90744, 90746-90747
**ENG**, 81406
**ENT**
See Ear, Nose, and Throat; Otorhinolaryngology, Diagnostic
Therapeutic
See Otorhinolaryngology
**Entamoeba Histolytica**
Antigen Detection
Enzyme Immunoassay, 87336, 87337

**Enterectomy**, 44126-44128, 44137
with Enterostomy, 44125
Donor, 44132, 44133
for Congenital Atresia, 44126-44128
Laparoscopic, 44202-44203
Partial, 44133
Resection, 44120, 44121
Transplanted Allograft, 44137
**Enterocele**
Repair
with Colporrhaphy, 57265
Abdominal Approach, 57270
Hysterectomy, 58263, 58270, 58280, 58292, 58294
Vaginal Approach, 57268, 57556
**Enterocystoplasty**, 51960
Camey, 50825
**Enteroenterostomy**, 44130
**Enterolysis**, 44005
Laparoscopic, 44180
**Enteropancreatostomy**
See Anastomosis, Pancreas to Intestines
**Enterorrhaphy**, 44602, 44603, 44615
**Enteroscopy**
Intestines, Small
Biopsy, 44361, 44377
Control of Bleeding, 44378
Destruction
Lesion, 44369
Tumor, 44369
Diagnostic, 44376
Exploration, 44360
Hemorrhage, 44366
Pelvic Pouch, 44385, 44386
Removal
Foreign Body, 44363
Lesion, 44364, 44365
Polyp, 44364, 44365
Tumor, 44364, 44365
Tube Placement, 44372
Tube Revision, 44373
via Stoma, 44380-44384 [44381]
Tumor, 44364-44365
**Enterostomy**
with Enterectomy
Intestine, Small, 44125
with Enteroenterostomy, 44130
with Proctectomy, 45119, 45397
Closure, 44227, 44620, 44625, 44626
Tube Placement, 44300
**Enterotomy**
Biopsy, 44020
Decompression, 44021
Excision of Lesion, 44110-44111
Exploration, 44020
Foreign Body Removal, 44020
Intestinal Stricturoplasty, 44615
**Enterovirus**
Antibody, 86658
Antigen Detection
Direct Fluorescence, 87265-87272, 87276, 87278, 87280, 87285-87290
**Entropion**
Repair, 67921-67924
Blepharoplasty
Excision Tarsal Wedge, 67923
Extensive, 67923
Suture, 67921
Thermocauterization, 67922
**Enucleation, Cyst, Ovarian**
See Cystectomy, Ovarian
**Enucleation**
Cyst
Mandible, 21040
Maxilla, 21030
Zygoma, 21030
Eye
with Implant, 65103
Muscles Attached, 65105
without Implant, 65101
Pleural, 32540
Prostate, 52649
Tumor, Benign
Mandible, 21040
Maxilla, 21030

**Enucleation** — continued
Tumor, Benign — continued
Zygoma, 21030
**Environmental Intervention**
for Psychiatric Patients, 90882
**Enzyme Activity**
Constituents, 88319
Detection, 87185
Incubation, 86977
Infectious Agent, 87905
Nonradioactive Substrate, 82657
Radioactive Substrate, 82658
**Enzyme, Angiotensin Converting**
See Angiotensin Converting Enzyme (ACE)
**Enzyme, Angiotensin–Forming**
See Renin
**EOG (Electro–Oculography)**, 92270
**Eosinocyte**
See Eosinophils
**Eosinophils**
Nasal Smear, 89190
**EPCAM**, 81403, 81436
**Epiandrosterone**, [80327, 80328]
**Epicondylitis**, 24357-24359
**Epidemic Parotitis**
See Mumps
**Epididymectomy**
with Excision Spermatocele, 54840
Bilateral, 54861
Unilateral, 54860
**Epididymis**
Abscess
Incision and Drainage, 54700
Anastomosis
to Vas Deferens
Bilateral, 54901
Unilateral, 54900
Biopsy, 54800, 54865
Epididymography, 74440
Excision
Bilateral, 54861
Unilateral, 54860
Exploration
Biopsy, 54865
Hematoma
Incision and Drainage, 54700
Lesion
Excision
Local, 54830
Spermatocele, 54840
Needle Biopsy, 54800
Repair, 54900, 54901
Spermatocele
Excision, 54840
Unlisted Procedures, Male Genital, 54699, 55899
X–ray with Contrast, 74440
**Epididymograms**, 55300
**Epididymography**, 74440
**Epididymoplasty**
See Repair, Epididymis
**Epididymovasostomy**
Bilateral, 54901
Unilateral, 54900
**Epidural**
With Disc Decompression, 62287
Analgesia
Continuous, 01967-01969
Drug Administration, 01996
Catheter
Insertion, 62350-62351
Removal, 62355
Clot or Blood Patch, 62273
Electrode
Insertion, 63650, 63655
Removal, 63661-63662
Injection, 0228T-0231T, 62281, 62282, 62320-62327, 64479-64484
Lysis, 62263, 62264
Neurolytic Substance, 62281-62282
**Epidurography**, 72275
**Epigastric**
Hernia Repair, 49570, 49572
Laparoscopic, 49652
**Epiglottidectomy**, 31420

© 2017 Optum360, LLC
CPT © 2017 American Medical Association. All Rights Reserved.

**Epiglottis — Established Patient**

Index

[Resequenced]

CPT © 2017 American Medical Association. All Rights Reserved.

© 2017 Optum360, LLC

Index

Excision — Excision

CPT © 2017 American Medical Association. All Rights Reserved.        © 2017 Optum360, LLC

CPT © 2017 American Medical Association. All Rights Reserved.    © 2017 Optum360, LLC

**Gastrointestinal Prophylaxis for NSAID Use Prescribed**, 4017F
**Gastrointestinal Tract**
  Imaging Intraluminal
    Colon, 0355T
    Distal Ileum, 0355T
    Esophagus Through Ileum, 91110
    Esophagus, 91111
  Reconstruction, 43360, 43361
  Transit and Pressure Measurements, 91112
  Upper
    Dilation, 43249
    X–ray, 74240-74245
      with Contrast, 74246-74249
      Guide Dilator, 74360
      Guide Intubation, 49440, 74340
**Gastrointestinal, Upper**
  Biopsy
    Endoscopy, 43239
  Dilation
    Endoscopy, 43245
    Esophagus, 43248
  Endoscopy
    Catheterization, 43241
    Destruction
      Lesion, *[43270]*
    Dilation, 43245
    Drainage
      Pseudocyst, 43240
    Exploration, 43235
    Hemorrhage, 43255
    Inject Varices, 43243
    Needle Biopsy, 43238, 43242
    Removal
      Foreign Body, 43247
      Lesion, 43250-43251
      Polyp, 43250-43251
      Tumor, 43250-43251
    Resection, Mucosa, 43254
    Stent Placement, *[43266]*
    Thermal Radiation, 43257
    Tube Placement, 43246
    Ultrasound, 43237, 43238, 43242, 43253, 76975
  Exploration
    Endoscopy, 43235
  Hemorrhage
    Endoscopic Control, 43255
  Injection
    Submucosal, 43236
    Varices, 43243
  Lesion
    Destruction, *[43270]*
  Ligation of Vein, 43244
  Needle Biopsy
    Endoscopy, 43238, 43242
  Removal
    Foreign body, 43247
    Lesion, 43250-43251
    Polyp, 43250-43251
    Tumor, 43250-43251
  Stent Placement, *[43266]*
  Tube Placement
    Endoscopy, 43237, 43238, 43246
  Ultrasound
    Endoscopy, 43237, 43238, 43242, 43259, 76975
**Gastrojejunostomy**, 43860, 43865
  with Duodenal Exclusion, 48547
  with Partial Gastrectomy, 43632
  with Vagotomy, 43825
  without Vagotomy, 43820
  Contrast Injection, 49465
  Conversion from Gastrostomy Tube, 49446
  Removal
    Obstructive Material, 49460
  Replacement
    Tube, 49452
  Revision, 43860
    with Vagotomy, 43865
**Gastroplasty**
  Collis, 43283, 43338
  Esophageal Lengthening Procedure, 43283, 43338
  Laparoscopic, 43283, 43644-43645

**Gastroplasty** — *continued*
  Restrictive for Morbid Obesity, 43842-43843, 43845-43848
    Other than Vertical Banded, 43843
  Wedge, 43283, 43338
**Gastrorrhaphy**, 43840
**Gastroschisis**, 49605
**Gastrostomy**
  with Pancreatic Drain, 48001
  with Pyloroplasty, 43640
  with Vagotomy, 43640
  Closure, 43870
  Laparoscopic
    Permanent, 43832
    Temporary, 43653
  Temporary, 43830
    Laparoscopic, 43653
    Neonatal, 43831
  Tube
    Change of, 43760
    Conversion to Gastro-jejunostomy Tube, 49446
    Directed Placement
      Endoscopic, 43246
      Percutaneous, 49440
    Insertion
      Endoscopic, 43246
      Percutaneous, 49440
    Percutaneous, 49440
    Removal
      Obstructive Material, 49460
    Replacement, 49450
    Repositioning, 43761
**Gastrotomy**, 43500, 43501, 43510
**Gaucher Disease Genomic Sequence Analysis**, 81412
**GBA**, 81251, 81412
**GCDH**, 81406
**GCH1**, 81405
**GCK**, 81406
**GDAP1**, 81405
**GDH**, 82965
**GE**
  Reflux, 78262
**Gel Diffusion**, 86331
**Gene Analysis**
  *See* Analysis, Gene
**Genioplasty**, 21120-21123
  Augmentation, 21120, 21123
  Osteotomy, 21121-21123
**Genitalia**
  Female
    Anesthesia, 00940-00952
  Male
    Anesthesia, 00920-00938
    Skin Graft
      Delay of Flap, 15620
      Full Thickness, 15240, 15241
      Pedicle Flap, 15574
      Split, 15120, 15121
      Tissue Transfer, Adjacent, 14040, 14041
**Genitourinary Sphincter, Artificial**
  *See* Prosthesis, Urethral Sphincter
**Genotype Analysis**
  *See* Analysis, Gene
**Gentamicin**, 80170
  Assay, 80170
**Gentiobiase**, 82963
**Genus: Human Cytomegalovirus Group**
  *See* Cytomegalovirus
**GERD**
  *See* Gastroesophageal Reflux Test
**German Measles**
  *See* Rubella
**Gestational Trophoblastic Tumor**
  *See* Hydatidiform Mole
**GFAP**, 81405
**GGT**, 82977
**GH**, 83003
**GH1**, 81404
**GHb**, 83036
**GHR**, 81405
**GHRHR**, 81405
**GI Tract**
  *See* Gastrointestinal Tract
  X–Rays, 74240-74249, 74340, 74360

**Giardia Lamblia**
  Antibody, 86674
**Giardia**
  Antigen Detection
    Enzyme Immunoassay, 87329
    Immunofluorescence, 87269
**Gibbons Stent**, 52332
**GIF**, 84307
**GIFT**, 58976
**Gill Operation**, 63012
**Gillies Approach**
  Fracture
    Zygomatic Arch, 21356
**Gingiva, Abscess**
  *See* Abscess
  Fracture
    *See* Abscess, Gums; Gums
    Zygomatic Arch
      *See* Abscess, Gums; Gums, Abscess
**Gingiva**
  *See* Gums
**Gingivectomy**, 41820
**Gingivoplasty**, 41872
**Girdlestone Laminectomy**
  *See* Laminectomy
**Girdlestone Procedure**
  Acetabulum, Reconstruction, 27120, 27122
**GJB1**, 81403, *[81448]*
**GJB2**, 81252-81253, 81430
**GJB6**, 81254
**Gla Protein (Bone)**
  *See* Osteocalcin
**GLA**, 81405
**Glabellar Frown Lines**
  Rhytidectomy, 15826
**Gland, Adrenal**
  *See* Adrenal Gland
**Gland, Bartholin's**
  *See* Bartholin's Gland
**Gland, Bulbourethral**
  *See* Bulbourethral Gland
**Gland, Lacrimal**
  *See* Lacrimal Gland
**Gland, Mammary**
  *See* Breast
**Gland, Parathyroid**
  *See* Parathyroid Gland
**Gland, Parotid**
  *See* Parotid Gland
**Gland, Pituitary**
  *See* Pituitary Gland
**Gland, Salivary**
  *See* Salivary Glands
**Gland, Sublingual**
  *See* Sublingual Gland
**Gland, Sweat**
  *See* Sweat Glands
**Gland, Thymus**
  *See* Thymus Gland
**Gland, Thyroid**
  *See* Thyroid Gland
**Gland**
  *See* Specific Gland
**Glasses**
  *See* Spectacle Services
**Glaucoma Drainage Implant**
  *See* Aqueous Shunt
**Glaucoma**
  Cryotherapy, 66720
  Cyclophotocoagulation, 66710, 66711
  Diathermy, 66700
  Fistulization of Sclera, 66150
**Glenn Procedure**, 33622, 33766-33767
**Glenohumeral Joint**
  Arthrotomy, 23040
    with Biopsy, 23100
    with Synovectomy, 23105
  Exploration, 23107
  Removal
    Foreign or Loose Body, 23107
**Glenoid Fossa**
  Reconstruction, 21255
**GLN**, 82127-82131
**Globulin, Corticosteroid–Binding**, 84449
**Globulin, Rh Immune**, 90384-90386

**Globulin, Thyroxine–Binding**, 84442
**Globulin**
  Antihuman, 86880-86886
  Immune, 90281-90399
  Sex Hormone Binding, 84270
**Glomerular Procoagulant Activity**
  *See* Thromboplastin
**Glomus Caroticum**
  *See* Carotid Body
**Glossectomies**, 41120-41155
**Glossectomy**, 41120-41155
**Glossopexy**, 41500
**Glossorrhaphy**
  *See* Suture, Tongue
**Glucagon**, 82943
  Tolerance Panel, 80422, 80424
  Tolerance Test, 82946
**Glucose Phosphate Isomerase Measurement**, 84087
**Glucose Phosphate Isomerase**, 84087
**Glucose**, 80422, 80424, 80430-80435, 95251 *[95249]*
  Blood Test, 82947-82950, 82962
  Body Fluid, 82945
  Hormone Panel, 80430
  Interstitial Fluid
    Continuous Monitoring, 95250-95251 *[95249]*
  Interstitial Sensor (implantable), 0446T-0448T
  Tolerance Test, 82951, 82952
**Glucose-6-Phosphatase, Catalytic Subunit Gene Analysis**, 81250
**Glucose–6–Phosphate**
  Dehydrogenase, 82955, 82960
**Glucosidase**, 82963
  Beta Acid Gene Analysis, 81251
**Glucuronide Androstanediol**, 82154
**GLUD1**, 81406
**Glue**
  Cornea Wound, 65286
  Sclera Wound, 65286
**Glukagon**
  *See* Glucagon
**Glutamate Dehydrogenase**, 82965
**Glutamate Pyruvate Transaminase**, 84460
**Glutamic Alanine Transaminase**, 84460
**Glutamic Aspartic Transaminase**, 84450
**Glutamic Dehydrogenase**, 82965
**Glutamine**, 82127-82131
**Glutamyltransferase, Gamma**, 82977
**Glutathione**, 82978
  Glutathione Reductase, 82979
**Glycanhydrolase, N–Acetylmuramide**
  *See* Lysozyme
**Glycated Hemoglobins**
  *See* Glycohemoglobin
**Glycated Protein**, 82985
**Glycerol, Phosphatidyl**
  *See* Phosphatidylglycerol
**Glycerol Phosphoglycerides**
  *See* Phosphatidylglycerol
**Glycerophosphatase**
  *See* Alkaline Phosphatase
**Glycinate, Theophylline Sodium**
  *See* Theophylline
**Glycocholic Acid**
  *See* Cholylglycine
**Glycohemoglobin**, 83036-83037
**Glycol, Ethylene**
  *See* Ethylene Glycol
**Glycols, Ethylene**
  *See* Ethylene Glycol
**Glycosaminoglycan**
  *See* Mucopolysaccharides
**GNAQ**, 81403
**GNE**, 81400, 81406
**Goeckerman Treatment**
  Photochemotherapy, 96910-96913
**Gold**
  Assay, *[80375]*
**Goldwaite Procedure**
  Reconstruction, Patella, for Instability, 27422
**Golfer's Elbow**, 24357-24359
**Gol–Vernet Operation**, 50120
**Gonadectomy, Female**
  *See* Oophorectomy

Index — Immunization — Incision and Drainage

*Index*

*Insertion — Integumentary System*

**Knee** — *continued*
Reconstruction — *continued*
Ligament, 27427-27429
Removal
Foreign Body, 27310, 27331, 27372
Loose Body, 27331
Prosthesis, 27488
Repair
Ligament, 27405-27409
Collateral and Cruciate, 27409
Collateral, 27405
Cruciate, 27407, 27409
Meniscus, 27403
Tendon, 27380, 27381
Replacement, 27447
Retinacular
Release, 27425
Strapping, 29530
Suture
Tendon, 27380, 27381
Transplantation
Chondrocytes, 27412
Meniscus, 29868
Osteochondral
Allograft, 27415, 29867
Autograft, 27412, 29866
Tumor, 27327-27328 *[27337, 27339]*, 27355-27358, 27364-27365 *[27329]*
Unlisted Services and Procedures, 27599
X–ray with Contrast
Angiography, 73706
Arthrography, 73580
X–ray, 73560-73564
Arthrography, 73580
Bilateral, 73565
**Kneecap**
Excision, 27350
Repair
Instability, 27420-27424
**Knock–Knee Repair**, 27455, 27457
**Kocher Operation**, 23650-23680
*See* Clavicle; Scapula; Shoulder, Dislocation, Closed Treatment
**Kocher Pylorectomy**
Gastrectomy, Partial, 43631
**Kock Pouch**, 44316
Formation, 50825
**Kock Procedure**, 44316
**KOH**
Hair, Nails, Tissue, Examination for Fungi, 87220
**Konno Procedure**, 33412
**Koop Inguinal Orchiopexy**, 54640
**KRAS**, 81275-81276, 81405
**Kraske Procedure**, 45116
**Krause Operation**
Gasserian Ganglion, Sensory Root, Decompression, 61450
**Kroenlein Procedure**, 67420
**Krukenberg Procedure**, 25915
**Krupin-Denver Valve**
Implant, 66180
Removal, 67120
Revision, 66185
**KS**, 83586, 83593
**KUB**, 74241, 74247, 74270, 74420
**Kuhlmann Test**, 96101-96103
**Kuhnt–Szymanowski Procedure**, 67917
**K–Wire Fixation**
Tongue, 41500
**Kyphectomy**
More than Two Segments, 22819
Up to Two Segments, 22818
**Kyphoplasty**, 22513-22515

---

## L

**L Ascorbic Acid**
*See* Ascorbic Acid
**L Aspartate 2 Oxoglutarate Aminotransferase**
*See* Transaminase, Glutamic Oxaloacetic
**L Glutamine**
*See* Glutamine
**L1CAM**, 81407
**Labial Adhesions**
Lysis, 56441

**Labyrinth**
*See* Ear, Inner
**Labyrinthectomy**
with Mastoidectomy, 69910
with Skull Base Surgery, 61596
Transcanal, 69905
**Labyrinthotomy**
with Skull Base Surgery, 61596
Inner Ear, 69949
Transcanal, 69801
**Laceration Repair**
*See* Repair, Laceration, Skin
**Lacrimal Duct**
Balloon, 68816
Canaliculi
Incision, 68899
Repair, 68700
Dilation, 68816
Exploration, 68810
with Anesthesia, 68811
Canaliculi, 68840
Stent, 68815
Insertion
Stent, 68815
Nasolacrimal Duct Probing, 68816
Removal
Dacryolith, 68530
Foreign Body, 68530
X–ray with Contrast, 70170
**Lacrimal Gland**
Biopsy, 68510
Close Fistula, 68770
Excision
Partial, 68505
Total, 68500
Fistulization, 68720
Incision and Drainage, 68400
Injection
X–ray, 68850
Nuclear Medicine
Tear Flow, 78660
Removal
Dacryolith, 68530
Foreign Body, 68530
Repair
Fistula, 68770
Tumor
Excision
with Osteotomy, 68550
without Closure, 68540
X–Ray, 70170
**Lacrimal Punctum**
Closure
by Plug, 68761
by Thermocauterization, Ligation or Laser Surgery, 68760
Dilation, 68801
Incision, 68440
Repair, 68705
**Lacrimal Sac**
Biopsy, 68525
Excision, 68520
Incision and Drainage, 68420
**Lacrimal System**
Unlisted Services and Procedures, 68899
**Lacryoaptography**
Nuclear, 78660
**Lactase Deficiency Breath Test**, 91065
**Lactate**, 83605
**Lactic Acid Measurement**
*See* Lactate
**Lactic Acid**, 83605
**Lactic Cytochrome Reductase**
*See* Lactic Dehydrogenase
**Lactic Dehydrogenase**, 83615, 83625
**Lactiferous Duct**
Excision, 19112
Exploration, 19110
**Lactoferrin**
Fecal, 83630-83631
**Lactogen, Human Placental**, 83632
**Lactogenic Hormone**
*See* Prolactin
**Lactose**
Urine, 83633
**Ladd Procedure**, 44055

**Lagophthalmos**
Repair, 67912
**Laki Lorand Factor**
*See* Fibrin Stabilizing Factor
**L–Alanine**
*See* Aminolevulinic Acid (ALA)
**LAMA2**, 81408
**LAMB2**, 81407
**Lamblia Intestinalis**
*See* Giardia Lamblia
**Lambrinudi Operation**
Arthrodesis, Foot Joints, 28730, 28735, 28740
**Lamellar Keratoplasties**
*See* Keratoplasty, Lamellar
**Laminaria**
Insertion, 59200
**Laminectomy**, 62351, 63001-63003, 63005-63011, 63015-63044, 63180-63200, 63265-63290, 63600-63655
with Facetectomy, 63045-63048
Decompression
Cervical, 63001, 63015
with Facetectomy and Foraminotomy, 63045, 63048
Neural Elements, 0274T
Laminotomy
Initial
Cervical, 63020
Each Additional Space, 63035
Lumbar, 63030
Reexploration
Cervical, 63040
Each Additional Interspace, 63043
Lumbar, 63042
Each Additional Interspace, 63044
Lumbar, 63005, 63017
with Facetectomy and Foraminotomy, 63047, 63048
Neural Elements, 0275T
Sacral, 63011
Thoracic, 63003, 63016
with Facetectomy and Foraminotomy, 63046, 63048
Neural Elements, 0274T
Excision
Lesion, 63250-63273
Neoplasm, 63275-63290
Lumbar, 22630, 63012
Surgical, 63170-63200
**Laminoplasty**
Cervical, 63050-63051
**Laminotomy**
Cervical, One Interspace, 63020
Lumbar, 63042
One Interspace, 62380, 63030
Each Additional, 63035
Re–exploration, Cervical, 63040
**Lamotrigine**
Assay, 80175
**LAMP2**, 81405
**Landboldt's Operation**, 67971, 67973, 67975
**Lane's Operation**, 44150
**Langerhans Islands**
*See* Islet Cell
**Language Evaluation**, 92521-92524
**Language Therapy**, 92507, 92508
**LAP**, 83670
**Laparoscopy**
Abdominal, 49320-49329
Surgical, 49321-49326
Adrenal Gland
Biopsy, 60650
Excision, 60650
Adrenalectomy, 60650
Appendectomy, 44970
Aspiration, 49322
Biopsy, 49321
Lymph Nodes, 38570
Ovary, 49321
Bladder
Repair
Sling Procedure, 51992
Urethral Suspension, 51990
Unlisted, 51999

**Laparoscopy** — *continued*
Cecostomy, 44188
Cholecystectomy, 47562-47564
Cholecystoenterostomy, 47570
Closure
Enterostomy, 44227
Colectomy
Partial, 44204-44208, 44213
Total, 44210-44212
Colostomy, 44188
Destruction
Lesion, 58662
Diagnostic, 49320
Drainage
Extraperitoneal Lymphocele, 49323
Ectopic Pregnancy, 59150
with Salpingectomy and/or Oophorectomy, 59151
Electrode
Implantation
Gastric
Antrum, 43647
Lesser Curvature, 43659
Removal
Gastric, 43648, 43659
Replacement
Gastric, 43647
Revision
Gastric, 43648, 43659
Enterectomy, 44202
Enterolysis, 44180
Enterostomy
Closure, 44227
Esophageal Lengthening, 43283
Esophagogastric Fundoplasty, 43280
Esophagomyotomy, 43279
Esophagus
Esophageal Lengthening, 43283
Esophageal Sphincter Augmentation, 43284
Removal, 43285
Esophagogastric Fundoplasty, 43280
Esophagomyotomy, 43279
Fimbrioplasty, 58672
Gastric Restrictive Procedures, 43644-43645, 43770-43774
Gastrostomy
Temporary, 43653
Graft Revision
Vaginal, 57426
Hernia Repair
Epigastric, 49652
Incarcerated or Strangulated, 49653
Incisional, 49654
Incarcerated or Strangulated, 49655
Recurrent, 49656
Incarcerated or Strangulated, 49657
Initial, 49650
Recurrent, 49651
Spigelian, 49652
Incarcerated or Strangulated, 49653
Umbilical, 49652
Incarcerated or Strangulated, 49653
Ventral, 49652
Incarcerated or Strangulated, 49653
Hysterectomy, 58541-58554, 58570-58575
Radical, 58548
Total, 58570-58575
Ileostomy, 44187
In Vitro Fertilization, 58976
Retrieve Oocyte, 58970
Transfer Embryo, 58974
Transfer Gamete, 58976
Incontinence Repair, 51990, 51992
Jejunostomy, 44186-44187
Kidney
Ablation, 50541-50542
Ligation
Veins, Spermatic, 55500

---

 CPT © 2017 American Medical Association. All Rights Reserved.

[Resequenced]

CPT © 2017 American Medical Association. All Rights Reserved.

© 2017 Optum360, LLC

**Lung — Maltose**

**Maxillectomy**, 31225, 31230
**Maxillofacial Fixation**
  Application
    Halo Type Appliance, 21100
**Maxillofacial Impressions**
  Auricular Prosthesis, 21086
  Definitive Obturator Prosthesis, 21080
  Facial Prosthesis, 21088
  Interim Obturator Prosthesis, 21079
  Mandibular Resection Prosthesis, 21081
  Nasal Prosthesis, 21087
  Oral Surgical Splint, 21085
  Orbital Prosthesis, 21077
  Palatal Augmentation Prosthesis, 21082
  Palatal Lift Prosthesis, 21083
  Speech Aid Prosthesis, 21084
  Surgical Obturator Prosthesis, 21076
**Maxillofacial Procedures**
  Unlisted Services and Procedures, 21299
**Maxillofacial Prosthetics**, 21076-21088
  Unlisted Services and Procedures, 21089
**Maydl Operation**, 45563, 50810
**Mayo Hernia Repair**, 49580-49587
**Mayo Operation**
  Varicose Vein Removal, 37700-37735, 37780,
    37785
**Maze Procedure**, 33254-33259, 33265-33266
**MBC**, 87181-87190
**MC4R**, 81403
**McBurney Operation**
  Hernia Repair, Inguinal, 49495-49500, 49505
    Incarcerated, 49496, 49501, 49507,
      49521
    Recurrent, 49520
    Sliding, 49525
**McCall Culdoplasty**, 57283
**McCannel Procedure**, 66682
**McCauley Procedure**, 28240
**MCCC1**, 81406
**MCCC2**, 81406
**McDonald Operation**, 57700
**McKeown Esophagectomy**, 43112
**McKissock Surgery**, 19318
**McIndoe Procedure**, 57291
**MCOLN1**, 81290, 81412
**McVay Operation**
  Hernia Repair, Inguinal, 49495-49500, 49505
    Incarcerated, 49496, 49501, 49507,
      49521
    Laparoscopic, 49650, 49651
    Recurrent, 49520
    Sliding, 49525
**MEA (Microwave Endometrial Ablation)**, 58563
**Measles, German**
  Antibody, 86756
  Vaccine, 90707, 90710
**Measles Immunization**, 90707, 90710
**Measles, Mumps, Rubella Vaccine**, 90707
**Measles Uncomplicated**
  Antibody, 86765
  Antigen Detection, 87283
**Measles Vaccine**, 90707, 90710
**Measurement**
  Ocular Blood Flow, 0198T
  Spirometric Forced Expiratory Flow, 94011-
    94012
**Meat Fibers**
  Feces, 89160
**Meatoplasty**, 69310
**Meatotomy**, 53020-53025
  Contact Laser Vaporization with/without
    Transurethral Resection of Prostate,
    52648
    with Cystourethroscopy, 52281
  Infant, 53025
  Non–Contact Laser Coagulation Prostate,
    52647
  Prostate
    Laser Coagulation, 52647
    Laser Vaporization, 52648
  Transurethral Electrosurgical Resection
    Prostate, 52601
  Ureter, 52290
  Urethral
    Cystourethroscopy, 52290-52305

**Meckel's Diverticulum**
  Excision, 44800
  Unlisted Services and Procedures, 44899
**MECP2**, 81302-81304
**MED12**, 81401
**Median Nerve Compression**
  Decompression, 64721
    Endoscopy, 29848
  Injection, 20526
**Median Nerve**
  Decompression, 64721
  Neuroplasty, 64721
  Release, 64721
  Repair
    Suture
      Motor, 64835
  Transposition, 64721
**Mediastinoscopy**
  with Biopsy, 39401-39402
  with Esophagogastric Fundoplasty, [43210]
**Mediastinotomy**
  Cervical Approach, 39000
  Transthoracic Approach, 39010
**Mediastinum**
  *See* Chest; Thorax
  Cyst
    Excision, 32662, 39200
  Endoscopy
    Biopsy, 39401-39402
    Esophagogastric Fundoplasty, [43210]
    Exploration, 39401
  Exploration, 39000, 39010
  Incision and Drainage, 39000, 39010
  Lymphadenectomy, 32674
  Needle Biopsy, 32405
  Removal
    Foreign Body, 39000, 39010
  Tumor
    Excision, 32662, 39220
  Unlisted Procedures, 39499
**Medical Disability Evaluation Services**, 99455,
  99456
**Medical Genetics**
  Counseling, 96040
**Medical Nutrition Therapy**, 97802-97804
**Medical Team Conference**, 99366-99368
**Medical Testimony**, 99075
**Medication Therapy Management**
  By a Pharmacist
    Initial Encounter, 99605-99606
    Subsequent Encounter, 99607
    Each Additional 15 Minutes, 99607
**Medicine, Preventive**
  *See* Preventive Medicine
**Medicine, Pulmonary**
  *See* Pulmonology
**MEFV**, 81402, 81404
**MEG (Magnetoencephalography)**, 95965-95967
**MEG3/DLK1**, 81401
**Meibomian Cyst**
  Excision, 67805
    Multiple
      Different Lids, 67805
      Same Lid, 67801
    Single, 67800
    Under Anesthesia, 67808
**Membrane, Mucous**
  *See* Mucosa
**Membrane, Tympanic**
  *See* Ear, Drum
**MEN1**, 81404-81405
**Menactra**, 90734
**MenB-4C**, [90620]
**MenB-FHbp**, [90621]
**Meninges**
  Tumor
    Excision, 61512, 61519
**Meningioma**
  Excision, 61512, 61519
  Tumor
    Excision, 61512, 61519
**Meningitis, Lymphocytic Benign**
  Antibody, 86727
**Meningocele Repair**, 63700, 63702

**Meningococcal Vaccine**
  Conjugate, Serogroups A, C, Y, MCV4, Men-
    ACWY, W-135, 90734
  Conjugate, Serogroups C & Y and Hemophilus
    Influenza B, 90644
  Polysaccharide, Any Groups, 90733
  Recombinant, 90620-90621
**Meningococcus**, 86741
**Meningomyelocele**
  Repair, 63704-63706
**Meniscal Temporal Lobectomy**, 61566
**Meniscectomy**
  Knee Joint, 27332, 27333
  Temporomandibular Joint, 21060
**Meniscus**
  Knee
    Excision, 27332, 27333
    Repair, 27403
    Transplantation, 29868
**Menomune**, 90733
**Mental Nerve**
  Avulsion, 64736
  Incision, 64736
  Transection, 64736
**Menveo**, 90734
**Meprobamate**, [80369, 80370]
**Mercury**, 83015, 83825
**Merskey Test**
  Fibrin Degradation Products, 85362-85379
**Mesencephalic Tract**
  Incision, 61480
  Section, 61480
**Mesencephalon**
  Tractotomy, 61480
**Mesenteric Arteries**
  *See* Artery, Mesenteric
**Mesentery**
  Lesion
    Excision, 44820
  Repair, 44850
  Suture, 44850
  Unlisted Services and Procedures, 44899
**Mesh Implantation**
  Closure of Necrotizing Soft Tissue Infection,
    49568
  Incisional or Ventral Hernia, 49568
  Vagina, 57267
**Mesh**
  Implantation
    Hernia, 49568
  Insertion
    Pelvic Floor, 57267
  Removal
    Abdominal Infected, 11008
**Metabisulfite Test**
  Red Blood Cell, Sickling, 85660
**Metabolic Panel**
  Calcium Ionized, 80047
  Calcium Total, 80048
  Comprehensive, 80053
**Metabolite**
  Cocaine, [80353]
  Thromboxane, 84431
**Metacarpal**
  Amputation, 26910
  Craterization, 26230
  Cyst
    Excision, 26200, 26205
  Diaphysectomy, 26230
  Excision, 26230
    Radical for Tumor, 26250
  Fracture
    with Manipulation, 26605, 26607
    without Manipulation, 26600
    Closed Treatment, 26605
      with Fixation, 26607
    Open Treatment, 26615
    Percutaneous Fixation, 26608
  Ostectomy
    Radical
      for Tumor, 26250
  Repair
    Lengthening, 26568
    Nonunion, 26546
    Osteotomy, 26565
  Saucerization, 26230

**Metacarpal** — *continued*
  Tumor
    Excision, 26200, 26205
**Metacarpophalangeal Joint**
  Arthrodesis, 26850, 26852
  Arthroplasty, 26530, 26531
  Arthroscopy
    Diagnostic, 29900
    Surgical, 29901, 29902
  Arthrotomy, 26075
  Biopsy
    Synovium, 26105
  Capsule
    Excision, 26520
    Incision, 26520
  Capsulodesis, 26516-26518
  Dislocation
    with Manipulation, 26340
    Closed Treatment, 26700
    Open Treatment, 26715
    Percutaneous Fixation, 26705, 26706
  Exploration, 26075
  Fracture
    with Manipulation, 26742
    Closed Treatment, 26740
    Open Treatment, 26746
  Fusion, 26516-26518, 26850, 26852
  Removal of Foreign Body, 26075
  Repair
    Collateral Ligament, 26540-26542
  Synovectomy, 26135
**Metadrenaline**, 83835
**Metals, Heavy**, 83015, 83018
**Metanephrine**, 83835
**Metatarsal**
  *See* Foot
  Amputation, 28810
  Condyle
    Excision, 28288
  Craterization, 28122
  Cyst
    Excision, 28104-28107
  Diaphysectomy, 28122
  Excision, 28110-28114, 28122, 28140
  Fracture
    Closed Treatment
      with Manipulation, 28475, 28476
      without Manipulation, 28470
    Open Treatment, 28485
    Percutaneous Fixation, 28476
  Free Osteocutaneous Flap with Microvascular
    Anastomosis, 20972
  Repair, 28322
    Lengthening, 28306, 28307
    Osteotomy, 28306-28309
  Saucerization, 28122
  Tumor
    Excision, 28104-28107, 28173
**Metatarsectomy**, 28140
**Metatarsophalangeal Joint**
  Arthrotomy, 28022, 28052
  Cheilectomy, 28289, 28291
  Dislocation, 28630, 28635, 28645
    Open Treatment, 28645
    Percutaneous Fixation, 28636
  Exploration, 28022
  Great Toe
    Arthrodesis, 28750
    Fusion, 28750
  Release, 28289, 28291
  Removal
    of Foreign Body, 28022
    of Loose Body, 28022
  Repair
    Hallux Rigidus, 28289, 28291
  Synovial
    Biopsy, 28052
    Excision, 28072
  Toe, 28270
**Methadone**, [80358]
**Methamphetamine**, [80359]
**Methbipyranone**, 80436
**Methemalbumin**, 83857
**Methemoglobin**, 83045, 83050, 84741
**Methenamine Silver Stain**, 88312
**Methopyrapone**, 80436

*[Resequenced]*     CPT © 2017 American Medical Association. All Rights Reserved.     © 2017 Optum360, LLC

CPT © 2017 American Medical Association. All Rights Reserved.            © 2017 Optum360, LLC

**Natural Ostium** — *continued*
  Sinus — *continued*
    Sphenoid, 31002
**Navicular**
  Arthroplasty
    with Implant, 25443
  Fracture
    with Manipulation, 25624
    Closed Treatment, 25622
    Open Treatment, 25628
  Repair, 25440
**Navigation**
  Computer Assisted, 20985, 61781-61783
**NDP**, 81403-81404
**NDUFA1**, 81404
**NDUFAF2**, 81404
**NDUFS1**, 81406
**NDUFS4**, 81404
**NDUFS7**, 81405
**NDUFS8**, 81405
**NDUFV1**, 81405
**Near-infrared**
  Spectroscopy Studies
    Lower Extremity Wound, 0493T
**NEB**, 81400, 81408
**Neck, Humerus**
  Fracture
    with Shoulder Dislocation
      Closed Treatment, 23680
      Open Treatment, 23675
**Neck Muscle**
  Division, Scalenus Anticus, 21700, 21705
    Sternocleidomastoid, 21720-21725
**Neck**
  Angiography, 70498, 70547-70549
  Artery
    Ligation, 37615
  Biopsy, 21550
  Bypass Graft, 35901
  CT Scan, 70490-70492, 70498
  Dissection, Radical
    *See* Radical Neck Dissection
  Exploration
    Blood Vessels, 35800
    Lymph Nodes, 38542
  Incision and Drainage
    Abscess, 21501, 21502
    Hematoma, 21501, 21502
  Lipectomy, Suction Assisted, 15876
  Magnetic Resonance Angiography (MRA), 70547-70549
  Magnetic Resonance Imaging (MRI), 70540-70543
  Nerve
    Graft, 64885, 64886
  Repair
    with Other Graft, 35261
    with Vein Graft, 35231
    Blood Vessel, 35201
  Rhytidectomy, 15825, 15828
  Skin Graft
    Delay of Flap, 15620
    Full Thickness, 15240, 15241
    Pedicle Flap, 15574
    Split, 15120, 15121
  Skin
    Revision, 15819
  Surgery, Unlisted, 21899
  Tissue Transfer, Adjacent, 14040, 14041
  Tumor, 21555-21558 *[21552, 21554]*
  Ultrasound Exam, 76536
  Unlisted Services and Procedures, 21899
  Urinary Bladder
    *See* Bladder, Neck
  Wound Exploration
    Penetrating, 20100
    X–ray, 70360
**Necropsy**
  Coroner Examination, 88045
  Forensic Examination, 88040
  Gross and Microscopic Examination, 88020-88029
  Gross Examination, 88000-88016
  Organ, 88037
  Regional, 88036
  Unlisted Services and Procedures, 88099

**Needle Biopsy**
  *See* Biopsy
  Abdomen Mass, 49180
  Bone Marrow, 38221
  Bone, 20220, 20225
  Breast, 19100
  Colon Sigmoid
    Endoscopy, 45342
  Colon
    Endoscopy, 45392
  CT Scan Guidance, 77012
  Epididymis, 54800
  Esophagus
    Endoscopy, 43232, 43238
  Fluoroscopic Guidance, 77002
  Gastrointestinal, Upper
    Endoscopy, 43238, 43242
  Kidney, 50200
  Liver, 47000, 47001
  Lung, 32405
  Lymph Node, 38505
  Mediastinum, 32405
  Muscle, 20206
  Pancreas, 48102
  Pleura, 32400
  Prostate, 55700
    with Fluorescence Spectroscopy, 0443T
  Retroperitoneal Mass, 49180
  Salivary Gland, 42400
  Spinal Cord, 62269
  Testis, 54500
  Thyroid Gland, 60100
  Transbronchial, 31629, 31633
**Needle Localization**
  Breast
    with Biopsy, 19081-19086
    with Lesion Excision, 19125, 19126
    Placement, 19281-19288
  Magnetic Resonance Guidance, 77021
**Needle Manometer Technique**, 20950
**Needle Wire**
  Introduction
    Trachea, 31730
  Placement
    Breast, 19281-19288
**Neer Procedure**, 23470
**NEFL**, 81405
**Negative Pressure Wound Therapy (NPWT)**, 97605-97608
**Neisseria Gonorrhoeae**, 87590-87592, 87850
**Neisseria Meningitidis**
  Antibody, 86741
**Neobladder**
  Construction, 51596
**Neonatal Alloimmune Thrombocytopenia [NAIT]**, *[81105, 81106, 81107, 81108, 81109, 81110, 81111, 81112]*
**Neonatal Critical Care**, 99468-99469
**Neonatal Intensive Care**
  *See* Newborn Care
  Initial, 99477-99480
  Subsequent, 99478-99480
**Neoplasm**
  See Tumor
**Neoplastic Growth**
  *See* Tumor
**Nephelometry**, 83883
**Nephrectomy**
  with Ureters, 50220-50236, 50546, 50548
  Donor, 50300, 50320, 50547
  Laparoscopic, 50545-50548
  Partial, 50240
    Laparoscopic, 50543
  Recipient, 50340
**Nephrolith**
  *See* Calculus, Removal, Kidney
**Nephrolithotomy**, 50060-50075
**Nephropexy**, 50400, 50405
**Nephroplasty**
  *See* Kidney, Repair
**Nephropyeloplasty**, 50400-50405, 50544
**Nephrorrhaphy**, 50500
**Nephroscopy**
  *See* Endoscopy, Kidney
**Nephrostogram**, *[50430, 50431]*

**Nephrostolithotomy**
  Percutaneous, 50080, 50081
**Nephrostomy Tract**
  Establishment, 50395
**Nephrostomy**
  Change Tube, *[50435]*
    with Drainage, 50400
  Closure, 53899
  Endoscopic, 50562-50570
    with Exploration, 50045
  Percutaneous, 52334
  X–ray with Contrast
    to Guide Dilation, 74485
**Nephrotomogram**
  *See* Nephrotomography
**Nephrotomography**, 74415
**Nephrotomy**, 50040, 50045
  with Exploration, 50045
**Nerve Conduction**
  Motor and/or Sensory, 95905-95913
**Nerve II, Cranial**
  *See* Optic Nerve
**Nerve Root**
  *See* Cauda Equina; Spinal Cord
  Decompression, 62380, 63020-63048, 63055-63103
  Incision, 63185, 63190
  Section, 63185, 63190
**Nerve Stimulation, Transcutaneous**
  *See* Application, Neurostimulation
**Nerve Teasing**, 88362
**Nerve V, Cranial**
  *See* Trigeminal Nerve
**Nerve VII, Cranial**
  *See* Facial Nerve
**Nerve X, Cranial**
  *See* Vagus Nerve
**Nerve XI, Cranial**
  *See* Accessory Nerve
**Nerve XII, Cranial**
  *See* Hypoglossal Nerve
**Nerve**
  Cranial
    *See* Cranial Nerve
  Facial
    *See* Facial Nerve
  Foot
    Incision, 28035
  Intercostal
    *See* Intercostal Nerve
  Median
    *See* Median Nerve
  Obturator
    *See* Obturator Nerve
  Peripheral
    *See* Peripheral Nerve
  Phrenic
    *See* Phrenic Nerve
  Sciatic
    *See* Sciatic Nerve
  Spinal
    *See* Spinal Nerve
  Tibial
    *See* Tibial Nerve
  Ulnar
    *See* Ulnar Nerve
  Vestibular
    *See* Vestibular Nerve
**Nerves**
  Anastomosis
    Facial to Hypoglossal, 64868
    Facial to Spinal Accessory, 64866
  Avulsion, 64732-64772
  Biopsy, 64795
  Cryoablation, Percutaneous, 0440T-0442T
  Decompression, 62380, 64702-64727
  Destruction, 64600-64681 *[64633, 64634, 64635, 64636]*
    Laryngeal, Recurrent, 31595
    Paravertebral Facet Joint, *[64633, 64634, 64635, 64636]*
  Foot
    Excision, 28055
    Incision, 28035
  Graft, 64885-64907

**Nerves** — *continued*
  Implantation
    Electrode, 64553-64581
    to Bone, 64787
    to Muscle, 64787
  Incision, 43640, 43641, 64732-64772
  Injection
    Anesthetic, 01991-01992, 64400-64530
    Neurolytic Agent, 64600-64681 *[64633, 64634, 64635, 64636]*
  Insertion
    Electrode, 64553-64581
  Lesion
    Excision, 64774-64792
  Neurofibroma
    Excision, 64788-64792
  Neurolemmoma
    Excision, 64788-64792
  Neurolytic
    Internal, 64727
  Neuroma
    Excision, 64774-64786
  Neuroplasty, 64702-64721
  Nuclear Medicine
    Unlisted Services and Procedures, 78699
  Removal
    Electrode, 64585
  Repair
    Graft, 64885-64911
    Microdissection
      with Surgical Microscope, 69990
    Suture, 64831-64876
  Spinal Accessory
    Incision, 63191
    Section, 63191
  Suture, 64831-64876
  Sympathectomy
    Excision, 64802-64818
  Transection, 43640, 43641, 64732-64772
  Transposition, 64718-64721
  Unlisted Services and Procedures, 64999
**Nervous System**
  Nuclear Medicine
    Unlisted Services and Procedures, 78699
**Nesidioblast**
  *See* Islet Cell
**Neurectasis**, 64999
**Neurectomy**
  Foot, 28055
  Gastrocnemius, 27326
  Hamstring Muscle, 27325
  Leg, Lower, 27326
  Leg, Upper, 27325
  Popliteal, 27326
  Tympanic, 69676
**Neuroendoscopy**
  Intracranial, 62160-62165
**Neurofibroma**
  Cutaneous Nerve
    Excision, 64788
  Extensive
    Destruction, 0419T-0420T
    Excision, 64792
  Peripheral Nerve
    Excision, 64790
**Neurolemmoma**
  Cutaneous Nerve
    Excision, 64788
  Extensive
    Excision, 64792
  Peripheral Nerve
    Excision, 64790
**Neurologic System**
  *See* Nervous System
**Neurology**
  Brain
    Cortex Magnetic Stimulation, 90867-90869
    Mapping, 96020
    Surface Electrode Stimulation, 95961-95962
  Central Motor
    Electrocorticogram
      Intraoperative, 95829
    Electroencephalogram (EEG)
      Brain Death, 95824

CPT © 2017 American Medical Association. All Rights Reserved.      © 2017 Optum360, LLC

**Pachymetry**
  Eye, 76514
**Packing**
  Nasal Hemorrhage, 30901-30906
**PAFAH1B1**, 81405-81406
**PAH**, 81406
**Pain Management**
  Epidural, 62350-62351, 62360-62362, 99601-99602
  Intrathecal, 62350-62351, 62360-62362, 99601-99602
  Intravenous Therapy, 96360-96368, 96374-96376
**Pain Therapy**, 0278T, 62350-62365
**Palatal Augmentation Prosthesis**, 21082
**Palatal Lift Prosthesis**, 21083
**Palate, Cleft**
  Repair, 42200-42225
  Rhinoplasty, 30460-30462
**Palate**
  Abscess
    Incision and Drainage, 42000
  Biopsy, 42100
  Excision, 42120, 42145
  Fracture
    Closed Treatment, 21421
    Open Treatment, 21422-21423
  Lesion
    Destruction, 42160
    Excision, 42104-42120
  Prosthesis
    Augmentation, 21082
    Impression, 42280
    Insertion, 42281
    Lift, 21089
  Reconstruction
    Lengthening, 42226-42227
  Repair
    Cleft Palate, 42200-42225
    Laceration, 42180-42182
    Vomer Flap, 42235
  Unlisted Services and Procedures, 42299
**Palatopharyngoplasty**, 42145
**Palatoplasty**, 42200-42225
**Palatoschisis**, 42200-42225
**PALB2**, 81406, 81432, [81448]
**Palm**
  Bursa
    Incision and Drainage, 26025-26030
  Fasciectomy, 26121-26125
  Fasciotomy, 26040-26045
  Tendon Sheath
    Excision, 26145
    Incision and Drainage, 26020
  Tendon
    Excision, 26170
**Palsy, Seventh Nerve**
  Graft/Repair, 15840-15845
**PAMG-1**, 84112
**P&P**, 85230
**Pancoast Tumor Resection**, 32503-32504
**Pancreas, Endocrine Only**
  Islet Cell
    Antibody, 86341
    Transplantation, 48160
**Pancreas**
  Anastomosis
    with Intestines, 48520-48540, 48548
  Anesthesia, 00794
  Biopsy, 48100
    Needle Biopsy, 48102
  Cyst
    Anastomosis, 48520-48540
    Repair, 48500
  Debridement
    Peripancreatic Tissue, 48105
  Excision
    Ampulla of Vater, 48148
    Duct, 48148
    Partial, 48140-48146, 48150-48154, 48160
    Peripancreatic Tissue, 48105
    Total, 48155-48160
  Lesion
    Excision, 48120
  Needle Biopsy, 48102

**Pancreas** — *continued*
  Placement
    Drains, 48000-48001
  Pseudocyst
    Drainage
      Open, 48510
  Removal Transplanted Allograft, 48556
  Removal
    Calculi (Stone), 48020
  Repair
    Cyst, 48500
  Resection, 48105
  Suture, 48545
  Transplantation, 48160, 48550, 48554-48556
    Allograft Preparation, 48550-48552
  Unlisted Services and Procedures, 48999
  X-ray with Contrast, 74300-74301
    Injection Procedure, 48400
**Pancreatectomy**
  with Transplantation, 48160
  Donor, 48550
  Partial, 48140-48146, 48150-48154, 48160
  Total, 48155-48160
**Pancreatic DNAse**
  *See* DNAse
**Pancreatic Duct**
  Destruction
    Calculi (Stone), 43265
    Tumor, [43278]
  Dilation
    Endoscopy, [43277]
  Drainage
    of Cyst, 48999
  Endoscopy
    Collection
      Specimen, 43260
    Destruction
      Calculi (Stone), 43265
      Tumor, [43278]
    Dilation, [43277]
    Removal
      Calculi (Stone), 43264
      Foreign Body, [43275]
      Stent, [43275, 43276]
    Sphincter Pressure, 43263
    Sphincterotomy, 43262
  Incision
    Sphincter, 43262
  Placement
    Stent, [43274]
  Removal
    Calculi (Stone), 43264
    Foreign Body, [43275]
    Stent, [43275, 43276]
  Tumor
    Destruction, [43278]
  X-ray with Contrast
    Guide Catheter, 74329-74330
**Pancreatic Elastase 1 (PE1)**, 82656
**Pancreatic Islet Cell AB**, 86341
**Pancreaticojejunostomy**, 48548
**Pancreatitis**
  Incision and Drainage, 48000
**Pancreatography**
  Injection Procedure, 48400
  Intraoperative, 74300-74301
**Pancreatojejunostomies**
  *See* Pancreaticojejunostomy
**Pancreatorrhaphy**, 48545
**Pancreatotomy**
  Sphincter, 43262
**Pancreozymin–Secretin Test**, 82938
**Panel**
  *See* Blood Tests; Organ or Disease Oriented panel
**Panniculectomy**, 15830
**Pap Smears**, 88141-88155, 88164-88167, 88174-88175
**PAP**, 88141-88167, 88174-88175
**Papilla Excision**, 46230 [46220]
**Papilla, Interdental**
  *See* Gums
**Papilloma**
  Destruction
    Anus, 46900-46924
    Penis, 54050-54065

**Papillotomy**, 43262
  Destruction
    Anus, 46900-46924
    Penis, 54050-54065
**PAPP D**, 83632
**Paracentesis**
  Abdomen, 49082-49083
  Eye
    Anterior Chamber
      with Diagnostic Aspiration of Aqueous, 65800
      with Removal of Blood, 65815
      with Removal Vitreous and or Discission of Anterior Hyaloid Membrane, 65810
**Paracervical Nerve**
  Injection
    Anesthetic, 64435
**Paraffin Bath Therapy**, 97018
**Paraganglioma, Medullary**, 80424
**Parainfluenza Virus**
  Antigen Detection
    Immunofluorescence, 87279
**Paralysis, Facial Nerve**
  Graft, 15840-15845
  Repair, 15840-15845
**Paralysis, Infantile**
  Polio
    Antibody, 86658
    Vaccine, 90713
**Paranasal Sinuses**
  *See* Sinus
**Parasites**
  Blood, 87206-87209
  Concentration, 87015
  Examination, 87169
  Smear, 87177
  Tissue, 87220
**Parasitic Worms**, 86682
**Paraspinous Block, Thoracic**, [64461, 64462, 64463]
**Parathormone**, 83970
**Parathyrin**, 83970
**Parathyroid Autotransplantation**, 60512
**Parathyroid Gland**
  Autotransplant, 60512
  Biopsy, 60699
  Excision, 60500-60502
  Exploration, 60500-60505
  Nuclear Medicine
    Imaging, 78070-78072
**Parathyroid Hormone Measurement**, 83970
**Parathyroid Hormone**, 83970
**Parathyroid Transplantation**, 60512
**Parathyroidectomy**, 60500-60505
**Para–Tyrosine**, 84510
**Paraurethral Gland**
  Abscess
    Incision and Drainage, 53060
**Paravertebral Nerve**
  Destruction, [64633, 64634, 64635, 64636]
  Injection
    Anesthetic, 64490-64495
    Neurolytic, [64633, 64634, 64635, 64636]
**Parietal Cell Vagotomies**, 43641
**Parietal Craniotomy**, 61556
**Paring**
  Skin Lesion
    Benign Hyperkeratotic
      More than Four Lesions, 11057
      Single Lesion, 11055
      Two to Four Lesions, 11056
**Park Posterior Anal Repair**, 46761
**PARK2**, 81405-81406
**Paronychia**
  Incision and Drainage, 10060-10061
**Parotid Duct**
  Diversion, 42507-42510
  Reconstruction, 42507-42510
**Parotid Gland**
  Abscess
    Incision and Drainage, 42300-42305
  Calculi (Stone)
    Excision, 42330, 42340
  Excision
    Partial, 42410-42415

**Parotid Gland** — *continued*
  Excision — *continued*
    Total, 42420-42426
  Tumor
    Excision, 42410-42426
**Parotidectomy**, 61590
**Parotitides, Epidemic**
  *See* Mumps
**Pars Abdominalis Aortae**
  *See* Aorta, Abdominal
**Partial Claviculectomy**, 23120, 23180
**Partial Colectomy**, 44140-44147, 44160, 44204-44208, 44213
**Partial Cystectomy**, 51550-51565
**Partial Esophagectomy**, 43116-43124
**Partial Gastrectomy**, 43631-43635, 43845
**Partial Glossectomy**, 41120-41135
**Partial Hepatectomy**, 47120, 47125-47130, 47140-47142
**Partial Mastectomies**, 19301-19302
  *See Also* Breast, Excision, Lesion
**Partial Nephrectomy**, 50240, 50543
**Partial Pancreatectomy**, 48140-48146, 48150, 48153-48154, 48160
**Partial Splenectomy**, 38101, 38120
**Partial Thromboplastin Time**, 85730-85732
**Partial Ureterectomy**, 50220, 50546
**Particle Agglutination**, 86403-86406
**Parvovirus**
  Antibody, 86747
**Patch**
  Allergy Tests, 95044
**Patella**
  *See Also* Knee
  Dislocation, 27560-27566
  Excision, 27350
    with Reconstruction, 27424
  Fracture, 27520-27524
  Reconstruction, 27437-27438
  Repair
    Chondromalacia, 27418
    Instability, 27420-27424
**Patellar Tendon Bearing (PTB) Cast**, 29435
**Patellectomy**, 27350, 27524, 27566
  with Reconstruction, 27424
**Patent Ductus Arteriosus**
  Closure, 93582
**Paternity Testing**, 86910-86911
**Patey's Operation**
  Mastectomy, Modified Radical, 19307
**Pathologic Dilatation**
  *See* Dilation
**Pathology**
  Clinical
    Consultation, 80500-80502
    Intraoperative, 88329-88334
  Molecular, 81400-81408
  Report Includes pT Category, pN Category, Gleason Score, Statement of Margin Status, 3267F
  Surgical
    Consultation, 88321-88325
    Intraoperative, 88329-88332
    Decalcification Procedure, 88311
    Electron Microscopy, 88348
    Gross and Micro Exam
      Level II, 88302
      Level III, 88304
      Level IV, 88305
      Level V, 88307
      Level VI, 88309
    Gross Exam
      Level I, 88300
    Histochemistry, 88319
    Immunocytochemistry, 88342, 88344, [88341]
    Immunofluorescence, 88346, [88350]
    In situ Hybridization, 88365, 88366, [88364]
    Morphometry
      Hybridization Techniques, 88367-88369 [88373, 88374], [88377]
    Nerve, 88356
    Skeletal Muscle, 88355
    Tumor, 88358, 88361

CPT © 2017 American Medical Association. All Rights Reserved.    © 2017 Optum360, LLC

Index

Perfusion, Intracranial Arterial — Phosphoglycerides, Glycerol

**Perfusion, Intracranial Arterial**
Percutaneous, 61645
Thrombolysis, 61624
**Perfusion Pump**
*See* Infusion Pump
**Perfusion**
Brain
Imaging, 0042T
Myocardial, 78451-78454
Imaging, 0439T, 78466-78469
Positron Emission Tomography (PET)
Myocardial Imaging, 78491-78492
Pulmonary, 78580, 78582, 78597-78598
**Pericardectomies**, 33030-33031
Endoscopic, 32659
**Pericardial Cyst**
*See* Cyst, Pericardial
Excision, 33050
Thoracoscopic, 32661
**Pericardial Sac**
Drainage, 32659
**Pericardial Window**
for Drainage, 33025
Thoracoscopic, 32659
**Pericardiectomy**
Complete, 33030-33031
Subtotal, 33030-33031
**Pericardiocentesis**, 33010-33011
Ultrasound Guidance, 76930
**Pericardiostomy**
Tube, 33015
**Pericardiotomy**
Removal
Clot/Foreign Body, 33020
via Thoracoscopy, 32658
**Pericardium**
Cyst
Excision, 32661, 33050
Excision, 32659, 33030-33031
Incision and Drainage, 33025
Incision, 33030-33031
with Tube, 33015
Removal
Clot, 33020
Foreign Body, 33020
Puncture Aspiration, 33010-33011
Removal
Clot
Endoscopic, 32658
Foreign Body
Endoscopic, 32658
Tumor
Excision, 32661, 33050
**Peridural Anesthesia**
*See* Anesthesia, Epidural
**Peridural Injection**, 62281-62282, 62320-62327, 64479-64484
**Perineal Prostatectomy**
Partial, 55801
Radical, 55810-55815
**Perineoplasty**, 56810
**Perineorrhaphy**
Repair
Rectocele, 57250
**Perineum**
Abscess
Incision and Drainage, 56405
Biopsy, 56605-56606
Colposcopy, 99170
Debridement
Infected, 11004, 11006
Removal
Prosthesis, 53442
Repair, 56810
X-ray with Contrast, 74775
**Perionychia**, 10060-10061
**Periorbital Region**
Reconstruction–Osteotomy
with Graft, 21267-21268
Repair–Osteotomy, 21260-21263
**Peripheral Artery Disease (PAD) Rehabilitation**, 93668
**Peripheral Blood Stem Cell Transplant**, 38240-38242

**Peripheral Nerve**
Repair/Suture
Major, 64856, 64859
**Periprostatic Placement Biodegradable Material**
Transperineal, 55874
**Periprosthetic Capsulotomy**
Breast, 19371
**Peristaltic Pumps**
*See* Infusion Pump
**Peritoneal Dialysis**, 4055F, 90945-90947
Kt/V Level, 3082F-3084F
Training
Counseling, 90989, 90993
**Peritoneal Free Air**, 49400
**Peritoneal Lavage**, 49084
**Peritoneoscopy**
Biopsy, 49321
Exploration, 49320
**Peritoneum**
Abscess
Incision and Drainage, 49020
Chemotherapy Administration, 96446
Endoscopy
Drainage
Lymphocele, 49323
Exchange
Drainage Catheter, 49423
Injection
Contrast
Via Catheter, 49424
Ligation
Shunt, 49428
Removal
Cannula
Catheter, 49422
Foreign Body, 49402
Shunt, 49429
Tumor
Resection, 58950-58954
Unlisted Services and Procedures, 49999
Venous Shunt, 49427
X-ray, 74190
**Persistent, Omphalomesenteric Duct**
Excision, 44800
**Persistent Truncus Arteriosus**
*See* Truncus Arteriosus
Repair, 33786
**Personal Care**
*See* Self Care
**Personality Test**, 96101-96103
Computer-Assisted, 96103
**Pertussis Immunization**, 90715, 90723
**Pessary**
Insertion, 57160
**Pesticides**
Chlorinated Hydrocarbons, 82441
**PET**
with Computed Tomography (CT)
Limited Area, 78814
Skull Base to Mid-thigh, 78815
Whole Body, 78816
Brain, 78608-78609
Heart, 78459
Limited Area, 78811
Myocardial Blood Flow
Absolute Quantitation, 0482T
Myocardial Imaging Perfusion Study, 78491-78492
Skull Base to Mid-thigh, 78812
Whole Body, 78813
**Petrous Temporal**
Excision
Apex, 69530
**Peyreva Procedure**, 51845
**Peyronie Disease**
with Graft, 54110-54112
Injection, 54200
Surgical Exposure, 54205
**PFG (Percutaneous Fluoroscopic Gastrostomy)**, 49440
**PFT (Pulmonary Function Test)**, 94010-94799
**PG**, 84081, 84150
**pH**
Blood Gases, 82800-82805
Body Fluid, Not Otherwise Specified, 83986
Exhaled Breath Condensate, 83987

**Phacoemulsification**
Removal
Extracapsular Cataract, 66982, 66984
Secondary Membranous Cataract, 66850
**Phagocytosis**
White Blood Cells, 86344
**Phalangectomy**
Toe, 28150
Partial, 28160
**Phalanges (Hand)**
*See Also* Finger, Bone
Incision, Bone Cortex, 26034
**Phalanx, Finger**
Craterization, 26235, 26236
Cyst
Excision, 26210, 26215
Diaphysectomy, 26235, 26236
Excision, 26235, 26236
Radical
for Tumor, 26260-26262
Fracture
Articular
with Manipulation, 26742
Closed Treatment, 26740
Open Treatment, 26746
Distal, 26755, 26756
Closed Treatment, 26750
Open Treatment, 26765
Percutaneous, 26756
Open Treatment, 26735
Distal, 26765
Percutaneous Fixation, 26756
Shaft, 26720-26727
Open Treatment, 26735
Incision and Drainage, 26034
Ostectomy
Radical
for Tumor, 26260-26262
Repair
Lengthening, 26568
Nonunion, 26546
Osteotomy, 26567
Saucerization, 26235, 26236
Thumb
Fracture
Shaft, 26720-26727
Tumor, 26115-26118 [26111, 26113], 26210-26215, 26260-26262
**Phalanx, Great Toe**
*See Also* Phalanx, Toe
Fracture
Closed Treatment, 28490
with Manipulation, 28495
Open Treatment, 28505
Percutaneous Skeletal Fixation, 28496
**Phalanx, Toe**
Condyle
Excision, 28126
Craterization, 28124
Cyst
Excision, 28108
Diaphysectomy, 28124
Excision, 28124, 28150-28160
Fracture
with Manipulation, 28515
without Manipulation, 28510
Open Treatment, 28525
Repair
Osteotomy, 28310, 28312
Saucerization, 28124
Tumor
Excision, 28108, 28175
**Pharmaceutic Preparations**
*See* Drug
**Pharmacotherapies**
*See* Chemotherapy
**Pharyngeal Tonsil**
Excision, 42830-42836
with Tonsils, 42820-42821
Unlisted Services/Procedures, 42999
**Pharyngectomy**
Partial, 42890
**Pharyngolaryngectomy**, 31390, 31395
**Pharyngoplasty**, 42950
**Pharyngorrhaphy**, 42900
**Pharyngostomy**, 42955

**Pharyngotomy**
*See* Incision, Pharynx
**Pharyngotympanic Tube**
Inflation
with Myringotomy, 69420-69421
**Pharynx**
*See Also* Nasopharynx; Throat
Biopsy, 42800-42806
Cineradiography, 70371, 74230
Creation
Stoma, 42955
Excision, 42145
with Larynx, 31390, 31395
Partial, 42890
Resection, 42892, 42894
Hemorrhage, 42960-42962
Lesion
Destruction, 42808
Excision, 42808
Reconstruction, 42950
Removal, Foreign Body, 42809
Repair
with Esophagus, 42953
Unlisted Services and Procedures, 42999
Video, 70371, 74230
X-ray, 70370, 74210
**Phencyclidine**, 83992
**Phenobarbital**, [80345]
Assay, 80184
**Phenothiazine**, [80342, 80343, 80344]
**Phenotype Analysis**
by Nucleic Acid
Infectious Agent
HIV-1 Drug Resistance, 87903, 87904
**Phenotype Prediction**
by Generic Database
HIV-1
Drug Susceptibility, 87900
Using Regularly Updated Genotypic Bioinformatics, 87900
**Phenylalanine**, 84030
**Phenylalanine–Tyrosine Ratio**, 84030
**Phenylketones**, 84035
**Phenylketonuria**, 84030
**Phenytoin**
Assay, 80185, 80186
**Pheochromocytoma**, 80424
**Pheresis**, 36511-36516
**PHEX**, 81406
**Phlebectasia**
with Tissue Excision, 37735-37760
Ablation, 36473-36479
Removal, 37718-37735, 37765-37785
**Phlebectomy**
Stab, 37765-37766
**Phlebographies**, 75820-75880, 75885, 75893, 78445, 78457-78458
Injection, 36005
**Phleborrhaphy**
Femoral, 37650
Iliac, 37660
**Phlebotomy**
Therapeutic, 99195
**Phonocardiogram**
Evaluation, 93799
Intracardiac, 93799
Tracing, 93799
**Phoria**
*See* Strabismus
**Phosphatase, Acid**, 84060
Blood, 84066
**Phosphatase**
Alkaline, 84075, 84080
Blood, 84078
Forensic Examination, 84061
**Phosphate, Pyridoxal**, 84207
**Phosphatidyl Glycerol**, 84081
**Phosphatidylcholine Cholinephosphohydrolase**
*See* Tissue Typing
**Phosphatidylglycerol**, 84081
**Phosphocreatine Phosphotransferase, ADP**, 82550-82552
**Phosphogluconate-6**
Dehydrogenase, 84085
**Phosphoglycerides, Glycerol**, 84081

 *[Resequenced]* CPT © 2017 American Medical Association. All Rights Reserved. © 2017 Optum360, LLC

CPT © 2017 American Medical Association. All Rights Reserved.　　　　　© 2017 Optum360, LLC

**Physician Quality Reporting System (PQRS)** —
*continued*
Tobacco
Cessation, 4000F-4001F
Use, 1035F-1036F
Transfer, 0581F-0584F
Treatment
Options, 4325F
Plan, 5050F
Tuberculosis, 3455F, 3510F
Tympanometry, 2035F
Urinary Incontinence, 0509F, 1090F-1091F
Vaccine
Hepatitis
A, 4155F
B, 4149F, 4157F
Influenza, 4037F
Pneumococcal, 4040F
Vein Thromboembolism, 4069F
Ventricle, 3019F-3020F, 3055F-3056F
Verification, 6100F
Vital Signs Documented and Reviewed, 2010F
Volume Overload, 1004F, 2002F
Warfarin Therapy, 4012F, 4300F-4301F
Warming
Intraoperative, 4250F
Weight Recorded, 2001F
Wound, 2050F
Culture, 4260F-4261F
Dressings, 4265F-4266F
**Physician Services**
Care Plan Oversight Services, 99339-99340,
99374-99380
Domiciliary Facility, 99339-99340
Extracorporeal Liver Assist System, 0405T
Home Health Agency Care, 99374
Home/Rest Home Care, 99339-99340
Hospice, 99377, 99378
Nursing Facility, 99379, 99380
Case Management Services, 99366-99368
Direction, Advanced Life Support, 99288
Online, 99444
Prolonged
with Direct Patient Contact, 99354-99357
Outpatient Office, 99354, 99355
with Direct Patient Services
Inpatient, 99356, 99357
without Direct Patient Contact, 99358,
99359
Standby, 99360
Supervision, Care Plan Oversight Services,
0405T, 99339-99340, 99374-99380
Team Conference, 99367
Telephone, 99441-99443
**Physiologic Recording of Tremor**, 95999
**PICC Line Insertion**, 36568-36569
**Pierce Ears**, 69090
**Piercing of Ear Lobe**, 69090
**PIK3CA**, 81404
**Piles**
*See* Hemorrhoids
**Pilon Fracture Treatment**, 27824
**Pilonidal Cyst**
Excision, 11770-11772
Incision and Drainage, 10080, 10081
**Pin**
*See Also* Wire
Insertion
Removal
Skeletal Traction, 20650
Prophylactic Treatment
Femur, 27187
Humerus, 24498
Shoulder, 23490, 23491
**Pinch Graft**, 15050
**Pineal Gland**
Excision
Partial, 60699
Total, 60699
Incision, 60699
**PINK1**, 81405
**Pinna**
*See* Ear, External
**Pinworms**
Examination, 87172
**Pirogoff Procedure**, 27888

**Pituitary Epidermoid Tumor**
*See* Craniopharyngioma
**Pituitary Fossa**
Exploration, 60699
**Pituitary Gland**
Excision, 61546, 61548
Incision, 60699
Tumor
Excision, 61546, 61548, 62165
**Pituitary Growth Hormone**
*See* Growth Hormone
**Pituitary Lactogenic Hormone**
*See* Prolactin
**Pituitectomy**
*See* Excision, Pituitary Gland
**PKD1**, 81407
**PKD2**, 81406
**PKHD1**, 81408
**PKLR**, 81405
**PKP**, 65730-65755
**PKP2**, 81406, 81439
**PKU**, 84030
**PL**, 80418, 84146
**PLA Codes**
*see* Proprietary Laboratory Analyses (PLA)
**Placement**
Adjustable Gastric Restrictive Device, 43770
Amniotic Membrane
Ocular Surface, 65778-65779
Aqueous Drainage Device, 0191T *[0253T,
0376T]*, 0449T-0450T, 0474T, 66179-
66185
Breast Localization Device
with Guidance
Mammographic, 19281-19282
MRI, 19287-19288
Stereotactic, 19283-19284
Ultrasound, 19285-19286
Bronchial Stent, 31636-31637
Catheter, Cardiac, 93503
*See Also* Catheterization, Cardiac
Catheter
Aneurysm Sac Pressure Sensor, 34701-
34708
Bile Duct, 47533-47540
Brain for Chemotherapy, 64999
Bronchus
for Intracavitary Radioelement Ap-
plication, 31643
*See* Catheterization
for Interstitial Radioelement Application
Breast, 19296-19298
Genitalia, 55920
Head/Neck, 41019
Muscle, 20555
Pelvic Organs, 55920
Prostate, 55875
Soft Tissue, 20555
Pleural, 32550
Renal Artery, 36251-36254
Cecostomy Tube, 44300, 49442
Colonic Stent, 45327, 45347, 45389
Dosimeter
Prostate, 55876
Drainage
Pancreas, 48001
Drug-eluting ocular Insert, 0444T-0445T
Duodenostomy Tube, 49441
Endovascular Prosthesis
Aorta, 33883-33886, 34701-34706
Fenestrated Endograft, 34841-34848
Iliac Artery, 34707-34711
Enterostomy Tube, 44300
Fiducial Markers
Duodenum/Jejunum, 43253
Esophagus, 43253
Intra-abdominal, 49411
Intra-pelvic, 49411
Intrathoracic, 32553
Prostate, 55876
Retroperitoneum, 49411
Stomach, 43253
Gastrostomy Tube, 43246, 49440
Guidance Catheter
Abscess, 75989
Specimen, 75989

**Placement** — *continued*
Interstitial Device
Bone, 0347T
Intra-abdominal, 49327, 49411-49412
Intra-pelvic, 49411
Intra-thoracic, 32553
Prostate, 55876
Retroperitoneum, 49411
Intrafacet Implant(s), 0219T-0222T
Intravascular Stent
Cervical Carotid Artery, 37215-37216
Innominate Artery, 37217-37218
Intracranial, 61635
Intrathoracic Common Carotid Artery,
37217-37218
IVC Filter, 37191
Jejunostomy Tube
Endoscopic, 44372
Percutaneous, 49441
Localization Device, Breast, 19281-19288
Nasogastric Tube, 43752
Needle Wire
Breast, 19281-19288
Needle
Bone, 36680
for Interstitial Radioelement Application
Genitalia, 55920
Head, 41019
Muscle, 20555
Neck, 41019
Pelvic Organs, 55920
Prostate, 55875
Soft Tissue, 20555
Head and/or Neck, 41019
Muscle or Soft Tissue
for Radioelement Application,
20555
Pelvic Organs and/or Genitalia, 55920
Prostate, 55875-55876
Orogastric Tube, 43752
Pharmacological Agent
Intravitreal Drug Delivery System, 67027
Pressure Sensor, 34701-34708
Prosthesis, Thoracic Aorta, 75958-75959
Radiation Delivery Device
Intracoronary Artery, *[92974]*
Intraocular, 0190T
Pleural Cavity, 32553
Therapy Applicator for IORT, 19294
Sensor, Wireless
Endovascular Repair, 34701-34708
Seton
Anal, 46020
Stereotactic Frame, 20660
Head Frame, 61800
Subconjunctival Retinal Prosthesis Receiver,
0100T
Tracheal Stent, 31631
Transcatheter
Extracranial, 0075T-0076T
Physiologic Sensor, 34701-34708
Ureteral Stent, 50693-50695, 50947
**Placenta**
Delivery, 59414
**Placental Villi**
*See* Chorionic Villus
**Placental**
Alpha Microglobulin-1, 84112
Lactogen, 83632
**Plafond Fracture Treatment**
Tibial, 27824
**Plagiocephaly**, 21175
**Planing**
Nose
Skin, 30120
**Plantar Digital Nerve**
Decompression, 64726
**Plantar Pressure Measurements**
Dynamic, 96001, 96004
**Plasma Prokallikrein**
*See* Fletcher Factor
**Plasma Protein–A, Pregnancy Associated
(PAPP–A)**, 84163
**Plasma Test**
Volume Determination, 78110-78111

**Plasma Thromboplastin**
Antecedent, 85270
Component, 85250
Frozen Preparation, 86927
**Plasma**
Frozen Preparation, 86927
Injection, 0232T
Volume Determination, 78110, 78111
**Plasmin Antiactivator**
*See* Alpha–2 Antiplasmin
**Plasmin**, 85400
**Plasminogen**, 85420, 85421
**Plasmodium**
Antibody, 86750
**Plastic Repair of Mouth**
*See* Mouth, Repair
**Plate, Bone**
*See* Bone Plate
**Platelet Cofactor I**
*See* Clotting Factor
**Platelet Test**
Survival Test, 78191
**Platelet Thromboplastin Antecedent**, 85270
**Platelet**
*See Also* Blood Cell Count; Complete Blood
Count
Aggregation, 85576
Antibody, 86022, 86023
Assay, 85055
Blood, 85025
Count, 85032, 85049
Neutralization, 85597
**Platysmal Flap**, 15825
**PLCE1**, 81407
**Pleoptic Training**, 92065
**Plethysmography**
Extremities, 93922, 93923
Lung Volume, 94726
Penis, 54240
**Pleura**
Biopsy, 32098, 32400
Decortication, 32320
Empyema
Excision, 32540
Excision, 32310, 32320
Endoscopic, 32656
Foreign Body
Removal, 32150, 32151
Incision, 32320
Needle Biopsy, 32400
Removal
Foreign Body, 32150, 32653
Repair, 32215
Thoracotomy, 32096-32098, 32100-32160
Unlisted Services and Procedures, 32999
**Pleural Cavity**
Catheterization, 32550
Chemotherapy Administration, 96440, 96446
Fusion, 32560
Incision
Empyema, 32035, 32036
Pneumothorax, 32551
Puncture and Drainage, 32554-32557
Thoracostomy, 32035, 32036
**Pleural Endoscopies**
*See* Thoracoscopy
**Pleural Scarification**
for Repeat Pneumothorax, 32215
**Pleural Tap**
*See* Thoracentesis
**Pleurectomy**
Anesthesia, 00542
Parietal, 32310, 32320
Endoscopic, 32656
**Pleuritis, Purulent**, 21501-21502
**Pleurodesis**
Agent for Pleurodesis, 32560
Endoscopic, 32650
**Pleurosclerosis, Chemical**
*See* Pleurodesis, Chemical
**Pleurosclerosis**
*See* Pleurodesis
**Plexectomy, Choroid**
*See* Choroid Plexus, Excision
**Plexus Brachialis**
*See* Brachial Plexus

**Pulmonology** — *continued*
  Unlisted Noninvasive Vascular Diagnostic
    Study, 93998
  Unlisted Services and Procedures, 94799
**Pulse Generator**
  Electronic Analysis, 95970-95979, 95980-95982
  Heart
    Insertion/Replacement, 33212, 33213
**Pulse Rate Increased**
  Heart
    Recording, 93609
**Pump, Infusion**
  *See* Infusion Pump
**Pump Services**
  Oxygenator/Heat Exchange, 99190-99192
**Pump Stomach for Poison**, 43753
**Pump**
  *See* Chemotherapy, Pump Services; Infusion
    Pump
**Punch Graft**, 15775, 15776
**Puncture Aspiration**
  Abscess
    Skin, 10160
  Bulla, 10160
  Cyst
    Breast, 19000, 19001
    Skin, 10160
  Hematoma, 10160
**Puncture**
  Artery, 36600
  Chest
    with Imaging Guidance, 32555, 32557
    without Imaging Guidance, 32554,
      32556
  Cisternal, 61050-61055
  Lumbar, 62270-62272
  Pericardium, 33010, 33011
  Pleural Cavity
    Drainage, 32556-32557
  Skull
    Drain Fluid, 61000-61020
      Cistern, 61050
    Inject Cistern, 61055
    Inject Ventricle, 61026
    Shunt
      Drainage of Fluid, 61070
      Injection, 61070
  Spinal Cord
    Diagnostic, 62270
    Drainage of Fluid, 62272
    Lumbar, 62270
  Spleen, 38999
  Tracheal
    Aspiration and/or Injection, 31612
**Puncturing**
  *See* Puncture
**Pupillometry, Quantitative**, 0341T
**Pure–Tone Audiometry**, 0208T-0209T, 92552,
  92553
**Pustules**
  Removal, 10040
**Putti–Platt Procedure**, 23450
**PUVA**, 96912, 96913
**PV**, 90713
**PVA (Percutaneous Vertebral Augmentation)**,
  22513-22515
**PVB (Paraspinous Vertebral Block), Thoracic**,
  *[64461, 64462, 64463]*
**Pyelogram**
  *See* Urography, Intravenous; Urography, Retro-
    grade
**Pyelography**, 74400, 74425
**Pyelolithotomy**, 50130
  Anatrophic, 50075
  Coagulum, 50130
**Pyeloplasty**, 50400, 50405, 50544
  Repair
    Horseshoe Kidney, 50540
  Secondary, 50405
**Pyeloscopy**
  with Cystourethroscopy, 52351
    Biopsy, 52354
    Destruction, 52354
    Lithotripsy, 52353
    Removal
      Calculus, 52352

**Pyeloscopy** — *continued*
  with Cystourethroscopy — *continued*
    Tumor Excision, 52355
**Pyelostolithotomy**
  Percutaneous, 50080, 50081
**Pyelostomy**, 50125, 50400, 50405
  Closure, 53899
**Pyelotomy**
  with Drainage, 50125
  with Removal Calculus, 50130
  Complicated, 50135
  Endoscopic, 50570
  Exploration, 50120
**Pyeloureteroplasty**, 50400, 50405, 50544
**PYGM**, 81401, 81406
**Pyloric Sphincter**
  Incision, 43520
  Reconstruction, 43800
**Pyloromyotomy**, 43520
**Pyloroplasty**, 43800
  with Vagotomy, 43640
**Pyothorax**
  Incision and Drainage, 21501, 21502
**Pyridoxal Phosphate**, 84207
**Pyrophosphate, Adenosine**, 82030
**Pyrophosphorylase, UDP Galactose**, 82775-82776
**Pyruvate**, 84210, 84220

---

### Q

**Q Fever ab**, 86638
**Q Fever**, 86000, 86638
**QSART**, 95923
**QST (Quantitative Sensory Testing)**, 0106T-0110T
**Quadrantectomy**, 19301-19302
**Quadriceps Repair**, 27430
**Qualifying Circumstances**
  Anesthesia, 99100, 99116, 99135, 99140
**Quantitative Carotid Atheroma Evaluation**, 93895
**Quantitative Carotid Intima Media Thickness**
  **Evaluation**, 93895
**Quantitative Pupillometry**, 0341T
**Quantitative Sensory Testing (QST)**
  Using Cooling Stimuli, 0108T
  Using Heat–Pain Stimuli, 0109T
  Using Other Stimuli, 0110T
  Using Touch Pressure Stimuli, 0106T
  Using Vibration Stimuli, 0107T
**Quick Test**
  Prothrombin Time, 85610, 85611
**Quinidine**
  Assay, 80194
**Quinine**, 84228

---

### R

**RA Factor**
  Qualitative, 86430
  Quantitative, 86431
**RAB7A**, 81405
**RabAvert**, 90675
**Rabies**
  Immune Globulin, 90375-90376
  Vaccine, 90675-90676
**Rachicentesis**, 62270-62272
**Radial Arteries**
  Aneurysm, 35045
  Embolectomy, 34111
  Sympathectomy, 64821
  Thrombectomy, 34111
**Radial Head, Subluxation**, 24640
**Radial Keratotomy**, 65771
**Radiation Physics**
  Consultation, 77336-77370
  Unlisted Services and Procedures, 77399
**Radiation Therapy**
  Consultation
    Radiation Physics, 77336-77370
  CT Scan Guidance, 77014
  Dose Plan, 77300, 77306-77331
    Brachytherapy, 77316-77318
    High-Dose Electronic Brachytherapy,
      0394T-0395T
    Intensity Modulation, 77301
    Teletherapy, 77306-77321
  Field Set–Up, 77280-77290
  Guidance for Localization, *[77387]*

**Radiation Therapy** — *continued*
  Intraoperative, 19294, 77469, *[77424, 77425]*
  Localization of Patient Movement, *[77387]*
  Multi-leaf Collimator Device Design and Con-
    struction, 77338
  Planning, 77261-77290, 77293-77331 *[77295]*
  Special, 77470
  Stereotactic, 77371-77373, 77432
    Body, 77373
    Cranial Lesion, 77371-77372, 77432
  Treatment Delivery
    => 1MeV Complex, 77412
    => 1MeV Intermediate, 77407
    => 1MeV Simple, 77402
    Beam Modulation, *[77385]*
    Guidance for Localization, *[77387]*
    High Energy Neutron, 77423
    Intensity Modulated Radiation (IMRT)
      Complex, *[77386]*
      Simple, *[77385]*
    Intraoperative, *[77424, 77425]*
    Proton Beam, 77520-77525
    Single, 77402
    Stereotactic
      Body, 77373
      Cranial Lesion(s), 77371-77372
    Superficial, 77401
    Three or More Areas, 77412
    Two Areas, 77407
    Weekly, 77427
  Treatment Device, 77332-77334
  Treatment Management
    Intraoperative, 77469
    One or Two Fractions Only, 77431
    Stereotactic
      Body, 77435
      Cerebral, 77432
    Unlisted Services and Procedures, 77499
    Weekly, 77427
**Radiation X**
  *See* X–Ray
**Radiation**
  Blood Products, 86945
**Radical Excision of Lymph Nodes**
  Axillary, 38740-38745
  Cervical, 38720-38724
  Suprahyoid, 38700
**Radical Mastectomies, Modified**, 19307
**Radical Neck Dissection**
  with Auditory Canal Surgery, 69155
  with Thyroidectomy, 60254
  with Tongue Excision, 41135, 41145, 41153,
    41155
  Laryngectomy, 31365-31368
  Pharyngolaryngectomy, 31390, 31395
**Radical Vaginal Hysterectomy**, 58285
**Radical Vulvectomy**, 56630-56640
**Radioactive Colloid Therapy**, 79300
**Radioactive Substance**
  Insertion
    Prostate, 55860
**Radiocarpal Joint**
  Arthrotomy, 25040
  Dislocation
    Closed Treatment, 25660
**Radiocinematographies**
  Esophagus, 74230
  Pharynx, 70371, 74230
  Speech Evaluation, 70371
  Swallowing Evaluation, 74230
  Unlisted Services and Procedures, 76120-76125
**Radio–Cobalt B12 Schilling Test**
  Vitamin B12 Absorption Study, 78270-78272
**Radioelement Substance**
  Catheter Placement
    Breast, 19296-19298
    Bronchus, 31643
    Head and/or Neck, 41019
    Muscle and/or Soft Tissue, 20555
    Pelvic Organs or Genitalia, 55920
    Prostate, 55875
  Catheterization, 55875
  Needle Placement
    Head and/or Neck, 41019
    Muscle and/or Soft Tissue, 20555
    Pelvic Organs and Genitalia, 55920

**Radioelement Substance** — *continued*
  Needle Placement — *continued*
    Prostate, 55875
**Radioelement**
  Application, 77761-77772
    with Ultrasound, 76965
    Surface, 77789
  Handling, 77790
  Infusion, 77750
  Placement *See* Radioelement Substance
**Radiography**
  *See* Radiology, Diagnostic; X–Ray
**Radioimmunosorbent Test**
  Gammaglobulin, Blood, 82784-82785
**Radioisotope Brachytherapy**
  *See* Brachytherapy
**Radioisotope Scan**
  *See* Nuclear Medicine
**Radiological Marker**
  Preoperative Placement
    Excision of Breast Lesion, 19125, 19126
**Radiology**
  *See Also* Nuclear Medicine, Radiation Therapy,
    X–Ray, Ultrasound
  Diagnostic
    Unlisted Services and Procedures, 76499
    Examination, 70030
      Stress Views, 77071
    Joint Survey, 77077
  Therapeutic
    Field Set–Up, 77280-77290
    Planning, 77261-77263, 77299
    Port Film, 77417
**Radionuclide Therapy**
  Heart, 79440
  Interstitial, 79300
  Intra–arterial, 79445
  Intra–articular, 79440
  Intracavitary, 79200
  Intravascular, 79101
  Intravenous Infusion, 79101, 79403
  Intravenous, 79101, 79403
  Oral, 79005
  Remote Afterloading, 77767-77768, 77770-
    77772
  Unlisted Services and Procedures, 79999
**Radionuclide Tomography, Single–Photon**
  **Emission–Computed**
  Abscess Localization, 78807
  Bone, 78320
  Brain, 78607
  Cerebrospinal Fluid, 78647
  Heart, 78451-78454
  Joint, 78320
  Kidney, 78710
  Liver, 78205
  Tumor Localization, 78803
**Radiopharmaceutical Therapy**
  Heart, 79440
  Interstitial, 79300
    Colloid Administration, 79300
  Intra-arterial Particulate, 79445
  Intra–articular, 79440
  Intracavitary, 79200
  Intravascular, 79101
  Intravenous, 78808, 79101, 79403
  Oral, 79005
  Unlisted Services and Procedures, 79999
**Radiostereometic Analysis**
  Lower Extremity, 0350T
  Placement Interstitial Device, 0347T
  Spine, 0348T
  Upper Extremity, 0349T
**Radiosurgery**
  Cranial Lesion, 61796-61799
  Spinal Lesion, 63620-63621
**Radiotherapeutic**
  *See* Radiation Therapy
**Radiotherapies**
  *See* Irradiation
**Radiotherapy, Surface**, 77789
**Radiotherapy**
  Afterloading, 77767-77768, 77770-77772
    Catheter Insertion, 19296-19298
    Planning, 77316-77318

---

**Reconstruction** — *continued*
  Parotid Duct
    Diversion, 42507-42510
  Patella, 27437, 27438
    Instability, 27420-27424
  Penis
    Angulation, 54360
    Chordee, 54300, 54304
    Complications, 54340-54348
    Epispadias, 54380-54390
    Hypospadias, 54332, 54352
      One Stage Distal with Urethroplasty, 54324-54328
      One Stage Perineal, 54336
  Periorbital Region
    Osteotomy with Graft, 21267, 21268
  Pharynx, 42950
  Pyloric Sphincter, 43800
  Radius, 24365, 25390-25393, 25441
    Arthroplasty
      with Implant, 24366
  Shoulder Joint
    with Implant, 23470, 23472
  Skull, 21172-21180
    Defect, 62140, 62141, 62145
  Sternum, 21740-21742
    with Thoracoscopy, 21743
  Stomach
    with Duodenum, 43810, 43850, 43855, 43865
    with Jejunum, 43820, 43825, 43860
    for Obesity, 43644-43645, 43845-43848
    Gastric Bypass, 43644-43846
    Roux-en-Y, 43644, 43846
  Superior-Lateral Orbital Rim and Forehead, 21172, 21175
  Supraorbital Rim and Forehead, 21179, 21180
  Symblepharon, 68335
  Temporomandibular Joint
    Arthroplasty, 21240-21243
  Throat, 42950
  Thumb
    from Finger, 26550
    Opponensplasty, 26490-26496
  Tibia
    Lengthening, 27715
    Tubercle, 27418
  Toe
    Angle Deformity, 28313
    Extra, 28344
    Hammertoe, 28285, 28286
    Macrodactyly, 28340, 28341
    Polydactylous, 26587
    Syndactyly, 28345
    Webbed Toe, 28345
  Tongue
    Frenum, 41520
  Trachea
    Carina, 31766
    Cervical, 31750
    Fistula, 31755
    Graft Repair, 31770
    Intrathoracic, 31760
  Trapezium, 25445
  Tympanic Membrane, 69620
  Ulna, 25390-25393, 25442
    Radioulnar, 25337
  Ureter, 50700
    with Intestines, 50840
  Urethra, 53410-53440, 53445
    Complications, 54340-54348
    Hypospadias
      Meatus, 53450, 53460
      One Stage Distal with Meatal Advancement, 54322
      One Stage Distal with Urethroplasty, 54324 54328
      Suture to Bladder, 51840, 51841
      Urethroplasty for Second Stage, 54308-54316
      Urethroplasty for Third Stage, 54318
  Uterus, 58540
  Vas Deferens, 55400
  Vena Cava, 34502
    with Resection, 37799

**Reconstruction** — *continued*
  Wound Repair, 13100-13160
  Wrist, 25332
    Capsulectomy, 25320
    Capsulorrhaphy, 25320
    Realign, 25335
  Zygomatic Arch, 21255
**Recording**
  Fetal Magnetic Cardiac Signal, 0475T-0478T
  Tremor, 95999
**Rectal Bleeding**
  Endoscopic Control, 45317
**Rectal Packing**, 45999
**Rectal Prolapse**
  Excision, 45130-45135
  Repair, 45900
**Rectal Sphincter**
  Dilation, 45910
**Rectocele**
  Repair, 45560
**Rectopexy**
  Laparoscopic, 45400-45402
  Open, 45540-45550
**Rectoplasty**, 45500-45505
**Rectorrhaphy**, 45540-45541, 45800-45825
**Rectovaginal Fistula**
  *See* Fistula, Rectovaginal
**Rectovaginal Hernia**
  *See* Rectocele
**Rectum**
  *See Also* Anus
  Abscess
    Incision and Drainage, 45005, 45020, 46040, 46060
  Biopsy, 45100
  Dilation
    Endoscopy, 45303
  Endoscopy
    Destruction
      Tumor, 45320
    Dilation, 45303
    Exploration, 45300
    Hemorrhage, 45317
    Removal
      Foreign Body, 45307
      Polyp, 45308-45315
      Tumor, 45308-45315
    Volvulus, 45321
  Excision
    with Colon, 45121
    Partial, 45111, 45113-45116, 45123
    Total, 45110, 45112, 45119, 45120
  Exploration
    Endoscopic, 45300
    Surgical, 45990
  Hemorrhage
    Endoscopic, 45317
  Injection
    Sclerosing Solution, 45520
  Laparoscopy, 45499
  Lesion
    Excision, 45108
  Manometry, 91122
  Prolapse
    Excision, 45130, 45135
  Removal
    Fecal Impaction, 45915
    Foreign Body, 45307, 45915
  Repair
    with Sigmoid Excision, 45550
    Fistula, 45800-45825, 46706-46707
    Injury, 45562, 45563
    Prolapse, 45505-45541, 45900
    Rectocele, 45560
    Stenosis, 45500
  Sensation, Tone, and Compliance Test, 91120
  Stricture
    Excision, 45150
  Suture
    Fistula, 45800-45825
    Prolapse, 45540, 45541
  Tumor
    Destruction, 45190, 45320
    Excision, 45160, 45171-45172
  Unlisted Services and Procedures, 45999

**Rectus Sheath Block**
  Bilateral, 64488-64489
  Unilateral, 64486-64487
**Red Blood Cell (RBC)**
  Antibody, 86850-86870
    Pretreatment, 86970-86972
  Count, 85032-85041
  Fragility
    Mechanical, 85547
    Osmotic, 85555, 85557
  Hematocrit, 85014
  Morphology, 85007
  Platelet Estimation, 85007
  Sedimentation Rate
    Automated, 85652
    Manual, 85651
  Sequestration, 78140
  Sickling, 85660
  Survival Test, 78130, 78135
  Volume Determination, 78120, 78121
**Red Blood Cell ab**, 86850-86870
**Reductase, Glutathione**, 82978
**Reductase, Lactic Cytochrome**, 83615, 83625
**Reduction**
  Blood Volume, 86960
  Dislocation
    Acromioclavicular
      Closed Treatment, 23545
      Open Treatment, 23550, 23552
    Ankle
      Closed Treatment, 27840, 27842
      Open Treatment, 27846, 27848
    Bennet's
      Closed Treatment, 26670, 26675
      Open Treatment, 26665, 26685, 26686
      Percutaneous Fixation, 26650, 26676
    Carpometacarpal
      Closed Treatment, 26641, 26645, 26670, 26675
      Open Treatment, 26665, 26685, 26686
      Percutaneous Fixation, 26650, 26676
    Clavicle
      Closed Treatment, 23540, 23545
      Open Treatment, 23550, 23552
    Elbow
      Closed Treatment, 24600, 24605, 24620, 24640
      Monteggia, 24620
      Open Treatment
        Acute, 24615
        Chronic, 24615
        Monteggia, 24635
        Periarticular, 24586, 24587
    Galeazzi
      Closed Treatment, 25520
      Open Treatment, 25525, 25526
        with Fracture
          Radial Shaft, 25525, 25526
        with Repair
          Triangular Cartilage, 25526
    Hip
      Post Arthroplasty
        Closed Treatment, 27265, 27266
      Spontaneous/Pathologic
        Closed Treatment, 27257
      Developmental/Congenital
        Closed Treatment, 27257
        Open Treatment, 27258
          with Femoral Shaft Shortening, 27259
      Open Treatment, 27258
        with Femoral Shaft Shortening, 27259
      Traumatic
        Closed Treatment, 27250, 27252

**Reduction** — *continued*
  Dislocation — *continued*
    Hip — *continued*
      Traumatic — *continued*
        Open Treatment, 27253, 27254
          Acetabular Wall, 27254
          Femoral Head, 27254
    Intercarpal
      Closed Treatment, 25660
      Open Treatment, 25670
    Interphalangeal Joint
      Foot/Toe
        Closed Treatment, 28660, 28665
        Open Treatment, 28675
        Percutaneous Fixation, 28666
      Hand/Finger
        Closed Treatment, 26770, 26775
        Open Treatment, 26785
        Percutaneous Fixation, 26776
    Knee
      Closed Treatment, 27550, 27552
      Open Treatment, 27556-27558
    Lunate
      Closed Treatment, 25690
      Open Treatment, 25695
    Metacarpophalangeal Joint
      Closed Treatment, 26700-26706
      Open Treatment, 26715
    Metatarsophalangeal Joint
      Closed Treatment, 28630, 28635
      Open Treatment, 28645
      Percutaneous Fixation, 28636
    Monteggia, 24635
    Odontoid
      Open Treatment, 22318, 22319
    Patella, Patellar
      Acute
        Closed Treatment, 27560, 27562
        Open Treatment, 27566
        Partial, 27566
        Total, 27566
      Recurrent, 27420-27424
        with Patellectomy, 27424
    Pelvic, Ring
      Closed Treatment, 27197-27198
      Open Treatment, 27217-27218
      Percutaneous Fixation, 27216
    Radiocarpal
      Closed Treatment, 25660
      Open Treatment, 25670
    Radio-ulnar Joint
      Closed Treatment, 25675
        with Radial Fracture, 25520
      Open Treatment, 25676
        with Radial Fracture, 25525, 25526
    Radius
      with Fracture
        Closed Treatment, 24620
        Open Treatment, 24635
      Closed Treatment, 24640
    Sacrum, 27218
    Shoulder
      Closed Treatment with Manipulation, 23650, 23655
        with Fracture of Greater Humeral Tuberosity, 23665
        with Surgical or Anatomical Neck Fracture, 23675
      Open Treatment, 23660
      Recurrent, 23450-23466
    Sternoclavicular
      Closed Treatment, 23525
      Open Treatment, 23530, 23532
    Talotarsal joint
      Closed Treatment, 28570, 28575
      Open Treatment, 28585
      Percutaneous Fixation, 28576
    Tarsal
      Closed Treatment, 28540, 28545
      Open Treatment, 28555

CPT © 2017 American Medical Association. All Rights Reserved.

© 2017 Optum360, LLC

Index

Reduction — Removal

CPT © 2017 American Medical Association. All Rights Reserved.

**Repair** — *continued*
  Periorbital Region
    Osteotomy, 21260-21263
  Peritoneum, 49999
  Phalanges
    Finger
      Lengthening, 26568
      Osteotomy, 26567
      Nonunion, 26546
    Toe
      Osteotomy, 28310, 28312
  Pharynx
    with Esophagus, 42953
  Pleura, 32215
  Prosthesis
    Penis, 54408
  Pseudarthrosis
    Tibia, 27727
  Pulmonary Artery, 33917, 33920, 33925-33926
    Reimplantation, 33788
  Pulmonary Valve, 33470-33474
  Pulmonary Venous
    Anomaly, 33724
    Stenosis, 33726
  Quadriceps, 27430
  Radius
    with Graft, 25405, 25420-25426
    Epiphyseal, 25450, 25455
    Malunion or Nonunion, 25400-25420
    Osteotomy, 25350, 25355, 25370, 25375
  Rectocele, 45560, 57250
  Rectovaginal Fistula, 57308
  Rectum
    with Sigmoid Excision, 45550
    Fistula, 45800-45825, 46706-46707,
      46715-46716, 46740, 46742
    Injury, 45562-45563
    Prolapse, 45505-45541, 45900
    Rectocele, 45560, 57250
    Stenosis, 45500
  Retinal Detachment, 67101-67113
  Rotator Cuff, 23410-23412, 23420, 29827
  Salivary Duct, 42500, 42505
    Fistula, 42600
  Scalenus Anticus, 21700, 21705
  Scapula
    Fixation, 23400
    Scapulopexy, 23400
  Sclera
    with Glue, 65286
    Reinforcement
      with Graft, 67255
      without Graft, 67250
    Staphyloma
      with Graft, 66225
      without Graft, 66220
    Wound
      Operative, 66250
      Tissue Glue, 65286
  Scrotum, 55175, 55180
  Septal Defect, 33813-33814
  Septum, Nasal, 30420
  Shoulder
    Capsule, 23450-23466
    Cuff, 23410, 23412
    Ligament Release, 23415
    Muscle Transfer, 23395, 23397
    Musculotendinous (Rotator) Cuff, 23410,
      23412
    Rotator Cuff, 23415, 23420
    Tendon, 23410, 23412, 23430, 23440
    Tenomyotomy, 23405, 23406
  Simple, Integumentary System, 12001-12021
  Sinus of Valsalva, 33702-33722
  Sinus
    Ethmoid
      Cerebrospinal Fluid Leak, 31290
      Meningocele, 63700, 63702
      Myelomeningocele, 63704, 63706
    Sphenoid
      Cerebrospinal Fluid Leak, 31291
  Skin
    *See Also* Repair, Laceration
    Wound
      Complex, 13100-13160
      Intermediate, 12031-12057

**Repair** — *continued*
  Skin — *continued*
    Wound — *continued*
      Simple, 12020, 12021
  Skull
    Cerebrospinal Fluid Leak, 62100
    Encephalocele, 62120
  SLAP Lesion, 29807
  Spectacles, 92370, 92371
    Prosthesis, 92371
  Sphincter, 53449
  Spica Cast, 29720
  Spinal Cord, 63700
    Cerebrospinal Fluid Leak, 63707, 63709
    Meningocele, 63700, 63702
    Myelomeningocele, 63704, 63706
  Spinal Meningocele, 63700-63702
  Spine
    Cervical Vertebra, 22510, 22512
    Lumbar Vertebra, 22511-22512, 22514-
      22515
    Osteotomy, 22210-22226
    Sacral Vertebra, 22511-22512
    Thoracic Vertebra, 22510, 22512, 22513,
      22515
  Spleen, 38115
  Stenosis
    Nasal Vestibular, 30465
    Pulmonary, 33782-33783
  Sternocleidomastoid, 21720, 21725
  Stomach
    Esophagogastrostomy, 43112, 43320
    Fistula, 43880
    Fundoplasty, 43325-43328
    Laceration, 43501, 43502
    Stoma, 43870
    Ulcer, 43501
  Symblepharon, 68330, 68335, 68340
  Syndactyly, 26560-26562
  Talus
    Osteotomy, 28302
  Tarsal, 28320
    Osteotomy, 28304, 28305
  Tear
    Lung, 32110
  Tendon
    Achilles, 27650, 27652, 27654
    Extensor, 26410, 26412, 26418, 26420,
      26426, 26428, 26433-26434,
      27664-27665
    Foot, 28208, 28210
    Flexor, 26350, 26352, 26356-26358,
      27658-27659
    Leg, 28200, 28202
    Foot, 28200, 28202, 28208, 28210
    Leg, 27658-27659, 27664-27665
    Peroneal, 27675-27676
    Profundus, 26370, 26372-26373
    Upper Arm or Elbow, 24341
  Testis
    Injury, 54670
    Suspension, 54620, 54640
    Torsion, 54600
  Tetralogy of Fallot, 33692, 33694, 33697
  Throat
    Pharyngoesophageal, 42953
    Wound, 42900
  Thumb
    Muscle, 26508
    Tendon, 26510
  Tibia, 27720-27725
    Epiphysis, 27477-27485, 27730-27742
    Osteotomy, 27455, 27457, 27705, 27709,
      27712
    Pseudarthrosis, 27727
  Toe(s)
    Bunion, 28289-28299 *[28295]*
    Macrodactyly, 26590
    Muscle, 28240
    Polydactylous, 26587
    Ruiz–Mora Procedure, 28286
    Tendon, 28240
    Webbed Toe, 28280, 28345
  Tongue, 41250-41252
    Fixation, 41500
    Laceration, 41250-41252

**Repair** — *continued*
  Tongue — *continued*
    Mechanical, 41500
    Suture, 41510
  Trachea
    Fistula, 31755
      with Plastic Repair, 31825
      without Plastic Repair, 31820
    Stenosis, 31780, 31781
    Stoma, 31613, 31614
      with Plastic Repair, 31825
      without Plastic Repair, 31820
    Scar, 31830
    Wound
      Cervical, 31800
      Intrathoracic, 31805
  Transposition
    Great Arteries, 33770-33771, 33774-
      33781
  Triangular Fibrocartilage, 29846
  Tricuspid Valve, 33463-33465
  Trigger Finger, 26055
  Truncus Arteriosus
    Rastelli Type, 33786
  Tunica Vaginalis
    Hydrocele, 55060
  Tympanic Membrane, 69450, 69610, 69635-
    69637, 69641-69646
  Ulcer, 43501
  Ulna
    with Graft, 25405, 25420
    Epiphyseal, 25450, 25455
    Malunion or Nonunion, 25400-25415
    Osteotomy, 25360, 25370, 25375, 25425,
      25426
  Umbilicus
    Omphalocele, 49600-49611
  Ureter
    Anastomosis, 50740-50825
    Continent Diversion, 50825
    Deligation, 50940
    Fistula, 50920, 50930
    Lysis Adhesions, 50715-50725
    Suture, 50900
    Urinary Undiversion, 50830
  Ureterocele, 51535
  Urethra
    with Replantation Penis, 54438
    Artificial Sphincter, 53449
    Diverticulum, 53240, 53400, 53405
    Fistula, 45820, 45825, 53400, 53405,
      53520
    Prostatic or Membranous Urethra, 53415,
      53420, 53425
    Stoma, 53520
    Stricture, 53400, 53405
    Urethrocele, 57230
    Wound, 53502-53515
  Urethral Sphincter, 57220
  Urinary Incontinence, 53431, 53440, 53445
  Uterus
    Anomaly, 58540
    Fistula, 51920, 51925
    Rupture, 58520, 59350
    Suspension, 58400, 58410
      Presacral Sympathectomy, 58410
  Vagina
    Anterior, 57240, 57289
      with Insertion of Mesh, 57267
      with Insertion of Prosthesis, 57267
    Cystocele, 57240, 57260
    Enterocele, 57265
    Episiotomy, 59300
    Fistula, 46715, 46716, 51900
      Rectovaginal, 57300-57307
      Transvesical and Vaginal Approach,
        57330
      Urethrovaginal, 57310, 57311
      Vaginoenteric, 58999
      Vesicovaginal, 57320, 57330
    Hysterectomy, 58267, 58293
    Incontinence, 57288
    Pereyra Procedure, 57289
    Postpartum, 59300
    Prolapse, 57282, 57284
    Rectocele, 57250, 57260

**Repair** — *continued*
  Vagina — *continued*
    Suspension, 57280-57284
      Laparoscopic, 57425
    Wound, 57200, 57210
  Vaginal Wall Prolapse
    Anterior, 57240, 57267, 57289
    Anteroposterior, 57260-57267
    Nonobstetrical, 57200
    Posterior, 57250, 57267
  Vas Deferens
    Suture, 55400
  Vein
    Angioplasty, *[37248, 37249]*
    Femoral, 34501
    Graft, 34520
    Pulmonary, 33730
    Transposition, 34510
  Ventricle, 33545, 33611-33612, 33782-33783
  Vulva
    Postpartum, 59300
  Wound Dehiscence
    Abdominal Wall, 49900
    Skin and Subcutaneous Tissue
      Complex, 13160
      Simple, 12020, 12021
  Wound
    Cardiac, 33300, 33305
    Complex, 13100-13160
    Extraocular Muscle, 65290
    Intermediate, 12031-12057
    Operative Wound Anterior Segment,
      66250
    Simple, 12001-12021
  Wrist, 25260, 25263, 25270, 25447
    Bones, 25440
    Carpal Bone, 25431
    Cartilage, 25107
    Muscles, 25260-25274
    Removal
      Implant, 25449
    Secondary, 25265, 25272, 25274
    Tendon, 25280-25316
    Sheath, 25275
    Total Replacement, 25446
**Repeat Surgeries**
  Carotid
    Thromboendarterectomy, 35390
  Coronary Artery Bypass
    Valve Procedure, 33530
  Distal Vessel Bypass, 35700
**Replacement**
  Adjustable Gastric Restrictive Device, 43773
  Aortic Valve, 33405-33413
    Transcatheter, 33361-33369
  Arthroplasty
    Hip, 27125-27138
    Knee, 0396T, 27447
    Spine, 22856-22857, 22861-22862
  Artificial Heart
    Intracorporeal, 33928-33929
  Cardio-Defibrillator, 33249, *[33262, 33263,*
    *33264]*
  Carotid Sinus Baroreflex Activation Device,
    0266T-0268T
  Cecostomy Tube, 49450
  Cerebrospinal Fluid Shunt, 62160, 62194,
    62225, 62230
  Chest Wall Respiratory Sensor Electrode or
    Electrode Array, 0467T
  Colonic Tube, 49450
  Contact Lens, 92326
    *See Also* Contact Lens Services
  Duodenostomy Tube, 49451
  Elbow
    Total, 24363
  Electrode
    Heart, 33210, 33211, 33216, 33217
    Stomach, 43647
  External Fixation, 20697
  Eye
    Drug Delivery System, 67121
  Gastro-jejunostomy Tube, 49452
  Gastrostomy Tube, 43760, 49450
  Hearing Aid
    Bone Conduction, 69710

**Replacement** — *continued*
  Heart
    Defibrillator
      Leads, 33249
    Hip, 27130, 27132
      Revision, 27134-27138
  Implant
    Bone
      for External Speech Processor/Cochlear Stimulator, 69717, 69718
  Intervertebral Disc
    Cervical Interspace, 0375T, 22856
    Lumbar Interspace, 0163T, 22862
  Intracardiac Ischemia Monitoring System, 0302T
    Device Only, 0304T
    Electrode Only, 0303T
  Jejunostomy Tube, 49451
  Knee
    Intraoperative Balance Sensor, 0396T
    Total, 27447
  Mitral Valve, 33430
  Nerve, 64726
  Neurostimulator
    Electrode, 63663-63664, 64569
    Pulse Generator/Receiver
      Intracranial, 61885
      Peripheral Nerve, 64590
      Spinal, 63685
  Ossicles
    with Prosthesis, 69633, 69637
  Ossicular Replacement, 69633, 69637
  Pacemaker, 33206-33208, *[33227, 33228, 33229]*
    Catheter, 33210
    Electrode, 33210, 33211, 33216, 33217
    Pulse Generator, 33212-33214 *[33221]*, 33224-33233 *[33227, 33228, 33229]*
  Pacing Cardioverter–Defibrillator
    Leads, 33243, 33244
    Pulse Generator Only, 33241
  Penile
    Prosthesis, 54410, 54411, 54416, 54417
  Prosthesis
    Skull, 62143
    Urethral Sphincter, 53448
  Pulmonary Valve, 33475
  Pulse Generator
    Brain, 61885
    Peripheral Nerve, 64590
    Spinal Cord, 63685
    Vagus Nerve Blocking Therapy, 0316T
  Receiver
    Brain, 61885
    Peripheral Nerve, 64590
    Spinal Cord, 63685
  Skin, 15002-15278
  Skull Plate, 62143
  Spinal Cord
    Reservoir, 62360
  Stent
    Ureteral, 50382, 50385
  Strut, 20697
  Subcutaneous Port for Gastric Restrictive Procedure, 43888
  Tissue Expanders
    Skin, 11970
  Total Replacement Heart System
    Intracorporeal, 33928-33929
  Total Replacement Hip, 27130-27132
  Tricuspid Valve, 33465
  Ureter
    with Intestines, 50840
    Electronic Stimulator, 53899
  Uterus
    Inverted, 59899
  Venous Access Device, 36582, 36583, 36585
    Catheter, 36578
  Venous Catheter
    Central, 36580, 36581, 36584
  Ventricular Assist Device, 0451T-0454T, 0459T, 33981-33983

**Replantation, Reimplantation**
  Adrenal Tissue, 60699

**Replantation, Reimplantation** — *continued*
  Arm, Upper, 20802
  Digit, 20816, 20822
  Foot, 20838
  Forearm, 20805
  Hand, 20808
  Penis, 54438
  Scalp, 17999
  Thumb, 20824, 20827

**Report Preparation**
  Extended, Medical, 99080
  Psychiatric, 90889

**Reposition**
  Toe to Hand, 26551-26556

**Repositioning**
  Canalith, 95992
  Central Venous Catheter, Previously Placed, 36597
  Defibrillator, *[33273]*
  Electrode
    Heart, 33215, 33226
  Gastrostomy Tube, 43761
  Intraocular Lens, 66825
  Intravascular Vena Cava Filter, 37192
  Tricuspid Valve, 33468
  Ventricular Assist Device, 0460T-0461T

**Reproductive Tissue**
  Preparation
    Thawing, 89354
  Storage, 89344

**Reprogramming**
  Infusion Pump, 62369-62370
  Peripheral Subcutaneous Field Stimulation
    Pulse Generator, 64999
  Shunt
    Brain, 62252

**Reptilase**
  Test, 85635
  Time, 85670-85675

**Resection**
  Abdomen, 51597
  Aortic Valve Stenosis, 33415
  Bladder Diverticulum, 52305
  Bladder Neck
    Transurethral, 52500
  Brain Lobe, 61323, 61537-61540
  Bullae, 32141
  Chest Wall, 19260-19272
  Cyst
    Mediastinal, 39200
  Diaphragm, 39560-39561
  Emphysematous Lung, 32672
  Endaural, 69905-69910
  Humeral Head, 23195
  Intestines, Small
    Laparoscopic, 44202-44203
  Lung, 32491, 32503-32504, 32672
  Mouth
    with Tongue Excision, 41153
  Myocardium
    Aneurysm, 33542
    Septal Defect, 33545
  Nasal Septum, Submucous, 30520
  Nose
    Septum, 30520
  Ovary, Wedge, 58920
  Palate, 42120
  Pancoast Tumor, 32503-32504
  Phalangeal Head
    Toe, 28153
  Prostate, Transurethral, 52601, 52630
  Radical
    Abdomen, 22904-22905, 51597
    Acetabulum, 27049 *[27059]*, 27076
    Ankle, 27615-27616, 27645-27647
    Arm, Lower, 24152, 25077-25078, 25170
    Arm, Upper, 23220, 24077-24079, 24150
    Back, 21935-21936
    Calcaneus, 27615-27616, 27647
    Elbow, 24077-24079, 24152
      Capsule Soft Tissue, 24149
    Face, 21015-21016
    Femur, 27364-27365 *[27329]*
    Fibula, 27615-27616, 27646
    Finger, 26117-26118, 26260-26262
    Flank, 21935-21936

**Resection** — *continued*
  Radical — *continued*
    Foot, 28046-28047, 28171-28173
    Forearm, 25077-25078, 25170
    Hand, 26117-26118, 26250
    Hip, 27049 *[27059]*, 27075-27078
    Humerus, 23220, 24077-24079
    Innominate, 27049 *[27059]*, 27077
    Ischial, 27049 *[27059]*, 27078
    Knee, 27364-27365 *[27329]*
    Lymph Node(s)
      Abdomen, 38747
      Axillary, 38740, 38745
      Cervical, 38720, 38724
      Groin Area, 38760, 38765
      Pelvic, 38770
      Retroperitoneal, 38780
      Suprahyoid, 38700
      Thoracic, 38746
    Metacarpal, 26117-26118, 26250
    Metatarsal, 28046-28047, 28173
    Mouth
      with Tongue Excision, 41150, 41155
    Neck, 21557-21558
    Ovarian Tumor
      with Radical Dissection for Debulking, 58952-58954
      with Total Abdominal Hysterectomy, 58951, 58953-58956
      Bilateral Salpingo–Oophorectomy–Omentectomy, 58950-58954
      Omentectomy, 58950-58956
    Pelvis, 27049 *[27059]*, 27075-27078
    Peritoneal Tumor
      with Radical Dissection for Debulking, 58952-58954
      Bilateral Salpingo–Oophorectomy–Omentectomy, 58952-58954
    Phalanges
      Fingers, 26117-26118, 26260-26262
      Toes, 28046-28047, 28175
    Radius, 24152, 25077-25078, 25170
    Scalp, 21015-21016
    Scapula, 23077-23078, 23210
    Shoulder, 23077-23078, 23220
    Sternum, 21557-21558, 21630-21632
    Talus, 27615-27616, 27647
    Tarsal, 28046-28047, 28171
    Thigh, 27364-27365 *[27329]*
    Thorax, 21557-21558
    Tibia, 27615-27616, 27645
    Tonsil, 42842-42845
    Ulna, 25077-25078, 25170
    Wrist, 25077-25078, 25115-25116, 25170
  Rhinectomy
    Partial, 30150
    Total, 30160
  Ribs, 19260-19272, 32900
  Synovial Membrane
    *See* Synovectomy
  Temporal Bone, 69535
  Thoracotomy Wedge, 32505-32507
  Thymus, 32673
  Tumor
    Fallopian Tube, 58957-58958
    Lung, 32503-32504
    Mediastinal, 39220
    Ovary, 58957-58958
    Pericardial, 33050
    Peritoneum, 58957-58958
  Ulna
    Arthrodesis
      Radioulnar Joint, 25830
  Ureterocele
    Ectopic, 52301
    Orthotopic, 52300
  Vena Cava
    with Reconstruction, 37799

**Residual Urine Collection**, 51701

**Resistance**
  Airway, 94728

**Resonance Spectroscopy, Magnetic**, 76390

**Respiration, Positive–Pressure**, 94660
**Respiratory Motion Management Simulation**, 77293
**Respiratory Pattern Recording**
  Preventive
    Infant, 94772
**Respiratory Syncytial Virus**
  Antibody, 86756
  Antigen Detection
    Direct Fluorescent Antibody, 87280
    Direct Optical Observation, 87807
    Enzyme Immunoassay, 87420
  Recombinant, 90378
**Response, Auditory Evoked**, 92585-92586
  *See Also* Audiologic Function Tests
**Rest Home Visit**
  Care Plan Oversight Services, 99339-99340
  Established Patient, 99334-99337
  New Patient, 99324-99328
**Restoration**
  Ventricular, 33548
**Resuscitation**
  Cardiac Massage via Thoracotomy, 32160
  Cardiopulmonary (CPR), 92950
  Newborn, 99460-99465
**RET**, 81404-81406
**Reticulocyte**
  Count, 85044-85045
**Retina**
  Computer-aided Animation and Analysis, 0380T
  Electrode Array, 0472T-0473T
  Examination, Macula/Fundus, Dilated, 2019F-2021F
    Communication of Findings for Diabetes Management, 5010F
  Incision
    Encircling Material, 67115
  Lesion
    Extensive
      Destruction, 67227-67228
    Localized
      Destruction, 67208-67218
  Polarization Scan, 0469T
  Repair
    Detachment
      with Vitrectomy, 67108, 67113
      by Scleral Buckling, 67107-67108
      Cryotherapy, 67101
      Injection of Air, 67110
      Photocoagulation, 67105
      Scleral Dissection, 67107
    Prophylaxis
      Detachment, 67141, 67145
  Retinal electrode array, 0472T-0473T
  Retinopathy
    Destruction
      Cryotherapy, Diathermy, 67227, 67229
      Photocoagulation, 67228-67229
      Preterm Infant, 67229
**Retinacular**
  Knee
    Release, 27425
**Retinopathy**
  Destruction/Treatment
    Cryotherapy, Diathermy, 67227, 67229
    Photocoagulation, 67228-67229
**Retinopexy, Pneumatic**, 67110
**Retraction, Clot**
  *See* Clot Retraction
**Retrocaval Ureter**
  Ureterolysis, 50725
**Retrograde Cholangiopancreatographies, Endoscopic**
  *See* Cholangiopancreatography
**Retrograde Cystourethrogram**
  *See* Urethrocystography, Retrograde
**Retrograde Pyelogram**
  *See* Urography, Retrograde
**Retroperitoneal Area**
  Abscess
    Incision and Drainage
      Open, 49060
  Biopsy, 49010

CPT © 2017 American Medical Association. All Rights Reserved.      © 2017 Optum360, LLC

**Sternoclavicular Joint** — *continued*
  Dislocation
    Closed Treatment
      with Manipulation, 23525
      without Manipulation, 23520
    Open Treatment, 23530-23532
      with Fascial Graft, 23532
**Sternocleidomastoid**
  Division, 21720-21725
**Sternotomy**
  Closure, 21750
**Sternum**
  Debridement, 21627
  Excision, 21620, 21630-21632
  Fracture
    Closed Treatment, 21820
    Open Treatment, 21825
  Ostectomy, 21620
  Radical Resection, 21630-21632
  Reconstruction, 21740-21742, 21750
    with Thoracoscopy, 21743
  X-Ray, 71120-71130
**Steroid-Binding Protein, Sex**, 84270
**Steroids**
  Anabolic
    *See* Androstenedione
  Injection
    Morton's Neuroma, 64455
    Paravertebral
      Facet Joint, 64490-64495
      Paraspinous Block, [64461, 64462, 64463]
    Plantar Common Digital Nerve, 64455
    Sympathetic Nerves, 64505-64530
    Transforaminal Epidural, 64479-64484
    Urethral Stricture, 52283
  Ketogenic
    Urine, 83582
**STG**, 15100-15121
**STH**, 83003
**Stimson's Method Reduction**, 23650, 23655
**Stimulating Antibody, Thyroid**, 84445
**Stimulation**
  Electric
    *See Also* Electrical Stimulation
    Brain Surface, 95961-95962
  Lymphocyte, 86353
  Spinal Cord
    Stereotaxis, 63610
  Transcutaneous Electric, 64550
**Stimulator, Long-Acting Thyroid**, 80438-80439
**Stimulators, Cardiac**, 33202-33213
  *See Also* Heart, Pacemaker
**Stimulus Evoked Response**, 51792
**STK11**, 81404-81405, 81432-81433, 81435-81436
**Stoffel Operation**
  Rhizotomy, 63185, 63190
**Stoma**
  Closure
    Intestines, 44620
  Creation
    Bladder, 51980
    Kidney, 50551-50561
    Stomach
      Neonatal, 43831
      Permanent, 43832
      Temporary, 43830, 43831
    Ureter, 50860
  Revision
    Colostomy, 44345
    Ileostomy
      Complicated, 44314
      Simple, 44312
    Ureter
      Endoscopy via, 50951-50961
**Stomach**
  Anastomosis
    with Duodenum, 43810, 43850-43855
    with Jejunum, 43820-43825, 43860-43865
  Biopsy, 43605
  Creation
    Stoma
      Permanent, 43832
      Temporary, 43830-43831
        Laparoscopic, 43653

**Stomach** — *continued*
  Electrode
    Implantation, 43647, 43881
    Removal/Revision, 43882
  Electrogastrography, 91132-91133
  Excision
    Partial, 43631-43635, 43845
    Total, 43620-43622
  Exploration, 43500
  Gastric Bypass, 43644-43645, 43846-43847
    Revision, 43848
  Gastric Restrictive Procedures, 43644-43645, 43770-43774, 43842-43848, 43886-43888
  Gastropexy, 43659, 43999
  Implantation
    Electrodes, 43647, 43881
  Incision, 43830-43832
    Exploration, 43500
    Pyloric Sphincter, 43520
    Removal
      Foreign Body, 43500
  Intubation, 43753-43756
  Laparoscopy, 43647-43648
  Nuclear Medicine
    Blood Loss Study, 78278
    Emptying Study, 78264-78266
    Imaging, 78261
    Protein Loss Study, 78282
    Reflux Study, 78262
    Vitamin B-12
      Absorption, 78270-78272
  Reconstruction
    for Obesity, 43644-43645, 43842-43847
    Roux-en-Y, 43644, 43846
  Removal
    Foreign Body, 43500
  Repair, 48547
    Fistula, 43880
    Fundoplasty, 43279-43282, 43325-43328
      Laparoscopic, 43280
    Laceration, 43501, 43502
    Stoma, 43870
    Ulcer, 43501
  Specimen Collection, 43754-43755
  Suture
    Fistula, 43880
    for Obesity, 43842, 43843
    Stoma, 43870
    Ulcer, 43840
    Wound, 43840
  Tumor
    Excision, 43610, 43611
  Ulcer
    Excision, 43610
  Unlisted Services and Procedures, 43659, 43999
**Stomatoplasty**
  Vestibule, 40840-40845
**Stone, Kidney**
  Removal, 50060-50081, 50130, 50561, 50580, 52352
**Stone**
  Calculi
    Bile Duct, 43264, 47420, 47425
      Percutaneous, 47554
    Bladder, 51050, 51310-52318, 52352
    Gallbladder, 47480
    Hepatic Duct, 47400
    Kidney, 50060-50081, 50130, 50561, 50580, 52352
    Pancreas, 48020
    Pancreatic Duct, 43264
    Salivary Gland, 42330-42340
    Ureter, 50610-50630, 50961, 50980, 51060, 51065, 52320-52330, 52352
    Urethra, 52310, 52315, 52352
**Stookey-Scarff Procedure**
  Ventriculocisternostomy, 62200
**Stool Blood**, 82270, 82272-82274
**Storage**
  Embryo, 89342
  Oocyte, 89346
  Reproductive Tissue, 89344
  Sperm, 89343

**STR**, 81265-81266
**Strabismus**
  Chemodenervation, 67345
  Repair
    Adjustable Sutures, 67335
    Extraocular Muscles, 67340
    One Horizontal Muscle, 67311
    One Vertical Muscle, 67314
    Posterior Fixation Suture Technique, 67334, 67335
    Previous Surgery not Involving Extraocular Muscles, 67331
    Release Extensive Scar Tissue, 67343
    Superior Oblique Muscle, 67318
    Transposition, 67320
    Two Horizontal Muscles, 67312
    Two or More Vertical Muscles, 67316
**Strapping**
  *See Also* Cast; Splint
  Ankle, 29540
  Chest, 29200
  Elbow, 29260
  Finger, 29280
  Foot, 29540
  Hand, 29280
  Hip, 29520
  Knee, 29530
  Shoulder, 29240
  Thorax, 29200
  Toes, 29550
  Unlisted Services and Procedures, 29799
  Unna Boot, 29580
  Wrist, 29260
**Strassman Procedure**, 58540
**Strayer Procedure**, 27687
**Strep Quick Test**, 86403
**Streptococcus, Group A**
  Antigen Detection
    Enzyme Immunoassay, 87430
    Nucleic Acid, 87650-87652
  Direct Optical Observation, 87880
**Streptococcus, Group B**
  by Immunoassay
    with Direct Optical Observation, 87802
**Streptococcus Pneumoniae Vaccine**
  *See* Vaccines
**Streptokinase, Antibody**, 86590
**Stress Tests**
  Cardiovascular, 93015-93024
    Echocardiography, 93350-93351
      with Contrast, 93352
    Multiple Gated Acquisition (MUGA), 78472, 78473
    Myocardial Perfusion Imaging, 0439T, 78451-78454
  Pulmonary, 94618-94621
    *See* Pulmonology, Diagnostic
**Stricture**
  Ureter, 50706
  Urethra
    Dilation, 52281
    Repair, 53400
**Strictureplasty**
  Intestines, 44615
**Stroboscopy**
  Larynx, 31579
**STS**, 86592-86593
**STSG**, 15100-15121
**Stuart-Prower Factor**, 85260
**Study**
  Color Vision, 92283
  Common Carotid Intima-media Thickness (IMT), 0126T
**Sturmdorf Procedure**, 57520
**STXBP1**, 81406
**Styloid Process**
  Fracture, 25645, 25650
  Radial
    Excision, 25230
**Styloidectomy**
  Radial, 25230
**Stypven Time**, 85612-85613
**Subacromial Bursa**
  Arthrocentesis, 20610-20611
**Subarachnoid Drug Administration**, 0186T, 01996

**Subclavian Arteries**
  Aneurysm, 35001-35002, 35021-35022
  Angioplasty, [37246, 37247]
  Bypass Graft, 35506, 35511-35516, 35526, 35606-35616, 35626, 35645
  Embolectomy, 34001-34101
  Thrombectomy, 34001-34101
  Thromboendarterectomy, 35301, 35311
  Transposition, 33889
  Unlisted Services/Procedures, 37799
**Subcutaneous Implantable Defibrillator Device**
  Electrophysiologic Evaluation, [33270]
  Insertion, [33270]
    Defibrillator Electrode, [33271]
    Implantable Defibrillator System and Electrode, [33270]
    Pulse Generator with Existing Electrode, 33240
  Interrogation Device Evaluation (In Person), [93261]
  Programming Device Evaluation (In Person), [93260]
  Removal
    Electrode Only, [33272]
    Pulse Generator Only, 33241
      with Replacement, [33262, 33263, 33264]
  Repositioning Electrode or Pulse Generator, [33273]
**Subcutaneous Mastectomies**, 19304
**Subcutaneous Tissue**
  Excision, 15830-15839, 15847
  Repair
    Complex, 13100-13160
    Intermediate, 12031-12057
    Simple, 12020, 12021
**Subcutaneous**
  Chemotherapy, 96401-96402
  Infusion, 96369-96371
  Injection, 96372
**Subdiaphragmatic Abscess**, 49040
**Subdural Electrode**
  Insertion, 61531-61533
  Removal, 61535
**Subdural Hematoma**, 61108, 61154
**Subdural Puncture**, 61105-61108
**Subdural Tap**, 61000, 61001
**Sublingual Gland**
  Abscess
    Incision and Drainage, 42310, 42320
  Calculi (Stone)
    Excision, 42330
  Cyst
    Drainage, 42409
    Excision, 42408
  Excision, 42450
**Subluxation**
  Elbow, 24640
**Submandibular Gland**
  Calculi (Stone)
    Excision, 42330, 42335
  Excision, 42440
**Submaxillary Gland**
  Abscess
    Incision and Drainage, 42310-42320
**Submental Fat Pad**
  Excision
    Excess Skin, 15838
**Submucous Resection of Nasal Septum**, 30520
**Subperiosteal Implant**
  Reconstruction
    Mandible, 21245, 21246
    Maxilla, 21245, 21246
**Subphrenic Abscess**, 49040
**Substance and/or Alcohol Abuse Screening and Intervention**, 99408-99409
**Substance S, Reichstein's**, 80436, 82634
**Substitute Skin Application**, 15271-15278
**Subtalar Joint Stabilization**, 0335T
**Subtrochanteric Fracture**
  with Implant, 27244-27245
  Closed Treatment, 27238
    with Manipulation, 27240
**Sucrose Hemolysis Test**, 85555-85557
**Suction Lipectomies**, 15876-15879

**Sudiferous Gland**
  Excision
    Axillary, 11450-11451
    Inguinal, 11462-11463
    Perianal, 11470-11471
    Perineal, 11470-11471
    Umbilical, 11470-11471
**Sugar Water Test**, 85555-85557
**Sugars**, 84375-84379
**Sugiura Procedure**
  Esophagus, Repair, Varices, 43401
**Sulfate**
  Chondroitin, 82485
  DHA, 82627
  Urine, 84392
**Sulfation Factor**, 84305
**Sulphates**
  Chondroitin, 82485
  DHA, 82627
  Urine, 84392
**Sumatran Mite Fever**, 86000
**Sunrise View X-Ray**, 73560-73564
**Superficial Musculoaponeurotic Systems (SMAS) Flap**
  Rhytidectomy, 15829
**Supernumerary Digit**
  Reconstruction, 26587
  Repair, 26587
**Supervision**
  Home Health Agency Patient, 99374-99375
**Supply**
  Chemotherapeutic Agent
    See Chemotherapy
  Educational Materials, 99071
  Low Vision Aids
    Fitting, 92354-92355
    Repair, 92370
  Materials, 99070
  Prosthesis
    Breast, 19396
**Suppositories, Vaginal**, 57160
  for Induced Abortion, 59855-59857
**Suppression**, 80400-80408
**Suppression/Testing**, 80400-80439
**Suppressor T Lymphocyte Marker**, 86360
**Suppurative Hidradenitis**
  Incision and Drainage, 10060-10061
**Suprachoroidal Injection**, 0465T
**Suprahyoid**
  Lymphadenectomy, 38700
**Supraorbital Nerve**
  Avulsion, 64732
  Incision, 64732
  Transection, 64732
**Supraorbital Rim and Forehead**
  Reconstruction, 21179-21180
**Suprapubic Prostatectomies**, 55821
**Suprarenal**
  Gland
    Biopsy, 60540-60545, 60650
    Excision, 60540-60545, 60650
    Exploration, 60540-60545, 60650
    Nuclear Medicine Imaging, 78075
  Vein
    Venography, 75840-75842
**Suprascapular Nerve**
  Injection
    Anesthetic, 64418
**Suprasellar Cyst**, 61545
**SURF1**, 81405
**Surface CD4 Receptor**, 86360
**Surface Radiotherapy**, 77789
**Surgeries**
  Breast–Conserving, 19120-19126, 19301
  Laser
    Anus, 46614, 46917
    Bladder/Urethra, 52214-52240
    Esophagus, 43227
    Lacrimal Punctum, 68760
    Lens, Posterior, 66821
    Lesion
      Mouth, 40820
      Nose, 30117-30118
      Penis, 54057
      Skin, 17000-17111, 17260-17286
    Myocardium, 33140-33141

**Surgeries** — *continued*
  Laser — *continued*
    Prostate, 52647-52648
    Spine, 62287
    Mohs, 17311-17315
    Repeat
      Cardiac Valve Procedure, 33530
      Carotid Thromboendarterectomy, 35390
      Coronary Artery Bypass, 33530
      Distal Vessel Bypass, 35700
**Surgical Correction**
  Uterus
    Inverted, 59899
**Surgical Services**
  Post–Operative Visit, 99024
**Surgical**
  Avulsion
    Nails, 11730-11732
    Nerve, 64732-64772
  Cartilage
    Excision, 21060
  Cataract Removal, 3073F, 66830, 66982-66984
  Collapse Therapy, Thoracoplasty, 32905-32906
  Diathermy
    Ciliary Body, 66700
    Lesions
      Benign, 17000-17111
      Malignant, 17260-17286
      Premalignant, 17000-17111
  Galvanism, 17380
  Incision
    See Incision
  Meniscectomy, 21060
  Microscopes, 69990
  Pathology
    See Pathology, Surgical
  Planing
    Nose
      Skin, 30120
  Pneumoperitoneum, 49400
  Preparation
    Cadaver Donor Lung(s), 0494T
  Removal, Eye
    with Implant, 65103-65105
    without Implant, 65101
  Revision
    Cardiac Valve Procedure, 33530
    Carotid Thromboendarterectomy, 35390
    Coronary Artery Bypass, 33530
    Distal Vessel Bypass, 35700
  Services
    Postoperative Visit, 99024
  Ventricular Restoration, 33548
**Surveillance**
  See Monitoring
**Suspension**
  Aorta, 33800
  Hyoid, 21685
  Kidney, 50400-50405
  Tongue Base, 41512
  Urethra, 51990, 57289
  Uterine, 58400-58410
  Vagina, 57280-57283, 57425
  Vesical Neck, 51845
**Suture**
  See Also Repair
  Abdomen, 49900
  Anus, 46999
  Aorta, 33320, 33321
  Bile Duct
    Wound, 47900
  Bladder
    Fistulization, 44660-44661, 45800-45805, 51880-51925
      Vesicouterine, 51920-51925
      Vesicovaginal, 51900
    Wound, 51860-51865
  Cervix, 57720
  Colon
    Diverticula, 44604-44605
    Fistula, 44650-44661
    Plication, 44680
    Stoma, 44620-44625
    Ulcer, 44604-44605
    Wound, 44604-44605

**Suture** — *continued*
  Esophagus
    Wound, 43410, 43415
  Eyelid, 67880
    with Transposition of Tarsal Plate, 67882
    Closure of, 67875
    Wound
      Full Thickness, 67935
      Partial Thickness, 67930
  Facial Nerve
    Intratemporal
      Lateral to Geniculate Ganglion, 69740
      Medial to Geniculate Ganglion, 69745
  Fallopian Tube
    Simple, 58999
  Foot
    Tendon, 28200-28210
  Gastroesophageal, 43405
  Great Vessel, 33320-33322
  Hemorrhoids, [46945], [46946]
  Hepatic Duct, 47765, 47802
  Intestines
    Large, 44604-44605
    Small, 44602-44603
      Fistula, 44640-44661
      Plication, 44680
      Stoma, 44620-44625
  Iris
    with Ciliary Body, 66682
  Kidney
    Fistula, 50520-50526
    Horseshoe, 50540
    Wound, 50500
  Leg, Lower
    Tendon, 27658-27665
  Leg, Upper
    Muscles, 27385, 27386
  Liver
    Wound, 47350-47361
  Mesentery, 44850
  Nerve, 64831-64876
  Pancreas, 48545
  Pharynx
    Wound, 42900
  Rectum
    Fistula, 45800-45825
    Prolapse, 45540, 45541
  Removal
    Anesthesia, 15850, 15851
  Spleen, 38115
  Stomach
    Fistula, 43880
    Laceration, 43501, 43502
    Stoma, 43870
    Ulcer, 43501, 43840
    Wound, 43840
  Tendon
    Foot, 28200-28210
    Knee, 27380, 27381
  Testis
    Injury, 54670
    Suspension, 54620, 54640
  Thoracic Duct
    Abdominal Approach, 38382
    Cervical Approach, 38380
    Thoracic Approach, 38381
  Throat
    Wound, 42900
  Tongue
    to Lip, 41510
  Trachea
    Fistula, 31825
      with Plastic Repair, 31825
      without Plastic Repair, 31820
    Stoma, 31825
      with Plastic Repair, 31825
      without Plastic Repair, 31820
    Wound
      Cervical, 31800
      Intrathoracic, 31805
  Ulcer, 44604-44605
  Ureter, 50900, 50940
    Deligation, 50940
    Fistula, 50920-50930

**Suture** — *continued*
  Urethra
    Fistula, 45820-45825, 53520
    Stoma, 53520
    to Bladder, 51840-51841
    Wound, 53502-53515
  Uterus
    Fistula, 51920-51925
    Rupture, 58520, 59350
    Suspension, 58400-58410
  Vagina
    Cystocele, 57240, 57260
    Enterocele, 57265
    Fistula
      Rectovaginal, 57300-57307
      Transvesical and Vaginal Approach, 57330
      Urethrovaginal, 57310-57311
      Vesicovaginal, 51900, 57320-57330
    Rectocele, 57250-57260
    Suspension, 57280-57283
    Wound, 57200-57210
  Vas Deferens, 55400
  Vein
    Femoral, 37650
    Iliac, 37660
    Vena Cava, 37619
  Wound, 44604-44605
    Skin
      Complex, 13100-13160
      Intermediate, 12031-12057
      Simple, 12020-12021
**SUZI (Sub-Zonal Insemination)**, 89280
**SVR (Surgical Ventricular Restoration)**, 33548
**Swallowing**
  Cine, 74230
  Evaluation, 92610-92613, 92616-92617
  Therapy, 92526
  Video, 74230
**Swan-Ganz Catheter Insertion**, 93503
**Swanson Procedure**
  Repair, Metatarsal, 28322
  Osteotomy, 28306-28309
**Sweat Collection**
  Iontophoresis, 89230
**Sweat Glands**
  Excision
    Axillary, 11450, 11451
    Inguinal, 11462, 11463
    Perianal, 11470, 11471
    Perineal, 11470, 11471
    Umbilical, 11470, 11471
**Sweat Test**
  Chloride, Blood, 82435
**Swenson Procedure**, 45120
**Syme Procedure**, 27888
**Sympathectomy**
  with Rib Excision, 21616
  Artery
    Digital, 64820
    Radial, 64821
    Superficial Palmar Arch, 64823
    Ulnar, 64822
  Cervical, 64802
  Cervicothoracic, 64804
  Digital Artery with Magnification, 64820
  Lumbar, 64818
  Presacral, 58410
  Renal, 0338T-0339T
  Thoracic, 32664
  Thoracolumbar, 64809
**Sympathetic Nerve**
  Excision, 64802-64818
  Injection
    Anesthetic, 64508, 64520-64530
**Sympathins**, 80424, 82382-82384
**Symphysiotomy**
  Horseshoe Kidney, 50540
**Symphysis, Pubic**, 27282
**Synagis**, 90378
**Syncytial Virus, Respiratory**
  Antibody, 86756
  Antigen Detection
    Direct Fluorescence, 87280
    Direct Optical Observation, 87807
    Enzyme Immunoassay, 87420

# T

Index

Thoracic — *Thyroxine*

CPT © 2017 American Medical Association. All Rights Reserved.          © 2017 Optum360, LLC

CPT © 2017 American Medical Association. All Rights Reserved.    © 2017 Optum360, LLC

**Ultrasound** — *continued*
  *See Also* Echocardiography; Echography
  Abdomen, 76700, 76705-76706
  Ablation
    Uterine Leiomyomata, 0071T-0072T, 0404T
  Arm, 76881-76882
  Artery
    Intracranial, 93886-93893
    Middle Cerebral, 76821
    Umbilical, 76820
  Bladder, 51798
  Bone Density Study, 76977
  Breast, 76641-76642
  Chest, 76604
  Colon
    Endoscopic, 45391-45392
  Colon–Sigmoid
    Endoscopic, 45341, 45342
  Computer Aided Surgical Navigation
    Intraoperative, 0054T-0055T
  Drainage
    Abscess, 75989
  Echoencephalography, 76506
  Esophagus
    Endoscopy, 43231, 43232
  Extremity, 76881-76882
  Eye, 76511-76513
    Biometry, 76514-76519
    Foreign Body, 76529
    Pachymetry, 76514
  Fetus, 76818, 76819
  Follow–Up, 76970
  for Physical Therapy, 97035
  Gastrointestinal, Upper
    Endoscopic, 43242, 43259
  Gastrointestinal, 76975
  Guidance
    Amniocentesis, 59001, 76946
    Amnioinfusion, 59070
    Arteriovenous Fistulae, 76936
    Chorionic Villus Sampling, 76945
    Cryosurgery, 55873
    Drainage
      Fetal Fluid, 59074
    Endometrial Ablation, 58356
    Esophagogastroduodenoscopy
      with Drainage Pseudocyst with Placement
        Catheters/Stents, 43240
      with Injection Diagnostic or Thera-peutic Substance, 43253
      Examination, 43237, 43259
      Fine Needle Aspiration/Biopsy, 43238, 43242
    Fetal Cordocentesis, 76941
    Fetal Transfusion, 76941
    Heart Biopsy, 76932
    Injection Facet Joint, 0213T-0218T
    Needle Biopsy, 43232, 43242, 45342, 76942
    Occlusion
      Umbilical Cord, 59072
    Ova Retrieval, 76948
    Pericardiocentesis, 76930
    Pseudoaneurysm, 76936
    Radioelement, 76965
    Shunt Placement
      Fetal, 59076
    Thoracentesis, 76942
    Uterine Fibroid Ablation, 0404T, 58674
    Vascular Access, 76937
  Head, 76506, 76536
  Heart
    Fetal, 76825
  Hips
    Infant, 76885, 76886
  Hysterosonography, 76831
  Intraoperative, 76998
  Intravascular
    Intraoperative, 37252-37253
  Kidney, 76770-76776
  Leg, 76881-76882
  Neck, 76536
  Needle or Catheter Insertion, 20555
  Pelvis, 76856, 76857

**Ultrasound** — *continued*
  Physical Therapy, 97035
  Pregnant Uterus, 76801-76817
  Prostate, 76872, 76873
  Rectal, 76872, 76873
  Retroperitoneal, 76770, 76775
  Screening Study, Abdomen, 76706
  Scrotum, 76870
  Sonohysterography, 76831
  Stimulation to Aid Bone Healing, 20979
  Umbilical Artery, 76820
  Unlisted Services and Procedures, 76999
  Uterus
    Tumor Ablation, 0071T-0072T
  Vagina, 76830
  Wound Treatment, 97610
**Ultraviolet A Therapy**, 96912
**Ultraviolet B Therapy**, 96910
**Ultraviolet Light Therapy**
  Dermatology, 96900
    Ultraviolet A, 96912
    Ultraviolet B, 96910
  for Physical Medicine, 97028
**Umbilectomy**, 49250
**Umbilical Cord**
  Occlusion, 59072
**Umbilical**
  Artery Ultrasound, 76820
  Hernia
    Repair, 49580-49587
      Omphalocele, 49600-49611
  Vein Catheterization, 36510
**Umbilicus**
  Excision, 49250
  Repair
    Hernia, 49580-49587
    Omphalocele, 49600-49611
**UMOD**, 81406
**Undescended Testicle**
  Exploration, 54550-54560
**Unguis**
  *See* Nails
**Unilateral Simple Mastectomy**, 19303
**Unlisted Services or Procedures**, 99499
  Abdomen, 22999, 49329, 49999
  Allergy
    Immunology, 95199
  Anal, 46999
  Anesthesia, 01999
  Arm, Upper, 24999
  Arthroscopy, 29999
  Autopsy, 88099
  Bile Duct, 47999
  Bladder, 53899
  Brachytherapy, 77799
  Breast, 19499
  Bronchi, 31899
  Cardiac, 33999
  Cardiovascular Studies, 93799
  Casting, 29799
  Cervix, 58999
  Chemistry Procedure, 84999
  Chemotherapy, 96549
  Chest, 32999
  Coagulation, 85999
  Colon, *[45399]*
  Conjunctiva Surgery, 68399
  Craniofacial, 21299
  CT Scan, 76497
  Cytogenetic Study, 88299
  Cytopathology, 88199
  Dermatology, 96999
  Dialysis, 90999
  Diaphragm, 39599
  Ear
    External, 69399
    Inner, 69949
    Middle, 69799
  Endocrine System, 60699
  Epididymis, 55899
  Esophagus, 43289, 43499
  Evaluation and Management Services, 99499
  Eye Muscle, 67399
  Eye Surgery
    Anterior Segment, 66999
    Posterior Segment, 67299

**Unlisted Services or Procedures** — *continued*
  Eyelid, 67999
  Fluoroscopy, 76496
  Forearm, 25999
  Gallbladder Surgery, 47999
  Gastroenterology Test, 91299
  Gum Surgery, 41899
  Hand, 26989
  Hemic System, 38999
  Hepatic Duct, 47999
  Hip Joint, 27299
  Hysteroscopy, 58579
  Immunization, 90749
  Immunology, 86849
  In Vivo, 88749
  Infusion, 96379
  Injection of Medication, 96379
  Injection, 96379
  Intestine, 44799
  Kidney, 53899
  Lacrimal System, 68899
  Laparoscopy, 38129, 38589, 43289, 43659, 44979, 47379, 47579, 49329, 49659, 50549, 50949, 54699, 55559, 58578, 58679, 59898, 60659
  Larynx, 31599
  Lip, 40799
  Liver, 47379, 47399
  Lungs, 32999
  Lymphatic System, 38999
  Magnetic Resonance, 76498
  Maxillofacial Prosthetics, 21089
  Maxillofacial, 21299
  Meckel's Diverticulum, 44899
  Mediastinum, 39499
  Mesentery Surgery, 44899
  Microbiology, 87999
  Molecular Pathology, 81479
  Mouth, 40899, 41599
  Musculoskeletal Surgery
    Abdominal Wall, 22999
    Neck, 21899
    Spine, 22899
    Thorax, 21899
  Musculoskeletal System, 20999
    Ankle, 27899
    Arm, Upper, 24999
    Elbow, 24999
    Head, 21499
    Knee, 27599
    Leg, Lower, 27899
    Leg, Upper, 27599
  Musculoskeletal, 25999, 26989
  Necropsy, 88099
  Nervous System Surgery, 64999
  Neurology
    Neuromuscular Testing, 95999
  Noninvasive Vascular Diagnostic Study, 93998
  Nose, 30999
  Nuclear Medicine, 78999
    Blood, 78199
    Bone, 78399
    Endocrine Procedure, 78099
    Genitourinary System, 78799
    Heart, 78499
    Hematopoietic System, 78199
    Lymphatic System, 78199
    Musculoskeletal System, 78399
    Nervous System, 78699
    Therapeutic, 79999
  Obstetric Care, 59898, 59899
  Omentum, 49329, 49999
  Ophthalmology, 92499
  Orbit, 67599
  Otorhinolaryngology, 92700
  Ovary, 58679, 58999
  Oviduct, 58679, 58999
  Palate, 42299
  Pancreas Surgery, 48999
  Pathology, 89240
  Pelvis, 27299
  Penis, 55899
  Peritoneum, 49329, 49999
  Pharynx, 42999
  Physical Therapy, 97039, 97139, 97799
  Pleura, 32999

**Unlisted Services or Procedures** — *continued*
  Pressure Ulcer, 15999
  Preventive Medicine, 99429
  Prostate, 55899
  Psychiatric, 90899
  Pulmonology, 94799
  Radiation Physics, 77399
  Radiation Therapy, 77499
    Planning, 77299
  Radiology, Diagnostic, 76499
  Radionuclide Therapy, 79999
  Radiopharmaceutical Therapy, 79999
  Rectum, 45999
  Reproductive Medicine Lab, 89398
  Salivary Gland, 42699
  Scrotum, 55899
  Seminal Vesicle, 54699, 55899
  Shoulder, 23929
  Sinuses, 31299
  Skin, 17999
  Small Intestine, 44799
  Special Services and Reports, 99199
  Spine, 22899
  Stomach, 43659, 43999
  Strapping, 29799
  Surgical Pathology, 88399
  Temporal Bone, 69979
  Testis, 54699, 55899
  Throat, 42999
  Toe, 28899
  Tongue, 41599
  Tonsil
    Adenoid, 42999
  Toxoid, 90749
  Trachea, 31899
  Transfusion, 86999
  Ultrasound, 76999
  Ureter, 50949
  Urinary System, 53899
  Uterus, 58578, 58579, 58999
  Uvula, 42299
  Vaccine, 90749
  Vagina, 58999
  Vas Deferens, 55899
  Vascular Endoscopy, 37501
  Vascular Injection, 36299
  Vascular Studies, 93799
  Vascular, 37799
  Wrist, 25999
**Unna Paste Boot**, 29580
  Removal, 29700
**UPD [uniparental disomy]**, 81402
**UPP (Urethral Pressure Profile)**, 51727, 51729
**Upper**
  Digestive System Endoscopy
    *See* Endoscopy, Gastrointestinal, Upper
  Extremity
    *See* Arm, Upper; Elbow; Humerus
  Gastrointestinal Bleeding
    Endoscopic Control, 43255
  Gastrointestinal Endoscopy, Biopsy, 43239
  GI Tract
    *See* Gastrointestinal Tract, Upper
**UPPP (Uvulopalatopharyngoplasty)**, 42145
**Urachal Cyst**
  Bladder
    Excision, 51500
**Urea Breath Test**, 78267, 78268, 83014
**Urea Nitrogen**, 84525
  Blood, 84520, 84525
  Clearance, 84545
  Quantitative, 84520
  Semiquantitative, 84525
  Urine, 84540
**Urecholine Supersensitivity Test**
  Cystometrogram, 51725, 51726
**Ureter**
  Anastomosis
    to Bladder, 50780-50785
    to Colon, 50810, 50815
    to Intestine, 50800, 50820, 50825
    to Kidney, 50740, 50750
    to Ureter, 50760, 50770
  Biopsy, 50606, 50955-50957, 50974-50976, 52007
  Catheterization, 52005

**Urethral** — *continued*
  Stenosis
    Dilation, 52281
    Stent
      Insertion, 52282, 53855
      Removal
        Bladder, 52310, 52315
        Urethra, 52310, 52315
  Stricture
    Dilation, 52281, 53600-53621
    Injection
      Steroids, 52283
  Syndrome
    Cystourethroscopy, 52285
**Urethrectomy**
  Total
    Female, 53210
    Male, 53215
**Urethrocele**
  Repair, 57230-57240
**Urethrocystography**, 74450, 74455
  Contrast and/or Chain, 51605
  Retrograde, 51610
  Voiding, 51600
**Urethrocystopexy**, 51840-51841
**Urethromeatoplasty**, 53450, 53460
**Urethropexy**, 51840, 51841
**Urethroplasty**, 46744, 46746
  First Stage, 53400
    Hypospadias, 54322-54328
  Reconstruction
    Female Urethra, 53430
    Male Anterior Urethra, 53410
    Prostatic
      Membranous Urethra
        First Stage, 53420
        One Stage, 53415
        Second Stage, 53425
  Second Stage, 53405
    Hypospadias, 54308-54316
  Third Stage
    Hypospadias, 54318
**Urethrorrhaphy**, 53502-53515
**Urethroscopy**, 52000-52315, 52320-52402
  Perineal, 53899
**Urethrostomy**, 53000, 53010
**Urethrotomy**, 53000, 53010
  with Cystourethroscopy
    Female, 52270
    Male, 52275
  Direct Vision
    with Cystourethroscopy, 52276
  Internal, 52601, 52647, 52648
**Uric Acid**
  Blood, 84550
  Other Source, 84560
  Urine, 84560
**Uridyltransferase, Galactose–1–Phosphate,**
  82775-82776
**Uridylyltransferase, Galactosephophate**, 82775-
  82776
**Urinalysis**, 81000-81099
  without Microscopy, 81002
  Automated, 81001, 81003
  Glass Test, 81020
  Microalbumin, 82043, 82044
  Microscopic, 81015
  Pregnancy Test, 81025
  Qualitative, 81005
  Routine, 81002
  Screen, 81007
  Semiquantitative, 81005
  Unlisted Services and Procedures, 81099
  Volume Measurement, 81050
**Urinary Bladder**
  *See* Bladder
**Urinary Catheter Irrigation**, 51700
**Urinary Sphincter, Artificial**
  Insertion, 53445
  Removal, 53446
    with Replacement, 53447-53448
  Repair, 53449
**Urinary Tract**
  X–ray with Contrast, 74400-74425
**Urine Sensitivity Test**, 87181-87190

**Urine**
  Albumin, 82043-82044
  Blood, 81000-81005
  Colony Count, 87086
  Pregnancy Test, 81025
  Tests, 81000-81099
**Urobilinogen**
  Feces, 84577
  Urine, 84578-84583
**Urodynamic Tests**
  Bladder Capacity
    Ultrasound, 51798
  Cystometrogram, 51725-51729
  Electromyography Studies
    Needle, 51785
    Rectal, *[51797]*
  Residual Urine
    Ultrasound, 51798
  Stimulus Evoked Response, 51792
  Urethra Pressure Profile, *[51797]*
  Uroflowmetry, 51736, 51741
  Voiding Pressure Studies
    Bladder, 51728-51729
    Intra–Abdominal, *[51797]*
**Uroflowmetry**, 51736, 51741
**Urography**
  Antegrade, 74425
  Infusion, 74410, 74415
  Intravenous, 74400-74415
  Retrograde, 74420
**Uroporphyrin**, 84120
**Urostomy**, 50727, 50728
**Urothromboplastin**
  Inhibition Test, 85347
  Inhibition, 85705
  Partial Time, 85730-85732
**USH1C**, 81407, 81430
**USH1G**, 81404, 81430
**USH2A**, 81408, 81430, 81434
**Uterine**
  Adhesion
    Lysis, 58559
  Cervix
    *See* Cervix
  Endoscopies
    *See* Endoscopy, Uterus
  Hemorrhage
    Postpartum, 59160
**Uterus**
  Ablation
    Endometrium, 58353-58356
    Tumor
      Radiofrequency, 58674
      Ultrasound Focused, 0071T-0072T
    Uterine Fibroid
      Transcervical, 0404T
  Biopsy
    Endometrium, 58100
    Endoscopy, 58558
  Catheterization
    X–ray, 58340
  Chromotubation, 58350
  Curettage, 58356
    Postpartum, 59160
  Dilation and Curettage, 58120
    Postpartum, 59160
  Ectopic Pregnancy
    Interstitial
      Partial Resection Uterus, 59136
      Total Hysterectomy, 59135
  Endoscopy
    Endometrial Ablation, 58563
    Exploration, 58555
    Surgery, 58558-58565
    Treatment, 58558-58565
  Excision
    Laparoscopic, 58550
      with Removal of Ovaries, 58552,
        58554
      Total, 58570-58573
    Partial, 58180
    Radical
      Laparoscopic, 58548
      Open, 58210, 58285

**Uterus** — *continued*
  Excision — *continued*
    Removal of Tubes and/or Ovaries, 58262,
      58263, 58291-58293, 58552,
      58554
    Sonohysterography, 76831
    Total, 58150-58152, 58200, 58953-58956
    Vaginal, 58260-58270, 58290-58294,
      58550-58554
      with Colpectomy, 58275, 58280
      with Colpo–Urethrocystopexy,
        58267
      with Repair of Enterocele, 58270,
        58294
  Hemorrhage
    Postpartum, 59160
  Hydatidiform Mole
    Excision, 59100
  Hydrotubation, 58350
  Hysterosalpingography, 74740
  Hysterosonography, 76831
  Incision
    Removal of Lesion, 59100
  Insertion
    Heyman Capsule
      for Brachytherapy, 58346
    Intrauterine Device, 58300
    Tandem
      for Brachytherapy, 57155
  Laparoscopy
    Tumor Ablation, 58674
    Unlisted, 58578
  Lesion
    Excision, 58545, 58546, 59100
  Reconstruction, 58540
  Removal
    Intrauterine Device (IUD), 58301
  Repair
    Fistula, 51920, 51925
    Rupture, 58520, 59350
    Suspension, 58400
      with Presacral Sympathectomy,
        58410
  Sonohysterography, 76831
  Suture
    Rupture, 59350
  Tumor
    Ablation
      Radiofrequency, 58674
      Ultrasound Focused, 0071T-0072T
    Excision
      Abdominal Approach, 58140,
        58146
      Vaginal Approach, 58145
  Unlisted Services and Procedures, 58578,
    58999
  X–ray with Contrast, 74740
**UTP Hexose 1 Phosphate Uridylyltransferase**,
  82775-82776
**UV Light Therapy**, 96900
**UVC**, 36510
**Uvula**
  Abscess
    Incision and Drainage, 42000
  Biopsy, 42100
  Excision, 42140, 42145
  Lesion
    Destruction, 42145
    Excision, 42104-42107
  Unlisted Services and Procedures, 42299
**Uvulectomy**, 42140
**Uvulopalatopharyngoplasty**, 42145
**Uvulopharyngoplasty**, 42145

**V**

**V, Cranial Nerve**
  Destruction, 64600-64610
  Injection
    Neurolytic, 64600-64610
**Vaccines**
  Adenovirus, 90476, 90477
  Anthrax, 90581
  Chicken Pox, 90716
  Cholera Injectable, *[90625]*
  Dengue, 90587

**Vaccines** — *continued*
  Diphtheria, Tetanus, Acellular Pertussis, and
    Poliovirus Inactivated (DTaP-IPV),
    90696
  Diphtheria, Tetanus, Acellular Pertussis,
    Hemophilus Influenza B, and Poliovirus
    Inactivated (DTaPp-IPV/Hib), 90698
  Diphtheria, Tetanus, Acellular Pertussis,
    Hemophilus Influenza B, Hepatitis B,
    and Poliovirus Inactivated
    (DTaP–IPV–Hib–HepB), 90697
  Diphtheria, Tetanus, Acellular Pertussis, Hep-
    atitis B, and Inactivated Poliovirus
    (DTaP–HepB–IPV), 90723
  Diphtheria, Tetanus, Acellular Pertussis (DTaP),
    90700
  Diphtheria, Tetanus, and Acellular Pertussis,
    (Tdap), 90715
  Diphtheria, Tetanus (DT), 90702
  Encephalitis, Japanese, 90738
  Hemophilus Influenza B, 90647-90648
  Hepatitis A and Hepatitis B, 90636
  Hepatitis A, 90632-90634
  Hepatitis B and Hemophilus Influenza B
    (HepB–Hib), 90748
  Hepatitis B, 90739-90747
  Human Papilloma Virus, 90649-90651
  Influenza, 90653-90668 *[90630, 90672, 90673]*,
    90682, 90685-90688, *[90674]*, *[90756]*
  Japanese Encephalitis, 90738
  Measles, Mumps and Rubella (MMR), 90707
  Measles, Mumps, Rubella and Varicella (MM-
    RV), 90710
  MenB-4C, *[90620]*
  MenB-FHbp, *[90621]*
  Meningococcal, 90620, 90621, 90733-90734,
    *[90644]*
  Pneumococcal, 90670, 90732
  Poliovirus, Inactivated
    Intramuscular, 90713
    Subcutaneous, 90713
  Rabies, 90675, 90676
  Rotavirus, 90680-90681
  Shingles, 90736, *[90750]*
  Tetanus and Diphtheria, 90702, 90714
  Tetanus, Diphtheria and Acellular Pertussis
    (Tdap), 90715
  Tuberculosis (BCG), 90585
  Typhoid, 90690-90691
  Unlisted Vaccine
    Toxoid, 90749
  Varicella (Chicken Pox), 90716
  Yellow Fever, 90717
  Zoster, 90736, *[90750]*
**Vagina**
  Abscess
    Incision and Drainage, 57010
  Amines Test, 82120
  Biopsy
    Colposcopy, 57421
    Endocervical, 57454
    Extensive, 57105
    Simple, 57100
  Closure, 57120
  Colposcopy, 57420-57421, 57455-57456,
    57461
  Construction
    with Graft, 57292
    without Graft, 57291
  Cyst
    Excision, 57135
  Dilation, 57400
  Endocervical
    Biopsy, 57454
    Exploration, 57452
  Excision
    Closure, 57120
    Complete
      with Removal of Paravaginal Tissue
        with Lymphadenectomy,
        57112
      with Removal of Paravaginal Tis-
        sue, 57111
      with Removal of Vaginal Wall,
        57110

CPT © 2017 American Medical Association. All Rights Reserved.     © 2017 Optum360, LLC

## 00100-00126 Anesthesia for Cleft Lip, Ear, ECT, Eyelid, and Salivary Gland Procedures

**CMS:** 100-04,12,140.1 Qualified Nonphysician Anesthetists; 100-04,12,140.3 Payment for Qualified Nonphysician Anesthetists; 100-04,12,140.3.3 Billing Modifiers; 100-04,12,140.3.4 General Billing Instructions; 100-04,12,140.4.1 Anesthesiologist/Qualified Nonphysican Anesthetist; 100-04,12,140.4.2 Anesthetist and Anesthesiologist in a Single Procedure; 100-04,12,140.4.3 Payment for Medical /Surgical Services by CRNAs; 100-04,12,140.4.4 Conversion Factors for Anesthesia Services; 100-04,4,250.3.2 Anesthesia in a Hospital Outpatient Setting

**00100** **Anesthesia for procedures on salivary glands, including biopsy**
🚑 0.00   ⚖ 0.00   **FUD** XXX   N 🖵
**AMA:** 2017,Jan,8; 2016,Jan,13; 2015,Jan,16; 2014,Aug,5; 2014,Jan,11; 2012,Jul,12-14; 2012,Jan,15-42

**00102** **Anesthesia for procedures involving plastic repair of cleft lip**
🚑 0.00   ⚖ 0.00   **FUD** XXX   N 🖵
**AMA:** 2017,Jan,8; 2016,Jan,13; 2015,Jan,16; 2014,Aug,5; 2014,Jan,11; 2012,Jul,12-14; 2012,Jan,15-42

**00103** **Anesthesia for reconstructive procedures of eyelid (eg, blepharoplasty, ptosis surgery)**
🚑 0.00   ⚖ 0.00   **FUD** XXX   N 🖵
**AMA:** 2017,Jan,8; 2016,Jan,13; 2015,Jan,16; 2014,Aug,5; 2014,Jan,11; 2012,Jul,12-14; 2012,Jan,15-42

**00104** **Anesthesia for electroconvulsive therapy**
🚑 0.00   ⚖ 0.00   **FUD** XXX   N 🖵
**AMA:** 2017,Jan,8; 2016,Jan,13; 2015,Jan,16; 2014,Aug,5; 2014,Jan,11; 2012,Jul,12-14; 2012,Jan,15-42

**00120** **Anesthesia for procedures on external, middle, and inner ear including biopsy; not otherwise specified**
🚑 0.00   ⚖ 0.00   **FUD** XXX   N 🖵
**AMA:** 2017,Jan,8; 2016,Jan,13; 2015,Jan,16; 2014,Aug,5; 2014,Jan,11; 2012,Jul,12-14; 2012,Jan,15-42

**00124** **otoscopy**
🚑 0.00   ⚖ 0.00   **FUD** XXX   N 🖵
**AMA:** 2017,Jan,8; 2016,Jan,13; 2015,Jan,16; 2014,Aug,5; 2014,Jan,11; 2012,Jul,12-14; 2012,Jan,15-42

**00126** **tympanotomy**
🚑 0.00   ⚖ 0.00   **FUD** XXX   N 🖵
**AMA:** 2017,Jan,8; 2016,Jan,13; 2015,Jan,16; 2014,Aug,5; 2014,Jan,11; 2012,Jul,12-14; 2012,Jan,15-42

## 00140-00148 Anesthesia for Eye Procedures

**CMS:** 100-04,12,140.1 Qualified Nonphysician Anesthetists; 100-04,12,140.3 Payment for Qualified Nonphysician Anesthetists; 100-04,12,140.3.3 Billing Modifiers; 100-04,12,140.3.4 General Billing Instructions; 100-04,12,140.4.1 Anesthesiologist/Qualified Nonphysican Anesthetist; 100-04,12,140.4.2 Anesthetist and Anesthesiologist in a Single Procedure; 100-04,12,140.4.3 Payment for Medical /Surgical Services by CRNAs; 100-04,12,140.4.4 Conversion Factors for Anesthesia Services; 100-04,4,250.3.2 Anesthesia in a Hospital Outpatient Setting

**00140** **Anesthesia for procedures on eye; not otherwise specified**
🚑 0.00   ⚖ 0.00   **FUD** XXX   N 🖵
**AMA:** 2017,Jan,8; 2016,Jan,13; 2015,Jan,16; 2014,Aug,5; 2014,Jan,11; 2012,Jul,12-14; 2012,Jan,15-42

**00142** **lens surgery**
🚑 0.00   ⚖ 0.00   **FUD** XXX   N 🖵
**AMA:** 2017,Jan,8; 2016,Jan,13; 2015,Jan,16; 2014,Aug,5; 2014,Jan,11; 2012,Jul,12-14; 2012,Jan,15-42

**00144** **corneal transplant**
🚑 0.00   ⚖ 0.00   **FUD** XXX   N 🖵
**AMA:** 2017,Jan,8; 2016,Jan,13; 2015,Jan,16; 2014,Aug,5; 2014,Jan,11; 2012,Jul,12-14; 2012,Jan,15-42

**00145** **vitreoretinal surgery**
🚑 0.00   ⚖ 0.00   **FUD** XXX   N 🖵
**AMA:** 2017,Jan,8; 2016,Jan,13; 2015,Jan,16; 2014,Aug,5; 2014,Jan,11; 2012,Jul,12-14; 2012,Jan,15-42

**00147** **iridectomy**
🚑 0.00   ⚖ 0.00   **FUD** XXX   N 🖵
**AMA:** 2017,Jan,8; 2016,Jan,13; 2015,Jan,16; 2014,Aug,5; 2014,Jan,11; 2012,Jul,12-14; 2012,Jan,15-42

**00148** **ophthalmoscopy**
🚑 0.00   ⚖ 0.00   **FUD** XXX   N 🖵
**AMA:** 2017,Jan,8; 2016,Jan,13; 2015,Jan,16; 2014,Aug,5; 2014,Jan,11; 2012,Jul,12-14; 2012,Jan,15-42

## 00160-00326 Anesthesia for Face and Head Procedures

**CMS:** 100-04,12,140.1 Qualified Nonphysician Anesthetists; 100-04,12,140.3 Payment for Qualified Nonphysician Anesthetists; 100-04,12,140.3.3 Billing Modifiers; 100-04,12,140.3.4 General Billing Instructions; 100-04,12,140.4.1 Anesthesiologist/Qualified Nonphysican Anesthetist; 100-04,12,140.4.2 Anesthetist and Anesthesiologist in a Single Procedure; 100-04,12,140.4.4 Conversion Factors for Anesthesia Services; 100-04,4,250.3.2 Anesthesia in a Hospital Outpatient Setting

**00160** **Anesthesia for procedures on nose and accessory sinuses; not otherwise specified**
🚑 0.00   ⚖ 0.00   **FUD** XXX   N 🖵
**AMA:** 2017,Jan,8; 2016,Jan,13; 2015,Jan,16; 2014,Aug,5; 2014,Jan,11; 2012,Jul,12-14; 2012,Jan,15-42

**00162** **radical surgery**
🚑 0.00   ⚖ 0.00   **FUD** XXX   N 🖵
**AMA:** 2017,Jan,8; 2016,Jan,13; 2015,Jan,16; 2014,Aug,5; 2014,Jan,11; 2012,Jul,12-14; 2012,Jan,15-42

**00164** **biopsy, soft tissue**
🚑 0.00   ⚖ 0.00   **FUD** XXX   N 🖵
**AMA:** 2017,Jan,8; 2016,Jan,13; 2015,Jan,16; 2014,Aug,5; 2014,Jan,11; 2012,Jul,12-14; 2012,Jan,15-42

**00170** **Anesthesia for intraoral procedures, including biopsy; not otherwise specified**
🚑 0.00   ⚖ 0.00   **FUD** XXX   N 🖵
**AMA:** 2017,Jan,8; 2016,Jan,13; 2015,Jan,16; 2014,Aug,5; 2014,Jan,11; 2012,Jul,12-14; 2012,Jan,15-42

**00172** **repair of cleft palate**
🚑 0.00   ⚖ 0.00   **FUD** XXX   N 🖵
**AMA:** 2017,Jan,8; 2016,Jan,13; 2015,Jan,16; 2014,Aug,5; 2014,Jan,11; 2012,Jul,12-14; 2012,Jan,15-42

**00174** **excision of retropharyngeal tumor**
🚑 0.00   ⚖ 0.00   **FUD** XXX   N 🖵
**AMA:** 2017,Jan,8; 2016,Jan,13; 2015,Jan,16; 2014,Aug,5; 2014,Jan,11; 2012,Jul,12-14; 2012,Jan,15-42

**00176** **radical surgery**
🚑 0.00   ⚖ 0.00   **FUD** XXX   C 🖵
**AMA:** 2017,Jan,8; 2016,Jan,13; 2015,Jan,16; 2014,Aug,5; 2014,Jan,11; 2012,Jul,12-14; 2012,Jan,15-42

**00190** **Anesthesia for procedures on facial bones or skull; not otherwise specified**
🚑 0.00   ⚖ 0.00   **FUD** XXX   N 🖵
**AMA:** 2017,Jan,8; 2016,Jan,13; 2015,Jan,16; 2014,Aug,5; 2014,Jan,11; 2012,Jul,12-14; 2012,Jan,15-42

**00192** **radical surgery (including prognathism)**
🚑 0.00   ⚖ 0.00   **FUD** XXX   C 🖵
**AMA:** 2017,Jan,8; 2016,Jan,13; 2015,Jan,16; 2014,Aug,5; 2014,Jan,11; 2012,Jul,12-14; 2012,Jan,15-42

**00210** **Anesthesia for intracranial procedures; not otherwise specified**
🚑 0.00   ⚖ 0.00   **FUD** XXX   N 🖵
**AMA:** 2017,Jan,8; 2016,Jan,13; 2015,Jan,16; 2014,Aug,5; 2014,Jan,11; 2012,Jul,12-14; 2012,Jan,15-42

**00211** **craniotomy or craniectomy for evacuation of hematoma**
🚑 0.00   ⚖ 0.00   **FUD** XXX   C 🖵
**AMA:** 2017,Jan,8; 2016,Jan,13; 2015,Jan,16; 2014,Aug,5; 2014,Jan,11; 2012,Jul,12-14; 2012,Jan,15-42

**00212** **subdural taps**
🚑 0.00   ⚖ 0.00   **FUD** XXX   N 🖵
**AMA:** 2017,Jan,8; 2016,Jan,13; 2015,Jan,16; 2014,Aug,5; 2014,Jan,11; 2012,Jul,12-14; 2012,Jan,15-42

**00214** **burr holes, including ventriculography**
🚑 0.00   ⚖ 0.00   **FUD** XXX   C 🖵
**AMA:** 2017,Jan,8; 2016,Jan,13; 2015,Jan,16; 2014,Aug,5; 2014,Jan,11; 2012,Jul,12-14; 2012,Jan,15-42

---

● New Code　▲ Revised Code　○ Reinstated　● New Web Release　▲ Revised Web Release　Unlisted　Not Covered　# Resequenced
⊘ AMA Mod 51 Exempt　⑨ Optum Mod 51 Exempt　⑨ Mod 63 Exempt　✐ Non-FDA Drug　★ Telemedicine　Ⓜ Maternity　Ⓐ Age Edit　✚ Add-on　**AMA:** CPT Asst

© 2017 Optum360, LLC　　CPT © 2017 American Medical Association. All Rights Reserved.　　**1**

| 00215 | **cranioplasty or elevation of depressed skull fracture, extradural (simple or compound)** |
|---|---|

🖪 0.00   ⚕ 0.00   **FUD** XXX

**AMA:** 2017,Jan,8; 2016,Jan,13; 2015,Jan,16; 2014,Aug,5; 2014,Jan,11; 2012,Jul,12-14; 2012,Jan,15-42

00216   **vascular procedures**

🖪 0.00   ⚕ 0.00   **FUD** XXX

**AMA:** 2017,Jan,8; 2016,Jan,13; 2015,Jan,16; 2014,Aug,5; 2014,Jan,11; 2012,Jul,12-14; 2012,Jan,15-42

00218   **procedures in sitting position**

🖪 0.00   ⚕ 0.00   **FUD** XXX

**AMA:** 2017,Jan,8; 2016,Jan,13; 2015,Jan,16; 2014,Aug,5; 2014,Jan,11; 2012,Jul,12-14; 2012,Jan,15-42

00220   **cerebrospinal fluid shunting procedures**

🖪 0.00   ⚕ 0.00   **FUD** XXX

**AMA:** 2017,Jan,8; 2016,Jan,13; 2015,Jan,16; 2014,Aug,5; 2014,Jan,11; 2012,Jul,12-14; 2012,Jan,15-42

00222   **electrocoagulation of intracranial nerve**

🖪 0.00   ⚕ 0.00   **FUD** XXX

**AMA:** 2017,Jan,8; 2016,Jan,13; 2015,Jan,16; 2014,Aug,5; 2014,Jan,11; 2012,Jul,12-14; 2012,Jan,15-42

00300   **Anesthesia for all procedures on the integumentary system, muscles and nerves of head, neck, and posterior trunk, not otherwise specified**

🖪 0.00   ⚕ 0.00   **FUD** XXX

**AMA:** 2017,Jan,8; 2016,Jan,13; 2015,Jan,16; 2014,Aug,5; 2014,Jan,11; 2012,Jul,12-14; 2012,Jan,15-42

00320   **Anesthesia for all procedures on esophagus, thyroid, larynx, trachea and lymphatic system of neck; not otherwise specified, age 1 year or older**

🖪 0.00   ⚕ 0.00   **FUD** XXX

**AMA:** 2017,Jan,8; 2016,Jan,13; 2015,Jan,16; 2014,Aug,5; 2014,Jan,11; 2012,Jul,12-14; 2012,Jan,15-42

00322   **needle biopsy of thyroid**

EXCLUDES   *Cervical spine and spinal cord procedures (00600, 00604, 00670)*

🖪 0.00   ⚕ 0.00   **FUD** XXX

**AMA:** 2017,Jan,8; 2016,Jan,13; 2015,Jan,16; 2014,Aug,5; 2014,Jan,11; 2012,Jul,12-14; 2012,Jan,15-42

00326   **Anesthesia for all procedures on the larynx and trachea in children younger than 1 year of age**   A

INCLUDES   Anesthesia for patient of extreme age, younger than 1 year and older than 70 (99100)

🖪 0.00   ⚕ 0.00   **FUD** XXX

**AMA:** 2017,Jan,8; 2016,Jan,13; 2015,Jan,16; 2014,Aug,5; 2014,Jan,11; 2012,Jul,12-14; 2012,Jan,15-42

## 00350-00352 Anesthesia for Neck Vessel Procedures

**CMS:** 100-04,12,140.1 Qualified Nonphysician Anesthetists; 100-04,12,140.3 Payment for Qualified Nonphysician Anesthetists; 100-04,12,140.3.3 Billing Modifiers; 100-04,12,140.3.4 General Billing Instructions; 100-04,12,140.4.1 Anesthesiologist/Qualified Nonphysican Anesthetist; 100-04,12,140.4.2 Anesthetist and Anesthesiologist in a Single Procedure; 100-04,12,140.4.3 Payment for Medical /Surgical Services by CRNAs; 100-04,12,140.4.4 Conversion Factors for Anesthesia Services; 100-04,4,250.3.2 Anesthesia in a Hospital Outpatient Setting

EXCLUDES   *Arteriography (01916)*

00350   **Anesthesia for procedures on major vessels of neck; not otherwise specified**

🖪 0.00   ⚕ 0.00   **FUD** XXX

**AMA:** 2017,Jan,8; 2016,Jan,13; 2015,Jan,16; 2014,Aug,5; 2014,Jan,11; 2012,Jul,12-14; 2012,Jan,15-42

00352   **simple ligation**

🖪 0.00   ⚕ 0.00   **FUD** XXX

**AMA:** 2017,Jan,8; 2016,Jan,13; 2015,Jan,16; 2014,Aug,5; 2014,Jan,11; 2012,Jul,12-14; 2012,Jan,15-42

## 00400-00529 Anesthesia for Chest/Pectoral Girdle Procedures

**CMS:** 100-04,12,140.1 Qualified Nonphysician Anesthetists; 100-04,12,140.3 Payment for Qualified Nonphysician Anesthetists; 100-04,12,140.3.3 Billing Modifiers; 100-04,12,140.3.4 General Billing Instructions; 100-04,12,140.4.1 Anesthesiologist/Qualified Nonphysican Anesthetist; 100-04,12,140.4.2 Anesthetist and Anesthesiologist in a Single Procedure; 100-04,12,140.4.3 Payment for Medical /Surgical Services by CRNAs; 100-04,12,140.4.4 Conversion Factors for Anesthesia Services; 100-04,4,250.3.2 Anesthesia in a Hospital Outpatient Setting

00400   **Anesthesia for procedures on the integumentary system on the extremities, anterior trunk and perineum; not otherwise specified**

🖪 0.00   ⚕ 0.00   **FUD** XXX

**AMA:** 2017,Jan,8; 2016,Jan,13; 2015,Jan,16; 2014,Aug,5; 2014,Jan,11; 2012,Jul,12-14; 2012,Jan,15-42

00402   **reconstructive procedures on breast (eg, reduction or augmentation mammoplasty, muscle flaps)**

🖪 0.00   ⚕ 0.00   **FUD** XXX

**AMA:** 2017,Jan,8; 2016,Jan,13; 2015,Jan,16; 2014,Aug,5; 2014,Jan,11; 2012,Jul,12-14; 2012,Jan,15-42

00404   **radical or modified radical procedures on breast**

🖪 0.00   ⚕ 0.00   **FUD** XXX

**AMA:** 2017,Jan,8; 2016,Jan,13; 2015,Jan,16; 2014,Aug,5; 2014,Jan,11; 2012,Jul,12-14; 2012,Jan,15-42

00406   **radical or modified radical procedures on breast with internal mammary node dissection**

🖪 0.00   ⚕ 0.00   **FUD** XXX

**AMA:** 2017,Jan,8; 2016,Jan,13; 2015,Jan,16; 2014,Aug,5; 2014,Jan,11; 2012,Jul,12-14; 2012,Jan,15-42

00410   **electrical conversion of arrhythmias**

🖪 0.00   ⚕ 0.00   **FUD** XXX

**AMA:** 2017,Jan,8; 2016,Jan,13; 2015,Jan,16; 2014,Aug,5; 2014,Jan,11; 2012,Jul,12-14; 2012,Jan,15-42

00450   **Anesthesia for procedures on clavicle and scapula; not otherwise specified**

🖪 0.00   ⚕ 0.00   **FUD** XXX

**AMA:** 2017,Jan,8; 2016,Jan,13; 2015,Jan,16; 2014,Aug,5; 2014,Jan,11; 2012,Jul,12-14; 2012,Jan,15-42

00454   **biopsy of clavicle**

🖪 0.00   ⚕ 0.00   **FUD** XXX

**AMA:** 2017,Jan,8; 2016,Jan,13; 2015,Jan,16; 2014,Aug,5; 2014,Jan,11; 2012,Jul,12-14; 2012,Jan,15-42

00470   **Anesthesia for partial rib resection; not otherwise specified**

🖪 0.00   ⚕ 0.00   **FUD** XXX

**AMA:** 2017,Jan,8; 2016,Jan,13; 2015,Jan,16; 2014,Aug,5; 2014,Jan,11; 2012,Jul,12-14; 2012,Jan,15-42

00472   **thoracoplasty (any type)**

🖪 0.00   ⚕ 0.00   **FUD** XXX

**AMA:** 2017,Jan,8; 2016,Jan,13; 2015,Jan,16; 2014,Aug,5; 2014,Jan,11; 2012,Jul,12-14; 2012,Jan,15-42

00474   **radical procedures (eg, pectus excavatum)**

🖪 0.00   ⚕ 0.00   **FUD** XXX

**AMA:** 2017,Jan,8; 2016,Jan,13; 2015,Jan,16; 2014,Aug,5; 2014,Jan,11; 2012,Jul,12-14; 2012,Jan,15-42

00500   **Anesthesia for all procedures on esophagus**

🖪 0.00   ⚕ 0.00   **FUD** XXX

**AMA:** 2017,Jan,8; 2016,Jan,13; 2015,Jan,16; 2014,Aug,5; 2014,Jan,11; 2012,Jul,12-14; 2012,Jan,15-42

00520   **Anesthesia for closed chest procedures; (including bronchoscopy) not otherwise specified**

🖪 0.00   ⚕ 0.00   **FUD** XXX

**AMA:** 2017,Jan,8; 2016,Jan,13; 2015,Jan,16; 2014,Aug,5; 2014,Jan,11; 2012,Jul,12-14; 2012,Jan,15-42

00522   **needle biopsy of pleura**

🖪 0.00   ⚕ 0.00   **FUD** XXX

**AMA:** 2017,Jan,8; 2016,Jan,13; 2015,Jan,16; 2014,Aug,5; 2014,Jan,11; 2012,Jul,12-14; 2012,Jan,15-42

2G/TC PC/TC Only   A2-Z3 ASC Payment   50 Bilateral   ♂ Male Only   ♀ Female Only   🖪 Facility RVU   ⚕ Non-Facility RVU   ▢ CCI
**FUD** Follow-up Days   **CMS:** IOM (Pub 100)   A-Y OPPSI   80/80 Surg Assist Allowed / w/Doc   Lab Crosswalk   Radiology Crosswalk   ✖ CLIA

2

CPT © 2017 American Medical Association. All Rights Reserved.   © 2017 Optum360, LLC

**00524**    **pneumocentesis**
🔧 0.00    ✂ 0.00    **FUD** XXX     C 🖥
**AMA:** 2017,Jan,8; 2016,Jan,13; 2015,Jan,16; 2014,Aug,5; 2014,Jan,11; 2012,Jul,12-14; 2012,Jan,15-42

**00528**    **mediastinoscopy and diagnostic thoracoscopy not utilizing 1 lung ventilation**
EXCLUDES   *Tracheobronchial reconstruction (00539)*
🔧 0.00    ✂ 0.00    **FUD** XXX     N 🖥
**AMA:** 2017,Jan,8; 2016,Jan,13; 2015,Jan,16; 2014,Aug,5; 2014,Jan,11; 2012,Jul,12-14; 2012,Jan,15-42

**00529**    **mediastinoscopy and diagnostic thoracoscopy utilizing 1 lung ventilation**
🔧 0.00    ✂ 0.00    **FUD** XXX     N 🖥
**AMA:** 2017,Jan,8; 2016,Jan,13; 2015,Jan,16; 2014,Aug,5; 2014,Jan,11; 2012,Jul,12-14; 2012,Jan,15-42

## 00530 Anesthesia for Cardiac Pacemaker Procedure

**CMS:** 100-03,10.6 Anesthesia in Cardiac Pacemaker Surgery; 100-04,12,140.1 Qualified Nonphysician Anesthetists; 100-04,12,140.3 Payment for Qualified Nonphysician Anesthetists; 100-04,12,140.3.3 Billing Modifiers; 100-04,12,140.3.4 General Billing Instructions; 100-04,12,140.4.1 Anesthesiologist/Qualified Nonphysican Anesthetist; 100-04,12,140.4.2 Anesthetist and Anesthesiologist in a Single Procedure; 100-04,12,140.4.3 Payment for Medical /Surgical Services by CRNAs; 100-04,12,140.4.4 Conversion Factors for Anesthesia Services; 100-04,4,250.3.2 Anesthesia in a Hospital Outpatient Setting

**00530**    **Anesthesia for permanent transvenous pacemaker insertion**
🔧 0.00    ✂ 0.00    **FUD** XXX     N 🖥
**AMA:** 2017,Jan,8; 2016,Jan,13; 2015,Jan,16; 2014,Aug,5; 2014,Jan,11; 2012,Jul,12-14; 2012,Jan,15-42

## 00532-00550 Anesthesia for Heart and Lung Procedures

**CMS:** 100-04,12,140.1 Qualified Nonphysician Anesthetists; 100-04,12,140.3 Payment for Qualified Nonphysician Anesthetists; 100-04,12,140.3.3 Billing Modifiers; 100-04,12,140.3.4 General Billing Instructions; 100-04,12,140.4.1 Anesthesiologist/Qualified Nonphysican Anesthetist; 100-04,12,140.4.2 Anesthetist and Anesthesiologist in a Single Procedure; 100-04,12,140.4.3 Payment for Medical /Surgical Services by CRNAs; 100-04,12,140.4.4 Conversion Factors for Anesthesia Services; 100-04,4,250.3.2 Anesthesia in a Hospital Outpatient Setting

**00532**    **Anesthesia for access to central venous circulation**
🔧 0.00    ✂ 0.00    **FUD** XXX     N 🖥
**AMA:** 2017,Jan,8; 2016,Jan,13; 2015,Jan,16; 2014,Aug,5; 2014,Jan,11; 2012,Jul,12-14; 2012,Jan,15-42

**00534**    **Anesthesia for transvenous insertion or replacement of pacing cardioverter-defibrillator**
EXCLUDES   *Transthoracic approach (00560)*
🔧 0.00    ✂ 0.00    **FUD** XXX     N 🖥
**AMA:** 2017,Jan,8; 2016,Jan,13; 2015,Jan,16; 2014,Aug,5; 2014,Jan,11; 2012,Jul,12-14; 2012,Jan,15-42

**00537**    **Anesthesia for cardiac electrophysiologic procedures including radiofrequency ablation**
🔧 0.00    ✂ 0.00    **FUD** XXX     N 🖥
**AMA:** 2017,Jan,8; 2016,Jan,13; 2015,Jan,16; 2014,Aug,5; 2014,Jan,11; 2012,Jul,12-14; 2012,Jan,15-42

**00539**    **Anesthesia for tracheobronchial reconstruction**
🔧 0.00    ✂ 0.00    **FUD** XXX     N 🖥
**AMA:** 2017,Jan,8; 2016,Jan,13; 2015,Jan,16; 2014,Aug,5; 2014,Jan,11; 2012,Jul,12-14; 2012,Jan,15-42

**00540**    **Anesthesia for thoracotomy procedures involving lungs, pleura, diaphragm, and mediastinum (including surgical thoracoscopy); not otherwise specified**
EXCLUDES   *Thoracic spine and spinal cord procedures via anterior transthoracic approach (00625-00626)*
🔧 0.00    ✂ 0.00    **FUD** XXX     C 🖥
**AMA:** 2017,Jan,8; 2016,Jan,13; 2015,Jan,16; 2014,Aug,5; 2014,Jan,11; 2012,Jul,12-14; 2012,Jan,15-42

**00541**    **utilizing 1 lung ventilation**
EXCLUDES   *Thoracic spine and spinal cord procedures via anterior transthoracic approach (00625-00626)*
🔧 0.00    ✂ 0.00    **FUD** XXX     N 🖥
**AMA:** 2017,Jan,8; 2016,Jan,13; 2015,Jan,16; 2014,Aug,5; 2014,Jan,11; 2012,Jul,12-14; 2012,Jan,15-42

**00542**    **decortication**
🔧 0.00    ✂ 0.00    **FUD** XXX     C 🖥
**AMA:** 2017,Jan,8; 2016,Jan,13; 2015,Jan,16; 2014,Aug,5; 2014,Jan,11; 2012,Jul,12-14; 2012,Jan,15-42

**00546**    **pulmonary resection with thoracoplasty**
🔧 0.00    ✂ 0.00    **FUD** XXX     C 🖥
**AMA:** 2017,Jan,8; 2016,Jan,13; 2015,Jan,16; 2014,Aug,5; 2014,Jan,11; 2012,Jul,12-14; 2012,Jan,15-42

**00548**    **intrathoracic procedures on the trachea and bronchi**
🔧 0.00    ✂ 0.00    **FUD** XXX     N 🖥
**AMA:** 2017,Jan,8; 2016,Jan,13; 2015,Jan,16; 2014,Aug,5; 2014,Jan,11; 2012,Jul,12-14; 2012,Jan,15-42

**00550**    **Anesthesia for sternal debridement**
🔧 0.00    ✂ 0.00    **FUD** XXX     N 🖥
**AMA:** 2017,Jan,8; 2016,Jan,13; 2015,Jan,16; 2014,Aug,5; 2014,Jan,11; 2012,Jul,12-14; 2012,Jan,15-42

## 00560-00580 Anesthesia for Open Heart Procedures

**CMS:** 100-04,12,140.1 Qualified Nonphysician Anesthetists; 100-04,12,140.3 Payment for Qualified Nonphysician Anesthetists; 100-04,12,140.3.3 Billing Modifiers; 100-04,12,140.3.4 General Billing Instructions; 100-04,12,140.4.1 Anesthesiologist/Qualified Nonphysican Anesthetist; 100-04,12,140.4.2 Anesthetist and Anesthesiologist in a Single Procedure; 100-04,12,140.4.3 Payment for Medical /Surgical Services by CRNAs; 100-04,12,140.4.4 Conversion Factors for Anesthesia Services; 100-04,4,250.3.2 Anesthesia in a Hospital Outpatient Setting

**00560**    **Anesthesia for procedures on heart, pericardial sac, and great vessels of chest; without pump oxygenator**
🔧 0.00    ✂ 0.00    **FUD** XXX     C 🖥
**AMA:** 2017,Jan,8; 2016,Jan,13; 2015,Jan,16; 2014,Aug,5; 2014,Jan,11; 2012,Jul,12-14; 2012,Jan,15-42

**00561**    **with pump oxygenator, younger than 1 year of age**   A
INCLUDES   Anesthesia complicated by utilization of controlled hypotension (99135)
Anesthesia complicated by utilization of total body hypothermia (99116)
Anesthesia for patient of extreme age, younger than 1 year and older than 70 (99100)
🔧 0.00    ✂ 0.00    **FUD** XXX     C 🖥
**AMA:** 2017,Jan,8; 2016,Jan,13; 2015,Jan,16; 2014,Aug,5; 2014,Jan,11; 2012,Jul,12-14; 2012,Jan,15-42

**00562**    **with pump oxygenator, age 1 year or older, for all noncoronary bypass procedures (eg, valve procedures) or for re-operation for coronary bypass more than 1 month after original operation**   A
🔧 0.00    ✂ 0.00    **FUD** XXX     C 🖥
**AMA:** 2017,Jan,8; 2016,Jan,13; 2015,Jan,16; 2014,Aug,5; 2014,Jan,11; 2012,Jul,12-14; 2012,Jan,15-42

**00563**    **with pump oxygenator with hypothermic circulatory arrest**
🔧 0.00    ✂ 0.00    **FUD** XXX     N 🖥
**AMA:** 2017,Jan,8; 2016,Jan,13; 2015,Jan,16; 2014,Aug,5; 2014,Jan,11; 2012,Jul,12-14; 2012,Jan,15-42

**00566**    **Anesthesia for direct coronary artery bypass grafting; without pump oxygenator**
🔧 0.00    ✂ 0.00    **FUD** XXX     N 🖥
**AMA:** 2017,Jan,8; 2016,Jan,13; 2015,Jan,16; 2014,Aug,5; 2014,Jan,11; 2012,Jul,12-14; 2012,Jan,15-42

**00567**    **with pump oxygenator**
🔧 0.00    ✂ 0.00    **FUD** XXX     C 🖥
**AMA:** 2017,Jan,8; 2016,Jan,13; 2015,Jan,16; 2014,Aug,5; 2014,Jan,11; 2012,Jul,12-14; 2012,Jan,15-42

**00580**    **Anesthesia for heart transplant or heart/lung transplant**
🔧 0.00    ✂ 0.00    **FUD** XXX     C 🖥
**AMA:** 2017,Jan,8; 2016,Jan,13; 2015,Jan,16; 2014,Aug,5; 2014,Jan,11; 2012,Jul,12-14; 2012,Jan,15-42

## 00600-00670 Anesthesia for Spinal Procedures

**CMS:** 100-04,12,140.1 Qualified Nonphysician Anesthetists; 100-04,12,140.3 Payment for Qualified Nonphysician Anesthetists; 100-04,12,140.3.3 Billing Modifiers; 100-04,12,140.3.4 General Billing Instructions; 100-04,12,140.4.1 Anesthesiologist/Qualified Nonphysican Anesthetist; 100-04,12,140.4.2 Anesthetist and Anesthesiologist in a Single Procedure; 100-04,12,140.4.3 Payment for Medical /Surgical Services by CRNAs; 100-04,12,140.4.4 Conversion Factors for Anesthesia Services; 100-04,4,250.3.2 Anesthesia in a Hospital Outpatient Setting

**00600** **Anesthesia for procedures on cervical spine and cord; not otherwise specified**

> EXCLUDES *Percutaneous image-guided spine and spinal cord anesthesia services (01935-01936)*

🔀 0.00 ⚕ 0.00 **FUD** XXX N 🖵

**AMA:** 2017,Jan,8; 2016,Jan,13; 2015,Jan,16; 2014,Aug,5; 2014,Jan,11; 2012,Jul,12-14; 2012,Jan,15-42

**00604** **procedures with patient in the sitting position**

🔀 0.00 ⚕ 0.00 **FUD** XXX C 🖵

**AMA:** 2017,Jan,8; 2016,Jan,13; 2015,Jan,16; 2014,Aug,5; 2014,Jan,11; 2012,Jul,12-14; 2012,Jan,15-42

**00620** **Anesthesia for procedures on thoracic spine and cord, not otherwise specified**

🔀 0.00 ⚕ 0.00 **FUD** XXX N 🖵

**AMA:** 2017,Jan,8; 2016,Jan,13; 2015,Jan,16; 2014,Aug,5; 2014,Jan,11; 2012,Jul,12-14; 2012,Jan,15-42

**00625** **Anesthesia for procedures on the thoracic spine and cord, via an anterior transthoracic approach; not utilizing 1 lung ventilation**

> EXCLUDES *Anesthesia services for thoracotomy procedures other than spine (00540-00541)*

🔀 0.00 ⚕ 0.00 **FUD** XXX N 🖵

**AMA:** 2017,Jan,8; 2016,Jan,13; 2015,Jan,16; 2014,Aug,5; 2014,Jan,11; 2012,Jul,12-14; 2012,Jan,15-42

**00626** **utilizing 1 lung ventilation**

> EXCLUDES *Anesthesia services for thoracotomy procedures other than spine (00540-00541)*

🔀 0.00 ⚕ 0.00 **FUD** XXX N 🖵

**AMA:** 2017,Jan,8; 2016,Jan,13; 2015,Jan,16; 2014,Aug,5; 2014,Jan,11; 2012,Jul,12-14; 2012,Jan,15-42

**00630** **Anesthesia for procedures in lumbar region; not otherwise specified**

🔀 0.00 ⚕ 0.00 **FUD** XXX N 🖵

**AMA:** 2017,Jan,8; 2016,Jan,13; 2015,Jan,16; 2014,Aug,5; 2014,Jan,11; 2012,Jul,12-14; 2012,Jan,15-42

**00632** **lumbar sympathectomy**

🔀 0.00 ⚕ 0.00 **FUD** XXX C 🖵

**AMA:** 2017,Jan,8; 2016,Jan,13; 2015,Jan,16; 2014,Aug,5; 2014,Jan,11; 2012,Jul,12-14; 2012,Jan,15-42

**00635** **diagnostic or therapeutic lumbar puncture**

🔀 0.00 ⚕ 0.00 **FUD** XXX N 🖵

**AMA:** 2017,Jan,8; 2016,Jan,13; 2015,Jan,16; 2014,Aug,5; 2014,Jan,11; 2012,Jul,12-14; 2012,Jan,15-42

**00640** **Anesthesia for manipulation of the spine or for closed procedures on the cervical, thoracic or lumbar spine**

🔀 0.00 ⚕ 0.00 **FUD** XXX N 🖵

**AMA:** 2017,Jan,8; 2016,Jan,13; 2015,Jan,16; 2014,Aug,5; 2014,Jan,11; 2012,Jul,12-14; 2012,Jan,15-42

**00670** **Anesthesia for extensive spine and spinal cord procedures (eg, spinal instrumentation or vascular procedures)**

🔀 0.00 ⚕ 0.00 **FUD** XXX C 🖵

**AMA:** 2017,Jan,8; 2016,Jan,13; 2015,Jan,16; 2014,Aug,5; 2014,Jan,11; 2012,Jul,12-14; 2012,Jan,15-42

## 00700-00882 Anesthesia for Abdominal Procedures

**CMS:** 100-04,12,140.1 Qualified Nonphysician Anesthetists; 100-04,12,140.3 Payment for Qualified Nonphysician Anesthetists; 100-04,12,140.3.3 Billing Modifiers; 100-04,12,140.3.4 General Billing Instructions; 100-04,12,140.4.1 Anesthesiologist/Qualified Nonphysican Anesthetist; 100-04,12,140.4.2 Anesthetist and Anesthesiologist in a Single Procedure; 100-04,12,140.4.3 Payment for Medical /Surgical Services by CRNAs; 100-04,12,140.4.4 Conversion Factors for Anesthesia Services; 100-04,4,250.3.2 Anesthesia in a Hospital Outpatient Setting

**00700** **Anesthesia for procedures on upper anterior abdominal wall; not otherwise specified**

🔀 0.00 ⚕ 0.00 **FUD** XXX N 🖵

**AMA:** 2017,Jan,8; 2016,Jan,13; 2015,Jan,16; 2014,Aug,5; 2014,Jan,11; 2012,Jul,12-14; 2012,Jan,15-42

**00702** **percutaneous liver biopsy**

🔀 0.00 ⚕ 0.00 **FUD** XXX N 🖵

**AMA:** 2017,Jan,8; 2016,Jan,13; 2015,Jan,16; 2014,Aug,5; 2014,Jan,11; 2012,Jul,12-14; 2012,Jan,15-42

**00730** **Anesthesia for procedures on upper posterior abdominal wall**

🔀 0.00 ⚕ 0.00 **FUD** XXX N 🖵

**AMA:** 2017,Jan,8; 2016,Jan,13; 2015,Jan,16; 2014,Aug,5; 2014,Jan,11; 2012,Jul,12-14; 2012,Jan,15-42

● **00731** **Anesthesia for upper gastrointestinal endoscopic procedures, endoscope introduced proximal to duodenum; not otherwise specified**

> EXCLUDES *Combination of upper and lower endoscopic gastrointestinal procedures (00813)*

● **00732** **endoscopic retrograde cholangiopancreatography (ERCP)**

> EXCLUDES *Combination of upper and lower endoscopic gastrointestinal procedures (00813)*

~~00740~~ ~~Anesthesia for upper gastrointestinal endoscopic procedures, endoscope introduced proximal to duodenum~~

To report. see 00731-00732

**00750** **Anesthesia for hernia repairs in upper abdomen; not otherwise specified**

🔀 0.00 ⚕ 0.00 **FUD** XXX N 🖵

**AMA:** 2017,Jan,8; 2016,Jan,13; 2015,Jan,16; 2014,Aug,5; 2014,Jan,11; 2012,Jul,12-14; 2012,Jan,15-42

**00752** **lumbar and ventral (incisional) hernias and/or wound dehiscence**

🔀 0.00 ⚕ 0.00 **FUD** XXX N 🖵

**AMA:** 2017,Jan,8; 2016,Jan,13; 2015,Jan,16; 2014,Aug,5; 2014,Jan,11; 2012,Jul,12-14; 2012,Jan,15-42

**00754** **omphalocele**

🔀 0.00 ⚕ 0.00 **FUD** XXX N 🖵

**AMA:** 2017,Jan,8; 2016,Jan,13; 2015,Jan,16; 2014,Aug,5; 2014,Jan,11; 2012,Jul,12-14; 2012,Jan,15-42

**00756** **transabdominal repair of diaphragmatic hernia**

🔀 0.00 ⚕ 0.00 **FUD** XXX N 🖵

**AMA:** 2017,Jan,8; 2016,Jan,13; 2015,Jan,16; 2014,Aug,5; 2014,Jan,11; 2012,Jul,12-14; 2012,Jan,15-42

**00770** **Anesthesia for all procedures on major abdominal blood vessels**

🔀 0.00 ⚕ 0.00 **FUD** XXX N 🖵

**AMA:** 2017,Jan,8; 2016,Jan,13; 2015,Jan,16; 2014,Aug,5; 2014,Jan,11; 2012,Jul,12-14; 2012,Jan,15-42

**00790** **Anesthesia for intraperitoneal procedures in upper abdomen including laparoscopy; not otherwise specified**

🔀 0.00 ⚕ 0.00 **FUD** XXX N 🖵

**AMA:** 2017,Jan,8; 2016,Jan,13; 2015,Jan,16; 2014,Aug,5; 2014,Jan,11; 2012,Jul,12-14; 2012,Jan,15-42

**00792** **partial hepatectomy or management of liver hemorrhage (excluding liver biopsy)**

🔀 0.00 ⚕ 0.00 **FUD** XXX C 🖵

**AMA:** 2017,Jan,8; 2016,Jan,13; 2015,Jan,16; 2014,Aug,5; 2014,Jan,11; 2012,Jul,12-14; 2012,Jan,15-42

26/TC PC/TC Only  A2-Z3 ASC Payment  50 Bilateral  ♂ Male Only  ♀ Female Only  🔀 Facility RVU  ⚕ Non-Facility RVU  🖵 CCI
FUD Follow-up Days  CMS: IOM (Pub 100)  A-Y OPPSI  80/80 Surg Assist Allowed / w/Doc  🔲 Lab Crosswalk  ▣ Radiology Crosswalk  ✖ CLIA

4
CPT © 2017 American Medical Association. All Rights Reserved.
© 2017 Optum360, LLC

| 00794 | pancreatectomy, partial or total (eg, Whipple procedure) |
|---|---|

    🚑 0.00    ✂ 0.00    **FUD** XXX    C 🖵

    **AMA:** 2017,Jan,8; 2016,Jan,13; 2015,Jan,16; 2014,Aug,5; 2014,Jan,11; 2012,Jul,12-14; 2012,Jan,15-42

**00796**    liver transplant (recipient)

    EXCLUDES   *Physiological support during liver harvest (01990)*

    🚑 0.00    ✂ 0.00    **FUD** XXX    C 🖵

    **AMA:** 2017,Jan,8; 2016,Jan,13; 2015,Jan,16; 2014,Aug,5; 2014,Jan,11; 2012,Jul,12-14; 2012,Jan,15-42

**00797**    gastric restrictive procedure for morbid obesity

    🚑 0.00    ✂ 0.00    **FUD** XXX    N 🖵

    **AMA:** 2017,Jan,8; 2016,Jan,13; 2015,Jan,16; 2014,Aug,5; 2014,Jan,11; 2012,Jul,12-14; 2012,Jan,15-42

**00800**    Anesthesia for procedures on lower anterior abdominal wall; not otherwise specified

    🚑 0.00    ✂ 0.00    **FUD** XXX    N 🖵

    **AMA:** 2017,Jan,8; 2016,Jan,13; 2015,Jan,16; 2014,Aug,5; 2014,Jan,11; 2012,Jul,12-14; 2012,Jan,15-42

**00802**    panniculectomy

    🚑 0.00    ✂ 0.00    **FUD** XXX    C 🖵

    **AMA:** 2017,Jan,8; 2016,Jan,13; 2015,Jan,16; 2014,Aug,5; 2014,Jan,11; 2012,Jul,12-14; 2012,Jan,15-42

~~00810~~    ~~Anesthesia for lower intestinal endoscopic procedures, endoscope introduced distal to duodenum~~

    To report, see 00811-00813

● **00811**    Anesthesia for lower intestinal endoscopic procedures, endoscope introduced distal to duodenum; not otherwise specified

● **00812**    screening colonoscopy

    INCLUDES   Anesthesia services for all screening colonoscopy irrespective of findings

● **00813**    Anesthesia for combined upper and lower gastrointestinal endoscopic procedures, endoscope introduced both proximal to and distal to the duodenum

**00820**    Anesthesia for procedures on lower posterior abdominal wall

    🚑 0.00    ✂ 0.00    **FUD** XXX    N 🖵

    **AMA:** 2017,Jan,8; 2016,Jan,13; 2015,Jan,16; 2014,Aug,5; 2014,Jan,11; 2012,Jul,12-14; 2012,Jan,15-42

**00830**    Anesthesia for hernia repairs in lower abdomen; not otherwise specified

    EXCLUDES   *Anesthesia for hernia repairs on infants one year old or less (00834, 00836)*

    🚑 0.00    ✂ 0.00    **FUD** XXX    N 🖵

    **AMA:** 2017,Jan,8; 2016,Jan,13; 2015,Jan,16; 2014,Aug,5; 2014,Jan,11; 2012,Jul,12-14; 2012,Jan,15-42

**00832**    ventral and incisional hernias

    EXCLUDES   *Anesthesia for hernia repairs on infants one year old or less (00834, 00836)*

    🚑 0.00    ✂ 0.00    **FUD** XXX    N 🖵

    **AMA:** 2017,Jan,8; 2016,Jan,13; 2015,Jan,16; 2014,Aug,5; 2014,Jan,11; 2012,Jul,12-14; 2012,Jan,15-42

**00834**    Anesthesia for hernia repairs in the lower abdomen not otherwise specified, younger than 1 year of age    A

    INCLUDES   Anesthesia for patient of extreme age, younger than 1 year and older than 70 (99100)

    🚑 0.00    ✂ 0.00    **FUD** XXX    N 🖵

    **AMA:** 2017,Jan,8; 2016,Jan,13; 2015,Jan,16; 2014,Aug,5; 2014,Jan,11; 2012,Jul,12-14; 2012,Jan,15-42

**00836**    Anesthesia for hernia repairs in the lower abdomen not otherwise specified, infants younger than 37 weeks gestational age at birth and younger than 50 weeks gestational age at time of surgery    A

    INCLUDES   Anesthesia for patient of extreme age, younger than 1 year and older than 70 (99100)

    🚑 0.00    ✂ 0.00    **FUD** XXX    N 🖵

    **AMA:** 2017,Jan,8; 2016,Jan,13; 2015,Jan,16; 2014,Aug,5; 2014,Jan,11; 2012,Jul,12-14; 2012,Jan,15-42

**00840**    Anesthesia for intraperitoneal procedures in lower abdomen including laparoscopy; not otherwise specified

    🚑 0.00    ✂ 0.00    **FUD** XXX    N 🖵

    **AMA:** 2017,Jan,8; 2016,Jan,13; 2015,Jan,16; 2014,Aug,5; 2014,Jan,11; 2012,Jul,12-14; 2012,Jan,15-42

**00842**    amniocentesis    M ♀

    🚑 0.00    ✂ 0.00    **FUD** XXX    N 🖵

    **AMA:** 2017,Jan,8; 2016,Jan,13; 2015,Jan,16; 2014,Aug,5; 2014,Jan,11; 2012,Jul,12-14; 2012,Jan,15-42

**00844**    abdominoperineal resection

    🚑 0.00    ✂ 0.00    **FUD** XXX    C 🖵

    **AMA:** 2017,Jan,8; 2016,Jan,13; 2015,Jan,16; 2014,Aug,5; 2014,Jan,11; 2012,Jul,12-14; 2012,Jan,15-42

**00846**    radical hysterectomy    ♀

    🚑 0.00    ✂ 0.00    **FUD** XXX    C 🖵

    **AMA:** 2017,Jan,8; 2016,Jan,13; 2015,Jan,16; 2014,Aug,5; 2014,Jan,11; 2012,Jul,12-14; 2012,Jan,15-42

**00848**    pelvic exenteration

    🚑 0.00    ✂ 0.00    **FUD** XXX    C 🖵

    **AMA:** 2017,Jan,8; 2016,Jan,13; 2015,Jan,16; 2014,Aug,5; 2014,Jan,11; 2012,Jul,12-14; 2012,Jan,15-42

**00851**    tubal ligation/transection    ♀

    🚑 0.00    ✂ 0.00    **FUD** XXX    N 🖵

    **AMA:** 2017,Jan,8; 2016,Jan,13; 2015,Jan,16; 2014,Oct,14; 2014,Aug,5; 2014,Jan,11; 2012,Jul,12-14; 2012,Jan,15-42

**00860**    Anesthesia for extraperitoneal procedures in lower abdomen, including urinary tract; not otherwise specified

    🚑 0.00    ✂ 0.00    **FUD** XXX    N 🖵

    **AMA:** 2017,Jan,8; 2016,Jan,13; 2015,Jan,16; 2014,Aug,5; 2014,Jan,11; 2012,Jul,12-14; 2012,Jan,15-42

**00862**    renal procedures, including upper one-third of ureter, or donor nephrectomy

    🚑 0.00    ✂ 0.00    **FUD** XXX    N 🖵

    **AMA:** 2017,Jan,8; 2016,Jan,13; 2015,Jan,16; 2014,Aug,5; 2014,Jan,11; 2012,Jul,12-14; 2012,Jan,15-42

**00864**    total cystectomy

    🚑 0.00    ✂ 0.00    **FUD** XXX    C 🖵

    **AMA:** 2017,Jan,8; 2016,Jan,13; 2015,Jan,16; 2014,Aug,5; 2014,Jan,11; 2012,Jul,12-14; 2012,Jan,15-42

**00865**    radical prostatectomy (suprapubic, retropubic)    ♂

    🚑 0.00    ✂ 0.00    **FUD** XXX    C 🖵

    **AMA:** 2017,Jan,8; 2016,Jan,13; 2015,Jan,16; 2014,Aug,5; 2014,Jan,11; 2012,Jul,12-14; 2012,Jan,15-42

**00866**    adrenalectomy

    🚑 0.00    ✂ 0.00    **FUD** XXX    C 🖵

    **AMA:** 2017,Jan,8; 2016,Jan,13; 2015,Jan,16; 2014,Aug,5; 2014,Jan,11; 2012,Jul,12-14; 2012,Jan,15-42

**00868**    renal transplant (recipient)

    EXCLUDES   *Anesthesia for donor nephrectomy (00862)*
                     *Physiological support during kidney harvest (01990)*

    🚑 0.00    ✂ 0.00    **FUD** XXX    C 🖵

    **AMA:** 2017,Jan,8; 2016,Jan,13; 2015,Jan,16; 2014,Aug,5; 2014,Jan,11; 2012,Jul,12-14; 2012,Jan,15-42

**00870**    cystolithotomy

    🚑 0.00    ✂ 0.00    **FUD** XXX    N 🖵

    **AMA:** 2017,Jan,8; 2016,Jan,13; 2015,Jan,16; 2014,Aug,5; 2014,Jan,11; 2012,Jul,12-14; 2012,Jan,15-42

● New Code    ▲ Revised Code    ○ Reinstated    ● New Web Release    ▲ Revised Web Release    Unlisted    Not Covered    # Resequenced

⊘ AMA Mod 51 Exempt    ⑨ Optum Mod 51 Exempt    ◎ Mod 63 Exempt    ✎ Non-FDA Drug    ★ Telemedicine    M Maternity    A Age Edit    + Add-on    **AMA:** CPT Asst

© 2017 Optum360, LLC    CPT © 2017 American Medical Association. All Rights Reserved.    5

**00872** **Anesthesia for lithotripsy, extracorporeal shock wave; with water bath**
🔲 0.00   🔲 0.00   **FUD** XXX                                    N 🔲
AMA: 2017,Jan,8; 2016,Jan,13; 2015,Jan,16; 2014,Aug,5; 2014,Jan,11; 2012,Jul,12-14; 2012,Jan,15-42

**00873** **without water bath**
🔲 0.00   🔲 0.00   **FUD** XXX                                    N 🔲
AMA: 2017,Jan,8; 2016,Jan,13; 2015,Jan,16; 2014,Aug,5; 2014,Jan,11; 2012,Jul,12-14; 2012,Jan,15-42

**00880** **Anesthesia for procedures on major lower abdominal vessels; not otherwise specified**
🔲 0.00   🔲 0.00   **FUD** XXX                                    N 🔲
AMA: 2017,Jan,8; 2016,Jan,13; 2015,Jan,16; 2014,Aug,5; 2014,Jan,11; 2012,Jul,12-14; 2012,Jan,15-42

**00882** **inferior vena cava ligation**
🔲 0.00   🔲 0.00   **FUD** XXX                                    C 🔲
AMA: 2017,Jan,8; 2016,Jan,13; 2015,Jan,16; 2014,Aug,5; 2014,Jan,11; 2012,Jul,12-14; 2012,Jan,15-42

## 00902-00952 Anesthesia for Genitourinary Procedures

**CMS:** 100-04,12,140.1 Qualified Nonphysician Anesthetists; 100-04,12,140.3 Payment for Qualified Nonphysician Anesthetists; 100-04,12,140.3.3 Billing Modifiers; 100-04,12,140.3.4 General Billing Instructions; 100-04,12,140.4.1 Anesthesiologist/Qualified Nonphysican Anesthetist; 100-04,12,140.4.2 Anesthetist and Anesthesiologist in a Single Procedure; 100-04,12,140.4.3 Payment for Medical /Surgical Services by CRNAs; 100-04,12,140.4.4 Conversion Factors for Anesthesia Services; 100-04,4,250.3.2 Anesthesia in a Hospital Outpatient Setting

EXCLUDES  *Procedures on perineal skin, muscles, and nerves (00300, 00400)*

**00902** **Anesthesia for; anorectal procedure**
🔲 0.00   🔲 0.00   **FUD** XXX                                    N 🔲
AMA: 2017,Jan,8; 2016,Jan,13; 2015,Jan,16; 2014,Aug,5; 2014,Jan,11; 2012,Jul,12-14; 2012,Jan,15-42

**00904** **radical perineal procedure**
🔲 0.00   🔲 0.00   **FUD** XXX                                    C 🔲
AMA: 2017,Jan,8; 2016,Jan,13; 2015,Jan,16; 2014,Aug,5; 2014,Jan,11; 2012,Jul,12-14; 2012,Jan,15-42

**00906** **vulvectomy**                                           ♀
🔲 0.00   🔲 0.00   **FUD** XXX                                    N 🔲
AMA: 2017,Jan,8; 2016,Jan,13; 2015,Jan,16; 2014,Aug,5; 2014,Jan,11; 2012,Jul,12-14; 2012,Jan,15-42

**00908** **perineal prostatectomy**                              ♂
🔲 0.00   🔲 0.00   **FUD** XXX                                    C 🔲
AMA: 2017,Jan,8; 2016,Jan,13; 2015,Jan,16; 2014,Aug,5; 2014,Jan,11; 2012,Jul,12-14; 2012,Jan,15-42

**00910** **Anesthesia for transurethral procedures (including urethrocystoscopy); not otherwise specified**
🔲 0.00   🔲 0.00   **FUD** XXX                                    N 🔲
AMA: 2017,Jan,8; 2016,Jan,13; 2015,Jan,16; 2014,Aug,5; 2014,Jan,11; 2012,Jul,12-14; 2012,Jan,15-42

**00912** **transurethral resection of bladder tumor(s)**
🔲 0.00   🔲 0.00   **FUD** XXX                                    N 🔲
AMA: 2017,Jan,8; 2016,Jan,13; 2015,Jan,16; 2014,Aug,5; 2014,Jan,11; 2012,Jul,12-14; 2012,Jan,15-42

**00914** **transurethral resection of prostate**                 ♂
🔲 0.00   🔲 0.00   **FUD** XXX                                    N 🔲
AMA: 2017,Jan,8; 2016,Jan,13; 2015,Jan,16; 2014,Aug,5; 2014,Jan,11; 2012,Jul,12-14; 2012,Jan,15-42

**00916** **post-transurethral resection bleeding**
🔲 0.00   🔲 0.00   **FUD** XXX                                    N 🔲
AMA: 2017,Jan,8; 2016,Jan,13; 2015,Jan,16; 2014,Aug,5; 2014,Jan,11; 2012,Jul,12-14; 2012,Jan,15-42

**00918** **with fragmentation, manipulation and/or removal of ureteral calculus**
🔲 0.00   🔲 0.00   **FUD** XXX                                    N 🔲
AMA: 2017,Jan,8; 2016,Jan,13; 2015,Jan,16; 2014,Aug,5; 2014,Jan,11; 2012,Jul,12-14; 2012,Jan,15-42

**00920** **Anesthesia for procedures on male genitalia (including open urethral procedures); not otherwise specified**   ♂
🔲 0.00   🔲 0.00   **FUD** XXX                                    N 🔲
AMA: 2017,Jan,8; 2016,Jan,13; 2015,Jan,16; 2014,Aug,5; 2014,Jan,11; 2012,Oct,14; 2012,Sep,16; 2012,Jul,12-14; 2012,Jan,15-42

**00921** **vasectomy, unilateral or bilateral**                  ♂
🔲 0.00   🔲 0.00   **FUD** XXX                                    N 🔲
AMA: 2017,Jan,8; 2016,Jan,13; 2015,Jan,16; 2014,Aug,5; 2014,Jan,11; 2012,Jul,12-14; 2012,Jan,15-42

**00922** **seminal vesicles**                                    ♂
🔲 0.00   🔲 0.00   **FUD** XXX                                    N 🔲
AMA: 2017,Jan,8; 2016,Jan,13; 2015,Jan,16; 2014,Aug,5; 2014,Jan,11; 2012,Jul,12-14; 2012,Jan,15-42

**00924** **undescended testis, unilateral or bilateral**         ♂
🔲 0.00   🔲 0.00   **FUD** XXX                                    N 🔲
AMA: 2017,Jan,8; 2016,Jan,13; 2015,Jan,16; 2014,Aug,5; 2014,Jan,11; 2012,Jul,12-14; 2012,Jan,15-42

**00926** **radical orchiectomy, inguinal**                       ♂
🔲 0.00   🔲 0.00   **FUD** XXX                                    N 🔲
AMA: 2017,Jan,8; 2016,Jan,13; 2015,Jan,16; 2014,Aug,5; 2014,Jan,11; 2012,Jul,12-14; 2012,Jan,15-42

**00928** **radical orchiectomy, abdominal**                      ♂
🔲 0.00   🔲 0.00   **FUD** XXX                                    N 🔲
AMA: 2017,Jan,8; 2016,Jan,13; 2015,Jan,16; 2014,Aug,5; 2014,Jan,11; 2012,Jul,12-14; 2012,Jan,15-42

**00930** **orchiopexy, unilateral or bilateral**                 ♂
🔲 0.00   🔲 0.00   **FUD** XXX                                    N 🔲
AMA: 2017,Jan,8; 2016,Jan,13; 2015,Jan,16; 2014,Aug,5; 2014,Jan,11; 2012,Jul,12-14; 2012,Jan,15-42

**00932** **complete amputation of penis**                        ♂
🔲 0.00   🔲 0.00   **FUD** XXX                                    C 🔲
AMA: 2017,Jan,8; 2016,Jan,13; 2015,Jan,16; 2014,Aug,5; 2014,Jan,11; 2012,Jul,12-14; 2012,Jan,15-42

**00934** **radical amputation of penis with bilateral inguinal lymphadenectomy**                                         ♂
🔲 0.00   🔲 0.00   **FUD** XXX                                    C 🔲
AMA: 2017,Jan,8; 2016,Jan,13; 2015,Jan,16; 2014,Aug,5; 2014,Jan,11; 2012,Jul,12-14; 2012,Jan,15-42

**00936** **radical amputation of penis with bilateral inguinal and iliac lymphadenectomy**                               ♂
🔲 0.00   🔲 0.00   **FUD** XXX                                    C 🔲
AMA: 2017,Jan,8; 2016,Jan,13; 2015,Jan,16; 2014,Aug,5; 2014,Jan,11; 2012,Jul,12-14; 2012,Jan,15-42

**00938** **insertion of penile prosthesis (perineal approach)**  ♂
🔲 0.00   🔲 0.00   **FUD** XXX                                    N 🔲
AMA: 2017,Jan,8; 2016,Jan,13; 2015,Jan,16; 2014,Aug,5; 2014,Jan,11; 2012,Jul,12-14; 2012,Jan,15-42

**00940** **Anesthesia for vaginal procedures (including biopsy of labia, vagina, cervix or endometrium); not otherwise specified**   ♀
🔲 0.00   🔲 0.00   **FUD** XXX                                    N 🔲
AMA: 2017,Jan,8; 2016,Jan,13; 2015,Jan,16; 2014,Aug,5; 2014,Jan,11; 2012,Jul,12-14; 2012,Jan,15-42

**00942** **colpotomy, vaginectomy, colporrhaphy, and open urethral procedures**                                          ♀
🔲 0.00   🔲 0.00   **FUD** XXX                                    N 🔲
AMA: 2017,Jan,8; 2016,Jan,13; 2015,Jan,16; 2014,Aug,5; 2014,Jan,11; 2012,Jul,12-14; 2012,Jan,15-42

**00944** **vaginal hysterectomy**                                ♀
🔲 0.00   🔲 0.00   **FUD** XXX                                    C 🔲
AMA: 2017,Jan,8; 2016,Jan,13; 2015,Jan,16; 2014,Aug,5; 2014,Jan,11; 2012,Jul,12-14; 2012,Jan,15-42

**00948** **cervical cerclage**                                   ♀
🔲 0.00   🔲 0.00   **FUD** XXX                                    N 🔲
AMA: 2017,Jan,8; 2016,Jan,13; 2015,Jan,16; 2014,Aug,5; 2014,Jan,11; 2012,Jul,12-14; 2012,Jan,15-42

| 26/TC PC/TC Only | 🔲-🔲 ASC Payment | 50 Bilateral | ♂ Male Only | ♀ Female Only | 🔲 Facility RVU | 🔲 Non-Facility RVU | 🔲 CCI |
| **FUD** Follow-up Days | **CMS:** IOM (Pub 100) | 🔲-🔲 OPPSI | 80/80 Surg Assist Allowed / w/Doc | | 🔲 Lab Crosswalk | 🔲 Radiology Crosswalk | 🔀 CLIA |

6                                   CPT © 2017 American Medical Association. All Rights Reserved.                      © 2017 Optum360, LLC

00950 culdoscopy ♀
🔲 0.00 🔲 0.00 **FUD** XXX 🔲🔲
**AMA:** 2017,Jan,8; 2016,Jan,13; 2015,Jan,16; 2014,Aug,5;
2014,Jan,11; 2012,Jul,12-14; 2012,Jan,15-42

00952 hysteroscopy and/or hysterosalpingography ♀
🔲 0.00 🔲 0.00 **FUD** XXX 🔲🔲
**AMA:** 2017,Jan,8; 2016,Jan,13; 2015,Jan,16; 2014,Aug,5;
2014,Jan,11; 2012,Jul,12-14; 2012,Jan,15-42

# 01112-01522 Anesthesia for Lower Extremity Procedures

**CMS:** 100-04,12,140.1 Qualified Nonphysician Anesthetists; 100-04,12,140.3 Payment for Qualified
Nonphysician Anesthetists; 100-04,12,140.3.3 Billing Modifiers; 100-04,12,140.3.4 General Billing Instructions;
100-04,12,140.4.1 Anesthesiologist/Qualified Nonphysican Anesthetist; 100-04,12,140.4.2 Anesthetist and
Anesthesiologist in a Single Procedure; 100-04,12,140.4.3 Payment for Medical /Surgical Services by CRNAs;
100-04,12,140.4.4 Conversion Factors for Anesthesia Services; 100-04,4,250.3.2 Anesthesia in a Hospital
Outpatient Setting

01112 Anesthesia for bone marrow aspiration and/or biopsy,
anterior or posterior iliac crest
🔲 0.00 🔲 0.00 **FUD** XXX 🔲🔲
**AMA:** 2017,Jan,8; 2016,Jan,13; 2015,Jan,16; 2014,Aug,5;
2014,Jan,11; 2012,Jul,12-14; 2012,Jan,15-42

01120 Anesthesia for procedures on bony pelvis
🔲 0.00 🔲 0.00 **FUD** XXX 🔲🔲
**AMA:** 2017,Jan,8; 2016,Jan,13; 2015,Jan,16; 2014,Aug,5;
2014,Jan,11; 2012,Jul,12-14; 2012,Jan,15-42

01130 Anesthesia for body cast application or revision
🔲 0.00 🔲 0.00 **FUD** XXX 🔲🔲
**AMA:** 2017,Jan,8; 2016,Jan,13; 2015,Jan,16; 2014,Aug,5;
2014,Jan,11; 2012,Jul,12-14; 2012,Jan,15-42

01140 Anesthesia for interpelviabdominal (hindquarter)
amputation
🔲 0.00 🔲 0.00 **FUD** XXX 🔲🔲
**AMA:** 2017,Jan,8; 2016,Jan,13; 2015,Jan,16; 2014,Aug,5;
2014,Jan,11; 2012,Jul,12-14; 2012,Jan,15-42

01150 Anesthesia for radical procedures for tumor of pelvis, except
hindquarter amputation
🔲 0.00 🔲 0.00 **FUD** XXX 🔲🔲
**AMA:** 2017,Jan,8; 2016,Jan,13; 2015,Jan,16; 2014,Aug,5;
2014,Jan,11; 2012,Jul,12-14; 2012,Jan,15-42

01160 Anesthesia for closed procedures involving symphysis pubis
or sacroiliac joint
🔲 0.00 🔲 0.00 **FUD** XXX 🔲🔲
**AMA:** 2017,Jan,8; 2016,Jan,13; 2015,Jan,16; 2014,Aug,5;
2014,Jan,11; 2012,Jul,12-14; 2012,Jan,15-42

01170 Anesthesia for open procedures involving symphysis pubis
or sacroiliac joint
🔲 0.00 🔲 0.00 **FUD** XXX 🔲🔲
**AMA:** 2017,Jan,8; 2016,Jan,13; 2015,Jan,16; 2014,Aug,5;
2014,Jan,11; 2012,Jul,12-14; 2012,Jan,15-42

01173 Anesthesia for open repair of fracture disruption of pelvis or
column fracture involving acetabulum
🔲 0.00 🔲 0.00 **FUD** XXX 🔲🔲
**AMA:** 2017,Jan,8; 2016,Jan,13; 2015,Jan,16; 2014,Aug,5;
2014,Jan,11; 2012,Jul,12-14; 2012,Jan,15-42

01180 ~~Anesthesia for obturator neurectomy; extrapelvic~~

01190 ~~intrapelvic~~

01200 Anesthesia for all closed procedures involving hip joint
🔲 0.00 🔲 0.00 **FUD** XXX 🔲🔲
**AMA:** 2017,Jan,8; 2016,Jan,13; 2015,Jan,16; 2014,Aug,5;
2014,Jan,11; 2012,Jul,12-14; 2012,Jan,15-42

01202 Anesthesia for arthroscopic procedures of hip joint
🔲 0.00 🔲 0.00 **FUD** XXX 🔲🔲
**AMA:** 2017,Jan,8; 2016,Jan,13; 2015,Jan,16; 2014,Aug,5;
2014,Jan,11; 2012,Jul,12-14; 2012,Jan,15-42

01210 Anesthesia for open procedures involving hip joint; not
otherwise specified
🔲 0.00 🔲 0.00 **FUD** XXX 🔲🔲
**AMA:** 2017,Jan,8; 2016,Jan,13; 2015,Jan,16; 2014,Aug,5;
2014,Jan,11; 2012,Jul,12-14; 2012,Jan,15-42

01212 hip disarticulation
🔲 0.00 🔲 0.00 **FUD** XXX 🔲🔲
**AMA:** 2017,Jan,8; 2016,Jan,13; 2015,Jan,16; 2014,Aug,5;
2014,Jan,11; 2012,Jul,12-14; 2012,Jan,15-42

01214 total hip arthroplasty
🔲 0.00 🔲 0.00 **FUD** XXX 🔲🔲
**AMA:** 2017,Jan,8; 2016,Jan,13; 2015,Jan,16; 2014,Aug,5;
2014,Jan,11; 2012,Jul,12-14; 2012,Jan,15-42

01215 revision of total hip arthroplasty
🔲 0.00 🔲 0.00 **FUD** XXX 🔲🔲
**AMA:** 2017,Jan,8; 2016,Jan,13; 2015,Jan,16; 2014,Aug,5;
2014,Jan,11; 2012,Jul,12-14; 2012,Jan,15-42

01220 Anesthesia for all closed procedures involving upper
two-thirds of femur
🔲 0.00 🔲 0.00 **FUD** XXX 🔲🔲
**AMA:** 2017,Jan,8; 2016,Jan,13; 2015,Jan,16; 2014,Aug,5;
2014,Jan,11; 2012,Jul,12-14; 2012,Jan,15-42

01230 Anesthesia for open procedures involving upper two-thirds
of femur; not otherwise specified
🔲 0.00 🔲 0.00 **FUD** XXX 🔲🔲
**AMA:** 2017,Jan,8; 2016,Jan,13; 2015,Jan,16; 2014,Aug,5;
2014,Jan,11; 2012,Jul,12-14; 2012,Jan,15-42

01232 amputation
🔲 0.00 🔲 0.00 **FUD** XXX 🔲🔲
**AMA:** 2017,Jan,8; 2016,Jan,13; 2015,Jan,16; 2014,Aug,5;
2014,Jan,11; 2012,Jul,12-14; 2012,Jan,15-42

01234 radical resection
🔲 0.00 🔲 0.00 **FUD** XXX 🔲🔲
**AMA:** 2017,Jan,8; 2016,Jan,13; 2015,Jan,16; 2014,Aug,5;
2014,Jan,11; 2012,Jul,12-14; 2012,Jan,15-42

01250 Anesthesia for all procedures on nerves, muscles, tendons,
fascia, and bursae of upper leg
🔲 0.00 🔲 0.00 **FUD** XXX 🔲🔲
**AMA:** 2017,Jan,8; 2016,Jan,13; 2015,Jan,16; 2014,Aug,5;
2014,Jan,11; 2012,Jul,12-14; 2012,Jan,15-42

01260 Anesthesia for all procedures involving veins of upper leg,
including exploration
🔲 0.00 🔲 0.00 **FUD** XXX 🔲🔲
**AMA:** 2017,Jan,8; 2016,Jan,13; 2015,Jan,16; 2014,Aug,5;
2014,Jan,11; 2012,Jul,12-14; 2012,Jan,15-42

01270 Anesthesia for procedures involving arteries of upper leg,
including bypass graft; not otherwise specified
🔲 0.00 🔲 0.00 **FUD** XXX 🔲🔲
**AMA:** 2017,Jan,8; 2016,Jan,13; 2015,Jan,16; 2014,Aug,5;
2014,Jan,11; 2012,Jul,12-14; 2012,Jan,15-42

01272 femoral artery ligation
🔲 0.00 🔲 0.00 **FUD** XXX 🔲🔲
**AMA:** 2017,Jan,8; 2016,Jan,13; 2015,Jan,16; 2014,Aug,5;
2014,Jan,11; 2012,Jul,12-14; 2012,Jan,15-42

01274 femoral artery embolectomy
🔲 0.00 🔲 0.00 **FUD** XXX 🔲🔲
**AMA:** 2017,Jan,8; 2016,Jan,13; 2015,Jan,16; 2014,Aug,5;
2014,Jan,11; 2012,Jul,12-14; 2012,Jan,15-42

01320 Anesthesia for all procedures on nerves, muscles, tendons,
fascia, and bursae of knee and/or popliteal area
🔲 0.00 🔲 0.00 **FUD** XXX 🔲🔲
**AMA:** 2017,Jan,8; 2016,Jan,13; 2015,Jan,16; 2014,Aug,5;
2014,Jan,11; 2012,Jul,12-14; 2012,Jan,15-42

01340 Anesthesia for all closed procedures on lower one-third of
femur
🔲 0.00 🔲 0.00 **FUD** XXX 🔲🔲
**AMA:** 2017,Jan,8; 2016,Jan,13; 2015,Jan,16; 2014,Aug,5;
2014,Jan,11; 2012,Jul,12-14; 2012,Jan,15-42

---

● New Code ▲ Revised Code ○ Reinstated ● New Web Release ▲ Revised Web Release Unlisted Not Covered # Resequenced
⊘ AMA Mod 51 Exempt ⑤ Optum Mod 51 Exempt ⑥③ Mod 63 Exempt ⁄ Non-FDA Drug ★ Telemedicine Ⓜ Maternity Ⓐ Age Edit + Add-on **AMA:** CPT Asst

© 2017 Optum360, LLC CPT © 2017 American Medical Association. All Rights Reserved.

| 01360 | Anesthesia for all open procedures on lower one-third of femur |
|---|---|

🔹 0.00   ⚕ 0.00   **FUD** XXX   N 🖵

**AMA:** 2017,Jan,8; 2016,Jan,13; 2015,Jan,16; 2014,Aug,5; 2014,Jan,11; 2012,Jul,12-14; 2012,Jan,15-42

| 01380 | Anesthesia for all closed procedures on knee joint |
|---|---|

🔹 0.00   ⚕ 0.00   **FUD** XXX   N 🖵

**AMA:** 2017,Jan,8; 2016,Jan,13; 2015,Jan,16; 2014,Aug,5; 2014,Jan,11; 2012,Jul,12-14; 2012,Jan,15-42

| 01382 | Anesthesia for diagnostic arthroscopic procedures of knee joint |
|---|---|

🔹 0.00   ⚕ 0.00   **FUD** XXX   N 🖵

**AMA:** 2017,Jan,8; 2016,Jan,13; 2015,Jan,16; 2014,Aug,5; 2014,Jan,11; 2012,Jul,12-14; 2012,Jan,15-42

| 01390 | Anesthesia for all closed procedures on upper ends of tibia, fibula, and/or patella |
|---|---|

🔹 0.00   ⚕ 0.00   **FUD** XXX   N 🖵

**AMA:** 2017,Jan,8; 2016,Jan,13; 2015,Jan,16; 2014,Aug,5; 2014,Jan,11; 2012,Jul,12-14; 2012,Jan,15-42

| 01392 | Anesthesia for all open procedures on upper ends of tibia, fibula, and/or patella |
|---|---|

🔹 0.00   ⚕ 0.00   **FUD** XXX   N 🖵

**AMA:** 2017,Jan,8; 2016,Jan,13; 2015,Jan,16; 2014,Aug,5; 2014,Jan,11; 2012,Jul,12-14; 2012,Jan,15-42

| 01400 | Anesthesia for open or surgical arthroscopic procedures on knee joint; not otherwise specified |
|---|---|

🔹 0.00   ⚕ 0.00   **FUD** XXX   N 🖵

**AMA:** 2017,Jan,8; 2016,Jan,13; 2015,Jan,16; 2014,Aug,5; 2014,Jan,11; 2012,Jul,12-14; 2012,Jan,15-42

| 01402 | total knee arthroplasty |
|---|---|

🔹 0.00   ⚕ 0.00   **FUD** XXX   C 🖵

**AMA:** 2017,Jan,8; 2016,Jan,13; 2015,Jan,16; 2014,Aug,5; 2014,Jan,11; 2012,Jul,12-14; 2012,Jan,15-42

| 01404 | disarticulation at knee |
|---|---|

🔹 0.00   ⚕ 0.00   **FUD** XXX   C 🖵

**AMA:** 2017,Jan,8; 2016,Jan,13; 2015,Jan,16; 2014,Aug,5; 2014,Jan,11; 2012,Jul,12-14; 2012,Jan,15-42

| 01420 | Anesthesia for all cast applications, removal, or repair involving knee joint |
|---|---|

🔹 0.00   ⚕ 0.00   **FUD** XXX   N 🖵

**AMA:** 2017,Jan,8; 2016,Jan,13; 2015,Jan,16; 2014,Aug,5; 2014,Jan,11; 2012,Jul,12-14; 2012,Jan,15-42

| 01430 | Anesthesia for procedures on veins of knee and popliteal area; not otherwise specified |
|---|---|

🔹 0.00   ⚕ 0.00   **FUD** XXX   N 🖵

**AMA:** 2017,Jan,8; 2016,Jan,13; 2015,Jan,16; 2014,Aug,5; 2014,Jan,11; 2012,Jul,12-14; 2012,Jan,15-42

| 01432 | arteriovenous fistula |
|---|---|

🔹 0.00   ⚕ 0.00   **FUD** XXX   N 🖵

**AMA:** 2017,Jan,8; 2016,Jan,13; 2015,Jan,16; 2014,Aug,5; 2014,Jan,11; 2012,Jul,12-14; 2012,Jan,15-42

| 01440 | Anesthesia for procedures on arteries of knee and popliteal area; not otherwise specified |
|---|---|

🔹 0.00   ⚕ 0.00   **FUD** XXX   N 🖵

**AMA:** 2017,Jan,8; 2016,Jan,13; 2015,Jan,16; 2014,Aug,5; 2014,Jan,11; 2012,Jul,12-14; 2012,Jan,15-42

| 01442 | popliteal thromboendarterectomy, with or without patch graft |
|---|---|

🔹 0.00   ⚕ 0.00   **FUD** XXX   C 🖵

**AMA:** 2017,Jan,8; 2016,Jan,13; 2015,Jan,16; 2014,Aug,5; 2014,Jan,11; 2012,Jul,12-14; 2012,Jan,15-42

| 01444 | popliteal excision and graft or repair for occlusion or aneurysm |
|---|---|

🔹 0.00   ⚕ 0.00   **FUD** XXX   C 🖵

**AMA:** 2017,Jan,8; 2016,Jan,13; 2015,Jan,16; 2014,Aug,5; 2014,Jan,11; 2012,Jul,12-14; 2012,Jan,15-42

| 01462 | Anesthesia for all closed procedures on lower leg, ankle, and foot |
|---|---|

🔹 0.00   ⚕ 0.00   **FUD** XXX   N 🖵

**AMA:** 2017,Jan,8; 2016,Jan,13; 2015,Jan,16; 2014,Aug,5; 2014,Jan,11; 2012,Jul,12-14; 2012,Jan,15-42

| 01464 | Anesthesia for arthroscopic procedures of ankle and/or foot |
|---|---|

🔹 0.00   ⚕ 0.00   **FUD** XXX   N 🖵

**AMA:** 2017,Jan,8; 2016,Jan,13; 2015,Jan,16; 2014,Aug,5; 2014,Jan,11; 2012,Jul,12-14; 2012,Jan,15-42

| 01470 | Anesthesia for procedures on nerves, muscles, tendons, and fascia of lower leg, ankle, and foot; not otherwise specified |
|---|---|

🔹 0.00   ⚕ 0.00   **FUD** XXX   N 🖵

**AMA:** 2017,Jan,8; 2016,Jan,13; 2015,Jan,16; 2014,Aug,5; 2014,Jan,11; 2012,Jul,12-14; 2012,Jan,15-42

| 01472 | repair of ruptured Achilles tendon, with or without graft |
|---|---|

🔹 0.00   ⚕ 0.00   **FUD** XXX   N 🖵

**AMA:** 2017,Jan,8; 2016,Jan,13; 2015,Jan,16; 2014,Aug,5; 2014,Jan,11; 2012,Jul,12-14; 2012,Jan,15-42

| 01474 | gastrocnemius recession (eg, Strayer procedure) |
|---|---|

🔹 0.00   ⚕ 0.00   **FUD** XXX   N 🖵

**AMA:** 2017,Jan,8; 2016,Jan,13; 2015,Jan,16; 2014,Aug,5; 2014,Jan,11; 2012,Jul,12-14; 2012,Jan,15-42

| 01480 | Anesthesia for open procedures on bones of lower leg, ankle, and foot; not otherwise specified |
|---|---|

🔹 0.00   ⚕ 0.00   **FUD** XXX   N 🖵

**AMA:** 2017,Jan,8; 2016,Jan,13; 2015,Jan,16; 2014,Aug,5; 2014,Jan,11; 2012,Jul,12-14; 2012,Jan,15-42

| 01482 | radical resection (including below knee amputation) |
|---|---|

🔹 0.00   ⚕ 0.00   **FUD** XXX   N 🖵

**AMA:** 2017,Jan,8; 2016,Jan,13; 2015,Jan,16; 2014,Aug,5; 2014,Jan,11; 2012,Jul,12-14; 2012,Jan,15-42

| 01484 | osteotomy or osteoplasty of tibia and/or fibula |
|---|---|

🔹 0.00   ⚕ 0.00   **FUD** XXX   N 🖵

**AMA:** 2017,Jan,8; 2016,Jan,13; 2015,Jan,16; 2014,Aug,5; 2014,Jan,11; 2012,Jul,12-14; 2012,Jan,15-42

| 01486 | total ankle replacement |
|---|---|

🔹 0.00   ⚕ 0.00   **FUD** XXX   C 🖵

**AMA:** 2017,Jan,8; 2016,Jan,13; 2015,Jan,16; 2014,Aug,5; 2014,Jan,11; 2012,Jul,12-14; 2012,Jan,15-42

| 01490 | Anesthesia for lower leg cast application, removal, or repair |
|---|---|

🔹 0.00   ⚕ 0.00   **FUD** XXX   N 🖵

**AMA:** 2017,Jan,8; 2016,Jan,13; 2015,Jan,16; 2014,Aug,5; 2014,Jan,11; 2012,Jul,12-14; 2012,Jan,15-42

| 01500 | Anesthesia for procedures on arteries of lower leg, including bypass graft; not otherwise specified |
|---|---|

🔹 0.00   ⚕ 0.00   **FUD** XXX   N 🖵

**AMA:** 2017,Jan,8; 2016,Jan,13; 2015,Jan,16; 2014,Aug,5; 2014,Jan,11; 2012,Jul,12-14; 2012,Jan,15-42

| 01502 | embolectomy, direct or with catheter |
|---|---|

🔹 0.00   ⚕ 0.00   **FUD** XXX   C 🖵

**AMA:** 2017,Jan,8; 2016,Jan,13; 2015,Jan,16; 2014,Aug,5; 2014,Jan,11; 2012,Jul,12-14; 2012,Jan,15-42

| 01520 | Anesthesia for procedures on veins of lower leg; not otherwise specified |
|---|---|

🔹 0.00   ⚕ 0.00   **FUD** XXX   N 🖵

**AMA:** 2017,Jan,8; 2016,Jan,13; 2015,Jan,16; 2014,Aug,5; 2014,Jan,11; 2012,Jul,12-14; 2012,Jan,15-42

| 01522 | venous thrombectomy, direct or with catheter |
|---|---|

🔹 0.00   ⚕ 0.00   **FUD** XXX   N 🖵

**AMA:** 2017,Jan,8; 2016,Jan,13; 2015,Jan,16; 2014,Aug,5; 2014,Jan,11; 2012,Jul,12-14; 2012,Jan,15-42

**26/16** PC/TC Only    **42-23** ASC Payment    **50** Bilateral    ♂ Male Only    ♀ Female Only    🔹 Facility RVU    ⚕ Non-Facility RVU    🖵 CCI
**FUD** Follow-up Days    **CMS:** IOM (Pub 100)    **A-Y** OPPSI    **80/80** Surg Assist Allowed / w/Doc    🔲 Lab Crosswalk    🔲 Radiology Crosswalk    ❌ CLIA

8

CPT © 2017 American Medical Association. All Rights Reserved.

© 2017 Optum360, LLC

## 01610-01682 Anesthesia for Shoulder Procedures

**CMS:** 100-04,12,140.1 Qualified Nonphysician Anesthetists; 100-04,12,140.3 Payment for Qualified Nonphysician Anesthetists; 100-04,12,140.3.3 Billing Modifiers; 100-04,12,140.3.4 General Billing Instructions; 100-04,12,140.4.1 Anesthesiologist/Qualified Nonphysican Anesthetist; 100-04,12,140.4.2 Anesthetist and Anesthesiologist in a Single Procedure; 100-04,12,140.4.3 Payment for Medical /Surgical Services by CRNAs; 100-04,12,140.4.4 Conversion Factors for Anesthesia Services; 100-04,4,250.3.2 Anesthesia in a Hospital Outpatient Setting

INCLUDES Acromioclavicular joint
Humeral head and neck
Shoulder joint
Sternoclavicular joint

**01610** **Anesthesia for all procedures on nerves, muscles, tendons, fascia, and bursae of shoulder and axilla**
0.00　0.00　**FUD** XXX　N ▣
**AMA:** 2017,Jan,8; 2016,Jan,13; 2015,Jan,16; 2014,Aug,5; 2014,Jan,11; 2012,Jul,12-14; 2012,Jan,15-42

**01620** **Anesthesia for all closed procedures on humeral head and neck, sternoclavicular joint, acromioclavicular joint, and shoulder joint**
0.00　0.00　**FUD** XXX　N ▣
**AMA:** 2017,Jan,8; 2016,Jan,13; 2015,Jan,16; 2014,Aug,5; 2014,Jan,11; 2012,Jul,12-14; 2012,Jan,15-42

**01622** **Anesthesia for diagnostic arthroscopic procedures of shoulder joint**
0.00　0.00　**FUD** XXX　N ▣
**AMA:** 2017,Jan,8; 2016,Jan,13; 2015,Jan,16; 2014,Aug,5; 2014,Jan,11; 2012,Jul,12-14; 2012,Jan,15-42

**01630** **Anesthesia for open or surgical arthroscopic procedures on humeral head and neck, sternoclavicular joint, acromioclavicular joint, and shoulder joint; not otherwise specified**
0.00　0.00　**FUD** XXX　N ▣
**AMA:** 2017,Jan,8; 2016,Jan,13; 2015,Jan,16; 2014,Aug,5; 2014,Jan,11; 2012,Jul,12-14; 2012,Jan,15-42

**01634** **shoulder disarticulation**
0.00　0.00　**FUD** XXX　C ▣
**AMA:** 2017,Jan,8; 2016,Jan,13; 2015,Jan,16; 2014,Aug,5; 2014,Jan,11; 2012,Jul,12-14; 2012,Jan,15-42

**01636** **interthoracoscapular (forequarter) amputation**
0.00　0.00　**FUD** XXX　C ▣
**AMA:** 2017,Jan,8; 2016,Jan,13; 2015,Jan,16; 2014,Aug,5; 2014,Jan,11; 2012,Jul,12-14; 2012,Jan,15-42

**01638** **total shoulder replacement**
0.00　0.00　**FUD** XXX　C ▣
**AMA:** 2017,Jan,8; 2016,Jan,13; 2015,Jan,16; 2014,Aug,5; 2014,Jan,11; 2012,Jul,12-14; 2012,Jan,15-42

**01650** **Anesthesia for procedures on arteries of shoulder and axilla; not otherwise specified**
0.00　0.00　**FUD** XXX　N ▣
**AMA:** 2017,Jan,8; 2016,Jan,13; 2015,Jan,16; 2014,Aug,5; 2014,Jan,11; 2012,Jul,12-14; 2012,Jan,15-42

**01652** **axillary-brachial aneurysm**
0.00　0.00　**FUD** XXX　C ▣
**AMA:** 2017,Jan,8; 2016,Jan,13; 2015,Jan,16; 2014,Aug,5; 2014,Jan,11; 2012,Jul,12-14; 2012,Jan,15-42

**01654** **bypass graft**
0.00　0.00　**FUD** XXX　C ▣
**AMA:** 2017,Jan,8; 2016,Jan,13; 2015,Jan,16; 2014,Aug,5; 2014,Jan,11; 2012,Jul,12-14; 2012,Jan,15-42

**01656** **axillary-femoral bypass graft**
0.00　0.00　**FUD** XXX　C ▣
**AMA:** 2017,Jan,8; 2016,Jan,13; 2015,Jan,16; 2014,Aug,5; 2014,Jan,11; 2012,Jul,12-14; 2012,Jan,15-42

**01670** **Anesthesia for all procedures on veins of shoulder and axilla**
0.00　0.00　**FUD** XXX　N ▣
**AMA:** 2017,Jan,8; 2016,Jan,13; 2015,Jan,16; 2014,Aug,5; 2014,Jan,11; 2012,Jul,12-14; 2012,Jan,15-42

**01680** **Anesthesia for shoulder cast application, removal or repair, not otherwise specified**
0.00　0.00　**FUD** XXX　N ▣
**AMA:** 2017,Jan,8; 2016,Jan,13; 2015,Jan,16; 2014,Aug,5; 2014,Jan,11; 2012,Jul,12-14; 2012,Jan,15-42

**01682** ~~shoulder spica~~

## 01710-01860 Anesthesia for Upper Extremity Procedures

**CMS:** 100-04,12,140.1 Qualified Nonphysician Anesthetists; 100-04,12,140.3 Payment for Qualified Nonphysician Anesthetists; 100-04,12,140.3.3 Billing Modifiers; 100-04,12,140.3.4 General Billing Instructions; 100-04,12,140.4.1 Anesthesiologist/Qualified Nonphysican Anesthetist; 100-04,12,140.4.2 Anesthetist and Anesthesiologist in a Single Procedure; 100-04,12,140.4.3 Payment for Medical /Surgical Services by CRNAs; 100-04,12,140.4.4 Conversion Factors for Anesthesia Services; 100-04,4,250.3.2 Anesthesia in a Hospital Outpatient Setting

**01710** **Anesthesia for procedures on nerves, muscles, tendons, fascia, and bursae of upper arm and elbow; not otherwise specified**
0.00　0.00　**FUD** XXX　N ▣
**AMA:** 2017,Jan,8; 2016,Jan,13; 2015,Jan,16; 2014,Aug,5; 2014,Jan,11; 2012,Jul,12-14; 2012,Jan,15-42

**01712** **tenotomy, elbow to shoulder, open**
0.00　0.00　**FUD** XXX　N ▣
**AMA:** 2017,Jan,8; 2016,Jan,13; 2015,Jan,16; 2014,Aug,5; 2014,Jan,11; 2012,Jul,12-14; 2012,Jan,15-42

**01714** **tenoplasty, elbow to shoulder**
0.00　0.00　**FUD** XXX　N ▣
**AMA:** 2017,Jan,8; 2016,Jan,13; 2015,Jan,16; 2014,Aug,5; 2014,Jan,11; 2012,Jul,12-14; 2012,Jan,15-42

**01716** **tenodesis, rupture of long tendon of biceps**
0.00　0.00　**FUD** XXX　N ▣
**AMA:** 2017,Jan,8; 2016,Jan,13; 2015,Jan,16; 2014,Aug,5; 2014,Jan,11; 2012,Jul,12-14; 2012,Jan,15-42

**01730** **Anesthesia for all closed procedures on humerus and elbow**
0.00　0.00　**FUD** XXX　N ▣
**AMA:** 2017,Jan,8; 2016,Jan,13; 2015,Jan,16; 2014,Aug,5; 2014,Jan,11; 2012,Jul,12-14; 2012,Jan,15-42

**01732** **Anesthesia for diagnostic arthroscopic procedures of elbow joint**
0.00　0.00　**FUD** XXX　N ▣
**AMA:** 2017,Jan,8; 2016,Jan,13; 2015,Jan,16; 2014,Aug,5; 2014,Jan,11; 2012,Jul,12-14; 2012,Jan,15-42

**01740** **Anesthesia for open or surgical arthroscopic procedures of the elbow; not otherwise specified**
0.00　0.00　**FUD** XXX　N ▣
**AMA:** 2017,Jan,8; 2016,Jan,13; 2015,Jan,16; 2014,Aug,5; 2014,Jan,11; 2012,Jul,12-14; 2012,Jan,15-42

**01742** **osteotomy of humerus**
0.00　0.00　**FUD** XXX　N ▣
**AMA:** 2017,Jan,8; 2016,Jan,13; 2015,Jan,16; 2014,Aug,5; 2014,Jan,11; 2012,Jul,12-14; 2012,Jan,15-42

**01744** **repair of nonunion or malunion of humerus**
0.00　0.00　**FUD** XXX　N ▣
**AMA:** 2017,Jan,8; 2016,Jan,13; 2015,Jan,16; 2014,Aug,5; 2014,Jan,11; 2012,Jul,12-14; 2012,Jan,15-42

**01756** **radical procedures**
0.00　0.00　**FUD** XXX　C ▣
**AMA:** 2017,Jan,8; 2016,Jan,13; 2015,Jan,16; 2014,Aug,5; 2014,Jan,11; 2012,Jul,12-14; 2012,Jan,15-42

**01758** **excision of cyst or tumor of humerus**
0.00　0.00　**FUD** XXX　N ▣
**AMA:** 2017,Jan,8; 2016,Jan,13; 2015,Jan,16; 2014,Aug,5; 2014,Jan,11; 2012,Jul,12-14; 2012,Jan,15-42

**01760** **total elbow replacement**
0.00　0.00　**FUD** XXX　N ▣
**AMA:** 2017,Jan,8; 2016,Jan,13; 2015,Jan,16; 2014,Aug,5; 2014,Jan,11; 2012,Jul,12-14; 2012,Jan,15-42

● New Code　▲ Revised Code　○ Reinstated　● New Web Release　▲ Revised Web Release　Unlisted　Not Covered　# Resequenced
⊘ AMA Mod 51 Exempt　⑤⑩ Optum Mod 51 Exempt　⊛ Mod 63 Exempt　⁄ Non-FDA Drug　★ Telemedicine　Ⓜ Maternity　Ⓐ Age Edit　+ Add-on　AMA: CPT Asst
© 2017 Optum360, LLC　　CPT © 2017 American Medical Association. All Rights Reserved.　　**9**

**01770**   **Anesthesia for procedures on arteries of upper arm and elbow; not otherwise specified**
📁 0.00    ✂ 0.00    **FUD** XXX    N 🖥
**AMA:** 2017,Jan,8; 2016,Jan,13; 2015,Jan,16; 2014,Aug,5; 2014,Jan,11; 2012,Jul,12-14; 2012,Jan,15-42

**01772**   **embolectomy**
📁 0.00    ✂ 0.00    **FUD** XXX    N 🖥
**AMA:** 2017,Jan,8; 2016,Jan,13; 2015,Jan,16; 2014,Aug,5; 2014,Jan,11; 2012,Jul,12-14; 2012,Jan,15-42

**01780**   **Anesthesia for procedures on veins of upper arm and elbow; not otherwise specified**
📁 0.00    ✂ 0.00    **FUD** XXX    N 🖥
**AMA:** 2017,Jan,8; 2016,Jan,13; 2015,Jan,16; 2014,Aug,5; 2014,Jan,11; 2012,Jul,12-14; 2012,Jan,15-42

**01782**   **phleborrhaphy**
📁 0.00    ✂ 0.00    **FUD** XXX    N 🖥
**AMA:** 2017,Jan,8; 2016,Jan,13; 2015,Jan,16; 2014,Aug,5; 2014,Jan,11; 2012,Jul,12-14; 2012,Jan,15-42

**01810**   **Anesthesia for all procedures on nerves, muscles, tendons, fascia, and bursae of forearm, wrist, and hand**
📁 0.00    ✂ 0.00    **FUD** XXX    N 🖥
**AMA:** 2017,Jan,8; 2016,Jan,13; 2015,Jan,16; 2014,Aug,5; 2014,Jan,11; 2012,Jul,12-14; 2012,Jan,15-42

**01820**   **Anesthesia for all closed procedures on radius, ulna, wrist, or hand bones**
📁 0.00    ✂ 0.00    **FUD** XXX    N 🖥
**AMA:** 2017,Jan,8; 2016,Jan,13; 2015,Jan,16; 2014,Aug,5; 2014,Jan,11; 2012,Jul,12-14; 2012,Jan,15-42

**01829**   **Anesthesia for diagnostic arthroscopic procedures on the wrist**
📁 0.00    ✂ 0.00    **FUD** XXX    N 🖥
**AMA:** 2017,Jan,8; 2016,Jan,13; 2015,Jan,16; 2014,Aug,5; 2014,Jan,11; 2012,Jul,12-14; 2012,Jan,15-42

**01830**   **Anesthesia for open or surgical arthroscopic/endoscopic procedures on distal radius, distal ulna, wrist, or hand joints; not otherwise specified**
📁 0.00    ✂ 0.00    **FUD** XXX    N 🖥
**AMA:** 2017,Jan,8; 2016,Jan,13; 2015,Jan,16; 2014,Aug,5; 2014,Jan,11; 2012,Jul,12-14; 2012,Jan,15-42

**01832**   **total wrist replacement**
📁 0.00    ✂ 0.00    **FUD** XXX    N 🖥
**AMA:** 2017,Jan,8; 2016,Jan,13; 2015,Jan,16; 2014,Aug,5; 2014,Jan,11; 2012,Jul,12-14; 2012,Jan,15-42

**01840**   **Anesthesia for procedures on arteries of forearm, wrist, and hand; not otherwise specified**
📁 0.00    ✂ 0.00    **FUD** XXX    N 🖥
**AMA:** 2017,Jan,8; 2016,Jan,13; 2015,Jan,16; 2014,Aug,5; 2014,Jan,11; 2012,Jul,12-14; 2012,Jan,15-42

**01842**   **embolectomy**
📁 0.00    ✂ 0.00    **FUD** XXX    N 🖥
**AMA:** 2017,Jan,8; 2016,Jan,13; 2015,Jan,16; 2014,Aug,5; 2014,Jan,11; 2012,Jul,12-14; 2012,Jan,15-42

**01844**   **Anesthesia for vascular shunt, or shunt revision, any type (eg, dialysis)**
📁 0.00    ✂ 0.00    **FUD** XXX    N 🖥
**AMA:** 2017,Jan,8; 2016,Jan,13; 2015,Jan,16; 2014,Aug,5; 2014,Jan,11; 2012,Jul,12-14; 2012,Jan,15-42

**01850**   **Anesthesia for procedures on veins of forearm, wrist, and hand; not otherwise specified**
📁 0.00    ✂ 0.00    **FUD** XXX    N 🖥
**AMA:** 2017,Jan,8; 2016,Jan,13; 2015,Jan,16; 2014,Aug,5; 2014,Jan,11; 2012,Jul,12-14; 2012,Jan,15-42

**01852**   **phleborrhaphy**
📁 0.00    ✂ 0.00    **FUD** XXX    N 🖥
**AMA:** 2017,Jan,8; 2016,Jan,13; 2015,Jan,16; 2014,Aug,5; 2014,Jan,11; 2012,Jul,12-14; 2012,Jan,15-42

**01860**   **Anesthesia for forearm, wrist, or hand cast application, removal, or repair**
📁 0.00    ✂ 0.00    **FUD** XXX    N 🖥
**AMA:** 2017,Jan,8; 2016,Jan,13; 2015,Jan,16; 2014,Aug,5; 2014,Jan,11; 2012,Jul,12-14; 2012,Jan,15-42

## 01916-01936 Anesthesia for Interventional Radiology Procedures

**CMS:** 100-04,12,140.1 Qualified Nonphysician Anesthetists; 100-04,12,140.3 Payment for Qualified Nonphysician Anesthetists; 100-04,12,140.3.3 Billing Modifiers; 100-04,12,140.3.4 General Billing Instructions; 100-04,12,140.4.1 Anesthesiologist/Qualified Nonphysican Anesthetist; 100-04,12,140.4.2 Anesthetist and Anesthesiologist in a Single Procedure; 100-04,12,140.4.3 Payment for Medical /Surgical Services by CRNAs; 100-04,12,140.4.4 Conversion Factors for Anesthesia Services; 100-04,4,250.3.2 Anesthesia in a Hospital Outpatient Setting

**01916**   **Anesthesia for diagnostic arteriography/venography**
*EXCLUDES* *Anesthesia for therapeutic interventional radiological procedures involving the arterial system (01924-01926)*
*Anesthesia for therapeutic interventional radiological procedures involving the venous/lymphatic system (01930-01933)*
📁 0.00    ✂ 0.00    **FUD** XXX    N 🖥
**AMA:** 2017,Jan,8; 2016,Jan,13; 2015,Jan,16; 2014,Aug,5; 2014,Jan,11; 2012,Jul,12-14; 2012,Jan,15-42

**01920**   **Anesthesia for cardiac catheterization including coronary angiography and ventriculography (not to include Swan-Ganz catheter)**
📁 0.00    ✂ 0.00    **FUD** XXX    N 🖥
**AMA:** 2017,Jan,8; 2016,Jan,13; 2015,Jan,16; 2014,Aug,5; 2014,Jan,11; 2012,Jul,12-14; 2012,Jan,15-42

**01922**   **Anesthesia for non-invasive imaging or radiation therapy**
📁 0.00    ✂ 0.00    **FUD** XXX    N 🖥
**AMA:** 2017,Jan,8; 2016,Jan,13; 2015,Jan,16; 2014,Aug,5; 2014,Jan,11; 2012,Jul,12-14; 2012,Jan,15-42

**01924**   **Anesthesia for therapeutic interventional radiological procedures involving the arterial system; not otherwise specified**
📁 0.00    ✂ 0.00    **FUD** XXX    N 🖥
**AMA:** 2017,Jan,8; 2016,Jan,13; 2015,Jan,16; 2014,Aug,5; 2014,Jan,11; 2012,Jul,12-14; 2012,Jan,15-42

**01925**   **carotid or coronary**
📁 0.00    ✂ 0.00    **FUD** XXX    N 🖥
**AMA:** 2017,Jan,8; 2016,Jan,13; 2015,Jan,16; 2014,Aug,5; 2014,Jan,11; 2012,Jul,12-14; 2012,Jan,15-42

**01926**   **intracranial, intracardiac, or aortic**
📁 0.00    ✂ 0.00    **FUD** XXX    N 🖥
**AMA:** 2017,Jan,8; 2016,Jan,13; 2015,Jan,16; 2014,Aug,5; 2014,Jan,11; 2012,Jul,12-14; 2012,Jan,15-42

**01930**   **Anesthesia for therapeutic interventional radiological procedures involving the venous/lymphatic system (not to include access to the central circulation); not otherwise specified**
📁 0.00    ✂ 0.00    **FUD** XXX    N 🖥
**AMA:** 2017,Jan,8; 2016,Jan,13; 2015,Jan,16; 2014,Aug,5; 2014,Jan,11; 2012,Jul,12-14; 2012,Jan,15-42

**01931**   **intrahepatic or portal circulation (eg, transvenous intrahepatic portosystemic shunt[s] [TIPS])**
📁 0.00    ✂ 0.00    **FUD** XXX    N 🖥
**AMA:** 2017,Jan,8; 2016,Jan,13; 2015,Jan,16; 2014,Aug,5; 2014,Jan,11; 2012,Jul,12-14; 2012,Jan,15-42

**01932**   **intrathoracic or jugular**
📁 0.00    ✂ 0.00    **FUD** XXX    N 🖥
**AMA:** 2017,Jan,8; 2016,Jan,13; 2015,Jan,16; 2014,Aug,5; 2014,Jan,11; 2012,Jul,12-14; 2012,Jan,15-42

**01933**   **intracranial**
📁 0.00    ✂ 0.00    **FUD** XXX    N 🖥
**AMA:** 2017,Jan,8; 2016,Jan,13; 2015,Jan,16; 2014,Aug,5; 2014,Jan,11; 2012,Jul,12-14; 2012,Jan,15-42

**01935**  Anesthesia for percutaneous image guided procedures on the spine and spinal cord; diagnostic
🔵 0.00   ⚕ 0.00   **FUD** XXX                              Ⓝ🔲
**AMA:** 2017,Jan,8; 2016,Jan,13; 2015,Jan,16; 2014,Aug,5; 2014,Jan,11; 2012,Jul,12-14; 2012,Jan,15-42

**01936**  therapeutic
🔵 0.00   ⚕ 0.00   **FUD** XXX                              Ⓝ🔲
**AMA:** 2017,Jan,8; 2016,Jan,13; 2015,Jan,16; 2014,Aug,5; 2014,Jan,11; 2012,Jul,12-14; 2012,Jan,15-42

## 01951-01953 Anesthesia for Burn Procedures

**CMS:** 100-04,12,140.1 Qualified Nonphysician Anesthetists; 100-04,12,140.3 Payment for Qualified Nonphysician Anesthetists; 100-04,12,140.3.3 Billing Modifiers; 100-04,12,140.3.4 General Billing Instructions; 100-04,12,140.4.1 Anesthesiologist/Qualified Nonphysican Anesthetist; 100-04,12,140.4.2 Anesthetist and Anesthesiologist in a Single Procedure; 100-04,12,140.4.3 Payment for Medical /Surgical Services by CRNAs; 100-04,12,140.4.4 Conversion Factors for Anesthesia Services; 100-04,4,250.3.2 Anesthesia in a Hospital Outpatient Setting

**01951**  Anesthesia for second- and third-degree burn excision or debridement with or without skin grafting, any site, for total body surface area (TBSA) treated during anesthesia and surgery; less than 4% total body surface area
🔵 0.00   ⚕ 0.00   **FUD** XXX                              Ⓝ🔲
**AMA:** 2017,Jan,8; 2016,Jan,13; 2015,Jan,16; 2014,Aug,5; 2014,Jan,11; 2012,Jul,12-14; 2012,Jan,15-42

**01952**  between 4% and 9% of total body surface area
🔵 0.00   ⚕ 0.00   **FUD** XXX                              Ⓝ🔲
**AMA:** 2017,Jan,8; 2016,Jan,13; 2015,Jan,16; 2014,Aug,5; 2014,Jan,11; 2012,Jul,12-14; 2012,Jan,15-42

**+ 01953**  each additional 9% total body surface area or part thereof (List separately in addition to code for primary procedure)
Code first (01952)
🔵 0.00   ⚕ 0.00   **FUD** XXX                              Ⓝ🔲
**AMA:** 2017,Jan,8; 2016,Jan,13; 2015,Jan,16; 2014,Aug,5; 2014,Jan,11; 2012,Jul,12-14; 2012,Jan,15-42

## 01958-01969 Anesthesia for Obstetric Procedures

**CMS:** 100-04,12,140.1 Qualified Nonphysician Anesthetists; 100-04,12,140.3 Payment for Qualified Nonphysician Anesthetists; 100-04,12,140.3.3 Billing Modifiers; 100-04,12,140.3.4 General Billing Instructions; 100-04,12,140.4.1 Anesthesiologist/Qualified Nonphysican Anesthetist; 100-04,12,140.4.2 Anesthetist and Anesthesiologist in a Single Procedure; 100-04,12,140.4.3 Payment for Medical /Surgical Services by CRNAs; 100-04,12,140.4.4 Conversion Factors for Anesthesia Services; 100-04,4,250.3.2 Anesthesia in a Hospital Outpatient Setting

**01958**  Anesthesia for external cephalic version procedure        Ⓜ
🔵 0.00   ⚕ 0.00   **FUD** XXX                              Ⓝ🔲
**AMA:** 2017,Jan,8; 2016,Jan,13; 2015,Jan,16; 2014,Aug,5; 2014,Jan,11; 2012,Jul,12-14; 2012,Jan,15-42

**01960**  Anesthesia for vaginal delivery only                    Ⓜ ♀
🔵 0.00   ⚕ 0.00   **FUD** XXX                              Ⓝ🔲
**AMA:** 2017,Jan,8; 2016,Jan,13; 2015,Jan,16; 2014,Aug,5; 2014,Jan,11; 2012,Jul,12-14; 2012,Jan,15-42

**01961**  Anesthesia for cesarean delivery only                   Ⓜ ♀
🔵 0.00   ⚕ 0.00   **FUD** XXX                              Ⓝ🔲
**AMA:** 2017,Jan,8; 2016,Jan,13; 2015,Jan,16; 2014,Aug,5; 2014,Jan,11; 2012,Jul,12-14; 2012,Jan,15-42

**01962**  Anesthesia for urgent hysterectomy following delivery    Ⓜ ♀
🔵 0.00   ⚕ 0.00   **FUD** XXX                              Ⓝ🔲
**AMA:** 2017,Jan,8; 2016,Jan,13; 2015,Jan,16; 2014,Aug,5; 2014,Jan,11; 2012,Jul,12-14; 2012,Jan,15-42

**01963**  Anesthesia for cesarean hysterectomy without any labor analgesia/anesthesia care        Ⓜ ♀
🔵 0.00   ⚕ 0.00   **FUD** XXX                              Ⓝ🔲
**AMA:** 2017,Jan,8; 2016,Jan,13; 2015,Jan,16; 2014,Aug,5; 2014,Jan,11; 2012,Jul,12-14; 2012,Jan,15-42

**01965**  Anesthesia for incomplete or missed abortion procedures        Ⓜ ♀
🔵 0.00   ⚕ 0.00   **FUD** XXX                              Ⓝ🔲
**AMA:** 2017,Jan,8; 2016,Jan,13; 2015,Jan,16; 2014,Aug,5; 2014,Jan,11; 2012,Jul,12-14; 2012,Jan,15-42

**01966**  Anesthesia for induced abortion procedures              Ⓜ ♀
🔵 0.00   ⚕ 0.00   **FUD** XXX                              Ⓝ🔲
**AMA:** 2017,Jan,8; 2016,Jan,13; 2015,Jan,16; 2014,Aug,5; 2014,Jan,11; 2012,Jul,12-14; 2012,Jan,15-42

**01967**  Neuraxial labor analgesia/anesthesia for planned vaginal delivery (this includes any repeat subarachnoid needle placement and drug injection and/or any necessary replacement of an epidural catheter during labor)        Ⓜ ♀
🔵 0.00   ⚕ 0.00   **FUD** XXX                              Ⓝ🔲
**AMA:** 2017,Jan,8; 2016,Jan,13; 2015,Jan,16; 2014,Oct,14; 2014,Aug,5; 2014,Jan,11; 2012,Jul,12-14; 2012,Jan,15-42

**+ 01968**  Anesthesia for cesarean delivery following neuraxial labor analgesia/anesthesia (List separately in addition to code for primary procedure performed)        Ⓜ ♀
Code first (01967)
🔵 0.00   ⚕ 0.00   **FUD** XXX                              Ⓝ🔲
**AMA:** 2017,Jan,8; 2016,Jan,13; 2015,Jan,16; 2014,Oct,14; 2014,Aug,5; 2014,Jan,11; 2012,Jul,12-14; 2012,Jan,15-42

**+ 01969**  Anesthesia for cesarean hysterectomy following neuraxial labor analgesia/anesthesia (List separately in addition to code for primary procedure performed)        Ⓜ ♀
Code first (01967)
🔵 0.00   ⚕ 0.00   **FUD** XXX                              Ⓝ🔲
**AMA:** 2017,Jan,8; 2016,Jan,13; 2015,Jan,16; 2014,Aug,5; 2014,Jan,11; 2012,Jul,12-14; 2012,Jan,15-42

## 01990-01999 Anesthesia Miscellaneous

**CMS:** 100-04,12,140.1 Qualified Nonphysician Anesthetists; 100-04,12,140.3 Payment for Qualified Nonphysician Anesthetists; 100-04,12,140.3.3 Billing Modifiers; 100-04,12,140.3.4 General Billing Instructions; 100-04,12,140.4.1 Anesthesiologist/Qualified Nonphysican Anesthetist; 100-04,12,140.4.2 Anesthetist and Anesthesiologist in a Single Procedure; 100-04,12,140.4.3 Payment for Medical /Surgical Services by CRNAs; 100-04,12,140.4.4 Conversion Factors for Anesthesia Services; 100-04,4,250.3.2 Anesthesia in a Hospital Outpatient Setting

**01990**  Physiological support for harvesting of organ(s) from brain-dead patient
🔵 0.00   ⚕ 0.00   **FUD** XXX                              Ⓒ🔲
**AMA:** 2017,Jan,8; 2016,Jan,13; 2015,Jan,16; 2014,Aug,5; 2014,Jan,11; 2012,Jul,12-14; 2012,Jan,15-42

**01991**  Anesthesia for diagnostic or therapeutic nerve blocks and injections (when block or injection is performed by a different physician or other qualified health care professional); other than the prone position
*EXCLUDES*  Bier block for pain management (64999)
Moderate Sedation (99151-99153, 99155-99157)
Pain management via intra-arterial or IV therapy (96373-96374)
Regional or local anesthesia of arms or legs for surgical procedure
🔵 0.00   ⚕ 0.00   **FUD** XXX                              Ⓝ🔲
**AMA:** 2017,Jan,8; 2016,Jan,13; 2015,Jan,16; 2014,Aug,5; 2014,Jan,11; 2012,Jul,12-14; 2012,Jan,15-42

**01992**  prone position
*EXCLUDES*  Bier block for pain management (64999)
Moderate sedation (99151-99153, 99155-99157)
Pain management via intra-arterial or IV therapy (96373-96374)
Regional or local anesthesia of arms or legs for surgical procedure
🔵 0.00   ⚕ 0.00   **FUD** XXX                              Ⓝ🔲
**AMA:** 2017,Jan,8; 2016,Jan,13; 2015,Jan,16; 2014,Aug,5; 2014,Jan,11; 2012,Jul,12-14; 2012,Jan,15-42

● New Code   ▲ Revised Code   ○ Reinstated   ● New Web Release   ▲ Revised Web Release   Unlisted   Not Covered   # Resequenced
⊘ AMA Mod 51 Exempt   ⑤ Optum Mod 51 Exempt   ⑥ Mod 63 Exempt   ✗ Non-FDA Drug   ★ Telemedicine   Ⓜ Maternity   Ⓐ Age Edit   + Add-on   **AMA:** CPT Asst
© 2017 Optum360, LLC                    CPT © 2017 American Medical Association. All Rights Reserved.                    11

**01996** **Daily hospital management of epidural or subarachnoid continuous drug administration**

> INCLUDES Continuous epidural or subarachnoid drug services performed after insertion of an epidural or subarachnoid catheter

🚑 0.00   ⚕ 0.00   **FUD** XXX    N 💬

**AMA:** 2017,Sep,6; 2017,Jan,8; 2016,Jan,13; 2015,May,10; 2015,Jan,16; 2014,Aug,5; 2014,Jan,11; 2012,Oct,14; 2012,Jul,3-6; 2012,Jul,12-14; 2012,Jan,15-42

**01999** **Unlisted anesthesia procedure(s)**

🚑 0.00   ⚕ 0.00   **FUD** XXX    N 💬

**AMA:** 2017,Jan,8; 2016,Jan,13; 2015,May,10; 2015,Jan,16; 2014,Aug,5; 2014,Aug,14; 2014,Jan,11; 2012,Jul,12-14; 2012,Jan,15-42

26/TC PC/TC Only    A2-Z3 ASC Payment    50 Bilateral    ♂ Male Only    ♀ Female Only    🚑 Facility RVU    ⚕ Non-Facility RVU    💬 CCI

**FUD** Follow-up Days    **CMS:** IOM (Pub 100)    A-Y OPPSI    80/80 Surg Assist Allowed / w/Doc    ◣ Lab Crosswalk    ✖ Radiology Crosswalk    ✖ CLIA

12    CPT © 2017 American Medical Association. All Rights Reserved.    © 2017 Optum360, LLC

## 10021-10022 Fine Needle Aspiration

EXCLUDES *Percutaneous localization clip placement during breast biopsy (19081-19086)*
*Percutaneous needle biopsy of:*
*Abdominal or retroperitoneal mass (49180)*
*Bone (20220, 20225)*
*Bone marrow (38220-38221)*
*Epididymis (54800)*
*Kidney (50200)*
*Liver (47000)*
*Lung or mediastinum (32405)*
*Lymph node (38505)*
*Muscle (20206)*
*Nucleus pulposus, paravertebral tissue, intervertebral disc (62267)*
*Pancreas (48102)*
*Pleura (32400)*
*Prostate (55700, 55706)*
*Salivary gland (42400)*
*Spinal cord (62269)*
*Testis (54500)*
*Thyroid (60100)*
*Soft tissue percutaneous fluid drainage by catheter using image guidance (10030)*
*Thyroid cyst (60300)*

**10021** **Fine needle aspiration; without imaging guidance**
(88172-88173)
🔲 2.00   🔲 3.47   **FUD** XXX   T P3 80 📖
**AMA:** 2017,Jan,8; 2016,Jan,13; 2015,Jan,16; 2014,Jan,11; 2012,Jan,15-42

**10022** **with imaging guidance**
(76942, 77002, 77012, 77021)
(88172-88173)
🔲 1.88   🔲 4.00   **FUD** XXX   T P3 80 📖
**AMA:** 2017,Jan,8; 2016,Jan,13; 2015,Jan,16; 2014,Jan,11; 2012,Jan,15-42

## 10030-10180 Treatment of Lesions: Skin and Subcutaneous Tissues

EXCLUDES *Excision benign lesion (11400-11471)*

**10030** **Image-guided fluid collection drainage by catheter (eg, abscess, hematoma, seroma, lymphocele, cyst), soft tissue (eg, extremity, abdominal wall, neck), percutaneous**
INCLUDES Radiologic guidance (75989, 76942, 77002-77003, 77012, 77021)
EXCLUDES *Percutaneous drainage with imaging guidance of:*
*Peritoneal or retroperitoneal collections (49406)*
*Visceral collections (49405)*
*Transvaginal or transrectal drainage with imaging guidance of:*
*Peritoneal or retroperitoneal collections (49407)*
Code also every instance of fluid collection drained using a separate catheter (10030)
🔲 4.47   🔲 19.8   **FUD** 000   T P2 80 📖
**AMA:** 2017,Aug,9; 2017,Jan,8; 2016,Jan,13; 2015,Jan,16; 2014,May,9; 2014,May,3; 2013,Nov,9

**10035** **Placement of soft tissue localization device(s) (eg, clip, metallic pellet, wire/needle, radioactive seeds), percutaneous, including imaging guidance; first lesion**
INCLUDES Radiologic guidance (76942, 77002-77003, 77012, 77021)
EXCLUDES *Sites with a more specific code descriptor, such as the breast*
*Use of code more than one time per site, regardless of the number of markers used*
Code also each additional target on the same or opposite side (10036)
🔲 2.57   🔲 15.2   **FUD** 000   T N1 80 50 📖
**AMA:** 2017,Jan,8; 2016,Jun,3

**+ 10036** **each additional lesion (List separately in addition to code for primary procedure)**
INCLUDES Radiologic guidance (76942, 77002, 77012, 77021)
EXCLUDES *Sites with a more specific code descriptor, such as the breast*
*Use of code more than one time per site, regardless of the number of markers used*
Code first (10035)
🔲 1.28   🔲 13.1   **FUD** ZZZ   N N1 80 📖
**AMA:** 2017,Jan,8; 2016,Jun,3

**10040** **Acne surgery (eg, marsupialization, opening or removal of multiple milia, comedones, cysts, pustules)**
🔲 2.53   🔲 2.89   **FUD** 010   Q1 N1 📖
**AMA:** 2017,Jan,8; 2016,Jan,13; 2015,Jan,16; 2014,Jan,11; 2012,Jan,15-42

**10060** **Incision and drainage of abscess (eg, carbuncle, suppurative hidradenitis, cutaneous or subcutaneous abscess, cyst, furuncle, or paronychia); simple or single**
🔲 2.78   🔲 3.33   **FUD** 010   T P3 📖
**AMA:** 2017,Jan,8; 2016,Jan,13; 2015,Jan,16; 2014,Jan,11; 2012,Oct,12; 2012,Sep,10; 2012,Jan,15-42

**10061** **complicated or multiple**
🔲 5.13   🔲 5.86   **FUD** 010   T P3 📖
**AMA:** 2017,Jan,8; 2016,Jan,13; 2015,Jan,16; 2014,Jan,11; 2012,Oct,12; 2012,Sep,10

**10080** **Incision and drainage of pilonidal cyst; simple**
🔲 2.94   🔲 5.08   **FUD** 010   T P3 📖
**AMA:** 2017,Jan,8; 2016,Jan,13; 2015,Jan,16; 2014,Jan,11

**10081** **complicated**
EXCLUDES *Excision of pilonidal cyst (11770-11772)*
🔲 4.85   🔲 7.63   **FUD** 010   T P3 📖
**AMA:** 2017,Jan,8; 2016,Jan,13; 2015,Jan,16; 2014,Jan,11

**10120** **Incision and removal of foreign body, subcutaneous tissues; simple**
🔲 2.95   🔲 4.32   **FUD** 010   T P3 📖
**AMA:** 2017,Jan,8; 2016,Jan,13; 2015,Jan,16; 2014,Jan,11; 2013,Dec,16; 2013,Apr,10-11; 2012,Oct,12; 2012,Sep,10

**10121** **complicated**
EXCLUDES *Debridement associated with a fracture or dislocation (11010-11012)*
*Exploration penetrating wound (20100-20103)*
🔲 5.31   🔲 7.77   **FUD** 010   J A2 📖
**AMA:** 2017,Jan,8; 2016,Jan,13; 2015,Jan,16; 2014,Jan,11; 2013,Dec,16; 2012,Oct,12; 2012,Sep,10

**10140** **Incision and drainage of hematoma, seroma or fluid collection**
(76942, 77002, 77012, 77021)
🔲 3.38   🔲 4.63   **FUD** 010   J P3 📖
**AMA:** 2017,Jan,8; 2016,Jan,13; 2015,Jan,16; 2014,Nov,5; 2014,Jan,11; 2012,Jan,15-42

Hematoma may be decompressed with a hemostat

Drain may be placed to allow further drainage

● New Code  ▲ Revised Code  ○ Reinstated  ● New Web Release  ▲ Revised Web Release  Unlisted  Not Covered  # Resequenced
⊘ AMA Mod 51 Exempt  ⑤ Optum Mod 51 Exempt  ⑥ Mod 63 Exempt  ✗ Non-FDA Drug  ★ Telemedicine  Ⓜ Maternity  Ⓐ Age Edit  + Add-on  **AMA:** CPT Asst
© 2017 Optum360, LLC        CPT © 2017 American Medical Association. All Rights Reserved.        **13**

**10160** Puncture aspiration of abscess, hematoma, bulla, or cyst

　(76942, 77002, 77012, 77021)

　2.74　　3.68　**FUD** 010　　　　　　T P3 🖵

**AMA:** 2017,Aug,9; 2017,Jan,8; 2016,Jan,13; 2015,Jan,16; 2014,Jan,11; 2012,Jan,15-42

**10180** Incision and drainage, complex, postoperative wound infection

　*EXCLUDES*　*Wound dehiscence (12020-12021, 13160)*

　5.12　　7.00　**FUD** 010　　　　　　J A2 🖵

**AMA:** 2017,Jan,8; 2016,Jan,13; 2015,Jan,16; 2014,Nov,5; 2014,Jan,11; 2012,Jan,15-42

## 11000-11012 Removal of Foreign Substances and Infected/Devitalized Tissue

*EXCLUDES*　Debridement of:
　*Burns (16000-16030)*
　*Deeper tissue (11042-11047 [11045, 11046])*
　*Nails (11720-11721)*
　*Skin only (97597-97598)*
　*Wounds (11042-11047 [11045, 11046])*
　*Dermabrasions (15780-15783)*
　*Pressure ulcer excision (15920-15999)*

**11000** Debridement of extensive eczematous or infected skin; up to 10% of body surface

　*EXCLUDES*　*Necrotizing soft tissue infection of:*
　　*Abdominal wall (11005-11006)*
　　*External genitalia and perineum (11004, 11006)*

　0.82　　1.54　**FUD** 000　　　　　　T P3 🖵

**AMA:** 2017,Jan,8; 2016,Jan,13; 2015,Jan,16; 2014,Jan,11; 2012,Oct,3-8

**+ 11001** each additional 10% of the body surface, or part thereof (List separately in addition to code for primary procedure)

　*EXCLUDES*　*Necrotizing soft tissue infection of:*
　　*Abdominal wall (11005-11006)*
　　*External genitalia and perineum (11004, 11006)*

　Code first (11000)

　0.41　　0.61　**FUD** ZZZ　　　　　　N N1 🖵

**AMA:** 2017,Jan,8; 2016,Jan,13; 2015,Jan,16; 2014,Jan,11; 2012,Oct,3-8

**11004** Debridement of skin, subcutaneous tissue, muscle and fascia for necrotizing soft tissue infection; external genitalia and perineum

　*EXCLUDES*　*Skin grafts or flaps (14000-14350, 15040-15770)*

　16.7　　16.7　**FUD** 000　　　　　　C 🖵

**AMA:** 2017,Jan,8; 2016,Jan,13; 2015,Jan,16; 2014,Jan,11; 2013,Oct,15; 2012,Oct,3-8; 2012,Jan,6-10

**11005** abdominal wall, with or without fascial closure

　*EXCLUDES*　*Skin grafts or flaps (14000-14350, 15040-15770)*

　22.6　　22.6　**FUD** 000　　　　　　C 80 🖵

**AMA:** 2017,Jan,8; 2016,Jan,13; 2015,Jan,16; 2014,Jan,11; 2013,Oct,15; 2012,Oct,3-8; 2012,Jan,6-10

**11006** external genitalia, perineum and abdominal wall, with or without fascial closure

　*EXCLUDES*　*Orchiectomy (54520)*
　　*Skin grafts or flaps (14000-14350, 15040-15770)*
　　*Testicular transplant (54680)*

　20.4　　20.4　**FUD** 000　　　　　　C 🖵

**AMA:** 2017,Jan,8; 2016,Jan,13; 2015,Jan,16; 2014,Jan,11; 2013,Oct,15; 2012,Oct,3-8; 2012,Jan,6-10

**+ 11008** Removal of prosthetic material or mesh, abdominal wall for infection (eg, for chronic or recurrent mesh infection or necrotizing soft tissue infection) (List separately in addition to code for primary procedure)

　*EXCLUDES*　*Debridement (11000-11001, 11010-11044 [11045, 11046])*
　　*Insertion of mesh (49568)*
　　*Skin grafts or flaps (14000-14350, 15040-15770)*

　Code first (10180, 11004-11006)

　7.97　　7.97　**FUD** ZZZ　　　　　　C 80 🖵

**AMA:** 2017,Jan,8; 2016,Jan,13; 2015,Jan,16; 2014,Jan,11; 2012,Oct,3-8; 2012,Jan,6-10

**11010** Debridement including removal of foreign material at the site of an open fracture and/or an open dislocation (eg, excisional debridement); skin and subcutaneous tissues

　8.20　　14.3　**FUD** 010　　　　　　T A2 🖵

**AMA:** 2017,Jan,8; 2016,Jan,13; 2015,Jan,16; 2014,Jan,11; 2012,Oct,3-8; 2012,Oct,13; 2012,Jan,15-42

**11011** skin, subcutaneous tissue, muscle fascia, and muscle

　8.65　　15.2　**FUD** 000　　　　　　T A2 🖵

**AMA:** 2017,Jan,8; 2016,Jan,13; 2015,Jan,16; 2014,Jan,11; 2012,Oct,13; 2012,Oct,3-8

**11012** skin, subcutaneous tissue, muscle fascia, muscle, and bone

　12.3　　20.2　**FUD** 000　　　　　　J A2 🖵

**AMA:** 2017,Jan,8; 2016,Jan,13; 2015,Jan,16; 2014,Jan,11; 2012,Oct,3-8; 2012,Oct,13; 2012,Jan,15-42

## 11042-11047 [11045, 11046] Removal of Infected/Devitalized Tissue

*INCLUDES*　Debridement reported by the size and depth
　Debridement reported for multiple wounds by adding the total surface area of wounds of the same depth
　Injuries, wounds, chronic ulcers, infections

*EXCLUDES*　Debridement of:
　*Burn (16020-16030)*
　*Eczematous or infected skin (11000-11001)*
　*Nails (11720-11721)*
　*Necrotizing soft tissue infection of external genitalia, perineum, or abdominal wall (11004-11006)*
　*Non-elective debridement/active care management of same wound (97597-97602)*
　*Dermabrasions (15780-15783)*
　*Excision of pressure ulcers (15920-15999)*
　Code also each additional single wound of different depths
　Code also modifier 59 for additional wound debridement
　Code also multiple wound groups of different depths

**11042** Debridement, subcutaneous tissue (includes epidermis and dermis, if performed); first 20 sq cm or less

　1.77　　3.30　**FUD** 000　　　　　　T A2 🖵

**AMA:** 2017,Jan,8; 2016,Oct,3; 2016,Aug,9; 2016,Feb,13; 2016,Jan,13; 2015,Jan,16; 2014,Nov,5; 2014,Jan,11; 2013,Oct,15; 2013,Sep,17; 2013,Feb,16-17; 2012,Oct,3-8; 2012,Oct,13; 2012,Mar,3; 2012,Jan,15-42; 2012,Jan,6-10

**+ # 11045** each additional 20 sq cm, or part thereof (List separately in addition to code for primary procedure)

　Code first (11042)

　0.75　　1.16　**FUD** ZZZ　　　　　　N N1 80 🖵

**AMA:** 2017,Jan,8; 2016,Oct,3; 2016,Aug,9; 2016,Jan,13; 2015,Jan,16; 2014,Nov,5; 2014,Jan,11; 2013,Feb,16-17; 2012,Oct,13; 2012,Oct,3-8; 2012,Mar,3; 2012,Jan,6-10

**11043** Debridement, muscle and/or fascia (includes epidermis, dermis, and subcutaneous tissue, if performed); first 20 sq cm or less

　4.48　　6.48　**FUD** 000　　　　　　T A2 🖵

**AMA:** 2017,Jan,8; 2016,Oct,3; 2016,Aug,9; 2016,Jan,13; 2015,Jan,16; 2014,Nov,5; 2014,Jan,11; 2013,Feb,16-17; 2012,Oct,13; 2012,Oct,3-8; 2012,Mar,3; 2012,Jan,6-10; 2012,Jan,15-42

26/TC PC/TC Only　　A2-Z3 ASC Payment　　50 Bilateral　　♂ Male Only　　♀ Female Only　　🔧 Facility RVU　　Non-Facility RVU　　🖵 CCI
**FUD** Follow-up Days　　**CMS:** IOM (Pub 100)　　A-Y OPPSI　　80/80 Surg Assist Allowed / w/Doc　　Lab Crosswalk　　Radiology Crosswalk　　CLIA
**14**　　　　　　　　　　　　　　　　　　　　CPT © 2017 American Medical Association. All Rights Reserved.　　　　　　　　　© 2017 Optum360, LLC

**+ #  11046**    **each additional 20 sq cm, or part thereof (List separately in addition to code for primary procedure)**

Code first (11043)

🔧 1.62    ⚖ 2.09    **FUD** ZZZ                    N  N1  80 📋

**AMA:** 2017,Jan,8; 2016,Oct,3; 2016,Aug,9; 2016,Jan,13; 2015,Jan,16; 2014,Nov,5; 2014,Jan,11; 2013,Feb,16-17; 2012,Oct,13; 2012,Oct,3-8; 2012,Mar,3; 2012,Jan,6-10

**11044**    **Debridement, bone (includes epidermis, dermis, subcutaneous tissue, muscle and/or fascia, if performed); first 20 sq cm or less**

🔧 6.65    ⚖ 8.94    **FUD** 000                    J  A2 📋

**AMA:** 2017,Jan,8; 2016,Oct,3; 2016,Aug,9; 2016,Jan,13; 2015,Jan,16; 2014,Nov,5; 2014,Jan,11; 2013,Feb,16-17; 2012,Oct,13; 2012,Oct,3-8; 2012,Mar,3; 2012,Jan,6-10; 2012,Jan,15-42

*11045*    **Resequenced code. See code following 11042.**

*11046*    **Resequenced code. See code following 11043.**

**+  11047**    **each additional 20 sq cm, or part thereof (List separately in addition to code for primary procedure)**

Code first (11044)

🔧 2.88    ⚖ 3.55    **FUD** ZZZ                    N  N1  80 📋

**AMA:** 2017,Jan,8; 2016,Oct,3; 2016,Aug,9; 2016,Jan,13; 2015,Jan,16; 2014,Nov,5; 2014,Jan,11; 2012,Oct,13; 2012,Oct,3-8; 2012,Mar,3; 2012,Jan,6-10; 2012,Jan,15-42

## 11055-11057 Excision Benign Hypertrophic Skin Lesions

**CMS:** 100-04,32,80.8 CSF Edits: Routine Foot Care

*EXCLUDES*    *Destruction (17000-17004)*

**11055**    **Paring or cutting of benign hyperkeratotic lesion (eg, corn or callus); single lesion**

🔧 0.46    ⚖ 1.35    **FUD** 000                    01  N1 📋

**AMA:** 2017,Jan,8; 2016,Jan,13; 2015,Jan,16; 2014,Jan,11; 2012,Jan,15-42

**11056**    **2 to 4 lesions**

🔧 0.65    ⚖ 1.65    **FUD** 000                    01  N1 📋

**AMA:** 2017,Jan,8; 2016,Jan,13; 2015,Jan,16; 2014,Jan,11; 2012,Jan,15-42

**11057**    **more than 4 lesions**

🔧 0.85    ⚖ 1.85    **FUD** 000                    T  P3 📋

**AMA:** 2017,Jan,8; 2016,Jan,13; 2015,Jan,16; 2014,Jan,11

## 11100-11101 Surgical Biopsy Skin and Mucous Membranes

*INCLUDES*    Attaining tissue for pathologic exam

*EXCLUDES*    *Biopsies performed during related procedures*
*Biopsy of:*
*Conjunctiva (68100)*
*Eyelid ([67810])*

**11100**    **Biopsy of skin, subcutaneous tissue and/or mucous membrane (including simple closure), unless otherwise listed; single lesion**

🔧 1.41    ⚖ 2.93    **FUD** 000                    T  P3 📋

**AMA:** 2017,Jan,8; 2016,Jan,13; 2015,Jan,16; 2014,Jan,11; 2013,Mar,6-7; 2013,Feb,16-17

**+  11101**    **each separate/additional lesion (List separately in addition to code for primary procedure)**

Code first (11100)

🔧 0.72    ⚖ 0.93    **FUD** ZZZ                    N  N1 📋

**AMA:** 2017,Jan,8; 2016,Jan,13; 2015,Jan,16; 2014,Jan,11; 2013,Mar,6-7; 2013,Feb,16-17

## 11200-11201 Skin Tag Removal - All Techniques

*INCLUDES*    Chemical destruction
Electrocauterization
Electrosurgical destruction
Ligature strangulation
Removal with or without local anesthesia
Sharp excision or scissoring

*EXCLUDES*    *Extensive or complicated secondary wound closure (13160)*

**11200**    **Removal of skin tags, multiple fibrocutaneous tags, any area; up to and including 15 lesions**

🔧 2.11    ⚖ 2.51    **FUD** 010                    01  N1 📋

**AMA:** 2017,Jan,8; 2016,Jan,13; 2015,Jan,16; 2014,Jan,11; 2012,Jan,15-42

**+  11201**    **each additional 10 lesions, or part thereof (List separately in addition to code for primary procedure)**

Code first (11200)

🔧 0.48    ⚖ 0.54    **FUD** ZZZ                    N  N1 📋

**AMA:** 2017,Jan,8; 2016,Jan,13; 2015,Jan,16; 2014,Jan,11; 2012,Jan,15-42

## 11300-11313 Skin Lesion Removal: Shaving

*INCLUDES*    Local anesthesia
Partial thickness excision by horizontal slicing
Wound cauterization

**11300**    **Shaving of epidermal or dermal lesion, single lesion, trunk, arms or legs; lesion diameter 0.5 cm or less**

🔧 1.02    ⚖ 2.78    **FUD** 000                    01  N1  80 📋

**AMA:** 2017,Jan,8; 2016,Jan,13; 2015,Jan,16; 2014,Jan,11; 2012,Jan,15-42

Shave excision of an elevated lesion; technique also used to biopsy

Elliptical excision is often used when tissue removal is larger than 4 mm or when deep pathology is suspected

A punch biopsy cuts a core of tissue as the tool is twisted downward

**11301**    **lesion diameter 0.6 to 1.0 cm**

🔧 1.55    ⚖ 3.42    **FUD** 000                    01  N1  80 📋

**AMA:** 2017,Jan,8; 2016,Jan,13; 2015,Jan,16; 2014,Jan,11; 2012,Jan,15-42

**11302**    **lesion diameter 1.1 to 2.0 cm**

🔧 1.82    ⚖ 4.03    **FUD** 000                    01  N1  80 📋

**AMA:** 2017,Jan,8; 2016,Jan,13; 2015,Jan,16; 2014,Jan,11; 2012,Jan,15-42

**11303**    **lesion diameter over 2.0 cm**

🔧 2.15    ⚖ 4.45    **FUD** 000                    01  N1  80 📋

**AMA:** 2017,Jan,8; 2016,Jan,13; 2015,Jan,16; 2014,Jan,11; 2012,Jan,15-42

**11305**    **Shaving of epidermal or dermal lesion, single lesion, scalp, neck, hands, feet, genitalia; lesion diameter 0.5 cm or less**

🔧 1.13    ⚖ 2.81    **FUD** 000                    01  N1  80 📋

**AMA:** 2017,Jan,8; 2016,Jan,13; 2015,Jan,16; 2014,Jan,11; 2012,Jan,15-42

**11306**    **lesion diameter 0.6 to 1.0 cm**

🔧 1.50    ⚖ 3.48    **FUD** 000                    01  N1  80 📋

**AMA:** 2017,Jan,8; 2016,Jan,13; 2015,Jan,16; 2014,Jan,11; 2012,Jan,15-42

**11307**    **lesion diameter 1.1 to 2.0 cm**

🔧 1.93    ⚖ 4.09    **FUD** 000                    T  P2  80 📋

**AMA:** 2017,Jan,8; 2016,Jan,13; 2015,Jan,16; 2014,Jan,11; 2012,Jan,15-42

**11308**    **lesion diameter over 2.0 cm**

🔧 2.12    ⚖ 4.29    **FUD** 000                    01  N1  80 📋

**AMA:** 2017,Jan,8; 2016,Jan,13; 2015,Jan,16; 2014,Jan,11; 2012,Jan,15-42

● New Code    ▲ Revised Code    ○ Reinstated    ● New Web Release    ▲ Revised Web Release    Unlisted    Not Covered    # Resequenced
⊘ AMA Mod 51 Exempt    ⑤ Optum Mod 51 Exempt    ⑤ Mod 63 Exempt    ✗ Non-FDA Drug    ★ Telemedicine    M Maternity    A Age Edit    + Add-on    AMA: CPT Asst
© 2017 Optum360, LLC                    CPT © 2017 American Medical Association. All Rights Reserved.                    15

**11310** Shaving of epidermal or dermal lesion, single lesion, face, ears, eyelids, nose, lips, mucous membrane; lesion diameter 0.5 cm or less

  🚑 1.37    ✂ 3.24   **FUD** 000        T P2 80 ▣

**AMA:** 2017,Jan,8; 2016,Jan,13; 2015,Jan,16; 2014,Jan,11; 2013,Mar,6-7; 2013,Feb,16-17; 2012,Jan,15-42

**11311** lesion diameter 0.6 to 1.0 cm

  🚑 1.89    ✂ 3.15   **FUD** 000        T P3 80 ▣

**AMA:** 2017,Jan,8; 2016,Jan,13; 2015,Jan,16; 2014,Jan,11; 2013,Mar,6-7; 2013,Feb,16-17; 2012,Jan,15-42

**11312** lesion diameter 1.1 to 2.0 cm

  🚑 2.26    ✂ 4.57   **FUD** 000        T P3 80 ▣

**AMA:** 2017,Jan,8; 2016,Jan,13; 2015,Jan,16; 2014,Jan,11; 2013,Mar,6-7; 2013,Feb,16-17; 2012,Jan,15-42

**11313** lesion diameter over 2.0 cm

  🚑 2.90    ✂ 5.30   **FUD** 000        T P3 80 ▣

**AMA:** 2017,Jan,8; 2016,Jan,13; 2015,Jan,16; 2014,Jan,11; 2013,Mar,6-7; 2013,Feb,16-17; 2012,Jan,15-42

## 11400-11446 Skin Lesion Removal: Benign

INCLUDES  Biopsy on same lesion
Cicatricial lesion excision
Full thickness removal including margins
Lesion measurement before excision at largest diameter plus margin
Local anesthesia
Simple, nonlayered closure

EXCLUDES  *Adjacent tissue transfer: report only adjacent tissue transfer (14000-14302)*
*Biopsy of eyelid ([67810])*
*Destruction:*
  *Benign lesions, any method (17110-17111)*
  *Cutaneous vascular proliferative lesions (17106-17108)*
  *Destruction of eyelid lesion (67850)*
  *Malignant lesions (17260-17286)*
  *Premalignant lesions (17000, 17003-17004)*
*Escharotomy (16035-16036)*
*Excision and reconstruction of eyelid (67961-67975)*
*Excision of chalazion (67800-67808)*
*Eyelid procedures involving more than skin (67800 and subsequent codes)*
*Laser fenestration for scars (0479T-0480T)*
*Shave removal (11300-11313)*
Code also complex closure (13100-13153)
Code also each separate lesion
Code also intermediate closure (12031-12057)
Code also modifier 22 if excision is complicated or unusual
Code also reconstruction (15002-15261, 15570-15770)

**11400** Excision, benign lesion including margins, except skin tag (unless listed elsewhere), trunk, arms or legs; excised diameter 0.5 cm or less

  🚑 2.31    ✂ 3.52   **FUD** 010        T P3 ▣

**AMA:** 2017,Jan,8; 2016,Apr,3; 2016,Jan,13; 2015,Jan,16; 2014,Mar,4; 2014,Mar,12; 2014,Jan,11; 2012,May,13; 2012,Jan,15-42

**11401** excised diameter 0.6 to 1.0 cm

  🚑 2.98    ✂ 4.23   **FUD** 010        T P3 ▣

**AMA:** 2017,Jan,8; 2016,Apr,3; 2016,Jan,13; 2015,Jan,16; 2014,Mar,4; 2014,Mar,12; 2014,Jan,11; 2012,May,13; 2012,Jan,15-42

**11402** excised diameter 1.1 to 2.0 cm

  🚑 3.27    ✂ 4.71   **FUD** 010        T P3 ▣

**AMA:** 2017,Jan,8; 2016,Apr,3; 2016,Jan,13; 2015,Jan,16; 2014,Mar,4; 2014,Mar,12; 2014,Jan,11; 2012,May,13; 2012,Jan,15-42

**11403** excised diameter 2.1 to 3.0 cm

  🚑 4.23    ✂ 5.45   **FUD** 010        T P3 ▣

**AMA:** 2017,Jan,8; 2016,Apr,3; 2016,Jan,13; 2015,Jan,16; 2014,Mar,4; 2014,Mar,12; 2014,Jan,11; 2012,May,13

**11404** excised diameter 3.1 to 4.0 cm

  🚑 4.66    ✂ 6.19   **FUD** 010        J A2 ▣

**AMA:** 2017,Jan,8; 2016,Apr,3; 2016,Jan,13; 2015,Jan,16; 2014,Mar,4; 2014,Mar,12; 2014,Jan,11; 2012,May,13; 2012,Jan,15-42

**11406** excised diameter over 4.0 cm

  🚑 7.09    ✂ 8.92   **FUD** 010        J A2 ▣

**AMA:** 2017,Jan,8; 2016,Apr,3; 2016,Jan,13; 2015,Jan,16; 2014,Mar,4; 2014,Mar,12; 2014,Jan,11; 2012,May,13; 2012,Jan,15-42

**11420** Excision, benign lesion including margins, except skin tag (unless listed elsewhere), scalp, neck, hands, feet, genitalia; excised diameter 0.5 cm or less

  🚑 2.34    ✂ 3.47   **FUD** 010        J P3 ▣

**AMA:** 2017,Jan,8; 2016,Apr,3; 2016,Jan,13; 2015,Jan,16; 2014,Mar,4; 2014,Mar,12; 2014,Jan,11; 2013,Jan,15-16; 2012,May,13; 2012,Jan,15-42

**11421** excised diameter 0.6 to 1.0 cm

  🚑 3.16    ✂ 4.44   **FUD** 010        T P3 ▣

**AMA:** 2017,Jan,8; 2016,Apr,3; 2016,Jan,13; 2015,Jan,16; 2014,Mar,4; 2014,Mar,12; 2014,Jan,11; 2013,Jan,15-16; 2012,May,13

**11422** excised diameter 1.1 to 2.0 cm

  🚑 3.89    ✂ 4.98   **FUD** 010        J P3 ▣

**AMA:** 2017,Jan,8; 2016,Apr,3; 2016,Jan,13; 2015,Jan,16; 2014,Mar,4; 2014,Mar,12; 2014,Jan,11; 2013,Jan,15-16; 2012,May,13; 2012,Mar,4-7

**11423** excised diameter 2.1 to 3.0 cm

  🚑 4.50    ✂ 5.72   **FUD** 010        J P3 ▣

**AMA:** 2017,Jan,8; 2016,Apr,3; 2016,Jan,13; 2015,Jan,16; 2014,Mar,4; 2014,Mar,12; 2014,Jan,11; 2013,Jan,15-16; 2012,May,13

**11424** excised diameter 3.1 to 4.0 cm

  🚑 5.17    ✂ 6.64   **FUD** 010        J A2 ▣

**AMA:** 2017,Jan,8; 2016,Apr,3; 2016,Jan,13; 2015,Jan,16; 2014,Mar,4; 2014,Mar,12; 2014,Jan,11; 2013,Jan,15-16; 2012,May,13

**11426** excised diameter over 4.0 cm

  🚑 7.90    ✂ 9.49   **FUD** 010        J A2 ▣

**AMA:** 2017,Jan,8; 2016,Apr,3; 2016,Jan,13; 2015,Jan,16; 2014,Mar,4; 2014,Mar,12; 2014,Jan,11; 2013,Jan,15-16; 2012,May,13

**11440** Excision, other benign lesion including margins, except skin tag (unless listed elsewhere), face, ears, eyelids, nose, lips, mucous membrane; excised diameter 0.5 cm or less

  🚑 2.94    ✂ 3.81   **FUD** 010        T P3 ▣

**AMA:** 2017,Jan,8; 2016,Apr,3; 2016,Jan,13; 2015,Jan,16; 2014,Mar,4; 2014,Mar,12; 2014,Jan,11; 2012,May,13; 2012,Jan,15-42

The physician removes a benign lesion from the external ear, nose, or mucous membranes

**11441** excised diameter 0.6 to 1.0 cm

  🚑 3.75    ✂ 4.76   **FUD** 010        T P3 ▣

**AMA:** 2017,Jan,8; 2016,Apr,3; 2016,Jan,13; 2015,Jan,16; 2014,Mar,4; 2014,Mar,12; 2014,Jan,11; 2012,May,13; 2012,Jan,15-42

26/TC PC/TC Only    A2-Z3 ASC Payment    50 Bilateral    ♂ Male Only    ♀ Female Only    🚑 Facility RVU    ✂ Non-Facility RVU    ▣ CCI
**FUD** Follow-up Days    **CMS:** IOM (Pub 100)    A-Y OPPSI    80/80 Surg Assist Allowed / w/Doc    ▪ Lab Crosswalk    ✚ Radiology Crosswalk    ✖ CLIA

**16**            CPT © 2017 American Medical Association. All Rights Reserved.        © 2017 Optum360, LLC

**11442** excised diameter 1.1 to 2.0 cm
📅 4.16  ⚖ 5.33  **FUD** 010  T P3 🏳
**AMA:** 2017,Jan,8; 2016,Apr,3; 2016,Jan,13; 2015,Jan,16; 2014,Mar,4; 2014,Mar,12; 2014,Jan,11; 2012,May,13; 2012,Jan,15-42

**11443** excised diameter 2.1 to 3.0 cm
📅 5.11  ⚖ 6.36  **FUD** 010  J P3 🏳
**AMA:** 2017,Jan,8; 2016,Apr,3; 2016,Jan,13; 2015,Jan,16; 2014,Mar,4; 2014,Mar,12; 2014,Jan,11; 2012,May,13

**11444** excised diameter 3.1 to 4.0 cm
📅 6.52  ⚖ 8.00  **FUD** 010  J A2 🏳
**AMA:** 2017,Jan,8; 2016,Apr,3; 2016,Jan,13; 2015,Jan,16; 2014,Mar,4; 2014,Mar,12; 2014,Jan,11; 2012,May,13

**11446** excised diameter over 4.0 cm
📅 9.36  ⚖ 11.1  **FUD** 010  J A2 🏳
**AMA:** 2017,Jan,8; 2016,Apr,3; 2016,Jan,13; 2015,Jan,16; 2014,Mar,4; 2014,Mar,12; 2014,Jan,11; 2012,May,13; 2012,Jan,15-42

## 11450-11471 Treatment of Hidradenitis: Excision and Repair

Code also closure by skin graft or flap (14000-14350, 15040-15770)

**11450** Excision of skin and subcutaneous tissue for hidradenitis, axillary; with simple or intermediate repair
📅 7.25  ⚖ 10.8  **FUD** 090  J A2 50 🏳
**AMA:** 2017,Jan,8; 2016,Aug,9; 2016,Jan,13; 2015,Jan,16; 2014,Jan,11; 2012,May,13

Hidradenitis is a disease process stemming from clogged specialized sweat glands, principally located in the axilla and groin areas

Hair shaft

Hair matrix

Sweat (eccrine gland)

Hidradenitis of the axilla

**11451** with complex repair
📅 9.34  ⚖ 13.8  **FUD** 090  J A2 80 50 🏳
**AMA:** 2017,Jan,8; 2016,Aug,9; 2016,Jan,13; 2015,Jan,16; 2014,Jan,11; 2012,May,13

**11462** Excision of skin and subcutaneous tissue for hidradenitis, inguinal; with simple or intermediate repair
📅 6.93  ⚖ 10.5  **FUD** 090  J A2 80 50 🏳
**AMA:** 2017,Jan,8; 2016,Aug,9; 2016,Jan,13; 2015,Jan,16; 2014,Jan,11; 2012,May,13

**11463** with complex repair
📅 9.39  ⚖ 13.9  **FUD** 090  J A2 80 50 🏳
**AMA:** 2017,Jan,8; 2016,Aug,9; 2016,Jan,13; 2015,Jan,16; 2014,Jan,11; 2012,May,13

**11470** Excision of skin and subcutaneous tissue for hidradenitis, perianal, perineal, or umbilical; with simple or intermediate repair
📅 8.05  ⚖ 11.7  **FUD** 090  J A2 🏳
**AMA:** 2017,Jan,8; 2016,Aug,9; 2016,Jan,13; 2015,Jan,16; 2014,Jan,11; 2012,May,13

**11471** with complex repair
📅 10.0  ⚖ 14.5  **FUD** 090  J A2 80 🏳
**AMA:** 2017,Jan,8; 2016,Aug,9; 2016,Jan,13; 2015,Jan,16; 2014,Jan,11; 2012,May,13

## 11600-11646 Skin Lesion Removal: Malignant

**INCLUDES** Biopsy on same lesion
Excision of additional margin at same operative session
Full thickness removal including margins
Lesion measurement before excision at largest diameter plus margin
Local anesthesia
Simple, nonlayered closure

**EXCLUDES** *Adjacent tissue transfer. Report only adjacent tissue transfer (14000-14302)*
*Destruction (17260-17286)*
*Excision of additional margin at subsequent operative session (11600-11646)*

Code also complex closure (13100-13153)
Code also each separate lesion
Code also intermediate closure (12031-12057)
Code also modifier 58 if re-excision is performed during postoperative period
Code also reconstruction (15002-15261, 15570-15770)

**11600** Excision, malignant lesion including margins, trunk, arms, or legs; excised diameter 0.5 cm or less
📅 3.43  ⚖ 5.46  **FUD** 010  T P3 🏳
**AMA:** 2017,Jan,8; 2016,Jan,13; 2015,Jan,16; 2014,Mar,4; 2014,Mar,12; 2014,Jan,11; 2012,Jul,12-14; 2012,May,13; 2012,Jan,15-42

**11601** excised diameter 0.6 to 1.0 cm
📅 4.29  ⚖ 6.50  **FUD** 010  T P3 🏳
**AMA:** 2017,Jan,8; 2016,Jan,13; 2015,Jan,16; 2014,Mar,4; 2014,Mar,12; 2014,Jan,11; 2012,May,13; 2012,Jul,12-14; 2012,Mar,4-7

**11602** excised diameter 1.1 to 2.0 cm
📅 4.71  ⚖ 7.05  **FUD** 010  T P2 🏳
**AMA:** 2017,Jan,8; 2016,Jan,13; 2015,Jan,16; 2014,Mar,4; 2014,Mar,12; 2014,Jan,11; 2012,May,13; 2012,Jul,12-14

**11603** excised diameter 2.1 to 3.0 cm
📅 5.65  ⚖ 8.06  **FUD** 010  T P3 🏳
**AMA:** 2017,Jan,8; 2016,Jan,13; 2015,Jan,16; 2014,Mar,4; 2014,Mar,12; 2014,Jan,11; 2012,May,13; 2012,Jul,12-14

**11604** excised diameter 3.1 to 4.0 cm
📅 6.22  ⚖ 8.96  **FUD** 010  T A2 🏳
**AMA:** 2017,Jan,8; 2016,Jan,13; 2015,Jan,16; 2014,Mar,4; 2014,Mar,12; 2014,Jan,11; 2012,May,13; 2012,Jul,12-14

**11606** excised diameter over 4.0 cm
📅 9.24  ⚖ 12.8  **FUD** 010  J A2 🏳
**AMA:** 2017,Jan,8; 2016,Jan,13; 2015,Jan,16; 2014,Mar,4; 2014,Mar,12; 2014,Jan,11; 2012,May,13; 2012,Jul,12-14

**11620** Excision, malignant lesion including margins, scalp, neck, hands, feet, genitalia; excised diameter 0.5 cm or less
📅 3.47  ⚖ 5.51  **FUD** 010  J P3 🏳
**AMA:** 2017,Jan,8; 2016,Jan,13; 2015,Jan,16; 2014,Mar,4; 2014,Mar,12; 2014,Jan,11; 2012,May,13; 2012,Jul,12-14

**11621** excised diameter 0.6 to 1.0 cm
📅 4.32  ⚖ 6.54  **FUD** 010  T P3 🏳
**AMA:** 2017,Jan,8; 2016,Jan,13; 2015,Jan,16; 2014,Mar,4; 2014,Mar,12; 2014,Jan,11; 2012,May,13

**11622** excised diameter 1.1 to 2.0 cm
📅 4.95  ⚖ 7.29  **FUD** 010  T P3 🏳
**AMA:** 2017,Jan,8; 2016,Jan,13; 2015,Jan,16; 2014,Mar,4; 2014,Mar,12; 2014,Jan,11; 2012,May,13

**11623** excised diameter 2.1 to 3.0 cm
📅 6.12  ⚖ 8.55  **FUD** 010  J P3 🏳
**AMA:** 2017,Jan,8; 2016,Jan,13; 2015,Jan,16; 2014,Mar,4; 2014,Mar,12; 2014,Jan,11; 2012,May,13

**11624** excised diameter 3.1 to 4.0 cm
📅 6.94  ⚖ 9.65  **FUD** 010  J A2 🏳
**AMA:** 2017,Jan,8; 2016,Jan,13; 2015,Jan,16; 2014,Mar,4; 2014,Mar,12; 2014,Jan,11; 2012,May,13

**11626** excised diameter over 4.0 cm
📅 8.50  ⚖ 11.6  **FUD** 010  J A2 🏳
**AMA:** 2017,Jan,8; 2016,Jan,13; 2015,Jan,16; 2014,Mar,4; 2014,Mar,12; 2014,Jan,11; 2012,May,13

---

● New Code  ▲ Revised Code  ○ Reinstated  ● New Web Release  ▲ Revised Web Release  Unlisted  Not Covered  # Resequenced
⊘ AMA Mod 51 Exempt  ⑨ Optum Mod 51 Exempt  ⑥ Mod 63 Exempt  ✗ Non-FDA Drug  ★ Telemedicine  Ⓜ Maternity  🅐 Age Edit  + Add-on  **AMA:** CPT Asst

© 2017 Optum360, LLC
CPT © 2017 American Medical Association. All Rights Reserved.

**Integumentary System**

**11640 — 11952**

**11640** Excision, malignant lesion including margins, face, ears, eyelids, nose, lips; excised diameter 0.5 cm or less
   *EXCLUDES* Eyelid excision involving more than skin (67800-67808, 67840-67850, 67961-67966)
   3.59   5.69   **FUD** 010                                 T P3
   **AMA:** 2017,Jan,8; 2016,Jan,13; 2015,Jan,16; 2014,Mar,12; 2014,Mar,4; 2014,Jan,11; 2012,May,13

**11641** excised diameter 0.6 to 1.0 cm
   *EXCLUDES* Eyelid excision involving more than skin (67800-67808, 67840-67850, 67961-67966)
   4.50   6.76   **FUD** 010                                 T P3
   **AMA:** 2017,Jan,8; 2016,Jan,13; 2015,Jan,16; 2014,Mar,12; 2014,Mar,4; 2014,Jan,11; 2012,May,13

**11642** excised diameter 1.1 to 2.0 cm
   *EXCLUDES* Eyelid excision involving more than skin (67800-67808, 67840-67850, 67961-67966)
   5.31   7.72   **FUD** 010                                 T P3
   **AMA:** 2017,Jan,8; 2016,Jan,13; 2015,Jan,16; 2014,Mar,4; 2014,Mar,12; 2014,Jan,11; 2012,May,13

**11643** excised diameter 2.1 to 3.0 cm
   *EXCLUDES* Eyelid excision involving more than skin (67800-67808, 67840-67850, 67961-67966)
   6.65   9.10   **FUD** 010                                 J P3
   **AMA:** 2017,Jan,8; 2016,Jan,13; 2015,Jan,16; 2014,Mar,12; 2014,Mar,4; 2014,Jan,11; 2012,May,13

**11644** excised diameter 3.1 to 4.0 cm
   *EXCLUDES* Eyelid excision involving more than skin (67800-67808, 67840-67850, 67961-67966)
   8.22   11.2   **FUD** 010                                 J A2
   **AMA:** 2017,Jan,8; 2016,Jan,13; 2015,Jan,16; 2014,Mar,4; 2014,Mar,12; 2014,Jan,11; 2012,May,13

**11646** excised diameter over 4.0 cm
   *EXCLUDES* Eyelid excision involving more than skin (67800-67808, 67840-67850, 67961-67966)
   11.4   14.6   **FUD** 010                                 J A2
   **AMA:** 2017,Jan,8; 2016,Jan,13; 2015,Jan,16; 2014,Mar,4; 2014,Mar,12; 2014,Jan,11; 2012,May,13; 2012,Jan,15-42

## 11719-11765 Nails and Supporting Structures

**CMS:** 100-02,15,290 Foot Care
   *EXCLUDES* Drainage of paronychia or onychia (10060-10061)

**11719** Trimming of nondystrophic nails, any number
   0.22   0.40   **FUD** 000                                 01 N1
   **AMA:** 2017,Jan,8; 2016,Jan,13; 2015,Jan,16; 2014,Jan,11

**11720** Debridement of nail(s) by any method(s); 1 to 5
   0.42   0.91   **FUD** 000                                 01 N1
   **AMA:** 2017,Jan,8; 2016,Jan,13; 2015,Jan,16; 2014,Jan,11

**11721** 6 or more
   0.71   1.27   **FUD** 000                                 01 N1
   **AMA:** 2017,Jan,8; 2016,Jan,13; 2015,Jan,16; 2014,Jan,11

**11730** Avulsion of nail plate, partial or complete, simple; single
   1.59   2.97   **FUD** 000                                 01 N1
   **AMA:** 2017,Jan,8; 2016,Jan,13; 2015,Jan,16; 2014,Jan,11; 2012,Jan,15-42

+ **11732** each additional nail plate (List separately in addition to code for primary procedure)
   Code first (11730)
   0.51   0.90   **FUD** ZZZ                                 N N1
   **AMA:** 2017,Jan,8; 2016,Jan,13; 2015,Jan,16; 2014,Jan,11

**11740** Evacuation of subungual hematoma
   0.93   1.40   **FUD** 000                                 01 N1
   **AMA:** 2017,Jan,8; 2016,Jan,13; 2015,Jan,16; 2014,Jan,11

**11750** Excision of nail and nail matrix, partial or complete (eg, ingrown or deformed nail), for permanent removal;
   *EXCLUDES* Skin graft (15050)
   3.24   4.34   **FUD** 010                                 T P3
   **AMA:** 2017,Jan,8; 2016,Jan,13; 2015,Jan,16; 2014,Jan,11

**11755** Biopsy of nail unit (eg, plate, bed, matrix, hyponychium, proximal and lateral nail folds) (separate procedure)
   2.22   3.77   **FUD** 000                                 T P3 80
   **AMA:** 2017,Jan,8; 2016,Jan,13; 2015,Jan,16; 2014,Jan,11; 2012,Jan,15-42

**11760** Repair of nail bed
   3.28   5.35   **FUD** 010                                 T G2
   **AMA:** 2017,Jan,8; 2016,Jan,13; 2015,Jan,16; 2014,Jan,11

**11762** Reconstruction of nail bed with graft
   5.23   7.90   **FUD** 010                                 T P3
   **AMA:** 2017,Jan,8; 2016,Jan,13; 2015,Jan,16; 2014,Jan,11

**11765** Wedge excision of skin of nail fold (eg, for ingrown toenail)
   *INCLUDES* Cotting's operation
   2.69   4.74   **FUD** 010                                 01 N1
   **AMA:** 2017,Jan,8; 2016,Jan,13; 2015,Jan,16; 2014,Jan,11

## 11770-11772 Treatment Pilonidal Cyst: Excision

   *EXCLUDES* Incision of pilonidal cyst (10080-10081)

**11770** Excision of pilonidal cyst or sinus; simple
   5.31   7.87   **FUD** 010                                 J A2

**11771** extensive
   12.4   16.3   **FUD** 090                                 J A2

**11772** complicated
   16.5   19.7   **FUD** 090                                 J A2
   **AMA:** 2017,Jan,8; 2016,Jan,13; 2015,Sep,12

## 11900-11901 Treatment of Lesions: Injection

   *EXCLUDES* Injection of local anesthesia performed preoperatively
   Injection of veins (36470-36471)
   Intralesional chemotherapy (96405-96406)

**11900** Injection, intralesional; up to and including 7 lesions
   0.90   1.58   **FUD** 000                                 01 N1
   **AMA:** 2017,Jan,8; 2016,Jan,13; 2015,Jan,16; 2014,Jan,11; 2013,Nov,14; 2012,Jan,15-42

**11901** more than 7 lesions
   1.40   1.99   **FUD** 000                                 01 N1
   **AMA:** 2017,Jan,8; 2016,Jan,13; 2015,Jan,16; 2014,Jan,11; 2012,Jan,15-42

## 11920-11971 Tattoos, Tissue Expanders, and Dermal Fillers

**CMS:** 100-02,16,10 Exclusions from Coverage; 100-02,16,120 Cosmetic Procedures; 100-02,16,180 Services Related to Noncovered Procedures

**11920** Tattooing, intradermal introduction of insoluble opaque pigments to correct color defects of skin, including micropigmentation; 6.0 sq cm or less
   3.27   4.83   **FUD** 000                                 T P3 80
   **AMA:** 2017,Jan,8; 2016,Aug,9

**11921** 6.1 to 20.0 sq cm
   3.85   5.61   **FUD** 000                                 T P3 80
   **AMA:** 2017,Jan,8; 2016,Aug,9

+ **11922** each additional 20.0 sq cm, or part thereof (List separately in addition to code for primary procedure)
   0.86   1.74   **FUD** ZZZ                                 N N1 80
   Code first (11921)

**11950** Subcutaneous injection of filling material (eg, collagen); 1 cc or less
   1.53   2.21   **FUD** 000                                 T P3 80
   **AMA:** 2017,Jan,8; 2016,Jan,13; 2015,Jan,16; 2014,Jan,11; 2012,Jun,15-16

**11951** 1.1 to 5.0 cc
   2.09   2.84   **FUD** 000                                 T P3 80
   **AMA:** 2017,Jan,8; 2016,Jan,13; 2015,Jan,16; 2014,Jan,11; 2012,Jun,15-16

**11952** 5.1 to 10.0 cc
   2.69   3.54   **FUD** 000                                 T P3 80
   **AMA:** 2017,Jan,8; 2016,Jan,13; 2015,Jan,16; 2014,Jan,11; 2012,Jun,15-16

| 26/TC PC/TC Only | A2-Z3 ASC Payment | 50 Bilateral | ♂ Male Only | ♀ Female Only | Facility RVU | Non-Facility RVU | CCI |
| **FUD** Follow-up Days | **CMS:** IOM (Pub 100) | A-Y OPPSI | 80/80 Surg Assist Allowed / w/Doc | | Lab Crosswalk | Radiology Crosswalk | CLIA |

**18**                         CPT © 2017 American Medical Association. All Rights Reserved.                    © 2017 Optum360, LLC

**11954** over 10.0 cc
  3.31  4.49  **FUD** 000  T P3 80 ▢
  **AMA:** 2017,Jan,8; 2016,Jan,13; 2015,Jan,16; 2014,Jan,11; 2012,Jun,15-16

**11960** Insertion of tissue expander(s) for other than breast, including subsequent expansion
  *EXCLUDES* Breast reconstruction with tissue expander(s) (19357)
  27.2  27.2  **FUD** 090  T A2 ▢
  **AMA:** 1991,Win,1

**11970** Replacement of tissue expander with permanent prosthesis
  17.5  17.5  **FUD** 090  J A2 50 ▢
  **AMA:** 2017,Jan,8; 2016,Jan,13; 2015,Jan,16; 2014,Jan,11; 2013,Jan,15-16

**11971** Removal of tissue expander(s) without insertion of prosthesis
  9.11  13.3  **FUD** 090  02 A2 80 50 ▢
  **AMA:** 2017,Jan,8; 2016,Jan,13; 2015,Jan,16; 2014,Jan,11; 2012,Jan,15-42

## 11976-11983 Drug Implantation

**11976** Removal, implantable contraceptive capsules  ♀
  2.70  4.05  **FUD** 000  02 P3 80 ▢
  **AMA:** 1992,Win,1; 1991,Win,1

**11980** Subcutaneous hormone pellet implantation (implantation of estradiol and/or testosterone pellets beneath the skin)
  1.62  2.67  **FUD** 000  01 N1 ▢
  **AMA:** 2017,Jan,8; 2016,Jan,13; 2015,Jan,16; 2014,Jan,11

**11981** Insertion, non-biodegradable drug delivery implant
  2.39  4.01  **FUD** XXX  01 N1 80 ▢
  **AMA:** 2017,Jan,8; 2016,Jan,13; 2015,Jan,16; 2014,Jan,11; 2012,Jan,15-42

**11982** Removal, non-biodegradable drug delivery implant
  2.90  4.55  **FUD** XXX  01 N1 80 ▢

**11983** Removal with reinsertion, non-biodegradable drug delivery implant
  5.06  6.42  **FUD** XXX  01 N1 80 ▢

## 12001-12021 Suturing of Superficial Wounds

*INCLUDES* Administration of local anesthesia
  Cauterization without closure
  Simple:
    Exploration nerves, blood vessels, tendons
    Vessel ligation, in wound
  Simple repair that involves:
    Routine debridement and decontamination
    Simple one layer closure
    Superficial tissues
    Sutures, staples, tissue adhesives
    Total length of several repairs in same code category

*EXCLUDES* Adhesive strips only, see appropriate E&M service
  Complex repair nerves, blood vessels, tendons (see appropriate anatomical section)
  Debridement:
    Performed separately, no closure (11042-11047 [11045, 11046])
    That requires:
      Comprehensive cleaning
      Removal of significant tissue
      Removal soft tissue and/or bone, no fracture/dislocation (11042-11047 [11045, 11046])
      Removal soft tissue and/or bone with open fracture/dislocation (11010-11012)
  Deep tissue repair (12031-13153)
  Major exploration (20100-20103)
  Repair of nerves, blood vessels, tendons (See appropriate anatomical section. These repairs include simple and intermediate closure. Report complex closure with modifier 59.)
  Secondary closure/dehiscence (13160)

Code also modifier 59 added to the less complicated procedure code if reporting more than one classification of wound repair

**12001** Simple repair of superficial wounds of scalp, neck, axillae, external genitalia, trunk and/or extremities (including hands and feet); 2.5 cm or less
  1.27  2.54  **FUD** 000  01 N1 ▢
  **AMA:** 2017,Jan,8; 2016,Jan,13; 2015,Jan,16; 2014,Jan,11; 2012,Mar,4-7; 2012,Jan,15-42

**12002** 2.6 cm to 7.5 cm
  1.68  3.08  **FUD** 000  01 N1 ▢
  **AMA:** 2017,Jan,8; 2016,Jan,13; 2015,Jan,16; 2014,Oct,14; 2014,Jan,11; 2012,Jan,15-42

**12004** 7.6 cm to 12.5 cm
  2.10  3.62  **FUD** 000  01 N1 ▢
  **AMA:** 2017,Jan,8; 2016,Jan,13; 2015,Jan,16; 2014,Jan,11; 2012,Jan,15-42

**12005** 12.6 cm to 20.0 cm
  2.73  4.57  **FUD** 000  01 A2 ▢
  **AMA:** 2017,Jan,8; 2016,Jan,13; 2015,Jan,16; 2014,Jan,11; 2012,Jan,15-42

**12006** 20.1 cm to 30.0 cm
  3.36  5.40  **FUD** 000  02 A2 ▢
  **AMA:** 2017,Jan,8; 2016,Jan,13; 2015,Jan,16; 2014,Jan,11; 2012,Jan,15-42

**12007** over 30.0 cm
  4.21  6.21  **FUD** 000  T A2 ▢
  **AMA:** 2017,Jan,8; 2016,Jan,13; 2015,Jan,16; 2014,Jan,11; 2012,Jan,15-42

**12011** Simple repair of superficial wounds of face, ears, eyelids, nose, lips and/or mucous membranes; 2.5 cm or less
  1.58  3.10  **FUD** 000  01 N1 ▢
  **AMA:** 2017,Jan,8; 2016,Nov,7; 2016,Jan,13; 2015,Jan,16; 2014,Jan,11; 2012,Jan,15-42

**12013** 2.6 cm to 5.0 cm
  1.66  3.23  **FUD** 000  01 N1 ▢
  **AMA:** 2017,Jan,8; 2016,Jan,13; 2015,Jan,16; 2014,Jan,11; 2012,Jan,15-42

**12014** 5.1 cm to 7.5 cm
  2.14  3.78  **FUD** 000  01 N1 ▢
  **AMA:** 2017,Jan,8; 2016,Jan,13; 2015,Jan,16; 2014,Jan,11; 2012,Jan,15-42

● New Code  ▲ Revised Code  ○ Reinstated  ● New Web Release  ▲ Revised Web Release  Unlisted  Not Covered  # Resequenced
⊘ AMA Mod 51 Exempt  ⑨ Optum Mod 51 Exempt  ㊿ Mod 63 Exempt  ✗ Non-FDA Drug  ★ Telemedicine  M Maternity  A Age Edit  + Add-on  AMA: CPT Asst

**Integumentary System** (side tab)

**12015 — 12057** (side tab)

**12015**    **7.6 cm to 12.5 cm**
🚗 2.70    ⚕ 4.58    **FUD** 000    [01] [02] [▢]
**AMA:** 2017,Jan,8; 2016,Jan,13; 2015,Jan,16; 2014,Jan,11; 2012,Jan,15-42

**12016**    **12.6 cm to 20.0 cm**
🚗 3.68    ⚕ 5.79    **FUD** 000    [01] [A2] [▢]
**AMA:** 2017,Jan,8; 2016,Jan,13; 2015,Jan,16; 2014,Jan,11; 2012,Jan,15-42

**12017**    **20.1 cm to 30.0 cm**
🚗 4.48    ⚕ 4.48    **FUD** 000    [01] [A2] [80] [▢]
**AMA:** 2017,Jan,8; 2016,Jan,13; 2015,Jan,16; 2014,Jan,11; 2012,Jan,15-42

**12018**    **over 30.0 cm**
🚗 5.07    ⚕ 5.07    **FUD** 000    [01] [A2] [80] [▢]
**AMA:** 2017,Jan,8; 2016,Jan,13; 2015,Jan,16; 2014,Jan,11; 2012,Jan,15-42

**12020**    **Treatment of superficial wound dehiscence; simple closure**
EXCLUDES    *Secondary closure major/complex wound or dehiscence (13160)*
🚗 5.41    ⚕ 7.96    **FUD** 010    [T] [A2] [▢]
**AMA:** 2017,Jan,8; 2016,Jan,13; 2015,Jan,16; 2014,Jan,11; 2012,Jan,15-42

**12021**    **with packing**
EXCLUDES    *Secondary closure major/complex wound or dehiscence (13160)*
🚗 3.94    ⚕ 4.61    **FUD** 010    [T] [A2] [▢]
**AMA:** 2017,Jan,8; 2016,Jan,13; 2015,Jan,16; 2014,Jan,11; 2012,Jan,15-42

## 12031-12057 Suturing of Intermediate Wounds

INCLUDES    Administration of local anesthesia
Intermediate repair that involves:
    Closure of contaminated single layer wound
    Layer closure (e.g., subcutaneous tissue, superficial fascia)
    Removal foreign material (e.g. gravel, glass)
    Routine debridement and decontamination
Simple:
    Exploration nerves, blood vessels, tendons in wound
    Vessel ligation, in wound
Total length of several repairs in same code category

EXCLUDES    Debridement:
    *Performed separately, no closure (11042-11047 [11045, 11046])*
    *That requires:*
        *Removal soft tissue and/or bone, no fracture/dislocation (11042-11047 [11045, 11046])*
        *Removal soft tissue/bone due to open fracture/dislocation (11010-11012)*
    *Major exploration (20100-20103)*
    *Repair of nerves, blood vessels, tendons (See appropriate anatomical section. These repairs include simple and intermediate closure. Report complex closure with modifier 59.)*
    *Secondary closure major/complex wound or dehiscence (13160)*
    *Wound repair involving more than layer closure*
Code also modifier 59 added to the less complicated procedure code if reporting more than one classification of wound repair

**12031**    **Repair, intermediate, wounds of scalp, axillae, trunk and/or extremities (excluding hands and feet); 2.5 cm or less**
🚗 4.41    ⚕ 6.74    **FUD** 010    [T] [P2] [▢]
**AMA:** 2017,Jan,8; 2016,Jan,13; 2015,Jan,16; 2014,Jan,11; 2012,Jan,15-42

**12032**    **2.6 cm to 7.5 cm**
🚗 5.62    ⚕ 8.61    **FUD** 010    [T] [P2] [▢]
**AMA:** 2017,Jan,8; 2016,Jan,13; 2015,Jan,16; 2014,Jan,11; 2012,Jan,15-42

**12034**    **7.6 cm to 12.5 cm**
🚗 5.98    ⚕ 8.86    **FUD** 010    [T] [A2] [▢]
**AMA:** 2017,Jan,8; 2016,Jan,13; 2015,Jan,16; 2014,Jan,11; 2012,Jan,15-42

**12035**    **12.6 cm to 20.0 cm**
🚗 6.91    ⚕ 10.8    **FUD** 010    [T] [A2] [▢]
**AMA:** 2017,Jan,8; 2016,Jan,13; 2015,Jan,16; 2014,Jan,11; 2012,Jan,15-42

**12036**    **20.1 cm to 30.0 cm**
🚗 8.03    ⚕ 11.9    **FUD** 010    [T] [A2] [▢]
**AMA:** 2017,Jan,8; 2016,Jan,13; 2015,Jan,16; 2014,Jan,11; 2012,Jan,15-42

**12037**    **over 30.0 cm**
🚗 9.47    ⚕ 13.6    **FUD** 010    [T] [A2] [80] [▢]
**AMA:** 2017,Jan,8; 2016,Jan,13; 2015,Jan,16; 2014,Jan,11; 2012,Jan,15-42

**12041**    **Repair, intermediate, wounds of neck, hands, feet and/or external genitalia; 2.5 cm or less**
🚗 4.34    ⚕ 6.73    **FUD** 010    [02] [P3] [▢]
**AMA:** 2017,Jan,8; 2016,Jan,13; 2015,Jan,16; 2014,Jan,11; 2013,Jan,15-16; 2012,Jan,15-42

**12042**    **2.6 cm to 7.5 cm**
🚗 5.79    ⚕ 8.21    **FUD** 010    [T] [P2] [▢]
**AMA:** 2017,Jan,8; 2016,Jan,13; 2015,Jan,16; 2014,Jan,11; 2013,Jan,15-16; 2012,Jan,15-42

**12044**    **7.6 cm to 12.5 cm**
🚗 6.19    ⚕ 10.1    **FUD** 010    [T] [A2] [▢]
**AMA:** 2017,Jan,8; 2016,Jan,13; 2015,Jan,16; 2014,Jan,11; 2013,Jan,15-16; 2012,Jan,15-42

**12045**    **12.6 cm to 20.0 cm**
🚗 7.76    ⚕ 11.3    **FUD** 010    [T] [A2] [▢]
**AMA:** 2017,Jan,8; 2016,Jan,13; 2015,Jan,16; 2014,Jan,11; 2013,Jan,15-16; 2012,Jan,15-42

**12046**    **20.1 cm to 30.0 cm**
🚗 8.90    ⚕ 13.5    **FUD** 010    [T] [A2] [80] [▢]
**AMA:** 2017,Jan,8; 2016,Jan,13; 2015,Jan,16; 2014,Jan,11; 2013,Jan,15-16; 2012,Jan,15-42

**12047**    **over 30.0 cm**
🚗 10.6    ⚕ 15.5    **FUD** 010    [T] [A2] [80] [▢]
**AMA:** 2017,Jan,8; 2016,Jan,13; 2015,Jan,16; 2014,Jan,11; 2013,Jan,15-16; 2012,Jan,15-42

**12051**    **Repair, intermediate, wounds of face, ears, eyelids, nose, lips and/or mucous membranes; 2.5 cm or less**
🚗 4.94    ⚕ 7.32    **FUD** 010    [T] [P2] [▢]
**AMA:** 2017,Jan,8; 2016,Jan,13; 2015,Jan,16; 2014,Jan,11; 2012,Jan,15-42

**12052**    **2.6 cm to 5.0 cm**
🚗 5.89    ⚕ 8.35    **FUD** 010    [T] [P2] [▢]
**AMA:** 2017,Jan,8; 2016,Jan,13; 2015,Jan,16; 2014,Jan,11; 2012,Jan,15-42

**12053**    **5.1 cm to 7.5 cm**
🚗 6.28    ⚕ 9.80    **FUD** 010    [T] [P2] [▢]
**AMA:** 2017,Jan,8; 2016,Jan,13; 2015,Jan,16; 2014,Jan,11; 2012,Jan,15-42

**12054**    **7.6 cm to 12.5 cm**
🚗 6.41    ⚕ 10.2    **FUD** 010    [02] [A2] [▢]
**AMA:** 2017,Jan,8; 2016,Jan,13; 2015,Jan,16; 2014,Jan,11; 2012,Jan,15-42

**12055**    **12.6 cm to 20.0 cm**
🚗 8.79    ⚕ 13.2    **FUD** 010    [T] [A2] [▢]
**AMA:** 2017,Jan,8; 2016,Jan,13; 2015,Jan,16; 2014,Jan,11; 2012,Jan,15-42

**12056**    **20.1 cm to 30.0 cm**
🚗 9.85    ⚕ 13.9    **FUD** 010    [02] [A2] [80] [▢]
**AMA:** 2017,Jan,8; 2016,Jan,13; 2015,Jan,16; 2014,Jan,11; 2012,Jan,15-42

**12057**    **over 30.0 cm**
🚗 11.2    ⚕ 15.4    **FUD** 010    [T] [A2] [80] [▢]
**AMA:** 2017,Jan,8; 2016,Jan,13; 2015,Jan,16; 2014,Jan,11; 2012,Jan,15-42

## 13100-13160 Suturing of Complicated Wounds

**INCLUDES** Creation of a limited defect for repair
Debridement complicated wounds/avulsions
More complicated than layered closure
Simple:
    Exploration nerves, vessels, tendons in wound
    Vessel ligation in wound
Total length of several repairs in same code category
Undermining, stents, retention sutures

**EXCLUDES** *Complex/secondary wound closure or dehiscence*
*Debridement of open fracture/dislocation (15002-15005)*
*Excision:*
    *Benign lesions (11400-11446)*
    *Malignant lesions (11600-11646)*
    *Extensive exploration (20100-20103)*
*Repair of nerves, blood vessel, tendons (See appropriate anatomical section. These repairs include simple and intermediate closure. Report complex closure with modifier 59.)*
*Surgical preparation of a wound bed (15002-15005)*
Code also modifier 59 added to the less complicated procedure code if reporting more than one classification of wound repair

**13100** **Repair, complex, trunk; 1.1 cm to 2.5 cm**

    **EXCLUDES** *Complex repair 1.0 cm or less (12001, 12031)*

    🚑 5.95    ⚖ 9.50    **FUD** 010      T A2 ▣

    **AMA:** 2017,Apr,9; 2017,Jan,8; 2016,Jan,13; 2015,Jan,16; 2014,Jan,11; 2012,Dec,6-8; 2012,Jan,6-10; 2012,Jan,15-42

**13101** **2.6 cm to 7.5 cm**

    🚑 7.32    ⚖ 11.2    **FUD** 010      T A2 ▣

    **AMA:** 2017,Apr,9; 2017,Jan,8; 2016,Jan,13; 2015,Jan,16; 2014,Jan,11; 2012,Dec,6-8; 2012,Jan,6-10; 2012,Jan,15-42

**+ 13102** **each additional 5 cm or less (List separately in addition to code for primary procedure)**

    Code first (13101)

    🚑 2.15    ⚖ 3.45    **FUD** ZZZ      N N1 ▣

    **AMA:** 2017,Apr,9; 2017,Jan,8; 2016,Jan,13; 2015,Jan,16; 2014,Jan,11; 2012,Dec,6-8; 2012,Jan,6-10; 2012,Jan,15-42

**13120** **Repair, complex, scalp, arms, and/or legs; 1.1 cm to 2.5 cm**

    **EXCLUDES** *Complex repair 1.0 cm or less (12001, 12031)*

    🚑 6.82    ⚖ 9.94    **FUD** 010      T A2 ▣

    **AMA:** 2017,Jan,8; 2016,Jan,13; 2015,Jan,16; 2014,Jan,11; 2012,Dec,6-8; 2012,Jan,6-10; 2012,Jan,15-42

**13121** **2.6 cm to 7.5 cm**

    🚑 7.73    ⚖ 12.1    **FUD** 010      T A2 ▣

    **AMA:** 2017,Jan,8; 2016,Jan,13; 2015,Jan,16; 2014,Jan,11; 2012,Dec,6-8; 2012,Jan,6-10; 2012,Jan,15-42

**+ 13122** **each additional 5 cm or less (List separately in addition to code for primary procedure)**

    Code first (13121)

    🚑 2.48    ⚖ 3.79    **FUD** ZZZ      N N1 ▣

    **AMA:** 2017,Jan,8; 2016,Jan,13; 2015,Jan,16; 2014,Jan,11; 2012,Dec,6-8; 2012,Jan,6-10; 2012,Jan,15-42

**13131** **Repair, complex, forehead, cheeks, chin, mouth, neck, axillae, genitalia, hands and/or feet; 1.1 cm to 2.5 cm**

    **EXCLUDES** *Complex repair 1.0 cm or less (12001, 12011, 12031, 12041, 12051)*

    🚑 7.23    ⚖ 10.9    **FUD** 010      T A2 ▣

    **AMA:** 2017,Apr,9; 2017,Jan,8; 2016,Jan,13; 2015,Jan,16; 2014,Jan,11; 2013,Jan,15-16; 2012,Dec,6-8; 2012,Jan,6-10; 2012,Jan,15-42

**13132** **2.6 cm to 7.5 cm**

    🚑 9.11    ⚖ 13.5    **FUD** 010      T A2 ▣

    **AMA:** 2017,Apr,9; 2017,Jan,8; 2016,Jan,13; 2015,Jan,16; 2014,Oct,14; 2014,Jan,11; 2013,Jan,15-16; 2012,Dec,6-8; 2012,Jan,15-42; 2012,Jan,6-10

**+ 13133** **each additional 5 cm or less (List separately in addition to code for primary procedure)**

    Code first (13132)

    🚑 3.81    ⚖ 5.09    **FUD** ZZZ      N N1 ▣

    **AMA:** 2017,Apr,9; 2017,Jan,8; 2016,Jan,13; 2015,Jan,16; 2014,Jan,11; 2013,Jan,15-16; 2012,Dec,6-8; 2012,Jan,15-42; 2012,Jan,6-10

**13151** **Repair, complex, eyelids, nose, ears and/or lips; 1.1 cm to 2.5 cm**

    **EXCLUDES** *Complex repair 1.0 cm or less (12011, 12051)*

    🚑 8.31    ⚖ 12.0    **FUD** 010      T A2 ▣

    **AMA:** 2017,Jan,8; 2016,Jan,13; 2015,Jan,16; 2014,May,3; 2014,Mar,12; 2014,Jan,11; 2012,Dec,6-8; 2012,Jan,15-42; 2012,Jan,6-10

**13152** **2.6 cm to 7.5 cm**

    🚑 10.0    ⚖ 14.4    **FUD** 010      T A2 ▣

    **AMA:** 2017,Jan,8; 2016,Jan,13; 2015,Jan,16; 2014,Oct,14; 2014,May,3; 2014,Mar,12; 2014,Jan,11; 2012,Dec,6-8; 2012,Jan,15-42; 2012,Jan,6-10

**+ 13153** **each additional 5 cm or less (List separately in addition to code for primary procedure)**

    Code first (13152)

    🚑 4.10    ⚖ 5.53    **FUD** ZZZ      N N1 ▣

    **AMA:** 2017,Jan,8; 2016,Jan,13; 2015,Jan,16; 2014,May,3; 2014,Mar,12; 2014,Jan,11; 2012,Dec,6-8; 2012,Jan,15-42; 2012,Jan,6-10

**13160** **Secondary closure of surgical wound or dehiscence, extensive or complicated**

    **EXCLUDES** *Packing or simple secondary wound closure (12020-12021)*

    🚑 23.0    ⚖ 23.0    **FUD** 090      T A2 ▣

    **AMA:** 2017,Jan,8; 2016,Jan,13; 2015,Jan,16; 2014,Jan,11; 2012,Dec,6-8; 2012,Jan,15-42

## 14000-14350 Reposition Contiguous Tissue

**INCLUDES** Excision (with or without lesion) with repair by adjacent tissue transfer or tissue rearrangement
Size of defect includes primary (due to excision) and secondary (due to flap design)
Z-plasty, W-plasty, VY-plasty, rotation flap, advancement flap, double pedicle flap, random island flap

**EXCLUDES** *Closure of wounds by undermining surrounding tissue without additional incisions (13100-13160)*
*Full thickness closure of:*
    *Eyelid (67930-67935, 67961-67975)*
    *Lip (40650-40654)*
Code also skin graft necessary to repair secondary defect (15040-15731)

**14000** **Adjacent tissue transfer or rearrangement, trunk; defect 10 sq cm or less**

    **INCLUDES** Burrow's operation

    **EXCLUDES** *Excision of lesion with repair by adjacent tissue transfer or tissue rearrangement (11400-11446, 11600-11646)*

    🚑 14.4    ⚖ 17.7    **FUD** 090      T A2 ▣

    **AMA:** 2017,Jan,8; 2016,Jan,13; 2015,Sep,12; 2015,Feb,10; 2015,Jan,16; 2014,Apr,10; 2014,Jan,11; 2012,Dec,6-8; 2012,Nov,13-14; 2012,May,13; 2012,Jan,6-10; 2012,Jan,15-42

Example of common Z-plasty. Lesion is removed with oval-shaped incision

Two additional incisions (a. and b.) intersect the area

Skin of each incision is reflected back

The flaps are then transposed and the repair is closed

An adjacent flap, or other rearrangement flap, is performed to repair a defect

● New Code    ▲ Revised Code    ○ Reinstated    ● New Web Release    ▲ Revised Web Release    Unlisted    Not Covered    # Resequenced

⊘ AMA Mod 51 Exempt    ⑤ Optum Mod 51 Exempt    ⑥③ Mod 63 Exempt    ✗ Non-FDA Drug    ★ Telemedicine    Ⓜ Maternity    Ⓐ Age Edit    + Add-on    **AMA:** CPT Asst

© 2017 Optum360, LLC      CPT © 2017 American Medical Association. All Rights Reserved.      **21**

**14001** defect 10.1 sq cm to 30.0 sq cm

EXCLUDES *Excision of lesion with repair by adjacent tissue transfer or tissue rearrangement (11400-11446, 11600-11646)*

📷 18.9   ⚕ 22.8   **FUD** 090   T A2 ▢

AMA: 2017,Jan,8; 2016,Jan,13; 2015,Feb,10; 2015,Jan,16; 2014,Apr,10; 2014,Jan,11; 2012,Dec,6-8; 2012,Nov,13-14; 2012,May,13; 2012,Jan,6-10; 2012,Jan,15-42

**14020** Adjacent tissue transfer or rearrangement, scalp, arms and/or legs; defect 10 sq cm or less

EXCLUDES *Excision of lesion with repair by adjacent tissue transfer or tissue rearrangement (11400-11446, 11600-11646)*

📷 16.3   ⚕ 19.8   **FUD** 090   T A2 ▢

AMA: 2017,Jan,8; 2016,Jan,13; 2015,Jan,16; 2014,Jan,11; 2012,Dec,6-8; 2012,Nov,13-14; 2012,May,13; 2012,Jan,15-42; 2012,Jan,6-10

**14021** defect 10.1 sq cm to 30.0 sq cm

EXCLUDES *Excision of lesion with repair by adjacent tissue transfer or tissue rearrangement (11400-11446, 11600-11646)*

📷 20.7   ⚕ 24.8   **FUD** 090   T A2 ▢

AMA: 2017,Jan,8; 2016,Jan,13; 2015,Jan,16; 2014,Jan,11; 2012,Dec,6-8; 2012,Nov,13-14; 2012,May,13; 2012,Jan,15-42; 2012,Jan,6-10

**14040** Adjacent tissue transfer or rearrangement, forehead, cheeks, chin, mouth, neck, axillae, genitalia, hands and/or feet; defect 10 sq cm or less

INCLUDES Krimer's palatoplasty

EXCLUDES *Excision of lesion with repair by adjacent tissue transfer or tissue rearrangement (11400-11446, 11600-11646)*

📷 18.2   ⚕ 21.6   **FUD** 090   T A2 ▢

AMA: 2017,Jan,8; 2016,Jan,13; 2015,Jan,16; 2014,Jan,11; 2012,Dec,6-8; 2012,Nov,13-14; 2012,May,13; 2012,Jan,15-42; 2012,Jan,6-10

**14041** defect 10.1 sq cm to 30.0 sq cm

EXCLUDES *Excision of lesion with repair by adjacent tissue transfer or tissue rearrangement (11400-11446, 11600-11646)*

📷 22.4   ⚕ 26.8   **FUD** 090   T A2 ▢

AMA: 2017,Jan,8; 2016,Jan,13; 2015,Jan,16; 2014,Jan,11; 2012,Dec,6-8; 2012,Nov,13-14; 2012,May,13; 2012,Jan,15-42; 2012,Jan,6-10

**14060** Adjacent tissue transfer or rearrangement, eyelids, nose, ears and/or lips; defect 10 sq cm or less

INCLUDES Denonvillier's operation

EXCLUDES *Excision of lesion with repair by adjacent tissue transfer or tissue rearrangement (11400-11446, 11600-11646)*

*Eyelid, full thickness (67961-67966)*

📷 19.4   ⚕ 22.1   **FUD** 090   T A2 ▢

AMA: 2017,Jan,8; 2016,Jan,13; 2015,Jan,16; 2014,Jan,11; 2012,Dec,6-8; 2012,Nov,13-14; 2012,Aug,13-14; 2012,May,13; 2012,Jan,15-42; 2012,Jan,6-10

**14061** defect 10.1 sq cm to 30.0 sq cm

EXCLUDES *Excision of lesion with repair by adjacent tissue transfer or tissue rearrangement (11400-11446, 11600-11646)*

*Eyelid, full thickness (67961 and subsequent codes)*

📷 24.0   ⚕ 28.9   **FUD** 090   T A2 ▢

AMA: 2017,Jan,8; 2016,Jan,13; 2015,Jan,16; 2014,Jan,11; 2012,Dec,6-8; 2012,Nov,13-14; 2012,May,13; 2012,Jan,15-42; 2012,Jan,6-10

**14301** Adjacent tissue transfer or rearrangement, any area; defect 30.1 sq cm to 60.0 sq cm

EXCLUDES *Excision of lesion with repair by adjacent tissue transfer or tissue rearrangement (11400-11446, 11600-11646)*

📷 25.4   ⚕ 30.7   **FUD** 090   T 62 80 ▢

AMA: 2017,Apr,9; 2017,Jan,8; 2016,Jan,13; 2015,Jan,16; 2014,Jan,11; 2012,Dec,6-8; 2012,Nov,13-14; 2012,May,13

+ **14302** each additional 30.0 sq cm, or part thereof (List separately in addition to code for primary procedure)

EXCLUDES *Excision of lesion with repair by adjacent tissue transfer or tissue rearrangement (11400-11446, 11600-11646)*

Code first (14301)

📷 6.40   ⚕ 6.40   **FUD** ZZZ   N N1 80 ▢

AMA: 2017,Jan,8; 2016,Jan,13; 2015,Jan,16; 2014,Jan,11; 2012,Dec,6-8; 2012,Nov,13-14; 2012,May,13

**14350** Filleted finger or toe flap, including preparation of recipient site

📷 19.7   ⚕ 19.7   **FUD** 090   T A2 80 ▢

AMA: 2017,Jan,8; 2016,Jan,13; 2015,Jan,16; 2014,Jan,11; 2012,Dec,6-8; 2012,May,13; 2012,Jan,15-42

## 15002-15005 Development of Base for Tissue Grafting

INCLUDES Add together the surface area of multiple wounds in the same anatomical locations as indicated in the code descriptor groups, such as face and scalp. Do not add together multiple wounds at different anatomical site groups such as trunk and face

Ankle or wrist if code description describes leg or arm

Cleaning and preparing a viable wound surface for grafting or negative pressure wound therapy used to heal the wound primarily

Code selection based on the defect size and location

Percentage applies to children younger than age 10

Removal of nonviable tissue in nonchronic wounds for primary healing

Square centimeters applies to children and adults age 10 or older

EXCLUDES *Chronic wound management on wounds left to heal by secondary intention (11042-11047 [11045, 11046], 97597-97598)*

*Necrotizing soft tissue infections for specific anatomical locations (11004-11008)*

**15002** Surgical preparation or creation of recipient site by excision of open wounds, burn eschar, or scar (including subcutaneous tissues), or incisional release of scar contracture, trunk, arms, legs; first 100 sq cm or 1% of body area of infants and children

EXCLUDES *Linear scar revision (13100-13153)*

📷 6.55   ⚕ 9.88   **FUD** 000   T A2 80 ▢

AMA: 2017,Jan,8; 2016,Jan,13; 2015,Jan,16; 2014,Mar,12; 2014,Jan,11; 2013,Feb,16-17; 2012,Dec,6-8; 2012,Oct,3-8; 2012,Oct,13; 2012,Jan,15-42; 2012,Jan,6-10

+ **15003** each additional 100 sq cm, or part thereof, or each additional 1% of body area of infants and children (List separately in addition to code for primary procedure)

Code first (15002)

📷 1.32   ⚕ 2.15   **FUD** ZZZ   N N1 80 ▢

AMA: 2017,Jan,8; 2016,Jan,13; 2015,Jan,16; 2014,Mar,12; 2014,Jan,11; 2013,Feb,16-17; 2012,Oct,13; 2012,Oct,3-8; 2012,Jan,15-42; 2012,Jan,6-10

**15004** Surgical preparation or creation of recipient site by excision of open wounds, burn eschar, or scar (including subcutaneous tissues), or incisional release of scar contracture, face, scalp, eyelids, mouth, neck, ears, orbits, genitalia, hands, feet and/or multiple digits; first 100 sq cm or 1% of body area of infants and children

📷 7.78   ⚕ 11.3   **FUD** 000   T A2 80 ▢

AMA: 2017,Jan,8; 2016,Jan,13; 2015,Jan,16; 2014,Mar,12; 2014,Jan,11; 2013,Feb,16-17; 2012,Oct,13; 2012,Oct,3-8; 2012,Jan,15-42; 2012,Jan,6-10

+ **15005** each additional 100 sq cm, or part thereof, or each additional 1% of body area of infants and children (List separately in addition to code for primary procedure)

Code first (15004)

📷 2.64   ⚕ 3.56   **FUD** ZZZ   N N1 80 ▢

AMA: 2017,Jan,8; 2016,Jan,13; 2015,Jan,16; 2014,Mar,12; 2014,Jan,11; 2013,Feb,16-17; 2012,Oct,13; 2012,Oct,3-8; 2012,Jan,15-42; 2012,Jan,6-10

| 26/TC PC/TC Only | A2-Z3 ASC Payment | 50 Bilateral | ♂ Male Only | ♀ Female Only | 📷 Facility RVU | ⚕ Non-Facility RVU | ▢ CCI |
| FUD Follow-up Days | CMS: IOM (Pub 100) | A-Y OPPSI | 80/80 Surg Assist Allowed / w/Doc | | N Lab Crosswalk | Radiology Crosswalk | X CLIA |

22    CPT © 2017 American Medical Association. All Rights Reserved.    © 2017 Optum360, LLC

## 15040 Obtain Autograft

INCLUDES  Ankle or wrist if code description describes leg or arm
Percentage applies to children younger than age 10
Square centimeters applies to children and adults age 10 or older

**15040**  **Harvest of skin for tissue cultured skin autograft, 100 sq cm or less**

🖥 3.68  ✂ 7.22  **FUD** 000                    T A2 ▣

**AMA:** 2017,Jan,8; 2016,Jan,13; 2015,Jan,16; 2014,Jan,11; 2012,Jan,6-10; 2012,Jan,15-42

## 15050 Pinch Graft

INCLUDES  Autologous skin graft harvest and application
Current graft removal
Fixation and anchoring skin graft
Simple cleaning

EXCLUDES  *Removal of devitalized tissue from wound(s), non-selective debridement, without anesthesia (97602)*

Code also graft or flap necessary to repair donor site

**15050**  **Pinch graft, single or multiple, to cover small ulcer, tip of digit, or other minimal open area (except on face), up to defect size 2 cm diameter**

🖥 12.7  ✂ 15.9  **FUD** 090                    T A2 ▣

**AMA:** 2017,Jan,8; 2016,Jun,8; 2016,Jan,13; 2015,Jan,16; 2014,Jan,11; 2012,Jan,6-10; 2012,Jan,15-42

## 15100-15261 Skin Grafts and Replacements

INCLUDES  Add together the surface area of multiple wounds in the same anatomical locations as indicated in the code description groups, such as face and scalp. Do not add together multiple wounds at different anatomical site groups such as trunk and face.
Ankle or wrist if code description describes leg or arm
Autologous skin graft harvest and application
Code selection based on recipient site location and size and type of graft
Current graft removal
Fixation and anchoring skin graft
Percentage applies to children younger than age 10
Simple cleaning
Simple tissue debridement
Square centimeters applies to children and adults age 10 or older

EXCLUDES  *Debridement without immediate primary closure, when wound is grossly contaminated and extensive cleaning is needed, or when necrotic or contaminated tissue is removed (11042-11047 [11045, 11046], 97597-97598)*
*Removal of devitalized tissue from wound(s), non-selective debridement, without anesthesia (97602)*

Code also graft or flap necessary to repair donor site
Code also primary procedure requiring skin graft for definitive closure

**15100**  **Split-thickness autograft, trunk, arms, legs; first 100 sq cm or less, or 1% of body area of infants and children (except 15050)**

🖥 20.5  ✂ 24.4  **FUD** 090                    T A2 ▣

**AMA:** 2017,Jan,8; 2016,Jun,8; 2016,Jan,13; 2015,Jan,16; 2014,Jan,11; 2012,Oct,3-8; 2012,Jan,6-10; 2012,Jan,15-42

+  **15101**  **each additional 100 sq cm, or each additional 1% of body area of infants and children, or part thereof (List separately in addition to code for primary procedure)**

Code first (15100)

🖥 3.21  ✂ 5.29  **FUD** ZZZ                    N N1 ▣

**AMA:** 2017,Jan,8; 2016,Jun,8; 2016,Jan,13; 2015,Jan,16; 2014,Jan,11; 2012,Oct,3-8; 2012,Jan,6-10; 2012,Jan,15-42

**15110**  **Epidermal autograft, trunk, arms, legs; first 100 sq cm or less, or 1% of body area of infants and children**

🖥 19.8  ✂ 22.6  **FUD** 090                    T A2 ▣

**AMA:** 2017,Jan,8; 2016,Jan,13; 2015,Jan,16; 2014,Jan,11; 2012,Oct,3-8; 2012,Jan,6-10; 2012,Jan,15-42

+  **15111**  **each additional 100 sq cm, or each additional 1% of body area of infants and children, or part thereof (List separately in addition to code for primary procedure)**

Code first (15110)

🖥 2.99  ✂ 3.31  **FUD** ZZZ                    N N1 ▣

**AMA:** 2017,Jan,8; 2016,Jan,13; 2015,Jan,16; 2014,Jan,11; 2012,Oct,3-8; 2012,Jan,6-10; 2012,Jan,15-42

**15115**  **Epidermal autograft, face, scalp, eyelids, mouth, neck, ears, orbits, genitalia, hands, feet, and/or multiple digits; first 100 sq cm or less, or 1% of body area of infants and children**

🖥 20.0  ✂ 22.8  **FUD** 090                    T A2 ▣

**AMA:** 2017,Jan,8; 2016,Jan,13; 2015,Jan,16; 2014,Jan,11; 2012,Oct,3-8; 2012,Jan,6-10; 2012,Jan,15-42

+  **15116**  **each additional 100 sq cm, or each additional 1% of body area of infants and children, or part thereof (List separately in addition to code for primary procedure)**

Code first (15115)

🖥 4.28  ✂ 4.68  **FUD** ZZZ                    N N1 ▣

**AMA:** 2017,Jan,8; 2016,Jan,13; 2015,Jan,16; 2014,Jan,11; 2012,Oct,3-8; 2012,Jan,6-10; 2012,Jan,15-42

**15120**  **Split-thickness autograft, face, scalp, eyelids, mouth, neck, ears, orbits, genitalia, hands, feet, and/or multiple digits; first 100 sq cm or less, or 1% of body area of infants and children (except 15050)**

EXCLUDES  *Other eyelid repair (67961-67975)*

🖥 20.0  ✂ 24.2  **FUD** 090                    T A2 ▣

**AMA:** 2017,Jan,8; 2016,Jun,8; 2016,Jan,13; 2015,Jan,16; 2014,Jan,11; 2012,Oct,3-8; 2012,Jan,6-10; 2012,Jan,15-42

+  **15121**  **each additional 100 sq cm, or each additional 1% of body area of infants and children, or part thereof (List separately in addition to code for primary procedure)**

EXCLUDES  *Other eyelid repair (67961-67975)*

Code first (15120)

🖥 3.85  ✂ 5.94  **FUD** ZZZ                    N N1 ▣

**AMA:** 2017,Jan,8; 2016,Jun,8; 2016,Jan,13; 2015,Jan,16; 2014,Jan,11; 2012,Oct,3-8; 2012,Jan,6-10; 2012,Jan,15-42

**15130**  **Dermal autograft, trunk, arms, legs; first 100 sq cm or less, or 1% of body area of infants and children**

🖥 16.0  ✂ 19.0  **FUD** 090                    T A2 ▣

**AMA:** 2017,Jan,8; 2016,Jan,13; 2015,Jan,16; 2014,Jan,11; 2012,Oct,3-8; 2012,Jan,6-10; 2012,Jan,15-42

+  **15131**  **each additional 100 sq cm, or each additional 1% of body area of infants and children, or part thereof (List separately in addition to code for primary procedure)**

Code first (15130)

🖥 2.37  ✂ 2.58  **FUD** ZZZ                    N N1 ▣

**AMA:** 2017,Jan,8; 2016,Jan,13; 2015,Jan,16; 2014,Jan,11; 2012,Oct,3-8; 2012,Jan,6-10; 2012,Jan,15-42

**15135**  **Dermal autograft, face, scalp, eyelids, mouth, neck, ears, orbits, genitalia, hands, feet, and/or multiple digits; first 100 sq cm or less, or 1% of body area of infants and children**

🖥 21.0  ✂ 23.9  **FUD** 090                    T A2 ▣

**AMA:** 2017,Jan,8; 2016,Jan,13; 2015,Jan,16; 2014,Jan,11; 2012,Oct,3-8; 2012,Jan,6-10; 2012,Jan,15-42

+  **15136**  **each additional 100 sq cm, or each additional 1% of body area of infants and children, or part thereof (List separately in addition to code for primary procedure)**

Code first (15135)

🖥 2.33  ✂ 2.48  **FUD** ZZZ                    N N1 ▣

**AMA:** 2017,Jan,8; 2016,Jan,13; 2015,Jan,16; 2014,Jan,11; 2012,Oct,3-8; 2012,Jan,6-10; 2012,Jan,15-42

**15150**  **Tissue cultured skin autograft, trunk, arms, legs; first 25 sq cm or less**

🖥 17.9  ✂ 19.5  **FUD** 090                    T A2 ▣

**AMA:** 2017,Jan,8; 2016,Jan,13; 2015,Jan,16; 2014,Jan,11; 2012,Oct,3-8; 2012,Jan,6-10; 2012,Jan,15-42

+  **15151**  **additional 1 sq cm to 75 sq cm (List separately in addition to code for primary procedure)**

EXCLUDES  *Grafts over 75 sq cm (15152)*
*Use of code more than one time per session*

Code first (15150)

🖥 3.20  ✂ 3.46  **FUD** ZZZ                    N N1 ▣

**AMA:** 2017,Jan,8; 2016,Jan,13; 2015,Jan,16; 2014,Jan,11; 2012,Oct,3-8; 2012,Jan,6-10; 2012,Jan,15-42

● New Code  ▲ Revised Code  ○ Reinstated  ● New Web Release  ▲ Revised Web Release  Unlisted  Not Covered  # Resequenced
⊘ AMA Mod 51 Exempt  ⑤ Optum Mod 51 Exempt  ⑥ Mod 63 Exempt  ✗ Non-FDA Drug  ★ Telemedicine  Ⓜ Maternity  Ⓐ Age Edit  + Add-on  **AMA:** CPT Asst
© 2017 Optum360, LLC                            CPT © 2017 American Medical Association. All Rights Reserved.                            23

**+ 15152** each additional 100 sq cm, or each additional 1% of body area of infants and children, or part thereof (List separately in addition to code for primary procedure)

Code first (15151)
🔧 3.98   🔪 4.23   **FUD** ZZZ    N N1 🖳

**AMA:** 2017,Jan,8; 2016,Jan,13; 2015,Jan,16; 2014,Jan,11; 2012,Oct,3-8; 2012,Jan,6-10; 2012,Jan,15-42

**15155** Tissue cultured skin autograft, face, scalp, eyelids, mouth, neck, ears, orbits, genitalia, hands, feet, and/or multiple digits; first 25 sq cm or less

🔧 19.0   🔪 20.4   **FUD** 090    T A2 🖳

**AMA:** 2017,Jan,8; 2016,Jan,13; 2015,Jan,16; 2014,Jan,11; 2012,Oct,3-8; 2012,Jan,6-10; 2012,Jan,15-42

**+ 15156** additional 1 sq cm to 75 sq cm (List separately in addition to code for primary procedure)

*EXCLUDES*   *Grafts over 75 sq cm (15157)*
     *Use of code more than one time per session*
Code first (15155)
🔧 4.44   🔪 4.68   **FUD** ZZZ    N N1 🖳

**AMA:** 2017,Jan,8; 2016,Jan,13; 2015,Jan,16; 2014,Jan,11; 2012,Oct,3-8; 2012,Jan,6-10; 2012,Jan,15-42

**+ 15157** each additional 100 sq cm, or each additional 1% of body area of infants and children, or part thereof (List separately in addition to code for primary procedure)

Code first (15156)
🔧 4.93   🔪 5.27   **FUD** ZZZ    N N1 🖳

**AMA:** 2017,Jan,8; 2016,Jan,13; 2015,Jan,16; 2014,Jan,11; 2012,Oct,3-8; 2012,Jan,6-10; 2012,Jan,15-42

**15200** Full thickness graft, free, including direct closure of donor site, trunk; 20 sq cm or less

🔧 19.3   🔪 23.6   **FUD** 090    T A2 🖳

**AMA:** 2017,Jan,8; 2016,Jun,8; 2016,Jan,13; 2015,Jan,16; 2014,Jan,11; 2012,Oct,3-8; 2012,Jan,15-42; 2012,Jan,6-10

**+ 15201** each additional 20 sq cm, or part thereof (List separately in addition to code for primary procedure)

Code first (15200)
🔧 2.27   🔪 4.16   **FUD** ZZZ    N N1 🖳

**AMA:** 2017,Jan,8; 2016,Jun,8; 2016,Jan,13; 2015,Jan,16; 2014,Jan,11; 2012,Oct,3-8; 2012,Jan,6-10; 2012,Jan,15-42

**15220** Full thickness graft, free, including direct closure of donor site, scalp, arms, and/or legs; 20 sq cm or less

🔧 17.7   🔪 21.9   **FUD** 090    T A2 🖳

**AMA:** 2017,Jan,8; 2016,Jun,8; 2016,Jan,13; 2015,Jan,16; 2014,Jan,11; 2012,Oct,3-8; 2012,Jan,6-10; 2012,Jan,15-42

**+ 15221** each additional 20 sq cm, or part thereof (List separately in addition to code for primary procedure)

Code first (15220)
🔧 2.07   🔪 3.88   **FUD** ZZZ    N N1 🖳

**AMA:** 2017,Jan,8; 2016,Jun,8; 2016,Jan,13; 2015,Jan,16; 2014,Jan,11; 2012,Oct,3-8; 2012,Jan,6-10; 2012,Jan,15-42

**15240** Full thickness graft, free, including direct closure of donor site, forehead, cheeks, chin, mouth, neck, axillae, genitalia, hands, and/or feet; 20 sq cm or less

*EXCLUDES*   *Fingertip graft (15050)*
     *Syndactyly repair fingers (26560-26562)*
🔧 23.0   🔪 26.6   **FUD** 090    T A2 🖳

**AMA:** 2017,Jan,8; 2016,Jun,8; 2016,Jan,13; 2015,Jan,16; 2014,Jan,11; 2012,Oct,3-8; 2012,Jan,15-42; 2012,Jan,6-10

**+ 15241** each additional 20 sq cm, or part thereof (List separately in addition to code for primary procedure)

Code first (15240)
🔧 3.22   🔪 5.25   **FUD** ZZZ    N N1 🖳

**AMA:** 2017,Jan,8; 2016,Jun,8; 2016,Jan,13; 2015,Jan,16; 2014,Jan,11; 2012,Oct,3-8; 2012,Jan,15-42; 2012,Jan,6-10

**15260** Full thickness graft, free, including direct closure of donor site, nose, ears, eyelids, and/or lips; 20 sq cm or less

*EXCLUDES*   *Other eyelid repair (67961-67975)*
🔧 24.7   🔪 28.8   **FUD** 090    T A2 🖳

**AMA:** 2017,Jan,8; 2016,Jun,8; 2016,Jan,13; 2015,Jan,16; 2014,Jan,11; 2012,Oct,3-8; 2012,Jan,6-10; 2012,Jan,15-42

**+ 15261** each additional 20 sq cm, or part thereof (List separately in addition to code for primary procedure)

*EXCLUDES*   *Other eyelid repair (67961-67975)*
Code first (15260)
🔧 4.05   🔪 6.12   **FUD** ZZZ    N N1 🖳

**AMA:** 2017,Jan,8; 2016,Jun,8; 2016,Jan,13; 2015,Jan,16; 2014,Jan,11; 2012,Oct,3-8; 2012,Jan,6-10; 2012,Jan,15-42

## 15271-15278 Skin Substitute Graft Application

*INCLUDES*   Add together the surface area of multiple wounds in the same anatomical locations as indicated in the code description groups, such as face and scalp. Do not add together multiple wounds at different anatomical site groups such as trunk and face.
Ankle or wrist if code description describes leg or arm
Code selection based on defect site location and size
Fixation and anchoring skin graft
Graft types include:
     Biological material used for tissue engineering (e.g.,scaffold) for growing skin
     Nonautologous human skin such as:
        Acellular
        Allograft
        Cellular
        Dermal
        Epidermal
        Homograft
     Nonhuman grafts
Percentage applies to children younger than age 10
Removing current graft
Simple cleaning
Simple tissue debridement
Square centimeters applies to children and adults age 10 or older

*EXCLUDES*   *Application of nongraft dressing*
*Injected skin substitutes*
*Removal of devitalized tissue from wound(s), non-selective debridement, without anesthesia (97602)*
*Skin application procedures, low cost (C5271-C5278)*
Code also biologic implant for soft tissue reinforcement (15777)
Code also primary procedure requiring skin graft for definitive closure
Code also supply of high cost skin substitute product (C9363, Q4101, Q4103-Q4110, Q4116, Q4122-Q4123, Q4126-Q4128, Q4131-Q4133, Q4137-Q4138, Q4140-Q4141, Q4147-Q4148, Q4151-Q4154, Q4156, Q4158-Q4161, Q4169, Q4173, Q4175)

**15271** Application of skin substitute graft to trunk, arms, legs, total wound surface area up to 100 sq cm; first 25 sq cm or less wound surface area

*EXCLUDES*   *Total wound area greater than or equal to 100 sq cm (15273-15274)*
🔧 2.44   🔪 3.98   **FUD** 000    T G2 🖳

**AMA:** 2017,Jan,8; 2016,Jan,13; 2015,Jan,16; 2014,Jun,14; 2014,Jan,11; 2013,Oct,15; 2012,Oct,3-8; 2012,Jan,6-10; 2012,Jan,15-42

**+ 15272** each additional 25 sq cm wound surface area, or part thereof (List separately in addition to code for primary procedure)

*EXCLUDES*   *Total wound area greater than or equal to 100 sq cm (15273-15274)*
Code first (15271)
🔧 0.50   🔪 0.77   **FUD** ZZZ    N N1 🖳

**AMA:** 2017,Jan,8; 2016,Jan,13; 2015,Jan,16; 2014,Jun,14; 2014,Jan,11; 2013,Oct,15; 2012,Oct,3-8; 2012,Jan,6-10; 2012,Jan,15-42

**15273** Application of skin substitute graft to trunk, arms, legs, total wound surface area greater than or equal to 100 sq cm; first 100 sq cm wound surface area, or 1% of body area of infants and children

*EXCLUDES*   *Total wound surface area up to 100 cm (15271-15272)*
🔧 5.87   🔪 8.54   **FUD** 000    T G2 🖳

**AMA:** 2017,Jan,8; 2016,Jan,13; 2015,Jan,16; 2014,Jun,14; 2014,Jan,11; 2013,Oct,15; 2013,Nov,14; 2012,Oct,3-8; 2012,Jan,6-10; 2012,Jan,15-42

+ **15274** each additional 100 sq cm wound surface area, or part thereof, or each additional 1% of body area of infants and children, or part thereof (List separately in addition to code for primary procedure)

> EXCLUDES Total wound surface area up to 100 cm (15271-15272)
> Code first (15273)
> 🚑 1.33  ⚕ 2.04  **FUD** ZZZ    N N1 ▣

> **AMA:** 2017,Jan,8; 2016,Jan,13; 2015,Jan,16; 2014,Jun,14; 2014,Jan,11; 2013,Oct,15; 2013,Nov,14; 2012,Oct,3-8; 2012,Jan,6-10; 2012,Jan,15-42

**15275** Application of skin substitute graft to face, scalp, eyelids, mouth, neck, ears, orbits, genitalia, hands, feet, and/or multiple digits, total wound surface area up to 100 sq cm; first 25 sq cm or less wound surface area

> EXCLUDES Total wound area greater than or equal to 100 sq cm (15277-15278)
> 🚑 2.76  ⚕ 4.23  **FUD** 000    T G2 ▣

> **AMA:** 2017,Jan,8; 2016,Jan,13; 2015,Jan,16; 2014,Jun,14; 2014,Jan,11; 2013,Oct,15; 2012,Oct,3-8; 2012,Jan,6-10; 2012,Jan,15-42

+ **15276** each additional 25 sq cm wound surface area, or part thereof (List separately in addition to code for primary procedure)

> EXCLUDES Total wound area greater than or equal to 100 sq cm (15277-15278)
> Code first (15275)
> 🚑 0.73  ⚕ 0.99  **FUD** ZZZ    N N1 ▣

> **AMA:** 2017,Jan,8; 2016,Jan,13; 2015,Jan,16; 2014,Jun,14; 2014,Jan,11; 2013,Oct,15; 2012,Oct,3-8; 2012,Jan,6-10; 2012,Jan,15-42

**15277** Application of skin substitute graft to face, scalp, eyelids, mouth, neck, ears, orbits, genitalia, hands, feet, and/or multiple digits, total wound surface area greater than or equal to 100 sq cm; first 100 sq cm wound surface area, or 1% of body area of infants and children

> EXCLUDES Total surface area up to 100 sq cm (15275-15276)
> 🚑 6.58  ⚕ 9.31  **FUD** 000    T G2 ▣

> **AMA:** 2017,Jan,8; 2016,Jan,13; 2015,Jan,16; 2014,Jun,14; 2014,Jan,11; 2013,Oct,15; 2013,Nov,14; 2012,Oct,3-8; 2012,Jan,6-10; 2012,Jan,15-42

+ **15278** each additional 100 sq cm wound surface area, or part thereof, or each additional 1% of body area of infants and children, or part thereof (List separately in addition to code for primary procedure)

> EXCLUDES Total surface area up to 100 sq cm (15275-15276)
> Code first (15277)
> 🚑 1.67  ⚕ 2.44  **FUD** ZZZ    N N1 ▣

> **AMA:** 2017,Jan,8; 2016,Jan,13; 2015,Jan,16; 2014,Jun,14; 2014,Jan,11; 2013,Oct,15; 2013,Nov,14; 2012,Oct,3-8; 2012,Jan,6-10; 2012,Jan,15-42

## 15570-15731 Wound Reconstruction: Skin Flaps

> INCLUDES Ankle or wrist if code description describes leg or arm
> Code based on recipient site when the flap is attached in the transfer or to a final site and is based on donor site when a tube is created for transfer later or when the flap is delayed prior to transfer
> Fixation and anchoring skin graft
> Simple tissue debridement
> Tube formation for later transfer

> EXCLUDES Contiguous tissue transfer flaps (14040-14041, 14060-14061, 14301-14302)
> Debridement without immediate primary closure (11042-11047 [11045, 11046], 97597-97598)
> Excision of:
> Benign lesion (11400-11471)
> Burn eschar or scar (15002-15005)
> Malignant lesion (11600-11646)
> Microvascular repair (15756-15758)
> Primary procedure--see appropriate anatomical site

> Code also application of extensive immobilization apparatus
> Code also repair of donor site with skin grafts or flaps

**15570** Formation of direct or tubed pedicle, with or without transfer; trunk

> INCLUDES Flaps without a vascular pedicle
> 🚑 21.1  ⚕ 26.0  **FUD** 090    T A2 ▣

> **AMA:** 2017,Jan,8; 2016,Jan,13; 2015,Jan,16; 2014,Jan,11; 2012,Dec,6-8; 2012,Jan,15-42

**Pedicle flap**

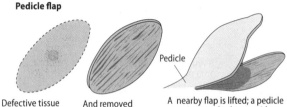

Defective tissue is identified | And removed | A nearby flap is lifted; a pedicle remains attached to provide an intact blood supply — Pedicle

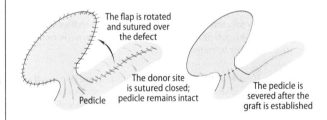

The flap is rotated and sutured over the defect | The donor site is sutured closed; pedicle remains intact — Pedicle | The pedicle is severed after the graft is established

**15572** scalp, arms, or legs

> INCLUDES Flaps without a vascular pedicle
> 🚑 21.5  ⚕ 25.3  **FUD** 090    T A2 ▣

> **AMA:** 2017,Jan,8; 2016,Jan,13; 2015,Jan,16; 2014,Jan,11; 2012,Dec,6-8; 2012,Jan,15-42

**15574** forehead, cheeks, chin, mouth, neck, axillae, genitalia, hands or feet

> INCLUDES Flaps without a vascular pedicle
> 🚑 22.0  ⚕ 25.9  **FUD** 090    T A2 ▣

> **AMA:** 2017,Jan,8; 2016,Jan,13; 2015,Jan,16; 2014,Jan,11; 2012,Dec,6-8; 2012,Jan,15-42

**15576** eyelids, nose, ears, lips, or intraoral

> INCLUDES Flaps without a vascular pedicle
> 🚑 19.3  ⚕ 22.9  **FUD** 090    T A2 ▣

> **AMA:** 2017,Jan,8; 2016,Jan,13; 2015,Jan,16; 2014,Jan,11; 2012,Dec,6-8; 2012,Jan,15-42

**15600** Delay of flap or sectioning of flap (division and inset); at trunk

> 🚑 5.92  ⚕ 9.14  **FUD** 090    T A2 80 ▣

> **AMA:** 2017,Jan,8; 2016,Jan,13; 2015,Jan,16; 2014,Jan,11; 2012,Dec,6-8

● New Code  ▲ Revised Code  ○ Reinstated  ● New Web Release  ▲ Revised Web Release  Unlisted  Not Covered  # Resequenced
⊘ AMA Mod 51 Exempt  ⑤ Optum Mod 51 Exempt  ⑥ Mod 63 Exempt  ✗ Non-FDA Drug  ★ Telemedicine  Ⓜ Maternity  Ⓐ Age Edit  + Add-on  **AMA:** CPT Asst

**15610** at scalp, arms, or legs

🚑 6.95    ⚕ 10.1    **FUD** 090     T A2 📮

**AMA:** 2017,Jan,8; 2016,Jan,13; 2015,Jan,16; 2014,Jan,11; 2012,Dec,6-8

**15620** at forehead, cheeks, chin, neck, axillae, genitalia, hands, or feet

🚑 9.32    ⚕ 12.4    **FUD** 090     T A2 📮

**AMA:** 2017,Jan,8; 2016,Jan,13; 2015,Jan,16; 2014,Jan,11; 2012,Dec,6-8

**15630** at eyelids, nose, ears, or lips

🚑 9.95    ⚕ 13.0    **FUD** 090     T A2 📮

**AMA:** 2017,Jan,8; 2016,Jan,13; 2015,Jan,16; 2014,Jan,11; 2012,Dec,6-8

**15650** Transfer, intermediate, of any pedicle flap (eg, abdomen to wrist, Walking tube), any location

> _EXCLUDES_  Defatting, revision, or rearranging of transferred pedicle flap or skin graft (13100-14302)
> Eyelids, ears, lips, and nose - refer to anatomical area

🚑 11.0    ⚕ 14.3    **FUD** 090     T A2 80 📮

**AMA:** 2017,Jan,8; 2016,Jan,13; 2015,Jan,16; 2014,Jan,11; 2012,Dec,6-8

● **15730** Midface flap (ie, zygomaticofacial flap) with preservation of vascular pedicle(s)

**15731** Forehead flap with preservation of vascular pedicle (eg, axial pattern flap, paramedian forehead flap)

> _EXCLUDES_  Muscle, myocutaneous, or fasciocutaneous flap of the head or neck (15733)

🚑 28.9    ⚕ 32.1    **FUD** 090     T A2 80 📮

**AMA:** 2017,Jan,8; 2016,Jan,13; 2015,Jan,16; 2014,Jan,11; 2012,Dec,6-8

## 15732-15738 Wound Reconstruction: Muscle Flaps

_INCLUDES_  Code based on donor site
_EXCLUDES_  Contiguous tissue transfer flaps (14040-14041, 14060-14061, 14301-14302)
Microvascular repair (15756-15758)
Code also application of extensive immobilization apparatus
Code also repair of donor site with skin grafts or flaps

~~15732~~  ~~Muscle, myocutaneous, or fasciocutaneous flap; head and neck (eg, temporalis, masseter muscle, sternocleidomastoid, levator scapulae)~~

To report, see 15733

● **15733** Muscle, myocutaneous, or fasciocutaneous flap; head and neck with named vascular pedicle (ie, buccinators, genioglossus, temporalis, masseter, sternocleidomastoid, levator scapulae)

> _INCLUDES_  Repair of extracranial defect by anterior pericranial flap on vascular pedicle (15731)

**15734** trunk

🚑 37.9    ⚕ 42.9    **FUD** 090     T A2 80 📮

**AMA:** 2017,Jan,8; 2016,Jan,13; 2015,Jan,16; 2014,Apr,10; 2014,Jan,11; 2013,Oct,15; 2012,Dec,6-8

**15736** upper extremity

🚑 32.7    ⚕ 37.6    **FUD** 090     T A2 📮

**AMA:** 2017,Jan,8; 2016,Jan,13; 2015,Jan,16; 2014,Jan,11; 2013,Mar,13; 2012,Dec,6-8

**15738** lower extremity

🚑 35.3    ⚕ 40.0    **FUD** 090     T A2 80 📮

**AMA:** 2017,Jan,8; 2016,Jan,13; 2015,Jan,16; 2014,Jan,11; 2012,Dec,6-8; 2012,Jan,15-42

## 15740-15758 Wound Reconstruction: Other

_INCLUDES_  Fixation and anchoring skin graft
Routine dressing
Simple tissue debridement
_EXCLUDES_  Adjacent tissue transfer (14000-14302)
Excision of:
  Benign lesion (11400-11471)
  Burn eschar or scar (15002-15005)
  Malignant lesion (11600-11646)
Flaps without addition of a vascular pedicle (15570-15576)
Primary procedure--see appropriate anatomical section
Skin graft for repair of donor site (15050-15278)
Code also repair of donor site with skin grafts or flaps (14000-14350, 15050-15278)

**15740** Flap; island pedicle requiring identification and dissection of an anatomically named axial vessel

> _EXCLUDES_  V-Y subcutaneous flaps, random island flaps, and other flaps from adjacent areas (14000-14302)

🚑 24.5    ⚕ 29.0    **FUD** 090     T A2 📮

**AMA:** 2017,Jan,8; 2016,Jan,13; 2015,Jan,16; 2014,Jan,11; 2012,Dec,6-8; 2012,Jan,15-42

**15750** neurovascular pedicle

> _EXCLUDES_  V-Y subcutaneous flaps, random island flaps, and other flaps from adjacent areas (14000-14302)

🚑 26.3    ⚕ 26.3    **FUD** 090     T A2 80 📮

**AMA:** 2010,Apr,3-4; 2002,Nov,5

**15756** Free muscle or myocutaneous flap with microvascular anastomosis

> _INCLUDES_  Operating microscope (69990)

🚑 66.8    ⚕ 66.8    **FUD** 090     C 80 📮

**AMA:** 2017,Jan,8; 2016,Feb,12; 2016,Jan,13; 2015,Jan,16; 2014,Jan,11

**15757** Free skin flap with microvascular anastomosis

> _INCLUDES_  Operating microscope (69990)

🚑 65.8    ⚕ 65.8    **FUD** 090     C 80 📮

**AMA:** 2017,Jan,8; 2016,Apr,8; 2016,Feb,12; 2016,Jan,13; 2015,Jan,16; 2014,Jan,11

**15758** Free fascial flap with microvascular anastomosis

> _INCLUDES_  Operating microscope (69990)

🚑 66.0    ⚕ 66.0    **FUD** 090     C 80 📮

**AMA:** 2017,Jan,8; 2016,Feb,12; 2016,Jan,13; 2015,Jan,16; 2014,Jan,11

## 15760-15770 Grafts Comprising Multiple Tissue Types

_INCLUDES_  Fixation and anchoring skin graft
Routine dressing
Simple tissue debridement
_EXCLUDES_  Adjacent tissue transfer (14000-14302)
Excision of:
  Benign lesion (11400-11471)
  Burn eschar or scar (15002-15005)
  Malignant lesion (11600-11646)
Flaps without addition of vascular pedicle (15570-15576)
Microvascular repair (15756-15758)
Primary procedure (see appropriate anatomical site)
Repair of donor site with skin grafts or flaps (14000-14350, 15050-15278)

**15760** Graft; composite (eg, full thickness of external ear or nasal ala), including primary closure, donor area

🚑 20.4    ⚕ 24.3    **FUD** 090     T A2 📮

**AMA:** 2017,Jan,8; 2016,Jan,13; 2015,Jan,16; 2014,Jan,11

**15770** derma-fat-fascia

🚑 19.1    ⚕ 19.1    **FUD** 090     T A2 80 📮

**AMA:** 2017,Jan,8; 2016,Jan,13; 2015,Jan,16; 2014,Jan,11

26/TC PC/TC Only    A2-Z3 ASC Payment    50 Bilateral    ♂ Male Only    ♀ Female Only    🚑 Facility RVU    ⚕ Non-Facility RVU    📮 CCI
**FUD** Follow-up Days    **CMS:** IOM (Pub 100)    A-Y OPPSI    80/80 Surg Assist Allowed / w/Doc    🔲 Lab Crosswalk    🔲 Radiology Crosswalk    ✖ CLIA

26

CPT © 2017 American Medical Association. All Rights Reserved.

© 2017 Optum360, LLC

## 15775-15839 Plastic, Reconstructive, and Aesthetic Surgery

**CMS:** 100-02,16,10 Exclusions from Coverage; 100-02,16,120 Cosmetic Procedures; 100-02,16,180 Services Related to Noncovered Procedures

**15775** **Punch graft for hair transplant; 1 to 15 punch grafts**
*EXCLUDES* *Strip transplant (15220)*
🔲 6.42 ⚕ 8.56 **FUD** 000 〔T〕〔A2〕〔80〕🔲
**AMA:** 2017,Jan,8; 2016,Jan,13; 2015,Jan,16; 2014,Jan,11

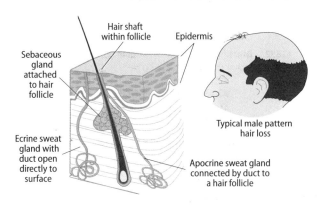

Hair shaft within follicle
Epidermis
Sebaceous gland attached to hair follicle
Ecrine sweat gland with duct open directly to surface
Apocrine sweat gland connected by duct to a hair follicle
Typical male pattern hair loss

**15776** **more than 15 punch grafts**
*EXCLUDES* *Strip transplant (15220)*
🔲 10.1 ⚕ 13.8 **FUD** 000 〔T〕〔A2〕〔80〕🔲
**AMA:** 2017,Jan,8; 2016,Jan,13; 2015,Jan,16; 2014,Jan,11

**+ 15777** **Implantation of biologic implant (eg, acellular dermal matrix) for soft tissue reinforcement (ie, breast, trunk) (List separately in addition to code for primary procedure)**
*EXCLUDES* *Application of skin substitute (high cost) to an external wound (15271-15278)*
*Application of skin substitute (low cost) to an external wound (C5271-C5278)*
*Mesh implantation for:*
*Open repair of ventral or incisional hernia (49560-49566) and (49568)*
*Repair of devitalized soft tissue infection (11004-11006) and (49568)*
*Repair of pelvic floor (57267)*
*Repair anorectal fistula with plug (46707)*
*Soft tissue reinforcement with biologic implants other than in the breast or trunk (17999)*
Code also supply of biologic implant
Code also synthetic or non-biological implant to reinforce abdominal wall (0437T)
Code first primary procedure
🔲 6.23 ⚕ 6.23 **FUD** ZZZ 〔N〕〔N1〕〔50〕🔲
**AMA:** 2017,Jan,8; 2016,Jan,13; 2015,Jan,16; 2014,Jan,11; 2013,Oct,15; 2012,Jan,6-10

**15780** **Dermabrasion; total face (eg, for acne scarring, fine wrinkling, rhytids, general keratosis)**
🔲 18.6 ⚕ 24.5 **FUD** 090 〔J〕〔P3〕〔80〕🔲
**AMA:** 2017,Jan,8; 2016,Jan,13; 2015,Jan,16; 2014,Jan,11; 2012,Jan,15-42

**15781** **segmental, face**
🔲 12.4 ⚕ 15.7 **FUD** 090 〔T〕〔P2〕🔲
**AMA:** 1997,Nov,1

**15782** **regional, other than face**
🔲 12.8 ⚕ 18.1 **FUD** 090 〔J〕〔P3〕〔80〕🔲
**AMA:** 1997,Nov,1

**15783** **superficial, any site (eg, tattoo removal)**
🔲 10.6 ⚕ 13.5 **FUD** 090 〔T〕〔P2〕〔80〕🔲
**AMA:** 2017,Jan,8; 2016,Jan,13; 2015,Jan,16; 2014,Jan,11

**15786** **Abrasion; single lesion (eg, keratosis, scar)**
🔲 3.91 ⚕ 6.96 **FUD** 010 〔Q1〕〔N1〕🔲
**AMA:** 1997,Nov,1

**+ 15787** **each additional 4 lesions or less (List separately in addition to code for primary procedure)**
Code first (15786)
🔲 0.49 ⚕ 1.40 **FUD** ZZZ 〔N〕〔N1〕🔲
**AMA:** 1997,Nov,1

**15788** **Chemical peel, facial; epidermal**
🔲 7.03 ⚕ 13.0 **FUD** 090 〔Q1〕〔N1〕🔲
**AMA:** 1997,Nov,1; 1993,Win,1

**15789** **dermal**
🔲 12.1 ⚕ 15.8 **FUD** 090 〔T〕〔P2〕🔲
**AMA:** 1997,Nov,1; 1993,Win,1

**15792** **Chemical peel, nonfacial; epidermal**
🔲 7.36 ⚕ 12.3 **FUD** 090 〔Q1〕〔N1〕〔80〕🔲
**AMA:** 1997,Nov,1; 1993,Win,1

**15793** **dermal**
🔲 10.5 ⚕ 14.0 **FUD** 090 〔Q1〕〔N1〕〔80〕🔲
**AMA:** 1997,Nov,1; 1993,Win,1

**15819** **Cervicoplasty**
🔲 22.7 ⚕ 22.7 **FUD** 090 〔T〕〔G2〕〔80〕🔲
**AMA:** 1997,Nov,1

**15820** **Blepharoplasty, lower eyelid;**
🔲 14.9 ⚕ 16.6 **FUD** 090 〔T〕〔A2〕〔80〕〔50〕🔲
**AMA:** 2017,Jan,8; 2016,Jan,13; 2015,Jan,16; 2014,Jan,11; 2012,Jan,15-42

**15821** **with extensive herniated fat pad**
🔲 15.4 ⚕ 17.2 **FUD** 090 〔T〕〔A2〕〔80〕〔50〕🔲
**AMA:** 2017,Jan,8; 2016,Jan,13; 2015,Jan,16; 2014,Jan,11

**15822** **Blepharoplasty, upper eyelid;**
🔲 11.1 ⚕ 12.6 **FUD** 090 〔T〕〔A2〕〔50〕🔲
**AMA:** 2017,Jan,8; 2016,Jan,13; 2015,Jan,16; 2014,Jan,11

**15823** **with excessive skin weighting down lid**
🔲 15.4 ⚕ 17.2 **FUD** 090 〔T〕〔A2〕〔50〕🔲
**AMA:** 2017,Jan,8; 2016,Jan,13; 2015,Jan,16; 2014,Jan,11

**15824** **Rhytidectomy; forehead**
*EXCLUDES* *Repair of brow ptosis (67900)*
🔲 0.00 ⚕ 0.00 **FUD** 000 〔T〕〔A2〕〔80〕〔50〕🔲
**AMA:** 2017,Apr,9

Frontalis (elevates brow)
Forehead rhytidectomy incision
A rhytidectomy is an excision to eliminate wrinkles. This procedure in the forehead region typically involves an incision just inside the scalp line. Skin and underlying tissues are then manipulated to eliminate wrinkles in the forehead
Procerus (wrinkles nose)
Corrugators (move brows medially)

**15825** **neck with platysmal tightening (platysmal flap, P-flap)**
🔲 0.00 ⚕ 0.00 **FUD** 000 〔T〕〔A2〕〔80〕〔50〕🔲
**AMA:** 2017,Apr,9

**15826** **glabellar frown lines**
🔲 0.00 ⚕ 0.00 **FUD** 000 〔T〕〔A2〕〔80〕〔50〕🔲
**AMA:** 1997,Nov,1

**15828** **cheek, chin, and neck**
🔲 0.00 ⚕ 0.00 **FUD** 000 〔T〕〔A2〕〔80〕〔50〕🔲
**AMA:** 1997,Nov,1

**15829** **superficial musculoaponeurotic system (SMAS) flap**
🔲 0.00 ⚕ 0.00 **FUD** 000 〔T〕〔A2〕〔80〕〔50〕🔲
**AMA:** 1997,Nov,1

---

● New Code ▲ Revised Code ○ Reinstated ● New Web Release ▲ Revised Web Release Unlisted Not Covered # Resequenced
⊘ AMA Mod 51 Exempt ⑤⑪ Optum Mod 51 Exempt ⑥③ Mod 63 Exempt ✗ Non-FDA Drug ★ Telemedicine Ⓜ Maternity ⒶAge Edit + Add-on **AMA:** CPT Asst

© 2017 Optum360, LLC CPT © 2017 American Medical Association. All Rights Reserved.

**Integumentary System**

**15830 — 15931**

15830 | **Excision, excessive skin and subcutaneous tissue (includes lipectomy); abdomen, infraumbilical panniculectomy**
- 📷 33.7  ✂ 33.7  **FUD** 090    J A2 80 ▭

EXCLUDES Adjacent tissue transfer, trunk (14302)
Complex wound repair, trunk (13100-13102)
Intermediate wound repair, trunk (12031-12032, 12034-12037)
Other abdominoplasty (17999)
Code also (15847)

15832 | **thigh**
- 📷 26.2  ✂ 26.2  **FUD** 090    J A2 80 50 ▭
- **AMA:** 1997,Nov,1

15833 | **leg**
- 📷 24.5  ✂ 24.5  **FUD** 090    J A2 80 50 ▭
- **AMA:** 1997,Nov,1

15834 | **hip**
- 📷 25.4  ✂ 25.4  **FUD** 090    J A2 80 50 ▭
- **AMA:** 1997,Nov,1

15835 | **buttock**
- 📷 26.2  ✂ 26.2  **FUD** 090    J A2 80 ▭
- **AMA:** 1997,Nov,1

15836 | **arm**
- 📷 22.6  ✂ 22.6  **FUD** 090    J A2 80 50 ▭
- **AMA:** 1997,Nov,1

15837 | **forearm or hand**
- 📷 20.4  ✂ 24.3  **FUD** 090    J G2 80 ▭
- **AMA:** 1997,Nov,1

15838 | **submental fat pad**
- 📷 16.3  ✂ 16.3  **FUD** 090    J G2 80 ▭
- **AMA:** 1998,Feb,1; 1997,Nov,1

15839 | **other area**
- 📷 21.1  ✂ 25.1  **FUD** 090    J A2 80 ▭
- **AMA:** 1997,Nov,1

## 15840-15845 Reanimation of the Paralyzed Face

INCLUDES Routine dressing and supplies
EXCLUDES Intravenous fluorescein evaluation of blood flow in graft or flap (15860)
Nerve:
Decompression (69720, 69725, 69955)
Pedicle transfer (64905, 64907)
Suture (64831-64876, 69740, 69745)
Code also repair of donor site with skin grafts or flaps

15840 | **Graft for facial nerve paralysis; free fascia graft (including obtaining fascia)**
- 📷 28.8  ✂ 28.8  **FUD** 090    T A2 ▭
- **AMA:** 1997,Nov,1

15841 | **free muscle graft (including obtaining graft)**
- 📷 45.7  ✂ 45.7  **FUD** 090    T A2 80 ▭
- **AMA:** 1997,Nov,1

15842 | **free muscle flap by microsurgical technique**
- INCLUDES Operating microscope (69990)
- 📷 70.1  ✂ 70.1  **FUD** 090    T G2 80 ▭
- **AMA:** 2016,Feb,12

15845 | **regional muscle transfer**
- 📷 28.5  ✂ 28.5  **FUD** 090    T A2 80 ▭
- **AMA:** 1998,Feb,1; 1997,Nov,1

## 15847 Removal of Excess Abdominal Tissue Add-on

**CMS:** 100-02,16,10 Exclusions from Coverage; 100-02,16,120 Cosmetic Procedures; 100-02,16,180 Services Related to Noncovered Procedures

+ 15847 | **Excision, excessive skin and subcutaneous tissue (includes lipectomy), abdomen (eg, abdominoplasty) (includes umbilical transposition and fascial plication) (List separately in addition to code for primary procedure)**
- 📷 0.00  ✂ 0.00  **FUD** YYY    N N1 80 ▭
- EXCLUDES Abdominal wall hernia repair (49491-49587)
Other abdominoplasty (17999)
Code first (15830)

## 15850-15852 Suture Removal/Dressing Change: Anesthesia Required

15850 | **Removal of sutures under anesthesia (other than local), same surgeon**
- 📷 1.19  ✂ 2.51  **FUD** XXX    T 62 ▭
- **AMA:** 2017,Jan,8; 2016,Jan,13; 2015,Jan,16; 2014,Jan,11

15851 | **Removal of sutures under anesthesia (other than local), other surgeon**
- 📷 1.31  ✂ 2.80  **FUD** 000    T P3 ▭
- **AMA:** 2017,Jan,8; 2016,Jan,13; 2015,Jan,16; 2014,Jan,11

15852 | **Dressing change (for other than burns) under anesthesia (other than local)**
- EXCLUDES Dressing change for burns (16020-16030)
- 📷 1.35  ✂ 1.35  **FUD** 000    Q1 N1 ▭
- **AMA:** 1997,Nov,1

## 15860 Injection for Vascular Flow Determination

15860 | **Intravenous injection of agent (eg, fluorescein) to test vascular flow in flap or graft**
- 📷 3.17  ✂ 3.17  **FUD** 000    Q1 N1 80 ▭
- **AMA:** 2002,May,7; 1997,Nov,1

## 15876-15879 Liposuction

**CMS:** 100-02,16,10 Exclusions from Coverage; 100-02,16,120 Cosmetic Procedures; 100-02,16,180 Services Related to Noncovered Procedures
EXCLUDES Obtaining tissue for adipose-derived regenerative cell therapy (0489T-0490T)

15876 | **Suction assisted lipectomy; head and neck**
- 📷 0.00  ✂ 0.00  **FUD** 000    T A2 80 ▭
- **AMA:** 1997,Nov,1

Cannula typically inserted through incision in front of ear

15877 | **trunk**
- 📷 0.00  ✂ 0.00  **FUD** 000    T A2 80 ▭
- **AMA:** 2017,Jan,8; 2016,Jan,13; 2015,Jan,16; 2014,Jan,11; 2012,Jan,15-42

15878 | **upper extremity**
- 📷 0.00  ✂ 0.00  **FUD** 000    T A2 80 50 ▭
- **AMA:** 1997,Nov,1

15879 | **lower extremity**
- 📷 0.00  ✂ 0.00  **FUD** 000    T A2 80 50 ▭
- **AMA:** 1997,Nov,1

## 15920-15999 Treatment of Decubitus Ulcers

Code also free skin graft to repair ulcer or donor site

15920 | **Excision, coccygeal pressure ulcer, with coccygectomy; with primary suture**
- 📷 17.8  ✂ 17.8  **FUD** 090    J A2 80 ▭
- **AMA:** 2011,May,3-5; 1997,Nov,1

15922 | **with flap closure**
- 📷 22.4  ✂ 22.4  **FUD** 090    T A2 80 ▭
- **AMA:** 2011,May,3-5; 1997,Nov,1

15931 | **Excision, sacral pressure ulcer, with primary suture;**
- 📷 19.7  ✂ 19.7  **FUD** 090    J A2
- **AMA:** 2011,May,3-5; 1997,Nov,1

| | | |
|---|---|---|
| **15933** | **with ostectomy** | |
| | 🚑 24.2  ✂ 24.2  **FUD** 090 | J A2 80 ▭ |
| | **AMA:** 2011,May,3-5; 1997,Nov,1 | |
| **15934** | **Excision, sacral pressure ulcer, with skin flap closure;** | |
| | 🚑 26.7  ✂ 26.7  **FUD** 090 | T A2 ▭ |
| | **AMA:** 2011,May,3-5; 1997,Nov,1 | |
| **15935** | **with ostectomy** | |
| | 🚑 31.6  ✂ 31.6  **FUD** 090 | T A2 80 ▭ |
| | **AMA:** 2011,May,3-5; 1997,Nov,1 | |
| **15936** | **Excision, sacral pressure ulcer, in preparation for muscle or myocutaneous flap or skin graft closure;** | |
| | Code also any defect repair with: | |
| | Muscle or myocutaneous flap (15734, 15738) | |
| | Split skin graft (15100-15101) | |
| | 🚑 25.5  ✂ 25.5  **FUD** 090 | T A2 ▭ |
| | **AMA:** 2011,May,3-5; 1998,Nov,1 | |
| **15937** | **with ostectomy** | |
| | Code also any defect repair with: | |
| | Muscle or myocutaneous flap (15734, 15738) | |
| | Split skin graft (15100-15101) | |
| | 🚑 29.6  ✂ 29.6  **FUD** 090 | T A2 ▭ |
| | **AMA:** 2011,May,3-5; 1998,Nov,1 | |
| **15940** | **Excision, ischial pressure ulcer, with primary suture;** | |
| | 🚑 20.0  ✂ 20.0  **FUD** 090 | J A2 ▭ |
| | **AMA:** 2011,May,3-5; 1997,Nov,1 | |
| **15941** | **with ostectomy (ischiectomy)** | |
| | 🚑 25.7  ✂ 25.7  **FUD** 090 | J A2 80 ▭ |
| | **AMA:** 2011,May,3-5; 1997,Nov,1 | |
| **15944** | **Excision, ischial pressure ulcer, with skin flap closure;** | |
| | 🚑 25.5  ✂ 25.5  **FUD** 090 | T A2 80 ▭ |
| | **AMA:** 2011,May,3-5; 1997,Nov,1 | |
| **15945** | **with ostectomy** | |
| | 🚑 28.2  ✂ 28.2  **FUD** 090 | T A2 80 ▭ |
| | **AMA:** 2011,May,3-5; 1997,Nov,1 | |
| **15946** | **Excision, ischial pressure ulcer, with ostectomy, in preparation for muscle or myocutaneous flap or skin graft closure** | |
| | Code also any defect repair with: | |
| | Muscle or myocutaneous flap (15734, 15738) | |
| | Split skin graft (15100-15101) | |
| | 🚑 47.0  ✂ 47.0  **FUD** 090 | T A2 ▭ |
| | **AMA:** 2017,Jan,8; 2016,Jan,13; 2015,Jan,16; 2014,Jan,11; 2012,Jan,15-42 | |
| **15950** | **Excision, trochanteric pressure ulcer, with primary suture;** | |
| | 🚑 16.9  ✂ 16.9  **FUD** 090 | J A2 ▭ |
| | **AMA:** 2011,May,3-5; 1997,Nov,1 | |
| **15951** | **with ostectomy** | |
| | 🚑 24.9  ✂ 24.9  **FUD** 090 | J A2 80 ▭ |
| | **AMA:** 2011,May,3-5; 1997,Nov,1 | |
| **15952** | **Excision, trochanteric pressure ulcer, with skin flap closure;** | |
| | 🚑 25.7  ✂ 25.7  **FUD** 090 | T A2 80 ▭ |
| | **AMA:** 2011,May,3-5; 1997,Nov,1 | |
| **15953** | **with ostectomy** | |
| | 🚑 28.5  ✂ 28.5  **FUD** 090 | T A2 ▭ |
| | **AMA:** 2011,May,3-5; 1997,Nov,1 | |
| **15956** | **Excision, trochanteric pressure ulcer, in preparation for muscle or myocutaneous flap or skin graft closure;** | |
| | Code also any defect repair with: | |
| | Muscle or myocutaneous flap (15734, 15738) | |
| | Split skin graft (15100-15101) | |
| | 🚑 33.0  ✂ 33.0  **FUD** 090 | T A2 ▭ |
| | **AMA:** 2011,May,3-5; 1998,Nov,1 | |
| **15958** | **with ostectomy** | |
| | Code also any defect repair with: | |
| | Muscle or myocutaneous flap (15734-15738) | |
| | Split skin graft (15100-15101) | |
| | 🚑 33.6  ✂ 33.6  **FUD** 090 | T A2 ▭ |
| | **AMA:** 2011,May,3-5; 1998,Nov,1 | |

| | | |
|---|---|---|
| **15999** | **Unlisted procedure, excision pressure ulcer** | |
| | 🚑 0.00  ✂ 0.00  **FUD** YYY | T 80 ▭ |
| | **AMA:** 2011,May,3-5; 1997,Nov,1 | |

## 16000-16036 Burn Care

| | |
|---|---|
| INCLUDES | Local care of burn surface only |
| EXCLUDES | Application of skin grafts including all services described in the following codes (15100-15777) |
| | E&M services |
| | Flaps (15570-15650) |
| | Laser fenestration for scars (0479T-0480T) |

| | | |
|---|---|---|
| **16000** | **Initial treatment, first degree burn, when no more than local treatment is required** | |
| | 🚑 1.32  ✂ 1.96  **FUD** 000 | Q1 N1 ▭ |
| | **AMA:** 2017,Jan,8; 2016,Jan,13; 2015,Jan,16; 2014,Jan,11; 2012,Oct,3-8 | |
| **16020** | **Dressings and/or debridement of partial-thickness burns, initial or subsequent; small (less than 5% total body surface area)** | |
| | INCLUDES  Wound coverage other than skin graft | |
| | 🚑 1.55  ✂ 2.32  **FUD** 000 | Q1 N1 ▭ |
| | **AMA:** 2017,Jan,8; 2016,Jan,13; 2015,Jan,16; 2014,Jan,11; 2012,Oct,3-8 | |
| **16025** | **medium (eg, whole face or whole extremity, or 5% to 10% total body surface area)** | |
| | INCLUDES  Wound coverage other than skin graft | |
| | 🚑 3.20  ✂ 4.19  **FUD** 000 | T A2 ▭ |
| | **AMA:** 2017,Jan,8; 2016,Jan,13; 2015,Jan,16; 2014,Jan,11; 2012,Oct,3-8; 2012,Jan,15-42 | |
| **16030** | **large (eg, more than 1 extremity, or greater than 10% total body surface area)** | |
| | INCLUDES  Wound coverage other than skin graft | |
| | 🚑 3.85  ✂ 5.28  **FUD** 000 | T A2 ▭ |
| | **AMA:** 2017,Jan,8; 2016,Jan,13; 2015,Jan,16; 2014,Jan,11; 2012,Oct,3-8; 2012,Jan,15-42 | |
| **16035** | **Escharotomy; initial incision** | |
| | EXCLUDES  Debridement or scraping of burn (16020-16030) | |
| | 🚑 5.60  ✂ 5.60  **FUD** 000 | T 02 ▭ |
| | **AMA:** 2017,Jan,8; 2016,Jan,13; 2015,Jan,16; 2014,Jan,11; 2012,Oct,3-8 | |
| **+ 16036** | **each additional incision (List separately in addition to code for primary procedure)** | |
| | EXCLUDES  Debridement or scraping of burn (16020-16030) | |
| | Code first (16035) | |
| | 🚑 2.35  ✂ 2.35  **FUD** ZZZ | C ▭ |
| | **AMA:** 2017,Jan,8; 2016,Jan,13; 2015,Jan,16; 2014,Jan,11; 2012,Oct,3-8 | |

---

● New Code    ▲ Revised Code    ○ Reinstated    ● New Web Release    ▲ Revised Web Release    Unlisted    Not Covered    # Resequenced
⊘ AMA Mod 51 Exempt    ⑤ Optum Mod 51 Exempt    ⑥³ Mod 63 Exempt    ⊬ Non-FDA Drug    ★ Telemedicine    Ⓜ Maternity    🄰 Age Edit    + Add-on    **AMA:** CPT Asst

© 2017 Optum360, LLC              CPT © 2017 American Medical Association. All Rights Reserved.                                                                    **29**

## 17000-17004 Destruction Any Method: Premalignant Lesion

**CMS:** 100-03,140.5 Laser Procedures

**EXCLUDES** Cryotherapy acne (17340)
Destruction of:
Benign lesions other than cutaneous vascular proliferative lesions (17110-17111)
Cutaneous vascular proliferative lesions (17106-17108)
Malignant lesions (17260-17286)
Plantar warts (17110-17111)
Destruction of lesion of:
Anus (46900-46917, 46924)
Conjunctiva (68135)
Eyelid (67850)
Penis (54050-54057, 54065)
Vagina (57061, 57065)
Vestibule of mouth (40820)
Vulva (56501, 56515)
Destruction or excision of skin tags (11200-11201)
Escharotomy (16035-16036)
Excision benign lesion (11400-11446)
Laser fenestration for scars (0479T-0480T)
Localized chemotherapy treatment see appropriate office visit service code
Paring or excision of benign hyperkeratotic lesion (11055-11057)
Shaving skin lesions (11300-11313)
Treatment of inflammatory skin disease via laser (96920-96922)

**17000** Destruction (eg, laser surgery, electrosurgery, cryosurgery, chemosurgery, surgical curettement), premalignant lesions (eg, actinic keratoses); first lesion
🚑 1.52   ♨ 1.89   **FUD** 010                      [01] [N1] 🖻
**AMA:** 2017,Jan,8; 2016,Apr,3; 2016,Jan,13; 2015,Jan,16; 2014,Jan,11; 2012,May,13; 2012,Mar,4-7; 2012,Jan,15-42

**+    17003** second through 14 lesions, each (List separately in addition to code for first lesion)
Code first (17000)
🚑 0.07   ♨ 0.16   **FUD** ZZZ                      [N] [N1] 🖻
**AMA:** 2017,Jan,8; 2016,Apr,3; 2016,Jan,13; 2015,Jan,16; 2014,Jan,11; 2012,May,13; 2012,Jan,15-42

**17004** Destruction (eg, laser surgery, electrosurgery, cryosurgery, chemosurgery, surgical curettement), premalignant lesions (eg, actinic keratoses), 15 or more lesions
**EXCLUDES** Use of code for destruction of less than 15 lesions (17000-17003)
🚑 2.86   ♨ 4.26   **FUD** 010                      ⊘ [T] [P3] 🖻
**AMA:** 2017,Jan,8; 2016,Apr,3; 2016,Jan,13; 2015,Jan,16; 2014,Jan,11; 2012,May,13; 2012,Jan,15-42

## 17106-17250 Destruction Any Method: Vascular Proliferative Lesion

**CMS:** 100-02,16,10 Exclusions from Coverage; 100-02,16,120 Cosmetic Procedures

**EXCLUDES** Destruction of lesion of:
Anus (46900-46917, 46924)
Conjunctiva (68135)
Eyelid (67850)
Penis (54050-54057, 54065)
Vagina (57061, 57065)
Vestibule of mouth (40820)
Vulva (56501, 56515)
Treatment of inflammatory skin disease via laser (96920-96922)

**17106** Destruction of cutaneous vascular proliferative lesions (eg, laser technique); less than 10 sq cm
🚑 7.96   ♨ 9.75   **FUD** 090                      [T] [P2] 🖻
**AMA:** 2017,Jan,8; 2016,Apr,3; 2016,Jan,13; 2015,Jan,16; 2014,Jan,11; 2012,May,13; 2012,Jan,15-42

**17107** 10.0 to 50.0 sq cm
🚑 9.94   ♨ 12.3   **FUD** 090                      [T] [P2] 🖻
**AMA:** 2017,Jan,8; 2016,Apr,3; 2016,Jan,13; 2015,Jan,16; 2014,Jan,11; 2012,May,13; 2012,Jan,15-42

**17108** over 50.0 sq cm
🚑 15.2   ♨ 18.3   **FUD** 090                      [T] [P3] [80] 🖻
**AMA:** 2017,Jan,8; 2016,Apr,3; 2016,Jan,13; 2015,Jan,16; 2014,Jan,11; 2012,May,13; 2012,Jan,15-42

**17110** Destruction (eg, laser surgery, electrosurgery, cryosurgery, chemosurgery, surgical curettement), of benign lesions other than skin tags or cutaneous vascular proliferative lesions; up to 14 lesions
🚑 2.00   ♨ 3.14   **FUD** 010                      [01] [N1] 🖻
**AMA:** 2017,Jan,8; 2016,Apr,3; 2016,Jan,13; 2015,Jan,16; 2014,Jan,11; 2012,May,13; 2012,Jan,15-42

**17111** 15 or more lesions
**EXCLUDES** Destruction of neurofibromas, 50-100 lesions (0419T-0420T)
🚑 2.46   ♨ 3.73   **FUD** 010                      [01] [N1] 🖻
**AMA:** 2017,Jan,8; 2016,Apr,3; 2016,Jan,13; 2015,Jan,16; 2014,Jan,11; 2012,May,13; 2012,Jan,15-42

▲    **17250** Chemical cauterization of granulation tissue (ie, proud flesh)
**EXCLUDES** Excision/removal codes for the same lesion
Chemical cauterization when applied for hemostasis of wound
Wound care management (97597-97598, 97602)
🚑 1.06   ♨ 2.24   **FUD** 000                      [01] [N1] 🖻
**AMA:** 2017,Jan,8; 2016,Jan,13; 2015,Jan,16; 2014,Jan,11; 2012,Dec,12; 2012,May,13; 2012,Jan,15-42

## 17260-17286 Destruction, Any Method: Malignant Lesion

**CMS:** 100-03,140.5 Laser Procedures

**EXCLUDES** Destruction of lesion of:
Anus (46900-46917, 46924)
Conjunctiva (68135)
Eyelid (67850)
Penis (54050-54057, 54065)
Vestibule of mouth (40820)
Vulva (56501-56515)
Localized chemotherapy treatment see appropriate office visit service code
Shaving skin lesion (11300-11313)
Treatment of inflammatory skin disease via laser (96920-96922)

**17260** Destruction, malignant lesion (eg, laser surgery, electrosurgery, cryosurgery, chemosurgery, surgical curettement), trunk, arms or legs; lesion diameter 0.5 cm or less
🚑 2.02   ♨ 2.69   **FUD** 010                      [01] [N1] 🖻
**AMA:** 2017,Jan,8; 2016,Jan,13; 2015,Jan,16; 2014,Jan,11; 2012,May,13

**17261** lesion diameter 0.6 to 1.0 cm
🚑 2.63   ♨ 4.06   **FUD** 010                      [01] [N1] 🖻
**AMA:** 2017,Jan,8; 2016,Jan,13; 2015,Jan,16; 2014,Jan,11; 2012,May,13

**17262** lesion diameter 1.1 to 2.0 cm
🚑 3.35   ♨ 4.96   **FUD** 010                      [01] [N1] 🖻
**AMA:** 2017,Jan,8; 2016,Jan,13; 2015,Jan,16; 2014,Jan,11; 2012,May,13

**17263** lesion diameter 2.1 to 3.0 cm
🚑 3.71   ♨ 5.42   **FUD** 010                      [01] [N1] 🖻
**AMA:** 2017,Jan,8; 2016,Jan,13; 2015,Jan,16; 2014,Jan,11; 2012,May,13

**17264** lesion diameter 3.1 to 4.0 cm
🚑 3.95   ♨ 5.79   **FUD** 010                      [T] [P3] 🖻
**AMA:** 2017,Jan,8; 2016,Jan,13; 2015,Jan,16; 2014,Jan,11; 2012,May,13

**17266** lesion diameter over 4.0 cm
🚑 4.65   ♨ 6.60   **FUD** 010                      [T] [P3] 🖻
**AMA:** 2017,Jan,8; 2016,Jan,13; 2015,Jan,16; 2014,Jan,11; 2012,May,13

**17270** Destruction, malignant lesion (eg, laser surgery, electrosurgery, cryosurgery, chemosurgery, surgical curettement), scalp, neck, hands, feet, genitalia; lesion diameter 0.5 cm or less
🚑 2.88   ♨ 4.27   **FUD** 010                      [T] [P2] 🖻
**AMA:** 2017,Jan,8; 2016,Jan,13; 2015,Jan,16; 2014,Jan,11; 2012,May,13

Integumentary System

17000 — 17270

**17271** lesion diameter 0.6 to 1.0 cm
　🔧 3.19　✂ 4.63　**FUD** 010　　T P2 ▣
　**AMA:** 2017,Jan,8; 2016,Jan,13; 2015,Jan,16; 2014,Jan,11;
　2012,May,13

**17272** lesion diameter 1.1 to 2.0 cm
　🔧 3.67　✂ 5.28　**FUD** 010　　Q1 N1 ▣
　**AMA:** 2017,Jan,8; 2016,Jan,13; 2015,Jan,16; 2014,Jan,11;
　2012,May,13

**17273** lesion diameter 2.1 to 3.0 cm
　🔧 4.16　✂ 5.90　**FUD** 010　　T P3 ▣
　**AMA:** 2017,Jan,8; 2016,Jan,13; 2015,Jan,16; 2014,Jan,11;
　2012,May,13

**17274** lesion diameter 3.1 to 4.0 cm
　🔧 5.09　✂ 6.98　**FUD** 010　　T P3 ▣
　**AMA:** 2017,Jan,8; 2016,Jan,13; 2015,Jan,16; 2014,Jan,11;
　2012,May,13

**17276** lesion diameter over 4.0 cm
　🔧 6.08　✂ 8.06　**FUD** 010　　T P3 ▣
　**AMA:** 2017,Jan,8; 2016,Jan,13; 2015,Jan,16; 2014,Jan,11;
　2012,May,13

**17280** Destruction, malignant lesion (eg, laser surgery,
electrosurgery, cryosurgery, chemosurgery, surgical
curettement), face, ears, eyelids, nose, lips, mucous
membrane; lesion diameter 0.5 cm or less
　🔧 2.62　✂ 4.00　**FUD** 010　　Q1 N1 ▣
　**AMA:** 2017,Jan,8; 2016,Jan,13; 2015,Jan,16; 2014,Jan,11;
　2012,May,13

**17281** lesion diameter 0.6 to 1.0 cm
　🔧 3.60　✂ 5.05　**FUD** 010　　T P3 ▣
　**AMA:** 2017,Jan,8; 2016,Jan,13; 2015,Jan,16; 2014,Jan,11;
　2012,May,13

**17282** lesion diameter 1.1 to 2.0 cm
　🔧 4.14　✂ 5.80　**FUD** 010　　T P3 ▣
　**AMA:** 2017,Jan,8; 2016,Jan,13; 2015,Jan,16; 2014,Jan,11;
　2012,May,13

**17283** lesion diameter 2.1 to 3.0 cm
　🔧 5.18　✂ 6.95　**FUD** 010　　T P3 ▣
　**AMA:** 2017,Jan,8; 2016,Jan,13; 2015,Jan,16; 2014,Jan,11;
　2012,May,13

**17284** lesion diameter 3.1 to 4.0 cm
　🔧 6.05　✂ 7.94　**FUD** 010　　T P3 ▣
　**AMA:** 2017,Jan,8; 2016,Jan,13; 2015,Jan,16; 2014,Jan,11;
　2012,May,13

**17286** lesion diameter over 4.0 cm
　🔧 8.11　✂ 10.1　**FUD** 010　　T P3 ▣
　**AMA:** 2017,Jan,8; 2016,Jan,13; 2015,Jan,16; 2014,Jan,11;
　2012,May,13

## 17311-17315 Mohs Surgery

**INCLUDES**　The following surgical/pathology services performed by the same physician
　or other qualified health care provider:
　Evaluation of skin margins by surgeon
　Pathology exam on Mohs surgery specimen (88302-88309)
　Routine frozen section stain (88314)
　Tumor removal, mapping, preparation, and examination of lesion

**EXCLUDES**　*Frozen section if no prior diagnosis determination has been performed (88331)*

Code also any special histochemical stain on a frozen section, nonroutine (with
　modifier 59) (88311-88314, 88342)
Code also biopsy (with modifier 59) if no prior diagnosis determination has been
　performed, if biopsy is indeterminate, or performed more than 90 days
　preoperatively (11100-11101)
Code also complex repair (13100-13160)
Code also flaps or grafts (14000-14350, 15050-15770)
Code also intermediate repair (12031-12057)
Code also simple repair (12001-12021)

**17311** Mohs micrographic technique, including removal of all gross
tumor, surgical excision of tissue specimens, mapping, color
coding of specimens, microscopic examination of specimens
by the surgeon, and histopathologic preparation including
routine stain(s) (eg, hematoxylin and eosin, toluidine blue),
head, neck, hands, feet, genitalia, or any location with surgery
directly involving muscle, cartilage, bone, tendon, major
nerves, or vessels; first stage, up to 5 tissue blocks
　🔧 10.9　✂ 18.7　**FUD** 000　　T P2 ▣
　**AMA:** 2017,Jan,8; 2016,Jan,13; 2015,Jan,16; 2014,Oct,14;
　2014,Feb,10; 2012,May,13

+ **17312** each additional stage after the first stage, up to 5 tissue
blocks (List separately in addition to code for primary
procedure)
　Code first (17311)
　🔧 5.82　✂ 11.0　**FUD** ZZZ　　N M1 ▣
　**AMA:** 2017,Jan,8; 2016,Jan,13; 2015,Jan,16; 2014,Oct,14;
　2014,Feb,10; 2012,May,13

**17313** Mohs micrographic technique, including removal of all gross
tumor, surgical excision of tissue specimens, mapping, color
coding of specimens, microscopic examination of specimens
by the surgeon, and histopathologic preparation including
routine stain(s) (eg, hematoxylin and eosin, toluidine blue),
of the trunk, arms, or legs; first stage, up to 5 tissue blocks
　🔧 9.81　✂ 17.5　**FUD** 000　　T P2 ▣
　**AMA:** 2017,Jan,8; 2016,Jan,13; 2015,Jan,16; 2014,Oct,14;
　2014,Feb,10; 2012,May,13

+ **17314** each additional stage after the first stage, up to 5 tissue
blocks (List separately in addition to code for primary
procedure)
　Code first (17313)
　🔧 5.40　✂ 10.5　**FUD** ZZZ　　N M1 ▣
　**AMA:** 2017,Jan,8; 2016,Jan,13; 2015,Jan,16; 2014,Oct,14;
　2014,Feb,10; 2012,May,13

+ **17315** Mohs micrographic technique, including removal of all gross
tumor, surgical excision of tissue specimens, mapping, color
coding of specimens, microscopic examination of specimens
by the surgeon, and histopathologic preparation including
routine stain(s) (eg, hematoxylin and eosin, toluidine blue),
each additional block after the first 5 tissue blocks, any stage
(List separately in addition to code for primary procedure)
　Code first (17311-17314)
　🔧 1.54　✂ 2.28　**FUD** ZZZ　　N M1 ▣
　**AMA:** 2017,Jan,8; 2016,Jan,13; 2015,Jan,16; 2014,Oct,14;
　2014,Feb,10; 2014,Jan,11; 2012,May,13

## 17340-17999 Treatment for Active Acne and Permanent Hair Removal

**CMS:** 100-02,16,10 Exclusions from Coverage; 100-02,16,120 Cosmetic Procedures

**17340** Cryotherapy ($CO_2$ slush, liquid N2) for acne
　🔧 1.40　✂ 1.47　**FUD** 010　　Q1 N1 ▣
　**AMA:** 2017,Jan,8; 2016,Jan,13; 2015,Jan,16; 2014,Jan,11;
　2012,May,13

---

● New Code　▲ Revised Code　○ Reinstated　● New Web Release　▲ Revised Web Release　Unlisted　Not Covered　# Resequenced
⊘ AMA Mod 51 Exempt　⑤ Optum Mod 51 Exempt　⑥ Mod 63 Exempt　✗ Non-FDA Drug　★ Telemedicine　Ⅿ Maternity　Ⓐ Age Edit　+ Add-on　**AMA:** CPT Asst
© 2017 Optum360, LLC　　　CPT © 2017 American Medical Association. All Rights Reserved.

**17360** Chemical exfoliation for acne (eg, acne paste, acid)

🖪 2.83 ⚕ 3.65 **FUD** 010 [01] [N1] [80] [▭]

**AMA:** 2017,Jan,8; 2016,Jan,13; 2015,Jan,16; 2014,Jan,11; 2012,May,13

**17380** Electrolysis epilation, each 30 minutes

EXCLUDES Actinotherapy (96900)

🖪 0.00 ⚕ 0.00 **FUD** 000 [T] [R2] [80] [▭]

**AMA:** 2017,Jan,8; 2016,Jan,13; 2015,Jan,16; 2014,Jan,11; 2012,May,13

**17999** Unlisted procedure, skin, mucous membrane and subcutaneous tissue

🖪 0.00 ⚕ 0.00 **FUD** YYY [01] [80]

**AMA:** 2017,Jan,8; 2016,May,13; 2016,Jan,13; 2015,Jan,16; 2014,Jan,11; 2013,Oct,15; 2012,May,13; 2012,Jan,15-42

## 19000-19030 Treatment of Breast Abscess and Cyst with Injection, Aspiration, Incision

**19000** Puncture aspiration of cyst of breast;

🔀 (76942, 77021)

🖪 1.26 ⚕ 3.20 **FUD** 000 [T] [P3] [▭]

**AMA:** 2017,Jan,8; 2016,Jan,13; 2015,Jan,16; 2014,Jan,11; 2013,Dec,16

+ **19001** each additional cyst (List separately in addition to code for primary procedure)

Code first (19000)

🔀 (76942, 77021)

🖪 0.63 ⚕ 0.77 **FUD** ZZZ [N] [N1] [▭]

**AMA:** 2017,Jan,8; 2016,Jan,13; 2015,Jan,16; 2014,Jan,11; 2013,Dec,16

**19020** Mastotomy with exploration or drainage of abscess, deep

🖪 8.78 ⚕ 13.4 **FUD** 090 [J] [A2] [50] [▭]

**AMA:** 2017,Jan,8; 2016,Jan,13; 2015,Jan,16; 2014,Dec,16; 2014,Dec,16; 2014,Jan,11

**19030** Injection procedure only for mammary ductogram or galactogram

🔀 (77053-77054)

🖪 2.25 ⚕ 4.69 **FUD** 000 [N] [N1] [50] [▭]

**AMA:** 2017,Jan,8; 2016,Jan,13; 2015,Jan,16; 2014,Jan,11

## 19081-19086 Breast Biopsy with Imaging Guidance

**CMS:** 100-03,220.13 Percutaneous Image-guided Breast Biopsy; 100-04,12,40.7 Bilateral Procedures; 100-04,13,80.1 Physician Presence; 100-04,13,80.2 S&I Multiple Procedure Reduction

INCLUDES Breast biopsy with placement of localization devices (19281-19288)
Fluoroscopic guidance for needle placement (77002)
Magnetic resonance guidance for needle placement (77021)
Radiological examination, surgical specimen (76098)
Ultrasonic guidance for needle placement (76942)

EXCLUDES Biopsy of breast without imaging guidance (19100-19101)
Lesion removal without concentration on surgical margins (19110-19126)
Open biopsy after placement of localization device (19101)
Partial mastectomy (19301-19302)
Placement of localization devices only (19281-19288)
Total mastectomy (19303-19307)
Code also additional biopsies performed with different imaging modalities

**19081** Biopsy, breast, with placement of breast localization device(s) (eg, clip, metallic pellet), when performed, and imaging of the biopsy specimen, when performed, percutaneous; first lesion, including stereotactic guidance

🖪 4.89 ⚕ 19.6 **FUD** 000 [J] [G2] [80] [50] [▭]

**AMA:** 2017,Jan,8; 2016,Jun,3; 2016,Jan,13; 2015,May,8; 2015,Mar,5; 2015,Jan,16; 2014,Jun,14; 2014,May,3

+ **19082** each additional lesion, including stereotactic guidance (List separately in addition to code for primary procedure)

Code first (19081)

🖪 2.46 ⚕ 16.2 **FUD** ZZZ [N] [N1] [80] [▭]

**AMA:** 2017,Jan,8; 2016,Jun,3; 2016,Jan,13; 2015,May,8; 2015,Mar,5; 2015,Jan,16; 2014,Jun,14; 2014,May,3

**19083** Biopsy, breast, with placement of breast localization device(s) (eg, clip, metallic pellet), when performed, and imaging of the biopsy specimen, when performed, percutaneous; first lesion, including ultrasound guidance

🖪 4.60 ⚕ 19.0 **FUD** 000 [J] [G2] [80] [50] [▭]

**AMA:** 2017,Jan,8; 2016,Jun,3; 2016,Jan,13; 2015,May,8; 2015,Mar,5; 2015,Jan,16; 2014,Jun,14; 2014,May,3

+ **19084** each additional lesion, including ultrasound guidance (List separately in addition to code for primary procedure)

Code first (19083)

🖪 2.29 ⚕ 15.5 **FUD** ZZZ [N] [N1] [80] [▭]

**AMA:** 2017,Jan,8; 2016,Jun,3; 2016,Jan,13; 2015,May,8; 2015,Mar,5; 2015,Jan,16; 2014,Jun,14; 2014,May,3

**19085** Biopsy, breast, with placement of breast localization device(s) (eg, clip, metallic pellet), when performed, and imaging of the biopsy specimen, when performed, percutaneous; first lesion, including magnetic resonance guidance

🖪 5.37 ⚕ 28.9 **FUD** 000 [J] [G2] [80] [50] [▭]

**AMA:** 2017,Jan,8; 2016,Jun,3; 2016,Jan,13; 2015,May,8; 2015,Mar,5; 2015,Jan,16; 2014,Jun,14; 2014,May,3

+ **19086** each additional lesion, including magnetic resonance guidance (List separately in addition to code for primary procedure)

Code first (19085)

🖪 2.67 ⚕ 23.1 **FUD** ZZZ [N] [N1] [80] [▭]

**AMA:** 2017,Jan,8; 2016,Jun,3; 2016,Jan,13; 2015,May,8; 2015,Mar,5; 2015,Jan,16; 2014,Jun,14; 2014,May,3

## 19100-19101 Breast Biopsy Without Imaging Guidance

EXCLUDES Biopsy of breast with imaging guidance (19081-19086)
Lesion removal without concentration on surgical margins (19110-19126)
Partial mastectomy (19301-19302)
Total mastectomy (19303-19307)

**19100** Biopsy of breast; percutaneous, needle core, not using imaging guidance (separate procedure)

EXCLUDES Fine needle aspiration:
With imaging guidance (10022)
Without imaging guidance (10021)

🖪 2.02 ⚕ 4.28 **FUD** 000 [J] [A2] [50] [▭]

**AMA:** 2017,Jan,8; 2016,Jan,13; 2015,Jan,16; 2014,May,3; 2014,Jan,11; 2012,Jan,15-42

Clavicle · Tail of Spence area · Deltoid · Brachialis · Parasternal nodes · Lateral nodes · Subscapular nodes · Axillary lymph nodes · Pectoral nodes · Central nodes · Lactiferous ducts and gland lobules · Latissimus dorsi muscle · Areola · Nipple

**19101** open, incisional

Code also placement of localization device with imaging guidance (19281-19288)

🖪 6.36 ⚕ 9.70 **FUD** 010 [J] [A2] [50] [▭]

**AMA:** 2017,Jan,8; 2016,Jan,13; 2015,Jan,16; 2014,May,3; 2014,Jan,11; 2012,Jan,15-42

26/TC PC/TC Only   A2-Z6 ASC Payment   50 Bilateral   ♂ Male Only   ♀ Female Only   🖪 Facility RVU   ⚕ Non-Facility RVU   ▭ CCI
FUD Follow-up Days   CMS: IOM (Pub 100)   A-Y OPPSI   80/80 Surg Assist Allowed / w/Doc   🔳 Lab Crosswalk   🔀 Radiology Crosswalk   ⊠ CLIA

32    CPT © 2017 American Medical Association. All Rights Reserved.    © 2017 Optum360, LLC

## 19105 Treatment of Fibroadenoma: Cryoablation

**CMS:** 100-04,13,80.1 Physician Presence; 100-04,13,80.2 S&I Multiple Procedure Reduction

INCLUDES Adjacent lesions treated with one cryoprobe
Ultrasound guidance (76940, 76942)

**19105**   **Ablation, cryosurgical, of fibroadenoma, including ultrasound guidance, each fibroadenoma**
    5.78   66.5   **FUD** 000     J P2 50
**AMA:** 2007,Mar,7-8

## 19110-19126 Excisional Procedures: Breast

INCLUDES Open removal of breast mass without concentration on surgical margins

**19110**   **Nipple exploration, with or without excision of a solitary lactiferous duct or a papilloma lactiferous duct**
    9.83   13.8   **FUD** 090     J A2 50
**AMA:** 2017,Jan,8; 2016,Jan,13; 2015,Jan,16; 2014,Jan,11

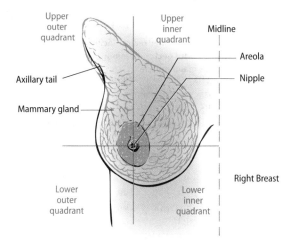

Upper outer quadrant / Upper inner quadrant / Midline / Areola / Nipple / Axillary tail / Mammary gland / Lower outer quadrant / Lower inner quadrant / Right Breast

**19112**   **Excision of lactiferous duct fistula**
    8.97   13.0   **FUD** 090     J A2 80 50
**AMA:** 2017,Jan,8; 2016,Jan,13; 2015,Jan,16; 2014,Jan,11

**19120**   **Excision of cyst, fibroadenoma, or other benign or malignant tumor, aberrant breast tissue, duct lesion, nipple or areolar lesion (except 19300), open, male or female, 1 or more lesions**
    11.8   14.0   **FUD** 090     J A2 50
**AMA:** 2017,Jan,8; 2016,Jan,13; 2015,Mar,5; 2015,Jan,16; 2014,Mar,13; 2014,Jan,11; 2012,Jan,15-42

**19125**   **Excision of breast lesion identified by preoperative placement of radiological marker, open; single lesion**
INCLUDES Intraoperative clip placement
    13.1   15.6   **FUD** 090     J A2 50
**AMA:** 2017,Jan,8; 2016,Jan,13; 2015,Mar,5; 2015,Jan,16; 2014,Jan,11; 2012,Jan,15-42

**+ 19126**   **each additional lesion separately identified by a preoperative radiological marker (List separately in addition to code for primary procedure)**
INCLUDES Intraoperative clip placement
Code first (19125)
    4.68   4.68   **FUD** ZZZ     N N1
**AMA:** 2017,Jan,8; 2016,Jan,13; 2015,Jan,16; 2014,Jan,11; 2012,Jan,15-42

## 19260-19272 Excisional Procedures: Chest Wall

EXCLUDES Resection of apical lung tumor (eg, Pancoast tumor), including chest wall resection, rib(s) resection(s), neurovascular dissection, when performed; without chest wall reconstruction(s) (32503-32504)
Thoracentesis, needle or catheter, aspiration of the pleural space; without imaging guidance (32554-32555)
Thoracotomy; with exploration (32100)
Tube thoracostomy, includes connection to drainage system (eg, water seal), when performed, open (separate procedure) (32551)

**19260**   **Excision of chest wall tumor including ribs**
    34.6   34.6   **FUD** 090     J 80
**AMA:** 2017,Jan,8; 2016,Jan,13; 2015,Jan,16; 2014,Jan,11; 2012,Oct,9-11; 2012,Sep,3-8

**19271**   **Excision of chest wall tumor involving ribs, with plastic reconstruction; without mediastinal lymphadenectomy**
    46.7   46.7   **FUD** 090     C 80
**AMA:** 2017,Jan,8; 2016,Jan,13; 2015,Jan,16; 2014,Jan,11; 2012,Oct,9-11; 2012,Sep,3-8

**19272**   **with mediastinal lymphadenectomy**
    51.2   51.2   **FUD** 090     C 80
**AMA:** 2017,Jan,8; 2016,Jan,13; 2015,Jan,16; 2014,Jan,11; 2012,Oct,9-11; 2012,Sep,3-8

## 19281-19288 Placement of Localization Markers

INCLUDES Placement of localization devices only
EXCLUDES Biopsy of breast without imaging guidance (19100-19101)
Fluoroscopic guidance for needle placement (77002)
Localization device placement with biopsy of breast (19081-19086)
Magnetic resonance guidance for needle placement (77021)
Ultrasonic guidance for needle placement (76942)
Code also open incisional breast biopsy when performed after localization device placement (19101)
Code also radiography of surgical specimen (76098)

**19281**   **Placement of breast localization device(s) (eg, clip, metallic pellet, wire/needle, radioactive seeds), percutaneous; first lesion, including mammographic guidance**
    2.93   6.82   **FUD** 000     Q1 N1 80 50
**AMA:** 2017,Jan,8; 2016,Jun,3; 2016,Jan,13; 2015,May,8; 2015,Jan,16; 2014,Jun,14; 2014,May,3

**+ 19282**   **each additional lesion, including mammographic guidance (List separately in addition to code for primary procedure)**
Code first (19281)
    1.47   4.73   **FUD** ZZZ     N N1 80
**AMA:** 2017,Jan,8; 2016,Jun,3; 2016,Jan,13; 2015,May,8; 2015,Jan,16; 2014,Jun,14; 2014,May,3

**19283**   **Placement of breast localization device(s) (eg, clip, metallic pellet, wire/needle, radioactive seeds), percutaneous; first lesion, including stereotactic guidance**
    2.96   7.70   **FUD** 000     Q1 N1 80 50
**AMA:** 2017,Jan,8; 2016,Jun,3; 2016,May,13; 2016,Jan,13; 2015,May,8; 2015,Jan,16; 2014,May,3

**+ 19284**   **each additional lesion, including stereotactic guidance (List separately in addition to code for primary procedure)**
Code first (19283)
    1.49   5.79   **FUD** ZZZ     N N1 80
**AMA:** 2017,Jan,8; 2016,Jun,3; 2016,May,13; 2016,Jan,13; 2015,May,8; 2015,Jan,16; 2014,May,3

**19285**   **Placement of breast localization device(s) (eg, clip, metallic pellet, wire/needle, radioactive seeds), percutaneous; first lesion, including ultrasound guidance**
    2.51   14.6   **FUD** 000     Q1 N1 80 50
**AMA:** 2017,Jan,8; 2016,Jun,3; 2016,May,13; 2016,Jan,13; 2015,May,8; 2015,Jan,16; 2014,May,3

**+ 19286**   **each additional lesion, including ultrasound guidance (List separately in addition to code for primary procedure)**
Code first (19285)
    1.26   12.7   **FUD** ZZZ     N N1 80
**AMA:** 2017,Jan,8; 2016,Jun,3; 2016,May,13; 2016,Jan,13; 2015,May,8; 2015,Jan,16; 2014,May,3

**Integumentary System** *(side tab)*
**19287 — 19342** *(side tab)*

**19287** Placement of breast localization device(s) (eg clip, metallic pellet, wire/needle, radioactive seeds), percutaneous; first lesion, including magnetic resonance guidance
🔷 3.75   ⚕ 24.5   **FUD** 000    01 N1 80 50 ▭
**AMA:** 2017,Jan,8; 2016,Jun,3; 2016,May,13; 2016,Jan,13; 2015,Jan,16; 2014,May,3

**+ 19288** each additional lesion, including magnetic resonance guidance (List separately in addition to code for primary procedure)
Code first (19287)
🔷 1.87   ⚕ 19.7   **FUD** ZZZ    N N1 80 ▭
**AMA:** 2017,Jan,8; 2016,Jun,3; 2016,May,13; 2016,Jan,13; 2015,Jan,16; 2014,May,3

## 19294-19298 Radioelement Application

**● + 19294** Preparation of tumor cavity, with placement of a radiation therapy applicator for intraoperative radiation therapy (IORT) concurrent with partial mastectomy (List separately in addition to code for primary procedure)
🔷 0.00   ⚕ 0.00   **FUD** 000
Code first (19301-19302)

**19296** Placement of radiotherapy afterloading expandable catheter (single or multichannel) into the breast for interstitial radioelement application following partial mastectomy, includes imaging guidance; on date separate from partial mastectomy
🔷 6.09   ⚕ 111.   **FUD** 000    J J8 80 50 ▭
**AMA:** 2017,Jan,8; 2016,Jan,13; 2015,Jan,16; 2014,Jan,11; 2012,Jan,15-42

**+ 19297** concurrent with partial mastectomy (List separately in addition to code for primary procedure)
Code first (19301-19302)
🔷 2.75   ⚕ 2.75   **FUD** ZZZ    N N1 80 ▭
**AMA:** 2017,Jan,8; 2016,Jan,13; 2015,Jan,16; 2014,Jan,11; 2012,Jan,15-42

**19298** Placement of radiotherapy after loading brachytherapy catheters (multiple tube and button type) into the breast for interstitial radioelement application following (at the time of or subsequent to) partial mastectomy, includes imaging guidance
🔷 9.07   ⚕ 27.8   **FUD** 000    J G2 80 50 ▭
**AMA:** 2017,Jan,8; 2016,Jan,13; 2015,Jan,16; 2014,Jan,11

## 19300-19307 Mastectomies: Partial, Simple, Radical

**CMS:** 100-04,12,40.7 Bilateral Procedures
INCLUDES   Intraoperative clip placement
EXCLUDES   Insertion of prosthesis (19340, 19342)

**19300** Mastectomy for gynecomastia            ♂
🔷 11.8   ⚕ 14.9   **FUD** 090    J A2 50 ▭
**AMA:** 2017,Jan,8; 2016,Jan,13; 2015,Jan,16; 2014,Mar,13; 2014,Jan,11

**19301** Mastectomy, partial (eg, lumpectomy, tylectomy, quadrantectomy, segmentectomy);
EXCLUDES   Insertion of radiotherapy afterloading balloon or brachytherapy catheters (19296-19298)
Tumor cavity preparation with intraoperative radiation therapy applicator (19294)
🔷 18.7   ⚕ 18.7   **FUD** 090    J A2 80 50 ▭
**AMA:** 2017,Jan,8; 2016,Jan,13; 2015,Mar,5; 2015,Jan,16; 2014,Jan,11; 2013,Nov,14; 2012,Jan,15-42

**19302** with axillary lymphadenectomy
EXCLUDES   Insertion of radiotherapy afterloading balloon or brachytherapy catheters (19296-19298)
Tumor cavity preparation with intraoperative radiation therapy applicator (19294)
🔷 25.9   ⚕ 25.9   **FUD** 090    J A2 80 50 ▭
**AMA:** 2017,Jan,8; 2016,Jan,13; 2015,Mar,5; 2015,Jan,16; 2014,Jan,11; 2012,Jan,15-42

**19303** Mastectomy, simple, complete
EXCLUDES   Gynecomastia (19300)
🔷 29.0   ⚕ 29.0   **FUD** 090    J A2 80 50 ▭
**AMA:** 2017,Jan,8; 2016,Jan,13; 2015,Mar,5; 2015,Jan,16; 2014,Jan,11

**19304** Mastectomy, subcutaneous
🔷 16.5   ⚕ 16.5   **FUD** 090    J A2 80 50 ▭
**AMA:** 2017,Jan,8; 2016,Jan,13; 2015,Jan,16; 2014,Jan,11; 2012,Jan,15-42

**19305** Mastectomy, radical, including pectoral muscles, axillary lymph nodes
🔷 32.5   ⚕ 32.5   **FUD** 090    C 80 50 ▭
**AMA:** 2017,Jan,8; 2016,Jan,13; 2015,Jan,16; 2014,Jan,11

**19306** Mastectomy, radical, including pectoral muscles, axillary and internal mammary lymph nodes (Urban type operation)
🔷 34.1   ⚕ 34.1   **FUD** 090    C 80 50 ▭
**AMA:** 2017,Jan,8; 2016,Jan,13; 2015,Jan,16; 2014,Jan,11

**19307** Mastectomy, modified radical, including axillary lymph nodes, with or without pectoralis minor muscle, but excluding pectoralis major muscle
🔷 34.4   ⚕ 34.4   **FUD** 090    J 80 50 ▭
**AMA:** 2017,Jan,8; 2016,Jan,13; 2015,Mar,5; 2015,Jan,16; 2014,Jan,11

## 19316-19499 Plastic, Reconstructive, and Aesthetic Breast Procedures

**CMS:** 100-03,140.2 Breast Reconstruction Following Mastectomy; 100-04,12,40.7 Bilateral Procedures
Code also biologic implant for tissue reinforcement (15777)

**19316** Mastopexy
🔷 22.1   ⚕ 22.1   **FUD** 090    J A2 80 50 ▭
**AMA:** 2017,Jan,8; 2016,Jan,13; 2015,Jan,16; 2014,Jan,11; 2012,Feb,11

**19318** Reduction mammaplasty
INCLUDES   Aries-Pitanguy mammaplasty
Biesenberger mammaplasty
🔷 31.7   ⚕ 31.7   **FUD** 090    J A2 80 50 ▭
**AMA:** 2017,Jan,8; 2016,Jan,13; 2015,Jan,16; 2014,Apr,10; 2014,Jan,11; 2012,Jan,15-42

**19324** Mammaplasty, augmentation; without prosthetic implant
🔷 14.2   ⚕ 14.2   **FUD** 090    J A2 80 50 ▭
**AMA:** 2017,Jan,8; 2016,Jan,13; 2015,Jan,16; 2014,Jan,11

**19325** with prosthetic implant
EXCLUDES   Flap or graft (15100-15650)
🔷 18.4   ⚕ 18.4   **FUD** 090    J G2 80 50 ▭
**AMA:** 2017,Jan,8; 2016,Jan,13; 2015,Jan,16; 2014,Jan,11

**19328** Removal of intact mammary implant
🔷 14.2   ⚕ 14.2   **FUD** 090    02 A2 50 ▭
**AMA:** 2017,Jan,8; 2016,Jan,13; 2015,Jan,16; 2014,Jan,11

**19330** Removal of mammary implant material
🔷 18.2   ⚕ 18.2   **FUD** 090    02 A2 50 ▭
**AMA:** 2017,Jan,8; 2016,Jan,13; 2015,Jan,16; 2014,Jan,11; 2012,Jan,15-42

**19340** Immediate insertion of breast prosthesis following mastopexy, mastectomy or in reconstruction
EXCLUDES   Supply of prosthetic implant (99070, L8030, L8039, L8600)
🔷 28.8   ⚕ 28.8   **FUD** 090    J A2 50 ▭
**AMA:** 2017,Jan,8; 2016,Jan,13; 2015,Dec,18; 2015,Jan,16; 2014,Jan,11; 2012,Jan,15-42

**19342** Delayed insertion of breast prosthesis following mastopexy, mastectomy or in reconstruction
EXCLUDES   Preparation of moulage for custom breast implant (19396)
🔷 26.5   ⚕ 26.5   **FUD** 090    J G2 80 50 ▭
**AMA:** 2017,Jan,8; 2016,Jan,13; 2015,Nov,10; 2015,Jan,16; 2014,Jan,11; 2013,Jan,15-16

---

26/TC PC/TC Only    A2-Z6 ASC Payment    50 Bilateral    ♂ Male Only    ♀ Female Only    🔷 Facility RVU    ⚕ Non-Facility RVU    ▭ CCI
**FUD** Follow-up Days    **CMS:** IOM (Pub 100)    A-Y OPPSI    80/80 Surg Assist Allowed / w/Doc    Lab Crosswalk    Radiology Crosswalk    ✖ CLIA

**34**                                      CPT © 2017 American Medical Association. All Rights Reserved.                 © 2017 Optum360, LLC

**19350**   **Nipple/areola reconstruction**
  🚑 19.3   ⚕ 23.5   **FUD** 090                        J A2 50 ▣
  **AMA:** 2017,Jan,8; 2016,Aug,9; 2016,Jan,13; 2015,Jan,16;
  2014,Jan,11; 2013,Jan,15-16; 2012,Jan,15-42

**19355**   **Correction of inverted nipples**
  🚑 16.3   ⚕ 19.9   **FUD** 090                        J A2 80 50 ▣
  **AMA:** 2017,Jan,8; 2016,Jan,13; 2015,Jan,16; 2014,Jan,11

**19357**   **Breast reconstruction, immediate or delayed, with tissue**
  **expander, including subsequent expansion**
  🚑 43.2   ⚕ 43.2   **FUD** 090                        J G2 80 50 ▣
  **AMA:** 2017,Jan,8; 2016,Jan,13; 2015,Feb,10; 2015,Jan,16;
  2014,Jan,11; 2013,Oct,15; 2012,Jan,15-42

**19361**   **Breast reconstruction with latissimus dorsi flap, without**
  **prosthetic implant**
  EXCLUDES   *Implant of prosthesis (19340)*
  🚑 45.3   ⚕ 45.3   **FUD** 090                        C 80 50 ▣
  **AMA:** 2017,Jan,8; 2016,Jan,13; 2015,Feb,10; 2015,Jan,16;
  2014,Jan,11

**19364**   **Breast reconstruction with free flap**
  INCLUDES   Closure of donor site
              Harvesting of skin graft
              Inset shaping of flap into breast
              Microvascular repair
              Operating microscope (69990)
  🚑 79.4   ⚕ 79.4   **FUD** 090                        C 80 50 ▣
  **AMA:** 2017,Jan,8; 2016,Feb,12; 2016,Jan,13; 2015,Feb,10;
  2015,Jan,16; 2014,Apr,10; 2014,Jan,11; 2013,Mar,13;
  2012,Jul,12-14; 2012,Jan,15-42

**19366**   **Breast reconstruction with other technique**
  INCLUDES   Operating microscope (69990)
  Code also implant of prosthesis if appropriate (19340, 19342)
  🚑 40.6   ⚕ 40.6   **FUD** 090                        J A2 80 50 ▣
  **AMA:** 2017,Jan,8; 2016,Jan,13; 2015,Feb,10; 2015,Jan,16;
  2014,Apr,10; 2014,Jan,11; 2012,Jan,15-42

**19367**   **Breast reconstruction with transverse rectus abdominis**
  **myocutaneous flap (TRAM), single pedicle, including closure**
  **of donor site;**
  🚑 51.5   ⚕ 51.5   **FUD** 090                        C 80 50 ▣
  **AMA:** 2017,Jan,8; 2016,Jan,13; 2015,Feb,10; 2015,Jan,16;
  2014,Jan,11

**19368**       **with microvascular anastomosis (supercharging)**
  INCLUDES   Operating microscope (69990)
  🚑 63.5   ⚕ 63.5   **FUD** 090                        C 80 50 ▣
  **AMA:** 2017,Jan,8; 2016,Feb,12; 2016,Jan,13; 2015,Feb,10;
  2015,Jan,16; 2014,Jan,11

**19369**   **Breast reconstruction with transverse rectus abdominis**
  **myocutaneous flap (TRAM), double pedicle, including closure**
  **of donor site**
  🚑 58.4   ⚕ 58.4   **FUD** 090                        C 80 50 ▣
  **AMA:** 2017,Jan,8; 2016,Jan,13; 2015,Feb,10; 2015,Jan,16;
  2014,Jan,11

**19370**   **Open periprosthetic capsulotomy, breast**
  🚑 19.7   ⚕ 19.7   **FUD** 090                        J A2 50 ▣
  **AMA:** 2017,Jan,8; 2016,Jan,13; 2015,Dec,18; 2015,Jan,16;
  2014,Jan,11

**19371**   **Periprosthetic capsulectomy, breast**
  🚑 22.5   ⚕ 22.5   **FUD** 090                        J A2 50 ▣
  **AMA:** 2017,Jan,8; 2016,Jan,13; 2015,Jan,16; 2014,Jan,11;
  2013,Jan,15-16; 2012,Jan,15-42

**19380**   **Revision of reconstructed breast**
  🚑 22.2   ⚕ 22.2   **FUD** 090                        J A2 50 ▣
  **AMA:** 2017,Jan,8; 2016,Jan,13; 2015,Dec,18; 2015,Jan,16;
  2014,Jan,11

**19396**   **Preparation of moulage for custom breast implant**
  🚑 4.21   ⚕ 8.32   **FUD** 000                        J G2 80 50 ▣
  **AMA:** 2017,Jan,8; 2016,Jan,13; 2015,Jan,16; 2014,Jan,11

**19499**   **Unlisted procedure, breast**
  🚑 0.00   ⚕ 0.00   **FUD** YYY                        J 80 50
  **AMA:** 2017,Jan,8; 2016,Dec,16; 2016,Jan,13; 2015,Mar,5;
  2015,Jan,16; 2014,Dec,16; 2014,Dec,16; 2014,Jan,11;
  2013,Nov,14; 2012,Jan,15-42

● New Code     ▲ Revised Code     ○ Reinstated     ● New Web Release     ▲ Revised Web Release     Unlisted     Not Covered     # Resequenced
⊘ AMA Mod 51 Exempt   ⑨ Optum Mod 51 Exempt   ⑥ Mod 63 Exempt   ✗ Non-FDA Drug   ★ Telemedicine   Ⓜ Maternity   Ⓐ Age Edit   + Add-on   **AMA:** CPT Asst
© 2017 Optum360, LLC                              CPT © 2017 American Medical Association. All Rights Reserved.                              35

## 20005 Incisional Treatment Soft Tissue Abscess

EXCLUDES Superficial incision and drainage (10040-10160)

20005 Incision and drainage of soft tissue abscess, subfascial (ie, involves the soft tissue below the deep fascia)
6.74   8.88   **FUD** 010
J 62

## 20100-20103 Exploratory Surgery of Traumatic Wound

INCLUDES Debridement
Expanded dissection of wound for exploration
Extraction of foreign material
Open examination
Tying or coagulation of small vessels

EXCLUDES Cutaneous/subcutaneous incision and drainage procedures (10060-10061)
Laparotomy (49000-49010)
Repair of major vessels of:
Abdomen (35221, 35251, 35281)
Chest (35211, 35216, 35241, 35246, 35271, 35276)
Extremity (35206-35207, 35226, 35236, 35256, 35266, 35286)
Neck (35201, 35231, 35261)
Thoracotomy (32100-32160)

20100 Exploration of penetrating wound (separate procedure); neck
17.5   17.5   **FUD** 010
T 80 50
**AMA:** 2017,Jan,8; 2016,Jan,13; 2015,Jan,16; 2014,Jan,11; 2012,Jan,15-42

20101 chest
6.01   12.7   **FUD** 010
T
**AMA:** 2017,Jan,8; 2016,Jan,13; 2015,Jan,16; 2014,Jan,11; 2012,Jan,15-42

20102 abdomen/flank/back
7.34   13.8   **FUD** 010
T
**AMA:** 2017,Jan,8; 2016,Jan,13; 2015,Jan,16; 2014,Jan,11; 2012,Jan,15-42

20103 extremity
10.0   16.6   **FUD** 010
T 62 80
**AMA:** 2017,Jan,8; 2016,Jan,13; 2015,Jan,16; 2014,Jan,11; 2012,Jan,15-42

## 20150 Epiphyseal Bar Resection

20150 Excision of epiphyseal bar, with or without autogenous soft tissue graft obtained through same fascial incision
27.1   27.1   **FUD** 090
J 62 80 50
**AMA:** 1996,Nov,1

## 20200-20206 Muscle Biopsy

EXCLUDES Removal of muscle tumor (see appropriate anatomic section)

20200 Biopsy, muscle; superficial
2.76   5.90   **FUD** 000
J A2

20205 deep
4.51   8.24   **FUD** 000
J A2

20206 Biopsy, muscle, percutaneous needle
EXCLUDES Fine needle aspiration (10021-10022)
(76942, 77002, 77012, 77021)
(88172-88173)
1.71   6.68   **FUD** 000
J A2
**AMA:** 2001,Jan,8

## 20220-20225 Percutaneous Bone Biopsy

EXCLUDES Bone marrow aspiration(s) or biopsy(ies) (38220-38222)

20220 Biopsy, bone, trocar, or needle; superficial (eg, ilium, sternum, spinous process, ribs)
(77002, 77012, 77021)
2.08   4.77   **FUD** 000
J A2
**AMA:** 2017,Jan,8; 2016,Jan,13; 2015,Jan,16; 2014,Jan,11

20225 deep (eg, vertebral body, femur)
EXCLUDES Percutaneous vertebroplasty (22510-22515)
Percutaneous sacral augmentation (sacroplasty) (0200T-0201T)
(77002, 77012, 77021)
3.13   14.8   **FUD** 000
J A2
**AMA:** 2017,Jan,8; 2016,Jan,13; 2015,Jan,8; 2015,Jan,16; 2014,Jan,11; 2012,Jun,10-11

## 20240-20251 Open Bone Biopsy

EXCLUDES Sequestrectomy or incision and drainage of bone abscess of:
Calcaneus (28120)
Carpal bone (25145)
Clavicle (23170)
Humeral head (23174)
Humerus (24134)
Olecranon process (24138)
Radius (24136, 25145)
Scapula (23172)
Skull (61501)
Talus (28120)
Ulna (24138, 24145)

20240 Biopsy, bone, open; superficial (eg, sternum, spinous process, rib, patella, olecranon process, calcaneus, tarsal, metatarsal, carpal, metacarpal, phalanx)
4.41   4.41   **FUD** 000
J A2
**AMA:** 2017,Jan,8; 2016,Jan,13; 2015,Jan,16; 2014,Jan,11; 2012,Jan,15-42

20245 deep (eg, humeral shaft, ischium, femoral shaft)
10.2   10.2   **FUD** 000
J A2
**AMA:** 2017,Jan,8; 2016,Jan,13; 2015,Jan,16; 2014,Jan,11

20250 Biopsy, vertebral body, open; thoracic
11.2   11.2   **FUD** 010
J A2
**AMA:** 2017,Jan,8; 2016,Jan,13; 2015,Jan,16; 2014,Jan,11

20251 lumbar or cervical
12.2   12.2   **FUD** 010
J A2 80
**AMA:** 2017,Jan,8; 2016,Jan,13; 2015,Jan,16; 2014,Jan,11

## 20500-20501 Injection Fistula/Sinus Tract

EXCLUDES Arthrography injection of:
Ankle (27648)
Elbow (24220)
Hip (27093, 27095)
Knee (27370)
Sacroiliac joint (27096)
Shoulder (23350)
Temporomandibular joint (TMJ) (21116)
Wrist (25246)
Autologous adipose-derived regenerative cells injection (0489T-0490T)

20500 Injection of sinus tract; therapeutic (separate procedure)
2.40   2.93   **FUD** 010
T P3
(76080)

20501 diagnostic (sinogram)
1.10   3.35   **FUD** 000
N N1
EXCLUDES Contrast injection or injections for radiological evaluation of existing gastrostomy, duodenostomy, jejunostomy, gastro-jejunostomy, or cecostomy (or other colonic) tube from percutaneous approach (49465)
(76080)

## 20520-20525 Foreign Body Removal

20520 Removal of foreign body in muscle or tendon sheath; simple
4.20   5.80   **FUD** 010
J P3

20525 deep or complicated
7.12   13.6   **FUD** 010
J A2

● New Code   ▲ Revised Code   ○ Reinstated   ● New Web Release   ▲ Revised Web Release   Unlisted   Not Covered   # Resequenced
⊘ AMA Mod 51 Exempt   ⑤ Optum Mod 51 Exempt   ⑥ Mod 63 Exempt   ✗ Non-FDA Drug   ★ Telemedicine   Ⓜ Maternity   Ⓐ Age Edit   ✚ Add-on   **AMA:** CPT Asst

## 20526-20553 Therapeutic Injections: Tendons, Trigger Points

**EXCLUDES**  *Autologous adipose-derived regenerative cells injection (0489T-0490T)*
*Platelet rich plasma (PRP) injections (0232T)*

**20526**  **Injection, therapeutic (eg, local anesthetic, corticosteroid), carpal tunnel**
  ⚙ 1.66  ⚖ 2.20  **FUD** 000  Ⓣ P3 50 ▢
  **AMA:** 2017,Jan,8; 2016,Jan,13; 2015,Jan,16; 2014,Jan,11; 2012,Jan,15-42

**20527**  **Injection, enzyme (eg, collagenase), palmar fascial cord (ie, Dupuytren's contracture)**
  **EXCLUDES**  *Post injection palmar fascial cord manipulation (26341)*
  ⚙ 1.92  ⚖ 2.40  **FUD** 000  Ⓣ P3 50 ▢
  **AMA:** 2017,Jan,8; 2016,Jan,13; 2015,Jan,16; 2014,Jan,11; 2012,Jul,8

**20550**  **Injection(s); single tendon sheath, or ligament, aponeurosis (eg, plantar "fascia")**
  **EXCLUDES**  *Autologous WBC injection (0481T)*
  *Platelet rich plasma injection (0232T)*
  *Morton's neuroma (64455, 64632)*
  ✖ (76942, 77002, 77021)
  ⚙ 1.13  ⚖ 1.50  **FUD** 000  Ⓣ P3 50 ▢
  **AMA:** 2017,Jan,8; 2016,Jan,13; 2015,Jan,16; 2014,Oct,9; 2014,Jan,11; 2012,Jul,8; 2012,Jan,15-42

**20551**  **single tendon origin/insertion**
  **EXCLUDES**  *Autologous WBC injection (0481T)*
  *Platelet rich plasma injection (0232T)*
  ✖ (76942, 77002, 77021)
  ⚙ 1.22  ⚖ 1.72  **FUD** 000  Ⓣ P3 ▢
  **AMA:** 2017,Jan,8; 2016,Jan,13; 2015,Jan,16; 2014,Oct,9; 2014,Jan,11; 2012,Jan,15-42

**20552**  **Injection(s); single or multiple trigger point(s), 1 or 2 muscle(s)**
  **EXCLUDES**  *Autologous WBC injection*
  *Platelet rich plasma injection*
  ✖ (76942, 77002, 77021)
  ⚙ 1.09  ⚖ 1.57  **FUD** 000  Ⓣ P3 ▢
  **AMA:** 2017,Jun,10; 2017,Jan,8; 2016,Jan,13; 2015,Jan,16; 2014,Oct,9; 2014,Jan,11; 2012,Apr,19; 2012,Jan,15-42

**20553**  **single or multiple trigger point(s), 3 or more muscles**
  ✖ (76942, 77002, 77021)
  ⚙ 1.24  ⚖ 1.81  **FUD** 000  Ⓣ P3 ▢
  **AMA:** 2017,Jun,10; 2017,Jan,8; 2016,Jan,13; 2015,Jan,16; 2014,Oct,9; 2014,Jan,11; 2012,Jan,15-42

## 20555 Placement of Catheters/Needles for Brachytherapy

**CMS:** 100-04,13,70.4 Clinical Brachytherapy
Code also interstitial radioelement application (77770-77772, 77778)

**20555**  **Placement of needles or catheters into muscle and/or soft tissue for subsequent interstitial radioelement application (at the time of or subsequent to the procedure)**
  **EXCLUDES**  *Interstitial radioelement:*
  *Devices placed into the breast (19296-19298)*
  *Placement of needle, catheters, or devices into muscle or soft tissue of the head and neck (41019)*
  *Placement of needles or catheters into pelvic organs or genitalia (55920)*
  *Placement of needles or catheters into prostate (55875)*
  ✖ (76942, 77002, 77012, 77021)
  ⚙ 9.40  ⚖ 9.40  **FUD** 000  Ⓙ R2 80 ▢
  **AMA:** 2017,Jan,8; 2016,Jan,13; 2015,Jan,16; 2014,Jan,11; 2012,Jan,15-42

## 20600-20611 Aspiration and/or Injection of Joint

**CMS:** 100-03,150.7 Prolotherapy, Joint Sclerotherapy, and Ligamentous Injections with Sclerosing Agents
**EXCLUDES**  *Autologous adipose-derived regenerative cells injection (0489T-0490T)*
*Ultrasonic guidance for needle placement (76942)*

**20600**  **Arthrocentesis, aspiration and/or injection, small joint or bursa (eg, fingers, toes); without ultrasound guidance**
  ✖ (77002, 77012, 77021)
  ⚙ 1.02  ⚖ 1.36  **FUD** 000  Ⓣ P3 50 ▢
  **AMA:** 2017,Aug,9; 2017,Jan,8; 2016,Jan,13; 2015,Nov,10; 2015,Feb,6; 2015,Jan,16; 2014,Jan,11

**20604**  **with ultrasound guidance, with permanent recording and reporting**
  **EXCLUDES**  *Autologous adipose-derived regenerative cells injection (0489T-0490T)*
  ✖ (77002, 77012, 77021)
  ⚙ 1.34  ⚖ 2.06  **FUD** 000  Ⓣ P3 50 ▢
  **AMA:** 2017,Jan,8; 2016,Jan,13; 2015,Jul,10; 2015,Feb,6

**20605**  **Arthrocentesis, aspiration and/or injection, intermediate joint or bursa (eg, temporomandibular, acromioclavicular, wrist, elbow or ankle, olecranon bursa); without ultrasound guidance**
  ✖ (77002, 77012, 77021)
  ⚙ 1.07  ⚖ 1.43  **FUD** 000  Ⓣ P3 50 ▢
  **AMA:** 2017,Aug,9; 2017,Jan,8; 2016,Jan,13; 2015,Nov,10; 2015,Feb,6; 2015,Jan,16; 2014,Jan,11

**20606**  **with ultrasound guidance, with permanent recording and reporting**
  ✖ (77002, 77012, 77021)
  ⚙ 1.52  ⚖ 2.28  **FUD** 000  Ⓣ P3 50 ▢
  **AMA:** 2017,Jan,8; 2016,Jan,13; 2015,Jul,10; 2015,Feb,6

**20610**  **Arthrocentesis, aspiration and/or injection, major joint or bursa (eg, shoulder, hip, knee, subacromial bursa); without ultrasound guidance**
  **EXCLUDES**  *Injection of contrast for knee arthrography (27370)*
  ✖ (77002, 77012, 77021)
  ⚙ 1.33  ⚖ 1.72  **FUD** 000  Ⓣ P3 50 ▢
  **AMA:** 2017,Apr,9; 2017,Jan,8; 2016,Jan,13; 2015,Nov,10; 2015,Aug,6; 2015,Feb,6; 2015,Jan,16; 2014,Dec,18; 2014,Jan,11; 2012,Jun,14; 2012,Mar,4-7; 2012,Jan,15-42

**20611**  **with ultrasound guidance, with permanent recording and reporting**
  **EXCLUDES**  *Injection of contrast for knee arthrography (27370)*
  ✖ (77002, 77012, 77021)
  ⚙ 1.77  ⚖ 2.59  **FUD** 000  Ⓣ P3 50 ▢
  **AMA:** 2017,Jan,8; 2016,Jan,13; 2015,Nov,10; 2015,Aug,6; 2015,Jul,10; 2015,Feb,6

## 20612-20615 Aspiration and/or Injection of Cyst

**EXCLUDES**  *Autologous adipose-derived regenerative cells injection*

**20612**  **Aspiration and/or injection of ganglion cyst(s) any location**
  ⚙ 1.20  ⚖ 1.72  **FUD** 000  Ⓣ P3 ▢
  Code also modifier 59 for multiple major joint aspirations or injections

**20615**  **Aspiration and injection for treatment of bone cyst**
  ⚙ 4.65  ⚖ 6.87  **FUD** 010  Ⓣ P3 ▢

## 20650-20697 Procedures Related to Bony Fixation

**20650**  **Insertion of wire or pin with application of skeletal traction, including removal (separate procedure)**
  ⚙ 4.53  ⚖ 5.95  **FUD** 010  Ⓙ A2 ▢

**20660**  **Application of cranial tongs, caliper, or stereotactic frame, including removal (separate procedure)**
  ⚙ 7.14  ⚖ 7.14  **FUD** 000  02 ▢
  **AMA:** 2017,Jan,8; 2016,Jan,13; 2015,Jan,16; 2014,Jan,11; 2012,Aug,14; 2012,Apr,11-13; 2012,Apr,13; 2012,Jan,15-42

**20661** Application of halo, including removal; cranial
   🚑 14.5      14.5   **FUD** 090           C ▣
   **AMA:** 2017,Jan,8; 2016,Jan,13; 2015,Jan,16; 2014,Jan,11; 2012,Aug,14

**20662** pelvic
   🚑 12.4      12.4   **FUD** 090        J R2 80 ▣

**20663** femoral
   🚑 13.0      13.0   **FUD** 090     J R2 80 50 ▣

**20664** Application of halo, including removal, cranial, 6 or more pins placed, for thin skull osteology (eg, pediatric patients, hydrocephalus, osteogenesis imperfecta)
   🚑 25.3      25.3   **FUD** 090           C ▣
   **AMA:** 2017,Jan,8; 2016,Jan,13; 2015,Jan,16; 2014,Jan,11; 2013,Aug,12; 2012,Aug,14

**20665** Removal of tongs or halo applied by another individual
   🚑 2.60      3.02   **FUD** 010     01 G2 80 ▣
   **AMA:** 2017,Jan,8; 2016,Jan,13; 2015,Jan,16; 2014,Jan,11; 2012,Apr,11-13

**20670** Removal of implant; superficial (eg, buried wire, pin or rod) (separate procedure)
   🚑 4.22      10.7   **FUD** 010        02 A2 ▣
   **AMA:** 2017,Jan,8; 2016,Jan,13; 2015,Jan,16; 2014,Jan,11; 2012,Apr,17-18; 2012,Jan,15-42

**20680** deep (eg, buried wire, pin, screw, metal band, nail, rod or plate)
   🚑 12.1      17.6   **FUD** 090     02 A2 80 ▣
   **AMA:** 2017,Jan,8; 2016,Nov,9; 2016,Jan,13; 2015,Nov,10; 2015,Jan,16; 2014,Mar,4; 2014,Jan,11; 2012,Oct,14; 2012,Sep,16; 2012,Jan,15-42

**20690** Application of a uniplane (pins or wires in 1 plane), unilateral, external fixation system
   🚑 17.1      17.1   **FUD** 090        J A2 ▣
   **AMA:** 2017,Jan,8; 2016,Jan,13; 2015,Jan,16; 2014,Jan,11; 2012,Jan,15-42

**20692** Application of a multiplane (pins or wires in more than 1 plane), unilateral, external fixation system (eg, Ilizarov, Monticelli type)
   🚑 32.1      32.1   **FUD** 090     J J8 80 ▣
   **AMA:** 2017,Jan,8; 2016,Jan,13; 2015,Jan,16; 2014,Jan,11; 2012,Jan,15-42

**20693** Adjustment or revision of external fixation system requiring anesthesia (eg, new pin[s] or wire[s] and/or new ring[s] or bar[s])
   🚑 12.7      12.7   **FUD** 090        J A2 ▣
   **AMA:** 2017,Jan,8; 2016,Jan,13; 2015,Jan,16; 2014,Jan,11; 2012,Jan,15-42

**20694** Removal, under anesthesia, of external fixation system
   🚑 9.70      12.1   **FUD** 090        02 A2 ▣
   **AMA:** 2017,Jan,8; 2016,Jan,13; 2015,Jan,16; 2014,Jan,11; 2012,Jan,15-42

**20696** Application of multiplane (pins or wires in more than 1 plane), unilateral, external fixation with stereotactic computer-assisted adjustment (eg, spatial frame), including imaging; initial and subsequent alignment(s), assessment(s), and computation(s) of adjustment schedule(s)
   *EXCLUDES* Application of multiplane external fixation system (20692)
               Application of multiplan external fixation system, with stereotactic computer-assisted adjustment (20696)
   🚑 34.7      34.7   **FUD** 090     J R2 80 ▣
   **AMA:** 2017,Jan,8; 2016,Jan,13; 2015,Jan,16; 2014,Jan,11

**20697** exchange (ie, removal and replacement) of strut, each
   *EXCLUDES* Application of multiplane external fixation system (20692)
               Exchange of strut for multiplane external fixation system (20697)
   🚑 59.7      59.7   **FUD** 000     ⊘ J P2 80 TC ▣
   **AMA:** 2017,Jan,8; 2016,Jan,13; 2015,Jan,16; 2014,Jan,11

## 20802-20838 Reimplantation Procedures
*EXCLUDES* Repair of incomplete amputation (see individual repair codes for bone(s), ligament(s), tendon(s), nerve(s), or blood vessel(s) and append modifier 52)

**20802** Replantation, arm (includes surgical neck of humerus through elbow joint), complete amputation
   🚑 79.7      79.7   **FUD** 090     C 80 50 ▣
   **AMA:** 1997,Apr,4

**20805** Replantation, forearm (includes radius and ulna to radial carpal joint), complete amputation
   🚑 90.1      90.1   **FUD** 090     C 80 50 ▣
   **AMA:** 1997,Apr,4

**20808** Replantation, hand (includes hand through metacarpophalangeal joints), complete amputation
   🚑 115.      115.   **FUD** 090     C 80 50 ▣
   **AMA:** 1997,Apr,4

**20816** Replantation, digit, excluding thumb (includes metacarpophalangeal joint to insertion of flexor sublimis tendon), complete amputation
   🚑 60.7      60.7   **FUD** 090        C 80 ▣
   **AMA:** 2017,Jan,8; 2016,Jan,13; 2015,Jan,16; 2014,Jan,11; 2012,Jan,15-42

**20822** Replantation, digit, excluding thumb (includes distal tip to sublimis tendon insertion), complete amputation
   🚑 51.6      51.6   **FUD** 090        J G2 80 ▣
   **AMA:** 1997,Apr,4

**20824** Replantation, thumb (includes carpometacarpal joint to MP joint), complete amputation
   🚑 56.3      56.3   **FUD** 090     C 80 50 ▣
   **AMA:** 1997,Apr,4

**20827** Replantation, thumb (includes distal tip to MP joint), complete amputation
   🚑 52.9      52.9   **FUD** 090     C 80 50 ▣
   **AMA:** 1997,Apr,4

**20838** Replantation, foot, complete amputation
   🚑 77.7      77.7   **FUD** 090     C 80 50 ▣
   **AMA:** 1997,Apr,4

## 20900-20926 Bone and Tissue Autografts
*EXCLUDES* Acquisition of autogenous bone, bone marrow, cartilage, tendon, fascia lata or other grafts through distinct incision unless included in the code description
               Bone graft procedures on the spine (20930-20938)

**20900** Bone graft, any donor area; minor or small (eg, dowel or button)
   🚑 5.46      11.8   **FUD** 000        J A2 80 ▣
   **AMA:** 2017,Jan,8; 2016,Jan,13; 2015,Jan,16; 2014,Jan,11; 2012,Jan,15-42

**20902** major or large
   🚑 8.24      8.24   **FUD** 000        J A2 80 ▣
   **AMA:** 2017,Jan,8; 2016,Jan,13; 2015,Jan,16; 2014,Jan,11; 2012,Jan,15-42

**20910** Cartilage graft; costochondral
   *EXCLUDES* Graft with ear cartilage (21235)
   🚑 12.9      12.9   **FUD** 090        T A2 60 ▣
   **AMA:** 2017,Jan,8; 2016,Jan,13; 2015,Jan,16; 2014,Jan,11; 2013,Jan,15-16

**20912** nasal septum
   *EXCLUDES* Graft with ear cartilage (21235)
   🚑 13.6      13.6   **FUD** 090        T A2 60 ▣
   **AMA:** 2002,Apr,13; 1999,Aug,5

**20920** Fascia lata graft; by stripper
   🚑 11.3      11.3   **FUD** 090          T A2 ▣
   **AMA:** 2017,Jan,8; 2016,Jan,13; 2015,Jan,16; 2014,Jan,11

**20922** by incision and area exposure, complex or sheet
   🚑 14.0      16.8   **FUD** 090        T A2 80 ▣
   **AMA:** 2017,Jan,8; 2016,Jan,13; 2015,Jan,16; 2014,Jan,11

---

● New Code   ▲ Revised Code   ○ Reinstated   ● New Web Release   ▲ Revised Web Release   Unlisted   Not Covered   # Resequenced
⊘ AMA Mod 51 Exempt   51 Optum Mod 51 Exempt   63 Mod 63 Exempt   ✗ Non-FDA Drug   ★ Telemedicine   M Maternity   A Age Edit   + Add-on   **AMA:** CPT Asst

© 2017 Optum360, LLC        CPT © 2017 American Medical Association. All Rights Reserved.

**20924**    Tendon graft, from a distance (eg, palmaris, toe extensor, plantaris)
       14.5    14.5    **FUD** 090      J A2 80 ▭
       **AMA:** 2005,Jan,7-13; 2002,Apr,13

**20926**    Tissue grafts, other (eg, paratenon, fat, dermis)
       EXCLUDES   Autologous adipose-derived regenerative cells injection (0489T-0490T)
               Platelet rich plasma injection (0232T)
       12.1    12.1    **FUD** 090      T A2 ▭
       **AMA:** 2017,Jan,8; 2016,Oct,11; 2016,Jan,13; 2015,Jan,16; 2014,Jan,11; 2012,Jun,15-16; 2012,Apr,14-16; 2012,Jan,15-42

## 20930-20939 Bone Allograft and Autograft of Spine

**+**   **20930**    Allograft, morselized, or placement of osteopromotive material, for spine surgery only (List separately in addition to code for primary procedure)
       Code first (22319, 22532-22533, 22548-22558, 22590-22612, 22630, 22633-22634, 22800-22812)
       0.00    0.00    **FUD** XXX      N N1 ▭
       **AMA:** 2017,Mar,7; 2017,Jan,8; 2016,Jan,13; 2015,Jan,16; 2014,Jan,11; 2013,Jul,3-5; 2012,Jun,10-11; 2012,Apr,14-16; 2012,Jan,15-42

**+**   **20931**    Allograft, structural, for spine surgery only (List separately in addition to code for primary procedure)
       Code first (22319, 22532-22533, 22548-22558, 22590-22612, 22630, 22633-22634, 22800-22812)
       3.29    3.29    **FUD** ZZZ      N N1 ▭
       **AMA:** 2017,Mar,7; 2017,Jan,8; 2016,Jan,13; 2015,Jan,16; 2014,Jan,11; 2013,Jul,3-5; 2012,Jun,10-11; 2012,Apr,14-16; 2012,Jan,15-42

**+**   **20936**    Autograft for spine surgery only (includes harvesting the graft); local (eg, ribs, spinous process, or laminar fragments) obtained from same incision (List separately in addition to code for primary procedure)
       Code first (22319, 22532-22533, 22548-22558, 22590-22612, 22630, 22633-22634, 22800-22812)
       0.00    0.00    **FUD** XXX      N N1 ▭
       **AMA:** 2017,Mar,7; 2017,Jan,8; 2016,Jan,13; 2015,Jan,16; 2014,Jan,11; 2013,Jul,3-5; 2012,Jun,10-11; 2012,Apr,14-16; 2012,Jan,15-42

**+**   **20937**    morselized (through separate skin or fascial incision) (List separately in addition to code for primary procedure)
       Code first (22319, 22532-22533, 22548-22558, 22590-22612, 22630, 22633-22634, 22800-22812)
       4.90    4.90    **FUD** ZZZ      N N1 80 ▭
       **AMA:** 2017,Mar,7; 2017,Jan,8; 2016,Jan,13; 2015,Jan,16; 2014,Jan,11; 2013,Jul,3-5; 2012,Jun,10-11; 2012,Apr,14-16; 2012,Jan,15-42

**+**   **20938**    structural, bicortical or tricortical (through separate skin or fascial incision) (List separately in addition to code for primary procedure)
       EXCLUDES   Bone marrow for bone grafting in spinal surgery (20939)
       Code first (22319, 22532-22533, 22548-22558, 22590-22612, 22630, 22633-22634, 22800-22812)
       5.42    5.42    **FUD** ZZZ      N N1 80 ▭
       **AMA:** 2017,Mar,7; 2017,Jan,8; 2016,Jan,13; 2015,Jan,16; 2014,Jan,11; 2013,Jul,3-5; 2012,May,11-12; 2012,Jun,10-11; 2012,Apr,14-16; 2012,Apr,11-13; 2012,Jan,15-42

**● +**   **20939**    Bone marrow aspiration for bone grafting, spine surgery only, through separate skin or fascial incision (List separately in addition to code for primary procedure)
       0.00    0.00    **FUD** 000
       EXCLUDES   Bone marrow aspiration for other than bone grafting in spinal surgery (20999)
               Diagnostic bone marrow aspiration (38220, 38222)
               Platelet rich plasma injection (0232T)
       Code first primary procedure (22319, 22532-22534, 22548, 22551-22552, 22554, 22556, 22558, 22590, 22595, 22600, 22610, 22612, 22630, 22633-22634, 22800, 22802, 22804, 22808, 22810, 22812)

## 20950 Measurement of Intracompartmental Pressure

**20950**    Monitoring of interstitial fluid pressure (includes insertion of device, eg, wick catheter technique, needle manometer technique) in detection of muscle compartment syndrome
       2.62    7.15    **FUD** 000      T 62 80 ▭
       **AMA:** 2017,Jan,8; 2016,Jan,13; 2015,Jan,16; 2014,Jan,11; 2012,Jan,15-42

## 20955-20973 Bone and Osteocutaneous Grafts

INCLUDES   Operating microscope (69990)

**20955**    Bone graft with microvascular anastomosis; fibula
       72.2    72.2    **FUD** 090      C 80 ▭
       **AMA:** 2017,Jan,8; 2016,Feb,12; 2016,Jan,13; 2015,Jan,16; 2014,Jan,11

**20956**    iliac crest
       76.7    76.7    **FUD** 090      C 80 ▭
       **AMA:** 2017,Jan,8; 2016,Feb,12; 2016,Jan,13; 2015,Jan,16; 2014,Jan,11

**20957**    metatarsal
       65.5    65.5    **FUD** 090      C 80 ▭
       **AMA:** 2017,Jan,8; 2016,Feb,12; 2016,Jan,13; 2015,Jan,16; 2014,Jan,11

**20962**    other than fibula, iliac crest, or metatarsal
       62.0    62.0    **FUD** 090      C 80 ▭
       **AMA:** 2016,Feb,12

**20969**    Free osteocutaneous flap with microvascular anastomosis; other than iliac crest, metatarsal, or great toe
       79.6    79.6    **FUD** 090      C 80 ▭
       **AMA:** 2017,Jan,8; 2016,Feb,12; 2016,Jan,13; 2015,Jan,16; 2014,Jan,11

**20970**    iliac crest
       83.0    83.0    **FUD** 090      C 80 ▭
       **AMA:** 2017,Jan,8; 2016,Feb,12; 2016,Jan,13; 2015,Jan,16; 2014,Jan,11

**20972**    metatarsal
       69.5    69.5    **FUD** 090      J 62 80 ▭
       **AMA:** 2017,Jan,8; 2016,Feb,12; 2016,Jan,13; 2015,Jan,16; 2014,Jan,11

**20973**    great toe with web space
       EXCLUDES   Wrap-around repair (26551)
       71.3    71.3    **FUD** 090      J A2 80 50 ▭
       **AMA:** 2017,Jan,8; 2016,Feb,12; 2016,Jan,13; 2015,Jan,16; 2014,Jan,11

## 20974-20979 Osteogenic Stimulation

**CMS:** 100-03,150.2 Osteogenic Stimulation

**20974**    Electrical stimulation to aid bone healing; noninvasive (nonoperative)
       1.46    2.20    **FUD** 000      ⊘ A
       **AMA:** 2017,Jan,8; 2016,Jan,13; 2015,Jan,16; 2014,Jan,11; 2012,Jan,15-42

**20975**    invasive (operative)
       5.16    5.16    **FUD** 000      ⊘ N N1 80 ▭
       **AMA:** 2002,Apr,13; 2000,Nov,8

**20979**    Low intensity ultrasound stimulation to aid bone healing, noninvasive (nonoperative)
       0.93    1.48    **FUD** 000      01 N1 ▭
       **AMA:** 2017,Jan,8; 2016,Jan,13; 2015,Jan,16; 2014,Jan,11; 2012,Jan,15-42

## 20982-20999 General Musculoskeletal Procedures

**20982**    Ablation therapy for reduction or eradication of 1 or more bone tumors (eg, metastasis) including adjacent soft tissue when involved by tumor extension, percutaneous, including imaging guidance when performed; radiofrequency
       EXCLUDES   Radiologic guidance (76940, 77002, 77013, 77022)
       10.6    48.3    **FUD** 000      J 62 50 ▭
       **AMA:** 2017,Jan,8; 2016,Jan,13; 2015,Sep,12; 2015,Jul,8

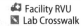

**20983**    **cryoablation**

> *EXCLUDES* *Radiologic guidance (76940, 77002, 77013, 77022)*
> 🚑 10.6    ⚕ 178.    **FUD** 000                          [J] [G2] [50] 📄
> **AMA:** 2017,Jan,8; 2016,Jan,13; 2015,Jul,8

**+    20985**    **Computer-assisted surgical navigational procedure for musculoskeletal procedures, image-less (List separately in addition to code for primary procedure)**

> *EXCLUDES* *Image guidance derived from intraoperative and preoperative obtained images (0054T-0055T)*
> *Stereotactic computer-assisted navigational procedure; cranial or intradural (61781-61783)*
> Code first primary procedure
> 🚑 4.26    ⚕ 4.26    **FUD** ZZZ                          [N] [N1] [80] 📄
> **AMA:** 2017,Jan,8; 2016,Jan,13; 2015,Jan,16; 2014,Jan,11

**20999**    **Unlisted procedure, musculoskeletal system, general**

> 🚑 0.00    ⚕ 0.00    **FUD** YYY                          [T] [80]
> **AMA:** 2017,Jan,8; 2016,Jan,13; 2015,Jul,8; 2015,Jan,16; 2014,Oct,9; 2014,Jan,11

## 21010 Temporomandibular Joint Arthrotomy

**21010**    **Arthrotomy, temporomandibular joint**

> *EXCLUDES* *Excision of foreign body from dentoalveolar site (41805-41806)*
> *Soft tissue (subfascial) abscess drainage (20005)*
> *Superficial abscess and hematoma drainage (10060-10061)*
> 🚑 21.7    ⚕ 21.7    **FUD** 090                          [J] [A2] [80] [50] 📄
> **AMA:** 2002,Apr,13

## 21011-21016 Excision Soft Tissue Tumors Face and Scalp

> *INCLUDES* Any necessary elevation of tissue planes or dissection
> Measurement of tumor and necessary margin at greatest diameter prior to excision
> Simple and intermediate repairs
> Types of excision:
> Fascial or subfascial soft tissue tumors: simple and marginal resection of tumors found either in or below the deep fascia, not including bone or excision of a substantial amount of normal tissue; primarily benign and intramuscular tumors
> Radical resection soft tissue tumor: wide resection of tumor involving substantial margins of normal tissue and may include tissue removal from one or more layers; most often malignant or aggressive benign
> Subcutaneous: simple and marginal resection of tumors in the subcutaneous tissue above the deep fascia; most often benign
> *EXCLUDES* *Complex repair*
> *Excision of benign cutaneous lesions (eg, sebaceous cyst) (11420-11426)*
> *Radical resection of cutaneous tumors (eg, melanoma) (11620-11646)*
> *Significant exploration of vessels or neuroplasty*

**21011**    **Excision, tumor, soft tissue of face or scalp, subcutaneous; less than 2 cm**

> 🚑 7.45    ⚕ 9.93    **FUD** 090                          [J] [P3] [80] 📄
> **AMA:** 2017,Jan,8; 2016,Jan,13; 2015,Jan,16; 2014,Jan,11

**21012**    **2 cm or greater**

> 🚑 9.75    ⚕ 9.75    **FUD** 090                          [J] [R2] [80] 📄
> **AMA:** 2017,Jan,8; 2016,Jan,13; 2015,Jan,16; 2014,Jan,11

**21013**    **Excision, tumor, soft tissue of face and scalp, subfascial (eg, subgaleal, intramuscular); less than 2 cm**

> 🚑 11.5    ⚕ 14.8    **FUD** 090                          [J] [P3] [80] 📄
> **AMA:** 2017,Jan,8; 2016,Jan,13; 2015,Jan,16; 2014,Jan,11

**21014**    **2 cm or greater**

> 🚑 15.0    ⚕ 15.0    **FUD** 090                          [J] [R2] [80] 📄
> **AMA:** 2017,Jan,8; 2016,Jan,13; 2015,Jan,16; 2014,Jan,11

**21015**    **Radical resection of tumor (eg, sarcoma), soft tissue of face or scalp; less than 2 cm**

> *EXCLUDES* *Removal of cranial tumor for osteomyelitis (61501)*
> 🚑 20.3    ⚕ 20.3    **FUD** 090                          [J] [G2] 📄
> **AMA:** 2017,Jan,8; 2016,Jan,13; 2015,Jan,16; 2014,Jan,11

**21016**    **2 cm or greater**

> 🚑 29.3    ⚕ 29.3    **FUD** 090                          [J] [G2] [80] 📄
> **AMA:** 2017,Jan,8; 2016,Jan,13; 2015,Jan,16; 2014,Jan,11

## 21025-21070 Procedures of Cranial and Facial Bones

> *INCLUDES* Any necessary elevation of tissue planes or dissection
> Measurement of tumor and necessary margins prior to excision
> Radical resection of bone tumor involves resection of the tumor (may include entire bone) and wide margins of normal tissue primarily for malignant or aggressive benign tumors
> Simple and intermediate repairs
> *EXCLUDES* *Complex repair*
> *Excision of soft tissue tumors, face and scalp (21011-21016)*
> *Radical resection of cutaneous tumors (e.g., melanoma) (11620-11646)*
> *Significant exploration of vessels, neuroplasty, reconstruction, or complex bone repair*

**21025**    **Excision of bone (eg, for osteomyelitis or bone abscess); mandible**

> 🚑 21.7    ⚕ 25.6    **FUD** 090                          [J] [A2] 📄
> **AMA:** 2017,Jan,8; 2016,Jan,13; 2015,Jan,16; 2014,Jan,11; 2012,Jan,15-42

**21026**    **facial bone(s)**

> 🚑 14.4    ⚕ 17.8    **FUD** 090                          [J] [A2] 📄
> **AMA:** 2002,Apr,13

**21029**    **Removal by contouring of benign tumor of facial bone (eg, fibrous dysplasia)**

> 🚑 18.4    ⚕ 22.1    **FUD** 090                          [J] [A2] [80] 📄
> **AMA:** 2002,Apr,13

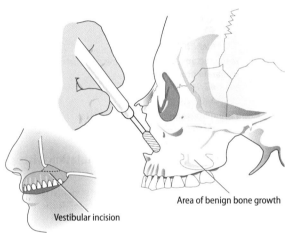

Area of benign bone growth

Vestibular incision

Burrs, files, and osteotomes used to remove bone

**21030**    **Excision of benign tumor or cyst of maxilla or zygoma by enucleation and curettage**

> 🚑 12.1    ⚕ 14.9    **FUD** 090                          [J] [P3] [50] 📄
> **AMA:** 2017,Jan,8; 2016,Jan,13; 2015,Jan,16; 2014,Jan,11

**21031**    **Excision of torus mandibularis**

> 🚑 8.57    ⚕ 11.4    **FUD** 090                          [J] [P3] [50] 📄
> **AMA:** 2002,Apr,13

**21032**    **Excision of maxillary torus palatinus**

> 🚑 8.45    ⚕ 11.5    **FUD** 090                          [J] [P3]
> **AMA:** 2002,Apr,13

**21034**    **Excision of malignant tumor of maxilla or zygoma**

> 🚑 33.4    ⚕ 37.8    **FUD** 090                          [J] [A2] [80] 📄
> **AMA:** 2017,Jan,8; 2016,Jan,13; 2015,Jan,16; 2014,Jan,11

**21040**    **Excision of benign tumor or cyst of mandible, by enucleation and/or curettage**

> *INCLUDES* Removal of benign tumor or cyst without osteotomy
> *EXCLUDES* *Removal of benign tumor or cyst with osteotomy (21046-21047)*
> 🚑 12.1    ⚕ 15.0    **FUD** 090                          [J] [A2] 📄
> **AMA:** 2017,Jan,8; 2016,Jan,13; 2015,Jan,16; 2014,Jan,11

**21044**    **Excision of malignant tumor of mandible;**

> 🚑 25.2    ⚕ 25.2    **FUD** 090                          [J] [A2] [80] 📄
> **AMA:** 2002,Apr,13

**Musculoskeletal System**

**21045   radical resection**
Code also bone graft procedure (21215)
35.3   35.3   **FUD** 090
C 80
**AMA:** 2002,Apr,13

**21046   Excision of benign tumor or cyst of mandible; requiring intra-oral osteotomy (eg, locally aggressive or destructive lesion[s])**
32.3   32.3   **FUD** 090
J A2 80
**AMA:** 2017,Jan,8; 2016,Jan,13; 2015,Jan,16; 2014,Jan,11

**21047   requiring extra-oral osteotomy and partial mandibulectomy (eg, locally aggressive or destructive lesion[s])**
38.0   38.0   **FUD** 090
J A2 80
**AMA:** 2017,Jan,8; 2016,Jan,13; 2015,Jan,16; 2014,Jan,11

**21048   Excision of benign tumor or cyst of maxilla; requiring intra-oral osteotomy (eg, locally aggressive or destructive lesion[s])**
33.2   33.2   **FUD** 090
J A2 80
**AMA:** 2017,Jan,8; 2016,Jan,13; 2015,Jan,16; 2014,Jan,11

**21049   requiring extra-oral osteotomy and partial maxillectomy (eg, locally aggressive or destructive lesion[s])**
34.7   34.7   **FUD** 090
J 80
**AMA:** 2017,Jan,8; 2016,Jan,13; 2015,Jan,16; 2014,Jan,11

**21050   Condylectomy, temporomandibular joint (separate procedure)**
24.0   24.0   **FUD** 090
J A2 80 50
**AMA:** 2002,Apr,13

**21060   Meniscectomy, partial or complete, temporomandibular joint (separate procedure)**
23.1   23.1   **FUD** 090
J A2 80 50
**AMA:** 2002,Apr,13

**21070   Coronoidectomy (separate procedure)**
17.5   17.5   **FUD** 090
J A2 80 50
**AMA:** 2002,Apr,13

## 21073 Temporomandibular Joint Manipulation with Anesthesia

**21073   Manipulation of temporomandibular joint(s) (TMJ), therapeutic, requiring an anesthesia service (ie, general or monitored anesthesia care)**
EXCLUDES   Closed treatment of TMJ dislocation (21480, 21485)
Manipulation of TMJ without general or MAC anesthesia (97140, 98925-98929, 98943)
7.41   11.4   **FUD** 090
T P3 80 50
**AMA:** 2017,Jan,8; 2016,Jan,13; 2015,Jan,16; 2014,Jan,11; 2012,Jan,15-42

## 21076-21089 Medical Impressions for Fabrication Maxillofacial Prosthesis

INCLUDES   Design, preparation, and professional services rendered by a physician or other qualified health care professional
EXCLUDES   Application or removal of caliper or tongs (20660, 20665)
Professional services rendered for outside laboratory designed and prepared prosthesis

**21076   Impression and custom preparation; surgical obturator prosthesis**
24.0   28.6   **FUD** 010
T P3 80
**AMA:** 2017,Jan,8; 2016,Jan,13; 2015,Jan,16; 2014,Jan,11; 2012,Jan,15-42

**21077   orbital prosthesis**
61.0   72.4   **FUD** 090
J P3 80 50
**AMA:** 2017,Jan,8; 2016,Jan,13; 2015,Jan,16; 2014,Jan,11

**21079   interim obturator prosthesis**
40.6   48.8   **FUD** 090
J P3
**AMA:** 2017,Jan,8; 2016,Jan,13; 2015,Jan,16; 2014,Jan,11

**21080   definitive obturator prosthesis**
45.2   54.8   **FUD** 090
J P3
**AMA:** 2017,Jan,8; 2016,Jan,13; 2015,Jan,16; 2014,Jan,11

**21081   mandibular resection prosthesis**
41.6   50.5   **FUD** 090
J P3 80 CLIA
**AMA:** 2017,Jan,8; 2016,Jan,13; 2015,Jan,16; 2014,Jan,11

**21082   palatal augmentation prosthesis**
38.8   47.6   **FUD** 090
J P3 80
**AMA:** 2017,Jan,8; 2016,Jan,13; 2015,Jan,16; 2014,Jan,11

**21083   palatal lift prosthesis**
36.1   45.4   **FUD** 090
J P3 80
**AMA:** 2017,Jan,8; 2016,Jan,13; 2015,Jan,16; 2014,Jan,11

**21084   speech aid prosthesis**
41.8   52.1   **FUD** 090
J P3 80
**AMA:** 2017,Jan,8; 2016,Jan,13; 2015,Jan,16; 2014,Jan,11

**21085   oral surgical splint**
16.4   21.8   **FUD** 010
T P2 80
**AMA:** 2017,Sep,14; 2017,Jan,8; 2016,Jan,13; 2015,Jan,16; 2014,Jan,11

**21086   auricular prosthesis**
45.1   53.8   **FUD** 090
J P3 80 50
**AMA:** 2017,Jan,8; 2016,Jan,13; 2015,Jan,16; 2014,Jan,11

**21087   nasal prosthesis**
44.8   53.5   **FUD** 090
J P3 80 50
**AMA:** 2017,Jan,8; 2016,Jan,13; 2015,Jan,16; 2014,Jan,11

**21088   facial prosthesis**
0.00   0.00   **FUD** 090
J P2 80 50
**AMA:** 2017,Jan,8; 2016,Jan,13; 2015,Jan,16; 2014,Jan,11

**21089   Unlisted maxillofacial prosthetic procedure**
0.00   0.00   **FUD** YYY
T
**AMA:** 2017,Jan,8; 2016,Jan,13; 2015,Jan,16; 2014,Jan,11; 2012,Jan,15-42

## 21100-21110 Application Fixation Device

**21100   Application of halo type appliance for maxillofacial fixation, includes removal (separate procedure)**
11.6   23.9   **FUD** 090
J A2 80
**AMA:** 2002,Apr,13

**21110   Application of interdental fixation device for conditions other than fracture or dislocation, includes removal**
EXCLUDES   Interdental fixation device removal by different provider (20670-20680)
19.4   23.1   **FUD** 090
Q2 P2
**AMA:** 2017,Jan,8; 2016,Jan,13; 2015,Jan,16; 2014,Jan,11; 2013,Dec,16; 2012,Jan,15-42

## 21116 Injection for TMJ Arthrogram

**CMS:** 100-02,15,150.1 Treatment of Temporomandibular Joint (TMJ) Syndrome; 100-04,13,80.1 Physician Presence; 100-04,13,80.2 S&I Multiple Procedure Reduction

**21116   Injection procedure for temporomandibular joint arthrography**
(70332)
1.28   4.19   **FUD** 000
N N1 50
**AMA:** 2017,Jan,8; 2016,May,13; 2016,Jan,13; 2015,Aug,6

## 21120-21299 Repair/Reconstruction Craniofacial Bones

EXCLUDES *Cranioplasty (21179-21180, 62120, 62140-62147)*

**21120** **Genioplasty; augmentation (autograft, allograft, prosthetic material)**
🔧 13.7  ⚖ 17.2  **FUD** 090  〔J〕〔J8〕▢
**AMA:** 2002,Apr,13

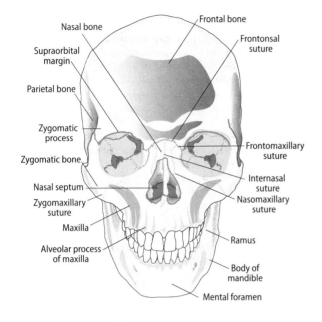

Nasal bone
Frontal bone
Frontonsal suture
Supraorbital margin
Parietal bone
Zygomatic process
Frontomaxillary suture
Zygomatic bone
Internasal suture
Nasal septum
Nasomaxillary suture
Zygomaxillary suture
Maxilla
Ramus
Alveolar process of maxilla
Body of mandible
Mental foramen

**21121** **sliding osteotomy, single piece**
🔧 19.4  ⚖ 23.1  **FUD** 090  〔J〕〔A2〕〔80〕▢
**AMA:** 2002,Apr,13

**21122** **sliding osteotomies, 2 or more osteotomies (eg, wedge excision or bone wedge reversal for asymmetrical chin)**
🔧 19.0  ⚖ 19.0  **FUD** 090  〔J〕〔A2〕〔80〕▢
**AMA:** 2002,Apr,13

**21123** **sliding, augmentation with interpositional bone grafts (includes obtaining autografts)**
🔧 26.0  ⚖ 26.0  **FUD** 090  〔J〕〔A2〕〔80〕▢
**AMA:** 2002,Apr,13

**21125** **Augmentation, mandibular body or angle; prosthetic material**
🔧 21.2  ⚖ 91.5  **FUD** 090  〔J〕〔A2〕〔80〕▢
**AMA:** 2002,Apr,13

**21127** **with bone graft, onlay or interpositional (includes obtaining autograft)**
🔧 25.7  ⚖ 125.  **FUD** 090  〔J〕〔A2〕〔80〕▢
**AMA:** 2002,Apr,13

**21137** **Reduction forehead; contouring only**
🔧 20.0  ⚖ 20.0  **FUD** 090  〔J〕〔62〕〔80〕▢
**AMA:** 2002,Apr,13

**21138** **contouring and application of prosthetic material or bone graft (includes obtaining autograft)**
🔧 26.4  ⚖ 26.4  **FUD** 090  〔J〕〔62〕〔80〕▢
**AMA:** 2002,Apr,13

**21139** **contouring and setback of anterior frontal sinus wall**
🔧 31.2  ⚖ 31.2  **FUD** 090  〔J〕〔62〕〔80〕▢
**AMA:** 2002,Apr,13

**21141** **Reconstruction midface, LeFort I; single piece, segment movement in any direction (eg, for Long Face Syndrome), without bone graft**
🔧 39.2  ⚖ 39.2  **FUD** 090  〔C〕〔80〕▢
**AMA:** 2002,Apr,13; 1995,Win,1

**21142** **2 pieces, segment movement in any direction, without bone graft**
🔧 41.5  ⚖ 41.5  **FUD** 090  〔C〕〔80〕▢
**AMA:** 2002,Apr,13; 1995,Win,1

**21143** **3 or more pieces, segment movement in any direction, without bone graft**
🔧 42.3  ⚖ 42.3  **FUD** 090  〔C〕〔80〕▢
**AMA:** 2002,Apr,13; 1995,Win,1

**21145** **single piece, segment movement in any direction, requiring bone grafts (includes obtaining autografts)**
🔧 46.2  ⚖ 46.2  **FUD** 090  〔C〕〔80〕▢
**AMA:** 2002,Apr,13; 1995,Win,1

**21146** **2 pieces, segment movement in any direction, requiring bone grafts (includes obtaining autografts) (eg, ungrafted unilateral alveolar cleft)**
🔧 48.1  ⚖ 48.1  **FUD** 090  〔C〕〔80〕▢
**AMA:** 2002,Apr,13; 1995,Win,1

**21147** **3 or more pieces, segment movement in any direction, requiring bone grafts (includes obtaining autografts) (eg, ungrafted bilateral alveolar cleft or multiple osteotomies)**
🔧 48.5  ⚖ 48.5  **FUD** 090  〔C〕〔80〕▢
**AMA:** 2002,Apr,13; 1995,Win,1

**21150** **Reconstruction midface, LeFort II; anterior intrusion (eg, Treacher-Collins Syndrome)**
🔧 50.1  ⚖ 50.1  **FUD** 090  〔J〕〔62〕〔80〕▢
**AMA:** 2002,Apr,13

**21151** **any direction, requiring bone grafts (includes obtaining autografts)**
🔧 58.1  ⚖ 58.1  **FUD** 090  〔C〕〔80〕▢
**AMA:** 2002,Apr,13

**21154** **Reconstruction midface, LeFort III (extracranial), any type, requiring bone grafts (includes obtaining autografts); without LeFort I**
🔧 54.3  ⚖ 54.3  **FUD** 090  〔C〕〔80〕▢
**AMA:** 2002,Apr,13

**21155** **with LeFort I**
🔧 60.3  ⚖ 60.3  **FUD** 090  〔C〕〔80〕▢
**AMA:** 2002,Apr,13

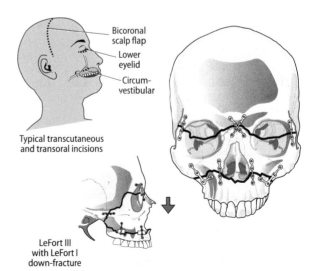

Bicoronal scalp flap
Lower eyelid
Circum-vestibular

Typical transcutaneous and transoral incisions

LeFort III with LeFort I down-fracture

**21159** **Reconstruction midface, LeFort III (extra and intracranial) with forehead advancement (eg, mono bloc), requiring bone grafts (includes obtaining autografts); without LeFort I**
🔧 75.7  ⚖ 75.7  **FUD** 090  〔C〕〔80〕▢
**AMA:** 2002,Apr,13

● New Code  ▲ Revised Code  ○ Reinstated  ● New Web Release  ▲ Revised Web Release  Unlisted  Not Covered  # Resequenced
⊘ AMA Mod 51 Exempt  ⑪ Optum Mod 51 Exempt  ⑥³ Mod 63 Exempt  ✗ Non-FDA Drug  ★ Telemedicine  Ⓜ Maternity  Ⓐ Age Edit  + Add-on  **AMA:** CPT Asst
© 2017 Optum360, LLC     CPT © 2017 American Medical Association. All Rights Reserved.     **43**

Musculoskeletal System

21160 — 21240

**21160** **with LeFort I**
78.4   78.4   **FUD** 090   C 80
AMA: 2002,Apr,13

**21172** **Reconstruction superior-lateral orbital rim and lower forehead, advancement or alteration, with or without grafts (includes obtaining autografts)**
EXCLUDES Frontal or parietal craniotomy for craniosynostosis (61556)
59.5   59.5   **FUD** 090   J 80
AMA: 2002,Apr,13

**21175** **Reconstruction, bifrontal, superior-lateral orbital rims and lower forehead, advancement or alteration (eg, plagiocephaly, trigonocephaly, brachycephaly), with or without grafts (includes obtaining autografts)**
EXCLUDES Bifrontal craniotomy for craniosynostosis (61557)
60.8   60.8   **FUD** 090   J 80
AMA: 2002,Apr,13

**21179** **Reconstruction, entire or majority of forehead and/or supraorbital rims; with grafts (allograft or prosthetic material)**
EXCLUDES Extensive craniotomy for numerous suture craniosynostosis (61558-61559)
39.3   39.3   **FUD** 090   C 80
AMA: 2002,Apr,13

**21180** **with autograft (includes obtaining grafts)**
EXCLUDES Extensive craniotomy for numerous suture craniosynostosis (61558-61559)
45.8   45.8   **FUD** 090   C 80
AMA: 2002,Apr,13

**21181** **Reconstruction by contouring of benign tumor of cranial bones (eg, fibrous dysplasia), extracranial**
21.3   21.3   **FUD** 090   J A2 80
AMA: 2002,Apr,13

**21182** **Reconstruction of orbital walls, rims, forehead, nasoethmoid complex following intra- and extracranial excision of benign tumor of cranial bone (eg, fibrous dysplasia), with multiple autografts (includes obtaining grafts); total area of bone grafting less than 40 sq cm**
EXCLUDES Removal of benign tumor of the skull (61563-61564)
57.0   57.0   **FUD** 090   C 80
AMA: 2002,May,7; 2002,Apr,13

**21183** **total area of bone grafting greater than 40 sq cm but less than 80 sq cm**
EXCLUDES Removal of benign tumor of the skull (61563-61564)
64.3   64.3   **FUD** 090   C 80
AMA: 2002,Apr,13

**21184** **total area of bone grafting greater than 80 sq cm**
EXCLUDES Removal of benign tumor of the skull (61563-61564)
78.7   78.7   **FUD** 090   C 80
AMA: 2002,Apr,13

**21188** **Reconstruction midface, osteotomies (other than LeFort type) and bone grafts (includes obtaining autografts)**
47.0   47.0   **FUD** 090   C 80
AMA: 2002,Apr,13

**21193** **Reconstruction of mandibular rami, horizontal, vertical, C, or L osteotomy; without bone graft**
34.0   34.0   **FUD** 090   J 80
AMA: 2017,Jan,8; 2016,Jan,13; 2015,Jan,16; 2014,Jan,11; 2012,Jan,15-42

**21194** **with bone graft (includes obtaining graft)**
42.7   42.7   **FUD** 090   C 80
AMA: 2017,Jan,8; 2016,Jan,13; 2015,Jan,16; 2014,Jan,11

**21195** **Reconstruction of mandibular rami and/or body, sagittal split; without internal rigid fixation**
38.0   38.0   **FUD** 090   J 80
AMA: 2017,Jan,8; 2016,Jan,13; 2015,Jan,16; 2014,Jan,11; 2012,Jan,15-42

**21196** **with internal rigid fixation**
42.9   42.9   **FUD** 090   C 80
AMA: 2017,Jan,8; 2016,Jan,13; 2015,Jan,16; 2014,Jan,11; 2012,Jan,15-42

**21198** **Osteotomy, mandible, segmental;**
EXCLUDES Total maxillary osteotomy (21141-21160)
33.7   33.7   **FUD** 090   J 62 80
AMA: 2017,Jan,8; 2016,Jan,13; 2015,Jan,16; 2014,Jan,11; 2013,Dec,16

**21199** **with genioglossus advancement**
EXCLUDES Total maxillary osteotomy (21141-21160)
29.1   29.1   **FUD** 090   J 62 80
AMA: 2017,Jan,8; 2016,Jan,13; 2015,Jan,16; 2014,Jan,11

**21206** **Osteotomy, maxilla, segmental (eg, Wassmund or Schuchard)**
35.1   35.1   **FUD** 090   J A2 80
AMA: 2002,Apr,13

**21208** **Osteoplasty, facial bones; augmentation (autograft, allograft, or prosthetic implant)**
24.3   52.8   **FUD** 090   J A2 80
AMA: 2002,Apr,13

**21209** **reduction**
17.8   23.3   **FUD** 090   J A2 80
AMA: 2002,Apr,13

**21210** **Graft, bone; nasal, maxillary or malar areas (includes obtaining graft)**
EXCLUDES Cleft palate procedures (42200-42225)
25.1   65.2   **FUD** 090   J A2
AMA: 2002,Apr,13

**21215** **mandible (includes obtaining graft)**
26.1   114.   **FUD** 090   J A2
AMA: 2002,Apr,13

**21230** **Graft; rib cartilage, autogenous, to face, chin, nose or ear (includes obtaining graft)**
EXCLUDES Augmentation of facial bones (21208)
21.4   21.4   **FUD** 090   J A2 80
AMA: 2002,Apr,13

**21235** **ear cartilage, autogenous, to nose or ear (includes obtaining graft)**
EXCLUDES Augmentation of facial bones (21208)
16.2   20.7   **FUD** 090   J A2
AMA: 2017,Jan,8; 2016,Jan,13; 2015,Jan,16; 2012,Jan,15-42

**21240** **Arthroplasty, temporomandibular joint, with or without autograft (includes obtaining graft)**
32.4   32.4   **FUD** 090   J A2 80 50
AMA: 2002,Apr,13; 1994,Win,1

TMJ syndrome is often related to stress and tooth-grinding; in other cases, arthritis, injury, poorly aligned teeth, or ill-fitting dentures may be the cause

Upper joint space
Lower joint space
Articular disc (meniscus)
Condyle
Mandible
Cutaway detail

**Cutaway view of temporomandibular joint (TMJ)**

Symptoms include facial pain and chewing problems; TMJ syndrome occurs more frequently in women

26/TC PC/TC Only | A2-Z3 ASC Payment | 50 Bilateral | ♂ Male Only | ♀ Female Only | Facility RVU | Non-Facility RVU | CCI
FUD Follow-up Days | CMS: IOM (Pub 100) | A-Y OPPSI | 80/80 Surg Assist Allowed / w/Doc | Lab Crosswalk | Radiology Crosswalk | CLIA
CPT © 2017 American Medical Association. All Rights Reserved. © 2017 Optum360, LLC

| | | |
|---|---|---|
| **21242** | **Arthroplasty, temporomandibular joint, with allograft** | |

29.8   29.8   **FUD** 090     J A2 80 50

**AMA:** 2002,Apr,13

**21243**   **Arthroplasty, temporomandibular joint, with prosthetic joint replacement**

49.5   49.5   **FUD** 090     J J8 80 50

**AMA:** 2002,Apr,13

**21244**   **Reconstruction of mandible, extraoral, with transosteal bone plate (eg, mandibular staple bone plate)**

30.7   30.7   **FUD** 090     J A2 80

**AMA:** 2004,Mar,7; 2002,Apr,13

**21245**   **Reconstruction of mandible or maxilla, subperiosteal implant; partial**

25.4   31.6   **FUD** 090     J A2 80

**AMA:** 2002,Apr,13

**21246**   **complete**

25.5   25.5   **FUD** 090     J A2 80

**AMA:** 2002,Apr,13

**21247**   **Reconstruction of mandibular condyle with bone and cartilage autografts (includes obtaining grafts) (eg, for hemifacial microsomia)**

44.2   44.2   **FUD** 090     C 80 50

**AMA:** 2002,Apr,13

**21248**   **Reconstruction of mandible or maxilla, endosteal implant (eg, blade, cylinder); partial**

*EXCLUDES*   *Midface reconstruction (21141-21160)*

26.2   32.0   **FUD** 090     J A2

**AMA:** 2002,Apr,13

**21249**   **complete**

*EXCLUDES*   *Midface reconstruction (21141-21160)*

37.1   43.6   **FUD** 090     J A2 80

**AMA:** 2002,Apr,13

**21255**   **Reconstruction of zygomatic arch and glenoid fossa with bone and cartilage (includes obtaining autografts)**

39.9   39.9   **FUD** 090     C 80 50

**AMA:** 2002,Apr,13

**21256**   **Reconstruction of orbit with osteotomies (extracranial) and with bone grafts (includes obtaining autografts) (eg, micro-ophthalmia)**

34.6   34.6   **FUD** 090     J 80 50

**AMA:** 2002,Apr,13

**21260**   **Periorbital osteotomies for orbital hypertelorism, with bone grafts; extracranial approach**

35.9   35.9   **FUD** 090     J 62 80

**AMA:** 2002,Apr,13

**21261**   **combined intra- and extracranial approach**

60.8   60.8   **FUD** 090     J 80

**AMA:** 2002,Apr,13

**21263**   **with forehead advancement**

56.1   56.1   **FUD** 090     J 80

**AMA:** 2002,Apr,13

Grafts

A frontal craniotomy is performed, the brain retracted, and the orbit approached from inside the skull; frontal bone is advanced and secured

Grafts are placed and the bony orbits realigned

Osteotomies are cut 360 degrees around the orbit; portions of nasal and ethmoid bones are removed

**21267**   **Orbital repositioning, periorbital osteotomies, unilateral, with bone grafts; extracranial approach**

45.6   45.6   **FUD** 090     J A2 80 50

**AMA:** 2002,Apr,13

**21268**   **combined intra- and extracranial approach**

50.1   50.1   **FUD** 090     C 80 50

**AMA:** 2002,Apr,13

**21270**   **Malar augmentation, prosthetic material**

*EXCLUDES*   *Augmentation procedure with bone graft (21210)*

20.8   27.7   **FUD** 090     J A2 80 50

**AMA:** 2002,Apr,13

**21275**   **Secondary revision of orbitocraniofacial reconstruction**

24.1   24.1   **FUD** 090     J J8 80

**AMA:** 2002,Apr,13

**21280**   **Medial canthopexy (separate procedure)**

*EXCLUDES*   *Reconstruction of canthus (67950)*

16.2   16.2   **FUD** 090     J A2 80 50

**AMA:** 2002,Apr,13

**21282**   **Lateral canthopexy**

10.8   10.8   **FUD** 090     J A2 50

**AMA:** 2002,Apr,13

**21295**   **Reduction of masseter muscle and bone (eg, for treatment of benign masseteric hypertrophy); extraoral approach**

5.33   5.33   **FUD** 090     T A2 80 50

**AMA:** 2002,Apr,13

**21296**   **intraoral approach**

12.7   12.7   **FUD** 090     J A2 80 50

**AMA:** 2002,Apr,13

**21299**   **Unlisted craniofacial and maxillofacial procedure**

0.00   0.00   **FUD** YYY     T 80

**AMA:** 2002,Apr,13; 1995,Win,1

## 21310-21499 Care of Fractures/Dislocations of the Cranial and Facial Bones

*EXCLUDES*   *Closed treatment of skull fracture, report with appropriate E&M service*
*Open treatment of skull fracture (62000-62010)*

**21310**   **Closed treatment of nasal bone fracture without manipulation**

0.78   3.77   **FUD** 000     T A2

**AMA:** 2002,Apr,13

● New Code   ▲ Revised Code   ○ Reinstated   ● New Web Release   ▲ Revised Web Release   Unlisted   Not Covered   # Resequenced
⊘ AMA Mod 51 Exempt   ⑩ Optum Mod 51 Exempt   ⊚ Mod 63 Exempt   ✗ Non-FDA Drug   ★ Telemedicine   M Maternity   A Age Edit   + Add-on   **AMA:** CPT Asst
© 2017 Optum360, LLC     CPT © 2017 American Medical Association. All Rights Reserved.     **45**

**21315** Closed treatment of nasal bone fracture; without stabilization
⚕ 4.34 ⚚ 7.86 **FUD** 010 T A2 ▢
AMA: 2002,Apr,13

**21320** with stabilization
⚕ 3.87 ⚚ 7.29 **FUD** 010 J A2 ▢
AMA: 2002,Apr,13

**21325** Open treatment of nasal fracture; uncomplicated
⚕ 13.5 ⚚ 13.5 **FUD** 090 J A2 80 ▢
AMA: 2002,Apr,13

**21330** complicated, with internal and/or external skeletal fixation
⚕ 16.4 ⚚ 16.4 **FUD** 090 J A2 80 ▢
AMA: 2002,Apr,13

**21335** with concomitant open treatment of fractured septum
⚕ 20.7 ⚚ 20.7 **FUD** 090 J A2 ▢
AMA: 2002,Apr,13

**21336** Open treatment of nasal septal fracture, with or without stabilization
⚕ 18.4 ⚚ 18.4 **FUD** 090 J A2 80 ▢
AMA: 2002,Apr,13

**21337** Closed treatment of nasal septal fracture, with or without stabilization
⚕ 8.47 ⚚ 11.5 **FUD** 090 J A2 80 ▢
AMA: 2002,Apr,13

**21338** Open treatment of nasoethmoid fracture; without external fixation
⚕ 21.5 ⚚ 21.5 **FUD** 090 J A2 80 ▢
AMA: 2002,Apr,13

**21339** with external fixation
⚕ 24.3 ⚚ 24.3 **FUD** 090 J A2 80 ▢
AMA: 2002,Apr,13

**21340** Percutaneous treatment of nasoethmoid complex fracture, with splint, wire or headcap fixation, including repair of canthal ligaments and/or the nasolacrimal apparatus
⚕ 23.0 ⚚ 23.0 **FUD** 090 J A2 80 ▢
AMA: 2002,Apr,13

**21343** Open treatment of depressed frontal sinus fracture
⚕ 34.9 ⚚ 34.9 **FUD** 090 C 80 ▢
AMA: 2002,Apr,13

**21344** Open treatment of complicated (eg, comminuted or involving posterior wall) frontal sinus fracture, via coronal or multiple approaches
⚕ 40.0 ⚚ 40.0 **FUD** 090 C 80 ▢
AMA: 2002,Apr,13

**21345** Closed treatment of nasomaxillary complex fracture (LeFort II type), with interdental wire fixation or fixation of denture or splint
⚕ 18.6 ⚚ 23.0 **FUD** 090 T A2 80 ▢
AMA: 2002,Apr,13

**21346** Open treatment of nasomaxillary complex fracture (LeFort II type); with wiring and/or local fixation
⚕ 26.0 ⚚ 26.0 **FUD** 090 J ▢
AMA: 2002,Apr,13

**21347** requiring multiple open approaches
⚕ 32.7 ⚚ 32.7 **FUD** 090 C 80 ▢
AMA: 2002,Apr,13

**21348** with bone grafting (includes obtaining graft)
⚕ 34.6 ⚚ 34.6 **FUD** 090 C 80 ▢
AMA: 2002,Apr,13

**21355** Percutaneous treatment of fracture of malar area, including zygomatic arch and malar tripod, with manipulation
⚕ 9.60 ⚚ 12.8 **FUD** 010 J A2 80 50 ▢
AMA: 2002,Apr,13

**21356** Open treatment of depressed zygomatic arch fracture (eg, Gillies approach)
⚕ 10.8 ⚚ 14.3 **FUD** 010 J A2 80 50 ▢
AMA: 2002,Apr,13

**21360** Open treatment of depressed malar fracture, including zygomatic arch and malar tripod
⚕ 15.5 ⚚ 15.5 **FUD** 090 J 62 80 50 ▢
AMA: 2002,Apr,13

**21365** Open treatment of complicated (eg, comminuted or involving cranial nerve foramina) fracture(s) of malar area, including zygomatic arch and malar tripod; with internal fixation and multiple surgical approaches
⚕ 32.0 ⚚ 32.0 **FUD** 090 J 80 50 ▢
AMA: 2002,Apr,13

**21366** with bone grafting (includes obtaining graft)
⚕ 32.6 ⚚ 32.6 **FUD** 090 C 80 50 ▢
AMA: 2002,Apr,13

**21385** Open treatment of orbital floor blowout fracture; transantral approach (Caldwell-Luc type operation)
⚕ 19.4 ⚚ 19.4 **FUD** 090 J 80 50 ▢
AMA: 2002,Apr,13

**21386** periorbital approach
⚕ 19.9 ⚚ 19.9 **FUD** 090 J 80 50 ▢
AMA: 2002,Apr,13

**21387** combined approach
⚕ 20.3 ⚚ 20.3 **FUD** 090 J 80 50 ▢
AMA: 2002,Apr,13

**21390** periorbital approach, with alloplastic or other implant
⚕ 22.8 ⚚ 22.8 **FUD** 090 J 62 80 50 ▢
AMA: 2003,Jan,1; 2002,Apr,13

**21395** periorbital approach with bone graft (includes obtaining graft)
⚕ 29.1 ⚚ 29.1 **FUD** 090 J 80 50 ▢
AMA: 2002,Apr,13

**21400** Closed treatment of fracture of orbit, except blowout; without manipulation
⚕ 4.48 ⚚ 5.50 **FUD** 090 T A2 80 50 ▢
AMA: 2002,Apr,13

**21401** with manipulation
⚕ 8.75 ⚚ 13.9 **FUD** 090 T A2 80 50 ▢
AMA: 2002,Apr,13

**21406** Open treatment of fracture of orbit, except blowout; without implant
⚕ 16.4 ⚚ 16.4 **FUD** 090 J 62 80 50 ▢
AMA: 2002,Apr,13

**21407** with implant
⚕ 18.5 ⚚ 18.5 **FUD** 090 J 62 80 50 ▢
AMA: 2002,Apr,13

**21408** with bone grafting (includes obtaining graft)
⚕ 25.7 ⚚ 25.7 **FUD** 090 J 80 50 ▢
AMA: 2002,Apr,13

**21421** Closed treatment of palatal or maxillary fracture (LeFort I type), with interdental wire fixation or fixation of denture or splint
⚕ 20.1 ⚚ 24.2 **FUD** 090 J A2 80 ▢
AMA: 2002,Apr,13

**21422** Open treatment of palatal or maxillary fracture (LeFort I type);
⚕ 19.5 ⚚ 19.5 **FUD** 090 C 80 ▢
AMA: 2002,Apr,13

**21423** complicated (comminuted or involving cranial nerve foramina), multiple approaches
⚕ 22.7 ⚚ 22.7 **FUD** 090 C 80 ▢
AMA: 2002,Apr,13

**21431** Closed treatment of craniofacial separation (LeFort III type) using interdental wire fixation of denture or splint
🔧 21.1 ✂ 21.1 **FUD** 090    C 80 ▣
**AMA:** 2002,Apr,13

**21432** Open treatment of craniofacial separation (LeFort III type); with wiring and/or internal fixation
🔧 19.5 ✂ 19.5 **FUD** 090    C 80 ▣
**AMA:** 2002,Apr,13

**21433** complicated (eg, comminuted or involving cranial nerve foramina), multiple surgical approaches
🔧 50.1 ✂ 50.1 **FUD** 090    C 80 ▣
**AMA:** 2002,Apr,13

**21435** complicated, utilizing internal and/or external fixation techniques (eg, head cap, halo device, and/or intermaxillary fixation)
EXCLUDES *Removal of internal or external fixation (20670)*
🔧 36.6 ✂ 36.6 **FUD** 090    C 80 ▣
**AMA:** 2002,Apr,13

**21436** complicated, multiple surgical approaches, internal fixation, with bone grafting (includes obtaining graft)
🔧 54.7 ✂ 54.7 **FUD** 090    C 80 ▣
**AMA:** 2002,Apr,13

**21440** Closed treatment of mandibular or maxillary alveolar ridge fracture (separate procedure)
🔧 13.5 ✂ 16.6 **FUD** 090    J P3 80 ▣
**AMA:** 2002,Apr,13

**21445** Open treatment of mandibular or maxillary alveolar ridge fracture (separate procedure)
🔧 18.0 ✂ 22.0 **FUD** 090    J A2 80 ▣
**AMA:** 2002,Apr,13

**21450** Closed treatment of mandibular fracture; without manipulation
🔧 14.2 ✂ 17.7 **FUD** 090    T A2 80 ▣
**AMA:** 2002,Apr,13

**21451** with manipulation
🔧 19.4 ✂ 23.6 **FUD** 090    T A2 80 ▣
**AMA:** 2002,Apr,13

**21452** Percutaneous treatment of mandibular fracture, with external fixation
🔧 9.69 ✂ 16.3 **FUD** 090    J A2 80 ▣
**AMA:** 2002,Apr,13

Comminuted fractures

Metal or acrylic bar

Rods and pins placed in drilled holes

**21453** Closed treatment of mandibular fracture with interdental fixation
🔧 22.5 ✂ 26.2 **FUD** 090    J A2 80 ▣
**AMA:** 2017,Jan,8; 2016,Jan,13; 2015,Jan,16; 2014,Jan,11; 2012,Jan,15-42

**21454** Open treatment of mandibular fracture with external fixation
🔧 16.6 ✂ 16.6 **FUD** 090    J A2 80 ▣
**AMA:** 2002,Apr,13

**21461** Open treatment of mandibular fracture; without interdental fixation
🔧 27.1 ✂ 61.3 **FUD** 090    J A2 ▣
**AMA:** 2002,Apr,13

**21462** with interdental fixation
🔧 30.2 ✂ 65.2 **FUD** 090    J A2 80 ▣
**AMA:** 2002,Apr,13

**21465** Open treatment of mandibular condylar fracture
🔧 27.1 ✂ 27.1 **FUD** 090    J A2 80 50 ▣
**AMA:** 2002,Apr,13

**21470** Open treatment of complicated mandibular fracture by multiple surgical approaches including internal fixation, interdental fixation, and/or wiring of dentures or splints
🔧 34.8 ✂ 34.8 **FUD** 090    J 80 ▣
**AMA:** 2017,Jan,8; 2016,Jan,13; 2015,Jan,16; 2014,Jan,11; 2012,Jan,15-42

**21480** Closed treatment of temporomandibular dislocation; initial or subsequent
🔧 0.92 ✂ 2.81 **FUD** 000    T A2 50 ▣
**AMA:** 2002,Apr,13

**21485** complicated (eg, recurrent requiring intermaxillary fixation or splinting), initial or subsequent
🔧 16.8 ✂ 20.0 **FUD** 090    T A2 80 50 ▣
**AMA:** 2002,Apr,13

**21490** Open treatment of temporomandibular dislocation
EXCLUDES *Interdental wiring (21497)*
🔧 26.4 ✂ 26.4 **FUD** 090    J A2 80 50 ▣
**AMA:** 2002,Apr,13

**21497** Interdental wiring, for condition other than fracture
🔧 17.7 ✂ 21.2 **FUD** 090    T A2 80 ▣
**AMA:** 2017,Jan,8; 2016,Jan,13; 2015,Jan,16; 2014,Jan,11; 2012,Jan,15-42

**21499** Unlisted musculoskeletal procedure, head
EXCLUDES *Unlisted procedures of craniofacial or maxillofacial areas (21299)*
🔧 0.00 ✂ 0.00 **FUD** YYY    T 80
**AMA:** 2002,Apr,13; 1995,Win,1

## 21501-21510 Surgical Incision for Drainage: Chest and Soft Tissues of Neck

EXCLUDES *Biopsy of the flank or back (21920-21925)*
*Simple incision and drainage of abscess or hematoma (10060, 10140)*
*Tumor removal of flank or back (21930-21936)*

**21501** Incision and drainage, deep abscess or hematoma, soft tissues of neck or thorax;
EXCLUDES *Deep incision and drainage of posterior spine (22010-22015)*
🔧 9.21 ✂ 12.9 **FUD** 090    J A2 ▣
**AMA:** 2017,Jan,8; 2016,Jan,13; 2015,Jan,16; 2014,Dec,16; 2014,Dec,16

**21502** with partial rib ostectomy
🔧 14.6 ✂ 14.6 **FUD** 090    J A2 80 ▣
**AMA:** 2002,Apr,13

**21510** Incision, deep, with opening of bone cortex (eg, for osteomyelitis or bone abscess), thorax
🔧 12.8 ✂ 12.8 **FUD** 090    C 80 ▣
**AMA:** 2002,Apr,13

## 21550 Soft Tissue Biopsy of Chest or Neck

EXCLUDES *Biopsy of bone (20220-20251)*
*Soft tissue needle biopsy (20206)*

**21550** Biopsy, soft tissue of neck or thorax
🔧 4.54 ✂ 7.49 **FUD** 010    J G2 ▣
**AMA:** 2002,Apr,13

● New Code ▲ Revised Code ○ Reinstated ● New Web Release ▲ Revised Web Release   Unlisted   Not Covered   # Resequenced
Ⓢ AMA Mod 51 Exempt ⑤ Optum Mod 51 Exempt ⑥ Mod 63 Exempt ⚲ Non-FDA Drug ★ Telemedicine Ⓜ Maternity Ⓐ Age Edit + Add-on **AMA:** CPT Asst
© 2017 Optum360, LLC    CPT © 2017 American Medical Association. All Rights Reserved.

## 21552-21558 [21552, 21554] Excision Soft Tissue Tumors Chest and Neck

INCLUDES    Any necessary elevation of tissue planes or dissection
Measurement of tumor and necessary margin at greatest diameter prior to excision
Resection without removal of significant normal tissue
Simple and intermediate repairs
Types of excision:
Fascial or subfascial soft tissue tumors: simple and marginal resection of tumors found either in or below the deep fascia, not involving bone or excision of a substantial amount of normal tissue; primarily benign and intramuscular tumors
Radical resection soft tissue tumor: wide resection of tumor, involving substantial margins of normal tissue and may involve tissue removal from one or more layers; most often malignant or aggressive benign
Subcutaneous: simple and marginal resection of tumors in the subcutaneous tissue above the deep fascia; most often benign

EXCLUDES    Complex repair
Excision of benign cutaneous lesions (eg, sebaceous cyst) (11400-11426)
Radical resection of cutaneous tumors (eg, melanoma) (11600-11626)
Significant exploration of the vessels or neuroplasty

**21552**    Resequenced code. See code following 21555.

**21554**    Resequenced code. See code following 21556.

**21555**    Excision, tumor, soft tissue of neck or anterior thorax, subcutaneous; less than 3 cm
🚑 8.80    ✋ 11.8    **FUD** 090    J 62 ▣
**AMA:** 2017,Jan,8; 2016,Jan,13; 2015,Jan,16; 2014,Jan,11; 2012,Jan,15-42

\#    **21552**    **3 cm or greater**
🚑 12.8    ✋ 12.8    **FUD** 090    J 62 80 ▣

**21556**    Excision, tumor, soft tissue of neck or anterior thorax, subfascial (eg, intramuscular); less than 5 cm
🚑 15.2    ✋ 15.2    **FUD** 090    J 62 ▣
**AMA:** 2002,Apr,13

\#    **21554**    **5 cm or greater**
🚑 21.0    ✋ 21.0    **FUD** 090    J 62 80 ▣

**21557**    Radical resection of tumor (eg, sarcoma), soft tissue of neck or anterior thorax; less than 5 cm
🚑 27.6    ✋ 27.6    **FUD** 090    J 62 80 ▣
**AMA:** 2017,Jan,8; 2016,Jan,13; 2015,Jan,16; 2014,Jan,11

**21558**    **5 cm or greater**
🚑 38.8    ✋ 38.8    **FUD** 090    J 62 80 ▣

## 21600-21632 Bony Resection Chest and Neck

**21600**    Excision of rib, partial
EXCLUDES    Extensive debridement (11044, 11047)
Extensive tumor removal (19260)
🚑 15.9    ✋ 15.9    **FUD** 090    J A2 80 ▣
**AMA:** 2017,Jan,8; 2016,Jan,13; 2015,Jan,16; 2014,Jan,11; 2013,Mar,13; 2012,Jul,12-14

**21610**    Costotransversectomy (separate procedure)
🚑 34.1    ✋ 34.1    **FUD** 090    J A2 80 ▣
**AMA:** 2002,Apr,13

**21615**    Excision first and/or cervical rib;
🚑 17.9    ✋ 17.9    **FUD** 090    C 80 50 ▣
**AMA:** 2017,Jan,8; 2016,Jan,13; 2015,Jan,16; 2014,Mar,13

**21616**    with sympathectomy
🚑 21.7    ✋ 21.7    **FUD** 090    C 80 50 ▣
**AMA:** 2002,Apr,13

**21620**    Ostectomy of sternum, partial
🚑 14.5    ✋ 14.5    **FUD** 090    C 80 ▣
**AMA:** 2002,Apr,13

**21627**    Sternal debridement
EXCLUDES    Debridement with sternotomy closure (21750)
🚑 15.5    ✋ 15.5    **FUD** 090    C 80 ▣
**AMA:** 2017,Jan,8; 2016,Jan,13; 2015,Jan,16; 2014,Jan,11

**21630**    Radical resection of sternum;
🚑 35.0    ✋ 35.0    **FUD** 090    C 80 ▣
**AMA:** 2002,Apr,13; 1994,Win,1

**21632**    with mediastinal lymphadenectomy
🚑 34.4    ✋ 34.4    **FUD** 090    C 80 ▣
**AMA:** 2002,Apr,13

## 21685-21750 Repair/Reconstruction Chest and Soft Tissues Neck

EXCLUDES    Biopsy of chest or neck (21550)
Repair of simple wounds (12001-12007)
Tumor removal of chest or neck (21552-21558 [21552, 21554])

**21685**    Hyoid myotomy and suspension
🚑 28.5    ✋ 28.5    **FUD** 090    J 62 80 ▣
**AMA:** 2017,Jan,8; 2016,Jan,13; 2015,Jan,16; 2014,Jan,11; 2012,Jan,15-42

**21700**    Division of scalenus anticus; without resection of cervical rib
🚑 10.6    ✋ 10.6    **FUD** 090    J A2 80 50 ▣
**AMA:** 2002,Apr,13

**21705**    with resection of cervical rib
🚑 15.9    ✋ 15.9    **FUD** 090    C 80 50 ▣
**AMA:** 2017,Jan,8; 2016,Jan,13; 2015,Jan,16; 2014,Mar,13

**21720**    Division of sternocleidomastoid for torticollis, open operation; without cast application
EXCLUDES    Transection of spinal accessory and cervical nerves (63191, 64722)
🚑 14.2    ✋ 14.2    **FUD** 090    J A2 80 ▣
**AMA:** 2002,Apr,13

**21725**    with cast application
EXCLUDES    Transection of spinal accessory and cervical nerves (63191, 64722)
🚑 15.5    ✋ 15.5    **FUD** 090    T A2 80 ▣
**AMA:** 2002,Apr,13

**21740**    Reconstructive repair of pectus excavatum or carinatum; open
🚑 29.7    ✋ 29.7    **FUD** 090    C 80 ▣
**AMA:** 2002,Apr,13

**21742**    minimally invasive approach (Nuss procedure), without thoracoscopy
🚑 0.00    ✋ 0.00    **FUD** 090    J 80 ▣
**AMA:** 2002,Apr,13

**21743**    minimally invasive approach (Nuss procedure), with thoracoscopy
🚑 0.00    ✋ 0.00    **FUD** 090    J 80 ▣
**AMA:** 2002,Apr,13

**21750**    Closure of median sternotomy separation with or without debridement (separate procedure)
🚑 19.7    ✋ 19.7    **FUD** 090    C 80 ▣
**AMA:** 2017,Jan,8; 2016,Jan,13; 2015,Jan,16; 2014,Jan,11

## 21811-21825 Fracture Care: Ribs and Sternum

EXCLUDES    E&M services for treatment of closed uncomplicated rib fractures

**21811**    Open treatment of rib fracture(s) with internal fixation, includes thoracoscopic visualization when performed, unilateral; 1-3 ribs
🚑 17.5    ✋ 17.5    **FUD** 000    J 80 50 ▣
**AMA:** 2017,Jan,8; 2016,Jan,13; 2015,Aug,3

**21812**    4-6 ribs
🚑 21.0    ✋ 21.0    **FUD** 000    J 80 50 ▣
**AMA:** 2017,Jan,8; 2016,Jan,13; 2015,Aug,3

**21813**    7 or more ribs
🚑 27.7    ✋ 27.7    **FUD** 000    J 80 50 ▣
**AMA:** 2017,Jan,8; 2016,Jan,13; 2015,Aug,3

**21820**    Closed treatment of sternum fracture
🚑 4.10    ✋ 4.00    **FUD** 090    T A2 ▣
**AMA:** 2002,Apr,13

| 26/TC PC/TC Only | A2-Z3 ASC Payment | 50 Bilateral | ♂ Male Only | ♀ Female Only | 🚑 Facility RVU | ✋ Non-Facility RVU | ▣ CCI |
| FUD Follow-up Days | CMS: IOM (Pub 100) | A-Y OPPSI | | | 80/80 Surg Assist Allowed / w/Doc | 🔬 Lab Crosswalk | 📷 Radiology Crosswalk | ✖ CLIA |

48    CPT © 2017 American Medical Association. All Rights Reserved.    © 2017 Optum360, LLC

**21825** Open treatment of sternum fracture with or without skeletal fixation

> EXCLUDES Treatment of sternoclavicular dislocation (23520-23532)
>
> 🔧 15.5 ⚕ 15.5 **FUD** 090 C 80 ▱
>
> **AMA:** 2002,Apr,13

## 21899 Unlisted Procedures of Chest or Neck

CMS: 100-04,4,180.3 Unlisted Service or Procedure

**21899** Unlisted procedure, neck or thorax

> 🔧 0.00 ⚕ 0.00 **FUD** YYY T 80
>
> **AMA:** 2017,Jan,8; 2016,Jan,13; 2015,Aug,3

## 21920-21925 Biopsy Soft Tissue of Back and Flank

EXCLUDES Soft tissue needle biopsy (20206)

**21920** Biopsy, soft tissue of back or flank; superficial

> 🔧 4.61 ⚕ 7.34 **FUD** 010 J P3 ▱
>
> **AMA:** 2002,Apr,13; 1993,Sum,25

**21925** deep

> 🔧 10.2 ⚕ 12.8 **FUD** 090 J A2 ▱
>
> **AMA:** 2002,Apr,13

## 21930-21936 Excision Soft Tissue Tumors Back or Flank

INCLUDES Any necessary elevation of tissue planes or dissection
Measurement of tumor and necessary margin at greatest diameter prior to excision
Simple and intermediate repairs
Types of excision:
    Fascial or subfascial soft tissue tumors: simple and marginal resection of tumors found either in or below the deep fascia, not involving bone or excision of a substantial amount of normal tissue; most often benign and intramuscular tumors
    Radical resection soft tissue tumor: wide resection of tumor, involving substantial margins of normal tissue and may include tissue removal from one or more layers; most often malignant or aggressive benign
    Subcutaneous: simple and marginal resection of tumors in the subcutaneous tissue above the deep fascia; most often benign

EXCLUDES Complex repair
Excision of benign cutaneous lesions (eg, sebaceous cyst) (11400-11406)
Radical resection of cutaneous tumors (eg, melanoma) (11600-11606)
Significant exploration of the vessels or neuroplasty

**21930** Excision, tumor, soft tissue of back or flank, subcutaneous; less than 3 cm

> 🔧 10.5 ⚕ 13.5 **FUD** 090 J G2 ▱
>
> **AMA:** 2017,Jan,8; 2016,Jan,13; 2015,Jan,16; 2014,Jan,11; 2012,Jan,15-42

**21931** 3 cm or greater

> 🔧 13.5 ⚕ 13.5 **FUD** 090 J G2 80 ▱

**21932** Excision, tumor, soft tissue of back or flank, subfascial (eg, intramuscular); less than 5 cm

> 🔧 19.0 ⚕ 19.0 **FUD** 090 J G2 80 ▱

**21933** 5 cm or greater

> 🔧 21.2 ⚕ 21.2 **FUD** 090 J G2 80 ▱

**21935** Radical resection of tumor (eg, sarcoma), soft tissue of back or flank; less than 5 cm

> 🔧 29.7 ⚕ 29.7 **FUD** 090 J G2 ▱
>
> **AMA:** 2002,Apr,13; 1990,Win,4

**21936** 5 cm or greater

> 🔧 40.8 ⚕ 40.8 **FUD** 090 J G2 80 ▱

## 22010-22015 Incision for Drainage of Deep Spinal Abscess

EXCLUDES Incision and drainage of hematoma (10060, 10140)
Injection:
    Chemonucleolysis (62292)
    Discography (62290-62291)
    Facet joint (64490-64495, [64633, 64634, 64635, 64636])
    Myelography (62284)
Needle/trocar biopsy (20220-20225)

**22010** Incision and drainage, open, of deep abscess (subfascial), posterior spine; cervical, thoracic, or cervicothoracic

> 🔧 27.5 ⚕ 27.5 **FUD** 090 C 80 ▱

**22015** lumbar, sacral, or lumbosacral

> 🔧 27.1 ⚕ 27.1 **FUD** 090 C ▱
>
> EXCLUDES Incision and drainage, complex, postoperative wound infection (10180)
> Incision and drainage, open, of deep abscess (subfascial), posterior spine; cervical, thoracic, or cervicothoracic (22010)
> Removal of posterior nonsegmental instrumentation (eg, Harrington rod) (22850)
> Removal of posterior segmental instrumentation (22852)

## 22100-22103 Partial Resection Vertebral Component

EXCLUDES Back or flank biopsy (21920-21925)
Bone biopsy (20220-20251)
Injection:
    Chemonucleolysis (62292)
    Discography (62290-62291)
    Facet joint (64490-64495, [64633, 64634, 64635, 64636])
    Myelography (62284)
Removal of tumor flank or back (21930)
Soft tissue needle biopsy (20206)
Spinal reconstruction with vertebral body prosthesis:
    Cervical (20931, 20938, 22554, 63081)
    Thoracic (20931, 20938, 22556, 63085, 63087)

**22100** Partial excision of posterior vertebral component (eg, spinous process, lamina or facet) for intrinsic bony lesion, single vertebral segment; cervical

> 🔧 26.6 ⚕ 26.6 **FUD** 090 J 80 ▱
>
> **AMA:** 2017,Mar,7; 2017,Jan,8; 2016,Jan,13; 2015,Jan,16; 2013,Jul,3-5

**22101** thoracic

> 🔧 24.5 ⚕ 24.5 **FUD** 090 J 80 ▱
>
> **AMA:** 2017,Mar,7; 2017,Jan,8; 2016,Jan,13; 2015,Jan,16; 2013,Jul,3-5

**22102** lumbar

> Code also posterior spinous process distraction device insertion, if applicable (22867-22870)
>
> 🔧 22.5 ⚕ 22.5 **FUD** 090 J G2 80 ▱
>
> **AMA:** 2017,Mar,7; 2017,Jan,8; 2016,Jan,13; 2015,Jan,16; 2013,Jul,3-5

+ **22103** each additional segment (List separately in addition to code for primary procedure)

> Code first (22100-22102)
>
> 🔧 4.08 ⚕ 4.08 **FUD** ZZZ N N1 80 ▱
>
> **AMA:** 2003,Jan,1; 2002,Apr,13

## 22110-22116 Partial Resection Vertebral Component without Decompression

EXCLUDES Back or flank biopsy (21920-21925)
Bone biopsy (20220-20251)
Bone grafting procedures (20930-20938)
Harvest bone graft (20931, 20938)
Injection:
    Chemonucleolysis (62292)
    Discography (62290-62291)
    Facet joint (64490-64495, [64633, 64634, 64635, 64636])
    Myelography (62284)
Osteotomy (22210-22226)
Removal of tumor flank or back (21930)
Restoration after vertebral body resection (22585, 63082, 63086, 63088, 63091)
Spinal restoration with graft:
    Cervical (20931, 20938, 22554, 63081)
    Lumbar (20931, 20938, 22558, 63087, 63090)
    Thoracic (20931, 20938, 22556, 63085, 63087)
Spinal restoration with prosthesis:
    Cervical (20931, 20938, 22554, 22853-22854 [22859], 63081)
    Lumbar (20931, 20938, 22558, 22853-22854 [22859], 63087, 63090)
    Thoracic (20931, 20938, 22556, 22853-22854 [22859], 63085, 63087)
Vertebral corpectomy (63081-63091)

**22110** Partial excision of vertebral body, for intrinsic bony lesion, without decompression of spinal cord or nerve root(s), single vertebral segment; cervical

> 🔧 30.2 ⚕ 30.2 **FUD** 090 C 80 ▱
>
> **AMA:** 2017,Mar,7; 2017,Jan,8; 2016,Jan,13; 2015,Jan,16; 2013,Jul,3-5

● New Code ▲ Revised Code ○ Reinstated ● New Web Release ▲ Revised Web Release Unlisted Not Covered # Resequenced
⊘ AMA Mod 51 Exempt ⑤ Optum Mod 51 Exempt ⑥³ Mod 63 Exempt ✗ Non-FDA Drug ★ Telemedicine M Maternity A Age Edit + Add-on AMA: CPT Asst
© 2017 Optum360, LLC CPT © 2017 American Medical Association. All Rights Reserved.

| | 22112 | **thoracic** | | | |
|---|---|---|---|---|---|
| | | 📓 31.9   ⚖ 31.9   **FUD** 090 | | | C 80 📄 |

**AMA:** 2017,Mar,7; 2017,Jan,8; 2016,Jan,13; 2015,Jan,16; 2013,Jul,3-5

| | 22114 | **lumbar** | | | |
|---|---|---|---|---|---|
| | | 📓 28.5   ⚖ 28.5   **FUD** 090 | | | C 80 📄 |

**AMA:** 2017,Mar,7; 2017,Jan,8; 2016,Jan,13; 2015,Jan,16; 2013,Jul,3-5

+ **22116** **each additional vertebral segment (List separately in addition to code for primary procedure)**

Code first (22110-22114)

📓 4.12   ⚖ 4.12   **FUD** ZZZ      C 80 📄

**AMA:** 2003,Feb,7; 2002,Apr,13

## 22206-22216 Spinal Osteotomy: Posterior/Posterolateral Approach

EXCLUDES  *Decompression of the spinal cord and/or nerve roots (63001-63308)*
*Injection:*
  *Chemonucleolysis (62292)*
  *Discography (62290-62292)*
  *Facet joint (64490-64495, [64633, 64634, 64635, 64636])*
  *Myelography (62284)*
  *Repair of vertebral fracture by the anterior approach, see appropriate arthrodesis, bone graft, instrumentation codes, and (63081-63091)*
Code also arthrodesis (22590-22632)
Code also bone grafting procedures (20930-20938)
Code also spinal instrumentation (22840-22855 [22859])

**22206** **Osteotomy of spine, posterior or posterolateral approach, 3 columns, 1 vertebral segment (eg, pedicle/vertebral body subtraction); thoracic**

EXCLUDES  *Osteotomy of spine, posterior or posterolateral approach, lumbar (22207)*
*Procedures performed at same level (22210-22226, 22830, 63001-63048, 63055-63066, 63075-63091, 63101-63103)*

📓 71.1   ⚖ 71.1   **FUD** 090      C 80 📄

**AMA:** 2017,Mar,7; 2017,Jan,8; 2016,Jan,13; 2015,Jan,16; 2014,Jan,11; 2013,Jul,3-5; 2012,Jan,15-42

**22207** **lumbar**

EXCLUDES  *Osteotomy of spine, posterior or posterolateral approach, thoracic (22206)*
*Procedures performed at the same level (22210-22226, 22830, 63001-63048, 63055-63066, 63075-63091, 63101-63103)*

📓 69.7   ⚖ 69.7   **FUD** 090      C 80 📄

**AMA:** 2017,Mar,7; 2017,Jan,8; 2016,Jan,13; 2015,Jan,16; 2014,Jan,11; 2013,Jul,3-5; 2012,Jan,15-42

+ **22208** **each additional vertebral segment (List separately in addition to code for primary procedure)**

EXCLUDES  *Procedures performed at the same level (22210-22226, 22830, 63001-63048, 63055-63066, 63075-63091, 63101-63103)*

Code first (22206, 22207)

📓 17.0   ⚖ 17.0   **FUD** ZZZ      C 80 📄

**AMA:** 2017,Jan,8; 2016,Jan,13; 2015,Jan,16; 2014,Jan,11; 2012,Jan,15-42

**22210** **Osteotomy of spine, posterior or posterolateral approach, 1 vertebral segment; cervical**

📓 51.9   ⚖ 51.9   **FUD** 090      C 80 📄

**AMA:** 2017,Mar,7; 2017,Jan,8; 2016,Jan,13; 2015,Jan,16; 2013,Jul,3-5

Patient is stabilized by halo and traction to correct cervical problem

Several sections may be removed

C-6
C-7
T-1

**Physician removes spinous processes, lamina**

| | 22212 | **thoracic** | | | |
|---|---|---|---|---|---|
| | | 📓 43.0   ⚖ 43.0   **FUD** 090 | | | C 80 📄 |

**AMA:** 2017,Mar,7; 2017,Jan,8; 2016,Jan,13; 2015,Jan,16; 2014,Jan,11; 2013,Jul,3-5

| | 22214 | **lumbar** | | | |
|---|---|---|---|---|---|
| | | 📓 43.1   ⚖ 43.1   **FUD** 090 | | | C 80 📄 |

**AMA:** 2017,Mar,7; 2017,Jan,8; 2016,Jan,13; 2015,Jan,16; 2014,Dec,16; 2014,Dec,16; 2014,Jan,11; 2013,Jul,3-5

+ **22216** **each additional vertebral segment (List separately in addition to primary procedure)**

Code first (22210-22214)

📓 10.6   ⚖ 10.6   **FUD** ZZZ      C 80 📄

**AMA:** 2017,Jan,8; 2016,Jan,13; 2015,Jan,16; 2014,Jan,11

## 22220-22226 Spinal Osteotomy: Anterior Approach

EXCLUDES  *Corpectomy (63081-63091)*
*Decompression of the spinal cord and/or nerve roots (63001-63308)*
*Injection:*
  *Chemonucleolysis (62292)*
  *Discography (62290-62291)*
  *Facet joint (64490-64495, [64633], [64634], [64635], [64636])*
  *Myelography (62284)*
*Needle/trocar biopsy (20220-20225)*
*Repair of vertebral fracture by the anterior approach, see appropriate arthrodesis, bone graft, instrumentation codes, and (63081-63091)*
Code also arthrodesis (22590-22632)
Code also bone grafting procedures (20930-20938)
Code also spinal instrumentation (22840-22855 [22859])

**22220** **Osteotomy of spine, including discectomy, anterior approach, single vertebral segment; cervical**

📓 46.3   ⚖ 46.3   **FUD** 090      C 80 📄

**AMA:** 2017,Mar,7; 2017,Jan,8; 2016,Jan,13; 2015,Jan,16; 2013,Jul,3-5

**22222** **thoracic**

📓 43.4   ⚖ 43.4   **FUD** 090      C 80 📄

**AMA:** 2017,Mar,7; 2017,Jan,8; 2016,Jan,13; 2015,Jan,16; 2014,Jan,11; 2013,Jul,3-5

**22224** **lumbar**

📓 45.8   ⚖ 45.8   **FUD** 090      C 80 📄

**AMA:** 2017,Mar,7; 2017,Jan,8; 2016,Jan,13; 2015,Jan,16; 2013,Jul,3-5

+ **22226** **each additional vertebral segment (List separately in addition to code for primary procedure)**

Code first (22220-22224)

📓 10.5   ⚖ 10.5   **FUD** ZZZ      C 80 📄

**AMA:** 2002,Feb,4; 2002,Apr,13

| 26/TC PC/TC Only | A2-A3 ASC Payment | 50 Bilateral | ♂ Male Only | ♀ Female Only | 📓 Facility RVU | ⚖ Non-Facility RVU | 📄 CCI |
|---|---|---|---|---|---|---|---|
| **FUD** Follow-up Days | **CMS:** IOM (Pub 100) | A-Y OPPSI | 80/80 Surg Assist Allowed / w/Doc | | 📋 Lab Crosswalk | 📋 Radiology Crosswalk | ❌ CLIA |

50

CPT © 2017 American Medical Association. All Rights Reserved.

© 2017 Optum360, LLC

## 22310-22315 Closed Treatment Vertebral Fractures

EXCLUDES    Injection:
            Chemonucleolysis (62292)
            Discography (62290-62291)
            Facet joint (64490-64495, [64633], [64634], [64635], [64636])
            Myelography (62284)
            Percutaneous vertebroplasty at same level (22510-22515)
Code also arthrodesis (22590-22632)
Code also bone grafting procedures (20930-20938)
Code also spinal instrumentation (22840-22855 [22859])

**22310**    **Closed treatment of vertebral body fracture(s), without manipulation, requiring and including casting or bracing**
             🗐 8.13    ⚒ 8.82    **FUD** 090                    T A2 ▯
             **AMA:** 2017,Mar,7; 2017,Jan,8; 2016,Jan,13; 2015,Jan,8; 2015,Jan,16; 2014,Jul,8; 2014,Jan,11; 2013,Jul,3-5; 2012,Jun,10-11; 2012,Jan,15-42

**22315**    **Closed treatment of vertebral fracture(s) and/or dislocation(s) requiring casting or bracing, with and including casting and/or bracing by manipulation or traction**
             EXCLUDES    Spinal manipulation (97140)
             🗐 22.2    ⚒ 25.3    **FUD** 090                    J A2 ▯
             **AMA:** 2017,Mar,7; 2017,Jan,8; 2016,Jan,13; 2015,Jan,8; 2015,Jan,16; 2014,Jan,11; 2013,Jul,3-5; 2012,Jun,10-11; 2012,Apr,11-13

## 22318-22319 Open Treatment Odontoid Fracture: Anterior Approach

EXCLUDES    Injection:
            Chemonucleolysis (62292)
            Discography (62290-62291)
            Facet joint (64490-64495, [64633, 64634, 64635, 64636])
            Myelography (62284)
            Needle/trocar biopsy (20220-20225)
Code also arthrodesis (22590-22632)
Code also bone grafting procedures (20930-20938)
Code also spinal instrumentation (22840-22855 [22859])

**22318**    **Open treatment and/or reduction of odontoid fracture(s) and or dislocation(s) (including os odontoideum), anterior approach, including placement of internal fixation; without grafting**
             🗐 47.7    ⚒ 47.7    **FUD** 090                    C 80 ▯
             **AMA:** 2017,Mar,7; 2017,Jan,8; 2016,Jan,13; 2015,Jan,16; 2014,Jan,11; 2013,Jul,3-5; 2012,Apr,11-13

**22319**    **with grafting**
             🗐 53.3    ⚒ 53.3    **FUD** 090                    C 80 ▯
             **AMA:** 2017,Mar,7; 2017,Jan,8; 2016,Jan,13; 2015,Jan,16; 2014,Jan,11; 2013,Jul,3-5; 2012,Apr,14-16

## 22325-22328 Open Treatment Vertebral Fractures: Posterior Approach

EXCLUDES    Corpectomy (63081-63091)
            Injection:
            Chemonucleolysis (62292)
            Discography (62290-62291)
            Facet joint (64490-64495, [64633], [64634], [64635], [64636])
            Myelography (62284)
            Needle/trocar biopsy (20220-20225)
            Spine decompression (63001-63091)
            Vertebral fracture care by arthrodesis (22548-22632)
            Vertebral fracture care frontal approach (63081-63091)
Code also arthrodesis (22548-22632)
Code also bone grafting procedures (20930-20938)
Code also spinal instrumentation (22840-22855 [22859])

**22325**    **Open treatment and/or reduction of vertebral fracture(s) and/or dislocation(s), posterior approach, 1 fractured vertebra or dislocated segment; lumbar**
             EXCLUDES    Percutaneous vertebral augmentation performed at same level (22514-22515)
                         Percutaneous vertebroplasty performed at same level (22511-22512)
             🗐 41.7    ⚒ 41.7    **FUD** 090                    C 80 ▯
             **AMA:** 2017,Aug,9; 2017,Mar,7; 2017,Jan,8; 2016,Jan,13; 2015,Jan,8; 2015,Jan,16; 2014,Jan,11; 2013,Jul,3-5; 2012,Jun,10-11

**22326**    **cervical**
             EXCLUDES    Percutaneous vertebroplasty performed at same level (22510, 22512)
             🗐 43.3    ⚒ 43.3    **FUD** 090                    C 80 ▯
             **AMA:** 2017,Mar,7; 2017,Jan,8; 2016,Jan,13; 2015,Jan,16; 2014,Jan,11; 2013,Jul,3-5

**22327**    **thoracic**
             EXCLUDES    Percutaneous vertebral augmentation performed at same level (22515)
                         Percutaneous vertebroplasty performed at same level (22510, 22512-22513)
             🗐 43.5    ⚒ 43.5    **FUD** 090                    C 80 ▯
             **AMA:** 2017,Mar,7; 2017,Jan,8; 2016,Jan,13; 2015,Jan,8; 2015,Jan,16; 2014,Jan,11; 2013,Jul,3-5; 2012,Jun,10-11

+ **22328**    **each additional fractured vertebra or dislocated segment (List separately in addition to code for primary procedure)**
             Code first (22325-22327)
             🗐 8.27    ⚒ 8.27    **FUD** ZZZ                    C 80 ▯
             **AMA:** 2002,Apr,13; 1997,Nov,1

## 22505 Spinal Manipulation with Anesthesia

EXCLUDES    Manipulation not requiring anesthesia (97140)

**22505**    **Manipulation of spine requiring anesthesia, any region**
             🗐 3.82    ⚒ 3.82    **FUD** 010                    J A2 ▯
             **AMA:** 2017,Jan,8; 2016,Jan,13; 2015,Jan,16; 2014,Jan,11; 2012,Jan,15-42

## 22510-22515 Percutaneous Vertebroplasty/Kyphoplasty

INCLUDES    Bone biopsy when applicable (20225)
            Radiological guidance
EXCLUDES    Closed treatment vertebral fractures (22310, 22315)
            Open treatment/reduction vertebral fractures (22325, 22327)
            Sacroplasty/augmentation (0200T-0201T)

**22510**    **Percutaneous vertebroplasty (bone biopsy included when performed), 1 vertebral body, unilateral or bilateral injection, inclusive of all imaging guidance; cervicothoracic**
             🗐 12.6    ⚒ 47.7    **FUD** 010                    J 62 ▯
             **AMA:** 2017,Jan,8; 2016,Jan,13; 2015,Jan,8

**22511**    **lumbosacral**
             🗐 11.8    ⚒ 47.3    **FUD** 010                    J 62 ▯
             **AMA:** 2017,Jan,8; 2016,Jan,13; 2015,Apr,8; 2015,Jan,8

+ **22512**    **each additional cervicothoracic or lumbosacral vertebral body (List separately in addition to code for primary procedure)**
             Code first (22510-22511)
             🗐 6.07    ⚒ 27.1    **FUD** ZZZ                    N M1 ▯
             **AMA:** 2017,Jan,8; 2016,Jan,13; 2015,Jan,8

**22513**    **Percutaneous vertebral augmentation, including cavity creation (fracture reduction and bone biopsy included when performed) using mechanical device (eg, kyphoplasty), 1 vertebral body, unilateral or bilateral cannulation, inclusive of all imaging guidance; thoracic**
             🗐 15.1    ⚒ 203.    **FUD** 010                    J 62 ▯
             **AMA:** 2017,Jan,8; 2016,Jan,13; 2015,Jan,8

**22514**    **lumbar**
             🗐 14.0    ⚒ 202.    **FUD** 010                    J 62 ▯
             **AMA:** 2017,Jan,8; 2016,Jan,13; 2015,Jan,8

+ **22515**    **each additional thoracic or lumbar vertebral body (List separately in addition to code for primary procedure)**
             Code first (22513-22514)
             🗐 6.54    ⚒ 123.    **FUD** ZZZ                    N M1 ▯
             **AMA:** 2017,Jan,8; 2016,Jan,13; 2015,Jan,8

**Musculoskeletal System**

**22526 — 22552**

## 22526-22527 Percutaneous Annuloplasty

**CMS:** 100-04,32,220.1 Thermal Intradiscal Procedures (TIPS)

INCLUDES Fluoroscopic guidance (77002, 77003)
EXCLUDES Needle/trocar biopsy (20220-20225)
Injection:
  Chemonucleolysis (62292)
  Discography (62290-62291)
  Facet joint (64490-64495, [64633], [64634], [64635], [64636])
  Myelography (62284)
Procedure performed by other methods (22899)

**22526** Percutaneous intradiscal electrothermal annuloplasty, unilateral or bilateral including fluoroscopic guidance; single level

🔧 9.72   ⚕ 65.6   **FUD** 010   E ▣

**AMA:** 2017,Jan,8; 2016,Jan,13; 2015,Jan,8; 2015,Jan,16; 2014,Jan,11; 2012,Jan,15-42

**+ 22527** 1 or more additional levels (List separately in addition to code for primary procedure)

Code first (22526)

🔧 4.60   ⚕ 55.3   **FUD** ZZZ   E ▣

**AMA:** 2017,Jan,8; 2016,Jan,13; 2015,Jan,16; 2015,Jan,8; 2014,Jan,11

## 22532-22534 Spinal Fusion: Lateral Extracavitary Approach

EXCLUDES Corpectomy (63101-63103)
Exploration of spinal fusion (22830)
Fracture care (22310-22328)
Injection:
  Chemonucleolysis (62292)
  Discography (62290-62291)
  Facet joint (64490-64495, [64633], [64634], [64635], [64636])
  Myelography (62284)
Laminectomy (63001-63017)
Needle/trocar biopsy (20220-20225)
Osteotomy (22206-22226)
Code also bone grafting procedures (20930-20938)
Code also spinal instrumentation (22840-22855 [22859])

**22532** Arthrodesis, lateral extracavitary technique, including minimal discectomy to prepare interspace (other than for decompression); thoracic

🔧 51.6   ⚕ 51.6   **FUD** 090   C 80 ▣

**AMA:** 2017,Mar,7; 2017,Feb,9; 2017,Jan,8; 2016,Jan,13; 2015,Jan,16; 2014,Jan,11; 2013,Jul,3-5; 2012,Apr,14-16

**22533** lumbar

🔧 48.1   ⚕ 48.1   **FUD** 090   C 80 ▣

**AMA:** 2017,Mar,7; 2017,Feb,9; 2017,Jan,8; 2016,Jan,13; 2015,Jan,16; 2014,Jan,11; 2013,Jul,3-5; 2012,Apr,14-16

**+ 22534** thoracic or lumbar, each additional vertebral segment (List separately in addition to code for primary procedure)

Code first (22532-22533)

🔧 10.5   ⚕ 10.5   **FUD** ZZZ   C 80 ▣

**AMA:** 2017,Feb,9

## 22548-22634 Spinal Fusion: Anterior and Posterior Approach

EXCLUDES Corpectomy (63081-63091)
Exploration of spinal fusion (22830)
Fracture care (22310-22328)
Facet joint arthrodesis (0219T-0222T)
Injection:
  Chemonucleolysis (62292)
  Discography (62290-62291)
  Facet joint (64490-64495, [64633], [64634], [64635], [64636])
  Myelography (62284)
Laminectomy (63001-63017)
Needle/trocar biopsy (20220-20225)
Osteotomy (22206-22226)
Code also bone grafting procedures (20930-20938)
Code also spinal instrumentation (22840-22855 [22859])

**22548** Arthrodesis, anterior transoral or extraoral technique, clivus-C1-C2 (atlas-axis), with or without excision of odontoid process

EXCLUDES Laminectomy or laminotomy with disc removal (63020-63042)

🔧 56.8   ⚕ 56.8   **FUD** 090   C 80 ▣

**AMA:** 2017,Mar,7; 2017,Jan,8; 2016,Jan,13; 2015,Jan,16; 2014,Jan,11; 2013,Jul,3-5; 2012,Apr,14-16; 2012,Jan,15-42

**22551** Arthrodesis, anterior interbody, including disc space preparation, discectomy, osteophytectomy and decompression of spinal cord and/or nerve roots; cervical below C2

INCLUDES Operating microscope (69990)

🔧 49.8   ⚕ 49.8   **FUD** 090   J J8 80 ▣

**AMA:** 2017,Mar,7; 2017,Jan,8; 2016,May,13; 2016,Feb,12; 2016,Jan,13; 2015,Jan,13; 2015,Jan,16; 2014,Jan,11; 2013,Jul,3-5; 2012,Apr,14-16; 2012,Jan,15-42

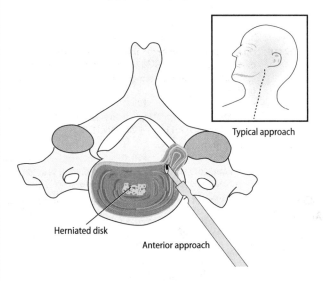

Typical approach

Herniated disk

Anterior approach

**+ 22552** cervical below C2, each additional interspace (List separately in addition to code for separate procedure)

INCLUDES Operating microscope (69990)

Code first (22551)

🔧 11.6   ⚕ 11.6   **FUD** ZZZ   N N1 80 ▣

**AMA:** 2017,Mar,7; 2017,Jan,8; 2016,Feb,12; 2016,Jan,13; 2015,Jan,16; 2014,Jan,11; 2013,Jul,3-5; 2012,Apr,14-16; 2012,Jan,15-42

**22554**    **Arthrodesis, anterior interbody technique, including minimal discectomy to prepare interspace (other than for decompression); cervical below C2**

> *EXCLUDES* *Anterior discectomy and interbody fusion during the same operative session (regardless if performed by multiple surgeons) (22551)*
> *Discectomy, anterior, with decompression of spinal cord and/or nerve root(s), cervical (even by separate individual) (63075-63076)*

🚑 36.4    ⚕ 36.4    **FUD** 090                        J J8 80 ▣

**AMA:** 2017,Mar,7; 2017,Jan,8; 2016,Jan,13; 2015,Apr,7; 2015,Jan,16; 2014,Jan,11; 2013,Jul,3-5; 2012,Apr,11-13; 2012,Apr,14-16; 2012,Jan,15-42

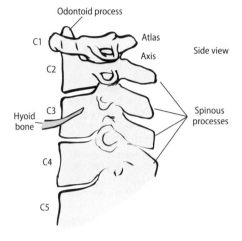

Odontoid process

C1 — Atlas — Axis — Side view

C2

Hyoid bone — C3 — Spinous processes

C4

C5

**22556**    **thoracic**

🚑 48.5    ⚕ 48.5    **FUD** 090                        C 80 ▣

**AMA:** 2017,Mar,7; 2017,Jan,8; 2016,Jan,13; 2015,Jan,16; 2014,Jan,11; 2013,Jul,3-5; 2012,Apr,14-16; 2012,Jan,15-42

**22558**    **lumbar**

> *EXCLUDES* *Arthrodesis using pre-sacral interbody technique (22586, 0195T)*

🚑 44.6    ⚕ 44.6    **FUD** 090                        C 80 ▣

**AMA:** 2017,Mar,7; 2017,Feb,9; 2017,Jan,8; 2016,Jan,13; 2015,Mar,9; 2015,Jan,16; 2014,Jan,11; 2013,Jul,3-5; 2012,Apr,14-16; 2012,Jan,15-42

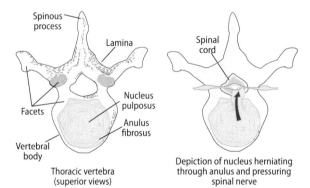

Spinous process

Lamina — Spinal cord

Facets — Nucleus pulposus

Vertebral body — Anulus fibrosus

Thoracic vertebra (superior views)

Depiction of nucleus herniating through anulus and pressuring spinal nerve

**+**    **22585**    **each additional interspace (List separately in addition to code for primary procedure)**

> *EXCLUDES* *Anterior discectomy and interbody fusion during the same operative session (regardless if performed by multiple surgeons) (22552)*
> *Discectomy, anterior, with decompression of spinal cord and/or nerve root(s), cervical (even by separate individual) (63075)*
> Code first (22554-22558)

🚑 9.61    ⚕ 9.61    **FUD** ZZZ                        N N1 80 ▣

**AMA:** 2017,Jan,8; 2016,Jan,13; 2015,Jan,16; 2014,Jan,11; 2012,Jan,15-42

**22586**    **Arthrodesis, pre-sacral interbody technique, including disc space preparation, discectomy, with posterior instrumentation, with image guidance, includes bone graft when performed, L5-S1 interspace**

🚑 55.4    ⚕ 55.4    **FUD** 090                        C 80 ▣

> *INCLUDES* Radiologic guidance (77002-77003, 77011-77012)
> *EXCLUDES* Allograft and autograft of spinal bone (20930-20938)
> *Epidurography, radiological supervision and interpretation (72275)*
> *Pelvic fixation, other than sacrum (22848)*
> *Posterior non-segmental instrumentation (22840)*

**22590**    **Arthrodesis, posterior technique, craniocervical (occiput-C2)**

> *EXCLUDES* *Posterior intrafacet implant insertion (0219T-0222T)*

🚑 46.0    ⚕ 46.0    **FUD** 090                        C 80 ▣

**AMA:** 2017,Mar,7; 2017,Jan,8; 2016,Jan,13; 2015,Jan,16; 2014,Jan,11; 2013,Jul,3-5; 2012,Apr,14-16

**Skull and cervical vertebrae; posterior view**

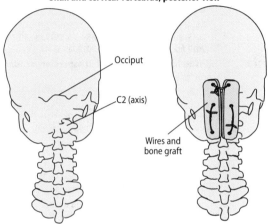

Occiput

C2 (axis)

Wires and bone graft

The physician fuses skull to C2 (axis) to stabilize cervical vertebrae; anchor holes are drilled in the occiput of the skull

**22595**    **Arthrodesis, posterior technique, atlas-axis (C1-C2)**

> *EXCLUDES* *Posterior intrafacet implant insertion (0219T-0222T)*

🚑 43.9    ⚕ 43.9    **FUD** 090                        C 80 ▣

**AMA:** 2017,Mar,7; 2017,Jan,8; 2016,Jan,13; 2015,Jan,16; 2014,Jan,11; 2013,Jul,3-5; 2012,Apr,11-13; 2012,Apr,14-16

**22600**    **Arthrodesis, posterior or posterolateral technique, single level; cervical below C2 segment**

> *EXCLUDES* *Posterior intrafacet implant insertion (0219T-0222T)*

🚑 37.5    ⚕ 37.5    **FUD** 090                        C 80 ▣

**AMA:** 2017,Mar,7; 2017,Jan,8; 2016,Jan,13; 2015,Jan,16; 2014,Jan,11; 2013,Jul,3-5; 2012,Jun,10-11; 2012,Apr,14-16

**22610**    **thoracic (with lateral transverse technique, when performed)**

> *EXCLUDES* *Posterior intrafacet implant insertion (0219T-0222T)*

🚑 36.7    ⚕ 36.7    **FUD** 090                        C 80 ▣

**AMA:** 2017,Mar,7; 2017,Jan,8; 2016,Jan,13; 2015,Jan,16; 2014,Jan,11; 2013,Jul,3-5; 2012,Jun,10-11; 2012,Apr,14-16

**22612**    **lumbar (with lateral transverse technique, when performed)**

> *EXCLUDES* *Arthrodesis performed at same interspace and segment (22630)*
> *Combined technique at the same interspace and segment (22633)*
> *Posterior intrafacet implant insertion (0219T-0222T)*

🚑 46.1    ⚕ 46.1    **FUD** 090                        J 62 80 ▣

**AMA:** 2017,Mar,7; 2017,Feb,9; 2017,Jan,8; 2016,Jan,13; 2015,Jan,16; 2014,Jan,11; 2013,Dec,14; 2013,Jul,3-5; 2012,Jun,10-11; 2012,Apr,14-16; 2012,Jan,3-5; 2012,Jan,15-42

● New Code      ▲ Revised Code      ○ Reinstated      ● New Web Release      ▲ Revised Web Release      Unlisted      Not Covered      # Resequenced
Ⓢ AMA Mod 51 Exempt      Ⓢ Optum Mod 51 Exempt      Ⓢ Mod 63 Exempt      ✗ Non-FDA Drug      ★ Telemedicine      Ⓜ Maternity      Ⓐ Age Edit      + Add-on      **AMA:** CPT Asst
© 2017 Optum360, LLC                          CPT © 2017 American Medical Association. All Rights Reserved.                          **53**

+ **22614** **each additional vertebral segment (List separately in addition to code for primary procedure)**

INCLUDES Additional level fusion arthrodesis posterior or posterolateral interbody

EXCLUDES *Additional level interbody arthrodesis combined posterolateral or posterior with posterior interbody arthrodesis (22634)*

*Additional level posterior interbody arthrodesis (22632)*

*Posterior intrafacet implant insertion (0219T-0222T)*

Code first (22600, 22610, 22612, 22630, 22633)

🚗 11.4   ⚕ 11.4   **FUD** ZZZ   N M1 80 ▭

**AMA:** 2017,Feb,9; 2017,Jan,8; 2016,Jan,13; 2015,Jan,16; 2014,Jan,11; 2013,Jul,3-5; 2012,Jun,10-11

**22630** **Arthrodesis, posterior interbody technique, including laminectomy and/or discectomy to prepare interspace (other than for decompression), single interspace; lumbar**

EXCLUDES *Arthrodesis performed at same interspace and segment (22612)*

*Combined technique (22612 and 22630) for same interspace and segment (22633)*

🚗 45.7   ⚕ 45.7   **FUD** 090   C 80 ▭

**AMA:** 2017,Mar,7; 2017,Feb,9; 2017,Jan,8; 2016,Jan,13; 2015,Jan,16; 2014,Jan,11; 2013,Jul,3-5; 2012,Jun,10-11; 2012,Apr,14-16; 2012,Jan,3-5; 2012,Jan,15-42

+ **22632** **each additional interspace (List separately in addition to code for primary procedure)**

INCLUDES Includes posterior interbody fusion arthrodesis, additional level

EXCLUDES *Additional level combined technique (22634)*

*Additional level posterior or posterolateral fusion (22614)*

Code first (22612, 22630, 22633)

🚗 9.43   ⚕ 9.43   **FUD** ZZZ   C 80 ▭

**AMA:** 2017,Feb,9; 2017,Jan,8; 2016,Jan,13; 2015,Jan,16; 2014,Jan,11; 2013,Jul,3-5; 2012,Jun,10-11

**22633** **Arthrodesis, combined posterior or posterolateral technique with posterior interbody technique including laminectomy and/or discectomy sufficient to prepare interspace (other than for decompression), single interspace and segment; lumbar**

EXCLUDES *Arthrodesis performed at same interspace and segment (22612, 22630)*

🚗 53.9   ⚕ 53.9   **FUD** 090   C 80 ▭

**AMA:** 2017,Mar,7; 2017,Feb,9; 2017,Jan,8; 2016,Oct,11; 2016,Jan,13; 2015,Jan,16; 2014,Jan,11; 2013,Jul,3-5; 2012,Jun,10-11; 2012,Jan,3-5; 2012,Jan,15-42

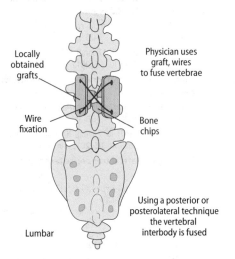

Locally obtained grafts

Physician uses graft, wires to fuse vertebrae

Wire fixation

Bone chips

Lumbar

Using a posterior or posterolateral technique the vertebral interbody is fused

+ **22634** **each additional interspace and segment (List separately in addition to code for primary procedure)**

Code first (22633)

🚗 14.5   ⚕ 14.5   **FUD** ZZZ   C 80 ▭

**AMA:** 2017,Mar,7; 2017,Feb,9; 2017,Jan,8; 2016,Jan,13; 2015,Jan,16; 2014,Jan,11; 2013,Jul,3-5; 2012,Jun,10-11; 2012,Jan,3-5; 2012,Jan,15-42

## 22800-22819 Procedures to Correct Anomalous Spinal Vertebrae

**CMS:** 100-03,150.2 Osteogenic Stimulation

EXCLUDES *Facet injection (64490-64495, [64633, 64634, 64635, 64636])*

Code also bone grafting procedures (20930-20938)

Code also spinal instrumentation (22840-22855 [22859])

**22800** **Arthrodesis, posterior, for spinal deformity, with or without cast; up to 6 vertebral segments**

🚗 39.2   ⚕ 39.2   **FUD** 090   C 80 ▭

**AMA:** 2017,Sep,14; 2017,Mar,7; 2017,Feb,9; 2017,Jan,8; 2016,Jan,13; 2015,Jan,16; 2014,Jan,11; 2013,Jul,3-5; 2012,Apr,14-16

**22802** **7 to 12 vertebral segments**

🚗 61.0   ⚕ 61.0   **FUD** 090   C 80 ▭

**AMA:** 2017,Sep,14; 2017,Mar,7; 2017,Feb,9; 2017,Jan,8; 2016,Jan,13; 2015,Jan,16; 2014,Jan,11; 2013,Jul,3-5; 2012,Apr,14-16; 2012,Jan,15-42

**22804** **13 or more vertebral segments**

🚗 70.5   ⚕ 70.5   **FUD** 090   C 80 ▭

**AMA:** 2017,Sep,14; 2017,Mar,7; 2017,Feb,9; 2017,Jan,8; 2016,Jan,13; 2015,Jan,16; 2014,Jan,11; 2013,Jul,3-5; 2012,Apr,14-16

**22808** **Arthrodesis, anterior, for spinal deformity, with or without cast; 2 to 3 vertebral segments**

INCLUDES Smith-Robinson arthrodesis

🚗 53.7   ⚕ 53.7   **FUD** 090   C 80 ▭

**AMA:** 2017,Sep,14; 2017,Mar,7; 2017,Jan,8; 2016,Jan,13; 2015,Jan,16; 2014,Jan,11; 2013,Jul,3-5; 2012,Apr,14-16

**22810** **4 to 7 vertebral segments**

🚗 59.5   ⚕ 59.5   **FUD** 090   C 80 ▭

**AMA:** 2017,Sep,14; 2017,Mar,7; 2017,Jan,8; 2016,Jan,13; 2015,Jan,16; 2014,Jan,11; 2013,Jul,3-5; 2012,Apr,14-16; 2012,Jan,15-42

**22812** **8 or more vertebral segments**

🚗 63.6   ⚕ 63.6   **FUD** 090   C 80 ▭

**AMA:** 2017,Sep,14; 2017,Mar,7; 2017,Jan,8; 2016,Jan,13; 2015,Jan,16; 2014,Jan,11; 2013,Jul,3-5; 2012,Apr,14-16

**22818** **Kyphectomy, circumferential exposure of spine and resection of vertebral segment(s) (including body and posterior elements); single or 2 segments**

EXCLUDES *Arthrodesis (22800-22804)*

🚗 63.5   ⚕ 63.5   **FUD** 090   C 80 ▭

**AMA:** 2017,Sep,14

26/TC PC/TC Only   M2-Z3 ASC Payment   50 Bilateral   ♂ Male Only   ♀ Female Only   🚗 Facility RVU   ⚕ Non-Facility RVU   ▭ CCI

**FUD** Follow-up Days   **CMS:** IOM (Pub 100)   A-Y OPPSI   80/80 Surg Assist Allowed / w/Doc   ⬛ Lab Crosswalk   ⬛ Radiology Crosswalk   ⬛ CLIA

CPT © 2017 American Medical Association. All Rights Reserved.   © 2017 Optum360, LLC

**22819 3 or more segments**

> EXCLUDES *Arthrodesis (22800-22804)*

🚑 79.4   ⚕ 79.4   **FUD** 090   [C] [80] [▣]

**AMA:** 2017,Sep,14

Excessively kyphotic thoracic spine may be caused by Scheuermann's disease or juvenile kyphosis

Excessive convexity in the thoracic region is known as kyphosis

Excessive concavity in the lumbar region is known as lordosis

Scoliosis is the lateral curvature of the spine; most commonly diagnosed during adolescence; occurrence is higher among females

## 22830 Surgical Exploration Previous Spinal Fusion

**CMS:** 100-03,150.2 Osteogenic Stimulation

> EXCLUDES *Arthrodesis (22532-22819)*
> *Bone grafting procedures (20930-20938)*
> *Facet injection (64490-64495, [64633, 64634, 64635, 64636])*
> *Instrumentation removal (22850, 22852, 22855)*
> *Spinal decompression (63001-63103)*
> Code also spinal instrumentation (22840-22855 [22859])

**22830 Exploration of spinal fusion**

🚑 23.5   ⚕ 23.5   **FUD** 090   [C] [80] [▣]

**AMA:** 2017,Jan,8; 2016,Jan,13; 2015,Jan,16; 2014,Jan,11; 2012,Jan,15-42

## 22840-22848 Posterior, Anterior, Pelvic Spinal Instrumentation

> INCLUDES Removal or revision of previously placed spinal instrumentation during same session as insertion of new instrumentation at levels including all or part of previously instrumented segments (22849, 22850, 22852, 22855)
> EXCLUDES *Arthrodesis (22532-22534, 22548-22812)*
> *Bone grafting procedures (20930-20938)*
> *Exploration of spinal fusion (22830)*
> *Fracture treatment (22325-22328)*
> *Use of more than one instrumentation code per incision*

**+ 22840 Posterior non-segmental instrumentation (eg, Harrington rod technique, pedicle fixation across 1 interspace, atlantoaxial transarticular screw fixation, sublaminar wiring at C1, facet screw fixation) (List separately in addition to code for primary procedure)**

> Code first (22100-22102, 22110-22114, 22206-22207, 22210-22214, 22220-22224, 22310-22327, 22532-22533, 22548-22558, 22590-22612, 22630, 22633-22634, 22800-22812, 63001-63030, 63040-63042, 63045-63047, 63050-63056, 63064, 63075, 63077, 63081, 63085, 63087, 63090, 63101-63102, 63170-63290, 63300-63307)

🚑 22.2   ⚕ 22.2   **FUD** ZZZ   [N] [N1] [80] [▣]

**AMA:** 2017,Jun,10; 2017,Feb,9; 2017,Jan,8; 2016,Jan,13; 2015,Jan,16; 2014,Oct,14; 2014,Jan,11; 2013,Dec,16; 2013,Jul,3-5; 2012,Jun,10-11; 2012,Apr,11-13; 2012,Jan,15-42

**+ 22841 Internal spinal fixation by wiring of spinous processes (List separately in addition to code for primary procedure)**

> Code first (22100-22102, 22110-22114, 22206-22207, 22210-22214, 22220-22224, 22310-22327, 22532-22533, 22548-22558, 22590-22612, 22630, 22633-22634, 22800-22812, 63001-63030, 63040-63042, 63045-63047, 63050-63056, 63064, 63075, 63077, 63081, 63085, 63087, 63090, 63101-63102, 63170-63290, 63300-63307)

🚑 0.00   ⚕ 0.00   **FUD** XXX   [C] [▣]

**AMA:** 2017,Feb,9; 2017,Jan,8; 2016,Jan,13; 2015,Jan,16; 2014,Jan,11; 2013,Jul,3-5; 2012,Jun,10-11

**+ 22842 Posterior segmental instrumentation (eg, pedicle fixation, dual rods with multiple hooks and sublaminar wires); 3 to 6 vertebral segments (List separately in addition to code for primary procedure)**

> Code first (22100-22102, 22110-22114, 22206-22207, 22210-22214, 22220-22224, 22310-22327, 22532-22533, 22548-22558, 22590-22612, 22630, 22633-22634, 22800-22812, 63001-63030, 63040-63042, 63045-63047, 63050-63056, 63064, 63075, 63077, 63081, 63085, 63087, 63090, 63101-63102, 63170-63290, 63300-63307)

🚑 22.3   ⚕ 22.3   **FUD** ZZZ   [N] [N1] [80] [▣]

**AMA:** 2017,Feb,9; 2017,Jan,8; 2016,Jan,13; 2015,Jan,16; 2014,Jan,11; 2013,Jul,3-5; 2012,Jun,10-11

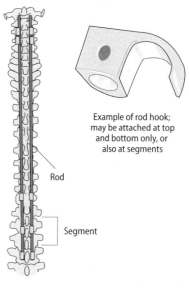

Example of rod hook; may be attached at top and bottom only, or also at segments

Rod

Segment

**+ 22843 7 to 12 vertebral segments (List separately in addition to code for primary procedure)**

> Code first (22100-22102, 22110-22114, 22206-22207, 22210-22214, 22220-22224, 22310-22327, 22532-22533, 22548-22558, 22590-22612, 22630, 22633-22634, 22800-22812, 63001-63030, 63040-63042, 63045-63047, 63050-63056, 63064, 63075, 63077, 63081, 63085, 63087, 63090, 63101-63102, 63170-63290, 63300-63307)

🚑 23.9   ⚕ 23.9   **FUD** ZZZ   [C] [80] [▣]

**AMA:** 2017,Jan,8; 2016,Jan,13; 2015,Jan,16; 2014,Jan,11; 2013,Jul,3-5; 2012,Jun,10-11

**+ 22844 13 or more vertebral segments (List separately in addition to code for primary procedure)**

> Code first (22100-22102, 22110-22114, 22206-22207, 22210-22214, 22220-22224, 22310-22327, 22532-22533, 22548-22558, 22590-22612, 22630, 22633-22634, 22800-22812, 63001-63030, 63040-63042, 63045-63047, 63050-63056, 63064, 63075, 63077, 63081, 63085, 63087, 63090, 63101-63102, 63170-63290, 63300-63307)

🚑 28.8   ⚕ 28.8   **FUD** ZZZ   [C] [80] [▣]

**AMA:** 2017,Jan,8; 2016,Jan,13; 2015,Jan,16; 2014,Jan,11; 2013,Jul,3-5; 2012,Jun,10-11

**+ 22845 Anterior instrumentation; 2 to 3 vertebral segments (List separately in addition to code for primary procedure)**

> INCLUDES Dwyer instrumentation technique
> Code first (22100-22102, 22110-22114, 22206-22207, 22210-22214, 22220-22224, 22310-22327, 22532-22533, 22548-22558, 22590-22612, 22630, 22633-22634, 22800-22812, 63001-63030, 63040-63042, 63045-63047, 63050-63056, 63064, 63075, 63077, 63081, 63085, 63087, 63090, 63101-63102, 63170-63290, 63300-63307)

🚑 21.4   ⚕ 21.4   **FUD** ZZZ   [N] [N1] [80] [▣]

**AMA:** 2017,Mar,7; 2017,Jan,8; 2016,May,13; 2016,Jan,13; 2015,Apr,7; 2015,Mar,9; 2015,Jan,16; 2015,Jan,13; 2014,Nov,14; 2014,Jan,11; 2013,Jul,3-5; 2012,Jun,10-11; 2012,Jan,15-42

---

● New Code   ▲ Revised Code   ○ Reinstated   ● New Web Release   ▲ Revised Web Release   Unlisted   Not Covered   # Resequenced
⊘ AMA Mod 51 Exempt   ⑧ Optum Mod 51 Exempt   ⑥ Mod 63 Exempt   ∕ Non-FDA Drug   ★ Telemedicine   Ⓜ Maternity   Ⓐ Age Edit   + Add-on   **AMA:** CPT Asst

© 2017 Optum360, LLC   CPT © 2017 American Medical Association. All Rights Reserved.

**+ 22846    4 to 7 vertebral segments (List separately in addition to code for primary procedure)**

INCLUDES    Dwyer instrumentation technique
Code first (22100-22102, 22110-22114, 22206-22207, 22210-22214, 22220-22224, 22310-22327, 22532-22533, 22548-22558, 22590-22612, 22630, 22633-22634, 22800-22812, 63001-63030, 63040-63042, 63045-63047, 63050-63056, 63064, 63075, 63077, 63081, 63085, 63087, 63090, 63101-63102, 63170-63290, 63300-63307)

🔪 22.2   ⚕ 22.2   **FUD** ZZZ                            C 80 ▭

**AMA:** 2017,Jan,8; 2016,May,13; 2016,Jan,13; 2015,Jan,16; 2014,Jan,11; 2013,Jul,3-5; 2012,Jun,10-11; 2012,Jan,15-42

**+ 22847    8 or more vertebral segments (List separately in addition to code for primary procedure)**

INCLUDES    Dwyer instrumentation technique
Code first (22100-22102, 22110-22114, 22206-22207, 22210-22214, 22220-22224, 22310-22327, 22532-22533, 22548-22558, 22590-22612, 22630, 22633-22634, 22800-22812, 63001-63030, 63040-63042, 63045-63047, 63050-63056, 63064, 63075, 63077, 63081, 63085, 63087, 63090, 63101-63102, 63170-63290, 63300-63307)

🔪 24.3   ⚕ 24.3   **FUD** ZZZ                            C 80 ▭

**AMA:** 2017,Jan,8; 2016,May,13; 2016,Jan,13; 2015,Jan,16; 2014,Jan,11; 2013,Jul,3-5; 2012,Jun,10-11; 2012,Jan,15-42

**+ 22848    Pelvic fixation (attachment of caudal end of instrumentation to pelvic bony structures) other than sacrum (List separately in addition to code for primary procedure)**

Code first (22100-22102, 22110-22114, 22206-22207, 22210-22214, 22220-22224, 22310-22327, 22532-22533, 22548-22558, 22590-22612, 22630, 22633-22634, 22800-22812, 63001-63030, 63040-63042, 63045-63047, 63050-63056, 63064, 63075, 63077, 63081, 63085, 63087, 63090, 63101-63102, 63170-63290, 63300-63307)

🔪 10.5   ⚕ 10.5   **FUD** ZZZ                            C 80 ▭

**AMA:** 2017,Jan,8; 2016,Jan,13; 2015,Jan,16; 2014,Jan,11; 2013,Jul,3-5; 2012,Jun,10-11

## 22849-22855 [22859] Miscellaneous Spinal Instrumentation

EXCLUDES    Arthrodesis (22532-22534, 22548-22812)
Bone grafting procedures (20930-20938)
Exploration of spinal fusion (22830)
Facet injection (64490-64495, [64633], [64634], [64635], [64636])
Fracture treatment (22325-22328)

**22849    Reinsertion of spinal fixation device**

INCLUDES    Removal of instrumentation at the same level (22850, 22852, 22855)

🔪 37.7   ⚕ 37.7   **FUD** 090                            C 80 ▭

**AMA:** 2017,Jun,10; 2017,Jan,8; 2016,May,13; 2016,Jan,13; 2015,Jan,16; 2014,Jan,11; 2013,Jul,3-5; 2012,Jun,10-11; 2012,Jan,15-42

**22850    Removal of posterior nonsegmental instrumentation (eg, Harrington rod)**

🔪 20.9   ⚕ 20.9   **FUD** 090                            C 80 ▭

**AMA:** 2017,Jun,10; 2017,Jan,8; 2016,May,13; 2016,Jan,13; 2015,Jan,16; 2014,Jan,11; 2013,Jul,3-5; 2012,Jun,10-11

**22852    Removal of posterior segmental instrumentation**

🔪 20.0   ⚕ 20.0   **FUD** 090                            C 80 ▭

**AMA:** 2017,Jun,10; 2017,Jan,8; 2016,Jan,13; 2015,Jan,16; 2014,Jan,11; 2012,Jun,10-11; 2012,Jan,15-42

**+ 22853    Insertion of interbody biomechanical device(s) (eg, synthetic cage, mesh) with integral anterior instrumentation for device anchoring (eg, screws, flanges), when performed, to intervertebral disc space in conjunction with interbody arthrodesis, each interspace (List separately in addition to code for primary procedure)**

Code also intervertebral bone device/graft application (20930-20931, 20936-20938)
Code also subsequent disc spaces undergoing device insertion when disc spaces are not connected (22853-22854, [22859])
Code first (22100-22102, 22110-22114, 22206-22207, 22210-22214, 22220-22224, 22310-22327, 22532-22533, 22548-22558, 22590-22612, 22630, 22633-22634, 22800-22812, 63001-63030, 63040, 63042, 63045-63047, 63050-63056, 63064, 63075, 63077, 63081, 63085, 63087, 63090, 63101-63102, 63170-63290, 63300-63307)

🔪 7.64   ⚕ 7.64   **FUD** ZZZ                            N N1 80 ▭

**AMA:** 2017,Aug,9; 2017,Mar,7

**+ 22854    Insertion of intervertebral biomechanical device(s) (eg, synthetic cage, mesh) with integral anterior instrumentation for device anchoring (eg, screws, flanges), when performed, to vertebral corpectomy(ies) (vertebral body resection, partial or complete) defect, in conjunction with interbody arthrodesis, each contiguous defect (List separately in addition to code for primary procedure)**

Code also intervertebral bone device/graft application (20930-20931, 20936-20938)
Code also subsequent disc spaces undergoing device insertion when disc spaces are not connected (22853-22854, [22859])
Code first (22100-22102, 22110-22114, 22206-22207, 22210-22214, 22220-22224, 22310-22327, 22532-22533, 22548-22558, 22590-22612, 22630, 22633-22634, 22800-22812, 63001-63030, 63040, 63042, 63045-63047, 63050-63056, 63064, 63075, 63077, 63081, 63085, 63087, 63090, 63101-63102, 63170-63290, 63300-63307)

🔪 9.89   ⚕ 9.89   **FUD** ZZZ                            N N1 80 ▭

**AMA:** 2017,Mar,7

**+ # 22859    Insertion of intervertebral biomechanical device(s) (eg, synthetic cage, mesh, methylmethacrylate) to intervertebral disc space or vertebral body defect without interbody arthrodesis, each contiguous defect (List separately in addition to code for primary procedure)**

Code also intervertebral bone device/graft application (20930-20931, 20936-20938)
Code also subsequent disc spaces undergoing device insertion when disc spaces are not connected (22853-22854, 22854)
Code first (22100-22102, 22110-22114, 22206-22207, 22210-22214, 22220-22224, 22310-22327, 22532-22533, 22548-22558, 22590-22612, 22630, 22633-22634, 22800-22812, 63001-63030, 63040-63042, 63045-63047, 63050-63056, 63064, 63075, 63077, 63081, 63085, 63087, 63090, 63101-63102, 63170-63290, 63300-63307)

🔪 9.89   ⚕ 9.89   **FUD** ZZZ                            N N1 80 ▭

**AMA:** 2017,Mar,7

**22855    Removal of anterior instrumentation**

🔪 32.1   ⚕ 32.1   **FUD** 090                            C 80 ▭

**AMA:** 2017,Jun,10; 2017,Jan,8; 2016,Jan,13; 2015,Jan,16; 2014,Jan,11; 2012,Jun,10-11

26/TC PC/TC Only    AZ-ZZ ASC Payment    50 Bilateral    ♂ Male Only    ♀ Female Only    🔪 Facility RVU    ⚕ Non-Facility RVU    ▭ CCI
**FUD** Follow-up Days    **CMS:** IOM (Pub 100)    A-Y OPPSI    80/80 Surg Assist Allowed / w/Doc    ▨ Lab Crosswalk    ▨ Radiology Crosswalk    ✖ CLIA
CPT © 2017 American Medical Association. All Rights Reserved.                              © 2017 Optum360, LLC

## 22856-22865 [22858] Artificial Disc Replacement

**EXCLUDES** *Fluoroscopy*
*Spinal decompression (63001-63048)*

**22856** **Total disc arthroplasty (artificial disc), anterior approach, including discectomy with end plate preparation (includes osteophytectomy for nerve root or spinal cord decompression and microdissection); single interspace, cervical**

**INCLUDES** Operating microscope (69990)
**EXCLUDES** *Application of intervertebral biomechanical device(s) at the same level (22853-22854, [22859])*
*Arthrodesis at the same level (22554)*
*Cervical total disc arthroplasty, 3 or more levels (0375T)*
*Discectomy at the same level (63075)*
*Insertion of instrumentation at the same level (22845)*
Code also ([22858])

🔧 47.6    ⚕ 47.6    **FUD** 090     J 80 ▣

**AMA:** 2017,Jan,8; 2016,Feb,12; 2016,Jan,13; 2015,Apr,7

+ # **22858** **second level, cervical (List separately in addition to code for primary procedure)**

**EXCLUDES** *Cervical total disc arthroplasty, 3 or more levels (0375T)*
Code first (22856)

🔧 14.6    ⚕ 14.6    **FUD** ZZZ     N 80 ▣

**AMA:** 2017,Jan,8; 2016,Feb,12; 2016,Jan,13; 2015,Apr,7

**22857** **Total disc arthroplasty (artificial disc), anterior approach, including discectomy to prepare interspace (other than for decompression), single interspace, lumbar**

**INCLUDES** Operating microscope (69990)
**EXCLUDES** *Application of intervertebral biomechanical device(s) at the same level (22853-22854, [22859])*
*Arthrodesis at the same level (22558)*
*Insertion of instrumentation at the same level (22845)*
*Retroperitoneal exploration (49010)*
Code also arthroplasty more than one interspace, when performed (0163T)

🔧 51.4    ⚕ 51.4    **FUD** 090     C 80 ▣

**AMA:** 2016,Feb,12

**22858** **Resequenced code. See code following 22856.**

**22859** **Resequenced code. See code following 22854.**

**22861** **Revision including replacement of total disc arthroplasty (artificial disc), anterior approach, single interspace; cervical**

**INCLUDES** Operating microscope (69990)
**EXCLUDES** *Procedures performed at the same level (22845, 22853-22854, [22859], 22864, 63075)*
*Revision of additional cervical arthroplasty (0098T)*

🔧 57.0    ⚕ 57.0    **FUD** 090     C 80 ▣

**AMA:** 2016,Feb,12

**22862** **lumbar**

**EXCLUDES** *Arthroplasty revision more than one interspace (0165T)*
*Procedures performed at the same level (22558, 22845, 22853-22854, [22859], 22865, 49010)*

🔧 61.7    ⚕ 61.7    **FUD** 090     C 80 ▣

**AMA:** 2017,Jan,8; 2016,Jan,13; 2015,Jan,16; 2014,Jan,11

**22864** **Removal of total disc arthroplasty (artificial disc), anterior approach, single interspace; cervical**

🔧 60.3    ⚕ 60.3    **FUD** 090     C 80 ▣

**INCLUDES** Operating microscope (69990)
**EXCLUDES** *Cervical total disc arthroplasty with additional interspace removal (0095T)*
*Revision of total disc arthroplasty (22861)*

**22865** **lumbar**

**EXCLUDES** *Arthroplasty more than one level (0164T)*
*Exploration, retroperitoneal area with or without biopsy(s) (49010)*

🔧 59.0    ⚕ 59.0    **FUD** 090     C 80 ▣

**AMA:** 2017,Jan,8; 2016,Jan,13; 2015,Jan,16; 2014,Jan,11

## 22867-22899 Spinal Distraction/Stabilization Device

**22867** **Insertion of interlaminar/interspinous process stabilization/distraction device, without fusion, including image guidance when performed, with open decompression, lumbar; single level**

**EXCLUDES** *Interlaminar/interspinous stabilization/distraction device insertion (22869, 22870)*
*Procedures at the same level (22532-22534, 22558, 22612, 22614, 22630, 22632-22634, 22800, 22802, 22804, 22840-22842, 22869-22870, 63005, 63012, 63017, 63030, 63035, 63042, 63044, 63047-63048, 77003)*

🔧 28.5    ⚕ 28.5    **FUD** 090     J J8 80 ▣

**AMA:** 2017,Feb,9

+ **22868** **second level (List separately in addition to code for primary procedure)**

**EXCLUDES** *Interlaminar/interspinous stabilization/distraction device insertion (22869-22870)*
*Procedures at the same level (22532-22534, 22558, 22612, 22614, 22630, 22632-22634, 22800, 22802, 22804, 22840-22842, 22869-22870, 63005, 63012, 63017, 63030, 63035, 63042, 63044, 63047-63048, 77003)*
Code first (22867)

🔧 7.14    ⚕ 7.14    **FUD** ZZZ     N N1 80 ▣

**AMA:** 2017,Feb,9

**22869** **Insertion of interlaminar/interspinous process stabilization/distraction device, without open decompression or fusion, including image guidance when performed, lumbar; single level**

🔧 15.7    ⚕ 15.7    **FUD** 090     J J8 80 ▣

**AMA:** 2017,Feb,9

+ **22870** **second level (List separately in addition to code for primary procedure)**

**EXCLUDES** *Procedures at the same level (22532-22534, 22558, 22612, 22614, 22630, 22632-22634, 22800, 22802, 22804, 22840-22842, 63005, 63012, 63017, 63030, 63035, 63042, 63044, 63047-63048, 77003)*
Code first (22869)

🔧 4.16    ⚕ 4.16    **FUD** ZZZ     N N1 80 ▣

**AMA:** 2017,Feb,9

**22899** **Unlisted procedure, spine**

🔧 0.00    ⚕ 0.00    **FUD** YYY     T 80

**AMA:** 2017,Feb,9; 2017,Jan,8; 2016,Jan,13; 2015,Jan,8; 2015,Jan,16; 2014,Oct,14; 2014,Jan,11; 2013,Dec,16; 2013,Dec,14; 2012,Dec,12; 2012,Oct,14; 2012,Sep,16; 2012,Jan,13-14; 2012,Jan,15-42

## 22900-22999 Musculoskeletal Procedures of Abdomen

**INCLUDES** Any necessary elevation of tissue planes or dissection
Measurement of tumor and necessary margin at greatest diameter prior to excision
Simple and intermediate repairs
Types of excision:
  Fascial or subfascial soft tissue tumors: simple and marginal resection of tumors found either in or below the deep fascia, not involving bone or excision of a substantial amount of normal tissue; primarily benign and intramuscular tumors
  Radical resection soft tissue tumor: wide resection of tumor involving substantial margins of normal tissue and may include tissue removal from one or more layers; most often malignant or aggressive benign
  Subcutaneous: simple and marginal resection of tumors in the subcutaneous tissue above the deep fascia; most often benign
**EXCLUDES** *Complex repair*
*Excision of benign cutaneous lesions (eg, sebaceous cyst) (11400-11406)*
*Radical resection of cutaneous tumors (eg, melanoma) (11600-11606)*
*Significant exploration of the vessels or neuroplasty*

**22900** **Excision, tumor, soft tissue of abdominal wall, subfascial (eg, intramuscular); less than 5 cm**

🔧 16.2    ⚕ 16.2    **FUD** 090     J 62 80 ▣

**AMA:** 2002,Apr,13

**22901** **5 cm or greater**

🔧 19.2    ⚕ 19.2    **FUD** 090     J 62 80 ▣

---

● New Code   ▲ Revised Code   ○ Reinstated   ● New Web Release   ▲ Revised Web Release   Unlisted   Not Covered   # Resequenced
⊘ AMA Mod 51 Exempt   ⑤ Optum Mod 51 Exempt   ⑥ Mod 63 Exempt   ✗ Non-FDA Drug   ★ Telemedicine   M Maternity   A Age Edit   + Add-on   **AMA:** CPT Asst
© 2017 Optum360, LLC    CPT © 2017 American Medical Association. All Rights Reserved.    **57**

**22902** Excision, tumor, soft tissue of abdominal wall, subcutaneous; less than 3 cm
 9.51  12.5  **FUD** 090  J G2 80

**22903** 3 cm or greater
 12.6  12.6  **FUD** 090  J G2 80

**22904** Radical resection of tumor (eg, sarcoma), soft tissue of abdominal wall; less than 5 cm
 30.3  30.3  **FUD** 090  J G2 80

**22905** 5 cm or greater
 38.4  38.4  **FUD** 090  J G2 80

**22999** Unlisted procedure, abdomen, musculoskeletal system
 0.00  0.00  **FUD** YYY  T 80
**AMA:** 2002,Apr,13

## 23000-23044 Surgical Incision Shoulder: Drainage, Foreign Body Removal, Contracture Release

**23000** Removal of subdeltoid calcareous deposits, open
*EXCLUDES* Arthroscopic removal calcium deposits of bursa (29999)
 10.5  16.5  **FUD** 090  J A2 80 50
**AMA:** 2002,Apr,13

**23020** Capsular contracture release (eg, Sever type procedure)
*EXCLUDES* Simple incision and drainage (10040-10160)
 19.8  19.8  **FUD** 090  J A2 80 50
**AMA:** 2002,Apr,13; 1998,Nov,1

**23030** Incision and drainage, shoulder area; deep abscess or hematoma
 7.36  12.6  **FUD** 010  J A2
**AMA:** 2002,Apr,13

**23031** infected bursa
 6.30  12.1  **FUD** 010  J A2 50
**AMA:** 2002,Apr,13

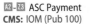

Acromion
Supraspinatus muscle and tendon
Scapula
Bursa
Head of humerus
Acromion
Clavicle
Glenoid cavity
Deltoid muscle
Teres major muscle
Coracoid process
Humerus
Scapula
Triceps

**Section of left shoulder**

The fibrous capsule enclosing the shoulder is thin and loose to allow freedom of movement; four rotator cuff muscles (supraspinatous, infraspinatous, teres minor, and scapularis) work together to hold the head of the humerus in the glenoid cavity

**23035** Incision, bone cortex (eg, osteomyelitis or bone abscess), shoulder area
 19.5  19.5  **FUD** 090  J A2 80 50
**AMA:** 2003,Jan,1; 2002,Apr,13

**23040** Arthrotomy, glenohumeral joint, including exploration, drainage, or removal of foreign body
 20.6  20.6  **FUD** 090  J A2 80 50
**AMA:** 2002,Apr,13; 1998,Nov,1

**23044** Arthrotomy, acromioclavicular, sternoclavicular joint, including exploration, drainage, or removal of foreign body
 16.3  16.3  **FUD** 090  J A2 50
**AMA:** 2002,Apr,13; 1998,Nov,1

## 23065-23066 Shoulder Biopsy
*EXCLUDES* Soft tissue needle biopsy (20206)

**23065** Biopsy, soft tissue of shoulder area; superficial
 4.83  6.21  **FUD** 010  J P3 50
**AMA:** 2002,Apr,13

**23066** deep
 10.2  15.9  **FUD** 090  J A2 50
**AMA:** 2002,Apr,13

## 23071-23078 [23071, 23073] Excision Soft Tissue Tumors of Shoulder

*INCLUDES* Any necessary elevation of tissue planes or dissection
Measurement of tumor and necessary margin at greatest diameter prior to excision
Simple and intermediate repairs
Types of excision:
  Fascial or subfascial soft tissue tumors: simple and marginal resection of tumors found either in or below the deep fascia, not involving bone or excision of a substantial amount of normal tissue; primarily benign and intramuscular tumors
  Radical resection soft tissue tumor: wide resection of tumor, involving substantial margins of normal tissue and may involve tissue removal from one or more layers; most often malignant or aggressive benign
  Subcutaneous: simple and marginal resection of tumors in the subcutaneous tissue above the deep fascia; most often benign

*EXCLUDES* Complex repair
Excision of benign cutaneous lesions (eg, sebaceous cyst) (11400-11406)
Radical resection of cutaneous tumors (eg, melanoma) (11600-11606)
Significant exploration of the vessels or neuroplasty

*23071* Resequenced code. See code following 23075.

*23073* Resequenced code. See code following 23076.

**23075** Excision, tumor, soft tissue of shoulder area, subcutaneous; less than 3 cm
 9.39  13.3  **FUD** 090  J G2 50
**AMA:** 2017,Jan,8; 2016,Jan,13; 2015,Jan,16; 2014,Jan,11

\# **23071** 3 cm or greater
 12.0  12.0  **FUD** 090  J G2 80 50
**AMA:** 2009,Oct,7,8&13

**23076** Excision, tumor, soft tissue of shoulder area, subfascial (eg, intramuscular); less than 5 cm
 15.5  15.5  **FUD** 090  J G2 50
**AMA:** 2017,Jan,8; 2016,Jan,13; 2015,Jan,16; 2014,Jan,11

\# **23073** 5 cm or greater
 20.0  20.0  **FUD** 090  J G2 80 50
**AMA:** 2009,Oct,7,8&13

**23077** Radical resection of tumor (eg, sarcoma), soft tissue of shoulder area; less than 5 cm
 32.9  32.9  **FUD** 090  J G2 80 50
**AMA:** 2002,Apr,13; 1990,Win,4

**23078** 5 cm or greater
 41.4  41.4  **FUD** 090  J G2 80 50

## 23100-23195 Bone and Joint Procedures of Shoulder

*INCLUDES* Acromioclavicular joint
Clavicle
Head and neck of humerus
Scapula
Shoulder joint
Sternoclavicular joint

**23100** Arthrotomy, glenohumeral joint, including biopsy
 14.3  14.3  **FUD** 090  J A2 80 50
**AMA:** 2002,Apr,13; 1998,Nov,1

**23101** Arthrotomy, acromioclavicular joint or sternoclavicular joint, including biopsy and/or excision of torn cartilage
 12.8  12.8  **FUD** 090  J A2 50
**AMA:** 2002,Apr,13; 1998,Nov,1

**23105** Arthrotomy; glenohumeral joint, with synovectomy, with or without biopsy
 18.2  18.2  **FUD** 090  J A2 80 50
**AMA:** 2002,Apr,13; 1998,Nov,1

26/TC PC/TC Only  A2-Z3 ASC Payment  50 Bilateral  ♂ Male Only  ♀ Female Only   Facility RVU   Non-Facility RVU   CCI
**FUD** Follow-up Days  **CMS:** IOM (Pub 100)  A-Y OPPSI  80/80 Surg Assist Allowed / w/Doc   Lab Crosswalk   Radiology Crosswalk   CLIA

CPT © 2017 American Medical Association. All Rights Reserved.                    © 2017 Optum360, LLC

**23106** sternoclavicular joint, with synovectomy, with or without biopsy
🚗 13.8 ⚕ 13.8 **FUD** 090   J A2 50 ▣
**AMA:** 2002,Apr,13; 1998,Nov,1

**23107** Arthrotomy, glenohumeral joint, with joint exploration, with or without removal of loose or foreign body
🚗 18.9 ⚕ 18.9 **FUD** 090   J A2 80 50 ▣
**AMA:** 2002,Apr,13

**23120** Claviculectomy; partial
INCLUDES Mumford operation
EXCLUDES Arthroscopic claviculectomy (29824)
🚗 16.7 ⚕ 16.7 **FUD** 090   J A2 80 50 ▣
**AMA:** 2017,Jan,8; 2016,Jan,13; 2015,Jan,16; 2014,Jan,11; 2012,Oct,14; 2012,Sep,16

**23125** total
🚗 19.9 ⚕ 19.9 **FUD** 090   J A2 80 50 ▣
**AMA:** 2003,Jan,1; 2002,Apr,13

**23130** Acromioplasty or acromionectomy, partial, with or without coracoacromial ligament release
🚗 17.4 ⚕ 17.4 **FUD** 090   J A2 50 ▣
**AMA:** 2017,Jan,8; 2016,Jan,13; 2015,Mar,7; 2015,Feb,10; 2015,Jan,16; 2014,Jan,11; 2012,Jan,15-42

**23140** Excision or curettage of bone cyst or benign tumor of clavicle or scapula;
🚗 15.4 ⚕ 15.4 **FUD** 090   J A2 50 ▣
**AMA:** 2002,Apr,13

**23145** with autograft (includes obtaining graft)
🚗 19.7 ⚕ 19.7 **FUD** 090   J A2 80 50 ▣
**AMA:** 2002,Apr,13

**23146** with allograft
🚗 17.6 ⚕ 17.6 **FUD** 090   J A2 80 50 ▣
**AMA:** 2002,Apr,13

**23150** Excision or curettage of bone cyst or benign tumor of proximal humerus;
🚗 18.9 ⚕ 18.9 **FUD** 090   J A2 80 50 ▣
**AMA:** 2002,Apr,13

**23155** with autograft (includes obtaining graft)
🚗 22.6 ⚕ 22.6 **FUD** 090   J A2 80 50 ▣
**AMA:** 2002,Apr,13

**23156** with allograft
🚗 19.2 ⚕ 19.2 **FUD** 090   J A2 80 50 ▣
**AMA:** 2002,Apr,13

**23170** Sequestrectomy (eg, for osteomyelitis or bone abscess), clavicle
🚗 16.0 ⚕ 16.0 **FUD** 090   J A2 50 ▣
**AMA:** 2002,Apr,13

**23172** Sequestrectomy (eg, for osteomyelitis or bone abscess), scapula
🚗 15.9 ⚕ 15.9 **FUD** 090   J A2 80 50 ▣
**AMA:** 2002,Apr,13

**23174** Sequestrectomy (eg, for osteomyelitis or bone abscess), humeral head to surgical neck
🚗 21.7 ⚕ 21.7 **FUD** 090   J A2 80 50 ▣
**AMA:** 2002,Apr,13

**23180** Partial excision (craterization, saucerization, or diaphysectomy) bone (eg, osteomyelitis), clavicle
🚗 19.0 ⚕ 19.0 **FUD** 090   J A2 50 ▣
**AMA:** 2002,Apr,13; 1998,Nov,1

**23182** Partial excision (craterization, saucerization, or diaphysectomy) bone (eg, osteomyelitis), scapula
🚗 18.8 ⚕ 18.8 **FUD** 090   J A2 80 50 ▣
**AMA:** 2002,Apr,13; 1998,Nov,1

**23184** Partial excision (craterization, saucerization, or diaphysectomy) bone (eg, osteomyelitis), proximal humerus
🚗 21.0 ⚕ 21.0 **FUD** 090   J A2 80 50 ▣
**AMA:** 2002,Apr,13; 1998,Nov,1

**23190** Ostectomy of scapula, partial (eg, superior medial angle)
🚗 16.4 ⚕ 16.4 **FUD** 090   J A2 80 50 ▣
**AMA:** 2002,Apr,13

**23195** Resection, humeral head
EXCLUDES Arthroplasty with replacement with implant (23470)
🚗 21.7 ⚕ 21.7 **FUD** 090   J A2 80 50 ▣
**AMA:** 2003,Jan,1; 2002,Apr,13

## 23200-23220 Radical Resection of Bone Tumors of Shoulder

INCLUDES Any necessary elevation of tissue planes or dissection
Excision of adjacent soft tissue during bone tumor resection (23071-23078 [23071, 23073])
Measurement of tumor and necessary margin at greatest diameter prior to excision
Radical resection of cutaneous tumors (e.g., melanoma)
Resection of the tumor (may include entire bone) and wide margins of normal tissues primarily for malignant or aggressive benign tumors
Simple and intermediate repairs
EXCLUDES Complex repair
Significant exploration of vessels, neuroplasty, reconstruction, or complex bone repair

**23200** Radical resection of tumor; clavicle
🚗 43.5 ⚕ 43.5 **FUD** 090   C 80 50 ▣
**AMA:** 2002,Apr,13

**23210** scapula
🚗 50.9 ⚕ 50.9 **FUD** 090   C 80 50 ▣
**AMA:** 2002,Apr,13

**23220** Radical resection of tumor, proximal humerus
🚗 56.1 ⚕ 56.1 **FUD** 090   C 80 50 ▣
**AMA:** 2002,Apr,13; 1998,Nov,1

## 23330-23335 Removal Implant/Foreign Body from Shoulder

EXCLUDES Bursal arthrocentesis or needling (20610)
K-wire or pin insertion (20650)
K-wire or pin removal (20670, 20680)

**23330** Removal of foreign body, shoulder; subcutaneous
🚗 4.43 ⚕ 7.05 **FUD** 010   T A2 80 50 ▣
**AMA:** 2017,Jan,8; 2016,Jan,13; 2015,Jan,16; 2014,Mar,4; 2014,Jan,11

**23333** deep (subfascial or intramuscular)
🚗 12.9 ⚕ 12.9 **FUD** 090   J 62 80 50 ▣
**AMA:** 2017,Jan,8; 2016,Jan,13; 2015,Jan,16; 2014,Mar,4

**23334** Removal of prosthesis, includes debridement and synovectomy when performed; humeral or glenoid component
EXCLUDES Foreign body removal (23330, 23333)
Prosthesis removal and replacement in same shoulder (eg, glenoid and/or humeral components) (23473-23474)
🚗 31.0 ⚕ 31.0 **FUD** 090   J 62 50 ▣
**AMA:** 2017,Jan,8; 2016,Jan,13; 2015,Jan,16; 2014,Mar,4

**23335** humeral and glenoid components (eg, total shoulder)
EXCLUDES Foreign body removal (23330, 23333)
Prosthesis removal and replacement in same shoulder (eg, glenoid and/or humeral components) (23473-23474)
🚗 36.9 ⚕ 36.9 **FUD** 090   C 50 ▣
**AMA:** 2017,Jan,8; 2016,Jan,13; 2015,Jan,16; 2014,Mar,4

## 23350 Injection for Shoulder Arthrogram

**23350** Injection procedure for shoulder arthrography or enhanced CT/MRI shoulder arthrography
EXCLUDES Shoulder biopsy (29805-29826)
(73040, 73201-73202, 73222-73223, 77002)
🚗 1.47 ⚕ 3.70 **FUD** 000   N N1 50 ▣
**AMA:** 2017,Jan,8; 2016,May,13; 2016,Jan,13; 2015,Aug,6; 2015,Jan,16; 2014,Jan,11

● New Code   ▲ Revised Code   ○ Reinstated   ● New Web Release   ▲ Revised Web Release   Unlisted   Not Covered   # Resequenced
⊘ AMA Mod 51 Exempt   ⑨ Optum Mod 51 Exempt   ⑥ Mod 63 Exempt   ⚡ Non-FDA Drug   ★ Telemedicine   Ⓜ Maternity   ⒶAge Edit   + Add-on   AMA: CPT Asst
© 2017 Optum360, LLC             CPT © 2017 American Medical Association. All Rights Reserved.

Musculoskeletal System

23395 — 23525

## 23395-23491 Repair/Reconstruction of Shoulder

**23395**   **Muscle transfer, any type, shoulder or upper arm; single**
 ⚙ 36.8   ✂ 36.8   **FUD** 090            J A2 80 ▣
 **AMA:** 2003,Jan,1; 2002,Apr,13

**23397**   **multiple**
 ⚙ 32.8   ✂ 32.8   **FUD** 090            J A2 80 ▣
 **AMA:** 2003,Jan,1; 2002,Apr,13

**23400**   **Scapulopexy (eg, Sprengels deformity or for paralysis)**
 ⚙ 27.1   ✂ 27.1   **FUD** 090            J A2 80 50 ▣
 **AMA:** 2003,Jan,1; 2002,Apr,13

**23405**   **Tenotomy, shoulder area; single tendon**
 ⚙ 17.8   ✂ 17.8   **FUD** 090            J A2 80 ▣
 **AMA:** 2002,Apr,13; 1998,Nov,1

**23406**   **multiple tendons through same incision**
 ⚙ 22.1   ✂ 22.1   **FUD** 090            J J8 80 ▣
 **AMA:** 2002,Apr,13; 1998,Nov,1

**23410**   **Repair of ruptured musculotendinous cuff (eg, rotator cuff) open; acute**
 *EXCLUDES*   *Arthroscopic repair (29827)*
 ⚙ 23.6   ✂ 23.6   **FUD** 090            J A2 80 50 ▣
 **AMA:** 2017,Jan,8; 2016,Jan,13; 2015,Jan,16; 2014,Jan,11; 2012,Jan,15-42

**23412**   **chronic**
 *EXCLUDES*   *Arthroscopic repair (29827)*
 ⚙ 24.4   ✂ 24.4   **FUD** 090            J A2 80 50 ▣
 **AMA:** 2017,Jan,8; 2016,Jan,13; 2015,Jun,10; 2015,Feb,10; 2015,Jan,16; 2014,Jan,11; 2012,Oct,14; 2012,Sep,16; 2012,Jan,15-42

**23415**   **Coracoacromial ligament release, with or without acromioplasty**
 *EXCLUDES*   *Arthroscopic repair (29826)*
 ⚙ 20.0   ✂ 20.0   **FUD** 090            J A2 50 ▣
 **AMA:** 2017,Jan,8; 2016,Jan,13; 2015,Mar,7

**23420**   **Reconstruction of complete shoulder (rotator) cuff avulsion, chronic (includes acromioplasty)**
 ⚙ 27.8   ✂ 27.8   **FUD** 090            J A2 80 50 ▣
 **AMA:** 2017,Jan,8; 2016,Jan,13; 2015,Jan,16; 2014,Jan,11; 2012,Jan,15-42

**23430**   **Tenodesis of long tendon of biceps**
 *EXCLUDES*   *Arthroscopic biceps tenodesis (29828)*
 ⚙ 21.4   ✂ 21.4   **FUD** 090            J A2 80 50 ▣
 **AMA:** 2002,Apr,13; 1994,Win,1

**23440**   **Resection or transplantation of long tendon of biceps**
 ⚙ 21.6   ✂ 21.6   **FUD** 090            J A2 80 50 ▣
 **AMA:** 2002,Apr,13; 1994,Win,1

**23450**   **Capsulorrhaphy, anterior; Putti-Platt procedure or Magnuson type operation**
 *EXCLUDES*   *Arthroscopic thermal capsulorrhaphy (29999)*
 ⚙ 27.3   ✂ 27.3   **FUD** 090            J A2 80 50 ▣
 **AMA:** 2002,Apr,13; 1998,Nov,1

**23455**   **with labral repair (eg, Bankart procedure)**
 *EXCLUDES*   *Arthroscopic repair (29806)*
 ⚙ 28.6   ✂ 28.6   **FUD** 090            J A2 80 50 ▣
 **AMA:** 2002,Apr,13; 1998,Nov,1

**23460**   **Capsulorrhaphy, anterior, any type; with bone block**
 *INCLUDES*   Bristow procedure
 ⚙ 31.2   ✂ 31.2   **FUD** 090            J A2 80 50 ▣
 **AMA:** 2002,Apr,13; 1994,Win,1

**23462**   **with coracoid process transfer**
 *EXCLUDES*   *Open thermal capsulorrhaphy (23929)*
 ⚙ 30.3   ✂ 30.3   **FUD** 090            J A2 80 50 ▣
 **AMA:** 2002,Apr,13

**23465**   **Capsulorrhaphy, glenohumeral joint, posterior, with or without bone block**
 *EXCLUDES*   *Sternoclavicular and acromioclavicular joint repair (23530, 23550)*
 ⚙ 31.9   ✂ 31.9   **FUD** 090            J G2 80 50 ▣
 **AMA:** 2002,Apr,13; 1998,Nov,1

**23466**   **Capsulorrhaphy, glenohumeral joint, any type multi-directional instability**
 ⚙ 32.1   ✂ 32.1   **FUD** 090            J A2 80 50 ▣
 **AMA:** 2002,Apr,13; 1998,Nov,1

**23470**   **Arthroplasty, glenohumeral joint; hemiarthroplasty**
 ⚙ 34.6   ✂ 34.6   **FUD** 090            J 80 50 ▣
 **AMA:** 2017,Jan,8; 2016,Jan,13; 2015,Jan,16; 2014,Mar,4

**23472**   **total shoulder (glenoid and proximal humeral replacement (eg, total shoulder))**
 *EXCLUDES*   *Proximal humerus osteotomy (24400)*
         *Removal of total shoulder components (23334-23335)*
 ⚙ 41.9   ✂ 41.9   **FUD** 090            C 80 50 ▣
 **AMA:** 2017,Jan,8; 2016,Jan,13; 2015,Jan,16; 2014,Mar,4; 2014,Jan,11; 2013,Mar,12; 2012,Jan,15-42

**23473**   **Revision of total shoulder arthroplasty, including allograft when performed; humeral or glenoid component**
 *EXCLUDES*   *Removal of prosthesis only (glenoid and/or humeral component) (23334-23335)*
 ⚙ 46.8   ✂ 46.8   **FUD** 090            J 80 50 ▣
 **AMA:** 2017,Jan,8; 2016,Jan,13; 2015,Jan,16; 2014,Mar,4; 2014,Jan,11; 2013,Mar,12; 2013,Feb,11-12

**23474**   **humeral and glenoid component**
 *EXCLUDES*   *Removal of prosthesis only (glenoid and/or humeral component) (23334-23335)*
 ⚙ 50.6   ✂ 50.6   **FUD** 090            C 80 50 ▣
 **AMA:** 2017,Jan,8; 2016,Jan,13; 2015,Jan,16; 2014,Mar,4; 2014,Jan,11; 2013,Mar,12; 2013,Feb,11-12

**23480**   **Osteotomy, clavicle, with or without internal fixation;**
 ⚙ 23.5   ✂ 23.5   **FUD** 090            J A2 50 ▣
 **AMA:** 2002,Apr,13

**23485**   **with bone graft for nonunion or malunion (includes obtaining graft and/or necessary fixation)**
 ⚙ 27.4   ✂ 27.4   **FUD** 090            J J8 80 50 ▣
 **AMA:** 2002,Apr,13

**23490**   **Prophylactic treatment (nailing, pinning, plating or wiring) with or without methylmethacrylate; clavicle**
 ⚙ 24.1   ✂ 24.1   **FUD** 090            J A2 80 50 ▣
 **AMA:** 2002,Apr,13

**23491**   **proximal humerus**
 ⚙ 29.0   ✂ 29.0   **FUD** 090            J G2 80 50 ▣
 **AMA:** 2002,Apr,13; 1998,Nov,1

## 23500-23680 Treatment of Shoulder Fracture/Dislocation

**23500**   **Closed treatment of clavicular fracture; without manipulation**
 ⚙ 6.31   ✂ 6.21   **FUD** 090            T A2 50 ▣
 **AMA:** 2002,Apr,13

**23505**   **with manipulation**
 ⚙ 9.43   ✂ 9.98   **FUD** 090            J A2 50 ▣
 **AMA:** 2002,Apr,13

**23515**   **Open treatment of clavicular fracture, includes internal fixation, when performed**
 ⚙ 20.6   ✂ 20.6   **FUD** 090            J A2 80 50 ▣
 **AMA:** 2017,Jan,8; 2016,Jan,13; 2015,Jan,16; 2014,Jan,11

**23520**   **Closed treatment of sternoclavicular dislocation; without manipulation**
 ⚙ 6.61   ✂ 6.51   **FUD** 090            J A2 80 50 ▣
 **AMA:** 2002,Apr,13

**23525**   **with manipulation**
 ⚙ 9.83   ✂ 10.6   **FUD** 090            T A2 80 50 ▣
 **AMA:** 2002,Apr,13

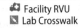

**23530** Open treatment of sternoclavicular dislocation, acute or chronic;
16.3 ⚕ 16.3 **FUD** 090  [J] [A2] [80] [50] [▣]
**AMA:** 2002,Apr,13

**23532** with fascial graft (includes obtaining graft)
17.7 ⚕ 17.7 **FUD** 090  [J] [A2] [80] [50] [▣]
**AMA:** 2002,Apr,13

**23540** Closed treatment of acromioclavicular dislocation; without manipulation
6.47 ⚕ 6.37 **FUD** 090  [T] [A2] [50] [▣]
**AMA:** 2002,Apr,13

**23545** with manipulation
8.72 ⚕ 9.57 **FUD** 090  [T] [A2] [80] [50] [▣]
**AMA:** 2002,Apr,13

**23550** Open treatment of acromioclavicular dislocation, acute or chronic;
16.0 ⚕ 16.0 **FUD** 090  [J] [A2] [80] [50] [▣]
**AMA:** 2002,Apr,13

**23552** with fascial graft (includes obtaining graft)
18.8 ⚕ 18.8 **FUD** 090  [J] [G2] [80] [50] [▣]
**AMA:** 2002,Apr,13

**23570** Closed treatment of scapular fracture; without manipulation
6.81 ⚕ 6.60 **FUD** 090  [T] [A2] [50] [▣]
**AMA:** 2002,Apr,13

**23575** with manipulation, with or without skeletal traction (with or without shoulder joint involvement)
10.6 ⚕ 11.3 **FUD** 090  [J] [A2] [80] [50] [▣]
**AMA:** 2002,Apr,13

**23585** Open treatment of scapular fracture (body, glenoid or acromion) includes internal fixation, when performed
28.1 ⚕ 28.1 **FUD** 090  [J] [A2] [80] [50] [▣]
**AMA:** 2017,Jan,8; 2016,Jan,13; 2015,Jan,16; 2014,Jan,11; 2012,Jan,15-42

**23600** Closed treatment of proximal humeral (surgical or anatomical neck) fracture; without manipulation
8.75 ⚕ 9.28 **FUD** 090  [T] [P2] [50] [▣]
**AMA:** 2002,Apr,13

**23605** with manipulation, with or without skeletal traction
12.0 ⚕ 13.1 **FUD** 090  [J] [A2] [50] [▣]
**AMA:** 2002,Apr,13

**23615** Open treatment of proximal humeral (surgical or anatomical neck) fracture, includes internal fixation, when performed, includes repair of tuberosity(s), when performed;
25.4 ⚕ 25.4 **FUD** 090  [J] [J8] [80] [50] [▣]
**AMA:** 2017,Jan,8; 2016,Jan,13; 2015,Jan,16; 2014,Jan,11

**23616** with proximal humeral prosthetic replacement
35.7 ⚕ 35.7 **FUD** 090  [J] [J8] [80] [50] [▣]
**AMA:** 2002,Apr,13

**23620** Closed treatment of greater humeral tuberosity fracture; without manipulation
7.29 ⚕ 7.65 **FUD** 090  [T] [P2] [50] [▣]
**AMA:** 2002,Apr,13; 1998,Nov,1

**23625** with manipulation
10.0 ⚕ 10.7 **FUD** 090  [J] [A2] [50] [▣]
**AMA:** 2002,Apr,13

**23630** Open treatment of greater humeral tuberosity fracture, includes internal fixation, when performed
22.4 ⚕ 22.4 **FUD** 090  [J] [A2] [80] [50] [▣]
**AMA:** 2002,Apr,13; 1998,Nov,1

**23650** Closed treatment of shoulder dislocation, with manipulation; without anesthesia
8.20 ⚕ 8.92 **FUD** 090  [T] [A2] [50] [▣]
**AMA:** 2002,Apr,13

**23655** requiring anesthesia
11.4 ⚕ 11.4 **FUD** 090  [J] [A2] [50] [▣]
**AMA:** 2002,Apr,13

**23660** Open treatment of acute shoulder dislocation
*EXCLUDES* *Chronic dislocation repair (23450-23466)*
16.6 ⚕ 16.6 **FUD** 090  [J] [A2] [80] [50] [▣]
**AMA:** 2017,Jan,8; 2016,Jan,13; 2015,Jan,16; 2014,Jan,11

**23665** Closed treatment of shoulder dislocation, with fracture of greater humeral tuberosity, with manipulation
11.2 ⚕ 12.1 **FUD** 090  [J] [A2] [50] [▣]
**AMA:** 2002,Apr,13; 1998,Nov,1

**23670** Open treatment of shoulder dislocation, with fracture of greater humeral tuberosity, includes internal fixation, when performed
25.1 ⚕ 25.1 **FUD** 090  [J] [A2] [80] [50] [▣]
**AMA:** 2002,Apr,13; 1998,Nov,1

**23675** Closed treatment of shoulder dislocation, with surgical or anatomical neck fracture, with manipulation
14.2 ⚕ 15.6 **FUD** 090  [J] [A2] [50] [▣]
**AMA:** 2002,Apr,13

**23680** Open treatment of shoulder dislocation, with surgical or anatomical neck fracture, includes internal fixation, when performed
26.6 ⚕ 26.6 **FUD** 090  [J] [A2] [80] [50] [▣]
**AMA:** 2002,Apr,13

## 23700-23929 Other/Unlisted Shoulder Procedures

**23700** Manipulation under anesthesia, shoulder joint, including application of fixation apparatus (dislocation excluded)
5.63 ⚕ 5.63 **FUD** 010  [J] [A2] [50] [▣]
**AMA:** 2017,Jan,8; 2016,Jan,13; 2015,Jun,10; 2015,Jan,16; 2014,Jan,11; 2012,Jan,15-42

**23800** Arthrodesis, glenohumeral joint;
29.2 ⚕ 29.2 **FUD** 090  [J] [G2] [80] [50] [▣]
**AMA:** 2002,Apr,13; 1998,Nov,1

**23802** with autogenous graft (includes obtaining graft)
36.8 ⚕ 36.8 **FUD** 090  [J] [G2] [80] [50] [▣]
**AMA:** 2002,Apr,13; 1998,Nov,1

**23900** Interthoracoscapular amputation (forequarter)
40.0 ⚕ 40.0 **FUD** 090  [C] [80] [▣]
**AMA:** 2002,Apr,13

**23920** Disarticulation of shoulder;
31.7 ⚕ 31.7 **FUD** 090  [C] [80] [50] [▣]
**AMA:** 2002,Apr,13

**23921** secondary closure or scar revision
13.3 ⚕ 13.3 **FUD** 090  [T] [A2] [50] [▣]
**AMA:** 2002,Apr,13

**23929** Unlisted procedure, shoulder
0.00 ⚕ 0.00 **FUD** YYY  [T] [80]
**AMA:** 2002,Apr,13

## 23930-24006 Surgical Incision Elbow/Upper Arm
*EXCLUDES* *Simple incision and drainage procedures (10040-10160)*

**23930** Incision and drainage, upper arm or elbow area; deep abscess or hematoma
6.22 ⚕ 10.1 **FUD** 010  [J] [A2] [50] [▣]
**AMA:** 2002,Apr,13

**23931** bursa
4.58 ⚕ 8.17 **FUD** 010  [J] [A2] [50] [▣]
**AMA:** 2002,Apr,13; 1998,Nov,1

**23935** Incision, deep, with opening of bone cortex (eg, for osteomyelitis or bone abscess), humerus or elbow
14.5 ⚕ 14.5 **FUD** 090  [J] [A2] [80] [50] [▣]
**AMA:** 2002,Apr,13

● New Code ▲ Revised Code ○ Reinstated ● New Web Release ▲ Revised Web Release Unlisted Not Covered # Resequenced
⊘ AMA Mod 51 Exempt ⑤ Optum Mod 51 Exempt ⑥ Mod 63 Exempt ✒ Non-FDA Drug ★ Telemedicine Ⓜ Maternity Ⓐ Age Edit + Add-on **AMA:** CPT Asst
© 2017 Optum360, LLC          CPT © 2017 American Medical Association. All Rights Reserved.          **61**

**Musculoskeletal System**

**24000 — 24149**

**24000** Arthrotomy, elbow, including exploration, drainage, or removal of foreign body
🚑 13.7　📐 13.7　**FUD** 090　　　J A2 80 50 ▣
**AMA:** 2002,Apr,13; 1998,Nov,1

**24006** Arthrotomy of the elbow, with capsular excision for capsular release (separate procedure)
🚑 20.4　📐 20.4　**FUD** 090　　　J A2 80 50 ▣
**AMA:** 2002,Apr,13; 1996,Nov,1

## 24065-24066 Biopsy of Elbow/Upper Arm

EXCLUDES *Soft tissue needle biopsy (20206)*

**24065** Biopsy, soft tissue of upper arm or elbow area; superficial
🚑 4.83　📐 7.31　**FUD** 010　　　J P3 50 ▣
**AMA:** 2002,Apr,13

**24066** deep (subfascial or intramuscular)
🚑 11.9　📐 17.8　**FUD** 090　　　J A2 50 ▣
**AMA:** 2002,Apr,13; 1998,Nov,1

## 24071-24079 [24071, 24073] Excision Soft Tissue Tumors Elbow/Upper Arm

INCLUDES Any necessary elevation of tissue planes or dissection
Measurement of tumor and necessary margin at greatest diameter prior to excision
Types of excision:
　　Fascial or subfascial soft tissue tumors: simple and marginal resection of tumors found either in or below the deep fascia, not involving bone or excision of a substantial amount of normal tissue; primarily benign and intramuscular tumors
　　Radical resection of soft tissue tumor: wide resection of tumor involving substantial margins of normal tissue and may involve tissue removal from one or more layers; most often malignant or aggressive tumors
　　Subcutaneous: simple and marginal resection of tumors found in the subcutaneous tissue above the deep fascia; most often benign

EXCLUDES *Complex repair*
*Excision of benign cutaneous lesion (eg, sebaceous cyst) (11400-11406)*
*Radical resection of cutaneous tumors (eg, melanoma) (11600-11606)*
*Significant exploration of vessels or neuroplasty*

**24071** Resequenced code. See code following 24075.

**24073** Resequenced code. See code following 24076.

**24075** Excision, tumor, soft tissue of upper arm or elbow area, subcutaneous; less than 3 cm
🚑 9.49　📐 14.0　**FUD** 090　　　J 62 50 ▣
**AMA:** 2002,Apr,13

\# **24071** 3 cm or greater
🚑 11.6　📐 11.6　**FUD** 090　　　J 62 80 50 ▣

**24076** Excision, tumor, soft tissue of upper arm or elbow area, subfascial (eg, intramuscular); less than 5 cm
🚑 15.6　📐 15.6　**FUD** 090　　　J 62 50 ▣
**AMA:** 2002,Apr,13

\# **24073** 5 cm or greater
🚑 19.9　📐 19.9　**FUD** 090　　　J 62 80 50 ▣

**24077** Radical resection of tumor (eg, sarcoma), soft tissue of upper arm or elbow area; less than 5 cm
🚑 29.8　📐 29.8　**FUD** 090　　　J 62 50 ▣
**AMA:** 2002,Apr,13; 1990,Win,4

**24079** 5 cm or greater
🚑 38.3　📐 38.3　**FUD** 090　　　J 02 80 50 ▣

## 24100-24149 Bone/Joint Procedures Upper Arm/Elbow

**24100** Arthrotomy, elbow; with synovial biopsy only
🚑 11.8　📐 11.8　**FUD** 090　　　J A2 80 50 ▣
**AMA:** 2002,Apr,13; 1994,Win,1

**24101** with joint exploration, with or without biopsy, with or without removal of loose or foreign body
🚑 14.2　📐 14.2　**FUD** 090　　　J A2 80 50 ▣
**AMA:** 2002,Apr,13

**24102** with synovectomy
🚑 17.6　📐 17.6　**FUD** 090　　　J A2 80 50 ▣
**AMA:** 2002,Apr,13; 1994,Win,1

**24105** Excision, olecranon bursa
🚑 10.0　📐 10.0　**FUD** 090　　　J A2 50 ▣
**AMA:** 2002,Apr,13

**24110** Excision or curettage of bone cyst or benign tumor, humerus;
🚑 16.7　📐 16.7　**FUD** 090　　　J A2 50 ▣
**AMA:** 2002,Apr,13

**24115** with autograft (includes obtaining graft)
🚑 20.8　📐 20.8　**FUD** 090　　　J A2 80 50 ▣
**AMA:** 2002,Apr,13

**24116** with allograft
🚑 24.8　📐 24.8　**FUD** 090　　　J A2 80 50 ▣
**AMA:** 2002,Apr,13

**24120** Excision or curettage of bone cyst or benign tumor of head or neck of radius or olecranon process;
🚑 15.1　📐 15.1　**FUD** 090　　　J A2 80 50 ▣
**AMA:** 2002,Apr,13

**24125** with autograft (includes obtaining graft)
🚑 17.6　📐 17.6　**FUD** 090　　　J A2 80 50 ▣
**AMA:** 2002,Apr,13

**24126** with allograft
🚑 18.4　📐 18.4　**FUD** 090　　　J A2 80 50 ▣
**AMA:** 2002,Apr,13

**24130** Excision, radial head
EXCLUDES *Radial head arthroplasty with implant (24366)*
🚑 14.5　📐 14.5　**FUD** 090　　　J A2 50 ▣
**AMA:** 2002,Apr,13

**24134** Sequestrectomy (eg, for osteomyelitis or bone abscess), shaft or distal humerus
🚑 21.4　📐 21.4　**FUD** 090　　　J A2 80 50 ▣
**AMA:** 2002,Apr,13

**24136** Sequestrectomy (eg, for osteomyelitis or bone abscess), radial head or neck
🚑 17.0　📐 17.0　**FUD** 090　　　J A2 50 ▣
**AMA:** 2002,Apr,13

**24138** Sequestrectomy (eg, for osteomyelitis or bone abscess), olecranon process
🚑 19.3　📐 19.3　**FUD** 090　　　J A2 80 50 ▣
**AMA:** 2002,Apr,13

**24140** Partial excision (craterization, saucerization, or diaphysectomy) bone (eg, osteomyelitis), humerus
🚑 20.1　📐 20.1　**FUD** 090　　　J A2 80 50 ▣
**AMA:** 2002,Apr,13; 1998,Nov,1

**24145** Partial excision (craterization, saucerization, or diaphysectomy) bone (eg, osteomyelitis), radial head or neck
🚑 16.7　📐 16.7　**FUD** 090　　　J A2 50 ▣
**AMA:** 2002,Apr,13; 1998,Nov,1

**24147** Partial excision (craterization, saucerization, or diaphysectomy) bone (eg, osteomyelitis), olecranon process
🚑 17.8　📐 17.8　**FUD** 090　　　J A2 50 ▣
**AMA:** 2002,Apr,13; 1998,Nov,1

**24149** Radical resection of capsule, soft tissue, and heterotopic bone, elbow, with contracture release (separate procedure)
EXCLUDES *Capsular and soft tissue release (24006)*
🚑 33.7　📐 33.7　**FUD** 090　　　J 62 80 50 ▣
**AMA:** 2002,Apr,13; 1996,Nov,1

| 26/TC PC/TC Only | A2-Z3 ASC Payment | 50 Bilateral | ♂ Male Only | ♀ Female Only | 🚑 Facility RVU | 📐 Non-Facility RVU | ▣ CCI |
| FUD Follow-up Days | CMS: IOM (Pub 100) | A-Y OPPSI | 80/80 Surg Assist Allowed / w/Doc | | 🔬 Lab Crosswalk | ☢ Radiology Crosswalk | ✖ CLIA |

62　　　　　　　　　　　　　　CPT © 2017 American Medical Association. All Rights Reserved.　　　　　　　　© 2017 Optum360, LLC

## 24150-24152 Radical Resection Bone Tumor Upper Arm

**INCLUDES** Any necessary elevation of tissue planes or dissection
Excision of adjacent soft tissue during bone tumor resection (24071-24079 [24071, 24073])
Measurement of tumor and necessary margin at greatest diameter prior to excision
Resection of the tumor (may include entire bone) and wide margins of normal tissue primarily for malignant or aggressive benign tumors
Simple and intermediate repairs

**EXCLUDES** Complex repair
Significant exploration of vessels, neuroplasty, reconstruction, or complex bone repair

**24150** **Radical resection of tumor, shaft or distal humerus**
🚑 44.9 ✂ 44.9 **FUD** 090 [J] [80] [50] ▢
**AMA:** 2003,Jan,1; 2002,Apr,13

**24152** **Radical resection of tumor, radial head or neck**
🚑 38.5 ✂ 38.5 **FUD** 090 [J] [G2] [80] [50] ▢
**AMA:** 2003,Jan,1; 2002,Apr,13

## 24155 Elbow Arthrectomy

**24155** **Resection of elbow joint (arthrectomy)**
🚑 24.5 ✂ 24.5 **FUD** 090 [J] [A2] [80] [50] ▢
**AMA:** 2002,Apr,13; 1996,Nov,1

## 24160-24201 Removal Implant/Foreign Body from Elbow/Upper Arm

**EXCLUDES** Bursal or joint arthrocentesis or needling (20605)
K-wire or pin insertion (20650)
K-wire or pin removal (20670, 20680)

**24160** **Removal of prosthesis, includes debridement and synovectomy when performed; humeral and ulnar components**
**INCLUDES** Prosthesis removal and replacement in same elbow (eg, humeral and/or ulnar component(s)) (24370-24371)
**EXCLUDES** Foreign body removal (24200-24201)
Hardware removal other than prosthesis (20680)
🚑 36.4 ✂ 36.4 **FUD** 090 [02] [A2] [50] ▢
**AMA:** 2017,Jan,8; 2016,Jan,13; 2015,Jan,16; 2014,Mar,4; 2014,Jan,11; 2013,Feb,11-12

**24164** **radial head**
**EXCLUDES** Foreign body removal (24200-24201)
Hardware removal other than prosthesis (20680)
🚑 20.9 ✂ 20.9 **FUD** 090 [02] [A2] [50] ▢
**AMA:** 2017,Jan,8; 2016,Jan,13; 2015,Jan,16; 2014,Mar,4

**24200** **Removal of foreign body, upper arm or elbow area; subcutaneous**
🚑 4.00 ✂ 5.89 **FUD** 010 [J] [P3] [80] [50] ▢
**AMA:** 2017,Jan,8; 2016,Jan,13; 2015,Jan,16; 2014,Mar,4

**24201** **deep (subfascial or intramuscular)**
🚑 10.4 ✂ 15.6 **FUD** 090 [J] [A2] [50] ▢
**AMA:** 2017,Jan,8; 2016,Jan,13; 2015,Jan,16; 2014,Mar,4

## 24220 Injection for Elbow Arthrogram

**24220** **Injection procedure for elbow arthrography**
**EXCLUDES** Injection tennis elbow (20550)
▦ (73085)
🚑 1.98 ✂ 4.51 **FUD** 000 [N] [N1] [80] [50] ▢
**AMA:** 2017,Jan,8; 2016,May,13; 2016,Jan,13; 2015,Aug,6

## 24300-24498 Repair/Reconstruction of Elbow/Upper Arm

**24300** **Manipulation, elbow, under anesthesia**
**EXCLUDES** External fixation (20690, 20692)
🚑 11.8 ✂ 11.8 **FUD** 090 [J] [G2] [50] ▢
**AMA:** 2002,Apr,13

**24301** **Muscle or tendon transfer, any type, upper arm or elbow, single (excluding 24320-24331)**
🚑 21.5 ✂ 21.5 **FUD** 090 [J] [A2] [80] ▢
**AMA:** 2002,Apr,13

**24305** **Tendon lengthening, upper arm or elbow, each tendon**
🚑 16.5 ✂ 16.5 **FUD** 090 [J] [A2] [80] ▢
**AMA:** 2002,Apr,13; 1998,Nov,1

**24310** **Tenotomy, open, elbow to shoulder, each tendon**
🚑 13.4 ✂ 13.4 **FUD** 090 [J] [A2] [80] ▢
**AMA:** 2002,Apr,13; 1998,Nov,1

**24320** **Tenoplasty, with muscle transfer, with or without free graft, elbow to shoulder, single (Seddon-Brookes type procedure)**
🚑 21.9 ✂ 21.9 **FUD** 090 [J] [A2] [80] ▢
**AMA:** 2002,Apr,13

**24330** **Flexor-plasty, elbow (eg, Steindler type advancement);**
🚑 20.5 ✂ 20.5 **FUD** 090 [J] [A2] [80] [50] ▢
**AMA:** 2002,Apr,13

**24331** **with extensor advancement**
🚑 22.3 ✂ 22.3 **FUD** 090 [J] [A2] [80] [50] ▢
**AMA:** 2002,Apr,13

**24332** **Tenolysis, triceps**
🚑 17.5 ✂ 17.5 **FUD** 090 [J] [G2] [50] ▢
**AMA:** 2002,Apr,13

**24340** **Tenodesis of biceps tendon at elbow (separate procedure)**
🚑 17.5 ✂ 17.5 **FUD** 090 [J] [A2] [80] [50] ▢
**AMA:** 2002,Apr,13; 1994,Win,1

**24341** **Repair, tendon or muscle, upper arm or elbow, each tendon or muscle, primary or secondary (excludes rotator cuff)**
🚑 21.4 ✂ 21.4 **FUD** 090 [J] [A2] [80] [50] ▢
**AMA:** 2002,Apr,13; 1996,Nov,1

**24342** **Reinsertion of ruptured biceps or triceps tendon, distal, with or without tendon graft**
🚑 22.2 ✂ 22.2 **FUD** 090 [J] [A2] [80] [50] ▢
**AMA:** 2017,Apr,9

**24343** **Repair lateral collateral ligament, elbow, with local tissue**
🚑 20.2 ✂ 20.2 **FUD** 090 [J] [G2] [80] [50] ▢
**AMA:** 2002,Apr,13

**24344** **Reconstruction lateral collateral ligament, elbow, with tendon graft (includes harvesting of graft)**
🚑 31.3 ✂ 31.3 **FUD** 090 [J] [G2] [80] [50] ▢
**AMA:** 2002,Apr,13

**24345** **Repair medial collateral ligament, elbow, with local tissue**
🚑 20.1 ✂ 20.1 **FUD** 090 [J] [A2] [80] [50] ▢
**AMA:** 2002,Apr,13

**24346** **Reconstruction medial collateral ligament, elbow, with tendon graft (includes harvesting of graft)**
🚑 31.5 ✂ 31.5 **FUD** 090 [J] [G2] [80] [50] ▢
**AMA:** 2002,Apr,13

**24357** **Tenotomy, elbow, lateral or medial (eg, epicondylitis, tennis elbow, golfer's elbow); percutaneous**
**EXCLUDES** Arthroscopy, elbow, surgical; debridement (29837-29838)
🚑 12.0 ✂ 12.0 **FUD** 090 [J] [G2] [80] [50] ▢
**AMA:** 2017,Jan,8; 2016,Jan,13; 2015,Jan,16; 2014,Jan,11

**24358** **debridement, soft tissue and/or bone, open**
**EXCLUDES** Arthroscopy, elbow, surgical; debridement (29837-29838)
🚑 14.9 ✂ 14.9 **FUD** 090 [J] [G2] [80] [50] ▢
**AMA:** 2017,Jan,8; 2016,Jan,13; 2015,Jan,16; 2014,Jan,11

**24359** **debridement, soft tissue and/or bone, open with tendon repair or reattachment**
**EXCLUDES** Arthroscopy, elbow, surgical; debridement (29837-29838)
🚑 18.9 ✂ 18.9 **FUD** 090 [J] [G2] [80] [50] ▢
**AMA:** 2017,Jan,8; 2016,Jan,13; 2015,Jan,16; 2014,Jan,11

**24360** **Arthroplasty, elbow; with membrane (eg, fascial)**
🚑 25.8 ✂ 25.8 **FUD** 090 [J] [A2] [80] [50] ▢
**AMA:** 2002,Apr,13; 1998,Nov,1

● New Code ▲ Revised Code ○ Reinstated ● New Web Release ▲ Revised Web Release Unlisted Not Covered # Resequenced
⊘ AMA Mod 51 Exempt ⑤ Optum Mod 51 Exempt ⑥³ Mod 63 Exempt ✗ Non-FDA Drug ★ Telemedicine Ⓜ Maternity ▢ Age Edit + Add-on AMA: CPT Asst
© 2017 Optum360, LLC CPT © 2017 American Medical Association. All Rights Reserved.

**24361** with distal humeral prosthetic replacement
🔧 28.8 ✂ 28.8 **FUD** 090 [J] [J8] [80] [50] [🖳]
**AMA:** 2002,Apr,13

**24362** with implant and fascia lata ligament reconstruction
🔧 30.5 ✂ 30.5 **FUD** 090 [J] [J8] [80] [50] [🖳]
**AMA:** 2002,Apr,13

**24363** with distal humerus and proximal ulnar prosthetic replacement (eg, total elbow)
EXCLUDES Total elbow implant revision (24370-24371)
🔧 41.9 ✂ 41.9 **FUD** 090 [J] [J8] [80] [50] [🖳]
**AMA:** 2017,Jan,8; 2016,Jan,13; 2015,Jan,16; 2014,Jan,11; 2013,Feb,11-12

**24365** Arthroplasty, radial head;
🔧 18.3 ✂ 18.3 **FUD** 090 [J] [J8] [80] [50] [🖳]
**AMA:** 2002,Apr,13

**24366** with implant
🔧 19.5 ✂ 19.5 **FUD** 090 [J] [J8] [80] [50] [🖳]
**AMA:** 2002,Apr,13

**24370** Revision of total elbow arthroplasty, including allograft when performed; humeral or ulnar component
EXCLUDES Prosthesis removal without replacement (eg, humeral and/or ulnar component/s) (24160)
🔧 44.7 ✂ 44.7 **FUD** 090 [J] [J8] [80] [50] [🖳]
**AMA:** 2017,Jan,8; 2016,Jan,13; 2015,Jan,16; 2014,Mar,4; 2013,Feb,11-12

**24371** humeral and ulnar component
EXCLUDES Prosthesis removal without replacement (eg, humeral and/or ulnar component/s) (24160)
🔧 51.4 ✂ 51.4 **FUD** 090 [J] [J8] [80] [50] [🖳]
**AMA:** 2017,Jan,8; 2016,Jan,13; 2015,Jan,16; 2014,Mar,4; 2013,Feb,11-12

**24400** Osteotomy, humerus, with or without internal fixation
🔧 23.5 ✂ 23.5 **FUD** 090 [J] [A2] [80] [50] [🖳]
**AMA:** 2017,Jan,8; 2016,Jan,13; 2015,Jan,16; 2014,Mar,4

**24410** Multiple osteotomies with realignment on intramedullary rod, humeral shaft (Sofield type procedure)
🔧 30.4 ✂ 30.4 **FUD** 090 [J] [G2] [80] [50] [🖳]
**AMA:** 2002,Apr,13

**24420** Osteoplasty, humerus (eg, shortening or lengthening) (excluding 64876)
🔧 28.3 ✂ 28.3 **FUD** 090 [J] [A2] [80] [50] [🖳]
**AMA:** 2002,Apr,13

**24430** Repair of nonunion or malunion, humerus; without graft (eg, compression technique)
🔧 30.4 ✂ 30.4 **FUD** 090 [J] [J8] [80] [50] [🖳]
**AMA:** 2002,Apr,13

**24435** with iliac or other autograft (includes obtaining graft)
🔧 30.9 ✂ 30.9 **FUD** 090 [J] [J8] [80] [50] [🖳]
**AMA:** 2002,Apr,13

**24470** Hemiepiphyseal arrest (eg, cubitus varus or valgus, distal humerus)
🔧 19.2 ✂ 19.2 **FUD** 090 [J] [A2] [80] [50] [🖳]
**AMA:** 2002,Apr,13; 1998,Nov,1

**24495** Decompression fasciotomy, forearm, with brachial artery exploration
🔧 15.3 ✂ 15.3 **FUD** 090 [J] [A2] [80] [50] [🖳]
**AMA:** 2002,Apr,13

**24498** Prophylactic treatment (nailing, pinning, plating or wiring), with or without methylmethacrylate, humeral shaft
🔧 24.8 ✂ 24.8 **FUD** 090 [J] [G2] [80] [50] [🖳]
**AMA:** 2002,Apr,13; 1998,Nov,1

## 24500-24685 Treatment of Fracture/Dislocation of Elbow/Upper Arm

INCLUDES Treatment for either closed or open fractures or dislocations

**24500** Closed treatment of humeral shaft fracture; without manipulation
🔧 9.29 ✂ 10.1 **FUD** 090 [T] [A2] [50] [🖳]
**AMA:** 2002,Apr,13

**24505** with manipulation, with or without skeletal traction
🔧 12.8 ✂ 14.2 **FUD** 090 [J] [A2] [50] [🖳]
**AMA:** 2002,Apr,13

**24515** Open treatment of humeral shaft fracture with plate/screws, with or without cerclage
🔧 25.1 ✂ 25.1 **FUD** 090 [J] [G2] [80] [50] [🖳]
**AMA:** 2002,Apr,13

**24516** Treatment of humeral shaft fracture, with insertion of intramedullary implant, with or without cerclage and/or locking screws
🔧 24.7 ✂ 24.7 **FUD** 090 [J] [G2] [80] [50] [🖳]
**AMA:** 2017,Jan,8; 2016,Jan,13; 2015,Jan,16; 2014,Jan,11

**24530** Closed treatment of supracondylar or transcondylar humeral fracture, with or without intercondylar extension; without manipulation
🔧 9.81 ✂ 10.8 **FUD** 090 [T] [A2] [50] [🖳]
**AMA:** 2002,Apr,13

**24535** with manipulation, with or without skin or skeletal traction
🔧 16.2 ✂ 17.5 **FUD** 090 [J] [A2] [50] [🖳]
**AMA:** 2002,Apr,13

**24538** Percutaneous skeletal fixation of supracondylar or transcondylar humeral fracture, with or without intercondylar extension
🔧 21.3 ✂ 21.3 **FUD** 090 [J] [A2] [50] [🖳]
**AMA:** 2017,Jan,8; 2016,Jan,13; 2015,Jan,16; 2014,Jan,11

**24545** Open treatment of humeral supracondylar or transcondylar fracture, includes internal fixation, when performed; without intercondylar extension
🔧 26.7 ✂ 26.7 **FUD** 090 [J] [J8] [80] [50] [🖳]
**AMA:** 2002,Apr,13

**24546** with intercondylar extension
🔧 29.9 ✂ 29.9 **FUD** 090 [J] [J8] [80] [50] [🖳]
**AMA:** 2002,Apr,13

**24560** Closed treatment of humeral epicondylar fracture, medial or lateral; without manipulation
🔧 8.18 ✂ 9.11 **FUD** 090 [T] [A2] [50] [🖳]
**AMA:** 2002,Apr,13

**24565** with manipulation
🔧 13.9 ✂ 15.1 **FUD** 090 [J] [A2] [50] [🖳]
**AMA:** 2002,Apr,13

**24566** Percutaneous skeletal fixation of humeral epicondylar fracture, medial or lateral, with manipulation
🔧 20.6 ✂ 20.6 **FUD** 090 [J] [A2] [50] [🖳]
**AMA:** 2002,Apr,13; 1993,Win,1

**24575** Open treatment of humeral epicondylar fracture, medial or lateral, includes internal fixation, when performed
🔧 21.0 ✂ 21.0 **FUD** 090 [J] [G2] [80] [50] [🖳]
**AMA:** 2002,Apr,13

**24576** Closed treatment of humeral condylar fracture, medial or lateral; without manipulation
🔧 8.69 ✂ 9.66 **FUD** 090 [T] [A2] [50] [🖳]
**AMA:** 2002,Apr,13

**24577** with manipulation
🔧 14.2 ✂ 15.5 **FUD** 090 [J] [A2] [50] [🖳]
**AMA:** 2002,Apr,13

26/TC PC/TC Only   A2-Z3 ASC Payment   50 Bilateral   ♂ Male Only   ♀ Female Only   🔧 Facility RVU   ✂ Non-Facility RVU   🖳 CCI
FUD Follow-up Days   CMS: IOM (Pub 100)   A-Y OPPSI   80/80 Surg Assist Allowed / w/Doc   ⬛ Lab Crosswalk   ⬛ Radiology Crosswalk   ⬛ CLIA
64   CPT © 2017 American Medical Association. All Rights Reserved.   © 2017 Optum360, LLC

**24579** Open treatment of humeral condylar fracture, medial or lateral, includes internal fixation, when performed

> *EXCLUDES* *Closed treatment without manipulation (24530, 24560, 24576, 24650, 24670)*
> *Repair with manipulation (24535, 24565, 24577, 24675)*

🚲 24.0   ⚕ 24.0   **FUD** 090    [J] [62] [80] [50] [▣]

**AMA:** 2002,Apr,13

**24582** Percutaneous skeletal fixation of humeral condylar fracture, medial or lateral, with manipulation

🚲 23.2   ⚕ 23.2   **FUD** 090    [J] [A2] [50] [▣]

**AMA:** 2002,Apr,13; 1993,Win,1

**24586** Open treatment of periarticular fracture and/or dislocation of the elbow (fracture distal humerus and proximal ulna and/or proximal radius);

🚲 31.1   ⚕ 31.1   **FUD** 090    [J] [G2] [80] [50] [▣]

**AMA:** 2002,Apr,13

**24587** with implant arthroplasty

> *EXCLUDES* *Distal humerus arthroplasty with implant (24361)*

🚲 31.1   ⚕ 31.1   **FUD** 090    [J] [J8] [80] [50] [▣]

**AMA:** 2002,Apr,13

**24600** Treatment of closed elbow dislocation; without anesthesia

🚲 9.49   ⚕ 10.3   **FUD** 090    [T] [A2] [50] [▣]

**AMA:** 2002,Apr,13

**24605** requiring anesthesia

🚲 13.4   ⚕ 13.4   **FUD** 090    [J] [A2] [50] [▣]

**AMA:** 2002,Apr,13

**24615** Open treatment of acute or chronic elbow dislocation

🚲 20.4   ⚕ 20.4   **FUD** 090    [J] [A2] [80] [50] [▣]

**AMA:** 2002,Apr,13

**24620** Closed treatment of Monteggia type of fracture dislocation at elbow (fracture proximal end of ulna with dislocation of radial head), with manipulation

🚲 15.7   ⚕ 15.7   **FUD** 090    [J] [A2] [80] [50] [▣]

**AMA:** 2002,Apr,13

**24635** Open treatment of Monteggia type of fracture dislocation at elbow (fracture proximal end of ulna with dislocation of radial head), includes internal fixation, when performed

🚲 19.3   ⚕ 19.3   **FUD** 090    [J] [A2] [80] [50] [▣]

**AMA:** 2002,Apr,13

**24640** Closed treatment of radial head subluxation in child, nursemaid elbow, with manipulation    [A]

🚲 2.45   ⚕ 3.33   **FUD** 010    [T] [P3] [80] [50] [▣]

**AMA:** 2002,Apr,13

**24650** Closed treatment of radial head or neck fracture; without manipulation

🚲 6.83   ⚕ 7.43   **FUD** 090    [T] [P2] [50] [▣]

**AMA:** 2002,Apr,13

**24655** with manipulation

🚲 11.3   ⚕ 12.4   **FUD** 090    [J] [A2] [50] [▣]

**AMA:** 2002,Apr,13

**24665** Open treatment of radial head or neck fracture, includes internal fixation or radial head excision, when performed;

🚲 18.7   ⚕ 18.7   **FUD** 090    [J] [A2] [80] [50] [▣]

**AMA:** 2002,Apr,13

**24666** with radial head prosthetic replacement

🚲 21.0   ⚕ 21.0   **FUD** 090    [J] [J8] [80] [50] [▣]

**AMA:** 2002,Apr,13

**24670** Closed treatment of ulnar fracture, proximal end (eg, olecranon or coronoid process[es]); without manipulation

🚲 7.47   ⚕ 8.26   **FUD** 090    [T] [A2] [50] [▣]

**AMA:** 2002,Apr,13

**24675** with manipulation

🚲 11.7   ⚕ 12.8   **FUD** 090    [J] [A2] [50] [▣]

**AMA:** 2002,Apr,13

**24685** Open treatment of ulnar fracture, proximal end (eg, olecranon or coronoid process[es]), includes internal fixation, when performed

> *EXCLUDES* *Arthrotomy, elbow (24100-24102)*

🚲 18.7   ⚕ 18.7   **FUD** 090    [J] [A2] [80] [50] [▣]

**AMA:** 2002,Apr,13

## 24800-24999 Other/Unlisted Elbow/Upper Arm Procedures

**24800** Arthrodesis, elbow joint; local

🚲 23.8   ⚕ 23.8   **FUD** 090    [J] [A2] [80] [50] [▣]

**AMA:** 2002,Apr,13; 1998,Nov,1

**24802** with autogenous graft (includes obtaining graft)

🚲 28.3   ⚕ 28.3   **FUD** 090    [J] [G2] [80] [50] [▣]

**AMA:** 2002,Apr,13; 1998,Nov,1

**24900** Amputation, arm through humerus; with primary closure

🚲 21.0   ⚕ 21.0   **FUD** 090    [C] [80] [50] [▣]

**AMA:** 2002,Apr,13

**24920** open, circular (guillotine)

🚲 20.7   ⚕ 20.7   **FUD** 090    [C] [80] [50] [▣]

**AMA:** 2002,Apr,13

**24925** secondary closure or scar revision

🚲 14.9   ⚕ 14.9   **FUD** 090    [J] [A2] [80] [50] [▣]

**AMA:** 2002,Apr,13

**24930** re-amputation

🚲 21.8   ⚕ 21.8   **FUD** 090    [C] [80] [50] [▣]

**AMA:** 2002,Apr,13

**24931** with implant

🚲 23.0   ⚕ 23.0   **FUD** 090    [C] [80] [50] [▣]

**AMA:** 2002,Apr,13

**24935** Stump elongation, upper extremity

🚲 27.9   ⚕ 27.9   **FUD** 090    [J] [80] [50] [▣]

**AMA:** 2002,Apr,13

**24940** Cineplasty, upper extremity, complete procedure

🚲 0.00   ⚕ 0.00   **FUD** 090    [C] [80] [50] [▣]

**AMA:** 2002,Apr,13

**24999** Unlisted procedure, humerus or elbow

🚲 0.00   ⚕ 0.00   **FUD** YYY    [T] [80] [50]

**AMA:** 2002,Apr,13

## 25000-25001 Incision Tendon Sheath of Wrist

**25000** Incision, extensor tendon sheath, wrist (eg, deQuervains disease)

> *EXCLUDES* *Carpal tunnel release (64721)*

🚲 9.61   ⚕ 9.61   **FUD** 090    [J] [A2] [50] [▣]

**AMA:** 2002,Apr,13; 1998,Nov,1

**25001** Incision, flexor tendon sheath, wrist (eg, flexor carpi radialis)

🚲 9.82   ⚕ 9.82   **FUD** 090    [J] [G2] [50] [▣]

**AMA:** 2002,Apr,13

## 25020-25025 Decompression Fasciotomy Forearm/Wrist

**25020** Decompression fasciotomy, forearm and/or wrist, flexor OR extensor compartment; without debridement of nonviable muscle and/or nerve

> *EXCLUDES* *Brachial artery exploration (24495)*
> *Superficial incision and drainage (10060-10160)*

🚲 16.4   ⚕ 16.4   **FUD** 090    [J] [A2] [50] [▣]

**AMA:** 2002,Apr,13

**25023** with debridement of nonviable muscle and/or nerve

> *EXCLUDES* *Debridement (11000-11044 [11045, 11046])*
> *Decompression fasciotomy with exploration brachial artery exploration (24495)*
> *Superficial incision and drainage (10060-10160)*

🚲 31.5   ⚕ 31.5   **FUD** 090    [J] [A2] [80] [50] [▣]

**AMA:** 2002,Apr,13

---

● New Code     ▲ Revised Code     ○ Reinstated     ● New Web Release     ▲ Revised Web Release     Unlisted     Not Covered     # Resequenced
⊘ AMA Mod 51 Exempt     ⑨ Optum Mod 51 Exempt     ⑥³ Mod 63 Exempt     ✗ Non-FDA Drug     ★ Telemedicine     Ⓜ Maternity     🄰 Age Edit     ✚ Add-on     AMA: CPT Asst

**Musculoskeletal System** *(side tab)*

**25024 — 25115** *(side tab)*

**25024**   **Decompression fasciotomy, forearm and/or wrist, flexor AND extensor compartment; without debridement of nonviable muscle and/or nerve**
     🖭 22.2   ⚕ 22.2   **FUD** 090      J A2 50 ▢
     **AMA:** 2002,Apr,13

**25025**   **with debridement of nonviable muscle and/or nerve**
     🖭 35.2   ⚕ 35.2   **FUD** 090      J A2 80 50 ▢
     **AMA:** 2002,Apr,13

## 25028-25040 Incision for Drainage/Foreign Body Removal

**25028**   **Incision and drainage, forearm and/or wrist; deep abscess or hematoma**
     🖭 14.9   ⚕ 14.9   **FUD** 090      J A2 50 ▢
     **AMA:** 2002,Apr,13

**25031**   **bursa**
     🖭 10.3   ⚕ 10.3   **FUD** 090      J A2 80 50 ▢
     **AMA:** 2002,Apr,13; 1998,Nov,1

**25035**   **Incision, deep, bone cortex, forearm and/or wrist (eg, osteomyelitis or bone abscess)**
     🖭 16.7   ⚕ 16.7   **FUD** 090      J A2 80 50 ▢
     **AMA:** 2002,Apr,13; 1998,Nov,1

**25040**   **Arthrotomy, radiocarpal or midcarpal joint, with exploration, drainage, or removal of foreign body**
     🖭 16.1   ⚕ 16.1   **FUD** 090      J A2 80 50 ▢
     **AMA:** 2002,Apr,13; 1994,Win,1

## 25065-25066 Biopsy Forearm/Wrist

**EXCLUDES** *Soft tissue needle biopsy (20206)*

**25065**   **Biopsy, soft tissue of forearm and/or wrist; superficial**
     🖭 4.69   ⚕ 7.22   **FUD** 010      J P3 50 ▢
     **AMA:** 2002,Apr,13

**25066**   **deep (subfascial or intramuscular)**
     🖭 10.3   ⚕ 10.3   **FUD** 090      J A2 50 ▢
     **AMA:** 2002,Apr,13; 1998,Nov,1

## 25071-25078 [25071, 25073] Excision Soft Tissue Tumors Forearm/Wrist

**INCLUDES** Any necessary elevation of tissue planes or dissection
     Measurement of tumor and necessary margin at greatest diameter prior to excision
     Simple and intermediate repairs
     Types of excision:
         Fascial or subfascial soft tissue tumors: simple and marginal resection of tumors found either in or below the deep fascia, not involving bone or excision of a substantial amount of normal tissue; primarily benign and intramuscular tumors
         Radical resection soft tissue tumor: wide resection of tumor involving substantial margins of normal tissue and may include tissue removal from one or more layers; most often malignant or aggressive benign
         Subcutaneous: simple and marginal resection of tumors in the subcutaneous tissue above the deep fascia; most often benign

**EXCLUDES** *Complex repair*
     *Excision of benign cutaneous lesions (eg, sebaceous cyst) (11400-11406)*
     *Radical resection of cutaneous tumors (eg, melanoma) (11600-11606)*
     *Significant exploration of vessels or neuroplasty*

**25071**   **Resequenced code. See code following 25075.**

**25073**   **Resequenced code. See code following 25076.**

**25075**   **Excision, tumor, soft tissue of forearm and/or wrist area, subcutaneous; less than 3 cm**
     🖭 9.08   ⚕ 13.6   **FUD** 090      J G2 50 ▢
     **AMA:** 2002,Apr,13

\#   **25071**   **3 cm or greater**
     🖭 12.2   ⚕ 12.2   **FUD** 090      J G2 80 50 ▢

**25076**   **Excision, tumor, soft tissue of forearm and/or wrist area, subfascial (eg, intramuscular); less than 3 cm**
     🖭 14.8   ⚕ 14.8   **FUD** 090      J G2 50 ▢
     **AMA:** 2002,Apr,13

\#   **25073**   **3 cm or greater**
     🖭 15.3   ⚕ 15.3   **FUD** 090      J G2 80 50 ▢

**25077**   **Radical resection of tumor (eg, sarcoma), soft tissue of forearm and/or wrist area; less than 3 cm**
     🖭 25.6   ⚕ 25.6   **FUD** 090      J G2 50 ▢
     **AMA:** 2002,Apr,13; 1990,Win,4

**25078**   **3 cm or greater**
     🖭 33.5   ⚕ 33.5   **FUD** 090      J G2 80 50 ▢

## 25085-25240 Procedures of Bones/Joints Lower Arm/Wrist

**25085**   **Capsulotomy, wrist (eg, contracture)**
     🖭 12.8   ⚕ 12.8   **FUD** 090      J A2 80 50 ▢
     **AMA:** 2002,Apr,13; 1998,Nov,1

**25100**   **Arthrotomy, wrist joint; with biopsy**
     🖭 9.65   ⚕ 9.65   **FUD** 090      J A2 80 50 ▢
     **AMA:** 2002,Apr,13; 2000,Dec,12

**25101**   **with joint exploration, with or without biopsy, with or without removal of loose or foreign body**
     🖭 11.5   ⚕ 11.5   **FUD** 090      J A2 80 50 ▢
     **AMA:** 2002,Apr,13

**25105**   **with synovectomy**
     🖭 13.8   ⚕ 13.8   **FUD** 090      J A2 80 50 ▢
     **AMA:** 2002,Apr,13; 2000,Dec,12

**25107**   **Arthrotomy, distal radioulnar joint including repair of triangular cartilage, complex**
     🖭 17.6   ⚕ 17.6   **FUD** 090      J A2 80 50 ▢
     **AMA:** 2002,Apr,13; 1998,Nov,1

**25109**   **Excision of tendon, forearm and/or wrist, flexor or extensor, each**
     🖭 15.4   ⚕ 15.4   **FUD** 090      J G2 50 ▢

**25110**   **Excision, lesion of tendon sheath, forearm and/or wrist**
     🖭 9.77   ⚕ 9.77   **FUD** 090      J A2 50 ▢
     **AMA:** 2002,Apr,13

**25111**   **Excision of ganglion, wrist (dorsal or volar); primary**
     **EXCLUDES** *Excision of ganglion hand or finger (26160)*
     🖭 9.16   ⚕ 9.16   **FUD** 090      J A2 50 ▢
     **AMA:** 2002,Apr,13

Synovial sheaths (blue) of the dorsum of right wrist, containing extensor tendons

Ganglion

Anatomical "snuffbox"

Anatomical "snuffbox"

Ganglions are round cystic swellings usually appearing on the dorsum of the wrist or hand; these swellings often communicate with the synovial sheath

Typical location of ganglion

**25112**   **recurrent**
     **EXCLUDES** *Excision of ganglion hand or finger (26160)*
     🖭 11.0   ⚕ 11.0   **FUD** 090      J A2 50 ▢
     **AMA:** 2002,Apr,13

**25115**   **Radical excision of bursa, synovia of wrist, or forearm tendon sheaths (eg, tenosynovitis, fungus, Tbc, or other granulomas, rheumatoid arthritis); flexors**
     **EXCLUDES** *Finger synovectomy (26145)*
     🖭 21.7   ⚕ 21.7   **FUD** 090      J A2 50 ▢
     **AMA:** 2017,Jan,8; 2016,Jan,13; 2015,Jan,16; 2012,Jun,15-16

| | | | | | |
|---|---|---|---|---|---|
| **26/TC** PC/TC Only | A2-Z3 ASC Payment | 50 Bilateral | ♂ Male Only | ♀ Female Only | 🖭 Facility RVU | ⚕ Non-Facility RVU | ▢ CCI |
| **FUD** Follow-up Days | **CMS:** IOM (Pub 100) | A-Y OPPSI | 80/80 Surg Assist Allowed / w/Doc | | 🔬 Lab Crosswalk | 🩻 Radiology Crosswalk | ✖ CLIA |

**66**                CPT © 2017 American Medical Association. All Rights Reserved.                © 2017 Optum360, LLC

**25116**     extensors, with or without transposition of dorsal retinaculum

     EXCLUDES   *Finger synovectomy (26145)*
     🚑 17.1   ⚖ 17.1   **FUD** 090     J A2 80 50 ▣
     **AMA:** 2002,Apr,13

**25118**     Synovectomy, extensor tendon sheath, wrist, single compartment;

     EXCLUDES   *Finger synovectomy (26145)*
     🚑 10.9   ⚖ 10.9   **FUD** 090     J A2 50 ▣
     **AMA:** 2017,Jan,8; 2016,Jan,13; 2015,Jun,10; 2015,Jan,16; 2014,Jan,11; 2012,Apr,17-18

**25119**     with resection of distal ulna

     EXCLUDES   *Finger synovectomy (26145)*
     🚑 14.1   ⚖ 14.1   **FUD** 090     J A2 80 50 ▣
     **AMA:** 2002,Apr,13

**25120**     Excision or curettage of bone cyst or benign tumor of radius or ulna (excluding head or neck of radius and olecranon process);

     EXCLUDES   *Removal of bone cyst or tumor of radial head, neck, or olecranon process (24120-24126)*
     🚑 14.2   ⚖ 14.2   **FUD** 090     J A2 80 50 ▣
     **AMA:** 2002,Apr,13

**25125**     with autograft (includes obtaining graft)

     🚑 16.8   ⚖ 16.8   **FUD** 090     J A2 80 50 ▣
     **AMA:** 2002,Apr,13

**25126**     with allograft

     🚑 16.8   ⚖ 16.8   **FUD** 090     J A2 80 50 ▣
     **AMA:** 2002,Apr,13

**25130**     Excision or curettage of bone cyst or benign tumor of carpal bones;

     🚑 12.7   ⚖ 12.7   **FUD** 090     J A2 80 50 ▣
     **AMA:** 2002,Apr,13

**25135**     with autograft (includes obtaining graft)

     🚑 16.0   ⚖ 16.0   **FUD** 090     J A2 80 50 ▣
     **AMA:** 2002,Apr,13

**25136**     with allograft

     🚑 13.8   ⚖ 13.8   **FUD** 090     J A2 80 50 ▣
     **AMA:** 2002,Apr,13

**25145**     Sequestrectomy (eg, for osteomyelitis or bone abscess), forearm and/or wrist

     🚑 14.8   ⚖ 14.8   **FUD** 090     J A2 80 50 ▣
     **AMA:** 2002,Apr,13

**25150**     Partial excision (craterization, saucerization, or diaphysectomy) of bone (eg, for osteomyelitis); ulna

     🚑 16.1   ⚖ 16.1   **FUD** 090     J A2 50 ▣
     **AMA:** 2002,Apr,13

**25151**     radius

     EXCLUDES   *Partial removal of radial head, neck, or olecranon process (24145, 24147)*
     🚑 16.7   ⚖ 16.7   **FUD** 090     J A2 80 50 ▣
     **AMA:** 2002,Apr,13

**25170**     Radical resection of tumor, radius or ulna

     INCLUDES   Any necessary elevation of tissue planes or dissection
         Excision of adjacent soft tissue during bone tumor resection (25071-25078 [25071, 25073])
         Measurement of tumor and necessary margin at greatest diameter prior to excision
         Resection of the tumor (may include entire bone) and wide margins of normal tissue primarily for malignant or aggressive benign tumors
         Resection without removal of significant normal tissue
         Simple and intermediate repairs
     EXCLUDES   *Complex repair*
         *Excision of adjacent soft tissue during bone tumor resection (25076-25078 [25073])*
         *Radical resection of cutaneous tumors (e.g., melanoma) (11600-11646)*
         *Significant exploration of vessels, neuroplasty, reconstruction, or complex bone repair*
     🚑 42.6   ⚖ 42.6   **FUD** 090     J 80 50 ▣
     **AMA:** 2003,Jan,1; 2002,Apr,13

**25210**     Carpectomy; 1 bone

     EXCLUDES   *Carpectomy with insertion of implant (25441-25445)*
     🚑 13.9   ⚖ 13.9   **FUD** 090     J A2 80 ▣
     **AMA:** 2002,Apr,13

**25215**     all bones of proximal row

     🚑 17.7   ⚖ 17.7   **FUD** 090     J A2 80 50 ▣
     **AMA:** 2002,Apr,13

**25230**     Radial styloidectomy (separate procedure)

     🚑 12.3   ⚖ 12.3   **FUD** 090     J A2 50 ▣
     **AMA:** 2002,Apr,13

**25240**     Excision distal ulna partial or complete (eg, Darrach type or matched resection)

     EXCLUDES   *Acquisition of fascia for interposition (20920, 20922)*
         *Implant replacement (25442)*
     🚑 12.2   ⚖ 12.2   **FUD** 090     J A2 80 50 ▣
     **AMA:** 2002,Apr,13; 1994,Win,1

## 25246 Injection for Wrist Arthrogram

**25246**     Injection procedure for wrist arthrography

     EXCLUDES   *Excision of superficial foreign body (20520)*
     ▦ (73115)
     🚑 2.17   ⚖ 4.59   **FUD** 000     N N1 50 ▣
     **AMA:** 2017,Jan,8; 2016,Jan,13; 2015,Aug,6

## 25248-25251 Removal Foreign Body of Wrist

EXCLUDES   *Excision of superficial foreign body (20520)*
     *K-wire, pin, or rod insertion (20650)*
     *K-wire, pin, or rod removal (20670, 20680)*

**25248**     Exploration with removal of deep foreign body, forearm or wrist

     🚑 11.7   ⚖ 11.7   **FUD** 090     J A2 50 ▣
     **AMA:** 2002,Apr,13; 1994,Win,1

**25250**     Removal of wrist prosthesis; (separate procedure)

     🚑 15.2   ⚖ 15.2   **FUD** 090     02 A2 80 50 ▣
     **AMA:** 2002,Apr,13

**25251**     complicated, including total wrist

     🚑 20.6   ⚖ 20.6   **FUD** 090     02 A2 80 50 ▣
     **AMA:** 2002,Apr,13

## 25259 Manipulation of Wrist with Anesthesia

**25259**     Manipulation, wrist, under anesthesia

     EXCLUDES   *Application external fixation (20690, 20692)*
     🚑 11.8   ⚖ 11.8   **FUD** 090     J 62 50 ▣
     **AMA:** 2017,Jan,8; 2016,Jan,13; 2015,Jan,16; 2014,Jan,11; 2012,Jan,15-42

## 25260-25492 Repair/Reconstruction of Forearm/Wrist

**25260**     Repair, tendon or muscle, flexor, forearm and/or wrist; primary, single, each tendon or muscle

     🚑 18.0   ⚖ 18.0   **FUD** 090     J A2 ▣
     **AMA:** 2002,Apr,13; 1996,Nov,1

● New Code    ▲ Revised Code    ○ Reinstated    ● New Web Release    ▲ Revised Web Release    Unlisted    Not Covered    # Resequenced
⊘ AMA Mod 51 Exempt    ⑨ Optum Mod 51 Exempt    ⑥⑨ Mod 63 Exempt    ⋌ Non-FDA Drug    ★ Telemedicine    M Maternity    A Age Edit    ✚ Add-on    **AMA:** CPT Asst
© 2017 Optum360, LLC      CPT © 2017 American Medical Association. All Rights Reserved.

**Musculoskeletal System**

**25263 — 25420**

**25263**    secondary, single, each tendon or muscle
      🔧 17.8   ✂ 17.8   **FUD** 090      J A2 80 ▭
      **AMA:** 2002,Apr,13; 1996,Nov,1

**25265**    secondary, with free graft (includes obtaining graft), each tendon or muscle
      🔧 21.4   ✂ 21.4   **FUD** 090      J A2 80 ▭
      **AMA:** 2002,Apr,13; 1996,Nov,1

**25270**    Repair, tendon or muscle, extensor, forearm and/or wrist; primary, single, each tendon or muscle
      🔧 14.0   ✂ 14.0   **FUD** 090      J A2 80 ▭
      **AMA:** 2002,Apr,13; 1996,Nov,1

**25272**    secondary, single, each tendon or muscle
      🔧 15.8   ✂ 15.8   **FUD** 090      J A2 80 ▭
      **AMA:** 2002,Apr,13; 1996,Nov,1

**25274**    secondary, with free graft (includes obtaining graft), each tendon or muscle
      🔧 18.9   ✂ 18.9   **FUD** 090      J A2 80 ▭
      **AMA:** 2002,Apr,13; 1996,Nov,1

**25275**    Repair, tendon sheath, extensor, forearm and/or wrist, with free graft (includes obtaining graft) (eg, for extensor carpi ulnaris subluxation)
      🔧 19.2   ✂ 19.2   **FUD** 090      J A2 80 50 ▭
      **AMA:** 2002,Apr,13

**25280**    Lengthening or shortening of flexor or extensor tendon, forearm and/or wrist, single, each tendon
      🔧 16.1   ✂ 16.1   **FUD** 090      J A2 80 ▭
      **AMA:** 2002,Apr,13

**25290**    Tenotomy, open, flexor or extensor tendon, forearm and/or wrist, single, each tendon
      🔧 12.4   ✂ 12.4   **FUD** 090      J A2 ▭
      **AMA:** 2002,Apr,13

**25295**    Tenolysis, flexor or extensor tendon, forearm and/or wrist, single, each tendon
      🔧 15.0   ✂ 15.0   **FUD** 090      J A2 ▭
      **AMA:** 2017,Jan,8; 2016,Jan,13; 2015,Jan,16; 2014,Jan,11; 2012,Jan,15-42

**25300**    Tenodesis at wrist; flexors of fingers
      🔧 19.5   ✂ 19.5   **FUD** 090      J A2 80 50 ▭
      **AMA:** 2002,Apr,13

**25301**    extensors of fingers
      🔧 18.4   ✂ 18.4   **FUD** 090      J A2 80 50 ▭
      **AMA:** 2002,Apr,13

**25310**    Tendon transplantation or transfer, flexor or extensor, forearm and/or wrist, single; each tendon
      🔧 17.7   ✂ 17.7   **FUD** 090      J A2 80 ▭
      **AMA:** 2017,Jan,8; 2016,Jan,13; 2015,Jan,16; 2014,Jan,11; 2012,Jan,15-42

**25312**    with tendon graft(s) (includes obtaining graft), each tendon
      🔧 20.5   ✂ 20.5   **FUD** 090      J A2 80 ▭
      **AMA:** 2002,Apr,13

**25315**    Flexor origin slide (eg, for cerebral palsy, Volkmann contracture), forearm and/or wrist;
      🔧 22.1   ✂ 22.1   **FUD** 090      J A2 80 50 ▭
      **AMA:** 2002,Apr,13; 1994,Win,1

**25316**    with tendon(s) transfer
      🔧 26.1   ✂ 26.1   **FUD** 090      J A2 80 50 ▭
      **AMA:** 2002,Apr,13; 1994,Win,1

**25320**    Capsulorrhaphy or reconstruction, wrist, open (eg, capsulodesis, ligament repair, tendon transfer or graft) (includes synovectomy, capsulotomy and open reduction) for carpal instability
      🔧 28.3   ✂ 28.3   **FUD** 090      J A2 80 50 ▭
      **AMA:** 2002,Apr,13; 1994,Win,1

**25332**    Arthroplasty, wrist, with or without interposition, with or without external or internal fixation
      *EXCLUDES*   *Acquiring fascia for interposition (20920, 20922)*
                *Arthroplasty with prosthesis (25441-25446)*
      🔧 24.1   ✂ 24.1   **FUD** 090      J A2 80 50 ▭
      **AMA:** 2017,Jan,8; 2016,Jan,13; 2015,Jan,16; 2014,Jan,11

**25335**    Centralization of wrist on ulna (eg, radial club hand)
      🔧 27.1   ✂ 27.1   **FUD** 090      J A2 80 50 ▭
      **AMA:** 2002,Apr,13

**25337**    Reconstruction for stabilization of unstable distal ulna or distal radioulnar joint, secondary by soft tissue stabilization (eg, tendon transfer, tendon graft or weave, or tenodesis) with or without open reduction of distal radioulnar joint
      *EXCLUDES*   *Acquiring fascia lata graft (20920, 20922)*
      🔧 25.5   ✂ 25.5   **FUD** 090      J A2 50 ▭
      **AMA:** 2002,Apr,13; 1994,Win,1

**25350**    Osteotomy, radius; distal third
      🔧 19.3   ✂ 19.3   **FUD** 090      J J8 80 50 ▭
      **AMA:** 2002,Apr,13

**25355**    middle or proximal third
      🔧 21.8   ✂ 21.8   **FUD** 090      J A2 80 50 ▭
      **AMA:** 2002,Apr,13

**25360**    Osteotomy; ulna
      🔧 18.7   ✂ 18.7   **FUD** 090      J A2 80 50 ▭
      **AMA:** 2002,Apr,13

**25365**    radius AND ulna
      🔧 26.3   ✂ 26.3   **FUD** 090      J A2 80 50 ▭
      **AMA:** 2002,Apr,13

**25370**    Multiple osteotomies, with realignment on intramedullary rod (Sofield type procedure); radius OR ulna
      🔧 28.9   ✂ 28.9   **FUD** 090      J A2 80 ▭
      **AMA:** 2002,Apr,13

**25375**    radius AND ulna
      🔧 27.4   ✂ 27.4   **FUD** 090      J A2 80 50 ▭
      **AMA:** 2002,Apr,13

**25390**    Osteoplasty, radius OR ulna; shortening
      🔧 22.1   ✂ 22.1   **FUD** 090      J A2 80 50 ▭
      **AMA:** 2003,Jan,1; 2002,Apr,13

**25391**    lengthening with autograft
      🔧 28.6   ✂ 28.6   **FUD** 090      J J8 80 50 ▭
      **AMA:** 2003,Jan,1; 2002,Apr,13

**25392**    Osteoplasty, radius AND ulna; shortening (excluding 64876)
      🔧 29.3   ✂ 29.3   **FUD** 090      J A2 80 50 ▭
      **AMA:** 2003,Jan,1; 2002,Apr,13

**25393**    lengthening with autograft
      🔧 32.2   ✂ 32.2   **FUD** 090      J A2 80 50 ▭
      **AMA:** 2003,Jan,1; 2002,Apr,13

**25394**    Osteoplasty, carpal bone, shortening
      🔧 22.5   ✂ 22.5   **FUD** 090      J G2 80 50 ▭
      **AMA:** 2002,Apr,13

**25400**    Repair of nonunion or malunion, radius OR ulna; without graft (eg, compression technique)
      🔧 23.0   ✂ 23.0   **FUD** 090      J A2 80 50 ▭
      **AMA:** 2002,Apr,13

**25405**    with autograft (includes obtaining graft)
      🔧 29.8   ✂ 29.8   **FUD** 090      J A2 80 50 ▭
      **AMA:** 2002,Apr,13

**25415**    Repair of nonunion or malunion, radius AND ulna; without graft (eg, compression technique)
      🔧 27.8   ✂ 27.8   **FUD** 090      J A2 80 50 ▭
      **AMA:** 2002,Apr,13

**25420**    with autograft (includes obtaining graft)
      🔧 33.4   ✂ 33.4   **FUD** 090      J J8 80 50 ▭
      **AMA:** 2003,Jan,1; 2002,Apr,13

26/TC PC/TC Only    A2-Z3 ASC Payment    50 Bilateral    ♂ Male Only    ♀ Female Only    🔧 Facility RVU    ✂ Non-Facility RVU    ▭ CCI
**FUD** Follow-up Days    **CMS:** IOM (Pub 100)    A-Y OPPSI    80/80 Surg Assist Allowed / w/Doc    Lab Crosswalk    Radiology Crosswalk    ❌ CLIA

**68**                     CPT © 2017 American Medical Association. All Rights Reserved.           © 2017 Optum360, LLC

**25425** Repair of defect with autograft; radius OR ulna
🔧 27.6 ⚕ 27.6 **FUD** 090 J J8 80 50 ▣
**AMA:** 2002,Apr,13

**25426** radius AND ulna
🔧 31.4 ⚕ 31.4 **FUD** 090 J J8 80 50 ▣
**AMA:** 2002,Apr,13

**25430** Insertion of vascular pedicle into carpal bone (eg, Hori procedure)
🔧 21.0 ⚕ 21.0 **FUD** 090 J G2 50 ▣
**AMA:** 2002,Apr,13

**25431** Repair of nonunion of carpal bone (excluding carpal scaphoid (navicular)) (includes obtaining graft and necessary fixation), each bone
🔧 22.6 ⚕ 22.6 **FUD** 090 J G2 80 50 ▣
**AMA:** 2002,Apr,13

**25440** Repair of nonunion, scaphoid carpal (navicular) bone, with or without radial styloidectomy (includes obtaining graft and necessary fixation)
🔧 22.0 ⚕ 22.0 **FUD** 090 J A2 80 50 ▣
**AMA:** 2002,May,7; 2002,Apr,13

**25441** Arthroplasty with prosthetic replacement; distal radius
🔧 26.8 ⚕ 26.8 **FUD** 090 J J8 80 50 ▣
**AMA:** 2017,Aug,9; 2017,Jan,8; 2016,Jan,13; 2015,Jan,16; 2014,Jan,11

**25442** distal ulna
🔧 23.1 ⚕ 23.1 **FUD** 090 J J8 80 50 ▣
**AMA:** 2017,Aug,9; 2017,Jan,8; 2016,Jan,13; 2015,Jan,16; 2014,Jan,11

**25443** scaphoid carpal (navicular)
🔧 22.2 ⚕ 22.2 **FUD** 090 J J8 80 50 ▣
**AMA:** 2017,Jan,8; 2016,Jan,13; 2015,Jan,16; 2014,Jan,11

**25444** lunate
🔧 23.4 ⚕ 23.4 **FUD** 090 J J8 80 50 ▣
**AMA:** 2017,Jan,8; 2016,Jan,13; 2015,Jan,16; 2014,Jan,11

**25445** trapezium
🔧 20.7 ⚕ 20.7 **FUD** 090 J J8 50 ▣
**AMA:** 2017,Jan,8; 2016,Jan,13; 2015,Jan,16; 2014,Jan,11

**25446** distal radius and partial or entire carpus (total wrist)
🔧 33.7 ⚕ 33.7 **FUD** 090 J J8 80 50 ▣
**AMA:** 2017,Jan,8; 2016,Jan,13; 2015,Jan,16; 2014,Jan,11

**25447** Arthroplasty, interposition, intercarpal or carpometacarpal joints
    *EXCLUDES* Wrist arthroplasty (25332)
🔧 23.7 ⚕ 23.7 **FUD** 090 J A2 80 50 ▣
**AMA:** 2017,Jan,8; 2016,Jan,13; 2015,Jan,16; 2014,Jan,11

**25449** Revision of arthroplasty, including removal of implant, wrist joint
🔧 29.6 ⚕ 29.6 **FUD** 090 J A2 80 50 ▣
**AMA:** 2002,Apr,13

**25450** Epiphyseal arrest by epiphysiodesis or stapling; distal radius OR ulna
🔧 14.8 ⚕ 14.8 **FUD** 090 J A2 50 ▣
**AMA:** 2002,Apr,13

**25455** distal radius AND ulna
🔧 20.8 ⚕ 20.8 **FUD** 090 J A2 50 ▣
**AMA:** 2002,Apr,13

**25490** Prophylactic treatment (nailing, pinning, plating or wiring) with or without methylmethacrylate; radius
🔧 20.6 ⚕ 20.6 **FUD** 090 J A2 80 50 ▣
**AMA:** 2002,Apr,13

**25491** ulna
🔧 21.2 ⚕ 21.2 **FUD** 090 J A2 80 50 ▣
**AMA:** 2002,Apr,13

**25492** radius AND ulna
🔧 26.0 ⚕ 26.0 **FUD** 090 J A2 80 50 ▣
**AMA:** 2002,Apr,13

## 25500-25695 Treatment of Fracture/Dislocation of Forearm/Wrist
Code also external fixation (20690)

**25500** Closed treatment of radial shaft fracture; without manipulation
🔧 7.14 ⚕ 7.77 **FUD** 090 T P2 50 ▣
**AMA:** 2002,Apr,13

**25505** with manipulation
🔧 13.0 ⚕ 14.2 **FUD** 090 J A2 50 ▣
**AMA:** 2003,May,7; 2002,Apr,13

**25515** Open treatment of radial shaft fracture, includes internal fixation, when performed
🔧 19.1 ⚕ 19.1 **FUD** 090 J A2 80 50 ▣
**AMA:** 2002,Apr,13

**25520** Closed treatment of radial shaft fracture and closed treatment of dislocation of distal radioulnar joint (Galeazzi fracture/dislocation)
🔧 15.3 ⚕ 16.1 **FUD** 090 J A2 50 ▣
**AMA:** 2002,Apr,13

**25525** Open treatment of radial shaft fracture, includes internal fixation, when performed, and closed treatment of distal radioulnar joint dislocation (Galeazzi fracture/ dislocation), includes percutaneous skeletal fixation, when performed
🔧 22.5 ⚕ 22.5 **FUD** 090 J A2 80 50 ▣
**AMA:** 2002,Apr,13

**25526** Open treatment of radial shaft fracture, includes internal fixation, when performed, and open treatment of distal radioulnar joint dislocation (Galeazzi fracture/ dislocation), includes internal fixation, when performed, includes repair of triangular fibrocartilage complex
🔧 27.3 ⚕ 27.3 **FUD** 090 J A2 80 50 ▣
**AMA:** 2002,Apr,13

**25530** Closed treatment of ulnar shaft fracture; without manipulation
🔧 6.75 ⚕ 7.44 **FUD** 090 T P2 50 ▣
**AMA:** 2002,Apr,13

**25535** with manipulation
🔧 12.8 ⚕ 13.9 **FUD** 090 T A2 50 ▣
**AMA:** 2010,Sep,6-7; 2002,Apr,13

**25545** Open treatment of ulnar shaft fracture, includes internal fixation, when performed
🔧 17.8 ⚕ 17.8 **FUD** 090 J A2 80 50 ▣
**AMA:** 2017,Jan,8; 2016,Jan,13; 2015,Jan,16; 2014,Jan,11

**25560** Closed treatment of radial and ulnar shaft fractures; without manipulation
🔧 7.15 ⚕ 7.89 **FUD** 090 T P2 50 ▣
**AMA:** 2002,Apr,13

**25565** with manipulation
🔧 13.3 ⚕ 14.7 **FUD** 090 J A2 50 ▣
**AMA:** 2002,Apr,13

**25574** Open treatment of radial AND ulnar shaft fractures, with internal fixation, when performed; of radius OR ulna
🔧 19.3 ⚕ 19.3 **FUD** 090 J A2 80 50 ▣
**AMA:** 2017,Jan,8; 2016,Jan,13; 2015,Jan,16; 2014,Jan,11

**25575** of radius AND ulna
🔧 25.8 ⚕ 25.8 **FUD** 090 J G2 80 50 ▣
**AMA:** 2002,Apr,13

**25600** Closed treatment of distal radial fracture (eg, Colles or Smith type) or epiphyseal separation, includes closed treatment of fracture of ulnar styloid, when performed; without manipulation
    *INCLUDES* Closed treatment of ulnar styloid fracture (25650)
🔧 8.82 ⚕ 9.32 **FUD** 090 T P2 50 ▣
**AMA:** 2017,Jan,8; 2016,Jan,13; 2015,Jan,16; 2014,Jan,11; 2013,Apr,10-11

---

● New Code ▲ Revised Code ○ Reinstated ● New Web Release ▲ Revised Web Release Unlisted Not Covered # Resequenced
⊘ AMA Mod 51 Exempt ⑤ Optum Mod 51 Exempt ⑥ Mod 63 Exempt ✗ Non-FDA Drug ★ Telemedicine Ⅿ Maternity ⚠ Age Edit + Add-on AMA: CPT Asst
© 2017 Optum360, LLC    CPT © 2017 American Medical Association. All Rights Reserved.

**25605** **with manipulation**
INCLUDES Closed treatment of ulnar styloid fracture (25650)
14.5  15.4  **FUD** 090  J A2 50
AMA: 2017,Jan,8; 2016,Jan,13; 2015,Jan,16; 2014,Jan,11; 2013,Apr,10-11

**25606** **Percutaneous skeletal fixation of distal radial fracture or epiphyseal separation**
EXCLUDES Closed treatment of ulnar styloid fracture (25650)
Open repair of ulnar styloid fracture (25652)
Percutaneous repair of ulnar styloid fracture (25651)
19.0  19.0  **FUD** 090  J A2 50
AMA: 2007,Oct,7-10

**25607** **Open treatment of distal radial extra-articular fracture or epiphyseal separation, with internal fixation**
EXCLUDES Closed treatment of ulnar styloid fracture (25650)
Open repair of ulnar styloid fracture (25652)
Percutaneous repair of ulnar styloid fracture (25651)
21.0  21.0  **FUD** 090  J J8 80 50
AMA: 2017,Jan,8; 2016,Jan,13; 2015,Jan,16; 2014,Jan,11; 2012,Nov,13-14

**25608** **Open treatment of distal radial intra-articular fracture or epiphyseal separation; with internal fixation of 2 fragments**
EXCLUDES Closed treatment of ulnar styloid fracture (25650)
Open repair of ulnar styloid fracture (25652)
Open treatment of distal radial intra-articular fracture or epiphyseal separation; with internal fixation of 3 or more fragments (25609)
Percutaneous repair of ulnar styloid fracture (25651)
23.6  23.6  **FUD** 090  J J8 80 50
AMA: 2017,Jan,8; 2016,Jan,13; 2015,Jan,16; 2014,Jan,11

**25609** **with internal fixation of 3 or more fragments**
EXCLUDES Closed treatment of ulnar styloid fracture (25650)
Open repair of ulnar styloid fracture (25652)
Percutaneous repair of ulnar styloid fracture (25651)
30.0  30.0  **FUD** 090  J J8 80 50
AMA: 2017,Jan,8; 2016,Jan,13; 2015,Jan,16; 2014,Jan,11; 2013,Dec,14; 2013,Mar,13

**25622** **Closed treatment of carpal scaphoid (navicular) fracture; without manipulation**
7.90  8.65  **FUD** 090  T P2 50
AMA: 2002,Apr,13

**25624** **with manipulation**
12.3  13.5  **FUD** 090  J A2 80 50
AMA: 2002,Apr,13

**25628** **Open treatment of carpal scaphoid (navicular) fracture, includes internal fixation, when performed**
20.6  20.6  **FUD** 090  J A2 80 50
AMA: 2002,Apr,13

**25630** **Closed treatment of carpal bone fracture (excluding carpal scaphoid [navicular]); without manipulation, each bone**
7.99  8.68  **FUD** 090  T P2 50
AMA: 2002,Apr,13

**25635** **with manipulation, each bone**
10.7  11.9  **FUD** 090  J A2 80 50
AMA: 2002,Apr,13

**25645** **Open treatment of carpal bone fracture (other than carpal scaphoid [navicular]), each bone**
16.1  16.1  **FUD** 090  J A2 80 50
AMA: 2002,Apr,13

**25650** **Closed treatment of ulnar styloid fracture**
EXCLUDES Closed treatment of distal radial fracture (25600, 25605)
Open treatment of distal radial extra-articular fracture or epiphyseal separation, with internal fixation (25607-25609)
8.52  9.07  **FUD** 090  T P2 50
AMA: 2017,Jan,8; 2016,Jan,13; 2015,Jan,16; 2014,Jan,11; 2013,Apr,10-11

**25651** **Percutaneous skeletal fixation of ulnar styloid fracture**
13.8  13.8  **FUD** 090  J G2 80 50
AMA: 2007,Oct,7-10; 2002,Apr,13

**25652** **Open treatment of ulnar styloid fracture**
17.8  17.8  **FUD** 090  J G2 50
AMA: 2017,Jan,8; 2016,Jan,13; 2015,Jan,16; 2014,Jan,11

**25660** **Closed treatment of radiocarpal or intercarpal dislocation, 1 or more bones, with manipulation**
11.7  11.7  **FUD** 090  T A2 80 50
AMA: 2002,Apr,13

**25670** **Open treatment of radiocarpal or intercarpal dislocation, 1 or more bones**
17.3  17.3  **FUD** 090  J A2 80 50
AMA: 2002,Apr,13

**25671** **Percutaneous skeletal fixation of distal radioulnar dislocation**
15.1  15.1  **FUD** 090  J A2 50
AMA: 2002,Apr,13

**25675** **Closed treatment of distal radioulnar dislocation with manipulation**
11.2  12.2  **FUD** 090  T A2 80 50
AMA: 2002,Apr,13

**25676** **Open treatment of distal radioulnar dislocation, acute or chronic**
18.0  18.0  **FUD** 090  J A2 80 50
AMA: 2002,Apr,13

**25680** **Closed treatment of trans-scaphoperilunar type of fracture dislocation, with manipulation**
13.7  13.7  **FUD** 090  T A2 80 50
AMA: 2002,Apr,13

**25685** **Open treatment of trans-scaphoperilunar type of fracture dislocation**
21.0  21.0  **FUD** 090  J A2 80 50
AMA: 2002,Apr,13

**25690** **Closed treatment of lunate dislocation, with manipulation**
13.5  13.5  **FUD** 090  J A2 80 50
AMA: 2002,Apr,13

**25695** **Open treatment of lunate dislocation**
18.1  18.1  **FUD** 090  J A2 80 50
AMA: 2002,Apr,13

## 25800-25830 Wrist Fusion

**25800** **Arthrodesis, wrist; complete, without bone graft (includes radiocarpal and/or intercarpal and/or carpometacarpal joints)**
21.0  21.0  **FUD** 090  J J8 80 50
AMA: 2002,Apr,13; 1998,Nov,1

**25805** **with sliding graft**
24.2  24.2  **FUD** 090  J A2 80 50
AMA: 2002,Apr,13

**25810** **with iliac or other autograft (includes obtaining graft)**
24.9  24.9  **FUD** 090  J G2 80 50
AMA: 2002,Apr,13

**25820** **Arthrodesis, wrist; limited, without bone graft (eg, intercarpal or radiocarpal)**
17.6  17.6  **FUD** 090  J A2 80 50
AMA: 2002,Apr,13; 1998,Nov,1

**25825** **with autograft (includes obtaining graft)**
21.7  21.7  **FUD** 090  J A2 80 50
AMA: 2017,Jan,8; 2016,Jan,13; 2015,Jan,16; 2014,Jan,11; 2012,Jul,12-14

**25830** **Arthrodesis, distal radioulnar joint with segmental resection of ulna, with or without bone graft (eg, Sauve-Kapandji procedure)**
27.0  27.0  **FUD** 090  J A2 80 50
AMA: 2002,Apr,13; 1998,Nov,1

## 25900-25999 Amputation Through Forearm/Wrist

**25900** **Amputation, forearm, through radius and ulna;**
    🔲 20.3   ⚖ 20.3   **FUD** 090     C 80 50 ▣
    **AMA:** 2002,Apr,13

**25905** **open, circular (guillotine)**
    🔲 20.1   ⚖ 20.1   **FUD** 090     C 80 50 ▣
    **AMA:** 2002,Apr,13

**25907** **secondary closure or scar revision**
    🔲 17.4   ⚖ 17.4   **FUD** 090     J A2 80 50 ▣
    **AMA:** 2002,Apr,13

**25909** **re-amputation**
    🔲 19.5   ⚖ 19.5   **FUD** 090     J 80 50 ▣
    **AMA:** 2002,Apr,13

**25915** **Krukenberg procedure**
    🔲 29.1   ⚖ 29.1   **FUD** 090     C 80 50 ▣
    **AMA:** 2002,Apr,13

**25920** **Disarticulation through wrist;**
    🔲 19.9   ⚖ 19.9   **FUD** 090     C 80 50 ▣
    **AMA:** 2002,Apr,13

**25922** **secondary closure or scar revision**
    🔲 14.6   ⚖ 14.6   **FUD** 090     J A2 80 50 ▣
    **AMA:** 2002,Apr,13

**25924** **re-amputation**
    🔲 19.0   ⚖ 19.0   **FUD** 090     C 80 50 ▣
    **AMA:** 2002,Apr,13

**25927** **Transmetacarpal amputation;**
    🔲 23.0   ⚖ 23.0   **FUD** 090     C 80 50 ▣
    **AMA:** 2002,Apr,13

**25929** **secondary closure or scar revision**
    🔲 16.3   ⚖ 16.3   **FUD** 090     T A2 80 50 ▣
    **AMA:** 2002,Apr,13

**25931** **re-amputation**
    🔲 20.7   ⚖ 20.7   **FUD** 090     J G2 50 ▣
    **AMA:** 2002,Apr,13

**25999** **Unlisted procedure, forearm or wrist**
    🔲 0.00   ⚖ 0.00   **FUD** YYY     T 80 50
    **AMA:** 2002,Apr,13

## 26010-26037 Incision Hand/Fingers

**26010** **Drainage of finger abscess; simple**
    🔲 3.92   ⚖ 7.51   **FUD** 010     T P2 ▣
    **AMA:** 2003,May,7; 2003,Sep,3

The six synovial sheaths (blue) of the dorsum of the wrist branch into nine extensor tendons

Extensor pollicis longus

Anatomical "snuffbox"

Extensor digitorum (five tendons)

Extensor retinaculum

Head of ulna

Fibrous sheaths

Synovium

Flexor tendons

Tendons typically join in a common synovial sheath

**26011** **complicated (eg, felon)**
    🔲 5.29   ⚖ 11.0   **FUD** 010     J A2 ▣
    **AMA:** 2002,Apr,13

**26020** **Drainage of tendon sheath, digit and/or palm, each**
    🔲 12.3   ⚖ 12.3   **FUD** 090     J A2 ▣
    **AMA:** 2002,Apr,13; 1998,Nov,1

**26025** **Drainage of palmar bursa; single, bursa**
    🔲 12.0   ⚖ 12.0   **FUD** 090     J A2 80 50 ▣
    **AMA:** 2002,Apr,13; 1998,Nov,1

**26030** **multiple bursa**
    🔲 14.1   ⚖ 14.1   **FUD** 090     J A2 80 50 ▣
    **AMA:** 2002,Apr,13; 1998,Nov,1

**26034** **Incision, bone cortex, hand or finger (eg, osteomyelitis or bone abscess)**
    🔲 15.4   ⚖ 15.4   **FUD** 090     J A2
    **AMA:** 2002,Apr,13; 1998,Nov,1

**26035** **Decompression fingers and/or hand, injection injury (eg, grease gun)**
    🔲 24.5   ⚖ 24.5   **FUD** 090     J G2 80 ▣
    **AMA:** 2002,Apr,13

**26037** **Decompressive fasciotomy, hand (excludes 26035)**
    **EXCLUDES** *Injection injury (26035)*
    🔲 16.2   ⚖ 16.2   **FUD** 090     J G2 80 50 ▣
    **AMA:** 2002,Apr,13

## 26040-26045 Incision Palmar Fascia

**EXCLUDES** *Enzyme injection fasciotomy (20527, 26341)*
*Fasciectomy (26121, 26123, 26125)*

**26040** **Fasciotomy, palmar (eg, Dupuytren's contracture); percutaneous**
    🔲 8.91   ⚖ 8.91   **FUD** 090     J A2 50 ▣
    **AMA:** 2017,Jan,8; 2016,Jan,13; 2015,Jan,16; 2014,Jan,11; 2012,Jan,15-42

**26045** **open, partial**
    🔲 13.4   ⚖ 13.4   **FUD** 090     J A2 50 ▣
    **AMA:** 2017,Jan,8; 2016,Jan,13; 2015,Jan,16; 2014,Jan,11; 2012,Jan,15-42

## 26055-26080 Incision Tendon/Joint of Fingers/Hand

**26055** **Tendon sheath incision (eg, for trigger finger)**
    🔲 8.86   ⚖ 15.8   **FUD** 090     J A2 ▣
    **AMA:** 2002,Apr,13; 1994,Win,1

**26060** **Tenotomy, percutaneous, single, each digit**
    **EXCLUDES** *Arthrocentesis (20610)*
    🔲 7.44   ⚖ 7.44   **FUD** 090     J A2 80 ▣
    **AMA:** 2002,Apr,13; 1996,Nov,1

**26070** **Arthrotomy, with exploration, drainage, or removal of loose or foreign body; carpometacarpal joint**
    🔲 9.02   ⚖ 9.02   **FUD** 090     J A2 50 ▣
    **AMA:** 2002,Apr,13; 1998,Nov,1

**26075** **metacarpophalangeal joint, each**
    🔲 9.52   ⚖ 9.52   **FUD** 090     J A2 50 ▣
    **AMA:** 2017,Jan,8; 2016,Jan,13; 2015,Jan,16; 2014,Jan,11; 2012,Oct,12; 2012,Sep,10

**26080** **interphalangeal joint, each**
    🔲 11.1   ⚖ 11.1   **FUD** 090     J A2
    **AMA:** 2017,Jan,8; 2016,Jan,13; 2015,Jan,16; 2014,Jan,11; 2012,Oct,12; 2012,Sep,10

## 26100-26110 Arthrotomy with Biopsy of Joint Hand/Fingers

**26100** **Arthrotomy with biopsy; carpometacarpal joint, each**
    🔲 9.27   ⚖ 9.27   **FUD** 090     J A2 80 50 ▣
    **AMA:** 2002,Apr,13; 1998,Nov,1

**26105** **metacarpophalangeal joint, each**
    🔲 9.54   ⚖ 9.54   **FUD** 090     J A2 80 50 ▣
    **AMA:** 2002,Apr,13; 1998,Nov,1

**26110** **interphalangeal joint, each**
    🔲 9.20   ⚖ 9.20   **FUD** 090     J A2
    **AMA:** 2002,Apr,13; 1994,Win,1

● New Code   ▲ Revised Code   ○ Reinstated   ● New Web Release   ▲ Revised Web Release   Unlisted   Not Covered   # Resequenced
⊘ AMA Mod 51 Exempt   ⑤ Optum Mod 51 Exempt   ⑥³ Mod 63 Exempt   ✗ Non-FDA Drug   ★ Telemedicine   Ⓜ Maternity   Ⓐ Age Edit   + Add-on   **AMA:** CPT Asst
© 2017 Optum360, LLC      CPT © 2017 American Medical Association. All Rights Reserved.      **71**

# 26111-26118 [26111, 26113] Excision Soft Tissue Tumors Fingers and Hand

**INCLUDES** Any necessary elevation of tissue planes or dissection
Measurement of tumor and necessary margin at greatest diameter prior to excision
Simple and intermediate repairs
Types of excision:
Fascial or subfascial soft tissue tumors: simple and marginal resection of tumors found either in or below the deep fascia, not involving bone or excision of a substantial amount of normal tissue; primarily benign and intramuscular tumors
Tumors of fingers and toes involving joint capsules, tendons and tendon sheaths
Radical resection soft tissue tumor: wide resection of tumor, involving substantial margins of normal tissue and may include tissue removal from one or more layers; most often malignant or aggressive benign
Tumors of fingers and toes adjacent to joints, tendons and tendon sheaths
Subcutaneous: simple and marginal resection of tumors found in the subcutaneous tissue above the deep fascia; most often benign

**EXCLUDES** Complex repair
Excision of benign cutaneous lesions (eg, sebaceous cyst) (11420-11426)
Radical resection of cutaneous tumors (eg, melanoma) (11620-11626)
Significant exploration of the vessels or neuroplasty

**26111** Resequenced code. See code following 26115.

**26113** Resequenced code. See code following 26116.

**26115** Excision, tumor or vascular malformation, soft tissue of hand or finger, subcutaneous; less than 1.5 cm
📋 9.52  ⚖ 14.3  **FUD** 090    J G2 ▣
**AMA:** 2002,Apr,13

\# **26111** 1.5 cm or greater
📋 11.9  ⚖ 11.9  **FUD** 090    J G2 80 ▣

**26116** Excision, tumor, soft tissue, or vascular malformation, of hand or finger, subfascial (eg, intramuscular); less than 1.5 cm
📋 15.1  ⚖ 15.1  **FUD** 090    J G2 ▣
**AMA:** 2017,Jan,8; 2016,Jan,13; 2015,Jan,16; 2014,Jan,11

\# **26113** 1.5 cm or greater
📋 15.7  ⚖ 15.7  **FUD** 090    J G2 80 ▣

**26117** Radical resection of tumor (eg, sarcoma), soft tissue of hand or finger; less than 3 cm
📋 21.4  ⚖ 21.4  **FUD** 090    J G2 ▣
**AMA:** 2002,Apr,13; 1990,Win,4

**26118** 3 cm or greater
📋 30.3  ⚖ 30.3  **FUD** 090    J G2 80 ▣

# 26121-26236 Procedures of Bones, Fascia, Joints and Tendons Hands and Fingers

**26121** Fasciectomy, palm only, with or without Z-plasty, other local tissue rearrangement, or skin grafting (includes obtaining graft)
**EXCLUDES** Enzyme injection fasciotomy (20527, 26341)
Fasciotomy (26040, 26045)
📋 17.1  ⚖ 17.1  **FUD** 090    J A2 50 ▣
**AMA:** 2017,Jan,8; 2016,Jan,13; 2015,Jan,16; 2014,Jan,11; 2012,Jan,15-42

**26123** Fasciectomy, partial palmar with release of single digit including proximal interphalangeal joint, with or without Z-plasty, other local tissue rearrangement, or skin grafting (includes obtaining graft);
**EXCLUDES** Enzyme injection fasciotomy (20527, 26341)
Fasciotomy (26040, 26045)
📋 23.9  ⚖ 23.9  **FUD** 090    J A2 50 ▣
**AMA:** 2017,Jan,8; 2016,Jan,13; 2015,Jan,16; 2014,Jan,11; 2012,Jan,15-42

\+ **26125** each additional digit (List separately in addition to code for primary procedure)
**EXCLUDES** Enzyme injection fasciotomy (20527, 26341)
Fasciotomy (26040, 26045)
Code first (26123)
📋 7.92  ⚖ 7.92  **FUD** ZZZ    N M1 ▣
**AMA:** 2017,Jan,8; 2016,Jan,13; 2015,Jan,16; 2014,Jan,11; 2012,Jan,15-42

**26130** Synovectomy, carpometacarpal joint
📋 13.2  ⚖ 13.2  **FUD** 090    J A2 50 ▣
**AMA:** 2002,Apr,13

**26135** Synovectomy, metacarpophalangeal joint including intrinsic release and extensor hood reconstruction, each digit
📋 15.7  ⚖ 15.7  **FUD** 090    J A2 80 ▣
**AMA:** 2002,Apr,13

**26140** Synovectomy, proximal interphalangeal joint, including extensor reconstruction, each interphalangeal joint
📋 14.4  ⚖ 14.4  **FUD** 090    J A2 ▣
**AMA:** 2002,Apr,13

**26145** Synovectomy, tendon sheath, radical (tenosynovectomy), flexor tendon, palm and/or finger, each tendon
**EXCLUDES** Wrist synovectomy (25115-25116)
📋 14.6  ⚖ 14.6  **FUD** 090    J A2 ▣
**AMA:** 2002,Apr,13; 1998,Nov,1

**26160** Excision of lesion of tendon sheath or joint capsule (eg, cyst, mucous cyst, or ganglion), hand or finger
**EXCLUDES** Trigger finger (26055)
Wrist ganglion removal (25111-25112)
📋 9.54  ⚖ 16.3  **FUD** 090    J A2 ▣
**AMA:** 2002,Apr,13

**26170** Excision of tendon, palm, flexor or extensor, single, each tendon
**EXCLUDES** Excision extensor tendon, with implantation of synthetic rod for delayed tendon graft, hand or finger, each rod (26415)
Excision flexor tendon, with implantation of synthetic rod for delayed tendon graft, hand or finger, each rod (26390)
📋 11.6  ⚖ 11.6  **FUD** 090    J A2 80 ▣
**AMA:** 2017,Jan,8; 2016,Jan,13; 2015,Jan,16; 2013,Jun,13

**26180** Excision of tendon, finger, flexor or extensor, each tendon
**EXCLUDES** Excision extensor tendon, with implantation of synthetic rod for delayed tendon graft, hand or finger, each rod (26390)
Excision flexor tendon, with implantation of synthetic rod for delayed tendon graft, hand or finger, each rod (26390)
📋 12.6  ⚖ 12.6  **FUD** 090    J A2 80 ▣
**AMA:** 2002,Apr,13; 1998,Nov,1

**26185** Sesamoidectomy, thumb or finger (separate procedure)
📋 15.5  ⚖ 15.5  **FUD** 090    J A2 80 50 ▣
**AMA:** 2002,Apr,13; 1996,Nov,1

**26200** Excision or curettage of bone cyst or benign tumor of metacarpal;
📋 12.8  ⚖ 12.8  **FUD** 090    J A2 80 ▣
**AMA:** 2002,Apr,13

**26205** with autograft (includes obtaining graft)
📋 17.0  ⚖ 17.0  **FUD** 090    J A2 ▣
**AMA:** 2002,Apr,13

**26210** Excision or curettage of bone cyst or benign tumor of proximal, middle, or distal phalanx of finger;
📋 12.6  ⚖ 12.6  **FUD** 090    J A2 ▣
**AMA:** 2002,Apr,13

**26215** with autograft (includes obtaining graft)
📋 16.0  ⚖ 16.0  **FUD** 090    J A2 ▣
**AMA:** 2002,Apr,13

26/TC PC/TC Only     A2-Z3 ASC Payment     50 Bilateral     ♂ Male Only     ♀ Female Only     📋 Facility RVU     ⚖ Non-Facility RVU     ▣ CCI
FUD Follow-up Days     CMS: IOM (Pub 100)     A-Y OPPSI     80/80 Surg Assist Allowed / w/Doc     🔲 Lab Crosswalk     📷 Radiology Crosswalk     ✖ CLIA
72                                    CPT © 2017 American Medical Association. All Rights Reserved.                              © 2017 Optum360, LLC

**26230** Partial excision (craterization, saucerization, or diaphysectomy) bone (eg, osteomyelitis); metacarpal
⚙ 14.3   ⚒ 14.3   **FUD** 090                    J A2 80 ▢
AMA: 2002,Apr,13; 1998,Nov,1

**26235** proximal or middle phalanx of finger
⚙ 14.0   ⚒ 14.0   **FUD** 090                    J A2 80 ▢
AMA: 2002,Apr,13

**26236** distal phalanx of finger
⚙ 12.6   ⚒ 12.6   **FUD** 090                    J A2 ▢
AMA: 2002,Apr,13

## 26250-26262 Radical Resection Bone Tumor of Hand/Finger

INCLUDES Any necessary elevation of tissue planes or dissection
Excision of adjacent soft tissue during bone tumor resection (26111-26118 [26111, 26113])
Measurement of tumor and necessary margin at greatest diameter prior to excision
Resection of the tumor (may include entire bone) and wide margins of normal tissue primarily for malignant or aggressive benign tumors
Simple and intermediate repairs
EXCLUDES Complex repair
Significant exploration of vessels, neuroplasty, reconstruction, or complex bone repair

**26250** Radical resection of tumor, metacarpal
⚙ 31.0   ⚒ 31.0   **FUD** 090                    J A2 80 ▢
AMA: 2002,Apr,13; 1998,Nov,1

**26260** Radical resection of tumor, proximal or middle phalanx of finger
⚙ 23.1   ⚒ 23.1   **FUD** 090                    J A2 80 ▢
AMA: 2002,Apr,13; 1998,Nov,1

**26262** Radical resection of tumor, distal phalanx of finger
⚙ 18.0   ⚒ 18.0   **FUD** 090                    J A2 80 ▢
AMA: 2002,Apr,13; 1998,Nov,1

## 26320 Implant Removal Hand/Finger

**26320** Removal of implant from finger or hand
EXCLUDES Excision of foreign body (20520, 20525)
⚙ 9.91   ⚒ 9.91   **FUD** 090                    02 A2 ▢
AMA: 2002,Apr,13

## 26340-26548 Repair/Reconstruction of Fingers and Hand

**26340** Manipulation, finger joint, under anesthesia, each joint
EXCLUDES Application external fixation (20690, 20692)
⚙ 9.51   ⚒ 9.51   **FUD** 090                    J 62 50 ▢
AMA: 2017,Jan,8; 2016,Jan,13; 2015,Jan,16; 2014,Jan,11; 2012,Jan,15-42

**26341** Manipulation, palmar fascial cord (ie, Dupuytren's cord), post enzyme injection (eg, collagenase), single cord
EXCLUDES Enzyme injection fasciotomy (20527)
Code also custom orthotic fabrication and/or fitting
⚙ 2.15   ⚒ 2.81   **FUD** 010                    T P3 50 ▢
AMA: 2017,Jan,8; 2016,Jan,13; 2015,Jan,16; 2014,Jan,11; 2012,Jul,8

**26350** Repair or advancement, flexor tendon, not in zone 2 digital flexor tendon sheath (eg, no man's land); primary or secondary without free graft, each tendon
⚙ 20.0   ⚒ 20.0   **FUD** 090                    J A2 ▢
AMA: 2002,Apr,13; 1998,Nov,1

**26352** secondary with free graft (includes obtaining graft), each tendon
⚙ 22.5   ⚒ 22.5   **FUD** 090                    J A2 80 ▢
AMA: 2002,Apr,13

**26356** Repair or advancement, flexor tendon, in zone 2 digital flexor tendon sheath (eg, no man's land); primary, without free graft, each tendon
⚙ 22.7   ⚒ 22.7   **FUD** 090                    J A2 ▢
AMA: 2017,Jan,8; 2016,Jan,13; 2015,Jan,16; 2014,Sep,13; 2014,Jan,11; 2012,Jan,15-42

**26357** secondary, without free graft, each tendon
⚙ 25.4   ⚒ 25.4   **FUD** 090                    J A2 80 ▢
AMA: 2002,Apr,13

**26358** secondary, with free graft (includes obtaining graft), each tendon
⚙ 27.9   ⚒ 27.9   **FUD** 090                    J A2 80 ▢
AMA: 2002,Apr,13

**26370** Repair or advancement of profundus tendon, with intact superficialis tendon; primary, each tendon
⚙ 21.3   ⚒ 21.3   **FUD** 090                    J A2 80 ▢
AMA: 2017,Jan,8; 2016,Jan,13; 2015,Jan,16; 2014,Jan,11; 2012,Jan,15-42

**26372** secondary with free graft (includes obtaining graft), each tendon
⚙ 24.3   ⚒ 24.3   **FUD** 090                    J A2 80 ▢
AMA: 2002,Apr,13; 1998,Nov,1

**26373** secondary without free graft, each tendon
⚙ 23.5   ⚒ 23.5   **FUD** 090                    J A2 80 ▢
AMA: 2002,Apr,13; 1998,Nov,1

**26390** Excision flexor tendon, with implantation of synthetic rod for delayed tendon graft, hand or finger, each rod
⚙ 23.6   ⚒ 23.6   **FUD** 090                    J A2 80 ▢
AMA: 2002,Apr,13; 1998,Nov,1

**26392** Removal of synthetic rod and insertion of flexor tendon graft, hand or finger (includes obtaining graft), each rod
⚙ 27.4   ⚒ 27.4   **FUD** 090                    J A2 80 ▢
AMA: 2002,Apr,13; 1998,Nov,1

**26410** Repair, extensor tendon, hand, primary or secondary; without free graft, each tendon
⚙ 15.9   ⚒ 15.9   **FUD** 090                    J A2 ▢
AMA: 2002,Apr,13; 1998,Nov,1

**26412** with free graft (includes obtaining graft), each tendon
⚙ 19.5   ⚒ 19.5   **FUD** 090                    J A2 80 ▢
AMA: 2002,Apr,13; 1998,Nov,1

**26415** Excision of extensor tendon, with implantation of synthetic rod for delayed tendon graft, hand or finger, each rod
⚙ 19.2   ⚒ 19.2   **FUD** 090                    J A2 80 ▢
AMA: 2002,Apr,13; 1998,Nov,1

**26416** Removal of synthetic rod and insertion of extensor tendon graft (includes obtaining graft), hand or finger, each rod
⚙ 24.4   ⚒ 24.4   **FUD** 090                    J A2 ▢
AMA: 2017,Jan,8; 2016,Jan,13; 2015,Jan,16; 2014,Jan,11

**26418** Repair, extensor tendon, finger, primary or secondary; without free graft, each tendon
⚙ 16.2   ⚒ 16.2   **FUD** 090                    J A2 ▢
AMA: 2017,Jan,8; 2016,Jan,13; 2015,Jan,16; 2014,Jan,11; 2012,Jan,15-42

**26420** with free graft (includes obtaining graft) each tendon
⚙ 19.9   ⚒ 19.9   **FUD** 090                    J A2 80 ▢
AMA: 2002,Apr,13

**26426** Repair of extensor tendon, central slip, secondary (eg, boutonniere deformity); using local tissue(s), including lateral band(s), each finger
⚙ 14.3   ⚒ 14.3   **FUD** 090                    J A2 ▢
AMA: 2002,Apr,13; 1998,Nov,1

**26428** with free graft (includes obtaining graft), each finger
⚙ 20.8   ⚒ 20.8   **FUD** 090                    J A2 80 ▢
AMA: 2002,Apr,13; 1998,Nov,1

**26432** Closed treatment of distal extensor tendon insertion, with or without percutaneous pinning (eg, mallet finger)
⚙ 14.0   ⚒ 14.0   **FUD** 090                    J A2 ▢
AMA: 2002,Apr,13; 1998,Nov,1

---

● New Code   ▲ Revised Code   ○ Reinstated   ● New Web Release   ▲ Revised Web Release   Unlisted   Not Covered   # Resequenced
Ⓢ AMA Mod 51 Exempt   Ⓢ Optum Mod 51 Exempt   ⓺ Mod 63 Exempt   ✗ Non-FDA Drug   ★ Telemedicine   Ⓜ Maternity   Ⓐ Age Edit   + Add-on   AMA: CPT Asst

**26433** Repair of extensor tendon, distal insertion, primary or secondary; without graft (eg, mallet finger)

*EXCLUDES* Trigger finger (26055)

🔧 14.9  ✂ 14.9  **FUD** 090  [J] [A2] [⬜]

AMA: 2002,Apr,13; 1998,Nov,1

**26434** with free graft (includes obtaining graft)

*EXCLUDES* Trigger finger (26055)

🔧 18.2  ✂ 18.2  **FUD** 090  [J] [A2] [80] [⬜]

AMA: 2002,Apr,13

**26437** Realignment of extensor tendon, hand, each tendon

🔧 17.5  ✂ 17.5  **FUD** 090  [J] [A2] [⬜]

AMA: 2002,Apr,13; 1998,Nov,1

**26440** Tenolysis, flexor tendon; palm OR finger, each tendon

🔧 17.4  ✂ 17.4  **FUD** 090  [J] [A2] [⬜]

AMA: 2017,Jan,8; 2016,Jan,13; 2015,Jun,10; 2015,Jan,16; 2014,Jan,11; 2012,Jan,15-42

**26442** palm AND finger, each tendon

🔧 27.2  ✂ 27.2  **FUD** 090  [J] [A2] [⬜]

AMA: 2002,Apr,13

**26445** Tenolysis, extensor tendon, hand OR finger, each tendon

🔧 16.2  ✂ 16.2  **FUD** 090  [J] [A2] [⬜]

AMA: 2017,Jan,8; 2016,Jan,13; 2015,Jan,16; 2014,Jan,11; 2012,Jan,15-42

**26449** Tenolysis, complex, extensor tendon, finger, including forearm, each tendon

🔧 19.8  ✂ 19.8  **FUD** 090  [J] [A2] [80] [⬜]

AMA: 2002,Apr,13; 1998,Nov,1

**26450** Tenotomy, flexor, palm, open, each tendon

🔧 11.4  ✂ 11.4  **FUD** 090  [J] [A2] [80] [⬜]

AMA: 2002,Apr,13; 1998,Nov,1

**26455** Tenotomy, flexor, finger, open, each tendon

🔧 11.3  ✂ 11.3  **FUD** 090  [J] [A2] [80] [⬜]

AMA: 2002,Apr,13; 1998,Nov,1

**26460** Tenotomy, extensor, hand or finger, open, each tendon

🔧 11.1  ✂ 11.1  **FUD** 090  [J] [A2] [⬜]

AMA: 2002,Apr,13; 1998,Nov,1

**26471** Tenodesis; of proximal interphalangeal joint, each joint

🔧 17.3  ✂ 17.3  **FUD** 090  [J] [A2] [80] [⬜]

AMA: 2002,Apr,13; 1998,Nov,1

**26474** of distal joint, each joint

🔧 16.9  ✂ 16.9  **FUD** 090  [J] [A2] [80] [⬜]

AMA: 2002,Apr,13; 1998,Nov,1

**26476** Lengthening of tendon, extensor, hand or finger, each tendon

🔧 16.2  ✂ 16.2  **FUD** 090  [J] [A2] [⬜]

AMA: 2002,Apr,13; 1998,Nov,1

**26477** Shortening of tendon, extensor, hand or finger, each tendon

🔧 16.4  ✂ 16.4  **FUD** 090  [J] [A2] [⬜]

AMA: 2002,Apr,13; 1998,Nov,1

**26478** Lengthening of tendon, flexor, hand or finger, each tendon

🔧 17.4  ✂ 17.4  **FUD** 090  [J] [A2] [80] [⬜]

AMA: 2017,Jan,8; 2016,Jan,13; 2015,Jan,16; 2014,Jan,11; 2013,Dec,16

**26479** Shortening of tendon, flexor, hand or finger, each tendon

🔧 17.3  ✂ 17.3  **FUD** 090  [J] [A2] [80] [⬜]

AMA: 2002,Apr,13; 1998,Nov,1

**26480** Transfer or transplant of tendon, carpometacarpal area or dorsum of hand; without free graft, each tendon

🔧 21.1  ✂ 21.1  **FUD** 090  [J] [A2] [80] [⬜]

AMA: 2017,Jan,8; 2016,Jan,13; 2015,Jan,16; 2014,Jan,11; 2013,Dec,16

**26483** with free tendon graft (includes obtaining graft), each tendon

🔧 23.7  ✂ 23.7  **FUD** 090  [J] [A2] [80] [⬜]

AMA: 2002,Apr,13

**26485** Transfer or transplant of tendon, palmar; without free tendon graft, each tendon

🔧 22.7  ✂ 22.7  **FUD** 090  [J] [A2] [80] [⬜]

AMA: 2002,Apr,13; 1998,Nov,1

**26489** with free tendon graft (includes obtaining graft), each tendon

🔧 26.3  ✂ 26.3  **FUD** 090  [J] [A2] [80] [⬜]

AMA: 2002,Apr,13

**26490** Opponensplasty; superficialis tendon transfer type, each tendon

*EXCLUDES* Thumb fusion (26820)

🔧 22.5  ✂ 22.5  **FUD** 090  [J] [A2] [80] [⬜]

AMA: 2002,Apr,13; 1998,Nov,1

**26492** tendon transfer with graft (includes obtaining graft), each tendon

*EXCLUDES* Thumb fusion (26820)

🔧 25.0  ✂ 25.0  **FUD** 090  [J] [A2] [80] [⬜]

AMA: 2002,Apr,13; 1998,Nov,1

**26494** hypothenar muscle transfer

*EXCLUDES* Thumb fusion (26820)

🔧 22.0  ✂ 22.0  **FUD** 090  [J] [A2] [80] [⬜]

AMA: 2002,Apr,13

**26496** other methods

*EXCLUDES* Thumb fusion (26820)

🔧 24.2  ✂ 24.2  **FUD** 090  [J] [A2] [80] [⬜]

AMA: 2002,Apr,13

**26497** Transfer of tendon to restore intrinsic function; ring and small finger

🔧 24.5  ✂ 24.5  **FUD** 090  [J] [A2] [80] [⬜]

AMA: 2002,Apr,13; 1998,Nov,1

**26498** all 4 fingers

🔧 32.1  ✂ 32.1  **FUD** 090  [J] [A2] [80] [⬜]

AMA: 2002,Apr,13

**26499** Correction claw finger, other methods

🔧 23.1  ✂ 23.1  **FUD** 090  [J] [A2] [80] [⬜]

AMA: 2002,Apr,13

**26500** Reconstruction of tendon pulley, each tendon; with local tissues (separate procedure)

🔧 17.6  ✂ 17.6  **FUD** 090  [J] [A2] [80] [⬜]

AMA: 2002,Apr,13; 1998,Nov,1

**26502** with tendon or fascial graft (includes obtaining graft) (separate procedure)

🔧 20.0  ✂ 20.0  **FUD** 090  [J] [A2] [80] [⬜]

AMA: 2002,Apr,13

**26508** Release of thenar muscle(s) (eg, thumb contracture)

🔧 17.7  ✂ 17.7  **FUD** 090  [J] [A2] [80] [50] [⬜]

AMA: 2002,Apr,13; 1998,Nov,1

**26510** Cross intrinsic transfer, each tendon

🔧 16.7  ✂ 16.7  **FUD** 090  [J] [A2] [80] [⬜]

AMA: 2002,Apr,13

**26516** Capsulodesis, metacarpophalangeal joint; single digit

🔧 19.7  ✂ 19.7  **FUD** 090  [J] [A2] [80] [50] [⬜]

AMA: 2002,Apr,13; 1998,Nov,1

**26517** 2 digits

🔧 22.0  ✂ 22.0  **FUD** 090  [J] [A2] [80] [50] [⬜]

AMA: 2002,Apr,13

**26518** 3 or 4 digits

🔧 23.3  ✂ 23.3  **FUD** 090  [J] [A2] [80] [50] [⬜]

AMA: 2002,Apr,13

**26/TC** PC/TC Only    **A2-Z3** ASC Payment    **50** Bilateral    ♂ Male Only    ♀ Female Only    🔧 Facility RVU    ✂ Non-Facility RVU    [⬜] CCI

**FUD** Follow-up Days    **CMS:** IOM (Pub 100)    **A-Y** OPPSI    **80/80** Surg Assist Allowed / w/Doc    🔲 Lab Crosswalk    🔲 Radiology Crosswalk    ❌ CLIA

74    CPT © 2017 American Medical Association. All Rights Reserved.    © 2017 Optum360, LLC

**26520**  **Capsulectomy or capsulotomy; metacarpophalangeal joint, each joint**
  EXCLUDES  *Carpometacarpal joint arthroplasty (25447)*
  🚑 18.3   ⚕ 18.3   **FUD** 090                    J A2 ▢
  **AMA:** 2002,Apr,13; 1998,Nov,1

**26525**  **interphalangeal joint, each joint**
  EXCLUDES  *Carpometacarpal joint arthroplasty (25447)*
  🚑 18.3   ⚕ 18.3   **FUD** 090                    J A2 ▢
  **AMA:** 2017,Jan,8; 2016,Jan,13; 2015,Jun,10; 2015,Jan,16; 2014,Jan,11; 2012,Jan,15-42

**26530**  **Arthroplasty, metacarpophalangeal joint; each joint**
  EXCLUDES  *Carpometacarpal joint arthroplasty (25447)*
  🚑 15.4   ⚕ 15.4   **FUD** 090                    J A2 80 ▢
  **AMA:** 2002,Apr,13; 1998,Nov,1

**26531**  **with prosthetic implant, each joint**
  EXCLUDES  *Carpometacarpal joint arthroplasty (25447)*
  🚑 17.8   ⚕ 17.8   **FUD** 090                    J J8 80 ▢
  **AMA:** 2017,Jan,8; 2016,Jan,13; 2015,Jan,16; 2014,Jan,11; 2012,Jan,15-42

**26535**  **Arthroplasty, interphalangeal joint; each joint**
  EXCLUDES  *Carpometacarpal joint arthroplasty (25447)*
  🚑 12.0   ⚕ 12.0   **FUD** 090                    J A2 ▢
  **AMA:** 2002,Apr,13; 1998,Nov,1

**26536**  **with prosthetic implant, each joint**
  EXCLUDES  *Carpometacarpal joint arthroplasty (25447)*
  🚑 19.9   ⚕ 19.9   **FUD** 090                    J A2 80 ▢
  **AMA:** 2002,Apr,13; 1998,Nov,1

**26540**  **Repair of collateral ligament, metacarpophalangeal or interphalangeal joint**
  🚑 18.5   ⚕ 18.5   **FUD** 090                    J A2 80 ▢
  **AMA:** 2002,Apr,13; 1996,Nov,1

**26541**  **Reconstruction, collateral ligament, metacarpophalangeal joint, single; with tendon or fascial graft (includes obtaining graft)**
  🚑 22.6   ⚕ 22.6   **FUD** 090                    J A2 80 ▢
  **AMA:** 2017,Jan,8; 2016,Jan,13; 2015,Jan,16; 2014,Jan,11

**26542**  **with local tissue (eg, adductor advancement)**
  🚑 19.1   ⚕ 19.1   **FUD** 090                    J A2 80 ▢
  **AMA:** 2017,Jan,8; 2016,Jan,13; 2015,Jan,16; 2014,Jan,11

**26545**  **Reconstruction, collateral ligament, interphalangeal joint, single, including graft, each joint**
  🚑 19.9   ⚕ 19.9   **FUD** 090                    J A2 80 ▢
  **AMA:** 2002,Apr,13

**26546**  **Repair non-union, metacarpal or phalanx (includes obtaining bone graft with or without external or internal fixation)**
  🚑 28.1   ⚕ 28.1   **FUD** 090                    J A2 80 50 ▢
  **AMA:** 2002,Apr,13; 1996,Nov,1

**26548**  **Repair and reconstruction, finger, volar plate, interphalangeal joint**
  🚑 21.3   ⚕ 21.3   **FUD** 090                    J A2 80 ▢
  **AMA:** 2002,Apr,13

## 26550-26556 Reconstruction Procedures with Finger and Toe Transplants

**26550**  **Pollicization of a digit**
  🚑 46.6   ⚕ 46.6   **FUD** 090                    J A2 80 50 ▢
  **AMA:** 2002,Apr,13

**26551**  **Transfer, toe-to-hand with microvascular anastomosis; great toe wrap-around with bone graft**
  INCLUDES  Operating microscope (69990)
  EXCLUDES  *Big toe with web space (20973)*
  🚑 95.7   ⚕ 95.7   **FUD** 090                    C 80 50 ▢
  **AMA:** 2017,Jan,8; 2016,Feb,12; 2016,Jan,13; 2015,Jan,16; 2014,Jan,11

**26553**  **other than great toe, single**
  INCLUDES  Operating microscope (69990)
  🚑 80.9   ⚕ 80.9   **FUD** 090                    C 80 50 ▢
  **AMA:** 2017,Jan,8; 2016,Feb,12; 2016,Jan,13; 2015,Jan,16; 2014,Jan,11

**26554**  **other than great toe, double**
  INCLUDES  Operating microscope (69990)
  🚑 94.7   ⚕ 94.7   **FUD** 090                    C 80 50 ▢
  **AMA:** 2017,Jan,8; 2016,Feb,12; 2016,Jan,13; 2015,Jan,16; 2014,Jan,11

**26555**  **Transfer, finger to another position without microvascular anastomosis**
  🚑 36.4   ⚕ 36.4   **FUD** 090                    J A2 80 ▢
  **AMA:** 2002,Apr,13; 1998,Nov,1

**26556**  **Transfer, free toe joint, with microvascular anastomosis**
  INCLUDES  Operating microscope (69990)
  EXCLUDES  *Big toe to hand transfer (20973)*
  🚑 97.6   ⚕ 97.6   **FUD** 090                    C 80 ▢
  **AMA:** 2017,Jan,8; 2016,Feb,12; 2016,Jan,13; 2015,Jan,16; 2014,Jan,11

## 26560-26596 Repair of Other Deformities of the Fingers/Hand

**26560**  **Repair of syndactyly (web finger) each web space; with skin flaps**
  🚑 16.3   ⚕ 16.3   **FUD** 090                    J A2 80 ▢
  **AMA:** 2002,Apr,13

**26561**  **with skin flaps and grafts**
  🚑 26.3   ⚕ 26.3   **FUD** 090                    J A2 80 ▢
  **AMA:** 2002,Apr,13

**26562**  **complex (eg, involving bone, nails)**
  🚑 37.8   ⚕ 37.8   **FUD** 090                    J A2 80 ▢
  **AMA:** 2002,Apr,13

**26565**  **Osteotomy; metacarpal, each**
  🚑 19.1   ⚕ 19.1   **FUD** 090                    J A2 80 ▢
  **AMA:** 2002,Apr,13; 1998,Nov,1

**26567**  **phalanx of finger, each**
  🚑 19.1   ⚕ 19.1   **FUD** 090                    J A2 80 ▢
  **AMA:** 2017,Jan,8; 2016,Jan,13; 2015,Jan,16; 2014,Jan,11; 2012,Apr,17-18

**26568**  **Osteoplasty, lengthening, metacarpal or phalanx**
  🚑 25.4   ⚕ 25.4   **FUD** 090                    J J8 80 ▢
  **AMA:** 2002,Apr,13; 1998,Nov,1

**26580**  **Repair cleft hand**
  INCLUDES  Barsky's procedure
  🚑 42.5   ⚕ 42.5   **FUD** 090                    J A2 80 50 ▢
  **AMA:** 2002,Apr,13

**26587**  **Reconstruction of polydactylous digit, soft tissue and bone**
  EXCLUDES  *Soft tissue removal only (11200)*
  🚑 28.7   ⚕ 28.7   **FUD** 090                    J A2 80 ▢
  **AMA:** 2017,Jan,8; 2016,Jan,13; 2015,Jan,16; 2014,Jan,11; 2012,Jan,15-42

**26590**  **Repair macrodactylia, each digit**
  🚑 37.3   ⚕ 37.3   **FUD** 090                    J A2 80 ▢
  **AMA:** 2017,Jan,8; 2016,Jan,13; 2015,Jan,16; 2014,Jan,11; 2012,Jan,15-42

**26591**  **Repair, intrinsic muscles of hand, each muscle**
  🚑 12.2   ⚕ 12.2   **FUD** 090                    J A2 80 ▢
  **AMA:** 2017,Jan,8; 2016,Jan,13; 2015,Jan,16; 2014,Jan,11; 2012,Jan,15-42

**26593**  **Release, intrinsic muscles of hand, each muscle**
  🚑 16.9   ⚕ 16.9   **FUD** 090                    J A2 ▢
  **AMA:** 2002,Apr,13; 1998,Nov,1

● New Code   ▲ Revised Code   ○ Reinstated   ● New Web Release   ▲ Revised Web Release   Unlisted   Not Covered   # Resequenced
⊘ AMA Mod 51 Exempt   ⑧ Optum Mod 51 Exempt   ⑥ Mod 63 Exempt   ∕ Non-FDA Drug   ★ Telemedicine   M Maternity   A Age Edit   + Add-on   AMA: CPT Asst
© 2017 Optum360, LLC                    CPT © 2017 American Medical Association. All Rights Reserved.                    **75**

**26596** Excision of constricting ring of finger, with multiple Z-plasties

> EXCLUDES Graft repair or scar contracture release (11042, 14040-14041, 15120, 15240)
>
> 🖵 21.4  ⚕ 21.4  **FUD** 090  J A2 80 🖵
>
> **AMA:** 2002,Apr,13

## 26600-26785 Treatment of Fracture/Dislocation of Fingers and Hand

> INCLUDES Closed, percutaneous, and open treatment of fractures or dislocations

**26600** Closed treatment of metacarpal fracture, single; without manipulation, each bone

> 🖵 7.86  ⚕ 8.35  **FUD** 090  T P2 🖵
>
> **AMA:** 2002,Apr,13

**26605** with manipulation, each bone

> 🖵 8.33  ⚕ 9.12  **FUD** 090  T A2 🖵
>
> **AMA:** 2002,Apr,13

**26607** Closed treatment of metacarpal fracture, with manipulation, with external fixation, each bone

> 🖵 13.0  ⚕ 13.0  **FUD** 090  J A2 80 🖵
>
> **AMA:** 2002,Apr,13

**26608** Percutaneous skeletal fixation of metacarpal fracture, each bone

> 🖵 13.6  ⚕ 13.6  **FUD** 090  J A2 80 🖵
>
> **AMA:** 2002,Apr,13

**26615** Open treatment of metacarpal fracture, single, includes internal fixation, when performed, each bone

> 🖵 16.4  ⚕ 16.4  **FUD** 090  J A2 🖵
>
> **AMA:** 2002,Apr,13

**26641** Closed treatment of carpometacarpal dislocation, thumb, with manipulation

> 🖵 9.73  ⚕ 10.6  **FUD** 090  T P2 80 50 🖵
>
> **AMA:** 2002,Apr,13

**26645** Closed treatment of carpometacarpal fracture dislocation, thumb (Bennett fracture), with manipulation

> 🖵 11.1  ⚕ 12.1  **FUD** 090  J A2 80 50 🖵
>
> **AMA:** 2002,Apr,13

**26650** Percutaneous skeletal fixation of carpometacarpal fracture dislocation, thumb (Bennett fracture), with manipulation

> 🖵 13.6  ⚕ 13.6  **FUD** 090  J A2 50 🖵
>
> **AMA:** 2002,Apr,13

**26665** Open treatment of carpometacarpal fracture dislocation, thumb (Bennett fracture), includes internal fixation, when performed

> 🖵 17.9  ⚕ 17.9  **FUD** 090  J A2 50 🖵
>
> **AMA:** 2002,Apr,13

**26670** Closed treatment of carpometacarpal dislocation, other than thumb, with manipulation, each joint; without anesthesia

> 🖵 8.76  ⚕ 9.64  **FUD** 090  T P2 80 🖵
>
> **AMA:** 2002,Apr,13

**26675** requiring anesthesia

> 🖵 11.8  ⚕ 12.8  **FUD** 090  J A2 80 🖵
>
> **AMA:** 2002,Apr,13

**26676** Percutaneous skeletal fixation of carpometacarpal dislocation, other than thumb, with manipulation, each joint

> 🖵 14.2  ⚕ 14.2  **FUD** 090  J A2 🖵
>
> **AMA:** 2002,Apr,13

**26685** Open treatment of carpometacarpal dislocation, other than thumb; includes internal fixation, when performed, each joint

> 🖵 16.4  ⚕ 16.4  **FUD** 090  J A2 🖵
>
> **AMA:** 2002,Apr,13

**26686** complex, multiple, or delayed reduction

> 🖵 17.8  ⚕ 17.8  **FUD** 090  J A2 80 🖵
>
> **AMA:** 2002,Apr,13

**26700** Closed treatment of metacarpophalangeal dislocation, single, with manipulation; without anesthesia

> 🖵 8.63  ⚕ 9.18  **FUD** 090  T P2 🖵
>
> **AMA:** 2002,Apr,13

**26705** requiring anesthesia

> 🖵 10.7  ⚕ 11.7  **FUD** 090  J A2 80 🖵
>
> **AMA:** 2002,Apr,13

**26706** Percutaneous skeletal fixation of metacarpophalangeal dislocation, single, with manipulation

> 🖵 12.5  ⚕ 12.5  **FUD** 090  J A2 🖵
>
> **AMA:** 2002,Apr,13

**26715** Open treatment of metacarpophalangeal dislocation, single, includes internal fixation, when performed

> 🖵 16.3  ⚕ 16.3  **FUD** 090  J A2 80 🖵
>
> **AMA:** 2002,Apr,13

**26720** Closed treatment of phalangeal shaft fracture, proximal or middle phalanx, finger or thumb; without manipulation, each

> 🖵 5.23  ⚕ 5.62  **FUD** 090  T P2 🖵
>
> **AMA:** 2002,Apr,13

**26725** with manipulation, with or without skin or skeletal traction, each

> 🖵 8.63  ⚕ 9.55  **FUD** 090  T P2 🖵
>
> **AMA:** 2002,Apr,13

**26727** Percutaneous skeletal fixation of unstable phalangeal shaft fracture, proximal or middle phalanx, finger or thumb, with manipulation, each

> 🖵 13.4  ⚕ 13.4  **FUD** 090  J A2 🖵
>
> **AMA:** 2002,Apr,13

**26735** Open treatment of phalangeal shaft fracture, proximal or middle phalanx, finger or thumb, includes internal fixation, when performed, each

> 🖵 17.0  ⚕ 17.0  **FUD** 090  J A2 🖵
>
> **AMA:** 2002,Apr,13

**26740** Closed treatment of articular fracture, involving metacarpophalangeal or interphalangeal joint; without manipulation, each

> 🖵 6.15  ⚕ 6.54  **FUD** 090  T P2 🖵
>
> **AMA:** 2002,Apr,13

**26742** with manipulation, each

> 🖵 9.53  ⚕ 10.5  **FUD** 090  J A2 🖵
>
> **AMA:** 2002,Apr,13

**26746** Open treatment of articular fracture, involving metacarpophalangeal or interphalangeal joint, includes internal fixation, when performed, each

> 🖵 21.2  ⚕ 21.2  **FUD** 090  J A2 🖵
>
> **AMA:** 2002,Apr,13

**26750** Closed treatment of distal phalangeal fracture, finger or thumb; without manipulation, each

> 🖵 5.23  ⚕ 5.21  **FUD** 090  T P2 🖵
>
> **AMA:** 2002,Apr,13

**26755** with manipulation, each

> 🖵 7.76  ⚕ 8.90  **FUD** 090  T G2 🖵
>
> **AMA:** 2002,Apr,13

**26756** Percutaneous skeletal fixation of distal phalangeal fracture, finger or thumb, each

> 🖵 11.9  ⚕ 11.9  **FUD** 090  J A2 80 🖵
>
> **AMA:** 2002,Apr,13

**26765** Open treatment of distal phalangeal fracture, finger or thumb, includes internal fixation, when performed, each

> 🖵 14.3  ⚕ 14.3  **FUD** 090  J A2 🖵
>
> **AMA:** 2002,Apr,13

**26770** Closed treatment of interphalangeal joint dislocation, single, with manipulation; without anesthesia

> 🖵 7.23  ⚕ 7.80  **FUD** 090  T G2 🖵
>
> **AMA:** 2002,Apr,13

| 26/TC PC/TC Only | A2-Z3 ASC Payment | 50 Bilateral | ♂ Male Only | ♀ Female Only | 🖵 Facility RVU | ⚕ Non-Facility RVU | 🖵 CCI |
| FUD Follow-up Days | CMS: IOM (Pub 100) | A-Y OPPSI | 80/80 Surg Assist Allowed / w/Doc | | 🖵 Lab Crosswalk | 🖵 Radiology Crosswalk | ✖ CLIA |

76

CPT © 2017 American Medical Association. All Rights Reserved.

© 2017 Optum360, LLC

**26775** requiring anesthesia
🔪 9.86 ⚕ 10.8 **FUD** 090 [T] [P2] [▢]
**AMA:** 2002,Apr,13

**26776** Percutaneous skeletal fixation of interphalangeal joint dislocation, single, with manipulation
🔪 12.6 ⚕ 12.6 **FUD** 090 [J] [A2] [▢]
**AMA:** 2002,Apr,13

**26785** Open treatment of interphalangeal joint dislocation, includes internal fixation, when performed, single
🔪 15.6 ⚕ 15.6 **FUD** 090 [J] [A2] [▢]
**AMA:** 2002,Apr,13

## 26820-26863 Fusion of Joint(s) of Fingers or Hand

**26820** Fusion in opposition, thumb, with autogenous graft (includes obtaining graft)
🔪 21.6 ⚕ 21.6 **FUD** 090 [J] [A2] [80] [50] [▢]
**AMA:** 2002,Apr,13

**26841** Arthrodesis, carpometacarpal joint, thumb, with or without internal fixation;
🔪 20.4 ⚕ 20.4 **FUD** 090 [J] [A2] [80] [50] [▢]
**AMA:** 2002,Apr,13

**26842** with autograft (includes obtaining graft)
🔪 22.1 ⚕ 22.1 **FUD** 090 [J] [A2] [80] [50] [▢]
**AMA:** 2002,Apr,13

**26843** Arthrodesis, carpometacarpal joint, digit, other than thumb, each;
🔪 20.7 ⚕ 20.7 **FUD** 090 [J] [A2] [80] [▢]
**AMA:** 2017,Jan,8; 2016,Jan,13; 2015,Jan,16; 2014,Jan,11; 2012,Jan,15-42

**26844** with autograft (includes obtaining graft)
🔪 23.1 ⚕ 23.1 **FUD** 090 [J] [A2] [80] [▢]
**AMA:** 2002,Apr,13

**26850** Arthrodesis, metacarpophalangeal joint, with or without internal fixation;
🔪 19.5 ⚕ 19.5 **FUD** 090 [J] [A2] [80] [▢]
**AMA:** 2002,Apr,13

**26852** with autograft (includes obtaining graft)
🔪 22.4 ⚕ 22.4 **FUD** 090 [J] [A2] [80] [▢]
**AMA:** 2002,Apr,13

**26860** Arthrodesis, interphalangeal joint, with or without internal fixation;
🔪 15.9 ⚕ 15.9 **FUD** 090 [J] [A2] [▢]
**AMA:** 2017,Jan,8; 2016,Jan,13; 2015,Jan,16; 2014,Jan,11; 2012,Jan,15-42

+ **26861** each additional interphalangeal joint (List separately in addition to code for primary procedure)
Code first (26860)
🔪 2.99 ⚕ 2.99 **FUD** ZZZ [N] [N1] [▢]
**AMA:** 2017,Jan,8; 2016,Jan,13; 2015,Jan,16; 2014,Jan,11; 2012,Jan,15-42

**26862** with autograft (includes obtaining graft)
🔪 20.4 ⚕ 20.4 **FUD** 090 [J] [A2] [80] [▢]
**AMA:** 2002,Apr,13

+ **26863** with autograft (includes obtaining graft), each additional joint (List separately in addition to code for primary procedure)
Code first (26862)
🔪 6.68 ⚕ 6.68 **FUD** ZZZ [N] [N1] [80] [▢]
**AMA:** 2002,Apr,13

## 26910-26989 Amputations and Unlisted Procedures Finger/Hand

**26910** Amputation, metacarpal, with finger or thumb (ray amputation), single, with or without interosseous transfer
**EXCLUDES** *Repositioning (26550, 26555)*
*Transmetacarpal amputation of hand (25927)*
🔪 20.3 ⚕ 20.3 **FUD** 090 [J] [A2] [▢]
**AMA:** 2002,Apr,13

**26951** Amputation, finger or thumb, primary or secondary, any joint or phalanx, single, including neurectomies; with direct closure
**EXCLUDES** *Repair necessitating flaps or grafts (15050-15758)*
*Transmetacarpal amputation of hand (25927)*
🔪 18.4 ⚕ 18.4 **FUD** 090 [J] [A2] [▢]
**AMA:** 2002,Apr,13

**26952** with local advancement flaps (V-Y, hood)
**EXCLUDES** *Repair necessitating flaps or grafts (15050-15758)*
*Transmetacarpal amputation of hand (25927)*
🔪 18.1 ⚕ 18.1 **FUD** 090 [J] [A2] [▢]
**AMA:** 2002,Apr,13

**26989** Unlisted procedure, hands or fingers
🔪 0.00 ⚕ 0.00 **FUD** YYY [T]
**AMA:** 2002,Apr,13

## 26990-26992 Incision for Drainage of Pelvis or Hip
**EXCLUDES** *Simple incision and drainage procedures (10040-10160)*

**26990** Incision and drainage, pelvis or hip joint area; deep abscess or hematoma
🔪 17.9 ⚕ 17.9 **FUD** 090 [J] [A2] [▢]
**AMA:** 2002,Apr,13

**26991** infected bursa
🔪 15.0 ⚕ 20.1 **FUD** 090 [J] [A2] [80] [▢]
**AMA:** 2002,Apr,13

**26992** Incision, bone cortex, pelvis and/or hip joint (eg, osteomyelitis or bone abscess)
🔪 27.5 ⚕ 27.5 **FUD** 090 [C] [80] [▢]
**AMA:** 2017,Jan,8; 2016,Jan,13; 2015,Jan,16; 2014,Jan,11; 2012,Oct,14; 2012,Jan,15-42

## 27000-27006 Tenotomy Procedures of Hip

**27000** Tenotomy, adductor of hip, percutaneous (separate procedure)
🔪 11.6 ⚕ 11.6 **FUD** 090 [J] [A2] [50] [▢]
**AMA:** 2002,Apr,13; 1998,Nov,1

**27001** Tenotomy, adductor of hip, open
🔪 15.5 ⚕ 15.5 **FUD** 090 [J] [A2] [80] [50] [▢]
**AMA:** 2002,Apr,13; 1998,Nov,1

**27003** Tenotomy, adductor, subcutaneous, open, with obturator neurectomy
🔪 16.7 ⚕ 16.7 **FUD** 090 [J] [A2] [80] [50] [▢]
**AMA:** 2002,Apr,13

**27005** Tenotomy, hip flexor(s), open (separate procedure)
🔪 20.7 ⚕ 20.7 **FUD** 090 [C] [80] [50] [Asst]
**AMA:** 2002,Apr,13; 1998,Nov,1

**27006** Tenotomy, abductors and/or extensor(s) of hip, open (separate procedure)
🔪 21.0 ⚕ 21.0 **FUD** 090 [J] [80] [50] [▢]
**AMA:** 2002,Apr,13; 1998,Nov,1

## 27025-27036 Surgical Incision of Hip

**27025** Fasciotomy, hip or thigh, any type
🔪 26.2 ⚕ 26.2 **FUD** 090 [C] [80] [50] [▢]
**AMA:** 2002,Apr,13

**27027** Decompression fasciotomy(ies), pelvic (buttock) compartment(s) (eg, gluteus medius-minimus, gluteus maximus, iliopsoas, and/or tensor fascia lata muscle), unilateral
🔪 25.5 ⚕ 25.5 **FUD** 090 [J] [80] [50] [▢]

**27030** Arthrotomy, hip, with drainage (eg, infection)
🔪 26.9 ⚕ 26.9 **FUD** 090 [C] [80] [50] [▢]
**AMA:** 2002,Apr,13; 1998,Nov,1

**27033** Arthrotomy, hip, including exploration or removal of loose or foreign body
🔪 27.9 ⚕ 27.9 **FUD** 090 [J] [A2] [80] [50] [▢]
**AMA:** 2017,Jan,8; 2016,Jan,13; 2015,Jan,16; 2014,Jan,11

**27035** Denervation, hip joint, intrapelvic or extrapelvic intra-articular branches of sciatic, femoral, or obturator nerves

> *EXCLUDES* *Transection of obturator nerve (64763, 64766)*
> 🚗 30.5   ⚖ 30.5   **FUD** 090          J A2 80 50 ▣
> **AMA:** 2017,Jan,8; 2016,Jan,13; 2015,Jan,16; 2014,Mar,13

**27036** Capsulectomy or capsulotomy, hip, with or without excision of heterotopic bone, with release of hip flexor muscles (ie, gluteus medius, gluteus minimus, tensor fascia latae, rectus femoris, sartorius, iliopsoas)

> 🚗 29.0   ⚖ 29.0   **FUD** 090          C 80 50 ▣
> **AMA:** 2002,Apr,13; 1996,Nov,1

## 27040-27041 Biopsy of Hip/Pelvis

> *EXCLUDES* *Soft tissue needle biopsy (20206)*

**27040** Biopsy, soft tissue of pelvis and hip area; superficial

> 🚗 5.74   ⚖ 9.82   **FUD** 010          J A2 50 ▣
> **AMA:** 2002,Apr,13

**27041** deep, subfascial or intramuscular

> 🚗 19.9   ⚖ 19.9   **FUD** 090          J A2 50 ▣
> **AMA:** 2002,Apr,13; 1998,Nov,1

## 27043-27049 [27043, 27045, 27059] Excision Soft Tissue Tumors Hip/ Pelvis

> *INCLUDES* Any necessary elevation of tissue planes or dissection
> Measurement of tumor and necessary margin at greatest diameter prior to excision
> Simple and intermediate repairs
> Types of excision:
> Fascial or subfascial soft tissue tumors: simple and marginal resection of tumors found either in or below the deep fascia, not involving bone or excision of a substantial amount of normal tissue; primarily benign and intramuscular tumors
> Radical resection of soft tissue tumor: wide resection of tumor involving substantial margins of normal tissue and may involve tissue removal from one or more layers; mostly malignant or aggressive benign,
> Subcutaneous: simple and marginal resection of tumors found in the subcutaneous tissue above the deep fascia; most often benign
> *EXCLUDES* *Complex repair*
> *Excision of benign cutaneous lesions (eg, sebaceous cyst) (11400-11406)*
> *Radical resection of cutaneous tumors (eg, melanoma) (11600-11606)*
> *Significant exploration of vessels, neuroplasty, reconstruction, or complex bone repair*

**27043** Resequenced code. See code following 27047.

**27045** Resequenced code. See code following 27048.

**27047** Excision, tumor, soft tissue of pelvis and hip area, subcutaneous; less than 3 cm

> 🚗 10.4   ⚖ 13.3   **FUD** 090          J 62 50 ▣
> **AMA:** 2002,Apr,13; 1998,Nov,1

\# **27043** 3 cm or greater

> 🚗 13.5   ⚖ 13.5   **FUD** 090          J 62 50 ▣

**27048** Excision, tumor, soft tissue of pelvis and hip area, subfascial (eg, intramuscular); less than 5 cm

> 🚗 17.6   ⚖ 17.6   **FUD** 090          J 62 80 50 ▣
> **AMA:** 2002,Apr,13

\# **27045** 5 cm or greater

> 🚗 21.5   ⚖ 21.5   **FUD** 090          J 62 80 50 ▣

**27049** Radical resection of tumor (eg, sarcoma), soft tissue of pelvis and hip area; less than 5 cm

> 🚗 38.3   ⚖ 38.3   **FUD** 090          J 62 80 50 ▣
> **AMA:** 2002,Apr,13; 1998,Nov,1

\# **27059** 5 cm or greater

> 🚗 52.3   ⚖ 52.3   **FUD** 090          J 62 80 50 ▣

## 27050-27071 Procedures of Bones and Joints of Hip and Pelvis

**27050** Arthrotomy, with biopsy; sacroiliac joint

> 🚗 11.0   ⚖ 11.0   **FUD** 090          J A2 80 50 ▣
> **AMA:** 2002,Apr,13; 1994,Win,1

**27052** hip joint

> 🚗 16.6   ⚖ 16.6   **FUD** 090          J A2 80 50 CLIA
> **AMA:** 2002,Apr,13

**27054** Arthrotomy with synovectomy, hip joint

> 🚗 19.6   ⚖ 19.6   **FUD** 090          C 80 50 ▣
> **AMA:** 2002,Apr,13; 1994,Win,1

**27057** Decompression fasciotomy(ies), pelvic (buttock) compartment(s) (eg, gluteus medius-minimus, gluteus maximus, iliopsoas, and/or tensor fascia lata muscle) with debridement of nonviable muscle, unilateral

> 🚗 29.1   ⚖ 29.1   **FUD** 090          J 80 50 ▣

**27059** Resequenced code. See code following 27049.

**27060** Excision; ischial bursa

> 🚗 13.2   ⚖ 13.2   **FUD** 090          J A2 50 ▣
> **AMA:** 2002,Apr,13

**27062** trochanteric bursa or calcification

> *EXCLUDES* *Arthrocentesis (20610)*
> 🚗 13.0   ⚖ 13.0   **FUD** 090          J A2 50 ▣
> **AMA:** 2002,Apr,13

**27065** Excision of bone cyst or benign tumor, wing of ilium, symphysis pubis, or greater trochanter of femur; superficial, includes autograft, when performed

> 🚗 14.8   ⚖ 14.8   **FUD** 090          J A2 80 50 ▣
> **AMA:** 2002,Apr,13

**27066** deep (subfascial), includes autograft, when performed

> 🚗 23.3   ⚖ 23.3   **FUD** 090          J A2 80 50 ▣
> **AMA:** 2002,Apr,13

**27067** with autograft requiring separate incision

> 🚗 29.4   ⚖ 29.4   **FUD** 090          J A2 80 50 ▣
> **AMA:** 2002,Apr,13

**27070** Partial excision, wing of ilium, symphysis pubis, or greater trochanter of femur, (craterization, saucerization) (eg, osteomyelitis or bone abscess); superficial

> 🚗 24.4   ⚖ 24.4   **FUD** 090          C 80 50 ▣
> **AMA:** 2002,Apr,13; 1998,Nov,1

**27071** deep (subfascial or intramuscular)

> 🚗 26.3   ⚖ 26.3   **FUD** 090          C 80 50 ▣
> **AMA:** 2002,Apr,13

## 27075-27078 Radical Resection Bone Tumor of Hip/Pelvis

> *INCLUDES* Any necessary elevation of tissue planes or dissection
> Excision of adjacent soft tissue during bone tumor resection (27043-27049 [27043, 27045, 27059])
> Measurement of tumor and necessary margin at greatest diameter prior to excision
> Resection of the tumor (may include entire bone) and wide margins of normal tissue primarily for malignant or aggressive benign tumors
> Simple and intermediate repairs
> *EXCLUDES* *Complex repair*
> *Significant exploration of vessels, neuroplasty, reconstruction, or complex bone repair*

**27075** Radical resection of tumor; wing of ilium, 1 pubic or ischial ramus or symphysis pubis

> 🚗 60.2   ⚖ 60.2   **FUD** 090          C 80 ▣
> **AMA:** 2002,Apr,13; 1994,Win,1

**27076** ilium, including acetabulum, both pubic rami, or ischium and acetabulum

> 🚗 72.9   ⚖ 72.9   **FUD** 090          C 80 ▣
> **AMA:** 2002,Apr,13

**27077** innominate bone, total

> 🚗 81.3   ⚖ 81.3   **FUD** 090          C 80 ▣
> **AMA:** 2002,Apr,13

**27078** ischial tuberosity and greater trochanter of femur

> 🚗 59.4   ⚖ 59.4   **FUD** 090          C 80 50 ▣
> **AMA:** 2002,Apr,13

| 26/TC PC/TC Only | A2-Z3 ASC Payment | 50 Bilateral | ♂ Male Only | ♀ Female Only | 🚗 Facility RVU | ⚖ Non-Facility RVU | ▣ CCI |
| FUD Follow-up Days | CMS: IOM (Pub 100) | A-Y OPPSI | 80/80 Surg Assist Allowed / w/Doc | | 🗎 Lab Crosswalk | 🗎 Radiology Crosswalk | ✖ CLIA |

78                                    CPT © 2017 American Medical Association. All Rights Reserved.                              © 2017 Optum360, LLC

## 27080 Excision of Coccyx

EXCLUDES *Surgical excision of decubitus ulcers (15920, 15922, 15931-15958)*

**27080** **Coccygectomy, primary**
🚗 14.6  ⚖ 14.6  **FUD** 090  J A2 80 ▢
**AMA:** 2002,Apr,13

## 27086-27091 Removal Foreign Body or Hip Prosthesis

**27086** **Removal of foreign body, pelvis or hip; subcutaneous tissue**
🚗 4.61  ⚖ 7.91  **FUD** 010  J A2 80 50 ▢
**AMA:** 2017,Jan,8; 2016,Jan,13; 2015,Jan,16; 2014,Jan,11

**27087** **deep (subfascial or intramuscular)**
🚗 17.7  ⚖ 17.7  **FUD** 090  J A2 80 50 ▢
**AMA:** 2002,Apr,13; 1998,Nov,1

A foreign body is removed from the pelvis or hip

**27090** **Removal of hip prosthesis; (separate procedure)**
🚗 23.8  ⚖ 23.8  **FUD** 090  C 80 50 ▢
**AMA:** 2002,Apr,13

**27091** **complicated, including total hip prosthesis, methylmethacrylate with or without insertion of spacer**
🚗 46.0  ⚖ 46.0  **FUD** 090  C 80 50 ▢
**AMA:** 2017,Jan,8; 2016,Jan,13; 2015,Jan,16; 2014,Jan,11

## 27093-27096 Injection for Arthrogram Hip/Sacroiliac Joint

**27093** **Injection procedure for hip arthrography; without anesthesia**
🔋 (73525)
🚗 2.02  ⚖ 5.32  **FUD** 000  N N1 50 ▢
**AMA:** 2017,Jan,8; 2016,Jan,13; 2015,Aug,6; 2015,Jan,16; 2014,Jan,11; 2012,Jun,14

**27095** **with anesthesia**
🔋 (73525)
🚗 2.40  ⚖ 6.91  **FUD** 000  N N1 50 ▢
**AMA:** 2017,Jan,8; 2016,Jan,13; 2016,Jan,11; 2015,Aug,6; 2015,Jan,16; 2014,Jan,11; 2012,Jun,14

**27096** **Injection procedure for sacroiliac joint, anesthetic/steroid, with image guidance (fluoroscopy or CT) including arthrography when performed**
INCLUDES Confirmation of intra-articular needle placement with CT or fluoroscopy
Fluoroscopic guidance (77002-77003)
EXCLUDES *Procedure performed without fluoroscopy or CT guidance (20552)*
🚗 2.40  ⚖ 4.52  **FUD** 000  B 50 ▢
**AMA:** 2017,Jan,8; 2016,Jan,13; 2015,Aug,6; 2015,Jan,16; 2014,Jan,11; 2012,Jan,3-5; 2012,Jan,15-42

## 27097-27187 Revision/Reconstruction Hip and Pelvis

INCLUDES Closed, open and percutaneous treatment of fractures and dislocations

**27097** **Release or recession, hamstring, proximal**
🚗 19.4  ⚖ 19.4  **FUD** 090  J A2 80 50 ▢
**AMA:** 2002,Apr,13; 1998,Nov,1

**27098** **Transfer, adductor to ischium**
🚗 18.3  ⚖ 18.3  **FUD** 090  J A2 80 50 ▢
**AMA:** 2002,Apr,13; 1998,Nov,1

**27100** **Transfer external oblique muscle to greater trochanter including fascial or tendon extension (graft)**
INCLUDES Eggers procedure
🚗 23.4  ⚖ 23.4  **FUD** 090  J A2 80 50 ▢
**AMA:** 2002,Apr,13

**27105** **Transfer paraspinal muscle to hip (includes fascial or tendon extension graft)**
🚗 24.9  ⚖ 24.9  **FUD** 090  J A2 80 50 ▢
**AMA:** 2002,Apr,13

**27110** **Transfer iliopsoas; to greater trochanter of femur**
🚗 27.8  ⚖ 27.8  **FUD** 090  J A2 80 50 ▢
**AMA:** 2002,May,7; 2002,Apr,13

**27111** **to femoral neck**
🚗 25.9  ⚖ 25.9  **FUD** 090  J A2 80 50 ▢
**AMA:** 2002,Apr,13

**27120** **Acetabuloplasty; (eg, Whitman, Colonna, Haygroves, or cup type)**
🚗 37.2  ⚖ 37.2  **FUD** 090  C 80 50 ▢
**AMA:** 2002,Apr,13

**27122** **resection, femoral head (eg, Girdlestone procedure)**
🚗 31.7  ⚖ 31.7  **FUD** 090  C 80 50 ▢
**AMA:** 2002,Apr,13; 1998,Nov,1

**27125** **Hemiarthroplasty, hip, partial (eg, femoral stem prosthesis, bipolar arthroplasty)**
EXCLUDES *Hip replacement following hip fracture (27236)*
🚗 32.6  ⚖ 32.6  **FUD** 090  C 80 50 ▢
**AMA:** 2017,Jan,8; 2016,Jan,13; 2015,Jan,16; 2014,Jan,11; 2012,Jan,15-42

Acetabulum remains intact

Prosthesis

**27130** **Arthroplasty, acetabular and proximal femoral prosthetic replacement (total hip arthroplasty), with or without autograft or allograft**

    🔹 39.1   🔧 39.1   **FUD** 090     C 80 50 ▣

    **AMA:** 2017,Jan,8; 2016,Jan,13; 2015,Jan,16; 2014,Jan,11; 2012,Jan,15-42

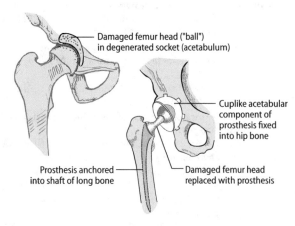

- Damaged femur head ("ball") in degenerated socket (acetabulum)
- Cuplike acetabular component of prosthesis fixed into hip bone
- Prosthesis anchored into shaft of long bone
- Damaged femur head replaced with prosthesis

**27132** **Conversion of previous hip surgery to total hip arthroplasty, with or without autograft or allograft**

    🔹 48.3   🔧 48.3   **FUD** 090     C 80 50 ▣

    **AMA:** 2017,Sep,14; 2017,Jan,8; 2016,Jan,13; 2015,Jan,16; 2014,Jan,11

**27134** **Revision of total hip arthroplasty; both components, with or without autograft or allograft**

    🔹 55.3   🔧 55.3   **FUD** 090     C 80 50 ▣

    **AMA:** 2017,Jan,8; 2016,Jan,13; 2015,Jan,16; 2014,Jan,11

**27137** **acetabular component only, with or without autograft or allograft**

    🔹 42.5   🔧 42.5   **FUD** 090     C 80 50 ▣

    **AMA:** 2017,Jan,8; 2016,Jan,13; 2015,Jan,16; 2014,Jan,11

**27138** **femoral component only, with or without allograft**

    🔹 44.1   🔧 44.1   **FUD** 090     C 80 50 ▣

    **AMA:** 2017,Jan,8; 2016,Jan,13; 2015,Jan,16; 2014,Jan,11

**27140** **Osteotomy and transfer of greater trochanter of femur (separate procedure)**

    🔹 25.6   🔧 25.6   **FUD** 090     C 80 50 ▣

    **AMA:** 2008,Dec,3-4; 2002,Apr,13

**27146** **Osteotomy, iliac, acetabular or innominate bone;**

    INCLUDES   Salter osteotomy

    🔹 36.7   🔧 36.7   **FUD** 090     C 80 50 ▣

    **AMA:** 2017,Jan,8; 2016,Jan,13; 2015,Jan,16; 2014,Jan,11; 2012,Jan,15-42

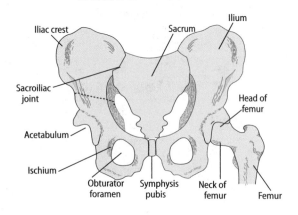

- Iliac crest
- Sacrum
- Ilium
- Sacroiliac joint
- Head of femur
- Acetabulum
- Ischium
- Obturator foramen
- Symphysis pubis
- Neck of femur
- Femur

**27147** **with open reduction of hip**

    INCLUDES   Pemberton osteotomy

    🔹 42.1   🔧 42.1   **FUD** 090     C 80 50 ▣

    **AMA:** 2008,Dec,3-4; 2002,Apr,13

- Ilium

Example of innominate osteotomy

Kirschner wires are drilled through the ilium and into lower fragment

- Greater trochanter
- Acetabulum
- Head of femur

Femoral head is reduced into the acetabulum

**27151** **with femoral osteotomy**

    🔹 45.9   🔧 45.9   **FUD** 090     C 80 50 ▣

    **AMA:** 2008,Dec,3-4; 2002,Apr,13

**27156** **with femoral osteotomy and with open reduction of hip**

    INCLUDES   Chiari osteotomy

    🔹 48.8   🔧 48.8   **FUD** 090     C 80 50 ▣

    **AMA:** 2008,Dec,3-4; 2002,Apr,13

**27158** **Osteotomy, pelvis, bilateral (eg, congenital malformation)**

    🔹 40.4   🔧 40.4   **FUD** 090     C 80 ▣

    **AMA:** 2008,Dec,3-4; 2002,Apr,13

**27161** **Osteotomy, femoral neck (separate procedure)**

    🔹 34.9   🔧 34.9   **FUD** 090     C 80 50 ▣

    **AMA:** 2008,Dec,3-4; 2002,Apr,13

**27165** **Osteotomy, intertrochanteric or subtrochanteric including internal or external fixation and/or cast**

    🔹 39.5   🔧 39.5   **FUD** 090     C 80 50 ▣

    **AMA:** 2017,Jan,8; 2016,Jan,13; 2015,Jan,16; 2014,Jan,11

**27170** **Bone graft, femoral head, neck, intertrochanteric or subtrochanteric area (includes obtaining bone graft)**

    🔹 33.8   🔧 33.8   **FUD** 090     C 80 50 ▣

    **AMA:** 2017,Jan,8; 2016,Jan,13; 2015,Jan,16; 2014,Jan,11

**27175** **Treatment of slipped femoral epiphysis; by traction, without reduction**

    🔹 18.8   🔧 18.8   **FUD** 090     C 80 50 ▣

    **AMA:** 2008,Dec,3-4; 2002,Apr,13

**27176** **by single or multiple pinning, in situ**

    🔹 26.4   🔧 26.4   **FUD** 090     C 80 50 ▣

    **AMA:** 2008,Dec,3-4; 2002,Apr,13

**27177** **Open treatment of slipped femoral epiphysis; single or multiple pinning or bone graft (includes obtaining graft)**

    🔹 32.1   🔧 32.1   **FUD** 090     C 80 50 ▣

    **AMA:** 2008,Dec,3-4; 2002,Apr,13

**27178** **closed manipulation with single or multiple pinning**

    🔹 23.0   🔧 23.0   **FUD** 090     C 80 50 ▣

    **AMA:** 2008,Dec,3-4; 2002,Apr,13

**27179** **osteoplasty of femoral neck (Heyman type procedure)**

    🔹 27.4   🔧 27.4   **FUD** 090     J 80 50 ▣

    **AMA:** 2008,Dec,3-4; 2002,Apr,13

**27181** **osteotomy and internal fixation**

    🔹 36.8   🔧 36.8   **FUD** 090     C 80 50 ▣

    **AMA:** 2008,Dec,3-4; 2002,Apr,13

26/TC PC/TC Only    A2-Z3 ASC Payment    50 Bilateral    ♂ Male Only    ♀ Female Only    🔹 Facility RVU    🔧 Non-Facility RVU    ▣ CCI

FUD Follow-up Days    CMS: IOM (Pub 100)    A-Y OPPSI    80/80 Surg Assist Allowed / w/Doc    🔲 Lab Crosswalk    🔲 Radiology Crosswalk    ✕ CLIA

80     CPT © 2017 American Medical Association. All Rights Reserved.     © 2017 Optum360, LLC

**27185** Epiphyseal arrest by epiphysiodesis or stapling, greater trochanter of femur
⚙ 20.6 ☒ 20.6 **FUD** 090 C 50 🔲
**AMA:** 2008,Dec,3-4; 2002,Apr,13

**27187** Prophylactic treatment (nailing, pinning, plating or wiring) with or without methylmethacrylate, femoral neck and proximal femur
⚙ 28.5 ☒ 28.5 **FUD** 090 C 80 50 🔲
**AMA:** 2017,Jan,8; 2016,Jan,13; 2015,Jan,16; 2014,Jan,11

# 27197-27269 Treatment of Fracture/Dislocation Hip/Pelvis

**27197** Closed treatment of posterior pelvic ring fracture(s), dislocation(s), diastasis or subluxation of the ilium, sacroiliac joint, and/or sacrum, with or without anterior pelvic ring fracture(s) and/or dislocation(s) of the pubic symphysis and/or superior/inferior rami, unilateral or bilateral; without manipulation
⚙ 3.35 ☒ 3.35 **FUD** 000 T J8 🔲
**AMA:** 2017,Jun,9

**27198** with manipulation, requiring more than local anesthesia (ie, general anesthesia, moderate sedation, spinal/epidural)
EXCLUDES Closed treatment anterior pelvic ring, pubic symphysis, inferior rami fracture/dislocation--see appropriate E&M codes
⚙ 8.54 ☒ 8.54 **FUD** 000 T J8 80 🔲
**AMA:** 2017,Jun,9

**27200** Closed treatment of coccygeal fracture
⚙ 5.38 ☒ 5.17 **FUD** 090 T P3 🔲
**AMA:** 2008,Dec,3-4; 2002,Apr,13

**27202** Open treatment of coccygeal fracture
⚙ 15.9 ☒ 15.9 **FUD** 090 J A2 80 🔲
**AMA:** 2008,Dec,3-4; 2002,Apr,13

**27215** Open treatment of iliac spine(s), tuberosity avulsion, or iliac wing fracture(s), unilateral, for pelvic bone fracture patterns that do not disrupt the pelvic ring, includes internal fixation, when performed
⚙ 17.9 ☒ 17.9 **FUD** 090 E 🔲
**AMA:** 2008,Dec,3-4; 2002,Apr,13

**27216** Percutaneous skeletal fixation of posterior pelvic bone fracture and/or dislocation, for fracture patterns that disrupt the pelvic ring, unilateral (includes ipsilateral ilium, sacroiliac joint and/or sacrum)
EXCLUDES Sacroiliac joint arthrodesis without fracture and/or dislocation, percutaneous or minimally invasive (27279)
⚙ 26.6 ☒ 26.6 **FUD** 090 E 🔲
**AMA:** 2017,Jan,8; 2016,Jan,13; 2015,Jan,16; 2014,Mar,4; 2013,Sep,17

**27217** Open treatment of anterior pelvic bone fracture and/or dislocation for fracture patterns that disrupt the pelvic ring, unilateral, includes internal fixation, when performed (includes pubic symphysis and/or ipsilateral superior/inferior rami)
⚙ 24.9 ☒ 24.9 **FUD** 090 E 🔲
**AMA:** 2008,Dec,3-4; 2002,Apr,13

**27218** Open treatment of posterior pelvic bone fracture and/or dislocation, for fracture patterns that disrupt the pelvic ring, unilateral, includes internal fixation, when performed (includes ipsilateral ilium, sacroiliac joint and/or sacrum)
EXCLUDES Sacroiliac joint arthrodesis without fracture and/or dislocation, percutaneous or minimally invasive (27279)
⚙ 34.5 ☒ 34.5 **FUD** 090 E 🔲
**AMA:** 2017,Jan,8; 2016,Jan,13; 2015,Jan,16; 2014,Mar,4

**27220** Closed treatment of acetabulum (hip socket) fracture(s); without manipulation
⚙ 15.0 ☒ 15.1 **FUD** 090 T 82 50 🔲
**AMA:** 2008,Dec,3-4; 2002,Apr,13

**27222** with manipulation, with or without skeletal traction
⚙ 28.0 ☒ 28.0 **FUD** 090 C 50 🔲
**AMA:** 2008,Dec,3-4; 2002,Apr,13

**27226** Open treatment of posterior or anterior acetabular wall fracture, with internal fixation
⚙ 30.4 ☒ 30.4 **FUD** 090 C 80 50 🔲
**AMA:** 2008,Dec,3-4; 2002,Apr,13

**27227** Open treatment of acetabular fracture(s) involving anterior or posterior (one) column, or a fracture running transversely across the acetabulum, with internal fixation
⚙ 47.9 ☒ 47.9 **FUD** 090 C 80 50 🔲
**AMA:** 2008,Dec,3-4; 2002,Apr,13

**27228** Open treatment of acetabular fracture(s) involving anterior and posterior (two) columns, includes T-fracture and both column fracture with complete articular detachment, or single column or transverse fracture with associated acetabular wall fracture, with internal fixation
⚙ 54.4 ☒ 54.4 **FUD** 090 C 80 50 🔲
**AMA:** 2008,Dec,3-4; 2002,Apr,13

**27230** Closed treatment of femoral fracture, proximal end, neck; without manipulation
⚙ 13.5 ☒ 13.6 **FUD** 090 T A2 50 🔲
**AMA:** 2008,Dec,3-4; 2002,Apr,13

**27232** with manipulation, with or without skeletal traction
⚙ 21.5 ☒ 21.5 **FUD** 090 C 50 🔲
**AMA:** 2008,Dec,3-4; 2002,Apr,13

**27235** Percutaneous skeletal fixation of femoral fracture, proximal end, neck
⚙ 26.1 ☒ 26.1 **FUD** 090 J 50 🔲
**AMA:** 2017,Jan,8; 2016,Jan,13; 2015,Jan,16; 2014,Jan,11

**27236** Open treatment of femoral fracture, proximal end, neck, internal fixation or prosthetic replacement
⚙ 34.4 ☒ 34.4 **FUD** 090 C 80 50 🔲
**AMA:** 2017,Jan,8; 2016,Nov,9; 2016,Jan,13; 2015,Jan,16; 2014,Jan,11; 2012,Jan,15-42

**27238** Closed treatment of intertrochanteric, peritrochanteric, or subtrochanteric femoral fracture; without manipulation
⚙ 13.1 ☒ 13.1 **FUD** 090 J A2 50 🔲
**AMA:** 2017,Jan,8; 2016,Jan,13; 2015,Jan,16; 2014,Jan,11

**27240** with manipulation, with or without skin or skeletal traction
⚙ 27.5 ☒ 27.5 **FUD** 090 C 50 🔲
**AMA:** 2017,Jan,8; 2016,Jan,13; 2015,Jan,16; 2014,Jan,11

**27244** Treatment of intertrochanteric, peritrochanteric, or subtrochanteric femoral fracture; with plate/screw type implant, with or without cerclage
⚙ 35.4 ☒ 35.4 **FUD** 090 C 80 50 🔲
**AMA:** 2017,Jan,8; 2016,Jan,13; 2015,Jan,16; 2014,Jan,11

**27245** with intramedullary implant, with or without interlocking screws and/or cerclage
⚙ 35.4 ☒ 35.4 **FUD** 090 C 80 50 🔲
**AMA:** 2017,Jan,8; 2016,Jan,13; 2015,Jan,16; 2014,Jan,11; 2013,Sep,17

**27246** Closed treatment of greater trochanteric fracture, without manipulation
⚙ 11.0 ☒ 11.0 **FUD** 090 T A2 50 🔲
**AMA:** 2008,Dec,3-4; 2002,Apr,13

**27248** Open treatment of greater trochanteric fracture, includes internal fixation, when performed
⚙ 21.3 ☒ 21.3 **FUD** 090 C 80 50 🔲
**AMA:** 2008,Dec,3-4; 2002,Apr,13

**27250** Closed treatment of hip dislocation, traumatic; without anesthesia
⚙ 5.19 ☒ 5.19 **FUD** 000 T A2 50 🔲
**AMA:** 2008,Dec,3-4; 2002,Apr,13

● New Code ▲ Revised Code ○ Reinstated ● New Web Release ▲ Revised Web Release Unlisted Not Covered # Resequenced
⊘ AMA Mod 51 Exempt ⑨ Optum Mod 51 Exempt ⊛ Mod 63 Exempt ⁄ Non-FDA Drug ★ Telemedicine Ⅿ Maternity Ⓐ Age Edit ✛ Add-on **AMA:** CPT Asst
© 2017 Optum360, LLC CPT © 2017 American Medical Association. All Rights Reserved. **81**

**Musculoskeletal System**

**27252 — 27324**

**27252** **requiring anesthesia**
🔧 21.7　✂ 21.7　**FUD** 090　　　　J A2 50 ▣
**AMA:** 2008,Dec,3-4; 2002,Apr,13

**27253** **Open treatment of hip dislocation, traumatic, without internal fixation**
🔧 27.1　✂ 27.1　**FUD** 090　　　　C 80 50 ▣
**AMA:** 2008,Dec,3-4; 2002,Apr,13

**27254** **Open treatment of hip dislocation, traumatic, with acetabular wall and femoral head fracture, with or without internal or external fixation**
*EXCLUDES* Acetabular fracture treatment (27226-27227)
🔧 36.5　✂ 36.5　**FUD** 090　　　　C 80 50 ▣
**AMA:** 2008,Dec,3-4; 2002,Apr,13

**27256** **Treatment of spontaneous hip dislocation (developmental, including congenital or pathological), by abduction, splint or traction; without anesthesia, without manipulation**
🔧 6.73　✂ 8.53　**FUD** 010　　　　T G2 80 50 ▣
**AMA:** 2008,Dec,3-4; 2002,Apr,13

**27257** **with manipulation, requiring anesthesia**
🔧 9.82　✂ 9.82　**FUD** 010　　　　J A2 80 50 ▣
**AMA:** 2008,Dec,3-4; 2002,Apr,13

**27258** **Open treatment of spontaneous hip dislocation (developmental, including congenital or pathological), replacement of femoral head in acetabulum (including tenotomy, etc);**
*INCLUDES* Lorenz's operation
🔧 31.9　✂ 31.9　**FUD** 090　　　　C 80 50 ▣
**AMA:** 2008,Dec,3-4; 2002,Apr,13

**27259** **with femoral shaft shortening**
🔧 44.8　✂ 44.8　**FUD** 090　　　　C 80 50 ▣
**AMA:** 2008,Dec,3-4; 2002,Apr,13

**27265** **Closed treatment of post hip arthroplasty dislocation; without anesthesia**
🔧 11.3　✂ 11.3　**FUD** 090　　　　T A2 50 ▣
**AMA:** 2008,Dec,3-4; 2002,Apr,13

**27266** **requiring regional or general anesthesia**
🔧 16.6　✂ 16.6　**FUD** 090　　　　J A2 50 ▣
**AMA:** 2008,Dec,3-4; 2002,Apr,13

**27267** **Closed treatment of femoral fracture, proximal end, head; without manipulation**
🔧 12.4　✂ 12.4　**FUD** 090　　　　J G2 80 50 ▣
**AMA:** 2017,Jan,8; 2016,Jan,13; 2015,Jan,16; 2014,Jan,11

**27268** **with manipulation**
🔧 15.2　✂ 15.2　**FUD** 090　　　　C 80 50 ▣
**AMA:** 2017,Jan,8; 2016,Jan,13; 2015,Jan,16; 2014,Jan,11

**27269** **Open treatment of femoral fracture, proximal end, head, includes internal fixation, when performed**
*EXCLUDES* Arthrotomy, hip (27033)
Open treatment of hip dislocation, traumatic, without internal fixation (27253)
🔧 35.8　✂ 35.8　**FUD** 090　　　　C 80 50 ▣
**AMA:** 2017,Jan,8; 2016,Jan,13; 2015,Jan,16; 2014,Jan,11

## 27275 Hip Manipulation with Anesthesia

**27275** **Manipulation, hip joint, requiring general anesthesia**
🔧 5.22　✂ 5.22　**FUD** 010　　　　J A2 ▣
**AMA:** 2017,Jan,8; 2016,May,13; 2016,Jan,13; 2016,Jan,11; 2015,Jan,16; 2014,Jan,11

## 27279-27286 Arthrodesis of Hip and Pelvis

**27279** **Arthrodesis, sacroiliac joint, percutaneous or minimally invasive (indirect visualization), with image guidance, includes obtaining bone graft when performed, and placement of transfixing device**
🔧 19.9　✂ 19.9　**FUD** 090　　　　J J8 80 50 ▣

**27280** **Arthrodesis, open, sacroiliac joint, including obtaining bone graft, including instrumentation, when performed**
*EXCLUDES* Sacroiliac joint arthrodesis without fracture and/or dislocation, percutaneous or minimally invasive (27279)
🔧 39.3　✂ 39.3　**FUD** 090　　　　C 80 50 ▣
**AMA:** 2017,Jan,8; 2016,Jan,13; 2015,Jan,16; 2014,Mar,4; 2014,Jan,11; 2013,Sep,17

**27282** **Arthrodesis, symphysis pubis (including obtaining graft)**
🔧 23.4　✂ 23.4　**FUD** 090　　　　C 80 ▣
**AMA:** 2008,Dec,3-4; 2002,Apr,13

**27284** **Arthrodesis, hip joint (including obtaining graft);**
🔧 42.7　✂ 42.7　**FUD** 090　　　　C 80 50 ▣
**AMA:** 2008,Dec,3-4; 2002,Apr,13

**27286** **with subtrochanteric osteotomy**
🔧 46.8　✂ 46.8　**FUD** 090　　　　C 80 50 ▣
**AMA:** 2017,Jan,8; 2016,Jan,13; 2015,Jan,16; 2014,Jan,11

## 27290-27299 Amputations and Unlisted Procedures of Hip and Pelvis

**27290** **Interpelviabdominal amputation (hindquarter amputation)**
*INCLUDES* Pean's amputation
🔧 46.4　✂ 46.4　**FUD** 090　　　　C 80 ▣
**AMA:** 2017,Jan,8; 2016,Jan,13; 2015,Jan,16; 2014,Jan,11

**27295** **Disarticulation of hip**
🔧 36.4　✂ 36.4　**FUD** 090　　　　C 80 50 ▣
**AMA:** 2017,Jan,8; 2016,Jan,13; 2015,Jan,16; 2014,Jan,11

**27299** **Unlisted procedure, pelvis or hip joint**
🔧 0.00　✂ 0.00　**FUD** YYY　　　　T 80 50
**AMA:** 2017,Jan,8; 2016,Jun,8; 2016,Jan,13; 2015,Jan,16; 2014,Mar,13; 2014,Jan,11; 2012,Nov,13-14; 2012,Oct,14; 2012,Jan,15-42

## 27301-27310 Incisional Procedures Femur or Knee
*EXCLUDES* Superficial incision and drainage (10040-10160)

**27301** **Incision and drainage, deep abscess, bursa, or hematoma, thigh or knee region**
🔧 14.4　✂ 19.1　**FUD** 090　　　　J A2 50 ▣
**AMA:** 2017,Jan,8; 2016,Jan,13; 2015,Jan,16; 2014,Jan,11

**27303** **Incision, deep, with opening of bone cortex, femur or knee (eg, osteomyelitis or bone abscess)**
🔧 18.3　✂ 18.3　**FUD** 090　　　　C 80 50 ▣
**AMA:** 2008,Dec,3-4; 2002,Apr,13

**27305** **Fasciotomy, iliotibial (tenotomy), open**
*EXCLUDES* Ober-Yount (gluteal-iliotibial) fasciotomy (27025)
🔧 13.7　✂ 13.7　**FUD** 090　　　　J A2 80 50 ▣
**AMA:** 2008,Dec,3-4; 2002,Apr,13

**27306** **Tenotomy, percutaneous, adductor or hamstring; single tendon (separate procedure)**
🔧 10.0　✂ 10.0　**FUD** 090　　　　J A2 80 50 ▣
**AMA:** 2017,Aug,9

**27307** **multiple tendons**
🔧 12.2　✂ 12.2　**FUD** 090　　　　J A2 80 50 ▣
**AMA:** 2017,Aug,9

**27310** **Arthrotomy, knee, with exploration, drainage, or removal of foreign body (eg, infection)**
🔧 20.9　✂ 20.9　**FUD** 090　　　　J A2 80 50 ▣
**AMA:** 2017,Jan,8; 2016,Jan,13; 2015,Jan,16; 2014,Jan,11

## 27323-27324 Biopsy Femur or Knee
*EXCLUDES* Soft tissue needle biopsy (20206)

**27323** **Biopsy, soft tissue of thigh or knee area; superficial**
🔧 5.13　✂ 7.73　**FUD** 010　　　　J A2 50 ▣
**AMA:** 2017,Jan,8; 2016,Jan,13; 2015,Jan,16; 2014,Jan,11

**27324** **deep (subfascial or intramuscular)**
🔧 11.4　✂ 11.4　**FUD** 090　　　　J A2 50 ▣
**AMA:** 2017,Jan,8; 2016,Jan,13; 2015,Jan,16; 2014,Jan,11

## 27325-27326 Neurectomy

**27325**    **Neurectomy, hamstring muscle**
    🖩 14.6   🔧 14.6   **FUD** 090    J A2 80 50 ▣

**27326**    **Neurectomy, popliteal (gastrocnemius)**
    🖩 14.3   🔧 14.3   **FUD** 090    J A2 80 50 ▣

## 27327-27329 [27337, 27339] Excision Soft Tissue Tumors Femur/ Knee

INCLUDES   Any necessary elevation of tissue planes or dissection
Measurement of tumor and necessary margin at greatest diameter prior
    to excision
Simple and intermediate repairs
Types of excision:
    Fascial or subfascial soft tissue tumors: simple and marginal resection
       of tumors found either in or below the deep fascia, not including
       bone or excision of a substantial amount of normal tissue; primarily
       benign and intramuscular tumors
    Radical resection of soft tissue tumor: wide resection of tumor involving
       substantial margins of normal tissue and may involve tissue
       removal from one or more layers; most often malignant or
       aggressive benign
    Subcutaneous: simple and marginal resection of tumors in the
       subcutaneous tissue above the deep fascia; most often benign

EXCLUDES   *Complex repair*
*Excision of benign cutaneous lesions (eg, sebaceous cyst) (11400-11406)*
*Radical resection of cutaneous tumors (eg, melanoma) (11600-11606)*
*Significant exploration of vessels or neuroplasty*

**27327**    **Excision, tumor, soft tissue of thigh or knee area, subcutaneous; less than 3 cm**
    🖩 9.02   🔧 13.1   **FUD** 090    J G2 50 ▣
    **AMA:** 2002,Apr,13

\#   **27337**    **3 cm or greater**
    🖩 12.0   🔧 12.0   **FUD** 090    J G2 80 50 ▣

**27328**    **Excision, tumor, soft tissue of thigh or knee area, subfascial (eg, intramuscular); less than 5 cm**
    🖩 17.8   🔧 17.8   **FUD** 090    J G2 50 ▣
    **AMA:** 2017,Jan,8; 2016,Nov,9

\#   **27339**    **5 cm or greater**
    🖩 21.7   🔧 21.7   **FUD** 090    J G2 80 50 ▣

*27329*    **Resequenced code. See code following 27360.**

## 27330-27360 Resection Procedures Thigh/Knee

**27330**    **Arthrotomy, knee; with synovial biopsy only**
    🖩 11.8   🔧 11.8   **FUD** 090    J A2 50 ▣
    **AMA:** 2017,Jan,8; 2016,Jan,13; 2015,Jan,16; 2014,Jan,11; 2012,Mar,9-10

**27331**    **including joint exploration, biopsy, or removal of loose or foreign bodies**
    🖩 13.6   🔧 13.6   **FUD** 090    J A2 80 50 ▣
    **AMA:** 2017,Jan,8; 2016,Jan,13; 2015,Jan,16; 2014,Jan,11; 2012,Nov,13-14

**27332**    **Arthrotomy, with excision of semilunar cartilage (meniscectomy) knee; medial OR lateral**
    🖩 18.4   🔧 18.4   **FUD** 090    J A2 80 50 ▣
    **AMA:** 2002,Apr,13; 1998,Nov,1

**Overhead view of right knee**

Labels: Lateral meniscus, Posterior cruciate ligament, Medial meniscus, Anterior horns, Posterior horns, Patellar ligament, Anterior cruciate ligament, Bucket handle tear, Radial tear, Meniscus

**27333**    **medial AND lateral**
    🖩 16.8   🔧 16.8   **FUD** 090    J A2 80 50 ▣
    **AMA:** 2017,Jan,8; 2016,Jan,13; 2015,Jan,16; 2014,Jan,11; 2012,Mar,9-10

**27334**    **Arthrotomy, with synovectomy, knee; anterior OR posterior**
    🖩 19.6   🔧 19.6   **FUD** 090    J A2 80 50 ▣
    **AMA:** 2002,Apr,13; 1998,Nov,1

**27335**    **anterior AND posterior including popliteal area**
    🖩 21.8   🔧 21.8   **FUD** 090    J A2 80 50 ▣
    **AMA:** 2002,Apr,13

*27337*    **Resequenced code. See code following 27327.**

*27339*    **Resequenced code. See code following 27328.**

**27340**    **Excision, prepatellar bursa**
    🖩 10.6   🔧 10.6   **FUD** 090    J A2 50 ▣
    **AMA:** 2002,Apr,13

**27345**    **Excision of synovial cyst of popliteal space (eg, Baker's cyst)**
    🖩 13.7   🔧 13.7   **FUD** 090    J A2 80 50 ▣
    **AMA:** 2002,Apr,13; 1998,Nov,1

**27347**    **Excision of lesion of meniscus or capsule (eg, cyst, ganglion), knee**
    🖩 15.1   🔧 15.1   **FUD** 090    J A2 80 50 ▣
    **AMA:** 2002,Apr,13; 1998,Nov,1

**27350**    **Patellectomy or hemipatellectomy**
    🖩 18.6   🔧 18.6   **FUD** 090    J A2 80 50 ▣
    **AMA:** 2002,Apr,13

**27355**    **Excision or curettage of bone cyst or benign tumor of femur;**
    🖩 17.3   🔧 17.3   **FUD** 090    J A2 80 50 ▣
    **AMA:** 2002,Apr,13

**27356**    **with allograft**
    🖩 21.1   🔧 21.1   **FUD** 090    J J8 80 50 ▣
    **AMA:** 2002,Apr,13

**27357**    **with autograft (includes obtaining graft)**
    🖩 23.3   🔧 23.3   **FUD** 090    J A2 80 50 ▣
    **AMA:** 2017,Jan,8; 2016,Jan,13; 2015,Jan,16; 2014,Jan,11; 2012,Jan,15-42

**Musculoskeletal System**

**27358 — 27415**

**+ 27358 with internal fixation (List in addition to code for primary procedure)**
Code first (27355-27357)
💰 8.08   ✄ 8.08   **FUD** ZZZ      N N1 80 🖵
**AMA:** 2002,Apr,13

**27360 Partial excision (craterization, saucerization, or diaphysectomy) bone, femur, proximal tibia and/or fibula (eg, osteomyelitis or bone abscess)**
💰 24.4   ✄ 24.4   **FUD** 090      J A2 80 50 🖵
**AMA:** 2002,Apr,13; 1998,Nov,1

## 27364-27365 [27329] Radical Resection Tumor Knee/Thigh

**INCLUDES**    Any necessary elevation of tissue planes or dissection
Excision of adjacent soft tissue during bone tumor resection
Measurement of tumor and necessary margin at greatest diameter prior to excision
Radical resection of bone tumor: resection of the tumor (may include entire bone) and wide margins of normal tissue primarily for malignant or aggressive benign tumors
Radical resection of soft tissue tumor: wide resection of tumor involving substantial margins of normal tissue that may include tissue removal from one or more layers; most often malignant or aggressive benign
Simple and intermediate repairs
**EXCLUDES**    *Complex repair*
*Radical resection of cutaneous tumors (eg, melanoma) (11600-11606)*
*Significant exploration of vessels, neuroplasty, reconstruction, or complex bone repair*

**# 27329 Radical resection of tumor (eg, sarcoma), soft tissue of thigh or knee area; less than 5 cm**
💰 29.9   ✄ 29.9   **FUD** 090      J G2 80 50 🖵
**AMA:** 2002,Apr,13; 1990,Win,4

**27364 5 cm or greater**
💰 45.0   ✄ 45.0   **FUD** 090      J G2 80 50 🖵

**27365 Radical resection of tumor, femur or knee**
**EXCLUDES**    *Soft tissue tumor excision thigh or knee area (27329, 27364)*
💰 59.5   ✄ 59.5   **FUD** 090      C 80 50 🖵
**AMA:** 2002,Apr,13; 1994,Win,1

## 27370 Injection for Arthrogram of Knee

**EXCLUDES**    *Arthrocentesis, aspiration and/or injection, knee (20610-20611)*
*Arthroscopy, knee (29871)*

**27370 Injection of contrast for knee arthrography**
🔲 (73580)
💰 1.46   ✄ 4.37   **FUD** 000      N N1 50 🖵
**AMA:** 2017,Jan,8; 2016,Jan,13; 2015,Aug,6; 2015,Feb,6

## 27372 Foreign Body Removal Femur or Knee

**EXCLUDES**    *Arthroscopic procedures (29870-29887)*
*Removal of knee prosthesis (27488)*

**27372 Removal of foreign body, deep, thigh region or knee area**
💰 11.5   ✄ 17.2   **FUD** 090      J A2 80 50 🖵
**AMA:** 2002,Apr,13

## 27380-27499 Repair/Reconstruction of Femur or Knee

**27380 Suture of infrapatellar tendon; primary**
💰 17.0   ✄ 17.0   **FUD** 090      J A2 80 50 🖵
**AMA:** 2002,Apr,13

**27381 secondary reconstruction, including fascial or tendon graft**
💰 22.9   ✄ 22.9   **FUD** 090      J A2 80 50 🖵
**AMA:** 2002,Apr,13

**27385 Suture of quadriceps or hamstring muscle rupture; primary**
💰 16.4   ✄ 16.4   **FUD** 090      J A2 80 50 🖵
**AMA:** 2017,Aug,9

**27386 secondary reconstruction, including fascial or tendon graft**
💰 23.7   ✄ 23.7   **FUD** 090      J A2 80 50 🖵
**AMA:** 2002,Apr,13

**27390 Tenotomy, open, hamstring, knee to hip; single tendon**
💰 12.6   ✄ 12.6   **FUD** 090      J A2 80 50 🖵
**AMA:** 2002,Apr,13; 1998,Nov,1

**27391 multiple tendons, 1 leg**
💰 16.4   ✄ 16.4   **FUD** 090      J A2 80 🖵
**AMA:** 2002,Apr,13; 1998,Nov,1

**27392 multiple tendons, bilateral**
💰 20.1   ✄ 20.1   **FUD** 090      J A2 80 🖵
**AMA:** 2002,Apr,13; 1998,Nov,1

**27393 Lengthening of hamstring tendon; single tendon**
💰 14.6   ✄ 14.6   **FUD** 090      A2 80 50 🖵
**AMA:** 2002,Apr,13; 1998,Nov,1

**27394 multiple tendons, 1 leg**
💰 18.2   ✄ 18.2   **FUD** 090      J A2 80 🖵
**AMA:** 2002,Apr,13; 1998,Nov,1

**27395 multiple tendons, bilateral**
💰 25.2   ✄ 25.2   **FUD** 090      J A2 80 🖵
**AMA:** 2002,Apr,13; 1998,Nov,1

**27396 Transplant or transfer (with muscle redirection or rerouting), thigh (eg, extensor to flexor); single tendon**
💰 17.5   ✄ 17.5   **FUD** 090      J A2 80 50 🖵
**AMA:** 2002,Apr,13; 1998,Nov,1

**27397 multiple tendons**
💰 26.0   ✄ 26.0   **FUD** 090      J J8 80 50 🖵
**AMA:** 2002,Apr,13; 1998,Nov,1

**27400 Transfer, tendon or muscle, hamstrings to femur (eg, Egger's type procedure)**
💰 19.6   ✄ 19.6   **FUD** 090      J A2 80 50 🖵
**AMA:** 2002,Apr,13; 1998,Nov,1

**27403 Arthrotomy with meniscus repair, knee**
**EXCLUDES**    *Arthroscopic treatment (29882)*
💰 18.3   ✄ 18.3   **FUD** 090      J A2 80 50 🖵
**AMA:** 2002,Apr,13; 1998,Nov,1

**27405 Repair, primary, torn ligament and/or capsule, knee; collateral**
💰 19.3   ✄ 19.3   **FUD** 090      J A2 80 50 🖵
**AMA:** 2017,Jan,8; 2016,Jan,13; 2015,Jan,16; 2014,Jan,11; 2012,Dec,12

**27407 cruciate**
**EXCLUDES**    *Reconstruction (27427)*
💰 22.2   ✄ 22.2   **FUD** 090      J J8 80 50 🖵
**AMA:** 2002,Apr,13; 1999,Nov,1

**27409 collateral and cruciate ligaments**
**EXCLUDES**    *Reconstruction (27427-27429)*
💰 27.7   ✄ 27.7   **FUD** 090      J A2 80 50 🖵
**AMA:** 2002,Apr,13; 1999,Nov,1

**27412 Autologous chondrocyte implantation, knee**
**EXCLUDES**    *Arthrotomy, knee (27331)*
*Manipulation of knee joint under general anesthesia (27570)*
*Obtaining chondrocytes (29870)*
*Tissue grafts, other (eg, paratenon, fat, dermis) (20926)*
💰 47.6   ✄ 47.6   **FUD** 090      J 80 50 🖵
**AMA:** 2002,Apr,13

**27415 Osteochondral allograft, knee, open**
**EXCLUDES**    *Arthroscopic procedure (29867)*
*Osteochondral autograft knee (27416)*
💰 39.6   ✄ 39.6   **FUD** 090      J J8 80 50 🖵
**AMA:** 2017,Jan,8; 2016,Jan,13; 2015,Jan,16; 2014,Jan,11; 2012,Jan,15-42

**27416** Osteochondral autograft(s), knee, open (eg, mosaicplasty) (includes harvesting of autograft[s])

> *EXCLUDES* *Procedures in the same compartment (29874, 29877, 29879, 29885-29887)*
> *Procedures performed at the same surgical session (27415, 29870-29871, 29875, 29884)*
> *Surgical arthroscopy of the knee with osteochondral autograft(s) (29866)*

🔧 28.2 ✂ 28.2 **FUD** 090 [J] [J8] [80] [50] ▣

**AMA:** 2017,Jan,8; 2016,Jan,13; 2015,Jan,16; 2014,Jan,11

**27418** Anterior tibial tubercleplasty (eg, Maquet type procedure)

🔧 23.6 ✂ 23.6 **FUD** 090 [J] [A2] [80] [50] ▣

**AMA:** 2017,Jan,8; 2016,Jan,13; 2015,Jan,16; 2014,Jan,11; 2012,Jan,15-42

**27420** Reconstruction of dislocating patella; (eg, Hauser type procedure)

🔧 21.3 ✂ 21.3 **FUD** 090 [J] [A2] [80] [50] ▣

**AMA:** 2017,Jan,8; 2016,Jan,13; 2015,Jan,16; 2014,Jan,11; 2012,Nov,13-14

Patella

Patella

Patellar ligament

Tuberosity is osteotomized

Attachment is shifted and fixed

**Patellar tendon insertion point is resected and shifted**

**27422** with extensor realignment and/or muscle advancement or release (eg, Campbell, Goldwaite type procedure)

🔧 21.3 ✂ 21.3 **FUD** 090 [J] [A2] [80] [50] ▣

**AMA:** 2017,Jan,8; 2016,Jan,13; 2015,Jan,16; 2014,Jan,11; 2012,Jan,15-42

**27424** with patellectomy

🔧 21.5 ✂ 21.5 **FUD** 090 [J] [A2] [80] [50] ▣

**AMA:** 2002,Apr,13; 1998,Nov,1

**27425** Lateral retinacular release, open

> *EXCLUDES* *Arthroscopic release (29873)*

🔧 12.8 ✂ 12.8 **FUD** 090 [J] [A2] [50] ▣

**AMA:** 2017,Jan,8; 2016,Jan,13; 2015,Nov,7; 2015,Jan,16; 2014,Jan,11; 2012,Jan,15-42

Lateral retinaculum

Patella

Medial retinaculum

Lateral and medial condyles

**Normal alignment**

**Poor alignment**

Iliotibial tract

Patella

Medial patellar retinaculum

Lateral patellar retinaculum is incised, decreasing lateral pull on patella

**27427** Ligamentous reconstruction (augmentation), knee; extra-articular

> *EXCLUDES* *Primary repair of ligament(s) (27405, 27407, 27409)*

🔧 20.4 ✂ 20.4 **FUD** 090 [J] [A2] [80] [50] ▣

**AMA:** 2017,Jan,8; 2016,Jan,13; 2015,Jan,16; 2014,Jan,11; 2012,Dec,12

**27428** intra-articular (open)

> *EXCLUDES* *Primary repair of ligament(s) (27405, 27407, 27409)*

🔧 31.9 ✂ 31.9 **FUD** 090 [J] [G2] [80] [50] ▣

**AMA:** 2017,Jan,8; 2016,Jan,13; 2015,Jan,16; 2014,Jan,11; 2012,Jan,15-42

**27429** intra-articular (open) and extra-articular

> *EXCLUDES* *Primary repair of ligament(s) (27405, 27407, 27409)*

🔧 35.7 ✂ 35.7 **FUD** 090 [J] [G2] [80] [50] ▣

**AMA:** 2017,Jan,8; 2016,Jan,13; 2015,Jan,16; 2014,Jan,11; 2012,Jan,15-42

**27430** Quadricepsplasty (eg, Bennett or Thompson type)

🔧 21.2 ✂ 21.2 **FUD** 090 [J] [A2] [80] [50] ▣

**AMA:** 2002,Apr,13; 1998,Nov,1

**27435** Capsulotomy, posterior capsular release, knee

🔧 23.1 ✂ 23.1 **FUD** 090 [J] [A2] [80] [50] ▣

**AMA:** 2002,Apr,13; 1998,Nov,1

**27437** Arthroplasty, patella; without prosthesis

🔧 19.0 ✂ 19.0 **FUD** 090 [J] [A2] [50] ▣

**AMA:** 2002,Apr,13

**27438** with prosthesis

🔧 24.1 ✂ 24.1 **FUD** 090 [J] [J8] [80] [50] ▣

**AMA:** 2002,Apr,13

**27440** Arthroplasty, knee, tibial plateau;

🔧 22.8 ✂ 22.8 **FUD** 090 [J] [J8] [80] [50] ▣

**AMA:** 2002,Apr,13

**27441** with debridement and partial synovectomy

🔧 23.7 ✂ 23.7 **FUD** 090 [J] [G2] [80] [50] ▣

**AMA:** 2002,Apr,13

**27442** Arthroplasty, femoral condyles or tibial plateau(s), knee;

🔧 25.0 ✂ 25.0 **FUD** 090 [J] [J8] [80] [50] ▣

**AMA:** 2017,Jan,8; 2016,Jun,8

**27443** with debridement and partial synovectomy

🔧 23.3 ✂ 23.3 **FUD** 090 [J] [G2] [80] [50] ▣

**AMA:** 2002,Apr,13

**27445** Arthroplasty, knee, hinge prosthesis (eg, Walldius type)

> *EXCLUDES* *Removal knee prosthesis (27488)*
> *Revision knee arthroplasty (27487)*

🔧 36.1 ✂ 36.1 **FUD** 090 [C] [80] [50] ▣

**AMA:** 2002,Apr,13; 1998,Nov,1

**27446** Arthroplasty, knee, condyle and plateau; medial OR lateral compartment

> *EXCLUDES* *Removal knee prosthesis (27488)*
> *Revision knee arthroplasty (27487)*

🔧 33.4 ✂ 33.4 **FUD** 090 [J] [J8] [80] [50] ▣

**AMA:** 2002,Apr,13

**27447** medial AND lateral compartments with or without patella resurfacing (total knee arthroplasty)

> *EXCLUDES* *Removal knee prosthesis (27488)*
> *Revision knee arthroplasty (27487)*

🔧 39.0 ✂ 39.0 **FUD** 090 [C] [80] [50] ▣

**AMA:** 2017,Jan,8; 2016,Jan,13; 2015,Jan,16; 2014,Jan,11

**27448** Osteotomy, femur, shaft or supracondylar; without fixation

🔧 22.1 ✂ 22.1 **FUD** 090 [C] [80] [50] ▣

**AMA:** 2002,Apr,13

**27450** with fixation

🔧 29.1 ✂ 29.1 **FUD** 090 [C] [80] [50] ▣

**AMA:** 2002,Apr,13

---

● New Code ▲ Revised Code ○ Reinstated ● New Web Release ▲ Revised Web Release Unlisted Not Covered # Resequenced

⊘ AMA Mod 51 Exempt ⑤ Optum Mod 51 Exempt ⑥ Mod 63 Exempt ✓ Non-FDA Drug ★ Telemedicine Ⅿ Maternity Ⓐ Age Edit + Add-on **AMA:** CPT Asst

© 2017 Optum360, LLC          CPT © 2017 American Medical Association. All Rights Reserved.

**27454** Osteotomy, multiple, with realignment on intramedullary rod, femoral shaft (eg, Sofield type procedure)
🔧 37.4   ✂ 37.4   **FUD** 090    C 80 50 ▣
**AMA:** 2002,Apr,13; 1998,Nov,1

**27455** Osteotomy, proximal tibia, including fibular excision or osteotomy (includes correction of genu varus [bowleg] or genu valgus [knock-knee]); before epiphyseal closure
🔧 27.0   ✂ 27.0   **FUD** 090    C 80 50 ▣
**AMA:** 2002,Apr,13

**27457** after epiphyseal closure
🔧 27.2   ✂ 27.2   **FUD** 090    C 80 50 ▣
**AMA:** 2002,Apr,13

**27465** Osteoplasty, femur; shortening (excluding 64876)
🔧 35.5   ✂ 35.5   **FUD** 090    C 80 50 ▣
**AMA:** 2002,Apr,13

**27466** lengthening
🔧 33.8   ✂ 33.8   **FUD** 090    C 80 50 ▣
**AMA:** 2002,Apr,13

**27468** combined, lengthening and shortening with femoral segment transfer
🔧 38.7   ✂ 38.7   **FUD** 090    C 80 50 ▣
**AMA:** 2002,Apr,13

**27470** Repair, nonunion or malunion, femur, distal to head and neck; without graft (eg, compression technique)
🔧 33.8   ✂ 33.8   **FUD** 090    C 80 50 ▣
**AMA:** 2002,Apr,13

**27472** with iliac or other autogenous bone graft (includes obtaining graft)
🔧 36.3   ✂ 36.3   **FUD** 090    C 80 50 ▣
**AMA:** 2002,Apr,13

**27475** Arrest, epiphyseal, any method (eg, epiphysiodesis); distal femur
🔧 19.0   ✂ 19.0   **FUD** 090    J 62 50 ▣
**AMA:** 2002,Apr,13; 2002,May,7

**27477** tibia and fibula, proximal
🔧 21.0   ✂ 21.0   **FUD** 090    J 50 ▣
**AMA:** 2002,May,7; 2002,Apr,13

**27479** combined distal femur, proximal tibia and fibula
🔧 26.5   ✂ 26.5   **FUD** 090    J J8 80 50 ▣
**AMA:** 2002,May,7; 2002,Apr,13

**27485** Arrest, hemiepiphyseal, distal femur or proximal tibia or fibula (eg, genu varus or valgus)
🔧 19.1   ✂ 19.1   **FUD** 090    J 50 ▣
**AMA:** 2002,Apr,13; 1998,Nov,1

**27486** Revision of total knee arthroplasty, with or without allograft; 1 component
🔧 40.5   ✂ 40.5   **FUD** 090    C 80 50 ▣
**AMA:** 2017,Jan,8; 2016,Jan,13; 2015,Jul,10; 2015,Jan,16; 2014,Jan,11; 2013,Dec,16

**27487** femoral and entire tibial component
🔧 50.7   ✂ 50.7   **FUD** 090    C 80 50 ▣
**AMA:** 2017,Jan,8; 2016,Jan,13; 2015,Jan,16; 2013,Jul,6

**27488** Removal of prosthesis, including total knee prosthesis, methylmethacrylate with or without insertion of spacer, knee
🔧 34.5   ✂ 34.5   **FUD** 090    C 80 50 ▣
**AMA:** 2017,Jan,8; 2016,Jan,13; 2015,Jan,16; 2013,Jul,6

**27495** Prophylactic treatment (nailing, pinning, plating, or wiring) with or without methylmethacrylate, femur
🔧 32.4   ✂ 32.4   **FUD** 090    C 80 50 ▣
**AMA:** 2002,Apr,13

**27496** Decompression fasciotomy, thigh and/or knee, 1 compartment (flexor or extensor or adductor);
🔧 15.4   ✂ 15.4   **FUD** 090    J A2 50 ▣
**AMA:** 2002,Apr,13

**27497** with debridement of nonviable muscle and/or nerve
🔧 16.5   ✂ 16.5   **FUD** 090    J A2 80 50 ▣ CLIA
**AMA:** 2002,Apr,13

**27498** Decompression fasciotomy, thigh and/or knee, multiple compartments;
🔧 18.6   ✂ 18.6   **FUD** 090    J A2 80 50 ▣
**AMA:** 2002,Apr,13

**27499** with debridement of nonviable muscle and/or nerve
🔧 19.8   ✂ 19.8   **FUD** 090    J A2 80 50 ▣
**AMA:** 2002,Apr,13

## 27500-27566 Treatment of Fracture/Dislocation of Femur/Knee

INCLUDES   Closed, percutaneous, and open treatment of fractures and dislocations

**27500** Closed treatment of femoral shaft fracture, without manipulation
🔧 13.7   ✂ 14.8   **FUD** 090    T A2 50 ▣
**AMA:** 2002,Apr,13

**27501** Closed treatment of supracondylar or transcondylar femoral fracture with or without intercondylar extension, without manipulation
🔧 14.3   ✂ 14.4   **FUD** 090    T A2 80 50 ▣
**AMA:** 2002,Apr,13

**27502** Closed treatment of femoral shaft fracture, with manipulation, with or without skin or skeletal traction
🔧 21.8   ✂ 21.8   **FUD** 090    J A2 50 ▣
**AMA:** 2017,Jan,8; 2016,Jan,13; 2015,Jan,16; 2014,Jan,11

**27503** Closed treatment of supracondylar or transcondylar femoral fracture with or without intercondylar extension, with manipulation, with or without skin or skeletal traction
🔧 22.9   ✂ 22.9   **FUD** 090    J A2 80 50 ▣
**AMA:** 2002,Apr,13

**27506** Open treatment of femoral shaft fracture, with or without external fixation, with insertion of intramedullary implant, with or without cerclage and/or locking screws
🔧 38.5   ✂ 38.5   **FUD** 090    C 80 50 ▣
**AMA:** 2017,Jan,8; 2016,Jan,13; 2015,Jan,16; 2014,Jan,11

**27507** Open treatment of femoral shaft fracture with plate/screws, with or without cerclage
🔧 28.0   ✂ 28.0   **FUD** 090    C 80 50 ▣
**AMA:** 2002,Apr,13

**27508** Closed treatment of femoral fracture, distal end, medial or lateral condyle, without manipulation
🔧 14.1   ✂ 15.0   **FUD** 090    T A2 50 ▣
**AMA:** 2002,Apr,13

**27509** Percutaneous skeletal fixation of femoral fracture, distal end, medial or lateral condyle, or supracondylar or transcondylar, with or without intercondylar extension, or distal femoral epiphyseal separation

🚑 18.4  ⚒ 18.4  **FUD** 090      J J8 80 50 ▭

AMA: 2002,Apr,13; 1993,Win,1

Pins are placed percutaneously

**27510** Closed treatment of femoral fracture, distal end, medial or lateral condyle, with manipulation

🚑 19.5  ⚒ 19.5  **FUD** 090      J A2 50 ▭

AMA: 2002,Apr,13

**27511** Open treatment of femoral supracondylar or transcondylar fracture without intercondylar extension, includes internal fixation, when performed

🚑 28.7  ⚒ 28.7  **FUD** 090      C 80 50 ▭

AMA: 2002,Apr,13; 1996,May,6

**27513** Open treatment of femoral supracondylar or transcondylar fracture with intercondylar extension, includes internal fixation, when performed

🚑 35.7  ⚒ 35.7  **FUD** 090      C 80 50 ▭

AMA: 2002,Apr,13

**27514** Open treatment of femoral fracture, distal end, medial or lateral condyle, includes internal fixation, when performed

🚑 27.8  ⚒ 27.8  **FUD** 090      C 80 50 ▭

AMA: 2002,Apr,13

**27516** Closed treatment of distal femoral epiphyseal separation; without manipulation

🚑 13.6  ⚒ 14.4  **FUD** 090      T A2 50 ▭

AMA: 2002,Apr,13

**27517** with manipulation, with or without skin or skeletal traction

🚑 18.3  ⚒ 18.3  **FUD** 090      J A2 80 50 ▭

AMA: 2002,Apr,13

**27519** Open treatment of distal femoral epiphyseal separation, includes internal fixation, when performed

🚑 25.7  ⚒ 25.7  **FUD** 090      C 80 50 ▭

AMA: 2002,Apr,13

**27520** Closed treatment of patellar fracture, without manipulation

🚑 8.40  ⚒ 9.19  **FUD** 090      T A2 50 ▭

AMA: 2002,Apr,13

**27524** Open treatment of patellar fracture, with internal fixation and/or partial or complete patellectomy and soft tissue repair

🚑 21.6  ⚒ 21.6  **FUD** 090      J G2 80 50 ▭

AMA: 2002,Apr,13

**27530** Closed treatment of tibial fracture, proximal (plateau); without manipulation

*EXCLUDES*  Arthroscopic repair (29855-29856)

🚑 7.98  ⚒ 8.59  **FUD** 090      T A2 50 ▭

AMA: 2002,Apr,13

**27532** with or without manipulation, with skeletal traction

*EXCLUDES*  Arthroscopic repair (29855-29856)

🚑 16.5  ⚒ 17.6  **FUD** 090      J A2 50 ▭

AMA: 2002,Apr,13

**27535** Open treatment of tibial fracture, proximal (plateau); unicondylar, includes internal fixation, when performed

*EXCLUDES*  Arthroscopic repair (29855-29856)

🚑 25.8  ⚒ 25.8  **FUD** 090      C 80 50 ▭

AMA: 2002,Apr,13

**27536** bicondylar, with or without internal fixation

*EXCLUDES*  Arthroscopic repair (29855-29856)

🚑 34.2  ⚒ 34.2  **FUD** 090      C 80 50 ▭

AMA: 2002,Apr,13

**27538** Closed treatment of intercondylar spine(s) and/or tuberosity fracture(s) of knee, with or without manipulation

*EXCLUDES*  Arthroscopic repair (29850-29851)

🚑 12.7  ⚒ 13.5  **FUD** 090      T A2 80 50 ▭

AMA: 2002,Apr,13

**27540** Open treatment of intercondylar spine(s) and/or tuberosity fracture(s) of the knee, includes internal fixation, when performed

🚑 23.3  ⚒ 23.3  **FUD** 090      C 80 50 ▭

AMA: 2002,Apr,13

**27550** Closed treatment of knee dislocation; without anesthesia

🚑 13.4  ⚒ 14.4  **FUD** 090      T A2 80 50 ▭

AMA: 2002,Apr,13

**27552** requiring anesthesia

🚑 17.9  ⚒ 17.9  **FUD** 090      J A2 80 50 ▭

AMA: 2002,Apr,13

**27556** Open treatment of knee dislocation, includes internal fixation, when performed; without primary ligamentous repair or augmentation/reconstruction

🚑 24.8  ⚒ 24.8  **FUD** 090      C 80 50 ▭

AMA: 2002,Apr,13

**27557** with primary ligamentous repair

🚑 29.4  ⚒ 29.4  **FUD** 090      C 80 50 ▭

AMA: 2002,Apr,13

**27558** with primary ligamentous repair, with augmentation/reconstruction

🚑 34.5  ⚒ 34.5  **FUD** 090      C 80 50 ▭

AMA: 2002,Apr,13

**27560** Closed treatment of patellar dislocation; without anesthesia

*EXCLUDES*  Recurrent dislocation (27420-27424)

🚑 9.46  ⚒ 10.2  **FUD** 090      T A2 50 ▭

AMA: 2002,Apr,13

**27562** requiring anesthesia

*EXCLUDES*  Recurrent dislocation (27420-27424)

🚑 13.6  ⚒ 13.6  **FUD** 090      T A2 80 50 ▭

AMA: 2002,Apr,13

**27566** Open treatment of patellar dislocation, with or without partial or total patellectomy

*EXCLUDES*  Recurrent dislocation (27420-27424)

🚑 25.5  ⚒ 25.5  **FUD** 090      J A2 80 50 ▭

AMA: 2002,Apr,13

● New Code    ▲ Revised Code    ○ Reinstated    ● New Web Release    ▲ Revised Web Release    Unlisted    Not Covered    # Resequenced
⊘ AMA Mod 51 Exempt    ⑤⑩ Optum Mod 51 Exempt    ⑥③ Mod 63 Exempt    ✗ Non-FDA Drug    ★ Telemedicine    Ⓜ Maternity    Ⓐ Age Edit    ✚ Add-on    AMA: CPT Asst
© 2017 Optum360, LLC                     CPT © 2017 American Medical Association. All Rights Reserved.                                    87

## 27570 Knee Manipulation with Anesthesia

**27570**   **Manipulation of knee joint under general anesthesia (includes application of traction or other fixation devices)**
🖫 4.33   ⚕ 4.33   **FUD** 010      J A2 50 ▣
**AMA:** 2017,Jan,8; 2016,Jan,13; 2015,Jan,16; 2014,Jan,11; 2012,Jan,15-42

## 27580 Knee Arthrodesis

**27580**   **Arthrodesis, knee, any technique**
INCLUDES   Albert's operation
🖫 41.3   ⚕ 41.3   **FUD** 090      C 80 50 ▣
**AMA:** 2002,Apr,13

## 27590-27599 Amputations and Unlisted Procedures at Femur or Knee

**27590**   **Amputation, thigh, through femur, any level;**
🖫 23.2   ⚕ 23.2   **FUD** 090      C 80 50 ▣
**AMA:** 2002,Apr,13

**27591**   **immediate fitting technique including first cast**
🖫 27.8   ⚕ 27.8   **FUD** 090      C 80 50 ▣
**AMA:** 2002,Apr,13

**27592**   **open, circular (guillotine)**
🖫 19.7   ⚕ 19.7   **FUD** 090      C 80 50 ▣
**AMA:** 2002,Apr,13

**27594**   **secondary closure or scar revision**
🖫 14.5   ⚕ 14.5   **FUD** 090      J A2 50 ▣
**AMA:** 2002,Apr,13

**27596**   **re-amputation**
🖫 20.9   ⚕ 20.9   **FUD** 090      C 50 ▣
**AMA:** 2002,Apr,13

**27598**   **Disarticulation at knee**
INCLUDES   Batch-Spittler-McFaddin operation
Callandar knee disarticulation
Gritti amputation
🖫 20.7   ⚕ 20.7   **FUD** 090      C 80 50 ▣
**AMA:** 2002,Apr,13

**27599**   **Unlisted procedure, femur or knee**
🖫 0.00   ⚕ 0.00   **FUD** YYY      T 80 50
**AMA:** 2017,Aug,9; 2017,Mar,10; 2017,Jan,8; 2016,Nov,9; 2016,Jun,8; 2016,Jan,13; 2015,Jan,16; 2015,Jan,13; 2014,Jan,11; 2014,Jan,9; 2012,Dec,12; 2012,Jan,15-42

## 27600-27602 Decompression Fasciotomy of Leg

EXCLUDES   Fasciotomy with debridement (27892-27894)
Simple incision and drainage (10140-10160)

**27600**   **Decompression fasciotomy, leg; anterior and/or lateral compartments only**
🖫 11.7   ⚕ 11.7   **FUD** 090      J A2 50 ▣
**AMA:** 2002,Apr,13

**27601**   **posterior compartment(s) only**
🖫 12.8   ⚕ 12.8   **FUD** 090      J A2 50 ▣
**AMA:** 2002,Apr,13

**27602**   **anterior and/or lateral, and posterior compartment(s)**
🖫 14.1   ⚕ 14.1   **FUD** 090      J A2 80 50 ▣
**AMA:** 2002,Apr,13

## 27603-27612 Incisional Procedures Lower Leg and Ankle

**27603**   **Incision and drainage, leg or ankle; deep abscess or hematoma**
🖫 11.1   ⚕ 15.1   **FUD** 090      J A2 50 ▣
**AMA:** 2002,Apr,13

**27604**   **infected bursa**
🖫 9.86   ⚕ 14.0   **FUD** 090      J A2 80 50 ▣
**AMA:** 2002,Apr,13

**27605**   **Tenotomy, percutaneous, Achilles tendon (separate procedure); local anesthesia**
🖫 5.32   ⚕ 9.79   **FUD** 010      J A2 80 50 ▣
**AMA:** 2002,Apr,13; 1998,Nov,1

**27606**   **general anesthesia**
🖫 8.10   ⚕ 8.10   **FUD** 010      J A2 50 ▣
**AMA:** 2002,Apr,13

**27607**   **Incision (eg, osteomyelitis or bone abscess), leg or ankle**
🖫 17.4   ⚕ 17.4   **FUD** 090      J A2 50 ▣
**AMA:** 2002,Apr,13; 1998,Nov,1

**27610**   **Arthrotomy, ankle, including exploration, drainage, or removal of foreign body**
🖫 18.6   ⚕ 18.6   **FUD** 090      J A2 50 ▣
**AMA:** 2002,Apr,13; 1998,Nov,1

**27612**   **Arthrotomy, posterior capsular release, ankle, with or without Achilles tendon lengthening**
EXCLUDES   Lengthening or shortening tendon (27685)
🖫 16.1   ⚕ 16.1   **FUD** 090      J A2 80 50 ▣
**AMA:** 2002,Apr,13; 1998,Nov,1

## 27613-27614 Biopsy Lower Leg and Ankle

EXCLUDES   Needle biopsy (20206)

**27613**   **Biopsy, soft tissue of leg or ankle area; superficial**
🖫 4.68   ⚕ 7.21   **FUD** 010      J P3 50 ▣
**AMA:** 2002,Apr,13

**27614**   **deep (subfascial or intramuscular)**
🖫 11.6   ⚕ 16.5   **FUD** 090      J A2 50 ▣
**AMA:** 2002,Apr,13; 1998,Nov,1

## 27615-27619 [27632, 27634] Excision Soft Tissue Tumors Lower Leg/Ankle

INCLUDES   Any necessary elevation of tissue planes or dissection
Measurement of tumor and necessary margin at greatest diameter prior to excision
Resection without removal of significant normal tissue
Simple and intermediate repairs
Types of excision:
     Fascial or subfascial soft tissue tumors: simple and marginal resection of most often benign and intramuscular tumors found either in or below the deep fascia, not involving bone
     Resection of the tumor (may include entire bone) and wide margins of normal tissue primarily for malignant or aggressive benign tumors
     Subcutaneous: simple and marginal resection of most often benign tumors found in the subcutaneous tissue above the deep fascia

EXCLUDES   Complex repair
Excision of benign cutaneous lesions (eg, sebaceous cyst) (11400-11406)
Radical resection of cutaneous tumors (eg, melanoma) (11600-11606)
Significant exploration of vessels or neuroplasty

**27615**   **Radical resection of tumor (eg, sarcoma), soft tissue of leg or ankle area; less than 5 cm**
🖫 29.4   ⚕ 29.4   **FUD** 090      J G2 80 50 ▣
**AMA:** 2002,Apr,13; 1990,Win,4

**27616**   **5 cm or greater**
🖫 36.6   ⚕ 36.6   **FUD** 090      J G2 80 50 ▣

**27618**   **Excision, tumor, soft tissue of leg or ankle area, subcutaneous; less than 3 cm**
🖫 8.87   ⚕ 12.8   **FUD** 090      J G2 50 ▣
**AMA:** 2017,Jan,8; 2016,Jan,13; 2015,Jan,16; 2014,Jan,11

\# **27632**   **3 cm or greater**
🖫 11.8   ⚕ 11.8   **FUD** 090      J G2 80 50 ▣

**27619**   **Excision, tumor, soft tissue of leg or ankle area, subfascial (eg, intramuscular); less than 5 cm**
🖫 13.4   ⚕ 13.4   **FUD** 090      J G2 50 ▣
**AMA:** 2002,Apr,13

\# **27634**   **5 cm or greater**
🖫 19.7   ⚕ 19.7   **FUD** 090      J G2 80 50 ▣

## 27620-27641 Bone and Joint Procedures Ankle/Leg

**27620**   **Arthrotomy, ankle, with joint exploration, with or without biopsy, with or without removal of loose or foreign body**
🖫 13.0   ⚕ 13.0   **FUD** 090      J A2 80 50 ▣
**AMA:** 2002,Apr,13

26/TC PC/TC Only    A2-Z3 ASC Payment    50 Bilateral    ♂ Male Only    ♀ Female Only    🖫 Facility RVU    ⚕ Non-Facility RVU    ▣ CCI
**FUD** Follow-up Days    **CMS:** IOM (Pub 100)    A-Y OPPSI    80/80 Surg Assist Allowed / w/Doc    🖫 Lab Crosswalk    🖫 Radiology Crosswalk    ❌ CLIA
**88**    CPT © 2017 American Medical Association. All Rights Reserved.          © 2017 Optum360, LLC

| **27625** | **Arthrotomy, with synovectomy, ankle;** |
|---|---|
| | 🔧 16.6   ✂ 16.6   **FUD** 090     J A2 80 50 🔲 |
| | **AMA:** 2002,Apr,13; 1998,Nov,1 |

| **27626** | **including tenosynovectomy** |
|---|---|
| | 🔧 17.3   ✂ 17.3   **FUD** 090     J A2 80 50 🔲 |
| | **AMA:** 2002,Apr,13 |

| **27630** | **Excision of lesion of tendon sheath or capsule (eg, cyst or ganglion), leg and/or ankle** |
|---|---|
| | 🔧 10.4   ✂ 15.9   **FUD** 090     J A2 50 🔲 |
| | **AMA:** 2002,Apr,13 |

**27632**  Resequenced code. See code following 27618.

**27634**  Resequenced code. See code following 27619.

| **27635** | **Excision or curettage of bone cyst or benign tumor, tibia or fibula;** |
|---|---|
| | 🔧 16.8   ✂ 16.8   **FUD** 090     J A2 50 🔲 |
| | **AMA:** 2017,Jan,8; 2016,Jan,13; 2015,Jan,16; 2014,Jan,11; 2012,Apr,17-18 |

| **27637** | **with autograft (includes obtaining graft)** |
|---|---|
| | 🔧 21.9   ✂ 21.9   **FUD** 090     J A2 80 50 🔲 |
| | **AMA:** 2002,Apr,13 |

| **27638** | **with allograft** |
|---|---|
| | 🔧 21.9   ✂ 21.9   **FUD** 090     J A2 80 50 🔲 |
| | **AMA:** 2002,Apr,13 |

| **27640** | **Partial excision (craterization, saucerization, or diaphysectomy), bone (eg, osteomyelitis); tibia** |
|---|---|
| | EXCLUDES   *Excision of exostosis (27635)* |
| | 🔧 23.9   ✂ 23.9   **FUD** 090     J A2 50 🔲 |
| | **AMA:** 2017,Jan,8; 2016,Jan,13; 2015,Jan,16; 2014,Jan,11; 2012,Apr,17-18 |

| **27641** | **fibula** |
|---|---|
| | EXCLUDES   *Excision of exostosis (27635)* |
| | 🔧 19.1   ✂ 19.1   **FUD** 090     J A2 50 🔲 |
| | **AMA:** 2002,Apr,13 |

## 27645-27647 Radical Resection Bone Tumor Ankle/Leg

INCLUDES   Any necessary elevation of tissue planes or dissection
Excision of adjacent soft tissue during bone tumor resection (27615-27619 [27632, 27634])
Measurement of tumor and necessary margin at greatest diameter prior to excision
Resection of the tumor (may include entire bone) and wide margins of normal tissue primarily for malignant or aggressive benign tumors
Simple and intermediate repairs

EXCLUDES   *Complex repair*
*Significant exploration of vessels, neuroplasty, reconstruction, or complex bone repair*

| **27645** | **Radical resection of tumor; tibia** |
|---|---|
| | 🔧 51.2   ✂ 51.2   **FUD** 090     C 80 50 🔲 |
| | **AMA:** 2002,Apr,13; 1994,Win,1 |

| **27646** | **fibula** |
|---|---|
| | 🔧 42.8   ✂ 42.8   **FUD** 090     C 80 50 🔲 |
| | **AMA:** 2002,Apr,13; 1994,Win,1 |

| **27647** | **talus or calcaneus** |
|---|---|
| | 🔧 29.5   ✂ 29.5   **FUD** 090     J A2 80 50 🔲 |
| | **AMA:** 2002,Apr,13; 1994,Win,1 |

## 27648 Injection for Ankle Arthrogram

EXCLUDES   *Arthroscopy (29894-29898)*

| **27648** | **Injection procedure for ankle arthrography** |
|---|---|
| | 📷 (73615) |
| | 🔧 1.52   ✂ 4.71   **FUD** 000     N N1 80 50 🔲 |
| | **AMA:** 2017,Jan,8; 2016,Jan,13; 2015,Aug,6 |

## 27650-27745 Repair/Reconstruction Lower Leg/Ankle

| **27650** | **Repair, primary, open or percutaneous, ruptured Achilles tendon;** |
|---|---|
| | 🔧 18.9   ✂ 18.9   **FUD** 090     J A2 80 50 🔲 |
| | **AMA:** 2017,Jan,8; 2016,Jan,13; 2015,Jan,16; 2014,Jul,5 |

| **27652** | **with graft (includes obtaining graft)** |
|---|---|
| | 🔧 19.6   ✂ 19.6   **FUD** 090     J A2 50 🔲 |
| | **AMA:** 2017,Jan,8; 2016,Jan,13; 2015,Jan,16; 2014,Jul,5 |

| **27654** | **Repair, secondary, Achilles tendon, with or without graft** |
|---|---|
| | 🔧 20.3   ✂ 20.3   **FUD** 090     J A2 80 50 🔲 |
| | **AMA:** 2017,Jan,8; 2016,Dec,16; 2016,Jan,13; 2015,Jan,16; 2014,Jul,5 |

| **27656** | **Repair, fascial defect of leg** |
|---|---|
| | 🔧 11.2   ✂ 17.7   **FUD** 090     J A2 80 50 🔲 |
| | **AMA:** 2002,Apr,13 |

| **27658** | **Repair, flexor tendon, leg; primary, without graft, each tendon** |
|---|---|
| | 🔧 10.7   ✂ 10.7   **FUD** 090     J A2 80 🔲 |
| | **AMA:** 2002,Apr,13; 1998,Nov,1 |

| **27659** | **secondary, with or without graft, each tendon** |
|---|---|
| | 🔧 13.7   ✂ 13.7   **FUD** 090     J A2 80 🔲 |
| | **AMA:** 2017,Jan,8; 2016,Jan,13; 2015,Jan,13 |

| **27664** | **Repair, extensor tendon, leg; primary, without graft, each tendon** |
|---|---|
| | 🔧 10.4   ✂ 10.4   **FUD** 090     J A2 80 🔲 |
| | **AMA:** 2017,Jan,8; 2016,Jan,13; 2015,Jan,13 |

| **27665** | **secondary, with or without graft, each tendon** |
|---|---|
| | 🔧 11.7   ✂ 11.7   **FUD** 090     J A2 80 🔲 |
| | **AMA:** 2002,Apr,13; 1998,Nov,1 |

| **27675** | **Repair, dislocating peroneal tendons; without fibular osteotomy** |
|---|---|
| | 🔧 14.0   ✂ 14.0   **FUD** 090     J A2 80 50 🔲 |
| | **AMA:** 2002,Apr,13; 1998,Nov,1 |

| **27676** | **with fibular osteotomy** |
|---|---|
| | 🔧 17.4   ✂ 17.4   **FUD** 090     J A2 80 50 🔲 |
| | **AMA:** 2002,Apr,13 |

| **27680** | **Tenolysis, flexor or extensor tendon, leg and/or ankle; single, each tendon** |
|---|---|
| | 🔧 12.3   ✂ 12.3   **FUD** 090     J A2 🔲 |
| | **AMA:** 2017,Jan,8; 2016,Jan,13; 2015,Jan,16; 2014,Jan,11 |

| **27681** | **multiple tendons (through separate incision[s])** |
|---|---|
| | 🔧 15.7   ✂ 15.7   **FUD** 090     J A2 50 🔲 |
| | **AMA:** 2002,Apr,13; 1998,Nov,1 |

| **27685** | **Lengthening or shortening of tendon, leg or ankle; single tendon (separate procedure)** |
|---|---|
| | 🔧 13.3   ✂ 19.0   **FUD** 090     J A2 80 50 🔲 |
| | **AMA:** 2017,Jan,8; 2016,Jan,13; 2015,Jan,16; 2014,Jan,11; 2012,Jan,15-42 |

| **27686** | **multiple tendons (through same incision), each** |
|---|---|
| | 🔧 16.0   ✂ 16.0   **FUD** 090     J A2 50 🔲 |
| | **AMA:** 2017,Jan,8; 2016,Jan,13; 2015,Jan,16; 2014,Jan,11; 2012,Jan,15-42 |

| **27687** | **Gastrocnemius recession (eg, Strayer procedure)** |
|---|---|
| | 🔧 13.0   ✂ 13.0   **FUD** 090     J A2 80 50 🔲 |
| | **AMA:** 2002,Apr,13 |

| **27690** | **Transfer or transplant of single tendon (with muscle redirection or rerouting); superficial (eg, anterior tibial extensors into midfoot)** |
|---|---|
| | INCLUDES   Toe extensors considered a single tendon with transplant into midfoot |
| | 🔧 18.1   ✂ 18.1   **FUD** 090     J A2 80 50 🔲 |
| | **AMA:** 2002,Apr,13; 1995,Win,1 |

| **27691** | **deep (eg, anterior tibial or posterior tibial through interosseous space, flexor digitorum longus, flexor hallucis longus, or peroneal tendon to midfoot or hindfoot)** |
|---|---|
| | INCLUDES   Barr procedure |
| | Toe extensors considered a single tendon with transplant into midfoot |
| | 🔧 21.4   ✂ 21.4   **FUD** 090     J A2 80 50 🔲 |
| | **AMA:** 2002,Apr,13; 1995,Win,1 |

**+ 27692** each additional tendon (List separately in addition to code for primary procedure)

INCLUDES Toe extensors considered a single tendon with transplant into midfoot

Code first (27690-27691)

🛠 3.03   ⚕ 3.03   **FUD** ZZZ   N N1 80 ▣

**AMA:** 2003,Feb,7; 2002,Apr,13

**27695** Repair, primary, disrupted ligament, ankle; collateral

🛠 13.7   ⚕ 13.7   **FUD** 090   J A2 50 ▣

**AMA:** 2017,Jan,8; 2016,Jan,13; 2015,Jan,16; 2014,Mar,13; 2014,Jan,11

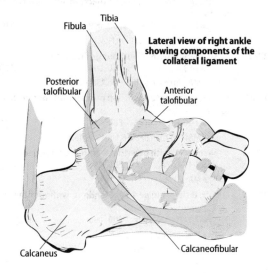

Fibula  Tibia

**Lateral view of right ankle showing components of the collateral ligament**

Posterior talofibular

Anterior talofibular

Calcaneus

Calcaneofibular

**27696** both collateral ligaments

🛠 15.8   ⚕ 15.8   **FUD** 090   J A2 50 ▣

**AMA:** 2017,Jan,8; 2016,Jan,13; 2015,Jan,16; 2014,Mar,13

**27698** Repair, secondary, disrupted ligament, ankle, collateral (eg, Watson-Jones procedure)

🛠 18.4   ⚕ 18.4   **FUD** 090   J A2 80 50 ▣

**AMA:** 2017,Jan,8; 2016,Jan,13; 2015,Jan,16; 2014,Mar,13

**27700** Arthroplasty, ankle;

🛠 17.5   ⚕ 17.5   **FUD** 090   J A2 80 50 ▣

**AMA:** 2002,Apr,13

**27702** with implant (total ankle)

🛠 27.7   ⚕ 27.7   **FUD** 090   C 80 50 ▣

**AMA:** 2002,Apr,13

**27703** revision, total ankle

🛠 31.9   ⚕ 31.9   **FUD** 090   C 80 50 ▣

**AMA:** 2002,Apr,13; 1998,Nov,1

**27704** Removal of ankle implant

🛠 16.5   ⚕ 16.5   **FUD** 090   02 A2 50 ▣

**AMA:** 2002,Apr,13

**27705** Osteotomy; tibia

EXCLUDES Genu varus or genu valgus repair (27455-27457)

🛠 21.7   ⚕ 21.7   **FUD** 090   J A2 80 50 ▣

**AMA:** 2002,Apr,13

**27707** fibula

EXCLUDES Genu varus or genu valgus repair (27455-27457)

🛠 11.4   ⚕ 11.4   **FUD** 090   J A2 50 ▣

**AMA:** 2002,Apr,13

**27709** tibia and fibula

EXCLUDES Genu varus or genu valgus repair (27455-27457)

🛠 33.7   ⚕ 33.7   **FUD** 090   J J8 80 50 ▣

**AMA:** 2002,Apr,13

**27712** multiple, with realignment on intramedullary rod (eg, Sofield type procedure)

EXCLUDES Genu varus or genu valgus repair (27455-27457)

🛠 31.8   ⚕ 31.8   **FUD** 090   C 80 50 ▣

**AMA:** 2002,Apr,13; 1998,Nov,1

**27715** Osteoplasty, tibia and fibula, lengthening or shortening

INCLUDES Anderson tibial lengthening

🛠 30.2   ⚕ 30.2   **FUD** 090   C 80 50 ▣

**AMA:** 2002,Apr,13; 1998,Nov,1

**27720** Repair of nonunion or malunion, tibia; without graft, (eg, compression technique)

🛠 25.1   ⚕ 25.1   **FUD** 090   J G2 80 50 ▣

**AMA:** 2002,Apr,13

**27722** with sliding graft

🛠 25.6   ⚕ 25.6   **FUD** 090   J 80 50 ▣

**AMA:** 2002,Apr,13

**27724** with iliac or other autograft (includes obtaining graft)

🛠 36.4   ⚕ 36.4   **FUD** 090   C 80 50 ▣

**AMA:** 2017,Jan,8; 2016,Jan,13; 2015,Jan,16; 2014,Jan,11; 2012,May,11-12

**27725** by synostosis, with fibula, any method

🛠 34.3   ⚕ 34.3   **FUD** 090   C 80 50 ▣

**AMA:** 2002,Apr,13

**27726** Repair of fibula nonunion and/or malunion with internal fixation

INCLUDES Osteotomy; fibula (27707)

🛠 27.7   ⚕ 27.7   **FUD** 090   J G2 50 ▣

**AMA:** 2017,Jan,8; 2016,Jan,13; 2015,Jan,16; 2014,Jan,11; 2012,Jan,15-42

**27727** Repair of congenital pseudarthrosis, tibia

🛠 25.6   ⚕ 25.6   **FUD** 090   C 80 50 ▣

**AMA:** 2002,Apr,13

**27730** Arrest, epiphyseal (epiphysiodesis), open; distal tibia

🛠 15.9   ⚕ 15.9   **FUD** 090   J A2 50 ▣

**AMA:** 2002,Apr,13; 1998,Nov,1

**27732** distal fibula

🛠 10.6   ⚕ 10.6   **FUD** 090   J A2 50 ▣

**AMA:** 2002,Apr,13

**27734** distal tibia and fibula

🛠 18.8   ⚕ 18.8   **FUD** 090   J A2 50 ▣

**AMA:** 2002,Apr,13

**27740** Arrest, epiphyseal (epiphysiodesis), any method, combined, proximal and distal tibia and fibula;

EXCLUDES Epiphyseal arrest of proximal tibia and fibula (27477)

🛠 19.9   ⚕ 19.9   **FUD** 090   J J8 80 50 ▣

**AMA:** 2002,Apr,13; 1998,Nov,1

**27742** and distal femur

EXCLUDES Epiphyseal arrest of proximal tibia and fibula (27477)

🛠 21.6   ⚕ 21.6   **FUD** 090   J A2 80 50 ▣

**AMA:** 2002,Apr,13

**27745** Prophylactic treatment (nailing, pinning, plating or wiring) with or without methylmethacrylate, tibia

🛠 21.7   ⚕ 21.7   **FUD** 090   J J8 80 50 ▣

**AMA:** 2002,Apr,13

## 27750-27848 Treatment of Fracture/Dislocation Lower Leg/Ankle

INCLUDES Treatment of open or closed fracture or dislocation

**27750** Closed treatment of tibial shaft fracture (with or without fibular fracture); without manipulation

🛠 9.06   ⚕ 9.87   **FUD** 090   T A2 50 ▣

**AMA:** 2017,Jan,8; 2016,Jan,13; 2015,Jan,16; 2014,Jan,11; 2012,Jan,15-42

**27752** with manipulation, with or without skeletal traction

🛠 14.1   ⚕ 15.3   **FUD** 090   J A2 50 ▣

**AMA:** 2017,Jan,8; 2016,Jan,13; 2015,Jan,16; 2014,Jan,11

26/TC PC/TC Only   A2-Z3 ASC Payment   50 Bilateral   ♂ Male Only   ♀ Female Only   🛠 Facility RVU   ⚕ Non-Facility RVU   ▣ CCI

FUD Follow-up Days   CMS: IOM (Pub 100)   A-Y OPPSI   80/80 Surg Assist Allowed / w/Doc   🔬 Lab Crosswalk   ☢ Radiology Crosswalk   ✖ CLIA

90   CPT © 2017 American Medical Association. All Rights Reserved.   © 2017 Optum360, LLC

**27756**  Percutaneous skeletal fixation of tibial shaft fracture (with or without fibular fracture) (eg, pins or screws)
🔧 16.5   ⚕ 16.5   **FUD** 090          [J] [A2] [80] [50] [📧]
AMA: 2017,Jan,8; 2016,Jan,13; 2015,Jan,16; 2014,Jan,11

**27758**  Open treatment of tibial shaft fracture (with or without fibular fracture), with plate/screws, with or without cerclage
🔧 25.6   ⚕ 25.6   **FUD** 090          [J] [A2] [80] [50] [📧]
AMA: 2017,Jan,8; 2016,Jan,13; 2015,Jan,16; 2014,Jan,11; 2012,Jan,15-42

**27759**  Treatment of tibial shaft fracture (with or without fibular fracture) by intramedullary implant, with or without interlocking screws and/or cerclage
🔧 28.7   ⚕ 28.7   **FUD** 090          [J] [G2] [80] [50] [📧]
AMA: 2017,Jan,8; 2016,Jan,13; 2015,Jan,16; 2014,Jan,11

**27760**  Closed treatment of medial malleolus fracture; without manipulation
🔧 8.65   ⚕ 9.47   **FUD** 090          [T] [A2] [50] [📧]
AMA: 2002,Apr,13; 1994,Sum,29

**27762**  with manipulation, with or without skin or skeletal traction
🔧 12.2   ⚕ 13.4   **FUD** 090          [J] [A2] [50] [📧]
AMA: 2002,Apr,13; 1994,Sum,29

**27766**  Open treatment of medial malleolus fracture, includes internal fixation, when performed
🔧 17.4   ⚕ 17.4   **FUD** 090          [J] [A2] [50] [📧]
AMA: 2002,Apr,13; 1994,Sum,29

**27767**  Closed treatment of posterior malleolus fracture; without manipulation
🔧 8.03   ⚕ 7.98   **FUD** 090          [T] [P2] [50] [📧]
> EXCLUDES Treatment of bimalleolar ankle fracture (27808-27814)
> Treatment of trimalleolar ankle fracture (27816-27823)

**27768**  with manipulation
🔧 12.5   ⚕ 12.5   **FUD** 090          [J] [G2] [50] [📧]
> EXCLUDES Treatment of bimalleolar ankle fracture (27808-27814)
> Treatment of trimalleolar ankle fracture (27816-27823)

**27769**  Open treatment of posterior malleolus fracture, includes internal fixation, when performed
🔧 20.7   ⚕ 20.7   **FUD** 090          [J] [G2] [50] [📧]
> EXCLUDES Treatment of bimalleolar ankle fracture (27808-27814)
> Treatment of trimalleolar ankle fracture (27816-27823)

**27780**  Closed treatment of proximal fibula or shaft fracture; without manipulation
🔧 7.94   ⚕ 8.71   **FUD** 090          [T] [A2] [50] [📧]
AMA: 2017,Jan,8; 2016,Jan,13; 2015,Jan,16; 2014,Jan,11

**27781**  with manipulation
🔧 11.2   ⚕ 12.1   **FUD** 090          [J] [A2] [50] [📧]
AMA: 2002,Apr,13

**27784**  Open treatment of proximal fibula or shaft fracture, includes internal fixation, when performed
🔧 20.5   ⚕ 20.5   **FUD** 090          [J] [A2] [50] [📧]
AMA: 2017,Jan,8; 2016,Jan,13; 2015,Jan,16; 2014,Jan,11; 2012,Jan,15-42

**27786**  Closed treatment of distal fibular fracture (lateral malleolus); without manipulation
🔧 8.15   ⚕ 8.99   **FUD** 090          [T] [A2] [50] [📧]
AMA: 2002,Apr,13

**27788**  with manipulation
🔧 10.9   ⚕ 11.9   **FUD** 090          [T] [A2] [50] [📧]
AMA: 2002,Apr,13

**27792**  Open treatment of distal fibular fracture (lateral malleolus), includes internal fixation, when performed
> EXCLUDES Repair of tibia and fibula shaft fracture (27750-27759)
🔧 18.7   ⚕ 18.7   **FUD** 090          [J] [A2] [50] [📧]
AMA: 2017,Jan,8; 2016,Jan,13; 2015,Jan,16; 2014,Jan,11

**27808**  Closed treatment of bimalleolar ankle fracture (eg, lateral and medial malleoli, or lateral and posterior malleoli or medial and posterior malleoli); without manipulation
🔧 8.55   ⚕ 9.51   **FUD** 090          [T] [A2] [50] [📧]
AMA: 2002,Apr,13

**27810**  with manipulation
🔧 12.0   ⚕ 13.2   **FUD** 090          [J] [A2] [50] [📧]
AMA: 2002,Apr,13

**27814**  Open treatment of bimalleolar ankle fracture (eg, lateral and medial malleoli, or lateral and posterior malleoli, or medial and posterior malleoli), includes internal fixation, when performed
🔧 22.1   ⚕ 22.1   **FUD** 090          [J] [A2] [80] [50] [📧]
AMA: 2017,Jan,8; 2016,Feb,13

**27816**  Closed treatment of trimalleolar ankle fracture; without manipulation
🔧 8.23   ⚕ 9.16   **FUD** 090          [T] [A2] [50] [📧]
AMA: 2002,Apr,13

**27818**  with manipulation
🔧 12.3   ⚕ 13.7   **FUD** 090          [J] [A2] [50] [📧]
AMA: 2002,Apr,13

**27822**  Open treatment of trimalleolar ankle fracture, includes internal fixation, when performed, medial and/or lateral malleolus; without fixation of posterior lip
🔧 24.6   ⚕ 24.6   **FUD** 090          [J] [A2] [80] [50] [📧]
AMA: 2002,Apr,13

**27823**  with fixation of posterior lip
🔧 27.9   ⚕ 27.9   **FUD** 090          [J] [G2] [80] [50] [📧]
AMA: 2002,Apr,13

**27824**  Closed treatment of fracture of weight bearing articular portion of distal tibia (eg, pilon or tibial plafond), with or without anesthesia; without manipulation
🔧 8.69   ⚕ 8.94   **FUD** 090          [T] [A2] [50] [📧]
AMA: 2002,Apr,13

**27825**  with skeletal traction and/or requiring manipulation
🔧 14.1   ⚕ 15.5   **FUD** 090          [J] [A2] [80] [50] [📧]
AMA: 2002,Apr,13

**27826**  Open treatment of fracture of weight bearing articular surface/portion of distal tibia (eg, pilon or tibial plafond), with internal fixation, when performed; of fibula only
🔧 24.4   ⚕ 24.4   **FUD** 090          [J] [A2] [80] [50] [📧]
AMA: 2002,Apr,13

**27827**  of tibia only
🔧 31.6   ⚕ 31.6   **FUD** 090          [J] [G2] [80] [50] [📧]
AMA: 2002,Apr,13

**27828**  of both tibia and fibula
🔧 37.8   ⚕ 37.8   **FUD** 090          [J] [G2] [80] [50] [📧]
AMA: 2017,Jan,8; 2016,Jan,13; 2015,Jan,16; 2014,Apr,10

**27829**  Open treatment of distal tibiofibular joint (syndesmosis) disruption, includes internal fixation, when performed
🔧 19.9   ⚕ 19.9   **FUD** 090          [J] [A2] [80] [50] [📧]
AMA: 2017,Jan,8; 2016,Feb,13; 2016,Jan,13; 2015,Jan,16; 2014,Jan,11; 2012,Jan,15-42

**27830**  Closed treatment of proximal tibiofibular joint dislocation; without anesthesia
🔧 10.0   ⚕ 10.7   **FUD** 090          [T] [A2] [80] [50] [📧]
AMA: 2002,Apr,13

**27831**  requiring anesthesia
🔧 10.8   ⚕ 10.8   **FUD** 090          [J] [A2] [80] [50] [📧]
AMA: 2002,Apr,13

**27832**  Open treatment of proximal tibiofibular joint dislocation, includes internal fixation, when performed, or with excision of proximal fibula
🔧 21.7   ⚕ 21.7   **FUD** 090          [J] [A2] [80] [50] [📧]
AMA: 2002,Apr,13

● New Code   ▲ Revised Code   ○ Reinstated   ● New Web Release   ▲ Revised Web Release   Unlisted   Not Covered   # Resequenced
⊘ AMA Mod 51 Exempt   ⑪ Optum Mod 51 Exempt   ⊛ Mod 63 Exempt   ✗ Non-FDA Drug   ★ Telemedicine   Ⓜ Maternity   🄰 Age Edit   + Add-on   **AMA:** CPT Asst

**27840** Closed treatment of ankle dislocation; without anesthesia
🔧 10.4  ✂ 10.4  **FUD** 090  T A2 50 ▣
AMA: 2002,Apr,13

**27842** requiring anesthesia, with or without percutaneous skeletal fixation
🔧 14.1  ✂ 14.1  **FUD** 090  J A2 50 ▣
AMA: 2002,Apr,13

**27846** Open treatment of ankle dislocation, with or without percutaneous skeletal fixation; without repair or internal fixation
*EXCLUDES* *Arthroscopy (29894-29898)*
🔧 20.9  ✂ 20.9  **FUD** 090  J A2 80 50 ▣
AMA: 2002,Apr,13

**27848** with repair or internal or external fixation
*EXCLUDES* *Arthroscopy (29894-29898)*
🔧 23.1  ✂ 23.1  **FUD** 090  J A2 80 50 ▣
AMA: 2002,Apr,13

## 27860 Ankle Manipulation with Anesthesia

**27860** Manipulation of ankle under general anesthesia (includes application of traction or other fixation apparatus)
🔧 4.96  ✂ 4.96  **FUD** 010  J A2 80 50 ▣
AMA: 2002,Apr,13

## 27870-27871 Arthrodesis Lower Leg/Ankle

**27870** Arthrodesis, ankle, open
*EXCLUDES* *Arthroscopic arthrodesis of ankle (29899)*
🔧 29.6  ✂ 29.6  **FUD** 090  J J8 80 50 ▣
AMA: 2002,Apr,13; 2001,Dec,3

**27871** Arthrodesis, tibiofibular joint, proximal or distal
🔧 19.6  ✂ 19.6  **FUD** 090  J J8 80 50 ▣
AMA: 2002,Apr,13

## 27880-27889 Amputations of Lower Leg/Ankle

**27880** Amputation, leg, through tibia and fibula;
*INCLUDES* Burgess amputation
🔧 26.6  ✂ 26.6  **FUD** 090  C 80 50 ▣
AMA: 2002,Apr,13

**27881** with immediate fitting technique including application of first cast
🔧 25.0  ✂ 25.0  **FUD** 090  C 80 50 ▣
AMA: 2002,Apr,13

**27882** open, circular (guillotine)
🔧 17.4  ✂ 17.4  **FUD** 090  C 80 50 ▣
AMA: 2002,Apr,13

**27884** secondary closure or scar revision
🔧 16.6  ✂ 16.6  **FUD** 090  J A2 50 ▣
AMA: 2002,Apr,13

**27886** re-amputation
🔧 19.0  ✂ 19.0  **FUD** 090  C 50 ▣
AMA: 2002,Apr,13

**27888** Amputation, ankle, through malleoli of tibia and fibula (eg, Syme, Pirogoff type procedures), with plastic closure and resection of nerves
🔧 19.8  ✂ 19.8  **FUD** 090  C 80 50 ▣
AMA: 2002,Apr,13; 1998,Nov,1

**27889** Ankle disarticulation
🔧 18.7  ✂ 18.7  **FUD** 090  J A2 50 ▣
AMA: 2002,Apr,13

## 27892-27899 Decompression Fasciotomy Lower Leg

*EXCLUDES* *Decompression fasciotomy without debridement (27600-27602)*

**27892** Decompression fasciotomy, leg; anterior and/or lateral compartments only, with debridement of nonviable muscle and/or nerve
🔧 15.9  ✂ 15.9  **FUD** 090  J A2 80 50 ▣
AMA: 2002,Apr,13

**27893** posterior compartment(s) only, with debridement of nonviable muscle and/or nerve
🔧 17.4  ✂ 17.4  **FUD** 090  J A2 80 50 ▣
AMA: 2002,Apr,13

**27894** anterior and/or lateral, and posterior compartment(s), with debridement of nonviable muscle and/or nerve
🔧 24.7  ✂ 24.7  **FUD** 090  J A2 80 50 ▣
AMA: 2002,Apr,13

**27899** Unlisted procedure, leg or ankle
🔧 0.00  ✂ 0.00  **FUD** YYY  T 80 50
AMA: 2017,Jan,8; 2016,Dec,16; 2016,Jan,13; 2015,Jan,16; 2014,Jan,11; 2012,Jan,15-42

## 28001-28008 Surgical Incision Foot/Toe

*EXCLUDES* *Simple incision and drainage (10060-10160)*

**28001** Incision and drainage, bursa, foot
🔧 4.87  ✂ 7.96  **FUD** 010  J P3 ▣
AMA: 2002,Apr,13; 1998,Nov,1

**28002** Incision and drainage below fascia, with or without tendon sheath involvement, foot; single bursal space
🔧 9.14  ✂ 12.7  **FUD** 010  J A2 ▣
AMA: 2002,Apr,13; 1998,Nov,1

**28003** multiple areas
🔧 16.1  ✂ 20.1  **FUD** 090  J A2 ▣
AMA: 2002,Apr,13; 1998,Nov,1

**28005** Incision, bone cortex (eg, osteomyelitis or bone abscess), foot
🔧 16.5  ✂ 16.5  **FUD** 090  J A2 ▣
AMA: 2002,Apr,13; 1998,Nov,1

**28008** Fasciotomy, foot and/or toe
*EXCLUDES* *Plantar fascia division (28250)*
*Plantar fasciectomy (28060, 28062)*
🔧 8.45  ✂ 12.4  **FUD** 090  J A2 50 ▣
AMA: 2002,Apr,13

## 28010-28011 Tenotomy/Toe

*EXCLUDES* *Open tenotomy (28230-28234)*
*Simple incision and drainage (10140-10160)*

**28010** Tenotomy, percutaneous, toe; single tendon
🔧 6.00  ✂ 6.66  **FUD** 090  J P3 ▣
AMA: 2002,Apr,13; 1998,Nov,1

**28011** multiple tendons
🔧 8.24  ✂ 9.22  **FUD** 090  J A2 ▣
AMA: 2002,Apr,13; 1998,Nov,1

## 28020-28024 Arthrotomy Foot/Toe

*EXCLUDES* *Simple incision and drainage (10140-10160)*

**28020** Arthrotomy, including exploration, drainage, or removal of loose or foreign body; intertarsal or tarsometatarsal joint
🔧 10.4  ✂ 15.5  **FUD** 090  J A2 ▣
AMA: 2002,Apr,13; 1998,Nov,1

**28022** metatarsophalangeal joint
🔧 9.31  ✂ 14.0  **FUD** 090  J A2 ▣
AMA: 2002,Apr,13

**28024** interphalangeal joint
🔧 8.74  ✂ 13.2  **FUD** 090  J A2 ▣
AMA: 2002,Apr,13

## 28035 Tarsal Tunnel Release

*EXCLUDES* *Other nerve decompression (64722)*
*Other neuroplasty (64704)*

**28035** Release, tarsal tunnel (posterior tibial nerve decompression)
🔧 10.2  ✂ 15.2  **FUD** 090  J A2 50 ▣
AMA: 2002,Apr,13; 1998,Nov,1

| 26/TC PC/TC Only | A2-Z3 ASC Payment | 50 Bilateral | ♂ Male Only | ♀ Female Only | 🔧 Facility RVU | ✂ Non-Facility RVU | ▣ CCI |
| FUD Follow-up Days | CMS: IOM (Pub 100) | A-Y OPPSI | 80/80 Surg Assist Allowed / w/Doc | | 🔲 Lab Crosswalk | 🔳 Radiology Crosswalk | ✖ CLIA |

92

CPT © 2017 American Medical Association. All Rights Reserved.
© 2017 Optum360, LLC

## 28039-28047 [28039, 28041] Excision Soft Tissue Tumors Foot/Toe

**INCLUDES**
Any necessary elevation of tissue planes or dissection
Measurement of tumor and necessary margin at greatest diameter prior to excision
Simple and intermediate repairs
Types of excision:
Fascial or subfascial soft tissue tumors: simple and marginal resection of tumors found either in or below the deep fascia, not involving bone or excision of a substantial amount of normal tissue; primarily benign and intramuscular tumors
Tumors of fingers and toes involving joint capsules, tendons and tendon sheaths
Radical resection soft tissue tumor: wide resection of tumor, involving substantial margins of normal tissue and may involve tissue removal from one or more layers; most often malignant or aggressive benign
Tumors of fingers and toes adjacent to joints, tendons and tendon sheaths
Subcutaneous: simple and marginal resection of tumors in the subcutaneous tissue above the deep fascia; most often benign

**EXCLUDES**
Complex repair
Excision of benign cutaneous lesions (eg, sebaceous cyst) (11420-11426)
Radical resection of cutaneous tumors (eg, melanoma) (11620-11626)
Significant exploration of vessels, neuroplasty, or reconstruction

**28039** Resequenced code. See code following 28043.

**28041** Resequenced code. See code following 28045.

**28043** Excision, tumor, soft tissue of foot or toe, subcutaneous; less than 1.5 cm
7.58  11.5  **FUD** 090  J G2 50
**AMA:** 2002,Apr,13; 1998,Nov,1

\# **28039** 1.5 cm or greater
10.0  14.6  **FUD** 090  J G2 80 50

**28045** Excision, tumor, soft tissue of foot or toe, subfascial (eg, intramuscular); less than 1.5 cm
10.0  14.3  **FUD** 090  J G2 80 50
**AMA:** 2002,Apr,13

\# **28041** 1.5 cm or greater
13.1  13.1  **FUD** 090  J G2 80 50

**28046** Radical resection of tumor (eg, sarcoma), soft tissue of foot or toe; less than 3 cm
20.9  20.9  **FUD** 090  J G2 50
**AMA:** 2002,Apr,13; 1990,Win,4

**28047** 3 cm or greater
30.6  30.6  **FUD** 090  J G2 80 50

## 28050-28160 Resection Procedures Foot/Toes

**28050** Arthrotomy with biopsy; intertarsal or tarsometatarsal joint
8.91  13.7  **FUD** 090  J A2 50
**AMA:** 2002,Apr,13; 1998,Nov,1

**28052** metatarsophalangeal joint
8.16  12.8  **FUD** 090  J A2 50
**AMA:** 2002,Apr,13

**28054** interphalangeal joint
6.92  11.1  **FUD** 090  J A2 80 50
**AMA:** 2002,Apr,13

**28055** Neurectomy, intrinsic musculature of foot
10.8  10.8  **FUD** 090  J A2 80 50

**28060** Fasciectomy, plantar fascia; partial (separate procedure)
**EXCLUDES** Plantar fasciotomy (28008, 28250)
10.2  14.9  **FUD** 090  J A2 50
**AMA:** 2017,Jan,8; 2016,Jan,13; 2015,Jan,16; 2014,Jan,11; 2012,Jan,15-42

**28062** radical (separate procedure)
**EXCLUDES** Plantar fasciotomy (28008, 28250)
11.7  16.9  **FUD** 090  J A2 50
**AMA:** 2002,Apr,13

**28070** Synovectomy; intertarsal or tarsometatarsal joint, each
10.3  15.5  **FUD** 090  J A2
**AMA:** 2002,Apr,13

**28072** metatarsophalangeal joint, each
9.60  14.7  **FUD** 090  J A2
**AMA:** 2002,Apr,13

**28080** Excision, interdigital (Morton) neuroma, single, each
10.5  15.1  **FUD** 090  J A2 80
**AMA:** 2017,Jan,8; 2016,Jan,13; 2015,Jan,16; 2014,Jan,11

**28086** Synovectomy, tendon sheath, foot; flexor
10.3  15.7  **FUD** 090  J A2 80 50
**AMA:** 2002,Apr,13

**28088** extensor
8.12  12.8  **FUD** 090  J A2 80 50
**AMA:** 2002,Apr,13

**28090** Excision of lesion, tendon, tendon sheath, or capsule (including synovectomy) (eg, cyst or ganglion); foot
8.87  13.5  **FUD** 090  J A2 50
**AMA:** 2002,Apr,13; 1998,Nov,1

**28092** toe(s), each
7.76  12.2  **FUD** 090  J A2
**AMA:** 2002,Apr,13; 1998,Nov,1

**28100** Excision or curettage of bone cyst or benign tumor, talus or calcaneus;
11.8  17.5  **FUD** 090  J A2 80 50
**AMA:** 2002,Apr,13

**28102** with iliac or other autograft (includes obtaining graft)
17.4  17.4  **FUD** 090  J A2 80 50
**AMA:** 2002,Apr,13

**28103** with allograft
11.4  11.4  **FUD** 090  J A2 80 50
**AMA:** 2002,Apr,13

**28104** Excision or curettage of bone cyst or benign tumor, tarsal or metatarsal, except talus or calcaneus;
10.1  15.2  **FUD** 090  J A2 80
**AMA:** 2002,May,7; 2002,Apr,13

**28106** with iliac or other autograft (includes obtaining graft)
12.3  12.3  **FUD** 090  J A2 80
**AMA:** 2002,May,7; 2002,Apr,13

**28107** with allograft
10.0  14.9  **FUD** 090  J A2 80
**AMA:** 2002,May,7; 2002,Apr,13

**28108** Excision or curettage of bone cyst or benign tumor, phalanges of foot
**EXCLUDES** Partial excision bone, toe (28124)
8.30  12.7  **FUD** 090  J A2
**AMA:** 2002,Apr,13

**28110** Ostectomy, partial excision, fifth metatarsal head (bunionette) (separate procedure)
8.34  13.3  **FUD** 090  J A2 50
**AMA:** 2017,Jan,8; 2016,Jan,13; 2015,Jan,16; 2014,Jan,11; 2012,Jan,15-42

**28111** Ostectomy, complete excision; first metatarsal head
9.39  14.2  **FUD** 090  J A2 50
**AMA:** 2002,Apr,13

**28112** other metatarsal head (second, third or fourth)
9.02  14.1  **FUD** 090  J A2 50
**AMA:** 2002,Apr,13

**28113** fifth metatarsal head
12.2  17.0  **FUD** 090  J A2 80 50
**AMA:** 2002,Apr,13

**28114** all metatarsal heads, with partial proximal phalangectomy, excluding first metatarsal (eg, Clayton type procedure)
24.1  31.0  **FUD** 090  J A2 80 50
**AMA:** 2002,Apr,13; 1998,Nov,1

**28116**   **Ostectomy, excision of tarsal coalition**
🟦 16.4   🔪 21.9   **FUD** 090          J A2 50 ▱
AMA: 2002,Apr,13

**28118**   **Ostectomy, calcaneus;**
🟦 11.8   🔪 17.0   **FUD** 090          J A2 80 50 ▱
AMA: 2017,Jan,8; 2016,Jan,13; 2015,Jan,16; 2015,Jan,13;
2014,Jan,11; 2012,Jan,15-42

**28119**   **for spur, with or without plantar fascial release**
🟦 10.3   🔪 15.1   **FUD** 090          J A2 50 ▱
AMA: 2017,Jan,8; 2016,Jan,13; 2015,Jan,16; 2014,Jan,11;
2012,Jan,15-42

**28120**   **Partial excision (craterization, saucerization, sequestrectomy, or diaphysectomy) bone (eg, osteomyelitis or bossing); talus or calcaneus**
INCLUDES   Barker operation
🟦 14.3   🔪 19.5   **FUD** 090          J A2 50 ▱
AMA: 2017,Jan,8; 2016,Jan,13; 2015,Jan,16; 2014,Jan,11;
2012,Jan,15-42

**28122**   **tarsal or metatarsal bone, except talus or calcaneus**
EXCLUDES   Hallux rigidus cheilectomy (28289)
           Partial removal of talus or calcaneus (28120)
🟦 12.6   🔪 17.3   **FUD** 090          J A2 80 50 ▱
AMA: 2002,Apr,13; 1998,Nov,1

**28124**   **phalanx of toe**
🟦 9.51   🔪 13.7   **FUD** 090          J P3 50 ▱
AMA: 2002,Apr,13

**28126**   **Resection, partial or complete, phalangeal base, each toe**
🟦 7.16   🔪 11.4   **FUD** 090          J A2 ▱
AMA: 2017,Jan,8; 2016,Jan,13; 2015,Mar,9

**28130**   **Talectomy (astragalectomy)**
INCLUDES   Whitman astragalectomy
EXCLUDES   Calcanectomy (28118)
🟦 18.5   🔪 18.5   **FUD** 090          J A2 80 50 ▱
AMA: 2002,Apr,13

**28140**   **Metatarsectomy**
🟦 12.6   🔪 17.2   **FUD** 090          J A2 ▱
AMA: 2002,Apr,13

**28150**   **Phalangectomy, toe, each toe**
🟦 8.07   🔪 12.3   **FUD** 090          J A2 ▱
AMA: 2002,Apr,13; 1998,Nov,1

**28153**   **Resection, condyle(s), distal end of phalanx, each toe**
🟦 7.58   🔪 11.8   **FUD** 090          J A2 ▱
AMA: 2017,Jan,8; 2016,Jan,13; 2015,Jan,16; 2014,Jan,11;
2012,Jan,15-42

**28160**   **Hemiphalangectomy or interphalangeal joint excision, toe, proximal end of phalanx, each**
🟦 7.74   🔪 12.1   **FUD** 090          J A2 ▱
AMA: 2002,Apr,13; 1998,Nov,1

## 28171-28175 Radical Resection Bone Tumor Foot/Toes

INCLUDES   Any necessary elevation of tissue planes or dissection
           Excision of adjacent soft tissue during bone tumor resection (28039-28047 [28039, 28041])
           Measurement of tumor and necessary margin at greatest diameter prior to excision
           Resection of the tumor (may include entire bone) and wide margins of normal tissue primarily for malignant or aggressive benign tumors
           Simple and intermediate repairs
EXCLUDES   Complex repair
           Radical tumor resection calcaneus or talus (27647)
           Significant exploration of vessels, neuroplasty, reconstruction, or complex bone repair

**28171**   **Radical resection of tumor; tarsal (except talus or calcaneus)**
🟦 24.4   🔪 24.4   **FUD** 090          J A2 80 ▱
AMA: 2002,Apr,13; 1994,Win,1

**28173**   **metatarsal**
🟦 21.8   🔪 21.8   **FUD** 090          J A2 ▱
AMA: 2002,Apr,13; 1994,Win,1

**28175**   **phalanx of toe**
🟦 14.1   🔪 14.1   **FUD** 090          J A2 CLIA
AMA: 2002,Apr,13

## 28190-28193 Foreign Body Removal: Foot

**28190**   **Removal of foreign body, foot; subcutaneous**
🟦 3.85   🔪 7.42   **FUD** 010          T P3 50 ▱
AMA: 2017,Jan,8; 2016,Jan,13; 2015,Jan,16; 2014,Jan,11;
2013,Dec,16

**28192**   **deep**
🟦 9.02   🔪 13.5   **FUD** 090          J A2 50 ▱
AMA: 2017,Jan,8; 2016,Jan,13; 2015,Jan,16; 2014,Jan,11;
2013,Dec,16

**28193**   **complicated**
🟦 10.6   🔪 15.3   **FUD** 090          J A2 50 ▱
AMA: 2002,Apr,13

## 28200-28360 [28295] Repair/Reconstruction of Foot/Toe

INCLUDES   Closed, open, and percutaneous treatment of fractures and dislocations

**28200**   **Repair, tendon, flexor, foot; primary or secondary, without free graft, each tendon**
🟦 9.27   🔪 14.1   **FUD** 090          J A2
AMA: 2017,Jan,8; 2016,Feb,15; 2016,Jan,13; 2015,Jan,16;
2014,Jul,5; 2014,Jan,11; 2012,Jan,15-42

**28202**   **secondary with free graft, each tendon (includes obtaining graft)**
🟦 12.2   🔪 17.1   **FUD** 090          J A2 80 ▱
AMA: 2002,Apr,13

**28208**   **Repair, tendon, extensor, foot; primary or secondary, each tendon**
🟦 9.03   🔪 13.7   **FUD** 090          J A2 ▱
AMA: 2002,Apr,13; 1998,Nov,1

**28210**   **secondary with free graft, each tendon (includes obtaining graft)**
🟦 11.9   🔪 16.8   **FUD** 090          J A2 80 ▱
AMA: 2002,Apr,13

**28220**   **Tenolysis, flexor, foot; single tendon**
🟦 8.72   🔪 13.0   **FUD** 090          J P3 50 ▱
AMA: 2002,Apr,13; 1998,Nov,1

**28222**   **multiple tendons**
🟦 10.0   🔪 14.6   **FUD** 090          J A2 50 ▱
AMA: 2002,Apr,13; 1998,Nov,1

**28225**   **Tenolysis, extensor, foot; single tendon**
🟦 7.52   🔪 11.9   **FUD** 090          J A2 50 ▱
AMA: 2002,Apr,13; 1998,Nov,1

**28226**   **multiple tendons**
🟦 9.12   🔪 14.1   **FUD** 090          J A2 50 ▱
AMA: 2002,Apr,13; 1998,Nov,1

**28230**   **Tenotomy, open, tendon flexor; foot, single or multiple tendon(s) (separate procedure)**
🟦 8.17   🔪 12.5   **FUD** 090          J P3 50 ▱
AMA: 2002,Apr,13; 1998,Nov,1

**28232**   **toe, single tendon (separate procedure)**
🟦 7.00   🔪 11.2   **FUD** 090          J P3 ▱
AMA: 2017,Jan,8; 2016,Jan,13; 2015,Mar,9

**28234**   **Tenotomy, open, extensor, foot or toe, each tendon**
EXCLUDES   Tendon transfer (27690-27691)
🟦 7.59   🔪 11.8   **FUD** 090          J A2 ▱
AMA: 2017,Jan,8; 2016,Jan,13; 2015,Jan,16; 2014,Jan,11

| 2G/TC PC/TC Only | A2-A3 ASC Payment | 50 Bilateral | ♂ Male Only | ♀ Female Only | 🟦 Facility RVU | 🔪 Non-Facility RVU | ▱ CCI |
| **FUD** Follow-up Days | **CMS:** IOM (Pub 100) | A-Y OPPSI | 80/80 Surg Assist Allowed / w/Doc | | 🟦 Lab Crosswalk | 🟥 Radiology Crosswalk | ✖ CLIA |

**94**                                                                    CPT © 2017 American Medical Association. All Rights Reserved.                                                                    © 2017 Optum360, LLC

**28238** Reconstruction (advancement), posterior tibial tendon with excision of accessory tarsal navicular bone (eg, Kidner type procedure)

> _EXCLUDES_ Extensor hallucis longus transfer with big toe fusion (28760)
> Jones procedure (28760)
> Subcutaneous tenotomy (28010-28011)
> Transfer or transplant of tendon with muscle redirection or rerouting (27690-27692)

14.0 19.3 **FUD** 090 J A2 80 50 ▣
**AMA:** 2002,Apr,13; 2002,May,7

**28240** Tenotomy, lengthening, or release, abductor hallucis muscle

8.53 13.0 **FUD** 090 J A2 50 ▣
**AMA:** 2002,Apr,13

**28250** Division of plantar fascia and muscle (eg, Steindler stripping) (separate procedure)

11.6 16.6 **FUD** 090 J A2 80 50 ▣
**AMA:** 2002,Apr,13; 1998,Nov,1

**28260** Capsulotomy, midfoot; medial release only (separate procedure)

14.8 20.0 **FUD** 090 J A2 80 50 ▣
**AMA:** 2002,Apr,13

**28261** with tendon lengthening

22.7 28.9 **FUD** 090 J A2 80 50 ▣
**AMA:** 2002,Apr,13

**28262** extensive, including posterior talotibial capsulotomy and tendon(s) lengthening (eg, resistant clubfoot deformity)

34.1 42.3 **FUD** 090 J A2 80 50 ▣
**AMA:** 2002,Apr,13; 1998,Nov,1

**28264** Capsulotomy, midtarsal (eg, Heyman type procedure)

19.3 25.2 **FUD** 090 J A2 80 50 ▣
**AMA:** 2002,Apr,13; 1998,Nov,1

**28270** Capsulotomy; metatarsophalangeal joint, with or without tenorrhaphy, each joint (separate procedure)

9.63 14.2 **FUD** 090 J A2 50 ▣
**AMA:** 2017,Jan,8; 2016,Jan,13; 2015,Jan,16; 2014,Sep,13; 2014,Jan,11; 2012,Jan,15-42

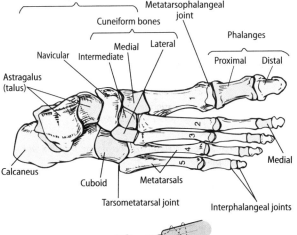

**Tenorrhaphy**

**28272** interphalangeal joint, each joint (separate procedure)

7.32 11.4 **FUD** 090 J P3 50 ▣
**AMA:** 2017,Jan,8; 2016,Jan,13; 2015,Jan,16; 2014,Jan,11; 2012,Jan,15-42

**28280** Syndactylization, toes (eg, webbing or Kelikian type procedure)

10.0 14.9 **FUD** 090 J A2 80 50 ▣
**AMA:** 2002,Apr,13; 1998,Nov,1

**28285** Correction, hammertoe (eg, interphalangeal fusion, partial or total phalangectomy)

10.8 15.4 **FUD** 090 J A2 50 ▣
**AMA:** 2017,Jan,8; 2016,Jun,8; 2016,Jan,13; 2015,Mar,9; 2015,Jan,16; 2014,Jan,11; 2012,Jan,15-42

**28286** Correction, cock-up fifth toe, with plastic skin closure (eg, Ruiz-Mora type procedure)

8.60 13.0 **FUD** 090 J A2 50 ▣
**AMA:** 2002,Apr,13; 1998,Nov,1

**28288** Ostectomy, partial, exostectomy or condylectomy, metatarsal head, each metatarsal head

12.3 17.4 **FUD** 090 J A2 ▣
**AMA:** 2002,Apr,13; 1998,Nov,1

**28289** Hallux rigidus correction with cheilectomy, debridement and capsular release of the first metatarsophalangeal joint; without implant

13.3 21.5 **FUD** 090 J A2 80 50 ▣
**AMA:** 2017,Jan,8; 2016,Dec,3; 2016,Jan,13; 2015,Sep,12; 2015,Jan,16; 2014,Jan,11

**28291** with implant

13.8 21.1 **FUD** 090 J J8 80 50 ▣
**AMA:** 2017,Jan,8; 2016,Dec,3

**28292** Correction, hallux valgus (bunionectomy), with sesamoidectomy, when performed; with resection of proximal phalanx base, when performed, any method

13.9 21.5 **FUD** 090 J A2 80 50 ▣
**AMA:** 2017,Jan,8; 2016,Dec,3; 2016,Jan,13; 2015,Jan,16; 2014,Jan,11; 2012,Jan,15-42

_28295_ Resequenced code. See code following 28296.

**28296** with distal metatarsal osteotomy, any method

14.8 26.3 **FUD** 090 J A2 80 50 ▣
**AMA:** 2017,Jan,8; 2016,Dec,3; 2016,Jan,13; 2015,Jan,16; 2014,Jan,11; 2013,Sep,17; 2012,Jan,15-42

# **28295** with proximal metatarsal osteotomy, any method

15.4 27.1 **FUD** 090 J J8 80 50 ▣
**AMA:** 2017,Jan,8; 2016,Dec,3

**28297** with first metatarsal and medial cuneiform joint arthrodesis, any method

17.3 30.2 **FUD** 090 J A2 80 50 ▣
**AMA:** 2017,Jan,8; 2016,Dec,3; 2016,Jan,13; 2015,Jan,16; 2014,Jan,11

**28298** with proximal phalanx osteotomy, any method

_INCLUDES_ Akin procedure

14.2 24.5 **FUD** 090 J A2 80 50 ▣
**AMA:** 2017,Jan,8; 2016,Dec,3; 2016,Jan,13; 2015,Jan,16; 2014,Jan,11; 2013,Oct,18

---

● New Code ▲ Revised Code ○ Reinstated ● New Web Release ▲ Revised Web Release Unlisted Not Covered # Resequenced
⊘ AMA Mod 51 Exempt ⑨ Optum Mod 51 Exempt ⑥ Mod 63 Exempt ⁄ Non-FDA Drug ★ Telemedicine M Maternity ▲ Age Edit + Add-on **AMA:** CPT Asst
© 2017 Optum360, LLC CPT © 2017 American Medical Association. All Rights Reserved. **95**

**28299** with double osteotomy, any method
To report, see (28899)
🔧 16.6   ⚕ 28.9   **FUD** 090   [J][A2][80][50][🔲]
**AMA:** 2017,Jan,8; 2016,Dec,3; 2016,Apr,8; 2016,Jan,13;
2015,Jan,16; 2014,Jan,11; 2013,Oct,18; 2013,Sep,17;
2012,Jan,15-42

Hallux valgus bunion

Medial eminence of metatarsal bone

Kirshner wires stabilize the osteotomies

A portion of the metatarsal head is resected

A wedge of the proximal phalanx is resected

**28300** Osteotomy; calcaneus (eg, Dwyer or Chambers type procedure), with or without internal fixation
🔧 18.7   ⚕ 18.7   **FUD** 090   [J][A2][80][50][🔲]
**AMA:** 2002,Apr,13; 1998,Nov,1

**28302** talus
🔧 20.5   ⚕ 20.5   **FUD** 090   [J][A2][80][50][🔲]
**AMA:** 2002,Apr,13

**28304** Osteotomy, tarsal bones, other than calcaneus or talus;
🔧 17.5   ⚕ 23.9   **FUD** 090   [J][A2][80][50][🔲]
**AMA:** 2002,Apr,13; 1998,Nov,1

**28305** with autograft (includes obtaining graft) (eg, Fowler type)
🔧 19.1   ⚕ 19.1   **FUD** 090   [J][J8][80][50][🔲]
**AMA:** 2002,Apr,13; 1998,Nov,1

**28306** Osteotomy, with or without lengthening, shortening or angular correction, metatarsal; first metatarsal
🔧 11.6   ⚕ 17.7   **FUD** 090   [J][A2][80][50][🔲]
**AMA:** 2017,Jan,8; 2016,Jan,13; 2015,Jan,16; 2014,Jan,11;
2012,Jan,15-42

**28307** first metatarsal with autograft (other than first toe)
🔧 12.6   ⚕ 19.2   **FUD** 090   [J][A2][80][50][🔲]
**AMA:** 2002,Apr,13; 1998,Nov,1

**28308** other than first metatarsal, each
🔧 10.8   ⚕ 16.3   **FUD** 090   [J][A2][80][50][🔲]
**AMA:** 2002,Apr,13; 1998,Nov,1

**28309** multiple (eg, Swanson type cavus foot procedure)
🔧 25.9   ⚕ 25.9   **FUD** 090   [J][A2][80][50][🔲]
**AMA:** 2017,Jan,8; 2016,Jan,13; 2015,Jan,16; 2014,Jan,11

**28310** Osteotomy, shortening, angular or rotational correction; proximal phalanx, first toe (separate procedure)
🔧 10.3   ⚕ 15.8   **FUD** 090   [J][A2][50][🔲]
**AMA:** 2017,Jan,8; 2016,Jan,13; 2015,Jan,16; 2013,Sep,17

**28312** other phalanges, any toe
🔧 9.18   ⚕ 14.7   **FUD** 090   [J][A2][🔲]
**AMA:** 2002,Apr,13

**28313** Reconstruction, angular deformity of toe, soft tissue procedures only (eg, overlapping second toe, fifth toe, curly toes)
🔧 10.2   ⚕ 15.2   **FUD** 090   [J][A2][🔲]
**AMA:** 2002,Apr,13; 1998,Nov,1

**28315** Sesamoidectomy, first toe (separate procedure)
🔧 9.39   ⚕ 13.9   **FUD** 090   [J][A2][50][🔲]
**AMA:** 2002,Apr,13

**28320** Repair, nonunion or malunion; tarsal bones
🔧 17.6   ⚕ 17.6   **FUD** 090   [J][A2][80][50][🔲]
**AMA:** 2002,Apr,13; 1998,Nov,1

**28322** metatarsal, with or without bone graft (includes obtaining graft)
🔧 16.6   ⚕ 22.7   **FUD** 090   [J][A2][80][🔲]
**AMA:** 2002,Apr,13

**28340** Reconstruction, toe, macrodactyly; soft tissue resection
🔧 11.9   ⚕ 16.7   **FUD** 090   [J][A2][🔲]
**AMA:** 2002,Apr,13

**28341** requiring bone resection
🔧 14.1   ⚕ 19.4   **FUD** 090   [J][A2][🔲]
**AMA:** 2002,Apr,13

**28344** Reconstruction, toe(s); polydactyly
🔧 10.2   ⚕ 16.1   **FUD** 090   [J][A2][50][🔲]
**AMA:** 2002,Apr,13

**28345** syndactyly, with or without skin graft(s), each web
🔧 10.6   ⚕ 15.3   **FUD** 090   [J][A2][80][🔲]
**AMA:** 2002,Apr,13

**28360** Reconstruction, cleft foot
🔧 26.5   ⚕ 26.5   **FUD** 090   [J][80][50][🔲]
**AMA:** 2002,Apr,13

## 28400-28675 Treatment of Fracture/Dislocation of Foot/Toe

**28400** Closed treatment of calcaneal fracture; without manipulation
🔧 6.49   ⚕ 7.10   **FUD** 090   [T][A2][50][🔲]
**AMA:** 2002,Apr,13

**28405** with manipulation
[INCLUDES]   Bohler reduction
🔧 10.2   ⚕ 11.2   **FUD** 090   [T][A2][80][50][🔲]
**AMA:** 2002,Apr,13

**28406** Percutaneous skeletal fixation of calcaneal fracture, with manipulation
🔧 14.9   ⚕ 14.9   **FUD** 090   [J][A2][80][50][🔲]
**AMA:** 2002,Apr,13

**28415** Open treatment of calcaneal fracture, includes internal fixation, when performed;
🔧 32.3   ⚕ 32.3   **FUD** 090   [J][A2][80][50][🔲]
**AMA:** 2002,Apr,13

**28420** with primary iliac or other autogenous bone graft (includes obtaining graft)
🔧 36.6   ⚕ 36.6   **FUD** 090   [J][J8][80][50][🔲]
**AMA:** 2002,Apr,13

**28430** Closed treatment of talus fracture; without manipulation
🔧 6.00   ⚕ 6.75   **FUD** 090   [T][P2][50][🔲]
**AMA:** 2002,Apr,13

**28435** with manipulation
🔧 8.23   ⚕ 9.20   **FUD** 090   [J][A2][80][50][🔲]
**AMA:** 2002,Apr,13

**28436** Percutaneous skeletal fixation of talus fracture, with manipulation
🔧 12.7   ⚕ 12.7   **FUD** 090   [J][J8][50][🔲]
**AMA:** 2002,Apr,13

**28445** Open treatment of talus fracture, includes internal fixation, when performed
🔧 30.6   ⚕ 30.6   **FUD** 090   [J][A2][80][50][🔲]
**AMA:** 2002,Apr,13

**28446** Open osteochondral autograft, talus (includes obtaining graft[s])
[INCLUDES]   Osteotomy; fibula (27707)
Osteotomy; tibia (27705)
[EXCLUDES]   *Arthroscopically aided osteochondral talus graft (29892)*
*Open osteochondral allograft or repairs with industrial grafts (28899)*
🔧 34.7   ⚕ 34.7   **FUD** 090   [J][02][80][50][🔲]
**AMA:** 2017,Jan,8; 2016,Jan,13; 2015,Jan,16; 2014,Jan,11

[26]/[TC] PC/TC Only   [A2]-[Z3] ASC Payment   [50] Bilateral   ♂ Male Only   ♀ Female Only   🔧 Facility RVU   ⚕ Non-Facility RVU   [🔲] CCI
**FUD** Follow-up Days   **CMS:** IOM (Pub 100)   [A]-[Y] OPPSI   [80]/[80] Surg Assist Allowed / w/Doc   ▪ Lab Crosswalk   ▪ Radiology Crosswalk   [X] CLIA

CPT © 2017 American Medical Association. All Rights Reserved.                    © 2017 Optum360, LLC

**28450**   **Treatment of tarsal bone fracture (except talus and calcaneus); without manipulation, each**
  🔷 5.50   ⚕ 6.17   **FUD** 090                    T P2 ▣
  AMA: 2017,Jan,8; 2016,Jan,13; 2015,Jan,16; 2014,Jan,11; 2012,Jan,15-42

**28455**       **with manipulation, each**
  🔷 7.40   ⚕ 8.23   **FUD** 090                    J P3 80 ▣
  AMA: 2002,Apr,13

**28456**   **Percutaneous skeletal fixation of tarsal bone fracture (except talus and calcaneus), with manipulation, each**
  🔷 9.02   ⚕ 9.02   **FUD** 090                    J A2 ▣
  AMA: 2002,Apr,13

**28465**   **Open treatment of tarsal bone fracture (except talus and calcaneus), includes internal fixation, when performed, each**
  🔷 18.0   ⚕ 18.0   **FUD** 090                    J A2 ▣
  AMA: 2002,Apr,13

**28470**   **Closed treatment of metatarsal fracture; without manipulation, each**
  🔷 5.84   ⚕ 6.25   **FUD** 090                    T P2 ▣
  AMA: 2002,Apr,13

**28475**       **with manipulation, each**
  🔷 6.50   ⚕ 7.31   **FUD** 090                    T P2 ▣
  AMA: 2002,Apr,13

**28476**   **Percutaneous skeletal fixation of metatarsal fracture, with manipulation, each**
  🔷 10.1   ⚕ 10.1   **FUD** 090                    J A2 80 ▣
  AMA: 2002,Apr,13

**28485**   **Open treatment of metatarsal fracture, includes internal fixation, when performed, each**
  🔷 15.5   ⚕ 15.5   **FUD** 090                    J A2 ▣
  AMA: 2002,Apr,13

**28490**   **Closed treatment of fracture great toe, phalanx or phalanges; without manipulation**
  🔷 3.58   ⚕ 4.16   **FUD** 090                    T P3 50 ▣
  AMA: 2002,Apr,13

**28495**       **with manipulation**
  🔷 4.30   ⚕ 5.10   **FUD** 090                    T P2 50 ▣
  AMA: 2002,Apr,13

**28496**   **Percutaneous skeletal fixation of fracture great toe, phalanx or phalanges, with manipulation**
  🔷 6.84   ⚕ 12.8   **FUD** 090                    J A2 50 ▣
  AMA: 2002,Apr,13

**28505**   **Open treatment of fracture, great toe, phalanx or phalanges, includes internal fixation, when performed**
  🔷 14.4   ⚕ 19.3   **FUD** 090                    J A2 50 ▣
  AMA: 2002,Apr,13

**28510**   **Closed treatment of fracture, phalanx or phalanges, other than great toe; without manipulation, each**
  🔷 3.44   ⚕ 3.54   **FUD** 090                    T P3 ▣
  AMA: 2002,Apr,13

**28515**       **with manipulation, each**
  🔷 4.09   ⚕ 4.63   **FUD** 090                    T P3 ▣
  AMA: 2002,Apr,13

**28525**   **Open treatment of fracture, phalanx or phalanges, other than great toe, includes internal fixation, when performed, each**
  🔷 11.4   ⚕ 16.2   **FUD** 090                    J A2 80 ▣
  AMA: 2002,Apr,13

**28530**   **Closed treatment of sesamoid fracture**
  🔷 2.93   ⚕ 3.30   **FUD** 090                    T P3 80 50 ▣
  AMA: 2002,Apr,13

**28531**   **Open treatment of sesamoid fracture, with or without internal fixation**
  🔷 5.24   ⚕ 9.90   **FUD** 090                    J A2 50 ▣
  AMA: 2002,Apr,13

**28540**   **Closed treatment of tarsal bone dislocation, other than talotarsal; without anesthesia**
  🔷 4.99   ⚕ 5.52   **FUD** 090                    T P2 80 50 ▣
  AMA: 2002,Apr,13

**28545**       **requiring anesthesia**
  🔷 7.52   ⚕ 8.47   **FUD** 090                    J J8 80 50 ▣
  AMA: 2002,Apr,13

**28546**   **Percutaneous skeletal fixation of tarsal bone dislocation, other than talotarsal, with manipulation**
  🔷 9.52   ⚕ 16.1   **FUD** 090                    J A2 80 50 ▣
  AMA: 2002,Apr,13

**28555**   **Open treatment of tarsal bone dislocation, includes internal fixation, when performed**
  🔷 19.2   ⚕ 25.3   **FUD** 090                    J A2 80 50 ▣
  AMA: 2002,Apr,13

**28570**   **Closed treatment of talotarsal joint dislocation; without anesthesia**
  🔷 4.37   ⚕ 5.16   **FUD** 090                    T P2 80 50 ▣
  AMA: 2002,Apr,13

**28575**       **requiring anesthesia**
  🔷 9.19   ⚕ 10.1   **FUD** 090                    J A2 80 50 ▣
  AMA: 2002,Apr,13

**28576**   **Percutaneous skeletal fixation of talotarsal joint dislocation, with manipulation**
  🔷 11.3   ⚕ 11.3   **FUD** 090                    J A2 80 50 ▣
  AMA: 2002,Apr,13

**28585**   **Open treatment of talotarsal joint dislocation, includes internal fixation, when performed**
  🔷 19.4   ⚕ 24.9   **FUD** 090                    J J8 80 50 ▣
  AMA: 2017,Jan,8; 2016,Jan,13; 2015,Jan,16; 2014,Jan,11; 2012,Jan,15-42

**28600**   **Closed treatment of tarsometatarsal joint dislocation; without anesthesia**
  🔷 5.44   ⚕ 6.34   **FUD** 090                    T P2 80 ▣
  AMA: 2002,Apr,13

**28605**       **requiring anesthesia**
  🔷 8.43   ⚕ 9.37   **FUD** 090                    T A2 80 ▣
  AMA: 2002,Apr,13

**28606**   **Percutaneous skeletal fixation of tarsometatarsal joint dislocation, with manipulation**
  🔷 11.3   ⚕ 11.3   **FUD** 090                    J A2 ▣
  AMA: 2002,Apr,13

**28615**   **Open treatment of tarsometatarsal joint dislocation, includes internal fixation, when performed**
  🔷 23.1   ⚕ 23.1   **FUD** 090                    J A2 80 ▣
  AMA: 2002,Apr,13

**28630**   **Closed treatment of metatarsophalangeal joint dislocation; without anesthesia**
  🔷 3.19   ⚕ 4.56   **FUD** 010                    T P3 80 ▣
  AMA: 2002,Apr,13

**28635**       **requiring anesthesia**
  🔷 3.80   ⚕ 5.05   **FUD** 010                    J A2 80 ▣
  AMA: 2002,Apr,13

**28636**   **Percutaneous skeletal fixation of metatarsophalangeal joint dislocation, with manipulation**
  🔷 6.45   ⚕ 10.0   **FUD** 010                    J A2 ▣
  AMA: 2002,Apr,13

**28645**   **Open treatment of metatarsophalangeal joint dislocation, includes internal fixation, when performed**
  🔷 13.9   ⚕ 18.9   **FUD** 090                    J A2 ▣
  AMA: 2017,Jan,8; 2016,Jan,13; 2015,Jan,16; 2014,Sep,13

**28660**   **Closed treatment of interphalangeal joint dislocation; without anesthesia**
  🔷 2.56   ⚕ 3.35   **FUD** 010                    T P3 ▣
  AMA: 2002,Apr,13

---

● New Code   ▲ Revised Code   ○ Reinstated   ● New Web Release   ▲ Revised Web Release   Unlisted   Not Covered   # Resequenced
⊘ AMA Mod 51 Exempt   ⊚ Optum Mod 51 Exempt   ⊛ Mod 63 Exempt   ✐ Non-FDA Drug   ★ Telemedicine   M Maternity   A Age Edit   + Add-on   AMA: CPT Asst

**Musculoskeletal System**

**28665 — 29065**

**28665**     requiring anesthesia
       🔧 3.79   ⚘ 4.46   **FUD** 010       T A2 80 ▣
AMA: 2002,Apr,13

**28666**     **Percutaneous skeletal fixation of interphalangeal joint dislocation, with manipulation**
       🔧 5.33   ⚘ 5.33   **FUD** 010       J A2 ▣
AMA: 2002,Apr,13

**28675**     **Open treatment of interphalangeal joint dislocation, includes internal fixation, when performed**
       🔧 11.8   ⚘ 16.8   **FUD** 090       J A2 ▣
AMA: 2002,Apr,13

## 28705-28760 Arthrodesis of Foot/Toe

**28705**     **Arthrodesis; pantalar**
       🔧 35.9   ⚘ 35.9   **FUD** 090       J J8 80 50 ▣
AMA: 2002,Apr,13

**28715**     **triple**
       🔧 27.0   ⚘ 27.0   **FUD** 090       J J8 80 50 ▣
AMA: 2002,Apr,13; 1998,Nov,1

**28725**     **subtalar**
       INCLUDES   Dunn arthrodesis
                   Grice arthrosis
       🔧 22.3   ⚘ 22.3   **FUD** 090       J G2 80 50 ▣
AMA: 2017,Jan,8; 2016,Jan,13; 2015,Jan,16; 2014,Jan,11; 2012,Jan,15-42

**28730**     **Arthrodesis, midtarsal or tarsometatarsal, multiple or transverse;**
       INCLUDES   Lambrinudi arthrodesis
       🔧 21.0   ⚘ 21.0   **FUD** 090       J J8 80 50 ▣
AMA: 2002,Apr,13

**28735**     **with osteotomy (eg, flatfoot correction)**
       🔧 22.5   ⚘ 22.5   **FUD** 090       J J8 80 50 ▣
AMA: 2002,Apr,13; 1998,Nov,1

**28737**     **Arthrodesis, with tendon lengthening and advancement, midtarsal, tarsal navicular-cuneiform (eg, Miller type procedure)**
       🔧 20.0   ⚘ 20.0   **FUD** 090       J J8 80 50 ▣
AMA: 2002,Apr,13; 2002,May,7

**28740**     **Arthrodesis, midtarsal or tarsometatarsal, single joint**
       🔧 17.9   ⚘ 24.4   **FUD** 090       J J8 80 ▣
AMA: 2017,Jan,8; 2016,Jan,13; 2015,Jan,16; 2014,Jan,11; 2012,Jan,15-42

**28750**     **Arthrodesis, great toe; metatarsophalangeal joint**
       🔧 16.9   ⚘ 23.3   **FUD** 090       J J8 80 50 ▣
AMA: 2017,Jan,8; 2016,Dec,3; 2016,Jan,13; 2015,Jan,16; 2014,Jan,11

**28755**     **interphalangeal joint**
       🔧 9.51   ⚘ 14.6   **FUD** 090       J A2 50 ▣
AMA: 2002,Apr,13

**28760**     **Arthrodesis, with extensor hallucis longus transfer to first metatarsal neck, great toe, interphalangeal joint (eg, Jones type procedure)**
       EXCLUDES   Hammer toe repair or interphalangeal fusion (28285)
       🔧 16.7   ⚘ 22.9   **FUD** 090       J A2 80 50 ▣
AMA: 2002,Apr,13; 1998,Nov,1

## 28800-28825 Amputation Foot/Toe

**28800**     **Amputation, foot; midtarsal (eg, Chopart type procedure)**
       🔧 15.5   ⚘ 15.5   **FUD** 090       C 80 50 ▣
AMA: 2002,Apr,13; 1998,Nov,1

**28805**     **transmetatarsal**
       🔧 21.1   ⚘ 21.1   **FUD** 090       J 80 50 ▣
AMA: 2002,Apr,13; 1997,May,4

**28810**     **Amputation, metatarsal, with toe, single**
       🔧 12.4   ⚘ 12.4   **FUD** 090       J A2 80 ▣
AMA: 2002,Apr,13

**28820**     **Amputation, toe; metatarsophalangeal joint**
       🔧 11.3   ⚘ 16.2   **FUD** 090       J A2 ▣
AMA: 2002,Apr,13; 1997,May,4

**28825**     **interphalangeal joint**
       🔧 10.6   ⚘ 15.5   **FUD** 090       J A2 ▣
AMA: 2002,Apr,13

## 28890-28899 Other/Unlisted Procedures Foot/Toe

**28890**     **Extracorporeal shock wave, high energy, performed by a physician or other qualified health care professional, requiring anesthesia other than local, including ultrasound guidance, involving the plantar fascia**
       EXCLUDES   Extracorporeal shock wave therapy of musculoskeletal system not otherwise specified (0101T-0102T)
       🔧 6.49   ⚘ 9.34   **FUD** 090       J P3 50 ▣
AMA: 2017,Jan,8; 2016,Jan,13; 2015,Jan,16; 2014,Jan,11; 2012,Jan,15-42

**28899**     **Unlisted procedure, foot or toes**
       🔧 0.00   ⚘ 0.00   **FUD** YYY       T 80
AMA: 2017,Sep,14; 2017,Jan,8; 2016,Dec,3; 2016,Jun,8; 2016,Jan,13; 2015,Nov,10; 2015,Jan,16; 2014,Jan,11; 2012,Jan,15-42

## 29000-29086 Casting: Arm/Shoulder/Torso

INCLUDES   Application of cast or strapping when provided as:
         An initial service to stabilize the fracture or injury without restorative treatment
         A replacement procedure
       Removal of cast
EXCLUDES   Cast or splint material
       E&M services provided as part of the initial service when restorative treatment is not provided
       Orthotic supervision and training (97760-97763)

**29000**     **Application of halo type body cast (see 20661-20663 for insertion)**
       🔧 5.22   ⚘ 8.59   **FUD** 000       T G2 80 ▣
AMA: 2017,Jan,8; 2016,Jan,13; 2015,Jan,16; 2014,Jan,11

**29010**     **Application of Risser jacket, localizer, body; only**
       🔧 3.98   ⚘ 6.25   **FUD** 000       T P2 80 ▣
AMA: 2017,Jan,8; 2016,Jan,13; 2015,Jan,16; 2014,Jan,11

**29015**     **including head**
       🔧 4.87   ⚘ 7.62   **FUD** 000       T P2 80 ▣
AMA: 2017,Jan,8; 2016,Jan,13; 2015,Jan,16; 2014,Jan,11

**29035**     **Application of body cast, shoulder to hips;**
       🔧 4.15   ⚘ 7.31   **FUD** 000       T P2 80 ▣
AMA: 2017,Jan,8; 2016,Jan,13; 2015,Jan,16; 2014,Jan,11

**29040**     **including head, Minerva type**
       🔧 4.19   ⚘ 6.45   **FUD** 000       T G2 80 ▣
AMA: 2017,Jan,8; 2016,Jan,13; 2015,Jan,16; 2014,Jan,11

**29044**     **including 1 thigh**
       🔧 4.41   ⚘ 7.14   **FUD** 000       T P2 80 ▣
AMA: 2017,Jan,8; 2016,Jan,13; 2015,Jan,16; 2014,Jan,11

**29046**     **including both thighs**
       🔧 4.76   ⚘ 7.47   **FUD** 000       T G2 80 ▣
AMA: 2017,Jan,8; 2016,Jan,13; 2015,Jan,16; 2014,Jan,11

**29049**     **Application, cast; figure-of-eight**
       🔧 1.62   ⚘ 2.10   **FUD** 000       T P3 80 ▣
AMA: 2017,Jan,8; 2016,Jan,13; 2015,Jan,16; 2014,Jan,11

**29055**     **shoulder spica**
       🔧 3.96   ⚘ 6.28   **FUD** 000       T P2 80 ▣
AMA: 2017,Jan,8; 2016,Jan,13; 2015,Jan,16; 2014,Jan,11

**29058**     **plaster Velpeau**
       🔧 2.70   ⚘ 3.51   **FUD** 000       T P3 80 ▣
AMA: 2017,Jan,8; 2016,Jan,13; 2015,Jan,16; 2014,Jan,11

**29065**     **shoulder to hand (long arm)**
       🔧 1.96   ⚘ 2.74   **FUD** 000       T P3 50 ▣
AMA: 2017,Jan,8; 2016,Jan,13; 2015,Jan,16; 2014,Jan,11

**29075** **elbow to finger (short arm)**
🔧 1.79 🔨 2.48 **FUD** 000 [T] [P3] [50] 🔲
**AMA:** 2017,Jan,8; 2016,Jan,13; 2015,Jan,16; 2014,Jan,11

**29085** **hand and lower forearm (gauntlet)**
🔧 1.95 🔨 2.73 **FUD** 000 [T] [P3] [50] 🔲
**AMA:** 2017,Jan,8; 2016,Jan,13; 2015,Jan,16; 2014,Jan,11;
2012,Jan,15-42

**29086** **finger (eg, contracture)**
🔧 1.43 🔨 2.17 **FUD** 000 [T] [P3] [50] 🔲
**AMA:** 2017,Jan,8; 2016,Jan,13; 2015,Jan,16; 2014,Jan,11

## 29105-29280 Splinting and Strapping: Torso/Upper Extremities

**INCLUDES** Application of splint or strapping when provided as:
An initial service to stabilize the fracture or dislocation
A replacement procedure

**EXCLUDES** *E&M services provided as part of the initial service when restorative treatment is not provided*
*Orthotic supervision and training (97760-97763)*
*Splinting and strapping material*

**29105** **Application of long arm splint (shoulder to hand)**
🔧 1.71 🔨 2.51 **FUD** 000 [T] [P3] [50] 🔲
**AMA:** 2017,Jan,8; 2016,Jan,13; 2015,Jan,16; 2014,Jan,11;
2012,Jan,15-42

**29125** **Application of short arm splint (forearm to hand); static**
🔧 1.13 🔨 1.84 **FUD** 000 [01] [N1] [50] 🔲
**AMA:** 2017,Jan,8; 2016,Jan,13; 2015,Jan,16; 2014,Jan,11

**29126** **dynamic**
🔧 1.38 🔨 2.16 **FUD** 000 [01] [N1] [50] 🔲
**AMA:** 2017,Jan,8; 2016,Jan,13; 2015,Jan,16; 2014,Jan,11

**29130** **Application of finger splint; static**
🔧 0.82 🔨 1.17 **FUD** 000 [01] [N1] [50] 🔲
**AMA:** 2017,Jan,8; 2016,Jan,13; 2015,Jan,16; 2014,Jan,11

**29131** **dynamic**
🔧 0.95 🔨 1.45 **FUD** 000 [01] [N1] [50] 🔲
**AMA:** 2017,Jan,8; 2016,Jan,13; 2015,Jan,16; 2014,Jan,11

**29200** **Strapping; thorax**
**EXCLUDES** *Strapping of low back (29799)*
🔧 0.52 🔨 0.85 **FUD** 000 [T] [P3]
**AMA:** 2017,Jan,8; 2016,Jan,13; 2015,Jan,16; 2014,Jan,11

**29240** **shoulder (eg, Velpeau)**
🔧 0.52 🔨 0.81 **FUD** 000 [01] [N1] [50] 🔲
**AMA:** 2017,Jan,8; 2016,Jan,13; 2015,Jan,16; 2014,Jan,11

**29260** **elbow or wrist**
🔧 0.56 🔨 0.82 **FUD** 000 [01] [N1] [50] 🔲
**AMA:** 2017,Jan,8; 2016,Jan,13; 2015,Jan,16; 2014,Jan,11

**29280** **hand or finger**
🔧 0.56 🔨 0.82 **FUD** 000 [01] [N1] [50] 🔲
**AMA:** 2017,Jan,8; 2016,Jan,13; 2015,Jan,16; 2014,Jan,11

## 29305-29450 Casting: Legs

**INCLUDES** Application of cast when provided as:
An initial service to stabilize the fracture or injury without restorative treatment
A replacement procedure
Removal of cast

**EXCLUDES** *Cast or splint materials*
*E&M services provided as part of the initial service when restorative treatment is not provided*
*Orthotic supervision and training (97760-97763)*

**29305** **Application of hip spica cast; 1 leg**
**EXCLUDES** *Hip spica cast thighs only (29046)*
🔧 4.56 🔨 7.01 **FUD** 000 [T] [P2] [80] 🔲
**AMA:** 2017,Jan,8; 2016,Jan,13; 2015,Jan,16; 2014,Jan,11

**29325** **1 and one-half spica or both legs**
**EXCLUDES** *Hip spica cast thighs only (29046)*
🔧 5.12 🔨 7.80 **FUD** 000 [T] [P2] [80] 🔲
**AMA:** 2017,Jan,8; 2016,Jan,13; 2015,Jan,16; 2014,Jan,11

**29345** **Application of long leg cast (thigh to toes);**
🔧 2.91 🔨 3.90 **FUD** 000 [T] [P3] [50] 🔲
**AMA:** 2017,Jan,8; 2016,Jan,13; 2015,Jan,16; 2014,Jan,11

**29355** **walker or ambulatory type**
🔧 3.07 🔨 4.03 **FUD** 000 [T] [P3] [50] 🔲
**AMA:** 2017,Jan,8; 2016,Jan,13; 2015,Jan,16; 2014,Jan,11

**29358** **Application of long leg cast brace**
🔧 2.99 🔨 4.59 **FUD** 000 [T] [P3] [50] 🔲
**AMA:** 2017,Jan,8; 2016,Jan,13; 2015,Jan,16; 2014,Jan,11

**29365** **Application of cylinder cast (thigh to ankle)**
🔧 2.52 🔨 3.51 **FUD** 000 [T] [P3] [50] 🔲
**AMA:** 2017,Jan,8; 2016,Jan,13; 2015,Jan,16; 2014,Jan,11

**29405** **Application of short leg cast (below knee to toes);**
🔧 1.73 🔨 2.34 **FUD** 000 [T] [P3] [50] 🔲
**AMA:** 2017,Jan,8; 2016,Jan,13; 2015,Jan,16; 2014,Jan,11

**29425** **walking or ambulatory type**
🔧 1.63 🔨 2.24 **FUD** 000 [T] [P3] [50] 🔲
**AMA:** 2017,Jan,8; 2016,Jan,13; 2015,Jan,16; 2014,Jan,11

**29435** **Application of patellar tendon bearing (PTB) cast**
🔧 2.40 🔨 3.36 **FUD** 000 [T] [P3] [50] 🔲
**AMA:** 2017,Jan,8; 2016,Jan,13; 2015,Jan,16; 2014,Jan,11

**29440** **Adding walker to previously applied cast**
🔧 0.83 🔨 1.25 **FUD** 000 [T] [P3] [50] 🔲
**AMA:** 2017,Jan,8; 2016,Jan,13; 2015,Jan,16; 2014,Jan,11

**29445** **Application of rigid total contact leg cast**
🔧 2.99 🔨 3.84 **FUD** 000 [T] [P3] [50] 🔲
**AMA:** 2017,Jan,8; 2016,Jan,13; 2015,Jan,16; 2014,Jan,11;
2012,Jan,15-42

**29450** **Application of clubfoot cast with molding or manipulation, long or short leg**
🔧 3.26 🔨 4.14 **FUD** 000 [T] [P3] [50] 🔲
**AMA:** 2017,Jan,8; 2016,Jan,13; 2015,Jan,16; 2014,Jan,11

## 29505-29584 Splinting and Strapping Ankle/Foot/Leg/Toes

**INCLUDES** Application of splinting and strapping when provided as:
An initial service to stabilize the fracture or injury without restorative treatment
A replacement procedure

**EXCLUDES** *E&M services provided as part of the initial service when restorative treatment is not provided*
*Orthotic supervision and training (97760-97763)*

**29505** **Application of long leg splint (thigh to ankle or toes)**
🔧 1.43 🔨 2.39 **FUD** 000 [T] [P3] [50] 🔲
**AMA:** 2017,Jan,8; 2016,Jan,13; 2015,Jan,16; 2014,Jan,11;
2012,Jan,15-42

**29515** **Application of short leg splint (calf to foot)**
🔧 1.43 🔨 2.06 **FUD** 000 [T] [P3] [50] 🔲
**AMA:** 2017,Jan,8; 2016,Jan,13; 2015,Jan,16; 2014,Jan,11

**29520** **Strapping; hip**
🔧 0.53 🔨 0.89 **FUD** 000 [01] [N1] [80] [50] 🔲
**AMA:** 2017,Jan,8; 2016,Jan,13; 2015,Jan,16; 2014,Jan,11

**29530** **knee**
🔧 0.52 🔨 0.81 **FUD** 000 [01] [N1] [50] 🔲
**AMA:** 2017,Jan,8; 2016,Jan,13; 2015,Jan,16; 2014,Jan,11

**29540** **ankle and/or foot**
**EXCLUDES** *Application of multi-layer compression system (29581)*
🔧 0.52 🔨 0.74 **FUD** 000 [T] [P3] [50] 🔲
**AMA:** 2017,Jan,8; 2016,Aug,3; 2016,Jan,13; 2015,Jan,16;
2014,Mar,4; 2014,Jan,11; 2012,Oct,14; 2012,Sep,16;
2012,Jan,15-42

**29550** **toes**
🔧 0.33 🔨 0.54 **FUD** 000 [01] [N1] [50] 🔲
**AMA:** 2017,Jan,8; 2016,Jan,13; 2015,Jan,16; 2014,Jan,11

---

● New Code ▲ Revised Code ○ Reinstated ● New Web Release ▲ Revised Web Release Unlisted Not Covered # Resequenced
⊘ AMA Mod 51 Exempt ⑨ Optum Mod 51 Exempt ⑨ Mod 63 Exempt ✎ Non-FDA Drug ★ Telemedicine Ⓜ Maternity Ⓐ Age Edit + Add-on **AMA:** CPT Asst

**29580    Unna boot**
EXCLUDES  *Application of multi-layer compression system (29581)*
🛏 1.02   ✂ 1.49   **FUD** 000                    T P3 50 ▣
**AMA:** 2017,Jan,8; 2016,Aug,3; 2016,Jan,13; 2015,Jan,16;
2014,Mar,4; 2014,Jan,11; 2012,Oct,14; 2012,Sep,16;
2012,Jan,15-42

**29581    Application of multi-layer compression system; leg (below knee), including ankle and foot**
EXCLUDES  *Endovenous ablation therapy of incompetent vein (36475-36476, 36478-36479)*
*Sclerosal injection for incompetent vein(s) (36468-36471)*
*Strapping (29540, 29580)*
🛏 0.37   ✂ 1.77   **FUD** 000                    T P3 80 50 ▣
**AMA:** 2017,Jan,8; 2016,Nov,3; 2016,Aug,3; 2016,Jan,13;
2015,Mar,9; 2015,Jan,16; 2014,Oct,6; 2014,Mar,4; 2014,Jan,11;
2013,Sep,17; 2012,Oct,14; 2012,Sep,16

**29582    ~~thigh and leg, including ankle and foot, when performed~~**

**29583    ~~upper arm and forearm~~**

**29584    upper arm, forearm, hand, and fingers**
🛏 0.45   ✂ 2.00   **FUD** 000                    T P3 80 50 ▣
**AMA:** 2017,Jan,8; 2016,Aug,3; 2016,Jan,13; 2015,Mar,9

## 29700-29799 Casting Services Other Than Application

INCLUDES  Casts applied by treating individual
Removal of casts applied by treating individual

**29700    Removal or bivalving; gauntlet, boot or body cast**
🛏 0.97   ✂ 1.80   **FUD** 000                    T P3 ▣
**AMA:** 2017,Jan,8; 2016,Jan,13; 2015,Jan,16; 2014,Jan,11

**29705    full arm or full leg cast**
🛏 1.36   ✂ 1.91   **FUD** 000                    T P3 50 ▣
**AMA:** 2017,Jan,8; 2016,Jan,13; 2015,Jan,16; 2014,Jan,11

**29710    shoulder or hip spica, Minerva, or Risser jacket, etc.**
🛏 2.40   ✂ 3.48   **FUD** 000                    T P3 80 50 ▣
**AMA:** 2017,Jan,8; 2016,Jan,13; 2015,Jan,16; 2014,Jan,11

**29720    Repair of spica, body cast or jacket**
🛏 1.28   ✂ 2.43   **FUD** 000                    T P3 ▣
**AMA:** 2017,Jan,8; 2016,Jan,13; 2015,Jan,16; 2014,Jan,11

**29730    Windowing of cast**
🛏 1.29   ✂ 1.84   **FUD** 000                    T P3 ▣
**AMA:** 2017,Jan,8; 2016,Jan,13; 2015,Jan,16; 2014,Jan,11

**29740    Wedging of cast (except clubfoot casts)**
🛏 2.03   ✂ 2.85   **FUD** 000                    T P3 ▣
**AMA:** 2017,Jan,8; 2016,Jan,13; 2015,Jan,16; 2014,Jan,11

**29750    Wedging of clubfoot cast**
🛏 1.98   ✂ 2.59   **FUD** 000                    T P3 80 50 ▣
**AMA:** 2017,Jan,8; 2016,Jan,13; 2015,Jan,16; 2014,Jan,11

**29799    Unlisted procedure, casting or strapping**
🛏 0.00   ✂ 0.00   **FUD** YYY                    T 80
**AMA:** 2017,Jan,8; 2016,Aug,3; 2016,Jan,13; 2015,Jan,16;
2014,Jan,11; 2012,Oct,14; 2012,Sep,16

## 29800-29999 [29914, 29915, 29916] Arthroscopic Procedures

INCLUDES  Diagnostic arthroscopy with surgical arthroscopy
Code also modifier 51 if arthroscopy is performed with arthrotomy

**29800    Arthroscopy, temporomandibular joint, diagnostic, with or without synovial biopsy (separate procedure)**
🛏 15.1   ✂ 15.1   **FUD** 090                    J A2 80 50 ▣
**AMA:** 2017,Jan,8; 2016,Jan,13; 2015,Jan,16; 2013,May,12

**29804    Arthroscopy, temporomandibular joint, surgical**
EXCLUDES  *Open surgery (21010)*
🛏 18.5   ✂ 18.5   **FUD** 090                    J A2 80 50 ▣
**AMA:** 2017,Jan,8; 2016,Jan,13; 2015,Jan,16; 2013,May,12

**29805    Arthroscopy, shoulder, diagnostic, with or without synovial biopsy (separate procedure)**
EXCLUDES  *Open surgery (23065-23066, 23100-23101)*
🛏 13.5   ✂ 13.5   **FUD** 090                    J A2 50 ▣
**AMA:** 2017,Jan,8; 2016,Jan,13; 2015,Jun,10; 2015,Jan,16;
2013,May,12

**29806    Arthroscopy, shoulder, surgical; capsulorrhaphy**
EXCLUDES  *Open surgery (23450-23466)*
*Thermal capsulorrhaphy (29999)*
🛏 30.5   ✂ 30.5   **FUD** 090                    J A2 50 ▣
**AMA:** 2017,Jan,8; 2016,Jan,13; 2015,Jul,10; 2015,Mar,7;
2015,Jan,16; 2013,May,12

**29807    repair of SLAP lesion**
🛏 29.8   ✂ 29.8   **FUD** 090                    J A2 50 ▣
**AMA:** 2017,Jan,8; 2016,Jan,13; 2015,Mar,7; 2015,Jan,16;
2013,May,12

**29819    with removal of loose body or foreign body**
EXCLUDES  *Open surgery (23040-23044, 23107)*
🛏 16.8   ✂ 16.8   **FUD** 090                    J A2 50 ▣
**AMA:** 2017,Jan,8; 2016,Jan,13; 2015,Mar,7; 2015,Jan,16;
2013,May,12

**29820    synovectomy, partial**
EXCLUDES  *Open surgery (23105)*
🛏 15.3   ✂ 15.3   **FUD** 090                    J A2 80 50 ▣
**AMA:** 2017,Jan,8; 2016,Jan,13; 2015,Mar,7; 2015,Jan,16;
2013,Jun,13; 2013,May,12

**29821    synovectomy, complete**
EXCLUDES  *Open surgery (23105)*
🛏 16.7   ✂ 16.7   **FUD** 090                    J A2 80 50 ▣
**AMA:** 2017,Jan,8; 2016,Jan,13; 2015,Mar,7; 2015,Jan,16;
2013,Jun,13; 2013,May,12

**29822    debridement, limited**
EXCLUDES  *Open surgery (see specific shoulder section)*
🛏 16.2   ✂ 16.2   **FUD** 090                    J A2 80 50 ▣
**AMA:** 2017,Jan,8; 2016,Jan,13; 2015,Mar,7; 2015,Jan,16;
2014,Jan,11; 2013,May,12; 2012,Oct,14; 2012,Sep,16;
2012,Apr,17-18

**29823    debridement, extensive**
EXCLUDES  *Open surgery (see specific shoulder section)*
🛏 17.7   ✂ 17.7   **FUD** 090                    J A2 80 50 ▣
**AMA:** 2017,Jan,8; 2016,Dec,16; 2016,Jan,13; 2015,Mar,7;
2015,Jan,16; 2014,Jan,11; 2013,May,12; 2012,Oct,14; 2012,Sep,16;
2012,Apr,17-18

**29824    distal claviculectomy including distal articular surface (Mumford procedure)**
INCLUDES  Mumford procedure
EXCLUDES  *Open surgery (23120)*
🛏 19.1   ✂ 19.1   **FUD** 090                    J A2 80 50 ▣
**AMA:** 2017,Jan,8; 2016,Jan,13; 2015,Mar,7; 2015,Jan,16;
2013,May,12

**29825    with lysis and resection of adhesions, with or without manipulation**
EXCLUDES  *Open surgery (see specific shoulder section)*
🛏 16.5   ✂ 16.5   **FUD** 090                    J A2 80 50 ▣
**AMA:** 2017,Jan,8; 2016,Jan,13; 2015,Mar,7; 2015,Jan,16;
2013,May,12

+ **29826    decompression of subacromial space with partial acromioplasty, with coracoacromial ligament (ie, arch) release, when performed (List separately in addition to code for primary procedure)**
EXCLUDES  *Open surgery (23130, 23415)*
Code first (29806-29825, 29827-29828)
🛏 5.10   ✂ 5.10   **FUD** ZZZ                    N N1 80 50 ▣
**AMA:** 2017,Jan,8; 2016,Jan,13; 2015,Mar,7; 2015,Jan,16;
2014,Jan,11; 2013,May,12; 2012,Oct,14; 2012,Sep,16

**29827** with rotator cuff repair

*EXCLUDES* *Distal clavicle excision (29824)*
*Open surgery or mini open repair (23412)*
*Subacromial decompression (29826)*

30.3   30.3   **FUD** 090   J A2 80 50 ▣

**AMA:** 2017,Jan,8; 2016,Jul,8; 2016,Jan,13; 2015,Mar,7; 2015,Jan,16; 2014,Jan,11; 2013,May,12; 2012,Jan,15-42

**29828** biceps tenodesis

*EXCLUDES* *Arthroscopy, shoulder, diagnostic, with or without synovial biopsy (29805)*
*Arthroscopy, shoulder, surgical; debridement, limited (29822)*
*Arthroscopy, shoulder, surgical; synovectomy, partial (29820)*
*Tenodesis of long tendon of biceps (23430)*

26.2   26.2   **FUD** 090   J G2 80 50 ▣

**AMA:** 2017,Jan,8; 2016,Jul,8; 2016,Jan,13; 2015,Mar,7; 2015,Jan,16; 2014,Jan,11; 2013,May,12; 2012,Jan,15-42

**29830** Arthroscopy, elbow, diagnostic, with or without synovial biopsy (separate procedure)

13.1   13.1   **FUD** 090   J A2 50 ▣

**AMA:** 2017,Jan,8; 2016,Jan,13; 2015,Jan,16; 2013,May,12

**29834** Arthroscopy, elbow, surgical; with removal of loose body or foreign body

13.9   13.9   **FUD** 090   J A2 80 50 ▣

**AMA:** 2017,Jan,8; 2016,Jan,13; 2015,Jan,16; 2013,May,12

**29835** synovectomy, partial

14.3   14.3   **FUD** 090   J A2 80 50 ▣

**AMA:** 2017,Jan,8; 2016,Jan,13; 2015,Jan,16; 2013,May,12

**29836** synovectomy, complete

16.4   16.4   **FUD** 090   J A2 80 50 ▣

**AMA:** 2017,Jan,8; 2016,Jan,13; 2015,Jan,16; 2013,May,12

**29837** debridement, limited

15.0   15.0   **FUD** 090   J A2 80 50 ▣

**AMA:** 2017,Jan,8; 2016,Jan,13; 2015,Jan,16; 2013,May,12

**29838** debridement, extensive

16.8   16.8   **FUD** 090   J A2 80 50 ▣

**AMA:** 2017,Jan,8; 2016,Jan,13; 2015,Jan,16; 2013,May,12

**29840** Arthroscopy, wrist, diagnostic, with or without synovial biopsy (separate procedure)

12.9   12.9   **FUD** 090   J A2 80 50 ▣

**AMA:** 2017,Jan,8; 2016,Jan,13; 2015,Jan,16; 2013,May,12

**29843** Arthroscopy, wrist, surgical; for infection, lavage and drainage

13.9   13.9   **FUD** 090   J A2 80 50 ▣

**AMA:** 2017,Jan,8; 2016,Jan,13; 2015,Jan,16; 2013,May,12

**29844** synovectomy, partial

14.2   14.2   **FUD** 090   J A2 80 50 ▣

**AMA:** 2017,Jan,8; 2016,Jan,13; 2015,Jan,16; 2013,May,12

**29845** synovectomy, complete

16.5   16.5   **FUD** 090   J A2 80 50 ▣

**AMA:** 2017,Jan,8; 2016,Jan,13; 2015,Jan,16; 2014,Jan,11; 2013,May,12; 2012,Jan,15-42

**29846** excision and/or repair of triangular fibrocartilage and/or joint debridement

14.9   14.9   **FUD** 090   J A2 80 50 ▣

**AMA:** 2017,Jan,8; 2016,Jan,13; 2015,Jan,16; 2014,Jan,11; 2013,May,12; 2012,Jan,15-42

**29847** internal fixation for fracture or instability

15.5   15.5   **FUD** 090   J A2 80 50 ▣

**AMA:** 2017,Jan,8; 2016,Jan,13; 2015,Jan,16; 2013,May,12

**29848** Endoscopy, wrist, surgical, with release of transverse carpal ligament

*EXCLUDES* *Open surgery (64721)*

14.6   14.6   **FUD** 090   J A2 50 ▣

**AMA:** 2017,Jan,6; 2017,Jan,8; 2016,Jan,13; 2015,Jul,10; 2015,Jan,16; 2014,Jan,11; 2013,May,12

**29850** Arthroscopically aided treatment of intercondylar spine(s) and/or tuberosity fracture(s) of the knee, with or without manipulation; without internal or external fixation (includes arthroscopy)

17.4   17.4   **FUD** 090   J A2 80 50 ▣

**AMA:** 2017,Jan,8; 2016,Jan,13; 2015,Jan,16; 2013,May,12

**29851** with internal or external fixation (includes arthroscopy)

*EXCLUDES* *Bone graft (20900, 20902)*

25.9   25.9   **FUD** 090   J A2 80 50 ▣

**AMA:** 2017,Jan,8; 2016,Jan,13; 2015,Jan,16; 2013,May,12

**29855** Arthroscopically aided treatment of tibial fracture, proximal (plateau); unicondylar, includes internal fixation, when performed (includes arthroscopy)

*EXCLUDES* *Bone graft (20900, 20902)*

22.5   22.5   **FUD** 090   J J8 80 50 ▣

**AMA:** 2017,Jan,8; 2016,Jan,13; 2015,Jan,16; 2013,May,12

**29856** bicondylar, includes internal fixation, when performed (includes arthroscopy)

*EXCLUDES* *Bone graft (20900, 20902)*

28.5   28.5   **FUD** 090   J J8 80 50 ▣

**AMA:** 2017,Jan,8; 2016,Jan,13; 2015,Jan,16; 2013,May,12

**29860** Arthroscopy, hip, diagnostic with or without synovial biopsy (separate procedure)

18.9   18.9   **FUD** 090   J A2 80 50 ▣

**AMA:** 2017,Jan,8; 2016,Jan,13; 2015,Jan,16; 2014,Jan,11; 2013,May,12

**29861** Arthroscopy, hip, surgical; with removal of loose body or foreign body

20.7   20.7   **FUD** 090   J A2 80 50 ▣

**AMA:** 2017,Jan,8; 2016,Jan,13; 2015,Jan,16; 2014,Jan,11; 2013,May,12

**29862** with debridement/shaving of articular cartilage (chondroplasty), abrasion arthroplasty, and/or resection of labrum

23.1   23.1   **FUD** 090   J A2 80 50 ▣

**AMA:** 2017,Jan,8; 2016,Jan,13; 2015,Jan,16; 2014,Jan,11; 2013,May,12

**29863** with synovectomy

23.1   23.1   **FUD** 090   J A2 80 50 ▣

**AMA:** 2017,Jan,8; 2016,Jan,13; 2015,Jan,16; 2014,Jan,11; 2013,May,12

\# **29914** with femoroplasty (ie, treatment of cam lesion)

28.5   28.5   **FUD** 090   J G2 80 50 ▣

**AMA:** 2017,Jan,8; 2016,Jan,13; 2015,Jan,16; 2014,Jan,11; 2012,Jan,15-42

\# **29915** with acetabuloplasty (ie, treatment of pincer lesion)

29.1   29.1   **FUD** 090   J G2 80 50 ▣

**AMA:** 2017,Jan,8; 2016,Jan,13; 2015,Jan,16; 2014,Jan,11; 2012,Jan,15-42

\# **29916** with labral repair

29.1   29.1   **FUD** 090   J G2 80 50 ▣

**AMA:** 2017,Jan,8; 2016,Jan,13; 2015,Jan,16; 2014,Jan,11; 2012,Jan,15-42

● New Code   ▲ Revised Code   ○ Reinstated   ● New Web Release   ▲ Revised Web Release   Unlisted   Not Covered   # Resequenced
⊘ AMA Mod 51 Exempt   ⑪ Optum Mod 51 Exempt   ⑬ Mod 63 Exempt   ✗ Non-FDA Drug   ★ Telemedicine   Ⓜ Maternity   Ⓐ Age Edit   + Add-on   **AMA:** CPT Asst
© 2017 Optum360, LLC   CPT © 2017 American Medical Association. All Rights Reserved.   **101**

**29866** **Arthroscopy, knee, surgical; osteochondral autograft(s) (eg, mosaicplasty) (includes harvesting of the autograft[s])**

EXCLUDES *Open osteochondral autograft of the knee (27416)*

*Procedures performed at the same surgical session (29870-29871, 29875, 29884)*

*Procedures performed in the same compartment (29874, 29877, 29879, 29885-29887)*

🚑 29.8    ✂ 29.8    **FUD** 090    [J] [02] [80] [50] [▭]

**AMA:** 2017,Jan,8; 2016,Jan,13; 2015,Jan,16; 2013,May,12

Cylindrical plugs of healthy bone are harvested, usually from a non-weight bearing area of the femur

The technique employs arthroscopy

Recipient holes are drilled and the grafts tamped into position

**29867** **osteochondral allograft (eg, mosaicplasty)**

EXCLUDES *Procedures performed at the same surgical session (27415, 27570, 29870-29871, 29875, 29884)*

*Procedures performed in the same compartment (29874, 29877, 29879, 29885-29887)*

🚑 36.9    ✂ 36.9    **FUD** 090    [J] [80] [50] [▭]

**AMA:** 2017,Jan,8; 2016,Jan,13; 2015,Jan,16; 2014,Jan,11; 2013,May,12; 2012,Jan,15-42

**29868** **meniscal transplantation (includes arthrotomy for meniscal insertion), medial or lateral**

EXCLUDES *Procedures performed at same surgical session (29870-29871, 29875, 29880, 29883-29884)*

*Procedures performed in same compartment (29874, 29877, 29881-29882)*

🚑 47.5    ✂ 47.5    **FUD** 090    [J] [80] [50] [▭]

**AMA:** 2017,Jan,8; 2016,Jan,13; 2015,Jan,16; 2013,May,12

**29870** **Arthroscopy, knee, diagnostic, with or without synovial biopsy (separate procedure)**

EXCLUDES *Open procedure (27412)*

🚑 11.8    ✂ 16.6    **FUD** 090    [J] [A2] [50] [▭]

**AMA:** 2017,Jan,8; 2016,Jan,13; 2015,Jan,16; 2014,Jan,11; 2013,May,12; 2012,Jan,15-42

**29871** **Arthroscopy, knee, surgical; for infection, lavage and drainage**

EXCLUDES *Injection of contrast for knee arthrography (27370)*

*Osteochondral graft (27412, 27415, 29866-29867)*

🚑 14.8    ✂ 14.8    **FUD** 090    [J] [A2] [50] [▭]

**AMA:** 2017,Jan,8; 2016,Jan,13; 2015,Aug,6; 2015,Jan,16; 2014,Jan,11; 2013,May,12

**29873** **with lateral release**

EXCLUDES *Open procedure (27425)*

🚑 15.0    ✂ 15.0    **FUD** 090    [J] [A2] [50] [▭]

**AMA:** 2017,Jan,8; 2016,Jan,13; 2015,Nov,7; 2015,Jan,16; 2014,Jan,11; 2013,May,12; 2012,Jan,15-42

**29874** **for removal of loose body or foreign body (eg, osteochondritis dissecans fragmentation, chondral fragmentation)**

🚑 15.4    ✂ 15.4    **FUD** 090    [J] [A2] [80] [50] [▭]

**AMA:** 2017,Jan,8; 2016,Jan,13; 2015,Jan,16; 2014,Jan,11; 2013,May,12

**29875** **synovectomy, limited (eg, plica or shelf resection) (separate procedure)**

🚑 14.2    ✂ 14.2    **FUD** 090    [J] [A2] [80] [50] [▭]

**AMA:** 2017,Jan,8; 2016,Jan,13; 2016,Jan,11; 2015,Jan,16; 2014,May,10; 2014,Jan,11; 2013,May,12

**29876** **synovectomy, major, 2 or more compartments (eg, medial or lateral)**

🚑 18.9    ✂ 18.9    **FUD** 090    [J] [A2] [50] [▭]

**AMA:** 2017,Jan,8; 2016,Jan,13; 2015,Jan,16; 2014,Jan,11; 2013,May,12

**29877** **debridement/shaving of articular cartilage (chondroplasty)**

EXCLUDES *Arthroscopy, knee, surgical; with meniscectomy (29880-29881)*

🚑 17.8    ✂ 17.8    **FUD** 090    [J] [A2] [80] [50] [▭]

**AMA:** 2017,Jan,8; 2016,Jan,13; 2015,Jan,16; 2014,Jan,11; 2013,May,12; 2012,Jan,15-42

**29879** **abrasion arthroplasty (includes chondroplasty where necessary) or multiple drilling or microfracture**

🚑 19.0    ✂ 19.0    **FUD** 090    [J] [A2] [80] [50] [▭]

**AMA:** 2017,Jan,8; 2016,Jan,13; 2015,Jan,16; 2014,Jan,11; 2013,May,12

**29880** **with meniscectomy (medial AND lateral, including any meniscal shaving) including debridement/shaving of articular cartilage (chondroplasty), same or separate compartment(s), when performed**

🚑 16.1    ✂ 16.1    **FUD** 090    [J] [A2] [80] [50] [▭]

**AMA:** 2017,Jan,8; 2016,Jan,13; 2015,Jan,16; 2014,Jan,11; 2013,May,12; 2012,Jan,3-5

**29881** **with meniscectomy (medial OR lateral, including any meniscal shaving) including debridement/shaving of articular cartilage (chondroplasty), same or separate compartment(s), when performed**

🚑 15.5    ✂ 15.5    **FUD** 090    [J] [A2] [80] [50] [▭]

**AMA:** 2017,Jan,8; 2016,Jan,13; 2016,Jan,11; 2015,Jan,16; 2014,May,10; 2014,Jan,11; 2013,May,12; 2012,Jan,3-5; 2012,Jan,15-42

**29882** **with meniscus repair (medial OR lateral)**

EXCLUDES *Meniscus transplant (29868)*

🚑 20.1    ✂ 20.1    **FUD** 090    [J] [A2] [50] [▭]

**AMA:** 2017,Jan,8; 2016,Jan,13; 2015,Jan,16; 2014,Jan,11; 2013,May,12; 2012,Jan,15-42

**29883** **with meniscus repair (medial AND lateral)**

EXCLUDES *Meniscus transplant (29868)*

🚑 24.3    ✂ 24.3    **FUD** 090    [J] [A2] [80] [50] [▭]

**AMA:** 2017,Jan,8; 2016,Jan,13; 2015,Jan,16; 2014,Jan,11; 2013,May,12; 2012,Jan,15-42

**29884** **with lysis of adhesions, with or without manipulation (separate procedure)**

🚑 17.6    ✂ 17.6    **FUD** 090    [J] [A2] [80] [50] [▭]

**AMA:** 2017,Jan,8; 2016,Jan,13; 2015,Jan,16; 2014,Jan,11; 2013,May,12; 2012,Jan,15-42

**29885** **drilling for osteochondritis dissecans with bone grafting, with or without internal fixation (including debridement of base of lesion)**

🚑 21.5    ✂ 21.5    **FUD** 090    [J] [A2] [80] [50] [▭]

**AMA:** 2017,Jan,8; 2016,Jan,13; 2015,Jan,16; 2014,Jan,11; 2013,May,12

**29886** **drilling for intact osteochondritis dissecans lesion**

🚑 18.2    ✂ 18.2    **FUD** 090    [J] [A2] [50] [▭]

**AMA:** 2017,Jan,8; 2016,Jan,13; 2015,Jan,16; 2014,Jan,11; 2013,May,12

26/TC PC/TC Only     A2-Z3 ASC Payment     50 Bilateral     ♂ Male Only     ♀ Female Only     🚑 Facility RVU     ✂ Non-Facility RVU     [▭] CCI
FUD Follow-up Days     CMS: IOM (Pub 100)     A-Y OPPSI     80/80 Surg Assist Allowed / w/Doc     🔲 Lab Crosswalk     🔲 Radiology Crosswalk     ❌ CLIA
CPT © 2017 American Medical Association. All Rights Reserved.

© 2017 Optum360, LLC

**29887** drilling for intact osteochondritis dissecans lesion with internal fixation
     21.2   21.2   **FUD** 090     J A2 80 50
     **AMA:** 2017,Jan,8; 2016,Jan,13; 2015,Jan,16; 2014,Jan,11; 2013,May,12

**29888** Arthroscopically aided anterior cruciate ligament repair/augmentation or reconstruction
     **EXCLUDES** Ligamentous reconstruction (augmentation), knee (27427-27429)
     28.3   28.3   **FUD** 090     J A2 80 50
     **AMA:** 2017,Jan,8; 2016,Nov,9; 2016,Jan,13; 2015,Jan,16; 2014,Jan,11; 2013,May,12; 2012,Jan,15-42

**29889** Arthroscopically aided posterior cruciate ligament repair/augmentation or reconstruction
     **EXCLUDES** Ligamentous reconstruction (augmentation), knee (27427-27429)
     35.2   35.2   **FUD** 090     J A2 80 50
     **AMA:** 2017,Jan,8; 2016,Jan,13; 2015,Jan,16; 2014,Jan,11; 2013,May,12; 2012,Jan,15-42

**29891** Arthroscopy, ankle, surgical, excision of osteochondral defect of talus and/or tibia, including drilling of the defect
     19.3   19.3   **FUD** 090     J A2 80 50
     **AMA:** 2017,Jan,8; 2016,Jan,13; 2015,Jan,16; 2013,May,12

**29892** Arthroscopically aided repair of large osteochondritis dissecans lesion, talar dome fracture, or tibial plafond fracture, with or without internal fixation (includes arthroscopy)
     18.6   18.6   **FUD** 090     J A2 80 50
     **AMA:** 2017,Jan,8; 2016,Jan,13; 2015,Jan,16; 2014,Jan,11; 2013,May,12

**29893** Endoscopic plantar fasciotomy
     12.2   17.6   **FUD** 090     J A2 50
     **AMA:** 2017,Jan,8; 2016,Jan,13; 2015,Jan,16; 2013,May,12

**29894** Arthroscopy, ankle (tibiotalar and fibulotalar joints), surgical; with removal of loose body or foreign body
     14.2   14.2   **FUD** 090     J A2 80 50
     **AMA:** 2017,Jan,8; 2016,Jan,13; 2015,Jan,16; 2013,May,12

**29895** synovectomy, partial
     13.7   13.7   **FUD** 090     J A2 80 50
     **AMA:** 2017,Jan,8; 2016,Jan,13; 2015,Jan,16; 2014,Jan,11; 2013,May,12; 2012,Jan,15-42

**29897** debridement, limited
     14.4   14.4   **FUD** 090     J A2 80 50
     **AMA:** 2017,Jan,8; 2016,Jan,13; 2015,Jan,16; 2013,May,12

**29898** debridement, extensive
     16.2   16.2   **FUD** 090     J A2 80 50
     **AMA:** 2017,Jan,8; 2016,Jan,13; 2015,Jan,16; 2013,May,12

**29899** with ankle arthrodesis
     **EXCLUDES** Open procedure (27870)
     29.9   29.9   **FUD** 090     J G2 80 50
     **AMA:** 2017,Jan,8; 2016,Jan,13; 2015,Jan,16; 2013,May,12

**29900** Arthroscopy, metacarpophalangeal joint, diagnostic, includes synovial biopsy
     **EXCLUDES** Arthroscopy, metacarpophalangeal joint, surgical (29901-29902)
     12.0   12.0   **FUD** 090     J A2 80 50
     **AMA:** 2017,Jan,8; 2016,Jan,13; 2015,Jan,16; 2013,May,12

**29901** Arthroscopy, metacarpophalangeal joint, surgical; with debridement
     15.1   15.1   **FUD** 090     J A2 80 50
     **AMA:** 2017,Jan,8; 2016,Jan,13; 2015,Jan,16; 2013,May,12

**29902** with reduction of displaced ulnar collateral ligament (eg, Stenar lesion)
     13.9   13.9   **FUD** 090     J A2 80 50
     **AMA:** 2017,Jan,8; 2016,Jan,13; 2015,Jan,16; 2013,May,12

**29904** Arthroscopy, subtalar joint, surgical; with removal of loose body or foreign body
     18.0   18.0   **FUD** 090     J G2 80 50
     **AMA:** 2017,Jan,8; 2016,Jan,13; 2015,Jan,16; 2013,May,12

**29905** with synovectomy
     19.5   19.5   **FUD** 090     J G2 80 50
     **AMA:** 2017,Jan,8; 2016,Jan,13; 2015,Jan,16; 2013,May,12

**29906** with debridement
     19.9   19.9   **FUD** 090     J G2 80 50
     **AMA:** 2017,Jan,8; 2016,Jan,13; 2015,Jan,16; 2013,May,12

**29907** with subtalar arthrodesis
     25.2   25.2   **FUD** 090     J G2 80 50
     **AMA:** 2017,Jan,8; 2016,Jan,13; 2015,Jan,16; 2013,May,12

*29914* Resequenced code. See code following 29863.

*29915* Resequenced code. See code following 29863.

*29916* Resequenced code. See code before 29866.

**29999** Unlisted procedure, arthroscopy
     0.00   0.00   **FUD** YYY     T 80 50
     **AMA:** 2017,Apr,9; 2017,Jan,8; 2016,Dec,16; 2016,Jan,13; 2015,Dec,16; 2015,Jan,16; 2014,Jan,11; 2013,May,12; 2012,Apr,17-18; 2012,Jan,15-42

● New Code   ▲ Revised Code   ○ Reinstated   ● New Web Release   ▲ Revised Web Release   Unlisted   Not Covered   # Resequenced
  AMA Mod 51 Exempt   Optum Mod 51 Exempt   Mod 63 Exempt   Non-FDA Drug   ★ Telemedicine   M Maternity   A Age Edit   + Add-on   **AMA:** CPT Asst

© 2017 Optum360, LLC    CPT © 2017 American Medical Association. All Rights Reserved.

## 30000-30115 I&D, Biopsy, Excision Procedures of the Nose

**30000** Drainage abscess or hematoma, nasal, internal approach

> *EXCLUDES* Incision and drainage (10060, 10140)

🚑 3.35  ⚕ 6.48  **FUD** 010        Ⓣ P2 80 🗔

**AMA:** 2005,May,13-14; 1994,Spr,24

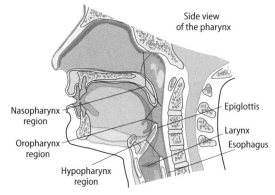

Side view
of the pharynx

Nasopharynx region
Oropharynx region
Hypopharynx region
Epiglottis
Larynx
Esophagus

The nasopharynx is the membranous passage above the level of the soft palate; the oropharynx is the region between the soft palate and the upper edge of the epiglottis; the hypopharynx is the region of the epiglottis to the juncture of the larynx and esophagus; the three regions are collectively known as the pharynx

**30020** Drainage abscess or hematoma, nasal septum

🚑 3.38  ⚕ 6.57  **FUD** 010        Ⓣ P3 🗔

> *EXCLUDES* Lateral rhinotomy incision (30118, 30320)

**30100** Biopsy, intranasal

🚑 1.96  ⚕ 3.98  **FUD** 000        Ⓣ P3 🗔

> *EXCLUDES* Superficial biopsy of nose (11100-11101)

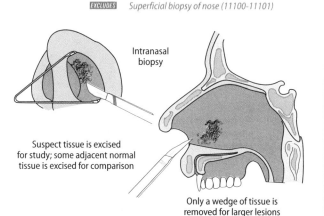

Intranasal biopsy

Suspect tissue is excised for study; some adjacent normal tissue is excised for comparison

Only a wedge of tissue is removed for larger lesions

**30110** Excision, nasal polyp(s), simple

🚑 3.70  ⚕ 6.51  **FUD** 010        Ⓣ P3 50 🗔

**30115** Excision, nasal polyp(s), extensive

🚑 12.2  ⚕ 12.2  **FUD** 090        Ⓙ A2 50 🗔

## 30117-30118 Destruction Procedures Nose

**CMS:** 100-03,140.5 Laser Procedures

**30117** Excision or destruction (eg, laser), intranasal lesion; internal approach

🚑 9.65  ⚕ 24.7  **FUD** 090        Ⓙ A2 🗔

**AMA:** 1990,Win,4

**30118** external approach (lateral rhinotomy)

🚑 21.8  ⚕ 21.8  **FUD** 090        Ⓙ A2 🗔

## 30120-30140 Excision Procedures Nose, Turbinate

**30120** Excision or surgical planing of skin of nose for rhinophyma

🚑 12.5  ⚕ 14.8  **FUD** 090        Ⓙ A2 🗔

**AMA:** 2017,Jan,8; 2016,Jan,13; 2015,Jan,16; 2014,Jan,11; 2012,Jan,15-42

**30124** Excision dermoid cyst, nose; simple, skin, subcutaneous

🚑 8.10  ⚕ 8.10  **FUD** 090        Ⓣ 82 🗔

**30125** complex, under bone or cartilage

🚑 17.1  ⚕ 17.1  **FUD** 090        Ⓙ A2 80 🗔

**30130** Excision inferior turbinate, partial or complete, any method

> *EXCLUDES* Ablation, soft tissue of inferior turbinates, unilateral or bilateral, any method (30801-30802)
> Excision middle/superior turbinate(s) (30999)
> Fracture nasal inferior turbinate(s), therapeutic (30930)

🚑 10.7  ⚕ 10.7  **FUD** 090        Ⓙ A2 50 🗔

**AMA:** 2017,Jan,8; 2016,Jan,13; 2015,Jan,16; 2014,Jan,11; 2012,Jan,15-42

**30140** Submucous resection inferior turbinate, partial or complete, any method

> *EXCLUDES* Ablation, soft tissue of inferior turbinates, unilateral or bilateral, any method (30801-30802)
> Endoscopic resection of concha bullosa of middle turbinate (31240)
> Fracture nasal inferior turbinate(s), therapeutic (30930)
> Submucous resection:
>   Nasal septum (30520)
>   Superior or middle turbinate (30999)

🚑 12.4  ⚕ 12.4  **FUD** 090        Ⓙ A2 50 🗔

**AMA:** 2017,Jan,8; 2016,Jan,13; 2015,Jan,16; 2014,Jan,11; 2012,Jan,15-42

## 30150-30160 Surgical Removal: Nose

> *EXCLUDES* Reconstruction and/or closure (primary or delayed primary intention) (13151-13160, 14060-14302, 15120-15121, 15260-15261, 15760, 20900-20912)

**30150** Rhinectomy; partial

🚑 21.8  ⚕ 21.8  **FUD** 090        Ⓙ A2 🗔

**30160** total

🚑 21.9  ⚕ 21.9  **FUD** 090        Ⓙ A2 80 🗔

## 30200-30320 Turbinate Injection, Removal Foreign Substance in the Nose

**30200** Injection into turbinate(s), therapeutic

🚑 1.69  ⚕ 3.19  **FUD** 000        Ⓣ P3 🗔

**AMA:** 2017,Jan,8; 2016,Jan,13; 2015,Jan,16; 2014,Jan,11; 2012,Jan,15-42

**30210** Displacement therapy (Proetz type)

🚑 2.83  ⚕ 4.23  **FUD** 010        Ⓣ P3 🗔

**AMA:** 2017,Jan,8; 2016,Jan,13; 2015,Jan,16; 2014,Jan,11; 2012,Jan,15-42

**30220** Insertion, nasal septal prosthesis (button)

🚑 3.55  ⚕ 8.55  **FUD** 010        Ⓣ A2 🗔

**30300** Removal foreign body, intranasal; office type procedure

🚑 3.01  ⚕ 5.04  **FUD** 010        Ⓞⓘ N1 🗔

**AMA:** 2017,Jan,8; 2016,Jan,13; 2015,Jan,16; 2014,Jan,11; 2012,Jan,13-14

**30310** requiring general anesthesia

🚑 5.85  ⚕ 5.85  **FUD** 010        Ⓙ A2 80 🗔

**30320** by lateral rhinotomy

🚑 12.8  ⚕ 12.8  **FUD** 090        Ⓣ A2 80 🗔

● New Code  ▲ Revised Code  ○ Reinstated  ● New Web Release  ▲ Revised Web Release  Unlisted  Not Covered  # Resequenced
Ⓢ AMA Mod 51 Exempt  Ⓢ Optum Mod 51 Exempt  Ⓢ Mod 63 Exempt  ✎ Non-FDA Drug  ★ Telemedicine  Ⓜ Maternity  Ⓐ Age Edit  ✚ Add-on  **AMA:** CPT Asst

© 2017 Optum360, LLC        CPT © 2017 American Medical Association. All Rights Reserved.        **105**

**Respiratory System**

## 30400-30630 Reconstruction or Repair of Nose

EXCLUDES　*Bone/tissue grafts (20900-20926, 21210)*

**30400** **Rhinoplasty, primary; lateral and alar cartilages and/or elevation of nasal tip**
　　🖩 28.6　　⚖ 28.6　　**FUD** 090　　　　　J A2 80 ▢

　　　INCLUDES　Carpue's operation
　　　EXCLUDES　*Reconstruction of columella (13151-13153)*

**30410** **complete, external parts including bony pyramid, lateral and alar cartilages, and/or elevation of nasal tip**
　　🖩 33.3　　⚖ 33.3　　**FUD** 090　　　　　J A2 80 ▢

**30420** **including major septal repair**
　　🖩 38.8　　⚖ 38.8　　**FUD** 090　　　　　J A2 ▢
　　**AMA:** 2017,Jan,8; 2016,Jul,8

**30430** **Rhinoplasty, secondary; minor revision (small amount of nasal tip work)**
　　🖩 24.2　　⚖ 24.2　　**FUD** 090　　　　　J A2 80 ▢

**30435** **intermediate revision (bony work with osteotomies)**
　　🖩 35.6　　⚖ 35.6　　**FUD** 090　　　　　J A2 80 ▢

**30450** **major revision (nasal tip work and osteotomies)**
　　🖩 42.3　　⚖ 42.3　　**FUD** 090　　　　　J A2 80 ▢

**30460** **Rhinoplasty for nasal deformity secondary to congenital cleft lip and/or palate, including columellar lengthening; tip only**
　　🖩 23.1　　⚖ 23.1　　**FUD** 090　　　　　J A2 80 ▢
　　**AMA:** 2017,Jan,8; 2016,Jan,13; 2015,Jan,16; 2014,Dec,18

Cleft lip and cleft palate are described according to length of cleft and whether bilateral or unilateral

Complete unilateral cleft lip

Hard palate
Soft palate

Isolated unilateral complete cleft of palate

Nasal cavity
Nasal septum

Bilateral complete cleft of lip and palate

**30462** **tip, septum, osteotomies**
　　🖩 40.0　　⚖ 40.0　　**FUD** 090　　　　　J A2 80 ▢
　　**AMA:** 2017,Jan,8; 2016,Jan,13; 2015,Jan,16; 2014,Dec,18

**30465** **Repair of nasal vestibular stenosis (eg, spreader grafting, lateral nasal wall reconstruction)**
　　🖩 27.8　　⚖ 27.8　　**FUD** 090　　　　　J A2 80 ▢
　　　INCLUDES　Bilateral procedure
　　　Code also modifier 52 for unilateral procedure

**30520** **Septoplasty or submucous resection, with or without cartilage scoring, contouring or replacement with graft**
　　　EXCLUDES　*Turbinate resection (30140)*
　　🖩 17.6　　⚖ 17.6　　**FUD** 090　　　　　J A2 ▢
　　**AMA:** 2017,Jan,8; 2016,Jan,13; 2015,Jul,10; 2015,Jan,16; 2014,Jan,11; 2012,Jan,15-42

**30540** **Repair choanal atresia; intranasal**
　　🖩 19.6　　⚖ 19.6　　**FUD** 090　　　　63 J A2 80 ▢

**30545** **transpalatine**
　　🖩 25.1　　⚖ 25.1　　**FUD** 090　　　　63 J A2 80 ▢

**30560** **Lysis intranasal synechia**
　　🖩 3.89　　⚖ 7.57　　**FUD** 010　　　　　T A2 ▢

**30580** **Repair fistula; oromaxillary (combine with 31030 if antrotomy is included)**
　　🖩 14.6　　⚖ 18.6　　**FUD** 090　　　　　J A2 ▢

**30600** **oronasal**
　　🖩 12.1　　⚖ 16.1　　**FUD** 090　　　　　J A2 80 ▢

**30620** **Septal or other intranasal dermatoplasty (does not include obtaining graft)**
　　🖩 17.7　　⚖ 17.7　　**FUD** 090　　　　　J A2 ▢

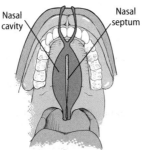

Retraction suture

Access incision for lateral rhinotomy

Diseased septal mucosa is excised and graft is placed

**30630** **Repair nasal septal perforations**
　　🖩 17.6　　⚖ 17.6　　**FUD** 090　　　　　J A2 80 ▢
　　**AMA:** 2017,Jan,8; 2016,Jan,13; 2015,Jan,16; 2014,Jan,11; 2012,Aug,13-14

## 30801-30802 Turbinate Destruction

EXCLUDES　*Ablation middle/superior turbinates (30999)*
　*Cautery to stop nasal bleeding (30901-30906)*
　*Excision inferior turbinate, partial or complete, any method (30130)*
　*Submucous resection inferior turbinate, partial or complete, any method (30140)*

**30801** **Ablation, soft tissue of inferior turbinates, unilateral or bilateral, any method (eg, electrocautery, radiofrequency ablation, or tissue volume reduction); superficial**
　　　EXCLUDES　*Submucosal ablation inferior turbinates (30802)*
　　🖩 3.87　　⚖ 6.47　　**FUD** 010　　　　　T A2 ▢
　　**AMA:** 2002,May,7; 1991,Win,1

**30802** **intramural (ie, submucosal)**
　　　EXCLUDES　*Superficial ablation inferior turbinates (30801)*
　　🖩 5.39　　⚖ 8.21　　**FUD** 010　　　　　T A2 ▢
　　**AMA:** 2017,Jan,8; 2016,Jan,13; 2015,Jan,16; 2014,Jan,11; 2012,Jan,15-42

## 30901-30920 Control Nose Bleed

**30901** **Control nasal hemorrhage, anterior, simple (limited cautery and/or packing) any method**
　　🖩 1.63　　⚖ 2.70　　**FUD** 000　　　　01 N1 50 ▢
　　**AMA:** 1990,Win,4

**30903** **Control nasal hemorrhage, anterior, complex (extensive cautery and/or packing) any method**
　　🖩 2.31　　⚖ 6.26　　**FUD** 000　　　　　T A2 50 ▢
　　**AMA:** 1990,Win,4

**30905** **Control nasal hemorrhage, posterior, with posterior nasal packs and/or cautery, any method; initial**
　　🖩 3.05　　⚖ 7.69　　**FUD** 000　　　　　T A2 ▢
　　**AMA:** 2017,Jan,8; 2016,Jan,13; 2015,Jan,16; 2014,Jan,11

**30906** **subsequent**
🚑 3.93 ⚕ 9.84 **FUD** 000 T A2 ▭
**AMA:** 2002,May,7

**30915** **Ligation arteries; ethmoidal**
🚑 16.3 ⚕ 16.3 **FUD** 090 T A2 ▭
EXCLUDES *External carotid artery (37600)*

**30920** **internal maxillary artery, transantral**
🚑 23.7 ⚕ 23.7 **FUD** 090 T A2 ▭
EXCLUDES *External carotid artery (37600)*

## 30930-30999 Other and Unlisted Procedures of Nose

**30930** **Fracture nasal inferior turbinate(s), therapeutic**
EXCLUDES *Excision inferior turbinate, partial or complete, any method (30130)*
*Fracture of superior or middle turbinate(s) (30999)*
*Submucous resection inferior turbinate, partial or complete, any method (30140)*
🚑 3.49 ⚕ 3.49 **FUD** 010 J A2 50 ▭
**AMA:** 2017,Jan,8; 2016,Jul,8; 2016,Jan,13; 2015,Jan,16; 2014,Jan,11; 2012,Jan,15-42

**30999** **Unlisted procedure, nose**
🚑 0.00 ⚕ 0.00 **FUD** YYY T 80
**AMA:** 2017,Jan,8; 2016,Jan,13; 2015,Jan,16; 2013,Feb,13

## 31000-31230 Opening Sinuses

**31000** **Lavage by cannulation; maxillary sinus (antrum puncture or natural ostium)**
🚑 3.01 ⚕ 5.21 **FUD** 010 T P2 50 ▭
**AMA:** 2017,Jan,8; 2016,Jan,13; 2015,Jan,16; 2014,Apr,10

Frontal sinus
Crista galli
Ethmoidal cells
Orbital cavity
Nostril
Superior, middle, and inferior conchae
Maxillary sinus
Caldwell-Luc approach

Frontal sinus
Posterior ethmoidal cells
Sphenoid sinus
Conchae (nasal cavity)
Hard palate

Schematic showing lateral wall of the nasal cavity (above) and coronal section showing nasal and paranasal sinuses (left)

**31002** **sphenoid sinus**
🚑 5.40 ⚕ 5.40 **FUD** 010 T R2 80 50 ▭

**31020** **Sinusotomy, maxillary (antrotomy); intranasal**
🚑 10.2 ⚕ 13.7 **FUD** 090 J A2 50 ▭

**31030** **radical (Caldwell-Luc) without removal of antrochoanal polyps**
🚑 15.0 ⚕ 19.5 **FUD** 090 J A2 50 ▭

**31032** **radical (Caldwell-Luc) with removal of antrochoanal polyps**
🚑 16.3 ⚕ 16.3 **FUD** 090 J A2 50 ▭

**31040** **Pterygomaxillary fossa surgery, any approach**
🚑 21.6 ⚕ 21.6 **FUD** 090 J R2 50 ▭
EXCLUDES *Transantral ligation internal maxillary artery (30920)*

**31050** **Sinusotomy, sphenoid, with or without biopsy;**
🚑 13.7 ⚕ 13.7 **FUD** 090 J A2 50 ▭

**31051** **with mucosal stripping or removal of polyp(s)**
🚑 18.2 ⚕ 18.2 **FUD** 090 J A2 50 ▭

**31070** **Sinusotomy frontal; external, simple (trephine operation)**
🚑 12.4 ⚕ 12.4 **FUD** 090 J A2 50 ▭
INCLUDES *Killian operation*
EXCLUDES *Intranasal frontal sinusotomy (31276)*

**31075** **transorbital, unilateral (for mucocele or osteoma, Lynch type)**
🚑 22.2 ⚕ 22.2 **FUD** 090 J A2 80 50 ▭

**31080** **obliterative without osteoplastic flap, brow incision (includes ablation)**
🚑 29.6 ⚕ 29.6 **FUD** 090 J A2 80 50 ▭
INCLUDES *Ridell sinusotomy*

**31081** **obliterative, without osteoplastic flap, coronal incision (includes ablation)**
🚑 42.5 ⚕ 42.5 **FUD** 090 J A2 80 50 ▭

**31084** **obliterative, with osteoplastic flap, brow incision**
🚑 33.7 ⚕ 33.7 **FUD** 090 J A2 80 50 ▭

**31085** **obliterative, with osteoplastic flap, coronal incision**
🚑 45.3 ⚕ 45.3 **FUD** 090 J A2 80 50 ▭

**31086** **nonobliterative, with osteoplastic flap, brow incision**
🚑 32.1 ⚕ 32.1 **FUD** 090 J A2 80 50 ▭

**31087** **nonobliterative, with osteoplastic flap, coronal incision**
🚑 30.9 ⚕ 30.9 **FUD** 090 J A2 80 50 ▭

**31090** **Sinusotomy, unilateral, 3 or more paranasal sinuses (frontal, maxillary, ethmoid, sphenoid)**
🚑 29.0 ⚕ 29.0 **FUD** 090 J A2 50 ▭
**AMA:** 1998,Nov,1; 1997,Nov,1

**31200** **Ethmoidectomy; intranasal, anterior**
🚑 16.2 ⚕ 16.2 **FUD** 090 J A2 50 ▭
**AMA:** 2017,Jan,8; 2016,Feb,10

**31201** **intranasal, total**
🚑 20.9 ⚕ 20.9 **FUD** 090 J A2 50 ▭
**AMA:** 2017,Jan,8; 2016,Feb,10

**31205** **extranasal, total**
🚑 25.5 ⚕ 25.5 **FUD** 090 J A2 80 50 ▭
**AMA:** 2017,Jan,8; 2016,Feb,10

**31225** **Maxillectomy; without orbital exenteration**
🚑 53.4 ⚕ 53.4 **FUD** 090 C 80 50 ▭

**31230** **with orbital exenteration (en bloc)**
🚑 58.8 ⚕ 58.8 **FUD** 090 C 80 50 ▭
EXCLUDES *Orbital exenteration without maxillectomy (65110-65114)*
*Skin grafts (15120-15121)*

## 31231-31235 Nasal Endoscopy, Diagnostic

INCLUDES *Complete sinus exam (e.g., nasal cavity, turbinates, sphenoethmoidal recess)*
*Code also stereotactic navigation, if performed (61782)*

**31231** **Nasal endoscopy, diagnostic, unilateral or bilateral (separate procedure)**
🚑 1.86 ⚕ 5.92 **FUD** 000 T P2 ▭
**AMA:** 2017,Jul,7; 2017,Jan,8; 2017,Jan,6; 2016,Dec,13; 2016,Feb,10; 2016,Jan,13; 2015,Jan,16; 2014,Jan,11

**31233** **Nasal/sinus endoscopy, diagnostic with maxillary sinusoscopy (via inferior meatus or canine fossa puncture)**
EXCLUDES *Nasal/sinus endoscopy, surgical; with dilation of maxillary sinus ostium (31295)*
🚑 3.91 ⚕ 7.42 **FUD** 000 T A2 80 50 ▭
**AMA:** 2017,Jan,8; 2016,Jan,13; 2015,Jan,16; 2014,Jan,11

**31235** **Nasal/sinus endoscopy, diagnostic with sphenoid sinusoscopy (via puncture of sphenoidal face or cannulation of ostium)**
EXCLUDES *Nasal/sinus endoscopy, surgical; with dilation of sphenoid sinus ostium (31297)*
🚑 4.62 ⚕ 8.47 **FUD** 000 J A2 80 50 ▭
**AMA:** 2017,Jan,8; 2016,Jan,13; 2015,Jan,16; 2014,Jan,11

---

● New Code ▲ Revised Code ○ Reinstated ● New Web Release ▲ Revised Web Release Unlisted Not Covered # Resequenced
⊘ AMA Mod 51 Exempt ⑤⓪ Optum Mod 51 Exempt ⑥③ Mod 63 Exempt ✗ Non-FDA Drug ★ Telemedicine Ⓜ Maternity Ⓐ Age Edit + Add-on **AMA:** CPT Asst

**Respiratory System**

**31237 — 31259**

## 31237-31253 Nasal Endoscopy, Surgical

| INCLUDES | Diagnostic nasal/sinus endoscopy |
| | Unilateral procedure |
| EXCLUDES | Frontal sinus exploration (31276) |
| | Maxillary antrostomy (31256) |
| | Osteomeatal complex (OMC) resection and/or partial (anterior) |
| | ethmoidectomy (31254) |
| | Removal of maxillary sinus tissue (31267) |
| | Total (anterior and posterior) ethmoidectomy (31255) |

Code also stereotactic navigation, if performed (61782)

**31237     Nasal/sinus endoscopy, surgical; with biopsy, polypectomy or debridement (separate procedure)**

🔧 4.61     ✂ 7.32     **FUD** 000     [J] [A2] [50] [💻]

AMA: 2017,Jan,8; 2016,Feb,10; 2016,Jan,13; 2015,Jan,16; 2015,Jan,13; 2014,Jan,11; 2012,Jan,15-42

**31238     with control of nasal hemorrhage**

EXCLUDES   Nasal/sinus endoscopy, surgical; with ligation of sphenopalatine artery, on the same side (31241)

🔧 4.83     ✂ 7.31     **FUD** 000     [J] [A2] [80] [50] [💻]

AMA: 2017,Jan,8; 2016,Jan,13; 2015,Jan,16; 2014,Jan,11

**31239     with dacryocystorhinostomy**

🔧 17.5     ✂ 17.5     **FUD** 010     [J] [A2] [80] [50] [💻]

AMA: 2017,Jan,8; 2016,Jan,13; 2015,Jan,16; 2014,Jan,11

**31240     with concha bullosa resection**

🔧 4.60     ✂ 4.60     **FUD** 000     [J] [A2] [80] [50] [💻]

AMA: 2017,Jan,8; 2016,Feb,10; 2016,Jan,13; 2015,Jan,16; 2014,Jan,11

● **31241     with ligation of sphenopalatine artery**

EXCLUDES   Nasal/sinus endoscopy, surgical; with control of nasal hemorrhage, on the same side (31238)

*31253*     **Resequenced code. See code following 31255.**

## 31254-31255 [31253, 31257, 31259] Nasal Endoscopy with Ethmoid Removal

| INCLUDES | Diagnostic nasal/sinus endoscopy |
| | Sinusotomy, when applicable |

Code also stereotactic navigation, if performed (61782)

▲ **31254     Nasal/sinus endoscopy, surgical with ethmoidectomy; partial (anterior)**

EXCLUDES   When performed on the same side:
Other total ethmoidectomy procedures (31253, 31255, [31257], [31259])
Placement of drug eluting stent (0406T-0407T)

🔧 7.82     ✂ 7.82     **FUD** 000     [J] [A2] [50] [💻]

AMA: 2017,Jan,8; 2016,Feb,10; 2016,Jan,13; 2015,Jan,16; 2014,Jan,11; 2012,Jan,15-42

▲ **31255     with ethmoidectomy, total (anterior and posterior)**

EXCLUDES   When performed on the same side:
Frontal sinus exploration (31276)
Other total ethmoidectomy procedures (31253, [31257], [31259])
Partial ethmoidectomy (31254)
Placement of drug eluting stent (0406T-0407T)
Sphenoidotomy (31287-31288)

🔧 11.4     ✂ 11.4     **FUD** 000     [J] [A2] [50] [💻]

AMA: 2017,Jan,8; 2016,Feb,10; 2016,Jan,13; 2015,Jan,16; 2014,Jan,11; 2012,Jan,15-42

● # **31253     total (anterior and posterior), including frontal sinus exploration, with removal of tissue from frontal sinus, when performed**

🔧 0.00     ✂ 0.00     **FUD** 000

EXCLUDES   When performed on the same side:
Biopsy, debridement, or polypectomy (31237)
Dilation of sinus (31296, 31298)
Frontal sinus exploration (31276)
Partial ethmoidectomy (31254)
Placement of drug eluting stent (0406T-0407T)
Total ethmoidectomy (31255)

● # **31257     total (anterior and posterior), including sphenoidotomy**

🔧 0.00     ✂ 0.00     **FUD** 000

EXCLUDES   When performed on the same side:
Biopsy, debridement, or polypectomy (31237)
Diagnostic sphenoid sinusocopy (31235)
Other total ethmoidectomy procedures (31255, [31259])
Partial ethmoidectomy (31254)
Placement of drug eluting stent (0406T-0407T)
Sinus dilation (31297-31298)
Sphenoidotomy (31287-31288)

● # **31259     total (anterior and posterior), including sphenoidotomy, with removal of tissue from the sphenoid sinus**

🔧 0.00     ✂ 0.00     **FUD** 000

EXCLUDES   When performed on the same side:
Biopsy, debridement, or polypectomy (31237)
Diagnostic sphenoid sinusocopy (31235)
Other total ethmoidectomy procedures (31255, [31257])
Partial ethmoidectomy (31254)
Placement of drug eluting stent (0406T-0407T)
Sinus dilation (31297-31298)
Sphenoidotomy (31287-31288)

[26]/[TC] PC/TC Only    [A2]-[Z3] ASC Payment    [50] Bilateral    ♂ Male Only    ♀ Female Only    🔧 Facility RVU    ✂ Non-Facility RVU    💻 CCI

**FUD** Follow-up Days    **CMS:** IOM (Pub 100)    [A]-[Y] OPPSI    [80]/[80] Surg Assist Allowed / w/Doc    📋 Lab Crosswalk    📋 Radiology Crosswalk    ✖ CLIA

**108**       CPT © 2017 American Medical Association. All Rights Reserved.       © 2017 Optum360, LLC

## 31256-31267 Nasal Endoscopy with Maxillary Procedures

INCLUDES    Diagnostic nasal/sinus endoscopy
Nasal/sinus endoscopy, surgical; with dilation of maxillary sinus ostium (31295)
Sinusotomy, when applicable
Code also stereotactic navigation, if performed (61782)

**31256    Nasal/sinus endoscopy, surgical, with maxillary antrostomy;**
Code also any combination of the following endoscopic procedures when performed in conjunction with maxillary antrostomy, regardless if polyps are removed:
Frontal sinus exploration (31276)
Sphenoidotomy, with or without removal of tissue; either (31287, 31288)
Total (anterior and posterior) ethmoidectomy (31255)

🔲 5.66    ⚕ 5.66    **FUD** 000    [J] [A2] [50] [▣]

**AMA:** 2017,Jan,8; 2016,Jan,13; 2015,Jan,16; 2014,Jan,11; 2013,Jun,13

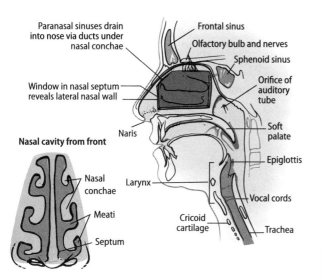

Paranasal sinuses drain into nose via ducts under nasal conchae

Frontal sinus

Olfactory bulb and nerves

Sphenoid sinus

Window in nasal septum reveals lateral nasal wall

Orifice of auditory tube

Naris

Soft palate

**Nasal cavity from front**

Nasal conchae

Larynx

Epiglottis

Meati

Vocal cords

Cricoid cartilage

Septum

Trachea

Frontal

Frontal
Ethmoid
Sphenoid
Maxillary

Ethmoid
Sphenoid

Maxillary

*31257*    **Resequenced code. See code following 31255.**

*31259*    **Resequenced code. See code following 31255.**

**31267    with removal of tissue from maxillary sinus**
Code also any combination of the following endoscopic procedures when performed in conjunction with maxillary antrostomy with removal of maxillary sinus tissue, regardless of whether polyps are removed:
Frontal sinus exploration (31276)
Sphenoidotomy, with or without removal of tissue; either (31287, 31288)
Total (anterior and posterior) ethmoidectomy (31255)

🔲 9.08    ⚕ 9.08    **FUD** 000    [J] [A2] [50] [▣]

**AMA:** 2017,Jan,8; 2016,Jan,13; 2015,Jan,16; 2014,Jan,11; 2012,Jan,15-42

## 31276 Nasal Endoscopy with Frontal Sinus Examination

INCLUDES    Diagnostic nasal/sinus endoscopy
Sinusotomy, when applicable
Unilateral procedure
EXCLUDES    Sinus dilation (31296, 31298)
Unilateral endoscopy two or more sinuses (31231-31235)
Code also any combination of the following endoscopic procedures when performed in conjunction with frontal sinus exploration, regardless of whether polyps are removed:
Antrostomy, with or without removal of maxillary sinus tissue; either (31256, 31267)
Other total ethmoidectomy procedures (31253, 31255)
Sphenoidotomy (31287, 31288)
Code also stereotactic navigation, if performed (61782)

▲    **31276    Nasal/sinus endoscopy, surgical, with frontal sinus exploration, including removal of tissue from frontal sinus, when performed**

🔲 14.4    ⚕ 14.4    **FUD** 000    [J] [A2] [50] [▣]

**AMA:** 2017,Jan,8; 2016,Jan,13; 2015,Jan,16; 2014,Jan,11; 2012,Jan,15-42

## 31287-31288 Nasal Endoscopy with Sphenoid Procedures

EXCLUDES    Other total ethmoidectomy procedures (31253, 31255, [31257], [31259])
Sinus dilation (31297-31298)
Code also stereotactic navigation, if performed (61782)

**31287    Nasal/sinus endoscopy, surgical, with sphenoidotomy;**
EXCLUDES    Sphenoidotomy with removal of tissue (31288)

🔲 6.64    ⚕ 6.64    **FUD** 000    [J] [A2] [80] [50] [▣]

**AMA:** 2017,Jan,8; 2016,Jan,13; 2015,Jan,16; 2014,Jan,11

**31288    with removal of tissue from the sphenoid sinus**
EXCLUDES    Sphenoidotomy without removal of tissue (31287)

🔲 7.70    ⚕ 7.70    **FUD** 000    [J] [A2] [80] [50] [▣]

**AMA:** 2017,Jan,8; 2016,Feb,10; 2016,Jan,13; 2015,Jan,16; 2014,Jan,11

## 31290-31294 Nasal Endoscopy with Repair and Decompression

INCLUDES    Diagnostic nasal/sinus endoscopy
Sinusotomy, when applicable
Code also stereotactic navigation, if performed (61782)

**31290    Nasal/sinus endoscopy, surgical, with repair of cerebrospinal fluid leak; ethmoid region**

🔲 33.0    ⚕ 33.0    **FUD** 010    [C] [80] [50] [▣]

**AMA:** 2017,Jan,8; 2016,Feb,10; 2016,Jan,13; 2015,Jan,16; 2014,Jan,11

**31291    sphenoid region**

🔲 35.2    ⚕ 35.2    **FUD** 010    [C] [80] [50] [▣]

**AMA:** 2017,Jan,8; 2016,Jan,13; 2015,Jan,16; 2014,Jan,11

**31292    Nasal/sinus endoscopy, surgical; with medial or inferior orbital wall decompression**

🔲 28.5    ⚕ 28.5    **FUD** 010    [J] [80] [50] [▣]

**AMA:** 2017,Jan,8; 2016,Jan,13; 2015,Jan,16; 2014,Jan,11

**31293    with medial orbital wall and inferior orbital wall decompression**

🔲 31.0    ⚕ 31.0    **FUD** 010    [J] [80] [50] [▣]

**AMA:** 2017,Jan,8; 2016,Jan,13; 2015,Jan,16; 2014,Jan,11

**31294    with optic nerve decompression**

🔲 35.9    ⚕ 35.9    **FUD** 010    [J] [80] [50] [▣]

**AMA:** 2017,Jan,8; 2016,Jan,13; 2015,Jan,16; 2014,Jan,11

## 31295-31298 Nasal Endoscopy with Sinus Ostia Dilation

INCLUDES    Any method of tissue displacement
Fluoroscopy, when performed
Code also stereotactic navigation, if performed (61782)

**31295    Nasal/sinus endoscopy, surgical; with dilation of maxillary sinus ostium (eg, balloon dilation), transnasal or via canine fossa**
EXCLUDES    When performed on the same side:
Maxillary antrostomy (31256-31267)
Maxillary sinusoscopy (31233)

🔲 4.69    ⚕ 57.3    **FUD** 000    [J] [P2] [80] [50] [▣]

**AMA:** 2017,Jan,8; 2016,Jan,13; 2015,Jan,16; 2014,Jan,11

● New Code    ▲ Revised Code    ○ Reinstated    ● New Web Release    ▲ Revised Web Release    Unlisted    Not Covered    # Resequenced
◌ AMA Mod 51 Exempt    ⑤ Optum Mod 51 Exempt    ⑥ Mod 63 Exempt    ✔ Non-FDA Drug    ★ Telemedicine    Ⅿ Maternity    Ⓐ Age Edit    + Add-on    AMA: CPT Asst
© 2017 Optum360, LLC    CPT © 2017 American Medical Association. All Rights Reserved.

**Respiratory System**

**31296 — 31511**

**31296** **with dilation of frontal sinus ostium (eg, balloon dilation)**

> EXCLUDES When performed on the same side:
> Frontal sinus exploration (31276)
> Sinus dilation (31297-31298)
> Total ethmoidectomy (31253)

🚑 5.62　🔪 58.4　**FUD** 000　　　　J P2 80 50 ▢

**AMA:** 2017,Jan,8; 2016,Jan,13; 2015,Jan,16; 2014,Jan,11

**31297** **with dilation of sphenoid sinus ostium (eg, balloon dilation)**

> EXCLUDES When performed on the same side:
> Diagnostic sphenoid sinusocopy (31235)
> Sinus dilation (31296, 31298)
> Sphenoidotomy (31287-31288)
> Total ethmoidectomy procedures ([31257], [31259])

🚑 4.60　🔪 57.4　**FUD** 000　　　　J P2 80 50 ▢

**AMA:** 2017,Jan,8; 2016,Jan,13; 2015,Jan,16; 2014,Jan,11

● **31298** **with dilation of frontal and sphenoid sinus ostia (eg, balloon dilation)**

> EXCLUDES When performed on the same side:
> Biopsy, debridement, or polypectomy (31237)
> Diagnostic sphenoid sinusocopy (31235)
> Dilation of frontal sinus only (31296)
> Dilation of sphenoid sinus only (31297)
> Frontal sinus exploration (31276)
> Other total ethmoidectomy procedures (31253, [31257], [31259])
> Sphenoidotomy (31287-31288)

## 31299 Unlisted Procedures of Accessory Sinuses

**CMS:** 100-04,4,180.3 Unlisted Service or Procedure

> EXCLUDES Hypophysectomy (61546, 61548)

**31299** **Unlisted procedure, accessory sinuses**

🚑 0.00　🔪 0.00　**FUD** YYY　　　　T 80

**AMA:** 2017,Jan,8; 2016,Feb,10; 2016,Jan,13; 2015,Jul,10; 2015,Jan,16; 2014,Jan,11; 2013,Jun,13; 2012,Jan,15-42

## 31300-31502 Procedures of the Larynx

**31300** **Laryngotomy (thyrotomy, laryngofissure), with removal of tumor or laryngocele, cordectomy**

🚑 37.3　🔪 37.3　**FUD** 090　　　　J A2 80 ▢

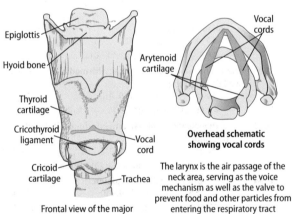

Epiglottis
Hyoid bone
Thyroid cartilage
Cricothyroid ligament
Cricoid cartilage
Vocal cords
Arytenoid cartilage
Vocal cord
Trachea

**Overhead schematic showing vocal cords**

The larynx is the air passage of the neck area, serving as the voice mechanism as well as the valve to prevent food and other particles from entering the respiratory tract

Frontal view of the major structures of the larynx

~~**31320**~~　~~**diagnostic**~~

**31360** **Laryngectomy; total, without radical neck dissection**

🚑 60.4　🔪 60.4　**FUD** 090　　　　C 80 ▢

**AMA:** 2017,Jan,8; 2016,Jan,13; 2015,Jan,16; 2014,Jan,11

**31365** **total, with radical neck dissection**

🚑 74.5　🔪 74.5　**FUD** 090　　　　C 80 ▢

**AMA:** 2017,Jan,8; 2016,Jan,13; 2015,Jan,16; 2014,Jan,11; 2012,Jan,15-42

**31367** **subtotal supraglottic, without radical neck dissection**

🚑 63.8　🔪 63.8　**FUD** 090　　　　C 80 ▢

**AMA:** 2017,Jan,8; 2016,Jan,13; 2015,Jan,16; 2014,Jan,11

**31368** **subtotal supraglottic, with radical neck dissection**

🚑 71.0　🔪 71.0　**FUD** 090　　　　C 80 ▢

**31370** **Partial laryngectomy (hemilaryngectomy); horizontal**

🚑 60.1　🔪 60.1　**FUD** 090　　　　C 80 ▢

**31375** **laterovertical**

🚑 57.0　🔪 57.0　**FUD** 090　　　　C 80 ▢

**31380** **anterovertical**

🚑 56.2　🔪 56.2　**FUD** 090　　　　C 80 ▢

**31382** **antero-latero-vertical**

🚑 61.8　🔪 61.8　**FUD** 090　　　　C 80 ▢

**31390** **Pharyngolaryngectomy, with radical neck dissection; without reconstruction**

🚑 83.1　🔪 83.1　**FUD** 090　　　　C 80 ▢

**31395** **with reconstruction**

🚑 87.8　🔪 87.8　**FUD** 090　　　　C 80 ▢

**31400** **Arytenoidectomy or arytenoidopexy, external approach**

🚑 28.1　🔪 28.1　**FUD** 090　　　　J A2 80 ▢

> EXCLUDES Endoscopic arytenoidectomy (31560)

**31420** **Epiglottidectomy**

🚑 23.7　🔪 23.7　**FUD** 090　　　　J A2 80 ▢

Epiglottis
Hyoid bone
Choanae
Parotid gland
Nasal septum
Root of tongue
Epiglottis
Aditus of larynx

**Posterior cutaway view**

**Plane of view**

**31500** **Intubation, endotracheal, emergency procedure**

> EXCLUDES Chest x-ray performed to confirm position of endotracheal tube

🚑 4.07　🔪 4.07　**FUD** 000　　　　⊘ T 62 ▢

**AMA:** 2017,Jan,8; 2016,Oct,8; 2016,May,3; 2016,Jan,13; 2015,Jan,16; 2014,Jan,11; 2012,Jan,15-42

**31502** **Tracheotomy tube change prior to establishment of fistula tract**

🚑 1.01　🔪 1.01　**FUD** 000　　　　T 62 ▢

**AMA:** 1990,Win,4

## 31505-31541 Endoscopy of the Larynx

**31505** **Laryngoscopy, indirect; diagnostic (separate procedure)**

🚑 1.41　🔪 2.34　**FUD** 000　　　　T P3 ▢

**AMA:** 2017,Jan,8; 2016,Jan,13; 2015,Jan,16; 2014,Jan,11

**31510** **with biopsy**

🚑 3.50　🔪 6.03　**FUD** 000　　　　J A2 80 ▢

**AMA:** 2017,Jan,8; 2016,Jan,13; 2015,Jan,16; 2014,Jan,11

**31511** **with removal of foreign body**

🚑 3.73　🔪 6.02　**FUD** 000　　　　T A2 ▢

**AMA:** 2017,Jan,8; 2016,Jan,13; 2015,Jan,16; 2014,Jan,11

26/TC PC/TC Only　　A2-Z3 ASC Payment　　50 Bilateral　　♂ Male Only　　♀ Female Only　　🚑 Facility RVU　　🔪 Non-Facility RVU　　▢ CCI
**FUD** Follow-up Days　　**CMS:** IOM (Pub 100)　　A-Y OPPSI　　80/80 Surg Assist Allowed / w/Doc　　🔬 Lab Crosswalk　　📻 Radiology Crosswalk　　✖ CLIA

110　　　　　　　　　　CPT © 2017 American Medical Association. All Rights Reserved.　　　　　　© 2017 Optum360, LLC

**31512** with removal of lesion
📋 3.74  ⚮ 5.87  **FUD** 000  `J A2 80 ▣`
AMA: 2017,Jan,8; 2016,Jan,13; 2015,Jan,16; 2014,Jan,11

**31513** with vocal cord injection
📋 3.80  ⚮ 3.80  **FUD** 000  `T A2 80 ▣`
AMA: 2017,Jan,8; 2016,Jan,13; 2015,Jan,16; 2014,Jan,11

**31515** Laryngoscopy direct, with or without tracheoscopy; for aspiration
📋 2.99  ⚮ 5.17  **FUD** 000  `T A2 ▣`
AMA: 1998,Nov,1; 1997,Nov,1

**31520** diagnostic, newborn  `A`
📋 4.51  ⚮ 4.51  **FUD** 000  `⊕ T 02 80 ▣`
AMA: 1998,Nov,1; 1997,Nov,1

**31525** diagnostic, except newborn
📋 4.61  ⚮ 7.20  **FUD** 000  `J A2 ▣`
AMA: 2017,Jan,8; 2016,Jan,13; 2015,Jan,16; 2014,Jan,11

**31526** diagnostic, with operating microscope or telescope
INCLUDES Operating microscope (69990)
📋 4.53  ⚮ 4.53  **FUD** 000  `J A2 ▣`
AMA: 2017,Jun,10; 2016,Feb,12

**31527** with insertion of obturator
📋 5.61  ⚮ 5.61  **FUD** 000  `J A2 80 ▣`
AMA: 1998,Nov,1; 1997,Nov,1

**31528** with dilation, initial
📋 4.17  ⚮ 4.17  **FUD** 000  `J A2 80 ▣`
AMA: 2002,May,7; 1998,Nov,1

**31529** with dilation, subsequent
📋 4.66  ⚮ 4.66  **FUD** 000  `J A2 80 ▣`
AMA: 2002,May,7; 1998,Nov,1

**31530** Laryngoscopy, direct, operative, with foreign body removal;
📋 5.71  ⚮ 5.71  **FUD** 000  `J A2 ▣`
AMA: 1998,Nov,1; 1997,Nov,1

**31531** with operating microscope or telescope
INCLUDES Operating microscope (69990)
📋 6.11  ⚮ 6.11  **FUD** 000  `J A2 80 ▣`
AMA: 2017,Jun,10; 2016,Feb,12

**31535** Laryngoscopy, direct, operative, with biopsy;
📋 5.46  ⚮ 5.46  **FUD** 000  `J A2 ▣`
AMA: 1998,Nov,1; 1997,Nov,1

**31536** with operating microscope or telescope
INCLUDES Operating microscope (69990)
📋 6.08  ⚮ 6.08  **FUD** 000  `J A2 ▣`
AMA: 2017,Jun,10; 2016,Feb,12

**31540** Laryngoscopy, direct, operative, with excision of tumor and/or stripping of vocal cords or epiglottis;
📋 6.98  ⚮ 6.98  **FUD** 000  `J A2 ▣`
AMA: 1998,Nov,1; 1997,Nov,1

**31541** with operating microscope or telescope
INCLUDES Operating microscope (69990)
📋 7.61  ⚮ 7.61  **FUD** 000  `J A2 ▣`
AMA: 2017,Jun,10; 2016,Feb,12

## 31545-31554 Endoscopy of Larynx with Reconstruction
INCLUDES Operating microscope (69990)
EXCLUDES Laryngoscopy, direct, operative, with excision of tumor and/or stripping of vocal cords or epiglottis (31540-31541)
Vocal cord reconstruction with allograft (31599)

**31545** Laryngoscopy, direct, operative, with operating microscope or telescope, with submucosal removal of non-neoplastic lesion(s) of vocal cord; reconstruction with local tissue flap(s)
📋 10.4  ⚮ 10.4  **FUD** 000  `J A2 50 ▣`
AMA: 2016,Feb,12

**31546** reconstruction with graft(s) (includes obtaining autograft)
EXCLUDES Tissue grafts, other (eg, paratenon, fat, dermis) (20926)
📋 15.8  ⚮ 15.8  **FUD** 000  `J A2 50 ▣`
AMA: 2017,Jan,8; 2016,Feb,12; 2016,Jan,13; 2015,Jan,16; 2014,Jan,11; 2012,Jan,15-42

*31551* Resequenced code. See code following 31580.

*31552* Resequenced code. See code following 31580.

*31553* Resequenced code. See code following 31580.

*31554* Resequenced code. See code following 31580.

## 31560-31571 Endoscopy of Larynx with Arytenoid Removal, Vocal Cord Injection

**31560** Laryngoscopy, direct, operative, with arytenoidectomy;
📋 9.03  ⚮ 9.03  **FUD** 000  `J A2 80 ▣`
AMA: 1998,Nov,1; 1997,Nov,1

**31561** with operating microscope or telescope
INCLUDES Operating microscope (69990)
📋 9.89  ⚮ 9.89  **FUD** 000  `J A2 80 ▣`
AMA: 2017,Jun,10; 2016,Feb,12

**31570** Laryngoscopy, direct, with injection into vocal cord(s), therapeutic;
📋 6.62  ⚮ 9.64  **FUD** 000  `J A2 ▣`
AMA: 2017,Jan,6; 2017,Jan,8; 2016,Jan,13; 2015,Jan,16; 2014,Jan,6

**31571** with operating microscope or telescope
INCLUDES Operating microscope (69990)
📋 7.21  ⚮ 7.21  **FUD** 000  `J A2 ▣`
AMA: 2017,Jun,10; 2017,Jan,6; 2017,Jan,8; 2016,Feb,12; 2016,Jan,13; 2015,Jan,16; 2014,Jan,11; 2014,Jan,6; 2012,Nov,13-14

## 31572-31579 [31572, 31573, 31574] Endoscopy of Larynx, Flexible Fiberoptic

EXCLUDES Evaluation by flexible fiberoptic endoscope:
Sensory assessment (92614-92615)
Swallowing (92612-92613)
Swallowing and sensory assessment (92616-92617)
Flexible fiberoptic endoscopic examination/testing by cine or video recording (92612-92617)

*31572* Resequenced code. See code following 31578.

*31573* Resequenced code. See code following 31578.

*31574* Resequenced code. See code following 31578.

**31575** Laryngoscopy, flexible; diagnostic
EXCLUDES Diagnostic nasal endoscopy not through additional endoscope (31231)
Procedures during same session (31572-31574, 31576-31578, 43197-43198, 92511, 92612, 92614, 92616)
📋 1.94  ⚮ 3.23  **FUD** 000  `T P3 ▣`
AMA: 2017,Jul,7; 2017,Apr,8; 2017,Jan,8; 2016,Dec,13

**31576** with biopsy(ies)
EXCLUDES Destruction or excision of lesion (31572, 31578)
📋 3.43  ⚮ 7.53  **FUD** 000  `J A2 ▣`
AMA: 2017,Jul,7; 2017,Apr,8; 2017,Jan,8; 2016,Dec,13

**31577** with removal of foreign body(s)
📋 3.87  ⚮ 7.80  **FUD** 000  `T A2 80 ▣`
AMA: 2017,Jul,7; 2017,Apr,8; 2017,Jan,8; 2016,Dec,13

**31578** with removal of lesion(s), non-laser
📋 4.30  ⚮ 8.57  **FUD** 000  `J A2 80 ▣`
AMA: 2017,Jul,7; 2017,Apr,8; 2017,Jan,8; 2016,Dec,13

# **31572** with ablation or destruction of lesion(s) with laser, unilateral
EXCLUDES Biopsy or excision of lesion (31576, 31578)
Swallowing evaluation or sensory testing (92612-92617)
📋 5.21  ⚮ 14.1  **FUD** 000  `J J8 80 50 ▣`
AMA: 2017,Jul,7; 2017,Apr,8; 2017,Jan,8; 2016,Dec,13

● New Code  ▲ Revised Code  ○ Reinstated  ● New Web Release  ▲ Revised Web Release  Unlisted  Not Covered  # Resequenced
⊘ AMA Mod 51 Exempt  ⑤ Optum Mod 51 Exempt  ⊛ Mod 63 Exempt  ／ Non-FDA Drug  ★ Telemedicine  M Maternity  A Age Edit  + Add-on  AMA: CPT Asst
© 2017 Optum360, LLC        CPT © 2017 American Medical Association. All Rights Reserved.        **111**

\# **31573** **with therapeutic injection(s) (eg, chemodenervation agent or corticosteroid, injected percutaneous, transoral, or via endoscope channel), unilateral**
🔧 4.30 ⚕ 7.53 **FUD** 000 J J8 80 50 ▢
**AMA:** 2017,Jul,7; 2017,Apr,8; 2017,Jan,8; 2016,Dec,13

\# **31574** **with injection(s) for augmentation (eg, percutaneous, transoral), unilateral**
🔧 4.30 ⚕ 29.1 **FUD** 000 J J8 80 50 ▢
**AMA:** 2017,Jul,7; 2017,Apr,8; 2017,Jan,8; 2016,Dec,13

**31579** **Laryngoscopy, flexible or rigid telescopic, with stroboscopy**
🔧 3.44 ⚕ 5.04 **FUD** 000 T P3 ▢
**AMA:** 2017,Jul,7; 2017,Apr,8; 2017,Jan,8; 2016,Dec,13

## 31580-31599 [31551, 31552, 31553, 31554] Larynx Reconstruction

**31580** **Laryngoplasty; for laryngeal web, with indwelling keel or stent insertion**
EXCLUDES *Keel or stent removal (31599)*
*Tracheostomy (31600-31601, 31603, 31605, 31610)*
*Treatment of laryngeal stenosis (31551-31554)*
🔧 35.7 ⚕ 35.7 **FUD** 090 J A2 80 ▢
**AMA:** 2017,Apr,5; 2017,Mar,10

\# **31551** **for laryngeal stenosis, with graft, without indwelling stent placement, younger than 12 years of age** A
EXCLUDES *Cartilage graft obtained through same incision*
*Procedure during same session (31552-31554, 31580)*
*Tracheostomy (31600-31601, 31603, 31605, 31610)*
🔧 40.7 ⚕ 40.7 **FUD** 090 J G2 80 ▢
**AMA:** 2017,Jul,7; 2017,Apr,5; 2017,Mar,10

\# **31552** **for laryngeal stenosis, with graft, without indwelling stent placement, age 12 years or older** A
EXCLUDES *Cartilage graft obtained through same incision*
*Procedure during same session (31551, 31553-31554, 31580)*
*Tracheostomy (31600-31601, 31603, 31605, 31610)*
🔧 41.1 ⚕ 41.1 **FUD** 090 J G2 80 ▢
**AMA:** 2017,Jul,7; 2017,Apr,5; 2017,Mar,10

\# **31553** **for laryngeal stenosis, with graft, with indwelling stent placement, younger than 12 years of age** A
EXCLUDES *Cartilage graft obtained through same incision*
*Procedure during same session (31551-31552, 31554, 31580)*
*Stent removal (31599)*
*Tracheostomy (31600-31601, 31603, 31605, 31610)*
🔧 44.9 ⚕ 44.9 **FUD** 090 J G2 80 ▢
**AMA:** 2017,Jul,7; 2017,Apr,5; 2017,Mar,10

\# **31554** **for laryngeal stenosis, with graft, with indwelling stent placement, age 12 years or older** A
EXCLUDES *Cartilage graft obtained through same incision*
*Procedure during same session (31551-31553, 31580)*
*Stent removal (31599)*
*Tracheostomy (31600-31601, 31603, 31605, 31610)*
🔧 47.2 ⚕ 47.2 **FUD** 090 J G2 80 ▢
**AMA:** 2017,Jul,7; 2017,Apr,5; 2017,Mar,10

**31584** **with open reduction and fixation of (eg, plating) fracture, includes tracheostomy, if performed**
EXCLUDES *Cartilage graft obtained through same incision*
🔧 39.6 ⚕ 39.6 **FUD** 090 J 80 ▢
**AMA:** 2017,Apr,5; 2017,Mar,10

**31587** **Laryngoplasty, cricoid split, without graft placement**
EXCLUDES *Tracheostomy (31600-31601, 31603, 31605, 31610)*
🔧 33.2 ⚕ 33.2 **FUD** 090 J 80 ▢
**AMA:** 2017,Apr,5; 2017,Mar,10

**31590** **Laryngeal reinnervation by neuromuscular pedicle**
🔧 24.9 ⚕ 24.9 **FUD** 090 J A2 80 ▢
**AMA:** 2017,Mar,10

**31591** **Laryngoplasty, medialization, unilateral**
🔧 29.8 ⚕ 29.8 **FUD** 090 J G2 80 ▢
**AMA:** 2017,Jul,7; 2017,Apr,5; 2017,Mar,10

**31592** **Cricotracheal resection**
EXCLUDES *Advancement or rotational flaps performed not requiring additional incision*
*Cartilage graft obtained through same incision*
*Tracheal stenosis excision/anastomosis (31780-31781)*
*Tracheostomy (31600-31601, 31603, 31605, 31610)*
🔧 48.3 ⚕ 48.3 **FUD** 090 J G2 80 ▢
**AMA:** 2017,Jul,7; 2017,Apr,5; 2017,Mar,10; 2017,Feb,14

**31595** **Section recurrent laryngeal nerve, therapeutic (separate procedure), unilateral**
🔧 21.6 ⚕ 21.6 **FUD** 090 J A2 80 50 ▢

Recurrent laryngeal nerve

Strap muscles retracted

Thyroid cartilage

Vocal cord

Cricoid cartilage

**31599** **Unlisted procedure, larynx**
🔧 0.00 ⚕ 0.00 **FUD** YYY T 80
**AMA:** 2017,Apr,5; 2017,Mar,10; 2017,Jan,8; 2017,Jan,6; 2016,Dec,13; 2016,Jan,13; 2015,Jan,16; 2014,Jan,11; 2012,Nov,13-14

## 31600-31610 Stoma Creation: Trachea

EXCLUDES *Aspiration of trachea, direct vision (31515)*
*Endotracheal intubation (31500)*

**31600** **Tracheostomy, planned (separate procedure);**
🔧 11.4 ⚕ 11.4 **FUD** 000 J ▢
**AMA:** 2017,Apr,5

**31601** **younger than 2 years** A
🔧 6.10 ⚕ 6.10 **FUD** 000 J 80 ▢
**AMA:** 2017,Apr,5

**31603** **Tracheostomy, emergency procedure; transtracheal**
🔧 6.44 ⚕ 6.44 **FUD** 000 T A2 ▢
**AMA:** 2017,Apr,5

**31605** **cricothyroid membrane**
🔧 5.32 ⚕ 5.32 **FUD** 000 T G2 ▢
**AMA:** 2017,Apr,5

**31610** **Tracheostomy, fenestration procedure with skin flaps**
🔧 20.3 ⚕ 20.3 **FUD** 090 J ▢
**AMA:** 2017,Apr,5

## 31611-31614 Procedures of the Trachea

**31611** **Construction of tracheoesophageal fistula and subsequent insertion of an alaryngeal speech prosthesis (eg, voice button, Blom-Singer prosthesis)**
🔧 15.3 ⚕ 15.3 **FUD** 090 J A2 80 ▢

**31612** **Tracheal puncture, percutaneous with transtracheal aspiration and/or injection**
EXCLUDES *Tracheal aspiration under direct vision (31515)*
🔧 1.39 ⚕ 2.37 **FUD** 000 J A2 80 ▢
**AMA:** 1994,Win,1

26/TC PC/TC Only   A2-Z3 ASC Payment   50 Bilateral   ♂ Male Only   ♀ Female Only   🔧 Facility RVU   ⚕ Non-Facility RVU   ▢ CCI
FUD Follow-up Days   CMS: IOM (Pub 100)   A-Y OPPSI   80/80 Surg Assist Allowed / w/Doc   🔬 Lab Crosswalk   📻 Radiology Crosswalk   ✖ CLIA

112   CPT © 2017 American Medical Association. All Rights Reserved.   © 2017 Optum360, LLC

| 31613 | Tracheostoma revision; simple, without flap rotation |
|---|---|

🚗 12.9     ♨ 12.9     **FUD** 090      J A2 ▣

| 31614 | complex, with flap rotation |
|---|---|

🚗 21.5     ♨ 21.5     **FUD** 090      J A2 ▣

## 31615 Endoscopy Through Tracheostomy

INCLUDES    Diagnostic bronchoscopy

EXCLUDES    *Endobronchial ultrasound [EBUS] guided biopsies of mediastinal or hilar lymph nodes (31652-31653)*
*Tracheoscopy (31515-31578)*
Code also endobronchial ultrasound [EBUS] during diagnostic/therapeutic peripheral lesion intervention (31654)

| 31615 | Tracheobronchoscopy through established tracheostomy incision |
|---|---|

🚗 3.31     ♨ 4.79     **FUD** 000      T A2 ▣

**AMA:** 2017,Jan,8; 2016,Jan,13; 2015,Jan,16; 2014,Jan,11; 2013,Mar,8-9; 2012,Nov,13-14

## 31622-31654 [31651] Endoscopy of Lung

INCLUDES    Diagnostic bronchoscopy with surgical bronchoscopy procedures
Fluoroscopic imaging guidance, when performed

| 31622 | Bronchoscopy, rigid or flexible, including fluoroscopic guidance, when performed; diagnostic, with cell washing, when performed (separate procedure) |
|---|---|

🚗 3.81     ♨ 6.86     **FUD** 000      J A2 ▣

**AMA:** 2017,Jan,8; 2016,Apr,5; 2016,Jan,13; 2015,Jan,16; 2014,Jan,11; 2013,Mar,8-9; 2012,Jan,15-42

| 31623 | with brushing or protected brushings |
|---|---|

🚗 3.87     ♨ 7.70     **FUD** 000      J A2 ▣

**AMA:** 2017,Jan,8; 2016,Apr,5; 2016,Jan,13; 2015,Jan,16; 2014,Jan,11; 2013,Mar,8-9; 2012,Jan,15-42

| 31624 | with bronchial alveolar lavage |
|---|---|

🚗 3.92     ♨ 7.20     **FUD** 000      J A2 ▣

**AMA:** 2017,Jun,10; 2017,Jan,8; 2016,Apr,5; 2016,Jan,13; 2015,Jan,16; 2014,Jan,11; 2013,Mar,8-9; 2012,Jan,15-42

| 31625 | with bronchial or endobronchial biopsy(s), single or multiple sites |
|---|---|

🚗 4.53     ♨ 9.43     **FUD** 000      J A2 ▣

**AMA:** 2017,Jan,8; 2016,Apr,5; 2016,Jan,13; 2015,Jan,16; 2014,Jan,11; 2013,Mar,8-9; 2012,Jan,15-42

| 31626 | with placement of fiducial markers, single or multiple |
|---|---|

Code also device

🚗 5.76     ♨ 23.9     **FUD** 000      J B2 80 ▣

**AMA:** 2017,Jun,10; 2017,Jan,8; 2016,Apr,5; 2016,Jan,13; 2015,Jun,6; 2015,Jan,16; 2014,Jan,11; 2013,Mar,8-9

| + 31627 | with computer-assisted, image-guided navigation (List separately in addition to code for primary procedure[s]) |
|---|---|

INCLUDES    3D reconstruction (76376-76377)
Code first (31615, 31622-31626, 31628-31631, 31635-31636, 31638-31643)

🚗 2.82     ♨ 39.6     **FUD** ZZZ      N N1 80 ▣

**AMA:** 2017,Jan,8; 2016,Jan,13; 2015,Jan,16; 2014,Jan,11; 2013,Mar,8-9

| 31628 | with transbronchial lung biopsy(s), single lobe |
|---|---|

INCLUDES    All biopsies taken from lobe

EXCLUDES    *Transbronchial biopsies by needle aspiration (31629, 31633)*
Code also transbronchial biopsies of additional lobe(s) (31632)

🚗 5.09     ♨ 10.0     **FUD** 000      J A2 ▣

**AMA:** 2017,Jun,10; 2017,Jan,8; 2016,Apr,5; 2016,Jan,13; 2015,Jan,16; 2014,Jan,11; 2013,Mar,8-9; 2012,Jan,15-42

| 31629 | with transbronchial needle aspiration biopsy(s), trachea, main stem and/or lobar bronchus(i) |
|---|---|

INCLUDES    All biopsies from same lobe or upper airway

EXCLUDES    *Transbronchial biopsies of lung (31628, 31632)*
Code also transbronchial needle biopsies of additional lobe(s) (31633)

🚗 5.42     ♨ 12.3     **FUD** 000      J A2 ▣

**AMA:** 2017,Jan,8; 2016,Apr,5; 2016,Jan,13; 2015,Jan,16; 2014,Jan,11; 2013,Mar,8-9; 2012,Jan,15-42

| 31630 | with tracheal/bronchial dilation or closed reduction of fracture |
|---|---|

🚗 5.78     ♨ 5.78     **FUD** 000      J A2 ▣

**AMA:** 2017,Jan,8; 2016,Jan,13; 2015,Jan,16; 2014,Jan,11; 2013,Mar,8-9

| 31631 | with placement of tracheal stent(s) (includes tracheal/bronchial dilation as required) |
|---|---|

EXCLUDES    *Bronchial stent placement (31636-31637)*
*Revision bronchial or tracheal stent (31638)*

🚗 6.63     ♨ 6.63     **FUD** 000      J A2 ▣

**AMA:** 2017,Jan,8; 2016,Jan,13; 2015,Jan,16; 2014,Jan,11; 2013,Mar,8-9

| + 31632 | with transbronchial lung biopsy(s), each additional lobe (List separately in addition to code for primary procedure) |
|---|---|

INCLUDES    All biopsies of additional lobe of lung
Code first (31628)

🚗 1.42     ♨ 1.84     **FUD** ZZZ      N N1 ▣

**AMA:** 2017,Jan,8; 2016,Jan,13; 2015,Jan,16; 2014,Jan,11; 2013,Mar,8-9

| + 31633 | with transbronchial needle aspiration biopsy(s), each additional lobe (List separately in addition to code for primary procedure) |
|---|---|

INCLUDES    All needle biopsies from another lobe or from trachea
Code first (31629)

🚗 1.83     ♨ 2.29     **FUD** ZZZ      N N1 ▣

**AMA:** 2017,Jan,8; 2016,Jan,13; 2015,Jan,16; 2014,Jan,11; 2013,Mar,8-9; 2012,Jan,15-42

| 31634 | with balloon occlusion, with assessment of air leak, with administration of occlusive substance (eg, fibrin glue), if performed |
|---|---|

EXCLUDES    *Bronchoscopy, rigid or flexible, including fluoroscopic guidance, when performed; with balloon occlusion, when performed, assessment of air leak, airway sizing, and insertion of bronchial valve(s), initial lobe (31647, [31651])*

🚗 5.61     ♨ 50.8     **FUD** 000      J B2 80 ▣

**AMA:** 2017,Jan,8; 2016,Jan,13; 2015,Jan,16; 2014,Jan,11; 2013,Mar,8-9

| 31635 | with removal of foreign body |
|---|---|

EXCLUDES    *Removal implanted bronchial valves (31648-31649)*

🚗 5.07     ♨ 7.96     **FUD** 000      J A2 ▣

**AMA:** 2017,Jan,8; 2016,Jan,13; 2015,Jan,16; 2014,Jan,11; 2013,Mar,8-9; 2012,Jan,15-42

| 31636 | with placement of bronchial stent(s) (includes tracheal/bronchial dilation as required), initial bronchus |
|---|---|

🚗 6.37     ♨ 6.37     **FUD** 000      J J8 ▣

**AMA:** 2017,Jan,8; 2016,Jan,13; 2015,Jan,16; 2014,Jan,11; 2013,Mar,8-9

| + 31637 | each additional major bronchus stented (List separately in addition to code for primary procedure) |
|---|---|

Code first (31636)

🚗 2.14     ♨ 2.14     **FUD** ZZZ      N N1 ▣

**AMA:** 2017,Jan,8; 2016,Jan,13; 2015,Jan,16; 2014,Jan,11; 2013,Mar,8-9

| 31638 | with revision of tracheal or bronchial stent inserted at previous session (includes tracheal/bronchial dilation as required) |
|---|---|

🚗 7.26     ♨ 7.26     **FUD** 000      J A2 ▣

**AMA:** 2017,Jan,8; 2016,Jan,13; 2015,Jan,16; 2014,Jan,11; 2013,Mar,8-9

| 31640 | with excision of tumor |
|---|---|

🚗 7.30     ♨ 7.30     **FUD** 000      J A2 ▣

**AMA:** 2017,Jan,8; 2016,Apr,5; 2016,Jan,13; 2015,Jan,16; 2014,Jan,11; 2013,Mar,8-9

---

● New Code    ▲ Revised Code    ○ Reinstated    ● New Web Release    ▲ Revised Web Release    Unlisted    Not Covered    # Resequenced
⊘ AMA Mod 51 Exempt    ⑨ Optum Mod 51 Exempt    ⊛ Mod 63 Exempt    ✂ Non-FDA Drug    ★ Telemedicine    M Maternity    A Age Edit    + Add-on    **AMA:** CPT Asst

© 2017 Optum360, LLC      CPT © 2017 American Medical Association. All Rights Reserved.

**31641** **with destruction of tumor or relief of stenosis by any method other than excision (eg, laser therapy, cryotherapy)**

Code also any photodynamic therapy via bronchoscopy (96570-96571)

7.45    7.45    **FUD** 000    J A2

**AMA:** 2017,Jan,8; 2016,Jan,13; 2015,Jan,16; 2014,Jan,11; 2013,Apr,8-9; 2013,Mar,8-9

**31643** **with placement of catheter(s) for intracavitary radioelement application**

Code also if appropriate (77761-77763, 77770-77772)

5.12    5.12    **FUD** 000    J A2

**AMA:** 2017,Jan,8; 2016,Apr,5; 2016,Jan,13; 2015,Jan,16; 2014,Jan,11; 2013,Mar,8-9

▲ **31645** **with therapeutic aspiration of tracheobronchial tree, initial (eg, drainage of lung abscess)**

EXCLUDES   Bedside aspiration of trachea, bronchi (31725)

4.31    7.25    **FUD** 000    J A2

**AMA:** 2017,Jan,8; 2016,Apr,5; 2016,Jan,13; 2015,Jan,16; 2014,Jan,11; 2013,Mar,8-9

▲ **31646** **with therapeutic aspiration of tracheobronchial tree, subsequent**

EXCLUDES   Bedside aspiration of trachea, bronchi (31725)

3.68    6.53    **FUD** 000    T A2

**AMA:** 2017,Jan,8; 2016,Apr,5; 2016,Jan,13; 2015,Jan,16; 2014,Jan,11; 2013,Mar,8-9

**31647** **with balloon occlusion, when performed, assessment of air leak, airway sizing, and insertion of bronchial valve(s), initial lobe**

6.10    6.10    **FUD** 000    J G2

**AMA:** 2017,Jan,8; 2016,Jan,13; 2015,Jan,16; 2014,Jan,11; 2013,Mar,8-9

+ # **31651** **with balloon occlusion, when performed, assessment of air leak, airway sizing, and insertion of bronchial valve(s), each additional lobe (List separately in addition to code for primary procedure[s])**

Code first (31647)

2.15    2.15    **FUD** ZZZ    N N1

**AMA:** 2017,Jan,8; 2016,Jan,13; 2015,Jan,16; 2014,Jan,11; 2013,Mar,8-9

**31648** **with removal of bronchial valve(s), initial lobe**

EXCLUDES   Removal with reinsertion bronchial valve during same session (31647 and 31648) and ([31651])

5.57    5.57    **FUD** 000    J G2

**AMA:** 2017,Jan,8; 2016,Jan,13; 2015,Jan,16; 2014,Jan,11; 2013,Mar,8-9

+ **31649** **with removal of bronchial valve(s), each additional lobe (List separately in addition to code for primary procedure)**

Code first (31648)

2.01    2.01    **FUD** ZZZ    02 G2

**AMA:** 2017,Jan,8; 2016,Jan,13; 2015,Jan,16; 2014,Jan,11; 2013,Mar,8-9

*31651*   **Resequenced code. See code following 31647.**

**31652** **with endobronchial ultrasound (EBUS) guided transtracheal and/or transbronchial sampling (eg, aspiration[s]/biopsy[ies]), one or two mediastinal and/or hilar lymph node stations or structures**

EXCLUDES   Procedures performed more than one time per session

6.42    23.4    **FUD** 000    J G2

**AMA:** 2017,Jan,8; 2016,Apr,5

**31653** **with endobronchial ultrasound (EBUS) guided transtracheal and/or transbronchial sampling (eg, aspiration[s]/biopsy[ies]), 3 or more mediastinal and/or hilar lymph node stations or structures**

EXCLUDES   Procedures performed more than one time per session

7.11    24.8    **FUD** 000    J G2

**AMA:** 2017,Jan,8; 2016,Apr,5

+ **31654** **with transendoscopic endobronchial ultrasound (EBUS) during bronchoscopic diagnostic or therapeutic intervention(s) for peripheral lesion(s) (List separately in addition to code for primary procedure[s])**

EXCLUDES   Endobronchial ultrasound [EBUS] for mediastinal/hilar lymph node station/adjacent structure access (31652-31653)
            Procedures performed more than one time per session

Code first (31622-31626, 31628-31629, 31640, 31643-31646)

1.96    3.59    **FUD** ZZZ    N N1

**AMA:** 2017,Jan,8; 2016,Apr,5

## 31660-31661 Bronchial Thermoplasty

INCLUDES   Fluoroscopic imaging guidance, when performed

**31660** **Bronchoscopy, rigid or flexible, including fluoroscopic guidance, when performed; with bronchial thermoplasty, 1 lobe**

5.66    5.66    **FUD** 000    J

**AMA:** 2017,Jan,8; 2016,Jan,13; 2015,Jan,16; 2014,Jan,11; 2013,Mar,8-9

**31661** **with bronchial thermoplasty, 2 or more lobes**

5.97    5.97    **FUD** 000    J

**AMA:** 2017,Jan,8; 2016,Jan,13; 2015,Jan,16; 2014,Jan,11; 2013,Mar,8-9

## 31717-31899 Respiratory Procedures

EXCLUDES   Endotracheal intubation (31500)
            Tracheal aspiration under direct vision (31515)

**31717** **Catheterization with bronchial brush biopsy**

3.12    7.39    **FUD** 000    T A2 CCI

**AMA:** 2017,Jan,8; 2016,Jan,13; 2015,Jan,16; 2014,Jan,11; 2012,Jan,15-42

**31720** **Catheter aspiration (separate procedure); nasotracheal**

1.50    1.50    **FUD** 000    01 N1

**AMA:** 1994,Win,1

**31725** **tracheobronchial with fiberscope, bedside**

2.25    2.25    **FUD** 000    C

**31730** **Transtracheal (percutaneous) introduction of needle wire dilator/stent or indwelling tube for oxygen therapy**

4.32    35.0    **FUD** 000    J A2

**AMA:** 1992,Win,1

**31750** **Tracheoplasty; cervical**

40.1    40.1    **FUD** 090    J A2 80

**31755** **tracheopharyngeal fistulization, each stage**

50.8    50.8    **FUD** 090    J A2 80

**31760** **intrathoracic**

40.2    40.2    **FUD** 090    C 80

**31766** **Carinal reconstruction**

51.6    51.6    **FUD** 090    C 80

**31770** **Bronchoplasty; graft repair**

38.6    38.6    **FUD** 090    C 80

EXCLUDES   Bronchoplasty done with lobectomy (32501)

**31775** **excision stenosis and anastomosis**

36.9    36.9    **FUD** 090    C 80

EXCLUDES   Bronchoplasty done with lobectomy (32501)

**31780** **Excision tracheal stenosis and anastomosis; cervical**

33.8    33.8    **FUD** 090    C 80

**AMA:** 2017,Apr,5; 2017,Feb,14

**31781** **cervicothoracic**

40.2    40.2    **FUD** 090    C 80

**AMA:** 2017,Apr,5; 2017,Feb,14

**31785** **Excision of tracheal tumor or carcinoma; cervical**

31.0    31.0    **FUD** 090    J 80

**AMA:** 2003,Jan,1

**31786** **thoracic**

43.1    43.1    **FUD** 090    C 80

**31800** **Suture of tracheal wound or injury; cervical**
  🔧 21.0   ✂ 21.0   **FUD** 090                    Ⓒ 80 ▢
  **AMA:** 1994,Win,1

**31805** **intrathoracic**
  🔧 23.6   ✂ 23.6   **FUD** 090                    Ⓒ 80 ▢

**31820** **Surgical closure tracheostomy or fistula; without plastic repair**
  🔧 9.36   ✂ 12.3   **FUD** 090                    Ⓙ A2 80 ▢
  *EXCLUDES*   *Tracheoesophageal fistula repair (43305, 43312)*

**31825** **with plastic repair**
  🔧 13.7   ✂ 17.0   **FUD** 090                    Ⓙ A2 80 ▢
  *EXCLUDES*   *Tracheoesophageal fistula repair (43305, 43312)*

**31830** **Revision of tracheostomy scar**
  🔧 9.82   ✂ 12.5   **FUD** 090                    Ⓙ A2 80 ▢

Any of a wide variety of scar revision techniques may be employed. A Z-plasty may be used to lengthen or realign the scar line. Revision also serves to neutralize contractures that occur along the scar line

Thyroid cartilage

Cricoid cartilage

1st ring
2nd ring
3rd ring

Tracheostomies typically enter at the second, third, or fourth ring

**Example of a common Z-plasty where flaps are rotated to break scar line**

A tracheostomy closure scar is revised, usually to make the scar less noticeable

**31899** **Unlisted procedure, trachea, bronchi**
  🔧 0.00   ✂ 0.00   **FUD** YYY                    Ⓣ 80
  **AMA:** 2017,Jan,8; 2016,Jan,13; 2015,Jan,16; 2014,May,10; 2014,Jan,11; 2013,Mar,8-9; 2012,Jan,15-42

## 32035-32036 Procedures for Empyema

*EXCLUDES*   *Wound exploration without thoracotomy for penetrating wound of chest (20101)*

**32035** **Thoracostomy; with rib resection for empyema**
  🔧 20.9   ✂ 20.9   **FUD** 090                    Ⓒ 80 50 ▢

**32036** **with open flap drainage for empyema**
  🔧 22.3   ✂ 22.3   **FUD** 090                    Ⓒ 80 50 ▢

## 32096-32098 Open Biopsy of Chest and Pleura

*INCLUDES*   Varying amounts of lung tissue excised for analysis
  Wedge technique with tissue obtained without precise consideration of margins
*EXCLUDES*   *Percutaneous needle biopsy of pleura, lung, and mediastinum (32400, 32405)*
  *Thoracoscopy with biopsy (32607-32609)*
  *Thoracoscopy with diagnostic wedge resection resulting in anatomic lung resection (32668)*
  *Thoracotomy with diagnostic wedge resection resulting in anatomic lung resection (32507)*

**32096** **Thoracotomy, with diagnostic biopsy(ies) of lung infiltrate(s) (eg, wedge, incisional), unilateral**
  *EXCLUDES*   *Procedure performed more than one time per lung*
    *Removal of lung (32440-32445, 32488)*
  Code also appropriate add-on code for the more extensive procedure at the same location if diagnostic wedge resection results in the need for further surgery (32507, 32668)
  🔧 23.3   ✂ 23.3   **FUD** 090                    Ⓒ 80 ▢
  **AMA:** 2017,Jan,8; 2016,Jan,13; 2015,Jan,16; 2014,Jan,11; 2012,Oct,9-11; 2012,Sep,3-8

**32097** **Thoracotomy, with diagnostic biopsy(ies) of lung nodule(s) or mass(es) (eg, wedge, incisional), unilateral**
  *EXCLUDES*   *Procedure performed more than one time per lung*
    *Removal of lung (32440-32445, 32488)*
  Code also appropriate add-on code for the more extensive procedure in the same location if diagnostic wedge resection results in the need for further surgery (32507, 32668)
  🔧 23.2   ✂ 23.2   **FUD** 090                    Ⓒ 80 ▢
  **AMA:** 2017,Jan,8; 2016,Jan,13; 2015,Jan,16; 2014,Jan,11; 2012,Oct,9-11; 2012,Sep,3-8

Right main bronchus
Upper bronchial lobe
Middle bronchial lobe
Mass
Lower bronchial lobe
Trachea
Left main bronchus

**32098** **Thoracotomy, with biopsy(ies) of pleura**
  🔧 22.0   ✂ 22.0   **FUD** 090                    Ⓒ 80 ▢
  **AMA:** 2017,Jan,8; 2016,Jan,13; 2015,Jan,16; 2014,Jan,11

## 32100-32160 Open Procedures: Chest

*INCLUDES*   Exploration of penetrating wound of chest
*EXCLUDES*   *Lung resection (32480-32504)*
  *Wound exploration without thoracotomy for penetrating wound of chest (20101)*

**32100** **Thoracotomy; with exploration**
  *EXCLUDES*   *Excision of chest wall tumor including ribs (19260, 19271-19272)*
    *Extracorporeal membrane oxygenation (ECMO)/extracorporeal life support (ECLS) (33955-33957, [33963, 33964])*
    *Resection of apical lung tumor (32503-32504)*
  🔧 23.4   ✂ 23.4   **FUD** 090                    Ⓒ 80 ▢
  **AMA:** 2017,Jan,8; 2016,Jan,13; 2015,Jul,3; 2015,Jan,16; 2014,Jan,11; 2013,Jan,6-8

**32110** **with control of traumatic hemorrhage and/or repair of lung tear**
  🔧 42.3   ✂ 42.3   **FUD** 090                    Ⓒ 80 ▢
  **AMA:** 2017,Jan,8; 2016,Jan,13; 2015,Jan,16; 2014,Jan,11

**32120** **for postoperative complications**
  🔧 25.2   ✂ 25.2   **FUD** 090                    Ⓒ 80 ▢

**32124** **with open intrapleural pneumonolysis**
  🔧 26.8   ✂ 26.8   **FUD** 090                    Ⓒ 80 ▢
  **AMA:** 2017,Jan,8; 2016,Jan,13; 2015,Jan,16; 2014,Jan,11

**32140** **with cyst(s) removal, includes pleural procedure when performed**
  🔧 28.5   ✂ 28.5   **FUD** 090                    Ⓒ 80 ▢
  **AMA:** 2017,Jan,8; 2016,Jan,13; 2015,Jan,16; 2014,Jan,11

**32141** **with resection-plication of bullae, includes any pleural procedure when performed**
  *EXCLUDES*   *Lung volume reduction (32491)*
  🔧 44.1   ✂ 44.1   **FUD** 090                    Ⓒ 80 ▢
  **AMA:** 2017,Jan,8; 2016,Jan,13; 2015,Jan,16; 2014,Jan,11

**32150** **with removal of intrapleural foreign body or fibrin deposit**
  🔧 29.0   ✂ 29.0   **FUD** 090                    Ⓒ 80 ▢
  **AMA:** 2017,Jan,8; 2016,Jan,13; 2015,Jan,16; 2014,Jan,11

● New Code   ▲ Revised Code   ○ Reinstated   ● New Web Release   ▲ Revised Web Release   Unlisted   Not Covered   # Resequenced
⊘ AMA Mod 51 Exempt   ⑤ Optum Mod 51 Exempt   ⑥ Mod 63 Exempt   ✎ Non-FDA Drug   ★ Telemedicine   Ⓜ Maternity   Ⓐ Age Edit   ✚ Add-on   AMA: CPT Asst

**32151**    **with removal of intrapulmonary foreign body**
🖐 29.0    ⚕ 29.0    **FUD** 090     C 80 ▢

**32160**    **with cardiac massage**
🖐 22.8    ⚕ 22.8    **FUD** 090     C 80 ▢

## 32200-32320 Open Procedures: Lung

**32200**    **Pneumonostomy, with open drainage of abscess or cyst**
> EXCLUDES   *Image-guided, percutaneous drainage (eg, abscess, cyst) of lungs/mediastinum via catheter (49405)*
> 🔬 (75989)
🖐 32.6    ⚕ 32.6    **FUD** 090     C 80 ▢
**AMA:** 2013,Nov,9

**32215**    **Pleural scarification for repeat pneumothorax**
🖐 23.0    ⚕ 23.0    **FUD** 090     C 80 50 ▢

**32220**    **Decortication, pulmonary (separate procedure); total**
🖐 45.8    ⚕ 45.8    **FUD** 090     C 80 50 ▢

**32225**    **partial**
🖐 28.7    ⚕ 28.7    **FUD** 090     C 80 50 ▢

**32310**    **Pleurectomy, parietal (separate procedure)**
🖐 26.4    ⚕ 26.4    **FUD** 090     C 80 ▢
**AMA:** 1994,Win,1

**32320**    **Decortication and parietal pleurectomy**
🖐 46.2    ⚕ 46.2    **FUD** 090     C 80 ▢
**AMA:** 1994,Fall,1

## 32400-32405 Lung Biopsy

> EXCLUDES   *Open lung biopsy (32096-32097)*
> *Open mediastinal biopsy (39000-39010)*
> *Thoracoscopic (VATS) biopsy of lung, pericardium, pleural or mediastinal space (32604-32609)*

**32400**    **Biopsy, pleura, percutaneous needle**
> EXCLUDES   *Fine needle aspiration (10021-10022)*
> 🔬 (76942, 77002, 77012, 77021)
🖐 2.52    ⚕ 4.30    **FUD** 000     J A2 ▢
**AMA:** 2017,Jan,8; 2016,Jan,13; 2015,Jan,16; 2014,Jan,11

**32405**    **Biopsy, lung or mediastinum, percutaneous needle**
> EXCLUDES   *Fine needle aspiration (10022)*
> 🔬 (76942, 77002, 77012, 77021)
🖐 2.64    ⚕ 11.0    **FUD** 000     J A2 ▢
**AMA:** 2017,Jan,8; 2016,Jan,13; 2015,Jan,16; 2014,Jan,11; 2012,Jan,15-42

## 32440-32501 Lung Resection

**32440**    **Removal of lung, pneumonectomy;**
> Code also excision of chest wall tumor (19260-19272)
🖐 45.2    ⚕ 45.2    **FUD** 090     C 80 ▢
**AMA:** 2017,Jan,8; 2016,Jan,13; 2015,Jan,16; 2014,Jan,11; 2012,Oct,9-11; 2012,Sep,3-8

Removal of entire lung

**32442**    **with resection of segment of trachea followed by broncho-tracheal anastomosis (sleeve pneumonectomy)**
> Code also excision of chest wall tumor (19260-19272)
🖐 89.1    ⚕ 89.1    **FUD** 090     C 80 ▢
**AMA:** 2017,Jun,10; 2017,Jan,8; 2016,Jan,13; 2015,Jan,16; 2014,Jan,11; 2012,Oct,9-11; 2012,Sep,3-8

**32445**    **extrapleural**
> Code also empyemectomy with extrapleural pneumonectomy (32540)
> Code also excision of chest wall tumor (19260-19272)
🖐 102.    ⚕ 102.    **FUD** 090     C 80 ▢
**AMA:** 2017,Jan,8; 2016,Jan,13; 2015,Jan,16; 2014,Jan,11; 2012,Oct,9-11; 2012,Sep,3-8

**32480**    **Removal of lung, other than pneumonectomy; single lobe (lobectomy)**
> EXCLUDES   *Lung removal with bronchoplasty (32501)*
> Code also decortication (32320)
> Code also excision of chest wall tumor (19260-19272)
🖐 42.7    ⚕ 42.7    **FUD** 090     C 80 ▢
**AMA:** 2017,Jan,8; 2016,Jan,13; 2015,Jan,16; 2014,Jan,11; 2012,Oct,9-11; 2012,Sep,3-8

**32482**    **2 lobes (bilobectomy)**
> EXCLUDES   *Lung removal with bronchoplasty (32501)*
> Code also decortication (32320)
> Code also excision of chest wall tumor (19260-19272)
🖐 45.7    ⚕ 45.7    **FUD** 090     C 80 ▢
**AMA:** 2017,Jan,8; 2016,Jan,13; 2015,Jan,16; 2014,Jan,11; 2012,Oct,9-11; 2012,Sep,3-8; 2012,Jan,15-42

**32484**    **single segment (segmentectomy)**
> EXCLUDES   *Lung removal with bronchoplasty (32501)*
> Code also decortication (32320)
> Code also excision of chest wall tumor (19260-19272)
🖐 41.5    ⚕ 41.5    **FUD** 090     C 80 ▢
**AMA:** 2017,Jan,8; 2016,Jan,13; 2015,Jan,16; 2014,Jan,11; 2012,Oct,9-11; 2012,Sep,3-8

**32486**    **with circumferential resection of segment of bronchus followed by broncho-bronchial anastomosis (sleeve lobectomy)**
> Code also decortication (32320)
> Code also excision of chest wall tumor (19260-19272)
🖐 68.1    ⚕ 68.1    **FUD** 090     C 80 ▢
**AMA:** 2017,Jun,10; 2017,Jan,8; 2016,Jan,13; 2015,Jan,16; 2014,Jan,11; 2012,Oct,9-11; 2012,Sep,3-8

**32488**    **with all remaining lung following previous removal of a portion of lung (completion pneumonectomy)**
> Code also decortication (32320)
> Code also excision of chest wall tumor (19260-19272)
🖐 69.5    ⚕ 69.5    **FUD** 090     C 80 ▢
**AMA:** 2017,Jan,8; 2016,Jan,13; 2015,Jan,16; 2014,Jan,11; 2012,Oct,9-11; 2012,Sep,3-8

**32491**    **with resection-plication of emphysematous lung(s) (bullous or non-bullous) for lung volume reduction, sternal split or transthoracic approach, includes any pleural procedure, when performed**
🖐 42.6    ⚕ 42.6    **FUD** 090     C 80 50 ▢
**AMA:** 2017,Jan,8; 2016,Jan,13; 2015,Jan,16; 2014,Jan,11

**+ 32501**    **Resection and repair of portion of bronchus (bronchoplasty) when performed at time of lobectomy or segmentectomy (List separately in addition to code for primary procedure)**
> INCLUDES   Plastic closure of bronchus, not closure of a resected end of bronchus
> Code first (32480-32484)
🖐 7.10    ⚕ 7.10    **FUD** ZZZ     C 80 ▢
**AMA:** 1995,Win,1

| 26/TC PC/TC Only | A2-Z3 ASC Payment | 50 Bilateral | ♂ Male Only | ♀ Female Only | 🖐 Facility RVU | ⚕ Non-Facility RVU | ▢ CCI |
| FUD Follow-up Days | CMS: IOM (Pub 100) | A-Y OPPSI | 80/80 Surg Assist Allowed / w/Doc | | 🔬 Lab Crosswalk | 🔬 Radiology Crosswalk | ✖ CLIA |

116       CPT © 2017 American Medical Association. All Rights Reserved.       © 2017 Optum360, LLC

## 32503-32504 Excision of Lung Neoplasm

EXCLUDES *Excision of chest wall tumor involving ribs (19260, 19271-19272)*
*Lung resection performed in conjunction with chest wall resection*
*Thoracentesis, needle or catheter, aspiration of the pleural space (32554-32555)*
*Thoracotomy; with exploration (32100)*
*Tube thoracostomy (32551)*

**32503** **Resection of apical lung tumor (eg, Pancoast tumor), including chest wall resection, rib(s) resection(s), neurovascular dissection, when performed; without chest wall reconstruction(s)**
52.3  52.3  **FUD** 090                                    C 80

AMA: 2012,Oct,9-11; 2012,Sep,3-8

**32504** **with chest wall reconstruction**
60.1  60.1  **FUD** 090                                    C 80

AMA: 2012,Oct,9-11; 2012,Sep,3-8

## 32505-32507 Thoracotomy with Wedge Resection

INCLUDES Wedge technique with tissue obtained with precise consideration of margins and complete resection

Code also resection of chest wall tumor with lung resection when performed (19260-19272)

**32505** **Thoracotomy; with therapeutic wedge resection (eg, mass, nodule), initial**

EXCLUDES *Removal of lung (32440, 32442, 32445, 32488)*

Code also a more extensive procedure of the lung when performed on the contralateral lung or different lobe with modifier 59 regardless of intraoperative pathology consultation
26.9  26.9  **FUD** 090                                    C 80

AMA: 2017,Jan,8; 2016,Jan,13; 2015,Jan,16; 2014,Jan,11; 2012,Oct,9-11; 2012,Sep,3-8

**+ 32506** **with therapeutic wedge resection (eg, mass or nodule), each additional resection, ipsilateral (List separately in addition to code for primary procedure)**

Code also a more extensive procedure of the lung when performed on the contralateral lung or different lobe with modifier 59

Code first (32505)
4.54  4.54  **FUD** ZZZ                                    C 80

AMA: 2017,Jan,8; 2016,Jan,13; 2015,Jan,16; 2014,Jan,11; 2012,Oct,9-11; 2012,Sep,3-8

**+ 32507** **with diagnostic wedge resection followed by anatomic lung resection (List separately in addition to code for primary procedure)**

INCLUDES Classification as a diagnostic wedge resection if intraoperative pathology consultation dictates more extensive resection in the same anatomical area

EXCLUDES *Diagnostic wedge resection by thoracoscopy (32668)*
*Therapeutic wedge resection (32505-32506, 32666-32667)*

Code first (32440, 32442, 32445, 32480-32488, 32503-32504)
4.54  4.54  **FUD** ZZZ                                    C 80

AMA: 2017,Jan,8; 2016,Jan,13; 2015,Jan,16; 2014,Jan,11; 2012,Oct,9-11; 2012,Sep,3-8

## 32540 Removal of Empyema

**32540** **Extrapleural enucleation of empyema (empyemectomy)**

EXCLUDES *Lung removal code when empyemectomy is performed with lobectomy (see appropriate lung removal code)*

Code also appropriate removal of lung code when done with lobectomy (32480-32488)
50.2  50.2  **FUD** 090                                    C 80

AMA: 1994,Fall,1

## 32550-32552 Chest Tube/Catheter

**32550** **Insertion of indwelling tunneled pleural catheter with cuff**

EXCLUDES *Procedures performed on same side of chest with (32554-32557)*

(75989)
6.05  20.2  **FUD** 000                                    J 62

AMA: 2017,Jan,8; 2016,Jan,13; 2015,Jan,16; 2014,May,3; 2014,Mar,13; 2014,Jan,11; 2012,Nov,3-5; 2012,Jan,15-42

**32551** **Tube thoracostomy, includes connection to drainage system (eg, water seal), when performed, open (separate procedure)**
4.56  4.56  **FUD** 000                                    T 50

AMA: 2017,Jun,10; 2017,Jan,8; 2016,Jan,13; 2015,Jan,16; 2014,May,3; 2014,Jan,11; 2012,Nov,3-5

**32552** **Removal of indwelling tunneled pleural catheter with cuff**
4.58  5.28  **FUD** 010                                    02 62 80

AMA: 2017,Jan,8; 2016,Jan,13; 2015,Jan,16; 2014,Jan,11; 2012,Nov,3-5; 2012,Jan,15-42

## 32553 Intrathoracic Placement Radiation Therapy Devices

EXCLUDES *Percutaneous placement of interstitial device(s) for radiation therapy guidance: intra-abdominal, intrapelvic, and/or retroperitoneal (49411)*

Code also device

**32553** **Placement of interstitial device(s) for radiation therapy guidance (eg, fiducial markers, dosimeter), percutaneous, intra-thoracic, single or multiple**

(76942, 77002, 77012, 77021)
5.25  14.8  **FUD** 000                                    S 62 80

AMA: 2017,Jan,8; 2016,Jun,3; 2016,Jan,13; 2015,Jun,6; 2015,Jan,16; 2014,Jan,11

## 32554-32557 Pleural Aspiration and Drainage

EXCLUDES *Chest x-ray performed to confirm position of chest tube, complications, adequacy of procedure*
*Open tube thoracostomy (32551)*
*Placement of indwelling tunneled pleural drainage catheter (cuffed) (32550)*
*Radiologic guidance (75989, 76942, 77002, 77012, 77021)*

**32554** **Thoracentesis, needle or catheter, aspiration of the pleural space; without imaging guidance**
2.59  5.74  **FUD** 000                                    T 62 50

AMA: 2017,Jan,8; 2016,Jan,13; 2015,Jan,16; 2014,Jan,11; 2013,Nov,9; 2012,Nov,3-5

**32555** **with imaging guidance**
3.25  8.24  **FUD** 000                                    T 62 50

AMA: 2017,Jan,8; 2016,Jan,13; 2015,Jan,16; 2014,Jan,11; 2013,Nov,9; 2012,Nov,3-5

**32556** **Pleural drainage, percutaneous, with insertion of indwelling catheter; without imaging guidance**
3.56  15.7  **FUD** 000                                    J 62 50

AMA: 2017,Jan,8; 2016,Jan,13; 2015,Jan,16; 2014,Jan,11; 2013,Nov,9; 2012,Nov,3-5

**32557** **with imaging guidance**
4.43  14.5  **FUD** 000                                    T 62 50

AMA: 2017,Jan,8; 2016,Jan,13; 2015,Jan,16; 2014,May,3; 2014,Jan,11; 2013,Nov,9; 2012,Nov,3-5

## 32560-32562 Instillation Drug/Chemical by Chest Tube

EXCLUDES *Insertion of chest tube (32551)*

**32560** **Instillation, via chest tube/catheter, agent for pleurodesis (eg, talc for recurrent or persistent pneumothorax)**
2.26  6.93  **FUD** 000                                    T

AMA: 2017,Jan,8; 2016,Jan,13; 2015,Jan,16; 2014,Jan,11

**32561** **Instillation(s), via chest tube/catheter, agent for fibrinolysis (eg, fibrinolytic agent for break up of multiloculated effusion); initial day**

EXCLUDES *Use of code more than one time on the date of initial treatment*
1.98  2.64  **FUD** 000                                    T 80

AMA: 2017,Jan,8; 2016,Jan,13; 2015,Jan,16; 2014,Jan,11

---

**32562** **subsequent day**

> *EXCLUDES* *Use of code more than one time on each day of subsequent treatment*

⚕ 1.78   ✂ 2.37   **FUD** 000   T 80 ▭

**AMA:** 2017,Jan,8; 2016,Jan,13; 2015,Jan,16; 2014,Jan,11

## 32601-32674 Thoracic Surgery: Video-Assisted (VATS)

> INCLUDES  Diagnostic thoracoscopy in surgical thoracoscopy

**32601** **Thoracoscopy, diagnostic (separate procedure); lungs, pericardial sac, mediastinal or pleural space, without biopsy**

⚕ 8.94   ✂ 8.94   **FUD** 000   J 80 ▭

**AMA:** 2017,Jan,8; 2016,Jan,13; 2015,Jan,16; 2014,Jan,11; 2013,Aug,13; 2012,Oct,9-11; 2012,Sep,3-8

**32604** **pericardial sac, with biopsy**

> *EXCLUDES* *Open biopsy of pericardium (39010)*

⚕ 14.0   ✂ 14.0   **FUD** 000   J 80 ▭

**AMA:** 2017,Jan,8; 2016,Jan,13; 2015,Jan,16; 2014,Jan,11; 2013,Aug,13; 2012,Oct,9-11; 2012,Sep,3-8

**32606** **mediastinal space, with biopsy**

⚕ 13.4   ✂ 13.4   **FUD** 000   J 80 ▭

**AMA:** 2017,Jan,8; 2016,Jan,13; 2015,Jan,16; 2014,Jan,11; 2013,Aug,13; 2012,Oct,9-11; 2012,Sep,3-8

**32607** **Thoracoscopy; with diagnostic biopsy(ies) of lung infiltrate(s) (eg, wedge, incisional), unilateral**

> *EXCLUDES* *Removal of lung (32440-32445, 32488)*
> *Thoracoscopy, surgical; with removal of lung (32671)*
> *Use of code more than one time per lung*

⚕ 8.94   ✂ 8.94   **FUD** 000   J 80 ▭

**AMA:** 2017,Jan,8; 2016,Jan,13; 2015,Jan,16; 2014,Jan,11; 2013,Aug,13; 2012,Oct,9-11; 2012,Sep,3-8

**32608** **with diagnostic biopsy(ies) of lung nodule(s) or mass(es) (eg, wedge, incisional), unilateral**

> *EXCLUDES* *Removal of lung (32440-32445, 32488)*
> *Thoracoscopy, surgical; with removal of lung (32671)*
> *Use of code more than one time per lung*

⚕ 10.9   ✂ 10.9   **FUD** 000   J 80 ▭

**AMA:** 2017,Jan,8; 2016,Jan,13; 2015,Jan,16; 2014,Jan,11; 2013,Aug,13; 2012,Oct,9-11; 2012,Sep,3-8

**32609** **with biopsy(ies) of pleura**

⚕ 7.50   ✂ 7.50   **FUD** 000   J 80 ▭

**AMA:** 2017,Jan,8; 2016,Jan,13; 2015,Jan,16; 2014,Jan,11; 2013,Aug,13; 2012,Oct,9-11; 2012,Sep,3-8

**32650** **Thoracoscopy, surgical; with pleurodesis (eg, mechanical or chemical)**

⚕ 19.2   ✂ 19.2   **FUD** 090   C 80 50 ▭

**AMA:** 2017,Jan,8; 2016,Jan,13; 2015,Jan,16; 2014,Jan,11; 2013,Aug,13

**32651** **with partial pulmonary decortication**

⚕ 31.7   ✂ 31.7   **FUD** 090   C 80 50 ▭

**AMA:** 2017,Jan,8; 2016,Jan,13; 2015,Jan,16; 2014,Jan,11; 2013,Aug,13

**32652** **with total pulmonary decortication, including intrapleural pneumonolysis**

⚕ 48.1   ✂ 48.1   **FUD** 090   C 80 50 ▭

**AMA:** 2017,Jan,8; 2016,Jan,13; 2015,Jan,16; 2014,Jan,11; 2013,Aug,13

**32653** **with removal of intrapleural foreign body or fibrin deposit**

⚕ 30.6   ✂ 30.6   **FUD** 090   C 80 ▭

**AMA:** 2017,Jan,8; 2016,Jan,13; 2015,Jan,16; 2014,Jan,11; 2013,Aug,13

**32654** **with control of traumatic hemorrhage**

⚕ 34.2   ✂ 34.2   **FUD** 090   C 80 50 ▭

**AMA:** 2017,Jan,8; 2016,Jan,13; 2015,Jan,16; 2014,Jan,11; 2013,Aug,13

**32655** **with resection-plication of bullae, includes any pleural procedure when performed**

> *EXCLUDES* *Thoracoscopic lung volume reduction surgery (32672)*

⚕ 27.6   ✂ 27.6   **FUD** 090   C 80 50 ▭

**AMA:** 2017,Jan,8; 2016,Jan,13; 2015,Jan,16; 2014,Jan,11; 2013,Aug,13; 2012,Jan,15-42

**32656** **with parietal pleurectomy**

⚕ 23.1   ✂ 23.1   **FUD** 090   C 80 50 ▭

**AMA:** 2017,Jan,8; 2016,Jan,13; 2015,Jan,16; 2014,Jan,11; 2013,Aug,13

**32658** **with removal of clot or foreign body from pericardial sac**

⚕ 20.6   ✂ 20.6   **FUD** 090   C 80 ▭

**AMA:** 2017,Jan,8; 2016,Jan,13; 2015,Jan,16; 2014,Jan,11; 2013,Aug,13

**32659** **with creation of pericardial window or partial resection of pericardial sac for drainage**

⚕ 21.1   ✂ 21.1   **FUD** 090   C 80 ▭

**AMA:** 2017,Jan,8; 2016,Jan,13; 2015,Jan,16; 2014,Jan,11; 2013,Aug,13

**32661** **with excision of pericardial cyst, tumor, or mass**

⚕ 23.1   ✂ 23.1   **FUD** 090   C 80 ▭

**AMA:** 2017,Jan,8; 2016,Jan,13; 2015,Jan,16; 2014,Jan,11; 2013,Aug,13

**32662** **with excision of mediastinal cyst, tumor, or mass**

⚕ 25.8   ✂ 25.8   **FUD** 090   C 80 ▭

**AMA:** 2017,Jan,8; 2016,Jan,13; 2015,Jan,16; 2014,Jan,11; 2013,Aug,13; 2012,Jan,15-42

**32663** **with lobectomy (single lobe)**

> *EXCLUDES* *Thoracoscopic segmentectomy (32669)*

⚕ 40.5   ✂ 40.5   **FUD** 090   C 80 ▭

**AMA:** 2017,Jan,8; 2016,Jan,13; 2015,Jan,16; 2014,Jan,11; 2013,Aug,13; 2012,Oct,9-11; 2012,Sep,3-8

**32664** **with thoracic sympathectomy**

⚕ 24.4   ✂ 24.4   **FUD** 090   C 80 50 ▭

**AMA:** 2017,Jan,8; 2016,Jan,13; 2015,Dec,16; 2015,Jan,16; 2014,Jan,11; 2013,Aug,13; 2012,Jan,15-42

**32665** **with esophagomyotomy (Heller type)**

> *EXCLUDES* *Exploratory thoracoscopy with and without biopsy (32601-32609)*

⚕ 35.7   ✂ 35.7   **FUD** 090   C 80 ▭

**AMA:** 2017,Jan,8; 2016,Jan,13; 2015,Jan,16; 2014,Jan,11; 2013,Aug,13

**32666** **with therapeutic wedge resection (eg, mass, nodule), initial unilateral**

> *EXCLUDES* *Removal of lung (32440-32445, 32488)*
> *Thoracoscopy, surgical; with removal of lung (32671)*
> Code also a more extensive procedure of the lung when performed on the contralateral lung or different lobe with modifier 59 regardless of pathology consultation

⚕ 25.2   ✂ 25.2   **FUD** 090   C 80 50 ▭

**AMA:** 2017,Jan,8; 2016,Jan,13; 2015,Jan,16; 2014,Jan,11; 2013,Aug,13; 2012,Oct,9-11; 2012,Sep,3-8

**+ 32667** **with therapeutic wedge resection (eg, mass or nodule), each additional resection, ipsilateral (List separately in addition to code for primary procedure)**

> *EXCLUDES* *Removal of lung (32440-32445, 32488)*
> *Thoracoscopy, surgical; with removal of lung (32671)*
> Code also a more extensive procedure of the lung when performed on the contralateral lung or different lobe with modifier 59 regardless of intraoperative pathology consultation
> Code first (32666)

⚕ 4.56   ✂ 4.56   **FUD** ZZZ   C 80 ▭

**AMA:** 2017,Jan,8; 2016,Jan,13; 2015,Jan,16; 2014,Jan,11; 2013,Aug,13; 2012,Oct,9-11; 2012,Sep,3-8

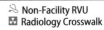

**+ 32668** **with diagnostic wedge resection followed by anatomic lung resection (List separately in addition to code for primary procedure)**

INCLUDES Classification as a diagnostic wedge resection if intraoperative pathology consultation dictates more extensive resection in the same anatomical area

Code first (32440-32488, 32503-32504, 32663, 32669-32671)

4.56  4.56  **FUD** ZZZ  C 80

**AMA:** 2017,Jan,8; 2016,Jan,13; 2015,Jan,16; 2014,Jan,11; 2013,Aug,13; 2012,Oct,9-11; 2012,Sep,3-8

**32669** **with removal of a single lung segment (segmentectomy)**

38.9  38.9  **FUD** 090  C 80

**AMA:** 2017,Jan,8; 2016,Jan,13; 2015,Jan,16; 2014,Jan,11; 2013,Aug,13; 2012,Oct,9-11; 2012,Sep,3-8

**32670** **with removal of two lobes (bilobectomy)**

46.4  46.4  **FUD** 090  C 80

**AMA:** 2017,Jan,8; 2016,Jan,13; 2015,Jan,16; 2014,Jan,11; 2013,Aug,13; 2012,Oct,9-11; 2012,Sep,3-8

**32671** **with removal of lung (pneumonectomy)**

51.4  51.4  **FUD** 090  C 80

**AMA:** 2017,Jan,8; 2016,Jan,13; 2015,Jan,16; 2014,Jan,11; 2013,Aug,13; 2012,Oct,9-11; 2012,Sep,3-8

**32672** **with resection-plication for emphysematous lung (bullous or non-bullous) for lung volume reduction (LVRS), unilateral includes any pleural procedure, when performed**

44.1  44.1  **FUD** 090  C 80

**AMA:** 2017,Jan,8; 2016,Jan,13; 2015,Jan,16; 2014,Jan,11; 2013,Aug,13; 2012,Oct,9-11; 2012,Sep,3-8

**32673** **with resection of thymus, unilateral or bilateral**

EXCLUDES Exploratory thoracoscopy with and without biopsy (32601-32609)
Open excision mediastinal cyst (39200)
Open excision mediastinal tumor (39220)
Open thymectomy (60520-60522)

35.2  35.2  **FUD** 090  C 80

**AMA:** 2017,Jan,8; 2016,Jan,13; 2015,Jan,16; 2014,Jan,11; 2013,Aug,13; 2012,Oct,9-11; 2012,Sep,3-8

**+ 32674** **with mediastinal and regional lymphadenectomy (List separately in addition to code for primary procedure)**

INCLUDES Mediastinal lymph nodes:
Left side:
Aortopulmonary window
Inferior pulmonary ligament
Paraesophageal
Subcarinal
Right side:
Inferior pulmonary ligament
Paraesophageal
Paratracheal
Subcarinal

EXCLUDES Mediastinal and regional lymphadenectomy by thoracotomy (38746)

Code first (19260, 31760, 31766, 31786, 32096-32200, 32220-32320, 32440-32491, 32503-32505, 32601-32663, 32666, 32669-32673, 32815, 33025, 33030, 33050-33130, 39200-39220, 39560-39561, 43101, 43112, 43117-43118, 43122-43123, 43287-43288, 43351, 60270, 60505)

6.27  6.27  **FUD** ZZZ  C 80

**AMA:** 2017,Jan,8; 2016,Jan,13; 2015,Jan,16; 2014,May,3; 2014,Jan,11; 2013,Aug,13; 2012,Oct,9-11; 2012,Sep,3-8

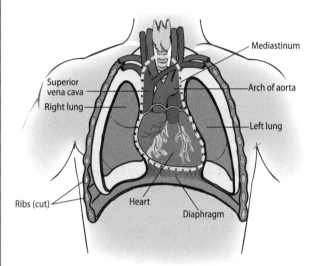

Mediastinum
Superior vena cava
Arch of aorta
Right lung
Left lung
Ribs (cut)
Heart
Diaphragm

## 32701 Target Delineation for Stereotactic Radiation Therapy

INCLUDES Collaboration between the radiation oncologist and surgeon
Correlation of tumor and contiguous body structures
Determination of borders and volume of tumor
Identification of fiducial markers
Verification of target when fiducial markers are not used

EXCLUDES Fiducial marker insertion (31626, 32553)
Procedure performed by same physician as radiation treatment management (77427-77499)
Radiation oncology services (77295, 77331, 77370, 77373, 77435)
Therapeutic radiology (77261-77799 [77295, 77385, 77386, 77387, 77424, 77425])

**32701** **Thoracic target(s) delineation for stereotactic body radiation therapy (SRS/SBRT), (photon or particle beam), entire course of treatment**

6.21  6.21  **FUD** XXX  B 80 26

**AMA:** 2017,Jan,8; 2016,Jan,13; 2015,Jun,6

## 32800-32820 Chest Repair and Reconstruction Procedures

**32800** **Repair lung hernia through chest wall**

27.3  27.3  **FUD** 090  C 80

**32810** **Closure of chest wall following open flap drainage for empyema (Clagett type procedure)**

25.8  25.8  **FUD** 090  C 80

**32815** **Open closure of major bronchial fistula**

80.8  80.8  **FUD** 090  C 80

**32820**    Major reconstruction, chest wall (posttraumatic)
    ⚙ 40.7    ⚕ 40.7    **FUD** 090    C 80

## 32850-32856 Lung Transplant Procedures

INCLUDES    Harvesting donor lung(s), cold preservation, preparation of donor lung(s), transplantation into recipient

EXCLUDES    *Assessment of marginal cadaver donor lungs (0494T-0496T)*
    *Repairs or resection of donor lung(s) (32491, 32505-32507, 35216, 35276)*

**32850**    Donor pneumonectomy(s) (including cold preservation), from cadaver donor
    ⚙ 0.00    ⚕ 0.00    **FUD** XXX    C
    **AMA:** 1993,Win,1

**32851**    Lung transplant, single; without cardiopulmonary bypass
    ⚙ 95.6    ⚕ 95.6    **FUD** 090    C 80
    **AMA:** 1993,Win,1

**32852**    with cardiopulmonary bypass
    ⚙ 104.    ⚕ 104.    **FUD** 090    C 80
    **AMA:** 1993,Win,1

**32853**    Lung transplant, double (bilateral sequential or en bloc); without cardiopulmonary bypass
    ⚙ 133.    ⚕ 133.    **FUD** 090    C 80
    **AMA:** 1993,Win,1

**32854**    with cardiopulmonary bypass
    ⚙ 141.    ⚕ 141.    **FUD** 090    C 80
    **AMA:** 1993,Win,1

**32855**    Backbench standard preparation of cadaver donor lung allograft prior to transplantation, including dissection of allograft from surrounding soft tissues to prepare pulmonary venous/atrial cuff, pulmonary artery, and bronchus; unilateral
    ⚙ 0.00    ⚕ 0.00    **FUD** XXX    C 80

**32856**    bilateral
    ⚙ 0.00    ⚕ 0.00    **FUD** XXX    C 80

## 32900-32997 Chest and Respiratory Procedures

**32900**    Resection of ribs, extrapleural, all stages
    ⚙ 40.7    ⚕ 40.7    **FUD** 090    C 80

**32905**    Thoracoplasty, Schede type or extrapleural (all stages);
    ⚙ 38.9    ⚕ 38.9    **FUD** 090    C 80

**32906**    with closure of bronchopleural fistula
    ⚙ 47.9    ⚕ 47.9    **FUD** 090    C 80
    EXCLUDES    *Open closure of bronchial fistula (32815)*
        *Resection first rib for thoracic compression (21615-21616)*

**32940**    Pneumonolysis, extraperiosteal, including filling or packing procedures
    ⚙ 35.8    ⚕ 35.8    **FUD** 090    C 80

**32960**    Pneumothorax, therapeutic, intrapleural injection of air
    ⚙ 2.68    ⚕ 3.66    **FUD** 000    T 62

*32994*    Resequenced code. See code following 32998.

**32997**    Total lung lavage (unilateral)
    EXCLUDES    *Broncho-alveolar lavage by bronchoscopy (31624)*
    ⚙ 9.88    ⚕ 9.88    **FUD** 000    C 50
    **AMA:** 2017,Jan,8; 2016,Jan,13; 2015,Jan,16; 2014,Jan,11

## 32998-32999 [32994] Destruction of Lung Neoplasm

▲ **32998**    Ablation therapy for reduction or eradication of 1 or more pulmonary tumor(s) including pleura or chest wall when involved by tumor extension, percutaneous, including imaging guidance when performed, unilateral; radiofrequency
    ⚙ 8.19    ⚕ 54.9    **FUD** 000    J 62 80 50

● # **32994**    cryoablation
    ⚙ 0.00    ⚕ 0.00    **FUD** 000

**32999**    Unlisted procedure, lungs and pleura
    ⚙ 0.00    ⚕ 0.00    **FUD** YYY    T
    **AMA:** 2017,Jan,8; 2016,Jan,13; 2015,Dec,16; 2015,Jun,6; 2015,Jan,16; 2014,Jan,11; 2012,Jan,15-42

26/TC PC/TC Only    A2-Z3 ASC Payment    50 Bilateral    ♂ Male Only    ♀ Female Only    ⚙ Facility RVU    ⚕ Non-Facility RVU    CCI
**FUD** Follow-up Days    **CMS:** IOM (Pub 100)    A-Y OPPSI    80/80 Surg Assist Allowed / w/Doc    Lab Crosswalk    Radiology Crosswalk    CLIA
CPT © 2017 American Medical Association. All Rights Reserved.

© 2017 Optum360, LLC

## 33010-33050 Procedures of the Pericardial Sac

EXCLUDES Surgical thoracoscopy (video-assisted thoracic surgery [VATS]) procedures of pericardium (32601, 32604, 32658-32659, 32661)

**33010** Pericardiocentesis; initial
🔲 (76930)
🔧 3.11 ⚬ 3.11 **FUD** 000 T A2 🖵
**AMA:** 2017,Jan,8; 2016,Sep,9; 2016,Jan,13; 2015,Feb,10

Fluid is drained by multi-port syringe

Trachea
Aorta
Sternum
Heart in pericardium
Diaphragm

A centesis syringe is inserted into the pericardial sac, either under fluoroscopic guidance or by use of anatomical landmarks, and excess fluid is removed

**33011** subsequent
🔲 (76930)
🔧 3.14 ⚬ 3.14 **FUD** 000 T A2 80 🖵
**AMA:** 2017,Jan,8; 2016,Sep,9; 2016,Jan,13; 2015,Feb,10; 2015,Jan,16; 2014,Jan,11

**33015** Tube pericardiostomy
🔧 14.8 ⚬ 14.8 **FUD** 090 C 🖵
**AMA:** 2017,Jan,8; 2016,Jan,13; 2015,Jan,16; 2014,Aug,14

**33020** Pericardiotomy for removal of clot or foreign body (primary procedure)
🔧 25.4 ⚬ 25.4 **FUD** 090 C 80 🖵
**AMA:** 1997,Nov,1

**33025** Creation of pericardial window or partial resection for drainage
EXCLUDES Surgical thoracoscopy (video-assisted thoracic surgery [VATS]) creation of pericardial window (32659)
🔧 23.1 ⚬ 23.1 **FUD** 090 C 80 🖵
**AMA:** 1997,Nov,1

**33030** Pericardiectomy, subtotal or complete; without cardiopulmonary bypass
INCLUDES Delorme pericardiectomy
🔧 58.1 ⚬ 58.1 **FUD** 090 C 80 🖵
**AMA:** 1997,Nov,1; 1994,Win,1

**33031** with cardiopulmonary bypass
🔧 71.6 ⚬ 71.6 **FUD** 090 C 80 🖵
**AMA:** 1997,Nov,1; 1994,Win,1

**33050** Resection of pericardial cyst or tumor
EXCLUDES Open biopsy of pericardium (39010)
Surgical thoracoscopy (video-assisted thoracic surgery [VATS]) resection of cyst, mass, or tumor of pericardium (32661)
🔧 28.9 ⚬ 28.9 **FUD** 090 C 80 🖵
**AMA:** 1997,Nov,1

## 33120-33130 Neoplasms of Heart

Code also removal of thrombus through a separate heart incision, when performed (33310-33315); append modifier 59 to (33315)

**33120** Excision of intracardiac tumor, resection with cardiopulmonary bypass
🔧 60.9 ⚬ 60.9 **FUD** 090 C 80 🖵
**AMA:** 2017,Jan,8; 2016,Jan,13; 2015,Jan,16; 2014,Jan,11

**33130** Resection of external cardiac tumor
🔧 40.0 ⚬ 40.0 **FUD** 090 C 80 🖵
**AMA:** 2017,Jan,8; 2016,Jan,13; 2015,Jan,16; 2014,Jan,11

## 33140-33141 Transmyocardial Revascularization

**33140** Transmyocardial laser revascularization, by thoracotomy; (separate procedure)
🔧 45.7 ⚬ 45.7 **FUD** 090 C 80 🖵
**AMA:** 2017,Jan,8; 2016,Jan,13; 2015,Jan,16; 2014,Jan,11; 2012,Jan,15-42

**+ 33141** performed at the time of other open cardiac procedure(s) (List separately in addition to code for primary procedure)
Code first (33390-33391, 33404-33496, 33510-33536, 33542)
🔧 3.83 ⚬ 3.83 **FUD** ZZZ C 80 🖵
**AMA:** 2017,Jan,8; 2016,Jan,13; 2015,Jan,16; 2014,Jan,11

## 33202-33203 Placement Epicardial Leads

INCLUDES Imaging guidance:
Fluoroscopy (76000-76001)
Ultrasound (76942, 76998, 93318)
Temporary pacemaker (33210-33211)
Code also insertion of pulse generator when performed by same physician/same surgical session (33212-33213, [33221], 33230-33231, 33240)

**33202** Insertion of epicardial electrode(s); open incision (eg, thoracotomy, median sternotomy, subxiphoid approach)
🔧 22.4 ⚬ 22.4 **FUD** 090 C 🖵
**AMA:** 2017,Jan,8; 2016,Aug,5; 2016,May,5; 2016,Jan,13; 2015,May,3; 2015,Jan,16; 2014,Nov,5; 2014,Jan,11; 2012,Jun,3-9

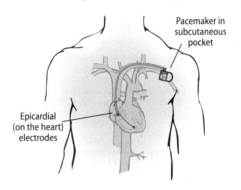

Pacemaker in subcutaneous pocket
Epicardial (on the heart) electrodes

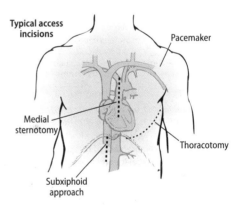

Typical access incisions
Medial sternotomy
Pacemaker
Thoracotomy
Subxiphoid approach

**33203** endoscopic approach (eg, thoracoscopy, pericardioscopy)
🔧 23.3 ⚬ 23.3 **FUD** 090 C 🖵
**AMA:** 2017,Jan,8; 2016,Aug,5; 2016,May,5; 2016,Jan,13; 2015,May,3; 2015,Jan,16; 2014,Nov,5; 2014,Jan,11; 2012,Jun,3-9

---

● New Code ▲ Revised Code ○ Reinstated ● New Web Release ▲ Revised Web Release Unlisted Not Covered # Resequenced
⊘ AMA Mod 51 Exempt ⑪ Optum Mod 51 Exempt ⑥ Mod 63 Exempt ✓ Non-FDA Drug ★ Telemedicine Ⓜ Maternity Ⓐ Age Edit + Add-on **AMA:** CPT Asst
© 2017 Optum360, LLC    CPT © 2017 American Medical Association. All Rights Reserved.

## 33206-33214 [33221] Pacemakers

**INCLUDES** Device evaluation (93279-93299 [93260, 93261])
Dual lead: device that paces and senses in two heart chambers
Imaging guidance:
Fluoroscopy (76000-76001)
Ultrasound (76942, 76998, 93318)
Multiple lead: device that paces and senses in three or more heart chambers
Radiological supervision and interpretation for pacemaker procedure
Single lead: device that paces and senses in one heart chamber
Skin pocket revision, when performed
If revision includes incision/drainage of a wound infection or hematoma code also (10140, 10180, 11042-11047 [11045, 11046])
Temporary pacemaker (33210-33211)

**EXCLUDES** Electrode repositioning:
*Left ventricle (33226)*
*Pacemaker (33215)*
*Insertion of lead for left ventricular (biventricular) pacing (33224-33225)*
*Leadless pacemaker systems (0387T-0391T)*

**33206 Insertion of new or replacement of permanent pacemaker with transvenous electrode(s); atrial**

**INCLUDES** Pulse generator insertion/transvenous electrode placement

**EXCLUDES** *Insertion of transvenous electrode (33216-33217)*
*Removal and replacement of pacemaker pulse generator (33227-33229)*

Code also removal of pacemaker pulse generator and electrodes when removal and replacement of pulse generator and electrodes is performed (33233, 33234, 33235)

🔲 13.0   ⚖ 13.0   **FUD** 090      J J8 ▢

**AMA:** 2017,Jan,8; 2016,Aug,5; 2016,May,5; 2016,Jan,13; 2015,May,3; 2015,Jan,16; 2014,Nov,5; 2014,Jan,11; 2013,Apr,10-11; 2012,Jun,3-9; 2012,Jan,15-42

**33207 ventricular**

**EXCLUDES** *Insertion of transvenous electrode (33216-33217)*
*Removal and replacement of pacemaker pulse generator (33227-33229)*

Code also removal of pacemaker pulse generator and electrodes when removal and replacement of pulse generator and electrodes is performed (33224, 33225, 33233)

🔲 13.9   ⚖ 13.9   **FUD** 090      J J8 ▢

**AMA:** 2017,Jan,8; 2016,Aug,5; 2016,May,5; 2016,Jan,13; 2015,May,3; 2015,Jan,16; 2014,Nov,5; 2014,Jan,11; 2013,Apr,10-11; 2012,Jun,3-9; 2012,Jan,15-42

**33208 atrial and ventricular**

**INCLUDES** Pulse generator insertion/transvenous electrode placement

**EXCLUDES** *Insertion of transvenous electrode (33216-33217)*
*Removal and replacement of pacemaker pulse generator (33227-33229)*

Code also removal of pacemaker pulse generator and electrodes when removal and replacement of pulse generator and electrodes is performed (33233, 33234, 33235)

🔲 15.1   ⚖ 15.1   **FUD** 090      J J8 ▢

**AMA:** 2017,Jan,8; 2016,Aug,5; 2016,May,5; 2016,Jan,13; 2015,May,3; 2015,Jan,16; 2014,Nov,5; 2014,Jan,11; 2013,Apr,10-11; 2012,Jun,3-9; 2012,Jan,15-42

**33210 Insertion or replacement of temporary transvenous single chamber cardiac electrode or pacemaker catheter (separate procedure)**

🔲 4.81   ⚖ 4.81   **FUD** 000      J G2 ▢

**AMA:** 2017,Jan,8; 2016,Aug,5; 2016,May,5; 2016,Jan,13; 2015,May,3; 2015,Jan,16; 2014,Nov,5; 2014,Jan,11; 2013,Jan,6-8; 2012,Jun,3-9

**33211 Insertion or replacement of temporary transvenous dual chamber pacing electrodes (separate procedure)**

🔲 4.92   ⚖ 4.92   **FUD** 000      J J8 ▢

**AMA:** 2017,Jan,8; 2016,Aug,5; 2016,May,5; 2016,Jan,13; 2015,May,3; 2015,Jan,16; 2014,Nov,5; 2014,Jan,11; 2012,Jun,3-9

**33212 Insertion of pacemaker pulse generator only; with existing single lead**

**EXCLUDES** *Insertion of a single transvenous electrode (33216-33217)*
*Removal and replacement of pacemaker pulse generator (33227-33229)*
*Removal of permanent pacemaker pulse generator only (33233)*

Code also placement of epicardial leads by same physician/same surgical session (33202-33203)

🔲 9.28   ⚖ 9.28   **FUD** 090      J J8 ▢

**AMA:** 2017,Jan,8; 2016,Aug,5; 2016,May,5; 2016,Jan,13; 2015,May,3; 2015,Jan,16; 2014,Nov,5; 2014,Jan,11; 2012,Jun,3-9; 2012,Jan,15-42

**33213 with existing dual leads**

**EXCLUDES** *Insertion of a single transvenous electrode (33216-33217)*
*Removal and replacement of pacemaker pulse generator (33227-33229)*
*Removal of permanent pacemaker pulse generator only (33233)*

Code also placement of epicardial leads by same physician/same surgical session (33202-33203)

🔲 9.71   ⚖ 9.71   **FUD** 090      J J8 ▢

**AMA:** 2017,Jan,8; 2016,Aug,5; 2016,May,5; 2016,Jan,13; 2015,May,3; 2015,Jan,16; 2014,Nov,5; 2014,Jan,11; 2012,Jun,3-9; 2012,Jan,15-42

**# 33221 with existing multiple leads**

**EXCLUDES** *Insertion of a single transvenous electrode (33216-33217)*
*Removal and replacement of pacemaker pulse generator (33227-33229)*
*Removal of permanent pacemaker pulse generator only (33233)*

Code also placement of epicardial leads by same physician/same surgical session (33202-33203)

🔲 10.4   ⚖ 10.4   **FUD** 090      J J8 ▢

**AMA:** 2017,Jan,8; 2016,Aug,5; 2016,May,5; 2016,Jan,13; 2015,May,3; 2015,Jan,16; 2014,Nov,5; 2014,Jan,11; 2012,Jun,3-9

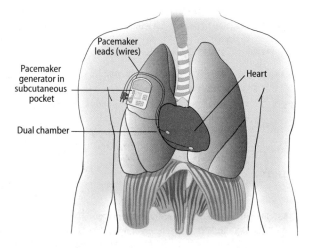

Pacemaker leads (wires)

Pacemaker generator in subcutaneous pocket

Heart

Dual chamber

**33214 Upgrade of implanted pacemaker system, conversion of single chamber system to dual chamber system (includes removal of previously placed pulse generator, testing of existing lead, insertion of new lead, insertion of new pulse generator)**

**EXCLUDES** *Insertion of a single transvenous electrode (33216-33217)*
*Removal and replacement of pacemaker pulse generator (33227-33229)*

🔲 13.8   ⚖ 13.8   **FUD** 090      J J8 80 ▢

**AMA:** 2017,Jan,8; 2016,Aug,5; 2016,May,5; 2016,Jan,13; 2015,May,3; 2015,Jan,16; 2014,Nov,5; 2014,Jan,11; 2012,Jun,3-9

## 33215-33249 [33227, 33228, 33229, 33230, 33231, 33262, 33263, 33264] Pacemakers/Implantable Defibrillator/Electrode Insertion/Replacement/Revision/Repair

**INCLUDES**  Device evaluation (93279-93299 [93260, 93261])
Dual lead: device that paces and senses in two heart chambers
Imaging guidance:
   Fluoroscopy (76000-76001)
   Ultrasound (76942, 76998, 93318)
Multiple lead: device that paces and senses in three or more heart chambers
Radiological supervision and interpretation for pacemaker or pacing cardioverter-defibrillator procedure
Single lead: device that paces and senses in one heart chamber
Skin pocket revision, when performed
   If revision includes incision/drainage of a wound infection or hematoma code also (10140, 10180, 11042-11047 [11045, 11046])
Temporary pacemaker (33210-33211)

**EXCLUDES**  Electrode repositioning:
   Left ventricle (33226)
   Pacemaker or implantable defibrillator (33215)
Insertion of lead for left ventricular (biventricular) pacing (33224-33225)
Removal of leadless pacemaker system (0388T)
Removal of subcutaneous implantable defibrillator electrode ([33272])
Testing of defibrillator threshold (DFT) during follow-up evaluation (93642-93644)
Testing of defibrillator threshold (DFT) during insertion/replacement (93640-93641)

**33215** Repositioning of previously implanted transvenous pacemaker or implantable defibrillator (right atrial or right ventricular) electrode
   🚑 9.01  ⚖ 9.01  **FUD** 090   [T][62][▢]
   **AMA:** 2017,Jan,8; 2016,Aug,5; 2016,May,5; 2016,Jan,13; 2015,May,3; 2015,Jan,16; 2014,Nov,5; 2014,Jan,11; 2012,Jun,3-9

**33216** Insertion of a single transvenous electrode, permanent pacemaker or implantable defibrillator
   **EXCLUDES**  Insertion or replacement of a lead for a cardiac venous system (33224-33225)
   Insertion or replacement of permanent implantable defibrillator generator or system (33249)
   Removal and replacement of permanent pacemaker or implantable defibrillator (33206-33208, 33212-33213, [33221], 33227-33229, 33230-33231, 33240, [33262, 33263, 33264])
   🚑 10.7  ⚖ 10.7  **FUD** 090   [J][J8][▢]
   **AMA:** 2017,Jan,8; 2016,Aug,5; 2016,May,5; 2016,Jan,13; 2015,May,3; 2015,Jan,16; 2014,Nov,5; 2014,Jan,11; 2012,Jun,3-9; 2012,Jan,15-42

**33217** Insertion of 2 transvenous electrodes, permanent pacemaker or implantable defibrillator
   **EXCLUDES**  Insertion or replacement of a lead for a cardiac venous system (33224-33225)
   Insertion or replacement of permanent implantable defibrillator generator or system (33249)
   Removal and replacement of permanent pacemaker or implantable defibrillator (33206-33208, 33212-33213, [33221], 33227-33229, 33230-33231, 33240, [33262, 33263, 33264])
   🚑 10.5  ⚖ 10.5  **FUD** 090   [J][J8][▢]
   **AMA:** 2017,Jan,8; 2016,Aug,5; 2016,May,5; 2016,Jan,13; 2015,May,3; 2015,Jan,16; 2014,Nov,5; 2014,Jan,11; 2012,Jun,3-9; 2012,Jan,15-42

**33218** Repair of single transvenous electrode, permanent pacemaker or implantable defibrillator
   Code also replacement of implantable defibrillator pulse generator, when performed ([33262, 33263, 33264])
   Code also replacement of pacemaker pulse generator, when performed (33227-33229)
   🚑 11.2  ⚖ 11.2  **FUD** 090   [T][62][▢]
   **AMA:** 2017,Jan,8; 2016,Aug,5; 2016,May,5; 2016,Jan,13; 2015,May,3; 2015,Jan,16; 2014,Nov,5; 2014,Jan,11; 2012,Jun,3-9; 2012,Jan,15-42

**33220** Repair of 2 transvenous electrodes for permanent pacemaker or implantable defibrillator
   Code also modifier 52 Reduced services, when one electrode of a two-chamber system is repaired
   Code also replacement of implantable defibrillator pulse generator, when performed ([33263, 33264])
   Code also replacement of pacemaker pulse generator, when performed (33228-33229)
   🚑 11.2  ⚖ 11.2  **FUD** 090   [T][62][▢]
   **AMA:** 2017,Jan,8; 2016,Aug,5; 2016,May,5; 2016,Jan,13; 2015,May,3; 2015,Jan,16; 2014,Nov,5; 2014,Jan,11; 2012,Jun,3-9; 2012,Jan,15-42

**33221** Resequenced code. See code following 33213.

**33222** Relocation of skin pocket for pacemaker
   **INCLUDES**  Formation of the new pocket
   Procedures related to the existing pocket:
      Accessing the pocket
      Incision/drainage of any abscess or hematoma (10140, 10180)
      Pocket closure (13100-13102)
   **EXCLUDES**  Debridement, subcutaneous tissue (11042-11047 [11045, 11046])
   Code also removal and replacement of an existing generator
   🚑 9.74  ⚖ 9.74  **FUD** 090   [T][A2][▢]
   **AMA:** 2017,Jan,8; 2016,Aug,5; 2016,May,5; 2016,Jan,13; 2015,May,3; 2015,Jan,16; 2014,Nov,5; 2014,Jan,11; 2012,Jun,3-9

**33223** Relocation of skin pocket for implantable defibrillator
   **INCLUDES**  Formation of the new pocket
   Procedures related to the existing pocket:
      Accessing the pocket
      Incision/drainage of any abscess or hematoma (10140, 10180)
      Pocket closure (13100-13102)
   **EXCLUDES**  Debridement, subcutaneous tissue (11042-11047 [11045, 11046])
   Code also removal and replacement of an existing generator
   🚑 11.8  ⚖ 11.8  **FUD** 090   [T][A2][80][▢]
   **AMA:** 2017,Jan,8; 2016,Aug,5; 2016,Jan,13; 2015,Jan,16; 2014,Nov,5; 2014,Jan,11; 2012,Jun,3-9

**33224** Insertion of pacing electrode, cardiac venous system, for left ventricular pacing, with attachment to previously placed pacemaker or implantable defibrillator pulse generator (including revision of pocket, removal, insertion, and/or replacement of existing generator)
   Code also placement of epicardial electrode when appropriate (33202-33203)
   🚑 15.0  ⚖ 15.0  **FUD** 000   [J][J8][▢]
   **AMA:** 2017,Jan,8; 2016,Aug,5; 2016,May,5; 2016,Jan,13; 2015,May,3; 2015,Jan,16; 2014,Nov,5; 2014,Jan,11; 2012,Jun,3-9; 2012,Jan,15-42

**+ 33225** Insertion of pacing electrode, cardiac venous system, for left ventricular pacing, at time of insertion of implantable defibrillator or pacemaker pulse generator (eg, for upgrade to dual chamber system) (List separately in addition to code for primary procedure)
   Code first (33206-33208, 33212-33213, [33221], 33214, 33216-33217, 33223, 33228-33229, 33230-33231, 33233, 33234-33235, 33240, [33263, 33264], 33249)
   Code first (33223) for relocation of pocket for implantable defibrillator
   Code first (33222) for relocation of pocket for pacemaker pulse generator
   🚑 13.6  ⚖ 13.6  **FUD** ZZZ   [N][N1][▢]
   **AMA:** 2017,Jan,8; 2016,Aug,5; 2016,May,5; 2016,Jan,13; 2015,May,3; 2015,Jan,16; 2014,Nov,5; 2014,Jan,11; 2012,Jun,3-9; 2012,Jan,15-42

**33226** Repositioning of previously implanted cardiac venous system (left ventricular) electrode (including removal, insertion and/or replacement of existing generator)
   🚑 14.4  ⚖ 14.4  **FUD** 000   [T][62][▢]
   **AMA:** 2017,Jan,8; 2016,Aug,5; 2016,May,5; 2016,Jan,13; 2015,May,3; 2015,Jan,16; 2014,Nov,5; 2014,Jan,11; 2012,Jun,3-9

---

● New Code   ▲ Revised Code   ○ Reinstated   ● New Web Release   ▲ Revised Web Release   Unlisted   Not Covered   # Resequenced
⊘ AMA Mod 51 Exempt   ⑤⓪ Optum Mod 51 Exempt   ⑥③ Mod 63 Exempt   ⚕ Non-FDA Drug   ★ Telemedicine   Ⓜ Maternity   🅰 Age Edit   + Add-on   **AMA:** CPT Asst
© 2017 Optum360, LLC          CPT © 2017 American Medical Association. All Rights Reserved.          **123**

*Cardiovascular, Hemic, and Lymphatic*

*33227 — 33241*

*33227* Resequenced code. See code following 33233.

*33228* Resequenced code. See code following 33233.

*33229* Resequenced code. See code before 33234.

*33230* Resequenced code. See code following 33240.

*33231* Resequenced code. See code before 33241.

**33233** **Removal of permanent pacemaker pulse generator only**

EXCLUDES *Removal and replacement of pacemaker pulse generator and transvenous electrode(s): code 33233 with (33206, 33207, 33208, 33234, 33235)*

*Removal of permanent pacemaker pulse generator with replacement of pacemaker pulse generator; single lead system (33227-33229)*

43 6.65 ⚕ 6.65 **FUD** 090 Q2 G2 □

**AMA:** 2017,Jan,8; 2016,Aug,5; 2016,May,5; 2016,Jan,13; 2015,Jan,16; 2014,Nov,5; 2014,Jan,11; 2012,Jun,3-9; 2012,Jan,15-42

# **33227** **Removal of permanent pacemaker pulse generator with replacement of pacemaker pulse generator; single lead system**

43 9.79 ⚕ 9.79 **FUD** 090 J J8 □

**AMA:** 2017,Jan,8; 2016,Aug,5; 2016,May,5; 2016,Jan,13; 2015,Jan,16; 2014,Nov,5; 2014,Jan,11; 2013,Apr,10-11; 2012,Jun,3-9

# **33228** **dual lead system**

43 10.2 ⚕ 10.2 **FUD** 090 J J8 □

**AMA:** 2017,Jan,8; 2016,Aug,5; 2016,May,5; 2016,Jan,13; 2015,Jan,16; 2014,Nov,5; 2014,Jan,11; 2013,Apr,10-11; 2012,Jun,3-9

# **33229** **multiple lead system**

43 10.8 ⚕ 10.8 **FUD** 090 J J8 □

**AMA:** 2017,Jan,8; 2016,Aug,5; 2016,May,5; 2016,Jan,13; 2015,Jan,16; 2014,Nov,5; 2014,Jan,11; 2013,Apr,10-11; 2012,Jun,3-9

**33234** **Removal of transvenous pacemaker electrode(s); single lead system, atrial or ventricular**

EXCLUDES *Removal and replacement of pacemaker pulse generator and transvenous electrode 33234 and 33233 and (33206, 33207, 33208)*

*Thoracotomy to remove electrodes (33238, 33243)*

Code also pacing electrode insertion in cardiac venous system for pacing of left ventricle during insertion of pulse generator (pacemaker or implantable defibrillator) when performed (33225)

43 14.0 ⚕ 14.0 **FUD** 090 Q2 G2 □

**AMA:** 2017,Jan,8; 2016,Aug,5; 2016,May,5; 2016,Jan,13; 2015,Jan,16; 2014,Nov,5; 2014,Jan,11; 2012,Oct,14; 2012,Jun,3-9

**33235** **dual lead system**

EXCLUDES *Removal and replacement of pacemaker pulse generator and transvenous electrode(s) 33235 and 33233 and (33206, 33207, 33208, 33233, 33235)*

*Thoracotomy to remove electrode(s) (33238, 33243)*

Code also pacing electrode insertion in cardiac venous system for pacing of left ventricle during insertion of pulse generator (pacemaker or implantable defibrillator) when performed (33225)

43 18.4 ⚕ 18.4 **FUD** 090 Q2 G2 □

**AMA:** 2017,Jan,8; 2016,Aug,5; 2016,May,5; 2016,Jan,13; 2015,Jan,16; 2014,Nov,5; 2014,Jan,11; 2013,Dec,14; 2012,Oct,14; 2012,Jun,3-9

**33236** **Removal of permanent epicardial pacemaker and electrodes by thoracotomy; single lead system, atrial or ventricular**

EXCLUDES *Removal of implantable defibrillator electrode(s) by thoracotomy (33243)*

*Removal of transvenous electrodes by thoracotomy (33238)*

*Removal of transvenous pacemaker electrodes, single or dual lead system; without thoracotomy (33234, 33235)*

43 22.7 ⚕ 22.7 **FUD** 090 C 80 □

**AMA:** 2017,Jan,8; 2016,Aug,5; 2016,May,5; 2016,Jan,13; 2015,Jan,16; 2014,Nov,5; 2014,Jan,11; 2012,Jun,3-9

**33237** **dual lead system**

EXCLUDES *Removal of implantable defibrillator electrode(s) by thoracotomy (33243)*

*Removal of transvenous electrodes by thoracotomy (33238)*

*Removal of transvenous pacemaker electrodes, single or dual lead system; without thoracotomy (33234, 33235)*

43 24.2 ⚕ 24.2 **FUD** 090 C 80 □

**AMA:** 2017,Jan,8; 2016,Aug,5; 2016,May,5; 2016,Jan,13; 2015,Jan,16; 2014,Nov,5; 2014,Jan,11; 2012,Jun,3-9

**33238** **Removal of permanent transvenous electrode(s) by thoracotomy**

EXCLUDES *Removal of implantable defibrillator electrode(s) by thoracotomy (33243)*

*Removal of transvenous pacemaker electrodes, single or dual lead system; without thoracotomy (33234, 33235)*

43 27.0 ⚕ 27.0 **FUD** 090 C 80 □

**AMA:** 2017,Jan,8; 2016,Aug,5; 2016,May,5; 2016,Jan,13; 2015,Jan,16; 2014,Nov,5; 2014,Jan,11; 2012,Jun,3-9

**33240** **Insertion of implantable defibrillator pulse generator only; with existing single lead**

EXCLUDES *Insertion of electrode (33216-33217, [33271])*

*Programming and interrogation of device (93260-93261)*

*Removal and replacement of implantable defibrillator pulse generator ([33262, 33263, 33264])*

Code also placement of epicardial leads by same physician/same surgical session as generator insertion (33202-33203)

43 10.5 ⚕ 10.5 **FUD** 090 J J8 □

**AMA:** 2017,Jan,8; 2016,Aug,5; 2016,Jan,13; 2015,Jan,16; 2014,Nov,5; 2014,Jan,11; 2012,Jun,3-9; 2012,Jan,15-42

# **33230** **with existing dual leads**

EXCLUDES *Insertion of a single transvenous electrode, permanent pacemaker or implantable defibrillator (33216-33217)*

*Removal and replacement of implantable defibrillator pulse generator ([33262, 33263, 33264])*

Code also placement of epicardial leads by same physician/same surgical session as generator insertion (33202-33203)

43 11.1 ⚕ 11.1 **FUD** 090 J J8 □

**AMA:** 2017,Jan,8; 2016,Aug,5; 2016,Jan,13; 2015,Jan,16; 2014,Nov,5; 2014,Jan,11; 2012,Jun,3-9

# **33231** **with existing multiple leads**

EXCLUDES *Insertion of a single transvenous electrode, permanent pacemaker or implantable defibrillator (33216-33217)*

*Removal and replacement of implantable defibrillator pulse generator ([33262, 33263, 33264])*

Code also placement of epicardial leads by same physician/same surgical session as generator placement (33202-33203)

43 11.6 ⚕ 11.6 **FUD** 090 J J8 □

**AMA:** 2017,Jan,8; 2016,Aug,5; 2016,Jan,13; 2015,Jan,16; 2014,Nov,5; 2014,Jan,11; 2012,Jun,3-9

**33241** **Removal of implantable defibrillator pulse generator only**

EXCLUDES *Insertion of implantable defibrillator pulse generator only (33230-33231, 33240)*

*Programming and interrogation of device (93260-93261)*

*Removal and replacement of implantable defibrillator pulse generator ([33262, 33263, 33264])*

Code also electrode removal by thoracotomy (33243)

Code also insertion of subcutaneous defibrillator system and removal of subcutaneous defibrillator lead, when performed ([33270], [33272])

Code also removal of defibrillator leads and insertion of defibrillator system, when performed (33243, 33244, 33249)

Code also transvenous removal of electrode(s) (33244)

43 6.23 ⚕ 6.23 **FUD** 090 Q2 G2 □

**AMA:** 2017,Jan,8; 2016,Aug,5; 2016,Jan,13; 2015,Jan,16; 2014,Nov,5; 2014,Jan,11; 2012,Jun,3-9

26/TC PC/TC Only  A2-Z3 ASC Payment  50 Bilateral  ♂ Male Only  ♀ Female Only  43 Facility RVU  ⚕ Non-Facility RVU  □ CCI

**FUD** Follow-up Days  **CMS:** IOM (Pub 100)  A-Y OPPSI  80/80 Surg Assist Allowed / w/Doc  🔬 Lab Crosswalk  ☢ Radiology Crosswalk  ✖ CLIA

124  CPT © 2017 American Medical Association. All Rights Reserved.  © 2017 Optum360, LLC

**#  33262  Removal of implantable defibrillator pulse generator with replacement of implantable defibrillator pulse generator; single lead system**

> EXCLUDES  *Insertion of electrode (33216-33217, [33271])*
> *Programming and interrogation of device (93260-93261)*
> *Removal of implantable defibrillator pulse generator only (33241)*
> *Repair of implantable defibrillator pulse generator and/or leads (33218, 33220)*

Code also electrode(s) removal by thoracotomy (33243)
Code also subcutaneous electrode removal ([33272])
Code also transvenous removal of electrode(s) (33244)

📷 10.8    ☑ 10.8    **FUD** 090                    J  J8  ▣

**AMA:** 2017,Jan,8; 2016,Aug,5; 2016,Jan,13; 2015,Jan,16; 2014,Nov,5; 2014,Jan,11; 2012,Jun,3-9

**#  33263  dual lead system**

> EXCLUDES  *Insertion of a single transvenous electrode, permanent pacemaker or implantable defibrillator (33216-33217)*
> *Removal of implantable defibrillator pulse generator only (33241)*
> *Repair of implantable defibrillator pulse generator and/or leads (33218, 33220)*

Code also removal of electrodes by thoracotomy (33243)
Code also subcutaneous electrode removal ([33272])
Code also transvenous removal of electrodes (33244)

📷 11.2    ☑ 11.2    **FUD** 090                    J  J8  ▣

**AMA:** 2017,Jan,8; 2016,Aug,5; 2016,Jan,13; 2015,Jan,16; 2014,Nov,5; 2014,Jan,11; 2013,Dec,16; 2012,Jun,3-9

**#  33264  multiple lead system**

> EXCLUDES  *Insertion of a single transvenous electrode, permanent pacemaker or implantable defibrillator (33216-33217)*
> *Removal of implantable defibrillator pulse generator only (33241)*
> *Repair of implantable defibrillator pulse generator and/or leads (33218, 33220)*

Code also removal of electrodes by thoracotomy (33243)
Code also subcutaneous electrode removal ([33272])
Code also transvenous removal of electrodes (33244)

📷 11.7    ☑ 11.7    **FUD** 090                    J  J8  ▣

**AMA:** 2017,Jan,8; 2016,Aug,5; 2016,Jan,13; 2015,Jan,16; 2014,Nov,5; 2014,Jan,11; 2013,Dec,16; 2012,Jun,3-9

**33243  Removal of single or dual chamber implantable defibrillator electrode(s); by thoracotomy**

> EXCLUDES  *Transvenous removal of defibrillator electrode(s) (33244)*

Code also removal of defibrillator generator and insertion/replacement of defibrillator system (generator and leads), when performed (33241, 33249)

📷 39.7    ☑ 39.7    **FUD** 090                    C  80  ▣

**AMA:** 2017,Jan,8; 2016,Aug,5; 2016,Jan,13; 2015,Jan,16; 2014,Nov,5; 2014,Jan,11; 2012,Jun,3-9

**33244  by transvenous extraction**

> EXCLUDES  *Thoracotomy to remove electrodes (33238, 33243)*

Code also removal of defibrillator generator and insertion/replacement of defibrillator system (generator and leads), when performed (33241, 33249)

📷 24.9    ☑ 24.9    **FUD** 090                    02  ▣

**AMA:** 2017,Jan,8; 2016,Aug,5; 2016,Jan,13; 2015,Jan,16; 2014,Nov,5; 2014,Jan,11; 2012,Jun,3-9

**33249  Insertion or replacement of permanent implantable defibrillator system, with transvenous lead(s), single or dual chamber**

> EXCLUDES  *Insertion of a single transvenous electrode, permanent pacemaker or implantable defibrillator (33216-33217)*

Code also removal of defibrillator generator and removal of leads (by thoracotomy or transvenous), when performed (33241, 33243, 33244)
Code also removal of defibrillator generator when upgrading from single to dual-chamber system (33241)

📷 26.6    ☑ 26.6    **FUD** 090                    J  J8  ▣

**AMA:** 2017,Jan,8; 2016,Aug,5; 2016,Jan,13; 2015,Jan,16; 2014,Nov,5; 2014,Jan,11; 2012,Jun,3-9

## [33270, 33271, 33272, 33273] Subcutaneous Implantable Defibrillator

> INCLUDES  Programming and interrogation of device (93260, 93261)
> EXCLUDES  *Defibrillation threshold testing (DFT) during subcutaneous defibrillator implant (93640-93641)*

**#  33270  Insertion or replacement of permanent subcutaneous implantable defibrillator system, with subcutaneous electrode, including defibrillation threshold evaluation, induction of arrhythmia, evaluation of sensing for arrhythmia termination, and programming or reprogramming of sensing or therapeutic parameters, when performed**

> EXCLUDES  *Electrophysiologic evaluation of subcutaneous implantable defibrillator (93644)*
> *Insertion of subcutaneous implantable defibrillator electrode ([33271])*

Code also removal of defibrillator generator and subcutaneous electrode, when performed (33241, [33272])

📷 17.1    ☑ 17.1    **FUD** 090                    J  J8  ▣

**AMA:** 2017,Jan,8; 2016,Aug,5; 2016,Jan,13; 2015,Jan,16; 2014,Nov,5

**#  33271  Insertion of subcutaneous implantable defibrillator electrode**

> EXCLUDES  *Insertion of implantable defibrillator pulse generator only (33240)*
> *Insertion or replacement of permanent subcutaneous implantable defibrillator system ([33270])*
> *Removal and replacement of implantable defibrillator pulse generator ([33262])*

📷 14.3    ☑ 14.3    **FUD** 090                    J  J8  ▣

**AMA:** 2017,Jan,8; 2016,Aug,5; 2016,Jan,13; 2015,Jan,16; 2014,Nov,5

**#  33272  Removal of subcutaneous implantable defibrillator electrode**

Code also removal defibrillator generator and insertion/replacement subcutaneous defibrillator system (generator and leads), when performed (33241, [33270])
Code also removal of defibrillator generator with replacement, when performed ([33262])
Code also removal of defibrillator generator (without replacement), when performed (33241)

📷 10.1    ☑ 10.1    **FUD** 090                    02  ▣

**AMA:** 2017,Jan,8; 2016,Aug,5; 2016,Jan,13; 2015,Jan,16; 2014,Nov,5

**#  33273  Repositioning of previously implanted subcutaneous implantable defibrillator electrode**

📷 11.8    ☑ 11.8    **FUD** 090                    T  62  ▣

**AMA:** 2017,Jan,8; 2016,Aug,5; 2016,Jan,13; 2015,Jan,16; 2014,Nov,5

Cardiovascular, Hemic, and Lymphatic

33262 — 33273

## 33250-33251 Surgical Ablation Arrhythmogenic Foci, Supraventricular

INCLUDES  Procedures using cryotherapy, laser, microwave, radiofrequency, and ultrasound

**33250** **Operative ablation of supraventricular arrhythmogenic focus or pathway (eg, Wolff-Parkinson-White, atrioventricular node re-entry), tract(s) and/or focus (foci); without cardiopulmonary bypass**

EXCLUDES  *Pacing and mapping during surgery by other provider (93631)*

🖫 42.1    ⚕ 42.1    **FUD** 090    C 80 ▢

**AMA:** 2017,Jan,8; 2016,Jan,13; 2015,Jan,16; 2014,Jan,11

**33251** **with cardiopulmonary bypass**

🖫 47.1    ⚕ 47.1    **FUD** 090    C 80 ▢

**AMA:** 2017,Jan,8; 2016,Jan,13; 2015,Jan,16; 2014,Jan,11

## 33254-33256 Surgical Ablation Arrhythmogenic Foci, Atrial (e.g., Maze)

INCLUDES  Excision or isolation of the left atrial appendage
Procedures using cryotherapy, laser, microwave, radiofrequency, and ultrasound

EXCLUDES  *Any procedure involving median sternotomy or cardiopulmonary bypass*
*Aortic valve procedures (33390-33391, 33404-33415)*
*Aortoplasty (33417)*
*Ascending aorta graft, with cardiopulmonary bypass (33860-33864)*
*Coronary artery bypass (33510-33516, 33517-33523, 33533-33536)*
*Excision of intracardiac tumor, resection with cardiopulmonary bypass (33120)*
*Mitral valve procedures (33418-33430)*
*Outflow tract augmentation (33478)*
*Prosthetic valve repair (33496)*
*Pulmonary artery embolectomy; with cardiopulmonary bypass (33910-33920)*
*Pulmonary valve procedures (33470-33476)*
*Repair aberrant coronary artery anatomy (33500-33507)*
*Repair aberrant heart anatomy (33600-33853)*
*Resection of external cardiac tumor (33130)*
*Temporary pacemaker (33210-33211)*
*Thoracotomy; with exploration (32100)*
*Transcatheter pulmonary valve implantation (33477)*
*Tricuspid valve procedures (33460-33468)*
*Tube thoracostomy, includes connection to drainage system (32551)*
*Ventricular reconstruction (33542-33548)*
*Ventriculomyotomy (33416)*

**33254** **Operative tissue ablation and reconstruction of atria, limited (eg, modified maze procedure)**

🖫 39.5    ⚕ 39.5    **FUD** 090    C 80 ▢

**AMA:** 2017,Jan,8; 2016,Jan,13; 2015,Jan,16; 2014,Jan,11

**33255** **Operative tissue ablation and reconstruction of atria, extensive (eg, maze procedure); without cardiopulmonary bypass**

🖫 47.6    ⚕ 47.6    **FUD** 090    C 80 ▢

**AMA:** 2017,Jan,8; 2016,Jan,13; 2015,Jan,16; 2014,Jan,11

**33256** **with cardiopulmonary bypass**

🖫 56.3    ⚕ 56.3    **FUD** 090    C 80 ▢

**AMA:** 2017,Jan,8; 2016,Jan,13; 2015,Jan,16; 2014,Jan,11

## 33257-33259 Surgical Ablation Arrhythmogenic Foci, Atrial, with Other Heart Procedure(s)

EXCLUDES  *Endoscopy, surgical; operative tissue ablation and reconstruction of atria, limited (33265-33266)*
*Operative tissue ablation and reconstruction of atria, limited (33254-33256)*
*Temporary pacemaker (33210-33211)*
*Tube thoracostomy, includes connection to drainage system (32551)*

+ **33257** **Operative tissue ablation and reconstruction of atria, performed at the time of other cardiac procedure(s), limited (eg, modified maze procedure) (List separately in addition to code for primary procedure)**

🖫 16.8    ⚕ 16.8    **FUD** ZZZ    C 80 ▢

Code first (33120-33130, 33250-33251, 33261, 33300-33335, 33390-33391, 33404-33496, 33500-33507, 33510-33516, 33533-33548, 33600-33619, 33641-33697, 33702-33732, 33735-33767, 33770-33814, 33840-33877, 33910-33922, 33925-33926, 33935, 33945, 33975-33980)

+ **33258** **Operative tissue ablation and reconstruction of atria, performed at the time of other cardiac procedure(s), extensive (eg, maze procedure), without cardiopulmonary bypass (List separately in addition to code for primary procedure)**

🖫 18.9    ⚕ 18.9    **FUD** ZZZ    C 80 ▢

Code first, if performed without cardiopulmonary bypass (33130, 33250, 33300, 33310, 33320-33321, 33330, 33390-33391, 33414-33417, 33420, 33470-33471, 33501-33503, 33510-33516, 33533-33536, 33690, 33735, 33737, 33800-33813, 33840-33852, 33915, 33925)

+ **33259** **Operative tissue ablation and reconstruction of atria, performed at the time of other cardiac procedure(s), extensive (eg, maze procedure), with cardiopulmonary bypass (List separately in addition to code for primary procedure)**

🖫 24.4    ⚕ 24.4    **FUD** ZZZ    C 80 ▢

Code first, if performed with cardiopulmonary bypass (33120, 33251, 33261, 33305, 33315, 33322, 33335, 33390-33391, 33404-33413, 33422-33468, 33474-33496, 33500, 33504-33507, 33510-33516, 33533-33548, 33600-33688, 33692-33722, 33730, 33732, 33736, 33750-33767, 33770-33781, 33786-33788, 33814, 33853, 33860-33877, 33910, 33916-33922, 33926, 33935, 33945, 33975-33980)

## 33261-33264 Surgical Ablation Arrhythmogenic Foci, Ventricular

**33261** **Operative ablation of ventricular arrhythmogenic focus with cardiopulmonary bypass**

🖫 47.1    ⚕ 47.1    **FUD** 090    C 80 ▢

**AMA:** 2017,Jan,8; 2016,Jan,13; 2015,Jan,16; 2014,Jan,11

Impulse centers that are causing arrhythmia are treated with ablation

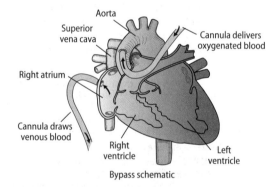

Bypass schematic

*33262* **Resequenced code. See code following 33241.**

*33263* **Resequenced code. See code following 33241.**

*33264* **Resequenced code. See code before 33243.**

## 33265-33273 Surgical Ablation Arrhythmogenic Foci, Endoscopic

EXCLUDES  *Insertion or replacement of temporary transvenous single chamber cardiac electrode or pacemaker catheter (separate procedure) (33210-33211)*
*Tube thoracostomy, includes connection to drainage system (32551)*

**33265** **Endoscopy, surgical; operative tissue ablation and reconstruction of atria, limited (eg, modified maze procedure), without cardiopulmonary bypass**

🖫 39.3    ⚕ 39.3    **FUD** 090    C 80 ▢

**AMA:** 2017,Jan,8; 2016,Jan,13; 2015,Jan,16; 2014,Jan,11

| 26/TC PC/TC Only | A2-Z3 ASC Payment | 50 Bilateral | ♂ Male Only | ♀ Female Only | 🖫 Facility RVU | ⚕ Non-Facility RVU | ▢ CCI |
| **FUD** Follow-up Days | **CMS:** IOM (Pub 100) | A-Y OPPSI | 80/80 Surg Assist Allowed / w/Doc | | ▧ Lab Crosswalk | ▧ Radiology Crosswalk | ✖ CLIA |

126

CPT © 2017 American Medical Association. All Rights Reserved.

© 2017 Optum360, LLC

**33266** operative tissue ablation and reconstruction of atria, extensive (eg, maze procedure), without cardiopulmonary bypass
📇 53.5   � 53.5   **FUD** 090   [C] [80] [▢]
**AMA:** 2017,Jan,8; 2016,Jan,13; 2015,Jan,16; 2014,Jan,11

**33270** Resequenced code. See code following 33249.

**33271** Resequenced code. See code following 33249.

**33272** Resequenced code. See code following 33249.

**33273** Resequenced code. See code following 33249.

## 33282-33284 Implantable Loop Recorder

**33282** Implantation of patient-activated cardiac event recorder
> INCLUDES   Initial programming of device
> EXCLUDES   Subsequent electronic analysis and/or reprogramming of device (93285, 93291, 93298-93299)
📇 6.53   ⚪ 6.53   **FUD** 090   [J] [J8] [▢]
**AMA:** 2017,Jan,8; 2016,Jan,13; 2015,Jan,16; 2014,Jan,11; 2012,Jan,15-42

**33284** Removal of an implantable, patient-activated cardiac event recorder
📇 5.74   ⚪ 5.74   **FUD** 090   [Q2] [G2] [▢]
**AMA:** 2017,Jan,8; 2016,Jan,13; 2015,Jan,16; 2014,Jan,11

## 33300-33315 Procedures for Injury of the Heart

> INCLUDES   Procedures with and without cardiopulmonary bypass
> EXCLUDES   Cardiac assist services (33946-33949, 33967-33983, 33990-33993)

**33300** Repair of cardiac wound; without bypass
📇 71.1   ⚪ 71.1   **FUD** 090   [C] [80] [▢]
**AMA:** 1997,Nov,1

**33305** with cardiopulmonary bypass
📇 119.   ⚪ 119.   **FUD** 090   [C] [80] [▢]
**AMA:** 1997,Nov,1

**33310** Cardiotomy, exploratory (includes removal of foreign body, atrial or ventricular thrombus); without bypass
> EXCLUDES   Other cardiac procedures unless separate incision into heart is necessary in order to remove thrombus
📇 34.2   ⚪ 34.2   **FUD** 090   [C] [80] [▢]
**AMA:** 1997,Nov,1

**33315** with cardiopulmonary bypass
> EXCLUDES   Other cardiac procedures unless separate incision into heart is necessary in order to remove thrombus
> Code also excision of thrombus with cardiopulmonary bypass and append modifier 59 if separate incision is required with (33120, 33130, 33420-33430, 33460-33468, 33496, 33542, 33545, 33641-33647, 33670, 33681, 33975-33980)
📇 55.5   ⚪ 55.5   **FUD** 090   [C] [80] [▢]
**AMA:** 2017,Jan,8; 2016,Jan,13; 2015,Jan,16; 2014,Jan,11; 2012,Jan,15-42

## 33320-33335 Procedures for Injury of the Aorta/Great Vessels

**33320** Suture repair of aorta or great vessels; without shunt or cardiopulmonary bypass
📇 30.8   ⚪ 30.8   **FUD** 090   [C] [80] [▢]
**AMA:** 2017,Jan,8; 2016,Jan,13; 2015,Jan,16; 2014,Jan,11

**33321** with shunt bypass
📇 34.5   ⚪ 34.5   **FUD** 090   [C] [80] [▢]
**AMA:** 1997,Nov,1; 1994,Win,1

**33322** with cardiopulmonary bypass
📇 40.2   ⚪ 40.2   **FUD** 090   [C] [80] [▢]
**AMA:** 2017,Jan,8; 2016,Jan,13; 2015,Jan,16; 2014,Jan,11

**33330** Insertion of graft, aorta or great vessels; without shunt, or cardiopulmonary bypass
📇 41.4   ⚪ 41.4   **FUD** 090   [C] [80] [▢]
**AMA:** 1997,Nov,1; 1994,Win,1

**33335** with cardiopulmonary bypass
📇 54.4   ⚪ 54.4   **FUD** 090   [C] [80] [▢]
**AMA:** 1997,Nov,1

## 33340 Closure Left Atrial Appendage

> EXCLUDES   Cardiac catheterization except for reasons other than closure left atrial appendage (93451-93453, 93456, 93458-93461, 93462, 93530-93533)

**33340** Percutaneous transcatheter closure of the left atrial appendage with endocardial implant, including fluoroscopy, transseptal puncture, catheter placement(s), left atrial angiography, left atrial appendage angiography, when performed, and radiological supervision and interpretation
📇 23.2   ⚪ 23.2   **FUD** 000   [C] [80] [▢]
**AMA:** 2017,Jul,3

## 33361-33369 Transcatheter Aortic Valve Replacement

**CMS:** 100-03,20.32 Transcatheter Aortic Valve Replacement (TAVR); 100-04,32,290.1.1 Coding Requirements for TAVR Services; 100-04,32,290.2 Claims Processing for TAVR/ Professional Claims; 100-04,32,290.3 Claims Processing TAVR Inpatient; 100-04,32,290.4 Payment of TAVR for MA Plan Participants

> INCLUDES   Access and implantation of the aortic valve (33361-33366)
> Access sheath placement
> Advancement of valve delivery system
> Arteriotomy closure
> Balloon aortic valvuloplasty
> Cardiac or open arterial approach
> Deployment of valve
> Percutaneous access
> Temporary pacemaker
> Valve repositioning when necessary
> Radiology procedures:
> Angiography during and after procedure
> Assessment of access site for closure
> Documentation of completion of the intervention
> Guidance for valve placement
> Supervision and interpretation
> EXCLUDES   Cardiac catheterization procedures included in the TAVR/TAVI service (93452-93453, 93458-93461, 93567)
> Percutaneous coronary interventional procedures
> Transvascular ventricular support (33967, 33970, 33973, 33975-33976, 33990-33993, 33999)

Code also cardiac catheterization services for purposes other than TAVR/TAVI

Code also diagnostic coronary angiography at a different session from the interventional procedure

Code also diagnostic coronary angiography at the same time as TAVR/TAVI when:
A previous study is available, but documentation states the patient's condition has changed since the previous study, visualization of the anatomy/pathology is inadequate, or a change occurs during the procedure warranting additional evaluation of an area outside the current target area
No previous catheter-based coronary angiography study is available, and a full diagnostic study is performed, with the decision to perform the intervention based on that study

Code also modifier 59 when diagnostic coronary angiography procedures are performed as separate and distinct procedural services on the same day or session as TAVR/TAVI

Code also modifier 62 as all TAVI/TAVR procedures require the work of two physicians

**33361** Transcatheter aortic valve replacement (TAVR/TAVI) with prosthetic valve; percutaneous femoral artery approach
> Code also cardiopulmonary bypass when performed (33367-33369)
📇 39.5   ⚪ 39.5   **FUD** 000   [C] [80] [▢]
**AMA:** 2017,Jan,8; 2016,Jan,13; 2015,Mar,9; 2015,Jan,16; 2014,Jul,8; 2014,Jan,11; 2014,Jan,5; 2013,Jan,6-8

**33362** open femoral artery approach
> Code also cardiopulmonary bypass when performed (33367-33369)
📇 43.2   ⚪ 43.2   **FUD** 000   [C] [80] [▢]
**AMA:** 2017,Jan,8; 2016,Jan,13; 2015,Mar,9; 2015,Jan,16; 2014,Jul,8; 2014,Jan,11; 2014,Jan,5; 2013,Jan,6-8

**33363** open axillary artery approach
> Code also cardiopulmonary bypass when performed (33367-33369)
📇 45.4   ⚪ 45.4   **FUD** 000   [C] [80] [▢]
**AMA:** 2017,Jan,8; 2016,Jan,13; 2015,Mar,9; 2015,Jan,16; 2014,Jul,8; 2014,Jan,11; 2014,Jan,5; 2013,Jan,6-8

**33364** open iliac artery approach
> Code also cardiopulmonary bypass when performed (33367-33369)
📇 47.1   ⚪ 47.1   **FUD** 000   [C] [80] [▢]
**AMA:** 2017,Jan,8; 2016,Jan,13; 2015,Mar,9; 2015,Jan,16; 2014,Jul,8; 2014,Jan,11; 2014,Jan,5; 2013,Jan,6-8

● New Code   ▲ Revised Code   ○ Reinstated   ● New Web Release   ▲ Revised Web Release   Unlisted   Not Covered   # Resequenced
⊘ AMA Mod 51 Exempt   ⑨ Optum Mod 51 Exempt   ⑥ Mod 63 Exempt   ✗ Non-FDA Drug   ★ Telemedicine   [M] Maternity   [A] Age Edit   + Add-on   **AMA:** CPT Asst

**33365**     **transaortic approach (eg, median sternotomy, mediastinotomy)**
      Code also cardiopulmonary bypass when performed (33367-33369)
      🔧 51.8    ✂ 51.8    **FUD** 000               C 80 ▭
      AMA: 2017,Jan,8; 2016,Jan,13; 2015,Mar,9; 2015,Jan,16; 2014,Jul,8; 2014,Jan,11; 2014,Jan,5; 2013,Jan,6-8

**33366**     **transapical exposure (eg, left thoracotomy)**
      Code also cardiopulmonary bypass when performed (33367-33369)
      🔧 56.1    ✂ 56.1    **FUD** 000               C 80 ▭
      AMA: 2017,Jan,8; 2016,Jan,13; 2015,Mar,9; 2015,Jan,16; 2014,Jul,8; 2014,Jan,5

+ **33367**    **cardiopulmonary bypass support with percutaneous peripheral arterial and venous cannulation (eg, femoral vessels) (List separately in addition to code for primary procedure)**
      EXCLUDES    Cardiopulmonary bypass support with open or central arterial and venous cannulation (33368-33369)
      Code first (33361-33366, 33418, 33477, 0483T-0484T)
      🔧 18.2    ✂ 18.2    **FUD** ZZZ               C 80 ▭
      AMA: 2017,Jan,8; 2016,Mar,5; 2016,Jan,13; 2015,Sep,3; 2015,Jan,16; 2013,Jan,6-8

+ **33368**    **cardiopulmonary bypass support with open peripheral arterial and venous cannulation (eg, femoral, iliac, axillary vessels) (List separately in addition to code for primary procedure)**
      EXCLUDES    Cardiopulmonary bypass support with percutaneous or central arterial and venous cannulation (33367, 33369)
      Code first (33361-33366, 33418, 33477, 0483T-0484T)
      🔧 21.7    ✂ 21.7    **FUD** ZZZ               C 80 ▭
      AMA: 2017,Jan,8; 2016,Mar,5; 2016,Jan,13; 2015,Sep,3; 2015,Jan,16; 2013,Jan,6-8

+ **33369**    **cardiopulmonary bypass support with central arterial and venous cannulation (eg, aorta, right atrium, pulmonary artery) (List separately in addition to code for primary procedure)**
      EXCLUDES    Cardiopulmonary bypass support with percutaneous or open arterial and venous cannulation (33367-33368)
      Code first (33361-33366, 33418, 33477, 0483T-0484T)
      🔧 28.7    ✂ 28.7    **FUD** ZZZ               C 80 ▭
      AMA: 2017,Jan,8; 2016,Mar,5; 2016,Jan,13; 2015,Sep,3; 2015,Jan,16; 2013,Jan,6-8

## 33390-33415 Aortic Valve Procedures

**33390**     **Valvuloplasty, aortic valve, open, with cardiopulmonary bypass; simple (ie, valvotomy, debridement, debulking, and/or simple commissural resuspension)**
      🔧 55.3    ✂ 55.3    **FUD** 090               C 80 ▭

**33391**     **complex (eg, leaflet extension, leaflet resection, leaflet reconstruction, or annuloplasty)**
      🔧 65.6    ✂ 65.6    **FUD** 090               C 80 ▭
      INCLUDES    Simple aortic valvuloplasty (33390)

**33404**     **Construction of apical-aortic conduit**
      🔧 50.9    ✂ 50.9    **FUD** 090               C 80 ▭
      AMA: 2017,Jan,8; 2016,Jan,13; 2015,Jan,16; 2014,Jan,11; 2012,Jan,15-42

**33405**     **Replacement, aortic valve, open, with cardiopulmonary bypass; with prosthetic valve other than homograft or stentless valve**
      🔧 65.8    ✂ 65.8    **FUD** 090               C 80 ▭
      AMA: 2017,Jan,8; 2016,Jan,13; 2015,Jan,16; 2014,Jan,11; 2013,Jan,6-8

**33406**     **with allograft valve (freehand)**
      🔧 83.5    ✂ 83.5    **FUD** 090               C 80 ▭
      AMA: 2017,Jan,8; 2016,Jan,13; 2015,Jan,16; 2014,Jan,11

**33410**     **with stentless tissue valve**
      🔧 73.8    ✂ 73.8    **FUD** 090               C 80 ▭
      AMA: 2017,Jan,8; 2016,Jan,13; 2015,Jan,16; 2014,Jan,11

**33411**     **Replacement, aortic valve; with aortic annulus enlargement, noncoronary sinus**
      🔧 97.4    ✂ 97.4    **FUD** 090               C 80 ▭
      AMA: 2017,Jan,8; 2016,Jan,13; 2015,Jan,16; 2014,Jan,11; 2012,Jan,15-42

Overhead schematic of major heart valves

**33412**     **with transventricular aortic annulus enlargement (Konno procedure)**
      🔧 92.1    ✂ 92.1    **FUD** 090               C 80 ▭
      AMA: 2017,Jan,8; 2016,Jan,13; 2015,Jan,16; 2014,Jan,11

**33413**     **by translocation of autologous pulmonary valve with allograft replacement of pulmonary valve (Ross procedure)**
      🔧 94.2    ✂ 94.2    **FUD** 090               C 80 ▭
      AMA: 2017,Jan,8; 2016,Jan,13; 2015,Jan,16; 2014,Jan,11

**33414**     **Repair of left ventricular outflow tract obstruction by patch enlargement of the outflow tract**
      🔧 62.7    ✂ 62.7    **FUD** 090               C 80 ▭
      AMA: 2017,Jan,8; 2016,Jan,13; 2015,Jan,16; 2014,Jan,11

**33415**     **Resection or incision of subvalvular tissue for discrete subvalvular aortic stenosis**
      🔧 59.0    ✂ 59.0    **FUD** 090               C 80 ▭
      AMA: 2017,Jan,8; 2016,Jan,13; 2015,Jan,16; 2014,Jan,11

## 33416 Ventriculectomy

**CMS:** 100-03,20.26 Partial Ventriculectomy
      EXCLUDES    Percutaneous transcatheter septal reduction therapy (93583)

**33416**     **Ventriculomyotomy (-myectomy) for idiopathic hypertrophic subaortic stenosis (eg, asymmetric septal hypertrophy)**
      🔧 58.9    ✂ 58.9    **FUD** 090               C 80 ▭
      AMA: 2017,Jan,8; 2016,Jan,13; 2015,Jan,16; 2014,Jan,11

## 33417 Repair of Supravalvular Stenosis by Aortoplasty

**33417**     **Aortoplasty (gusset) for supravalvular stenosis**
      🔧 48.5    ✂ 48.5    **FUD** 090               C 80 ▭
      AMA: 2017,Jan,8; 2016,Jan,13; 2015,Jan,16; 2014,Jan,11

26/TC PC/TC Only      A2-Z3 ASC Payment      50 Bilateral      ♂ Male Only      ♀ Female Only      🔧 Facility RVU      ✂ Non-Facility RVU      ▭ CCI
FUD Follow-up Days    CMS: IOM (Pub 100)      A-Y OPPSI      80/80 Surg Assist Allowed / w/Doc      🔲 Lab Crosswalk      ✚ Radiology Crosswalk      ✖ CLIA
**128**                              CPT © 2017 American Medical Association. All Rights Reserved.                    © 2017 Optum360, LLC

## 33418-33419 Transcatheter Mitral Valve Procedures

INCLUDES  Access sheath placement
Advancement of valve delivery system
Deployment of valve
Radiology procedures:
Angiography during and after procedure
Documentation of completion of the intervention
Guidance for valve placement
Supervision and interpretation
Valve repositioning when necessary
EXCLUDES  *Cardiac catheterization services for purposes other than TMVR*
*Diagnostic angiography at different session from interventional procedure*
*Percutaneous approach through the coronary sinus for TMVR (0345T)*
*Percutaneous coronary interventional procedures*
*Transcatheter TMVI by percutaneous or transthoracic approach (0483T-0484T)*
Code also cardiopulmonary bypass:
Central (33369)
Open peripheral (33368)
Percutaneous peripheral (33367)
Code also diagnostic coronary angiography and cardiac catheterization procedures when:
No previous study available and full diagnostic study performed
Previous study inadequate or patient's clinical indication for the study changed prior to or during the procedure
Use modifier 59 with cardiac catheterization procedures when on same day or same session as TMVR
Code also transvascular ventricular support:
Balloon pump (33967, 33970, 33973)
Ventricular assist device (33990-33993)

33418  **Transcatheter mitral valve repair, percutaneous approach, including transseptal puncture when performed; initial prosthesis**
Code also left heart catheterization when performed by transapical puncture (93462)
🔧 52.4  ✂ 52.4  **FUD** 090          C 80 ▣
**AMA:** 2017,Jan,8; 2016,Jan,13; 2015,Sep,3

+  33419  **additional prosthesis(es) during same session (List separately in addition to code for primary procedure)**
EXCLUDES  *Procedures performed more than one time per session*
Code first (33418)
🔧 12.3  ✂ 12.3  **FUD** ZZZ          N N1 80 ▣
**AMA:** 2017,Jan,8; 2016,Jan,13; 2015,Sep,3

## 33420-33430 Mitral Valve Procedures

Code also removal of thrombus through a separate heart incision, when performed (33310-33315); append modifier 59 to (33315)

33420  **Valvotomy, mitral valve; closed heart**
🔧 42.4  ✂ 42.4  **FUD** 090          C ▣
**AMA:** 2017,Jan,8; 2016,Jan,13; 2015,Sep,3; 2015,Jan,16; 2014,Jan,11

33422  **open heart, with cardiopulmonary bypass**
🔧 48.4  ✂ 48.4  **FUD** 090          C 80 ▣
**AMA:** 2017,Jan,8; 2016,Jan,13; 2015,Sep,3; 2015,Jan,16; 2014,Jan,11

33425  **Valvuloplasty, mitral valve, with cardiopulmonary bypass;**
🔧 79.2  ✂ 79.2  **FUD** 090          C 80 ▣
**AMA:** 2017,Jan,8; 2016,Jan,13; 2015,Sep,3; 2015,Jan,16; 2014,Jan,11; 2012,Jan,15-42

33426  **with prosthetic ring**
🔧 69.1  ✂ 69.1  **FUD** 090          C 80 ▣
**AMA:** 2017,Jan,8; 2016,Jan,13; 2015,Sep,3; 2015,Jan,16; 2014,Jan,11

33427  **radical reconstruction, with or without ring**
🔧 70.9  ✂ 70.9  **FUD** 090          C 80 ▣
**AMA:** 2017,Jan,8; 2016,Jan,13; 2015,Sep,3; 2015,Jan,16; 2014,Jan,11

33430  **Replacement, mitral valve, with cardiopulmonary bypass**
🔧 81.2  ✂ 81.2  **FUD** 090          C 80 ▣
**AMA:** 2017,Jan,8; 2016,Jan,13; 2015,Sep,3; 2015,Jan,16; 2014,Jan,11

## 33460-33468 Tricuspid Valve Procedures

Code also removal of thrombus through a separate heart incision, when performed (33310-33315); append modifier 59 to (33315)

33460  **Valvectomy, tricuspid valve, with cardiopulmonary bypass**
🔧 70.4  ✂ 70.4  **FUD** 090          C 80 ▣
**AMA:** 2017,Jan,8; 2016,Jan,13; 2015,Jan,16; 2014,Jan,11

33463  **Valvuloplasty, tricuspid valve; without ring insertion**
🔧 89.7  ✂ 89.7  **FUD** 090          C 80 ▣
**AMA:** 2017,Jan,8; 2016,Jan,13; 2015,Jan,16; 2014,Jan,11

33464  **with ring insertion**
🔧 70.8  ✂ 70.8  **FUD** 090          C 80 ▣
**AMA:** 2017,Jan,8; 2016,Jan,13; 2015,Jan,16; 2014,Jan,11

33465  **Replacement, tricuspid valve, with cardiopulmonary bypass**
🔧 80.0  ✂ 80.0  **FUD** 090          C 80 ▣
**AMA:** 2017,Jan,8; 2016,Jan,13; 2015,Jan,16; 2014,Jan,11

33468  **Tricuspid valve repositioning and plication for Ebstein anomaly**
🔧 71.4  ✂ 71.4  **FUD** 090          C 80 ▣
**AMA:** 2017,Jan,8; 2016,Jan,13; 2015,Jan,16; 2014,Jan,11

## 33470-33474 Pulmonary Valvotomy

INCLUDES  Brock's operation
Code also the concurrent ligation/takedown of a systemic-to-pulmonary artery shunt (33924)

33470  **Valvotomy, pulmonary valve, closed heart; transventricular**
🔧 37.7  ✂ 37.7  **FUD** 090          63 C 80 ▣
**AMA:** 2017,Jan,8; 2016,Jan,13; 2015,Jan,16; 2014,Jan,11

33471  **via pulmonary artery**
EXCLUDES  *Percutaneous valvuloplasty of pulmonary valve (92990)*
🔧 40.3  ✂ 40.3  **FUD** 090          C 80 ▣
**AMA:** 2017,Jan,8; 2016,Jan,13; 2015,Jan,16; 2014,Jan,11

33474  **Valvotomy, pulmonary valve, open heart, with cardiopulmonary bypass**
🔧 63.4  ✂ 63.4  **FUD** 090          C 80 ▣
**AMA:** 2007,Mar,1-3; 2005,Feb,13-16

## 33475-33476 Other Procedures Pulmonary Valve

Code also the concurrent ligation/takedown of a systemic-to-pulmonary artery shunt (33924)

33475  **Replacement, pulmonary valve**
🔧 67.6  ✂ 67.6  **FUD** 090          C 80 ▣
**AMA:** 2017,Jan,8; 2016,Jan,13; 2015,Jan,16; 2014,Jan,11

33476  **Right ventricular resection for infundibular stenosis, with or without commissurotomy**
INCLUDES  Brock's operation
🔧 44.3  ✂ 44.3  **FUD** 090          C 80 ▣
**AMA:** 2017,Jan,8; 2016,Jan,13; 2015,Jan,16; 2014,Jan,11

## 33477 Transcatheter Pulmonary Valve Implantation

**INCLUDES** Cardiac catheterization, contrast injection, angiography, fluoroscopic guidance and the supervision and interpretation for device placement
Percutaneous balloon angioplasty within the treatment area
Valvuloplasty or stent insertion in pulmonary valve conduit (37236-37237, 92997-92998)
Pre-, intra-, and post-operative hemodynamic measurements

**EXCLUDES** Balloon pump insertion (33967, 33970, 33973)
Cardiopulmonary bypass performed in the same session (33367-33369)
Extracorporeal membrane oxygenation (ECMO) (33946-33959 [33962, 33963, 33964, 33965, 33966, 33969, 33984, 33985, 33986, 33987, 33988, 33989])
Fluoroscopy (76000-76001)
Injection procedure during cardiac catheterization (93563, 93566-93568)
Percutaneous cardiac intervention procedures, when performed
Procedures performed more than one time per session
Right heart catheterization (93451, 93453-93461, 93530-93533)
Ventricular assist device (VAD) (33990-33993)
Code also the concurrent ligation/takedown of a systemic-to-pulmonary artery shunt (33924)

**33477** Transcatheter pulmonary valve implantation, percutaneous approach, including pre-stenting of the valve delivery site, when performed
📇 38.0 ⚖ 38.0 **FUD** 000 C 80 ▭
**AMA:** 2017,Jan,8; 2016,Aug,9; 2016,Mar,5

## 33478 Outflow Tract Augmentation

Code also for cavopulmonary anastamosis to a second superior vena cava (33768)
Code also the concurrent ligation/takedown of a systemic-to-pulmonary artery shunt (33924)

**33478** Outflow tract augmentation (gusset), with or without commissurotomy or infundibular resection
📇 45.8 ⚖ 45.8 **FUD** 090 C 80 ▭
**AMA:** 2017,Jan,8; 2016,Jan,13; 2015,Jan,16; 2014,Jan,11

## 33496 Prosthetic Valve Repair

Code also removal of thrombus through a separate heart incision, when performed (33310-33315); append modifier 59 to (33315)
Code also reoperation if performed (33530)

**33496** Repair of non-structural prosthetic valve dysfunction with cardiopulmonary bypass (separate procedure)
📇 48.5 ⚖ 48.5 **FUD** 090 C 80 ▭
**AMA:** 2017,Jan,8; 2016,Jan,13; 2015,Jan,16; 2014,Jan,11

## 33500-33507 Repair Aberrant Coronary Artery Anatomy

**INCLUDES** Angioplasty and/or endarterectomy

**33500** Repair of coronary arteriovenous or arteriocardiac chamber fistula; with cardiopulmonary bypass
📇 45.3 ⚖ 45.3 **FUD** 090 C 80 ▭
**AMA:** 2007,Mar,1-3; 1997,Nov,1

**33501** without cardiopulmonary bypass
📇 32.3 ⚖ 32.3 **FUD** 090 C 80 ▭
**AMA:** 2007,Mar,1-3; 1997,Nov,1

**33502** Repair of anomalous coronary artery from pulmonary artery origin; by ligation
📇 37.1 ⚖ 37.1 **FUD** 090 63 C 80 ▭
**AMA:** 2007,Mar,1-3; 1997,Nov,1

**33503** by graft, without cardiopulmonary bypass
📇 38.6 ⚖ 38.6 **FUD** 090 63 C 80 ▭
**AMA:** 2007,Mar,1-3; 1997,Nov,1

**33504** by graft, with cardiopulmonary bypass
📇 42.6 ⚖ 42.6 **FUD** 090 C 80 ▭
**AMA:** 2007,Mar,1-3; 1997,Nov,1

**33505** with construction of intrapulmonary artery tunnel (Takeuchi procedure)
📇 60.1 ⚖ 60.1 **FUD** 090 63 C 80 ▭
**AMA:** 2007,Mar,1-3; 1997,Nov,1

**33506** by translocation from pulmonary artery to aorta
📇 59.9 ⚖ 59.9 **FUD** 090 63 C 80 ▭
**AMA:** 2007,Mar,1-3; 1997,Nov,1

**33507** Repair of anomalous (eg, intramural) aortic origin of coronary artery by unroofing or translocation
📇 50.2 ⚖ 50.2 **FUD** 090 C 80 ▭
**AMA:** 2017,Jan,8; 2016,Jan,13; 2015,Jan,16; 2014,Jan,11

## 33508 Endoscopic Harvesting of Venous Graft

**INCLUDES** Diagnostic endoscopy
**EXCLUDES** Harvesting of vein of upper extremity (35500)
Code first (33510-33523)

+ **33508** Endoscopy, surgical, including video-assisted harvest of vein(s) for coronary artery bypass procedure (List separately in addition to code for primary procedure)
📇 0.47 ⚖ 0.47 **FUD** ZZZ N M1 80 ▭
**AMA:** 1997,Nov,1

## 33510-33516 Coronary Artery Bypass: Venous Grafts

**INCLUDES** Obtaining saphenous vein grafts
Venous bypass grafting only
**EXCLUDES** Arterial bypass (33533-33536)
Combined arterial-venous bypass (33517-33523, 33533-33536)
Obtaining vein graft:
Femoropopliteal vein (35572)
Upper extremity vein (35500)
Percutaneous ventricular assist devices (33990-33993)
Code also modifier 80 when assistant at surgery obtains grafts

**33510** Coronary artery bypass, vein only; single coronary venous graft
📇 56.0 ⚖ 56.0 **FUD** 090 C 80 ▭
**AMA:** 2017,Jan,8; 2016,Jan,13; 2015,Jan,16; 2014,Aug,14; 2014,Jan,11; 2012,Apr,3-9; 2012,Jan,15-42

**33511** 2 coronary venous grafts
📇 61.6 ⚖ 61.6 **FUD** 090 C 80 ▭
**AMA:** 2017,Jan,8; 2016,Jan,13; 2015,Jan,16; 2014,Aug,14; 2014,Jan,11; 2012,Apr,3-9

**33512** 3 coronary venous grafts
📇 70.0 ⚖ 70.0 **FUD** 090 C 80 ▭
**AMA:** 2017,Jan,8; 2016,Jan,13; 2015,Jan,16; 2014,Aug,14; 2014,Jan,11; 2012,Apr,3-9

**33513** 4 coronary venous grafts
📇 72.1 ⚖ 72.1 **FUD** 090 C 80 ▭
**AMA:** 2017,Jan,8; 2016,Jan,13; 2015,Jan,16; 2014,Aug,14; 2014,Jan,11; 2012,Apr,3-9

**33514** 5 coronary venous grafts
📇 76.1 ⚖ 76.1 **FUD** 090 C 80 ▭
**AMA:** 2017,Jan,8; 2016,Jan,13; 2015,Jan,16; 2014,Aug,14; 2014,Jan,11; 2012,Apr,3-9

**33516** 6 or more coronary venous grafts
📇 79.7 ⚖ 79.7 **FUD** 090 C 80 ▭
**AMA:** 2017,Jan,8; 2016,Jan,13; 2015,Jan,16; 2014,Aug,14; 2014,Jan,11; 2012,Apr,3-9

## 33517-33523 Coronary Artery Bypass: Venous AND Arterial Grafts

**INCLUDES** Obtaining saphenous vein grafts
**EXCLUDES** Obtaining arterial graft:
Upper extremity (35600)
Obtaining vein graft:
Femoropopliteal vein graft (35572)
Upper extremity (35500)
Percutaneous ventricular assist devices (33990-33993)
Code also modifier 80 when assistant at surgery obtains grafts
Code first (33533-33536)

+ **33517** Coronary artery bypass, using venous graft(s) and arterial graft(s); single vein graft (List separately in addition to code for primary procedure)
📇 5.45 ⚖ 5.45 **FUD** ZZZ C 80 ▭
**AMA:** 2017,Jan,8; 2016,Jan,13; 2015,Jan,16; 2014,Jan,11; 2012,Apr,3-9

| 26/TC PC/TC Only | A2-Z3 ASC Payment | 50 Bilateral | ♂ Male Only | ♀ Female Only | 📇 Facility RVU | ⚖ Non-Facility RVU | ▭ CCI |
| FUD Follow-up Days | CMS: IOM (Pub 100) | A-Y OPPSI | 80/80 Surg Assist Allowed / w/Doc | | 🔬 Lab Crosswalk | ☢ Radiology Crosswalk | ✖ CLIA |

130
CPT © 2017 American Medical Association. All Rights Reserved.
© 2017 Optum360, LLC

+ **33518** **2 venous grafts (List separately in addition to code for primary procedure)**
🚑 11.9    🔪 11.9    **FUD** ZZZ    [C] [80] 🔲
**AMA:** 2017,Jan,8; 2016,Jan,13; 2015,Jan,16; 2014,Jan,11; 2012,Apr,3-9

+ **33519** **3 venous grafts (List separately in addition to code for primary procedure)**
🚑 15.8    🔪 15.8    **FUD** ZZZ    [C] [80] 🔲
**AMA:** 2017,Jan,8; 2016,Jan,13; 2015,Jan,16; 2014,Jan,11; 2012,Apr,3-9

+ **33521** **4 venous grafts (List separately in addition to code for primary procedure)**
🚑 18.9    🔪 18.9    **FUD** ZZZ    [C] [80] 🔲
**AMA:** 2017,Jan,8; 2016,Jan,13; 2015,Jan,16; 2014,Jan,11; 2012,Apr,3-9

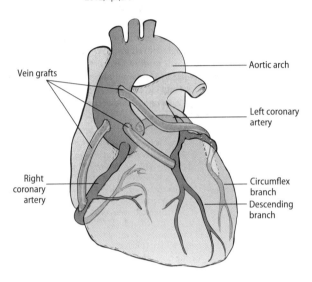

Vein grafts
Aortic arch
Left coronary artery
Right coronary artery
Circumflex branch
Descending branch

+ **33522** **5 venous grafts (List separately in addition to code for primary procedure)**
🚑 21.3    🔪 21.3    **FUD** ZZZ    [C] [80] 🔲
**AMA:** 2017,Jan,8; 2016,Jan,13; 2015,Jan,16; 2014,Jan,11; 2012,Apr,3-9

+ **33523** **6 or more venous grafts (List separately in addition to code for primary procedure)**
🚑 24.1    🔪 24.1    **FUD** ZZZ    [C] [80] 🔲
**AMA:** 2017,Jan,8; 2016,Jan,13; 2015,Jan,16; 2014,Jan,11; 2012,Apr,3-9

## 33530 Reoperative Coronary Artery Bypass Graft or Valve Procedure

*EXCLUDES*   *Percutaneous ventricular assist devices (33990-33993)*
Code first (33390-33391, 33404-33496, 33510-33536, 33863)

+ **33530** **Reoperation, coronary artery bypass procedure or valve procedure, more than 1 month after original operation (List separately in addition to code for primary procedure)**
🚑 15.2    🔪 15.2    **FUD** ZZZ    [C] [80] 🔲
**AMA:** 2017,Jan,8; 2016,Jan,13; 2015,Jan,16; 2014,Jan,11; 2012,Apr,3-9; 2012,Jan,15-42

## 33533-33536 Coronary Artery Bypass: Arterial Grafts

*INCLUDES*   Obtaining arterial graft (eg, epigastric, internal mammary, gastroepiploic and others)
*EXCLUDES*   *Obtaining arterial graft:*
    *Upper extremity (35600)*
  *Obtaining venous graft:*
    *Femoropopliteal vein (35572)*
    *Upper extremity (35500)*
  *Percutaneous ventricular assist devices (33990-33993)*
  *Venous bypass (33510-33516)*
Code also for combined arterial venous grafts (33517-33523)
Code also modifier 80 when assistant at surgery obtains grafts

**33533** **Coronary artery bypass, using arterial graft(s); single arterial graft**
🚑 54.2    🔪 54.2    **FUD** 090    [C] [80] 🔲
**AMA:** 2017,Jan,8; 2016,Jan,13; 2015,Jan,16; 2014,Nov,14; 2014,Jan,11; 2012,Apr,3-9

**33534** **2 coronary arterial grafts**
🚑 63.8    🔪 63.8    **FUD** 090    [C] [80] 🔲
**AMA:** 2017,Jan,8; 2016,Jan,13; 2015,Jan,16; 2014,Jan,11; 2012,Apr,3-9

**33535** **3 coronary arterial grafts**
🚑 71.2    🔪 71.2    **FUD** 090    [C] [80] 🔲
**AMA:** 2017,Jan,8; 2016,Jan,13; 2015,Jan,16; 2014,Jan,11; 2012,Apr,3-9

**33536** **4 or more coronary arterial grafts**
🚑 76.7    🔪 76.7    **FUD** 090    [C] [80] 🔲
**AMA:** 2017,Jan,8; 2016,Jan,13; 2015,Jan,16; 2014,Nov,14; 2014,Jan,11; 2012,Apr,3-9

## 33542-33548 Ventricular Reconstruction

**33542** **Myocardial resection (eg, ventricular aneurysmectomy)**
Code also removal of thrombus through a separate heart incision, when performed (33310-33315); append modifier 59 to (33315)
🚑 76.1    🔪 76.1    **FUD** 090    [C] [80] 🔲
**AMA:** 2017,Jan,8; 2016,Jan,13; 2015,Jan,16; 2014,Jan,11

**33545** **Repair of postinfarction ventricular septal defect, with or without myocardial resection**
Code also removal of thrombus through a separate heart incision, when performed (33310-33315); append modifier 59 to (33315)
🚑 89.9    🔪 89.9    **FUD** 090    [C] [80] 🔲
**AMA:** 2017,Jan,8; 2016,Jan,13; 2015,Jan,16; 2014,Jan,11

**33548** **Surgical ventricular restoration procedure, includes prosthetic patch, when performed (eg, ventricular remodeling, SVR, SAVER, Dor procedures)**
*EXCLUDES*   *Batista procedure or pachopexy (33999)*
  *Cardiotomy, exploratory (33310, 33315)*
  *Temporary pacemaker (33210-33211)*
  *Tube thoracostomy (32551)*
🚑 86.1    🔪 86.1    **FUD** 090    [C] [80] 🔲
**AMA:** 2017,Jan,8; 2016,Jan,13; 2015,Jan,16; 2014,Jan,11; 2012,Jan,15-42

## 33572 Endarterectomy with CABG (LAD, RCA, Cx)

Code first (33510-33516, 33533-33536)

+ **33572** **Coronary endarterectomy, open, any method, of left anterior descending, circumflex, or right coronary artery performed in conjunction with coronary artery bypass graft procedure, each vessel (List separately in addition to primary procedure)**
🚑 6.69    🔪 6.69    **FUD** ZZZ    [C] [80] 🔲
**AMA:** 1997,Nov,1; 1994,Win,1

## 33600-33622 Repair Aberrant Heart Anatomy

**33600** **Closure of atrioventricular valve (mitral or tricuspid) by suture or patch**
🚑 50.0    🔪 50.0    **FUD** 090    [C] [80] 🔲
**AMA:** 2017,Jan,8; 2016,Jan,13; 2015,Jan,16; 2014,Jan,11

● New Code   ▲ Revised Code   ○ Reinstated   ● New Web Release   ▲ Revised Web Release   Unlisted   Not Covered   # Resequenced
⊘ AMA Mod 51 Exempt   ⑤⓪ Optum Mod 51 Exempt   ⑥③ Mod 63 Exempt   ✔ Non-FDA Drug   ★ Telemedicine   Ⓜ Maternity   Ⓐ Age Edit   + Add-on   **AMA:** CPT Asst
© 2017 Optum360, LLC    CPT © 2017 American Medical Association. All Rights Reserved.    **131**

**33602** Closure of semilunar valve (aortic or pulmonary) by suture or patch

Code also the concurrent ligation/takedown of a systemic-to-pulmonary artery shunt (33924)

🔧 48.5    ✂ 48.5    **FUD** 090    C 80 ▢

**AMA:** 2007,Mar,1-3; 1997,Nov,1

**33606** Anastomosis of pulmonary artery to aorta (Damus-Kaye-Stansel procedure)

Code also the concurrent ligation/takedown of a systemic-to-pulmonary artery shunt (33924)

🔧 51.8    ✂ 51.8    **FUD** 090    C 80 ▢

**AMA:** 2007,Mar,1-3; 1997,Nov,1

**33608** Repair of complex cardiac anomaly other than pulmonary atresia with ventricular septal defect by construction or replacement of conduit from right or left ventricle to pulmonary artery

EXCLUDES  *Unifocalization of arborization anomalies of pulmonary artery (33925, 33926)*

Code also the concurrent ligation/takedown of a systemic-to-pulmonary artery shunt (33924)

🔧 52.4    ✂ 52.4    **FUD** 090    C 80 ▢

**AMA:** 2007,Mar,1-3; 1997,Nov,1

**33610** Repair of complex cardiac anomalies (eg, single ventricle with subaortic obstruction) by surgical enlargement of ventricular septal defect

Code also the concurrent ligation/takedown of a systemic-to-pulmonary artery shunt (33924)

🔧 51.7    ✂ 51.7    **FUD** 090    63 C 80 ▢

**AMA:** 2007,Mar,1-3; 2002,May,7

**33611** Repair of double outlet right ventricle with intraventricular tunnel repair;

Code also the concurrent ligation/takedown of a systemic-to-pulmonary artery shunt (33924)

🔧 56.9    ✂ 56.9    **FUD** 090    63 C 80 ▢

**AMA:** 2007,Mar,1-3; 1997,Nov,1

**33612** with repair of right ventricular outflow tract obstruction

Code also the concurrent ligation/takedown of a systemic-to-pulmonary artery shunt (33924)

🔧 58.4    ✂ 58.4    **FUD** 090    C 80 ▢

**AMA:** 2007,Mar,1-3; 1997,Nov,1

**33615** Repair of complex cardiac anomalies (eg, tricuspid atresia) by closure of atrial septal defect and anastomosis of atria or vena cava to pulmonary artery (simple Fontan procedure)

Code also the concurrent ligation/takedown of a systemic-to-pulmonary artery shunt (33924)

🔧 58.2    ✂ 58.2    **FUD** 090    C 80 ▢

**AMA:** 2007,Mar,1-3; 1997,Nov,1

**33617** Repair of complex cardiac anomalies (eg, single ventricle) by modified Fontan procedure

Code also cavopulmonary anastomosis to a second superior vena cava (33768)

Code also the concurrent ligation/takedown of a systemic-to-pulmonary artery shunt (33924)

🔧 63.0    ✂ 63.0    **FUD** 090    C 80 ▢

**AMA:** 2007,Mar,1-3; 1997,Nov,1

**33619** Repair of single ventricle with aortic outflow obstruction and aortic arch hypoplasia (hypoplastic left heart syndrome) (eg, Norwood procedure)

🔧 79.4    ✂ 79.4    **FUD** 090    63 C 80 ▢

**AMA:** 2017,Jan,8; 2016,Jul,3; 2016,Jan,13; 2015,Jan,16; 2014,Jan,11; 2012,May,14-15

**33620** Application of right and left pulmonary artery bands (eg, hybrid approach stage 1)

EXCLUDES  *Banding of main pulmonary artery related to septal defect (33690)*

Code also transthoracic insertion of catheter for stent placement with removal of catheter and closure when performed during same session (33621)

🔧 48.1    ✂ 48.1    **FUD** 090    C 80 ▢

**AMA:** 2017,Jan,8; 2016,Jul,3; 2016,Jan,13; 2015,Jan,16; 2014,Jan,11; 2012,May,14-15

**33621** Transthoracic insertion of catheter for stent placement with catheter removal and closure (eg, hybrid approach stage 1)

Code also application of right and left pulmonary artery bands when performed during same session (33620)

Code also stent placement (37236)

🔧 27.1    ✂ 27.1    **FUD** 090    C 80 ▢

**AMA:** 2017,Jan,8; 2016,Jul,3; 2016,Jan,13; 2015,Jan,16; 2014,Jan,11; 2012,May,14-15

**33622** Reconstruction of complex cardiac anomaly (eg, single ventricle or hypoplastic left heart) with palliation of single ventricle with aortic outflow obstruction and aortic arch hypoplasia, creation of cavopulmonary anastomosis, and removal of right and left pulmonary bands (eg, hybrid approach stage 2, Norwood, bidirectional Glenn, pulmonary artery debanding)

EXCLUDES  *Excision of coarctation of aorta (33840, 33845, 33851)*

*Repair of hypoplastic or interrupted aortic arch (33853)*

*Repair of patent ductus arteriosus (33822)*

*Repair of pulmonary artery stenosis by reconstruction with patch or graft (33917)*

*Repair of single ventricle with aortic outflow obstruction and aortic arch hypoplasia (33619)*

*Shunt; superior vena cava to pulmonary artery for flow to both lungs (33767)*

Code also anastomosis, cavopulmonary, second superior vena cava for bilateral bidirectional Glenn procedure (33768)

Code also the concurrent ligation/takedown of a systemic-to-pulmonary artery shunt (33924)

🔧 106.    ✂ 106.    **FUD** 090    C 80 ▢

**AMA:** 2017,Jan,8; 2016,Jul,3; 2016,Jan,13; 2015,Jan,16; 2014,Jan,11; 2012,May,14-15

## 33641-33645 Closure of Defect: Atrium

Code also removal of thrombus through a separate heart incision, when performed (33310-33315); append modifier 59 to (33315)

**33641** Repair atrial septal defect, secundum, with cardiopulmonary bypass, with or without patch

🔧 47.8    ✂ 47.8    **FUD** 090    C 80 ▢

**AMA:** 2017,Jan,8; 2016,Jan,13; 2015,Jan,16; 2014,Jan,11; 2012,Jan,15-42

**33645** Direct or patch closure, sinus venosus, with or without anomalous pulmonary venous drainage

EXCLUDES  *Repair of isolated partial anomalous pulmonary venous return (33724)*

*Repair of pulmonary venous stenosis (33726)*

🔧 50.4    ✂ 50.4    **FUD** 090    C 80 ▢

**AMA:** 2007,Mar,1-3; 1997,Nov,1

## 33647 Closure of Septal Defect: Atrium AND Ventricle

EXCLUDES  *Tricuspid atresia repair procedures (33615)*

Code also removal of thrombus through a separate heart incision, when performed (33310-33315); append modifier 59 to (33315)

**33647** Repair of atrial septal defect and ventricular septal defect, with direct or patch closure

🔧 53.0    ✂ 53.0    **FUD** 090    63 C 80 ▢

**AMA:** 2007,Mar,1-3; 1997,Nov,1

## 33660-33670 Closure of Defect: Atrioventricular Canal

**33660** Repair of incomplete or partial atrioventricular canal (ostium primum atrial septal defect), with or without atrioventricular valve repair

🔧 51.2    ✂ 51.2    **FUD** 090    C 80 ▢

**AMA:** 2007,Mar,1-3; 1997,Nov,1

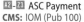 PC/TC Only
**FUD** Follow-up Days
A2-Z3 ASC Payment
**CMS:** IOM (Pub 100)
50 Bilateral
A-Y OPPSI
♂ Male Only
80/80 Surg Assist Allowed / w/Doc
♀ Female Only
🔧 Facility RVU
🧪 Lab Crosswalk
✂ Non-Facility RVU
Radiology Crosswalk
▢ CCI
✖ CLIA

132

CPT © 2017 American Medical Association. All Rights Reserved.

© 2017 Optum360, LLC

**33665** Repair of intermediate or transitional atrioventricular canal, with or without atrioventricular valve repair
  57.3  57.3  **FUD** 090
  [C] [80] [⌐]
  **AMA:** 2007,Mar,1-3; 1997,Nov,1

**33670** Repair of complete atrioventricular canal, with or without prosthetic valve
  Code also removal of thrombus through a separate heart incision, when performed (33310-33315); append modifier 59 to (33315)
  57.5  57.5  **FUD** 090
  [63] [C] [80] [⌐]
  **AMA:** 2007,Mar,1-3; 1997,Nov,1

## 33675-33677 Closure of Multiple Septal Defects: Ventricle

EXCLUDES  Closure of single ventricular septal defect (33681, 33684, 33688)
  Insertion or replacement of temporary transvenous single chamber cardiac electrode or pacemaker catheter (33210)
  Percutaneous closure (93581)
  Thoracentesis (32554-32555)
  Thoracotomy (32100)
  Tube thoracostomy (32551)

**33675** Closure of multiple ventricular septal defects;
  57.5  57.5  **FUD** 090
  [C] [80] [⌐]
  **AMA:** 2017,Jan,8; 2016,Jan,13; 2015,Jan,16; 2014,Jan,11

**33676** with pulmonary valvotomy or infundibular resection (acyanotic)
  62.3  62.3  **FUD** 090
  [C] [80] [⌐]
  **AMA:** 2017,Jan,8; 2016,Jan,13; 2015,Jan,16; 2014,Jan,11

**33677** with removal of pulmonary artery band, with or without gusset
  64.7  64.7  **FUD** 090
  [C] [80] [⌐]
  **AMA:** 2017,Jan,8; 2016,Jan,13; 2015,Jan,16; 2014,Jan,11

## 33681-33688 Closure of Septal Defect: Ventricle

EXCLUDES  Repair of pulmonary vein that requires creating an atrial septal defect (33724)

**33681** Closure of single ventricular septal defect, with or without patch;
  Code also removal of thrombus through a separate heart incision, when performed (33310-33315); append modifier 59 to (33315)
  53.5  53.5  **FUD** 090
  [C] [80] [⌐]
  **AMA:** 2017,Jan,8; 2016,Jan,13; 2015,Jan,16; 2014,Jan,11

**33684** with pulmonary valvotomy or infundibular resection (acyanotic)
  Code also concurrent ligation/takedown of a systemic-to-pulmonary artery shunt if performed (33924)
  55.1  55.1  **FUD** 090
  [C] [80] [⌐]
  **AMA:** 2007,Mar,1-3; 1997,Nov,1

**33688** with removal of pulmonary artery band, with or without gusset
  Code also the concurrent ligation/takedown of a systemic-to-pulmonary artery shunt if performed (33924)
  58.1  58.1  **FUD** 090
  [C] [80] [⌐]
  **AMA:** 2007,Mar,1-3; 1997,Nov,1

## 33690 Reduce Pulmonary Overcirculation in Septal Defects

EXCLUDES  Left and right pulmonary artery banding in a single ventricle (33620)

**33690** Banding of pulmonary artery
  34.9  34.9  **FUD** 090
  [63] [C] [80] [⌐]
  **AMA:** 2017,Jan,8; 2016,Jan,13; 2015,Jan,16; 2014,Jan,11; 2012,May,14-15

## 33692-33697 Repair of Defects of Tetralogy of Fallot

Code also the concurrent ligation/takedown of a systemic-to-pulmonary artery shunt (33924)

**33692** Complete repair tetralogy of Fallot without pulmonary atresia;
  60.3  60.3  **FUD** 090
  [C] [80] [⌐]
  **AMA:** 2007,Mar,1-3; 1997,Nov,1

**33694** with transannular patch
  56.9  56.9  **FUD** 090
  [63] [C] [80] [⌐]
  **AMA:** 2007,Mar,1-3; 1997,Nov,1

**33697** Complete repair tetralogy of Fallot with pulmonary atresia including construction of conduit from right ventricle to pulmonary artery and closure of ventricular septal defect
  59.9  59.9  **FUD** 090
  [C] [80] [⌐]
  **AMA:** 2017,Jan,8; 2016,Jan,13; 2015,Jan,16; 2014,Jan,11

## 33702-33722 Repair Anomalies Sinus of Valsalva

**33702** Repair sinus of Valsalva fistula, with cardiopulmonary bypass;
  45.0  45.0  **FUD** 090
  [C] [80] [⌐]
  **AMA:** 2017,Jan,8; 2016,Jan,13; 2015,Jan,16; 2014,Jan,11

**33710** with repair of ventricular septal defect
  59.8  59.8  **FUD** 090
  [C] [80] [⌐]
  **AMA:** 2007,Mar,1-3; 1997,Nov,1

**33720** Repair sinus of Valsalva aneurysm, with cardiopulmonary bypass
  45.0  45.0  **FUD** 090
  [C] [80] [⌐]
  **AMA:** 2007,Mar,1-3; 1997,Nov,1

**33722** Closure of aortico-left ventricular tunnel
  47.3  47.3  **FUD** 090
  [C] [80] [⌐]
  **AMA:** 2017,Jan,8; 2016,Jan,13; 2015,Jan,16; 2014,Jan,11

## 33724-33732 Repair Aberrant Pulmonary Venous Connection

**33724** Repair of isolated partial anomalous pulmonary venous return (eg, Scimitar Syndrome)
  EXCLUDES  Temporary pacemaker (33210-33211)
    Tube thoracostomy (32551)
  44.8  44.8  **FUD** 090
  [C] [80] [⌐]
  **AMA:** 2017,Jan,8; 2016,Jan,13; 2015,Jan,16; 2014,Jan,11

**33726** Repair of pulmonary venous stenosis
  EXCLUDES  Temporary pacemaker (33210-33211)
    Tube thoracostomy (32551)
  59.3  59.3  **FUD** 090
  [C] [80] [⌐]
  **AMA:** 2017,Jan,8; 2016,Jan,13; 2015,Jan,16; 2014,Jan,11

**33730** Complete repair of anomalous pulmonary venous return (supracardiac, intracardiac, or infracardiac types)
  EXCLUDES  Partial anomalous pulmonary venous return (33724)
    Repair of pulmonary venous stenosis (33726)
  58.4  58.4  **FUD** 090
  [63] [C] [80] [⌐]
  **AMA:** 2017,Jan,8; 2016,Jan,13; 2015,Jan,16; 2014,Jan,11

**33732** Repair of cor triatriatum or supravalvular mitral ring by resection of left atrial membrane
  48.0  48.0  **FUD** 090
  [63] [C] [80] [⌐]
  **AMA:** 2017,Jan,8; 2016,Jan,13; 2015,Jan,16; 2014,Jan,11

## 33735-33737 Creation of Atrial Septal Defect

Code also the concurrent ligation/takedown of a systemic-to-pulmonary artery shunt (33924)

**33735** Atrial septectomy or septostomy; closed heart (Blalock-Hanlon type operation)
  37.7  37.7  **FUD** 090
  [63] [C] [80] [⌐]
  **AMA:** 2017,Jan,8; 2016,Jan,13; 2015,Jan,16; 2014,Jan,11

**33736** open heart with cardiopulmonary bypass
  40.9  40.9  **FUD** 090
  [63] [C] [80] [⌐]
  **AMA:** 2007,Mar,1-3; 1997,Nov,1

**33737** open heart, with inflow occlusion
  EXCLUDES  Atrial septectomy/septostomy:
    Blade method (92993)
    Transvenous balloon method (92992)
  37.7  37.7  **FUD** 090
  [C] [80] [⌐]
  **AMA:** 2007,Mar,1-3; 1997,Nov,1

## 33750-33767 Systemic Vessel to Pulmonary Artery Shunts

Code also the concurrent ligation/takedown of a systemic-to-pulmonary artery shunt (33924)

**33750** Shunt; subclavian to pulmonary artery (Blalock-Taussig type operation)
  38.5  38.5  **FUD** 090
  [63] [C] [80] [⌐]
  **AMA:** 2007,Mar,1-3; 1997,Nov,1

---

● New Code  ▲ Revised Code  ○ Reinstated  ● New Web Release  ▲ Revised Web Release  Unlisted  Not Covered  # Resequenced
⊘ AMA Mod 51 Exempt  ⑤ Optum Mod 51 Exempt  ⑥③ Mod 63 Exempt  ✗ Non-FDA Drug  ★ Telemedicine  Ⓜ Maternity  Ⓐ Age Edit  + Add-on  **AMA:** CPT Asst

© 2017 Optum360, LLC  CPT © 2017 American Medical Association. All Rights Reserved.

**33755**     **ascending aorta to pulmonary artery (Waterston type operation)**
    🚑 40.0     ⚕ 40.0     **FUD** 090                         ⑥③ C 80 ▭
    **AMA:** 2007,Mar,1-3; 1997,Nov,1

**33762**     **descending aorta to pulmonary artery (Potts-Smith type operation)**
    🚑 39.1     ⚕ 39.1     **FUD** 090                         ⑥③ C 80 ▭
    **AMA:** 2007,Mar,1-3; 1997,Nov,1

**33764**     **central, with prosthetic graft**
    🚑 38.3     ⚕ 38.3     **FUD** 090                         C 80 ▭
    **AMA:** 2007,Mar,1-3; 1997,Nov,1

**33766**     **superior vena cava to pulmonary artery for flow to 1 lung (classical Glenn procedure)**
    🚑 40.7     ⚕ 40.7     **FUD** 090                         C 80 ▭
    **AMA:** 2007,Mar,1-3; 1997,Nov,1

**33767**     **superior vena cava to pulmonary artery for flow to both lungs (bidirectional Glenn procedure)**
    🚑 41.4     ⚕ 41.4     **FUD** 090                         C 80 ▭
    **AMA:** 2017,Jan,8; 2016,Jul,3

## 33768 Cavopulmonary Anastomosis to Decrease Volume Load

> **EXCLUDES**  Temporary pacemaker (33210-33211)
>                     Tube thoracostomy (32551)
> Code first (33478, 33617, 33622, 33767)

**+**   **33768**     **Anastomosis, cavopulmonary, second superior vena cava (List separately in addition to primary procedure)**
    🚑 12.9     ⚕ 12.9     **FUD** ZZZ                         C 80 ▭
    **AMA:** 2017,Jan,8; 2016,Jul,3; 2016,Jan,13; 2015,Jan,16; 2014,Jan,11

## 33770-33783 Repair Aberrant Anatomy: Transposition Great Vessels

> Code also the concurrent ligation/takedown of a systemic-to-pulmonary artery shunt (33924)

**33770**     **Repair of transposition of the great arteries with ventricular septal defect and subpulmonary stenosis; without surgical enlargement of ventricular septal defect**
    🚑 65.3     ⚕ 65.3     **FUD** 090                         C 80 ▭
    **AMA:** 2017,Jan,8; 2016,Jan,13; 2015,Jan,16; 2014,Jan,11

**33771**     **with surgical enlargement of ventricular septal defect**
    🚑 67.3     ⚕ 67.3     **FUD** 090                         C 80 ▭
    **AMA:** 2007,Mar,1-3; 1997,Nov,1

**33774**     **Repair of transposition of the great arteries, atrial baffle procedure (eg, Mustard or Senning type) with cardiopulmonary bypass;**
    🚑 52.4     ⚕ 52.4     **FUD** 090                         C 80 ▭
    **AMA:** 2007,Mar,1-3; 1997,Nov,1

**33775**     **with removal of pulmonary band**
    🚑 56.7     ⚕ 56.7     **FUD** 090                         C 80 ▭
    **AMA:** 2007,Mar,1-3; 1997,Nov,1

**33776**     **with closure of ventricular septal defect**
    🚑 59.9     ⚕ 59.9     **FUD** 090                         C 80 ▭
    **AMA:** 2007,Mar,1-3; 1997,Nov,1

**33777**     **with repair of subpulmonic obstruction**
    🚑 55.1     ⚕ 55.1     **FUD** 090                         C 80 ▭
    **AMA:** 2007,Mar,1-3; 1997,Nov,1

**33778**     **Repair of transposition of the great arteries, aortic pulmonary artery reconstruction (eg, Jatene type);**
    🚑 68.5     ⚕ 68.5     **FUD** 090                         ⑥③ C 80 ▭
    **AMA:** 2007,Mar,1-3; 1997,Nov,1

**33779**     **with removal of pulmonary band**
    🚑 71.8     ⚕ 71.8     **FUD** 090                         C 80 ▭
    **AMA:** 2007,Mar,1-3; 1997,Nov,1

**33780**     **with closure of ventricular septal defect**
    🚑 73.1     ⚕ 73.1     **FUD** 090                         C 80 ▭
    **AMA:** 2007,Mar,1-3; 1997,Nov,1

**33781**     **with repair of subpulmonic obstruction**
    🚑 71.5     ⚕ 71.5     **FUD** 090                         C 80 ▭
    **AMA:** 2017,Jan,8; 2016,Jan,13; 2015,Jan,16; 2014,Jan,11

**33782**     **Aortic root translocation with ventricular septal defect and pulmonary stenosis repair (ie, Nikaidoh procedure); without coronary ostium reimplantation**
    🚑 94.2     ⚕ 94.2     **FUD** 090                         C 80 ▭

> **EXCLUDES**  Closure of single ventricular septal defect (33681)
>                     Repair of complex cardiac anomaly other than pulmonary atresia (33608)
>                     Repair of pulmonary atresia with ventricular septal defect (33920)
>                     Repair of transposition of the great arteries (33770-33771, 33778, 33780)
>                     Replacement, aortic valve (33412-33413)

**33783**     **with reimplantation of 1 or both coronary ostia**
    🚑 101.     ⚕ 101.     **FUD** 090                         C 80 ▭

## 33786-33788 Repair Aberrant Anatomy: Truncus Arteriosus

**33786**     **Total repair, truncus arteriosus (Rastelli type operation)**
> Code also the concurrent ligation/takedown of a systemic-to-pulmonary artery shunt (33924)

    🚑 70.1     ⚕ 70.1     **FUD** 090                         ⑥③ C 80 ▭
    **AMA:** 2017,Jan,8; 2016,Jan,13; 2015,Jan,16; 2014,Jan,11

**33788**     **Reimplantation of an anomalous pulmonary artery**
> **EXCLUDES**  Pulmonary artery banding (33690)

    🚑 46.9     ⚕ 46.9     **FUD** 090                         C 80 ▭
    **AMA:** 2017,Jan,8; 2016,Jan,13; 2015,Jan,16; 2014,Jan,11

## 33800-33853 Repair Aberrant Anatomy: Aorta

**33800**     **Aortic suspension (aortopexy) for tracheal decompression (eg, for tracheomalacia) (separate procedure)**
    🚑 28.7     ⚕ 28.7     **FUD** 090                         C 80 ▭
    **AMA:** 2017,Jan,8; 2016,Jan,13; 2015,Jan,16; 2014,Jan,11

**33802**     **Division of aberrant vessel (vascular ring);**
    🚑 31.5     ⚕ 31.5     **FUD** 090                         C 80 ▭
    **AMA:** 2007,Mar,1-3; 1997,Nov,1

**33803**     **with reanastomosis**
    🚑 33.5     ⚕ 33.5     **FUD** 090                         C 80 ▭
    **AMA:** 2007,Mar,1-3; 1997,Nov,1

**33813**     **Obliteration of aortopulmonary septal defect; without cardiopulmonary bypass**
    🚑 37.7     ⚕ 37.7     **FUD** 090                         C 80 ▭
    **AMA:** 2007,Mar,1-3; 1997,Nov,1

**33814**     **with cardiopulmonary bypass**
    🚑 44.3     ⚕ 44.3     **FUD** 090                         C 80 ▭
    **AMA:** 2007,Mar,1-3; 1997,Nov,1

**33820**     **Repair of patent ductus arteriosus; by ligation**
> **EXCLUDES**  Percutaneous transcatheter closure patent ductus arteriosus (93582)

    🚑 28.2     ⚕ 28.2     **FUD** 090                         C 80 ▭
    **AMA:** 2017,Jan,8; 2016,Jan,13; 2015,Jan,16; 2014,Jan,11

**33822**     **by division, younger than 18 years**                         A
> **EXCLUDES**  Percutaneous transcatheter closure patent ductus arteriosus (93582)

    🚑 31.1     ⚕ 31.1     **FUD** 090                         C 80 ▭
    **AMA:** 2017,Jan,8; 2016,Jul,3; 2016,Jan,13; 2015,Jan,16; 2014,Jan,11

**33824**     **by division, 18 years and older**
> **EXCLUDES**  Percutaneous closure patent ductus arteriosus (93582)

    🚑 34.3     ⚕ 34.3     **FUD** 090                         C 80 ▭
    **AMA:** 2007,Mar,1-3; 1997,Nov,1

**33840**     **Excision of coarctation of aorta, with or without associated patent ductus arteriosus; with direct anastomosis**
    🚑 37.6     ⚕ 37.6     **FUD** 090                         C 80 ▭
    **AMA:** 2017,Jan,8; 2016,Jul,3

| 26/TC PC/TC Only | AZ-Z3 ASC Payment | 50 Bilateral | ♂ Male Only | ♀ Female Only | 🚑 Facility RVU | ⚕ Non-Facility RVU | ▭ CCI |
| **FUD** Follow-up Days | **CMS:** IOM (Pub 100) | A-Y OPPSI | 80/80 Surg Assist Allowed / w/Doc | | 🔬 Lab Crosswalk | ➕ Radiology Crosswalk | ✖ CLIA |

134                                              CPT © 2017 American Medical Association. All Rights Reserved.                                    © 2017 Optum360, LLC

**33845** with graft
🔧 38.8 ⚒ 38.8 **FUD** 090 C 80 ▭
**AMA:** 2017,Jan,8; 2016,Jul,3

**33851** repair using either left subclavian artery or prosthetic material as gusset for enlargement
🔧 38.7 ⚒ 38.7 **FUD** 090 C 80 ▭
**AMA:** 2017,Jan,8; 2016,Jul,3

**33852** Repair of hypoplastic or interrupted aortic arch using autogenous or prosthetic material; without cardiopulmonary bypass
EXCLUDES *Hypoplastic left heart syndrome repair by excision of coarctation of aorta (33619)*
🔧 40.7 ⚒ 40.7 **FUD** 090 C 80 ▭
**AMA:** 2007,Mar,1-3; 1997,Nov,1

**33853** with cardiopulmonary bypass
EXCLUDES *Hypoplastic left heart syndrome repair by excision of coarctation of aorta (33619)*
🔧 53.4 ⚒ 53.4 **FUD** 090 C 80 ▭
**AMA:** 2017,Jan,8; 2016,Jul,3; 2016,Jan,13; 2015,Jan,16; 2014,Jan,11

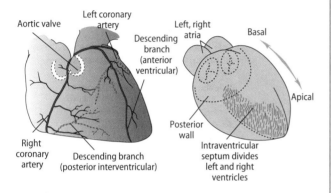

## 33860-33877 Aortic Graft Procedures

**33860** Ascending aorta graft, with cardiopulmonary bypass, includes valve suspension, when performed
🔧 93.2 ⚒ 93.2 **FUD** 090 C 80 ▭
**AMA:** 2017,Jan,8; 2016,Jan,13; 2015,Jan,16; 2014,Jan,11

**33863** Ascending aorta graft, with cardiopulmonary bypass, with aortic root replacement using valved conduit and coronary reconstruction (eg, Bentall)
INCLUDES Ascending aorta graft, with cardiopulmonary bypass, includes valve suspension, when performed (33860)
EXCLUDES *Replacement, aortic valve, with cardiopulmonary bypass (33405-33406, 33410-33413)*
🔧 91.5 ⚒ 91.5 **FUD** 090 C 80 ▭
**AMA:** 2017,Jan,8; 2016,Jan,13; 2015,Jan,16; 2014,Jan,11; 2012,Jan,15-42

**33864** Ascending aorta graft, with cardiopulmonary bypass with valve suspension, with coronary reconstruction and valve-sparing aortic root remodeling (eg, David Procedure, Yacoub Procedure)
INCLUDES Ascending aorta graft with cardiopulmonary bypass (33860-33863)
🔧 93.7 ⚒ 93.7 **FUD** 090 C 80 ▭
**AMA:** 2017,Jan,8; 2016,Jan,13; 2015,Jan,16; 2014,Jan,11; 2012,Jan,15-42

**33870** Transverse arch graft, with cardiopulmonary bypass
🔧 73.3 ⚒ 73.3 **FUD** 090 C 80 ▭
**AMA:** 1997,Nov,1

**33875** Descending thoracic aorta graft, with or without bypass
🔧 79.6 ⚒ 79.6 **FUD** 090 C 80 ▭
**AMA:** 1997,Nov,1

**33877** Repair of thoracoabdominal aortic aneurysm with graft, with or without cardiopulmonary bypass
🔧 105. ⚒ 105. **FUD** 090 C 80 ▭
**AMA:** 1997,Nov,1

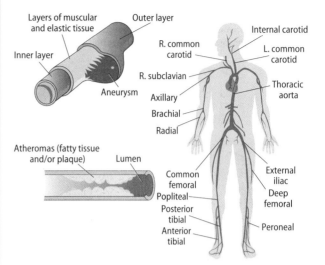

## 33880-33891 Endovascular Repair Aortic Aneurysm: Thoracic

INCLUDES Balloon angioplasty
Deployment of stent
Introduction, manipulation, placement, and deployment of the device
EXCLUDES *Additional interventional procedures provided during the endovascular repair*
*Carotid-carotid bypass (33891)*
*Guidewire and catheter insertion (36140, 36200-36218)*
*Open exposure of artery/subsequent closure ([34812], 34714-34716 [34820, 34833, 34834], [34820], [34833, 34834])*
*Subclavian to carotid artery transposition (33889)*
*Substantial artery repair/replacement (35226, 35286)*

**33880** Endovascular repair of descending thoracic aorta (eg, aneurysm, pseudoaneurysm, dissection, penetrating ulcer, intramural hematoma, or traumatic disruption); involving coverage of left subclavian artery origin, initial endoprosthesis plus descending thoracic aortic extension(s), if required, to level of celiac artery origin
INCLUDES Placement of distal extensions in distal thoracic aorta
EXCLUDES *Proximal extensions*
🔧 (75956)
🔧 52.5 ⚒ 52.5 **FUD** 090 C 80 ▭
**AMA:** 2017,Jan,8; 2016,Jan,13; 2015,Jan,16; 2014,Jan,11

**33881** not involving coverage of left subclavian artery origin, initial endoprosthesis plus descending thoracic aortic extension(s), if required, to level of celiac artery origin
INCLUDES Placement of distal extensions in distal thoracic aorta
EXCLUDES *Procedure where the placement of extension includes coverage of left subclavian artery origin (33880)*
*Proximal extensions*
🔧 (75957)
🔧 45.1 ⚒ 45.1 **FUD** 090 C 80 ▭
**AMA:** 2017,Jan,8; 2016,Jan,13; 2015,Jan,16; 2014,Jan,11

**33883** Placement of proximal extension prosthesis for endovascular repair of descending thoracic aorta (eg, aneurysm, pseudoaneurysm, dissection, penetrating ulcer, intramural hematoma, or traumatic disruption); initial extension
EXCLUDES *Procedure where the placement of extension includes coverage of left subclavian artery origin (33880)*
🔧 (75958)
🔧 32.7 ⚒ 32.7 **FUD** 090 C 80 ▭
**AMA:** 2017,Jan,8; 2016,Jan,13; 2015,Jan,16; 2014,Jan,11

● New Code ▲ Revised Code ○ Reinstated ● New Web Release ▲ Revised Web Release Unlisted Not Covered # Resequenced
⊘ AMA Mod 51 Exempt ⑤ Optum Mod 51 Exempt ⑥ Mod 63 Exempt ✗ Non-FDA Drug ★ Telemedicine Ⓜ Maternity Ⓐ Age Edit + Add-on **AMA:** CPT Asst
© 2017 Optum360, LLC CPT © 2017 American Medical Association. All Rights Reserved. **135**

**+ 33884** **each additional proximal extension (List separately in addition to code for primary procedure)**
Code first (33883)
⚡ (75958)
🚑 12.0   ⚖ 12.0   **FUD** ZZZ                C 80 ▣
**AMA:** 2017,Jan,8; 2016,Jan,13; 2015,Jan,16; 2014,Jan,11

**33886** **Placement of distal extension prosthesis(s) delayed after endovascular repair of descending thoracic aorta**
INCLUDES   All modules deployed
EXCLUDES   *Endovascular repair of descending thoracic aorta (33880, 33881)*
⚡ (75959)
🚑 28.1   ⚖ 28.1   **FUD** 090                C 80 ▣
**AMA:** 2017,Jan,8; 2016,Jan,13; 2015,Jan,16; 2014,Jan,11

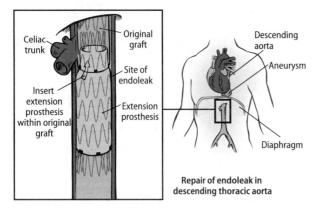

Repair of endoleak in descending thoracic aorta

**33889** **Open subclavian to carotid artery transposition performed in conjunction with endovascular repair of descending thoracic aorta, by neck incision, unilateral**
EXCLUDES   *Transposition and/or reimplantation; subclavian to carotid artery (35694)*
🚑 23.0   ⚖ 23.0   **FUD** 000              C 80 50 ▣
**AMA:** 2017,Jan,8; 2016,Jan,13; 2015,Jan,16; 2014,Jan,11

**33891** **Bypass graft, with other than vein, transcervical retropharyngeal carotid-carotid, performed in conjunction with endovascular repair of descending thoracic aorta, by neck incision**
EXCLUDES   *Bypass graft (35509, 35601)*
🚑 28.6   ⚖ 28.6   **FUD** 000              C 80 50 ▣
**AMA:** 2017,Jan,8; 2016,Jan,13; 2015,Jan,16; 2014,Jan,11

## 33910-33926 Surgical Procedures of Pulmonary Artery

**33910** **Pulmonary artery embolectomy; with cardiopulmonary bypass**
🚑 76.5   ⚖ 76.5   **FUD** 090                C 80 ▣
**AMA:** 2017,Jan,8; 2016,Jan,13; 2015,Jan,16; 2014,Jan,11

**33915** **without cardiopulmonary bypass**
🚑 36.9   ⚖ 36.9   **FUD** 090                C 80 ▣
**AMA:** 2017,Jan,8; 2016,Jan,13; 2015,Jan,16; 2014,Jan,11

**33916** **Pulmonary endarterectomy, with or without embolectomy, with cardiopulmonary bypass**
🚑 122.   ⚖ 122.   **FUD** 090                C 80 ▣
**AMA:** 2017,Jan,8; 2016,Jan,13; 2015,Jan,16; 2014,Jan,11

**33917** **Repair of pulmonary artery stenosis by reconstruction with patch or graft**
Code also the concurrent ligation/takedown of a systemic-to-pulmonary artery shunt (33924)
🚑 42.4   ⚖ 42.4   **FUD** 090                C 80 ▣
**AMA:** 2017,Jan,8; 2016,Jul,3; 2016,Jan,13; 2015,Jan,16; 2014,Jan,11

**33920** **Repair of pulmonary atresia with ventricular septal defect, by construction or replacement of conduit from right or left ventricle to pulmonary artery**
EXCLUDES   *Repair of complicated cardiac anomalies by creating/replacing conduit from ventricle to pulmonary artery (33608)*
Code also the concurrent ligation/takedown of a systemic-to-pulmonary artery shunt (33924)
🚑 55.5   ⚖ 55.5   **FUD** 090                C 80 ▣
**AMA:** 2017,Jan,8; 2016,Jan,13; 2015,Jan,16; 2014,Jan,11

**33922** **Transection of pulmonary artery with cardiopulmonary bypass**
Code also the concurrent ligation/takedown of a systemic-to-pulmonary artery shunt (33924)
🚑 40.4   ⚖ 40.4   **FUD** 090            ⊛ C 80 ▣
**AMA:** 1997,Nov,1; 1995,Win,1

**+ 33924** **Ligation and takedown of a systemic-to-pulmonary artery shunt, performed in conjunction with a congenital heart procedure (List separately in addition to code for primary procedure)**
Code first (33470-33478, 33600-33617, 33622, 33684-33688, 33692-33697, 33735-33767, 33770-33783, 33786, 33917, 33920-33922, 33925-33926, 33935, 33945)
🚑 8.35   ⚖ 8.35   **FUD** ZZZ                C 80 ▣
**AMA:** 1997,Nov,1; 1995,Win,1

**33925** **Repair of pulmonary artery arborization anomalies by unifocalization; without cardiopulmonary bypass**
🚑 50.1   ⚖ 50.1   **FUD** 090                C 80 ▣
Code also the concurrent ligation/takedown of a systemic-to-pulmonary artery shunt (33924)

**33926** **with cardiopulmonary bypass**
🚑 74.6   ⚖ 74.6   **FUD** 090                C 80 ▣
Code also the concurrent ligation/takedown of a systemic-to-pulmonary artery shunt (33924)

## 33927-33945 Heart and Heart-Lung Transplants

INCLUDES   Backbench work to prepare the donor heart and/or lungs for transplantation (33933, 33944)
Harvesting of donor organs with cold preservation (33930, 33940)
Transplantation of heart and/or lungs into recipient (33935, 33945)

● **33927** **Implantation of a total replacement heart system (artificial heart) with recipient cardiectomy**
EXCLUDES   *Implantation ventricular assist device:*
*Extracorporeal (33975-33976)*
*Intracorporeal (33979)*
*Percutaneous (33990-33991)*

● **33928** **Removal and replacement of total replacement heart system (artificial heart)**
EXCLUDES   *Replacement or revision elements of artificial heart (33999)*

● + **33929** **Removal of a total replacement heart system (artificial heart) for heart transplantation (List separately in addition to code for primary procedure)**
🚑 0.00   ⚖ 0.00   **FUD** 000
Code first (33945)

**33930** **Donor cardiectomy-pneumonectomy (including cold preservation)**
🚑 0.00   ⚖ 0.00   **FUD** XXX                C ▣
**AMA:** 1997,Nov,1

**33933** **Backbench standard preparation of cadaver donor heart/lung allograft prior to transplantation, including dissection of allograft from surrounding soft tissues to prepare aorta, superior vena cava, inferior vena cava, and trachea for implantation**
🚑 0.00   ⚖ 0.00   **FUD** XXX                C 80 ▣
**AMA:** 1997,Nov,1

**33935** **Heart-lung transplant with recipient cardiectomy-pneumonectomy**
　　Code also the concurrent ligation/takedown of a systemic-to-pulmonary artery shunt (33924)
　　🛒 144.　　✂ 144.　　**FUD** 090　　C 80 ▣
　　**AMA:** 1997,Nov,1

**33940** **Donor cardiectomy (including cold preservation)**
　　🛒 0.00　　✂ 0.00　　**FUD** XXX　　C ▣
　　**AMA:** 2017,Jan,8; 2016,Jan,13; 2015,Jan,16; 2014,Jan,11

**33944** **Backbench standard preparation of cadaver donor heart allograft prior to transplantation, including dissection of allograft from surrounding soft tissues to prepare aorta, superior vena cava, inferior vena cava, pulmonary artery, and left atrium for implantation**
　　EXCLUDES　*Procedures performed on donor heart (33300, 33310, 33320, 33390, 33463-33464, 33510, 33641, 35216, 35276, 35685)*
　　🛒 0.00　　✂ 0.00　　**FUD** XXX　　C 80 ▣
　　**AMA:** 1997,Nov,1

**33945** **Heart transplant, with or without recipient cardiectomy**
　　Code also the concurrent ligation/takedown of a systemic-to-pulmonary artery shunt (33924)
　　🛒 141.　　✂ 141.　　**FUD** 090　　C 80 ▣
　　**AMA:** 1997,May,4; 1997,Nov,1

# 33946-33959 [33962, 33963, 33964, 33965, 33966, 33969, 33984, 33985, 33986, 33987, 33988, 33989] Extracorporeal Circulatory and Respiratory Support

INCLUDES　Cannula repositioning and cannula insertion performed during same procedure
　　Multiple physician and nonphysician team collaboration
　　Veno-arterial ECMO/ECLS for heart and lung support
　　Veno-venous ECMO/ECLS for lung support
Code also extensive arterial repair/replacement (35266, 35286, 35371, 35665)
Code also overall daily management services needed to manage a patient; report the appropriate observation, hospital inpatient, or critical care E/M codes

**33946** **Extracorporeal membrane oxygenation (ECMO)/extracorporeal life support (ECLS) provided by physician; initiation, veno-venous**
　　EXCLUDES　*Daily ECMO/ECLS veno-venous management on day of initial service (33948)*
　　　*Repositioning of ECMO/ECLS cannula on day of initial service (33957-33959 [33962, 33963, 33964])*
　　Code also cannula insertion (33951-33956)
　　🛒 8.97　　✂ 8.97　　**FUD** XXX　　63 C ▣
　　**AMA:** 2017,Jan,8; 2016,Mar,5; 2016,Jan,13; 2015,Jul,3

**33947** **initiation, veno-arterial**
　　EXCLUDES　*Daily ECMO/ECLS veno-arterial management on day of initial service (33949)*
　　　*Repositioning of ECMO/ECLS cannula on day of initial service (33957-33959 [33962, 33963, 33964])*
　　Code also cannula insertion (33951-33956)
　　🛒 9.96　　✂ 9.96　　**FUD** XXX　　63 C ▣
　　**AMA:** 2017,Jan,8; 2016,Mar,5; 2016,Jan,13; 2015,Jul,3

**33948** **daily management, each day, veno-venous**
　　EXCLUDES　*ECMO/ECLS initiation, veno-venous (33946)*
　　🛒 6.94　　✂ 6.94　　**FUD** XXX　　63 C ▣
　　**AMA:** 2017,Jan,8; 2016,Mar,5; 2016,Jan,13; 2015,Jul,3

**33949** **daily management, each day, veno-arterial**
　　EXCLUDES　*ECMO/ECLS initiation, veno-arterial (33947)*
　　🛒 6.80　　✂ 6.80　　**FUD** XXX　　63 C ▣
　　**AMA:** 2017,Jan,8; 2016,Mar,5; 2016,Jan,13; 2015,Jul,3

**33951** **insertion of peripheral (arterial and/or venous) cannula(e), percutaneous, birth through 5 years of age (includes fluoroscopic guidance, when performed)** ▣A
　　INCLUDES　Cannula replacement in same vessel
　　　Cannula repositioning during same episode of care
　　Code also cannula removal if new cannula inserted in different vessel with ([33965, 33966, 33969, 33984, 33985, 33986])
　　Code also ECMO/ECLS initiation or daily management (33946-33947, 33948-33949)
　　🛒 12.4　　✂ 12.4　　**FUD** 000　　C 80 ▣
　　**AMA:** 2017,Jan,8; 2016,Mar,5; 2016,Jan,13; 2015,Jul,3

**33952** **insertion of peripheral (arterial and/or venous) cannula(e), percutaneous, 6 years and older (includes fluoroscopic guidance, when performed)** ▣A
　　INCLUDES　Cannula replacement in same vessel
　　　Cannula repositioning during same episode of care
　　Code also cannula removal if new cannula inserted in different vessel with ([33965, 33966, 33969, 33984, 33985, 33986])
　　Code also ECMO/ECLS initiation or daily management (33946-33947, 33948-33949)
　　🛒 12.4　　✂ 12.4　　**FUD** 000　　C 80 ▣
　　**AMA:** 2017,Jan,8; 2016,Mar,5; 2016,Jan,13; 2015,Jul,3

**33953** **insertion of peripheral (arterial and/or venous) cannula(e), open, birth through 5 years of age** ▣A
　　INCLUDES　Cannula replacement in same vessel
　　　Cannula repositioning during same episode of care
　　EXCLUDES　*Open artery exposure for delivery/deployment of endovascular prosthesis ([34812], 34714-34716 [34820, 34833, 34834], [34820])*
　　Code also cannula removal if new cannula inserted in different vessel with ([33965, 33966, 33969, 33984, 33985, 33986])
　　Code also ECMO/ECLS initiation or daily management (33496-33947, 33948-33949)
　　🛒 13.9　　✂ 13.9　　**FUD** 000　　C 80 ▣
　　**AMA:** 2017,Jan,8; 2016,Mar,5; 2016,Jan,13; 2015,Jul,3

**33954** **insertion of peripheral (arterial and/or venous) cannula(e), open, 6 years and older** ▣A
　　INCLUDES　Cannula replacement in same vessel
　　　Cannula repositioning during same episode of care
　　EXCLUDES　*Open artery exposure for delivery/deployment of endovascular prosthesis ([34812], 34714-34716 [34820, 34833, 34834], [34820])*
　　Code also cannula removal if new cannula inserted in different vessel with ([33965, 33966, 33969, 33984, 33985, 33986])
　　Code also ECMO/ECLS initiation or daily management (33946-33947, 33948-33949)
　　🛒 13.9　　✂ 13.9　　**FUD** 000　　C 80 ▣
　　**AMA:** 2017,Jan,8; 2016,Mar,5; 2016,Jan,13; 2015,Jul,3

**33955** **insertion of central cannula(e) by sternotomy or thoracotomy, birth through 5 years of age** ▣A
　　INCLUDES　Cannula replacement in same vessel
　　　Cannula repositioning during same episode of care
　　EXCLUDES　*Mediastinotomy (39010)*
　　　*Thoracotomy (32100)*
　　Code also cannula removal if new cannula inserted in different vessel with ([33965, 33966, 33969, 33984, 33985, 33986])
　　Code also ECMO/ECLS initiation or daily management (33946-33947, 33948-33949)
　　🛒 24.3　　✂ 24.3　　**FUD** 000　　C 80 ▣
　　**AMA:** 2017,Jan,8; 2016,Mar,5; 2016,Jan,13; 2015,Jul,3

● New Code　▲ Revised Code　○ Reinstated　● New Web Release　▲ Revised Web Release　Unlisted　Not Covered　# Resequenced
⊘ AMA Mod 51 Exempt　⑤⑪ Optum Mod 51 Exempt　63 Mod 63 Exempt　✗ Non-FDA Drug　★ Telemedicine　Ⓜ Maternity　▣A Age Edit　+ Add-on　**AMA:** CPT Asst
© 2017 Optum360, LLC　　CPT © 2017 American Medical Association. All Rights Reserved.

**33956**　　**insertion of central cannula(e) by sternotomy or thoracotomy, 6 years and older** 　A

> INCLUDES　　Cannula replacement in same vessel
> Cannula repositioning during same episode of care
> EXCLUDES　　*Mediastinotomy (39010)*
> *Thoracotomy (32100)*
> Code also cannula removal if new cannula inserted in different vessel with ([33965, 33966, 33969, 33984, 33985, 33986])
> Code also ECMO/ECLS initiation or daily management (33946-33947, 33948-33949)

　🔾 24.2　　⚕ 24.2　　**FUD** 000　　C 80 ▭

**AMA:** 2017,Jan,8; 2016,Mar,5; 2016,Jan,13; 2015,Jul,3

**33957**　　**reposition peripheral (arterial and/or venous) cannula(e), percutaneous, birth through 5 years of age (includes fluoroscopic guidance, when performed)** 　A

> INCLUDES　　Fluoroscopic guidance
> EXCLUDES　　*ECMO/ECLS initiation, veno-arterial (33947)*
> *ECMO/ECLS initiation, veno-venous (33946)*
> *ECMO/ECLS insertion of cannula (33951-33956)*
> *Percutaneous access and closure femoral artery for endograft delivery (34713)*

　🔾 5.43　　⚕ 5.43　　**FUD** 000　　C 80 ▭

**AMA:** 2017,Jan,8; 2016,Mar,5; 2016,Jan,13; 2015,Jul,3

**33958**　　**reposition peripheral (arterial and/or venous) cannula(e), percutaneous, 6 years and older (includes fluoroscopic guidance, when performed)** 　A

> INCLUDES　　Fluoroscopic guidance
> EXCLUDES　　*ECMO/ECLS initiation, veno-arterial (33947)*
> *ECMO/ECLS initiation, veno-venous (33946)*
> *ECMO/ECLS insertion of cannula (33951-33956)*
> *Percutaneous access and closure femoral artery for endograft delivery (34713)*

　🔾 5.30　　⚕ 5.30　　**FUD** 000　　C 80 ▭

**AMA:** 2017,Jan,8; 2016,Mar,5; 2016,Jan,13; 2015,Jul,3

**33959**　　**reposition peripheral (arterial and/or venous) cannula(e), open, birth through 5 years of age (includes fluoroscopic guidance, when performed)** 　A

> INCLUDES　　Fluoroscopic guidance
> EXCLUDES　　*ECMO/ECLS initiation, veno-arterial (33947)*
> *ECMO/ECLS initiation, veno-venous (33946)*
> *ECMO/ECLS insertion of cannula (33951-33956)*
> *Open artery exposure for delivery/deployment of endovascular prosthesis ([34812], 34714-34716 [34820, 34833, 34834])*

　🔾 6.88　　⚕ 6.88　　**FUD** 000　　C 80 ▭

**AMA:** 2017,Jan,8; 2016,Mar,5; 2016,Jan,13; 2015,Jul,3

\#　**33962**　　**reposition peripheral (arterial and/or venous) cannula(e), open, 6 years and older (includes fluoroscopic guidance, when performed)** 　A

> INCLUDES　　Fluoroscopic guidance
> EXCLUDES　　*ECMO/ECLS initiation, veno-arterial (33947)*
> *ECMO/ECLS initiation, veno-venous (33946)*
> *ECMO/ECLS insertion of cannula (33951-33956)*
> *Open artery exposure for delivery/deployment of endovascular prosthesis ([34812], 34714-34716 [34820, 34833, 34834])*

　🔾 6.88　　⚕ 6.88　　**FUD** 000　　C 80 ▭

**AMA:** 2017,Jan,8; 2016,Mar,5; 2016,Jan,13; 2015,Jul,3

\#　**33963**　　**reposition of central cannula(e) by sternotomy or thoracotomy, birth through 5 years of age (includes fluoroscopic guidance, when performed)** 　A

> INCLUDES　　Fluoroscopic guidance
> EXCLUDES　　*ECMO/ECLS initiation, veno-arterial (33947)*
> *ECMO/ECLS initiation, veno-venous (33946)*
> *ECMO/ECLS insertion of cannula (33951-33956)*
> *Open artery exposure for delivery/deployment of endovascular prosthesis ([34812], 34714-34716 [34820, 34833, 34834])*

　🔾 13.7　　⚕ 13.7　　**FUD** 000　　C 80 ▭

**AMA:** 2017,Jan,8; 2016,Mar,5; 2016,Jan,13; 2015,Jul,3

---

\#　**33964**　　**reposition central cannula(e) by sternotomy or thoracotomy, 6 years and older (includes fluoroscopic guidance, when performed)** 　A

> INCLUDES　　Fluoroscopic guidance
> EXCLUDES　　*ECMO/ECLS initiation, veno-arterial (33947)*
> *ECMO/ECLS initiation, veno-venous (33946)*
> *ECMO/ECLS insertion of cannula (33951-33956)*
> *Mediastinotomy (39010)*
> *Thoracotomy (32100)*

　🔾 14.0　　⚕ 14.0　　**FUD** 000　　C 80 ▭

**AMA:** 2017,Jan,8; 2016,Mar,5; 2016,Jan,13; 2015,Jul,3

\#　**33965**　　**removal of peripheral (arterial and/or venous) cannula(e), percutaneous, birth through 5 years of age** 　A

> Code also extensive arterial repair/replacement, when performed (35266, 35286, 35371, 35665)
> Code also new cannula insertion into different vessel (33951-33956)

　🔾 5.43　　⚕ 5.43　　**FUD** 000　　C 80 ▭

**AMA:** 2017,Jan,8; 2016,Mar,5; 2016,Jan,13; 2015,Jul,3

\#　**33966**　　**removal of peripheral (arterial and/or venous) cannula(e), percutaneous, 6 years and older** 　A

> Code also extensive arterial repair/replacement, when performed (35266, 35286, 35371, 35665)
> Code also new cannula insertion into different vessel (33951-33956)

　🔾 6.91　　⚕ 6.91　　**FUD** 000　　C 80 ▭

**AMA:** 2017,Jan,8; 2016,Mar,5; 2016,Jan,13; 2015,Jul,3

\#　**33969**　　**removal of peripheral (arterial and/or venous) cannula(e), open, birth through 5 years of age** 　A

> EXCLUDES　　*Open artery exposure for delivery/deployment of endovascular prosthesis ([34812], 34714-34716 [34820, 34833, 34834])*
> *Repair blood vessel (35201, 35206, 35211, 35216, 35226)*
> Code also extensive arterial repair/replacement, when performed (35266, 35286, 35371, 35665)
> Code also new cannula insertion into different vessel (33951-33956)

　🔾 8.04　　⚕ 8.04　　**FUD** 000　　C 80 ▭

**AMA:** 2017,Jan,8; 2016,Mar,5; 2016,Jan,13; 2015,Jul,3

\#　**33984**　　**removal of peripheral (arterial and/or venous) cannula(e), open, 6 years and older** 　A

> EXCLUDES　　*Open artery exposure for delivery/deployment of endovascular prosthesis ([34812], 34714-34716 [34820, 34833, 34834])*
> *Repair blood vessel (35201, 35206, 35211, 35216, 35226)*

　🔾 8.35　　⚕ 8.35　　**FUD** 000　　C 80 ▭

**AMA:** 2017,Jan,8; 2016,Mar,5; 2016,Jan,13; 2015,Jul,3

\#　**33985**　　**removal of central cannula(e) by sternotomy or thoracotomy, birth through 5 years of age** 　A

> EXCLUDES　　*Repair blood vessel (35201, 35206, 35211, 35216, 35226)*
> Code also extensive arterial repair/replacement, when performed (35266, 35286, 35371, 35665)
> Code also new cannula insertion into different vessel (33951-33956)

　🔾 15.0　　⚕ 15.0　　**FUD** 000　　C 80 ▭

**AMA:** 2017,Jan,8; 2016,Mar,5; 2016,Jan,13; 2015,Jul,3

\#　**33986**　　**removal of central cannula(e) by sternotomy or thoracotomy, 6 years and older** 　A

> EXCLUDES　　*Repair blood vessel (35201, 35206, 35211, 35216, 35226)*
> Code also extensive arterial repair/replacement, when performed (35266, 35286, 35371, 35665)
> Code also new cannula insertion into different vessel (33951-33956)

　🔾 15.2　　⚕ 15.2　　**FUD** 000　　C 80 ▭

**AMA:** 2017,Jan,8; 2016,Mar,5; 2016,Jan,13; 2015,Jul,3

---

| 26/TC PC/TC Only | A2-Z3 ASC Payment | 50 Bilateral | ♂ Male Only | ♀ Female Only | 🔾 Facility RVU | ⚕ Non-Facility RVU | ▭ CCI |
| FUD Follow-up Days | CMS: IOM (Pub 100) | A-Y OPPSI | 80/80 Surg Assist Allowed / w/Doc | | 🔬 Lab Crosswalk | ☢ Radiology Crosswalk | ✖ CLIA |

138　　　　　　　　　　　　　　　　　　CPT © 2017 American Medical Association. All Rights Reserved.　　　　　　　　　　　© 2017 Optum360, LLC

**+ # 33987** **Arterial exposure with creation of graft conduit (eg, chimney graft) to facilitate arterial perfusion for ECMO/ECLS (List separately in addition to code for primary procedure)**

> EXCLUDES Open artery exposure for delivery/deployment of endovascular prosthesis ([34812], 34714-34716 [34820, 34833, 34834])
>
> Code first (33953-33956)
>
> 🖐 6.12    ✂ 6.12    **FUD** ZZZ    C 80 ▭
>
> **AMA:** 2017,Jan,8; 2016,Mar,5; 2016,Jan,13; 2015,Jul,3

**# 33988** **Insertion of left heart vent by thoracic incision (eg, sternotomy, thoracotomy) for ECMO/ECLS**

> 🖐 22.8    ✂ 22.8    **FUD** 000    C 80 ▭
>
> **AMA:** 2017,Jan,8; 2016,Mar,5; 2016,Jan,13; 2015,Jul,3

**# 33989** **Removal of left heart vent by thoracic incision (eg, sternotomy, thoracotomy) for ECMO/ECLS**

> 🖐 14.4    ✂ 14.4    **FUD** 000    C 80 ▭
>
> **AMA:** 2017,Jan,8; 2016,Mar,5; 2016,Jan,13; 2015,Jul,3

# 33962-33999 Mechanical Circulatory Support

*33962*    Resequenced code. See code following 33959.

*33963*    Resequenced code. See code following 33959.

*33964*    Resequenced code. See code following 33959.

*33965*    Resequenced code. See code following 33959.

*33966*    Resequenced code. See code following 33959.

**33967**    **Insertion of intra-aortic balloon assist device, percutaneous**

> 🖐 7.56    ✂ 7.56    **FUD** 000    C 80 ▭
>
> **AMA:** 2017,Jan,8; 2016,Mar,5; 2016,Jan,13; 2015,Sep,3; 2015,Jul,3; 2015,Jan,16; 2014,Jan,11; 2013,Mar,10-11; 2012,Jan,15-42

**33968**    **Removal of intra-aortic balloon assist device, percutaneous**

> EXCLUDES Removal of implantable aortic couterpulsation ventricular assist system (0455T-0458T)
>
> 🖐 0.98    ✂ 0.98    **FUD** 000    C ▭
>
> **AMA:** 2017,Jan,8; 2016,Mar,5; 2016,Jan,13; 2015,Jul,3; 2015,Jan,16; 2014,Jan,11; 2012,Jan,15-42

*33969*    Resequenced code. See code following 33959.

**33970**    **Insertion of intra-aortic balloon assist device through the femoral artery, open approach**

> EXCLUDES Insertion/replacement implantable aortic counterpulsation ventricular assist system (0451T-0454T)
>
> Percutaneous insertion of intra-aortic balloon assist device (33967)
>
> 🖐 10.3    ✂ 10.3    **FUD** 000    C 80 ▭
>
> **AMA:** 2017,Jan,8; 2016,Mar,5; 2016,Jan,13; 2015,Sep,3; 2015,Jul,3; 2015,Jan,16; 2014,Jan,11; 2013,Mar,10-11

**33971**    **Removal of intra-aortic balloon assist device including repair of femoral artery, with or without graft**

> EXCLUDES Removal of implantable aortic counterpulsation ventricular assist system (0455T-0458T)
>
> 🖐 20.6    ✂ 20.6    **FUD** 090    C ▭
>
> **AMA:** 2017,Jan,8; 2016,Mar,5; 2016,Jan,13; 2015,Jul,3; 2015,Jan,16; 2014,Jan,11

**33973**    **Insertion of intra-aortic balloon assist device through the ascending aorta**

> EXCLUDES Insertion/replacement of implantable aortic counterpulsation ventricular assist system (0451T-0454T)
>
> 🖐 15.0    ✂ 15.0    **FUD** 000    C 80 ▭
>
> **AMA:** 2017,Jan,8; 2016,Mar,5; 2016,Jan,13; 2015,Sep,3; 2015,Jul,3; 2015,Jan,16; 2014,Jan,11; 2013,Mar,10-11

**33974**    **Removal of intra-aortic balloon assist device from the ascending aorta, including repair of the ascending aorta, with or without graft**

> EXCLUDES Removal of implantable aortic counterpulsation ventricular assist system (0455T-0458T)
>
> 🖐 25.9    ✂ 25.9    **FUD** 090    C ▭
>
> **AMA:** 2017,Jan,8; 2016,Mar,5; 2016,Jan,13; 2015,Jul,3; 2015,Jan,16; 2014,Jan,11

**33975**    **Insertion of ventricular assist device; extracorporeal, single ventricle**

> INCLUDES Insertion of the new pump with de-airing, connection, and initiation
>
> Removal of the old pump with replacement of the entire ventricular assist device system, including pump(s) and cannulas
>
> Transthoracic approach
>
> EXCLUDES Percutaneous approach (33990-33991)
>
> Code also removal of thrombus through a separate heart incision, when performed (33310-33315); append modifier 59 to (33315)
>
> 🖐 38.1    ✂ 38.1    **FUD** XXX    C 80 ▭
>
> **AMA:** 2017,Jan,8; 2016,Mar,5; 2016,Jan,13; 2015,Jul,3; 2015,Jan,16; 2014,Jan,11; 2013,Mar,10-11; 2012,Jan,15-42

**33976**    **extracorporeal, biventricular**

> INCLUDES Insertion of the new pump with de-airing, connection, and initiation
>
> Removal with replacement of the entire ventricular assist device system, including pump(s) and cannulas
>
> Transthoracic approach
>
> EXCLUDES Percutaneous approach (33990-33991)
>
> Code also removal of thrombus through a separate heart incision, when performed (33310-33315); append modifier 59 to (33315)
>
> 🖐 46.4    ✂ 46.4    **FUD** XXX    C 80 ▭
>
> **AMA:** 2017,Jan,8; 2016,Mar,5; 2016,Jan,13; 2015,Jul,3; 2015,Jan,16; 2014,Jan,11; 2013,Mar,10-11; 2012,Jan,15-42

**33977**    **Removal of ventricular assist device; extracorporeal, single ventricle**

> INCLUDES Removal of the entire device and the cannulas
>
> EXCLUDES Removal of ventricular assist device when performed at the same time of insertion of a new device
>
> Code also removal of thrombus through a separate heart incision, when performed (33310-33315); append modifier 59 to (33315)
>
> 🖐 32.8    ✂ 32.8    **FUD** XXX    C 80 ▭
>
> **AMA:** 2017,Jan,8; 2016,Mar,5; 2016,Jan,13; 2015,Jul,3; 2015,Jan,16; 2014,Jan,11; 2013,Mar,10-11; 2012,Jan,15-42

**33978**    **extracorporeal, biventricular**

> INCLUDES Removal of the entire device and the cannulas
>
> EXCLUDES Removal of ventricular assist device when performed at the same time of insertion of a new device
>
> Code also removal of thrombus through a separate heart incision, when performed (33310-33315); append modifier 59 to (33315)
>
> 🖐 38.8    ✂ 38.8    **FUD** XXX    C 80 ▭
>
> **AMA:** 2017,Jan,8; 2016,Mar,5; 2016,Jan,13; 2015,Jul,3; 2015,Jan,16; 2014,Jan,11; 2013,Mar,10-11; 2012,Jan,15-42

**33979** Insertion of ventricular assist device, implantable intracorporeal, single ventricle

INCLUDES New pump insertion with connection, de-airing, and initiation
Removal with replacement of the entire ventricular assist device system, including pump(s) and cannulas
Transthoracic approach

EXCLUDES Insertion/replacement of implantable aortic counterpulsation ventricular assist system (0451T-0454T)
Percutaneous approach (33990-33991)

Code also removal of thrombus through a separate heart incision, when performed (33310-33315); append modifier 59 to (33315)

⚕ 56.8  ⚖ 56.8  **FUD** XXX  C 80 ▢

**AMA:** 2017,Jan,8; 2016,Mar,5; 2016,Jan,13; 2015,Jul,3; 2015,Jan,16; 2014,Jan,11; 2013,Mar,10-11; 2012,Jan,15-42

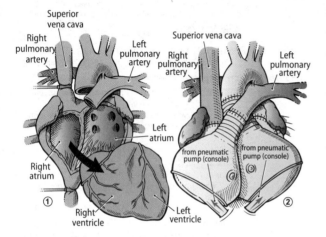

**33980** Removal of ventricular assist device, implantable intracorporeal, single ventricle

INCLUDES Removal of the entire device and the cannulas

EXCLUDES Removal of implantable aortic counterpulsation ventricular assist system (0455T-0458T)
Removal of ventricular assist device when performed at the same time of insertion of a new device

Code also removal of thrombus through a separate heart incision, when performed (33310-33315); append modifier 59 to (33315)

⚕ 51.9  ⚖ 51.9  **FUD** XXX  C 80 ▢

**AMA:** 2017,Jan,8; 2016,Mar,5; 2016,Jan,13; 2015,Jul,3; 2015,Jan,16; 2014,Jan,11; 2013,Mar,10-11

**33981** Replacement of extracorporeal ventricular assist device, single or biventricular, pump(s), single or each pump

INCLUDES Insertion of the new pump with de-airing, connection, and initiation
Removal of the old pump

⚕ 24.1  ⚖ 24.1  **FUD** XXX  C 80 ▢

**AMA:** 2017,Jan,8; 2016,Mar,5; 2016,Jan,13; 2015,Jul,3; 2015,Jan,16; 2014,Jan,11

**33982** Replacement of ventricular assist device pump(s); implantable intracorporeal, single ventricle, without cardiopulmonary bypass

INCLUDES New pump insertion with connection, de-airing, and initiation
Removal of the old pump

⚕ 57.0  ⚖ 57.0  **FUD** XXX  C 80 ▢

**AMA:** 2017,Jan,8; 2016,Mar,5; 2016,Jan,13; 2015,Jul,3; 2015,Jan,16; 2014,Jan,11

**33983** implantable intracorporeal, single ventricle, with cardiopulmonary bypass

Removal of the old pump

EXCLUDES Insertion/replacement of implantable aortic counterpulsation ventricular assist system (0451T-0454T)
Percutaneous transseptal approach (33999)

⚕ 67.4  ⚖ 67.4  **FUD** XXX  C 80 ▢

**AMA:** 2017,Jan,8; 2016,Mar,5; 2016,Jan,13; 2015,Jul,3; 2015,Jan,16; 2014,Jan,11

**33984** Resequenced code. See code following 33959.
**33985** Resequenced code. See code following 33959.
**33986** Resequenced code. See code following 33959.
**33987** Resequenced code. See code following 33959.
**33988** Resequenced code. See code following 33959.
**33989** Resequenced code. See code following 33959.

**33990** Insertion of ventricular assist device, percutaneous including radiological supervision and interpretation; arterial access only

INCLUDES Initial insertion and replacement of percutaneous ventricular assist device

EXCLUDES Extensive artery repair/replacement (35226, 35286)
Insertion/replacement of implantable aortic counterpulsation ventricular assist system (0451T-0454T)
Open arterial approach to aid insertion of percutaneous ventricular assist device, when used ([34812], 34714-34716 [34820, 34833, 34834], [34820])
Removal of percutaneous ventricular assist device at time of replacement of the entire system (33992)
Transthoracic approach (33975-33976)

⚕ 12.4  ⚖ 12.4  **FUD** XXX  C 80 ▢

**AMA:** 2017,Jan,8; 2016,Mar,5; 2016,Jan,13; 2015,Sep,3; 2015,Jan,16; 2014,Oct,14; 2014,Jan,11; 2013,Mar,10-11

**33991** both arterial and venous access, with transseptal puncture

INCLUDES Initial insertion as well as replacement of percutaneous ventricular assist device

EXCLUDES Extensive artery repair/replacement (35226, 35286)
Insertion/replacement of implantable aortic counterpulsation ventricular assist system (0451T-0454T)
Open arterial approach to aid with insertion of percutaneous ventricular assist device, when performed ([34812], 34714-34716 [34820, 34833, 34834])
Removal of percutaneous ventricular assist device at time of replacement of the entire system (33992)
Transthoracic approach (33975-33976)

⚕ 18.1  ⚖ 18.1  **FUD** XXX  C 80 ▢

**AMA:** 2017,Jan,8; 2016,Mar,5; 2016,Jan,13; 2015,Sep,3; 2015,Jan,16; 2014,Jan,11; 2013,Mar,10-11

**33992** Removal of percutaneous ventricular assist device at separate and distinct session from insertion

INCLUDES Removal of device and cannulas

EXCLUDES Removal of implantable aortic counterpulsation ventricular assist system (0455T-0458T)

Code also modifier 59 when percutaneous ventricular assist device is removed on the same day as the insertion, but at a different session

⚕ 5.84  ⚖ 5.84  **FUD** XXX  C 80 ▢

**AMA:** 2017,Jan,8; 2016,Mar,5; 2016,Jan,13; 2015,Sep,3; 2015,Jan,16; 2014,Jan,11; 2013,Mar,10-11

CPT © 2017 American Medical Association. All Rights Reserved.  © 2017 Optum360, LLC

**33993** Repositioning of percutaneous ventricular assist device with imaging guidance at separate and distinct session from insertion

> EXCLUDES *Repositioning of a percutaneous ventricular assist device without image guidance*
> *Repositioning of device/electrode (0460T-0461T)*
> *Repositioning of the percutaneous ventricular assist device at the same session as the insertion (33990-33991)*
> *Skin pocket relocation with replacement implantable aortic counterpulsation ventricular assist device and electrodes (0459T)*
>
> Code also modifier 59 when percutaneous ventricular assist device is repositioned using imaging guidance on the same day as the insertion, but at a different session

🔪 5.10   ✂ 5.10   **FUD** XXX   [C] [80] [▭]

**AMA:** 2017,Jan,8; 2016,Mar,5; 2016,Jan,13; 2015,Sep,3; 2015,Jan,16; 2014,Jan,11; 2013,Mar,10-11

**33999** Unlisted procedure, cardiac surgery

🔪 0.00   ✂ 0.00   **FUD** YYY   [T] [80]

**AMA:** 2017,Jan,8; 2016,May,5; 2016,Jan,13; 2015,Jan,16; 2014,Dec,16; 2014,Dec,16; 2014,Jan,11; 2013,Dec,14; 2013,Mar,10-11; 2013,Feb,13; 2012,Jan,15-42

## 34001-34530 Surgical Revascularization: Veins and Arteries

INCLUDES Repair of blood vessel
Surgeon's component of operative arteriogram

**34001** Embolectomy or thrombectomy, with or without catheter; carotid, subclavian or innominate artery, by neck incision

🔪 28.3   ✂ 28.3   **FUD** 090   [C] [80] [50] [▭]

**AMA:** 1997,Nov,1

Major arteries of the arm: Subclavian artery, Axillary artery, Brachial, Superior ulnar collateral, Radial artery, Posterior ulnar recurrent, Ulnar artery, Common interosseous. Major arteries of the leg: Aorto-femoral artery, Femoral and deep femoral branches, Popliteal artery, Peroneal artery, Anterior tibial artery, Posterior tibial artery. Arteries (red) are usually accompanied by at least one vein (blue)

**34051** innominate, subclavian artery, by thoracic incision

🔪 25.9   ✂ 25.9   **FUD** 090   [C] [80] [50] [▭]

**AMA:** 1997,Nov,1

**34101** axillary, brachial, innominate, subclavian artery, by arm incision

🔪 17.5   ✂ 17.5   **FUD** 090   [T] [80] [50] [▭]

**AMA:** 1997,Nov,1

**34111** radial or ulnar artery, by arm incision

🔪 17.5   ✂ 17.5   **FUD** 090   [T] [80] [50] [▭]

**AMA:** 1997,Nov,1

**34151** renal, celiac, mesentery, aortoiliac artery, by abdominal incision

🔪 41.0   ✂ 41.0   **FUD** 090   [C] [80] [50] [▭]

**AMA:** 1997,Nov,1

**34201** femoropopliteal, aortoiliac artery, by leg incision

🔪 30.2   ✂ 30.2   **FUD** 090   [T] [80] [50] [▭]

**AMA:** 2017,Jan,8; 2016,Jan,13; 2015,Jan,16; 2014,Jan,11; 2012,Jan,15-42

**34203** popliteal-tibio-peroneal artery, by leg incision

🔪 27.9   ✂ 27.9   **FUD** 090   [T] [80] [50] [▭]

**AMA:** 1997,Nov,1

**34401** Thrombectomy, direct or with catheter; vena cava, iliac vein, by abdominal incision

🔪 42.6   ✂ 42.6   **FUD** 090   [C] [80] [50] [▭]

**AMA:** 1997,Nov,1

**34421** vena cava, iliac, femoropopliteal vein, by leg incision

🔪 21.2   ✂ 21.2   **FUD** 090   [T] [80] [50] [▭]

**AMA:** 2017,Jan,8; 2016,Jan,13; 2015,Jan,16; 2014,Jan,11

**34451** vena cava, iliac, femoropopliteal vein, by abdominal and leg incision

🔪 47.7   ✂ 47.7   **FUD** 090   [C] [80] [50] [▭]

**AMA:** 1997,Nov,1

**34471** subclavian vein, by neck incision

🔪 31.8   ✂ 31.8   **FUD** 090   [T] [50] [▭]

**AMA:** 1997,Nov,1

**34490** axillary and subclavian vein, by arm incision

🔪 17.8   ✂ 17.8   **FUD** 090   [T] [62] [50] [▭]

**AMA:** 1997,Nov,1

**34501** Valvuloplasty, femoral vein

🔪 26.2   ✂ 26.2   **FUD** 090   [T] [80] [50] [▭]

**AMA:** 1997,Nov,1

**34502** Reconstruction of vena cava, any method

🔪 44.8   ✂ 44.8   **FUD** 090   [C] [80] [▭]

**AMA:** 1997,Nov,1

**34510** Venous valve transposition, any vein donor

🔪 34.8   ✂ 34.8   **FUD** 090   [T] [80] [50] [▭]

**AMA:** 1997,Nov,1

**34520** Cross-over vein graft to venous system

🔪 30.8   ✂ 30.8   **FUD** 090   [T] [80] [50] [▭]

**AMA:** 1997,Nov,1

**34530** Saphenopopliteal vein anastomosis

🔪 27.8   ✂ 27.8   **FUD** 090   [T] [80] [50] [▭]

**AMA:** 1997,Nov,1

## 34701-34713 Abdominal Aorta and Iliac Artery Repairs

INCLUDES Treatment with a covered stent for conditions such as:
Aneurysm
Aortic dissection
Arteriovenous malformation
Pseudoaneurysm
Trauma
Treatment zones:
Infrarenal aorta (34701-34702)
Infrarenal and both common iliac arteries (34705-34706)
Infrarenal and ipsilateral common iliac artery (34703-34704)
Section of iliac artery containing the endograft (34707-34708)

● **34701** Endovascular repair of infrarenal aorta by deployment of an aorto-aortic tube endograft including pre-procedure sizing and device selection, all nonselective catheterization(s), all associated radiological supervision and interpretation, all endograft extension(s) placed in the aorta from the level of the renal arteries to the aortic bifurcation, and all angioplasty/stenting performed from the level of the renal arteries to the aortic bifurcation; for other than rupture (eg, for aneurysm, pseudoaneurysm, dissection, penetrating ulcer)

> INCLUDES Nonselective catheterization
>
> EXCLUDES *Revascularization aorta for occlusive disease with covered stent (37236-37237)*
>
> Code also decompressive laparotomy for treatment abdominal compartment syndrome (49000)
> Code also intravascular ultrasound when performed (37252-37253)
> Code also percutaneous closure of artery when endograft is delivered through a sheath 12 French or larger (34713)
> Code also selective catheterization of arteries outside target treatment zone

● 34702   **for rupture including temporary aortic and/or iliac balloon occlusion, when performed (eg, for aneurysm, pseudoaneurysm, dissection, penetrating ulcer, traumatic disruption)**

INCLUDES   Nonselective catheterization

Code also decompressive laparotomy for treatment abdominal compartment syndrome (49000)

Code also intravascular ultrasound when performed (37252-37253)

Code also percutaneous closure of artery when endograft is delivered through a sheath 12 French or larger (34713)

Code also selective catheterization of arteries outside target treatment zone

● 34703   **Endovascular repair of infrarenal aorta and/or iliac artery(ies) by deployment of an aorto-uni-iliac endograft including pre-procedure sizing and device selection, all nonselective catheterization(s), all associated radiological supervision and interpretation, all endograft extension(s) placed in the aorta from the level of the renal arteries to the iliac bifurcation, and all angioplasty/stenting performed from the level of the renal arteries to the iliac bifurcation; for other than rupture (eg, for aneurysm, pseudoaneurysm, dissection, penetrating ulcer)**

INCLUDES   Endograft extensions ending in the common iliac arteries

Nonselective catheterization

Code also intravascular ultrasound when performed (37252-37253)

Code also percutaneous closure of artery when endograft is delivered through a sheath 12 French or larger (34713)

Code also selective catheterization of arteries outside target treatment zone

● 34704   **for rupture including temporary aortic and/or iliac balloon occlusion, when performed (eg, for aneurysm, pseudoaneurysm, dissection, penetrating ulcer, traumatic disruption)**

INCLUDES   Endograft extensions ending in the common iliac arteries

Nonselective catheterization

Code also decompressive laparotomy for treatment abdominal compartment syndrome (49000)

Code also intravascular ultrasound when performed (37252-37253)

Code also percutaneous closure of artery when endograft is delivered through a sheath 12 French or larger (34713)

Code also selective catheterization of arteries outside target treatment zone

● 34705   **Endovascular repair of infrarenal aorta and/or iliac artery(ies) by deployment of an aorto-bi-iliac endograft including pre-procedure sizing and device selection, all nonselective catheterization(s), all associated radiological supervision and interpretation, all endograft extension(s) placed in the aorta from the level of the renal arteries to the iliac bifurcation, and all angioplasty/stenting performed from the level of the renal arteries to the iliac bifurcation; for other than rupture (eg, for aneurysm, pseudoaneurysm, dissection, penetrating ulcer)**

INCLUDES   Endograft extensions ending in the common iliac arteries

Nonselective catheterization

Code also intravascular ultrasound when performed (37252-37253)

Code also percutaneous closure of artery when endograft is delivered through a sheath 12 French or larger (34713)

Code also selective catheterization of arteries outside target treatment zone

● 34706   **for rupture including temporary aortic and/or iliac balloon occlusion, when performed (eg, for aneurysm, pseudoaneurysm, dissection, penetrating ulcer, traumatic disruption)**

INCLUDES   Endograft extensions ending in the common iliac arteries

Nonselective catheterization

Code also decompressive laparotomy for treatment abdominal compartment syndrome (49000)

Code also intravascular ultrasound when performed (37252-37253)

Code also percutaneous closure of artery when endograft is delivered through a sheath 12 French or larger (34713)

Code also selective catheterization of arteries outside target treatment zone

● 34707   **Endovascular repair of iliac artery by deployment of an ilio-iliac tube endograft including pre-procedure sizing and device selection, all nonselective catheterization(s), all associated radiological supervision and interpretation, and all endograft extension(s) proximally to the aortic bifurcation and distally to the iliac bifurcation, and treatment zone angioplasty/stenting, when performed, unilateral; for other than rupture (eg, for aneurysm, pseudoaneurysm, dissection, arteriovenous malformation)**

INCLUDES   Endograft extensions ending in the common iliac arteries

Nonselective catheterization

EXCLUDES   *Revascularization aorta for occlusive disease with covered stent (37236-37237)*

*Revascularization iliac artery for occlusive disease with covered stent (37221, 37223)*

Code also intravascular ultrasound when performed (37252-37253)

Code also percutaneous closure of artery when endograft is delivered through a sheath 12 French or larger (34713)

Code also selective catheterization of arteries outside target treatment zone

● 34708   **for rupture including temporary aortic and/or iliac balloon occlusion, when performed (eg, for aneurysm, pseudoaneurysm, dissection, arteriovenous malformation, traumatic disruption)**

INCLUDES   Endograft extensions ending in the common iliac arteries

Nonselective catheterization

Code also decompressive laparotomy for treatment abdominal compartment syndrome (49000)

Code also intravascular ultrasound when performed (37252-37253)

Code also percutaneous closure of artery when endograft is delivered through a sheath 12 French or larger (34713)

Code also selective catheterization of arteries outside target treatment zone

● + 34709   **Placement of extension prosthesis(es) distal to the common iliac artery(ies) or proximal to the renal artery(ies) for endovascular repair of infrarenal abdominal aortic or iliac aneurysm, false aneurysm, dissection, penetrating ulcer, including pre-procedure sizing and device selection, all nonselective catheterization(s), all associated radiological supervision and interpretation, and treatment zone angioplasty/stenting, when performed, per vessel treated (List separately in addition to code for primary procedure)**

🖾 0.00   🖾 0.00   **FUD** 000

EXCLUDES   *Placement of covered stent (37236-37237)*

*Use of code more than one time for each vessel treated*

Code first (34701-34708)

● 34710 **Delayed placement of distal or proximal extension prosthesis for endovascular repair of infrarenal abdominal aortic or iliac aneurysm, false aneurysm, dissection, endoleak, or endograft migration, including pre-procedure sizing and device selection, all nonselective catheterization(s), all associated radiological supervision and interpretation, and treatment zone angioplasty/stenting, when performed; initial vessel treated**

    EXCLUDES *Fenestrated endograft repair (34841-34848)*
        *Initial endovascular repair by endograft (34701-34709)*
        Code also decompressive laparotomy for treatment abdominal compartment syndrome (49000)

● + 34711 **each additional vessel treated (List separately in addition to code for primary procedure)**

    🚑 0.00    ✄ 0.00    **FUD** 000

    EXCLUDES *Fenestrated endograft repair (34841-34848)*
        *Initial endovascular repair by endograft (34701-34709)*
        Code also decompressive laparotomy for treatment abdominal compartment syndrome (49000)
        Code first (34710)

● 34712 **Transcatheter delivery of enhanced fixation device(s) to the endograft (eg, anchor, screw, tack) and all associated radiological supervision and interpretation**

    EXCLUDES *Use of code more than one time per procedure*

● + 34713 **Percutaneous access and closure of femoral artery for delivery of endograft through a large sheath (12 French or larger), including ultrasound guidance, when performed, unilateral (List separately in addition to code for primary procedure)**

    🚑 0.00    ✄ 0.00    **FUD** 000

    INCLUDES Unilateral procedure
    EXCLUDES *Endovascular revascularization procedures (37221, 37223, 37236-37237)*
        *Ultrasound imaging guidance*
        *Use of code for closure after delivery of endograft using a sheath size less than 12 French*
        Code first (33880-33881, 33883-33884, 34701-34708, 34841-34848)

## 34714-34834 [34812, 34820, 34833, 34834] Open Exposure for Endovascular Prosthesis Delivery

    INCLUDES Balloon angioplasty/stent deployment within the target treatment zone
        Introduction, manipulation, placement, and deployment of the device
        Open exposure of femoral or iliac artery/subsequent closure
        Thromboendarterectomy at site of aneurysm
    EXCLUDES *Additional interventional procedures outside of target treatment zone*
        *Guidewire and catheter insertion (36140, 36200, 36245-36248)*
        *Substantial artery repair/replacement (35226, 35286)*

▲ + # 34812 **Open femoral artery exposure for delivery of endovascular prosthesis, by groin incision, unilateral (List separately in addition to code for primary procedure)**

    INCLUDES Unilateral procedure
    EXCLUDES *ECMO/ECLS insertion, removal or repositioning (33953-33954, 33959, [33962], [33969], [33984], [33987])*
        *Repair of femoral artery (35226, 35286)*
        Code first (33880-33881, 33883-33884, 33886, 33990-33991, 34701-34708, 34841-34848, 0254T)

    🚑 9.88    ✄ 9.88    **FUD** 000      C 80 50 ▱

    **AMA:** 2017,Jan,8; 2016,Jan,13; 2015,Jul,3; 2015,Jan,16; 2014,Jan,11; 2013,Dec,8; 2013,Mar,10-11; 2012,Apr,3-9; 2012,Jan,15-42

● + 34714 **Open femoral artery exposure with creation of conduit for delivery of endovascular prosthesis or for establishment of cardiopulmonary bypass, by groin incision, unilateral (List separately in addition to code for primary procedure)**

    🚑 0.00    ✄ 0.00    **FUD** 000

    INCLUDES Unilateral procedure
    EXCLUDES *Delivery of endovascular prosthesis via open femoral artery ([34812])*
        *ECMO/ECLS insertion, removal or repositioning on same side (33953-33954, 33959, [33962], [33969], [33984])*
        *Transcatheter aortic valve replacement via open axillary artery (33362)*
    Code first (32852, 32854, 33031, 33120, 33251, 33256, 33259, 33261, 33305, 33315, 33322, 33335, 33390-33391, 33404-33417, 33422, 33425-33427, 33430, 33460, 33463-33465, 33468, 33474-33476, 33478, 33496, 33500, 33502, 33504-33507, 33510-33516, 33533-33536, 33542, 33545, 33548, 33600-33688, 33692, 33694, 33702, 33710, 33720, 33722, 33724, 33726, 33730, 33732, 33736, 33750, 33755, 33762, 33764, 33766-33767, 33770-33783, 33786, 33788, 33802-33803, 33814, 33820, 33822, 33824, 33840, 33845, 33851, 33853, 33860, 33863-33864, 33870, 33875, 33877, 33880-33881, 33883-33884, 33886, 33910, 33916-33917, 33920, 33922, 33926, 33935, 33945, 33975-33980, 33983, 33990-33991, 34701-34708, 34841-34848, 0254T)

▲ + # 34820 **Open iliac artery exposure for delivery of endovascular prosthesis or iliac occlusion during endovascular therapy, by abdominal or retroperitoneal incision, unilateral (List separately in addition to code for primary procedure)**

    INCLUDES Unilateral procedure
    Code first (33880-33881, 33883-33884, 33886, 33990-33991, 34701-34708, 34841-34848, 0254T)

    🚑 14.3    ✄ 14.3    **FUD** 000      C 80 50 ▱

    **AMA:** 2017,Jan,8; 2016,Jan,13; 2015,Jul,3; 2015,Jan,16; 2014,Jan,11; 2012,Apr,3-9; 2012,Jan,15-42

▲ + # 34833 **Open iliac artery exposure with creation of conduit for delivery of endovascular prosthesis or for establishment of cardiopulmonary bypass, by abdominal or retroperitoneal incision, unilateral (List separately in addition to code for primary procedure)**

    INCLUDES Unilateral procedure
    EXCLUDES *Delivery of endovascular prosthesis via open iliac artery ([34820])*
        *ECMO/ECLS insertion, removal or repositioning on same side (33953-33954, 33959, [33962], [33969], [33984])*
        *Transcatheter aortic valve replacement via open iliac artery (33364)*
    Code first (32852, 32854, 33031, 33256, 33259, 33261, 33305, 33315, 33322, 33335, 33390-33391, 33404-33417, 33422, 33425-33427, 33430, 33460, 33463-33465, 33468, 33474-33476, 33478, 33496, 33500, 33502, 33504-33514, 33516, 33533-33536, 33542, 33545, 33548, 33600-33688, 33692, 33694, 33697, 33702, 33710, 33720, 33722, 33724, 33726, 33730, 33732, 33736, 33750, 33755, 33762, 33764, 33766-33767, 33770-33783, 33786, 33788, 33802-33803, 33814, 33820, 33822, 33824, 33840, 33845, 33851, 33853, 33860, 33863-33864, 33870, 33875, 33877, 33880-33881, 33883-33884, 33886, 33910, 33916-33917, 33920, 33922, 33926, 33935, 33945, 33975-33980, 33983, 33990-33991, 34701-34708, 34841-34848, 0254T)

    🚑 17.8    ✄ 17.8    **FUD** 000      C 80 50 ▱

    **AMA:** 2017,Jan,8; 2016,Jan,13; 2015,Jul,3; 2015,Jan,16; 2014,Jan,11; 2012,Jan,15-42

**▲ + # 34834** **Open brachial artery exposure for delivery of endovascular prosthesis, unilateral (List separately in addition to code for primary procedure)**

INCLUDES Unilateral procedure

EXCLUDES ECMO/ECLS insertion, removal or repositioning (33953-33954, 33959, [33962], [33969], [33984])

Code first (33880-33881, 33883-33884, 33886, 33990-33991, 34701-34708, 34841-34848, 0254T)

🚗 7.97  ✂ 7.97  **FUD** 000  C 80 50 ▭

**AMA:** 2017,Jan,8; 2016,Jan,13; 2015,Jul,3; 2015,Jan,16; 2014,Jan,11

**● + 34715** **Open axillary/subclavian artery exposure for delivery of endovascular prosthesis by infraclavicular or supraclavicular incision, unilateral (List separately in addition to code for primary procedure)**

🚗 0.00  ✂ 0.00  **FUD** 000

INCLUDES Unilateral procedure

EXCLUDES ECMO/ECLS insertion, removal or repositioning on same side (33953-33954, 33959, [33962], [33969], [33984])

Implantation or replacement of aortic counterpulsation ventricular assist system (0451T-0452T, 0455T-0456T)

Transcatheter aortic valve replacement via open axillary artery (33363)

Code first (33880-33881, 33883-33884, 33886, 33990-33991, 34701-34708, 34841-34848, 0254T)

**● + 34716** **Open axillary/subclavian artery exposure with creation of conduit for delivery of endovascular prosthesis or for establishment of cardiopulmonary bypass, by infraclavicular or supraclavicular incision, unilateral (List separately in addition to code for primary procedure)**

🚗 0.00  ✂ 0.00  **FUD** 000

INCLUDES Unilateral procedure

EXCLUDES ECMO/ECLS insertion, removal or repositioning on same side (33953-33954, 33959, [33962], [33969], [33984])

Implantation or replacement of aortic counterpulsation ventricular assist system (0451T-0452T, 0455T-0456T)

Code first (32852, 32854, 33031, 33256, 33259, 33261, 33305, 33315, 33322, 33335, 33390-33391, 33404-33417, 33422, 33425-33427, 33430, 33460, 33463-33465, 33468, 33474-33476, 33478, 33496, 33500, 33502, 33504-33514, 33516, 33533-33536, 33542, 33545, 33548, 33600-33688, 33692, 33694, 33697, 33702-33722, 33724, 33726, 33730, 33732, 33736, 33750, 33755, 33762, 33764, 33766-33767, 33770-33783)

**34800** ~~Endovascular repair of infrarenal abdominal aortic aneurysm or dissection; using aorto-aortic tube prosthesis~~

To report, see 34701-34708

**34802** ~~using modular bifurcated prosthesis (1 docking limb)~~

To report, see 34701-34708

**34803** ~~using modular bifurcated prosthesis (2 docking limbs)~~

To report, see 34701-34708

**34804** ~~using unibody bifurcated prosthesis~~

To report, see 34701-34708

**34805** ~~using aorto-uniiliac or aorto-unifemoral prosthesis~~

To report, see 34701-34708

**34806** ~~Transcatheter placement of wireless physiologic sensor in aneurysmal sac during endovascular repair, including radiological supervision and interpretation, instrument calibration, and collection of pressure data (List separately in addition to code for primary procedure)~~

To report, see 34701-34708

**+ 34808** **Endovascular placement of iliac artery occlusion device (List separately in addition to code for primary procedure)**

Code first (34701-34702, 34707-34710, 34813, 34841-34844)

🚗 6.08  ✂ 6.08  **FUD** ZZZ  C 80 ▭

**AMA:** 2017,Jan,8; 2016,Jan,13; 2015,Jan,16; 2014,Jan,11; 2012,Apr,3-9

**34812** Resequenced code. See code following 34713.

**+ 34813** **Placement of femoral-femoral prosthetic graft during endovascular aortic aneurysm repair (List separately in addition to code for primary procedure)**

EXCLUDES Grafting of femoral artery (35521, 35533, 35539, 35540, 35556, 35558, 35566, 35621, 35646, 35654-35661, 35666, 35700)

Code first ([34812])

🚗 6.92  ✂ 6.92  **FUD** ZZZ  C 80 ▭

**AMA:** 2017,Jan,8; 2016,Jan,13; 2015,Jan,16; 2014,Jan,11; 2012,Apr,3-9

**34820** Resequenced code. See code following 34714.

**34825** ~~Placement of proximal or distal extension prosthesis for endovascular repair of infrarenal abdominal aortic or iliac aneurysm, false aneurysm, or dissection; initial vessel~~

To report, see 34709-34711

**34826** ~~each additional vessel (List separately in addition to code for primary procedure)~~

To report, see 34709-34711

**34830** **Open repair of infrarenal aortic aneurysm or dissection, plus repair of associated arterial trauma, following unsuccessful endovascular repair; tube prosthesis**

🚗 52.7  ✂ 52.7  **FUD** 090  C 80 ▭

**AMA:** 2017,Jan,8; 2016,Jan,13; 2015,Jan,16; 2014,Jan,11; 2012,Jan,15-42

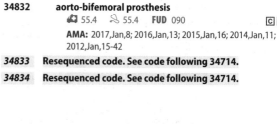

A tube prosthesis is placed and any associated arterial trauma is repaired

**34831** **aorto-bi-iliac prosthesis**

🚗 55.7  ✂ 55.7  **FUD** 090  C 80 ▭

**AMA:** 2017,Jan,8; 2016,Jan,13; 2015,Jan,16; 2014,Jan,11; 2012,Jan,15-42

**34832** **aorto-bifemoral prosthesis**

🚗 55.4  ✂ 55.4  **FUD** 090  C 80 ▭

**AMA:** 2017,Jan,8; 2016,Jan,13; 2015,Jan,16; 2014,Jan,11; 2012,Jan,15-42

**34833** Resequenced code. See code following 34714.

**34834** Resequenced code. See code following 34714.

## 34839-34848 Repair Visceral Aorta with Fenestrated Endovascular Grafts

**INCLUDES**  Balloon angioplasty before and after deployment of graft
Angiography
Fluoroscopic guidance
Guidewire and catheter insertion of vessels in the target treatment zone
Radiologic supervision and interpretation
Visceral aorta (34841-34844)
Visceral aorta and associated infrarenal abdominal aorta (34845-34848)

**EXCLUDES**  *Catheterization of:*
  *Arterial families outside treatment zone*
  *Hypogastric arteries*
*Distal extension prosthesis terminating in the common femoral, external iliac, or internal iliac artery (34709-34711, 0254T)*
*Insertion of bare metal or covered intravascular stents in visceral branches in the target treatment zone (37236-37237)*
*Interventional procedures outside treatment zone*
*Open exposure of access vessels (34713-34716 [34812, 34820, 34833, 34834])*
*Repair of abdominal aortic aneurysm without a fenestrated graft (34701-34708)*
*Substantial artery repair (35226, 35286)*
Code also associated endovascular repair of descending thoracic aorta (33880-33886, 75956-75959)

**34839**  **Physician planning of a patient-specific fenestrated visceral aortic endograft requiring a minimum of 90 minutes of physician time**

🚑 0.00   ✂ 0.00   **FUD** YYY         B 80 ▭

**EXCLUDES**  *3D rendering with interpretation and reporting of imaging (76376-76377)*
*Endovascular repair procedure on day of or day after planning (34701-34706, 34841-34848)*
*Planning on day of or day before endovascular repair procedure*
*Total planning time of less than 90 minutes*

**34841**  **Endovascular repair of visceral aorta (eg, aneurysm, pseudoaneurysm, dissection, penetrating ulcer, intramural hematoma, or traumatic disruption) by deployment of a fenestrated visceral aortic endograft and all associated radiological supervision and interpretation, including target zone angioplasty, when performed; including one visceral artery endoprosthesis (superior mesenteric, celiac or renal artery)**

**EXCLUDES**  *Endovascular repair of aorta (34701-34706, 34845-34848)*
*Physician planning of a patient-specific fenestrated visceral aortic endograft (34839)*

🚑 0.00   ✂ 0.00   **FUD** YYY         C 80 ▭

**AMA:** 2017,Jul,3; 2017,Jan,8; 2016,Jan,13; 2015,Jan,16; 2014,Jan,11; 2013,Dec,8

**34842**     **including two visceral artery endoprostheses (superior mesenteric, celiac and/or renal artery[s])**

**INCLUDES**  Repairs extending from the visceral aorta to one or more of the four visceral artery origins to the level of the infrarenal aorta

**EXCLUDES**  *Endovascular repair of aorta (34701-34706, 34845-34848)*
*Physician planning of a patient-specific fenestrated visceral aortic endograft (34839)*

🚑 0.00   ✂ 0.00   **FUD** YYY         C 80 ▭

**AMA:** 2017,Jul,3; 2017,Jan,8; 2016,Jan,13; 2015,Jan,16; 2014,Jan,11; 2013,Dec,8

**34843**     **including three visceral artery endoprostheses (superior mesenteric, celiac and/or renal artery[s])**

**INCLUDES**  Repairs extending from the visceral aorta to one or more of the four visceral artery origins to the level of the infrarenal aorta

**EXCLUDES**  *Endovascular repair of aorta (34701-34706, 34845-34848)*
*Physician planning of a patient-specific fenestrated visceral aortic endograft (34839)*

🚑 0.00   ✂ 0.00   **FUD** YYY         C 80 ▭

**AMA:** 2017,Jul,3; 2017,Jan,8; 2016,Jan,13; 2015,Jan,16; 2014,Jan,11; 2013,Dec,8

**34844**     **including four or more visceral artery endoprostheses (superior mesenteric, celiac and/or renal artery[s])**

**INCLUDES**  Repairs extending from the visceral aorta to one or more of the four visceral artery origins to the level of the infrarenal aorta

**EXCLUDES**  *Endovascular repair of aorta (34701-34706, 34845-34848)*
*Physician planning of a patient-specific fenestrated visceral aortic endograft (34839)*

🚑 0.00   ✂ 0.00   **FUD** YYY         C 80 ▭

**AMA:** 2017,Jul,3; 2017,Jan,8; 2016,Jan,13; 2015,Jan,16; 2014,Jan,11; 2013,Dec,8

**34845**  **Endovascular repair of visceral aorta and infrarenal abdominal aorta (eg, aneurysm, pseudoaneurysm, dissection, penetrating ulcer, intramural hematoma, or traumatic disruption) with a fenestrated visceral aortic endograft and concomitant unibody or modular infrarenal aortic endograft and all associated radiological supervision and interpretation, including target zone angioplasty, when performed; including one visceral artery endoprosthesis (superior mesenteric, celiac or renal artery)**

**INCLUDES**  Placement of device and extensions into the common iliac arteries
Repairs extending from the visceral aorta into the common iliac arteries

**EXCLUDES**  *Direct repair aneurysm (35081, 35102)*
*Endovascular repair of aorta (34701-34706, 34841-34848)*
*Physician planning of a patient-specific fenestrated visceral aortic endograft (34839)*
Code also iliac artery revascularization when performed outside zone of target treatment (37220-37223)

🚑 0.00   ✂ 0.00   **FUD** YYY         C 80 ▭

**AMA:** 2017,Jul,3; 2017,Jan,8; 2016,Jan,13; 2015,Jan,16; 2014,Jan,11; 2013,Dec,8

**34846**     **including two visceral artery endoprostheses (superior mesenteric, celiac and/or renal artery[s])**

**INCLUDES**  Placement of device and extensions into the common iliac arteries
Repairs extending from the visceral aorta into the common iliac arteries

**EXCLUDES**  *Direct repair aneurysm (35081, 35102)*
*Endovascular repair of aorta (34701-34706, 34841-34844)*
*Physician planning of a patient-specific fenestrated visceral aortic endograft (34839)*
Code also iliac artery revascularization when performed outside zone of target treatment (37220-37223)

🚑 0.00   ✂ 0.00   **FUD** YYY         C 80 ▭

**AMA:** 2017,Jul,3; 2017,Jan,8; 2016,Jan,13; 2015,Jan,16; 2014,Jan,11; 2013,Dec,8

**34847**     **including three visceral artery endoprostheses (superior mesenteric, celiac and/or renal artery[s])**

**INCLUDES**  Placement of device and extensions into the common iliac arteries
Repairs extending from the visceral aorta into the common iliac arteries

**EXCLUDES**  *Direct repair aneurysm (35081, 35102)*
*Endovascular repair of aorta (34701-34706, 34841-34844)*
*Physician planning of a patient-specific fenestrated visceral aortic endograft (34839)*
Code also iliac artery revascularization when performed outside zone of target treatment (37220-37223)

🚑 0.00   ✂ 0.00   **FUD** YYY         C 80 ▭

**AMA:** 2017,Jul,3; 2017,Jan,8; 2016,Jan,13; 2015,Jan,16; 2014,Jan,11; 2013,Dec,8

**34848** including four or more visceral artery endoprostheses (superior mesenteric, celiac and/or renal artery[s])

> **INCLUDES** Placement of device and extensions into the common iliac arteries
>
> Repairs extending from the visceral aorta into the common iliac arteries
>
> **EXCLUDES** Direct repair aneurysm (35081, 35102)
>
> Endovascular repair of aorta (34701-34706, 34841-34844)
>
> Physician planning of a patient-specific fenestrated visceral aortic endograft (34839)
>
> Code also iliac artery revascularization when performed outside zone of target treatment (37220-37223)

🔲 0.00   ⚖ 0.00   **FUD** YYY    C 80 ▣

**AMA:** 2017,Aug,9; 2017,Jul,3; 2017,Jan,8; 2016,Jul,6; 2016,Jan,13; 2015,Jan,16; 2014,Jan,11; 2013,Dec,8

## 34900 Endovascular Stent Grafting Iliac Artery

**34900** ~~Endovascular repair of iliac artery (eg, aneurysm, pseudoaneurysm, arteriovenous malformation, trauma) using ilio-iliac tube endoprosthesis~~

> To report, see 34707-34708

## 35001-35152 Repair Aneurysm, False Aneurysm, Related Arterial Disease

> **INCLUDES** Endarterectomy procedures
>
> **EXCLUDES** Endovascular repairs of:
>
> Abdominal aortic aneurysm (34701-34716 [34812, 34820, 34833, 34834])
>
> Thoracic aortic aneurysm (33880-33891)
>
> Intracranial aneurysms (61697-61710)
>
> Open repairs thoracic aortic aneurysm (33860-33875)
>
> Repairs related to occlusive disease only (35201-35286)

**35001** Direct repair of aneurysm, pseudoaneurysm, or excision (partial or total) and graft insertion, with or without patch graft; for aneurysm and associated occlusive disease, carotid, subclavian artery, by neck incision

🔲 32.6   ⚖ 32.6   **FUD** 090    C 80 50 ▣

**AMA:** 2002,May,7; 2000,Dec,1

**35002** for ruptured aneurysm, carotid, subclavian artery, by neck incision

🔲 33.5   ⚖ 33.5   **FUD** 090    C 80 50 ▣

**AMA:** 2002,May,7; 1997,Nov,1

**35005** for aneurysm, pseudoaneurysm, and associated occlusive disease, vertebral artery

🔲 32.9   ⚖ 32.9   **FUD** 090    C 80 50 ▣

**AMA:** 2002,May,7; 1997,Nov,1

An incision is made in the back of the neck to directly approach an aneurysm or false aneurysm of the vertebral artery. The artery is either repaired directly or excised with a graft

Graft repair

Vertebral artery

Subclavian artery

**35011** for aneurysm and associated occlusive disease, axillary-brachial artery, by arm incision

🔲 29.4   ⚖ 29.4   **FUD** 090    T 80 50 ▣

**AMA:** 2002,May,7; 1997,Nov,1

**35013** for ruptured aneurysm, axillary-brachial artery, by arm incision

🔲 36.7   ⚖ 36.7   **FUD** 090    C 80 50 ▣

**AMA:** 2002,May,7; 1997,Nov,1

**35021** for aneurysm, pseudoaneurysm, and associated occlusive disease, innominate, subclavian artery, by thoracic incision

🔲 36.1   ⚖ 36.1   **FUD** 090    C 80 50 ▣

**AMA:** 2002,May,7; 1997,Nov,1

**35022** for ruptured aneurysm, innominate, subclavian artery, by thoracic incision

🔲 41.7   ⚖ 41.7   **FUD** 090    C 80 50 ▣

**AMA:** 2002,May,7; 1997,Nov,1

**35045** for aneurysm, pseudoaneurysm, and associated occlusive disease, radial or ulnar artery

🔲 28.9   ⚖ 28.9   **FUD** 090    T 80 50 ▣

**AMA:** 2002,May,7; 1997,Nov,1

**35081** for aneurysm, pseudoaneurysm, and associated occlusive disease, abdominal aorta

🔲 51.1   ⚖ 51.1   **FUD** 090    C 80 ▣

**AMA:** 2017,Jan,8; 2016,Jan,13; 2015,Jan,16; 2014,Jan,11; 2013,Dec,8; 2012,Jan,15-42

**35082** for ruptured aneurysm, abdominal aorta

🔲 64.3   ⚖ 64.3   **FUD** 090    C 80 ▣

**AMA:** 2002,May,7; 1997,Nov,1

**35091** for aneurysm, pseudoaneurysm, and associated occlusive disease, abdominal aorta involving visceral vessels (mesenteric, celiac, renal)

🔲 52.5   ⚖ 52.5   **FUD** 090    C 80 50 ▣

**AMA:** 2017,Jan,8; 2016,Jan,13; 2015,Jan,16; 2014,Jan,11

**35092** for ruptured aneurysm, abdominal aorta involving visceral vessels (mesenteric, celiac, renal)

🔲 76.3   ⚖ 76.3   **FUD** 090    C 80 50 ▣

**AMA:** 2002,May,7; 1997,Nov,1

**35102** for aneurysm, pseudoaneurysm, and associated occlusive disease, abdominal aorta involving iliac vessels (common, hypogastric, external)

🔲 55.2   ⚖ 55.2   **FUD** 090    C 80 50 ▣

**AMA:** 2017,Jan,8; 2016,Jan,13; 2015,Jan,16; 2014,Jan,11; 2013,Dec,8

**35103** for ruptured aneurysm, abdominal aorta involving iliac vessels (common, hypogastric, external)

🔲 65.9   ⚖ 65.9   **FUD** 090    C 80 50 ▣

**AMA:** 2002,May,7; 1997,Nov,1

**35111** for aneurysm, pseudoaneurysm, and associated occlusive disease, splenic artery

🔲 38.8   ⚖ 38.8   **FUD** 090    C 80 50 ▣

**AMA:** 2002,May,7; 1997,Nov,1

**35112** for ruptured aneurysm, splenic artery

🔲 55.2   ⚖ 55.2   **FUD** 090    C 80 50 ▣

**AMA:** 2002,May,7; 1997,Nov,1

**35121** for aneurysm, pseudoaneurysm, and associated occlusive disease, hepatic, celiac, renal, or mesenteric artery

🔲 48.4   ⚖ 48.4   **FUD** 090    C 80 50 ▣

**AMA:** 2002,May,7; 1997,Nov,1

**35122** for ruptured aneurysm, hepatic, celiac, renal, or mesenteric artery

🔲 63.2   ⚖ 63.2   **FUD** 090    C 80 50 ▣

**AMA:** 2002,May,7; 1997,Nov,1

**35131** for aneurysm, pseudoaneurysm, and associated occlusive disease, iliac artery (common, hypogastric, external)

🔲 40.7   ⚖ 40.7   **FUD** 090    C 80 50 ▣

**AMA:** 2017,Jan,8; 2016,Jan,13; 2015,Jan,16; 2014,Jan,11

---

| 26/TC PC/TC Only | A2-Z3 ASC Payment | 50 Bilateral | ♂ Male Only | ♀ Female Only | 🔲 Facility RVU | ⚖ Non-Facility RVU | ▣ CCI |
|---|---|---|---|---|---|---|---|
| **FUD** Follow-up Days | **CMS:** IOM (Pub 100) | A-Y OPPSI | 80/80 Surg Assist Allowed / w/Doc | | 🔳 Lab Crosswalk | 🔀 Radiology Crosswalk | ✖ CLIA |

CPT © 2017 American Medical Association. All Rights Reserved.

© 2017 Optum360, LLC

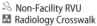

**35132** for ruptured aneurysm, iliac artery (common, hypogastric, external)
  🔧 47.9   ✂ 47.9   **FUD** 090   C 80 50 ▣
  **AMA:** 2002,May,7; 1997,Nov,1

**35141** for aneurysm, pseudoaneurysm, and associated occlusive disease, common femoral artery (profunda femoris, superficial femoral)
  🔧 32.4   ✂ 32.4   **FUD** 090   C 80 50 ▣
  **AMA:** 2002,May,7; 1997,Nov,1

**35142** for ruptured aneurysm, common femoral artery (profunda femoris, superficial femoral)
  🔧 38.7   ✂ 38.7   **FUD** 090   C 80 50 ▣
  **AMA:** 2002,May,7; 1997,Nov,1

**35151** for aneurysm, pseudoaneurysm, and associated occlusive disease, popliteal artery
  🔧 36.3   ✂ 36.3   **FUD** 090   C 80 50 ▣
  **AMA:** 2002,May,7; 1997,Nov,1

**35152** for ruptured aneurysm, popliteal artery
  🔧 40.7   ✂ 40.7   **FUD** 090   C 80 50 ▣
  **AMA:** 2002,May,7; 1997,Nov,1

## 35180-35190 Surgical Repair Arteriovenous Fistula

**35180** Repair, congenital arteriovenous fistula; head and neck
  🔧 27.8   ✂ 27.8   **FUD** 090   T 80 ▣
  **AMA:** 2017,Jan,8; 2016,Jan,13; 2015,Jan,16; 2014,Jan,11; 2012,Jan,15-42

**35182** thorax and abdomen
  🔧 52.0   ✂ 52.0   **FUD** 090   C 80 ▣
  **AMA:** 2017,Jan,8; 2016,Jan,13; 2015,Jan,16; 2014,Jan,11; 2012,Jan,15-42

**35184** extremities
  🔧 32.8   ✂ 32.8   **FUD** 090   T 80 ▣
  **AMA:** 2017,Jan,8; 2016,Jan,13; 2015,Jan,16; 2014,Jan,11; 2012,Jan,15-42

**35188** Repair, acquired or traumatic arteriovenous fistula; head and neck
  🔧 31.1   ✂ 31.1   **FUD** 090   T A2 80 ▣
  **AMA:** 2017,Jan,8; 2016,Jan,13; 2015,Jan,16; 2014,Jan,11; 2012,Jan,15-42

**35189** thorax and abdomen
  🔧 46.5   ✂ 46.5   **FUD** 090   C 80 ▣
  **AMA:** 2017,Jan,8; 2016,Jan,13; 2015,Jan,16; 2014,Jan,11; 2012,Jan,15-42

**35190** extremities
  🔧 22.2   ✂ 22.2   **FUD** 090   T 80 ▣
  **AMA:** 2017,Jan,8; 2016,Jan,13; 2015,Jan,16; 2014,Jan,11; 2012,Jan,15-42

## 35201-35286 Surgical Repair Artery or Vein

EXCLUDES Arteriovenous fistula repair (35180-35190)
Primary open vascular procedures

**35201** Repair blood vessel, direct; neck
  EXCLUDES Removal ECMO/ECLS of cannula ([33969, 33984, 33985, 33986])
  🔧 27.6   ✂ 27.6   **FUD** 090   T 80 50 ▣
  **AMA:** 2017,Jan,8; 2016,Jan,13; 2015,Jul,3; 2015,Jan,16; 2014,Mar,8

**35206** upper extremity
  EXCLUDES Removal ECMO/ECLS of cannula ([33969, 33984, 33985, 33986])
  🔧 22.7   ✂ 22.7   **FUD** 090   T 80 50 ▣
  **AMA:** 2017,Jan,8; 2016,Jan,13; 2015,Jul,3; 2015,Jan,16; 2014,Apr,10; 2014,Jan,11; 2012,Apr,3-9

**35207** hand, finger
  🔧 21.8   ✂ 21.8   **FUD** 090   T A2 50 ▣
  **AMA:** 2012,Apr,3-9

**35211** intrathoracic, with bypass
  EXCLUDES Removal ECMO/ECLS of cannula ([33969, 33984, 33985, 33986])
  🔧 40.0   ✂ 40.0   **FUD** 090   C 80 50 ▣
  **AMA:** 2015,Jul,3; 2012,Apr,3-9

**35216** intrathoracic, without bypass
  EXCLUDES Removal ECMO/ECLS of cannula ([33969, 33984, 33985, 33986])
  🔧 59.5   ✂ 59.5   **FUD** 090   C 80 50 ▣
  **AMA:** 2017,Jan,8; 2016,Jan,13; 2015,Jan,16; 2014,Jan,11; 2012,Apr,3-9

**35221** intra-abdominal
  🔧 42.6   ✂ 42.6   **FUD** 090   C 80 50 ▣
  **AMA:** 2012,Apr,3-9

**35226** lower extremity
  EXCLUDES Removal ECMO/ECLS of cannula ([33969, 33984, 33985, 33986])
  🔧 24.4   ✂ 24.4   **FUD** 090   T 80 50 ▣
  **AMA:** 2017,Aug,10; 2017,Jul,3; 2017,Jan,8; 2016,Jul,6; 2016,Jan,13; 2015,Jul,3; 2015,Jan,16; 2014,Jan,11; 2013,Dec,8; 2013,Mar,10-11; 2012,Apr,3-9

**35231** Repair blood vessel with vein graft; neck
  🔧 36.0   ✂ 36.0   **FUD** 090   T 80 50 ▣
  **AMA:** 2012,Apr,3-9

**35236** upper extremity
  🔧 28.7   ✂ 28.7   **FUD** 090   T 80 50 ▣
  **AMA:** 2017,Jan,8; 2016,Jan,13; 2015,Jan,16; 2014,Jan,11; 2012,Apr,3-9

**35241** intrathoracic, with bypass
  🔧 40.0   ✂ 40.0   **FUD** 090   C 80 50 ▣
  **AMA:** 2012,Apr,3-9

**35246** intrathoracic, without bypass
  🔧 45.8   ✂ 45.8   **FUD** 090   C 80 50 ▣
  **AMA:** 2012,Apr,3-9

**35251** intra-abdominal
  🔧 50.0   ✂ 50.0   **FUD** 090   C 80 50 ▣
  **AMA:** 2012,Apr,3-9

**35256** lower extremity
  🔧 29.8   ✂ 29.8   **FUD** 090   T 80 50 ▣
  **AMA:** 2012,Apr,3-9

**35261** Repair blood vessel with graft other than vein; neck
  🔧 31.1   ✂ 31.1   **FUD** 090   T 80 50 ▣
  **AMA:** 2012,Apr,3-9

**35266** upper extremity
  🔧 25.3   ✂ 25.3   **FUD** 090   T 80 50 ▣
  **AMA:** 2017,Jan,8; 2016,Jan,13; 2015,Jan,16; 2014,Jan,11; 2012,Apr,3-9

**35271** intrathoracic, with bypass
  🔧 40.3   ✂ 40.3   **FUD** 090   C 80 50 ▣
  **AMA:** 2012,Apr,3-9

**35276** intrathoracic, without bypass
  🔧 42.5   ✂ 42.5   **FUD** 090   C 80 50 ▣
  **AMA:** 2012,Apr,3-9

**35281** intra-abdominal
  🔧 47.2   ✂ 47.2   **FUD** 090   C 80 50 ▣
  **AMA:** 2012,Apr,3-9

**35286** lower extremity
  🔧 27.3   ✂ 27.3   **FUD** 090   T 80 50 ▣
  **AMA:** 2017,Aug,10; 2017,Jul,3; 2017,Jan,8; 2016,Jul,6; 2016,Jan,13; 2015,Jan,16; 2014,Jan,11; 2013,Dec,8; 2013,Mar,10-11; 2012,Apr,3-9

● New Code   ▲ Revised Code   ○ Reinstated   ● New Web Release   ▲ Revised Web Release   Unlisted   Not Covered   # Resequenced
⊘ AMA Mod 51 Exempt   ⑤① Optum Mod 51 Exempt   ⑥③ Mod 63 Exempt   ✗ Non-FDA Drug   ★ Telemedicine   Ⓜ Maternity   Ⓐ Age Edit   + Add-on   **AMA:** CPT Asst
© 2017 Optum360, LLC   CPT © 2017 American Medical Association. All Rights Reserved.   147

**Cardiovascular, Hemic, and Lymphatic**

**35301 — 35506**

## 35301-35372 Surgical Thromboendarterectomy Peripheral and Visceral Arteries

**INCLUDES** Obtaining saphenous or arm vein for graft
Thrombectomy/embolectomy

**EXCLUDES** *Coronary artery bypass procedures (33510-33536, 33572)*
*Thromboendarterectomy for vascular occlusion on a different vessel during the same session*

**35301** **Thromboendarterectomy, including patch graft, if performed; carotid, vertebral, subclavian, by neck incision**
🔹 33.1　✂ 33.1　**FUD** 090　　　© 80 50 ▭

**AMA:** 2017,Jan,8; 2016,Jan,13; 2015,Jan,16; 2014,Jan,11

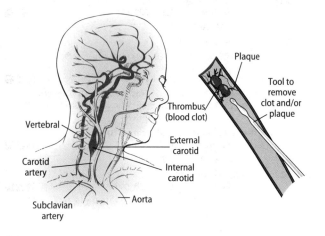

Plaque

Tool to remove clot and/or plaque

Thrombus (blood clot)

Vertebral

External carotid

Carotid artery

Internal carotid

Subclavian artery

Aorta

**35302** **superficial femoral artery**
**EXCLUDES** *Revascularization, endovascular, open or percutaneous, femoral, popliteal artery(s) (37225, 37227)*
🔹 32.9　✂ 32.9　**FUD** 090　　　© 80 50 ▭
**AMA:** 2017,Jan,8; 2016,Jan,13; 2015,Jan,16; 2014,Jan,11

**35303** **popliteal artery**
**EXCLUDES** *Revascularization, endovascular, open or percutaneous, femoral, popliteal artery(s) (37225, 37227)*
🔹 36.3　✂ 36.3　**FUD** 090　　　© 80 50 ▭
**AMA:** 2017,Jan,8; 2016,Jan,13; 2015,Jan,16; 2014,Jan,11

**35304** **tibioperoneal trunk artery**
**EXCLUDES** *Revascularization, endovascular, open or percutaneous, tibial/peroneal artery (37229, 37231, 37233, 37235)*
🔹 37.7　✂ 37.7　**FUD** 090　　　© 80 50 ▭
**AMA:** 2017,Jan,8; 2016,Jan,13; 2015,Jan,16; 2014,Jan,11

**35305** **tibial or peroneal artery, initial vessel**
**EXCLUDES** *Revascularization, endovascular, open or percutaneous, tibial/peroneal artery (37229, 37231, 37233, 37235)*
🔹 36.0　✂ 36.0　**FUD** 090　　　© 80 50 ▭
**AMA:** 2017,Jan,8; 2016,Jan,13; 2015,Jan,16; 2014,Jan,11; 2012,Jan,15-42

**+ 35306** **each additional tibial or peroneal artery (List separately in addition to code for primary procedure)**
**EXCLUDES** *Revascularization, endovascular, open or percutaneous, tibial/peroneal artery (37229, 37231, 37233, 37235)*
Code first (35305)
🔹 13.0　✂ 13.0　**FUD** ZZZ　　　© 80 ▭
**AMA:** 2017,Jan,8; 2016,Jan,13; 2015,Jan,16; 2014,Jan,11

**35311** **subclavian, innominate, by thoracic incision**
🔹 45.5　✂ 45.5　**FUD** 090　　　© 80 50 ▭
**AMA:** 1997,Nov,1

**35321** **axillary-brachial**
🔹 26.1　✂ 26.1　**FUD** 090　　　Ⓣ 80 50 ▭
**AMA:** 1997,Nov,1

**35331** **abdominal aorta**
🔹 42.5　✂ 42.5　**FUD** 090　　　© 80 50 ▭
**AMA:** 1997,Nov,1

**35341** **mesenteric, celiac, or renal**
🔹 40.1　✂ 40.1　**FUD** 090　　　© 80 50 ▭
**AMA:** 1997,Nov,1

**35351** **iliac**
🔹 37.5　✂ 37.5　**FUD** 090　　　© 80 50 ▭
**AMA:** 1997,Nov,1

**35355** **iliofemoral**
🔹 30.3　✂ 30.3　**FUD** 090　　　© 80 50 ▭
**AMA:** 1997,Nov,1

**35361** **combined aortoiliac**
🔹 44.6　✂ 44.6　**FUD** 090　　　© 80 50 ▭
**AMA:** 1997,Nov,1

**35363** **combined aortoiliofemoral**
🔹 51.7　✂ 51.7　**FUD** 090　　　© 80 50 ▭
**AMA:** 1997,Nov,1

**35371** **common femoral**
🔹 24.0　✂ 24.0　**FUD** 090　　　© 80 50 ▭
**AMA:** 2017,Aug,10; 2017,Jul,3; 2017,Jan,8; 2016,Jan,13; 2015,Jan,16; 2014,Jan,11; 2012,Apr,3-9

**35372** **deep (profunda) femoral**
🔹 28.7　✂ 28.7　**FUD** 090　　　© 80 50 ▭
**AMA:** 2017,Jan,8; 2016,Jan,13; 2015,Jan,16; 2014,Jan,11

## 35390 Surgical Thromboendarterectomy: Carotid Reoperation

Code first (35301)

**+ 35390** **Reoperation, carotid, thromboendarterectomy, more than 1 month after original operation (List separately in addition to code for primary procedure)**
🔹 4.68　✂ 4.68　**FUD** ZZZ　　　© 80 ▭
**AMA:** 1997,Nov,1; 1993,Win,1

## 35400 Endoscopic Visualization of Vessels

Code first the therapeutic intervention

**+ 35400** **Angioscopy (noncoronary vessels or grafts) during therapeutic intervention (List separately in addition to code for primary procedure)**
🔹 4.37　✂ 4.37　**FUD** ZZZ　　　© 80 ▭
**AMA:** 1997,Dec,1; 1997,Nov,1

## 35500 Obtain Arm Vein for Graft

**EXCLUDES** *Endoscopic harvest (33508)*
*Harvesting of multiple vein segments (35682, 35683)*
Code first (33510-33536, 35556, 35566, 35570-35571, 35583-35587)

**+ 35500** **Harvest of upper extremity vein, 1 segment, for lower extremity or coronary artery bypass procedure (List separately in addition to code for primary procedure)**
🔹 9.36　✂ 9.36　**FUD** ZZZ　　　Ⓝ 80 ▭
**AMA:** 2017,Jan,8; 2016,Jan,13; 2015,Jan,16; 2014,Jan,11; 2012,Apr,3-9

## 35501-35571 Arterial Bypass Using Vein Grafts

**INCLUDES** Obtaining saphenous vein grafts

**EXCLUDES** *Obtaining multiple vein segments (35682, 35683)*
*Obtaining vein grafts, upper extremity or femoropopliteal (35500, 35572)*
*Treatment of different sites with different bypass procedures during the same operative session*

**35501** **Bypass graft, with vein; common carotid-ipsilateral internal carotid**
🔹 43.9　✂ 43.9　**FUD** 090　　　© 80 50 ▭
**AMA:** 2017,Jan,8; 2016,Jan,13; 2015,Jan,16; 2014,Jan,11; 2012,Apr,3-9

**35506** **carotid-subclavian or subclavian-carotid**
🔹 37.4　✂ 37.4　**FUD** 090　　　© 80 50 ▭
**AMA:** 2017,Jan,8; 2016,Jan,13; 2015,Jan,16; 2014,Jan,11

**35508**     **carotid-vertebral**

INCLUDES     Endoscopic procedure

🚑 39.1   ⚗ 39.1   **FUD** 090                    C 80 50 ▣

**AMA:** 1999,Mar,6; 1999,Apr,11

**35509**     **carotid-contralateral carotid**

🚑 41.3   ⚗ 41.3   **FUD** 090                    C 80 50 ▣

**AMA:** 2017,Jan,8; 2016,Jan,13; 2015,Jan,16; 2014,Jan,11;
2012,Jan,15-42

**35510**     **carotid-brachial**

🚑 35.9   ⚗ 35.9   **FUD** 090                    C 80 50 ▣

**AMA:** 2017,Jan,8; 2016,Jan,13; 2015,Jan,16; 2014,Jan,11;
2012,Jan,15-42

**35511**     **subclavian-subclavian**

🚑 35.7   ⚗ 35.7   **FUD** 090                    C 80 50 ▣

**AMA:** 2017,Jan,8; 2016,Jan,13; 2015,Jan,16; 2014,Jan,11

**35512**     **subclavian-brachial**

🚑 40.2   ⚗ 40.2   **FUD** 090                    C 80 50 ▣

**AMA:** 2017,Jan,8; 2016,Jan,13; 2015,Jan,16; 2014,Jan,11

**35515**     **subclavian-vertebral**

🚑 42.4   ⚗ 42.4   **FUD** 090                    C 80 50 ▣

**AMA:** 1999,Mar,6; 1999,Apr,11

**35516**     **subclavian-axillary**

🚑 35.7   ⚗ 35.7   **FUD** 090                    C 80 50 ▣

**AMA:** 1999,Mar,6; 1999,Apr,11

**35518**     **axillary-axillary**

🚑 34.0   ⚗ 34.0   **FUD** 090                    C 80 50 ▣

**AMA:** 2017,Jan,8; 2016,Jan,13; 2015,Jan,16; 2014,Jan,11

**35521**     **axillary-femoral**

EXCLUDES     Synthetic graft (35621)

🚑 35.9   ⚗ 35.9   **FUD** 090                    C 80 50 ▣

**AMA:** 2017,Jan,8; 2016,Jan,13; 2015,Jan,16; 2014,Jan,11;
2012,Apr,3-9

**35522**     **axillary-brachial**

🚑 35.4   ⚗ 35.4   **FUD** 090                    C 80 50 ▣

**AMA:** 2017,Jan,8; 2016,Jan,13; 2015,Jan,16; 2014,Jan,11

**35523**     **brachial-ulnar or -radial**

🚑 37.5   ⚗ 37.5   **FUD** 090                    C 80 50 ▣

EXCLUDES     Bypass graft using synthetic conduit (37799)
Bypass graft, with vein; brachial-brachial (35525)
Distal revascularization and interval ligation (DRIL),
   upper extremity hemodialysis access (steal
   syndrome) (36838)
Harvest of upper extremity vein, 1 segment, for lower
   extremity or coronary artery bypass procedure
   (35500)
Repair blood vessel, direct; upper extremity (35206)

**35525**     **brachial-brachial**

🚑 33.6   ⚗ 33.6   **FUD** 090                    C 80 50 ▣

**AMA:** 2017,Jan,8; 2016,Jan,13; 2015,Jan,16; 2014,Jan,11

**35526**     **aortosubclavian, aortoinnominate, or aortocarotid**

EXCLUDES     Synthetic graft (35626)

🚑 49.4   ⚗ 49.4   **FUD** 090                    C 80 50 ▣

**AMA:** 1999,Mar,6; 1999,Apr,11

**35531**     **aortoceliac or aortomesenteric**

🚑 59.4   ⚗ 59.4   **FUD** 090                    C 80 50 ▣

**AMA:** 1999,Mar,6; 1999,Apr,11

**35533**     **axillary-femoral-femoral**

EXCLUDES     Synthetic graft (35654)

🚑 43.9   ⚗ 43.9   **FUD** 090                    C 80 50 ▣

**AMA:** 2012,Apr,3-9

**35535**     **hepatorenal**

🚑 56.1   ⚗ 56.1   **FUD** 090                    C 80 50 ▣

EXCLUDES     Bypass graft (35536, 35560, 35631, 35636)
Harvest of upper extremity vein, 1 segment, for lower
   extremity or coronary artery bypass procedure
   (35500)
Repair blood vessel (35221, 35251, 35281)

**35536**     **splenorenal**

🚑 50.4   ⚗ 50.4   **FUD** 090                    C 80 50 ▣

**AMA:** 2017,Jan,8; 2016,Jan,13; 2015,Jan,16; 2014,Jan,11;
2012,Jan,15-42

**35537**     **aortoiliac**

EXCLUDES     Bypass graft, with vein; aortobi-iliac (35538)
Synthetic graft (35637)

🚑 69.6   ⚗ 69.6   **FUD** 090                    C 80 ▣

**AMA:** 2017,Jan,8; 2016,Jan,13; 2015,Jan,16; 2014,Jan,11;
2012,Apr,3-9

**35538**     **aortobi-iliac**

EXCLUDES     Bypass graft, with vein; aortoiliac (35537)
Synthetic graft (35638)

🚑 68.9   ⚗ 68.9   **FUD** 090                    C 80 ▣

**AMA:** 2017,Jan,8; 2016,Jan,13; 2015,Jan,16; 2014,Jan,11;
2012,Apr,3-9

Blockage in lower aorta
Aorta
Common iliac
Femoral
Femoral arteries (bilateral graft shown)

**35539**     **aortofemoral**

EXCLUDES     Bypass graft, with vein; aortobifemoral (35540)
Synthetic graft (35647)

🚑 65.3   ⚗ 65.3   **FUD** 090                    C 80 50 ▣

**AMA:** 2017,Jan,8; 2016,Jan,13; 2015,Jan,16; 2014,Jan,11;
2012,Apr,3-9

**35540**     **aortobifemoral**

EXCLUDES     Bypass graft, with vein; aortofemoral (35539)
Synthetic graft (35646)

🚑 75.1   ⚗ 75.1   **FUD** 090                    C 50 ▣

**AMA:** 2017,Jan,8; 2016,Jan,13; 2015,Jan,16; 2014,Jan,11;
2012,Apr,3-9

**35556**     **femoral-popliteal**

🚑 41.0   ⚗ 41.0   **FUD** 090                    C 80 50 ▣

**AMA:** 2017,Jan,8; 2016,Jan,13; 2015,Jan,16; 2014,Jan,11;
2012,Apr,3-9

**35558**     **femoral-femoral**

🚑 36.1   ⚗ 36.1   **FUD** 090                    C 80 50 ▣

**AMA:** 2012,Apr,3-9

**35560**     **aortorenal**

🚑 50.0   ⚗ 50.0   **FUD** 090                    C 80 50 ▣

**AMA:** 2017,Jan,8; 2016,Jan,13; 2015,Jan,16; 2014,Jan,11;
2012,Jan,15-42

**35563**     **ilioiliac**

🚑 43.9   ⚗ 43.9   **FUD** 090                    C 80 50 ▣

**AMA:** 1999,Mar,6; 1999,Apr,11

**35565**     **iliofemoral**

🚑 39.0   ⚗ 39.0   **FUD** 090                    C 80 50 ▣

**AMA:** 2012,Apr,3-9

**35566**     **femoral-anterior tibial, posterior tibial, peroneal artery
or other distal vessels**

🚑 49.0   ⚗ 49.0   **FUD** 090                    C 80 50 ▣

**AMA:** 2017,Jan,8; 2016,Jan,13; 2015,Jan,16; 2014,Jan,11;
2012,Apr,3-9

● New Code   ▲ Revised Code   ○ Reinstated   ● New Web Release   ▲ Revised Web Release   Unlisted   Not Covered   # Resequenced
⊘ AMA Mod 51 Exempt   Ⓢ Optum Mod 51 Exempt   Ⓖ Mod 63 Exempt   ⁄ Non-FDA Drug   ★ Telemedicine   Ⓜ Maternity   Ⓐ Age Edit   ✛ Add-on   **AMA:** CPT Asst

© 2017 Optum360, LLC                    CPT © 2017 American Medical Association. All Rights Reserved.                    **149**

**35570** tibial-tibial, peroneal-tibial, or tibial/peroneal trunk-tibial

*EXCLUDES* *Repair of blood vessel with graft (35256, 35286)*

🔷 44.3   ⚕ 44.3   **FUD** 090   C 80 50 ▣

**AMA:** 2017,Jan,8; 2016,Jan,13; 2015,Jan,16; 2014,Jan,11; 2012,Apr,3-9

**35571** popliteal-tibial, -peroneal artery or other distal vessels

🔷 38.9   ⚕ 38.9   **FUD** 090   C 80 50 ▣

**AMA:** 2017,Jan,8; 2016,Jan,13; 2015,Jan,16; 2014,Jan,11; 2012,Apr,3-9

## 35572 Obtain Femoropopliteal Vein for Graft

Code first (33510-33523, 33533-33536, 34502, 34520, 35001-35002, 35011-35022, 35102-35103, 35121-35152, 35231-35256, 35501-35587, 35879-35907)

+ **35572** Harvest of femoropopliteal vein, 1 segment, for vascular reconstruction procedure (eg, aortic, vena caval, coronary, peripheral artery) (List separately in addition to code for primary procedure)

🔷 10.1   ⚕ 10.1   **FUD** ZZZ   N N1 80 ▣

**AMA:** 2017,Jan,8; 2016,Jan,13; 2015,Jan,16; 2014,Jan,11; 2012,Jan,15-42

## 35583-35587 Lower Extremity Revascularization: In-situ Vein Bypass

*INCLUDES* Obtaining saphenous vein grafts

*EXCLUDES* *Obtaining multiple vein segments (35682, 35683)*
*Obtaining vein graft, upper extremity or femoropopliteal (35500, 35572)*

**35583** In-situ vein bypass; femoral-popliteal

Code also aortobifemoral bypass graft other than vein for aortobifemoral bypass using synthetic conduit and femoral-popliteal bypass with vein conduit in situ (35646)

Code also concurrent aortofemoral bypass for aortofemoral bypass graft with synthetic conduit and femoral-popliteal bypass with vein conduit in-situ (35647)

Code also concurrent aortofemoral bypass (vein) for an aortofemoral bypass using a vein conduit or a femoral-popliteal bypass with vein conduit in-situ (35539)

🔷 42.4   ⚕ 42.4   **FUD** 090   C 80 50 ▣

**AMA:** 2017,Jan,8; 2016,Jan,13; 2015,Jan,16; 2014,Jan,11; 2012,Apr,3-9

**35585** femoral-anterior tibial, posterior tibial, or peroneal artery

🔷 49.2   ⚕ 49.2   **FUD** 090   C 80 50 ▣

**AMA:** 2017,Jan,8; 2016,Jan,13; 2015,Jan,16; 2014,Jan,11; 2012,Apr,3-9

**35587** popliteal-tibial, peroneal

🔷 40.1   ⚕ 40.1   **FUD** 090   C 80 50 ▣

**AMA:** 2017,Jan,8; 2016,Jan,13; 2015,Jan,16; 2014,Jan,11; 2012,Apr,3-9

## 35600 Obtain Arm Artery for Coronary Bypass

*EXCLUDES* *Transposition and/or reimplantation of arteries (35691-35695)*

Code first (33533-33536)

+ **35600** Harvest of upper extremity artery, 1 segment, for coronary artery bypass procedure (List separately in addition to code for primary procedure)

🔷 7.43   ⚕ 7.43   **FUD** ZZZ   C 80 ▣

**AMA:** 2017,Jan,8; 2016,Jan,13; 2015,Jan,16; 2014,Jan,11; 2012,Jan,15-42

Median

Ulnar

Radial

An upper extremity artery or segment is harvested for a coronary artery bypass procedure

## 35601-35671 Arterial Bypass: Grafts Other Than Veins

*EXCLUDES* *Transposition and/or reimplantation of arteries (35691-35695)*

**35601** Bypass graft, with other than vein; common carotid-ipsilateral internal carotid

*EXCLUDES* *Open transcervical common carotid-common carotid bypass with endovascular repair of descending thoracic aorta (33891)*

🔷 41.1   ⚕ 41.1   **FUD** 090   C 80 50 ▣

**AMA:** 2017,Jan,8; 2016,Jan,13; 2015,Jan,16; 2014,Jan,11

**35606** carotid-subclavian

*EXCLUDES* *Open subclavian to carotid artery transposition performed with endovascular thoracic aneurysm repair via neck incision (33889)*

🔷 34.4   ⚕ 34.4   **FUD** 090   C 80 50 ▣

**AMA:** 1997,Nov,1

**35612** subclavian-subclavian

🔷 31.2   ⚕ 31.2   **FUD** 090   C 80 50 ▣

**AMA:** 1997,Nov,1

**35616** subclavian-axillary

🔷 32.4   ⚕ 32.4   **FUD** 090   C 80 50 ▣

**AMA:** 1997,Nov,1

**35621** axillary-femoral

🔷 32.2   ⚕ 32.2   **FUD** 090   C 80 50 ▣

**AMA:** 2017,Jan,8; 2016,Jan,13; 2015,Jan,16; 2014,Jan,11; 2012,Apr,3-9

**35623** axillary-popliteal or -tibial

🔷 38.7   ⚕ 38.7   **FUD** 090   C 80 50 ▣

**AMA:** 2012,Apr,3-9

**35626** aortosubclavian, aortoinnominate, or aortocarotid

🔷 46.0   ⚕ 46.0   **FUD** 090   C 80 50 ▣

**AMA:** 1997,Nov,1

**35631** **aortoceliac, aortomesenteric, aortorenal**
  🔪 54.3   ✂ 54.3   **FUD** 090   C 80 50 ▣
  **AMA:** 1997,Nov,1

Vena cava and renal veins — Celiac trunk — Abdominal aorta — Superior mesenteric — Renal — Synthetic graft — Abdominal aorta as it exits diaphragm — Blockage

**35632** **ilio-celiac**
  🔪 52.9   ✂ 52.9   **FUD** 090   C 80 50 ▣
  *EXCLUDES* Bypass graft (35531, 35631)
    Repair of blood vessel (35221, 35251, 35281)

**35633** **ilio-mesenteric**
  🔪 58.8   ✂ 58.8   **FUD** 090   C 80 50 ▣
  *EXCLUDES* Bypass graft (35531, 35631)
    Repair of blood vessel (35221, 35251, 35281)

**35634** **iliorenal**
  🔪 52.8   ✂ 52.8   **FUD** 090   C 80 50 ▣
  *EXCLUDES* Bypass graft (35536, 35560, 35631)
    Repair of blood vessel (35221, 35251, 35281)

**35636** **splenorenal (splenic to renal arterial anastomosis)**
  🔪 47.6   ✂ 47.6   **FUD** 090   C 80 50 ▣
  **AMA:** 1997,Nov,1; 1994,Win,1

**35637** **aortoiliac**
  *EXCLUDES* Bypass graft (35638, 35646)
  🔪 50.9   ✂ 50.9   **FUD** 090   C 80 ▣
  **AMA:** 2017,Jan,8; 2016,Jan,13; 2015,Jan,16; 2014,Jan,11;
  2012,Jan,15-42

**35638** **aortobi-iliac**
  *EXCLUDES* Bypass graft (35637, 35646)
    Open placement of aorto-bi-iliac prosthesis after a failed
      endovascular repair (34831)
  🔪 51.7   ✂ 51.7   **FUD** 090   C 80 ▣
  **AMA:** 2017,Jan,8; 2016,Jan,13; 2015,Jan,16; 2014,Jan,11;
  2012,Jan,15-42

**35642** **carotid-vertebral**
  🔪 32.1   ✂ 32.1   **FUD** 090   C 80 50 ▣
  **AMA:** 1997,Nov,1

**35645** **subclavian-vertebral**
  🔪 30.5   ✂ 30.5   **FUD** 090   C 80 50 ▣
  **AMA:** 1997,Nov,1

**35646** **aortobifemoral**
  *EXCLUDES* Bypass graft using vein graft (35540)
    Open placement of aortobifemoral prosthesis after a
      failed endovascular repair (34832)
  🔪 50.3   ✂ 50.3   **FUD** 090   C 80 ▣
  **AMA:** 2017,Jan,8; 2016,Jan,13; 2015,Jan,16; 2014,Jan,11;
  2012,Apr,3-9

**35647** **aortofemoral**
  *EXCLUDES* Bypass graft using vein graft (35539)
  🔪 45.6   ✂ 45.6   **FUD** 090   C 80 50 ▣
  **AMA:** 2017,Jan,8; 2016,Jan,13; 2015,Jan,16; 2014,Jan,11

**35650** **axillary-axillary**
  🔪 31.9   ✂ 31.9   **FUD** 090   C 80 50 ▣
  **AMA:** 1997,Nov,1

**35654** **axillary-femoral-femoral**
  🔪 40.2   ✂ 40.2   **FUD** 090   C 80 ▣
  **AMA:** 2017,Jan,8; 2016,Jan,13; 2015,Jan,16; 2014,Jan,11;
  2012,Apr,3-9

**35656** **femoral-popliteal**
  🔪 31.8   ✂ 31.8   **FUD** 090   C 80 50 ▣
  **AMA:** 2017,Jan,8; 2016,Jan,13; 2015,Jan,16; 2014,Jan,11;
  2012,Apr,3-9

**35661** **femoral-femoral**
  🔪 31.8   ✂ 31.8   **FUD** 090   C 80 50 ▣
  **AMA:** 2017,Jan,8; 2016,Jan,13; 2015,Jan,16; 2014,Jan,11;
  2012,Apr,3-9

**35663** **ilioiliac**
  🔪 36.6   ✂ 36.6   **FUD** 090   C 80 50 ▣
  **AMA:** 1997,Nov,1

**35665** **iliofemoral**
  🔪 34.4   ✂ 34.4   **FUD** 090   C 80 50 ▣
  **AMA:** 2017,Jan,8; 2016,Jan,13; 2015,Jan,16; 2014,Jan,11

**35666** **femoral-anterior tibial, posterior tibial, or peroneal
artery**
  🔪 37.1   ✂ 37.1   **FUD** 090   C 80 50 ▣
  **AMA:** 2017,Jan,8; 2016,Jan,13; 2015,Jan,16; 2014,Jan,11;
  2012,Apr,3-9

**35671** **popliteal-tibial or -peroneal artery**
  🔪 32.7   ✂ 32.7   **FUD** 090   C 80 50 ▣
  **AMA:** 2012,Apr,3-9

## 35681-35683 Arterial Bypass Using Combination Synthetic and Donor Graft

  *INCLUDES* Acquiring multiple segments of vein from sites other than the extremity
    for which the arterial bypass is performed
    Anastomosis of vein segments to creat bypass graft conduits

+ **35681** **Bypass graft; composite, prosthetic and vein (List separately
in addition to code for primary procedure)**
  *EXCLUDES* Bypass graft (35682, 35683)
    Code first primary procedure
  🔪 2.36   ✂ 2.36   **FUD** ZZZ   C 80 ▣
  **AMA:** 2017,Jan,8; 2016,Jan,13; 2015,Jan,16; 2014,Jan,11;
  2012,Jan,15-42

+ **35682** **autogenous composite, 2 segments of veins from 2
locations (List separately in addition to code for primary
procedure)**
  *EXCLUDES* Bypass graft (35681, 35683)
    Code first (35556, 35566, 35570-35571, 35583-35587)
  🔪 10.3   ✂ 10.3   **FUD** ZZZ   C 80 ▣
  **AMA:** 2017,Jan,8; 2016,Jan,13; 2015,Jan,16; 2014,Jan,11;
  2012,Jan,15-42

+ **35683** **autogenous composite, 3 or more segments of vein from
2 or more locations (List separately in addition to code for
primary procedure)**
  *EXCLUDES* Bypass graft (35681-35682)
    Code first (35556, 35566, 35570-35571, 35583-35587)
  🔪 11.9   ✂ 11.9   **FUD** ZZZ   C 80 ▣
  **AMA:** 2017,Jan,8; 2016,Jan,13; 2015,Jan,16; 2014,Jan,11;
  2012,Jan,15-42

## 35685-35686 Supplemental Procedures

  *INCLUDES* Additional procedures that may be needed with a bypass graft to increase
    the patency of the graft
  *EXCLUDES* Composite grafts (35681-35683)

+ **35685** **Placement of vein patch or cuff at distal anastomosis of bypass
graft, synthetic conduit (List separately in addition to code
for primary procedure)**
  *INCLUDES* Connection of a segment of vein (cuff or patch)
    between the distal portion of the synthetic graft
    and the native artery
    Code first (35656, 35666, 35671)
  🔪 5.83   ✂ 5.83   **FUD** ZZZ   N 80 ▣
  **AMA:** 2017,Jan,8; 2016,Jan,13; 2015,Jan,16; 2014,Jan,11

**+** **35686** **Creation of distal arteriovenous fistula during lower extremity bypass surgery (non-hemodialysis) (List separately in addition to code for primary procedure)**

INCLUDES Creation of a fistula between the peroneal or tibial artery and vein at or past the site of the distal anastomosis

Code first (35556, 35566, 35570-35571, 35583-35587, 35623, 35656, 35666, 35671)

🚗 4.70 ⚕ 4.70 **FUD** ZZZ N 80 ▣

**AMA:** 2017,Jan,8; 2016,Jan,13; 2015,Jan,16; 2014,Jan,11; 2012,Apr,3-9

## 35691-35697 Arterial Translocation

**CMS:** 100-03,160.8 Electroencephalographic Monitoring During Cerebral Vasculature Surgery

**35691** **Transposition and/or reimplantation; vertebral to carotid artery**

🚗 27.5 ⚕ 27.5 **FUD** 090 C 80 50 ▣

**AMA:** 1997,Nov,1; 1993,Win,1

**35693** **vertebral to subclavian artery**

🚗 24.4 ⚕ 24.4 **FUD** 090 C 80 50 ▣

**AMA:** 1997,Nov,1; 1994,Sum,29

**35694** **subclavian to carotid artery**

EXCLUDES Subclavian to carotid artery transposition procedure (open) with concurrent repair of descending thoracic aorta (endovascular) (33889)

🚗 28.9 ⚕ 28.9 **FUD** 090 C 80 50 ▣

**AMA:** 1997,Nov,1; 1993,Win,1

**35695** **carotid to subclavian artery**

🚗 30.5 ⚕ 30.5 **FUD** 090 C 80 50 ▣

**AMA:** 1997,Nov,1; 1993,Win,1

**+** **35697** **Reimplantation, visceral artery to infrarenal aortic prosthesis, each artery (List separately in addition to code for primary procedure)**

EXCLUDES Repair of thoracoabdominal aortic aneurysm with graft (33877)

Code first primary procedure

🚗 4.33 ⚕ 4.33 **FUD** ZZZ C 80 ▣

**AMA:** 1997,Nov,1

## 35700 Reoperative Bypass Lower Extremities

Code first (35556, 35566, 35570-35571, 35583, 35585, 35587, 35656, 35666, 35671)

**+** **35700** **Reoperation, femoral-popliteal or femoral (popliteal)-anterior tibial, posterior tibial, peroneal artery, or other distal vessels, more than 1 month after original operation (List separately in addition to code for primary procedure)**

🚗 4.48 ⚕ 4.48 **FUD** ZZZ C 80 ▣

**AMA:** 2017,Jan,8; 2016,Jan,13; 2015,Jan,16; 2014,Jan,11; 2012,Apr,3-9

## 35701-35761 Arterial Exploration without Repair

**35701** **Exploration (not followed by surgical repair), with or without lysis of artery; carotid artery**

🚗 16.4 ⚕ 16.4 **FUD** 090 C 80 50 ▣

**AMA:** 1997,Nov,1

**35721** **femoral artery**

🚗 13.4 ⚕ 13.4 **FUD** 090 C 80 50 ▣

**AMA:** 2017,Jan,8; 2016,Jan,13; 2015,Jan,16; 2014,Jan,11

**35741** **popliteal artery**

🚗 14.9 ⚕ 14.9 **FUD** 090 C 80 50 ▣

**AMA:** 1997,Nov,1

**35761** **other vessels**

🚗 11.3 ⚕ 11.3 **FUD** 090 T G2 80 50 ▣

**AMA:** 1997,Nov,1

## 35800-35860 Arterial Exploration for Postoperative Complication

INCLUDES Return to the operating room for postoperative hemorrhage

**35800** **Exploration for postoperative hemorrhage, thrombosis or infection; neck**

🚗 20.8 ⚕ 20.8 **FUD** 090 C 80 ▣

**AMA:** 1997,Nov,1

**35820** **chest**

🚗 58.4 ⚕ 58.4 **FUD** 090 C 80 ▣

**AMA:** 1997,Nov,1

**35840** **abdomen**

🚗 34.6 ⚕ 34.6 **FUD** 090 C 80 ▣

**AMA:** 1997,May,4; 1997,Nov,1

**35860** **extremity**

🚗 24.5 ⚕ 24.5 **FUD** 090 T 80 ▣

**AMA:** 2017,Jan,8; 2016,Jan,13; 2015,Jan,16; 2014,Apr,10

## 35870 Repair Secondary Aortoenteric Fistula

**35870** **Repair of graft-enteric fistula**

🚗 36.4 ⚕ 36.4 **FUD** 090 C 80 ▣

**AMA:** 1997,Nov,1

## 35875-35876 Removal of Thrombus from Graft

EXCLUDES Thrombectomy dialysis fistula or graft (36831, 36833)
Thrombectomy with blood vessel repair, lower extremity, vein graft (35256)
Thrombectomy with blood vessel repair, lower extremity, with/without patch angioplasty (35226)

**35875** **Thrombectomy of arterial or venous graft (other than hemodialysis graft or fistula);**

🚗 17.4 ⚕ 17.4 **FUD** 090 T A2 ▣

**AMA:** 2017,Jan,8; 2016,Jan,13; 2015,Jan,16; 2014,Jan,11; 2012,Jan,15-42

**35876** **with revision of arterial or venous graft**

🚗 27.7 ⚕ 27.7 **FUD** 090 T A2 80 ▣

**AMA:** 1999,Mar,6; 1999,Nov,1

## 35879-35884 Revision Lower Extremity Bypass Graft

EXCLUDES Removal of infected graft (35901-35907)
Revascularization following removal of infected graft(s)
Thrombectomy dialysis fistula or graft (36831, 36833)
Thrombectomy with blood vessel repair, lower extremity, vein graft (35256)
Thrombectomy with blood vessel repair, lower extremity, with/without patch angioplasty (35226)
Thrombectomy with graft revision (35876)

**35879** **Revision, lower extremity arterial bypass, without thrombectomy, open; with vein patch angioplasty**

🚗 27.0 ⚕ 27.0 **FUD** 090 T 80 50 ▣

**AMA:** 2017,Jan,8; 2016,Jan,13; 2015,Jan,16; 2014,Jan,11

**35881** **with segmental vein interposition**

EXCLUDES Revision of femoral anastomosis of synthetic arterial bypass graft (35883-35884)

🚗 29.9 ⚕ 29.9 **FUD** 090 T 80 50 ▣

**AMA:** 2017,Jan,8; 2016,Jan,13; 2015,Jan,16; 2014,Jan,11

**35883** **Revision, femoral anastomosis of synthetic arterial bypass graft in groin, open; with nonautogenous patch graft (eg, Dacron, ePTFE, bovine pericardium)**

EXCLUDES Reoperation, femoral-popliteal or femoral (popliteal)-anterior tibial, posterior tibial, peroneal artery, or other distal vessels (35700)
Revision, femoral anastomosis of synthetic arterial bypass graft in groin, open; with autogenous vein patch graft (35884)
Thrombectomy of arterial or venous graft (35875)

🚗 35.4 ⚕ 35.4 **FUD** 090 T 80 50 ▣

**AMA:** 2017,Jan,8; 2016,Jan,13; 2015,Jan,16; 2014,Jan,11; 2012,Jan,15-42

**35884** **with autogenous vein patch graft**

EXCLUDES Reoperation, femoral-popliteal or femoral (popliteal)-anterior tibial, posterior tibial, peroneal artery, or other distal vessels (35700)
Revision, femoral anastomosis of synthetic arterial bypass graft in groin, open; with autogenous vein patch graft (35883)
Thrombectomy of arterial or venous graft (35875-35876)

🚗 36.3 ⚕ 36.3 **FUD** 090 T 80 50 ▣

**AMA:** 2017,Jan,8; 2016,Jan,13; 2015,Jan,16; 2014,Jan,11; 2012,Jan,15-42

---

26/TC PC/TC Only     ASC Payment    50 Bilateral    ♂ Male Only    ♀ Female Only    🚗 Facility RVU    ⚕ Non-Facility RVU    ▣ CCI

**FUD** Follow-up Days    **CMS:** IOM (Pub 100)     OPPSI    80/80 Surg Assist Allowed / w/Doc     Lab Crosswalk    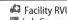 Radiology Crosswalk    ✖ CLIA

CPT © 2017 American Medical Association. All Rights Reserved.      © 2017 Optum360, LLC

## 35901-35907 Removal of Infected Graft

**35901** **Excision of infected graft; neck**
🔧 14.4 ✂ 14.4 **FUD** 090 ⬚ C 80 🔲
**AMA:** 1997,Nov,1; 1993,Win,1

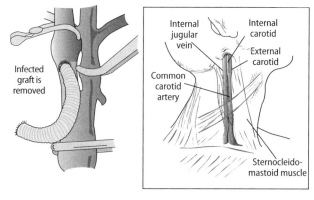

The physician removes an infected graft from the neck and repairs the blood vessel.
If a new graft is placed, report the appropriate revascularization code

**35903** **extremity**
🔧 16.4 ✂ 16.4 **FUD** 090 ⬚ T 80 🔲
**AMA:** 1997,Nov,1; 1993,Win,1

**35905** **thorax**
🔧 51.8 ✂ 51.8 **FUD** 090 ⬚ C 80 🔲
**AMA:** 1997,Nov,1; 1993,Win,1

**35907** **abdomen**
🔧 56.0 ✂ 56.0 **FUD** 090 ⬚ C 80 🔲
**AMA:** 1997,Nov,1; 1993,Win,1

## 36000 Intravenous Access Established

INCLUDES Venous access for phlebotomy, prophylactic intravenous access, infusion therapy, chemotherapy, hydration, transfusion, drug administration, etc. which is included in the work value of the primary procedure

**36000** **Introduction of needle or intracatheter, vein**
🔧 0.27 ✂ 0.73 **FUD** XXX ⬚ N N1 🔲
**AMA:** 2017,Jan,8; 2016,Nov,3; 2016,Jan,13; 2015,Jan,16; 2014,Oct,6; 2014,Sep,13; 2014,May,4; 2014,Jan,11; 2012,Jan,15-42

## 36002 Injection Treatment of Pseudoaneurysm

INCLUDES Insertion of needle or catheter, local anesthesia, injection of contrast, power injections, and all pre- and postinjection care provided
EXCLUDES Arteriotomy site sealant
Compression repair pseudoaneurysm, ultrasound guided (76936)
Medications, contrast material, catheters

**36002** **Injection procedures (eg, thrombin) for percutaneous treatment of extremity pseudoaneurysm**
📋 (76942, 77002, 77012, 77021)
🔧 3.09 ✂ 4.60 **FUD** 000 ⬚ T 62 50 🔲
**AMA:** 2017,Jan,8; 2016,Nov,3; 2016,Jan,13; 2015,Jan,16; 2014,Oct,6; 2014,Jan,11; 2013,Nov,6

## 36005-36015 Insertion Needle or Intracatheter: Venous

INCLUDES Insertion of needle/catheter, local anesthesia, injection of contrast, power injections, all pre- and postinjection care
EXCLUDES Medications, contrast materials, catheters
Code also catheterization of second order vessels (or higher) supplied by the same first order branch, same vascular family (36012)
Code also each vascular family (e.g., bilateral procedures are separate vascular families)

**36005** **Injection procedure for extremity venography (including introduction of needle or intracatheter)**
📋 (75820, 75822)
🔧 1.40 ✂ 9.15 **FUD** 000 ⬚ N N1 80 50 🔲
**AMA:** 2017,Jan,8; 2016,Nov,3; 2016,Jul,6; 2016,Jan,13; 2015,Jan,16; 2014,Oct,6

**36010** **Introduction of catheter, superior or inferior vena cava**
🔧 3.19 ✂ 13.7 **FUD** XXX ⬚ N N1 50 🔲
**AMA:** 2017,Feb,14; 2017,Jan,8; 2016,Jul,6; 2016,Jan,13; 2015,Jan,16; 2014,Jan,11; 2012,Apr,3-9; 2012,Jan,15-42

**36011** **Selective catheter placement, venous system; first order branch (eg, renal vein, jugular vein)**
🔧 4.57 ✂ 23.4 **FUD** XXX ⬚ N N1 50 🔲
**AMA:** 2017,Jan,8; 2016,Jul,6; 2016,Jan,13; 2015,Jan,16; 2014,Jan,11; 2012,Apr,3-9

**36012** **second order, or more selective, branch (eg, left adrenal vein, petrosal sinus)**
🔧 5.05 ✂ 24.1 **FUD** XXX ⬚ N N1 50 🔲
**AMA:** 2017,Jan,8; 2016,Jul,6; 2016,Jan,13; 2015,Jan,16; 2014,Jan,11; 2012,Apr,3-9

**36013** **Introduction of catheter, right heart or main pulmonary artery**
🔧 3.58 ✂ 21.8 **FUD** XXX ⬚ N N1 🔲
**AMA:** 2017,Jan,8; 2016,Jul,6; 2016,Jan,13; 2015,Jan,16; 2014,Jan,11; 2012,Jan,15-42

**36014** **Selective catheter placement, left or right pulmonary artery**
🔧 4.39 ✂ 22.6 **FUD** XXX ⬚ N N1 50 🔲
**AMA:** 2017,Jan,8; 2016,Jul,6; 2016,Jan,13; 2015,Jan,16; 2014,Jan,11

**36015** **Selective catheter placement, segmental or subsegmental pulmonary artery**
EXCLUDES Placement of Swan Ganz/other flow directed catheter for monitoring (93503)
Selective blood sampling, specific organs (36500)
🔧 4.98 ✂ 24.4 **FUD** XXX ⬚ N N1 50 🔲
**AMA:** 2017,Jan,8; 2016,Jul,6; 2016,Jan,13; 2015,Jan,16; 2014,Jan,11; 2012,Mar,9-10

## 36100-36218 Insertion Needle or Intracatheter: Arterial

INCLUDES Introduction of the catheter and catheterization of all lesser order vessels used for the approach
Local anesthesia, placement of catheter/needle, injection of contrast, power injections, all pre- and postinjection care
EXCLUDES Angiography (36222-36228, 75600-75774)
Angioplasty ([37246, 37247])
Chemotherapy injections (96401-96549)
Injection procedures for cardiac catheterizations (93455, 93457, 93459, 93461, 93530-93533, 93564)
Internal mammary artery angiography without left heart catheterization (36216, 36217)
Medications, contrast, catheters
Transcatheter interventions (37200, [37211], [37213, 37214], 37236-37239, 37241-37244, 61624, 61626)
Code also additional first order or higher catheterization for vascular families if the vascular family is supplied by a first order vessel that is different from one already coded
Code also catheterization of second and third order vessels supplied by the same first order branch, same vascular family (36218, 36248)

**36100** **Introduction of needle or intracatheter, carotid or vertebral artery**
🔧 4.47 ✂ 13.5 **FUD** XXX ⬚ N N1 50 🔲
**AMA:** 2000,Oct,4; 1998,Apr,1

**36120** ~~Introduction of needle or intracatheter; retrograde brachial artery~~

▲ **36140** **Introduction of needle or intracatheter, upper or lower extremity artery**
EXCLUDES Arteriovenous cannula insertion (36810-36821)
🔧 2.63 ✂ 11.9 **FUD** XXX ⬚ N N1 🔲
**AMA:** 2017,Jan,8; 2016,Jan,13; 2015,Jan,16; 2014,Jan,11; 2012,Jan,15-42

**36160** **Introduction of needle or intracatheter, aortic, translumbar**
🔧 3.60 ✂ 13.9 **FUD** XXX ⬚ N N1 🔲
**AMA:** 2017,Jan,8; 2016,Jan,13; 2015,Jan,16; 2014,Jan,11

● New Code ▲ Revised Code ○ Reinstated ● New Web Release ▲ Revised Web Release Unlisted Not Covered # Resequenced
⊘ AMA Mod 51 Exempt ⑩ Optum Mod 51 Exempt ⑬ Mod 63 Exempt ⁄ Non-FDA Drug ★ Telemedicine Ⓜ Maternity Ⓐ Age Edit + Add-on AMA: CPT Asst
© 2017 Optum360, LLC CPT © 2017 American Medical Association. All Rights Reserved. **153**

**36200** **Introduction of catheter, aorta**

*EXCLUDES* *Nonselective angiography of the extracranial carotid and/or cerebral vessels and cervicocerebral arch (36221)*

⚙ 4.09  ⚕ 15.9  **FUD** 000  N N1 50 ▣

**AMA:** 2017,Mar,3; 2017,Jan,8; 2016,Jul,6; 2016,Jan,13; 2015,Jan,16; 2014,Jan,11; 2013,Feb,16-17; 2012,Apr,3-9; 2012,Jan,15-42

**36215** **Selective catheter placement, arterial system; each first order thoracic or brachiocephalic branch, within a vascular family**

*INCLUDES* Introduction of catheter into the aorta (36200)

*EXCLUDES* *Placement of catheter for coronary angiography (93454-93461)*

⚙ 6.81  ⚕ 31.8  **FUD** XXX  N N1 ▣

**AMA:** 2017,Mar,3; 2017,Jan,8; 2016,Jul,6; 2016,Jan,13; 2015,Jan,16; 2014,Jan,11; 2012,Apr,3-9; 2012,Jan,15-42

**36216** **initial second order thoracic or brachiocephalic branch, within a vascular family**

⚙ 7.90  ⚕ 32.9  **FUD** XXX  N N1 ▣

**AMA:** 2017,Jan,8; 2016,Jul,6; 2016,Jan,13; 2015,Jan,16; 2014,Jan,11; 2013,Nov,14; 2012,Apr,3-9

**36217** **initial third order or more selective thoracic or brachiocephalic branch, within a vascular family**

⚙ 9.40  ⚕ 53.8  **FUD** XXX  N N1 ▣

**AMA:** 2017,Jan,8; 2016,Jul,6; 2016,Jan,13; 2015,Jan,16; 2014,Jan,11; 2012,Apr,3-9

**+ 36218** **additional second order, third order, and beyond, thoracic or brachiocephalic branch, within a vascular family (List in addition to code for initial second or third order vessel as appropriate)**

Code also transcatheter therapy procedures (37200, [37211], [37213, 37214], 37236-37239, 37241-37244, 61624, 61626)
Code first (36216-36217, 36225-36226)

⚙ 1.51  ⚕ 5.27  **FUD** ZZZ  N N1 ▣

**AMA:** 2017,Jan,8; 2016,Jul,6; 2016,Jan,13; 2015,Jan,16; 2014,Jan,11; 2013,May,3-5; 2012,Apr,3-9

## 36221-36228 Diagnostic Studies: Aortic Arch/Carotid/Vertebral Arteries

*INCLUDES* Accessing the vessel
Arterial contrast injection that includes arterial, capillary, and venous phase imaging, when performed
Arteriotomy closure (pressure or closure device)
Catheter placement
Radiologic supervision and interpretation
Reporting of selective catheter placement based on intensity of services in the following hierarchy:
36226>36225
36224>36223>36222

*EXCLUDES* *3D rendering when performed (76376-76377)*
*Interventional procedures*
*Transcatheter intravascular stent placement of common carotid or innominate artery on the same side (37217)*
*Ultrasound guidance (76937)*

Code also diagnostic angiography of upper extremities/other vascular beds during the same session, if performed (75774)

**36221** **Non-selective catheter placement, thoracic aorta, with angiography of the extracranial carotid, vertebral, and/or intracranial vessels, unilateral or bilateral, and all associated radiological supervision and interpretation, includes angiography of the cervicocerebral arch, when performed**

*EXCLUDES* *Selective catheter placement, common carotid or innominate artery (36222-36226)*
*Transcatheter intravascular stent placement of common carotid or innominate artery on the same side (37217)*

⚙ 5.88  ⚕ 29.2  **FUD** 000  02 N1 ▣

**AMA:** 2017,Jan,8; 2016,Mar,3; 2016,Jan,13; 2015,Nov,3; 2015,May,7; 2015,Jan,16; 2014,Mar,8; 2014,Jan,11; 2013,Oct,18; 2013,Jun,12; 2013,May,3-5; 2013,Feb,16-17

**36222** **Selective catheter placement, common carotid or innominate artery, unilateral, any approach, with angiography of the ipsilateral extracranial carotid circulation and all associated radiological supervision and interpretation, includes angiography of the cervicocerebral arch, when performed**

*INCLUDES* Unilateral catheterization of artery

*EXCLUDES* *Transcatheter placement of intravascular stent(s) (37215-37218)*

Code also modifier 59 when different territories on both sides of the body are being studied

⚙ 8.22  ⚕ 34.1  **FUD** 000  02 N1 50 ▣

**AMA:** 2017,Jan,8; 2016,Mar,3; 2016,Jan,13; 2015,Nov,3; 2015,Nov,10; 2015,May,7; 2015,Jan,16; 2014,Mar,8; 2014,Jan,11; 2013,Oct,18; 2013,Nov,14; 2013,Jun,12; 2013,May,3-5; 2013,Feb,16-17

**36223** **Selective catheter placement, common carotid or innominate artery, unilateral, any approach, with angiography of the ipsilateral intracranial carotid circulation and all associated radiological supervision and interpretation, includes angiography of the extracranial carotid and cervicocerebral arch, when performed**

*INCLUDES* Unilateral catheterization of artery

*EXCLUDES* *Transcatheter placement of intravascular stent(s) (37215-37218)*

Code also modifier 59 when different territories on both sides of the body are being studied

⚙ 9.08  ⚕ 41.9  **FUD** 000  02 N1 50 ▣

**AMA:** 2017,Jan,8; 2016,Mar,3; 2016,Jan,13; 2015,Nov,3; 2015,Jan,16; 2014,Mar,8; 2014,Jan,11; 2013,Oct,18; 2013,Jun,12; 2013,May,3-5; 2013,Feb,16-17

**36224** **Selective catheter placement, internal carotid artery, unilateral, with angiography of the ipsilateral intracranial carotid circulation and all associated radiological supervision and interpretation, includes angiography of the extracranial carotid and cervicocerebral arch, when performed**

*INCLUDES* Unilateral catheterization of artery

*EXCLUDES* *Transcatheter placement of intravascular stent(s) (37215-37218)*

Code also modifier 59 when different territories on both sides of the body are being studied

⚙ 10.3  ⚕ 53.3  **FUD** 000  02 N1 50 ▣

**AMA:** 2017,Jan,8; 2016,Mar,3; 2016,Jan,13; 2015,Nov,3; 2015,Jan,16; 2014,Mar,8; 2014,Jan,11; 2013,Oct,18; 2013,Jun,12; 2013,May,3-5; 2013,Feb,16-17

**36225** **Selective catheter placement, subclavian or innominate artery, unilateral, with angiography of the ipsilateral vertebral circulation and all associated radiological supervision and interpretation, includes angiography of the cervicocerebral arch, when performed**

*EXCLUDES* *Transcatheter placement of intravascular stent(s) (37217)*

⚙ 9.04  ⚕ 40.3  **FUD** 000  02 N1 50 ▣

**AMA:** 2017,Jan,8; 2016,Mar,3; 2016,Jan,13; 2015,Nov,3; 2015,Jan,16; 2014,Mar,8; 2014,Jan,11; 2013,Oct,18; 2013,Nov,14; 2013,Jun,12; 2013,May,3-5

**36226** **Selective catheter placement, vertebral artery, unilateral, with angiography of the ipsilateral vertebral circulation and all associated radiological supervision and interpretation, includes angiography of the cervicocerebral arch, when performed**

*EXCLUDES* *Transcatheter placement of intravascular stent(s) (37217)*

⚙ 10.1  ⚕ 50.6  **FUD** 000  02 N1 50 ▣

**AMA:** 2017,Jan,8; 2016,Mar,3; 2016,Jan,13; 2015,Nov,3; 2015,Jan,16; 2014,Mar,8; 2013,Oct,18; 2013,Jun,12; 2013,May,3-5

**+ 36227** Selective catheter placement, external carotid artery, unilateral, with angiography of the ipsilateral external carotid circulation and all associated radiological supervision and interpretation (List separately in addition to code for primary procedure)

INCLUDES   Unilateral catheter placement/diagnostic imaging of ipsilateral external carotid circulation

EXCLUDES   *Transcatheter placement of intravascular stent(s) (37217)*

Code first (36222-36224)

🚑 3.38   ⚕ 7.20   **FUD** ZZZ   N M1 50 ▭

**AMA:** 2017,Jan,8; 2016,Jan,13; 2015,Nov,10; 2015,Jan,16; 2014,Mar,8; 2014,Jan,11; 2013,Oct,18; 2013,Jun,12; 2013,May,3-5; 2013,Feb,16-17

**+ 36228** Selective catheter placement, each intracranial branch of the internal carotid or vertebral arteries, unilateral, with angiography of the selected vessel circulation and all associated radiological supervision and interpretation (eg, middle cerebral artery, posterior inferior cerebellar artery) (List separately in addition to code for primary procedure)

INCLUDES   Unilateral catheter placement/imaging of initial and each additional intracranial branch of internal carotid or vertebral arteries

EXCLUDES   *Procedure performed more than 2 times per side*

Code first (36223-36226)

🚑 6.92   ⚕ 36.2   **FUD** ZZZ   N M1 50 ▭

**AMA:** 2017,Jan,8; 2016,Jan,13; 2015,Nov,3; 2015,Jan,16; 2014,Jan,11; 2013,Oct,18; 2013,Jun,12; 2013,May,3-5; 2013,Feb,16-17

## 36245-36254 Catheter Placement: Arteries of the Lower Body

INCLUDES   Introduction of the catheter and catheterization of all lesser order vessels used for the approach

Local anesthesia, placement of catheter/needle, injection of contrast, power injections

EXCLUDES   *Angiography (36222-36228, 75600-75774)*

*Chemotherapy injections (96401-96549)*

*Injection procedures for cardiac catheterizations (93455, 93457, 93459, 93461, 93530-93533, 93564)*

*Internal mammary artery angiography without left heart catheterization (36216-36217)*

*Medications, contrast, catheters*

*Transcatheter procedures (37200, [37211], [37213, 37214], 37236-37239, 37241-37244, 61624, 61626)*

Code also additional first order or higher catheterization for vascular families if the vascular family is supplied by a first order vessel that is different from one already coded

Code also catheterization of second and third order vessels supplied by the same first order branch, same vascular family (36218, 36248)

🔳 (75600-75774)

**36245** Selective catheter placement, arterial system; each first order abdominal, pelvic, or lower extremity artery branch, within a vascular family

🚑 6.98   ⚕ 36.9   **FUD** XXX   N M1 50 ▭

**AMA:** 2017,Jan,8; 2016,Jul,6; 2016,Jan,13; 2015,Jan,16; 2014,Jan,11; 2013,Nov,14; 2012,Apr,3-9; 2012,Jan,15-42

**36246** initial second order abdominal, pelvic, or lower extremity artery branch, within a vascular family

🚑 7.46   ⚕ 23.3   **FUD** 000   N M1 50 ▭

**AMA:** 2017,Jan,8; 2016,Jul,6; 2016,Jan,13; 2015,Jan,16; 2014,Jan,11; 2013,Nov,14; 2012,Apr,3-9; 2012,Jan,15-42

**36247** initial third order or more selective abdominal, pelvic, or lower extremity artery branch, within a vascular family

🚑 8.87   ⚕ 42.4   **FUD** 000   N M1 50 ▭

**AMA:** 2017,Jan,8; 2016,Jul,6; 2016,Jan,13; 2015,Jan,16; 2014,Jan,11; 2013,Nov,14; 2012,Apr,3-9; 2012,Jan,15-42

**+ 36248** additional second order, third order, and beyond, abdominal, pelvic, or lower extremity artery branch, within a vascular family (List in addition to code for initial second or third order vessel as appropriate)

Code first (36246, 36247)

🚑 1.43   ⚕ 4.33   **FUD** ZZZ   N M1 ▭

**AMA:** 2017,Jan,8; 2016,Jul,6; 2016,Jan,13; 2015,Jan,16; 2014,Jan,11; 2012,Apr,3-9; 2012,Jan,15-42

**36251** Selective catheter placement (first-order), main renal artery and any accessory renal artery(s) for renal angiography, including arterial puncture and catheter placement(s), fluoroscopy, contrast injection(s), image postprocessing, permanent recording of images, and radiological supervision and interpretation, including pressure gradient measurements when performed, and flush aortogram when performed; unilateral

INCLUDES   Closure device placement at vascular access site

EXCLUDES   *Transcatheter renal sympathetic denervation, percutaneous approach (0338T-0339T)*

🚑 7.74   ⚕ 38.9   **FUD** 000   02 M1 ▭

**AMA:** 2017,Jan,8; 2016,Jan,13; 2015,Jan,16; 2014,Jan,11; 2013,Nov,14; 2012,Aug,13-14; 2012,Apr,3-9; 2012,Jan,15-42

**36252** bilateral

INCLUDES   Closure device placement at vascular access site

EXCLUDES   *Transcatheter renal sympathetic denervation, percutaneous approach (0338T-0339T)*

🚑 10.5   ⚕ 42.1   **FUD** 000   02 M1 ▭

**AMA:** 2017,Jan,8; 2016,Jan,13; 2015,Jan,16; 2014,Jan,11; 2012,Apr,3-9; 2012,Jan,15-42

**36253** Superselective catheter placement (one or more second order or higher renal artery branches) renal artery and any accessory renal artery(s) for renal angiography, including arterial puncture, catheterization, fluoroscopy, contrast injection(s), image postprocessing, permanent recording of images, and radiological supervision and interpretation, including pressure gradient measurements when performed, and flush aortogram when performed; unilateral

INCLUDES   Closure device placement at vascular access site

EXCLUDES   *Procedure performed on same kidney with (36251)*

*Transcatheter renal sympathetic denervation, percutaneous approach (0338T-0339T)*

🚑 10.5   ⚕ 62.4   **FUD** 000   02 M1 ▭

**AMA:** 2017,Jan,8; 2016,Jan,13; 2015,Jan,16; 2014,Jan,11; 2013,Nov,14; 2012,Aug,13-14; 2012,Apr,3-9; 2012,Jan,15-42

**36254** bilateral

INCLUDES   Closure device placement at vascular access site

EXCLUDES   *Selective catheter placement (first-order), main renal artery and any accessory renal artery(s) for renal angiography (36252)*

*Transcatheter renal sympathetic denervation, percutaneous approach (0338T-0339T)*

🚑 12.3   ⚕ 60.6   **FUD** 000   02 M1 ▭

**AMA:** 2017,Jan,8; 2016,Jan,13; 2015,Jan,16; 2014,Jan,11; 2012,Aug,13-14; 2012,Apr,3-9; 2012,Jan,15-42

## 36260-36299 Implanted Infusion Pumps: Intra-arterial

**36260** Insertion of implantable intra-arterial infusion pump (eg, for chemotherapy of liver)

🚑 18.4   ⚕ 18.4   **FUD** 090   T J8 ▭

**AMA:** 2017,Jan,8; 2016,Jan,13; 2015,Jan,16; 2014,Jan,11

**36261** Revision of implanted intra-arterial infusion pump

🚑 9.39   ⚕ 9.39   **FUD** 090   T J8 80 ▭

**AMA:** 2000,Oct,4; 1997,Nov,1

**36262** Removal of implanted intra-arterial infusion pump

🚑 8.66   ⚕ 8.66   **FUD** 090   02 62 ▭

**AMA:** 2000,Oct,4; 1997,Nov,1

**36299** Unlisted procedure, vascular injection

🚑 0.00   ⚕ 0.00   **FUD** YYY   N 80

**AMA:** 2000,Oct,4; 1997,Nov,1

---

● New Code  ▲ Revised Code  ○ Reinstated  ● New Web Release  ▲ Revised Web Release  Unlisted  Not Covered  # Resequenced
◎ AMA Mod 51 Exempt  ⑤ Optum Mod 51 Exempt  63 Mod 63 Exempt  ✗ Non-FDA Drug  ★ Telemedicine  M Maternity  A Age Edit  + Add-on  **AMA:** CPT Asst

**Cardiovascular, Hemic, and Lymphatic**

**36400 — 36466**

## 36400-36425 Specimen Collection: Phlebotomy

**EXCLUDES** Collection of specimen from:
A completely implantable device (36591)
An established catheter (36592)

**36400** Venipuncture, younger than age 3 years, necessitating the skill of a physician or other qualified health care professional, not to be used for routine venipuncture; femoral or jugular vein    A
0.52    0.77    **FUD** XXX    N N1
AMA: 2017,Jan,8; 2016,Jan,13; 2015,Jan,16; 2014,May,4; 2014,Jan,11

**36405** scalp vein    A
0.47    0.73    **FUD** XXX    N N1
AMA: 2017,Jan,8; 2016,Jan,13; 2015,Jan,16; 2014,May,4; 2014,Jan,11

**36406** other vein    A
0.26    0.53    **FUD** XXX    N N1
AMA: 2017,Jan,8; 2016,Jan,13; 2015,Jan,16; 2014,May,4; 2014,Jan,11

**36410** Venipuncture, age 3 years or older, necessitating the skill of a physician or other qualified health care professional (separate procedure), for diagnostic or therapeutic purposes (not to be used for routine venipuncture)    A
0.27    0.48    **FUD** XXX    N N1
AMA: 2017,Jan,8; 2016,Nov,3; 2016,Jan,13; 2015,Jan,16; 2014,Oct,6; 2014,Jan,11; 2013,Sep,17; 2012,Jan,15-42

**36415** Collection of venous blood by venipuncture
0.00    0.00    **FUD** XXX    63 Q
AMA: 2017,Jan,8; 2016,Jan,13; 2015,Jan,16; 2014,May,4; 2014,Jan,11; 2012,Jan,15-42

**36416** Collection of capillary blood specimen (eg, finger, heel, ear stick)
0.00    0.00    **FUD** XXX    N N1
AMA: 2008,Apr,-9; 2003,Feb,7

**36420** Venipuncture, cutdown; younger than age 1 year    A
1.56    1.56    **FUD** XXX    63 01 N1 80
AMA: 2017,Jan,8; 2016,Jan,13; 2015,Jan,16; 2014,Jan,11

**36425** age 1 or over    A
**EXCLUDES** Endovenous ablation therapy of incompetent vein, extremity (36475-36476, 36478-36479)
1.16    1.16    **FUD** XXX    01 N1
AMA: 2017,Jan,8; 2016,Nov,3; 2016,Jan,13; 2015,Jan,16; 2014,Oct,6

## 36430-36460 Transfusions

**CMS:** 100-01,3,20.5 Blood Deductibles; 100-03,110.16 Transfusion in Kidney Transplants; 100-03,110.7 Blood Transfusions; 100-03,110.8 Blood Platelet Transfusions

**36430** Transfusion, blood or blood components
**EXCLUDES** Infant partial exchange transfusion (36456)
0.99    0.99    **FUD** XXX    S P3
AMA: 2017,Jul,3; 2017,Jan,8; 2016,Jan,13; 2015,Jan,16; 2014,Jan,11; 2012,Jan,15-42

**36440** Push transfusion, blood, 2 years or younger    A
**EXCLUDES** Infant partial exchange transfusion (36456)
1.57    1.57    **FUD** XXX    S R2 80
AMA: 2017,Jul,3; 2017,Jan,8; 2016,Jan,13; 2015,Jan,16; 2014,Jan,11

**36450** Exchange transfusion, blood; newborn    A
**EXCLUDES** Infant partial exchange transfusion (36456)
5.40    5.40    **FUD** XXX    63 S R2 80
AMA: 2017,Jul,3

**36455** other than newborn    A
3.71    3.71    **FUD** XXX    S 62
AMA: 2003,Apr,7; 1997,Nov,1

---

**36456** Partial exchange transfusion, blood, plasma or crystalloid necessitating the skill of a physician or other qualified health care professional, newborn    A
**EXCLUDES** Transfusions of other types (36430-36450)
3.09    3.09    **FUD** XXX    63 S 80
AMA: 2017,Jul,3

**36460** Transfusion, intrauterine, fetal    A ♀
(76941)
9.95    9.95    **FUD** XXX    63 S 80
AMA: 2003,Apr,7; 1997,Nov,1

## 36465-36471 [36465, 36466] Destruction Spider Veins

**INCLUDES** All supplies, equipment, compression stockings or bandages when performed in the physician office

**EXCLUDES** Multi-layer compression system applied to leg (29581)
Use of code more than one time for each extremity treated
Vascular embolization and occlusion (37241-37244)
Vascular embolization vein in same operative field (37241)

**36465** Resequenced code. See code following 36471.

**36466** Resequenced code. See code following 36471.

▲ **36468** Injection(s) of sclerosant for spider veins (telangiectasia), limb or trunk
(76942)
0.00    0.00    **FUD** 000    01 N1 80
AMA: 2017,Jan,8; 2016,Nov,3; 2016,Jan,13; 2015,Apr,10; 2015,Jan,16; 2014,Oct,6; 2014,Aug,14; 2013,Nov,6

▲ **36470** Injection of sclerosant; single incompetent vein (other than telangiectasia)
**EXCLUDES** Injection of foam sclerosant with ultrasound guidance for compression maneuvers (36465-36466)
(76942)
2.40    4.19    **FUD** 010    T P3 50
AMA: 2017,Jan,8; 2016,Nov,3; 2016,Jan,13; 2015,Nov,10; 2015,Apr,10; 2015,Jan,16; 2014,Oct,6; 2014,Aug,14; 2013,Nov,6

▲ **36471** multiple incompetent veins (other than telangiectasia), same leg
**EXCLUDES** Injection of foam sclerosant with ultrasound guidance for compression maneuvers (36465-36466)
(76942)
2.90    4.97    **FUD** 010    T P3 50
AMA: 2017,Jan,8; 2016,Nov,3; 2016,Jan,13; 2015,Nov,10; 2015,Aug,8; 2015,Apr,10; 2015,Jan,16; 2014,Oct,6; 2014,Aug,14; 2013,Nov,6

● # **36465** Injection of non-compounded foam sclerosant with ultrasound compression maneuvers to guide dispersion of the injectate, inclusive of all imaging guidance and monitoring; single incompetent extremity truncal vein (eg, great saphenous vein, accessory saphenous vein)
0.00    0.00    **FUD** 000
**EXCLUDES** Ablation of vein using chemical adhesive ([36482, 36483])
Injection of foam sclerosant without ultrasound guidance for compression maneuvers (36470-36471)
Vascular embolization vein in same operative field (37241)

● # **36466** multiple incompetent truncal veins (eg, great saphenous vein, accessory saphenous vein), same leg
0.00    0.00    **FUD** 000
**EXCLUDES** Ablation of vein using chemical adhesive ([36482, 36483])
Injection of foam sclerosant without ultrasound guidance for compression maneuvers (36470-36471)
Use of code more than one time for each extremity
Vascular embolization vein in same operative field (37241)

---

26/TC PC/TC Only    A2-Z3 ASC Payment    50 Bilateral    ♂ Male Only    ♀ Female Only    Facility RVU    Non-Facility RVU    CCI
**FUD** Follow-up Days    **CMS:** IOM (Pub 100)    A-Y OPPSI    80/80 Surg Assist Allowed / w/Doc    Lab Crosswalk    Radiology Crosswalk    CLIA
CPT © 2017 American Medical Association. All Rights Reserved.        © 2017 Optum360, LLC

## 36473-36479 [36482, 36483] Vein Ablation

INCLUDES Compression system of lower extremities (29581)
Venous access/injections (36000-36410, 36425)
Radiological guidance (76000-76001, 76937, 76942, 76998, 77002)
Patient monitoring

EXCLUDES *Duplex scans (93970-93971)*
*Transcatheter embolization (75894)*
*Vascular embolization vein in same operative field (37241)*

**36473** Endovenous ablation therapy of incompetent vein, extremity, inclusive of all imaging guidance and monitoring, percutaneous, mechanochemical; first vein treated

INCLUDES Local anesthesia

EXCLUDES *Laser ablation incompetent vein (36478-36479)*
*Radiofrequency ablation incompetent vein (36475-36476)*

📅 5.01  ⚕ 42.4  FUD 000  T P2 50 ▣

AMA: 2017,Jan,8; 2016,Nov,3

+ **36474** subsequent vein(s) treated in a single extremity, each through separate access sites (List separately in addition to code for primary procedure)

INCLUDES Local anesthesia

EXCLUDES *Laser ablation incompetent vein (36478-36479)*
*Radiofrequency ablation incompetent vein (36475-36476)*
*Use of code more than one time per extremity*

Code first (36473)

📅 2.51  ⚕ 7.77  FUD ZZZ  N N1 50 ▣

AMA: 2017,Jan,8; 2016,Nov,3

**36475** Endovenous ablation therapy of incompetent vein, extremity, inclusive of all imaging guidance and monitoring, percutaneous, radiofrequency; first vein treated

INCLUDES Tumescent anesthesia

EXCLUDES *Ablation of vein using chemical adhesive ([36482, 36483])*
*Endovenous ablation therapy of incompetent vein (36478-36479)*

📅 8.16  ⚕ 43.0  FUD 000  T A2 50 ▣

AMA: 2017,Jan,8; 2016,Nov,3; 2016,Aug,3; 2016,Jan,13; 2015,Apr,10; 2015,Jan,16; 2014,Oct,6; 2014,Aug,14; 2014,Mar,4; 2014,Jan,11; 2013,Nov,6; 2012,Jan,15-42

+ **36476** subsequent vein(s) treated in a single extremity, each through separate access sites (List separately in addition to code for primary procedure)

INCLUDES Tumescent anesthesia

EXCLUDES *Ablation of vein using chemical adhesive ([36482, 36483])*
*Endovenous ablation therapy of incompetent vein (36478-36479)*
*Use of code more than one time per extremity*
*Vascular embolization or occlusion (37242-37244)*

Code first (36475)

📅 3.97  ⚕ 8.39  FUD ZZZ  N N1 50 ▣

AMA: 2017,Jan,8; 2016,Nov,3; 2016,Aug,3; 2016,Jan,13; 2015,Apr,10; 2015,Jan,16; 2014,Oct,6; 2014,Aug,14; 2014,Mar,4; 2014,Jan,11; 2013,Nov,6; 2012,Jan,15-42

**36478** Endovenous ablation therapy of incompetent vein, extremity, inclusive of all imaging guidance and monitoring, percutaneous, laser; first vein treated

INCLUDES Tumescent anesthesia

EXCLUDES *Ablation of vein using chemical adhesive ([36482, 36483])*
*Endovenous ablation therapy of incompetent vein (36475-36476)*

📅 8.11  ⚕ 34.1  FUD 000  T A2 50 ▣

AMA: 2017,Jan,8; 2016,Nov,3; 2016,Aug,3; 2016,Jan,13; 2015,Apr,10; 2015,Jan,16; 2014,Oct,6; 2014,Aug,14; 2014,Mar,4; 2014,Jan,11; 2013,Nov,6; 2012,Jul,12-14

+ **36479** subsequent vein(s) treated in a single extremity, each through separate access sites (List separately in addition to code for primary procedure)

INCLUDES Tumescent anesthesia

EXCLUDES *Ablation of vein using chemical adhesive ([36482, 36483])*
*Endovenous ablation therapy of incompetent vein (36475-36476)*
*Vascular embolization or occlusion (37241)*

Code first (36478)

📅 3.99  ⚕ 8.81  FUD ZZZ  N N1 50 ▣

AMA: 2017,Jan,8; 2016,Nov,3; 2016,Aug,3; 2016,Jan,13; 2015,Apr,10; 2015,Jan,16; 2014,Oct,6; 2014,Aug,14; 2014,Mar,4; 2014,Jan,11; 2013,Nov,6; 2012,Jul,12-14; 2012,Jan,15-42

● # **36482** Endovenous ablation therapy of incompetent vein, extremity, by transcatheter delivery of a chemical adhesive (eg, cyanoacrylate) remote from the access site, inclusive of all imaging guidance and monitoring, percutaneous; first vein treated

📅 0.00  ⚕ 0.00  FUD 000

INCLUDES Local anesthesia

EXCLUDES *Laser ablation incompetent vein (36478-36479)*
*Radiofrequency ablation incompetent vein (36475-36476)*

● + # **36483** subsequent vein(s) treated in a single extremity, each through separate access sites (List separately in addition to code for primary procedure)

📅 0.00  ⚕ 0.00  FUD 000

INCLUDES Local anesthesia

EXCLUDES *Laser ablation incompetent vein (36478-36479)*
*Radiofrequency ablation incompetent vein (36475-36476)*
*Use of code more than one time per extremity*

Code first ([36482])

## 36481-36510 Other Venous Catheterization Procedures

EXCLUDES *Collection of a specimen from:*
*A completely implantable device (36591)*
*An established catheter (36592)*

**36481** Percutaneous portal vein catheterization by any method

🔲 (75885, 75887)

📅 9.78  ⚕ 55.6  FUD 000  N N1 ▣

AMA: 2017,Jan,8; 2016,Jan,13; 2015,Jan,16; 2014,Jan,11; 2012,Jan,15-42

*36482* Resequenced code. See code following 36479.

*36483* Resequenced code. See code following 36479.

**36500** Venous catheterization for selective organ blood sampling

EXCLUDES *Inferior or superior vena cava catheterization (36010)*

🔲 (75893)

📅 5.30  ⚕ 5.30  FUD 000  N N1 ▣

AMA: 2014,Jan,11

**36510** Catheterization of umbilical vein for diagnosis or therapy, newborn  A

EXCLUDES *Collection of a specimen from:*
*Capillary blood (36416)*
*Venipuncture (36415)*

📅 1.62  ⚕ 2.47  FUD 000  63 N N1 80 ▣

AMA: 2017,Jan,8; 2016,May,3; 2016,Jan,13; 2015,Jan,16; 2014,Jan,11

## 36511-36516 Apheresis

CMS: 100-03,110.14 Apheresis (Therapeutic Pheresis); 100-04,4,231.9 Billing for Pheresis and Apheresis Services

EXCLUDES *Collection of a specimen for therapeutic treatment from:*
*A completely implantable device (36591)*
*An established catheter (36592)*

**36511** Therapeutic apheresis; for white blood cells

📅 2.69  ⚕ 2.69  FUD 000  S 62 ▣

AMA: 2017,Jan,8; 2016,Jan,13; 2015,Jan,16; 2014,Jan,11; 2013,Oct,3

---

● New Code  ▲ Revised Code  ○ Reinstated  ● New Web Release  ▲ Revised Web Release  Unlisted  Not Covered  # Resequenced
⊘ AMA Mod 51 Exempt  ⑨ Optum Mod 51 Exempt  63 Mod 63 Exempt  ✗ Non-FDA Drug  ★ Telemedicine  M Maternity  A Age Edit  + Add-on  AMA: CPT Asst

© 2017 Optum360, LLC                    CPT © 2017 American Medical Association. All Rights Reserved.

**36512** **for red blood cells**
🚑 2.72   📐 2.72   **FUD** 000    S G2 📠
**AMA:** 2017,Jan,8; 2016,Jan,13; 2015,Jan,16; 2014,Jan,11; 2013,Oct,3

**36513** **for platelets**
EXCLUDES   *Collection of platelets from donors*
🚑 2.80   📐 2.80   **FUD** 000    S G2 📠
**AMA:** 2017,Jan,8; 2016,Jan,13; 2015,Jan,16; 2014,Jan,11; 2013,Oct,3; 2012,Jan,15-42

**36514** **for plasma pheresis**
🚑 2.69   📐 15.3   **FUD** 000    S G2 📠
**AMA:** 2017,Jan,8; 2016,Jan,13; 2015,Jan,16; 2014,Jan,11; 2013,Oct,3

**36515** ~~**with extracorporeal immunoadsorption and plasma reinfusion**~~
To report, see 36516

▲ **36516** **with extracorporeal immunoadsorption, selective adsorption or selective filtration and plasma reinfusion**
Code also modifier 26 for professional evaluation
🚑 2.02   📐 59.5   **FUD** 000    S P2 📠
**AMA:** 2017,Jan,8; 2016,Jan,13; 2015,Jan,16; 2014,Jan,11; 2013,Oct,3

## 36522 Extracorporeal Photopheresis

**CMS:** 100-03,110.4 Extracorporeal Photopheresis; 100-04,32,190 Billing for Extracorporeal Photopheresis; 100-04,32,190.2 Extracorporeal Photopheresis; 100-04,32,190.3 Medicare Denial Codes; 100-04,4,231.9 Billing for Pheresis and Apheresis Services

**36522** **Photopheresis, extracorporeal**
🚑 2.95   📐 40.2   **FUD** 000    S G2 📠
**AMA:** 2017,Jan,8; 2016,Jan,13; 2015,Jan,16; 2014,Jan,11; 2013,Oct,3; 2012,Jan,15-42

## 36555-36571 Placement of Implantable Venous Access Device

INCLUDES   Devices accessed by an exposed catheter, or a subcutaneous port or pump
Devices inserted via cutdown or percutaneous access:
  Centrally (eg, femoral, jugular, subclavian veins, or inferior vena cava)
  Peripherally (eg, basilic or cephalic)
Devices terminating in the brachiocephalic (innominate), iliac, or subclavian veins, vena cava, or right atrium
Venous access obtained by cutdown or percutaneously with any size catheter
EXCLUDES   *Maintenance/refilling of implantable pump/reservoir (96522)*
Code also removal of central venous access device (if code available) when a new device is placed through a separate venous access
🔄 (76937, 77001)

**36555** **Insertion of non-tunneled centrally inserted central venous catheter; younger than 5 years of age**   A
EXCLUDES   *Peripheral insertion (36568)*
🚑 3.07   📐 5.83   **FUD** 000    T A2 📠
**AMA:** 2017,Jan,8; 2016,Jan,13; 2015,Jan,16; 2014,Jan,11

A non-tunneled centrally inserted CVC is inserted

**36556** **age 5 years or older**   A
EXCLUDES   *Peripheral insertion (36569)*
🚑 3.48   📐 6.64   **FUD** 000    T A2 📠
**AMA:** 2017,Jan,8; 2016,Jan,13; 2015,Jan,16; 2014,Jan,11

**36557** **Insertion of tunneled centrally inserted central venous catheter, without subcutaneous port or pump; younger than 5 years of age**   A
🚑 9.08   📐 26.1   **FUD** 010    T A2 80 50 📠
**AMA:** 2017,Jan,8; 2016,Jan,13; 2015,Jan,16; 2014,Jan,11

Tunneled portion

A tunneled centrally inserted CVC is inserted

**36558** **age 5 years or older**   A
EXCLUDES   *Peripheral insertion (36571)*
🚑 7.63   📐 20.3   **FUD** 010    T A2 80 50 📠
**AMA:** 2017,Jan,8; 2016,Jan,13; 2015,Jan,16; 2015,Jan,13; 2014,Jan,11

**36560** **Insertion of tunneled centrally inserted central venous access device, with subcutaneous port; younger than 5 years of age**   A
EXCLUDES   *Peripheral insertion (36570)*
🚑 9.88   📐 28.5   **FUD** 010    T A2 80 50 📠
**AMA:** 2017,Jan,8; 2016,Jan,13; 2015,Jan,16; 2014,Jan,11; 2012,Jan,15-42

**36561** **age 5 years or older**   A
EXCLUDES   *Peripheral insertion (36571)*
🚑 9.85   📐 30.9   **FUD** 010    T A2 80 50 📠
**AMA:** 2017,Jan,8; 2016,Jan,13; 2015,Jan,16; 2014,Jan,11; 2012,Jan,15-42

**36563** **Insertion of tunneled centrally inserted central venous access device with subcutaneous pump**  
🚑 10.6   📐 34.9   **FUD** 010    T A2 80
**AMA:** 2017,Jan,8; 2016,Jan,13; 2015,Jan,16; 2014,Jan,11

**36565** **Insertion of tunneled centrally inserted central venous access device, requiring 2 catheters via 2 separate venous access sites; without subcutaneous port or pump (eg, Tesio type catheter)**  
🚑 9.70   📐 25.1   **FUD** 010    T A2 80 50 📠
**AMA:** 2017,Jan,8; 2016,Jan,13; 2015,Jan,16; 2014,Jan,11

**36566** **with subcutaneous port(s)**
🚑 10.8   📐 153.   **FUD** 010    T A2 80 50 📠
**AMA:** 2017,Jan,8; 2016,Jan,13; 2015,Jan,16; 2014,Jan,11

**36568** **Insertion of peripherally inserted central venous catheter (PICC), without subcutaneous port or pump; younger than 5 years of age**   A
EXCLUDES   *Centrally inserted placement (36555)*
  *PICC line removal with codes for removal of tunneled central venous catheters; report appropriate E&M code*
🚑 2.46   📐 7.03   **FUD** 000    T A2 📠
**AMA:** 2017,Jan,8; 2016,Jan,13; 2015,Jan,16; 2014,Jan,11; 2012,Nov,13-14; 2012,Jan,15-42

26/TC PC/TC Only    A2-Z3 ASC Payment    50 Bilateral    ♂ Male Only    ♀ Female Only    🚑 Facility RVU    📐 Non-Facility RVU    📠 CCI
**FUD** Follow-up Days    **CMS:** IOM (Pub 100)    A-Y OPPSI    80/80 Surg Assist Allowed / w/Doc    🔬 Lab Crosswalk    🔄 Radiology Crosswalk    ❌ CLIA
  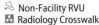

CPT © 2017 American Medical Association. All Rights Reserved.      © 2017 Optum360, LLC

**36569** **age 5 years or older** [A]

> EXCLUDES Centrally inserted placement (36556)
> PICC line removal with codes for removal of tunneled central venous catheters; report appropriate E&M code
>
> 2.65   7.10   **FUD** 000    [T] [A2] [▭]
>
> **AMA:** 2017,Jan,8; 2016,Jan,13; 2015,Jan,16; 2014,Sep,13; 2014,Jan,11; 2013,Sep,17; 2012,Nov,13-14; 2012,Jan,15-42

**36570** **Insertion of peripherally inserted central venous access device, with subcutaneous port; younger than 5 years of age** [A]

> EXCLUDES Centrally inserted placement (36560)
>
> 9.16   35.0   **FUD** 010    [T] [A2] [80] [50] [▭]
>
> **AMA:** 2017,Jan,8; 2016,Jan,13; 2015,Jan,16; 2014,Jan,11; 2012,Jan,15-42

**36571** **age 5 years or older** [A]

> EXCLUDES Centrally inserted placement (36561)
>
> 8.98   34.4   **FUD** 010    [T] [A2] [80] [50] [▭]
>
> **AMA:** 2017,Jan,8; 2016,Jan,13; 2015,Jan,16; 2014,Jan,11; 2012,Jan,15-42

## 36575-36590 Repair, Removal, and Replacement Implantable Venous Access Device

EXCLUDES Mechanical removal obstructive material, pericatheter/intraluminal (36595, 36596)

Code also a frequency of two for procedures involving both catheters from a multicatheter device

**36575** **Repair of tunneled or non-tunneled central venous access catheter, without subcutaneous port or pump, central or peripheral insertion site**

> INCLUDES Repair of the device without replacing any parts
>
> 1.01   4.71   **FUD** 000    [T] [A2] [80] [▭]
>
> **AMA:** 2017,Jan,8; 2016,Jan,13; 2015,Jan,16; 2014,Jan,11

**36576** **Repair of central venous access device, with subcutaneous port or pump, central or peripheral insertion site**

> INCLUDES Repair of the device without replacing any parts
>
> 5.34   8.96   **FUD** 010    [T] [A2] [80] [▭]
>
> **AMA:** 2017,Jan,8; 2016,Jan,13; 2015,Jan,16; 2014,Jan,11

**36578** **Replacement, catheter only, of central venous access device, with subcutaneous port or pump, central or peripheral insertion site**

> INCLUDES Partial replacement (catheter only)
> EXCLUDES Total replacement of the entire device using the same venous access sites (36582-36583)
>
> 5.88   12.7   **FUD** 010    [T] [A2] [80] [▭]
>
> **AMA:** 2017,Jan,8; 2016,Jan,13; 2015,Jan,16; 2014,Jan,11

**36580** **Replacement, complete, of a non-tunneled centrally inserted central venous catheter, without subcutaneous port or pump, through same venous access**

> INCLUDES Complete replacement (replace all components/same access site)
>
> 1.93   6.07   **FUD** 000    [T] [A2] [▭]
>
> **AMA:** 2017,Jan,8; 2016,Jan,13; 2015,Jan,16; 2014,Jan,11

**36581** **Replacement, complete, of a tunneled centrally inserted central venous catheter, without subcutaneous port or pump, through same venous access**

> INCLUDES Complete replacement (replace all components/same access site)
> EXCLUDES Removal of old device and insertion of new device using a separate venous access site
>
> 5.31   19.9   **FUD** 010    [T] [A2] [80] [▭]
>
> **AMA:** 2017,Jan,8; 2016,Jan,13; 2015,Jan,16; 2014,Jan,11

**36582** **Replacement, complete, of a tunneled centrally inserted central venous access device, with subcutaneous port, through same venous access**

> INCLUDES Complete replacement (replace all components/same access site)
> EXCLUDES Removal of old device and insertion of new device using a separate venous access site
>
> 8.45   28.6   **FUD** 010    [T] [A2] [80] [▭]
>
> **AMA:** 2017,Jan,8; 2016,Jan,13; 2015,Jan,16; 2014,Jan,11

**36583** **Replacement, complete, of a tunneled centrally inserted central venous access device, with subcutaneous pump, through same venous access**

> INCLUDES Complete replacement (replace all components/same access site)
> EXCLUDES Removal of old device and insertion of new device using a separate venous access site
>
> 9.38   35.4   **FUD** 010    [T] [J8] [80] [▭]
>
> **AMA:** 2017,Jan,8; 2016,Jan,13; 2015,Jan,16; 2014,Jan,11

**36584** **Replacement, complete, of a peripherally inserted central venous catheter (PICC), without subcutaneous port or pump, through same venous access**

> INCLUDES Complete replacement (replace all components/same access site)
>
> 1.92   5.81   **FUD** 000    [T] [A2] [▭]
>
> **AMA:** 2017,Jan,8; 2016,Jan,13; 2015,Jan,16; 2014,Jan,11

**36585** **Replacement, complete, of a peripherally inserted central venous access device, with subcutaneous port, through same venous access**

> INCLUDES Complete replacement (replace all components/same access site)
>
> 7.92   30.5   **FUD** 010    [T] [A2] [80] [▭]
>
> **AMA:** 2017,Jan,8; 2016,Jan,13; 2015,Jan,16; 2014,Jan,11

**36589** **Removal of tunneled central venous catheter, without subcutaneous port or pump**

> INCLUDES Complete removal/all components
> EXCLUDES Non-tunneled central venous catheter removal; report appropriate E&M code
>
> 3.97   4.69   **FUD** 010    [02] [A2] [80] [▭]
>
> **AMA:** 2017,Jan,8; 2016,Jan,13; 2015,Nov,10; 2015,Jan,16; 2014,Jan,11

**36590** **Removal of tunneled central venous access device, with subcutaneous port or pump, central or peripheral insertion**

> INCLUDES Complete removal/all components
> EXCLUDES Non-tunneled central venous catheter removal; report appropriate E&M code
>
> 5.53   6.35   **FUD** 010    [02] [A2] [80] [▭]
>
> **AMA:** 2017,Jan,8; 2016,Jan,13; 2015,Jan,16; 2014,Jan,11; 2012,Jan,15-42

## 36591-36592 Obtain Blood Specimen from Implanted Device or Catheter

EXCLUDES Use of code with any other service except laboratory services

**36591** **Collection of blood specimen from a completely implantable venous access device**

> EXCLUDES Collection of:
> Capillary blood specimen (36416)
> Venous blood specimen by venipuncture (36415)
>
> 0.67   0.67   **FUD** XXX    [Q1] [M1] [80] [TC] [▭]
>
> **AMA:** 2017,Jan,8; 2016,Jan,13; 2015,Jan,16; 2014,May,4; 2014,Jan,11; 2012,Jan,15-42

**36592** **Collection of blood specimen using established central or peripheral catheter, venous, not otherwise specified**

> EXCLUDES Collection of blood from an established arterial catheter (37799)
>
> 0.75   0.75   **FUD** XXX    [Q1] [M1] [80] [TC] [▭]
>
> **AMA:** 2017,Jan,8; 2016,Jan,13; 2015,Jan,16; 2014,Jan,11; 2012,Jan,15-42

---

● New Code   ▲ Revised Code   ○ Reinstated   ● New Web Release   ▲ Revised Web Release   Unlisted   Not Covered   # Resequenced
⊘ AMA Mod 51 Exempt   ⑨ Optum Mod 51 Exempt   ⑥ Mod 63 Exempt   ✗ Non-FDA Drug   ★ Telemedicine   M Maternity   A Age Edit   + Add-on   AMA: CPT Asst
© 2017 Optum360, LLC    CPT © 2017 American Medical Association. All Rights Reserved.

## 36593-36596 Restore Patency of Occluded Catheter or Device

EXCLUDES   *Venous catheterization (36010-36012)*

**36593**   **Declotting by thrombolytic agent of implanted vascular access device or catheter**
🔌 0.89   ⚖ 0.89   **FUD** XXX                                    T P3 80 TC 🖥

AMA: 2017,Jan,8; 2016,Jan,13; 2015,Jan,16; 2014,Jan,11; 2013,Feb,3-6; 2012,Jan,15-42

**36595**   **Mechanical removal of pericatheter obstructive material (eg, fibrin sheath) from central venous device via separate venous access**

EXCLUDES   *Declotting by thrombolytic agent (36593)*
🔀 (75901)
🔌 5.32   ⚖ 16.6   **FUD** 000                                       T P3 🖥

AMA: 2017,Jan,8; 2016,Jan,13; 2015,Jan,16; 2014,Jan,11

**36596**   **Mechanical removal of intraluminal (intracatheter) obstructive material from central venous device through device lumen**

EXCLUDES   *Declotting by thrombolytic agent (36593)*
🔀 (75902)
🔌 1.29   ⚖ 3.74   **FUD** 000                                       T G2 🖥

AMA: 2017,Jan,8; 2016,Jan,13; 2015,Jan,16; 2014,Jan,11

## 36597-36598 Repositioning or Assessment of In Situ Venous Access Device

**36597**   **Repositioning of previously placed central venous catheter under fluoroscopic guidance**
🔀 (76000)
🔌 1.77   ⚖ 3.61   **FUD** 000                                       T G2 🖥

AMA: 2017,Jan,8; 2016,Jan,13; 2015,Jan,16; 2014,Sep,5; 2014,Jan,11

**36598**   **Contrast injection(s) for radiologic evaluation of existing central venous access device, including fluoroscopy, image documentation and report**

EXCLUDES   *Complete venography studies (75820, 75825, 75827)*
*Fluoroscopy (76000)*
*Mechanical removal of pericatheter obstructive material (36595-36596)*
🔌 1.07   ⚖ 3.15   **FUD** 000                                   T P3 80 50 🖥

AMA: 2014,Jan,11

## 36600-36660 Insertion Needle or Catheter: Artery

**36600**   **Arterial puncture, withdrawal of blood for diagnosis**

EXCLUDES   *Critical care services*
🔌 0.44   ⚖ 0.89   **FUD** XXX                                     Q1 N1 🖥

AMA: 2017,Jan,8; 2016,Jan,13; 2015,Jan,16; 2014,May,4; 2014,Jan,11

**36620**   **Arterial catheterization or cannulation for sampling, monitoring or transfusion (separate procedure); percutaneous**
🔌 1.47   ⚖ 1.47   **FUD** 000                                      ⊘ N N1 🖥

AMA: 2017,Jan,8; 2016,Jan,13; 2015,Jan,16; 2014,Jan,11

**36625**      **cutdown**
🔌 3.02   ⚖ 3.02   **FUD** 000                                         N N1 🖥

AMA: 2017,Jan,8; 2016,Jan,13; 2015,Jan,16; 2014,Jan,11

**36640**   **Arterial catheterization for prolonged infusion therapy (chemotherapy), cutdown**

EXCLUDES   *Intraarterial chemotherapy (96420-96425)*
*Transcatheter embolization (75894)*
🔌 3.31   ⚖ 3.31   **FUD** 000                                         T A2 🖥

AMA: 2017,Jan,8; 2016,Jan,13; 2015,Jan,16; 2014,Jan,11

**36660**   **Catheterization, umbilical artery, newborn, for diagnosis or therapy**                                                  A
🔌 2.13   ⚖ 2.13   **FUD** 000                               ⑥③ C 80 🖥

AMA: 2017,Jan,8; 2016,Jan,13; 2015,Jan,16; 2014,Jan,11

## 36680 Percutaneous Placement of Catheter/Needle into Bone Marrow Cavity

**36680**   **Placement of needle for intraosseous infusion**
🔌 1.69   ⚖ 1.69   **FUD** 000                                     Q1 N1 80 🖥

AMA: 2017,Jan,8; 2016,Jan,13; 2015,Jan,16; 2014,Jan,11; 2012,Jan,15-42

## 36800-36821 Vascular Access for Hemodialysis

**36800**   **Insertion of cannula for hemodialysis, other purpose (separate procedure); vein to vein**
🔌 3.57   ⚖ 3.57   **FUD** 000                                         T A2 🖥

AMA: 2017,Jan,8; 2016,Jan,13; 2015,Jan,16; 2014,Jan,11

**36810**      **arteriovenous, external (Scribner type)**
🔌 6.26   ⚖ 6.26   **FUD** 000                                         T A2 🖥

AMA: 2017,Jan,8; 2016,Jan,13; 2015,Jan,16; 2014,Jan,11

**36815**      **arteriovenous, external revision, or closure**
🔌 4.00   ⚖ 4.00   **FUD** 000                                         T A2 🖥

AMA: 2017,Jan,8; 2016,Jan,13; 2015,Jan,16; 2014,Jan,11

**36818**   **Arteriovenous anastomosis, open; by upper arm cephalic vein transposition**

INCLUDES   Two incisions in the upper arm; a medial incision over the brachial artery and a lateral incision for exposure of a portion of the cephalic vein

EXCLUDES   *When performed unilaterally with:*
*Arteriovenous anastomosis, open (36819-36820)*
*Creation of arteriovenous fistula by other than direct arteriovenous anastomosis (36830)*
Code also modifier 50 or 59, as appropriate, for a bilateral procedure
🔌 20.3   ⚖ 20.3   **FUD** 090                                     T A2 80 🖥

AMA: 2017,Mar,3; 2017,Jan,8; 2016,Mar,10; 2016,Jan,13; 2015,Jan,16; 2014,Jan,11

**36819**      **by upper arm basilic vein transposition**

EXCLUDES   *When performed unilaterally with:*
*Arteriovenous anastomosis, open (36818, 36820-36821)*
*Creation of arteriovenous fistula by other than direct arteriovenous anastomosis (36830)*
Code also modifier 50 or 59, as appropriate, for bilateral procedure
🔌 21.4   ⚖ 21.4   **FUD** 090                                     T A2 80 🖥

AMA: 2017,Mar,3; 2017,Jan,8; 2016,Jan,13; 2015,Jan,16; 2014,Jan,11

**36820**      **by forearm vein transposition**
🔌 21.4   ⚖ 21.4   **FUD** 090                               T A2 80 50 🖥

AMA: 2017,Mar,3; 2017,Jan,8; 2016,Jan,13; 2015,Jan,16; 2014,Jan,11

**36821**      **direct, any site (eg, Cimino type) (separate procedure)**
🔌 19.4   ⚖ 19.4   **FUD** 090                                     T A2 80 🖥

AMA: 2017,Mar,3; 2017,Jan,8; 2016,Jan,13; 2015,Aug,8; 2015,Jan,16; 2014,Jan,11

## 36823 Vascular Access for Extracorporeal Circulation

INCLUDES   Chemotherapy perfusion
EXCLUDES   *Chemotherapy administration (96409-96425)*
*Maintenance for extracorporeal circulation (33946-33949)*

**36823**   **Insertion of arterial and venous cannula(s) for isolated extracorporeal circulation including regional chemotherapy perfusion to an extremity, with or without hyperthermia, with removal of cannula(s) and repair of arteriotomy and venotomy sites**
🔌 40.2   ⚖ 40.2   **FUD** 090                                          C 🖥

AMA: 2017,Mar,3; 2014,Jan,11

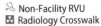

## 36825-36835 Permanent Vascular Access Procedures

**36825** **Creation of arteriovenous fistula by other than direct arteriovenous anastomosis (separate procedure); autogenous graft**

> *EXCLUDES* *Direct arteriovenous (AV) anastomosis (36821)*
>
> 🔃 23.4   ⚬ 23.4   **FUD** 090   [T] [A2] [80] 🔲
>
> **AMA:** 2017,Mar,3; 2017,Jan,8; 2016,Jan,13; 2015,Jan,16; 2014,Jan,11

Artery and vein connected by a vein graft in an end-to-side manner, creating an arteriovenous fistula

Radial artery

Radial artery

Basilic vein

Graft

Basilic vein

Artery and vein connected by a synthetic graft

**36830** **nonautogenous graft (eg, biological collagen, thermoplastic graft)**

> *EXCLUDES* *Direct arteriovenous (AV) anastomosis (36821)*
>
> 🔃 19.5   ⚬ 19.5   **FUD** 090   [T] [A2] [80] 🔲
>
> **AMA:** 2017,Mar,3; 2017,Jan,8; 2016,Jan,13; 2015,Jan,16; 2014,Jan,11

**36831** **Thrombectomy, open, arteriovenous fistula without revision, autogenous or nonautogenous dialysis graft (separate procedure)**

> 🔃 18.0   ⚬ 18.0   **FUD** 090   [T] [A2] [80] 🔲
>
> **AMA:** 2017,Mar,3; 2017,Jan,8; 2016,Jan,13; 2015,Jan,16; 2014,Jan,11; 2012,Jan,15-42

**36832** **Revision, open, arteriovenous fistula; without thrombectomy, autogenous or nonautogenous dialysis graft (separate procedure)**

> *INCLUDES* *Revision of an arteriovenous access fistula or graft*
>
> 🔃 22.1   ⚬ 22.1   **FUD** 090   [T] [A2] [80] 🔲
>
> **AMA:** 2017,Mar,3; 2017,Jan,8; 2016,Jan,13; 2015,Jan,16; 2014,Jan,11; 2012,Jan,15-42

**36833** **with thrombectomy, autogenous or nonautogenous dialysis graft (separate procedure)**

> *EXCLUDES* *Hemodialysis circuit procedures (36901-36906)*
>
> 🔃 23.7   ⚬ 23.7   **FUD** 090   [T] [A2] [80] 🔲
>
> **AMA:** 2017,Mar,3; 2017,Jan,8; 2016,Jan,13; 2015,Jan,16; 2014,Jan,11; 2012,Jan,15-42

**36835** **Insertion of Thomas shunt (separate procedure)**

> 🔃 14.3   ⚬ 14.3   **FUD** 090   [T] [A2] 🔲
>
> **AMA:** 2014,Jan,11

## 36838 DRIL Procedure for Ischemic Steal Syndrome

> *EXCLUDES* *Bypass graft, with vein (35512, 35522-35523)*
> *Ligation (37607, 37618)*
> *Revision, open, arteriovenous fistula (36832)*

**36838** **Distal revascularization and interval ligation (DRIL), upper extremity hemodialysis access (steal syndrome)**

> 🔃 33.5   ⚬ 33.5   **FUD** 090   [T] [80] [50] 🔲
>
> **AMA:** 2014,Jan,11

## 36860-36861 Restore Patency of Occluded Cannula or Arteriovenous Fistula

**36860** **External cannula declotting (separate procedure); without balloon catheter**

> 📷 (76000)
>
> 🔃 3.20   ⚬ 5.95   **FUD** 000   [T] [A2] 🔲
>
> **AMA:** 2017,Jan,8; 2016,Jan,13; 2015,Jan,16; 2014,Jan,11

**36861** **with balloon catheter**

> 📷 (76000)
>
> 🔃 3.91   ⚬ 3.91   **FUD** 000   [T] [A2] 🔲
>
> **AMA:** 2017,Jan,8; 2016,Jan,13; 2015,Jan,16; 2014,Jan,11

## 36901-36909 Hemodialysis Circuit Procedures

> *EXCLUDES* *Arteriography to assess inflow to hemodialysis circuit when performed (76937)*

**36901** **Introduction of needle(s) and/or catheter(s), dialysis circuit, with diagnostic angiography of the dialysis circuit, including all direct puncture(s) and catheter placement(s), injection(s) of contrast, all necessary imaging from the arterial anastomosis and adjacent artery through entire venous outflow including the inferior or superior vena cava, fluoroscopic guidance, radiological supervision and interpretation and image documentation and report;**

> *INCLUDES* Access
> Catheter advancement (e.g., imaging of accessory veins, assess all sections of circuit)
> Contrast injection
>
> *EXCLUDES* *Balloon angioplasty of peripheral segment (36902)*
> *Open revision with thrombectomy of arteriovenous fistula (36833)*
> *Percutaneous transluminal procedures of peripheral segment (36904-36906)*
> *Stent placement in peripheral segment (36903)*
> *Use of code more than one time per procedure*
>
> 🔃 4.21   ⚬ 16.1   **FUD** 000   [T] [P2] 🔲
>
> **AMA:** 2017,Mar,3

**36902** **with transluminal balloon angioplasty, peripheral dialysis segment, including all imaging and radiological supervision and interpretation necessary to perform the angioplasty**

> *EXCLUDES* *Open revision with thrombectomy of arteriovenous fistula (36833)*
> *Percutaneous transluminal procedures of peripheral segment (36904-36906)*
> *Stent placement in peripheral segment (36903)*
> *Use of code more than one time per procedure*
>
> 🔃 6.27   ⚬ 34.4   **FUD** 000   [J] [J8] 🔲
>
> **AMA:** 2017,Jul,3; 2017,Mar,3

**36903** **with transcatheter placement of intravascular stent(s), peripheral dialysis segment, including all imaging and radiological supervision and interpretation necessary to perform the stenting, and all angioplasty within the peripheral dialysis segment**

> *INCLUDES* Balloon angioplasty of peripheral segment (36902)
>
> *EXCLUDES* *Central hemodialysis circuit procedures (36907-36908)*
> *Open revision with thrombectomy of arteriovenous fistula (36833)*
> *Percutaneous transluminal procedures of peripheral segment (36904-36906)*
> *Use of code more than one time per procedure*
>
> 🔃 8.58   ⚬ 157.   **FUD** 000   [J] [J8] 🔲
>
> **AMA:** 2017,Jul,3; 2017,Mar,3

**36904** **Percutaneous transluminal mechanical thrombectomy and/or infusion for thrombolysis, dialysis circuit, any method, including all imaging and radiological supervision and interpretation, diagnostic angiography, fluoroscopic guidance, catheter placement(s), and intraprocedural pharmacological thrombolytic injection(s);**

> *EXCLUDES* *Open thrombectomy of arteriovenous fistula with/without revision (36831, 36833)*
> *Use of code more than one time per procedure*
>
> 🔃 9.88   ⚬ 50.1   **FUD** 000   [J] [J8] 🔲
>
> **AMA:** 2017,Jul,3; 2017,Mar,3

● New Code   ▲ Revised Code   ○ Reinstated   ● New Web Release   ▲ Revised Web Release   Unlisted   Not Covered   # Resequenced
⊘ AMA Mod 51 Exempt   ⑤ Optum Mod 51 Exempt   ⑥ Mod 63 Exempt   ✗ Non-FDA Drug   ★ Telemedicine   Ⓜ Maternity   🄰 Age Edit   + Add-on   **AMA:** CPT Asst
© 2017 Optum360, LLC                     CPT © 2017 American Medical Association. All Rights Reserved.                     **161**

**36905** with transluminal balloon angioplasty, peripheral dialysis segment, including all imaging and radiological supervision and interpretation necessary to perform the angioplasty

INCLUDES　Percutaneous mechanical thrombectomy (36904)

EXCLUDES　*Use of code more than one time per procedure*

🚗 12.4　　✂ 64.2　　**FUD** 000　　　　　　J J8 ▣

**AMA:** 2017,Jul,3; 2017,Mar,3

**36906** with transcatheter placement of intravascular stent(s), peripheral dialysis segment, including all imaging and radiological supervision and interpretation necessary to perform the stenting, and all angioplasty within the peripheral dialysis circuit

INCLUDES　Percutaneous transluminal balloon angioplasty (36905)

Percutaneous transluminal thrombectomy (36904)

EXCLUDES　*Hemodialysis circuit procedures provided by catheter or needle access (36901-36903)*

*Use of code more than one time per procedure*

Code also balloon angioplasty of central veins, when performed (36907)

Code also stent placement in central veins, when performed (36908)

🚗 14.4　　✂ 191.　　**FUD** 000　　　　　　J J8 ▣

**AMA:** 2017,Jul,3; 2017,Mar,3

+ **36907** Transluminal balloon angioplasty, central dialysis segment, performed through dialysis circuit, including all imaging and radiological supervision and interpretation required to perform the angioplasty (List separately in addition to code for primary procedure)

INCLUDES　All central hemodialysis segment angiography

EXCLUDES　*Angiography with stent placement (36908)*

Code first (36818-36833, 36901-36906)

🚗 3.61　　✂ 20.5　　**FUD** ZZZ　　　　　　N N1 ▣

**AMA:** 2017,Jul,3; 2017,Mar,3

▲ + **36908** Transcatheter placement of intravascular stent(s), central dialysis segment, performed through dialysis circuit, including all imaging and radiological supervision and interpretation required to perform the stenting, and all angioplasty in the central dialysis segment (List separately in addition to code for primary procedure)

INCLUDES　All central hemodialysis segment stent(s) placed

Ballooon angioplasty central dialysis segment (36907)

Code first when performed (36818-36833, 36901-36906)

🚗 5.41　　✂ 75.8　　**FUD** ZZZ　　　　　　N N1 ▣

**AMA:** 2017,Jul,3; 2017,Mar,3

+ **36909** Dialysis circuit permanent vascular embolization or occlusion (including main circuit or any accessory veins), endovascular, including all imaging and radiological supervision and interpretation necessary to complete the intervention (List separately in addition to code for primary procedure)

INCLUDES　All embolization/occlusion procedures performed in the hemodialysis circuit

EXCLUDES　*Banding/ligation of arteriovenous fistula (37607)*

*Use of code more than one time per day*

Code first (36901-36906)

🚗 5.14　　✂ 55.3　　**FUD** ZZZ　　　　　　N N1 ▣

**AMA:** 2017,Mar,3

## 37140-37181 Open Decompression of Portal Circulation

EXCLUDES　*Peritoneal-venous shunt (49425)*

**37140** Venous anastomosis, open; portocaval

🚗 67.1　　✂ 67.1　　**FUD** 090　　　　　　C ▣

**AMA:** 2014,Jan,11

**37145** renoportal

🚗 62.3　　✂ 62.3　　**FUD** 090　　　　　　C 80 ▣

**AMA:** 2014,Jan,11

**37160** caval-mesenteric

🚗 64.1　　✂ 64.1　　**FUD** 090　　　　　　C 80 ▣

**AMA:** 2014,Jan,11

**37180** splenorenal, proximal

🚗 61.6　　✂ 61.6　　**FUD** 090　　　　　　C 80 ▣

**AMA:** 2014,Jan,11

**37181** splenorenal, distal (selective decompression of esophagogastric varices, any technique)

EXCLUDES　*Percutaneous procedure (37182)*

🚗 62.4　　✂ 62.4　　**FUD** 090　　　　　　C 80 ▣

**AMA:** 2014,Jan,11

## 37182-37183 Transvenous Decompression of Portal Circulation

INCLUDES　Percutaneous transhepatic portography (75885, 75887)

**37182** Insertion of transvenous intrahepatic portosystemic shunt(s) (TIPS) (includes venous access, hepatic and portal vein catheterization, portography with hemodynamic evaluation, intrahepatic tract formation/dilatation, stent placement and all associated imaging guidance and documentation)

EXCLUDES　*Open procedure (37140)*

🚗 24.0　　✂ 24.0　　**FUD** 000　　　　　　C 80 ▣

**AMA:** 2017,Jan,8; 2016,Jan,13; 2015,Jan,16; 2014,Jan,11; 2013,Sep,17; 2012,Jan,15-42

**37183** Revision of transvenous intrahepatic portosystemic shunt(s) (TIPS) (includes venous access, hepatic and portal vein catheterization, portography with hemodynamic evaluation, intrahepatic tract recanulization/dilatation, stent placement and all associated imaging guidance and documentation)

EXCLUDES　*Arteriovenous (AV) aneurysm repair (36832)*

🚗 11.0　　✂ 164.　　**FUD** 000　　　　　　J 80 ▣

**AMA:** 2017,Jan,8; 2016,Jan,13; 2015,Jan,16; 2014,Jan,11; 2012,Jan,15-42

## 37184-37188 Removal of Thrombus from Vessel: Percutaneous

INCLUDES　Fluoroscopic guidance (76000-76001)

Injection(s) of thrombolytics during the procedure

Postprocedure evaluation

Pretreatment planning

EXCLUDES　*Continuous infusion of thrombolytics prior to and after the procedure ([37211, 37212, 37213, 37214])*

*Diagnostic studies*

*Intracranial arterial mechanical thrombectomy or infusion (61645)*

*Mechanical thrombectomy, coronary (92973)*

*Other interventions performed percutaneously (e.g., balloon angioplasty)*

*Placement of catheters*

*Radiological supervision/interpretation*

**37184** Primary percutaneous transluminal mechanical thrombectomy, noncoronary, non-intracranial, arterial or arterial bypass graft, including fluoroscopic guidance and intraprocedural pharmacological thrombolytic injection(s); initial vessel

EXCLUDES　*Intracranial arterial mechanical thrombectomy (61645)*

*Mechanical thrombectomy for embolus/thrombus complicating another percutaneous interventional procedure (37186)*

*Mechanical thrombectomy of another vascular family/separate access site, append modifier 51 to code, as appropriate*

*Therapeutic, prophylactic, or diagnostic injection (96374)*

🚗 13.1　　✂ 62.9　　**FUD** 000　　　　　　T J8 50 ▣

**AMA:** 2017,Jan,8; 2016,Jul,6; 2016,Mar,3; 2016,Jan,13; 2015,Nov,3; 2015,Apr,10; 2015,Jan,16; 2014,Jan,11; 2013,Feb,3-6

| | | | | | |
|---|---|---|---|---|---|
| 26/TC PC/TC Only | A2-Z3 ASC Payment  | 50 Bilateral 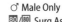 | ♂ Male Only | ♀ Female Only | 🚗 Facility RVU　　✂ Non-Facility RVU　　▣ CCI |
| FUD Follow-up Days | CMS: IOM (Pub 100) | A-Y OPPSI | 80/80 Surg Assist Allowed / w/Doc 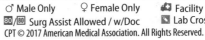 | | 🔬 Lab Crosshwalk　　📻 Radiology Crosswalk　　✖ CLIA |

**162**
CPT © 2017 American Medical Association. All Rights Reserved.　　　　© 2017 Optum360, LLC

**+ 37185** second and all subsequent vessel(s) within the same vascular family (List separately in addition to code for primary mechanical thrombectomy procedure)

INCLUDES Treatment of second and all succeeding vessel(s) in same vascular family

EXCLUDES *Intravenous drug injections administered subsequent to an initial service*
*Mechanical thrombectomy for treating of embolus/thrombus complicating another percutaneous interventional procedure (37186)*
*Mechanical thrombectomy of another vascular family/separate access site, append modifier 51 to code as appropriate*
*Therapeutic, prophylactic, or diagnostic injection (96375)*

Code first (37184)

🔧 4.92 ⚕ 20.0 **FUD** ZZZ    N N1 🔲

**AMA:** 2017,Jan,8; 2016,Jul,6; 2016,Jan,13; 2015,Nov,3; 2015,Apr,10; 2015,Jan,16; 2014,Jan,11; 2013,Feb,3-6

**+ 37186** Secondary percutaneous transluminal thrombectomy (eg, nonprimary mechanical, snare basket, suction technique), noncoronary, non-intracranial, arterial or arterial bypass graft, including fluoroscopic guidance and intraprocedural pharmacological thrombolytic injections, provided in conjunction with another percutaneous intervention other than primary mechanical thrombectomy (List separately in addition to code for primary procedure)

INCLUDES Removal of small emboli/thrombi prior to or after another percutaneous procedure

EXCLUDES *Primary percutaneous transluminal mechanical thrombectomy, noncoronary, non-intracranial (37184-37185)*
*Therapeutic, prophylactic, or diagnostic injection (96375)*

Code first primary procedure

🔧 7.22 ⚕ 37.8 **FUD** ZZZ    N N1 🔲

**AMA:** 2017,Jan,8; 2016,Jul,6; 2016,Jan,13; 2015,Nov,3; 2015,Jan,16; 2014,Jan,11; 2013,Feb,3-6; 2012,Jan,15-42

**37187** Percutaneous transluminal mechanical thrombectomy, vein(s), including intraprocedural pharmacological thrombolytic injections and fluoroscopic guidance

INCLUDES Secondary or subsequent intravenous injection after another initial service

EXCLUDES *Therapeutic, prophylactic, or diagnostic injection (96375)*

🔧 11.4 ⚕ 55.8 **FUD** 000    T G2 50 🔲

**AMA:** 2017,Jan,8; 2016,Jul,6; 2016,Mar,3; 2016,Jan,13; 2015,Nov,3; 2015,Jan,16; 2014,Jan,11; 2013,Feb,3-6

**37188** Percutaneous transluminal mechanical thrombectomy, vein(s), including intraprocedural pharmacological thrombolytic injections and fluoroscopic guidance, repeat treatment on subsequent day during course of thrombolytic therapy

EXCLUDES *Therapeutic, prophylactic, or diagnostic injection (96375)*

🔧 8.14 ⚕ 47.6 **FUD** 000    T G2 50 🔲

**AMA:** 2017,Jan,8; 2016,Jul,6; 2016,Mar,3; 2016,Jan,13; 2015,Nov,3; 2015,Jan,16; 2014,Jan,11; 2013,Feb,3-6

## 37191-37193 Vena Cava Filters

**37191** Insertion of intravascular vena cava filter, endovascular approach including vascular access, vessel selection, and radiological supervision and interpretation, intraprocedural roadmapping, and imaging guidance (ultrasound and fluoroscopy), when performed

EXCLUDES *Open ligation of inferior vena cava via laparotomy or retroperitoneal approach (37619)*

🔧 6.58 ⚕ 72.6 **FUD** 000    T 🔲

**AMA:** 2017,Feb,14; 2017,Jan,8; 2016,May,11; 2016,Jan,13; 2015,Jan,16; 2014,Jan,11; 2013,Feb,3-6; 2012,Apr,3-9

**37192** Repositioning of intravascular vena cava filter, endovascular approach including vascular access, vessel selection, and radiological supervision and interpretation, intraprocedural roadmapping, and imaging guidance (ultrasound and fluoroscopy), when performed

EXCLUDES *Insertion of intravascular vena cava filter (37191)*

🔧 10.5 ⚕ 45.3 **FUD** 000    T 🔲

**AMA:** 2017,Jan,8; 2016,May,11; 2016,Jan,13; 2015,Jan,16; 2014,Jan,11; 2013,Feb,3-6; 2012,Apr,3-9

**37193** Retrieval (removal) of intravascular vena cava filter, endovascular approach including vascular access, vessel selection, and radiological supervision and interpretation, intraprocedural roadmapping, and imaging guidance (ultrasound and fluoroscopy), when performed

EXCLUDES *Transcatheter retrieval, percutaneous, of intravascular foreign body (37197)*

🔧 10.2 ⚕ 43.3 **FUD** 000    T 🔲

**AMA:** 2017,Jan,8; 2016,May,11; 2016,Jan,13; 2015,Jan,16; 2014,Jan,11; 2013,Feb,3-6; 2012,Apr,3-9

## 37195 Intravenous Cerebral Thrombolysis

**37195** Thrombolysis, cerebral, by intravenous infusion

🔧 0.00 ⚕ 0.00 **FUD** XXX    T 80 🔲

**AMA:** 2014,Jan,11

## 37197-37214 [37211, 37212, 37213, 37214] Transcatheter Procedures: Infusions, Biopsy, Foreign Body Removal

**37197** Transcatheter retrieval, percutaneous, of intravascular foreign body (eg, fractured venous or arterial catheter), includes radiological supervision and interpretation, and imaging guidance (ultrasound or fluoroscopy), when performed

EXCLUDES *Percutaneous vena cava filter retrieval (37193)*
*Removal leadless pacemaker system (0388T)*

🔧 8.82 ⚕ 40.8 **FUD** 000    T G2 🔲

**AMA:** 2017,Feb,14; 2017,Jan,8; 2016,May,11; 2016,Jan,13; 2015,Jan,16; 2014,Jan,11; 2013,Feb,3-6

**37200** Transcatheter biopsy

📷 (75970)

🔧 6.37 ⚕ 6.37 **FUD** 000    T G2 🔲

**AMA:** 2014,Jan,11

**# 37211** Transcatheter therapy, arterial infusion for thrombolysis other than coronary or intracranial, any method, including radiological supervision and interpretation, initial treatment day

INCLUDES Catheter exchange or position change
E&M services on the day of and related to thrombolysis
First day of transcatheter thrombolytic infusion
Fluoroscopic guidance
Follow-up arteriography or venography
Radiologic supervision and interpretation

EXCLUDES *Angiography through existing catheter for follow-up study for transcatheter therapy, embolization or infusion, other than for thrombolysis (75898)*
*Catheter placement*
*Declotting of implanted catheter or vascular access device by thrombolytic agent (36593)*
*Diagnostic studies*
*Intracranial arterial mechanical thrombectomy or infusion (61645)*
*Percutaneous interventions*
*Procedure performed more than one time per date of service*
*Ultrasound guidance (76937)*

Code also significant, separately identifiable E&M service on the day of thrombolysis using modifier 25

🔧 11.2 ⚕ 11.2 **FUD** 000    T G2 50 🔲

**AMA:** 2017,Jan,8; 2016,Jul,6; 2016,Mar,3; 2016,Jan,13; 2015,Nov,3; 2015,Jan,16; 2014,Jan,11; 2013,Feb,3-6

**# 37212** Transcatheter therapy, venous infusion for thrombolysis, any method, including radiological supervision and interpretation, initial treatment day

INCLUDES Catheter position change or exchange
E&M services on the day of and related to thrombolysis
First day of transcatheter thrombolytic infusion
Fluoroscopic guidance
Follow-up arteriography or venography
Initiation and completion of thrombolysis on same date of service
Radiologic supervision and interpretation

EXCLUDES *Angiography through existing catheter for follow-up study for transcatheter therapy, embolization or infusion, other than for thrombolysis (75898)*
*Catheter placement*
*Declotting of implanted catheter or vascular access device by thrombolytic agent (36593)*
*Diagnostic studies*
*Percutaneous interventions*
*Procedure performed more than one time per date of service*
*Ultrasound guidance (76937)*

Code also significant, separately identifiable E&M service on the same day as thrombolysis using modifier 25

🚑 9.82   ⚕ 9.82   **FUD** 000   T 02 50 🖵

**AMA:** 2017,Jan,8; 2016,Jul,6; 2016,Mar,3; 2016,Jan,13; 2015,Nov,3; 2015,Jan,16; 2014,Jan,11; 2013,Feb,3-6

**# 37213** Transcatheter therapy, arterial or venous infusion for thrombolysis other than for coronary, any method, including radiological supervision and interpretation, continued treatment on subsequent day during course of thrombolytic therapy, including follow-up catheter contrast injection, position change, or exchange, when performed;

INCLUDES Continued thrombolytic infusions on subsequent days besides the initial and last days of treatment
E&M services on the day of and related to the thrombolysis
Fluoroscopic guidance
Radiologic supervision and interpretation

EXCLUDES *Angiography through existing catheter for follow-up study for transcatheter therapy, embolization or infusion, other than for thrombolysis (75898)*
*Catheter placement*
*Declotting of implanted catheter or vascular access device by thrombolytic agent (36593)*
*Diagnostic studies*
*Percutaneous interventions*
*Procedure performed more than one time per date of service*
*Ultrasound guidance (76937)*

Code also significant, separately identifiable E&M services not related to the thrombolysis using modifier 25

🚑 6.83   ⚕ 6.83   **FUD** 000   T 🖵

**AMA:** 2017,Jan,8; 2016,Jul,6; 2016,Mar,3; 2016,Jan,13; 2015,Nov,3; 2015,Jan,16; 2014,Jan,11; 2013,Feb,3-6

**# 37214** cessation of thrombolysis including removal of catheter and vessel closure by any method

INCLUDES E&M services on the day of and related to the thrombolysis
Fluoroscopic guidance
Last day of transcatheter thrombolytic infusions
Radiologic supervision and interpretation

EXCLUDES *Angiography through existing catheter for follow-up study for transcatheter therapy, embolization or infusion, other than for thrombolysis (75898)*
*Catheter placement*
*Declotting of implanted catheter or vascular access device by thrombolytic agent (36593)*
*Diagnostic studies*
*Percutaneous interventions*
*Procedure performed more than one time per date of service*
*Ultrasound guidance (76937)*

Code also significant, separately identifiable E&M service not related to thrombolysis using modifier 25

🚑 3.59   ⚕ 3.59   **FUD** 000   T 🖵

**AMA:** 2017,Jan,8; 2016,Jul,6; 2016,Mar,3; 2016,Jan,13; 2015,Nov,3; 2015,Jan,16; 2014,Jan,11; 2013,Feb,3-6

*37211* **Resequenced code. See code following 37200.**

*37212* **Resequenced code. See code following 37200.**

*37213* **Resequenced code. See code following 37200.**

*37214* **Resequenced code. See code following 37200.**

## 37215-37216 Stenting of Cervical Carotid Artery with/without Insertion Distal Embolic Protection Device

INCLUDES Carotid stenting, if required
Ipsilateral cerebral and cervical carotid diagnostic imaging/supervision and interpretation
Ipsilateral selective carotid catheterization

EXCLUDES *Carotid catheterization and imaging, if carotid stenting not required*
*Selective catheter placement, common carotid or innominate artery (36222-36224)*
*Transcatheter placement extracranial vertebral artery stents, open or percutaneous (0075T, 0076T)*

**37215** Transcatheter placement of intravascular stent(s), cervical carotid artery, open or percutaneous, including angioplasty, when performed, and radiological supervision and interpretation; with distal embolic protection

🚑 29.0   ⚕ 29.0   **FUD** 090   C 80 50 🖵

**AMA:** 2017,Jul,3; 2017,Jan,8; 2016,Jan,13; 2015,Jan,16; 2014,Mar,8; 2014,Jan,11; 2013,Feb,3-6

Balloon is advanced to the affected portion of artery

Balloon is inflated, which activates the stent

The catheter is withdrawn

Temporal artery

External carotid

Internal carotid

Common carotid (cervical)

Clot filitering stent

| 26/TC PC/TC Only | A2-Z3 ASC Payment | 50 Bilateral | ♂ Male Only | ♀ Female Only | 🚑 Facility RVU | ⚕ Non-Facility RVU | 🖵 CCI |
| FUD Follow-up Days | CMS: IOM (Pub 100) | A-Y OPPSI | 80/80 Surg Assist Allowed / w/Doc | | 🔬 Lab Crosswalk | 🔴 Radiology Crosswalk | ❌ CLIA |

**164**
CPT © 2017 American Medical Association. All Rights Reserved.
© 2017 Optum360, LLC

**37216** without distal embolic protection

⚙ 0.00  ⚒ 0.00  **FUD** 090  E 🖥

**AMA:** 2017,Jul,3; 2017,Jan,8; 2016,Jan,13; 2015,Jan,16; 2014,Mar,8; 2014,Jan,11; 2013,Feb,3-6

## 37217-37218 Stenting of Intrathoracic Carotid Artery/Innominate Artery

INCLUDES  Access to vessel (open)
Arteriotomy closure by suture
Catheterization of the vessel (selective)
Imaging during and after the procedure
Radiological supervision and interpretation

EXCLUDES  *Transcatheter insertion extracranial vertebral artery stents, open or percutaneous (0075T-0076T)*
*Transcatheter insertion intracranial stents (61635)*
*Transcatheter insertion intravascular cervical carotid artery stents, open or percutaneous (37215-37216)*

**37217** Transcatheter placement of intravascular stent(s), intrathoracic common carotid artery or innominate artery by retrograde treatment, open ipsilateral cervical carotid artery exposure, including angioplasty, when performed, and radiological supervision and interpretation

EXCLUDES  *Services performed on the same side:*
*Non-selective catheter placement, thoracic aorta (36221-36227)*
*Repair blood vessel, direct; neck (35201)*
*Transluminal balloon angioplasty ([37246, 37247])*
Code also revascularization of carotid artery, when performed (33891, 35301, 35509-35510, 35601, 35606)

⚙ 32.1  ⚒ 32.1  **FUD** 090  C 80 50 🖥

**AMA:** 2017,Jul,3; 2017,Jan,8; 2016,Jan,13; 2015,May,7; 2015,Jan,16; 2014,Mar,8; 2014,Jan,11

**37218** Transcatheter placement of intravascular stent(s), intrathoracic common carotid artery or innominate artery, open or percutaneous antegrade approach, including angioplasty, when performed, and radiological supervision and interpretation

EXCLUDES  *Selective catheter placement, common carotid or innominate artery (36222-36224)*

⚙ 23.8  ⚒ 23.8  **FUD** 090  C 80 50 🖥

**AMA:** 2017,Jul,3; 2017,Jan,8; 2016,Jan,13; 2015,May,7

## 37220-37235 Endovascular Revascularization Lower Extremities

INCLUDES  Percutaneous and open interventional and associated procedures for lower extremity occlusive disease; unilateral
Accessing the vessel
Arteriotomy closure by suturing of puncture or pressure with application of arterial closure device
Atherectomy (e.g., directional, laser, rotational)
Balloon angioplasty (e.g., cryoplasty, cutting balloon, low-profile)
Catheterization of the vessel (selective)
Embolic protection
Imaging once procedure is complete
Radiological supervision and interpretation of intervention(s)
Stenting (e.g., bare metal, balloon-expandable, covered, drug-eluting, self-expanding)
Transversing of the lesion
Reporting the most comprehensive treatment in a given vessel according to the following hierarchy:
1. Stent and atherectomy
2. Atherectomy
3. Stent
4. PTA
Revascularization procedures for three arterial vascular territories:
Femoral/popliteal vascular territory including the common, deep, and superficial femoral arteries, and the popliteal artery (one extremity = a single vessel) (37224-37227)
Iliac vascular territory: common iliac, external iliac, internal iliac (37220-37223)
Tibial/peroneal territory: includes anterior tibial, peroneal artery, posterior tibial (37228-37235)

EXCLUDES  *Assignment of more than one code from this family for each lower extremity vessel treated*
*Assignment of more than one code when multiple vessels are treated in the femoral/popliteal territory (report the most complex service for more than one lesion in the territory); when a contiguous lesion that spans from one territory to another can be opened with a single procedure; or when more than one stent is deployed in the same vessel*
*Extensive repair or replacement of artery (35226, 35286)*
*Mechanical thrombectomy and/or thrombolysis*
Code also add-on codes for different vessels, but not different lesions in the same vessel; and for multiple territories in the same leg
Code also modifier 59 for a bilateral procedure
Code first one primary code for the initial service in each leg

**37220** Revascularization, endovascular, open or percutaneous, iliac artery, unilateral, initial vessel; with transluminal angioplasty

Code also only when transluminal angioplasty is performed outside the treatment target zone of (34701-34711, 34845-34848, 0254T)

⚙ 11.7  ⚒ 86.7  **FUD** 000  J 62 50 🖥

**AMA:** 2017,Jul,3; 2017,Jan,8; 2016,Jul,8; 2016,Jan,13; 2015,Jan,16; 2014,Jan,11; 2013,Dec,8

**37221** with transluminal stent placement(s), includes angioplasty within the same vessel, when performed

Code also only when transluminal angioplasty is performed outside the treatment target zone of (34701-34711, 34845-34848, 0254T)

⚙ 14.5  ⚒ 128.  **FUD** 000  J J8 80 50 🖥

**AMA:** 2017,Jul,3; 2017,Jan,8; 2016,Jul,8; 2016,Jul,6; 2016,Jan,13; 2015,Jan,16; 2015,Jan,13; 2014,Jan,11; 2013,Dec,8; 2012,Apr,3-9; 2012,Jan,15-42

+ **37222** Revascularization, endovascular, open or percutaneous, iliac artery, each additional ipsilateral iliac vessel; with transluminal angioplasty (List separately in addition to code for primary procedure)

Code also only when transluminal angioplasty is performed outside the treatment target zone of (34701-34711, 34845-34848, 0254T)
Code first (37220-37221)

⚙ 5.48  ⚒ 24.3  **FUD** ZZZ  N 11 80 50 🖥

**AMA:** 2017,Jul,3; 2017,Jan,8; 2016,Jul,8; 2016,Jan,13; 2015,Jan,16; 2014,Jan,11; 2013,Dec,8

**Cardiovascular, Hemic, and Lymphatic**

**37223 — 37248**

+ **37223** with transluminal stent placement(s), includes angioplasty within the same vessel, when performed (List separately in addition to code for primary procedure)

> Code also only when transluminal angioplasty is performed outside the treatment target zone of (34701-34711, 34845-34848, 0254T)
>
> Code first (37221)
>
> 6.28   72.1   **FUD** ZZZ    N N1 80 50
>
> **AMA:** 2017,Jul,3; 2017,Jan,8; 2016,Jul,8; 2016,Jul,6; 2016,Jan,13; 2015,Jan,16; 2014,Jan,11; 2013,Dec,8; 2012,Apr,3-9

**37224** Revascularization, endovascular, open or percutaneous, femoral, popliteal artery(s), unilateral; with transluminal angioplasty

> 13.0   105.   **FUD** 000    J J8 80 50
>
> **AMA:** 2017,Jul,3; 2017,Jan,8; 2016,Jul,8; 2016,Jan,13; 2015,Jan,16; 2014,Jan,11; 2012,Jan,15-42

**37225** with atherectomy, includes angioplasty within the same vessel, when performed

> 17.7   308.   **FUD** 000    J J8 80 50
>
> **AMA:** 2017,Jul,3; 2017,Jan,8; 2016,Jul,8; 2016,Jan,13; 2015,Jan,16; 2014,Jan,11

**37226** with transluminal stent placement(s), includes angioplasty within the same vessel, when performed

> 15.3   252.   **FUD** 000    J J8 80 50
>
> **AMA:** 2017,Jul,3; 2017,Jan,8; 2016,Jul,8; 2016,Jul,6; 2016,Jan,13; 2015,Jan,16; 2014,Jan,11; 2012,Jan,15-42

**37227** with transluminal stent placement(s) and atherectomy, includes angioplasty within the same vessel, when performed

> 21.4   417.   **FUD** 000    J J8 80 50
>
> **AMA:** 2017,Jul,3; 2017,Jan,8; 2016,Jul,8; 2016,Jan,13; 2015,Jan,16; 2014,Jan,11

**37228** Revascularization, endovascular, open or percutaneous, tibial, peroneal artery, unilateral, initial vessel; with transluminal angioplasty

> 15.9   150.   **FUD** 000    J G2 80 50
>
> **AMA:** 2017,Jul,3; 2017,Jan,8; 2016,Jul,8; 2016,Jan,13; 2015,Jan,16; 2014,Jan,11

**37229** with atherectomy, includes angioplasty within the same vessel, when performed

> 20.7   303.   **FUD** 000    J J8 80 50
>
> **AMA:** 2017,Jul,3; 2017,Jan,8; 2016,Jul,8; 2016,Jan,13; 2015,Jan,16; 2014,Jan,11; 2012,Apr,3-9

**37230** with transluminal stent placement(s), includes angioplasty within the same vessel, when performed

> 20.5   232.   **FUD** 000    J J8 80 50
>
> **AMA:** 2017,Jul,3; 2017,Jan,8; 2016,Jul,8; 2016,Jul,6; 2016,Jan,13; 2015,Jan,16; 2014,Jan,11; 2012,Apr,3-9

**37231** with transluminal stent placement(s) and atherectomy, includes angioplasty within the same vessel, when performed

> 22.2   375.   **FUD** 000    J J8 80 50
>
> **AMA:** 2017,Jul,3; 2017,Jan,8; 2016,Jul,8; 2016,Jul,6; 2016,Jan,13; 2015,Jan,16; 2014,Jan,11; 2012,Apr,3-9

+ **37232** Revascularization, endovascular, open or percutaneous, tibial/peroneal artery, unilateral, each additional vessel; with transluminal angioplasty (List separately in addition to code for primary procedure)

> Code first (37228-37231)
>
> 5.94   33.6   **FUD** ZZZ    N N1 80 50
>
> **AMA:** 2017,Jul,3; 2017,Jan,8; 2016,Jul,8; 2016,Jan,13; 2015,Jan,16; 2014,Jan,11; 2012,Apr,3-9

+ **37233** with atherectomy, includes angioplasty within the same vessel, when performed (List separately in addition to code for primary procedure)

> Code first (37229, 37231)
>
> 9.65   40.6   **FUD** ZZZ    N N1 80 50
>
> **AMA:** 2017,Jul,3; 2017,Jan,8; 2016,Jul,8; 2016,Jan,13; 2015,Jan,16; 2014,Jan,11; 2012,Apr,3-9

+ **37234** with transluminal stent placement(s), includes angioplasty within the same vessel, when performed (List separately in addition to code for primary procedure)

> Code first (37229-37231)
>
> 8.36   110.   **FUD** ZZZ    N N1 80 50
>
> **AMA:** 2017,Jul,3; 2017,Jan,8; 2016,Jul,8; 2016,Jul,6; 2016,Jan,13; 2015,Jan,16; 2014,Jan,11; 2012,Apr,3-9

+ **37235** with transluminal stent placement(s) and atherectomy, includes angioplasty within the same vessel, when performed (List separately in addition to code for primary procedure)

> Code first (37231)
>
> 11.5   118.   **FUD** ZZZ    N N1 80 50
>
> **AMA:** 2017,Jul,3; 2017,Jan,8; 2016,Jul,8; 2016,Jul,6; 2016,Jan,13; 2015,Jan,16; 2014,Jan,11

## [37246, 37247, 37248, 37249] Transluminal Balloon Angioplasty

> **INCLUDES** Open and percutaneous balloon angioplasty
> Radiological supervision and interpretation (37220-37235)
>
> **EXCLUDES** Angioplasty of other vessels:
>    Aortic/visceral arteries (with endovascular repair) (34841-34848)
>    Coronary artery (92920-92944)
>    Intracranial artery (61630, 61635)
>    Performed in a hemodialysis circuit (36901-36909)
>    Percutaneous removal of thrombus/infusion of thrombolytics (37184-37188, [37211, 37212, 37213, 37214])
>    Pulmonary artery (92997-92998)
>    Use of codes more than one time for all services performed in a single vessel or treatable with one angioplasty procedure
> Code also angioplasty of different vessel, when performed ([37247], [37249])
> Code also extensive repair or replacement of artery, when performed (35226, 35286)
> Code also intravascular ultrasound, when performed (37252-37253)

\# **37246** Transluminal balloon angioplasty (except lower extremity artery(ies) for occlusive disease, intracranial, coronary, pulmonary, or dialysis circuit), open or percutaneous, including all imaging and radiological supervision and interpretation necessary to perform the angioplasty within the same artery; initial artery

> **EXCLUDES** Intravascular stent placement except lower extremities (37236-37237)
> Revascularization lower extremities (37220-37235)
> Stent placement:
>    Cervical carotid artery (37215-37216)
>    Intrathoracic carotid or innominate artery (37217-37218)
>
> Code first (37239)
>
> 10.2   60.6   **FUD** 000    J J8 50
>
> **AMA:** 2017,Aug,10; 2017,Jul,3

+ \# **37247** each additional artery (List separately in addition to code for primary procedure)

> **EXCLUDES** Intravascular stent placement except lower extremities (37236-37237)
> Revascularization lower extremities (37220-37235)
> Stent placement:
>    Cervical carotid artery (37215-37216)
>    Intrathoracic carotid or innominate artery (37217-37218)
>
> Code first ([37246])
>
> 5.10   24.5   **FUD** ZZZ    N N1 50
>
> **AMA:** 2017,Aug,10; 2017,Jul,3

\# **37248** Transluminal balloon angioplasty (except dialysis circuit), open or percutaneous, including all imaging and radiological supervision and interpretation necessary to perform the angioplasty within the same vein; initial vein

> **EXCLUDES** Placement of intravascular (venous) stent in same vein, same session as (37238-37239)
>
> 8.85   41.9   **FUD** 000    J J8 50
>
> **AMA:** 2017,Aug,10; 2017,Jul,3; 2017,Mar,3

| 26/TC PC/TC Only | A2-Z3 ASC Payment | 50 Bilateral | ♂ Male Only | ♀ Female Only | Facility RVU | Non-Facility RVU | CCI |
| FUD Follow-up Days | CMS: IOM (Pub 100) | A-Y OPPSI | 80/80 Surg Assist Allowed / w/Doc | | Lab Crosswalk | Radiology Crosswalk | CLIA |

166          CPT © 2017 American Medical Association. All Rights Reserved.          © 2017 Optum360, LLC

**+ # 37249** **each additional vein (List separately in addition to code for primary procedure)**

> EXCLUDES *Placement of intravascular (venous) stent in same vein, same session as (37238-37239)*
>
> Code first (37239)

📷 4.34  ⚕ 17.9  **FUD** ZZZ  Ⓝ M1 50 📄

AMA: 2017,Aug,10; 2017,Jul,3; 2017,Mar,3

## 37236-37239 Endovascular Revascularization Excluding Lower Extremities

> INCLUDES Arteriotomy closure by suturing of a puncture, pressure or application of arterial closure device
> Balloon angioplasty
>   Post-dilation after stent deployment
>   Predilation performed as primary or secondary angioplasty
>   Treatment of lesion inside same vessel but outside of stented portion
>   Treatment using different-sized balloons to accomplish the procedure
> Endovascular revascularization of arteries and veins other than carotid, coronary, extracranial, intracranial, lower extremities
> Imaging once procedure is complete
> Radiological supervision and interpretation
> Stent placement provided as the only treatment
>
> EXCLUDES *Angioplasty in an unrelated vessel*
> *Extensive repair or replacement of an artery (35226, 35286)*
> *Insertion of multiple stents in a single vessel using more than one code*
> *Intravascular ultrasound (37252-37253)*
> *Mechanical thrombectomy (37184-37188)*
> *Selective and nonselective catheterization (36005, 36010-36015, 36200, 36215-36218, 36245-36248)*
> *Stent placement in:*
>   *Arteries of the lower extremities for occlusive disease (37221, 37223, 37226-37227, 37230-37231, 37234-37235)*
>   *Cervical carotid artery (37215-37216)*
>   *Extracranial vertebral (0075T-0076T)*
>   *Hemodialysis circuit (36903, 36905, 36908)*
>   *Intracoronary (92928-92929, 92933-92934, 92937-92938, 92941, 92943-92944)*
>   *Intracranial (61635)*
>   *Intrathoracic common carotid or innominate artery, retrograde or antegrade approach (37218)*
>   *Visceral arteries with fenestrated aortic repair (34841-34848)*
> *Thrombolytic therapy ([37211, 37212, 37213, 37214])*
> *Ultrasound guidance (76937)*
>
> Code also add-on codes for different vessels treated during the same operative session

**37236** **Transcatheter placement of an intravascular stent(s) (except lower extremity artery(s) for occlusive disease, cervical carotid, extracranial vertebral or intrathoracic carotid, intracranial, or coronary), open or percutaneous, including radiological supervision and interpretation and including all angioplasty within the same vessel, when performed; initial artery**

> EXCLUDES *Procedures in the same target treatment zone with (34841-34848)*

📷 12.9  ⚕ 111.  **FUD** 000  J 62 80 50 📄

AMA: 2017,Jul,3; 2017,Jan,8; 2016,Jul,3; 2016,Jul,6; 2016,Mar,5; 2016,Jan,13; 2015,May,7; 2015,Jan,16; 2014,Jan,11; 2013,Dec,8

**+ 37237** **each additional artery (List separately in addition to code for primary procedure)**

> EXCLUDES *Procedures in the same target treatment zone with (34841-34848)*
>
> Code first (37236)

📷 6.25  ⚕ 68.3  **FUD** ZZZ  Ⓝ M1 80 50 📄

AMA: 2017,Jul,3; 2017,Jan,8; 2016,Jul,6; 2016,Mar,5; 2016,Jan,13; 2015,Jan,16; 2014,Jan,11; 2013,Dec,8

**37238** **Transcatheter placement of an intravascular stent(s), open or percutaneous, including radiological supervision and interpretation and including angioplasty within the same vessel, when performed; initial vein**

📷 8.76  ⚕ 116.  **FUD** 000  J J8 80 50 📄

AMA: 2017,Jul,3; 2017,Mar,3; 2017,Jan,8; 2016,Jul,6; 2016,Jun,8; 2014,Jan,11

**+ 37239** **each additional vein (List separately in addition to code for primary procedure)**

> Code first (37238)

📷 4.42  ⚕ 56.7  **FUD** ZZZ  Ⓝ M1 80 50 📄

AMA: 2017,Jul,3; 2017,Mar,3; 2017,Jan,8; 2016,Jul,6; 2014,Jan,11

## 37241-37249 Therapeutic Vascular Embolization/Occlusion

> INCLUDES Embolization or occlusion of arteries, lymphatics, and veins except for head/neck and central nervous system
> Imaging once procedure is complete
> Intraprocedural guidance
> Radiological supervision and interpretation
> Roadmapping
> Stent placement provided as support for embolization
>
> EXCLUDES *Embolization code assigned more than once per operative field*
> *Head, neck, or central nervous system embolization (61624, 61626, 61710)*
> *Multiple codes for indications that overlap, code only the indication needing the most immediate attention*
> *Stent deployment as primary management of aneurysm, pseudoaneurysm, or vascular extravasation*
> *Vein destruction with sclerosing solution (36468-36471)*
>
> Code also additional embolization procedure(s) and the appropriate modifiers (eg, modifier 59) when embolization procedures are performed in multiple operative fields
> Code also diagnostic angiography and catheter placement using modifier 59 when appropriate

**37241** **Vascular embolization or occlusion, inclusive of all radiological supervision and interpretation, intraprocedural roadmapping, and imaging guidance necessary to complete the intervention; venous, other than hemorrhage (eg, congenital or acquired venous malformations, venous and capillary hemangiomas, varices, varicoceles)**

> EXCLUDES *Embolization of side branch(s) of an outflow vein from a hemodialysis access (36909)*
> *Procedure in same operative field with:*
>   *Endovenous ablation therapy of incompetent vein (36475-36479)*
>   *Injection of sclerosing solution; single vein (36470-36471)*
>   *Transcatheter embolization procedures (75894, 75898)*
>   *Vein destruction (36468-36479)*

📷 12.9  ⚕ 134.  **FUD** 000  J 62 📄

AMA: 2017,Mar,3; 2017,Jan,8; 2016,Nov,3; 2016,Jan,13; 2015,Nov,3; 2015,Aug,8; 2015,Apr,10; 2015,Jan,16; 2014,Oct,6; 2014,Aug,14; 2014,Jan,11; 2013,Nov,6; 2013,Nov,14

**37242** **arterial, other than hemorrhage or tumor (eg, congenital or acquired arterial malformations, arteriovenous malformations, arteriovenous fistulas, aneurysms, pseudoaneurysms)**

> EXCLUDES *Percutaneous treatment of pseudoaneurysm of an extremity (36002)*

📷 14.0  ⚕ 210.  **FUD** 000  J 62 📄

AMA: 2017,Jan,8; 2016,Jan,13; 2015,Nov,3; 2015,Jan,16; 2014,Oct,6; 2014,Jan,11; 2013,Nov,6; 2013,Nov,14

**37243** **for tumors, organ ischemia, or infarction**

> INCLUDES Embolization of uterine fibroids (37244)
>
> EXCLUDES *Procedure in same operative field:*
>   *Angiography (75898)*
>   *Transcatheter embolization in same operative field (75894)*
>
> Code also chemotherapy when provided with embolization procedure (96420-96425)
> Code also injection of radioisotopes when provided with embolization procedure (79445)

📷 16.5  ⚕ 273.  **FUD** 000  J 62 📄

AMA: 2017,Jan,8; 2016,Jan,13; 2015,Nov,3; 2015,Jan,16; 2014,Oct,6; 2014,Jan,11; 2013,Nov,6; 2013,Nov,14

**37244** **for arterial or venous hemorrhage or lymphatic extravasation**

> INCLUDES Embolization of uterine arteries for hemorrhage

📷 19.5  ⚕ 190.  **FUD** 000  J 📄

AMA: 2017,Jan,8; 2016,Jan,13; 2015,Nov,3; 2015,Jan,16; 2014,Oct,6; 2014,Aug,14; 2014,Jan,11; 2013,Nov,6; 2013,Nov,14

*37246* **Resequenced code. See code following 37235.**

*37247* **Resequenced code. See code following 37235.**

*37248* **Resequenced code. See code following 37235.**

*37249* **Resequenced code. See code following 37235.**

---

## 37252-37253 Intravascular Ultrasound: Noncoronary

**INCLUDES** Manipulation and repositioning of the transducer prior to and after therapeutic interventional procedures

**EXCLUDES** Selective or non-selective catheter placement for access (36005-36248)
Transcatheter procedures (37200, 37236-37239, 37241-37244, 61624, 61626)
Vena cava filter procedures (37191-37193, 37197)

Code first (33361-33369, 33477, 33880-33886, 34701-34711, 34841-34848, 36010-36015, 36100-36218, 36221-36228, 36245-36248, 36251-36254, 36481, 36555-36571, 36578, 36580-36585, 36595, 36901-36909, 37184-37188, 37200, 37211-37218 [37211, 37212, 37213, 37214], 37220-37235)

**+  37252**  **Intravascular ultrasound (noncoronary vessel) during diagnostic evaluation and/or therapeutic intervention, including radiological supervision and interpretation; initial noncoronary vessel (List separately in addition to code for primary procedure)**
Code first primary procedure
🖩 2.69   ⚕ 39.0   **FUD** ZZZ   [N] [N1] [80] 🔲
**AMA:** 2017,Aug,10; 2017,Mar,3; 2017,Jan,8; 2016,Jul,6; 2016,May,11

**+  37253**  **each additional noncoronary vessel (List separately in addition to code for primary procedure)**
Code first (37252)
🖩 2.17   ⚕ 5.88   **FUD** ZZZ   [N] [N1] [80] 🔲
**AMA:** 2017,Aug,10; 2017,Mar,3; 2017,Jan,8; 2016,Jul,6; 2016,May,11

## 37500-37501 Vascular Endoscopic Procedures

**INCLUDES** Diagnostic endoscopy
**EXCLUDES** Open procedure (37760)

**37500**  **Vascular endoscopy, surgical, with ligation of perforator veins, subfascial (SEPS)**
🖩 18.8   ⚕ 18.8   **FUD** 090   [T] [A2] [50] 🔲
**AMA:** 2017,Jan,8; 2016,Jan,13; 2015,Jan,16; 2014,Jan,11

**37501**  **Unlisted vascular endoscopy procedure**
🖩 0.00   ⚕ 0.00   **FUD** YYY   [T] [50]
**AMA:** 2014,Jan,11

## 37565-37606 Ligation Procedures: Jugular Vein, Carotid Arteries

**CMS:** 100-03,160.8 Electroencephalographic Monitoring During Cerebral Vasculature Surgery

**EXCLUDES** Arterial balloon occlusion, endovascular, temporary (61623)
Suture of arteries and veins (35201-35286)
Transcatheter arterial embolization/occlusion, permanent (61624-61626)
Treatment of intracranial aneurysm (61703)

**37565**  **Ligation, internal jugular vein**
🖩 21.3   ⚕ 21.3   **FUD** 090   [T] [80] [50] 🔲
**AMA:** 2014,Jan,11

**37600**  **Ligation; external carotid artery**
🖩 20.6   ⚕ 20.6   **FUD** 090   [T] [80] 🔲
**AMA:** 2014,Jan,11

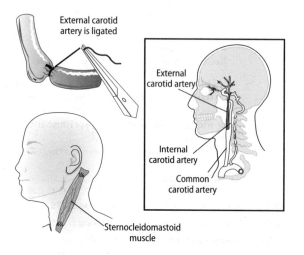

External carotid artery is ligated

External carotid artery

Internal carotid artery

Common carotid artery

Sternocleidomastoid muscle

**37605**  **internal or common carotid artery**
🖩 23.0   ⚕ 23.0   **FUD** 090   [T] [80] 🔲
**AMA:** 2014,Jan,11

**37606**  **internal or common carotid artery, with gradual occlusion, as with Selverstone or Crutchfield clamp**
🖩 15.0   ⚕ 15.0   **FUD** 090   [T] [80] 🔲
**AMA:** 2014,Jan,11

## 37607-37609 Ligation Hemodialysis Angioaccess or Temporal Artery

**EXCLUDES** Suture of arteries and veins (35201-35286)

**37607**  **Ligation or banding of angioaccess arteriovenous fistula**
🖩 10.9   ⚕ 10.9   **FUD** 090   [T] [A2] 🔲
**AMA:** 2014,Jan,11

**37609**  **Ligation or biopsy, temporal artery**
🖩 5.99   ⚕ 8.84   **FUD** 010   [J] [A2] [50] 🔲
**AMA:** 2014,Jan,11

## 37615-37618 Arterial Ligation, Major Vessel, for Injury/Rupture

**EXCLUDES** Suture of arteries and veins (35201-35286)

**37615**  **Ligation, major artery (eg, post-traumatic, rupture); neck**
**INCLUDES** Touroff ligation
🖩 14.7   ⚕ 14.7   **FUD** 090   [T] [80] 🔲
**AMA:** 2014,Jan,11

**37616**  **chest**
**INCLUDES** Bardenheuer operation
🖩 31.9   ⚕ 31.9   **FUD** 090   [C] [80] 🔲
**AMA:** 2014,Jan,11

**37617**  **abdomen**
🖩 38.9   ⚕ 38.9   **FUD** 090   [C] [80] 🔲
**AMA:** 2017,Jan,8; 2016,Jan,13; 2015,Jan,16; 2014,Jan,11; 2013,Aug,13

**37618**  **extremity**
🖩 11.1   ⚕ 11.1   **FUD** 090   [C] [80] 🔲
**AMA:** 2014,Jan,11

## 37619 Ligation Inferior Vena Cava

**EXCLUDES** Suture of arteries and veins (35201-35286)
Endovascular delivery of inferior vena cava filter (37191)

**37619**  **Ligation of inferior vena cava**
🖩 47.9   ⚕ 47.9   **FUD** 090   [T] [80] 🔲
**AMA:** 2017,Jan,8; 2016,Jan,13; 2015,Jan,16; 2014,Jan,11; 2012,Apr,3-9

## 37650-37660 Venous Ligation, Femoral and Common Iliac

**EXCLUDES** Suture of arteries and veins (35201-35286)

**37650**  **Ligation of femoral vein**
🖩 13.5   ⚕ 13.5   **FUD** 090   [T] [A2] [50] 🔲
**AMA:** 2014,Jan,11

**37660**  **Ligation of common iliac vein**
🖩 37.7   ⚕ 37.7   **FUD** 090   [C] [80] [50] 🔲
**AMA:** 2014,Jan,11

## 37700-37785 Treatment of Varicose Veins of Legs

**EXCLUDES** Suture of arteries and veins (35201-35286)

**37700**  **Ligation and division of long saphenous vein at saphenofemoral junction, or distal interruptions**
**INCLUDES** Babcock operation
**EXCLUDES** Ligation, division, and stripping of vein (37718, 37722)
🖩 7.23   ⚕ 7.23   **FUD** 090   [T] [A2] [50] 🔲
**AMA:** 2017,Jan,8; 2016,Jan,13; 2015,Jan,16; 2014,Jan,11; 2012,Jan,15-42

**37718**  **Ligation, division, and stripping, short saphenous vein**
**EXCLUDES** Ligation, division, and stripping of vein (37700, 37735, 37780)
🖩 12.6   ⚕ 12.6   **FUD** 090   [T] [A2] [50] 🔲
**AMA:** 2017,Jan,8; 2014,Jan,11

[26]/[TC] PC/TC Only   [A2]-[23] ASC Payment   [50] Bilateral   ♂ Male Only   ♀ Female Only   🖩 Facility RVU   ⚕ Non-Facility RVU   🔲 CCI
**FUD** Follow-up Days   **CMS:** IOM (Pub 100)   [A]-[Y] OPPSI   [80]/[80] Surg Assist Allowed / w/Doc   🔲 Lab Crosswalk   🔲 Radiology Crosswalk   ❌ CLIA

168   CPT © 2017 American Medical Association. All Rights Reserved.   © 2017 Optum360, LLC

**37722** Ligation, division, and stripping, long (greater) saphenous veins from saphenofemoral junction to knee or below

> EXCLUDES *Ligation, division, and stripping of vein (37700, 37718, 37735)*

🚑 13.9 ⚕ 13.9 **FUD** 090 　　　　T A2 50 ▣

**AMA:** 2017,Jan,8; 2014,Jan,11

**37735** Ligation and division and complete stripping of long or short saphenous veins with radical excision of ulcer and skin graft and/or interruption of communicating veins of lower leg, with excision of deep fascia

> EXCLUDES *Ligation, division, and stripping of vein (37700, 37718, 37722, 37780)*

🚑 17.0 ⚕ 17.0 **FUD** 090 　　　　T A2 50 ▣

**AMA:** 2017,Jan,8; 2016,Jan,13; 2015,Jan,16; 2014,Jan,11

**37760** Ligation of perforator veins, subfascial, radical (Linton type), including skin graft, when performed, open,1 leg

> EXCLUDES *Duplex scan of extremity veins (93971)*
> *Ligation of subfascial perforator veins, endoscopic (37500)*
> *Ultrasonic guidance (76937, 76942, 76998)*

🚑 17.9 ⚕ 17.9 **FUD** 090 　　　　T A2 50 ▣

**AMA:** 2017,Jan,8; 2016,Jan,13; 2015,Jan,16; 2014,Jan,11

**37761** Ligation of perforator vein(s), subfascial, open, including ultrasound guidance, when performed, 1 leg

> EXCLUDES *Duplex scan of extremity veins (93971)*
> *Ligation of subfascial perforator veins, endoscopic (37500)*
> *Ultrasonic guidance (76937, 76942, 76998)*

🚑 16.0 ⚕ 16.0 **FUD** 090 　　　　T R2 80 50 ▣

**AMA:** 2017,Jan,8; 2016,Jan,13; 2015,Jan,16; 2014,Jan,11

**37765** Stab phlebectomy of varicose veins, 1 extremity; 10-20 stab incisions

> EXCLUDES *Fewer than 10 incisions (37799)*
> *More than 20 incisions (37766)*

🚑 13.0 ⚕ 18.6 **FUD** 090 　　　　T P3 50 ▣

**AMA:** 2017,Jan,8; 2016,Nov,3; 2016,Jan,13; 2015,Jan,16; 2014,Oct,6; 2014,Jan,11

**37766** more than 20 incisions

> EXCLUDES *Fewer than 10 incisions (37799)*
> *10-20 incisions (37765)*

🚑 15.9 ⚕ 22.1 **FUD** 090 　　　　T P3 50 ▣

**AMA:** 2017,Jan,8; 2016,Nov,3; 2016,Jan,13; 2015,Jan,16; 2014,Oct,6; 2014,Jan,11; 2013,Sep,17

**37780** Ligation and division of short saphenous vein at saphenopopliteal junction (separate procedure)

🚑 7.31 ⚕ 7.31 **FUD** 090 　　　　T A2 50 ▣

**AMA:** 2017,Jan,8; 2016,Jan,13; 2015,Jan,16; 2014,Jan,11; 2012,Jan,15-42

**37785** Ligation, division, and/or excision of varicose vein cluster(s), 1 leg

🚑 7.63 ⚕ 10.2 **FUD** 090 　　　　T A2 50 ▣

**AMA:** 2017,Jan,8; 2016,Jan,13; 2015,Jan,16; 2014,Jan,11; 2012,Jan,15-42

## 37788-37790 Treatment of Vascular Disease of the Penis

**37788** Penile revascularization, artery, with or without vein graft ♂

🚑 36.5 ⚕ 36.5 **FUD** 090 　　　　C 80 ▣

**AMA:** 2014,Jan,11

**37790** Penile venous occlusive procedure

🚑 14.0 ⚕ 14.0 **FUD** 090 　　　　J A2 80 ▣

**AMA:** 2014,Jan,11

## 37799 Unlisted Vascular Surgery Procedures

**CMS:** 100-04,32,161 Intracranial Percutaneous Transluminal Angioplasty (PTA) With Stenting; 100-04,4,180.3 Unlisted Service or Procedure

**37799** Unlisted procedure, vascular surgery

🚑 0.00 ⚕ 0.00 **FUD** YYY 　　　　T 80

**AMA:** 2017,Jan,8; 2016,Nov,3; 2016,Jan,13; 2015,Apr,10; 2015,Jan,16; 2014,Oct,6; 2014,Aug,14; 2014,Mar,8; 2014,Jan,11; 2013,Nov,14; 2012,Jan,15-42

## 38100-38200 Splenic Procedures

**38100** Splenectomy; total (separate procedure)

🚑 33.4 ⚕ 33.4 **FUD** 090 　　　　C 80 ▣

**AMA:** 2017,Jan,8; 2016,Jan,13; 2015,Jan,16; 2014,Jan,11; 2012,Oct,3-8; 2012,Sep,11-13

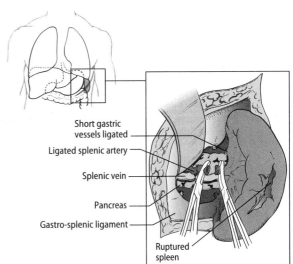

Short gastric vessels ligated
Ligated splenic artery
Splenic vein
Pancreas
Gastro-splenic ligament
Ruptured spleen

**38101** partial (separate procedure)

🚑 33.4 ⚕ 33.4 **FUD** 090 　　　　C 80 ▣

**AMA:** 2017,Jan,8; 2016,Jan,13; 2015,Jan,16; 2014,Jan,11; 2012,Oct,3-8; 2012,Sep,11-13

➕ **38102** total, en bloc for extensive disease, in conjunction with other procedure (List in addition to code for primary procedure)

> Code first primary procedure

🚑 7.62 ⚕ 7.62 **FUD** ZZZ 　　　　C 80 ▣

**AMA:** 2017,Jan,8; 2016,Jan,13; 2015,Jan,16; 2014,Jan,11; 2012,Oct,3-8; 2012,Sep,11-13

**38115** Repair of ruptured spleen (splenorrhaphy) with or without partial splenectomy

🚑 36.7 ⚕ 36.7 **FUD** 090 　　　　C 80 ▣

**AMA:** 2017,Jan,8; 2016,Jan,13; 2015,Jan,16; 2014,Jan,11; 2012,Oct,3-8; 2012,Sep,11-13

**38120** Laparoscopy, surgical, splenectomy

> INCLUDES *Diagnostic laparoscopy (49320)*

🚑 30.4 ⚕ 30.4 **FUD** 090 　　　　J 80 ▣

**AMA:** 2017,Jan,8; 2016,Jan,13; 2015,Jan,16; 2014,Jan,11; 2012,Oct,3-8; 2012,Sep,11-13

**38129** Unlisted laparoscopy procedure, spleen

🚑 0.00 ⚕ 0.00 **FUD** YYY 　　　　J 80

**AMA:** 2017,Jan,8; 2016,Jan,13; 2015,Jan,16; 2014,Jan,11; 2012,Oct,3-8; 2012,Sep,11-13

**38200** Injection procedure for splenoportography

> ⚡ (75810)

🚑 3.92 ⚕ 3.92 **FUD** 000 　　　　N N1 80 ▣

**AMA:** 2014,Jan,11

● New Code　▲ Revised Code　○ Reinstated　● New Web Release　▲ Revised Web Release　Unlisted　Not Covered　# Resequenced
⊘ AMA Mod 51 Exempt　⑧ Optum Mod 51 Exempt　⑱ Mod 63 Exempt　✐ Non-FDA Drug　★ Telemedicine　Ⓜ Maternity　Ⓐ Age Edit　+ Add-on　**AMA:** CPT Asst
© 2017 Optum360, LLC　　　CPT © 2017 American Medical Association. All Rights Reserved.　　　**169**

Cardiovascular, Hemic, and Lymphatic

38204 — 38232

## 38204-38215 Hematopoietic Stem Cell Preparation

**CMS:** 100-03,110.23 Stem Cell Transplantation; 100-04,3,90.3 Stem Cell Transplantation; 100-04,3,90.3.1 Allogeneic Stem Cell Transplantation; 100-04,3,90.3.3 Billing for Allogeneic Stem Cell Transplants; 100-04,32,90 Billing for Stem Cell Transplantation; 100-04,32,90.2.1 Coding for Stem Cell Transplantation; 100-04,4,231.10 Billing for Autologous Stem Cell Transplants; 100-04,4,231.11 Billing for Allogeneic Stem Cell Transplants

INCLUDES Preservation, preparation, purification of stem cells before transplant or reinfusion

EXCLUDES *Procedure performed more than one time per day*

**38204** **Management of recipient hematopoietic progenitor cell donor search and cell acquisition**

🚑 3.04 ⚖ 3.04 **FUD** XXX [N] [N1] [📷]

**AMA:** 2017,Jan,8; 2016,Jan,13; 2015,Jan,16; 2014,Jan,11; 2013,Oct,3

**38205** **Blood-derived hematopoietic progenitor cell harvesting for transplantation, per collection; allogeneic**

🚑 2.40 ⚖ 2.40 **FUD** 000 [B] [80] [📷]

**AMA:** 2017,Jan,8; 2016,Jan,13; 2015,Jan,16; 2014,Jan,11; 2013,Oct,3

**38206** **autologous**

🚑 2.40 ⚖ 2.40 **FUD** 000 [S] [G2] [80] [📷]

**AMA:** 2017,Jan,8; 2016,Jan,13; 2015,Jan,16; 2014,Jan,11; 2013,Oct,3

**38207** **Transplant preparation of hematopoietic progenitor cells; cryopreservation and storage**

EXCLUDES *Flow cytometry (88182, 88184-88189)*

🔬 (88240)

🚑 1.35 ⚖ 1.35 **FUD** XXX [S] [📷]

**AMA:** 2017,Jan,8; 2016,Jan,13; 2015,Jan,16; 2014,Jan,11; 2013,Oct,3

**38208** **thawing of previously frozen harvest, without washing, per donor**

EXCLUDES *Flow cytometry (88182, 88184-88189)*

🔬 (88241)

🚑 0.86 ⚖ 0.86 **FUD** XXX [S] [📷]

**AMA:** 2017,Jan,8; 2016,Jan,13; 2015,Jan,16; 2014,Jan,11; 2013,Oct,3

**38209** **thawing of previously frozen harvest, with washing, per donor**

EXCLUDES *Flow cytometry (88182, 88184-88189)*

🚑 0.36 ⚖ 0.36 **FUD** XXX [S] [📷]

**AMA:** 2017,Jan,8; 2016,Jan,13; 2015,Jan,16; 2014,Jan,11; 2013,Oct,3

**38210** **specific cell depletion within harvest, T-cell depletion**

EXCLUDES *Flow cytometry (88182, 88184-88189)*

🚑 2.38 ⚖ 2.38 **FUD** XXX [S] [📷]

**AMA:** 2017,Jan,8; 2016,Jan,13; 2015,Jan,16; 2014,Jan,11; 2013,Oct,3

**38211** **tumor cell depletion**

EXCLUDES *Flow cytometry (88182, 88184-88189)*

🚑 2.16 ⚖ 2.16 **FUD** XXX [S] [📷]

**AMA:** 2017,Jan,8; 2016,Jan,13; 2015,Jan,16; 2014,Jan,11; 2013,Oct,3

**38212** **red blood cell removal**

EXCLUDES *Flow cytometry (88182, 88184-88189)*

🚑 1.43 ⚖ 1.43 **FUD** XXX [S] [📷]

**AMA:** 2017,Jan,8; 2016,Jan,13; 2015,Jan,16; 2014,Jan,11; 2013,Oct,3

**38213** **platelet depletion**

EXCLUDES *Flow cytometry (88182, 88184-88189)*

🚑 0.36 ⚖ 0.36 **FUD** XXX [S] [📷]

**AMA:** 2017,Jan,8; 2016,Jan,13; 2015,Jan,16; 2014,Jan,11; 2013,Oct,3

**38214** **plasma (volume) depletion**

EXCLUDES *Flow cytometry (88182, 88184-88189)*

🚑 1.23 ⚖ 1.23 **FUD** XXX [S] [📷]

**AMA:** 2017,Jan,8; 2016,Jan,13; 2015,Jan,16; 2014,Jan,11; 2013,Oct,3

**38215** **cell concentration in plasma, mononuclear, or buffy coat layer**

EXCLUDES *Flow cytometry (88182, 88184-88189)*

🚑 1.43 ⚖ 1.43 **FUD** XXX [S] [📷]

**AMA:** 2017,Jan,8; 2016,Jan,13; 2015,Jan,16; 2014,Jan,11; 2013,Oct,3

## 38220-38232 Bone Marrow Procedures

**CMS:** 100-03,110.23 Stem Cell Transplantation; 100-04,3,90.3 Stem Cell Transplantation; 100-04,32,90 Billing for Stem Cell Transplantation; 100-04,4,231.11 Billing for Allogeneic Stem Cell Transplants

▲ **38220** **Diagnostic bone marrow; aspiration(s)**

EXCLUDES *Aspiration of bone marrow for spinal graft (20939)*
*Bone marrow biopsy (38221)*
*Bone marrow for platelet rich stem cell injection (0232T)*
Code also biopsy bone marrow during same session (38222)

🚑 1.78 ⚖ 4.77 **FUD** XXX [J] [P3] [80] [50] [📷]

**AMA:** 2017,Jan,8; 2016,Jan,13; 2015,Mar,9; 2015,Jan,16; 2014,Jan,11; 2013,Oct,3; 2012,May,11-12; 2012,Apr,14-16; 2012,Jan,15-42

▲ **38221** **biopsy(ies)**

EXCLUDES *Aspiration and biopsy during same session (38220)*
*Aspiration of bone marrow (38220)*

🔬 (88305)

🚑 2.15 ⚖ 4.77 **FUD** XXX [J] [P3] [80] [50] [📷]

**AMA:** 2017,Jan,8; 2016,Jan,13; 2015,Mar,9; 2014,Jan,11; 2012,May,11-12

● **38222** **biopsy(ies) and aspiration(s)**

EXCLUDES *Aspiration of bone marrow only (38221)*
*Biopsy of bone marrow only (38220)*

🔬 (88305)

**38230** **Bone marrow harvesting for transplantation; allogeneic**

EXCLUDES *Aspiration of bone marrow for platelet rich stem cell injection (0232T)*
*Harvesting of blood-derived hematopoietic progenitor cells for transplant (allogeneic) (38205)*

🚑 5.73 ⚖ 5.73 **FUD** 000 [S] [G2] [80] [📷]

**AMA:** 2017,Jan,8; 2016,Jan,13; 2015,Jan,16; 2014,Jan,11; 2013,Oct,3; 2012,May,11-12

**38232** **autologous**

EXCLUDES *Aspiration of bone marrow (38220, 38222)*
*Aspiration of bone marrow for platelet rich stem cell injection (0232T)*
*Aspiration of bone marrow for spinal graft (20939)*
*Harvesting of blood-derived peripheral stem cells for transplant (allogenic/autologous) (38205-38206)*

🚑 5.65 ⚖ 5.65 **FUD** 000 [S] [J8] [80] [📷]

**AMA:** 2017,Jan,8; 2016,Jan,13; 2015,Jan,16; 2014,Jan,11; 2013,Oct,3; 2012,May,11-12

## 38240-38243 [38243] Hematopoietic Progenitor Cell Transplantation

**CMS:** 100-03,110.23 Stem Cell Transplantation; 100-04,3,90.3 Stem Cell Transplantation; 100-04,3,90.3.1 Allogeneic Stem Cell Transplantation; 100-04,3,90.3.2 Autologous Stem Cell Transplantation (AuSCT); 100-04,3,90.3.3 Billing for Allogeneic Stem Cell Transplants; 100-04,32,90 Billing for Stem Cell Transplantation; 100-04,32,90.2 Allogeneic Stem Cell Transplantation; 100-04,32,90.2.1 Coding for Stem Cell Transplantation; 100-04,32,90.3 Autologous Stem Cell Transplantation; 100-04,32,90.4 Edits Stem Cell Transplant; 100-04,32,90.6 Clinical Trials for Stem Cell Transplant for Myelodysplastic Syndrome (; 100-04,4,231.10 Billing for Autologous Stem Cell Transplants; 100-04,4,231.11 Billing for Allogeneic Stem Cell Transplants

INCLUDES  Evaluation of patient prior to, during, and after the infusion
Management of uncomplicated adverse reactions such as hives or nausea
Monitoring of physiological parameters
Physician presence during the infusion
Supervision of clinical staff

EXCLUDES  *Administration of fluids for the transplant or for incidental hydration separately*
*Concurrent administration of medications with the infusion for the transplant*
*Cryopreservation, freezing, and storage of hematopoietic progenitor cells for transplant (38207)*
*Human leukocyte antigen (HLA) testing (81379-81383, 86812-86821)*
*Modification, treatment, processing of hematopoietic progenitor cell specimens for transplant (38210-38215)*
*Thawing and expansion of hematopoietic progenitor cells for transplant (38208-38209)*

Code also administration of medications and/or fluids not related to the transplant with modifier 59
Code also E&M service for the treatment of more complicated adverse reactions after the infusion, as appropriate
Code also separately identifiable E&M service on the same date, using modifier 25 as appropriate (99211-99215, 99217-99220, [99224, 99225, 99226], 99221-99223, 99231-99239, 99471-99472, 99475-99476)

**38240**  **Hematopoietic progenitor cell (HPC); allogeneic transplantation per donor**

EXCLUDES  *Allogeneic lymphocyte infusions on same date of service with (38242)*
*Hematopoietic progenitor cell (HPC); HPC boost on same date of service with ([38243])*

🔲 6.46  🔲 6.46  **FUD** XXX    J 80 🔲

**AMA:** 2017,Jan,8; 2016,Jan,13; 2015,Jan,16; 2014,Jan,11; 2013,Oct,3

**38241**  **autologous transplantation**

🔲 4.83  🔲 4.83  **FUD** XXX    S 62 80 🔲

**AMA:** 2017,Jan,8; 2016,Jan,13; 2015,Jan,16; 2014,Jan,11; 2013,Oct,3

\# **38243**  **HPC boost**

EXCLUDES  *Allogeneic lymphocyte infusions on same date of service with (38242)*
*Hematopoietic progenitor cell (HPC); allogeneic transplantation per donor on same date of service with (38240)*

🔲 3.42  🔲 3.42  **FUD** 000    S R2 80 🔲

**AMA:** 2017,Jan,8; 2016,Jan,13; 2015,Feb,10; 2015,Jan,16; 2014,Jan,11; 2013,Oct,3; 2013,Jun,13

**38242**  **Allogeneic lymphocyte infusions**

EXCLUDES  *Aspiration of bone marrow (38220, 38222)*
*Aspiration of bone marrow for platelet rich stem cell injection (0232T)*
*Aspiration of bone marrow for spinal graft (20939)*
*Hematopoietic progenitor cell (HPC); allogeneic transplantation per donor on same date of service with (38240)*
*Hematopoietic progenitor cell (HPC); HPC boost on same date of service with ([38243])*

🔲 (81379-81383, 86812-86813, 86816-86817, 86821)

🔲 3.42  🔲 3.42  **FUD** 000    S R2 80 🔲

**AMA:** 2017,Jan,8; 2016,Jan,13; 2015,Jan,16; 2014,Jan,11; 2013,Oct,3; 2013,Jun,13

*38243*  **Resequenced code. See code following 38241.**

## 38300-38382 Incision Lymphatic Vessels

**38300**  **Drainage of lymph node abscess or lymphadenitis; simple**

🔲 5.23  🔲 7.74  **FUD** 010    J A2 🔲

**AMA:** 2014,Jan,11

**38305**  **extensive**

🔲 13.2  🔲 13.2  **FUD** 090    J A2 🔲

**AMA:** 2014,Jan,11

**38308**  **Lymphangiotomy or other operations on lymphatic channels**

🔲 12.8  🔲 12.8  **FUD** 090    J A2 80 🔲

**AMA:** 2014,Jan,11

**38380**  **Suture and/or ligation of thoracic duct; cervical approach**

🔲 16.1  🔲 16.1  **FUD** 090    C 80 🔲

**AMA:** 2014,Jan,11

**38381**  **thoracic approach**

🔲 23.2  🔲 23.2  **FUD** 090    C 80 🔲

**AMA:** 2014,Jan,11

**38382**  **abdominal approach**

🔲 19.4  🔲 19.4  **FUD** 090    C 80 🔲

**AMA:** 2014,Jan,11

## 38500-38555 Biopsy/Excision Lymphatic Vessels

EXCLUDES  *Injection for sentinel node identification (38792)*
*Percutaneous needle biopsy retroperitoneal mass (49180)*

**38500**  **Biopsy or excision of lymph node(s); open, superficial**

EXCLUDES  *Lymphadenectomy (38700-38780)*

🔲 7.34  🔲 9.49  **FUD** 010    J A2 50 🔲

**AMA:** 2017,Jan,8; 2016,Jan,13; 2015,Jan,16; 2014,Jan,11; 2012,Jun,15-16; 2012,Jan,15-42

**38505**  **by needle, superficial (eg, cervical, inguinal, axillary)**

EXCLUDES  *Fine needle aspiration (10021-10022)*

🔲 (76942, 77002, 77012, 77021)

🔲 2.06  🔲 3.59  **FUD** 000    J A2 50 🔲

**AMA:** 2017,Jan,8; 2016,Jan,13; 2015,Jan,16; 2014,Jan,11; 2012,Jan,15-42

**38510**  **open, deep cervical node(s)**

🔲 12.1  🔲 14.8  **FUD** 010    J A2 50 🔲

**AMA:** 2017,Jan,8; 2016,Jan,13; 2015,Jan,16; 2014,Jan,11; 2012,Jun,15-16; 2012,Jan,15-42

**38520**  **open, deep cervical node(s) with excision scalene fat pad**

🔲 13.3  🔲 13.3  **FUD** 090    J A2 50 🔲

**AMA:** 2017,Jan,8; 2016,Jan,13; 2015,Jan,16; 2014,Jan,11; 2012,Jan,15-42

**38525**  **open, deep axillary node(s)**

🔲 12.6  🔲 12.6  **FUD** 090    J A2 50 🔲

**AMA:** 2017,Jan,8; 2016,Jan,13; 2015,Mar,5; 2015,Jan,16; 2014,Apr,10; 2014,Jan,11; 2012,Jan,15-42

**38530**  **open, internal mammary node(s)**

EXCLUDES  *Fine needle aspiration (10022)*
*Lymphadenectomy (38720-38746)*

🔲 15.9  🔲 15.9  **FUD** 090    J A2 80 50 🔲

**AMA:** 2017,Jan,8; 2016,Jan,13; 2015,Jan,16; 2014,Apr,10; 2014,Jan,11

**38542**  **Dissection, deep jugular node(s)**

EXCLUDES  *Complete cervical lymphadenectomy (38720)*

🔲 14.9  🔲 14.9  **FUD** 090    J A2 80 50 🔲

**AMA:** 2017,Jan,8; 2016,Jan,13; 2015,Jan,16; 2014,Jan,11

**38550**  **Excision of cystic hygroma, axillary or cervical; without deep neurovascular dissection**

🔲 14.5  🔲 14.5  **FUD** 090    J A2 80 🔲

**AMA:** 2014,Jan,11

**38555**  **with deep neurovascular dissection**

🔲 29.3  🔲 29.3  **FUD** 090    J A2 80 🔲

**AMA:** 2014,Jan,11

● New Code  ▲ Revised Code  ○ Reinstated  ● New Web Release  ▲ Revised Web Release  Unlisted  Not Covered  # Resequenced
⊘ AMA Mod 51 Exempt  ⑨ Optum Mod 51 Exempt  ㉚ Mod 63 Exempt  ✗ Non-FDA Drug  ★ Telemedicine  Ⓜ Maternity  Ⓐ Age Edit  + Add-on  AMA: CPT Asst
© 2017 Optum360, LLC

## 38562-38564 Limited Lymphadenectomy: Staging

**38562** **Limited lymphadenectomy for staging (separate procedure); pelvic and para-aortic**

> **EXCLUDES** Prostatectomy (55812, 55842)
> Radioactive substance inserted into prostate (55862)

> 🔧 20.3    ✂ 20.3    **FUD** 090    Ⓒ 80 ▭

> **AMA:** 2017,Jan,8; 2016,Jan,13; 2015,Jan,16; 2014,Jan,11; 2012,Jan,15-42

**38564** **retroperitoneal (aortic and/or splenic)**

> 🔧 20.2    ✂ 20.2    **FUD** 090    Ⓒ 80 ▭

> **AMA:** 2014,Jan,11

## 38570-38589 Laparoscopic Lymph Node Procedures

> **INCLUDES** Diagnostic laparoscopy (49320)
> **EXCLUDES** Laparoscopy with draining of lymphocele to peritoneal cavity (49323)
> Limited lymphadenectomy:
>   Pelvic (38562)
>   Retroperitoneal (38564)

**38570** **Laparoscopy, surgical; with retroperitoneal lymph node sampling (biopsy), single or multiple**

> 🔧 14.5    ✂ 14.5    **FUD** 010    J A2 80 ▭

> **AMA:** 2017,Jan,8; 2016,Jan,13; 2015,Jan,16; 2014,Jan,11

**38571** **with bilateral total pelvic lymphadenectomy**

> 🔧 19.3    ✂ 19.3    **FUD** 010    J A2 80 ▭

> **AMA:** 2017,Jan,8; 2016,Jan,13; 2015,Jan,16; 2014,Jan,11

**38572** **with bilateral total pelvic lymphadenectomy and peri-aortic lymph node sampling (biopsy), single or multiple**

> **EXCLUDES** Lymphocele drainage into peritoneal cavity (49323)

> 🔧 27.1    ✂ 27.1    **FUD** 010    J A2 80 ▭

> **AMA:** 2017,Jan,8; 2016,Jan,13; 2015,Jan,16; 2015,Jan,13; 2014,Jan,11

● **38573** **with bilateral total pelvic lymphadenectomy and peri-aortic lymph node sampling, peritoneal washings, peritoneal biopsy(ies), omentectomy, and diaphragmatic washings, including diaphragmatic and other serosal biopsy(ies), when performed**

> **EXCLUDES** Laparoscopy abdomen, diagnostic (separate procedure)(49320)
> Laparoscopic hysterectomy procedures (58541-58554)
> Laparoscopic omentopexy (separate procedure) (49326)
> Laparoscopy unlisted (38589)
> Laparoscopy without omentectomy (38570-38572)
> Lymphadenectomy for staging (38562-38564)
> Omentectomy (separate procedure) (49255)
> Pelvic lymphadenectomy of external iliac, hypogastric, and obturator nodes (38770)
> Retroperitoneal lymphadenectomy of aortic, pelvic, and renal nodes (separate procedure)(38780)

**38589** **Unlisted laparoscopy procedure, lymphatic system**

> 🔧 0.00    ✂ 0.00    **FUD** YYY    J 80 50

> **AMA:** 2017,Jan,8; 2016,Jan,13; 2015,Jan,16; 2014,Jan,11

## 38700-38780 Lymphadenectomy Procedures

> **INCLUDES** Lymph node biopsy/excision (38500)
> **EXCLUDES** Excision of lymphedematous skin and subcutaneous tissue (15004-15005)
> Limited lymphadenectomy
>   Pelvic (38562)
>   Retroperitoneal (38564)
> Repair of lymphedematous skin and tissue (15570-15650)

**38700** **Suprahyoid lymphadenectomy**

> 🔧 23.1    ✂ 23.1    **FUD** 090    J 62 80 50 ▭

> **AMA:** 2017,Jan,8; 2016,Jan,13; 2015,Jan,16; 2014,Jan,11

**38720** **Cervical lymphadenectomy (complete)**

> 🔧 38.7    ✂ 38.7    **FUD** 090    J 80 50 ▭

> **AMA:** 2017,Jan,8; 2016,Jan,13; 2015,Jan,16; 2014,Jan,11; 2012,Jan,15-42

**38724** **Cervical lymphadenectomy (modified radical neck dissection)**

> 🔧 41.8    ✂ 41.8    **FUD** 090    Ⓒ 80 50 ▭

> **AMA:** 2017,Jan,8; 2016,Jan,13; 2015,Jan,16; 2014,Jan,11; 2012,Dec,3-5; 2012,Jan,15-42

**38740** **Axillary lymphadenectomy; superficial**

> 🔧 20.0    ✂ 20.0    **FUD** 090    J A2 80 50 ▭

> **AMA:** 2017,Jan,8; 2016,Jan,13; 2015,Jan,16; 2014,Apr,10; 2014,Jan,11

**38745** **complete**

> 🔧 25.3    ✂ 25.3    **FUD** 090    J A2 80 50 ▭

> **AMA:** 2014,Jan,11

+ **38746** **Thoracic lymphadenectomy by thoracotomy, mediastinal and regional lymphadenectomy (List separately in addition to code for primary procedure)**

> **INCLUDES** Left side
>   Aortopulmonary window
>   Inferior pulmonary ligament
>   Paraesophageal
>   Subcarinal
> Right side
>   Inferior pulmonary ligament
>   Paraesophageal
>   Paratracheal
>   Subcarinal

> **EXCLUDES** Thoracoscopic mediastinal and regional lymphadenectomy (32674)
> Code first primary procedure (19260, 31760, 31766, 31786, 32096-32200, 32220-32320, 32440-32491, 32503-32505, 33025, 33030, 33050-33130, 39200-39220, 39560-39561, 43101, 43112, 43117-43118, 43122-43123, 43351, 60270, 60505)

> 🔧 6.25    ✂ 6.25    **FUD** ZZZ    Ⓒ 80 ▭

> **AMA:** 2017,Jan,8; 2016,Jan,13; 2015,Jan,16; 2014,May,3; 2014,Jan,11; 2012,Oct,9-11; 2012,Sep,3-8

Parasternal nodes

Central nodes

+ **38747** **Abdominal lymphadenectomy, regional, including celiac, gastric, portal, peripancreatic, with or without para-aortic and vena caval nodes (List separately in addition to code for primary procedure)**

> Code first primary procedure
> 🔧 7.75    ✂ 7.75    **FUD** ZZZ    Ⓒ 80 ▭

> **AMA:** 2014,Jan,11

**38760** **Inguinofemoral lymphadenectomy, superficial, including Cloquet's node (separate procedure)**

> 🔧 24.3    ✂ 24.3    **FUD** 090    J A2 80 50 ▭

> **AMA:** 2017,Jan,8; 2016,Jan,13; 2015,Jan,16; 2014,Jan,11; 2012,Jan,15-42

**38765** Inguinofemoral lymphadenectomy, superficial, in continuity with pelvic lymphadenectomy, including external iliac, hypogastric, and obturator nodes (separate procedure)
37.4    37.4    **FUD** 090    C 80 50
**AMA:** 2017,Jan,8; 2016,Jan,13; 2015,Jan,16; 2014,Jan,11; 2012,Jan,15-42

**38770** Pelvic lymphadenectomy, including external iliac, hypogastric, and obturator nodes (separate procedure)
23.3    23.3    **FUD** 090    C 80 50
**AMA:** 2014,Jan,11

**38780** Retroperitoneal transabdominal lymphadenectomy, extensive, including pelvic, aortic, and renal nodes (separate procedure)
29.6    29.6    **FUD** 090    C 80
**AMA:** 2014,Jan,11

## 38790-38999 Cannulation/Injection/Other Procedures

**38790** Injection procedure; lymphangiography
(75801-75807)
2.40    2.40    **FUD** 000    N N1 50
**AMA:** 2014,Jan,11

**38792** radioactive tracer for identification of sentinel node
*EXCLUDES* Sentinel node excision (38500-38542)
Sentinel node(s) identification (mapping) intraoperative with nonradioactive dye injection (38900)
(78195)
1.15    1.15    **FUD** 000    01 N1 50
**AMA:** 2017,Jan,8; 2016,Jan,13; 2015,Mar,5; 2015,Jan,16; 2014,Jan,11

**38794** Cannulation, thoracic duct
8.66    8.66    **FUD** 090    N N1 80
**AMA:** 2014,Jan,11

+ **38900** Intraoperative identification (eg, mapping) of sentinel lymph node(s) includes injection of non-radioactive dye, when performed (List separately in addition to code for primary procedure)
*EXCLUDES* Injection of tracer for sentinel node identification (38792)
Code first (19302, 19307, 38500, 38510, 38520, 38525, 38530, 38542, 38740, 38745)
4.01    4.01    **FUD** ZZZ    N N1 80 50
**AMA:** 2017,Jan,8; 2016,Jan,13; 2015,Mar,5; 2014,Jan,11

**38999** Unlisted procedure, hemic or lymphatic system
0.00    0.00    **FUD** YYY    S 80
**AMA:** 2017,Jan,8; 2016,Jan,13; 2015,Jan,16; 2014,Jan,11; 2012,Jan,15-42

## 39000-39499 Surgical Procedures: Mediastinum

**39000** Mediastinotomy with exploration, drainage, removal of foreign body, or biopsy; cervical approach
14.3    14.3    **FUD** 090    C 80
**AMA:** 2014,Jan,11

**39010** transthoracic approach, including either transthoracic or median sternotomy
*EXCLUDES* ECMO/ECLS insertion or reposition of cannula (33955-33956, [33963, 33964])
Video-assisted thoracic surgery (VATS) pericardial biopsy (32604)
22.8    22.8    **FUD** 090    C 80
**AMA:** 2017,Jan,8; 2016,Jan,13; 2015,Jul,3; 2015,Jan,16; 2014,Jan,11; 2014,Jan,5; 2013,Jan,6-8

**39200** Resection of mediastinal cyst
25.2    25.2    **FUD** 090    C 80
**AMA:** 2014,Jan,11; 2012,Oct,9-11; 2012,Sep,3-8

**39220** Resection of mediastinal tumor
*EXCLUDES* Thymectomy (60520)
Thyroidectomy, substernal (60270)
Video-assisted thoracic surgery (VATS) resection cyst, mass, or tumor of mediastinum (32662)
32.8    32.8    **FUD** 090    C 80
**AMA:** 2014,Jan,11; 2012,Oct,9-11; 2012,Sep,3-8

**39401** Mediastinoscopy; includes biopsy(ies) of mediastinal mass (eg, lymphoma), when performed
9.02    9.02    **FUD** 000    J
**AMA:** 2017,Jan,8; 2016,Jun,4

**39402** with lymph node biopsy(ies) (eg, lung cancer staging)
11.7    11.7    **FUD** 000    J
**AMA:** 2017,Jan,8; 2016,Jun,4

**39499** Unlisted procedure, mediastinum
0.00    0.00    **FUD** YYY    C 80
**AMA:** 2014,Jan,11

## 39501-39599 Surgical Procedures: Diaphragm

*EXCLUDES* Esophagogastric fundoplasty, with fundic patch (43325)
Repair of diaphragmatic (esophageal) hernias:
Laparoscopic with fundoplication (43280-43282)
Laparotomy (43332-43333)
Thoracoabdominal (43336-43337)
Thoracotomy (43334-43335)

**39501** Repair, laceration of diaphragm, any approach
24.5    24.5    **FUD** 090    C 80
**AMA:** 2017,Jan,8; 2016,Jan,13; 2015,Jan,16; 2014,Dec,16; 2014,Dec,16; 2014,Jan,11

**39503** Repair, neonatal diaphragmatic hernia, with or without chest tube insertion and with or without creation of ventral hernia    A
172.    172.    **FUD** 090    63 C 80
**AMA:** 2017,Jan,8; 2016,Jan,13; 2015,Jan,16; 2014,Jan,11; 2012,Feb,3-7

Trachea

Lungs

Diaphragm

A defect of the diaphragm can allow abdominal contents to herniate into the thoracic cavity

**39540** Repair, diaphragmatic hernia (other than neonatal), traumatic; acute
25.1    25.1    **FUD** 090    C 80
**AMA:** 2017,Jan,8; 2016,Jan,13; 2015,Jan,16; 2014,Jan,11

**39541** chronic
27.3    27.3    **FUD** 090    C 80
**AMA:** 2017,Jan,8; 2016,Jan,13; 2015,Jan,16; 2014,Jan,11

**39545** Imbrication of diaphragm for eventration, transthoracic or transabdominal, paralytic or nonparalytic
25.6    25.6    **FUD** 090    C 80
**AMA:** 2017,Jan,8; 2016,Jan,13; 2015,Jan,16; 2014,Jan,11

**39560** Resection, diaphragm; with simple repair (eg, primary suture)

      🚑 23.1   ⚕ 23.1   **FUD** 090      C 80 ▭

      **AMA:** 2017,Jan,8; 2016,Jan,13; 2015,Jan,16; 2014,Jan,11

**39561** with complex repair (eg, prosthetic material, local muscle flap)

      🚑 35.9   ⚕ 35.9   **FUD** 090      C 80 ▭

      **AMA:** 2017,Jan,8; 2016,Jan,13; 2015,Jan,16; 2014,Jan,11

**39599** Unlisted procedure, diaphragm

      🚑 0.00   ⚕ 0.00   **FUD** YYY      C 80

      **AMA:** 2014,Jan,11

| | | | | | | | |
|---|---|---|---|---|---|---|---|
| 26/TC PC/TC Only | A2-Z3 ASC Payment | 50 Bilateral | ♂ Male Only | ♀ Female Only | 🚑 Facility RVU | ⚕ Non-Facility RVU | ▭ CCI |
| **FUD** Follow-up Days | **CMS:** IOM (Pub 100) | A-Y OPPSI | 80/80 Surg Assist Allowed / w/Doc | | ◼ Lab Crosswalk | ⬚ Radiology Crosswalk | ✖ CLIA |

**174**

CPT © 2017 American Medical Association. All Rights Reserved.

© 2017 Optum360, LLC

# 40490-40799 Resection and Repair Procedures of the Lips

EXCLUDES Procedures on the skin of lips-see integumenary section codes

**40490** **Biopsy of lip**
📋 2.13 ⚕ 3.69 **FUD** 000 T P3 🖿
**AMA:** 2014,Jan,11

**40500** **Vermilionectomy (lip shave), with mucosal advancement**
📋 10.5 ⚕ 14.5 **FUD** 090 J A2 🖿
**AMA:** 2014,Jan,11

**40510** **Excision of lip; transverse wedge excision with primary closure**
EXCLUDES Excision of mucous lesions (40810-40816)
📋 10.3 ⚕ 13.9 **FUD** 090 J A2 🖿
**AMA:** 2014,Jan,11

**40520** **V-excision with primary direct linear closure**
EXCLUDES Excision of mucous lesions (40810-40816)
📋 10.3 ⚕ 14.0 **FUD** 090 J A2 🖿
**AMA:** 2014,Jan,11

**40525** **full thickness, reconstruction with local flap (eg, Estlander or fan)**
📋 15.9 ⚕ 15.9 **FUD** 090 J A2 🖿
**AMA:** 2014,Jan,11

**40527** **full thickness, reconstruction with cross lip flap (Abbe-Estlander)**
INCLUDES Cleft lip repair with cross lip pedicle flap (Abbe-Estlander type), without pedicle sectioning and insertion
EXCLUDES Cleft lip repair with cross lip pedicle flap (Abbe-Estlander type), with pedicle sectioning and insertion (40761)
📋 18.0 ⚕ 18.0 **FUD** 090 J A2 80 🖿
**AMA:** 2014,Jan,11

**40530** **Resection of lip, more than one-fourth, without reconstruction**
EXCLUDES Reconstruction (13131-13153)
📋 11.6 ⚕ 15.4 **FUD** 090 J A2 🖿
**AMA:** 2014,Jan,11

**40650** **Repair lip, full thickness; vermilion only**
📋 8.63 ⚕ 12.5 **FUD** 090 T A2 80 🖿
**AMA:** 2017,Jan,8; 2016,Nov,7; 2016,Jan,13; 2015,Jan,16; 2014,Jan,11; 2012,Jan,15-42

**40652** **up to half vertical height**
📋 10.2 ⚕ 14.1 **FUD** 090 T A2 80 🖿
**AMA:** 2017,Jan,8; 2016,Nov,7; 2016,Jan,13; 2015,Jan,16; 2014,Jan,11; 2012,Jan,15-42

**40654** **over one-half vertical height, or complex**
📋 12.3 ⚕ 16.4 **FUD** 090 T A2 🖿
**AMA:** 2017,Jan,8; 2016,Nov,7; 2014,Jan,11

**40700** **Plastic repair of cleft lip/nasal deformity; primary, partial or complete, unilateral**
EXCLUDES Cleft lip repair with cross lip pedicle flap (Abbe-Estlander type):
With pedicle sectioning and insertion (40761)
Without pedicle sectioning and insertion (40527)
Rhinoplasty for nasal deformity secondary to congenital cleft lip (30460, 30462)
📋 29.2 ⚕ 29.2 **FUD** 090 J A2 80 🖿
**AMA:** 2017,Jan,8; 2016,Jan,13; 2015,Jan,16; 2014,Dec,18; 2014,Jan,11

**40701** **primary bilateral, 1-stage procedure**
EXCLUDES Cleft lip repair with cross lip pedicle flap (Abbe-Estlander type):
With pedicle sectioning and insertion (40761)
Without pedicle sectioning and insertion (40527)
Rhinoplasty for nasal deformity secondary to congenital cleft lip (30460, 30462)
📋 34.6 ⚕ 34.6 **FUD** 090 J A2 80 🖿
**AMA:** 2017,Jan,8; 2016,Jan,13; 2015,Jan,16; 2014,Dec,18; 2014,Jan,11

Bilateral cleft lip

Cleft margins on both sides are incised

Margins are closed, correcting cleft

**40702** **primary bilateral, 1 of 2 stages**
EXCLUDES Cleft lip repair with cross lip pedicle flap (Abbe-Estlander type):
With pedicle sectioning and insertion (40761)
Without pedicle sectioning and insertion (40527)
Rhinoplasty for nasal deformity secondary to congenital cleft lip (30460, 30462)
📋 26.0 ⚕ 26.0 **FUD** 090 J R2 80 🖿
**AMA:** 2017,Jan,8; 2016,Jan,13; 2015,Jan,16; 2014,Dec,18; 2014,Jan,11

**40720** **secondary, by recreation of defect and reclosure**
EXCLUDES Cleft lip repair with cross lip pedicle flap (Abbe-Estlander type):
With pedicle sectioning and insertion (40761)
Without pedicle sectioning and insertion (40527)
Rhinoplasty for nasal deformity secondary to congenital cleft lip (30460, 30462)
📋 28.8 ⚕ 28.8 **FUD** 090 J A2 80 50 🖿
**AMA:** 2017,Jan,8; 2016,Jan,13; 2015,Jan,16; 2014,Dec,18; 2014,Jan,11

**40761** **with cross lip pedicle flap (Abbe-Estlander type), including sectioning and inserting of pedicle**
EXCLUDES Cleft lip repair with cross lip pedicle flap (Abbe-Estlander type) without sectioning and insertion of pedicle (40527)
Cleft palate repair (42200-42225)
Other reconstructive procedures (14060-14061, 15120-15261, 15574, 15576, 15630)
📋 28.0 ⚕ 28.0 **FUD** 090 J A2 🖿
**AMA:** 2014,Jan,11

**40799** **Unlisted procedure, lips**
📋 0.00 ⚕ 0.00 **FUD** YYY T 80
**AMA:** 2014,Jan,11

# 40800-40819 Incision and Resection of Buccal Cavity

INCLUDES Mucosal/submucosal tissue of lips/cheeks
Oral cavity outside the dentoalveolar structures

**40800** **Drainage of abscess, cyst, hematoma, vestibule of mouth; simple**
📋 3.85 ⚕ 6.16 **FUD** 010 T P3 🖿
**AMA:** 2014,Jan,11

**40801** **complicated**
📋 6.51 ⚕ 9.13 **FUD** 010 T A2 🖿
**AMA:** 2014,Jan,11

**40804** Removal of embedded foreign body, vestibule of mouth; simple
    🔹 3.31   ⚕ 5.31   **FUD** 010   [01] [N1] [80] [▢]
    **AMA:** 2014,Jan,11

**40805** complicated
    🔹 6.81   ⚕ 9.33   **FUD** 010   [T] [P3] [80] [▢]
    **AMA:** 2014,Jan,11

**40806** Incision of labial frenum (frenotomy)
    🔹 0.96   ⚕ 3.02   **FUD** 000   [T] [P3] [80] [▢]
    **AMA:** 2014,Jan,11

**40808** Biopsy, vestibule of mouth
    🔹 3.16   ⚕ 5.39   **FUD** 010   [T] [P3] [▢]
    **AMA:** 2014,Jan,11

**40810** Excision of lesion of mucosa and submucosa, vestibule of mouth; without repair
    🔹 3.72   ⚕ 5.97   **FUD** 010   [J] [P3] [▢]
    **AMA:** 2014,Jan,11

**40812** with simple repair
    🔹 5.78   ⚕ 8.38   **FUD** 010   [J] [P3] [▢]
    **AMA:** 2014,Jan,11

**40814** with complex repair
    🔹 8.93   ⚕ 11.2   **FUD** 090   [J] [A2] [▢]
    **AMA:** 2014,Jan,11

**40816** complex, with excision of underlying muscle
    🔹 9.25   ⚕ 11.6   **FUD** 090   [J] [A2] [▢]
    **AMA:** 2014,Jan,11

**40818** Excision of mucosa of vestibule of mouth as donor graft
    🔹 7.98   ⚕ 10.4   **FUD** 090   [T] [A2] [80] [▢]
    **AMA:** 2014,Jan,11

**40819** Excision of frenum, labial or buccal (frenumectomy, frenulectomy, frenectomy)
    🔹 7.02   ⚕ 9.18   **FUD** 090   [T] [A2] [80] [▢]
    **AMA:** 2014,Jan,11

## 40820 Destruction of Lesion of Buccal Cavity

**CMS:** 100-03,140.5 Laser Procedures
INCLUDES   Mucosal/submucosal tissue of lips/cheeks
           Oral cavity outside the dentoalveolar structures

**40820** Destruction of lesion or scar of vestibule of mouth by physical methods (eg, laser, thermal, cryo, chemical)
    🔹 5.04   ⚕ 7.69   **FUD** 010   [J] [P3] [▢]
    **AMA:** 2014,Jan,11

## 40830-40899 Repair Procedures of the Buccal Cavity

INCLUDES   Mucosal/submucosal tissue of lips/cheeks
           Oral cavity outside the dentoalveolar structures
EXCLUDES   Skin grafts (15002-15630)

**40830** Closure of laceration, vestibule of mouth; 2.5 cm or less
    🔹 4.85   ⚕ 7.76   **FUD** 010   [T] [62] [80] [▢]
    **AMA:** 2014,Jan,11

**40831** over 2.5 cm or complex
    🔹 6.58   ⚕ 9.78   **FUD** 010   [T] [A2] [80] [▢]
    **AMA:** 2014,Jan,11

**40840** Vestibuloplasty; anterior
    🔹 18.2   ⚕ 23.3   **FUD** 090   [J] [A2] [80] [▢]
    **AMA:** 2014,Jan,11

**40842** posterior, unilateral
    🔹 18.8   ⚕ 23.6   **FUD** 090   [J] [A2] [80] [▢]
    **AMA:** 2014,Jan,11

**40843** posterior, bilateral
    🔹 24.8   ⚕ 31.3   **FUD** 090   [J] [A2] [80] [▢]
    **AMA:** 2014,Jan,11

**40844** entire arch
    🔹 30.4   ⚕ 37.2   **FUD** 090   [J] [A2] [80] [▢]
    **AMA:** 2014,Jan,11

**40845** complex (including ridge extension, muscle repositioning)
    🔹 35.5   ⚕ 42.1   **FUD** 090   [J] [A2] [80] [▢]
    **AMA:** 2014,Jan,11

**40899** Unlisted procedure, vestibule of mouth
    🔹 0.00   ⚕ 0.00   **FUD** YYY   [T] [80]
    **AMA:** 2014,Jan,11

## 41000-41018 Surgical Incision of Floor of Mouth or Tongue

EXCLUDES   Frenoplasty (41520)

**41000** Intraoral incision and drainage of abscess, cyst, or hematoma of tongue or floor of mouth; lingual
    🔹 3.27   ⚕ 4.69   **FUD** 010   [T] [P3] [▢]
    **AMA:** 2014,Jan,11

A small incision is made in the floor of the mouth; the cyst is opened and the fluid is drained

Cyst and line of incision

**41005** sublingual, superficial
    🔹 3.63   ⚕ 6.55   **FUD** 010   [T] [A2] [80] [▢]
    **AMA:** 2014,Jan,11

**41006** sublingual, deep, supramylohyoid
    🔹 7.89   ⚕ 11.2   **FUD** 090   [T] [A2] [80] [▢]
    **AMA:** 2014,Jan,11

**41007** submental space
    🔹 7.65   ⚕ 11.0   **FUD** 090   [T] [A2] [80] [▢]
    **AMA:** 2014,Jan,11

**41008** submandibular space
    🔹 7.92   ⚕ 11.0   **FUD** 090   [J] [A2] [80] [▢]
    **AMA:** 2014,Jan,11

**41009** masticator space
    🔹 8.60   ⚕ 11.7   **FUD** 090   [T] [A2] [80] [▢]
    **AMA:** 2014,Jan,11

**41010** Incision of lingual frenum (frenotomy)
    🔹 3.11   ⚕ 5.77   **FUD** 010   [T] [A2] [80] [▢]
    **AMA:** 2017,Sep,14; 2014,Jan,11

**41015** Extraoral incision and drainage of abscess, cyst, or hematoma of floor of mouth; sublingual
    🔹 10.2   ⚕ 13.2   **FUD** 090   [T] [A2] [80] [▢]
    **AMA:** 2014,Jan,11

**41016** submental
    🔹 10.3   ⚕ 12.8   **FUD** 090   [J] [A2] [80] [▢]
    **AMA:** 2014,Jan,11

**41017** submandibular
    🔹 10.3   ⚕ 12.9   **FUD** 090   [J] [A2] [80] [▢]
    **AMA:** 2014,Jan,11

**41018** masticator space
    🔹 12.0   ⚕ 14.7   **FUD** 090   [T] [A2] [80] [▢]
    **AMA:** 2014,Jan,11

# 41019 Placement of Devices for Brachytherapy

**EXCLUDES** *Application of interstitial radioelements (77770-77772, 77778)*
*Intracranial brachytherapy radiation sources with stereotactic insertion (61770)*

**41019** Placement of needles, catheters, or other device(s) into the head and/or neck region (percutaneous, transoral, or transnasal) for subsequent interstitial radioelement application

📷 (76942, 77002, 77012, 77021)

🔧 13.6 ✂ 13.6 **FUD** 000  [J] [G2] [80] [▧]

**AMA:** 2017,Jan,8; 2016,Jan,13; 2015,Jan,16; 2014,Jan,11

# 41100-41599 Resection and Repair of the Tongue

**41100** Biopsy of tongue; anterior two-thirds

🔧 3.13 ✂ 4.85 **FUD** 010  [T] [P3] [▧]

**AMA:** 2014,Jan,11

Anterior (front) two-thirds of tongue makes up most of the easily visible portions

Anterior two-thirds

Lesion and elliptical incision

**41105** posterior one-third

🔧 3.26 ✂ 4.94 **FUD** 010  [J] [P3] [▧]

**AMA:** 2014,Jan,11

**41108** Biopsy of floor of mouth

🔧 2.64 ✂ 4.28 **FUD** 010  [J] [P3] [▧]

**AMA:** 2014,Jan,11

**41110** Excision of lesion of tongue without closure

🔧 3.82 ✂ 6.12 **FUD** 010  [J] [P3] [▧]

**AMA:** 2014,Jan,11

**41112** Excision of lesion of tongue with closure; anterior two-thirds

🔧 7.40 ✂ 9.71 **FUD** 090  [J] [A2] [▧]

**AMA:** 2014,Jan,11

**41113** posterior one-third

🔧 8.19 ✂ 10.6 **FUD** 090  [J] [A2] [▧]

**AMA:** 2014,Jan,11

**41114** with local tongue flap

**INCLUDES** Excision lesion of tongue with closure anterior/posterior two-thirds (41112-41113)

🔧 18.4 ✂ 18.4 **FUD** 090  [J] [A2] [80] [▧]

**AMA:** 2014,Jan,11

**41115** Excision of lingual frenum (frenectomy)

🔧 4.21 ✂ 7.10 **FUD** 090  [T] [P3] [80] [▧]

**AMA:** 2017,Sep,14; 2014,Jan,11

**41116** Excision, lesion of floor of mouth

🔧 6.42 ✂ 9.59 **FUD** 090  [J] [A2] [▧]

**AMA:** 2014,Jan,11

**41120** Glossectomy; less than one-half tongue

🔧 31.3 ✂ 31.3 **FUD** 090  [J] [A2] [80] [▧]

**AMA:** 2017,Jan,8; 2016,Jan,13; 2015,Jan,16; 2014,Jan,11

**41130** hemiglossectomy

🔧 38.5 ✂ 38.5 **FUD** 090  [C] [80] [▧]

**AMA:** 2017,Jan,8; 2016,Jan,13; 2015,Jan,16; 2014,Jan,11

**41135** partial, with unilateral radical neck dissection

🔧 63.4 ✂ 63.4 **FUD** 090  [C] [80] [▧]

**AMA:** 2017,Jan,8; 2016,Jan,13; 2015,Jan,16; 2014,Jan,11

**41140** complete or total, with or without tracheostomy, without radical neck dissection

**INCLUDES** Regnoli's excision

🔧 63.9 ✂ 63.9 **FUD** 090  [C] [80] [▧]

**AMA:** 2017,Jan,8; 2016,Jan,13; 2015,Jan,16; 2014,Jan,11

**41145** complete or total, with or without tracheostomy, with unilateral radical neck dissection

🔧 80.8 ✂ 80.8 **FUD** 090  [C] [80] [▧]

**AMA:** 2017,Jan,8; 2016,Jan,13; 2015,Jan,16; 2014,Jan,11

**41150** composite procedure with resection floor of mouth and mandibular resection, without radical neck dissection

🔧 64.2 ✂ 64.2 **FUD** 090  [C] [80] [▧]

**AMA:** 2017,Jan,8; 2016,Jan,13; 2015,Jan,16; 2014,Jan,11

**41153** composite procedure with resection floor of mouth, with suprahyoid neck dissection

🔧 69.8 ✂ 69.8 **FUD** 090  [C] [80] [▧]

**AMA:** 2017,Jan,8; 2016,Jan,13; 2015,Jan,16; 2014,Jan,11

**41155** composite procedure with resection floor of mouth, mandibular resection, and radical neck dissection (Commando type)

🔧 88.0 ✂ 88.0 **FUD** 090  [C] [80] [▧]

**AMA:** 2017,Jan,8; 2016,Jan,13; 2015,Jan,16; 2014,Jan,11; 2012,Jan,15-42

**41250** Repair of laceration 2.5 cm or less; floor of mouth and/or anterior two-thirds of tongue

🔧 4.46 ✂ 7.71 **FUD** 010  [Q1] [N1] [80] [▧]

**AMA:** 2014,Jan,11

**41251** posterior one-third of tongue

🔧 5.27 ✂ 8.28 **FUD** 010  [T] [A2] [80] [▧]

**AMA:** 2014,Jan,11

**41252** Repair of laceration of tongue, floor of mouth, over 2.6 cm or complex

🔧 6.15 ✂ 9.16 **FUD** 010  [T] [A2] [80] [▧]

**AMA:** 2014,Jan,11

**41500** Fixation of tongue, mechanical, other than suture (eg, K-wire)

🔧 13.0 ✂ 13.0 **FUD** 090  [J] [A2] [80] [▧]

**AMA:** 2017,Jan,8; 2016,Jan,13; 2015,Jan,16; 2014,Jan,11

**41510** Suture of tongue to lip for micrognathia (Douglas type procedure)

🔧 12.3 ✂ 12.3 **FUD** 090  [J] [A2] [80] [▧]

**AMA:** 2017,Jan,8; 2016,Jan,13; 2015,Jan,16; 2014,Jan,11

**41512** Tongue base suspension, permanent suture technique

**EXCLUDES** *Mechanical fixation of tongue, other than suture (41500)*
*Suture tongue to lip for micrognathia (41510)*

🔧 19.1 ✂ 19.1 **FUD** 090  [J] [G2] [80] [▧]

**AMA:** 2017,Jan,8; 2016,Jan,13; 2015,Jan,16; 2014,Jan,11; 2012,Aug,13-14

**41520** Frenoplasty (surgical revision of frenum, eg, with Z-plasty)

**EXCLUDES** *Frenotomy (40806, 41010)*

🔧 7.52 ✂ 10.2 **FUD** 090  [J] [A2] [80] [▧]

**AMA:** 2017,Sep,14; 2014,Jan,11

**41530** Submucosal ablation of the tongue base, radiofrequency, 1 or more sites, per session

🔧 10.8 ✂ 28.1 **FUD** 000  [J] [P3] [80] [▧]

**AMA:** 2017,Jan,8; 2016,Jan,13; 2015,Jan,16; 2014,Jan,11

**41599** Unlisted procedure, tongue, floor of mouth

🔧 0.00 ✂ 0.00 **FUD** YYY  [T] [80]

**AMA:** 2017,Jan,8; 2016,Jan,13; 2015,Jan,16; 2014,Jan,11; 2012,Jan,15-42

● New Code    ▲ Revised Code    ○ Reinstated    ● New Web Release    ▲ Revised Web Release    Unlisted    Not Covered    # Resequenced
⊘ AMA Mod 51 Exempt    Ⓢ Optum Mod 51 Exempt    ⑥③ Mod 63 Exempt    ✗ Non-FDA Drug    ★ Telemedicine    Ⓜ Maternity    Ⓐ Age Edit    ✚ Add-on    AMA: CPT Asst
© 2017 Optum360, LLC                    CPT © 2017 American Medical Association. All Rights Reserved.

Digestive System

41800 — 42182

## 41800-41899 Procedures of the Teeth and Supporting Structures

**41800** **Drainage of abscess, cyst, hematoma from dentoalveolar structures**
🚑 4.31  ⚕ 7.98  **FUD** 010  〔01〕〔N1〕▢
**AMA:** 2014,Jan,11

**41805** **Removal of embedded foreign body from dentoalveolar structures; soft tissues**
🚑 4.98  ⚕ 7.15  **FUD** 010  〔T〕〔P3〕〔80〕▢
**AMA:** 2014,Jan,11

**41806** **bone**
🚑 7.59  ⚕ 10.2  **FUD** 010  〔T〕〔P3〕〔80〕▢
**AMA:** 2014,Jan,11

**41820** **Gingivectomy, excision gingiva, each quadrant**
🚑 0.00  ⚕ 0.00  **FUD** 000  〔J〕〔R2〕〔80〕▢
**AMA:** 2014,Jan,11

Gingival recession

Excessive mucosal growth

Gingivitis is an inflammatory response to bacteria on the teeth; it is characterized by tender, red, swollen gums and can lead to gingival recession

**41821** **Operculectomy, excision pericoronal tissues**
🚑 0.00  ⚕ 0.00  **FUD** 000  〔T〕〔G2〕〔80〕▢
**AMA:** 2014,Jan,11

**41822** **Excision of fibrous tuberosities, dentoalveolar structures**
🚑 5.42  ⚕ 9.12  **FUD** 010  〔T〕〔P3〕〔80〕▢
**AMA:** 2014,Jan,11

**41823** **Excision of osseous tuberosities, dentoalveolar structures**
🚑 9.78  ⚕ 13.3  **FUD** 090  〔J〕〔P3〕〔80〕▢
**AMA:** 2014,Jan,11

**41825** **Excision of lesion or tumor (except listed above), dentoalveolar structures; without repair**
*EXCLUDES* *Lesion destruction nonexcisional (41850)*
🚑 3.57  ⚕ 6.15  **FUD** 010  〔J〕〔P3〕▢
**AMA:** 2014,Jan,11

**41826** **with simple repair**
*EXCLUDES* *Lesion destruction nonexcisional (41850)*
🚑 6.25  ⚕ 9.18  **FUD** 010  〔J〕〔P3〕▢
**AMA:** 2014,Jan,11

**41827** **with complex repair**
*EXCLUDES* *Lesion destruction nonexcisional (41850)*
🚑 9.04  ⚕ 12.8  **FUD** 090  〔J〕〔A2〕▢
**AMA:** 2014,Jan,11

**41828** **Excision of hyperplastic alveolar mucosa, each quadrant (specify)**
🚑 6.28  ⚕ 8.95  **FUD** 010  〔J〕〔P3〕〔80〕▢
**AMA:** 2014,Jan,11

**41830** **Alveolectomy, including curettage of osteitis or sequestrectomy**
🚑 8.32  ⚕ 11.4  **FUD** 010  〔J〕〔P3〕〔80〕▢
**AMA:** 2014,Jan,11

**41850** **Destruction of lesion (except excision), dentoalveolar structures**
🚑 0.00  ⚕ 0.00  **FUD** 000  〔T〕〔R2〕〔80〕▢
**AMA:** 2014,Jan,11

**41870** **Periodontal mucosal grafting**
🚑 0.00  ⚕ 0.00  **FUD** 000  〔J〕〔G2〕〔80〕▢
**AMA:** 2014,Jan,11

**41872** **Gingivoplasty, each quadrant (specify)**
🚑 7.70  ⚕ 10.9  **FUD** 090  〔J〕〔P3〕〔80〕▢
**AMA:** 2014,Jan,11

**41874** **Alveoloplasty, each quadrant (specify)**
*EXCLUDES* *Fracture reduction (21421-21490)*
*Laceration closure (40830-40831)*
*Maxilla osteotomy, segmental (21206)*
🚑 7.55  ⚕ 11.0  **FUD** 090  〔J〕〔P3〕〔80〕▢
**AMA:** 2014,Jan,11

**41899** **Unlisted procedure, dentoalveolar structures**
🚑 0.00  ⚕ 0.00  **FUD** YYY  〔T〕〔80〕
**AMA:** 2014,Jan,11

## 42000-42299 Procedures of the Palate and Uvula

**42000** **Drainage of abscess of palate, uvula**
🚑 3.03  ⚕ 4.61  **FUD** 010  〔T〕〔A2〕〔80〕▢
**AMA:** 2014,Jan,11

**42100** **Biopsy of palate, uvula**
🚑 3.18  ⚕ 4.34  **FUD** 010  〔T〕〔P3〕▢
**AMA:** 2014,Jan,11

**42104** **Excision, lesion of palate, uvula; without closure**
🚑 4.05  ⚕ 6.23  **FUD** 010  〔J〕〔P3〕▢
**AMA:** 2014,Jan,11

**42106** **with simple primary closure**
🚑 5.23  ⚕ 7.95  **FUD** 010  〔J〕〔P3〕▢
**AMA:** 2014,Jan,11

**42107** **with local flap closure**
*EXCLUDES* *Mucosal graft (40818)*
*Skin graft (14040-14302)*
🚑 10.0  ⚕ 13.3  **FUD** 090  〔J〕〔A2〕▢
**AMA:** 2014,Jan,11

**42120** **Resection of palate or extensive resection of lesion**
*EXCLUDES* *Palate reconstruction using extraoral tissue (14040-14302, 15050, 15120, 15240, 15576)*
🚑 29.5  ⚕ 29.5  **FUD** 090  〔J〕〔A2〕〔80〕▢
**AMA:** 2014,Jan,11

**42140** **Uvulectomy, excision of uvula**
🚑 4.47  ⚕ 7.26  **FUD** 090  〔J〕〔A2〕▢
**AMA:** 2014,Jan,11

**42145** **Palatopharyngoplasty (eg, uvulopalatopharyngoplasty, uvulopharyngoplasty)**
*EXCLUDES* *Excision of maxillary torus palatinus (21032)*
*Excision of torus mandibularis (21031)*
🚑 20.3  ⚕ 20.3  **FUD** 090  〔J〕〔A2〕▢
**AMA:** 2017,Jan,8; 2016,Jan,13; 2015,Jan,16; 2014,Jan,11; 2012,Jan,15-42

**42160** **Destruction of lesion, palate or uvula (thermal, cryo or chemical)**
🚑 4.27  ⚕ 6.70  **FUD** 010  〔J〕〔P3〕〔80〕▢
**AMA:** 2017,Jan,8; 2016,Jan,13; 2015,Jan,16; 2014,Jan,11; 2012,Jan,15-42

**42180** **Repair, laceration of palate; up to 2 cm**
🚑 5.30  ⚕ 7.01  **FUD** 010  〔T〕〔A2〕〔80〕▢
**AMA:** 2014,Jan,11

**42182** **over 2 cm or complex**
🚑 7.40  ⚕ 9.22  **FUD** 010  〔J〕〔A2〕〔80〕▢
**AMA:** 2014,Jan,11

| 26/TC PC/TC Only | A2-Z3 ASC Payment | 50 Bilateral | ♂ Male Only | ♀ Female Only | 🚑 Facility RVU | ⚕ Non-Facility RVU | ▢ CCI |
| FUD Follow-up Days | CMS: IOM (Pub 100) | A-Y OPPSI | 80/80 Surg Assist Allowed / w/Doc | | 🔬 Lab Crosswalk | ☢ Radiology Crosswalk | ✖ CLIA |

178    CPT © 2017 American Medical Association. All Rights Reserved.    © 2017 Optum360, LLC

**42200**  **Palatoplasty for cleft palate, soft and/or hard palate only**
⚕ 24.6    ⚭ 24.6    **FUD** 090    J A2 80 ▣
**AMA:** 2017,Jan,8; 2016,Jan,13; 2015,Mar,9; 2015,Jan,16; 2014,Jul,8; 2014,Jan,11

**42205**  **Palatoplasty for cleft palate, with closure of alveolar ridge; soft tissue only**
⚕ 26.3    ⚭ 26.3    **FUD** 090    J A2 80 ▣
**AMA:** 2014,Jan,11

**42210**  **with bone graft to alveolar ridge (includes obtaining graft)**
⚕ 30.0    ⚭ 30.0    **FUD** 090    J A2 80 ▣
**AMA:** 2014,Jan,11

**42215**  **Palatoplasty for cleft palate; major revision**
⚕ 20.9    ⚭ 20.9    **FUD** 090    J A2 80 ▣
**AMA:** 2014,Jan,11

**42220**  **secondary lengthening procedure**
⚕ 15.2    ⚭ 15.2    **FUD** 090    J A2 80 ▣
**AMA:** 2014,Jan,11

**42225**  **attachment pharyngeal flap**
⚕ 25.2    ⚭ 25.2    **FUD** 090    J G2 80 ▣
**AMA:** 2017,Jan,8; 2016,Jan,13; 2015,Jan,16; 2014,Jan,11; 2012,Jan,15-42

**42226**  **Lengthening of palate, and pharyngeal flap**
⚕ 26.1    ⚭ 26.1    **FUD** 090    J A2 80 ▣
**AMA:** 2014,Jan,11

**42227**  **Lengthening of palate, with island flap**
⚕ 24.6    ⚭ 24.6    **FUD** 090    J G2 80 ▣
**AMA:** 2014,Jan,11

**42235**  **Repair of anterior palate, including vomer flap**
EXCLUDES    Oronasal fistula repair (30600)
⚕ 21.0    ⚭ 21.0    **FUD** 090    J A2 80 ▣
**AMA:** 2017,Jan,8; 2016,Jan,13; 2015,Mar,9; 2015,Jan,16; 2014,Jul,8; 2014,Jan,11

**42260**  **Repair of nasolabial fistula**
EXCLUDES    Cleft lip repair (40700-40761)
⚕ 20.1    ⚭ 24.2    **FUD** 090    J A2 80 ▣
**AMA:** 2014,Jan,11

**42280**  **Maxillary impression for palatal prosthesis**
⚕ 3.23    ⚭ 4.74    **FUD** 010    T P3 80 ▣
**AMA:** 2014,Jan,11

**42281**  **Insertion of pin-retained palatal prosthesis**
⚕ 4.36    ⚭ 5.89    **FUD** 010    J G2 80 ▣
**AMA:** 2014,Jan,11

**42299**  **Unlisted procedure, palate, uvula**
⚕ 0.00    ⚭ 0.00    **FUD** YYY    T 80
**AMA:** 2017,Jan,8; 2016,Jan,13; 2015,Jan,16; 2014,Jul,8; 2014,Jan,11; 2012,Jan,15-42

## 42300-42699 Procedures of the Salivary Ducts and Glands

**42300**  **Drainage of abscess; parotid, simple**
⚕ 4.41    ⚭ 6.01    **FUD** 010    T A2 ▣
**AMA:** 2014,Jan,11

**42305**  **parotid, complicated**
⚕ 12.4    ⚭ 12.4    **FUD** 090    J A2 80 ▣
**AMA:** 2014,Jan,11

**42310**  **Drainage of abscess; submaxillary or sublingual, intraoral**
⚕ 3.58    ⚭ 4.63    **FUD** 010    T A2 80 ▣
**AMA:** 2014,Jan,11

**42320**  **submaxillary, external**
⚕ 5.04    ⚭ 7.13    **FUD** 010    T A2 80 ▣
**AMA:** 2014,Jan,11

**42330**  **Sialolithotomy; submandibular (submaxillary), sublingual or parotid, uncomplicated, intraoral**
⚕ 4.77    ⚭ 6.68    **FUD** 010    J P3 ▣
**AMA:** 2014,Jan,11

**42335**  **submandibular (submaxillary), complicated, intraoral**
⚕ 7.45    ⚭ 10.7    **FUD** 090    J P3 ▣
**AMA:** 2014,Jan,11

**42340**  **parotid, extraoral or complicated intraoral**
⚕ 9.75    ⚭ 13.4    **FUD** 090    J A2 80 50 ▣
**AMA:** 2014,Jan,11

**42400**  **Biopsy of salivary gland; needle**
EXCLUDES    Fine needle aspiration (10021-10022)
🖥 (76942, 77002, 77012, 77021)
🖥 (88172-88173)
⚕ 1.59    ⚭ 3.02    **FUD** 000    T P3 ▣
**AMA:** 2014,Jan,11

**42405**  **incisional**
🖥 (76942, 77002, 77012, 77021)
⚕ 6.54    ⚭ 8.59    **FUD** 010    J A2 ▣
**AMA:** 2014,Jan,11

**42408**  **Excision of sublingual salivary cyst (ranula)**
⚕ 9.45    ⚭ 13.0    **FUD** 090    J A2 80 ▣
**AMA:** 2014,Jan,11

**42409**  **Marsupialization of sublingual salivary cyst (ranula)**
⚕ 6.42    ⚭ 9.58    **FUD** 090    J A2 80 ▣
**AMA:** 2014,Jan,11

**42410**  **Excision of parotid tumor or parotid gland; lateral lobe, without nerve dissection**
EXCLUDES    Facial nerve suture or graft (64864, 64865, 69740, 69745)
⚕ 17.9    ⚭ 17.9    **FUD** 090    J A2 80 50 ▣
**AMA:** 2014,Jan,11

**42415**  **lateral lobe, with dissection and preservation of facial nerve**
EXCLUDES    Facial nerve suture or graft (64864, 64865, 69740, 69745)
⚕ 30.4    ⚭ 30.4    **FUD** 090    J A2 80 50 ▣
**AMA:** 2014,Jan,11

**42420**  **total, with dissection and preservation of facial nerve**
EXCLUDES    Facial nerve suture or graft (64864, 64865, 69740, 69745)
⚕ 34.1    ⚭ 34.1    **FUD** 090    J A2 80 50 ▣
**AMA:** 2014,Jan,11

**42425**  **total, en bloc removal with sacrifice of facial nerve**
EXCLUDES    Facial nerve suture or graft (64864, 64865, 69740, 69745)
⚕ 24.1    ⚭ 24.1    **FUD** 090    J A2 80 50 ▣
**AMA:** 2014,Jan,11

**42426**  **total, with unilateral radical neck dissection**
EXCLUDES    Facial nerve suture or graft (64864, 64865, 69740, 69745)
⚕ 38.9    ⚭ 38.9    **FUD** 090    C 80 50 ▣
**AMA:** 2017,Jan,8; 2016,Jan,13; 2015,Jan,16; 2014,Jan,11

**42440**  **Excision of submandibular (submaxillary) gland**
⚕ 11.8    ⚭ 11.8    **FUD** 090    J A2 80 50 ▣
**AMA:** 2014,Jan,11

**42450**  **Excision of sublingual gland**
⚕ 10.3    ⚭ 13.0    **FUD** 090    J A2 80 ▣
**AMA:** 2014,Jan,11

**42500**  **Plastic repair of salivary duct, sialodochoplasty; primary or simple**
⚕ 9.89    ⚭ 12.4    **FUD** 090    J A2 80 ▣
**AMA:** 2014,Jan,11

**42505**  **secondary or complicated**
⚕ 13.0    ⚭ 15.9    **FUD** 090    J A2 ▣
**AMA:** 2014,Jan,11

**42507**  **Parotid duct diversion, bilateral (Wilke type procedure);**
⚕ 14.4    ⚭ 14.4    **FUD** 090    J A2 80 ▣
**AMA:** 2014,Jan,11

● New Code    ▲ Revised Code    ○ Reinstated    ● New Web Release    ▲ Revised Web Release    Unlisted    Not Covered    # Resequenced
⊘ AMA Mod 51 Exempt    ⑤⓪ Optum Mod 51 Exempt    ⑥③ Mod 63 Exempt    ⁄ Non-FDA Drug    ★ Telemedicine    Ⓜ Maternity    Ⓐ Age Edit    + Add-on    AMA: CPT Asst
© 2017 Optum360, LLC    CPT © 2017 American Medical Association. All Rights Reserved.    179

**42509** with excision of both submandibular glands
⚙ 24.3  ⚖ 24.3  **FUD** 090  [J] [A2] [80] [▢]
**AMA:** 2014,Jan,11

**42510** with ligation of both submandibular (Wharton's) ducts
⚙ 18.6  ⚖ 18.6  **FUD** 090  [J] [A2] [80] [▢]
**AMA:** 2014,Jan,11

**42550** Injection procedure for sialography
📷 (70390)
⚙ 1.83  ⚖ 3.87  **FUD** 000  [N] [N1] [▢]
**AMA:** 2014,Jan,11

**42600** Closure salivary fistula
⚙ 9.91  ⚖ 13.5  **FUD** 090  [J] [A2] [80] [▢]
**AMA:** 2014,Jan,11

**42650** Dilation salivary duct
⚙ 1.70  ⚖ 2.40  **FUD** 000  [T] [P3] [▢]
**AMA:** 2014,Jan,11

**42660** Dilation and catheterization of salivary duct, with or without injection
⚙ 2.60  ⚖ 3.70  **FUD** 000  [T] [P3] [80] [▢]
**AMA:** 2014,Jan,11

**42665** Ligation salivary duct, intraoral
⚙ 6.01  ⚖ 9.08  **FUD** 090  [J] [A2] [80] [▢]
**AMA:** 2014,Jan,11

**42699** Unlisted procedure, salivary glands or ducts
⚙ 0.00  ⚖ 0.00  **FUD** YYY  [T] [80]
**AMA:** 2014,Jan,11

## 42700-42999 Procedures of the Adenoids/Throat/Tonsils

**42700** Incision and drainage abscess; peritonsillar
⚙ 3.91  ⚖ 5.44  **FUD** 010  [T] [A2] [▢]
**AMA:** 2014,Jan,11

**42720** retropharyngeal or parapharyngeal, intraoral approach
⚙ 11.3  ⚖ 13.0  **FUD** 010  [J] [A2] [80] [▢]
**AMA:** 2014,Jan,11

**42725** retropharyngeal or parapharyngeal, external approach
⚙ 23.7  ⚖ 23.7  **FUD** 090  [J] [A2] [80] [▢]
**AMA:** 2014,Jan,11

**42800** Biopsy; oropharynx
*EXCLUDES* Laryngoscopy with biopsy (31510, 31535-31536, 31576)
⚙ 3.23  ⚖ 4.55  **FUD** 010  [J] [P3] [▢]
**AMA:** 2014,Jan,11

**42804** nasopharynx, visible lesion, simple
*EXCLUDES* Laryngoscopy with biopsy (31510, 31535-31536)
⚙ 3.26  ⚖ 5.60  **FUD** 010  [J] [A2] [▢]
**AMA:** 2014,Jan,11

**42806** nasopharynx, survey for unknown primary lesion
*EXCLUDES* Laryngoscopy with biopsy (31510, 31535-31536)
⚙ 3.80  ⚖ 6.29  **FUD** 010  [J] [A2] [▢]
**AMA:** 2014,Jan,11

**42808** Excision or destruction of lesion of pharynx, any method
⚙ 4.68  ⚖ 6.52  **FUD** 010  [J] [A2] [▢]
**AMA:** 2014,Jan,11

**42809** Removal of foreign body from pharynx
⚙ 3.53  ⚖ 5.76  **FUD** 010  [01] [N1] [▢]
**AMA:** 2014,Jan,11

Choanae
Nasopharynx
Parotid gland
Nasal septum
Oropharynx
Submandibular gland
Root of tongue
Laryngopharynx
Epiglottis
Esophagus
Trachea
Plane of view

A foreign body is removed from the pharynx

**42810** Excision branchial cleft cyst or vestige, confined to skin and subcutaneous tissues
⚙ 8.33  ⚖ 11.1  **FUD** 090  [J] [A2] [80] [50] [▢]
**AMA:** 2014,Jan,11

**42815** Excision branchial cleft cyst, vestige, or fistula, extending beneath subcutaneous tissues and/or into pharynx
⚙ 16.1  ⚖ 16.1  **FUD** 090  [J] [A2] [80] [50] [▢]
**AMA:** 2014,Jan,11

**42820** Tonsillectomy and adenoidectomy; younger than age 12  [A]
⚙ 8.32  ⚖ 8.32  **FUD** 090  [J] [A2] [80] [▢]
**AMA:** 2017,Jan,8; 2016,Jan,13; 2015,Jan,16; 2014,Jan,11; 2012,Jan,15-42

**42821** age 12 or over  [A]
⚙ 8.68  ⚖ 8.68  **FUD** 090  [J] [A2] [80] [▢]
**AMA:** 2017,Jan,8; 2016,Jan,13; 2015,Jan,16; 2014,Jan,11; 2012,Jan,15-42

**42825** Tonsillectomy, primary or secondary; younger than age 12  [A]
⚙ 7.55  ⚖ 7.55  **FUD** 090  [J] [A2] [80] [▢]
**AMA:** 2017,Jan,8; 2016,Jan,13; 2015,Jan,16; 2014,Jan,11; 2012,Jan,15-42

**42826** age 12 or over  [A]
⚙ 7.25  ⚖ 7.25  **FUD** 090  [J] [A2] [▢]
**AMA:** 2017,Jan,8; 2016,Jan,13; 2015,Jan,16; 2014,Jan,11; 2012,Jan,15-42

**42830** Adenoidectomy, primary; younger than age 12  [A]
⚙ 5.97  ⚖ 5.97  **FUD** 090  [J] [A2] [80] [▢]
**AMA:** 2017,Jan,8; 2016,Jan,13; 2015,Jan,16; 2014,Jan,11

**42831** age 12 or over  [A]
⚙ 6.45  ⚖ 6.45  **FUD** 090  [J] [A2] [80] [▢]
**AMA:** 2017,Jan,8; 2016,Jan,13; 2015,Jan,16; 2014,Jan,11

**42835** Adenoidectomy, secondary; younger than age 12  [A]
⚙ 5.24  ⚖ 5.24  **FUD** 090  [J] [A2] [80] [▢]
**AMA:** 2017,Jan,8; 2016,Jan,13; 2015,Jan,16; 2014,Jan,11

**42836** age 12 or over  [A]
⚙ 6.94  ⚖ 6.94  **FUD** 090  [J] [A2] [80] [▢]
**AMA:** 2017,Jan,8; 2016,Jan,13; 2015,Jan,16; 2014,Jan,11; 2012,Jan,15-42

**42842** Radical resection of tonsil, tonsillar pillars, and/or retromolar trigone; without closure
🚑 29.4  ⚕ 29.4  **FUD** 090  `J` `80` 🖥
**AMA:** 2017,Jan,8; 2016,Jan,13; 2015,Jan,16; 2014,Jan,11

**42844** closure with local flap (eg, tongue, buccal)
🚑 40.5  ⚕ 40.5  **FUD** 090  `J` `80` 🖥
**AMA:** 2017,Jan,8; 2016,Jan,13; 2015,Jan,16; 2014,Jan,11

**42845** closure with other flap
Code also closure with other flap(s)
Code also radical neck dissection when combined (38720)
🚑 65.0  ⚕ 65.0  **FUD** 090  `C` `80` 🖥
**AMA:** 2017,Jan,8; 2016,Jan,13; 2015,Jan,16; 2014,Jan,11

**42860** Excision of tonsil tags
🚑 5.42  ⚕ 5.42  **FUD** 090  `J` `A2` `80` 🖥
**AMA:** 2014,Jan,11

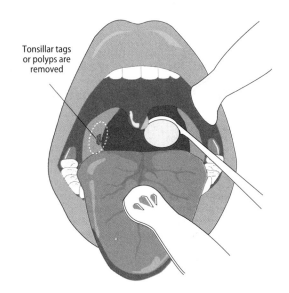

Tonsillar tags or polyps are removed

**42870** Excision or destruction lingual tonsil, any method (separate procedure)
*EXCLUDES* *Nasopharynx resection (juvenile angiofibroma) by transzygomatic/bicoronal approach (61586, 61600)*
🚑 17.3  ⚕ 17.3  **FUD** 090  `J` `A2` `80` 🖥
**AMA:** 2014,Jan,11

**42890** Limited pharyngectomy
Code also radical neck dissection when combined (38720)
🚑 41.7  ⚕ 41.7  **FUD** 090  `J` `A2` `80` 🖥
**AMA:** 2014,Jan,11

**42892** Resection of lateral pharyngeal wall or pyriform sinus, direct closure by advancement of lateral and posterior pharyngeal walls
Code also radical neck dissection when combined (38720)
🚑 55.1  ⚕ 55.1  **FUD** 090  `J` `A2` `80` 🖥
**AMA:** 2017,Jan,8; 2016,Jan,13; 2015,Jan,16; 2014,Jan,11

**42894** Resection of pharyngeal wall requiring closure with myocutaneous or fasciocutaneous flap or free muscle, skin, or fascial flap with microvascular anastomosis
*EXCLUDES* *Flap used for reconstruction (15730, 15733-15734, 15756-15758)*
Code also radical neck dissection when combined (38720)
🚑 69.2  ⚕ 69.2  **FUD** 090  `C` `80` 🖥
**AMA:** 2017,Jan,8; 2016,Jan,13; 2015,Jan,16; 2014,Jan,11; 2012,Jan,15-42

**42900** Suture pharynx for wound or injury
🚑 9.76  ⚕ 9.76  **FUD** 010  `T` `A2` `80` 🖥
**AMA:** 2014,Jan,11

**42950** Pharyngoplasty (plastic or reconstructive operation on pharynx)
*EXCLUDES* *Pharyngeal flap (42225)*
🚑 23.7  ⚕ 23.7  **FUD** 090  `J` `A2` `80` 🖥
**AMA:** 2017,Jan,8; 2016,Apr,8; 2014,Jan,11

**42953** Pharyngoesophageal repair
Code also closure using myocutaneous or other flap
🚑 28.5  ⚕ 28.5  **FUD** 090  `C` `80` 🖥
**AMA:** 2014,Jan,11

**42955** Pharyngostomy (fistulization of pharynx, external for feeding)
🚑 22.1  ⚕ 22.1  **FUD** 090  `T` `A2` `80` 🖥
**AMA:** 2014,Jan,11

**42960** Control oropharyngeal hemorrhage, primary or secondary (eg, post-tonsillectomy); simple
🚑 4.91  ⚕ 4.91  **FUD** 010  `T` `A2` `80` 🖥
**AMA:** 2014,Jan,11

**42961** complicated, requiring hospitalization
🚑 12.1  ⚕ 12.1  **FUD** 090  `C` `80` 🖥
**AMA:** 2014,Jan,11

**42962** with secondary surgical intervention
🚑 15.0  ⚕ 15.0  **FUD** 090  `J` `A2` 🖥
**AMA:** 2014,Jan,11

**42970** Control of nasopharyngeal hemorrhage, primary or secondary (eg, postadenoidectomy); simple, with posterior nasal packs, with or without anterior packs and/or cautery
🚑 11.8  ⚕ 11.8  **FUD** 090  `T` `R2` 🖥
**AMA:** 2014,Jan,11

**42971** complicated, requiring hospitalization
🚑 13.2  ⚕ 13.2  **FUD** 090  `C` `80` 🖥
**AMA:** 2014,Jan,11

**42972** with secondary surgical intervention
🚑 14.7  ⚕ 14.7  **FUD** 090  `J` `A2` `80` 🖥
**AMA:** 2014,Jan,11

**42999** Unlisted procedure, pharynx, adenoids, or tonsils
🚑 0.00  ⚕ 0.00  **FUD** YYY  `T` `80`
**AMA:** 2017,Jan,8; 2016,Jan,13; 2015,Jan,16; 2014,Feb,11; 2014,Jan,11

## 43020-43135 Incision/Resection of Esophagus
*EXCLUDES* *Gastrointestinal reconstruction for previous esophagectomy (43360-43361)*
*Gastrotomy with intraluminal tube insertion (43510)*

**43020** Esophagotomy, cervical approach, with removal of foreign body
*EXCLUDES* *Laparotomy with esophageal intubation (43510)*
🚑 15.4  ⚕ 15.4  **FUD** 090  `T` `80` 🖥
**AMA:** 2014,Jan,11

**43030** Cricopharyngeal myotomy
*EXCLUDES* *Laparotomy with esophageal intubation (43510)*
🚑 14.9  ⚕ 14.9  **FUD** 090  `J` `62` `80` 🖥
**AMA:** 2014,Jan,11

**43045** Esophagotomy, thoracic approach, with removal of foreign body
*EXCLUDES* *Laparotomy with esophageal intubation (43510)*
🚑 37.7  ⚕ 37.7  **FUD** 090  `C` `80` 🖥
**AMA:** 2014,Jan,11

**43100** Excision of lesion, esophagus, with primary repair; cervical approach
*EXCLUDES* *Wide excision of malignant lesion of cervical esophagus, with total laryngectomy:*
*With radical neck dissection (31365, 43107, 43116, 43124)*
*Without radical neck dissection (31360, 43107, 43116, 43124)*
🚑 17.9  ⚕ 17.9  **FUD** 090  `C` `80` 🖥
**AMA:** 2014,Jan,11

● New Code  ▲ Revised Code  ○ Reinstated  ● New Web Release  ▲ Revised Web Release  Unlisted  Not Covered  # Resequenced
⊘ AMA Mod 51 Exempt  ⑤ Optum Mod 51 Exempt  ⑥⑤ Mod 63 Exempt  ⁄ Non-FDA Drug  ★ Telemedicine  Ⓜ Maternity  Ⓐ Age Edit  + Add-on  **AMA:** CPT Asst
© 2017 Optum360, LLC          CPT © 2017 American Medical Association. All Rights Reserved.          **181**

**Digestive System**

**43101 — 43192**

**43101** **thoracic or abdominal approach**

EXCLUDES *Wide excision of malignant lesion of cervical esophagus with total laryngectomy:*
*With radical neck dissection (31365, 43107, 43116, 43124)*
*Without radical neck dissection (31360, 43107, 43116, 43124)*

🚑 30.8　⚕ 30.8　**FUD** 090　　　　　C 80 ▢

AMA: 2017,Jan,8; 2016,Jan,13; 2015,Jan,16; 2014,Jan,11

**43107** **Total or near total esophagectomy, without thoracotomy; with pharyngogastrostomy or cervical esophagogastrostomy, with or without pyloroplasty (transhiatal)**

🚑 74.1　⚕ 74.1　**FUD** 090　　　　　C 80 ▢

AMA: 2014,Jan,11

**43108** **with colon interposition or small intestine reconstruction, including intestine mobilization, preparation and anastomosis(es)**

🚑 135.　⚕ 135.　**FUD** 090　　　　　C 80 ▢

AMA: 2014,Jan,11

▲ **43112** **Total or near total esophagectomy, with thoracotomy; with pharyngogastrostomy or cervical esophagogastrostomy, with or without pyloroplasty (ie, McKeown esophagectomy or tri-incisional esophagectomy)**

🚑 78.3　⚕ 78.3　**FUD** 090　　　　　C 80 ▢

AMA: 2017,Jan,8; 2016,Jan,13; 2015,Jan,16; 2014,Jan,11; 2013,Aug,13

**43113** **with colon interposition or small intestine reconstruction, including intestine mobilization, preparation, and anastomosis(es)**

🚑 126.　⚕ 126.　**FUD** 090　　　　　C 80 ▢

AMA: 2014,Jan,11

**43116** **Partial esophagectomy, cervical, with free intestinal graft, including microvascular anastomosis, obtaining the graft and intestinal reconstruction**

INCLUDES Operating microscope (69990)

EXCLUDES *Free jejunal graft with microvascular anastomosis done by a different physician (43496)*
Code also modifier 52 if intestinal or free jejunal graft with microvascular anastomosis is done by another physician

🚑 152.　⚕ 152.　**FUD** 090　　　　　C 80 ▢

AMA: 2016,Feb,12; 2014,Jan,11

**43117** **Partial esophagectomy, distal two-thirds, with thoracotomy and separate abdominal incision, with or without proximal gastrectomy; with thoracic esophagogastrostomy, with or without pyloroplasty (Ivor Lewis)**

EXCLUDES *Esophagogastrectomy (lower third) and vagotomy (43122)*
*Total esophagectomy with gastropharyngostomy (43107, 43124)*

🚑 71.6　⚕ 71.6　**FUD** 090　　　　　C 80 ▢

AMA: 2014,Jan,11

**43118** **with colon interposition or small intestine reconstruction, including intestine mobilization, preparation, and anastomosis(es)**

EXCLUDES *Esophagogastrectomy (lower third) and vagotomy (43122)*
*Total esophagectomy with gastropharyngostomy (43107, 43124)*

🚑 109.　⚕ 109.　**FUD** 090　　　　　C 80 ▢

AMA: 2014,Jan,11

**43121** **Partial esophagectomy, distal two-thirds, with thoracotomy only, with or without proximal gastrectomy, with thoracic esophagogastrostomy, with or without pyloroplasty**

🚑 82.8　⚕ 82.8　**FUD** 090　　　　　C 80 ▢

AMA: 2014,Jan,11

**43122** **Partial esophagectomy, thoracoabdominal or abdominal approach, with or without proximal gastrectomy; with esophagogastrostomy, with or without pyloroplasty**

🚑 74.3　⚕ 74.3　**FUD** 090　　　　　C 80 ▢

AMA: 2014,Jan,11

**43123** **with colon interposition or small intestine reconstruction, including intestine mobilization, preparation, and anastomosis(es)**

🚑 136.　⚕ 136.　**FUD** 090　　　　　C 80 ▢

AMA: 2014,Jan,11

**43124** **Total or partial esophagectomy, without reconstruction (any approach), with cervical esophagostomy**

🚑 111.　⚕ 111.　**FUD** 090　　　　　C 80 ▢

AMA: 2017,Jan,8; 2016,Jan,13; 2015,Jan,16; 2014,Jan,11

**43130** **Diverticulectomy of hypopharynx or esophagus, with or without myotomy; cervical approach**

EXCLUDES *Diverticulectomy hypopharynx or cervical esophagus, endoscopic (43180)*

🚑 22.6　⚕ 22.6　**FUD** 090　　　　J 62 80 ▢

AMA: 2017,Jan,8; 2016,Jan,13; 2015,Jan,16; 2014,Jan,11; 2012,Jan,15-42

**43135** **thoracic approach**

EXCLUDES *Diverticulectomy hypopharynx or cervical esophagus, endoscopic (43180)*

🚑 43.0　⚕ 43.0　**FUD** 090　　　　　C 80 ▢

AMA: 2017,Jan,8; 2016,Jan,13; 2015,Jan,16; 2014,Jan,11; 2012,Jan,15-42

## 43180-43233 [43211, 43212, 43213, 43214] Endoscopic Procedures: Esophagus

INCLUDES Control of bleeding as a result of endoscopic procedure during same operative session
Diagnostic endoscopy with surgical endoscopy
Examination of upper esophageal sphincter (cricopharyngeus muscle) to/including the gastroesophageal junction
Retroflexion examination of proximal region of stomach

**43180** **Esophagoscopy, rigid, transoral with diverticulectomy of hypopharynx or cervical esophagus (eg, Zenker's diverticulum), with cricopharyngeal myotomy, includes use of telescope or operating microscope and repair, when performed**

INCLUDES Operating microscope (69990)

EXCLUDES *Esophagogastroduodenoscopy, flexible, transoral; with esophagogastric fundoplasty (43210)*
*Open diverticulectomy hypopharynx or esophagus (43130-43135)*

🚑 15.8　⚕ 15.8　**FUD** 090　　　　J 62 ▢

AMA: 2017,Jan,8; 2016,Feb,12; 2016,Jan,13; 2015,Nov,8

**43191** **Esophagoscopy, rigid, transoral; diagnostic, including collection of specimen(s) by brushing or washing when performed (separate procedure)**

EXCLUDES *Esophagogastroduodenoscopy, flexible, transoral; with esophagogastric fundoplasty (43210)*
*Esophagoscopy, flexible, transnasal (43197-43198)*
*Esophagoscopy, flexible, transoral (43200)*
*Esophagoscopy, rigid, transoral (43192-43196)*

🚑 4.47　⚕ 4.47　**FUD** 000　　　　J 62 ▢

AMA: 2017,Jan,8; 2016,Jan,13; 2015,Nov,8; 2015,Jan,16; 2014,Feb,9; 2014,Jan,11; 2013,Dec,3

**43192** **with directed submucosal injection(s), any substance**

EXCLUDES *Esophagoscopy, flexible, transnasal; with biopsy, single or multiple (43197-43198)*
*Esophagoscopy, flexible, transoral (43201)*
*Esophagoscopy, rigid or flexible, diagnostic (43191)*
*Injection sclerosis of esophageal varices:*
*Flexible, transoral (43204)*
*Rigid, transoral (43499)*

🚑 4.92　⚕ 4.92　**FUD** 000　　　　J 62 ▢

AMA: 2017,Jan,8; 2016,Jan,13; 2015,Jan,16; 2014,Feb,9; 2014,Jan,11; 2013,Dec,3

**43193** **with biopsy, single or multiple**

*EXCLUDES* *Esophagoscopy, flexible, transnasal; with biopsy, single or multiple (43197-43198)*

*Esophagoscopy, rigid or flexible, diagnostic (43191, 43197)*

*Flexible, transoral (43202)*

🚑 4.91 ⚕ 4.91 **FUD** 000 [J] [B2] [▢]

**AMA:** 2017,Jan,8; 2016,Jan,13; 2015,Jan,16; 2014,Feb,9; 2014,Jan,11; 2013,Dec,3

**43194** **with removal of foreign body(s)**

*EXCLUDES* *Esophagoscopy, flexible, transnasal; with biopsy, single or multiple (43198)*

*Esophagoscopy, rigid or flexible, diagnostic (43191, 43197)*

*Flexible, transoral (43215)*

▦ (76000)

🚑 5.61 ⚕ 5.61 **FUD** 000 [J] [B2] [▢]

**AMA:** 2017,Jan,8; 2016,Jan,13; 2015,Jan,16; 2014,Feb,9; 2014,Jan,11; 2013,Dec,3

**43195** **with balloon dilation (less than 30 mm diameter)**

*EXCLUDES* *Dilation of esophagus:*
  *Flexible, with balloon diameter 30 mm or larger (43214, 43233)*
  *Flexible, with balloon diameter less than 30 mm (43220)*
  *Without endoscopic visualization (43450-43453)*
*Esophagoscopy, flexible, transnasal; with biopsy, single or multiple (43198)*
*Esophagoscopy, rigid or flexible, diagnostic (43191, 43197)*

▦ (74360)

🚑 5.36 ⚕ 5.36 **FUD** 000 [J] [B2] [▢]

**AMA:** 2017,Jan,8; 2016,Jan,13; 2015,Jan,16; 2014,Feb,9; 2014,Jan,11; 2013,Dec,3

**43196** **with insertion of guide wire followed by dilation over guide wire**

*EXCLUDES* *Esophagoscopy, flexible, transnasal; with biopsy, single or multiple (43198)*

*Esophagoscopy, rigid or flexible, diagnostic (43191, 43197)*

*Flexible, transoral (43226)*

▦ (74360)

🚑 5.72 ⚕ 5.72 **FUD** 000 [J] [B2] [▢]

**AMA:** 2017,Jan,8; 2016,Jan,13; 2015,Jan,16; 2014,Feb,9; 2014,Jan,11; 2013,Dec,3

**43197** **Esophagoscopy, flexible, transnasal; diagnostic, including collection of specimen(s) by brushing or washing, when performed (separate procedure)**

*EXCLUDES* *Esophagogastroduodenoscopy, flexible, transoral (43235-43259 [43233, 43266, 43270])*

*Esophagoscopy, flexible, transnasal; with biopsy, single or multiple (43198)*

*Flexible, transoral (43200-43232 [43211, 43212, 43213, 43214])*

*Laryngoscopy, flexible fiberoptic; diagnostic (31575)*

*Nasal endoscopy, diagnostic, unless different type of endoscope used (31231)*

*Nasopharyngoscopy with endoscope (92511)*

*Rigid, transoral (43191-43196)*

🚑 2.41 ⚕ 5.37 **FUD** 000 [T] [P3] [▢]

**AMA:** 2017,Jul,7; 2017,Jan,8; 2016,Dec,13; 2016,Sep,6; 2016,Jan,13; 2015,Nov,8; 2015,Jan,16; 2014,Feb,9; 2014,Jan,11; 2013,Dec,3

**43198** **with biopsy, single or multiple**

*EXCLUDES* *Esophagogastroduodenoscopy, flexible, transoral (43235-43259 [43233, 43266, 43270])*

*Flexible, transoral (43200-43232 [43211, 43212, 43213, 43214])*

*Laryngoscopy, flexible fiberoptic; diagnostic (31575)*

*Nasal endoscopy, diagnostic, unless different type of endoscope used (31231)*

*Nasopharyngoscopy with endoscope (92511)*

*Rigid, transoral (43191-43197)*

🚑 2.88 ⚕ 5.95 **FUD** 000 [T] [P3] [▢]

**AMA:** 2017,Jul,7; 2017,Jan,8; 2016,Dec,13; 2016,Sep,6; 2016,Jan,13; 2015,Jan,16; 2014,Feb,9; 2014,Jan,11; 2013,Dec,3

**43200** **Esophagoscopy, flexible, transoral; diagnostic, including collection of specimen(s) by brushing or washing, when performed (separate procedure)**

*EXCLUDES* *Esophagoscopy, flexible, transoral (43201-43232 [43211, 43212, 43213, 43214])*

*Flexible, transnasal (43197-43198)*

*Rigid, transoral (43191)*

*Upper gastrointestinal endoscopy (43235)*

🚑 2.56 ⚕ 6.15 **FUD** 000 [T] [A2] [▢]

**AMA:** 2017,Jan,8; 2016,Jan,13; 2015,Nov,8; 2015,Jan,16; 2014,Feb,9; 2014,Jan,11; 2013,Dec,3; 2013,Feb,16-17; 2013,Jan,11-12; 2012,Jan,15-42

**43201** **with directed submucosal injection(s), any substance**

*EXCLUDES* *Esophagoscopy, flexible, transnasal (43197-43198)*

*Esophagoscopy, flexible, transoral on the same lesion (43200, 43204, 43211, 43227)*

*Injection sclerosis of esophageal varices:*
  *Flexible, transoral (43204)*
  *Rigid, transoral (43192, 43499)*

🚑 3.02 ⚕ 6.28 **FUD** 000 [J] [A2] [▢]

**AMA:** 2017,Jan,8; 2016,Jan,13; 2015,Jan,16; 2014,Feb,9; 2014,Jan,11; 2013,Dec,3; 2013,Jan,11-12

**43202** **with biopsy, single or multiple**

*EXCLUDES* *Esophagoscopy, flexible, transoral; diagnostic (43200)*

*Esophagoscopy, flexible, transoral on same lesion (43211)*

*Flexible, transnasal (43197-43198)*

*Rigid, transoral (43193)*

🚑 3.03 ⚕ 8.72 **FUD** 000 [J] [A2] [▢]

**AMA:** 2017,Jan,8; 2016,Jan,13; 2015,Jan,16; 2014,Feb,9; 2014,Jan,11; 2013,Dec,3; 2013,Jan,11-12

**43204** **with injection sclerosis of esophageal varices**

*EXCLUDES* *Band ligation non-variceal bleeding (43227)*

*Esophagoscopy, flexible, transnasal or transoral; diagnostic (43197-43198, 43200)*

*Esophagoscopy, flexible, transoral; with control of bleeding, any method on the same lesion (43227)*

*Esophagoscopy, flexible, transoral; with directed submucosal injection(s), any substance on the same lesion (43201)*

*Rigid, transoral (43499)*

🚑 3.99 ⚕ 3.99 **FUD** 000 [J] [A2] [▢]

**AMA:** 2017,Jan,8; 2016,Jan,13; 2015,Jan,16; 2014,Feb,9; 2014,Jan,11; 2013,Dec,3; 2013,Jan,11-12

**43205** **with band ligation of esophageal varices**

*EXCLUDES* *Band ligation non-variceal bleeding on the same lesion (43227)*

*Esophagoscopy, flexible, transnasal or transoral; diagnostic (43197-43198, 43200)*

🚑 4.15 ⚕ 4.15 **FUD** 000 [J] [A2] [▢]

**AMA:** 2017,Jan,8; 2016,Jan,13; 2015,Jan,16; 2014,Feb,9; 2014,Jan,11; 2013,Dec,3; 2013,Jan,11-12

● New Code   ▲ Revised Code   ○ Reinstated   ● New Web Release   ▲ Revised Web Release   Unlisted   Not Covered   # Resequenced
⊘ AMA Mod 51 Exempt   ⑨ Optum Mod 51 Exempt   ⊛ Mod 63 Exempt   ✗ Non-FDA Drug   ★ Telemedicine   Ⓜ Maternity   🅐 Age Edit   + Add-on   **AMA:** CPT Asst

**43206** **with optical endomicroscopy**

EXCLUDES *Esophagoscopy, flexible, transnasal or transoral; diagnostic (43197-43198, 43200)*

*Optical endomicroscopic image(s), interpretation and report (88375)*

Code also contrast agent

🖭 3.92 ⚕ 7.56 **FUD** 000 J G2 ▣

**AMA:** 2017,Jan,8; 2016,Jan,13; 2015,Jan,16; 2014,Feb,9; 2014,Jan,11; 2013,Dec,3; 2013,Aug,5; 2013,Jan,11-12

*43210* **Resequenced code. See code following 43259.**

*43211* **Resequenced code. See code following 43217.**

*43212* **Resequenced code. See code following 43217.**

*43213* **Resequenced code. See code following 43220.**

*43214* **Resequenced code. See code following 43220.**

**43215** **with removal of foreign body(s)**

EXCLUDES *Esophagoscopy, flexible, transnasal or transoral; diagnostic (43197-43198, 43200)*

*Rigid, transoral (43194)*

*Upper gastrointestinal endoscopy (43247)*

🖭 (76000)

🖭 4.16 ⚕ 10.2 **FUD** 000 J A2 ▣

**AMA:** 2017,Jan,8; 2016,Jan,13; 2015,Jan,16; 2014,Feb,9; 2014,Jan,11; 2013,Dec,3; 2013,Jan,11-12

**43216** **with removal of tumor(s), polyp(s), or other lesion(s) by hot biopsy forceps**

EXCLUDES *Esophagoscopy, flexible, transnasal or transoral; diagnostic (43197-43198, 43200)*

*Removal by snare technique (43217)*

🖭 3.95 ⚕ 10.1 **FUD** 000 J A2 ▣

**AMA:** 2017,Jan,8; 2016,Jan,13; 2015,Jan,16; 2014,Feb,9; 2014,Jan,11; 2013,Dec,3; 2013,Jan,11-12

**43217** **with removal of tumor(s), polyp(s), or other lesion(s) by snare technique**

EXCLUDES *Esophagoscopy, flexible, transnasal or transoral; diagnostic (43197-43198, 43200)*

*Esophagoscopy, flexible, transoral; with endoscopic mucosal resection on the same lesion (43211)*

*Upper gastrointestinal endoscopy with snare technique (43251)*

🖭 4.72 ⚕ 10.7 **FUD** 000 J A2 ▣

**AMA:** 2017,Jan,8; 2016,Jan,13; 2015,Jan,16; 2014,Feb,9; 2014,Jan,11; 2013,Dec,3; 2013,Jan,11-12

\# **43211** **with endoscopic mucosal resection**

EXCLUDES *Esophagoscopy, flexible, transnasal or transoral; diagnostic (43197-43198, 43200)*

*Esophagoscopy, flexible, transoral; with directed submucosal injection(s) (43201-43202)*

*Esophagoscopy, flexible, transoral; with removal of tumor(s), polyp(s), or other lesion(s) by snare technique (43217)*

🖭 6.93 ⚕ 6.93 **FUD** 000 J G2 ▣

**AMA:** 2017,Jan,8; 2016,Jan,13; 2015,Jan,16; 2014,Feb,9; 2014,Jan,11; 2013,Dec,3

\# **43212** **with placement of endoscopic stent (includes pre- and post-dilation and guide wire passage, when performed)**

EXCLUDES *Esophagogastroduodenoscopy, flexible, transoral; with insertion of intraluminal tube or catheter (43241)*

*Esophagoscopy, flexible, transnasal or transoral; diagnostic (43197-43198, 43200)*

*Esophagoscopy, flexible, transoral; with insertion of guide wire followed by passage of dilator(s) over guide wire (43226)*

*Esophagoscopy, flexible, transoral; with transendoscopic balloon dilation (43220)*

🖭 (74360)

🖭 5.58 ⚕ 5.58 **FUD** 000 J J8 ▣

**AMA:** 2017,Jan,8; 2016,Jan,13; 2015,Jan,16; 2014,Feb,9; 2014,Jan,11; 2013,Dec,3

**43220** **with transendoscopic balloon dilation (less than 30 mm diameter)**

EXCLUDES *Dilation of esophagus:*

*Rigid, with balloon diameter 30 mm or larger (43214)*

*Rigid, with balloon diameter less than 30mm (43195)*

*Without endoscopic visualization (43450, 43453)*

*Esophagoscopy, flexible, transnasal; diagnostic (43197-43198)*

*Esophagoscopy, flexible, transoral (43200, 43212, 43226, 43229)*

🖭 (74360)

🖭 3.46 ⚕ 30.4 **FUD** 000 J A2 ▣

**AMA:** 2017,Jan,8; 2016,Jan,13; 2015,Jan,16; 2014,Feb,9; 2014,Jan,11; 2013,Dec,3; 2013,Jan,11-12; 2012,Jan,15-42

\# **43213** **with dilation of esophagus, by balloon or dilator, retrograde (includes fluoroscopic guidance, when performed)**

INCLUDES *Fluoroscopy (76000-76001)*

EXCLUDES *Esophagoscopy, flexible, transnasal or transoral; diagnostic (43197-43198, 43200)*

*Intraluminal dilation of strictures and/or obstructions (eg, esophagus), radiological supervision and interpretation (74360)*

Code also each additional stricture treated in same operative session with modifier 59 and (43213)

🖭 7.59 ⚕ 32.6 **FUD** 000 J G2 ▣

**AMA:** 2017,Jan,8; 2016,Jan,13; 2015,Jan,16; 2014,Feb,9; 2014,Jan,11; 2013,Dec,3

\# **43214** **with dilation of esophagus with balloon (30 mm diameter or larger) (includes fluoroscopic guidance, when performed)**

INCLUDES *Fluoroscopy (76000-76001)*

EXCLUDES *Esophagoscopy, flexible, transnasal or transoral; diagnostic (43197-43198, 43200)*

*Intraluminal dilation of strictures and/or obstructions (eg, esophagus), radiological supervision and interpretation (74360)*

🖭 5.65 ⚕ 5.65 **FUD** 000 J G2 ▣

**AMA:** 2017,Jan,8; 2016,Jan,13; 2015,Jan,16; 2014,Feb,9; 2014,Jan,11; 2013,Dec,3

**43226** **with insertion of guide wire followed by passage of dilator(s) over guide wire**

EXCLUDES *Esophagoscopy, flexible, transnasal or transoral; diagnostic (43197-43198, 43200)*

*Esophagoscopy, flexible, transoral; with ablation of tumor(s), polyp(s), or other lesion(s) on the same lesion (43229)*

*Esophagoscopy, flexible, transoral; with placement of endoscopic stent (43212)*

*Esophagoscopy, flexible, transoral; with transendoscopic balloon dilation (43220)*

*Rigid, transoral (43196)*

🖭 (74360)

🖭 3.83 ⚕ 9.02 **FUD** 000 J A2 ▣

**AMA:** 2017,Jan,8; 2016,Jan,13; 2015,Jan,16; 2014,Feb,9; 2014,Jan,11; 2013,Dec,3; 2013,Jan,11-12

**43227** **with control of bleeding, any method**

EXCLUDES *Esophagoscopy, flexible, transnasal or transoral; diagnostic (43197-43198, 43200)*

*Esophagoscopy, flexible, transoral; with directed submucosal injection(s) on the same lesion (43201)*

*Esophagoscopy, flexible, transoral; with injection sclerosis of esophageal varices on the same lesion (43204-43205)*

🖭 4.85 ⚕ 17.8 **FUD** 000 J A2 ▣

**AMA:** 2017,Jan,8; 2016,Jan,13; 2015,Jan,16; 2014,Feb,9; 2014,Feb,11; 2014,Jan,11; 2013,Dec,3; 2013,Jan,11-12

A2-Z3 ASC Payment
CMS: IOM (Pub 100)
50 Bilateral
A-Y OPPSI
♂ Male Only
80/80 Surg Assist Allowed / w/Doc
♀ Female Only
🖭 Facility RVU
⚕ Non-Facility RVU
▣ CCI
🖭 Lab Crosswalk
🖭 Radiology Crosswalk
✖ CLIA
CPT © 2017 American Medical Association. All Rights Reserved.
© 2017 Optum360, LLC

**43229** **with ablation of tumor(s), polyp(s), or other lesion(s) (includes pre- and post-dilation and guide wire passage, when performed)**

> EXCLUDES
> Esophagoscopy, flexible, transnasal or transoral; diagnostic (43197-43198, 43200)
> Esophagoscopy, flexible, transoral; with insertion of guide wire followed by passage of dilator(s) over guide wire on the same lesion (43226)
> Esophagoscopy, flexible, transoral; with transendoscopic balloon dilation on the same lesion (43220)
>
> Code also esophagoscopic photodynamic therapy, when performed (96570-96571)

  5.80    18.3    **FUD** 000    J G2

**AMA:** 2017,Jan,8; 2016,Jan,13; 2015,Jan,16; 2014,Feb,9; 2014,Jan,11; 2013,Dec,3

**43231** **with endoscopic ultrasound examination**

> INCLUDES
> Gastrointestinal endoscopic ultrasound, supervision and interpretation (76975)
>
> EXCLUDES
> Esophagoscopy, flexible, transnasal or transoral; diagnostic (43197-43198, 43200, 76975)
> Esophagoscopy, flexible, transoral; with transendoscopic ultrasound-guided intramural or transmural fine needle aspiration/biopsy(s) (43232)
> Procedure performed more than one time per operative session

  4.70    9.52    **FUD** 000    J A2

**AMA:** 2017,Jan,8; 2016,Jan,13; 2015,Jan,16; 2014,Feb,9; 2014,Jan,11; 2013,Dec,3; 2013,Jan,11-12

**43232** **with transendoscopic ultrasound-guided intramural or transmural fine needle aspiration/biopsy(s)**

> EXCLUDES
> Esophagoscopy, flexible, transnasal or transoral; diagnostic (43197-43198, 43200)
> Esophagoscopy, flexible, transoral; with endoscopic ultrasound examination (43231)
> Gastrointestinal endoscopic ultrasound, supervision and interpretation (76975)
> Procedure performed more than one time per operative session
> Ultrasonic guidance (76942)

  5.81    11.4    **FUD** 000    J A2

**AMA:** 2017,Jan,8; 2016,Jan,13; 2015,Jan,16; 2014,Feb,9; 2014,Jan,11; 2013,Dec,3; 2013,Jan,11-12; 2012,Jan,15-42

**43233** **Resequenced code. See code following 43249.**

## 43235-43259 [43210, 43233, 43266, 43270] Endoscopic Procedures: Esophagogastroduodenoscopy (EGD)

> INCLUDES
> Control of bleeding as result of the endoscopic procedure during same operative session
> Diagnostic endoscopy with surgical endoscopy
>
> EXCLUDES
> Exam of jejunum distal to the anastomosis in surgically altered stomach, including post-gastroenterostomy (Billroth II) and gastric bypass (43235-43259 [43233, 43266, 43270])
> Exam of upper esophageal sphincter (cricopharyngeus muscle) to/including gastroesophageal junction and/or retroflexion exam of proximal region of stomach (43197-43232 [43211, 43212, 43213, 43214])
>
> Code also modifier 52 when duodenum is not examined either deliberately or due to significant issues and repeat procedure will not be performed
> Code also modifier 53 when duodenum is not examined either deliberately or due to significant issues and repeat procedure is planned

**43235** **Esophagogastroduodenoscopy, flexible, transoral; diagnostic, including collection of specimen(s) by brushing or washing, when performed (separate procedure)**

> EXCLUDES
> Endoscopy of small intestine (44360-44379)
> Esophagogastroduodenoscopy, flexible, transoral; with esophagogastric fundoplasty (43210)
> Esophagoscopy, flexible, transnasal; diagnostic (43197-43198)
> Procedure performed with surgical endoscopy (43236-43259 [43233, 43266, 43270])

  3.61    7.28    **FUD** 000    T A2

**AMA:** 2017,Jul,10; 2017,Jan,8; 2016,Jan,13; 2015,Nov,8; 2015,Jan,16; 2014,Jan,11; 2013,Dec,3; 2013,Jan,11-12; 2012,Jan,15-42

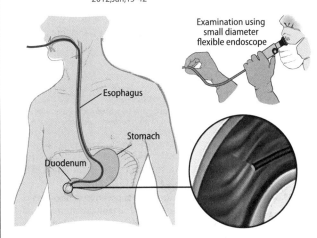

Examination using small diameter flexible endoscope

Esophagus

Stomach

Duodenum

**43236** **with directed submucosal injection(s), any substance**

> EXCLUDES
> Endoscopy of small intestine (44360-44379)
> Esophagogastroduodenoscopy, flexible, transoral; with control of bleeding, any method (43255)
> Esophagogastroduodenoscopy, flexible, transoral; with endoscopic mucosal resection on the same lesion (43254)
> Esophagogastroduodenoscopy, flexible, transoral; with injection sclerosis of esophageal/gastric varices on the same lesion (43243)
> Esophagoscopy, flexible, transnasal or transoral; diagnostic (43197-43198, 43235)
> Injection sclerosis of varices, esophageal/gastric (43243)

  4.07    9.34    **FUD** 000    T A2

**AMA:** 2017,Jan,8; 2016,Jan,13; 2015,Jan,16; 2014,Jan,11; 2013,Dec,3; 2013,Jan,11-12

● New Code    ▲ Revised Code    ○ Reinstated    ● New Web Release    ▲ Revised Web Release    Unlisted    Not Covered    # Resequenced
⊘ AMA Mod 51 Exempt    ⑤ Optum Mod 51 Exempt    ⑥③ Mod 63 Exempt    ✗ Non-FDA Drug    ★ Telemedicine    Ⓜ Maternity    Ⓐ Age Edit    ✛ Add-on    **AMA:** CPT Asst
© 2017 Optum360, LLC      CPT © 2017 American Medical Association. All Rights Reserved.      **185**

**43237** **with endoscopic ultrasound examination limited to the esophagus, stomach or duodenum, and adjacent structures**

INCLUDES  Gastrointestinal endoscopic ultrasound, supervision and interpretation (76975)

EXCLUDES  *Endoscopy of small intestine (44360-44379)*
*Esophagogastroduodenoscopy, flexible, transoral (43235, 43238, 43242, 43253, 43259)*
*Esophagoscopy, flexible, transnasal; diagnostic (43197-43198)*
*Procedure performed more than one time per operative session*

♣ 5.75    ⚕ 5.75    **FUD** 000          J A2 🖵

**AMA:** 2017,Jan,8; 2016,Jan,13; 2016,Jan,11; 2015,Jan,16; 2014,Jan,11; 2013,Dec,3; 2013,Jan,11-12

**43238** **with transendoscopic ultrasound-guided intramural or transmural fine needle aspiration/biopsy(s), (includes endoscopic ultrasound examination limited to the esophagus, stomach or duodenum, and adjacent structures)**

INCLUDES  Gastrointestinal endoscopic ultrasound, supervision and interpretation (76975)
Ultrasonic guidance (76942)

EXCLUDES  *Endoscopy of small intestine (44360-44379)*
*Esophagogastroduodenoscopy, flexible, transoral (43235, 43237, 43242)*
*Esophagoscopy, flexible, transnasal (43197-43198)*
*Procedure performed more than one time per operative session*

♣ 6.85    ⚕ 6.85    **FUD** 000          J A2 🖵

**AMA:** 2017,Jan,8; 2016,Jan,13; 2015,Jan,16; 2014,Jan,11; 2013,Dec,3; 2013,Jan,11-12

**43239** **with biopsy, single or multiple**

EXCLUDES  *Endoscopy of small intestine (44360-44379)*
*Esophagogastroduodenoscopy, flexible, transoral; diagnostic (43235)*
*Esophagogastroduodenoscopy, flexible, transoral; with endoscopic mucosal resection on the same lesion (43254)*
*Esophagoscopy, flexible, transnasal (43197-43198)*

♣ 4.08    ⚕ 9.73    **FUD** 000          T A2 🖵

**AMA:** 2017,Jan,8; 2016,Jan,13; 2015,Jan,16; 2014,Jan,11; 2013,Dec,3; 2013,Jan,11-12; 2012,Jan,15-42

**43240** **with transmural drainage of pseudocyst (includes placement of transmural drainage catheter[s]/stent[s], when performed, and endoscopic ultrasound, when performed)**

EXCLUDES  *Endoscopic pancreatic necrosectomy (48999)*
*Endoscopy of small intestine (44360-44379)*
*Esophagogastroduodenoscopy, flexible, transoral (43235, 43242, [43266], 43259)*
*Esophagogastroduodenoscopy, flexible, transoral; with transendoscopic ultrasound-guided transmural injection of diagnostic or therapeutic substance(s) on the same lesion (43253)*
*Esophagoscopy, flexible, transnasal (43197-43198)*
*Procedure performed more than one time per operative session*

♣ 11.5    ⚕ 11.5    **FUD** 000          J A2 🖵

**AMA:** 2017,Jan,8; 2016,Jan,13; 2015,Jan,16; 2014,Jan,11; 2013,Dec,3; 2013,Jan,11-12

**43241** **with insertion of intraluminal tube or catheter**

EXCLUDES  *Endoscopy of small intestine (44360-44379)*
*Esophagogastroduodenoscopy, flexible, transoral (43235, [43266])*
*Esophagoscopy, flexible, transnasal or transoral (43197-43198, 43212)*
*Tube placement:*
   *Enteric, non-endoscopic (44500, 74340)*
   *Naso or oro-gastric requiring professional skill and fluoroscopic guidance (43752)*

♣ 4.19    ⚕ 4.19    **FUD** 000          J A2 🖵

**AMA:** 2017,Jan,8; 2016,Jan,13; 2015,Jan,16; 2014,Jan,11; 2013,Dec,3; 2013,Jan,11-12

**43242** **with transendoscopic ultrasound-guided intramural or transmural fine needle aspiration/biopsy(s) (includes endoscopic ultrasound examination of the esophagus, stomach, and either the duodenum or a surgically altered stomach where the jejunum is examined distal to the anastomosis)**

INCLUDES  Gastrointestinal endoscopic ultrasound, supervision and interpretation (76975)
Ultrasonic guidance (76942)

EXCLUDES  *Endoscopy of small intestine (44360-44379)*
*Esophagogastroduodenoscopy, flexible, transoral (43235, 43237-43238, 43240, 43259)*
*Esophagoscopy, flexible, transnasal (43197-43198)*
*Procedure performed more than one time per operative session*
*Transmural fine needle biopsy/aspiration with ultrasound guidance, transendoscopic, esophagus/stomach/duodenum/neighboring structure (43238)*

🔬 88172-88173

♣ 7.73    ⚕ 7.73    **FUD** 000          J A2 🖵

**AMA:** 2017,Jan,8; 2016,Jan,13; 2015,Jan,16; 2014,Jan,11; 2013,Dec,3; 2013,Jan,11-12

**43243** **with injection sclerosis of esophageal/gastric varices**

EXCLUDES  *Endoscopy of small intestine (44360-44379)*
*Esophagogastroduodenoscopy, flexible, transoral; diagnostic (43235)*
*Esophagogastroduodenoscopy, flexible, transoral with on the same lesion (43236, 43255)*
*Esophagoscopy, flexible, transnasal (43197-43198)*

♣ 6.97    ⚕ 6.97    **FUD** 000          J A2 🖵

**AMA:** 2017,Jan,8; 2016,Jan,13; 2015,Jan,16; 2014,Jan,11; 2013,Dec,3; 2013,Jan,11-12

**43244** **with band ligation of esophageal/gastric varices**

EXCLUDES  *Band ligation, non-variceal bleeding (43255)*
*Endoscopy of small intestine (44360-44379)*
*Esophagogastroduodenoscopy, flexible, transoral (43235, 43255)*
*Esophagoscopy, flexible, transnasal (43197-43198)*

♣ 7.22    ⚕ 7.22    **FUD** 000          J A2 🖵

**AMA:** 2017,Jan,8; 2016,Jan,13; 2015,Jan,16; 2014,Jan,11; 2013,Dec,3; 2013,Jan,11-12; 2012,Jan,15-42

**43245** **with dilation of gastric/duodenal stricture(s) (eg, balloon, bougie)**

EXCLUDES  *Endoscopy of small intestine (44360-44379)*
*Esophagogastroduodenoscopy, flexible, transoral (43235, [43266])*
*Esophagoscopy, flexible, transnasal (43197-43198)*

📻 (74360)

♣ 5.16    ⚕ 15.6    **FUD** 000          J A2 🖵

**AMA:** 2017,Jan,8; 2016,Jan,13; 2015,Jan,16; 2014,Jan,11; 2013,Dec,3; 2013,Jan,11-12; 2012,Jan,15-42

**43246** **with directed placement of percutaneous gastrostomy tube**

> EXCLUDES Endoscopy of small intestine (44360-44372, 44376-44379)
> Esophagogastroduodenoscopy, flexible, transoral; diagnostic (43235)
> Esophagoscopy, flexible, transnasal (43197-43198)
> Gastrostomy tube replacement without endoscopy or imaging (43760)
> Percutaneous insertion of gastrostomy tube, nonendoscopic (49440)

5.88  5.88  **FUD** 000  [J] [A2] [80] [▭]

**AMA:** 2017,Jan,8; 2016,Jan,13; 2015,Jan,16; 2014,Jan,11; 2013,Dec,3; 2013,May,12; 2013,Jan,11-12; 2012,Jan,15-42

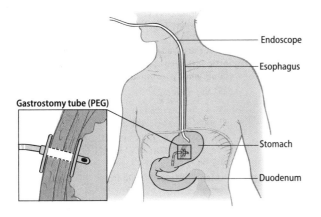

Endoscope
Esophagus
Gastrostomy tube (PEG)
Stomach
Duodenum

**43247** **with removal of foreign body(s)**

> EXCLUDES Endoscopy of small intestine (44360-44379)
> Esophagogastroduodenoscopy, flexible, transoral; diagnostic (43235)
> Esophagoscopy, flexible, transnasal (43197-43198)

(76000)

5.20  9.94  **FUD** 000  [T] [A2] [▭]

**AMA:** 2017,Jan,8; 2016,Jan,13; 2015,Jan,16; 2014,Jan,11; 2013,Dec,3; 2013,Jan,11-12; 2012,Jan,15-42

**43248** **with insertion of guide wire followed by passage of dilator(s) through esophagus over guide wire**

> EXCLUDES Endoscopy of small intestine (44360-44379)
> Esophagogastroduodenoscopy, flexible, transoral (43235, [43266], [43270])
> Esophagoscopy, flexible, transnasal (43197-43198)

(74360)

4.88  9.95  **FUD** 000  [T] [A2] [▭]

**AMA:** 2017,Jul,10; 2017,Jan,8; 2016,Jan,13; 2015,Jan,16; 2014,Jan,11; 2013,Dec,3; 2013,Jan,11-12; 2012,Jan,15-42

**43249** **with transendoscopic balloon dilation of esophagus (less than 30 mm diameter)**

> EXCLUDES Endoscopy of small intestine (44360-44379)
> Esophagogastroduodenoscopy, flexible, transoral (43235, [43266], [43270])
> Esophagoscopy, flexible, transnasal (43197-43198)

(74360)

4.52  28.8  **FUD** 000  [J] [A2] [▭]

**AMA:** 2017,Jan,8; 2016,Jan,13; 2015,Jan,16; 2014,Jan,11; 2013,Dec,3; 2013,Jan,11-12

**# 43233** **with dilation of esophagus with balloon (30 mm diameter or larger) (includes fluoroscopic guidance, when performed)**

6.69  6.69  **FUD** 000  [J] [G2] [▭]

**AMA:** 2017,Jan,8; 2016,Jan,13; 2015,Jan,16; 2014,Jan,11; 2013,Dec,3

**43250** **with removal of tumor(s), polyp(s), or other lesion(s) by hot biopsy forceps**

> EXCLUDES Endoscopy of small intestine (44360-44379)
> Esophagogastroduodenoscopy, flexible, transoral (43235)
> Esophagoscopy, flexible, transnasal (43197-43198)

5.00  11.2  **FUD** 000  [J] [A2] [▭]

**AMA:** 2017,Jan,8; 2016,Jan,13; 2015,Jan,16; 2014,Jan,11; 2013,Dec,3; 2013,Jan,11-12; 2012,Jan,15-42

**43251** **with removal of tumor(s), polyp(s), or other lesion(s) by snare technique**

> EXCLUDES Endoscopic mucosal resection when performed on same lesion (43254)
> Endoscopy of small intestine (44360-44379)
> Esophagogastroduodenoscopy, flexible, transoral (43235)
> Esophagoscopy, flexible, transnasal (43197-43198)

5.76  12.5  **FUD** 000  [J] [A2] [▭]

**AMA:** 2017,Jan,8; 2016,Jan,13; 2015,Jan,16; 2014,Jan,11; 2013,Dec,3; 2013,Jan,11-12; 2012,Jan,15-42

**43252** **with optical endomicroscopy**

> EXCLUDES Endoscopy of small intestine (44360-44379)
> Esophagogastroduodenoscopy, flexible, transoral (43235)
> Esophagoscopy, flexible, transnasal (43197-43198)
> Optical endomicroscopic image(s), interpretation and report (88375)

Code also contrast agent

4.95  8.58  **FUD** 000  [J] [G2] [▭]

**AMA:** 2017,Jan,8; 2016,Jan,13; 2015,Jan,16; 2014,Jan,11; 2013,Dec,3; 2013,Aug,5; 2013,Jan,11-12

**43253** **with transendoscopic ultrasound-guided transmural injection of diagnostic or therapeutic substance(s) (eg, anesthetic, neurolytic agent) or fiducial marker(s) (includes endoscopic ultrasound examination of the esophagus, stomach, and either the duodenum or a surgically altered stomach where the jejunum is examined distal to the anastomosis)**

> INCLUDES Gastrointestinal endoscopic ultrasound, supervision and interpretation (76975)
> Ultrasonic guidance (76942)
> EXCLUDES Endoscopy of small intestine (44360-44379)
> Esophagogastroduodenoscopy, flexible, transoral (43235, 43237, 43259)
> Esophagogastroduodenoscopy, flexible, transoral; with transmural drainage of pseudocyst on the same lesion with (43240)
> Esophagoscopy, flexible, transnasal (43197-43198)
> Procedure performed more than one time per operative session
> Transmural fine needle biopsy/aspiration with ultrasound guidance, transendoscopic, esophagus/stomach/duodenum/neighboring structures (43238, 43242)

7.73  7.73  **FUD** 000  [J] [G2] [▭]

**AMA:** 2017,Jan,8; 2016,Jan,13; 2015,Jan,16; 2014,Jan,11; 2013,Dec,3

**43254** **with endoscopic mucosal resection**

> EXCLUDES Endoscopy of small intestine (44360-44379)
> Esophagogastroduodenoscopy, flexible, transoral; diagnostic (43235)
> Esophagogastroduodenoscopy, flexible, transoral on the same lesion (43236, 43239, 43251)
> Esophagoscopy, flexible, transnasal (43197-43198)

7.96  7.96  **FUD** 000  [J] [G2] [▭]

**AMA:** 2017,Jan,8; 2016,Jan,13; 2015,Jan,16; 2014,Jan,11; 2013,Dec,3

**Digestive System**

**43255 — 43261**

| | **43255** | **with control of bleeding, any method** |
|---|---|---|

EXCLUDES Endoscopy of small intestine (44360-44379)
Esophagogastroduodenoscopy, flexible, transoral (43235)
Esophagogastroduodenoscopy, flexible, transoral on the same lesion (43236, 43243-43244)
Esophagoscopy, flexible, transnasal (43197-43198)

🚑 5.91   ⚖ 18.8   **FUD** 000   [J] [A2] ▭

**AMA:** 2017,Jan,8; 2016,Jan,13; 2015,Jan,16; 2014,Jan,11; 2013,Dec,3; 2013,Jan,11-12

# **43266** **with placement of endoscopic stent (includes pre- and post-dilation and guide wire passage, when performed)**

🚑 6.42   ⚖ 6.42   **FUD** 000   [J] [J8] ▭

**AMA:** 2017,Jan,8; 2016,Jan,13; 2015,Jan,16; 2014,Jan,11; 2013,Dec,3

**43257** **with delivery of thermal energy to the muscle of lower esophageal sphincter and/or gastric cardia, for treatment of gastroesophageal reflux disease**

EXCLUDES Endoscopy small intestine (44360-44379)
Esophageal lesion ablation (43229, [43270])
Esophagogastroduodenoscopy, flexible, transoral; diagnostic (43235)
Esophagoscopy, flexible, transnasal (43197-43198)

🚑 6.83   ⚖ 6.83   **FUD** 000   [J] [A2] ▭

**AMA:** 2017,Jan,8; 2016,Jan,13; 2015,Jan,16; 2014,Jan,11; 2013,Dec,3; 2013,Jan,11-12

# **43270** **with ablation of tumor(s), polyp(s), or other lesion(s) (includes pre- and post-dilation and guide wire passage, when performed)**

🚑 6.61   ⚖ 18.9   **FUD** 000   [J] [G2] ▭

**AMA:** 2017,Jan,8; 2016,Jan,13; 2015,Jan,16; 2014,Jan,11; 2013,Dec,3

**43259** **with endoscopic ultrasound examination, including the esophagus, stomach, and either the duodenum or a surgically altered stomach where the jejunum is examined distal to the anastomosis**

INCLUDES Gastrointestinal endoscopic ultrasound, supervision and interpretation (76975)
EXCLUDES Endoscopy of small intestine (44360-44379)
Esophagogastroduodenoscopy, flexible, transoral (43235, 43237, 43240, 43242, 43253)
Esophagoscopy, flexible, transnasal (43197-43198)
Procedure performed more than one time per operative session

🚑 6.65   ⚖ 6.65   **FUD** 000   [J] [A2] ▭

**AMA:** 2017,Jan,8; 2016,Jan,13; 2016,Jan,11; 2015,Jan,16; 2014,Jan,11; 2013,Dec,3; 2013,Jan,11-12

# **43210** **with esophagogastric fundoplasty, partial or complete, includes duodenoscopy when performed**

🚑 12.6   ⚖ 12.6   **FUD** 000   [J] [G2] ▭

**AMA:** 2017,Jan,8; 2016,Jan,13; 2015,Nov,8

## **43260-43278 [43274, 43275, 43276, 43277, 43278]**
## **Endoscopic Procedures: ERCP**

INCLUDES Diagnostic endoscopy with surgical endoscopy
Pancreaticobiliary system:
Biliary tree (right and left hepatic ducts, cystic duct/gallbladder, and common bile ducts)
Pancreas (major and minor ducts)
EXCLUDES ERCP via Roux-en-Y anatomy (for instance post-gastric or bariatric bypass or post total gastrectomy) or via gastrostomy (open or laparoscopic) (47999, 48999)
Optical endomicroscopy of biliary tract and pancreas, report one time per session (0397T)
Percutaneous biliary catheter procedures (47490-47544)
Code also appropriate endoscopy of each anatomic site examined
Code also sphincteroplasty or ductal stricture dilation, when performed prior to the debris/stone removal from the duct ([43277])
Code also the appropriate ERCP procedure when performed on altered postoperative anatomy (i.e. Billroth II gastroenterostomy)
🔀 (74328-74330)

**43260** **Endoscopic retrograde cholangiopancreatography (ERCP); diagnostic, including collection of specimen(s) by brushing or washing, when performed (separate procedure)**

EXCLUDES Endoscopic retrograde cholangiopancreatography (ERCP) (43261-43270 [43274, 43275, 43276, 43277, 43278])

🚑 9.48   ⚖ 9.48   **FUD** 000   [J] [A2] ▭

**AMA:** 2017,Jan,8; 2016,Jan,13; 2015,Dec,3; 2015,Jan,16; 2014,Jan,11; 2013,Dec,3; 2013,Jan,11-12; 2012,Jan,15-42; 2012,Jan,11-12

**43261** **with biopsy, single or multiple**

EXCLUDES Endoscopic retrograde cholangiopancreatography (ERCP); diagnostic (43260)
Percutaneous endoluminal biopsy of biliary tree (47543)

🚑 9.96   ⚖ 9.96   **FUD** 000   [J] [A2] ▭

**AMA:** 2017,Jan,8; 2016,Jan,13; 2015,Dec,3; 2015,Jan,16; 2014,Jan,11; 2013,Dec,3; 2013,Jan,11-12; 2012,Jan,15-42

**43262    with sphincterotomy/papillotomy**

> EXCLUDES    Endoscopic retrograde cholangiopancreatography (ERCP) (43260, [43277])
> Endoscopic retrograde cholangiopancreatography (ERCP) with placement or exchange of stent in the same location ([43274])
> Endoscopic retrograde cholangiopancreatography (ERCP) with removal foreign body in the same location ([43276])
> Esophagogastroduodenoscopy, flexible, transoral with ablation of tumor(s), polyp(s), or other lesion(s) in the same location ([43270])
> Percutaneous balloon dilation biliary duct or ampulla (47542)

Code also procedure performed with sphincterotomy (43261, 43263-43265, [43275], [43278])

🖥 10.5    ⚲ 10.5    **FUD** 000    Ⓙ Ⓐ₂ 🖵

**AMA:** 2017,Jan,8; 2016,Jan,13; 2015,Dec,3; 2015,Jan,16; 2014,Jan,11; 2013,Dec,3; 2013,Jan,11-12; 2012,Jan,15-42

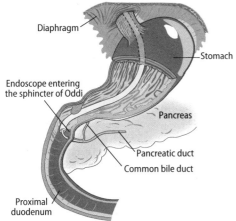

Diaphragm

Stomach

Endoscope entering the sphincter of Oddi

Pancreas

Pancreatic duct

Common bile duct

Proximal duodenum

An endoscope is fed through the stomach and into the duodenum Usually a smaller sub-scope is fed up the sphincter of Oddi and into the ducts that drain the pancreas and the gallbladder (common bile)

**43263    with pressure measurement of sphincter of Oddi**

> EXCLUDES    Endoscopic retrograde cholangiopancreatography (ERCP); diagnostic (43260)
> Procedure performed more than one time per session

🖥 10.5    ⚲ 10.5    **FUD** 000    Ⓙ Ⓐ₂ 🖵

**AMA:** 2017,Jan,8; 2016,Jan,13; 2015,Jan,16; 2014,Jan,11; 2013,Dec,3; 2013,Jan,11-12

**43264    with removal of calculi/debris from biliary/pancreatic duct(s)**

> INCLUDES    Incidental dilation due to passage of instrument
> EXCLUDES    Endoscopic retrograde cholangiopancreatography (ERCP) (43260, 43265)
> Findings without debris or calculi, even if balloon was used
> Percutaneous calculus/debris removal (47544)

Code also sphincteroplasty when dilation is necessary in order to access the area of debris/stones ([43277])

🖥 10.7    ⚲ 10.7    **FUD** 000    Ⓙ Ⓐ₂ 🖵

**AMA:** 2017,Jan,8; 2016,Jan,13; 2015,Dec,3; 2015,Jan,16; 2014,Jan,11; 2013,Dec,3; 2013,Jan,11-12; 2012,Jan,15-42

**43265    with destruction of calculi, any method (eg, mechanical, electrohydraulic, lithotripsy)**

> INCLUDES    Incidental dilation due to passage of instrument
> Stone removal when in the same ductal system
> EXCLUDES    Endoscopic retrograde cholangiopancreatography (ERCP) (43260, 43264)
> Findings without debris or calculi, even if balloon was used
> Percutaneous calculus/debris removal (47544)

Code also sphincteroplasty when dilation is necessary in order to access the area of debris/stones ([43277])

🖥 12.7    ⚲ 12.7    **FUD** 000    Ⓙ Ⓐ₂ 🖵

**AMA:** 2017,Jan,8; 2016,Jan,13; 2015,Dec,3; 2015,Jan,16; 2014,Jan,11; 2013,Dec,3; 2013,Jan,11-12

**#    43274    with placement of endoscopic stent into biliary or pancreatic duct, including pre- and post-dilation and guide wire passage, when performed, including sphincterotomy, when performed, each stent**

> INCLUDES    Balloon dilation when in the same duct
> Tube placement for naso-pancreatic or naso-biliary drainage
> EXCLUDES    Percutaneous placement biliary stent (47538-47540)
> Procedures for stent placement or exchange in the same duct (43262, [43275], [43276], [43277])

Code also for each additional stent placement in different ducts or side by side in same duct in same session/day, using modifier 59 with ([43274])

🖥 13.6    ⚲ 13.6    **FUD** 000    Ⓙ ₲₂ 🖵

**AMA:** 2017,Jan,8; 2016,Jan,13; 2015,Jan,16; 2014,Jan,11; 2013,Dec,3

**#    43275    with removal of foreign body(s) or stent(s) from biliary/pancreatic duct(s)**

> EXCLUDES    Endoscopic retrograde cholangiopancreatography (ERCP) (43260, [43274], [43276])
> Pancreatic or biliary duct stent removal without ERCP (43247)
> Percutaneous calculus/debris removal (47544)
> Procedure performed more than one time per session

🖥 11.0    ⚲ 11.0    **FUD** 000    Ⓙ ₲₂ 🖵

**AMA:** 2017,Jan,8; 2016,Jan,13; 2015,Jan,16; 2014,Jan,11; 2013,Dec,3

**#    43276    with removal and exchange of stent(s), biliary or pancreatic duct, including pre- and post-dilation and guide wire passage, when performed, including sphincterotomy, when performed, each stent exchanged**

> INCLUDES    Balloon dilation when in the same duct
> Stent placement or exchange of one stent
> EXCLUDES    Endoscopic retrograde cholangiopancreatography (ERCP) (43260, [43275])
> Procedures for stent insertion or exchange of stent in same duct (43262, [43274])

Code also each additional stent exchanged in same session/day, using modifier 59 with ([43276])

🖥 14.1    ⚲ 14.1    **FUD** 000    Ⓙ ₲₂ 🖵

**AMA:** 2017,Jan,8; 2016,Jan,13; 2015,Jan,16; 2014,Jan,11; 2013,Dec,3

**43266    Resequenced code. See code following 43255.**

**43270    Resequenced code. See code following 43257.**

● New Code    ▲ Revised Code    ○ Reinstated    ● New Web Release    ▲ Revised Web Release    Unlisted    Not Covered    # Resequenced
⊘ AMA Mod 51 Exempt    ⑩ Optum Mod 51 Exempt    ㊿ Mod 63 Exempt    ✖ Non-FDA Drug    ★ Telemedicine    Ⓜ Maternity    Ⓐ Age Edit    + Add-on    **AMA:** CPT Asst
© 2017 Optum360, LLC                    CPT © 2017 American Medical Association. All Rights Reserved.                    **189**

**43277 — 43284**

Digestive System

**#** **43277** **with trans-endoscopic balloon dilation of biliary/pancreatic duct(s) or of ampulla (sphincteroplasty), including sphincterotomy, when performed, each duct**

> EXCLUDES Endoscopic retrograde cholangiopancreatography (ERCP) (43260, 43262, [43274], [43276])
> Endoscopic retrograde cholangiopancreatography (ERCP); with ablation of tumor(s), polyp(s), or other lesion(s) for the same lesion ([43278])
> Percutaneous dilation biliary duct/ampulla (47542)
> Removal of stone/debris, dilation incidental to instrument passage (43264-43265)

Code also both right and left hepatic duct (bilateral) balloon dilation, using ([43277]) and append modifier 59 to second procedure

Code also each additional balloon dilation in different ducts or side by side in same duct in same session/day, using modifier 59 with ([43277])

Code also same session sphincterotomy without sphincteroplasty in different duct, using modifier 59 with (43262)

> 📠 11.1 ⚕ 11.1 **FUD** 000 [J] [62] 🔲

**AMA:** 2017,Jan,8; 2016,Jan,13; 2015,Dec,3; 2015,Jan,16; 2014,Jan,11; 2013,Dec,3

**#** **43278** **with ablation of tumor(s), polyp(s), or other lesion(s), including pre- and post-dilation and guide wire passage, when performed**

> EXCLUDES Ampullectomy (43254)
> Endoscopic retrograde cholangiopancreatography (ERCP); diagnostic (43260)
> Endoscopic retrograde cholangiopancreatography (ERCP); with trans-endoscopic balloon dilation of biliary/pancreatic duct(s) or of ampulla (sphincteroplasty) on the same lesion with ([43277])

> 📠 12.7 ⚕ 12.7 **FUD** 000 [J] [62] 🔲

**AMA:** 2017,Jan,8; 2016,Jan,13; 2015,Jan,16; 2014,Jan,11; 2013,Dec,3

**+** **43273** **Endoscopic cannulation of papilla with direct visualization of pancreatic/common bile duct(s) (List separately in addition to code(s) for primary procedure)**

> 📠 3.52 ⚕ 3.52 **FUD** ZZZ [N] [N1] [80] 🔲

**AMA:** 2017,Jan,8; 2016,Jan,13; 2015,Jan,16; 2014,Jan,11; 2013,Dec,3; 2013,Jan,11-12; 2012,Jan,15-42

**43274** Resequenced code. See code following 43265.

**43275** Resequenced code. See code following 43265.

**43276** Resequenced code. See code following 43265.

**43277** Resequenced code. See code before 43273.

**43278** Resequenced code. See code before 43273.

## 43279-43289 Laparoscopic Procedures of Esophagus

> INCLUDES Diagnostic laparoscopy with surgical laparoscopy (49320)

**43279** **Laparoscopy, surgical, esophagomyotomy (Heller type), with fundoplasty, when performed**

> EXCLUDES Esophagomyotomy, open method (43330-43331)
> Laparoscopy, surgical, esophagogastric fundoplasty (43280)

> 📠 37.4 ⚕ 37.4 **FUD** 090 [C] [80] 🔲

**AMA:** 2017,Aug,6; 2017,Jan,8; 2016,Jan,13; 2015,Jan,16; 2014,Jan,11; 2013,Jan,11-12; 2012,Feb,3-7

**43280** **Laparoscopy, surgical, esophagogastric fundoplasty (eg, Nissen, Toupet procedures)**

> EXCLUDES Esophagogastric fundoplasty, open method (43327-43328)
> Esophagogastroduodenoscopy fundoplasty, transoral (43210)
> Laparoscopy, surgical, esophageal sphincter augmentation (43284-43285)
> Laparoscopy, surgical, esophagomyotomy (43279)
> Laparoscopy, surgical, fundoplasty (43281-43282)

> 📠 31.3 ⚕ 31.3 **FUD** 090 [J] [80] 🔲

**AMA:** 2017,Aug,6; 2017,Jan,8; 2016,Jan,13; 2015,Nov,8; 2015,Jan,16; 2014,Dec,16; 2014,Dec,16; 2014,Jan,11; 2013,Jan,11-12; 2012,Feb,3-7

Esophagus

Diaphragm

Fundus of stomach

Normal stomach          After surgery

**43281** **Laparoscopy, surgical, repair of paraesophageal hernia, includes fundoplasty, when performed; without implantation of mesh**

> EXCLUDES Dilation of esophagus (43450, 43453)
> Implantation of mesh or other prosthesis (49568)
> Laparoscopy, surgical, esophagogastric fundoplasty (43280)
> Transabdominal repair of paraesophageal hiatal hernia (43332-43333)
> Transthoracic repair of diaphragmatic hernia (43334-43335)

> 📠 44.7 ⚕ 44.7 **FUD** 090 [J] [80] 🔲

**AMA:** 2017,Aug,6; 2017,Jan,8; 2016,Jan,13; 2015,Jan,16; 2014,Dec,16; 2014,Dec,16; 2014,Jan,11; 2013,Jan,11-12; 2012,Feb,3-7

**43282** **with implantation of mesh**

> EXCLUDES Dilation of esophagus (43450, 43453)
> Laparoscopy, surgical, esophagogastric fundoplasty (43280)
> Transabdominal paraesophageal hernia repair (43332-43333)
> Transthoracic paraesophageal hernia repair (43334-43335)

> 📠 50.3 ⚕ 50.3 **FUD** 090 [C] [80] 🔲

**AMA:** 2017,Aug,6; 2017,Jan,8; 2016,Aug,9; 2016,Jan,13; 2015,Jan,16; 2014,Dec,16; 2014,Dec,16; 2014,Jan,11; 2013,Jan,11-12; 2012,Feb,3-7

**+** **43283** **Laparoscopy, surgical, esophageal lengthening procedure (eg, Collis gastroplasty or wedge gastroplasty) (List separately in addition to code for primary procedure)**

> Code first (43280-43282)

> 📠 4.61 ⚕ 4.61 **FUD** ZZZ [C] [80] 🔲

**AMA:** 2017,Jan,8; 2016,Jan,13; 2015,Jan,16; 2014,Jan,11; 2013,Jan,11-12; 2012,Feb,3-7

**43284** **Laparoscopy, surgical, esophageal sphincter augmentation procedure, placement of sphincter augmentation device (ie, magnetic band), including cruroplasty when performed**

> EXCLUDES Performed during the same session (43279-43282)

> 📠 18.7 ⚕ 18.7 **FUD** 090 [J] [J8] [80] 🔲

**AMA:** 2017,Aug,6

| 43285 | **Removal of esophageal sphincter augmentation device** |
|---|---|

🚗 19.0   ⚕ 19.0   **FUD** 090   02 J8 80 ▣

**AMA:** 2017,Aug,6

● **43286** **Esophagectomy, total or near total, with laparoscopic mobilization of the abdominal and mediastinal esophagus and proximal gastrectomy, with laparoscopic pyloric drainage procedure if performed, with open cervical pharyngogastrostomy or esophagogastrostomy (ie, laparoscopic transhiatal esophagectomy)**

● **43287** **Esophagectomy, distal two-thirds, with laparoscopic mobilization of the abdominal and lower mediastinal esophagus and proximal gastrectomy, with laparoscopic pyloric drainage procedure if performed, with separate thoracoscopic mobilization of the middle and upper mediastinal esophagus and thoracic esophagogastrostomy (ie, laparoscopic thoracoscopic esophagectomy, Ivor Lewis esophagectomy)**

**EXCLUDES** *Right tube thoracostomy (32551)*

● **43288** **Esophagectomy, total or near total, with thoracoscopic mobilization of the upper, middle, and lower mediastinal esophagus, with separate laparoscopic proximal gastrectomy, with laparoscopic pyloric drainage procedure if performed, with open cervical pharyngogastrostomy or esophagogastrostomy (ie, thoracoscopic, laparoscopic and cervical incision esophagectomy, McKeown esophagectomy, tri-incisional esophagectomy)**

**EXCLUDES** *Right tube thoracostomy (32551)*

**43289** **Unlisted laparoscopy procedure, esophagus**

🚗 0.00   ⚕ 0.00   **FUD** YYY   J 80 50

**AMA:** 2017,Jan,8; 2016,Jan,13; 2015,Jan,16; 2014,Dec,16; 2014,Dec,16; 2014,Jan,11; 2013,Jan,11-12

## 43300-43425 Open Esophageal Repair Procedures

**43300** **Esophagoplasty (plastic repair or reconstruction), cervical approach; without repair of tracheoesophageal fistula**

🚗 17.8   ⚕ 17.8   **FUD** 090   C 80 ▣

**AMA:** 2014,Jan,11; 2013,Jan,11-12

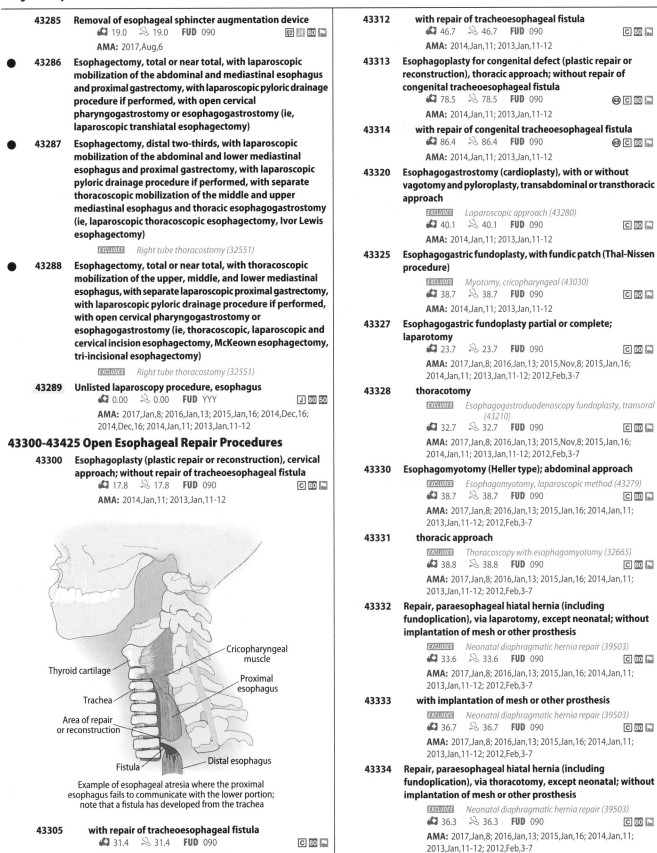

Thyroid cartilage
Trachea
Area of repair or reconstruction
Fistula
Cricopharyngeal muscle
Proximal esophagus
Distal esophagus

Example of esophageal atresia where the proximal esophagus fails to communicate with the lower portion; note that a fistula has developed from the trachea

**43305** **with repair of tracheoesophageal fistula**

🚗 31.4   ⚕ 31.4   **FUD** 090   C 80 ▣

**AMA:** 2014,Jan,11; 2013,Jan,11-12

**43310** **Esophagoplasty (plastic repair or reconstruction), thoracic approach; without repair of tracheoesophageal fistula**

🚗 42.7   ⚕ 42.7   **FUD** 090   C 80 ▣

**AMA:** 2014,Jan,11; 2013,Jan,11-12

**43312** **with repair of tracheoesophageal fistula**

🚗 46.7   ⚕ 46.7   **FUD** 090   C 80 ▣

**AMA:** 2014,Jan,11; 2013,Jan,11-12

**43313** **Esophagoplasty for congenital defect (plastic repair or reconstruction), thoracic approach; without repair of congenital tracheoesophageal fistula**

🚗 78.5   ⚕ 78.5   **FUD** 090   63 C 80 ▣

**AMA:** 2014,Jan,11; 2013,Jan,11-12

**43314** **with repair of congenital tracheoesophageal fistula**

🚗 86.4   ⚕ 86.4   **FUD** 090   63 C 80 ▣

**AMA:** 2014,Jan,11; 2013,Jan,11-12

**43320** **Esophagogastrostomy (cardioplasty), with or without vagotomy and pyloroplasty, transabdominal or transthoracic approach**

**EXCLUDES** *Laparoscopic approach (43280)*

🚗 40.1   ⚕ 40.1   **FUD** 090   C 80 ▣

**AMA:** 2014,Jan,11; 2013,Jan,11-12

**43325** **Esophagogastric fundoplasty, with fundic patch (Thal-Nissen procedure)**

**EXCLUDES** *Myotomy, cricopharyngeal (43030)*

🚗 38.7   ⚕ 38.7   **FUD** 090   C 80 ▣

**AMA:** 2014,Jan,11; 2013,Jan,11-12

**43327** **Esophagogastric fundoplasty partial or complete; laparotomy**

🚗 23.7   ⚕ 23.7   **FUD** 090   C 80 ▣

**AMA:** 2017,Jan,8; 2016,Jan,13; 2015,Nov,8; 2015,Jan,16; 2014,Jan,11; 2013,Jan,11-12; 2012,Feb,3-7

**43328** **thoracotomy**

**EXCLUDES** *Esophagogastroduodenoscopy fundoplasty, transoral (43210)*

🚗 32.7   ⚕ 32.7   **FUD** 090   C 80 ▣

**AMA:** 2017,Jan,8; 2016,Jan,13; 2015,Nov,8; 2015,Jan,16; 2014,Jan,11; 2013,Jan,11-12; 2012,Feb,3-7

**43330** **Esophagomyotomy (Heller type); abdominal approach**

**EXCLUDES** *Esophagomyotomy, laparoscopic method (43279)*

🚗 38.7   ⚕ 38.7   **FUD** 090   C 80 ▣

**AMA:** 2017,Jan,8; 2016,Jan,13; 2015,Jan,16; 2014,Jan,11; 2013,Jan,11-12; 2012,Feb,3-7

**43331** **thoracic approach**

**EXCLUDES** *Thoracoscopy with esophagomyotomy (32665)*

🚗 38.8   ⚕ 38.8   **FUD** 090   C 80 ▣

**AMA:** 2017,Jan,8; 2016,Jan,13; 2015,Jan,16; 2014,Jan,11; 2013,Jan,11-12; 2012,Feb,3-7

**43332** **Repair, paraesophageal hiatal hernia (including fundoplication), via laparotomy, except neonatal; without implantation of mesh or other prosthesis**

**EXCLUDES** *Neonatal diaphragmatic hernia repair (39503)*

🚗 33.6   ⚕ 33.6   **FUD** 090   C 80 ▣

**AMA:** 2017,Jan,8; 2016,Jan,13; 2015,Jan,16; 2014,Jan,11; 2013,Jan,11-12; 2012,Feb,3-7

**43333** **with implantation of mesh or other prosthesis**

**EXCLUDES** *Neonatal diaphragmatic hernia repair (39503)*

🚗 36.7   ⚕ 36.7   **FUD** 090   C 80 ▣

**AMA:** 2017,Jan,8; 2016,Jan,13; 2015,Jan,16; 2014,Jan,11; 2013,Jan,11-12; 2012,Feb,3-7

**43334** **Repair, paraesophageal hiatal hernia (including fundoplication), via thoracotomy, except neonatal; without implantation of mesh or other prosthesis**

**EXCLUDES** *Neonatal diaphragmatic hernia repair (39503)*

🚗 36.3   ⚕ 36.3   **FUD** 090   C 80 ▣

**AMA:** 2017,Jan,8; 2016,Jan,13; 2015,Jan,16; 2014,Jan,11; 2013,Jan,11-12; 2012,Feb,3-7

**43335** **with implantation of mesh or other prosthesis**

**EXCLUDES** *Neonatal diaphragmatic hernia repair (39503)*

🚗 38.9   ⚕ 38.9   **FUD** 090   C 80 ▣

**AMA:** 2017,Jan,8; 2016,Jan,13; 2015,Jan,16; 2014,Jan,11; 2013,Jan,11-12; 2012,Feb,3-7

**Digestive System**

**43336 — 43499**

**43336**    **Repair, paraesophageal hiatal hernia, (including fundoplication), via thoracoabdominal incision, except neonatal; without implantation of mesh or other prosthesis**
EXCLUDES    *Neonatal diaphragmatic hernia repair (39503)*
43.7    43.7    **FUD** 090                            C 80
**AMA:** 2017,Jan,8; 2016,Jan,13; 2015,Jan,16; 2014,Jan,11; 2013,Jan,11-12; 2012,Feb,3-7

**43337**    **with implantation of mesh or other prosthesis**
EXCLUDES    *Neonatal diaphragmatic hernia repair (39503)*
47.1    47.1    **FUD** 090                            C 80
**AMA:** 2017,Jan,8; 2016,Jan,13; 2015,Jan,16; 2014,Jan,11; 2013,Jan,11-12; 2012,Feb,3-7

+ **43338**    **Esophageal lengthening procedure (eg, Collis gastroplasty or wedge gastroplasty) (List separately in addition to code for primary procedure)**
Code first (43280, 43327-43337)
3.38    3.38    **FUD** ZZZ                            C 80
**AMA:** 2017,Jan,8; 2016,Jan,13; 2015,Jan,16; 2014,Jan,11; 2013,Jan,11-12; 2012,Feb,3-7

**43340**    **Esophagojejunostomy (without total gastrectomy); abdominal approach**
39.6    39.6    **FUD** 090                            C 80
**AMA:** 2014,Jan,11; 2013,Jan,11-12

**43341**    **thoracic approach**
40.7    40.7    **FUD** 090                            C 80
**AMA:** 2014,Jan,11; 2013,Jan,11-12

**43351**    **Esophagostomy, fistulization of esophagus, external; thoracic approach**
39.9    39.9    **FUD** 090                            C 80
**AMA:** 2014,Jan,11; 2013,Jan,11-12

**43352**    **cervical approach**
31.0    31.0    **FUD** 090                            C 80
**AMA:** 2014,Jan,11; 2013,Jan,11-12

**43360**    **Gastrointestinal reconstruction for previous esophagectomy, for obstructing esophageal lesion or fistula, or for previous esophageal exclusion; with stomach, with or without pyloroplasty**
68.5    68.5    **FUD** 090                            C 80
**AMA:** 2014,Jan,11; 2013,Jan,11-12

**43361**    **with colon interposition or small intestine reconstruction, including intestine mobilization, preparation, and anastomosis(es)**
74.8    74.8    **FUD** 090                            C 80
**AMA:** 2014,Jan,11; 2013,Jan,11-12

**43400**    **Ligation, direct, esophageal varices**
43.1    43.1    **FUD** 090                            C 80
**AMA:** 2014,Jan,11; 2013,Jan,11-12

**43401**    **Transection of esophagus with repair, for esophageal varices**
42.7    42.7    **FUD** 090                            C 80
**AMA:** 2014,Jan,11; 2013,Jan,11-12

**43405**    **Ligation or stapling at gastroesophageal junction for pre-existing esophageal perforation**
44.3    44.3    **FUD** 090                            C 80
**AMA:** 2014,Jan,11; 2013,Jan,11-12

**43410**    **Suture of esophageal wound or injury; cervical approach**
30.4    30.4    **FUD** 090                            C 80
**AMA:** 2017,Jan,8; 2016,Jan,13; 2015,Jan,16; 2014,Jan,11; 2013,Jan,11-12

**43415**    **transthoracic or transabdominal approach**
74.5    74.5    **FUD** 090                            C 80
**AMA:** 2014,Jan,11; 2013,Jan,11-12

**43420**    **Closure of esophagostomy or fistula; cervical approach**
EXCLUDES    *Paraesophageal hiatal hernia repair:*
*Transabdominal (43332-43333)*
*Transthoracic (43334-43335)*
29.3    29.3    **FUD** 090                            J 80
**AMA:** 2014,Jan,11; 2013,Jan,11-12

**43425**    **transthoracic or transabdominal approach**
EXCLUDES    *Paraesophageal hiatal hernia repair:*
*Transabdominal (43332-43333)*
*Transthoracic (43334-43335)*
42.2    42.2    **FUD** 090                            C 80
**AMA:** 2014,Jan,11; 2013,Jan,11-12

## 43450-43453 Esophageal Dilation

**43450**    **Dilation of esophagus, by unguided sound or bougie, single or multiple passes**
(74220, 74360)
2.33    4.46    **FUD** 000                            T A2
**AMA:** 2017,Jul,10; 2017,Jan,8; 2016,Jan,13; 2015,Jan,16; 2014,Jan,11; 2013,Dec,3; 2013,Jan,11-12; 2012,Jan,15-42

**43453**    **Dilation of esophagus, over guide wire**
EXCLUDES    *Dilation performed with direct visualization (43195, 43226)*
*Endoscopic dilation by dilator or balloon:*
*Balloon diameter 30 mm or larger (43214, 43233)*
*Balloon diameter less than 30 mm (43195, 43220, 43249)*
(74220, 74360)
2.52    25.7    **FUD** 000                            J A2
**AMA:** 2017,Jan,8; 2016,Jan,13; 2015,Jan,16; 2014,Jan,11; 2013,Dec,3; 2013,Jan,11-12; 2012,Jan,15-42

## 43460-43499 Other/Unlisted Esophageal Procedures

**43460**    **Esophagogastric tamponade, with balloon (Sengstaken type)**
EXCLUDES    *Removal of foreign body of the esophagus with balloon catheter (43499, 74235)*
(74220)
6.26    6.26    **FUD** 000                            C
**AMA:** 2014,Jan,11; 2013,Jan,11-12

Esophagus
Esophageal balloon
Inferior esophageal sphincter
Diaphragm
Fundus of stomach
Gastric balloon and aspiration tube

Inflated cuff
Endotracheal tube

An inflated endotracheal cuff may be used to protect the trachea from collapse

Gastric aspiration tube
Tube to gastric balloon
Tube to esophageal balloon

Cutaway view of Sengstaken-type esophagogastric tamponade with balloons inflated

**43496**    **Free jejunum transfer with microvascular anastomosis**
INCLUDES    Operating microscope (69990)
0.00    0.00    **FUD** 090                            C 80
**AMA:** 2017,Jan,8; 2016,Feb,12; 2016,Jan,13; 2015,Jan,16; 2014,Jan,11; 2013,Jan,11-12

**43499**    **Unlisted procedure, esophagus**
0.00    0.00    **FUD** YYY                            T
**AMA:** 2017,Jan,8; 2016,Jan,13; 2015,Nov,10; 2015,Nov,8; 2015,Jan,16; 2014,Jan,11; 2013,Dec,3; 2013,Mar,13; 2013,Jan,11-12; 2012,Jan,15-42

## 43500-43641 Open Gastric Incisional and Resection Procedures

**43500**  **Gastrotomy; with exploration or foreign body removal**
🚜 22.7  ✀ 22.7  **FUD** 090                              Ⓒ 80 ▭
AMA: 2014,Jan,11; 2013,Jan,11-12

**43501**  **with suture repair of bleeding ulcer**
🚜 39.0  ✀ 39.0  **FUD** 090                              Ⓒ 80 ▭
AMA: 2014,Jan,11; 2013,Jan,11-12

**43502**  **with suture repair of pre-existing esophagogastric laceration (eg, Mallory-Weiss)**
🚜 43.6  ✀ 43.6  **FUD** 090                              Ⓒ 80 ▭
AMA: 2014,Jan,11; 2013,Jan,11-12

**43510**  **with esophageal dilation and insertion of permanent intraluminal tube (eg, Celestin or Mousseaux-Barbin)**
🚜 26.8  ✀ 26.8  **FUD** 090                              Ⓣ 80 ▭
AMA: 2014,Jan,11; 2013,Jan,11-12

**43520**  **Pyloromyotomy, cutting of pyloric muscle (Fredet-Ramstedt type operation)**
🚜 19.8  ✀ 19.8  **FUD** 090                         ⊛ Ⓒ 80 ▭
AMA: 2014,Jan,11; 2013,Jan,11-12

**43605**  **Biopsy of stomach, by laparotomy**
🚜 24.3  ✀ 24.3  **FUD** 090                              Ⓒ 80 ▭
AMA: 2014,Jan,11; 2013,Jan,11-12

**43610**  **Excision, local; ulcer or benign tumor of stomach**
🚜 28.3  ✀ 28.3  **FUD** 090                              Ⓒ 80 ▭
AMA: 2014,Jan,11; 2013,Jan,11-12

**43611**  **malignant tumor of stomach**
🚜 35.4  ✀ 35.4  **FUD** 090                              Ⓒ 80 ▭
AMA: 2014,Jan,11; 2013,Jan,11-12

**43620**  **Gastrectomy, total; with esophagoenterostomy**
🚜 57.0  ✀ 57.0  **FUD** 090                              Ⓒ 80 ▭
AMA: 2014,Jan,11; 2013,Jan,11-12

**43621**  **with Roux-en-Y reconstruction**
🚜 65.8  ✀ 65.8  **FUD** 090                              Ⓒ 80 ▭
AMA: 2014,Jan,11; 2013,Jan,11-12

**43622**  **with formation of intestinal pouch, any type**
🚜 66.5  ✀ 66.5  **FUD** 090                              Ⓒ 80 ▭
AMA: 2014,Jan,11; 2013,Jan,11-12

**43631**  **Gastrectomy, partial, distal; with gastroduodenostomy**
INCLUDES  Billroth operation
🚜 42.0  ✀ 42.0  **FUD** 090                              Ⓒ 80 ▭
AMA: 2014,Jan,11; 2013,Jan,11-12

**43632**  **with gastrojejunostomy**
INCLUDES  Polya anastomosis
🚜 58.9  ✀ 58.9  **FUD** 090                              Ⓒ 80 ▭
AMA: 2014,Jan,11; 2013,Jan,11-12

**43633**  **with Roux-en-Y reconstruction**
🚜 55.7  ✀ 55.7  **FUD** 090                              Ⓒ 80 ▭
AMA: 2014,Jan,11; 2013,Jan,11-12

**43634**  **with formation of intestinal pouch**
🚜 61.4  ✀ 61.4  **FUD** 090                              Ⓒ 80 ▭
AMA: 2014,Jan,11; 2013,Jan,11-12

+ **43635**  **Vagotomy when performed with partial distal gastrectomy (List separately in addition to code[s] for primary procedure)**
Code first as appropriate (43631-43634)
🚜 3.28  ✀ 3.28  **FUD** ZZZ                              Ⓒ 80 ▭
AMA: 2014,Jan,11; 2013,Jan,11-12

**43640**  **Vagotomy including pyloroplasty, with or without gastrostomy; truncal or selective**
EXCLUDES  Pyloroplasty (43800)
            Vagotomy (64755, 64760)
🚜 34.1  ✀ 34.1  **FUD** 090                              Ⓒ 80 ▭
AMA: 2014,Jan,11; 2013,Jan,11-12

**43641**  **parietal cell (highly selective)**
EXCLUDES  Upper gastrointestinal endoscopy (43235-43259 [43233, 43266, 43270])
🚜 34.5  ✀ 34.5  **FUD** 090                              Ⓒ 80 ▭
AMA: 2014,Jan,11; 2013,Jan,11-12

## 43644-43645 Laparoscopic Gastric Bypass with Small Bowel Resection

**CMS:** 100-03,100.1 Bariatric Surgery for Treatment Co-morbid Conditions Due to Morbid Obesity; 100-04,32,150.1 Bariatric Surgery: Treatment of Co-Morbid Conditions Due to Morbid Obesity; 100-04,32,150.2 HCPCS Procedure Codes for Bariatric Surgery; 100-04,32,150.5 ICD Diagnosis Codes for BMI ≥35; 100-04,32,150.6 Bariatric Surgery Claims Guidance

INCLUDES  Diagnostic laparoscopy (49320)
EXCLUDES  Endoscopy, upper gastrointestinal, (esophagus/stomach/duodenum/jejunum) (43235-43259 [43233, 43266, 43270])

**43644**  **Laparoscopy, surgical, gastric restrictive procedure; with gastric bypass and Roux-en-Y gastroenterostomy (roux limb 150 cm or less)**
EXCLUDES  Roux limb less than 150 cm (43846)
            Roux limb greater than 150 cm (43645)
🚜 50.2  ✀ 50.2  **FUD** 090                              Ⓒ 80 ▭
AMA: 2014,Jan,11; 2013,Jan,11-12

**43645**  **with gastric bypass and small intestine reconstruction to limit absorption**
EXCLUDES  Roux limb less than 150 cm (43847)
🚜 53.5  ✀ 53.5  **FUD** 090                              Ⓒ 80 ▭
AMA: 2017,Jan,8; 2016,Jan,13; 2015,Jan,16; 2014,Jan,11; 2013,Jan,11-12

## 43647-43659 Other and Unlisted Laparoscopic Gastric Procedures

INCLUDES  Diagnostic laparoscopy (49320)
EXCLUDES  Endoscopy, upper gastrointestinal, (esophagus/stomach/duodenum/jejunum) (43235-43259 [43233, 43266, 43270])

**43647**  **Laparoscopy, surgical; implantation or replacement of gastric neurostimulator electrodes, antrum**
EXCLUDES  Electronic analysis/programming gastric neurostimulator (95980-95982)
            Insertion gastric neurostimulator pulse generator (64590)
            Laparoscopy with implantation, removal, or revision of gastric neurostimulator electrodes on the lesser curvature of the stomach (43659)
            Open method (43881)
            Vagus nerve blocking pulse generator and/or neurostimulator electrode array implantation, reprogramming, replacement, revision, or removal at the esophagogastric junction performed laparoscopically (0312T-0317T)
🚜 0.00  ✀ 0.00  **FUD** YYY                              Ⓙ 80 ▭
AMA: 2017,Jan,8; 2016,Jan,13; 2015,Jan,16; 2014,Jan,11; 2013,Jan,11-12; 2012,Jan,15-42

**43648**  **revision or removal of gastric neurostimulator electrodes, antrum**
EXCLUDES  Electronic analysis/programming gastric neurostimulator (95980-95982)
            Laparoscopy with implantation, removal, or revision of gastric neurostimulator electrodes on the lesser curvature of the stomach (43659)
            Open method (43882)
            Revision/removal gastric neurostimulator pulse generator (64595)
            Vagus nerve blocking pulse generator and/or neurostimulator electrode array implantation, reprogramming, replacement, revision, or removal at the esophagogastric junction performed laparoscopically (0312T-0317T)
🚜 0.00  ✀ 0.00  **FUD** YYY                              Ⓙ 80 ▭
AMA: 2017,Jan,8; 2016,Jan,13; 2015,Jan,16; 2014,Jan,11; 2013,Jan,11-12

---

● New Code   ▲ Revised Code   ○ Reinstated   ● New Web Release   ▲ Revised Web Release   Unlisted   Not Covered   # Resequenced
⊘ AMA Mod 51 Exempt   ⑤ Optum Mod 51 Exempt   ⊛ Mod 63 Exempt   ✗ Non-FDA Drug   ★ Telemedicine   Ⓜ Maternity   Ⓐ Age Edit   + Add-on   AMA: CPT Asst

© 2017 Optum360, LLC   CPT © 2017 American Medical Association. All Rights Reserved.

**Digestive System**

**43651 — 43774**

**43651** **Laparoscopy, surgical; transection of vagus nerves, truncal**
🚑 18.8  ⚖ 18.8  **FUD** 090  [J] [80] ▣
**AMA:** 2017,Jan,8; 2016,Jan,13; 2015,Jan,16; 2014,Jan,11; 2013,Jan,11-12

**43652** **transection of vagus nerves, selective or highly selective**
🚑 22.1  ⚖ 22.1  **FUD** 090  [J] [80] ▣
**AMA:** 2017,Jan,8; 2016,Jan,13; 2015,Jan,16; 2014,Jan,11; 2013,Jan,11-12

**43653** **gastrostomy, without construction of gastric tube (eg, Stamm procedure) (separate procedure)**
🚑 16.5  ⚖ 16.5  **FUD** 090  [J] [A2] [80] ▣
**AMA:** 2017,Jan,8; 2016,Jan,13; 2015,Jan,16; 2014,Jan,11; 2013,Jan,11-12

**43659** **Unlisted laparoscopy procedure, stomach**
🚑 0.00  ⚖ 0.00  **FUD** YYY  [J] [80] [50]
**AMA:** 2017,Jan,8; 2016,Jan,13; 2015,Jan,16; 2014,Jan,11; 2013,Jun,13; 2013,Feb,13; 2013,Jan,11-12; 2012,Jan,15-42

## 43752-43761 Nonsurgical Gastric Tube Procedures

**43752** **Naso- or oro-gastric tube placement, requiring physician's skill and fluoroscopic guidance (includes fluoroscopy, image documentation and report)**
EXCLUDES  *Critical care services (99291-99292)*
*Initial inpatient neonatal/pediatric critical care, per day (99468-99469, 99471-99472)*
*Percutaneous insertion of gastrostomy tube (43246, 49440)*
*Placement of enteric tube (44500, 74340)*
*Subsequent intensive care, per day, for low birth weight infant (99478-99479)*
🚑 1.18  ⚖ 1.18  **FUD** 000  [Q1] [G2] ▣
**AMA:** 2017,Jan,8; 2016,Jan,13; 2015,Jan,16; 2014,May,4; 2014,Jan,11; 2013,Jan,11-12; 2012,Jan,15-42

**43753** **Gastric intubation and aspiration(s) therapeutic, necessitating physician's skill (eg, for gastrointestinal hemorrhage), including lavage if performed**
🚑 0.63  ⚖ 0.63  **FUD** 000  [Q1] [N1] [80] ▣
**AMA:** 2017,Jan,8; 2016,Jan,13; 2015,Jan,16; 2014,May,4; 2014,Jan,11; 2013,Jan,11-12

**43754** **Gastric intubation and aspiration, diagnostic; single specimen (eg, acid analysis)**
EXCLUDES  *Analysis of gastic acid (82930)*
*Naso- or oro-gastric tube placement using fluoroscopic guidance (43752)*
🚑 1.02  ⚖ 3.48  **FUD** 000  [Q1] [N1] [80] ▣
**AMA:** 2017,Jan,8; 2016,Jan,13; 2015,Jan,16; 2014,Jan,11; 2013,Jan,11-12

**43755** **collection of multiple fractional specimens with gastric stimulation, single or double lumen tube (gastric secretory study) (eg, histamine, insulin, pentagastrin, calcium, secretin), includes drug administration**
EXCLUDES  *Analysis of gastic acid (82930)*
*Naso- or oro-gastric tube placement using fluoroscopic guidance (43752)*
Code also drugs or substances administered
🚑 1.74  ⚖ 3.92  **FUD** 000  [S] [G2] [80] ▣
**AMA:** 2017,Jan,8; 2016,Jan,13; 2015,Jan,16; 2014,Jan,11; 2013,Jan,11-12

**43756** **Duodenal intubation and aspiration, diagnostic, includes image guidance; single specimen (eg, bile study for crystals or afferent loop culture)**
Code also drugs or substances administered
🔬 (89049-89240)
🚑 1.47  ⚖ 5.74  **FUD** 000  [Q1] [G2] [80] ▣
**AMA:** 2017,Jan,8; 2016,Jan,13; 2015,Jan,16; 2014,Jan,11; 2013,Jan,11-12

**43757** **collection of multiple fractional specimens with pancreatic or gallbladder stimulation, single or double lumen tube, includes drug administration**
Code also drugs or substances administered
🔬 (89049-89240)
🚑 2.25  ⚖ 8.26  **FUD** 000  [T] [G2] [80] ▣
**AMA:** 2017,Jan,8; 2016,Jan,13; 2015,Jan,16; 2014,Jan,11; 2013,Jan,11-12

**43760** **Change of gastrostomy tube, percutaneous, without imaging or endoscopic guidance**
EXCLUDES  *Endoscopic placement of gastrostomy tube (43246)*
*Gastrostomy tube replacement using fluoroscopy (49450)*
🚑 1.36  ⚖ 13.9  **FUD** 000  [T] [A2] ▣
**AMA:** 2017,Jan,8; 2016,Jan,13; 2015,Jan,16; 2014,Jan,11; 2013,Jan,11-12; 2012,Jan,15-42

**43761** **Repositioning of a naso- or oro-gastric feeding tube, through the duodenum for enteric nutrition**
EXCLUDES  *Conversion of gastrostomy tube to gastro-jejunostomy tube, percutaneous (49446)*
*Gastrostomy tube converted endoscopically to jejunostomy tube (44373)*
*Introduction of long gastrointestinal tube into the duodenum (44500)*
📷 (76000)
🚑 2.98  ⚖ 3.36  **FUD** 000  [T] [A2] ▣
**AMA:** 2017,Jan,8; 2016,Jan,13; 2015,Jan,16; 2014,Jan,11; 2013,Jan,11-12

## 43770-43775 Laparoscopic Bariatric Procedures

**CMS:** 100-03,100.1 Bariatric Surgery for Treatment Co-morbid Conditions Due to Morbid Obesity; 100-04,32,150.1 Bariatric Surgery: Treatment of Co-Morbid Conditions Due to Morbid Obesity; 100-04,32,150.2 HCPCS Procedure Codes for Bariatric Surgery; 100-04,32,150.5 ICD Diagnosis Codes for BMI ≥35; 100-04,32,150.6 Bariatric Surgery Claims Guidance

INCLUDES  *Diagnostic laparoscopy (49320)*
*Stomach/duodenum/jejunum/ileum*
*Subsequent band adjustments (change of the gastric band component diameter by injection/aspiration of fluid through the subcutaneous port component) during the postoperative period*

**43770** **Laparoscopy, surgical, gastric restrictive procedure; placement of adjustable gastric restrictive device (eg, gastric band and subcutaneous port components)**
Code also modifier 52 for placement of individual component
🚑 32.4  ⚖ 32.4  **FUD** 090  [J] [80] ▣
**AMA:** 2017,Jan,8; 2016,Jan,13; 2015,Jan,16; 2014,Jan,11; 2013,Jan,11-12; 2012,Jan,15-42

**43771** **revision of adjustable gastric restrictive device component only**
🚑 36.8  ⚖ 36.8  **FUD** 090  [C] [80] ▣
**AMA:** 2017,Jan,8; 2016,Jan,13; 2015,Jan,16; 2014,Jan,11; 2013,Jan,11-12

**43772** **removal of adjustable gastric restrictive device component only**
🚑 27.4  ⚖ 27.4  **FUD** 090  [C] [80] ▣
**AMA:** 2017,Jan,8; 2016,Jan,13; 2015,Jan,16; 2014,Jan,11; 2013,Jan,11-12

**43773** **removal and replacement of adjustable gastric restrictive device component only**
EXCLUDES  *Laparoscopy, surgical, gastric restrictive procedure; removal of adjustable gastric restrictive device component only (43772)*
🚑 36.9  ⚖ 36.9  **FUD** 090  [C] [80] ▣
**AMA:** 2017,Jan,8; 2016,Jan,13; 2015,Jan,16; 2014,Jan,11; 2013,Jan,11-12

**43774** **removal of adjustable gastric restrictive device and subcutaneous port components**
EXCLUDES  *Removal/replacement of subcutaneous port components and gastric band (43659)*
🚑 27.7  ⚖ 27.7  **FUD** 090  [C] [80] ▣
**AMA:** 2017,Jan,8; 2016,Jan,13; 2015,Jan,16; 2014,Jan,11; 2013,Jan,11-12; 2012,Jan,15-42

**43775** **longitudinal gastrectomy (ie, sleeve gastrectomy)**

> *EXCLUDES* *Open gastric restrictive procedure for morbid obesity, without gastric bypass, other than vertical-banded gastroplasty (43843)*
> *Vagus nerve blocking pulse generator and/or neurostimulator electrode array implantation, reprogramming, replacement, revision, or removal at the esophagogastric junction performed laparoscopically (0312T-0317T)*

🔧 31.9   ⚕ 31.9   **FUD** 090   Ⓒ 80 ▣

**AMA:** 2014,Jan,11; 2013,Jan,11-12

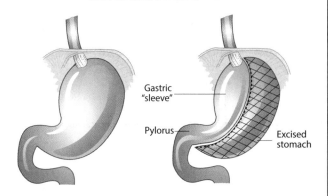

Gastric "sleeve"

Pylorus

Excised stomach

## 43800-43840 Open Gastric Incisional/Repair/Resection Procedures

**43800** **Pyloroplasty**
> *EXCLUDES* *Vagotomy with pyloroplasty (43640)*

🔧 26.9   ⚕ 26.9   **FUD** 090   Ⓒ 80 ▣

**AMA:** 2014,Jan,11; 2013,Jan,11-12

**43810** **Gastroduodenostomy**

🔧 29.3   ⚕ 29.3   **FUD** 090   Ⓒ 80 ▣

**AMA:** 2014,Jan,11; 2013,Jan,11-12

**43820** **Gastrojejunostomy; without vagotomy**

🔧 38.8   ⚕ 38.8   **FUD** 090   Ⓒ 80 ▣

**AMA:** 2014,Jan,11; 2013,Jan,11-12

**43825** **with vagotomy, any type**

🔧 37.4   ⚕ 37.4   **FUD** 090   Ⓒ 80 ▣

**AMA:** 2014,Jan,11; 2013,Jan,11-12

**43830** **Gastrostomy, open; without construction of gastric tube (eg, Stamm procedure) (separate procedure)**

🔧 20.2   ⚕ 20.2   **FUD** 090   Ⓙ 80 ▣

**AMA:** 2017,Jan,8; 2016,Jan,13; 2015,Jan,16; 2014,Jan,11; 2013,Jan,11-12

**43831** **neonatal, for feeding**   Ⓐ
> *EXCLUDES* *Change of gastrostomy tube (43760)*

🔧 16.2   ⚕ 16.2   **FUD** 090   63 Ⓣ 80 ▣

**AMA:** 2017,Jan,8; 2016,Jan,13; 2015,Jan,16; 2014,Jan,11; 2013,Jan,11-12

**43832** **with construction of gastric tube (eg, Janeway procedure)**
> *EXCLUDES* *Endoscopic placement of percutaneous gastrostomy tube (43246)*

🔧 30.0   ⚕ 30.0   **FUD** 090   Ⓒ 80 ▣

**AMA:** 2017,Jan,8; 2016,Jan,13; 2015,Jan,16; 2014,Jan,11; 2013,Jan,11-12

**43840** **Gastrorrhaphy, suture of perforated duodenal or gastric ulcer, wound, or injury**

🔧 39.3   ⚕ 39.3   **FUD** 090   Ⓒ 80 ▣

**AMA:** 2014,Jan,11; 2013,Jan,11-12

## 43842-43848 Open Bariatric Procedures for Morbid Obesity

**CMS:** 100-03,100.1 Bariatric Surgery for Treatment Co-morbid Conditions Due to Morbid Obesity; 100-04,32,150.1 Bariatric Surgery: Treatment of Co-Morbid Conditions Due to Morbid Obesity; 100-04,32,150.2 HCPCS Procedure Codes for Bariatric Surgery; 100-04,32,150.5 ICD Diagnosis Codes for BMI ≥35; 100-04,32,150.6 Bariatric Surgery Claims Guidance

**43842** **Gastric restrictive procedure, without gastric bypass, for morbid obesity; vertical-banded gastroplasty**

🔧 34.4   ⚕ 34.4   **FUD** 090   Ⓔ ▣

**AMA:** 2017,Jan,8; 2016,Jan,13; 2015,Jan,16; 2014,Jan,11; 2013,Jan,11-12

Surgical staples partition off a portion of stomach

Synthetic ring

The stomach is surgically restricted to treat morbid obesity; a vertical-banded partitioning technique gives the patient a sensation of fullness, thus decreasing daily caloric intake

**43843** **other than vertical-banded gastroplasty**
> *EXCLUDES* *Laparoscopic longitudinal gastrectomy (e.g., sleeve gastrectomy) (43775)*

🔧 36.8   ⚕ 36.8   **FUD** 090   Ⓒ 80 ▣

**AMA:** 2017,Jan,8; 2016,Jan,13; 2015,Jan,16; 2014,Jan,11; 2013,Jan,11-12

**43845** **Gastric restrictive procedure with partial gastrectomy, pylorus-preserving duodenoileostomy and ileoileostomy (50 to 100 cm common channel) to limit absorption (biliopancreatic diversion with duodenal switch)**
> *EXCLUDES* *Enteroenterostomy, anastomosis of intestine (44130)*
> *Exploratory laparotomy, exploratory celiotomy (49000)*
> *Gastrectomy, partial, distal; with Roux-en-Y reconstruction (43633)*
> *Gastric restrictive procedure, with gastric bypass for morbid obesity; with small intestine reconstruction (43847)*

🔧 56.8   ⚕ 56.8   **FUD** 090   Ⓒ 80 ▣

**AMA:** 2017,Jan,8; 2016,Jan,13; 2015,Jan,16; 2014,Jan,11; 2013,Jan,11-12

**43846** **Gastric restrictive procedure, with gastric bypass for morbid obesity; with short limb (150 cm or less) Roux-en-Y gastroenterostomy**
> *EXCLUDES* *Performed laparoscopically (43644)*
> *Roux limb more than 150 cm (43847)*

🔧 46.9   ⚕ 46.9   **FUD** 090   Ⓒ 80 ▣

**AMA:** 2017,Jan,8; 2016,Jan,13; 2015,Jan,16; 2014,Jan,11; 2013,Jan,11-12

**43847** **with small intestine reconstruction to limit absorption**
> *EXCLUDES* *Performed laparoscopically (43645)*

🔧 51.4   ⚕ 51.4   **FUD** 090   Ⓒ 80 ▣

**AMA:** 2017,Jan,8; 2016,Jan,13; 2015,Jan,16; 2014,Jan,11; 2013,Jan,11-12

● New Code   ▲ Revised Code   ○ Reinstated   ● New Web Release   ▲ Revised Web Release   Unlisted   Not Covered   # Resequenced
Ⓢ AMA Mod 51 Exempt   Ⓢ Optum Mod 51 Exempt   63 Mod 63 Exempt   ⁄ Non-FDA Drug   ★ Telemedicine   Ⓜ Maternity   Ⓐ Age Edit   + Add-on   AMA: CPT Asst
© 2017 Optum360, LLC          CPT © 2017 American Medical Association. All Rights Reserved.          195

**43848** Revision, open, of gastric restrictive procedure for morbid obesity, other than adjustable gastric restrictive device (separate procedure)

> EXCLUDES *Gastric restrictive port procedures (43886-43888)*
> *Procedures for adjustable gastric restrictive devices (43770-43774)*

🛏 55.7  ⚕ 55.7  **FUD** 090  C 80 ▭

**AMA:** 2017,Jan,8; 2016,Jan,13; 2015,Jan,16; 2014,Jan,11; 2013,Jan,11-12

## 43850-43882 Open Gastric Procedures: Closure/Implantation/Replacement/Revision

**43850** Revision of gastroduodenal anastomosis (gastroduodenostomy) with reconstruction; without vagotomy

🛏 46.7  ⚕ 46.7  **FUD** 090  C 80 ▭

**AMA:** 2014,Jan,11; 2013,Jan,11-12

**43855** with vagotomy

🛏 48.4  ⚕ 48.4  **FUD** 090  C 80 ▭

**AMA:** 2014,Jan,11; 2013,Jan,11-12

**43860** Revision of gastrojejunal anastomosis (gastrojejunostomy) with reconstruction, with or without partial gastrectomy or intestine resection; without vagotomy

🛏 47.4  ⚕ 47.4  **FUD** 090  C 80 ▭

**AMA:** 2014,Jan,11; 2013,Jan,11-12

**43865** with vagotomy

🛏 49.0  ⚕ 49.0  **FUD** 090  C 80 ▭

**AMA:** 2014,Jan,11; 2013,Jan,11-12

**43870** Closure of gastrostomy, surgical

🛏 20.5  ⚕ 20.5  **FUD** 090  J A2 80 ▭

**AMA:** 2014,Jan,11; 2013,Jan,11-12

**43880** Closure of gastrocolic fistula

🛏 46.3  ⚕ 46.3  **FUD** 090  C 80 ▭

**AMA:** 2014,Jan,11; 2013,Jan,11-12

**43881** Implantation or replacement of gastric neurostimulator electrodes, antrum, open

> EXCLUDES *Electronic analysis and programming (95980-95982)*
> *Implantation/removal/revision gastric neurostimulator electrodes, lesser curvature or vagal trunk (EGJ):*
> *Laparoscopically (43659)*
> *Open, lesser curvature (43999)*
> *Implantation/replacement performed laparoscopically (43647)*
> *Insertion of gastric neurostimulator pulse generator (64590)*
> *Vagus nerve blocking pulse generator and/or neurostimulator electrode array implantation, reprogramming, replacement, revision, or removal at the esophagogastric junction performed laparoscopically (0312T-0317T)*

🛏 0.00  ⚕ 0.00  **FUD** YYY  C 80 ▭

**AMA:** 2017,Jan,8; 2016,Jan,13; 2015,Jan,16; 2014,Jan,11; 2013,Jan,11-12

**43882** Revision or removal of gastric neurostimulator electrodes, antrum, open

> EXCLUDES *Electronic analysis and programming (95980-95982)*
> *Implantation/removal/revision gastric neurostimulator electrodes, lesser curvature or vagal trunk (EGJ):*
> *Laparoscopic (43659)*
> *Open, lesser curvature (43999)*
> *Revision/removal gastric neurostimulator electrodes, antrum, performed laparoscopically (43648)*
> *Revision/removal gastric neurostimulator pulse generator (64595)*
> *Vagus nerve blocking pulse generator and/or neurostimulator electrode array implantation, reprogramming, replacement, revision, or removal at the esophagogastric junction performed laparoscopically (0312T-0317T)*

🛏 0.00  ⚕ 0.00  **FUD** YYY  C 80 ▭

**AMA:** 2017,Jan,8; 2016,Jan,13; 2015,Jan,16; 2014,Jan,11; 2013,Jan,11-12

## 43886-43999 Bariatric Procedures: Removal/Replacement/Revision Port Components

**CMS:** 100-04,32,150.1 Bariatric Surgery: Treatment of Co-Morbid Conditions Due to Morbid Obesity; 100-04,32,150.2 HCPCS Procedure Codes for Bariatric Surgery; 100-04,32,150.5 ICD Diagnosis Codes for BMI ≥35; 100-04,32,150.6 Bariatric Surgery Claims Guidance

**43886** Gastric restrictive procedure, open; revision of subcutaneous port component only

🛏 10.4  ⚕ 10.4  **FUD** 090  T 62 80 ▭

**AMA:** 2017,Jan,8; 2016,Jan,13; 2015,Jan,16; 2014,Jan,11; 2013,Jan,11-12

**43887** removal of subcutaneous port component only

> EXCLUDES *Gastric band and subcutaneous port components:*
> *Removal and replacement performed laparoscopically (43659)*
> *Removal performed laparoscopically (43774)*

🛏 9.43  ⚕ 9.43  **FUD** 090  Q2 62 80 ▭

**AMA:** 2017,Jan,8; 2016,Jan,13; 2015,Jan,16; 2014,Jan,11; 2013,Jan,11-12

**43888** removal and replacement of subcutaneous port component only

> EXCLUDES *Gastric band and subcutaneous port components:*
> *Removal and replacement performed laparoscopically (43659)*
> *Removal performed laparoscopically (43774)*
> *Gastric restrictive procedure, open; removal of subcutaneous port component only (43887)*

🛏 13.2  ⚕ 13.2  **FUD** 090  T 62 80 ▭

**AMA:** 2017,Jan,8; 2016,Jan,13; 2015,Jan,16; 2014,Jan,11; 2013,Jan,11-12

**43999** Unlisted procedure, stomach

🛏 0.00  ⚕ 0.00  **FUD** YYY  T 80

**AMA:** 2017,Jan,8; 2016,Jan,13; 2015,Jan,16; 2014,Jan,11; 2013,Feb,13; 2013,Jan,11-12; 2012,Jan,15-42

## 44005-44130 Incisional and Resection Procedures of Bowel

**44005** Enterolysis (freeing of intestinal adhesion) (separate procedure)

> EXCLUDES *Enterolysis performed laparoscopically (44180)*
> *Excision of ileoanal reservoir with ileostomy (45136)*

🛏 31.7  ⚕ 31.7  **FUD** 090  C 80 ▭

**AMA:** 2017,Jan,8; 2016,Jan,13; 2015,Jan,16; 2014,Jan,11; 2013,Jan,11-12; 2012,Jan,15-42

**44010** Duodenotomy, for exploration, biopsy(s), or foreign body removal

🛏 25.0  ⚕ 25.0  **FUD** 090  C 80 ▭

**AMA:** 2014,Jan,11; 2013,Jan,11-12

The duodenum is surgically accessed and explored A foreign body may be removed and/or a biopsy specimen taken

| | | | | | | |
|---|---|---|---|---|---|---|
| 26/TC PC/TC Only | A2-23 ASC Payment | 50 Bilateral | ♂ Male Only | ♀ Female Only | 🛏 Facility RVU | ⚕ Non-Facility RVU | ▭ CCI |
| FUD Follow-up Days | CMS: IOM (Pub 100) | A-Y OPPSI | 80/80 Surg Assist Allowed / w/Doc | | 🔬 Lab Crosswalk | ☢ Radiology Crosswalk | ❌ CLIA |

196  CPT © 2017 American Medical Association. All Rights Reserved.  © 2017 Optum360, LLC

**+ 44015** Tube or needle catheter jejunostomy for enteral alimentation, intraoperative, any method (List separately in addition to primary procedure)

　　Code first the primary procedure
　　🔧 4.14　🔪 4.14　**FUD** ZZZ　　Ⓒ 80 ▢
　　**AMA:** 2017,Jan,8; 2016,Jan,13; 2015,Jan,16; 2014,Jan,11; 2013,Jan,11-12; 2012,Jan,15-42

**44020** Enterotomy, small intestine, other than duodenum; for exploration, biopsy(s), or foreign body removal

　　🔧 28.1　🔪 28.1　**FUD** 090　　Ⓒ 80 ▢
　　**AMA:** 2014,Jan,11; 2013,Jan,11-12

**44021** for decompression (eg, Baker tube)

　　🔧 28.2　🔪 28.2　**FUD** 090　　Ⓒ 80 ▢
　　**AMA:** 2014,Jan,11; 2013,Jan,11-12

**44025** Colotomy, for exploration, biopsy(s), or foreign body removal

　　INCLUDES　Amussat's operation
　　EXCLUDES　Intestine exteriorization (Mikulicz resection with crushing of spur) (44602-44605)
　　🔧 28.4　🔪 28.4　**FUD** 090　　Ⓒ 80 ▢
　　**AMA:** 2014,Jan,11; 2013,Jan,11-12

**44050** Reduction of volvulus, intussusception, internal hernia, by laparotomy

　　🔧 27.0　🔪 27.0　**FUD** 090　　Ⓒ 80 ▢
　　**AMA:** 2014,Jan,11; 2013,Jan,11-12

**44055** Correction of malrotation by lysis of duodenal bands and/or reduction of midgut volvulus (eg, Ladd procedure)

　　🔧 43.2　🔪 43.2　**FUD** 090　　㊿ Ⓒ 80 ▢
　　**AMA:** 2014,Jan,11; 2013,Jan,11-12

**44100** Biopsy of intestine by capsule, tube, peroral (1 or more specimens)

　　🔧 3.17　🔪 3.17　**FUD** 000　　Ⓣ A2 ▢
　　**AMA:** 2014,Jan,11; 2013,Jan,11-12

**44110** Excision of 1 or more lesions of small or large intestine not requiring anastomosis, exteriorization, or fistulization; single enterotomy

　　🔧 24.6　🔪 24.6　**FUD** 090　　Ⓒ 80 ▢
　　**AMA:** 2014,Jan,11; 2013,Jan,11-12

**44111** multiple enterotomies

　　🔧 28.4　🔪 28.4　**FUD** 090　　Ⓒ 80 ▢
　　**AMA:** 2014,Jan,11; 2013,Jan,11-12

**44120** Enterectomy, resection of small intestine; single resection and anastomosis

　　EXCLUDES　Excision of ileoanal reservoir with ileostomy (45136)
　　🔧 35.4　🔪 35.4　**FUD** 090　　Ⓒ 80 ▢
　　**AMA:** 2017,Jan,8; 2016,Jan,13; 2015,Jan,16; 2014,Jan,11; 2013,Jan,11-12

**+ 44121** each additional resection and anastomosis (List separately in addition to code for primary procedure)

　　Code first (44120)
　　🔧 7.04　🔪 7.04　**FUD** ZZZ　　Ⓒ 80 ▢
　　**AMA:** 2014,Jan,11; 2013,Jan,11-12

**44125** with enterostomy

　　🔧 34.2　🔪 34.2　**FUD** 090　　Ⓒ 80 ▢
　　**AMA:** 2014,Jan,11; 2013,Jan,11-12

**44126** Enterectomy, resection of small intestine for congenital atresia, single resection and anastomosis of proximal segment of intestine; without tapering

　　🔧 70.6　🔪 70.6　**FUD** 090　　㊿ Ⓒ 80 ▢
　　**AMA:** 2014,Jan,11; 2013,Jan,11-12

**44127** with tapering

　　🔧 80.2　🔪 80.2　**FUD** 090　　㊿ Ⓒ 80 ▢
　　**AMA:** 2014,Jan,11; 2013,Jan,11-12

**+ 44128** each additional resection and anastomosis (List separately in addition to code for primary procedure)

　　Code first single resection of small intestine (44126, 44127)
　　🔧 7.12　🔪 7.12　**FUD** ZZZ　　㊿ Ⓒ 80 ▢
　　**AMA:** 2014,Jan,11; 2013,Jan,11-12

**44130** Enteroenterostomy, anastomosis of intestine, with or without cutaneous enterostomy (separate procedure)

　　🔧 38.0　🔪 38.0　**FUD** 090　　Ⓒ 80 ▢
　　**AMA:** 2014,Jan,11; 2013,Jan,11-12

## 44132-44137 Intestine Transplant Procedures

**CMS:** 100-03,260.5 Intestinal and Multi-Visceral Transplantation; 100-04,3,90.6 Intestinal and Multi-Visceral Transplants

**44132** Donor enterectomy (including cold preservation), open; from cadaver donor

　　INCLUDES　Graft:
　　　　　　　　Cold preservation
　　　　　　　　Harvest
　　EXCLUDES　Preparation/reconstruction of backbench intestinal graft (44715, 44720-44721)
　　🔧 0.00　🔪 0.00　**FUD** XXX　　Ⓒ 80 ▢
　　**AMA:** 2014,Jan,11; 2013,Jan,11-12

**44133** partial, from living donor

　　INCLUDES　Donor care
　　　　　　　　Graft:
　　　　　　　　Cold preservation
　　　　　　　　Harvest
　　EXCLUDES　Preparation/reconstruction of backbench intestinal graft (44715, 44720-44721)
　　🔧 0.00　🔪 0.00　**FUD** XXX　　Ⓒ 80 ▢
　　**AMA:** 2014,Jan,11; 2013,Jan,11-12

**44135** Intestinal allotransplantation; from cadaver donor

　　INCLUDES　Allograft transplantation
　　　　　　　　Recipient care
　　🔧 0.00　🔪 0.00　**FUD** XXX　　Ⓒ 80 ▢
　　**AMA:** 2014,Jan,11; 2013,Jan,11-12

**44136** from living donor

　　INCLUDES　Allograft transplantation
　　　　　　　　Recipient care
　　🔧 0.00　🔪 0.00　**FUD** XXX　　Ⓒ 80 ▢
　　**AMA:** 2014,Jan,11; 2013,Jan,11-12

**44137** Removal of transplanted intestinal allograft, complete

　　EXCLUDES　Partial removal of transplant allograft (44120-44121, 44140)
　　🔧 0.00　🔪 0.00　**FUD** XXX　　Ⓒ 80 ▢
　　**AMA:** 2014,Jan,11; 2013,Jan,11-12

## 44139-44160 Colon Resection Procedures

**+ 44139** Mobilization (take-down) of splenic flexure performed in conjunction with partial colectomy (List separately in addition to primary procedure)

　　Code first partial colectomy (44140-44147)
　　🔧 3.53　🔪 3.53　**FUD** ZZZ　　Ⓒ 80 ▢
　　**AMA:** 2014,Jan,11; 2013,Jan,11-12

**44140** Colectomy, partial; with anastomosis

　　EXCLUDES　Laparoscopic method (44204)
　　🔧 38.8　🔪 38.8　**FUD** 090　　Ⓒ 80 ▢
　　**AMA:** 2017,Jan,8; 2016,Jan,13; 2015,Jan,16; 2014,Jan,11; 2013,Jan,11-12

**44141** with skin level cecostomy or colostomy

　　🔧 52.9　🔪 52.9　**FUD** 090　　Ⓒ 80 ▢
　　**AMA:** 2017,Jan,8; 2016,Jan,13; 2015,Jan,16; 2014,Jan,11; 2013,Jan,11-12

**44143** with end colostomy and closure of distal segment (Hartmann type procedure)

　　EXCLUDES　Laparoscopic method (44206)
　　🔧 48.2　🔪 48.2　**FUD** 090　　Ⓒ 80 ▢
　　**AMA:** 2017,Jan,8; 2016,Jan,13; 2015,Jan,16; 2014,Jan,11; 2013,Jan,11-12

● New Code　▲ Revised Code　○ Reinstated　● New Web Release　▲ Revised Web Release　Unlisted　Not Covered　# Resequenced
⊘ AMA Mod 51 Exempt　⑨ Optum Mod 51 Exempt　㊿ Mod 63 Exempt　✗ Non-FDA Drug　★ Telemedicine　Ⓜ Maternity　Ⓐ Age Edit　+ Add-on　**AMA:** CPT Asst
© 2017 Optum360, LLC　　　　　CPT © 2017 American Medical Association. All Rights Reserved.

**Digestive System**

**44144 — 44208**

**44144**     with resection, with colostomy or ileostomy and creation of mucofistula
    🚑 51.3    ⚗ 51.3    **FUD** 090                    C 80 ▣
    **AMA:** 2017,Jan,8; 2016,Jan,13; 2015,Jan,16; 2014,Jan,11; 2013,Jan,11-12

**44145**     with coloproctostomy (low pelvic anastomosis)
    EXCLUDES    *Laparoscopic method (44207)*
    🚑 48.0    ⚗ 48.0    **FUD** 090                    C 80 ▣
    **AMA:** 2014,Jan,11; 2013,Jan,11-12

**44146**     with coloproctostomy (low pelvic anastomosis), with colostomy
    EXCLUDES    *Laparoscopic method (44208)*
    🚑 61.5    ⚗ 61.5    **FUD** 090                    C 80 ▣
    **AMA:** 2017,Jan,8; 2016,Jan,13; 2015,Jan,16; 2014,Jan,11; 2013,Jan,11-12

**44147**     abdominal and transanal approach
    🚑 56.3    ⚗ 56.3    **FUD** 090                    C 80 ▣
    **AMA:** 2017,Jan,8; 2016,Jan,13; 2015,Jan,16; 2014,Jan,11; 2013,Jan,11-12

**44150**     Colectomy, total, abdominal, without proctectomy; with ileostomy or ileoproctostomy
    INCLUDES    Lane's operation
    EXCLUDES    *Laparoscopic method (44210)*
    🚑 54.1    ⚗ 54.1    **FUD** 090                    C 80 ▣
    **AMA:** 2014,Jan,11; 2013,Jan,11-12

**44151**     with continent ileostomy
    🚑 61.8    ⚗ 61.8    **FUD** 090                    C 80 ▣
    **AMA:** 2014,Jan,11; 2013,Jan,11-12

**44155**     Colectomy, total, abdominal, with proctectomy; with ileostomy
    INCLUDES    Miles' colectomy
    EXCLUDES    *Laparoscopic method (44212)*
    🚑 60.4    ⚗ 60.4    **FUD** 090                    C 80 ▣
    **AMA:** 2014,Jan,11; 2013,Jan,11-12

**44156**     with continent ileostomy
    🚑 65.7    ⚗ 65.7    **FUD** 090                    C 80 ▣
    **AMA:** 2014,Jan,11; 2013,Jan,11-12

**44157**     with ileoanal anastomosis, includes loop ileostomy, and rectal mucosectomy, when performed
    🚑 62.5    ⚗ 62.5    **FUD** 090                    C 80 ▣
    **AMA:** 2014,Jan,11; 2013,Jan,11-12

**44158**     with ileoanal anastomosis, creation of ileal reservoir (S or J), includes loop ileostomy, and rectal mucosectomy, when performed
    EXCLUDES    *Laparoscopic method (44211)*
    🚑 64.7    ⚗ 64.7    **FUD** 090                    C 80 ▣
    **AMA:** 2014,Jan,11; 2013,Jan,11-12

**44160**     Colectomy, partial, with removal of terminal ileum with ileocolostomy
    EXCLUDES    *Laparoscopic method (44205)*
    🚑 35.9    ⚗ 35.9    **FUD** 090                    C 80 ▣
    **AMA:** 2017,Jan,8; 2016,Jan,13; 2015,Jan,16; 2014,Jan,11; 2013,Jan,11-12

## 44180 Laparoscopic Enterolysis
    INCLUDES    Diagnostic laparoscopy (49320)
    EXCLUDES    *Laparoscopic salpingolysis/ovariolysis (58660)*

**44180**     Laparoscopy, surgical, enterolysis (freeing of intestinal adhesion) (separate procedure)
    🚑 26.6    ⚗ 26.6    **FUD** 090                    J 80 ▣
    **AMA:** 2017,Jan,8; 2016,Jan,13; 2015,Jan,16; 2014,Jan,11; 2013,Jan,11-12

## 44186-44238 Laparoscopic Enterostomy Procedures
    INCLUDES    Diagnostic laparoscopy (49320)

**44186**     Laparoscopy, surgical; jejunostomy (eg, for decompression or feeding)
    🚑 18.8    ⚗ 18.8    **FUD** 090                    J 80 ▣
    **AMA:** 2017,Jan,8; 2016,Jan,13; 2015,Jan,16; 2014,Jan,11; 2013,Jan,11-12

**44187**     ileostomy or jejunostomy, non-tube
    EXCLUDES    *Open method (44310)*
    🚑 32.0    ⚗ 32.0    **FUD** 090                    C 80 ▣
    **AMA:** 2017,Jan,8; 2016,Jan,13; 2015,Jan,16; 2014,Jan,11; 2013,Jan,11-12

**44188**     Laparoscopy, surgical, colostomy or skin level cecostomy
    EXCLUDES    *Laparoscopy, surgical, appendectomy (44970)*
                *Open method (44320)*
    🚑 35.5    ⚗ 35.5    **FUD** 090                    C 80 ▣
    **AMA:** 2017,Jan,8; 2016,Jan,13; 2015,Jan,16; 2014,Jan,11; 2013,Jan,11-12; 2012,Jan,15-42

**44202**     Laparoscopy, surgical; enterectomy, resection of small intestine, single resection and anastomosis
    EXCLUDES    *Open method (44120)*
    🚑 40.1    ⚗ 40.1    **FUD** 090                    C 80 ▣
    **AMA:** 2017,Jan,8; 2016,Jan,13; 2015,Jan,16; 2014,Jan,11; 2013,Jan,11-12

**+ 44203**     each additional small intestine resection and anastomosis (List separately in addition to code for primary procedure)
    EXCLUDES    *Open method (44121)*
    Code first single resection of small intestine (44202)
    🚑 7.01    ⚗ 7.01    **FUD** ZZZ                    C 80 ▣
    **AMA:** 2017,Jan,8; 2016,Jan,13; 2015,Jan,16; 2014,Jan,11; 2013,Jan,11-12

**44204**     colectomy, partial, with anastomosis
    EXCLUDES    *Open method (44140)*
    🚑 44.6    ⚗ 44.6    **FUD** 090                    C 80 ▣
    **AMA:** 2017,Jan,8; 2016,Jan,13; 2015,Jan,16; 2014,Jan,11; 2013,Jan,11-12; 2012,Jan,15-42

**44205**     colectomy, partial, with removal of terminal ileum with ileocolostomy
    EXCLUDES    *Open method (44160)*
    🚑 38.8    ⚗ 38.8    **FUD** 090                    C 80 ▣
    **AMA:** 2017,Jan,8; 2016,Jan,13; 2015,Jan,16; 2014,Jan,11; 2013,Jan,11-12

**44206**     colectomy, partial, with end colostomy and closure of distal segment (Hartmann type procedure)
    EXCLUDES    *Open method (44143)*
    🚑 50.8    ⚗ 50.8    **FUD** 090                    C 80 ▣
    **AMA:** 2017,Jan,8; 2016,Jan,13; 2015,Jan,16; 2014,Jan,11; 2013,Jan,11-12

**44207**     colectomy, partial, with anastomosis, with coloproctostomy (low pelvic anastomosis)
    EXCLUDES    *Open method (44145)*
    🚑 52.8    ⚗ 52.8    **FUD** 090                    C 80 ▣
    **AMA:** 2017,Jan,8; 2016,Jan,13; 2015,Jan,16; 2014,Jan,11; 2013,Jan,11-12

**44208**     colectomy, partial, with anastomosis, with coloproctostomy (low pelvic anastomosis) with colostomy
    EXCLUDES    *Open method (44146)*
    🚑 57.6    ⚗ 57.6    **FUD** 090                    C 80 ▣
    **AMA:** 2017,Jan,8; 2016,Jan,13; 2015,Jan,16; 2014,Jan,11; 2013,Jan,11-12

**44210** colectomy, total, abdominal, without proctectomy, with ileostomy or ileoproctostomy

> EXCLUDES Open method (44150)
> 51.6  51.6  **FUD** 090
> C 80
> **AMA:** 2017,Jan,8; 2016,Jan,13; 2015,Jan,16; 2014,Jan,11; 2013,Jan,11-12

**44211** colectomy, total, abdominal, with proctectomy, with ileoanal anastomosis, creation of ileal reservoir (S or J), with loop ileostomy, includes rectal mucosectomy, when performed

> EXCLUDES Open method (44157-44158)
> 63.4  63.4  **FUD** 090
> C 80
> **AMA:** 2017,Jan,8; 2016,Jan,13; 2015,Jan,16; 2014,Jan,11; 2013,Jan,11-12

**44212** colectomy, total, abdominal, with proctectomy, with ileostomy

> EXCLUDES Open method (44155)
> 59.3  59.3  **FUD** 090
> C 80
> **AMA:** 2017,Jan,8; 2016,Jan,13; 2015,Jan,16; 2014,Jan,11; 2013,Jan,11-12

**+ 44213** Laparoscopy, surgical, mobilization (take-down) of splenic flexure performed in conjunction with partial colectomy (List separately in addition to primary procedure)

> EXCLUDES Open method (44139)
> Code first partial colectomy (44204-44208)
> 5.48  **FUD** ZZZ
> C 80
> **AMA:** 2017,Jan,8; 2016,Jan,13; 2015,Jan,16; 2014,Jan,11; 2013,Jan,11-12; 2012,Jan,15-42

**44227** Laparoscopy, surgical, closure of enterostomy, large or small intestine, with resection and anastomosis

> EXCLUDES Open method (44625-44626)
> 48.3  48.3  **FUD** 090
> C 80
> **AMA:** 2017,Jan,8; 2016,Jan,13; 2015,Jan,16; 2014,Jan,11; 2013,Jan,11-12

**44238** Unlisted laparoscopy procedure, intestine (except rectum)

> 0.00  0.00  **FUD** YYY
> J 80 50
> **AMA:** 2017,Jul,10; 2017,Jan,8; 2016,Jan,13; 2015,Jan,16; 2014,Jan,11; 2013,Jan,11-12

## 44300-44346 Open Enterostomy Procedures

**44300** Placement, enterostomy or cecostomy, tube open (eg, for feeding or decompression) (separate procedure)

> EXCLUDES Intraoperative lavage, colon (44701)
> Other gastrointestinal tube(s) placed percutaneously with fluoroscopic imaging guidance (49441-49442)
> 24.3  24.3  **FUD** 090
> C 80
> **AMA:** 2017,Jan,8; 2016,Jan,13; 2015,Jan,16; 2014,Jan,11; 2013,Jan,11-12; 2012,Jan,15-42

**44310** Ileostomy or jejunostomy, non-tube

> EXCLUDES Colectomy, partial; with resection, with colostomy or ileostomy and creation of mucofistula (44144)
> Colectomy, total, abdominal (44150-44151, 44155-44156)
> Excision of ileoanal reservoir with ileostomy (45136)
> Laparoscopic method (44187)
> Proctectomy (45113, 45119)
> 30.2  30.2  **FUD** 090
> C 80
> **AMA:** 2017,Jan,8; 2016,Jan,13; 2015,Jan,16; 2014,Jan,11; 2013,Jan,11-12; 2012,Jan,15-42

**44312** Revision of ileostomy; simple (release of superficial scar) (separate procedure)

> 17.0  17.0  **FUD** 090
> T A2 80
> **AMA:** 2014,Jan,11; 2013,Jan,11-12

**44314** complicated (reconstruction in-depth) (separate procedure)

> 29.0  29.0  **FUD** 090
> C 80
> **AMA:** 2014,Jan,11; 2013,Jan,11-12

**44316** Continent ileostomy (Kock procedure) (separate procedure)

> EXCLUDES Fiberoptic evaluation (44385)
> 41.1  41.1  **FUD** 090
> C 80
> **AMA:** 2014,Jan,11; 2013,Jan,11-12

**44320** Colostomy or skin level cecostomy;

> EXCLUDES Closure of fistula (45805, 45825, 57307)
> Colectomy, partial (44141, 44144, 44146)
> Exploration, repair, and presacral drainage (45563)
> Laparoscopic method (44188)
> Pelvic exenteration (45126, 51597, 58240)
> Proctectomy (45110, 45119)
> Suture of large intestine (44605)
> Ureterosigmoidostomy (50810)
> 34.8  34.8  **FUD** 090
> C 80
> **AMA:** 2017,Jan,8; 2016,Jan,13; 2015,Jan,16; 2014,Jan,11; 2013,Jan,11-12

**44322** with multiple biopsies (eg, for congenital megacolon) (separate procedure)

> 28.8  28.8  **FUD** 090
> C 80
> **AMA:** 2014,Jan,11; 2013,Jan,11-12

**44340** Revision of colostomy; simple (release of superficial scar) (separate procedure)

> 18.0  18.0  **FUD** 090
> T A2
> **AMA:** 2014,Jan,11; 2013,Jan,11-12

**44345** complicated (reconstruction in-depth) (separate procedure)

> 30.4  30.4  **FUD** 090
> C 80
> **AMA:** 2014,Jan,11; 2013,Jan,11-12

**44346** with repair of paracolostomy hernia (separate procedure)

> 34.2  34.2  **FUD** 090
> C 80
> **AMA:** 2017,Jan,8; 2016,Jan,13; 2015,Jan,16; 2014,Jan,11; 2013,Jan,11-12; 2012,Jan,15-42

Skin

Herniations that have formed around the site of a colostomy are repaired

The colon is mobilized, trimmed if necessary, and a new stoma is often created

## 44360-44379 Endoscopy of Small Intestine

> INCLUDES Control of bleeding as a result of endoscopic procedure during same operative session
> EXCLUDES Esophagogastroduodenoscopy, flexible, transoral (43235-43259 [43233, 43266, 43270])
> Retrograde exam through anus/colon stoma (44799)

**44360** Small intestinal endoscopy, enteroscopy beyond second portion of duodenum, not including ileum; diagnostic, including collection of specimen(s) by brushing or washing, when performed (separate procedure)

> EXCLUDES Small intestinal endoscopy, enteroscopy (44376-44379)
> 4.23  4.23  **FUD** 000
> J A2
> **AMA:** 2017,Jan,8; 2016,Jan,13; 2015,Jan,16; 2014,Nov,3; 2014,Jan,11; 2013,Dec,3; 2013,Jan,11-12; 2012,Jan,15-42

**44361** with biopsy, single or multiple

> EXCLUDES Small intestinal endoscopy, enteroscopy (44376-44379)
> 4.67  4.67  **FUD** 000
> J A2
> **AMA:** 2014,Nov,3; 2014,Jan,11; 2013,Dec,3; 2013,Jan,11-12

**44363**   with removal of foreign body(s)
> EXCLUDES *Small intestinal endoscopy, enteroscopy (44376-44379)*
> 🔧 5.64   ✂ 5.64   **FUD** 000   [J] [A2] [80] [▭]
>
> **AMA:** 2014,Nov,3; 2014,Jan,11; 2013,Dec,3; 2013,Jan,11-12

**44364**   with removal of tumor(s), polyp(s), or other lesion(s) by snare technique
> EXCLUDES *Small intestinal endoscopy, enteroscopy (44376-44379)*
> 🔧 6.01   ✂ 6.01   **FUD** 000   [J] [A2] [80] [▭]
>
> **AMA:** 2014,Nov,3; 2014,Jan,11; 2013,Dec,3; 2013,Jan,11-12

**44365**   with removal of tumor(s), polyp(s), or other lesion(s) by hot biopsy forceps or bipolar cautery
> EXCLUDES *Small intestinal endoscopy, enteroscopy (44376-44379)*
> 🔧 5.30   ✂ 5.30   **FUD** 000   [J] [A2] [80] [▭]
>
> **AMA:** 2014,Nov,3; 2014,Jan,11; 2013,Dec,3; 2013,Jan,11-12

**44366**   with control of bleeding (eg, injection, bipolar cautery, unipolar cautery, laser, heater probe, stapler, plasma coagulator)
> EXCLUDES *Small intestinal endoscopy, enteroscopy (44376-44379)*
> 🔧 7.06   ✂ 7.06   **FUD** 000   [J] [A2] [▭]
>
> **AMA:** 2017,Jan,8; 2016,Jan,13; 2015,Jan,16; 2014,Nov,3; 2014,Jan,11; 2013,Dec,3; 2013,Jan,11-12

**44369**   with ablation of tumor(s), polyp(s), or other lesion(s) not amenable to removal by hot biopsy forceps, bipolar cautery or snare technique
> EXCLUDES *Small intestinal endoscopy, enteroscopy (44376-44379)*
> 🔧 7.24   ✂ 7.24   **FUD** 000   [J] [A2] [80] [▭]
>
> **AMA:** 2014,Nov,3; 2014,Jan,11; 2013,Dec,3; 2013,Jan,11-12

**44370**   with transendoscopic stent placement (includes predilation)
> EXCLUDES *Small intestinal endoscopy, enteroscopy (44376-44379)*
> 🔧 7.84   ✂ 7.84   **FUD** 000   [J] [J8] [80] [▭]
>
> **AMA:** 2017,Jan,8; 2016,Jan,13; 2015,Jan,16; 2014,Nov,3; 2014,Jan,11; 2013,Dec,3; 2013,Jan,11-12

**44372**   with placement of percutaneous jejunostomy tube
> EXCLUDES *Small intestinal endoscopy, enteroscopy (44376-44379)*
> 🔧 7.07   ✂ 7.07   **FUD** 000   [J] [A2] [▭]
>
> **AMA:** 2017,Jan,8; 2016,Jan,13; 2015,Jan,16; 2014,Nov,3; 2014,Jan,11; 2013,Dec,3; 2013,Jan,11-12

**44373**   with conversion of percutaneous gastrostomy tube to percutaneous jejunostomy tube
> EXCLUDES *Jejunostomy, fiberoptic, through stoma (43235)*
> *Small intestinal endoscopy, enteroscopy (44376-44379)*
> 🔧 5.65   ✂ 5.65   **FUD** 000   [J] [A2] [▭]
>
> **AMA:** 2017,Jan,8; 2016,Jan,13; 2015,Jan,16; 2014,Nov,3; 2014,Jan,11; 2013,Dec,3; 2013,Jan,11-12

**44376**   Small intestinal endoscopy, enteroscopy beyond second portion of duodenum, including ileum; diagnostic, with or without collection of specimen(s) by brushing or washing (separate procedure)
> EXCLUDES *Small intestinal endoscopy, enteroscopy (44360-44373)*
> 🔧 8.36   ✂ 8.36   **FUD** 000   [J] [A2] [80] [▭]
>
> **AMA:** 2017,Jan,8; 2016,Jan,13; 2015,Jan,16; 2014,Nov,3; 2014,Jan,11; 2013,Dec,3; 2013,Jan,11-12

**44377**   with biopsy, single or multiple
> EXCLUDES *Small intestinal endoscopy, enteroscopy (44360-44373)*
> 🔧 8.81   ✂ 8.81   **FUD** 000   [J] [A2] [80] [▭]
>
> **AMA:** 2017,Jan,8; 2016,Jan,13; 2015,Jan,16; 2014,Nov,3; 2014,Jan,11; 2013,Dec,3; 2013,Jan,11-12

**44378**   with control of bleeding (eg, injection, bipolar cautery, unipolar cautery, laser, heater probe, stapler, plasma coagulator)
> EXCLUDES *Small intestinal endoscopy, enteroscopy (44360-44373)*
> 🔧 11.3   ✂ 11.3   **FUD** 000   [J] [A2] [80] [▭]
>
> **AMA:** 2017,Jan,8; 2016,Jan,13; 2015,Jan,16; 2014,Nov,3; 2014,Jan,11; 2013,Dec,3; 2013,Jan,11-12; 2012,Apr,17-18

**44379**   with transendoscopic stent placement (includes predilation)
> EXCLUDES *Small intestinal endoscopy, enteroscopy (44360-44373)*
> 🔧 12.0   ✂ 12.0   **FUD** 000   [J] [A2] [80] [▭]
>
> **AMA:** 2017,Jan,8; 2016,Jan,13; 2015,Jan,16; 2014,Nov,3; 2014,Jan,11; 2013,Dec,3; 2013,Jan,11-12

## 44380-44384 [44381] Ileoscopy Via Stoma

> INCLUDES Control of bleeding as result of endoscopic procedure during same operative session
> EXCLUDES *Computed tomographic colonography (74261-74263)*

Code also exam of nonfunctional distal colon/rectum, when performed, with:
   Anoscopy (46600, 46604-46606, 46608-46615)
   Proctosigmoidoscopy (45300-45327)
   Sigmoidoscopy (45330-45347 [45346])

**44380**   Ileoscopy, through stoma; diagnostic, including collection of specimen(s) by brushing or washing, when performed (separate procedure)
> EXCLUDES *Ileoscopy, through stoma (44382-44384 [44381])*
> 🔧 1.65   ✂ 4.77   **FUD** 000   [T] [A2] [▭]
>
> **AMA:** 2017,Jan,8; 2016,Jan,13; 2015,Jan,16; 2014,Dec,3; 2014,Nov,3; 2014,Jan,11; 2013,Dec,3; 2013,Jan,11-12

*44381*   **Resequenced code. See code following 44382.**

**44382**   with biopsy, single or multiple
> EXCLUDES *Ileoscopy, through stoma; diagnostic (44380)*
> 🔧 2.15   ✂ 7.43   **FUD** 000   [T] [A2] [▭]
>
> **AMA:** 2017,Jan,8; 2016,Jan,13; 2015,Jan,16; 2014,Dec,3; 2014,Nov,3; 2014,Jan,11; 2013,Dec,3; 2013,Jan,11-12

# **44381**   with transendoscopic balloon dilation
> EXCLUDES *Ileoscopy, through stoma (44380, 44384)*
> Code also each additional stricture dilated in same session, using modifier 59 with (44381)
> 🔧 (74360)
> 🔧 2.49   ✂ 26.5   **FUD** 000   [J] [G2] [▭]
>
> **AMA:** 2017,Jan,8; 2016,Jan,13; 2015,Jan,16; 2014,Dec,3; 2014,Nov,3

**44384**   with placement of endoscopic stent (includes pre- and post-dilation and guide wire passage, when performed)
> EXCLUDES *Ileoscopy, through stoma (44380-44381)*
> 🔧 (74360)
> 🔧 4.48   ✂ 4.48   **FUD** 000   [J] [G2] [▭]
>
> **AMA:** 2017,Jan,8; 2016,Jan,13; 2015,Jan,16; 2014,Dec,3; 2014,Nov,3

## 44385-44386 Endoscopy of Small Intestinal Pouch

> INCLUDES Control of bleeding as result of the endoscopic procedure during same operative session
> EXCLUDES *Computed tomographic colonography (74261-74263)*

**44385**   Endoscopic evaluation of small intestinal pouch (eg, Kock pouch, ileal reservoir [S or J]); diagnostic, including collection of specimen(s) by brushing or washing, when performed (separate procedure)
> EXCLUDES *Endoscopic evaluation of small intestinal pouch (44386)*
> 🔧 2.11   ✂ 5.42   **FUD** 000   [T] [A2] [▭]
>
> **AMA:** 2017,Jan,8; 2016,Jan,13; 2015,Jan,16; 2014,Dec,3; 2014,Nov,3; 2014,Jan,11; 2013,Dec,3; 2013,Jan,11-12

**44386**   with biopsy, single or multiple
> EXCLUDES *Endoscopic evaluation of small intestinal pouch (44385)*
> 🔧 2.61   ✂ 8.10   **FUD** 000   [T] [A2] [▭]
>
> **AMA:** 2017,Jan,8; 2016,Jan,13; 2015,Jan,16; 2014,Dec,3; 2014,Nov,3; 2014,Jan,11; 2013,Dec,3; 2013,Jan,11-12

26/TC PC/TC Only   A2-Z3 ASC Payment   50 Bilateral   ♂ Male Only   ♀ Female Only   🔧 Facility RVU   ✂ Non-Facility RVU   ▭ CCI
FUD Follow-up Days   CMS: IOM (Pub 100)   A-Y OPPSI   80/80 Surg Assist Allowed / w/Doc   🔧 Lab Crosswalk   🔧 Radiology Crosswalk   ✖ CLIA
CPT © 2017 American Medical Association. All Rights Reserved.

© 2017 Optum360, LLC

## 44388-44408 [44401] Colonoscopy Via Stoma

INCLUDES    Control of bleeding as result of endoscopic procedure during same operative session

EXCLUDES    *Colonoscopy via rectum (45378, 45392-45393 [45390, 45398])*

*Computed tomographic colonography (74261-74263)*

Code also exam of nonfunctional distal colon/rectum, when performed, with:
Anoscopy (46600, 46604-46606, 46608-46615)
Proctosigmoidoscopy (45300-45327)
Sigmoidoscopy (45330-45347 [45346])

**44388**    **Colonoscopy through stoma; diagnostic, including collection of specimen(s) by brushing or washing, when performed (separate procedure)**

EXCLUDES    *Colonoscopy through stoma (44389-44408 [44401])*

Code also modifier 53 when planned total colonoscopy cannot be completed

4.59    8.21    **FUD** 000      T A2

**AMA:** 2017,Jan,8; 2016,Jan,13; 2015,Jan,16; 2014,Dec,3; 2014,Nov,3; 2014,Jan,11; 2013,Dec,3; 2013,Jan,11-12; 2012,Jan,15-42

**44389**    **with biopsy, single or multiple**

EXCLUDES    *Colonoscopy through stoma; diagnostic (44388)*

*Colonoscopy through stoma; with endoscopic mucosal resection on the same lesion (44403)*

Code also modifier 52 when colonoscope fails to reach the junction of the small intestine

5.05    10.7    **FUD** 000      T A2

**AMA:** 2017,Jan,8; 2016,Jan,13; 2015,Jan,16; 2014,Dec,3; 2014,Nov,3; 2014,Jan,11; 2013,Dec,3; 2013,Jan,11-12

**44390**    **with removal of foreign body(s)**

EXCLUDES    *Colonoscopy through stoma; diagnostic (44388)*

Code also modifier 52 when colonoscope fails to reach the junction of the small intestine

(76000)

6.20    10.6    **FUD** 000      T A2

**AMA:** 2017,Jan,8; 2016,Jan,13; 2015,Jan,16; 2014,Dec,3; 2014,Nov,3; 2014,Jan,11; 2013,Dec,3; 2013,Jan,11-12

**44391**    **with control of bleeding, any method**

EXCLUDES    *Colonoscopy through stoma; diagnostic (44388)*

*Colonoscopy through stoma; with directed submucosal injection(s) on the same lesion (44404)*

Code also modifier 52 when colonoscope fails to reach the junction of the small intestine

6.77    19.6    **FUD** 000      T A2

**AMA:** 2017,Jan,8; 2016,Jan,13; 2015,Jan,16; 2014,Dec,3; 2014,Nov,3; 2014,Jan,11; 2013,Dec,3; 2013,Jan,11-12

**44392**    **with removal of tumor(s), polyp(s), or other lesion(s) by hot biopsy forceps**

EXCLUDES    *Colonoscopy through stoma; diagnostic (44388)*

Code also modifier 52 when colonoscope fails to reach the junction of the small intestine

5.82    9.96    **FUD** 000      T A2

**AMA:** 2017,Jan,8; 2016,Jan,13; 2015,Jan,16; 2014,Dec,3; 2014,Nov,3; 2014,Jan,11; 2013,Dec,3; 2013,Jan,11-12

**# 44401**    **with ablation of tumor(s), polyp(s), or other lesion(s) (includes pre-and post-dilation and guide wire passage, when performed)**

EXCLUDES    *Colonoscopy through stoma; diagnostic (44388)*

*Colonoscopy through stoma; with transendoscopic balloon dilation on the same lesion (44405)*

Code also modifier 52 when colonoscope fails to reach the junction of the small intestine

7.12    90.0    **FUD** 000      T 62

**AMA:** 2017,Jan,8; 2016,Jan,13; 2015,Jan,16; 2014,Dec,3; 2014,Nov,3

**44394**    **with removal of tumor(s), polyp(s), or other lesion(s) by snare technique**

EXCLUDES    *Colonoscopy through stoma; diagnostic (44388)*

*Colonoscopy through stoma; with endoscopic mucosal resection on the same lesion (44403)*

Code also modifier 52 when colonoscope fails to reach the junction of the small intestine

6.63    11.4    **FUD** 000      T A2

**AMA:** 2017,Jan,8; 2016,Jan,13; 2015,Jan,16; 2014,Dec,3; 2014,Nov,3; 2014,Jan,11; 2013,Dec,3; 2013,Jan,11-12

*44401*    **Resequenced code. See code following 44392.**

**44402**    **with endoscopic stent placement (including pre- and post-dilation and guide wire passage, when performed)**

EXCLUDES    *Colonoscopy through stoma (44388, 44405)*

Code also modifier 52 when colonoscope fails to reach the junction of the small intestine

(74360)

7.65    7.65    **FUD** 000      J J8

**AMA:** 2017,Jan,8; 2016,Jan,13; 2015,Jan,16; 2014,Dec,3; 2014,Nov,3

**44403**    **with endoscopic mucosal resection**

EXCLUDES    *Colonoscopy through stoma; diagnostic (44388)*

*Colonoscopy through stoma on the same lesion (44389, 44394, 44404)*

Code also modifier 52 when colonoscope fails to reach the junction of the small intestine

8.92    8.92    **FUD** 000      T 62

**AMA:** 2017,Jan,8; 2016,Jan,13; 2015,Jan,16; 2014,Dec,3; 2014,Nov,3

**44404**    **with directed submucosal injection(s), any substance**

EXCLUDES    *Colonoscopy through stoma; diagnostic (44388)*

*Colonoscopy through stoma on the same lesion (44391, 44403)*

Code also modifier 52 when colonoscope fails to reach the junction of the small intestine

5.05    10.2    **FUD** 000      T 62

**AMA:** 2017,Jan,8; 2016,Jan,13; 2015,Jan,16; 2014,Dec,3; 2014,Nov,3

**44405**    **with transendoscopic balloon dilation**

EXCLUDES    *Colonoscopy through stoma (44388, [44401], 44402)*

Code also each additional stricture dilated in same session, using modifier 59 with (44405)

Code also modifier 52 when colonoscope fails to reach the junction of the small intestine

(74360)

5.38    15.3    **FUD** 000      T 62

**AMA:** 2017,Jan,8; 2016,Jan,13; 2015,Jan,16; 2014,Dec,3; 2014,Nov,3

**44406**    **with endoscopic ultrasound examination, limited to the sigmoid, descending, transverse, or ascending colon and cecum and adjacent structures**

INCLUDES    Gastrointestinal endoscopic ultrasound, supervision and interpretation (76975)

EXCLUDES    *Colonoscopy through stoma (44388, 44407)*

*Procedure performed more than one time per operative session*

Code also modifier 52 when colonoscope fails to reach the junction of the small intestine

6.75    6.75    **FUD** 000      T 62

**AMA:** 2017,Jan,8; 2016,Jan,13; 2015,Jan,16; 2014,Dec,3; 2014,Nov,3

● New Code    ▲ Revised Code    ○ Reinstated    ● New Web Release    ▲ Revised Web Release    Unlisted    Not Covered    # Resequenced
⊘ AMA Mod 51 Exempt    50 Optum Mod 51 Exempt    63 Mod 63 Exempt    ⁄ Non-FDA Drug    ★ Telemedicine    M Maternity    A Age Edit    + Add-on    AMA: CPT Asst
© 2017 Optum360, LLC      CPT © 2017 American Medical Association. All Rights Reserved.

**Digestive System**

**44407 — 44721**

**44407** **with transendoscopic ultrasound guided intramural or transmural fine needle aspiration/biopsy(s), includes endoscopic ultrasound examination limited to the sigmoid, descending, transverse, or ascending colon and cecum and adjacent structures**

> INCLUDES　Gastrointestinal endoscopic ultrasound, supervision and interpretation (76975)
> Ultrasonic guidance (76942)
> EXCLUDES　*Colonoscopy through stoma (44388, 44406)*
> *Procedure performed more than one time per operative session*
> Code also modifier 52 when colonoscope fails to reach the junction of the small intestine

🖩 8.09　⚕ 8.09　**FUD** 000　　　　T 62 🔲

**AMA:** 2017,Jan,8; 2016,Jan,13; 2015,Jan,16; 2014,Dec,3; 2014,Nov,3

**44408** **with decompression (for pathologic distention) (eg, volvulus, megacolon), including placement of decompression tube, when performed**

> EXCLUDES　*Colonoscopy through stoma; diagnostic (44388)*
> *Procedure performed more than one time per operative session*

🖩 6.81　⚕ 6.81　**FUD** 000　　　　T 62 🔲

**AMA:** 2017,Jan,8; 2016,Jan,13; 2015,Jan,16; 2014,Dec,3; 2014,Nov,3

## 44500 Gastrointestinal Intubation

**44500** **Introduction of long gastrointestinal tube (eg, Miller-Abbott) (separate procedure)**

> EXCLUDES　*Placement of oro- or naso-gastric tube (43752)*
> 🔧 *(74340)*

🖩 0.56　⚕ 0.56　**FUD** 000　　　⊘ T 62 80 🔲

**AMA:** 2017,Jan,8; 2016,Sep,9; 2016,Jan,13; 2015,Jan,16; 2014,Jan,11; 2013,Dec,3; 2013,Jan,11-12

## 44602-44680 Open Repair Procedures of Intestines

**44602** **Suture of small intestine (enterorrhaphy) for perforated ulcer, diverticulum, wound, injury or rupture; single perforation**

🖩 40.9　⚕ 40.9　**FUD** 090　　　　C 80 🔲

**AMA:** 2014,Jan,11; 2013,Dec,3; 2013,Jan,11-12

**44603** **multiple perforations**

🖩 47.0　⚕ 47.0　**FUD** 090　　　　C 80 🔲

**AMA:** 2014,Jan,11; 2013,Dec,3; 2013,Jan,11-12

**44604** **Suture of large intestine (colorrhaphy) for perforated ulcer, diverticulum, wound, injury or rupture (single or multiple perforations); without colostomy**

🖩 30.6　⚕ 30.6　**FUD** 090　　　　C 80 🔲

**AMA:** 2014,Jan,11; 2013,Dec,3; 2013,Jan,11-12

**44605** **with colostomy**

🖩 37.7　⚕ 37.7　**FUD** 090　　　　C 80 🔲

**AMA:** 2014,Jan,11; 2013,Dec,3; 2013,Jan,11-12

**44615** **Intestinal stricturoplasty (enterotomy and enterorrhaphy) with or without dilation, for intestinal obstruction**

🖩 31.1　⚕ 31.1　**FUD** 090　　　　C 80 🔲

**AMA:** 2014,Jan,11; 2013,Dec,3; 2013,Jan,11-12

**44620** **Closure of enterostomy, large or small intestine;**

> EXCLUDES　*Laparoscopic method (44227)*

🖩 25.1　⚕ 25.1　**FUD** 090　　　　C 80 🔲

**AMA:** 2014,Jan,11; 2013,Dec,3; 2013,Jan,11-12

**44625** **with resection and anastomosis other than colorectal**

> EXCLUDES　*Laparoscopic method (44227)*

🖩 29.4　⚕ 29.4　**FUD** 090　　　　C 80 🔲

**AMA:** 2014,Jan,11; 2013,Dec,3; 2013,Jan,11-12

**44626** **with resection and colorectal anastomosis (eg, closure of Hartmann type procedure)**

> EXCLUDES　*Laparoscopic method (44227)*

🖩 46.5　⚕ 46.5　**FUD** 090　　　　C 80 🔲

**AMA:** 2014,Jan,11; 2013,Dec,3; 2013,Jan,11-12

**44640** **Closure of intestinal cutaneous fistula**

🖩 40.6　⚕ 40.6　**FUD** 090　　　　C 80 🔲

**AMA:** 2014,Jan,11; 2013,Dec,3; 2013,Jan,11-12

**44650** **Closure of enteroenteric or enterocolic fistula**

🖩 41.9　⚕ 41.9　**FUD** 090　　　　C 80 🔲

**AMA:** 2014,Jan,11; 2013,Dec,3; 2013,Jan,11-12

**44660** **Closure of enterovesical fistula; without intestinal or bladder resection**

> EXCLUDES　*Closure of fistula:*
> *Gastrocolic (43880)*
> *Rectovesical (45800, 45805)*
> *Renocolic (50525-50526)*

🖩 38.7　⚕ 38.7　**FUD** 090　　　　C 80 🔲

**AMA:** 2014,Jan,11; 2013,Dec,3; 2013,Jan,11-12

**44661** **with intestine and/or bladder resection**

> EXCLUDES　*Closure of fistula:*
> *Gastrocolic (43880)*
> *Rectovesical (45800, 45805)*
> *Renocolic (50525-50526)*

🖩 44.9　⚕ 44.9　**FUD** 090　　　　C 80 🔲

**AMA:** 2014,Jan,11; 2013,Dec,3; 2013,Jan,11-12

**44680** **Intestinal plication (separate procedure)**

> INCLUDES　Noble intestinal plication

🖩 30.9　⚕ 30.9　**FUD** 090　　　　C 80 🔲

**AMA:** 2014,Jan,11; 2013,Dec,3; 2013,Jan,11-12

## 44700-44705 Other Intestinal Procedures

**44700** **Exclusion of small intestine from pelvis by mesh or other prosthesis, or native tissue (eg, bladder or omentum)**

> EXCLUDES　*Therapeutic radiation clinical treatment (77261-77799 [77295, 77385, 77386, 77387, 77424, 77425])*

🖩 29.4　⚕ 29.4　**FUD** 090　　　　C 80 🔲

**AMA:** 2014,Jan,11; 2013,Dec,3; 2013,Jan,11-12

+ **44701** **Intraoperative colonic lavage (List separately in addition to code for primary procedure)**

> EXCLUDES　*Appendectomy (44950-44960)*
> Code first as appropriate (44140, 44145, 44150, 44604)

🖩 4.89　⚕ 4.89　**FUD** ZZZ　　　N N1 80 🔲

**AMA:** 2014,Jan,11; 2013,Dec,3; 2013,Jan,11-12

**44705** **Preparation of fecal microbiota for instillation, including assessment of donor specimen**

> EXCLUDES　*Fecal instillation by enema or oro-nasogastric tube (44799)*
> *Therapeutic enema (74283)*

🖩 0.00　⚕ 0.00　**FUD** XXX　　　　B 🔲

**AMA:** 2017,Jan,8; 2016,Jan,13; 2015,Jan,16; 2014,Jan,11; 2013,Dec,3; 2013,May,12; 2013,Jan,11-12

## 44715-44799 Backbench Transplant Procedures

**CMS:** 100-04,3,90.6 Intestinal and Multi-Visceral Transplants

**44715** **Backbench standard preparation of cadaver or living donor intestine allograft prior to transplantation, including mobilization and fashioning of the superior mesenteric artery and vein**

> INCLUDES　Mobilization/fashioning of superior mesenteric vein/artery

🖩 0.00　⚕ 0.00　**FUD** XXX　　　　C 80 🔲

**AMA:** 2014,Jan,11; 2013,Dec,3; 2013,Jan,11-12

**44720** **Backbench reconstruction of cadaver or living donor intestine allograft prior to transplantation; venous anastomosis, each**

🖩 8.82　⚕ 8.82　**FUD** XXX　　　　C 80 🔲

**AMA:** 2014,Jan,11; 2013,Dec,3; 2013,Jan,11-12

**44721** **arterial anastomosis, each**

🖩 11.1　⚕ 11.1　**FUD** XXX　　　　C 80 🔲

**AMA:** 2017,Jan,8; 2016,Jan,13; 2015,Jan,16; 2014,Jan,11; 2013,Dec,3; 2013,Jan,11-12

**44799** Unlisted procedure, small intestine

> EXCLUDES *Unlisted colon procedure (45399)*
> *Unlisted intestinal procedure performed laparoscopically (44238)*
> *Unlisted rectal procedure (45499, 45999)*

🚑 0.00 ⚕ 0.00 **FUD** YYY     T

**AMA:** 2017,Jan,8; 2016,Jan,13; 2015,Jan,16; 2014,Nov,3; 2014,Jan,11; 2013,Dec,3; 2013,May,12; 2013,Jan,11-12; 2012,Jan,15-42

## 44800-44899 Meckel's Diverticulum and Mesentery Procedures

**44800** Excision of Meckel's diverticulum (diverticulectomy) or omphalomesenteric duct

🚑 22.1 ⚕ 22.1 **FUD** 090     C 80

**AMA:** 2014,Jan,11; 2013,Dec,3; 2013,Jan,11-12

**44820** Excision of lesion of mesentery (separate procedure)

> EXCLUDES *Resection of intestine (44120-44128, 44140-44160)*

🚑 24.2 ⚕ 24.2 **FUD** 090     C 80

**AMA:** 2014,Jan,11; 2013,Dec,3; 2013,Jan,11-12

**44850** Suture of mesentery (separate procedure)

> EXCLUDES *Internal hernia repair/reduction (44050)*

🚑 21.7 ⚕ 21.7 **FUD** 090     C 80

**AMA:** 2014,Jan,11; 2013,Dec,3; 2013,Jan,11-12

**44899** Unlisted procedure, Meckel's diverticulum and the mesentery

🚑 0.00 ⚕ 0.00 **FUD** YYY     C 80

**AMA:** 2014,Jan,11; 2013,Dec,3; 2013,Jan,11-12

## 44900-44979 Open and Endoscopic Appendix Procedures

**44900** Incision and drainage of appendiceal abscess, open

> EXCLUDES *Image guided percutaneous catheter drainage (49406)*

🚑 22.2 ⚕ 22.2 **FUD** 090     C 80

**AMA:** 2014,Jan,11; 2013,Nov,9; 2013,Dec,3; 2013,Jan,11-12

**44950** Appendectomy;

> INCLUDES Battle's operation
> EXCLUDES *Procedure performed with other intra-abdominal procedure(s) when appendectomy is incidental*

🚑 18.5 ⚕ 18.5 **FUD** 090     J 80

**AMA:** 2017,Jan,8; 2016,Jan,13; 2015,Jan,16; 2014,Jan,11; 2013,Dec,3; 2013,Jan,11-12

Cecum

Swollen and inflamed appendix

+ **44955** when done for indicated purpose at time of other major procedure (not as separate procedure) (List separately in addition to code for primary procedure)

Code first primary procedure

🚑 2.44 ⚕ 2.44 **FUD** ZZZ     N 80

**AMA:** 2017,Jan,8; 2016,Jan,13; 2015,Jan,16; 2014,Jan,11; 2013,Dec,3; 2013,Jan,11-12; 2012,Jan,13-14

**44960** for ruptured appendix with abscess or generalized peritonitis

> INCLUDES Battle's operation

🚑 25.3 ⚕ 25.3 **FUD** 090     C 80

**AMA:** 2017,Jan,8; 2016,Jan,13; 2015,Jan,16; 2014,Jan,11; 2013,Dec,3; 2013,Jan,11-12

**44970** Laparoscopy, surgical, appendectomy

> INCLUDES Diagnostic laparoscopy

🚑 17.3 ⚕ 17.3 **FUD** 090     J 80

**AMA:** 2017,Jan,8; 2016,Jan,13; 2015,Mar,3; 2015,Jan,16; 2014,Jan,11; 2013,Dec,3; 2013,Jan,11-12; 2012,Jan,15-42

**44979** Unlisted laparoscopy procedure, appendix

🚑 0.00 ⚕ 0.00 **FUD** YYY     J 80 50

**AMA:** 2017,Jan,8; 2016,Jan,13; 2015,Jan,16; 2014,Jan,11; 2013,Dec,3; 2013,Jan,11-12; 2012,Jan,13-14

## 45000-45190 Open and Transrectal Procedures of Rectum

**45000** Transrectal drainage of pelvic abscess

> EXCLUDES *Image guided transrectal catheter drainage (49407)*

🚑 12.2 ⚕ 12.2 **FUD** 090     T A2

**AMA:** 2014,Jan,11; 2013,Nov,9; 2013,Dec,3; 2013,Jan,11-12

**45005** Incision and drainage of submucosal abscess, rectum

🚑 4.66 ⚕ 7.86 **FUD** 010     T A2

**AMA:** 2014,Jan,11; 2013,Dec,3; 2013,Jan,11-12

**45020** Incision and drainage of deep supralevator, pelvirectal, or retrorectal abscess

> EXCLUDES *Incision and drainage of perianal, ischiorectal, intramural abscess (46050, 46060)*

🚑 16.5 ⚕ 16.5 **FUD** 090     J A2

**AMA:** 2014,Jan,11; 2013,Dec,3; 2013,Jan,11-12

**45100** Biopsy of anorectal wall, anal approach (eg, congenital megacolon)

> EXCLUDES *Biopsy performed endoscopically (45305)*

🚑 8.64 ⚕ 8.64 **FUD** 090     J A2

**AMA:** 2014,Jan,11; 2013,Dec,3; 2013,Jan,11-12

**45108** Anorectal myomectomy

🚑 10.5 ⚕ 10.5 **FUD** 090     J A2

**AMA:** 2014,Jan,11; 2013,Dec,3; 2013,Jan,11-12

**45110** Proctectomy; complete, combined abdominoperineal, with colostomy

> EXCLUDES *Laparoscopic method (45395)*

🚑 53.5 ⚕ 53.5 **FUD** 090     C 80

**AMA:** 2014,Jan,11; 2013,Dec,3; 2013,Jan,11-12

**45111** partial resection of rectum, transabdominal approach

> INCLUDES Luschka proctectomy

🚑 31.4 ⚕ 31.4 **FUD** 090     C 80

**AMA:** 2014,Jan,11; 2013,Dec,3; 2013,Jan,11-12

**45112** Proctectomy, combined abdominoperineal, pull-through procedure (eg, colo-anal anastomosis)

> EXCLUDES *Proctectomy for colo-anal anastomosis with creation of colonic pouch or reservoir (45119)*

🚑 54.4 ⚕ 54.4 **FUD** 090     C 80

**AMA:** 2014,Jan,11; 2013,Dec,3; 2013,Jan,11-12

**45113** Proctectomy, partial, with rectal mucosectomy, ileoanal anastomosis, creation of ileal reservoir (S or J), with or without loop ileostomy

🚑 56.0 ⚕ 56.0 **FUD** 090     C 80

**AMA:** 2014,Jan,11; 2013,Dec,3; 2013,Jan,11-12

**45114** Proctectomy, partial, with anastomosis; abdominal and transsacral approach

🚑 52.3 ⚕ 52.3 **FUD** 090     C 80

**AMA:** 2014,Jan,11; 2013,Dec,3; 2013,Jan,11-12

**45116** transsacral approach only (Kraske type)

🚑 46.8 ⚕ 46.8 **FUD** 090     C 80

**AMA:** 2014,Jan,11; 2013,Dec,3; 2013,Jan,11-12

**45119** Proctectomy, combined abdominoperineal pull-through procedure (eg, colo-anal anastomosis), with creation of colonic reservoir (eg, J-pouch), with diverting enterostomy when performed

> EXCLUDES *Laparoscopic method (45397)*

🚑 56.4 ⚕ 56.4 **FUD** 090     C 80

**AMA:** 2017,Jan,8; 2016,Jan,13; 2015,Jan,16; 2014,Jan,11; 2013,Dec,3; 2013,Jan,11-12

● New Code ▲ Revised Code ○ Reinstated ● New Web Release ▲ Revised Web Release Unlisted Not Covered # Resequenced
⊘ AMA Mod 51 Exempt ⑤ Optum Mod 51 Exempt ⑥ Mod 63 Exempt ✗ Non-FDA Drug ★ Telemedicine Ⓜ Maternity Ⓐ Age Edit + Add-on **AMA:** CPT Asst
© 2017 Optum360, LLC     CPT © 2017 American Medical Association. All Rights Reserved.

**45120** Proctectomy, complete (for congenital megacolon), abdominal and perineal approach; with pull-through procedure and anastomosis (eg, Swenson, Duhamel, or Soave type operation)

🔹 45.9  ⚕ 45.9  **FUD** 090  [C] [80] [▭]

**AMA:** 2014,Jan,11; 2013,Dec,3; 2013,Jan,11-12

**45121** with subtotal or total colectomy, with multiple biopsies

🔹 48.1  ⚕ 48.1  **FUD** 090  [C] [80] [▭]

**AMA:** 2014,Jan,11; 2013,Dec,3; 2013,Jan,11-12

**45123** Proctectomy, partial, without anastomosis, perineal approach

🔹 32.4  ⚕ 32.4  **FUD** 090  [C] [80] [▭]

**AMA:** 2014,Jan,11; 2013,Dec,3; 2013,Jan,11-12

**45126** Pelvic exenteration for colorectal malignancy, with proctectomy (with or without colostomy), with removal of bladder and ureteral transplantations, and/or hysterectomy, or cervicectomy, with or without removal of tube(s), with or without removal of ovary(s), or any combination thereof

🔹 80.9  ⚕ 80.9  **FUD** 090  [C] [80] [▭]

**AMA:** 2014,Jan,11; 2013,Dec,3; 2013,Jan,11-12

**45130** Excision of rectal procidentia, with anastomosis; perineal approach

[INCLUDES]  Altemeier procedure

🔹 31.5  ⚕ 31.5  **FUD** 090  [C] [80] [▭]

**AMA:** 2014,Jan,11; 2013,Dec,3; 2013,Jan,11-12

**45135** abdominal and perineal approach

[INCLUDES]  Altemeier procedure

🔹 39.5  ⚕ 39.5  **FUD** 090  [C] [80] [▭]

**AMA:** 2014,Jan,11; 2013,Dec,3; 2013,Jan,11-12

**45136** Excision of ileoanal reservoir with ileostomy

Enterolysis (44005)
Ileostomy or jejunostomy, non-tube (44310)

🔹 55.3  ⚕ 55.3  **FUD** 090  [C] [80] [▭]

**AMA:** 2014,Jan,11; 2013,Dec,3; 2013,Jan,11-12

**45150** Division of stricture of rectum

🔹 10.4  ⚕ 10.4  **FUD** 090  [T] [A2] [80] [▭]

**AMA:** 2014,Jan,11; 2013,Dec,3; 2013,Jan,11-12

**45160** Excision of rectal tumor by proctotomy, transsacral or transcoccygeal approach

🔹 29.5  ⚕ 29.5  **FUD** 090  [J] [A2] [80] [▭]

**AMA:** 2014,Jan,11; 2013,Dec,3; 2013,Jan,11-12

**45171** Excision of rectal tumor, transanal approach; not including muscularis propria (ie, partial thickness)

[EXCLUDES]  Transanal destruction of rectal tumor (45190)
Transanal endoscopic microsurgical tumor excision (TEMS) (0184T)

🔹 17.3  ⚕ 17.3  **FUD** 090  [J] [B2] [80] [▭]

**AMA:** 2017,Jan,8; 2016,Jan,13; 2015,Jan,16; 2014,Jan,11; 2013,Dec,3; 2013,Jan,11-12

**45172** including muscularis propria (ie, full thickness)

[EXCLUDES]  Transanal destruction of rectal tumor (45190)
Transanal endoscopic microsurgical tumor excision (TEMS) (0184T)

🔹 23.4  ⚕ 23.4  **FUD** 090  [J] [B2] [80] [▭]

**AMA:** 2017,Jan,8; 2016,Jan,13; 2015,Jan,16; 2014,Jan,11; 2013,Dec,3; 2013,Jan,11-12

**45190** Destruction of rectal tumor (eg, electrodesiccation, electrosurgery, laser ablation, laser resection, cryosurgery) transanal approach

[EXCLUDES]  Transanal endoscopic microsurgical tumor excision (TEMS) (0184T)
Transanal excision of rectal tumor (45171-45172)

🔹 20.1  ⚕ 20.1  **FUD** 090  [J] [A2] [▭]

**AMA:** 2017,Jan,8; 2016,Jan,13; 2015,Jan,16; 2014,Jan,11; 2013,Dec,3; 2013,Jan,11-12

## 45300-45327 Rigid Proctosigmoidoscopy Procedures

[INCLUDES]  Control of bleeding as result of the endoscopic procedure during same operative session
Exam of:
 Entire rectum
 Portion of sigmoid colon

[EXCLUDES]  Computed tomographic colonography (74261-74263)

Code also examination of colon through stoma:
 Colonoscopy via stoma (44388-44408 [44401])
 Ileoscopy via stoma (44380-44384 [44381])

**45300** Proctosigmoidoscopy, rigid; diagnostic, with or without collection of specimen(s) by brushing or washing (separate procedure)

📡 (74360)

🔹 1.57  ⚕ 3.51  **FUD** 000  [T] [P3] [▭]

**AMA:** 2017,Jan,8; 2016,Jan,13; 2015,Jan,16; 2014,Jan,11; 2013,Dec,3; 2013,Jan,11-12

**45303** with dilation (eg, balloon, guide wire, bougie)

📡 (74360)

🔹 2.52  ⚕ 25.6  **FUD** 000  [T] [P2] [▭]

**AMA:** 2017,Jan,8; 2016,Jan,13; 2015,Jan,16; 2014,Jan,11; 2013,Dec,3; 2013,Jan,11-12

**45305** with biopsy, single or multiple

🔹 2.13  ⚕ 4.06  **FUD** 000  [T] [A2] [▭]

**AMA:** 2017,Jan,8; 2016,Jan,13; 2015,Jan,16; 2014,Jan,11; 2013,Dec,3; 2013,Jan,11-12

**45307** with removal of foreign body

🔹 2.83  ⚕ 4.74  **FUD** 000  [J] [A2] [80] [▭]

**AMA:** 2017,Jan,8; 2016,Jan,13; 2015,Jan,16; 2014,Jan,11; 2013,Dec,3; 2013,Jan,11-12

**45308** with removal of single tumor, polyp, or other lesion by hot biopsy forceps or bipolar cautery

🔹 2.44  ⚕ 4.55  **FUD** 000  [J] [A2] [▭]

**AMA:** 2017,Jan,8; 2016,Jan,13; 2015,Jan,16; 2014,Jan,11; 2013,Dec,3; 2013,Jan,11-12

Hot biopsy forceps or cautery

Rectal tumor

Rectal polyp

Sigmoid flexure

Rigid scope

Sigmoid

A rigid proctosigmoid procedure of the rectum and sigmoid is performed

**45309** with removal of single tumor, polyp, or other lesion by snare technique

🔹 2.60  ⚕ 4.74  **FUD** 000  [T] [A2] [▭]

**AMA:** 2017,Jan,8; 2016,Jan,13; 2015,Jan,16; 2014,Jan,11; 2013,Dec,3; 2013,Jan,11-12

**45315** with removal of multiple tumors, polyps, or other lesions by hot biopsy forceps, bipolar cautery or snare technique

🔹 3.06  ⚕ 5.15  **FUD** 000  [T] [A2] [▭]

**AMA:** 2017,Jan,8; 2016,Jan,13; 2015,Jan,16; 2014,Jan,11; 2013,Dec,3; 2013,Jan,11-12

[26]/[TC] PC/TC Only  [A2]-[Z3] ASC Payment  [50] Bilateral  ♂ Male Only  ♀ Female Only  🔹 Facility RVU  ⚕ Non-Facility RVU  [▭] CCI
**FUD** Follow-up Days  **CMS:** IOM (Pub 100)  [A]-[Y] OPPSI  [80]/[80] Surg Assist Allowed / w/Doc  📡 Lab Crosswalk  📡 Radiology Crosswalk  ❌ CLIA
204  CPT © 2017 American Medical Association. All Rights Reserved.  © 2017 Optum360, LLC

**45317**     **with control of bleeding (eg, injection, bipolar cautery, unipolar cautery, laser, heater probe, stapler, plasma coagulator)**

🚑 3.26   ⚓ 5.20   **FUD** 000                    Ⓣ A2 ▢

**AMA:** 2017,Jan,8; 2016,Jan,13; 2015,Jan,16; 2014,Jan,11; 2013,Dec,3; 2013,Jan,11-12

**45320**     **with ablation of tumor(s), polyp(s), or other lesion(s) not amenable to removal by hot biopsy forceps, bipolar cautery or snare technique (eg, laser)**

🚑 3.03   ⚓ 5.05   **FUD** 000                    Ⓙ A2 ▢

**AMA:** 2017,Jan,8; 2016,Jan,13; 2015,Jan,16; 2014,Jan,11; 2013,Dec,3; 2013,Jan,11-12

**45321**     **with decompression of volvulus**

🚑 2.95   ⚓ 2.95   **FUD** 000                    Ⓙ A2 ▢

**AMA:** 2017,Jan,8; 2016,Jan,13; 2015,Jan,16; 2014,Jan,11; 2013,Dec,3; 2013,Jan,11-12

**45327**     **with transendoscopic stent placement (includes predilation)**

🚑 3.30   ⚓ 3.30   **FUD** 000                    Ⓙ A2 ▢

**AMA:** 2017,Jan,8; 2016,Jan,13; 2015,Jan,16; 2014,Jan,11; 2013,Dec,3; 2013,Jan,11-12

## 45330-45350 [45346] Flexible Sigmoidoscopy Procedures

INCLUDES    Control of bleeding as result of the endoscopic procedure during same operative session
            Exam of:
            Entire rectum
            Entire sigmoid colon
            Portion of descending colon (when performed)
EXCLUDES    *Computed tomographic colonography (74261-74263)*
Code also examination of colon through stoma when appropriate:
    Colonoscopy (44388-44408 [44401])
    Ileoscopy (44380-44384 [44381])

**45330**     **Sigmoidoscopy, flexible; diagnostic, including collection of specimen(s) by brushing or washing, when performed (separate procedure)**

EXCLUDES    *Sigmoidoscopy, flexible (45331-45350 [45346])*

🚑 1.64   ⚓ 4.74   **FUD** 000                    Ⓣ P3 ▢

**AMA:** 2017,Jan,8; 2016,Feb,13; 2016,Jan,13; 2015,Sep,12; 2015,Jan,16; 2014,Dec,3; 2014,Dec,18; 2014,Jan,11; 2013,Dec,3; 2013,Jan,11-12; 2012,Jan,15-42

**45331**     **with biopsy, single or multiple**

EXCLUDES    *Sigmoidoscopy, flexible; with endoscopic mucosal resection on the same lesion (45349)*

🚑 2.11   ⚓ 7.27   **FUD** 000                    Ⓣ A2 ▢

**AMA:** 2017,Jan,8; 2016,Feb,13; 2016,Jan,13; 2015,Jan,16; 2014,Dec,3; 2014,Dec,18; 2014,Jan,11; 2013,Dec,3; 2013,Jan,11-12; 2012,Jan,15-42

**45332**     **with removal of foreign body(s)**

EXCLUDES    *Sigmoidoscopy, flexible; diagnostic (45330)*
⊞ (76000)

🚑 3.09   ⚓ 7.13   **FUD** 000                    Ⓣ A2 ▢

**AMA:** 2017,Jan,8; 2016,Feb,13; 2016,Jan,13; 2015,Jan,16; 2014,Dec,3; 2014,Dec,18; 2014,Jan,11; 2013,Dec,3; 2013,Jan,11-12

**45333**     **with removal of tumor(s), polyp(s), or other lesion(s) by hot biopsy forceps**

EXCLUDES    *Sigmoidoscopy, flexible; diagnostic (45330)*

🚑 2.76   ⚓ 8.33   **FUD** 000                    Ⓣ A2 ▢

**AMA:** 2017,Jan,8; 2016,Feb,13; 2016,Jan,13; 2015,Jan,16; 2014,Dec,3; 2014,Dec,18; 2014,Jan,11; 2013,Dec,3; 2013,Jan,11-12

**45334**     **with control of bleeding, any method**

EXCLUDES    *Sigmoidoscopy, flexible; diagnostic (45330)*
            *Sigmoidoscopy, flexible; with band ligation on the same lesion (45350)*
            *Sigmoidoscopy, flexible; with directed submucosal injection on the same lesion (45335)*

🚑 3.46   ⚓ 15.6   **FUD** 000                    Ⓣ A2 ▢

**AMA:** 2017,Jan,8; 2016,Feb,13; 2016,Jan,13; 2015,Jan,16; 2014,Dec,3; 2014,Dec,18; 2014,Jan,11; 2013,Dec,3; 2013,Jan,11-12; 2012,Jan,15-42

**45335**     **with directed submucosal injection(s), any substance**

EXCLUDES    *Sigmoidoscopy, flexible; diagnostic (45330)*
            *Sigmoidoscopy, flexible; with control of bleeding on the same lesion (45334)*
            *Sigmoidoscopy, flexible; with endoscopic mucosal resection on the same lesion (45349)*

🚑 1.95   ⚓ 6.63   **FUD** 000                    Ⓣ A2 ▢

**AMA:** 2017,Jan,8; 2016,Feb,13; 2016,Jan,13; 2015,Jan,16; 2014,Dec,3; 2014,Dec,18; 2014,Jan,11; 2013,Dec,3; 2013,Jan,11-12; 2012,Jan,15-42

**45337**     **with decompression (for pathologic distention) (eg, volvulus, megacolon), including placement of decompression tube, when performed**

EXCLUDES    *Procedure performed more than one time per operative session*
            *Sigmoidoscopy, flexible; diagnostic (45330)*

🚑 3.39   ⚓ 3.39   **FUD** 000                    Ⓣ A2 ▢

**AMA:** 2017,Jan,8; 2016,Feb,13; 2016,Jan,13; 2015,Jan,16; 2014,Dec,3; 2014,Dec,18; 2014,Jan,11; 2013,Dec,3; 2013,Jan,11-12

**45338**     **with removal of tumor(s), polyp(s), or other lesion(s) by snare technique**

EXCLUDES    *Sigmoidoscopy, flexible; diagnostic (45330)*
            *Sigmoidoscopy, flexible; with endoscopic mucosal resection on the same lesion (45349)*

🚑 3.54   ⚓ 7.63   **FUD** 000                    Ⓣ A2 ▢

**AMA:** 2017,Jan,8; 2016,Feb,13; 2016,Jan,13; 2015,Jan,16; 2014,Dec,3; 2014,Dec,18; 2014,Jan,11; 2013,Dec,3; 2013,Jan,11-12

\#   **45346**     **with ablation of tumor(s), polyp(s), or other lesion(s) (includes pre- and post-dilation and guide wire passage, when performed)**

EXCLUDES    *Sigmoidoscopy, flexible; diagnostic (45330)*
            *Sigmoidoscopy, flexible; with transendoscopic balloon dilation on the same lesion (45340)*

🚑 4.72   ⚓ 86.5   **FUD** 000                    Ⓣ G2 ▢

**AMA:** 2017,Jan,8; 2016,Feb,13; 2016,Jan,13; 2015,Jan,16; 2014,Dec,3

**45340**     **with transendoscopic balloon dilation**

EXCLUDES    *Sigmoidoscopy, flexible (45330, [45346], 45347)*
Code also each additional stricture dilated in same session, using modifier 59 with (45340)
⊞ (74360)

🚑 2.28   ⚓ 12.2   **FUD** 000                    Ⓣ A2 ▢

**AMA:** 2017,Jan,8; 2016,Feb,13; 2016,Jan,13; 2015,Jan,16; 2014,Dec,18; 2014,Dec,3; 2014,Jan,11; 2013,Dec,3; 2013,Jan,11-12

**45341**     **with endoscopic ultrasound examination**

INCLUDES    Ultrasound, transrectal (76872)
EXCLUDES    *Gastrointestinal endoscopic ultrasound, supervision and interpretation (76975)*
            *Procedure performed more than one time per operative session*
            *Sigmoidoscopy, flexible (45330, 45342)*

🚑 3.64   ⚓ 3.64   **FUD** 000                    Ⓣ A2 ▢

**AMA:** 2017,Jan,8; 2016,Feb,13; 2016,Jan,13; 2015,Jan,16; 2014,Dec,3; 2014,Dec,18; 2014,Jan,11; 2013,Dec,3; 2013,Jan,11-12

● New Code   ▲ Revised Code   ○ Reinstated   ● New Web Release   ▲ Revised Web Release   Unlisted   Not Covered   # Resequenced
⊘ AMA Mod 51 Exempt   ⑨ Optum Mod 51 Exempt   ⑨ Mod 63 Exempt   ✗ Non-FDA Drug   ★ Telemedicine   Ⓜ Maternity   Ⓐ Age Edit   + Add-on   **AMA:** CPT Asst
© 2017 Optum360, LLC                        CPT © 2017 American Medical Association. All Rights Reserved.

## Digestive System

**45342** **with transendoscopic ultrasound guided intramural or transmural fine needle aspiration/biopsy(s)**

INCLUDES Gastrointestinal endoscopic ultrasound, supervision and interpretation (76975)
Ultrasonic guidance (76942)
Ultrasound, transrectal (76872)

EXCLUDES Sigmoidoscopy, flexible (45330, 45341)
Procedure performed more than one time per operative session

⬛ 4.99   ⬛ 4.99   **FUD** 000   T A2 ▭

**AMA:** 2017,Jan,8; 2016,Feb,13; 2016,Jan,13; 2015,Jan,16; 2014,Dec,3; 2014,Dec,18; 2014,Jan,11; 2013,Dec,3; 2013,Jan,11-12

**45346** **Resequenced code. See code following 45338.**

**45347** **with placement of endoscopic stent (includes pre- and post-dilation and guide wire passage, when performed)**

EXCLUDES Sigmoidoscopy, flexible (45330, 45340)
⬛ (74360)
⬛ 4.54   ⬛ 4.54   **FUD** 000   J J8 ▭

**AMA:** 2017,Jan,8; 2016,Feb,13; 2016,Jan,13; 2015,Jan,16; 2014,Dec,3

**45349** **with endoscopic mucosal resection**

EXCLUDES Procedure performed on the same lesion with (45331, 45335, 45338, 45350)
Sigmoidoscopy, flexible; diagnostic (45330)
⬛ 5.83   ⬛ 5.83   **FUD** 000   T G2 ▭

**AMA:** 2017,Jan,8; 2016,Jan,13; 2015,Jan,16; 2014,Dec,3

**45350** **with band ligation(s) (eg, hemorrhoids)**

EXCLUDES Hemorrhoidectomy, internal, by rubber band ligation (46221)
Procedure performed more than one time per operative session
Sigmoidoscopy, flexible; diagnostic (45330)
Sigmoidoscopy, flexible; with control of bleeding, same lesion (45334)
Sigmoidoscopy, flexible; with endoscopic mucosal resection (45349)
⬛ 2.96   ⬛ 14.8   **FUD** 000   T G2 ▭

**AMA:** 2017,Jan,8; 2016,Jan,13; 2015,Jan,16; 2014,Dec,3

## 45378-45393 [45388, 45390, 45398] Flexible and Rigid Colonoscopy Procedures

INCLUDES Control of bleeding as result of the endoscopic procedure during same operative session
Exam of:
Entire colon (rectum to cecum)
Terminal ileum (when performed)

EXCLUDES Computed tomographic colonography (74261-74263)
Code also modifier 53 (physician), or 73, 74 (facility) for an incomplete colonoscopy

**45378** **Colonoscopy, flexible; diagnostic, including collection of specimen(s) by brushing or washing, when performed (separate procedure)**

EXCLUDES Colonoscopy, flexible (45379-45393 [45388, 45390, 45398])
Decompression for pathological distention (45393)
Code also modifier 53 (physician), or 73, 74 (facility) for an incomplete colonoscopy
⬛ 5.44   ⬛ 8.99   **FUD** 000   T A2 ▭

**AMA:** 2017,Sep,14; 2017,Jan,8; 2016,Jan,13; 2015,Sep,12; 2015,Jan,16; 2014,Dec,3; 2014,Nov,3; 2014,Jan,11; 2013,Dec,3; 2013,Jan,11-12; 2012,Jan,15-42

**45379** **with removal of foreign body(s)**

EXCLUDES Colonoscopy, flexible; diagnostic (45378)
Code also modifier 52 when colonoscope fails to reach the junction of the small intestine
⬛ (76000)
⬛ 7.03   ⬛ 11.6   **FUD** 000   T A2 ▭

**AMA:** 2017,Jan,8; 2016,Jan,13; 2015,Jan,16; 2014,Dec,3; 2014,Jan,11; 2013,Dec,3; 2013,Jan,11-12

**45380** **with biopsy, single or multiple**

EXCLUDES Colonoscopy, flexible; diagnostic (45378)
Colonoscopy, flexible; with endoscopic mucosal resection on the same lesion (45390)
Code also modifier 52 when colonoscope fails to reach the junction of the small intestine
⬛ 5.90   ⬛ 11.5   **FUD** 000   T A2 ▭

**AMA:** 2017,Jan,8; 2016,Jan,13; 2015,Jan,16; 2014,Dec,3; 2014,Jan,11; 2013,Dec,3; 2013,Jan,11-12; 2012,Jan,15-42

**45381** **with directed submucosal injection(s), any substance**

EXCLUDES Colonoscopy, flexible; diagnostic (45378)
Colonoscopy, flexible; with control of bleeding on the same lesion (45382)
Colonoscopy, flexible; with endoscopic mucosal resection on the same lesion (45390)
Code also modifier 52 when colonoscope fails to reach the junction of the small intestine
⬛ 5.90   ⬛ 10.9   **FUD** 000   T A2 ▭

**AMA:** 2017,Jan,6; 2017,Jan,8; 2016,Jan,13; 2015,Jan,16; 2014,Dec,3; 2014,Jan,11; 2013,Dec,3; 2013,Jan,11-12; 2012,Jan,15-42

**45382** **with control of bleeding, any method**

EXCLUDES Colonoscopy, flexible; diagnostic (45378)
Colonoscopy, flexible; with band ligation on the same lesion ([45398])
Colonoscopy, flexible; with directed submucosal injection on the same lesion (45381)
Code also modifier 52 when colonoscope fails to reach the junction of the small intestine
⬛ 7.62   ⬛ 20.4   **FUD** 000   T A2 ▭

**AMA:** 2017,Jan,8; 2016,Jan,13; 2015,Jan,16; 2014,Dec,3; 2014,Jan,11; 2013,Dec,3; 2013,Jan,11-12

**# 45388** **with ablation of tumor(s), polyp(s), or other lesion(s) (includes pre- and post-dilation and guide wire passage, when performed)**

EXCLUDES Colonoscopy, flexible (45378, 45386)
Code also modifier 53 (physician), or 73, 74 (facility) for an incomplete colonoscopy
⬛ 7.96   ⬛ 90.9   **FUD** 000   T G2 ▭

**AMA:** 2017,Jan,8; 2016,Jan,13; 2015,Jan,16; 2014,Dec,3

**45384** **with removal of tumor(s), polyp(s), or other lesion(s) by hot biopsy forceps**

EXCLUDES Colonoscopy, flexible; diagnostic (45378)
Code also modifier 52 when colonoscope fails to reach the junction of the small intestine
⬛ 6.71   ⬛ 12.7   **FUD** 000   T A2 ▭

**AMA:** 2017,Jan,8; 2016,Jan,13; 2015,Jun,10; 2015,Jan,16; 2014,Dec,3; 2014,Jan,11; 2013,Dec,3; 2013,Jan,11-12; 2012,Jan,15-42

**45385** **with removal of tumor(s), polyp(s), or other lesion(s) by snare technique**

EXCLUDES Colonoscopy, flexible; diagnostic (45378)
Colonoscopy, flexible; with endoscopic mucosal resection on the same lesion (45390)
⬛ 7.48   ⬛ 12.0   **FUD** 000   T A2 ▭

**AMA:** 2017,Jan,6; 2017,Jan,8; 2016,Jan,13; 2015,Jan,16; 2014,Dec,3; 2014,Jan,11; 2013,Dec,3; 2013,Jan,11-12; 2012,Jan,15-42

**45386** **with transendoscopic balloon dilation**

EXCLUDES Colonoscopy, flexible (45378, [45388], 45389)
Code also each additional stricture dilated in same operative session, using modifier 59 with (45386)
⬛ (74360)
⬛ 6.23   ⬛ 16.6   **FUD** 000   T A2 ▭

**AMA:** 2017,Jan,8; 2016,Jan,13; 2015,Jan,16; 2014,Dec,3; 2014,Jan,11; 2013,Dec,3; 2013,Jan,11-12

**45388** **Resequenced code. See code following 45382.**

26/TC PC/TC Only   A2-Z3 ASC Payment   50 Bilateral   ♂ Male Only   ♀ Female Only   ⬛ Facility RVU   ⬛ Non-Facility RVU   ▭ CCI
FUD Follow-up Days   CMS: IOM (Pub 100)   A-Y OPPSI   80/80 Surg Assist Allowed / w/Doc   ⬛ Lab Crosswalk   ⬛ Radiology Crosswalk   ❌ CLIA
CPT © 2017 American Medical Association. All Rights Reserved.          © 2017 Optum360, LLC

**45389**    **with endoscopic stent placement (includes pre- and post-dilation and guide wire passage, when performed)**

EXCLUDES    *Colonoscopy, flexible (45378, 45386)*

    (74360)

    8.53    8.53    **FUD** 000    J J8

AMA: 2017,Jan,8; 2016,Jan,13; 2015,Jan,16; 2014,Dec,3

*45390*    **Resequenced code. See code following 45392.**

**45391**    **with endoscopic ultrasound examination limited to the rectum, sigmoid, descending, transverse, or ascending colon and cecum, and adjacent structures**

INCLUDES    Gastrointestinal endoscopic ultrasound, supervision and interpretation (76975)
    Ultrasound, transrectal (76872)

EXCLUDES    *Colonoscopy, flexible (45378, 45392)*
    *Procedure performed more than one time per operative session*

    7.58    7.58    **FUD** 000    T A2

AMA: 2017,Jan,8; 2016,Jan,13; 2015,Jan,16; 2014,Dec,3; 2014,Jan,11; 2013,Dec,3; 2013,Jan,11-12

**45392**    **with transendoscopic ultrasound guided intramural or transmural fine needle aspiration/biopsy(s), includes endoscopic ultrasound examination limited to the rectum, sigmoid, descending, transverse, or ascending colon and cecum, and adjacent structures**

INCLUDES    Gastrointestinal endoscopic ultrasound, supervision and interpretation (76975)
    Ultrasonic guidance (76942)
    Ultrasound, transrectal (76872)

EXCLUDES    *Colonoscopy, flexible (45378, 45391)*
    *Procedure performed more than one time per operative session*

    8.94    8.94    **FUD** 000    T A2

AMA: 2017,Jan,8; 2016,Jan,13; 2015,Jan,16; 2014,Dec,3; 2014,Jan,11; 2013,Dec,3; 2013,Jan,11-12

\# **45390**    **with endoscopic mucosal resection**

EXCLUDES    *Colonoscopy, flexible; diagnostic (45378)*
    *Colonoscopy, flexible; with band ligation on the same lesion ([45398])*
    *Colonoscopy, flexible; with biopsy on the same lesion (45380-45381)*
    *Colonoscopy, flexible; with removal of tumor(s), polyp(s), or other lesion(s) by snare technique on the same lesion (45385)*

    9.77    9.77    **FUD** 000    T G2

AMA: 2017,Jan,6; 2017,Jan,8; 2016,Jan,13; 2015,Jan,16; 2014,Dec,3

**45393**    **with decompression (for pathologic distention) (eg, volvulus, megacolon), including placement of decompression tube, when performed**

EXCLUDES    *Colonoscopy, flexible; diagnostic (45378)*
    *Procedure performed more than one time per operative session*

    7.43    7.43    **FUD** 000    T G2

AMA: 2017,Jan,8; 2016,Jan,13; 2015,Jan,16; 2014,Dec,3

\# **45398**    **with band ligation(s) (eg, hemorrhoids)**

EXCLUDES    *Bleeding control by band ligation (45382)*
    *Colonoscopy, flexible (45378, 45390)*
    *Hemorrhoidectomy, internal, by rubber band ligation (46221)*
    *Procedure performed more than one time per operative session*
    Code also modifier 52 when colonoscope fails to reach the junction of the small intestine

    6.90    19.0    **FUD** 000    T G2

AMA: 2017,Sep,14; 2017,Jan,8; 2016,Jan,13; 2015,Jan,16; 2014,Dec,3

## 45395-45499 Laparoscopic Procedures of Rectum

INCLUDES    Diagnostic laparoscopy

**45395**    **Laparoscopy, surgical; proctectomy, complete, combined abdominoperineal, with colostomy**

EXCLUDES    *Open method (45110)*

    57.3    57.3    **FUD** 090    C 80

AMA: 2017,Jan,8; 2016,Jan,13; 2015,Jan,16; 2014,Jan,11; 2013,Jan,11-12

**45397**    **proctectomy, combined abdominoperineal pull-through procedure (eg, colo-anal anastomosis), with creation of colonic reservoir (eg, J-pouch), with diverting enterostomy, when performed**

EXCLUDES    *Open method (45119)*

    62.4    62.4    **FUD** 090    C 80

AMA: 2017,Jan,8; 2016,Jan,13; 2015,Jan,16; 2014,Jan,11; 2013,Jan,11-12; 2012,Jan,15-42

*45398*    **Resequenced code. See code following 45393.**

*45399*    **Resequenced code. See code before 45990.**

**45400**    **Laparoscopy, surgical; proctopexy (for prolapse)**

EXCLUDES    *Open method (45540-45541)*

    33.0    33.0    **FUD** 090    C 80

AMA: 2017,Jan,8; 2016,Jan,13; 2015,Jan,16; 2014,Jan,11; 2013,Jan,11-12

**45402**    **proctopexy (for prolapse), with sigmoid resection**

EXCLUDES    *Open method (45550)*

    44.0    44.0    **FUD** 090    C 80

AMA: 2017,Jan,8; 2016,Jan,13; 2015,Jan,16; 2014,Jan,11; 2013,Jan,11-12

**45499**    **Unlisted laparoscopy procedure, rectum**

EXCLUDES    *Unlisted rectal procedure performed via open technique (45999)*

    0.00    0.00    **FUD** YYY    J 80

AMA: 2014,Jan,11; 2013,Jan,11-12

## 45500-45825 Open Repairs of Rectum

**45500**    **Proctoplasty; for stenosis**

    15.0    15.0    **FUD** 090    J A2 80

AMA: 2014,Jan,11; 2013,Jan,11-12

**45505**    **for prolapse of mucous membrane**

    17.1    17.1    **FUD** 090    J A2

AMA: 2017,Jan,8; 2016,Jan,13; 2015,Mar,9; 2015,Jan,16; 2014,Jan,11; 2013,Oct,18; 2013,Jan,11-12

**45520**    **Perirectal injection of sclerosing solution for prolapse**

    1.17    4.42    **FUD** 000    01 N1

AMA: 2017,Jan,8; 2016,Jan,13; 2015,Jan,16; 2014,Jan,11; 2013,Jan,11-12; 2012,Jan,15-42

**45540**    **Proctopexy (eg, for prolapse); abdominal approach**

EXCLUDES    *Laparoscopic method (45400)*

    30.6    30.6    **FUD** 090    C 80

AMA: 2014,Jan,11; 2013,Jan,11-12

**45541**    **perineal approach**

    27.3    27.3    **FUD** 090    J G2 80

AMA: 2014,Jan,11; 2013,Jan,11-12

**45550**    **with sigmoid resection, abdominal approach**

INCLUDES    Frickman proctopexy

EXCLUDES    *Laparoscopic method (45402)*

    42.3    42.3    **FUD** 090    C 80

AMA: 2014,Jan,11; 2013,Jan,11-12

● New Code    ▲ Revised Code    ○ Reinstated    ● New Web Release    ▲ Revised Web Release    Unlisted    Not Covered    # Resequenced
⊘ AMA Mod 51 Exempt    ⑤ Optum Mod 51 Exempt    ⊚ Mod 63 Exempt    ∕ Non-FDA Drug    ★ Telemedicine    Ⓜ Maternity    Ⓐ Age Edit    + Add-on    AMA: CPT Asst
© 2017 Optum360, LLC                          CPT © 2017 American Medical Association. All Rights Reserved.                          207

**Digestive System**

**45560**    **Repair of rectocele (separate procedure)**

> EXCLUDES   *Posterior colporrhaphy with rectocele repair (57250)*

   19.8    19.8   **FUD** 090      J A2 80

**AMA:** 2014,Jan,11; 2013,Jan,11-12

Urethra             Posterior vaginal wall

The posterior wall of the vagina is opened directly over the rectocele; the walls of both structures are repaired; a rectocele is a herniated protrusion of part of the rectum into the vagina

**45562**    **Exploration, repair, and presacral drainage for rectal injury;**

   32.5    32.5   **FUD** 090      C 80

**AMA:** 2014,Jan,11; 2013,Jan,11-12

**45563**    **with colostomy**

> INCLUDES   Maydl colostomy

   47.5    47.5   **FUD** 090      C 80

**AMA:** 2014,Jan,11; 2013,Jan,11-12

**45800**    **Closure of rectovesical fistula;**

   34.8    34.8   **FUD** 090      C 80

**AMA:** 2014,Jan,11; 2013,Jan,11-12

**45805**    **with colostomy**

   41.5    41.5   **FUD** 090      C 80

**AMA:** 2014,Jan,11; 2013,Jan,11-12

**45820**    **Closure of rectourethral fistula;**

> EXCLUDES   *Closure of fistula, rectovaginal (57300-57308)*

   32.6    32.6   **FUD** 090      C 80

**AMA:** 2014,Jan,11; 2013,Jan,11-12

**45825**    **with colostomy**

> EXCLUDES   *Closure of fistula, rectovaginal (57300-57308)*

   41.4    41.4   **FUD** 090      C 80

**AMA:** 2014,Jan,11; 2013,Jan,11-12

## 45900-45999 [45399] Closed Procedures of Rectum With Anesthesia

**45900**    **Reduction of procidentia (separate procedure) under anesthesia**

   5.85    5.85   **FUD** 010      T A2 80

**AMA:** 2014,Jan,11; 2013,Jan,11-12

**45905**    **Dilation of anal sphincter (separate procedure) under anesthesia other than local**

   4.87    4.87   **FUD** 010      T A2

**AMA:** 2014,Jan,11; 2013,Jan,11-12

**45910**    **Dilation of rectal stricture (separate procedure) under anesthesia other than local**

   5.59    5.59   **FUD** 010      T A2

**AMA:** 2014,Jan,11; 2013,Jan,11-12

**45915**    **Removal of fecal impaction or foreign body (separate procedure) under anesthesia**

   6.54    9.48   **FUD** 010      T A2

**AMA:** 2017,Jan,8; 2016,Jan,13; 2015,Jan,16; 2014,Jan,11; 2013,Jan,11-12; 2012,Jan,15-42

\#   **45399**    **Unlisted procedure, colon**

   0.00    0.00   **FUD** XXX      T

**AMA:** 2017,Jan,8; 2016,Jan,13; 2015,Jan,16; 2014,Dec,3; 2014,Nov,3

**45990**    **Anorectal exam, surgical, requiring anesthesia (general, spinal, or epidural), diagnostic**

> INCLUDES   Diagnostic:
> Anoscopy
> Proctoscopy, rigid
> Exam:
> Pelvic (when performed)
> Perineal, external
> Rectal, digital

> EXCLUDES   *Anogenital examination (99170)*
> *Anoscopy; diagnostic (46600)*
> *Pelvic examination under anesthesia (57410)*
> *Proctosigmoidoscopy, rigid (45300-45327)*

   3.12    3.12   **FUD** 000      J A2 80

**AMA:** 2017,Jan,8; 2016,Jan,13; 2015,Jan,16; 2014,Jan,11; 2013,Jan,11-12; 2012,Jan,15-42

**45999**    **Unlisted procedure, rectum**

> EXCLUDES   *Unlisted rectal procedure performed laparoscopically (45499)*

   0.00    0.00   **FUD** YYY      T 80

**AMA:** 2017,Jan,8; 2016,Jan,13; 2015,Jan,16; 2014,Jan,11; 2013,Jan,11-12

## 46020-46083 Surgical Incision of Anus

> EXCLUDES   *Cryosurgical destruction of hemorrhoid(s) (46999)*
> *Fistulotomy, subcutaneous (46270)*
> *Hemorrhoidopexy ([46947])*
> *Injection of hemorrhoid(s) (46500)*
> *Thermal energy destruction of internal hemorrhoid(s) (46930)*

**46020**    **Placement of seton**

> EXCLUDES   *Anoscopy; diagnostic (46600)*
> *Incision and drainage of ischiorectal or intramural abscess (46060)*
> *Ligation, hemorrhoidal vascular bundle (0249T)*
> *Surgical anal fistula treatment (46280)*

   6.75    7.92   **FUD** 010      J A2

**AMA:** 2014,Jan,11; 2013,Jan,11-12

**46030**    **Removal of anal seton, other marker**

   2.61    3.98   **FUD** 010      T A2 80

**AMA:** 2014,Jan,11; 2013,Jan,11-12

**46040**    **Incision and drainage of ischiorectal and/or perirectal abscess (separate procedure)**

   11.9    15.3   **FUD** 090      T A2

**AMA:** 2014,Jan,11; 2013,Jan,11-12

**46045**    **Incision and drainage of intramural, intramuscular, or submucosal abscess, transanal, under anesthesia**

   12.5    12.5   **FUD** 090      J A2

**AMA:** 2014,Jan,11; 2013,Jan,11-12

**46050**    **Incision and drainage, perianal abscess, superficial**

> EXCLUDES   *Incision and drainage abscess:*
> *Ischiorectal/intramural (46060)*
> *Supralevator/pelvirectal/retrorectal (45020)*

   2.81    5.75   **FUD** 010      T A2

**AMA:** 2014,Jan,11; 2013,Jan,11-12

**46060**    **Incision and drainage of ischiorectal or intramural abscess, with fistulectomy or fistulotomy, submuscular, with or without placement of seton**

> EXCLUDES   *Incision and drainage abscess:*
> *Supralevator/pelvirectal/retrorectal (45020)*
> *Placement of seton (46020)*

   13.7    13.7   **FUD** 090      J A2

**AMA:** 2014,Jan,11; 2013,Jan,11-12

**46070**    **Incision, anal septum (infant)**      A

> EXCLUDES   *Anoplasty (46700-46705)*

   6.53    6.53   **FUD** 090      63 J A2 80

**AMA:** 2014,Jan,11; 2013,Jan,11-12

**46080**    **Sphincterotomy, anal, division of sphincter (separate procedure)**

   4.61    7.10   **FUD** 010      J A2

**AMA:** 2014,Jan,11; 2013,Jan,11-12

| 26/TC PC/TC Only | A2-Z3 ASC Payment | 50 Bilateral | ♂ Male Only | ♀ Female Only | Facility RVU | Non-Facility RVU | CCI |
| FUD Follow-up Days | CMS: IOM (Pub 100) | A-Y OPPSI | 80/80 Surg Assist Allowed / w/Doc | | Lab Crosswalk | Radiology Crosswalk | CLIA |

CPT © 2017 American Medical Association. All Rights Reserved.

208                                                    © 2017 Optum360, LLC

Digestive System     45560 — 46080

**46083**  Incision of thrombosed hemorrhoid, external
📇 3.07   ☒ 5.04   **FUD** 010                    T P2
**AMA:** 2017,Jan,8; 2016,Jan,13; 2015,Jan,16; 2014,Jan,11; 2013,Jan,11-12; 2012,Jan,15-42

## 46200-46262 [46220, 46320, 46945, 46946] Anal Resection and Hemorrhoidectomies

EXCLUDES  *Cryosurgical destruction of hemorrhoid(s) (46999)*
*Hemorrhoidopexy ([46947])*
*Injection of hemorrhoid(s) (46500)*
*Thermal energy destruction of internal hemorrhoid(s) (46930)*

**46200**  Fissurectomy, including sphincterotomy, when performed
📇 9.38   ☒ 12.7   **FUD** 090                    J A2
**AMA:** 2014,Jan,11; 2013,Jan,11-12

*46220*  Resequenced code. See code before 46230.

**46221**  Hemorrhoidectomy, internal, by rubber band ligation(s)
EXCLUDES  *Colonoscopy or sigmoidoscopy, flexible; with band ligation (45350, [45398])*
*Ligation of hemorrhoidal vascular bundles including ultrasound guidance (0249T)*
📇 5.48   ☒ 7.66   **FUD** 010                    T P3
**AMA:** 2017,Sep,14; 2017,Jan,8; 2016,Jan,13; 2015,Apr,10; 2015,Jan,16; 2014,Dec,3; 2014,Jan,11; 2013,Jan,11-12

\#   **46945**  Hemorrhoidectomy, internal, by ligation other than rubber band; single hemorrhoid column/group
EXCLUDES  *Other hemorrhoid procedures:*
*Destruction (46930)*
*Excision (46250-46262)*
*Injection sclerosing solution (46500)*
*Ligation, hemorrhoidal vascular bundle (0249T)*
📇 6.50   ☒ 8.83   **FUD** 090                    J P3
**AMA:** 2017,Jan,8; 2016,Jan,13; 2015,Apr,10; 2014,Jan,11; 2013,Jan,11-12

\#   **46946**  2 or more hemorrhoid columns/groups
EXCLUDES  *Ligation, hemorrhoidal vascular bundle (0249T)*
📇 6.48   ☒ 8.96   **FUD** 090                    J A2
**AMA:** 2017,Jan,8; 2016,Jan,13; 2015,Apr,10; 2014,Jan,11; 2013,Jan,11-12

\#   **46220**  Excision of single external papilla or tag, anus
📇 3.42   ☒ 5.88   **FUD** 010                    T A2
**AMA:** 2014,Jan,11; 2013,Jan,11-12

**46230**  Excision of multiple external papillae or tags, anus
📇 4.98   ☒ 7.81   **FUD** 010                    J A2
**AMA:** 2014,Jan,11; 2013,Jan,11-12

\#   **46320**  Excision of thrombosed hemorrhoid, external
📇 3.20   ☒ 5.25   **FUD** 010                    T P3
**AMA:** 2014,Jan,11; 2013,Jan,11-12

**46250**  Hemorrhoidectomy, external, 2 or more columns/groups
EXCLUDES  *Hemorrhoidectomy, external, single column/group (46999)*
*Ligation, hemorrhoidal vascular bundle (0249T)*
📇 9.08   ☒ 13.2   **FUD** 090                    J A2
**AMA:** 2014,Jan,11; 2013,Jan,11-12

**46255**  Hemorrhoidectomy, internal and external, single column/group;
EXCLUDES  *Ligation, hemorrhoidal vascular bundle (0249T)*
📇 10.2   ☒ 14.4   **FUD** 090                    J A2
**AMA:** 2017,Jan,8; 2016,Jan,13; 2015,Jan,16; 2014,Oct,14; 2014,Jan,11; 2013,Jan,11-12

**46257**  with fissurectomy
EXCLUDES  *Ligation, hemorrhoidal vascular bundle (0249T)*
📇 12.1   ☒ 12.1   **FUD** 090                    J A2
**AMA:** 2014,Jan,11; 2013,Jan,11-12

**46258**  with fistulectomy, including fissurectomy, when performed
EXCLUDES  *Ligation, hemorrhoidal vascular bundle (0249T)*
📇 13.3   ☒ 13.3   **FUD** 090                    J A2 80
**AMA:** 2014,Jan,11; 2013,Jan,11-12

**46260**  Hemorrhoidectomy, internal and external, 2 or more columns/groups;
INCLUDES  Whitehead hemorrhoidectomy
EXCLUDES  *Ligation, hemorrhoidal vascular bundle (0249T)*
📇 13.7   ☒ 13.7   **FUD** 090                    J A2
**AMA:** 2014,Jan,11; 2013,Jan,11-12

**46261**  with fissurectomy
EXCLUDES  *Ligation, hemorrhoidal vascular bundle (0249T)*
📇 15.0   ☒ 15.0   **FUD** 090                    J A2
**AMA:** 2014,Jan,11; 2013,Jan,11-12

**46262**  with fistulectomy, including fissurectomy, when performed
EXCLUDES  *Ligation, hemorrhoidal vascular bundle (0249T)*
📇 15.9   ☒ 15.9   **FUD** 090                    J A2
**AMA:** 2017,Jan,8; 2016,Jan,13; 2015,Jan,16; 2014,Jan,11; 2013,Jan,11-12

## 46270-46320 Resection of Anal Fistula

**46270**  Surgical treatment of anal fistula (fistulectomy/fistulotomy); subcutaneous
📇 11.2   ☒ 14.5   **FUD** 090                    J A2
**AMA:** 2014,Jan,11; 2013,Jan,11-12

**46275**  intersphincteric
📇 11.9   ☒ 15.4   **FUD** 090                    J A2
**AMA:** 2014,Jan,11; 2013,Jan,11-12

**46280**  transsphincteric, suprasphincteric, extrasphincteric or multiple, including placement of seton, when performed
EXCLUDES  *Placement of seton (46020)*
📇 13.5   ☒ 13.5   **FUD** 090                    J A2
**AMA:** 2014,Jan,11; 2013,Jan,11-12

**46285**  second stage
📇 11.9   ☒ 15.3   **FUD** 090                    J A2
**AMA:** 2014,Jan,11; 2013,Jan,11-12

**46288**  Closure of anal fistula with rectal advancement flap
📇 15.8   ☒ 15.8   **FUD** 090                    J A2
**AMA:** 2014,Jan,11; 2013,Jan,11-12

*46320*  Resequenced code. See code following 46230.

## 46500 Other Hemorrhoid Procedures

EXCLUDES  *Anoscopic injection of bulking agent, submucosal, for fecal incontinence (0377T)*

**46500**  Injection of sclerosing solution, hemorrhoids
📇 3.55   ☒ 5.36   **FUD** 010                    T P3
**AMA:** 2017,Jan,8; 2016,Jan,13; 2015,Jan,16; 2014,Jan,11; 2013,Jan,11-12

A sclerosing agent is injected into the tissues underlying hemorrhoids

*Labels: Internal hemorrhoids; Internal anal sphincter; External hemorrhoids; External anal sphincter; Dentate line*

● New Code   ▲ Revised Code   ○ Reinstated   ● New Web Release   ▲ Revised Web Release   Unlisted   Not Covered   # Resequenced
☒ AMA Mod 51 Exempt   ⑤ Optum Mod 51 Exempt   ⑥ Mod 63 Exempt   ∕ Non-FDA Drug   ★ Telemedicine   Ⓜ Maternity   Ⓐ Age Edit   + Add-on   **AMA:** CPT Asst
© 2017 Optum360, LLC                    CPT © 2017 American Medical Association. All Rights Reserved.

**Digestive System**

**46505 — 46740**

## 46505 Chemodenervation Anal Sphincter

EXCLUDES Chemodenervation of:
Extremity muscles (64642-64645)
Muscles/facial nerve (64612)
Neck muscles (64616)
Other peripheral nerve/branch (64640)
Pudendal nerve (64630)
Trunk muscles (64646-64647)
Code also drug(s)/substance(s) given

**46505** Chemodenervation of internal anal sphincter
🔧 6.87 ⚕ 8.16 **FUD** 010 T G2 50 ▢
**AMA:** 2017,Jan,8; 2016,Jan,13; 2015,Jan,16; 2014,Jan,11;
2013,Jan,11-12

## 46600-46615 Anoscopic Procedures

EXCLUDES Delivery of thermal energy via anoscope to the muscle of the anal canal
(46999)
Injection of bulking agent, submucosal, for fecal incontinence (0377T)

**46600** Anoscopy; diagnostic, including collection of specimen(s) by
brushing or washing, when performed (separate
procedure)
EXCLUDES Excision of rectal tumor, transanal endoscopic
microsurgical approach (ie, TEMS) (0184T)
High-resolution anoscopy (HRA), diagnostic (46601)
Ligation, hemorrhoidal vascular bundle (0249T)
Surgical incision of anus (46020-46762 [46220, 46320,
46945, 46946, 46947])
🔧 1.18 ⚕ 2.52 **FUD** 000 01 N1 ▢
**AMA:** 2017,Jan,8; 2016,Jan,13; 2015,Jan,16; 2014,Jan,11;
2013,Jan,11-12; 2012,Jan,15-42

**46601** diagnostic, with high-resolution magnification (HRA) (eg,
colposcope, operating microscope) and chemical agent
enhancement, including collection of specimen(s) by
brushing or washing, when performed
INCLUDES Operating microscope (69990)
🔧 2.72 ⚕ 3.89 **FUD** 000 01 N1 ▢
**AMA:** 2016,Feb,12

**46604** with dilation (eg, balloon, guide wire, bougie)
🔧 1.93 ⚕ 17.6 **FUD** 000 T P2 ▢
**AMA:** 2017,Jan,8; 2016,Jan,13; 2015,Jan,16; 2014,Jan,11;
2013,Jan,11-12

**46606** with biopsy, single or multiple
EXCLUDES High resolution anoscopy (HRA) with biopsy (46607)
🔧 2.20 ⚕ 6.44 **FUD** 000 T P3 ▢
**AMA:** 2017,Jan,8; 2016,Jan,13; 2015,Jan,16; 2014,Jan,11;
2013,Jan,11-12

**46607** with high-resolution magnification (HRA) (eg, colposcope,
operating microscope) and chemical agent enhancement,
with biopsy, single or multiple
INCLUDES Operating microscope (69990)
🔧 3.68 ⚕ 5.49 **FUD** 000 T G2 ▢
**AMA:** 2016,Feb,12

**46608** with removal of foreign body
🔧 2.42 ⚕ 6.68 **FUD** 000 T A2 ▢
**AMA:** 2017,Jan,8; 2016,Jan,13; 2015,Jan,16; 2014,Jan,11;
2013,Jan,11-12

**46610** with removal of single tumor, polyp, or other lesion by
hot biopsy forceps or bipolar cautery
🔧 2.36 ⚕ 6.49 **FUD** 000 J A2 ▢
**AMA:** 2017,Jan,8; 2016,Jan,13; 2015,Jan,16; 2014,Jan,11;
2013,Jan,11-12

**46611** with removal of single tumor, polyp, or other lesion by
snare technique
🔧 2.36 ⚕ 5.03 **FUD** 000 T A2 ▢
**AMA:** 2017,Jan,8; 2016,Jan,13; 2015,Jan,16; 2014,Jan,11;
2013,Jan,11-12

**46612** with removal of multiple tumors, polyps, or other lesions
by hot biopsy forceps, bipolar cautery or snare
technique
🔧 2.66 ⚕ 7.10 **FUD** 000 J A2 ▢
**AMA:** 2017,Jan,8; 2016,Jan,13; 2015,Jan,16; 2014,Jan,11;
2013,Jan,11-12

**46614** with control of bleeding (eg, injection, bipolar cautery,
unipolar cautery, laser, heater probe, stapler, plasma
coagulator)
🔧 1.87 ⚕ 3.66 **FUD** 000 T P3 ▢
**AMA:** 2017,Jan,8; 2016,Jan,13; 2015,Jan,16; 2014,Jan,11;
2013,Jan,11-12

**46615** with ablation of tumor(s), polyp(s), or other lesion(s) not
amenable to removal by hot biopsy forceps, bipolar
cautery or snare technique
🔧 2.68 ⚕ 4.09 **FUD** 000 J A2 ▢
**AMA:** 2017,Jan,8; 2016,Jan,13; 2015,Jan,16; 2014,Jan,11;
2013,Jan,11-12

## 46700-46762 [46947] Anal Repairs and Stapled Hemorrhoidopexy

**46700** Anoplasty, plastic operation for stricture; adult
🔧 18.8 ⚕ 18.8 **FUD** 090 J A2 ▢
**AMA:** 2014,Jan,11; 2013,Jan,11-12

**46705** infant A
EXCLUDES Anal septum incision (46070)
🔧 14.4 ⚕ 14.4 **FUD** 090 63 C 80 ▢
**AMA:** 2014,Jan,11; 2013,Jan,11-12

**46706** Repair of anal fistula with fibrin glue
🔧 5.04 ⚕ 5.04 **FUD** 010 J A2 ▢
**AMA:** 2014,Jan,11; 2013,Jan,11-12

**46707** Repair of anorectal fistula with plug (eg, porcine small
intestine submucosa [SIS])
🔧 13.5 ⚕ 13.5 **FUD** 090 J G2 80 ▢
**AMA:** 2017,Jan,8; 2016,Jan,13; 2015,Jan,16; 2014,Jan,11;
2013,Oct,15; 2013,Jan,11-12; 2012,Jan,6-10

**46710** Repair of ileoanal pouch fistula/sinus (eg, perineal or vaginal),
pouch advancement; transperineal approach
🔧 30.1 ⚕ 30.1 **FUD** 090 C 80 ▢
**AMA:** 2017,Jan,8; 2016,Jan,13; 2015,Jan,16; 2014,Jan,11;
2013,Jan,11-12

**46712** combined transperineal and transabdominal approach
🔧 61.1 ⚕ 61.1 **FUD** 090 C 80 ▢
**AMA:** 2017,Jan,8; 2016,Jan,13; 2015,Jan,16; 2014,Jan,11;
2013,Jan,11-12

**46715** Repair of low imperforate anus; with anoperineal fistula
(cut-back procedure)
🔧 15.6 ⚕ 15.6 **FUD** 090 63 C 80 ▢
**AMA:** 2014,Jan,11; 2013,Jan,11-12

**46716** with transposition of anoperineal or anovestibular
fistula
🔧 31.9 ⚕ 31.9 **FUD** 090 63 C 80 ▢
**AMA:** 2014,Jan,11; 2013,Jan,11-12

**46730** Repair of high imperforate anus without fistula; perineal or
sacroperineal approach
🔧 52.6 ⚕ 52.6 **FUD** 090 63 C 80 ▢
**AMA:** 2014,Jan,11; 2013,Jan,11-12

**46735** combined transabdominal and sacroperineal
approaches
🔧 60.9 ⚕ 60.9 **FUD** 090 63 C 80 ▢
**AMA:** 2014,Jan,11; 2013,Jan,11-12

**46740** Repair of high imperforate anus with rectourethral or
rectovaginal fistula; perineal or sacroperineal approach
🔧 58.7 ⚕ 58.7 **FUD** 090 63 C 80 ▢
**AMA:** 2014,Jan,11; 2013,Jan,11-12

**46742**  **combined transabdominal and sacroperineal approaches**
⚙ 78.6  ⚖ 78.6  **FUD** 090  ⑨ C 80 ▣
**AMA:** 2014,Jan,11; 2013,Jan,11-12

**46744**  **Repair of cloacal anomaly by anorectovaginoplasty and urethroplasty, sacroperineal approach**  ♀
⚙ 102.  ⚖ 102.  **FUD** 090  ⑨ C 80 ▣
**AMA:** 2014,Jan,11; 2013,Jan,11-12

**46746**  **Repair of cloacal anomaly by anorectovaginoplasty and urethroplasty, combined abdominal and sacroperineal approach;**  ♀
⚙ 103.  ⚖ 103.  **FUD** 090  C 80 ▣
**AMA:** 2014,Jan,11; 2013,Jan,11-12

**46748**  **with vaginal lengthening by intestinal graft or pedicle flaps**  ♀
⚙ 114.  ⚖ 114.  **FUD** 090  C 80 ▣
**AMA:** 2014,Jan,11; 2013,Jan,11-12

**46750**  **Sphincteroplasty, anal, for incontinence or prolapse; adult**
⚙ 21.7  ⚖ 21.7  **FUD** 090  J A2 80 ▣
**AMA:** 2014,Jan,11; 2013,Jan,11-12

**46751**  **child**  A
⚙ 17.1  ⚖ 17.1  **FUD** 090  C 80 ▣
**AMA:** 2014,Jan,11; 2013,Jan,11-12

**46753**  **Graft (Thiersch operation) for rectal incontinence and/or prolapse**
⚙ 16.6  ⚖ 16.6  **FUD** 090  J A2 ▣
**AMA:** 2014,Jan,11; 2013,Jan,11-12

**46754**  **Removal of Thiersch wire or suture, anal canal**
⚙ 6.54  ⚖ 8.43  **FUD** 010  J A2 80 ▣
**AMA:** 2014,Jan,11; 2013,Jan,11-12

**46760**  **Sphincteroplasty, anal, for incontinence, adult; muscle transplant**
⚙ 31.9  ⚖ 31.9  **FUD** 090  J A2 80 ▣
**AMA:** 2014,Jan,11; 2013,Jan,11-12

**46761**  **levator muscle imbrication (Park posterior anal repair)**
⚙ 26.6  ⚖ 26.6  **FUD** 090  J A2 80 ▣
**AMA:** 2014,Jan,11; 2013,Jan,11-12

**46762**  **implantation artificial sphincter**
EXCLUDES  *Anoscopic injection of bulking agent, submucosal, for fecal incontinence (0377T)*
⚙ 26.3  ⚖ 26.3  **FUD** 090  J J8 80 ▣
**AMA:** 2014,Jan,11; 2013,Jan,11-12

\# **46947**  **Hemorrhoidopexy (eg, for prolapsing internal hemorrhoids) by stapling**
⚙ 11.0  ⚖ 11.0  **FUD** 090  J A2 ▣
**AMA:** 2017,Jan,8; 2016,Jan,13; 2015,Jan,16; 2014,Jan,11; 2013,Jan,11-12; 2012,Jan,15-42

## 46900-46999 Destruction Procedures: Anus

**46900**  **Destruction of lesion(s), anus (eg, condyloma, papilloma, molluscum contagiosum, herpetic vesicle), simple; chemical**
⚙ 3.95  ⚖ 6.91  **FUD** 010  T P2 ▣
**AMA:** 2014,Jan,11; 2013,Jan,11-12

**46910**  **electrodesiccation**
⚙ 3.85  ⚖ 7.32  **FUD** 010  T P3 ▣
**AMA:** 2014,Jan,11; 2013,Jan,11-12

**46916**  **cryosurgery**
⚙ 4.13  ⚖ 6.57  **FUD** 010  T P2 ▣
**AMA:** 2014,Jan,11; 2013,Jan,11-12

**46917**  **laser surgery**
⚙ 3.82  ⚖ 12.9  **FUD** 010  J A2 ▣
**AMA:** 2014,Jan,11; 2013,Jan,11-12

**46922**  **surgical excision**
⚙ 3.90  ⚖ 7.62  **FUD** 010  J A2 ▣
**AMA:** 2014,Jan,11; 2013,Jan,11-12

**46924**  **Destruction of lesion(s), anus (eg, condyloma, papilloma, molluscum contagiosum, herpetic vesicle), extensive (eg, laser surgery, electrosurgery, cryosurgery, chemosurgery)**
⚙ 5.29  ⚖ 15.1  **FUD** 010  J A2 ▣
**AMA:** 2014,Jan,11; 2013,Jan,11-12

**46930**  **Destruction of internal hemorrhoid(s) by thermal energy (eg, infrared coagulation, cautery, radiofrequency)**
EXCLUDES  *Other hemorrhoid procedures:*
*Cryosurgery destruction (46999)*
*Excision ([46320], 46250-46262)*
*Hemorrhoidopexy ([46947])*
*Incision (46083)*
*Injection sclerosing solution (46500)*
*Ligation (46221, [46945, 46946])*
⚙ 4.22  ⚖ 5.87  **FUD** 090  T P3 80 ▣
**AMA:** 2017,Jan,8; 2016,Jul,8; 2016,Jan,13; 2015,Apr,10; 2014,Jan,11; 2013,Jan,11-12

**46940**  **Curettage or cautery of anal fissure, including dilation of anal sphincter (separate procedure); initial**
⚙ 4.22  ⚖ 6.53  **FUD** 010  J P3 ▣
**AMA:** 2014,Jan,11; 2013,Jan,11-12

**46942**  **subsequent**
⚙ 3.79  ⚖ 6.17  **FUD** 010  T P3 80 ▣
**AMA:** 2014,Jan,11; 2013,Jan,11-12

*46945*  **Resequenced code. See code following 46221.**

*46946*  **Resequenced code. See code following 46221.**

*46947*  **Resequenced code. See code following 46762.**

**46999**  **Unlisted procedure, anus**
⚙ 0.00  ⚖ 0.00  **FUD** YYY  T 80
**AMA:** 2017,Jan,8; 2016,Jan,13; 2015,Apr,10; 2015,Jan,16; 2014,Jan,11; 2013,Jan,11-12

## 47000-47001 Needle Biopsy of Liver
EXCLUDES  *Fine needle aspiration (10021, 10022)*

**47000**  **Biopsy of liver, needle; percutaneous**
🔧 (76942, 77002, 77012, 77021)
🔬 (88172-88173)
⚙ 2.61  ⚖ 8.70  **FUD** 000  J A2 ▣
**AMA:** 2017,Jan,8; 2016,Jan,13; 2015,Jan,16; 2014,Jan,11; 2013,Jan,11-12; 2012,Jan,15-42

+ **47001**  **when done for indicated purpose at time of other major procedure (List separately in addition to code for primary procedure)**
Code first primary procedure
🔧 (76942, 77002)
🔬 (88172-88173)
⚙ 3.03  ⚖ 3.03  **FUD** ZZZ  N N1 ▣
**AMA:** 2017,Jan,8; 2016,Jan,13; 2015,Jan,16; 2014,Jan,11; 2013,Jan,11-12; 2012,Jan,15-42

## 47010-47130 Open Incisional and Resection Procedures of Liver

**47010**  **Hepatotomy, for open drainage of abscess or cyst, 1 or 2 stages**
EXCLUDES  *Image guided percutaneous catheter drainage (49505)*
⚙ 34.9  ⚖ 34.9  **FUD** 090  C 80 ▣
**AMA:** 2014,Jan,11; 2013,Nov,9; 2013,Jan,11-12

**47015**  **Laparotomy, with aspiration and/or injection of hepatic parasitic (eg, amoebic or echinococcal) cyst(s) or abscess(es)**
⚙ 33.6  ⚖ 33.6  **FUD** 090  C 80 ▣
**AMA:** 2014,Jan,11; 2013,Jan,11-12

**47100**  **Biopsy of liver, wedge**
⚙ 24.4  ⚖ 24.4  **FUD** 090  C 80 ▣
**AMA:** 2014,Jan,11; 2013,Jan,11-12

● New Code   ▲ Revised Code   ○ Reinstated   ● New Web Release   ▲ Revised Web Release   Unlisted   Not Covered   # Resequenced
⊘ AMA Mod 51 Exempt   ⑨ Optum Mod 51 Exempt   ⑥ Mod 63 Exempt   ✗ Non-FDA Drug   ★ Telemedicine   M Maternity   A Age Edit   + Add-on   AMA: CPT Asst
© 2017 Optum360, LLC   CPT © 2017 American Medical Association. All Rights Reserved.

**47120** Hepatectomy, resection of liver; partial lobectomy
🗍 67.5  ⚕ 67.5  **FUD** 090  [C] [80] [▭]
**AMA:** 2017,Jan,8; 2016,Oct,11; 2016,Jan,13; 2015,Jan,16; 2014,Sep,13; 2014,Jan,11; 2013,Jan,11-12; 2012,Jan,15-42

**47122** trisegmentectomy
🗍 99.4  ⚕ 99.4  **FUD** 090  [C] [80] [▭]
**AMA:** 2014,Jan,11; 2013,Jan,11-12

**47125** total left lobectomy
🗍 89.1  ⚕ 89.1  **FUD** 090  [C] [80] [▭]
**AMA:** 2014,Jan,11; 2013,Jan,11-12

**47130** total right lobectomy
🗍 95.7  ⚕ 95.7  **FUD** 090  [C] [80] [▭]
**AMA:** 2014,Jan,11; 2013,Jan,11-12

## 47133-47147 Liver Transplant Procedures

**CMS:** 100-03,260.1 Adult Liver Transplantation; 100-03,260.2 Pediatric Liver Transplantation; 100-04,3,90.4 Liver Transplants; 100-04,3,90.4.1 Standard Liver Acquisition Charge; 100-04,3,90.4.2 Billing for Liver Transplant and Acquisition Services; 100-04,3,90.6 Intestinal and Multi-Visceral Transplants

**47133** Donor hepatectomy (including cold preservation), from cadaver donor
[INCLUDES] Graft:
Cold preservation
Harvest
🗍 0.00  ⚕ 0.00  **FUD** XXX  [C] [▭]
**AMA:** 2014,Jan,11; 2013,Jan,11-12

**47135** Liver allotransplantation, orthotopic, partial or whole, from cadaver or living donor, any age
[INCLUDES] Partial/whole recipient hepatectomy
Partial/whole transplant of allograft
Recipient care
🗍 155.  ⚕ 155.  **FUD** 090  [C] [80] [▭]
**AMA:** 2017,Jan,8; 2016,Jan,13; 2015,Jan,16; 2014,Jan,11; 2013,Jan,11-12; 2012,Jan,15-42

**47140** Donor hepatectomy (including cold preservation), from living donor; left lateral segment only (segments II and III)
[INCLUDES] Donor care
Graft:
Cold preservation
Harvest
🗍 96.8  ⚕ 96.8  **FUD** 090  [C] [80] [▭]
**AMA:** 2017,Jan,8; 2016,Jan,13; 2015,Jan,16; 2014,Jan,11; 2013,Jan,11-12; 2012,Jan,15-42

**47141** total left lobectomy (segments II, III and IV)
[INCLUDES] Donor care
Graft:
Cold preservation
Harvest
🗍 123.  ⚕ 123.  **FUD** 090  [C] [80] [▭]
**AMA:** 2014,Jan,11; 2013,Jan,11-12

**47142** total right lobectomy (segments V, VI, VII and VIII)
[INCLUDES] Donor care
Graft:
Cold preservation
Harvest
🗍 135.  ⚕ 135.  **FUD** 090  [C] [80] [▭]
**AMA:** 2014,Jan,11; 2013,Jan,11-12

**47143** Backbench standard preparation of cadaver donor whole liver graft prior to allotransplantation, including cholecystectomy, if necessary, and dissection and removal of surrounding soft tissues to prepare the vena cava, portal vein, hepatic artery, and common bile duct for implantation; without trisegment or lobe split
[EXCLUDES] Cholecystectomy (47600, 47610)
Hepatectomy (47120-47125)
🗍 0.00  ⚕ 0.00  **FUD** XXX  [C] [80] [▭]
**AMA:** 2017,Jan,8; 2016,Jan,13; 2015,Jan,16; 2014,Jan,11; 2013,Jan,11-12

**47144** with trisegment split of whole liver graft into 2 partial liver grafts (ie, left lateral segment [segments II and III] and right trisegment [segments I and IV through VIII])
[EXCLUDES] Cholecystectomy (47600, 47610)
Hepatectomy (47120-47125)
🗍 0.00  ⚕ 0.00  **FUD** 090  [C] [80] [▭]
**AMA:** 2014,Jan,11; 2013,Jan,11-12

**47145** with lobe split of whole liver graft into 2 partial liver grafts (ie, left lobe [segments II, III, and IV] and right lobe [segments I and V through VIII])
[EXCLUDES] Cholecystectomy (47600, 47610)
Hepatectomy (47120-47125)
🗍 0.00  ⚕ 0.00  **FUD** XXX  [C] [80] [▭]
**AMA:** 2014,Jan,11; 2013,Jan,11-12

**47146** Backbench reconstruction of cadaver or living donor liver graft prior to allotransplantation; venous anastomosis, each
[EXCLUDES] Cholecystectomy (47600, 47610)
Hepatectomy (47120-47125)
🗍 9.59  ⚕ 9.59  **FUD** XXX  [C] [80] [▭]
**AMA:** 2014,Jan,11; 2013,Jan,11-12

**47147** arterial anastomosis, each
[EXCLUDES] Cholecystectomy (47600, 47610)
Hepatectomy (47120-47125)
🗍 11.1  ⚕ 11.1  **FUD** XXX  [C] [80] [▭]
**AMA:** 2014,Jan,11; 2013,Jan,11-12

## 47300-47362 Open Repair of Liver

**47300** Marsupialization of cyst or abscess of liver
🗍 32.7  ⚕ 32.7  **FUD** 090  [C] [80] [▭]
**AMA:** 2014,Jan,11; 2013,Jan,11-12

Anterior abdominal skin    Hepatic cyst

**Cutaway view of liver**

**Marsupialization of cyst**

A liver cyst or abscess is marsupialized; this method involves surgical access to the cyst and making an incision into it; the edges of the cyst are sutured to the abdominal wall and drainage, open or closed, is placed into the cyst

**47350** Management of liver hemorrhage; simple suture of liver wound or injury
🗍 39.6  ⚕ 39.6  **FUD** 090  [C] [80] [▭]
**AMA:** 2014,Jan,11; 2013,Jan,11-12

**47360** complex suture of liver wound or injury, with or without hepatic artery ligation
🗍 53.6  ⚕ 53.6  **FUD** 090  [C] [80] [▭]
**AMA:** 2014,Jan,11; 2013,Jan,11-12

**47361** exploration of hepatic wound, extensive debridement, coagulation and/or suture, with or without packing of liver
🗍 87.9  ⚕ 87.9  **FUD** 090  [C] [80] [▭]
**AMA:** 2014,Jan,11; 2013,Jan,11-12

| [26]/[1C] PC/TC Only | [A2]-[Z3] ASC Payment | [50] Bilateral | ♂ Male Only | ♀ Female Only | 🗍 Facility RVU | ⚕ Non-Facility RVU | [▭] CCI |
| FUD Follow-up Days | CMS: IOM (Pub 100) | [A]-[Y] OPPSI | [80]/[80] Surg Assist Allowed / w/Doc | | [▨] Lab Crosswalk | [▨] Radiology Crosswalk | [✖] CLIA |

CPT © 2017 American Medical Association. All Rights Reserved.

212                                                                                          © 2017 Optum360, LLC

47362     re-exploration of hepatic wound for removal of packing
     42.0   42.0   **FUD** 090     C 80
     **AMA:** 2014,Jan,11; 2013,Jan,11-12

## 47370-47379 Laparoscopic Ablation Liver Tumors

INCLUDES   Diagnostic laparoscopy (49320)

47370     **Laparoscopy, surgical, ablation of 1 or more liver tumor(s); radiofrequency**
     (76940)
     36.1   36.1   **FUD** 090     J 80
     **AMA:** 2017,Jan,8; 2016,Jan,13; 2015,Jan,16; 2014,Jan,11; 2013,Jan,11-12

47371     **cryosurgical**
     (76940)
     35.9   35.9   **FUD** 090     J 80
     **AMA:** 2014,Jan,11; 2013,Jan,11-12

47379     **Unlisted laparoscopic procedure, liver**
     0.00   0.00   **FUD** YYY     J 80
     **AMA:** 2017,Jan,8; 2016,Jan,13; 2015,Jan,16; 2014,Dec,18; 2014,Jan,11; 2013,Jan,11-12; 2012,Jan,15-42

## 47380-47399 Open/Percutaneous Ablation Liver Tumors

47380     **Ablation, open, of 1 or more liver tumor(s); radiofrequency**
     (76940)
     41.7   41.7   **FUD** 090     C 80
     **AMA:** 2017,Jan,8; 2016,Jan,13; 2015,Jan,16; 2014,Jan,11; 2013,Jan,11-12

47381     **cryosurgical**
     (76940)
     40.0   40.0   **FUD** 090     C 80
     **AMA:** 2014,Jan,11; 2013,Jan,11-12

47382     **Ablation, 1 or more liver tumor(s), percutaneous, radiofrequency**
     (76940, 77013, 77022)
     21.8   137.   **FUD** 010     J 62
     **AMA:** 2017,Jan,8; 2016,Jan,13; 2015,Jan,16; 2014,Jan,11; 2013,Jan,11-12

47383     **Ablation, 1 or more liver tumor(s), percutaneous, cryoablation**
     (76940, 77013, 77022)
     13.1   192.   **FUD** 010     J 62
     **AMA:** 2017,Jan,8; 2016,Jan,13; 2015,Jan,16; 2014,Dec,18

47399     **Unlisted procedure, liver**
     0.00   0.00   **FUD** YYY     T
     **AMA:** 2017,Mar,10; 2017,Jan,8; 2016,Jan,13; 2015,Jan,16; 2014,Dec,18; 2014,Jan,11; 2013,Jan,11-12

## 47400-47490 Biliary Tract Procedures

47400     **Hepaticotomy or hepaticostomy with exploration, drainage, or removal of calculus**
     61.8   61.8   **FUD** 090     C 80
     **AMA:** 2014,Jan,11; 2013,Jan,11-12

47420     **Choledochotomy or choledochostomy with exploration, drainage, or removal of calculus, with or without cholecystotomy; without transduodenal sphincterotomy or sphincteroplasty**
     38.8   38.8   **FUD** 090     C 80
     **AMA:** 2014,Jan,11; 2013,Jan,11-12

47425     **with transduodenal sphincterotomy or sphincteroplasty**
     37.8   37.8   **FUD** 090     C 80
     **AMA:** 2014,Jan,11; 2013,Jan,11-12

47460     **Transduodenal sphincterotomy or sphincteroplasty, with or without transduodenal extraction of calculus (separate procedure)**
     36.4   36.4   **FUD** 090     C 80
     **AMA:** 2014,Jan,11; 2013,Jan,11-12

47480     **Cholecystotomy or cholecystostomy, open, with exploration, drainage, or removal of calculus (separate procedure)**
     EXCLUDES   *Percutaneous cholecystostomy (47490)*
     25.3   25.3   **FUD** 090     C 80
     **AMA:** 2017,Jan,8; 2016,Jan,13; 2015,Jan,16; 2014,Jan,11; 2013,Jan,11-12; 2012,Jan,15-42

47490     **Cholecystostomy, percutaneous, complete procedure, including imaging guidance, catheter placement, cholecystogram when performed, and radiological supervision and interpretation**
     INCLUDES   Radiological guidance (75989, 76942, 77002, 77012, 77021)
     EXCLUDES   *Injection procedure for cholangiography (47531-47532)*
       *Open cholecystostomy (47480)*
     9.57   9.57   **FUD** 010     J
     **AMA:** 2017,Jan,8; 2016,Jan,13; 2015,Dec,3; 2015,Jan,16; 2014,Jan,11; 2013,Nov,9; 2013,Jan,11-12; 2012,Jan,15-42

Percutaneous catheter passed through liver to gallbladder

Common hepatic duct
Gallstone impacted in cystic duct
Inflamed thick walled gallbladder

## 47531-47532 Injection/Insertion Procedures of Biliary Tract

INCLUDES   Contrast material injection
     Radiologic supervision and interpretation
EXCLUDES   *Intraoperative cholangiography (74300-74301)*
     *Procedures performed via the same access (47490, 47533-47541)*

47531     **Injection procedure for cholangiography, percutaneous, complete diagnostic procedure including imaging guidance (eg, ultrasound and/or fluoroscopy) and all associated radiological supervision and interpretation; existing access**
     2.06   8.88   **FUD** 000     02 N1
     **AMA:** 2017,Jan,8; 2015,Dec,3

47532     **new access (eg, percutaneous transhepatic cholangiogram)**
     6.23   22.7   **FUD** 000     02 N1
     **AMA:** 2017,Jan,8; 2015,Dec,3

## 47533-47544 Percutaneous Procedures of the Biliary Tract

47533     **Placement of biliary drainage catheter, percutaneous, including diagnostic cholangiography when performed, imaging guidance (eg, ultrasound and/or fluoroscopy), and all associated radiological supervision and interpretation; external**
     EXCLUDES   *Conversion to internal-external drainage catheter (47535)*
       *Percutaneous placement stent in bile duct (47538)*
       *Placement stent into bile duct, new access (47540)*
       *Replacement existing internal drainage catheter (47536)*
     7.82   35.1   **FUD** 000     J 62
     **AMA:** 2017,Jan,8; 2015,Dec,3

● New Code    ▲ Revised Code    ○ Reinstated    ● New Web Release    ▲ Revised Web Release    Unlisted    Not Covered    # Resequenced
⊘ AMA Mod 51 Exempt    ⑨ Optum Mod 51 Exempt    ⑨ Mod 63 Exempt    ✗ Non-FDA Drug    ★ Telemedicine    M Maternity    A Age Edit    + Add-on    **AMA:** CPT Asst
© 2017 Optum360, LLC      CPT © 2017 American Medical Association. All Rights Reserved.      **213**

**47534** internal-external

       *EXCLUDES* *Conversion to external only drainage catheter (47536)*
       *Percutaneous placement stent in bile duct (47538)*
       *Placement stent into bile duct, new access (47540)*

    10.8    41.8   **FUD** 000         J 62 🖵

**AMA:** 2017,Jan,8; 2015,Dec,3

**47535** Conversion of external biliary drainage catheter to
internal-external biliary drainage catheter, percutaneous,
including diagnostic cholangiography when performed,
imaging guidance (eg, fluoroscopy), and all associated
radiological supervision and interpretation

    5.80    28.8   **FUD** 000         J 62 🖵

**AMA:** 2017,Jan,8; 2015,Dec,3

**47536** Exchange of biliary drainage catheter (eg, external,
internal-external, or conversion of internal-external to
external only), percutaneous, including diagnostic
cholangiography when performed, imaging guidance (eg,
fluoroscopy), and all associated radiological supervision and
interpretation

       *INCLUDES* Exchange of one drainage catheter
       *EXCLUDES* *Placement of stent(s) into a bile duct, percutaneous (47538)*
       Code also exchange of additional catheters in same session with
         modifier 59 (47536)

    3.88    19.5   **FUD** 000         J 62 🖵

**AMA:** 2017,Jan,8; 2015,Dec,3

**47537** Removal of biliary drainage catheter, percutaneous, requiring
fluoroscopic guidance (eg, with concurrent indwelling biliary
stents), including diagnostic cholangiography when
performed, imaging guidance (eg, fluoroscopy), and all
associated radiological supervision and interpretation

       *EXCLUDES* *Placement of stent(s) into a bile duct via the same access (47538)*
       *Removal without use of fluoroscopic guidance; report*
       *with appropriate E&M service code*

    2.82    10.4   **FUD** 000         02 62 🖵

**AMA:** 2017,Jan,8; 2015,Dec,3

**47538** Placement of stent(s) into a bile duct, percutaneous, including
diagnostic cholangiography, imaging guidance (eg,
fluoroscopy and/or ultrasound), balloon dilation, catheter
exchange(s) and catheter removal(s) when performed, and
all associated radiological supervision and interpretation;
existing access

       *EXCLUDES* *Drainage catheter inserted following stent placement*
       *(47536)*
       *Procedures performed via the same access*
       *(47536-47537)*
       *Treatment of same lesion in same operative session*
       *([43277], 47542, 47555-47556)*
       Code also multiple stents placed during same session when:
         (47538-47540)
         Serial stents placed within the same bile duct;
         Stent placement via two or more percutaneous access sites
           or the space between two other stents
         Two or more stents inserted through the same percutaneous
           access

    6.90    122.   **FUD** 000         J 62 🖵

**AMA:** 2017,Jan,8; 2016,Mar,10; 2015,Dec,3

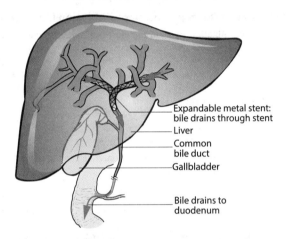

Expandable metal stent:
bile drains through stent
Liver
Common
bile duct
Gallbladder

Bile drains to
duodenum

**47539** new access, without placement of separate biliary drainage
catheter

       *EXCLUDES* *Treatment of same lesion in same session ([43277],*
       *47542, 47555-47556)*
       Code also multiple stents placed during same session when:
         (47538-47540)
         Serial stents placed within the same bile duct
         Stent placement via two or more percutaneous access sites
           or the space between two other stents
         Two or more stents inserted through the same percutaneous
           access

    12.5    135.   **FUD** 000         J 62 🖵

**AMA:** 2017,Jan,8; 2016,Mar,10; 2015,Dec,3

**47540** new access, with placement of separate biliary drainage
catheter (eg, external or internal-external)

       *EXCLUDES* *Procedure performed via the same access (47533-47534)*
       *Treatment of same lesion in same session ([43277],*
       *47542, 47555-47556)*
       Code also multiple stents placed during same session when:
         (47538-47540)
         Serial stents placed within the same bile duct;
         Stent placement via two or more percutaneous access sites
           or the space between two other stents;
         Two or more stents inserted through the same percutaneous
           access

    12.9    138.   **FUD** 000         J 62 🖵

**AMA:** 2017,Jan,8; 2016,Mar,10; 2015,Dec,3

26/TC PC/TC Only    A2-Z3 ASC Payment    50 Bilateral    ♂ Male Only    ♀ Female Only    Facility RVU    Non-Facility RVU    🖵 CCI
**FUD** Follow-up Days    **CMS:** IOM (Pub 100)    A-Y OPPSI    80/80 Surg Assist Allowed / w/Doc    Lab Crosswalk    Radiology Crosswalk    ✖ CLIA

CPT © 2017 American Medical Association. All Rights Reserved.          © 2017 Optum360, LLC

**47541** Placement of access through the biliary tree and into small bowel to assist with an endoscopic biliary procedure (eg, rendezvous procedure), percutaneous, including diagnostic cholangiography when performed, imaging guidance (eg, ultrasound and/or fluoroscopy), and all associated radiological supervision and interpretation, new access

> *EXCLUDES* *Access through biliary tree into small bowel for endoscopic biliary procedure (47535-47537)*
> *Conversion, exchange, or removal of external biliary drainage catheter (47535-47537)*
> *Injection procedure for cholangiography (47531-47532)*
> *Placement of biliary drainage catheter (47533-47534)*
> *Placement of stent(s) into a bile duct (47538-47540)*
> *Procedure performed when previous catheter access exists*

📋 9.75  ✂ 33.3  **FUD** 000  [J] [G2] [▭]

**AMA:** 2017,Jan,8; 2015,Dec,3

**+ 47542** Balloon dilation of biliary duct(s) or of ampulla (sphincteroplasty), percutaneous, including imaging guidance (eg, fluoroscopy), and all associated radiological supervision and interpretation, each duct (List separately in addition to code for primary procedure)

> *EXCLUDES* *Biliary endoscopy, with dilation of biliary duct stricture (47555-47556)*
> *Endoscopic balloon dilation ([43277], 47555-47556)*
> *Endoscopic retrograde cholangiopancreatography (ERCP) (43262, [43277])*
> *Placement of stent(s) into a bile duct (47538-47540)*
> *Procedure performed with balloon used to remove calculi, debris, sludge without dilation (47544)*
> Code also one additional dilation code when more than one dilation performed in same session, using modifier 59 with (47542)
> Code first (47531-47537, 47541)

📋 3.97  ✂ 13.1  **FUD** ZZZ  [N] [N1] [▭]

**AMA:** 2017,Jan,8; 2015,Dec,3

**+ 47543** Endoluminal biopsy(ies) of biliary tree, percutaneous, any method(s) (eg, brush, forceps, and/or needle), including imaging guidance (eg, fluoroscopy), and all associated radiological supervision and interpretation, single or multiple (List separately in addition to code for primary procedure)

> *EXCLUDES* *Endoscopic biopsy (46261, 47553)*
> *Endoscopic brushings (43260, 47552)*
> *Procedure performed more than one time per session*
> Code first (47531-47540)

📋 4.65  ✂ 16.3  **FUD** ZZZ  [N] [N1] [▭]

**AMA:** 2017,Jan,8; 2015,Dec,3

**+ 47544** Removal of calculi/debris from biliary duct(s) and/or gallbladder, percutaneous, including destruction of calculi by any method (eg, mechanical, electrohydraulic, lithotripsy) when performed, imaging guidance (eg, fluoroscopy), and all associated radiological supervision and interpretation (List separately in addition to code for primary procedure)

> *EXCLUDES* *Device deployment without findings of calculi/debris*
> *Endoscopic calculi removal/destruction (43264-43265, 47554)*
> *Endoscopic retrograde cholangiopancreatography (ERCP); with removal of calculi/debris from biliary/pancreatic duct(s) (43264)*
> *Procedures with removal of incidental debris (47531-47543)*
> Code first when debris removal not incidental, as appropriate (47531-47540)

📋 4.71  ✂ 30.8  **FUD** ZZZ  [N] [N1] [▭]

**AMA:** 2017,Jan,8; 2015,Dec,3

## 47550-47556 Endoscopic Procedures of the Biliary Tract

*INCLUDES* Diagnostic endoscopy (49320)

*EXCLUDES* *Endoscopic retrograde cholangiopancreatography (ERCP) (43260-43265, [43274], [43275], [43276], [43277], [43278], 74328-74330, 74363)*

**+ 47550** Biliary endoscopy, intraoperative (choledochoscopy) (List separately in addition to code for primary procedure)

> Code first primary procedure

📋 4.81  ✂ 4.81  **FUD** ZZZ  [C] [80] [▭]

**AMA:** 2014,Jan,11; 2013,Jan,11-12

**47552** Biliary endoscopy, percutaneous via T-tube or other tract; diagnostic, with collection of specimen(s) by brushing and/or washing, when performed (separate procedure)

📋 8.99  ✂ 8.99  **FUD** 000  [J] [A2] [▭]

**AMA:** 2017,Jan,8; 2016,Jan,13; 2015,Dec,3; 2015,Jan,16; 2014,Jan,11; 2013,Jan,11-12; 2012,Jan,15-42

**47553** with biopsy, single or multiple

📋 8.93  ✂ 8.93  **FUD** 000  [J] [A2] [▭]

**AMA:** 2017,Jan,8; 2016,Jan,13; 2015,Dec,3; 2015,Jan,16; 2014,Jan,11; 2013,Jan,11-12; 2012,Jan,15-42

**47554** with removal of calculus/calculi

📋 13.7  ✂ 13.7  **FUD** 000  [J] [A2] [▭]

**AMA:** 2017,Jan,8; 2016,Jan,13; 2015,Dec,3; 2015,Jan,16; 2014,Jan,11; 2013,Jan,11-12; 2012,Jan,15-42

**47555** with dilation of biliary duct stricture(s) without stent

> 🔧 (74363)

📋 10.6  ✂ 10.6  **FUD** 000  [J] [A2] [▭]

**AMA:** 2017,Jan,8; 2016,Jan,13; 2015,Dec,3; 2015,Jan,16; 2014,Jan,11; 2013,Jan,11-12; 2012,Jan,15-42

**47556** with dilation of biliary duct stricture(s) with stent

> 🔧 (74363)

📋 12.0  ✂ 12.0  **FUD** 000  [J] [J8] [▭]

**AMA:** 2017,Jan,8; 2016,Jan,13; 2015,Dec,3; 2015,Jan,16; 2014,Jan,11; 2013,Jan,11-12; 2012,Jan,15-42

## 47562-47579 Laparoscopic Gallbladder Procedures

*INCLUDES* Diagnostic laparoscopy (49320)

**47562** Laparoscopy, surgical; cholecystectomy

📋 19.0  ✂ 19.0  **FUD** 090  [J] [G2] [80] [▭]

**AMA:** 2017,Jan,8; 2016,Jan,13; 2015,Jan,16; 2014,Jan,11; 2013,Jan,11-12; 2012,Jan,15-42

**47563** cholecystectomy with cholangiography

> *EXCLUDES* *Percutaneous cholangiography (47531-47532)*
> Code also intraoperative radiology supervision and interpretation (74300-74301)

📋 20.6  ✂ 20.6  **FUD** 090  [J] [G2] [80] [▭]

**AMA:** 2017,Jan,8; 2016,Jan,13; 2015,Jan,16; 2014,Jan,11; 2013,Jan,11-12; 2012,Jan,15-42

**47564** cholecystectomy with exploration of common duct

📋 32.2  ✂ 32.2  **FUD** 090  [J] [G2] [80] [▭]

**AMA:** 2017,Jan,8; 2016,Jan,13; 2015,Jan,16; 2014,Jan,11; 2013,Jan,11-12; 2012,Jan,15-42

**47570** cholecystoenterostomy

📋 22.4  ✂ 22.4  **FUD** 090  [C] [80] [▭]

**AMA:** 2017,Jan,8; 2016,Jan,13; 2015,Jan,16; 2014,Jan,11; 2013,Jan,11-12

**47579** Unlisted laparoscopy procedure, biliary tract

📋 0.00  ✂ 0.00  **FUD** YYY  [J] [80] [50]

**AMA:** 2017,Jan,8; 2016,Jan,13; 2015,Jan,16; 2014,Jan,11; 2013,Jan,11-12

## 47600-47620 Open Gallbladder Procedures

**47600** Cholecystectomy;

> *EXCLUDES* *Laparoscopic method (47562-47564)*

📋 30.9  ✂ 30.9  **FUD** 090  [C] [80] [▭]

**AMA:** 2017,Jan,8; 2016,Jan,13; 2015,Jan,16; 2014,Jan,11; 2013,Jan,11-12

---

● New Code  ▲ Revised Code  ○ Reinstated  ● New Web Release  ▲ Revised Web Release  Unlisted  Not Covered  # Resequenced
⊘ AMA Mod 51 Exempt  ⑤ Optum Mod 51 Exempt  ⑥ Mod 63 Exempt  ✗ Non-FDA Drug  ★ Telemedicine  Ⓜ Maternity  Ⓐ Age Edit  + Add-on  **AMA:** CPT Asst

**47605**    with cholangiography
> *EXCLUDES*   *Laparoscopic method (47563-47564)*
> 🔹 32.5   🔹 32.5   **FUD** 090     [C][80][▭]
> **AMA:** 2017,Jan,8; 2016,Jan,13; 2015,Jan,16; 2014,Jan,11; 2013,Jan,11-12; 2012,Jan,15-42

**47610**    **Cholecystectomy with exploration of common duct;**
> *EXCLUDES*   *Laparoscopic method (47564)*
> Code also biliary endoscopy when performed in conjunction with cholecystectomy with exploration of common duct (47550)
> 🔹 36.3   🔹 36.3   **FUD** 090     [C][80][▭]
> **AMA:** 2017,Jan,8; 2016,Jan,13; 2015,Jan,16; 2014,Jan,11; 2013,Jan,11-12; 2012,Jan,15-42

**47612**    with choledochoenterostomy
> 🔹 36.7   🔹 36.7   **FUD** 090     [C][80][▭]
> **AMA:** 2014,Jan,11; 2013,Jan,11-12

**47620**    with transduodenal sphincterotomy or sphincteroplasty, with or without cholangiography
> 🔹 39.6   🔹 39.6   **FUD** 090     [C][80][▭]
> **AMA:** 2014,Jan,11; 2013,Jan,11-12

## 47700-47999 Open Resection and Repair of Biliary Tract

**47700**    **Exploration for congenital atresia of bile ducts, without repair, with or without liver biopsy, with or without cholangiography**
> 🔹 30.0   🔹 30.0   **FUD** 090     [63][C][80][▭]
> **AMA:** 2014,Jan,11; 2013,Jan,11-12

**47701**    **Portoenterostomy (eg, Kasai procedure)**
> 🔹 49.4   🔹 49.4   **FUD** 090     [63][C][80][▭]
> **AMA:** 2014,Jan,11; 2013,Jan,11-12

**47711**    **Excision of bile duct tumor, with or without primary repair of bile duct; extrahepatic**
> *EXCLUDES*   *Anastomosis (47760-47800)*
> 🔹 45.0   🔹 45.0   **FUD** 090     [C][80][▭]
> **AMA:** 2014,Jan,11; 2013,Jan,11-12

**47712**    intrahepatic
> *EXCLUDES*   *Anastomosis (47760-47800)*
> 🔹 57.7   🔹 57.7   **FUD** 090     [C][80][▭]
> **AMA:** 2014,Jan,11; 2013,Jan,11-12

**47715**    **Excision of choledochal cyst**
> 🔹 38.3   🔹 38.3   **FUD** 090     [C][80][▭]
> **AMA:** 2017,Jan,8; 2016,Jan,13; 2015,Jan,16; 2014,Jan,11; 2013,Jan,11-12; 2012,Jan,15-42

**47720**    **Cholecystoenterostomy; direct**
> *EXCLUDES*   *Laparoscopic method (47570)*
> 🔹 33.0   🔹 33.0   **FUD** 090     [C][80][▭]
> **AMA:** 2017,Jan,8; 2016,Jan,13; 2015,Jan,16; 2014,Jan,11; 2013,Jan,11-12

**47721**    with gastroenterostomy
> 🔹 39.1   🔹 39.1   **FUD** 090     [C][80][▭]
> **AMA:** 2014,Jan,11; 2013,Jan,11-12

**47740**    Roux-en-Y
> 🔹 37.8   🔹 37.8   **FUD** 090     [C][80][▭]
> **AMA:** 2014,Jan,11; 2013,Jan,11-12

**47741**    Roux-en-Y with gastroenterostomy
> 🔹 42.0   🔹 42.0   **FUD** 090     [C][80][▭]
> **AMA:** 2014,Jan,11; 2013,Jan,11-12

**47760**    **Anastomosis, of extrahepatic biliary ducts and gastrointestinal tract**
> 🔹 65.3   🔹 65.3   **FUD** 090     [C][80][▭]
> **AMA:** 2014,Jan,11; 2013,Jan,11-12

**47765**    **Anastomosis, of intrahepatic ducts and gastrointestinal tract**
> *INCLUDES*   *Longmire anastomosis*
> 🔹 88.1   🔹 88.1   **FUD** 090     [C][80][▭]
> **AMA:** 2014,Jan,11; 2013,Jan,11-12

**47780**    **Anastomosis, Roux-en-Y, of extrahepatic biliary ducts and gastrointestinal tract**
> 🔹 71.7   🔹 71.7   **FUD** 090     [C][80][▭]
> **AMA:** 2014,Jan,11; 2013,Jan,11-12

**47785**    **Anastomosis, Roux-en-Y, of intrahepatic biliary ducts and gastrointestinal tract**
> 🔹 94.0   🔹 94.0   **FUD** 090     [C][80][▭]
> **AMA:** 2014,Jan,11; 2013,Jan,11-12

**47800**    **Reconstruction, plastic, of extrahepatic biliary ducts with end-to-end anastomosis**
> 🔹 45.6   🔹 45.6   **FUD** 090     [C][80][▭]
> **AMA:** 2014,Jan,11; 2013,Jan,11-12

**47801**    **Placement of choledochal stent**
> 🔹 29.0   🔹 29.0   **FUD** 090     [C][80][▭]
> **AMA:** 2017,Jan,8; 2016,Jan,13; 2015,Jan,16; 2014,Jan,11; 2013,Jan,11-12; 2012,Jan,15-42

**47802**    **U-tube hepaticoenterostomy**
> 🔹 44.1   🔹 44.1   **FUD** 090     [C][80][▭]
> **AMA:** 2014,Jan,11; 2013,Jan,11-12

**47900**    **Suture of extrahepatic biliary duct for pre-existing injury (separate procedure)**
> 🔹 39.7   🔹 39.7   **FUD** 090     [C][80][▭]
> **AMA:** 2014,Jan,11; 2013,Jan,11-12

**47999**    **Unlisted procedure, biliary tract**
> 🔹 0.00   🔹 0.00   **FUD** YYY     [T]
> **AMA:** 2017,Jan,8; 2016,Jan,13; 2015,Jan,16; 2014,Jan,11; 2013,Jan,11-12; 2012,Jan,15-42

## 48000-48548 Open Procedures of the Pancreas

> *EXCLUDES*   *Peroral pancreatic procedures performed endoscopically (43260-43265, [43274], [43275], [43276], [43277], [43278])*

**48000**    **Placement of drains, peripancreatic, for acute pancreatitis;**
> 🔹 54.0   🔹 54.0   **FUD** 090     [C][80][▭]
> **AMA:** 2014,Jan,11; 2013,Jan,11-12

Head   Neck   Body   Tail
Common bile duct
Accessory pancreatic duct
Duodenum
Spleen
Pancreatic duct (of Wirsung)
Uncinate process
Superior mesenteric artery
Superior mesenteric vein

**48001**    with cholecystostomy, gastrostomy, and jejunostomy
> 🔹 67.0   🔹 67.0   **FUD** 090     [C][80][▭]
> **AMA:** 2014,Jan,11; 2013,Jan,11-12

**48020**    **Removal of pancreatic calculus**
> 🔹 33.6   🔹 33.6   **FUD** 090     [C][80][▭]
> **AMA:** 2014,Jan,11; 2013,Jan,11-12

| | | | | | |
|---|---|---|---|---|---|
| 26/TC PC/TC Only | A2-Z3 ASC Payment | 50 Bilateral | ♂ Male Only | ♀ Female Only | 🔹 Facility RVU   🔹 Non-Facility RVU   ▭ CCI |
| FUD Follow-up Days | CMS: IOM (Pub 100) | A-Y OPPSI | 80/80 Surg Assist Allowed / w/Doc | | 🔹 Lab Crosswalk   🔹 Radiology Crosswalk   ⊠ CLIA |

216      CPT © 2017 American Medical Association. All Rights Reserved.      © 2017 Optum360, LLC

**48100** **Biopsy of pancreas, open (eg, fine needle aspiration, needle core biopsy, wedge biopsy)**
    25.7    25.7    **FUD** 090      C 80
    **AMA:** 2014,Jan,11; 2013,Jan,11-12

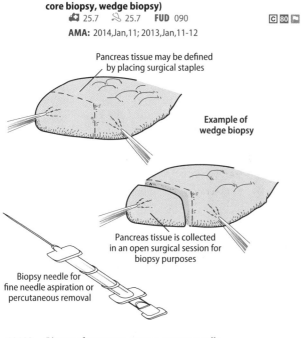

Pancreas tissue may be defined by placing surgical staples

Example of wedge biopsy

Pancreas tissue is collected in an open surgical session for biopsy purposes

Biopsy needle for fine needle aspiration or percutaneous removal

**48102** **Biopsy of pancreas, percutaneous needle**
    *EXCLUDES*    *Aspiration, fine needle (10022)*
    (76942, 77002, 77012, 77021)
    (88172-88173)
    7.01    15.1    **FUD** 010      J A2
    **AMA:** 2014,Jan,11; 2013,Jan,11-12

**48105** **Resection or debridement of pancreas and peripancreatic tissue for acute necrotizing pancreatitis**
    82.5    82.5    **FUD** 090      C 80
    **AMA:** 2014,Jan,11; 2013,Jan,11-12

**48120** **Excision of lesion of pancreas (eg, cyst, adenoma)**
    32.0    32.0    **FUD** 090      C 80
    **AMA:** 2014,Jan,11; 2013,Jan,11-12

**48140** **Pancreatectomy, distal subtotal, with or without splenectomy; without pancreaticojejunostomy**
    45.3    45.3    **FUD** 090      C 80
    **AMA:** 2017,Jul,10; 2014,Jan,11; 2013,Jan,11-12

**48145** **with pancreaticojejunostomy**
    47.0    47.0    **FUD** 090      C 80
    **AMA:** 2014,Jan,11; 2013,Jan,11-12

**48146** **Pancreatectomy, distal, near-total with preservation of duodenum (Child-type procedure)**
    54.2    54.2    **FUD** 090      C 80
    **AMA:** 2014,Jan,11; 2013,Jan,11-12

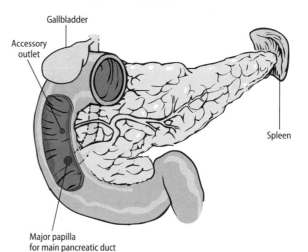

Gallbladder

Accessory outlet

Spleen

Major papilla for main pancreatic duct

**48148** **Excision of ampulla of Vater**
    36.0    36.0    **FUD** 090      C 80
    **AMA:** 2014,Jan,11; 2013,Jan,11-12

**48150** **Pancreatectomy, proximal subtotal with total duodenectomy, partial gastrectomy, choledochoenterostomy and gastrojejunostomy (Whipple-type procedure); with pancreatojejunostomy**
    90.2    90.2    **FUD** 090      C 80
    **AMA:** 2017,Jan,8; 2016,Jan,13; 2015,Dec,16; 2014,Jan,11; 2013,Jan,11-12

**48152** **without pancreatojejunostomy**
    83.6    83.6    **FUD** 090      C 80
    **AMA:** 2014,Jan,11; 2013,Jan,11-12

**48153** **Pancreatectomy, proximal subtotal with near-total duodenectomy, choledochoenterostomy and duodenojejunostomy (pylorus-sparing, Whipple-type procedure); with pancreatojejunostomy**
    89.7    89.7    **FUD** 090      C 80
    **AMA:** 2014,Jan,11; 2013,Jan,11-12

**48154** **without pancreatojejunostomy**
    83.6    83.6    **FUD** 090      C 80
    **AMA:** 2014,Jan,11; 2013,Jan,11-12

**48155** **Pancreatectomy, total**
    52.6    52.6    **FUD** 090      C 80
    **AMA:** 2014,Jan,11; 2013,Jan,11-12

**48160** **Pancreatectomy, total or subtotal, with autologous transplantation of pancreas or pancreatic islet cells**
    0.00    0.00    **FUD** XXX      E
    **AMA:** 2014,Jan,11; 2013,Jan,11-12

**+ 48400** **Injection procedure for intraoperative pancreatography (List separately in addition to code for primary procedure)**
    Code first primary procedure
    (74300-74301)
    3.10    3.10    **FUD** ZZZ      C 80
    **AMA:** 2017,Jan,8; 2016,Jan,13; 2015,Jan,16; 2014,Jan,11; 2013,Jan,11-12; 2012,Jan,15-42

**48500** **Marsupialization of pancreatic cyst**
    32.7    32.7    **FUD** 090      C 80
    **AMA:** 2014,Jan,11; 2013,Jan,11-12

**48510** **External drainage, pseudocyst of pancreas, open**
    *EXCLUDES*    *Image guided percutaneous catheter drainage (49405)*
    31.5    31.5    **FUD** 090      C 80
    **AMA:** 2014,Jan,11; 2013,Nov,9; 2013,Jan,11-12

**48520** **Internal anastomosis of pancreatic cyst to gastrointestinal tract; direct**
🚑 31.6  ⚕ 31.6  **FUD** 090  Ⓒ 80 ▣
**AMA:** 2014,Jan,11; 2013,Jan,11-12

**48540** **Roux-en-Y**
🚑 37.9  ⚕ 37.9  **FUD** 090  Ⓒ 80 ▣
**AMA:** 2014,Jan,11; 2013,Jan,11-12

**48545** **Pancreatorrhaphy for injury**
🚑 38.9  ⚕ 38.9  **FUD** 090  Ⓒ 80 ▣
**AMA:** 2014,Jan,11; 2013,Jan,11-12

**48547** **Duodenal exclusion with gastrojejunostomy for pancreatic injury**
🚑 51.7  ⚕ 51.7  **FUD** 090  Ⓒ 80 ▣
**AMA:** 2014,Jan,11; 2013,Jan,11-12

**48548** **Pancreaticojejunostomy, side-to-side anastomosis (Puestow-type operation)**
🚑 48.0  ⚕ 48.0  **FUD** 090  Ⓒ 80 ▣
**AMA:** 2014,Jan,11; 2013,Jan,11-12

## 48550-48999 Pancreas Transplant Procedures

**CMS:** 100-03,260.3 Pancreas Transplants; 100-04,3,90.5 Pancreas Transplants with Kidney Transplants; 100-04,3,90.5.1 Pancreas Transplants Alone

**48550** **Donor pancreatectomy (including cold preservation), with or without duodenal segment for transplantation**
INCLUDES   Graft:
Cold preservation
Harvest (with or without duodenal segment)
🚑 0.00  ⚕ 0.00  **FUD** XXX  Ⓔ ▣
**AMA:** 2017,Jan,8; 2016,Jan,13; 2015,Jan,16; 2014,Jan,11; 2013,Jan,11-12

**48551** **Backbench standard preparation of cadaver donor pancreas allograft prior to transplantation, including dissection of allograft from surrounding soft tissues, splenectomy, duodenotomy, ligation of bile duct, ligation of mesenteric vessels, and Y-graft arterial anastomoses from iliac artery to superior mesenteric artery and to splenic artery**
EXCLUDES   Biopsy of pancreas (48100-48102)
Bypass graft, with vein (35531, 35563)
Duodenotomy (44010)
Endoscopic procedures of the biliary tract (47550-47556)
Excision of lesion of mesentery (44820)
Excision of lesion of pancreas (48120)
Pancreatorrhaphy for injury (48545)
Placement of vein patch or cuff at distal anastomosis of bypass graft (35685)
Resection or debridement of pancreas (48105)
Splenectomy (38100-38102)
Suture of mesentery (44850)
Transduodenal sphincterotomy, sphincteroplasty (47460)
🚑 0.00  ⚕ 0.00  **FUD** XXX  Ⓒ 80 ▣
**AMA:** 2014,Jan,11; 2013,Jan,11-12

**48552** **Backbench reconstruction of cadaver donor pancreas allograft prior to transplantation, venous anastomosis, each**
EXCLUDES   Biopsy of pancreas (48100-48102)
Bypass graft, with vein (35531, 35563)
Duodenotomy (44010)
Endoscopic procedures of the biliary tract (47550-47556)
Excision of lesion of mesentery (44820)
Excision of lesion of pancreas (48120)
Pancreatorrhaphy for injury (48545)
Placement of vein patch or cuff at distal anastomosis of bypass graft (35685)
Resection or debridement of pancreas (48105)
Splenectomy (38100-38102)
Suture of mesentery (44850)
Transduodenal sphincterotomy, sphincteroplasty (47460)
🚑 6.81  ⚕ 6.81  **FUD** XXX  Ⓒ 80 ▣
**AMA:** 2014,Jan,11; 2013,Jan,11-12

**48554** **Transplantation of pancreatic allograft**
INCLUDES   Allograft transplant
Recipient care
🚑 73.8  ⚕ 73.8  **FUD** 090  Ⓒ 80 ▣
**AMA:** 2014,Jan,11; 2013,Jan,11-12

**48556** **Removal of transplanted pancreatic allograft**
🚑 36.6  ⚕ 36.6  **FUD** 090  Ⓒ 80 ▣
**AMA:** 2014,Jan,11; 2013,Jan,11-12

**48999** **Unlisted procedure, pancreas**
🚑 0.00  ⚕ 0.00  **FUD** YYY  Ⓣ 80
**AMA:** 2017,Jan,8; 2016,Jan,13; 2015,Jan,16; 2014,Jan,11; 2013,Feb,13; 2013,Jan,11-12; 2012,Jan,15-42

## 49000-49084 Exploratory and Drainage Procedures: Abdomen/Peritoneum

**49000** **Exploratory laparotomy, exploratory celiotomy with or without biopsy(s) (separate procedure)**
EXCLUDES   Exploration of penetrating wound without laparotomy (20102)
🚑 22.2  ⚕ 22.2  **FUD** 090  Ⓒ 80 ▣
**AMA:** 2017,Jan,8; 2016,Jan,13; 2015,Jan,16; 2014,Jan,11; 2013,Jan,11-12; 2012,Oct,3-8; 2012,Sep,11-13; 2012,Jan,15-42

**49002** **Reopening of recent laparotomy**
EXCLUDES   Hepatic wound re-exploration for packing removal (47362)
🚑 30.2  ⚕ 30.2  **FUD** 090  Ⓒ 80 ▣
**AMA:** 2017,Jan,8; 2016,Jan,13; 2015,Jan,16; 2014,Jan,11; 2013,Jan,11-12

**49010** **Exploration, retroperitoneal area with or without biopsy(s) (separate procedure)**
EXCLUDES   Exploration of penetrating wound without laparotomy (20102)
🚑 27.0  ⚕ 27.0  **FUD** 090  Ⓒ 80 ▣
**AMA:** 2014,Jan,11; 2013,Jan,11-12

**49020** **Drainage of peritoneal abscess or localized peritonitis, exclusive of appendiceal abscess, open**
EXCLUDES   Appendiceal abscess (44900)
Image guided percutaneous catheter drainage of abscess/peritonitis via catheter (49406)
Image-guided transrectal/transvaginal drainage of peritoneal abscess via catheter (49407)
🚑 46.0  ⚕ 46.0  **FUD** 090  Ⓒ 80 ▣
**AMA:** 2014,Jan,11; 2013,Nov,9; 2013,Jan,11-12

**49040** **Drainage of subdiaphragmatic or subphrenic abscess, open**
EXCLUDES   Image-guided percutaneous drainage of subdiaphragmatic/subphrenic abscess via catheter (49406)
🚑 28.9  ⚕ 28.9  **FUD** 090  Ⓒ 80 ▣
**AMA:** 2014,Jan,11; 2013,Nov,9; 2013,Jan,11-12

**49060** **Drainage of retroperitoneal abscess, open**
EXCLUDES   Image-guided percutaneous drainage of retroperitoneal abscess via catheter (49406)
Transrectal/transvaginal image-guided drainage of retroperitoneal abscess via catheter (49407)
🚑 31.8  ⚕ 31.8  **FUD** 090  Ⓒ ▣
**AMA:** 2017,Jan,8; 2016,Jan,13; 2015,Jan,16; 2014,Jan,11; 2013,Nov,9; 2013,Jan,11-12; 2012,Jan,15-42

**49062** **Drainage of extraperitoneal lymphocele to peritoneal cavity, open**
EXCLUDES   Drainage of lymphocele to peritoneal cavity, laparoscopic (49323)
Image-guided percutaneous drainage of retroperitoneal lymphocele via catheter (49406)
🚑 21.4  ⚕ 21.4  **FUD** 090  Ⓒ 80 ▣
**AMA:** 2017,Jan,8; 2016,Jan,13; 2015,Jan,16; 2014,Jan,11; 2013,Jan,11-12; 2012,Jan,15-42

26/TC PC/TC Only   A2-Z3 ASC Payment   50 Bilateral   ♂ Male Only   ♀ Female Only   🚑 Facility RVU   ⚕ Non-Facility RVU   ▣ CCI
FUD Follow-up Days   CMS: IOM (Pub 100)   A-Y OPPSI   80/80 Surg Assist Allowed / w/Doc   Ⓛ Lab Crosswalk   Ⓡ Radiology Crosswalk   ☒ CLIA
CPT © 2017 American Medical Association. All Rights Reserved.

© 2017 Optum360, LLC

**49082** Abdominal paracentesis (diagnostic or therapeutic); without imaging guidance

   🚗 2.15    ⚕ 5.48    **FUD** 000      [T] [62] 🖼

   **AMA:** 2017,Jan,8; 2016,Jan,13; 2015,Jan,16; 2014,Jan,11; 2013,Nov,9; 2013,Jan,11-12; 2012,Dec,9-10

**49083** with imaging guidance

   [INCLUDES] Radiological guidance (76942, 77002, 77012, 77021)

   [EXCLUDES] *Image-guided percutaneous drainage of retroperitoneal abscess via catheter (49406)*

   🚗 3.15    ⚕ 8.36    **FUD** 000      [T] [62] 🖼

   **AMA:** 2017,Jan,8; 2016,Jan,13; 2015,Jan,16; 2014,Mar,13; 2014,Jan,11; 2013,Nov,9; 2013,Jan,11-12; 2012,Dec,9-10

**49084** Peritoneal lavage, including imaging guidance, when performed

   [INCLUDES] Radiological guidance (76942, 77002, 77012, 77021)

   [EXCLUDES] *Image-guided percutaneous drainage of retroperitoneal abscess via catheter (49406)*

   🚗 3.15    ⚕ 3.15    **FUD** 000      [T] [62] 🖼

   **AMA:** 2017,Jan,8; 2016,Jan,13; 2015,Jan,16; 2014,Jan,11; 2013,Nov,9; 2013,Jan,11-12; 2012,Dec,9-10

## 49180 Biopsy of Mass: Abdomen/Retroperitoneum

[EXCLUDES] *Aspiration, fine needle (10021, 10022)*
*Lysis of intestinal adhesions (44005)*

**49180** Biopsy, abdominal or retroperitoneal mass, percutaneous needle

   📷 (76942, 77002, 77012, 77021)

   🔬 (88172-88173)

   🚗 2.48    ⚕ 4.64    **FUD** 000      [J] [A2] 🖼

   **AMA:** 2017,Jan,8; 2016,Jan,13; 2015,Jan,16; 2014,Jan,11; 2013,Jan,11-12

## 49185 Sclerotherapy of a Fluid Collection

**49185** Sclerotherapy of a fluid collection (eg, lymphocele, cyst, or seroma), percutaneous, including contrast injection(s), sclerosant injection(s), diagnostic study, imaging guidance (eg, ultrasound, fluoroscopy) and radiological supervision and interpretation when performed

   [INCLUDES] Multiple lesions treated via same access

   [EXCLUDES] *Contrast injection for assessment of abscess or cyst (49424)*
   *Pleurodesis (32560)*
   *Radiologic examination, abscess, fistula or sinus tract stud (76080)*
   *Sclerosis of veins/endovenous ablation of incompetent veins of extremity (36468, 36470-36471, 36475-36476, 36478-36479)*
   *Sclerotherapy of lymphatic/vascular malformation (37241)*

   Code also access or drainage via needle or catheter (10030, 10160, 49405-49407, 50390)
   Code also existing catheter exchange pre- or post-sclerosant injection (49423, 75984)
   Code also modifier 59 for treatment of multiple lesions in same session via separate access

   🚗 3.54    ⚕ 27.7    **FUD** 000      [T] 🖼

   **AMA:** 2017,Jan,8; 2016,Mar,10

## 49203-49205 Open Destruction or Excision: Abdominal Tumors

[EXCLUDES] *Ablation, open, 1 or more renal mass lesion(s), cryosurgical*
*Biopsy of kidney or ovary (50205, 58900)*
*Cryoablation of renal tumor (50250, 50593)*
*Excision of perinephric cyst (50290)*
*Excision of presacral or sacrococcygeal tumor (49215)*
*Exploration, renal or retroperitoneal area (49010, 50010)*
*Exploratory laparotomy (49000)*
*Laparotomy, for staging or restaging of ovarian, tubal, or primary peritoneal malignancy (58960)*
*Nephrectomy (50225, 50236)*
*Oophorectomy (58940-58958)*
*Ovarian cystectomy (58925)*
*Pelvic or retroperitoneal lymphadenectomy (38770, 38780)*
*Primary, recurrent ovarian, uterine, or tubal resection (58957-58958)*
*Wedge resection or bisection of ovary (58920)*

Code also colectomy (44140)
Code also nephrectomy (50220, 50240)
Code also vena caval resection with reconstruction (37799)
Code also small bowel resection (44120)

**49203** Excision or destruction, open, intra-abdominal tumors, cysts or endometriomas, 1 or more peritoneal, mesenteric, or retroperitoneal primary or secondary tumors; largest tumor 5 cm diameter or less

   🚗 34.6    ⚕ 34.6    **FUD** 090      [C] [80] 🖼

   **AMA:** 2017,Jan,8; 2016,Jan,13; 2015,Jan,16; 2014,Jan,11; 2013,Jan,11-12

**49204** largest tumor 5.1-10.0 cm diameter

   🚗 44.4    ⚕ 44.4    **FUD** 090      [C] [80] 🖼

   **AMA:** 2017,Jan,8; 2016,Jan,13; 2015,Jan,16; 2014,Jan,11; 2013,Jan,11-12

**49205** largest tumor greater than 10.0 cm diameter

   🚗 51.0    ⚕ 51.0    **FUD** 090      [C] [80] 🖼

   **AMA:** 2017,Jan,8; 2016,Jan,13; 2015,Jan,16; 2014,Jan,11; 2013,Jan,11-12

## 49215 Resection Presacral/Sacrococcygeal Tumor

**49215** Excision of presacral or sacrococcygeal tumor

   🚗 64.3    ⚕ 64.3    **FUD** 090      [63] [C] [80] 🖼

   **AMA:** 2014,Jan,11; 2013,Jan,11-12

## 49220-49255 Other Open Abdominal Procedures

[EXCLUDES] *Lysis of intestinal adhesions (44005)*

**49220** Staging laparotomy for Hodgkins disease or lymphoma (includes splenectomy, needle or open biopsies of both liver lobes, possibly also removal of abdominal nodes, abdominal node and/or bone marrow biopsies, ovarian repositioning)

   🚗 28.1    ⚕ 28.1    **FUD** 090      [C] [80] 🖼

   **AMA:** 2014,Jan,11; 2013,Jan,11-12

**49250** Umbilectomy, omphalectomy, excision of umbilicus (separate procedure)

   🚗 17.0    ⚕ 17.0    **FUD** 090      [J] [A2] 🖼

   **AMA:** 2014,Jan,11; 2013,Jan,11-12

**49255** Omentectomy, epiploectomy, resection of omentum (separate procedure)

   🚗 22.8    ⚕ 22.8    **FUD** 090      [C] [80] 🖼

   **AMA:** 2017,Jan,8; 2016,Jan,13; 2015,Jan,16; 2014,Jan,11; 2013,Jan,11-12

## 49320-49329 Laparoscopic Procedures of the Abdomen/Peritoneum/Omentum

[INCLUDES] Diagnostic laparoscopy (49320)

[EXCLUDES] *Fulguration/excision of lesions of ovary/pelvic viscera/peritoneal surface, performed laparoscopically (58662)*

**49320** Laparoscopy, abdomen, peritoneum, and omentum, diagnostic, with or without collection of specimen(s) by brushing or washing (separate procedure)

   🚗 9.41    ⚕ 9.41    **FUD** 010      [J] [A2] [80] 🖼

   **AMA:** 2017,Apr,7; 2017,Jan,8; 2016,Jan,13; 2015,Dec,16; 2015,Jan,16; 2014,Jan,11; 2013,Jan,11-12; 2012,Jan,15-42

---

● New Code    ▲ Revised Code    ○ Reinstated    ⬤ New Web Release    ▲ Revised Web Release    Unlisted    Not Covered    # Resequenced
⊘ AMA Mod 51 Exempt    ⑤ Optum Mod 51 Exempt    ⑥ Mod 63 Exempt    ⁄ Non-FDA Drug    ★ Telemedicine    Ⓜ Maternity    Ⓐ Age Edit    + Add-on    **AMA:** CPT Asst

© 2017 Optum360, LLC      CPT © 2017 American Medical Association. All Rights Reserved.

**Digestive System**

**49321 — 49412**

**49321** **Laparoscopy, surgical; with biopsy (single or multiple)**
🔪 9.97   ✂ 9.97   **FUD** 010   Ⓙ A2 80 ▣
**AMA:** 2017,Jan,8; 2016,Jan,13; 2015,Jan,16; 2014,Jan,11; 2013,Jan,11-12

**49322** **with aspiration of cavity or cyst (eg, ovarian cyst) (single or multiple)**
🔪 10.6   ✂ 10.6   **FUD** 010   Ⓙ A2 80 ▣
**AMA:** 2017,Jan,8; 2016,Jan,13; 2015,Jan,16; 2014,Jan,11; 2013,Jan,11-12

**49323** **with drainage of lymphocele to peritoneal cavity**
EXCLUDES   *Open drainage of lymphocele to peritoneal cavity (49062)*
🔪 18.4   ✂ 18.4   **FUD** 090   Ⓙ 80 ▣
**AMA:** 2017,Jan,8; 2016,Jan,13; 2015,Jan,16; 2014,Jan,11; 2013,Jan,11-12; 2012,Jan,15-42

**49324** **with insertion of tunneled intraperitoneal catheter**
EXCLUDES   *Open approach (49421)*
Code also insertion of subcutaneous extension to intraperitoneal cannula with remote chest exit site, when appropriate (49435)
🔪 11.2   ✂ 11.2   **FUD** 010   Ⓙ G2 80 ▣
**AMA:** 2014,Jan,11; 2013,Jan,11-12

**49325** **with revision of previously placed intraperitoneal cannula or catheter, with removal of intraluminal obstructive material if performed**
🔪 12.0   ✂ 12.0   **FUD** 010   Ⓙ G2 80 ▣
**AMA:** 2014,Jan,11; 2013,Jan,11-12

**+** **49326** **with omentopexy (omental tacking procedure) (List separately in addition to code for primary procedure)**
Code first laparoscopy with permanent intraperitoneal cannula or catheter insertion or revision of previously placed catheter/cannula (49324, 49325)
🔪 5.49   ✂ 5.49   **FUD** ZZZ   Ⓝ N1 80 ▣
**AMA:** 2014,Jan,11; 2013,Jan,11-12

**+** **49327** **with placement of interstitial device(s) for radiation therapy guidance (eg, fiducial markers, dosimeter), intra-abdominal, intrapelvic, and/or retroperitoneum, including imaging guidance, if performed, single or multiple (List separately in addition to code for primary procedure)**
EXCLUDES   *Open approach (49412)*
*Percutaneous approach (49411)*
Code first laparoscopic abdominal, pelvic or retroperitoneal procedures
🔪 3.80   ✂ 3.80   **FUD** ZZZ   Ⓝ N1 80 ▣
**AMA:** 2014,Jan,11; 2013,Jan,11-12

**49329** **Unlisted laparoscopy procedure, abdomen, peritoneum and omentum**
🔪 0.00   ✂ 0.00   **FUD** YYY   Ⓙ 80 50
**AMA:** 2017,Jan,8; 2016,Jan,13; 2015,Jan,16; 2014,Jan,11; 2013,Oct,18; 2013,Jan,11-12; 2012,Jan,15-42

## 49400-49436 Peritoneal and Visceral Procedures: Drainage/Insertion/Modifications/Removal

**49400** **Injection of air or contrast into peritoneal cavity (separate procedure)**
📷 (74190)
🔪 2.70   ✂ 3.85   **FUD** 000   Ⓝ N1 ▣
**AMA:** 2017,Jan,8; 2016,Jan,13; 2015,Jan,16; 2014,Jan,11; 2013,Jan,11-12; 2012,Jan,15-42

**49402** **Removal of peritoneal foreign body from peritoneal cavity**
EXCLUDES   *Enterolysis (44005)*
*Percutaneous or open drainage or lavage (49020, 49040, 49082-49084, 49406)*
*Percutaneous tunneled intraperitoneal catheter insertion without subcutaneous port (49418)*
🔪 24.7   ✂ 24.7   **FUD** 090   Ⓙ A2 ▣
**AMA:** 2014,Jan,11; 2013,Jan,11-12

**49405** **Image-guided fluid collection drainage by catheter (eg, abscess, hematoma, seroma, lymphocele, cyst); visceral (eg, kidney, liver, spleen, lung/mediastinum), percutaneous**
INCLUDES   Radiological guidance (75989, 76942, 77002-77003, 77012, 77021)
EXCLUDES   *Open drainage (47010, 48510, 50020)*
*Percutaneous cholecystostomy (47490)*
*Percutaneous pleural drainage (32556-32557)*
*Pneumonostomy (32200)*
*Thoracentesis (32554-32555)*
Code also each individual collection drained per separate catheter
🔪 5.77   ✂ 22.9   **FUD** 000   Ⓙ ▣
**AMA:** 2017,Jan,8; 2016,Jan,13; 2015,Jan,16; 2014,May,9; 2014,Jan,11; 2013,Nov,9

**49406** **peritoneal or retroperitoneal, percutaneous**
INCLUDES   Radiological guidance (75989, 76942, 77002-77003, 77012, 77021)
EXCLUDES   *Diagnostic or therapeutic percutaneous abdominal paracentesis (49082-49083)*
*Open peritoneal/retroperitoneal drainage (44900, 49020-49062, 49084, 50020, 58805, 58822)*
*Open transrectal drainage pelvic abscess (45000)*
*Percutaneous tunneled intraperitoneal catheter insertion without subcutaneous port (49418)*
*Transrectal/transvaginal image-guided peritoneal/retroperitoneal drainage via catheter (49407)*
Code also each individual collection drained per separate catheter
🔪 5.77   ✂ 22.9   **FUD** 000   Ⓙ G2 ▣
**AMA:** 2017,Jan,8; 2016,Jan,13; 2015,Jan,16; 2014,May,9; 2014,Jan,11; 2013,Nov,9

**49407** **peritoneal or retroperitoneal, transvaginal or transrectal**
INCLUDES   Radiological guidance (75989, 76942, 77002-77003, 77012, 77021)
EXCLUDES   *Image guided percutaneous catheter drainage of soft tissue (eg, abdominal wall, neck, extremity) (10030)*
*Open transrectal/transvaginal drainage (45000, 58800, 58820)*
*Percutaneous pleural drainage (32556-32557)*
*Peritoneal drainage or lavage, open or percutaneous (49020, 49040, 49060)*
*Thoracentesis (32554-32555)*
Code also each individual collection drained per separate catheter
🔪 6.14   ✂ 18.6   **FUD** 000   Ⓙ G2 ▣
**AMA:** 2017,Jan,8; 2016,Jan,13; 2015,Jan,16; 2014,May,9; 2014,Jan,11; 2013,Nov,9

**49411** **Placement of interstitial device(s) for radiation therapy guidance (eg, fiducial markers, dosimeter), percutaneous, intra-abdominal, intra-pelvic (except prostate), and/or retroperitoneum, single or multiple**
EXCLUDES   *Placement (percutaneous) of interstitial device(s) for intrathoracic radiation therapy guidance (32553)*
Code also supply of device
📷 (76942, 77002, 77012, 77021)
🔪 5.35   ✂ 13.7   **FUD** 000   Ⓢ P3 80 ▣
**AMA:** 2017,Jan,8; 2016,Jun,3; 2016,Jan,13; 2015,Jan,16; 2014,Jan,11; 2013,Jan,11-12

**+** **49412** **Placement of interstitial device(s) for radiation therapy guidance (eg, fiducial markers, dosimeter), open, intra-abdominal, intrapelvic, and/or retroperitoneum, including image guidance, if performed, single or multiple (List separately in addition to code for primary procedure)**
EXCLUDES   *Laparoscopic approach (49327)*
*Percutaneous approach (49411)*
Code first open abdominal, pelvic or retroperitoneal procedure(s)
🔪 2.39   ✂ 2.39   **FUD** ZZZ   Ⓒ 80 ▣
**AMA:** 2014,Jan,11; 2013,Jan,11-12

26/TC PC/TC Only       A2-Z3 ASC Payment       50 Bilateral       ♂ Male Only       ♀ Female Only       🔪 Facility RVU       ✂ Non-Facility RVU       ▣ CCI
FUD Follow-up Days   CMS: IOM (Pub 100)   A-Y OPPSI       80/80 Surg Assist Allowed / w/Doc       🔬 Lab Crosswalk       📷 Radiology Crosswalk       ✖ CLIA
220                                               CPT © 2017 American Medical Association. All Rights Reserved.                                       © 2017 Optum360, LLC

**49418** Insertion of tunneled intraperitoneal catheter (eg, dialysis, intraperitoneal chemotherapy instillation, management of ascites), complete procedure, including imaging guidance, catheter placement, contrast injection when performed, and radiological supervision and interpretation, percutaneous

🔧 5.95 ♻ 38.7 **FUD** 000 J 62 80 ▭

**AMA:** 2014,Jan,11; 2013,Nov,9; 2013,Jan,11-12

**49419** Insertion of tunneled intraperitoneal catheter, with subcutaneous port (ie, totally implantable)

*EXCLUDES* Removal of catheter/cannula (49422)

🔧 12.8 ♻ 12.8 **FUD** 090 T A2 ▭

**AMA:** 2014,Jan,11; 2013,Jan,11-12

**49421** Insertion of tunneled intraperitoneal catheter for dialysis, open

*EXCLUDES* Laparoscopic approach (49324)

Code also insertion of subcutaneous extension to intraperitoneal cannula with remote chest exit site, when appropriate (49435)

🔧 6.67 ♻ 6.67 **FUD** 000 J 62 ▭

**AMA:** 2017,Jan,8; 2016,Jan,13; 2015,Jan,16; 2014,Jan,11; 2013,Jan,11-12; 2012,Jan,15-42

**49422** Removal of tunneled intraperitoneal catheter

*EXCLUDES* Removal temporary catheter or cannula (Use appropriate E&M code)

🔧 11.0 ♻ 11.0 **FUD** 000 02 A2 ▭

**AMA:** 2014,Jan,11; 2013,Jan,11-12

**49423** Exchange of previously placed abscess or cyst drainage catheter under radiological guidance (separate procedure)

✖ (75984)

🔧 2.08 ♻ 15.5 **FUD** 000 J 62 80 ▭

**AMA:** 2017,Jan,8; 2016,Jan,13; 2015,Jan,16; 2014,Jan,11; 2013,Jan,11-12

**49424** Contrast injection for assessment of abscess or cyst via previously placed drainage catheter or tube (separate procedure)

✖ (76080)

🔧 1.11 ♻ 4.14 **FUD** 000 N N1 80 ▭

**AMA:** 2017,Jan,8; 2016,Jan,13; 2015,Jan,16; 2014,Jan,11; 2013,Jan,11-12; 2012,Jan,15-42

**49425** Insertion of peritoneal-venous shunt

🔧 20.8 ♻ 20.8 **FUD** 090 C 80 ▭

**AMA:** 2014,Jan,11; 2013,Jan,11-12

**49426** Revision of peritoneal-venous shunt

*EXCLUDES* Shunt patency test (78291)

🔧 17.6 ♻ 17.6 **FUD** 090 J A2 ▭

**AMA:** 2014,Jan,11; 2013,Jan,11-12

**49427** Injection procedure (eg, contrast media) for evaluation of previously placed peritoneal-venous shunt

✖ (75809, 78291)

🔧 1.33 ♻ 1.33 **FUD** 000 N N1 80 ▭

**AMA:** 2014,Jan,11; 2013,Jan,11-12

**49428** Ligation of peritoneal-venous shunt

🔧 13.2 ♻ 13.2 **FUD** 010 C ▭

**AMA:** 2014,Jan,11; 2013,Jan,11-12

**49429** Removal of peritoneal-venous shunt

🔧 13.3 ♻ 13.3 **FUD** 010 02 82 ▭

**AMA:** 2014,Jan,11; 2013,Jan,11-12

**+ 49435** Insertion of subcutaneous extension to intraperitoneal cannula or catheter with remote chest exit site (List separately in addition to code for primary procedure)

Code first permanent insertion of intraperitoneal catheter/cannula (49324, 49421)

🔧 3.47 ♻ 3.47 **FUD** ZZZ N N1 80 ▭

**AMA:** 2014,Jan,11; 2013,Jan,11-12

**49436** Delayed creation of exit site from embedded subcutaneous segment of intraperitoneal cannula or catheter

🔧 5.39 ♻ 5.39 **FUD** 010 J 62 80 ▭

**AMA:** 2014,Jan,11; 2013,Jan,11-12

## 49440-49442 Insertion of Percutaneous Gastrointestinal Tube

*EXCLUDES* Naso- or oro-gastric tube placement (43752)

**49440** Insertion of gastrostomy tube, percutaneous, under fluoroscopic guidance including contrast injection(s), image documentation and report

*INCLUDES* Needle placement with fluoroscopic guidance (77002)

Code also gastrostomy to gastro-jejunostomy tube conversion with initial gastrostomy tube insertion, when performed (49446)

🔧 6.03 ♻ 27.5 **FUD** 010 J 62 80 ▭

**AMA:** 2017,Jan,8; 2016,Jan,13; 2015,Jan,16; 2014,Dec,18; 2014,Sep,5; 2014,Jan,11; 2013,Jan,11-12; 2012,Jan,15-42

**49441** Insertion of duodenostomy or jejunostomy tube, percutaneous, under fluoroscopic guidance including contrast injection(s), image documentation and report

*EXCLUDES* Gastrostomy tube to gastrojejunostomy tube conversion (49446)

🔧 7.04 ♻ 31.0 **FUD** 010 J 62 80 ▭

**AMA:** 2017,Jan,8; 2016,Jan,13; 2015,Jan,16; 2014,Dec,18; 2014,Sep,5; 2014,Jan,11; 2013,Jan,11-12; 2012,Jan,15-42

**49442** Insertion of cecostomy or other colonic tube, percutaneous, under fluoroscopic guidance including contrast injection(s), image documentation and report

🔧 6.07 ♻ 25.8 **FUD** 010 T 62 80 ▭

**AMA:** 2017,Jan,8; 2016,Jan,13; 2015,Jan,16; 2014,Dec,18; 2014,Sep,5; 2014,Jan,11; 2013,Jan,11-12; 2012,Jan,15-42

## 49446 Percutaneous Conversion: Gastrostomy to Gastro-jejunostomy Tube

*EXCLUDES* Code also initial gastrostomy tube insertion (49440) when conversion is performed at the same time

**49446** Conversion of gastrostomy tube to gastro-jejunostomy tube, percutaneous, under fluoroscopic guidance including contrast injection(s), image documentation and report

🔧 4.35 ♻ 26.4 **FUD** 000 J 62 80 ▭

**AMA:** 2017,Jan,8; 2016,Jan,13; 2015,Jan,16; 2014,Sep,5; 2014,Jan,11; 2013,Jan,11-12; 2012,Jan,15-42

## 49450-49452 Replacement Gastrointestinal Tube

*EXCLUDES* Placement of new tube whether gastrostomy, jejunostomy, duodenostomy, gastro-jejunostomy, or cecostomy at different percutaneous site (49440-49442)

**49450** Replacement of gastrostomy or cecostomy (or other colonic) tube, percutaneous, under fluoroscopic guidance including contrast injection(s), image documentation and report

*EXCLUDES* Change of gastrostomy tube, percutaneous, without imaging or endoscopic guidance (43760)

🔧 1.94 ♻ 18.8 **FUD** 000 T 62 80 ▭

**AMA:** 2017,Jan,8; 2016,Jan,13; 2015,Jan,16; 2014,Sep,5; 2014,Jan,11; 2013,Dec,16; 2013,Jan,11-12; 2012,Jan,15-42

**49451** Replacement of duodenostomy or jejunostomy tube, percutaneous, under fluoroscopic guidance including contrast injection(s), image documentation and report

🔧 2.63 ♻ 20.6 **FUD** 000 T 62 80 ▭

**AMA:** 2017,Jan,8; 2016,Jan,13; 2015,Jan,16; 2014,Dec,18; 2014,Sep,5; 2014,Jan,11; 2013,Jan,11-12; 2012,Jan,15-42

**49452** Replacement of gastro-jejunostomy tube, percutaneous, under fluoroscopic guidance including contrast injection(s), image documentation and report

🔧 4.05 ♻ 25.5 **FUD** 000 T 62 80 ▭

**AMA:** 2017,Jan,8; 2016,Jan,13; 2015,Jan,16; 2014,Sep,5; 2014,Jan,11; 2013,Jan,11-12; 2012,Jan,15-42

---

● New Code  ▲ Revised Code  ○ Reinstated  ● New Web Release  ▲ Revised Web Release  Unlisted  Not Covered  # Resequenced
Ⓢ AMA Mod 51 Exempt  ⑤ Optum Mod 51 Exempt  ⑥ Mod 63 Exempt  ✗ Non-FDA Drug  ★ Telemedicine  Ⓜ Maternity  Ⓐ Age Edit  + Add-on  **AMA:** CPT Asst

**Digestive System**

## 49460-49465 Removal of Obstruction/Injection for Contrast Through Gastrointestinal Tube

**49460** Mechanical removal of obstructive material from gastrostomy, duodenostomy, jejunostomy, gastro-jejunostomy, or cecostomy (or other colonic) tube, any method, under fluoroscopic guidance including contrast injection(s), if performed, image documentation and report

INCLUDES   Contrast injection (49465)

EXCLUDES   *Replacement of gastrointestinal tube (49450-49452)*

🚑 1.39   🩺 20.8   **FUD** 000    T 02 80 ▢

**AMA:** 2017,Jan,8; 2016,Jan,13; 2015,Jan,16; 2014,Sep,5; 2014,Jan,11; 2013,Jan,11-12

**49465** Contrast injection(s) for radiological evaluation of existing gastrostomy, duodenostomy, jejunostomy, gastro-jejunostomy, or cecostomy (or other colonic) tube, from a percutaneous approach including image documentation and report

EXCLUDES   *Mechanical removal of obstructive material from gastrointestinal tube (49460)*

          *Replacement of gastrointestinal tube (49450-49452)*

🚑 0.90   🩺 4.66   **FUD** 000    Q1 02 80 ▢

**AMA:** 2017,Jan,8; 2016,Jan,13; 2015,Jan,16; 2014,Sep,5; 2014,Jan,11; 2013,Jan,11-12

## 49491-49492 Inguinal Hernia Repair on Premature Infant

INCLUDES   Hernia repairs done on preterm infants younger than or equal to 50 weeks postconception age but younger than 6 months of age since birth

         Initial repair: no previous repair required

         Mesh or other prosthesis

EXCLUDES   *Abdominal wall debridement (11042, 11043)*

         *Intra-abdominal hernia repair/reduction (44050)*

Code also repair or excision of testicle(s), intestine, ovaries if performed (44120, 54520, 58940)

**49491** Repair, initial inguinal hernia, preterm infant (younger than 37 weeks gestation at birth), performed from birth up to 50 weeks postconception age, with or without hydrocelectomy; reducible    A

🚑 22.6   🩺 22.6   **FUD** 090    63 J 80 50 ▢

**AMA:** 2017,Jan,8; 2016,Jan,13; 2015,Jan,16; 2014,Jan,11; 2013,Jan,11-12; 2012,Jan,15-42

**49492** incarcerated or strangulated    A

🚑 27.7   🩺 27.7   **FUD** 090    63 J 80 50 ▢

**AMA:** 2017,Jan,8; 2016,Jan,13; 2015,Jan,16; 2014,Jan,11; 2013,Jan,11-12

## 49495-49557 Hernia Repair: Femoral/Inguinal /Lumbar

INCLUDES   Initial repair: no previous repair required

         Mesh or other prosthesis

         Recurrent repair: required previous repair(s)

EXCLUDES   *Abdominal wall debridement (11042, 11043)*

         *Intra-abdominal hernia repair/reduction (44050)*

Code also repair or excision of testicle(s), intestine, ovaries if performed (44120, 54520, 58940)

**49495** Repair, initial inguinal hernia, full term infant younger than age 6 months, or preterm infant older than 50 weeks postconception age and younger than age 6 months at the time of surgery, with or without hydrocelectomy; reducible    A

INCLUDES   Hernia repairs done on preterm infants older than 50 weeks postconception age and younger than 6 months

🚑 10.9   🩺 10.9   **FUD** 090    63 J A2 80 50 ▢

**AMA:** 2017,Jan,8; 2016,Jan,13; 2015,Jan,16; 2014,Jan,11; 2013,Jan,11-12; 2012,Jan,15-42

**49496** incarcerated or strangulated    A

INCLUDES   Hernia repairs done on preterm infants older than 50 weeks postconception age and younger than 6 months

🚑 15.6   🩺 15.6   **FUD** 090    63 J A2 80 50 ▢

**AMA:** 2017,Jan,8; 2016,Jan,13; 2015,Jan,16; 2014,Jan,11; 2013,Jan,11-12; 2012,Jan,15-42

**49500** Repair initial inguinal hernia, age 6 months to younger than 5 years, with or without hydrocelectomy; reducible    A

INCLUDES   Repairs performed on patients 6 months to younger than 5 years old

🚑 11.3   🩺 11.3   **FUD** 090    J A2 80 50 ▢

**AMA:** 2017,Jan,8; 2016,Jan,13; 2015,Jan,16; 2014,Nov,14; 2014,Jan,11; 2013,Jan,11-12; 2012,Jan,15-42

**49501** incarcerated or strangulated    A

INCLUDES   Repairs performed on patients 6 months to younger than 5 years old

🚑 17.5   🩺 17.5   **FUD** 090    J A2 80 50 ▢

**AMA:** 2017,Jan,8; 2016,Jan,13; 2015,Jan,16; 2014,Jan,11; 2013,Jan,11-12; 2012,Jan,15-42

**49505** Repair initial inguinal hernia, age 5 years or older; reducible    A

INCLUDES   MacEwen hernia repair

Code also when performed:

     Excision of hydrocele (55040)

     Excision of spermatocele (54840)

     Simple orchiectomy (54520)

🚑 15.0   🩺 15.0   **FUD** 090    J A2 80 50 ▢

**AMA:** 2017,Jan,8; 2016,Jan,13; 2015,Jan,16; 2014,Jan,11; 2013,Jan,11-12; 2012,Jan,15-42

**49507** incarcerated or strangulated    A

Code also when performed:

     Excision of hydrocele (55040)

     Excision of spermatocele (54840)

     Simple orchiectomy (54520)

🚑 16.9   🩺 16.9   **FUD** 090    J A2 80 50 CLIA

**AMA:** 2017,Jan,8; 2016,Jan,13; 2015,Jan,16; 2014,Jan,11; 2013,Jan,11-12; 2012,Jan,15-42

**49520** Repair recurrent inguinal hernia, any age; reducible    A

🚑 18.2   🩺 18.2   **FUD** 090    J A2 80 50 ▢

**AMA:** 2017,Jan,8; 2016,Jan,13; 2015,Jan,16; 2014,Jan,11; 2013,Jan,11-12; 2012,Jan,15-42

**49521** incarcerated or strangulated    A

🚑 20.7   🩺 20.7   **FUD** 090    J A2 80 50 ▢

**AMA:** 2017,Jan,8; 2016,Jan,13; 2015,Jan,16; 2014,Jan,11; 2013,Jan,11-12; 2012,Jan,15-42

**49525** Repair inguinal hernia, sliding, any age    A

EXCLUDES   *Inguinal hernia repair, incarcerated/strangulated (49496, 49501, 49507, 49521)*

🚑 16.5   🩺 16.5   **FUD** 090    J A2 80 50 ▢

**AMA:** 2017,Jan,8; 2016,Jan,13; 2015,Jan,16; 2014,Jan,11; 2013,Jan,11-12; 2012,Jan,15-42

Peritoneal lining is forced through a defect in the inguinal wall

A peritoneal sac is created

Sliding inguinal hernia

Anterior inguinal wall

Spermatic cord

Inguinal ligament

Femoral sheath

Because the bowel is attached to the peritoneum, it is pulled through the abdominal defect as well

**49540** Repair lumbar hernia

🚑 19.4   🩺 19.4   **FUD** 090    J A2 80 50 ▢

**AMA:** 2017,Jan,8; 2016,Jan,13; 2015,Jan,16; 2014,Jan,11; 2013,Jan,11-12

| 26/TC PC/TC Only | A2-Z3 ASC Payment | 50 Bilateral | ♂ Male Only | ♀ Female Only | 🚑 Facility RVU | 🩺 Non-Facility RVU | ▢ CCI |
| FUD Follow-up Days | CMS: IOM (Pub 100) | A-Y OPPSI | 80/80 Surg Assist Allowed / w/Doc | | 🔬 Lab Crosswalk | ☢ Radiology Crosswalk | ✖ CLIA |

222                    CPT © 2017 American Medical Association. All Rights Reserved.              © 2017 Optum360, LLC

**49550** Repair initial femoral hernia, any age; reducible
📅 16.6   ⚕ 16.6   **FUD** 090    Ⓙ A2 80 50 ▢
**AMA:** 2017,Jan,8; 2016,Jan,13; 2015,Jan,16; 2014,Jan,11; 2013,Jan,11-12

**49553** incarcerated or strangulated
📅 18.2   ⚕ 18.2   **FUD** 090    Ⓙ A2 80 50 ▢
**AMA:** 2017,Jan,8; 2016,Jan,13; 2015,Jan,16; 2014,Jan,11; 2013,Jan,11-12

**49555** Repair recurrent femoral hernia; reducible
📅 17.2   ⚕ 17.2   **FUD** 090    Ⓙ A2 80 50 ▢
**AMA:** 2017,Jan,8; 2016,Jan,13; 2015,Jan,16; 2014,Jan,11; 2013,Jan,11-12

**49557** incarcerated or strangulated
📅 20.9   ⚕ 20.9   **FUD** 090    Ⓙ A2 80 50 ▢
**AMA:** 2017,Jan,8; 2016,Jan,13; 2015,Jan,16; 2014,Jan,11; 2013,Jan,11-12

## 49560-49568 Hernia Repair: Incisional/Ventral

INCLUDES   Initial repair: no previous repair required
   Recurrent repair: required previous repair(s)
EXCLUDES   *Abdominal wall debridement (11042, 11043)*
   *Intra-abdominal hernia repair/reduction (44050)*
Code also repair or excision of testicle(s), intestine, ovaries if performed (44120, 54520, 58940)

**49560** Repair initial incisional or ventral hernia; reducible
Code also implantation of mesh or other prosthesis if performed (49568)
📅 21.3   ⚕ 21.3   **FUD** 090    Ⓙ A2 80 50 ▢
**AMA:** 2017,Jan,8; 2016,Jan,13; 2015,Jan,16; 2014,Jan,11; 2013,Oct,15; 2013,Jan,11-12; 2012,Jan,6-10

**49561** incarcerated or strangulated
Code also implantation of mesh or other prosthesis if performed (49568)
📅 26.9   ⚕ 26.9   **FUD** 090    Ⓙ A2 80 50 ▢
**AMA:** 2017,Jan,8; 2016,Jan,13; 2015,Jan,16; 2014,Jan,11; 2013,Oct,15; 2013,Jan,11-12; 2012,Jan,6-10

**49565** Repair recurrent incisional or ventral hernia; reducible
Code also implantation of mesh or other prosthesis if performed (49568)
📅 22.2   ⚕ 22.2   **FUD** 090    Ⓙ A2 80 50 ▢
**AMA:** 2017,Jan,8; 2016,Jan,13; 2015,Jan,16; 2014,Jan,11; 2013,Oct,15; 2013,Jan,11-12; 2012,Jan,6-10

**49566** incarcerated or strangulated
Code also implantation of mesh or other prosthesis if performed (49568)
📅 27.1   ⚕ 27.1   **FUD** 090    Ⓙ A2 80 50 ▢
**AMA:** 2017,Jan,8; 2016,Jan,13; 2015,Jan,16; 2014,Jan,11; 2013,Oct,15; 2013,Jan,11-12; 2012,Jan,6-10

**+ 49568** Implantation of mesh or other prosthesis for open incisional or ventral hernia repair or mesh for closure of debridement for necrotizing soft tissue infection (List separately in addition to code for the incisional or ventral hernia repair)
Code first (11004-11006, 49560-49566)
📅 7.76   ⚕ 7.76   **FUD** ZZZ    N M1 80 ▢
**AMA:** 2017,Jan,8; 2016,Jan,13; 2015,Jan,16; 2014,Jan,11; 2013,Oct,15; 2013,Jan,11-12; 2012,Jan,15-42; 2012,Jan,6-10

## 49570-49590 Hernia Repair: Epigastric/Lateral Ventral/Umbilical

INCLUDES   Mesh or other prosthesis
EXCLUDES   *Abdominal wall debridement (11042, 11043)*
   *Intra-abdominal hernia repair/reduction (44050)*
Code also repair or excision of testicle(s), intestine, ovaries if performed (44120, 54520, 58940)

**49570** Repair epigastric hernia (eg, preperitoneal fat); reducible (separate procedure)
📅 12.0   ⚕ 12.0   **FUD** 090    Ⓙ A2 80 50 ▢
**AMA:** 2017,Jan,8; 2016,Jan,13; 2015,Jan,16; 2014,Jan,11; 2013,Jan,11-12

**49572** incarcerated or strangulated
📅 14.9   ⚕ 14.9   **FUD** 090    Ⓙ A2 80 50 ▢
**AMA:** 2017,Jan,8; 2016,Jan,13; 2015,Jan,16; 2014,Jan,11; 2013,Jan,11-12

**49580** Repair umbilical hernia, younger than age 5 years; reducible    A
📅 9.46   ⚕ 9.46   **FUD** 090    Ⓙ A2 80 ▢
**AMA:** 2017,Jan,8; 2016,Jan,13; 2015,Jan,16; 2014,Jan,11; 2013,Jan,11-12

**49582** incarcerated or strangulated    A
📅 13.3   ⚕ 13.3   **FUD** 090    Ⓙ A2 80 ▢
**AMA:** 2017,Jan,8; 2016,Jan,13; 2015,Jan,16; 2014,Jan,11; 2013,Jan,11-12

**49585** Repair umbilical hernia, age 5 years or older; reducible    A
INCLUDES   Mayo hernia repair
📅 12.8   ⚕ 12.8   **FUD** 090    Ⓙ A2 80 ▢
**AMA:** 2017,Jan,8; 2016,Jan,13; 2015,Jan,16; 2014,Jan,11; 2013,Jan,11-12

**49587** incarcerated or strangulated    A
📅 13.7   ⚕ 13.7   **FUD** 090    Ⓙ A2 80 ▢
**AMA:** 2017,Jan,8; 2016,Jan,13; 2015,Jan,16; 2014,Jan,11; 2013,Jan,11-12

**49590** Repair spigelian hernia
📅 16.5   ⚕ 16.5   **FUD** 090    Ⓙ A2 80 50 ▢
**AMA:** 2017,Jan,8; 2016,Jan,13; 2015,Jan,16; 2014,Jan,11; 2013,Jan,11-12

## 49600-49611 Repair Birth Defect Abdominal Wall: Omphalocele/Gastroschisis

INCLUDES   Mesh or other prosthesis
EXCLUDES   *Abdominal wall debridement (11042, 11043)*
   *Intra-abdominal hernia repair/reduction (44050)*
   *Repair of:*
    *Diaphragmatic or hiatal hernia (39503, 43332-43337)*
    *Omentum (49999)*

**49600** Repair of small omphalocele, with primary closure
📅 19.0   ⚕ 19.0   **FUD** 090    63 Ⓙ A2 80 ▢
**AMA:** 2017,Jan,8; 2016,Jan,13; 2015,Jan,16; 2014,Jan,11; 2013,Jan,11-12

**49605** Repair of large omphalocele or gastroschisis; with or without prosthesis
📅 143.   ⚕ 143.   **FUD** 090    63 C 80 ▢
**AMA:** 2017,Jan,8; 2016,Jan,13; 2015,Jan,16; 2014,Jan,11; 2013,Jan,11-12

**49606** with removal of prosthesis, final reduction and closure, in operating room
📅 32.8   ⚕ 32.8   **FUD** 090    63 C 80 ▢
**AMA:** 2017,Jan,8; 2016,Jan,13; 2015,Jan,16; 2014,Jan,11; 2013,Jan,11-12

**49610** Repair of omphalocele (Gross type operation); first stage
📅 18.8   ⚕ 18.8   **FUD** 090    63 C 80 ▢
**AMA:** 2017,Jan,8; 2016,Jan,13; 2015,Jan,16; 2014,Jan,11; 2013,Jan,11-12

**49611** second stage
📅 16.1   ⚕ 16.1   **FUD** 090    63 C 80 ▢
**AMA:** 2017,Jan,8; 2016,Jan,13; 2015,Jan,16; 2014,Jan,11; 2013,Jan,11-12; 2012,Jan,15-42

## 49650-49659 Laparoscopic Hernia Repair

INCLUDES   Diagnostic laparoscopy (49320)

**49650** Laparoscopy, surgical; repair initial inguinal hernia
📅 12.3   ⚕ 12.3   **FUD** 090    Ⓙ A2 80 50 ▢
**AMA:** 2017,Jan,8; 2016,Jan,13; 2015,Jan,16; 2014,Jul,5; 2014,Jan,11; 2013,Jan,11-12

**49651** repair recurrent inguinal hernia
📅 16.0   ⚕ 16.0   **FUD** 090    Ⓙ A2 80 50 ▢
**AMA:** 2017,Jan,8; 2016,Jan,13; 2015,Jan,16; 2014,Jan,11; 2013,Jan,11-12

**49652** Laparoscopy, surgical, repair, ventral, umbilical, spigelian or epigastric hernia (includes mesh insertion, when performed); reducible

INCLUDES Laparoscopy, surgical, enterolysis (44180)
EXCLUDES *Implantation of mesh or other prosthesis (49568)*
🔧 21.5  ✂ 21.5  **FUD** 090  J 62 80 50 ▣
**AMA:** 2014,Jan,11; 2013,Jan,11-12

**49653** incarcerated or strangulated
INCLUDES Laparoscopy, surgical, enterolysis (44180)
EXCLUDES *Implantation of mesh or other prosthesis (49568)*
🔧 26.8  ✂ 26.8  **FUD** 090  J 62 80 50 ▣
**AMA:** 2014,Jan,11; 2013,Jan,11-12

**49654** Laparoscopy, surgical, repair, incisional hernia (includes mesh insertion, when performed); reducible
INCLUDES Laparoscopy, surgical, enterolysis (44180)
EXCLUDES *Implantation of mesh or other prosthesis (49568)*
🔧 24.4  ✂ 24.4  **FUD** 090  J 62 80 50 ▣
**AMA:** 2014,Jan,11; 2013,Jan,11-12

**49655** incarcerated or strangulated
INCLUDES Laparoscopy, surgical, enterolysis (44180)
EXCLUDES *Implantation of mesh or other prosthesis (49568)*
🔧 29.8  ✂ 29.8  **FUD** 090  J 62 80 50 ▣
**AMA:** 2014,Jan,11; 2013,Jan,11-12

**49656** Laparoscopy, surgical, repair, recurrent incisional hernia (includes mesh insertion, when performed); reducible
INCLUDES Laparoscopy, surgical, enterolysis (44180)
EXCLUDES *Implantation of mesh or other prosthesis (49568)*
🔧 26.5  ✂ 26.5  **FUD** 090  J 62 80 50 ▣
**AMA:** 2014,Jan,11; 2013,Jan,11-12

**49657** incarcerated or strangulated
INCLUDES Laparoscopy, surgical, enterolysis (44180)
EXCLUDES *Implantation of mesh or other prosthesis (49568)*
🔧 38.2  ✂ 38.2  **FUD** 090  J 62 80 50 ▣
**AMA:** 2014,Jan,11; 2013,Jan,11-12

**49659** Unlisted laparoscopy procedure, hernioplasty, herniorrhaphy, herniotomy
🔧 0.00  ✂ 0.00  **FUD** YYY  J 80 50 ▣
**AMA:** 2017,Jul,10; 2017,Jan,8; 2016,Jan,13; 2015,Jan,16; 2014,Dec,16; 2014,Dec,16; 2014,Jul,5; 2014,Jan,11; 2013,Jan,11-12; 2012,Jan,15-42

## 49900 Surgical Repair Abdominal Wall

EXCLUDES *Abdominal wall debridement (11042, 11043)*
*Suture of ruptured diaphragm (39540-39541)*

**49900** Suture, secondary, of abdominal wall for evisceration or dehiscence
🔧 23.5  ✂ 23.5  **FUD** 090  C 80 ▣
**AMA:** 2017,Jan,8; 2016,Jan,13; 2015,Jan,16; 2014,Jan,11; 2013,Jan,11-12

## 49904-49999 Harvesting of Omental Flap

**49904** Omental flap, extra-abdominal (eg, for reconstruction of sternal and chest wall defects)
INCLUDES Harvest and transfer
EXCLUDES *Omental flap harvest by second surgeon: both surgeons report code with modifier 62*
🔧 41.0  ✂ 41.0  **FUD** 090  C ▣
**AMA:** 2014,Jan,11; 2013,Jan,11-12

+ **49905** Omental flap, intra-abdominal (List separately in addition to code for primary procedure)
EXCLUDES *Exclusion of small intestine from pelvis by mesh or other prosthesis, or native tissue (44700)*
Code first primary procedure
🔧 10.2  ✂ 10.2  **FUD** ZZZ  C 80 ▣
**AMA:** 2017,Jan,8; 2016,Jan,13; 2015,Jan,16; 2014,Jan,11; 2013,Jan,11-12; 2012,Jan,15-42

**49906** Free omental flap with microvascular anastomosis
INCLUDES Operating microscope (69990)
🔧 0.00  ✂ 0.00  **FUD** 090  C ▣
**AMA:** 2017,Jan,8; 2016,Feb,12; 2016,Jan,13; 2015,Jan,16; 2014,Jan,11; 2013,Jan,11-12

**49999** Unlisted procedure, abdomen, peritoneum and omentum
🔧 0.00  ✂ 0.00  **FUD** YYY  T
**AMA:** 2017,Jan,8; 2016,Jan,13; 2015,Jan,16; 2014,Jan,9; 2014,Jan,11; 2013,Jan,11-12; 2012,Jan,15-42

26/TC PC/TC Only    A2-Z3 ASC Payment    50 Bilateral    ♂ Male Only    ♀ Female Only    🔧 Facility RVU    ✂ Non-Facility RVU    ▣ CCI
FUD Follow-up Days    CMS: IOM (Pub 100)    A-Y OPPSI    80/80 Surg Assist Allowed / w/Doc    🔬 Lab Crosswalk    ✚ Radiology Crosswalk    ✖ CLIA
224    CPT © 2017 American Medical Association. All Rights Reserved.    © 2017 Optum360, LLC

## 50010-50045 Kidney Procedures for Exploration or Drainage

*EXCLUDES* *Donor nephrectomy performed laparoscopically (50547)*
*Retroperitoneal*
*Abscess drainage (49060)*
*Exploration (49010)*
*Tumor/cyst excision (49203-49205)*

**50010** **Renal exploration, not necessitating other specific procedures**

*EXCLUDES* *Laparoscopic ablation of mass lesions of kidney (50542)*

📋 21.3 🔪 21.3 **FUD** 090 C 80 50 🏳

**AMA:** 2014,Jan,11

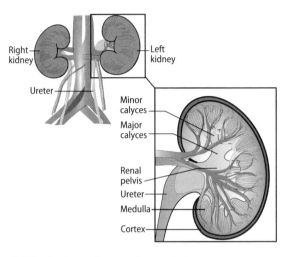

Right kidney
Left kidney
Ureter
Minor calyces
Major calyces
Renal pelvis
Ureter
Medulla
Cortex

**50020** **Drainage of perirenal or renal abscess, open**

*EXCLUDES* *Image-guided percutaneous of perirenal or renal abscess (49405)*

📋 29.3 🔪 29.3 **FUD** 090 J 🏳

**AMA:** 2017,Jan,8; 2016,Jan,13; 2015,Jan,16; 2014,May,9; 2014,Jan,11; 2013,Nov,9

**50040** **Nephrostomy, nephrotomy with drainage**

📋 26.7 🔪 26.7 **FUD** 090 C 50 🏳

**AMA:** 2017,Jan,8; 2016,Jan,13; 2015,Jan,16; 2014,Jan,11

**50045** **Nephrotomy, with exploration**

*EXCLUDES* *Renal endoscopy through nephrotomy (50570-50580)*

📋 27.1 🔪 27.1 **FUD** 090 C 80 50 🏳

**AMA:** 2017,Jan,8; 2016,Jan,13; 2015,Jan,16; 2014,Jan,11

## 50060-50081 Treatment of Kidney Stones

**CMS:** 100-03,230.1 NCD for Treatment of Kidney Stones

*EXCLUDES* *Retroperitoneal:*
*Abscess drainage (49060)*
*Exploration (49010)*
*Tumor/cyst excision (49203-49205)*

**50060** **Nephrolithotomy; removal of calculus**

📋 32.9 🔪 32.9 **FUD** 090 C 80 50 🏳

**AMA:** 2017,Jan,8; 2016,Jan,13; 2015,Jan,16; 2014,Jan,11

**50065** **secondary surgical operation for calculus**

📋 34.9 🔪 34.9 **FUD** 090 C 80 50 🏳

**AMA:** 2017,Jan,8; 2016,Jan,13; 2015,Jan,16; 2014,Jan,11

**50070** **complicated by congenital kidney abnormality**

📋 35.8 🔪 35.8 **FUD** 090 C 80 50 🏳

**AMA:** 2017,Jan,8; 2016,Jan,13; 2015,Jan,16; 2014,Jan,11

**50075** **removal of large staghorn calculus filling renal pelvis and calyces (including anatrophic pyelolithotomy)**

📋 42.1 🔪 42.1 **FUD** 090 C 80 50 🏳

**AMA:** 2017,Jan,8; 2016,Jan,13; 2015,Jan,16; 2014,Jan,11

**50080** **Percutaneous nephrostolithotomy or pyelostolithotomy, with or without dilation, endoscopy, lithotripsy, stenting, or basket extraction; up to 2 cm**

*EXCLUDES* *Nephrostomy without nephrostolithotomy (50040, 50395, 52334)*

📷 (76000, 76001)

📋 25.1 🔪 25.1 **FUD** 090 J 62 50 🏳

**AMA:** 2017,Jan,8; 2016,Jan,13; 2015,Jan,16; 2014,Jan,11; 2012,Jan,15-42

**50081** **over 2 cm**

*EXCLUDES* *Nephrostomy without nephrostolithotomy (50040, 50395, 52334)*

📷 (76000, 76001)

📋 36.8 🔪 36.8 **FUD** 090 J 62 80 50 🏳

**AMA:** 2017,Jan,8; 2016,Jan,13; 2015,Jan,16; 2014,Jan,11; 2012,Jan,15-42

## 50100 Repair of Anomalous Vessels of the Kidney

*EXCLUDES* *Retroperitoneal:*
*Abscess drainage (49060)*
*Exploration (49010)*
*Tumor/cyst excision (49203-49205)*

**50100** **Transection or repositioning of aberrant renal vessels (separate procedure)**

📋 31.7 🔪 31.7 **FUD** 090 C 80 50 🏳

**AMA:** 2017,Jan,8; 2016,Jan,13; 2015,Jan,16; 2014,Jan,11

## 50120-50135 Procedures of Renal Pelvis

*EXCLUDES* *Retroperitoneal:*
*Abscess drainage (49060)*
*Exploration (49010)*
*Tumor/cyst excision (49203-49205)*

**50120** **Pyelotomy; with exploration**

*INCLUDES* Gol-Vernet pyelotomy

*EXCLUDES* *Renal endoscopy through pyelotomy (50570-50580)*

📋 27.8 🔪 27.8 **FUD** 090 C 80 50 🏳

**AMA:** 2017,Jan,8; 2016,Jan,13; 2015,Jan,16; 2014,Jan,11

**50125** **with drainage, pyelostomy**

📋 29.6 🔪 29.6 **FUD** 090 C 80 50 🏳

**AMA:** 2017,Jan,8; 2016,Jan,13; 2015,Jan,16; 2014,Jan,11

**50130** **with removal of calculus (pyelolithotomy, pelviolithotomy, including coagulum pyelolithotomy)**

📋 29.8 🔪 29.8 **FUD** 090 C 80 50 🏳

**AMA:** 2017,Jan,8; 2016,Jan,13; 2015,Jan,16; 2014,Jan,11

**50135** **complicated (eg, secondary operation, congenital kidney abnormality)**

📋 32.4 🔪 32.4 **FUD** 090 C 80 50 🏳

**AMA:** 2017,Jan,8; 2016,Jan,13; 2015,Jan,16; 2014,Jan,11

## 50200-50205 Biopsy of Kidney

*EXCLUDES* *Laparoscopic renal mass lesion ablation (50542)*
*Retroperitoneal tumor/cyst excision (49203-49205)*

**50200** **Renal biopsy; percutaneous, by trocar or needle**

*EXCLUDES* *Fine needle aspiration (10022)*

📷 (76942, 77002, 77012, 77021)

🔬 (88172-88173)

📋 3.75 🔪 15.2 **FUD** 000 J A2 50 🏳

**AMA:** 2017,Jan,8; 2016,Jan,13; 2015,Jan,16; 2014,Jan,11

**50205** **by surgical exposure of kidney**

📋 21.8 🔪 21.8 **FUD** 090 C 80 50 🏳

**AMA:** 2017,Jan,8; 2016,Jan,13; 2015,Jan,16; 2014,Jan,11

## 50220-50240 Nephrectomy Procedures

*EXCLUDES* *Laparoscopic renal mass lesion ablation (50542)*
*Retroperitoneal tumor/cyst excision (49203-49205)*

**50220** **Nephrectomy, including partial ureterectomy, any open approach including rib resection;**

📋 30.2 🔪 30.2 **FUD** 090 C 80 50 🏳

**AMA:** 2017,Jan,8; 2016,Jan,13; 2015,Jan,16; 2014,Jan,11

---

● New Code ▲ Revised Code ○ Reinstated ● New Web Release ▲ Revised Web Release Unlisted Not Covered # Resequenced
⊘ AMA Mod 51 Exempt ⑤ Optum Mod 51 Exempt ⓔ Mod 63 Exempt ✗ Non-FDA Drug ★ Telemedicine Ⓜ Maternity Ⓐ Age Edit + Add-on **AMA:** CPT Asst
© 2017 Optum360, LLC CPT © 2017 American Medical Association. All Rights Reserved.

**50225**     **complicated because of previous surgery on same kidney**

 34.7     ⚕ 34.7     **FUD** 090          C 80 50 ▣

**AMA:** 2017,Jan,8; 2016,Jan,13; 2015,Jan,16; 2014,Jan,11

**50230**     **radical, with regional lymphadenectomy and/or vena caval thrombectomy**

*EXCLUDES*     *Vena caval resection with reconstruction (37799)*

 37.0     ⚕ 37.0     **FUD** 090          C 80 50 ▣

**AMA:** 2017,Jan,8; 2016,Jan,13; 2015,Jan,16; 2014,Jan,11

**50234**     **Nephrectomy with total ureterectomy and bladder cuff; through same incision**

 37.6     ⚕ 37.6     **FUD** 090          C 80 50 ▣

**AMA:** 2017,Jan,8; 2016,Jan,13; 2015,Jan,16; 2014,Jan,11

**50236**     **through separate incision**

 42.4     ⚕ 42.4     **FUD** 090          C 80 50 ▣

**AMA:** 2017,Jan,8; 2016,Jan,13; 2015,Jan,16; 2014,Jan,11

**50240**     **Nephrectomy, partial**

*EXCLUDES*     *Laparoscopic partial nephrectomy (50543)*

 38.2     ⚕ 38.2     **FUD** 090          C 80 50 ▣

**AMA:** 2017,Jan,8; 2016,Jan,13; 2015,Jan,16; 2014,Jan,11

## 50250-50290 Open Removal Kidney Lesions

*EXCLUDES*     *Open destruction or excision intra-abdominal tumors (49203-49205)*

**50250**     **Ablation, open, 1 or more renal mass lesion(s), cryosurgical, including intraoperative ultrasound guidance and monitoring, if performed**

*EXCLUDES*     *Laparoscopic renal mass lesion ablation (50542)*
*Percutaneous renal tumor ablation (50592-50593)*

 34.9     ⚕ 34.9     **FUD** 090          C 80 ▣

**AMA:** 2017,Jan,8; 2016,Jan,13; 2015,Jan,16; 2014,Jan,11; 2012,Jan,15-42

**50280**     **Excision or unroofing of cyst(s) of kidney**

*EXCLUDES*     *Renal cyst laparoscopic ablation (50541)*

 27.7     ⚕ 27.7     **FUD** 090          C 80 50 ▣

**AMA:** 2017,Jan,8; 2016,Jan,13; 2015,Jan,16; 2014,Jan,11

**50290**     **Excision of perinephric cyst**

 25.9     ⚕ 25.9     **FUD** 090          C 80 ▣

**AMA:** 2017,Jan,8; 2016,Jan,13; 2015,Jan,16; 2014,Jan,11

## 50300-50380 Kidney Transplant Procedures

**CMS:** 100-04,3,90.1 Kidney Transplant - General; 100-04,3,90.1.1 Standard Kidney Acquisition Charge; 100-04,3,90.1.2 Billing for Kidney Transplant and Acquisition Services; 100-04,3,90.5 Pancreas Transplants with Kidney Transplants

*EXCLUDES*     *Dialysis procedures (90935-90999)*
*Lymphocele drainage to peritoneal cavity performed laparoscopically (49323)*

**50300**     **Donor nephrectomy (including cold preservation); from cadaver donor, unilateral or bilateral**

*INCLUDES*     Graft:
Cold preservation
Harvesting

*EXCLUDES*     *Donor nephrectomy performed laparoscopically (50547)*

 0.00     ⚕ 0.00     **FUD** XXX          C ▣

**AMA:** 2017,Jan,8; 2016,Jan,13; 2015,Jan,16; 2014,Jan,11

**50320**     **open, from living donor**

*INCLUDES*     Donor care
Graft:
Cold preservation
Harvesting

*EXCLUDES*     *Donor nephrectomy performed laparoscopically (50547)*

 43.4     ⚕ 43.4     **FUD** 090          C 80 50 ▣

**AMA:** 2017,Jan,8; 2016,Jan,13; 2015,Jan,16; 2014,Jan,11

**50323**     **Backbench standard preparation of cadaver donor renal allograft prior to transplantation, including dissection and removal of perinephric fat, diaphragmatic and retroperitoneal attachments, excision of adrenal gland, and preparation of ureter(s), renal vein(s), and renal artery(s), ligating branches, as necessary**

*EXCLUDES*     *Adrenalectomy (60540, 60545)*

 0.00     ⚕ 0.00     **FUD** XXX          C 80 ▣

**AMA:** 2017,Jan,8; 2016,Jan,13; 2015,Jan,16; 2014,Jan,11

**50325**     **Backbench standard preparation of living donor renal allograft (open or laparoscopic) prior to transplantation, including dissection and removal of perinephric fat and preparation of ureter(s), renal vein(s), and renal artery(s), ligating branches, as necessary**

 0.00     ⚕ 0.00     **FUD** XXX          C 80 ▣

**AMA:** 2014,Jan,11

**50327**     **Backbench reconstruction of cadaver or living donor renal allograft prior to transplantation; venous anastomosis, each**

 6.30     ⚕ 6.30     **FUD** XXX          C 80 ▣

**AMA:** 2014,Jan,11

**50328**     **arterial anastomosis, each**

 5.52     ⚕ 5.52     **FUD** XXX          C 80 ▣

**AMA:** 2014,Jan,11

**50329**     **ureteral anastomosis, each**

 5.21     ⚕ 5.21     **FUD** XXX          C 80 ▣

**AMA:** 2014,Jan,11

**50340**     **Recipient nephrectomy (separate procedure)**

 27.3     ⚕ 27.3     **FUD** 090          C 80 50 ▣

**AMA:** 2014,Jan,11

**50360**     **Renal allotransplantation, implantation of graft; without recipient nephrectomy**

*INCLUDES*     Allograft transplantation
Recipient care
Code also backbench work (50323, 50325, 50327-50329)
Code also donor nephrectomy (cadaver or living donor) (50300, 50320, 50547)

 70.0     ⚕ 70.0     **FUD** 090          C 80 ▣

**AMA:** 2014,Jan,11

**50365**     **with recipient nephrectomy**

*INCLUDES*     Allograft transplantation
Recipient care

 82.6     ⚕ 82.6     **FUD** 090          C 80 50 ▣

**AMA:** 2017,Jan,8; 2016,Jan,13; 2015,Jan,16; 2014,Jan,11

**50370**     **Removal of transplanted renal allograft**

 34.7     ⚕ 34.7     **FUD** 090          C 80 ▣

**AMA:** 2014,Jan,11

**50380**     **Renal autotransplantation, reimplantation of kidney**

*INCLUDES*     Reimplantation of autograft

*EXCLUDES*     *Secondary procedures:*
*Nephrolithotomy (50060-50075)*
*Partial nephrectomy (50240, 50543)*

 55.5     ⚕ 55.5     **FUD** 090          C 80 ▣

**AMA:** 2017,Jan,8; 2016,Jan,13; 2015,Jan,16; 2014,Jan,11

## 50382-50386 Removal With/Without Replacement Internal Ureteral Stent

*INCLUDES*     Radiological supervision and interpretation

**50382**     **Removal (via snare/capture) and replacement of internally dwelling ureteral stent via percutaneous approach, including radiological supervision and interpretation**

*EXCLUDES*     *Introduction of guide into renal pelvis and/or ureter with dilation (50395)*
*Removal and replacement of an internally dwelling ureteral stent using a transurethral approach (50385)*

 7.48     ⚕ 31.5     **FUD** 000          J 62 50 ▣

**AMA:** 2017,Jan,8; 2016,Jan,13; 2016,Jan,3; 2015,Jan,16; 2014,Jan,11

---

26/TC PC/TC Only          A2-Z3 ASC Payment          50 Bilateral          ♂ Male Only          ♀ Female Only           Facility RVU          ⚕ Non-Facility RVU          ▣ CCI
**FUD** Follow-up Days          **CMS:** IOM (Pub 100)          A-Y OPPSI          80/80 Surg Assist Allowed / w/Doc           Lab Crosswalk           Radiology Crosswalk          ✖ CLIA

226                                        CPT © 2017 American Medical Association. All Rights Reserved.                                        © 2017 Optum360, LLC

**50384** Removal (via snare/capture) of internally dwelling ureteral stent via percutaneous approach, including radiological supervision and interpretation

> *EXCLUDES* *Introduction of guide into renal pelvis and/or ureter with dilation (50395)*
> *Removal of an internally dwelling ureteral stent using a transurethral approach (50386)*

🔧 6.75　⚕ 24.7　**FUD** 000　　　02 62 50 ▣

**AMA:** 2017,Jan,8; 2016,Jan,13; 2016,Jan,3; 2015,Jan,16; 2014,Jan,11

**50385** Removal (via snare/capture) and replacement of internally dwelling ureteral stent via transurethral approach, without use of cystoscopy, including radiological supervision and interpretation

🔧 6.36　⚕ 30.6　**FUD** 000　　　J 62 80 50 ▣

**AMA:** 2017,Jan,8; 2016,Jan,13; 2016,Jan,3; 2015,Jan,16; 2014,Jan,11

**50386** Removal (via snare/capture) of internally dwelling ureteral stent via transurethral approach, without use of cystoscopy, including radiological supervision and interpretation

🔧 4.75　⚕ 19.5　**FUD** 000　　　02 P3 80 50 ▣

**AMA:** 2017,Jan,8; 2016,Jan,13; 2016,Jan,3; 2015,Jan,16; 2014,Jan,11

## 50387 Remove/Replace Accessible Ureteral Stent

> *EXCLUDES* *Removal and replacement of ureteral stent through ureterostomy tube or ileal conduit (50688)*
> *Removal without replacement of externally accessible ureteral stent without fluoroscopic guidance, report with appropriate E&M code*

**50387** Removal and replacement of externally accessible nephroureteral catheter (eg, external/internal stent) requiring fluoroscopic guidance, including radiological supervision and interpretation

🔧 2.46　⚕ 13.9　**FUD** 000　　　J 62 80 50 ▣

**AMA:** 2017,Jan,8; 2016,Mar,10; 2016,Jan,13; 2016,Jan,3; 2015,Oct,5; 2015,Jan,16; 2014,Jan,11; 2012,Mar,9-10

## 50389-50396 [50430, 50431, 50432, 50433, 50434, 50435] Percutaneous and Injection Procedures With/Without Indwelling Tube/Catheter Access

**50389** Removal of nephrostomy tube, requiring fluoroscopic guidance (eg, with concurrent indwelling ureteral stent)

> *EXCLUDES* *Nephrostomy tube removal without fluoroscopic guidance, report with appropriate E&M code*

🔧 1.57　⚕ 8.44　**FUD** 000　　　02 62 50 ▣

**AMA:** 2017,Jan,8; 2016,Jan,13; 2016,Jan,3; 2015,Oct,5; 2015,Jan,16; 2014,Jan,11

**50390** Aspiration and/or injection of renal cyst or pelvis by needle, percutaneous

> *EXCLUDES* *Antegrade nephrostogram/pyelogram ([50430, 50431])*
> 🔳 *(74425, 74470, 76942, 77002, 77012, 77021)*

🔧 2.79　⚕ 2.79　**FUD** 000　　　T A2 50 ▣

**AMA:** 2017,Jan,8; 2016,Jan,13; 2015,Oct,5; 2015,Jan,16; 2014,Jan,11

**50391** Instillation(s) of therapeutic agent into renal pelvis and/or ureter through established nephrostomy, pyelostomy or ureterostomy tube (eg, anticarcinogenic or antifungal agent)

> Code also therapeutic agent

🔧 2.83　⚕ 3.49　**FUD** 000　　　T P3 50 ▣

**AMA:** 2017,Jan,8; 2016,Jan,13; 2015,Oct,5; 2015,Jan,16; 2014,Jan,11

**50395** Introduction of guide into renal pelvis and/or ureter with dilation to establish nephrostomy tract, percutaneous

> *EXCLUDES* *Percutaneous nephrostolithotomy (50080-50081)*
> *Placement of nephrostomy catheter ([50432, 50433])*
> *Removal, replacement internally dwelling ureteral stent (50382, 50384)*
> *Renal endoscopy (50551-50561)*
> *Retrograde percutaneous nephrostomy (52334)*
> 🔳 *(74485)*

🔧 5.16　⚕ 5.16　**FUD** 000　　　J A2 50 ▣

**AMA:** 2017,Jan,8; 2016,Jan,13; 2015,Oct,5; 2015,Jan,16; 2014,Jan,11; 2012,Jan,15-42

**50396** Manometric studies through nephrostomy or pyelostomy tube, or indwelling ureteral catheter

> 🔳 *(74425)*

🔧 3.39　⚕ 3.39　**FUD** 000　　　T A2 80 50 ▣

**AMA:** 2017,Jan,8; 2016,Jan,13; 2015,Jan,16; 2014,Jan,11

\# **50430** Injection procedure for antegrade nephrostogram and/or ureterogram, complete diagnostic procedure including imaging guidance (eg, ultrasound and fluoroscopy) and all associated radiological supervision and interpretation; new access

> *INCLUDES* Renal pelvis and associated ureter as a single element
> *EXCLUDES* *Procedure performed for same renal collecting system/ureter ([50432, 50433, 50434, 50435], 50693-50695, 74425)*

🔧 4.46　⚕ 12.9　**FUD** 000　　　02 N1 80 50 ▣

**AMA:** 2017,Jan,8; 2016,Jan,3; 2016,Jan,13; 2015,Oct,5

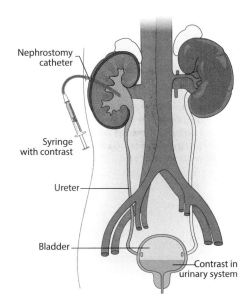

Nephrostomy catheter

Syringe with contrast

Ureter

Bladder

Contrast in urinary system

\# **50431** existing access

> *INCLUDES* Renal pelvis and associated ureter as a single element
> *EXCLUDES* *Procedure performed for same renal collecting system/ureter ([50432, 50433, 50434, 50435], 50693-50695, 74425)*

🔧 1.92　⚕ 4.63　**FUD** 000　　　02 N1 50 ▣

**AMA:** 2017,Jan,8; 2016,Jan,3; 2016,Jan,13; 2015,Oct,5

● New Code　　▲ Revised Code　　○ Reinstated　　● New Web Release　　　▲ Revised Web Release　　Unlisted　　Not Covered　　# Resequenced
⊘ AMA Mod 51 Exempt　　⑤¹ Optum Mod 51 Exempt　　⑥³ Mod 63 Exempt　　✗ Non-FDA Drug　　★ Telemedicine　　Ⓜ Maternity　　🄰 Age Edit　　✚ Add-on　　**AMA:** CPT Asst
© 2017 Optum360, LLC　　　　　CPT © 2017 American Medical Association. All Rights Reserved.　　　　　**227**

**# 50432**   **Placement of nephrostomy catheter, percutaneous, including diagnostic nephrostogram and/or ureterogram when performed, imaging guidance (eg, ultrasound and/or fluoroscopy) and all associated radiological supervision and interpretation**

> INCLUDES  Renal pelvis and associated ureter as a single element
> EXCLUDES  *Procedure performed for same renal collecting system/ureter ([50430, 50431], [50433], 50694-50695, 74425)*
> *Procedure performed with dilation of nephrostomy tube tract (50395)*

🚑 6.02   ⚕ 21.9   **FUD** 000                 Ⓙ 62 50 ▭

**AMA:** 2017,Jan,8; 2016,Jan,3; 2016,Jan,13; 2015,Oct,5

Kidney
Major calyces
Renal pelvis
Percutaneous nephrostomy tube
Catheter bag

**# 50433**   **Placement of nephroureteral catheter, percutaneous, including diagnostic nephrostogram and/or ureterogram when performed, imaging guidance (eg, ultrasound and/or fluoroscopy) and all associated radiological supervision and interpretation, new access**

> INCLUDES  Renal pelvis and associated ureter as a single element
> EXCLUDES  *Dilation of nephroureteral catheter tract (50395)*
> *Nephroureteral catheter removal/replacement (50387)*
> *Procedures performed for same renal collecting system/ureter ([50430, 50431, 50432], 50693-50695, 74425)*

🚑 7.51   ⚕ 30.0   **FUD** 000                 Ⓙ 62 50 ▭

**AMA:** 2017,Jan,8; 2016,Jan,3; 2016,Jan,13; 2015,Oct,5

**# 50434**   **Convert nephrostomy catheter to nephroureteral catheter, percutaneous, including diagnostic nephrostogram and/or ureterogram when performed, imaging guidance (eg, ultrasound and/or fluoroscopy) and all associated radiological supervision and interpretation, via pre-existing nephrostomy tract**

> INCLUDES  Renal pelvis and associated ureter as a single element
> EXCLUDES  *Procedure performed for same renal collecting system/ureter ([50430, 50431], [50435], 50684, 50693, 74425)*

🚑 5.68   ⚕ 23.5   **FUD** 000                 Ⓣ 62 50 ▭

**AMA:** 2017,Jan,8; 2016,Jan,3; 2016,Jan,13; 2015,Oct,5

**# 50435**   **Exchange nephrostomy catheter, percutaneous, including diagnostic nephrostogram and/or ureterogram when performed, imaging guidance (eg, ultrasound and/or fluoroscopy) and all associated radiological supervision and interpretation**

> INCLUDES  Renal pelvis and associated ureter as a single element
> EXCLUDES  *Procedure performed for same renal collecting system/ureter ([50430, 50431], [50434], 50693, 74425)*
> *Removal nephrostomy catheter that requires fluoroscopic guidance (50389)*

🚑 2.93   ⚕ 13.3   **FUD** 000                 Ⓣ 62 50 ▭

**AMA:** 2017,Jan,8; 2016,Jan,3; 2016,Jan,13; 2015,Oct,5

## 50400-50540 Open Surgical Procedures of Kidney

**50400**   **Pyeloplasty (Foley Y-pyeloplasty), plastic operation on renal pelvis, with or without plastic operation on ureter, nephropexy, nephrostomy, pyelostomy, or ureteral splinting; simple**

> EXCLUDES  *Laparoscopic pyeloplasty (50544)*

🚑 33.4   ⚕ 33.4   **FUD** 090                 Ⓒ 80 50 ▭

**AMA:** 2017,Jan,8; 2016,Jan,13; 2015,Jan,16; 2014,Jan,11

**50405**   **complicated (congenital kidney abnormality, secondary pyeloplasty, solitary kidney, calycoplasty)**

> EXCLUDES  *Laparoscopic pyeloplasty (50544)*

🚑 40.4   ⚕ 40.4   **FUD** 090                 Ⓒ 80 50 ▭

**AMA:** 2017,Jan,8; 2016,Jan,13; 2015,Jan,16; 2014,Jan,11

*50430*   Resequenced code. See code following 50396.

*50431*   Resequenced code. See code following 50396.

*50432*   Resequenced code. See code following 50396.

*50433*   Resequenced code. See code following 50396.

*50434*   Resequenced code. See code following 50396.

*50435*   Resequenced code. See code following 50396.

**50500**   **Nephrorrhaphy, suture of kidney wound or injury**

🚑 33.4   ⚕ 33.4   **FUD** 090                 Ⓒ 80 ▭

**AMA:** 2014,Jan,11

Periaortic lymph nodes
Adrenal gland
Kidney
Major renal vessels
Aorta
Upper ureter
Renal pelvis
Bladder
Glomerulus
Capillaries
Vein
Artery
Bowman's capsule
Collecting tubule
Schematic of nephron

**50520**   **Closure of nephrocutaneous or pyelocutaneous fistula**

🚑 29.7   ⚕ 29.7   **FUD** 090                 Ⓒ 80 ▭

**AMA:** 2014,Jan,11

**50525**   **Closure of nephrovisceral fistula (eg, renocolic), including visceral repair; abdominal approach**

🚑 45.8   ⚕ 45.8   **FUD** 090                 Ⓒ 80 ▭

**AMA:** 2014,Jan,11

**50526**   **thoracic approach**

🚑 42.7   ⚕ 42.7   **FUD** 090                 Ⓒ 80 ▭

**AMA:** 2014,Jan,11

**50540** **Symphysiotomy for horseshoe kidney with or without pyeloplasty and/or other plastic procedure, unilateral or bilateral (1 operation)**
 32.9  32.9  **FUD** 090  C 80
**AMA:** 2014,Jan,11

## 50541-50549 Laparoscopic Surgical Procedures of the Kidney

INCLUDES  Diagnostic laparoscopy (49320)
EXCLUDES  Laparoscopic drainage of lymphocele to peritoneal cavity (49323)

**50541** **Laparoscopy, surgical; ablation of renal cysts**
 26.5  26.5  **FUD** 090  J 80 50
**AMA:** 2017,Jan,8; 2016,Jan,13; 2015,Jan,16; 2014,Jan,11

**50542** **ablation of renal mass lesion(s), including intraoperative ultrasound guidance and monitoring, when performed**
EXCLUDES  Open ablation of renal mass lesions (50250)
Percutaneous ablation of renal tumors (50592-50593)
 33.6  33.6  **FUD** 090  J 80 50
**AMA:** 2017,Jan,8; 2016,Jan,13; 2015,Jan,16; 2014,Jan,11; 2012,Jan,15-42

**50543** **partial nephrectomy**
EXCLUDES  Partial nephrectomy, open approach (50240)
 42.9  42.9  **FUD** 090  J 80 50
**AMA:** 2017,Jan,8; 2016,Jan,13; 2015,Jan,16; 2014,Jan,11

**50544** **pyeloplasty**
 36.0  36.0  **FUD** 090  J 80 50
**AMA:** 2017,Jan,8; 2016,Jan,13; 2015,Jan,16; 2014,Jan,11

**50545** **radical nephrectomy (includes removal of Gerota's fascia and surrounding fatty tissue, removal of regional lymph nodes, and adrenalectomy)**
EXCLUDES  Radical nephrectomy, open approach (50230)
 38.7  38.7  **FUD** 090  C 80 50
**AMA:** 2017,Jan,8; 2016,Jan,13; 2015,Jan,16; 2014,Jan,11

**50546** **nephrectomy, including partial ureterectomy**
 34.7  34.7  **FUD** 090  C 80 50
**AMA:** 2017,Jan,8; 2016,Jan,13; 2015,Jan,16; 2014,Jan,11

**50547** **donor nephrectomy (including cold preservation), from living donor**
INCLUDES  Donor care
Graft:
 Cold preservation
 Harvesting
EXCLUDES  Backbench reconstruction renal allograft prior to transplantation (50327-50329)
Backbench standard preparation of living donor renal allograft prior to transplantation (50325)
Donor nephrectomy, open approach (50320)
 46.5  46.5  **FUD** 090  C 80 50
**AMA:** 2017,Jan,8; 2016,Jan,13; 2015,Jan,16; 2014,Jan,11

**50548** **nephrectomy with total ureterectomy**
EXCLUDES  Nephrectomy, open approach (50234, 50236)
 38.9  38.9  **FUD** 090  C 80 50
**AMA:** 2017,Jan,8; 2016,Jan,13; 2015,Jan,16; 2014,Jan,11

**50549** **Unlisted laparoscopy procedure, renal**
 0.00  0.00  **FUD** YYY  J 80 50
**AMA:** 2017,Jan,8; 2016,Jan,13; 2015,Jan,16; 2014,Jan,11; 2012,Jan,15-42

## 50551-50562 Endoscopic Procedures of Kidney via Established Nephrostomy/Pyelostomy Access

**50551** **Renal endoscopy through established nephrostomy or pyelostomy, with or without irrigation, instillation, or ureteropyelography, exclusive of radiologic service;**
 8.53  10.3  **FUD** 000  J A2 80 50
**AMA:** 2017,Jan,8; 2016,Jan,13; 2015,Jan,16; 2014,Jan,11

**50553** **with ureteral catheterization, with or without dilation of ureter**
EXCLUDES  Image-guided ureter dilation without endoscopic guidance (50706)
 9.06  11.0  **FUD** 000  J A2 50
**AMA:** 2017,Jan,8; 2016,Jan,13; 2016,Jan,3; 2015,Jan,16; 2014,Jan,11

**50555** **with biopsy**
EXCLUDES  Image-guided biopsy ureter/renal pelvis without endoscopic guidance (50606)
 9.88  11.8  **FUD** 000  J A2 50
**AMA:** 2017,Jan,8; 2016,Jan,13; 2016,Jan,3; 2015,Jan,16; 2014,Jan,11

**50557** **with fulguration and/or incision, with or without biopsy**
 10.0  12.0  **FUD** 000  J A2 50
**AMA:** 2017,Jan,8; 2016,Jan,13; 2015,Jan,16; 2014,Jan,11

**50561** **with removal of foreign body or calculus**
 11.4  13.6  **FUD** 000  J A2 80 50
**AMA:** 2017,Jan,8; 2016,Jan,13; 2015,Jan,16; 2014,Jan,11

**50562** **with resection of tumor**
 16.8  16.8  **FUD** 090  J 63 80
**AMA:** 2017,Jan,8; 2016,Jan,13; 2015,Jan,16; 2014,Jan,11

## 50570-50580 Endoscopic Procedures of Kidney via Nephrotomy/Pyelotomy Access

Code also if provided service is significant and identifiable (50045, 50120)

**50570** **Renal endoscopy through nephrotomy or pyelotomy, with or without irrigation, instillation, or ureteropyelography, exclusive of radiologic service;**
 14.2  14.2  **FUD** 000  J 63 80 50
**AMA:** 2017,Jan,8; 2016,Jan,13; 2015,Jan,16; 2014,Jan,11

**50572** **with ureteral catheterization, with or without dilation of ureter**
EXCLUDES  Image-guided ureter dilation without endoscopic guidance (50706)
 15.4  15.4  **FUD** 000  T 63 80 50
**AMA:** 2017,Jan,8; 2016,Jan,13; 2016,Jan,3; 2015,Jan,16; 2014,Jan,11

**50574** **with biopsy**
EXCLUDES  Image-guide ureter/renal pelvis biopsy without endoscopic guidance (50606)
 16.3  16.3  **FUD** 000  T 63 80 50
**AMA:** 2017,Jan,8; 2016,Jan,13; 2016,Jan,3; 2015,Jan,16; 2014,Jan,11

**50575** **with endopyelotomy (includes cystoscopy, ureteroscopy, dilation of ureter and ureteral pelvic junction, incision of ureteral pelvic junction and insertion of endopyelotomy stent)**
 20.7  20.7  **FUD** 000  J 63 50
**AMA:** 2017,Jan,8; 2016,Jan,13; 2015,Jan,16; 2014,Jan,11; 2012,Jan,15-42

**50576** **with fulguration and/or incision, with or without biopsy**
 16.3  16.3  **FUD** 000  J 63 80 50
**AMA:** 2017,Jan,8; 2016,Jan,13; 2015,Jan,16; 2014,Jan,11

**50580** **with removal of foreign body or calculus**
 17.6  17.6  **FUD** 000  J 63 80 50
**AMA:** 2017,Jan,8; 2016,Jan,13; 2015,Jan,16; 2014,Jan,11

● New Code   ▲ Revised Code   ○ Reinstated   ● New Web Release   ▲ Revised Web Release   Unlisted   Not Covered   # Resequenced
⊘ AMA Mod 51 Exempt   ⑤ Optum Mod 51 Exempt   ⑥③ Mod 63 Exempt   ✗ Non-FDA Drug   ★ Telemedicine   Ⓜ Maternity   Ⓐ Age Edit   + Add-on   AMA: CPT Asst

## 50590-50593 Noninvasive and Minimally Invasive Procedures of the Kidney

**50590**    **Lithotripsy, extracorporeal shock wave**
     16.3    20.6    **FUD** 090      J G2 50
     **AMA:** 2017,Jan,8; 2016,Jan,13; 2015,Jan,16; 2014,Jan,11; 2012,Jan,15-42

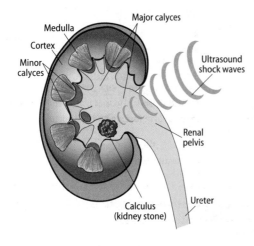

Labels in figure: Medulla, Cortex, Minor calyces, Major calyces, Ultrasound shock waves, Renal pelvis, Ureter, Calculus (kidney stone)

**50592**    **Ablation, 1 or more renal tumor(s), percutaneous, unilateral, radiofrequency**
     (76940, 77013, 77022)
     10.0    35.0    **FUD** 010      J G2 50
     **AMA:** 2014,Jan,11

**50593**    **Ablation, renal tumor(s), unilateral, percutaneous, cryotherapy**
     (76940, 77013, 77022)
     13.4    128.    **FUD** 010      J G2 80 50
     **AMA:** 2014,Jan,11

## 50600-50940 Open and Injection Procedures of Ureter

**50600**    **Ureterotomy with exploration or drainage (separate procedure)**
     Code also ureteral endoscopy through ureterotomy when procedures constitute a significant identifiable service (50970-50980)
     27.2    27.2    **FUD** 090      C 80 50
     **AMA:** 2014,Jan,11

**50605**    **Ureterotomy for insertion of indwelling stent, all types**
     28.5    28.5    **FUD** 090      C 80 50
     **AMA:** 2017,Jan,8; 2016,Jan,13; 2015,Jan,16; 2014,Jan,11; 2012,Apr,17-18; 2012,Jan,15-42

**+ 50606**    **Endoluminal biopsy of ureter and/or renal pelvis, non-endoscopic, including imaging guidance (eg, ultrasound and/or fluoroscopy) and all associated radiological supervision and interpretation (List separately in addition to code for primary procedure)**
     INCLUDES   Renal pelvis and associated ureter as a single element
     EXCLUDES   *Procedure performed for same renal collecting system/associated ureter with (50555, 50574, 50955, 50974, 52007, 74425)*
     Code first (50382-50389, [50430, 50431, 50432, 50433, 50434, 50435], 50684, 50688, 50690, 50693-50695, 51610)
     4.54    19.9    **FUD** ZZZ      N N1 50
     **AMA:** 2017,Jan,8; 2016,Jan,3

**50610**    **Ureterolithotomy; upper one-third of ureter**
     EXCLUDES   *Cystotomy with calculus basket extraction of ureteral calculus (51065)*
           *Transvesical ureterolithotomy (51060)*
           *Ureteral calculus manipulation/extraction performed endoscopically (50080-50081, 50561, 50961, 50980, 52320-52330, 52352-52353, [52356])*
           *Ureterolithotomy performed laparoscopically (50945)*
     27.9    27.9    **FUD** 090      C 80 50
     **AMA:** 2017,Jan,8; 2016,Jan,13; 2015,Jan,16; 2014,Jan,11

**50620**    **middle one-third of ureter**
     EXCLUDES   *Cystotomy with calculus basket extraction of ureteral calculus (51065)*
           *Transvesical ureterolithotomy (51060)*
           *Ureteral calculus manipulation/extraction performed endoscopically (50080-50081, 50561, 50961, 50980, 52320-52330, 52352-52353, [52356])*
           *Ureterolithotomy performed laparoscopically (50945)*
     26.0    26.0    **FUD** 090      C 80 50
     **AMA:** 2017,Jan,8; 2016,Jan,13; 2015,Jan,16; 2014,Jan,11

**50630**    **lower one-third of ureter**
     EXCLUDES   *Cystotomy with calculus basket extraction of ureteral calculus (51065)*
           *Transvesical ureterolithotomy (51060)*
           *Ureteral calculus manipulation/extraction performed endoscopically (50080-50081, 50561, 50961, 50980, 52320-52330, 52352-52353, [52356])*
           *Ureterolithotomy performed laparoscopically (50945)*
     25.9    25.9    **FUD** 090      C 80 50
     **AMA:** 2017,Jan,8; 2016,Jan,13; 2015,Jan,16; 2014,May,3; 2014,Jan,11

**50650**    **Ureterectomy, with bladder cuff (separate procedure)**
     EXCLUDES   *Ureterocele (51535, 52300)*
     29.9    29.9    **FUD** 090      C 80 50
     **AMA:** 2014,Jan,11

**50660**    **Ureterectomy, total, ectopic ureter, combination abdominal, vaginal and/or perineal approach**
     EXCLUDES   *Ureterocele (51535, 52300) .*
     33.4    33.4    **FUD** 090      C 80
     **AMA:** 2014,Jan,11

**50684**    **Injection procedure for ureterography or ureteropyelography through ureterostomy or indwelling ureteral catheter**
     EXCLUDES   *Placement of nephroureteral catheter ([50433, 50434])*
           *Placement of ureteral stent (50693-50695)*
     (74425)
     1.46    3.03    **FUD** 000      N N1 50
     **AMA:** 2017,Jan,8; 2016,Jan,3; 2015,Oct,5; 2014,Jan,11

**50686**    **Manometric studies through ureterostomy or indwelling ureteral catheter**
     2.59    4.19    **FUD** 000      S P2 80
     **AMA:** 2014,Jan,11

**50688**    **Change of ureterostomy tube or externally accessible ureteral stent via ileal conduit**
     (75984)
     2.29    2.29    **FUD** 010      J A2
     **AMA:** 2017,Jan,8; 2016,Jan,3; 2014,Jan,11

**50690**    **Injection procedure for visualization of ileal conduit and/or ureteropyelography, exclusive of radiologic service**
     (74425)
     2.04    2.82    **FUD** 000      N N1
     **AMA:** 2017,Jan,8; 2016,Jan,3; 2014,Jan,11

**50693** Placement of ureteral stent, percutaneous, including diagnostic nephrostogram and/or ureterogram when performed, imaging guidance (eg, ultrasound and/or fluoroscopy), and all associated radiological supervision and interpretation; pre-existing nephrostomy tract

INCLUDES Renal pelvis and associated ureter as a single element
EXCLUDES Procedure performed for the same renal collecting system/ureter ([50430, 50431, 50432, 50433, 50434, 50435], 50684, 74425)

5.96 28.0 **FUD** 000 [J][62][50][□]

**AMA:** 2017,Jan,8; 2016,Jan,3; 2016,Jan,13; 2015,Oct,5

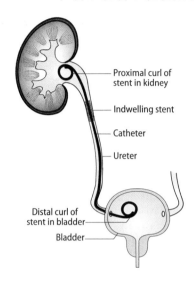

- Proximal curl of stent in kidney
- Indwelling stent
- Catheter
- Ureter
- Distal curl of stent in bladder
- Bladder

**50694** new access, without separate nephrostomy catheter

INCLUDES Renal pelvis and associated ureter as a single element
EXCLUDES Procedure performed for the same renal collecting system/ureter ([50430, 50431, 50432, 50433, 50434, 50435], 50684, 74425)

7.80 30.7 **FUD** 000 [J][62][50][□]

**AMA:** 2017,Jan,8; 2016,Jan,3; 2016,Jan,13; 2015,Oct,5

**50695** new access, with separate nephrostomy catheter

INCLUDES Placement of separate ureteral stent and nephrostomy catheter into a ureter/associated renal pelvis through a new access
Renal pelvis and associated ureter as a single element
EXCLUDES Procedure performed for the same renal collecting system/ureter ([50430, 50431, 50432, 50433, 50434, 50435], 50684, 74425)

10.0 37.7 **FUD** 000 [J][62][50][□]

**AMA:** 2017,Jan,8; 2016,Jan,3; 2016,Jan,13; 2015,Oct,5

**50700** Ureteroplasty, plastic operation on ureter (eg, stricture)

26.6 26.6 **FUD** 090 [C][80][50][□]

**AMA:** 2014,Jan,11

+ **50705** Ureteral embolization or occlusion, including imaging guidance (eg, ultrasound and/or fluoroscopy) and all associated radiological supervision and interpretation (List separately in addition to code for primary procedure)

INCLUDES Renal pelvis and associated ureter as a single element
Code also when performed:
additional catheter insertions
diagnostic pyelography/ureterography
other interventions
Code first (50382-50389, [50430, 50431, 50432, 50433, 50434, 50435], 50684, 50688, 50690, 50693-50695, 51610)

5.79 54.9 **FUD** ZZZ [N][M1][50][□]

**AMA:** 2017,Jan,8; 2016,Jan,3

+ **50706** Balloon dilation, ureteral stricture, including imaging guidance (eg, ultrasound and/or fluoroscopy) and all associated radiological supervision and interpretation (List separately in addition to code for primary procedure)

INCLUDES Dilation of nephrostomy, ureters, or urethra (74485)
Renal pelvis and associated ureter as a single element
EXCLUDES Cystourethroscopy (52341, 52344-52345)
Renal endoscopy (50553, 50572)
Ureteral endoscopy (50953, 50972)
Code also when performed:
additional catheter insertions
diagnostic pyelography/ureterography
other interventions
Code first (50382-50389, [50430, 50431, 50432, 50433, 50435], 50684, 50688, 50690, 50693-50695, 51610)

5.46 28.3 **FUD** ZZZ [N][M1][50][□]

**AMA:** 2017,Jan,8; 2016,Jan,3

**50715** Ureterolysis, with or without repositioning of ureter for retroperitoneal fibrosis

35.3 35.3 **FUD** 090 [C][80][50][□]

**AMA:** 2014,Jan,11

**50722** Ureterolysis for ovarian vein syndrome ♀

30.3 30.3 **FUD** 090 [C][80]

**AMA:** 2014,Jan,11

**50725** Ureterolysis for retrocaval ureter, with reanastomosis of upper urinary tract or vena cava

32.5 32.5 **FUD** 090 [C][80][□]

**AMA:** 2014,Jan,11

**50727** Revision of urinary-cutaneous anastomosis (any type urostomy);

14.6 14.6 **FUD** 090 [J][62][80][□]

**AMA:** 2014,Jan,11

**50728** with repair of fascial defect and hernia

20.1 20.1 **FUD** 090 [C][80][□]

**AMA:** 2014,Jan,11

**50740** Ureteropyelostomy, anastomosis of ureter and renal pelvis

35.1 35.1 **FUD** 090 [C][80][50][□]

**AMA:** 2017,Jan,8; 2016,Jan,13; 2015,Jan,16; 2014,Jan,11

**50750** Ureterocalycostomy, anastomosis of ureter to renal calyx

33.1 33.1 **FUD** 090 [C][80][50][□]

**AMA:** 2017,Jan,8; 2016,Jan,13; 2015,Jan,16; 2014,Jan,11

**50760** Ureteroureterostomy

32.5 32.5 **FUD** 090 [C][80][50][□]

**AMA:** 2017,Jan,8; 2016,Jan,13; 2015,Jan,16; 2014,Jan,11

**50770** Transureteroureterostomy, anastomosis of ureter to contralateral ureter

33.9 33.9 **FUD** 090 [C][80]

**AMA:** 2014,Jan,11

**50780** Ureteroneocystostomy; anastomosis of single ureter to bladder

INCLUDES Minor procedures to prevent vesicoureteral reflux
EXCLUDES Cystourethroplasty with ureteroneocystostomy (51820)

32.0 32.0 **FUD** 090 [C][80][50][□]

**AMA:** 2017,Jan,8; 2016,Jan,13; 2015,Jan,16; 2014,Jan,11

**50782** anastomosis of duplicated ureter to bladder

INCLUDES Minor procedures to prevent vesicoureteral reflux

34.4 34.4 **FUD** 090 [C][80][50][□]

**AMA:** 2017,Jan,8; 2016,Jan,13; 2015,Jan,16; 2014,Jan,11

**50783** with extensive ureteral tailoring

INCLUDES Minor procedures to prevent vesicoureteral reflux

32.7 32.7 **FUD** 090 [C][80][50][□]

**AMA:** 2017,Jan,8; 2016,Jan,13; 2015,Jan,16; 2014,Jan,11

**50785** with vesico-psoas hitch or bladder flap

INCLUDES Minor procedures to prevent vesicoureteral reflux

35.0 35.0 **FUD** 090 [C][80][50][□]

**AMA:** 2017,Jan,8; 2016,Jan,13; 2015,Jan,16; 2014,Jan,11

● New Code ▲ Revised Code ○ Reinstated ● New Web Release ▲ Revised Web Release Unlisted Not Covered # Resequenced
⊘ AMA Mod 51 Exempt ⑤ Optum Mod 51 Exempt ⑥³ Mod 63 Exempt ✗ Non-FDA Drug ★ Telemedicine [M] Maternity [A] Age Edit + Add-on **AMA:** CPT Asst
© 2017 Optum360, LLC CPT © 2017 American Medical Association. All Rights Reserved. 231

**50800**   **Ureteroenterostomy, direct anastomosis of ureter to intestine**

    *EXCLUDES*   *Cystectomy with ureterosigmoidostomy/ureteroileal conduit (51580-51595)*

    🔧 26.6   ⚕ 26.6   **FUD** 090     Ⓒ 80 50 🔲

    **AMA:** 2017,Jan,8; 2016,Jan,13; 2015,Jan,16; 2014,Jan,11

**50810**   **Ureterosigmoidostomy, with creation of sigmoid bladder and establishment of abdominal or perineal colostomy, including intestine anastomosis**

    *EXCLUDES*   *Cystectomy with ureterosigmoidostomy/ureteroileal conduit (51580-51595)*

    🔧 39.5   ⚕ 39.5   **FUD** 090     Ⓒ 80 🔲

    **AMA:** 2017,Jan,8; 2016,Jan,13; 2015,Jan,16; 2014,Jan,11

**50815**   **Ureterocolon conduit, including intestine anastomosis**

    *EXCLUDES*   *Cystectomy with ureterosigmoidostomy/ureteroileal conduit (51580-51595)*

    🔧 35.4   ⚕ 35.4   **FUD** 090     Ⓒ 80 50 🔲

    **AMA:** 2017,Jan,8; 2016,Jan,13; 2015,Jan,16; 2014,Jan,11

**50820**   **Ureteroileal conduit (ileal bladder), including intestine anastomosis (Bricker operation)**

    *EXCLUDES*   *Cystectomy with ureterosigmoidostomy/ureteroileal conduit (51580-51595)*

    🔧 38.0   ⚕ 38.0   **FUD** 090     Ⓒ 80 50 🔲

    **AMA:** 2017,Jan,8; 2016,Jan,13; 2015,Jan,16; 2014,Jan,11

**50825**   **Continent diversion, including intestine anastomosis using any segment of small and/or large intestine (Kock pouch or Camey enterocystoplasty)**

    🔧 47.9   ⚕ 47.9   **FUD** 090     Ⓒ 80 🔲

    **AMA:** 2017,Jan,8; 2016,Jan,13; 2015,Jan,16; 2014,Jan,11

**50830**   **Urinary undiversion (eg, taking down of ureteroileal conduit, ureterosigmoidostomy or ureteroenterostomy with ureteroureterostomy or ureteroneocystostomy)**

    🔧 52.5   ⚕ 52.5   **FUD** 090     Ⓒ 80 🔲

    **AMA:** 2017,Jan,8; 2016,Jan,13; 2015,Jan,16; 2014,Jan,11

**50840**   **Replacement of all or part of ureter by intestine segment, including intestine anastomosis**

    🔧 35.5   ⚕ 35.5   **FUD** 090     Ⓒ 80 50 🔲

    **AMA:** 2017,Jan,8; 2016,Jan,13; 2015,Jan,16; 2014,Jan,11

**50845**   **Cutaneous appendico-vesicostomy**

    *INCLUDES*   Mitrofanoff operation

    🔧 36.1   ⚕ 36.1   **FUD** 090     Ⓒ 80 🔲

    **AMA:** 2014,Jan,11

**50860**   **Ureterostomy, transplantation of ureter to skin**

    🔧 27.5   ⚕ 27.5   **FUD** 090     Ⓒ 80 50 🔲

    **AMA:** 2014,Jan,11

**50900**   **Ureterorrhaphy, suture of ureter (separate procedure)**

    🔧 24.8   ⚕ 24.8   **FUD** 090     Ⓒ 80 50 🔲

    **AMA:** 2014,Jan,11

**50920**   **Closure of ureterocutaneous fistula**

    🔧 26.4   ⚕ 26.4   **FUD** 090     Ⓒ 80 🔲

    **AMA:** 2014,Jan,11

**50930**   **Closure of ureterovisceral fistula (including visceral repair)**

    🔧 31.8   ⚕ 31.8   **FUD** 090     Ⓒ 80 🔲

    **AMA:** 2014,Jan,11

**50940**   **Deligation of ureter**

    *EXCLUDES*   *Ureteroplasty/ureterolysis (50700-50860)*

    🔧 25.5   ⚕ 25.5   **FUD** 090     Ⓒ 80 50 🔲

    **AMA:** 2014,Jan,11

## 50945-50949 Laparoscopic Procedures of Ureter

    *INCLUDES*   Diagnostic laparoscopy (49320)

    *EXCLUDES*   *Ureteroneocystostomy, open approach (50780-50785)*

**50945**   **Laparoscopy, surgical; ureterolithotomy**

    🔧 28.2   ⚕ 28.2   **FUD** 090     Ⓙ 80 50 🔲

    **AMA:** 2017,Jan,8; 2016,Jan,13; 2015,Jan,16; 2014,Jan,11; 2012,Jan,15-42

**50947**   **ureteroneocystostomy with cystoscopy and ureteral stent placement**

    🔧 40.1   ⚕ 40.1   **FUD** 090     Ⓙ A2 80 50 🔲

    **AMA:** 2017,Jan,8; 2016,Jan,13; 2015,Jan,16; 2014,Jan,11

**50948**   **ureteroneocystostomy without cystoscopy and ureteral stent placement**

    🔧 36.9   ⚕ 36.9   **FUD** 090     Ⓙ A2 80 50 🔲

    **AMA:** 2017,Jan,8; 2016,Jan,13; 2015,Jan,16; 2014,Jan,11

**50949**   **Unlisted laparoscopy procedure, ureter**

    🔧 0.00   ⚕ 0.00   **FUD** YYY     Ⓙ 80 50

    **AMA:** 2017,Jan,8; 2016,Jan,13; 2015,Jan,16; 2014,Jan,11

## 50951-50961 Endoscopic Procedures of Ureter via Established Ureterostomy Access

**50951**   **Ureteral endoscopy through established ureterostomy, with or without irrigation, instillation, or ureteropyelography, exclusive of radiologic service;**

    🔧 8.88   ⚕ 10.8   **FUD** 000     Ⓙ A2 80 50 🔲

    **AMA:** 2017,Jan,8; 2016,Jan,13; 2015,Jan,16; 2014,Jan,11; 2012,Jan,15-42

**50953**   **with ureteral catheterization, with or without dilation of ureter**

    *EXCLUDES*   *Image-guided ureter dilation without endoscopic guidance (50706)*

    🔧 9.43   ⚕ 11.4   **FUD** 000     Ⓙ A2 80 50 🔲

    **AMA:** 2017,Jan,8; 2016,Jan,13; 2016,Jan,3; 2015,Jan,16; 2014,Jan,11

**50955**   **with biopsy**

    *EXCLUDES*   *Image-guided biopsy of ureter and/or renal pelvis without endoscopic guidance (50606)*

    🔧 10.2   ⚕ 12.2   **FUD** 000     Ⓙ A2 80 50 🔲

    **AMA:** 2017,Jan,8; 2016,Jan,13; 2016,Jan,3; 2015,Jan,16; 2014,Jan,11

**50957**   **with fulguration and/or incision, with or without biopsy**

    🔧 10.2   ⚕ 12.3   **FUD** 000     Ⓙ A2 80 50 🔲

    **AMA:** 2017,Jan,8; 2016,Jan,13; 2015,Jan,16; 2014,Jan,11

**50961**   **with removal of foreign body or calculus**

    🔧 9.19   ⚕ 11.1   **FUD** 000     Ⓙ A2 80 50 🔲

    **AMA:** 2017,Jan,8; 2016,Jan,13; 2015,Jan,16; 2014,Jan,11; 2012,Jan,15-42

## 50970-50980 Endoscopic Procedures of Ureter via Ureterotomy

    *EXCLUDES*   *Ureterotomy (50600)*

**50970**   **Ureteral endoscopy through ureterotomy, with or without irrigation, instillation, or ureteropyelography, exclusive of radiologic service;**

    🔧 10.7   ⚕ 10.7   **FUD** 000     Ⓣ A2 80 50 🔲

    **AMA:** 2017,Jan,8; 2016,Jan,13; 2015,Jan,16; 2014,Jan,11

**50972**   **with ureteral catheterization, with or without dilation of ureter**

    *EXCLUDES*   *Image-guided ureter dilation without endoscopic guidance (50706)*

    🔧 10.3   ⚕ 10.3   **FUD** 000     Ⓣ A2 80 50 🔲

    **AMA:** 2017,Jan,8; 2016,Jan,13; 2016,Jan,3; 2015,Jan,16; 2014,Jan,11

**50974**   **with biopsy**

    *EXCLUDES*   *Image-guided biopsy of ureter and/or renal pelvis without endoscopic guidance (50606)*

    🔧 13.7   ⚕ 13.7   **FUD** 000     Ⓙ A2 80 50 🔲

    **AMA:** 2017,Jan,8; 2016,Jan,13; 2016,Jan,3; 2015,Jan,16; 2014,Jan,11

**50976**   **with fulguration and/or incision, with or without biopsy**

    🔧 13.5   ⚕ 13.5   **FUD** 000     Ⓙ A2 80 50 🔲

    **AMA:** 2017,Jan,8; 2016,Jan,13; 2015,Jan,16; 2014,Jan,11

**50980**   **with removal of foreign body or calculus**

    🔧 10.3   ⚕ 10.3   **FUD** 000     Ⓙ A2 80 50 🔲

    **AMA:** 2017,Jan,8; 2016,Jan,13; 2015,Jan,16; 2014,Jan,11

---

26/TC PC/TC Only    A2-A3 ASC Payment    50 Bilateral    ♂ Male Only    ♀ Female Only    🔧 Facility RVU    ⚕ Non-Facility RVU    🔲 CCI
**FUD** Follow-up Days    **CMS:** IOM (Pub 100)    A-Y OPPSI    80/80 Surg Assist Allowed / w/Doc    🔳 Lab Crosswalk    🔳 Radiology Crosswalk    ❌ CLIA

CPT © 2017 American Medical Association. All Rights Reserved.      © 2017 Optum360, LLC

## 51020-51080 Open Incisional Procedures of Bladder

**51020**  **Cystotomy or cystostomy; with fulguration and/or insertion of radioactive material**
13.5  13.5  **FUD** 090  [J] [A2] [80] [▭]
**AMA:** 2014,Jan,11

**51030**  **with cryosurgical destruction of intravesical lesion**
13.5  13.5  **FUD** 090  [J] [A2] [80] [▭]
**AMA:** 2014,Jan,11

**51040**  **Cystostomy, cystotomy with drainage**
8.35  8.35  **FUD** 090  [J] [A2] [80] [▭]
**AMA:** 2014,Jan,11

**51045**  **Cystotomy, with insertion of ureteral catheter or stent (separate procedure)**
14.1  14.1  **FUD** 090  [J] [A2] [80] [▭]
**AMA:** 2014,Jan,11

**51050**  **Cystolithotomy, cystotomy with removal of calculus, without vesical neck resection**
13.6  13.6  **FUD** 090  [J] [A2] [80] [▭]
**AMA:** 2014,Jan,11

**51060**  **Transvesical ureterolithotomy**
16.7  16.7  **FUD** 090  [J] [80] [▭]
**AMA:** 2014,Jan,11

**51065**  **Cystotomy, with calculus basket extraction and/or ultrasonic or electrohydraulic fragmentation of ureteral calculus**
16.7  16.7  **FUD** 090  [J] [A2] [80] [▭]
**AMA:** 2014,Jan,11

**51080**  **Drainage of perivesical or prevesical space abscess**
EXCLUDES  *Image-guided percutaneous catheter drainage (49406)*
11.8  11.8  **FUD** 090  [J] [A2] [80] [▭]
**AMA:** 2014,Jan,11

## 51100-51102 Bladder Aspiration Procedures

**51100**  **Aspiration of bladder; by needle**
(76942, 77002, 77012)
1.13  1.76  **FUD** 000  [T] [P3] [▭]
**AMA:** 2017,Jan,8; 2016,Jan,13; 2015,Jan,16; 2014,Jan,11

Pubic bone

Bladder

Uterus

Rectum

**51101**  **by trocar or intracatheter**
(76942, 77002, 77012)
1.50  3.52  **FUD** 000  [S] [P3] [▭]
**AMA:** 2017,Jan,8; 2016,Jan,13; 2015,Jan,16; 2014,Jan,11

**51102**  **with insertion of suprapubic catheter**
(76942, 77002, 77012)
4.18  6.48  **FUD** 000  [J] [A2] [▭]
**AMA:** 2017,Jan,8; 2016,Jan,13; 2015,Jan,16; 2014,Jan,11

## 51500-51597 Open Excisional Procedures of Bladder

**51500**  **Excision of urachal cyst or sinus, with or without umbilical hernia repair**
18.4  18.4  **FUD** 090  [J] [A2] [80] [▭]
**AMA:** 2014,Jan,11

**51520**  **Cystotomy; for simple excision of vesical neck (separate procedure)**
17.2  17.2  **FUD** 090  [J] [A2] [80] [▭]
**AMA:** 2014,Jan,11

**51525**  **for excision of bladder diverticulum, single or multiple (separate procedure)**
EXCLUDES  *Transurethral resection (52305)*
24.8  24.8  **FUD** 090  [C] [80] [▭]
**AMA:** 2014,Jan,11

**51530**  **for excision of bladder tumor**
EXCLUDES  *Transurethral resection (52234-52240, 52305)*
23.0  23.0  **FUD** 090  [C] [80] [▭]
**AMA:** 2014,Jan,11

**51535**  **Cystotomy for excision, incision, or repair of ureterocele**
EXCLUDES  *Transurethral excision (52300)*
22.5  22.5  **FUD** 090  [J] [82] [80] [50] [▭]
**AMA:** 2014,Jan,11

**51550**  **Cystectomy, partial; simple**
27.8  27.8  **FUD** 090  [C] [80] [▭]
**AMA:** 2014,Jan,11

**51555**  **complicated (eg, postradiation, previous surgery, difficult location)**
36.6  36.6  **FUD** 090  [C] [80] [▭]
**AMA:** 2014,Jan,11

**51565**  **Cystectomy, partial, with reimplantation of ureter(s) into bladder (ureteroneocystostomy)**
37.5  37.5  **FUD** 090  [C] [80] [▭]
**AMA:** 2014,Jan,11

**51570**  **Cystectomy, complete; (separate procedure)**
42.7  42.7  **FUD** 090  [C] [80] [▭]
**AMA:** 2014,Jan,11

**51575**  **with bilateral pelvic lymphadenectomy, including external iliac, hypogastric, and obturator nodes**
52.6  52.6  **FUD** 090  [C] [80] [▭]
**AMA:** 2014,Jan,11

**51580**  **Cystectomy, complete, with ureterosigmoidostomy or ureterocutaneous transplantations;**
55.5  55.5  **FUD** 090  [C] [80] [▭]
**AMA:** 2014,Jan,11

**51585**  **with bilateral pelvic lymphadenectomy, including external iliac, hypogastric, and obturator nodes**
61.1  61.1  **FUD** 090  [C] [80] [▭]
**AMA:** 2014,Jan,11

**51590**  **Cystectomy, complete, with ureteroileal conduit or sigmoid bladder, including intestine anastomosis;**
55.9  55.9  **FUD** 090  [C] [80] [▭]
**AMA:** 2014,Jan,11

**51595**  **with bilateral pelvic lymphadenectomy, including external iliac, hypogastric, and obturator nodes**
63.2  63.2  **FUD** 090  [C] [80] [▭]
**AMA:** 2014,Jan,11

**51596**  **Cystectomy, complete, with continent diversion, any open technique, using any segment of small and/or large intestine to construct neobladder**
68.0  68.0  **FUD** 090  [C] [80] [▭]
**AMA:** 2014,Jan,11

● New Code  ▲ Revised Code  ○ Reinstated  ● New Web Release  ▲ Revised Web Release  Unlisted  Not Covered  # Resequenced
⊘ AMA Mod 51 Exempt  ⑤ Optum Mod 51 Exempt  ⑥ Mod 63 Exempt  ✗ Non-FDA Drug  ★ Telemedicine  Ⓜ Maternity  Ⓐ Age Edit  + Add-on  **AMA:** CPT Asst
© 2017 Optum360, LLC                        CPT © 2017 American Medical Association. All Rights Reserved.

**Urinary System**

**51597** | Pelvic exenteration, complete, for vesical, prostatic or urethral malignancy, with removal of bladder and ureteral transplantations, with or without hysterectomy and/or abdominoperineal resection of rectum and colon and colostomy, or any combination thereof
EXCLUDES *Pelvic exenteration for gynecologic malignancy (58240)*
📋 66.2   ✂ 66.2   **FUD** 090                      C 80 📠
**AMA:** 2014,Jan,11

## 51600-51720 Injection/Insertion/Instillation Procedures of Bladder

**51600** | Injection procedure for cystography or voiding urethrocystography
📺 (74430, 74455)
📋 1.28   ✂ 5.22   **FUD** 000                      N N1 📠
**AMA:** 2014,Jan,11

**51605** | Injection procedure and placement of chain for contrast and/or chain urethrocystography
📺 (74430)
📋 1.11   ✂ 1.11   **FUD** 000                      N N1 📠
**AMA:** 2014,Jan,11

**51610** | Injection procedure for retrograde urethrocystography
📺 (74450)
📋 1.86   ✂ 3.04   **FUD** 000                      N N1 📠
**AMA:** 2017,Jan,8; 2016,Jan,3; 2014,Jan,11

**51700** | Bladder irrigation, simple, lavage and/or instillation
📋 1.04   ✂ 2.07   **FUD** 000                      T P3 📠
**AMA:** 2014,Jan,11

**51701** | Insertion of non-indwelling bladder catheter (eg, straight catheterization for residual urine)
EXCLUDES *Catheterization for specimen collection (P9612)*
*Insertion of catheter as an inclusive component of another procedure*
📋 0.74   ✂ 1.35   **FUD** 000                      Q1 N1 📠
**AMA:** 2017,Jan,8; 2016,Jan,13; 2015,Jan,16; 2014,Jan,11; 2012,Jan,15-42

**51702** | Insertion of temporary indwelling bladder catheter; simple (eg, Foley)
EXCLUDES *Focused ultrasound ablation of uterine leiomyomata (0071T-0072T)*
*Insertion of catheter as an inclusive component of another procedure*
📋 0.74   ✂ 1.79   **FUD** 000                      Q1 N1 📠
**AMA:** 2017,Jan,8; 2016,Jan,13; 2015,Jan,16; 2014,May,3; 2014,Jan,11; 2012,Jan,15-42

**51703** | complicated (eg, altered anatomy, fractured catheter/balloon)
📋 2.22   ✂ 3.56   **FUD** 000                      S P2 📠
**AMA:** 2017,Jan,8; 2016,Jan,13; 2015,Jan,16; 2014,Jan,11

**51705** | Change of cystostomy tube; simple
📋 1.50   ✂ 2.59   **FUD** 000                      T P3 📠
**AMA:** 2017,Jan,8; 2016,Jan,13; 2015,Jan,16; 2014,Jan,11; 2012,Jan,15-42

**51710** | complicated
📺 (75984)
📋 2.31   ✂ 3.67   **FUD** 000                      T A2 📠
**AMA:** 2017,Jan,8; 2016,Jan,13; 2015,Jan,16; 2014,Jan,11

**51715** | Endoscopic injection of implant material into the submucosal tissues of the urethra and/or bladder neck
EXCLUDES *Injection of bulking agent (submucosal) for fecal incontinence, via anoscope (0377T)*
📋 5.77   ✂ 8.31   **FUD** 000                      J A2 80 📠
**AMA:** 2014,Jan,11

**51720** | Bladder instillation of anticarcinogenic agent (including retention time)
Code also bacillus Calmette-Guerin vaccine (BCG) (90586)
📋 1.86   ✂ 2.51   **FUD** 000                      T P3 📠
**AMA:** 2017,Jan,8; 2016,Jan,13; 2015,Jan,16; 2014,Jan,11; 2012,Jan,15-42

## 51725-51798 [51797] Uroflowmetric Evaluations

INCLUDES Equipment
Fees for services of technician
Medications
Supplies
Code also modifier 26 if physician/other qualified health care professional provides only interpretation of results and/or operates the equipment

**51725** | Simple cystometrogram (CMG) (eg, spinal manometer)
📋 5.32   ✂ 5.32   **FUD** 000                      T P3 80 📠
**AMA:** 2017,Jan,8; 2016,Jan,13; 2015,Jan,16; 2014,Jan,11

**51726** | Complex cystometrogram (ie, calibrated electronic equipment);
📋 7.49   ✂ 7.49   **FUD** 000                      T A2 📠
**AMA:** 2017,Jan,8; 2016,Jan,13; 2015,Jan,16; 2014,Jan,11

**51727** | with urethral pressure profile studies (ie, urethral closure pressure profile), any technique
📋 8.85   ✂ 8.85   **FUD** 000                      T P3 80 📠
**AMA:** 2017,Jan,8; 2016,Jan,13; 2015,Jan,16; 2014,Jan,11

**51728** | with voiding pressure studies (ie, bladder voiding pressure), any technique
📋 8.95   ✂ 8.95   **FUD** 000                      T P3 80 📠
**AMA:** 2017,Jan,8; 2016,Jan,13; 2015,Jan,16; 2014,Jan,11

**51729** | with voiding pressure studies (ie, bladder voiding pressure) and urethral pressure profile studies (ie, urethral closure pressure profile), any technique
📋 9.67   ✂ 9.67   **FUD** 000                      T P3 80 📠
**AMA:** 2017,Jan,8; 2016,Jan,13; 2015,Jan,16; 2014,Jan,11

**+ # 51797** | Voiding pressure studies, intra-abdominal (ie, rectal, gastric, intraperitoneal) (List separately in addition to code for primary procedure)
Code first (51728-51729)
📋 3.18   ✂ 3.18   **FUD** ZZZ                      N N1 80 📠
**AMA:** 2017,Jan,8; 2016,Jan,13; 2015,Jan,16; 2014,Jan,11; 2012,Jan,15-42

**51736** | Simple uroflowmetry (UFR) (eg, stop-watch flow rate, mechanical uroflowmeter)
📋 0.44   ✂ 0.44   **FUD** XXX                      Q1 N1 80 📠
**AMA:** 2017,Jan,8; 2016,Jan,13; 2015,Jan,16; 2014,Jan,11

**51741** | Complex uroflowmetry (eg, calibrated electronic equipment)
📋 0.45   ✂ 0.45   **FUD** XXX                      Q1 N1 📠
**AMA:** 2017,Jan,8; 2016,Jan,13; 2015,Jan,16; 2014,Sep,13; 2014,Jan,11

**51784** | Electromyography studies (EMG) of anal or urethral sphincter, other than needle, any technique
EXCLUDES *Stimulus evoked response (51792)*
📋 1.97   ✂ 1.97   **FUD** XXX                      S P3 📠
**AMA:** 2017,Jan,8; 2016,Jan,13; 2015,Jan,16; 2014,Sep,13; 2014,Feb,11; 2014,Jan,11

**51785** | Needle electromyography studies (EMG) of anal or urethral sphincter, any technique
📋 7.52   ✂ 7.52   **FUD** XXX                      T A2 80 📠
**AMA:** 2017,Jan,8; 2016,Jan,13; 2015,Jan,16; 2014,Jan,11; 2012,Jan,15-42

**51792** | Stimulus evoked response (eg, measurement of bulbocavernosus reflex latency time)
EXCLUDES *Electromyography studies (EMG) of anal or urethral sphincter (51784)*
📋 6.01   ✂ 6.01   **FUD** 000                      Q1 N1 80 📠
**AMA:** 2017,Jan,8; 2016,Jan,13; 2015,Jan,16; 2014,Feb,11; 2014,Jan,11

**51797** | Resequenced code. See code following 51729.

| 51798 | Measurement of post-voiding residual urine and/or bladder capacity by ultrasound, non-imaging |
|---|---|

🔧 0.55   📐 0.55   **FUD** XXX    Q1 N1 80 TC 🖵

**AMA:** 2017,Jan,8; 2016,Jan,13; 2015,Jan,16; 2014,Jan,11

## 51800-51980 Open Repairs Urinary System

| 51800 | Cystoplasty or cystourethroplasty, plastic operation on bladder and/or vesical neck (anterior Y-plasty, vesical fundus resection), any procedure, with or without wedge resection of posterior vesical neck |
|---|---|

🔧 30.2   📐 30.2   **FUD** 090    C 80 🖵

**AMA:** 2014,Jan,11

| 51820 | Cystourethroplasty with unilateral or bilateral ureteroneocystostomy |
|---|---|

🔧 33.9   📐 33.9   **FUD** 090    C 80 🖵

**AMA:** 2014,Jan,11

| 51840 | Anterior vesicourethropexy, or urethropexy (eg, Marshall-Marchetti-Krantz, Burch); simple |
|---|---|

*EXCLUDES*   Pereyra type urethropexy (57289)

🔧 18.9   📐 18.9   **FUD** 090    C 80 🖵

**AMA:** 2017,Jan,8; 2016,Jan,13; 2015,Jan,16; 2014,Jan,11; 2012,Aug,13-14; 2012,Jan,15-42

| 51841 | complicated (eg, secondary repair) |
|---|---|

*EXCLUDES*   Pereyra type urethropexy (57289)

🔧 22.5   📐 22.5   **FUD** 090    C 80 🖵

**AMA:** 2017,Jan,8; 2016,Jan,13; 2015,Jan,16; 2014,Jan,11; 2012,Aug,13-14

| 51845 | Abdomino-vaginal vesical neck suspension, with or without endoscopic control (eg, Stamey, Raz, modified Pereyra) ♀ |
|---|---|

🔧 16.8   📐 16.8   **FUD** 090    J 80 🖵

**AMA:** 2017,Jan,8; 2016,Jan,13; 2015,Jan,16; 2014,Jan,11

| 51860 | Cystorrhaphy, suture of bladder wound, injury or rupture; simple |
|---|---|

🔧 21.5   📐 21.5   **FUD** 090    J 80 🖵

**AMA:** 2014,Jan,11

| 51865 | complicated |
|---|---|

🔧 25.8   📐 25.8   **FUD** 090    C 80 🖵

**AMA:** 2014,Jan,11

| 51880 | Closure of cystostomy (separate procedure) |
|---|---|

🔧 13.5   📐 13.5   **FUD** 090    J A2 80 🖵

**AMA:** 2014,Jan,11

Lower ureter

Cystostomy

Bladder

Bladder

**Physician removes a cystostomy tube**

| 51900 | Closure of vesicovaginal fistula, abdominal approach ♀ |
|---|---|

*EXCLUDES*   Vesicovaginal fistula closure, vaginal approach (57320-57330)

🔧 24.2   📐 24.2   **FUD** 090    C 80 🖵

**AMA:** 2014,Jan,11

| 51920 | Closure of vesicouterine fistula; ♀ |
|---|---|

*EXCLUDES*   Enterovesical fistula closure (44660-44661)
Rectovesical fistula closure (45800-45805)

🔧 22.6   📐 22.6   **FUD** 090    C 80 🖵

**AMA:** 2014,Jan,11

| 51925 | with hysterectomy ♀ |
|---|---|

*EXCLUDES*   Enterovesical fistula closure (44660-44661)
Rectovesical fistula closure (45800-45805)

🔧 29.7   📐 29.7   **FUD** 090    C 80 🖵

**AMA:** 2014,Jan,11

| 51940 | Closure, exstrophy of bladder |
|---|---|

*EXCLUDES*   Epispadias reconstruction with exstrophy of bladder (54390)

🔧 47.8   📐 47.8   **FUD** 090    C 80 🖵

**AMA:** 2014,Jan,11

| 51960 | Enterocystoplasty, including intestinal anastomosis |
|---|---|

🔧 40.0   📐 40.0   **FUD** 090    C 80 🖵

**AMA:** 2014,Jan,11

| 51980 | Cutaneous vesicostomy |
|---|---|

🔧 20.6   📐 20.6   **FUD** 090    C 80 🖵

**AMA:** 2014,Jan,11

## 51990-51999 Laparoscopic Procedures of Urinary System

**CMS:** 100-03,230.10 Incontinence Control Devices

*INCLUDES*   Diagnostic laparoscopy (49320)

| 51990 | Laparoscopy, surgical; urethral suspension for stress incontinence |
|---|---|

🔧 21.6   📐 21.6   **FUD** 090    J 80 🖵

**AMA:** 2017,Jan,8; 2016,Jan,13; 2015,Jan,16; 2014,Jan,11; 2012,Aug,13-14; 2012,Mar,9-10

| 51992 | sling operation for stress incontinence (eg, fascia or synthetic) |
|---|---|

*EXCLUDES*   Removal/revision of sling for stress incontinence (57287)
Sling operation for stress incontinence, open approach (57288)

🔧 24.2   📐 24.2   **FUD** 090    J A2 80 🖵

**AMA:** 2017,Jan,8; 2016,Jan,13; 2015,Jan,16; 2014,Jan,11; 2012,Aug,13-14; 2012,Mar,9-10

| 51999 | Unlisted laparoscopy procedure, bladder |
|---|---|

🔧 0.00   📐 0.00   **FUD** YYY    J 80

**AMA:** 2014,Jan,11

## 52000-52318 Endoscopic Procedures via Urethra: Bladder and Urethra

*INCLUDES*   Diagnostic and therapeutic endoscopy of bowel segments utilized as replacements for native bladder

| 52000 | Cystourethroscopy (separate procedure) |
|---|---|

*EXCLUDES*   Cystourethroscopy (52001, 52320, 52325, 52327, 52330, 52332, 52334, 52341-52343, [52356], 57240, 57260, 57265)

🔧 2.94   📐 4.68   **FUD** 000    T A2 🖵

**AMA:** 2017,Jan,8; 2016,Jan,13; 2015,Jan,16; 2014,May,3; 2014,Jan,11; 2013,Mar,13; 2012,Jan,15-42

| 52001 | Cystourethroscopy with irrigation and evacuation of multiple obstructing clots |
|---|---|

*INCLUDES*   Cystourethroscopy (separate procedure) (52000)

🔧 8.32   📐 10.6   **FUD** 000    J A2 🖵

**AMA:** 2014,Jan,11

● New Code   ▲ Revised Code   ○ Reinstated   ● New Web Release   ▲ Revised Web Release   Unlisted   Not Covered   # Resequenced
⊘ AMA Mod 51 Exempt   ⑨ Optum Mod 51 Exempt   ⑥₃ Mod 63 Exempt   ✗ Non-FDA Drug   ★ Telemedicine   Ⓜ Maternity   Ⓐ Age Edit   + Add-on   **AMA:** CPT Asst
© 2017 Optum360, LLC     CPT © 2017 American Medical Association. All Rights Reserved.     **235**

**Urinary System**

**52005** **Cystourethroscopy, with ureteral catheterization, with or without irrigation, instillation, or ureteropyelography, exclusive of radiologic service;**

INCLUDES Howard test

⚕ 3.86 ☌ 7.58 **FUD** 000 J A2 ▣

**AMA:** 2017,Jan,8; 2016,Jan,13; 2015,Jan,16; 2014,Jan,11; 2012,Jan,15-42

**52007** **with brush biopsy of ureter and/or renal pelvis**

EXCLUDES Image-guided ureter/renal pelvis biopsy without endoscopic guidance (50606)

⚕ 4.80 ☌ 12.6 **FUD** 000 J A2 50 ▣

**AMA:** 2017,Jan,8; 2016,Jan,13; 2016,Jan,3; 2015,Jan,16; 2014,Jan,11

**52010** **Cystourethroscopy, with ejaculatory duct catheterization, with or without irrigation, instillation, or duct radiography, exclusive of radiologic service** ♂

✖ (74440)

⚕ 4.80 ☌ 10.4 **FUD** 000 T A2 ▣

**AMA:** 2017,Jan,8; 2016,Jan,13; 2015,Jan,16; 2014,Jan,11

**52204** **Cystourethroscopy, with biopsy(s)**

⚕ 4.10 ☌ 10.5 **FUD** 000 J A2 ▣

**AMA:** 2017,Jan,8; 2016,May,12; 2016,Jan,13; 2015,Jan,16; 2014,Jan,11; 2012,Jan,15-42

**52214** **Cystourethroscopy, with fulguration (including cryosurgery or laser surgery) of trigone, bladder neck, prostatic fossa, urethra, or periurethral glands**

Code also modifier 78 when performed by same physician:
During postoperative period (52601, 52630)
During the postoperative period of a related surgical procedure
For postoperative bleeding

⚕ 5.11 ☌ 18.7 **FUD** 000 J A2 ▣

**AMA:** 2017,Jan,8; 2016,May,12; 2016,Jan,13; 2015,Jan,16; 2014,Jan,11

**52224** **Cystourethroscopy, with fulguration (including cryosurgery or laser surgery) or treatment of MINOR (less than 0.5 cm) lesion(s) with or without biopsy**

⚕ 5.91 ☌ 19.6 **FUD** 000 J A2 ▣

**AMA:** 2017,Jan,8; 2016,May,12; 2016,Jan,13; 2015,Jan,16; 2014,Jan,11; 2012,Jan,15-42

**52234** **Cystourethroscopy, with fulguration (including cryosurgery or laser surgery) and/or resection of; SMALL bladder tumor(s) (0.5 up to 2.0 cm)**

EXCLUDES Bladder tumor excision through cystotomy (51530)

⚕ 7.13 ☌ 7.13 **FUD** 000 J A2 ▣

**AMA:** 2017,Jan,8; 2016,May,12; 2016,Jan,13; 2015,Jan,16; 2014,Jan,11; 2012,Jan,15-42

**52235** **MEDIUM bladder tumor(s) (2.0 to 5.0 cm)**

EXCLUDES Bladder tumor excision through cystotomy (51530)

⚕ 8.36 ☌ 8.36 **FUD** 000 J A2 ▣

**AMA:** 2017,Jan,8; 2016,May,12; 2016,Jan,13; 2015,Jan,16; 2014,Jan,11

**52240** **LARGE bladder tumor(s)**

EXCLUDES Bladder tumor excision through cystotomy (51530)

⚕ 11.3 ☌ 11.3 **FUD** 000 J A2 ▣

**AMA:** 2017,Jan,8; 2016,May,12; 2016,Jan,13; 2015,Jan,16; 2014,Jan,11

**52250** **Cystourethroscopy with insertion of radioactive substance, with or without biopsy or fulguration**

⚕ 6.93 ☌ 6.93 **FUD** 000 J A2 ▣

**AMA:** 2017,Jan,8; 2016,Jan,13; 2015,Jan,16; 2014,Jan,11

**52260** **Cystourethroscopy, with dilation of bladder for interstitial cystitis; general or conduction (spinal) anesthesia**

⚕ 6.09 ☌ 6.09 **FUD** 000 J A2 ▣

**AMA:** 2017,Jan,8; 2016,Jan,13; 2015,Jan,16; 2014,Jan,11; 2012,Jan,15-42

**52265** **local anesthesia**

⚕ 4.70 ☌ 10.4 **FUD** 000 J P3 ▣

**AMA:** 2017,Jan,8; 2016,Jan,13; 2015,Jan,16; 2014,Jan,11

**52270** **Cystourethroscopy, with internal urethrotomy; female** ♀

⚕ 5.27 ☌ 10.1 **FUD** 000 J A2 ▣

**AMA:** 2017,Jan,8; 2016,Jan,13; 2015,Jan,16; 2014,Jan,11

**52275** **male** ♂

⚕ 7.20 ☌ 13.6 **FUD** 000 J A2 ▣

**AMA:** 2017,Jan,8; 2016,Jan,13; 2015,Jan,16; 2014,Jan,11

**52276** **Cystourethroscopy with direct vision internal urethrotomy**

⚕ 7.67 ☌ 7.67 **FUD** 000 J A2 ▣

**AMA:** 2017,Jan,8; 2016,Jan,13; 2015,Jan,16; 2014,Jan,11; 2012,Jan,15-42

**52277** **Cystourethroscopy, with resection of external sphincter (sphincterotomy)**

⚕ 9.36 ☌ 9.36 **FUD** 000 J A2 80 ▣

**AMA:** 2017,Jan,8; 2016,Jan,13; 2015,Jan,16; 2014,Jan,11

**52281** **Cystourethroscopy, with calibration and/or dilation of urethral stricture or stenosis, with or without meatotomy, with or without injection procedure for cystography, male or female**

EXCLUDES Urethral delivery therapeutic drug (0499T)

⚕ 4.41 ☌ 7.78 **FUD** 000 J A2 ▣

**AMA:** 2017,Jan,8; 2016,Jan,13; 2015,Jan,16; 2014,Jan,11; 2012,Jan,15-42

**52282** **Cystourethroscopy, with insertion of permanent urethral stent**

EXCLUDES Placement of temporary prostatic urethral stent (53855)

⚕ 9.75 ☌ 9.75 **FUD** 000 J A2 ▣

**AMA:** 2017,Jan,8; 2016,Jan,13; 2015,Jun,5; 2015,Jan,16; 2014,Jan,11

**52283** **Cystourethroscopy, with steroid injection into stricture**

⚕ 5.83 ☌ 7.93 **FUD** 000 J A2 ▣

**AMA:** 2017,Jan,8; 2016,Jan,13; 2015,Mar,9; 2015,Jan,16; 2014,Jan,11

**52285** **Cystourethroscopy for treatment of the female urethral syndrome with any or all of the following: urethral meatotomy, urethral dilation, internal urethrotomy, lysis of urethrovaginal septal fibrosis, lateral incisions of the bladder neck, and fulguration of polyp(s) of urethra, bladder neck, and/or trigone** ♀

⚕ 5.67 ☌ 8.00 **FUD** 000 J A2 ▣

**AMA:** 2017,Jan,8; 2016,Jan,13; 2015,Jan,16; 2014,Jan,11

**52287** **Cystourethroscopy, with injection(s) for chemodenervation of the bladder**

Code also supply of chemodenervation agent

⚕ 4.90 ☌ 8.88 **FUD** 000 J G2 ▣

**AMA:** 2014,Jan,11

**52290** **Cystourethroscopy; with ureteral meatotomy, unilateral or bilateral**

⚕ 7.06 ☌ 7.06 **FUD** 000 J A2 ▣

**AMA:** 2017,Jan,8; 2016,Jan,13; 2015,Jan,16; 2014,Jan,11

**52300** **with resection or fulguration of orthotopic ureterocele(s), unilateral or bilateral**

⚕ 8.12 ☌ 8.12 **FUD** 000 J A2 80 ▣

**AMA:** 2017,Jan,8; 2016,Jan,13; 2015,Jan,16; 2014,Jan,11

**52301** **with resection or fulguration of ectopic ureterocele(s), unilateral or bilateral**

⚕ 8.40 ☌ 8.40 **FUD** 000 J A2 80 ▣

**AMA:** 2017,Jan,8; 2016,Jan,13; 2015,Jan,16; 2014,Jan,11

**52305** **with incision or resection of orifice of bladder diverticulum, single or multiple**

⚕ 8.08 ☌ 8.08 **FUD** 000 J A2 ▣

**AMA:** 2017,Jan,8; 2016,Jan,13; 2015,Jan,16; 2014,Jan,11

26/TC PC/TC Only | A2-Z3 ASC Payment | 50 Bilateral | ♂ Male Only | ♀ Female Only | ⚕ Facility RVU | ☌ Non-Facility RVU | ▣ CCI
FUD Follow-up Days | CMS: IOM (Pub 100) | A-Y OPPSI | 80/80 Surg Assist Allowed / w/Doc | ▣ Lab Crosswalk | ✖ Radiology Crosswalk | ✖ CLIA

CPT © 2017 American Medical Association. All Rights Reserved. | © 2017 Optum360, LLC

52310    Cystourethroscopy, with removal of foreign body, calculus, or ureteral stent from urethra or bladder (separate procedure); simple
> Code also modifier 58 for removal of a self-retaining, indwelling ureteral stent
> 🔧 4.39    ✂ 6.95    **FUD** 000    Ⓙ A2 🖥
> **AMA:** 2017,Jan,8; 2016,Jan,13; 2015,Jun,5; 2015,Jan,16; 2014,Jan,11

52315    complicated
> Code also modifier 58 for removal of a self-retaining, indwelling ureteral stent
> 🔧 7.95    ✂ 11.8    **FUD** 000    Ⓙ A2 🖥
> **AMA:** 2017,Jan,8; 2016,Jan,13; 2015,Jan,16; 2014,Jan,11

52317    Litholapaxy: crushing or fragmentation of calculus by any means in bladder and removal of fragments; simple or small (less than 2.5 cm)
> 🔧 10.0    ✂ 22.9    **FUD** 000    Ⓙ A2 🖥
> **AMA:** 2017,Jan,8; 2016,Jan,13; 2015,Jan,16; 2014,Jan,11; 2012,Feb,11

52318    complicated or large (over 2.5 cm)
> 🔧 13.7    ✂ 13.7    **FUD** 000    Ⓙ A2 🖥
> **AMA:** 2017,Jan,8; 2016,Jan,13; 2015,Jan,16; 2014,Jan,11; 2012,Feb,11

## 52320-52356 [52356] Endoscopic Procedures via Urethra: Renal Pelvis and Ureter

INCLUDES  Diagnostic cystourethroscopy when performed with therapeutic cystourethroscopy
Insertion/removal of temporary ureteral catheter (52005)
EXCLUDES  *Self-retaining/indwelling ureteral stent removal by cystourethroscope, with modifier 58 if appropriate (52310, 52315)*
Code also the insertion of an indwelling stent performed in addition to other procedures within this section (52332)

52320    Cystourethroscopy (including ureteral catheterization); with removal of ureteral calculus
> INCLUDES  Cystourethroscopy (separate procedure) (52000)
> 🔧 7.15    ✂ 7.15    **FUD** 000    Ⓙ A2 50 🖥
> **AMA:** 2017,Jan,8; 2016,Jan,13; 2015,Jan,16; 2014,Jan,11; 2012,Jan,15-42

52325    with fragmentation of ureteral calculus (eg, ultrasonic or electro-hydraulic technique)
> INCLUDES  Cystourethroscopy (separate procedure) (52000)
> 🔧 9.30    ✂ 9.30    **FUD** 000    Ⓙ A2 50 🖥
> **AMA:** 2017,Jan,8; 2016,Jan,13; 2015,Jan,16; 2014,Jan,11; 2012,Jan,15-42

52327    with subureteric injection of implant material
> INCLUDES  Cystourethroscopy (separate procedure) (52000)
> 🔧 7.59    ✂ 7.59    **FUD** 000    Ⓙ A2 50 🖥
> **AMA:** 2017,Jan,8; 2016,Jan,13; 2015,Jan,16; 2014,Jan,11

52330    with manipulation, without removal of ureteral calculus
> INCLUDES  Cystourethroscopy (separate procedure) (52000)
> 🔧 7.64    ✂ 14.0    **FUD** 000    Ⓙ A2 50 🖥
> **AMA:** 2017,Jan,8; 2016,Jan,13; 2015,Jan,16; 2014,May,3; 2014,Jan,11; 2012,Jan,15-42

52332    Cystourethroscopy, with insertion of indwelling ureteral stent (eg, Gibbons or double-J type)
> INCLUDES  Cystourethroscopy (separate procedure) (52000)
> EXCLUDES  *Cystourethroscopy, with ureteroscopy and/or pyeloscopy; with lithotripsy when performed on the same side with (52353, [52356])*
> 🔧 4.51    ✂ 13.9    **FUD** 000    Ⓙ A2 50 🖥
> **AMA:** 2017,Jan,8; 2016,Jan,13; 2015,Jan,16; 2014,May,3; 2014,Jan,11; 2012,Jan,15-42

52334    Cystourethroscopy with insertion of ureteral guide wire through kidney to establish a percutaneous nephrostomy, retrograde
> INCLUDES  Cystourethroscopy (separate procedure) (52000)
> EXCLUDES  *Cystourethroscopy with incision/fulguration/resection of congenital posterior urethral valves/obstructive hypertrophic mucosal folds (52400)*
> *Cystourethroscopy with pyeloscopy and/or ureteroscopy (52351-52353 [52356])*
> *Nephrostomy tract establishment only (50395)*
> *Percutaneous nephrolithotomy (50080, 50081)*
> 🔧 7.40    ✂ 7.40    **FUD** 000    Ⓙ A2 50 🖥
> **AMA:** 2017,Jan,8; 2016,Jan,13; 2015,Jan,16; 2014,May,3; 2014,Jan,11

52341    Cystourethroscopy; with treatment of ureteral stricture (eg, balloon dilation, laser, electrocautery, and incision)
> INCLUDES  Diagnostic cystourethroscopy (52351)
> EXCLUDES  *Balloon dilation with imaging guidance (50706)*
> *Cystourethroscpy, separate procedure (52000)*
> 📷 (74485)
> 🔧 8.23    ✂ 8.23    **FUD** 000    Ⓙ A2 50 🖥
> **AMA:** 2017,Jan,8; 2016,Jan,13; 2016,Jan,3; 2015,Jan,16; 2014,Jan,11

52342    with treatment of ureteropelvic junction stricture (eg, balloon dilation, laser, electrocautery, and incision)
> INCLUDES  Diagnostic cystourethroscopy (52351)
> EXCLUDES  *Balloon dilation with imaging guidance (50706)*
> *Cystourethroscopy (separate procedure) (52000)*
> 📷 (74485)
> 🔧 8.96    ✂ 8.96    **FUD** 000    Ⓙ A2 50 🖥
> **AMA:** 2017,Jan,8; 2016,Jan,13; 2015,Jan,16; 2014,Jan,11; 2012,Jan,15-42

52343    with treatment of intra-renal stricture (eg, balloon dilation, laser, electrocautery, and incision)
> INCLUDES  Diagnostic cystourethroscopy (52351)
> EXCLUDES  *Balloon dilation with imaging guidance (50706)*
> *Cystourethroscopy (separate procedure) (52000)*
> 📷 (74485)
> 🔧 9.96    ✂ 9.96    **FUD** 000    Ⓙ A2 50 🖥
> **AMA:** 2017,Jan,8; 2016,Jan,13; 2015,Jan,16; 2014,May,3; 2014,Jan,11

52344    Cystourethroscopy with ureteroscopy; with treatment of ureteral stricture (eg, balloon dilation, laser, electrocautery, and incision)
> INCLUDES  Diagnostic cystourethroscopy (52351)
> EXCLUDES  *Balloon dilation, ureteral stricture (50706)*
> *Cystourethroscopy with transurethral resection or incision of ejaculatory ducts (52402)*
> 📷 (74485)
> 🔧 10.7    ✂ 10.7    **FUD** 000    Ⓙ A2 50 🖥
> **AMA:** 2017,Jan,8; 2016,Jan,13; 2016,Jan,3; 2015,Jan,16; 2014,Jan,11

52345    with treatment of ureteropelvic junction stricture (eg, balloon dilation, laser, electrocautery, and incision)
> INCLUDES  Diagnostic cystourethroscopy (52351)
> EXCLUDES  *Balloon dilation, ureteral stricture (50706)*
> *Cystourethroscopy with transurethral resection or incision of ejaculatory ducts (52402)*
> 📷 (74485)
> 🔧 11.4    ✂ 11.4    **FUD** 000    Ⓙ A2 80 50 🖥
> **AMA:** 2017,Jan,8; 2016,Jan,13; 2016,Jan,3; 2015,Jan,16; 2014,Jan,11

● New Code    ▲ Revised Code    ○ Reinstated    ● New Web Release    ▲ Revised Web Release    Unlisted    Not Covered    # Resequenced
⊘ AMA Mod 51 Exempt    ⑤⓪ Optum Mod 51 Exempt    ⑥③ Mod 63 Exempt    ✓ Non-FDA Drug    ★ Telemedicine    🖥 Maternity    🅰 Age Edit    ✛ Add-on    **AMA:** CPT Asst
© 2017 Optum360, LLC    CPT © 2017 American Medical Association. All Rights Reserved.    **237**

**52346** **with treatment of intra-renal stricture (eg, balloon dilation, laser, electrocautery, and incision)**

INCLUDES Diagnostic cystourethroscopy (52351)

EXCLUDES *Balloon dilation with imaging guidance (50706)*

*Cystourethroscopy with transurethral resection or incision of ejaculatory ducts (52402)*

(74485)

12.9 ⚲ 12.9 **FUD** 000 J A2 80 50 ▢

**AMA:** 2017,Jan,8; 2016,Jan,13; 2015,Jan,16; 2014,May,3; 2014,Jan,11

**52351** **Cystourethroscopy, with ureteroscopy and/or pyeloscopy; diagnostic**

EXCLUDES *Cystourethroscopy (52341-52346, 52352-52353 [52356])*

8.77 ⚲ 8.77 **FUD** 000 J A2 ▢

**AMA:** 2017,Jan,8; 2016,Jan,13; 2015,Jan,16; 2014,May,3; 2014,Jan,11

**52352** **with removal or manipulation of calculus (ureteral catheterization is included)**

INCLUDES Diagnostic cystourethroscopy (52351)

10.2 ⚲ 10.2 **FUD** 000 J A2 50 ▢

**AMA:** 2017,Jan,8; 2016,Jan,13; 2015,Jan,16; 2014,Jan,11; 2012,Jan,15-42

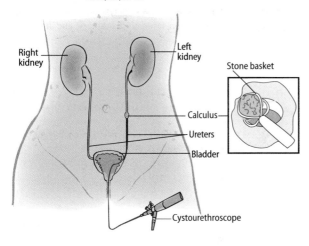

Right kidney — Left kidney — Stone basket — Calculus — Ureters — Bladder — Cystourethroscope

**52353** **with lithotripsy (ureteral catheterization is included)**

INCLUDES Diagnostic cystourethroscopy (52351)

EXCLUDES *Cystourethroscopy when performed on the same side (52332, [52356])*

11.3 ⚲ 11.3 **FUD** 000 J A2 50 ▢

**AMA:** 2017,Jan,8; 2016,Jan,13; 2015,Jan,16; 2014,May,3; 2014,Jan,11; 2012,Jan,15-42

\# **52356** **with lithotripsy including insertion of indwelling ureteral stent (eg, Gibbons or double-J type)**

INCLUDES Diagnostic cystourethroscopy (52351)

EXCLUDES *Cystourethroscopy when performed on the same side with (52332, 52353)*

*Cystourethroscopy (separate procedure) (52000)*

12.0 ⚲ 12.0 **FUD** 000 J 82 50 ▢

**AMA:** 2017,Jan,8; 2016,Jan,13; 2015,Jan,16; 2014,May,3; 2014,Jan,11

**52354** **with biopsy and/or fulguration of ureteral or renal pelvic lesion**

INCLUDES Diagnostic cystourethroscopy (52351)

EXCLUDES *Image guided biopsy without endoscopic guidance (50606)*

12.0 ⚲ 12.0 **FUD** 000 J A2 50 ▢

**AMA:** 2017,Jan,8; 2016,Jan,13; 2015,Jan,16; 2014,May,3; 2014,Jan,11

**52355** **with resection of ureteral or renal pelvic tumor**

INCLUDES Diagnostic cystourethroscopy (52351)

13.5 ⚲ 13.5 **FUD** 000 J A2 50 ▢

**AMA:** 2017,Jan,8; 2016,Jan,13; 2015,Jan,16; 2014,May,3; 2014,Jan,11

*52356* **Resequenced code. See code following 52353.**

## 52400-52700 Endoscopic Procedures via Urethra: Prostate and Vesical Neck

**52400** **Cystourethroscopy with incision, fulguration, or resection of congenital posterior urethral valves, or congenital obstructive hypertrophic mucosal folds**

13.8 ⚲ 13.8 **FUD** 090 J A2 ▢

**AMA:** 2017,Jan,8; 2016,Jan,13; 2015,Jan,16; 2014,Jan,11

**52402** **Cystourethroscopy with transurethral resection or incision of ejaculatory ducts** ♂

7.73 ⚲ 7.73 **FUD** 000 J A2 ▢

**AMA:** 2014,Jan,11

**52441** **Cystourethroscopy, with insertion of permanent adjustable transprostatic implant; single implant**

6.56 ⚲ 35.2 **FUD** 000 B ▢

**AMA:** 2017,Jan,8; 2016,Jan,13; 2015,Jun,5

+ **52442** **each additional permanent adjustable transprostatic implant (List separately in addition to code for primary procedure)**

EXCLUDES *Permanent urethral stent insertion (52282)*

*Removal of stent, calculus or foreign body (implant) (52310)*

*Temporary prostatic urethral stent insertion (53855)*

Code first (52441)

1.75 ⚲ 26.9 **FUD** ZZZ B ▢

**AMA:** 2017,Jan,8; 2016,Jan,13; 2015,Jun,5

**52450** **Transurethral incision of prostate** ♂

13.5 ⚲ 13.5 **FUD** 090 J A2 ▢

**AMA:** 2017,Jan,8; 2016,Jan,13; 2015,Jun,5; 2015,Jan,16; 2014,Jan,11; 2012,Jan,15-42

**52500** **Transurethral resection of bladder neck (separate procedure)**

14.0 ⚲ 14.0 **FUD** 090 J A2 ▢

**AMA:** 2017,Jan,8; 2016,Jan,13; 2015,Jan,16; 2014,Jan,11; 2012,Jan,15-42

**52601** **Transurethral electrosurgical resection of prostate, including control of postoperative bleeding, complete (vasectomy, meatotomy, cystourethroscopy, urethral calibration and/or dilation, and internal urethrotomy are included)** ♂

INCLUDES Stage 1 of partial transurethral resection of prostate

EXCLUDES *Ablation by waterjet (0421T)*

*Excision of prostate (55801-55845)*

*Transurethral fulguration of prostate (52214)*

Code also modifier 58 for stage 2 partial transurethral resection of prostate

24.4 ⚲ 24.4 **FUD** 090 J A2 ▢

**AMA:** 2017,Jan,8; 2016,Jan,13; 2015,Jun,5; 2015,Jan,16; 2014,Jan,11; 2012,Jan,15-42

**52630** **Transurethral resection; residual or regrowth of obstructive prostate tissue including control of postoperative bleeding, complete (vasectomy, meatotomy, cystourethroscopy, urethral calibration and/or dilation, and internal urethrotomy are included)** ♂

EXCLUDES *Ablation by waterjet (0421T)*

*Excision of prostate (55801-55845)*

Code also modifier 78 when performed by same physician within the postoperative period of a related procedure

11.5 ⚲ 11.5 **FUD** 090 J A2 ▢

**AMA:** 2017,Jan,8; 2016,Jan,13; 2015,Jan,16; 2014,Jan,11

26/TC PC/TC Only   A2-Z3 ASC Payment   50 Bilateral   ♂ Male Only   ♀ Female Only   ⚙ Facility RVU   ⚲ Non-Facility RVU   ▢ CCI

**FUD** Follow-up Days   **CMS:** IOM (Pub 100)   A-Y OPPSI   80/80 Surg Assist Allowed / w/Doc   ▨ Lab Crosswalk   ▧ Radiology Crosswalk   ✖ CLIA

238    CPT © 2017 American Medical Association. All Rights Reserved.    © 2017 Optum360, LLC

**52640** of postoperative bladder neck contracture
EXCLUDES *Excision of prostate (55801-55845)*
⊞ 9.09  ⊠ 9.09  **FUD** 090      J A2 ▭
AMA: 2017,Jan,8; 2016,Jan,13; 2015,Jan,16; 2014,Jan,11

**52647** Laser coagulation of prostate, including control of postoperative bleeding, complete (vasectomy, meatotomy, cystourethroscopy, urethral calibration and/or dilation, and internal urethrotomy are included if performed) ♂
⊞ 18.6  ⊠ 50.6  **FUD** 090      J A2 ▭
AMA: 2017,Jan,8; 2016,Jan,13; 2015,Jan,16; 2014,Jan,11; 2012,Jan,15-42

**52648** Laser vaporization of prostate, including control of postoperative bleeding, complete (vasectomy, meatotomy, cystourethroscopy, urethral calibration and/or dilation, internal urethrotomy and transurethral resection of prostate are included if performed) ♂
⊞ 19.9  ⊠ 52.1  **FUD** 090      J A2 ▭
AMA: 2017,Jan,8; 2016,Jan,13; 2015,Jun,5; 2015,Jan,16; 2014,Jan,11; 2012,Jan,15-42

**52649** Laser enucleation of the prostate with morcellation, including control of postoperative bleeding, complete (vasectomy, meatotomy, cystourethroscopy, urethral calibration and/or dilation, internal urethrotomy and transurethral resection of prostate are included if performed) ♂
INCLUDES  Cystourethroscopy (52000, 52276, 52281)
Laser coagulation of prostate (52647-52648)
Meatotomy (53020)
Transurethral resection of prostate (52601)
Vasectomy (55250)
⊞ 23.7  ⊠ 23.7  **FUD** 090      J G2 80 ▭
AMA: 2017,Jan,8; 2016,Jan,13; 2015,Jun,5; 2014,Jan,11

**52700** Transurethral drainage of prostatic abscess ♂
EXCLUDES *Litholapaxy (52317, 52318)*
⊞ 12.7  ⊠ 12.7  **FUD** 090      J A2 80 ▭
AMA: 2017,Jan,8; 2016,Jan,13; 2015,Jan,16; 2014,Jan,11

Bladder
Prostate
Urethra

## 53000-53520 Open Surgical Procedures of Urethra
EXCLUDES  *Endoscopic procedures; cystoscopy, urethroscopy, cystourethroscopy (52000-52700 [52356])*
*Urethrocystography injection procedure (51600-51610)*

**53000** Urethrotomy or urethrostomy, external (separate procedure); pendulous urethra
⊞ 4.26  ⊠ 4.26  **FUD** 010      J A2 ▭
AMA: 2014,Jan,11

**53010** perineal urethra, external
⊞ 8.50  ⊠ 8.50  **FUD** 090      J A2 ▭
AMA: 2014,Jan,11

**53020** Meatotomy, cutting of meatus (separate procedure); except infant
⊞ 2.81  ⊠ 2.81  **FUD** 000      J A2 ▭
AMA: 2014,Jan,11

**53025** infant  Ⓐ
⊞ 2.07  ⊠ 2.07  **FUD** 000      ⓷ J R2 80 ▭
AMA: 2014,Jan,11

**53040** Drainage of deep periurethral abscess
EXCLUDES  *Incision and drainage of subcutaneous abscess (10060-10061)*
⊞ 11.3  ⊠ 11.3  **FUD** 090      J A2 80 ▭
AMA: 2014,Jan,11

**53060** Drainage of Skene's gland abscess or cyst
⊞ 4.74  ⊠ 5.27  **FUD** 010      J P3 ▭
AMA: 2014,Jan,11

**53080** Drainage of perineal urinary extravasation; uncomplicated (separate procedure)
⊞ 12.1  ⊠ 12.1  **FUD** 090      J A2 ▭
AMA: 2014,Jan,11

**53085** complicated
⊞ 19.0  ⊠ 19.0  **FUD** 090      J G2 80 ▭
AMA: 2014,Jan,11

**53200** Biopsy of urethra
⊞ 4.12  ⊠ 4.49  **FUD** 000      J A2 ▭
AMA: 2014,Jan,11

**53210** Urethrectomy, total, including cystostomy; female ♀
⊞ 22.4  ⊠ 22.4  **FUD** 090      J A2 80 ▭
AMA: 2014,Jan,11

**53215** male ♂
⊞ 26.8  ⊠ 26.8  **FUD** 090      J A2 80 ▭
AMA: 2014,Jan,11

**53220** Excision or fulguration of carcinoma of urethra
⊞ 13.2  ⊠ 13.2  **FUD** 090      J A2 80 ▭
AMA: 2014,Jan,11

**53230** Excision of urethral diverticulum (separate procedure); female ♀
⊞ 17.4  ⊠ 17.4  **FUD** 090      J A2 80 ▭
AMA: 2014,Jan,11

**53235** male ♂
⊞ 18.3  ⊠ 18.3  **FUD** 090      J A2 80 ▭
AMA: 2014,Jan,11

**53240** Marsupialization of urethral diverticulum, male or female
⊞ 12.2  ⊠ 12.2  **FUD** 090      J A2 ▭
AMA: 2014,Jan,11

**53250** Excision of bulbourethral gland (Cowper's gland)
⊞ 11.8  ⊠ 11.8  **FUD** 090      J A2 ▭
AMA: 2014,Jan,11

**53260** Excision or fulguration; urethral polyp(s), distal urethra
EXCLUDES  *Endoscopic method (52214, 52224)*
⊞ 5.18  ⊠ 5.77  **FUD** 010      J A2 ▭
AMA: 2014,Jan,11

**53265** urethral caruncle
EXCLUDES  *Endoscopic method (52214, 52224)*
⊞ 5.36  ⊠ 6.25  **FUD** 010      J A2 ▭
AMA: 2014,Jan,11

**53270** Skene's glands
EXCLUDES  *Endoscopic method (52214, 52224)*
⊞ 5.31  ⊠ 5.92  **FUD** 010      J A2 ▭
AMA: 2014,Jan,11

**53275** urethral prolapse
EXCLUDES  *Endoscopic method (52214, 52224)*
⊞ 7.60  ⊠ 7.60  **FUD** 010      J A2 ▭
AMA: 2014,Jan,11

● New Code  ▲ Revised Code  ○ Reinstated  ● New Web Release  ▲ Revised Web Release  Unlisted  Not Covered  # Resequenced
⊘ AMA Mod 51 Exempt  ⑨ Optum Mod 51 Exempt  ㊻ Mod 63 Exempt  ✔ Non-FDA Drug  ★ Telemedicine  Ⓜ Maternity  Ⓐ Age Edit  + Add-on  AMA: CPT Asst
© 2017 Optum360, LLC          CPT © 2017 American Medical Association. All Rights Reserved.          239

**53400** Urethroplasty; first stage, for fistula, diverticulum, or stricture (eg, Johannsen type)

EXCLUDES    Hypospadias repair (54300-54352)
🔧 23.1    ✂ 23.1    **FUD** 090    J A2 80 📧
**AMA:** 2014,Jan,11

**53405** second stage (formation of urethra), including urinary diversion

EXCLUDES    Hypospadias repair (54300-54352)
🔧 25.3    ✂ 25.3    **FUD** 090    J A2 80 📧
**AMA:** 2014,Jan,11

**53410** Urethroplasty, 1-stage reconstruction of male anterior urethra    ♂

EXCLUDES    Hypospadias repair (54300-54352)
🔧 28.2    ✂ 28.2    **FUD** 090    J A2 80 📧
**AMA:** 2014,Jan,11

**53415** Urethroplasty, transpubic or perineal, 1-stage, for reconstruction or repair of prostatic or membranous urethra    ♂

🔧 32.6    ✂ 32.6    **FUD** 090    C 80 📧
**AMA:** 2014,Jan,11

**53420** Urethroplasty, 2-stage reconstruction or repair of prostatic or membranous urethra; first stage    ♂

🔧 24.3    ✂ 24.3    **FUD** 090    J A2 📧
**AMA:** 2014,Jan,11

**53425** second stage    ♂

🔧 27.0    ✂ 27.0    **FUD** 090    J A2 80 📧
**AMA:** 2014,Jan,11

**53430** Urethroplasty, reconstruction of female urethra    ♀

🔧 27.9    ✂ 27.9    **FUD** 090    J A2 80 📧
**AMA:** 2014,Jan,11

**53431** Urethroplasty with tubularization of posterior urethra and/or lower bladder for incontinence (eg, Tenago, Leadbetter procedure)

🔧 33.3    ✂ 33.3    **FUD** 090    J A2 80 📧
**AMA:** 2014,Jan,11

**53440** Sling operation for correction of male urinary incontinence (eg, fascia or synthetic)    ♂

🔧 21.7    ✂ 21.7    **FUD** 090    J J8 80 📧
**AMA:** 2014,Jan,11

**53442** Removal or revision of sling for male urinary incontinence (eg, fascia or synthetic)    ♂

🔧 22.5    ✂ 22.5    **FUD** 090    J A2 80 📧
**AMA:** 2014,Jan,11

**53444** Insertion of tandem cuff (dual cuff)

🔧 22.8    ✂ 22.8    **FUD** 090    J J8 80 📧
**AMA:** 2014,Jan,11

**53445** Insertion of inflatable urethral/bladder neck sphincter, including placement of pump, reservoir, and cuff

🔧 21.7    ✂ 21.7    **FUD** 090    J J8 80 📧
**AMA:** 2014,Jan,11

**53446** Removal of inflatable urethral/bladder neck sphincter, including pump, reservoir, and cuff

🔧 18.5    ✂ 18.5    **FUD** 090    02 A2 80 📧
**AMA:** 2014,Jan,11

**53447** Removal and replacement of inflatable urethral/bladder neck sphincter including pump, reservoir, and cuff at the same operative session

🔧 23.3    ✂ 23.3    **FUD** 090    J J8 80 📧
**AMA:** 2014,Jan,11

**53448** Removal and replacement of inflatable urethral/bladder neck sphincter including pump, reservoir, and cuff through an infected field at the same operative session including irrigation and debridement of infected tissue

INCLUDES    Debridement (11042, 11043)
🔧 37.0    ✂ 37.0    **FUD** 090    C 80 📧
**AMA:** 2014,Jan,11

**53449** Repair of inflatable urethral/bladder neck sphincter, including pump, reservoir, and cuff

🔧 17.6    ✂ 17.6    **FUD** 090    J A2 80 📧
**AMA:** 2014,Jan,11

**53450** Urethromeatoplasty, with mucosal advancement

EXCLUDES    Meatotomy (53020, 53025)
🔧 11.7    ✂ 11.7    **FUD** 090    J A2 📧
**AMA:** 2017,Jan,8; 2016,Jan,13; 2015,Jan,16; 2014,Jan,11; 2012,Oct,14; 2012,Sep,16

**53460** Urethromeatoplasty, with partial excision of distal urethral segment (Richardson type procedure)

🔧 13.2    ✂ 13.2    **FUD** 090    J A2 80 📧
**AMA:** 2014,Jan,11

**53500** Urethrolysis, transvaginal, secondary, open, including cystourethroscopy (eg, postsurgical obstruction, scarring)

INCLUDES    Cystourethroscopy (separate procedure) (52000)
EXCLUDES    Retropubic approach (53899)
🔧 21.6    ✂ 21.6    **FUD** 090    J 80 📧
**AMA:** 2017,Jan,8; 2016,Jan,13; 2015,Jan,16; 2014,Jan,11

**53502** Urethrorrhaphy, suture of urethral wound or injury, female    ♀

🔧 14.0    ✂ 14.0    **FUD** 090    J A2 📧
**AMA:** 2014,Jan,11

**53505** Urethrorrhaphy, suture of urethral wound or injury; penile    ♂

🔧 14.0    ✂ 14.0    **FUD** 090    J A2 80 📧
**AMA:** 2014,Jan,11

**53510** perineal    ♂

🔧 18.2    ✂ 18.2    **FUD** 090    J A2 80 📧
**AMA:** 2014,Jan,11

**53515** prostatomembranous    ♂

🔧 22.8    ✂ 22.8    **FUD** 090    J A2 80 📧
**AMA:** 2014,Jan,11

**53520** Closure of urethrostomy or urethrocutaneous fistula, male (separate procedure)    ♂

EXCLUDES    Closure of fistula:
Urethrorectal (45820, 45825)
Urethrovaginal (57310)
🔧 16.0    ✂ 16.0    **FUD** 090    J A2 📧
**AMA:** 2014,Jan,11

## 53600-53665 Urethral Dilation

EXCLUDES    Endoscopic procedures; cystoscopy, urethroscopy, cystourethroscopy (52000-52700 [52356])
Urethral catheterization (51701-51703)
Urethrocystography injection procedure (51600-51610)
📷 (74485)

**53600** Dilation of urethral stricture by passage of sound or urethral dilator, male; initial    ♂

🔧 1.84    ✂ 2.38    **FUD** 000    T P3 📧
**AMA:** 2014,Jan,11

**53601** subsequent    ♂

🔧 1.55    ✂ 2.32    **FUD** 000    01 N1 📧
**AMA:** 2014,Jan,11

**53605** Dilation of urethral stricture or vesical neck by passage of sound or urethral dilator, male, general or conduction (spinal) anesthesia ♂

EXCLUDES *Procedure performed under local anesthesia (53600-53601, 53620-53621)*

📋 1.87   ⚖ 1.87   **FUD** 000   J A2 ▭

**AMA:** 2014,Jan,11

**53620** Dilation of urethral stricture by passage of filiform and follower, male; initial ♂

📋 2.53   ⚖ 3.33   **FUD** 000   T P3 ▭

**AMA:** 2014,Jan,11

**53621** subsequent ♂

📋 2.09   ⚖ 3.12   **FUD** 000   T P3 ▭

**AMA:** 2014,Jan,11

**53660** Dilation of female urethra including suppository and/or instillation; initial ♀

📋 1.21   ⚖ 2.01   **FUD** 000   S P3 ▭

**AMA:** 2014,Jan,11

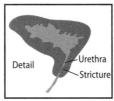

Urethra

Sound

Detail   Urethra
         Stricture

**Physician passes a dilator through a stricture in the urethra**

**53661** subsequent ♀

📋 1.17   ⚖ 1.98   **FUD** 000   Q1 N1 ▭

**AMA:** 2014,Jan,11

**53665** Dilation of female urethra, general or conduction (spinal) anesthesia ♀

EXCLUDES *Procedure performed under local anesthesia (53660-53661)*

📋 1.12   ⚖ 1.12   **FUD** 000   J A2 ▭

**AMA:** 2014,Jan,11

## 53850-53899 Transurethral Procedures

EXCLUDES *Endoscopic procedures; cystoscopy, urethroscopy, cystourethroscopy (52000-52700 [52356])*

**53850** Transurethral destruction of prostate tissue; by microwave thermotherapy ♂

🔬 (81020)

📋 17.5   ⚖ 58.9   **FUD** 090   J P2 ▭

**AMA:** 2017,Jan,8; 2016,Jan,13; 2015,Jun,5; 2015,Jan,16; 2014,Jan,11

**53852** by radiofrequency thermotherapy ♂

🔬 (81020)

📋 17.9   ⚖ 54.3   **FUD** 090   J P3 ▭

**AMA:** 2017,Jan,8; 2016,Jan,13; 2015,Jun,5; 2015,Jan,16; 2014,Jan,11

**53855** Insertion of a temporary prostatic urethral stent, including urethral measurement ♂

EXCLUDES *Permanent urethral stent insertion (52282)*

📋 2.39   ⚖ 22.0   **FUD** 000   J P3 80 ▭

**AMA:** 2017,Jan,8; 2016,Jan,13; 2015,Jun,5; 2015,Jan,16; 2014,Jan,11

**53860** Transurethral radiofrequency micro-remodeling of the female bladder neck and proximal urethra for stress urinary incontinence ♀

📋 6.50   ⚖ 44.5   **FUD** 090   J P2 80 ▭

**AMA:** 2014,Jan,11

**53899** Unlisted procedure, urinary system

📋 0.00   ⚖ 0.00   **FUD** YYY   T 80

**AMA:** 2017,Jan,8; 2016,Jan,13; 2015,Jun,5; 2015,Mar,9; 2015,Jan,16; 2014,Jan,11; 2012,Jan,15-42

**Genital System**

## 54000-54015 Procedures of Penis: Incisional

EXCLUDES *Debridement of abdominal perineal gangrene (11004-11006)*

**54000** **Slitting of prepuce, dorsal or lateral (separate procedure); newborn** A ♂
🔹 3.12　 ⚎ 4.23　 **FUD** 010　　　　 ⑥³ J A2 80 ▭
AMA: 2014,Jan,11

**54001** **except newborn** ♂
🔹 4.00　 ⚎ 5.28　 **FUD** 010　　　　 J A2 ▭
AMA: 2014,Jan,11

**54015** **Incision and drainage of penis, deep** ♂
EXCLUDES *Abscess, skin/subcutaneous (10060-10160)*
🔹 8.89　 ⚎ 8.89　 **FUD** 010　　　 J A2 80 ▭
AMA: 2014,Jan,11

Urethra

Hematoma
or abscess

Hematoma
or abscess

A postoperative drain may be
placed. Sutures are required
to repair the operative site

The physician incises the penis
to drain an abscess or hematoma

## 54050-54065 Destruction of Penis Lesions: Multiple Methods

EXCLUDES *Excision/destruction other lesions (11420-11426, 11620-11626, 17000-17250, 17270-17276)*

**54050** **Destruction of lesion(s), penis (eg, condyloma, papilloma, molluscum contagiosum, herpetic vesicle), simple; chemical** ♂
🔹 3.05　 ⚎ 3.79　 **FUD** 010　　　 01 N1 ▭
AMA: 2014,Jan,11

**54055** **electrodesiccation** ♂
🔹 2.67　 ⚎ 3.39　 **FUD** 010　　　 T P3 ▭
AMA: 2014,Jan,11

**54056** **cryosurgery** ♂
🔹 3.19　 ⚎ 4.05　 **FUD** 010　　　 01 N1 ▭
AMA: 2014,Jan,11

**54057** **laser surgery** ♂
🔹 2.74　 ⚎ 3.89　 **FUD** 010　　　 T A2 ▭
AMA: 2014,Jan,11

**54060** **surgical excision** ♂
🔹 3.76　 ⚎ 5.13　 **FUD** 010　　　 T A2 ▭
AMA: 2014,Jan,11

**54065** **Destruction of lesion(s), penis (eg, condyloma, papilloma, molluscum contagiosum, herpetic vesicle), extensive (eg, laser surgery, electrosurgery, cryosurgery, chemosurgery)** ♂
🔹 4.98　 ⚎ 6.25　 **FUD** 010　　　 T A2 ▭
AMA: 2014,Jan,11

## 54100-54115 Procedures of Penis: Excisional

**54100** **Biopsy of penis; (separate procedure)** ♂
🔹 3.64　 ⚎ 5.66　 **FUD** 000　　　 J A2 ▭
AMA: 2017,Jan,8; 2016,Jan,13; 2015,Jan,16; 2014,Jan,11

**54105** **deep structures** ♂
🔹 6.15　 ⚎ 7.57　 **FUD** 010　　　 J A2 ▭
AMA: 2014,Jan,11

**54110** **Excision of penile plaque (Peyronie disease);** ♂
🔹 18.0　 ⚎ 18.0　 **FUD** 090　　 J A2 80 ▭
AMA: 2014,Jan,11

**54111** **with graft to 5 cm in length** ♂
🔹 23.3　 ⚎ 23.3　 **FUD** 090　　 J A2 80 ▭
AMA: 2017,Jan,8; 2016,Jan,13; 2015,Jan,16; 2014,Jan,11; 2012,Jan,15-42

**54112** **with graft greater than 5 cm in length** ♂
🔹 27.0　 ⚎ 27.0　 **FUD** 090　　 J A2 80 ▭
AMA: 2014,Jan,11

**54115** **Removal foreign body from deep penile tissue (eg, plastic implant)** ♂
🔹 12.3　 ⚎ 13.0　 **FUD** 090　　 J A2 80 ▭
AMA: 2014,Jan,11

## 54120-54135 Amputation of Penis

EXCLUDES *Lymphadenectomy (separate procedure) (38760-38770)*

**54120** **Amputation of penis; partial** ♂
🔹 18.2　 ⚎ 18.2　 **FUD** 090　　 J A2 80 ▭
AMA: 2014,Jan,11

**54125** **complete** ♂
🔹 23.5　 ⚎ 23.5　 **FUD** 090　　 C 80 ▭
AMA: 2014,Jan,11

**54130** **Amputation of penis, radical; with bilateral inguinofemoral lymphadenectomy** ♂
🔹 34.4　 ⚎ 34.4　 **FUD** 090　　 C 80 ▭
AMA: 2014,Jan,11

**54135** **in continuity with bilateral pelvic lymphadenectomy, including external iliac, hypogastric and obturator nodes** ♂
🔹 43.7　 ⚎ 43.7　 **FUD** 090　　 C 80 ▭
AMA: 2014,Jan,11

## 54150-54164 Circumcision Procedures

**54150** **Circumcision, using clamp or other device with regional dorsal penile or ring block** ♂
Code also modifier 52 when performed without dorsal penile or ring block
🔹 2.83　 ⚎ 4.42　 **FUD** 000　 ⑥³ J A2 80 ▭
AMA: 2017,Jan,8; 2016,Jan,13; 2015,Jan,16; 2014,Jan,11; 2012,Jan,15-42

**54160** **Circumcision, surgical excision other than clamp, device, or dorsal slit; neonate (28 days of age or less)** A ♂
🔹 4.16　 ⚎ 6.28　 **FUD** 010　 ⑥³ J A2 ▭
AMA: 2017,Jan,8; 2016,Jan,13; 2015,Jan,16; 2014,Jan,11; 2012,Jan,15-42

**54161** **older than 28 days of age** A ♂
🔹 5.68　 ⚎ 5.68　 **FUD** 010　　 J A2 ▭
AMA: 2017,Jan,8; 2016,Jan,13; 2015,Jan,16; 2014,Jan,11; 2012,Jan,15-42

**54162** **Lysis or excision of penile post-circumcision adhesions** ♂
🔹 5.73　 ⚎ 7.35　 **FUD** 010　　 J A2 ▭
AMA: 2014,Jan,11

**54163** **Repair incomplete circumcision** ♂
🔹 6.31　 ⚎ 6.31　 **FUD** 010　　 J A2 ▭
AMA: 2014,Jan,11

**54164** **Frenulotomy of penis** ♂
EXCLUDES *Circumcision (54150-54163)*
🔹 5.59　 ⚎ 5.59　 **FUD** 010　　 J A2 ▭
AMA: 2014,Jan,11

## 54200-54250 Evaluation and Treatment of Erectile Abnormalities

**54200** **Injection procedure for Peyronie disease;** ♂
🔹 2.41　 ⚎ 3.06　 **FUD** 010　　 T P3 ▭
AMA: 2014,Jan,11

| 26/TC PC/TC Only | A2-Z3 ASC Payment | 50 Bilateral | ♂ Male Only | ♀ Female Only | 🔹 Facility RVU | ⚎ Non-Facility RVU | ▭ CCI |
| FUD Follow-up Days | CMS: IOM (Pub 100) | A-Y OPPSI | 80/80 Surg Assist Allowed / w/Doc | | 🔲 Lab Crosswalk | 🔶 Radiology Crosswalk | ❌ CLIA |

242　　　　　　　　　　　　　　　 CPT © 2017 American Medical Association. All Rights Reserved.　　　　　　　　　 © 2017 Optum360, LLC

Genital System

54000 — 54200

**54205** with surgical exposure of plaque ♂
🔧 15.3 📊 15.3 **FUD** 090 [J] [A2] [80] 🔲
**AMA:** 2014,Jan,11

**54220** Irrigation of corpora cavernosa for priapism ♂
🔧 3.88 📊 5.85 **FUD** 000 [T] [A2] 🔲
**AMA:** 2014,Jan,11

**54230** Injection procedure for corpora cavernosography ♂
🔀 (74445)
🔧 2.30 📊 2.77 **FUD** 000 [N] [N1] 🔲
**AMA:** 2014,Jan,11

**54231** Dynamic cavernosometry, including intracavernosal injection of vasoactive drugs (eg, papaverine, phentolamine) ♂
🔧 3.37 📊 4.02 **FUD** 000 [J] [P3] 🔲
**AMA:** 2014,Jan,11

**54235** Injection of corpora cavernosa with pharmacologic agent(s) (eg, papaverine, phentolamine) ♂
🔧 2.12 📊 2.59 **FUD** 000 [T] [P3] 🔲
**AMA:** 2017,Jan,8; 2016,Jan,13; 2015,Jan,16; 2014,Jan,11; 2012,Jan,15-42

**54240** Penile plethysmography ♂
🔧 2.98 📊 2.98 **FUD** 000 [S] [P3] [80] 🔲
**AMA:** 2014,Jan,11

**54250** Nocturnal penile tumescence and/or rigidity test ♂
🔧 3.48 📊 3.48 **FUD** 000 [T] [P3] [80] 🔲
**AMA:** 2014,Jan,11

## 54300-54390 Hypospadias Repair and Related Procedures

EXCLUDES Other urethroplasties (53400-53430)
Revascularization of penis (37788)

**54300** Plastic operation of penis for straightening of chordee (eg, hypospadias), with or without mobilization of urethra ♂
🔧 18.5 📊 18.5 **FUD** 090 [J] [A2] [80] 🔲
**AMA:** 2017,Jan,8; 2016,Jan,13; 2015,Jan,16; 2014,Dec,16; 2014,Dec,16; 2014,Jan,11

**54304** Plastic operation on penis for correction of chordee or for first stage hypospadias repair with or without transplantation of prepuce and/or skin flaps ♂
🔧 21.6 📊 21.6 **FUD** 090 [J] [A2] [80] 🔲
**AMA:** 2014,Jan,11

Chordee

Urethra Penis

Urethral opening

The foreskin is used in either a free graft or a flap graft to cover the ventral skin defects created to correct the chordee

**54308** Urethroplasty for second stage hypospadias repair (including urinary diversion); less than 3 cm ♂
🔧 20.6 📊 20.6 **FUD** 090 [J] [A2] [80] 🔲
**AMA:** 2014,Jan,11

**54312** greater than 3 cm ♂
🔧 24.7 📊 24.7 **FUD** 090 [J] [A2] [80] 🔲
**AMA:** 2014,Jan,11

**54316** Urethroplasty for second stage hypospadias repair (including urinary diversion) with free skin graft obtained from site other than genitalia ♂
🔧 30.1 📊 30.1 **FUD** 090 [J] [A2] [80] 🔲
**AMA:** 2014,Jan,11

**54318** Urethroplasty for third stage hypospadias repair to release penis from scrotum (eg, third stage Cecil repair) ♂
🔧 20.5 📊 20.5 **FUD** 090 [J] [A2] [80] 🔲
**AMA:** 2014,Jan,11

**54322** 1-stage distal hypospadias repair (with or without chordee or circumcision); with simple meatal advancement (eg, Magpi, V-flap) ♂
🔧 22.3 📊 22.3 **FUD** 090 [J] [A2] [80] 🔲
**AMA:** 2014,Jan,11

**54324** with urethroplasty by local skin flaps (eg, flip-flap, prepucial flap) ♂
INCLUDES Browne's operation
🔧 27.9 📊 27.9 **FUD** 090 [J] [A2] [80] 🔲
**AMA:** 2014,Jan,11

**54326** with urethroplasty by local skin flaps and mobilization of urethra ♂
🔧 27.3 📊 27.3 **FUD** 090 [J] [A2] [80] 🔲
**AMA:** 2014,Jan,11

**54328** with extensive dissection to correct chordee and urethroplasty with local skin flaps, skin graft patch, and/or island flap ♂
EXCLUDES Urethroplasty/straightening of chordee (54308)
🔧 27.6 📊 27.6 **FUD** 090 [J] [A2] [80] 🔲
**AMA:** 2017,Jan,8; 2016,Jan,13; 2015,Jan,16; 2014,Jan,11; 2012,Jan,15-42

**54332** 1-stage proximal penile or penoscrotal hypospadias repair requiring extensive dissection to correct chordee and urethroplasty by use of skin graft tube and/or island flap ♂
🔧 30.5 📊 30.5 **FUD** 090 [J] [80] 🔲
**AMA:** 2017,Jan,8; 2016,Jan,13; 2015,Jan,16; 2014,Jan,11; 2012,Jan,15-42

**54336** 1-stage perineal hypospadias repair requiring extensive dissection to correct chordee and urethroplasty by use of skin graft tube and/or island flap ♂
🔧 34.3 📊 34.3 **FUD** 090 [J] [80] 🔲
**AMA:** 2017,Jan,8; 2016,Jan,13; 2015,Jan,16; 2014,Jan,11; 2012,Jan,15-42

**54340** Repair of hypospadias complications (ie, fistula, stricture, diverticula); by closure, incision, or excision, simple ♂
🔧 16.3 📊 16.3 **FUD** 090 [J] [A2] [80] 🔲
**AMA:** 2014,Jan,11

**54344** requiring mobilization of skin flaps and urethroplasty with flap or patch graft ♂
🔧 27.3 📊 27.3 **FUD** 090 [J] [A2] [80] 🔲
**AMA:** 2014,Jan,11

**54348** requiring extensive dissection and urethroplasty with flap, patch or tubed graft (includes urinary diversion) ♂
🔧 29.3 📊 29.3 **FUD** 090 [J] [A2] [80] 🔲
**AMA:** 2014,Jan,11

**54352** Repair of hypospadias cripple requiring extensive dissection and excision of previously constructed structures including re-release of chordee and reconstruction of urethra and penis by use of local skin as grafts and island flaps and skin brought in as flaps or grafts ♂
🔧 40.9 📊 40.9 **FUD** 090 [J] [A2] [80] 🔲
**AMA:** 2014,Jan,11

**54360** Plastic operation on penis to correct angulation ♂
🔧 20.8   ✂ 20.8   **FUD** 090   J A2 80 ▣
**AMA:** 2014,Jan,11

**54380** Plastic operation on penis for epispadias distal to external sphincter; ♂
[INCLUDES] Lowsley's operation
🔧 23.0   ✂ 23.0   **FUD** 090   J A2 80 ▣
**AMA:** 2014,Jan,11

**54385** with incontinence ♂
🔧 28.0   ✂ 28.0   **FUD** 090   J A2 80 ▣
**AMA:** 2014,Jan,11

**54390** with exstrophy of bladder ♂
🔧 35.8   ✂ 35.8   **FUD** 090   C 80 ▣
**AMA:** 2014,Jan,11

## 54400-54417 Procedures to Treat Impotence

**CMS:** 100-03,230.4 Diagnosis and Treatment of Impotence
[EXCLUDES] Other urethroplasties (53400-53430)
Revascularization of penis (37788)

**54400** Insertion of penile prosthesis; non-inflatable (semi-rigid) ♂
[EXCLUDES] Replacement/removal penile prosthesis (54415, 54416)
🔧 15.2   ✂ 15.2   **FUD** 090   J J8 ▣
**AMA:** 2014,Jan,11

**54401** inflatable (self-contained) ♂
[EXCLUDES] Replacement/removal penile prosthesis (54415, 54416)
🔧 18.9   ✂ 18.9   **FUD** 090   J J8 ▣
**AMA:** 2014,Jan,11

**54405** Insertion of multi-component, inflatable penile prosthesis, including placement of pump, cylinders, and reservoir ♂
Code also modifier 52 for reduced services
🔧 23.3   ✂ 23.3   **FUD** 090   J J8 80 ▣
**AMA:** 2014,Jan,11

**54406** Removal of all components of a multi-component, inflatable penile prosthesis without replacement of prosthesis ♂
Code also modifier 52 for reduced services
🔧 21.1   ✂ 21.1   **FUD** 090   02 A2 80 ▣
**AMA:** 2014,Jan,11

**54408** Repair of component(s) of a multi-component, inflatable penile prosthesis ♂
🔧 22.8   ✂ 22.8   **FUD** 090   J A2 80 ▣
**AMA:** 2014,Jan,11

**54410** Removal and replacement of all component(s) of a multi-component, inflatable penile prosthesis at the same operative session ♂
🔧 24.8   ✂ 24.8   **FUD** 090   J J8 80 ▣
**AMA:** 2014,Jan,11

**54411** Removal and replacement of all components of a multi-component inflatable penile prosthesis through an infected field at the same operative session, including irrigation and debridement of infected tissue ♂
[INCLUDES] Debridement (11042, 11043)
Code also modifier 52 for reduced services
🔧 29.6   ✂ 29.6   **FUD** 090   J 80 ▣
**AMA:** 2014,Jan,11

**54415** Removal of non-inflatable (semi-rigid) or inflatable (self-contained) penile prosthesis, without replacement of prosthesis ♂
🔧 15.2   ✂ 15.2   **FUD** 090   02 A2 80 ▣
**AMA:** 2014,Jan,11

**54416** Removal and replacement of non-inflatable (semi-rigid) or inflatable (self-contained) penile prosthesis at the same operative session ♂
🔧 20.5   ✂ 20.5   **FUD** 090   J J8 80 ▣
**AMA:** 2014,Jan,11

**54417** Removal and replacement of non-inflatable (semi-rigid) or inflatable (self-contained) penile prosthesis through an infected field at the same operative session, including irrigation and debridement of infected tissue ♂
[INCLUDES] Debridement (11042, 11043)
🔧 25.9   ✂ 25.9   **FUD** 090   J 80 ▣
**AMA:** 2014,Jan,11

## 54420-54450 Other Procedures of the Penis

[EXCLUDES] Other urethroplasties (53400-53430)
Revascularization of penis (37788)

**54420** Corpora cavernosa-saphenous vein shunt (priapism operation), unilateral or bilateral ♂
🔧 20.3   ✂ 20.3   **FUD** 090   J A2 80 ▣
**AMA:** 2014,Jan,11

**54430** Corpora cavernosa-corpus spongiosum shunt (priapism operation), unilateral or bilateral ♂
🔧 18.4   ✂ 18.4   **FUD** 090   C 80 ▣
**AMA:** 2014,Jan,11

Cross section of penis

The physician creates a communication between the corpus cavernosum and the corpus spongiosum

**54435** Corpora cavernosa-glans penis fistulization (eg, biopsy needle, Winter procedure, rongeur, or punch) for priapism ♂
🔧 12.0   ✂ 12.0   **FUD** 090   J A2 ▣
**AMA:** 2014,Jan,11

**54437** Repair of traumatic corporeal tear(s) ♂
🔧 19.5   ✂ 19.5   **FUD** 090   J 62 80 ▣
[EXCLUDES] Urethral repair (53410, 53415)

**54438** Replantation, penis, complete amputation including urethral repair ♂
🔧 38.9   ✂ 38.9   **FUD** 090   C 80 ▣
[EXCLUDES] Replantation/repair of corporeal tear in incomplete amputation penis (54437)
Replantation/urethral repair in incomplete amputation penis (53410-53415)

**54440** Plastic operation of penis for injury ♂
🔧 0.00   ✂ 0.00   **FUD** 090   J A2 80 ▣
**AMA:** 2014,Jan,11

**54450** Foreskin manipulation including lysis of preputial adhesions and stretching ♂
🔧 1.67   ✂ 2.01   **FUD** 000   T A2 ▣
**AMA:** 2014,Jan,11

## 54500-54560 Testicular Procedures: Incisional

[EXCLUDES] Debridement of abdominal perineal gangrene (11004-11006)

**54500** Biopsy of testis, needle (separate procedure) ♂
[EXCLUDES] Fine needle aspiration (10021, 10022)
(88172-88173)
🔧 2.16   ✂ 2.16   **FUD** 000   J A2 80 50 ▣
**AMA:** 2014,Jan,11

| 26/TC PC/TC Only | A2-Z3 ASC Payment | 50 Bilateral | ♂ Male Only | ♀ Female Only | 🔧 Facility RVU | ✂ Non-Facility RVU | ▣ CCI |
| **FUD** Follow-up Days | **CMS:** IOM (Pub 100) | A-Y OPPSI | 80/80 Surg Assist Allowed / w/Doc | | 🔬 Lab Crosswalk | ☢ Radiology Crosswalk | ✖ CLIA |

244

CPT © 2017 American Medical Association. All Rights Reserved.

© 2017 Optum360, LLC

**54505** Biopsy of testis, incisional (separate procedure) ♂
Code also when combined with epididymogram, seminal vesiculogram or vasogram (55300)
🚑 6.06    ⚘ 6.06    **FUD** 010    J A2 80 50 ▭
**AMA:** 2017,Jan,8; 2016,Jan,13; 2015,Jan,16; 2014,Jan,11

**54512** Excision of extraparenchymal lesion of testis ♂
🚑 15.6    ⚘ 15.6    **FUD** 090    J A2 50 ▭
**AMA:** 2017,Jan,8; 2016,Jan,13; 2015,Jan,16; 2014,Jan,11; 2012,Jan,15-42

**54520** Orchiectomy, simple (including subcapsular), with or without testicular prosthesis, scrotal or inguinal approach ♂
INCLUDES Huggins' orchiectomy
EXCLUDES Lymphadenectomy, radical retroperitoneal (38780)
Code also hernia repair if performed (49505, 49507)
🚑 9.42    ⚘ 9.42    **FUD** 090    J A2 50 ▭
**AMA:** 2017,Jan,8; 2016,Jan,13; 2015,Jan,16; 2014,Jan,11

**54522** Orchiectomy, partial ♂
EXCLUDES Lymphadenectomy, radical retroperitoneal (38780)
🚑 17.0    ⚘ 17.0    **FUD** 090    J A2 80 50 ▭
**AMA:** 2017,Jan,8; 2016,Jan,13; 2015,Jan,16; 2014,Jan,11

**54530** Orchiectomy, radical, for tumor; inguinal approach ♂
EXCLUDES Lymphadenectomy, radical retroperitoneal (38780)
🚑 14.5    ⚘ 14.5    **FUD** 090    J A2 80 50 ▭
**AMA:** 2017,Jan,8; 2016,Jan,13; 2015,Jan,16; 2014,Jan,11

**54535** with abdominal exploration ♂
EXCLUDES Lymphadenectomy, radical retroperitoneal (38780)
🚑 21.7    ⚘ 21.7    **FUD** 090    J 80 50 ▭
**AMA:** 2017,Jan,8; 2016,Jan,13; 2015,Jan,16; 2014,Jan,11

**54550** Exploration for undescended testis (inguinal or scrotal area) ♂
🚑 14.3    ⚘ 14.3    **FUD** 090    J A2 80 50 ▭
**AMA:** 2017,Mar,10; 2017,Jan,8; 2016,Jan,13; 2015,Jan,16; 2014,Jan,11

**54560** Exploration for undescended testis with abdominal exploration ♂
🚑 20.7    ⚘ 20.7    **FUD** 090    J 63 80 50 ▭
**AMA:** 2017,Jan,8; 2016,Jan,13; 2015,Jan,16; 2014,Jan,11

## 54600-54699 Open and Laparoscopic Testicular Procedures

**54600** Reduction of torsion of testis, surgical, with or without fixation of contralateral testis ♂
🚑 13.1    ⚘ 13.1    **FUD** 090    J A2 50 ▭
**AMA:** 2017,Jan,8; 2016,Jan,13; 2015,Jan,16; 2014,Jan,11; 2012,Jan,15-42

Normal testes          Torsion of testis

**54620** Fixation of contralateral testis (separate procedure) ♂
🚑 8.66    ⚘ 8.66    **FUD** 010    J A2 50 ▭
**AMA:** 2014,Jan,11

**54640** Orchiopexy, inguinal approach, with or without hernia repair ♂
INCLUDES Bevan's operation
Koop inguinal orchiopexy
Prentice orchiopexy
EXCLUDES Repair inguinal hernia with inguinal orchiopexy (49495-49525)
🚑 13.8    ⚘ 13.8    **FUD** 090    J A2 80 50 ▭
**AMA:** 2017,Mar,10; 2017,Jan,8; 2016,Jan,13; 2015,Jan,16; 2014,Jan,11; 2012,Jan,15-42

**54650** Orchiopexy, abdominal approach, for intra-abdominal testis (eg, Fowler-Stephens) ♂
EXCLUDES Laparoscopic orchiopexy (54692)
🚑 20.9    ⚘ 20.9    **FUD** 090    J 80 50 ▭
**AMA:** 2017,Jan,8; 2016,Jan,13; 2015,Jan,16; 2014,Jan,11

**54660** Insertion of testicular prosthesis (separate procedure) ♂
🚑 10.5    ⚘ 10.5    **FUD** 090    J A2 80 50 ▭
**AMA:** 2017,Jan,8; 2016,Jan,13; 2015,Jan,16; 2014,Jan,11

**54670** Suture or repair of testicular injury ♂
🚑 11.8    ⚘ 11.8    **FUD** 090    J A2 80 50 ▭
**AMA:** 2017,Jan,8; 2016,Jan,13; 2015,Jan,16; 2014,Jan,11

**54680** Transplantation of testis(es) to thigh (because of scrotal destruction) ♂
🚑 23.1    ⚘ 23.1    **FUD** 090    J A2 80 50 ▭
**AMA:** 2017,Jan,8; 2016,Jan,13; 2015,Jan,16; 2014,Jan,11

**54690** Laparoscopy, surgical; orchiectomy ♂
INCLUDES Diagnostic laparoscopy (49320)
🚑 19.0    ⚘ 19.0    **FUD** 090    J A2 80 50 ▭
**AMA:** 2017,Jan,8; 2016,Jan,13; 2015,Jan,16; 2014,Jan,11

**54692** orchiopexy for intra-abdominal testis ♂
INCLUDES Diagnostic laparoscopy (49320)
🚑 23.0    ⚘ 23.0    **FUD** 090    J 63 50 ▭
**AMA:** 2017,Jan,8; 2016,Jan,13; 2015,Jan,16; 2014,Jan,11

**54699** Unlisted laparoscopy procedure, testis ♂
🚑 0.00    ⚘ 0.00    **FUD** YYY    J 80 50
**AMA:** 2017,Jan,8; 2016,Jan,13; 2015,Jan,16; 2014,Jan,11

## 54700-54901 Open Procedures of the Epididymis

**54700** Incision and drainage of epididymis, testis and/or scrotal space (eg, abscess or hematoma) ♂
EXCLUDES Debridement of genitalia for necrotizing soft tissue infection (11004-11006)
🚑 6.17    ⚘ 6.17    **FUD** 010    J A2 50 ▭
**AMA:** 2017,Jan,8; 2016,Jan,13; 2015,Jan,16; 2014,Jan,11

**54800** Biopsy of epididymis, needle ♂
EXCLUDES Fine needle aspiration (10021, 10022)
�768 88172-88173
🚑 3.85    ⚘ 3.85    **FUD** 000    J A2 80 50 ▭
**AMA:** 2017,Jan,8; 2016,Jan,13; 2015,Jan,16; 2014,Jan,11

**54830** Excision of local lesion of epididymis ♂
🚑 10.7    ⚘ 10.7    **FUD** 090    J A2 80 50 ▭
**AMA:** 2017,Jan,8; 2016,Jan,13; 2015,Jan,16; 2014,Jan,11

**54840** Excision of spermatocele, with or without epididymectomy ♂
🚑 9.27    ⚘ 9.27    **FUD** 090    J A2 50 ▭
**AMA:** 2017,Jan,8; 2016,Jan,13; 2015,Jan,16; 2014,Jan,11

**54860** Epididymectomy; unilateral ♂
🚑 12.0    ⚘ 12.0    **FUD** 090    J A2
**AMA:** 2014,Jan,11

**54861** bilateral ♂
🚑 16.3    ⚘ 16.3    **FUD** 090    J A2 80
**AMA:** 2014,Jan,11

**54865** Exploration of epididymis, with or without biopsy ♂
🚑 10.3    ⚘ 10.3    **FUD** 090    J A2 80
**AMA:** 2014,Jan,11

**54900** Epididymovasostomy, anastomosis of epididymis to vas deferens; unilateral ♂

   *EXCLUDES* *Operating microscope (69990)*

   🔷 24.1   24.1   **FUD** 090    J A2 80 CCI

   **AMA:** 2017,Jan,8; 2016,Jan,13; 2015,Jan,16; 2014,Jan,11; 2012,Jan,15-42

**54901** bilateral ♂

   *EXCLUDES* *Operating microscope (69990)*

   🔷 30.5   30.5   **FUD** 090    J A2 80 CCI

   **AMA:** 2017,Jan,8; 2016,Jan,13; 2015,Jan,16; 2014,Jan,11; 2012,Jan,15-42

## 55000-55180 Procedures of the Tunica Vaginalis and Scrotum

**55000** Puncture aspiration of hydrocele, tunica vaginalis, with or without injection of medication ♂

   🔷 2.46   3.35   **FUD** 000    T P3 50 CCI

   **AMA:** 2014,Jan,11

Testicle
Scrotum

Normal    Noncommunicating hydrocele    Communicating hydrocele    Hydrocele of the cord

**55040** Excision of hydrocele; unilateral ♂

   *EXCLUDES* *Repair of hernia with hydrocelectomy (49495-49501)*

   🔷 9.76   9.76   **FUD** 090    J A2 CCI

   **AMA:** 2017,Jan,8; 2016,Jan,13; 2015,Jan,16; 2014,Jan,11

**55041** bilateral ♂

   *EXCLUDES* *Repair of hernia with hydrocelectomy (49495-49501)*

   🔷 14.7   14.7   **FUD** 090    J A2 CCI

   **AMA:** 2014,Jan,11

**55060** Repair of tunica vaginalis hydrocele (Bottle type) ♂

   🔷 10.9   10.9   **FUD** 090    J A2 80 50 CCI

   **AMA:** 2017,Jan,8; 2016,Jan,13; 2015,Jan,16; 2014,Nov,14; 2014,Jan,11

**55100** Drainage of scrotal wall abscess ♂

   *EXCLUDES* *Debridement of genitalia for necrotizing soft tissue infection (11004-11006)*

   *Incision and drainage of scrotal space (54700)*

   🔷 4.78   6.16   **FUD** 010    J A2 CCI

   **AMA:** 2014,Jan,11

**55110** Scrotal exploration ♂

   🔷 11.2   11.2   **FUD** 090    J A2 CCI

   **AMA:** 2014,Jan,11

**55120** Removal of foreign body in scrotum ♂

   🔷 10.3   10.3   **FUD** 090    J A2 80 CCI

   **AMA:** 2014,Jan,11

**55150** Resection of scrotum ♂

   *EXCLUDES* *Lesion excision of skin of scrotum (11420-11426, 11620-11626)*

   🔷 14.2   14.2   **FUD** 090    J A2 80 CCI

   **AMA:** 2014,Jan,11

**55175** Scrotoplasty; simple ♂

   🔷 10.5   10.5   **FUD** 090    J A2 80 CCI

   **AMA:** 2017,Jan,8; 2016,Jan,13; 2015,Jan,16; 2014,Dec,16; 2014,Dec,16; 2014,Jan,11

**55180** complicated ♂

   🔷 19.8   19.8   **FUD** 090    J A2 80 CCI

   **AMA:** 2014,Jan,11

## 55200-55680 Procedures of Other Male Genital Ducts and Glands

**55200** Vasotomy, cannulization with or without incision of vas, unilateral or bilateral (separate procedure) ♂

   🔷 7.90   12.3   **FUD** 090    J A2 80 CCI

   **AMA:** 2014,Jan,11

**55250** Vasectomy, unilateral or bilateral (separate procedure), including postoperative semen examination(s) ♂

   🔷 6.58   11.0   **FUD** 090    J A2 CCI

   **AMA:** 2017,Jan,8; 2016,Jan,13; 2015,Jan,16; 2014,Jan,11; 2012,Jan,15-42

**55300** Vasotomy for vasograms, seminal vesiculograms, or epididymograms, unilateral or bilateral ♂

   Code also biopsy of testis and modifier 51 when combined (54505)

   📷 (74440)

   🔷 5.43   5.43   **FUD** 000    N N1 80 CCI

   **AMA:** 2014,Jan,11

**55400** Vasovasostomy, vasovasorrhaphy ♂

   *EXCLUDES* *Operating microscope (69990)*

   🔷 14.3   14.3   **FUD** 090    J A2 80 50 CCI

   **AMA:** 2017,Jan,8; 2016,Jan,13; 2015,Jan,16; 2014,Jan,11; 2012,Jan,15-42

**55450** ~~Ligation (percutaneous) of vas deferens, unilateral or bilateral (separate procedure)~~

   To report., see 55250

**55500** Excision of hydrocele of spermatic cord, unilateral (separate procedure) ♂

   🔷 11.4   11.4   **FUD** 090    J A2 80 50 CCI

   **AMA:** 2017,Jan,8; 2016,Jan,13; 2015,Jan,16; 2014,Jan,11

**55520** Excision of lesion of spermatic cord (separate procedure) ♂

   🔷 13.0   13.0   **FUD** 090    J A2 80 50 CCI

   **AMA:** 2017,Jan,8; 2016,Jan,13; 2015,Jan,16; 2014,Jan,11; 2012,Jan,15-42

**55530** Excision of varicocele or ligation of spermatic veins for varicocele; (separate procedure) ♂

   🔷 10.1   10.1   **FUD** 090    J A2 50 CCI

   **AMA:** 2017,Jan,8; 2016,Jan,13; 2015,Jan,16; 2014,Jan,11

**55535** abdominal approach ♂

   🔷 12.4   12.4   **FUD** 090    J A2 80 50 CCI

   **AMA:** 2017,Jan,8; 2016,Jan,13; 2015,Jan,16; 2014,Jan,11

**55540** with hernia repair ♂

   🔷 15.9   15.9   **FUD** 090    J A2 50 CCI

   **AMA:** 2017,Jan,8; 2016,Jan,13; 2015,Jan,16; 2014,Jan,11

**55550** Laparoscopy, surgical, with ligation of spermatic veins for varicocele ♂

   *INCLUDES* *Diagnostic laparoscopy (49320)*

   🔷 12.3   12.3   **FUD** 090    J A2 80 50 CCI

   **AMA:** 2017,Jan,8; 2016,Jan,13; 2015,Jan,16; 2014,Jan,11

**55559** Unlisted laparoscopy procedure, spermatic cord ♂

   🔷 0.00   0.00   **FUD** YYY    J 80 50

   **AMA:** 2017,Jan,8; 2016,Jan,13; 2015,Jan,16; 2014,Jan,11

**55600** Vesiculotomy; ♂

   🔷 12.1   12.1   **FUD** 090    J R2 80 50 CCI

   **AMA:** 2014,Jan,11

**55605** complicated ♂

   🔷 15.7   15.7   **FUD** 090    C 80 50 CCI

   **AMA:** 2014,Jan,11

26/TC PC/TC Only    A2-Z3 ASC Payment    50 Bilateral    ♂ Male Only    ♀ Female Only    🔷 Facility RVU    Non-Facility RVU    CCI

FUD Follow-up Days    CMS: IOM (Pub 100)    A-Y OPPSI    80/80 Surg Assist Allowed / w/Doc    Lab Crosswalk    Radiology Crosswalk    CLIA

CPT © 2017 American Medical Association. All Rights Reserved.     © 2017 Optum360, LLC

| 55650 | **Vesiculectomy, any approach** | ♂ |
|---|---|---|
| | 20.7  20.7  **FUD** 090 | C 80 50 |
| | **AMA:** 2014,Jan,11 | |

| 55680 | **Excision of Mullerian duct cyst** | ♂ |
|---|---|---|
| | EXCLUDES  Injection procedure (52010, 55300) | |
| | 10.5  10.5  **FUD** 090 | J A2 80 50 |
| | **AMA:** 2014,Jan,11 | |

## 55700-55725 Procedures of Prostate: Incisional

| 55700 | **Biopsy, prostate; needle or punch, single or multiple, any approach** | ♂ |
|---|---|---|
| | EXCLUDES  Fine needle aspiration (10021, 10022) | |
| | Needle biopsy of prostate, saturation sampling for prostate mapping (55706) | |
| | (76942, 77002, 77012, 77021) | |
| | (88172-88173) | |
| | 3.79  7.06  **FUD** 000 | J A2 |
| | **AMA:** 2017,Jan,8; 2016,Jan,13; 2015,Jan,16; 2014,Jan,11 | |

| 55705 | **incisional, any approach** | ♂ |
|---|---|---|
| | 7.69  7.69  **FUD** 010 | J A2 |
| | **AMA:** 2014,Jan,11 | |

| 55706 | **Biopsies, prostate, needle, transperineal, stereotactic template guided saturation sampling, including imaging guidance** | ♂ |
|---|---|---|
| | EXCLUDES  Biopsy, prostate; needle or punch (55700) | |
| | 10.7  10.7  **FUD** 010 | J 62 80 |
| | **AMA:** 2017,Jan,8; 2016,Jan,13; 2015,Jan,16; 2014,Jan,11; 2012,Jan,15-42 | |

| 55720 | **Prostatotomy, external drainage of prostatic abscess, any approach; simple** | ♂ |
|---|---|---|
| | EXCLUDES  Drainage of prostatic abscess, transurethral (52700) | |
| | 13.0  13.0  **FUD** 090 | J A2 80 |
| | **AMA:** 2014,Jan,11 | |

| 55725 | **complicated** | ♂ |
|---|---|---|
| | EXCLUDES  Drainage of prostatic abscess, transurethral (52700) | |
| | 18.8  18.8  **FUD** 090 | J A2 80 |
| | **AMA:** 2014,Jan,11 | |

## 55801-55845 Open Prostatectomy

EXCLUDES  Limited pelvic lymphadenectomy for staging (separate procedure) (38562)
Node dissection, independent (38770-38780)
Transurethral prostate
Destruction (53850-53852)
Resection (52601-52640)

| 55801 | **Prostatectomy, perineal, subtotal (including control of postoperative bleeding, vasectomy, meatotomy, urethral calibration and/or dilation, and internal urethrotomy)** | ♂ |
|---|---|---|
| | 31.6  31.6  **FUD** 090 | C 80 |
| | **AMA:** 2014,Jan,11 | |

| 55810 | **Prostatectomy, perineal radical;** | ♂ |
|---|---|---|
| | INCLUDES  Walsh modified radical prostatectomy | |
| | 37.8  37.8  **FUD** 090 | C 80 |
| | **AMA:** 2014,Jan,11 | |

| 55812 | **with lymph node biopsy(s) (limited pelvic lymphadenectomy)** | ♂ |
|---|---|---|
| | 47.8  47.8  **FUD** 090 | C 80 |
| | **AMA:** 2014,Jan,11 | |

| 55815 | **with bilateral pelvic lymphadenectomy, including external iliac, hypogastric and obturator nodes** | ♂ |
|---|---|---|
| | EXCLUDES  When performed on separate days, report: (38770, 55810) | |
| | Pelvic lymphadenectomy, bilateral, and append modifier 50 (38770) | |
| | Perineal radical prostatectomy (55810) | |
| | 51.1  51.1  **FUD** 090 | C 80 |
| | **AMA:** 2014,Jan,11 | |

| 55821 | **Prostatectomy (including control of postoperative bleeding, vasectomy, meatotomy, urethral calibration and/or dilation, and internal urethrotomy); suprapubic, subtotal, 1 or 2 stages** | ♂ |
|---|---|---|
| | 25.2  25.2  **FUD** 090 | C 80 |
| | **AMA:** 2014,Jan,11 | |

| 55831 | **retropubic, subtotal** | ♂ |
|---|---|---|
| | 27.3  27.3  **FUD** 090 | C 80 |
| | **AMA:** 2014,Jan,11 | |

| 55840 | **Prostatectomy, retropubic radical, with or without nerve sparing;** | ♂ |
|---|---|---|
| | EXCLUDES  Prostatectomy, radical retropubic, performed laparoscopically (55866) | |
| | 33.8  33.8  **FUD** 090 | C 80 |
| | **AMA:** 2014,Jan,11 | |

| 55842 | **with lymph node biopsy(s) (limited pelvic lymphadenectomy)** | ♂ |
|---|---|---|
| | EXCLUDES  Prostatectomy, retropubic radical, performed laparoscopically (55866) | |
| | 33.8  33.8  **FUD** 090 | C 80 |
| | **AMA:** 2014,Jan,11 | |

| 55845 | **with bilateral pelvic lymphadenectomy, including external iliac, hypogastric, and obturator nodes** | ♂ |
|---|---|---|
| | EXCLUDES  Prostatectomy, retropubic radical, performed laparoscopically (55866) | |
| | When performed on separate days, report: (38770, 55840) | |
| | Pelvic lymphadenectomy, bilateral, and append modifier 50 (38770) | |
| | Radical prostatectomy, retropubic, with or without nerve sparing (55840) | |
| | 39.4  39.4  **FUD** 090 | C 80 |
| | **AMA:** 2014,Jan,11 | |

## 55860-55865 Prostate Exposure for Radiation Source Application

| 55860 | **Exposure of prostate, any approach, for insertion of radioactive substance;** | ♂ |
|---|---|---|
| | EXCLUDES  Interstitial radioelement application (77770-77772, 77778) | |
| | 25.2  25.2  **FUD** 090 | J 62 |
| | **AMA:** 2014,Jan,11 | |

| 55862 | **with lymph node biopsy(s) (limited pelvic lymphadenectomy)** | ♂ |
|---|---|---|
| | 32.4  32.4  **FUD** 090 | C 80 |
| | **AMA:** 2014,Jan,11 | |

| 55865 | **with bilateral pelvic lymphadenectomy, including external iliac, hypogastric and obturator nodes** | ♂ |
|---|---|---|
| | 38.5  38.5  **FUD** 090 | C 80 |
| | **AMA:** 2014,Jan,11 | |

● New Code  ▲ Revised Code  ○ Reinstated  ● New Web Release  ▲ Revised Web Release  Unlisted  Not Covered  # Resequenced
⊘ AMA Mod 51 Exempt  ⑨ Optum Mod 51 Exempt  ⑥ Mod 63 Exempt  ✗ Non-FDA Drug  ★ Telemedicine  M Maternity  A Age Edit  + Add-on  **AMA:** CPT Asst
© 2017 Optum360, LLC  CPT © 2017 American Medical Association. All Rights Reserved.  **247**

## 55866 Laparoscopic Prostatectomy

**55866**    **Laparoscopy, surgical prostatectomy, retropubic radical, including nerve sparing, includes robotic assistance, when performed** ♂

> INCLUDES    Diagnostic laparoscopy (49320)
>
> EXCLUDES    Open method (55840)
>
> 🚑 41.7   ⚕ 41.7   **FUD** 090     C 80 CCI
>
> **AMA:** 2017,Jan,8; 2016,Jan,13; 2015,Jan,16; 2014,Jan,11; 2012,Mar,9-10

## 55870-55899 Miscellaneous Prostate Procedures

**55870**    **Electroejaculation** ♂

> EXCLUDES    Artificial insemination (58321-58322)
>
> 🚑 4.12   ⚕ 5.04   **FUD** 000     T P3 CCI
>
> **AMA:** 2014,Jan,11

**55873**    **Cryosurgical ablation of the prostate (includes ultrasonic guidance and monitoring)** ♂

> 🚑 22.0   ⚕ 200.   **FUD** 090     J J8 CCI
>
> **AMA:** 2017,Jan,8; 2016,Jan,13; 2015,Sep,12; 2015,Jan,16; 2014,Jan,11

● **55874**    **Transperineal placement of biodegradable material, peri-prostatic, single or multiple injection(s), including image guidance, when performed**

> INCLUDES    Utrasound guidance (76942)

**55875**    **Transperineal placement of needles or catheters into prostate for interstitial radioelement application, with or without cystoscopy** ♂

> Code also interstitial radioelement application (77770-77772, 77778)
>
> 📷 (76965)
>
> 🚑 22.0   ⚕ 22.0   **FUD** 090     Q3 A2 80 CCI
>
> **AMA:** 2017,Jan,8; 2016,Jan,13; 2015,Jan,16; 2014,Jan,11

**55876**    **Placement of interstitial device(s) for radiation therapy guidance (eg, fiducial markers, dosimeter), prostate (via needle, any approach), single or multiple** ♂

> Code also supply of device
>
> 📷 (76942, 77002, 77012, 77021)
>
> 🚑 2.91   ⚕ 3.88   **FUD** 000     S P3 CCI
>
> **AMA:** 2017,Jan,8; 2016,Jun,3; 2016,Jan,13; 2015,Jan,16; 2014,Jan,11; 2012,Jan,15-42

**55899**    **Unlisted procedure, male genital system** ♂

> 🚑 0.00   ⚕ 0.00   **FUD** YYY     T 80
>
> **AMA:** 2017,Jan,6; 2017,Jan,8; 2016,Jan,13; 2015,Jun,5; 2015,Jan,16; 2014,Jan,11

## 55920 Insertion Brachytherapy Catheters/Needles Pelvis/Genitalia, Male/Female

**55920**    **Placement of needles or catheters into pelvic organs and/or genitalia (except prostate) for subsequent interstitial radioelement application**

> EXCLUDES    Insertion of Heyman capsules for purposes of brachytherapy (58346)
>
>           Insertion of vaginal ovoids and/or uterine tandems for purposes of brachytherapy (57155)
>
>           Placement of catheters or needles, prostate (55875)
>
> 🚑 12.9   ⚕ 12.9   **FUD** 000     J G2 80 CCI
>
> **AMA:** 2017,Jan,8; 2016,Jan,13; 2015,Jan,16; 2014,Jan,11

## 55970-55980 Transsexual Surgery

**CMS:** 100-02,16,10 Exclusions from Coverage; 100-02,16,180 Services Related to Noncovered Procedures

**55970**    **Intersex surgery; male to female** ♂

> 🚑 0.00   ⚕ 0.00   **FUD** YYY     J CCI
>
> **AMA:** 2014,Jan,11

**55980**    **female to male** ♀

> 🚑 0.00   ⚕ 0.00   **FUD** YYY     J CCI
>
> **AMA:** 2014,Jan,11

## 56405-56420 Incision and Drainage of Abscess

> EXCLUDES    Incision and drainage Skene's gland cyst/abscess (53060)
>
>           Incision and drainage subcutaneous abscess/cyst/furuncle (10040, 10060, 10061)

**56405**    **Incision and drainage of vulva or perineal abscess** ♀

> 🚑 3.09   ⚕ 3.11   **FUD** 010     T P3 CCI
>
> **AMA:** 2014,Jan,11

**56420**    **Incision and drainage of Bartholin's gland abscess** ♀

> 🚑 2.60   ⚕ 3.44   **FUD** 010     T P3 CCI
>
> **AMA:** 2014,Jan,11

## 56440-56442 Other Female Genital Incisional Procedures

> EXCLUDES    Incision and drainage subcutaneous abscess/cyst/furuncle (10040, 10060, 10061)

**56440**    **Marsupialization of Bartholin's gland cyst** ♀

> 🚑 5.19   ⚕ 5.19   **FUD** 010     J A2 CCI
>
> **AMA:** 2014,Jan,11

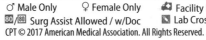

Bartholin's gland abscess · Vaginal orifice · Perineum · Anus

**56441**    **Lysis of labial adhesions** ♀

> 🚑 3.95   ⚕ 4.09   **FUD** 010     J A2 80 CCI
>
> **AMA:** 2014,Jan,11

**56442**    **Hymenotomy, simple incision** ♀

> 🚑 1.36   ⚕ 1.36   **FUD** 000     J A2 80 CCI
>
> **AMA:** 2014,Jan,11

## 56501-56515 Destruction of Vulvar Lesions, Any Method

> EXCLUDES    Excision/fulguration/destruction
>
>           Skene's glands (53270)
>
>           Urethral caruncle (53265)

**56501**    **Destruction of lesion(s), vulva; simple (eg, laser surgery, electrosurgery, cryosurgery, chemosurgery)** ♀

> 🚑 3.28   ⚕ 3.72   **FUD** 010     T P3 CCI
>
> **AMA:** 2014,Jan,11

**56515**    **extensive (eg, laser surgery, electrosurgery, cryosurgery, chemosurgery)** ♀

> 🚑 5.75   ⚕ 6.45   **FUD** 010     T A2 CCI
>
> **AMA:** 2014,Jan,11

## 56605-56606 Vulvar and Perineal Biopsies

> EXCLUDES    Excision local lesion (11420-11426, 11620-11626)

**56605**    **Biopsy of vulva or perineum (separate procedure); 1 lesion** ♀

> 🚑 1.73   ⚕ 2.34   **FUD** 000     T P3 CCI
>
> **AMA:** 2017,Jan,8; 2016,Jan,13; 2015,Jan,16; 2014,Jan,11

+ **56606**    **each separate additional lesion (List separately in addition to code for primary procedure)** ♀

> Code first (56605)
>
> 🚑 0.86   ⚕ 1.08   **FUD** ZZZ     N N1 CCI
>
> **AMA:** 2014,Jan,11

26/TC PC/TC Only    A2-Z6 ASC Payment    50 Bilateral    ♂ Male Only    ♀ Female Only    🚑 Facility RVU    ⚕ Non-Facility RVU    CCI

**FUD** Follow-up Days    **CMS:** IOM (Pub 100)    A-Y OPPSI    80/80 Surg Assist Allowed / w/Doc    Lab Crosswalk    📷 Radiology Crosswalk    CLIA

CPT © 2017 American Medical Association. All Rights Reserved.

## 56620-56640 Vulvectomy Procedures

INCLUDES Removal of:
Greater than 80% of the vulvar area - complete procedure
Less than 80% of the vulvar area - partial procedure
Skin and deep subcutaneous tissue - radical procedure
Skin and superficial subcutaneous tissues - simple procedure

EXCLUDES *Skin graft (15004-15005, 15120-15121, 15240-15241)*

**56620** **Vulvectomy simple; partial** ♀
🚗 14.9    ⚕ 14.9    **FUD** 090    J A2 80 ▢
**AMA:** 2017,Jan,8; 2016,Jan,13; 2015,Jan,16; 2014,Jan,11; 2013,Dec,14

**56625** **complete** ♀
🚗 18.1    ⚕ 18.1    **FUD** 090    J A2 80 ▢
**AMA:** 2014,Jan,11

**56630** **Vulvectomy, radical, partial;** ♀
🚗 26.7    ⚕ 26.7    **FUD** 090    C 80 ▢
**AMA:** 2014,Jan,11

**56631** **with unilateral inguinofemoral lymphadenectomy** ♀
INCLUDES Bassett's operation
🚗 34.0    ⚕ 34.0    **FUD** 090    C 80 ▢
**AMA:** 2014,Jan,11

**56632** **with bilateral inguinofemoral lymphadenectomy** ♀
INCLUDES Bassett's operation
🚗 39.7    ⚕ 39.7    **FUD** 090    C 80 ▢
**AMA:** 2014,Jan,11

**56633** **Vulvectomy, radical, complete;** ♀
INCLUDES Bassett's operation
🚗 34.9    ⚕ 34.9    **FUD** 090    C 80 ▢
**AMA:** 2014,Jan,11

**56634** **with unilateral inguinofemoral lymphadenectomy** ♀
INCLUDES Bassett's operation
🚗 37.4    ⚕ 37.4    **FUD** 090    C 80 ▢
**AMA:** 2014,Jan,11

**56637** **with bilateral inguinofemoral lymphadenectomy** ♀
INCLUDES Bassett's operation
🚗 43.6    ⚕ 43.6    **FUD** 090    C 80 ▢
**AMA:** 2014,Jan,11

**56640** **Vulvectomy, radical, complete, with inguinofemoral, iliac, and pelvic lymphadenectomy** ♀
INCLUDES Bassett's operation
EXCLUDES *Lymphadenectomy (38760-38780)*
🚗 43.9    ⚕ 43.9    **FUD** 090    C 80 50 ▢
**AMA:** 2014,Jan,11

## 56700-56740 Other Excisional Procedures: External Female Genitalia

**56700** **Partial hymenectomy or revision of hymenal ring** ♀
🚗 5.34    ⚕ 5.34    **FUD** 010    J A2 80 ▢
**AMA:** 2014,Jan,11

**56740** **Excision of Bartholin's gland or cyst** ♀
EXCLUDES *Excision/fulguration/marsupialization:*
*Skene's glands (53270)*
*Urethral carcinoma (53220)*
*Urethral caruncle (53265)*
*Urethral diverticulum (53230, 53240)*
🚗 8.58    ⚕ 8.58    **FUD** 010    J A2 50 ▢
**AMA:** 2014,Jan,11

## 56800-56810 Repair/Reconstruction External Female Genitalia

EXCLUDES *Repair of urethra for mucosal prolapse (53275)*

**56800** **Plastic repair of introitus** ♀
INCLUDES Emmet's operation
🚗 6.86    ⚕ 6.86    **FUD** 010    J A2 80 ▢
**AMA:** 2014,Jan,11

**56805** **Clitoroplasty for intersex state** ♀
🚗 36.1    ⚕ 36.1    **FUD** 090    J 62 80 ▢
**AMA:** 2014,Jan,11

**56810** **Perineoplasty, repair of perineum, nonobstetrical (separate procedure)** ♀
INCLUDES Emmet's operation
EXCLUDES *Genitalia wound repair (12001-12007, 12041-12047, 13131-13133)*
*Introitus plastic repair (56800)*
*Sphincteroplasty, anal (46750-46751)*
*Vaginal/perineum recent injury repair, nonobstetrical (57210)*
🚗 7.41    ⚕ 7.41    **FUD** 010    J A2 80 ▢
**AMA:** 2014,Jan,11

## 56820-56821 Vulvar Colposcopy with/without Biopsy

EXCLUDES *Colposcopic procedures and/or examinations:*
*Cervix (57452-57461)*
*Vagina (57420-57421)*

**56820** **Colposcopy of the vulva;** ♀
🚗 2.49    ⚕ 3.20    **FUD** 000    T P3 ▢
**AMA:** 2017,Jan,8; 2016,Jan,13; 2015,Jan,16; 2014,Jan,11

**56821** **with biopsy(s)** ♀
🚗 3.32    ⚕ 4.21    **FUD** 000    T P3 ▢
**AMA:** 2017,Jan,8; 2016,Jan,13; 2015,Jan,16; 2014,Jan,11

## 57000-57023 Incisional Procedures: Vagina

**57000** **Colpotomy; with exploration** ♀
🚗 5.25    ⚕ 5.25    **FUD** 010    J A2 80 ▢
**AMA:** 2017,Jan,8; 2016,Jan,13; 2015,Jan,16; 2014,Jan,11

**57010** **with drainage of pelvic abscess** ♀
INCLUDES Laroyenne operation
🚗 12.3    ⚕ 12.3    **FUD** 090    J A2 80 ▢
**AMA:** 2014,Jan,11

**57020** **Colpocentesis (separate procedure)** ♀
🚗 2.30    ⚕ 2.63    **FUD** 000    J A2 80 ▢
**AMA:** 2014,Jan,11

Speculum  Bladder  Fluid in pelvis

Vagina  Rectum

**The physician aspirates matter from the pelvis through a needle inserted through the vaginal wall**

**57022** **Incision and drainage of vaginal hematoma; obstetrical/postpartum** ♀
🚗 4.89    ⚕ 4.89    **FUD** 010    J R2 80 ▢
**AMA:** 2014,Jan,11

**57023** **non-obstetrical (eg, post-trauma, spontaneous bleeding)** ♀
🚗 8.80    ⚕ 8.80    **FUD** 010    J A2 80 ▢
**AMA:** 2014,Jan,11

**Genital System** *(side tab)*

**57061 — 57260** *(side tab)*

## 57061-57065 Destruction of Vaginal Lesions, Any Method

**CMS:** 100-03,140.5 Laser Procedures

**57061**    Destruction of vaginal lesion(s); simple (eg, laser surgery, electrosurgery, cryosurgery, chemosurgery) ♀
     2.80    3.22   **FUD** 010      J P3
     **AMA:** 2017,Jan,8; 2016,Jan,13; 2015,Jan,16; 2014,Jan,11; 2012,Jan,15-42

**57065**    extensive (eg, laser surgery, electrosurgery, cryosurgery, chemosurgery) ♀
     4.98    5.56   **FUD** 010      J A2
     **AMA:** 2017,Jan,8; 2016,Jan,13; 2015,Jan,16; 2014,Jan,11; 2012,Jan,15-42

## 57100-57135 Excisional Procedures: Vagina

**57100**    Biopsy of vaginal mucosa; simple (separate procedure) ♀
     1.93    2.55   **FUD** 000      T P3
     **AMA:** 2014,Jan,11

**57105**    extensive, requiring suture (including cysts) ♀
     3.61    3.88   **FUD** 010      J A2
     **AMA:** 2014,Jan,11

**57106**    Vaginectomy, partial removal of vaginal wall; ♀
     14.1    14.1   **FUD** 090      J 80
     **AMA:** 2017,Jan,8; 2016,Jan,13; 2015,Jan,16; 2014,Jan,11

**57107**    with removal of paravaginal tissue (radical vaginectomy) ♀
     41.7    41.7   **FUD** 090      J 80
     **AMA:** 2017,Jan,8; 2016,Jan,13; 2015,Jan,16; 2014,Jan,11

**57109**    with removal of paravaginal tissue (radical vaginectomy) with bilateral total pelvic lymphadenectomy and para-aortic lymph node sampling (biopsy) ♀
     50.6    50.6   **FUD** 090      J 80
     **AMA:** 2017,Jan,8; 2016,Jan,13; 2015,Jan,16; 2014,Jan,11

**57110**    Vaginectomy, complete removal of vaginal wall; ♀
     25.4    25.4   **FUD** 090      C 80
     **AMA:** 2017,Jan,8; 2016,Jan,13; 2015,Jan,16; 2014,Jan,11

**57111**    with removal of paravaginal tissue (radical vaginectomy) ♀
     46.2    46.2   **FUD** 090      C 80
     **AMA:** 2017,Jan,8; 2016,Jan,13; 2015,Jan,16; 2014,Jan,11

**57112**    with removal of paravaginal tissue (radical vaginectomy) with bilateral total pelvic lymphadenectomy and para-aortic lymph node sampling (biopsy) ♀
     51.7    51.7   **FUD** 090      C 80
     **AMA:** 2017,Jan,8; 2016,Jan,13; 2015,Jan,16; 2014,Jan,11

**57120**    Colpocleisis (Le Fort type) ♀
     14.4    14.4   **FUD** 090      J 62 80
     **AMA:** 2014,Jan,11

**57130**    Excision of vaginal septum ♀
     4.51    5.02   **FUD** 010      J A2 80
     **AMA:** 2014,Jan,11

**57135**    Excision of vaginal cyst or tumor ♀
     4.94    5.46   **FUD** 010      J A2
     **AMA:** 2014,Jan,11

## 57150-57180 Irrigation/Insertion/Introduction Vaginal Medication or Supply

**57150**    Irrigation of vagina and/or application of medicament for treatment of bacterial, parasitic, or fungoid disease ♀
     0.83    1.28   **FUD** 000      Q1 N1
     **AMA:** 2014,Jan,11

**57155**    Insertion of uterine tandem and/or vaginal ovoids for clinical brachytherapy ♀
     **EXCLUDES** *Insertion of radioelement sources or ribbons (77761-77763, 77770-77772)*
     *The placement of needles or catheters into the pelvic organs and/or genitalia (except for the prostate) for interstitial radioelement application (55920)*
     7.98    10.3   **FUD** 000      J A2
     **AMA:** 2017,Jan,8; 2016,Jan,13; 2015,Jan,16; 2014,Jan,11

**57156**    Insertion of a vaginal radiation afterloading apparatus for clinical brachytherapy ♀
     4.21    5.65   **FUD** 000      T 62 80
     **AMA:** 2014,Jan,11

**57160**    Fitting and insertion of pessary or other intravaginal support device ♀
     1.34    2.17   **FUD** 000      T P3
     **AMA:** 2017,Jan,8; 2016,Jan,13; 2015,Jan,16; 2014,Jan,11; 2012,Jan,15-42

**57170**    Diaphragm or cervical cap fitting with instructions ♀
     1.39    1.73   **FUD** 000      T P3 80
     **AMA:** 2014,Jan,11

**57180**    Introduction of any hemostatic agent or pack for spontaneous or traumatic nonobstetrical vaginal hemorrhage (separate procedure) ♀
     3.00    3.98   **FUD** 010      T A2
     **AMA:** 2017,Jan,8; 2016,Jan,13; 2015,Jan,16; 2014,Jan,11

## 57200-57335 Vaginal Repair and Reconstruction

**EXCLUDES** *Marshall-Marchetti-Kranz type urethral suspension, abdominal approach (51840-51841)*
*Urethral suspension performed laparoscopically (51990)*

**57200**    Colporrhaphy, suture of injury of vagina (nonobstetrical) ♀
     8.62    8.62   **FUD** 090      J A2 80
     **AMA:** 2014,Jan,11

**57210**    Colpoperineorrhaphy, suture of injury of vagina and/or perineum (nonobstetrical) ♀
     10.4    10.4   **FUD** 090      J A2 80
     **AMA:** 2014,Jan,11

**57220**    Plastic operation on urethral sphincter, vaginal approach (eg, Kelly urethral plication) ♀
     9.09    9.09   **FUD** 090      J A2 80
     **AMA:** 2014,Jan,11

**57230**    Plastic repair of urethrocele ♀
     11.2    11.2   **FUD** 090      J A2 80
     **AMA:** 2014,Jan,11

▲ **57240**    Anterior colporrhaphy, repair of cystocele with or without repair of urethrocele, including cystourethroscopy, when performed ♀
     **EXCLUDES** *Cystourethroscopy (52000)*
     19.1    19.1   **FUD** 090      J A2 80
     **AMA:** 2017,Jan,8; 2016,Jan,13; 2015,Jan,16; 2014,Jan,11

**57250**    Posterior colporrhaphy, repair of rectocele with or without perineorrhaphy ♀
     **EXCLUDES** *Rectocele repair (separate procedure) without posterior colporrhaphy (45560)*
     19.2    19.2   **FUD** 090      J A2 80
     **AMA:** 2017,Jan,8; 2016,Jan,13; 2015,Jan,16; 2014,Jan,11; 2012,Jan,15-42

▲ **57260**    Combined anteroposterior colporrhaphy, including cystourethroscopy, when performed ♀
     **EXCLUDES** *Cystourethroscopy (52000)*
     23.6    23.6   **FUD** 090      J A2 80
     **AMA:** 2017,Jan,8; 2016,Jan,13; 2015,Jan,16; 2014,Jan,11

**Genital System**

**57265 — 57410**

▲ **57265** **with enterocele repair** ♀
  EXCLUDES *Cystourethroscopy (52000)*
  🔧 25.9 ⚕ 25.9 **FUD** 090 [J] [A2] [80] [▭]
  **AMA:** 2017,Jan,8; 2016,Jan,13; 2015,Jan,16; 2014,Jan,11

+ **57267** **Insertion of mesh or other prosthesis for repair of pelvic floor defect, each site (anterior, posterior compartment), vaginal approach (List separately in addition to code for primary procedure)** ♀
  Code first (45560, 57240-57265, 57285)
  🔧 7.31 ⚕ 7.31 **FUD** ZZZ [N] [N1] [80] [▭]
  **AMA:** 2017,Jan,8; 2016,Jan,13; 2015,Jan,16; 2014,Jan,11; 2013,Oct,15; 2012,Jan,15-42; 2012,Jan,6-10

**57268** **Repair of enterocele, vaginal approach (separate procedure)** ♀
  🔧 13.7 ⚕ 13.7 **FUD** 090 [J] [A2] [80] [▭]
  **AMA:** 2017,Jan,8; 2016,Jan,13; 2015,Jan,16; 2014,Jan,11

**57270** **Repair of enterocele, abdominal approach (separate procedure)** ♀
  🔧 22.8 ⚕ 22.8 **FUD** 090 [C] [80] [▭]
  **AMA:** 2017,Jan,8; 2016,Jan,13; 2015,Jan,16; 2014,Jan,11

**57280** **Colpopexy, abdominal approach** ♀
  🔧 27.1 ⚕ 27.1 **FUD** 090 [C] [80] [▭]
  **AMA:** 2017,Jan,8; 2016,Jan,13; 2015,Jan,16; 2014,Jan,11

**57282** **Colpopexy, vaginal; extra-peritoneal approach (sacrospinous, iliococcygeus)** ♀
  🔧 14.2 ⚕ 14.2 **FUD** 090 [J] [80] [▭]
  **AMA:** 2017,Jan,8; 2016,Jan,13; 2015,Jan,16; 2014,Jan,11

**57283** **intra-peritoneal approach (uterosacral, levator myorrhaphy)** ♀
  EXCLUDES *Excision of cervical stump (57556)*
  *Vaginal hysterectomy (58263, 58270, 58280, 58292, 58294)*
  🔧 19.5 ⚕ 19.5 **FUD** 090 [J] [80] [▭]
  **AMA:** 2017,Jan,8; 2016,Jan,13; 2015,Jan,16; 2014,Jan,11; 2012,Jan,15-42

**57284** **Paravaginal defect repair (including repair of cystocele, if performed); open abdominal approach** ♀
  EXCLUDES *Anterior colporrhaphy (57240)*
  *Anterior vesicourethropexy (51840-51841)*
  *Combined anteroposterior colporrhaphy (57260-57265)*
  *Hysterectomy (58152, 58267)*
  *Laparoscopy, surgical; urethral suspension for stress incontinence (51990)*
  🔧 23.2 ⚕ 23.2 **FUD** 090 [J] [80] [▭]
  **AMA:** 2017,Jan,8; 2016,Jan,13; 2015,Jan,16; 2014,Jan,11; 2012,Jan,15-42

**57285** **vaginal approach** ♀
  EXCLUDES *Anterior colporrhaphy (57240)*
  *Combined anteroposterior colporrhaphy (57260-57265)*
  *Laparoscopy, surgical; urethral suspension for stress incontinence (51990)*
  *Vaginal hysterectomy (58267)*
  🔧 19.1 ⚕ 19.1 **FUD** 090 [J] [80] [▭]
  **AMA:** 2017,Jan,8; 2016,Jan,13; 2015,Jan,16; 2014,Jan,11

**57287** **Removal or revision of sling for stress incontinence (eg, fascia or synthetic)** ♀
  🔧 19.4 ⚕ 19.4 **FUD** 090 [02] [62] [80] [▭]
  **AMA:** 2017,Jan,8; 2016,Jan,13; 2015,Jan,16; 2014,Jan,11; 2012,Jan,15-42

**57288** **Sling operation for stress incontinence (eg, fascia or synthetic)** ♀
  INCLUDES *Millin-Read operation*
  EXCLUDES *Sling operation for stress incontinence performed laparoscopically (51992)*
  🔧 20.4 ⚕ 20.4 **FUD** 090 [J] [A2] [80] [▭]
  **AMA:** 2017,Jan,8; 2016,Jan,13; 2015,Jan,16; 2014,Jan,11; 2012,Jan,15-42

**57289** **Pereyra procedure, including anterior colporrhaphy** ♀
  🔧 21.0 ⚕ 21.0 **FUD** 090 [J] [A2] [80] [▭]
  **AMA:** 2017,Jan,8; 2016,Jan,13; 2015,Jan,16; 2014,Jan,11

**57291** **Construction of artificial vagina; without graft** ♀
  INCLUDES *McIndoe vaginal construction*
  🔧 15.0 ⚕ 15.0 **FUD** 090 [J] [A2] [80] [▭]
  **AMA:** 2014,Jan,11

**57292** **with graft** ♀
  🔧 23.2 ⚕ 23.2 **FUD** 090 [J] [80] [▭]
  **AMA:** 2014,Jan,11

**57295** **Revision (including removal) of prosthetic vaginal graft; vaginal approach** ♀
  EXCLUDES *Laparoscopic approach (57426)*
  🔧 13.5 ⚕ 13.5 **FUD** 090 [J] [62] [80] [▭]
  **AMA:** 2014,Jan,11

**57296** **open abdominal approach** ♀
  EXCLUDES *Laparoscopic approach (57426)*
  🔧 26.6 ⚕ 26.6 **FUD** 090 [C] [80] [▭]
  **AMA:** 2014,Jan,11

**57300** **Closure of rectovaginal fistula; vaginal or transanal approach** ♀
  🔧 16.0 ⚕ 16.0 **FUD** 090 [J] [A2] [80] [▭]
  **AMA:** 2014,Jan,11

**57305** **abdominal approach** ♀
  🔧 26.8 ⚕ 26.8 **FUD** 090 [C] [80] [▭]
  **AMA:** 2014,Jan,11

**57307** **abdominal approach, with concomitant colostomy** ♀
  🔧 30.2 ⚕ 30.2 **FUD** 090 [C] [80] [▭]
  **AMA:** 2014,Jan,11

**57308** **transperineal approach, with perineal body reconstruction, with or without levator plication** ♀
  🔧 18.1 ⚕ 18.1 **FUD** 090 [C] [80] [▭]
  **AMA:** 2014,Jan,11

**57310** **Closure of urethrovaginal fistula;** ♀
  🔧 13.3 ⚕ 13.3 **FUD** 090 [J] [62] [80] [▭]
  **AMA:** 2014,Jan,11

**57311** **with bulbocavernosus transplant** ♀
  🔧 15.0 ⚕ 15.0 **FUD** 090 [C] [80] [▭]
  **AMA:** 2014,Jan,11

**57320** **Closure of vesicovaginal fistula; vaginal approach** ♀
  EXCLUDES *Cystostomy, concomitant (51020-51040, 51101-51102)*
  🔧 15.2 ⚕ 15.2 **FUD** 090 [J] [62] [80] [▭]
  **AMA:** 2014,Jan,11

**57330** **transvesical and vaginal approach** ♀
  EXCLUDES *Vesicovaginal fistula closure, abdominal approach (51900)*
  🔧 21.5 ⚕ 21.5 **FUD** 090 [J] [80] [▭]
  **AMA:** 2014,Jan,11

**57335** **Vaginoplasty for intersex state** ♀
  🔧 35.6 ⚕ 35.6 **FUD** 090 [J] [80] [▭]
  **AMA:** 2014,Jan,11

## 57400-57415 Treatment of Vaginal Disorders Under Anesthesia

**57400** **Dilation of vagina under anesthesia (other than local)** ♀
  🔧 3.85 ⚕ 3.85 **FUD** 000 [J] [A2] [80] [▭]
  **AMA:** 2014,Jan,11

**57410** **Pelvic examination under anesthesia (other than local)** ♀
  🔧 3.08 ⚕ 3.08 **FUD** 000 [J] [A2] [▭]
  **AMA:** 2017,Jan,8; 2016,Jan,13; 2015,Jan,16; 2014,Jan,11

---

● New Code  ▲ Revised Code  ○ Reinstated  ● New Web Release  ▲ Revised Web Release  Unlisted  Not Covered  # Resequenced
⊘ AMA Mod 51 Exempt  ⑤⑦ Optum Mod 51 Exempt  ⑥③ Mod 63 Exempt  ✗ Non-FDA Drug  ★ Telemedicine  Ⓜ Maternity  Ⓐ Age Edit  + Add-on  **AMA:** CPT Asst

**57415** Removal of impacted vaginal foreign body (separate procedure) under anesthesia (other than local) ♀

> EXCLUDES Removal of impacted vaginal foreign body without anesthesia, report with appropriate E&M code

🔧 4.56 ⚕ 4.56 **FUD** 010 [J] [A2] [80] 🖥

**AMA:** 2014,Jan,11

## 57420-57426 Endoscopic Vaginal Procedures

**57420** Colposcopy of the entire vagina, with cervix if present; ♀

> EXCLUDES Colposcopic procedures and/or examinations:
> Cervix (57452-57461)
> Vulva (56820-56821)
> Code also endometrial sampling (biopsy) performed at the same time as colposcopy (58110)
> Code also modifier 51 for colposcopic procedures of different sites, as appropriate

🔧 2.64 ⚕ 3.36 **FUD** 000 [T] [P3] 🖥

**AMA:** 2017,Jan,8; 2016,Jan,13; 2015,Jan,16; 2014,Jan,11

**57421** with biopsy(s) of vagina/cervix ♀

> EXCLUDES Colposcopic procedures and/or examinations:
> Cervix (57452-57461)
> Vulva (56820-56821)
> Code also endometrial sampling (biopsy) performed at the same time as colposcopy (58110)
> Code also modifier 51 for colposcopic procedures of multiple sites, as appropriate

🔧 3.56 ⚕ 4.48 **FUD** 000 [T] [P3] 🖥

**AMA:** 2017,Jan,8; 2016,Jan,13; 2015,Jan,16; 2014,Jan,11; 2012,Jan,15-42

**57423** Paravaginal defect repair (including repair of cystocele, if performed), laparoscopic approach ♀

> EXCLUDES Anterior colporrhaphy (57240)
> Anterior vesicourethropexy (51840-51841)
> Combined anteroposterior colporrhaphy (57260)
> Diagnostic laparoscopy (49320)
> Hysterectomy (58152, 58267)
> Laparoscopy, surgical; urethral suspension for stress incontinence (51990)

🔧 25.9 ⚕ 25.9 **FUD** 090 [J] [80] 🖥

**AMA:** 2017,Jan,8; 2016,Jan,13; 2015,Jan,16; 2014,Jan,11

**57425** Laparoscopy, surgical, colpopexy (suspension of vaginal apex) ♀

🔧 27.6 ⚕ 27.6 **FUD** 090 [J] [80] 🖥

**AMA:** 2014,Jan,11

**57426** Revision (including removal) of prosthetic vaginal graft, laparoscopic approach ♀

> EXCLUDES Open abdominal approach (57296)
> Vaginal approach (57295)

🔧 23.9 ⚕ 23.9 **FUD** 090 [J] [G2] [80] 🖥

**AMA:** 2014,Jan,11

## 57452-57461 Endoscopic Cervical Procedures

> EXCLUDES Colposcopic procedures and/or examinations:
> Vagina (57420-57421)
> Vulva (56820-56821)
> Code also endometrial sampling (biopsy) performed at the same time as colposcopy (58110)

**57452** Colposcopy of the cervix including upper/adjacent vagina; ♀

🔧 2.64 ⚕ 3.10 **FUD** 000 [T] [P3] 🖥

**AMA:** 2017,Jan,8; 2016,Jan,13; 2015,Jan,16; 2014,Jan,11

Speculum — 
Light beam — 
— Uterus
— Cervix
— Vagina
Colposcope

**57454** with biopsy(s) of the cervix and endocervical curettage ♀

> INCLUDES Colposcopy of the cervix (57452)

🔧 3.88 ⚕ 4.34 **FUD** 000 [T] [P3] 🖥

**AMA:** 2017,Jan,8; 2016,Jan,13; 2015,Jan,16; 2014,Jan,11; 2012,Jan,15-42

**57455** with biopsy(s) of the cervix ♀

> INCLUDES Colposcopy of the cervix (57452)

🔧 3.17 ⚕ 4.05 **FUD** 000 [T] [P3] 🖥

**AMA:** 2017,Jan,8; 2016,Jan,13; 2015,Jan,16; 2014,Jan,11

**57456** with endocervical curettage ♀

> INCLUDES Colposcopy of the cervix (57452)
> EXCLUDES Colposcopy of the cervix including upper/adjacent vagina; with loop electrode conization of the cervix (57461)

🔧 2.95 ⚕ 3.82 **FUD** 000 [T] [P3] 🖥

**AMA:** 2017,Jan,8; 2016,Jan,13; 2015,Jan,16; 2014,Jan,11; 2012,Jan,15-42

**57460** with loop electrode biopsy(s) of the cervix ♀

> INCLUDES Colposcopy of the cervix (57452)

🔧 4.64 ⚕ 8.00 **FUD** 000 [J] [P3] 🖥

**AMA:** 2017,Jan,8; 2016,Jan,13; 2015,Jan,16; 2014,Jan,11; 2012,Jan,15-42

**57461** with loop electrode conization of the cervix ♀

> INCLUDES Colposcopy of the cervix (57452)
> EXCLUDES Colposcopy of the cervix including upper/adjacent vagina; with endocervical curettage (57456)

🔧 5.36 ⚕ 9.06 **FUD** 000 [J] [P3] 🖥

**AMA:** 2017,Jan,8; 2016,Jan,13; 2015,Jan,16; 2014,Jan,11; 2012,Jan,15-42

## 57500-57556 Cervical Procedures: Multiple Techniques

> EXCLUDES Radical surgical procedures (58200-58240)

**57500** Biopsy of cervix, single or multiple, or local excision of lesion, with or without fulguration (separate procedure) ♀

🔧 2.17 ⚕ 3.62 **FUD** 000 [T] [P3] 🖥

**AMA:** 2014,Jan,11

**57505** Endocervical curettage (not done as part of a dilation and curettage) ♀

🔧 2.63 ⚕ 2.90 **FUD** 010 [T] [P3] 🖥

**AMA:** 2017,Jan,8; 2016,Jan,13; 2015,Jan,16; 2014,Jan,11; 2012,Jan,15-42

[26]/[TC] PC/TC Only   [A2]-[Z3] ASC Payment   [50] Bilateral   ♂ Male Only   ♀ Female Only   🔧 Facility RVU   ⚕ Non-Facility RVU   🖥 CCI
**FUD** Follow-up Days   **CMS:** IOM (Pub 100)   [A]-[Y] OPPSI   [80]/[80] Surg Assist Allowed / w/Doc   🧪 Lab Crosswalk   ⊞ Radiology Crosswalk   ⊠ CLIA

252   CPT © 2017 American Medical Association. All Rights Reserved.   © 2017 Optum360, LLC

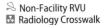

**57510**   **Cautery of cervix; electro or thermal**   ♀
   🚗 3.29   ⚕ 3.72   **FUD** 010   J P3 ▭
   **AMA:** 2014,Jan,11

**57511**   **cryocautery, initial or repeat**   ♀
   🚗 3.76   ⚕ 4.11   **FUD** 010   T P3 ▭
   **AMA:** 2014,Jan,11

**57513**   **laser ablation**   ♀
   🚗 3.82   ⚕ 4.12   **FUD** 010   J A2 ▭
   **AMA:** 2014,Jan,11

**57520**   **Conization of cervix, with or without fulguration, with or without dilation and curettage, with or without repair; cold knife or laser**
   EXCLUDES   *Dilation and curettage, diagnostic/therapeutic, nonobstetrical (58120)*
   🚗 7.87   ⚕ 8.75   **FUD** 090   J A2 ▭
   **AMA:** 2017,Jan,8; 2016,Jan,13; 2015,Jan,16; 2014,Jan,11

**57522**   **loop electrode excision**   ♀
   🚗 6.93   ⚕ 7.48   **FUD** 090   J A2 ▭
   **AMA:** 2017,Jan,8; 2016,Jan,13; 2015,Jan,16; 2014,Jan,11; 2012,Jan,15-42

**57530**   **Trachelectomy (cervicectomy), amputation of cervix (separate procedure)**   ♀
   🚗 9.90   ⚕ 9.90   **FUD** 090   J A2 80 ▭
   **AMA:** 2014,Jan,11

**57531**   **Radical trachelectomy, with bilateral total pelvic lymphadenectomy and para-aortic lymph node sampling biopsy, with or without removal of tube(s), with or without removal of ovary(s)**   ♀
   EXCLUDES   *Radical hysterectomy (58210)*
   🚗 52.9   ⚕ 52.9   **FUD** 090   C 80 ▭
   **AMA:** 2014,Jan,11

**57540**   **Excision of cervical stump, abdominal approach;**   ♀
   🚗 24.0   ⚕ 24.0   **FUD** 090   C 80 ▭
   **AMA:** 2014,Jan,11

**57545**   **with pelvic floor repair**   ♀
   🚗 23.7   ⚕ 23.7   **FUD** 090   C 80 ▭
   **AMA:** 2014,Jan,11

**57550**   **Excision of cervical stump, vaginal approach;**   ♀
   🚗 11.5   ⚕ 11.5   **FUD** 090   J A2 80 ▭
   **AMA:** 2014,Jan,11

**57555**   **with anterior and/or posterior repair**   ♀
   🚗 17.1   ⚕ 17.1   **FUD** 090   J 80 ▭
   **AMA:** 2014,Jan,11

**57556**   **with repair of enterocele**   ♀
   EXCLUDES   *Insertion of hemostatic agent/pack for spontaneous/traumatic nonobstetrical vaginal hemorrhage (57180)*
   *Intrauterine device insertion (58300)*
   🚗 16.0   ⚕ 16.0   **FUD** 090   J A2 80 ▭
   **AMA:** 2014,Jan,11

## 57558-57800 Cervical Procedures: Dilation, Suturing, or Instrumentation

**57558**   **Dilation and curettage of cervical stump**   ♀
   EXCLUDES   *Radical surgical procedures (58200-58240)*
   🚗 3.22   ⚕ 3.52   **FUD** 010   J A2 ▭
   **AMA:** 2014,Jan,11

**57700**   **Cerclage of uterine cervix, nonobstetrical**   ♀
   INCLUDES   McDonald cerclage
   Shirodker operation
   🚗 8.91   ⚕ 8.91   **FUD** 090   J A2 80 ▭
   **AMA:** 2014,Jan,11

**57720**   **Trachelorrhaphy, plastic repair of uterine cervix, vaginal approach**   ♀
   INCLUDES   Emmet operation
   🚗 8.74   ⚕ 8.74   **FUD** 090   J A2 80 ▭
   **AMA:** 2014,Jan,11

**57800**   **Dilation of cervical canal, instrumental (separate procedure)**   ♀
   🚗 1.39   ⚕ 1.72   **FUD** 000   J P3 ▭
   **AMA:** 2014,Jan,11

## 58100-58120 Procedures Involving the Endometrium

**58100**   **Endometrial sampling (biopsy) with or without endocervical sampling (biopsy), without cervical dilation, any method (separate procedure)**   ♀
   EXCLUDES   *Endocervical curettage only (57505)*
   *Endometrial sampling (biopsy) performed in conjunction with colposcopy (58110)*
   🚗 2.50   ⚕ 3.10   **FUD** 000   T P3 ▭
   **AMA:** 2014,Jan,11

+   **58110**   **Endometrial sampling (biopsy) performed in conjunction with colposcopy (List separately in addition to code for primary procedure)**   ♀
   Code first colposcopy (57420-57421, 57452-57461)
   🚗 1.17   ⚕ 1.36   **FUD** ZZZ   N N1 80 ▭
   **AMA:** 2017,Jan,8; 2016,Jan,13; 2015,Jan,16; 2014,Jan,11

**58120**   **Dilation and curettage, diagnostic and/or therapeutic (nonobstetrical)**   ♀
   EXCLUDES   *Postpartum hemorrhage (59160)*
   🚗 6.24   ⚕ 7.34   **FUD** 010   J A2 ▭
   **AMA:** 2017,Jan,8; 2016,Jan,13; 2015,Jan,16; 2014,Jan,11; 2012,Jan,15-42

Uterus
Endometrial lining
Curette
Cervix and cervical canal
Vaginal canal
Dilator expands cervical opening

## 58140-58146 Myomectomy Procedures

**58140**   **Myomectomy, excision of fibroid tumor(s) of uterus, 1 to 4 intramural myoma(s) with total weight of 250 g or less and/or removal of surface myomas; abdominal approach**   ♀
   🚗 26.1   ⚕ 26.1   **FUD** 090   C 80 ▭
   **AMA:** 2017,Jan,8; 2016,Jan,13; 2015,Jan,16; 2014,Jan,11; 2012,Jan,15-42

**58145**   **vaginal approach**   ♀
   🚗 15.6   ⚕ 15.6   **FUD** 090   J A2 80 ▭
   **AMA:** 2014,Jan,11

**58146**   **Myomectomy, excision of fibroid tumor(s) of uterus, 5 or more intramural myomas and/or intramural myomas with total weight greater than 250 g, abdominal approach**   ♀
   EXCLUDES   *Hysterectomy (58150-58240)*
   *Myomectomy procedures (58140-58145)*
   🚗 32.7   ⚕ 32.7   **FUD** 090   C 80 ▭
   **AMA:** 2017,Jan,8; 2016,Jan,13; 2015,Jan,16; 2014,Jan,11; 2012,Jan,15-42

## 58150-58294 Abdominal and Vaginal Hysterectomies

**CMS:** 100-03,230.3 Sterilization

*EXCLUDES* Destruction/excision of endometriomas, open method (49203-49205, 58957-58958)
Paracentesis (49082-49083)
Pelvic laparotomy (49000)
Secondary closure disruption or evisceration of abdominal wall (49900)

**58150** Total abdominal hysterectomy (corpus and cervix), with or without removal of tube(s), with or without removal of ovary(s); ♀
🚑 29.0  ⚕ 29.0  **FUD** 090  [C] [80] 🔲
**AMA:** 2017,Jan,8; 2016,Jan,13; 2015,Jan,16; 2014,Jan,11; 2012,Jan,15-42

**58152** with colpo-urethrocystopexy (eg, Marshall-Marchetti-Krantz, Burch) ♀
*EXCLUDES* Urethrocystopexy without hysterectomy (51840-51841)
🚑 35.5  ⚕ 35.5  **FUD** 090  [C] [80] 🔲
**AMA:** 2017,Jan,8; 2016,Jan,13; 2015,Jan,16; 2014,Jan,11

**58180** Supracervical abdominal hysterectomy (subtotal hysterectomy), with or without removal of tube(s), with or without removal of ovary(s) ♀
🚑 27.4  ⚕ 27.4  **FUD** 090  [C] [80] 🔲
**AMA:** 2014,Jan,11

**58200** Total abdominal hysterectomy, including partial vaginectomy, with para-aortic and pelvic lymph node sampling, with or without removal of tube(s), with or without removal of ovary(s) ♀
🚑 39.4  ⚕ 39.4  **FUD** 090  [C] [80] 🔲
**AMA:** 2014,Jan,11

**58210** Radical abdominal hysterectomy, with bilateral total pelvic lymphadenectomy and para-aortic lymph node sampling (biopsy), with or without removal of tube(s), with or without removal of ovary(s) ♀
*INCLUDES* Wertheim hysterectomy
*EXCLUDES* Chemotherapy (96401-96549)
Hysterectomy, radical, with transposition of ovary(s) (58825)
🚑 53.2  ⚕ 53.2  **FUD** 090  [C] [80] 🔲
**AMA:** 2017,Jan,8; 2016,Jan,13; 2015,Jan,16; 2014,Jan,11; 2012,May,14-15

**58240** Pelvic exenteration for gynecologic malignancy, with total abdominal hysterectomy or cervicectomy, with or without removal of tube(s), with or without removal of ovary(s), with removal of bladder and ureteral transplantations, and/or abdominoperineal resection of rectum and colon and colostomy, or any combination thereof ♀
*EXCLUDES* Chemotherapy (96401-96549)
Pelvic exenteration for male genital malignancy or lower urinary tract (51597)
🚑 83.7  ⚕ 83.7  **FUD** 090  [C] [80] 🔲
**AMA:** 2014,Jan,11

**58260** Vaginal hysterectomy, for uterus 250 g or less; ♀
🚑 23.4  ⚕ 23.4  **FUD** 090  [J] [62] [80] 🔲
**AMA:** 2017,Jan,8; 2016,Jan,13; 2015,Jan,16; 2014,Jan,11

**58262** with removal of tube(s), and/or ovary(s) ♀
🚑 26.1  ⚕ 26.1  **FUD** 090  [J] [62] [80] 🔲
**AMA:** 2014,Jan,11

**58263** with removal of tube(s), and/or ovary(s), with repair of enterocele ♀
🚑 28.0  ⚕ 28.0  **FUD** 090  [J] [80] 🔲
**AMA:** 2014,Jan,11

**58267** with colpo-urethrocystopexy (Marshall-Marchetti-Krantz type, Pereyra type) with or without endoscopic control ♀
🚑 29.7  ⚕ 29.7  **FUD** 090  [C] [80] 🔲
**AMA:** 2017,Jan,8; 2016,Jan,13; 2015,Jan,16; 2014,Jan,11

**58270** with repair of enterocele ♀
*EXCLUDES* Vaginal hysterectomy with repair of enterocele and removal of tubes and/or ovaries (58263)
🚑 25.0  ⚕ 25.0  **FUD** 090  [J] [80] 🔲
**AMA:** 2014,Jan,11

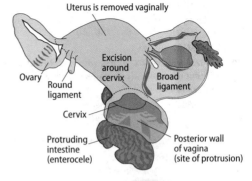

Uterus is removed vaginally
Ovary
Round ligament
Excision around cervix
Cervix
Broad ligament
Protruding intestine (enterocele)
Posterior wall of vagina (site of protrusion)

Repair of enterocele
Posterior vaginal wall

**58275** Vaginal hysterectomy, with total or partial vaginectomy; ♀
🚑 27.9  ⚕ 27.9  **FUD** 090  [C] [80] 🔲
**AMA:** 2014,Jan,11

**58280** with repair of enterocele ♀
🚑 29.8  ⚕ 29.8  **FUD** 090  [C] [80] 🔲
**AMA:** 2014,Jan,11

**58285** Vaginal hysterectomy, radical (Schauta type operation) ♀
🚑 41.0  ⚕ 41.0  **FUD** 090  [C] [80] 🔲
**AMA:** 2017,Jan,8; 2016,Jan,13; 2015,Jan,16; 2014,Jan,11

**58290** Vaginal hysterectomy, for uterus greater than 250 g; ♀
🚑 32.6  ⚕ 32.6  **FUD** 090  [J] [80] 🔲
**AMA:** 2014,Jan,11

**58291** with removal of tube(s) and/or ovary(s) ♀
🚑 35.2  ⚕ 35.2  **FUD** 090  [J] [80] 🔲
**AMA:** 2014,Jan,11

**58292** with removal of tube(s) and/or ovary(s), with repair of enterocele ♀
🚑 37.1  ⚕ 37.1  **FUD** 090  [J] [80] 🔲
**AMA:** 2014,Jan,11

**58293** with colpo-urethrocystopexy (Marshall-Marchetti-Krantz type, Pereyra type) with or without endoscopic control ♀
🚑 38.6  ⚕ 38.6  **FUD** 090  [C] [80] 🔲
**AMA:** 2014,Jan,11

**58294** with repair of enterocele ♀
🚑 34.4  ⚕ 34.4  **FUD** 090  [J] [80] 🔲
**AMA:** 2014,Jan,11

## 58300-58323 Contraception and Reproduction Procedures

**58300** Insertion of intrauterine device (IUD) ♀
*EXCLUDES* Insertion and/or removal of implantable contraceptive capsules (11976, 11981-11983)
🚑 1.54  ⚕ 2.06  **FUD** XXX  [E] 🔲
**AMA:** 2017,Jan,8; 2016,Jan,13; 2015,Jan,16; 2014,Jan,11; 2012,Jan,15-42

[26]/[TC] PC/TC Only  [A2]-[Z3] ASC Payment  [50] Bilateral  ♂ Male Only  ♀ Female Only  🚑 Facility RVU  ⚕ Non-Facility RVU  🔲 CCI
**FUD** Follow-up Days  **CMS:** IOM (Pub 100)  [A]-[Y] OPPSI  [80]/[80] Surg Assist Allowed / w/Doc  🧪 Lab Crosswalk  ☢ Radiology Crosswalk  ✖ CLIA

CPT © 2017 American Medical Association. All Rights Reserved.  © 2017 Optum360, LLC

Genital System

58150 — 58300

**58301** Removal of intrauterine device (IUD) ♀

    EXCLUDES *Insertion and/or removal of implantable contraceptive capsules (11976, 11981-11983)*

    🖫 1.93   ⚕ 2.69   **FUD** 000    02 P3 80 ▢

    **AMA:** 2017,Jan,8; 2016,Jan,13; 2015,Jan,16; 2014,Jan,11; 2012,Jan,15-42

**58321** Artificial insemination; intra-cervical ♀

    🖫 1.39   ⚕ 2.18   **FUD** 000    T P3 80 ▢

    **AMA:** 2014,Jan,11

**58322** intra-uterine ♀

    🖫 1.67   ⚕ 2.43   **FUD** 000    T P3 80 ▢

    **AMA:** 2014,Jan,11

**58323** Sperm washing for artificial insemination ♀

    🖫 0.34   ⚕ 0.43   **FUD** 000    T P3 80 ▢

    **AMA:** 2014,Jan,11

## 58340-58350 Fallopian Tube Patency and Brachytherapy Procedures

**58340** Catheterization and introduction of saline or contrast material for saline infusion sonohysterography (SIS) or hysterosalpingography ♀

    🔀 (74740, 76831)

    🖫 1.66   ⚕ 3.38   **FUD** 000    N N1 ▢

    **AMA:** 2017,Jan,8; 2016,Jan,13; 2015,Jan,16; 2014,Jan,11; 2012,Jan,15-42

**58345** Transcervical introduction of fallopian tube catheter for diagnosis and/or re-establishing patency (any method), with or without hysterosalpingography ♀

    🔀 (74742)

    🖫 7.89   ⚕ 7.89   **FUD** 010    J R2 80 50 ▢

    **AMA:** 2017,Jan,8; 2016,Jan,13; 2015,Jan,16; 2014,Jan,11; 2012,Jan,15-42

**58346** Insertion of Heyman capsules for clinical brachytherapy ♀

    EXCLUDES *Insertion of radioelement sources or ribbons (77761-77763, 77770-77772)*

    *The placement of needles or catheters into the pelvic organs and/or genitalia (except for the prostate) for interstitial radioelement application (55920)*

    🖫 13.0   ⚕ 13.0   **FUD** 090    J A2 ▢

    **AMA:** 2017,Jan,8; 2016,Jan,13; 2015,Jan,16; 2014,Jan,11

**58350** Chromotubation of oviduct, including materials ♀

    🖫 2.24   ⚕ 2.74   **FUD** 010    J A2 50 ▢

    **AMA:** 2017,Jan,8; 2016,Jan,13; 2015,Jan,16; 2014,Jan,11; 2012,Jan,15-42

## 58353-58356 Ablation of Endometrium

    EXCLUDES *Destruction/excision of endometriomas, open method (49203-49205)*

**58353** Endometrial ablation, thermal, without hysteroscopic guidance ♀

    EXCLUDES *Endometrial ablation performed hysteroscopically (58563)*

    🖫 6.22   ⚕ 28.4   **FUD** 010    J A2 ▢

    **AMA:** 2017,Jan,8; 2016,Jan,13; 2015,Jan,16; 2014,Jan,11; 2012,Jan,15-42

**58356** Endometrial cryoablation with ultrasonic guidance, including endometrial curettage, when performed ♀

    EXCLUDES *Dilation and curettage (58120)*

    *Endometrial biopsy (58100)*

    *Hysterosalpingography (58340)*

    *Ultrasound (76700, 76856)*

    🖫 9.82   ⚕ 53.2   **FUD** 010    J P3 80 ▢

    **AMA:** 2014,Jan,11

## 58400-58540 Uterine Repairs: Vaginal and Abdominal

**58400** Uterine suspension, with or without shortening of round ligaments, with or without shortening of sacrouterine ligaments; (separate procedure) ♀

    INCLUDES Alexander's operation

           Baldy-Webster operation

           Manchester colporrhaphy

    EXCLUDES *Anastomosis of tubes to uterus (58752)*

    🖫 12.5   ⚕ 12.5   **FUD** 090    C 80 ▢

    **AMA:** 2014,Jan,11

**58410** with presacral sympathectomy ♀

    INCLUDES Alexander's operation

    EXCLUDES *Anastomosis of tubes to uterus (58752)*

    🖫 22.9   ⚕ 22.9   **FUD** 090    C 80 ▢

    **AMA:** 2017,Jan,8; 2016,Jan,13; 2015,Jan,16; 2014,Jan,11; 2012,Jan,15-42

**58520** Hysterorrhaphy, repair of ruptured uterus (nonobstetrical) ♀

    🖫 23.8   ⚕ 23.8   **FUD** 090    C 80 ▢

    **AMA:** 2014,Jan,11

**58540** Hysteroplasty, repair of uterine anomaly (Strassman type) ♀

    INCLUDES Strassman type

    EXCLUDES *Vesicouterine fistula closure (51920)*

    🖫 25.5   ⚕ 25.5   **FUD** 090    C 80 ▢

    **AMA:** 2014,Jan,11

## 58541-58554 [58674] Laparoscopic Procedures of the Uterus

    INCLUDES Diagnostic laparoscopy

    EXCLUDES *Hysteroscopy (58555-58565)*

\# **58674** Laparoscopy, surgical, ablation of uterine fibroid(s) including intraoperative ultrasound guidance and monitoring, radiofrequency ♀

    INCLUDES Intraoperative ultrasound (76998)

    EXCLUDES *Laparoscopy (49320, 58541-58554, 58570-58573)*

    🖫 23.2   ⚕ 23.2   **FUD** 090    J J8 80 ▢

    **AMA:** 2017,Apr,7; 2017,Feb,14

**58541** Laparoscopy, surgical, supracervical hysterectomy, for uterus 250 g or less; ♀

    EXCLUDES *Colpotomy (57000)*

    *Hysteroscopy (58561)*

    *Laparoscopy (49320, 58545-58546, 58661, 58670-58671)*

    *Myomectomy procedures (58140-58146)*

    *Pelvic examination under anesthesia (57410)*

    *Treatment of nonobstetrical vaginal hemorrhage (57180)*

    🖫 20.3   ⚕ 20.3   **FUD** 090    J G2 80 ▢

    **AMA:** 2017,Apr,7; 2017,Jan,8; 2016,Jan,13; 2015,Jan,16; 2014,Jan,11

**58542** with removal of tube(s) and/or ovary(s) ♀

    EXCLUDES *Colpotomy (57000)*

    *Hysteroscopy (58561)*

    *Laparoscopy (49320, 58545-58546, 58661, 58670-58671)*

    *Myomectomy procedures (58140-58146)*

    *Pelvic examination under anesthesia (57410)*

    *Treatment of nonobstetrical vaginal hemorrhage (57180)*

    🖫 23.2   ⚕ 23.2   **FUD** 090    J G2 80 ▢

    **AMA:** 2017,Apr,7; 2017,Jan,8; 2016,Jan,13; 2015,Jan,16; 2014,Jan,11

● New Code   ▲ Revised Code   ○ Reinstated   ● New Web Release   ▲ Revised Web Release   Unlisted   Not Covered   # Resequenced
⊘ AMA Mod 51 Exempt   ⑤ Optum Mod 51 Exempt   ⊚ Mod 63 Exempt   ✗ Non-FDA Drug   ★ Telemedicine   Ⅿ Maternity   Ⓐ Age Edit   + Add-on   **AMA:** CPT Asst

**Genital System** *(left margin, rotated)*

**58543 — 58562** *(left margin, rotated)*

**58543** **Laparoscopy, surgical, supracervical hysterectomy, for uterus greater than 250 g;** ♀

> **EXCLUDES**  Colpotomy (57000)
> Hysteroscopy (58561)
> Laparoscopy (49320, 58545-58546, 58661, 58670-58671)
> Myomectomy procedures (58140-58146)
> Pelvic examination under anesthesia (57410)
> Treatment of nonobstetrical vaginal hemorrhage (57180)

🚑 23.4   ⚗ 23.4   **FUD** 090   J G2 80 ▣

**AMA:** 2017,Apr,7; 2017,Jan,8; 2016,Jan,13; 2015,Jan,16; 2014,Jan,11

**58544** **with removal of tube(s) and/or ovary(s)** ♀

> **EXCLUDES**  Colpotomy (57000)
> Hysteroscopy (58561)
> Laparoscopy (49320, 58545-58546, 58661, 58670-58671)
> Myomectomy procedures (58140-58146)
> Pelvic examination under anesthesia (57410)
> Treatment of nonobstetrical vaginal hemorrhage (57180)

🚑 25.6   ⚗ 25.6   **FUD** 090   J G2 80 ▣

**AMA:** 2017,Apr,7; 2017,Jan,8; 2016,Jan,13; 2015,Jan,16; 2014,Jan,11

**58545** **Laparoscopy, surgical, myomectomy, excision; 1 to 4 intramural myomas with total weight of 250 g or less and/or removal of surface myomas** ♀

🚑 25.7   ⚗ 25.7   **FUD** 090   J A2 80 ▣

**AMA:** 2017,Apr,7; 2014,Jan,11

**58546** **5 or more intramural myomas and/or intramural myomas with total weight greater than 250 g** ♀

🚑 31.8   ⚗ 31.8   **FUD** 090   J A2 80 ▣

**AMA:** 2017,Apr,7; 2017,Jan,8; 2016,Jan,13; 2015,Jan,16; 2014,Jan,11; 2012,Jan,15-42

**58548** **Laparoscopy, surgical, with radical hysterectomy, with bilateral total pelvic lymphadenectomy and para-aortic lymph node sampling (biopsy), with removal of tube(s) and ovary(s), if performed** ♀

> **EXCLUDES**  Laparoscopy (38570-38572, 58550-58554)
> Radical hysterectomy (58210, 58285)

🚑 54.8   ⚗ 54.8   **FUD** 090   C 80 ▣

**AMA:** 2017,Apr,7; 2017,Jan,8; 2016,Jan,13; 2015,Sep,12; 2015,Jan,16; 2014,Jan,11

**58550** **Laparoscopy, surgical, with vaginal hysterectomy, for uterus 250 g or less;** ♀

> **EXCLUDES**  Colpotomy (57000)
> Hysteroscopy (58561)
> Laparoscopy (49320, 58546, 58661, 58670-58671)
> Myomectomy procedures (58140-58146)
> Pelvic examination under anesthesia (57410)
> Treatment of nonobstetrical vaginal hemorrhage (57180)

🚑 25.0   ⚗ 25.0   **FUD** 090   J A2 80 ▣

**AMA:** 2017,Apr,7; 2017,Jan,8; 2016,Jan,13; 2015,Jan,16; 2014,Jan,11

**58552** **with removal of tube(s) and/or ovary(s)** ♀

> **EXCLUDES**  Colpotomy (57000)
> Hysteroscopy (58561)
> Laparoscopy (49320, 58545-58546, 58661, 58670-58671)
> Myomectomy procedures (58140-58146)
> Pelvic examination under anesthesia (57410)
> Treatment of nonobstetrical vaginal hemorrhage (57180)

🚑 28.1   ⚗ 28.1   **FUD** 090   J G2 80 ▣

**AMA:** 2017,Apr,7; 2017,Jan,8; 2016,Jan,13; 2015,Jan,16; 2014,Jan,11

**58553** **Laparoscopy, surgical, with vaginal hysterectomy, for uterus greater than 250 g;** ♀

> **EXCLUDES**  Colpotomy (57000)
> Hysteroscopy (58561)
> Laparoscopy (49320, 58545-58546, 58661, 58670-58671)
> Myomectomy procedures (58140-58146)
> Pelvic examination under anesthesia (57410)
> Treatment of nonobstetrical vaginal hemorrhage (57180)

🚑 32.3   ⚗ 32.3   **FUD** 090   J G2 80 ▣

**AMA:** 2017,Apr,7; 2014,Jan,11

**58554** **with removal of tube(s) and/or ovary(s)** ♀

> **EXCLUDES**  Colpotomy (57000)
> Hysteroscopy (58561)
> Laparoscopy (49320, 58546, 58661, 58670-58671)
> Myomectomy procedures (58140-58146)
> Pelvic examination under anesthesia (57410)
> Treatment of nonobstetrical vaginal hemorrhage (57180)

🚑 37.7   ⚗ 37.7   **FUD** 090   J G2 80 ▣

**AMA:** 2017,Apr,7; 2014,Jan,11

## 58555-58565 Hysteroscopy

> **INCLUDES**  Diagnostic hysteroscopy (58555)
> **EXCLUDES**  Laparoscopy (58541-58554, 58570-58578)

**58555** **Hysteroscopy, diagnostic (separate procedure)** ♀

🚑 4.40   ⚗ 7.60   **FUD** 000   J A2 80 ▣

**AMA:** 2017,Jan,8; 2016,Jan,13; 2015,Jan,16; 2014,Jan,11

Labels: Hysteroscope, Bladder, Uterus, Ovary, Spine, Vagina, Cervix

**58558** **Hysteroscopy, surgical; with sampling (biopsy) of endometrium and/or polypectomy, with or without D & C** ♀

🚑 6.72   ⚗ 38.5   **FUD** 000   J A2 ▣

**AMA:** 2017,Jan,8; 2016,Jan,13; 2015,Jan,16; 2014,Jan,11; 2012,Jan,15-42

**58559** **with lysis of intrauterine adhesions (any method)** ♀

🚑 8.28   ⚗ 8.28   **FUD** 000   J A2 ▣

**AMA:** 2017,Jan,8; 2016,Jan,13; 2015,Jan,16; 2014,Jan,11

**58560** **with division or resection of intrauterine septum (any method)** ♀

🚑 9.07   ⚗ 9.07   **FUD** 000   J A2 80 ▣

**AMA:** 2017,Jan,8; 2016,Jan,13; 2015,Jan,16; 2014,Jan,11

**58561** **with removal of leiomyomata** ♀

🚑 12.5   ⚗ 12.5   **FUD** 000   J A2 80 ▣

**AMA:** 2017,Jan,8; 2016,Jan,13; 2015,Jan,16; 2014,Jan,11

**58562** **with removal of impacted foreign body** ♀

🚑 6.64   ⚗ 9.64   **FUD** 000   J A2 ▣

**AMA:** 2017,Jan,8; 2016,Jan,13; 2015,Jan,16; 2014,Jan,11; 2012,Jan,15-42

26/TC PC/TC Only   A2-Z3 ASC Payment   50 Bilateral   ♂ Male Only   ♀ Female Only   🚑 Facility RVU   ⚗ Non-Facility RVU   ▣ CCI
FUD Follow-up Days   CMS: IOM (Pub 100)   A-Y OPPSI   80/80 Surg Assist Allowed / w/Doc   ▨ Lab Crosswalk   ✚ Radiology Crosswalk   ✖ CLIA

256

CPT © 2017 American Medical Association. All Rights Reserved.

© 2017 Optum360, LLC

**58563** with endometrial ablation (eg, endometrial resection, electrosurgical ablation, thermoablation) ♀

🔳 7.82  ✂ 44.9  **FUD** 000  [J] [A2] [80] 🖵

**AMA:** 2017,Jan,8; 2016,Jan,13; 2015,Jan,16; 2015,Jan,13; 2014,Jan,11; 2012,Feb,11; 2012,Jan,15-42

**58565** with bilateral fallopian tube cannulation to induce occlusion by placement of permanent implants ♀

EXCLUDES  Diagnostic hysteroscopy (58555)
Dilation of cervical canal (57800)

Code also modifier 52 when a unilateral procedure is performed

🔳 12.3  ✂ 53.1  **FUD** 090  [J] [A2] 🖵

**AMA:** 2017,Jan,8; 2016,Jan,13; 2015,Jan,16; 2014,Jan,11; 2012,Feb,11; 2012,Jan,15-42

## 58570-58579 Other Uterine Endoscopy

INCLUDES  Diagnostic laparoscopy
EXCLUDES  Hysteroscopy (58555-58565)

**58570** Laparoscopy, surgical, with total hysterectomy, for uterus 250 g or less; ♀

EXCLUDES  Colpotomy (57000)
Hysteroscopy (58561)
Laparoscopy (49320, 58545-58546, 58661, 58670-58671)
Myomectomy procedures (58140-58146)
Pelvic examination under anesthesia (57410)
Total abdominal hysterectomy (58150)
Treatment of nonobstetrical vaginal hemorrhage (57180)

🔳 22.1  ✂ 22.1  **FUD** 090  [J] [62] [80] 🖵

**AMA:** 2017,Apr,7; 2014,Jan,11

**58571** with removal of tube(s) and/or ovary(s) ♀

EXCLUDES  Colpotomy (57000)
Hysteroscopy (58561)
Laparoscopy (49320, 58545-58546, 58661, 58670-58671)
Myomectomy procedures (58140-58146)
Pelvic examination under anesthesia (57410)
Total abdominal hysterectomy (58150)
Treatment of nonobstetrical vaginal hemorrhage (57180)

🔳 25.6  ✂ 25.6  **FUD** 090  [J] [62] [80] 🖵

**AMA:** 2017,Apr,7; 2017,Jan,8; 2016,Jan,13; 2015,Jan,16; 2014,Jan,11; 2012,Aug,13-14; 2012,May,14-15

**58572** Laparoscopy, surgical, with total hysterectomy, for uterus greater than 250 g; ♀

EXCLUDES  Colpotomy (57000)
Hysteroscopy (58561)
Laparoscopy (49320, 58545-58546, 58661, 58670-58671)
Myomectomy procedures (58140-58146)
Pelvic examination under anesthesia (57410)
Total abdominal hysterectomy (58150)
Treatment of nonobstetrical vaginal hemorrhage (57180)

🔳 29.0  ✂ 29.0  **FUD** 090  [J] [80] 🖵

**AMA:** 2017,Apr,7; 2014,Jan,11

**58573** with removal of tube(s) and/or ovary(s) ♀

EXCLUDES  Colpotomy (57000)
Hysteroscopy (58561)
Laparoscopy (49320, 58545-58546, 58661, 58670-58671)
Myomectomy procedures (58140-58146)
Pelvic examination under anesthesia (57410)
Total abdominal hysterectomy (58150)
Treatment of nonobstetrical vaginal hemorrhage (57180)

🔳 34.7  ✂ 34.7  **FUD** 090  [J] [62] [80] 🖵

**AMA:** 2017,Apr,7; 2017,Jan,8; 2016,Jan,13; 2015,Jan,16; 2014,Jan,11; 2012,Aug,13-14; 2012,May,14-15

● **58575** Laparoscopy, surgical, total hysterectomy for resection of malignancy (tumor debulking), with omentectomy including salpingo-oophorectomy, unilateral or bilateral, when performed

EXCLUDES  Laparoscopy (49320-49321, 58570-58573, 58661)
Omentectomy (49255)

**58578** Unlisted laparoscopy procedure, uterus ♀

🔳 0.00  ✂ 0.00  **FUD** YYY  [J] [80] [50]

**AMA:** 2017,Jan,8; 2016,Jan,13; 2015,Jan,16; 2014,Jan,11; 2012,Jan,15-42

**58579** Unlisted hysteroscopy procedure, uterus ♀

🔳 0.00  ✂ 0.00  **FUD** YYY  [T] [80] [50]

**AMA:** 2017,Jan,8; 2016,Jan,13; 2015,Jan,16; 2014,Jan,11

## 58600-58615 Sterilization by Tubal Interruption

**CMS:** 100-03,230.3 Sterilization
EXCLUDES  Destruction/excision of endometriomas, open method (49203-49205)

**58600** Ligation or transection of fallopian tube(s), abdominal or vaginal approach, unilateral or bilateral ♀

INCLUDES  Madlener operation

🔳 10.3  ✂ 10.3  **FUD** 090  [J] [62] [80] 🖵

**AMA:** 2017,Jan,8; 2016,Jan,13; 2015,Jan,16; 2014,Jan,11

**58605** Ligation or transection of fallopian tube(s), abdominal or vaginal approach, postpartum, unilateral or bilateral, during same hospitalization (separate procedure) ♀

EXCLUDES  Laparoscopic methods (58670-58671)

🔳 9.33  ✂ 9.33  **FUD** 090  [C] [80] 🖵

**AMA:** 2017,Jan,8; 2016,Jan,13; 2015,Jan,16; 2014,Jan,11

+ **58611** Ligation or transection of fallopian tube(s) when done at the time of cesarean delivery or intra-abdominal surgery (not a separate procedure) (List separately in addition to code for primary procedure) ♀

Code first primary procedure

🔳 2.19  ✂ 2.19  **FUD** ZZZ  [C] [80] 🖵

**AMA:** 2014,Jan,11

**58615** Occlusion of fallopian tube(s) by device (eg, band, clip, Falope ring) vaginal or suprapubic approach ♀

EXCLUDES  Laparoscopic method (58671)
Lysis of adnexal adhesions (58740)

🔳 7.07  ✂ 7.07  **FUD** 010  [J] [62] [80] 🖵

**AMA:** 2017,Jan,8; 2016,Jan,13; 2015,Jan,16; 2014,Jan,11

## 58660-58679 Endoscopic Procedures Fallopian Tubes and/or Ovaries

**CMS:** 100-03,230.3 Sterilization
INCLUDES  Diagnostic laparoscopy (49320)
EXCLUDES  Laparoscopy with biopsy of fallopian tube or ovary (49321)
Laparoscopy with ovarian cyst aspiration (49322)

**58660** Laparoscopy, surgical; with lysis of adhesions (salpingolysis, ovariolysis) (separate procedure) ♀

🔳 19.1  ✂ 19.1  **FUD** 090  [J] [A2] [80] 🖵

**AMA:** 2017,Jan,8; 2016,Jan,13; 2015,Jan,16; 2014,Jan,11; 2012,Jan,15-42

**58661** with removal of adnexal structures (partial or total oophorectomy and/or salpingectomy) ♀

🔳 18.5  ✂ 18.5  **FUD** 010  [J] [A2] [80] [50] 🖵

**AMA:** 2017,Jan,8; 2016,Jan,13; 2015,Jan,16; 2014,Jan,11; 2012,Jan,15-42

**58662** with fulguration or excision of lesions of the ovary, pelvic viscera, or peritoneal surface by any method ♀

🔳 20.2  ✂ 20.2  **FUD** 090  [J] [A2] [80] 🖵

**AMA:** 2017,Jan,8; 2016,Jan,13; 2015,Jan,16; 2014,Jan,11

**58670** with fulguration of oviducts (with or without transection) ♀

🔳 10.3  ✂ 10.3  **FUD** 090  [J] [A2] 🖵

**AMA:** 2017,Jan,8; 2016,Jan,13; 2015,Jan,16; 2014,Jan,11

---

● New Code  ▲ Revised Code  ○ Reinstated  ⦿ New Web Release  ▲ Revised Web Release  Unlisted  Not Covered  # Resequenced
⊘ AMA Mod 51 Exempt  ⑤ Optum Mod 51 Exempt  ⑥③ Mod 63 Exempt  ⊁ Non-FDA Drug  ★ Telemedicine  Ⓜ Maternity  Ⓐ Age Edit  + Add-on  **AMA:** CPT Asst

**Genital System**

**58671 — 58943**

| 58671 | with occlusion of oviducts by device (eg, band, clip, or Falope ring) ♀ |
| | 🚑 10.3   ⚕ 10.3   **FUD** 090   J A2 |
| | **AMA:** 2017,Jan,8; 2016,Jan,13; 2015,Jan,16; 2014,Jan,11 |

| 58672 | with fimbrioplasty ♀ |
| | 🚑 20.8   ⚕ 20.8   **FUD** 090   J A2 80 50 |
| | **AMA:** 2017,Jan,8; 2016,Jan,13; 2015,Jan,16; 2014,Jan,11 |

| 58673 | with salpingostomy (salpingoneostomy) ♀ |
| | 🚑 22.6   ⚕ 22.6   **FUD** 090   J A2 80 50 |
| | **AMA:** 2017,Jan,8; 2016,Jan,13; 2015,Jan,16; 2014,Jan,11; 2012,Jan,15-42 |

| *58674* | **Resequenced code. See code before 58541.** |

| *58679* | Unlisted laparoscopy procedure, oviduct, ovary ♀ |
| | 🚑 0.00   ⚕ 0.00   **FUD** YYY   J 80 50 |
| | **AMA:** 2017,Jan,8; 2016,Jan,13; 2015,Jan,16; 2014,Jan,11 |

## 58700-58770 Open Procedures Fallopian Tubes, with/without Ovaries

*EXCLUDES*   Destruction/excision of endometriomas, open method (49203-49205, 58957-58958)

| 58700 | Salpingectomy, complete or partial, unilateral or bilateral (separate procedure) ♀ |
| | 🚑 22.2   ⚕ 22.2   **FUD** 090   C 80 |
| | **AMA:** 2014,Jan,11 |

| 58720 | Salpingo-oophorectomy, complete or partial, unilateral or bilateral (separate procedure) ♀ |
| | 🚑 21.0   ⚕ 21.0   **FUD** 090   C 80 |
| | **AMA:** 2017,Jan,8; 2016,Jan,13; 2015,Jan,16; 2014,Jan,11; 2012,Jan,15-42 |

| 58740 | Lysis of adhesions (salpingolysis, ovariolysis) ♀ |
| | *EXCLUDES*   Excision/fulguration of lesions performed laparoscopically (58662) |
| | Laparoscopic method (58660) |
| | 🚑 25.2   ⚕ 25.2   **FUD** 090   C 80 |
| | **AMA:** 2017,Jan,8; 2016,Jan,13; 2015,Jan,16; 2014,Jan,11 |

| 58750 | Tubotubal anastomosis ♀ |
| | 🚑 27.4   ⚕ 27.4   **FUD** 090   C 80 50 |
| | **AMA:** 2014,Jan,11 |

Occluded section of tube is excised

Tube ends are sutured

Ovary

| 58752 | Tubouterine implantation ♀ |
| | 🚑 25.8   ⚕ 25.8   **FUD** 090   C 80 50 |
| | **AMA:** 2014,Jan,11 |

| 58760 | Fimbrioplasty ♀ |
| | *EXCLUDES*   Laparoscopic method (58672) |
| | 🚑 22.9   ⚕ 22.9   **FUD** 090   C 80 50 |
| | **AMA:** 2017,Jan,8; 2016,Jan,13; 2015,Jan,16; 2014,Jan,11 |

| 58770 | Salpingostomy (salpingoneostomy) ♀ |
| | *EXCLUDES*   Laparoscopic method (58673) |
| | 🚑 24.8   ⚕ 24.8   **FUD** 090   J 80 50 |
| | **AMA:** 2017,Jan,8; 2016,Jan,13; 2015,Jan,16; 2014,Jan,11 |

## 58800-58925 Open Procedures: Ovary

**CMS:** 100-03,230.3 Sterilization

*EXCLUDES*   Destruction/excision of endometriomas, open method (49203-49205, 58957-58958)

| 58800 | Drainage of ovarian cyst(s), unilateral or bilateral (separate procedure); vaginal approach ♀ |
| | 🚑 8.43   ⚕ 8.98   **FUD** 090   J A2 |
| | **AMA:** 2014,Jan,11; 2013,Nov,9 |

| 58805 | abdominal approach ♀ |
| | 🚑 11.5   ⚕ 11.5   **FUD** 090   J G2 80 |
| | **AMA:** 2014,Jan,11; 2013,Nov,9 |

| 58820 | Drainage of ovarian abscess; vaginal approach, open ♀ |
| | *EXCLUDES*   Transrectal fluid drainage using catheter, image guided (49407) |
| | 🚑 9.29   ⚕ 9.29   **FUD** 090   J A2 80 50 |
| | **AMA:** 2014,Jan,11; 2013,Nov,9 |

| 58822 | abdominal approach ♀ |
| | *EXCLUDES*   Transrectal fluid drainage using catheter, image guided (49407) |
| | 🚑 19.8   ⚕ 19.8   **FUD** 090   C 80 50 |
| | **AMA:** 2014,Jan,11; 2013,Nov,9 |

| 58825 | Transposition, ovary(s) ♀ |
| | 🚑 21.5   ⚕ 21.5   **FUD** 090   C 80 |
| | **AMA:** 2014,Jan,11 |

| 58900 | Biopsy of ovary, unilateral or bilateral (separate procedure) ♀ |
| | *EXCLUDES*   Laparoscopy with biopsy of fallopian tube or ovary (49321) |
| | 🚑 11.7   ⚕ 11.7   **FUD** 090   J A2 80 |
| | **AMA:** 2017,Jan,8; 2016,Jan,13; 2015,Jan,16; 2014,Jan,11 |

| 58920 | Wedge resection or bisection of ovary, unilateral or bilateral ♀ |
| | 🚑 21.5   ⚕ 21.5   **FUD** 090   J 80 |
| | **AMA:** 2014,Jan,11 |

| 58925 | Ovarian cystectomy, unilateral or bilateral ♀ |
| | 🚑 21.3   ⚕ 21.3   **FUD** 090   J 80 |
| | **AMA:** 2014,Jan,11 |

## 58940-58960 Removal Ovary(s) with/without Multiple Procedures for Malignancy

**CMS:** 100-03,230.3 Sterilization

*EXCLUDES*   Chemotherapy (96401-96549)
Destruction/excision of tumors, cysts, or endometriomas, open method (49203-49205)

| 58940 | Oophorectomy, partial or total, unilateral or bilateral; ♀ |
| | *EXCLUDES*   Oophorectomy with tumor debulking for ovarian malignancy (58952) |
| | 🚑 15.0   ⚕ 15.0   **FUD** 090   C 80 |
| | **AMA:** 2017,Jan,8; 2016,Jan,13; 2015,Jan,16; 2014,Jan,11 |

| 58943 | for ovarian, tubal or primary peritoneal malignancy, with para-aortic and pelvic lymph node biopsies, peritoneal washings, peritoneal biopsies, diaphragmatic assessments, with or without salpingectomy(s), with or without omentectomy ♀ |
| | 🚑 33.7   ⚕ 33.7   **FUD** 090   C 80 |
| | **AMA:** 2014,Jan,11 |

**58950**    Resection (initial) of ovarian, tubal or primary peritoneal malignancy with bilateral salpingo-oophorectomy and omentectomy; ♀

    *EXCLUDES*  *Resection/tumor debulking of recurrent ovarian/tubal/primary peritoneal/uterine malignancy (58957-58958)*

    🚑 32.5  ✂ 32.5  **FUD** 090  C 80 ▣

    **AMA:** 2014,Jan,11

**58951**    with total abdominal hysterectomy, pelvic and limited para-aortic lymphadenectomy ♀

    *EXCLUDES*  *Resection/tumor debulking of recurrent ovarian/tubal/primary peritoneal/uterine malignancy (58957-58958)*

    🚑 41.9  ✂ 41.9  **FUD** 090  C 80 ▣

    **AMA:** 2017,Jan,8; 2016,Jan,13; 2015,Jan,16; 2014,Jan,11; 2012,Jan,15-42

**58952**    with radical dissection for debulking (ie, radical excision or destruction, intra-abdominal or retroperitoneal tumors) ♀

    *EXCLUDES*  *Resection/tumor debulking of recurrent ovarian/tubal/primary peritoneal/uterine malignancy (58957-58958)*

    🚑 47.4  ✂ 47.4  **FUD** 090  C 80 ▣

    **AMA:** 2017,Jan,8; 2016,Jan,13; 2015,Jan,16; 2014,Jan,11; 2012,Jan,15-42

**58953**    Bilateral salpingo-oophorectomy with omentectomy, total abdominal hysterectomy and radical dissection for debulking; ♀

    🚑 58.6  ✂ 58.6  **FUD** 090  C 80 ▣

    **AMA:** 2017,Jan,8; 2016,Jan,13; 2015,Jan,16; 2014,May,10; 2014,Jan,11

**58954**    with pelvic lymphadenectomy and limited para-aortic lymphadenectomy ♀

    🚑 63.7  ✂ 63.7  **FUD** 090  C 80 ▣

    **AMA:** 2017,Jan,8; 2016,Jan,13; 2015,Jan,16; 2014,Jan,11

**58956**    Bilateral salpingo-oophorectomy with total omentectomy, total abdominal hysterectomy for malignancy ♀

    *EXCLUDES*  *Biopsy of ovary (58900)*
        *Hysterectomy (58150, 58180, 58262-58263)*
        *Laparoscopy (58550, 58661)*
        *Omentectomy (49255)*
        *Oophorectomy (58940)*
        *Ovarian cystectomy (58925)*
        *Resection of malignancy (58957-58958)*
        *Salpingectomy salpingo-oophorectomy, (58700, 58720)*

    🚑 39.8  ✂ 39.8  **FUD** 090  C 80 ▣

    **AMA:** 2017,Jan,8; 2016,Jan,13; 2015,Jan,16; 2014,May,10; 2014,Jan,11

**58957**    Resection (tumor debulking) of recurrent ovarian, tubal, primary peritoneal, uterine malignancy (intra-abdominal, retroperitoneal tumors), with omentectomy, if performed; ♀

    *EXCLUDES*  *Biopsy of ovary (58900-58960)*
        *Destruction, excision cysts, endometriomas, or tumors (49203-49215)*
        *Enterolysis (44005)*
        *Exploratory laparotomy (49000)*
        *Lymphadenectomy (38770, 38780)*
        *Omentectomy (49255)*

    🚑 45.8  ✂ 45.8  **FUD** 090  C 80 ▣

    **AMA:** 2014,Jan,11

**58958**    with pelvic lymphadenectomy and limited para-aortic lymphadenectomy ♀

    *EXCLUDES*  *Biopsy of ovary (58900-58960)*
        *Destruction, excision cysts, endometriomas, or tumors (49203-49215)*
        *Enterolysis (44005)*
        *Exploratory laparotomy (49000)*
        *Lymphadenectomy (38770, 38780)*
        *Omentectomy (49255)*

    🚑 50.5  ✂ 50.5  **FUD** 090  C 80 ▣

    **AMA:** 2014,Jan,11

**58960**    Laparotomy, for staging or restaging of ovarian, tubal, or primary peritoneal malignancy (second look), with or without omentectomy, peritoneal washing, biopsy of abdominal and pelvic peritoneum, diaphragmatic assessment with pelvic and limited para-aortic lymphadenectomy ♀

    *EXCLUDES*  *Resection of malignancy (58957-58958)*

    🚑 27.8  ✂ 27.8  **FUD** 090  C 80 ▣

    **AMA:** 2014,Jan,11

## 58970-58999 Procedural Components: In Vitro Fertilization

**58970**    Follicle puncture for oocyte retrieval, any method  M ♀

    🔀 (76948)

    🚑 5.69  ✂ 6.32  **FUD** 000  T A2 80 ▣

    **AMA:** 2014,Jan,11

**58974**    Embryo transfer, intrauterine  M ♀

    🚑 0.00  ✂ 0.00  **FUD** 000  T A2 80 ▣

    **AMA:** 2014,Jan,11

**58976**    Gamete, zygote, or embryo intrafallopian transfer, any method  M ♀

    *EXCLUDES*  *Adnexal procedures performed laparoscopically (58660-58673)*

    🚑 6.22  ✂ 7.18  **FUD** 000  T A2 80 ▣

    **AMA:** 2017,Jan,8; 2016,Jan,13; 2015,Jan,16; 2014,Jan,11

**58999**    Unlisted procedure, female genital system (nonobstetrical) ♀

    🚑 0.00  ✂ 0.00  **FUD** YYY  T

    **AMA:** 2017,Jan,8; 2016,Jan,13; 2015,Jan,16; 2014,Jan,11; 2012,Jan,15-42

## 59000-59001 Aspiration of Amniotic Fluid

*EXCLUDES*  *Intrauterine fetal transfusion (36460)*
    *Unlisted fetal invasive procedure (59897)*

**59000**    Amniocentesis; diagnostic  M ♀

    🔀 (76946)

    🚑 2.35  ✂ 3.60  **FUD** 000  T P3 ▣

    **AMA:** 2017,Jan,8; 2016,Jan,13; 2015,Jan,16; 2014,Jan,11

**59001**    therapeutic amniotic fluid reduction (includes ultrasound guidance)  M ♀

    🚑 5.21  ✂ 5.21  **FUD** 000  T R2 ▣

    **AMA:** 2017,Jan,8; 2016,Jan,13; 2015,Jan,16; 2014,Jan,11

## 59012-59076 Fetal Testing and Treatment

*EXCLUDES*  *Intrauterine fetal transfusion (36460)*
    *Unlisted fetal invasive procedures (59897)*

**59012**    Cordocentesis (intrauterine), any method  M ♀

    🔀 (76941)

    🚑 5.89  ✂ 5.89  **FUD** 000  T G2 80 ▣

    **AMA:** 2014,Jan,11

**59015**    Chorionic villus sampling, any method  M ♀

    🔀 (76945)

    🚑 3.85  ✂ 4.49  **FUD** 000  T P3 80 ▣

    **AMA:** 2017,Jan,8; 2016,Jan,13; 2015,Jan,16; 2014,Jan,11

**59020**    Fetal contraction stress test  M ♀

    🚑 2.03  ✂ 2.03  **FUD** 000  T P3 80 ▣

    **AMA:** 2017,Jan,8; 2016,Jan,13; 2015,Jan,16; 2014,Jan,11

---

● New Code   ▲ Revised Code   ○ Reinstated   ● New Web Release   ▲ Revised Web Release   Unlisted   Not Covered   # Resequenced
⊘ AMA Mod 51 Exempt   ⑨ Optum Mod 51 Exempt   ㊿ Mod 63 Exempt   ✒ Non-FDA Drug   ★ Telemedicine   M Maternity   A Age Edit   + Add-on   **AMA:** CPT Asst

© 2017 Optum360, LLC    CPT © 2017 American Medical Association. All Rights Reserved.

**59025** **Fetal non-stress test**  M ♀
 1.38   1.38  **FUD** 000  T P3 80 ▢
 **AMA:** 2017,Jan,8; 2016,Jan,13; 2015,Jan,16; 2014,Jan,11;
 2012,Jan,15-42

**59030** **Fetal scalp blood sampling**  M ♀
 Code also modifier 76 or 77, as appropriate, for repeat fetal scalp
 blood sampling
 2.89   2.89  **FUD** 000  T 80 ▢
 **AMA:** 2014,Jan,11

**59050** **Fetal monitoring during labor by consulting physician (ie, non-attending physician) with written report; supervision and interpretation**  M ♀
 1.39   1.39  **FUD** XXX  M 80 ▢
 **AMA:** 2014,Jan,11

**59051** **interpretation only**  M ♀
 1.23   1.23  **FUD** XXX  B 80 ▢
 **AMA:** 2014,Jan,11

**59070** **Transabdominal amnioinfusion, including ultrasound guidance**  M ♀
 8.86   11.5  **FUD** 000  T 62 80 ▢
 **AMA:** 2017,Jan,8; 2016,Jan,13; 2015,Jan,16; 2014,Jan,11;
 2012,Jan,15-42

**59072** **Fetal umbilical cord occlusion, including ultrasound guidance**  M ♀
 13.5   13.5  **FUD** 000  T 62 ▢
 **AMA:** 2017,Jan,8; 2016,Jan,13; 2015,Jan,16; 2014,Jan,11;
 2012,Jan,15-42

**59074** **Fetal fluid drainage (eg, vesicocentesis, thoracocentesis, paracentesis), including ultrasound guidance**  M ♀
 8.73   11.0  **FUD** 000  T 62 80 ▢
 **AMA:** 2017,Jan,8; 2016,Jan,13; 2015,Jan,16; 2014,Jan,11;
 2012,Jan,15-42

**59076** **Fetal shunt placement, including ultrasound guidance**  M ♀
 13.5   13.5  **FUD** 000  T 62 80 ▢
 **AMA:** 2017,Jan,8; 2016,Jan,13; 2015,Jan,16; 2014,Jan,11;
 2012,Jan,15-42

## 59100-59151 Tubal Pregnancy/Hysterotomy Procedures

**CMS:** 100-03,230.3 Sterilization

**59100** **Hysterotomy, abdominal (eg, for hydatidiform mole, abortion)**  M ♀
 Code also ligation of fallopian tubes when performed at the
 same time as hysterotomy (58611)
 22.6   22.6  **FUD** 090  J R2 80 ▢
 **AMA:** 2014,Jan,11

**59120** **Surgical treatment of ectopic pregnancy; tubal or ovarian, requiring salpingectomy and/or oophorectomy, abdominal or vaginal approach**  M ♀
 22.8   22.8  **FUD** 090  C 80 ▢
 **AMA:** 2014,Jan,11

**59121** **tubal or ovarian, without salpingectomy and/or oophorectomy**  M ♀
 22.9   22.9  **FUD** 090  C 80 ▢
 **AMA:** 2014,Jan,11

**59130** **abdominal pregnancy**  M ♀
 26.8   26.8  **FUD** 090  C 80 ▢
 **AMA:** 2014,Jan,11

**59135** **interstitial, uterine pregnancy requiring total hysterectomy**  M ♀
 23.9   23.9  **FUD** 090  C 80 ▢
 **AMA:** 2014,Jan,11

**59136** **interstitial, uterine pregnancy with partial resection of uterus**  M ♀
 25.4   25.4  **FUD** 090  C 80 ▢
 **AMA:** 2014,Jan,11

**59140** **cervical, with evacuation**  M ♀
 10.6   10.6  **FUD** 090  C 80 ▢
 **AMA:** 2014,Jan,11

**59150** **Laparoscopic treatment of ectopic pregnancy; without salpingectomy and/or oophorectomy**  M ♀
 22.1   22.1  **FUD** 090  J 62 80 ▢
 **AMA:** 2017,Jan,8; 2016,Jan,13; 2015,Jan,16; 2014,Jan,11

**59151** **with salpingectomy and/or oophorectomy**  M ♀
 21.6   21.6  **FUD** 090  J 62 80 ▢
 **AMA:** 2014,Jan,11

## 59160-59200 Procedures of Uterus Prior To/After Delivery

**59160** **Curettage, postpartum**  M ♀
 5.01   5.85  **FUD** 010  J A2 80 ▢
 **AMA:** 2017,Jan,8; 2016,Jan,13; 2015,Jan,16; 2014,Jan,11;
 2012,Jan,15-42

**59200** **Insertion of cervical dilator (eg, laminaria, prostaglandin) (separate procedure)**  M ♀
 *EXCLUDES* *Fetal transfusion, intrauterine (36460)*
 *Hypertonic solution/prostaglandin introduction for*
 *labor initiation (59850-59857)*
 1.30   2.06  **FUD** 000  T P3 ▢
 **AMA:** 2017,Jan,8; 2016,Jan,13; 2015,Jan,16; 2014,Jan,11

## 59300-59350 Postpartum Vaginal/Cervical/Uterine Repairs

*EXCLUDES* *Nonpregnancy-related cerclage (57700)*

**59300** **Episiotomy or vaginal repair, by other than attending**  ♀
 4.28   5.53  **FUD** 000  J P3 80 ▢
 **AMA:** 2014,Jan,11

**59320** **Cerclage of cervix, during pregnancy; vaginal**  M ♀
 4.43   4.43  **FUD** 000  J A2 80 ▢
 **AMA:** 2017,Jan,8; 2016,Jan,13; 2015,Jan,16; 2014,Jan,11;
 2012,Jan,15-42

Uterine cavity · Cervix · Vaginal canal · Cerclage sutures · Amniotic sac · Uterus at term · Cervix · Vagina · Pubic bone

**59325** **abdominal**  M ♀
 7.04   7.04  **FUD** 000  C 80 ▢
 **AMA:** 2017,Jan,8; 2016,Jan,13; 2015,Jan,16; 2014,Jan,11;
 2012,Jan,15-42

**59350** **Hysterorrhaphy of ruptured uterus**  M ♀
 7.98   7.98  **FUD** 000  C 80 ▢
 **AMA:** 2014,Jan,11

Genital System

59025 — 59350

## 59400-59410 Vaginal Delivery: Comprehensive and Component Services

**CMS:** 100-02,15,180 Nurse-Midwife (CNM) Services; 100-02,15,20.1 Physician Expense for Surgery, Childbirth, and Treatment for Infertility

> **INCLUDES** Care provided for an uncomplicated pregnancy including delivery as well as antepartum and postpartum care:
> Admission history
> Admission to hospital
> Artificial rupture of membranes
> Management of uncomplicated labor
> Physical exam
> Vaginal delivery with or without episiotomy or forceps
>
> **EXCLUDES** Medical complications of pregnancy, labor, and delivery:
> Cardiac problems
> Diabetes
> Hyperemesis
> Hypertension
> Neurological problems
> Premature rupture of membranes
> Pre-term labor
> Toxemia
> Trauma
> Newborn circumcision (54150, 54160)
> Services incidental to or unrelated to the pregnancy

**59400** Routine obstetric care including antepartum care, vaginal delivery (with or without episiotomy, and/or forceps) and postpartum care Ⓜ♀

> **INCLUDES** Fetal heart tones
> Hospital/office visits following cesarean section or vaginal delivery
> Initial/subsequent history
> Physical exams
> Recording of weight/blood pressures
> Routine chemical urinalysis
> Routine prenatal visits:
> Each month up to 28 weeks gestation
> Every other week from 29 to 36 weeks gestation
> Weekly from 36 weeks until delivery

🚑 60.2　⚬ 60.2　**FUD** MMM　Ⓑ🖪

**AMA:** 2017,Jan,8; 2016,Jan,13; 2015,Jan,16; 2014,Jan,11; 2012,Jan,15-42

**59409** Vaginal delivery only (with or without episiotomy and/or forceps); Ⓜ♀

> **EXCLUDES** Inpatient management after delivery/discharge services (99217-99239 [99224, 99225, 99226])

🚑 23.5　⚬ 23.5　**FUD** MMM　Ⓙ⑳🖪

**AMA:** 2017,Jan,8; 2016,Jan,13; 2015,Jan,16; 2014,Jan,11; 2012,Jan,15-42

**59410** including postpartum care Ⓜ♀

> **INCLUDES** Hospital/office visits following cesarean section or vaginal delivery

🚑 30.1　⚬ 30.1　**FUD** MMM　Ⓑ🖪

**AMA:** 2014,Jan,11

## 59412-59414 Other Maternity Services

**CMS:** 100-02,15,180 Nurse-Midwife (CNM) Services; 100-02,15,20.1 Physician Expense for Surgery, Childbirth, and Treatment for Infertility

**59412** External cephalic version, with or without tocolysis Ⓜ♀

> Code also delivery code(s)

🚑 2.99　⚬ 2.99　**FUD** MMM　Ⓙ⑥②⑳🖪

**AMA:** 2014,Jan,11

Complete breech presentation at term

The physician feels for the baby's head and bottom externally

Turning the baby by applying external pressure

Baby is in cephalic presentation, engaged for normal delivery

**59414** Delivery of placenta (separate procedure) Ⓜ♀

🚑 2.67　⚬ 2.67　**FUD** MMM　Ⓙ⑥②⑳🖪

**AMA:** 2017,Jan,8; 2016,Jan,13; 2015,Jan,16; 2014,Jan,11; 2012,Jan,15-42

## 59425-59430 Prenatal and Postpartum Visits

**CMS:** 100-02,15,180 Nurse-Midwife (CNM) Services; 100-02,15,20.1 Physician Expense for Surgery, Childbirth, and Treatment for Infertility

> **INCLUDES** Physician/other qualified health care professional providing all or a portion of antepartum/postpartum care, but no delivery due to:
> Referral to another physician for delivery
> Termination of pregnancy by abortion
>
> **EXCLUDES** Antepartum care, 1-3 visits, report with appropriate E&M service code
> Medical complications of pregnancy, labor, and delivery:
> Cardiac problems
> Diabetes
> Hyperemesis
> Hypertension
> Neurological problems
> Premature rupture of membranes
> Pre-term labor
> Toxemia
> Trauma
> Newborn circumcision (54150, 54160)
> Services incidental to or unrelated to the pregnancy

**59425** Antepartum care only; 4-6 visits Ⓜ♀

> **INCLUDES** Fetal heart tones
> Initial/subsequent history
> Physical exams
> Recording of weight/blood pressures
> Routine chemical urinalysis
> Routine prenatal visits:
> Each month up to 28 weeks gestation
> Every other week from 29 to 36 weeks gestation
> Weekly from 36 weeks until delivery

🚑 10.3　⚬ 13.0　**FUD** MMM　Ⓑ⑳🖪

**AMA:** 2017,Jan,8; 2016,Jan,13; 2015,Jan,16; 2014,Jan,11; 2012,Jan,15-42

● New Code　▲ Revised Code　○ Reinstated　● New Web Release　▲ Revised Web Release　Unlisted　Not Covered　# Resequenced
⊘ AMA Mod 51 Exempt　⑤ Optum Mod 51 Exempt　⑥ Mod 63 Exempt　✗ Non-FDA Drug　★ Telemedicine　Ⓜ Maternity　Ⓐ Age Edit　+ Add-on　**AMA:** CPT Asst
© 2017 Optum360, LLC　　CPT © 2017 American Medical Association. All Rights Reserved.　　**261**

**Genital System**

**59426 — 59610**

**59426** **7 or more visits** Ⓜ ♀

INCLUDES Biweekly visits to 36 weeks gestation
Fetal heart tones
Initial/subsequent history
Monthly visits up to 28 weeks gestation
Physical exams
Recording of weight/blood pressures
Routine chemical urinalysis
Weekly visits until delivery

🔲 18.2 ⚖ 23.4 **FUD** MMM Ⓑ 80 🔲

**AMA:** 2017,Jan,8; 2016,Jan,13; 2015,Jan,16; 2014,Jan,11; 2012,Jan,15-42

**59430** **Postpartum care only (separate procedure)** Ⓜ ♀

INCLUDES Office/other outpatient visits following cesarean section or vaginal delivery

🔲 4.03 ⚖ 5.31 **FUD** MMM Ⓑ 🔲

**AMA:** 2017,Jan,8; 2016,Jan,13; 2015,Jan,16; 2014,Jan,11; 2012,Jan,15-42

## 59510-59525 Cesarean Section Delivery: Comprehensive and Components of Care

**CMS:** 100-02,15,20.1 Physician Expense for Surgery, Childbirth, and Treatment for Infertility

INCLUDES Classic cesarean section
Low cervical cesarean section

EXCLUDES Infant standby attendance (99360)
Medical complications of pregnancy, labor, and delivery:
  Cardiac problems
  Diabetes
  Hyperemesis
  Hypertension
  Neurological problems
  Premature rupture of membranes
  Pre-term labor
  Toxemia
  Trauma
Newborn circumcision (54150, 54160)
Services incidental to or unrelated to the pregnancy
Vaginal delivery after prior cesarean section (59610-59614)

**59510** **Routine obstetric care including antepartum care, cesarean delivery, and postpartum care** Ⓜ ♀

INCLUDES Admission history
Admission to hospital
Cesarean delivery
Fetal heart tones
Hospital/office visits following cesarean section
Initial/subsequent history
Management of uncomplicated labor
Physical exam
Recording of weight/blood pressures
Routine chemical urinalysis
Routine prenatal visits:
  Each month up to 28 weeks gestation
  Every other week 29 to 36 weeks gestation
  Weekly from 36 weeks until delivery

EXCLUDES Medical problems complicating labor and delivery

🔲 66.9 ⚖ 66.9 **FUD** MMM Ⓑ 🔲

**AMA:** 2017,Jan,8; 2016,Jan,13; 2015,Jan,16; 2014,Jan,11; 2013,Mar,13; 2012,Jan,15-42

Body of uterus
Tube
Classical
Low vertical
Low transverse
Pubic bone
Amniotic sac
Uterus at term
Cervix
Vagina

Types of Cesarean section are classified by uterine incision

**59514** **Cesarean delivery only;** Ⓜ ♀

INCLUDES Admission history
Admission to hospital
Cesarean delivery
Management of uncomplicated labor
Physical exam

EXCLUDES Inpatient management after delivery/discharge services (99217-99239 [99224, 99225, 99226])
Medical problems complicating labor and delivery

🔲 26.5 ⚖ 26.5 **FUD** MMM Ⓒ 80 🔲

**AMA:** 2017,Jan,8; 2016,Jan,13; 2015,Jan,16; 2014,Jan,11; 2013,Mar,13; 2012,Jan,15-42

**59515** **including postpartum care** Ⓜ ♀

INCLUDES Admission history
Admission to hospital
Cesarean delivery
Hospital/office visits following cesarean section or vaginal delivery
Management of uncomplicated labor
Physical exam

EXCLUDES Medical problems complicating labor and delivery

🔲 36.5 ⚖ 36.5 **FUD** MMM Ⓑ 🔲

**AMA:** 2017,Jan,8; 2016,Jan,13; 2015,Jan,16; 2014,Jan,11; 2013,Mar,13

**+ 59525** **Subtotal or total hysterectomy after cesarean delivery (List separately in addition to code for primary procedure)** Ⓜ ♀

Code first cesarean delivery (59510, 59514, 59515, 59618, 59620, 59622)

🔲 14.1 ⚖ 14.1 **FUD** ZZZ Ⓒ 80 🔲

**AMA:** 2014,Jan,11

## 59610-59614 Vaginal Delivery After Prior Cesarean Section: Comprehensive and Components of Care

**CMS:** 100-02,15,180 Nurse-Midwife (CNM) Services; 100-02,15,20.1 Physician Expense for Surgery, Childbirth, and Treatment for Infertility

INCLUDES Admission history
Admission to hospital
Management of uncomplicated labor
Patients with previous cesarean delivery who present with the expectation of a vaginal delivery
Physical exam
Successful vaginal delivery after previous cesarean delivery (VBAC)
Vaginal delivery with or without episiotomy or forceps

EXCLUDES Elective cesarean delivery (59510, 59514, 59515)
Medical complications of pregnancy, labor, and delivery:
  Cardiac problems
  Diabetes
  Hyperemesis
  Hypertension
  Neurological problems
  Premature rupture of membranes
  Pre-term labor
  Toxemia
  Trauma
Newborn circumcision (54150, 54160)
Services incidental to or unrelated to the pregnancy

**59610** **Routine obstetric care including antepartum care, vaginal delivery (with or without episiotomy, and/or forceps) and postpartum care, after previous cesarean delivery** Ⓜ ♀

INCLUDES Fetal heart tones
Hospital/office visits following cesarean section or vaginal delivery
Initial/subsequent history
Physical exams
Recording of weight/blood pressures
Routine chemical urinalysis
Routine prenatal visits:
  Each month up to 28 weeks gestation
  Every other week 29 to 36 weeks gestation
  Weekly from 36 weeks until delivery

🔲 63.4 ⚖ 63.4 **FUD** MMM Ⓑ 80 🔲

**AMA:** 2017,Jan,8; 2016,Jan,13; 2015,Jan,16; 2014,Jan,11

 PC/TC Only    ASC Payment    Bilateral   ♂ Male Only   ♀ Female Only    Facility RVU    Non-Facility RVU    CCI
**FUD** Follow-up Days   **CMS:** IOM (Pub 100)    OPPSI   80/80 Surg Assist Allowed / w/Doc    Lab Crosswalk   Radiology Crosswalk   ❌ CLIA

262
CPT © 2017 American Medical Association. All Rights Reserved.     © 2017 Optum360, LLC

| 59612 | Vaginal delivery only, after previous cesarean delivery (with or without episiotomy and/or forceps);    M ♀ |

EXCLUDES Inpatient management after delivery/discharge services (99217-99239 [99224, 99225, 99226])

🔧 26.6   ⚖ 26.6   **FUD** MMM    J 80 ▭

**AMA:** 2017,Jan,8; 2016,Jan,13; 2015,Jan,16; 2014,Jan,11

| 59614 | including postpartum care     M ♀ |

INCLUDES Hospital/office visits following cesarean section or vaginal delivery

🔧 33.0   ⚖ 33.0   **FUD** MMM    B 80 ▭

**AMA:** 2017,Jan,8; 2016,Jan,13; 2015,Jan,16; 2014,Jan,11

## 59618-59622 Cesarean Section After Attempted Vaginal Birth/Prior C-Section

**CMS:** 100-02,15,20.1 Physician Expense for Surgery, Childbirth, and Treatment for Infertility

INCLUDES Admission history
Admission to hospital
Cesarean delivery
Cesarean delivery following an unsuccessful vaginal delivery attempt after previous cesarean delivery
Management of uncomplicated labor
Patients with previous cesarean delivery who present with the expectation of a vaginal delivery
Physical exam

EXCLUDES Elective cesarean delivery (59510, 59514, 59515)
Medical complications of pregnancy, labor, and delivery:
  Cardiac problems
  Diabetes
  Hyperemesis
  Hypertension
  Neurological problems
  Premature rupture of membranes
  Pre-term labor
  Toxemia
  Trauma
Newborn circumcision (54150, 54160)
Services incidental to or unrelated to the pregnancy

| 59618 | Routine obstetric care including antepartum care, cesarean delivery, and postpartum care, following attempted vaginal delivery after previous cesarean delivery    M ♀ |

INCLUDES Fetal heart tones
Hospital/office visits following cesarean section or vaginal delivery
Initial/subsequent history
Physical exams
Recording of weight/blood pressures
Routine chemical urinalysis
Routine prenatal visits:
  Each month up to 28 weeks gestation
  Every two weeks 29 to 36 weeks gestation
  Weekly from 36 weeks until delivery

🔧 67.8   ⚖ 67.8   **FUD** MMM    B 80 ▭

**AMA:** 2017,Jan,8; 2016,Jan,13; 2015,Jan,16; 2014,Jan,11

| 59620 | Cesarean delivery only, following attempted vaginal delivery after previous cesarean delivery;    M ♀ |

EXCLUDES Inpatient management after delivery/discharge services (99217-99239 [99224, 99225, 99226])

🔧 27.1   ⚖ 27.1   **FUD** MMM    C 80 ▭

**AMA:** 2017,Jan,8; 2016,Jan,13; 2015,Jan,16; 2014,Jan,11

| 59622 | including postpartum care    M ♀ |

INCLUDES Hospital/office visits following cesarean section or vaginal delivery

🔧 37.2   ⚖ 37.2   **FUD** MMM    B 80 ▭

**AMA:** 2017,Jan,8; 2016,Jan,13; 2015,Jan,16; 2014,Jan,11

## 59812-59830 Treatment of Miscarriage

**CMS:** 100-02,15,20.1 Physician Expense for Surgery, Childbirth, and Treatment for Infertility

EXCLUDES Medical treatment of spontaneous complete abortion, any trimester (99201-99233 [99224, 99225, 99226])

| 59812 | Treatment of incomplete abortion, any trimester, completed surgically    M ♀ |

INCLUDES Surgical treatment of spontaneous abortion

🔧 8.54   ⚖ 9.17   **FUD** 090    J A2 ▭

**AMA:** 2017,Jan,8; 2016,Jan,13; 2015,Jan,16; 2014,Jan,11

| 59820 | Treatment of missed abortion, completed surgically; first trimester    M ♀ |

🔧 10.2   ⚖ 10.9   **FUD** 090    J A2 ▭

**AMA:** 2017,Jan,8; 2016,Jan,13; 2015,Jan,16; 2014,Jan,11

| 59821 | second trimester    M ♀ |

🔧 10.3   ⚖ 11.0   **FUD** 090    J A2 80 ▭

**AMA:** 2017,Jan,8; 2016,Jan,13; 2015,Jan,16; 2014,Jan,11

| 59830 | Treatment of septic abortion, completed surgically    M ♀ |

🔧 12.6   ⚖ 12.6   **FUD** 090    C 80 ▭

**AMA:** 2017,Jan,8; 2016,Jan,13; 2015,Jan,16; 2014,Jan,11

## 59840-59866 Elective Abortions

**CMS:** 100-02,1,90 Termination of Pregnancy; 100-02,15,20.1 Physician Expense for Surgery, Childbirth, and Treatment for Infertility; 100-03,140.1 Abortion; 100-04,3,100.1 Billing for Abortion Services

| 59840 | Induced abortion, by dilation and curettage    M ♀ |

🔧 5.99   ⚖ 6.24   **FUD** 010    J A2 80 ▭

**AMA:** 2017,Jan,8; 2016,Jan,13; 2015,Jan,16; 2014,Jan,11; 2012,Jan,15-42

| 59841 | Induced abortion, by dilation and evacuation    M ♀ |

🔧 10.4   ⚖ 11.0   **FUD** 010    J A2 80 ▭

**AMA:** 2017,Jan,8; 2016,Jan,13; 2015,Jan,16; 2014,Jan,11

| 59850 | Induced abortion, by 1 or more intra-amniotic injections (amniocentesis-injections), including hospital admission and visits, delivery of fetus and secundines;    M ♀ |

EXCLUDES Cervical dilator insertion (59200)

🔧 10.9   ⚖ 10.9   **FUD** 090    C 80 ▭

**AMA:** 2017,Jan,8; 2016,Jan,13; 2015,Jan,16; 2014,Jan,11

| 59851 | with dilation and curettage and/or evacuation    M ♀ |

EXCLUDES Cervical dilator insertion (59200)

🔧 11.5   ⚖ 11.5   **FUD** 090    C 80 ▭

**AMA:** 2017,Jan,8; 2016,Jan,13; 2015,Jan,16; 2014,Jan,11

| 59852 | with hysterotomy (failed intra-amniotic injection)    M ♀ |

EXCLUDES Cervical dilator insertion (59200)

🔧 14.4   ⚖ 14.4   **FUD** 090    C 80 ▭

**AMA:** 2017,Jan,8; 2016,Jan,13; 2015,Jan,16; 2014,Jan,11

| 59855 | Induced abortion, by 1 or more vaginal suppositories (eg, prostaglandin) with or without cervical dilation (eg, laminaria), including hospital admission and visits, delivery of fetus and secundines;    M ♀ |

🔧 12.0   ⚖ 12.0   **FUD** 090    C 80 ▭

**AMA:** 2014,Jan,11

| 59856 | with dilation and curettage and/or evacuation    M ♀ |

🔧 14.1   ⚖ 14.1   **FUD** 090    C 80 ▭

**AMA:** 2014,Jan,11

| 59857 | with hysterotomy (failed medical evacuation)    M ♀ |

🔧 14.8   ⚖ 14.8   **FUD** 090    C 80 ▭

**AMA:** 2014,Jan,11

| 59866 | Multifetal pregnancy reduction(s) (MPR)    M ♀ |

🔧 6.22   ⚖ 6.22   **FUD** 000    T 62 80 ▭

**AMA:** 2014,Jan,11

## 59870-59899 Miscellaneous Obstetrical Procedures

**CMS:** 100-02,15,20.1 Physician Expense for Surgery, Childbirth, and Treatment for Infertility

| 59870 | Uterine evacuation and curettage for hydatidiform mole    M ♀ |

🔧 13.6   ⚖ 13.6   **FUD** 090    J A2 80 ▭

**AMA:** 2017,Jan,8; 2016,Jan,13; 2015,Jan,16; 2014,Jan,11; 2012,Jan,15-42

| 59871 | Removal of cerclage suture under anesthesia (other than local)    M ♀ |

🔧 3.89   ⚖ 3.89   **FUD** 000    02 A2 80 ▭

**AMA:** 2017,Jan,8; 2016,Jan,13; 2015,Jan,16; 2014,Jan,11

| 59897 | Unlisted fetal invasive procedure, including ultrasound guidance, when performed    ♀ |

🔧 0.00   ⚖ 0.00   **FUD** YYY    T ▭

**AMA:** 2014,Jan,11

---

● New Code    ▲ Revised Code    ○ Reinstated    ● New Web Release    ▲ Revised Web Release    Unlisted    Not Covered    # Resequenced
⊘ AMA Mod 51 Exempt    ⑤ Optum Mod 51 Exempt    63 Mod 63 Exempt    ∕ Non-FDA Drug    ★ Telemedicine    M Maternity    A Age Edit    + Add-on    **AMA:** CPT Asst

**59898** Unlisted laparoscopy procedure, maternity care and delivery  M ♀
    ⚙ 0.00  ⚙ 0.00  **FUD** YYY  J 80 50
    **AMA:** 2017,Jan,8; 2016,Jan,13; 2015,Jan,16; 2014,Jan,11

**59899** Unlisted procedure, maternity care and delivery  M ♀
    ⚙ 0.00  ⚙ 0.00  **FUD** YYY  T 80
    **AMA:** 2017,Jan,8; 2016,Jan,13; 2015,Jan,16; 2014,Jan,11; 2013,Oct,3; 2012,Jan,15-42

# 60000 I&D of Infected Thyroglossal Cyst

**60000** Incision and drainage of thyroglossal duct cyst, infected

🔧 4.09 ⚗ 4.54 **FUD** 010    T A2 80 ▣

**AMA:** 2014,Jan,11

# 60100 Core Needle Biopsy: Thyroid

**EXCLUDES** *Fine needle aspiration (10021-10022)*

**60100** Biopsy thyroid, percutaneous core needle

📷 (76942, 77002, 77012, 77021)

🔬 (88172-88173)

🔧 2.28 ⚗ 3.22 **FUD** 000    T P3 ▣

**AMA:** 2017,Jan,8; 2016,Jan,13; 2015,Jan,16; 2014,Jan,11; 2012,Jan,15-42

# 60200 Surgical Removal Thyroid Cyst or Mass; Division of Isthmus

**60200** Excision of cyst or adenoma of thyroid, or transection of isthmus

🔧 19.0 ⚗ 19.0 **FUD** 090    J A2 80 ▣

**AMA:** 2017,Jan,8; 2016,Jan,13; 2015,Jan,16; 2014,Jan,11; 2012,Dec,3-5

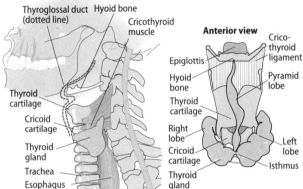

**Lateral view**

Thyroglossal duct (dotted line)
Hyoid bone
Cricothyroid muscle
Thyroid cartilage
Cricoid cartilage
Thyroid gland
Trachea
Esophagus

**Anterior view**

Crico-thyroid ligament
Epiglottis
Hyoid bone
Thyroid cartilage
Right lobe
Cricoid cartilage
Thyroid gland
Pyramid lobe
Left lobe
Isthmus

# 60210-60225 Subtotal Thyroidectomy

**60210** Partial thyroid lobectomy, unilateral; with or without isthmusectomy

🔧 20.3 ⚗ 20.3 **FUD** 090    J G2 80 ▣

**AMA:** 2017,Jan,8; 2016,Jan,13; 2015,Jan,16; 2014,Jan,11; 2012,Dec,3-5; 2012,Jan,15-42

**60212** with contralateral subtotal lobectomy, including isthmusectomy

🔧 29.0 ⚗ 29.0 **FUD** 090    J G2 80 ▣

**AMA:** 2017,Jan,8; 2016,Jan,13; 2015,Jan,16; 2014,Jan,11; 2012,Dec,3-5

**60220** Total thyroid lobectomy, unilateral; with or without isthmusectomy

🔧 20.3 ⚗ 20.3 **FUD** 090    J G2 80 ▣

**AMA:** 2017,Jan,8; 2016,Jan,13; 2015,Jan,16; 2014,Jan,11; 2012,Dec,3-5; 2012,Jan,15-42

**60225** with contralateral subtotal lobectomy, including isthmusectomy

🔧 26.8 ⚗ 26.8 **FUD** 090    J G2 80 ▣

**AMA:** 2017,Jan,8; 2016,Jan,13; 2015,Jan,16; 2014,Jan,11; 2012,Dec,3-5

# 60240-60271 Complete Thyroidectomy Procedures

**60240** Thyroidectomy, total or complete

**EXCLUDES** *Subtotal or partial thyroidectomy (60271)*

🔧 26.4 ⚗ 26.4 **FUD** 090    J G2 80 ▣

**AMA:** 2017,Jan,8; 2016,Jan,13; 2015,Jan,16; 2014,Jan,11; 2012,Dec,3-5

**60252** Thyroidectomy, total or subtotal for malignancy; with limited neck dissection

🔧 38.0 ⚗ 38.0 **FUD** 090    J 80 ▣

**AMA:** 2017,Jan,8; 2016,Jan,13; 2015,Jan,16; 2014,Jan,11; 2012,Dec,3-5; 2012,Jan,15-42

**60254** with radical neck dissection

🔧 48.0 ⚗ 48.0 **FUD** 090    C 80 ▣

**AMA:** 2017,Jan,8; 2016,Jan,13; 2015,Jan,16; 2014,Jan,11; 2012,Dec,3-5; 2012,Jan,15-42

**60260** Thyroidectomy, removal of all remaining thyroid tissue following previous removal of a portion of thyroid

🔧 31.4 ⚗ 31.4 **FUD** 090    J 80 50 ▣

**AMA:** 2017,Jan,8; 2016,Jan,13; 2015,Jan,16; 2014,Jan,11; 2012,Dec,3-5; 2012,Jan,15-42

**60270** Thyroidectomy, including substernal thyroid; sternal split or transthoracic approach

🔧 39.5 ⚗ 39.5 **FUD** 090    C 80 ▣

**AMA:** 2017,Jan,8; 2016,Jan,13; 2015,Jan,16; 2014,Jan,11; 2012,Dec,3-5

**60271** cervical approach

🔧 30.4 ⚗ 30.4 **FUD** 090    J 80 ▣

**AMA:** 2017,Jan,8; 2016,Jan,13; 2015,Jan,16; 2014,Jan,11; 2012,Dec,3-5

# 60280-60300 Treatment of Cyst/Sinus of Thyroid

**60280** Excision of thyroglossal duct cyst or sinus;

**EXCLUDES** *Thyroid ultrasound (76536)*

🔧 12.6 ⚗ 12.6 **FUD** 090    J A2 80 ▣

**AMA:** 2014,Jan,11

**60281** recurrent

**EXCLUDES** *Thyroid ultrasound (76536)*

🔧 16.9 ⚗ 16.9 **FUD** 090    J A2 80 ▣

**AMA:** 2014,Jan,11

**60300** Aspiration and/or injection, thyroid cyst

**EXCLUDES** *Fine needle aspiration (10021-10022)*

📷 (76942, 77012)

🔧 1.44 ⚗ 3.36 **FUD** 000    T P3 ▣

**AMA:** 2014,Jan,11

# 60500-60512 Parathyroid Procedures

**60500** Parathyroidectomy or exploration of parathyroid(s);

🔧 27.8 ⚗ 27.8 **FUD** 090    J G2 80 ▣

**AMA:** 2017,Jan,8; 2016,Jan,13; 2015,Jan,16; 2014,Jan,11; 2012,Dec,3-5

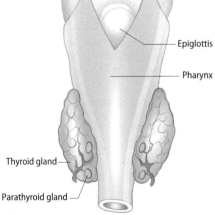

Epiglottis
Pharynx
Thyroid gland
Parathyroid gland

**Posterior view of pharynx, thyroid glands, and parathyroid glands**

**60502** re-exploration

🔧 37.1 ⚗ 37.1 **FUD** 090    J 80 ▣

**AMA:** 2017,Jan,8; 2016,Jan,13; 2015,Jan,16; 2014,Jan,11; 2012,Dec,3-5

---

● New Code   ▲ Revised Code   ○ Reinstated   ● New Web Release   ▲ Revised Web Release   Unlisted   Not Covered   # Resequenced
⊘ AMA Mod 51 Exempt   ⑤⓪ Optum Mod 51 Exempt   ⓺⓷ Mod 63 Exempt   ✗ Non-FDA Drug   ★ Telemedicine   Ⓜ Maternity   Ⓐ Age Edit   ✚ Add-on   **AMA:** CPT Asst

© 2017 Optum360, LLC    CPT © 2017 American Medical Association. All Rights Reserved.

**60505** with mediastinal exploration, sternal split or transthoracic approach

    🚗 39.9    ⚕ 39.9    **FUD** 090      C 80 ▣

    **AMA:** 2017,Jan,8; 2016,Jan,13; 2015,Jan,16; 2014,Jan,11; 2012,Dec,3-5

**+ 60512** Parathyroid autotransplantation (List separately in addition to code for primary procedure)

    Code first (60212, 60225, 60240, 60252, 60254, 60260, 60270-60271, 60500, 60502, 60505)

    🚗 7.03    ⚕ 7.03    **FUD** ZZZ      N 80 ▣

    **AMA:** 2017,Jan,6; 2017,Jan,8; 2016,Jan,13; 2015,Jan,16; 2014,Jan,11; 2012,Dec,3-5; 2012,Jan,15-42

## 60520-60522 Thymus Procedures

EXCLUDES    Surgical thoracoscopy (video-assisted thoracic surgery (VATS) thymectomy (32673)

**60520** Thymectomy, partial or total; transcervical approach (separate procedure)

    🚗 30.1    ⚕ 30.1    **FUD** 090      J 80 ▣

    **AMA:** 2014,Jan,11; 2012,Oct,9-11; 2012,Sep,3-8

**60521** sternal split or transthoracic approach, without radical mediastinal dissection (separate procedure)

    🚗 32.4    ⚕ 32.4    **FUD** 090      C 80 ▣

    **AMA:** 2017,Jan,8; 2016,Jan,13; 2015,Jan,16; 2014,Jan,11; 2012,Oct,9-11; 2012,Sep,3-8; 2012,Jan,15-42

**60522** sternal split or transthoracic approach, with radical mediastinal dissection (separate procedure)

    🚗 39.4    ⚕ 39.4    **FUD** 090      C 80 ▣

    **AMA:** 2014,Jan,11; 2012,Oct,9-11; 2012,Sep,3-8

## 60540-60545 Adrenal Gland Procedures

EXCLUDES    Laparoscopic approach (60650)
    Removal of remote or disseminated pheochromocytoma (49203-49205)
    Standard backbench preparation of cadaver donor (50323)

**60540** Adrenalectomy, partial or complete, or exploration of adrenal gland with or without biopsy, transabdominal, lumbar or dorsal (separate procedure);

    🚗 30.7    ⚕ 30.7    **FUD** 090      C 80 50 ▣

    **AMA:** 2014,Jan,11

**60545** with excision of adjacent retroperitoneal tumor

    🚗 35.2    ⚕ 35.2    **FUD** 090      C 80 50 ▣

    **AMA:** 2014,Jan,11

## 60600-60605 Carotid Body Procedures

**60600** Excision of carotid body tumor; without excision of carotid artery

    🚗 40.1    ⚕ 40.1    **FUD** 090      C 80 ▣

    **AMA:** 2014,Jan,11

**60605** with excision of carotid artery

    🚗 55.9    ⚕ 55.9    **FUD** 090      C 80 ▣

    **AMA:** 2017,Sep,13; 2016,Nov,8; 2016,Oct,10; 2016,Sep,8; 2016,Jul,10; 2014,Jan,11

## 60650-60699 Laparoscopic and Unlisted Procedures

INCLUDES    Diagnostic laparoscopy (49320)

**60650** Laparoscopy, surgical, with adrenalectomy, partial or complete, or exploration of adrenal gland with or without biopsy, transabdominal, lumbar or dorsal

    EXCLUDES    Peritoneoscopy performed as separate procedure (49320)

    🚗 34.5    ⚕ 34.5    **FUD** 090      C 80 50 ▣

    **AMA:** 2017,Jan,8; 2016,Jan,13; 2015,Jan,16; 2014,Jan,11

**60659** Unlisted laparoscopy procedure, endocrine system

    🚗 0.00    ⚕ 0.00    **FUD** YYY      J 80 50

    **AMA:** 2017,Jan,8; 2016,Jan,13; 2015,Jan,16; 2014,Jan,11

**60699** Unlisted procedure, endocrine system

    🚗 0.00    ⚕ 0.00    **FUD** YYY      J 80

    **AMA:** 2017,Jan,8; 2016,Jan,13; 2015,Jan,16; 2014,Jan,11; 2012,Jan,15-42

Nervous System

61000 — 61253

# 61000-61253 Transcranial Access via Puncture, Burr Hole, Twist Hole, or Trephine

*EXCLUDES* Injection for:
Cerebral angiography (36100-36218)

**61000** Subdural tap through fontanelle, or suture, infant, unilateral or bilateral; initial ⒜

*EXCLUDES* Injection for:
Pneumoencephalography (61055)
Ventriculography (61026, 61120)

🚑 3.28 ⚕ 3.28 **FUD** 000 Ⓣ Ⓡ2 🖥

**AMA:** 2014,Jan,11

**Overhead view of newborn skull**

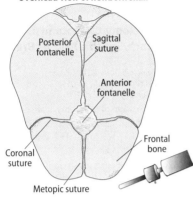

Posterior fontanelle
Sagittal suture
Anterior fontanelle
Coronal suture
Frontal bone
Metopic suture

An initial tap through to the subdural level is performed on an infant via a fontanelle or suture, either unilateral or bilateral

**61001** subsequent taps ⒜

🚑 2.42 ⚕ 2.42 **FUD** 000 Ⓣ Ⓡ2 🖥

**AMA:** 2014,Jan,11

**61020** Ventricular puncture through previous burr hole, fontanelle, suture, or implanted ventricular catheter/reservoir; without injection

🚑 2.94 ⚕ 2.94 **FUD** 000 Ⓣ A2 🖥

**AMA:** 2014,Jan,11

**61026** with injection of medication or other substance for diagnosis or treatment

*INCLUDES* Injection for ventriculography

🚑 3.02 ⚕ 3.02 **FUD** 000 Ⓣ A2 🖥

**AMA:** 2014,Jan,11

**61050** Cisternal or lateral cervical (C1-C2) puncture; without injection (separate procedure)

🚑 2.48 ⚕ 2.48 **FUD** 000 Ⓣ A2 80 🖥

**AMA:** 2014,Jan,11

**61055** with injection of medication or other substance for diagnosis or treatment

*INCLUDES* Injection for pneumoencephalography

*EXCLUDES* Myelography via lumbar injection (62302-62305)
Radiology procedures except when furnished by a different provider

🚑 3.52 ⚕ 3.52 **FUD** 000 Ⓣ A2 🖥

**AMA:** 2014,Sep,3; 2014,Jan,11

**61070** Puncture of shunt tubing or reservoir for aspiration or injection procedure

📷 (75809)

🚑 1.66 ⚕ 1.66 **FUD** 000 Ⓣ A2 🖥

**AMA:** 2017,Jan,8; 2016,Jan,13; 2015,Jan,16; 2014,Jan,11; 2012,Jan,15-42

**61105** Twist drill hole for subdural or ventricular puncture

🚑 12.9 ⚕ 12.9 **FUD** 090 Ⓒ 80 🖥

**AMA:** 2014,Jan,11

**61107** Twist drill hole(s) for subdural, intracerebral, or ventricular puncture; for implanting ventricular catheter, pressure recording device, or other intracerebral monitoring device

Code also intracranial neuroendoscopic ventricular catheter insertion or reinsertion, when performed (62160)

🚑 9.27 ⚕ 9.27 **FUD** 000 ⊘ Ⓒ 🖥

**AMA:** 2014,Jan,11

**61108** for evacuation and/or drainage of subdural hematoma

🚑 26.4 ⚕ 26.4 **FUD** 090 Ⓒ 🖥

**AMA:** 2014,Jan,11

**61120** Burr hole(s) for ventricular puncture (including injection of gas, contrast media, dye, or radioactive material)

*INCLUDES* Includes: Injection for ventriculography

🚑 21.8 ⚕ 21.8 **FUD** 090 Ⓒ 80 🖥

**AMA:** 2014,Jan,11

**61140** Burr hole(s) or trephine; with biopsy of brain or intracranial lesion

🚑 36.9 ⚕ 36.9 **FUD** 090 Ⓒ 80 🖥

**AMA:** 2014,Jan,11

**61150** with drainage of brain abscess or cyst

🚑 39.7 ⚕ 39.7 **FUD** 090 Ⓒ 🖥

**AMA:** 2014,Jan,11

**61151** with subsequent tapping (aspiration) of intracranial abscess or cyst

🚑 29.2 ⚕ 29.2 **FUD** 090 Ⓒ 🖥

**AMA:** 2014,Jan,11

**61154** Burr hole(s) with evacuation and/or drainage of hematoma, extradural or subdural

🚑 37.2 ⚕ 37.2 **FUD** 090 Ⓒ 80 50 🖥

**AMA:** 2014,Jan,11

**61156** Burr hole(s); with aspiration of hematoma or cyst, intracerebral

🚑 36.5 ⚕ 36.5 **FUD** 090 Ⓒ 80 🖥

**AMA:** 2014,Jan,11

**61210** for implanting ventricular catheter, reservoir, EEG electrode(s), pressure recording device, or other cerebral monitoring device (separate procedure)

Code also intracranial neuroendoscopic ventricular catheter insertion or reinsertion, when performed (62160)

🚑 10.9 ⚕ 10.9 **FUD** 000 Ⓒ 🖥

**AMA:** 2017,Jan,8; 2016,Jan,13; 2015,Jan,16; 2014,Jan,11; 2012,Jan,15-42

**61215** Insertion of subcutaneous reservoir, pump or continuous infusion system for connection to ventricular catheter

*EXCLUDES* Chemotherapy (96450)
Refilling and maintenance of implantable infusion pump (95990)

🚑 14.8 ⚕ 14.8 **FUD** 090 Ⓙ A2 🖥

**AMA:** 2017,Jan,8; 2016,Jan,13; 2015,Jan,16; 2014,Jan,11

**61250** Burr hole(s) or trephine, supratentorial, exploratory, not followed by other surgery

*EXCLUDES* Burr hole or trephine followed by craniotomy at same operative session (61304-61321)

🚑 24.2 ⚕ 24.2 **FUD** 090 Ⓒ 80 50 🖥

**AMA:** 2014,Jan,11

**61253** Burr hole(s) or trephine, infratentorial, unilateral or bilateral

*EXCLUDES* Burr hole or trephine followed by craniotomy at same operative session (61304-61321)

🚑 23.4 ⚕ 23.4 **FUD** 090 Ⓒ 80 🖥

**AMA:** 2017,Jan,8; 2016,Jan,13; 2015,Jan,16; 2014,Jan,11; 2012,Jan,15-42

**Nervous System**

## 61304-61323 Craniectomy/Craniotomy: By Indication/Specific Area of Brain

*EXCLUDES*  Injection for:
> *Cerebral angiography (36100-36218)*
> *Pneumoencephalography (61055)*
> *Ventriculography (61026, 61120)*

### 61304   Craniectomy or craniotomy, exploratory; supratentorial

> *EXCLUDES*  *Other craniectomy/craniotomy procedures when performed at the same anatomical site and during the same surgical encounter*

🖪 47.9   ⚕ 47.9   **FUD** 090                 C 80 ▭

**AMA:** 2014,Jan,11

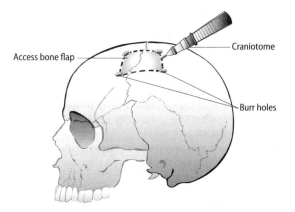

Access bone flap — Craniotome

Burr holes

### 61305   infratentorial (posterior fossa)

> *EXCLUDES*  *Other craniectomy/craniotomy procedures when performed at the same anatomical site and during the same surgical encounter*

🖪 59.2   ⚕ 59.2   **FUD** 090                 C 80 ▭

**AMA:** 2014,Jan,11

### 61312   Craniectomy or craniotomy for evacuation of hematoma, supratentorial; extradural or subdural

🖪 61.0   ⚕ 61.0   **FUD** 090                 C 80 ▭

**AMA:** 2017,Jan,8; 2016,Jan,13; 2015,Jan,16; 2014,Jan,11

### 61313   intracerebral

🖪 58.1   ⚕ 58.1   **FUD** 090                 C 80 ▭

**AMA:** 2014,Jan,11

### 61314   Craniectomy or craniotomy for evacuation of hematoma, infratentorial; extradural or subdural

🖪 53.6   ⚕ 53.6   **FUD** 090                 C 80 ▭

**AMA:** 2014,Jan,11

### 61315   intracerebellar

🖪 60.7   ⚕ 60.7   **FUD** 090                 C 80 ▭

**AMA:** 2014,Jan,11

+ ### 61316   Incision and subcutaneous placement of cranial bone graft (List separately in addition to code for primary procedure)

> Code first (61304, 61312-61313, 61322-61323, 61340, 61570-61571, 61680-61705)

🖪 2.62   ⚕ 2.62   **FUD** ZZZ                 C ▭

**AMA:** 2014,Jan,11

### 61320   Craniectomy or craniotomy, drainage of intracranial abscess; supratentorial

🖪 55.7   ⚕ 55.7   **FUD** 090                 C 80 ▭

**AMA:** 2014,Jan,11

### 61321   infratentorial

🖪 62.0   ⚕ 62.0   **FUD** 090                 C 80 ▭

**AMA:** 2014,Jan,11

### 61322   Craniectomy or craniotomy, decompressive, with or without duraplasty, for treatment of intracranial hypertension, without evacuation of associated intraparenchymal hematoma; without lobectomy

> *EXCLUDES*  *Craniectomy or craniotomy for evacuation of hematoma (61313)*
> *Subtemporal decompression (61340)*

🖪 69.8   ⚕ 69.8   **FUD** 090                 C 80 ▭

**AMA:** 2014,Jan,11

### 61323   with lobectomy

> *EXCLUDES*  *Craniectomy or craniotomy for evacuation of hematoma (61313)*
> *Subtemporal decompression (61340)*

🖪 70.7   ⚕ 70.7   **FUD** 090                 C 80 ▭

**AMA:** 2014,Jan,11

## 61330-61530 Craniectomy/Craniotomy/Decompression Brain By Surgical Approach/Specific Area of Brain

*EXCLUDES*  Injection for:
> *Cerebral angiography (36100-36218)*
> *Pneumoencephalography (61055)*
> *Ventriculography (61026, 61120)*

### 61330   Decompression of orbit only, transcranial approach

> *INCLUDES*  Naffziger operation

🖪 51.5   ⚕ 51.5   **FUD** 090                 J 02 80 50 ▭

**AMA:** 2014,Jan,11

### 61332   Exploration of orbit (transcranial approach); with biopsy

🖪 49.3   ⚕ 49.3   **FUD** 090                 C 80 50 ▭

**AMA:** 2014,Jan,11

### 61333   with removal of lesion

🖪 52.2   ⚕ 52.2   **FUD** 090                 C 80 50 ▭

**AMA:** 2014,Jan,11

### 61340   Subtemporal cranial decompression (pseudotumor cerebri, slit ventricle syndrome)

> *EXCLUDES*  *Decompression craniotomy or craniectomy for intracranial hypertension, without hematoma removal (61322-61323)*

🖪 42.6   ⚕ 42.6   **FUD** 090                 C 80 50 ▭

**AMA:** 2014,Jan,11

### 61343   Craniectomy, suboccipital with cervical laminectomy for decompression of medulla and spinal cord, with or without dural graft (eg, Arnold-Chiari malformation)

🖪 64.4   ⚕ 64.4   **FUD** 090                 C 80 ▭

**AMA:** 2014,Jan,11

### 61345   Other cranial decompression, posterior fossa

> *EXCLUDES*  *Kroenlein procedure (67445)*
> *Orbital decompression using a lateral wall approach (67445)*

🖪 59.7   ⚕ 59.7   **FUD** 090                 C 80 ▭

**AMA:** 2014,Jan,11

### 61450   Craniectomy, subtemporal, for section, compression, or decompression of sensory root of gasserian ganglion

> *INCLUDES*  Frazier-Spiller procedure
> Hartley-Krause
> Krause decompression
> Taarnhoj procedure

🖪 56.7   ⚕ 56.7   **FUD** 090                 C 80 ▭

**AMA:** 2014,Jan,11

### 61458   Craniectomy, suboccipital; for exploration or decompression of cranial nerves

> *INCLUDES*  Jannetta decompression

🖪 58.9   ⚕ 58.9   **FUD** 090                 C 80 ▭

**AMA:** 2014,Jan,11

**61460**     **for section of 1 or more cranial nerves**
        60.4     60.4     **FUD** 090     C 80
        **AMA:** 2014,Jan,11

Olfactory nerve (I)
Optic nerve (II)
Oculomotor nerve (III)
Trochlear nerve (IV)
Trigeminal nerve (V)
Abducens nerve (VI)
Pons
Facial nerve (VII)
Vestibulocochlear nerve (VIII)
Glossopharyngeal nerve (IX)
Vagus nerve (X)
Hypoglossal nerve (XII)
Accessory nerve (XI)

**61480**     **for mesencephalic tractotomy or pedunculotomy**
        57.2     57.2     **FUD** 090     C 80
        **AMA:** 2014,Jan,11

**61500**     **Craniectomy; with excision of tumor or other bone lesion of skull**
        38.4     38.4     **FUD** 090     C 80
        **AMA:** 2017,Jan,8; 2016,Jan,13; 2015,Jan,16; 2014,Jan,11; 2014,Jan,9

**61501**     **for osteomyelitis**
        33.3     33.3     **FUD** 090     C 80
        **AMA:** 2017,Jan,8; 2016,Jan,13; 2015,Jan,16; 2014,Jan,11; 2014,Jan,9

**61510**     **Craniectomy, trephination, bone flap craniotomy; for excision of brain tumor, supratentorial, except meningioma**
        64.0     64.0     **FUD** 090     C 80
        **AMA:** 2014,Jan,11

**61512**     **for excision of meningioma, supratentorial**
        74.7     74.7     **FUD** 090     C 80
        **AMA:** 2014,Jan,11

**61514**     **for excision of brain abscess, supratentorial**
        55.7     55.7     **FUD** 090     C 80
        **AMA:** 2014,Jan,11

**61516**     **for excision or fenestration of cyst, supratentorial**
        EXCLUDES     Craniopharyngioma (61545)
                Pituitary tumor removal (61546, 61548)
        54.4     54.4     **FUD** 090     C 80
        **AMA:** 2014,Jan,11

+ **61517**   **Implantation of brain intracavitary chemotherapy agent (List separately in addition to code for primary procedure)**
        EXCLUDES     Intracavity radioelement source or ribbon implantation (77770-77772)
        Code first (61510, 61518)
        2.58     2.58     **FUD** ZZZ     C
        **AMA:** 2014,Jan,11

**61518**     **Craniectomy for excision of brain tumor, infratentorial or posterior fossa; except meningioma, cerebellopontine angle tumor, or midline tumor at base of skull**
        80.8     80.8     **FUD** 090     C 80
        **AMA:** 2014,Jan,11

**61519**     **meningioma**
        86.3     86.3     **FUD** 090     C 80
        **AMA:** 2014,Jan,11

**61520**     **cerebellopontine angle tumor**
        110.     110.     **FUD** 090     C 80
        **AMA:** 2014,Jan,11

Central sulcus
Parietal lobe
Frontal lobe
Occipital lobe
Lateral sulcus
Cerebellum
Temporal lobe
Pons
Medulla oblongata

**61521**     **midline tumor at base of skull**
        93.3     93.3     **FUD** 090     C 80
        **AMA:** 2017,Jan,8; 2016,Jan,13; 2015,Jan,16; 2014,Jan,11

**61522**     **Craniectomy, infratentorial or posterior fossa; for excision of brain abscess**
        64.5     64.5     **FUD** 090     C 80
        **AMA:** 2014,Jan,11

**61524**     **for excision or fenestration of cyst**
        61.1     61.1     **FUD** 090     C 80
        **AMA:** 2014,Jan,11

**61526**     **Craniectomy, bone flap craniotomy, transtemporal (mastoid) for excision of cerebellopontine angle tumor;**
        107.     107.     **FUD** 090     C
        **AMA:** 2017,Jan,8; 2016,Jan,13; 2015,Jan,16; 2014,Jan,11

**61530**     **combined with middle/posterior fossa craniotomy/craniectomy**
        89.9     89.9     **FUD** 090     C
        **AMA:** 2014,Jan,11

## 61531-61545 Procedures for Seizures/Implanted Electrodes/Choroid Plexus/Craniopharyngioma

EXCLUDES     Craniotomy for:
            Multiple subpial transections during procedure (61567)
            Selective amygdalohippocampectomy (61566)
        Injection for:
            Cerebral angiography (36100-36218)
            Pneumoencephalography (61055)
            Ventriculography (61026, 61120)

**61531**     **Subdural implantation of strip electrodes through 1 or more burr or trephine hole(s) for long-term seizure monitoring**
        EXCLUDES     Continuous EEG observation (95950-95954)
                Craniotomy for intracranial arteriovenous malformation removal (61680-61692)
                Stereotactic insertion of electrodes (61760)
        35.2     35.2     **FUD** 090     C 80
        **AMA:** 2014,Jan,11

**61533**     **Craniotomy with elevation of bone flap; for subdural implantation of an electrode array, for long-term seizure monitoring**
        EXCLUDES     Continuous EEG observation (95950-95954)
        44.4     44.4     **FUD** 090     C 80
        **AMA:** 2014,Jan,11

**61534**     **for excision of epileptogenic focus without electrocorticography during surgery**
        48.4     48.4     **FUD** 090     C 80
        **AMA:** 2014,Jan,11

● New Code     ▲ Revised Code     ○ Reinstated     ● New Web Release     ▲ Revised Web Release     Unlisted     Not Covered     # Resequenced
⊘ AMA Mod 51 Exempt     ⑤⓪ Optum Mod 51 Exempt     ⑥③ Mod 63 Exempt     ✗ Non-FDA Drug     ★ Telemedicine     Ⓜ Maternity     Ⓐ Age Edit     + Add-on     **AMA:** CPT Asst
© 2017 Optum360, LLC     CPT © 2017 American Medical Association. All Rights Reserved.     **269**

**61535**   for removal of epidural or subdural electrode array, without excision of cerebral tissue (separate procedure)

    📷 28.8   ✂ 28.8   **FUD** 090   [C][80][CCI]

    **AMA:** 2014,Jan,11

**61536**   for excision of cerebral epileptogenic focus, with electrocorticography during surgery (includes removal of electrode array)

    📷 75.1   ✂ 75.1   **FUD** 090   [C][80][CCI]

    **AMA:** 2014,Jan,11

**61537**   for lobectomy, temporal lobe, without electrocorticography during surgery

    📷 72.7   ✂ 72.7   **FUD** 090   [C][80][CCI]

    **AMA:** 2014,Jan,11

**61538**   for lobectomy, temporal lobe, with electrocorticography during surgery

    📷 78.4   ✂ 78.4   **FUD** 090   [C][80][CCI]

    **AMA:** 2014,Jan,11

**61539**   for lobectomy, other than temporal lobe, partial or total, with electrocorticography during surgery

    📷 69.6   ✂ 69.6   **FUD** 090   [C][80][CCI]

    **AMA:** 2014,Jan,11

**61540**   for lobectomy, other than temporal lobe, partial or total, without electrocorticography during surgery

    📷 63.4   ✂ 63.4   **FUD** 090   [C][80][CCI]

    **AMA:** 2014,Jan,11

**61541**   for transection of corpus callosum

    📷 63.3   ✂ 63.3   **FUD** 090   [C][80][CCI]

    **AMA:** 2014,Jan,11

**61543**   for partial or subtotal (functional) hemispherectomy

    📷 61.3   ✂ 61.3   **FUD** 090   [C][80][CCI]

    **AMA:** 2014,Jan,11

**61544**   for excision or coagulation of choroid plexus

    📷 56.1   ✂ 56.1   **FUD** 090   [C][80][CCI]

    **AMA:** 2014,Jan,11

**61545**   for excision of craniopharyngioma

    📷 93.9   ✂ 93.9   **FUD** 090   [C][80][CCI]

    **AMA:** 2014,Jan,11

## 61546-61548 Removal Pituitary Gland/Tumor

EXCLUDES   Injection for:
    Cerebral angiography (36100-36218)
    Pneumoencephalography (61055)
    Ventriculography (61026, 61120)

**61546**   Craniotomy for hypophysectomy or excision of pituitary tumor, intracranial approach

    📷 67.7   ✂ 67.7   **FUD** 090   [C][80][CCI]

    **AMA:** 2014,Jan,11

**61548**   Hypophysectomy or excision of pituitary tumor, transnasal or transseptal approach, nonstereotactic

    INCLUDES   Operating microscope (69990)

    📷 46.0   ✂ 46.0   **FUD** 090   [C][80][CCI]

    **AMA:** 2016,Feb,12; 2014,Jan,11

## 61550-61559 Craniosynostosis Procedures

EXCLUDES   Injection for:
    Cerebral angiography (36100-36218)
    Pneumoencephalography (61055)
    Ventriculography (61026, 61120)
    Orbital hypertelorism reconstruction (21260-21263)
    Reconstruction (21172-21180)

**61550**   Craniectomy for craniosynostosis; single cranial suture

    📷 34.8   ✂ 34.8   **FUD** 090   [C][80][CCI]

    **AMA:** 2017,Jan,8; 2016,Jan,13; 2015,Jan,16; 2014,Jan,11; 2012,Feb,11

**61552**   multiple cranial sutures

    📷 33.5   ✂ 33.5   **FUD** 090   [C][80][CCI]

    **AMA:** 2017,Jan,8; 2016,Jan,13; 2015,Jan,16; 2014,Jan,11; 2012,Feb,11

**61556**   Craniotomy for craniosynostosis; frontal or parietal bone flap

    📷 45.3   ✂ 45.3   **FUD** 090   [C][80][CCI]

    **AMA:** 2017,Jan,8; 2016,Jan,13; 2015,Jan,16; 2014,Jan,11; 2012,Feb,11

**61557**   bifrontal bone flap

    📷 49.5   ✂ 49.5   **FUD** 090   [C][80][CCI]

    **AMA:** 2017,Jan,8; 2016,Jan,13; 2015,Jan,16; 2014,Jan,11; 2012,Feb,11

**61558**   Extensive craniectomy for multiple cranial suture craniosynostosis (eg, cloverleaf skull); not requiring bone grafts

    📷 55.3   ✂ 55.3   **FUD** 090   [C][80][CCI]

    **AMA:** 2017,Jan,8; 2016,Jan,13; 2015,Jan,16; 2014,Jan,11; 2012,Feb,11

**61559**   recontouring with multiple osteotomies and bone autografts (eg, barrel-stave procedure) (includes obtaining grafts)

    📷 66.9   ✂ 66.9   **FUD** 090   [C][80][CCI]

    **AMA:** 2017,Jan,8; 2016,Jan,13; 2015,Jan,16; 2014,Jan,11; 2012,Feb,11

## 61563-61564 Removal Cranial Bone Tumor With/Without Optic Nerve Decompression

EXCLUDES   Injection for:
    Cerebral angiography (36100-36218)
    Pneumoencephalography (61055)
    Ventriculography (61026, 61120)
    Reconstruction (21181-21183)

**61563**   Excision, intra and extracranial, benign tumor of cranial bone (eg, fibrous dysplasia); without optic nerve decompression

    📷 57.9   ✂ 57.9   **FUD** 090   [C][80][CCI]

    **AMA:** 2014,Jan,11

**61564**   with optic nerve decompression

    📷 66.9   ✂ 66.9   **FUD** 090   [C][80][50][CCI]

    **AMA:** 2014,Jan,11

## 61566-61567 Craniotomy for Seizures

EXCLUDES   Injection for:
    Cerebral angiography (36100-36218)
    Pneumoencephalography (61055)
    Ventriculography (61026, 61120)

**61566**   Craniotomy with elevation of bone flap; for selective amygdalohippocampectomy

    📷 66.3   ✂ 66.3   **FUD** 090   [C][80][CCI]

    **AMA:** 2014,Jan,11

**61567**   for multiple subpial transections, with electrocorticography during surgery

    📷 69.4   ✂ 69.4   **FUD** 090   [C][80][CCI]

    **AMA:** 2014,Jan,11

## 61570-61571 Removal of Foreign Body from Brain

EXCLUDES   Injection for:
    Cerebral angiography (36100-36218)
    Pneumoencephalography (61055)
    Ventriculography (61026, 61120)
    Sequestrectomy for osteomyelitis (61501)

**61570**   Craniectomy or craniotomy; with excision of foreign body from brain

    📷 53.9   ✂ 53.9   **FUD** 090   [C][80][CCI]

    **AMA:** 2014,Jan,11

**61571**   with treatment of penetrating wound of brain

    📷 58.6   ✂ 58.6   **FUD** 090   [C][80][CCI]

    **AMA:** 2014,Jan,11

26/TC PC/TC Only   A2-Z3 ASC Payment   50 Bilateral   ♂ Male Only   ♀ Female Only   📷 Facility RVU   ✂ Non-Facility RVU   CCI
**FUD** Follow-up Days   **CMS:** IOM (Pub 100)   A-Y OPPSI   80/80 Surg Assist Allowed / w/Doc   Lab Crosswalk   Radiology Crosswalk   CLIA
270    CPT © 2017 American Medical Association. All Rights Reserved.    © 2017 Optum360, LLC

## 61575-61576 Transoral Approach Posterior Cranial Fossa/Upper Cervical Cord

EXCLUDES Arthrodesis (22548)
Injection for:
Cerebral angiography (36100-36218)
Pneumoencephalography (61055)
Ventriculography (61026, 61120)

**61575** Transoral approach to skull base, brain stem or upper spinal cord for biopsy, decompression or excision of lesion;
🔲 72.9 🔲 72.9 **FUD** 090 C 80 ▣
**AMA:** 2014,Jan,11

**61576** requiring splitting of tongue and/or mandible (including tracheostomy)
🔲 98.6 🔲 98.6 **FUD** 090 C 80 ▣
**AMA:** 2014,Jan,11

## 61580-61598 Surgical Approach: Cranial Fossae

EXCLUDES Definitive surgery (61600-61616)
Dural repair and/or reconstruction (61618-61619)
Injection for:
Cerebral angiography (36100-36218)
Pneumoencephalography (61055)
Ventriculography (61026, 61120)
Primary closure (15730, 15733, 15756-15758)

**61580** Craniofacial approach to anterior cranial fossa; extradural, including lateral rhinotomy, ethmoidectomy, sphenoidectomy, without maxillectomy or orbital exenteration
🔲 71.4 🔲 71.4 **FUD** 090 C 50 ▣
**AMA:** 2017,Jan,8; 2016,Jan,13; 2015,Jan,16; 2014,Jan,11

**61581** extradural, including lateral rhinotomy, orbital exenteration, ethmoidectomy, sphenoidectomy and/or maxillectomy
🔲 76.4 🔲 76.4 **FUD** 090 C 50 ▣
**AMA:** 2017,Jan,8; 2016,Jan,13; 2015,Jan,16; 2014,Jan,11

**61582** extradural, including unilateral or bifrontal craniotomy, elevation of frontal lobe(s), osteotomy of base of anterior cranial fossa
🔲 87.6 🔲 87.6 **FUD** 090 C 80 ▣
**AMA:** 2017,Jan,8; 2016,Jan,13; 2015,Jan,16; 2014,Jan,11

**61583** intradural, including unilateral or bifrontal craniotomy, elevation or resection of frontal lobe, osteotomy of base of anterior cranial fossa
🔲 84.4 🔲 84.4 **FUD** 090 C 80 ▣
**AMA:** 2017,Jan,8; 2016,Jan,13; 2015,Jan,16; 2014,Jan,11

**61584** Orbitocranial approach to anterior cranial fossa, extradural, including supraorbital ridge osteotomy and elevation of frontal and/or temporal lobe(s); without orbital exenteration
🔲 82.8 🔲 82.8 **FUD** 090 C 80 50 ▣
**AMA:** 2017,Jan,8; 2016,Jan,13; 2015,Jan,16; 2014,Jan,11

**61585** with orbital exenteration
🔲 92.5 🔲 92.5 **FUD** 090 C 80 50 ▣
**AMA:** 2017,Jan,8; 2016,Jan,13; 2015,Jan,16; 2014,Jan,11

**61586** Bicoronal, transzygomatic and/or LeFort I osteotomy approach to anterior cranial fossa with or without internal fixation, without bone graft
🔲 69.1 🔲 69.1 **FUD** 090 C 80 ▣
**AMA:** 2014,Jan,11

**61590** Infratemporal pre-auricular approach to middle cranial fossa (parapharyngeal space, infratemporal and midline skull base, nasopharynx), with or without disarticulation of the mandible, including parotidectomy, craniotomy, decompression and/or mobilization of the facial nerve and/or petrous carotid artery
🔲 87.9 🔲 87.9 **FUD** 090 C 80 50 ▣
**AMA:** 2017,Jan,8; 2016,Jan,13; 2015,Jan,16; 2014,Jan,11

**61591** Infratemporal post-auricular approach to middle cranial fossa (internal auditory meatus, petrous apex, tentorium, cavernous sinus, parasellar area, infratemporal fossa) including mastoidectomy, resection of sigmoid sinus, with or without decompression and/or mobilization of contents of auditory canal or petrous carotid artery
🔲 89.1 🔲 89.1 **FUD** 090 C 80 50 ▣
**AMA:** 2017,Jan,8; 2016,Jan,13; 2015,Jan,16; 2014,Jan,11

**61592** Orbitocranial zygomatic approach to middle cranial fossa (cavernous sinus and carotid artery, clivus, basilar artery or petrous apex) including osteotomy of zygoma, craniotomy, extra- or intradural elevation of temporal lobe
🔲 92.6 🔲 92.6 **FUD** 090 C 80 50 ▣
**AMA:** 2017,Jan,8; 2016,Jan,13; 2015,Jan,16; 2014,Jan,11

**61595** Transtemporal approach to posterior cranial fossa, jugular foramen or midline skull base, including mastoidectomy, decompression of sigmoid sinus and/or facial nerve, with or without mobilization
🔲 67.9 🔲 67.9 **FUD** 090 C 50 ▣
**AMA:** 2017,Jan,8; 2016,Jan,13; 2015,Jan,16; 2014,Jan,11

**61596** Transcochlear approach to posterior cranial fossa, jugular foramen or midline skull base, including labyrinthectomy, decompression, with or without mobilization of facial nerve and/or petrous carotid artery
🔲 70.4 🔲 70.4 **FUD** 090 C 80 50 ▣
**AMA:** 2017,Jan,8; 2016,Jan,13; 2015,Jan,16; 2014,Jan,11

**61597** Transcondylar (far lateral) approach to posterior cranial fossa, jugular foramen or midline skull base, including occipital condylectomy, mastoidectomy, resection of C1-C3 vertebral body(s), decompression of vertebral artery, with or without mobilization
🔲 83.2 🔲 83.2 **FUD** 090 C 80 50 ▣
**AMA:** 2017,Jan,8; 2016,Jan,13; 2015,Jan,16; 2014,Jan,11

**61598** Transpetrosal approach to posterior cranial fossa, clivus or foramen magnum, including ligation of superior petrosal sinus and/or sigmoid sinus
🔲 81.6 🔲 81.6 **FUD** 090 C 80 ▣
**AMA:** 2017,Jan,8; 2016,Jan,13; 2015,Jan,16; 2014,Jan,11

## 61600-61616 Definitive Procedures: Cranial Fossae

EXCLUDES Dural repair and/or reconstruction (61618-61619)
Injection for:
Cerebral angiography (36100-36218)
Pneumoencephalography (61055)
Ventriculography (61026, 61120)
Primary closure (15730, 15733, 15756-15758)
Surgical approach (61580-61598)

**61600** Resection or excision of neoplastic, vascular or infectious lesion of base of anterior cranial fossa; extradural
🔲 61.4 🔲 61.4 **FUD** 090 C 80 ▣
**AMA:** 2017,Jan,8; 2016,Jan,13; 2015,Jan,16; 2014,Jan,11

**61601** intradural, including dural repair, with or without graft
🔲 69.8 🔲 69.8 **FUD** 090 C 80 ▣
**AMA:** 2017,Jan,8; 2016,Jan,13; 2015,Jan,16; 2014,Jan,11

**61605** Resection or excision of neoplastic, vascular or infectious lesion of infratemporal fossa, parapharyngeal space, petrous apex; extradural
🔲 62.4 🔲 62.4 **FUD** 090 C 80 ▣
**AMA:** 2017,Jan,8; 2016,Jan,13; 2015,Jan,16; 2014,Jan,11

**61606** intradural, including dural repair, with or without graft
🔲 86.2 🔲 86.2 **FUD** 090 C 80 ▣
**AMA:** 2017,Jan,8; 2016,Jan,13; 2015,Jan,16; 2014,Jan,11

**61607** Resection or excision of neoplastic, vascular or infectious lesion of parasellar area, cavernous sinus, clivus or midline skull base; extradural
🔲 78.2 🔲 78.2 **FUD** 090 C 80 ▣
**AMA:** 2017,Jan,8; 2016,Jan,13; 2015,Jan,16; 2014,Jan,11

● New Code ▲ Revised Code ○ Reinstated ● New Web Release ▲ Revised Web Release Unlisted Not Covered # Resequenced
⊗ AMA Mod 51 Exempt ⑤ Optum Mod 51 Exempt ⑥ Mod 63 Exempt ✗ Non-FDA Drug ★ Telemedicine ▣ Maternity ⒶAge Edit ✚ Add-on **AMA:** CPT Asst
© 2017 Optum360, LLC CPT © 2017 American Medical Association. All Rights Reserved. 271

**Nervous System**

**61608** — **61626**

**61608**  intradural, including dural repair, with or without graft
🚑 94.9  ✂ 94.9  **FUD** 090  C 80 💬
**AMA:** 2017,Jan,8; 2016,Jan,13; 2015,Jan,16; 2014,Jan,11

\+ **61610**  Transection or ligation, carotid artery in cavernous sinus, with repair by anastomosis or graft (List separately in addition to code for primary procedure)
Code first (61605-61608)
🚑 48.0  ✂ 48.0  **FUD** ZZZ  C 80 💬
**AMA:** 2017,Jan,8; 2016,Jan,13; 2015,Jan,16; 2014,Jan,11

\+ **61611**  Transection or ligation, carotid artery in petrous canal; without repair (List separately in addition to code for primary procedure)
Code first (61605-61608)
🚑 11.2  ✂ 11.2  **FUD** ZZZ  C 80 💬
**AMA:** 2017,Jan,8; 2016,Jan,13; 2015,Jan,16; 2014,Jan,11

\+ **61612**  with repair by anastomosis or graft (List separately in addition to code for primary procedure)
Code first (61605-61608)
🚑 34.6  ✂ 34.6  **FUD** ZZZ  C 80 💬
**AMA:** 2017,Jan,8; 2016,Jan,13; 2015,Jan,16; 2014,Jan,11

**61613**  Obliteration of carotid aneurysm, arteriovenous malformation, or carotid-cavernous fistula by dissection within cavernous sinus
🚑 94.1  ✂ 94.1  **FUD** 090  C 80 50 💬
**AMA:** 2017,Jan,8; 2016,Jan,13; 2015,Jan,16; 2014,Jan,11

**61615**  Resection or excision of neoplastic, vascular or infectious lesion of base of posterior cranial fossa, jugular foramen, foramen magnum, or C1-C3 vertebral bodies; extradural
🚑 71.6  ✂ 71.6  **FUD** 090  C 80 💬
**AMA:** 2017,Jan,8; 2016,Jan,13; 2015,Jan,16; 2014,Jan,11

**61616**  intradural, including dural repair, with or without graft
🚑 97.0  ✂ 97.0  **FUD** 090  C 80 💬
**AMA:** 2017,Jan,8; 2016,Jan,13; 2015,Jan,16; 2014,Jan,11

## 61618-61619 Reconstruction Post-Surgical Cranial Fossae Defects

EXCLUDES  Definitive surgery (61600-61616)
Injection for:
Cerebral angiography (36100-36218)
Pneumoencephalography (61055)
Ventriculography (61026, 61120)
Primary closure (15730, 15733, 15756-15758)
Surgical approach (61580-61598)

**61618**  Secondary repair of dura for cerebrospinal fluid leak, anterior, middle or posterior cranial fossa following surgery of the skull base; by free tissue graft (eg, pericranium, fascia, tensor fascia lata, adipose tissue, homologous or synthetic grafts)
🚑 37.7  ✂ 37.7  **FUD** 090  C 80 💬
**AMA:** 2017,Jan,8; 2016,Jan,13; 2015,Jan,16; 2014,Jan,11; 2012,Jan,15-42

**61619**  by local or regionalized vascularized pedicle flap or myocutaneous flap (including galea, temporalis, frontalis or occipitalis muscle)
🚑 41.6  ✂ 41.6  **FUD** 090  C 80 💬
**AMA:** 2017,Jan,8; 2016,Jan,13; 2015,Jan,16; 2014,Jan,11; 2012,Jan,15-42

## 61623-61651 Neurovascular Interventional Procedures

**61623**  Endovascular temporary balloon arterial occlusion, head or neck (extracranial/intracranial) including selective catheterization of vessel to be occluded, positioning and inflation of occlusion balloon, concomitant neurological monitoring, and radiologic supervision and interpretation of all angiography required for balloon occlusion and to exclude vascular injury post occlusion
EXCLUDES  Diagnostic angiography of target artery just before temporary occlusion; report only radiological supervision and interpretation
Selective catheterization and angiography of artery besides the target artery; report catheterization and radiological supervision and interpretation codes as appropriate
🚑 16.6  ✂ 16.6  **FUD** 000  J 💬
**AMA:** 2017,Jan,8; 2016,Jan,13; 2015,Jan,16; 2014,Jan,11

Pericallosal artery
Posterior cerebral artery
Superior cerebellar artery
Right anterior cerebral artery
Basilar artery
Left vertebral artery

**61624**  Transcatheter permanent occlusion or embolization (eg, for tumor destruction, to achieve hemostasis, to occlude a vascular malformation), percutaneous, any method; central nervous system (intracranial, spinal cord)
EXCLUDES  Non-central nervous system transcatheter occlusion or embolization other than head or neck (37241-37244)
🔀 (75894)
🚑 33.4  ✂ 33.4  **FUD** 000  C 💬
**AMA:** 2017,Jan,8; 2016,Jan,13; 2015,Jan,16; 2014,Jan,11; 2013,Nov,6; 2012,Jan,15-42

**61626**  non-central nervous system, head or neck (extracranial, brachiocephalic branch)
EXCLUDES  Non-central nervous system transcatheter occlusion or embolization other than head or neck (37241-37244)
🔀 (75894)
🚑 25.0  ✂ 25.0  **FUD** 000  J 💬
**AMA:** 2017,Jan,8; 2016,Jan,13; 2015,Jan,16; 2014,Jan,11; 2013,Nov,6

26/TC PC/TC Only   A2-Z3 ASC Payment   50 Bilateral   ♂ Male Only   ♀ Female Only   🚑 Facility RVU   ✂ Non-Facility RVU   💬 CCI
**FUD** Follow-up Days   **CMS:** IOM (Pub 100)   A-Y OPPSI   80/80 Surg Assist Allowed / w/Doc   🔲 Lab Crosswalk   🔀 Radiology Crosswalk   ❌ CLIA
272                                      CPT © 2017 American Medical Association. All Rights Reserved.                      © 2017 Optum360, LLC

**61630**  **Balloon angioplasty, intracranial (eg, atherosclerotic stenosis), percutaneous**

INCLUDES Diagnostic arteriogram if stent or angioplasty is necessary

Radiology services for arteriography of target vascular family

Selective catheterization of the target vascular family

EXCLUDES *Diagnostic arteriogram if stent or angioplasty is not necessary (use applicable code for selective catheterization and radiology services)*

*Percutaneous arterial transluminal mechanical thrombectomy and/or infusion for thrombolysis performed in the same vascular territory (61645)*

🚑 39.1   ⚖ 39.1   **FUD** XXX                C 80 ▣

**AMA:** 2017,Jul,3; 2017,Apr,9; 2017,Jan,8; 2016,Mar,3; 2016,Jan,13; 2015,Nov,3; 2015,Jan,16; 2014,Jan,11

**61635**  **Transcatheter placement of intravascular stent(s), intracranial (eg, atherosclerotic stenosis), including balloon angioplasty, if performed**

INCLUDES Diagnostic arteriogram if stent or angioplasty is necessary

Radiology services for arteriography of target vascular family

Selective catheterization of the target vascular family

EXCLUDES *Diagnostic arteriogram if stent or angioplasty is not necessary (use applicable code for selective catheterization and radiology services)*

*Percutaneous arterial transluminal thrombectomy in same vascular territory (61645)*

🚑 41.7   ⚖ 41.7   **FUD** XXX                C 80 ▣

**AMA:** 2017,Jul,3; 2017,Jan,8; 2016,Mar,3; 2016,Jan,13; 2015,Nov,3; 2015,Jan,16; 2014,Mar,8; 2014,Jan,11

**61640**  **Balloon dilatation of intracranial vasospasm, percutaneous; initial vessel**

INCLUDES Angiography after dilation of vessel

Fluoroscopic guidance

Injection of contrast material

Roadmapping

Selective catheterization of target vessel

Vessel analysis

EXCLUDES *Endovascular intracranial prolonged administration of pharmacologic agent performed in the same vascular territory (61650-61651)*

🚑 14.0   ⚖ 14.0   **FUD** 000                E ▣

**AMA:** 2017,Jan,8; 2016,Mar,3; 2016,Jan,13; 2015,Nov,3; 2015,Jan,16; 2014,May,10; 2014,Jan,11

+ **61641**    **each additional vessel in same vascular family (List separately in addition to code for primary procedure)**

INCLUDES Angiography after dilation of vessel

Fluoroscopic guidance

Injection of contrast material

Roadmapping

Selective catheterization of target vessel

Vessel analysis

Code first (61640)

🚑 4.92   ⚖ 4.92   **FUD** ZZZ                E ▣

**AMA:** 2017,Jan,8; 2016,Mar,3; 2016,Jan,13; 2015,Nov,3; 2015,Jan,16; 2014,May,10; 2014,Jan,11

+ **61642**    **each additional vessel in different vascular family (List separately in addition to code for primary procedure)**

INCLUDES Angiography after dilation of vessel

Fluoroscopic guidance

Injection of contrast material

Roadmapping

Selective catheterization of target vessel

Vessel analysis

EXCLUDES *Endovascular intracranial prolonged administration of pharmacologic agent performed in the same vascular territory (61650-61651)*

Code first (61640)

🚑 9.84   ⚖ 9.84   **FUD** ZZZ                E ▣

**AMA:** 2017,Jan,8; 2016,Mar,3; 2016,Jan,13; 2015,Nov,3; 2015,Jan,16; 2014,May,10; 2014,Jan,11

**61645**  **Percutaneous arterial transluminal mechanical thrombectomy and/or infusion for thrombolysis, intracranial, any method, including diagnostic angiography, fluoroscopic guidance, catheter placement, and intraprocedural pharmacological thrombolytic injection(s)**

INCLUDES Interventions performed in an intracranial artery including:

Angiography with radiologic supervision and interpretation (diagnostic and subsequent)

Closure of arteriotomy by any method

Fluoroscopy

Patient monitoring

Procedures performed in vascular territories:

Left carotid

Right carotid

Vertebro-basilar

EXCLUDES *Procedure performed in the same vascular target area:*

*Balloon angioplasty, intracranial (61630)*

*Diagnostic studies: aortic arch, carotid, and vertebral arteries (36221-36228)*

*Endovascular intracranial prolonged administration of pharmacologic agent (61650-61651)*

*Transcatheter placement of intravascular stent (61635)*

*Transluminal thrombectomy (37184, 37186)*

*Use of code more than one time for treatment of each intracranial vascular territory*

*Venous thrombectomy or thrombolysis (37187-37188, [37212], [37214])*

🚑 22.7   ⚖ 22.7   **FUD** 000                C 80 50 ▣

**AMA:** 2017,Jan,8; 2016,Mar,3; 2016,Jan,13; 2015,Dec,18; 2015,Nov,3

**61650**  **Endovascular intracranial prolonged administration of pharmacologic agent(s) other than for thrombolysis, arterial, including catheter placement, diagnostic angiography, and imaging guidance; initial vascular territory**

INCLUDES Interventions performed in an intracranial artery, including:

Angiography with radiologic supervision and interpretation (diagnostic and subsequent)

Closure of arteriotomy by any method

Fluoroscopy

Patient monitoring

Procedures performed in vascular territories:

Left carotid

Right carotid

Vertebro-basilar

Prolonged (at least 10 minutes) arterial administration of non-thrombolytic agents

EXCLUDES *Procedure performed in the same vascular target area:*

*Balloon dilatation of intracranial vasospasm (61640-61642)*

*Chemotherapy administration (96420-96425)*

*Diagnostic studies: aortic arch, carotid, and vertebral arteries (36221-36228)*

*Transluminal thrombectomy (37184, 37186, 61645)*

*Treatment of an iatrogenic condition*

*Use of code more than one time for treatment of each intracranial vascular territory*

*Venous thrombectomy or thrombolysis*

🚑 15.5   ⚖ 15.5   **FUD** 000                C ▣

**AMA:** 2017,Jan,8; 2016,Mar,3; 2016,Jan,13; 2015,Nov,3

---

● New Code      ▲ Revised Code      ○ Reinstated      ● New Web Release      ▲ Revised Web Release      Unlisted      Not Covered      # Resequenced
⊘ AMA Mod 51 Exempt   ⑪ Optum Mod 51 Exempt   ⑬ Mod 63 Exempt   ✗ Non-FDA Drug   ★ Telemedicine   Ⓜ Maternity   Ⓐ Age Edit   + Add-on   **AMA:** CPT Asst

**61651 — 61710**

**Nervous System**

**+ 61651** **each additional vascular territory (List separately in addition to code for primary procedure)**

> INCLUDES Interventions performed in an intracranial artery including:
> Angiography with radiologic supervision and interpretation (diagnostic and subsequent)
> Closure of arteriotomy by any method
> Fluoroscopy
> Patient monitoring
> Procedures performed in vascular territories:
> Left carotid
> Right carotid
> Vertebro-basilar
> Prolonged (at least 10 minutes) arterial administration of non-thrombolytic agents

> EXCLUDES *Procedure performed in the same vascular target area:*
> *Balloon dilatation of intracranial vasospasm (61640-61642)*
> *Chemotherapy administration (96420-96425)*
> *Diagnostic studies: aortic arch, carotid, and vertebral arteries (36221-36228)*
> *Transluminal thrombectomy (37184, 37186, 61645)*
> *Treatment of an iatrogenic condition*
> *Use of code more than two times for treatment of the two remaining intracranial vascular territory(ies)*
> *Venous thrombectomy or thrombolysis*

Code first (61650)

📟 6.62  ⚖ 6.62  **FUD** ZZZ          C 🖵

**AMA:** 2017,Jan,8; 2016,Mar,3; 2016,Jan,13; 2015,Nov,3

## 61680-61692 Surgical Treatment of Arteriovenous Malformation of the Brain

INCLUDES Craniotomy

**61680** **Surgery of intracranial arteriovenous malformation; supratentorial, simple**

📟 66.3  ⚖ 66.3  **FUD** 090          C 80 🖵

**AMA:** 2014,Jan,11

**61682** **supratentorial, complex**

📟 122.  ⚖ 122.  **FUD** 090          C 80 🖵

**AMA:** 2017,Jan,8; 2016,Jan,13; 2015,Jan,16; 2014,Jan,11; 2013,Jun,13

**61684** **infratentorial, simple**

📟 83.9  ⚖ 83.9  **FUD** 090          C 80 🖵

**AMA:** 2014,Jan,11

**61686** **infratentorial, complex**

📟 132.  ⚖ 132.  **FUD** 090          C 80 🖵

**AMA:** 2017,Jan,8; 2016,Jan,13; 2015,Jan,16; 2014,Jan,11; 2013,Jun,13

**61690** **dural, simple**

📟 63.9  ⚖ 63.9  **FUD** 090          C 80 🖵

**AMA:** 2014,Jan,11

**61692** **dural, complex**

📟 107.  ⚖ 107.  **FUD** 090          C 80 🖵

**AMA:** 2017,Jan,8; 2016,Jan,13; 2015,Jan,16; 2014,Jan,11; 2013,Jun,13

## 61697-61703 Surgical Treatment Brain Aneurysm

INCLUDES Craniotomy

**61697** **Surgery of complex intracranial aneurysm, intracranial approach; carotid circulation**

> INCLUDES Aneurysms bigger than 15 mm
> Calcification of the aneurysm neck
> Inclusion of normal vessels in aneurysm neck
> Surgery needing temporary vessel occlusion, trapping, or cardiopulmonary bypass to treat aneurysm

📟 123.  ⚖ 123.  **FUD** 090          C 80 🖵

**AMA:** 2014,Jan,11

**61698** **vertebrobasilar circulation**

> INCLUDES Aneurysm bigger than 15 mm
> Calcification of aneurysm neck
> Inclusion of normal vessels into aneurysm neck
> Surgery needing temporary vessel occlusion, trapping, or cardiopulmonary bypass to treat aneurysm

📟 136.  ⚖ 136.  **FUD** 090          C 80 🖵

**AMA:** 2014,Jan,11

**61700** **Surgery of simple intracranial aneurysm, intracranial approach; carotid circulation**

📟 100.  ⚖ 100.  **FUD** 090          C 80 🖵

**AMA:** 2017,Jan,8; 2016,Jan,13; 2015,Jan,16; 2014,Jan,11; 2012,Jan,15-42

**61702** **vertebrobasilar circulation**

📟 117.  ⚖ 117.  **FUD** 090          C 80 🖵

**AMA:** 2014,Jan,11

Berry aneurysm

Berry aneurysms form at the site of a weakness in an arterial wall, often at a junction

Common sites of berry aneurysms in the circle of Willis arteries

Anterior communicating artery 40%

34%

Internal carotid

4%  20%

Posterior communicating artery

Basilar artery

**61703** **Surgery of intracranial aneurysm, cervical approach by application of occluding clamp to cervical carotid artery (Selverstone-Crutchfield type)**

> EXCLUDES *Cervical approach for direct ligation of carotid artery (37600-37606)*

📟 36.0  ⚖ 36.0  **FUD** 090          C 80 🖵

**AMA:** 2014,Jan,11

## 61705-61710 Other Procedures for Aneurysm, Arteriovenous Malformation, and Carotid-Cavernous Fistula

INCLUDES Craniotomy

**61705** **Surgery of aneurysm, vascular malformation or carotid-cavernous fistula; by intracranial and cervical occlusion of carotid artery**

📟 76.8  ⚖ 76.8  **FUD** 090          C 80 🖵

**AMA:** 2014,Jan,11

**61708** **by intracranial electrothrombosis**

> EXCLUDES *Ligation or gradual occlusion of internal or common carotid artery (37605-37606)*

📟 67.9  ⚖ 67.9  **FUD** 090          C 80 🖵

**AMA:** 2014,Jan,11

**61710** **by intra-arterial embolization, injection procedure, or balloon catheter**

📟 62.5  ⚖ 62.5  **FUD** 090          C 80 🖵

**AMA:** 2017,Jan,8; 2016,Jan,13; 2015,Jan,16; 2014,Jan,11; 2013,Nov,6

**26/TC** PC/TC Only  **92-Z3** ASC Payment  **50** Bilateral  ♂ Male Only  ♀ Female Only  📟 Facility RVU  ⚖ Non-Facility RVU  🖵 CCI
**FUD** Follow-up Days  **CMS:** IOM (Pub 100)  **A-Y** OPPSI  **80/80** Surg Assist Allowed / w/Doc  🧪 Lab Crosswalk  ⬛ Radiology Crosswalk  ❌ CLIA

**274**

CPT © 2017 American Medical Association. All Rights Reserved.

© 2017 Optum360, LLC

## 61711 Extracranial-Intracranial Bypass

**CMS:** 100-02,16,10 Exclusions from Coverage; 100-03,20.2 Extracranial-intracranial (EC-IC) Arterial Bypass Surgery

INCLUDES    Craniotomy
EXCLUDES    *Carotid or vertebral thromboendarterectomy (35301)*
Code also operating microscope when appropriate (69990)

**61711    Anastomosis, arterial, extracranial-intracranial (eg, middle cerebral/cortical) arteries**
76.6    76.6    **FUD** 090    C 80
**AMA:** 2014,Jan,11

## 61720-61791 Stereotactic Procedures of the Brain

**61720    Creation of lesion by stereotactic method, including burr hole(s) and localizing and recording techniques, single or multiple stages; globus pallidus or thalamus**
37.4    37.4    **FUD** 090    J
**AMA:** 2017,Jan,8; 2016,Jan,13; 2015,Jan,16; 2014,Jul,8; 2014,Jan,11

**61735    subcortical structure(s) other than globus pallidus or thalamus**
46.8    46.8    **FUD** 090    C
**AMA:** 2014,Jul,8; 2014,Jan,11

**61750    Stereotactic biopsy, aspiration, or excision, including burr hole(s), for intracranial lesion;**
41.3    41.3    **FUD** 090    C
**AMA:** 2017,Jan,8; 2016,Jan,13; 2015,Jan,16; 2014,Jul,8; 2014,Jan,11

**61751    with computed tomography and/or magnetic resonance guidance**
(70450, 70460, 70470, 70551-70553)
40.5    40.5    **FUD** 090    C
**AMA:** 2017,Jan,8; 2016,Jan,13; 2015,Jan,16; 2014,Jul,8; 2014,Jan,11; 2012,Jan,15-42

**61760    Stereotactic implantation of depth electrodes into the cerebrum for long-term seizure monitoring**
46.3    46.3    **FUD** 090    C
**AMA:** 2014,Jul,8; 2014,Jan,11

**61770    Stereotactic localization, including burr hole(s), with insertion of catheter(s) or probe(s) for placement of radiation source**
47.8    47.8    **FUD** 090    J 62
**AMA:** 2017,Jan,8; 2016,Jan,13; 2015,Jan,16; 2014,Jul,8; 2014,Jan,11

**+    61781    Stereotactic computer-assisted (navigational) procedure; cranial, intradural (List separately in addition to code for primary procedure)**
EXCLUDES    *Creation of lesion by stereotactic method (61720-61791)*
*Extradural stereotactic computer-assisted procedure for same surgical session by same individual (61782)*
*Radiation treatment delivery, stereotactic radiosurgery (SRS) (77371-77373)*
*Stereotactic implantation of neurostimulator electrode array (61863-61868)*
*Stereotactic radiation treatment management (77432)*
*Stereotactic radiosurgery (61796-61799)*
*Ventriculocisternostomy (62201)*
Code first primary procedure
6.96    6.96    **FUD** ZZZ    N M 80
**AMA:** 2017,Jan,8; 2016,Jan,13; 2015,Jan,16; 2014,Sep,13; 2014,Jul,8; 2014,Jan,11

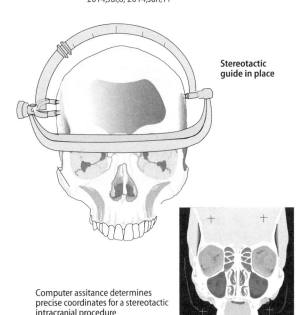

Stereotactic guide in place

Computer assitance determines precise coordinates for a stereotactic intracranial procedure

CT or MRI scan

**+    61782    cranial, extradural (List separately in addition to code for primary procedure)**
EXCLUDES    *Intradural stereotactic computer-assisted procedure for same surgical session by same individual (61781)*
*Stereotactic radiosurgery (61796-61799)*
Code first primary procedure
5.07    5.07    **FUD** ZZZ    N M 80
**AMA:** 2017,Jan,8; 2016,Jan,13; 2015,Jan,16; 2014,Jul,8; 2014,Jan,11

**+    61783    spinal (List separately in addition to code for primary procedure)**
EXCLUDES    *Stereotactic radiosurgery (61796-61799, 63620-63621)*
Code first primary procedure
6.83    6.83    **FUD** ZZZ    N M 80
**AMA:** 2017,Jan,8; 2016,Jan,13; 2015,Jan,16; 2014,Jul,8; 2014,Jan,11

**61790    Creation of lesion by stereotactic method, percutaneous, by neurolytic agent (eg, alcohol, thermal, electrical, radiofrequency); gasserian ganglion**
25.7    25.7    **FUD** 090    J A2 50
**AMA:** 2014,Jul,8; 2014,Jan,11

**61791    trigeminal medullary tract**
32.0    32.0    **FUD** 090    J A2 80 50
**AMA:** 2017,Jan,8; 2016,Jan,13; 2015,Jan,16; 2014,Jul,8; 2014,Jan,11

● New Code    ▲ Revised Code    ○ Reinstated    ● New Web Release    ▲ Revised Web Release    Unlisted    Not Covered    # Resequenced
⊘ AMA Mod 51 Exempt    ⑨ Optum Mod 51 Exempt    ⑥⑨ Mod 63 Exempt    ✗ Non-FDA Drug    ★ Telemedicine    M Maternity    A Age Edit    + Add-on    AMA: CPT Asst
© 2017 Optum360, LLC    CPT © 2017 American Medical Association. All Rights Reserved.    275

**Nervous System**

**61796 — 61868**

## 61796-61800 Stereotactic Radiosurgery (SRS): Brain

INCLUDES Planning, dosimetry, targeting, positioning or blocking performed by the neurosurgeon

EXCLUDES Application of cranial tongs, caliper, or stereotactic frame (20660)
Intensity modulated beam delivery plan and treatment (77301, 77385-77386)
Radiation treatment management and radiosurgery by the same provider (77427-77435)
Sterotactic body radiation therapy (77373, 77435)
Sterotactic radiosurgery more than once per lesion per treatment course
Treatment planning, physics and dosimetry, and treatment delivery performed by the radiation oncologist

**61796** **Stereotactic radiosurgery (particle beam, gamma ray, or linear accelerator); 1 simple cranial lesion**

INCLUDES Lesions < 3.5 cm

EXCLUDES Stereotactic computer-assisted proceudres (61781-61783)
Stereotactic radiosurgery (61798)
Treatment of complex lesions: (61798-61799)
Arteriovenous malformations (AVM)
Brainstem lesions
Cavernous sinus/parasellar/petroclival tumors, glomus tumors, pituitary tumors, and tumors of pineal region
Lesions located <= 5 mm from the optic nerve, chasm, or tract
Schwannomas
Code also stereotactic headframe application, when performed (61800)

⚙ 29.8 ◇ 29.8 **FUD** 090 B 80 ▣

**AMA:** 2017,Jan,8; 2016,Jan,13; 2015,Jun,6; 2015,Jan,16; 2014,Jul,8; 2014,Jan,11; 2012,Apr,11-13

+ **61797** **each additional cranial lesion, simple (List separately in addition to code for primary procedure)**

INCLUDES Lesions < 3.5 cm

EXCLUDES Stereotactic computer-assisted procedures (61781-61783)
Treatment of complex lesions: (61798-61799)
Arteriovenous malformations (AVM)
Brainstem lesion
Cavernous sinus/parasellar/petroclival tumors, glomus tumors, pituitary tumor, tumors of pineal region
Lesions located <= 5 mm from the optic nerve, chasm, or tract
Schwannomas
Use of code for additional stereotactic radiosurgery more than four times in total per treatment course when used alone or in combination with (61799)
Code first (61796, 61798)

⚙ 6.52 ◇ 6.52 **FUD** ZZZ B 80 ▣

**AMA:** 2017,Jan,8; 2016,Jan,13; 2015,Jun,6; 2015,Jan,16; 2014,Jul,8; 2014,Jan,11; 2012,Apr,11-13

**61798** **1 complex cranial lesion**

INCLUDES All therapeutic lesion creation procedures
Treatment of complex lesions:
Arteriovenous malformations (AVM)
Brainstem lesions
Cavernous sinus, parasellar, petroclival, glomus, pineal region, and pituitary tumors
Lesions located <= 5 mm from the optic nerve, chasm, or tract
Lesions >= 3.5 cm
Schwannomas
Treatment of multiple lesions as long as one is complex

EXCLUDES Stereotactic computer-assisted procedures (61781-61783)
Stereotactic radiosurgery (61796)
Code also stereotactic headframe application, when performed (61800)

⚙ 40.6 ◇ 40.6 **FUD** 090 B 80 ▣

**AMA:** 2017,Jan,8; 2016,Jan,13; 2015,Jun,6; 2015,Jan,16; 2014,Jul,8; 2014,Jan,11; 2012,Apr,11-13

+ **61799** **each additional cranial lesion, complex (List separately in addition to code for primary procedure)**

INCLUDES All therapeutic lesion creation procedures
Treatment of complex lesions:
Arteriovenous malformations (AVM)
Brainstem lesions
Cavernous sinus, parasellar, petroclival, glomus, pineal region, and pituitary tumors
Lesions located <= 5 mm from the optic nerve, chasm, or tract
Lesions >= 3.5 cm
Schwannomas

EXCLUDES Stereotactic computer-assisted procedures (61781-61783)
Use of code for additional stereotactic radiosurgery more than four times in total per treatment course when used alone or in combination with (61797)
Code first (61798)

⚙ 9.02 ◇ 9.02 **FUD** ZZZ B 80 ▣

**AMA:** 2017,Jan,8; 2016,Jan,13; 2015,Jun,6; 2015,Jan,16; 2014,Jul,8; 2014,Jan,11; 2012,Apr,11-13

+ **61800** **Application of stereotactic headframe for stereotactic radiosurgery (List separately in addition to code for primary procedure)**

Code first (61796, 61798)

⚙ 4.55 ◇ 4.55 **FUD** ZZZ B 80 ▣

**AMA:** 2017,Jan,8; 2016,Jan,13; 2015,Jun,6; 2015,Jan,16; 2014,Jan,11; 2012,Apr,11-13

## 61850-61888 Intracranial Neurostimulation

INCLUDES Microelectrode recording by operating surgeon

EXCLUDES Electronic analysis and reprogramming of neurostimulator pulse generator (95970-95975)
Neurophysiological mapping by another physician/qualified health care professional (95961-95962)

**61850** **Twist drill or burr hole(s) for implantation of neurostimulator electrodes, cortical**

⚙ 28.8 ◇ 28.8 **FUD** 090 C 80 ▣

**AMA:** 2017,Jan,8; 2016,Jan,13; 2015,Jan,16; 2014,Jan,11

**61860** **Craniectomy or craniotomy for implantation of neurostimulator electrodes, cerebral, cortical**

⚙ 45.5 ◇ 45.5 **FUD** 090 C 80 ▣

**AMA:** 2017,Jan,8; 2016,Jan,13; 2015,Jan,16; 2014,Jan,11

**61863** **Twist drill, burr hole, craniotomy, or craniectomy with stereotactic implantation of neurostimulator electrode array in subcortical site (eg, thalamus, globus pallidus, subthalamic nucleus, periventricular, periaqueductal gray), without use of intraoperative microelectrode recording; first array**

⚙ 44.1 ◇ 44.1 **FUD** 090 C 80 50 ▣

**AMA:** 2017,Jan,8; 2016,Jan,13; 2015,Jan,16; 2014,Jul,8; 2014,Jan,11; 2012,Jan,15-42

+ **61864** **each additional array (List separately in addition to primary procedure)**

Code first (61863)

⚙ 8.41 ◇ 8.41 **FUD** ZZZ C 80 ▣

**AMA:** 2014,Jul,8; 2014,Jan,11

**61867** **Twist drill, burr hole, craniotomy, or craniectomy with stereotactic implantation of neurostimulator electrode array in subcortical site (eg, thalamus, globus pallidus, subthalamic nucleus, periventricular, periaqueductal gray), with use of intraoperative microelectrode recording; first array**

⚙ 67.0 ◇ 67.0 **FUD** 090 C 80 50 ▣

**AMA:** 2014,Jul,8; 2014,Jan,11

+ **61868** **each additional array (List separately in addition to primary procedure)**

Code first (61867)

⚙ 14.7 ◇ 14.7 **FUD** ZZZ C 80 ▣

**AMA:** 2017,Jan,8; 2016,Jan,13; 2015,Jan,16; 2014,Jul,8; 2014,Jan,11

**61870** Craniectomy for implantation of neurostimulator electrodes, cerebellar, cortical
    30.1   30.1  **FUD** 090    C 80
    **AMA:** 2014,Jan,11

**61880** Revision or removal of intracranial neurostimulator electrodes
    16.5   16.5  **FUD** 090    02 62 80 50
    **AMA:** 2014,Jan,11

**61885** Insertion or replacement of cranial neurostimulator pulse generator or receiver, direct or inductive coupling; with connection to a single electrode array
    EXCLUDES  *Percutaneous procedure to place cranial nerve neurostimulator electrode(s) (64553)*
        *Revision or replacement cranial nerve neurostimulator electrode array (64569)*
    14.9   14.9  **FUD** 090    J J8 80 50
    **AMA:** 2017,Jan,8; 2016,Jan,13; 2015,Jan,16; 2014,Jan,11; 2012,Jan,15-42

**61886** with connection to 2 or more electrode arrays
    EXCLUDES  *Percutaneous procedure to place cranial nerve neurostimulator electrode(s) (64553)*
        *Revision or replacement cranial nerve neurostimulator electrode array (64569)*
    24.6   24.6  **FUD** 090    J J8 80
    **AMA:** 2017,Jan,8; 2016,Jan,13; 2015,Jan,16; 2014,Jan,11; 2012,Jan,15-42

**61888** Revision or removal of cranial neurostimulator pulse generator or receiver
    EXCLUDES  *Insertion or replacement of cranial neurostimulator pulse generator or receiver (61885-61886)*
    11.5   11.5  **FUD** 010    J J8 50
    **AMA:** 2017,Jan,8; 2016,Jan,13; 2015,Jan,16; 2014,Jan,11; 2012,Jan,15-42

## 62000-62148 Repair of Skull and/or Cerebrospinal Fluid Leaks

**62000** Elevation of depressed skull fracture; simple, extradural
    28.0   28.0  **FUD** 090    J
    **AMA:** 2014,Jan,11

**62005** compound or comminuted, extradural
    36.9   36.9  **FUD** 090    C 80
    **AMA:** 2014,Jan,11

**62010** with repair of dura and/or debridement of brain
    44.8   44.8  **FUD** 090    C 80
    **AMA:** 2014,Jan,11

**62100** Craniotomy for repair of dural/cerebrospinal fluid leak, including surgery for rhinorrhea/otorrhea
    EXCLUDES  *Repair of spinal fluid leak (63707, 63709)*
    46.3   46.3  **FUD** 090    C 80
    **AMA:** 2014,Jan,11

**62115** Reduction of craniomegalic skull (eg, treated hydrocephalus); not requiring bone grafts or cranioplasty
    37.8   37.8  **FUD** 090    C 80
    **AMA:** 2014,Jan,11

**62117** requiring craniotomy and reconstruction with or without bone graft (includes obtaining grafts)
    57.8   57.8  **FUD** 090    C 80
    **AMA:** 2014,Jan,11

**62120** Repair of encephalocele, skull vault, including cranioplasty
    47.9   47.9  **FUD** 090    C 80
    **AMA:** 2014,Jan,11

**62121** Craniotomy for repair of encephalocele, skull base
    46.1   46.1  **FUD** 090    C 80
    **AMA:** 2014,Jan,11

**62140** Cranioplasty for skull defect; up to 5 cm diameter
    30.2   30.2  **FUD** 090    C 80
    **AMA:** 2017,Jan,8; 2016,Jan,13; 2015,Jan,16; 2014,Jan,11; 2014,Jan,9

**62141** larger than 5 cm diameter
    33.3   33.3  **FUD** 090    C 80
    **AMA:** 2017,Jan,8; 2016,Jan,13; 2015,Jan,16; 2014,Jan,11; 2014,Jan,9

**62142** Removal of bone flap or prosthetic plate of skull
    25.9   25.9  **FUD** 090    C 80
    **AMA:** 2017,Jan,8; 2016,Jan,13; 2015,Jan,16; 2014,Jan,11; 2014,Jan,9

**62143** Replacement of bone flap or prosthetic plate of skull
    30.5   30.5  **FUD** 090    C 80
    **AMA:** 2017,Jan,8; 2016,Jan,13; 2015,Jan,16; 2014,Jan,11; 2014,Jan,9

**62145** Cranioplasty for skull defect with reparative brain surgery
    41.4   41.4  **FUD** 090    C 80
    **AMA:** 2017,Jan,8; 2016,Jan,13; 2015,Jan,16; 2014,Jan,11; 2014,Jan,9

**62146** Cranioplasty with autograft (includes obtaining bone grafts); up to 5 cm diameter
    35.0   35.0  **FUD** 090    C 80
    **AMA:** 2017,Jan,8; 2016,Jan,13; 2015,Jan,16; 2014,Jan,11; 2014,Jan,9

**62147** larger than 5 cm diameter
    41.6   41.6  **FUD** 090    C 80
    **AMA:** 2017,Jan,8; 2016,Jan,13; 2015,Jan,16; 2014,Jan,11; 2014,Jan,9

**+ 62148** Incision and retrieval of subcutaneous cranial bone graft for cranioplasty (List separately in addition to code for primary procedure)
    Code first (62140-62147)
    3.74   3.74  **FUD** ZZZ    C
    **AMA:** 2014,Jan,11

## 62160-62165 Neuroendoscopic Brain Procedures

INCLUDES  Diagnostic endoscopy

**+ 62160** Neuroendoscopy, intracranial, for placement or replacement of ventricular catheter and attachment to shunt system or external drainage (List separately in addition to code for primary procedure)
    Code first (61107, 61210, 62220-62230, 62258)
    5.63   5.63  **FUD** ZZZ    N N1
    **AMA:** 2017,Jan,8; 2016,Jan,13; 2015,Jan,16; 2014,Jan,11; 2012,Dec,12; 2012,Jan,15-42

**62161** Neuroendoscopy, intracranial; with dissection of adhesions, fenestration of septum pellucidum or intraventricular cysts (including placement, replacement, or removal of ventricular catheter)
    44.4   44.4  **FUD** 090    C 80
    **AMA:** 2014,Jan,11

**62162** with fenestration or excision of colloid cyst, including placement of external ventricular catheter for drainage
    55.4   55.4  **FUD** 090    C 80
    **AMA:** 2014,Jan,11

**62163** with retrieval of foreign body
    36.0   36.0  **FUD** 090    C 80
    **AMA:** 2014,Jan,11

**62164** with excision of brain tumor, including placement of external ventricular catheter for drainage
    60.9   60.9  **FUD** 090    C 80
    **AMA:** 2014,Jan,11

**62165** with excision of pituitary tumor, transnasal or trans-sphenoidal approach
    44.8   44.8  **FUD** 090    C 80
    **AMA:** 2014,Jan,11

## 62180-62258 Cerebrospinal Fluid Diversion Procedures

**62180** Ventriculocisternostomy (Torkildsen type operation)
    47.1   47.1  **FUD** 090    C 80
    **AMA:** 2014,Jan,11

---

● New Code   ▲ Revised Code   ○ Reinstated   ● New Web Release   ▲ Revised Web Release   Unlisted   Not Covered   # Resequenced
⊘ AMA Mod 51 Exempt   ⑩ Optum Mod 51 Exempt   ⑬ Mod 63 Exempt   ✗ Non-FDA Drug   ★ Telemedicine   M Maternity   A Age Edit   + Add-on   **AMA:** CPT Asst
© 2017 Optum360, LLC    CPT © 2017 American Medical Association. All Rights Reserved.    277

**62190** **Creation of shunt; subarachnoid/subdural-atrial, -jugular, -auricular**
       20.9    20.9    **FUD** 090      C
       **AMA:** 2014,Jan,11

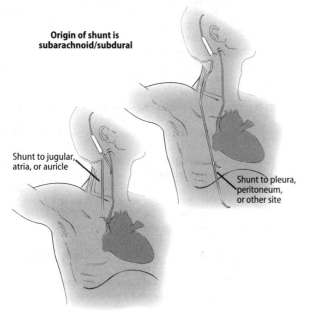

Origin of shunt is subarachnoid/subdural

Shunt to jugular, atria, or auricle

Shunt to pleura, peritoneum, or other site

**62192** **subarachnoid/subdural-peritoneal, -pleural, other terminus**
       28.6    28.6    **FUD** 090      C 80
       **AMA:** 2014,Jan,11

**62194** **Replacement or irrigation, subarachnoid/subdural catheter**
       12.9    12.9    **FUD** 010      J A2 80
       **AMA:** 2017,Jan,8; 2016,Jan,13; 2015,Jan,16; 2014,Jan,11

**62200** **Ventriculocisternostomy, third ventricle;**
       INCLUDES    Dandy ventriculocisternostomy
       39.6    39.6    **FUD** 090      C 80
       **AMA:** 2014,Jan,11

**62201** **stereotactic, neuroendoscopic method**
       EXCLUDES    *Intracranial neuroendoscopic surgery (62161-62165)*
       35.2    35.2    **FUD** 090      C
       **AMA:** 2017,Jan,8; 2016,Jan,13; 2015,Jan,16; 2014,Jul,8; 2014,Jan,11; 2012,Jan,15-42

**62220** **Creation of shunt; ventriculo-atrial, -jugular, -auricular**
       Code also intracranial neuroendoscopic ventricular catheter insertion, when performed (62160)
       30.2    30.2    **FUD** 090      C 80
       **AMA:** 2014,Jan,11

**62223** **ventriculo-peritoneal, -pleural, other terminus**
       Code also intracranial neuroendoscopic ventricular catheter insertion, when performed (62160)
       30.5    30.5    **FUD** 090      C 80
       **AMA:** 2014,Jan,11

**62225** **Replacement or irrigation, ventricular catheter**
       Code also intracranial neuroendoscopic ventricular catheter insertion, when performed (62160)
       14.7    14.7    **FUD** 090      J A2
       **AMA:** 2017,Jan,8; 2016,Jan,13; 2015,Jan,16; 2014,Jan,11; 2012,Jan,15-42

**62230** **Replacement or revision of cerebrospinal fluid shunt, obstructed valve, or distal catheter in shunt system**
       Code also intracranial neuroendoscopic ventricular catheter insertion, when performed (62160)
       Code also when proximal catheter and valve are replaced (62225)
       24.6    24.6    **FUD** 090      J A2 80
       **AMA:** 2017,Jan,8; 2016,Jan,13; 2015,Jan,16; 2014,Jan,11; 2012,Dec,12; 2012,Jan,15-42

**62252** **Reprogramming of programmable cerebrospinal shunt**
       2.46    2.46    **FUD** XXX      S P3 80
       **AMA:** 2014,Jan,11

**62256** **Removal of complete cerebrospinal fluid shunt system; without replacement**
       EXCLUDES    *Reprogramming cerebrospinal fluid (CSF) shunt (62252)*
       17.5    17.5    **FUD** 090      C 80
       **AMA:** 2014,Jan,11

**62258** **with replacement by similar or other shunt at same operation**
       EXCLUDES    *Aspiration or irrigation of shunt reservoir (61070)*
                           *Reprogramming of a cerebrospinal fluid (CSF) shunt (62252)*
       Code also intracranial neuroendoscopic ventricular catheter insertion, when performed (62160)
       32.7    32.7    **FUD** 090      C 80
       **AMA:** 2017,Jan,8; 2016,Jan,13; 2015,Jan,16; 2014,Jan,11; 2012,Jan,15-42

## 62263-62264 Lysis of Epidural Lesions with Injection of Solution/Mechanical Methods

   INCLUDES    Epidurography (72275)
               Fluoroscopic guidance (77003)
               Percutaneous mechanical lysis

**62263** **Percutaneous lysis of epidural adhesions using solution injection (eg, hypertonic saline, enzyme) or mechanical means (eg, catheter) including radiologic localization (includes contrast when administered), multiple adhesiolysis sessions; 2 or more days**
       INCLUDES    All adhesiolysis treatments, injections, and infusions during course of treatment
               Percutaneous epidural catheter insertion and removal for neurolytic agent injections during a series of treatment sessions
       EXCLUDES    *Procedure performed more than one time for the complete series spanning two or more treatment days*
       9.30    17.1    **FUD** 010      T A2
       **AMA:** 2017,Jan,8; 2016,Jan,13; 2015,Jan,16; 2014,Jan,11; 2012,Jun,12-13; 2012,Jan,15-42

**62264** **1 day**
       INCLUDES    Multiple treatment sessions performed on the same day
       EXCLUDES    *Percutaneous lysis of epidural adhesions using solution injection, 2 or more days (62263)*
       6.82    11.9    **FUD** 010      T A2
       **AMA:** 2017,Jan,8; 2016,Jan,13; 2015,Jan,16; 2014,Jan,11; 2012,Jun,12-13; 2012,Jan,15-42

## 62267-62269 Percutaneous Procedures of Spinal Cord

**62267** **Percutaneous aspiration within the nucleus pulposus, intervertebral disc, or paravertebral tissue for diagnostic purposes**
       EXCLUDES    *Bone biopsy (20225)*
                      *Decompression of intervertebral disc (62287)*
                      *Fine needle aspiration (10022)*
                      *Injection for discography (62290-62291)*
       Code also fluoroscopic guidance (77003)
       4.60    7.09    **FUD** 000      T 62 80
       **AMA:** 2017,Feb,12; 2017,Jan,8; 2016,Jan,13; 2015,Jan,16; 2014,Jan,11; 2012,Jul,3-6

26/TC PC/TC Only    A2-Z3 ASC Payment    50 Bilateral    ♂ Male Only    ♀ Female Only    Facility RVU    Non-Facility RVU    CCI
**FUD** Follow-up Days    **CMS:** IOM (Pub 100)    A-Y OPPSI    80/80 Surg Assist Allowed / w/Doc    Lab Crosswalk    Radiology Crosswalk    CLIA
CPT © 2017 American Medical Association. All Rights Reserved.

© 2017 Optum360, LLC

**62268** Percutaneous aspiration, spinal cord cyst or syrinx
(76942, 77002, 77012)
7.47    7.47    **FUD** 000                                T A2 ▢

**AMA:** 2014,Jan,11

**62269** Biopsy of spinal cord, percutaneous needle
EXCLUDES    Fine needle aspiration (10021-10022)
(76942, 77002, 77012)
(88172-88173)
7.72    7.72    **FUD** 000                                J A2 80 ▢

**AMA:** 2014,Jan,11

## 62270-62272 Spinal Puncture, Subarachnoid Space, Diagnostic/Therapeutic
Code also fluoroscopic guidance (77003)

**62270** Spinal puncture, lumbar, diagnostic
2.25    4.51    **FUD** 000                                T A2 ▢

**AMA:** 2017,Jan,8; 2016,Jan,13; 2015,Jan,16; 2014,Sep,3; 2014,Jan,11; 2012,Mar,4-7

Common position to access vertebral interspace

**62272** Spinal puncture, therapeutic, for drainage of cerebrospinal fluid (by needle or catheter)
2.43    5.74    **FUD** 000                                T A2 ▢

**AMA:** 2017,Jan,8; 2016,Jan,13; 2015,Jan,16; 2014,Jan,11; 2013,Dec,14

## 62273 Epidural Blood Patch
**CMS:** 100-03,10.5 NCD for Autogenous Epidural Blood Graft (10.5)
EXCLUDES    Injection of diagnostic or therapeutic material (62320-62327)
Code also fluoroscopic guidance (77003)

**62273** Injection, epidural, of blood or clot patch
3.26    4.90    **FUD** 000                                T A2 ▢

**AMA:** 2017,Jan,8; 2016,Jan,13; 2015,Jan,16; 2014,Jan,11

## 62280-62282 Neurolysis
INCLUDES    Contrast injection during fluoroscopic guidance/localization
EXCLUDES    Injection of diagnostic or therapeutic material only (62320-62327)
Code also fluoroscopic guidance and localization unless a formal contrast study is performed (77003)

**62280** Injection/infusion of neurolytic substance (eg, alcohol, phenol, iced saline solutions), with or without other therapeutic substance; subarachnoid
4.61    8.57    **FUD** 010                                T A2 ▢

**AMA:** 2017,Jan,8; 2016,Jan,13; 2015,Jan,16; 2014,Jan,11; 2012,Jun,12-13

**62281** epidural, cervical or thoracic
4.51    6.87    **FUD** 010                                T A2 ▢

**AMA:** 2017,Jan,8; 2016,Jan,13; 2015,Jan,16; 2014,Jan,11; 2012,Jun,12-13

**62282** epidural, lumbar, sacral (caudal)
4.21    8.43    **FUD** 010                                T A2 ▢

**AMA:** 2017,Jan,8; 2016,Jan,13; 2015,Jan,16; 2014,Jan,11; 2012,Jun,12-13; 2012,Jan,15-42

## 62284-62294 Injection/Aspiration of Spine, Diagnostic/Therapeutic

**62284** Injection procedure for myelography and/or computed tomography, lumbar
EXCLUDES    Injection at C1-C2 (61055)
Myelography (62302-62305, 72240, 72255, 72265, 72270)
Code also fluoroscopic guidance (77003)
2.53    5.32    **FUD** 000                                N N1 ▢

**AMA:** 2017,Jan,8; 2016,Jan,13; 2015,Jan,16; 2014,Sep,3; 2014,Jan,11; 2012,Jan,15-42

**62287** Decompression procedure, percutaneous, of nucleus pulposus of intervertebral disc, any method utilizing needle based technique to remove disc material under fluoroscopic imaging or other form of indirect visualization, with discography and/or epidural injection(s) at the treated level(s), when performed, single or multiple levels, lumbar
INCLUDES    Endoscopic approach
EXCLUDES    Injection for discography (62290)
Injection of diagnostic or therapeutic substance(s) (62322)
Lumbar discography (72295)
Percutaneous aspiration, diagnostic (62267)
Percutaneous decompression of nucleus pulposus of an intervertebral disc, non-needle based technique (0274T-0275T)
Radiological guidance (77003, 77012)
16.5    16.5    **FUD** 090                                J A2 ▢

**AMA:** 2017,Feb,12; 2017,Jan,8; 2016,Jan,13; 2015,Mar,9; 2015,Jan,16; 2014,Apr,10; 2014,Jan,11; 2012,Oct,14; 2012,Jul,3-6; 2012,Jan,15-42

**62290** Injection procedure for discography, each level; lumbar
(72295)
4.91    9.36    **FUD** 000                                N N1 ▢

**AMA:** 2017,Feb,12; 2017,Jan,8; 2016,Jan,13; 2015,Jan,16; 2014,Jan,11; 2012,Jul,3-6; 2012,Jan,15-42

**62291** cervical or thoracic
(72285)
4.88    9.41    **FUD** 000                                N N1 ▢

**AMA:** 2017,Jan,8; 2016,Jan,13; 2015,Jan,16; 2014,Jan,11

● New Code    ▲ Revised Code    ○ Reinstated    ● New Web Release    ▲ Revised Web Release    Unlisted    Not Covered    # Resequenced
⊘ AMA Mod 51 Exempt    ⑤ Optum Mod 51 Exempt    ⑥ Mod 63 Exempt    ✗ Non-FDA Drug    ★ Telemedicine    🅼 Maternity    🄰 Age Edit    + Add-on    **AMA:** CPT Asst
© 2017 Optum360, LLC                        CPT © 2017 American Medical Association. All Rights Reserved.                        279

**Nervous System** *(side tab)*

**62292 — 62367** *(side tab)*

**62292** **Injection procedure for chemonucleolysis, including discography, intervertebral disc, single or multiple levels, lumbar**
🚑 16.6    ⚓ 16.6    **FUD** 090      J A2 80 🖵
AMA: 2017,Jan,8; 2016,Jan,13; 2015,Jan,16; 2014,Jan,11; 2012,Jan,15-42

**62294** **Injection procedure, arterial, for occlusion of arteriovenous malformation, spinal**
🚑 27.8    ⚓ 27.8    **FUD** 090      T A2 🖵
AMA: 2014,Jan,11

## 62302-62305 Myelography

EXCLUDES   *C1-C2 injection (61055)*
*Lumbar myelogram furnished by other providers (62284, 72240, 72255, 72265, 72270)*

**62302** **Myelography via lumbar injection, including radiological supervision and interpretation; cervical**
🚑 3.55    ⚓ 6.90    **FUD** 000      Q2 N1 🖵
EXCLUDES   *Myelography (62303-62305)*

**62303** **thoracic**
🚑 3.58    ⚓ 7.11    **FUD** 000      Q2 N1 🖵
EXCLUDES   *Myelography (62302, 62304-62305)*

**62304** **lumbosacral**
🚑 3.48    ⚓ 6.81    **FUD** 000      Q2 N1 🖵
EXCLUDES   *Myelography (62302-62303, 62305)*

**62305** **2 or more regions (eg, lumbar/thoracic, cervical/thoracic, lumbar/cervical, lumbar/thoracic/cervical)**
🚑 3.64    ⚓ 7.41    **FUD** 000      Q2 N1 🖵
EXCLUDES   *Myelography (62302-62305)*

## 62320-62327 Injection/Infusion Diagnostic/Therapeutic Material

EXCLUDES   *Epidurography (72275)*
*Transforaminal epidural injection (64479-64484)*
*Use of code more than one time even when catheter tip or injected drug travels into a different area of the spine*

**62320** **Injection(s), of diagnostic or therapeutic substance(s) (eg, anesthetic, antispasmodic, opioid, steroid, other solution), not including neurolytic substances, including needle or catheter placement, interlaminar epidural or subarachnoid, cervical or thoracic; without imaging guidance**
🚑 2.94    ⚓ 4.75    **FUD** 000      T 62 🖵
AMA: 2017,Sep,6

**62321** **with imaging guidance (ie, fluoroscopy or CT)**
INCLUDES   Radiologic guidance (76942, 77003, 77012)
🚑 3.17    ⚓ 7.06    **FUD** 000      T 62 🖵
AMA: 2017,Sep,6

**62322** **Injection(s), of diagnostic or therapeutic substance(s) (eg, anesthetic, antispasmodic, opioid, steroid, other solution), not including neurolytic substances, including needle or catheter placement, interlaminar epidural or subarachnoid, lumbar or sacral (caudal); without imaging guidance**
🚑 2.53    ⚓ 4.43    **FUD** 000      T 62 🖵
AMA: 2017,Sep,6; 2017,Feb,12

**62323** **with imaging guidance (ie, fluoroscopy or CT)**
INCLUDES   Radiologic guidance (76942, 77003, 77012)
🚑 2.89    ⚓ 6.93    **FUD** 000      T 62 🖵
AMA: 2017,Sep,6

**62324** **Injection(s), including indwelling catheter placement, continuous infusion or intermittent bolus, of diagnostic or therapeutic substance(s) (eg, anesthetic, antispasmodic, opioid, steroid, other solution), not including neurolytic substances, interlaminar epidural or subarachnoid, cervical or thoracic; without imaging guidance**
Code also hospital management of continuous infusion of drug, epidural or subarachnoid (01996)
🚑 2.68    ⚓ 4.15    **FUD** 000      T 62 🖵
AMA: 2017,Sep,6

**62325** **with imaging guidance (ie, fluoroscopy or CT)**
INCLUDES   Radiologic guidance (76942, 77003, 77012)
Code also hospital management of continuous infusion of drug, epidural or subarachnoid (01996)
🚑 3.08    ⚓ 6.26    **FUD** 000      T 62 🖵
AMA: 2017,Sep,6

**62326** **Injection(s), including indwelling catheter placement, continuous infusion or intermittent bolus, of diagnostic or therapeutic substance(s) (eg, anesthetic, antispasmodic, opioid, steroid, other solution), not including neurolytic substances, interlaminar epidural or subarachnoid, lumbar or sacral (caudal); without imaging guidance**
Code also hospital management of continuous infusion of drug, epidural or subarachnoid (01996)
🚑 2.63    ⚓ 4.36    **FUD** 000      T 62 🖵
AMA: 2017,Sep,6

**62327** **with imaging guidance (ie, fluoroscopy or CT)**
INCLUDES   Radiologic guidance (76942, 77003, 77012)
Code also hospital management of continuous infusion of drug, epidural or subarachnoid (01996)
🚑 2.80    ⚓ 6.38    **FUD** 000      T 62 🖵
AMA: 2017,Sep,6

## 62350-62370 Procedures Related to Epidural and Intrathecal Catheters

EXCLUDES   *Epidural blood patch (62273)*
*Injection epidural/subarachnoid diagnostic/therapeutic drugs (62320-62327)*
*Injection for lumbar computed tomography/myelography (62284)*
*Injection/infusion neurolytic substances (62280-62282)*
*Spinal puncture (62270-62272)*

**62350** **Implantation, revision or repositioning of tunneled intrathecal or epidural catheter, for long-term medication administration via an external pump or implantable reservoir/infusion pump; without laminectomy**
🚑 11.5    ⚓ 11.5    **FUD** 010      J A2 🖵
AMA: 2017,Jan,8; 2016,Jan,13; 2015,Jan,16; 2014,Jan,11

**62351** **with laminectomy**
🚑 24.9    ⚓ 24.9    **FUD** 090      J 80 🖵
AMA: 2017,Jan,8; 2016,Jan,13; 2015,Jan,16; 2014,Jan,11

**62355** **Removal of previously implanted intrathecal or epidural catheter**
🚑 7.72    ⚓ 7.72    **FUD** 010      Q2 A2 80 🖵
AMA: 2014,Jan,11

**62360** **Implantation or replacement of device for intrathecal or epidural drug infusion; subcutaneous reservoir**
🚑 8.92    ⚓ 8.92    **FUD** 010      J J8 80 🖵
AMA: 2014,Jan,11

**62361** **nonprogrammable pump**
🚑 12.2    ⚓ 12.2    **FUD** 010      J J8 80 🖵
AMA: 2014,Jan,11

**62362** **programmable pump, including preparation of pump, with or without programming**
🚑 11.1    ⚓ 11.1    **FUD** 010      J J6 80 🖵
AMA: 2017,Jan,8; 2016,Jan,13; 2015,Jan,16; 2014,Jan,11; 2012,Jan,15-42

**62365** **Removal of subcutaneous reservoir or pump, previously implanted for intrathecal or epidural infusion**
🚑 8.60    ⚓ 8.60    **FUD** 010      Q2 A2 80 🖵
AMA: 2014,Jan,11

**62367** **Electronic analysis of programmable, implanted pump for intrathecal or epidural drug infusion (includes evaluation of reservoir status, alarm status, drug prescription status); without reprogramming or refill**
🚑 0.73    ⚓ 1.17    **FUD** XXX      S P3 🖵
AMA: 2017,Jan,8; 2016,Jan,13; 2015,Jan,16; 2014,Jan,11; 2012,Aug,10-12; 2012,Jul,3-6

| 26/TC PC/TC Only | A2-Z3 ASC Payment | 50 Bilateral | ♂ Male Only | ♀ Female Only | 🚑 Facility RVU | ⚓ Non-Facility RVU | 🖵 CCI |
| FUD Follow-up Days | CMS: IOM (Pub 100) | A-Y OPPSI | 80/80 Surg Assist Allowed / w/Doc | | 🔬 Lab Crosswalk | 📻 Radiology Crosswalk | ⊗ CLIA |

**280**
CPT © 2017 American Medical Association. All Rights Reserved.
© 2017 Optum360, LLC

**62368**     **with reprogramming**
  1.01    1.60   **FUD** XXX                          S P3
  **AMA:** 2017,Jan,8; 2016,Jan,13; 2015,Jan,16; 2014,Jan,11;
  2012,Aug,10-12; 2012,Jul,3-6; 2012,Jan,15-42

**62369**     **with reprogramming and refill**
  1.02    3.36   **FUD** XXX                          S P3
  **AMA:** 2017,Jan,8; 2016,Jan,13; 2015,Jan,16; 2014,Jan,11;
  2012,Aug,10-12; 2012,Jul,3-6

**62370**     **with reprogramming and refill (requiring skill of a
              physician or other qualified health care professional)**
  1.33    3.55   **FUD** XXX                          S P3
  **AMA:** 2017,Jan,8; 2016,Jan,13; 2015,Jan,16; 2014,Jan,11;
  2012,Aug,10-12; 2012,Jul,3-6

## 62380 Endoscopic Decompression/Laminectomy/Laminotomy

EXCLUDES   Open decompression (63030, 63056)
           Percutaneous decompression (62267, 0274T-0275T)
Code also operating microscope, when applicable (69990)

**62380**     **Endoscopic decompression of spinal cord, nerve root(s),
              including laminotomy, partial facetectomy, foraminotomy,
              discectomy and/or excision of herniated intervertebral disc,
              1 interspace, lumbar**
  0.00    0.00   **FUD** 090                   J J8 80 50
  **AMA:** 2017,Feb,12

## 63001-63048 Posterior Midline Approach: Laminectomy/Laminotomy/Decompression

INCLUDES   Endoscopic assistance through open and direct visualization
EXCLUDES   Arthrodesis (22590-22614)
           Percutaneous decompression (62287, 0274T, 0275T)
Code also operating microscope, when applicable (69990)

**63001**     **Laminectomy with exploration and/or decompression of
              spinal cord and/or cauda equina, without facetectomy,
              foraminotomy or discectomy (eg, spinal stenosis), 1 or 2
              vertebral segments; cervical**
  36.2    36.2   **FUD** 090                   J 62 80
  **AMA:** 2017,Mar,7; 2017,Jan,8; 2016,Jan,13; 2015,Jan,16;
  2014,Jan,11; 2013,Jul,3-5; 2012,Jul,3-6; 2012,Jan,15-42

**63003**     **thoracic**
  36.1    36.1   **FUD** 090                   J 62 80
  **AMA:** 2017,Mar,7; 2017,Jan,8; 2016,Jan,13; 2015,Jan,16;
  2014,Jan,11; 2013,Jul,3-5; 2012,Jul,3-6; 2012,Jan,15-42

**63005**     **lumbar, except for spondylolisthesis**
  34.4    34.4   **FUD** 090                   J 62 80
  **AMA:** 2017,Mar,7; 2017,Feb,9; 2017,Jan,8; 2016,Jan,13;
  2015,Jan,16; 2014,Jan,11; 2013,Dec,16; 2013,Jul,3-5; 2012,Jul,3-6;
  2012,Jan,15-42

**63011**     **sacral**
  31.7    31.7   **FUD** 090                   J 80
  **AMA:** 2017,Mar,7; 2017,Jan,8; 2016,Jan,13; 2015,Jan,16;
  2014,Jan,11; 2013,Jul,3-5; 2012,Jan,15-42

**63012**     **Laminectomy with removal of abnormal facets and/or pars
              inter-articularis with decompression of cauda equina and
              nerve roots for spondylolisthesis, lumbar (Gill type
              procedure)**
  34.6    34.6   **FUD** 090                   J 80
  **AMA:** 2017,Mar,7; 2017,Feb,9; 2017,Jan,8; 2016,Jan,13;
  2015,Jan,16; 2014,Jan,11; 2013,Jul,3-5; 2012,Jan,15-42

**63015**     **Laminectomy with exploration and/or decompression of
              spinal cord and/or cauda equina, without facetectomy,
              foraminotomy or discectomy (eg, spinal stenosis), more than
              2 vertebral segments; cervical**
  43.3    43.3   **FUD** 090                   J 80
  **AMA:** 2017,Mar,7; 2017,Jan,8; 2016,Jan,13; 2015,Jan,16;
  2014,Jan,11; 2013,Jul,3-5; 2012,Jan,15-42

**63016**     **thoracic**
  44.5    44.5   **FUD** 090                   J 80
  **AMA:** 2017,Mar,7; 2017,Jan,8; 2016,Jan,13; 2015,Jan,16;
  2014,Jan,11; 2013,Jul,3-5; 2012,Jan,15-42

**63017**     **lumbar**
  36.6    36.6   **FUD** 090                   J 80
  **AMA:** 2017,Mar,7; 2017,Feb,9; 2017,Jan,8; 2016,Jan,13;
  2015,Jan,16; 2014,Jan,11; 2013,Jul,3-5; 2012,Jan,15-42

Nerve root problems
in C5 through C7
cause paralysis
of the upper limb

C1 to C4

C5 to C7

Atlas
(C1)

Axis
(C2)

The specialized atlas allows for rotary
motion, which turns the head

**63020**     **Laminotomy (hemilaminectomy), with decompression of
              nerve root(s), including partial facetectomy, foraminotomy
              and/or excision of herniated intervertebral disc; 1 interspace,
              cervical**
  33.8    33.8   **FUD** 090                   J 62 80 50
  **AMA:** 2017,Mar,7; 2017,Jan,8; 2016,Jan,13; 2015,Jan,16;
  2014,Jan,11; 2013,Jul,3-5; 2012,Dec,12; 2012,Jul,3-6;
  2012,Jan,15-42

**63030**     **1 interspace, lumbar**
  28.2    28.2   **FUD** 090                   J 62 80 50
  **AMA:** 2017,Mar,7; 2017,Feb,9; 2017,Feb,12; 2017,Jan,8;
  2016,May,13; 2016,Jan,13; 2015,Jan,16; 2014,Jan,11; 2013,Dec,16;
  2013,Jul,3-5; 2012,Dec,12; 2012,Jul,3-6; 2012,Jan,15-42

+ **63035**   **each additional interspace, cervical or lumbar (List
              separately in addition to code for primary procedure)**
  Code first (63020-63030)
  5.61    5.61   **FUD** ZZZ                   N 80 50
  **AMA:** 2017,Feb,9; 2017,Jan,8; 2016,Jan,13; 2015,Jan,16;
  2014,Jan,11; 2012,Jul,3-6; 2012,Jan,15-42

**63040**     **Laminotomy (hemilaminectomy), with decompression of
              nerve root(s), including partial facetectomy, foraminotomy
              and/or excision of herniated intervertebral disc,
              reexploration, single interspace; cervical**
  40.5    40.5   **FUD** 090                   J 80 50
  **AMA:** 2017,Mar,7; 2017,Jan,8; 2016,Jan,13; 2015,Jan,16;
  2014,Jan,11; 2013,Jul,3-5; 2012,Jan,15-42

**63042**     **lumbar**
  37.6    37.6   **FUD** 090                   J 62 80 50
  **AMA:** 2017,Mar,7; 2017,Feb,9; 2017,Jan,8; 2016,Jan,13;
  2015,Jan,16; 2014,Jan,11; 2013,Jul,3-5; 2012,Jan,15-42

+ **63043**   **each additional cervical interspace (List separately in
              addition to code for primary procedure)**
  Code first (63040)
  0.00    0.00   **FUD** ZZZ                   N 80 50
  **AMA:** 2017,Jan,8; 2016,Jan,13; 2015,Jan,16; 2014,Jan,11;
  2012,Jan,15-42

+ **63044**   **each additional lumbar interspace (List separately in
              addition to code for primary procedure)**
  Code first (63042)
  0.00    0.00   **FUD** ZZZ                   N M 80 50
  **AMA:** 2017,Feb,9; 2017,Jan,8; 2016,Jan,13; 2015,Jan,16;
  2014,Jan,11; 2012,Jan,15-42

---

● New Code      ▲ Revised Code      ○ Reinstated      ● New Web Release      ▲ Revised Web Release      Unlisted      Not Covered      # Resequenced
Ø AMA Mod 51 Exempt   Ⓢ Optum Mod 51 Exempt   Ⓢ Mod 63 Exempt   ✗ Non-FDA Drug   ★ Telemedicine   M Maternity   A Age Edit   + Add-on   AMA: CPT Asst

**Nervous System**

**63045 — 63082**

**63045** **Laminectomy, facetectomy and foraminotomy (unilateral or bilateral with decompression of spinal cord, cauda equina and/or nerve root[s], [eg, spinal or lateral recess stenosis]), single vertebral segment; cervical**
    🔧 37.5    ✂ 37.5    **FUD** 090    J 62 80 ▣
    **AMA:** 2017,Mar,7; 2017,Jan,8; 2016,Jan,13; 2015,Jan,16; 2014,Jan,11; 2013,Jul,3-5; 2012,Dec,12; 2012,Jan,15-42

**63046** **thoracic**
    🔧 35.5    ✂ 35.5    **FUD** 090    J 62 80 ▣
    **AMA:** 2017,Mar,7; 2017,Jan,8; 2016,Jan,13; 2015,Jan,16; 2014,Jan,11; 2013,Jul,3-5; 2012,Dec,12; 2012,Jan,15-42

**63047** **lumbar**
    🔧 32.0    ✂ 32.0    **FUD** 090    J 62 80 ▣
    **AMA:** 2017,Mar,7; 2017,Feb,9; 2017,Feb,12; 2017,Jan,8; 2016,Oct,11; 2016,Jan,13; 2015,Jan,16; 2014,Dec,16; 2014,Dec,16; 2014,Jan,11; 2013,Dec,16; 2013,Jul,3-5; 2012,Dec,12; 2012,Jan,15-42

+ **63048** **each additional segment, cervical, thoracic, or lumbar (List separately in addition to code for primary procedure)**
    Code first (63045-63047)
    🔧 6.19    ✂ 6.19    **FUD** ZZZ    N 80 ▣
    **AMA:** 2017,Feb,9; 2017,Jan,8; 2016,Jan,13; 2015,Jan,16; 2014,Jan,11; 2012,Dec,12; 2012,Jan,15-42

## 63050-63051 Cervical Laminoplasty: Posterior Midline Approach

EXCLUDES    *Procedure performed on the same vertebral segment(s) (22600, 22614, 22840-22842, 63001, 63015, 63045, 63048, 63295)*

**63050** **Laminoplasty, cervical, with decompression of the spinal cord, 2 or more vertebral segments;**
    🔧 43.7    ✂ 43.7    **FUD** 090    C 80 ▣
    **AMA:** 2017,Mar,7; 2017,Jan,8; 2016,Jan,13; 2015,Jan,16; 2014,Jan,11; 2013,Jul,3-5

**63051** **with reconstruction of the posterior bony elements (including the application of bridging bone graft and non-segmental fixation devices [eg, wire, suture, mini-plates], when performed)**
    🔧 49.7    ✂ 49.7    **FUD** 090    C 80 ▣
    **AMA:** 2017,Mar,7; 2017,Jan,8; 2016,Jan,13; 2015,Jan,16; 2014,Jan,11; 2013,Jul,3-5

## 63055-63066 Spinal Cord/Nerve Root Decompression: Costovertebral or Transpedicular Approach

**63055** **Transpedicular approach with decompression of spinal cord, equina and/or nerve root(s) (eg, herniated intervertebral disc), single segment; thoracic**
    🔧 47.5    ✂ 47.5    **FUD** 090    J 62 80 ▣
    **AMA:** 2017,Mar,7; 2017,Jan,8; 2016,Jan,13; 2015,Jan,16; 2014,Jan,11; 2013,Jul,3-5

**63056** **lumbar (including transfacet, or lateral extraforaminal approach) (eg, far lateral herniated intervertebral disc)**
    🔧 43.2    ✂ 43.2    **FUD** 090    J 62 80 ▣
    **AMA:** 2017,Mar,7; 2017,Feb,12; 2017,Jan,8; 2016,Jan,13; 2015,Jan,16; 2014,Jan,11; 2014,Jan,9; 2013,Jul,3-5; 2012,Jul,3-6; 2012,Jan,15-42

+ **63057** **each additional segment, thoracic or lumbar (List separately in addition to code for primary procedure)**
    Code first (63055-63056)
    🔧 9.37    ✂ 9.37    **FUD** ZZZ    N 80 ▣
    **AMA:** 2017,Jan,8; 2016,Jan,13; 2015,Jan,16; 2014,Jan,11

**63064** **Costovertebral approach with decompression of spinal cord or nerve root(s) (eg, herniated intervertebral disc), thoracic; single segment**
    EXCLUDES  *Laminectomy with intraspinal thoracic lesion removal (63266, 63271, 63276, 63281, 63286)*
    🔧 51.7    ✂ 51.7    **FUD** 090    J 80 ▣
    **AMA:** 2017,Mar,7; 2017,Jan,8; 2016,Jan,13; 2015,Jan,16; 2014,Jan,11; 2013,Jul,3-5

+ **63066** **each additional segment (List separately in addition to code for primary procedure)**
    EXCLUDES  *Laminectomy with intraspinal thoracic lesion removal (63266, 63271, 63276, 63281, 63286)*
    Code first (63064)
    🔧 6.08    ✂ 6.08    **FUD** ZZZ    N 80 ▣
    **AMA:** 2014,Jan,11

## 63075-63078 Discectomy: Anterior or Anterolateral Approach

INCLUDES    Operating microscope (69990)

**63075** **Discectomy, anterior, with decompression of spinal cord and/or nerve root(s), including osteophytectomy; cervical, single interspace**
    EXCLUDES  *Anterior cervical discectomy and anterior interbody fusion at same level during same operative session (22551)*
    *Anterior interbody arthrodesis (even by another provider) (22554)*
    🔧 39.4    ✂ 39.4    **FUD** 090    J 80 ▣
    **AMA:** 2017,Mar,7; 2017,Jan,8; 2016,Feb,12; 2016,Jan,13; 2015,Apr,7; 2015,Jan,16; 2014,Jan,11; 2013,Jul,3-5; 2012,Jan,15-42

+ **63076** **cervical, each additional interspace (List separately in addition to code for primary procedure)**
    EXCLUDES  *Anterior cervical discectomy and anterior interbody fusion at same level during same operative session (22552)*
    *Anterior interbody arthrodesis (even by another provider) (22554)*
    Code first (63075)
    🔧 7.26    ✂ 7.26    **FUD** ZZZ    N 80 ▣
    **AMA:** 2017,Jan,8; 2016,Feb,12; 2016,Jan,13; 2015,Jan,16; 2014,Jan,11; 2012,Jan,15-42

**63077** **thoracic, single interspace**
    🔧 43.4    ✂ 43.4    **FUD** 090    C 80 ▣
    **AMA:** 2017,Mar,7; 2017,Jan,8; 2016,Feb,12; 2016,Jan,13; 2015,Jan,16; 2014,Jan,11; 2013,Jul,3-5; 2012,Jan,15-42

+ **63078** **thoracic, each additional interspace (List separately in addition to code for primary procedure)**
    Code first (63077)
    🔧 5.67    ✂ 5.67    **FUD** ZZZ    C 80 ▣
    **AMA:** 2017,Jan,8; 2016,Feb,12; 2016,Jan,13; 2015,Jan,16; 2014,Jan,11; 2012,Jan,15-42

## 63081-63091 Vertebral Corpectomy, All Levels, Anterior Approach

INCLUDES    Disc removal at the level below and/or above vertebral segment
    Partial removal:
        Cervical: Removal of ≥ 1/2 of vertebral body
        Lumbar: Removal of ≥ 1/3 of vertebral body
        Thoracic: Removal of ≥ 1/3 of vertebral body
EXCLUDES    *Arthrodesis (22548-22812)*
Code also reconstruction (20930-20938, 22548-22812, 22840-22855 [22859])

**63081** **Vertebral corpectomy (vertebral body resection), partial or complete, anterior approach with decompression of spinal cord and/or nerve root(s); cervical, single segment**
    EXCLUDES  *Transoral approach (61575-61576)*
    🔧 51.1    ✂ 51.1    **FUD** 090    C 80 ▣
    **AMA:** 2017,Mar,7; 2017,Jan,8; 2016,Apr,8; 2016,Jan,13; 2015,Jun,10; 2015,Jan,16; 2014,Jan,11; 2013,Jul,3-5

+ **63082** **cervical, each additional segment (List separately in addition to code for primary procedure)**
    EXCLUDES  *Transoral approach (61575-61576)*
    Code first (63081)
    🔧 7.80    ✂ 7.80    **FUD** ZZZ    C 80 ▣
    **AMA:** 2017,Jan,8; 2016,Apr,8; 2016,Jan,13; 2015,Jan,16; 2014,Jan,11

| 26/TC PC/TC Only | A2-Z3 ASC Payment | 50 Bilateral | ♂ Male Only | ♀ Female Only | 🔧 Facility RVU | ✂ Non-Facility RVU | ▣ CCI |
| FUD Follow-up Days | CMS: IOM (Pub 100) | A-Y OPPSI | 80/80 Surg Assist Allowed / w/Doc | | ▦ Lab Crosswalk | ▨ Radiology Crosswalk | ✖ CLIA |

282
CPT © 2017 American Medical Association. All Rights Reserved.
© 2017 Optum360, LLC

**63085** Vertebral corpectomy (vertebral body resection), partial or complete, transthoracic approach with decompression of spinal cord and/or nerve root(s); thoracic, single segment
🔧 55.8 ✂ 55.8 **FUD** 090 [C] [80] [▣]
**AMA:** 2017,Mar,7; 2017,Jan,8; 2016,Apr,8; 2016,Jan,13; 2015,Jan,16; 2014,Jan,11; 2013,Jul,3-5

**+ 63086** thoracic, each additional segment (List separately in addition to code for primary procedure)
Code first (63085)
🔧 5.58 ✂ 5.58 **FUD** ZZZ [C] [80] [▣]
**AMA:** 2017,Jan,8; 2016,Apr,8; 2016,Jan,13; 2015,Jan,16; 2014,Jan,11

**63087** Vertebral corpectomy (vertebral body resection), partial or complete, combined thoracolumbar approach with decompression of spinal cord, cauda equina or nerve root(s), lower thoracic or lumbar; single segment
🔧 70.2 ✂ 70.2 **FUD** 090 [C] [80] [▣]
**AMA:** 2017,Mar,7; 2017,Jan,8; 2016,Apr,8; 2016,Jan,13; 2015,Jan,16; 2014,Jan,11; 2013,Jul,3-5

**+ 63088** each additional segment (List separately in addition to code for primary procedure)
Code first (63087)
🔧 7.61 ✂ 7.61 **FUD** ZZZ [C] [80] [▣]
**AMA:** 2017,Jan,8; 2016,Apr,8; 2016,Jan,13; 2015,Jan,16; 2014,Jan,11

**63090** Vertebral corpectomy (vertebral body resection), partial or complete, transperitoneal or retroperitoneal approach with decompression of spinal cord, cauda equina or nerve root(s), lower thoracic, lumbar, or sacral; single segment
🔧 56.8 ✂ 56.8 **FUD** 090 [C] [80] [▣]
**AMA:** 2017,Mar,7; 2017,Jan,8; 2016,Apr,8; 2016,Jan,13; 2015,Jan,16; 2014,Jan,11; 2013,Jul,3-5

**+ 63091** each additional segment (List separately in addition to code for primary procedure)
Code first (63090)
🔧 5.18 ✂ 5.18 **FUD** ZZZ [C] [80] [▣]
**AMA:** 2017,Jan,8; 2016,Apr,8; 2016,Jan,13; 2015,Jan,16; 2014,Jan,11

## 63101-63103 Corpectomy: Lateral Extracavitary Approach

INCLUDES Partial removal:
Cervical: Removal of ≥ 1/2 of vertebral body
Lumbar: Removal of ≥ 1/3 of vertebral body
Thoracic: Removal of ≥ 1/3 of vertebral body

**63101** Vertebral corpectomy (vertebral body resection), partial or complete, lateral extracavitary approach with decompression of spinal cord and/or nerve root(s) (eg, for tumor or retropulsed bone fragments); thoracic, single segment
🔧 67.5 ✂ 67.5 **FUD** 090 [C] [80] [▣]
**AMA:** 2017,Mar,7; 2017,Jan,8; 2016,Jan,13; 2015,Jan,16; 2014,Jan,11; 2013,Jul,3-5

**63102** lumbar, single segment
🔧 66.2 ✂ 66.2 **FUD** 090 [C] [80] [▣]
**AMA:** 2017,Mar,7; 2017,Jan,8; 2016,Jan,13; 2015,Jan,16; 2014,Jan,11; 2013,Jul,3-5

**+ 63103** thoracic or lumbar, each additional segment (List separately in addition to code for primary procedure)
Code first (63101-63102)
🔧 8.57 ✂ 8.57 **FUD** ZZZ [C] [80] [▣]
**AMA:** 2014,Jan,11

## 63170-63295 Laminectomies

**63170** Laminectomy with myelotomy (eg, Bischof or DREZ type), cervical, thoracic, or thoracolumbar
🔧 46.9 ✂ 46.9 **FUD** 090 [C] [80] [▣]
**AMA:** 2017,Mar,7; 2017,Jan,8; 2016,Jan,13; 2015,Jan,16; 2014,Jan,11; 2013,Jul,3-5

**63172** Laminectomy with drainage of intramedullary cyst/syrinx; to subarachnoid space
🔧 41.3 ✂ 41.3 **FUD** 090 [C] [80] [▣]
**AMA:** 2017,Mar,7; 2017,Jan,8; 2016,Jan,13; 2015,Jan,16; 2014,Jan,11; 2013,Jul,3-5

**63173** to peritoneal or pleural space
🔧 50.0 ✂ 50.0 **FUD** 090 [C] [80] [▣]
**AMA:** 2017,Mar,7; 2017,Jan,8; 2016,Jan,13; 2015,Jan,16; 2014,Jan,11; 2013,Jul,3-5

**63180** Laminectomy and section of dentate ligaments, with or without dural graft, cervical; 1 or 2 segments
🔧 39.0 ✂ 39.0 **FUD** 090 [C] [80] [▣]
**AMA:** 2017,Mar,7; 2017,Jan,8; 2016,Jan,13; 2015,Jan,16; 2014,Jan,11; 2013,Jul,3-5

**63182** more than 2 segments
🔧 48.0 ✂ 48.0 **FUD** 090 [C] [80] [▣]
**AMA:** 2017,Mar,7; 2017,Jan,8; 2016,Jan,13; 2015,Jan,16; 2014,Jan,11; 2013,Jul,3-5

**63185** Laminectomy with rhizotomy; 1 or 2 segments
INCLUDES Dana rhizotomy
Stoffel rhizotomy
🔧 33.2 ✂ 33.2 **FUD** 090 [C] [80] [▣]
**AMA:** 2017,Mar,7; 2017,Jan,8; 2016,Jan,13; 2015,Jan,16; 2014,Jan,11; 2013,Jul,3-5

**63190** more than 2 segments
🔧 37.2 ✂ 37.2 **FUD** 090 [C] [80] [▣]
**AMA:** 2017,Mar,7; 2017,Jan,8; 2016,Jan,13; 2015,Jan,16; 2014,Jan,11; 2013,Jul,3-5

**63191** Laminectomy with section of spinal accessory nerve
EXCLUDES Division of sternocleidomastoid muscle for torticollis (21720)
🔧 36.8 ✂ 36.8 **FUD** 090 [C] [80] [50] [▣]
**AMA:** 2017,Mar,7; 2017,Jan,8; 2016,Jan,13; 2015,Jan,16; 2014,Jan,11; 2013,Jul,3-5

**63194** Laminectomy with cordotomy, with section of 1 spinothalamic tract, 1 stage; cervical
🔧 40.6 ✂ 40.6 **FUD** 090 [C] [80] [▣]
**AMA:** 2017,Mar,7; 2017,Jan,8; 2016,Jan,13; 2015,Jan,16; 2014,Jan,11; 2013,Jul,3-5

**63195** thoracic
🔧 36.7 ✂ 36.7 **FUD** 090 [C] [80] [▣]
**AMA:** 2017,Mar,7; 2017,Jan,8; 2016,Jan,13; 2015,Jan,16; 2014,Jan,11; 2013,Jul,3-5

**63196** Laminectomy with cordotomy, with section of both spinothalamic tracts, 1 stage; cervical
🔧 40.8 ✂ 40.8 **FUD** 090 [C] [80] [▣]
**AMA:** 2017,Mar,7; 2017,Jan,8; 2016,Jan,13; 2015,Jan,16; 2014,Jan,11; 2013,Jul,3-5

**63197** thoracic
🔧 40.9 ✂ 40.9 **FUD** 090 [C] [80] [▣]
**AMA:** 2017,Mar,7; 2017,Jan,8; 2016,Jan,13; 2015,Jan,16; 2014,Jan,11; 2013,Jul,3-5

**63198** Laminectomy with cordotomy with section of both spinothalamic tracts, 2 stages within 14 days; cervical
INCLUDES Keen laminectomy
🔧 48.1 ✂ 48.1 **FUD** 090 [C] [80] [▣]
**AMA:** 2017,Mar,7; 2017,Jan,8; 2016,Jan,13; 2015,Jan,16; 2014,Jan,11; 2013,Jul,3-5

**63199** thoracic
🔧 50.4 ✂ 50.4 **FUD** 090 [C] [80] [▣]
**AMA:** 2017,Mar,7; 2017,Jan,8; 2016,Jan,13; 2015,Jan,16; 2014,Jan,11; 2013,Jul,3-5

**63200** Laminectomy, with release of tethered spinal cord, lumbar
🔧 44.9 ✂ 44.9 **FUD** 090 [C] [80] [▣]
**AMA:** 2017,Mar,7; 2017,Jan,8; 2016,Jan,13; 2015,Jan,16; 2014,Jan,11; 2013,Jul,3-5

● New Code ▲ Revised Code ○ Reinstated ● New Web Release ▲ Revised Web Release Unlisted Not Covered # Resequenced
⊘ AMA Mod 51 Exempt ⑪ Optum Mod 51 Exempt ⑬ Mod 63 Exempt ✗ Non-FDA Drug ★ Telemedicine Ⓜ Maternity ▲ Age Edit + Add-on **AMA:** CPT Asst
© 2017 Optum360, LLC CPT © 2017 American Medical Association. All Rights Reserved.

**63250** Laminectomy for excision or occlusion of arteriovenous malformation of spinal cord; cervical

🚗 87.6   ✂ 87.6   **FUD** 090   Ⓒ 80 ▢

**AMA:** 2017,Mar,7; 2017,Jan,8; 2016,Jan,13; 2015,Jan,16; 2014,Jan,11; 2013,Jul,3-5

Cervical
C₁ to C₇

Thoracic
T₁ to T₁₂

Lumbar
L₁ to L₅

Sacrum

Dura mater

Nerve roots

Pia mater

Arachnoid

White matter

Gray matter

**Schematic of spinal cord layers**

**63251** thoracic

🚗 88.7   ✂ 88.7   **FUD** 090   Ⓒ 80 ▢

**AMA:** 2017,Mar,7; 2017,Jan,8; 2016,Jan,13; 2015,Jan,16; 2014,Jan,11; 2013,Jul,3-5

**63252** thoracolumbar

🚗 89.0   ✂ 89.0   **FUD** 090   Ⓒ 80 ▢

**AMA:** 2017,Mar,7; 2017,Jan,8; 2016,Jan,13; 2015,Jan,16; 2014,Jan,11; 2013,Jul,3-5

**63265** Laminectomy for excision or evacuation of intraspinal lesion other than neoplasm, extradural; cervical

🚗 48.7   ✂ 48.7   **FUD** 090   Ⓒ 80 ▢

**AMA:** 2017,Mar,7; 2017,Jan,8; 2016,Jan,13; 2015,Jan,16; 2014,Jan,11; 2013,Jul,3-5

**63266** thoracic

🚗 50.2   ✂ 50.2   **FUD** 090   Ⓒ 80 ▢

**AMA:** 2017,Mar,7; 2014,Jan,11; 2013,Jul,3-5

**63267** lumbar

🚗 39.9   ✂ 39.9   **FUD** 090   Ⓒ 80 ▢

**AMA:** 2017,Mar,7; 2017,Jan,8; 2016,Jan,13; 2015,Jan,16; 2014,Jan,11; 2013,Jul,3-5

**63268** sacral

🚗 40.7   ✂ 40.7   **FUD** 090   Ⓒ 80 ▢

**AMA:** 2017,Mar,7; 2017,Jan,8; 2016,Jan,13; 2015,Jan,16; 2014,Jan,11; 2013,Jul,3-5

**63270** Laminectomy for excision of intraspinal lesion other than neoplasm, intradural; cervical

🚗 60.9   ✂ 60.9   **FUD** 090   Ⓒ 80 ▢

**AMA:** 2017,Mar,7; 2017,Jan,8; 2016,Jan,13; 2015,Jan,16; 2014,Jan,11; 2013,Jul,3-5

**63271** thoracic

🚗 60.4   ✂ 60.4   **FUD** 090   Ⓒ 80 ▢

**AMA:** 2017,Mar,7; 2017,Jan,8; 2016,Jan,13; 2015,Jan,16; 2014,Jan,11; 2013,Jul,3-5

**63272** lumbar

🚗 55.2   ✂ 55.2   **FUD** 090   Ⓒ 80 ▢

**AMA:** 2017,Mar,7; 2017,Jan,8; 2016,Jan,13; 2015,Jan,16; 2014,Jan,11; 2013,Jul,3-5

**63273** sacral

🚗 53.6   ✂ 53.6   **FUD** 090   Ⓒ 80 ▢

**AMA:** 2017,Mar,7; 2017,Jan,8; 2016,Jan,13; 2015,Jan,16; 2014,Jan,11; 2013,Jul,3-5

**63275** Laminectomy for biopsy/excision of intraspinal neoplasm; extradural, cervical

🚗 52.6   ✂ 52.6   **FUD** 090   Ⓒ 80 ▢

**AMA:** 2017,Mar,7; 2017,Jan,8; 2016,Jan,13; 2015,Jan,16; 2014,Jan,11; 2013,Jul,3-5

**63276** extradural, thoracic

🚗 52.3   ✂ 52.3   **FUD** 090   Ⓒ 80 ▢

**AMA:** 2017,Mar,7; 2017,Jan,8; 2016,Jan,13; 2015,Jan,16; 2014,Jan,11; 2013,Jul,3-5

**63277** extradural, lumbar

🚗 45.2   ✂ 45.2   **FUD** 090   Ⓒ 80 ▢

**AMA:** 2017,Mar,7; 2017,Jan,8; 2016,Jan,13; 2015,Jan,16; 2014,Jan,11; 2013,Jul,3-5

**63278** extradural, sacral

🚗 46.2   ✂ 46.2   **FUD** 090   Ⓒ 80 ▢

**AMA:** 2017,Mar,7; 2017,Jan,8; 2016,Jan,13; 2015,Jan,16; 2014,Jan,11; 2013,Jul,3-5

**63280** intradural, extramedullary, cervical

🚗 61.8   ✂ 61.8   **FUD** 090   Ⓒ 80 ▢

**AMA:** 2017,Mar,7; 2017,Jan,8; 2016,Jan,13; 2015,Jan,16; 2014,Jan,11; 2013,Jul,3-5

**63281** intradural, extramedullary, thoracic

🚗 61.3   ✂ 61.3   **FUD** 090   Ⓒ 80 ▢

**AMA:** 2017,Mar,7; 2017,Jan,8; 2016,Jan,13; 2015,Jan,16; 2014,Jan,11; 2013,Jul,3-5

**63282** intradural, extramedullary, lumbar

🚗 57.6   ✂ 57.6   **FUD** 090   Ⓒ 80 ▢

**AMA:** 2017,Mar,7; 2017,Jan,8; 2016,Jan,13; 2015,Jan,16; 2014,Jan,11; 2013,Jul,3-5

**63283** intradural, sacral

🚗 55.3   ✂ 55.3   **FUD** 090   Ⓒ 80 ▢

**AMA:** 2017,Mar,7; 2017,Jan,8; 2016,Jan,13; 2015,Jan,16; 2014,Jan,11; 2013,Jul,3-5

**63285** intradural, intramedullary, cervical

🚗 77.2   ✂ 77.2   **FUD** 090   Ⓒ 80 ▢

**AMA:** 2017,Mar,7; 2017,Jan,8; 2016,Jan,13; 2015,Jan,16; 2014,Jan,11; 2013,Jul,3-5

**63286** intradural, intramedullary, thoracic

🚗 75.2   ✂ 75.2   **FUD** 090   Ⓒ 80 ▢

**AMA:** 2017,Mar,7; 2017,Jan,8; 2016,Jan,13; 2015,Jan,16; 2014,Jan,11; 2013,Jul,3-5

**63287** intradural, intramedullary, thoracolumbar

🚗 81.0   ✂ 81.0   **FUD** 090   Ⓒ 80 ▢

**AMA:** 2017,Mar,7; 2017,Jan,8; 2016,Jan,13; 2015,Jan,16; 2014,Jan,11; 2013,Jul,3-5

**63290** combined extradural-intradural lesion, any level

*EXCLUDES* *Drainage intramedullary cyst or syrinx (63172-63173)*

🚗 81.9   ✂ 81.9   **FUD** 090   Ⓒ 80 ▢

**AMA:** 2017,Mar,7; 2017,Jan,8; 2016,Jan,13; 2015,Jan,16; 2014,Jan,11; 2013,Jul,3-5

+ **63295** Osteoplastic reconstruction of dorsal spinal elements, following primary intraspinal procedure (List separately in addition to code for primary procedure)

*EXCLUDES* *Procedure performed at the same vertebral segment(s) (22590-22614, 22840-22844, 63050-63051)*

Code first (63172-63173, 63185, 63190, 63200-63290)

🚗 9.82   ✂ 9.82   **FUD** ZZZ   Ⓒ 80 ▢

**AMA:** 2014,Jan,11

## 63300-63308 Vertebral Corpectomy for Intraspinal Lesion: Anterior/Anterolateral Approach

INCLUDES  Partial removal:
Cervical: Removal of ≥ 1/2 of vertebral body
Lumbar: Removal of ≥ 1/3 of vertebral body
Thoracic: Removal of ≥ 1/3 of vertebral body

EXCLUDES  *Arthrodesis (22548-22585)*
*Spinal reconstruction (20930-20938)*

**63300**  **Vertebral corpectomy (vertebral body resection), partial or complete, for excision of intraspinal lesion, single segment; extradural, cervical**
53.5  53.5  **FUD** 090   C 80
**AMA:** 2017,Mar,7; 2017,Jan,8; 2016,Jan,13; 2015,Jan,16; 2014,Jan,11; 2013,Jul,3-5

**63301**  **extradural, thoracic by transthoracic approach**
60.6  60.6  **FUD** 090   C 80
**AMA:** 2017,Mar,7; 2017,Jan,8; 2016,Jan,13; 2015,Jan,16; 2014,Jan,11; 2013,Jul,3-5

**63302**  **extradural, thoracic by thoracolumbar approach**
63.1  63.1  **FUD** 090   C 80
**AMA:** 2017,Mar,7; 2017,Jan,8; 2016,Jan,13; 2015,Jan,16; 2014,Jan,11; 2013,Jul,3-5

**63303**  **extradural, lumbar or sacral by transperitoneal or retroperitoneal approach**
66.0  66.0  **FUD** 090   C 80
**AMA:** 2017,Mar,7; 2017,Jan,8; 2016,Jan,13; 2015,Jan,16; 2014,Jan,11; 2013,Jul,3-5

**63304**  **intradural, cervical**
67.9  67.9  **FUD** 090   C 80
**AMA:** 2017,Mar,7; 2017,Jan,8; 2016,Jan,13; 2015,Jan,16; 2014,Jan,11; 2013,Jul,3-5

**63305**  **intradural, thoracic by transthoracic approach**
70.4  70.4  **FUD** 090   C 80
**AMA:** 2017,Mar,7; 2017,Jan,8; 2016,Jan,13; 2015,Jan,16; 2014,Jan,11; 2013,Jul,3-5

**63306**  **intradural, thoracic by thoracolumbar approach**
60.4  60.4  **FUD** 090   C 80
**AMA:** 2017,Mar,7; 2017,Jan,8; 2016,Jan,13; 2015,Jan,16; 2014,Jan,11; 2013,Jul,3-5

**63307**  **intradural, lumbar or sacral by transperitoneal or retroperitoneal approach**
63.3  63.3  **FUD** 090   C 80
**AMA:** 2017,Mar,7; 2017,Jan,8; 2016,Jan,13; 2015,Jan,16; 2014,Jan,11; 2013,Jul,3-5

**+  63308**  **each additional segment (List separately in addition to codes for single segment)**
Code first (63300-63307)
9.47  9.47  **FUD** ZZZ   C 80
**AMA:** 2014,Jan,11

## 63600-63615 Stereotactic Procedures of the Spinal Cord

**63600**  **Creation of lesion of spinal cord by stereotactic method, percutaneous, any modality (including stimulation and/or recording)**
25.7  25.7  **FUD** 090   J A2 80
**AMA:** 2014,Jan,11

**63610**  **Stereotactic stimulation of spinal cord, percutaneous, separate procedure not followed by other surgery**
12.9  12.9  **FUD** 000   J A2 80
**AMA:** 2014,Jan,11

**63615**  **Stereotactic biopsy, aspiration, or excision of lesion, spinal cord**
36.4  36.4  **FUD** 090   J R2
**AMA:** 2014,Jan,11

## 63620-63621 Stereotactic Radiosurgery (SRS): Spine

INCLUDES  Computer assisted planning
Planning dosimetry, targeting, positioning, or blocking by neurosurgeon

EXCLUDES  *Arteriovenous malformations (see Radiation Oncology Section)*
*Intensity modulated beam delivery plan and treatment (77301, 77385-77386)*
*Radiation treatment management by the same provider (77427-77432)*
*Stereotactic body radiation therapy (77373, 77435)*
*Stereotactic computer-assisted procedures (61781-61783)*
*Treatment planning, physics, dosimetry, treatment delivery and management provided by the radiation oncologist (77261-77790 [77295, 77385, 77386, 77387, 77424, 77425])*

**63620**  **Stereotactic radiosurgery (particle beam, gamma ray, or linear accelerator); 1 spinal lesion**
EXCLUDES  *Use of code more than one time per treatment course*
32.8  32.8  **FUD** 090   B 80
**AMA:** 2017,Jan,8; 2016,Jan,13; 2015,Jun,6; 2015,Jan,16; 2014,Jan,11

**+  63621**  **each additional spinal lesion (List separately in addition to code for primary procedure)**
EXCLUDES  *Use of code more than one time per lesion*
*Use of code more than two times per entire treatment course*
Code first (63620)
7.41  7.41  **FUD** ZZZ   B 80
**AMA:** 2017,Jan,8; 2016,Jan,13; 2015,Jun,6; 2015,Jan,16; 2014,Jan,11

## 63650-63688 Spinal Neurostimulation

INCLUDES  Complex and simple neurostimulators
EXCLUDES  *Analysis and programming of neurostimulator pulse generator (95970-95975)*

**63650**  **Percutaneous implantation of neurostimulator electrode array, epidural**
INCLUDES  The following are components of a neurostimulator system:
Collection of contacts of which four or more provide the electrical stimulation in the epidural space
Contacts on a catheter-type lead (array)
Extension
External controller
Implanted neurostimulator
11.8  37.2  **FUD** 010   J J8
**AMA:** 2017,Jan,8; 2016,Jan,11; 2016,Jan,13; 2015,Dec,18; 2015,Jan,16; 2014,Jan,11; 2013,Oct,18; 2012,Jan,15-42

**63655**  **Laminectomy for implantation of neurostimulator electrodes, plate/paddle, epidural**
INCLUDES  The following are components of a neurostimulator system:
Collection of contacts of which four or more provide the electrical stimulation in the epidural space
Contacts on a plate or paddle-shaped surface for systems placed by open exposure
Extension
External controller
Implanted neurostimulator
24.0  24.0  **FUD** 090   J J8 80
**AMA:** 2017,Jan,8; 2016,Jan,13; 2015,Jan,16; 2014,Jan,11; 2012,Jan,15-42

## 63661 Removal of spinal neurostimulator electrode percutaneous array(s), including fluoroscopy, when performed

INCLUDES The following are components of a neurostimulator system:
Collection of contacts of which four or more provide the electrical stimulation in the epidural space
Contacts on a catheter-type lead (array)
Extension
External controller
Implanted neurostimulator

EXCLUDES Use of code when removing or replacing a temporary array placed percutaneously for an external generator

🔧 9.27  ✂ 16.5  **FUD** 010  02 62 80 ▢

**AMA:** 2017,Jan,8; 2016,Jan,13; 2015,Jan,16; 2014,Jan,11

## 63662 Removal of spinal neurostimulator electrode plate/paddle(s) placed via laminotomy or laminectomy, including fluoroscopy, when performed

INCLUDES The following are components of a neurostimulator system:
Collection of contacts of which four or more provide the electrical stimulation in the epidural space
Contacts on a plate or paddle-shaped surface for systems placed by open exposure
Extension
External controller
Implanted neurostimulator

🔧 24.3  ✂ 24.3  **FUD** 090  02 02 80 ▢

**AMA:** 2017,Jan,8; 2016,Jan,13; 2015,Jan,16; 2014,Jan,11

## 63663 Revision including replacement, when performed, of spinal neurostimulator electrode percutaneous array(s), including fluoroscopy, when performed

INCLUDES The following are components of a neurostimulator system:
Collection of contacts of which four or more provide the electrical stimulation in the epidural space
Contacts on a catheter-type lead (array)
Extension
External controller
Implanted neurostimulator

EXCLUDES Removal of spinal neurostimulator electrode percutaneous array(s), plate/paddle(s) at same level (63661-63662)
Use of code when removing or replacing a temporary array placed percutaneously for an external generator

🔧 12.9  ✂ 22.3  **FUD** 010  J J8 80 ▢

**AMA:** 2017,Jan,8; 2016,Jan,13; 2015,Jan,16; 2014,Jan,11

## 63664 Revision including replacement, when performed, of spinal neurostimulator electrode plate/paddle(s) placed via laminotomy or laminectomy, including fluoroscopy, when performed

INCLUDES The following are components of a neurostimulator system:
Collection of contacts of which four or more provide the electrical stimulation in the epidural space
Contacts on a plate or paddle-shaped surface for systems placed by open exposure
Extension
External controller
Implanted neurostimulator

EXCLUDES Removal of spinal neurostimulator electrode percutaneous array(s), plate/paddle(s) (63661-63662)

🔧 25.1  ✂ 25.1  **FUD** 090  J J8 80 ▢

**AMA:** 2017,Jan,8; 2016,Jan,13; 2015,Jan,16; 2014,Jan,11

## 63685 Insertion or replacement of spinal neurostimulator pulse generator or receiver, direct or inductive coupling

EXCLUDES Use of code for insertion/replacement with code for revision/removal (63688)

🔧 10.5  ✂ 10.5  **FUD** 010  J J8 80 ▢

**AMA:** 2017,Jan,8; 2016,Jan,13; 2015,Jan,16; 2014,Jan,11; 2012,Jan,15-42

## 63688 Revision or removal of implanted spinal neurostimulator pulse generator or receiver

EXCLUDES Use of code for revision/removal with code for insertion/replacement (63685)

🔧 10.7  ✂ 10.7  **FUD** 010  02 A2 ▢

**AMA:** 2017,Jan,8; 2016,Jan,13; 2015,Jan,16; 2014,Jan,11

# 63700-63706 Repair Congenital Neural Tube Defects

EXCLUDES Complex skin repair (see appropriate integumentary closure code)

## 63700 Repair of meningocele; less than 5 cm diameter

🔧 33.4  ✂ 33.4  **FUD** 090  63 C 80 ▢

**AMA:** 2014,Jan,11

Most children with severe spina bifida also have hydrocephalus, which is excessive fluid in the skull

Cervical
Thoracic
Lumbar

A fluid-filled herniation that protrudes is spina bifida cystica, or meningocele

If nerves protrude into the defect, it is called rachischisis, or meningomyelocele

Dura mater
Spinal cord
Vertebra

## 63702 larger than 5 cm diameter

🔧 37.1  ✂ 37.1  **FUD** 090  63 C 80 ▢

**AMA:** 2014,Jan,11

## 63704 Repair of myelomeningocele; less than 5 cm diameter

🔧 42.2  ✂ 42.2  **FUD** 090  63 C 80 ▢

**AMA:** 2014,Jan,11

## 63706 larger than 5 cm diameter

🔧 50.7  ✂ 50.7  **FUD** 090  63 C 80 ▢

**AMA:** 2014,Jan,11

# 63707-63710 Repair Dural Cerebrospinal Fluid Leak

## 63707 Repair of dural/cerebrospinal fluid leak, not requiring laminectomy

🔧 26.7  ✂ 26.7  **FUD** 090  C 80 ▢

**AMA:** 2014,Jan,11

## 63709 Repair of dural/cerebrospinal fluid leak or pseudomeningocele, with laminectomy

🔧 32.0  ✂ 32.0  **FUD** 090  C 80 ▢

**AMA:** 2014,Jan,11

## 63710 Dural graft, spinal

EXCLUDES Laminectomy and section of dentate ligament (63180, 63182)

🔧 31.4  ✂ 31.4  **FUD** 090  C 80 ▢

**AMA:** 2014,Jan,11

26/TC PC/TC Only       A2-Z3 ASC Payment       50 Bilateral       ♂ Male Only       ♀ Female Only       🔧 Facility RVU       ✂ Non-Facility RVU       ▢ CCI
**FUD** Follow-up Days   **CMS:** IOM (Pub 100)   A-Y OPPSI       80/80 Surg Assist Allowed / w/Doc   📋 Lab Crosswalk   📋 Radiology Crosswalk   ✗ CLIA

CPT © 2017 American Medical Association. All Rights Reserved.                    © 2017 Optum360, LLC

## 63740-63746 Cerebrospinal Fluid (CSF) Shunt: Lumbar

EXCLUDES  Placement of subarachnoid catheter with reservoir and/or pump:
Not requiring laminectomy (62350, 62360-62362)
With laminectomy (62351, 62360-62362)

**63740** Creation of shunt, lumbar, subarachnoid-peritoneal, -pleural, or other; including laminectomy
🔧 27.2  ⚖ 27.2  **FUD** 090      C 80 📅
AMA: 2014,Jan,11

**63741** percutaneous, not requiring laminectomy
🔧 19.6  ⚖ 19.6  **FUD** 090      J 80 📅
AMA: 2014,Jan,11

**63744** Replacement, irrigation or revision of lumbosubarachnoid shunt
🔧 19.2  ⚖ 19.2  **FUD** 090      J A2 80 📅
AMA: 2014,Jan,11

**63746** Removal of entire lumbosubarachnoid shunt system without replacement
🔧 17.6  ⚖ 17.6  **FUD** 090      Q2 A2 80 📅
AMA: 2014,Jan,11

## 64400-64463 Nerve Blocks

EXCLUDES  Epidural or subarachnoid injection (62320-62327)
Nerve destruction (62280-62282, 64600-64681 [64633, 64634, 64635, 64636])

**64400** Injection, anesthetic agent; trigeminal nerve, any division or branch
🔧 2.05  ⚖ 3.63  **FUD** 000      T P3 50 📅
AMA: 2017,Jan,8; 2016,Jan,13; 2015,Jan,16; 2014,Jan,11; 2013,Jan,13-14; 2012,Jan,15-42

**64402** facial nerve
🔧 2.32  ⚖ 3.81  **FUD** 000      01 N1 50 📅
AMA: 2017,Jan,8; 2016,Jan,13; 2015,Jan,16; 2014,Jan,11; 2013,Jan,13-14; 2012,Jan,15-42

**64405** greater occipital nerve
🔧 1.81  ⚖ 2.86  **FUD** 000      T P3 50 📅
AMA: 2017,Jan,8; 2016,Oct,11; 2016,Jan,13; 2015,Jan,16; 2014,Jan,11; 2013,Jan,13-14; 2012,Jan,15-42

**64408** vagus nerve
🔧 2.49  ⚖ 3.38  **FUD** 000      T P3 80 50 📅
AMA: 2017,Jan,8; 2016,Jan,13; 2015,Jan,16; 2014,Jan,11; 2013,Jan,13-14; 2012,Jan,15-42

**64410** phrenic nerve
🔧 2.17  ⚖ 3.85  **FUD** 000      T A2 80 50 📅
AMA: 2017,Jan,8; 2016,Jan,13; 2015,Jan,16; 2014,Jan,11; 2013,Jan,13-14; 2012,Jan,15-42

**64413** cervical plexus
🔧 2.33  ⚖ 3.62  **FUD** 000      T P3 50 📅
AMA: 2017,Jan,8; 2016,Jan,13; 2015,Jan,16; 2014,Jan,11; 2013,Jan,13-14; 2012,Jan,15-42

**64415** brachial plexus, single
🔧 1.86  ⚖ 3.32  **FUD** 000      T A2 50 📅
AMA: 2017,Jan,8; 2016,Jan,13; 2015,Jan,16; 2014,Jan,11; 2013,Jan,13-14; 2012,Jan,15-42

**64416** brachial plexus, continuous infusion by catheter (including catheter placement)
EXCLUDES  Management of epidural or subarachnoid continuous drug administration (01996)
🔧 2.26  ⚖ 2.26  **FUD** 000      T 62 50 📅
AMA: 2017,Jan,8; 2016,Jan,13; 2015,Jan,16; 2014,Jan,11; 2013,Jan,13-14; 2012,Jan,15-42

**64417** axillary nerve
🔧 2.01  ⚖ 3.63  **FUD** 000      T A2 50 📅
AMA: 2017,Jan,8; 2016,Jan,13; 2015,Jan,16; 2014,Jan,11; 2013,Jan,13-14; 2012,Jan,15-42

**64418** suprascapular nerve
🔧 2.19  ⚖ 4.12  **FUD** 000      T P3 50 📅
AMA: 2017,Jan,8; 2016,Jan,13; 2015,Jan,16; 2014,Jan,11; 2013,Jan,13-14; 2012,Jan,15-42

**64420** intercostal nerve, single
🔧 1.94  ⚖ 3.15  **FUD** 000      T A2 📅
AMA: 2017,Jan,8; 2016,Jan,9; 2016,Jan,13; 2015,Jun,3; 2015,Jan,16; 2014,Jan,11; 2013,Jan,13-14; 2012,Jan,15-42

**64421** intercostal nerves, multiple, regional block
🔧 2.63  ⚖ 4.25  **FUD** 000      T A2 50 📅
AMA: 2017,Jan,8; 2016,Jan,9; 2016,Jan,13; 2015,Jun,3; 2015,Jan,16; 2014,Jan,11; 2013,Jan,13-14; 2012,Jan,15-42

**64425** ilioinguinal, iliohypogastric nerves
🔧 2.68  ⚖ 3.74  **FUD** 000      T P3 50 📅
AMA: 2017,Jan,8; 2016,Jan,13; 2015,Jun,3; 2015,Jan,16; 2014,Jan,11; 2013,Jan,13-14; 2012,Jan,15-42

**64430** pudendal nerve
🔧 2.33  ⚖ 3.90  **FUD** 000      T A2 50 📅
AMA: 2017,Jan,8; 2016,Jan,13; 2015,Jan,16; 2014,Jan,11; 2013,Jan,13-14; 2012,Jan,15-42

**64435** paracervical (uterine) nerve                              ♀
🔧 2.38  ⚖ 3.84  **FUD** 000      T P3 50 📅
AMA: 2017,Jan,8; 2016,Jan,13; 2015,Jan,16; 2014,Jan,11; 2013,Jan,13-14; 2012,Feb,11; 2012,Jan,15-42

**64445** sciatic nerve, single
EXCLUDES  Use of code more than one time per encounter even when multiple areas are injected around sciatic nerve
🔧 2.07  ⚖ 3.84  **FUD** 000      T P3 50 📅
AMA: 2017,Jan,8; 2016,Jan,13; 2015,Jan,16; 2014,Jan,11; 2013,Jan,13-14; 2012,Apr,19

**64446** sciatic nerve, continuous infusion by catheter (including catheter placement)
EXCLUDES  Management of epidural or subarachnoid continuous drug administration (01996)
🔧 2.26  ⚖ 2.26  **FUD** 000      T 62 50 📅
AMA: 2017,Jan,8; 2016,Jan,13; 2015,Jan,16; 2014,Jan,11; 2013,Jan,13-14

**64447** femoral nerve, single
EXCLUDES  Management of epidural or subarachnoid continuous drug administration (01996)
🔧 1.90  ⚖ 3.38  **FUD** 000      T P3 50 📅
AMA: 2017,Jan,8; 2016,Jan,13; 2015,Sep,12; 2015,Jan,16; 2014,Dec,16; 2014,Dec,16; 2014,Nov,14; 2014,Jan,11; 2013,Jan,13-14

**64448** femoral nerve, continuous infusion by catheter (including catheter placement)
EXCLUDES  Management of epidural or subarachnoid continuous drug administration (01996)
🔧 2.04  ⚖ 2.04  **FUD** 000      T 62 50 📅
AMA: 2017,Jan,8; 2016,Jan,13; 2015,Sep,12; 2015,Jan,16; 2014,Dec,16; 2014,Dec,16; 2014,Nov,14; 2014,Jan,11; 2013,Jan,13-14

**64449** lumbar plexus, posterior approach, continuous infusion by catheter (including catheter placement)
EXCLUDES  Management of epidural or subarachnoid continuous drug administration (01996)
🔧 2.40  ⚖ 2.40  **FUD** 000      T 62 50 📅
AMA: 2017,Jan,8; 2016,Jan,13; 2015,Jan,16; 2014,Jan,11; 2013,Jan,13-14

**64450** other peripheral nerve or branch
EXCLUDES  Morton's neuroma (64455, 64632)
Use of code more than one time per encounter when multiple injections are required to block nerve and branches
🔧 1.30  ⚖ 2.27  **FUD** 000      T P3 50 📅
AMA: 2017,Jan,8; 2016,Oct,11; 2016,Jan,13; 2015,Nov,10; 2015,Sep,12; 2015,Jun,3; 2015,Jan,16; 2014,Jan,11; 2013,Jan,13-14; 2012,Jan,15-42

● New Code   ▲ Revised Code   ○ Reinstated   ● New Web Release   ▲ Revised Web Release   Unlisted   Not Covered   # Resequenced
⊘ AMA Mod 51 Exempt   ⑤ Optum Mod 51 Exempt   ⑥③ Mod 63 Exempt   ✗ Non-FDA Drug   ★ Telemedicine   Ⓜ Maternity   🅰 Age Edit   + Add-on   AMA: CPT Asst
© 2017 Optum360, LLC                    CPT © 2017 American Medical Association. All Rights Reserved.                    287

**64455** Injection(s), anesthetic agent and/or steroid, plantar common digital nerve(s) (eg, Morton's neuroma)

> EXCLUDES  *Destruction by neurolytic agent; plantar common digital nerve (64632)*
>
> 🔧 1.00   ⚖ 1.36   **FUD** 000   [T] [P3] [80] [50]
>
> **AMA:** 2017,Jan,8; 2016,Jan,13; 2015,Jan,16; 2014,Jan,11; 2013,Nov,14; 2013,Jan,13-14; 2012,Sep,14-15; 2012,Sep,14-15

*64461* Resequenced code. See code following 64484.

*64462* Resequenced code. See code following 64484.

*64463* Resequenced code. See code following 64484.

## 64479-64484 Transforaminal Injection

> INCLUDES  Imaging guidance (fluoroscopy or CT) and contrast injection
>
> EXCLUDES  *Epidural or subarachnoid injection (62320-62327)*
> *Nerve destruction (62280-62282, 64600-64681 [64633, 64634, 64635, 64636])*

**64479** Injection(s), anesthetic agent and/or steroid, transforaminal epidural, with imaging guidance (fluoroscopy or CT); cervical or thoracic, single level

> INCLUDES  Transforaminal epidural injection at T12-L1 level
>
> EXCLUDES  *Transforaminal epidural injection using ultrasonic guidance (0228T)*
>
> 🔧 3.79   ⚖ 6.65   **FUD** 000   [T] [A2] [50]
>
> **AMA:** 2017,Jan,8; 2016,Jan,9; 2016,Jan,13; 2015,Jan,16; 2014,Jan,11; 2012,Jul,3-6; 2012,Jan,15-42

**Thoracic vertebra (superior view)**

Labels: Spinous process, Transverse costal facet, Lamina, Superior articular facets, Pedicle, Superior costal facet, Vertebral body, Spinous process, Superior articular facets, Vertebral body

**Superior view of C7**

+ **64480** cervical or thoracic, each additional level (List separately in addition to code for primary procedure)

> EXCLUDES  *Transforaminal epidural injection at T12-L1 level*
> *Transforaminal epidural injection using ultrasonic guidance (0229T)*
> Code first (64479)
>
> 🔧 1.82   ⚖ 3.19   **FUD** ZZZ   [N] [N1] [50]
>
> **AMA:** 2017,Jan,8; 2016,Jan,9; 2016,Jan,13; 2015,Jan,16; 2014,Jan,11; 2012,Jul,3-6; 2012,Jan,15-42

**64483** lumbar or sacral, single level

> EXCLUDES  *Transforaminal epidural injection using ultrasonic guidance (0230T)*
>
> 🔧 3.21   ⚖ 6.17   **FUD** 000   [T] [A2] [50]
>
> **AMA:** 2017,Jan,8; 2016,Oct,11; 2016,Jan,9; 2016,Jan,13; 2015,Jan,16; 2014,Jan,11; 2012,May,14-15; 2012,Jul,3-6

+ **64484** lumbar or sacral, each additional level (List separately in addition to code for primary procedure)

> EXCLUDES  *Transforaminal epidural injection using ultrasonic guidance (0231T)*
> Code first (64483)
>
> 🔧 1.49   ⚖ 2.48   **FUD** ZZZ   [N] [N1] [50]
>
> **AMA:** 2017,Jan,8; 2016,Jan,9; 2016,Jan,13; 2015,Jan,16; 2014,Jan,11; 2012,Jul,3-6; 2012,Jan,15-42

## [64461, 64462, 64463] Paravertebral Blocks

> INCLUDES  Radiological guidance (76942, 77002-77003)
>
> EXCLUDES  *Injection of:*
> *Anesthetic agent (64420-64421, 64479-64480)*
> *Diagnostic or therapeutic substance (62320, 62324, 64490-64492)*

\# **64461** Paravertebral block (PVB) (paraspinous block), thoracic; single injection site (includes imaging guidance, when performed)

> 🔧 2.50   ⚖ 4.21   **FUD** 000   [T] [P3] [50]
>
> **AMA:** 2017,Jan,8; 2016,Jan,9

+ \# **64462** second and any additional injection site(s) (includes imaging guidance, when performed) (List separately in addition to code for primary procedure)

> EXCLUDES  *Procedure performed more than one time per day*
> Code first (64461)
>
> 🔧 1.57   ⚖ 2.39   **FUD** ZZZ   [N] [N1] [50]
>
> **AMA:** 2017,Jan,8; 2016,Jan,9

\# **64463** continuous infusion by catheter (includes imaging guidance, when performed)

> 🔧 2.57   ⚖ 4.72   **FUD** 000   [T] [P3] [50]
>
> **AMA:** 2017,Jan,8; 2016,Jan,9

## 64486-64489 Transversus Abdominis Plane (TAP) Block

**64486** Transversus abdominis plane (TAP) block (abdominal plane block, rectus sheath block) unilateral; by injection(s) (includes imaging guidance, when performed)

> 🔧 1.79   ⚖ 3.45   **FUD** 000   [N] [N1] [50]
>
> **AMA:** 2017,Jan,8; 2016,Jan,13; 2015,Jun,3

**64487** by continuous infusion(s) (includes imaging guidance, when performed)

> 🔧 1.94   ⚖ 3.82   **FUD** 000   [N] [N1] [50]
>
> **AMA:** 2017,Jan,8; 2016,Jan,13; 2015,Jun,3

**64488** Transversus abdominis plane (TAP) block (abdominal plane block, rectus sheath block) bilateral; by injections (includes imaging guidance, when performed)

> 🔧 2.12   ⚖ 3.96   **FUD** 000   [N] [N1]
>
> **AMA:** 2017,Jan,8; 2016,Jan,13; 2015,Jun,3

**64489** by continuous infusions (includes imaging guidance, when performed)

> 🔧 2.26   ⚖ 5.06   **FUD** 000   [N] [N1]
>
> **AMA:** 2017,Jan,8; 2016,Jan,13; 2015,Jun,3

## 64490-64495 Paraspinal Nerve Injections

> INCLUDES  Image guidance (CT or fluoroscopy) and any contrast injection
>
> EXCLUDES  *Injection without imaging (20552-20553)*
> *Ultrasonic guidance (0213T-0218T)*

**64490** Injection(s), diagnostic or therapeutic agent, paravertebral facet (zygapophyseal) joint (or nerves innervating that joint) with image guidance (fluoroscopy or CT), cervical or thoracic; single level

> INCLUDES  Injection of T12-L1 joint and nerves that innervate that joint
>
> 🔧 3.05   ⚖ 5.35   **FUD** 000   [T] [62] [80] [50]
>
> **AMA:** 2017,Jan,8; 2016,Jan,9; 2016,Jan,13; 2015,Jan,16; 2014,Jan,11; 2012,Oct,14; 2012,Jun,10-11; 2012,Jan,15-42

+ **64491** second level (List separately in addition to code for primary procedure)

> Code first (64490)
>
> 🔧 1.73   ⚖ 2.65   **FUD** ZZZ   [N] [N1] [80] [50]
>
> **AMA:** 2017,Jan,8; 2016,Jan,9; 2016,Jan,13; 2015,Jan,16; 2014,Jan,11; 2012,Oct,14; 2012,Jun,10-11; 2012,Jan,15-42

+ **64492** third and any additional level(s) (List separately in addition to code for primary procedure)

> EXCLUDES  *Procedure performed more than one time per day*
> Code also when appropriate (64491)
> Code first (64490)
>
> 🔧 1.75   ⚖ 2.66   **FUD** ZZZ   [N] [N1] [80] [50]
>
> **AMA:** 2017,Jan,8; 2016,Jan,9; 2016,Jan,13; 2015,Jan,16; 2014,Jan,11; 2012,Oct,14; 2012,Jun,10-11; 2012,Jan,15-42

| [26]/[TC] PC/TC Only | [A2]-[Z3] ASC Payment | [50] Bilateral | ♂ Male Only | ♀ Female Only | 🔧 Facility RVU | ⚖ Non-Facility RVU | CCI |
| **FUD** Follow-up Days | **CMS:** IOM (Pub 100) | [A]-[Y] OPPSI | [80]/[80] Surg Assist Allowed / w/Doc | | [Lab] Lab Crosswalk | [Rad] Radiology Crosswalk | [X] CLIA |

288                        CPT © 2017 American Medical Association. All Rights Reserved.                        © 2017 Optum360, LLC

**64493**     Injection(s), diagnostic or therapeutic agent, paravertebral facet (zygapophyseal) joint (or nerves innervating that joint) with image guidance (fluoroscopy or CT), lumbar or sacral; single level
2.60    4.85    **FUD** 000    T G2 80 50
**AMA:** 2017,Jan,8; 2016,Jan,13; 2015,Jan,16; 2014,Jan,11; 2012,Oct,14; 2012,Jun,10-11; 2012,Jan,15-42

+    **64494**     second level (List separately in addition to code for primary procedure)
Code first (64493)
1.49    2.44    **FUD** ZZZ    N N1 80 50
**AMA:** 2017,Jan,8; 2016,Jan,13; 2015,Jan,16; 2014,Jan,11; 2012,Oct,14; 2012,Jun,10-11

+    **64495**     third and any additional level(s) (List separately in addition to code for primary procedure)
    *EXCLUDES*    *Procedure performed more than one time per day*
Code also when appropriate (64494)
Code first (64493)
1.51    2.45    **FUD** ZZZ    N N1 80 50
**AMA:** 2017,Jan,8; 2016,Jan,13; 2015,Jan,16; 2014,Jan,11; 2012,Oct,14; 2012,Jun,10-11

## 64505-64530 Sympathetic Nerve Blocks

**64505**     Injection, anesthetic agent; sphenopalatine ganglion
2.52    3.01    **FUD** 000    T P3 50
**AMA:** 2017,Jan,8; 2016,Jan,13; 2015,Jan,16; 2014,Jul,8; 2014,Jan,11; 2013,Jan,13-14; 2012,Jan,15-42

**64508**     carotid sinus (separate procedure)
2.06    1.71    **FUD** 000    T P3 80 50
**AMA:** 2017,Jan,8; 2016,Jan,13; 2015,Jan,16; 2014,Jan,11; 2013,Jan,13-14

**64510**     stellate ganglion (cervical sympathetic)
2.10    3.59    **FUD** 000    T A2 50
**AMA:** 2017,Jan,8; 2016,Jan,13; 2015,Jan,16; 2014,Jan,11; 2013,Jan,13-14

**64517**     superior hypogastric plexus
3.56    5.27    **FUD** 000    T A2
**AMA:** 2017,Jan,8; 2016,Jan,13; 2015,Jan,16; 2014,Jan,11; 2013,Jan,13-14; 2012,Jan,15-42

**64520**     lumbar or thoracic (paravertebral sympathetic)
2.32    5.25    **FUD** 000    T A2 50
**AMA:** 2017,Jan,8; 2016,Jan,13; 2015,Jan,16; 2014,Jan,11; 2013,Jan,13-14; 2012,Jan,15-42

**64530**     celiac plexus, with or without radiologic monitoring
    *EXCLUDES*    *Transmural anesthetic injection with transendoscopic ultrasound-guidance (43253)*
2.62    5.35    **FUD** 000    T A2
**AMA:** 2017,Jan,8; 2016,Jan,13; 2015,Jan,16; 2014,Jan,11; 2013,Jan,13-14; 2012,Jan,15-42

## 64550 Transcutaneous Electrical Nerve Stimulation

**CMS:** 100-03,10.2 Transcutaneous Electrical Nerve Stimulation (TENS) for Acute Postoperative Pain
    *INCLUDES*    Application to any body area
    *EXCLUDES*    *Analysis and programming neurostimulator pulse generator (95970-95975)*
    *Implantation of electrode array(s), either trial or permanent, with pulse generator for peripheral subcutaneous field stimulation (64999)*

▲    **64550**     Application of surface (transcutaneous) neurostimulator (eg, TENS unit)
0.25    0.45    **FUD** 000    A
**AMA:** 2017,Jan,8; 2016,Jan,13; 2015,Jan,16; 2014,Jan,11; 2012,Jan,15-42

## 64553-64570 Electrical Nerve Stimulation: Insertion/Replacement/Removal/Revision

    *INCLUDES*    Simple and complex neurostimulators
    *EXCLUDES*    *Analysis and programming of neurostimulator pulse generator (95970-95975)*

**64553**     Percutaneous implantation of neurostimulator electrode array; cranial nerve
    *INCLUDES*    Temporary and permanent percutaneous array placement
    *EXCLUDES*    *Open procedure (61885-61886)*
    *Percutaneous electrical stimulation of peripheral nerve with needle or needle electrodes (64999)*
4.35    5.77    **FUD** 010    J J8 80
**AMA:** 2017,Jan,8; 2016,Jan,13; 2015,Jan,16; 2014,Jan,11

**64555**     peripheral nerve (excludes sacral nerve)
    *INCLUDES*    Temporary and permanent percutaneous array placement
    *EXCLUDES*    *Percutaneous electrical stimulation of a cranial nerve with needle or needle electrodes (64999)*
    *Posterior tibial neurostimulation (64566)*
4.38    5.99    **FUD** 010    J J8
**AMA:** 2017,Jan,8; 2016,Feb,13; 2016,Jan,13; 2015,Jan,16; 2015,Jan,13; 2014,Jan,11; 2012,Jan,15-42

**64561**     sacral nerve (transforaminal placement) including image guidance, if performed
    *INCLUDES*    Temporary and permanent percutaneous array placement
    *EXCLUDES*    *Percutaneous electrical stimulation or neuromodulation with needle or needle electrodes (64999)*
8.74    23.4    **FUD** 010    J J8 50
**AMA:** 2017,Jan,8; 2016,Jan,13; 2015,Jan,16; 2014,Sep,5; 2014,Jan,11; 2012,Dec,12

**64565**     ~~neuromuscular~~

**64566**     Posterior tibial neurostimulation, percutaneous needle electrode, single treatment, includes programming
    *EXCLUDES*    *Electronic analysis of implanted neurostimulator pulse generator system (95970-95972)*
    *Percutaneous implantation of neurostimulator electrode array; peripheral nerve (64555)*
0.87    3.61    **FUD** 000    T P3 80
**AMA:** 2017,Jan,8; 2016,Jan,13; 2015,Jan,16; 2014,Jan,11

**64568**     Incision for implantation of cranial nerve (eg, vagus nerve) neurostimulator electrode array and pulse generator
    *EXCLUDES*    *Insertion chest wall respiratory sensor electrode or array with pulse generator connection (0466T)*
    *Insertion, replacement of cranial neurostimulator pulse generator or receiver (61885-61886)*
    *Removal of neurostimulator electrode array and pulse generator (64570)*
18.8    18.8    **FUD** 090    J J8 80 50
**AMA:** 2017,Jan,8; 2016,Nov,6; 2016,Jan,13; 2015,Jan,16; 2014,Jan,11; 2012,Jan,15-42

**64569**     Revision or replacement of cranial nerve (eg, vagus nerve) neurostimulator electrode array, including connection to existing pulse generator
    *EXCLUDES*    *Removal of neurostimulator electrode array and pulse generator (64570)*
    *Replacement of pulse generator (61885)*
    *Revision or replacement chest wall respiratory sensor electrode with pulse generator connection (0467T)*
    *Revision, removal pulse generator (61888)*
22.7    22.7    **FUD** 090    J J8 80 50
**AMA:** 2017,Jan,8; 2016,Nov,6; 2016,Jan,13; 2015,Jan,16; 2014,Jan,11

● New Code    ▲ Revised Code    ○ Reinstated    ● New Web Release    ▲ Revised Web Release    Unlisted    Not Covered    # Resequenced
⊘ AMA Mod 51 Exempt    ⑨ Optum Mod 51 Exempt    ⑥③ Mod 63 Exempt    ✗ Non-FDA Drug    ★ Telemedicine    M Maternity    A Age Edit    + Add-on    AMA: CPT Asst
© 2017 Optum360, LLC                                    CPT © 2017 American Medical Association. All Rights Reserved.                                    **289**

Nervous System

64570 — 64612

**64570** Removal of cranial nerve (eg, vagus nerve) neurostimulator electrode array and pulse generator

> **EXCLUDES** *Laparoscopic revision, replacement, removal, or implantation of vagus nerve blocking neurostimulator pulse generator and/or electrode array at the esophagogastric junction (0312T-0317T)*
> *Removal of chest wall respiratory sensor electrode or array (0468T)*
> *Revision, removal pulse generator (61888)*

🚚 19.0   ⚕ 19.0   **FUD** 090   [Q2] [G2] [80] [50] [▣]

**AMA:** 2017,Jan,8; 2016,Nov,6; 2016,Jan,13; 2015,Jan,16; 2014,Jan,11

## 64575-64595 Implantation/Revision/Removal Neurostimulators: Incisional

**INCLUDES** Simple and complex neurostimulators
**EXCLUDES** *Analysis and programming neurostimulator pulse generator (95970-95975)*

**64575** Incision for implantation of neurostimulator electrode array; peripheral nerve (excludes sacral nerve)

🚚 9.22   ⚕ 9.22   **FUD** 090   [J] [J8] [▣]

**AMA:** 2014,Jan,11

**64580** neuromuscular

🚚 8.69   ⚕ 8.69   **FUD** 090   [J] [J8] [80] [▣]

**AMA:** 2014,Jan,11

**64581** sacral nerve (transforaminal placement)

🚚 19.1   ⚕ 19.1   **FUD** 090   [J] [J8] [▣]

**AMA:** 2017,Jan,8; 2016,Jan,13; 2015,Jan,16; 2014,Sep,5; 2014,Jan,11; 2012,Dec,12

**64585** Revision or removal of peripheral neurostimulator electrode array

🚚 4.12   ⚕ 6.98   **FUD** 010   [Q2] [A2] [▣]

**AMA:** 2014,Jan,11

**64590** Insertion or replacement of peripheral or gastric neurostimulator pulse generator or receiver, direct or inductive coupling

> **EXCLUDES** *Revision, removal of neurostimulator pulse generator (64595)*

🚚 4.63   ⚕ 7.56   **FUD** 010   [J] [J8] [▣]

**AMA:** 2017,Jan,8; 2016,Jan,13; 2015,Jan,16; 2015,Jan,13; 2014,Jan,11; 2012,Dec,12; 2012,Jan,15-42

**64595** Revision or removal of peripheral or gastric neurostimulator pulse generator or receiver

> **EXCLUDES** *Insertion, replacement of neurostimulator pulse generator (64590)*

🚚 3.63   ⚕ 7.00   **FUD** 010   [Q2] [A2] [▣]

**AMA:** 2017,Jan,8; 2016,Jan,13; 2015,Jan,16; 2014,Jan,11; 2012,Jan,15-42

## 64600-64610 Chemical Denervation Trigeminal Nerve

**INCLUDES** Injection of therapeutic medication
**EXCLUDES** *The following chemodenervation procedures:*
> *Anal sphincter (46505)*
> *Bladder (52287)*
> *Muscle electrical stimulation or EMG with needle guidance (95873, 95874)*
> *Strabismus that involves the extraocular muscles (67345)*
> *Treatments that do not destroy the target nerve (64999)*
Code also chemodenervation agent

**64600** Destruction by neurolytic agent, trigeminal nerve; supraorbital, infraorbital, mental, or inferior alveolar branch

🚚 6.34   ⚕ 11.1   **FUD** 010   [T] [A2] [▣]

**AMA:** 2017,Jan,8; 2016,Jan,13; 2015,Jan,16; 2014,Jan,11; 2012,Sep,14-15; 2012,Sep,14-15

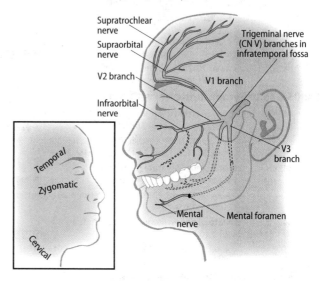

**64605** second and third division branches at foramen ovale

🚚 9.96   ⚕ 17.3   **FUD** 010   [J] [A2] [80] [50] [▣]

**AMA:** 2017,Jan,8; 2016,Jan,13; 2015,Jan,16; 2014,Jan,11; 2012,Sep,14-15; 2012,Sep,14-15

**64610** second and third division branches at foramen ovale under radiologic monitoring

🚚 14.2   ⚕ 21.3   **FUD** 010   [J] [A2] [50] [▣]

**AMA:** 2017,Apr,9; 2017,Jan,8; 2016,Jan,13; 2015,Jan,16; 2014,Jan,11; 2012,Sep,14-15; 2012,Sep,14-15

## 64611-64617 Chemical Denervation Procedures Head and Neck

**INCLUDES** Injection of therapeutic medication
**EXCLUDES** *Electromyography or muscle electric stimulation guidance (95873-95874)*
> *Nerve destruction of:*
> *Anal sphincter (46505)*
> *Bladder (52287)*
> *Extraocular muscles to treat strabismus (67345)*
> *Treatments that do not destroy the target nerve (64999)*

**64611** Chemodenervation of parotid and submandibular salivary glands, bilateral

> Code also modifier 52 for injection of fewer than four salivary glands

🚚 2.97   ⚕ 3.37   **FUD** 010   [T] [P3] [80] [▣]

**AMA:** 2017,Jan,8; 2016,Jan,13; 2015,Jan,16; 2014,Jan,11; 2012,Sep,14-15; 2012,Sep,14-15

**64612** Chemodenervation of muscle(s); muscle(s) innervated by facial nerve, unilateral (eg, for blepharospasm, hemifacial spasm)

🚚 3.35   ⚕ 3.73   **FUD** 010   [T] [P3] [50] [▣]

**AMA:** 2017,Jan,8; 2016,Jan,13; 2015,Jan,16; 2014,May,5; 2014,Jan,6; 2014,Jan,11; 2013,Dec,10; 2013,Apr,5-6; 2012,Sep,14-15; 2012,Sep,14-15; 2012,Jan,15-42

**64615**     **muscle(s) innervated by facial, trigeminal, cervical spinal and accessory nerves, bilateral (eg, for chronic migraine)**

> *EXCLUDES*   *Chemodenervation (64612, 64616-64617, 64642-64647)*
> *Procedure performed more than one time per session*
> Code also any guidance by muscle electrical stimulation or needle electromyography but report only once (95873-95874)
> 🚑 3.62    ⚕ 4.16    **FUD** 010                    T P3 🖪

> **AMA:** 2017,Jan,8; 2016,Jan,13; 2015,Jan,16; 2014,Jan,11; 2014,Jan,6; 2013,Apr,5-6

**64616**     **neck muscle(s), excluding muscles of the larynx, unilateral (eg, for cervical dystonia, spasmodic torticollis)**

> Code also guidance by muscle electrical stimulation or needle electromyography, but report only once (95873-95874)
> 🚑 3.18    ⚕ 3.65    **FUD** 010                    T P3 50 🖪

> **AMA:** 2017,Jan,8; 2016,Jan,13; 2015,Jan,16; 2014,May,5; 2014,Jan,11; 2014,Jan,6

**64617**     **larynx, unilateral, percutaneous (eg, for spasmodic dysphonia), includes guidance by needle electromyography, when performed**

> *EXCLUDES*   *Chemodenervation of larynx via direct laryngoscopy (31570-31571)*
> *Diagnostic needle electromyography of larynx (95865)*
> *Electrical stimulation guidance for chemodenervation (95873-95874)*
> 🚑 3.41    ⚕ 5.12    **FUD** 010                    T P3 50 🖪

> **AMA:** 2017,Jan,8; 2016,Jan,13; 2015,Jan,16; 2014,Jan,11; 2014,Jan,6

## 64620-64640 [64633, 64634, 64635, 64636] Chemical Denervation Intercostal, Facet Joint, Plantar, and Pudendal Nerve(s)

> *INCLUDES*   Injection of therapeutic medication

**64620**     **Destruction by neurolytic agent, intercostal nerve**

> 🚑 4.91    ⚕ 5.80    **FUD** 010                    T A2 🖪

> **AMA:** 2017,Jan,8; 2016,Jan,13; 2015,Jan,16; 2014,Jan,6; 2014,Jan,11; 2012,Sep,14-15; 2012,Sep,14-15

\#   **64633**     **Destruction by neurolytic agent, paravertebral facet joint nerve(s), with imaging guidance (fluoroscopy or CT); cervical or thoracic, single facet joint**

> *INCLUDES*   Paravertebral facet destruction of T12-L1 joint or nerve(s) that innervate that joint
> Radiological guidance (77003, 77012)
> *EXCLUDES*   *Denervation performed using chemical, low grade thermal, or pulsed radiofrequency methods (64999)*
> *Destruction of paravertebral facet joint nerve(s) without imaging guidance (64999)*
> 🚑 6.47    ⚕ 11.8    **FUD** 010                    J 62 50 🖪

> **AMA:** 2017,Jan,8; 2016,Jan,13; 2015,Feb,9; 2015,Jan,16; 2014,Jan,11; 2013,Apr,10-11; 2012,Sep,14-15; 2012,Sep,14-15; 2012,Jul,3-6; 2012,Jun,10-11

\+ \#   **64634**     **cervical or thoracic, each additional facet joint (List separately in addition to code for primary procedure)**

> *INCLUDES*   Radiological guidance (77003, 77012)
> *EXCLUDES*   *Denervation performed using chemical, low grade thermal, or pulsed radiofrequency methods (64999)*
> *Destruction of paravertebral facet joint nerve(s) without imaging guidance (64999)*
> Code first ([64633])
> 🚑 1.96    ⚕ 5.32    **FUD** ZZZ                    N N1 50 🖪

> **AMA:** 2017,Jan,8; 2016,Jan,13; 2015,Feb,9; 2015,Jan,16; 2014,Jan,11; 2013,Apr,10-11; 2012,Sep,14-15; 2012,Sep,14-15; 2012,Jul,3-6; 2012,Jun,10-11

\#   **64635**     **lumbar or sacral, single facet joint**

> *INCLUDES*   Radiological guidance (77003, 77012)
> *EXCLUDES*   *Denervation performed using chemical, low grade thermal, or pulsed radiofrequency methods (64999)*
> *Destruction of individual nerves, sacroiliac joint, by neurolytic agent (64640)*
> *Destruction of paravertebral facet joint nerve(s) without imaging guidance (64999)*
> 🚑 6.38    ⚕ 11.7    **FUD** 010                    J 62 50 🖪

> **AMA:** 2017,Jan,8; 2016,Jan,13; 2015,Feb,9; 2015,Jan,16; 2014,Jan,11; 2013,Apr,10-11; 2012,Sep,14-15; 2012,Sep,14-15; 2012,Jul,3-6; 2012,Jun,10-11

\+ \#   **64636**     **lumbar or sacral, each additional facet joint (List separately in addition to code for primary procedure)**

> *INCLUDES*   Radiological guidance (77003, 77012)
> *EXCLUDES*   *Denervation performed using chemical, low grade thermal, or pulsed radiofrequency methods (64999)*
> *Destruction of individual nerves, sacroiliac joint, by neurolytic agent (64640)*
> *Destruction of paravertebral facet joint nerve(s) without imaging guidance (64999)*
> Code first ([64635])
> 🚑 1.71    ⚕ 4.84    **FUD** ZZZ                    N N1 50 🖪

> **AMA:** 2017,Jan,8; 2016,Jan,13; 2015,Feb,9; 2015,Jan,16; 2014,Jan,11; 2013,Apr,10-11; 2012,Sep,14-15; 2012,Sep,14-15; 2012,Jul,3-6; 2012,Jun,10-11

**64630**     **Destruction by neurolytic agent; pudendal nerve**

> 🚑 5.50    ⚕ 6.58    **FUD** 010                    T A2 80 🖪

> **AMA:** 2017,Jan,8; 2016,Jan,13; 2015,Jan,16; 2014,Jan,11; 2012,Sep,14-15; 2012,Sep,14-15

**64632**     **plantar common digital nerve**

> *EXCLUDES*   *Injection(s), anesthetic agent and/or steroid (64455)*
> 🚑 1.97    ⚕ 2.43    **FUD** 010                    T P3 80 50 🖪

> **AMA:** 2017,Jan,8; 2016,Jan,13; 2015,Jul,10; 2015,Jan,16; 2014,Jan,11; 2013,Nov,14; 2013,Jan,13-14; 2012,Sep,14-15; 2012,Sep,14-15

*64633*     Resequenced code. See code following 64620.

*64634*     Resequenced code. See code following 64620.

*64635*     Resequenced code. See code following 64620.

*64636*     Resequenced code. See code before 64630.

**64640**     **other peripheral nerve or branch**

> *INCLUDES*   Neurolytic destruction of nerves of sacroiliac joint
> 🚑 2.66    ⚕ 3.75    **FUD** 010                    T P3 50 🖪

> **AMA:** 2017,Jan,8; 2016,Jan,13; 2015,Jan,16; 2014,Jan,11; 2012,Sep,14-15; 2012,Sep,14-15; 2012,Jun,15-16; 2012,Jan,15-42

## 64642-64645 Chemical Denervation Extremity Muscles

> *INCLUDES*   Trunk muscles include erector spine, obliques, paraspinal, and rectus abdominus. The rest of the muscles are considered neck, head or extremity muscles
> *EXCLUDES*   *Chemodenervation with needle-guided electromyography or with guidance provided by muscle electrical stimulation (95873-95874)*
> *Procedure performed more than once per extremity*
> Code also other extremities when appropriate, up to a total of 4 units per patient (if all extremities are injected) (64642-64645)

**64642**     **Chemodenervation of one extremity; 1-4 muscle(s)**

> *EXCLUDES*   *Use of more than one base code per session (64642)*
> 🚑 3.15    ⚕ 4.06    **FUD** 000                    T P3 🖪

> **AMA:** 2017,Jan,8; 2016,Jan,13; 2015,Jan,16; 2014,Oct,14; 2014,Jan,11; 2014,Jan,6

\+   **64643**     **each additional extremity, 1-4 muscle(s) (List separately in addition to code for primary procedure)**

> Code first (64642, 64644)
> 🚑 2.09    ⚕ 2.65    **FUD** ZZZ                    N N1 🖪

> **AMA:** 2017,Jan,8; 2016,Jan,13; 2015,Jan,16; 2014,Oct,14; 2014,Jan,11; 2014,Jan,6

---

● New Code     ▲ Revised Code     ○ Reinstated     ● New Web Release     ▲ Revised Web Release     Unlisted     Not Covered     # Resequenced
⊘ AMA Mod 51 Exempt     ⑤ Optum Mod 51 Exempt     ⑥ Mod 63 Exempt     ⊁ Non-FDA Drug     ★ Telemedicine     Ⓜ Maternity     Ⓐ Age Edit     + Add-on     AMA: CPT Asst

© 2017 Optum360, LLC                         CPT © 2017 American Medical Association. All Rights Reserved.

**Nervous System**

**64644 — 64742**

**64644**    Chemodenervation of one extremity; 5 or more muscles
🚑 3.44   ⚕ 4.67   **FUD** 000                            T P3 ▯
**AMA:** 2017,Jan,8; 2016,Jan,13; 2015,Jan,16; 2014,Oct,14; 2014,Jan,11; 2014,Jan,6

**+    64645**    each additional extremity, 5 or more muscles (List separately in addition to code for primary procedure)
Code first (64644)
🚑 2.42   ⚕ 3.28   **FUD** ZZZ                            N N1 ▯
**AMA:** 2017,Jan,8; 2016,Jan,13; 2015,Jan,16; 2014,Oct,14; 2014,Jan,11; 2014,Jan,6

## 64646-64647 Chemical Denervation Trunk Muscles
EXCLUDES    *Procedure performed more than once per session*

**64646**    Chemodenervation of trunk muscle(s); 1-5 muscle(s)
🚑 3.37   ⚕ 4.26   **FUD** 000                            T P3 ▯
**AMA:** 2017,Jan,8; 2016,Jan,13; 2015,Jan,16; 2014,Jan,11; 2014,Jan,6

**64647**    6 or more muscles
🚑 3.99   ⚕ 5.08   **FUD** 000                            T P3 ▯
**AMA:** 2017,Jan,8; 2016,Jan,13; 2015,Jan,16; 2014,Jan,11; 2014,Jan,6

## 64650-64653 Chemical Denervation Eccrine Glands
INCLUDES    Injection of therapeutic medication
EXCLUDES    *Bladder chemodenervation (52287)*
            *Chemodenervation of extremities (64999)*
Code also drugs or other substances used

**64650**    Chemodenervation of eccrine glands; both axillae
🚑 1.22   ⚕ 2.21   **FUD** 000                            T P3 80 ▯
**AMA:** 2017,Jan,8; 2016,Jan,13; 2015,Jan,16; 2014,Jan,11; 2012,Sep,14-15; 2012,Sep,14-15

**64653**    other area(s) (eg, scalp, face, neck), per day
🚑 1.56   ⚕ 2.69   **FUD** 000                            T P3 80 ▯
**AMA:** 2017,Jan,8; 2016,Jan,13; 2015,Jan,16; 2014,Jan,11; 2012,Sep,14-15; 2012,Sep,14-15

## 64680-64681 Neurolysis: Celiac Plexus, Superior Hypogastric Plexus
INCLUDES    Injection of therapeutic medication

**64680**    Destruction by neurolytic agent, with or without radiologic monitoring; celiac plexus
EXCLUDES    *Transmural neurolytic agent injection with transendoscopic ultrasound guidance (43253)*
🚑 4.73   ⚕ 8.69   **FUD** 010                            T A2 ▯
**AMA:** 2017,Jan,8; 2016,Jan,13; 2015,Jan,16; 2014,Jan,11; 2012,Sep,14-15; 2012,Sep,14-15; 2012,Jan,15-42

**64681**    superior hypogastric plexus
🚑 7.83   ⚕ 14.9   **FUD** 010                            T A2 ▯
**AMA:** 2017,Jan,8; 2016,Jan,13; 2015,Jan,16; 2014,Jan,11; 2012,Sep,14-15; 2012,Sep,14-15; 2012,Jan,15-42

## 64702-64727 Decompression and/or Transposition of Nerve
INCLUDES    External neurolysis and/or transposition to repair or restore a nerve
            Neuroplasty with nerve wrapping
            Surgical decompression/freeing of nerve from scar tissue
EXCLUDES    *Facial nerve decompression (69720)*
            *Percutaneous neurolysis (62263-62264, 62280-62282)*

**64702**    Neuroplasty; digital, 1 or both, same digit
🚑 14.3   ⚕ 14.3   **FUD** 090                            J A2 ▯
**AMA:** 2017,Jan,8; 2016,Jan,13; 2015,Jan,16; 2014,Jan,11; 2012,Jan,15-42

**64704**    nerve of hand or foot
🚑 9.16   ⚕ 9.16   **FUD** 090                            J A2 80 ▯
**AMA:** 2017,Jan,8; 2016,Jan,13; 2015,Jan,16; 2014,Jan,11; 2012,Jan,15-42

**64708**    Neuroplasty, major peripheral nerve, arm or leg, open; other than specified
🚑 14.3   ⚕ 14.3   **FUD** 090                            J 02 80 ▯
**AMA:** 2017,Jan,8; 2016,Jan,13; 2015,Jan,16; 2014,Jan,11; 2012,Jun,12-13; 2012,Jan,15-42

**64712**    sciatic nerve
🚑 16.7   ⚕ 16.7   **FUD** 090                            J 02 80 50 ▯
**AMA:** 2017,Jan,8; 2016,Jan,13; 2015,Jan,16; 2014,Jan,11; 2012,Jun,12-13; 2012,Jan,15-42

**64713**    brachial plexus
🚑 22.1   ⚕ 22.1   **FUD** 090                            J 02 80 50 ▯
**AMA:** 2017,Jan,8; 2016,Jan,13; 2015,Jan,16; 2014,Jan,11; 2013,May,12; 2012,Jun,12-13; 2012,Jan,15-42

**64714**    lumbar plexus
🚑 20.4   ⚕ 20.4   **FUD** 090                            J 02 80 50 ▯
**AMA:** 2017,Jan,8; 2016,Jan,13; 2015,Jan,16; 2014,Jan,11; 2013,Dec,16; 2012,Jun,12-13; 2012,Jan,15-42

**64716**    Neuroplasty and/or transposition; cranial nerve (specify)
🚑 15.3   ⚕ 15.3   **FUD** 090                            J A2 80 ▯
**AMA:** 2017,Jan,8; 2016,Jan,13; 2015,Jan,16; 2014,Jan,11; 2012,Jan,15-42

**64718**    ulnar nerve at elbow
🚑 16.9   ⚕ 16.9   **FUD** 090                            J A2 80 50 ▯
**AMA:** 2017,Jan,8; 2016,Jan,13; 2015,Jan,16; 2014,Jan,11; 2012,Jan,15-42

**64719**    ulnar nerve at wrist
🚑 11.4   ⚕ 11.4   **FUD** 090                            J A2 50 ▯
**AMA:** 2017,Jan,8; 2016,Jan,13; 2015,Jan,16; 2014,Jan,11; 2012,Jan,15-42

**64721**    median nerve at carpal tunnel
EXCLUDES    *Arthroscopic procedure (29848)*
🚑 12.2   ⚕ 12.3   **FUD** 090                            J A2 50 ▯
**AMA:** 2017,Jan,8; 2016,Jan,13; 2015,Jul,10; 2015,Jan,16; 2014,Jan,11; 2013,Dec,14; 2012,Oct,14; 2012,Sep,16; 2012,Jun,15-16; 2012,Jan,15-42

**64722**    Decompression; unspecified nerve(s) (specify)
🚑 10.4   ⚕ 10.4   **FUD** 090                            J A2 80 ▯
**AMA:** 2017,Jan,8; 2016,Jan,13; 2015,Jan,16; 2014,Jan,11; 2012,Jan,15-42

**64726**    plantar digital nerve
🚑 7.83   ⚕ 7.83   **FUD** 090                            J A2 ▯
**AMA:** 2017,Jan,8; 2016,Jan,13; 2015,Jan,16; 2014,Jan,11; 2012,Jan,15-42

**+    64727**    Internal neurolysis, requiring use of operating microscope (List separately in addition to code for neuroplasty) (Neuroplasty includes external neurolysis)
INCLUDES    Operating microscope (69990)
Code first neuroplasty (64702-64721)
🚑 5.35   ⚕ 5.35   **FUD** ZZZ                            N N1 ▯
**AMA:** 2017,Jan,8; 2016,Feb,12; 2016,Jan,13; 2015,Jan,16; 2014,Jan,11; 2012,Jun,12-13; 2012,Jan,15-42

## 64732-64772 Surgical Avulsion/Transection of Nerve
EXCLUDES    *Stereotactic lesion of gasserian ganglion (61790)*

**64732**    Transection or avulsion of; supraorbital nerve
🚑 10.8   ⚕ 10.8   **FUD** 090                            J A2 80 50 ▯
**AMA:** 2017,Jan,8; 2016,Jan,13; 2015,Jan,16; 2014,Jan,11

**64734**    infraorbital nerve
🚑 14.5   ⚕ 14.5   **FUD** 090                            J A2 80 50 ▯
**AMA:** 2014,Jan,11

**64736**    mental nerve
🚑 11.1   ⚕ 11.1   **FUD** 090                            J A2 80 50 ▯
**AMA:** 2014,Jan,11

**64738**    inferior alveolar nerve by osteotomy
🚑 13.2   ⚕ 13.2   **FUD** 090                            J A2 80 50 ▯
**AMA:** 2014,Jan,11

**64740**    lingual nerve
🚑 12.9   ⚕ 12.9   **FUD** 090                            J A2 80 50 ▯
**AMA:** 2014,Jan,11

**64742**    facial nerve, differential or complete
🚑 13.0   ⚕ 13.0   **FUD** 090                            J A2 80 50 ▯
**AMA:** 2014,Jan,11

| 26/TC PC/TC Only | A2-Z3 ASC Payment | 50 Bilateral | ♂ Male Only | ♀ Female Only | 🚑 Facility RVU | ⚕ Non-Facility RVU | ▯ CCI |
| FUD Follow-up Days | CMS: IOM (Pub 100) | A-Y OPPSI | 80/80 Surg Assist Allowed / w/Doc | | 🧪 Lab Crosswalk | 📻 Radiology Crosswalk | ✖ CLIA |

292                                  CPT © 2017 American Medical Association. All Rights Reserved.                    © 2017 Optum360, LLC

| 64744 | **greater occipital nerve** |
|---|---|
| | 🔧 14.1   ⚕ 14.1   **FUD** 090     J A2 80 50 ▢ |
| | **AMA:** 2014,Jan,11 |

| 64746 | **phrenic nerve** |
|---|---|
| | EXCLUDES  *Section of recurrent unilateral laryngeal nerve (31595)* |
| | 🔧 12.2   ⚕ 12.2   **FUD** 090     J A2 80 50 ▢ |
| | **AMA:** 2014,Jan,11 |

| 64755 | **vagus nerves limited to proximal stomach (selective proximal vagotomy, proximal gastric vagotomy, parietal cell vagotomy, supra- or highly selective vagotomy)** |
|---|---|
| | EXCLUDES  *Laparoscopic procedure (43652)* |
| | 🔧 25.2   ⚕ 25.2   **FUD** 090     C 80 ▢ |
| | **AMA:** 2017,Jan,8; 2016,Jan,13; 2015,Jan,16; 2014,Jan,11 |

| 64760 | **vagus nerve (vagotomy), abdominal** |
|---|---|
| | EXCLUDES  *Laparoscopic procedure (43651)* |
| | 🔧 14.2   ⚕ 14.2   **FUD** 090     C 80 ▢ |
| | **AMA:** 2017,Jan,8; 2016,Jan,13; 2015,Jan,16; 2014,Jan,11 |

| 64763 | **Transection or avulsion of obturator nerve, extrapelvic, with or without adductor tenotomy** |
|---|---|
| | 🔧 13.8   ⚕ 13.8   **FUD** 090     J 62 80 50 ▢ |
| | **AMA:** 2014,Jan,11 |

| 64766 | **Transection or avulsion of obturator nerve, intrapelvic, with or without adductor tenotomy** |
|---|---|
| | 🔧 16.2   ⚕ 16.2   **FUD** 090     J J8 80 50 ▢ |
| | **AMA:** 2014,Jan,11 |

| 64771 | **Transection or avulsion of other cranial nerve, extradural** |
|---|---|
| | 🔧 17.2   ⚕ 17.2   **FUD** 090     J A2 80 ▢ |
| | **AMA:** 2014,Jan,11 |

| 64772 | **Transection or avulsion of other spinal nerve, extradural** |
|---|---|
| | EXCLUDES  *Removal of tender scar and soft tissue including neuroma if necessary (11400-11446, 13100-13153)* |
| | 🔧 16.2   ⚕ 16.2   **FUD** 090     J A2 80 ▢ |
| | **AMA:** 2017,Jan,8; 2016,Jan,13; 2015,Apr,10; 2014,Jan,11 |

## 64774-64823 Excisional Nerve Procedures

EXCLUDES  *Morton neuroma excision (28080)*

| 64774 | **Excision of neuroma; cutaneous nerve, surgically identifiable** |
|---|---|
| | 🔧 11.9   ⚕ 11.9   **FUD** 090     J A2 ▢ |
| | **AMA:** 2014,Jan,11 |

| 64776 | **digital nerve, 1 or both, same digit** |
|---|---|
| | 🔧 11.1   ⚕ 11.1   **FUD** 090     J A2 80 ▢ |
| | **AMA:** 2014,Jan,11 |

| + 64778 | **digital nerve, each additional digit (List separately in addition to code for primary procedure)** |
|---|---|
| | Code first (64776) |
| | 🔧 4.09   ⚕ 4.09   **FUD** ZZZ     N N1 ▢ |
| | **AMA:** 2014,Jan,11 |

| 64782 | **hand or foot, except digital nerve** |
|---|---|
| | 🔧 13.0   ⚕ 13.0   **FUD** 090     J A2 ▢ |
| | **AMA:** 2014,Jan,11 |

| + 64783 | **hand or foot, each additional nerve, except same digit (List separately in addition to code for primary procedure)** |
|---|---|
| | Code first (64782) |
| | 🔧 6.41   ⚕ 6.41   **FUD** ZZZ     N N1 ▢ |
| | **AMA:** 2014,Jan,11 |

| 64784 | **major peripheral nerve, except sciatic** |
|---|---|
| | 🔧 20.9   ⚕ 20.9   **FUD** 090     J A2 80 ▢ |
| | **AMA:** 2014,Jan,11 |

| 64786 | **sciatic nerve** |
|---|---|
| | 🔧 31.2   ⚕ 31.2   **FUD** 090     J A2 80 50 ▢ |
| | **AMA:** 2014,Jan,11 |

| + 64787 | **Implantation of nerve end into bone or muscle (List separately in addition to neuroma excision)** |
|---|---|
| | Code also, when appropriate (64774-64786) |
| | 🔧 7.03   ⚕ 7.03   **FUD** ZZZ     N N1 80 ▢ |
| | **AMA:** 2014,Jan,11 |

| 64788 | **Excision of neurofibroma or neurolemmoma; cutaneous nerve** |
|---|---|
| | 🔧 11.4   ⚕ 11.4   **FUD** 090     J A2 ▢ |
| | **AMA:** 2017,Jan,8; 2016,Apr,3; 2014,Jan,11 |

| 64790 | **major peripheral nerve** |
|---|---|
| | 🔧 24.4   ⚕ 24.4   **FUD** 090     J A2 80 ▢ |
| | **AMA:** 2017,Jan,8; 2016,Apr,3; 2014,Jan,11 |

| 64792 | **extensive (including malignant type)** |
|---|---|
| | EXCLUDES  *Destruction neurofibroma of skin (0419T-0420T)* |
| | 🔧 31.2   ⚕ 31.2   **FUD** 090     J A2 80 ▢ |
| | **AMA:** 2017,Jan,8; 2016,Apr,3; 2014,Jan,11 |

| 64795 | **Biopsy of nerve** |
|---|---|
| | 🔧 5.61   ⚕ 5.61   **FUD** 000     J A2 ▢ |
| | **AMA:** 2014,Jan,11 |

| 64802 | **Sympathectomy, cervical** |
|---|---|
| | 🔧 18.5   ⚕ 18.5   **FUD** 090     J A2 80 50 ▢ |
| | **AMA:** 2014,Jan,11 |

| 64804 | **Sympathectomy, cervicothoracic** |
|---|---|
| | 🔧 25.8   ⚕ 25.8   **FUD** 090     J 80 50 ▢ |
| | **AMA:** 2014,Jan,11 |

| 64809 | **Sympathectomy, thoracolumbar** |
|---|---|
| | INCLUDES  Leriche sympathectomy |
| | 🔧 26.1   ⚕ 26.1   **FUD** 090     C 80 50 ▢ |
| | **AMA:** 2014,Jan,11 |

| 64818 | **Sympathectomy, lumbar** |
|---|---|
| | 🔧 16.4   ⚕ 16.4   **FUD** 090     C 80 50 ▢ |
| | **AMA:** 2014,Jan,11 |

| 64820 | **Sympathectomy; digital arteries, each digit** |
|---|---|
| | INCLUDES  Operating microscope (69990) |
| | 🔧 20.3   ⚕ 20.3   **FUD** 090     J 62 |
| | **AMA:** 2017,Jan,8; 2016,Feb,12; 2016,Jan,13; 2015,Jan,16; 2014,Jan,11; 2012,Jan,15-42 |

| 64821 | **radial artery** |
|---|---|
| | INCLUDES  Operating microscope (69990) |
| | 🔧 19.8   ⚕ 19.8   **FUD** 090     J A2 50 ▢ |
| | **AMA:** 2016,Feb,12; 2014,Jan,11 |

| 64822 | **ulnar artery** |
|---|---|
| | INCLUDES  Operating microscope (69990) |
| | 🔧 19.8   ⚕ 19.8   **FUD** 090     J 62 50 ▢ |
| | **AMA:** 2016,Feb,12; 2014,Jan,11 |

| 64823 | **superficial palmar arch** |
|---|---|
| | INCLUDES  Operating microscope (69990) |
| | 🔧 22.6   ⚕ 22.6   **FUD** 090     J 62 50 ▢ |
| | **AMA:** 2016,Feb,12; 2014,Jan,11 |

## 64831-64907 Nerve Repair: Suture and Nerve Grafts

| 64831 | **Suture of digital nerve, hand or foot; 1 nerve** |
|---|---|
| | 🔧 19.7   ⚕ 19.7   **FUD** 090     J A2 50 ▢ |
| | **AMA:** 2017,Jan,8; 2016,Jan,13; 2015,Jan,16; 2014,Sep,13; 2014,Jan,11 |

| + 64832 | **each additional digital nerve (List separately in addition to code for primary procedure)** |
|---|---|
| | Code first (64831) |
| | 🔧 9.78   ⚕ 9.78   **FUD** ZZZ     N N1 80 ▢ |
| | **AMA:** 2017,Jan,8; 2016,Jan,13; 2015,Jan,16; 2014,Jan,11 |

| 64834 | **Suture of 1 nerve; hand or foot, common sensory nerve** |
|---|---|
| | 🔧 21.4   ⚕ 21.4   **FUD** 090     J A2 80 50 ▢ |
| | **AMA:** 2014,Jan,11 |

| 64835 | **median motor thenar** |
|---|---|
| | 🔧 23.2   ⚕ 23.2   **FUD** 090     J A2 80 50 ▢ |
| | **AMA:** 2014,Jan,11 |

---

● New Code     ▲ Revised Code     ○ Reinstated     ● New Web Release     ▲ Revised Web Release     Unlisted     Not Covered     # Resequenced
⊘ AMA Mod 51 Exempt     ⑤ Optum Mod 51 Exempt     ⑥ Mod 63 Exempt     ⁄ Non-FDA Drug     ★ Telemedicine     Ⓜ Maternity     Ⓐ Age Edit     + Add-on     **AMA:** CPT Asst
© 2017 Optum360, LLC                          CPT © 2017 American Medical Association. All Rights Reserved.                          293

**64836**   **ulnar motor**
    🚑 23.7   ⚖ 23.7   **FUD** 090                    Ⓙ A2 80 50 ▣
    AMA: 2014,Jan,11

**+  64837**   **Suture of each additional nerve, hand or foot (List separately in addition to code for primary procedure)**
    Code first (64834-64836)
    🚑 11.0   ⚖ 11.0   **FUD** ZZZ                    Ⓝ N1 80 ▣
    AMA: 2014,Jan,11

**64840**   **Suture of posterior tibial nerve**
    🚑 28.0   ⚖ 28.0   **FUD** 090                    Ⓙ A2 80 50 ▣
    AMA: 2014,Jan,11

**64856**   **Suture of major peripheral nerve, arm or leg, except sciatic; including transposition**
    🚑 29.1   ⚖ 29.1   **FUD** 090                    Ⓙ A2 ▣
    AMA: 2014,Jan,11

**64857**   **without transposition**
    🚑 30.4   ⚖ 30.4   **FUD** 090                    Ⓙ A2 80 ▣
    AMA: 2014,Jan,11

**64858**   **Suture of sciatic nerve**
    🚑 33.7   ⚖ 33.7   **FUD** 090                    Ⓙ A2 80 50 ▣
    AMA: 2014,Jan,11

**+  64859**   **Suture of each additional major peripheral nerve (List separately in addition to code for primary procedure)**
    Code first (64856-64857)
    🚑 7.27   ⚖ 7.27   **FUD** ZZZ                    Ⓝ N1 80 ▣
    AMA: 2014,Jan,11

**64861**   **Suture of; brachial plexus**
    🚑 36.0   ⚖ 36.0   **FUD** 090                    Ⓙ A2 80 50 ▣
    AMA: 2014,Jan,11

**64862**   **lumbar plexus**
    🚑 40.1   ⚖ 40.1   **FUD** 090                    Ⓙ A2 80 50 ▣
    AMA: 2014,Jan,11

**64864**   **Suture of facial nerve; extracranial**
    🚑 25.3   ⚖ 25.3   **FUD** 090                    Ⓙ A2 80 ▣
    AMA: 2014,Jan,11

**64865**   **infratemporal, with or without grafting**
    🚑 32.1   ⚖ 32.1   **FUD** 090                    Ⓙ A2 80 ▣
    AMA: 2014,Jan,11

**64866**   **Anastomosis; facial-spinal accessory**
    🚑 32.9   ⚖ 32.9   **FUD** 090                    Ⓒ 80 ▣
    AMA: 2014,Jan,11

**64868**   **facial-hypoglossal**
    INCLUDES   Korte-Ballance anastomosis
    🚑 29.7   ⚖ 29.7   **FUD** 090                    Ⓒ 80 ▣
    AMA: 2014,Jan,11

**+  64872**   **Suture of nerve; requiring secondary or delayed suture (List separately in addition to code for primary neurorrhaphy)**
    Code first (64831-64865)
    🚑 3.39   ⚖ 3.39   **FUD** ZZZ                    Ⓝ N1 80 ▣
    AMA: 2014,Jan,11

**+  64874**   **requiring extensive mobilization, or transposition of nerve (List separately in addition to code for nerve suture)**
    Code first (64831-64865)
    🚑 4.76   ⚖ 4.76   **FUD** ZZZ                    Ⓝ N1 80 ▣
    AMA: 2014,Jan,11

**+  64876**   **requiring shortening of bone of extremity (List separately in addition to code for nerve suture)**
    Code first (64831-64865)
    🚑 5.12   ⚖ 5.12   **FUD** ZZZ                    Ⓝ N1 80 ▣
    AMA: 2014,Jan,11

**64885**   **Nerve graft (includes obtaining graft), head or neck; up to 4 cm in length**
    🚑 32.7   ⚖ 32.7   **FUD** 090                    Ⓙ A2 80 ▣
    AMA: 2017,Jan,8; 2016,Jan,13; 2015,Jan,16; 2014,Jan,11; 2012,Jan,15-42

**64886**   **more than 4 cm length**
    🚑 37.4   ⚖ 37.4   **FUD** 090                    Ⓙ A2 80 CCI
    AMA: 2017,Jan,8; 2016,Jan,13; 2015,Jan,16; 2014,Jan,11; 2012,Jan,15-42

**64890**   **Nerve graft (includes obtaining graft), single strand, hand or foot; up to 4 cm length**
    🚑 31.4   ⚖ 31.4   **FUD** 090                    Ⓙ J8 80 ▣
    AMA: 2017,Jan,8; 2016,Jan,13; 2015,Aug,8; 2015,Apr,10; 2014,Jan,11

**64891**   **more than 4 cm length**
    🚑 33.2   ⚖ 33.2   **FUD** 090                    Ⓙ J8 80 ▣
    AMA: 2014,Jan,11

**64892**   **Nerve graft (includes obtaining graft), single strand, arm or leg; up to 4 cm length**
    🚑 30.1   ⚖ 30.1   **FUD** 090                    Ⓙ A2 80 ▣
    AMA: 2014,Jan,11

**64893**   **more than 4 cm length**
    🚑 32.8   ⚖ 32.8   **FUD** 090                    Ⓙ J8 80 ▣
    AMA: 2014,Jan,11

**64895**   **Nerve graft (includes obtaining graft), multiple strands (cable), hand or foot; up to 4 cm length**
    🚑 38.7   ⚖ 38.7   **FUD** 090                    Ⓙ A2 80 ▣
    AMA: 2017,Jan,8; 2016,Jan,13; 2015,Jan,16; 2014,Jan,11

**64896**   **more than 4 cm length**
    🚑 41.5   ⚖ 41.5   **FUD** 090                    Ⓙ A2 80 ▣
    AMA: 2017,Jan,8; 2016,Jan,13; 2015,Jan,16; 2014,Jan,11

**64897**   **Nerve graft (includes obtaining graft), multiple strands (cable), arm or leg; up to 4 cm length**
    🚑 37.0   ⚖ 37.0   **FUD** 090                    Ⓙ J8 80 ▣
    AMA: 2017,Jan,8; 2016,Jan,13; 2015,Jan,16; 2014,Jan,11

**64898**   **more than 4 cm length**
    🚑 42.8   ⚖ 42.8   **FUD** 090                    Ⓙ A2 80 ▣
    AMA: 2017,Jan,8; 2016,Jan,13; 2015,Jan,16; 2014,Jan,11

**+  64901**   **Nerve graft, each additional nerve; single strand (List separately in addition to code for primary procedure)**
    Code first (64885-64893)
    🚑 16.1   ⚖ 16.1   **FUD** ZZZ                    Ⓝ N1 80 ▣
    AMA: 2017,Jan,8; 2016,Jan,13; 2015,Jan,16; 2014,Jan,11

**+  64902**   **multiple strands (cable) (List separately in addition to code for primary procedure)**
    Code first (64885-64886, 64895-64898)
    🚑 18.8   ⚖ 18.8   **FUD** ZZZ                    Ⓝ N1 80 ▣
    AMA: 2017,Jan,8; 2016,Jan,13; 2015,Jan,16; 2014,Jan,11

**64905**   **Nerve pedicle transfer; first stage**
    🚑 29.8   ⚖ 29.8   **FUD** 090                    Ⓙ A2 80 ▣
    AMA: 2014,Jan,11

**64907**   **second stage**
    🚑 38.3   ⚖ 38.3   **FUD** 090                    Ⓙ A2 80 ▣
    AMA: 2014,Jan,11

## 64910-64999 Nerve Repair: Synthetic and Vein Grafts

64910     **Nerve repair; with synthetic conduit or vein allograft (eg, nerve tube), each nerve**

     INCLUDES    Operating microscope (69990)

     23.6    23.6    **FUD** 090      J 62 80

     **AMA:** 2017,Jan,8; 2016,Jan,13; 2015,Aug,8; 2015,Apr,10; 2015,Jan,16; 2014,Jan,11

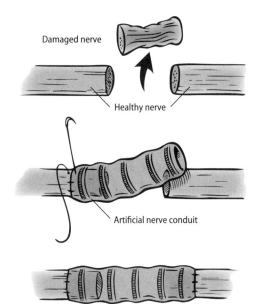

Damaged nerve

Healthy nerve

Artificial nerve conduit

A synthetic "bridge" is affixed to each end of a severed nerve with sutures
The procedure is performed using an operating microscope

64911     **with autogenous vein graft (includes harvest of vein graft), each nerve**

     INCLUDES    Operating microscope (69990)

     29.2    29.2    **FUD** 090      J 80

     **AMA:** 2017,Jan,8; 2016,Jan,13; 2015,Jan,16; 2014,Jan,11

●   64912     **with nerve allograft, each nerve, first strand (cable)**

     INCLUDES    Operating microscope (69990)

● +   64913     **with nerve allograft, each additional strand (List separately in addition to code for primary procedure)**

     0.00    0.00    **FUD** 000

     INCLUDES    Operating microscope (69990)

     Code first (64912)

64999     **Unlisted procedure, nervous system**

     0.00    0.00    **FUD** YYY      T 80

     **AMA:** 2017,Jan,8; 2016,Nov,6; 2016,Oct,11; 2016,Feb,13; 2016,Jan,13; 2015,Oct,9; 2015,Aug,8; 2015,Jul,10; 2015,Apr,10; 2015,Feb,9; 2015,Jan,16; 2014,Jul,8; 2014,Feb,11; 2014,Jan,9; 2014,Jan,8; 2014,Jan,11; 2013,Dec,14; 2013,Nov,14; 2013,Jun,13; 2013,Apr,5-6; 2013,Apr,10-11; 2012,Dec,12; 2012,Sep,14-15; 2012,Oct,14; 2012,Sep,16; 2012,Sep,14-15; 2012,May,14-15; 2012,Feb,11; 2012,Jan,13-14; 2012,Jan,15-42

● New Code   ▲ Revised Code   ○ Reinstated   ● New Web Release   ▲ Revised Web Release   Unlisted   Not Covered   # Resequenced
⊘ AMA Mod 51 Exempt   ⑨ Optum Mod 51 Exempt   ⓢ Mod 63 Exempt   ✗ Non-FDA Drug   ★ Telemedicine   Ⓜ Maternity   Ⓐ Age Edit   + Add-on   **AMA:** CPT Asst

## 65091-65093 Surgical Removal of Eyeball Contents

INCLUDES Operating microscope (69990)

**65091** **Evisceration of ocular contents; without implant**
🔧 18.0 ⚕ 18.0 **FUD** 090 J A2 80 50 ▣
**AMA:** 2016,Feb,12; 2014,Jan,11

Conjunctiva
Sclera

Muscles are severed at their attachment to the eyeball

Evisceration involves removal of the contents of the eyeball: the vitreous; retina; choroid; lens; iris; and ciliary muscle. Only the scleral shell remains. A temporary or permanent implant is usually inserted

Enucleation involves severing the extraorbital muscles and optic nerve with removal of the eyeball. An implant is usually inserted and, if permanent, may involve attachment to the severed extraorbital muscles

**65093** **with implant**
🔧 17.7 ⚕ 17.7 **FUD** 090 J A2 50 ▣
**AMA:** 2016,Feb,12; 2014,Jan,11

## 65101-65105 Surgical Removal of Eyeball

INCLUDES Operating microscope (69990)
EXCLUDES Conjunctivoplasty following enucleation (68320-68328)

**65101** **Enucleation of eye; without implant**
🔧 20.9 ⚕ 20.9 **FUD** 090 J A2 50 ▣
**AMA:** 2016,Feb,12; 2014,Jan,11

**65103** **with implant, muscles not attached to implant**
🔧 21.8 ⚕ 21.8 **FUD** 090 J A2 50 ▣
**AMA:** 2016,Feb,12; 2014,Jan,11

**65105** **with implant, muscles attached to implant**
🔧 24.0 ⚕ 24.0 **FUD** 090 J A2 80 50 ▣
**AMA:** 2016,Feb,12; 2014,Jan,11

## 65110-65114 Surgical Removal of Orbital Contents

INCLUDES Operating microscope (69990)
EXCLUDES Free full thickness graft (15260-15261)
Repair more extensive than skin (67930-67975)
Skin graft (15120-15121)

**65110** **Exenteration of orbit (does not include skin graft), removal of orbital contents; only**
🔧 34.6 ⚕ 34.6 **FUD** 090 J A2 80 50 ▣
**AMA:** 2016,Feb,12; 2014,Jan,11

**65112** **with therapeutic removal of bone**
🔧 40.2 ⚕ 40.2 **FUD** 090 J A2 80 50 ▣
**AMA:** 2016,Feb,12; 2014,Jan,11

**65114** **with muscle or myocutaneous flap**
🔧 41.9 ⚕ 41.9 **FUD** 090 J A2 80 50 ▣
**AMA:** 2016,Feb,12; 2014,Jan,11

## 65125-65175 Implant Procedures: Insertion, Removal, and Revision

INCLUDES Operating microscope (69990)
EXCLUDES Orbital implant insertion outside muscle cone (67550)
Orbital implant removal or revision outside muscle cone (67560)

**65125** **Modification of ocular implant with placement or replacement of pegs (eg, drilling receptacle for prosthesis appendage) (separate procedure)**
🔧 8.19 ⚕ 12.7 **FUD** 090 J 62 50 ▣
**AMA:** 2016,Feb,12; 2014,Jan,11

**65130** **Insertion of ocular implant secondary; after evisceration, in scleral shell**
🔧 20.6 ⚕ 20.6 **FUD** 090 J A2 50 ▣
**AMA:** 2016,Feb,12; 2014,Jan,11

**65135** **after enucleation, muscles not attached to implant**
🔧 21.0 ⚕ 21.0 **FUD** 090 J A2 50 ▣
**AMA:** 2016,Feb,12; 2014,Jan,11

**65140** **after enucleation, muscles attached to implant**
🔧 22.8 ⚕ 22.8 **FUD** 090 J A2 50 ▣
**AMA:** 2016,Feb,12; 2014,Jan,11

**65150** **Reinsertion of ocular implant; with or without conjunctival graft**
🔧 16.3 ⚕ 16.3 **FUD** 090 J A2 80 50 ▣
**AMA:** 2016,Feb,12; 2014,Jan,11

**65155** **with use of foreign material for reinforcement and/or attachment of muscles to implant**
🔧 23.9 ⚕ 23.9 **FUD** 090 J A2 50 ▣
**AMA:** 2016,Feb,12; 2014,Jan,11

**65175** **Removal of ocular implant**
🔧 18.6 ⚕ 18.6 **FUD** 090 J A2 50 ▣
**AMA:** 2016,Feb,12; 2014,Jan,11

## 65205-65265 Foreign Body Removal By Area of Eye

INCLUDES Operating microscope (69990)
EXCLUDES Removal:
Anterior segment implant (65920)
Ocular implant (65175)
Orbital implant outside muscle cone (67560)
Posterior segment implant (67120)
Removal of foreign body:
Eyelid (67938)
Lacrimal system (68530)
Orbit:
Lateral approach (67430)
Frontal approach (67413)

**65205** **Removal of foreign body, external eye; conjunctival superficial**
🔄 (70030, 76529)
🔧 1.25 ⚕ 1.59 **FUD** 000 Q1 N1 50 ▣
**AMA:** 2017,Jan,8; 2016,Feb,12; 2016,Jan,13; 2015,Jan,16; 2014,Jan,11; 2013,Oct,18; 2012,Jan,15-42

**65210** **conjunctival embedded (includes concretions), subconjunctival, or scleral nonperforating**
🔄 (70030, 76529)
🔧 1.51 ⚕ 1.94 **FUD** 000 Q1 N1 50 ▣
**AMA:** 2016,Feb,12; 2014,Jan,11

**65220** **corneal, without slit lamp**
EXCLUDES Repair of corneal wound with foreign body (65275)
🔄 (70030, 76529)
🔧 1.21 ⚕ 1.65 **FUD** 000 Q1 N1 50 ▣
**AMA:** 2017,Jan,8; 2016,Feb,12; 2016,Jan,13; 2015,Jan,16; 2014,Jan,11; 2012,Jan,15-42

**65222** **corneal, with slit lamp**
EXCLUDES Repair of corneal wound with foreign body (65275)
🔄 (70030, 76529)
🔧 1.48 ⚕ 1.89 **FUD** 000 Q1 N1 50 ▣
**AMA:** 2017,Jan,8; 2016,Feb,12; 2016,Jan,13; 2015,Jan,16; 2014,Jan,11; 2012,Jan,15-42

**65235** **Removal of foreign body, intraocular; from anterior chamber of eye or lens**
🔄 (70030, 76529)
🔧 20.1 ⚕ 20.1 **FUD** 090 J A2 80 50 ▣
**AMA:** 2017,Jan,8; 2016,Feb,12; 2016,Jan,13; 2015,Jan,16; 2014,Jan,11

**65260** **from posterior segment, magnetic extraction, anterior or posterior route**
🔄 (70030, 76529)
🔧 27.2 ⚕ 27.2 **FUD** 090 J A2 80 50 ▣
**AMA:** 2016,Feb,12; 2014,Jan,11

● New Code ▲ Revised Code ○ Reinstated ● New Web Release ▲ Revised Web Release Unlisted Not Covered # Resequenced
⊘ AMA Mod 51 Exempt ⑤ Optum Mod 51 Exempt ⑥ Mod 63 Exempt ✗ Non-FDA Drug ★ Telemedicine Ⓜ Maternity ⒶAge Edit + Add-on **AMA:** CPT Asst
© 2017 Optum360, LLC     CPT © 2017 American Medical Association. All Rights Reserved.

**65265**    from posterior segment, nonmagnetic extraction
📷 (70030, 76529)
💲 30.6    ✂ 30.6    **FUD** 090    [J] [A2] [80] [50] 🔲
**AMA:** 2016,Feb,12; 2014,Jan,11

## 65270-65290 Laceration Repair External Eye

**INCLUDES**  Conjunctival flap
Operating microscope (69990)
Restoration of anterior chamber with air or saline injection
**EXCLUDES**  Repair:
Ciliary body or iris (66680)
Eyelid laceration (12011-12018, 12051-12057, 13151-13160, 67930, 67935)
Lacrimal system injury (68700)
Surgical wound (66250)
Treatment of orbit fracture (21385-21408)

**65270**    Repair of laceration; conjunctiva, with or without nonperforating laceration sclera, direct closure
💲 3.98    ✂ 7.50    **FUD** 010    [J] [A2] [80] [50] 🔲
**AMA:** 2017,Jan,8; 2016,Feb,12; 2016,Jan,13; 2015,Jan,16; 2014,Jan,11; 2012,Aug,9

**65272**    conjunctiva, by mobilization and rearrangement, without hospitalization
💲 9.95    ✂ 14.2    **FUD** 090    [J] [A2] [50] 🔲
**AMA:** 2016,Feb,12; 2014,Jan,11

**65273**    conjunctiva, by mobilization and rearrangement, with hospitalization
💲 10.8    ✂ 10.8    **FUD** 090    [C] [50] 🔲
**AMA:** 2016,Feb,12; 2014,Jan,11

**65275**    cornea, nonperforating, with or without removal foreign body
💲 13.0    ✂ 16.3    **FUD** 090    [J] [A2] [80] [50] 🔲
**AMA:** 2016,Feb,12; 2014,Jan,11

**65280**    cornea and/or sclera, perforating, not involving uveal tissue
**EXCLUDES**  Procedure performed for surgical wound repair
💲 19.0    ✂ 19.0    **FUD** 090    [J] [A2] [80] [50] 🔲
**AMA:** 2017,Jan,8; 2016,Feb,12; 2016,Jan,13; 2015,Jan,16; 2014,Jan,11; 2012,Aug,9

**65285**    cornea and/or sclera, perforating, with reposition or resection of uveal tissue
**EXCLUDES**  Procedure performed for surgical wound repair
💲 31.4    ✂ 31.4    **FUD** 090    [J] [A2] [50] 🔲
**AMA:** 2017,Jan,8; 2016,Feb,12; 2016,Jan,13; 2015,Jan,16; 2014,Jan,11; 2012,Aug,9

**65286**    application of tissue glue, wounds of cornea and/or sclera
💲 14.0    ✂ 19.9    **FUD** 090    [J] [P3] [50] 🔲
**AMA:** 2017,Jan,8; 2016,Feb,12; 2016,Jan,13; 2015,Jan,16; 2014,Jan,11

**65290**    Repair of wound, extraocular muscle, tendon and/or Tenon's capsule
💲 13.9    ✂ 13.9    **FUD** 090    [J] [A2] [50] 🔲
**AMA:** 2016,Feb,12; 2014,Jan,11

## 65400-65600 Removal Corneal Lesions

**INCLUDES**  Operating microscope (69990)

**65400**    Excision of lesion, cornea (keratectomy, lamellar, partial), except pterygium
💲 17.1    ✂ 19.2    **FUD** 090    [T] [A2] [50] 🔲
**AMA:** 2017,Jan,8; 2016,Feb,12; 2016,Jan,13; 2015,Jan,16; 2014,Jan,11

**65410**    Biopsy of cornea
💲 2.97    ✂ 4.04    **FUD** 000    [J] [A2] [80] [50] 🔲
**AMA:** 2017,Jan,8; 2016,Feb,12; 2016,Jan,13; 2015,Jan,16; 2014,Jan,11

**65420**    Excision or transposition of pterygium; without graft
💲 10.7    ✂ 14.5    **FUD** 090    [J] [A2] [50] 🔲
**AMA:** 2017,Jan,8; 2016,Feb,12; 2016,Jan,13; 2015,Jan,16; 2014,Jan,11; 2012,Jan,15-42

The conjunctiva is subject to numerous acute and chronic irritations and disorders

Conjunctiva
Cornea
Lens
Posterior chamber
Iris
Anterior chamber
Pterygium

**65426**    with graft
💲 13.5    ✂ 18.4    **FUD** 090    [J] [A2] [50] 🔲
**AMA:** 2017,Jan,8; 2016,Feb,12; 2016,Jan,13; 2015,Jan,16; 2014,Jan,11

**65430**    Scraping of cornea, diagnostic, for smear and/or culture
💲 2.94    ✂ 3.23    **FUD** 000    [01] [N1] [50] 🔲
**AMA:** 2016,Feb,12; 2014,Jan,11

**65435**    Removal of corneal epithelium; with or without chemocauterization (abrasion, curettage)
**EXCLUDES**  Collagen cross-linking of cornea (0402T)
💲 1.98    ✂ 2.26    **FUD** 000    [T] [P3] [50] 🔲
**AMA:** 2017,Jan,8; 2016,Feb,12; 2016,Jan,13; 2015,Jan,16; 2014,Jan,11; 2012,Jan,15-42

**65436**    with application of chelating agent (eg, EDTA)
💲 10.5    ✂ 10.9    **FUD** 090    [J] [P3] [50] 🔲
**AMA:** 2016,Feb,12; 2014,Jan,11

**65450**    Destruction of lesion of cornea by cryotherapy, photocoagulation or thermocauterization
💲 9.11    ✂ 9.20    **FUD** 090    [T] [G2] [50] 🔲
**AMA:** 2016,Feb,12; 2014,Jan,11

**65600**    Multiple punctures of anterior cornea (eg, for corneal erosion, tattoo)
💲 9.76    ✂ 11.1    **FUD** 090    [J] [P3] [50] 🔲
**AMA:** 2016,Feb,12; 2014,Jan,11

## 65710-65757 Corneal Transplants

**CMS:** 100-03,80.7 Refractive Keratoplasty
**INCLUDES**  Operating microscope (69990)
**EXCLUDES**  Computerized corneal topography (92025)
Processing, preserving, and transporting corneal tissue (V2785)

**65710**    Keratoplasty (corneal transplant); anterior lamellar
**INCLUDES**  Use and preparation of fresh or preserved graft
**EXCLUDES**  Refractive keratoplasty surgery (65760-65767)
💲 31.3    ✂ 31.3    **FUD** 090    [J] [A2] [80] [50] 🔲
**AMA:** 2017,Jan,8; 2016,Feb,12; 2016,Jan,13; 2015,Jan,16; 2014,Jan,11; 2012,Aug,9

**65730**    penetrating (except in aphakia or pseudophakia)
**INCLUDES**  Use and preparation of fresh or preserved graft
**EXCLUDES**  Refractive keratoplasty surgery (65760-65767)
💲 34.7    ✂ 34.7    **FUD** 090    [J] [A2] [80] [50] 🔲
**AMA:** 2017,Jan,8; 2016,Feb,12; 2016,Jan,13; 2015,Jan,16; 2014,Jan,11; 2012,Aug,9; 2012,Jan,15-42

**65750**    penetrating (in aphakia)
**INCLUDES**  Use and preparation of fresh or preserved graft
**EXCLUDES**  Refractive keratoplasty surgery (65760-65767)
💲 34.9    ✂ 34.9    **FUD** 090    [J] [A2] [80] [50] 🔲
**AMA:** 2017,Jan,8; 2016,Feb,12; 2016,Jan,13; 2015,Jan,16; 2014,Jan,11; 2012,Aug,9

**65755** penetrating (in pseudophakia)

INCLUDES Use and preparation of fresh or preserved graft

EXCLUDES Refractive keratoplasty surgery (65760-65767)

🚗 34.7 ⚒ 34.7 **FUD** 090  [J] [A2] [80] [50] 🔲

**AMA:** 2017,Jan,8; 2016,Feb,12; 2016,Jan,13; 2015,Jan,16; 2014,Jan,11; 2012,Aug,9

**65756** endothelial

EXCLUDES Refractive keratoplasty surgery (65760-65767)

Code also donor material

Code also if appropriate (65757)

🚗 33.5 ⚒ 33.5 **FUD** 090  [J] [62] [80] [50] 🔲

**AMA:** 2017,Jan,8; 2016,Feb,12; 2016,Jan,13; 2015,Jan,16; 2014,Jan,11; 2012,Jan,15-42

+ **65757** Backbench preparation of corneal endothelial allograft prior to transplantation (List separately in addition to code for primary procedure)

Code first (65756)

🚗 0.00 ⚒ 0.00 **FUD** ZZZ  [N] [N1] [80] 🔲

**AMA:** 2017,Jan,8; 2016,Feb,12; 2016,Jan,13; 2015,Jan,16; 2014,Aug,14; 2014,Jan,11; 2012,Jan,15-42

## 65760-65785 Corneal Refractive Procedures

**CMS:** 100-03,80.7 Refractive Keratoplasty

INCLUDES Operating microscope (69990)

EXCLUDES Unlisted corneal procedures (66999)

**65760** Keratomileusis

EXCLUDES Computerized corneal topography (92025)

🚗 0.00 ⚒ 0.00 **FUD** XXX  [E] 🔲

**AMA:** 2016,Feb,12; 2014,Jan,11

**65765** Keratophakia

EXCLUDES Computerized corneal topography (92025)

🚗 0.00 ⚒ 0.00 **FUD** XXX  [E] 🔲

**AMA:** 2016,Feb,12; 2014,Jan,11

**65767** Epikeratoplasty

EXCLUDES Computerized corneal topography (92025)

🚗 0.00 ⚒ 0.00 **FUD** XXX  [E] 🔲

**AMA:** 2016,Feb,12; 2014,Jan,11

**65770** Keratoprosthesis

EXCLUDES Computerized corneal topography (92025)

🚗 39.7 ⚒ 39.7 **FUD** 090  [J] [J8] [80] [50] 🔲

**AMA:** 2016,Feb,12; 2014,Jan,11

**65771** Radial keratotomy

EXCLUDES Computerized corneal topography (92025)

🚗 0.00 ⚒ 0.00 **FUD** XXX  [E] 🔲

**AMA:** 2016,Feb,12; 2014,Jan,11

**65772** Corneal relaxing incision for correction of surgically induced astigmatism

🚗 11.5 ⚒ 12.7 **FUD** 090  [T] [A2] [50] 🔲

**AMA:** 2016,Feb,12; 2014,Jan,11

**65775** Corneal wedge resection for correction of surgically induced astigmatism

EXCLUDES Fitting of contact lens to treat disease (92071-92072)

🚗 15.6 ⚒ 15.6 **FUD** 090  [J] [A2] [50] 🔲

**AMA:** 2017,Jan,8; 2016,Feb,12; 2016,Jan,13; 2015,Jan,16; 2014,Jan,11; 2012,Aug,9

**65778** Placement of amniotic membrane on the ocular surface; without sutures

EXCLUDES Ocular surface reconstruction (65780)

Removal of corneal epithelium (65435)

Scraping of cornea, diagnostic (65430)

Use of tissue glue to place amniotic membrane (66999)

🚗 1.63 ⚒ 40.1 **FUD** 000  [02] [N1] [80] [50] 🔲

**AMA:** 2017,Jan,8; 2016,Feb,12; 2016,Jan,13; 2015,Jan,16; 2014,May,5; 2014,Jan,11

**65779** single layer, sutured

EXCLUDES Ocular surface reconstruction (65430, 65435, 65780)

Removal of corneal epithelium (65435)

Scraping of cornea, diagnostic (65430)

Use of tissue glue to place amniotic membrane (66999)

🚗 4.32 ⚒ 33.9 **FUD** 000  [02] [N1] [80] [50] 🔲

**AMA:** 2017,Jan,8; 2016,Feb,12; 2016,Jan,13; 2015,Jan,16; 2014,May,5; 2014,Jan,11

**65780** Ocular surface reconstruction; amniotic membrane transplantation, multiple layers

🚗 18.8 ⚒ 18.8 **FUD** 090  [J] [A2] [50] 🔲

**AMA:** 2017,Jan,8; 2016,Feb,12; 2016,Jan,13; 2015,Jan,16; 2014,May,5; 2014,Jan,11; 2012,Jan,15-42

**65781** limbal stem cell allograft (eg, cadaveric or living donor)

🚗 37.8 ⚒ 37.8 **FUD** 090  [J] [A2] [80] [50] 🔲

**AMA:** 2017,Jan,8; 2016,Feb,12; 2016,Jan,13; 2015,Jan,16; 2014,Jan,11

**65782** limbal conjunctival autograft (includes obtaining graft)

EXCLUDES Conjunctival allograft harvest from a living donor (68371)

🚗 32.6 ⚒ 32.6 **FUD** 090  [J] [A2] [50] 🔲

**AMA:** 2017,Jan,8; 2016,Feb,12; 2016,Jan,13; 2015,Jan,16; 2014,Jan,11; 2012,Jan,15-42

**65785** Implantation of intrastromal corneal ring segments

🚗 11.0 ⚒ 59.7 **FUD** 090  [J] [P2] [50] 🔲

**AMA:** 2016,Feb,12

## 65800-66030 Anterior Segment Procedures

INCLUDES Operating microscope (69990)

EXCLUDES Unlisted procedures of anterior segment (66999)

**65800** Paracentesis of anterior chamber of eye (separate procedure); with removal of aqueous

EXCLUDES Insertion of ocular telescope prosthesis (0308T)

🚗 2.60 ⚒ 3.37 **FUD** 000  [J] [A2] [50] 🔲

**AMA:** 2017,Jan,8; 2016,Feb,12; 2016,Jan,13; 2015,Jan,16; 2014,Jan,11; 2013,Mar,6-7; 2012,Nov,10

**65810** with removal of vitreous and/or discission of anterior hyaloid membrane, with or without air injection

EXCLUDES Insertion of ocular telescope prosthesis (0308T)

🚗 13.1 ⚒ 13.1 **FUD** 090  [J] [A2] [50] 🔲

**AMA:** 2017,Jan,8; 2016,Feb,12; 2016,Jan,13; 2015,Jan,16; 2014,Jan,11; 2012,Nov,10

**65815** with removal of blood, with or without irrigation and/or air injection

EXCLUDES Injection only (66020-66030)

Insertion of ocular telescope prosthesis (0308T)

Removal of blood clot only (65930)

🚗 13.5 ⚒ 18.0 **FUD** 090  [J] [A2] [50] 🔲

**AMA:** 2017,Jan,8; 2016,Feb,12; 2016,Jan,13; 2015,Jan,16; 2014,Jan,11; 2012,Nov,10

**65820** Goniotomy

INCLUDES Barkan's operation

Code also ophthalmic endoscope if used (69990)

🚗 21.1 ⚒ 21.1 **FUD** 090  [63] [J] [A2] [80] [50] 🔲

**AMA:** 2017,Jan,8; 2016,Feb,12; 2016,Jan,13; 2015,Jan,16; 2014,Jan,11

**65850** Trabeculotomy ab externo

🚗 23.7 ⚒ 23.7 **FUD** 090  [J] [A2] [50] 🔲

**AMA:** 2016,Feb,12; 2014,Jan,11

**65855** Trabeculoplasty by laser surgery

EXCLUDES Severing adhesions of anterior segment (65860-65880)

Trabeculectomy ab externo (66170)

Code also modifier 22 Increased procedural services, or 52 Reduced services, as appropriate, for re-treatment after several months for advancing disease

🚗 5.90 ⚒ 6.92 **FUD** 010  [T] [P3] [50] 🔲

**AMA:** 2017,Jan,8; 2016,Feb,12; 2016,Jan,13; 2015,Jan,16; 2014,Jan,11; 2012,Jan,15-42

● New Code  ▲ Revised Code  ○ Reinstated  ● New Web Release  ▲ Revised Web Release  Unlisted  Not Covered  # Resequenced
⊘ AMA Mod 51 Exempt  ⑤ Optum Mod 51 Exempt  ⑥ Mod 63 Exempt  ∕ Non-FDA Drug  ★ Telemedicine  Ⓜ Maternity  Ⓐ Age Edit  + Add-on  AMA: CPT Asst

**65860** Severing adhesions of anterior segment, laser technique (separate procedure)

    ⚙ 7.19   ✂ 8.73   **FUD** 090   [T] [P3] [80] [50] [▱]

    **AMA:** 2016,Feb,12; 2014,Jan,11

**65865** Severing adhesions of anterior segment of eye, incisional technique (with or without injection of air or liquid) (separate procedure); goniosynechiae

    *EXCLUDES*   *Laser trabeculectomy (65855)*

    ⚙ 13.4   ✂ 13.4   **FUD** 090   [J] [A2] [50] [▱]

    **AMA:** 2016,Feb,12; 2014,Jan,11

**65870** anterior synechiae, except goniosynechiae

    ⚙ 16.7   ✂ 16.7   **FUD** 090   [J] [A2] [50] [▱]

    **AMA:** 2016,Feb,12; 2014,Jan,11

**65875** posterior synechiae

    Code also ophthalmic endoscope if used (66990)

    ⚙ 17.8   ✂ 17.8   **FUD** 090   [J] [A2] [50] [▱]

    **AMA:** 2017,Jan,8; 2016,Feb,12; 2016,Jan,13; 2015,Jan,16; 2014,Jan,11

**65880** corneovitreal adhesions

    *EXCLUDES*   *Laser procedure (66821)*

    ⚙ 18.8   ✂ 18.8   **FUD** 090   [J] [A2] [50] [▱]

    **AMA:** 2016,Feb,12; 2014,Jan,11

**65900** Removal of epithelial downgrowth, anterior chamber of eye

    ⚙ 27.3   ✂ 27.3   **FUD** 090   [J] [A2] [80] [50] [▱]

    **AMA:** 2016,Feb,12; 2014,Jan,11

**65920** Removal of implanted material, anterior segment of eye

    Code also ophthalmic endoscope if used (66990)

    ⚙ 22.3   ✂ 22.3   **FUD** 090   [J] [A2] [50] [▱]

    **AMA:** 2017,Jan,8; 2016,Feb,12; 2016,Jan,13; 2015,Jan,16; 2014,Jan,11

**65930** Removal of blood clot, anterior segment of eye

    ⚙ 18.0   ✂ 18.0   **FUD** 090   [J] [A2] [50] [▱]

    **AMA:** 2016,Feb,12; 2014,Jan,11

**66020** Injection, anterior chamber of eye (separate procedure); air or liquid

    *EXCLUDES*   *Insertion of ocular telescope prosthesis (0308T)*

    ⚙ 3.72   ✂ 5.27   **FUD** 010   [J] [A2] [50] [▱]

    **AMA:** 2017,Jan,8; 2016,Feb,12; 2016,Jan,13; 2015,Jan,16; 2014,Jan,11; 2012,Nov,10

**66030** medication

    *EXCLUDES*   *Insertion of ocular telescope prosthesis (0308T)*

    ⚙ 3.14   ✂ 4.69   **FUD** 010   [J] [A2] [50] [▱]

    **AMA:** 2016,Feb,12; 2014,Jan,11; 2012,Nov,10

## 66130 Excision Scleral Lesion

  *INCLUDES*   Operating microscope (69990)

  *EXCLUDES*   *Intraocular foreign body removal (65235)*

                *Surgery on posterior sclera (67250, 67255)*

**66130** Excision of lesion, sclera

    ⚙ 16.1   ✂ 19.7   **FUD** 090   [J] [A2] [80] [50] [▱]

    **AMA:** 2016,Feb,12; 2014,Jan,11

## 66150-66185 Procedures for Glaucoma

  *INCLUDES*   Operating microscope (69990)

  *EXCLUDES*   *Intraocular foreign body removal (65235)*

                *Surgery on posterior sclera (67250, 67255)*

**66150** Fistulization of sclera for glaucoma; trephination with iridectomy

    ⚙ 24.8   ✂ 24.8   **FUD** 090   [J] [A2] [50] [▱]

    **AMA:** 2016,Feb,12; 2014,Jan,11

**66155** thermocauterization with iridectomy

    ⚙ 24.8   ✂ 24.8   **FUD** 090   [J] [A2] [50] [▱]

    **AMA:** 2016,Feb,12; 2014,Jan,11

**66160** sclerectomy with punch or scissors, with iridectomy

    *INCLUDES*   Knapp's operation

    ⚙ 27.9   ✂ 27.9   **FUD** 090   [J] [A2] [50] [▱]

    **AMA:** 2016,Feb,12; 2014,Jan,11

**66170** trabeculectomy ab externo in absence of previous surgery

    *EXCLUDES*   *Repair of surgical wound (66250)*

                *Trabeculectomy ab externo (65850)*

    ⚙ 31.0   ✂ 31.0   **FUD** 090   [J] [A2] [80] [50] [▱]

    **AMA:** 2017,Jan,8; 2016,Feb,12; 2016,Jan,13; 2015,Jan,16; 2014,Jan,11; 2012,Dec,12

**66172** trabeculectomy ab externo with scarring from previous ocular surgery or trauma (includes injection of antifibrotic agents)

    ⚙ 33.7   ✂ 33.7   **FUD** 090   [J] [A2] [80] [50] [▱]

    **AMA:** 2017,Jan,8; 2016,Feb,12; 2016,Jan,13; 2015,Jan,16; 2014,Jan,11; 2012,Dec,12

**66174** Transluminal dilation of aqueous outflow canal; without retention of device or stent

    ⚙ 26.8   ✂ 26.8   **FUD** 090   [J] [A2] [80] [50] [▱]

    **AMA:** 2016,Feb,12; 2014,Jan,11

**66175** with retention of device or stent

    ⚙ 28.1   ✂ 28.1   **FUD** 090   [J] [A2] [80] [50] [▱]

    **AMA:** 2016,Feb,12; 2014,Jan,11

**66179** Aqueous shunt to extraocular equatorial plate reservoir, external approach; without graft

    ⚙ 30.5   ✂ 30.5   **FUD** 090   [J] [G2] [80] [50] [▱]

    **AMA:** 2017,Jan,8; 2016,Feb,12; 2016,Jan,13; 2015,Jan,10

**66180** with graft

    *EXCLUDES*   *Scleral reinforcement (67255)*

    ⚙ 32.2   ✂ 32.2   **FUD** 090   [J] [A2] [80] [50] [▱]

    **AMA:** 2017,Jan,8; 2016,Feb,12; 2016,Jan,13; 2015,Jan,10; 2015,Jan,16; 2014,Jan,11; 2012,Jun,15-16

**66183** Insertion of anterior segment aqueous drainage device, without extraocular reservoir, external approach

    ⚙ 29.1   ✂ 29.1   **FUD** 090   [J] [G2] [80] [50] [▱]

    **AMA:** 2017,Jan,8; 2016,Feb,12; 2016,Jan,13; 2015,Jan,16; 2014,May,5; 2014,Jan,11

**66184** Revision of aqueous shunt to extraocular equatorial plate reservoir; without graft

    ⚙ 22.2   ✂ 22.2   **FUD** 090   [J] [G2] [80] [50] [▱]

    **AMA:** 2017,Jan,8; 2016,Feb,12; 2016,Jan,13; 2015,Jan,10

**66185** with graft

    *EXCLUDES*   *Implanted shunt removal (67120)*

                *Scleral reinforcement (67255)*

    ⚙ 23.9   ✂ 23.9   **FUD** 090   [J] [A2] [80] [50] [▱]

    **AMA:** 2017,Jan,8; 2016,Feb,12; 2016,Jan,13; 2015,Jan,10; 2014,Jan,11

## 66220-66225 Staphyloma Repair

  *INCLUDES*   Operating microscope (69990)

  *EXCLUDES*   *Scleral procedures with retinal procedures (67101-67228)*

                *Scleral reinforcement (67250, 67255)*

**66220** Repair of scleral staphyloma; without graft

    ⚙ 20.1   ✂ 20.1   **FUD** 090   [J] [A2] [80] [50] [▱]

    **AMA:** 2016,Feb,12; 2014,Jan,11

**66225** with graft

    ⚙ 26.4   ✂ 26.4   **FUD** 090   [J] [A2] [50] [▱]

    **AMA:** 2016,Feb,12; 2014,Jan,11

## 66250 Anterior Segment Operative Wound Revision or Repair

  *INCLUDES*   Operating microscope (69990)

  *EXCLUDES*   *Unlisted procedures of anterior sclera (66999)*

**66250** Revision or repair of operative wound of anterior segment, any type, early or late, major or minor procedure

    ⚙ 15.8   ✂ 21.1   **FUD** 090   [J] [A2] [50] [▱]

    **AMA:** 2017,Jan,8; 2016,Feb,12; 2016,Jan,13; 2015,Jan,16; 2014,Jan,11; 2012,Jan,15-42

| [26]/[TC] PC/TC Only | [A2]-[Z3] ASC Payment | [50] Bilateral | ♂ Male Only | ♀ Female Only | ⚙ Facility RVU | ✂ Non-Facility RVU | [▱] CCI |
| --- | --- | --- | --- | --- | --- | --- | --- |
| **FUD** Follow-up Days | **CMS:** IOM (Pub 100) | [A]-[Y] OPPSI | | | [80]/[80] Surg Assist Allowed / w/Doc | [▨] Lab crosswalk | [▨] Radiology crosswalk | [✕] CLIA |

300                    CPT © 2017 American Medical Association. All Rights Reserved.         © 2017 Optum360, LLC

## 66500-66505 Iridotomy With/Without Transfixion

INCLUDES Operating microscope (69990)
EXCLUDES *Photocoagulation iridotomy (66761)*

**66500** **Iridotomy by stab incision (separate procedure); except transfixion**
  10.0    10.0    **FUD** 090    [J] [A2] [50] [▢]
  **AMA:** 2016,Feb,12; 2014,Jan,11

**66505** **with transfixion as for iris bombe**
  11.0    11.0    **FUD** 090    [J] [A2] [50] [▢]
  **AMA:** 2016,Feb,12; 2014,Jan,11

## 66600-66635 Iridectomy Procedures

INCLUDES Operating microscope (69990)
EXCLUDES *Insertion of ocular telescope prosthesis (0308T)*
  *Photocoagulation coreoplasty (66762)*

**66600** **Iridectomy, with corneoscleral or corneal section; for removal of lesion**
  23.5    23.5    **FUD** 090    [J] [A2] [50] [▢]
  **AMA:** 2016,Feb,12; 2014,Jan,11

**66605** **with cyclectomy**
  29.9    29.9    **FUD** 090    [J] [A2] [50] [▢]
  **AMA:** 2016,Feb,12; 2014,Jan,11

**66625** **peripheral for glaucoma (separate procedure)**
  12.1    12.1    **FUD** 090    [J] [A2] [50] [▢]
  **AMA:** 2016,Feb,12; 2014,Jan,11

**66630** **sector for glaucoma (separate procedure)**
  16.1    16.1    **FUD** 090    [J] [A2] [50] [▢]
  **AMA:** 2016,Feb,12; 2014,Jan,11

**66635** **optical (separate procedure)**
  16.2    16.2    **FUD** 090    [J] [A2] [50] [▢]
  **AMA:** 2016,Feb,12; 2014,Jan,11

## 66680-66770 Other Procedures of the Uveal Tract

INCLUDES Operating microscope (69990)
EXCLUDES *Unlisted procedures of ciliary body or iris (66999)*

**66680** **Repair of iris, ciliary body (as for iridodialysis)**
  EXCLUDES *Resection or repositioning of uveal tissue for perforating laceration of cornea and/or sclera (65285)*
  14.6    14.6    **FUD** 090    [J] [A2] [50] [▢]
  **AMA:** 2016,Feb,12; 2014,Jan,11

**66682** **Suture of iris, ciliary body (separate procedure) with retrieval of suture through small incision (eg, McCannel suture)**
  18.0    18.0    **FUD** 090    [J] [A2] [50] [▢]
  **AMA:** 2016,Feb,12; 2014,Jan,11

**66700** **Ciliary body destruction; diathermy**
  INCLUDES Heine's operation
  11.1    12.7    **FUD** 090    [J] [A2] [80] [50] [▢]
  **AMA:** 2016,Feb,12; 2014,Jan,11

**66710** **cyclophotocoagulation, transscleral**
  11.1    12.4    **FUD** 090    [J] [A2] [50] [▢]
  **AMA:** 2017,Jan,8; 2016,Feb,12; 2016,Jan,13; 2015,Jan,16; 2014,Jan,11; 2012,Jan,15-42

**66711** **cyclophotocoagulation, endoscopic**
  18.2    18.2    **FUD** 090    [J] [A2] [50] [▢]
  **AMA:** 2017,Jan,8; 2016,Feb,12; 2016,Jan,13; 2015,Jan,16; 2014,Jan,11; 2012,Jan,15-42

**66720** **cryotherapy**
  11.6    13.0    **FUD** 090    [J] [A2] [50] [▢]
  **AMA:** 2016,Feb,12; 2014,Jan,11

**66740** **cyclodialysis**
  11.1    12.3    **FUD** 090    [J] [A2] [50] [▢]
  **AMA:** 2016,Feb,12; 2014,Jan,11

**66761** **Iridotomy/iridectomy by laser surgery (eg, for glaucoma) (per session)**
  EXCLUDES *Insertion of ocular telescope prosthesis (0308T)*
  6.69    8.37    **FUD** 010    [T] [P3] [50] [▢]
  **AMA:** 2017,Jan,8; 2016,Feb,12; 2016,Jan,13; 2015,Jan,16; 2014,Jan,11

**66762** **Iridoplasty by photocoagulation (1 or more sessions) (eg, for improvement of vision, for widening of anterior chamber angle)**
  12.0    13.4    **FUD** 090    [T] [P2] [50] [▢]
  **AMA:** 2017,Jan,8; 2016,Feb,12; 2016,Jan,13; 2015,Jan,16; 2014,Jan,11

**66770** **Destruction of cyst or lesion iris or ciliary body (nonexcisional procedure)**
  EXCLUDES Excision:
    *Epithelial downgrowth (65900)*
    *Iris, ciliary body lesion (66600-66605)*
  13.7    14.9    **FUD** 090    [T] [P2] [50] [▢]
  **AMA:** 2016,Feb,12; 2014,Jan,11

## 66820-66825 Post-Cataract Surgery Procedures

INCLUDES Operating microscope (69990)

**66820** **Discission of secondary membranous cataract (opacified posterior lens capsule and/or anterior hyaloid); stab incision technique (Ziegler or Wheeler knife)**
  11.1    11.1    **FUD** 090    [J] [62] [50] [▢]
  **AMA:** 2016,Feb,12; 2014,Jan,11

Cataract
Iris
Lens

Artificial lens
Cornea
Opaque lens capsule
Iris

An after-cataract is a cataract that develops in a lens tissue that remains after most of the lens has already been removed

**66821** **laser surgery (eg, YAG laser) (1 or more stages)**
  8.81    9.33    **FUD** 090    [T] [A2] [50] [▢]
  **AMA:** 2016,Feb,12; 2014,Jan,11

**66825** **Repositioning of intraocular lens prosthesis, requiring an incision (separate procedure)**
  EXCLUDES *Insertion of ocular telescope prosthesis (0308T)*
  21.5    21.5    **FUD** 090    [J] [A2] [80] [50] [▢]
  **AMA:** 2016,Feb,12; 2014,Jan,11

● New Code    ▲ Revised Code    ○ Reinstated    ● New Web Release    ▲ Revised Web Release    Unlisted    Not Covered    # Resequenced
⊘ AMA Mod 51 Exempt    ⑤ Optum Mod 51 Exempt    ⑥⑨ Mod 63 Exempt    ⁄ Non-FDA Drug    ★ Telemedicine    Ⓜ Maternity    Ⓐ Age Edit    + Add-on    **AMA:** CPT Asst
© 2017 Optum360, LLC    CPT © 2017 American Medical Association. All Rights Reserved.    **301**

## 66830-66940 Cataract Extraction; Without Insertion Intraocular Lens

**CMS:** 100-03,80.10 Phacoemulsification Procedure--Cataract Extraction

INCLUDES Anterior and/or posterior capsulotomy
Enzymatic zonulysis
Iridectomy/iridotomy
Lateral canthotomy
Medications
Operating microscope (69990)
Subconjunctival injection
Subtenon injection
Use of viscoelastic material

EXCLUDES *Removal of intralenticular foreign body without lens excision (65235)*
*Repair of surgical laceration (66250)*

**66830** **Removal of secondary membranous cataract (opacified posterior lens capsule and/or anterior hyaloid) with corneo-scleral section, with or without iridectomy (iridocapsulotomy, iridocapsulectomy)**

INCLUDES Graefe's operation

🚑 20.2 ✂ 20.2 **FUD** 090 J A2 50 ▢

**AMA:** 2016,Feb,12; 2014,Jan,11

A congenital keyhole pupil is also called a coloboma of the iris

**66840** **Removal of lens material; aspiration technique, 1 or more stages**

INCLUDES Fukala's operation

🚑 19.7 ✂ 19.7 **FUD** 090 J A2 50 ▢

**AMA:** 2017,Jan,8; 2016,Sep,9; 2016,Jun,6; 2016,Apr,8; 2016,Feb,12; 2016,Jan,13; 2015,Jan,16; 2014,Jan,11; 2012,Jan,15-42

**66850** **phacofragmentation technique (mechanical or ultrasonic) (eg, phacoemulsification), with aspiration**

🚑 22.4 ✂ 22.4 **FUD** 090 J A2 50 ▢

**AMA:** 2017,Jan,8; 2016,Jun,6; 2016,Feb,12; 2016,Jan,13; 2015,Jan,16; 2014,Jan,11; 2012,Jan,15-42

**66852** **pars plana approach, with or without vitrectomy**

🚑 23.9 ✂ 23.9 **FUD** 090 J A2 80 50 ▢

**AMA:** 2017,Jan,8; 2016,Jun,6; 2016,Feb,12; 2016,Jan,13; 2015,Jan,16; 2014,Jan,11; 2012,Jan,15-42

**66920** **intracapsular**

🚑 21.3 ✂ 21.3 **FUD** 090 J A2 80 50 ▢

**AMA:** 2017,Jan,8; 2016,Feb,12; 2016,Jan,13; 2015,Jan,16; 2014,Jan,11; 2012,Jan,15-42

**66930** **intracapsular, for dislocated lens**

🚑 24.2 ✂ 24.2 **FUD** 090 J A2 80 50 ▢

**AMA:** 2017,Jan,8; 2016,Feb,12; 2016,Jan,13; 2015,Jan,16; 2014,Jan,11; 2012,Jan,15-42

**66940** **extracapsular (other than 66840, 66850, 66852)**

🚑 22.1 ✂ 22.1 **FUD** 090 J A2 80 50 ▢

**AMA:** 2017,Jan,8; 2016,Jun,6; 2016,Feb,12; 2016,Jan,13; 2015,Jan,16; 2014,Jan,11; 2012,Jan,15-42

## 66982-66984 Cataract Extraction: With Insertion Intraocular Lens

**CMS:** 100-03,80.10 Phacoemulsification Procedure--Cataract Extraction; 100-04,32,120.2 PC-IOL and A-C IOL Billing

INCLUDES Anterior or posterior capsulotomy
Enzymatic zonulysis
Iridectomy/iridotomy
Lateral canthotomy
Medications
Operating microscope (69990)
Subconjunctival injection
Subtenon injection
Use of viscoelastic material

EXCLUDES *Implanted material removal from the anterior segment (65920)*
*Insertion of ocular telescope prosthesis (0308T)*
*Ocular telescope prosthesis insertion with lens removal (0308T)*
*Secondary fixation (66682)*
*Supply of intraocular lens*

**66982** **Extracapsular cataract removal with insertion of intraocular lens prosthesis (1-stage procedure), manual or mechanical technique (eg, irrigation and aspiration or phacoemulsification), complex, requiring devices or techniques not generally used in routine cataract surgery (eg, iris expansion device, suture support for intraocular lens, or primary posterior capsulorrhexis) or performed on patients in the amblyogenic developmental stage**

🔀 (76519)

🚑 22.5 ✂ 22.5 **FUD** 090 J A2 50 ▢

**AMA:** 2017,Jan,8; 2016,Mar,10; 2016,Feb,12; 2016,Jan,13; 2015,Jan,16; 2014,Jan,11; 2013,Mar,6-7; 2012,Jan,15-42

**66983** **Intracapsular cataract extraction with insertion of intraocular lens prosthesis (1 stage procedure)**

🔀 (76519)

🚑 21.0 ✂ 21.0 **FUD** 090 J A2 50 ▢

**AMA:** 2017,Jan,8; 2016,Feb,12; 2016,Jan,13; 2015,Jan,16; 2014,Jan,11; 2013,Mar,6-7; 2012,Jan,15-42

**66984** **Extracapsular cataract removal with insertion of intraocular lens prosthesis (1 stage procedure), manual or mechanical technique (eg, irrigation and aspiration or phacoemulsification)**

EXCLUDES *Complex extracapsular cataract removal (66982)*

🔀 (76519)

🚑 18.1 ✂ 18.1 **FUD** 090 J A2 50 ▢

**AMA:** 2017,Jan,8; 2016,Feb,12; 2016,Jan,13; 2015,Jan,16; 2014,Jan,11; 2013,Mar,6-7; 2012,Jan,15-42

## 66985-66986 Secondary Insertion or Replacement of Intraocular Lens

**CMS:** 100-03,80.10 Phacoemulsification Procedure--Cataract Extraction; 100-03,80.12 Intraocular Lenses (IOLs); 100-04,32,120.2 PC-IOL and A-C IOL Billing

INCLUDES Operating microscope (69990)

EXCLUDES *Implanted material removal from the anterior segment (65920)*
*Insertion of ocular telescope prosthesis (0308T)*
*Secondary fixation (66682)*
*Supply of intraocular lens*
Code also ophthalmic endoscope if used (66990)

**66985** **Insertion of intraocular lens prosthesis (secondary implant), not associated with concurrent cataract removal**

EXCLUDES *Insertion of lens at the time of cataract procedure (66982-66984)*

🔀 (76519)

🚑 21.8 ✂ 21.8 **FUD** 090 J A2 50 ▢

**AMA:** 2017,Jan,8; 2016,Feb,12; 2016,Jan,13; 2015,Jan,16; 2014,Jan,11; 2013,Mar,6-7; 2012,Jan,15-42

**66986** **Exchange of intraocular lens**

🔀 (76519)

🚑 25.7 ✂ 25.7 **FUD** 090 J A2 50 ▢

**AMA:** 2017,Jan,8; 2016,Feb,12; 2016,Jan,13; 2015,Jan,16; 2014,Jan,11

26/TC PC/TC Only    A2-Z3 ASC Payment    50 Bilateral    ♂ Male Only    ♀ Female Only    🚑 Facility RVU    ✂ Non-Facility RVU    ▢ CCI
**FUD** Follow-up Days    **CMS:** IOM (Pub 100)    A-Y OPPSI    80/80 Surg Assist Allowed / w/Doc    Lab crosswalk    🔀 Radiology crosswalk    🗙 CLIA

302

CPT © 2017 American Medical Association. All Rights Reserved.      © 2017 Optum360, LLC

## 66990-66999 Ophthalmic Endoscopy

INCLUDES    Operating microscope (69990)

+    **66990**    **Use of ophthalmic endoscope (List separately in addition to code for primary procedure)**
Code first (65820, 65875, 65920, 66985-66986, 67036, 67039-67043, 67113)
🚗 2.57    ⚕ 2.57    **FUD** ZZZ                                 N M1 ▣
**AMA:** 2017,Jan,8; 2016,Sep,5; 2016,Feb,12; 2016,Jan,13; 2015,Jan,16; 2014,Jan,11; 2012,Jan,15-42

**66999**    **Unlisted procedure, anterior segment of eye**
🚗 0.00    ⚕ 0.00    **FUD** YYY                                 J 80 50
**AMA:** 2017,Jan,8; 2016,Apr,8; 2016,Feb,12; 2016,Jan,13; 2015,Jan,16; 2014,Jan,11

## 67005-67015 Vitrectomy: Partial and Subtotal

INCLUDES    Operating microscope (69990)

**67005**    **Removal of vitreous, anterior approach (open sky technique or limbal incision); partial removal**
EXCLUDES    *Anterior chamber vitrectomy by paracentesis (65810)*
*Severing of corneovitreal adhesions (65880)*
🚗 13.3    ⚕ 13.3    **FUD** 090                                 J A2 50 ▣
**AMA:** 2017,Jan,8; 2016,Feb,12; 2016,Jan,13; 2015,Jan,16; 2014,Jan,11

**67010**    **subtotal removal with mechanical vitrectomy**
EXCLUDES    *Anterior chamber vitrectomy by paracentesis (65810)*
*Severing of corneovitreal adhesions (65880)*
🚗 15.3    ⚕ 15.3    **FUD** 090                                 J A2 50 ▣
**AMA:** 2017,Jan,8; 2016,Feb,12; 2016,Jan,13; 2015,Jan,16; 2014,Jan,11

**67015**    **Aspiration or release of vitreous, subretinal or choroidal fluid, pars plana approach (posterior sclerotomy)**
🚗 16.4    ⚕ 16.4    **FUD** 090                                 J A2 50 ▣
**AMA:** 2017,Jan,8; 2016,Sep,5; 2016,Jun,6; 2016,Feb,12; 2014,Jan,11

## 67025-67028 Intravitreal Injection/Implantation

INCLUDES    Operating microscope (69990)

**67025**    **Injection of vitreous substitute, pars plana or limbal approach (fluid-gas exchange), with or without aspiration (separate procedure)**
🚗 17.9    ⚕ 20.5    **FUD** 090                                 J A2 50 ▣
**AMA:** 2016,Feb,12; 2014,Jan,11

**67027**    **Implantation of intravitreal drug delivery system (eg, ganciclovir implant), includes concomitant removal of vitreous**
EXCLUDES    *Removal of drug delivery system (67121)*
🚗 24.1    ⚕ 24.1    **FUD** 090                                 J A2 80 50 ▣
**AMA:** 2017,Jan,8; 2016,Feb,12; 2016,Jan,13; 2015,Jan,16; 2014,Jan,11; 2012,Jan,15-42

**67028**    **Intravitreal injection of a pharmacologic agent (separate procedure)**
🚗 2.85    ⚕ 2.89    **FUD** 000                                 S P3 50 ▣
**AMA:** 2017,Jan,8; 2016,Feb,12; 2016,Jan,13; 2015,Jan,16; 2014,Jan,11; 2012,Oct,14

## 67030-67031 Incision of Vitreous Strands/Membranes

INCLUDES    Operating microscope (69990)

**67030**    **Discission of vitreous strands (without removal), pars plana approach**
🚗 15.0    ⚕ 15.0    **FUD** 090                                 J A2 50 ▣
**AMA:** 2016,Feb,12; 2014,Jan,11

**67031**    **Severing of vitreous strands, vitreous face adhesions, sheets, membranes or opacities, laser surgery (1 or more stages)**
🚗 10.1    ⚕ 11.0    **FUD** 090                                 T A2 50 ▣
**AMA:** 2016,Feb,12; 2014,Jan,11

## 67036-67043 Pars Plana Mechanical Vitrectomy

INCLUDES    Operating microscope (69990)
EXCLUDES    *Foreign body removal (65260, 65265)*
*Lens removal (66850)*
*Unlisted vitreal procedures (67299)*
*Vitrectomy in retinal detachment (67108, 67113)*
Code also ophthalmic endoscope if used (66990)

**67036**    **Vitrectomy, mechanical, pars plana approach;**
Code also placement of intraocular radiation source applicator (0190T)
🚗 25.5    ⚕ 25.5    **FUD** 090                                 J A2 80 50
**AMA:** 2017,Jan,8; 2016,Sep,5; 2016,Feb,12; 2016,Jan,13; 2015,Jan,16; 2014,Jan,11

**67039**    **with focal endolaser photocoagulation**
🚗 27.3    ⚕ 27.3    **FUD** 090                                 J A2 80 50 ▣
**AMA:** 2017,Jan,8; 2016,Sep,5; 2016,Feb,12; 2016,Jan,13; 2015,Jan,16; 2014,Jan,11; 2012,Jan,15-42

**67040**    **with endolaser panretinal photocoagulation**
🚗 29.5    ⚕ 29.5    **FUD** 090                                 J A2 80 50 ▣
**AMA:** 2017,Jan,8; 2016,Sep,5; 2016,Feb,12; 2016,Jan,13; 2015,Jan,16; 2014,Jan,11; 2012,Jan,15-42

**67041**    **with removal of preretinal cellular membrane (eg, macular pucker)**
🚗 32.6    ⚕ 32.6    **FUD** 090                                 J 62 80 50 ▣
**AMA:** 2017,Jan,8; 2016,Sep,5; 2016,Feb,12; 2016,Jan,13; 2015,Jan,16; 2014,Jan,11

**67042**    **with removal of internal limiting membrane of retina (eg, for repair of macular hole, diabetic macular edema), includes, if performed, intraocular tamponade (ie, air, gas or silicone oil)**
🚗 32.6    ⚕ 32.6    **FUD** 090                                 J 62 80 50 ▣
**AMA:** 2017,Jan,8; 2016,Sep,5; 2016,Feb,12; 2016,Jan,13; 2015,Jan,16; 2014,Jan,11

**67043**    **with removal of subretinal membrane (eg, choroidal neovascularization), includes, if performed, intraocular tamponade (ie, air, gas or silicone oil) and laser photocoagulation**
🚗 34.5    ⚕ 34.5    **FUD** 090                                 J 62 80 50 ▣
**AMA:** 2017,Jan,8; 2016,Sep,5; 2016,Feb,12; 2016,Jan,13; 2015,Jan,16; 2014,Jan,11

## 67101-67115 Detached Retina Repair

INCLUDES    Operating microscope (69990)
Primary technique when cryotherapy and/or diathermy and/or photocoagulation are used in combination

**67101**    **Repair of retinal detachment, including drainage of subretinal fluid when performed; cryotherapy**
🚗 8.07    ⚕ 9.28    **FUD** 010                                 J P3 50 ▣
**AMA:** 2017,Feb,14; 2017,Jan,8; 2016,Sep,5; 2016,Jun,6; 2016,Feb,12; 2016,Jan,13; 2015,Jan,16; 2014,Jan,11

Optic nerve

Vitreous

Optic disc

Choroid

Sclera

Retina

Posterior chamber    Pars plana

● New Code    ▲ Revised Code    ○ Reinstated    ● New Web Release    ▲ Revised Web Release    Unlisted    Not Covered    # Resequenced
⊘ AMA Mod 51 Exempt    ⑤ Optum Mod 51 Exempt    ⊛ Mod 63 Exempt    ✗ Non-FDA Drug    ★ Telemedicine    M Maternity    ⚠ Age Edit    + Add-on    **AMA:** CPT Asst
© 2017 Optum360, LLC                              CPT © 2017 American Medical Association. All Rights Reserved.                              **303**

**Eye, Ocular Adnexa, and Ear**

**67105 — 67229**

| | |
|---|---|

**67105**      photocoagulation
🚗 7.80   ✂ 8.40   **FUD** 010                    T P3 50
**AMA:** 2017,Feb,14; 2017,Jan,8; 2016,Sep,5; 2016,Jun,6; 2016,Feb,12; 2016,Jan,13; 2015,Jan,16; 2014,Jan,11

**67107**   Repair of retinal detachment; scleral buckling (such as lamellar scleral dissection, imbrication or encircling procedure), including, when performed, implant, cryotherapy, photocoagulation, and drainage of subretinal fluid
INCLUDES    Gonin's operation
🚗 32.1   ✂ 32.1   **FUD** 090          J 62 80 50
**AMA:** 2017,Jan,8; 2016,Sep,5; 2016,Jun,6; 2016,Feb,12; 2014,Jan,11

**67108**   with vitrectomy, any method, including, when performed, air or gas tamponade, focal endolaser photocoagulation, cryotherapy, drainage of subretinal fluid, scleral buckling, and/or removal of lens by same technique
🚗 34.0   ✂ 34.0   **FUD** 090          J 62 80 50
**AMA:** 2017,Jan,8; 2016,Sep,5; 2016,Jun,6; 2016,Feb,12; 2016,Jan,13; 2015,Jan,16; 2014,Jan,11; 2012,Mar,9-10; 2012,Jan,15-42

**67110**   by injection of air or other gas (eg, pneumatic retinopexy)
🚗 23.0   ✂ 24.8   **FUD** 090          J P3 50
**AMA:** 2017,Jan,8; 2016,Sep,5; 2016,Jun,6; 2016,Feb,12; 2014,Jan,11

**67113**   Repair of complex retinal detachment (eg, proliferative vitreoretinopathy, stage C-1 or greater, diabetic traction retinal detachment, retinopathy of prematurity, retinal tear of greater than 90 degrees), with vitrectomy and membrane peeling, including, when performed, air, gas, or silicone oil tamponade, cryotherapy, endolaser photocoagulation, drainage of subretinal fluid, scleral buckling, and/or removal of lens
EXCLUDES    Vitrectomy for other than retinal detachment, pars plana approach (67036-67043)
Code also ophthalmic endoscope if used (66990)
🚗 38.0   ✂ 38.0   **FUD** 090          J 62 80 50
**AMA:** 2017,Jan,8; 2016,Sep,5; 2016,Jun,6; 2016,Feb,12; 2016,Jan,13; 2015,Jan,16; 2014,Jan,11

**67115**   Release of encircling material (posterior segment)
🚗 14.1   ✂ 14.1   **FUD** 090          J A2 50
**AMA:** 2016,Feb,12; 2014,Jan,11

## 67120-67121 Removal of Previously Implanted Prosthetic Device
INCLUDES    Operating microscope (69990)
EXCLUDES    Foreign body removal (65260, 65265)
Removal of implanted material anterior segment (65920)

**67120**   Removal of implanted material, posterior segment; extraocular
🚗 15.8   ✂ 18.6   **FUD** 090          J A2 50
**AMA:** 2016,Feb,12; 2014,Jan,11

**67121**   intraocular
🚗 25.7   ✂ 25.7   **FUD** 090          J A2 80 50
**AMA:** 2016,Feb,12; 2014,Jan,11

## 67141-67145 Retinal Detachment: Preventative Procedures
INCLUDES    Operating microscope (69990)
Treatment at one or more sessions that may occur at different encounters
EXCLUDES    Procedure performed more than one time during a defined period of treatment

**67141**   Prophylaxis of retinal detachment (eg, retinal break, lattice degeneration) without drainage, 1 or more sessions; cryotherapy, diathermy
🚗 13.8   ✂ 14.8   **FUD** 090          T A2 50
**AMA:** 2017,Jan,8; 2016,Sep,5; 2016,Feb,12; 2016,Jan,13; 2015,Jan,16; 2014,Jan,11

**67145**   photocoagulation (laser or xenon arc)
🚗 14.1   ✂ 14.9   **FUD** 090          T P2 50
**AMA:** 2017,Jan,8; 2016,Sep,5; 2016,Feb,12; 2016,Jan,13; 2015,Jan,16; 2014,Jan,11

## 67208-67218 Destruction of Retinal Lesions
INCLUDES    Operating microscope (69990)
Treatment at one or more sessions that may occur at different encounters
EXCLUDES    Procedure performed more than one time during a defined period of treatment
Unlisted retinal procedures (67299)

**67208**   Destruction of localized lesion of retina (eg, macular edema, tumors), 1 or more sessions; cryotherapy, diathermy
🚗 16.4   ✂ 16.9   **FUD** 090          T P2 50
**AMA:** 2017,Jan,8; 2016,Feb,12; 2016,Jan,13; 2015,Jan,16; 2014,Jan,11

**67210**   photocoagulation
🚗 14.1   ✂ 14.6   **FUD** 090          T P2 50
**AMA:** 2017,Jan,8; 2016,Feb,12; 2016,Jan,13; 2015,Jan,16; 2014,Jan,11; 2012,Jan,3-5

**67218**   radiation by implantation of source (includes removal of source)
🚗 39.2   ✂ 39.2   **FUD** 090          J A2 50
**AMA:** 2017,Jan,8; 2016,Feb,12; 2016,Jan,13; 2015,Jan,16; 2014,Jan,11

## 67220-67225 Destruction of Choroidal Lesions
INCLUDES    Operating microscope (69990)

**67220**   Destruction of localized lesion of choroid (eg, choroidal neovascularization); photocoagulation (eg, laser), 1 or more sessions
INCLUDES    Treatment at one or more sessions that may occur at different encounters
EXCLUDES    Procedure performed more than one time during a defined period of treatment
🚗 14.1   ✂ 15.1   **FUD** 090          T P2 50
**AMA:** 2017,Jan,8; 2016,Feb,12; 2016,Jan,13; 2015,Jan,16; 2014,Jan,11; 2012,Jan,3-5; 2012,Jan,15-42

**67221**   photodynamic therapy (includes intravenous infusion)
🚗 6.07   ✂ 8.12   **FUD** 000          T P3
**AMA:** 2017,Jan,8; 2016,Feb,12; 2016,Jan,13; 2015,Jan,16; 2014,Jan,11; 2012,Jan,15-42

\+ **67225**   photodynamic therapy, second eye, at single session (List separately in addition to code for primary eye treatment)
Code first (67221)
🚗 0.80   ✂ 0.84   **FUD** ZZZ                    N N1
**AMA:** 2017,Jan,8; 2016,Feb,12; 2016,Jan,13; 2015,Jan,16; 2014,Jan,11; 2012,Jan,15-42

## 67227-67229 Destruction Retinopathy
INCLUDES    Operating microscope (69990)
EXCLUDES    Unlisted retinal procedures (67299)

**67227**   Destruction of extensive or progressive retinopathy (eg, diabetic retinopathy), cryotherapy, diathermy
🚗 7.29   ✂ 8.21   **FUD** 010          J 62 50
**AMA:** 2017,Jan,8; 2016,Feb,12; 2016,Jan,13; 2015,Jan,16; 2014,Jan,11; 2012,Jan,15-42

**67228**   Treatment of extensive or progressive retinopathy (eg, diabetic retinopathy), photocoagulation
🚗 8.72   ✂ 9.65   **FUD** 010          T P3 50
**AMA:** 2017,Jan,8; 2016,Feb,12; 2016,Jan,13; 2015,Jan,16; 2014,Jan,11

**67229**   Treatment of extensive or progressive retinopathy, 1 or more sessions, preterm infant (less than 37 weeks gestation at birth), performed from birth up to 1 year of age (eg, retinopathy of prematurity), photocoagulation or cryotherapy
INCLUDES    Treatment at one or more sessions that may occur at different encounters
EXCLUDES    Procedure performed more than one time during a defined period of treatment
🚗 33.0   ✂ 33.0   **FUD** 090          T R2 50
**AMA:** 2017,Jan,8; 2016,Feb,12; 2016,Jan,13; 2015,Jan,16; 2014,Jan,11

 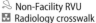

## 67250-67255 Reinforcement of Posterior Sclera

INCLUDES  Operating microscope (69990)
EXCLUDES  Removal of lesion of sclera (66130)
          Repair scleral staphyloma (66220, 66225)

**67250**  **Scleral reinforcement (separate procedure); without graft**
    22.1    22.1  **FUD** 090     J A2 50 🗅
    **AMA:** 2016,Feb,12; 2014,Jan,11

**67255**  **with graft**
    EXCLUDES  *Aqueous shunt to extraocular equatorial plate reservoir (66180)*
           *Revision of aqueous shunt to extraocular equatorial plate reservoir; with graft (66185)*
    19.3    19.3  **FUD** 090     J A2 80 50 🗅
    **AMA:** 2017,Jan,8; 2016,Feb,12; 2016,Jan,13; 2015,Jan,16; 2015,Jan,10; 2014,Jan,11; 2012,Jun,15-16

## 67299 Unlisted Posterior Segment Procedure

CMS: 100-04,4,180.3 Unlisted Service or Procedure
INCLUDES  Operating microscope (69990)

**67299**  **Unlisted procedure, posterior segment**
    0.00    0.00  **FUD** YYY     J 80 50 🗅
    **AMA:** 2017,Jan,8; 2016,Feb,12; 2016,Jan,13; 2015,Jan,16; 2014,Jan,11; 2012,Jan,15-42

## 67311-67334 Strabismus Procedures on Extraocular Muscles

INCLUDES  Operating microscope (69990)
Code also adjustable sutures (67335)

**67311**  **Strabismus surgery, recession or resection procedure; 1 horizontal muscle**
    16.9    16.9  **FUD** 090     J A2 50 🗅
    **AMA:** 2017,Jan,6; 2017,Jan,8; 2016,Feb,12; 2016,Jan,13; 2015,Jan,16; 2014,Jan,11; 2012,Jan,15-42

Superior oblique
Superior rectus
Lateral rectus
Inferior oblique
Inferior rectus
Medial rectus (not shown)

**Muscles of the eyeball (right eye shown)**

**67312**  **2 horizontal muscles**
    20.1    20.1  **FUD** 090     J A2 50 🗅
    **AMA:** 2017,Jan,8; 2016,Feb,12; 2016,Jan,13; 2015,Jan,16; 2014,Jan,11; 2012,Jan,15-42

**67314**  **1 vertical muscle (excluding superior oblique)**
    19.0    19.0  **FUD** 090     J A2 50 🗅
    **AMA:** 2017,Jan,8; 2016,Feb,12; 2016,Jan,13; 2015,Jan,16; 2014,Jan,11

**67316**  **2 or more vertical muscles (excluding superior oblique)**
    22.7    22.7  **FUD** 090     J A2 80 50 🗅
    **AMA:** 2017,Jan,8; 2016,Feb,12; 2016,Jan,13; 2015,Jan,16; 2014,Jan,11

**67318**  **Strabismus surgery, any procedure, superior oblique muscle**
    20.0    20.0  **FUD** 090     J A2 50 🗅
    **AMA:** 2017,Jan,8; 2016,Feb,12; 2016,Jan,13; 2015,Jan,16; 2014,Jan,11

**+ 67320**  **Transposition procedure (eg, for paretic extraocular muscle), any extraocular muscle (specify) (List separately in addition to code for primary procedure)**
    Code first (67311-67318)
    9.17    9.17  **FUD** ZZZ     N M1 🗅
    **AMA:** 2017,Jan,8; 2016,Feb,12; 2016,Jan,13; 2015,Jan,16; 2014,Jan,11

**+ 67331**  **Strabismus surgery on patient with previous eye surgery or injury that did not involve the extraocular muscles (List separately in addition to code for primary procedure)**
    Code first (67311-67318)
    8.71    8.71  **FUD** ZZZ     N M1 50 🗅
    **AMA:** 2017,Jan,8; 2016,Feb,12; 2016,Jan,13; 2015,Jan,16; 2014,Jan,11

**+ 67332**  **Strabismus surgery on patient with scarring of extraocular muscles (eg, prior ocular injury, strabismus or retinal detachment surgery) or restrictive myopathy (eg, dysthyroid ophthalmopathy) (List separately in addition to code for primary procedure)**
    Code first (67311-67318)
    9.45    9.45  **FUD** ZZZ     N M1 50 🗅
    **AMA:** 2017,Jan,8; 2016,Feb,12; 2016,Jan,13; 2015,Jan,16; 2014,Jan,11

**+ 67334**  **Strabismus surgery by posterior fixation suture technique, with or without muscle recession (List separately in addition to code for primary procedure)**
    Code first (67311-67318)
    8.58    8.58  **FUD** ZZZ     N M1 50 🗅
    **AMA:** 2017,Jan,8; 2016,Feb,12; 2016,Jan,13; 2015,Jan,16; 2014,Jan,11

## 67335-67399 Other Procedures of Extraocular Muscles

INCLUDES  Operating microscope (69990)

**+ 67335**  **Placement of adjustable suture(s) during strabismus surgery, including postoperative adjustment(s) of suture(s) (List separately in addition to code for specific strabismus surgery)**
    Code first (67311-67334)
    4.23    4.23  **FUD** ZZZ     N M1 50 🗅
    **AMA:** 2017,Jan,8; 2016,Feb,12; 2016,Jan,13; 2015,Jan,16; 2014,Jan,11

**+ 67340**  **Strabismus surgery involving exploration and/or repair of detached extraocular muscle(s) (List separately in addition to code for primary procedure)**
    INCLUDES  Hummelsheim operation
    Code first (67311-67334)
    10.2    10.2  **FUD** ZZZ     N M1 80 🗅
    **AMA:** 2017,Jan,8; 2016,Feb,12; 2016,Jan,13; 2015,Jan,16; 2014,Jan,11

**67343**  **Release of extensive scar tissue without detaching extraocular muscle (separate procedure)**
    Code also if these procedures are performed on other than the affected muscle (67311-67340)
    18.5    18.5  **FUD** 090     J A2 50 🗅
    **AMA:** 2017,Jan,8; 2016,Feb,12; 2016,Jan,13; 2015,Jan,16; 2014,Jan,11

**67345**  **Chemodenervation of extraocular muscle**
    EXCLUDES  *Nerve destruction for blepharospasm and other neurological disorders (64612, 64616)*
    6.20    6.87  **FUD** 010     T P3 50 🗅
    **AMA:** 2017,Jan,8; 2016,Feb,12; 2016,Jan,13; 2015,Jan,16; 2014,May,5; 2014,Jan,11; 2013,Dec,10; 2012,Jan,15-42

**67346**  **Biopsy of extraocular muscle**
    EXCLUDES  *Repair laceration extraocular muscle, tendon, or Tenon's capsule (65290)*
    5.51    5.51  **FUD** 000     J A2 80 50 🗅
    **AMA:** 2016,Feb,12; 2014,Jan,11

**67399**  **Unlisted procedure, extraocular muscle**
    0.00    0.00  **FUD** YYY     T 80 50
    **AMA:** 2017,Jul,10; 2016,Feb,12; 2014,Jan,11

---

● New Code  ▲ Revised Code  ○ Reinstated  ● New Web Release  ▲ Revised Web Release  Unlisted  Not Covered  # Resequenced
Ⓢ AMA Mod 51 Exempt  Ⓢ Optum Mod 51 Exempt  Ⓢ Mod 63 Exempt  ✗ Non-FDA Drug  ★ Telemedicine  M Maternity  A Age Edit  + Add-on  AMA: CPT Asst

**Eye, Ocular Adnexa, and Ear** *(side tab)*

**67400 — 67808** *(side tab)*

## 67400-67415 Frontal Orbitotomy

INCLUDES    Operating microscope (69990)

**67400**    **Orbitotomy without bone flap (frontal or transconjunctival approach); for exploration, with or without biopsy**
     26.3    26.3    **FUD** 090        J A2 50
     **AMA:** 2016,Feb,12; 2014,Jan,11

**67405**    **with drainage only**
     22.4    22.4    **FUD** 090        J A2 50
     **AMA:** 2017,Jan,8; 2016,Feb,12; 2016,Jan,13; 2015,Jan,16; 2014,Jan,11; 2012,Jan,15-42

**67412**    **with removal of lesion**
     24.0    24.0    **FUD** 090        J A2 50
     **AMA:** 2016,Feb,12; 2014,Jan,11

**67413**    **with removal of foreign body**
     24.1    24.1    **FUD** 090        J A2 80 50
     **AMA:** 2016,Feb,12; 2014,Jan,11

**67414**    **with removal of bone for decompression**
     37.6    37.6    **FUD** 090        G2 80 50
     **AMA:** 2017,Jan,8; 2016,Feb,12; 2016,Jan,13; 2015,Jan,16; 2014,Jan,11; 2012,Jan,15-42

**67415**    **Fine needle aspiration of orbital contents**
     EXCLUDES   Decompression optic nerve (67570)
                Exenteration, enucleation, and repair (65101-65175)
     2.99    2.99    **FUD** 000        J A2 80 50
     **AMA:** 2016,Feb,12; 2014,Jan,11

## 67420-67450 Lateral Orbitotomy

INCLUDES    Operating microscope (69990)
EXCLUDES    Orbital implant (67550, 67560)
            Surgical removal of all or some of the orbital contents or repair after removal (65091-65175)
            Transcranial approach orbitotomy (61330-61333)

**67420**    **Orbitotomy with bone flap or window, lateral approach (eg, Kroenlein); with removal of lesion**
     45.8    45.8    **FUD** 090        J A2 80 50
     **AMA:** 2016,Feb,12; 2014,Jan,11

**67430**    **with removal of foreign body**
     35.0    35.0    **FUD** 090        J A2 80 50
     **AMA:** 2016,Feb,12; 2014,Jan,11

**67440**    **with drainage**
     34.1    34.1    **FUD** 090        J A2 80 50
     **AMA:** 2016,Feb,12; 2014,Jan,11

**67445**    **with removal of bone for decompression**
     EXCLUDES   Decompression optic nerve sheath (67570)
     39.7    39.7    **FUD** 090        J A2 80 50
     **AMA:** 2016,Feb,12; 2014,Jan,11

**67450**    **for exploration, with or without biopsy**
     35.4    35.4    **FUD** 090        J A2 80 50
     **AMA:** 2016,Feb,12; 2014,Jan,11

## 67500-67515 Eye Injections

INCLUDES    Operating microscope (69990)

**67500**    **Retrobulbar injection; medication (separate procedure, does not include supply of medication)**
     2.04    2.22    **FUD** 000        T G2 50
     **AMA:** 2017,Jan,8; 2016,Feb,12; 2016,Jan,13; 2015,Jan,16; 2014,Jan,11; 2012,Nov,10

**67505**    **alcohol**
     2.30    2.51    **FUD** 000        T P3 50
     **AMA:** 2016,Feb,12; 2014,Jan,11

**67515**    **Injection of medication or other substance into Tenon's capsule**
     EXCLUDES   Subconjunctival injection (68200)
     2.54    2.75    **FUD** 000        T P3 50
     **AMA:** 2017,Jan,8; 2016,Feb,12; 2016,Jan,13; 2015,Jan,16; 2014,Jan,11; 2012,Nov,10

## 67550-67560 Orbital Implant

INCLUDES    Operating microscope (69990)
EXCLUDES    Fracture repair malar area, orbit (21355-21408)
            Ocular implant inside muscle cone (65093-65105, 65130-65175)

**67550**    **Orbital implant (implant outside muscle cone); insertion**
     27.3    27.3    **FUD** 090        J A2 50
     **AMA:** 2016,Feb,12; 2014,Jan,11

**67560**    **removal or revision**
     27.9    27.9    **FUD** 090        J A2 80 50
     **AMA:** 2016,Feb,12; 2014,Jan,11

## 67570-67599 Other and Unlisted Orbital Procedures

INCLUDES    Operating microscope (69990)

**67570**    **Optic nerve decompression (eg, incision or fenestration of optic nerve sheath)**
     33.0    33.0    **FUD** 090        J A2 80 50
     **AMA:** 2016,Feb,12; 2014,Jan,11

**67599**    **Unlisted procedure, orbit**
     0.00    0.00    **FUD** YYY        T 80 50
     **AMA:** 2016,Feb,12; 2014,Jan,11

## 67700-67715 [67810] Incisional Procedures of Eyelids

INCLUDES    Operating microscope (69990)

**67700**    **Blepharotomy, drainage of abscess, eyelid**
     3.30    7.56    **FUD** 010        T P2 50
     **AMA:** 2017,Jan,8; 2016,Feb,12; 2016,Jan,13; 2015,Jan,16; 2014,Jan,11; 2013,Mar,6-7

**67710**    **Severing of tarsorrhaphy**
     2.75    6.29    **FUD** 010        T P3 50
     **AMA:** 2017,Jan,8; 2016,Feb,12; 2016,Jan,13; 2015,Jan,16; 2014,Jan,11; 2013,Mar,6-7

**67715**    **Canthotomy (separate procedure)**
     EXCLUDES   Canthoplasty (67950)
            Symblepharon division (68340)
     3.07    6.75    **FUD** 010        J A2 50
     **AMA:** 2017,Jan,8; 2016,Feb,12; 2016,Jan,13; 2015,Jan,16; 2014,Jan,11; 2013,Mar,6-7

**#**    **67810**    **Incisional biopsy of eyelid skin including lid margin**
     EXCLUDES   Biopsy of eyelid skin (11100-11101, 11310-11313)
     2.06    4.87    **FUD** 000        T P3 50
     **AMA:** 2017,Jan,8; 2016,Feb,12; 2016,Jan,13; 2015,Jan,16; 2014,Jan,11; 2013,Mar,6-7; 2013,Feb,16-17; 2012,Jan,15-42

## 67800-67808 Excision of Chalazion (Meibomian Cyst)

INCLUDES    Lesion removal requiring more than skin:
            Lid margin
            Palpebral conjunctiva
            Tarsus
       Operating microscope (69990)
EXCLUDES    Blepharoplasty, graft, or reconstructive procedures (67930-67975)
            Excision/destruction skin lesion of eyelid (11310-11313, 11440-11446, 11640-11646, 17000-17004)

**67800**    **Excision of chalazion; single**
     2.94    3.58    **FUD** 010        T P3
     **AMA:** 2017,Jan,8; 2016,Feb,12; 2016,Jan,13; 2015,Jan,16; 2014,Jan,11; 2013,Mar,6-7; 2012,Jan,15-42

**67801**    **multiple, same lid**
     3.78    4.58    **FUD** 010        T P3
     **AMA:** 2016,Feb,12; 2014,Jan,11; 2013,Mar,6-7

**67805**    **multiple, different lids**
     4.67    5.69    **FUD** 010        T P3
     **AMA:** 2017,Jan,8; 2016,Feb,12; 2016,Jan,13; 2015,Jan,16; 2014,Jan,11; 2013,Mar,6-7; 2012,Jan,15-42

**67808**    **under general anesthesia and/or requiring hospitalization, single or multiple**
     10.4    10.4    **FUD** 090        J A2
     **AMA:** 2016,Feb,12; 2014,Jan,11; 2013,Mar,6-7

## 67810-67850 Other Eyelid Procedures

INCLUDES   Operating microscope (69990)

**67810**     Resequenced code. See code following 67715.

**67820**     Correction of trichiasis; epilation, by forceps only

      1.51   1.42  **FUD** 000     Q1 N1 50

      **AMA:** 2017,Jan,8; 2016,Feb,12; 2016,Jan,13; 2015,Jan,16; 2014,Jan,11; 2012,Jan,15-42

**67825**     epilation by other than forceps (eg, by electrosurgery, cryotherapy, laser surgery)

      3.44   3.63  **FUD** 010     T P3 50

      **AMA:** 2017,Jan,8; 2016,Feb,12; 2016,Jan,13; 2015,Jan,16; 2014,Jan,11; 2012,Jan,15-42

**67830**     incision of lid margin

      3.91   7.49  **FUD** 010     T A2 50

      **AMA:** 2016,Feb,12; 2014,Jan,11

**67835**     incision of lid margin, with free mucous membrane graft

      12.4   12.4  **FUD** 090     J A2 80 50

      **AMA:** 2016,Feb,12; 2014,Jan,11

**67840**     Excision of lesion of eyelid (except chalazion) without closure or with simple direct closure

      EXCLUDES   *Eyelid resection and reconstruction (67961, 67966)*

      4.49   7.76  **FUD** 010     T P3 50

      **AMA:** 2016,Feb,12; 2014,Jan,11

**67850**     Destruction of lesion of lid margin (up to 1 cm)

      EXCLUDES   *Mohs micro procedures (17311-17315)*
               *Topical chemotherapy (99201-99215)*

      3.87   6.08  **FUD** 010     T P3 50

      **AMA:** 2016,Feb,12; 2014,Jan,11

## 67875-67882 Suturing of the Eyelids

INCLUDES   Operating microscope (69990)
EXCLUDES   *Canthoplasty (67950)*
           *Canthotomy (67715)*
           *Severing of tarsorrhaphy (67710)*

**67875**     Temporary closure of eyelids by suture (eg, Frost suture)

      2.77   4.84  **FUD** 000     T G2 50

      **AMA:** 2016,Feb,12; 2014,Jan,11

**67880**     Construction of intermarginal adhesions, median tarsorrhaphy, or canthorrhaphy;

      10.4   12.9  **FUD** 090     J A2 50

      **AMA:** 2016,Feb,12; 2014,Jan,11

**67882**     with transposition of tarsal plate

      13.3   15.9  **FUD** 090     J A2 50

      **AMA:** 2016,Feb,12; 2014,Jan,11

## 67900-67912 Repair of Ptosis/Retraction Eyelids, Eyebrows

INCLUDES   Operating microscope (69990)

**67900**     Repair of brow ptosis (supraciliary, mid-forehead or coronal approach)

      EXCLUDES   *Forehead rhytidectomy (15824)*

      14.4   18.1  **FUD** 090     J A2 50

      **AMA:** 2017,Jan,8; 2016,Feb,12; 2016,Jan,13; 2015,Jan,16; 2014,Jan,11; 2012,Jan,15-42

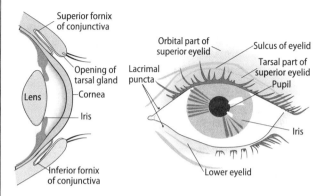

Superior fornix of conjunctiva — Orbital part of superior eyelid — Sulcus of eyelid — Tarsal part of superior eyelid — Pupil — Opening of tarsal gland — Lacrimal puncta — Cornea — Lens — Iris — Iris — Inferior fornix of conjunctiva — Lower eyelid

**67901**     Repair of blepharoptosis; frontalis muscle technique with suture or other material (eg, banked fascia)

      16.3   21.3  **FUD** 090     J A2 50

      **AMA:** 2017,Jul,10; 2017,Jan,8; 2016,Feb,12; 2016,Jan,13; 2015,Jan,16; 2014,Jan,11

**67902**     frontalis muscle technique with autologous fascial sling (includes obtaining fascia)

      20.5   20.5  **FUD** 090     J A2 50

      **AMA:** 2017,Jan,8; 2016,Feb,12; 2016,Jan,13; 2015,Jan,16; 2014,Jan,11

**67903**     (tarso) levator resection or advancement, internal approach

      13.7   16.7  **FUD** 090     J A2 50

      **AMA:** 2017,Jan,8; 2016,Feb,12; 2016,Jan,13; 2015,Jan,16; 2014,Jan,11

**67904**     (tarso) levator resection or advancement, external approach

      INCLUDES   Everbusch's operation

      16.9   20.7  **FUD** 090     J A2 50

      **AMA:** 2017,Jan,8; 2016,Feb,12; 2016,Jan,13; 2015,Jan,16; 2014,Jan,11

**67906**     superior rectus technique with fascial sling (includes obtaining fascia)

      14.4   14.4  **FUD** 090     J A2 50

      **AMA:** 2017,Jan,8; 2016,Feb,12; 2016,Jan,13; 2015,Jan,16; 2014,Jan,11

**67908**     conjunctivo-tarso-Muller's muscle-levator resection (eg, Fasanella-Servat type)

      12.0   13.9  **FUD** 090     J A2 50

      **AMA:** 2017,Jan,8; 2016,Feb,12; 2016,Jan,13; 2015,Jan,16; 2014,Jan,11

**67909**     Reduction of overcorrection of ptosis

      12.4   15.1  **FUD** 090     J A2 50

      **AMA:** 2017,Jan,8; 2016,Feb,12; 2016,Jan,13; 2015,Jan,16; 2014,Jan,11

**67911**     Correction of lid retraction

      EXCLUDES   *Graft harvest (20920, 20922, 20926)*
               *Mucous membrane graft repair of trichiasis (67835)*

      15.9   15.9  **FUD** 090     J A2 50

      **AMA:** 2017,Jan,8; 2016,Feb,12; 2016,Jan,13; 2015,Jan,16; 2014,Jan,11

**67912** **Correction of lagophthalmos, with implantation of upper eyelid lid load (eg, gold weight)**
🚑 13.9   ⚖ 24.8   **FUD** 090                    J A2 50 ▣
**AMA:** 2017,Jan,8; 2016,Feb,12; 2016,Jan,13; 2015,Jan,16; 2014,Jan,11; 2012,Jan,15-42

## 67914-67924 Repair Ectropion/Entropion
INCLUDES  Operating microscope (69990)
EXCLUDES  Cicatricial ectropion or entropion with scar excision or graft (67961-67966)

**67914** **Repair of ectropion; suture**
INCLUDES  Canthoplasty (67950)
🚑 9.29   ⚖ 13.2   **FUD** 090                    J A2 50 ▣
**AMA:** 2017,Jan,8; 2016,Feb,12; 2016,Jan,13; 2015,Jan,16; 2014,Jan,11

**67915** **thermocauterization**
🚑 5.60   ⚖ 8.24   **FUD** 090                    J P3 50 ▣
**AMA:** 2017,Jan,8; 2016,Feb,12; 2016,Jan,13; 2015,Jan,16; 2014,Jan,11

**67916** **excision tarsal wedge**
🚑 12.2   ⚖ 16.7   **FUD** 090                    J A2 50 ▣
**AMA:** 2017,Jan,8; 2016,Feb,12; 2016,Jan,13; 2015,Jan,16; 2014,Jan,11; 2012,Jan,15-42

**67917** **extensive (eg, tarsal strip operations)**
EXCLUDES  Repair of everted punctum (68705)
🚑 13.0   ⚖ 17.0   **FUD** 090                    J A2 50 ▣
**AMA:** 2017,Jan,8; 2016,Feb,12; 2016,Jan,13; 2015,Jan,16; 2014,Jan,11; 2012,Jan,15-42

**67921** **Repair of entropion; suture**
🚑 8.80   ⚖ 12.9   **FUD** 090                    J A2 50 ▣
**AMA:** 2017,Jan,8; 2016,Feb,12; 2016,Jan,13; 2015,Jan,16; 2014,Jan,11

**67922** **thermocauterization**
🚑 5.60   ⚖ 8.17   **FUD** 090                    J P3 50 ▣
**AMA:** 2017,Jan,8; 2016,Feb,12; 2016,Jan,13; 2015,Jan,16; 2014,Jan,11

**67923** **excision tarsal wedge**
🚑 12.2   ⚖ 16.7   **FUD** 090                    J A2 50 ▣
**AMA:** 2017,Jan,8; 2016,Feb,12; 2016,Jan,13; 2015,Jan,16; 2014,Jan,11

**67924** **extensive (eg, tarsal strip or capsulopalpebral fascia repairs operation)**
INCLUDES  Canthoplasty (67950)
🚑 13.0   ⚖ 17.8   **FUD** 090                    J A2 50 ▣
**AMA:** 2017,Jan,8; 2016,Feb,12; 2016,Jan,13; 2015,Jan,16; 2014,Jan,11

## 67930-67935 Repair Eyelid Wound
INCLUDES  Operating microscope (69990)
Repairs involving more than skin:
Lid margin
Palpebral conjunctiva
Tarsus
EXCLUDES  Blepharoplasty for entropion or ectropion (67916-67917, 67923-67924)
Correction of lid retraction and blepharoptosis (67901-67911)
Free graft (15120-15121, 15260-15261)
Graft preparation (15004)
Plastic repair of lacrimal canaliculi (68700)
Removal of eyelid lesion (67800 [67810], 67840-67850)
Repair involving skin of eyelid (12011-12018, 12051-12057, 13151-13153)
Repair of blepharochalasis (15820-15823)
Skin adjacent tissue transfer (14060-14061)
Tarsorrhaphy, canthorrhaphy (67880, 67882)

**67930** **Suture of recent wound, eyelid, involving lid margin, tarsus, and/or palpebral conjunctiva direct closure; partial thickness**
🚑 6.83   ⚖ 10.3   **FUD** 010                    J P3 50 ▣
**AMA:** 2016,Feb,12; 2014,Jan,11

**67935** **full thickness**
🚑 12.5   ⚖ 16.8   **FUD** 090                    J A2 50 ▣
**AMA:** 2016,Feb,12; 2014,Jan,11

## 67938-67999 Eyelid Reconstruction/Repair/Removal Deep Foreign Body
INCLUDES  Operating microscope (69990)
EXCLUDES  Blepharoplasty for entropion or ectropion (67916-67917, 67923-67924)
Correction of lid retraction and blepharoptosis (67901-67911)
Free graft (15120-15121, 15260-15261)
Graft preparation (15004)
Plastic repair of lacrimal canaliculi (68700)
Removal of eyelid lesion (67800-67808, 67840-67850)
Repair involving skin of eyelid (12011-12018, 12051-12057, 13151-13153)
Repair of blepharochalasis (15820-15823)
Skin adjacent tissue transfer (14060-14061)
Tarsorrhaphy, canthorrhaphy (67880, 67882)

**67938** **Removal of embedded foreign body, eyelid**
🚑 3.30   ⚖ 6.87   **FUD** 010                    T P2 50 ▣
**AMA:** 2017,Jan,8; 2016,Feb,12; 2016,Jan,13; 2015,Jan,16; 2014,May,5; 2014,Jan,11

**67950** **Canthoplasty (reconstruction of canthus)**
🚑 13.1   ⚖ 16.1   **FUD** 090                    J A2 50 ▣
**AMA:** 2016,Feb,12; 2014,Jan,11

**67961** **Excision and repair of eyelid, involving lid margin, tarsus, conjunctiva, canthus, or full thickness, may include preparation for skin graft or pedicle flap with adjacent tissue transfer or rearrangement; up to one-fourth of lid margin**
INCLUDES  Canthoplasty (67950)
EXCLUDES  Delay flap (15630)
Flap attachment (15650)
Free skin grafts (15120-15121, 15260-15261)
Tubed pedicle flap preparation (15576)
🚑 12.9   ⚖ 16.2   **FUD** 090              J A2 80 50 ▣
**AMA:** 2017,Jan,8; 2016,Feb,12; 2016,Jan,13; 2015,Jan,16; 2014,Jan,11

**67966** **over one-fourth of lid margin**
INCLUDES  Canthoplasty (67950)
EXCLUDES  Delay flap (15630)
Flap attachment (15650)
Free skin grafts (15120-15121, 15260-15261)
Tubed pedicle flap preparation (15576)
🚑 18.6   ⚖ 21.7   **FUD** 090                    J A2 50 ▣
**AMA:** 2017,Jan,8; 2016,Feb,12; 2016,Jan,13; 2015,Jan,16; 2014,Jan,11; 2012,Nov,13-14

**67971** **Reconstruction of eyelid, full thickness by transfer of tarsoconjunctival flap from opposing eyelid; up to two-thirds of eyelid, 1 stage or first stage**
INCLUDES  Dupuy-Dutemp reconstruction
Landboldt's operation
🚑 20.5   ⚖ 20.5   **FUD** 090                    J A2 50 ▣
**AMA:** 2016,Feb,12; 2014,Jan,11

**67973** **total eyelid, lower, 1 stage or first stage**
INCLUDES  Landboldt's operation
🚑 26.4   ⚖ 26.4   **FUD** 090              J A2 80 50 ▣
**AMA:** 2016,Feb,12; 2014,Jan,11

**67974** **total eyelid, upper, 1 stage or first stage**
INCLUDES  Landboldt's operation
🚑 26.3   ⚖ 26.3   **FUD** 090              J A2 80 50 ▣
**AMA:** 2016,Feb,12; 2014,Jan,11

**67975** **second stage**
INCLUDES  Landboldt's operation
🚑 19.4   ⚖ 19.4   **FUD** 090                    J A2 50 ▣
**AMA:** 2016,Feb,12; 2014,Jan,11

**67999** **Unlisted procedure, eyelids**
🚑 0.00   ⚖ 0.00   **FUD** YYY                    T 80 50
**AMA:** 2017,Jul,10; 2017,Jan,8; 2016,Feb,12; 2016,Jan,13; 2015,Jan,16; 2014,Jan,11; 2012,Jan,15-42

26/TC PC/TC Only     A2-Z3 ASC Payment     50 Bilateral     ♂ Male Only     ♀ Female Only     🚑 Facility RVU     ⚖ Non-Facility RVU     ▣ CCI
FUD Follow-up Days     CMS: IOM (Pub 100)     A-Y OPPSI     80/80 Surg Assist Allowed / w/Doc     ▣ Lab crosswalk     ▣ Radiology crosswalk     ☒ CLIA
CPT © 2017 American Medical Association. All Rights Reserved.

© 2017 Optum360, LLC

## 68020-68200 Conjunctival Biopsy/Injection/Treatment of Lesions

INCLUDES Operating microscope (69990)
EXCLUDES Foreign body removal (65205-65265)

**68020** **Incision of conjunctiva, drainage of cyst**
⚙ 3.13 ✂ 3.38 **FUD** 010 ⬚T ⬚P3 ⬚50 ⬚
AMA: 2016,Feb,12; 2014,Jan,11

**68040** **Expression of conjunctival follicles (eg, for trachoma)**
EXCLUDES *Automated evacuation meibomian glands with heat/pressure (0207T)*
⚙ 1.43 ✂ 1.75 **FUD** 000 ⬚T ⬚P3 ⬚50 ⬚
AMA: 2017,Jan,8; 2016,Feb,12; 2016,Jan,13; 2015,Jan,16; 2014,May,5; 2014,Jan,11

**68100** **Biopsy of conjunctiva**
⚙ 2.77 ✂ 4.79 **FUD** 000 ⬚J ⬚P3 ⬚50 ⬚
AMA: 2016,Feb,12; 2014,Jan,11

**68110** **Excision of lesion, conjunctiva; up to 1 cm**
⚙ 4.21 ✂ 6.36 **FUD** 010 ⬚J ⬚P3 ⬚50 ⬚
AMA: 2017,Jan,6; 2016,Feb,12; 2014,Jan,11

**68115** **over 1 cm**
⚙ 5.22 ✂ 8.78 **FUD** 010 ⬚J ⬚A2 ⬚50 ⬚
AMA: 2016,Feb,12; 2014,Jan,11

**68130** **with adjacent sclera**
⚙ 11.6 ✂ 15.2 **FUD** 090 ⬚J ⬚A2 ⬚50 ⬚
AMA: 2016,Feb,12; 2014,Jan,11

**68135** **Destruction of lesion, conjunctiva**
⚙ 4.28 ✂ 4.43 **FUD** 010 ⬚J ⬚P3 ⬚50 ⬚
AMA: 2016,Feb,12; 2014,Jan,11

**68200** **Subconjunctival injection**
EXCLUDES *Retrobulbar or Tenon's capsule injection (67500-67515)*
⚙ 0.99 ✂ 1.17 **FUD** 000 ⬚01 ⬚N1 ⬚50 ⬚
AMA: 2017,Jan,8; 2016,Feb,12; 2016,Jan,13; 2015,Jan,16; 2014,Jan,11; 2012,Nov,10; 2012,Jan,15-42

## 68320-68340 Conjunctivoplasty Procedures

INCLUDES Operating microscope (69990)
EXCLUDES Conjunctival foreign body removal (65205, 65210)
Laceration repair (65270-65273)

**68320** **Conjunctivoplasty; with conjunctival graft or extensive rearrangement**
⚙ 15.2 ✂ 20.4 **FUD** 090 ⬚J ⬚A2 ⬚50 ⬚
AMA: 2017,Jan,8; 2016,Feb,12; 2016,Jan,13; 2015,Jan,16; 2014,Jan,11; 2012,Jan,15-42

**68325** **with buccal mucous membrane graft (includes obtaining graft)**
⚙ 18.6 ✂ 18.6 **FUD** 090 ⬚J ⬚A2 ⬚50 ⬚
AMA: 2016,Feb,12; 2014,Jan,11

**68326** **Conjunctivoplasty, reconstruction cul-de-sac; with conjunctival graft or extensive rearrangement**
⚙ 18.3 ✂ 18.3 **FUD** 090 ⬚J ⬚A2 ⬚50 ⬚
AMA: 2016,Feb,12; 2014,Jan,11

**68328** **with buccal mucous membrane graft (includes obtaining graft)**
⚙ 20.1 ✂ 20.1 **FUD** 090 ⬚J ⬚A2 ⬚80 ⬚50 ⬚
AMA: 2016,Feb,12; 2014,Jan,11

**68330** **Repair of symblepharon; conjunctivoplasty, without graft**
⚙ 13.0 ✂ 17.0 **FUD** 090 ⬚J ⬚A2 ⬚80 ⬚50 ⬚
AMA: 2016,Feb,12; 2014,Jan,11

**68335** **with free graft conjunctiva or buccal mucous membrane (includes obtaining graft)**
⚙ 18.3 ✂ 18.3 **FUD** 090 ⬚J ⬚A2 ⬚50 ⬚
AMA: 2016,Feb,12; 2014,Jan,11

**68340** **division of symblepharon, with or without insertion of conformer or contact lens**
⚙ 11.3 ✂ 15.3 **FUD** 090 ⬚J ⬚A2 ⬚80 ⬚50 ⬚
AMA: 2016,Feb,12; 2014,Jan,11

## 68360-68399 Conjunctival Flaps and Unlisted Procedures

INCLUDES Operating microscope (69990)

**68360** **Conjunctival flap; bridge or partial (separate procedure)**
EXCLUDES *Conjunctival flap for injury (65280, 65285)*
*Conjunctival foreign body removal (65205, 65210)*
*Surgical wound repair (66250)*
⚙ 11.6 ✂ 15.0 **FUD** 090 ⬚J ⬚A2 ⬚50 ⬚
AMA: 2016,Feb,12; 2014,Jan,11

**68362** **total (such as Gunderson thin flap or purse string flap)**
EXCLUDES *Conjunctival flap for injury (65280, 65285)*
*Conjunctival foreign body removal (65205, 65210)*
*Surgical wound repair (66250)*
⚙ 18.6 ✂ 18.6 **FUD** 090 ⬚J ⬚A2 ⬚50 ⬚
AMA: 2017,Jan,8; 2016,Feb,12; 2016,Jan,13; 2015,Jan,16; 2014,Jan,11

**68371** **Harvesting conjunctival allograft, living donor**
⚙ 11.7 ✂ 11.7 **FUD** 010 ⬚J ⬚A2 ⬚50 ⬚
AMA: 2017,Jan,8; 2016,Feb,12; 2016,Jan,13; 2015,Jan,16; 2014,Jan,11

**68399** **Unlisted procedure, conjunctiva**
⚙ 0.00 ✂ 0.00 **FUD** YYY ⬚T ⬚80 ⬚50 ⬚
AMA: 2017,Jan,8; 2016,Feb,12; 2016,Jan,13; 2015,Jan,16; 2014,Jan,11

## 68400-68899 Nasolacrimal System Procedures

INCLUDES Operating microscope (69990)

**68400** **Incision, drainage of lacrimal gland**
⚙ 3.74 ✂ 8.00 **FUD** 010 ⬚T ⬚P3 ⬚50 ⬚
AMA: 2016,Feb,12; 2014,Jan,11

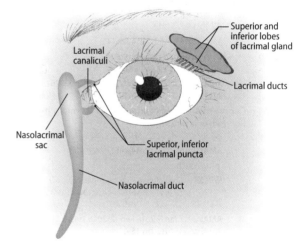

Superior and inferior lobes of lacrimal gland

Lacrimal canaliculi

Lacrimal ducts

Nasolacrimal sac

Superior, inferior lacrimal puncta

Nasolacrimal duct

**68420** **Incision, drainage of lacrimal sac (dacryocystotomy or dacryocystostomy)**
⚙ 4.78 ✂ 9.05 **FUD** 010 ⬚J ⬚P3 ⬚50 ⬚
AMA: 2016,Feb,12; 2014,Jan,11

**68440** **Snip incision of lacrimal punctum**
⚙ 2.80 ✂ 2.88 **FUD** 010 ⬚T ⬚P3 ⬚50 ⬚
AMA: 2016,Feb,12; 2014,Jan,11

**68500** **Excision of lacrimal gland (dacryoadenectomy), except for tumor; total**
⚙ 27.7 ✂ 27.7 **FUD** 090 ⬚J ⬚A2 ⬚50 ⬚
AMA: 2016,Feb,12; 2014,Jan,11

**68505** **partial**
⚙ 27.4 ✂ 27.4 **FUD** 090 ⬚J ⬚A2 ⬚50 ⬚
AMA: 2016,Feb,12; 2014,Jan,11

**68510** **Biopsy of lacrimal gland**
⚙ 8.29 ✂ 12.5 **FUD** 000 ⬚J ⬚A2 ⬚80 ⬚50 ⬚
AMA: 2016,Feb,12; 2014,Jan,11

● New Code ▲ Revised Code ○ Reinstated ● New Web Release ▲ Revised Web Release Unlisted Not Covered # Resequenced
⊘ AMA Mod 51 Exempt ⑤ Optum Mod 51 Exempt ⑥③ Mod 63 Exempt ✗ Non-FDA Drug ★ Telemedicine Ⓜ Maternity Ⓐ Age Edit + Add-on **AMA:** CPT Asst
© 2017 Optum360, LLC CPT © 2017 American Medical Association. All Rights Reserved. **309**

**68520** **Excision of lacrimal sac (dacryocystectomy)**
🚑 19.4   ⚕ 19.4   **FUD** 090   [J] [A2] [80] [50] [▢]
**AMA:** 2016,Feb,12; 2014,Jan,11

**68525** **Biopsy of lacrimal sac**
🚑 7.52   ⚕ 7.52   **FUD** 000   [J] [A2] [50] [▢]
**AMA:** 2016,Feb,12; 2014,Jan,11

**68530** **Removal of foreign body or dacryolith, lacrimal passages**
[INCLUDES] Meller's excision
🚑 7.32   ⚕ 12.0   **FUD** 010   [T] [P2] [50] [▢]
**AMA:** 2016,Feb,12; 2014,Jan,11

**68540** **Excision of lacrimal gland tumor; frontal approach**
🚑 26.3   ⚕ 26.3   **FUD** 090   [J] [A2] [50] [▢]
**AMA:** 2016,Feb,12; 2014,Jan,11

**68550** **involving osteotomy**
🚑 31.5   ⚕ 31.5   **FUD** 090   [J] [A2] [50] [▢]
**AMA:** 2016,Feb,12; 2014,Jan,11

**68700** **Plastic repair of canaliculi**
🚑 17.1   ⚕ 17.1   **FUD** 090   [J] [A2] [50] [▢]
**AMA:** 2016,Feb,12; 2014,Jan,11

**68705** **Correction of everted punctum, cautery**
🚑 4.72   ⚕ 6.68   **FUD** 010   [T] [P2] [50] [▢]
**AMA:** 2017,Jan,8; 2016,Feb,12; 2016,Jan,13; 2015,Jan,16; 2014,Jan,11

**68720** **Dacryocystorhinostomy (fistulization of lacrimal sac to nasal cavity)**
🚑 21.4   ⚕ 21.4   **FUD** 090   [J] [A2] [80] [50] [▢]
**AMA:** 2017,Jan,8; 2016,Feb,12; 2016,Jan,13; 2015,Jan,16; 2014,Jan,11; 2012,Jan,15-42

**68745** **Conjunctivorhinostomy (fistulization of conjunctiva to nasal cavity); without tube**
🚑 21.5   ⚕ 21.5   **FUD** 090   [J] [A2] [80] [50] [▢]
**AMA:** 2016,Feb,12; 2014,Jan,11

**68750** **with insertion of tube or stent**
🚑 22.3   ⚕ 22.3   **FUD** 090   [J] [A2] [80] [50] [▢]
**AMA:** 2017,Jan,8; 2016,Feb,12; 2016,Jan,13; 2015,Jan,16; 2014,Jan,11; 2012,Jan,15-42

**68760** **Closure of the lacrimal punctum; by thermocauterization, ligation, or laser surgery**
🚑 4.14   ⚕ 5.68   **FUD** 010   [T] [P3] [50] [▢]
**AMA:** 2016,Feb,12; 2014,Jan,11

**68761** **by plug, each**
[EXCLUDES] Drug-eluting lacrimal implant (0356T)
Drug-eluting ocular insert (0444T-0445T)
🚑 3.37   ⚕ 4.17   **FUD** 010   [T] [P3] [80] [50] [▢]
**AMA:** 2017,Jan,8; 2016,Feb,12; 2016,Jan,13; 2015,Jan,16; 2014,Jan,11; 2012,Jan,15-42

**68770** **Closure of lacrimal fistula (separate procedure)**
🚑 17.8   ⚕ 17.8   **FUD** 090   [J] [A2] [80] [50] [▢]
**AMA:** 2016,Feb,12; 2014,Jan,11

**68801** **Dilation of lacrimal punctum, with or without irrigation**
🚑 2.24   ⚕ 2.50   **FUD** 010   [01] [N1] [50] [▢]
**AMA:** 2016,Feb,12; 2014,Jan,11

**68810** **Probing of nasolacrimal duct, with or without irrigation;**
[EXCLUDES] Ophthalmological exam under anesthesia (92018)
🚑 3.62   ⚕ 4.45   **FUD** 010   [T] [A2] [50] [▢]
**AMA:** 2017,Jan,8; 2016,Feb,12; 2016,Jan,13; 2015,Jan,16; 2014,Jan,11

**68811** **requiring general anesthesia**
[EXCLUDES] Ophthalmological exam under anesthesia (92018)
🚑 3.87   ⚕ 3.87   **FUD** 010   [J] [A2] [50] [▢]
**AMA:** 2017,Jan,8; 2016,Feb,12; 2016,Jan,13; 2015,Jan,16; 2014,Jan,11; 2012,Jan,15-42

**68815** **with insertion of tube or stent**
[EXCLUDES] Drug eluting ocular insert (0444T-0445T)
Drug eluting lacrimal implant
Ophthalmological exam under anesthesia (92018)
🚑 6.29   ⚕ 11.2   **FUD** 010   [J] [A2] [50] [▢]
**AMA:** 2017,Jan,8; 2016,Feb,12; 2016,Jan,13; 2015,Jan,16; 2014,Jan,11; 2012,Jan,15-42

**68816** **with transluminal balloon catheter dilation**
[EXCLUDES] Probing of nasolacrimal duct (68810-68811, 68815)
🚑 4.63   ⚕ 18.2   **FUD** 010   [J] [G2] [50] [▢]
**AMA:** 2017,Jan,8; 2016,Feb,12; 2016,Jan,13; 2015,Jan,16; 2014,Jan,11

**68840** **Probing of lacrimal canaliculi, with or without irrigation**
🚑 3.30   ⚕ 3.61   **FUD** 010   [T] [P3] [50] [▢]
**AMA:** 2016,Feb,12; 2014,Jan,11

**68850** **Injection of contrast medium for dacryocystography**
📠 (70170, 78660)
🚑 1.61   ⚕ 1.75   **FUD** 000   [N] [N1] [50] [▢]
**AMA:** 2017,Jan,8; 2016,Feb,12; 2016,Jan,13; 2015,Jan,16; 2014,Jan,11; 2012,Jan,15-42

**68899** **Unlisted procedure, lacrimal system**
🚑 0.00   ⚕ 0.00   **FUD** YYY   [T] [80] [50]
**AMA:** 2014,Jan,11

## 69000-69020 Treatment External Abscess/Hematoma

**69000** **Drainage external ear, abscess or hematoma; simple**
🚑 3.40   ⚕ 5.32   **FUD** 010   [T] [P3] [50] [▢]
**AMA:** 2017,Jan,8; 2016,Jan,13; 2015,Jan,16; 2014,Jan,11; 2012,Jan,15-42

An incision is made to drain the contents of an abscess or hematoma

**69005** **complicated**
🚑 4.48   ⚕ 6.10   **FUD** 010   [J] [P3] [50] [▢]
**AMA:** 2014,Jan,11

**69020** **Drainage external auditory canal, abscess**
🚑 4.06   ⚕ 6.58   **FUD** 010   [T] [P3] [50] [▢]
**AMA:** 2017,Jan,8; 2016,Jan,13; 2015,Jan,16; 2014,Jan,11; 2012,Jan,15-42

## 69090 Cosmetic Ear Piercing
**CMS:** 100-02,16,10 Exclusions from Coverage; 100-02,16,120 Cosmetic Procedures

**69090** **Ear piercing**
🚑 0.00   ⚕ 0.00   **FUD** XXX   [E] [▢]
**AMA:** 2014,Jan,11

## 69100-69222 External Ear/Auditory Canal Procedures

EXCLUDES *Reconstruction of ear (see integumentary section codes)*

**69100** **Biopsy external ear**
📋 1.41 ♨ 2.86 **FUD** 000 [T] [P3]
**AMA:** 2014,Jan,11

**69105** **Biopsy external auditory canal**
📋 1.82 ♨ 3.97 **FUD** 000 [T] [P3] [50] 🔲
**AMA:** 2014,Jan,11

**69110** **Excision external ear; partial, simple repair**
📋 9.28 ♨ 13.0 **FUD** 090 [J] [A2] [50] 🔲
**AMA:** 2014,Jan,11

**69120** **complete amputation**
📋 11.6 ♨ 11.6 **FUD** 090 [J] [A2] 🔲
**AMA:** 2014,Jan,11

**69140** **Excision exostosis(es), external auditory canal**
📋 24.9 ♨ 24.9 **FUD** 090 [J] [A2] [80] [50] 🔲
**AMA:** 2014,Jan,11

**69145** **Excision soft tissue lesion, external auditory canal**
📋 7.12 ♨ 11.2 **FUD** 090 [J] [A2] [50] 🔲
**AMA:** 2014,Jan,11

**69150** **Radical excision external auditory canal lesion; without neck dissection**
EXCLUDES *Skin graft (15004-15261)*
*Temporal bone resection (69535)*
📋 29.9 ♨ 29.9 **FUD** 090 [J] [A2]
**AMA:** 2014,Jan,11

**69155** **with neck dissection**
EXCLUDES *Skin graft (15004-15261)*
*Temporal bone resection (69535)*
📋 47.7 ♨ 47.7 **FUD** 090 [C] [80] 🔲
**AMA:** 2014,Jan,11

**69200** **Removal foreign body from external auditory canal; without general anesthesia**
📋 1.36 ♨ 2.35 **FUD** 000 [01] [N1] [50] 🔲
**AMA:** 2014,Jan,11

**69205** **with general anesthesia**
📋 2.90 ♨ 2.90 **FUD** 010 [J] [A2] [50] 🔲
**AMA:** 2017,Jan,8; 2016,Jan,13; 2015,Jan,16; 2014,Jan,11; 2013,Apr,10-11

**69209** **Removal impacted cerumen using irrigation/lavage, unilateral**
EXCLUDES *Removal impacted cerumen using instrumentation (69210)*
*Removal of nonimpacted cerumen (see appropriate E&M code(s)) (99201-99233 [99224, 99225, 99226], 99241-99255, 99281-99285, 99304-99318, 99324-99337, 99341-99350)*
📋 0.36 ♨ 0.36 **FUD** 000 [01] [N1] [50] 🔲
**AMA:** 2017,Jan,8; 2016,Mar,10; 2016,Feb,13; 2016,Jan,7

**69210** **Removal impacted cerumen requiring instrumentation, unilateral**
EXCLUDES *Removal of impacted cerumen using irrigation or lavage (69209)*
*Removal of nonimpacted cerumen (see appropriate E&M code(s)) (99201-99233 [99224, 99225, 99226], 99241-99255, 99281-99285, 99304-99318, 99324-99337, 99341-99350)*
📋 0.94 ♨ 1.39 **FUD** 000 [01] [N1]
**AMA:** 2017,Jan,8; 2016,Mar,10; 2016,Feb,13; 2016,Jan,13; 2016,Jan,7; 2015,Jan,16; 2014,Nov,14; 2014,Jan,11; 2013,Oct,14; 2012,Jan,15-42

**69220** **Debridement, mastoidectomy cavity, simple (eg, routine cleaning)**
📋 1.48 ♨ 2.56 **FUD** 000 [01] [N1] [50] 🔲
**AMA:** 2014,Jan,11

**69222** **Debridement, mastoidectomy cavity, complex (eg, with anesthesia or more than routine cleaning)**
📋 3.90 ♨ 6.22 **FUD** 010 [T] [P3] [50] 🔲
**AMA:** 2014,Jan,11

## 69300 Plastic Surgery for Prominent Ears

CMS: 100-02,16,120 Cosmetic Procedures; 100-02,16,180 Services Related to Noncovered Procedures
EXCLUDES *Suture of laceration of external ear (12011-14302)*

**69300** **Otoplasty, protruding ear, with or without size reduction**
📋 13.1 ♨ 16.8 **FUD** YYY [J] [A2] [80] [50] 🔲
**AMA:** 2014,Jan,11

## 69310-69399 Reconstruction Auditory Canal: Postaural Approach

EXCLUDES *Suture of laceration of external ear (12011-14302)*

**69310** **Reconstruction of external auditory canal (meatoplasty) (eg, for stenosis due to injury, infection) (separate procedure)**
📋 31.1 ♨ 31.1 **FUD** 090 [J] [A2] [50] 🔲
**AMA:** 2017,Jan,8; 2016,Jan,13; 2015,Jan,16; 2014,Jul,8; 2014,Jan,11; 2014,Jan,9

**69320** **Reconstruction external auditory canal for congenital atresia, single stage**
EXCLUDES *Other reconstruction surgery with graft (13151-15760, 21230-21235)*
*Tympanoplasty (69631, 69641)*
📋 43.5 ♨ 43.5 **FUD** 090 [J] [A2] [80] [50] 🔲
**AMA:** 2014,Jan,11

**69399** **Unlisted procedure, external ear**
EXCLUDES *Otoscopy under general anesthesia (92502)*
📋 0.00 ♨ 0.00 **FUD** YYY [T] [80]
**AMA:** 2014,Jan,11

## 69420-69450 Ear Drum Procedures

**69420** **Myringotomy including aspiration and/or eustachian tube inflation**
📋 3.44 ♨ 5.42 **FUD** 010 [T] [P2] [50] 🔲
**AMA:** 2017,Jan,8; 2016,Jan,13; 2015,Jan,16; 2014,Jan,11

**69421** **Myringotomy including aspiration and/or eustachian tube inflation requiring general anesthesia**
📋 4.25 ♨ 4.25 **FUD** 010 [J] [A2] [50] 🔲
**AMA:** 2017,Jan,8; 2016,Jan,13; 2015,Jan,16; 2014,Jan,11

**69424** **Ventilating tube removal requiring general anesthesia**
EXCLUDES *Cochlear device implantation (69930)*
*Eardrum repair (69610-69646)*
*Foreign body removal (69205)*
*Implantation, replacement of electromagnetic bone conduction hearing device in temporal bone (69710-69745)*
*Labyrinth procedures (69801-69915)*
*Mastoid obliteration (69670)*
*Myringotomy (69420-69421)*
*Polyp, glomus tumor removal (69535-69554)*
*Removal impacted cerumen requiring instrumentation (69210)*
*Repair of window (69666-69667)*
*Revised mastoidectomy (69601-69605)*
*Stapes procedures (69650-69662)*
*Transmastoid excision (69501-69530)*
*Tympanic neurectomy (69676)*
*Tympanostomy, tympanolysis (69433-69450)*
📋 1.78 ♨ 3.61 **FUD** 000 [02] [P3] [50] 🔲
**AMA:** 2017,Jan,8; 2016,Jan,13; 2015,Jan,16; 2014,Jan,11; 2012,Jan,15-42

● New Code ▲ Revised Code ○ Reinstated ● New Web Release ▲ Revised Web Release Unlisted Not Covered # Resequenced
⊘ AMA Mod 51 Exempt ⑤ Optum Mod 51 Exempt ⊚ Mod 63 Exempt ✗ Non-FDA Drug ★ Telemedicine Ⓜ Maternity Ⓐ Age Edit + Add-on **AMA:** CPT Asst
© 2017 Optum360, LLC CPT © 2017 American Medical Association. All Rights Reserved.

**Eye, Ocular Adnexa, and Ear**

**69433 — 69633**

**69433** **Tympanostomy (requiring insertion of ventilating tube), local or topical anesthesia**
🔧 3.78  ✂ 5.74  **FUD** 010  T P3 50 ▭
AMA: 2017,Jan,8; 2016,Jan,13; 2015,Jan,16; 2014,Jan,11

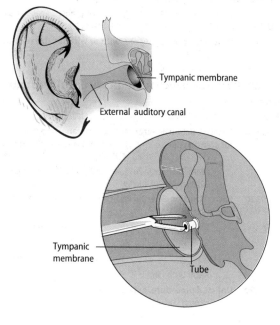

Tympanic membrane

External auditory canal

Tympanic membrane

Tube

**69436** **Tympanostomy (requiring insertion of ventilating tube), general anesthesia**
🔧 4.58  ✂ 4.58  **FUD** 010  T A2 50 ▭
AMA: 2017,Jan,8; 2016,Jan,13; 2015,Jan,16; 2014,Jan,11; 2012,May,14-15

**69440** **Middle ear exploration through postauricular or ear canal incision**
EXCLUDES  Atticotomy (69601-69605)
🔧 19.6  ✂ 19.6  **FUD** 090  J A2 50 ▭
AMA: 2014,Jan,11

**69450** **Tympanolysis, transcanal**
🔧 15.5  ✂ 15.5  **FUD** 090  J A2 80 50 ▭
AMA: 2014,Jan,11

## 69501-69530 Transmastoid Excision
EXCLUDES  Mastoidectomy cavity debridement (69220, 69222)
Skin graft (15004-15770)

**69501** **Transmastoid antrotomy (simple mastoidectomy)**
🔧 20.9  ✂ 20.9  **FUD** 090  J A2 50 ▭
AMA: 2017,Jan,8; 2016,Jan,13; 2015,Jan,16; 2014,Jan,11

**69502** **Mastoidectomy; complete**
🔧 27.9  ✂ 27.9  **FUD** 090  J A2 80 50 ▭
AMA: 2017,Jan,8; 2016,Jan,13; 2015,Jan,16; 2014,Jan,11

**69505** **modified radical**
🔧 34.3  ✂ 34.3  **FUD** 090  J A2 80 50 ▭
AMA: 2017,Jan,8; 2016,Jan,13; 2015,Jan,16; 2014,Jan,11

**69511** **radical**
🔧 35.2  ✂ 35.2  **FUD** 090  J A2 80 50 ▭
AMA: 2017,Jan,8; 2016,Jan,13; 2015,Jan,16; 2014,Jan,11

**69530** **Petrous apicectomy including radical mastoidectomy**
🔧 47.7  ✂ 47.7  **FUD** 090  J A2 80 50 ▭
AMA: 2014,Jan,11

## 69535-69554 Polyp and Glomus Tumor Removal

**69535** **Resection temporal bone, external approach**
EXCLUDES  Middle fossa approach (69950-69970)
🔧 77.1  ✂ 77.1  **FUD** 090  C 50 ▭
AMA: 2014,Jan,11

**69540** **Excision aural polyp**
🔧 3.62  ✂ 5.92  **FUD** 010  T P3 50 ▭
AMA: 2014,Jan,11

**69550** **Excision aural glomus tumor; transcanal**
🔧 29.7  ✂ 29.7  **FUD** 090  J A2 80 50 ▭
AMA: 2014,Jan,11

**69552** **transmastoid**
🔧 44.5  ✂ 44.5  **FUD** 090  J A2 80 50 ▭
AMA: 2014,Jan,11

**69554** **extended (extratemporal)**
🔧 72.1  ✂ 72.1  **FUD** 090  C 80 50 ▭
AMA: 2014,Jan,11

## 69601-69605 Revised Mastoidectomy
EXCLUDES  Skin graft (15120-15121, 15260-15261)

**69601** **Revision mastoidectomy; resulting in complete mastoidectomy**
🔧 29.9  ✂ 29.9  **FUD** 090  J A2 80 50 ▭
AMA: 2017,Jan,8; 2016,Jan,13; 2015,Jan,16; 2014,Jan,11

**69602** **resulting in modified radical mastoidectomy**
🔧 31.2  ✂ 31.2  **FUD** 090  J A2 80 50 ▭
AMA: 2017,Jan,8; 2016,Jan,13; 2015,Jan,16; 2014,Jan,11

**69603** **resulting in radical mastoidectomy**
🔧 36.2  ✂ 36.2  **FUD** 090  J A2 80 50 ▭
AMA: 2017,Jan,8; 2016,Jan,13; 2015,Jan,16; 2014,Jan,11

**69604** **resulting in tympanoplasty**
EXCLUDES  Secondary tympanoplasty following mastoidectomy (69631-69632)
🔧 31.8  ✂ 31.8  **FUD** 090  J A2 50 ▭
AMA: 2017,Jan,8; 2016,Jan,13; 2015,Jan,16; 2014,Jan,11

**69605** **with apicectomy**
🔧 47.9  ✂ 47.9  **FUD** 090  J A2 80 50 ▭
AMA: 2014,Jan,11

## 69610-69646 Eardrum Repair with/without Other Procedures

**69610** **Tympanic membrane repair, with or without site preparation of perforation for closure, with or without patch**
🔧 8.34  ✂ 10.9  **FUD** 010  J P3 50 ▭
AMA: 2017,Jan,8; 2016,Jan,13; 2015,May,10; 2015,Apr,10; 2015,Jan,16; 2014,Jan,11; 2012,Jan,15-42

**69620** **Myringoplasty (surgery confined to drumhead and donor area)**
🔧 13.9  ✂ 19.7  **FUD** 090  J A2 50 ▭
AMA: 2017,Jan,8; 2016,Jan,13; 2015,May,10; 2015,Apr,10; 2015,Jan,16; 2014,Jan,11; 2012,Jan,15-42

**69631** **Tympanoplasty without mastoidectomy (including canalplasty, atticotomy and/or middle ear surgery), initial or revision; without ossicular chain reconstruction**
🔧 25.2  ✂ 25.2  **FUD** 090  J A2 50 ▭
AMA: 2017,Jan,8; 2016,Jan,13; 2015,Jan,16; 2014,Jan,11; 2012,Dec,11; 2012,Jan,15-42

**69632** **with ossicular chain reconstruction (eg, postfenestration)**
🔧 30.8  ✂ 30.8  **FUD** 090  J A2 50 ▭
AMA: 2017,Jan,8; 2016,Jan,13; 2015,Jan,16; 2014,Jan,11

**69633** **with ossicular chain reconstruction and synthetic prosthesis (eg, partial ossicular replacement prosthesis [PORP], total ossicular replacement prosthesis [TORP])**
🔧 29.8  ✂ 29.8  **FUD** 090  J A2 50 ▭
AMA: 2017,Jan,8; 2016,Jan,13; 2015,Jan,16; 2014,Jan,11

**69635** Tympanoplasty with antrotomy or mastoidotomy (including canalplasty, atticotomy, middle ear surgery, and/or tympanic membrane repair); without ossicular chain reconstruction
🔪 35.3  ✂ 35.3  **FUD** 090  J A2 50 ▣
AMA: 2017,Jan,8; 2016,Jan,13; 2015,Jan,16; 2014,Jan,11

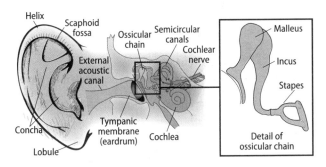

Helix, Scaphoid fossa, Ossicular chain, Semicircular canals, Cochlear nerve, External acoustic canal, Concha, Tympanic membrane (eardrum), Cochlea, Lobule, Malleus, Incus, Stapes, Detail of ossicular chain

**69636** with ossicular chain reconstruction
🔪 39.4  ✂ 39.4  **FUD** 090  J A2 80 50 ▣
AMA: 2017,Jan,8; 2016,Jan,13; 2015,Jan,16; 2014,Jan,11

**69637** with ossicular chain reconstruction and synthetic prosthesis (eg, partial ossicular replacement prosthesis [PORP], total ossicular replacement prosthesis [TORP])
🔪 40.0  ✂ 40.0  **FUD** 090  J A2 80 50 ▣
AMA: 2017,Jan,8; 2016,Jan,13; 2015,Jan,16; 2014,Jan,11

**69641** Tympanoplasty with mastoidectomy (including canalplasty, middle ear surgery, tympanic membrane repair); without ossicular chain reconstruction
🔪 29.7  ✂ 29.7  **FUD** 090  J A2 50 ▣
AMA: 2017,Jan,8; 2016,Jan,13; 2015,Jan,16; 2014,Jan,11

**69642** with ossicular chain reconstruction
🔪 38.1  ✂ 38.1  **FUD** 090  J A2 50 ▣
AMA: 2017,Jan,8; 2016,Jan,13; 2015,Jan,16; 2014,Jan,11

**69643** with intact or reconstructed wall, without ossicular chain reconstruction
🔪 34.9  ✂ 34.9  **FUD** 090  J A2 50 ▣
AMA: 2017,Jan,8; 2016,Jan,13; 2015,Jan,16; 2014,Jan,11

**69644** with intact or reconstructed canal wall, with ossicular chain reconstruction
🔪 42.2  ✂ 42.2  **FUD** 090  J A2 50 ▣
AMA: 2017,Jan,8; 2016,Jan,13; 2015,Jan,16; 2014,Jan,11

**69645** radical or complete, without ossicular chain reconstruction
🔪 41.5  ✂ 41.5  **FUD** 090  J A2 50 ▣
AMA: 2017,Jan,8; 2016,Jan,13; 2015,Jan,16; 2014,Jan,11

**69646** radical or complete, with ossicular chain reconstruction
🔪 44.1  ✂ 44.1  **FUD** 090  J A2 80 50 ▣
AMA: 2017,Jan,8; 2016,Jan,13; 2015,Jan,16; 2014,Jan,11

## 69650-69662 Stapes Procedures

**69650** Stapes mobilization
🔪 23.0  ✂ 23.0  **FUD** 090  J A2 50 ▣
AMA: 2014,Jan,11

**69660** Stapedectomy or stapedotomy with reestablishment of ossicular continuity, with or without use of foreign material;
🔪 26.5  ✂ 26.5  **FUD** 090  J A2 50 ▣
AMA: 2014,Jan,11

**69661** with footplate drill out
🔪 34.4  ✂ 34.4  **FUD** 090  J A2 80 50 ▣
AMA: 2014,Jan,11

**69662** Revision of stapedectomy or stapedotomy
🔪 33.2  ✂ 33.2  **FUD** 090  J A2 50 ▣
AMA: 2014,Jan,11

## 69666-69700 Other Inner Ear Procedures

**69666** Repair oval window fistula
🔪 23.2  ✂ 23.2  **FUD** 090  J A2 80 50 ▣
AMA: 2014,Jan,11

**69667** Repair round window fistula
🔪 23.2  ✂ 23.2  **FUD** 090  J A2 80 50 ▣
AMA: 2014,Jan,11

**69670** Mastoid obliteration (separate procedure)
🔪 27.1  ✂ 27.1  **FUD** 090  J A2 80 50 ▣
AMA: 2014,Jan,11

**69676** Tympanic neurectomy
🔪 23.7  ✂ 23.7  **FUD** 090  J A2 50 ▣
AMA: 2014,Jan,11

**69700** Closure postauricular fistula, mastoid (separate procedure)
🔪 19.8  ✂ 19.8  **FUD** 090  T A2 50 ▣
AMA: 2014,Jan,11

## 69710-69718 Procedures Related to Hearing Aids/Auditory Implants
**CMS:** 100-02,16,100 Hearing Devices

**69710** Implantation or replacement of electromagnetic bone conduction hearing device in temporal bone
INCLUDES  Removal of existing device when performing replacement procedure
🔪 0.00  ✂ 0.00  **FUD** XXX  E ▣
AMA: 2014,Jan,11

**69711** Removal or repair of electromagnetic bone conduction hearing device in temporal bone
🔪 24.6  ✂ 24.6  **FUD** 090  J A2 80 50 ▣
AMA: 2014,Jan,11

**69714** Implantation, osseointegrated implant, temporal bone, with percutaneous attachment to external speech processor/cochlear stimulator; without mastoidectomy
🔪 30.8  ✂ 30.8  **FUD** 090  J J8 50 ▣
AMA: 2017,Jan,8; 2016,Jan,13; 2015,Jan,16; 2014,Jan,11; 2013,Oct,18

**69715** with mastoidectomy
🔪 39.5  ✂ 39.5  **FUD** 090  J J8 50 ▣
AMA: 2014,Jan,11

**69717** Replacement (including removal of existing device), osseointegrated implant, temporal bone, with percutaneous attachment to external speech processor/cochlear stimulator; without mastoidectomy
🔪 32.4  ✂ 32.4  **FUD** 090  J J8 50 ▣
AMA: 2014,Jan,11

**69718** with mastoidectomy
🔪 38.4  ✂ 38.4  **FUD** 090  J G2 50 ▣
AMA: 2014,Jan,11

## 69720-69799 Procedures of the Facial Nerve
EXCLUDES  Extracranial suture of facial nerve (64864)

**69720** Decompression facial nerve, intratemporal; lateral to geniculate ganglion
🔪 34.8  ✂ 34.8  **FUD** 090  J A2 80 50 ▣
AMA: 2014,Jan,11

**69725** including medial to geniculate ganglion
🔪 53.8  ✂ 53.8  **FUD** 090  J 80 50 ▣
AMA: 2014,Jan,11

**69740** Suture facial nerve, intratemporal, with or without graft or decompression; lateral to geniculate ganglion
🔪 34.2  ✂ 34.2  **FUD** 090  J A2 80 50 ▣
AMA: 2014,Jan,11

**69745** including medial to geniculate ganglion
🔪 33.5  ✂ 33.5  **FUD** 090  J A2 80 50 ▣
AMA: 2014,Jan,11

● New Code  ▲ Revised Code  ○ Reinstated  ● New Web Release  ▲ Revised Web Release  Unlisted  Not Covered  # Resequenced
⊘ AMA Mod 51 Exempt  ⑧ Optum Mod 51 Exempt  ⑥ Mod 63 Exempt  ✗ Non-FDA Drug  ★ Telemedicine  Ⓜ Maternity  Ⓐ Age Edit  + Add-on  **AMA:** CPT Asst

**69799** Unlisted procedure, middle ear
🔧 0.00 ⚕ 0.00 **FUD** YYY ☐T☐ 80 50
**AMA:** 2017,Jan,8; 2016,Jan,13; 2015,Jan,16; 2014,Jan,11

## 69801-69915 Procedures of the Labyrinth

**69801** Labyrinthotomy, with perfusion of vestibuloactive drug(s), transcanal
> EXCLUDES *Myringotomy, tympanostomy on the same ear (69420-69421, 69433, 69436)*
> *Procedure performed more than one time per day*
🔧 3.62 ⚕ 5.56 **FUD** 000 ☐T☐ P3 80 50 ☐
**AMA:** 2017,Jan,8; 2016,Jan,13; 2015,Jan,16; 2014,Jan,11; 2012,Jan,15-42

**69805** Endolymphatic sac operation; without shunt
🔧 30.1 ⚕ 30.1 **FUD** 090 ☐J☐ A2 80 50 ☐
**AMA:** 2014,Jan,11

**69806** with shunt
🔧 27.0 ⚕ 27.0 **FUD** 090 ☐J☐ A2 50 ☐
**AMA:** 2014,Jan,11

**69820** ~~Fenestration semicircular canal~~

**69840** ~~Revision fenestration operation~~

**69905** Labyrinthectomy; transcanal
🔧 26.2 ⚕ 26.2 **FUD** 090 ☐J☐ A2 50 ☐
**AMA:** 2014,Jan,11

**69910** with mastoidectomy
🔧 29.3 ⚕ 29.3 **FUD** 090 ☐J☐ A2 80 50 ☐
**AMA:** 2014,Jan,11

**69915** Vestibular nerve section, translabyrinthine approach
> EXCLUDES *Transcranial approach (69950)*
🔧 45.4 ⚕ 45.4 **FUD** 090 ☐J☐ A2 80 50 ☐
**AMA:** 2014,Jan,11

## 69930-69949 Cochlear Implantation

**CMS:** 100-02,16,100 Hearing Devices

**69930** Cochlear device implantation, with or without mastoidectomy
🔧 35.0 ⚕ 35.0 **FUD** 090 ☐J☐ J8 80 50 ☐
**AMA:** 2014,Jan,11

The internal coil is secured to the temporal bone and an electrode is fed through the round window into the cochlea

**69949** Unlisted procedure, inner ear
🔧 0.00 ⚕ 0.00 **FUD** YYY ☐T☐ 80 50
**AMA:** 2014,Jan,11

## 69950-69979 Inner Ear Procedures via Craniotomy

> EXCLUDES *External approach (69535)*

**69950** Vestibular nerve section, transcranial approach
🔧 52.0 ⚕ 52.0 **FUD** 090 ☐C☐ 80 50 ☐
**AMA:** 2014,Jan,11

**69955** Total facial nerve decompression and/or repair (may include graft)
🔧 56.5 ⚕ 56.5 **FUD** 090 ☐J☐ 80 50 ☐
**AMA:** 2014,Jan,11

**69960** Decompression internal auditory canal
🔧 55.1 ⚕ 55.1 **FUD** 090 ☐J☐ 80 50 ☐
**AMA:** 2014,Jan,11

**69970** Removal of tumor, temporal bone
🔧 61.4 ⚕ 61.4 **FUD** 090 ☐J☐ 80 50 ☐
**AMA:** 2014,Jan,11

**69979** Unlisted procedure, temporal bone, middle fossa approach
🔧 0.00 ⚕ 0.00 **FUD** YYY ☐T☐ 80 50
**AMA:** 2017,Jan,8; 2016,Jan,13; 2015,Jan,16; 2014,Sep,13; 2014,Jan,11

## 69990 Operating Microscope

> EXCLUDES *Magnifying loupes*
> *Use of code with (15756-15758, 15842, 19364, 19368, 20955-20962, 20969-20973, 22551-22552, 22856-22861 [22858], 26551-26554, 26556, 31526, 31531, 31536, 31541, 31545-31546, 31561, 31571, 43116, 43180, 43496, 46601, 46607, 49906, 61548, 63075-63078, 64727, 64820-64823, 65091-68850 [67810], 0184T, 0308T, 0402T)*

+ **69990** Microsurgical techniques, requiring use of operating microscope (List separately in addition to code for primary procedure)
Code first primary procedure
🔧 6.43 ⚕ 6.43 **FUD** ZZZ ☐N☐ N1 80 ☐
**AMA:** 2017,Jan,8; 2016,Feb,12; 2016,Jan,13; 2015,Jan,16; 2014,Sep,13; 2014,Apr,10; 2014,Jan,11; 2014,Jan,8; 2013,Oct,14; 2012,Dec,12; 2012,Jun,12-13; 2012,Mar,9-10; 2012,Jan,15-42

| 26/TC PC/TC Only | A2-Z3 ASC Payment | 50 Bilateral | ♂ Male Only | ♀ Female Only | 🔧 Facility RVU | ⚕ Non-Facility RVU | ☐ CCI |
|---|---|---|---|---|---|---|---|
| **FUD** Follow-up Days | **CMS:** IOM (Pub 100) | A-Y OPPSI | 80/80 Surg Assist Allowed / w/Doc | | 🔲 Lab crosswalk | 🔲 Radiology crosswalk | ☒ CLIA |

314
CPT © 2017 American Medical Association. All Rights Reserved.
© 2017 Optum360, LLC

# 70010-70015 Radiography: Neurodiagnostic

**70010** Myelography, posterior fossa, radiological supervision and interpretation

    📷 1.90    ⚖ 1.90    **FUD** XXX    02 N1 80 ▭

    **AMA:** 2017,Jan,8; 2016,Jan,13; 2015,Jan,16; 2014,Jan,11; 2012,Feb,9-10

**70015** Cisternography, positive contrast, radiological supervision and interpretation

    📷 4.40    ⚖ 4.40    **FUD** XXX    02 N1 80 ▭

    **AMA:** 2014,Jan,11; 2012,Feb,9-10

# 70030-70390 Radiography: Head, Neck, Orofacial Structures

**INCLUDES**  Minimum number of views or more views when needed to adequately complete the study

    Radiographs that have to be repeated during the encounter due to substandard quality; only one unit of service is reported

**EXCLUDES**  *Obtaining more films after review of initial films, based on the discretion of the radiologist, an order for the test, and a change in the patient's condition*

**70030** Radiologic examination, eye, for detection of foreign body

    📷 0.78    ⚖ 0.78    **FUD** XXX    01 N1 80 ▭

    **AMA:** 2014,Jan,11; 2012,Feb,9-10

**70100** Radiologic examination, mandible; partial, less than 4 views

    📷 0.93    ⚖ 0.93    **FUD** XXX    01 N1 80 ▭

    **AMA:** 2014,Jan,11; 2012,Feb,9-10

**70110** complete, minimum of 4 views

    📷 1.07    ⚖ 1.07    **FUD** XXX    01 N1 80 ▭

    **AMA:** 2014,Jan,11; 2012,Feb,9-10

**70120** Radiologic examination, mastoids; less than 3 views per side

    📷 0.95    ⚖ 0.95    **FUD** XXX    01 N1 80 ▭

    **AMA:** 2014,Jan,11; 2012,Feb,9-10

**70130** complete, minimum of 3 views per side

    📷 1.54    ⚖ 1.54    **FUD** XXX    01 N1 80 ▭

    **AMA:** 2014,Jan,11; 2012,Feb,9-10

**70134** Radiologic examination, internal auditory meati, complete

    📷 1.46    ⚖ 1.46    **FUD** XXX    01 N1 80 ▭

    **AMA:** 2014,Jan,11; 2012,Feb,9-10

**70140** Radiologic examination, facial bones; less than 3 views

    📷 0.84    ⚖ 0.84    **FUD** XXX    01 N1 80 ▭

    **AMA:** 2014,Jan,11; 2012,Feb,9-10

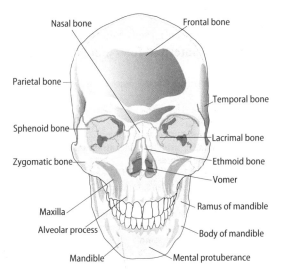

**70150** complete, minimum of 3 views

    📷 1.17    ⚖ 1.17    **FUD** XXX    01 N1 80 ▭

    **AMA:** 2014,Jan,11; 2012,Feb,9-10

**70160** Radiologic examination, nasal bones, complete, minimum of 3 views

    📷 0.92    ⚖ 0.92    **FUD** XXX    01 N1 80 ▭

    **AMA:** 2014,Jan,11; 2012,Feb,9-10

**70170** Dacryocystography, nasolacrimal duct, radiological supervision and interpretation

    **EXCLUDES**  *Injection of contrast (68850)*

    📷 0.00    ⚖ 0.00    **FUD** XXX    02 N1 80 ▭

    **AMA:** 2014,Jan,11; 2012,Feb,9-10

**70190** Radiologic examination; optic foramina

    📷 1.00    ⚖ 1.00    **FUD** XXX    01 N1 80 ▭

    **AMA:** 2014,Jan,11; 2012,Feb,9-10

**70200** orbits, complete, minimum of 4 views

    📷 1.19    ⚖ 1.19    **FUD** XXX    01 N1 80 ▭

    **AMA:** 2014,Jan,11; 2012,Feb,9-10

**70210** Radiologic examination, sinuses, paranasal, less than 3 views

    📷 0.84    ⚖ 0.84    **FUD** XXX    01 N1 80 ▭

    **AMA:** 2014,Jan,11; 2012,Feb,9-10

**70220** Radiologic examination, sinuses, paranasal, complete, minimum of 3 views

    📷 1.06    ⚖ 1.06    **FUD** XXX    01 N1 80 ▭

    **AMA:** 2014,Jan,11; 2012,Feb,9-10

**70240** Radiologic examination, sella turcica

    📷 0.85    ⚖ 0.85    **FUD** XXX    01 N1 80 ▭

    **AMA:** 2014,Jan,11; 2012,Feb,9-10

**70250** Radiologic examination, skull; less than 4 views

    📷 1.02    ⚖ 1.02    **FUD** XXX    01 N1 80 ▭

    **AMA:** 2014,Jan,11; 2012,Feb,9-10

**70260** complete, minimum of 4 views

    📷 1.29    ⚖ 1.29    **FUD** XXX    01 N1 80 ▭

    **AMA:** 2014,Jan,11; 2012,Feb,9-10

**70300** Radiologic examination, teeth; single view

    📷 0.42    ⚖ 0.42    **FUD** XXX    01 N1 80 ▭

    **AMA:** 2014,Jan,11; 2012,Feb,9-10

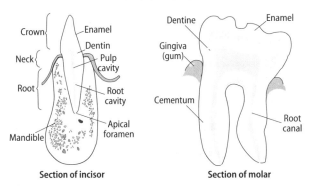

Section of incisor        Section of molar

**70310** partial examination, less than full mouth

    📷 1.02    ⚖ 1.02    **FUD** XXX    01 N1 80 ▭

    **AMA:** 2014,Jan,11; 2012,Feb,9-10

● New Code  ▲ Revised Code  ○ Reinstated  ● New Web Release  ▲ Revised Web Release  Unlisted  Not Covered  # Resequenced

⚖ AMA Mod 51 Exempt  ⑤ Optum Mod 51 Exempt  ⑥ Mod 63 Exempt  ✗ Non-FDA Drug  ★ Telemedicine  M Maternity  A Age Edit  + Add-on  **AMA:** CPT Asst

© 2017 Optum360, LLC    CPT © 2017 American Medical Association. All Rights Reserved.    **315**

Radiology

70320 — 70498

**70320** **complete, full mouth**
📠 1.50 ⚕ 1.50 **FUD** XXX
[01] [N1] [80] [▯]
AMA: 2014,Jan,11; 2012,Feb,9-10

**70328** **Radiologic examination, temporomandibular joint, open and closed mouth; unilateral**
📠 0.86 ⚕ 0.86 **FUD** XXX
[01] [N1] [80] [▯]
AMA: 2014,Jan,11; 2012,Feb,9-10

**70330** **bilateral**
📠 1.36 ⚕ 1.36 **FUD** XXX
[01] [N1] [80] [▯]
AMA: 2017,Jan,8; 2016,Jan,13; 2015,Jan,16; 2014,Jan,11; 2012,Feb,9-10; 2012,Jan,15-42

**70332** **Temporomandibular joint arthrography, radiological supervision and interpretation**
[INCLUDES] Fluoroscopic guidance (77002)
📠 2.26 ⚕ 2.26 **FUD** XXX
[02] [N1] [80] [▯]
AMA: 2017,Jan,8; 2016,Jan,13; 2015,Jan,16; 2014,Jan,11; 2012,Feb,9-10; 2012,Jan,15-42

**70336** **Magnetic resonance (eg, proton) imaging, temporomandibular joint(s)**
📠 9.08 ⚕ 9.08 **FUD** XXX
[03] [Z2] [80] [▯]
AMA: 2017,Jan,8; 2016,Jan,13; 2015,Aug,6; 2015,Jan,16; 2014,Jan,11; 2012,Feb,9-10; 2012,Jan,15-42

**70350** **Cephalogram, orthodontic**
📠 0.56 ⚕ 0.56 **FUD** XXX
[01] [N1] [80] [▯]
AMA: 2017,Jan,8; 2016,Jan,13; 2015,Jan,16; 2014,Jan,11; 2012,Aug,13-14; 2012,Feb,9-10

**70355** **Orthopantogram (eg, panoramic x-ray)**
📠 0.59 ⚕ 0.59 **FUD** XXX
[01] [N1] [80] [▯]
AMA: 2014,Jan,11; 2012,Feb,9-10

**70360** **Radiologic examination; neck, soft tissue**
📠 0.79 ⚕ 0.79 **FUD** XXX
[01] [N1] [80] [▯]
AMA: 2014,Jan,11; 2012,Feb,9-10

**70370** **pharynx or larynx, including fluoroscopy and/or magnification technique**
📠 2.17 ⚕ 2.17 **FUD** XXX
[01] [N1] [80] [▯]
AMA: 2014,Jan,11; 2012,Feb,9-10

**70371** **Complex dynamic pharyngeal and speech evaluation by cine or video recording**
[EXCLUDES] Laryngeal computed tomography (70490-70492)
📠 2.54 ⚕ 2.54 **FUD** XXX
[01] [N1] [80] [▯]
AMA: 2017,Jan,8; 2016,Jan,13; 2015,Jan,16; 2014,Jul,5; 2014,Jan,11; 2012,Feb,9-10

**70380** **Radiologic examination, salivary gland for calculus**
📠 1.01 ⚕ 1.01 **FUD** XXX
[01] [N1] [80] [▯]
AMA: 2014,Jan,11; 2012,Feb,9-10

**70390** **Sialography, radiological supervision and interpretation**
📠 2.64 ⚕ 2.64 **FUD** XXX
[02] [N1] [80] [▯]
AMA: 2014,Jan,11; 2012,Feb,9-10

## 70450-70492 Computerized Tomography: Head, Neck, Face

**CMS:** 100-04,4,250.16 Multiple Procedure Payment Reduction: Certain Diagnostic Imaging Procedures Rendered by Physicians
[INCLUDES] Imaging using tomographic technique enhanced by computer imaging to create a cross-sectional plane of the body
[EXCLUDES] 3D rendering (76376-76377)

**70450** **Computed tomography, head or brain; without contrast material**
📠 3.28 ⚕ 3.28 **FUD** XXX
[03] [Z2] [80] [▯]
AMA: 2017,Jan,8; 2016,Jan,13; 2015,Jan,16; 2014,Jan,11; 2012,Feb,9-10; 2012,Jan,15-42

**70460** **with contrast material(s)**
📠 4.58 ⚕ 4.58 **FUD** XXX
[03] [Z3] [80] [▯]
AMA: 2017,Jan,8; 2016,Jan,13; 2015,Jan,16; 2014,Jan,11; 2012,Feb,9-10; 2012,Jan,15-42

**70470** **without contrast material, followed by contrast material(s) and further sections**
📠 5.42 ⚕ 5.42 **FUD** XXX
[03] [Z2] [80] [▯]
AMA: 2017,Jan,8; 2016,Jan,13; 2015,Jan,16; 2014,Jan,11; 2012,Feb,9-10; 2012,Jan,15-42

**70480** **Computed tomography, orbit, sella, or posterior fossa or outer, middle, or inner ear; without contrast material**
📠 6.58 ⚕ 6.58 **FUD** XXX
[03] [Z2] [80] [▯]
AMA: 2017,Jan,8; 2016,Jan,13; 2015,Jan,16; 2014,Jan,11; 2012,Feb,9-10; 2012,Jan,15-42

**70481** **with contrast material(s)**
📠 7.78 ⚕ 7.78 **FUD** XXX
[03] [Z2] [80] [▯]
AMA: 2017,Jan,8; 2016,Jan,13; 2015,Jan,16; 2014,Jan,11; 2012,Feb,9-10; 2012,Jan,15-42

**70482** **without contrast material, followed by contrast material(s) and further sections**
📠 8.49 ⚕ 8.49 **FUD** XXX
[03] [Z2] [80] [▯]
AMA: 2014,Jan,11; 2012,Feb,9-10

**70486** **Computed tomography, maxillofacial area; without contrast material**
📠 3.93 ⚕ 3.93 **FUD** XXX
[03] [Z2] [80] [▯]
AMA: 2017,Jan,8; 2016,Jan,13; 2015,Jan,16; 2014,Jan,11; 2012,Feb,9-10; 2012,Jan,15-42

**70487** **with contrast material(s)**
📠 4.73 ⚕ 4.73 **FUD** XXX
[03] [Z3] [80] [▯]
AMA: 2014,Jan,11; 2012,Feb,9-10

**70488** **without contrast material, followed by contrast material(s) and further sections**
📠 5.77 ⚕ 5.77 **FUD** XXX
[03] [Z3] [80] [▯]
AMA: 2014,Jan,11; 2012,Feb,9-10

**70490** **Computed tomography, soft tissue neck; without contrast material**
[EXCLUDES] CT of the cervical spine (72125)
📠 5.45 ⚕ 5.45 **FUD** XXX
[03] [Z2] [80] [▯]
AMA: 2014,Jan,11; 2012,Feb,9-10

**70491** **with contrast material(s)**
[EXCLUDES] CT of the cervical spine (72126)
📠 6.65 ⚕ 6.65 **FUD** XXX
[03] [Z2] [80] [▯]
AMA: 2014,Jan,11; 2012,Feb,9-10

**70492** **without contrast material followed by contrast material(s) and further sections**
[EXCLUDES] CT of the cervical spine (72125-72127)
📠 7.84 ⚕ 7.84 **FUD** XXX
[03] [Z2] [80] [▯]
AMA: 2014,Jan,11; 2012,Feb,9-10

## 70496-70498 Computerized Tomographic Angiography: Head and Neck

**CMS:** 100-04,4,250.16 Multiple Procedure Payment Reduction: Certain Diagnostic Imaging Procedures Rendered by Physicians
[INCLUDES] Use of computed tomography to visualize arterial and venous vessels of the body

**70496** **Computed tomographic angiography, head, with contrast material(s), including noncontrast images, if performed, and image postprocessing**
📠 8.28 ⚕ 8.28 **FUD** XXX
[03] [Z2] [80] [▯]
AMA: 2017,Jan,8; 2016,Jan,13; 2015,Jan,16; 2014,Jan,11; 2012,Feb,9-10

**70498** **Computed tomographic angiography, neck, with contrast material(s), including noncontrast images, if performed, and image postprocessing**
📠 8.26 ⚕ 8.26 **FUD** XXX
[03] [Z2] [80] [▯]
AMA: 2017,Jan,8; 2016,Jan,13; 2015,Jan,16; 2014,Jan,11; 2012,Feb,9-10

## 70540-70543 Magnetic Resonance Imaging: Face, Neck, Orbits

**CMS:** 100-04,4,250.16 Multiple Procedure Payment Reduction: Certain Diagnostic Imaging Procedures Rendered by Physicians

INCLUDES   Application of an external magnetic field that forces alignment of hydrogen atom nuclei in soft tissues which converts to sets of tomographic images that can be displayed as three-dimensional images

EXCLUDES   *Magnetic resonance angiography head/neck (70544-70549)*
*Procedure performed more than one time per session*

**70540**   **Magnetic resonance (eg, proton) imaging, orbit, face, and/or neck; without contrast material(s)**
     8.53    8.53   **FUD** XXX      Q3 Z2 80 ▢
     **AMA:** 2017,Jan,8; 2016,Jan,13; 2015,Jan,16; 2014,Jan,11; 2012,Feb,9-10; 2012,Jan,15-42

**70542**   **with contrast material(s)**
     9.58    9.58   **FUD** XXX      Q3 Z2 80 ▢
     **AMA:** 2017,Jan,8; 2016,Jan,13; 2015,Jan,16; 2014,Jan,11; 2012,Feb,9-10; 2012,Jan,15-42

**70543**   **without contrast material(s), followed by contrast material(s) and further sequences**
     11.7    11.7   **FUD** XXX      Q3 Z2 80 ▢
     **AMA:** 2017,Jan,8; 2016,Jan,13; 2015,Jan,16; 2014,Jan,11; 2012,Feb,9-10; 2012,Jan,15-42

## 70544-70549 Magnetic Resonance Angiography: Head and Neck

**CMS:** 100-04,13,40.1.1 Magnetic Resonance Angiography; 100-04,13,40.1.2 HCPCS Coding Requirements; 100-04,4,250.16 Multiple Procedure Payment Reduction: Certain Diagnostic Imaging Procedures Rendered by Physicians

INCLUDES   Use of magnetic fields and radio waves to produce detailed cross-sectional images of internal body structures

EXCLUDES   *Use of code with the following unless a separate diagnostic MRI is performed (70551-70553)*

**70544**   **Magnetic resonance angiography, head; without contrast material(s)**
     11.0    11.0   **FUD** XXX      Q3 Z2 80 ▢
     **AMA:** 2017,Jan,8; 2016,Jan,13; 2015,Jan,16; 2014,Jan,11; 2012,Feb,9-10

**70545**   **with contrast material(s)**
     10.9    10.9   **FUD** XXX      Q3 Z2 80 ▢
     **AMA:** 2017,Jan,8; 2016,Jan,13; 2015,Jan,16; 2014,Jan,11; 2012,Feb,9-10

**70546**   **without contrast material(s), followed by contrast material(s) and further sequences**
     16.8    16.8   **FUD** XXX      Q3 Z2 80 ▢
     **AMA:** 2017,Jan,8; 2016,Jan,13; 2015,Jan,16; 2014,Jan,11; 2012,Feb,9-10

**70547**   **Magnetic resonance angiography, neck; without contrast material(s)**
     11.1    11.1   **FUD** XXX      Q3 Z2 80 ▢
     **AMA:** 2017,Jan,8; 2016,Jan,13; 2015,Jan,16; 2014,Jan,11; 2012,Feb,9-10

**70548**   **with contrast material(s)**
     11.6    11.6   **FUD** XXX      Q3 Z2 80 ▢
     **AMA:** 2017,Jan,8; 2016,Jan,13; 2015,Jan,16; 2014,Jan,11; 2012,Feb,9-10

**70549**   **without contrast material(s), followed by contrast material(s) and further sequences**
     16.9    16.9   **FUD** XXX      Q3 Z2 80 ▢
     **AMA:** 2017,Jan,8; 2016,Jan,13; 2015,Jan,16; 2014,Jan,11; 2012,Feb,9-10

## 70551-70553 Magnetic Resonance Imaging: Brain and Brain Stem

**CMS:** 100-04,4,200.3.2 Multi-Source Photon Stereotactic Radiosurgery Planning and Delivery; 100-04,4,250.16 Multiple Procedure Payment Reduction: Certain Diagnostic Imaging Procedures Rendered by Physicians

INCLUDES   Application of an external magnetic field that forces alignment of hydrogen atom nuclei in soft tissues which converts to sets of tomographic images that can be displayed as three-dimensional images

EXCLUDES   *Magnetic spectroscopy (76390)*

**70551**   **Magnetic resonance (eg, proton) imaging, brain (including brain stem); without contrast material**
     6.52    6.52   **FUD** XXX      Q3 Z2 80 ▢
     **AMA:** 2017,Jan,8; 2016,Jan,13; 2015,Jan,16; 2014,Jan,11; 2012,Feb,9-10; 2012,Jan,15-42

**70552**   **with contrast material(s)**
     9.04    9.04   **FUD** XXX      Q3 Z2 80 ▢
     **AMA:** 2017,Jan,8; 2016,Jan,13; 2015,Jan,16; 2014,Jan,11; 2012,Feb,9-10; 2012,Jan,15-42

**70553**   **without contrast material, followed by contrast material(s) and further sequences**
     10.6    10.6   **FUD** XXX      Q3 Z2 80 ▢
     **AMA:** 2017,Jan,8; 2016,Jan,13; 2015,Jan,16; 2014,Jan,11; 2012,Feb,9-10; 2012,Jan,15-42

## 70554-70555 Magnetic Resonance Imaging: Brain Mapping

INCLUDES   Neuroimaging technique using MRI to identify and map signals related to brain activity

EXCLUDES   *Use of code with the following unless a separate diagnostic MRI is performed (70551-70553)*

**70554**   **Magnetic resonance imaging, brain, functional MRI; including test selection and administration of repetitive body part movement and/or visual stimulation, not requiring physician or psychologist administration**

     EXCLUDES   *Functional brain mapping (96020)*
          *Testing performed by a physician or psychologist (70555)*
     12.6    12.6   **FUD** XXX      Q3 Z2 80 ▢
     **AMA:** 2017,Jan,8; 2016,Jan,13; 2015,Jan,16; 2014,Jan,11; 2012,Feb,9-10; 2012,Jan,15-42

**70555**   **requiring physician or psychologist administration of entire neurofunctional testing**

     EXCLUDES   *Testing performed by a technologist, nonphysician, or nonpsychologist (70554)*
     Code also (96020)
     0.00    0.00   **FUD** XXX      S Z2 80 ▢
     **AMA:** 2017,Jan,8; 2016,Jan,13; 2015,Jan,16; 2014,Jan,11; 2012,Feb,9-10

## 70557-70559 Magnetic Resonance Imaging: Intraoperative

EXCLUDES   *Intracranial lesion stereotaxic biopsy with magnetic resonance guidance (61751, 77021-77022)*
*Procedures performed more than one time per surgical encounter*
*Use of codes unless a separate report is generated*
Code also stereotactic biopsy, aspiration, or excision, when performed with magnetic resonance imaging (61751)

**70557**   **Magnetic resonance (eg, proton) imaging, brain (including brain stem and skull base), during open intracranial procedure (eg, to assess for residual tumor or residual vascular malformation); without contrast material**
     0.00    0.00   **FUD** XXX      S Z2 80 ▢
     **AMA:** 2014,Jan,11; 2012,Feb,9-10

**70558**   **with contrast material(s)**
     0.00    0.00   **FUD** XXX      S Z2 80 ▢
     **AMA:** 2014,Jan,11; 2012,Feb,9-10

**70559**   **without contrast material(s), followed by contrast material(s) and further sequences**
     0.00    0.00   **FUD** XXX      S Z2 80 ▢
     **AMA:** 2014,Jan,11; 2012,Feb,9-10

## 71010-71130 Radiography: Thorax

~~**71010**~~   ~~Radiologic examination, chest; single view, frontal~~
     To report, see 71045

---

Radiology

**71015** ~~stereo, frontal~~

    To report, see 71045

**71020** ~~Radiologic examination, chest, 2 views, frontal and lateral;~~

    To report, see 71046

**71021** ~~with apical lordotic procedure~~

    To report, see 71047

**71022** ~~with oblique projections~~

    To report, see 71047-71048

**71023** ~~with fluoroscopy~~

    To report, see 71046, 76000-76001

**71030** ~~Radiologic examination, chest, complete, minimum of 4 views;~~

    To report, see 71048

**71034** ~~with fluoroscopy~~

    To report, see 71048, 76000-76001

**71035** ~~Radiologic examination, chest, special views (eg, lateral decubitus, Bucky studies)~~

    To report, see 71046-71048

● **71045** Radiologic examination, chest; single view

    *EXCLUDES* *Acute abdomen series that includes a view of the chest (74022)*

    *Remotely performed CAD (0175T)*

    Code also concurrent computer-aided detection (CAD) (0174T)

● **71046** 2 views

    *EXCLUDES* *Acute abdomen series that includes a view of the chest (74022)*

    *Remotely performed CAD (0175T)*

    Code also concurrent computer-aided detection (CAD) (0174T)

● **71047** 3 views

    *EXCLUDES* *Acute abdomen series that includes a view of the chest (74022)*

    *Remotely performed CAD (0175T)*

    Code also concurrent computer-aided detection (CAD) (0174T)

● **71048** 4 or more views

    *EXCLUDES* *Acute abdomen series that includes a view of the chest (74022)*

    *Remotely performed CAD (0175T)*

    Code also concurrent computer-aided detection (CAD) (0174T)

**71100** Radiologic examination, ribs, unilateral; 2 views

    📷 0.93   📷 0.93   **FUD** XXX    Q1 N1 80 🖵

    **AMA:** 2014,Jan,11; 2012,Feb,9-10

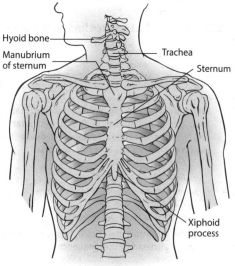

Hyoid bone

Manubrium of sternum

Trachea

Sternum

Xiphoid process

**71101** including posteroanterior chest, minimum of 3 views

    📷 1.03   📷 1.03   **FUD** XXX    Q1 N1 80 🖵

    **AMA:** 2014,Jan,11; 2012,Feb,9-10

**71110** Radiologic examination, ribs, bilateral; 3 views

    📷 1.06   📷 1.06   **FUD** XXX    Q1 N1 80 🖵

    **AMA:** 2014,Jan,11; 2012,Feb,9-10

**71111** including posteroanterior chest, minimum of 4 views

    📷 1.36   📷 1.36   **FUD** XXX    Q1 N1 80 🖵

    **AMA:** 2014,Jan,11; 2012,Feb,9-10

**71120** Radiologic examination; sternum, minimum of 2 views

    📷 0.83   📷 0.83   **FUD** XXX    Q1 N1 80 🖵

    **AMA:** 2014,Jan,11; 2012,Feb,9-10

**71130** sternoclavicular joint or joints, minimum of 3 views

    📷 1.01   📷 1.01   **FUD** XXX    Q1 N1 80 🖵

    **AMA:** 2014,Jan,11; 2012,Feb,9-10

## 71250-71270 Computerized Tomography: Thorax

**CMS:** 100-04,4,250.16 Multiple Procedure Payment Reduction: Certain Diagnostic Imaging Procedures Rendered by Physicians

*INCLUDES* Imaging using tomographic technique enhanced by computer imaging to create a cross-sectional plane of the body

*EXCLUDES* *3D rendering (76376-76377)*

    *CT of the heart (75571-75574)*

**71250** Computed tomography, thorax; without contrast material

    📷 5.10   📷 5.10   **FUD** XXX    Q3 ZZ 80 🖵

    **AMA:** 2017,Jan,8; 2016,Jan,13; 2015,Jan,16; 2014,Jan,11; 2012,Feb,9-10; 2012,Jan,15-42

**71260** with contrast material(s)

    📷 6.48   📷 6.48   **FUD** XXX    Q3 ZZ 80 🖵

    **AMA:** 2017,Jan,8; 2016,Jan,13; 2015,Jan,16; 2014,Jan,11; 2012,Feb,9-10; 2012,Jan,15-42

**71270** without contrast material, followed by contrast material(s) and further sections

    📷 7.76   📷 7.76   **FUD** XXX    Q3 ZZ 80 🖵

    **AMA:** 2017,Jan,8; 2016,Jan,13; 2015,Jan,16; 2014,Jan,11; 2012,Feb,9-10; 2012,Jan,15-42

## 71275 Computerized Tomographic Angiography: Thorax

**CMS:** 100-04,4,250.16 Multiple Procedure Payment Reduction: Certain Diagnostic Imaging Procedures Rendered by Physicians

*INCLUDES* Multiple rapid thin section CT scans to create cross-sectional images of bones, organs and tissues

*EXCLUDES* *CT angiography of coronary arteries that includes calcification score and/or cardiac morphology (75574)*

**71275** Computed tomographic angiography, chest (noncoronary), with contrast material(s), including noncontrast images, if performed, and image postprocessing

    📷 8.48   📷 8.48   **FUD** XXX    Q3 ZZ 80 🖵

    **AMA:** 2017,Jan,8; 2016,Jan,13; 2015,Jan,16; 2014,Jan,11; 2012,Feb,9-10; 2012,Jan,15-42

## 71550-71552 Magnetic Resonance Imaging: Thorax

**CMS:** 100-04,4,250.16 Multiple Procedure Payment Reduction: Certain Diagnostic Imaging Procedures Rendered by Physicians

*INCLUDES* Application of an external magnetic field that forces alignment of hydrogen atom nuclei in soft tissues which converts to sets of tomographic images that can be displayed as three-dimensional images

*EXCLUDES* *MRI of the breast (77058-77059)*

**71550** Magnetic resonance (eg, proton) imaging, chest (eg, for evaluation of hilar and mediastinal lymphadenopathy); without contrast material(s)

    📷 11.7   📷 11.7   **FUD** XXX    Q3 ZZ 80 🖵

    **AMA:** 2017,Jan,8; 2016,Jan,13; 2015,Jan,16; 2014,Jan,11; 2012,Feb,9-10; 2012,Jan,15-42

**71551** with contrast material(s)

    📷 13.0   📷 13.0   **FUD** XXX    Q3 ZZ 80 🖵

    **AMA:** 2017,Jan,8; 2016,Jan,13; 2015,Jan,16; 2014,Jan,11; 2012,Feb,9-10; 2012,Jan,15-42

**71552** without contrast material(s), followed by contrast material(s) and further sequences

    📷 16.3   📷 16.3   **FUD** XXX    Q3 ZZ 80 🖵

    **AMA:** 2017,Jan,8; 2016,Jan,13; 2015,Jan,16; 2014,Jan,11; 2012,Feb,9-10; 2012,Jan,15-42

**26/TC** PC/TC Only   **A2-Z3** ASC Payment   **50** Bilateral   ♂ Male Only   ♀ Female Only   📷 Facility RVU   Non-Facility RVU   🖵 CCI
**FUD** Follow-up Days   **CMS:** IOM (Pub 100)   **A-Y** OPPSI   **80/80** Surg Assist Allowed / w/Doc   Lab Crosswalk   Radiology Crosswalk   **X** CLIA

318     CPT © 2017 American Medical Association. All Rights Reserved.     © 2017 Optum360, LLC

## 71555 Magnetic Resonance Angiography: Thorax

**CMS:** 100-04,13,40.1.1 Magnetic Resonance Angiography; 100-04,13,40.1.2 HCPCS Coding Requirements; 100-04,4,250.16 Multiple Procedure Payment Reduction: Certain Diagnostic Imaging Procedures Rendered by Physicians

**71555** **Magnetic resonance angiography, chest (excluding myocardium), with or without contrast material(s)**
🚗 11.2  ⚕ 11.2  **FUD** XXX    B 80 📷
**AMA:** 2017,Jan,8; 2016,Jan,13; 2015,Jan,16; 2014,Jan,11; 2012,Feb,9-10

## 72020-72120 Radiography: Spine

**INCLUDES**  Minimum number of views or more views when needed to adequately complete the study
Radiographs that have to be repeated during the encounter due to substandard quality; only one unit of service is reported

**EXCLUDES**  *Obtaining more films after review of initial films, based on the discretion of the radiologist, an order for the test, and a change in the patient's condition*

**72020** **Radiologic examination, spine, single view, specify level**
**EXCLUDES**  *Single view of entire thoracic and lumbar spine (72081)*
🚗 0.62  ⚕ 0.62  **FUD** XXX    01 N1 80 📷
**AMA:** 2017,Jan,8; 2016,Sep,4; 2016,Jan,13; 2015,Oct,9; 2015,Jan,16; 2014,Jan,11; 2013,Jul,10; 2012,Feb,9-10

**72040** **Radiologic examination, spine, cervical; 2 or 3 views**
🚗 0.93  ⚕ 0.93  **FUD** XXX    01 N1 80 📷
**AMA:** 2017,Jan,8; 2016,Jan,13; 2015,Jan,16; 2014,Jan,11; 2013,Jul,10; 2012,Feb,9-10

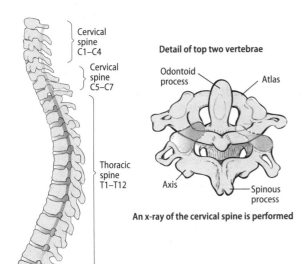

Cervical spine C1–C4
Cervical spine C5–C7
Thoracic spine T1–T12

**Detail of top two vertebrae**

Odontoid process
Atlas
Axis
Spinous process

**An x-ray of the cervical spine is performed**

**72050** **4 or 5 views**
🚗 1.28  ⚕ 1.28  **FUD** XXX    01 N1 80 📷
**AMA:** 2014,Jan,11; 2012,Feb,9-10

**72052** **6 or more views**
🚗 1.58  ⚕ 1.58  **FUD** XXX    01 N1 80 📷
**AMA:** 2014,Jan,11; 2012,Feb,9-10

**72070** **Radiologic examination, spine; thoracic, 2 views**
🚗 0.96  ⚕ 0.96  **FUD** XXX    01 N1 80 📷
**AMA:** 2017,Jan,8; 2016,Jan,13; 2015,Jan,16; 2014,Jan,11; 2012,Feb,9-10

**72072** **thoracic, 3 views**
🚗 0.97  ⚕ 0.97  **FUD** XXX    01 N1 80 📷
**AMA:** 2017,Jan,8; 2016,Jan,13; 2015,Jan,16; 2014,Jan,11; 2012,Feb,9-10

**72074** **thoracic, minimum of 4 views**
🚗 1.10  ⚕ 1.10  **FUD** XXX    01 N1 80 📷
**AMA:** 2017,Jan,8; 2016,Jan,13; 2015,Jan,16; 2014,Jan,11; 2012,Feb,9-10

**72080** **thoracolumbar junction, minimum of 2 views**
**EXCLUDES**  *Single view of thoracolumbar junction (72020)*
🚗 0.86  ⚕ 0.86  **FUD** XXX    01 N1 80 📷
**AMA:** 2017,Jan,8; 2016,Sep,4; 2016,Jan,13; 2015,Oct,9; 2015,Jan,16; 2014,Jan,11; 2012,Feb,9-10

**72081** **Radiologic examination, spine, entire thoracic and lumbar, including skull, cervical and sacral spine if performed (eg, scoliosis evaluation); one view**
🚗 1.10  ⚕ 1.10  **FUD** XXX    01 N1 80 📷
**AMA:** 2017,Jan,8; 2016,Sep,4

**72082** **2 or 3 views**
🚗 1.76  ⚕ 1.76  **FUD** XXX    01 N1 80 📷
**AMA:** 2017,Jan,8; 2016,Sep,4

**72083** **4 or 5 views**
🚗 1.91  ⚕ 1.91  **FUD** XXX    S Z3 80 📷
**AMA:** 2017,Jan,8; 2016,Sep,4

**72084** **minimum of 6 views**
🚗 2.27  ⚕ 2.27  **FUD** XXX    S Z3 80 📷
**AMA:** 2017,Jan,8; 2016,Sep,4

**72100** **Radiologic examination, spine, lumbosacral; 2 or 3 views**
🚗 0.99  ⚕ 0.99  **FUD** XXX    01 N1 80 📷
**AMA:** 2017,Jan,8; 2016,Jan,13; 2015,Jan,16; 2014,Jan,11; 2012,Feb,9-10

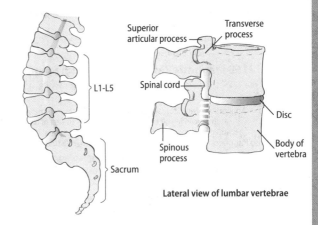

L1-L5
Sacrum

Superior articular process
Transverse process
Spinal cord
Disc
Body of vertebra
Spinous process

**Lateral view of lumbar vertebrae**

**72110** **minimum of 4 views**
🚗 1.38  ⚕ 1.38  **FUD** XXX    01 N1 80 📷
**AMA:** 2017,Jan,8; 2016,Jan,13; 2015,Jan,16; 2014,Jan,11; 2012,Feb,9-10

**72114** **complete, including bending views, minimum of 6 views**
🚗 1.75  ⚕ 1.75  **FUD** XXX    01 N1 80 📷
**AMA:** 2014,Jan,11; 2012,Feb,9-10

**72120** **bending views only, 2 or 3 views**
🚗 1.14  ⚕ 1.14  **FUD** XXX    01 N1 80 📷
**AMA:** 2017,Jan,8; 2016,Aug,7; 2014,Jan,11; 2012,Feb,9-10

## 72125-72133 Computerized Tomography: Spine

**CMS:** 100-04,12,20.4.7 Services Not Meeting National Electrical Manufacturers Association (NEMA) Standard; 100-04,4,20.6.12 Use of HCPCS Modifier – CT; 100-04,4,250.16 Multiple Procedure Payment Reduction: Certain Diagnostic Imaging Procedures Rendered by Physicians

**INCLUDES**  Imaging using tomographic technique enhanced by computer imaging to create a cross-sectional plane of the body

**EXCLUDES**  *3D rendering (76376-76377)*
Code also intrathecal injection procedure when performed (61055, 62284)

**72125** **Computed tomography, cervical spine; without contrast material**
🚗 5.22  ⚕ 5.22  **FUD** XXX    03 Z2 80 📷
**AMA:** 2014,Jan,11; 2012,Feb,9-10

**72126** **with contrast material**
🚗 6.45  ⚕ 6.45  **FUD** XXX    03 Z3 80 📷
**AMA:** 2017,Jan,8; 2016,Jan,13; 2015,Jan,16; 2014,Jan,11; 2012,Feb,9-10

Radiology

721297—72191

**72127** without contrast material, followed by contrast material(s) and further sections
🚗 7.62   ⚕ 7.62   **FUD** XXX   [Q3] [Z2] [80] [▭]
**AMA:** 2014,Jan,11; 2012,Feb,9-10

**72128** Computed tomography, thoracic spine; without contrast material
🚗 5.10   ⚕ 5.10   **FUD** XXX   [Q3] [Z2] [80] [▭]
**AMA:** 2014,Jan,11; 2012,Feb,9-10

**72129** with contrast material
🚗 6.48   ⚕ 6.48   **FUD** XXX   [Q3] [Z2] [80] [▭]
**AMA:** 2017,Jan,8; 2016,Jan,13; 2015,Jan,16; 2014,Jan,11; 2012,Feb,9-10

**72130** without contrast material, followed by contrast material(s) and further sections
🚗 7.65   ⚕ 7.65   **FUD** XXX   [Q3] [Z2] [80] [▭]
**AMA:** 2014,Jan,11; 2012,Feb,9-10

**72131** Computed tomography, lumbar spine; without contrast material
🚗 5.08   ⚕ 5.08   **FUD** XXX   [Q3] [Z2] [80] [▭]
**AMA:** 2014,Jan,11; 2012,Feb,9-10

**72132** with contrast material
🚗 6.44   ⚕ 6.44   **FUD** XXX   [Q3] [Z3] [80] [▭]
**AMA:** 2017,Jan,8; 2016,Jan,13; 2015,Jan,16; 2014,Jan,11; 2012,Feb,9-10

**72133** without contrast material, followed by contrast material(s) and further sections
🚗 7.61   ⚕ 7.61   **FUD** XXX   [Q3] [Z2] [80] [▭]
**AMA:** 2014,Jan,11; 2012,Feb,9-10

## 72141-72158 Magnetic Resonance Imaging: Spine

**CMS:** 100-04,4,250.16 Multiple Procedure Payment Reduction: Certain Diagnostic Imaging Procedures Rendered by Physicians

[INCLUDES] Application of an external magnetic field that forces alignment of hydrogen atom nuclei in soft tissues which converts to sets of tomographic images that can be displayed as three-dimensional images
Code also intrathecal injection procedure when performed (61055, 62284)

**72141** Magnetic resonance (eg, proton) imaging, spinal canal and contents, cervical; without contrast material
🚗 6.34   ⚕ 6.34   **FUD** XXX   [Q3] [Z2] [80] [▭]
**AMA:** 2017,Jan,8; 2016,Jan,13; 2015,Jan,16; 2014,Jun,14; 2014,Jan,11; 2012,Feb,9-10

**72142** with contrast material(s)
[EXCLUDES] MRI of cervical spinal canal performed without contrast followed by repeating the study with contrast (72156)
🚗 9.18   ⚕ 9.18   **FUD** XXX   [Q3] [Z2] [80] [▭]
**AMA:** 2017,Jan,8; 2016,Jan,13; 2015,Jan,16; 2014,Jan,11; 2012,Feb,9-10

**72146** Magnetic resonance (eg, proton) imaging, spinal canal and contents, thoracic; without contrast material
🚗 6.35   ⚕ 6.35   **FUD** XXX   [Q3] [Z2] [80] [▭]
**AMA:** 2017,Jan,8; 2016,Jan,13; 2015,Jan,16; 2014,Jun,14; 2014,Jan,11; 2012,Feb,9-10

**72147** with contrast material(s)
[EXCLUDES] MRI of thoracic spinal canal performed without contrast followed by repeating the study with contrast (72157)
🚗 9.12   ⚕ 9.12   **FUD** XXX   [Q3] [Z2] [80] [▭]
**AMA:** 2017,Jan,8; 2016,Jan,13; 2015,Jan,16; 2014,Jan,11; 2012,Feb,9-10; 2012,Jan,15-42

**72148** Magnetic resonance (eg, proton) imaging, spinal canal and contents, lumbar; without contrast material
🚗 6.32   ⚕ 6.32   **FUD** XXX   [Q3] [Z2] [80] [▭]
**AMA:** 2017,Jan,8; 2016,Jan,13; 2015,Jan,16; 2014,Jun,14; 2014,Jan,11; 2012,Feb,9-10; 2012,Jan,15-42

**72149** with contrast material(s)
[EXCLUDES] MRI of lumbar spinal canal performed without contrast followed by repeating the study with contrast (72158)
🚗 9.08   ⚕ 9.08   **FUD** XXX   [Q3] [Z2] [80] [▭]
**AMA:** 2014,Jan,11; 2012,Feb,9-10

**72156** Magnetic resonance (eg, proton) imaging, spinal canal and contents, without contrast material, followed by contrast material(s) and further sequences; cervical
🚗 10.7   ⚕ 10.7   **FUD** XXX   [Q3] [Z2] [80] [▭]
**AMA:** 2014,Jan,11; 2012,Feb,9-10

**72157** thoracic
🚗 10.7   ⚕ 10.7   **FUD** XXX   [Q3] [Z2] [80] [▭]
**AMA:** 2014,Jan,11; 2012,Feb,9-10

**72158** lumbar
🚗 10.6   ⚕ 10.6   **FUD** XXX   [Q3] [Z2] [80] [▭]
**AMA:** 2014,Jan,11; 2012,Feb,9-10

Spinal cord — Body of column

Spinous process

**Superior view of thoracic spine and surrounding paraspinal muscles**

## 72159 Magnetic Resonance Angiography: Spine

**CMS:** 100-04,13,40.1.1 Magnetic Resonance Angiography; 100-04,13,40.1.2 HCPCS Coding Requirements; 100-04,4,250.16 Multiple Procedure Payment Reduction: Certain Diagnostic Imaging Procedures Rendered by Physicians

**72159** Magnetic resonance angiography, spinal canal and contents, with or without contrast material(s)
🚗 11.7   ⚕ 11.7   **FUD** XXX   [B] [80] [▭]
**AMA:** 2017,Jan,8; 2016,Jan,13; 2015,Jan,16; 2014,Jan,11; 2012,Feb,9-10

## 72170-72190 Radiography: Pelvis

[INCLUDES] Minimum number of views or more views when needed to adequately complete the study
Radiographs that have to be repeated during the encounter due to substandard quality; only one unit of service is reported
[EXCLUDES] A second interpretation by the requesting physician (included in E&M service)
Combined CT or CT angiography of abdomen and pelvis (74174, 74176-74178)
Obtaining more films after review of initial films, based on the discretion of the radiologist, an order for the test, and a change in the patient's condition
Pelvimetry (74710)

**72170** Radiologic examination, pelvis; 1 or 2 views
🚗 0.90   ⚕ 0.90   **FUD** XXX   [Q1] [N1] [80] [▭]
**AMA:** 2017,Jan,8; 2016,Aug,7; 2016,Jun,5; 2016,Jan,13; 2015,Jan,16; 2014,Jan,11; 2012,Feb,9-10; 2012,Jan,15-42

**72190** complete, minimum of 3 views
🚗 1.07   ⚕ 1.07   **FUD** XXX   [Q1] [N1] [80] [▭]
**AMA:** 2016,Jun,5; 2014,Jan,11; 2012,Feb,9-10

## 72191 Computerized Tomographic Angiography: Pelvis

**CMS:** 100-04,4,250.16 Multiple Procedure Payment Reduction: Certain Diagnostic Imaging Procedures Rendered by Physicians
[EXCLUDES] Computed tomographic angiography (73706, 74174-74175, 75635)

**72191** Computed tomographic angiography, pelvis, with contrast material(s), including noncontrast images, if performed, and image postprocessing
🚗 8.64   ⚕ 8.64   **FUD** XXX   [Q3] [Z2] [80] [▭]
**AMA:** 2017,Jan,8; 2016,Jan,13; 2015,Jan,16; 2014,Jan,11; 2012,Feb,9-10

[26]/[TC] PC/TC Only   [A8]-[Z8] ASC Payment   [50] Bilateral   ♂ Male Only   ♀ Female Only   🚗 Facility RVU   ⚕ Non-Facility RVU   [▭] CCI
**FUD** Follow-up Days   **CMS:** IOM (Pub 100)   [A]-[Y] OPPSI   [80]/[80] Surg Assist Allowed / w/Doc   [▨] Lab Crosswalk   [▤] Radiology Crosswalk   [✗] CLIA
CPT © 2017 American Medical Association. All Rights Reserved.

© 2017 Optum360, LLC

## 72192-72194 Computerized Tomography: Pelvis

**CMS:** 100-04,4,250.16 Multiple Procedure Payment Reduction: Certain Diagnostic Imaging Procedures Rendered by Physicians

*EXCLUDES*   *3D rendering (76376-76377)*
*Combined CT of abdomen and pelvis (74176-74178)*
*CT colonography, diagnostic (74261-74262)*
*CT colonography, screening (74263)*

**72192**   **Computed tomography, pelvis; without contrast material**
  4.13   4.13   **FUD** XXX    03 Z2 80 □
**AMA:** 2017,Jan,8; 2016,Jan,13; 2015,Jan,16; 2014,Jan,11; 2012,Oct,12; 2012,Feb,9-10; 2012,Jan,15-42

**72193**   **with contrast material(s)**
  6.38   6.38   **FUD** XXX    03 Z2 80 □
**AMA:** 2017,Jan,8; 2016,Jan,13; 2015,Jan,16; 2014,Jan,11; 2012,Oct,12; 2012,Feb,9-10

**72194**   **without contrast material, followed by contrast material(s) and further sections**
  7.34   7.34   **FUD** XXX    03 Z2 80 □
**AMA:** 2017,Jan,8; 2016,Jan,13; 2015,Jan,16; 2014,Jan,11; 2012,Oct,12; 2012,Feb,9-10; 2012,Jan,15-42

## 72195-72197 Magnetic Resonance Imaging: Pelvis

**CMS:** 100-04,4,250.16 Multiple Procedure Payment Reduction: Certain Diagnostic Imaging Procedures Rendered by Physicians

*INCLUDES*   Application of an external magnetic field that forces alignment of hydrogen atom nuclei in soft tissues which converts to sets of tomographic images that can be displayed as three-dimensional images

*EXCLUDES*   *Magnetic resonance imaging of fetus(es) (74712-74713)*

**72195**   **Magnetic resonance (eg, proton) imaging, pelvis; without contrast material(s)**
  10.5   10.5   **FUD** XXX    03 Z2 80 □
**AMA:** 2017,Jan,8; 2016,Jun,5; 2016,Jan,13; 2015,Jan,16; 2014,Jun,14; 2014,Jan,11; 2012,Feb,9-10; 2012,Jan,15-42

**72196**   **with contrast material(s)**
  11.5   11.5   **FUD** XXX    03 Z2 80 □
**AMA:** 2017,Jan,8; 2016,Jun,5; 2016,Jan,13; 2015,Jan,16; 2014,Jan,11; 2012,Feb,9-10; 2012,Jan,15-42

**72197**   **without contrast material(s), followed by contrast material(s) and further sequences**
  14.2   14.2   **FUD** XXX    03 Z2 80 □
**AMA:** 2017,Jan,8; 2016,Jun,5; 2016,Jan,13; 2015,Jan,16; 2014,Jan,11; 2012,Feb,9-10

## 72198 Magnetic Resonance Angiography: Pelvis

**CMS:** 100-04,13,40.1.1 Magnetic Resonance Angiography; 100-04,13,40.1.2 HCPCS Coding Requirements; 100-04,4,250.16 Multiple Procedure Payment Reduction: Certain Diagnostic Imaging Procedures Rendered by Physicians

*INCLUDES*   Use of magnetic fields and radio waves to produce detailed cross-sectional images of the arteries and veins

**72198**   **Magnetic resonance angiography, pelvis, with or without contrast material(s)**
  11.3   11.3   **FUD** XXX    B 80 □
**AMA:** 2017,Jan,8; 2016,Jan,13; 2015,Jan,16; 2014,Jan,11; 2012,Feb,9-10

## 72200-72220 Radiography: Pelvisacral

*INCLUDES*   Minimum number of views or more views when needed to adequately complete the study
Radiographs that have to be repeated during the encounter due to substandard quality; only one unit of service is reported

*EXCLUDES*   *Obtaining more films after review of initial films, based on the discretion of the radiologist, an order for the test, and a change in the patient's condition*
*Second interpretation by the requesting physician (included in E&M service)*

**72200**   **Radiologic examination, sacroiliac joints; less than 3 views**
  0.80   0.80   **FUD** XXX    01 N1 80 □
**AMA:** 2014,Jan,11; 2012,Feb,9-10

**72202**   **3 or more views**
  0.93   0.93   **FUD** XXX    01 N1 80 □
**AMA:** 2014,Jan,11; 2012,Feb,9-10

**72220**   **Radiologic examination, sacrum and coccyx, minimum of 2 views**
  0.79   0.79   **FUD** XXX    01 N1 80 □
**AMA:** 2014,Jan,11; 2012,Feb,9-10

## 72240-72270 Myelography with Contrast: Spinal Cord

**CMS:** 100-04,13,30.1.3.1 Payment for Low Osmolar Contrast Material

*EXCLUDES*   *Injection procedure for myelography (62284)*
*Myelography (62302-62305)*
Code also injection at C1-C2 for complete myelography (61055)

**72240**   **Myelography, cervical, radiological supervision and interpretation**
  2.78   2.78   **FUD** XXX    02 N1 80 □
**AMA:** 2017,Jan,8; 2016,Jan,13; 2015,Jan,16; 2014,Sep,3; 2014,Jan,11; 2012,Feb,9-10

**72255**   **Myelography, thoracic, radiological supervision and interpretation**
  2.79   2.79   **FUD** XXX    02 N1 80 □
**AMA:** 2017,Jan,8; 2016,Jan,13; 2015,Jan,16; 2014,Sep,3; 2014,Jan,11; 2012,Feb,9-10

**72265**   **Myelography, lumbosacral, radiological supervision and interpretation**
  2.61   2.61   **FUD** XXX    02 N1 80 □
**AMA:** 2017,Jan,8; 2016,Jan,13; 2015,Jan,16; 2014,Sep,3; 2014,Jan,11; 2012,Feb,9-10

**72270**   **Myelography, 2 or more regions (eg, lumbar/thoracic, cervical/thoracic, lumbar/cervical, lumbar/thoracic/cervical), radiological supervision and interpretation**
  3.60   3.60   **FUD** XXX    02 N1 80 □
**AMA:** 2017,Jan,8; 2016,Jan,13; 2015,Jan,16; 2014,Sep,3; 2014,Jan,11; 2012,Feb,9-10

## 72275 Radiography: Epidural Space

*INCLUDES*   Epidurogram, documentation of images, formal written report
Fluoroscopic guidance (77003)

*EXCLUDES*   *Arthrodesis (22586, 0195T-0196T)*
*Second interpretation by the requesting physician (included in E&M service)*
Code also injection procedure as appropriate (62280-62282, 62320-62327, 64479-64480, 64483-64484)

**72275**   **Epidurography, radiological supervision and interpretation**
  3.26   3.26   **FUD** XXX    N N1 80 □
**AMA:** 2017,Jan,8; 2016,Jan,13; 2015,Jan,16; 2014,Jan,11; 2012,Jul,3-6; 2012,Jun,12-13; 2012,Feb,9-10; 2012,Jan,15-42

## 72285 Radiography: Intervertebral Disc (Cervical/Thoracic)

**CMS:** 100-04,13,30.1.3.1 Payment for Low Osmolar Contrast Material
Code also discography injection procedure (62291)

**72285**   **Discography, cervical or thoracic, radiological supervision and interpretation**
  3.19   3.19   **FUD** XXX    02 N1 80 □
**AMA:** 2017,Jan,8; 2016,Jan,13; 2015,Jan,16; 2014,Jan,11; 2012,Feb,9-10

## 72295 Radiography: Intervertebral Disc (Lumbar)

**CMS:** 100-04,13,30.1.3.1 Payment for Low Osmolar Contrast Material
Code also discography injection procedure (62290)

**72295**   **Discography, lumbar, radiological supervision and interpretation**
  2.76   2.76   **FUD** XXX    02 N1 80 □
**AMA:** 2017,Feb,12; 2017,Jan,8; 2016,Jan,13; 2015,Jan,16; 2014,Jan,11; 2012,Jul,3-6; 2012,Feb,9-10; 2012,Jan,15-42

## 73000-73085 Radiography: Shoulder and Upper Arm

**INCLUDES** Minimum number of views or more views when needed to adequately complete the study
Radiographs that have to be repeated during the encounter due to substandard quality; only one unit of service is reported

**EXCLUDES** *Obtaining more films after review of initial films, based on the discretion of the radiologist, an order for the test, and a change in the patient's condition*
*Second interpretation by the requesting physician (included in E&M service)*
*Stress views of upper body joint(s), when performed (77071)*

**73000** **Radiologic examination; clavicle, complete**
0.78  0.78  **FUD** XXX  01 N1 80
**AMA:** 2014,Jan,11; 2012,Feb,9-10

**Radiograph**

- Gold wedding band absorbs all x-rays (white)
- Air allows all rays to reach film (black)
- Soft tissues absorb part of rays and will vary in gray intensity
- Calcium in bone absorbs most of rays and is nearly white

X-ray beam

Film

**Posterioranterior (PA) chest study; lateral views also common**

**73010** **scapula, complete**
0.85  0.85  **FUD** XXX  01 N1 80
**AMA:** 2014,Jan,11; 2012,Feb,9-10

**73020** **Radiologic examination, shoulder; 1 view**
0.65  0.65  **FUD** XXX  01 N1 80
**AMA:** 2014,Jan,11; 2012,Feb,9-10

**73030** **complete, minimum of 2 views**
0.82  0.82  **FUD** XXX  01 N1 80
**AMA:** 2014,Jan,11; 2012,Feb,9-10

**73040** **Radiologic examination, shoulder, arthrography, radiological supervision and interpretation**
**INCLUDES** Fluoroscopic guidance (77002)
Code also arthrography injection procedure (23350)
2.82  2.82  **FUD** XXX  02 N1 80
**AMA:** 2017,Jan,8; 2016,Jan,13; 2015,Jan,16; 2014,Jan,11; 2012,Feb,9-10; 2012,Jan,15-42

**73050** **Radiologic examination; acromioclavicular joints, bilateral, with or without weighted distraction**
1.00  1.00  **FUD** XXX  01 N1 80
**AMA:** 2014,Jan,11; 2012,Feb,9-10

**73060** **humerus, minimum of 2 views**
0.82  0.82  **FUD** XXX  01 N1 80
**AMA:** 2014,Jan,11; 2012,Feb,9-10

**73070** **Radiologic examination, elbow; 2 views**
0.77  0.77  **FUD** XXX  01 N1 80
**AMA:** 2017,Jan,8; 2016,Jan,13; 2015,Jan,16; 2014,Jan,11; 2012,Feb,9-10

**73080** **complete, minimum of 3 views**
0.88  0.88  **FUD** XXX  01 N1 80
**AMA:** 2014,Jan,11; 2012,Feb,9-10

**73085** **Radiologic examination, elbow, arthrography, radiological supervision and interpretation**
**INCLUDES** Fluoroscopic guidance (77002)
Code also arthrography injection procedure (24220)
2.70  2.70  **FUD** XXX  02 N1 80
**AMA:** 2017,Jan,8; 2016,Jan,13; 2015,Jan,16; 2014,Jan,11; 2012,Feb,9-10

## 73090-73140 Radiography: Forearm and Hand

**INCLUDES** Minimum number of views or more views when needed to adequately complete the study
Radiographs that have to be repeated during the encounter due to substandard quality; only one unit of service is reported

**EXCLUDES** *Obtaining more films after review of initial films, based on the discretion of the radiologist, an order for the test, and a change in the patient's condition*
*Second interpretation by the requesting physician (included in E&M service)*
*Stress views of upper body joint(s), when performed (77071)*

**73090** **Radiologic examination; forearm, 2 views**
0.73  0.73  **FUD** XXX  01 N1 80
**AMA:** 2017,Jan,8; 2016,Jan,13; 2015,Jan,16; 2014,Jan,11; 2012,Feb,9-10

**73092** **upper extremity, infant, minimum of 2 views**  A
0.78  0.78  **FUD** XXX  01 N1 80
**AMA:** 2014,Jan,11; 2012,Feb,9-10

**73100** **Radiologic examination, wrist; 2 views**
0.82  0.82  **FUD** XXX  01 N1 80
**AMA:** 2017,Jan,8; 2016,Jan,13; 2015,Jan,16; 2014,Jan,11; 2012,Feb,9-10

**73110** **complete, minimum of 3 views**
1.00  1.00  **FUD** XXX  01 N1 80
**AMA:** 2017,Jan,8; 2016,Jan,13; 2015,Jan,16; 2014,Jan,11; 2012,Feb,9-10; 2012,Jan,15-42

**73115** **Radiologic examination, wrist, arthrography, radiological supervision and interpretation**
**INCLUDES** Fluoroscopic guidance (77002)
Code also arthrography injection procedure (25246)
3.00  3.00  **FUD** XXX  02 N1 80
**AMA:** 2017,Jan,8; 2016,Jan,13; 2015,Jan,16; 2014,Jan,11; 2012,Feb,9-10

**73120** **Radiologic examination, hand; 2 views**
0.74  0.74  **FUD** XXX  01 N1 80
**AMA:** 2014,Jan,11; 2012,Feb,9-10

**73130** **minimum of 3 views**
0.87  0.87  **FUD** XXX  01 N1 80
**AMA:** 2014,Jan,11; 2012,Feb,9-10

**73140** **Radiologic examination, finger(s), minimum of 2 views**
0.89  0.89  **FUD** XXX  01 N1 80
**AMA:** 2017,Jan,8; 2016,Jan,13; 2015,Jan,16; 2014,Jan,11; 2012,Feb,9-10

## 73200-73202 Computerized Tomography: Shoulder, Arm, Hand

**CMS:** 100-04,4,250.16 Multiple Procedure Payment Reduction: Certain Diagnostic Imaging Procedures Rendered by Physicians

**INCLUDES** Imaging using tomographic technique enhanced by computer imaging to create a cross-sectional plane of the body
Intravascular, intrathecal, or intra-articular contrast materials when noted in code descriptor

**EXCLUDES** *3D rendering (76376-76377)*

**73200** **Computed tomography, upper extremity; without contrast material**
5.07  5.07  **FUD** XXX  03 Z2 80
**AMA:** 2017,Jan,8; 2016,Jan,13; 2015,Jan,16; 2014,Jan,11; 2012,Feb,9-10; 2012,Jan,15-42

**73201** **with contrast material(s)**
6.28  6.28  **FUD** XXX  03 Z2 80
**AMA:** 2017,Jan,8; 2016,Jan,13; 2015,Aug,6; 2015,Jan,16; 2014,Jan,11; 2012,Feb,9-10; 2012,Jan,15-42

73202      **without contrast material, followed by contrast material(s) and further sections**
     7.82    7.82    **FUD** XXX    Ⓠ3 Ⓩ2 ⑧0 ▣
     **AMA:** 2014,Jan,11; 2012,Feb,9-10

## 73206 Computerized Tomographic Angiography: Shoulder, Arm, and Hand

**CMS:** 100-04,4,250.16 Multiple Procedure Payment Reduction: Certain Diagnostic Imaging Procedures Rendered by Physicians

INCLUDES    Intravascular, intrathecal, or intra-articular contrast materials when noted in code descriptor
     Multiple rapid thin section CT scans to create cross-sectional images of the arteries and veins

73206      **Computed tomographic angiography, upper extremity, with contrast material(s), including noncontrast images, if performed, and image postprocessing**
     9.27    9.27    **FUD** XXX    Ⓠ3 Ⓩ2 ⑧0 ▣
     **AMA:** 2017,Jan,8; 2016,Jan,13; 2015,Jan,16; 2014,Jan,11; 2012,Feb,9-10

## 73218-73223 Magnetic Resonance Imaging: Shoulder, Arm, Hand

**CMS:** 100-04,4,250.16 Multiple Procedure Payment Reduction: Certain Diagnostic Imaging Procedures Rendered by Physicians

INCLUDES    Application of an external magnetic field that forces alignment of hydrogen atom nuclei in soft tissues which converts to sets of tomographic images that can be displayed as three-dimensional images
     Intravascular, intrathecal, or intra-articular contrast materials when noted in code descriptor

73218      **Magnetic resonance (eg, proton) imaging, upper extremity, other than joint; without contrast material(s)**
     10.3    10.3    **FUD** XXX    Ⓠ3 Ⓩ2 ⑧0 ▣
     **AMA:** 2017,Jan,8; 2016,Jan,13; 2015,Jan,16; 2014,Jan,11; 2012,Feb,9-10; 2012,Jan,15-42

73219      **with contrast material(s)**
     11.3    11.3    **FUD** XXX    Ⓠ3 Ⓩ2 ⑧0 ▣
     **AMA:** 2017,Jan,8; 2016,Jan,13; 2015,Jan,16; 2014,Jan,11; 2012,Feb,9-10; 2012,Jan,15-42

73220      **without contrast material(s), followed by contrast material(s) and further sequences**
     14.1    14.1    **FUD** XXX    Ⓠ3 Ⓩ2 ⑧0 ▣
     **AMA:** 2017,Jan,8; 2016,Jan,13; 2015,Jan,16; 2014,Jan,11; 2012,Feb,9-10

73221      **Magnetic resonance (eg, proton) imaging, any joint of upper extremity; without contrast material(s)**
     6.70    6.70    **FUD** XXX    Ⓠ3 Ⓩ2 ⑧0 ▣
     **AMA:** 2017,Jan,8; 2016,Jan,13; 2015,Jan,16; 2014,Jan,11; 2012,Feb,9-10; 2012,Jan,15-42

73222      **with contrast material(s)**
     10.6    10.6    **FUD** XXX    Ⓠ3 Ⓩ3 ⑧0 ▣
     **AMA:** 2017,Jan,8; 2016,Jan,13; 2015,Aug,6; 2015,Jan,16; 2014,Jan,11; 2012,Feb,9-10

73223      **without contrast material(s), followed by contrast material(s) and further sequences**
     13.2    13.2    **FUD** XXX    Ⓠ3 Ⓩ2 ⑧0 ▣
     **AMA:** 2017,Jan,8; 2016,Jan,13; 2015,Jan,16; 2014,Jan,11; 2012,Feb,9-10

## 73225 Magnetic Resonance Angiography: Shoulder, Arm, Hand

**CMS:** 100-04,13,40.1.1 Magnetic Resonance Angiography; 100-04,4,250.16 Multiple Procedure Payment Reduction: Certain Diagnostic Imaging Procedures Rendered by Physicians

INCLUDES    Intravascular, intrathecal, or intra-articular contrast materials when noted in code descriptor
     Use of magnetic fields and radio waves to produce detailed cross-sectional images of the arteries and veins

73225      **Magnetic resonance angiography, upper extremity, with or without contrast material(s)**
     11.5    11.5    **FUD** XXX    Ⓑ ⑧0 ▣
     **AMA:** 2017,Jan,8; 2016,Jan,13; 2015,Jan,16; 2014,Jan,11; 2012,Feb,9-10

## 73501-73552 Radiography: Pelvic Region and Thigh

EXCLUDES    *Stress views of lower body joint(s), when performed (77071)*

73501      **Radiologic examination, hip, unilateral, with pelvis when performed; 1 view**
     0.84    0.84    **FUD** XXX    Ⓠ1 Ⓝ1 ⑧0 ▣
     **AMA:** 2017,Jan,8; 2016,Aug,7; 2016,Jun,8; 2016,Jan,13; 2015,Oct,9

73502      **2-3 views**
     1.17    1.17    **FUD** XXX    Ⓠ1 Ⓝ1 ⑧0 ▣
     **AMA:** 2017,Jan,8; 2016,Aug,7; 2016,Jun,8; 2016,Jan,13; 2015,Oct,9

73503      **minimum of 4 views**
     1.46    1.46    **FUD** XXX    Ⓠ1 Ⓝ1 ⑧0 ▣
     **AMA:** 2017,Jan,8; 2016,Aug,7; 2016,Jun,8; 2016,Jan,13; 2015,Oct,9

73521      **Radiologic examination, hips, bilateral, with pelvis when performed; 2 views**
     1.12    1.12    **FUD** XXX    Ⓠ1 Ⓝ1 ⑧0 ▣
     **AMA:** 2017,Jan,8; 2016,Aug,7; 2016,Jun,8; 2016,Jan,13; 2015,Oct,9

73522      **3-4 views**
     1.38    1.38    **FUD** XXX    Ⓠ1 Ⓝ1 ⑧0 ▣
     **AMA:** 2017,Jan,8; 2016,Aug,7; 2016,Jun,8; 2016,Jan,13; 2015,Oct,9

73523      **minimum of 5 views**
     1.60    1.60    **FUD** XXX    Ⓢ Ⓝ1 ⑧0 ▣
     **AMA:** 2017,Jan,8; 2016,Aug,7; 2016,Jun,8; 2016,Jan,13; 2015,Oct,9

73525      **Radiologic examination, hip, arthrography, radiological supervision and interpretation**
     INCLUDES    Fluoroscopic guidance (77002)
     2.87    2.87    **FUD** XXX    Ⓠ2 Ⓝ1 ⑧0 ▣
     **AMA:** 2017,Jan,8; 2016,Nov,10; 2016,Aug,7; 2016,Jan,13; 2015,Jan,16; 2014,Jan,11; 2012,Jun,14; 2012,Feb,9-10

73551      **Radiologic examination, femur; 1 view**
     0.79    0.79    **FUD** XXX    Ⓠ1 Ⓝ1 ⑧0 ▣
     **AMA:** 2017,Jan,8; 2016,Aug,7

73552      **minimum 2 views**
     0.92    0.92    **FUD** XXX    Ⓠ1 Ⓝ1 ⑧0 ▣
     **AMA:** 2017,Jan,8; 2016,Aug,7

## 73560-73660 Radiography: Lower Leg, Ankle, and Foot

EXCLUDES    *Stress views of lower body joint(s), when performed (77071)*

73560      **Radiologic examination, knee; 1 or 2 views**
     0.87    0.87    **FUD** XXX    Ⓠ1 Ⓝ1 ⑧0 ▣
     **AMA:** 2017,Jan,8; 2016,Jan,13; 2015,May,10; 2015,Feb,10; 2014,Jan,11; 2012,Feb,9-10

73562      **3 views**
     1.01    1.01    **FUD** XXX    Ⓠ1 Ⓝ1 ⑧0 ▣
     **AMA:** 2014,Jan,11; 2012,Feb,9-10

73564      **complete, 4 or more views**
     1.12    1.12    **FUD** XXX    Ⓠ1 Ⓝ1 ⑧0 ▣
     **AMA:** 2017,Jan,8; 2016,Jan,13; 2015,May,10; 2015,Feb,10; 2015,Jan,16; 2014,Jan,11; 2012,Feb,9-10; 2012,Jan,15-42

73565      **both knees, standing, anteroposterior**
     1.01    1.01    **FUD** XXX    Ⓠ1 Ⓝ1 ⑧0 ▣
     **AMA:** 2017,Jan,8; 2016,Jan,13; 2015,May,10; 2015,Feb,10; 2014,Jan,11; 2012,Feb,9-10

73580      **Radiologic examination, knee, arthrography, radiological supervision and interpretation**
     INCLUDES    Fluoroscopic guidance (77002)
     3.21    3.21    **FUD** XXX    Ⓠ2 Ⓝ1 ⑧0 ▣
     **AMA:** 2017,Jan,8; 2016,Jan,13; 2015,Aug,6; 2015,Jan,16; 2014,Jan,11; 2012,Feb,9-10

● New Code    ▲ Revised Code    ○ Reinstated    ● New Web Release    ▲ Revised Web Release    Unlisted    Not Covered    # Resequenced
⊘ AMA Mod 51 Exempt    ⑤ Optum Mod 51 Exempt    ⑥③ Mod 63 Exempt    ✗ Non-FDA Drug    ★ Telemedicine    Ⓜ Maternity    Ⓐ Age Edit    ✛ Add-on    **AMA:** CPT Asst
© 2017 Optum360, LLC      CPT © 2017 American Medical Association. All Rights Reserved.      323

73590　Radiologic examination; tibia and fibula, 2 views
    📷 0.81　⚖ 0.81　**FUD** XXX　[01] [N1] [80] [▭]
    **AMA:** 2017,Jan,8; 2016,Jan,13; 2015,Jan,16; 2014,Jan,11; 2012,Feb,9-10

73592　lower extremity, infant, minimum of 2 views　[A]
    📷 0.78　⚖ 0.78　**FUD** XXX　[01] [N1] [80] [▭]
    **AMA:** 2014,Jan,11; 2012,Feb,9-10

73600　Radiologic examination, ankle; 2 views
    📷 0.84　⚖ 0.84　**FUD** XXX　[01] [N1] [80] [▭]
    **AMA:** 2017,Jan,8; 2016,Jan,13; 2015,Jan,16; 2014,Jan,11; 2012,Feb,9-10

73610　complete, minimum of 3 views
    📷 0.89　⚖ 0.89　**FUD** XXX　[01] [N1] [80] [▭]
    **AMA:** 2017,Jan,8; 2016,Jan,13; 2015,Jan,16; 2014,Jan,11; 2012,Feb,9-10

73615　Radiologic examination, ankle, arthrography, radiological supervision and interpretation
    INCLUDES　Fluoroscopic guidance (77002)
    📷 2.97　⚖ 2.97　**FUD** XXX　[02] [N1] [80] [▭]
    **AMA:** 2017,Jan,8; 2016,Jan,13; 2015,Jan,16; 2014,Jan,11; 2012,Feb,9-10

73620　Radiologic examination, foot; 2 views
    📷 0.73　⚖ 0.73　**FUD** XXX　[01] [N1] [80] [▭]
    **AMA:** 2017,Jan,8; 2016,Jan,13; 2015,Jan,16; 2014,Jan,11; 2012,Feb,9-10

73630　complete, minimum of 3 views
    📷 0.82　⚖ 0.82　**FUD** XXX　[01] [N1] [80] [▭]
    **AMA:** 2014,Jan,11; 2012,Feb,9-10

73650　Radiologic examination; calcaneus, minimum of 2 views
    📷 0.76　⚖ 0.76　**FUD** XXX　[01] [N1] [80] [▭]
    **AMA:** 2014,Jan,11; 2012,Feb,9-10

73660　toe(s), minimum of 2 views
    📷 0.79　⚖ 0.79　**FUD** XXX　[01] [N1] [80] [▭]
    **AMA:** 2014,Jan,11; 2012,Feb,9-10

## 73700-73702 Computerized Tomography: Leg, Ankle, and Foot

**CMS:** 100-04,4,250.16 Multiple Procedure Payment Reduction: Certain Diagnostic Imaging Procedures Rendered by Physicians
EXCLUDES　3D rendering (76376-76377)

73700　Computed tomography, lower extremity; without contrast material
    📷 5.08　⚖ 5.08　**FUD** XXX　[03] [Z2] [80] [▭]
    **AMA:** 2017,Jan,8; 2016,Jan,13; 2015,Jan,16; 2014,Jan,11; 2012,Feb,9-10; 2012,Jan,15-42

73701　with contrast material(s)
    📷 6.38　⚖ 6.38　**FUD** XXX　[03] [Z2] [80] [▭]
    **AMA:** 2017,Jan,8; 2016,Jan,13; 2015,Jan,16; 2014,Jan,11; 2012,Feb,9-10

73702　without contrast material, followed by contrast material(s) and further sections
    📷 7.73　⚖ 7.73　**FUD** XXX　[03] [Z2] [80] [▭]
    **AMA:** 2017,Jan,8; 2016,Jan,13; 2015,Jan,16; 2014,Jan,11; 2012,Feb,9-10

## 73706 Computerized Tomographic Angiography: Leg, Ankle, and Foot

**CMS:** 100-04,4,250.16 Multiple Procedure Payment Reduction: Certain Diagnostic Imaging Procedures Rendered by Physicians
EXCLUDES　CT angiography for aorto-iliofemoral runoff (75635)

73706　Computed tomographic angiography, lower extremity, with contrast material(s), including noncontrast images, if performed, and image postprocessing
    📷 10.0　⚖ 10.0　**FUD** XXX　[03] [Z2] [80] [▭]
    **AMA:** 2017,Jan,8; 2016,Jan,13; 2015,Jan,16; 2014,Jan,11; 2012,Feb,9-10; 2012,Jan,15-42

## 73718-73723 Magnetic Resonance Imaging: Leg, Ankle, and Foot

**CMS:** 100-04,4,250.16 Multiple Procedure Payment Reduction: Certain Diagnostic Imaging Procedures Rendered by Physicians

73718　Magnetic resonance (eg, proton) imaging, lower extremity other than joint; without contrast material(s)
    📷 10.2　⚖ 10.2　**FUD** XXX　[03] [Z2] [80] [▭]
    **AMA:** 2017,Jan,8; 2016,Jan,13; 2015,Jan,16; 2014,Jan,11; 2012,Feb,9-10

73719　with contrast material(s)
    📷 11.4　⚖ 11.4　**FUD** XXX　[03] [Z2] [80] [▭]
    **AMA:** 2017,Jan,8; 2016,Jan,13; 2015,Jan,16; 2014,Jan,11; 2012,Feb,9-10

73720　without contrast material(s), followed by contrast material(s) and further sequences
    📷 14.1　⚖ 14.1　**FUD** XXX　[03] [Z2] [80] [▭]
    **AMA:** 2017,Jan,8; 2016,Jan,13; 2015,Jan,16; 2014,Jan,11; 2012,Feb,9-10

73721　Magnetic resonance (eg, proton) imaging, any joint of lower extremity; without contrast material
    📷 6.69　⚖ 6.69　**FUD** XXX　[03] [Z2] [80] [▭]
    **AMA:** 2017,Jan,8; 2016,Jan,13; 2015,Jan,16; 2014,Jan,11; 2012,Feb,9-10; 2012,Jan,15-42

73722　with contrast material(s)
    📷 10.7　⚖ 10.7　**FUD** XXX　[03] [Z3] [80] [▭]
    **AMA:** 2017,Jan,8; 2016,Jan,13; 2015,Aug,6; 2015,Jan,16; 2014,Jan,11; 2012,Feb,9-10

73723　without contrast material(s), followed by contrast material(s) and further sequences
    📷 13.2　⚖ 13.2　**FUD** XXX　[03] [Z2] [80] [▭]
    **AMA:** 2017,Jan,8; 2016,Jan,13; 2015,Jan,16; 2014,Jan,11; 2012,Feb,9-10

## 73725 Magnetic Resonance Angiography: Leg, Ankle, and Foot

**CMS:** 100-04,13,40.1.2 HCPCS Coding Requirements; 100-04,4,250.16 Multiple Procedure Payment Reduction: Certain Diagnostic Imaging Procedures Rendered by Physicians

73725　Magnetic resonance angiography, lower extremity, with or without contrast material(s)
    📷 11.3　⚖ 11.3　**FUD** XXX　[B] [80] [▭]
    **AMA:** 2017,Jan,8; 2016,Jan,13; 2015,Jan,16; 2014,Jan,11; 2012,Feb,9-10

## 74000-74022 Radiography: Abdomen--General

74000　~~Radiologic examination, abdomen; single anteroposterior view~~
    To report, see 74018

74010　~~anteroposterior and additional oblique and cone views~~
    To report, see 74019, 74021

● 74018　Radiologic examination, abdomen; 1 view

● 74019　2 views

74020　~~complete, including decubitus and/or erect views~~
    To report, see 74019, 74021

● 74021　3 or more views

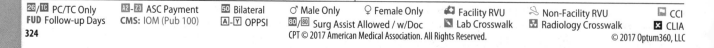

[26]/[TC] PC/TC Only　[A2]-[Z3] ASC Payment　[50] Bilateral　♂ Male Only　♀ Female Only　📷 Facility RVU　⚖ Non-Facility RVU　[▭] CCI
**FUD** Follow-up Days　**CMS:** IOM (Pub 100)　[A]-[Y] OPPSI　[80]/[80] Surg Assist Allowed / w/Doc　Lab Crosswalk　Radiology Crosswalk　CLIA

324　CPT © 2017 American Medical Association. All Rights Reserved.　© 2017 Optum360, LLC

74022   **Radiologic examination, abdomen; complete acute abdomen series, including supine, erect, and/or decubitus views, single view chest**
    📷 1.26    🔬 1.26    **FUD** XXX      01 N1 80 🖵
    **AMA:** 2016,Jun,5; 2014,Jan,11; 2012,Feb,9-10

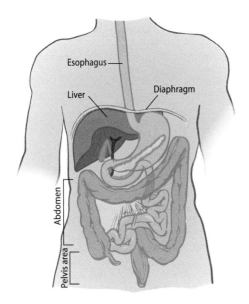

## 74150-74170 Computerized Tomography: Abdomen–General

**CMS:** 100-04,4,250.16 Multiple Procedure Payment Reduction: Certain Diagnostic Imaging Procedures Rendered by Physicians

    *EXCLUDES*   *3D rendering (76376-76377)*
        *Combined CT of abdomen and pelvis (74176-74178)*
        *CT colonography, diagnostic (74261-74262)*
        *CT colonography, screening (74263)*

74150   **Computed tomography, abdomen; without contrast material**
    📷 4.23    🔬 4.23    **FUD** XXX      03 Z2 80 🖵
    **AMA:** 2017,Jan,8; 2016,Jun,5; 2016,Jan,13; 2015,Jan,16; 2014,Jan,11; 2012,Oct,12; 2012,Feb,9-10; 2012,Jan,15-42

74160   **with contrast material(s)**
    📷 6.52    🔬 6.52    **FUD** XXX      03 Z2 80 🖵
    **AMA:** 2017,Jan,8; 2016,Jun,5; 2016,Jan,13; 2015,Jan,16; 2014,Jan,11; 2012,Oct,12; 2012,Feb,9-10

74170   **without contrast material, followed by contrast material(s) and further sections**
    📷 7.41    🔬 7.41    **FUD** XXX      03 Z2 80 🖵
    **AMA:** 2017,Jan,8; 2016,Jun,5; 2016,Jan,13; 2015,Jan,16; 2014,Jan,11; 2012,Oct,12; 2012,Feb,9-10

## 74174-74175 Computerized Tomographic Angiography: Abdomen and Pelvis

**CMS:** 100-04,4,250.16 Multiple Procedure Payment Reduction: Certain Diagnostic Imaging Procedures Rendered by Physicians

    *EXCLUDES*   *CT angiography for aorto-iliofemoral runoff (75635)*
        *CT angiography, lower extremity (73706)*
        *CT angiography, pelvis (72191)*

74174   **Computed tomographic angiography, abdomen and pelvis, with contrast material(s), including noncontrast images, if performed, and image postprocessing**
      *EXCLUDES*   *3D rendering (76376-76377)*
          *Computed tomographic angiography abdomen (74175)*
    📷 10.9    🔬 10.9    **FUD** XXX      S Z2 80 🖵
    **AMA:** 2014,Jan,11; 2012,Feb,9-10

74175   **Computed tomographic angiography, abdomen, with contrast material(s), including noncontrast images, if performed, and image postprocessing**
    📷 8.67    🔬 8.67    **FUD** XXX      03 Z2 80 🖵
    **AMA:** 2017,Jan,8; 2016,Jan,13; 2015,Jan,16; 2014,Jan,11; 2012,Feb,9-10; 2012,Jan,15-42

## 74176-74178 Computerized Tomography: Abdomen and Pelvis

**CMS:** 100-04,4,250.16 Multiple Procedure Payment Reduction: Certain Diagnostic Imaging Procedures Rendered by Physicians

    *EXCLUDES*   *Computed tomography of abdomen or pelvis alone (72192-72194, 74150-74170)*
        *Procedure performed more than one time for each combined examination of the abdomen and pelvis*

74176   **Computed tomography, abdomen and pelvis; without contrast material**
    📷 5.68    🔬 5.68    **FUD** XXX      03 Z3 🖵
    **AMA:** 2017,Jan,8; 2016,Jan,13; 2015,Jan,16; 2014,Jan,11; 2012,Feb,9-10

74177   **with contrast material(s)**
    📷 8.79    🔬 8.79    **FUD** XXX      03 Z2 🖵
    **AMA:** 2017,Jan,8; 2016,Jan,13; 2015,Jan,16; 2014,Jan,11; 2012,Feb,9-10

74178   **without contrast material in one or both body regions, followed by contrast material(s) and further sections in one or both body regions**
    📷 9.98    🔬 9.98    **FUD** XXX      03 Z2 🖵
    **AMA:** 2017,Jan,8; 2016,Jan,13; 2015,Jan,16; 2014,Jan,11; 2012,Feb,9-10

## 74181-74183 Magnetic Resonance Imaging: Abdomen–General

**CMS:** 100-04,4,250.16 Multiple Procedure Payment Reduction: Certain Diagnostic Imaging Procedures Rendered by Physicians

74181   **Magnetic resonance (eg, proton) imaging, abdomen; without contrast material(s)**
    📷 9.39    🔬 9.39    **FUD** XXX      03 Z2 80 🖵
    **AMA:** 2017,Jan,8; 2016,Jan,13; 2015,Jan,16; 2014,Jan,11; 2012,Feb,9-10; 2012,Jan,15-42

74182   **with contrast material(s)**
    📷 12.8    🔬 12.8    **FUD** XXX      03 Z2 80 🖵
    **AMA:** 2017,Jan,8; 2016,Jan,13; 2015,Jan,16; 2014,Jan,11; 2012,Feb,9-10; 2012,Jan,15-42

74183   **without contrast material(s), followed by with contrast material(s) and further sequences**
    📷 14.3    🔬 14.3    **FUD** XXX      03 Z2 80 🖵
    **AMA:** 2017,Jan,8; 2016,Jan,13; 2015,Jan,16; 2014,Jan,11; 2012,Feb,9-10

## 74185 Magnetic Resonance Angiography: Abdomen–General

**CMS:** 100-04,13,40.1.1 Magnetic Resonance Angiography; 100-04,13,40.1.2 HCPCS Coding Requirements; 100-04,4,250.16 Multiple Procedure Payment Reduction: Certain Diagnostic Imaging Procedures Rendered by Physicians

74185   **Magnetic resonance angiography, abdomen, with or without contrast material(s)**
    📷 11.3    🔬 11.3    **FUD** XXX      B 80 🖵
    **AMA:** 2017,Jan,8; 2016,Jan,13; 2015,Jan,16; 2014,Jan,11; 2012,Feb,9-10

## 74190 Peritoneography

74190   **Peritoneogram (eg, after injection of air or contrast), radiological supervision and interpretation**
      *EXCLUDES*   *Computed tomography, pelvis or abdomen (72192, 74150)*
    Code also injection procedure (49400)
    📷 0.00    🔬 0.00    **FUD** XXX      02 N1 80 🖵
    **AMA:** 2017,Jan,8; 2016,Jan,13; 2015,Jan,16; 2014,Jan,11; 2012,Feb,9-10; 2012,Jan,15-42

## 74210-74235 Radiography: Throat and Esophagus

EXCLUDES Percutaneous placement of gastrostomy tube, endoscopic (43246)
Percutaneous placement of gastrostomy tube, fluoroscopic guidance (49440)

**74210** Radiologic examination; pharynx and/or cervical esophagus
⚕ 2.19 ⚗ 2.19 **FUD** XXX 〔01〕〔N1〕〔80〕〔▭〕
AMA: 2014,Jan,11; 2012,Feb,9-10

**74220** esophagus
⚕ 2.49 ⚗ 2.49 **FUD** XXX 〔01〕〔N1〕〔80〕〔▭〕
AMA: 2014,Jan,11; 2012,Feb,9-10

**74230** Swallowing function, with cineradiography/videoradiography
⚕ 3.61 ⚗ 3.61 **FUD** XXX 〔01〕〔N1〕〔80〕〔▭〕
AMA: 2017,Jan,8; 2016,Jan,13; 2015,Jan,16; 2014,Jul,5;
2014,Jan,11; 2012,Feb,9-10

**74235** Removal of foreign body(s), esophageal, with use of balloon catheter, radiological supervision and interpretation
Code also procedure (43499)
⚕ 0.00 ⚗ 0.00 **FUD** XXX 〔N〕〔N1〕〔80〕〔▭〕
AMA: 2014,Jan,11; 2012,Feb,9-10

## 74240-74283 Radiography: Intestines

EXCLUDES Percutaneous placement of gastrostomy tube, endoscopic (43246)
Percutaneous placement of gastrostomy tube, fluoroscopic guidance (49440)

**74240** Radiologic examination, gastrointestinal tract, upper; with or without delayed images, without KUB
⚕ 3.18 ⚗ 3.18 **FUD** XXX 〔01〕〔Z2〕〔80〕〔▭〕
AMA: 2017,Jan,8; 2016,Sep,7; 2014,Jan,11; 2012,Feb,9-10

**74241** with or without delayed images, with KUB
⚕ 3.32 ⚗ 3.32 **FUD** XXX 〔01〕〔Z2〕〔80〕〔▭〕
AMA: 2017,Jan,8; 2016,Sep,7; 2014,Jan,11; 2012,Feb,9-10

**74245** with small intestine, includes multiple serial images
⚕ 4.83 ⚗ 4.83 **FUD** XXX 〔S〕〔Z2〕〔80〕〔▭〕
AMA: 2017,Jan,8; 2016,Sep,7; 2014,Jan,11; 2012,Feb,9-10

**74246** Radiological examination, gastrointestinal tract, upper, air contrast, with specific high density barium, effervescent agent, with or without glucagon; with or without delayed images, without KUB
INCLUDES Moynihan test
⚕ 3.58 ⚗ 3.58 **FUD** XXX 〔01〕〔Z2〕〔80〕〔▭〕
AMA: 2017,Jan,8; 2016,Sep,7; 2014,Jan,11; 2012,Feb,9-10

**74247** with or without delayed images, with KUB
⚕ 3.99 ⚗ 3.99 **FUD** XXX 〔01〕〔Z2〕〔80〕〔▭〕
AMA: 2017,Jan,8; 2016,Sep,7; 2014,Jan,11; 2012,Feb,9-10

**74249** with small intestine follow-through
⚕ 5.18 ⚗ 5.18 **FUD** XXX 〔S〕〔Z2〕〔80〕〔▭〕
AMA: 2014,Jan,11; 2012,Feb,9-10

**74250** Radiologic examination, small intestine, includes multiple serial images;
⚕ 2.93 ⚗ 2.93 **FUD** XXX 〔01〕〔Z2〕〔80〕〔▭〕
AMA: 2017,Jan,8; 2016,Sep,7; 2014,Jan,11; 2012,Feb,9-10

**74251** via enteroclysis tube
⚕ 11.8 ⚗ 11.8 **FUD** XXX 〔S〕〔Z2〕〔80〕〔▭〕
AMA: 2017,Jan,8; 2016,Sep,7; 2014,Jan,11; 2012,Feb,9-10

**74260** Duodenography, hypotonic
⚕ 9.66 ⚗ 9.66 **FUD** XXX 〔01〕〔N1〕〔80〕〔▭〕
AMA: 2014,Jan,11; 2012,Feb,9-10

**74261** Computed tomographic (CT) colonography, diagnostic, including image postprocessing; without contrast material
EXCLUDES 3D rendering (76376-76377)
Computed tomography of abdomen or pelvis alone (72192-72194, 74150-74170)
Screening computed tomographic (CT) colonography (74263)
⚕ 13.7 ⚗ 13.7 **FUD** XXX 〔03〕〔Z2〕〔80〕〔▭〕
AMA: 2017,Jan,8; 2016,Jan,13; 2015,Jan,16; 2014,Jan,11;
2012,Feb,9-10

**74262** with contrast material(s) including non-contrast images, if performed
EXCLUDES 3D rendering (76376-76377)
Computed tomography of abdomen or pelvis alone (72192-72194, 74150-74170)
Screening computed tomographic (CT) colonography (74263)
⚕ 15.3 ⚗ 15.3 **FUD** XXX 〔03〕〔Z2〕〔80〕〔▭〕
AMA: 2017,Jan,8; 2016,Jan,13; 2015,Jan,16; 2014,Jan,11;
2012,Feb,9-10

**74263** Computed tomographic (CT) colonography, screening, including image postprocessing
EXCLUDES 3D rendering (76376-76377)
Computed tomographic (CT) colonography (74261-74262)
Computed tomography of abdomen or pelvis alone (72192-72194, 74150-74170)
⚕ 21.2 ⚗ 21.2 **FUD** XXX 〔E〕〔▭〕
AMA: 2017,Jan,8; 2016,Jan,13; 2015,Jan,16; 2014,Jan,11;
2012,Feb,9-10

**74270** Radiologic examination, colon; contrast (eg, barium) enema, with or without KUB
⚕ 4.23 ⚗ 4.23 **FUD** XXX 〔01〕〔N1〕〔80〕〔▭〕
AMA: 2017,Jan,8; 2016,Jan,13; 2015,Jan,16; 2014,Jan,11;
2012,Feb,9-10; 2012,Jan,15-42

**74280** air contrast with specific high density barium, with or without glucagon
⚕ 6.02 ⚗ 6.02 **FUD** XXX 〔S〕〔Z2〕〔80〕〔▭〕
AMA: 2014,Jan,11; 2012,Feb,9-10

**74283** Therapeutic enema, contrast or air, for reduction of intussusception or other intraluminal obstruction (eg, meconium ileus)
⚕ 5.90 ⚗ 5.90 **FUD** XXX 〔S〕〔Z2〕〔80〕〔▭〕
AMA: 2014,Jan,11; 2012,Feb,9-10

## 74290-74330 Radiography: Biliary Tract

**74290** Cholecystography, oral contrast
⚕ 1.98 ⚗ 1.98 **FUD** XXX 〔01〕〔N1〕〔80〕〔▭〕
AMA: 2014,Jan,11; 2012,Feb,9-10

**74300** Cholangiography and/or pancreatography; intraoperative, radiological supervision and interpretation
⚕ 0.00 ⚗ 0.00 **FUD** XXX 〔N〕〔N1〕〔80〕〔▭〕
AMA: 2017,Jan,8; 2016,Jan,13; 2015,Dec,3; 2015,Jan,16;
2014,Jan,11; 2012,Feb,9-10; 2012,Jan,15-42

**+ 74301** additional set intraoperative, radiological supervision and interpretation (List separately in addition to code for primary procedure)
Code first (74300)
⚕ 0.00 ⚗ 0.00 **FUD** ZZZ 〔N〕〔N1〕〔80〕〔▭〕
AMA: 2015,Dec,3; 2014,Jan,11; 2012,Feb,9-10

**74328** Endoscopic catheterization of the biliary ductal system, radiological supervision and interpretation
Code also ERCP (43260-43270 [43274, 43275, 43276, 43277, 43278])
⚕ 0.00 ⚗ 0.00 **FUD** XXX 〔N〕〔N1〕〔80〕〔▭〕
AMA: 2017,Jan,8; 2016,Jan,13; 2015,Jan,16; 2014,Jan,11;
2012,Feb,9-10; 2012,Jan,15-42

**74329** Endoscopic catheterization of the pancreatic ductal system, radiological supervision and interpretation
Code also ERCP (43260-43270 [43274, 43275, 43276, 43277, 43278])
⚕ 0.00 ⚗ 0.00 **FUD** XXX 〔N〕〔N1〕〔80〕〔▭〕
AMA: 2014,Jan,11; 2012,Feb,9-10

**74330** Combined endoscopic catheterization of the biliary and pancreatic ductal systems, radiological supervision and interpretation
Code also ERCP (43260-43270 [43274, 43275, 43276, 43277, 43278])
⚕ 0.00 ⚗ 0.00 **FUD** XXX 〔N〕〔N1〕〔80〕〔▭〕
AMA: 2014,Jan,11; 2012,Feb,9-10

26/TC PC/TC Only
FUD Follow-up Days
A2-Z3 ASC Payment
CMS: IOM (Pub 100)
50 Bilateral
A-Y OPPSI
♂ Male Only
80/80 Surg Assist Allowed / w/Doc
♀ Female Only
⚕ Facility RVU
⚗ Non-Facility RVU
🔲 Lab Crosswalk
▦ Radiology Crosswalk
▭ CCI
✖ CLIA
326
CPT © 2017 American Medical Association. All Rights Reserved.
© 2017 Optum360, LLC

## 74340-74363 Radiography: Bilidigestive Intubation

**EXCLUDES** *Percutaneous insertion of gastrostomy tube, endoscopic (43246)*
*Percutaneous placement of gastrostomy tube, fluoroscopic guidance (49440)*

**74340** Introduction of long gastrointestinal tube (eg, Miller-Abbott), including multiple fluoroscopies and images, radiological supervision and interpretation
Code also placement of tube (44500)
🔵 0.00   ⚖ 0.00   **FUD** XXX      N N1 80 ▢
**AMA:** 2017,Jan,8; 2016,Sep,9; 2014,Jan,11; 2012,Feb,9-10

**74355** Percutaneous placement of enteroclysis tube, radiological supervision and interpretation
**INCLUDES** Fluoroscopic guidance (77002)
🔵 0.00   ⚖ 0.00   **FUD** XXX      N N1 80 ▢
**AMA:** 2017,Jan,8; 2016,Jan,13; 2015,Jan,16; 2014,Jan,11; 2012,Feb,9-10

**74360** Intraluminal dilation of strictures and/or obstructions (eg, esophagus), radiological supervision and interpretation
**EXCLUDES** *Esophagogastroduodenoscopy, flexible, transoral; with dilation of esophagus (43233)*
*Esophagoscopy, flexible, transoral; with dilation of esophagus (43213-43214)*
🔵 0.00   ⚖ 0.00   **FUD** XXX      N N1 80 ▢
**AMA:** 2017,Jan,8; 2016,Jan,13; 2015,Jan,16; 2014,Jan,11; 2012,Feb,9-10

**74363** Percutaneous transhepatic dilation of biliary duct stricture with or without placement of stent, radiological supervision and interpretation
**EXCLUDES** *Surgical procedure (47555-47556)*
🔵 0.00   ⚖ 0.00   **FUD** XXX      N N1 80 ▢
**AMA:** 2014,Jan,11; 2012,Feb,9-10

## 74400-74775 Radiography: Urogenital

**74400** Urography (pyelography), intravenous, with or without KUB, with or without tomography
🔵 3.11   ⚖ 3.11   **FUD** XXX      S Z2 80 ▢
**AMA:** 2014,Jan,11; 2012,Feb,9-10

**74410** Urography, infusion, drip technique and/or bolus technique;
🔵 3.07   ⚖ 3.07   **FUD** XXX      S Z2 80 ▢
**AMA:** 2014,Jan,11; 2012,Feb,9-10

**74415** with nephrotomography
🔵 3.85   ⚖ 3.85   **FUD** XXX      S Z2 80 ▢
**AMA:** 2014,Jan,11; 2012,Feb,9-10

**74420** Urography, retrograde, with or without KUB
🔵 0.00   ⚖ 0.00   **FUD** XXX      S Z2 80 ▢
**AMA:** 2017,Jan,8; 2016,Jan,13; 2015,Jan,16; 2014,Jan,11; 2012,Feb,9-10; 2012,Jan,15-42

**74425** Urography, antegrade (pyelostogram, nephrostogram, loopogram), radiological supervision and interpretation
**EXCLUDES** *Injection for antegrade nephrostogram and/or ureterogram ([50430, 50431, 50432, 50433, 50434, 50435])*
*Ureteral stent placement (50693-50695)*
🔵 0.00   ⚖ 0.00   **FUD** XXX      Q2 N1 80 ▢
**AMA:** 2017,Jan,8; 2016,Jan,13; 2016,Jan,3; 2015,Oct,5; 2015,Jan,16; 2014,Jan,11; 2012,Feb,9-10

Nephrostomy catheter

Syringe with contrast

Ureter

Bladder

Contrast in urinary system

**Nephrostogram**

**74430** Cystography, minimum of 3 views, radiological supervision and interpretation
🔵 1.07   ⚖ 1.07   **FUD** XXX      Q2 N1 80 ▢
**AMA:** 2014,Jan,11; 2012,Feb,9-10

**74440** Vasography, vesiculography, or epididymography, radiological supervision and interpretation ♂
🔵 2.29   ⚖ 2.29   **FUD** XXX      Q2 N1 80 ▢
**AMA:** 2014,Jan,11; 2012,Feb,9-10

**74445** Corpora cavernosography, radiological supervision and interpretation ♂
**INCLUDES** Needle placement with fluoroscopic guidance (77002)
🔵 0.00   ⚖ 0.00   **FUD** XXX      Q2 N1 80 ▢
**AMA:** 2017,Jan,8; 2016,Jan,13; 2015,Jan,16; 2014,Jan,11; 2012,Feb,9-10

**74450** Urethrocystography, retrograde, radiological supervision and interpretation
🔵 0.00   ⚖ 0.00   **FUD** XXX      Q2 N1 80 ▢
**AMA:** 2014,Jan,11; 2012,Feb,9-10

**74455** Urethrocystography, voiding, radiological supervision and interpretation
🔵 2.31   ⚖ 2.31   **FUD** XXX      Q2 N1 80 ▢
**AMA:** 2014,Jan,11; 2012,Feb,9-10

**74470** Radiologic examination, renal cyst study, translumbar, contrast visualization, radiological supervision and interpretation
**INCLUDES** Needle placement with fluoroscopic guidance (77002)
🔵 0.00   ⚖ 0.00   **FUD** XXX      Q2 N1 80 ▢
**AMA:** 2017,Jan,8; 2016,Jan,13; 2015,Jan,16; 2014,Jan,11; 2012,Feb,9-10

● New Code   ▲ Revised Code   ○ Reinstated   ● New Web Release   ▲ Revised Web Release   Unlisted   Not Covered   # Resequenced
⊘ AMA Mod 51 Exempt   ⑨ Optum Mod 51 Exempt   ⑨ Mod 63 Exempt   ✗ Non-FDA Drug   ★ Telemedicine   Ⓜ Maternity   🄰 Age Edit   + Add-on   **AMA:** CPT Asst
© 2017 Optum360, LLC                    CPT © 2017 American Medical Association. All Rights Reserved.                    **327**

**74485** **Dilation of nephrostomy, ureters, or urethra, radiological supervision and interpretation**

> EXCLUDES Change of pyelostomy/nephrostomy tube ([50435])
> Ureter dilation without radiologic guidance (52341, 52344)

📇 2.59   ⅏ 2.59   **FUD** XXX    02 N1 80 ▣

**AMA:** 2017,Jan,8; 2016,Jan,13; 2016,Jan,3; 2015,Oct,5; 2015,Jan,16; 2014,Jan,11; 2012,Feb,9-10; 2012,Jan,15-42

**74710** **Pelvimetry, with or without placental localization** ♀

> EXCLUDES Imaging procedures on abdomen and pelvis
> (72170-72190, 74018-74019, 74021-74022, 74150-74170)

📇 1.04   ⅏ 1.04   **FUD** XXX    01 N1 80 ▣

**AMA:** 2014,Jan,11; 2012,Feb,9-10

**74712** **Magnetic resonance (eg, proton) imaging, fetal, including placental and maternal pelvic imaging when performed; single or first gestation** ♀

> EXCLUDES Imaging of maternal pelvis or placenta without fetal imaging (72195-72197)

📇 13.5   ⅏ 13.5   **FUD** XXX    S Z2 80 ▣

**AMA:** 2017,Jan,8; 2016,Jun,5

**+ 74713** **each additional gestation (List separately in addition to code for primary procedure)** ⚥

> EXCLUDES Imaging of maternal pelvis or placenta without fetal imaging (72195-72197)
> Code first (74712)

📇 6.58   ⅏ 6.58   **FUD** ZZZ    N N1 80 ▣

**AMA:** 2017,Jan,8; 2016,Jun,5

**74740** **Hysterosalpingography, radiological supervision and interpretation** ♀

> EXCLUDES Imaging procedures on abdomen and pelvis
> (72170-72190, 74018-74022, 74150, 74160, 74170)
> Code also injection of saline/contrast (58340)

📇 2.11   ⅏ 2.11   **FUD** XXX    02 N1 80 ▣

**AMA:** 2017,Jan,8; 2016,Jan,13; 2015,Jan,16; 2014,Jan,11; 2012,Feb,9-10; 2012,Jan,15-42

Tube

Ovary

Delivery apparatus

Uterus

Cervix

Vaginal canal

Hysterosalpingography (imaging of the uterus and tubes) is performed. Report for radiological supervision and interpretation

**74742** **Transcervical catheterization of fallopian tube, radiological supervision and interpretation** ♀

> EXCLUDES Imaging procedures on abdomen and pelvis
> (72170-72190, 74018-74019, 74021-74022, 74150-74170)
> Code also (58345)

📇 0.00   ⅏ 0.00   **FUD** XXX    N N1 80 ▣

**AMA:** 2017,Jan,8; 2016,Jan,13; 2015,Jan,16; 2014,Jan,11; 2012,Feb,9-10

**74775** **Perineogram (eg, vaginogram, for sex determination or extent of anomalies)** M ♀

> EXCLUDES Imaging procedures on abdomen and pelvis
> (72170-72190, 74018-74019, 74021-74022, 74150-74170)

📇 0.00   ⅏ 0.00   **FUD** XXX    S Z2 80 ▣

**AMA:** 2014,Jan,11; 2012,Feb,9-10

## 75557-75565 Magnetic Resonance Imaging: Heart Structure and Physiology

> INCLUDES Physiologic evaluation of cardiac function
> EXCLUDES 3D rendering (76376-76377)
> Cardiac catheterization procedures (93451-93572)
> Use of more than one code in this group per session
> Code also separate vascular injection (36000-36299)

**75557** **Cardiac magnetic resonance imaging for morphology and function without contrast material;**

📇 9.04   ⅏ 9.04   **FUD** XXX    03 Z2 80 ▣

**AMA:** 2017,Jan,8; 2016,Jan,13; 2015,Jan,16; 2014,Jan,11; 2012,Feb,9-10

**75559** **with stress imaging**

> INCLUDES Pharmacologic wall motion stress evaluation without contrast
> Code also stress testing when performed (93015-93018)

📇 12.3   ⅏ 12.3   **FUD** XXX    03 Z2 80 ▣

**AMA:** 2017,Jan,8; 2016,Jan,13; 2015,Jan,16; 2014,Jan,11; 2012,Feb,9-10

**75561** **Cardiac magnetic resonance imaging for morphology and function without contrast material(s), followed by contrast material(s) and further sequences;**

📇 12.0   ⅏ 12.0   **FUD** XXX    03 Z2 80 ▣

**AMA:** 2017,Jan,8; 2016,Jan,13; 2015,Jan,16; 2014,Jan,11; 2012,Feb,9-10

**75563** **with stress imaging**

> INCLUDES Pharmacologic perfusion stress evaluation with contrast
> Code also stress testing when performed (93015-93018)

📇 14.3   ⅏ 14.3   **FUD** XXX    03 Z2 80 ▣

**AMA:** 2017,Jan,8; 2016,Jan,13; 2015,Jan,16; 2014,Jan,11; 2012,Feb,9-10

**+ 75565** **Cardiac magnetic resonance imaging for velocity flow mapping (List separately in addition to code for primary procedure)**

> Code first (75557, 75559, 75561, 75563)

📇 1.55   ⅏ 1.55   **FUD** ZZZ    N N1 80 ▣

**AMA:** 2017,Jan,8; 2016,Jan,13; 2015,Jan,16; 2014,Jan,11; 2012,Feb,9-10

## 75571-75574 Computed Tomographic Imaging: Heart

**CMS:** 100-04,12,20.4.7 Services Not Meeting National Electrical Manufacturers Association (NEMA) Standard; 100-04,4,20.6.12 Use of HCPCS Modifier – CT; 100-04,4,250.16 Multiple Procedure Payment Reduction: Certain Diagnostic Imaging Procedures Rendered by Physicians

> EXCLUDES 3D rendering (76376-76377)
> Use of more than one code in this group per session

**75571** **Computed tomography, heart, without contrast material, with quantitative evaluation of coronary calcium**

📇 2.85   ⅏ 2.85   **FUD** XXX    01 N1 80 ▣

**AMA:** 2017,Jan,8; 2016,Jan,13; 2015,Jan,16; 2014,Jan,11; 2012,Feb,9-10

26/TC PC/TC Only    A2-Z3 ASC Payment    50 Bilateral    ♂ Male Only    ♀ Female Only    📇 Facility RVU    ⅏ Non-Facility RVU    ▣ CCI
**FUD** Follow-up Days    **CMS:** IOM (Pub 100)    A-Y OPPSI    80/80 Surg Assist Allowed / w/Doc    Lab Crosswalk    Radiology Crosswalk    CLIA

328    CPT © 2017 American Medical Association. All Rights Reserved.    © 2017 Optum360, LLC

**75572** Computed tomography, heart, with contrast material, for evaluation of cardiac structure and morphology (including 3D image postprocessing, assessment of cardiac function, and evaluation of venous structures, if performed)

    8.01    8.01   **FUD** XXX        S Z2 80 ▭

    **AMA:** 2017,Jan,8; 2016,Jan,13; 2015,Jan,16; 2014,Jan,11; 2012,Feb,9-10

**75573** Computed tomography, heart, with contrast material, for evaluation of cardiac structure and morphology in the setting of congenital heart disease (including 3D image postprocessing, assessment of LV cardiac function, RV structure and function and evaluation of venous structures, if performed)

    11.0    11.0   **FUD** XXX        S Z2 80 ▭

    **AMA:** 2017,Jan,8; 2016,Jan,13; 2015,Jan,16; 2014,Jan,11; 2012,Feb,9-10

**75574** Computed tomographic angiography, heart, coronary arteries and bypass grafts (when present), with contrast material, including 3D image postprocessing (including evaluation of cardiac structure and morphology, assessment of cardiac function, and evaluation of venous structures, if performed)

    11.8    11.8   **FUD** XXX        S Z2 80 ▭

    **AMA:** 2017,Jan,8; 2016,Jan,13; 2015,Jan,16; 2014,Jan,11; 2012,Feb,9-10

## 75600-75774 Radiography: Arterial

**INCLUDES**   Diagnostic angiography specifically included in the interventional code description
The following diagnostic procedures with interventional supervision and interpretation:
Angiography
Contrast injection
Fluoroscopic guidance for intervention
Post-angioplasty/atherectomy/stent angiography
Roadmapping
Vessel measurement

**EXCLUDES**   *Catheterization codes for diagnostic angiography of lower extremity when an access site other than the site used for the therapy is required*
*Diagnostic angiogram during a separate encounter from the interventional procedure*
*Diagnostic angiography with interventional procedure if:*
  *1. No previous catheter-based angiogram is accessible and a complete diagnostic procedure is performed and the decision to proceed with an interventional procedure is based on the diagnostic service, OR*
  *2. The previous diagnostic angiogram is accessible but the documentation in the medical record specifies that:*
    *A. the patient's condition has changed*
    *B. there is insufficient imaging of the patient's anatomy and/or disease, OR*
    *C. there is a clinical change during the procedure that necessitates a new examination away from the site of the intervention*
  *3. Modifier 59 is appended to the code(s) for the diagnostic radiological supervision and interpretation service to indicate the guidelines were met*
*Intra-arterial procedures (36100-36248)*
*Intravenous procedures (36000, 36005-36015)*

**75600** Aortography, thoracic, without serialography, radiological supervision and interpretation

    **EXCLUDES**   *Supravalvular aortography (93567)*

    5.58    5.58   **FUD** XXX        Q2 N1 80 ▭

    **AMA:** 2014,Jan,11; 2012,Feb,9-10

**75605** Aortography, thoracic, by serialography, radiological supervision and interpretation

    **EXCLUDES**   *Supravalvular aortography (93567)*

    3.90    3.90   **FUD** XXX        Q2 N1 80 ▭

    **AMA:** 2017,Jan,8; 2016,Jan,13; 2015,Jan,16; 2014,Jan,11; 2013,Jan,6-8; 2012,Feb,9-10; 2012,Jan,15-42

**75625** Aortography, abdominal, by serialography, radiological supervision and interpretation

    **EXCLUDES**   *Supravalvular aortography (93567)*

    3.88    3.88   **FUD** XXX        Q2 N1 80 ▭

    **AMA:** 2017,Jan,8; 2016,Jan,13; 2015,Jan,16; 2014,Jan,11; 2013,Feb,16-17; 2013,Jan,6-8; 2012,Feb,9-10; 2012,Jan,15-42

**75630** Aortography, abdominal plus bilateral iliofemoral lower extremity, catheter, by serialography, radiological supervision and interpretation

    **EXCLUDES**   *Supravalvular aortography (93567)*

    4.81    4.81   **FUD** XXX        Q2 N1 80 ▭

    **AMA:** 2017,Jan,8; 2016,Jan,13; 2015,Jan,16; 2014,Jan,11; 2012,Feb,9-10; 2012,Jan,15-42

**75635** Computed tomographic angiography, abdominal aorta and bilateral iliofemoral lower extremity runoff, with contrast material(s), including noncontrast images, if performed, and image postprocessing

    **EXCLUDES**   *3D rendering (76376-76377)*
            *Computed tomographic angiography, abdomen, lower extremity, pelvis (72191, 73706, 74174-74175)*

    10.7    10.7   **FUD** XXX        Q2 N1 80 ▭

    **AMA:** 2017,Jan,8; 2016,Jan,13; 2015,Jan,16; 2014,Jan,11; 2012,Feb,9-10; 2012,Jan,15-42

**75658** ~~Angiography, brachial, retrograde, radiological supervision and interpretation~~

    To report, see 75710

**75705** Angiography, spinal, selective, radiological supervision and interpretation

    6.99    6.99   **FUD** XXX        Q2 N1 80 ▭

    **AMA:** 2014,Jan,11; 2012,Feb,9-10

**75710** Angiography, extremity, unilateral, radiological supervision and interpretation

    4.58    4.58   **FUD** XXX        Q2 N1 80 ▭

    **AMA:** 2017,Mar,3; 2017,Jan,8; 2016,Jan,13; 2015,Jan,16; 2014,Jan,11; 2012,Feb,9-10; 2012,Jan,15-42

**75716** Angiography, extremity, bilateral, radiological supervision and interpretation

    5.27    5.27   **FUD** XXX        Q2 N1 80 ▭

    **AMA:** 2017,Jan,8; 2016,Jan,13; 2015,Jan,16; 2014,Jan,11; 2012,Feb,9-10; 2012,Jan,15-42

**75726** Angiography, visceral, selective or supraselective (with or without flush aortogram), radiological supervision and interpretation

    **EXCLUDES**   *Selective angiography, each additional visceral vessel examined after basic examination (75774)*

    4.22    4.22   **FUD** XXX        Q2 N1 80 ▭

    **AMA:** 2014,Jan,11; 2012,Feb,9-10

**75731** Angiography, adrenal, unilateral, selective, radiological supervision and interpretation

    4.85    4.85   **FUD** XXX        Q2 N1 80 ▭

    **AMA:** 2014,Jan,11; 2012,Feb,9-10

**75733** Angiography, adrenal, bilateral, selective, radiological supervision and interpretation

    5.25    5.25   **FUD** XXX        Q2 N1 80 ▭

    **AMA:** 2014,Jan,11; 2012,Feb,9-10

**75736** Angiography, pelvic, selective or supraselective, radiological supervision and interpretation

    4.52    4.52   **FUD** XXX        Q2 N1 80 ▭

    **AMA:** 2014,Jan,11; 2012,Feb,9-10

**75741** Angiography, pulmonary, unilateral, selective, radiological supervision and interpretation

    4.26    4.26   **FUD** XXX        Q2 N1 80 ▭

    **AMA:** 2017,Jan,8; 2016,Jan,13; 2015,Jan,16; 2014,Jan,11; 2013,Jan,6-8; 2012,Feb,9-10; 2012,Mar,9-10

**75743** Angiography, pulmonary, bilateral, selective, radiological supervision and interpretation

    4.77    4.77   **FUD** XXX        Q2 N1 80 ▭

    **AMA:** 2017,Jan,8; 2016,Jan,13; 2015,Jan,16; 2014,Jan,11; 2013,Jan,6-8; 2012,Feb,9-10

● New Code    ▲ Revised Code    ○ Reinstated    ● New Web Release    ▲ Revised Web Release    Unlisted    Not Covered    # Resequenced
⊘ AMA Mod 51 Exempt    ⑨ Optum Mod 51 Exempt    ⑥③ Mod 63 Exempt    ✗ Non-FDA Drug    ★ Telemedicine    Ⅿ Maternity    Ⓐ Age Edit    + Add-on    **AMA:** CPT Asst
© 2017 Optum360, LLC        CPT © 2017 American Medical Association. All Rights Reserved.        329

Radiology

75746 — 75880

**75746** **Angiography, pulmonary, by nonselective catheter or venous injection, radiological supervision and interpretation**

> EXCLUDES   Nonselective injection procedure or catheter introduction with cardiac cath (93568)
>
> 🔲 4.33   ◇ 4.33   **FUD** XXX   02 N1 80 🖵
>
> **AMA:** 2014,Jan,11; 2012,Feb,9-10

**75756** **Angiography, internal mammary, radiological supervision and interpretation**

> EXCLUDES   Internal mammary angiography with cardiac cath (93455, 93457, 93459, 93461, 93564)
>
> 🔲 4.80   ◇ 4.80   **FUD** XXX   02 N1 80 🖵
>
> **AMA:** 2017,Jan,8; 2016,Jan,13; 2015,Jan,16; 2014,Jan,11; 2012,Feb,9-10

**+ 75774** **Angiography, selective, each additional vessel studied after basic examination, radiological supervision and interpretation (List separately in addition to code for primary procedure)**

> EXCLUDES   Angiography (75600-75756)
>            Cardiac cath procedures (93452-93462, 93531-93533, 93563-93568)
>            Catheterizations (36215-36248)
>            Dialysis circuit angiography (current access), use modifier 52 with (36901)
>            Nonselective catheter placement, thoracic aorta (36221-36228)
>
> Code also diagnostic angiography of upper extremities and other vascular beds (except cervicocerebral vessels), when appropriate
> Code first initial vessel
>
> 🔲 2.44   ◇ 2.44   **FUD** ZZZ   N N1 80 🖵
>
> **AMA:** 2017,Jan,8; 2016,Jan,13; 2015,Jan,16; 2014,Jan,11; 2013,Oct,18; 2013,Jun,12; 2013,May,3-5; 2013,Feb,16-17; 2012,Feb,9-10; 2012,Jan,15-42

## 75801-75893 Radiography: Lymphatic and Venous

INCLUDES   Diagnostic venography specifically included in the interventional code description
The following diagnostic procedures with interventional supervision and interpretation:
Contrast injection
Fluoroscopic guidance for intervention
Post-angioplasty/venography
Roadmapping
Venography
Vessel measurement

EXCLUDES   Diagnostic venogram during a separate encounter from the interventional procedure
Diagnostic venography with interventional procedure if:
1. No previous catheter-based venogram is accessible and a complete diagnostic procedure is performed and the decision to proceed with an interventional procedure is based on the diagnostic service, OR
2. The previous diagnostic venogram is accessible but the documentation in the medical record specifies that:
   A. The patient's condition has changed
   B. There is insufficient imaging of the patient's anatomy and/or disease, OR
   C. There is a clinical change during the procedure that necessitates a new examination away from the site of the intervention
Intravenous procedures (36000-36015, 36400-36510)
Lymphatic injection procedures (38790)

**75801** **Lymphangiography, extremity only, unilateral, radiological supervision and interpretation**

> 🔲 0.00   ◇ 0.00   **FUD** XXX   02 N1 80 🖵
>
> **AMA:** 2014,Jan,11; 2012,Feb,9-10

**75803** **Lymphangiography, extremity only, bilateral, radiological supervision and interpretation**

> 🔲 0.00   ◇ 0.00   **FUD** XXX   02 N1 80 🖵
>
> **AMA:** 2014,Jan,11; 2012,Feb,9-10

**75805** **Lymphangiography, pelvic/abdominal, unilateral, radiological supervision and interpretation**

> 🔲 0.00   ◇ 0.00   **FUD** XXX   02 N1 80 🖵
>
> **AMA:** 2014,Jan,11; 2012,Feb,9-10

**75807** **Lymphangiography, pelvic/abdominal, bilateral, radiological supervision and interpretation**

> 🔲 0.00   ◇ 0.00   **FUD** XXX   02 N1 80 🖵
>
> **AMA:** 2014,Jan,11; 2012,Feb,9-10

**75809** **Shuntogram for investigation of previously placed indwelling nonvascular shunt (eg, LeVeen shunt, ventriculoperitoneal shunt, indwelling infusion pump), radiological supervision and interpretation**

> Code also surgical procedure (49427, 61070)
>
> 🔲 2.79   ◇ 2.79   **FUD** XXX   02 N1 80 🖵
>
> **AMA:** 2017,Jan,8; 2016,Jan,13; 2015,Jan,16; 2014,Jan,11; 2012,Feb,9-10; 2012,Jan,15-42

**75810** **Splenoportography, radiological supervision and interpretation**

> 🔲 0.00   ◇ 0.00   **FUD** XXX   02 N1 80 🖵
>
> **AMA:** 2017,Jan,8; 2016,Jan,13; 2015,Jan,16; 2014,Jan,11; 2012,Feb,9-10

**75820** **Venography, extremity, unilateral, radiological supervision and interpretation**

> 🔲 3.26   ◇ 3.26   **FUD** XXX   02 N1 80 🖵
>
> **AMA:** 2017,Jan,8; 2016,May,5; 2016,Jan,13; 2015,May,3; 2015,Jan,16; 2014,Jan,11; 2012,Feb,9-10; 2012,Jan,15-42

**75822** **Venography, extremity, bilateral, radiological supervision and interpretation**

> 🔲 3.87   ◇ 3.87   **FUD** XXX   02 N1 80 🖵
>
> **AMA:** 2014,Jan,11; 2012,Feb,9-10

**75825** **Venography, caval, inferior, with serialography, radiological supervision and interpretation**

> 🔲 3.83   ◇ 3.83   **FUD** XXX   02 N1 80 🖵
>
> **AMA:** 2017,Feb,14; 2017,Jan,8; 2016,Jan,13; 2015,Jan,16; 2014,Jan,11; 2012,Feb,9-10; 2012,Jan,15-42

**75827** **Venography, caval, superior, with serialography, radiological supervision and interpretation**

> 🔲 3.91   ◇ 3.91   **FUD** XXX   02 N1 80 🖵
>
> **AMA:** 2017,Jan,8; 2016,Jan,13; 2015,Jan,16; 2014,Jan,11; 2012,Feb,9-10

**75831** **Venography, renal, unilateral, selective, radiological supervision and interpretation**

> 🔲 3.96   ◇ 3.96   **FUD** XXX   02 N1 80 🖵
>
> **AMA:** 2014,Jan,11; 2012,Feb,9-10

**75833** **Venography, renal, bilateral, selective, radiological supervision and interpretation**

> 🔲 4.66   ◇ 4.66   **FUD** XXX   02 N1 80 🖵
>
> **AMA:** 2014,Jan,11; 2012,Feb,9-10

**75840** **Venography, adrenal, unilateral, selective, radiological supervision and interpretation**

> 🔲 4.22   ◇ 4.22   **FUD** XXX   02 N1 80 🖵
>
> **AMA:** 2014,Jan,11; 2012,Feb,9-10

**75842** **Venography, adrenal, bilateral, selective, radiological supervision and interpretation**

> 🔲 5.07   ◇ 5.07   **FUD** XXX   02 N1 80 🖵
>
> **AMA:** 2014,Jan,11; 2012,Feb,9-10

**75860** **Venography, venous sinus (eg, petrosal and inferior sagittal) or jugular, catheter, radiological supervision and interpretation**

> 🔲 4.06   ◇ 4.06   **FUD** XXX   02 N1 80 🖵
>
> **AMA:** 2014,Jan,11; 2012,Feb,9-10

**75870** **Venography, superior sagittal sinus, radiological supervision and interpretation**

> 🔲 4.22   ◇ 4.22   **FUD** XXX   02 N1 80 🖵
>
> **AMA:** 2014,Jan,11; 2012,Feb,9-10

**75872** **Venography, epidural, radiological supervision and interpretation**

> 🔲 4.39   ◇ 4.39   **FUD** XXX   02 N1 80 🖵
>
> **AMA:** 2014,Jan,11; 2012,Feb,9-10

**75880** **Venography, orbital, radiological supervision and interpretation**

> 🔲 4.15   ◇ 4.15   **FUD** XXX   02 N1 80 🖵
>
> **AMA:** 2014,Jan,11; 2012,Feb,9-10

**75885**  **Percutaneous transhepatic portography with hemodynamic evaluation, radiological supervision and interpretation**
  4.42   4.42   **FUD** XXX   [Q2] [N1] [80] [icon]
  **AMA:** 2017,Jan,8; 2016,Jan,13; 2015,Jan,16; 2014,Jan,11; 2012,Feb,9-10; 2012,Jan,15-42

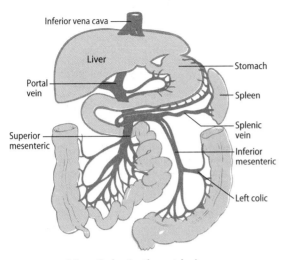

Inferior vena cava — 
Liver
Portal vein
Superior mesenteric
Stomach
Spleen
Splenic vein
Inferior mesenteric
Left colic

**Schematic showing the portal vein**

**75887**  **Percutaneous transhepatic portography without hemodynamic evaluation, radiological supervision and interpretation**
  4.47   4.47   **FUD** XXX   [Q2] [N1] [80] [icon]
  **AMA:** 2017,Jan,8; 2016,Jan,13; 2015,Jan,16; 2014,Jan,11; 2012,Feb,9-10; 2012,Jan,15-42

**75889**  **Hepatic venography, wedged or free, with hemodynamic evaluation, radiological supervision and interpretation**
  4.06   4.06   **FUD** XXX   [Q2] [N1] [80] [icon]
  **AMA:** 2014,Jan,11; 2012,Feb,9-10

**75891**  **Hepatic venography, wedged or free, without hemodynamic evaluation, radiological supervision and interpretation**
  4.11   4.11   **FUD** XXX   [Q2] [N1] [80] [icon]
  **AMA:** 2014,Jan,11; 2012,Feb,9-10

**75893**  **Venous sampling through catheter, with or without angiography (eg, for parathyroid hormone, renin), radiological supervision and interpretation**
  Code also surgical procedure (36500)
  3.36   3.36   **FUD** XXX   [Q2] [N1] [80] [icon]
  **AMA:** 2014,Jan,11; 2012,Feb,9-10

## 75894-75902 Transcatheter Procedures

**INCLUDES** The following diagnostic procedures with interventional supervision and interpretation:
  Angiography/venography
  Completion angiography/venography except for those services allowed by (75898)
  Contrast injection
  Fluoroscopic guidance for intervention
  Roadmapping
  Vessel measurement
**EXCLUDES** Diagnostic angiography/venography performed at the same session as transcatheter therapy unless it is specifically included in the code descriptor or is excluded in the venography/angiography notes (75600-75893)

**75894**  **Transcatheter therapy, embolization, any method, radiological supervision and interpretation**
  **EXCLUDES** Endovenous ablation therapy of incompetent vein (36478-36479)
  Transluminal balloon angioplasty (36475-36476)
  Vascular embolization or occlusion (37241-37244)
  0.00   0.00   **FUD** XXX   [N] [N1] [80] [icon]
  **AMA:** 2017,Jan,8; 2016,Nov,3; 2016,Jan,13; 2015,Jan,16; 2014,Oct,6; 2014,Jan,11; 2013,Nov,14; 2013,Nov,6; 2012,Feb,9-10; 2012,Apr,3-9

**75898**  **Angiography through existing catheter for follow-up study for transcatheter therapy, embolization or infusion, other than for thrombolysis**
  **EXCLUDES** Noncoronary thrombolysis infusion ([37211, 37212, 37213, 37214], 61645)
  Percutaneous arterial transluminal mechanical thrombectomy (61645)
  Prolonged endovascular intracranial administration of pharmacologic agent(s) (61650-61651)
  Transcatheter therapy, arterial infusion for thrombolysis ([37211, 37212, 37213, 37214])
  Vascular embolization or occlusion (37241-37244)
  0.00   0.00   **FUD** XXX   [Q2] [N1] [80] [icon]
  **AMA:** 2017,Jan,8; 2016,Jan,13; 2015,Nov,3; 2015,Jan,16; 2014,Oct,6; 2014,Jan,11; 2013,Nov,14; 2013,Nov,6; 2012,Feb,9-10; 2012,Jan,15-42

**75901**  **Mechanical removal of pericatheter obstructive material (eg, fibrin sheath) from central venous device via separate venous access, radiologic supervision and interpretation**
  **EXCLUDES** Venous catheterization (36010-36012)
  Code also surgical procedure (36595)
  5.00   5.00   **FUD** XXX   [N] [N1] [80] [icon]
  **AMA:** 2017,Jan,8; 2016,Jan,13; 2015,Jan,16; 2014,Jan,11; 2012,Feb,9-10

**75902**  **Mechanical removal of intraluminal (intracatheter) obstructive material from central venous device through device lumen, radiologic supervision and interpretation**
  **EXCLUDES** Venous catheterization (36010-36012)
  Code also surgical procedure (36596)
  2.04   2.04   **FUD** XXX   [N] [N1] [80] [icon]
  **AMA:** 2017,Jan,8; 2016,Jan,13; 2015,Jan,16; 2014,Jan,11; 2012,Feb,9-10

## 75952-75959 Endovascular Aneurysm Repair

**INCLUDES** The following diagnostic procedures with interventional supervision and interpretation:
  Angiography/venography
  Completion angiography/venography except for those services allowed by (75898)
  Contrast injection
  Fluoroscopic guidance for intervention
  Injection procedure only for transcatheter therapy or biopsy (36100-36299)
  Percutaneous needle biopsy
    Pancreas (48102)
    Retroperitoneal lymph node/mass (49180)
  Roadmapping
  Vessel measurement
**EXCLUDES** Diagnostic angiography/venography performed at the same session as transcatheter therapy unless it is specifically included in the code descriptor (75600-75893)
  Radiological supervision and interpretation for transluminal angioplasty in:
  Femoral/popliteal arteries (37224-37227)
  Iliac artery (37220-37223)
  Tibial/peroneal artery (37228-37235)

**75952**  ~~Endovascular repair of infrarenal abdominal aortic aneurysm or dissection, radiological supervision and interpretation~~
  To report, see 34701-34711, 0254T

**75953**  ~~Placement of proximal or distal extension prosthesis for endovascular repair of infrarenal aortic or iliac artery aneurysm, pseudoaneurysm, or dissection, radiological supervision and interpretation~~
  To report, see 34701-34711, 0254T

**75954**  ~~Endovascular repair of iliac artery aneurysm, pseudoaneurysm, arteriovenous malformation, or trauma, using ilio-iliac tube endoprosthesis, radiological supervision and interpretation~~
  To report, see 34701-34711, 0254T

● New Code   ▲ Revised Code   ○ Reinstated   ● New Web Release   ▲ Revised Web Release   Unlisted   Not Covered   # Resequenced
⊘ AMA Mod 51 Exempt   ⑤ Optum Mod 51 Exempt   ⊚ Mod 63 Exempt   ⊁ Non-FDA Drug   ★ Telemedicine   Ⓜ Maternity   🅐 Age Edit   + Add-on   AMA: CPT Asst

**75956** Endovascular repair of descending thoracic aorta (eg, aneurysm, pseudoaneurysm, dissection, penetrating ulcer, intramural hematoma, or traumatic disruption); involving coverage of left subclavian artery origin, initial endoprosthesis plus descending thoracic aortic extension(s), if required, to level of celiac artery origin, radiological supervision and interpretation

Code also endovascular graft implantation (33880)

🚑 0.00   🔧 0.00   **FUD** XXX    C 80 🖥

**AMA:** 2017,Jan,8; 2016,Jan,13; 2015,Jan,16; 2014,Jan,11; 2012,Feb,9-10

**75957** not involving coverage of left subclavian artery origin, initial endoprosthesis plus descending thoracic aortic extension(s), if required, to level of celiac artery origin, radiological supervision and interpretation

Code also endovascular graft implantation (33881)

🚑 0.00   🔧 0.00   **FUD** XXX    C 80 🖥

**AMA:** 2017,Jan,8; 2016,Jan,13; 2015,Jan,16; 2014,Jan,11; 2012,Feb,9-10

**75958** Placement of proximal extension prosthesis for endovascular repair of descending thoracic aorta (eg, aneurysm, pseudoaneurysm, dissection, penetrating ulcer, intramural hematoma, or traumatic disruption), radiological supervision and interpretation

Code also placement of each additional proximal extension(s) (75958)

Code also proximal endovascular extension implantation (33883-33884)

🚑 0.00   🔧 0.00   **FUD** XXX    C 80 🖥

**AMA:** 2017,Jan,8; 2016,Jan,13; 2015,Jan,16; 2014,Jan,11; 2012,Feb,9-10

**75959** Placement of distal extension prosthesis(s) (delayed) after endovascular repair of descending thoracic aorta, as needed, to level of celiac origin, radiological supervision and interpretation

INCLUDES   Corresponding services for placement of distal thoracic endovascular extension(s) placed during procedure following the principal procedure

EXCLUDES   *Endovascular repair of descending thoracic aorta (75956-75957)*

*Use of code more than one time no matter how many modules are deployed*

Code also placement of distal endovascular extension (33886)

🚑 0.00   🔧 0.00   **FUD** XXX    C 80 🖥

**AMA:** 2017,Jan,8; 2016,Jan,13; 2015,Jan,16; 2014,Jan,11; 2012,Feb,9-10

## 75970 Percutaneous Transluminal Angioplasty

INCLUDES   The following diagnostic procedures with interventional supervision and interpretation:

Angiography/venography

Completion angiography/venography except for those services allowed by (75898)

Contrast injection

Fluoroscopic guidance for intervention

Roadmapping

Vessel measurement

EXCLUDES   *Diagnostic angiography/venography performed at the same session as transcatheter therapy unless it is specifically included in the code descriptor (75600-75893)*

*Injection procedure only for transcatheter therapy or biopsy (36100-36299)*

*Percutaneous needle biopsy (48102)*

*Pancreas (48102)*

*Retroperitoneal lymph node/mass (49180)*

*Radiological supervision and interpretation for transluminal balloon angioplasty in:*

*Femoral/popliteal arteries (37224-37227)*

*Iliac artery (37220-37223)*

*Tibial/peroneal artery (37228-37235)*

*Transcatheter renal/ureteral biopsy (52007)*

**75970** Transcatheter biopsy, radiological supervision and interpretation

🚑 0.00   🔧 0.00   **FUD** XXX    N N1 80 🖥

**AMA:** 2014,Jan,11; 2012,Feb,9-10

## 75984-75989 Percutaneous Drainage

**75984** Change of percutaneous tube or drainage catheter with contrast monitoring (eg, genitourinary system, abscess), radiological supervision and interpretation

EXCLUDES   *Change only of nephrostomy/pyelostomy tube ([50435])*

*Cholecystostomy, percutaneous (47490)*

*Introduction procedure only for percutaneous biliary drainage (47531-47544)*

*Nephrostolithotomy/pyelostolithotomy, percutaneous (50080-50081)*

*Percutaneous replacement of gastrointestinal tube using fluoroscopic guidance (49450-49452)*

*Removal and/or replacement of internal ureteral stent using transurethral approach (50385-50386)*

🚑 2.99   🔧 2.99   **FUD** XXX    N N1 80 🖥

**AMA:** 2014,Jan,11; 2012,Feb,9-10

**75989** Radiological guidance (ie, fluoroscopy, ultrasound, or computed tomography), for percutaneous drainage (eg, abscess, specimen collection), with placement of catheter, radiological supervision and interpretation

INCLUDES   Imaging guidance

EXCLUDES   *Cholecystostomy (47490)*

*Image-guided fluid collection drainage by catheter (10030, 49405-49407)*

*Thoracentesis (32554-32557)*

🚑 3.42   🔧 3.42   **FUD** XXX    N N1 80 🖥

**AMA:** 2017,Jan,8; 2016,Jan,13; 2015,Dec,3; 2015,Jan,16; 2014,May,9; 2014,Jan,11; 2013,Nov,9; 2012,Nov,3-5; 2012,Feb,9-10; 2012,Jan,15-42

## 76000-76140 Miscellaneous Techniques

EXCLUDES   *Arthrography:*

*Ankle (73615)*

*Elbow (73085)*

*Hip (73525)*

*Knee (73580)*

*Shoulder (73040)*

*Wrist (73115)*

*CT cerebral perfusion test (0042T)*

▲ **76000** Fluoroscopy (separate procedure), up to 1 hour physician or other qualified health care professional time

EXCLUDES   *Extracorporeal membrane oxygenation (ECMO)/extracorporeal life support (ECLS) (33957-33959, [33962, 33963, 33964])*

🚑 1.34   🔧 1.34   **FUD** XXX    S Z3 80 🖥

**AMA:** 2017,Jan,8; 2016,Nov,3; 2016,Aug,5; 2016,May,5; 2016,May,13; 2016,Mar,5; 2016,Jan,11; 2016,Jan,13; 2015,Nov,3; 2015,Sep,3; 2015,May,3; 2015,Jan,16; 2014,Dec,3; 2014,Nov,5; 2014,Oct,6; 2014,Sep,5; 2014,Jan,11; 2013,Sep,17; 2013,Mar,10-11; 2013,Feb,3-6; 2012,Feb,9-10; 2012,Jan,15-42

**76001** Fluoroscopy, physician or other qualified health care professional time more than 1 hour, assisting a nonradiologic physician or other qualified health care professional (eg, nephrostolithotomy, ERCP, bronchoscopy, transbronchial biopsy)

EXCLUDES   *Extracorporeal membrane oxygenation (ECMO)/extracorporeal life support (ECLS) (33957-33959, [33962, 33963, 33964])*

🚑 0.00   🔧 0.00   **FUD** XXX    N N1 80 🖥

**AMA:** 2017,Jan,8; 2016,Nov,3; 2016,Mar,5; 2016,Jan,13; 2015,Nov,3; 2015,Sep,3; 2015,Jan,16; 2014,Oct,6; 2014,Sep,5; 2014,Jan,11; 2013,Mar,10-11; 2013,Feb,3-6; 2012,Feb,9-10; 2012,Jan,15-42

**76010** Radiologic examination from nose to rectum for foreign body, single view, child    A

🚑 0.74   🔧 0.74   **FUD** XXX    01 N1 80 🖥

**AMA:** 2017,Jan,8; 2016,Jan,13; 2015,Jan,16; 2014,Jan,11; 2012,Feb,9-10; 2012,Jan,15-42

26/TC PC/TC Only   A2-Z3 ASC Payment   50 Bilateral   ♂ Male Only   ♀ Female Only   🚑 Facility RVU   🔧 Non-Facility RVU   🖥 CCI

FUD Follow-up Days   CMS: IOM (Pub 100)   A-Y OPPSI   80/80 Surg Assist Allowed / w/Doc   Lab Crosswalk   Radiology Crosswalk   CLIA

332    CPT © 2017 American Medical Association. All Rights Reserved.    © 2017 Optum360, LLC

Radiology

75956 — 76010

| 76080 | Radiologic examination, abscess, fistula or sinus tract study, radiological supervision and interpretation |
|---|---|

EXCLUDES Contrast injections, radiology evaluation, and guidance via fluoroscopy of gastrostomy, duodenostomy, jejunostomy, gastro-jejunostomy, or cecostomy tube (49465)

1.56  1.56  **FUD** XXX  [02] [N1] [80] [▭]

**AMA:** 2017,Jan,8; 2016,Jan,13; 2015,Jan,16; 2014,Jan,11; 2012,Feb,9-10; 2012,Jan,15-42

| 76098 | Radiological examination, surgical specimen |
|---|---|

EXCLUDES Breast biopsy with placement of breast localization device(s) (19081-19086)

0.47  0.47  **FUD** XXX  [02] [N1] [80] [▭]

**AMA:** 2012,Feb,9-10

| 76100 | Radiologic examination, single plane body section (eg, tomography), other than with urography |
|---|---|

2.59  2.59  **FUD** XXX  [01] [N1] [80] [▭]

**AMA:** 2012,Feb,9-10

| 76101 | Radiologic examination, complex motion (ie, hypercycloidal) body section (eg, mastoid polytomography), other than with urography; unilateral |
|---|---|

EXCLUDES Nephrotomography (74415)
Panoramic x-ray (70355)
Procedure performed more than one time per day

3.72  3.72  **FUD** XXX  [01] [Z2] [80] [▭]

**AMA:** 2012,Feb,9-10

| 76102 | bilateral |
|---|---|

EXCLUDES Nephrotomography (74415)
Panoramic x-ray (70355)
Procedure performed more than one time per day

4.85  4.85  **FUD** XXX  [S] [Z2] [80] [▭]

**AMA:** 2012,Feb,9-10

| 76120 | Cineradiography/videoradiography, except where specifically included |
|---|---|

2.39  2.39  **FUD** XXX  [01] [N1] [80] [▭]

**AMA:** 2017,Jan,8; 2016,Jan,13; 2015,Jan,16; 2014,Jan,11; 2012,Feb,9-10

| + | 76125 | Cineradiography/videoradiography to complement routine examination (List separately in addition to code for primary procedure) |
|---|---|---|

Code first primary procedure

0.00  0.00  **FUD** ZZZ  [N] [N1] [80] [▭]

**AMA:** 2017,Jan,8; 2016,Jan,13; 2015,Jan,16; 2014,Jan,11; 2012,Feb,9-10

| 76140 | Consultation on X-ray examination made elsewhere, written report |
|---|---|

0.00  0.00  **FUD** XXX  [E] [▭]

**AMA:** 2017,Jan,8; 2016,Jan,13; 2015,Jan,16; 2014,Jan,11; 2012,Feb,9-10; 2012,Jan,15-42

## 76376-76377 Three-dimensional Manipulation

INCLUDES Concurrent physician supervision of image postprocessing
3D manipulation of volumetric data set
Rendering of image

EXCLUDES Arthrography:
Ankle (73615)
Elbow (73085)
Hip (73525)
Knee (73580)
Shoulder (73040)
Wrist (73115)
Cardiac magnetic resonance imaging (75557, 75559, 75561, 75563, 75565)
Computer-aided detection of MRI data for lesion, breast MRI (0159T)
Computed tomographic angiography (70496, 70498, 71275, 72191, 73206, 73706, 74174-74175, 74261-74263, 75571, 75574, 75635)
CT cerebral perfusion test (0042T)
Digital breast tomosynthesis (77061-77063)
Echocardiography, transesophageal (TEE) for guidance (93355)
Magnetic resonance angiography (70544-70549, 71555, 72198, 73225, 73725, 74185)
Nuclear radiology procedures (78012-78999)
Physician planning of a patient-specific fenestrated visceral aortic endograft (34839)
Code also base imaging procedure(s)

| 76376 | 3D rendering with interpretation and reporting of computed tomography, magnetic resonance imaging, ultrasound, or other tomographic modality with image postprocessing under concurrent supervision; not requiring image postprocessing on an independent workstation |
|---|---|

EXCLUDES 3D rendering (76377)
Bronchoscopy, with computer-assisted, image-guided navigation (31627)

0.66  0.66  **FUD** XXX  [N] [N1] [80] [▭]

**AMA:** 2017,Jan,8; 2016,Apr,8; 2016,Jan,13; 2015,Jan,16; 2014,Jan,11; 2013,Jun,12; 2013,May,3-5; 2012,Feb,9-10; 2012,Jan,15-42

| 76377 | requiring image postprocessing on an independent workstation |
|---|---|

EXCLUDES 3D rendering (76376)

2.02  2.02  **FUD** XXX  [N] [N1] [80] [▭]

**AMA:** 2017,Jan,8; 2016,Apr,8; 2016,Jan,13; 2015,Jan,16; 2014,Jan,11; 2013,Jun,12; 2013,May,3-5; 2012,Feb,9-10; 2012,Jan,15-42

## 76380 Computerized Tomography: Delimited

EXCLUDES Arthrography:
Ankle (73615)
Elbow (73085)
Hip (73525)
Knee (73580)
Shoulder (73040)
Wrist (73115)
CT cerebral perfusion test (0042T)

| 76380 | Computed tomography, limited or localized follow-up study |
|---|---|

4.12  4.12  **FUD** XXX  [01] [N1] [80] [▭]

**AMA:** 2017,Jan,8; 2016,Jan,13; 2015,Jan,16; 2014,Jan,11; 2012,Feb,9-10

## 76390 Magnetic Resonance Spectroscopy

**CMS:** 100-03,220.2.1 Magnetic Resonance Spectroscopy

EXCLUDES Arthrography:
Ankle (73615)
Elbow (73085)
Hip (73525)
Knee (73580)
Shoulder (73040)
Wrist (73115)
CT cerebral perfusion test (0042T)

| 76390 | Magnetic resonance spectroscopy |
|---|---|

EXCLUDES MRI

12.5  12.5  **FUD** XXX  [E] [▭]

**AMA:** 2012,Feb,9-10

● New Code  ▲ Revised Code  ○ Reinstated  ● New Web Release  ▲ Revised Web Release  Unlisted  Not Covered  # Resequenced
⊘ AMA Mod 51 Exempt  ⑤ Optum Mod 51 Exempt  ⊛ Mod 63 Exempt  ✗ Non-FDA Drug  ★ Telemedicine  Ⓜ Maternity  Ⓐ Age Edit  + Add-on  AMA: CPT Asst
© 2017 Optum360, LLC  CPT © 2017 American Medical Association. All Rights Reserved.  333

**Radiology** *(left margin)*

**76496 — 76642** *(left margin)*

## 76496-76499 Unlisted Radiology Procedures

**76496** Unlisted fluoroscopic procedure (eg, diagnostic, interventional)
🚑 0.00  ⚕ 0.00  **FUD** XXX  [Q1] [N1] [80] [CCI]
**AMA:** 2012,Feb,9-10

**76497** Unlisted computed tomography procedure (eg, diagnostic, interventional)
🚑 0.00  ⚕ 0.00  **FUD** XXX  [Q1] [N1] [80] [CCI]
**AMA:** 2017,Jan,8; 2016,Jan,13; 2015,Jan,16; 2014,Jan,11; 2012,Feb,9-10; 2012,Jan,15-42

**76498** Unlisted magnetic resonance procedure (eg, diagnostic, interventional)
🚑 0.00  ⚕ 0.00  **FUD** XXX  [S] [Z2] [80] [CCI]
**AMA:** 2017,Jan,8; 2016,Jan,13; 2015,Jan,16; 2014,Jan,11; 2012,Feb,9-10; 2012,Jan,15-42

**76499** Unlisted diagnostic radiographic procedure
🚑 0.00  ⚕ 0.00  **FUD** XXX  [Q1] [N1] [80]
**AMA:** 2017,Jan,8; 2016,Dec,15; 2016,Jul,8; 2016,Jan,13; 2015,Jan,16; 2014,Jan,11; 2013,Dec,16; 2012,Feb,9-10; 2012,Jan,15-42

## 76506 Ultrasound: Brain

INCLUDES Required permanent documentation of ultrasound images except when diagnostic purpose is biometric measurement
Written documentation
EXCLUDES *Noninvasive vascular studies, diagnostic (93880-93990)*
*Ultrasound exam that does not include thorough assessment of organ or site, recorded image, and written report*

**76506** Echoencephalography, real time with image documentation (gray scale) (for determination of ventricular size, delineation of cerebral contents, and detection of fluid masses or other intracranial abnormalities), including A-mode encephalography as secondary component where indicated
🚑 3.36  ⚕ 3.36  **FUD** XXX  [Q1] [N1] [80] [CCI]
**AMA:** 2017,Jan,8; 2016,Jan,13; 2015,Jan,16; 2014,Jan,11; 2012,Feb,9-10

## 76510-76529 Ultrasound: Eyes

INCLUDES Required permanent documentation of ultrasound images except when diagnostic purpose is biometric measurement
Written documentation

**76510** Ophthalmic ultrasound, diagnostic; B-scan and quantitative A-scan performed during the same patient encounter
🚑 4.80  ⚕ 4.80  **FUD** XXX  [Q1] [N1] [80] [CCI]
**AMA:** 2017,Jan,8; 2016,Jan,13; 2015,Jan,16; 2014,Jan,11; 2012,Feb,9-10

**76511** quantitative A-scan only
🚑 2.88  ⚕ 2.88  **FUD** XXX  [Q1] [N1] [80] [CCI]
**AMA:** 2017,Jan,8; 2016,Jan,13; 2015,Jan,16; 2014,Jan,11; 2012,Feb,9-10

**76512** B-scan (with or without superimposed non-quantitative A-scan)
🚑 2.62  ⚕ 2.62  **FUD** XXX  [Q1] [N1] [80] [CCI]
**AMA:** 2017,Jan,8; 2016,Jan,13; 2015,Jan,16; 2014,Jan,11; 2012,Feb,9-10

**76513** anterior segment ultrasound, immersion (water bath) B-scan or high resolution biomicroscopy
EXCLUDES *Computerized ophthalmic testing other than by ultrasound (92132-92134)*
🚑 2.69  ⚕ 2.69  **FUD** XXX  [Q1] [N1] [80] [CCI]
**AMA:** 2017,Jan,8; 2016,Jan,13; 2015,Jan,16; 2014,Jan,11; 2013,Apr,7; 2012,Feb,9-10; 2012,Jan,15-42

**76514** corneal pachymetry, unilateral or bilateral (determination of corneal thickness)
INCLUDES Biometric measurement for which permanent documentation of images is not required
EXCLUDES *Collagen cross-linking of cornea (0402T)*
🚑 0.43  ⚕ 0.43  **FUD** XXX  [Q1] [N1] [80] [CCI]
**AMA:** 2017,Jan,8; 2016,Feb,12; 2016,Jan,13; 2015,Jan,16; 2014,Jan,11; 2012,Feb,9-10; 2012,Jan,15-42

**76516** Ophthalmic biometry by ultrasound echography, A-scan;
INCLUDES Biometric measurement for which permanent documentation of images is not required
🚑 2.22  ⚕ 2.22  **FUD** XXX  [Q1] [N1] [80] [CCI]
**AMA:** 2017,Jan,8; 2016,Jan,13; 2015,Jan,16; 2014,Jan,11; 2012,Feb,9-10; 2012,Jan,15-42

**76519** with intraocular lens power calculation
INCLUDES Biometric measurement for which permanent documentation of images is not required
Written prescription that satisfies requirement for written report
EXCLUDES *Partial coherence interferometry (92136)*
🚑 2.39  ⚕ 2.39  **FUD** XXX  [Q1] [N1] [80] [CCI]
**AMA:** 2017,Jan,8; 2016,Jan,13; 2015,Jan,16; 2014,Jan,11; 2012,Feb,9-10; 2012,Jan,15-42

**76529** Ophthalmic ultrasonic foreign body localization
🚑 2.23  ⚕ 2.23  **FUD** XXX  [Q1] [N1] [80] [CCI]
**AMA:** 2017,Jan,8; 2016,Jan,13; 2015,Jan,16; 2014,Jan,11; 2012,Feb,9-10

## 76536-76800 Ultrasound: Neck, Thorax, Abdomen, and Spine

INCLUDES Required permanent documentation of ultrasound images except when diagnostic purpose is biometric measurement
Written documentation
EXCLUDES *Focused ultrasound ablation of uterine leiomyomata (0071T-0072T)*
*Ultrasound exam that does not include thorough assessment of organ or site, recorded image, and written report*

**76536** Ultrasound, soft tissues of head and neck (eg, thyroid, parathyroid, parotid), real time with image documentation
🚑 3.31  ⚕ 3.31  **FUD** XXX  [Q1] [N1] [80] [CCI]
**AMA:** 2017,Jan,8; 2016,Jan,13; 2015,Jan,16; 2014,Jan,11; 2012,Feb,9-10

**76604** Ultrasound, chest (includes mediastinum), real time with image documentation
🚑 2.51  ⚕ 2.51  **FUD** XXX  [Q1] [N1] [80] [CCI]
**AMA:** 2017,Jan,8; 2016,Jan,13; 2015,Jan,16; 2014,Jan,11; 2012,Nov,3-5; 2012,Feb,9-10

**76641** Ultrasound, breast, unilateral, real time with image documentation, including axilla when performed; complete
INCLUDES Complete examination of all four quadrants, retroareolar region, and axilla when performed
EXCLUDES *Procedure performed more than one time per breast per session*
🚑 3.05  ⚕ 3.05  **FUD** XXX  [Q1] [N1] [80] [50] [CCI]
**AMA:** 2017,Jan,8; 2016,Jan,13; 2015,Aug,8

**76642** limited
🚑 2.51  ⚕ 2.51  **FUD** XXX  [Q1] [N1] [80] [50] [CCI]
INCLUDES Examination not including all of the elements in complete examination
EXCLUDES *Procedure performed more than one time per breast per session*

[26]/[TC] PC/TC Only  [A2]-[Z6] ASC Payment  [50] Bilateral  ♂ Male Only  ♀ Female Only  🚑 Facility RVU  ⚕ Non-Facility RVU  [CCI] CCI
**FUD** Follow-up Days  **CMS:** IOM (Pub 100)  [A]-[Y] OPPSI  [80]/[80] Surg Assist Allowed / w/Doc  [L] Lab Crosswalk  [R] Radiology Crosswalk  [X] CLIA
CPT © 2017 American Medical Association. All Rights Reserved.
© 2017 Optum360, LLC

**76700** Ultrasound, abdominal, real time with image documentation; complete

    INCLUDES  Real time scans of:
- Common bile duct
- Gall bladder
- Inferior vena cava
- Kidneys
- Liver
- Pancreas
- Spleen
- Upper abdominal aorta

  3.48   3.48  **FUD** XXX  Q3 Z2 80

**AMA:** 2017,Jan,8; 2016,Jan,13; 2015,Jan,16; 2014,Jan,11; 2012,Feb,9-10

**76705** limited (eg, single organ, quadrant, follow-up)

  2.60   2.60  **FUD** XXX  Q3 Z2 80

**AMA:** 2017,Jan,8; 2016,Jan,13; 2015,Jan,16; 2014,Jan,11; 2012,Dec,9-10; 2012,Feb,9-10; 2012,Mar,9-10; 2012,Jan,15-42

**76706** Ultrasound, abdominal aorta, real time with image documentation, screening study for abdominal aortic aneurysm (AAA)

    EXCLUDES  *Diagnostic ultrasound of aorta (76770-76775)*
    *Duplex scan of aorta (93978-93979)*

  2.66   2.66  **FUD** XXX  S 80

**AMA:** 2017,Sep,11

**76770** Ultrasound, retroperitoneal (eg, renal, aorta, nodes), real time with image documentation; complete

    INCLUDES  Complete assessment of kidneys and bladder if history indicates urinary pathology

Real time scans of:
- Abdominal aorta
- Common iliac artery origins
- Inferior vena cava
- Kidneys

  3.22   3.22  **FUD** XXX  Q3 Z2 80

**AMA:** 2017,Jan,8; 2016,Jan,13; 2015,Jan,16; 2014,Jan,11; 2012,Feb,9-10

**76775** limited

  1.66   1.66  **FUD** XXX  Q1 N1 80

**AMA:** 2017,Jan,8; 2016,Jan,13; 2015,Jan,16; 2014,Jan,11; 2012,Feb,9-10; 2012,Jan,15-42

**76776** Ultrasound, transplanted kidney, real time and duplex Doppler with image documentation

    EXCLUDES  *Abdominal/pelvic/scrotal contents/retroperitoneal duplex scan (93975-93976)*
    *Transplanted kidney ultrasound without duplex doppler (76775)*

  4.46   4.46  **FUD** XXX  Q3 Z2 80

**AMA:** 2017,Jan,8; 2016,Jan,13; 2015,Jan,16; 2014,Jan,11; 2012,Feb,9-10

**76800** Ultrasound, spinal canal and contents

  4.06   4.06  **FUD** XXX  Q1 N1 80

**AMA:** 2017,Jan,8; 2016,Jan,13; 2015,Jan,16; 2014,Jan,11; 2012,Feb,9-10; 2012,Jan,15-42

## 76801-76802 Ultrasound: Pregnancy Less Than 14 Weeks

  INCLUDES  Determination of the number of gestational sacs and fetuses
Gestational sac/fetal measurement appropriate for gestational age (younger than 14 weeks 0 days)
Inspection of the maternal uterus and adnexa
Quality analysis of amniotic fluid volume/gestational sac shape
Visualization of fetal and placental anatomic formation
Written documentation of each component of exam

  EXCLUDES  *Focused ultrasound ablation of uterine leiomyomata (0071T-0072T)*
*Ultrasound exam that does not include thorough assessment of organ or site, recorded image, and written report*

**76801** Ultrasound, pregnant, real time with image documentation, fetal and maternal evaluation, first trimester (< 14 weeks 0 days), transabdominal approach; single or first gestation  M ♀

    EXCLUDES  *Fetal nuchal translucency measurement, first trimester (76813)*

  3.52   3.52  **FUD** XXX  S Z2 80

**AMA:** 2017,Jan,8; 2016,Jan,13; 2015,Jan,16; 2014,Jan,11; 2012,Feb,9-10; 2012,Jan,15-42

**+ 76802** each additional gestation (List separately in addition to code for primary procedure)  M ♀

    EXCLUDES  *Fetal nuchal translucency measurement, first trimester (76814)*

Code first (76801)
  1.84   1.84  **FUD** ZZZ  N N1 80

**AMA:** 2017,Jan,8; 2016,Jan,13; 2015,Jan,16; 2014,Jan,11; 2012,Feb,9-10; 2012,Jan,15-42

## 76805-76810 Ultrasound: Pregnancy of 14 Weeks or More

  INCLUDES  Determination of the number of gestational/chorionic sacs and fetuses
Evaluation of:
- Amniotic fluid
- Four chambered heart
- Intracranial, spinal, abdominal anatomy
- Placenta location
- Umbilical cord insertion site

Examination of maternal adnexa if visible
Gestational sac/fetal measurement appropriate for gestational age (older than or equal to 14 weeks 0 days)
Written documentation of each component of exam

  EXCLUDES  *Focused ultrasound ablation of uterine leiomyomata (0071T-0072T)*
*Ultrasound exam that does not include thorough assessment of organ or site, recorded image, and written report*

**76805** Ultrasound, pregnant uterus, real time with image documentation, fetal and maternal evaluation, after first trimester (> or = 14 weeks 0 days), transabdominal approach; single or first gestation  M ♀

  4.06   4.06  **FUD** XXX  S Z2 80

**AMA:** 2017,Jan,8; 2016,Jan,13; 2015,Jan,16; 2014,Jan,11; 2012,Feb,9-10

**+ 76810** each additional gestation (List separately in addition to code for primary procedure)  M ♀

Code first (76805)
  2.66   2.66  **FUD** ZZZ  N N1 80

**AMA:** 2017,Jan,8; 2016,Jan,13; 2015,Jan,16; 2014,Jan,11; 2012,Feb,9-10

**Radiology** *(side margin)*

**76811 — 76828** *(side margin)*

## 76811-76812 Ultrasound: Pregnancy, with Additional Studies of Fetus

**INCLUDES** Determination of the number of gestational/chorionic sacs and fetuses
Evaluation of:
Abdominal organ specific anatomy
Amniotic fluid
Chest anatomy
Face
Fetal brain/ventricles
Four chambered heart
Heart/outflow tracts and chest anatomy
Intracranial, spinal, abdominal anatomy
Limbs including number, length, and architecture
Other fetal anatomy as indicated
Placenta location
Umbilical cord insertion site
Examination of maternal adnexa if visible
Gestational sac/fetal measurement appropriate for gestational age (older than or equal to 14 weeks 0 days)
Written documentation of each component of exam, including reason for nonvisualization, when applicable

**EXCLUDES** *Focused ultrasound ablation of uterine leiomyomata (0071T-0072T)*
*Ultrasound exam that does not include thorough assessment organ or site, recorded image, and written report*

**76811** Ultrasound, pregnant uterus, real time with image documentation, fetal and maternal evaluation plus detailed fetal anatomic examination, transabdominal approach; single or first gestation  Ⓜ ♀
🚑 5.24  ⚕ 5.24  **FUD** XXX  Ⓢ Ⓩ2 80 🖳
**AMA:** 2017,Jan,8; 2016,Jan,13; 2015,Jan,16; 2014,Jan,11; 2012,Feb,9-10

**+ 76812** each additional gestation (List separately in addition to code for primary procedure)  Ⓜ ♀
Code first (76811)
🚑 5.87  ⚕ 5.87  **FUD** ZZZ  Ⓝ Ⓝ1 80 🖳
**AMA:** 2017,Jan,8; 2016,Jan,13; 2015,Jan,16; 2014,Jan,11; 2012,Feb,9-10

## 76813-76828 Ultrasound: Other Fetal Evaluations

**INCLUDES** Required permanent documentation of ultrasound images except when diagnostic purpose is biometric measurement
Written documentation

**EXCLUDES** *Focused ultrasound ablation of uterine leiomyomata (0071T-0072T)*
*Ultrasound exam that does not include thorough assessment of organ or site, recorded image, and written report*

**76813** Ultrasound, pregnant uterus, real time with image documentation, first trimester fetal nuchal translucency measurement, transabdominal or transvaginal approach; single or first gestation  Ⓜ ♀
🚑 3.49  ⚕ 3.49  **FUD** XXX  Ⓠ1 Ⓝ1 80 🖳
**AMA:** 2017,Jan,8; 2016,Jan,13; 2015,Jan,16; 2014,Jan,11; 2012,Feb,9-10

**+ 76814** each additional gestation (List separately in addition to code for primary procedure)  Ⓜ ♀
Code first (76813)
🚑 2.32  ⚕ 2.32  **FUD** XXX  Ⓝ Ⓝ1 80 🖳
**AMA:** 2017,Jan,8; 2016,Jan,13; 2015,Jan,16; 2014,Jan,11; 2012,Feb,9-10

**76815** Ultrasound, pregnant uterus, real time with image documentation, limited (eg, fetal heart beat, placental location, fetal position and/or qualitative amniotic fluid volume), 1 or more fetuses  Ⓜ ♀
**INCLUDES** Exam concentrating on one or more elements
Reporting only one time per exam, instead of per element
**EXCLUDES** *Fetal nuchal translucency measurement, first trimester (76813-76814)*
🚑 2.42  ⚕ 2.42  **FUD** XXX  Ⓠ1 Ⓝ1 80 🖳
**AMA:** 2017,Jan,8; 2016,Jan,13; 2015,Jan,16; 2014,Jan,11; 2012,Feb,9-10; 2012,Jan,15-42

**76816** Ultrasound, pregnant uterus, real time with image documentation, follow-up (eg, re-evaluation of fetal size by measuring standard growth parameters and amniotic fluid volume, re-evaluation of organ system(s) suspected or confirmed to be abnormal on a previous scan), transabdominal approach, per fetus  Ⓜ ♀
**INCLUDES** Re-evaluation of fetal size, interval growth, or aberrancies noted on a prior ultrasound
Code also modifier 59 for examination of each additional fetus in a multiple pregnancy
🚑 3.31  ⚕ 3.31  **FUD** XXX  Ⓠ1 Ⓝ1 80 🖳
**AMA:** 2017,Jan,8; 2016,Jan,13; 2015,Jan,16; 2014,Jan,11; 2012,Feb,9-10; 2012,Jan,15-42

**76817** Ultrasound, pregnant uterus, real time with image documentation, transvaginal  Ⓜ ♀
**EXCLUDES** *Transvaginal ultrasound, non-obstetrical (76830)*
Code also transabdominal obstetrical ultrasound, if performed
🚑 2.78  ⚕ 2.78  **FUD** XXX  Ⓠ1 Ⓝ1 80 🖳
**AMA:** 2017,Jan,8; 2016,Jan,13; 2015,Jan,16; 2014,Jan,11; 2012,Feb,9-10; 2012,Jan,15-42

**76818** Fetal biophysical profile; with non-stress testing  Ⓜ ♀
Code also modifier 59 for each additional fetus
🚑 3.53  ⚕ 3.53  **FUD** XXX  Ⓢ Ⓩ2 80 🖳
**AMA:** 2017,Jan,8; 2016,Jan,13; 2015,Jan,16; 2014,Jan,11; 2012,Feb,9-10; 2012,Jan,15-42

**76819** without non-stress testing  Ⓜ ♀
**EXCLUDES** *Amniotic fluid index without non-stress test (76815)*
Code also modifier 59 for each additional fetus
🚑 2.58  ⚕ 2.58  **FUD** XXX  Ⓢ Ⓩ3 80 🖳
**AMA:** 2017,Jan,8; 2016,Jan,13; 2015,Jan,16; 2014,Jan,11; 2012,Feb,9-10; 2012,Jan,15-42

**76820** Doppler velocimetry, fetal; umbilical artery  Ⓜ
🚑 1.38  ⚕ 1.38  **FUD** XXX  Ⓠ1 Ⓝ1 80 🖳
**AMA:** 2017,Jan,8; 2016,Jul,8; 2016,Jan,13; 2015,Jan,16; 2014,Jan,11; 2012,Feb,9-10

**76821** middle cerebral artery  Ⓜ
🚑 2.66  ⚕ 2.66  **FUD** XXX  Ⓠ1 Ⓝ1 80 🖳
**AMA:** 2017,Jan,8; 2016,Jan,13; 2015,Jan,16; 2014,Jan,11; 2012,Feb,9-10

**76825** Echocardiography, fetal, cardiovascular system, real time with image documentation (2D), with or without M-mode recording;  Ⓜ ♀
🚑 7.93  ⚕ 7.93  **FUD** XXX  Ⓢ Ⓩ3 80 🖳
**AMA:** 2017,Sep,14; 2017,Jan,8; 2016,Jan,13; 2015,Jan,16; 2014,Jan,11; 2012,Feb,9-10

**76826** follow-up or repeat study  Ⓜ ♀
🚑 4.66  ⚕ 4.66  **FUD** XXX  Ⓢ Ⓩ2 80 🖳
**AMA:** 2017,Sep,14; 2012,Feb,9-10

**76827** Doppler echocardiography, fetal, pulsed wave and/or continuous wave with spectral display; complete  Ⓜ ♀
🚑 2.16  ⚕ 2.16  **FUD** XXX  Ⓠ1 Ⓝ1 80 🖳
**AMA:** 2017,Jan,8; 2016,Jan,13; 2015,Jan,16; 2014,Jan,11; 2012,Feb,9-10

**76828** follow-up or repeat study  Ⓜ ♀
**EXCLUDES** *Color mapping (93325)*
🚑 1.54  ⚕ 1.54  **FUD** XXX  Ⓠ1 Ⓝ1 80 🖳
**AMA:** 2017,Jan,8; 2016,Jan,13; 2015,Jan,16; 2014,Jan,11; 2012,Feb,9-10

## 76830-76873 Ultrasound: Male and Female Genitalia

INCLUDES Required permanent documentation of ultrasound images except when diagnostic purpose is biometric measurement
Written documentation

EXCLUDES *Focused ultrasound ablation of uterine leiomyomata (0071T-0072T)*
*Ultrasound exam that does not include thorough assessment of organ or site, recorded image, and written report*

### 76830 Ultrasound, transvaginal ♀

EXCLUDES *Transvaginal ultrasound, obstetric (76817)*
Code also transabdominal non-obstetrical ultrasound, if performed

🚑 3.48    ⚕ 3.48    **FUD** XXX                    S Z2 80 🖃

**AMA:** 2017,Jan,8; 2016,Jan,13; 2015,Jan,16; 2014,Jan,11; 2012,Feb,9-10; 2012,Jan,15-42

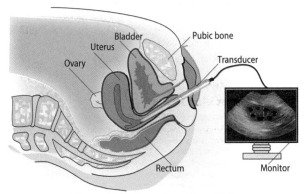

**Ultrasound is performed in real time with image documentation by a transvaginal approach**

### 76831 Saline infusion sonohysterography (SIS), including color flow Doppler, when performed ♀

Code also saline introduction for saline infusion sonohysterography (58340)

🚑 3.41    ⚕ 3.41    **FUD** XXX                    Q3 Z3 80 🖃

**AMA:** 2017,Jan,8; 2016,Jan,13; 2015,Jan,16; 2014,Jan,11; 2012,Feb,9-10; 2012,Jan,15-42

### 76856 Ultrasound, pelvic (nonobstetric), real time with image documentation; complete

INCLUDES Total examination of the female pelvic anatomy which includes:
Bladder measurement
Description and measurement of the uterus and adnexa
Description of any pelvic pathology
Measurement of the endometrium
Total examination of the male pelvis which includes:
Bladder measurement
Description of any pelvic pathology
Evaluation of prostate and seminal vesicles

🚑 3.14    ⚕ 3.14    **FUD** XXX                    Q3 Z2 80 🖃

**AMA:** 2017,Jan,8; 2016,Aug,9; 2016,Jan,13; 2015,Jan,16; 2014,Jan,11; 2012,Feb,9-10; 2012,Jan,15-42

### 76857 limited or follow-up (eg, for follicles)

INCLUDES Focused evaluation limited to:
Evaluation of one or more elements listed in 76856 and/or
Reevaluation of one or more pelvic aberrances noted on a prior ultrasound
Urinary bladder alone

EXCLUDES *Bladder volume or post-voided residual measurement without imaging the bladder (51798)*
*Urinary bladder and kidneys (76770)*

🚑 1.37    ⚕ 1.37    **FUD** XXX                    Q3 Z3 80 🖃

**AMA:** 2017,Jan,8; 2016,Jan,13; 2015,Jan,16; 2014,Jan,11; 2012,Feb,9-10; 2012,Jan,15-42

### 76870 Ultrasound, scrotum and contents ♂

🚑 1.94    ⚕ 1.94    **FUD** XXX                    Q1 N1 80 🖃

**AMA:** 2012,Feb,9-10

### 76872 Ultrasound, transrectal;

EXCLUDES *Colonoscopy (45391-45392)*
*Ligation, hemorrhoidal vascular bundle(s) (0249T)*
*Sigmoidoscopy (45341-45342)*
*Transurethral prostate ablation (0421T)*

🚑 2.70    ⚕ 2.70    **FUD** XXX                    S Z2 80 🖃

**AMA:** 2017,Jan,8; 2016,Jan,13; 2015,Jan,16; 2014,Jan,11; 2012,Feb,9-10

### 76873 prostate volume study for brachytherapy treatment planning (separate procedure) ♂

🚑 4.86    ⚕ 4.86    **FUD** XXX                    S Z2 80 🖃

**AMA:** 2017,Jan,8; 2016,Jan,13; 2015,Jan,16; 2014,Jan,11; 2012,Feb,9-10

## 76881-76886 Ultrasound: Extremities

EXCLUDES *Doppler studies of the extremities (93925-93926, 93930-93931, 93970-93971)*

▲ ### 76881 Ultrasound, complete joint (ie, joint space and peri-articular soft tissue structures) real-time with image documentation

INCLUDES Real time scans of a specific joint including assessment of:
Joint space
Muscles
Other soft tissue
Tendons
Required permanent documentation of images
Stress manipulations and dynamic imaging when performed
Written documentation including an explanation of any components of the joint that cannot be visualized

🚑 3.36    ⚕ 3.36    **FUD** XXX                    S Z2 🖃

**AMA:** 2017,Jan,8; 2016,Sep,9; 2012,Feb,9-10

▲ ### 76882 Ultrasound, limited, joint or other nonvascular extremity structure(s) (eg, joint space, peri-articular tendon[s], muscle[s], nerve[s], other soft tissue structure[s], or soft tissue mass[es]), real-time with image documentation

INCLUDES Limited examination of a joint or for evaluation of an extremity for a mass or other abnormality not requiring all of the components of a complete joint evaluation (76881)
Real time scans of a specific joint including assessment of:
Joint space
Muscles
Other soft tissue
Tendons
Required permanent documentation of images
Written documentation containing a description of all of the components of the joint visualized

🚑 1.02    ⚕ 1.02    **FUD** XXX                    Q1 N1 🖃

**AMA:** 2017,Jan,8; 2016,Sep,9; 2012,Feb,9-10

### 76885 Ultrasound, infant hips, real time with imaging documentation; dynamic (requiring physician or other qualified health care professional manipulation) 🅰

🚑 4.17    ⚕ 4.17    **FUD** XXX                    Q1 N1 80 🖃

**AMA:** 2012,Feb,9-10

### 76886 limited, static (not requiring physician or other qualified health care professional manipulation) 🅰

🚑 3.10    ⚕ 3.10    **FUD** XXX                    Q1 N1 80 🖃

**AMA:** 2012,Feb,9-10

## 76930-76970 Imaging Guidance: Ultrasound

INCLUDES Required permanent documentation of ultrasound images except when diagnostic purpose is biometric measurement
Written documentation

EXCLUDES *Focused ultrasound ablation of uterine leiomyomata (0071T-0072T)*
*Ultrasound exam that does not include thorough assessment of organ or site, recorded image, and written report*

### 76930 Ultrasonic guidance for pericardiocentesis, imaging supervision and interpretation

🚑 0.00    ⚕ 0.00    **FUD** XXX                    N N1 80 🖃

**AMA:** 2017,Jan,8; 2016,Sep,9; 2012,Feb,9-10

● New Code    ▲ Revised Code    ○ Reinstated    ● New Web Release    ▲ Revised Web Release    Unlisted    Not Covered    # Resequenced
⊘ AMA Mod 51 Exempt    ⑤ Optum Mod 51 Exempt    ⑥ Mod 63 Exempt    ✎ Non-FDA Drug    ★ Telemedicine    Ⓜ Maternity    🅰 Age Edit    + Add-on    **AMA:** CPT Asst
© 2017 Optum360, LLC                    CPT © 2017 American Medical Association. All Rights Reserved.                    337

**Radiology**

**76932** Ultrasonic guidance for endomyocardial biopsy, imaging supervision and interpretation
🔲 0.00 　 0.00 　**FUD** YYY 　　　N N1 80 📺
**AMA:** 2012,Feb,9-10

**76936** Ultrasound guided compression repair of arterial pseudoaneurysm or arteriovenous fistulae (includes diagnostic ultrasound evaluation, compression of lesion and imaging)
🔲 7.74 　 7.74 　**FUD** XXX 　　　S Z2 80 📺
**AMA:** 2012,Feb,9-10

**+ 76937** Ultrasound guidance for vascular access requiring ultrasound evaluation of potential access sites, documentation of selected vessel patency, concurrent realtime ultrasound visualization of vascular needle entry, with permanent recording and reporting (List separately in addition to code for primary procedure)

　INCLUDES　Ultrasonic guidance (76942)
　EXCLUDES　*Extremity venous noninvasive vascular diagnostic study performed separately from venous access guidance (93970-93971)*
　　　*Insertion of intravascular vena cava filter (37191-37193)*
　　　*Ligation perforator veins (37760-37761)*
Code first primary procedure
🔲 0.89 　 0.89 　**FUD** ZZZ 　　　N N1 80 📺
**AMA:** 2017,Aug,10; 2017,Jul,3; 2017,Mar,3; 2017,Jan,8; 2016,Nov,3; 2016,Jul,6; 2016,Jan,13; 2015,Jul,10; 2015,Jan,16; 2014,Oct,6; 2014,Jan,11; 2013,Sep,17; 2013,Jun,12; 2013,May,3-5; 2013,Feb,3-6; 2012,Apr,3-9; 2012,Feb,9-10

**76940** Ultrasound guidance for, and monitoring of, parenchymal tissue ablation

　EXCLUDES　*Ablation (20982-20983, 32994, 32998, 47370-47383, 50250, 50542, 50592-50593)*
　　　*Ultrasound guidance:*
　　　*Intraoperative (76998)*
　　　*Needle placement (76942)*
🔲 0.00 　 0.00 　**FUD** YYY 　　　N N1 80 📺
**AMA:** 2017,Jan,8; 2016,Jan,13; 2015,Jul,8; 2015,Jan,16; 2014,Jan,11; 2012,Feb,9-10

**76941** Ultrasonic guidance for intrauterine fetal transfusion or cordocentesis, imaging supervision and interpretation　　　　　　　M ♀
Code also surgical procedure (36460, 59012)
🔲 0.00 　 0.00 　**FUD** XXX 　　　N N1 80 📺
**AMA:** 2012,Feb,9-10

**76942** Ultrasonic guidance for needle placement (eg, biopsy, aspiration, injection, localization device), imaging supervision and interpretation

　EXCLUDES　*Arthrocentesis (20604, 20606, 20611)*
　　　*Breast biopsy with placement of localization device(s) (19083)*
　　　*Esophagogastroduodenoscopy (43237, 43242)*
　　　*Esophagoscopy (43232)*
　　　*Gastrointestinal endoscopic ultrasound (76975)*
　　　*Image-guided fluid collection drainage by catheter (10030)*
　　　*Injection procedures (27096, 64479-64484, 0228T-0229T, 0231T-0232T)*
　　　*Ligation (37760-37761, 0249T)*
　　　*Paravertebral facet joint injections (64490-64491, 64493-64494, 0213T-0218T)*
　　　*Placement of breast localization device(s) (19285)*
　　　*Sigmoidoscopy (45341-45342)*
　　　*Thoracentesis (32554-32557)*
🔲 1.71 　 1.71 　**FUD** XXX 　　　N N1 80 📺
**AMA:** 2017,Sep,6; 2017,Jun,10; 2017,Jan,8; 2016,Nov,3; 2016,Jun,3; 2016,Jan,9; 2016,Jan,13; 2015,Dec,3; 2015,Nov,10; 2015,Aug,8; 2015,Feb,6; 2015,Jan,16; 2014,Oct,6; 2014,Jan,11; 2013,Dec,3; 2013,Nov,9; 2012,Dec,9-10; 2012,Nov,3-5; 2012,Feb,9-10; 2012,Jan,15-42

**76945** Ultrasonic guidance for chorionic villus sampling, imaging supervision and interpretation　　　　　M ♀
Code also surgical procedure (59015)
🔲 0.00 　 0.00 　**FUD** XXX 　　　N N1 80 📺
**AMA:** 2012,Feb,9-10

**76946** Ultrasonic guidance for amniocentesis, imaging supervision and interpretation　　　　　　　　M ♀
🔲 0.93 　 0.93 　**FUD** XXX 　　　N N1 80 📺
**AMA:** 2012,Feb,9-10

**76948** Ultrasonic guidance for aspiration of ova, imaging supervision and interpretation　　　　　　　M ♀
🔲 2.03 　 2.03 　**FUD** XXX 　　　N N1 80 📺
**AMA:** 2012,Feb,9-10

**76965** Ultrasonic guidance for interstitial radioelement application
🔲 2.58 　 2.58 　**FUD** XXX 　　　N N1 80 📺
**AMA:** 2012,Feb,9-10

**76970** Ultrasound study follow-up (specify)
🔲 2.62 　 2.62 　**FUD** XXX 　　　Q1 N1 80 📺
**AMA:** 2012,Feb,9-10

## 76975 Endoscopic Ultrasound

**CMS:** 100-04,12,30.1 Upper Gastrointestinal Endoscopy Including Endoscopic Ultrasound (EUS)
　INCLUDES　Required permanent documentation of ultrasound images except when diagnostic purpose is biometric measurement
　　　Written documentation
　EXCLUDES　*Focused ultrasound ablation of uterine leiomyomata (0071T-0072T)*
　　　*Ultrasound exam that does not include thorough assessment of organ or site, recorded image, and written report*

**76975** Gastrointestinal endoscopic ultrasound, supervision and interpretation
　INCLUDES　Ultrasonic guidance (76942)
　EXCLUDES　*Colonoscopy (44406-44407, 45391-45392)*
　　　*Esophagogastroduodenoscopy (43237-43238, 43240, 43242, 43259)*
　　　*Esophagoscopy (43231-43232)*
　　　*Sigmoidoscopy (45341-45342)*
🔲 0.00 　 0.00 　**FUD** XXX 　　　Q2 N1 80 📺
**AMA:** 2017,Jan,8; 2016,Jan,13; 2015,Jan,16; 2014,Jan,11; 2013,Dec,3; 2012,Feb,9-10

## 76977 Bone Density Measurements: Ultrasound

**CMS:** 100-02,15,80.5.5 Frequency Standards
　INCLUDES　Required permanent documentation of ultrasound images except when diagnostic purpose is biometric measurement
　　　Written documentation
　EXCLUDES　*Ultrasound exam that does not include thorough assessment of organ or site, recorded image, and written report*

**76977** Ultrasound bone density measurement and interpretation, peripheral site(s), any method
🔲 0.21 　 0.21 　**FUD** XXX 　　　S Z3 80 📺
**AMA:** 2012,Feb,9-10

## 76998-76999 Imaging Guidance During Surgery: Ultrasound

　INCLUDES　Required permanent documentation of ultrasound images except when diagnostic purpose is biometric measurement
　　　Written documentation
　EXCLUDES　*Focused ultrasound ablation of uterine leiomyomata (0071T-0072T)*
　　　*Ultrasound exam that does not include thorough assessment of organ or site, recorded image, and written report*

**76998** Ultrasonic guidance, intraoperative
　EXCLUDES　*Ablation (47370-47371, 47380-47382, 76940)*
　　　*Endovenous ablation therapy of incompetent vein (36475, 36479)*
　　　*Ligation (37760-37761, 0249T)*
🔲 0.00 　 0.00 　**FUD** XXX 　　　N N1 80 📺
**AMA:** 2017,Apr,7; 2017,Jan,8; 2016,Nov,3; 2016,Jan,13; 2015,Aug,8; 2015,Jan,16; 2014,Oct,6; 2014,Jan,11; 2014,Jan,5; 2013,Jan,6-8; 2012,Feb,9-10

Radiology

76932 — 76998

**76999** Unlisted ultrasound procedure (eg, diagnostic, interventional)

🚑 0.00 ⚕ 0.00 **FUD** XXX [Q1] [N1] [80]

**AMA:** 2017,Jan,8; 2016,Jan,13; 2015,Jan,16; 2014,Jan,11; 2012,Feb,9-10

## 77001-77022 Imaging Guidance Techniques

+ **77001** Fluoroscopic guidance for central venous access device placement, replacement (catheter only or complete), or removal (includes fluoroscopic guidance for vascular access and catheter manipulation, any necessary contrast injections through access site or catheter with related venography radiologic supervision and interpretation, and radiographic documentation of final catheter position) (List separately in addition to code for primary procedure)

INCLUDES   Fluoroscopic guidance for needle placement (77002)

EXCLUDES   Any procedure codes that include fluoroscopic guidance in the code descriptor

Extracorporeal membrane oxygenation (ECMO)/extracorporeal life support (ECLS) (33957-33959, [33962, 33963, 33964])

Formal extremity venography performed separately from venous access and interpreted separately (36005, 75820, 75822, 75825, 75827)

Code first primary procedure

🚑 2.38 ⚕ 2.38 **FUD** ZZZ [N] [N1] [80] 🖥

**AMA:** 2017,Jan,8; 2016,Jan,13; 2015,Jan,16; 2014,Jan,11; 2012,Feb,9-10; 2012,Jan,15-42

+ **77002** Fluoroscopic guidance for needle placement (eg, biopsy, aspiration, injection, localization device) (List separately in addition to code for primary procedure)

EXCLUDES   Ablation therapy (20982-20983)

Any procedure codes that include fluoroscopic guidance in the code descriptor:

Corpora cavernosography (74445)

Insertion of gastrostomy tube (49440)

Placement of enteroclysis tube (74355)

Radiological guidance for percutaneous drainage by catheter (75989)

Renal cyst study (74470)

Shuntogram (75809-75810)

Transhepatic portography (75885, 75887)

Arthrography procedure(s) (70332, 73040, 73085, 73115, 73525, 73580, 73615)

Biopsy, breast, with placement of breast localization device(s) (19081-19086)

Image-guided fluid collection drainage by catheter (10030)

Placement of breast localization device(s) (19281-19288)

Platelet rich plasma injection(s) (0232T)

Thoracentesis (32554-32557)

Code first surgical procedure (10022, 10160, 20206, 20220, 20225, 20525-20526, 20550-20555, 20600, 20605, 20610, 20612, 20615, 21116, 21550, 23350, 24220, 25246, 27093-27095, 27370, 27648, 32400-32405, 32553, 36002, 38220-38221, 38505, 38794, 41019, 42400-42405, 47000-47001, 48102, 49180, 49411, 50200, 50390, 51100-51102, 55700, 55876, 60100, 62268-62269, 64505-64508, 64600-64605)

🚑 2.63 ⚕ 2.63 **FUD** ZZZ [N] [N1] [80] 🖥

**AMA:** 2017,Jun,10; 2017,Jan,8; 2016,Sep,9; 2016,Aug,7; 2016,Jun,3; 2016,Jan,13; 2016,Jan,9; 2015,Dec,3; 2015,Aug,6; 2015,Jul,8; 2015,Feb,6; 2015,Feb,10; 2015,Jan,16; 2014,Jan,11; 2013,Nov,9; 2012,Dec,9-10; 2012,Nov,3-5; 2012,Jun,14; 2012,Feb,11; 2012,Feb,9-10; 2012,Apr,19; 2012,Jan,15-42

+ **77003** Fluoroscopic guidance and localization of needle or catheter tip for spine or paraspinous diagnostic or therapeutic injection procedures (epidural or subarachnoid) (List separately in addition to code for primary procedure)

EXCLUDES   Any procedure codes that include fluoroscopic guidance in the code descriptor

Arthrodesis (22586, 0195T-0196T)

Image-guided fluid collection drainage by catheter (10030)

Injection of medication (subarachnoid/interlaminar epidural) (62320-62327)

Code first primary procedure (61050-61055, 62267, 62270-62273, 62280-62284, 64510, 64517, 64520, 64610, 96450)

🚑 2.66 ⚕ 2.66 **FUD** ZZZ [N] [N1] [80] 🖥

**AMA:** 2017,Sep,6; 2017,Feb,12; 2017,Feb,9; 2017,Jan,8; 2016,Jan,11; 2016,Jan,9; 2016,Jan,13; 2015,Jan,16; 2014,Jan,11; 2013,Nov,9; 2013,Dec,14; 2012,Sep,14-15; 2012,Sep,14-15; 2012,Jul,3-6; 2012,Jun,12-13; 2012,Feb,9-10; 2012,Jan,15-42

**77011** Computed tomography guidance for stereotactic localization

EXCLUDES   Arthrodesis (22586, 0195T-0196T)

🚑 6.33 ⚕ 6.33 **FUD** XXX [N] [N1] 🖥

**AMA:** 2017,Jan,8; 2016,Jan,13; 2015,Jan,16; 2014,Jan,11; 2012,Feb,9-10

**77012** Computed tomography guidance for needle placement (eg, biopsy, aspiration, injection, localization device), radiological supervision and interpretation

EXCLUDES   Arthrodesis (22586, 0195T-0196T)

Autologous white blood cell concentrate (0481T)

Destruction of paravertebral facet joint nerve by neurolysis ([64633, 64634, 64635, 64636])

Image-guided fluid collection drainage by catheter (10030)

Injection, paravertebral facet joint (64490-64495)

Platelet rich plasma injection(s) (0232T)

Sacroiliac joint arthrography (27096)

Thoracentesis (32554-32557)

Transforaminal epidural needle placement/injection (64479-64480, 64483-64484)

🚑 3.51 ⚕ 3.51 **FUD** XXX [N] [N1] 🖥

**AMA:** 2017,Sep,6; 2017,Feb,12; 2017,Jan,8; 2016,Jun,3; 2016,Jan,13; 2015,Dec,3; 2015,Feb,6; 2015,Jan,16; 2014,Jan,11; 2013,Nov,9; 2012,Dec,9-10; 2012,Nov,3-5; 2012,Sep,14-15; 2012,Sep,14-15; 2012,Jul,3-6; 2012,Feb,9-10; 2012,Jan,15-42

**77013** Computed tomography guidance for, and monitoring of, parenchymal tissue ablation

EXCLUDES   Ablation therapy (20982-20983, 32994, 32998, 47382-47383, 50592-50593)

🚑 0.00 ⚕ 0.00 **FUD** XXX [N] [N1] [80] 🖥

**AMA:** 2017,Jan,8; 2016,Jan,13; 2015,Jul,8; 2015,Jan,16; 2014,Jan,11; 2012,Feb,9-10

**77014** Computed tomography guidance for placement of radiation therapy fields

Code also placement of interstitial device(s) for radiation therapy guidance (31627, 32553, 49411, 55876)

🚑 3.35 ⚕ 3.35 **FUD** XXX [N] [N1] 🖥

**AMA:** 2017,Jan,8; 2016,Feb,3; 2016,Jan,13; 2015,Apr,10; 2015,Jan,16; 2014,Jan,11; 2012,Feb,9-10

● New Code   ▲ Revised Code   ○ Reinstated   ● New Web Release   ▲ Revised Web Release   Unlisted   Not Covered   # Resequenced
⊘ AMA Mod 51 Exempt   ⑤ Optum Mod 51 Exempt   ⑥³ Mod 63 Exempt   ✗ Non-FDA Drug   ★ Telemedicine   Ⓜ Maternity   Ⓐ Age Edit   + Add-on   AMA: CPT Asst
© 2017 Optum360, LLC   CPT © 2017 American Medical Association. All Rights Reserved.   339

**77021** **Magnetic resonance guidance for needle placement (eg, for biopsy, needle aspiration, injection, or placement of localization device) radiological supervision and interpretation**

> *EXCLUDES* Autologous white blood cell concentrate (0481T)
> Biopsy, breast, with placement of breast localization device(s) (19085)
> Image-guided fluid collection drainage by catheter (10030)
> Placement of breast localization device(s) (19287)
> Platelet rich plasma injection(s) (0232T)
> Surgical procedure
> Thoracentesis (32554-32557)

🚗 11.3   🔧 11.3   **FUD** XXX                          [N] [N1] [🖵]

**AMA:** 2017,Jun,10; 2017,Jan,8; 2016,Jun,3; 2016,Jan,13; 2015,Dec,3; 2015,Feb,6; 2015,Jan,16; 2014,Jan,11; 2013,Nov,9; 2012,Dec,9-10; 2012,Nov,3-5; 2012,Feb,9-10

**77022** **Magnetic resonance guidance for, and monitoring of, parenchymal tissue ablation**

> *EXCLUDES* Ablation:
> Percutaneous radiofrequency (32994, 32998, 47382-47383, 50592-50593)
> Reduction or eradication of 1 or more bone tumors (20982-20983)
> Uterine leiomyomata by focused ablation (0071T-0072T)

🚗 0.00   🔧 0.00   **FUD** XXX                          [N] [N1] [80] [🖵]

**AMA:** 2017,Jan,8; 2016,Nov,3; 2016,Jan,13; 2015,Jul,8; 2015,Jan,16; 2014,Oct,6; 2014,Jan,11; 2012,Feb,9-10

## 77053-77067 Radiography: Breast

**77053** **Mammary ductogram or galactogram, single duct, radiological supervision and interpretation**

> Code also injection procedure (19030)

🚗 1.66   🔧 1.66   **FUD** XXX                          [02] [N1] [🖵]

**AMA:** 2017,Jan,8; 2016,Jan,13; 2015,Jan,16; 2014,Jan,11; 2012,Feb,9-10

**77054** **Mammary ductogram or galactogram, multiple ducts, radiological supervision and interpretation**

🚗 2.19   🔧 2.19   **FUD** XXX                          [02] [N1] [🖵]

**AMA:** 2017,Jan,8; 2016,Jan,13; 2015,Jan,16; 2014,Jan,11; 2012,Feb,9-10

**77058** **Magnetic resonance imaging, breast, without and/or with contrast material(s); unilateral**

🚗 15.2   🔧 15.2   **FUD** XXX                          [B] [🖵]

**AMA:** 2017,Jan,8; 2016,Jan,13; 2015,Jan,16; 2014,Jan,11; 2012,Feb,9-10

**77059** **bilateral**

🚗 15.1   🔧 15.1   **FUD** XXX                          [B] [🖵]

**AMA:** 2017,Jan,8; 2016,Jan,13; 2015,Jan,16; 2014,Jan,11; 2012,Feb,9-10

**77061** **Digital breast tomosynthesis; unilateral**

🚗 0.00   🔧 0.00   **FUD** XXX                          [E] [🖵]

> *EXCLUDES* 3D rendering (76376-76377)
> Screening mammography (77067)

**77062** **bilateral**

> *EXCLUDES* 3D rendering (76376-76377)
> Screening mammography (77067)

🚗 0.00   🔧 0.00   **FUD** XXX                          [E] [🖵]

**AMA:** 2017,Jan,8; 2016,Dec,15

**+ 77063** **Screening digital breast tomosynthesis, bilateral (List separately in addition to code for primary procedure)**

> *EXCLUDES* 3D rendering (76376-76377)
> Diagnostic mammography (77065-77066)

> Code first (77067)

🚗 1.57   🔧 1.57   **FUD** ZZZ                          [A] [🖵]

**AMA:** 2017,Jan,8; 2016,Dec,15

**77065** **Diagnostic mammography, including computer-aided detection (CAD) when performed; unilateral**

🚗 3.76   🔧 3.76   **FUD** XXX                          [B] [🖵]

**AMA:** 2017,Jan,8; 2016,Dec,15

**77066** **bilateral**

🚗 4.77   🔧 4.77   **FUD** XXX                          [B] [🖵]

**AMA:** 2017,Jan,8; 2016,Dec,15

**77067** **Screening mammography, bilateral (2-view study of each breast), including computer-aided detection (CAD) when performed**

> *EXCLUDES* Breast scan, electrical impedance (76499)

🚗 3.85   🔧 3.85   **FUD** XXX                          [B] [🖵]

**AMA:** 2017,Jan,8; 2016,Dec,15

## 77071-77086 [77085, 77086] Additional Evaluations of Bones and Joints

**77071** **Manual application of stress performed by physician or other qualified health care professional for joint radiography, including contralateral joint if indicated**

> Code also interpretation of stressed images according to anatomical site and number of views

🚗 1.37   🔧 1.37   **FUD** XXX                  [01] [N1] [80] [26] [🖵]

**AMA:** 2017,Jan,8; 2016,Jan,13; 2015,Jan,16; 2014,Jan,11; 2012,Feb,9-10

**77072** **Bone age studies**

🚗 0.65   🔧 0.65   **FUD** XXX                  [01] [N1] [80] [🖵]

**AMA:** 2017,Jan,8; 2016,Jan,13; 2015,Jan,16; 2014,Jan,11; 2012,Feb,9-10

**77073** **Bone length studies (orthoroentgenogram, scanogram)**

🚗 1.01   🔧 1.01   **FUD** XXX                  [01] [N1] [80] [🖵]

**AMA:** 2017,Jan,8; 2016,Jan,13; 2015,Jan,16; 2014,Jan,11; 2012,Feb,9-10

**77074** **Radiologic examination, osseous survey; limited (eg, for metastases)**

🚗 1.82   🔧 1.82   **FUD** XXX                  [01] [N1] [80] [🖵]

**AMA:** 2017,Jan,8; 2016,Jan,13; 2015,Jan,16; 2014,Jan,11; 2012,Feb,9-10

**77075** **complete (axial and appendicular skeleton)**

🚗 2.46   🔧 2.46   **FUD** XXX                  [01] [N1] [80] [🖵]

**AMA:** 2017,Jan,8; 2016,Jan,13; 2015,Jan,16; 2014,Jan,11; 2012,Feb,9-10

**77076** **Radiologic examination, osseous survey, infant**

🚗 2.73   🔧 2.73   **FUD** XXX                  [01] [N1] [80] [🖵]

**AMA:** 2017,Jan,8; 2016,Jan,13; 2015,Jan,16; 2014,Jan,11; 2012,Feb,9-10

**77077** **Joint survey, single view, 2 or more joints (specify)**

🚗 1.05   🔧 1.05   **FUD** XXX                  [01] [N1] [80] [🖵]

**AMA:** 2017,Jan,8; 2016,Jan,13; 2015,Jan,16; 2014,Jan,11; 2012,Feb,9-10

**77078** **Computed tomography, bone mineral density study, 1 or more sites, axial skeleton (eg, hips, pelvis, spine)**

🚗 3.23   🔧 3.23   **FUD** XXX                  [S] [Z2] [80] [🖵]

**AMA:** 2017,Jan,8; 2016,Jan,13; 2015,Jan,16; 2014,Jan,11; 2012,Feb,9-10

**77080** **Dual-energy X-ray absorptiometry (DXA), bone density study, 1 or more sites; axial skeleton (eg, hips, pelvis, spine)**

> *EXCLUDES* Dual-energy x-ray absorptiometry (DXA), bone density study ([77085])
> Vertebral fracture assessment via dual-energy x-ray absorptiometry (DXA) ([77086])

🚗 1.16   🔧 1.16   **FUD** XXX                  [S] [Z3] [80] [🖵]

**AMA:** 2017,Jan,8; 2016,Jan,13; 2015,Jan,16; 2014,Jan,11; 2012,Feb,9-10

**77081** **appendicular skeleton (peripheral) (eg, radius, wrist, heel)**

🚗 0.79   🔧 0.79   **FUD** XXX                  [S] [Z3] [80] [🖵]

**AMA:** 2017,Jan,8; 2016,Jan,13; 2015,Jan,16; 2014,Jan,11; 2012,Feb,9-10

| 26/TC PC/TC Only | A2-Z3 ASC Payment | 50 Bilateral | ♂ Male Only | ♀ Female Only | 🚗 Facility RVU | 🔧 Non-Facility RVU | 🖵 CCI |
| FUD Follow-up Days | CMS: IOM (Pub 100) | A-Y OPPSI | 80/80 Surg Assist Allowed / w/Doc | | 🔬 Lab Crosswalk | 📷 Radiology Crosswalk | ✖ CLIA |

**340**
CPT © 2017 American Medical Association. All Rights Reserved.                    © 2017 Optum360, LLC

Radiology

77021 — 77081

# 77085 axial skeleton (eg, hips, pelvis, spine), including vertebral fracture assessment

\# 77085

📖 1.58   ⚕ 1.58   **FUD** XXX   [01] [N1] [80] 🖵

**EXCLUDES** *Dual-energy x-ray absorptiometry (DXA), bone density study (77080)*
*Vertebral fracture assessment via dual-energy x-ray absorptiometry (DXA) ([77086])*

\# 77086 **Vertebral fracture assessment via dual-energy X-ray absorptiometry (DXA)**

📖 1.00   ⚕ 1.00   **FUD** XXX   [01] [N1] [80] 🖵

**EXCLUDES** *Dual-energy x-ray absorptiometry (DXA), bone density study (77080)*
*Therapy performed more than one time for treatment to a specific area*
*Vertebral fracture assessment via dual-energy X-ray absorptiometry (DXA) ([77085])*

77084 **Magnetic resonance (eg, proton) imaging, bone marrow blood supply**

📖 11.0   ⚕ 11.0   **FUD** XXX   [S] [Z2] [80] 🖵

**AMA:** 2017,Jan,8; 2016,Jan,13; 2015,Jan,16; 2014,Jan,11; 2012,Feb,9-10

77085 **Resequenced code. See code following 77081.**

77086 **Resequenced code. See code before 77084.**

## 77261-77263 Therapeutic Radiology: Treatment Planning

**INCLUDES** Determination of:
Appropriate treatment devices
Number and size of treatment ports
Treatment method
Treatment time/dosage
Treatment volume
Interpretation of special testing
Tumor localization
**EXCLUDES** *Brachytherapy (0394T-0395T)*
*Radiation treatment delivery, superficial (77401)*

77261 **Therapeutic radiology treatment planning; simple**

**INCLUDES** Planning for single treatment area included in a single port or simple parallel opposed ports with simple or no blocking

📖 2.16   ⚕ 2.16   **FUD** XXX   [B] [80] [26] 🖵

**AMA:** 2017,Jan,8; 2016,Feb,3; 2016,Jan,13; 2015,Jan,16; 2014,Jan,11; 2012,Feb,9-10

77262 **intermediate**

**INCLUDES** Planning for three or more converging ports, two separate treatment sites, multiple blocks, or special time dose constraints

📖 3.21   ⚕ 3.21   **FUD** XXX   [B] [80] [26] 🖵

**AMA:** 2017,Jan,8; 2016,Feb,3; 2016,Jan,13; 2015,Jan,16; 2014,Jan,11; 2012,Feb,9-10

77263 **complex**

**INCLUDES** Planning for very complex blocking, custom shielding blocks, tangential ports, special wedges or compensators, three or more separate treatment areas, rotational or special beam considerations, combination of treatment modalities

📖 4.71   ⚕ 4.71   **FUD** XXX   [B] [80] [26] 🖵

**AMA:** 2017,Jan,8; 2016,Feb,3; 2016,Jan,13; 2015,Jan,16; 2014,Jan,11; 2012,Feb,9-10

## 77280-77299 Radiation Therapy Simulation

77280 **Therapeutic radiology simulation-aided field setting; simple**

**INCLUDES** Simulation of a single treatment site

📖 7.77   ⚕ 7.77   **FUD** XXX   [S] [Z2] [80] 🖵

**AMA:** 2017,Jan,8; 2016,Jan,13; 2015,Apr,10; 2015,Jan,16; 2014,Jan,11; 2013,Nov,11; 2012,Feb,9-10; 2012,Jan,15-42

77285 **intermediate**

**INCLUDES** Two different treatment sites

📖 12.3   ⚕ 12.3   **FUD** XXX   [S] [Z2] [80] 🖵

**AMA:** 2017,Jan,8; 2016,Jan,13; 2015,Apr,10; 2015,Jan,16; 2014,Jan,11; 2013,Nov,11; 2012,Feb,9-10

77290 **complex**

**INCLUDES** Brachytherapy
Complex blocking
Contrast material
Custom shielding blocks
Hyperthermia probe verification
Rotation, arc or particle therapy
Simulation to ≥ 3 treatment sites

📖 14.6   ⚕ 14.6   **FUD** XXX   [S] [Z2] [80] 🖵

**AMA:** 2017,Jan,8; 2016,Sep,9; 2016,Jan,13; 2015,Apr,10; 2015,Jan,16; 2014,Jan,11; 2013,Nov,11; 2012,Feb,9-10; 2012,Jan,15-42

+ 77293 **Respiratory motion management simulation (List separately in addition to code for primary procedure)**

Code first (77295, 77301)

📖 13.2   ⚕ 13.2   **FUD** ZZZ   [N] [N1] [80] 🖵

**AMA:** 2017,Jan,8; 2016,Jan,13; 2015,Dec,16; 2013,Nov,11

77295 **Resequenced code. See code before 77300.**

77299 **Unlisted procedure, therapeutic radiology clinical treatment planning**

📖 0.00   ⚕ 0.00   **FUD** XXX   [S] [Z2] [80] 🖵

**AMA:** 2017,Jan,8; 2016,Jan,13; 2015,Jan,16; 2014,Jan,11; 2013,Nov,11; 2012,Feb,9-10; 2012,Jan,15-42

## 77300-77370 [77295] Radiation Physics Services

**CMS:** 100-04,13,70.5 Radiation Physics Services

\# 77295 **3-dimensional radiotherapy plan, including dose-volume histograms**

📖 13.9   ⚕ 13.9   **FUD** XXX   [S] [Z3] [80] 🖵

**AMA:** 2017,Jan,8; 2016,Jan,13; 2015,Dec,16; 2015,Jun,6; 2015,Jan,16; 2014,Jan,11; 2013,Nov,11; 2012,Feb,9-10

77300 **Basic radiation dosimetry calculation, central axis depth dose calculation, TDF, NSD, gap calculation, off axis factor, tissue inhomogeneity factors, calculation of non-ionizing radiation surface and depth dose, as required during course of treatment, only when prescribed by the treating physician**

**EXCLUDES** *Brachytherapy (77316-77318, 77767-77772, 0394T-0395T)*
*Teletherapy plan (77306-77307, 77321)*

📖 1.89   ⚕ 1.89   **FUD** XXX   [S] [Z3] [80] 🖵

**AMA:** 2017,Jan,8; 2016,Jan,13; 2015,Jan,16; 2014,Jan,11; 2013,Nov,11; 2012,Feb,9-10; 2012,Jan,15-42

77301 **Intensity modulated radiotherapy plan, including dose-volume histograms for target and critical structure partial tolerance specifications**

📖 55.4   ⚕ 55.4   **FUD** XXX   [S] [Z2] [80] 🖵

**AMA:** 2017,Jan,8; 2016,Jan,13; 2015,Jan,16; 2014,Jan,11; 2013,Nov,11; 2012,Feb,9-10; 2012,Jan,15-42

77306 **Teletherapy isodose plan; simple (1 or 2 unmodified ports directed to a single area of interest), includes basic dosimetry calculation(s)**

**EXCLUDES** *Brachytherapy (0394T-0395T)*
*Radiation dosimetry calculation (77300)*
*Radiation treatment delivery (77401)*
*Therapy performed more than one time for treatment to a specific area*

📖 4.24   ⚕ 4.24   **FUD** XXX   [S] [Z3] [80] 🖵

**AMA:** 2017,Jan,8; 2016,Feb,3

77307 **complex (multiple treatment areas, tangential ports, the use of wedges, blocking, rotational beam, or special beam considerations), includes basic dosimetry calculation(s)**

**EXCLUDES** *Brachytherapy (0394T-0395T)*
*Radiation dosimetry calculation (77300)*
*Radiation treatment delivery (77401)*
*Therapy performed more than one time for treatment to a specific area*

📖 8.20   ⚕ 8.20   **FUD** XXX   [S] [Z3] [80] 🖵

**AMA:** 2017,Jan,8; 2016,Feb,3

● New Code   ▲ Revised Code   ○ Reinstated   ● New Web Release   ▲ Revised Web Release   Unlisted   Not Covered   # Resequenced
⊘ AMA Mod 51 Exempt   ⑧ Optum Mod 51 Exempt   ⑥ Mod 63 Exempt   ⁄ Non-FDA Drug   ★ Telemedicine   Ⓜ Maternity   ⒜ Age Edit   + Add-on   **AMA:** CPT Asst
© 2017 Optum360, LLC   CPT © 2017 American Medical Association. All Rights Reserved.   341

**Radiology**

**77316** **Brachytherapy isodose plan; simple (calculation[s] made from 1 to 4 sources, or remote afterloading brachytherapy, 1 channel), includes basic dosimetry calculation(s)**

EXCLUDES Brachytherapy (0394T-0395T)
Radiation dosimetry calculation (77300)
Radiation treatment delivery (77401)

5.35 5.35 **FUD** XXX ⑤ ⦾ ⑧⓪ ▭

**AMA:** 2017,Jan,8; 2016,Feb,3

**77317** **intermediate (calculation[s] made from 5 to 10 sources, or remote afterloading brachytherapy, 2-12 channels), includes basic dosimetry calculation(s)**

EXCLUDES Brachytherapy (0394T-0395T)
Radiation dosimetry calculation (77300)
Radiation treatment delivery (77401)

6.97 6.97 **FUD** XXX ⑤ ⦾ ⑧⓪ ▭

**AMA:** 2017,Jan,8

**77318** **complex (calculation[s] made from over 10 sources, or remote afterloading brachytherapy, over 12 channels), includes basic dosimetry calculation(s)**

EXCLUDES Brachytherapy (0394T-0395T)
Radiation dosimetry calculation (77300)
Radiation treatment delivery (77401)

10.0 10.0 **FUD** XXX ⑤ ⦾ ⑧⓪ ▭

**AMA:** 2017,Jan,8; 2016,Feb,3

**77321** **Special teletherapy port plan, particles, hemibody, total body**

2.64 2.64 **FUD** XXX ⑤ ⦾ ⑧⓪ ▭

**AMA:** 2017,Jan,8; 2016,Jan,13; 2015,Jan,16; 2014,Jan,11; 2013,Nov,11; 2012,Feb,9-10

**77331** **Special dosimetry (eg, TLD, microdosimetry) (specify), only when prescribed by the treating physician**

1.82 1.82 **FUD** XXX ⑤ ⦾ ⑧⓪ ▭

**AMA:** 2017,Jan,8; 2016,Jan,13; 2015,Jun,6; 2015,Jan,16; 2014,Jan,11; 2013,Nov,11; 2012,Feb,9-10

**77332** **Treatment devices, design and construction; simple (simple block, simple bolus)**

EXCLUDES Brachytherapy (0394T-0395T)
Radiation treatment delivery (77401)

1.91 1.91 **FUD** XXX ⑤ ⦾ ⑧⓪ ▭

**AMA:** 2017,Jan,8; 2016,Feb,3; 2016,Jan,13; 2015,Jan,16; 2014,Jan,11; 2013,Nov,11; 2012,Feb,9-10; 2012,Jan,15-42

**77333** **intermediate (multiple blocks, stents, bite blocks, special bolus)**

EXCLUDES Brachytherapy (0394T-0395T)
Radiation treatment delivery (77401)

2.74 2.74 **FUD** XXX ⑤ ⦾ ⑧⓪ ▭

**AMA:** 2017,Jan,8; 2016,Feb,3; 2016,Jan,13; 2015,Jan,16; 2014,Jan,11; 2013,Nov,11; 2012,Feb,9-10

**77334** **complex (irregular blocks, special shields, compensators, wedges, molds or casts)**

EXCLUDES Brachytherapy (0394T-0395T)
Radiation treatment delivery (77401)

3.71 3.71 **FUD** XXX ⑤ ⦾ ⑧⓪ ▭

**AMA:** 2017,Jan,8; 2016,Sep,9; 2016,Feb,3; 2016,Jan,13; 2015,Dec,16; 2015,Jan,16; 2014,Jan,11; 2013,Nov,11; 2012,Feb,9-10; 2012,Jan,15-42

**77336** **Continuing medical physics consultation, including assessment of treatment parameters, quality assurance of dose delivery, and review of patient treatment documentation in support of the radiation oncologist, reported per week of therapy**

EXCLUDES Brachytherapy (0394T-0395T)
Radiation treatment delivery (77401)

2.25 2.25 **FUD** XXX ⑤ ⦾ ⑧⓪ ⓣⓒ ▭

**AMA:** 2017,Jan,8; 2016,Feb,3; 2016,Jan,13; 2015,Jan,16; 2014,Jan,11; 2013,Nov,11; 2012,Feb,9-10

**77338** **Multi-leaf collimator (MLC) device(s) for intensity modulated radiation therapy (IMRT), design and construction per IMRT plan**

EXCLUDES Immobilization in IMRT treatment (77332-77334)
Intensity modulated radiation treatment delivery (IMRT) (77385)
Use of code more than one time per IMRT plan

14.4 14.4 **FUD** XXX ⑤ ⦾ ⑧⓪ ▭

**AMA:** 2017,Jan,8; 2016,Jan,13; 2015,Jan,16; 2014,Jan,11; 2013,Nov,11; 2012,Feb,9-10; 2012,Jan,15-42

**77370** **Special medical radiation physics consultation**

3.46 3.46 **FUD** XXX ⑤ ⦾ ⑧⓪ ⓣⓒ ▭

**AMA:** 2017,Jan,8; 2016,Feb,3; 2016,Jan,13; 2015,Jun,6; 2015,Jan,16; 2014,Jan,11; 2013,Nov,11; 2012,Feb,9-10; 2012,Jan,15-42

## 77371-77399 Stereotactic Radiosurgery (SRS) Planning and Delivery

**CMS:** 100-04,13,70.5 Radiation Physics Services

**77371** **Radiation treatment delivery, stereotactic radiosurgery (SRS), complete course of treatment of cranial lesion(s) consisting of 1 session; multi-source Cobalt 60 based**

EXCLUDES Guidance with computed tomography for radiation therapy field placement (77014)

0.00 0.00 **FUD** XXX ⓙ ⑧⓪ ⓣⓒ ▭

**AMA:** 2017,Jan,8; 2016,Jan,13; 2015,Jan,16; 2014,Jul,8; 2014,Jan,11; 2012,Feb,9-10

**77372** **linear accelerator based**

EXCLUDES Guidance with computed tomography for radiation therapy field placement (77014)
Radiation treatment supervision (77432)

30.4 30.4 **FUD** XXX ⓙ ⑧⓪ ⓣⓒ ▭

**AMA:** 2017,Jan,8; 2016,Jan,13; 2015,Jan,16; 2014,Jul,8; 2014,Jan,11; 2012,Feb,9-10

**77373** **Stereotactic body radiation therapy, treatment delivery, per fraction to 1 or more lesions, including image guidance, entire course not to exceed 5 fractions**

EXCLUDES Guidance with computed tomography for radiation therapy field placement (77014)
Intensity modulated radiation treatment delivery (IMRT) (77385-77386)
Radiation treatment delivery (77401-77402, 77407, 77412)
Single fraction cranial lesion(s) (77371-77372)

38.6 38.6 **FUD** XXX ⑤ ⑧⓪ ⓣⓒ ▭

**AMA:** 2017,Jan,8; 2016,Jan,13; 2015,Jun,6; 2015,Jan,16; 2014,Jul,8; 2014,Jan,11; 2012,Feb,9-10

**77385** **Resequenced code. See code following 77417.**

**77386** **Resequenced code. See code following 77417.**

**77387** **Resequenced code. See code following 77417.**

**77399** **Unlisted procedure, medical radiation physics, dosimetry and treatment devices, and special services**

0.00 0.00 **FUD** XXX ⑤ ⦾ ⑧⓪ ▭

**AMA:** 2017,Jan,8; 2016,Jan,13; 2015,Jan,16; 2014,Jan,11; 2012,Feb,9-10

## 77401-77417 [77385, 77386, 77387, 77424, 77425] Radiation Treatment

INCLUDES Technical component and assorted energy levels

**77401** **Radiation treatment delivery, superficial and/or ortho voltage, per day**

EXCLUDES Continuing medical physics consultation (77336)
Isodose plan:
Brachytherapy (77316-77318)
Teletherapy (77306-77307)
Management of:
Intraoperative radiation treatment (77469-77470)
Radiation therapy (77431-77432)
Radiation treatment (77427)
Stereotactic body radiation therapy (77435)
Stereotactic body radiation therapy, treatment delivery (77373)
Unlisted procedure, therapeutic radiology treatment management (77499)
Therapeutic radiology treatment planning (77261-77263)
Treatment devices, design and construction (77332-77334)
Code also E&M services when performed alone, as appropriate
🔧 0.70 ⚖ 0.70 **FUD** XXX [S][Z3][80][TC][▯]
**AMA:** 2017,Jan,8; 2016,Feb,3; 2016,Jan,13; 2015,Dec,14; 2015,Jan,16; 2014,Jan,11; 2012,Feb,9-10

**77402** **Radiation treatment delivery, ≥1 MeV; simple1 MeV; simple**

EXCLUDES Stereotactic body radiation therapy, treatment delivery (77373)
🔧 0.00 ⚖ 0.00 **FUD** XXX [S][Z2][80][TC][▯]
**AMA:** 2017,Jan,8; 2016,Jun,9; 2016,Mar,7; 2016,Feb,3; 2016,Jan,13; 2015,Dec,14; 2015,Jan,16; 2014,Jan,11; 2012,Feb,9-10

**77407** **intermediate**

EXCLUDES Stereotactic body radiation therapy, treatment delivery (77373)
🔧 0.00 ⚖ 0.00 **FUD** XXX [S][Z2][80][TC][▯]
**AMA:** 2017,Jan,8; 2016,Jun,9; 2016,Mar,7; 2016,Feb,3; 2016,Jan,13; 2015,Dec,14; 2015,Jan,16; 2014,Jan,11; 2012,Feb,9-10

**77412** **complex**

EXCLUDES Stereotactic body radiation therapy, treatment delivery (77373)
🔧 0.00 ⚖ 0.00 **FUD** XXX [S][Z2][80][TC][▯]
**AMA:** 2017,Jan,8; 2016,Jun,9; 2016,Mar,7; 2016,Feb,3; 2016,Jan,13; 2015,Dec,14; 2015,Jan,16; 2014,Jan,11; 2012,Feb,9-10

**77417** **Therapeutic radiology port image(s)**

EXCLUDES Intensity modulated treatment planning (77301)
🔧 0.31 ⚖ 0.31 **FUD** XXX [N][N1][80][TC][▯]
**AMA:** 2017,Jan,8; 2016,Jan,13; 2015,Dec,14; 2015,Jan,16; 2014,Jan,11; 2012,Feb,9-10; 2012,Jan,15-42

\# **77385** **Intensity modulated radiation treatment delivery (IMRT), includes guidance and tracking, when performed; simple**

EXCLUDES Radiation treatment delivery, stereotactic radiosurgery (SRS) (77371-77373)
Code also modifier 26 for professional component tracking and guidance with (77387)
🔧 0.00 ⚖ 0.00 **FUD** XXX [S][Z2][80][TC]
**AMA:** 2017,Jan,8; 2016,Feb,3

\# **77386** **complex**

EXCLUDES Radiation treatment delivery, stereotactic radiosurgery (SRS) (77371-77373)
Code also modifier 26 for professional component tracking and guidance with (77387)
🔧 0.00 ⚖ 0.00 **FUD** XXX [S][Z2][80][TC]
**AMA:** 2017,Jan,8; 2016,Feb,3

\# **77387** **Guidance for localization of target volume for delivery of radiation treatment delivery, includes intrafraction tracking, when performed**

EXCLUDES Guidance with computed tomography for radiation therapy field placement (77014)
Intensity modulated radiation treatment delivery (IMRT) (77385)
Radiation treatment delivery, stereotactic radiosurgery (SRS) (77371-77373)
🔧 0.00 ⚖ 0.00 **FUD** XXX [N][N1][80]
**AMA:** 2017,Jan,8; 2016,Feb,3; 2016,Jan,13; 2015,Dec,16; 2015,Dec,14

\# **77424** **Intraoperative radiation treatment delivery, x-ray, single treatment session**

🔧 0.00 ⚖ 0.00 **FUD** XXX [J][Z2][▯]
**AMA:** 2017,Jan,8; 2016,Jan,13; 2015,Dec,14; 2012,Feb,9-10

\# **77425** **Intraoperative radiation treatment delivery, electrons, single treatment session**

🔧 0.00 ⚖ 0.00 **FUD** XXX [J][Z2][▯]
**AMA:** 2017,Jan,8; 2016,Jan,13; 2015,Dec,14; 2015,Jan,16; 2014,Jan,11; 2012,Feb,9-10

## 77422-77425 Neutron Therapy

**77422** ~~High energy neutron radiation treatment delivery; single treatment area using a single port or parallel-opposed ports with no blocks or simple blocking~~

**77423** **High energy neutron radiation treatment delivery, 1 or more isocenter(s) with coplanar or non-coplanar geometry with blocking and/or wedge, and/or compensator(s)**

🔧 0.00 ⚖ 0.00 **FUD** XXX [S][Z3][80][TC][▯]
**AMA:** 2017,Jan,8; 2016,Jan,13; 2015,Dec,14; 2015,Jan,16; 2014,Jan,11; 2012,Feb,9-10

**77424** Resequenced code. See code following 77417.

**77425** Resequenced code. See code following 77417.

## 77427-77499 Radiation Therapy Management

INCLUDES Assessment of patient for medical evaluation and management (at least one per treatment management service) that includes:
Coordination of care/treatment
Evaluation of patient's response to treatment
Review of:
Dose delivery
Dosimetry
Lab tests
Patient treatment set-up
Port film
Treatment parameters
X-rays
Units of five fractions or treatment sessions regardless of time. Two or more fractions performed on the same day can be counted separately provided there is a distinct break in service between sessions and the fractions are of the character usually furnished on different days.
EXCLUDES High dose rate electronic brachytherapy (0394T-0395T)
Radiation treatment delivery (77401)

**77427** **Radiation treatment management, 5 treatments**

INCLUDES 3 or 4 fractions beyond a multiple of five at the end of a treatment period
EXCLUDES Use of code separately when one or two more fractions are provided beyond a multiple of five at the end of a course of treatment
🔧 5.27 ⚖ 5.27 **FUD** XXX [B][26][▯]
**AMA:** 2017,Jan,8; 2016,Feb,3; 2016,Jan,13; 2015,Jun,6; 2015,Jan,16; 2014,Jan,11; 2012,Feb,9-10

**77431** **Radiation therapy management with complete course of therapy consisting of 1 or 2 fractions only**

EXCLUDES Use of code when used to fill in the last week of a protracted therapy course
🔧 2.90 ⚖ 2.90 **FUD** XXX [B][80][26][▯]
**AMA:** 2017,Jan,8; 2016,Feb,3; 2016,Jan,13; 2015,Jun,6; 2015,Jan,16; 2014,Jan,11; 2012,Feb,9-10

● New Code  ▲ Revised Code  ○ Reinstated  ● New Web Release  ▲ Revised Web Release  Unlisted  Not Covered  # Resequenced
⊗ AMA Mod 51 Exempt  ⑤ Optum Mod 51 Exempt  ⑥³ Mod 63 Exempt  ✗ Non-FDA Drug  ★ Telemedicine  Ⓜ Maternity  Ⓐ Age Edit  + Add-on  AMA: CPT Asst
© 2017 Optum360, LLC  CPT © 2017 American Medical Association. All Rights Reserved.  343

**Radiology** *(side tab)*

**77432 — 77761** *(side tab)*

**77432**   **Stereotactic radiation treatment management of cranial lesion(s) (complete course of treatment consisting of 1 session)**

> INCLUDES   Guidance for localization of target volume for radiation delivery (professional component)
>
> EXCLUDES   *Stereotactic body radiation therapy treatment (77432, 77435)*
>
>   *Stereotactic radiosurgery by same physician (61796-61800)*
>
> Code also technical component of guidance for localization of target volume by appending modifier TC to (77387)

  🔧 11.8   ✂ 11.8   **FUD** XXX   [B] [80] [26] ▢

**AMA:** 2017,Jan,8; 2016,Feb,3; 2016,Jan,13; 2015,Dec,14; 2015,Dec,16; 2015,Jun,6; 2015,Jan,16; 2014,Jul,8; 2014,Jan,11; 2012,Feb,9-10; 2012,Jan,15-42

**77435**   **Stereotactic body radiation therapy, treatment management, per treatment course, to 1 or more lesions, including image guidance, entire course not to exceed 5 fractions**

> INCLUDES   Guidance for localization of target volume for radiation delivery (professional component)
>
> EXCLUDES   *Radiation treatment management (77435)*
>
>   *Stereotactic radiosurgery by same physician (32701, 63620-63621)*
>
> Code also technical component of guidance for localization of target volume by appending modifier TC to (77387)

  🔧 17.8   ✂ 17.8   **FUD** XXX   [N] [11] [80] [26] ▢

**AMA:** 2017,Jan,8; 2016,Feb,3; 2016,Jan,13; 2015,Dec,14; 2015,Jun,6; 2015,Jan,16; 2014,Jan,11; 2012,Feb,9-10; 2012,Jan,15-42

**77469**   **Intraoperative radiation treatment management**

> EXCLUDES   *Medical E&M services provided outside of the intraoperative treatment management*

  🔧 9.12   ✂ 9.12   **FUD** XXX   [B] [80] ▢

**AMA:** 2017,Jan,8; 2016,Feb,3; 2015,Jun,6; 2012,Feb,9-10

**77470**   **Special treatment procedure (eg, total body irradiation, hemibody radiation, per oral or endocavitary irradiation)**

> EXCLUDES   *Daily or weekly patient management*
>
>   *Intraoperative radiation treatment delivery and management ([77424, 77425], 77469)*
>
>   *Procedure performed more than one time per course of therapy*

  🔧 4.09   ✂ 4.09   **FUD** XXX   [S] [Z3] [80] ▢

**AMA:** 2017,Jan,8; 2016,Feb,3; 2016,Jan,13; 2015,Jun,6; 2015,Jan,16; 2014,Jan,11; 2012,Feb,9-10

**77499**   **Unlisted procedure, therapeutic radiology treatment management**

  🔧 0.00   ✂ 0.00   **FUD** XXX   [B] [80] ▢

**AMA:** 2017,Jan,8; 2016,Feb,3; 2016,Jan,13; 2015,Jun,6; 2015,Jan,16; 2014,Jan,11; 2012,Feb,9-10

## 77520-77525 Proton Therapy

> EXCLUDES   *High dose rate electronic brachytherapy, per fraction (0394T-0395T)*

**77520**   **Proton treatment delivery; simple, without compensation**

> INCLUDES   Single treatment site using:
>
>   Single nontangential/oblique port

  🔧 0.00   ✂ 0.00   **FUD** XXX   [S] [Z2] [80] [TC] ▢

**AMA:** 2017,Jan,8; 2016,Jan,13; 2015,Jan,16; 2014,Jan,11; 2012,Feb,9-10

**77522**   **simple, with compensation**

> INCLUDES   Single treatment site using:
>
>   Custom block with compensation
>
>   Single nontangential/oblique port

  🔧 0.00   ✂ 0.00   **FUD** XXX   [S] [Z2] [80] [TC] ▢

**AMA:** 2012,Feb,9-10

---

**77523**   **intermediate**

> INCLUDES   One or more treatment sites using:
>
>   One or more tangential/oblique ports with custom blocks and compensators OR
>
>   Two or more ports with custom blocks and compensators

  🔧 0.00   ✂ 0.00   **FUD** XXX   [S] [Z2] [80] [TC] ▢

**AMA:** 2017,Jan,8; 2016,Jan,13; 2015,Jan,16; 2014,Jan,11; 2012,Feb,9-10

**77525**   **complex**

> INCLUDES   One or more treatment sites using:
>
>   Two or more ports with matching or patching fields and custom blocks and compensators

  🔧 0.00   ✂ 0.00   **FUD** XXX   [S] [Z2] [80] [TC] ▢

**AMA:** 2012,Feb,9-10

## 77600-77620 Hyperthermia Treatment

**CMS:** 100-03,110.1 Hyperthermia for Treatment of Cancer

> INCLUDES   Interstitial insertion of temperature sensors
>
> Management during the course of therapy
>
> Normal follow-up care for three months after completion
>
> Physics planning
>
> Use of heat generating devices
>
> EXCLUDES   *Initial E&M service*
>
> *Radiation therapy treatment (77371-77373, 77401-77412, 77423)*

**77600**   **Hyperthermia, externally generated; superficial (ie, heating to a depth of 4 cm or less)**

  🔧 11.7   ✂ 11.7   **FUD** XXX   [S] [Z2] [80] ▢

**AMA:** 2017,Jan,8; 2016,Jan,13; 2015,Jan,16; 2014,Jan,11; 2013,Dec,16; 2012,Feb,9-10

**77605**   **deep (ie, heating to depths greater than 4 cm)**

  🔧 22.0   ✂ 22.0   **FUD** XXX   [S] [Z2] [80] ▢

**AMA:** 2017,Jan,8; 2016,Jan,13; 2015,Jan,16; 2014,Jan,11; 2013,Dec,16; 2012,Feb,9-10

**77610**   **Hyperthermia generated by interstitial probe(s); 5 or fewer interstitial applicators**

  🔧 24.3   ✂ 24.3   **FUD** XXX   [S] [Z2] [80] ▢

**AMA:** 2017,Jan,8; 2016,Jan,13; 2015,Jan,16; 2014,Jan,11; 2013,Dec,16; 2012,Feb,9-10

**77615**   **more than 5 interstitial applicators**

  🔧 29.0   ✂ 29.0   **FUD** XXX   [S] [Z2] [80] ▢

**AMA:** 2017,Jan,8; 2016,Jan,13; 2015,Jan,16; 2014,Jan,11; 2013,Dec,16; 2012,Feb,9-10

**77620**   **Hyperthermia generated by intracavitary probe(s)**

  🔧 13.1   ✂ 13.1   **FUD** XXX   [S] [Z2] [80] ▢

**AMA:** 2016,Jan,13; 2015,Jan,16; 2014,Jan,11; 2013,Dec,16; 2012,Feb,9-10

## 77750-77799 Brachytherapy

**CMS:** 100-04,13,70.4 Clinical Brachytherapy; 100-04,4,61.4.4 Billing for Brachytherapy Source Supervision, Handling and Loading Costs

> INCLUDES   Hospital admission and daily visits
>
> EXCLUDES   *Placement of:*
>
>   *Heyman capsules (58346)*
>
>   *Ovoids and tandems (57155)*

**77750**   **Infusion or instillation of radioelement solution (includes 3-month follow-up care)**

> EXCLUDES   *Monoclonal antibody infusion (79403)*
>
>   *Nonantibody radiopharmaceutical therapy infusion without follow-up care (79101)*

  🔧 10.5   ✂ 10.5   **FUD** 090   [S] [Z2] [80] ▢

**AMA:** 2017,Jan,8; 2016,Jan,13; 2015,Jan,16; 2014,Jan,11; 2012,Feb,9-10

**77761**   **Intracavitary radiation source application; simple**

> INCLUDES   One to four sources/ribbons
>
> EXCLUDES   *High dose rate electronic brachytherapy (0394T-0395T)*

  🔧 11.1   ✂ 11.1   **FUD** 090   [S] [Z3] [80] ▢

**AMA:** 2017,Jan,8; 2016,Jan,13; 2015,Jan,16; 2014,Jan,11; 2012,Feb,9-10; 2012,Jan,15-42

---

[26]/[TC] PC/TC Only    [A2]-[Z3] ASC Payment    [50] Bilateral    ♂ Male Only    ♀ Female Only    🔧 Facility RVU    ✂ Non-Facility RVU    ▢ CCI

**FUD** Follow-up Days    **CMS:** IOM (Pub 100)    [A]-[Y] OPPSI    [80]/[80] Surg Assist Allowed / w/Doc    🔲 Lab Crosswalk    ❌ Radiology Crosswalk    ❌ CLIA

**344**                  CPT © 2017 American Medical Association. All Rights Reserved.               © 2017 Optum360, LLC

**77762** **intermediate**

INCLUDES    Five to ten sources/ribbons

EXCLUDES    *High dose rate electronic brachytherapy (0394T-0395T)*

🚗 14.8   👤 14.8   **FUD** 090                    S Z3 80 ▭

AMA: 2017,Jan,8; 2016,Jan,13; 2015,Jan,16; 2014,Jan,11; 2012,Feb,9-10

**77763** **complex**

INCLUDES    More than ten sources/ribbons

EXCLUDES    *High dose rate electronic brachytherapy (0394T-0395T)*

🚗 20.8   👤 20.8   **FUD** 090                    S Z3 80 ▭

AMA: 2017,Jan,8; 2016,Jan,13; 2015,Jan,16; 2014,Jan,11; 2012,Feb,9-10

**77767** **Remote afterloading high dose rate radionuclide skin surface brachytherapy, includes basic dosimetry, when performed; lesion diameter up to 2.0 cm or 1 channel**

🚗 6.38   👤 6.38   **FUD** XXX                    S Z2 80 ▭

EXCLUDES    *Basic radiation dosimetry calculation (77300)*
*High dose rate electronic brachytherapy (0394T-0395T)*
*Superficial non-brachytherapy superficial treatment delivery (77401)*

**77768** **lesion diameter over 2.0 cm and 2 or more channels, or multiple lesions**

🚗 10.0   👤 10.0   **FUD** XXX                    S Z2 80 ▭

EXCLUDES    *Basic radiation dosimetry calculation (77300)*
*High dose rate electronic brachytherapy (0394T-0395T)*
*Superficial non-brachytherapy superficial treatment delivery (77401)*

**77770** **Remote afterloading high dose rate radionuclide interstitial or intracavitary brachytherapy, includes basic dosimetry, when performed; 1 channel**

🚗 9.10   👤 9.10   **FUD** XXX                    S Z3 80 ▭

EXCLUDES    *Basic radiation dosimetry calculation (77300)*
*High dose rate electronic brachytherapy (0394T-0395T)*
*Superficial non-brachytherapy superficial treatment delivery (77401)*

**77771** **2-12 channels**

🚗 16.9   👤 16.9   **FUD** XXX                    S Z2 80 ▭

EXCLUDES    *Basic radiation dosimetry calculation (77300)*
*High dose rate electronic brachytherapy (0394T-0395T)*
*Superficial non-brachytherapy superficial treatment delivery (77401)*

**77772** **over 12 channels**

🚗 25.9   👤 25.9   **FUD** XXX                    S Z2 80 ▭

EXCLUDES    *Basic radiation dosimetry calculation (77300)*
*High dose rate electronic brachytherapy (0394T-0395T)*
*Superficial non-brachytherapy superficial treatment delivery (77401)*

**77778** **Interstitial radiation source application, complex, includes supervision, handling, loading of radiation source, when performed**

INCLUDES    More than ten sources/ribbons

EXCLUDES    *High dose rate electronic brachytherapy (0394T-0395T)*
*Supervision, handling, loading of radiation source (77790)*

🚗 23.3   👤 23.3   **FUD** 000                    Q3 Z3 80 ▭

AMA: 2017,Jan,8; 2016,Jan,13; 2015,Jan,16; 2014,Jan,11; 2012,Feb,9-10

**77789** **Surface application of low dose rate radionuclide source**

EXCLUDES    *High dose rate electronic brachytherapy (0394T-0395T)*
*Radiation treatment delivery, superficial and/or ortho voltage (77401)*
*Remote afterloading high dose rate radionuclide skin surface brachytherapy (77767-77768)*

🚗 3.37   👤 3.37   **FUD** 000                    S Z3 80 ▭

AMA: 2017,Jan,8; 2016,Jan,13; 2015,Jan,16; 2014,Jan,11; 2012,Feb,9-10

**77790** **Supervision, handling, loading of radiation source**

EXCLUDES    *Interstitial radiation source application, complex (77778)*

🚗 0.42   👤 0.42   **FUD** XXX              N N1 80 TC ▭

AMA: 2017,Jan,8; 2016,Jan,13; 2015,Jan,16; 2014,Jan,11; 2012,Feb,9-10

**77799** **Unlisted procedure, clinical brachytherapy**

🚗 0.00   👤 0.00   **FUD** XXX                    S Z2 80

AMA: 2017,Jan,8; 2016,Jan,13; 2015,Jan,16; 2014,Jan,11; 2012,Feb,9-10

## 78012-78099 Nuclear Radiology: Thyroid, Parathyroid, Adrenal

EXCLUDES    *Diagnostic services (see appropriate sections)*
*Follow-up care (see appropriate section)*
Code also radiopharmaceutical(s) and/or drug(s) supplied

**78012** **Thyroid uptake, single or multiple quantitative measurement(s) (including stimulation, suppression, or discharge, when performed)**

🚗 2.35   👤 2.35   **FUD** XXX                    S Z2 80 ▭

AMA: 2017,Jan,8; 2016,Jan,13; 2015,Jan,16; 2013,Jun,9-11

**78013** **Thyroid imaging (including vascular flow, when performed);**

🚗 5.59   👤 5.59   **FUD** XXX                    S Z2 80 ▭

AMA: 2017,Jan,8; 2016,Jan,13; 2015,Jan,16; 2013,Jun,9-11

**78014** **with single or multiple uptake(s) quantitative measurement(s) (including stimulation, suppression, or discharge, when performed)**

🚗 7.07   👤 7.07   **FUD** XXX                    S Z2 80 ▭

AMA: 2017,Jan,8; 2016,Jan,13; 2015,Jan,16; 2013,Jun,9-11

**78015** **Thyroid carcinoma metastases imaging; limited area (eg, neck and chest only)**

🚗 6.49   👤 6.49   **FUD** XXX                    S Z2 80 ▭

AMA: 2017,Jan,8; 2016,Jan,13; 2015,Jan,16; 2014,Jan,11; 2012,Feb,9-10

**78016** **with additional studies (eg, urinary recovery)**

🚗 8.31   👤 8.31   **FUD** XXX                    S Z2 80 ▭

AMA: 2017,Jan,8; 2016,Jan,13; 2015,Jan,16; 2014,Jan,11; 2012,Feb,9-10

**78018** **whole body**

🚗 9.16   👤 9.16   **FUD** XXX                    S Z2 80 ▭

AMA: 2017,Jan,8; 2016,Jan,13; 2015,Jan,16; 2014,Jan,11; 2012,Feb,9-10

+ **78020** **Thyroid carcinoma metastases uptake (List separately in addition to code for primary procedure)**

Code first (78018)

🚗 2.43   👤 2.43   **FUD** ZZZ                    N N1 80 ▭

AMA: 2017,Jan,8; 2016,Jan,13; 2015,Jan,16; 2014,Jan,11; 2012,Feb,9-10; 2012,Jan,15-42

**78070** **Parathyroid planar imaging (including subtraction, when performed);**

🚗 8.78   👤 8.78   **FUD** XXX                    S Z2 80 ▭

AMA: 2017,Jan,8; 2016,Dec,9; 2016,Dec,16; 2016,Jan,13; 2015,Jan,16; 2014,Jan,11; 2012,Feb,9-10

**78071** **with tomographic (SPECT)**

🚗 10.4   👤 10.4   **FUD** XXX                    S Z2 80 ▭

AMA: 2017,Jan,8; 2016,Dec,16; 2016,Dec,9

**78072** **with tomographic (SPECT), and concurrently acquired computed tomography (CT) for anatomical localization**

🚗 12.0   👤 12.0   **FUD** XXX                    S Z2 80 ▭

AMA: 2017,Jan,8; 2016,Dec,16; 2016,Dec,9

**78075** **Adrenal imaging, cortex and/or medulla**

🚗 12.9   👤 12.9   **FUD** XXX                    S Z2 80 ▭

AMA: 2017,Jan,8; 2016,Jan,13; 2015,Jan,16; 2014,Jan,11; 2012,Feb,9-10

● New Code   ▲ Revised Code   ○ Reinstated   ● New Web Release   ▲ Revised Web Release   Unlisted   Not Covered   # Resequenced
Ⓢ AMA Mod 51 Exempt   ⑤ Optum Mod 51 Exempt   ⑥ Mod 63 Exempt   ✗ Non-FDA Drug   ★ Telemedicine   M Maternity   A Age Edit   + Add-on   AMA: CPT Asst

© 2017 Optum360, LLC                    CPT © 2017 American Medical Association. All Rights Reserved.

**78099** Unlisted endocrine procedure, diagnostic nuclear
medicine

   0.00    0.00    **FUD** XXX     S Z2 80

   **AMA:** 2017,Jan,8; 2016,Dec,9; 2016,Jan,13; 2015,Jan,16;
2014,Jan,11; 2012,Feb,9-10

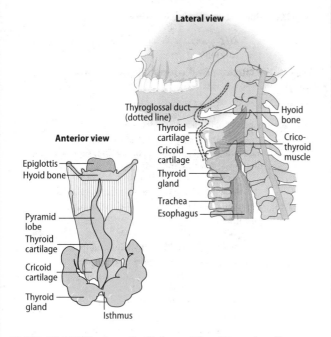

Lateral view

Anterior view

## 78102-78199 Nuclear Radiology: Blood Forming Organs

EXCLUDES Diagnostic services (see appropriate sections)
Follow-up care (see appropriate section)
Radioimmunoassays (82009-84999 [82652])
Code also radiopharmaceutical(s) and/or drug(s) supplied

**78102** Bone marrow imaging; limited area

   4.98    4.98    **FUD** XXX     S Z2 80

   **AMA:** 2017,Jan,8; 2016,Jan,13; 2015,Jan,16; 2014,Jan,11;
2012,Feb,9-10

**78103** multiple areas

   6.42    6.42    **FUD** XXX     S Z2 80

   **AMA:** 2012,Feb,9-10

**78104** whole body

   7.17    7.17    **FUD** XXX     S Z2 80

   **AMA:** 2012,Feb,9-10

**78110** Plasma volume, radiopharmaceutical volume-dilution
technique (separate procedure); single sampling

   2.92    2.92    **FUD** XXX     S Z2 80

   **AMA:** 2012,Feb,9-10

**78111** multiple samplings

   2.78    2.78    **FUD** XXX     S Z2 80

   **AMA:** 2012,Feb,9-10

**78120** Red cell volume determination (separate procedure); single
sampling

   2.74    2.74    **FUD** XXX     S Z2 80

   **AMA:** 2012,Feb,9-10

**78121** multiple samplings

   3.04    3.04    **FUD** XXX     S Z2 80

   **AMA:** 2012,Feb,9-10

**78122** Whole blood volume determination, including separate
measurement of plasma volume and red cell volume
(radiopharmaceutical volume-dilution technique)

   2.81    2.81    **FUD** XXX     S Z2 80

   **AMA:** 2012,Feb,9-10

**78130** Red cell survival study;

   4.89    4.89    **FUD** XXX     S Z2 80

   **AMA:** 2012,Feb,9-10

---

**78135** differential organ/tissue kinetics (eg, splenic and/or
hepatic sequestration)

   10.3    10.3    **FUD** XXX     S Z2 80

   **AMA:** 2012,Feb,9-10

**78140** Labeled red cell sequestration, differential organ/tissue (eg,
splenic and/or hepatic)

   4.04    4.04    **FUD** XXX     S Z2 80

   **AMA:** 2012,Feb,9-10

**78185** Spleen imaging only, with or without vascular flow

   EXCLUDES Liver imaging (78215-78216)

   6.18    6.18    **FUD** XXX     S Z2 80

   **AMA:** 2012,Feb,9-10

~~**78190** Kinetics, study of platelet survival, with or without differential
organ/tissue localization~~

**78191** Platelet survival study

   4.89    4.89    **FUD** XXX     S Z2 80

   **AMA:** 2012,Feb,9-10

**78195** Lymphatics and lymph nodes imaging

   EXCLUDES Sentinel node identification without scintigraphy
(38792)
Sentinel node removal (38500-38542)

   10.4    10.4    **FUD** XXX     S Z2 80

   **AMA:** 2017,Jan,8; 2016,Jan,13; 2015,Jan,16; 2014,Jan,11;
2012,Feb,9-10

**78199** Unlisted hematopoietic, reticuloendothelial and lymphatic
procedure, diagnostic nuclear medicine

   0.00    0.00    **FUD** XXX     S Z2 80

   **AMA:** 2017,Jan,8; 2016,Jan,13; 2015,Jan,16; 2014,Jan,11;
2012,Feb,9-10

## 78201-78299 Nuclear Radiology: Digestive System

EXCLUDES Diagnostic services (see appropriate sections)
Follow-up care (see appropriate section)
Code also radiopharmaceutical(s) and/or drug(s) supplied

**78201** Liver imaging; static only

   EXCLUDES Spleen imaging only (78185)

   5.52    5.52    **FUD** XXX     S Z2 80

   **AMA:** 2017,Jan,8; 2016,Jan,13; 2015,Jan,16; 2014,Jan,11;
2012,Feb,9-10

**78202** with vascular flow

   EXCLUDES Spleen imaging only (78185)

   5.85    5.85    **FUD** XXX     S Z2 80

   **AMA:** 2012,Feb,9-10

**78205** Liver imaging (SPECT);

   6.17    6.17    **FUD** XXX     S Z2 80

   **AMA:** 2012,Feb,9-10

**78206** with vascular flow

   10.0    10.0    **FUD** XXX     S Z2 80

   **AMA:** 2012,Feb,9-10

**78215** Liver and spleen imaging; static only

   5.68    5.68    **FUD** XXX     S Z2 80

   **AMA:** 2012,Feb,9-10

**78216** with vascular flow

   3.70    3.70    **FUD** XXX     S Z2 80

   **AMA:** 2012,Feb,9-10

**78226** Hepatobiliary system imaging, including gallbladder when
present;

   9.68    9.68    **FUD** XXX     S Z2 80

   **AMA:** 2012,Feb,9-10

**78227** with pharmacologic intervention, including quantitative
measurement(s) when performed

   13.1    13.1    **FUD** XXX     S Z2 80

   **AMA:** 2012,Feb,9-10

**78230** Salivary gland imaging;

   5.11    5.11    **FUD** XXX     S Z2 80

   **AMA:** 2012,Feb,9-10

26/TC PC/TC Only    A2-Z ASC Payment    50 Bilateral    ♂ Male Only    ♀ Female Only    Facility RVU    Non-Facility RVU    CCI
FUD Follow-up Days    CMS: IOM (Pub 100)    A-Y OPPSI    80/80 Surg Assist Allowed / w/Doc    Lab Crosswalk    Radiology Crosswalk    CLIA
346

CPT © 2017 American Medical Association. All Rights Reserved.      © 2017 Optum360, LLC

| 78231 | with serial images |
|---|---|
| | 📷 3.76    ⅀ 3.76    **FUD** XXX        S Z2 80 ▱ |
| | **AMA:** 2012,Feb,9-10 |

**78232** Salivary gland function study
📷 2.92    ⅀ 2.92    **FUD** XXX        S Z2 80 ▱
**AMA:** 2012,Feb,9-10

**78258** Esophageal motility
📷 6.58    ⅀ 6.58    **FUD** XXX        S Z2 80 ▱
**AMA:** 2012,Feb,9-10

**78261** Gastric mucosa imaging
📷 7.18    ⅀ 7.18    **FUD** XXX        S Z2 80 ▱
**AMA:** 2012,Feb,9-10

**78262** Gastroesophageal reflux study
📷 7.09    ⅀ 7.09    **FUD** XXX        S Z2 80 ▱
**AMA:** 2017,Jan,8; 2016,Jan,13; 2015,Dec,11; 2012,Feb,9-10

**78264** Gastric emptying imaging study (eg, solid, liquid, or both);
EXCLUDES   Procedure performed more than one time per study
📷 9.84    ⅀ 9.84    **FUD** XXX        S Z2 80 ▱
**AMA:** 2017,Jan,8; 2016,Jan,13; 2015,Dec,11; 2012,Feb,9-10

**78265** with small bowel transit
EXCLUDES   Procedure performed more than one time per study
📷 11.6    ⅀ 11.6    **FUD** XXX        S Z2 80 ▱
**AMA:** 2017,Jan,8; 2015,Dec,11

**78266** with small bowel and colon transit, multiple days
EXCLUDES   Procedure performed more than one time per study
📷 13.8    ⅀ 13.8    **FUD** XXX        S Z2 80 ▱
**AMA:** 2017,Jan,8; 2015,Dec,11

**78267** Urea breath test, C-14 (isotopic); acquisition for analysis
EXCLUDES   Breath hydrogen/methane test (91065)
📷 0.00    ⅀ 0.00    **FUD** XXX        A ▱
**AMA:** 2017,Jan,8; 2016,Jan,13; 2015,Jan,16; 2014,Jan,11; 2012,Feb,9-10

**78268** analysis
EXCLUDES   Breath hydrogen/methane test (91065)
📷 0.00    ⅀ 0.00    **FUD** XXX        A ▱
**AMA:** 2017,Jan,8; 2016,Jan,13; 2015,Jan,16; 2014,Jan,11; 2012,Feb,9-10

**78270** Vitamin B-12 absorption study (eg, Schilling test); without intrinsic factor
📷 2.96    ⅀ 2.96    **FUD** XXX        S Z2 80 ▱
**AMA:** 2012,Feb,9-10

**78271** with intrinsic factor
📷 2.62    ⅀ 2.62    **FUD** XXX        S Z2 80 ▱
**AMA:** 2012,Feb,9-10

**78272** Vitamin B-12 absorption studies combined, with and without intrinsic factor
📷 2.86    ⅀ 2.86    **FUD** XXX        S Z2 80 ▱
**AMA:** 2012,Feb,9-10

**78278** Acute gastrointestinal blood loss imaging
📷 10.1    ⅀ 10.1    **FUD** XXX        S Z2 80 ▱
**AMA:** 2012,Feb,9-10

**78282** Gastrointestinal protein loss
📷 0.00    ⅀ 0.00    **FUD** XXX        S Z2 80 ▱
**AMA:** 2012,Feb,9-10

**78290** Intestine imaging (eg, ectopic gastric mucosa, Meckel's localization, volvulus)
📷 9.71    ⅀ 9.71    **FUD** XXX        S Z2 80 ▱
**AMA:** 2012,Feb,9-10

**78291** Peritoneal-venous shunt patency test (eg, for LeVeen, Denver shunt)
Code also (49427)
📷 7.48    ⅀ 7.48    **FUD** XXX        S Z2 80 ▱
**AMA:** 2012,Feb,9-10

**78299** Unlisted gastrointestinal procedure, diagnostic nuclear medicine
📷 0.00    ⅀ 0.00    **FUD** XXX        S Z2 80
**AMA:** 2017,Jan,8; 2016,Jan,13; 2015,Jan,16; 2014,Jan,11; 2012,Feb,9-10

## 78300-78399 Nuclear Radiology: Bones and Joints

EXCLUDES   Diagnostic services (see appropriate sections)
Follow-up care (see appropriate section)
Code also radiopharmaceutical(s) and/or drug(s) supplied

**78300** Bone and/or joint imaging; limited area
📷 5.30    ⅀ 5.30    **FUD** XXX        S Z2 80 ▱
**AMA:** 2017,Jan,8; 2016,Jan,13; 2015,Jan,16; 2014,Jan,11; 2012,Feb,9-10; 2012,Jan,15-42

**78305** multiple areas
📷 6.78    ⅀ 6.78    **FUD** XXX        S Z2 80 ▱
**AMA:** 2017,Jan,8; 2016,Jan,13; 2015,Jan,16; 2014,Jan,11; 2012,Feb,9-10

**78306** whole body
📷 7.35    ⅀ 7.35    **FUD** XXX        S Z2 80 ▱
**AMA:** 2017,Jan,8; 2016,Jan,13; 2015,Jan,16; 2014,Jan,11; 2012,Feb,9-10; 2012,Jan,15-42

**78315** 3 phase study
📷 10.1    ⅀ 10.1    **FUD** XXX        S Z2 80 ▱
**AMA:** 2017,Jan,8; 2016,Jan,13; 2015,Jan,16; 2014,Jan,11; 2012,Feb,9-10; 2012,Jan,15-42

**78320** tomographic (SPECT)
📷 6.67    ⅀ 6.67    **FUD** XXX        S Z2 80 ▱
**AMA:** 2017,Jan,8; 2016,Jan,13; 2015,Jan,16; 2014,Jan,11; 2012,Feb,9-10; 2012,Jan,15-42

**78350** Bone density (bone mineral content) study, 1 or more sites; single photon absorptiometry
📷 0.93    ⅀ 0.93    **FUD** XXX        E ▱
**AMA:** 2012,Feb,9-10

**78351** dual photon absorptiometry, 1 or more sites
📷 0.44    ⅀ 0.44    **FUD** XXX        E ▱
**AMA:** 2012,Feb,9-10

**78399** Unlisted musculoskeletal procedure, diagnostic nuclear medicine
📷 0.00    ⅀ 0.00    **FUD** XXX        S Z2 80
**AMA:** 2017,Jan,8; 2016,Jan,13; 2015,Jan,16; 2014,Jan,11; 2012,Feb,9-10

## 78414-78499 Nuclear Radiology: Heart and Vascular

EXCLUDES   Diagnostic services (see appropriate sections)
Follow-up care (see appropriate section)
Code also radiopharmaceutical(s) and/or drug(s) supplied

**78414** Determination of central c-v hemodynamics (non-imaging) (eg, ejection fraction with probe technique) with or without pharmacologic intervention or exercise, single or multiple determinations
📷 0.00    ⅀ 0.00    **FUD** XXX        S Z2 80 ▱
**AMA:** 2017,Jan,8; 2016,Jan,13; 2015,Jan,16; 2014,Jan,11; 2012,Feb,9-10

**78428** Cardiac shunt detection
📷 5.29    ⅀ 5.29    **FUD** XXX        S Z2 80 ▱
**AMA:** 2017,Jan,8; 2016,Jan,13; 2015,Jan,16; 2014,Jan,11; 2012,Feb,9-10

**78445** Non-cardiac vascular flow imaging (ie, angiography, venography)
📷 5.31    ⅀ 5.31    **FUD** XXX        S Z2 80 ▱
**AMA:** 2017,Jan,8; 2016,Jan,13; 2015,Jan,16; 2014,Jan,11; 2012,Feb,9-10

Radiology

78231 — 78445

**78451** **Myocardial perfusion imaging, tomographic (SPECT) (including attenuation correction, qualitative or quantitative wall motion, ejection fraction by first pass or gated technique, additional quantification, when performed); single study, at rest or stress (exercise or pharmacologic)**
Code also stress testing when performed (93015-93018)
9.92    9.92    **FUD** XXX          S Z2 80 ▭
**AMA:** 2017,Jan,8; 2016,Jan,13; 2015,Jan,16; 2014,Jan,11; 2012,Feb,9-10; 2012,Jan,15-42

**78452** **multiple studies, at rest and/or stress (exercise or pharmacologic) and/or redistribution and/or rest reinjection**
Code also stress testing when performed (93015-93018)
13.7    13.7    **FUD** XXX          S Z2 80 ▭
**AMA:** 2017,Jan,8; 2016,Jan,13; 2015,Jan,16; 2014,Jan,11; 2012,Feb,9-10; 2012,Jan,15-42

**78453** **Myocardial perfusion imaging, planar (including qualitative or quantitative wall motion, ejection fraction by first pass or gated technique, additional quantification, when performed); single study, at rest or stress (exercise or pharmacologic)**
Code also stress testing when performed (93015-93018)
8.87    8.87    **FUD** XXX          S Z2 80 ▭
**AMA:** 2017,Jan,8; 2016,Jan,13; 2015,Jan,16; 2014,Jan,11; 2012,Feb,9-10

**78454** **multiple studies, at rest and/or stress (exercise or pharmacologic) and/or redistribution and/or rest reinjection**
Code also stress testing when performed (93015-93018)
12.7    12.7    **FUD** XXX          S Z2 80 ▭
**AMA:** 2017,Jan,8; 2016,Jan,13; 2015,Jan,16; 2014,Jan,11; 2012,Feb,9-10

**78456** **Acute venous thrombosis imaging, peptide**
9.34    9.34    **FUD** XXX          S Z2 ▭
**AMA:** 2017,Jan,8; 2016,Jan,13; 2015,Jan,16; 2014,Jan,11; 2012,Feb,9-10

**78457** **Venous thrombosis imaging, venogram; unilateral**
5.13    5.13    **FUD** XXX          S Z2 80 ▭
**AMA:** 2017,Jan,8; 2016,Jan,13; 2015,Jan,16; 2014,Jan,11; 2012,Feb,9-10

**78458** **bilateral**
5.98    5.98    **FUD** XXX          S Z2 80 ▭
**AMA:** 2017,Jan,8; 2016,Jan,13; 2015,Jan,16; 2014,Jan,11; 2012,Feb,9-10

**78459** **Myocardial imaging, positron emission tomography (PET), metabolic evaluation**
EXCLUDES    *Myocardial perfusion studies (78491-78492)*
0.00    0.00    **FUD** XXX          S Z2 80 ▭
**AMA:** 2017,Jan,8; 2016,Jan,13; 2015,Jan,16; 2014,Jan,11; 2012,Feb,9-10

**78466** **Myocardial imaging, infarct avid, planar; qualitative or quantitative**
5.71    5.71    **FUD** XXX          S Z2 80 ▭
**AMA:** 2012,Feb,9-10

**78468** **with ejection fraction by first pass technique**
5.67    5.67    **FUD** XXX          S Z2 80 ▭
**AMA:** 2017,Jan,8; 2016,Jan,13; 2015,Jan,16; 2014,Jan,11; 2012,Feb,9-10

**78469** **tomographic SPECT with or without quantification**
EXCLUDES    *Myocardial sympathetic innervation imaging (0331T-0332T)*
6.63    6.63    **FUD** XXX          S Z2 80 ▭
**AMA:** 2017,Jan,8; 2016,Jan,13; 2015,Jan,16; 2014,Jan,11; 2012,Feb,9-10

**78472** **Cardiac blood pool imaging, gated equilibrium; planar, single study at rest or stress (exercise and/or pharmacologic), wall motion study plus ejection fraction, with or without additional quantitative processing**
EXCLUDES    *Cardiac blood pool imaging (78481, 78483, 78494)*
*Myocardial perfusion imaging (78451-78454)*
*Right ventricular ejection fraction by first pass technique (78496)*
Code also stress testing when performed (93015-93018)
6.68    6.68    **FUD** XXX          S Z2 80 ▭
**AMA:** 2017,Jan,8; 2016,Jan,13; 2015,Jan,16; 2014,Jan,11; 2012,Feb,9-10

**78473** **multiple studies, wall motion study plus ejection fraction, at rest and stress (exercise and/or pharmacologic), with or without additional quantification**
EXCLUDES    *Cardiac blood pool imaging (78481, 78483, 78494)*
*Myocardial perfusion imaging (78451-78454)*
Code also stress testing when performed (93015-93018)
8.42    8.42    **FUD** XXX          S Z2 80 ▭
**AMA:** 2017,Jan,8; 2016,Jan,13; 2015,Jan,16; 2014,Jan,11; 2012,Feb,9-10

**78481** **Cardiac blood pool imaging (planar), first pass technique; single study, at rest or with stress (exercise and/or pharmacologic), wall motion study plus ejection fraction, with or without quantification**
EXCLUDES    *Myocardial perfusion imaging (78451-78454)*
Code also stress testing when performed (93015-93018)
5.09    5.09    **FUD** XXX          S Z2 80 ▭
**AMA:** 2017,Jan,8; 2016,Jan,13; 2015,Jan,16; 2014,Jan,11; 2012,Feb,9-10

**78483** **multiple studies, at rest and with stress (exercise and/or pharmacologic), wall motion study plus ejection fraction, with or without quantification**
EXCLUDES    *Blood flow studies of the brain (78610)*
*Myocardial perfusion imaging (78451-78454)*
Code also stress testing when performed (93015-93018)
7.06    7.06    **FUD** XXX          S Z2 80 ▭
**AMA:** 2017,Jan,8; 2016,Jan,13; 2015,Jan,16; 2014,Jan,11; 2012,Feb,9-10

**78491** **Myocardial imaging, positron emission tomography (PET), perfusion; single study at rest or stress**
Code also stress testing when performed (93015-93018)
0.00    0.00    **FUD** XXX          S Z2 80 ▭
**AMA:** 2017,Jan,8; 2016,Jan,13; 2015,Jan,16; 2014,Jan,11; 2012,Feb,9-10

**78492** **multiple studies at rest and/or stress**
Code also stress testing when performed (93015-93018)
0.00    0.00    **FUD** XXX          S Z2 80 ▭
**AMA:** 2017,Jan,8; 2016,Jan,13; 2015,Jan,16; 2014,Jan,11; 2012,Feb,9-10

**78494** **Cardiac blood pool imaging, gated equilibrium, SPECT, at rest, wall motion study plus ejection fraction, with or without quantitative processing**
6.54    6.54    **FUD** XXX          S Z2 80 ▭
**AMA:** 2017,Jan,8; 2016,Jan,13; 2015,Jan,16; 2014,Jan,11; 2012,Feb,9-10

+ **78496** **Cardiac blood pool imaging, gated equilibrium, single study, at rest, with right ventricular ejection fraction by first pass technique (List separately in addition to code for primary procedure)**
Code first (78472)
1.27    1.27    **FUD** ZZZ          N N1 80 ▭
**AMA:** 2017,Jan,8; 2016,Jan,13; 2015,Jan,16; 2014,Jan,11; 2012,Feb,9-10; 2012,Jan,15-42

**78499** **Unlisted cardiovascular procedure, diagnostic nuclear medicine**
0.00    0.00    **FUD** XXX          S Z2 80
**AMA:** 2017,Jan,8; 2016,Jan,13; 2015,Jan,16; 2014,Jan,11; 2012,Feb,9-10

## 78579-78599 Nuclear Radiology: Lungs

EXCLUDES  Diagnostic services (see appropriate sections)
Follow-up care (see appropriate sections)
Code also radiopharmaceutical(s) and/or drug(s) supplied

**78579**  **Pulmonary ventilation imaging (eg, aerosol or gas)**
EXCLUDES  Procedure performed more than one time per imaging session
🚑 5.44  ⚷ 5.44  **FUD** XXX  [S] [72] [80] [▭]
**AMA:** 2012,Feb,9-10

**78580**  **Pulmonary perfusion imaging (eg, particulate)**
EXCLUDES  Myocardial perfusion imaging (78451-78454)
Procedure performed more than one time per imaging session
🚑 6.99  ⚷ 6.99  **FUD** XXX  [S] [72] [80] [▭]
**AMA:** 2017,Jan,8; 2016,Jan,13; 2015,Jan,16; 2014,Jan,11; 2012,Feb,9-10

**78582**  **Pulmonary ventilation (eg, aerosol or gas) and perfusion imaging**
EXCLUDES  Myocardial perfusion imaging (78451-78454)
Procedure performed more than one time per imaging session
🚑 9.79  ⚷ 9.79  **FUD** XXX  [S] [72] [80] [▭]
**AMA:** 2012,Feb,9-10

**78597**  **Quantitative differential pulmonary perfusion, including imaging when performed**
EXCLUDES  Myocardial perfusion imaging (78451-78454)
Procedure performed more than one time per imaging session
🚑 5.90  ⚷ 5.90  **FUD** XXX  [S] [72] [80] [▭]
**AMA:** 2012,Feb,9-10

**78598**  **Quantitative differential pulmonary perfusion and ventilation (eg, aerosol or gas), including imaging when performed**
EXCLUDES  Myocardial perfusion imaging (78451-78454)
Procedure performed more than one time per imaging session
🚑 8.95  ⚷ 8.95  **FUD** XXX  [S] [72] [80] [▭]
**AMA:** 2012,Feb,9-10

**78599**  **Unlisted respiratory procedure, diagnostic nuclear medicine**
🚑 0.00  ⚷ 0.00  **FUD** XXX  [S] [72] [80]
**AMA:** 2017,Jan,8; 2016,Jan,13; 2015,Jan,16; 2014,Jan,11; 2012,Feb,9-10

## 78600-78650 Nuclear Radiology: Brain/Cerebrospinal Fluid

EXCLUDES  Diagnostic services (see appropriate sections)
Follow-up care (see appropriate section)
Code also radiopharmaceutical(s) and/or drug(s) supplied

**78600**  **Brain imaging, less than 4 static views;**
🚑 5.42  ⚷ 5.42  **FUD** XXX  [S] [72] [80] [▭]
**AMA:** 2017,Jan,8; 2016,Jan,13; 2015,Jan,16; 2014,Jan,11; 2012,Feb,9-10

X-ray beam

Linear focal plane

Schematic of frontal coronal CT section of skull

**78601**  **with vascular flow**
🚑 6.28  ⚷ 6.28  **FUD** XXX  [S] [72] [80] [▭]
**AMA:** 2012,Feb,9-10

**78605**  **Brain imaging, minimum 4 static views;**
🚑 5.86  ⚷ 5.86  **FUD** XXX  [S] [72] [80] [▭]
**AMA:** 2012,Feb,9-10

**78606**  **with vascular flow**
🚑 9.65  ⚷ 9.65  **FUD** XXX  [S] [72] [80] [▭]
**AMA:** 2012,Feb,9-10

**78607**  **Brain imaging, tomographic (SPECT)**
🚑 10.2  ⚷ 10.2  **FUD** XXX  [S] [72] [80] [▭]
**AMA:** 2012,Feb,9-10

**78608**  **Brain imaging, positron emission tomography (PET); metabolic evaluation**
🚑 0.00  ⚷ 0.00  **FUD** XXX  [S] [72] [80] [▭]
**AMA:** 2012,Feb,9-10

**78609**  **perfusion evaluation**
🚑 2.12  ⚷ 2.12  **FUD** XXX  [E] [▭]
**AMA:** 2012,Feb,9-10

**78610**  **Brain imaging, vascular flow only**
🚑 5.12  ⚷ 5.12  **FUD** XXX  [S] [72] [80] [▭]
**AMA:** 2012,Feb,9-10

**78630**  **Cerebrospinal fluid flow, imaging (not including introduction of material); cisternography**
Code also injection procedure (61000-61070, 62270-62327)
🚑 9.91  ⚷ 9.91  **FUD** XXX  [S] [72] [80] [▭]
**AMA:** 2012,Feb,9-10

**78635**  **ventriculography**
Code also injection procedure (61000-61070, 62270-62294)
🚑 10.0  ⚷ 10.0  **FUD** XXX  [S] [72] [80] [▭]
**AMA:** 2012,Feb,9-10

**78645**  **shunt evaluation**
Code also injection procedure (61000-61070, 62270-62294)
🚑 9.49  ⚷ 9.49  **FUD** XXX  [S] [72] [80] [▭]
**AMA:** 2012,Feb,9-10

**78647**  **tomographic (SPECT)**
🚑 10.3  ⚷ 10.3  **FUD** XXX  [S] [72] [80] [▭]
**AMA:** 2012,Feb,9-10

**78650**  **Cerebrospinal fluid leakage detection and localization**
Code also injection procedure (61000-61070, 62270-62294)
🚑 9.69  ⚷ 9.69  **FUD** XXX  [S] [72] [80] [▭]
**AMA:** 2012,Feb,9-10

## 78660-78699 Nuclear Radiology: Lacrimal Duct System

Code also radiopharmaceutical(s) and/or drug(s) supplied

**78660**  **Radiopharmaceutical dacryocystography**
🚑 5.25  ⚷ 5.25  **FUD** XXX  [S] [72] [80] [▭]
**AMA:** 2012,Feb,9-10

**78699**  **Unlisted nervous system procedure, diagnostic nuclear medicine**
🚑 0.00  ⚷ 0.00  **FUD** XXX  [S] [72] [80]
**AMA:** 2017,Jan,8; 2016,Jan,13; 2015,Jan,16; 2014,Jan,11; 2012,Feb,9-10

## 78700-78725 Nuclear Radiology: Renal Anatomy and Function

EXCLUDES  Diagnostic services (see appropriate sections)
Follow-up care (see appropriate section)
Renal endoscopy with insertion of radioactive substances (77778)
Code also radiopharmaceutical(s) and/or drug(s) supplied

**78700**  **Kidney imaging morphology;**
🚑 5.01  ⚷ 5.01  **FUD** XXX  [S] [72] [80] [▭]
**AMA:** 2017,Jan,8; 2016,Jan,13; 2015,Jan,16; 2014,Jan,11; 2012,Feb,9-10

**78701**  **with vascular flow**
🚑 6.18  ⚷ 6.18  **FUD** XXX  [S] [72] [80] [▭]
**AMA:** 2012,Feb,9-10

● New Code  ▲ Revised Code  ○ Reinstated  ● New Web Release  ▲ Revised Web Release  Unlisted  Not Covered  # Resequenced
⊗ AMA Mod 51 Exempt  ⑤⓪ Optum Mod 51 Exempt  ⊚ Mod 63 Exempt  ✗ Non-FDA Drug  ★ Telemedicine  Ⓜ Maternity  Ⓐ Age Edit  + Add-on  AMA: CPT Asst
© 2017 Optum360, LLC  CPT © 2017 American Medical Association. All Rights Reserved.  **349**

**78707** with vascular flow and function, single study without pharmacological intervention
🚗 6.80 ⚖ 6.80 **FUD** XXX
[S] [Z2] [80] [▭]
**AMA:** 2017,Jan,8; 2016,Jan,13; 2015,Jan,16; 2014,Jan,11; 2012,Feb,9-10

**78708** with vascular flow and function, single study, with pharmacological intervention (eg, angiotensin converting enzyme inhibitor and/or diuretic)
🚗 5.13 ⚖ 5.13 **FUD** XXX
[S] [Z2] [80] [▭]
**AMA:** 2017,Jan,8; 2016,Jan,13; 2015,Jan,16; 2014,Jan,11; 2012,Feb,9-10

**78709** with vascular flow and function, multiple studies, with and without pharmacological intervention (eg, angiotensin converting enzyme inhibitor and/or diuretic)
🚗 10.6 ⚖ 10.6 **FUD** XXX
[S] [Z2] [80] [▭]
**AMA:** 2017,Jan,8; 2016,Jan,13; 2015,Jan,16; 2014,Jan,11; 2012,Feb,9-10

**78710** tomographic (SPECT)
🚗 5.87 ⚖ 5.87 **FUD** XXX
[S] [Z2] [80] [▭]
**AMA:** 2017,Jan,8; 2016,Jan,13; 2015,Jan,16; 2014,Jan,11; 2012,Feb,9-10

**78725** Kidney function study, non-imaging radioisotopic study
🚗 3.11 ⚖ 3.11 **FUD** XXX
[S] [Z2] [80] [▭]
**AMA:** 2012,Feb,9-10

## 78730-78799 Nuclear Radiology: Urogenital
**EXCLUDES** Diagnostic services (see appropriate sections)
Follow-up care (see appropriate section)
Code also radiopharmaceutical(s) and/or drug(s) supplied

+ **78730** Urinary bladder residual study (List separately in addition to code for primary procedure)
**EXCLUDES** Measurement of postvoid residual urine and/or bladder capacity using ultrasound (51798)
Ultrasound imaging of the bladder only with measurement of postvoid residual urine (76857)
Code first (78740)
🚗 2.06 ⚖ 2.06 **FUD** ZZZ
[N] [N1] [80] [▭]
**AMA:** 2017,Jan,8; 2016,Jan,13; 2015,Jan,16; 2014,Jan,11; 2012,Feb,9-10

**78740** Ureteral reflux study (radiopharmaceutical voiding cystogram)
**EXCLUDES** Catheterization (51701-51703)
Code also urinary bladder residual study (78730)
🚗 6.40 ⚖ 6.40 **FUD** XXX
[S] [Z2] [80] [▭]
**AMA:** 2012,Feb,9-10

**78761** Testicular imaging with vascular flow ♂
🚗 6.24 ⚖ 6.24 **FUD** XXX
[S] [Z2] [80] [▭]
**AMA:** 2017,Jan,8; 2016,Jan,13; 2015,Jan,16; 2014,Jan,11; 2012,Feb,9-10

**78799** Unlisted genitourinary procedure, diagnostic nuclear medicine
🚗 0.00 ⚖ 0.00 **FUD** XXX
[S] [Z2] [80]
**AMA:** 2017,Jan,8; 2016,Jan,13; 2015,Jan,16; 2014,Jan,11; 2012,Feb,9-10

## 78800-78804 Nuclear Radiology: Tumor Localization
Code also radiopharmaceutical(s) and/or drug(s) supplied

**78800** Radiopharmaceutical localization of tumor or distribution of radiopharmaceutical agent(s); limited area
**INCLUDES** Ocular radiophosphorus tumor identification
**EXCLUDES** Specific organ (see appropriate site)
🚗 5.63 ⚖ 5.63 **FUD** XXX
[S] [Z2] [80] [▭]
**AMA:** 2017,Jan,8; 2016,Jan,13; 2015,Jan,16; 2014,Jan,11; 2012,Feb,9-10; 2012,Jan,15-42

**78801** multiple areas
🚗 7.68 ⚖ 7.68 **FUD** XXX
[S] [Z2] [80] [▭]
**AMA:** 2017,Jan,8; 2016,Jan,13; 2015,Jan,16; 2014,Jan,11; 2012,Feb,9-10; 2012,Jan,15-42

**78802** whole body, single day imaging
🚗 9.47 ⚖ 9.47 **FUD** XXX
[S] [Z2] [80] [▭]
**AMA:** 2012,Feb,9-10

**78803** tomographic (SPECT)
🚗 9.99 ⚖ 9.99 **FUD** XXX
[S] [Z2] [80] [▭]
**AMA:** 2017,Jan,8; 2016,Dec,9; 2016,Dec,16; 2016,Jan,13; 2015,Oct,9; 2012,Feb,9-10

**78804** whole body, requiring 2 or more days imaging
🚗 16.5 ⚖ 16.5 **FUD** XXX
[S] [Z2] [80] [▭]
**AMA:** 2012,Feb,9-10

## 78805-78807 Nuclear Radiology: Inflammation and Infection
**EXCLUDES** Imaging bone infectious or inflammatory disease with bone imaging radiopharmaceutical (78300, 78805-78306)
Code also radiopharmaceutical(s) and/or drug(s) supplied

**78805** Radiopharmaceutical localization of inflammatory process; limited area
🚗 5.35 ⚖ 5.35 **FUD** XXX
[S] [Z2] [80] [▭]
**AMA:** 2017,Jan,8; 2016,Jan,13; 2015,Jan,16; 2014,Jan,11; 2012,Feb,9-10

**78806** whole body
🚗 9.75 ⚖ 9.75 **FUD** XXX
[S] [Z2] [80] [▭]
**AMA:** 2017,Jan,8; 2016,Jan,13; 2015,Jan,16; 2014,Jan,11; 2012,Feb,9-10

**78807** tomographic (SPECT)
🚗 10.0 ⚖ 10.0 **FUD** XXX
[S] [Z2] [80] [▭]
**AMA:** 2012,Feb,9-10

## 78808 Intravenous Injection for Radiopharmaceutical Localization
Code also radiopharmaceutical(s) and/or drug(s) supplied

**78808** Injection procedure for radiopharmaceutical localization by non-imaging probe study, intravenous (eg, parathyroid adenoma)
**EXCLUDES** Identification of sentinel node (38792)
🚗 1.28 ⚖ 1.28 **FUD** XXX
[Q1] [N1] [80] [▭]
**AMA:** 2017,Jan,8; 2016,Dec,9; 2012,Feb,9-10

## 78811-78999 Nuclear Radiology: Diagnosis, Staging, Restaging or Monitoring Cancer
**CMS:** 100-03,220.6.17 Positron Emission Tomography (FDG) for Oncologic Conditions; 100-03,220.6.19 NaF-18 PET to Identify Bone Metastasis of Cancer; 100-03,220.6.9 FDG PET for Refractory Seizures; 100-04,13,60 Positron Emission Tomography (PET) Scans - General Information; 100-04,13,60.13 Billing for PET Scans for Specific Indications of Cervical Cancer; 100-04,13,60.15 Billing for CMS-Approved Clinical Trials for PET Scans; 100-04,13,60.16 Billing and Coverage for PET Scans; 100-04,13,60.17 Billing and Coverage Changes for PET Scans for Cervical Cancer; 100-04,13,60.18 Billing and Coverage for PET (NaF-18) Scans to Identify Bone Metastasis; 100-04,13,60.2 Use of Gamma Cameras, Full and Partial Ring PET Scanners; 100-04,13,60.3 PET Scan Qualifying Conditions; 100-04,13,60.3.1 Appropriate Codes for PET Scans; 100-04,13,60.3.2 Tracer Codes Required for PET Scans
**EXCLUDES** CT scan performed for other than attenuation correction and anatomical localization (report with the appropriate site-specific CT code and modifier 59)
Ocular radiophosphorus tumor identification (78800)
PET brain scan (78608-78609)
PET myocardial imaging (78459, 78491-78492)
Procedure performed more than one time per imaging session
Code also radiopharmaceutical(s) and/or drug(s) supplied

**78811** Positron emission tomography (PET) imaging; limited area (eg, chest, head/neck)
🚗 0.00 ⚖ 0.00 **FUD** XXX
[S] [Z2] [80] [▭]
**AMA:** 2017,Jan,8; 2016,Jan,13; 2015,Jan,16; 2014,Jan,11; 2012,Feb,9-10

**78812** skull base to mid-thigh
🚗 0.00 ⚖ 0.00 **FUD** XXX
[S] [Z2] [80] [▭]
**AMA:** 2017,Jan,8; 2016,Jan,13; 2015,Jan,16; 2014,Jan,11; 2013,Feb,16-17; 2012,Feb,9-10

**78813** whole body
🚗 0.00 ⚖ 0.00 **FUD** XXX
[S] [Z2] [80] [▭]
**AMA:** 2017,Jan,8; 2016,Jan,13; 2015,Jan,16; 2014,Jan,11; 2013,Feb,16-17; 2012,Feb,9-10

26/TC PC/TC Only    A2-Z3 ASC Payment    50 Bilateral    ♂ Male Only    ♀ Female Only    🚗 Facility RVU    ⚖ Non-Facility RVU    ▭ CCI
FUD Follow-up Days    CMS: IOM (Pub 100)    A-Y OPPSI    80/80 Surg Assist Allowed / w/Doc    Lab Crosswalk    Radiology Crosswalk    CLIA

   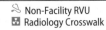

350      CPT © 2017 American Medical Association. All Rights Reserved.      © 2017 Optum360, LLC

**78814** Positron emission tomography (PET) with concurrently acquired computed tomography (CT) for attenuation correction and anatomical localization imaging; limited area (eg, chest, head/neck)

    🚑 0.00    ⚕ 0.00    **FUD** XXX        [S] [Z2] [80] [▭]

    **AMA:** 2017,Jan,8; 2016,Jan,13; 2015,Jan,16; 2014,Jan,11; 2013,Feb,16-17; 2012,Feb,9-10; 2012,Jan,15-42

**78815** skull base to mid-thigh

    🚑 0.00    ⚕ 0.00    **FUD** XXX        [S] [Z2] [80] [▭]

    **AMA:** 2017,Jan,8; 2016,Jan,13; 2015,Jan,16; 2014,Jan,11; 2013,Feb,16-17; 2012,Feb,9-10; 2012,Jan,15-42

**78816** whole body

    🚑 0.00    ⚕ 0.00    **FUD** XXX        [S] [Z2] [80] [▭]

    **AMA:** 2017,Jan,8; 2016,Jan,13; 2015,Jan,16; 2014,Jan,11; 2013,Feb,16-17; 2012,Feb,9-10; 2012,Jan,15-42

**78999** Unlisted miscellaneous procedure, diagnostic nuclear medicine

    🚑 0.00    ⚕ 0.00    **FUD** XXX        [S] [Z2] [80]

    **AMA:** 2017,Jan,8; 2016,Dec,9; 2016,Dec,16; 2016,Jan,13; 2015,Oct,9; 2015,Jan,16; 2014,Jan,11; 2012,Feb,9-10

# 79005-79999 Systemic Radiopharmaceutical Therapy

*EXCLUDES* *Imaging guidance*
*Injection into artery, body cavity, or joint (see appropriate injection codes)*
*Radiological supervision and interpretation*

**79005** Radiopharmaceutical therapy, by oral administration

    *EXCLUDES* *Monoclonal antibody treatment (79403)*
    🚑 3.90    ⚕ 3.90    **FUD** XXX        [S] [Z3] [80] [▭]

    **AMA:** 2017,Jan,8; 2016,Jan,13; 2015,Jan,16; 2014,Jan,11; 2012,Feb,9-10

**79101** Radiopharmaceutical therapy, by intravenous administration

    *EXCLUDES* *Administration of nonantibody radioelement solution including follow-up care (77750)*
    *Hydration infusion (96360)*
    *Intravenous injection, IV push (96374-96375, 96409)*
    *Radiolabeled monoclonal antibody IV infusion (79403)*
    *Venipuncture (36400, 36410)*
    🚑 4.09    ⚕ 4.09    **FUD** XXX        [S] [Z3] [80] [▭]

    **AMA:** 2017,Jan,8; 2016,Jan,13; 2015,Jan,16; 2014,Jan,11; 2012,Feb,9-10

**79200** Radiopharmaceutical therapy, by intracavitary administration

    🚑 3.99    ⚕ 3.99    **FUD** XXX        [S] [Z3] [80] [▭]

    **AMA:** 2017,Jan,8; 2016,Jan,13; 2015,Jan,16; 2014,Jan,11; 2012,Feb,9-10

**79300** Radiopharmaceutical therapy, by interstitial radioactive colloid administration

    🚑 0.00    ⚕ 0.00    **FUD** XXX        [S] [Z2] [80] [▭]

    **AMA:** 2017,Jan,8; 2016,Jan,13; 2015,Jan,16; 2014,Jan,11; 2012,Feb,9-10

**79403** Radiopharmaceutical therapy, radiolabeled monoclonal antibody by intravenous infusion

    *EXCLUDES* *Intravenous radiopharmaceutical therapy (79101)*
    🚑 5.47    ⚕ 5.47    **FUD** XXX        [S] [Z3] [80] [▭]

    **AMA:** 2017,Jan,8; 2016,Jan,13; 2015,Jan,16; 2014,Jan,11; 2012,Feb,9-10

**79440** Radiopharmaceutical therapy, by intra-articular administration

    🚑 4.21    ⚕ 4.21    **FUD** XXX        [S] [Z3] [80] [▭]

    **AMA:** 2017,Jan,8; 2016,Jan,13; 2015,Jan,16; 2014,Jan,11; 2012,Feb,9-10

**79445** Radiopharmaceutical therapy, by intra-arterial particulate administration

    *EXCLUDES* *Intra-arterial injections (96373, 96420)*
    *Procedural and radiological supervision and interpretation for angiographic and interventional procedures before intra-arterial radiopharmaceutical therapy*
    🚑 0.00    ⚕ 0.00    **FUD** XXX        [S] [Z2] [80] [▭]

    **AMA:** 2017,Jan,8; 2016,Jan,13; 2015,Jan,16; 2014,Jan,11; 2013,Nov,6; 2012,Feb,9-10

**79999** Radiopharmaceutical therapy, unlisted procedure

    🚑 0.00    ⚕ 0.00    **FUD** XXX        [S] [Z2] [80]

    **AMA:** 2017,Jan,8; 2016,Jan,13; 2015,Jan,16; 2014,Jan,11; 2012,Feb,9-10

## 80047-80081 [80081] Multi-test Laboratory Panels

INCLUDES Groups of specified tests that may be reported as a panel

EXCLUDES *Reporting two or more panel codes that include the same tests; report the panel with the highest number of tests in common to meet the definition of the panel code*

Code also individual tests that are not part of the panel, when appropriate

### 80047 Basic metabolic panel (Calcium, ionized)

INCLUDES Calcium, ionized (82330)
Carbon dioxide (bicarbonate) (82374)
Chloride (82435)
Creatinine (82565)
Glucose (82947)
Potassium (84132)
Sodium (84295)
Urea nitrogen (BUN) (84520)

🚑 0.00   ⚕ 0.00   **FUD** XXX   ☒ Ⓠ ▢

**AMA:** 2017,Jan,8; 2016,Jan,13; 2015,Jan,16; 2014,Jan,11; 2013,Apr,10-11

### 80048 Basic metabolic panel (Calcium, total)

INCLUDES Calcium, total (82310)
Carbon dioxide (bicarbonate) (82374)
Chloride (82435)
Creatinine (82565)
Glucose (82947)
Potassium (84132)
Sodium (84295)
Urea nitrogen (BUN) (84520)

🚑 0.00   ⚕ 0.00   **FUD** XXX   ☒ Ⓠ ▢

**AMA:** 2017,Jan,8; 2016,Jan,13; 2015,Jan,16; 2014,Jan,11

### 80050 General health panel

INCLUDES Complete blood count (CBC), automated, with:
Manual differential WBC count
Blood smear with manual differential AND complete (CBC), automated (85007, 85027)
Manual differential WBC count, buffy coat AND complete (CBC), automated (85009, 85027)
OR
Automated differential WBC count
Automated differential WBC count AND complete (CBC), automated/automated differential WBC count (85004, 85025)
Automated differential WBC count AND complete (CBC), automated (85004, 85027)
Comprehensive metabolic profile (80053)
Thyroid stimulating hormone (84443)

🚑 0.00   ⚕ 0.00   **FUD** XXX   Ⓔ

**AMA:** 2017,Jan,8; 2016,Jan,13; 2015,Jan,16; 2014,Jan,11; 2012,Jan,15-42

### 80051 Electrolyte panel

INCLUDES Carbon dioxide (bicarbonate) (82374)
Chloride (82435)
Potassium (84132)
Sodium (84295)

🚑 0.00   ⚕ 0.00   **FUD** XXX   ☒ Ⓠ ▢

**AMA:** 2017,Jan,8; 2016,Jan,13; 2015,Jan,16; 2014,Jan,11; 2012,Jan,15-42

### 80053 Comprehensive metabolic panel

INCLUDES Albumin (82040)
Bilirubin, total (82247)
Calcium, total (82310)
Carbon dioxide (bicarbonate) (82374)
Chloride (82435)
Creatinine (82565)
Glucose (82947)
Phosphatase, alkaline (84075)
Potassium (84132)
Protein, total (84155)
Sodium (84295)
Transferase, alanine amino (ALT) (SGPT) (84460)
Transferase, aspartate amino (AST) (SGOT) (84450)
Urea nitrogen (BUN) (84520)

🚑 0.00   ⚕ 0.00   **FUD** XXX   ☒ Ⓠ ▢

**AMA:** 2017,Jan,8; 2016,Jan,13; 2015,Jan,16; 2014,Jan,11; 2013,Apr,10-11; 2012,Jan,15-42

### 80055 Obstetric panel                               Ⓜ ♀

INCLUDES Complete blood count (CBC), automated, with:
Manual differential WBC count
Blood smear with manual differential AND complete (CBC), automated (85007, 85027)
Manual differential WBC count, buffy coat AND complete (CBC), automated (85009, 85027)
OR
Automated differential WBC count
Automated differential WBC count AND complete (CBC), automated/automated differential WBC count (85004, 85025)
Automated differential WBC count AND complete (CBC), automated (85004, 85027)
Blood typing, ABO and Rh (86900-86901)
Hepatitis B surface antigen (HBsAg) (87340)
RBC antibody screen, each serum technique (86850)
Rubella antibody (86762)
Syphilis test, non-treponemal antibody qualitative (86592)

EXCLUDES *Use of code when syphilis screening is provided using a treponemal antibody approach. Instead, assign individual codes for tests performed in the OB panel (86780)*

🚑 0.00   ⚕ 0.00   **FUD** XXX   Ⓔ

**AMA:** 2017,Jan,8; 2016,Jan,13; 2015,Jan,16; 2014,Jan,11; 2012,Jan,15-42

### # 80081 Obstetric panel (includes HIV testing)          ♀

INCLUDES Complete blood count (CBC), automated, with:
Manual differential WBC count
Blood smear with manual differential AND complete (CBC), automated (85007, 85027)
Manual differential WBC count, buffy count AND complete (CBC), automated (85009, 85027)
OR
Automated differential WBC count
Automated differential WBC count AND complete (CBC), automated/automated differential WBC count (85004, 85025)
Automated differential WBC count AND complete (CBC), automated (85004, 85027)
Blood typing, ABO and Rh (86900-86901)
Hepatitis B surface antigen (HBsAg) (87340)
HIV-1 antigens, with HIV-1 and HIV-2 antibodies, single result (87389)
RBC antibody screen, each serum technique (86850)
Rubella antibody (86762)
Syphilis test, non-treponemal antibody qualitative (86592)

EXCLUDES *Use of code when syphilis screening is provided using a treponemal antibody approach. Instead, assign individual codes for tests performed in the OB panel (86780)*

🚑 0.00   ⚕ 0.00   **FUD** XXX   Ⓠ ▢

**AMA:** 2017,Jan,8; 2016,Jan,13

### 80061 Lipid panel

INCLUDES  Cholesterol, serum, total (82465)
Lipoprotein, direct measurement, high density cholesterol (HDL cholesterol) (83718)
Triglycerides (84478)

🖥 0.00   ⚗ 0.00   **FUD** XXX   🅧 Ⓐ ▭

**AMA:** 2017,Sep,11; 2017,Jan,8; 2016,Jan,13; 2015,Jan,16; 2014,Jan,11; 2012,Jan,15-42

### 80069 Renal function panel

INCLUDES  Albumin (82040)
Calcium, total (82310)
Carbon dioxide (bicarbonate) (82374)
Chloride (82435)
Creatinine (82565)
Glucose (82947)
Phosphorus inorganic (phosphate) (84100)
Potassium (84132)
Sodium (84295)
Urea nitrogen (BUN) (84520)

🖥 0.00   ⚗ 0.00   **FUD** XXX   🅧 Ⓠ ▭

**AMA:** 2017,Jan,8; 2016,Jan,13; 2015,Jan,16; 2014,Jan,11; 2012,Jan,15-42

### 80074 Acute hepatitis panel

INCLUDES  Hepatitis A antibody (HAAb) IgM (86709)
Hepatitis B core antibody (HBcAb), IgM (86705)
Hepatitis B surface antigen (HBsAg) (87340)
Hepatitis C antibody (86803)

🖥 0.00   ⚗ 0.00   **FUD** XXX   Ⓠ ▭

**AMA:** 2017,Jan,8; 2016,Jan,13; 2015,Jan,16; 2014,Jan,11; 2012,Jan,15-42

### 80076 Hepatic function panel

INCLUDES  Albumin (82040)
Bilirubin, direct (82248)
Bilirubin, total (82247)
Phosphatase, alkaline (84075)
Protein, total (84155)
Transferase, alanine amino (ALT) (SGPT) (84460)
Transferase, aspartate amino (AST) (SGOT) (84450)

🖥 0.00   ⚗ 0.00   **FUD** XXX   Ⓠ ▭

**AMA:** 2017,Jan,8; 2016,Jan,13; 2015,Jan,16; 2014,Jan,11; 2012,Jan,15-42

*80081*  Resequenced code. See code following 80055.

## [80305, 80306, 80307] Nonspecific Drug Screening

INCLUDES  All testing procedures provided despite the number of tests performed per modality
EXCLUDES  *Confirmatory drug testing ([80320, 80321, 80322, 80323, 80324, 80325, 80326, 80327, 80328, 80329, 80330, 80331, 80332, 80333, 80334, 80335, 80336, 80337, 80338, 80339, 80340, 80341, 80342, 80343, 80344, 80345, 80346, 80347, 80348, 80349, 80350, 80351, 80352, 80353, 80354, 80355, 80356, 80357, 80358, 80359, 80360, 80361, 80362, 80363, 80364, 80365, 80366, 80367, 80368, 80369, 80370, 80371, 80372, 80373, 80374, 80375, 80376, 80377, 83992], [83992])*
*Validation testing*

▲ # **80305**  Drug test(s), presumptive, any number of drug classes, any number of devices or procedures; capable of being read by direct optical observation only (eg, utilizing immunoassay [eg, dipsticks, cups, cards, or cartridges]), includes sample validation when performed, per date of service

🖥 0.00   ⚗ 0.00   **FUD** XXX   🅧 Ⓠ ▭

**AMA:** 2017,Mar,6

▲ # **80306**  read by instrument assisted direct optical observation (eg, utilizing immunoassay [eg, dipsticks, cups, cards, or cartridges]), includes sample validation when performed, per date of service

🖥 0.00   ⚗ 0.00   **FUD** XXX   Ⓠ ▭

**AMA:** 2017,Mar,6

▲ # **80307**  by instrument chemistry analyzers (eg, utilizing immunoassay [eg, EIA, ELISA, EMIT, FPIA, IA, KIMS, RIA]), chromatography (eg, GC, HPLC), and mass spectrometry either with or without chromatography, (eg, DART, DESI, GC-MS, GC-MS/MS, LC-MS, LC-MS/MS, LDTD, MALDI, TOF) includes sample validation when performed, per date of service

🖥 0.00   ⚗ 0.00   **FUD** XXX   Ⓠ ▭

**AMA:** 2017,Mar,6

## [80320, 80321, 80322, 80323, 80324, 80325, 80326, 80327, 80328, 80329, 80330, 80331, 80332, 80333, 80334, 80335, 80336, 80337, 80338, 80339, 80340, 80341, 80342, 80343, 80344, 80345, 80346, 80347, 80348, 80349, 80350, 80351, 80352, 80353, 80354, 80355, 80356, 80357, 80358, 80359, 80360, 80361, 80362, 80363, 80364, 80365, 80366, 80367, 80368, 80369, 80370, 80371, 80372, 80373, 80374, 80375, 80376, 80377, 83992] Confirmatory Drug Testing

INCLUDES  Antihistamine drug tests ([80375, 80376, 80377])
Detection of specific drugs using methods other than immunoassay or enzymatic technique
EXCLUDES  *Metabolites separate from the code for the drug except when a distinct code is available*

# **80320  Alcohols**

🖥 0.00   ⚗ 0.00   **FUD** XXX   Ⓑ

**AMA:** 2017,Jan,8; 2016,Jan,13; 2015,Apr,3

# **80321  Alcohol biomarkers; 1 or 2**

🖥 0.00   ⚗ 0.00   **FUD** XXX   Ⓑ

**AMA:** 2015,Apr,3

# **80322  3 or more**

🖥 0.00   ⚗ 0.00   **FUD** XXX   Ⓑ

**AMA:** 2015,Apr,3

# **80323  Alkaloids, not otherwise specified**

🖥 0.00   ⚗ 0.00   **FUD** XXX   Ⓑ

**AMA:** 2015,Apr,3

# **80324  Amphetamines; 1 or 2**

🖥 0.00   ⚗ 0.00   **FUD** XXX   Ⓑ

**AMA:** 2015,Apr,3

# **80325  3 or 4**

🖥 0.00   ⚗ 0.00   **FUD** XXX   Ⓑ

**AMA:** 2015,Apr,3

# **80326  5 or more**

🖥 0.00   ⚗ 0.00   **FUD** XXX   Ⓑ

**AMA:** 2015,Apr,3

# **80327  Anabolic steroids; 1 or 2**

🖥 0.00   ⚗ 0.00   **FUD** XXX   Ⓑ

**AMA:** 2015,Apr,3

# **80328  3 or more**

🖥 0.00   ⚗ 0.00   **FUD** XXX   Ⓑ

**AMA:** 2015,Apr,3

# **80329  Analgesics, non-opioid; 1 or 2**

🖥 0.00   ⚗ 0.00   **FUD** XXX   Ⓑ

**AMA:** 2015,Apr,3

# **80330  3-5**

🖥 0.00   ⚗ 0.00   **FUD** XXX   Ⓑ

**AMA:** 2015,Apr,3

# **80331  6 or more**

🖥 0.00   ⚗ 0.00   **FUD** XXX   Ⓑ

**AMA:** 2015,Apr,3

# **80332  Antidepressants, serotonergic class; 1 or 2**

🖥 0.00   ⚗ 0.00   **FUD** XXX   Ⓑ

**AMA:** 2015,Apr,3

26/TC PC/TC Only   A2-A8 ASC Payment   50 Bilateral   ♂ Male Only   ♀ Female Only   🖥 Facility RVU   ⚗ Non-Facility RVU   ▭ CCI
FUD Follow-up Days   CMS: IOM (Pub 100)   A-Y OPPSI   80/80 Surg Assist Allowed / w/Doc   🔲 Lab Crosswalk   🔲 Radiology Crosswalk   🅧 CLIA
CPT © 2017 American Medical Association. All Rights Reserved.   © 2017 Optum360, LLC

| # | 80333 | 3-5 |
|---|---|---|
| | | 🚑 0.00  🔪 0.00  **FUD** XXX  Ⓑ |
| | | **AMA:** 2015,Apr,3 |

| # | 80334 | 6 or more |
|---|---|---|
| | | 🚑 0.00  🔪 0.00  **FUD** XXX  Ⓑ |
| | | **AMA:** 2015,Apr,3 |

| # | 80335 | Antidepressants, tricyclic and other cyclicals; 1 or 2 |
|---|---|---|
| | | 🚑 0.00  🔪 0.00  **FUD** XXX  Ⓑ |
| | | **AMA:** 2015,Apr,3 |

| # | 80336 | 3-5 |
|---|---|---|
| | | 🚑 0.00  🔪 0.00  **FUD** XXX  Ⓑ |
| | | **AMA:** 2015,Apr,3 |

| # | 80337 | 6 or more |
|---|---|---|
| | | 🚑 0.00  🔪 0.00  **FUD** XXX  Ⓑ |
| | | **AMA:** 2015,Apr,3 |

| # | 80338 | Antidepressants, not otherwise specified |
|---|---|---|
| | | 🚑 0.00  🔪 0.00  **FUD** XXX  Ⓑ |
| | | **AMA:** 2015,Apr,3 |

| # | 80339 | Antiepileptics, not otherwise specified; 1-3 |
|---|---|---|
| | | 🚑 0.00  🔪 0.00  **FUD** XXX  Ⓑ |
| | | **AMA:** 2015,Apr,3 |

| # | 80340 | 4-6 |
|---|---|---|
| | | 🚑 0.00  🔪 0.00  **FUD** XXX  Ⓑ |
| | | **AMA:** 2015,Apr,3 |

| # | 80341 | 7 or more |
|---|---|---|
| | | 🚑 0.00  🔪 0.00  **FUD** XXX  Ⓑ |
| | | **AMA:** 2015,Apr,3 |

| # | 80342 | Antipsychotics, not otherwise specified; 1-3 |
|---|---|---|
| | | 🚑 0.00  🔪 0.00  **FUD** XXX  Ⓑ |
| | | **AMA:** 2015,Apr,3 |

| # | 80343 | 4-6 |
|---|---|---|
| | | 🚑 0.00  🔪 0.00  **FUD** XXX  Ⓑ |
| | | **AMA:** 2015,Apr,3 |

| # | 80344 | 7 or more |
|---|---|---|
| | | 🚑 0.00  🔪 0.00  **FUD** XXX  Ⓑ |
| | | **AMA:** 2015,Apr,3 |

| # | 80345 | Barbiturates |
|---|---|---|
| | | 🚑 0.00  🔪 0.00  **FUD** XXX  Ⓑ |
| | | **AMA:** 2015,Apr,3 |

| # | 80346 | Benzodiazepines; 1-12 |
|---|---|---|
| | | 🚑 0.00  🔪 0.00  **FUD** XXX  Ⓑ |
| | | **AMA:** 2015,Apr,3 |

| # | 80347 | 13 or more |
|---|---|---|
| | | 🚑 0.00  🔪 0.00  **FUD** XXX  Ⓑ |
| | | **AMA:** 2015,Apr,3 |

| # | 80348 | Buprenorphine |
|---|---|---|
| | | 🚑 0.00  🔪 0.00  **FUD** XXX  Ⓑ |
| | | **AMA:** 2015,Apr,3 |

| # | 80349 | Cannabinoids, natural |
|---|---|---|
| | | 🚑 0.00  🔪 0.00  **FUD** XXX  Ⓑ |
| | | **AMA:** 2015,Apr,3 |

| # | 80350 | Cannabinoids, synthetic; 1-3 |
|---|---|---|
| | | 🚑 0.00  🔪 0.00  **FUD** XXX  Ⓑ |
| | | **AMA:** 2015,Apr,3 |

| # | 80351 | 4-6 |
|---|---|---|
| | | 🚑 0.00  🔪 0.00  **FUD** XXX  Ⓑ |
| | | **AMA:** 2015,Apr,3 |

| # | 80352 | 7 or more |
|---|---|---|
| | | 🚑 0.00  🔪 0.00  **FUD** XXX  Ⓑ |
| | | **AMA:** 2015,Apr,3 |

| # | 80353 | Cocaine |
|---|---|---|
| | | 🚑 0.00  🔪 0.00  **FUD** XXX  Ⓑ |
| | | **AMA:** 2015,Apr,3 |

| # | 80354 | Fentanyl |
|---|---|---|
| | | 🚑 0.00  🔪 0.00  **FUD** XXX  Ⓑ |
| | | **AMA:** 2015,Apr,3 |

| # | 80355 | Gabapentin, non-blood |
|---|---|---|
| | | 🚑 0.00  🔪 0.00  **FUD** XXX  Ⓑ |
| | | **AMA:** 2017,Jan,8; 2016,Jan,13; 2015,Apr,3 |

| # | 80356 | Heroin metabolite |
|---|---|---|
| | | 🚑 0.00  🔪 0.00  **FUD** XXX  Ⓑ |
| | | **AMA:** 2015,Apr,3 |

| # | 80357 | Ketamine and norketamine |
|---|---|---|
| | | 🚑 0.00  🔪 0.00  **FUD** XXX  Ⓑ |
| | | **AMA:** 2015,Apr,3 |

| # | 80358 | Methadone |
|---|---|---|
| | | 🚑 0.00  🔪 0.00  **FUD** XXX  Ⓑ |
| | | **AMA:** 2015,Apr,3 |

| # | 80359 | Methylenedioxyamphetamines (MDA, MDEA, MDMA) |
|---|---|---|
| | | 🚑 0.00  🔪 0.00  **FUD** XXX  Ⓑ |
| | | **AMA:** 2015,Apr,3 |

| # | 80360 | Methylphenidate |
|---|---|---|
| | | 🚑 0.00  🔪 0.00  **FUD** XXX  Ⓑ |
| | | **AMA:** 2015,Apr,3 |

| # | 80361 | Opiates, 1 or more |
|---|---|---|
| | | 🚑 0.00  🔪 0.00  **FUD** XXX  Ⓑ |
| | | **AMA:** 2015,Apr,3 |

| # | 80362 | Opioids and opiate analogs; 1 or 2 |
|---|---|---|
| | | 🚑 0.00  🔪 0.00  **FUD** XXX  Ⓑ |
| | | **AMA:** 2015,Apr,3 |

| # | 80363 | 3 or 4 |
|---|---|---|
| | | 🚑 0.00  🔪 0.00  **FUD** XXX  Ⓑ |
| | | **AMA:** 2015,Apr,3 |

| # | 80364 | 5 or more |
|---|---|---|
| | | 🚑 0.00  🔪 0.00  **FUD** XXX  Ⓑ |
| | | **AMA:** 2015,Apr,3 |

| # | 80365 | Oxycodone |
|---|---|---|
| | | 🚑 0.00  🔪 0.00  **FUD** XXX  Ⓑ |
| | | **AMA:** 2015,Apr,3 |

| # | 83992 | Phencyclidine (PCP) |
|---|---|---|
| | | 🚑 0.00  🔪 0.00  **FUD** XXX  Ⓑ |
| | | **AMA:** 2017,Jan,8; 2016,Jan,13; 2015,Jun,10; 2015,Apr,3 |

| # | 80366 | Pregabalin |
|---|---|---|
| | | 🚑 0.00  🔪 0.00  **FUD** XXX  Ⓑ |
| | | **AMA:** 2015,Apr,3 |

| # | 80367 | Propoxyphene |
|---|---|---|
| | | 🚑 0.00  🔪 0.00  **FUD** XXX  Ⓑ |
| | | **AMA:** 2015,Apr,3 |

| # | 80368 | Sedative hypnotics (non-benzodiazepines) |
|---|---|---|
| | | 🚑 0.00  🔪 0.00  **FUD** XXX  Ⓑ |
| | | **AMA:** 2015,Apr,3 |

| # | 80369 | Skeletal muscle relaxants; 1 or 2 |
|---|---|---|
| | | 🚑 0.00  🔪 0.00  **FUD** XXX  Ⓑ |
| | | **AMA:** 2015,Apr,3 |

| # | 80370 | 3 or more |
|---|---|---|
| | | 🚑 0.00  🔪 0.00  **FUD** XXX  Ⓑ |
| | | **AMA:** 2015,Apr,3 |

| # | 80371 | Stimulants, synthetic |
|---|---|---|
| | | 🚑 0.00  🔪 0.00  **FUD** XXX  Ⓑ |
| | | **AMA:** 2015,Apr,3 |

| # | 80372 | Tapentadol |
|---|---|---|
| | | 🚑 0.00  🔪 0.00  **FUD** XXX  Ⓑ |
| | | **AMA:** 2015,Apr,3 |

| # | 80373 | Tramadol |
|---|---|---|
| | | 🚑 0.00  🔪 0.00  **FUD** XXX  Ⓑ |
| | | **AMA:** 2015,Apr,3 |

---

● New Code   ▲ Revised Code   ○ Reinstated   ● New Web Release   ▲ Revised Web Release   Unlisted   Not Covered   # Resequenced
Ⓢ AMA Mod 51 Exempt   Ⓢ Optum Mod 51 Exempt   ⑥③ Mod 63 Exempt   ✚ Non-FDA Drug   ★ Telemedicine   Ⓜ Maternity   Ⓐ Age Edit   ✚ Add-on   **AMA:** CPT Asst

| # | 80374 | **Stereoisomer (enantiomer) analysis, single drug class** | | | |
|---|---|---|---|---|---|

# | 80374 | **Stereoisomer (enantiomer) analysis, single drug class**
Code also index drug analysis if appropriate
🚑 0.00　🔪 0.00　**FUD** XXX　　　　B
**AMA:** 2015,Apr,3

# | 80375 | **Drug(s) or substance(s), definitive, qualitative or quantitative, not otherwise specified; 1-3**
🚑 0.00　🔪 0.00　**FUD** XXX　　　　B
**AMA:** 2017,Jan,8; 2016,Jan,13; 2015,Apr,3

# | 80376 | **4-6**
🚑 0.00　🔪 0.00　**FUD** XXX　　　　B
**AMA:** 2017,Jan,8; 2016,Jan,13; 2015,Apr,3

# | 80377 | **7 or more**
🚑 0.00　🔪 0.00　**FUD** XXX　　　　B
**AMA:** 2017,Jan,8; 2016,Jan,13; 2015,Apr,3

## 80150-80377 [80164, 80165, 80171] Therapeutic Drug Levels

INCLUDES　Testing of drug and metabolite(s) in primary code
Tests on specimens from blood and blood components, and spinal fluid

80150　**Amikacin**
🚑 0.00　🔪 0.00　**FUD** XXX　　　　Q
**AMA:** 2017,Jan,8; 2016,Jan,13; 2015,Apr,3; 2015,Jan,16; 2014,Jan,11; 2012,Jan,15-42

80155　**Caffeine**
🚑 0.00　🔪 0.00　**FUD** XXX　　　　Q
**AMA:** 2015,Apr,3; 2014,Jan,11

80156　**Carbamazepine; total**
🚑 0.00　🔪 0.00　**FUD** XXX　　　　Q
**AMA:** 2017,Jan,8; 2016,Jan,13; 2015,Apr,3; 2015,Jan,16; 2014,Jan,11

80157　**free**
🚑 0.00　🔪 0.00　**FUD** XXX　　　　Q
**AMA:** 2017,Jan,8; 2016,Jan,13; 2015,Apr,3; 2015,Jan,16; 2014,Jan,11

80158　**Cyclosporine**
🚑 0.00　🔪 0.00　**FUD** XXX　　　　Q
**AMA:** 2017,Jan,8; 2016,Jan,13; 2015,Apr,3; 2015,Jan,16; 2014,Jan,11

80159　**Clozapine**
🚑 0.00　🔪 0.00　**FUD** XXX　　　　Q
**AMA:** 2015,Apr,3; 2014,Jan,11

80162　**Digoxin; total**
🚑 0.00　🔪 0.00　**FUD** XXX　　　　Q
**AMA:** 2017,Jan,8; 2016,Jan,13; 2015,Apr,3; 2015,Jan,16; 2014,Jan,11

80163　**free**
🚑 0.00　🔪 0.00　**FUD** XXX　　　　Q
**AMA:** 2017,Jan,8; 2016,Jan,13; 2015,Apr,3

*80164*　**Resequenced code. See code following 80201.**

*80165*　**Resequenced code. See code following 80201.**

80168　**Ethosuximide**
🚑 0.00　🔪 0.00　**FUD** XXX　　　　Q
**AMA:** 2017,Jan,8; 2016,Jan,13; 2015,Apr,3; 2015,Jan,16; 2014,Jan,11

80169　**Everolimus**
🚑 0.00　🔪 0.00　**FUD** XXX　　　　Q
**AMA:** 2015,Apr,3; 2014,Jan,11

# | 80171 | **Gabapentin, whole blood, serum, or plasma**
🚑 0.00　🔪 0.00　**FUD** XXX　　　　Q
**AMA:** 2017,Jan,8; 2016,Jan,13; 2015,Apr,3; 2014,Jan,11

80170　**Gentamicin**
🚑 0.00　🔪 0.00　**FUD** XXX　　　　Q
**AMA:** 2017,Jan,8; 2016,Jan,13; 2015,Apr,3; 2015,Jan,16; 2014,Jan,11

*80171*　**Resequenced code. See code following 80169.**

80173　**Haloperidol**
🚑 0.00　🔪 0.00　**FUD** XXX　　　　Q
**AMA:** 2017,Jan,8; 2016,Jan,13; 2015,Apr,3; 2015,Jan,16; 2014,Jan,11

80175　**Lamotrigine**
🚑 0.00　🔪 0.00　**FUD** XXX　　　　Q
**AMA:** 2015,Apr,3; 2014,Jan,11

80176　**Lidocaine**
🚑 0.00　🔪 0.00　**FUD** XXX　　　　Q
**AMA:** 2017,Jan,8; 2016,Jan,13; 2015,Apr,3; 2015,Jan,16; 2014,Jan,11

80177　**Levetiracetam**
🚑 0.00　🔪 0.00　**FUD** XXX　　　　Q
**AMA:** 2015,Apr,3; 2014,Jan,11

80178　**Lithium**
🚑 0.00　🔪 0.00　**FUD** XXX　　　　X Q
**AMA:** 2017,Jan,8; 2016,Jan,13; 2015,Apr,3; 2015,Jan,16; 2014,Jan,11

80180　**Mycophenolate (mycophenolic acid)**
🚑 0.00　🔪 0.00　**FUD** XXX　　　　Q
**AMA:** 2015,Apr,3; 2014,Jan,11

80183　**Oxcarbazepine**
🚑 0.00　🔪 0.00　**FUD** XXX　　　　Q
**AMA:** 2015,Apr,3; 2014,Jan,11

80184　**Phenobarbital**
🚑 0.00　🔪 0.00　**FUD** XXX　　　　Q
**AMA:** 2017,Jan,8; 2016,Jan,13; 2015,Apr,3; 2015,Jan,16; 2014,Jan,11

80185　**Phenytoin; total**
🚑 0.00　🔪 0.00　**FUD** XXX　　　　Q
**AMA:** 2017,Jan,8; 2016,Jan,13; 2015,Apr,3; 2015,Jan,16; 2014,Jan,11

80186　**free**
🚑 0.00　🔪 0.00　**FUD** XXX　　　　Q
**AMA:** 2017,Jan,8; 2016,Jan,13; 2015,Apr,3; 2015,Jan,16; 2014,Jan,11

80188　**Primidone**
🚑 0.00　🔪 0.00　**FUD** XXX　　　　Q
**AMA:** 2017,Jan,8; 2016,Jan,13; 2015,Apr,3; 2015,Jan,16; 2014,Jan,11

80190　**Procainamide;**
🚑 0.00　🔪 0.00　**FUD** XXX　　　　Q
**AMA:** 2017,Jan,8; 2016,Jan,13; 2015,Apr,3; 2015,Jan,16; 2014,Jan,11

80192　**with metabolites (eg, n-acetyl procainamide)**
🚑 0.00　🔪 0.00　**FUD** XXX　　　　Q ⬜
**AMA:** 2017,Jan,8; 2016,Jan,13; 2015,Apr,3; 2015,Jan,16; 2014,Jan,11

80194　**Quinidine**
🚑 0.00　🔪 0.00　**FUD** XXX　　　　Q
**AMA:** 2017,Jan,8; 2016,Jan,13; 2015,Apr,3; 2015,Jan,16; 2014,Jan,11

80195　**Sirolimus**
🚑 0.00　🔪 0.00　**FUD** XXX　　　　Q
**AMA:** 2017,Jan,8; 2016,Jan,13; 2015,Apr,3; 2015,Jan,16; 2014,Jan,11

80197　**Tacrolimus**
🚑 0.00　🔪 0.00　**FUD** XXX　　　　Q
**AMA:** 2017,Jan,8; 2016,Jan,13; 2015,Apr,3; 2015,Jan,16; 2014,Jan,11

80198　**Theophylline**
🚑 0.00　🔪 0.00　**FUD** XXX　　　　Q
**AMA:** 2017,Jan,8; 2016,Jan,13; 2015,Apr,3; 2015,Jan,16; 2014,Jan,11

80199　**Tiagabine**
🚑 0.00　🔪 0.00　**FUD** XXX　　　　Q
**AMA:** 2015,Apr,3; 2014,Jan,11

---

26/TC PC/TC Only　　42-Z3 ASC Payment　　50 Bilateral　　♂ Male Only　　♀ Female Only　　🚑 Facility RVU　　🔪 Non-Facility RVU　　⬜ CCI
**FUD** Follow-up Days　　**CMS:** IOM (Pub 100)　　A-Y OPPSI　　80/80 Surg Assist Allowed / w/Doc　　🔲 Lab Crosswalk　　❌ Radiology Crosswalk　　❌ CLIA

CPT © 2017 American Medical Association. All Rights Reserved.　　　　© 2017 Optum360, LLC

**80200** **Tobramycin**
🔲 0.00    ⅍ 0.00    **FUD** XXX    [Q]
**AMA:** 2017,Jan,8; 2016,Jan,13; 2015,Apr,3; 2015,Jan,16; 2014,Jan,11

**80201** **Topiramate**
🔲 0.00    ⅍ 0.00    **FUD** XXX    [Q]
**AMA:** 2017,Jan,8; 2016,Jan,13; 2015,Apr,3; 2015,Jan,16; 2014,Jan,11

# **80164** **Valproic acid (dipropylacetic acid); total**
🔲 0.00    ⅍ 0.00    **FUD** XXX    [Q]
**AMA:** 2017,Jan,8; 2016,Jan,13; 2015,Apr,3; 2015,Jan,16; 2014,Jan,11

# **80165** **free**
🔲 0.00    ⅍ 0.00    **FUD** XXX    [Q]
**AMA:** 2017,Jan,8; 2016,Jan,13; 2015,Apr,3

**80202** **Vancomycin**
🔲 0.00    ⅍ 0.00    **FUD** XXX    [Q]
**AMA:** 2017,Jan,8; 2016,Jan,13; 2015,Apr,3; 2015,Jan,16; 2014,Jan,11; 2012,Jan,15-42

**80203** **Zonisamide**
🔲 0.00    ⅍ 0.00    **FUD** XXX    [Q]
**AMA:** 2015,Apr,3; 2014,Jan,11

**80299** **Quantitation of therapeutic drug, not elsewhere specified**
🔲 0.00    ⅍ 0.00    **FUD** XXX    [Q]
**AMA:** 2017,Jan,8; 2016,Jan,13; 2015,Apr,3; 2015,Jan,16; 2014,Jan,11; 2012,Jan,15-42

*80305* Resequenced code. See code before 80150.

*80306* Resequenced code. See code before 80150.

*80307* Resequenced code. See code before 80150.

*80320* Resequenced code. See code before 80150.

*80321* Resequenced code. See code before 80150.

*80322* Resequenced code. See code before 80150.

*80323* Resequenced code. See code before 80150.

*80324* Resequenced code. See code before 80150.

*80325* Resequenced code. See code before 80150.

*80326* Resequenced code. See code before 80150.

*80327* Resequenced code. See code before 80150.

*80328* Resequenced code. See code before 80150.

*80329* Resequenced code. See code before 80150.

*80330* Resequenced code. See code before 80150.

*80331* Resequenced code. See code before 80150.

*80332* Resequenced code. See code before 80150.

*80333* Resequenced code. See code before 80150.

*80334* Resequenced code. See code before 80150.

*80335* Resequenced code. See code before 80150.

*80336* Resequenced code. See code before 80150.

*80337* Resequenced code. See code before 80150.

*80338* Resequenced code. See code before 80150.

*80339* Resequenced code. See code before 80150.

*80340* Resequenced code. See code before 80150.

*80341* Resequenced code. See code before 80150.

*80342* Resequenced code. See code before 80150.

*80343* Resequenced code. See code before 80150.

*80344* Resequenced code. See code before 80150.

*80345* Resequenced code. See code before 80150.

*80346* Resequenced code. See code before 80150.

*80347* Resequenced code. See code before 80150.

*80348* Resequenced code. See code before 80150.

*80349* Resequenced code. See code before 80150.

*80350* Resequenced code. See code before 80150.

*80351* Resequenced code. See code before 80150.

*80352* Resequenced code. See code before 80150.

*80353* Resequenced code. See code before 80150.

*80354* Resequenced code. See code before 80150.

*80355* Resequenced code. See code before 80150.

*80356* Resequenced code. See code before 80150.

*80357* Resequenced code. See code before 80150.

*80358* Resequenced code. See code before 80150.

*80359* Resequenced code. See code before 80150.

*80360* Resequenced code. See code before 80150.

*80361* Resequenced code. See code before 80150.

*80362* Resequenced code. See code before 80150.

*80363* Resequenced code. See code before 80150.

*80364* Resequenced code. See code before 80150.

*80365* Resequenced code. See code before 80150.

*80366* Resequenced code. See code before 80150.

*80367* Resequenced code. See code before 80150.

*80368* Resequenced code. See code before 80150.

*80369* Resequenced code. See code before 80150.

*80370* Resequenced code. See code before 80150.

*80371* Resequenced code. See code before 80150.

*80372* Resequenced code. See code before 80150.

*80373* Resequenced code. See code before 80150.

*80374* Resequenced code. See code before 80150.

*80375* Resequenced code. See code before 80150.

*80376* Resequenced code. See code before 80150.

*80377* Resequenced code. See code before 80150.

## 80400-80439 Stimulation and Suppression Test Panels

**EXCLUDES** *Administration of evocative or suppressive material (96365-96368, 96372, 96374-96376, C8957)*
*Evocative or suppression test substances, as applicable*
*Physician monitoring and attendance during test (see E&M services)*

**80400** **ACTH stimulation panel; for adrenal insufficiency**
**INCLUDES** Cortisol x 2 (82533)
🔲 0.00    ⅍ 0.00    **FUD** XXX    [Q][M]
**AMA:** 2017,Jan,8; 2016,Jan,13; 2015,Jan,16; 2014,Jan,11

**80402** **for 21 hydroxylase deficiency**
**INCLUDES** 17 hydroxyprogesterone X 2 (83498)
Cortisol x 2 (82533)
🔲 0.00    ⅍ 0.00    **FUD** XXX    [Q][M]
**AMA:** 2014,Jan,11

**80406** **for 3 beta-hydroxydehydrogenase deficiency**
**INCLUDES** 17 hydroxypregnenolone x 2 (84143)
Cortisol x 2 (82533)
🔲 0.00    ⅍ 0.00    **FUD** XXX    [Q][M]
**AMA:** 2014,Jan,11

**80408** **Aldosterone suppression evaluation panel (eg, saline infusion)**
**INCLUDES** Aldosterone x 2 (82088)
Renin x 2 (84244)
🔲 0.00    ⅍ 0.00    **FUD** XXX    [Q][M]
**AMA:** 2014,Jan,11

**80410** **Calcitonin stimulation panel (eg, calcium, pentagastrin)**
**INCLUDES** Calcitonin x 3 (82308)
🔲 0.00    ⅍ 0.00    **FUD** XXX    [Q][M]
**AMA:** 2014,Jan,11

---

● New Code    ▲ Revised Code    ○ Reinstated    ● New Web Release    ▲ Revised Web Release    Unlisted    Not Covered    # Resequenced
⊘ AMA Mod 51 Exempt    ⑨ Optum Mod 51 Exempt    ⊚ Mod 63 Exempt    ✓ Non-FDA Drug    ★ Telemedicine    Ⓜ Maternity    Ⓐ Age Edit    ＋ Add-on    **AMA:** CPT Asst

© 2017 Optum360, LLC    CPT © 2017 American Medical Association. All Rights Reserved.

**80412** Corticotropic releasing hormone (CRH) stimulation panel
INCLUDES Adrenocorticotropic hormone (ACTH) x 6 (82024)
Cortisol x 6 (82533)
0.00   0.00   **FUD** XXX
AMA: 2014,Jan,11

**80414** Chorionic gonadotropin stimulation panel; testosterone response
INCLUDES Testosterone x 2 on three pooled blood samples (84403)
0.00   0.00   **FUD** XXX
AMA: 2014,Jan,11

**80415** estradiol response
INCLUDES Estradiol x 2 on three pooled blood samples (82670)
0.00   0.00   **FUD** XXX
AMA: 2014,Jan,11

**80416** Renal vein renin stimulation panel (eg, captopril)
INCLUDES Renin x 6 (84244)
0.00   0.00   **FUD** XXX
AMA: 2014,Jan,11

**80417** Peripheral vein renin stimulation panel (eg, captopril)
INCLUDES Renin x 2 (84244)
0.00   0.00   **FUD** XXX
AMA: 2014,Jan,11

**80418** Combined rapid anterior pituitary evaluation panel
INCLUDES Adrenocorticotropic hormone (ACTH) x 4 (82024)
Cortisol x 4 (82533)
Follicle stimulating hormone (FSH) x 4 (83001)
Human growth hormone x 4 (83003)
Luteinizing hormone (LH) x 4 (83002)
Prolactin x 4 (84146)
Thyroid stimulating hormone (TSH) x 4 (84443)
0.00   0.00   **FUD** XXX
AMA: 2014,Jan,11

**80420** Dexamethasone suppression panel, 48 hour
INCLUDES Cortisol x 2 (82533)
Free cortisol, urine x 2 (82530)
Volume measurement for timed collection x 2 (81050)
EXCLUDES Single dose dexamethasone (82533)
0.00   0.00   **FUD** XXX
AMA: 2014,Jan,11

**80422** Glucagon tolerance panel; for insulinoma
INCLUDES Glucose x 3 (82947)
Insulin x 3 (83525)
0.00   0.00   **FUD** XXX
AMA: 2014,Jan,11

**80424** for pheochromocytoma
INCLUDES Catecholamines, fractionated x 2 (82384)
0.00   0.00   **FUD** XXX
AMA: 2014,Jan,11

**80426** Gonadotropin releasing hormone stimulation panel
INCLUDES Follicle stimulating hormone (FSH) x 4 (83001)
Luteinizing hormone (LH) x 4 (83002)
0.00   0.00   **FUD** XXX
AMA: 2014,Jan,11

**80428** Growth hormone stimulation panel (eg, arginine infusion, l-dopa administration)
INCLUDES Human growth hormone (HGH) x 4 (83003)
0.00   0.00   **FUD** XXX
AMA: 2014,Jan,11

**80430** Growth hormone suppression panel (glucose administration)
INCLUDES Glucose x 3 (82947)
Human growth hormone (HGH) x 4 (83003)
0.00   0.00   **FUD** XXX
AMA: 2014,Jan,11

**80432** Insulin-induced C-peptide suppression panel
INCLUDES C-peptide x 5 (84681)
Glucose x 5 (82947)
Insulin (83525)
0.00   0.00   **FUD** XXX
AMA: 2014,Jan,11

**80434** Insulin tolerance panel; for ACTH insufficiency
INCLUDES Cortisol x 5 (82533)
Glucose x 5 (82947)
0.00   0.00   **FUD** XXX
AMA: 2014,Jan,11

**80435** for growth hormone deficiency
INCLUDES Glucose x 5 (82947)
Human growth hormone (HGH) x 5 (83003)
0.00   0.00   **FUD** XXX
AMA: 2014,Jan,11

**80436** Metyrapone panel
INCLUDES 11 deoxycortisol x 2 (82634)
Cortisol x 2 (82533)
0.00   0.00   **FUD** XXX
AMA: 2014,Jan,11

**80438** Thyrotropin releasing hormone (TRH) stimulation panel; 1 hour
INCLUDES Thyroid stimulating hormone (TSH) x 3 (84443)
0.00   0.00   **FUD** XXX
AMA: 2014,Jan,11

**80439** 2 hour
INCLUDES Thyroid stimulating hormone (TSH) x 4 (84443)
0.00   0.00   **FUD** XXX
AMA: 2014,Jan,11

## 80500-80502 Consultation By Clinical Pathologist

INCLUDES Pharmacokinetic consultations
Written report by pathologist for tests requiring additional medical judgment and requested by a physician or other qualified health care professional
EXCLUDES Consultations that include patient examination
Use of code when a medical interpretive assessment is not provided

**80500** Clinical pathology consultation; limited, without review of patient's history and medical records
0.57   0.66   **FUD** XXX
AMA: 2017,Jan,8; 2016,Jan,13; 2015,Jan,16; 2014,Jan,11

**80502** comprehensive, for a complex diagnostic problem, with review of patient's history and medical records
2.01   2.09   **FUD** XXX
AMA: 2017,Jan,8; 2016,Jan,13; 2015,Jan,16; 2014,Jan,11

## 81000-81099 Urine Tests

**81000** Urinalysis, by dip stick or tablet reagent for bilirubin, glucose, hemoglobin, ketones, leukocytes, nitrite, pH, protein, specific gravity, urobilinogen, any number of these constituents; non-automated, with microscopy
0.00   0.00   **FUD** XXX
AMA: 2017,Jan,8; 2016,Jan,13; 2015,Jan,16; 2014,Jan,11

**81001** automated, with microscopy
0.00   0.00   **FUD** XXX
AMA: 2014,Jan,11

**81002** non-automated, without microscopy
INCLUDES Mosenthal test
0.00   0.00   **FUD** XXX
AMA: 2017,Jan,8; 2016,Jan,13; 2015,Jan,16; 2014,Jan,11

**81003** automated, without microscopy
0.00   0.00   **FUD** XXX
AMA: 2017,Jan,8; 2016,Jan,13; 2015,Jan,16; 2014,Jan,11

---

**81005**   **Urinalysis; qualitative or semiquantitative, except immunoassays**

> INCLUDES   Benedict test for dextrose
>
> EXCLUDES   *Immunoassay, qualitative or semiquantitative (83518)*
> *Microalbumin (82043-82044)*
> *Nonimmunoassay reagent strip analysis (81000, 81002)*

> 🔲 0.00    ⚕ 0.00    **FUD** XXX                                        Q 🖭

> **AMA:** 2017,Jan,8; 2016,Jan,13; 2015,Jan,16; 2014,Jan,11

**81007**   **bacteriuria screen, except by culture or dipstick**

> EXCLUDES   *Culture (87086-87088)*
> *Dipstick (81000, 81002)*

> 🔲 0.00    ⚕ 0.00    **FUD** XXX                                        ⊠ Q 🖭

> **AMA:** 2014,Jan,11

**81015**   **microscopic only**

> EXCLUDES   *Sperm evaluation for retrograde ejaculation (89331)*

> 🔲 0.00    ⚕ 0.00    **FUD** XXX                                        Q

> **AMA:** 2014,Jan,11

**81020**   **2 or 3 glass test**

> INCLUDES   Valentine's test

> 🔲 0.00    ⚕ 0.00    **FUD** XXX                                        Q 🖭

> **AMA:** 2014,Jan,11

**81025**   **Urine pregnancy test, by visual color comparison methods**                                        Ⓜ ♀

> 🔲 0.00    ⚕ 0.00    **FUD** XXX                                        ⊠ Q

> **AMA:** 2017,Jan,8; 2016,Jan,13; 2015,Jan,16; 2014,Jan,11

**81050**   **Volume measurement for timed collection, each**

> 🔲 0.00    ⚕ 0.00    **FUD** XXX                                        Q

> **AMA:** 2014,Jan,11

**81099**   **Unlisted urinalysis procedure**

> 🔲 0.00    ⚕ 0.00    **FUD** XXX                                        Q

> **AMA:** 2017,Jan,8; 2016,Jan,13; 2015,Jan,16; 2014,Jan,11

## 81105-81364 [81105, 81106, 81107, 81108, 81109, 81110, 81111, 81112, 81120, 81121, 81161, 81162, 81230, 81231, 81238, 81269, 81283, 81287, 81288, 81334] Gene Analysis: Tier 1 Procedures

> INCLUDES   All analytical procedures in the evaluation such as:
> Amplification
> Cell lysis
> Detection
> Digestion
> Extraction
> Nucleic acid stabilization
> Code selection based on specific gene being reviewed
> Evaluation of constitutional or somatic gene variations
> Evaluation of the presence of gene variants using the common gene variant name
> Examples of proteins or diseases in the code description that are not all inclusive
> Generally all the listed gene variants in the code description would be tested but lists are not all inclusive
> Gene specific and genomic testing
> Genes described using Human Genome Organization (HUGO) approved names
> Qualitative results unless otherwise stated
> Tier 1 molecular pathology codes (81200-81355 [81105, 81106, 81107, 81108, 81109, 81110, 81111, 81112, 81120, 81121, 81161, 81162, 81230, 81231, 81238, 81269, 81283, 81287, 81288, 81334])
>
> EXCLUDES   *Full gene sequencing using separate gene variant assessment codes unless it is specifically stated in the code description*
> *In situ hybridization analyses (88271-88275, 88365-88368 [88364, 88373, 88374])*
> *Microbial identification (87149-87153, 87471-87801 [87623, 87624, 87625], 87900-87904 [87906, 87910, 87912])*
> *Other related gene variants not listed in code*
> *Tier 1 molecular pathology codes (81370-81383)*
> *Tier 2 codes (81400-81408)*
> *Unlisted molecular pathology procedures ([81479])*
> Code also modifier 26 when only interpretation and report are performed
> Code also services required before cell lysis

**81105**   **Resequenced code. See code following 81269.**

**81106**   **Resequenced code. See code following 81269.**

**81107**   **Resequenced code. See code following 81269.**

**81108**   **Resequenced code. See code following 81269.**

**81109**   **Resequenced code. See code following 81269.**

**81110**   **Resequenced code. See code following 81269.**

**81111**   **Resequenced code. See code following 81269.**

**81112**   **Resequenced code. See code following 81269.**

**81120**   **Resequenced code. See code following 81269.**

**81121**   **Resequenced code. See code following 81269.**

**81161**   **Resequenced code. See code before 81232.**

**81162**   **Resequenced code. See code following 81211.**

**81170**   **ABL1 (ABL proto-oncogene 1, non-receptor tyrosine kinase) (eg, acquired imatinib tyrosine kinase inhibitor resistance), gene analysis, variants in the kinase domain**

> 🔲 0.00    ⚕ 0.00    **FUD** XXX                                        A 🖭

> **AMA:** 2017,Jan,8; 2016,Aug,9

● **81175**   **ASXL1 (additional sex combs like 1, transcriptional regulator) (eg, myelodysplastic syndrome, myeloproliferative neoplasms, chronic myelomonocytic leukemia), gene analysis; full gene sequence**

● **81176**       **targeted sequence analysis (eg, exon 12)**

**81200**   **ASPA (aspartoacylase) (eg, Canavan disease) gene analysis, common variants (eg, E285A, Y231X)**

> 🔲 0.00    ⚕ 0.00    **FUD** XXX                                        A 🖭

> **AMA:** 2017,Jan,8; 2016,Aug,9; 2016,Jan,13; 2015,Jan,16; 2014,Jan,11; 2013,Sep,3-12; 2012,May,3-10

**81201**   **APC (adenomatous polyposis coli) (eg, familial adenomatosis polyposis [FAP], attenuated FAP) gene analysis; full gene sequence**

> 🔲 0.00    ⚕ 0.00    **FUD** XXX                                        A 🖭

> **AMA:** 2017,Jan,8; 2016,Aug,9; 2016,Jan,13; 2015,Jan,16; 2014,Jan,11; 2013,Sep,3-12

**81202**       **known familial variants**

> 🔲 0.00    ⚕ 0.00    **FUD** XXX                                        A 🖭

> **AMA:** 2017,Jan,8; 2016,Aug,9; 2016,Jan,13; 2015,Jan,16; 2014,Jan,11; 2013,Sep,3-12

**81203**       **duplication/deletion variants**

> 🔲 0.00    ⚕ 0.00    **FUD** XXX                                        A 🖭

> **AMA:** 2017,Jan,8; 2016,Aug,9; 2016,Jan,13; 2015,Jan,16; 2014,Jan,11; 2013,Sep,3-12

**81205**   **BCKDHB (branched-chain keto acid dehydrogenase E1, beta polypeptide) (eg, maple syrup urine disease) gene analysis, common variants (eg, R183P, G278S, E422X)**

> 🔲 0.00    ⚕ 0.00    **FUD** XXX                                        A 🖭

> **AMA:** 2017,Jan,8; 2016,Aug,9; 2016,Jan,13; 2015,Jan,16; 2014,Jan,11; 2013,Sep,3-12; 2012,May,3-10

**81206**   **BCR/ABL1 (t(9;22)) (eg, chronic myelogenous leukemia) translocation analysis; major breakpoint, qualitative or quantitative**

> 🔲 0.00    ⚕ 0.00    **FUD** XXX                                        A 🖭

> **AMA:** 2017,Jan,8; 2016,Aug,9; 2016,Jan,13; 2015,Jan,16; 2014,Jan,11; 2013,Sep,3-12; 2012,May,3-10

**81207**       **minor breakpoint, qualitative or quantitative**

> 🔲 0.00    ⚕ 0.00    **FUD** XXX                                        A 🖭

> **AMA:** 2017,Jan,8; 2016,Aug,9; 2016,Jan,13; 2015,Jan,16; 2014,Jan,11; 2013,Sep,3-12; 2012,May,3-10

**81208**       **other breakpoint, qualitative or quantitative**

> 🔲 0.00    ⚕ 0.00    **FUD** XXX                                        A 🖭

> **AMA:** 2017,Jan,8; 2016,Aug,9; 2016,Jan,13; 2015,Jan,16; 2014,Jan,11; 2013,Sep,3-12; 2012,May,3-10

**81209**   **BLM (Bloom syndrome, RecQ helicase-like) (eg, Bloom syndrome) gene analysis, 2281del6ins7 variant**

> 🔲 0.00    ⚕ 0.00    **FUD** XXX                                        A 🖭

> **AMA:** 2017,Jan,8; 2016,Aug,9; 2016,Jan,13; 2015,Jan,16; 2014,Jan,11; 2013,Sep,3-12; 2012,May,3-10

● New Code     ▲ Revised Code     ○ Reinstated     ● New Web Release     ▲ Revised Web Release     Unlisted     Not Covered     # Resequenced
⊘ AMA Mod 51 Exempt     ⑪ Optum Mod 51 Exempt     ⑬ Mod 63 Exempt     ✗ Non-FDA Drug     ★ Telemedicine     Ⓜ Maternity     A Age Edit     ✚ Add-on     **AMA:** CPT Asst
© 2017 Optum360, LLC                                CPT © 2017 American Medical Association. All Rights Reserved.                                **359**

**81210** **BRAF (B-Raf proto-oncogene, serine/threonine kinase) (eg, colon cancer, melanoma), gene analysis, V600 variant(s)**
🔧 0.00   ⚖ 0.00   **FUD** XXX   🅰️▢
AMA: 2017,Jan,8; 2016,Aug,9; 2016,Jan,13; 2015,Jan,16; 2014,Jan,11; 2013,Sep,3-12; 2012,May,3-10

**81211** **BRCA1, BRCA2 (breast cancer 1 and 2) (eg, hereditary breast and ovarian cancer) gene analysis; full sequence analysis and common duplication/deletion variants in BRCA1 (ie, exon 13 del 3.835kb, exon 13 dup 6kb, exon 14-20 del 26kb, exon 22 del 510bp, exon 8-9 del 7.1kb)**
EXCLUDES   *BRCA1, BRCA2 (breast cancer 1 and 2) (81162)*
🔧 0.00   ⚖ 0.00   **FUD** XXX   🅰️▢
AMA: 2017,Jan,8; 2016,Aug,9; 2016,Jan,13; 2015,Jan,16; 2014,Jan,11; 2013,Sep,3-12; 2012,May,3-10

\#   **81162** **full sequence analysis and full duplication/deletion analysis**
EXCLUDES   *BRCA1, BRCA2 (breast cancer 1 and 2) (81211, 81213-81214)*
*BRCA2 (breast cancer 2) (81216)*
🔧 0.00   ⚖ 0.00   **FUD** XXX   🅰️▢
AMA: 2017,Jan,8; 2016,Aug,9

**81212** **185delAG, 5385insC, 6174delT variants**
🔧 0.00   ⚖ 0.00   **FUD** XXX   🅰️▢
AMA: 2017,Jan,8; 2016,Aug,9; 2016,Jan,13; 2015,Jan,16; 2014,Jan,11; 2013,Sep,3-12; 2012,May,3-10

**81213** **uncommon duplication/deletion variants**
EXCLUDES   *BRCA1, BRCA2 (breast cancer 1 and 2) (81162)*
🔧 0.00   ⚖ 0.00   **FUD** XXX   🅰️▢
AMA: 2017,Jan,8; 2016,Aug,9; 2016,Jan,13; 2015,Jan,16; 2014,Jan,11; 2013,Sep,3-12; 2012,May,3-10

**81214** **BRCA1 (breast cancer 1) (eg, hereditary breast and ovarian cancer) gene analysis; full sequence analysis and common duplication/deletion variants (ie, exon 13 del 3.835kb, exon 13 dup 6kb, exon 14-20 del 26kb, exon 22 del 510bp, exon 8-9 del 7.1kb)**
EXCLUDES   *BRCA1 with BRCA2 full sequence testing (81162, 81211)*
🔧 0.00   ⚖ 0.00   **FUD** XXX   🅰️▢
AMA: 2017,Jan,8; 2016,Aug,9; 2016,Jan,13; 2015,Jan,16; 2014,Jan,11; 2013,Sep,3-12; 2012,May,3-10

**81215** **known familial variant**
🔧 0.00   ⚖ 0.00   **FUD** XXX   🅰️▢
AMA: 2017,Jan,8; 2016,Aug,9; 2016,Jan,13; 2015,Jan,16; 2014,Jan,11; 2013,Sep,3-12; 2012,May,3-10

**81216** **BRCA2 (breast cancer 2) (eg, hereditary breast and ovarian cancer) gene analysis; full sequence analysis**
EXCLUDES   *BRCA1 with BRCA2 full sequence testing (81162, 81211)*
🔧 0.00   ⚖ 0.00   **FUD** XXX   🅰️▢
AMA: 2017,Jan,8; 2016,Aug,9; 2016,Jan,13; 2015,Jan,16; 2014,Jan,11; 2013,Sep,3-12; 2012,May,3-10

**81217** **known familial variant**
🔧 0.00   ⚖ 0.00   **FUD** XXX   🅰️▢
AMA: 2017,Jan,8; 2016,Aug,9; 2016,Jan,13; 2015,Jan,16; 2014,Jan,11; 2013,Sep,3-12; 2012,May,3-10

**81218** **CEBPA (CCAAT/enhancer binding protein [C/EBP], alpha) (eg, acute myeloid leukemia), gene analysis, full gene sequence**
🔧 0.00   ⚖ 0.00   **FUD** XXX   🅰️▢
AMA: 2017,Jan,8; 2016,Aug,9

**81219** **CALR (calreticulin) (eg, myeloproliferative disorders), gene analysis, common variants in exon 9**
🔧 0.00   ⚖ 0.00   **FUD** XXX   🅰️▢
AMA: 2017,Jan,8; 2016,Aug,9

**81220** **CFTR (cystic fibrosis transmembrane conductance regulator) (eg, cystic fibrosis) gene analysis; common variants (eg, ACMG/ACOG guidelines)**
EXCLUDES   *CFTR (cystic fibrosis transmembrane conductance regulator) (81224)*
🔧 0.00   ⚖ 0.00   **FUD** XXX   🅰️▢
AMA: 2017,Jan,8; 2016,Aug,9; 2016,Jan,13; 2015,Jan,16; 2014,Jan,11; 2013,Sep,3-12; 2012,May,3-10

**81221** **known familial variants**
🔧 0.00   ⚖ 0.00   **FUD** XXX   🅰️▢
AMA: 2017,Jan,8; 2016,Aug,9; 2016,Jan,13; 2015,Jan,16; 2014,Jan,11; 2013,Sep,3-12; 2012,May,3-10

**81222** **duplication/deletion variants**
🔧 0.00   ⚖ 0.00   **FUD** XXX   🅰️▢
AMA: 2017,Jan,8; 2016,Aug,9; 2016,Jan,13; 2015,Jan,16; 2014,Jan,11; 2013,Sep,3-12; 2012,May,3-10

**81223** **full gene sequence**
🔧 0.00   ⚖ 0.00   **FUD** XXX   🅰️▢
AMA: 2017,Jan,8; 2016,Aug,9; 2016,Jan,13; 2015,Jan,16; 2014,Jan,11; 2013,Sep,3-12; 2012,May,3-10

**81224** **intron 8 poly-T analysis (eg, male infertility)**
🔧 0.00   ⚖ 0.00   **FUD** XXX   🅰️▢
AMA: 2017,Jan,8; 2016,Aug,9; 2016,Jan,13; 2015,Jan,16; 2014,Jan,11; 2013,Sep,3-12; 2012,May,3-10

**81225** **CYP2C19 (cytochrome P450, family 2, subfamily C, polypeptide 19) (eg, drug metabolism), gene analysis, common variants (eg, *2, *3, *4, *8, *17)**
🔧 0.00   ⚖ 0.00   **FUD** XXX   🅰️▢
AMA: 2017,Jan,8; 2016,Aug,9; 2016,Jan,13; 2015,Jan,16; 2014,Jan,11; 2013,Sep,3-12; 2012,May,3-10

**81226** **CYP2D6 (cytochrome P450, family 2, subfamily D, polypeptide 6) (eg, drug metabolism), gene analysis, common variants (eg, *2, *3, *4, *5, *6, *9, *10, *17, *19, *29, *35, *41, *1XN, *2XN, *4XN)**
🔧 0.00   ⚖ 0.00   **FUD** XXX   🅰️▢
AMA: 2017,Jan,8; 2016,Aug,9; 2016,Jan,13; 2015,Jan,16; 2014,Jan,11; 2013,Sep,3-12; 2012,May,3-10

**81227** **CYP2C9 (cytochrome P450, family 2, subfamily C, polypeptide 9) (eg, drug metabolism), gene analysis, common variants (eg, *2, *3, *5, *6)**
🔧 0.00   ⚖ 0.00   **FUD** XXX   🅰️▢
AMA: 2017,Jan,8; 2016,Aug,9; 2016,Jan,13; 2015,Jan,16; 2014,Jan,11; 2013,Sep,3-12; 2012,May,3-10

● \#   **81230** **CYP3A4 (cytochrome P450 family 3 subfamily A member 4) (eg, drug metabolism), gene analysis, common variant(s) (eg, *2, *22)**
🔧 0.00   ⚖ 0.00   **FUD** 000

● \#   **81231** **CYP3A5 (cytochrome P450 family 3 subfamily A member 5) (eg, drug metabolism), gene analysis, common variants (eg, *2, *3, *4, *5, *6, *7)**
🔧 0.00   ⚖ 0.00   **FUD** 000

**81228** **Cytogenomic constitutional (genome-wide) microarray analysis; interrogation of genomic regions for copy number variants (eg, bacterial artificial chromosome [BAC] or oligo-based comparative genomic hybridization [CGH] microarray analysis)**
EXCLUDES   *Cytogenomic constitutional microarray analysis (genome-wide) (81229)*
*Cytogenomic constitutional microarray analysis (not genome-wide), report code for targeted analysis or unlisted molecular pathology (81405, [81479])*
*Molecular cytogenetics (88271)*
*Use of code with analyte-specific procedures when the analytes are included in the microarray analysis*
🔧 0.00   ⚖ 0.00   **FUD** XXX   🅰️▢
AMA: 2017,Apr,3; 2017,Jan,8; 2016,Aug,9; 2016,Jan,13; 2015,Jan,16; 2014,Jan,11; 2013,Sep,3-12; 2012,May,3-10

| 26/🔟 PC/TC Only | 🔢-🔢 ASC Payment | 🔟 Bilateral | ♂ Male Only | ♀ Female Only | 🔧 Facility RVU | ⚖ Non-Facility RVU | ▢ CCI |
| **FUD** Follow-up Days | **CMS:** IOM (Pub 100) | 🅰️-🆈 OPPSI | 80/80 Surg Assist Allowed / w/Doc | | 🔲 Lab Crosswalk | 🔲 Radiology Crosswalk | ❌ CLIA |

360

CPT © 2017 American Medical Association. All Rights Reserved.
© 2017 Optum360, LLC

**81229** interrogation of genomic regions for copy number and single nucleotide polymorphism (SNP) variants for chromosomal abnormalities

EXCLUDES *Cytogenomic constitutional microarray analysis (genome-wide) (81228)*

*Cytogenomic constitutional microarray analysis (not genome-wide), report code for targeted analysis or unlisted molecular pathology (81405, [81479])*

*Fetal chromosome analysis using maternal blood ([81479], 81420-81422)*

*Molecular cytogenetics (88271)*

*Use of code with analyte-specific procedures when the analytes are included in the microarray analysis*

0.00   0.00   **FUD** XXX

**AMA:** 2017,Apr,3; 2017,Jan,8; 2016,Aug,9; 2016,Jan,13; 2015,Jan,16; 2014,Jan,11; 2013,Sep,3-12; 2012,May,3-10

**81230** Resequenced code. See code following 81227.

**81231** Resequenced code. See code before 81228.

\# **81161** *DMD (dystrophin) (eg, Duchenne/Becker muscular dystrophy) deletion analysis, and duplication analysis, if performed*

0.00   0.00   **FUD** XXX

**AMA:** 2017,Jan,8; 2016,Aug,9; 2014,Jan,11

● **81232** *DPYD (dihydropyrimidine dehydrogenase) (eg, 5-fluorouracil/5-FU and capecitabine drug metabolism), gene analysis, common variant(s) (eg, *2A, *4, *5, *6)*

**81235** *EGFR (epidermal growth factor receptor) (eg, non-small cell lung cancer) gene analysis, common variants (eg, exon 19 LREA deletion, L858R, T790M, G719A, G719S, L861Q)*

0.00   0.00   **FUD** XXX

**AMA:** 2017,Jan,8; 2016,Aug,9; 2016,Jan,13; 2015,Jan,16; 2014,Jan,11; 2013,Sep,3-12

**81238** Resequenced code. See code following 81241.

**81240** *F2 (prothrombin, coagulation factor II) (eg, hereditary hypercoagulability) gene analysis, 20210G>A variant*

0.00   0.00   **FUD** XXX

**AMA:** 2017,Jan,8; 2016,Aug,9; 2016,Jan,13; 2015,Jan,16; 2014,Jan,11; 2013,Sep,3-12; 2012,May,3-10

**81241** *F5 (coagulation factor V) (eg, hereditary hypercoagulability) gene analysis, Leiden variant*

0.00   0.00   **FUD** XXX

**AMA:** 2017,Jan,8; 2016,Aug,9; 2016,Jan,13; 2015,Jan,16; 2014,Jan,11; 2013,Sep,3-12; 2012,May,3-10

● \# **81238** *F9 (coagulation factor IX) (eg, hemophilia B), full gene sequence*

0.00   0.00   **FUD** 000

**81242** *FANCC (Fanconi anemia, complementation group C) (eg, Fanconi anemia, type C) gene analysis, common variant (eg, IVS4+4A>T)*

0.00   0.00   **FUD** XXX

**AMA:** 2017,Jan,8; 2016,Aug,9; 2016,Jan,13; 2015,Jan,16; 2014,Jan,11; 2013,Sep,3-12; 2012,May,3-10

**81243** *FMR1 (fragile X mental retardation 1) (eg, fragile X mental retardation) gene analysis; evaluation to detect abnormal (eg, expanded) alleles*

INCLUDES Testing for detection and characterization of abnormal alleles using a single assay such as PCR

0.00   0.00   **FUD** XXX

**AMA:** 2017,Jan,8; 2016,Aug,9; 2016,Jan,13; 2015,Jan,16; 2014,Jan,11; 2013,Sep,3-12; 2012,May,3-10

**81244** characterization of alleles (eg, expanded size and methylation status)

EXCLUDES *Testing for detection and characterization of abnormal alleles using a single assay such as PCR (81243)*

0.00   0.00   **FUD** XXX

**AMA:** 2017,Jan,8; 2016,Aug,9; 2016,Jan,13; 2015,Jan,16; 2014,Jan,11; 2013,Sep,3-12; 2012,May,3-10

**81245** *FLT3 (fms-related tyrosine kinase 3) (eg, acute myeloid leukemia), gene analysis; internal tandem duplication (ITD) variants (ie, exons 14, 15)*

0.00   0.00   **FUD** XXX

**AMA:** 2017,Jan,8; 2016,Aug,9; 2016,Jan,13; 2015,Jan,16; 2015,Jan,3; 2014,Jan,11; 2013,Sep,3-12; 2012,May,3-10

**81246** tyrosine kinase domain (TKD) variants (eg, D835, I836)

0.00   0.00   **FUD** XXX

**AMA:** 2017,Jan,8; 2016,Aug,9; 2016,Jan,13; 2015,Jan,3

● **81247** *G6PD (glucose-6-phosphate dehydrogenase) (eg, hemolytic anemia, jaundice), gene analysis; common variant(s) (eg, A, A-)*

● **81248** known familial variant(s)

● **81249** full gene sequence

**81250** *G6PC (glucose-6-phosphatase, catalytic subunit) (eg, Glycogen storage disease, type 1a, von Gierke disease) gene analysis, common variants (eg, R83C, Q347X)*

0.00   0.00   **FUD** XXX

**AMA:** 2017,Jan,8; 2016,Aug,9; 2016,Jan,13; 2015,Jan,16; 2014,Jan,11; 2013,Sep,3-12; 2012,May,3-10

**81251** *GBA (glucosidase, beta, acid) (eg, Gaucher disease) gene analysis, common variants (eg, N370S, 84GG, L444P, IVS2+1G>A)*

0.00   0.00   **FUD** XXX

**AMA:** 2017,Jan,8; 2016,Aug,9; 2016,Jan,13; 2015,Jan,16; 2014,Jan,11; 2013,Sep,3-12; 2012,May,3-10

**81252** *GJB2 (gap junction protein, beta 2, 26kDa, connexin 26) (eg, nonsyndromic hearing loss) gene analysis; full gene sequence*

0.00   0.00   **FUD** XXX

**AMA:** 2017,Jan,8; 2016,Aug,9; 2016,Jan,13; 2015,Jan,16; 2014,Jan,11; 2013,Sep,3-12

**81253** known familial variants

0.00   0.00   **FUD** XXX

**AMA:** 2017,Jan,8; 2016,Aug,9; 2016,Jan,13; 2015,Jan,16; 2014,Jan,11; 2013,Sep,3-12

**81254** *GJB6 (gap junction protein, beta 6, 30kDa, connexin 30) (eg, nonsyndromic hearing loss) gene analysis, common variants (eg, 309kb [del(GJB6-D13S1830)] and 232kb [del(GJB6-D13S1854)])*

0.00   0.00   **FUD** XXX

**AMA:** 2017,Jan,8; 2016,Aug,9; 2016,Jan,13; 2015,Jan,16; 2014,Jan,11; 2013,Sep,3-12

**81255** *HEXA (hexosaminidase A [alpha polypeptide]) (eg, Tay-Sachs disease) gene analysis, common variants (eg, 1278insTATC, 1421+1G>C, G269S)*

0.00   0.00   **FUD** XXX

**AMA:** 2017,Jan,8; 2016,Aug,9; 2016,Jan,13; 2015,Jan,16; 2014,Jan,11; 2013,Sep,3-12; 2012,May,3-10

**81256** *HFE (hemochromatosis) (eg, hereditary hemochromatosis) gene analysis, common variants (eg, C282Y, H63D)*

0.00   0.00   **FUD** XXX

**AMA:** 2017,Jan,8; 2016,Aug,9; 2016,Jan,13; 2015,Jan,16; 2014,Jan,11; 2013,Sep,3-12; 2012,May,3-10

▲ **81257** *HBA1/HBA2 (alpha globin 1 and alpha globin 2) (eg, alpha thalassemia, Hb Bart hydrops fetalis syndrome, HbH disease), gene analysis; common deletions or variant (eg, Southeast Asian, Thai, Filipino, Mediterranean, alpha3.7, alpha4.2, alpha20.5, Constant Spring)*

0.00   0.00   **FUD** XXX

**AMA:** 2017,Jan,8; 2016,Aug,9; 2016,Jan,13; 2015,Jan,16; 2014,Jan,11; 2013,Sep,3-12; 2012,May,3-10

● **81258** known familial variant

● **81259** full gene sequence

● \# **81269** duplication/deletion variants

0.00   0.00   **FUD** 000

● New Code   ▲ Revised Code   ○ Reinstated   ● New Web Release   ▲ Revised Web Release   Unlisted   Not Covered   \# Resequenced
○ AMA Mod 51 Exempt   ⑤ Optum Mod 51 Exempt   ⑥ Mod 63 Exempt   ⊘ Non-FDA Drug   ★ Telemedicine   Ⓜ Maternity   Ⓐ Age Edit   + Add-on   AMA: CPT Asst
© 2017 Optum360, LLC          CPT © 2017 American Medical Association. All Rights Reserved.

● # **81105** *Human Platelet Antigen 1 genotyping (HPA-1), ITGB3 (integrin, beta 3 [platelet glycoprotein IIIa], antigen CD61 [GPIIIa]) (eg, neonatal alloimmune thrombocytopenia [NAIT], post-transfusion purpura), gene analysis, common variant, HPA-1a/b (L33P)*
    🖧 0.00   ✎ 0.00   **FUD** 000

● # **81106** *Human Platelet Antigen 2 genotyping (HPA-2), GP1BA (glycoprotein Ib [platelet], alpha polypeptide [GPIba]) (eg, neonatal alloimmune thrombocytopenia [NAIT], post-transfusion purpura), gene analysis, common variant, HPA-2a/b (T145M)*
    🖧 0.00   ✎ 0.00   **FUD** 000

● # **81107** *Human Platelet Antigen 3 genotyping (HPA-3), ITGA2B (integrin, alpha 2b [platelet glycoprotein IIb of IIb/IIIa complex], antigen CD41 [GPIIb]) (eg, neonatal alloimmune thrombocytopenia [NAIT], post-transfusion purpura), gene analysis, common variant, HPA-3a/b (I843S)*
    🖧 0.00   ✎ 0.00   **FUD** 000

● # **81108** *Human Platelet Antigen 4 genotyping (HPA-4), ITGB3 (integrin, beta 3 [platelet glycoprotein IIIa], antigen CD61 [GPIIIa]) (eg, neonatal alloimmune thrombocytopenia [NAIT], post-transfusion purpura), gene analysis, common variant, HPA-4a/b (R143Q)*
    🖧 0.00   ✎ 0.00   **FUD** 000

● # **81109** *Human Platelet Antigen 5 genotyping (HPA-5), ITGA2 (integrin, alpha 2 [CD49B, alpha 2 subunit of VLA-2 receptor] [GPIa]) (eg, neonatal alloimmune thrombocytopenia [NAIT], post-transfusion purpura), gene analysis, common variant (eg, HPA-5a/b (K505E))*
    🖧 0.00   ✎ 0.00   **FUD** 000

● # **81110** *Human Platelet Antigen 6 genotyping (HPA-6w), ITGB3 (integrin, beta 3 [platelet glycoprotein IIIa, antigen CD61] [GPIIIa]) (eg, neonatal alloimmune thrombocytopenia [NAIT], post-transfusion purpura), gene analysis, common variant, HPA-6a/b (R489Q)*
    🖧 0.00   ✎ 0.00   **FUD** 000

● # **81111** *Human Platelet Antigen 9 genotyping (HPA-9w), ITGA2B (integrin, alpha 2b [platelet glycoprotein IIb of IIb/IIIa complex, antigen CD41] [GPIIb]) (eg, neonatal alloimmune thrombocytopenia [NAIT], post-transfusion purpura), gene analysis, common variant, HPA-9a/b (V837M)*
    🖧 0.00   ✎ 0.00   **FUD** 000

● # **81112** *Human Platelet Antigen 15 genotyping (HPA-15), CD109 (CD109 molecule) (eg, neonatal alloimmune thrombocytopenia [NAIT], post-transfusion purpura), gene analysis, common variant, HPA-15a/b (S682Y)*
    🖧 0.00   ✎ 0.00   **FUD** 000

● # **81120** *IDH1 (isocitrate dehydrogenase 1 [NADP+], soluble) (eg, glioma), common variants (eg, R132H, R132C)*
    🖧 0.00   ✎ 0.00   **FUD** 000

● # **81121** *IDH2 (isocitrate dehydrogenase 2 [NADP+], mitochondrial) (eg, glioma), common variants (eg, R140W, R172M)*
    🖧 0.00   ✎ 0.00   **FUD** 000

● # **81283** *IFNL3 (interferon, lambda 3) (eg, drug response), gene analysis, rs12979860 variant*
    🖧 0.00   ✎ 0.00   **FUD** 000

**81260** *IKBKAP (inhibitor of kappa light polypeptide gene enhancer in B-cells, kinase complex-associated protein) (eg, familial dysautonomia) gene analysis, common variants (eg, 2507+6T>C, R696P)*
    🖧 0.00   **FUD** XXX    Ⓐ ▭
    **AMA:** 2017,Jan,8; 2016,Aug,9; 2016,Jan,13; 2015,Jan,16; 2014,Jan,11; 2013,Sep,3-12; 2012,May,3-10

**81261** *IGH@ (Immunoglobulin heavy chain locus) (eg, leukemias and lymphomas, B-cell), gene rearrangement analysis to detect abnormal clonal population(s); amplified methodology (eg, polymerase chain reaction)*
    🖧 0.00   ✎ 0.00   **FUD** XXX    Ⓐ ▭
    **AMA:** 2017,Jan,8; 2016,Aug,9; 2016,Jan,13; 2015,Jan,16; 2014,Jan,11; 2013,Sep,3-12; 2012,May,3-10

**81262** **direct probe methodology (eg, Southern blot)**
    🖧 0.00   ✎ 0.00   **FUD** XXX    Ⓐ ▭
    **AMA:** 2017,Jan,8; 2016,Aug,9; 2016,Jan,13; 2015,Jan,16; 2014,Jan,11; 2013,Sep,3-12; 2012,May,3-10

**81263** *IGH@ (Immunoglobulin heavy chain locus) (eg, leukemia and lymphoma, B-cell), variable region somatic mutation analysis*
    🖧 0.00   ✎ 0.00   **FUD** XXX    Ⓐ ▭
    **AMA:** 2017,Jan,8; 2016,Aug,9; 2016,Jan,13; 2015,Jan,16; 2014,Jan,11; 2013,Sep,3-12; 2012,May,3-10

**81264** *IGK@ (Immunoglobulin kappa light chain locus) (eg, leukemia and lymphoma, B-cell), gene rearrangement analysis, evaluation to detect abnormal clonal population(s)*
    **EXCLUDES** *Immunoglobulin kappa deleting element (IGKDEL) analysis ([81479])*
       *Immunoglobulin lambda gene (IGL@) rearrangement ([81479])*
    🖧 0.00   ✎ 0.00   **FUD** XXX    Ⓐ ▭
    **AMA:** 2017,Jan,8; 2016,Aug,9; 2016,Jan,13; 2015,Jan,16; 2014,Jan,11; 2013,Sep,3-12; 2012,May,3-10

**81265** **Comparative analysis using Short Tandem Repeat (STR) markers; patient and comparative specimen (eg, pre-transplant recipient and donor germline testing, post-transplant non-hematopoietic recipient germline [eg, buccal swab or other germline tissue sample] and donor testing, twin zygosity testing, or maternal cell contamination of fetal cells)**
    Code also the following codes for chimerism testing if comparative short tandem repeat (STR) analysis of recipient (using buccal swab or other germline tissue sample) and donor are performed after hematopoietic stem cell transplantation (81266-81268)
    🖧 0.00   ✎ 0.00   **FUD** XXX    Ⓐ ▭
    **AMA:** 2017,Jan,8; 2016,Aug,9; 2016,Jan,13; 2015,Jan,16; 2014,Jan,11; 2013,Sep,3-12; 2012,May,3-10

+ **81266** **each additional specimen (eg, additional cord blood donor, additional fetal samples from different cultures, or additional zygosity in multiple birth pregnancies) (List separately in addition to code for primary procedure)**
    Code also the following codes for chimerism testing if comparative short tandem repeat (STR) analysis of recipient (using buccal swab or other germline tissue sample) and donor are performed after hematopoietic stem cell transplantation (81267-81268)
    Code first (81265)
    🖧 0.00   ✎ 0.00   **FUD** XXX    Ⓐ ▭
    **AMA:** 2017,Jan,8; 2016,Aug,9; 2016,Jan,13; 2015,Jan,16; 2014,Jan,11; 2013,Sep,3-12; 2012,May,3-10

**81267** **Chimerism (engraftment) analysis, post transplantation specimen (eg, hematopoietic stem cell), includes comparison to previously performed baseline analyses; without cell selection**
    Code also the following codes for chimerism testing if comparative short tandem repeat (STR) analysis of recipient (using buccal swab or other germline tissue sample) and donor are performed after hematopoietic stem cell transplantation (81265-81266, 81268)
    🖧 0.00   ✎ 0.00   **FUD** XXX    Ⓐ ▭
    **AMA:** 2017,Jan,8; 2016,Aug,9; 2016,Jan,13; 2015,Jan,16; 2014,Jan,11; 2013,Sep,3-12; 2012,May,3-10

**81268** with cell selection (eg, CD3, CD33), each cell type

Code also the following codes for chimerism testing if comparative short tandem repeat (STR) analysis of recipient (using buccal swab or other germline tissue sample) and donor are performed after hematopoietic stem cell transplantation (81265-81267)

⚫ 0.00   ⚗ 0.00   **FUD** XXX   Ⓐ▢

**AMA:** 2017,Jan,8; 2016,Aug,9; 2016,Jan,13; 2015,Jan,16; 2014,Jan,11; 2013,Sep,3-12; 2012,May,3-10

*81269* **Resequenced code. See code following 81259.**

**81270** *JAK2 (Janus kinase 2) (eg, myeloproliferative disorder) gene analysis, p.Val617Phe (V617F) variant*

⚫ 0.00   ⚗ 0.00   **FUD** XXX   Ⓐ▢

**AMA:** 2017,Jan,8; 2016,Aug,9; 2016,Jan,13; 2015,Jan,16; 2014,Jan,11; 2013,Sep,3-12; 2012,May,3-10

**81272** *KIT (v-kit Hardy-Zuckerman 4 feline sarcoma viral oncogene homolog) (eg, gastrointestinal stromal tumor [GIST], acute myeloid leukemia, melanoma), gene analysis, targeted sequence analysis (eg, exons 8, 11, 13, 17, 18)*

⚫ 0.00   ⚗ 0.00   **FUD** XXX   Ⓐ▢

**AMA:** 2017,Jan,8; 2016,Aug,9

**81273** *KIT (v-kit Hardy-Zuckerman 4 feline sarcoma viral oncogene homolog) (eg, mastocytosis), gene analysis, D816 variant*

⚫ 0.00   ⚗ 0.00   **FUD** XXX   Ⓐ▢

**AMA:** 2017,Jan,8; 2016,Aug,9

**81275** *KRAS (Kirsten rat sarcoma viral oncogene homolog) (eg, carcinoma) gene analysis; variants in exon 2 (eg, codons 12 and 13)*

⚫ 0.00   ⚗ 0.00   **FUD** XXX   Ⓐ▢

**AMA:** 2017,Jan,8; 2016,Aug,9; 2016,Jan,13; 2015,Jan,16; 2014,Jan,11; 2013,Sep,3-12; 2012,May,3-10

**81276** additional variant(s) (eg, codon 61, codon 146)

⚫ 0.00   ⚗ 0.00   **FUD** XXX   Ⓐ▢

**AMA:** 2017,Jan,8; 2016,Aug,9

*81283* **Resequenced code. See code following 81269.**

*81287* **Resequenced code. See code following 81290.**

*81288* **Resequenced code. See code following 81292.**

**81290** *MCOLN1 (mucolipin 1) (eg, Mucolipidosis, type IV) gene analysis, common variants (eg, IVS3-2A>G, del6.4kb)*

⚫ 0.00   ⚗ 0.00   **FUD** XXX   Ⓐ▢

**AMA:** 2017,Jan,8; 2016,Aug,9; 2016,Jan,13; 2015,Jan,16; 2014,Jan,11; 2013,Sep,3-12; 2012,May,3-10

\# **81287** *MGMT (O-6-methylguanine-DNA methyltransferase) (eg, glioblastoma multiforme), methylation analysis*

⚫ 0.00   ⚗ 0.00   **FUD** XXX   Ⓐ▢

**AMA:** 2017,Jan,8; 2016,Aug,9; 2014,Jan,11

**81291** *MTHFR (5,10-methylenetetrahydrofolate reductase) (eg, hereditary hypercoagulability) gene analysis, common variants (eg, 677T, 1298C)*

⚫ 0.00   ⚗ 0.00   **FUD** XXX   Ⓐ▢

**AMA:** 2017,Jan,8; 2016,Aug,9; 2016,Jan,13; 2015,Jan,16; 2014,Jan,11; 2013,Sep,3-12; 2012,May,3-10

**81292** *MLH1 (mutL homolog 1, colon cancer, nonpolyposis type 2) (eg, hereditary non-polyposis colorectal cancer, Lynch syndrome) gene analysis; full sequence analysis*

⚫ 0.00   ⚗ 0.00   **FUD** XXX   Ⓐ▢

**AMA:** 2017,Jan,8; 2016,Aug,9; 2016,Jan,13; 2015,Jan,16; 2015,Jan,3; 2014,Jan,11; 2013,Sep,3-12; 2012,May,3-10

\# **81288** promoter methylation analysis

⚫ 0.00   ⚗ 0.00   **FUD** XXX   Ⓐ▢

**AMA:** 2017,Jan,8; 2016,Aug,9; 2016,Jan,13; 2015,Jan,3

**81293** known familial variants

⚫ 0.00   ⚗ 0.00   **FUD** XXX   Ⓐ▢

**AMA:** 2017,Jan,8; 2016,Aug,9; 2016,Jan,13; 2015,Jan,16; 2014,Jan,11; 2013,Sep,3-12; 2012,May,3-10

**81294** duplication/deletion variants

⚫ 0.00   ⚗ 0.00   **FUD** XXX   Ⓐ▢

**AMA:** 2017,Jan,8; 2016,Aug,9; 2016,Jan,13; 2015,Jan,16; 2014,Jan,11; 2013,Sep,3-12; 2012,May,3-10

**81295** *MSH2 (mutS homolog 2, colon cancer, nonpolyposis type 1) (eg, hereditary non-polyposis colorectal cancer, Lynch syndrome) gene analysis; full sequence analysis*

⚫ 0.00   ⚗ 0.00   **FUD** XXX   Ⓐ▢

**AMA:** 2017,Jan,8; 2016,Aug,9; 2016,Jan,13; 2015,Jan,16; 2014,Jan,11; 2013,Sep,3-12; 2012,May,3-10

**81296** known familial variants

⚫ 0.00   ⚗ 0.00   **FUD** XXX   Ⓐ▢

**AMA:** 2017,Jan,8; 2016,Aug,9; 2016,Jan,13; 2015,Jan,16; 2014,Jan,11; 2013,Sep,3-12; 2012,May,3-10

**81297** duplication/deletion variants

⚫ 0.00   ⚗ 0.00   **FUD** XXX   Ⓐ▢

**AMA:** 2017,Jan,8; 2016,Aug,9; 2016,Jan,13; 2015,Jan,16; 2014,Jan,11; 2013,Sep,3-12; 2012,May,3-10

**81298** *MSH6 (mutS homolog 6 [E. coli]) (eg, hereditary non-polyposis colorectal cancer, Lynch syndrome) gene analysis; full sequence analysis*

⚫ 0.00   ⚗ 0.00   **FUD** XXX   Ⓐ▢

**AMA:** 2017,Jan,8; 2016,Aug,9; 2016,Jan,13; 2015,Jan,16; 2014,Jan,11; 2013,Sep,3-12; 2012,May,3-10

**81299** known familial variants

⚫ 0.00   ⚗ 0.00   **FUD** XXX   Ⓐ▢

**AMA:** 2017,Jan,8; 2016,Aug,9; 2016,Jan,13; 2015,Jan,16; 2014,Jan,11; 2013,Sep,3-12; 2012,May,3-10

**81300** duplication/deletion variants

⚫ 0.00   ⚗ 0.00   **FUD** XXX   Ⓐ▢

**AMA:** 2017,Jan,8; 2016,Aug,9; 2016,Jan,13; 2015,Jan,16; 2014,Jan,11; 2013,Sep,3-12; 2012,May,3-10

**81301** Microsatellite instability analysis (eg, hereditary non-polyposis colorectal cancer, Lynch syndrome) of markers for mismatch repair deficiency (eg, BAT25, BAT26), includes comparison of neoplastic and normal tissue, if performed

⚫ 0.00   ⚗ 0.00   **FUD** XXX   Ⓐ▢

**AMA:** 2017,Jan,8; 2016,Aug,9; 2016,Jan,13; 2015,Jan,16; 2014,Jan,11; 2013,Sep,3-12; 2012,May,3-10

**81302** *MECP2 (methyl CpG binding protein 2) (eg, Rett syndrome) gene analysis; full sequence analysis*

⚫ 0.00   ⚗ 0.00   **FUD** XXX   Ⓐ▢

**AMA:** 2017,Jan,8; 2016,Aug,9; 2016,Jan,13; 2015,Jan,16; 2014,Jan,11; 2013,Sep,3-12; 2012,May,3-10

**81303** known familial variant

⚫ 0.00   ⚗ 0.00   **FUD** XXX   Ⓐ▢

**AMA:** 2017,Jan,8; 2016,Aug,9; 2016,Jan,13; 2015,Jan,16; 2014,Jan,11; 2013,Sep,3-12; 2012,May,3-10

**81304** duplication/deletion variants

⚫ 0.00   ⚗ 0.00   **FUD** XXX   Ⓐ▢

**AMA:** 2017,Jan,8; 2016,Aug,9; 2016,Jan,13; 2015,Jan,16; 2014,Jan,11; 2013,Sep,3-12; 2012,May,3-10

**81310** *NPM1 (nucleophosmin) (eg, acute myeloid leukemia) gene analysis, exon 12 variants*

⚫ 0.00   ⚗ 0.00   **FUD** XXX   Ⓐ▢

**AMA:** 2017,Jan,8; 2016,Aug,9; 2016,Jan,13; 2015,Jan,16; 2014,Jan,11; 2013,Sep,3-12; 2012,May,3-10

**81311** *NRAS (neuroblastoma RAS viral [v-ras] oncogene homolog) (eg, colorectal carcinoma), gene analysis, variants in exon 2 (eg, codons 12 and 13) and exon 3 (eg, codon 61)*

⚫ 0.00   ⚗ 0.00   **FUD** XXX   Ⓐ▢

**AMA:** 2017,Jan,8; 2016,Aug,9

**81313** *PCA3/KLK3 (prostate cancer antigen 3 [non-protein coding]/kallikrein-related peptidase 3 [prostate specific antigen]) ratio (eg, prostate cancer)*

⚫ 0.00   ⚗ 0.00   **FUD** XXX   Ⓐ▢

**AMA:** 2017,Jan,8; 2016,Aug,9; 2016,Jan,13; 2015,Jan,3

---

⚫ New Code   ▲ Revised Code   ◯ Reinstated   ⚫ New Web Release   ▲ Revised Web Release   Unlisted   Not Covered   \# Resequenced
⊘ AMA Mod 51 Exempt   ⑨ Optum Mod 51 Exempt   ⑥ Mod 63 Exempt   ∕ Non-FDA Drug   ★ Telemedicine   Ⓜ Maternity   Ⓐ Age Edit   ✛ Add-on   **AMA:** CPT Asst

81314    *PDGFRA (platelet-derived growth factor receptor, alpha polypeptide) (eg, gastrointestinal stromal tumor [GIST]), gene analysis, targeted sequence analysis (eg, exons 12, 18)*
     0.00    0.00    **FUD** XXX    A ▣
     **AMA:** 2017,Jan,8; 2016,Aug,9

81315    *PML/RARalpha, (t(15;17)), (promyelocytic leukemia/retinoic acid receptor alpha) (eg, promyelocytic leukemia) translocation analysis; common breakpoints (eg, intron 3 and intron 6), qualitative or quantitative*
     INCLUDES    Intron 3 and 6 (and exon 6 if performed) testing
     0.00    0.00    **FUD** XXX    A ▣
     **AMA:** 2017,Jan,8; 2016,Aug,9; 2016,Jan,13; 2015,Jan,16; 2014,Jan,11; 2013,Sep,3-12; 2012,May,3-10

81316    single breakpoint (eg, intron 3, intron 6 or exon 6), qualitative or quantitative
     EXCLUDES    *Intron 3 and 6 (and exon 6 if performed) testing (81315)*
         *Use of more than one unit of this code for testing intron 6 and exon 6 without intron 3 (81316)*
     0.00    0.00    **FUD** XXX    A ▣
     **AMA:** 2017,Jan,8; 2016,Aug,9; 2016,Jan,13; 2015,Jan,16; 2014,Jan,11; 2013,Sep,3-12; 2012,May,3-10

81317    *PMS2 (postmeiotic segregation increased 2 [S. cerevisiae]) (eg, hereditary non-polyposis colorectal cancer, Lynch syndrome) gene analysis; full sequence analysis*
     0.00    0.00    **FUD** XXX    A ▣
     **AMA:** 2017,Jan,8; 2016,Aug,9; 2016,Jan,13; 2015,Jan,16; 2014,Jan,11; 2013,Sep,3-12; 2012,May,3-10

81318    known familial variants
     0.00    0.00    **FUD** XXX    A ▣
     **AMA:** 2017,Jan,8; 2016,Aug,9; 2016,Jan,13; 2015,Jan,16; 2014,Jan,11; 2013,Sep,3-12; 2012,May,3-10

81319    duplication/deletion variants
     0.00    0.00    **FUD** XXX    A ▣
     **AMA:** 2017,Jan,8; 2016,Aug,9; 2016,Jan,13; 2015,Jan,16; 2014,Jan,11; 2013,Sep,3-12; 2012,May,3-10

81321    *PTEN (phosphatase and tensin homolog) (eg, Cowden syndrome, PTEN hamartoma tumor syndrome) gene analysis; full sequence analysis*
     0.00    0.00    **FUD** XXX    A ▣
     **AMA:** 2017,Jan,8; 2016,Aug,9; 2016,Jan,13; 2015,Jan,16; 2014,Jan,11; 2013,Sep,3-12

81322    known familial variant
     0.00    0.00    **FUD** XXX    A ▣
     **AMA:** 2017,Jan,8; 2016,Aug,9; 2016,Jan,13; 2015,Jan,16; 2014,Jan,11; 2013,Sep,3-12

81323    duplication/deletion variant
     0.00    0.00    **FUD** XXX    A ▣
     **AMA:** 2017,Jan,8; 2016,Aug,9; 2016,Jan,13; 2015,Jan,16; 2014,Jan,11; 2013,Sep,3-12

81324    *PMP22 (peripheral myelin protein 22) (eg, Charcot-Marie-Tooth, hereditary neuropathy with liability to pressure palsies) gene analysis; duplication/deletion analysis*
     0.00    0.00    **FUD** XXX    A ▣
     **AMA:** 2017,Jan,8; 2016,Aug,9; 2016,Jan,13; 2015,Jan,16; 2014,Jan,11; 2013,Sep,3-12

81325    full sequence analysis
     0.00    0.00    **FUD** XXX    A ▣
     **AMA:** 2017,Jan,8; 2016,Aug,9; 2016,Jan,13; 2015,Jan,16; 2014,Jan,11; 2013,Sep,3-12

81326    known familial variant
     0.00    0.00    **FUD** XXX    A ▣
     **AMA:** 2017,Jan,8; 2016,Aug,9; 2016,Jan,13; 2015,Jan,16; 2014,Jan,11; 2013,Sep,3-12

● # 81334    *RUNX1 (runt related transcription factor 1) (eg, acute myeloid leukemia, familial platelet disorder with associated myeloid malignancy), gene analysis, targeted sequence analysis (eg, exons 3-8)*
     0.00    0.00    **FUD** 000

81327    *SEPT9 (Septin9) (eg, colorectal cancer) methylation analysis*
     0.00    0.00    **FUD** XXX    A ▣

● 81328    *SLCO1B1 (solute carrier organic anion transporter family, member 1B1) (eg, adverse drug reaction), gene analysis, common variant(s) (eg, *5)*

81330    *SMPD1 (sphingomyelin phosphodiesterase 1, acid lysosomal) (eg, Niemann-Pick disease, Type A) gene analysis, common variants (eg, R496L, L302P, fsP330)*
     0.00    0.00    **FUD** XXX    A ▣
     **AMA:** 2017,Jan,8; 2016,Aug,9; 2016,Jan,13; 2015,Jan,16; 2014,Jan,11; 2013,Sep,3-12; 2012,May,3-10

81331    *SNRPN/UBE3A (small nuclear ribonucleoprotein polypeptide N and ubiquitin protein ligase E3A) (eg, Prader-Willi syndrome and/or Angelman syndrome), methylation analysis*
     0.00    0.00    **FUD** XXX    A ▣
     **AMA:** 2017,Jan,8; 2016,Aug,9; 2016,Jan,13; 2015,Jan,16; 2014,Jan,11; 2013,Sep,3-12; 2012,May,3-10

81332    *SERPINA1 (serpin peptidase inhibitor, clade A, alpha-1 antiproteinase, antitrypsin, member 1) (eg, alpha-1-antitrypsin deficiency), gene analysis, common variants (eg, *S and *Z)*
     0.00    0.00    **FUD** XXX    A ▣
     **AMA:** 2017,Jan,8; 2016,Aug,9; 2016,Jan,13; 2015,Jan,16; 2014,Jan,11; 2013,Sep,3-12; 2012,May,3-10

*81334*    **Resequenced code. See code following 81326.**

● 81335    *TPMT (thiopurine S-methyltransferase) (eg, drug metabolism), gene analysis, common variants (eg, *2, *3)*

81340    *TRB@ (T cell antigen receptor, beta) (eg, leukemia and lymphoma), gene rearrangement analysis to detect abnormal clonal population(s); using amplification methodology (eg, polymerase chain reaction)*
     0.00    0.00    **FUD** XXX    A ▣
     **AMA:** 2017,Jan,8; 2016,Aug,9; 2016,Jan,13; 2015,Jan,16; 2014,Jan,11; 2013,Sep,3-12; 2012,May,3-10

81341    using direct probe methodology (eg, Southern blot)
     0.00    0.00    **FUD** XXX    A ▣
     **AMA:** 2017,Jan,8; 2016,Aug,9; 2016,Jan,13; 2015,Jan,16; 2014,Jan,11; 2013,Sep,3-12; 2012,May,3-10

81342    *TRG@ (T cell antigen receptor, gamma) (eg, leukemia and lymphoma), gene rearrangement analysis, evaluation to detect abnormal clonal population(s)*
     EXCLUDES    *T cell antigen alpha [TRA@] gene arrangement testing ([81479])*
         *T cell antigen delta [TRD@] gene arrangement testing (81402)*
     0.00    0.00    **FUD** XXX    A ▣
     **AMA:** 2017,Jan,8; 2016,Aug,9; 2016,Jan,13; 2015,Jan,16; 2014,Jan,11; 2013,Sep,3-12; 2012,May,3-10

● 81346    *TYMS (thymidylate synthetase) (eg, 5-fluorouracil/5-FU drug metabolism), gene analysis, common variant(s) (eg, tandem repeat variant)*

81350    *UGT1A1 (UDP glucuronosyltransferase 1 family, polypeptide A1) (eg, irinotecan metabolism), gene analysis, common variants (eg, *28, *36, *37)*
     0.00    0.00    **FUD** XXX    A ▣
     **AMA:** 2017,Jan,8; 2016,Aug,9; 2016,Jan,13; 2015,Jan,16; 2014,Jan,11; 2013,Sep,3-12; 2012,May,3-10

81355    *VKORC1 (vitamin K epoxide reductase complex, subunit 1) (eg, warfarin metabolism), gene analysis, common variant(s) (eg, -1639G>A, c.173+1000C>T)*
     0.00    0.00    **FUD** XXX    A ▣
     **AMA:** 2017,Jan,8; 2016,Aug,9; 2016,Jan,13; 2015,Jan,16; 2014,Jan,11; 2013,Sep,3-12; 2012,May,3-10

26/TC PC/TC Only    A2-Z3 ASC Payment    50 Bilateral    ♂ Male Only    ♀ Female Only    🔧 Facility RVU    Non-Facility RVU    ▣ CCI
**FUD** Follow-up Days    **CMS:** IOM (Pub 100)    A-Y OPPSI    80/80 Surg Assist Allowed / w/Doc    Lab Crosswalk    Radiology Crosswalk    ✖ CLIA
364      CPT © 2017 American Medical Association. All Rights Reserved.      © 2017 Optum360, LLC

● **81361** *HBB (hemoglobin, subunit beta)* **(eg, sickle cell anemia, beta thalassemia, hemoglobinopathy); common variant(s) (eg, HbS, HbC, HbE)**

● **81362** **known familial variant(s)**

● **81363** **duplication/deletion variant(s)**

● **81364** **full gene sequence**

## 81370-81383 Human Leukocyte Antigen (HLA) Testing

INCLUDES Additional testing that must be performed to resolve ambiguous allele combinations for high-resolution typing
All analytical procedures in the evaluation such as:
  Amplification
  Cell lysis
  Detection
  Digestion
  Extraction
  Nucleic acid stabilization
Analysis to identify human leukocyte antigen (HLA) alleles and allele groups connected to specific diseases and individual response to drug therapy in addition to other clinical uses
Code selection based on specific gene being reviewed
Evaluation of the presence of gene variants using the common gene variant name
Examples of proteins or diseases in the code description that are not all inclusive
Generally all the listed gene variants in the code description would be tested but lists are not all inclusive
Genes described using Human Genome Organization (HUGO) approved names
High-resolution typing resolves the common well-defined (CWD) alleles and is usually identified by at least four-digits. There are some instances when high-resolution typing may include some ambiguities for rare alleles, and those may be reported as a string of alleles or an NMDP code
Histocompatibility antigen testing
Intermediate resolution HLA testing is identified by a string of alleles or a National Marrow Donor Program (NMDP) code
Low and intermediate resolution are considered low resolution for code assignment
Low-resolution HLA type reporting is identified by two-digit HLA name
Multiple variant alleles or allele groups that can be identified by typing
One or more HLA genes in specific clinical circumstances
Qualitative results unless otherwise stated
Typing performed to determine the compatibility of recipients and potential donors undergoing solid organ or hematopoietic stem cell pretransplantation testing

EXCLUDES *Full gene sequencing using separate gene variant assessment codes unless it is specifically stated in the code description*
*HLA antigen typing by nonmolecular pathology methods (86812-86821)*
*In situ hybridization analyses (88271-88275, 88368-88375 [88377])*
*Microbial identification (87149-87153, 87471-87801 [87623, 87624, 87625], 87900-87904 [87906, 87910, 87912])*
*Other related gene variants not listed in code*
*Tier 1 molecular pathology codes (81200-81355 [81105, 81106, 81107, 81108, 81109, 81110, 81111, 81112, 81120, 81121, 81161, 81162, 81230, 81231, 81238, 81269, 81283, 81287, 81288, 81334])*
*Tier 2 and unlisted mocular pathology procedures (81400-81408, [81479])*
Code also modifier 26 when only interpretation and report are performed
Code also services required before cell lysis

**81370** **HLA Class I and II typing, low resolution (eg, antigen equivalents);** *HLA-A, -B, -C, -DRB1/3/4/5, and -DQB1*
🚗 0.00 ⚖ 0.00 **FUD** XXX A 🖼
**AMA:** 2017,Jan,8; 2016,Aug,9; 2016,Jan,13; 2015,Jan,16; 2014,Jan,11; 2013,Sep,3-12; 2012,May,3-10; 2012,Jun,15-16

**81371** *HLA-A, -B, and -DRB1* **(eg, verification typing)**
🚗 0.00 ⚖ 0.00 **FUD** XXX A 🖼
**AMA:** 2017,Jan,8; 2016,Aug,9; 2016,Jan,13; 2015,Jan,16; 2014,Jan,11; 2013,Sep,3-12; 2012,May,3-10; 2012,Jun,15-16

**81372** **HLA Class I typing, low resolution (eg, antigen equivalents); complete** *(ie, HLA-A, -B, and -C)*
EXCLUDES *Class I and II low-resolution HLA typing for HLA-A, -B, -C, -DRB1/3/4/5, and -DQB1 (81370)*
🚗 0.00 ⚖ 0.00 **FUD** XXX A 🖼
**AMA:** 2017,Jan,8; 2016,Aug,9; 2016,Jan,13; 2015,Jan,16; 2014,Jan,11; 2013,Sep,3-12; 2012,May,3-10; 2012,Jun,15-16

**81373** **one locus** *(eg, HLA-A, -B, or -C),* **each**
EXCLUDES *A complete Class 1 (HLA-A, -B, and -C) low-resolution typing (81372)*
*Reporting the presence or absence of a single antigen equivalent using low-resolution methodology (81374)*
🚗 0.00 ⚖ 0.00 **FUD** XXX A 🖼
**AMA:** 2017,Jan,8; 2016,Aug,9; 2016,Jan,13; 2015,Jan,16; 2014,Jan,11; 2013,Sep,3-12; 2012,May,3-10; 2012,Jun,15-16

**81374** **one antigen equivalent** *(eg, B\*27),* **each**
EXCLUDES *Testing for the presence or absence of more than 2 antigen equivalents at a locus, use the following code for each locus test (81373)*
🚗 0.00 ⚖ 0.00 **FUD** XXX A 🖼
**AMA:** 2017,Jan,8; 2016,Aug,9; 2016,Jan,13; 2015,Jan,16; 2014,Jan,11; 2013,Sep,3-12; 2012,May,3-10; 2012,Jun,15-16

**81375** **HLA Class II typing, low resolution (eg, antigen equivalents);** *HLA-DRB1/3/4/5 and -DQB1*
EXCLUDES *Class I and II low-resolution HLA typing for HLA-A, -B, -C, -DRB 1/3/4/5, and DQB1 (81370)*
🚗 0.00 ⚖ 0.00 **FUD** XXX A 🖼
**AMA:** 2017,Jan,8; 2016,Aug,9; 2016,Jan,13; 2015,Jan,16; 2014,Jan,11; 2013,Sep,3-12; 2012,May,3-10; 2012,Jun,15-16

**81376** **one locus** *(eg, HLA-DRB1, -DRB3/4/5, -DQB1, -DQA1, -DPB1, or -DPA1),* **each**
INCLUDES Low-resolution typing, HLA-DRB1/3/4/5 reported as a single locus
EXCLUDES *Low-resolution typing for HLA-DRB1/3/4/5 and -DQB1 (81375)*
🚗 0.00 ⚖ 0.00 **FUD** XXX A 🖼
**AMA:** 2017,Jan,8; 2016,Aug,9; 2016,Jan,13; 2015,Jan,16; 2014,Jan,11; 2013,Sep,3-12; 2012,May,3-10; 2012,Jun,15-16

**81377** **one antigen equivalent, each**
EXCLUDES *Testing for presence or absence of more than two antigen equivalents at a locus (81376)*
🚗 0.00 ⚖ 0.00 **FUD** XXX A 🖼
**AMA:** 2017,Jan,8; 2016,Aug,9; 2016,Jan,13; 2015,Jan,16; 2014,Jan,11; 2013,Sep,3-12; 2012,May,3-10; 2012,Jun,15-16

**81378** **HLA Class I and II typing, high resolution (ie, alleles or allele groups),** *HLA-A, -B, -C, and -DRB1*
🚗 0.00 ⚖ 0.00 **FUD** XXX A 🖼
**AMA:** 2017,Jan,8; 2016,Aug,9; 2016,Jan,13; 2015,Jan,16; 2014,Jan,11; 2013,Sep,3-12; 2012,May,3-10; 2012,Jun,15-16

**81379** **HLA Class I typing, high resolution (ie, alleles or allele groups); complete (ie,** *HLA-A, -B, and -C)*
🚗 0.00 ⚖ 0.00 **FUD** XXX A 🖼
**AMA:** 2017,Jan,8; 2016,Aug,9; 2016,Jan,13; 2015,Jan,16; 2014,Jan,11; 2013,Sep,3-12; 2012,May,3-10; 2012,Jun,15-16

**81380** **one locus (eg,** *HLA-A, -B, or -C),* **each**
EXCLUDES *Complete Class I high-resolution typing for HLA-A, -B, and -C (81379)*
*Testing for presence or absence of a single allele or allele group using high-resolution methodology (81381)*
🚗 0.00 ⚖ 0.00 **FUD** XXX A 🖼
**AMA:** 2017,Jan,8; 2016,Aug,9; 2016,Jan,13; 2015,Jan,16; 2014,Jan,11; 2013,Sep,3-12; 2012,May,3-10; 2012,Jun,15-16

**81381** **one allele or allele group (eg,** *B\*57:01P),* **each**
EXCLUDES *Testing for the presence or absence of more than two alleles or allele groups of locus, report the following code for each locus (81380)*
🚗 0.00 ⚖ 0.00 **FUD** XXX A 🖼
**AMA:** 2017,Jan,8; 2016,Aug,9; 2016,Jan,13; 2015,Jan,16; 2014,Jan,11; 2013,Sep,3-12; 2012,May,3-10; 2012,Jun,15-16

● New Code ▲ Revised Code ○ Reinstated ● New Web Release ▲ Revised Web Release Unlisted Not Covered # Resequenced
⊘ AMA Mod 51 Exempt ⑤ Optum Mod 51 Exempt ⑥ Mod 63 Exempt ⊬ Non-FDA Drug ★ Telemedicine Ⓜ Maternity A Age Edit + Add-on **AMA:** CPT Asst
© 2017 Optum360, LLC CPT © 2017 American Medical Association. All Rights Reserved.

**Pathology and Laboratory**

**81382 — 81401**

**81382**    **HLA Class II typing, high resolution (ie, alleles or allele groups); one locus (eg, HLA-DRB1, -DRB3/4/5, -DQB1, -DQA1, -DPB1, or -DPA1), each**

> INCLUDES   Typing of one or all of the DRB3/4/5 genes is regarded as one locus
>
> EXCLUDES   *Testing for just the presence or absence of a single allele or allele group using high-resolution methodology (81383)*

🖪 0.00    🔾 0.00    **FUD** XXX       Ⓐ 🖵

**AMA:** 2017,Jan,8; 2016,Jan,13; 2015,Jan,16; 2014,Jan,11; 2013,Sep,3-12; 2012,May,3-10; 2012,Jun,15-16

**81383**    **one allele or allele group (eg, HLA-DQB1\*06:02P), each**

> EXCLUDES   *For testing for the presence or absence of more than two alleles or allele groups at a locus, report the following code for each locus (81382)*

🖪 0.00    🔾 0.00    **FUD** XXX       Ⓐ 🖵

**AMA:** 2017,Jan,8; 2016,Jan,13; 2015,Jan,16; 2014,Jan,11; 2013,Sep,3-12; 2012,May,3-10; 2012,Jun,15-16

## 81400-81408 [81479] Molecular Pathology Tier 2 Procedures

> INCLUDES   All analytical procedures in the evaluation such as:
>      Amplification
>      Cell lysis
>      Detection
>      Digestion
>      Extraction
>      Nucleic acid stabilization
> Code selection based on specific gene being reviewed
> Codes that are arranged by level of technical resources and work involved
> Evaluation of the presence of a gene variant using the common gene variant name
> Examples of proteins or diseases in the code description (not all inclusive)
> Generally all the listed gene variants in the code description would be tested but lists are not all inclusive
> Genes described using the Human Genome Organization (HUGO) approved names
> Histocompatibility testing
> Qualitative results unless otherwise stated
> Specific analytes listed after the code description to use for selecting the appropriate molecular pathology procedure
> Targeted genomic testing (81410-81471 [81448])
> Testing for diseases that are more rare
>
> EXCLUDES   *Full gene sequencing using separate gene variant assessment codes unless it is specifically stated in the code description*
> *In situ hybridization analyses (88271-88275, 88365-88368 [88364, 88373, 88374])*
> *Microbial identification (87149-87153, 87471-87801 [87623, 87624, 87625], 87900-87904 [87906, 87910, 87912])*
> *Other related gene variants not listed in code*
> *Tier 1 molecular pathology (81200-81383 [81105, 81106, 81107, 81108, 81109, 81110, 81111, 81112, 81120, 81121, 81161, 81162, 81230, 81231, 81238, 81269, 81283, 81287, 81288, 81334])*
> *Unlisted molecular pathology procedures ([81479])*

Code also services required before cell lysis
Code also modifier 26 when only interpretation and report are performed

▲   **81400**    **Molecular pathology procedure, Level 1 (eg, identification of single germline variant [eg, SNP] by techniques such as restriction enzyme digestion or melt curve analysis)**

*ACADM (acyl-CoA dehydrogenase, C-4 to C-12 straight chain, MCAD) (eg, medium chain acyl dehydrogenase deficiency), K304E variant*

*ACE (angiotensin converting enzyme) (eg, hereditary blood pressure regulation), insertion/deletion variant*

*AGTR1 (angiotensin II receptor, type 1) (eg, essential hypertension), 1166A>C variant*

*BCKDHA (branched chain keto acid dehydrogenase E1, alpha polypeptide) (eg, maple syrup urine disease, type 1A), Y438N variant*

*CCR5 (chemokine C-C motif receptor 5) (eg, HIV resistance), 32-bp deletion mutation/794 825del32 deletion*

*CLRN1 (clarin 1) (eg, Usher syndrome, type 3), N48K variant*

*F2 (coagulation factor 2) (eg, hereditary hypercoagulability), 1199G>A variant*

*F5 (coagulation factor V) (eg, hereditary hypercoagulability), HR2 variant*

*F7 (coagulation factor VII [serum prothrombin conversion accelerator]) (eg, hereditary hypercoagulability), R353Q variant*

*F13B (coagulation factor XIII, B polypeptide) (eg, hereditary hypercoagulability), V34L variant*

*FGB (fibrinogen beta chain) (eg, hereditary ischemic heart disease), -455G>A variant*

*FGFR1 (fibroblast growth factor receptor 1) (eg, Pfeiffer syndrome type 1, craniosynostosis), P252R variant*

*FGFR3 (fibroblast growth factor receptor 3) (eg, Muenke syndrome), P250R variant*

*FKTN (fukutin) (eg, Fukuyama congenital muscular dystrophy), retrotransposon insertion variant*

*GNE (glucosamine [UDP-N-acetyl]-2 -epimerase/N-acetylmannosamine kinase) (eg, inclusion body myopathy 2 [IBM2], Nonaka myopathy), M712T variant*

*IVD (isovaleryl-CoA dehydrogenase) (eg, isovaleric acidemia), A282V variant*

*LCT (lactase-phlorizin hydrolase) (eg, lactose intolerance), 13910 C>T variant*

*NEB (nebulin) (eg, nemaline myopathy 2), exon 55 deletion variant*

*PCDH15 (protocadherin-related 15) (eg, Usher syndrome type 1F), R245X variant*

*SERPINE1 (serpine peptidase inhibitor clade E, member 1, plasminogen activator inhibitor -1, PAI-1) (eg, thrombophilia), 4G variant*

*SHOC2 (soc-2 suppressor of clear homolog) (eg, Noonan-like syndrome with loose anagen hair), S2G variant*

*SMN1 (survival of motor neuron 1, telomeric) (eg, spinal muscular atrophy), exon 7 deletion*

*SRY (sex determining region Y) (eg, 46,XX testicular disorder of sex development, gonadal dysgenesis), gene analysis*

*TOR1A (torsin family 1, member A [torsin A]) (eg, early-onset primary dystonia [DYT1]), 907_909delGAG (904_906delGAG) variant*

🖪 0.00    🔾 0.00    **FUD** XXX       Ⓐ 🖵

**AMA:** 2017,Jan,8; 2016,Aug,9; 2016,Jan,13; 2015,Jan,16; 2015,Jan,3; 2014,Jan,11; 2013,Sep,3-12; 2013,Jul,11-12; 2012,May,3-10

▲   **81401**    **Molecular pathology procedure, Level 2 (eg, 2-10 SNPs, 1 methylated variant, or 1 somatic variant [typically using nonsequencing target variant analysis], or detection of a dynamic mutation disorder/triplet repeat)**

*ABCC8 (ATP-binding cassette, sub-family C [CFTR/MRP], member 8) (eg, familial hyperinsulinism), common variants (eg, c.3898-9G>A [c.3992-9G>A], F1388del)*

*ABL1 (ABL proto oncogene 1, non-receptor tyrosine kinase) (eg, acquired imatinib resistance), T315I variant*

*ACADM (acyl-CoA dehydrogenase, C-4 to C-12 straight chain, MCAD) (eg, medium chain acyl dehydrogenase deficiency), common variants (eg, K304E, Y42H)*

*ADRB2 (adrenergic beta-2 receptor surface) (eg, drug metabolism), common variants (eg, G16R, Q27E)*

*AFF2 (AF4/FMR2 family, member 2 [FMR2]) (eg, fragile X mental retardation 2 [FRAXE]), evaluation to detect abnormal (eg, expanded) alleles*

*APOB (apolipoprotein B) (eg, familial hypercholesterolemia type B), common variants (eg, R3500Q, R3500W)*

*APOE (apolipoprotein E) (eg, hyperlipoproteinemia type III, cardiovascular disease, Alzheimer disease), common variants (eg, \*2, \*3, \*4)*

*AR (androgen receptor) (eg, spinal and bulbar muscular atrophy, Kennedy disease, X chromosome inactivation), characterization of alleles (eg, expanded size or methylation status)*

*ATN1 (atrophin 1) (eg, dentatorubral-pallidoluysian atrophy), evaluation to detect abnormal (eg, expanded) alleles*

---

| 26/TC PC/TC Only | A2-Z3 ASC Payment | 50 Bilateral | ♂ Male Only | ♀ Female Only | 🖪 Facility RVU | 🔾 Non-Facility RVU | 🖵 CCI |
| --- | --- | --- | --- | --- | --- | --- | --- |
| **FUD** Follow-up Days | **CMS:** IOM (Pub 100) | Ⓐ-Ⓨ OPPSI | 80/80 Surg Assist Allowed / w/Doc | | 🖹 Lab Crosswalk | 🖸 Radiology Crosswalk | ❌ CLIA |

366              CPT © 2017 American Medical Association. All Rights Reserved.            © 2017 Optum360, LLC

*ATXN1 (ataxin 1) (eg, spinocerebellar ataxia), evaluation to detect abnormal (eg, expanded) alleles*

*ATXN2 (ataxin 2) (eg, spinocerebellar ataxia), evaluation to detect abnormal (eg, expanded) alleles*

*ATXN3 (ataxin 3) (eg, spinocerebellar ataxia, Machado-Joseph disease), evaluation to detect abnormal (eg, expanded) alleles*

*ATXN7 (ataxin 7) (eg, spinocerebellar ataxia), evaluation to detect abnormal (eg, expanded) alleles*

*ATXN8OS (ATXN8 opposite strand [non-protein coding]) (eg, spinocerebellar ataxia), evaluation to detect abnormal (eg, expanded) alleles*

*ATXN10 (ataxin 10) (eg, spinocerebellar ataxia), evaluation to detect abnormal (eg, expanded) alleles*

*CACNA1A (calcium channel, voltage-dependent, P/Q type, alpha 1A subunit) (eg, spinocerebellar ataxia), evaluation to detect abnormal (eg, expanded) alleles*

*CBFB/MYH11 (inv(16)) (eg, acute myeloid leukemia), qualitative, and quantitative, if performed*

*CBS (cystathionine-beta-synthase) (eg, homocystinuria, cystathionine beta-synthase deficiency), common variants (eg, I278T, G307S)*

*CCND1/IGH (BCL1/IgH, t(11;14)) (eg, mantle cell lymphoma) translocation analysis, major breakpoint, qualitative and quantitative, if performed*

*CFH/ARMS2 (complement factor H/age-related maculopathy susceptibility 2) (eg, macular degeneration), common variants (eg, Y402H [CFH], A69S [ARMS2])*

*CNBP (CCHC-type zinc finger, nucleic acid binding protein) (eg, myotonic dystrophy type 2), evaluation to detect abnormal (eg, expanded) alleles*

*CSTB (cystatin B [stefin B]) (eg, Unverricht-Lundborg disease), evaluation to detect abnormal (eg, expanded) alleles*

*DEK/NUP214 (t(6;9))(eg, acute myeloid leukemia), translocation analysis, qualitative, and quantitative, if performed*

*DMPK (dystrophia myotonica-protein kinase) (eg, myotonic dystrophy, type 1), evaluation to detect abnormal (eg, expanded) alleles*

*E2A/PBX1 (t(1;19)) (eg, acute lymphocytic leukemia), translocation analysis, qualitative, and quantitative, if performed*

*EML4/ALK (inv(2)) (eg, non-small cell lung cancer), translocation or inversion analysis*

*ETV6/NTRK3 (t(12;15)) (eg, congenital/infantile fibrosarcoma), translocation analysis, qualitative, and quantitative, if performed*

*ETV6/RUNX1 (t(12;21)) (eg, acute lymphocytic leukemia), translocation analysis, qualitative and quantitative, if performed*

*EWSR1/ATF1 (t(12;22)) (eg, clear cell sarcoma), translocation analysis, qualitative, and quantitative, if performed*

*EWSR1/ERG (t(21;22)) (eg, Ewing sarcoma/peripheral neuroectodermal tumor), translocation analysis, qualitative and quantitative, if performed*

*EWSR1/FLI1 (t(11;22)) (eg, Ewing sarcoma/peripheral neuroectodermal tumor), translocation analysis, qualitative and quantitative, if performed*

*EWSR1/WT1 (t(11;22)) (eg, desmoplastic small round cell tumor), translocation analysis, qualitative and quantitative, if performed*

*F11 (coagulation factor XI) (eg, coagulation disorder), common variants (eg, E117X [Type II], F283L [Type III], IVS14del14, and IVS14+1G>A [Type I])*

*FGFR3 (fibroblast growth factor receptor 3) (eg, achondroplasia, hypochondroplasia), common variants (eg, 1138G>A, 1138G>C, 1620C>A, 1620C>G)*

*FIP1L1/PDGFRA (del[4q12]) (eg, imatinib-sensitive chronic eosinophilic leukemia), qualitative and quantitative, if performed*

*FLG (filaggrin) (eg, ichthyosis vulgaris), common variants (eg, R501X, 2282del4, R2447X, S3247X, 3702delG)*

*FOXO1/PAX3 (t(2;13)) (eg, alveolar rhabdomyosarcoma), translocation analysis, qualitative and quantitative, if performed*

*FOXO1/PAX7 (t(1;13)) (eg, alveolar rhabdomyosarcoma), translocation analysis, qualitative and quantitative, if performed*

*FUS/DDIT3 (t(12;16)) (eg, myxoid liposarcoma), translocation analysis, qualitative, and quantitative, if performed*

*FXN (frataxin) (eg, Friedreich ataxia), evaluation to detect abnormal (expanded) alleles*

*GALC (galactosylceramidase) (eg, Krabbe disease), common variants (eg, c.857G>A, 30-kb deletion)*

*GALT (galactose-1-phosphate uridylyltransferase) (eg, galactosemia), common variants (eg, Q188R, S135L, K285N, T138M, L195P, Y209C, IVS2-2A>G, P171S, del5kb, N314D, L218L/N314D)*

*H19 (imprinted maternally expressed transcript [non-protein coding]) (eg, Beckwith-Wiedemann syndrome), methylation analysis*

*HTT (huntingtin) (eg, Huntington disease), evaluation to detect abnormal (eg, expanded) alleles*

*IGH@/BCL2 (t(14;18)) (eg, follicular lymphoma), translocation and analysis; single breakpoint (eg) major breakpoint region [MBR] or minor cluster region [mcr]), qualitative or quantitative(When both MBR and mcr breakpoints are performed, use 81402)*

*KCNQ10T1 (KCNQ1 overlapping transcript 1 [non-protein coding]) (e.g, Beckwith-Wiedemann syndrome), methylation analysis*

*LINC00518 (long intergenic non-protein coding RNA 518) (eg, melanoma), expression analysis*

*LRRK2 (leucine-rich repeat kinase 2) (eg, Parkinson disease), common variants (eg, R1441G, G2019S, I2020T)*

*MED12 (mediator complex subunit 12) (eg, FG syndrome type 1, Lujan syndrome), common variants (eg, R961W, N1007S)*

*MEG3/DLK1 (maternally expressed 3 [non-protein coding]/delta-like 1 homolog [Drosophila]) (eg, intrauterine growth retardation), methylation analysis*

*MLL/AFF1 (t(4;11)) (eg acute lymphoblastic leukemia), translocation analysis, qualitative and quantitative, if performed*

*MLL/MLLT3 (t(9;11)) (eg, acute myeloid leukemia) translocation analysis, qualitative and quantitative, if performed*

*MT-RNR1 (mitochondrially encoded 12S RNA) (eg, nonsyndromic hearing loss), common variants (eg, m.1555>G, m1494C>T)*

*MUTYH (mutY homolog [E.coli]) (eg, MYH-associated polyposis), common variants (eg, Y165C, G382D)*

*MT-ATP6 (mitochondrially encoded ATP synthase 6) (eg, neuropathy with ataxia and retinitis pigmentosa [NARP], Leigh syndrome), common variants (eg, m.8993T>G, m.8993T>C)*

*MT-ND4, MT-ND6 (mitochondrially encoded NADH dehydrogenase 4, mitochondrially encoded NADH dehydrogenase 6) (eg, Leber hereditary optic neuropathy [LHON]), common variants (eg m.11778G>A, m3460G>A, m14484T>C)*

*MT-ND5 (mitochondrially encoded tRNA leucine 1 [UUA/G], mitochondrially encoded NADH dehydrogenase 5) (eg, mitochondrial encephalopathy with lactic acidosis and stroke-like episodes [MELAS]), common variants (eg, m.3243A>G, m.3271T>C, m.3252A>G, m.13513G>A)*

*MT-TK (mitochondrially encoded tRNA lysine) (eg, myoclonic epilepsy with ragged-red fibers [MERRF]), common variants (eg, m8344A>G, m.8356T>C)*

*MT-TL1 (mitochondrially encoded tRNA leucine 1[UUA/G]) (eg, diabetes and hearing loss), common variants (eg, m.3243A>G, m.14709 T>C) MT-TL1*

*MT-TS1, MT-RNR1 (mitochondrially encoded tRNA serine 1 [UCN], mitochondrially encoded 12S RNA) (eg, nonsyndromic sensorineural deafness [including aminoglycoside-induced nonsyndromic deafness]) common variants (eg, m.7445A>G, m.1555A>G)*

---

● New Code    ▲ Revised Code    ○ Reinstated    ● New Web Release    ▲ Revised Web Release    Unlisted    Not Covered    # Resequenced
⊘ AMA Mod 51 Exempt    ⑤ Optum Mod 51 Exempt    ⊛ Mod 63 Exempt    ✗ Non-FDA Drug    ★ Telemedicine    Ⓜ Maternity    Ⓐ Age Edit    + Add-on    **AMA:** CPT Asst

*NOD2 (nucleotide-binding oligomerization domain containing 2) (eg, Crohn's disease, Blau syndrome), common variants (eg, SNP 8, SNP 12, SNP 13)*

*NPM/ALK (t(2;5)) (eg, anaplastic large cell lymphoma), translocation analysis*

*PABPN1 (poly[A] binding protein, nuclear 1) (eg, oculopharyngeal muscular dystrophy), evaluation to detect abnormal (eg, expanded) alleles*

*PAX8/PPARG (t(2;3) (q13;p25)) (eg, follicular thyroid carcinoma), translocation analysis*

*PPP2R2B (protein phosphatase 2, regulatory subunit B, beta) (eg, spinocerebellar ataxia), evaluation to detect abnormal (eg, expanded) alleles*

*PRAME (preferentially expressed antigen in melanoma)(eg, melanoma), expression analysis*

*PRSS1 (protease, serine, 1 [trypsin 1]) (eg, hereditary pancreatitis), common variants (eg, N29I, A16V, R122H)*

*PYGM (phosphorylase, glycogen, muscle) (eg, glycogen storage disease type V, McArdle disease), common variants (eg, R50X, G205S)*

*RUNX1/RUNX1T1 (t(8;21)) (eg, acute myeloid leukemia) translocation analysis, qualitative and quantitative, if performed*

*SMN1/SMN2 (survival of motor neuron 1, telomeric/survival of motor neuron 2, centromeric) (eg, spinal muscular atrophy), dosage analysis (eg, carrier testing)*

*SMN1/SMN2 duplication/deletion analysis*

*SS18/SSX1 (t(X;18)) (eg, synovial sarcoma), translocation analysis, qualitative and quantitative, if performed*

*SS18/SSX2 (t(X;18)) (eg, synovial sarcoma), translocation analysis, qualitative and quantitative, if performed*

*TBP (TATA box binding protein) (eg, spinocerebellar ataxia), evaluation to detect abnormal (eg, expanded) alleles*

*VWF (von Willebrand factor) (eg, von Willebrand disease type 2N), common variants (eg, T791M, R816W, R854Q)*

   📣 0.00   ⚕ 0.00   **FUD** XXX   🅰️🖵

**AMA:** 2017,Jan,8; 2016,Aug,9; 2016,Jan,13; 2015,Jan,16; 2015,Jan,3; 2014,Jan,11; 2013,Sep,3-12; 2013,Jul,11-12; 2012,May,3-10

**81402** **Molecular pathology procedure, Level 3 (eg, >10 SNPs, 2-10 methylated variants, or 2-10 somatic variants [typically using non-sequencing target variant analysis], immunoglobulin and T-cell receptor gene rearrangements, duplication/deletion variants of 1 exon, loss of heterozygosity [LOH], uniparental disomy [UPD])**

*Chromosome 1p-/19q- (eg, glial tumors), deletion analysis*

*Chromosome 18q- (eg, D18S55, D18S58, D18S61, D18S64, and D18S69) (eg, colon cancer), allelic imbalance assessment (ie, loss of heterozygosity)*

*COL1A1/PDGFB (t(17;22)) (eg, dermatofibrosarcoma protuberans), translocation analysis, multiple breakpoints, qualitative, and quantitative, if performed*

*CYP21A2 (cytochrome P450, family 21, subfamily A, polypeptide 2) (eg, congenital adrenal hyperplasia, 21-hydroxylase deficiency), common variants (eg, IVS2-13G, P30L, I172N, exon 6 mutation cluster [I235N, V236E, M238K], V281L, L307FfsX6, Q318X, R356W, P453S, G110VfsX21, 30-kb deletion variant)*

*ESR1/PGR (receptor 1/progesterone receptor) ratio (eg, breast cancer)*

*IGH@/BCL2 (t(14;18)) (eg, follicular lymphoma), translocation analysis; major breakpoint region (MBR) and minor cluster region (mcr) breakpoints, qualitative or quantitative*

*MEFV (Mediterranean fever) (eg, familial Mediterranean fever), common variants (eg, E148Q, P369S, F479L, M680I, I692del, M694V, M694I, K695R, V726A, A744S, R761H)*

*MPL (myeloproliferative leukemia virus oncogene, thrombopoietin receptor, TPOR) (eg, myeloproliferative disorder), common variants (eg, W515A, W515K, W515L, W515R)*

*TRD@ (T cell antigen receptor, delta) (eg, leukemia and lymphoma), gene rearrangement analysis, evaluation to detect abnormal clonal population*

*Uniparental disomy (UPD) (eg, Russell-Silver syndrome, Prader-Willi/Angelman syndrome), short tandem repeat (STR) analysis*

   📣 0.00   ⚕ 0.00   **FUD** XXX   🅰️🖵

**AMA:** 2017,Jan,8; 2016,Aug,9; 2016,Jan,13; 2015,Jan,16; 2015,Jan,3; 2014,Jan,11; 2013,Sep,3-12; 2013,Jul,11-12; 2012,May,3-10

▲ **81403** **Molecular pathology procedure, Level 4 (eg, analysis of single exon by DNA sequence analysis, analysis of >10 amplicons using multiplex PCR in 2 or more independent reactions, mutation scanning or duplication/deletion variants of 2-5 exons)**

*ANG (angiogenin, ribonuclease, RNase A family, 5) (eg, amyotrophic lateral sclerosis), full gene sequence*

*ARX (aristaless-related homeobox) (eg, X-linked lissencephaly with ambiguous genitalia, X-linked mental retardation), duplication/deletion analysis*

*CEL (carboxyl ester lipase [bile salt-stimulated lipase]) (eg, maturity-onset diabetes of the young [MODY]), targeted sequence analysis of exon 11 (eg, c.1785delC, c.1686delT)*

*CTNNB1 (catenin [cadherin-associated protein], beta 1, 88kDa) (eg, desmoid tumors), targeted sequence analysis (eg, exon 3)*

*DAZ/SRY (deleted in azoospermia and sex determining region Y) (eg, male infertility), common deletions (eg, AZFa, AZFb, AZFc, AZFd)*

*DNMT3A (DNA [cytosine-5-]-methyltransferase 3 alpha) (eg, acute myeloid leukemia), targeted sequence analysis (eg, exon 23)*

*EPCAM (epithelial cell adhesion molecule) (eg, Lynch syndrome), duplication/deletion analysis*

*F8 (coagulation factor VIII) (eg, hemophilia A), inversion analysis, intron 1 and intron 22A*

*F12 (coagulation factor XII [Hageman factor]) (eg, angioedema, hereditary, type III; factor XII deficiency), targeted sequence analysis of exon 9*

*FGFR3 (fibroblast growth factor receptor 3) (eg, isolated craniosynostosis), targeted sequence analysis (eg, exon 7)*

*(For targeted sequence analysis of multiple FGFR3 exons, use 81404) (81404)*

*GJB1 (gap junction protein, beta 1) (eg, Charcot-Marie-Tooth X-linked), full gene sequence*

*GNAQ (guanine nucleotide-binding protein G[q] subunit alpha) (eg, uveal melanoma), common variants (eg, R183, Q209)*

*HRAS (v-Ha-ras Harvey rat sarcoma viral oncogene homolog) (eg, Costello syndrome), exon 2 sequence*

*Human erythrocyte antigen gene analyses (eg, SLC14A1 [Kidd blood group], BCAM [Lutheran blood group], ICAM4 [Landsteiner-Wiener blood group], SLC4A1 [Diego blood group], AQP1 [Colton blood group], ERMAP [Scianna blood group], RHCE [Rh blood group, CcEe antigens], KEL [Kell blood group], DARC [Duffy blood group], GYPA, GYPB, GYPE [MNS blood group], ART4 [Dombrock blood group]) (eg, sickle-cell disease, thalassemia, hemolytic transfusion reactions, hemolytic disease of the fetus or newborn), common variants*

*JAK2 (Janus kinase 2) (eg, myeloproliferative disorder), exon 12 sequence and exon 13 sequence, if performed*

*KCNC3 (potassium voltage-gated channel, Shaw-related subfamily, member 3) (eg, spinocerebellar ataxia), targeted sequence analysis (eg, exon 2)*

*KCNJ2 (potassium inwardly-rectifying channel, subfamily J, member 2) (eg, Andersen-Tawil syndrome), full gene sequence*

*KCNJ11 (potassium inwardly-rectifying channel, subfamily J, member 11) (eg, familial hyperinsulinism), full gene sequence*

*Killer cell immunoglobulin-like receptor (KIR) gene family (eg, hematopoietic stem cell transplantation), genotyping of KIR family genes*

*Known familial variant, not otherwise specified, for gene listed in Tier 1 or Tier 2, or identified during a genomic sequencing procedure, DNA sequence analysis, each variant exon*

*(For a known familial variant that is considered a common variant, use specific common variant Tier 1 or Tier 2 code)*

*MC4R (melanocortin 4 receptor) (eg, obesity), full gene sequence*

*MICA (MHC class I polypeptide-related sequence A) (eg, solid organ transplantation), common variants (eg, *001, *002)*

*MPL (myeloproliferative leukemia virus oncogene, thrombopoietin receptor, TPOR) (eg, myeloproliferative disorder), exon 10 sequence*

*MT-RNR1 (mitochondrially encoded 12S RNA) (eg, nonsyndromic hearing loss), full gene sequence*

*MT-TS1 (mitochondrially encoded tRNA serine 1) (eg, nonsyndromic hearing loss), full gene sequence*

*NDP (Norrie disease [pseudoglioma]) (eg, Norrie disease), duplication/deletion analysis*

*NHLRC1 (NHL repeat containing 1) (eg, progressive myoclonus epilepsy), full gene sequence*

*PHOX2B (paired-like homeobox 2b) (eg, congenital central hypoventilation syndrome), duplication/deletion analysis*

*PLN (phospholamban) (eg, dilated cardiomyopathy, hypertrophic cardiomyopathy), full gene sequence*

*RHD (Rh blood group, D antigen) (eg, hemolytic disease of the fetus and newborn, Rh maternal/fetal compatibility), deletion analysis (eg, exons 4, 5, and 7, pseudogene)*

*RHD (Rh blood group, D antigen) (eg, hemolytic disease of the fetus and newborn, Rh maternal/fetal compatibility), deletion analysis (eg, exons 4, 5, and 7, pseudogene), performed on cell-free fetal DNA in maternal blood*

*(For human erythrocyte gene analysis of RHD, use a separate unit of 81403)*

*SH2D1A (SH2 domain containing 1A) (eg, X-linked lymphoproliferative syndrome), duplication/deletion analysis*

*SMN1 (survival of motor neuron 1, telomeric) (eg, spinal muscular atrophy), known familial sequence variant(s)*

*TWIST1 (twist homolog 1 [Drosophila]) (eg, Saethre-Chotzen syndrome), duplication/deletion analysis*

*UBA1 (ubiquitin-like modifier activating enzyme 1) (eg, spinal muscular atrophy, X-linked), targeted sequence analysis (eg, exon 15)*

*VHL (von Hippel-Lindau tumor suppressor) (eg, von Hippel-Lindau familial cancer syndrome), deletion/duplication analysis*

*VWF (von Willebrand factor) (eg, von Willebrand disease types 2A, 2B, 2M), targeted sequence analysis (eg, exon 28)*

     🚑 0.00    ⚕ 0.00    **FUD** XXX     A ▯

**AMA:** 2017,Jan,8; 2016,Aug,9; 2016,Jan,13; 2015,Jan,16; 2015,Jan,3; 2014,Jan,11; 2013,Sep,3-12; 2013,Jul,11-12; 2012,May,3-10

▲ **81404** **Molecular pathology procedure, Level 5 (eg, analysis of 2-5 exons by DNA sequence analysis, mutation scanning or duplication/deletion variants of 6-10 exons, or characterization of a dynamic mutation disorder/triplet repeat by Southern blot analysis)**

*ACADS (acyl-CoA dehydrogenase, C-2 to C-3 short chain) (eg, short chain acyl-CoA dehydrogenase deficiency), targeted sequence analysis (eg, exons 5 and 6)*

*AFF2 (AF4/FMR2 family, member 2 [FMR2]) (eg, fragile X mental retardation 2 [FRAXE]), characterization of alleles (eg, expanded size and methylation status)*

*AQP2 (aquaporin 2 [collecting duct]) (eg, nephrogenic diabetes insipidus), full gene sequence*

*ARX (aristaless related homeobox) (eg, X-linked lissencephaly with ambiguous genitalia, X-linked mental retardation), full gene sequence*

*AVPR2 (arginine vasopressin receptor 2) (eg, nephrogenic diabetes insipidus), full gene sequence*

*BBS10 (Bardet-Biedl syndrome 10) (eg, Bardet-Biedl syndrome), full gene sequence*

*BTD (biotinidase) (eg, biotinidase deficiency), full gene sequence*

*C10orf2 (chromosome 10 open reading frame 2) (eg, mitochondrial DNA depletion syndrome), full gene sequence*

*CAV3 (caveolin 3) (eg, CAV3-related distal myopathy, limb-girdle muscular dystrophy type 1C), full gene sequence*

*CD40LG (CD40 ligand) (eg, X-linked hyper IgM syndrome), full gene sequence*

*CDKN2A (cyclin-dependent kinase inhibitor 2A) (eg, CDKN2A-related cutaneous malignant melanoma, familial atypical mole-malignant melanoma syndrome), full gene sequence*

*CLRN1 (clarin 1) (eg, Usher syndrome, type 3), full gene sequence*

*COX6B1 (cytochrome c oxidase subunit VIb polypeptide 1) (eg, mitochondrial respiratory chain complex IV deficiency), full gene sequence*

*CPT2 (carnitine palmitoyltransferase 2) (eg, carnitine palmitoyltransferase II deficiency), full gene sequence*

*CRX (cone-rod homeobox) (eg, cone-rod dystrophy 2, Leber congenital amaurosis), full gene sequence*

*CSTB (cystatin B [stefin B]) (eg, Unverricht-Lundborg disease), full gene sequence*

*CYP1B1 (cytochrome P450, family 1, subfamily B, polypeptide 1) (eg, primary congenital glaucoma), full gene sequence*

*DMPK (dystrophia myotonica-protein kinase) (eg, myotonic dystrophy type 1), characterization of abnormal (eg, expanded) alleles*

*EGR2 (early growth response 2) (eg, Charcot-Marie-Tooth), full gene sequence*

*EMD (emerin) (eg, Emery-Dreifuss muscular dystrophy), duplication/deletion analysis*

*EPM2A (epilepsy, progressive myoclonus type 2A, Lafora disease [laforin]) (eg, progressive myoclonus epilepsy), full gene sequence*

*FGF23 (fibroblast growth factor 23) (eg, hypophosphatemic rickets), full gene sequence*

*FGFR2 (fibroblast growth factor receptor 2) (eg, craniosynostosis, Apert syndrome, Crouzon syndrome), targeted sequence analysis (eg, exons 8, 10)*

*FGFR3 (fibroblast growth factor receptor 3) (eg, achondroplasia, hypochondroplasia), targeted sequence analysis (eg, exons 8, 11, 12, 13)*

*FHL1 (four and a half LIM domains 1) (eg, Emery-Dreifuss muscular dystrophy), full gene sequence*

*FKRP (Fukutin related protein) (eg, congenital muscular dystrophy type 1C [MDC1C], limb-girdle muscular dystrophy [LGMD] type 2I), full gene sequence*

*FOXG1 (forkhead box G1) (eg, Rett syndrome), full gene sequence*

*FSHMD1A (facioscapulohumeral muscular dystrophy 1A) (eg, facioscapulohumeral muscular dystrophy), evaluation to detect abnormal (eg, deleted) alleles*

*FSHMD1A (facioscapulohumeral muscular dystrophy 1A) (eg, facioscapulohumeral muscular dystrophy), characterization of haplotype(s) (ie, chromosome 4A and 4B haplotypes)*

*FXN (frataxin) (eg, Friedreich ataxia), full gene sequence*

● New Code    ▲ Revised Code    ○ Reinstated    ● New Web Release    ▲ Revised Web Release    Unlisted    Not Covered    # Resequenced

⊘ AMA Mod 51 Exempt    ⑩ Optum Mod 51 Exempt    ⊚ Mod 63 Exempt    ⁄ Non-FDA Drug    ★ Telemedicine    Ⓜ Maternity    Ⓐ Age Edit    + Add-on    **AMA:** CPT Asst

© 2017 Optum360, LLC      CPT © 2017 American Medical Association. All Rights Reserved.

GH1 (growth hormone 1) (eg, growth hormone deficiency), full gene sequence

GP1BB (glycoprotein Ib [platelet], beta polypeptide) (eg, Bernard-Soulier syndrome type B), full gene sequence

(For common deletion variants of alpha globin 1 and alpha globin 2 genes, use 81257)

HNF1B (HNF1 homeobox B) (eg, maturity-onset diabetes of the young [MODY]), duplication/deletion analysis

HRAS (v-Ha-ras Harvey rat sarcoma viral oncogene homolog) (eg, Costello syndrome), full gene sequence

HSD3B2 (hydroxy-delta-5-steroid dehydrogenase, 3 beta- and steroid delta-isomerase 2) (eg, 3-beta-hydroxysteroid dehydrogenase type II deficiency), full gene sequence

HSD11B2 (hydroxysteroid [11-beta] dehydrogenase 2) (eg, mineralocorticoid excess syndrome), full gene sequence

HSPB1 (heat shock 27kDa protein 1) (eg, Charcot-Marie-Tooth disease), full gene sequence

INS (insulin) (eg, diabetes mellitus), full gene sequence

KCNJ1 (potassium inwardly-rectifying channel, subfamily J, member 1) (eg, Bartter syndrome), full gene sequence

KCNJ10 (potassium inwardly-rectifying channel, subfamily J, member 10) (eg, SeSAME syndrome, EAST syndrome, sensorineural hearing loss), full gene sequence

LITAF (lipopolysaccharide-induced TNF factor) (eg, Charcot-Marie-Tooth), full gene sequence

MEFV (Mediterranean fever) (eg, familial Mediterranean fever), full gene sequence

MEN1 (multiple endocrine neoplasia I) (eg, multiple endocrine neoplasia type 1, Wermer syndrome), duplication/deletion analysis

MMACHC (methylmalonic aciduria [cobalamin deficiency] cblC type, with homocystinuria) (eg, methylmalonic acidemia and homocystinuria), full gene sequence

MPV17 (MpV17 mitochondrial inner membrane protein) (eg, mitochondrial DNA depletion syndrome), duplication/deletion analysis

NDP (Norrie disease [pseudoglioma]) (eg, Norrie disease), full gene sequence

NDUFA1 (NADH dehydrogenase [ubiquinone] 1 alpha subcomplex, 1, 7.5kDa) (eg, Leigh syndrome, mitochondrial complex I deficiency), full gene sequence

NDUFAF2 (NADH dehydrogenase [ubiquinone] 1 alpha subcomplex, assembly factor 2) (eg, Leigh syndrome, mitochondrial complex I deficiency), full gene sequence

NDUFS4 (NADH dehydrogenase [ubiquinone] Fe-S protein 4, 18kDa [NADH-coenzyme Q reductase]) (eg, Leigh syndrome, mitochondrial complex I deficiency), full gene sequence

NIPA1 (non-imprinted in Prader-Willi/Angelman syndrome 1) (eg, spastic paraplegia), full gene sequence

NLGN4X (neuroligin 4, X-linked) (eg, autism spectrum disorders), duplication/deletion analysis

NPC2 (Niemann-Pick disease, type C2 [epididymal secretory protein E1]) (eg, Niemann-Pick disease type C2), full gene sequence

NR0B1 (nuclear receptor subfamily 0, group B, member 1) (eg, congenital adrenal hypoplasia), full gene sequence

PDX1 (pancreatic and duodenal homeobox 1) (eg, maturity-onset diabetes of the young [MODY]), full gene sequence

PHOX2B (paired-like homeobox 2b) (eg, congenital central hypoventilation syndrome), full gene sequence

PIK3CA (phosphatidylinositol-4,5-bisphosphate 3-kinase, catalytic subunit alpha) (eg, colorectal cancer), targeted sequence analysis (eg, exons 9 and 20)

PLP1 (proteolipid protein 1) (eg, Pelizaeus-Merzbacher disease, spastic paraplegia), duplication/deletion analysis

PQBP1 (polyglutamine binding protein 1) (eg, Renpenning syndrome), duplication/deletion analysis

PRNP (prion protein) (eg, genetic prion disease), full gene sequence

PROP1 (PROP paired-like homeobox 1) (eg, combined pituitary hormone deficiency), full gene sequence

PRPH2 (peripherin 2 [retinal degeneration, slow]) (eg, retinitis pigmentosa), full gene sequence

PRSS1 (protease, serine, 1 [trypsin 1]) (eg, hereditary pancreatitis), full gene sequence

RAF1 (v-raf-1 murine leukemia viral oncogene homolog 1) (eg, LEOPARD syndrome), targeted sequence analysis (eg, exons 7, 12, 14, 17)

RET (ret proto-oncogene) (eg, multiple endocrine neoplasia, type 2B and familial medullary thyroid carcinoma), common variants (eg, M918T, 2647_2648delinsTT, A883F)

RHO (rhodopsin) (eg, retinitis pigmentosa), full gene sequence

RP1 (retinitis pigmentosa 1) (eg, retinitis pigmentosa), full gene sequence

SCN1B (sodium channel, voltage-gated, type I, beta) (eg, Brugada syndrome), full gene sequence

SCO2 (SCO cytochrome oxidase deficient homolog 2 [SCO1L]) (eg, mitochondrial respiratory chain complex IV deficiency), full gene sequence

SDHC (succinate dehydrogenase complex, subunit C, integral membrane protein, 15kDa) (eg, hereditary paraganglioma-pheochromocytoma syndrome), duplication/deletion analysis

SDHD (succinate dehydrogenase complex, subunit D, integral membrane protein) (eg, hereditary paraganglioma), full gene sequence

SGCG (sarcoglycan, gamma [35kDa dystrophin-associated glycoprotein]) (eg, limb-girdle muscular dystrophy), duplication/deletion analysis

SH2D1A (SH2 domain containing 1A) (eg, X-linked lymphoproliferative syndrome), full gene sequence

SLC16A2 (solute carrier family 16, member 2 [thyroid hormone transporter]) (eg, specific thyroid hormone cell transporter deficiency, Allan-Herndon-Dudley syndrome), duplication/deletion analysis

SLC25A20 (solute carrier family 25 [carnitine/acylcarnitine translocase], member 20) (eg, carnitine-acylcarnitine translocase deficiency), duplication/deletion analysis

SLC25A4 (solute carrier family 25 [mitochondrial carrier; adenine nucleotide translocation], member 4) (eg, progressive external ophthalmoplegia), full gene sequence

SOD1 (superoxide dismutase 1, soluble) (eg, amyotrophic lateral sclerosis), full gene sequence

SPINK1 (serine peptidase inhibitor, Kazal type 1) (eg, hereditary pancreatitis), full gene sequence

STK11 (serine/threonine kinase 11) (eg, Peutz-Jeghers syndrome), duplication/deletion analysis

TACO1 (translational activator of mitochondrial encoded cytochrome c oxidase I) (eg, mitochondrial respiratory chain complex IV deficiency), full gene sequence

THAP1 (THAP domain containing, apoptosis associated protein 1) (eg, torsion dystonia), full gene sequence

TOR1A (torsin family 1, member A [torsin A]) (eg, torsion dystonia), full gene sequence

TP53 (tumor protein 53) (eg, tumor samples), targeted sequence analysis of 2-5 exons

TTPA (tocopherol [alpha] transfer protein) (eg, ataxia), full gene sequence

Pathology and Laboratory

*TTR (transthyretin) (eg, familial transthyretin amyloidosis), full gene sequence*

*TWIST1 (twist homolog 1 [Drosophila]) (eg, Saethre-Chotzen syndrome), full gene sequence*

*TYR (tyrosinase [oculocutaneous albinism IA]) (eg, oculocutaneous albinism IA), full gene sequence*

*USH1G (Usher syndrome 1G [autosomal recessive]) (eg, Usher syndrome, type 1), full gene sequence*

*VWF (von Willebrand factor) (eg, von Willebrand disease type 1C), targeted sequence analysis (eg, exons 26, 27, 37)*

*VHL (von Hippel-Lindau tumor suppressor) (eg, von Hippel-Lindau familial cancer syndrome), full gene sequence*

*ZEB2 (zinc finger E-box binding homeobox 2) (eg, Mowat-Wilson syndrome), duplication/deletion analysis*

*ZNF41 (zinc finger protein 41) (eg, X-linked mental retardation 89), full gene sequence*

      🖧 0.00    � 0.00   **FUD** XXX        A 📷

**AMA:** 2017,Jan,8; 2016,Aug,9; 2016,Jan,13; 2015,Jan,16; 2015,Jan,3; 2014,Jan,11; 2013,Sep,3-12; 2013,Jul,11-12; 2012,May,3-10

▲   **81405**   **Molecular pathology procedure, Level 6 (eg, analysis of 6-10 exons by DNA sequence analysis, mutation scanning or duplication/deletion variants of 11-25 exons, regionally targeted cytogenomic array analysis)**

*ABCD1 (ATP-binding cassette, sub-family D [ALD], member 1) (eg, adrenoleukodystrophy), full gene sequence*

*ACADS (acyl-CoA dehydrogenase, C-2 to C-3 short chain) (eg, short chain acyl-CoA dehydrogenase deficiency), full gene sequence*

*ACTA2 (actin, alpha 2, smooth muscle, aorta) (eg, thoracic aortic aneurysms and aortic dissections), full gene sequence*

*ACTC1 (actin, alpha, cardiac muscle 1) (eg, familial hypertrophic cardiomyopathy), full gene sequence*

*ANKRD1 (ankyrin repeat domain 1) (eg, dilated cardiomyopathy), full gene sequence*

*APTX (aprataxin) (eg, ataxia with oculomotor apraxia 1), full gene sequence*

*AR (androgen receptor) (eg, androgen insensitivity syndrome), full gene sequence*

*ARSA (arylsulfatase A) (eg, arylsulfatase A deficiency), full gene sequence*

*BCKDHA (branched chain keto acid dehydrogenase E1, alpha polypeptide) (eg, maple syrup urine disease, type 1A), full gene sequence*

*BCS1L (BCS1-like [S. cerevisiae]) (eg, Leigh syndrome, mitochondrial complex III deficiency, GRACILE syndrome), full gene sequence*

*BMPR2 (bone morphogenetic protein receptor, type II [serine/threonine kinase]) (eg, heritable pulmonary arterial hypertension), duplication/deletion analysis*

*CASQ2 (calsequestrin 2 [cardiac muscle]) (eg, catecholaminergic polymorphic ventricular tachycardia), full gene sequence*

*CASR (calcium-sensing receptor) (eg, hypocalcemia), full gene sequence*

*CDKL5 (cyclin-dependent kinase-like 5) (eg, early infantile epileptic encephalopathy), duplication/deletion analysis*

*CHRNA4 (cholinergic receptor, nicotinic, alpha 4) (eg, nocturnal frontal lobe epilepsy), full gene sequence*

*CHRNB2 (cholinergic receptor, nicotinic, beta 2 [neuronal]) (eg, nocturnal frontal lobe epilepsy), full gene sequence*

*COX10 (COX10 homolog, cytochrome c oxidase assembly protein) (eg, mitochondrial respiratory chain complex IV deficiency), full gene sequence*

*COX15 (COX15 homolog, cytochrome c oxidase assembly protein) (eg, mitochondrial respiratory chain complex IV deficiency), full gene sequence*

*CPOX (coproporphyrinogen oxidase) (eg, hereditary coproporphyria), full gene sequence*

*CTRC (chymotrypsin C) (eg, hereditary pancreatitis), full gene sequence*

*CYP11B1 (cytochrome P450, family 11, subfamily B, polypeptide 1) (eg, congenital adrenal hyperplasia), full gene sequence*

*CYP17A1 (cytochrome P450, family 17, subfamily A, polypeptide 1) (eg, congenital adrenal hyperplasia), full gene sequence*

*CYP21A2 (cytochrome P450, family 21, subfamily A, polypeptide2) (eg, steroid 21-hydroxylase isoform, congenital adrenal hyperplasia), full gene sequence*

*Cytogenomic constitutional targeted microarray analysis of chromosome 22q13 by interrogation of genomic regions for copy number and single nucleotide polymorphism (SNP) variants for chromosomal abnormalities*

*(When performing genome-wide cytogenomic constitutional microarray analysis, see 81228, 81229) (81228-81229)*

*(Do not report analyte-specific molecular pathology procedures separately when the specific analytes are included as part of the microarray analysis of chromosome 22q13)*

*(Do not report 88271 when performing cytogenomic microarray analysis)*

*DBT (dihydrolipoamide branched chain transacylase E2) (eg, maple syrup urine disease, type 2), duplication/deletion analysis*

*DCX (doublecortin) (eg, X-linked lissencephaly), full gene sequence*

*DES (desmin) (eg, myofibrillar myopathy), full gene sequence*

*DFNB59 (deafness, autosomal recessive 59) (eg, autosomal recessive nonsyndromic hearing impairment), full gene sequence*

*DGUOK (deoxyguanosine kinase) (eg, hepatocerebral mitochondrial DNA depletion syndrome), full gene sequence*

*DHCR7 (7-dehydrocholesterol reductase) (eg, Smith-Lemli-Opitz syndrome), full gene sequence*

*EIF2B2 (eukaryotic translation initiation factor 2B, subunit 2 beta, 39kDa) (eg, leukoencephalopathy with vanishing white matter), full gene sequence*

*EMD (emerin) (eg, Emery-Dreifuss muscular dystrophy), full gene sequence*

*ENG (endoglin) (eg, hereditary hemorrhagic telangiectasia, type 1), duplication/deletion analysis*

*EYA1 (eyes absent homolog 1 [Drosophila]) (eg, branchio-oto-renal [BOR] spectrum disorders), duplication/deletion analysis*

*FGFR1 (fibroblast growth factor receptor 1) (eg, Kallmann syndrome 2), full gene sequence*

*FH (fumarate hydratase) (eg, fumarate hydratase deficiency, hereditary leiomyomatosis with renal cell cancer), full gene sequence*

*FKTN (fukutin) (eg, limb-girdle muscular dystrophy [LGMD] type 2M or 2L), full gene sequence*

*FTSJ1 (FtsJ RNA methyltransferase homolog 1 [E. coli]) (eg, X-linked mental retardation 9), duplication/deletion analysis*

*GABRG2 (gamma-aminobutyric acid [GABA] A receptor, gamma 2) (eg, generalized epilepsy with febrile seizures), full gene sequence*

*GCH1 (GTP cyclohydrolase 1) (eg, autosomal dominant dopa-responsive dystonia), full gene sequence*

*GDAP1 (ganglioside-induced differentiation-associated protein 1) (eg, Charcot-Marie-Tooth disease), full gene sequence*

*GFAP (glial fibrillary acidic protein) (eg, Alexander disease), full gene sequence*

*GHR (growth hormone receptor) (eg, Laron syndrome), full gene sequence*

**81404 — 81405**

---

● New Code   ▲ Revised Code   ○ Reinstated   ● New Web Release   ▲ Revised Web Release   Unlisted   Not Covered   # Resequenced
⊘ AMA Mod 51 Exempt   ⑤ Optum Mod 51 Exempt   ◉ Mod 63 Exempt   ✗ Non-FDA Drug   ★ Telemedicine   Ⓜ Maternity   A Age Edit   + Add-on   **AMA:** CPT Asst
© 2017 Optum360, LLC          CPT © 2017 American Medical Association. All Rights Reserved.       **371**

GHRHR (growth hormone releasing hormone receptor) (eg, growth hormone deficiency), full gene sequence

GLA (galactosidase, alpha) (eg, Fabry disease), full gene sequence

HNF1A (HNF1 homeobox A) (eg, maturity-onset diabetes of the young [MODY]), full gene sequence

HNF1B (HNF1 homeobox B) (eg, maturity-onset diabetes of the young [MODY]), full gene sequence

HTRA1 (HtrA serine peptidase 1) (eg, macular degeneration), full gene sequence

IDS (iduronate 2-sulfatase) (eg, mucopolysaccharidosis, type II), full gene sequence

IL2RG (interleukin 2 receptor, gamma) (eg, X-linked severe combined immunodeficiency), full gene sequence

ISPD (isoprenoid synthase domain containing) (eg, muscle-eye-brain disease, Walker-Warburg syndrome), full gene sequence

KRAS (Kirsten rat sarcoma viral oncogene homolog) (eg, Noonan syndrome), full gene sequence

LAMP2 (lysosomal-associated membrane protein 2) (eg, Danon disease), full gene sequence

LDLR (low density lipoprotein receptor) (eg, familial hypercholesterolemia), duplication/deletion analysis

MEN1 (multiple endocrine neoplasia I) (eg, multiple endocrine neoplasia type 1, Wermer syndrome), full gene sequence

MMAA (methylmalonic aciduria [cobalamin deficiency] type A) (eg, MMAA-related methylmalonic acidemia), full gene sequence

MMAB (methylmalonic aciduria [cobalamin deficiency] type B) (eg, MMAA-related methylmalonic acidemia), full gene sequence

MPI (mannose phosphate isomerase) (eg, congenital disorder of glycosylation 1b), full gene sequence

MPV17 (MpV17 mitochondrial inner membrane protein) (eg, mitochondrial DNA depletion syndrome), full gene sequence

MPZ (myelin protein zero) (eg, Charcot-Marie-Tooth), full gene sequence

MTM1 (myotubularin 1) (eg, X-linked centronuclear myopathy), duplication/deletion analysis

MYL2 (myosin, light chain 2, regulatory, cardiac, slow) (eg, familial hypertrophic cardiomyopathy), full gene sequence

MYL3 (myosin, light chain 3, alkali, ventricular, skeletal, slow) (eg, familial hypertrophic cardiomyopathy), full gene sequence

MYOT (myotilin) (eg, limb-girdle muscular dystrophy), full gene sequence

NDUFS7 (NADH dehydrogenase [ubiquinone] Fe-S protein 7, 20kDa [NADH-coenzyme Q reductase]) (eg, Leigh syndrome, mitochondrial complex I deficiency), full gene sequence

NDUFS8 (NADH dehydrogenase [ubiquinone] Fe-S protein 8, 23kDa [NADH-coenzyme Q reductase]) (eg, Leigh syndrome, mitochondrial complex I deficiency), full gene sequence

NDUFV1 (NADH dehydrogenase [ubiquinone] flavoprotein 1, 51kDa) (eg, Leigh syndrome, mitochondrial complex I deficiency), full gene sequence

NEFL (neurofilament, light polypeptide) (eg, Charcot-Marie-Tooth), full gene sequence

NF2 (neurofibromin 2 [merlin]) (eg, neurofibromatosis, type 2), duplication/deletion analysis

NLGN3 (neuroligin 3) (eg, autism spectrum disorders), full gene sequence

NLGN4X (neuroligin 4, X-linked) (eg, autism spectrum disorders), full gene sequence

NPHP1 (nephronophthisis 1 [juvenile]) (eg, Joubert syndrome), deletion analysis, and duplication analysis, if performed

NPHS2 (nephrosis 2, idiopathic, steroid-resistant [podocin]) (eg, steroid-resistant nephrotic syndrome), full gene sequence

NSD1 (nuclear receptor binding SET domain protein 1) (eg, Sotos syndrome), duplication/deletion analysis

OTC (ornithine carbamoyltransferase) (eg, ornithine transcarbamylase deficiency), full gene sequence

PAFAH1B1 (platelet-activating factor acetylhydrolase 1b, regulatory subunit 1 [45kDa]) (eg, lissencephaly, Miller-Dieker syndrome), duplication/deletion analysis

PARK2 (Parkinson protein 2, E3 ubiquitin protein ligase [parkin]) (eg, Parkinson disease), duplication/deletion analysis

PCCA (propionyl CoA carboxylase, alpha polypeptide) (eg, propionic acidemia, type 1), duplication/deletion analysis

PCDH19 (protocadherin 19) (eg, epileptic encephalopathy), full gene sequence

PDHA1 (pyruvate dehydrogenase [lipoamide] alpha 1) (eg, lactic acidosis), duplication/deletion analysis

PDHB (pyruvate dehydrogenase [lipoamide] beta) (eg, lactic acidosis), full gene sequence

PINK1 (PTEN induced putative kinase 1) (eg, Parkinson disease), full gene sequence

PKLR (pyruvate kinase, liver and RBC) (eg, pyruvate kinase deficiency), full gene sequence

PLP1 (proteolipid protein 1) (eg, Pelizaeus-Merzbacher disease, spastic paraplegia), full gene sequence

POU1F1 (POU class 1 homeobox 1) (eg, combined pituitary hormone deficiency), full gene sequence

PQBP1 (polyglutamine binding protein 1) (eg, Renpenning syndrome), full gene sequence

PRX (periaxin) (eg, Charcot-Marie-Tooth disease), full gene sequence

PSEN1 (presenilin 1) (eg, Alzheimer's disease), full gene sequence

RAB7A (RAB7A, member RAS oncogene family) (eg, Charcot-Marie-Tooth disease), full gene sequence

RAI1 (retinoic acid induced 1) (eg, Smith-Magenis syndrome), full gene sequence

REEP1 (receptor accessory protein 1) (eg, spastic paraplegia), full gene sequence

RET (ret proto-oncogene) (eg, multiple endocrine neoplasia, type 2A and familial medullary thyroid carcinoma), targeted sequence analysis (eg, exons 10, 11, 13-16)

RPS19 (ribosomal protein S19) (eg, Diamond-Blackfan anemia), full gene sequence

RRM2B (ribonucleotide reductase M2 B [TP53 inducible]) (eg, mitochondrial DNA depletion), full gene sequence

SCO1 (SCO cytochrome oxidase deficient homolog 1) (eg, mitochondrial respiratory chain complex IV deficiency), full gene sequence

SDHB (succinate dehydrogenase complex, subunit B, iron sulfur) (eg, hereditary paraganglioma), full gene sequence

SDHC (succinate dehydrogenase complex, subunit C, integral membrane protein, 15kDa) (eg, hereditary paraganglioma-pheochromocytoma syndrome), full gene sequence

SGCA (sarcoglycan, alpha [50kDa dystrophin-associated glycoprotein]) (eg, limb-girdle muscular dystrophy), full gene sequence

SGCB (sarcoglycan, beta [43kDa dystrophin-associated glycoprotein]) (eg, limb-girdle muscular dystrophy), full gene sequence

SGCD (sarcoglycan, delta [35kDa dystrophin-associated glycoprotein]) (eg, limb-girdle muscular dystrophy), full gene sequence

SGCE (sarcoglycan, epsilon) (eg, myoclonic dystonia), duplication/deletion analysis

SGCG (sarcoglycan, gamma [35kDa dystrophin-associated glycoprotein]) (eg, limb-girdle muscular dystrophy), full gene sequence

SHOC2 (soc-2 suppressor of clear homolog) (eg, Noonan-like syndrome with loose anagen hair), full gene sequence

26/TC PC/TC Only    A2-Z3 ASC Payment    50 Bilateral    ♂ Male Only    ♀ Female Only    Facility RVU    Non-Facility RVU    CCI

FUD Follow-up Days    CMS: IOM (Pub 100)    A-Y OPPSI    80/80 Surg Assist Allowed / w/Doc    Lab Crosswalk    Radiology Crosswalk    CLIA

372

CPT © 2017 American Medical Association. All Rights Reserved.      © 2017 Optum360, LLC

*SHOX (short stature homeobox) (eg, Langer mesomelic dysplasia), full gene sequence*

*SIL1 (SIL1 homolog, endoplasmic reticulum chaperone [S. cerevisiae]) (eg, ataxia), full gene sequence*

*SLC2A1 (solute carrier family 2 [facilitated glucose transporter], member 1) (eg, glucose transporter type 1 [GLUT 1] deficiency syndrome), full gene sequence*

*SLC16A2 (solute carrier family 16, member 2 [thyroid hormone transporter]) (eg, specific thyroid hormone cell transporter deficiency, Allan-Herndon-Dudley syndrome), full gene sequence*

*SLC22A5 (solute carrier family 22 [organic cation/carnitine transporter], member 5) (eg, systemic primary carnitine deficiency), full gene sequence*

*SLC25A20 (solute carrier family 25 [carnitine/acylcarnitine translocase], member 20) (eg, carnitine-acylcarnitine translocase deficiency), full gene sequence*

*SMAD4 (SMAD family member 4) (eg, hemorrhagic telangiectasia syndrome, juvenile polyposis), duplication/deletion analysis*

*SMN1 (survival of motor neuron 1, telomeric) (eg, spinal muscular atrophy), full gene sequence*

*SPAST (spastin) (eg, spastic paraplegia), duplication/deletion analysis*

*SPG7 (spastic paraplegia 7 [pure and complicated autosomal recessive]) (eg, spastic paraplegia), duplication/deletion analysis*

*SPRED1 (sprouty-related, EVH1 domain containing 1) (eg, Legius syndrome), full gene sequence*

*STAT3 (signal transducer and activator of transcription 3 [acute-phase response factor]) (eg, autosomal dominant hyper-IgE syndrome), targeted sequence analysis (eg, exons 12, 13, 14, 16, 17, 20, 21)*

*STK11 (serine/threonine kinase 11) (eg, Peutz-Jeghers syndrome), full gene sequence*

*SURF1 (surfeit 1) (eg, mitochondrial respiratory chain complex IV deficiency), full gene sequence*

*TARDBP (TAR DNA binding protein) (eg, amyotrophic lateral sclerosis), full gene sequence*

*TBX5 (T-box 5) (eg, Holt-Oram syndrome), full gene sequence*

*TCF4 (transcription factor 4) (eg, Pitt-Hopkins syndrome), duplication/deletion analysis*

*TGFBR1 (transforming growth factor, beta receptor 1) (eg, Marfan syndrome), full gene sequence*

*TGFBR2 (transforming growth factor, beta receptor 2) (eg, Marfan syndrome), full gene sequence*

*THRB (thyroid hormone receptor, beta) (eg, thyroid hormone resistance, thyroid hormone beta receptor deficiency), full gene sequence or targeted sequence analysis of >5 exons*

*TK2 (thymidine kinase 2, mitochondrial) (eg, mitochondrial DNA depletion syndrome), full gene sequence*

*TNNC1 (troponin C type 1 [slow]) (eg, hypertrophic cardiomyopathy or dilated cardiomyopathy), full gene sequence*

*TNNI3 (troponin I, type 3 [cardiac]) (eg, familial hypertrophic cardiomyopathy), full gene sequence*

*TP53 (tumor protein 53) (eg, Li-Fraumeni syndrome, tumor samples), full gene sequence or targeted sequence analysis of >5 exons*

*TPM1 (tropomyosin 1 [alpha]) (eg, familial hypertrophic cardiomyopathy), full gene sequence*

*TSC1 (tuberous sclerosis 1) (eg, tuberous sclerosis), duplication/deletion analysis*

*TYMP (thymidine phosphorylase) (eg, mitochondrial DNA depletion syndrome), full gene sequence*

*VWF (von Willebrand factor) (eg, von Willebrand disease type 2N), targeted sequence analysis (eg, exons 18-20, 23-25)*

*WT1 (Wilms tumor 1) (eg, Denys-Drash syndrome, familial Wilms tumor), full gene sequence*

*ZEB2 (zinc finger E-box binding homeobox 2) (eg, Mowat-Wilson syndrome), full gene sequence*

📷 0.00   ⚕ 0.00   **FUD** XXX   🅰 💾

**AMA:** 2017,Jan,8; 2016,Aug,9; 2016,Jan,13; 2015,Jan,16; 2015,Jan,3; 2014,Jan,11; 2013,Sep,3-12; 2013,Jul,11-12; 2012,May,3-10

▲ **81406**   **Molecular pathology procedure, Level 7 (eg, analysis of 11-25 exons by DNA sequence analysis, mutation scanning or duplication/deletion variants of 26-50 exons, cytogenomic array analysis for neoplasia)**

*ACADVL (acyl-CoA dehydrogenase, very long chain) (eg, very long chain acyl-coenzyme A dehydrogenase deficiency), full gene sequence*

*ACTN4 (actinin, alpha 4) (eg, focal segmental glomerulosclerosis), full gene sequence*

*AFG3L2 (AFG3 ATPase family gene 3-like 2 [S. cerevisiae]) (eg, spinocerebellar ataxia), full gene sequence*

*AIRE (autoimmune regulator) (eg, autoimmune polyendocrinopathy syndrome type 1), full gene sequence*

*ALDH7A1 (aldehyde dehydrogenase 7 family, member A1) (eg, pyridoxine-dependent epilepsy), full gene sequence*

*ANO5 (anoctamin 5) (eg, limb-girdle muscular dystrophy), full gene sequence*

*ANOS1 (anosim-1) (eg, Kallmann syndrome 1), full gene sequence*

*APP (amyloid beta [A4] precursor protein) (eg, Alzheimer's disease), full gene sequence*

*ASS1 (argininosuccinate synthase 1) (eg, citrullinemia type I), full gene sequence*

*ATL1 (atlastin GTPase 1) (eg, spastic paraplegia), full gene sequence*

*ATP1A2 (ATPase, Na+/K+ transporting, alpha 2 polypeptide) (eg, familial hemiplegic migraine), full gene sequence*

*ATP7B (ATPase, Cu++ transporting, beta polypeptide) (eg, Wilson disease), full gene sequence*

*BBS1 (Bardet-Biedl syndrome 1) (eg, Bardet-Biedl syndrome), full gene sequence*

*BBS2 (Bardet-Biedl syndrome 2) (eg, Bardet-Biedl syndrome), full gene sequence*

*BCKDHB (branched-chain keto acid dehydrogenase E1, beta polypeptide) (eg, maple syrup urine disease, type 1B), full gene sequence*

*BEST1 (bestrophin 1) (eg, vitelliform macular dystrophy), full gene sequence*

*BMPR2 (bone morphogenetic protein receptor, type II [serine/threonine kinase]) (eg, heritable pulmonary arterial hypertension), full gene sequence*

*BRAF (B-Raf proto-oncogene, serine/threonine kinase) (eg, Noonan syndrome), full gene sequence*

*BSCL2 (Berardinelli-Seip congenital lipodystrophy 2 [seipin]) (eg, Berardinelli-Seip congenital lipodystrophy), full gene sequence*

*BTK (Bruton agammaglobulinemia tyrosine kinase) (eg, X-linked agammaglobulinemia), full gene sequence*

*CACNB2 (calcium channel, voltage-dependent, beta 2 subunit) (eg, Brugada syndrome), full gene sequence*

*CAPN3 (calpain 3) (eg, limb-girdle muscular dystrophy [LGMD] type 2A, calpainopathy), full gene sequence*

*CBS (cystathionine-beta-synthase) (eg, homocystinuria, cystathionine beta-synthase deficiency), full gene sequence*

*CDH1 (cadherin 1, type 1, E-cadherin [epithelial]) (eg, hereditary diffuse gastric cancer), full gene sequence*

*CDKL5 (cyclin-dependent kinase-like 5) (eg, early infantile epileptic encephalopathy), full gene sequence*

*CLCN1 (chloride channel 1, skeletal muscle) (eg, myotonia congenita), full gene sequence*

● New Code   ▲ Revised Code   ○ Reinstated   ● New Web Release   ▲ Revised Web Release   Unlisted   Not Covered   # Resequenced
⊘ AMA Mod 51 Exempt   ⑤ Optum Mod 51 Exempt   ⑥ Mod 63 Exempt   ✗ Non-FDA Drug   ★ Telemedicine   Ⓜ Maternity   🅰 Age Edit   + Add-on   **AMA:** CPT Asst
© 2017 Optum360, LLC   CPT © 2017 American Medical Association. All Rights Reserved.   **373**

CLCNKB (chloride channel, voltage-sensitive Kb) (eg, Bartter syndrome 3 and 4b), full gene sequence

CNTNAP2 (contactin-associated protein-like 2) (eg, Pitt-Hopkins-like syndrome 1), full gene sequence

COL6A2 (collagen, type VI, alpha 2) (eg, collagen type VI-related disorders), duplication/deletion analysis

CPT1A (carnitine palmitoyltransferase 1A [liver]) (eg, carnitine palmitoyltransferase 1A [CPT1A] deficiency), full gene sequence

CRB1 (crumbs homolog 1 [Drosophila]) (eg, Leber congenital amaurosis), full gene sequence

CREBBP (CREB binding protein) (eg, Rubinstein-Taybi syndrome), duplication/deletion analysis

Cytogenomic microarray analysis, neoplasia (eg, interrogation of copy number, and loss-of-heterozygosity via single nucleotide polymorphism [SNP]-based comparative genomic hybridization [CGH] microarray analysis)

(Do not report analyte-specific molecular pathology procedures separately when the specific analytes are included as part of the cytogenomic microarray analysis for neoplasia)

(Do not report 88271 when performing cytogenomic microarray analysis) (88271)

DBT (dihydrolipoamide branched chain transacylase E2) (eg, maple syrup urine disease, type 2), full gene sequence

DLAT (dihydrolipoamide S-acetyltransferase) (eg, pyruvate dehydrogenase E2 deficiency), full gene sequence

DLD (dihydrolipoamide dehydrogenase) (eg, maple syrup urine disease, type III), full gene sequence

DSC2 (desmocollin) (eg, arrhythmogenic right ventricular dysplasia/cardiomyopathy 11), full gene sequence

DSG2 (desmoglein 2) (eg, arrhythmogenic right ventricular dysplasia/cardiomyopathy 10), full gene sequence

DSP (desmoplakin) (eg, arrhythmogenic right ventricular dysplasia/cardiomyopathy 8), full gene sequence

EFHC1 (EF-hand domain [C-terminal] containing 1) (eg, juvenile myoclonic epilepsy), full gene sequence

EIF2B3 (eukaryotic translation initiation factor 2B, subunit 3 gamma, 58kDa) (eg, leukoencephalopathy with vanishing white matter), full gene sequence

EIF2B4 (eukaryotic translation initiation factor 2B, subunit 4 delta, 67kDa) (eg, leukoencephalopathy with vanishing white matter), full gene sequence

EIF2B5 (eukaryotic translation initiation factor 2B, subunit 5 epsilon, 82kDa) (eg, childhood ataxia with central nervous system hypomyelination/vanishing white matter), full gene sequence

ENG (endoglin) (eg, hereditary hemorrhagic telangiectasia, type 1), full gene sequence

EYA1 (eyes absent homolog 1 [Drosophila]) (eg, branchio-oto-renal [BOR] spectrum disorders), full gene sequence

F8 (coagulation factor VIII) (eg, hemophilia A), duplication/deletion analysis

FAH (fumarylacetoacetate hydrolase [fumarylacetoacetase]) (eg, tyrosinemia, type 1), full gene sequence

FASTKD2 (FAST kinase domains 2) (eg, mitochondrial respiratory chain complex IV deficiency), full gene sequence

FIG4 (FIG4 homolog, SAC1 lipid phosphatase domain containing [S. cerevisiae]) (eg, Charcot-Marie-Tooth disease), full gene sequence

FTSJ1 (FtsJ RNA methyltransferase homolog 1 [E. coli]) (eg, X-linked mental retardation 9), full gene sequence

FUS (fused in sarcoma) (eg, amyotrophic lateral sclerosis), full gene sequence

GAA (glucosidase, alpha; acid) (eg, glycogen storage disease type II [Pompe disease]), full gene sequence

GALC (galactosylceramidase) (eg, Krabbe disease), full gene sequence

GALT (galactose-1-phosphate uridylyltransferase) (eg, galactosemia), full gene sequence

GARS (glycyl-tRNA synthetase) (eg, Charcot-Marie-Tooth disease), full gene sequence

GCDH (glutaryl-CoA dehydrogenase) (eg, glutaricacidemia type 1), full gene sequence

GCK (glucokinase [hexokinase 4]) (eg, maturity-onset diabetes of the young [MODY]), full gene sequence

GLUD1 (glutamate dehydrogenase 1) (eg, familial hyperinsulinism), full gene sequence

GNE (glucosamine [UDP-N-acetyl]-2-epimerase/N-acetylmannosamine kinase) (eg, inclusion body myopathy 2 [IBM2], Nonaka myopathy), full gene sequence

GRN (granulin) (eg, frontotemporal dementia), full gene sequence

HADHA (hydroxyacyl-CoA dehydrogenase/3-ketoacyl-CoA thiolase/enoyl-CoA hydratase [trifunctional protein] alpha subunit) (eg, long chain acyl-coenzyme A dehydrogenase deficiency), full gene sequence

HADHB (hydroxyacyl-CoA dehydrogenase/3-ketoacyl-CoA thiolase/enoyl-CoA hydratase [trifunctional protein], beta subunit) (eg, trifunctional protein deficiency), full gene sequence

HEXA (hexosaminidase A, alpha polypeptide) (eg, Tay-Sachs disease), full gene sequence

HLCS (HLCS holocarboxylase synthetase) (eg, holocarboxylase synthetase deficiency), full gene sequence

HMBS (hydroxymethylbilane synthase) (eg, acute intermittent porphyria), full gene sequence

HNF4A (hepatocyte nuclear factor 4, alpha) (eg, maturity-onset diabetes of the young [MODY]), full gene sequence

IDUA (iduronidase, alpha-L-) (eg, mucopolysaccharidosis type I), full gene sequence

INF2 (inverted formin, FH2 and WH2 domain containing) (eg, focal segmental glomerulosclerosis), full gene sequence

IVD (isovaleryl-CoA dehydrogenase) (eg, isovaleric acidemia), full gene sequence

JAG1 (jagged 1) (eg, Alagille syndrome), duplication/deletion analysis

JUP (junction plakoglobin) (eg, arrhythmogenic right ventricular dysplasia/cardiomyopathy 11), full gene sequence

KCNH2 (potassium voltage-gated channel, subfamily H [eag-related], member 2) (eg, short QT syndrome, long QT syndrome), full gene sequence

KCNQ1 (potassium voltage-gated channel, KQT-like subfamily, member 1) (eg, short QT syndrome, long QT syndrome), full gene sequence

KCNQ2 (potassium voltage-gated channel, KQT-like subfamily, member 2) (eg, epileptic encephalopathy), full gene sequence

LDB3 (LIM domain binding 3) (eg, familial dilated cardiomyopathy, myofibrillar myopathy), full gene sequence

LDLR (low density lipoprotein receptor) (eg, familial hypercholesterolemia), full gene sequence

LEPR (leptin receptor(eg, obesity with hypogonadism), full gene sequence

LHCGR (luteinizing hormone/choriogonadotropin receptor) (eg, precocious male puberty), full gene sequence

LMNA (lamin A/C) (eg, Emery-Dreifuss muscular dystrophy [EDMD1, 2 and 3] limb-girdle muscular dystrophy [LGMD] type 1B, dilated cardiomyopathy [CMD1A], familial partial lipodystrophy [FPLD2]), full gene sequence

LRP5 (low density lipoprotein receptor-related protein 5) (eg, osteopetrosis), full gene sequence

| 26/TC | PC/TC Only | A2-Z3 | ASC Payment | 50 | Bilateral | ♂ Male Only | ♀ Female Only | Facility RVU | Non-Facility RVU | CCI |
|---|---|---|---|---|---|---|---|---|---|---|
| FUD | Follow-up Days | CMS: | IOM (Pub 100) | A-Y | OPPSI | 80/80 Surg Assist Allowed / w/Doc | | Lab Crosswalk | Radiology Crosswalk | CLIA |

374

CPT © 2017 American Medical Association. All Rights Reserved.

© 2017 Optum360, LLC

*MAP2K1 (mitogen-activated protein kinase 1) (eg, cardiofaciocutaneous syndrome), full gene sequence*

*MAP2K2 (mitogen-activated protein kinase 2) (eg, cardiofaciocutaneous syndrome), full gene sequence*

*MAPT (microtubule-associated protein tau) (eg, frontotemporal dementia), full gene sequence*

*MCCC1 (methylcrotonoyl-CoA carboxylase 1 [alpha]) (eg, 3-methylcrotonyl-CoA carboxylase deficiency), full gene sequence*

*MCCC2 (methylcrotonoyl-CoA carboxylase 2 [beta]) (eg, 3-methylcrotonyl carboxylase deficiency), full gene sequence*

*MFN2 (mitofusin 2) (eg, Charcot-Marie-Tooth disease), full gene sequence*

*MTM1 (myotubularin 1) (eg, X-linked centronuclear myopathy), full gene sequence*

*MUT (methylmalonyl CoA mutase) (eg, methylmalonic acidemia), full gene sequence*

*MUTYH (mutY homolog [E. coli]) (eg, MYH-associated polyposis), full gene sequence*

*NDUFS1 (NADH dehydrogenase [ubiquinone] Fe-S protein 1, 75kDa [NADH-coenzyme Q reductase]) (eg, Leigh syndrome, mitochondrial complex I deficiency), full gene sequence*

*NF2 (neurofibromin 2 [merlin]) (eg, neurofibromatosis, type 2), full gene sequence*

*NOTCH3 (notch 3) (eg, cerebral autosomal dominant arteriopathy with subcortical infarcts and leukoencephalopathy [CADASIL]), targeted sequence analysis (eg, exons 1-23)*

*NPC1 (Niemann-Pick disease, type C1) (eg, Niemann-Pick disease), full gene sequence*

*NPHP1 (nephronophthisis 1 [juvenile]) (eg, Joubert syndrome), full gene sequence*

*NSD1 (nuclear receptor binding SET domain protein 1) (eg, Sotos syndrome), full gene sequence*

*OPA1 (optic atrophy 1) (eg, optic atrophy), duplication/deletion analysis*

*OPTN (optineurin) (eg, amyotrophic lateral sclerosis), full gene sequence*

*PAFAH1B1 (platelet-activating factor acetylhydrolase 1b, regulatory subunit 1 [45kDa]) (eg, lissencephaly, Miller-Dieker syndrome), full gene sequence*

*PAH (phenylalanine hydroxylase) (eg, phenylketonuria), full gene sequence*

*PALB2 (partner and localizer of BRCA2) (eg, breast and pancreatic cancer), full gene sequence*

*PARK2 (Parkinson protein 2, E3 ubiquitin protein ligase [parkin]) (eg, Parkinson disease), full gene sequence*

*PAX2 (paired box 2) (eg, renal coloboma syndrome), full gene sequence*

*PC (pyruvate carboxylase) (eg, pyruvate carboxylase deficiency), full gene sequence*

*PCCA (propionyl CoA carboxylase, alpha polypeptide) (eg, propionic acidemia, type 1), full gene sequence*

*PCCB (propionyl CoA carboxylase, beta polypeptide) (eg, propionic acidemia), full gene sequence*

*PCDH15 (protocadherin-related 15) (eg, Usher syndrome type 1F), duplication/deletion analysis*

*PCSK9 (proprotein convertase subtilisin/kexin type 9) (eg familial hypercholesterolemia), full gene sequence*

*PDHA1 (pyruvate dehydrogenase [lipoamide] alpha 1) (eg, lactic acidosis), full gene sequence*

*PDHX (pyruvate dehydrogenase complex, component X) (eg, lactic acidosis), full gene sequence*

*PHEX (phosphate-regulating endopeptidase homolog, X-linked) (eg, hypophosphatemic rickets), full gene sequence*

*PKD2 (polycystic kidney disease 2 [autosomal dominant]) (eg, polycystic kidney disease), full gene sequence*

*PKP2 (plakophilin 2) (eg, arrhythmogenic right ventricular dysplasia/cardiomyopathy 9), full gene sequence*

*PNKD (eg, paroxysmal nonkinesigenic dyskinesia), full gene sequence*

*POLG (polymerase [DNA directed], gamma) (eg, Alpers-Huttenlocher syndrome, autosomal dominant progressive external ophthalmoplegia), full gene sequence*

*POMGNT1 (protein O-linked mannose beta1, 2-N acetylglucosaminyltransferase) (eg, muscle-eye-brain disease, Walker-Warburg syndrome), full gene sequence*

*POMT1 (protein-O-mannosyltransferase 1) (eg, limb-girdle muscular dystrophy [LGMD] type 2K, Walker-Warburg syndrome), full gene sequence*

*POMT2 (protein-O-mannosyltransferase 2) (eg, limb-girdle muscular dystrophy [LGMD] type 2N, Walker-Warburg syndrome), full gene sequence*

*PPOX (protoporphyrinogen oxidase) (eg, variegate porphyria), full gene sequence*

*PRKAG2 (protein kinase, AMP-activated, gamma 2 non-catalytic subunit) (eg, familial hypertrophic cardiomyopathy with Wolff-Parkinson-White syndrome, lethal congenital glycogen storage disease of heart), full gene sequence*

*PRKCG (protein kinase C, gamma) (eg, spinocerebellar ataxia), full gene sequence*

*PSEN2 (presenilin 2[Alzheimer's disease 4]) (eg, Alzheimer's disease), full gene sequence*

*PTPN11 (protein tyrosine phosphatase, non-receptor type 11) (eg, Noonan syndrome, LEOPARD syndrome), full gene sequence*

*PYGM (phosphorylase, glycogen, muscle) (eg, glycogen storage disease type V, McArdle disease), full gene sequence*

*RAF1 (v-raf-1 murine leukemia viral oncogene homolog 1) (eg, LEOPARD syndrome), full gene sequence*

*RET (ret proto-oncogene) (eg, Hirschsprung disease), full gene sequence*

*RPE65 (retinal pigment epithelium-specific protein 65kDa) (eg, retinitis pigmentosa, Leber congenital amaurosis), full gene sequence*

*RYR1 (ryanodine receptor 1, skeletal) (eg, malignant hyperthermia), targeted sequence analysis of exons with functionally-confirmed mutations*

*SCN4A (sodium channel, voltage-gated, type IV, alpha subunit) (eg, hyperkalemic periodic paralysis), full gene sequence*

*SCNN1A (sodium channel, nonvoltage-gated 1 alpha) (eg, pseudohypoaldosteronism), full gene sequence*

*SCNN1B (sodium channel, nonvoltage-gated 1, beta) (eg, Liddle syndrome, pseudohypoaldosteronism), full gene sequence*

*SCNN1G (sodium channel, nonvoltage-gated 1, gamma) (eg, Liddle syndrome, pseudohypoaldosteronism), full gene sequence*

*SDHA (succinate dehydrogenase complex, subunit A, flavoprotein [Fp]) (eg, Leigh syndrome, mitochondrial complex II deficiency), full gene sequence*

*SETX (senataxin) (eg, ataxia), full gene sequence*

*SGCE (sarcoglycan, epsilon) (eg, myoclonic dystonia), full gene sequence*

*SH3TC2 (SH3 domain and tetratricopeptide repeats 2) (eg, Charcot-Marie-Tooth disease), full gene sequence*

*SLC9A6 (solute carrier family 9 [sodium/hydrogen exchanger], member 6) (eg, Christianson syndrome), full gene sequence*

*SLC26A4 (solute carrier family 26, member 4) (eg, Pendred syndrome), full gene sequence*

---

● New Code  ▲ Revised Code  ○ Reinstated  ● New Web Release  ▲ Revised Web Release  Unlisted  Not Covered  # Resequenced
⊘ AMA Mod 51 Exempt  ⑪ Optum Mod 51 Exempt  ⑥ Mod 63 Exempt  ✗ Non-FDA Drug  ★ Telemedicine  Ⓜ Maternity  Ⓐ Age Edit  ✚ Add-on  **AMA:** CPT Asst

*SLC37A4 (solute carrier family 37 [glucose-6-phosphate transporter], member 4) (eg, glycogen storage disease type Ib), full gene sequence*

*SMAD4 (SMAD family member 4) (eg, hemorrhagic telangiectasia syndrome, juvenile polyposis), full gene sequence*

*SOS1 (son of sevenless homolog 1) (eg, Noonan syndrome, gingival fibromatosis), full gene sequence*

*SPAST (spastin) (eg, spastic paraplegia), full gene sequence*

*SPG7 (spastic paraplegia 7 [pure and complicated autosomal recessive]) (eg, spastic paraplegia), full gene sequence*

*STXBP1 (syntaxin-binding protein 1) (eg, epileptic encephalopathy), full gene sequence*

*TAZ (tafazzin) (eg, methylglutaconic aciduria type 2, Barth syndrome), full gene sequence*

*TCF4 (transcription factor 4) (eg, Pitt-Hopkins syndrome), full gene sequence*

*TH (tyrosine hydroxylase) (eg, Segawa syndrome), full gene sequence*

*TMEM43 (transmembrane protein 43) (eg, arrhythmogenic right ventricular cardiomyopathy), full gene sequence*

*TNNT2 (troponin T, type 2 [cardiac]) (eg, familial hypertrophic cardiomyopathy), full gene sequence*

*TRPC6 (transient receptor potential cation channel, subfamily C, member 6) (eg, focal segmental glomerulosclerosis), full gene sequence*

*TSC1 (tuberous sclerosis 1) (eg, tuberous sclerosis), full gene sequence*

*TSC2 (tuberous sclerosis 2) (eg, tuberous sclerosis), duplication/deletion analysis*

*UBE3A (ubiquitin protein ligase E3A) (eg, Angelman syndrome) full gene sequence*

*UMOD (uromodulin) (eg, glomerulocystic kidney disease with hyperuricemia and isosthenuria), full gene sequence*

*VWF (von Willebrand factor) (von Willebrand disease type 2A), extended targeted sequence analysis (eg, exons 11-16, 24-26, 51, 52)*

*WAS (Wiskott-Aldrich syndrome [eczema-thrombocytopenia]) (eg, Wiskott-Aldrich syndrome), full gene sequence*

⚒ 0.00   ✂ 0.00   **FUD** XXX   🅰 🖼

**AMA:** 2017,Apr,9; 2017,Jan,8; 2016,Aug,9; 2016,Jan,13; 2015,Jan,16; 2015,Jan,3; 2014,Jan,11; 2013,Sep,3-12; 2013,Jul,11-12; 2012,May,3-10

**81407    Molecular pathology procedure, Level 8 (eg, analysis of 26-50 exons by DNA sequence analysis, mutation scanning or duplication/deletion variants of >50 exons, sequence analysis of multiple genes on one platform)**

*ABCC8 (ATP-binding cassette, sub-family C [CFTR/MRP], member 8) (eg, familial hyperinsulinism), full gene sequence*

*AGL (amylo-alpha-1, 6-glucosidase, 4-alpha-glucanotransferase) (eg, glycogen storage disease type III), full gene sequence*

*AHI1 (Abelson helper integration site 1) (eg, Joubert syndrome), full gene sequence*

*ASPM (asp [abnormal spindle] homolog, microcephaly associated [Drosophila]) (eg, primary microcephaly), full gene sequence*

*CACNA1A (calcium channel, voltage-dependent, P/Q type, alpha 1A subunit) (eg, familial hemiplegic migraine), full gene sequence*

*CHD7 (chromodomain helicase DNA binding protein 7) (eg, CHARGE syndrome), full gene sequence*

*COL4A4 (collagen, type IV, alpha 4) (eg, Alport syndrome), full gene sequence*

*COL4A5 (collagen, type IV, alpha 5) (eg, Alport syndrome), duplication/deletion analysis*

*COL6A1 (collagen, type VI, alpha 1) (eg, collagen type VI-related disorders), full gene sequence*

*COL6A2 (collagen, type VI, alpha 2) (eg, collagen type VI-related disorders), full gene sequence*

*COL6A3 (collagen, type VI, alpha 3) (eg, collagen type VI-related disorders), full gene sequence*

*CREBBP (CREB binding protein) (eg, Rubinstein-Taybi syndrome), full gene sequence*

*F8 (coagulation factor VIII) (eg, hemophilia A), full gene sequence*

*JAG1 (jagged 1) (eg, Alagille syndrome), full gene sequence*

*KDM5C (lysine [K]-specific demethylase 5C) (eg, X-linked mental retardation), full gene sequence*

*KIAA0196 (KIAA0196) (eg, spastic paraplegia), full gene sequence*

*L1CAM (L1 cell adhesion molecule) (eg, MASA syndrome, X-linked hydrocephaly), full gene sequence*

*LAMB2 (laminin, beta 2 [laminin S]) (eg, Pierson syndrome), full gene sequence*

*MYBPC3 (myosin binding protein C, cardiac) (eg, familial hypertrophic cardiomyopathy), full gene sequence*

*MYH6 (myosin, heavy chain 6, cardiac muscle, alpha) (eg, familial dilated cardiomyopathy), full gene sequence*

*MYH7 (myosin, heavy chain 7, cardiac muscle, beta) (eg, familial hypertrophic cardiomyopathy, Liang distal myopathy), full gene sequence*

*MYO7A (myosin VIIA) (eg, Usher syndrome, type 1), full gene sequence*

*NOTCH1 (notch 1) (eg, aortic valve disease), full gene sequence*

*NPHS1 (nephrosis 1, congenital, Finnish type [nephrin]) (eg, congenital Finnish nephrosis), full gene sequence*

*OPA1 (optic atrophy 1) (eg, optic atrophy), full gene sequence*

*PCDH15 (protocadherin-related 15) (eg, Usher syndrome, type 1), full gene sequence*

*PKD1 (polycystic kidney disease 1 [autosomal dominant]) (eg, polycystic kidney disease), full gene sequence*

*PLCE1 (phospholipase C, epsilon 1) (eg, nephrotic syndrome type 3), full gene sequence*

*SCN1A (sodium channel, voltage-gated, type 1, alpha subunit) (eg, generalized epilepsy with febrile seizures), full gene sequence*

*SCN5A (sodium channel, voltage-gated, type V, alpha subunit) (eg, familial dilated cardiomyopathy), full gene sequence*

*SLC12A1 (solute carrier family 12 [sodium/potassium/chloride transporters], member 1) (eg, Bartter syndrome), full gene sequence*

*SLC12A3 (solute carrier family 12 [sodium/chloride transporters], member 3) (eg, Gitelman syndrome), full gene sequence*

*SPG11 (spastic paraplegia 11 [autosomal recessive]) (eg, spastic paraplegia), full gene sequence*

*SPTBN2 (spectrin, beta, non-erythrocytic 2) (eg, spinocerebellar ataxia), full gene sequence*

*TMEM67 (transmembrane protein 67) (eg, Joubert syndrome), full gene sequence*

*TSC2 (tuberous sclerosis 2) (eg, tuberous sclerosis), full gene sequence*

*USH1C (Usher syndrome 1C [autosomal recessive, severe]) (eg, Usher syndrome, type 1), full gene sequence*

*VPS13B (vacuolar protein sorting 13 homolog B [yeast]) (eg, Cohen syndrome), duplication/deletion analysis*

*WDR62 (WD repeat domain 62) (eg, primary autosomal recessive microcephaly), full gene sequence*

⚒ 0.00   ✂ 0.00   **FUD** XXX   🅰 🖼

**AMA:** 2017,Jan,8; 2016,Aug,9; 2016,Jan,13; 2015,Jan,16; 2015,Jan,3; 2014,Jan,11; 2013,Sep,3-12; 2013,Jul,11-12; 2012,May,3-10

**81408    Molecular pathology procedure, Level 9 (eg, analysis of >50 exons in a single gene by DNA sequence analysis)**

*ABCA4 (ATP-binding cassette, sub-family A [ABC1], member 4) (eg, Stargardt disease, age-related macular degeneration), full gene sequence*

CPT © 2017 American Medical Association. All Rights Reserved.    © 2017 Optum360, LLC

*ATM (ataxia telangiectasia mutated) (eg, ataxia telangiectasia), full gene sequence*

*CDH23 (cadherin-related 23) (eg, Usher syndrome, type 1), full gene sequence*

*CEP290 (centrosomal protein 290kDa) (eg, Joubert syndrome), full gene sequence*

*COL1A1 (collagen, type I, alpha 1) (eg, osteogenesis imperfecta, type I), full gene sequence*

*COL1A2 (collagen, type I, alpha 2) (eg, osteogenesis imperfecta, type I), full gene sequence*

*COL4A1 (collagen, type IV, alpha 1) (eg, brain small-vessel disease with hemorrhage), full gene sequence*

*COL4A3 (collagen, type IV, alpha 3 [Goodpasture antigen]) (eg, Alport syndrome), full gene sequence*

*COL4A5 (collagen, type IV, alpha 5) (eg, Alport syndrome), full gene sequence*

*DMD (dystrophin) (eg, Duchenne/Becker muscular dystrophy), full gene sequence*

*DYSF (dysferlin, limb girdle muscular dystrophy 2B [autosomal recessive]) (eg, limb-girdle muscular dystrophy), full gene sequence*

*FBN1 (fibrillin 1) (eg, Marfan syndrome), full gene sequence*

*ITPR1 (inositol 1,4,5-trisphosphate receptor, type 1) (eg, spinocerebellar ataxia), full gene sequence*

*LAMA2 (laminin, alpha 2) (eg, congenital muscular dystrophy), full gene sequence*

*LRRK2 (leucine-rich repeat kinase 2) (eg, Parkinson disease), full gene sequence*

*MYH11 (myosin, heavy chain 11, smooth muscle) (eg, thoracic aortic aneurysms and aortic dissections), full gene sequence*

*NEB (nebulin) (eg, nemaline myopathy 2), full gene sequence*

*NF1 (neurofibromin 1) (eg, neurofibromatosis, type 1), full gene sequence*

*PKHD1 (polycystic kidney and hepatic disease 1) (eg, autosomal recessive polycystic kidney disease), full gene sequence*

*RYR1 (ryanodine receptor 1, skeletal) (eg, malignant hyperthermia), full gene sequence*

*RYR2 (ryanodine receptor 2 [cardiac]) (eg, catecholaminergic polymorphic ventricular tachycardia, arrhythmogenic right ventricular dysplasia), full gene sequence or targeted sequence analysis of > 50 exons*

*USH2A (Usher syndrome 2A [autosomal recessive, mild]) (eg, Usher syndrome, type 2), full gene sequence*

*VPS13B (vacuolar protein sorting 13 homolog B [yeast]) (eg, Cohen syndrome), full gene sequence*

*VWF (von Willebrand factor) (eg, von Willebrand disease types 1 and 3), full gene sequence*

🔢 0.00   ⚕ 0.00   **FUD** XXX   🅰️ 🖥️

**AMA:** 2017,Jan,8; 2016,Aug,9; 2016,Jan,13; 2015,Jan,16; 2015,Jan,3; 2014,Jan,11; 2013,Sep,3-12; 2013,Jul,11-12; 2012,May,3-10

**#    81479    Unlisted molecular pathology procedure**

🔢 0.00   ⚕ 0.00   **FUD** XXX   🅰️

**AMA:** 2017,Apr,9; 2017,Jan,8; 2016,Sep,9; 2016,Aug,9; 2016,Apr,4; 2016,Jan,13; 2015,Jan,16; 2015,Jan,3; 2014,Jan,11; 2013,Sep,3-12; 2013,Jul,11-12

## 81410-81479 [81448] Genomic Sequencing

EXCLUDES   *In situ hybridization analyses (88271-88275, 88365-88368 [88364, 88373, 88374])*
   *Microbial identification (87149-87153, 87471-87801 [87623, 87624, 87625], 87900-87904 [87906, 87910, 87912])*

**81410    Aortic dysfunction or dilation (eg, Marfan syndrome, Loeys Dietz syndrome, Ehler Danlos syndrome type IV, arterial tortuosity syndrome); genomic sequence analysis panel, must include sequencing of at least 9 genes, including *FBN1, TGFBR1, TGFBR2, COL3A1, MYH11, ACTA2, SLC2A10, SMAD3,* and *MYLK***

🔢 0.00   ⚕ 0.00   **FUD** XXX   🅰️ 🖥️

**AMA:** 2017,Jan,8; 2016,Jan,13; 2015,Jan,3

**81411    duplication/deletion analysis panel, must include analyses for *TGFBR1, TGFBR2, MYH11, and COL3A1***

🔢 0.00   ⚕ 0.00   **FUD** XXX   🅰️ 🖥️

**AMA:** 2017,Jan,8; 2016,Jan,13; 2015,Jan,3

**81412    Ashkenazi Jewish associated disorders (eg, Bloom syndrome, Canavan disease, cystic fibrosis, familial dysautonomia, Fanconi anemia group C, Gaucher disease, Tay-Sachs disease), genomic sequence analysis panel, must include sequencing of at least 9 genes, including *ASPA, BLM, CFTR, FANCC, GBA, HEXA, IKBKAP, MCOLN1,* and *SMPD1***

🔢 0.00   ⚕ 0.00   **FUD** XXX   🅰️ 🖥️

**AMA:** 2017,Jan,8; 2016,Apr,4

**81413    Cardiac ion channelopathies (eg, Brugada syndrome, long QT syndrome, short QT syndrome, catecholaminergic polymorphic ventricular tachycardia); genomic sequence analysis panel, must include sequencing of at least 10 genes, including ANK2, CASQ2, CAV3, KCNE1, KCNE2, KCNH2, KCNJ2, KCNQ1, RYR2, and SCN5A**

EXCLUDES   *Evaluation of cardiomyopathy (81439)*

🔢 0.00   ⚕ 0.00   **FUD** XXX   🅰️ 🖥️

**AMA:** 2017,Apr,3

**81414    duplication/deletion gene analysis panel, must include analysis of at least 2 genes, including KCNH2 and KCNQ1**

EXCLUDES   *Evaluation of cardiomyopathy (81439)*

🔢 0.00   ⚕ 0.00   **FUD** XXX   🅰️ 🖥️

**AMA:** 2017,Apr,3

**81415    Exome (eg, unexplained constitutional or heritable disorder or syndrome); sequence analysis**

🔢 0.00   ⚕ 0.00   **FUD** XXX   🅰️ 🖥️

**AMA:** 2017,Jan,8; 2016,Jan,13; 2015,Jan,3

**+    81416    sequence analysis, each comparator exome (eg, parents, siblings) (List separately in addition to code for primary procedure)**

Code first (81415)

🔢 0.00   ⚕ 0.00   **FUD** XXX   🅰️ 🖥️

**AMA:** 2017,Jan,8; 2016,Jan,13; 2015,Jan,3

**81417    re-evaluation of previously obtained exome sequence (eg, updated knowledge or unrelated condition/syndrome)**

EXCLUDES   *Microarray assessment (81228-81229)*
   *Results that are incidental*

🔢 0.00   ⚕ 0.00   **FUD** XXX   🅰️ 🖥️

**AMA:** 2017,Jan,8; 2016,Jan,13; 2015,Jan,3

**81420    Fetal chromosomal aneuploidy (eg, trisomy 21, monosomy X) genomic sequence analysis panel, circulating cell-free fetal DNA in maternal blood, must include analysis of chromosomes 13, 18, and 21**   Ⓜ

EXCLUDES   *Genome-wide microarray analysis (81228-81229)*
   *Molecular cytogenetics (88271)*

🔢 0.00   ⚕ 0.00   **FUD** XXX   🅰️ 🖥️

**AMA:** 2017,Jan,8; 2016,Jan,13; 2015,Dec,18; 2015,Jan,3

**Pathology and Laboratory**

**81422 — 81450**

**81422**  Fetal chromosomal microdeletion(s) genomic sequence analysis (eg, DiGeorge syndrome, Cri-du-chat syndrome), circulating cell-free fetal DNA in maternal blood
*EXCLUDES* *Genome-wide microarray analysis (81228-81229)*
*Molecular cytogenetics (88271)*
0.00   0.00   **FUD** XXX   A ▯
**AMA:** 2017,Apr,3

**81425**  Genome (eg, unexplained constitutional or heritable disorder or syndrome); sequence analysis
0.00   0.00   **FUD** XXX   A ▯
**AMA:** 2017,Jan,8; 2016,Jan,13; 2015,Jan,3

+ **81426**  sequence analysis, each comparator genome (eg, parents, siblings) (List separately in addition to code for primary procedure)
Code first (81425)
0.00   0.00   **FUD** XXX   A ▯
**AMA:** 2017,Jan,8; 2016,Jan,13; 2015,Jan,3

**81427**  re-evaluation of previously obtained genome sequence (eg, updated knowledge or unrelated condition/syndrome)
*EXCLUDES* *Genome-wide microarray analysis (81228-81229)*
*Results that are incidental*
0.00   0.00   **FUD** XXX   A ▯
**AMA:** 2017,Jan,8; 2016,Jan,13; 2015,Jan,3

**81430**  Hearing loss (eg, nonsyndromic hearing loss, Usher syndrome, Pendred syndrome); genomic sequence analysis panel, must include sequencing of at least 60 genes, including *CDH23, CLRN1, GJB2, GPR98, MTRNR1, MYO7A, MYO15A, PCDH15, OTOF, SLC26A4, TMC1, TMPRSS3, USH1C, USH1G, USH2A,* and *WFS1*
0.00   0.00   **FUD** XXX   A ▯
**AMA:** 2017,Jan,8; 2016,Jan,13; 2015,Jan,3; 2012,May,3-10

**81431**  duplication/deletion analysis panel, must include copy number analyses for *STRC* and *DFNB1* deletions in *GJB2* and *GJB6* genes
0.00   0.00   **FUD** XXX   A ▯
**AMA:** 2017,Jan,8; 2016,Jan,13; 2015,Jan,3

▲ **81432**  Hereditary breast cancer-related disorders (eg, hereditary breast cancer, hereditary ovarian cancer, hereditary endometrial cancer); genomic sequence analysis panel, must include sequencing of at least 10 genes, always including *BRCA1, BRCA2, CDH1, MLH1, MSH2, MSH6, PALB2, PTEN, STK11,* and *TP53*
0.00   0.00   **FUD** XXX   A ▯
**AMA:** 2017,Jan,8; 2016,Apr,4

**81433**  duplication/deletion analysis panel, must include analyses for *BRCA1, BRCA2, MLH1, MSH2,* and *STK11*
0.00   0.00   **FUD** XXX   A ▯
**AMA:** 2017,Jan,8; 2016,Apr,4

**81434**  Hereditary retinal disorders (eg, retinitis pigmentosa, Leber congenital amaurosis, cone-rod dystrophy), genomic sequence analysis panel, must include sequencing of at least 15 genes, including *ABCA4, CNGA1, CRB1, EYS, PDE6A, PDE6B, PRPF31, PRPH2, RDH12, RHO, RP1, RP2, RPE65, RPGR,* and *USH2A*
0.00   0.00   **FUD** XXX   A ▯
**AMA:** 2017,Jan,8; 2016,Apr,4

**81435**  Hereditary colon cancer disorders (eg, Lynch syndrome, PTEN hamartoma syndrome, Cowden syndrome, familial adenomatosis polyposis); genomic sequence analysis panel, must include sequencing of at least 10 genes, including *APC, BMPR1A, CDH1, MLH1, MSH2, MSH6, MUTYH, PTEN, SMAD4,* and *STK11*
0.00   0.00   **FUD** XXX   A ▯
**AMA:** 2017,Jan,8; 2016,Apr,4; 2016,Jan,13; 2015,Jan,3

**81436**  duplication/deletion analysis panel, must include analysis of at least 5 genes, including *MLH1, MSH2, EPCAM, SMAD4,* and *STK11*
0.00   0.00   **FUD** XXX   A ▯
**AMA:** 2017,Jan,8; 2016,Apr,4; 2016,Jan,13; 2015,Jan,3

**81437**  Hereditary neuroendocrine tumor disorders (eg, medullary thyroid carcinoma, parathyroid carcinoma, malignant pheochromocytoma or paraganglioma); genomic sequence analysis panel, must include sequencing of at least 6 genes, including *MAX, SDHB, SDHC, SDHD, TMEM127,* and *VHL*
0.00   0.00   **FUD** XXX   A ▯
**AMA:** 2017,Jan,8; 2016,Apr,4

**81438**  duplication/deletion analysis panel, must include analyses for *SDHB, SDHC, SDHD,* and *VHL*
0.00   0.00   **FUD** XXX   A ▯
**AMA:** 2017,Jan,8; 2016,Apr,4

● # **81448**  Hereditary peripheral neuropathies (eg, Charcot-Marie-Tooth, spastic paraplegia), genomic sequence analysis panel, must include sequencing of at least 5 peripheral neuropathy-related genes (eg, *BSCL2, GJB1, MFN2, MPZ, REEP1, SPAST, SPG11, SPTLC1*)
0.00   0.00   **FUD** 000

▲ **81439**  Hereditary cardiomyopathy (eg, hypertrophic cardiomyopathy, dilated cardiomyopathy, arrhythmogenic right ventricular cardiomyopathy), genomic sequence analysis panel, must include sequencing of at least 5 cardiomyopathy-related genes (eg, *DSG2, MYBPC3, MYH7, PKP2, TTN*)
*EXCLUDES* *Genetic tests of cardiac ion channelopathies*
*(81413-81414)*
0.00   0.00   **FUD** XXX   A ▯
**AMA:** 2017,Apr,3

**81440**  Nuclear encoded mitochondrial genes (eg, neurologic or myopathic phenotypes), genomic sequence panel, must include analysis of at least 100 genes, including *BCS1L, C10orf2, COQ2, COX10, DGUOK, MPV17, OPA1, PDSS2, POLG, POLG2, RRM2B, SCO1, SCO2, SLC25A4, SUCLA2, SUCLG1, TAZ, TK2,* and *TYMP*
0.00   0.00   **FUD** XXX   A ▯
**AMA:** 2017,Jan,8; 2016,Jan,13; 2015,Jan,3

**81442**  Noonan spectrum disorders (eg, Noonan syndrome, cardio-facio-cutaneous syndrome, Costello syndrome, LEOPARD syndrome, Noonan-like syndrome), genomic sequence analysis panel, must include sequencing of at least 12 genes, including *BRAF, CBL, HRAS, KRAS, MAP2K1, MAP2K2, NRAS, PTPN11, RAF1, RIT1, SHOC2,* and *SOS1*
0.00   0.00   **FUD** XXX   A ▯
**AMA:** 2017,Jan,8; 2016,Apr,4

**81445**  Targeted genomic sequence analysis panel, solid organ neoplasm, DNA analysis, and RNA analysis when performed, 5-50 genes (eg, *ALK, BRAF, CDKN2A, EGFR, ERBB2, KIT, KRAS, NRAS, MET, PDGFRA, PDGFRB, PGR, PIK3CA, PTEN, RET*), interrogation for sequence variants and copy number variants or rearrangements, if performed
*EXCLUDES* *Microarray copy number assessment (81406)*
0.00   0.00   **FUD** XXX   A ▯
**AMA:** 2017,Jan,8; 2016,Apr,4; 2016,Jan,13; 2015,Jan,3

*81448*  Resequenced code. See code following 81438.

**81450**  Targeted genomic sequence analysis panel, hematolymphoid neoplasm or disorder, DNA analysis, and RNA analysis when performed, 5-50 genes (eg, *BRAF, CEBPA, DNMT3A, EZH2, FLT3, IDH1, IDH2, JAK2, KRAS, KIT, MLL, NRAS, NPM1, NOTCH1*), interrogation for sequence variants, and copy number variants or rearrangements, or isoform expression or mRNA expression levels, if performed
*EXCLUDES* *Microarray copy number assessment (81406)*
0.00   0.00   **FUD** XXX   A ▯
**AMA:** 2017,Jan,8; 2016,Apr,4; 2016,Jan,13; 2015,Jan,3

**81455** Targeted genomic sequence analysis panel, solid organ or hematolymphoid neoplasm, DNA analysis, and RNA analysis when performed, 51 or greater genes (eg, *ALK, BRAF, CDKN2A, CEBPA, DNMT3A, EGFR, ERBB2, EZH2, FLT3, IDH1, IDH2, JAK2, KIT, KRAS, MLL, NPM1, NRAS, MET, NOTCH1, PDGFRA, PDGFRB, PGR, PIK3CA, PTEN, RET*), interrogation for sequence variants and copy number variants or rearrangements, if performed

EXCLUDES *Microarray copy number assessment (81406)*
🔧 0.00  ⚖ 0.00  **FUD** XXX  Ⓐ🖼
**AMA:** 2017,Jan,8; 2016,Apr,4; 2016,Jan,13; 2015,Jan,3

**81460** Whole mitochondrial genome (eg, Leigh syndrome, mitochondrial encephalomyopathy, lactic acidosis, and stroke-like episodes [MELAS], myoclonic epilepsy with ragged-red fibers [MERFF], neuropathy, ataxia, and retinitis pigmentosa [NARP], Leber hereditary optic neuropathy [LHON]), genomic sequence, must include sequence analysis of entire mitochondrial genome with heteroplasmy detection

🔧 0.00  ⚖ 0.00  **FUD** XXX  Ⓐ🖼
**AMA:** 2017,Jan,8; 2016,Jan,13; 2015,Jan,3

**81465** Whole mitochondrial genome large deletion analysis panel (eg, Kearns-Sayre syndrome, chronic progressive external ophthalmoplegia), including heteroplasmy detection, if performed

🔧 0.00  ⚖ 0.00  **FUD** XXX  Ⓐ🖼
**AMA:** 2017,Jan,8; 2016,Jan,13; 2015,Jan,3

**81470** X-linked intellectual disability (XLID) (eg, syndromic and non-syndromic XLID); genomic sequence analysis panel, must include sequencing of at least 60 genes, including *ARX, ATRX, CDKL5, FGD1, FMR1, HUWE1, IL1RAPL, KDM5C, L1CAM, MECP2, MED12, MID1, OCRL, RPS6KA3,* and *SLC16A2*

🔧 0.00  ⚖ 0.00  **FUD** XXX  Ⓐ🖼
**AMA:** 2017,Jan,8; 2016,Jan,13; 2015,Jan,3

**81471** duplication/deletion gene analysis, must include analysis of at least 60 genes, including *ARX, ATRX, CDKL5, FGD1, FMR1, HUWE1, IL1RAPL, KDM5C, L1CAM, MECP2, MED12, MID1, OCRL, RPS6KA3,* and *SLC16A2*

🔧 0.00  ⚖ 0.00  **FUD** XXX  Ⓐ🖼
**AMA:** 2017,Jan,8; 2016,Jan,13; 2015,Jan,3

*81479* Resequenced code. See code following 81408.

## 81490-81599 Multianalyte Assays

INCLUDES Procedures using results of multiple assay panels (eg, molecular pathology, fluorescent in situ hybridization, non-nucleic acid-based) and other patient information to perform algorithmic analysis
Required analytical services (eg, amplification, cell lysis, detection, digestion, extraction, hybridization, nucleic acid stabilization) and algorithmic analysis
EXCLUDES *Genomic resequencing tests (81410-81471 [81448])*
*In situ hybridization analyses (88271-88275, 88365-88368 [88364, 88373, 88374])*
*Microbial identification (87149-87153, 87471-87801 [87623, 87624, 87625], 87900-87904 [87906, 87910, 87912])*
*Multianalyte assays with algorithmic analyses without a Category 1 code (0001M-0004M, 0006M-0009M)*
Code also procedures performed prior to cell lysis (eg, microdissection) (88380-88381)

**81490** Autoimmune (rheumatoid arthritis), analysis of 12 biomarkers using immunoassays, utilizing serum, prognostic algorithm reported as a disease activity score

🔧 0.00  ⚖ 0.00  **FUD** XXX  Ⓠ🖼
EXCLUDES *C-reactive protein (86140)*

**81493** Coronary artery disease, mRNA, gene expression profiling by real-time RT-PCR of 23 genes, utilizing whole peripheral blood, algorithm reported as a risk score

🔧 0.00  ⚖ 0.00  **FUD** XXX  Ⓐ🖼

**81500** Oncology (ovarian), biochemical assays of two proteins (CA-125 and HE4), utilizing serum, with menopausal status, algorithm reported as a risk score ♀

EXCLUDES *Human epididymis protein 4 (HE4) (86305)*
*Immunoassay for tumor antigen, quantitative; CA 125 (86304)*
🔧 0.00  ⚖ 0.00  **FUD** XXX  Ⓔ🖼
**AMA:** 2015,Jan,3; 2014,Jan,11

**81503** Oncology (ovarian), biochemical assays of five proteins (CA-125, apolipoprotein A1, beta-2 microglobulin, transferrin, and pre-albumin), utilizing serum, algorithm reported as a risk score ♀

EXCLUDES *Apolipoprotein (82172)*
*Beta-2 microglobulin (82232)*
*Immunoassay for tumor antigen, quantitative; CA 125 (86304)*
*Prealbumin (84134)*
*Transferrin (84466)*
🔧 0.00  ⚖ 0.00  **FUD** XXX  Ⓠ🖼
**AMA:** 2015,Jan,3; 2014,Jan,11

**81504** Oncology (tissue of origin), microarray gene expression profiling of > 2000 genes, utilizing formalin-fixed paraffin-embedded tissue, algorithm reported as tissue similarity scores

🔧 0.00  ⚖ 0.00  **FUD** XXX  Ⓐ🖼
**AMA:** 2015,Jan,3; 2014,Jan,11

**81506** Endocrinology (type 2 diabetes), biochemical assays of seven analytes (glucose, HbA1c, insulin, hs-CRP, adiponectin, ferritin, interleukin 2-receptor alpha), utilizing serum or plasma, algorithm reporting a risk score

EXCLUDES *C-reactive protein; high sensitivity (hsCRP) (86141)*
*Ferritin (82728)*
*Glucose (82947)*
*Hemoglobin; glycosylated (A1C) (83036)*
*Immunoassay for analyte other than infectious agent antibody or infectious agent antigen (83520)*
*Insulin; total (83525)*
*Unlisted chemistry procedure (84999)*
🔧 0.00  ⚖ 0.00  **FUD** XXX  Ⓔ🖼
**AMA:** 2015,Jan,3; 2014,Jan,11

**81507** Fetal aneuploidy (trisomy 21, 18, and 13) DNA sequence analysis of selected regions using maternal plasma, algorithm reported as a risk score for each trisomy ♀

EXCLUDES *Genome-wide microarray analysis (81228-81229)*
*Molecular cytogenetics (88271)*
🔧 0.00  ⚖ 0.00  **FUD** XXX  Ⓐ🖼
**AMA:** 2015,Jan,3; 2014,Jan,11

**81508** Fetal congenital abnormalities, biochemical assays of two proteins (PAPP-A, hCG [any form]), utilizing maternal serum, algorithm reported as a risk score ♀

EXCLUDES *Gonadotropin, chorionic (hCG) (84702)*
*Pregnancy-associated plasma protein-A (PAPP-A) (84163)*
🔧 0.00  ⚖ 0.00  **FUD** XXX  Ⓔ🖼
**AMA:** 2015,Jan,3; 2014,Jan,11

**81509** Fetal congenital abnormalities, biochemical assays of three proteins (PAPP-A, hCG [any form], DIA), utilizing maternal serum, algorithm reported as a risk score ♀

EXCLUDES *Gonadotropin, chorionic (hCG) (84702)*
*Inhibin A (86336)*
*Pregnancy-associated plasma protein-A (PAPP-A) (84163)*
🔧 0.00  ⚖ 0.00  **FUD** XXX  Ⓔ🖼
**AMA:** 2015,Jan,3; 2014,Jan,11

● New Code  ▲ Revised Code  ○ Reinstated  ● New Web Release  ▲ Revised Web Release  Unlisted  Not Covered  # Resequenced
⊘ AMA Mod 51 Exempt  ⑨ Optum Mod 51 Exempt  ㊿ Mod 63 Exempt  ⚡ Non-FDA Drug  ★ Telemedicine  Ⓜ Maternity  Ⓐ Age Edit  ✛ Add-on  **AMA:** CPT Asst
© 2017 Optum360, LLC  CPT © 2017 American Medical Association. All Rights Reserved.  **379**

**81510** Fetal congenital abnormalities, biochemical assays of three analytes (AFP, uE3, hCG [any form]), utilizing maternal serum, algorithm reported as a risk score ♀

> EXCLUDES Alpha-fetoprotein (AFP) (82105)
> Estriol (82677)
> Gonadotropin, chorionic (hCG) (84702)

🔲 0.00 ⚖ 0.00 **FUD** XXX E 🖵

AMA: 2015,Jan,3; 2014,Jan,11

**81511** Fetal congenital abnormalities, biochemical assays of four analytes (AFP, uE3, hCG [any form], DIA) utilizing maternal serum, algorithm reported as a risk score (may include additional results from previous biochemical testing) ♀

> EXCLUDES Alpha-fetoprotein (AFP) (82105)
> Estriol (82677)
> Gonadotropin, chorionic (hCG) (84702)
> Inhibin A (86336)

🔲 0.00 ⚖ 0.00 **FUD** XXX E 🖵

AMA: 2015,Jan,3; 2014,Jan,11

**81512** Fetal congenital abnormalities, biochemical assays of five analytes (AFP, uE3, total hCG, hyperglycosylated hCG, DIA) utilizing maternal serum, algorithm reported as a risk score ♀

> EXCLUDES Alpha-fetoprotein (AFP) (82105)
> Estriol (82677)
> Gonadotropin, chorionic (hCG) (84702)
> Inhibin A (86336)

🔲 0.00 ⚖ 0.00 **FUD** XXX E 🖵

AMA: 2015,Jan,3; 2014,Jan,11

**81519** Oncology (breast), mRNA, gene expression profiling by real-time RT-PCR of 21 genes, utilizing formalin-fixed paraffin embedded tissue, algorithm reported as recurrence score

🔲 0.00 ⚖ 0.00 **FUD** XXX A 🖵

AMA: 2017,Jan,8; 2016,Jan,13; 2015,Jan,3

● **81520** Oncology (breast), mRNA gene expression profiling by hybrid capture of 58 genes (50 content and 8 housekeeping), utilizing formalin-fixed paraffin-embedded tissue, algorithm reported as a recurrence risk score

● **81521** Oncology (breast), mRNA, microarray gene expression profiling of 70 content genes and 465 housekeeping genes, utilizing fresh frozen or formalin-fixed paraffin-embedded tissue, algorithm reported as index related to risk of distant metastasis

**81525** Oncology (colon), mRNA, gene expression profiling by real-time RT-PCR of 12 genes (7 content and 5 housekeeping), utilizing formalin-fixed paraffin-embedded tissue, algorithm reported as a recurrence score

🔲 0.00 ⚖ 0.00 **FUD** XXX A 🖵

**81528** Oncology (colorectal) screening, quantitative real-time target and signal amplification of 10 DNA markers (*KRAS* mutations, promoter methylation of *NDRG4* and *BMP3*) and fecal hemoglobin, utilizing stool, algorithm reported as a positive or negative result

🔲 0.00 ⚖ 0.00 **FUD** XXX A 🖵

> EXCLUDES Blood, occult, by fecal hemoglobin (82274)
> KRAS (Kirsten rat sarcoma viral oncogene homolog) (81275)

**81535** Oncology (gynecologic), live tumor cell culture and chemotherapeutic response by DAPI stain and morphology, predictive algorithm reported as a drug response score; first single drug or drug combination

🔲 0.00 ⚖ 0.00 **FUD** XXX Q 🖵

+ **81536** each additional single drug or drug combination (List separately in addition to code for primary procedure)

🔲 0.00 ⚖ 0.00 **FUD** XXX Q 🖵

Code first (81535)

**81538** Oncology (lung), mass spectrometric 8-protein signature, including amyloid A, utilizing serum, prognostic and predictive algorithm reported as good versus poor overall survival

🔲 0.00 ⚖ 0.00 **FUD** XXX Q 🖵

**81539** Oncology (high-grade prostate cancer), biochemical assay of four proteins (Total PSA, Free PSA, Intact PSA, and human kallikrein-2 [hK2]), utilizing plasma or serum, prognostic algorithm reported as a probability score ♂

🔲 0.00 ⚖ 0.00 **FUD** XXX Q 🖵

AMA: 2017,Apr,3

**81540** Oncology (tumor of unknown origin), mRNA, gene expression profiling by real-time RT-PCR of 92 genes (87 content and 5 housekeeping) to classify tumor into main cancer type and subtype, utilizing formalin-fixed paraffin-embedded tissue, algorithm reported as a probability of a predicted main cancer type and subtype

🔲 0.00 ⚖ 0.00 **FUD** XXX A 🖵

● **81541** Oncology (prostate), mRNA gene expression profiling by real-time RT-PCR of 46 genes (31 content and 15 housekeeping), utilizing formalin-fixed paraffin-embedded tissue, algorithm reported as a disease-specific mortality risk score

**81545** Oncology (thyroid), gene expression analysis of 142 genes, utilizing fine needle aspirate, algorithm reported as a categorical result (eg, benign or suspicious)

🔲 0.00 ⚖ 0.00 **FUD** XXX A 🖵

● **81551** Oncology (prostate), promoter methylation profiling by real-time PCR of 3 genes (*GSTP1, APC, RASSF1*), utilizing formalin-fixed paraffin-embedded tissue, algorithm reported as a likelihood of prostate cancer detection on repeat biopsy

**81595** Cardiology (heart transplant), mRNA, gene expression profiling by real-time quantitative PCR of 20 genes (11 content and 9 housekeeping), utilizing subfraction of peripheral blood, algorithm reported as a rejection risk score

🔲 0.00 ⚖ 0.00 **FUD** XXX A 🖵

**81599** Unlisted multianalyte assay with algorithmic analysis

> INCLUDES MAAA services not reportable with (81490-81595, 0001M-0004M, 0006M-0009M)

🔲 0.00 ⚖ 0.00 **FUD** XXX E

AMA: 2015,Jan,3; 2014,Jan,11

## 82009-82030 Chemistry: Acetaldehyde—Adenosine

INCLUDES Clinical information not requested by the ordering physician
Mathematically calculated results
Quantitative analysis unless otherwise specified
Specimens from any source unless otherwise specified

EXCLUDES Analytes from nonrequested laboratory analysis
Calculated results that represent a score or probability that was derived by algorithm
Drug testing ([80305, 80306, 80307], [80324, 80325, 80326, 80327, 80328, 80329, 80330, 80331, 80332, 80333, 80334, 80335, 80336, 80337, 80338, 80339, 80340, 80341, 80342, 80343, 80344, 80345, 80346, 80347, 80348, 80349, 80350, 80351, 80352, 80353, 80354, 80355, 80356, 80357, 80358, 80359, 80360, 80361, 80362, 80363, 80364, 80365, 80366, 80367, 80368, 80369, 80370, 80371, 80372, 80373, 80374, 80375, 80376, 80377, 83992])
Organ or disease panels (80048-80076 [80081])
Therapeutic drug assays (80150-80299 [80164, 80165, 80171])

**82009** Ketone body(s) (eg, acetone, acetoacetic acid, beta-hydroxybutyrate); qualitative

🔲 0.00 ⚖ 0.00 **FUD** XXX Q

AMA: 2017,Jan,8; 2016,Jan,13; 2015,Jun,10; 2015,Apr,3; 2015,Jan,16; 2014,Jan,11

**82010** quantitative

🔲 0.00 ⚖ 0.00 **FUD** XXX ✖ Q

AMA: 2017,Jan,8; 2016,Jan,13; 2015,Jun,10; 2015,Apr,3; 2015,Jan,16; 2014,Jan,11

26/TC PC/TC Only  A2-Z3 ASC Payment  50 Bilateral  ♂ Male Only  ♀ Female Only  🔲 Facility RVU  ⚖ Non-Facility RVU  🖵 CCI
**FUD** Follow-up Days  CMS: IOM (Pub 100)  A-Y OPPSI  80/80 Surg Assist Allowed / w/Doc  🔲 Lab Crosswalk  ✖ Radiology Crosswalk  ✖ CLIA
**380**  CPT © 2017 American Medical Association. All Rights Reserved.  © 2017 Optum360, LLC

**82013 Acetylcholinesterase**

EXCLUDES Acid phosphatase (84060-84066)
Gastric acid analysis (82930)

0.00  0.00  **FUD** XXX  [Q]

**AMA:** 2015,Jun,10; 2015,Apr,3; 2014,Jan,11

**82016 Acylcarnitines; qualitative, each specimen**

0.00  0.00  **FUD** XXX  [Q]

**AMA:** 2015,Jun,10; 2015,Apr,3; 2014,Jan,11

**82017 quantitative, each specimen**

EXCLUDES Carnitine (82379)

0.00  0.00  **FUD** XXX  [Q][⊡]

**AMA:** 2015,Jun,10; 2015,Apr,3; 2014,Jan,11

**82024 Adrenocorticotropic hormone (ACTH)**

0.00  0.00  **FUD** XXX  [Q][⊡]

**AMA:** 2015,Jun,10; 2015,Apr,3; 2014,Jan,11

**82030 Adenosine, 5-monophosphate, cyclic (cyclic AMP)**

0.00  0.00  **FUD** XXX  [Q]

**AMA:** 2015,Jun,10; 2015,Apr,3; 2014,Jan,11

## 82040-82045 [82042] Chemistry: Albumin

INCLUDES Clinical information not requested by the ordering physician
Mathematically calculated results
Quantitative analysis unless otherwise specified
Specimens from any other sources unless otherwise specified

EXCLUDES Analytes from nonrequested laboratory analysis
Calculated results that represent a score or probability that was derived by algorithm
Drug testing ([80305, 80306, 80307], [80324, 80325, 80326, 80327, 80328, 80329, 80330, 80331, 80332, 80333, 80334, 80335, 80336, 80337, 80338, 80339, 80340, 80341, 80342, 80343, 80344, 80345, 80346, 80347, 80348, 80349, 80350, 80351, 80352, 80353, 80354, 80355, 80356, 80357, 80358, 80359, 80360, 80361, 80362, 80363, 80364, 80365, 80366, 80367, 80368, 80369, 80370, 80371, 80372, 80373, 80374, 80375, 80376, 80377, 83992])
Organ or disease panels (80048-80076 [80081])
Therapeutic drug assays (80150-80299 [80164, 80165, 80171])

**82040 Albumin; serum, plasma or whole blood**

0.00  0.00  **FUD** XXX  [X][Q]

**AMA:** 2017,Jan,8; 2016,Jan,13; 2015,Jun,10; 2015,Apr,3; 2015,Jan,16; 2014,Jan,11

*82042* **Resequenced code. See code following 82045.**

▲ **82043 urine (eg, microalbumin), quantitative**

0.00  0.00  **FUD** XXX  [X][Q][⊡]

**AMA:** 2017,Jan,8; 2016,Jan,13; 2015,Jun,10; 2015,Apr,3; 2015,Jan,16; 2014,Jan,11

▲ **82044 urine (eg, microalbumin), semiquantitative (eg, reagent strip assay)**

EXCLUDES Prealbumin (84134)

0.00  0.00  **FUD** XXX  [X][Q]

**AMA:** 2017,Jan,8; 2016,Jan,13; 2015,Jun,10; 2015,Apr,3; 2015,Jan,16; 2014,Jan,11; 2012,Jan,15-42

**82045 ischemia modified**

0.00  0.00  **FUD** XXX  [Q]

**AMA:** 2015,Jun,10; 2015,Apr,3

▲ # **82042 other source, quantitative, each specimen**

0.00  0.00  **FUD** XXX  [Q]

**AMA:** 2015,Jun,10; 2015,Apr,3; 2014,Jan,11

## 82075-82107 Chemistry: Alcohol—Alpha-fetoprotein (AFP)

INCLUDES Clinical information not requested by the ordering physician
Mathematically calculated results
Quantitative analysis unless otherwise specified
Specimens from any source unless otherwise specified

EXCLUDES Analytes from nonrequested laboratory analysis
Calculated results that represent a score or probability that was derived by algorithm
Drug testing ([80305, 80306, 80307], [80324, 80325, 80326, 80327, 80328, 80329, 80330, 80331, 80332, 80333, 80334, 80335, 80336, 80337, 80338, 80339, 80340, 80341, 80342, 80343, 80344, 80345, 80346, 80347, 80348, 80349, 80350, 80351, 80352, 80353, 80354, 80355, 80356, 80357, 80358, 80359, 80360, 80361, 80362, 80363, 80364, 80365, 80366, 80367, 80368, 80369, 80370, 80371, 80372, 80373, 80374, 80375, 80376, 80377, 83992])
Organ or disease panels (80048-80076 [80081])
Therapeutic drug assays (80150-80299 [80164, 80165, 80171])

**82075 Alcohol (ethanol), breath**

0.00  0.00  **FUD** XXX  [Q]

**AMA:** 2015,Jun,10; 2015,Apr,3

**82085 Aldolase**

0.00  0.00  **FUD** XXX  [Q]

**AMA:** 2015,Jun,10; 2015,Apr,3

**82088 Aldosterone**

0.00  0.00  **FUD** XXX  [Q][⊡]

**AMA:** 2015,Jun,10; 2015,Apr,3

**82103 Alpha-1-antitrypsin; total**

0.00  0.00  **FUD** XXX  [Q]

**AMA:** 2015,Jun,10; 2015,Apr,3

**82104 phenotype**

0.00  0.00  **FUD** XXX  [Q]

**AMA:** 2015,Jun,10; 2015,Apr,3

**82105 Alpha-fetoprotein (AFP); serum**

0.00  0.00  **FUD** XXX  [Q][⊡]

**AMA:** 2015,Jun,10; 2015,Apr,3

**82106 amniotic fluid** [M]

0.00  0.00  **FUD** XXX  [Q][⊡]

**AMA:** 2015,Jun,10; 2015,Apr,3

**82107 AFP-L3 fraction isoform and total AFP (including ratio)**

0.00  0.00  **FUD** XXX  [Q][⊡]

**AMA:** 2015,Jun,10; 2015,Apr,3

## 82108 Chemistry: Aluminum

**CMS:** 100-02,11,20.2 ESRD Laboratory Services

INCLUDES Clinical information not requested by the ordering physician
Mathematically calculated results
Quantitative analysis unless otherwise specified
Specimens from any source unless otherwise specified

EXCLUDES Analytes from nonrequested laboratory analysis
Calculated results that represent a score or probability that was derived by algorithm
Drug testing ([80305, 80306, 80307], [80324, 80325, 80326, 80327, 80328, 80329, 80330, 80331, 80332, 80333, 80334, 80335, 80336, 80337, 80338, 80339, 80340, 80341, 80342, 80343, 80344, 80345, 80346, 80347, 80348, 80349, 80350, 80351, 80352, 80353, 80354, 80355, 80356, 80357, 80358, 80359, 80360, 80361, 80362, 80363, 80364, 80365, 80366, 80367, 80368, 80369, 80370, 80371, 80372, 80373, 80374, 80375, 80376, 80377, 83992])
Organ or disease panels (80048-80076 [80081])
Therapeutic drug assays (80150-80299 [80164, 80165, 80171])

**82108 Aluminum**

0.00  0.00  **FUD** XXX  [Q]

**AMA:** 2015,Jun,10; 2015,Apr,3

● New Code  ▲ Revised Code  ○ Reinstated  ● New Web Release  ▲ Revised Web Release  Unlisted  Not Covered  # Resequenced
⊘ AMA Mod 51 Exempt  ⑤① Optum Mod 51 Exempt  ⑥③ Mod 63 Exempt  ∕ Non-FDA Drug  ★ Telemedicine  M Maternity  A Age Edit  + Add-on  **AMA:** CPT Asst
© 2017 Optum360, LLC  CPT © 2017 American Medical Association. All Rights Reserved.  381

## 82120-82261 Chemistry: Amines—Biotinidase

**INCLUDES** Clinical information not requested by the ordering physician
Mathematically calculated results
Quantitative analysis unless otherwise specified
Specimens from any source unless otherwise specified

**EXCLUDES** *Analytes from nonrequested laboratory analysis*
*Calculated results that represent a score or probability that was derived by algorithm*
*Drug testing ([80305, 80306, 80307], [80324, 80325, 80326, 80327, 80328, 80329, 80330, 80331, 80332, 80333, 80334, 80335, 80336, 80337, 80338, 80339, 80340, 80341, 80342, 80343, 80344, 80345, 80346, 80347, 80348, 80349, 80350, 80351, 80352, 80353, 80354, 80355, 80356, 80357, 80358, 80359, 80360, 80361, 80362, 80363, 80364, 80365, 80366, 80367, 80368, 80369, 80370, 80371, 80372, 80373, 80374, 80375, 80376, 80377, 83992])*
*Organ or disease panels (80048-80076 [80081])*
*Therapeutic drug assays (80150-80299 [80164, 80165, 80171])*

**82120** **Amines, vaginal fluid, qualitative** ♀

**EXCLUDES** *Combined pH and amines test for vaginitis (82120, 83986)*

📠 0.00   📐 0.00   **FUD** XXX    ☒ ⊡

**AMA:** 2017,Jan,8; 2016,Jan,13; 2015,Jun,10; 2015,Apr,3; 2015,Jan,16; 2014,Jan,11

**82127** **Amino acids; single, qualitative, each specimen**

📠 0.00   📐 0.00   **FUD** XXX    ⊡

**AMA:** 2015,Jun,10; 2015,Apr,3

**82128** **multiple, qualitative, each specimen**

📠 0.00   📐 0.00   **FUD** XXX    ⊡ ⊡

**AMA:** 2015,Jun,10; 2015,Apr,3

**82131** **single, quantitative, each specimen**

**INCLUDES** Van Slyke method

📠 0.00   📐 0.00   **FUD** XXX    ⊡ ⊡

**AMA:** 2017,Jan,8; 2016,Jan,13; 2015,Jun,10; 2015,Apr,3; 2015,Jan,16; 2014,Jan,11; 2012,Jan,15-42

**82135** **Aminolevulinic acid, delta (ALA)**

📠 0.00   📐 0.00   **FUD** XXX    ⊡

**AMA:** 2015,Jun,10; 2015,Apr,3

**82136** **Amino acids, 2 to 5 amino acids, quantitative, each specimen**

📠 0.00   📐 0.00   **FUD** XXX    ⊡ ⊡

**AMA:** 2015,Jun,10; 2015,Apr,3

**82139** **Amino acids, 6 or more amino acids, quantitative, each specimen**

📠 0.00   📐 0.00   **FUD** XXX    ⊡ ⊡

**AMA:** 2015,Jun,10; 2015,Apr,3

**82140** **Ammonia**

📠 0.00   📐 0.00   **FUD** XXX    ⊡

**AMA:** 2015,Jun,10; 2015,Apr,3

**82143** **Amniotic fluid scan (spectrophotometric)** Ⓜ ♀

**EXCLUDES** *L/S ratio (83661)*

📠 0.00   📐 0.00   **FUD** XXX    ⊡

**AMA:** 2015,Jun,10; 2015,Apr,3

**82150** **Amylase**

📠 0.00   📐 0.00   **FUD** XXX    ☒ ⊡

**AMA:** 2015,Jun,10; 2015,Apr,3

**82154** **Androstanediol glucuronide**

📠 0.00   📐 0.00   **FUD** XXX    ⊡

**AMA:** 2017,Jan,8; 2016,Jan,13; 2015,Jun,10; 2015,Apr,3; 2015,Jan,16; 2014,Jan,11

**82157** **Androstenedione**

📠 0.00   📐 0.00   **FUD** XXX    ⊡

**AMA:** 2015,Jun,10; 2015,Apr,3

**82160** **Androsterone**

📠 0.00   📐 0.00   **FUD** XXX    ⊡

**AMA:** 2015,Jun,10; 2015,Apr,3

**82163** **Angiotensin II**

📠 0.00   📐 0.00   **FUD** XXX    ⊡

**AMA:** 2015,Jun,10; 2015,Apr,3

**82164** **Angiotensin I - converting enzyme (ACE)**

📠 0.00   📐 0.00   **FUD** XXX    ⊡

**AMA:** 2015,Jun,10; 2015,Apr,3

**82172** **Apolipoprotein, each**

📠 0.00   📐 0.00   **FUD** XXX    ⊡

**AMA:** 2015,Jun,10; 2015,Apr,3

**82175** **Arsenic**

**EXCLUDES** *Heavy metal screening (83015)*

📠 0.00   📐 0.00   **FUD** XXX    ⊡

**AMA:** 2015,Jun,10; 2015,Apr,3

**82180** **Ascorbic acid (Vitamin C), blood**

📠 0.00   📐 0.00   **FUD** XXX    ⊡ ⊡

**AMA:** 2015,Jun,10; 2015,Apr,3

**82190** **Atomic absorption spectroscopy, each analyte**

📠 0.00   📐 0.00   **FUD** XXX    ⊡

**AMA:** 2015,Jun,10; 2015,Apr,3

**82232** **Beta-2 microglobulin**

📠 0.00   📐 0.00   **FUD** XXX    ⊡

**AMA:** 2015,Jun,10; 2015,Apr,3

**82239** **Bile acids; total**

📠 0.00   📐 0.00   **FUD** XXX    ⊡

**AMA:** 2015,Jun,10; 2015,Apr,3

**82240** **cholylglycine**

**EXCLUDES** *Bile pigments, urine (81000-81005)*

📠 0.00   📐 0.00   **FUD** XXX    ⊡

**AMA:** 2015,Jun,10; 2015,Apr,3

**82247** **Bilirubin; total**

**INCLUDES** Van Den Bergh test

📠 0.00   📐 0.00   **FUD** XXX    ☒ ⊡

**AMA:** 2017,Jan,8; 2016,Jan,13; 2015,Jun,10; 2015,Apr,3; 2015,Jan,16; 2014,Jan,11; 2012,Jan,15-42

**82248** **direct**

📠 0.00   📐 0.00   **FUD** XXX    ⊡

**AMA:** 2017,Jan,8; 2016,Jan,13; 2015,Jun,10; 2015,Apr,3; 2015,Jan,16; 2014,Jan,11; 2012,Jan,15-42

**82252** **feces, qualitative**

📠 0.00   📐 0.00   **FUD** XXX    ⊡

**AMA:** 2015,Jun,10; 2015,Apr,3

**82261** **Biotinidase, each specimen**

📠 0.00   📐 0.00   **FUD** XXX    ⊡

**AMA:** 2015,Jun,10; 2015,Apr,3

## 82270-82274 Chemistry: Occult Blood

**CMS:** 100-04,16,70.8 CLIA Waived Tests; 100-04,18,60 Colorectal Cancer Screening

**INCLUDES** Clinical information not requested by the ordering physician
Mathematically calculated results
Quantitative analysis unless otherwise specified
Specimens from any source unless otherwise specified

**EXCLUDES** *Analytes from nonrequested laboratory analysis*
*Calculated results that represent a score or probability that was derived by algorithm*
*Drug testing ([80305, 80306, 80307], [80324, 80325, 80326, 80327, 80328, 80329, 80330, 80331, 80332, 80333, 80334, 80335, 80336, 80337, 80338, 80339, 80340, 80341, 80342, 80343, 80344, 80345, 80346, 80347, 80348, 80349, 80350, 80351, 80352, 80353, 80354, 80355, 80356, 80357, 80358, 80359, 80360, 80361, 80362, 80363, 80364, 80365, 80366, 80367, 80368, 80369, 80370, 80371, 80372, 80373, 80374, 80375, 80376, 80377, 83992])*
*Organ or disease panels (80048-80076 [80081])*
*Therapeutic drug assays (80150-80299 [80164, 80165, 80171])*

**82270** **Blood, occult, by peroxidase activity (eg, guaiac), qualitative; feces, consecutive collected specimens with single determination, for colorectal neoplasm screening (ie, patient was provided 3 cards or single triple card for consecutive collection)**

**INCLUDES** Day test

📠 0.00   📐 0.00   **FUD** XXX    ☒ Ⓐ ⊡

**AMA:** 2017,Jan,8; 2016,Jan,13; 2015,Jun,10; 2015,Apr,3; 2015,Jan,16; 2014,Jan,11; 2012,Jan,15-42

| 82271 | other sources |
|---|---|
| | ⊕ 0.00   ⅌ 0.00   **FUD** XXX   ☒ Ⓠ |
| | **AMA:** 2015,Jun,10; 2015,Apr,3 |

| 82272 | **Blood, occult, by peroxidase activity (eg, guaiac), qualitative, feces, 1-3 simultaneous determinations, performed for other than colorectal neoplasm screening** |
|---|---|
| | ⊕ 0.00   ⅌ 0.00   **FUD** XXX   ☒ Ⓠ |
| | **AMA:** 2017,Jan,8; 2016,Jan,13; 2015,Jun,10; 2015,Apr,3; 2015,Jan,16; 2014,Jan,11; 2012,Jan,15-42 |

| 82274 | **Blood, occult, by fecal hemoglobin determination by immunoassay, qualitative, feces, 1-3 simultaneous determinations** |
|---|---|
| | ⊕ 0.00   ⅌ 0.00   **FUD** XXX   ☒ Ⓠ ▱ |
| | **AMA:** 2015,Jun,10; 2015,Apr,3 |

## 82286-82308 [82652] Chemistry: Bradykinin—Calcitonin

**INCLUDES**  Clinical information not requested by the ordering physician
Mathematically calculated results
Quantitative analysis unless otherwise specified
Specimens from any source unless otherwise specified

**EXCLUDES**  *Analytes from nonrequested laboratory analysis*
*Calculated results that represent a score or probability that was derived by algorithm*
*Drug testing ([80305, 80306, 80307], [80324, 80325, 80326, 80327, 80328, 80329, 80330, 80331, 80332, 80333, 80334, 80335, 80336, 80337, 80338, 80339, 80340, 80341, 80342, 80343, 80344, 80345, 80346, 80347, 80348, 80349, 80350, 80351, 80352, 80353, 80354, 80355, 80356, 80357, 80358, 80359, 80360, 80361, 80362, 80363, 80364, 80365, 80366, 80367, 80368, 80369, 80370, 80371, 80372, 80373, 80374, 80375, 80376, 80377, 83992])*
*Organ or disease panels (80048-80076 [80081])*
*Therapeutic drug assays (80150-80299 [80164, 80165, 80171])*

| 82286 | **Bradykinin** |
|---|---|
| | ⊕ 0.00   ⅌ 0.00   **FUD** XXX   Ⓠ |
| | **AMA:** 2015,Jun,10; 2015,Apr,3 |

| 82300 | **Cadmium** |
|---|---|
| | ⊕ 0.00   ⅌ 0.00   **FUD** XXX   Ⓠ |
| | **AMA:** 2015,Jun,10; 2015,Apr,3 |

| 82306 | **Vitamin D; 25 hydroxy, includes fraction(s), if performed** |
|---|---|
| | ⊕ 0.00   ⅌ 0.00   **FUD** XXX   Ⓠ ▱ |
| | **AMA:** 2015,Jun,10; 2015,Apr,3 |

| # 82652 | **1, 25 dihydroxy, includes fraction(s), if performed** |
|---|---|
| | ⊕ 0.00   ⅌ 0.00   **FUD** XXX   Ⓠ ▱ |
| | **AMA:** 2015,Jun,10; 2015,Apr,3 |

| 82308 | **Calcitonin** |
|---|---|
| | ⊕ 0.00   ⅌ 0.00   **FUD** XXX   Ⓠ ▱ |
| | **AMA:** 2015,Jun,10; 2015,Apr,3 |

## 82310-82373 Chemistry: Calcium, total; Carbohydrate Deficient Transferrin

**INCLUDES**  Clinical information not requested by the ordering physician
Mathematically calculated results
Quantitative analysis unless otherwise specified
Specimens from any source unless otherwise specified

**EXCLUDES**  *Analytes from nonrequested laboratory analysis*
*Calculated results that represent a score or probability that was derived by algorithm*
*Drug testing ([80305, 80306, 80307], [80324, 80325, 80326, 80327, 80328, 80329, 80330, 80331, 80332, 80333, 80334, 80335, 80336, 80337, 80338, 80339, 80340, 80341, 80342, 80343, 80344, 80345, 80346, 80347, 80348, 80349, 80350, 80351, 80352, 80353, 80354, 80355, 80356, 80357, 80358, 80359, 80360, 80361, 80362, 80363, 80364, 80365, 80366, 80367, 80368, 80369, 80370, 80371, 80372, 80373, 80374, 80375, 80376, 80377, 83992])*
*Organ or disease panels (80048-80076 [80081])*
*Therapeutic drug assays (80150-80299 [80164, 80165, 80171])*

| 82310 | **Calcium; total** |
|---|---|
| | ⊕ 0.00   ⅌ 0.00   **FUD** XXX   ☒ Ⓠ ▱ |
| | **AMA:** 2017,Jan,8; 2016,Jan,13; 2015,Jun,10; 2015,Apr,3; 2015,Jan,16; 2014,Jan,11 |

| 82330 | **ionized** |
|---|---|
| | ⊕ 0.00   ⅌ 0.00   **FUD** XXX   ☒ Ⓠ |
| | **AMA:** 2017,Jan,8; 2016,Jan,13; 2015,Jun,10; 2015,Apr,3; 2015,Jan,16; 2014,Jan,11; 2013,Apr,10-11 |

| 82331 | **after calcium infusion test** |
|---|---|
| | ⊕ 0.00   ⅌ 0.00   **FUD** XXX   Ⓠ ▱ |
| | **AMA:** 2015,Jun,10; 2015,Apr,3 |

| 82340 | **urine quantitative, timed specimen** |
|---|---|
| | ⊕ 0.00   ⅌ 0.00   **FUD** XXX   Ⓠ |
| | **AMA:** 2015,Jun,10; 2015,Apr,3 |

| 82355 | **Calculus; qualitative analysis** |
|---|---|
| | ⊕ 0.00   ⅌ 0.00   **FUD** XXX   Ⓠ ▱ |
| | **AMA:** 2015,Jun,10; 2015,Apr,3 |

| 82360 | **quantitative analysis, chemical** |
|---|---|
| | ⊕ 0.00   ⅌ 0.00   **FUD** XXX   Ⓠ ▱ |
| | **AMA:** 2015,Jun,10; 2015,Apr,3 |

| 82365 | **infrared spectroscopy** |
|---|---|
| | ⊕ 0.00   ⅌ 0.00   **FUD** XXX   Ⓠ ▱ |
| | **AMA:** 2015,Jun,10; 2015,Apr,3 |

| 82370 | **X-ray diffraction** |
|---|---|
| | ⊕ 0.00   ⅌ 0.00   **FUD** XXX   Ⓠ ▱ |
| | **AMA:** 2015,Jun,10; 2015,Apr,3 |

| 82373 | **Carbohydrate deficient transferrin** |
|---|---|
| | ⊕ 0.00   ⅌ 0.00   **FUD** XXX   Ⓠ |
| | **AMA:** 2015,Jun,10; 2015,Apr,3 |

## 82374 Chemistry: Carbon Dioxide

**CMS:** 100-02,11,20.2 ESRD Laboratory Services; 100-02,11,30.2.2 Automated Multi-Channel Chemistry (AMCC) Tests; 100-04,16,40.6.1 Automated Multi-Channel Chemistry (AMCC) Tests for ESRD Beneficiaries; 100-04,16,70.8 CLIA Waived Tests; 100-04,16,90.2 Organ or Disease Oriented Panels

**INCLUDES**  Clinical information not requested by the ordering physician
Mathematically calculated results
Quantitative analysis unless otherwise specified
Specimens from any source unless otherwise specified

**EXCLUDES**  *Analytes from nonrequested laboratory analysis*
*Calculated results that represent a score or probability that was derived by algorithm*
*Drug testing ([80305, 80306, 80307], [80324, 80325, 80326, 80327, 80328, 80329, 80330, 80331, 80332, 80333, 80334, 80335, 80336, 80337, 80338, 80339, 80340, 80341, 80342, 80343, 80344, 80345, 80346, 80347, 80348, 80349, 80350, 80351, 80352, 80353, 80354, 80355, 80356, 80357, 80358, 80359, 80360, 80361, 80362, 80363, 80364, 80365, 80366, 80367, 80368, 80369, 80370, 80371, 80372, 80373, 80374, 80375, 80376, 80377, 83992])*
*Organ or disease panels (80048-80076 [80081])*
*Therapeutic drug assays (80150-80299 [80164, 80165, 80171])*

| 82374 | **Carbon dioxide (bicarbonate)** |
|---|---|
| | **EXCLUDES** *Blood gases (82803)* |
| | ⊕ 0.00   ⅌ 0.00   **FUD** XXX   ☒ Ⓠ |
| | **AMA:** 2017,Jan,8; 2016,Jan,13; 2015,Jun,10; 2015,Apr,3; 2015,Jan,16; 2014,Jan,11; 2013,Apr,10-11 |

## 82375-82376 Chemistry: Carboxyhemoglobin (Carbon Monoxide)

**INCLUDES**  Clinical information not requested by the ordering physician
Mathematically calculated results
Specimens from any source unless otherwise specified

**EXCLUDES**  *Analytes from nonrequested laboratory analysis*
*Calculated results that represent a score or probability that was derived by algorithm*
*Drug testing ([80305, 80306, 80307], [80324, 80325, 80326, 80327, 80328, 80329, 80330, 80331, 80332, 80333, 80334, 80335, 80336, 80337, 80338, 80339, 80340, 80341, 80342, 80343, 80344, 80345, 80346, 80347, 80348, 80349, 80350, 80351, 80352, 80353, 80354, 80355, 80356, 80357, 80358, 80359, 80360, 80361, 80362, 80363, 80364, 80365, 80366, 80367, 80368, 80369, 80370, 80371, 80372, 80373, 80374, 80375, 80376, 80377, 83992])*
*Organ or disease panels (80048-80076 [80081])*
*Transcutaneous measurement of carboxyhemoglobin (88740)*

| 82375 | **Carboxyhemoglobin; quantitative** |
|---|---|
| | ⊕ 0.00   ⅌ 0.00   **FUD** XXX   Ⓠ ▱ |
| | **AMA:** 2017,Jan,8; 2016,Jan,13; 2015,Jun,10; 2015,Apr,3; 2015,Jan,16; 2014,Jan,11 |

| 82376 | **qualitative** |
|---|---|
| | ⊕ 0.00   ⅌ 0.00   **FUD** XXX   Ⓠ ▱ |
| | **AMA:** 2015,Jun,10; 2015,Apr,3 |

● New Code   ▲ Revised Code   ○ Reinstated   ● New Web Release   ▲ Revised Web Release   Unlisted   Not Covered   # Resequenced
⊘ AMA Mod 51 Exempt   ⑤⑪ Optum Mod 51 Exempt   ⑥⑨ Mod 63 Exempt   ✗ Non-FDA Drug   ★ Telemedicine   Ⓜ Maternity   Ⓐ Age Edit   + Add-on   **AMA:** CPT Asst
© 2017 Optum360, LLC                    CPT © 2017 American Medical Association. All Rights Reserved.

## 82378 Chemistry: Carcinoembryonic Antigen (CEA)

**CMS:** 100-03,190.26 Carcinoembryonic Antigen (CEA)

INCLUDES Clinical information not requested by the ordering physician

EXCLUDES *Analytes from nonrequested laboratory analysis*
*Calculated results that represent a score or probability that was derived by algorithm*

### 82378    **Carcinoembryonic antigen (CEA)**
 0.00     0.00    **FUD** XXX                                            Q

**AMA:** 2017,Jan,8; 2016,Jan,13; 2015,Jun,10; 2015,Apr,3; 2015,Jan,16; 2014,Jan,11; 2012,Jan,15-42

## 82379-82415 Chemistry: Carnitine—Chloramphenicol

INCLUDES Clinical information not requested by the ordering physician
Mathematically calculated results
Quantitative analysis unless otherwise specified
Specimens from any source unless otherwise specified

EXCLUDES *Analytes from nonrequested laboratory analysis*
*Calculated results that represent a score or probability that was derived by algorithm*
*Drug testing ([80305, 80306, 80307], [80324, 80325, 80326, 80327, 80328, 80329, 80330, 80331, 80332, 80333, 80334, 80335, 80336, 80337, 80338, 80339, 80340, 80341, 80342, 80343, 80344, 80345, 80346, 80347, 80348, 80349, 80350, 80351, 80352, 80353, 80354, 80355, 80356, 80357, 80358, 80359, 80360, 80361, 80362, 80363, 80364, 80365, 80366, 80367, 80368, 80369, 80370, 80371, 80372, 80373, 80374, 80375, 80376, 80377, 83992])*
*Organ or disease panels (80048-80076 [80081])*
*Therapeutic drug assays (80150-80299 [80164, 80165, 80171])*

### 82379    **Carnitine (total and free), quantitative, each specimen**
EXCLUDES *Acylcarnitine (82016-82017)*
 0.00     0.00    **FUD** XXX                                            Q

**AMA:** 2015,Jun,10; 2015,Apr,3

### 82380    **Carotene**
 0.00     0.00    **FUD** XXX                                            Q

**AMA:** 2015,Jun,10; 2015,Apr,3

### 82382    **Catecholamines; total urine**
 0.00     0.00    **FUD** XXX                                            Q

**AMA:** 2015,Jun,10; 2015,Apr,3

### 82383    **blood**
 0.00     0.00    **FUD** XXX                                            Q

**AMA:** 2015,Jun,10; 2015,Apr,3

### 82384    **fractionated**
EXCLUDES *Urine metabolites (83835, 84585)*
 0.00     0.00    **FUD** XXX                                         Q

**AMA:** 2015,Jun,10; 2015,Apr,3

### 82387    **Cathepsin-D**
 0.00     0.00    **FUD** XXX                                            Q

**AMA:** 2015,Jun,10; 2015,Apr,3

### 82390    **Ceruloplasmin**
 0.00     0.00    **FUD** XXX                                            Q

**AMA:** 2015,Jun,10; 2015,Apr,3

### 82397    **Chemiluminescent assay**
 0.00     0.00    **FUD** XXX                                            Q

**AMA:** 2017,Jan,8; 2016,Jan,13; 2015,Jun,10; 2015,Apr,3; 2015,Jan,16; 2014,Jan,11

### 82415    **Chloramphenicol**
 0.00     0.00    **FUD** XXX                                            Q

**AMA:** 2015,Jun,10; 2015,Apr,3

## 82435-82438 Chemistry: Chloride

INCLUDES Clinical information not requested by the ordering physician
Mathematically calculated results
Quantitative analysis unless otherwise specified
Specimens from any source unless otherwise specified

EXCLUDES *Analytes from nonrequested laboratory analysis*
*Calculated results that represent a score or probability that was derived by algorithm*
*Organ or disease panels (80048-80076 [80081])*
*Therapeutic drug assays (80150-80299 [80164, 80165, 80171])*

### 82435    **Chloride; blood**
 0.00     0.00    **FUD** XXX                                         X  Q

**AMA:** 2017,Jan,8; 2016,Jan,13; 2015,Jun,10; 2015,Apr,3; 2015,Jan,16; 2014,Jan,11; 2013,Apr,10-11

### 82436    **urine**
 0.00     0.00    **FUD** XXX                                            Q

**AMA:** 2015,Jun,10; 2015,Apr,3

### 82438    **other source**
EXCLUDES *Sweat collections by iontophoresis (89230)*
 0.00     0.00    **FUD** XXX                                            Q

**AMA:** 2017,Jan,8; 2016,Jan,13; 2015,Jun,10; 2015,Apr,3; 2015,Jan,16; 2014,Jan,11

## 82441 Chemistry: Chlorinated Hydrocarbons

INCLUDES Clinical information not requested by the ordering physician
Mathematically calculated results
Quantitative analysis unless otherwise specified
Specimens from any source unless otherwise specified

EXCLUDES *Analytes from nonrequested laboratory analysis*
*Calculated results that represent a score or probability that was derived by algorithm*

### 82441    **Chlorinated hydrocarbons, screen**
 0.00     0.00    **FUD** XXX                                         Q

**AMA:** 2015,Jun,10; 2015,Apr,3

## 82465 Chemistry: Cholesterol, Total

**CMS:** 100-03,190.23 Lipid Testing; 100-04,16,40.6.1 Automated Multi-Channel Chemistry (AMCC) Tests for ESRD Beneficiaries; 100-04,16,70.8 CLIA Waived Tests; 100-04,16,90.2 Organ or Disease Oriented Panels

INCLUDES Clinical information not requested by the ordering physician
Mathematically calculated results
Quantitative analysis unless otherwise specified

EXCLUDES *Analytes from nonrequested laboratory analysis*
*Calculated results that represent a score or probability that was derived by algorithm*
*Organ or disease panels (80048-80076 [80081])*

### 82465    **Cholesterol, serum or whole blood, total**
EXCLUDES *High density lipoprotein (HDL) (83718)*
 0.00     0.00    **FUD** XXX                                         X  A

**AMA:** 2017,Jan,8; 2016,Jan,13; 2015,Jun,10; 2015,Apr,3; 2015,Jan,16; 2014,Jan,11; 2012,Jan,15-42

## 82480-82507 Chemistry: Cholinesterase—Citrate

INCLUDES Clinical information not requested by the ordering physician
Mathematically calculated results
Quantitative analysis unless otherwise specified
Specimens from any source unless otherwise specified

EXCLUDES *Analytes from nonrequested laboratory analysis*
*Calculated results that represent a score or probability that was derived by algorithm*
*Drug testing ([80305, 80306, 80307], [80324, 80325, 80326, 80327, 80328, 80329, 80330, 80331, 80332, 80333, 80334, 80335, 80336, 80337, 80338, 80339, 80340, 80341, 80342, 80343, 80344, 80345, 80346, 80347, 80348, 80349, 80350, 80351, 80352, 80353, 80354, 80355, 80356, 80357, 80358, 80359, 80360, 80361, 80362, 80363, 80364, 80365, 80366, 80367, 80368, 80369, 80370, 80371, 80372, 80373, 80374, 80375, 80376, 80377, 83992])*
*Organ or disease panels (80048-80076 [80081])*
*Therapeutic drug assays (80150-80299 [80164, 80165, 80171])*

### 82480    **Cholinesterase; serum**
 0.00     0.00    **FUD** XXX                                            Q

**AMA:** 2015,Jun,10; 2015,Apr,3

### 82482    **RBC**
 0.00     0.00    **FUD** XXX                                            Q

**AMA:** 2015,Jun,10; 2015,Apr,3

### 82485    **Chondroitin B sulfate, quantitative**
 0.00     0.00    **FUD** XXX                                            Q

**AMA:** 2015,Jun,10; 2015,Apr,3

### 82495    **Chromium**
 0.00     0.00    **FUD** XXX                                            Q

**AMA:** 2015,Jun,10; 2015,Apr,3

### 82507    **Citrate**
 0.00     0.00    **FUD** XXX                                            Q

**AMA:** 2015,Jun,10; 2015,Apr,3

## 82523 Chemistry: Collagen Crosslinks, Any Method

**CMS:** 100-03,190.19 NCD for Collagen Crosslinks, Any Method; 100-04,16,70.8 CLIA Waived Tests

INCLUDES  Clinical information not requested by the ordering physician
Mathematically calculated results
Quantitative analysis unless otherwise specified
Specimens from any source unless otherwise specified

EXCLUDES  *Analytes from nonrequested laboratory analysis*
*Calculated results that represent a score or probability that was derived by algorithm*
*Organ or disease panels (80048-80076 [80081])*
*Therapeutic drug assays (80150-80299 [80164, 80165, 80171])*

**82523    Collagen cross links, any method**
🚑 0.00    ✂ 0.00    **FUD** XXX                    ☒ Q

AMA: 2015,Jun,10; 2015,Apr,3

## 82525-82735 Chemistry: Copper—Fluoride

INCLUDES  Clinical information not requested by the ordering physician
Mathematically calculated results
Quantitative analysis unless otherwise specified
Specimens from any source unless otherwise specified

EXCLUDES  *Analytes from nonrequested laboratory analysis*
*Calculated results that represent a score or probability that was derived by algorithm*
*Drug testing ([80305, 80306, 80307], [80324, 80325, 80326, 80327, 80328, 80329, 80330, 80331, 80332, 80333, 80334, 80335, 80336, 80337, 80338, 80339, 80340, 80341, 80342, 80343, 80344, 80345, 80346, 80347, 80348, 80349, 80350, 80351, 80352, 80353, 80354, 80355, 80356, 80357, 80358, 80359, 80360, 80361, 80362, 80363, 80364, 80365, 80366, 80367, 80368, 80369, 80370, 80371, 80372, 80373, 80374, 80375, 80376, 80377, 83992])*
*Organ or disease panels (80048-80076 [80081])*
*Therapeutic drug assays (80150-80299 [80164, 80165, 80171])*

**82525    Copper**
🚑 0.00    ✂ 0.00    **FUD** XXX                    Q

AMA: 2015,Jun,10; 2015,Apr,3

**82528    Corticosterone**
INCLUDES  Porter-Silber test
🚑 0.00    ✂ 0.00    **FUD** XXX                    Q

AMA: 2015,Jun,10; 2015,Apr,3

**82530    Cortisol; free**
🚑 0.00    ✂ 0.00    **FUD** XXX                    Q ▭

AMA: 2017,Jan,8; 2016,Jan,13; 2015,Jun,10; 2015,Apr,3;
2015,Jan,16; 2014,Jan,11

**82533        total**
🚑 0.00    ✂ 0.00    **FUD** XXX                    Q ▭

AMA: 2017,Jan,8; 2016,Jan,13; 2015,Jun,10; 2015,Apr,3;
2015,Jan,16; 2014,Jan,11

**82540    Creatine**
🚑 0.00    ✂ 0.00    **FUD** XXX                    Q

AMA: 2015,Jun,10; 2015,Apr,3

**82542    Column chromatography, includes mass spectrometry, if performed (eg, HPLC, LC, LC/MS, LC/MS-MS, GC, GC/MS-MS, GC/MS, HPLC/MS), non-drug analyte(s) not elsewhere specified, qualitative or quantitative, each specimen**
EXCLUDES  *Procedure performed more than one time per specimen*
🚑 0.00    ✂ 0.00    **FUD** XXX                    Q

AMA: 2017,Jan,8; 2016,Jan,13; 2015,Jun,10; 2015,Apr,3

**82550    Creatine kinase (CK), (CPK); total**
🚑 0.00    ✂ 0.00    **FUD** XXX                    ☒ Q ▭

AMA: 2017,Jan,8; 2016,Jan,13; 2015,Jun,10; 2015,Apr,3;
2015,Jan,16; 2014,Jan,11

**82552        isoenzymes**
🚑 0.00    ✂ 0.00    **FUD** XXX                    Q ▭

AMA: 2017,Jan,8; 2016,Jan,13; 2015,Jun,10; 2015,Apr,3;
2015,Jan,16; 2014,Jan,11

**82553        MB fraction only**
🚑 0.00    ✂ 0.00    **FUD** XXX                    Q ▭

AMA: 2017,Jan,8; 2016,Jan,13; 2015,Jun,10; 2015,Apr,3;
2015,Jan,16; 2014,Jan,11

**82554        isoforms**
🚑 0.00    ✂ 0.00    **FUD** XXX                    Q ▭

AMA: 2017,Jan,8; 2016,Jan,13; 2015,Jun,10; 2015,Apr,3;
2015,Jan,16; 2014,Jan,11

**82565    Creatinine; blood**
🚑 0.00    ✂ 0.00    **FUD** XXX                    ☒ Q

AMA: 2017,Jan,8; 2016,Jan,13; 2015,Jun,10; 2015,Apr,3;
2015,Jan,16; 2014,Jan,11; 2013,Apr,10-11

**82570        other source**
🚑 0.00    ✂ 0.00    **FUD** XXX                    ☒ Q

AMA: 2015,Jun,10; 2015,Apr,3

**82575        clearance**
INCLUDES  Holten test
🚑 0.00    ✂ 0.00    **FUD** XXX                    Q ▭

AMA: 2015,Jun,10; 2015,Apr,3

**82585    Cryofibrinogen**
🚑 0.00    ✂ 0.00    **FUD** XXX                    Q

AMA: 2015,Jun,10; 2015,Apr,3

**82595    Cryoglobulin, qualitative or semi-quantitative (eg, cryocrit)**
EXCLUDES  *Quantitative, cryoglobulin (82784-82785)*
🚑 0.00    ✂ 0.00    **FUD** XXX                    Q

AMA: 2015,Jun,10; 2015,Apr,3

**82600    Cyanide**
🚑 0.00    ✂ 0.00    **FUD** XXX                    Q

AMA: 2015,Jun,10; 2015,Apr,3

**82607    Cyanocobalamin (Vitamin B-12);**
🚑 0.00    ✂ 0.00    **FUD** XXX                    Q ▭

AMA: 2015,Jun,10; 2015,Apr,3

**82608        unsaturated binding capacity**
🚑 0.00    ✂ 0.00    **FUD** XXX                    Q

AMA: 2015,Jun,10; 2015,Apr,3

**82610    Cystatin C**
🚑 0.00    ✂ 0.00    **FUD** XXX                    Q

AMA: 2017,Jan,8; 2016,Jan,13; 2015,Jun,10; 2015,Apr,3;
2015,Jan,16; 2014,Jan,11; 2012,Jan,15-42

**82615    Cystine and homocystine, urine, qualitative**
🚑 0.00    ✂ 0.00    **FUD** XXX                    Q

AMA: 2015,Jun,10; 2015,Apr,3

**82626    Dehydroepiandrosterone (DHEA)**
EXCLUDES  *Anabolic steroids ([80327, 80328])*
🚑 0.00    ✂ 0.00    **FUD** XXX                    Q

AMA: 2017,Jan,8; 2016,Jan,13; 2015,Jun,10; 2015,Apr,3;
2015,Jan,16; 2014,Jan,11

**82627    Dehydroepiandrosterone-sulfate (DHEA-S)**
🚑 0.00    ✂ 0.00    **FUD** XXX                    Q

AMA: 2017,Jan,8; 2016,Jan,13; 2015,Jun,10; 2015,Apr,3;
2015,Jan,16; 2014,Jan,11

**82633    Desoxycorticosterone, 11-**
🚑 0.00    ✂ 0.00    **FUD** XXX                    Q

AMA: 2015,Jun,10; 2015,Apr,3

**82634    Deoxycortisol, 11-**
🚑 0.00    ✂ 0.00    **FUD** XXX                    Q ▭

AMA: 2015,Jun,10; 2015,Apr,3

**82638    Dibucaine number**
🚑 0.00    ✂ 0.00    **FUD** XXX                    Q

AMA: 2015,Jun,10; 2015,Apr,3

*82652*    **Resequenced code. See code following 82306.**

**82656    Elastase, pancreatic (EL-1), fecal, qualitative or semi-quantitative**
🚑 0.00    ✂ 0.00    **FUD** XXX                    Q

AMA: 2017,Jan,8; 2016,Jan,13; 2015,Apr,3;
2015,Jan,16; 2014,Jan,11; 2012,Jan,15-42

---

● New Code    ▲ Revised Code    ○ Reinstated    ● New Web Release    ▲ Revised Web Release    Unlisted    Not Covered    # Resequenced
⊘ AMA Mod 51 Exempt    ⑤ Optum Mod 51 Exempt    ⑥ Mod 63 Exempt    ✗ Non-FDA Drug    ★ Telemedicine    Ⓜ Maternity    Ⓐ Age Edit    ✛ Add-on    **AMA:** CPT Asst
© 2017 Optum360, LLC                    CPT © 2017 American Medical Association. All Rights Reserved.                    **385**

**82657** Enzyme activity in blood cells, cultured cells, or tissue, not elsewhere specified; nonradioactive substrate, each specimen
   🛒 0.00   ⚖ 0.00   **FUD** XXX   🅠
   **AMA:** 2015,Jun,10; 2015,Apr,3

**82658** radioactive substrate, each specimen
   🛒 0.00   ⚖ 0.00   **FUD** XXX   🅠
   **AMA:** 2015,Jun,10; 2015,Apr,3

**82664** Electrophoretic technique, not elsewhere specified
   🛒 0.00   ⚖ 0.00   **FUD** XXX   🅠
   **AMA:** 2015,Jun,10; 2015,Apr,3

**82668** Erythropoietin
   🛒 0.00   ⚖ 0.00   **FUD** XXX   🅠
   **AMA:** 2015,Jun,10; 2015,Apr,3

**82670** Estradiol
   🛒 0.00   ⚖ 0.00   **FUD** XXX   🅠 ▣
   **AMA:** 2015,Jun,10; 2015,Apr,3

**82671** Estrogens; fractionated
   *EXCLUDES*  *Estrogen receptor assay (84233)*
   🛒 0.00   ⚖ 0.00   **FUD** XXX   🅠
   **AMA:** 2015,Jun,10; 2015,Apr,3

**82672** total
   *EXCLUDES*  *Estrogen receptor assay (84233)*
   🛒 0.00   ⚖ 0.00   **FUD** XXX   🅠
   **AMA:** 2015,Jun,10; 2015,Apr,3

**82677** Estriol
   🛒 0.00   ⚖ 0.00   **FUD** XXX   🅠
   **AMA:** 2015,Jun,10; 2015,Apr,3

**82679** Estrone
   🛒 0.00   ⚖ 0.00   **FUD** XXX   ❌ 🅠
   **AMA:** 2015,Jun,10; 2015,Apr,3

**82693** Ethylene glycol
   🛒 0.00   ⚖ 0.00   **FUD** XXX   🅠
   **AMA:** 2015,Jun,10; 2015,Apr,3

**82696** Etiocholanolone
   *EXCLUDES*  *Fractionation of ketosteroids (83593)*
   🛒 0.00   ⚖ 0.00   **FUD** XXX   🅠
   **AMA:** 2015,Jun,10; 2015,Apr,3

**82705** Fat or lipids, feces; qualitative
   🛒 0.00   ⚖ 0.00   **FUD** XXX   🅠
   **AMA:** 2015,Jun,10; 2015,Apr,3

**82710** quantitative
   🛒 0.00   ⚖ 0.00   **FUD** XXX   🅠
   **AMA:** 2015,Jun,10; 2015,Apr,3

**82715** Fat differential, feces, quantitative
   🛒 0.00   ⚖ 0.00   **FUD** XXX   🅠
   **AMA:** 2015,Jun,10; 2015,Apr,3

**82725** Fatty acids, nonesterified
   🛒 0.00   ⚖ 0.00   **FUD** XXX   🅠
   **AMA:** 2015,Jun,10; 2015,Apr,3

**82726** Very long chain fatty acids
   *EXCLUDES*  *Long-chain (C20-22) omega-3 fatty acids in red blood cell (RBC) membranes (0111T)*
   🛒 0.00   ⚖ 0.00   **FUD** XXX   🅠
   **AMA:** 2015,Jun,10; 2015,Apr,3

**82728** Ferritin
   🛒 0.00   ⚖ 0.00   **FUD** XXX   🅠
   **AMA:** 2015,Jun,10; 2015,Apr,3

**82731** Fetal fibronectin, cervicovaginal secretions, semi-quantitative    Ⓜ ♀
   🛒 0.00   ⚖ 0.00   **FUD** XXX   🅠
   **AMA:** 2015,Jun,10; 2015,Apr,3

**82735** Fluoride
   🛒 0.00   ⚖ 0.00   **FUD** XXX   🅠
   **AMA:** 2015,Jun,10; 2015,Apr,3

## 82746-82941 Chemistry: Folic Acid—Gastrin

*INCLUDES*  Clinical information not requested by the ordering physician
Mathematically calculated results
Quantitative analysis unless otherwise specified
Specimens from any source unless otherwise specified

*EXCLUDES*  *Analytes from nonrequested laboratory analysis*
*Calculated results that represent a score or probability that was derived by algorithm*
*Drug testing ([80305, 80306, 80307], [80324, 80325, 80326, 80327, 80328, 80329, 80330, 80331, 80332, 80333, 80334, 80335, 80336, 80337, 80338, 80339, 80340, 80341, 80342, 80343, 80344, 80345, 80346, 80347, 80348, 80349, 80350, 80351, 80352, 80353, 80354, 80355, 80356, 80357, 80358, 80359, 80360, 80361, 80362, 80363, 80364, 80365, 80366, 80367, 80368, 80369, 80370, 80371, 80372, 80373, 80374, 80375, 80376, 80377, 83992])*
*Organ or disease panels (80048-80076 [80081])*
*Therapeutic drug assays (80150-80299 [80164, 80165, 80171])*

**82746** Folic acid; serum
   🛒 0.00   ⚖ 0.00   **FUD** XXX   🅠
   **AMA:** 2015,Jun,10; 2015,Apr,3

**82747** RBC
   🛒 0.00   ⚖ 0.00   **FUD** XXX   🅠
   **AMA:** 2015,Jun,10; 2015,Apr,3

**82757** Fructose, semen
   *EXCLUDES*  *Fructosamine (82985)*
      *Fructose, TLC screen (84375)*
   🛒 0.00   ⚖ 0.00   **FUD** XXX   🅠
   **AMA:** 2015,Jun,10; 2015,Apr,3

**82759** Galactokinase, RBC
   🛒 0.00   ⚖ 0.00   **FUD** XXX   🅠
   **AMA:** 2015,Jun,10; 2015,Apr,3

**82760** Galactose
   🛒 0.00   ⚖ 0.00   **FUD** XXX   🅠
   **AMA:** 2015,Jun,10; 2015,Apr,3

**82775** Galactose-1-phosphate uridyl transferase; quantitative
   🛒 0.00   ⚖ 0.00   **FUD** XXX   🅠
   **AMA:** 2015,Jun,10; 2015,Apr,3

**82776** screen
   🛒 0.00   ⚖ 0.00   **FUD** XXX   🅠
   **AMA:** 2015,Jun,10; 2015,Apr,3

**82777** Galectin-3
   🛒 0.00   ⚖ 0.00   **FUD** XXX   🅠
   **AMA:** 2015,Jun,10; 2015,Apr,3

**82784** Gammaglobulin (immunoglobulin); IgA, IgD, IgG, IgM, each
   *INCLUDES*  Farr test
   🛒 0.00   ⚖ 0.00   **FUD** XXX   🅠 ▣
   **AMA:** 2017,Jan,8; 2016,Jan,13; 2015,Jun,10; 2015,Apr,3; 2015,Jan,16; 2014,Jan,11; 2012,Jan,15-42

**82785** IgE
   *INCLUDES*  Farr test
   *EXCLUDES*  *Allergen specific, IgE (86003, 86005)*
   🛒 0.00   ⚖ 0.00   **FUD** XXX   🅠 ▣
   **AMA:** 2017,Jan,8; 2016,Jan,13; 2015,Jun,10; 2015,Apr,3; 2015,Jan,16; 2014,Jan,11

**82787** immunoglobulin subclasses (eg, IgG1, 2, 3, or 4), each
   *EXCLUDES*  *Gamma-glutamyltransferase (GGT) (82977)*
   🛒 0.00   ⚖ 0.00   **FUD** XXX   🅠 ▣
   **AMA:** 2015,Jun,10; 2015,Apr,3

**82800** Gases, blood, pH only
   🛒 0.00   ⚖ 0.00   **FUD** XXX   🅠 ▣
   **AMA:** 2015,Jun,10; 2015,Apr,3

**82803** Gases, blood, any combination of pH, pCO2, pO2, CO2, HCO3 (including calculated O2 saturation);
   *INCLUDES*  Two or more of the listed analytes
   🛒 0.00   ⚖ 0.00   **FUD** XXX   🅠 ▣
   **AMA:** 2015,Jun,10; 2015,Apr,3

---

| 26/TC PC/TC Only | A2-Z3 ASC Payment | 50 Bilateral | ♂ Male Only | ♀ Female Only | 🛒 Facility RVU | ⚖ Non-Facility RVU | ▣ CCI |
| FUD Follow-up Days | CMS: IOM (Pub 100) | A-Y OPPSI | 80/80 Surg Assist Allowed / w/Doc | | ⚕ Lab Crosswalk | ✚ Radiology Crosswalk | ❌ CLIA |

386     CPT © 2017 American Medical Association. All Rights Reserved.     © 2017 Optum360, LLC

**82805**     **with O2 saturation, by direct measurement, except pulse oximetry**
         🔪 0.00    ⚕ 0.00    **FUD** XXX                         ⬚⬚
         **AMA:** 2015,Jun,10; 2015,Apr,3

**82810**     **Gases, blood, O2 saturation only, by direct measurement, except pulse oximetry**
         EXCLUDES    *Pulse oximetry (94760)*
         🔪 0.00    ⚕ 0.00    **FUD** XXX                         ⬚⬚
         **AMA:** 2015,Jun,10; 2015,Apr,3

**82820**     **Hemoglobin-oxygen affinity (pO2 for 50% hemoglobin saturation with oxygen)**
         🔪 0.00    ⚕ 0.00    **FUD** XXX                         ⬚⬚
         **AMA:** 2015,Jun,10; 2015,Apr,3

**82930**     **Gastric acid analysis, includes pH if performed, each specimen**
         🔪 0.00    ⚕ 0.00    **FUD** XXX                         ⬚⬚
         **AMA:** 2017,Jan,8; 2016,Jan,13; 2015,Jun,10; 2015,Apr,3; 2015,Jan,16; 2014,Jan,11

**82938**     **Gastrin after secretin stimulation**
         🔪 0.00    ⚕ 0.00    **FUD** XXX                         ⬚
         **AMA:** 2015,Jun,10; 2015,Apr,3

**82941**     **Gastrin**
         EXCLUDES    *Qualitative column chromotography report specific analyte or (82542)*
         🔪 0.00    ⚕ 0.00    **FUD** XXX                         ⬚
         **AMA:** 2015,Jun,10; 2015,Apr,3

## 82943-82962 Chemistry: Glucagon—Glucose Testing

**CMS:** 100-03,190.20 Blood Glucose Testing
INCLUDES    Clinical information not requested by the ordering physician
         Mathematically calculated results
         Quantitative analysis unless otherwise specified
         Specimens from any source unless otherwise specified
EXCLUDES    *Analytes from nonrequested laboratory analysis*
         *Calculated results that represent a score or probability that was derived by algorithm*
         *Organ or disease panels (80048-80076 [80081])*
         *Therapeutic drug assays (80150-80299 [80164, 80165, 80171])*
Code also glucose administration injection (96374)

**82943**     **Glucagon**
         🔪 0.00    ⚕ 0.00    **FUD** XXX                         ⬚
         **AMA:** 2015,Jun,10; 2015,Apr,3

**82945**     **Glucose, body fluid, other than blood**
         🔪 0.00    ⚕ 0.00    **FUD** XXX                         ⬚⬚
         **AMA:** 2015,Jun,10; 2015,Apr,3

**82946**     **Glucagon tolerance test**
         🔪 0.00    ⚕ 0.00    **FUD** XXX                         ⬚
         **AMA:** 2015,Jun,10; 2015,Apr,3

**82947**     **Glucose; quantitative, blood (except reagent strip)**
         🔪 0.00    ⚕ 0.00    **FUD** XXX                      ☒⬚⬚
         **AMA:** 2017,Jan,8; 2016,Jan,13; 2015,Jun,10; 2015,Apr,3; 2015,Jan,16; 2014,Jan,11; 2013,Apr,10-11

**82948**     **blood, reagent strip**
         🔪 0.00    ⚕ 0.00    **FUD** XXX                         ⬚⬚
         **AMA:** 2017,Jan,8; 2016,Jan,13; 2015,Jun,10; 2015,Apr,3; 2015,Jan,16; 2014,Jan,11; 2012,Jan,15-42

**82950**     **post glucose dose (includes glucose)**
         🔪 0.00    ⚕ 0.00    **FUD** XXX                      ☒⬚⬚
         **AMA:** 2017,Jan,8; 2016,Jan,13; 2015,Jun,10; 2015,Apr,3; 2015,Jan,16; 2014,Jan,11; 2012,Jan,15-42

**82951**     **tolerance test (GTT), 3 specimens (includes glucose)**
         🔪 0.00    ⚕ 0.00    **FUD** XXX                      ☒⬚⬚
         **AMA:** 2017,Jan,8; 2016,Jan,13; 2015,Jun,10; 2015,Apr,3; 2015,Jan,16; 2014,Jan,11; 2012,Jan,15-42

**+ 82952**    **tolerance test, each additional beyond 3 specimens (List separately in addition to code for primary procedure)**
         Code first (82951)
         🔪 0.00    ⚕ 0.00    **FUD** XXX                      ☒⬚⬚
         **AMA:** 2017,Jan,8; 2016,Jan,13; 2015,Jun,10; 2015,Apr,3; 2015,Jan,16; 2014,Jan,11; 2012,Jan,15-42

**82955**     **Glucose-6-phosphate dehydrogenase (G6PD); quantitative**
         🔪 0.00    ⚕ 0.00    **FUD** XXX                         ⬚
         **AMA:** 2015,Jun,10; 2015,Apr,3

**82960**     **screen**
         🔪 0.00    ⚕ 0.00    **FUD** XXX                         ⬚
         **AMA:** 2015,Jun,10; 2015,Apr,3

**82962**     **Glucose, blood by glucose monitoring device(s) cleared by the FDA specifically for home use**
         🔪 0.00    ⚕ 0.00    **FUD** XXX                      ☒⬚⬚
         **AMA:** 2017,Jan,8; 2016,Jan,13; 2015,Jun,10; 2015,Apr,3; 2015,Jan,16; 2014,Jan,11; 2012,Jan,15-42

## 82963-83690 Chemistry: Glucosidase—Lipase

INCLUDES    Clinical information not requested by the ordering physician
         Mathematically calculated results
         Quantitative analysis unless otherwise specified
         Specimens from any source unless otherwise specified
EXCLUDES    *Analytes from nonrequested laboratory analysis*
         *Calculated results that represent a score or probability that was derived by algorithm*
         *Drug testing ([80305, 80306, 80307], [80324, 80325, 80326, 80327, 80328, 80329, 80330, 80331, 80332, 80333, 80334, 80335, 80336, 80337, 80338, 80339, 80340, 80341, 80342, 80343, 80344, 80345, 80346, 80347, 80348, 80349, 80350, 80351, 80352, 80353, 80354, 80355, 80356, 80357, 80358, 80359, 80360, 80361, 80362, 80363, 80364, 80365, 80366, 80367, 80368, 80369, 80370, 80371, 80372, 80373, 80374, 80375, 80376, 80377, 83992])*
         *Organ or disease panels (80048-80076 [80081])*
         *Therapeutic drug assays (80150-80299 [80164, 80165, 80171])*

**82963**     **Glucosidase, beta**
         🔪 0.00    ⚕ 0.00    **FUD** XXX                         ⬚
         **AMA:** 2015,Jun,10; 2015,Apr,3

**82965**     **Glutamate dehydrogenase**
         🔪 0.00    ⚕ 0.00    **FUD** XXX                         ⬚
         **AMA:** 2015,Jun,10; 2015,Apr,3

**82977**     **Glutamyltransferase, gamma (GGT)**
         🔪 0.00    ⚕ 0.00    **FUD** XXX                      ☒⬚
         **AMA:** 2017,Jan,8; 2016,Jan,13; 2015,Jun,10; 2015,Apr,3; 2015,Jan,16; 2014,Jan,11

**82978**     **Glutathione**
         🔪 0.00    ⚕ 0.00    **FUD** XXX                         ⬚
         **AMA:** 2015,Jun,10; 2015,Apr,3

**82979**     **Glutathione reductase, RBC**
         🔪 0.00    ⚕ 0.00    **FUD** XXX                         ⬚
         **AMA:** 2015,Jun,10; 2015,Apr,3

**82985**     **Glycated protein**
         EXCLUDES    *Gonadotropin chorionic (hCG) (84702-84703)*
         🔪 0.00    ⚕ 0.00    **FUD** XXX                      ☒⬚⬚
         **AMA:** 2017,Jan,8; 2016,Jan,13; 2015,Jun,10; 2015,Apr,3; 2015,Jan,16; 2014,Jan,11

**83001**     **Gonadotropin; follicle stimulating hormone (FSH)**
         🔪 0.00    ⚕ 0.00    **FUD** XXX                      ☒⬚⬚
         **AMA:** 2015,Jun,10; 2015,Apr,3

**83002**     **luteinizing hormone (LH)**
         EXCLUDES    *Luteinizing releasing factor (LRH) (83727)*
         🔪 0.00    ⚕ 0.00    **FUD** XXX                      ☒⬚⬚
         **AMA:** 2015,Jun,10; 2015,Apr,3

**83003**     **Growth hormone, human (HGH) (somatotropin)**
         EXCLUDES    *Antibody to human growth hormone (86277)*
         🔪 0.00    ⚕ 0.00    **FUD** XXX                         ⬚⬚
         **AMA:** 2015,Jun,10; 2015,Apr,3

**83006** **Growth stimulation expressed gene 2 (ST2, Interleukin 1 receptor like-1)**
🔧 0.00   ✂ 0.00   **FUD** XXX   ⬛
AMA: 2015,Jun,10; 2015,Apr,3

**83009** **Helicobacter pylori, blood test analysis for urease activity, non-radioactive isotope (eg, C-13)**
EXCLUDES   *H. pylori, breath test analysis for urease activity (83013-83014)*
🔧 0.00   ✂ 0.00   **FUD** XXX   ⬛ 🖥
AMA: 2015,Jun,10; 2015,Apr,3

**83010** **Haptoglobin; quantitative**
🔧 0.00   ✂ 0.00   **FUD** XXX   ⬛
AMA: 2015,Jun,10; 2015,Apr,3

**83012** **phenotypes**
🔧 0.00   ✂ 0.00   **FUD** XXX   ⬛
AMA: 2015,Jun,10; 2015,Apr,3

**83013** **Helicobacter pylori; breath test analysis for urease activity, non-radioactive isotope (eg, C-13)**
🔧 0.00   ✂ 0.00   **FUD** XXX   ⬛ 🖥
AMA: 2017,Jan,8; 2016,Jan,13; 2015,Jun,10; 2015,Apr,3; 2015,Jan,16; 2014,Jan,11

**83014** **drug administration**
EXCLUDES   *H. pylori:*
*Blood test analysis for urease activity (83009)*
*Enzyme immunoassay (87339)*
*Liquid scintillation counter (78267-78268)*
*Stool (87338)*
🔧 0.00   ✂ 0.00   **FUD** XXX   ⬛ 🖥
AMA: 2017,Jan,8; 2016,Jan,13; 2015,Jun,10; 2015,Apr,3; 2015,Jan,16; 2014,Jan,11

**83015** **Heavy metal (eg, arsenic, barium, beryllium, bismuth, antimony, mercury); qualitative, any number of analytes**
INCLUDES   Reinsch test
🔧 0.00   ✂ 0.00   **FUD** XXX   ⬛
AMA: 2015,Jun,10; 2015,Apr,3

**83018** **quantitative, each, not elsewhere specified**
EXCLUDES   *Evaluation of a known heavy metal with a specific code*
🔧 0.00   ✂ 0.00   **FUD** XXX   ⬛
AMA: 2015,Jun,10; 2015,Apr,3

**83020** **Hemoglobin fractionation and quantitation; electrophoresis (eg, A2, S, C, and/or F)**
🔧 0.00   ✂ 0.00   **FUD** XXX   ⬛ 🖥
AMA: 2015,Jun,10; 2015,Apr,3

**83021** **chromatography (eg, A2, S, C, and/or F)**
EXCLUDES   *Analysis of glycosylated (A1c) hemoglobin by chromatography or electrophoresis without an identified hemoglobin variant (83036)*
🔧 0.00   ✂ 0.00   **FUD** XXX   ⬛ 🖥
AMA: 2017,Jan,8; 2016,Jan,13; 2015,Jun,10; 2015,Apr,3; 2015,Jan,16; 2014,Jan,11

**83026** **Hemoglobin; by copper sulfate method, non-automated**
🔧 0.00   ✂ 0.00   **FUD** XXX   ❌ ⬛
AMA: 2015,Jun,10; 2015,Apr,3

**83030** **F (fetal), chemical**
🔧 0.00   ✂ 0.00   **FUD** XXX   ⬛ 🖥
AMA: 2015,Jun,10; 2015,Apr,3

**83033** **F (fetal), qualitative**
🔧 0.00   ✂ 0.00   **FUD** XXX   ⬛ 🖥
AMA: 2015,Jun,10; 2015,Apr,3

**83036** **glycosylated (A1C)**
EXCLUDES   *Analysis of glycosylated (A1c) hemoglobin by chromatography or electrophoresis without an identified hemoglobin variant (83021)*
*Detection of hemoglobin, fecal, by immunoassay (82274)*
🔧 0.00   ✂ 0.00   **FUD** XXX   ❌ ⬛
AMA: 2017,Jan,8; 2016,Jan,13; 2015,Jun,10; 2015,Apr,3; 2015,Jan,16; 2014,Jan,11

**83037** **glycosylated (A1C) by device cleared by FDA for home use**
🔧 0.00   ✂ 0.00   **FUD** XXX   ❌ ⬛ 🖥
AMA: 2017,Jan,8; 2016,Jan,13; 2015,Jun,10; 2015,Apr,3; 2015,Jan,16; 2014,Jan,11; 2012,Jan,15-42

**83045** **methemoglobin, qualitative**
🔧 0.00   ✂ 0.00   **FUD** XXX   ⬛
AMA: 2015,Jun,10; 2015,Apr,3

**83050** **methemoglobin, quantitative**
EXCLUDES   *Transcutaneous methemoglobin test (88741)*
🔧 0.00   ✂ 0.00   **FUD** XXX   ⬛ 🖥
AMA: 2017,Jan,8; 2016,Jan,13; 2015,Jun,10; 2015,Apr,3; 2015,Jan,16; 2014,Jan,11

**83051** **plasma**
🔧 0.00   ✂ 0.00   **FUD** XXX   ⬛
AMA: 2015,Jun,10; 2015,Apr,3

**83060** **sulfhemoglobin, quantitative**
🔧 0.00   ✂ 0.00   **FUD** XXX   ⬛
AMA: 2015,Jun,10; 2015,Apr,3

**83065** **thermolabile**
🔧 0.00   ✂ 0.00   **FUD** XXX   ⬛
AMA: 2015,Jun,10; 2015,Apr,3

**83068** **unstable, screen**
🔧 0.00   ✂ 0.00   **FUD** XXX   ⬛ 🖥
AMA: 2015,Jun,10; 2015,Apr,3

**83069** **urine**
🔧 0.00   ✂ 0.00   **FUD** XXX   ⬛
AMA: 2015,Jun,10; 2015,Apr,3

**83070** **Hemosiderin, qualitative**
EXCLUDES   *Qualitative column chromotography report specific analyte or (82542)*
🔧 0.00   ✂ 0.00   **FUD** XXX   ⬛
AMA: 2015,Jun,10; 2015,Apr,3

**83080** **b-Hexosaminidase, each assay**
🔧 0.00   ✂ 0.00   **FUD** XXX   ⬛
AMA: 2015,Jun,10; 2015,Apr,3

**83088** **Histamine**
🔧 0.00   ✂ 0.00   **FUD** XXX   ⬛
AMA: 2015,Jun,10; 2015,Apr,3

**83090** **Homocysteine**
🔧 0.00   ✂ 0.00   **FUD** XXX   ⬛ 🖥
AMA: 2017,Jan,8; 2016,Jan,13; 2015,Jun,10; 2015,Apr,3; 2015,Jan,16; 2014,Jan,11; 2012,Jan,15-42

**83150** **Homovanillic acid (HVA)**
🔧 0.00   ✂ 0.00   **FUD** XXX   ⬛
AMA: 2015,Jun,10; 2015,Apr,3

**83491** **Hydroxycorticosteroids, 17- (17-OHCS)**
EXCLUDES   *Cortisol (82530, 82533)*
*Deoxycortisol (82634)*
🔧 0.00   ✂ 0.00   **FUD** XXX   ⬛
AMA: 2015,Jun,10; 2015,Apr,3

**83497** **Hydroxyindolacetic acid, 5-(HIAA)**
EXCLUDES   *Urine qualitative test (81005)*
🔧 0.00   ✂ 0.00   **FUD** XXX   ⬛
AMA: 2015,Jun,10; 2015,Apr,3

**83498** **Hydroxyprogesterone, 17-d**
🔧 0.00   ✂ 0.00   **FUD** XXX   ⬛ 🖥
AMA: 2015,Jun,10; 2015,Apr,3

**83499** ~~**Hydroxyprogesterone, 20-**~~

**83500** **Hydroxyproline; free**
🔧 0.00   ✂ 0.00   **FUD** XXX   ⬛
AMA: 2015,Jun,10; 2015,Apr,3

**83505** **total**
🔧 0.00   ✂ 0.00   **FUD** XXX   ⬛
AMA: 2015,Jun,10; 2015,Apr,3

| 26/TC PC/TC Only | A2-Z3 ASC Payment | 50 Bilateral | ♂ Male Only | ♀ Female Only | 🔧 Facility RVU | ✂ Non-Facility RVU | 🖥 CCI |
| FUD Follow-up Days | CMS: IOM (Pub 100) | A-Y OPPSI | 80/80 Surg Assist Allowed / w/Doc | | 🖥 Lab Crosswalk | ⊞ Radiology Crosswalk | ❌ CLIA |

388                    CPT © 2017 American Medical Association. All Rights Reserved.                    © 2017 Optum360, LLC

**83516** Immunoassay for analyte other than infectious agent antibody or infectious agent antigen; qualitative or semiquantitative, multiple step method
🔲 0.00   🔲 0.00   **FUD** XXX   ☒ Q 🔲
**AMA:** 2015,Jun,10; 2015,Apr,3

**83518** qualitative or semiquantitative, single step method (eg, reagent strip)
🔲 0.00   🔲 0.00   **FUD** XXX   ☒ Q
**AMA:** 2015,Jun,10; 2015,Apr,3

**83519** quantitative, by radioimmunoassay (eg, RIA)
🔲 0.00   🔲 0.00   **FUD** XXX   Q 🔲
**AMA:** 2017,Jan,8; 2016,Jan,13; 2015,Jun,10; 2015,Apr,3; 2015,Jan,16; 2014,Jan,11

**83520** quantitative, not otherwise specified
🔲 0.00   🔲 0.00   **FUD** XXX   Q 🔲
**AMA:** 2015,Jun,10; 2015,Apr,3

**83525** Insulin; total
EXCLUDES   *Proinsulin (84206)*
🔲 0.00   🔲 0.00   **FUD** XXX   Q 🔲
**AMA:** 2015,Jun,10; 2015,Apr,3

**83527** free
🔲 0.00   🔲 0.00   **FUD** XXX   Q
**AMA:** 2017,Jan,8; 2016,Jan,13; 2015,Jun,10; 2015,Apr,3; 2015,Jan,16; 2014,Jan,11

**83528** Intrinsic factor
EXCLUDES   *Intrinsic factor antibodies (86340)*
🔲 0.00   🔲 0.00   **FUD** XXX   Q
**AMA:** 2015,Jun,10; 2015,Apr,3

**83540** Iron
🔲 0.00   🔲 0.00   **FUD** XXX   Q
**AMA:** 2017,Jan,8; 2016,Jan,13; 2015,Jun,10; 2015,Apr,3; 2015,Jan,16; 2014,Jan,11

**83550** Iron binding capacity
🔲 0.00   🔲 0.00   **FUD** XXX   Q
**AMA:** 2015,Jun,10; 2015,Apr,3

**83570** Isocitric dehydrogenase (IDH)
🔲 0.00   🔲 0.00   **FUD** XXX   Q
**AMA:** 2015,Jun,10; 2015,Apr,3

**83582** Ketogenic steroids, fractionation
🔲 0.00   🔲 0.00   **FUD** XXX   Q
**AMA:** 2015,Jun,10; 2015,Apr,3

**83586** Ketosteroids, 17- (17-KS); total
🔲 0.00   🔲 0.00   **FUD** XXX   Q
**AMA:** 2015,Jun,10; 2015,Apr,3

**83593** fractionation
🔲 0.00   🔲 0.00   **FUD** XXX   Q
**AMA:** 2015,Jun,10; 2015,Apr,3

**83605** Lactate (lactic acid)
🔲 0.00   🔲 0.00   **FUD** XXX   ☒ Q
**AMA:** 2015,Jun,10; 2015,Apr,3

**83615** Lactate dehydrogenase (LD), (LDH);
🔲 0.00   🔲 0.00   **FUD** XXX   Q
**AMA:** 2017,Jan,8; 2016,Jan,13; 2015,Jun,10; 2015,Apr,3; 2015,Jan,16; 2014,Jan,11

**83625** isoenzymes, separation and quantitation
🔲 0.00   🔲 0.00   **FUD** XXX   Q 🔲
**AMA:** 2017,Jan,8; 2016,Jan,13; 2015,Jun,10; 2015,Apr,3; 2015,Jan,16; 2014,Jan,11

**83630** Lactoferrin, fecal; qualitative
🔲 0.00   🔲 0.00   **FUD** XXX   Q
**AMA:** 2017,Jan,8; 2016,Jan,13; 2015,Jun,10; 2015,Apr,3; 2015,Jan,16; 2014,Jan,11

**83631** quantitative
🔲 0.00   🔲 0.00   **FUD** XXX   Q 🔲
**AMA:** 2017,Jan,8; 2016,Jan,13; 2015,Jun,10; 2015,Apr,3; 2015,Jan,16; 2014,Jan,11; 2012,Jan,15-42

**83632** Lactogen, human placental (HPL) human chorionic somatomammotropin   M
🔲 0.00   🔲 0.00   **FUD** XXX   Q
**AMA:** 2015,Jun,10; 2015,Apr,3

**83633** Lactose, urine, qualitative
🔲 0.00   🔲 0.00   **FUD** XXX   Q
**AMA:** 2015,Jun,10; 2015,Apr,3

**83655** Lead
🔲 0.00   🔲 0.00   **FUD** XXX   ☒ Q
**AMA:** 2015,Jun,10; 2015,Apr,3

**83661** Fetal lung maturity assessment; lecithin sphingomyelin (L/S) ratio   M
🔲 0.00   🔲 0.00   **FUD** XXX   Q 🔲
**AMA:** 2017,Jan,8; 2016,Jan,13; 2015,Jun,10; 2015,Apr,3; 2015,Jan,16; 2014,Jan,11

**83662** foam stability test   M
🔲 0.00   🔲 0.00   **FUD** XXX   Q 🔲
**AMA:** 2015,Jun,10; 2015,Apr,3

**83663** fluorescence polarization   M
🔲 0.00   🔲 0.00   **FUD** XXX   Q 🔲
**AMA:** 2015,Jun,10; 2015,Apr,3

**83664** lamellar body density   M
EXCLUDES   *Phosphatidylglycerol (84081)*
🔲 0.00   🔲 0.00   **FUD** XXX   Q 🔲
**AMA:** 2015,Jun,10; 2015,Apr,3

**83670** Leucine aminopeptidase (LAP)
🔲 0.00   🔲 0.00   **FUD** XXX   Q
**AMA:** 2015,Jun,10; 2015,Apr,3

**83690** Lipase
🔲 0.00   🔲 0.00   **FUD** XXX   Q
**AMA:** 2015,Jun,10; 2015,Apr,3

# 83695-83727 Chemistry: Lipoprotein—Luteinizing Releasing Factor

INCLUDES   Clinical information not requested by the ordering physician
Mathematically calculated results
Quantitative analysis unless otherwise specified
Specimens from any source unless otherwise specified
EXCLUDES   *Analytes from nonrequested laboratory analysis*
*Calculated results that represent a score or probability that was derived by algorithm*
*Organ or disease panels (80048-80076 [80081])*
*Therapeutic drug assays (80150-80299 [80164, 80165, 80171])*

**83695** Lipoprotein (a)
🔲 0.00   🔲 0.00   **FUD** XXX   Q 🔲
**AMA:** 2017,Jan,8; 2016,Jan,13; 2015,Jun,10; 2015,Apr,3; 2015,Jan,16; 2014,Jan,11

**83698** Lipoprotein-associated phospholipase A2 (Lp-PLA2)
EXCLUDES   *Secretory type II phospholipase A2 (sPLA2-IIA) (0423T)*
🔲 0.00   🔲 0.00   **FUD** XXX   Q
**AMA:** 2015,Jun,10; 2015,Apr,3

**83700** Lipoprotein, blood; electrophoretic separation and quantitation
🔲 0.00   🔲 0.00   **FUD** XXX   Q 🔲
**AMA:** 2017,Jan,8; 2016,Jan,13; 2015,Jun,10; 2015,Apr,3; 2015,Jan,16; 2014,Jan,11

**83701** high resolution fractionation and quantitation of lipoproteins including lipoprotein subclasses when performed (eg, electrophoresis, ultracentrifugation)
🔲 0.00   🔲 0.00   **FUD** XXX   Q 🔲
**AMA:** 2017,Jan,8; 2016,Jan,13; 2015,Jun,10; 2015,Apr,3; 2015,Jan,16; 2014,Jan,11

**83704** quantitation of lipoprotein particle number(s) (eg, by nuclear magnetic resonance spectroscopy), includes lipoprotein particle subclass(es), when performed
🔲 0.00   🔲 0.00   **FUD** XXX   Q 🔲
**AMA:** 2017,Jan,8; 2016,Jan,13; 2015,Jun,10; 2015,Apr,3; 2015,Jan,16; 2014,Jan,11

● New Code   ▲ Revised Code   ○ Reinstated   ● New Web Release   ▲ Revised Web Release   Unlisted   Not Covered   # Resequenced
🚫 AMA Mod 51 Exempt   Ⓢ Optum Mod 51 Exempt   Ⓢ Mod 63 Exempt   ⊁ Non-FDA Drug   ★ Telemedicine   Ⓜ Maternity   Ⓐ Age Edit   ✛ Add-on   **AMA:** CPT Asst
© 2017 Optum360, LLC          CPT © 2017 American Medical Association. All Rights Reserved.

**83718**  **Lipoprotein, direct measurement; high density cholesterol (HDL cholesterol)**
   🔶 0.00    ⚖ 0.00    **FUD** XXX                    ❌ 🅐 ▯

   **AMA:** 2017,Jan,8; 2016,Jan,13; 2015,Jun,10; 2015,Apr,3; 2015,Jan,16; 2014,Jan,11; 2013,Feb,3-6; 2012,Jan,15-42

**83719**  **VLDL cholesterol**
   🔶 0.00    ⚖ 0.00    **FUD** XXX                    ▯ ▯

   **AMA:** 2017,Jan,8; 2016,Jan,13; 2015,Jun,10; 2015,Apr,3; 2015,Jan,16; 2014,Jan,11; 2013,Feb,3-6; 2012,Jan,15-42

**83721**  **LDL cholesterol**
   *EXCLUDES*  *Fractionation by high resolution electrophoresis or ultracentrifugation (83701)*
             *Lipoprotein particle numbers and subclasses analysis by nuclear magnetic resonance spectroscopy (83704)*
   🔶 0.00    ⚖ 0.00    **FUD** XXX                    ❌ ▯ ▯

   **AMA:** 2017,Jan,8; 2016,Jan,13; 2015,Jun,10; 2015,Apr,3; 2015,Jan,16; 2014,Jan,11; 2013,Feb,3-6; 2012,Jan,15-42

**83727**  **Luteinizing releasing factor (LRH)**
   🔶 0.00    ⚖ 0.00    **FUD** XXX                    ▯

   **AMA:** 2015,Jun,10; 2015,Apr,3

## 83735-83885 Chemistry: Magnesium—Nickel

*INCLUDES*  Clinical information not requested by the ordering physician
           Mathematically calculated results
           Quantitative analysis unless otherwise specified
           Specimens from any source unless otherwise specified

*EXCLUDES*  *Analytes from nonrequested laboratory analysis*
           *Calculated results that represent a score or probability that was derived by algorithm*
           *Organ or disease panels (80048-80076 [80081])*
           *Therapeutic drug assays (80150-80299 [80164, 80165, 80171])*

**83735**  **Magnesium**
   🔶 0.00    ⚖ 0.00    **FUD** XXX                    ▯

   **AMA:** 2015,Jun,10; 2015,Apr,3

**83775**  **Malate dehydrogenase**
   🔶 0.00    ⚖ 0.00    **FUD** XXX                    ▯

   **AMA:** 2015,Jun,10; 2015,Apr,3

**83785**  **Manganese**
   🔶 0.00    ⚖ 0.00    **FUD** XXX                    ▯

   **AMA:** 2015,Jun,10; 2015,Apr,3

**83789**  **Mass spectrometry and tandem mass spectrometry (eg, MS, MS/MS, MALDI, MS-TOF, QTOF), non-drug analyte(s) not elsewhere specified, qualitative or quantitative, each specimen**
   *EXCLUDES*  *Procedure performed more than one time per specimen*
   🔶 0.00    ⚖ 0.00    **FUD** XXX                    ▯ ▯

   **AMA:** 2015,Jun,10; 2015,Apr,3

**83825**  **Mercury, quantitative**
   *EXCLUDES*  *Mercury screen (83015)*
   🔶 0.00    ⚖ 0.00    **FUD** XXX                    ▯

   **AMA:** 2015,Jun,10; 2015,Apr,3

**83835**  **Metanephrines**
   *EXCLUDES*  *Catecholamines (82382-82384)*
   🔶 0.00    ⚖ 0.00    **FUD** XXX                    ▯

   **AMA:** 2015,Jun,10; 2015,Apr,3

**83857**  **Methemalbumin**
   🔶 0.00    ⚖ 0.00    **FUD** XXX                    ▯

   **AMA:** 2015,Jun,10; 2015,Apr,3

**83861**  **Microfluidic analysis utilizing an integrated collection and analysis device, tear osmolarity**
   Code also when performed on both eyes 83861 X 2
   🔶 0.00    ⚖ 0.00    **FUD** XXX                    ❌ ▯ ▯

   **AMA:** 2015,Jun,10; 2015,Apr,3

**83864**  **Mucopolysaccharides, acid, quantitative**
   🔶 0.00    ⚖ 0.00    **FUD** XXX                    ▯

   **AMA:** 2015,Jun,10; 2015,Apr,3

**83872**  **Mucin, synovial fluid (Ropes test)**
   🔶 0.00    ⚖ 0.00    **FUD** XXX                    ▯

   **AMA:** 2015,Jun,10; 2015,Apr,3

**83873**  **Myelin basic protein, cerebrospinal fluid**
   *EXCLUDES*  *Oligoclonal bands (83916)*
   🔶 0.00    ⚖ 0.00    **FUD** XXX                    ▯

   **AMA:** 2015,Jun,10; 2015,Apr,3

**83874**  **Myoglobin**
   🔶 0.00    ⚖ 0.00    **FUD** XXX                    ▯

   **AMA:** 2017,Jan,8; 2016,Jan,13; 2015,Jun,10; 2015,Apr,3; 2015,Jan,16; 2014,Jan,11

**83876**  **Myeloperoxidase (MPO)**
   🔶 0.00    ⚖ 0.00    **FUD** XXX                    ▯ ▯

   **AMA:** 2015,Jun,10; 2015,Apr,3

**83880**  **Natriuretic peptide**
   🔶 0.00    ⚖ 0.00    **FUD** XXX                    ❌ ▯

   **AMA:** 2017,Jan,8; 2016,Jan,13; 2015,Jun,10; 2015,Apr,3; 2015,Jan,16; 2014,Jan,11

**83883**  **Nephelometry, each analyte not elsewhere specified**
   🔶 0.00    ⚖ 0.00    **FUD** XXX                    ▯

   **AMA:** 2015,Jun,10; 2015,Apr,3

**83885**  **Nickel**
   🔶 0.00    ⚖ 0.00    **FUD** XXX                    ▯

   **AMA:** 2015,Jun,10; 2015,Apr,3

## 83915-84066 Chemistry: Nucleotidase 5'- —Phosphatase (Acid)

*INCLUDES*  Clinical information not requested by the ordering physician
           Mathematically calculated results
           Quantitative analysis unless otherwise specified
           Specimens from any source unless otherwise specified

*EXCLUDES*  *Analytes from nonrequested laboratory analysis*
           *Calculated results that represent a score or probability that was derived by algorithm*
           *Drug testing ([80305, 80306, 80307], [80324, 80325, 80326, 80327, 80328, 80329, 80330, 80331, 80332, 80333, 80334, 80335, 80336, 80337, 80338, 80339, 80340, 80341, 80342, 80343, 80344, 80345, 80346, 80347, 80348, 80349, 80350, 80351, 80352, 80353, 80354, 80355, 80356, 80357, 80358, 80359, 80360, 80361, 80362, 80363, 80364, 80365, 80366, 80367, 80368, 80369, 80370, 80371, 80372, 80373, 80374, 80375, 80376, 80377, 83992])*
           *Organ or disease panels (80048-80076 [80081])*
           *Therapeutic drug assays (80150-80299 [80164, 80165, 80171])*

**83915**  **Nucleotidase 5'-**
   🔶 0.00    ⚖ 0.00    **FUD** XXX                    ▯

   **AMA:** 2015,Jun,10; 2015,Apr,3

**83916**  **Oligoclonal immune (oligoclonal bands)**
   🔶 0.00    ⚖ 0.00    **FUD** XXX                    ▯ ▯

   **AMA:** 2015,Jun,10; 2015,Apr,3

**83918**  **Organic acids; total, quantitative, each specimen**
   🔶 0.00    ⚖ 0.00    **FUD** XXX                    ▯ ▯

   **AMA:** 2017,Jan,8; 2016,Jan,13; 2015,Jun,10; 2015,Apr,3; 2015,Jan,16; 2014,Jan,11; 2012,Jan,15-42

**83919**  **qualitative, each specimen**
   🔶 0.00    ⚖ 0.00    **FUD** XXX                    ▯

   **AMA:** 2015,Jun,10; 2015,Apr,3

**83921**  **Organic acid, single, quantitative**
   🔶 0.00    ⚖ 0.00    **FUD** XXX                    ▯ ▯

   **AMA:** 2015,Jun,10; 2015,Apr,3

**83930**  **Osmolality; blood**
   *EXCLUDES*  *Tear osmolarity (83861)*
   🔶 0.00    ⚖ 0.00    **FUD** XXX                    ▯

   **AMA:** 2015,Jun,10; 2015,Apr,3

**83935**  **urine**
   *EXCLUDES*  *Tear osmolarity (83861)*
   🔶 0.00    ⚖ 0.00    **FUD** XXX                    ▯

   **AMA:** 2015,Jun,10; 2015,Apr,3

| 26/TC PC/TC Only | A2-Z3 ASC Payment | 50 Bilateral | ♂ Male Only | ♀ Female Only | 🔶 Facility RVU | ⚖ Non-Facility RVU | ▯ CCI |
| **FUD** Follow-up Days | **CMS:** IOM (Pub 100) | A-Y OPPSI | 80/80 Surg Assist Allowed / w/Doc | | 🔲 Lab Crosswalk | ➕ Radiology Crosswalk | ❌ CLIA |

**390**                            CPT © 2017 American Medical Association. All Rights Reserved.                    © 2017 Optum360, LLC

**83937** **Osteocalcin (bone g1a protein)**
0.00   0.00   **FUD** XXX   [Q]
**AMA:** 2017,Jan,8; 2016,Jan,13; 2015,Jun,10; 2015,Apr,3; 2015,Jan,16; 2014,Jan,11

**83945** **Oxalate**
0.00   0.00   **FUD** XXX   [Q]
**AMA:** 2015,Jun,10; 2015,Apr,3

**83950** **Oncoprotein; HER-2/neu**
EXCLUDES   Tissue (88342, 88365)
0.00   0.00   **FUD** XXX   [Q][▢]
**AMA:** 2015,Jun,10; 2015,Apr,3

**83951** **des-gamma-carboxy-prothrombin (DCP)**
0.00   0.00   **FUD** XXX   [Q][▢]
**AMA:** 2015,Jun,10; 2015,Apr,3

**83970** **Parathormone (parathyroid hormone)**
0.00   0.00   **FUD** XXX   [Q]
**AMA:** 2015,Jun,10; 2015,Apr,3

**83986** **pH; body fluid, not otherwise specified**
EXCLUDES   Blood pH (82800, 82803)
0.00   0.00   **FUD** XXX   [X][Q]
**AMA:** 2017,Jan,8; 2016,May,13; 2016,Jan,13; 2015,Jun,10; 2015,Apr,3; 2015,Jan,16; 2013,Sep,13-14

**83987** **exhaled breath condensate**
0.00   0.00   **FUD** XXX   [Q][▢]
**AMA:** 2015,Jun,10; 2015,Apr,3

**83992** *Resequenced code. See code following 80365.*

**83993** **Calprotectin, fecal**
0.00   0.00   **FUD** XXX   [Q]
**AMA:** 2017,Jan,8; 2016,Jan,13; 2015,Jun,10; 2015,Apr,3; 2015,Jan,16; 2014,Jan,11

**84030** **Phenylalanine (PKU), blood**
INCLUDES   Guthrie test
EXCLUDES   Phenylalanine-tyrosine ratio (84030, 84510)
0.00   0.00   **FUD** XXX   [Q]
**AMA:** 2015,Jun,10; 2015,Apr,3

**84035** **Phenylketones, qualitative**
0.00   0.00   **FUD** XXX   [Q]
**AMA:** 2015,Jun,10; 2015,Apr,3

**84060** **Phosphatase, acid; total**
0.00   0.00   **FUD** XXX   [Q]
**AMA:** 2015,Jun,10; 2015,Apr,3

**84061**   ~~forensic examination~~

**84066**   **prostatic**
0.00   0.00   **FUD** XXX   [Q]
**AMA:** 2015,Jun,10; 2015,Apr,3

## 84075-84080 Chemistry: Phosphatase (Alkaline)

**CMS:** 100-03,160.17 Payment for L-Dopa /Associated Inpatient Hospital Services
INCLUDES   Clinical information not requested by the ordering physician
Mathematically calculated results
Quantitative analysis unless otherwise specified
Specimens from any source unless otherwise specified
EXCLUDES   Analytes from nonrequested laboratory analysis
Calculated results that represent a score or probability that was derived by algorithm
Organ or disease panels (80048-80076 [80081])

**84075** **Phosphatase, alkaline;**
0.00   0.00   **FUD** XXX   [X][Q]
**AMA:** 2017,Jan,8; 2016,Jan,13; 2015,Jun,10; 2015,Apr,3; 2015,Jan,16; 2014,Jan,11

**84078** **heat stable (total not included)**
0.00   0.00   **FUD** XXX   [Q]
**AMA:** 2015,Jun,10; 2015,Apr,3

**84080** **isoenzymes**
0.00   0.00   **FUD** XXX   [Q][▢]
**AMA:** 2015,Jun,10; 2015,Apr,3

## 84081-84150 Chemistry: Phosphatidylglycerol—Prostaglandin

INCLUDES   Clinical information not requested by the ordering physician
Mathematically calculated results
Quantitative analysis unless otherwise specified
Specimens from any source unless otherwise specified
EXCLUDES   Analytes from nonrequested laboratory analysis
Calculated results that represent a score or probability that was derived by algorithm
Organ or disease panels (80048-80076 [80081])
Therapeutic drug assays (80150-80299 [80164, 80165, 80171])

**84081** **Phosphatidylglycerol**
0.00   0.00   **FUD** XXX   [Q]
**AMA:** 2015,Jun,10; 2015,Apr,3

**84085** **Phosphogluconate, 6-, dehydrogenase, RBC**
0.00   0.00   **FUD** XXX   [Q]
**AMA:** 2015,Jun,10; 2015,Apr,3

**84087** **Phosphohexose isomerase**
0.00   0.00   **FUD** XXX   [Q]
**AMA:** 2015,Jun,10; 2015,Apr,3

**84100** **Phosphorus inorganic (phosphate);**
0.00   0.00   **FUD** XXX   [Q]
**AMA:** 2017,Jan,8; 2016,Jan,13; 2015,Jun,10; 2015,Apr,3; 2015,Jan,16; 2014,Jan,11

**84105** **urine**
0.00   0.00   **FUD** XXX   [Q]
**AMA:** 2015,Jun,10; 2015,Apr,3

**84106** **Porphobilinogen, urine; qualitative**
0.00   0.00   **FUD** XXX   [Q]
**AMA:** 2015,Jun,10; 2015,Apr,3

**84110** **quantitative**
0.00   0.00   **FUD** XXX   [Q]
**AMA:** 2015,Jun,10; 2015,Apr,3

**84112** **Evaluation of cervicovaginal fluid for specific amniotic fluid protein(s) (eg, placental alpha microglobulin-1 [PAMG-1], placental protein 12 [PP12], alpha-fetoprotein), qualitative, each specimen**   ♀
0.00   0.00   **FUD** XXX   [Q][▢]
**AMA:** 2015,Jun,10; 2015,Apr,3

**84119** **Porphyrins, urine; qualitative**
0.00   0.00   **FUD** XXX   [Q]
**AMA:** 2015,Jun,10; 2015,Apr,3

**84120** **quantitation and fractionation**
0.00   0.00   **FUD** XXX   [Q]
**AMA:** 2015,Jun,10; 2015,Apr,3

**84126** **Porphyrins, feces, quantitative**
0.00   0.00   **FUD** XXX   [Q]
**AMA:** 2015,Jun,10; 2015,Apr,3

**84132** **Potassium; serum, plasma or whole blood**
0.00   0.00   **FUD** XXX   [X][Q]
**AMA:** 2017,Jan,8; 2016,Jan,13; 2015,Jun,10; 2015,Apr,3; 2015,Jan,16; 2014,Jan,11; 2013,Apr,10-11

**84133** **urine**
0.00   0.00   **FUD** XXX   [Q]
**AMA:** 2015,Jun,10; 2015,Apr,3

**84134** **Prealbumin**
EXCLUDES   Microalbumin (82043-82044)
0.00   0.00   **FUD** XXX   [Q]
**AMA:** 2015,Jun,10; 2015,Apr,3

**84135** **Pregnanediol**   ♀
0.00   0.00   **FUD** XXX   [Q]
**AMA:** 2015,Jun,10; 2015,Apr,3

**84138** **Pregnanetriol**   ♀
0.00   0.00   **FUD** XXX   [Q]
**AMA:** 2015,Jun,10; 2015,Apr,3

● New Code   ▲ Revised Code   ○ Reinstated   ● New Web Release   ▲ Revised Web Release   Unlisted   Not Covered   # Resequenced
⊘ AMA Mod 51 Exempt   ⑨ Optum Mod 51 Exempt   ⊚ Mod 63 Exempt   ✗ Non-FDA Drug   ★ Telemedicine   Ⓜ Maternity   Ⓐ Age Edit   + Add-on   **AMA:** CPT Asst
© 2017 Optum360, LLC   CPT © 2017 American Medical Association. All Rights Reserved.   391

84140 **Pregnenolone**
🖰 0.00   ⚖ 0.00   **FUD** XXX   回
**AMA:** 2017,Jan,8; 2016,Jan,13; 2015,Jun,10; 2015,Apr,3; 2015,Jan,16; 2014,Jan,11

84143 **17-hydroxypregnenolone**
🖰 0.00   ⚖ 0.00   **FUD** XXX   回
**AMA:** 2017,Jan,8; 2016,Jan,13; 2015,Jun,10; 2015,Apr,3; 2015,Jan,16; 2014,Jan,11

84144 **Progesterone**
EXCLUDES   *Progesterone receptor assay (84234)*
🖰 0.00   ⚖ 0.00   **FUD** XXX   回
**AMA:** 2015,Jun,10; 2015,Apr,3

84145 **Procalcitonin (PCT)**
🖰 0.00   ⚖ 0.00   **FUD** XXX   回 ▣
**AMA:** 2015,Jun,10; 2015,Apr,3

84146 **Prolactin**
🖰 0.00   ⚖ 0.00   **FUD** XXX   回 ▣
**AMA:** 2015,Jun,10; 2015,Apr,3

84150 **Prostaglandin, each**
🖰 0.00   ⚖ 0.00   **FUD** XXX   回
**AMA:** 2015,Jun,10; 2015,Apr,3

## 84152-84154 Chemistry: Prostate Specific Antigen

**CMS:** 100-03,190.31 Prostate Specific Antigen (PSA); 100-03,210.1 Prostate Cancer Screening Tests

INCLUDES   Clinical information not requested by the ordering physician
Mathematically calculated results
Quantitative analysis unless otherwise specified

EXCLUDES   *Analytes from nonrequested laboratory analysis*
*Calculated results that represent a score or probability that was derived by algorithm*

84152 **Prostate specific antigen (PSA); complexed (direct measurement)**   ♂
🖰 0.00   ⚖ 0.00   **FUD** XXX   回
**AMA:** 2015,Jun,10; 2015,Apr,3

84153 **total**   ♂
🖰 0.00   ⚖ 0.00   **FUD** XXX   回
**AMA:** 2017,Jan,8; 2016,Jan,13; 2015,Jun,10; 2015,Apr,3; 2015,Jan,16; 2014,Jan,11; 2012,Jan,15-42

84154 **free**   ♂
🖰 0.00   ⚖ 0.00   **FUD** XXX   回
**AMA:** 2017,Jan,8; 2016,Jan,13; 2015,Jun,10; 2015,Apr,3; 2015,Jan,16; 2014,Jan,11; 2012,Jan,15-42

## 84155-84157 Chemistry: Protein, Total (Not by Refractometry)

INCLUDES   Clinical information not requested by the ordering physician
Mathematically calculated results

EXCLUDES   *Analytes from nonrequested laboratory analysis*
*Calculated results that represent a score or probability that was derived by algorithm*
*Organ or disease panels (80048-80076 [80081])*

84155 **Protein, total, except by refractometry; serum, plasma or whole blood**
🖰 0.00   ⚖ 0.00   **FUD** XXX   ✖ 回 ▣
**AMA:** 2017,Jan,8; 2016,Jan,13; 2015,Jun,10; 2015,Apr,3; 2015,Jan,16; 2014,Jan,11

84156 **urine**
🖰 0.00   ⚖ 0.00   **FUD** XXX   回
**AMA:** 2015,Jun,10; 2015,Apr,3

84157 **other source (eg, synovial fluid, cerebrospinal fluid)**
🖰 0.00   ⚖ 0.00   **FUD** XXX   回
**AMA:** 2015,Jun,10; 2015,Apr,3

## 84160-84432 Chemistry: Protein, Total (Refractometry)—Thyroglobulin

INCLUDES   Clinical information not requested by the ordering physician
Mathematically calculated results
Quantitative analysis unless otherwise specified
Specimens from any source unless otherwise specified

EXCLUDES   *Analytes from nonrequested laboratory analysis*
*Calculated results that represent a score or probability that was derived by algorithm*
*Drug testing ([80305, 80306, 80307], [80324, 80325, 80326, 80327, 80328, 80329, 80330, 80331, 80332, 80333, 80334, 80335, 80336, 80337, 80338, 80339, 80340, 80341, 80342, 80343, 80344, 80345, 80346, 80347, 80348, 80349, 80350, 80351, 80352, 80353, 80354, 80355, 80356, 80357, 80358, 80359, 80360, 80361, 80362, 80363, 80364, 80365, 80366, 80367, 80368, 80369, 80370, 80371, 80372, 80373, 80374, 80375, 80376, 80377, 83992])*
*Organ or disease panels (80048-80076 [80081])*
*Therapeutic drug assays (80150-80299 [80164, 80165, 80171])*

84160 **Protein, total, by refractometry, any source**
EXCLUDES   *Dipstick urine protein (81000-81003)*
🖰 0.00   ⚖ 0.00   **FUD** XXX   回 ▣
**AMA:** 2015,Jun,10; 2015,Apr,3

84163 **Pregnancy-associated plasma protein-A (PAPP-A)**   ♀
🖰 0.00   ⚖ 0.00   **FUD** XXX   回
**AMA:** 2015,Jun,10; 2015,Apr,3

84165 **Protein; electrophoretic fractionation and quantitation, serum**
🖰 0.00   ⚖ 0.00   **FUD** XXX   回 ▣
**AMA:** 2015,Jun,10; 2015,Apr,3

84166 **electrophoretic fractionation and quantitation, other fluids with concentration (eg, urine, CSF)**
🖰 0.00   ⚖ 0.00   **FUD** XXX   回 ▣
**AMA:** 2015,Jun,10; 2015,Apr,3

84181 **Western Blot, with interpretation and report, blood or other body fluid**
🖰 0.00   ⚖ 0.00   **FUD** XXX   回 ▣
**AMA:** 2015,Jun,10; 2015,Apr,3

84182 **Western Blot, with interpretation and report, blood or other body fluid, immunological probe for band identification, each**
EXCLUDES   *Western Blot tissue testing (88371)*
🖰 0.00   ⚖ 0.00   **FUD** XXX   回 ▣
**AMA:** 2015,Jun,10; 2015,Apr,3

84202 **Protoporphyrin, RBC; quantitative**
🖰 0.00   ⚖ 0.00   **FUD** XXX   回
**AMA:** 2015,Jun,10; 2015,Apr,3

84203 **screen**
🖰 0.00   ⚖ 0.00   **FUD** XXX   回
**AMA:** 2015,Jun,10; 2015,Apr,3

84206 **Proinsulin**
🖰 0.00   ⚖ 0.00   **FUD** XXX   回
**AMA:** 2015,Jun,10; 2015,Apr,3

84207 **Pyridoxal phosphate (Vitamin B-6)**
🖰 0.00   ⚖ 0.00   **FUD** XXX   回 ▣
**AMA:** 2015,Jun,10; 2015,Apr,3

84210 **Pyruvate**
🖰 0.00   ⚖ 0.00   **FUD** XXX   回
**AMA:** 2015,Jun,10; 2015,Apr,3

84220 **Pyruvate kinase**
🖰 0.00   ⚖ 0.00   **FUD** XXX   回
**AMA:** 2015,Jun,10; 2015,Apr,3

84228 **Quinine**
🖰 0.00   ⚖ 0.00   **FUD** XXX   回
**AMA:** 2017,Jan,8; 2016,Jan,13; 2015,Jun,10; 2015,Apr,3

84233 **Receptor assay; estrogen**
🖰 0.00   ⚖ 0.00   **FUD** XXX   回 ▣
**AMA:** 2015,Jun,10; 2015,Apr,3

| 26/TC PC/TC Only | A2-Z3 ASC Payment | 50 Bilateral | ♂ Male Only | ♀ Female Only | 🖰 Facility RVU | ⚖ Non-Facility RVU | ▣ CCI |
| FUD Follow-up Days | CMS: IOM (Pub 100) | A-Y OPPSI | 80/80 Surg Assist Allowed / w/Doc | | 🖰 Lab Crosswalk | Radiology Crosswalk | ✖ CLIA |

392

CPT © 2017 American Medical Association. All Rights Reserved.

© 2017 Optum360, LLC

| 84234 | **progesterone** |
|---|---|
| | ⚕ 0.00 ☷ 0.00 **FUD** XXX ▣▢ |
| | **AMA:** 2015,Jun,10; 2015,Apr,3 |

| 84235 | **endocrine, other than estrogen or progesterone (specify hormone)** |
|---|---|
| | ⚕ 0.00 ☷ 0.00 **FUD** XXX ▣▢ |
| | **AMA:** 2015,Jun,10; 2015,Apr,3 |

| 84238 | **non-endocrine (specify receptor)** |
|---|---|
| | ⚕ 0.00 ☷ 0.00 **FUD** XXX ▣▢ |
| | **AMA:** 2017,Jan,8; 2016,Jan,13; 2015,Jun,10; 2015,Apr,3; 2015,Jan,16; 2014,Jan,11; 2012,Jan,15-42 |

| 84244 | **Renin** |
|---|---|
| | ⚕ 0.00 ☷ 0.00 **FUD** XXX ▣▢ |
| | **AMA:** 2015,Jun,10; 2015,Apr,3 |

| 84252 | **Riboflavin (Vitamin B-2)** |
|---|---|
| | ⚕ 0.00 ☷ 0.00 **FUD** XXX ▣▢ |
| | **AMA:** 2015,Jun,10; 2015,Apr,3 |

| 84255 | **Selenium** |
|---|---|
| | ⚕ 0.00 ☷ 0.00 **FUD** XXX ▣ |
| | **AMA:** 2015,Jun,10; 2015,Apr,3 |

| 84260 | **Serotonin** |
|---|---|
| | EXCLUDES *Urine metabolites (HIAA) (83497)* |
| | ⚕ 0.00 ☷ 0.00 **FUD** XXX ▣ |
| | **AMA:** 2015,Jun,10; 2015,Apr,3 |

| 84270 | **Sex hormone binding globulin (SHBG)** |
|---|---|
| | ⚕ 0.00 ☷ 0.00 **FUD** XXX ▣ |
| | **AMA:** 2017,Jan,8; 2016,Jan,13; 2015,Jun,10; 2015,Apr,3; 2015,Jan,16; 2014,Jan,11 |

| 84275 | **Sialic acid** |
|---|---|
| | ⚕ 0.00 ☷ 0.00 **FUD** XXX ▣ |
| | **AMA:** 2015,Jun,10; 2015,Apr,3 |

| 84285 | **Silica** |
|---|---|
| | ⚕ 0.00 ☷ 0.00 **FUD** XXX ▣ |
| | **AMA:** 2015,Jun,10; 2015,Apr,3 |

| 84295 | **Sodium; serum, plasma or whole blood** |
|---|---|
| | ⚕ 0.00 ☷ 0.00 **FUD** XXX ✗▣ |
| | **AMA:** 2017,Jan,8; 2016,Jan,13; 2015,Jun,10; 2015,Apr,3; 2015,Jan,16; 2014,Jan,11; 2013,Apr,10-11 |

| 84300 | **urine** |
|---|---|
| | ⚕ 0.00 ☷ 0.00 **FUD** XXX ▣ |
| | **AMA:** 2015,Jun,10; 2015,Apr,3 |

| 84302 | **other source** |
|---|---|
| | ⚕ 0.00 ☷ 0.00 **FUD** XXX ▣ |
| | **AMA:** 2017,Jan,8; 2016,Jan,13; 2015,Jun,10; 2015,Apr,3; 2015,Jan,16; 2014,Jan,11 |

| 84305 | **Somatomedin** |
|---|---|
| | ⚕ 0.00 ☷ 0.00 **FUD** XXX ▣ |
| | **AMA:** 2017,Jan,8; 2016,Jan,13; 2015,Jun,10; 2015,Apr,3; 2015,Jan,16; 2014,Jan,11 |

| 84307 | **Somatostatin** |
|---|---|
| | ⚕ 0.00 ☷ 0.00 **FUD** XXX ▣ |
| | **AMA:** 2017,Jan,8; 2016,Jan,13; 2015,Jun,10; 2015,Apr,3; 2015,Jan,16; 2014,Jan,11 |

| 84311 | **Spectrophotometry, analyte not elsewhere specified** |
|---|---|
| | ⚕ 0.00 ☷ 0.00 **FUD** XXX ▣ |
| | **AMA:** 2015,Jun,10; 2015,Apr,3 |

| 84315 | **Specific gravity (except urine)** |
|---|---|
| | EXCLUDES *Urine specific gravity (81000-81003)* |
| | ⚕ 0.00 ☷ 0.00 **FUD** XXX ▣ |
| | **AMA:** 2015,Jun,10; 2015,Apr,3 |

| 84375 | **Sugars, chromatographic, TLC or paper chromatography** |
|---|---|
| | ⚕ 0.00 ☷ 0.00 **FUD** XXX ▣ |
| | **AMA:** 2015,Jun,10; 2015,Apr,3 |

| 84376 | **Sugars (mono-, di-, and oligosaccharides); single qualitative, each specimen** |
|---|---|
| | ⚕ 0.00 ☷ 0.00 **FUD** XXX ▣ |
| | **AMA:** 2017,Jan,8; 2016,Jan,13; 2015,Jun,10; 2015,Apr,3; 2015,Jan,16; 2014,Jan,11 |

| 84377 | **multiple qualitative, each specimen** |
|---|---|
| | ⚕ 0.00 ☷ 0.00 **FUD** XXX ▣▢ |
| | **AMA:** 2017,Jan,8; 2016,Jan,13; 2015,Jun,10; 2015,Apr,3; 2015,Jan,16; 2014,Jan,11 |

| 84378 | **single quantitative, each specimen** |
|---|---|
| | ⚕ 0.00 ☷ 0.00 **FUD** XXX ▣▢ |
| | **AMA:** 2015,Jun,10; 2015,Apr,3 |

| 84379 | **multiple quantitative, each specimen** |
|---|---|
| | ⚕ 0.00 ☷ 0.00 **FUD** XXX ▣▢ |
| | **AMA:** 2017,Jan,8; 2016,Jan,13; 2015,Jun,10; 2015,Apr,3; 2015,Jan,16; 2014,Jan,11 |

| 84392 | **Sulfate, urine** |
|---|---|
| | ⚕ 0.00 ☷ 0.00 **FUD** XXX ▣ |
| | **AMA:** 2015,Jun,10; 2015,Apr,3 |

| 84402 | **Testosterone; free** |
|---|---|
| | EXCLUDES *Anabolic steroids ([80327, 80328])* |
| | ⚕ 0.00 ☷ 0.00 **FUD** XXX ▣ |
| | **AMA:** 2015,Jun,10; 2015,Apr,3 |

| 84403 | **total** |
|---|---|
| | EXCLUDES *Anabolic steroids ([80327, 80328])* |
| | ⚕ 0.00 ☷ 0.00 **FUD** XXX ▣▢ |
| | **AMA:** 2015,Jun,10; 2015,Apr,3 |

| 84410 | **bioavailable, direct measurement (eg, differential precipitation)** |
|---|---|
| | ⚕ 0.00 ☷ 0.00 **FUD** XXX ▣▢ |

| 84425 | **Thiamine (Vitamin B-1)** |
|---|---|
| | ⚕ 0.00 ☷ 0.00 **FUD** XXX ▣▢ |
| | **AMA:** 2015,Jun,10; 2015,Apr,3 |

| 84430 | **Thiocyanate** |
|---|---|
| | ⚕ 0.00 ☷ 0.00 **FUD** XXX ▣ |
| | **AMA:** 2015,Jun,10; 2015,Apr,3 |

| 84431 | **Thromboxane metabolite(s), including thromboxane if performed, urine** |
|---|---|
| | Code also for determination of concurrent urine creatinine (82570) |
| | ⚕ 0.00 ☷ 0.00 **FUD** XXX ▣ |
| | **AMA:** 2015,Jun,10; 2015,Apr,3 |

| 84432 | **Thyroglobulin** |
|---|---|
| | EXCLUDES *Thyroglobulin antibody (86800)* |
| | ⚕ 0.00 ☷ 0.00 **FUD** XXX ▣ |
| | **AMA:** 2017,Jan,8; 2016,Jan,13; 2015,Jun,10; 2015,Apr,3; 2015,Jan,16; 2014,Jan,11 |

## 84436-84445 Chemistry: Thyroid Tests

**CMS:** 100-03,190.22 Thyroid Testing

INCLUDES Clinical information not requested by the ordering physician
Mathematically calculated results
Quantitative analysis unless otherwise specified
Specimens from any source unless otherwise specified

EXCLUDES *Analytes from nonrequested laboratory analysis*
*Calculated results that represent a score or probability that was derived by algorithm*
*Organ or disease panels (80048-80076 [80081])*
*Therapeutic drug assays (80150-80299 [80164, 80165, 80171])*

| 84436 | **Thyroxine; total** |
|---|---|
| | ⚕ 0.00 ☷ 0.00 **FUD** XXX ▣▢ |
| | **AMA:** 2017,Jan,8; 2016,Jan,13; 2015,Jun,10; 2015,Apr,3; 2015,Jan,16; 2014,Jan,11 |

| 84437 | **requiring elution (eg, neonatal)** |
|---|---|
| | ⚕ 0.00 ☷ 0.00 **FUD** XXX ▣ |
| | **AMA:** 2015,Jun,10; 2015,Apr,3 |

| 84439 | **free** |
|---|---|
| | ⚕ 0.00 ☷ 0.00 **FUD** XXX ▣▢ |
| | **AMA:** 2015,Jun,10; 2015,Apr,3 |

84442 **Thyroxine binding globulin (TBG)**
⏣ 0.00   ⚕ 0.00   **FUD** XXX   Ⓠ
**AMA:** 2015,Jun,10; 2015,Apr,3

84443 **Thyroid stimulating hormone (TSH)**
⏣ 0.00   ⚕ 0.00   **FUD** XXX   ☒ Ⓠ ▢
**AMA:** 2015,Jun,10; 2015,Apr,3

84445 **Thyroid stimulating immune globulins (TSI)**
⏣ 0.00   ⚕ 0.00   **FUD** XXX   Ⓠ ▢
**AMA:** 2017,Jan,8; 2016,Jan,13; 2015,Jun,10; 2015,Apr,3;
2015,Jan,16; 2014,Jan,11

## 84446-84449 Chemistry: Tocopherol Alpha—Transcortin

INCLUDES   Clinical information not requested by the ordering physician
Mathematically calculated results
Quantitative analysis unless otherwise specified
Specimens from any source unless otherwise specified
EXCLUDES   *Analytes from nonrequested laboratory analysis*
*Calculated results that represent a score or probability that was derived by algorithm*
*Organ or disease panels (80048-80076 [80081])*
*Therapeutic drug assays (80150-80299 [80164, 80165, 80171])*

84446 **Tocopherol alpha (Vitamin E)**
⏣ 0.00   ⚕ 0.00   **FUD** XXX   Ⓠ ▢
**AMA:** 2015,Jun,10; 2015,Apr,3

84449 **Transcortin (cortisol binding globulin)**
⏣ 0.00   ⚕ 0.00   **FUD** XXX   Ⓠ
**AMA:** 2017,Jan,8; 2016,Jan,13; 2015,Jun,10; 2015,Apr,3;
2015,Jan,16; 2014,Jan,11

## 84450-84460 Chemistry: Transferase

**CMS:** 100-02,11,30.2.2 Automated Multi-Channel Chemistry (AMCC) Tests; 100-03,160.17 Payment for L-Dopa /Associated Inpatient Hospital Services; 100-04,16,40.6.1 Automated Multi-Channel Chemistry (AMCC) Tests for ESRD Beneficiaries; 100-04,16,70.8 CLIA Waived Tests

INCLUDES   Clinical information not requested by the ordering physician
Mathematically calculated results
Quantitative analysis unless otherwise specified
EXCLUDES   *Analytes from nonrequested laboratory analysis*
*Calculated results that represent a score or probability that was derived by algorithm*

84450 **Transferase; aspartate amino (AST) (SGOT)**
⏣ 0.00   ⚕ 0.00   **FUD** XXX   ☒ Ⓠ
**AMA:** 2017,Jan,8; 2016,Jan,13; 2015,Jun,10; 2015,Apr,3;
2015,Jan,16; 2014,Jan,11

84460 **alanine amino (ALT) (SGPT)**
⏣ 0.00   ⚕ 0.00   **FUD** XXX   ☒ Ⓠ
**AMA:** 2017,Jan,8; 2016,Jan,13; 2015,Jun,10; 2015,Apr,3;
2015,Jan,16; 2014,Jan,11

## 84466 Chemistry: Transferrin

**CMS:** 100-02,11,20.2 ESRD Laboratory Services; 100-03,190.18 Serum Iron Studies

INCLUDES   Clinical information not requested by the ordering physician
Mathematically calculated results
Quantitative analysis unless otherwise specified
EXCLUDES   *Analytes from nonrequested laboratory analysis*
*Calculated results that represent a score or probability that was derived by algorithm*

84466 **Transferrin**
EXCLUDES   *Iron binding capacity (83550)*
⏣ 0.00   ⚕ 0.00   **FUD** XXX   Ⓠ ▢
**AMA:** 2017,Jan,8; 2016,Jan,13; 2015,Jun,10; 2015,Apr,3;
2015,Jan,16; 2014,Jan,11

## 84478 Chemistry: Triglycerides

**CMS:** 100-02,11,30.2.2 Automated Multi-Channel Chemistry (AMCC) Tests; 100-03,190.23 Lipid Testing; 100-04,16,70.8 CLIA Waived Tests; 100-04,16,90.2 Organ or Disease Oriented Panels

INCLUDES   Clinical information not requested by the ordering physician
Mathematically calculated results
EXCLUDES   *Analytes from nonrequested laboratory analysis*
*Calculated results that represent a score or probability that was derived by algorithm*
*Organ or disease panels (80048-80076 [80081])*

84478 **Triglycerides**
⏣ 0.00   ⚕ 0.00   **FUD** XXX   ☒ Ⓐ ▢
**AMA:** 2017,Jan,8; 2016,Jan,13; 2015,Jun,10; 2015,Apr,3;
2015,Jan,16; 2014,Jan,11; 2012,Jan,15-42

## 84479-84482 Chemistry: Thyroid Hormone—Triiodothyronine

**CMS:** 100-03,190.22 Thyroid Testing

INCLUDES   Clinical information not requested by the ordering physician
Mathematically calculated results
Quantitative analysis unless otherwise specified
Specimens from any source unless otherwise specified
EXCLUDES   *Analytes from nonrequested laboratory analysis*
*Calculated results that represent a score or probability that was derived by algorithm*
*Organ or disease panels (80048-80076 [80081])*

84479 **Thyroid hormone (T3 or T4) uptake or thyroid hormone binding ratio (THBR)**
⏣ 0.00   ⚕ 0.00   **FUD** XXX   Ⓠ ▢
**AMA:** 2017,Jan,8; 2016,Jan,13; 2015,Jun,10; 2015,Apr,3;
2015,Jan,16; 2014,Jan,11

84480 **Triiodothyronine T3; total (TT-3)**
⏣ 0.00   ⚕ 0.00   **FUD** XXX   Ⓠ ▢
**AMA:** 2015,Jun,10; 2015,Apr,3

84481 **free**
⏣ 0.00   ⚕ 0.00   **FUD** XXX   Ⓠ ▢
**AMA:** 2015,Jun,10; 2015,Apr,3

84482 **reverse**
⏣ 0.00   ⚕ 0.00   **FUD** XXX   Ⓠ ▢
**AMA:** 2017,Jan,8; 2016,Jan,13; 2015,Jun,10; 2015,Apr,3;
2015,Jan,16; 2014,Jan,11

## 84484-84512 Chemistry: Troponin (Quantitative)—Troponin (Qualitative)

INCLUDES   Clinical information not requested by the ordering physician
Mathematically calculated results
Specimens from any source unless otherwise specified
EXCLUDES   *Analytes from nonrequested laboratory analysis*
*Calculated results that represent a score or probability that was derived by algorithm*
*Organ or disease panels*

84484 **Troponin, quantitative**
EXCLUDES   *Qualitative troponin assay (84512)*
⏣ 0.00   ⚕ 0.00   **FUD** XXX   Ⓠ
**AMA:** 2017,Jan,8; 2016,Jan,13; 2015,Jun,10; 2015,Apr,3;
2015,Jan,16; 2014,Jan,11

84485 **Trypsin; duodenal fluid**
⏣ 0.00   ⚕ 0.00   **FUD** XXX   Ⓠ
**AMA:** 2015,Jun,10; 2015,Apr,3

84488 **feces, qualitative**
⏣ 0.00   ⚕ 0.00   **FUD** XXX   Ⓠ
**AMA:** 2015,Jun,10; 2015,Apr,3

84490 **feces, quantitative, 24-hour collection**
⏣ 0.00   ⚕ 0.00   **FUD** XXX   Ⓠ
**AMA:** 2015,Jun,10; 2015,Apr,3

84510 **Tyrosine**
EXCLUDES   *Urate crystal identification (89060)*
⏣ 0.00   ⚕ 0.00   **FUD** XXX   Ⓠ
**AMA:** 2015,Jun,10; 2015,Apr,3

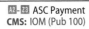 PC/TC Only
**FUD** Follow-up Days
**CMS:** IOM (Pub 100)
 ASC Payment
Ⓐ-Ⓨ OPPSI
 Bilateral
 Surg Assist Allowed / w/Doc
♂ Male Only
♀ Female Only
 Facility RVU
Lab Crosswalk
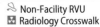 Non-Facility RVU
Radiology Crosswalk
▢ CCI
☒ CLIA

394

CPT © 2017 American Medical Association. All Rights Reserved.
© 2017 Optum360, LLC

Pathology and Laboratory

| 84512 | Troponin, qualitative |
|---|---|

EXCLUDES    *Quantitative troponin assay (84484)*
🔲 0.00   ⚬ 0.00   **FUD** XXX                              ☒ Ⓠ

**AMA:** 2017,Jan,8; 2016,Jan,13; 2015,Jun,10; 2015,Apr,3;
2015,Jan,16; 2014,Jan,11

## 84520-84525 Chemistry: Urea Nitrogen (Blood)

**CMS:** 100-03,160.17 Payment for L-Dopa /Associated Inpatient Hospital Services

INCLUDES    Clinical information not requested by the ordering physician
Mathematically calculated results
EXCLUDES    *Analytes from nonrequested laboratory analysis*
*Calculated results that represent a score or probability that was derived by*
*algorithm*
*Organ or disease panels (80048-80076 [80081])*

| 84520 | Urea nitrogen; quantitative |
|---|---|

🔲 0.00   ⚬ 0.00   **FUD** XXX                              ☒ Ⓠ

**AMA:** 2017,Jan,8; 2016,Jan,13; 2015,Jun,10; 2015,Apr,3;
2015,Jan,16; 2014,Jan,11; 2013,Apr,10-11

| 84525 | semiquantitative (eg, reagent strip test) |
|---|---|

INCLUDES    Patterson's test
🔲 0.00   ⚬ 0.00   **FUD** XXX                              Ⓠ

**AMA:** 2017,Jan,8; 2016,Jan,13; 2015,Jun,10; 2015,Apr,3;
2015,Jan,16; 2014,Jan,11

## 84540-84630 Chemistry: Urea Nitrogen (Urine)—Zinc

INCLUDES    Clinical information not requested by the ordering physician
Mathematically calculated results
Quantitative analysis unless otherwise specified
Specimens from any source unless otherwise specified
EXCLUDES    *Analytes from nonrequested laboratory analysis*
*Calculated results that represent a score or probability that was derived by*
*algorithm*
*Organ or disease panels (80048-80076 [80081])*
*Therapeutic drug assays (80150-80299 [80164, 80165, 80171])*

| 84540 | Urea nitrogen, urine |
|---|---|

🔲 0.00   ⚬ 0.00   **FUD** XXX                              Ⓠ

**AMA:** 2015,Jun,10; 2015,Apr,3

| 84545 | Urea nitrogen, clearance |
|---|---|

🔲 0.00   ⚬ 0.00   **FUD** XXX                              Ⓠ

**AMA:** 2015,Jun,10; 2015,Apr,3

| 84550 | Uric acid; blood |
|---|---|

🔲 0.00   ⚬ 0.00   **FUD** XXX                              ☒ Ⓠ

**AMA:** 2017,Jan,8; 2016,Jan,13; 2015,Jun,10; 2015,Apr,3;
2015,Jan,16; 2014,Jan,11

| 84560 | other source |
|---|---|

🔲 0.00   ⚬ 0.00   **FUD** XXX                              Ⓠ

**AMA:** 2015,Jun,10; 2015,Apr,3

| 84577 | Urobilinogen, feces, quantitative |
|---|---|

🔲 0.00   ⚬ 0.00   **FUD** XXX                              Ⓠ

**AMA:** 2015,Jun,10; 2015,Apr,3

| 84578 | Urobilinogen, urine; qualitative |
|---|---|

🔲 0.00   ⚬ 0.00   **FUD** XXX                              Ⓠ

**AMA:** 2015,Jun,10; 2015,Apr,3

| 84580 | quantitative, timed specimen |
|---|---|

🔲 0.00   ⚬ 0.00   **FUD** XXX                              Ⓠ 🖭

**AMA:** 2015,Jun,10; 2015,Apr,3

| 84583 | semiquantitative |
|---|---|

🔲 0.00   ⚬ 0.00   **FUD** XXX                              Ⓠ

**AMA:** 2015,Jun,10; 2015,Apr,3

| 84585 | Vanillylmandelic acid (VMA), urine |
|---|---|

🔲 0.00   ⚬ 0.00   **FUD** XXX                              Ⓠ

**AMA:** 2015,Jun,10; 2015,Apr,3

| 84586 | Vasoactive intestinal peptide (VIP) |
|---|---|

🔲 0.00   ⚬ 0.00   **FUD** XXX                              Ⓠ

**AMA:** 2017,Jan,8; 2016,Jan,13; 2015,Jun,10; 2015,Apr,3;
2015,Jan,16; 2014,Jan,11

| 84588 | Vasopressin (antidiuretic hormone, ADH) |
|---|---|

🔲 0.00   ⚬ 0.00   **FUD** XXX                              Ⓠ

**AMA:** 2015,Jun,10; 2015,Apr,3

| 84590 | Vitamin A |
|---|---|

🔲 0.00   ⚬ 0.00   **FUD** XXX                              Ⓠ 🖭

**AMA:** 2015,Jun,10; 2015,Apr,3

| 84591 | Vitamin, not otherwise specified |
|---|---|

🔲 0.00   ⚬ 0.00   **FUD** XXX                              Ⓠ

**AMA:** 2015,Jun,10; 2015,Apr,3

| 84597 | Vitamin K |
|---|---|

🔲 0.00   ⚬ 0.00   **FUD** XXX                              Ⓠ 🖭

**AMA:** 2015,Jun,10; 2015,Apr,3

| 84600 | Volatiles (eg, acetic anhydride, diethylether) |
|---|---|

EXCLUDES    *Carbon tetrachloride, dichloroethane, dichloromethane*
*(82441)*
*Isopropyl alcohol and methanol ([80320])*
🔲 0.00   ⚬ 0.00   **FUD** XXX                              Ⓠ

**AMA:** 2015,Jun,10; 2015,Apr,3

| 84620 | Xylose absorption test, blood and/or urine |
|---|---|

EXCLUDES    *Administration (99070)*
🔲 0.00   ⚬ 0.00   **FUD** XXX                              Ⓠ 🖭

**AMA:** 2015,Jun,10; 2015,Apr,3

| 84630 | Zinc |
|---|---|

🔲 0.00   ⚬ 0.00   **FUD** XXX                              Ⓠ

**AMA:** 2015,Jun,10; 2015,Apr,3

## 84681-84999 Other and Unlisted Chemistry Tests

INCLUDES    Clinical information not requested by the ordering physician
Mathematically calculated results
Quantitative analysis unless otherwise specified
Specimens from any source unless otherwise specified
EXCLUDES    *Analytes from nonrequested laboratory analysis*
*Calculated results that represent a score or probability that was derived by*
*algorithm*
*Confirmational testing of a not otherwise specified drug ([80375, 80376,*
*80377], 80299)*
*Organ or disease panels (80048-80076 [80081])*

| 84681 | C-peptide |
|---|---|

🔲 0.00   ⚬ 0.00   **FUD** XXX                              Ⓠ 🖭

**AMA:** 2015,Jun,10; 2015,Apr,3

| 84702 | Gonadotropin, chorionic (hCG); quantitative |
|---|---|

🔲 0.00   ⚬ 0.00   **FUD** XXX                              Ⓠ 🖭

**AMA:** 2015,Jun,10; 2015,Apr,3

| 84703 | qualitative |
|---|---|

EXCLUDES    *Urine pregnancy test by visual color comparison (81025)*
🔲 0.00   ⚬ 0.00   **FUD** XXX                              ☒ Ⓠ

**AMA:** 2015,Jun,10; 2015,Apr,3

| 84704 | free beta chain |
|---|---|

🔲 0.00   ⚬ 0.00   **FUD** XXX                              Ⓠ

**AMA:** 2017,Jan,8; 2016,Jan,13; 2015,Jun,10; 2015,Apr,3;
2015,Jan,16; 2014,Jan,11; 2012,Jan,15-42

| 84830 | Ovulation tests, by visual color comparison methods for human luteinizing hormone |
|---|---|

♀
🔲 0.00   ⚬ 0.00   **FUD** XXX                              ☒ Ⓠ

**AMA:** 2017,Jan,8; 2016,Jan,13; 2015,Jun,10; 2015,Apr,3

| 84999 | Unlisted chemistry procedure |
|---|---|

🔲 0.00   ⚬ 0.00   **FUD** XXX                              Ⓠ

**AMA:** 2017,Jan,8; 2016,Jan,13; 2015,Apr,3; 2015,Jan,16;
2014,Jan,11; 2012,Jan,15-42

## 85002 Bleeding Time Test

EXCLUDES    *Agglutinins (86000, 86156-86157)*
*Antiplasmin (85410)*
*Antithrombin III (85300-85301)*
*Blood banking procedures (86850-86999)*

| 85002 | Bleeding time |
|---|---|

🔲 0.00   ⚬ 0.00   **FUD** XXX                              Ⓠ

**AMA:** 2017,Jan,8; 2016,Jan,13; 2015,Jan,16; 2014,Jan,11

● New Code   ▲ Revised Code   ○ Reinstated   ● New Web Release   ▲ Revised Web Release   Unlisted   Not Covered   # Resequenced
⊘ AMA Mod 51 Exempt   ⑧ Optum Mod 51 Exempt   ⑥ Mod 63 Exempt   ✗ Non-FDA Drug   ★ Telemedicine   Ⓜ Maternity   Ⓐ Age Edit   ✚ Add-on   **AMA:** CPT Asst
© 2017 Optum360, LLC               CPT © 2017 American Medical Association. All Rights Reserved.

## 85004-85049 Blood Counts

**CMS:** 100-03,190.15 Blood Counts

*EXCLUDES*  Agglutinins (86000, 86156-86157)
Antiplasmin (85410)
Antithrombin III (85300-85301)
Blood banking procedures (86850-86999)

**85004**  **Blood count; automated differential WBC count**
🚑 0.00  🔬 0.00  **FUD** XXX  Ⓠ ▣

**AMA:** 2017,Jan,8; 2016,Jan,13; 2015,Jan,16; 2014,Jan,11; 2012,Jan,15-42

**85007**  **blood smear, microscopic examination with manual differential WBC count**
🚑 0.00  🔬 0.00  **FUD** XXX  Ⓠ ▣

**AMA:** 2017,Jan,8; 2016,Jan,13; 2015,Jan,16; 2014,Jan,11; 2012,Jan,15-42

**85008**  **blood smear, microscopic examination without manual differential WBC count**
*EXCLUDES*  Cell count other fluids (eg, CSF) (89050-89051)
🚑 0.00  🔬 0.00  **FUD** XXX  Ⓠ ▣

**AMA:** 2017,Jan,8; 2016,Jan,13; 2015,Jan,16; 2014,Jan,11; 2012,Jan,15-42

**85009**  **manual differential WBC count, buffy coat**
*EXCLUDES*  Eosinophils, nasal smear (89190)
🚑 0.00  🔬 0.00  **FUD** XXX  Ⓠ ▣

**AMA:** 2017,Jan,8; 2016,Jan,13; 2015,Jan,16; 2014,Jan,11; 2012,Jan,15-42

**85013**  **spun microhematocrit**
🚑 0.00  🔬 0.00  **FUD** XXX  ☒ Ⓠ ▣

**AMA:** 2005,Aug,7-8; 2005,Jul,11-12

**85014**  **hematocrit (Hct)**
🚑 0.00  🔬 0.00  **FUD** XXX  ☒ Ⓠ ▣

**AMA:** 2017,Jan,8; 2016,Jan,13; 2015,Jan,16; 2014,Jan,11

**85018**  **hemoglobin (Hgb)**
*EXCLUDES*  Immunoassay, hemoglobin, fecal (82274)
Other hemoglobin determination (83020-83069)
Transcutaneous hemoglobin measurement (88738)
🚑 0.00  🔬 0.00  **FUD** XXX  ☒ Ⓠ ▣

**AMA:** 2017,Jan,8; 2016,Jan,13; 2015,Jan,16; 2014,Jan,11

**85025**  **complete (CBC), automated (Hgb, Hct, RBC, WBC and platelet count) and automated differential WBC count**
🚑 0.00  🔬 0.00  **FUD** XXX  Ⓠ ▣

**AMA:** 2017,Jan,8; 2016,Jan,13; 2015,Jan,16; 2014,Jan,11; 2012,Jan,15-42

**85027**  **complete (CBC), automated (Hgb, Hct, RBC, WBC and platelet count)**
🚑 0.00  🔬 0.00  **FUD** XXX  Ⓠ ▣

**AMA:** 2017,Jan,8; 2016,Jan,13; 2015,Jan,16; 2014,Jan,11

**85032**  **manual cell count (erythrocyte, leukocyte, or platelet) each**
🚑 0.00  🔬 0.00  **FUD** XXX  Ⓠ ▣

**AMA:** 2017,Jan,8; 2016,Jan,13; 2015,Jan,16; 2014,Jan,11; 2012,Jan,15-42

**85041**  **red blood cell (RBC), automated**
*EXCLUDES*  Complete blood count (85025, 85027)
🚑 0.00  🔬 0.00  **FUD** XXX  Ⓠ ▣

**AMA:** 2017,Jan,8; 2016,Jan,13; 2015,Jan,16; 2014,Jan,11

**85044**  **reticulocyte, manual**
🚑 0.00  🔬 0.00  **FUD** XXX  Ⓠ

**AMA:** 2017,Jan,8; 2016,Jan,13; 2015,Jan,16; 2014,Jan,11

**85045**  **reticulocyte, automated**
🚑 0.00  🔬 0.00  **FUD** XXX  Ⓠ ▣

**AMA:** 2017,Jan,8; 2016,Jan,13; 2015,Jan,16; 2014,Jan,11

**85046**  **reticulocytes, automated, including 1 or more cellular parameters (eg, reticulocyte hemoglobin content [CHr], immature reticulocyte fraction [IRF], reticulocyte volume [MRV], RNA content), direct measurement**
🚑 0.00  🔬 0.00  **FUD** XXX  Ⓠ ▣

**AMA:** 2005,Aug,7-8; 2005,Jul,11-12

**85048**  **leukocyte (WBC), automated**
🚑 0.00  🔬 0.00  **FUD** XXX  Ⓠ ▣

**AMA:** 2017,Jan,8; 2016,Jan,13; 2015,Jan,16; 2014,Jan,11

**85049**  **platelet, automated**
🚑 0.00  🔬 0.00  **FUD** XXX  Ⓠ ▣

**AMA:** 2005,Aug,7-8; 2005,Jul,11-12

## 85055-85705 Coagulopathy Testing

*EXCLUDES*  Agglutinins (86000, 86156-86157)
Antiplasmin (85410)
Antithrombin III (85300-85301)
Blood banking procedures (86850-86999)

**85055**  **Reticulated platelet assay**
🚑 0.00  🔬 0.00  **FUD** XXX  Ⓠ

**AMA:** 2005,Aug,7-8; 2005,Jul,11-12

**85060**  **Blood smear, peripheral, interpretation by physician with written report**
🚑 0.71  🔬 0.71  **FUD** XXX  Ⓑ ⑧⓪

**AMA:** 2005,Aug,7-8; 2005,Jul,11-12

**85097**  **Bone marrow, smear interpretation**
*EXCLUDES*  Bone biopsy (20220, 20225, 20240, 20245, 20250-20251)
Special stains (88312-88313)
🚑 1.43  🔬 2.57  **FUD** XXX  ⓪② ⑧⓪

**AMA:** 2017,Jan,8; 2016,Jan,13; 2015,Jan,16; 2014,Jan,11; 2012,Jan,15-42

**85130**  **Chromogenic substrate assay**
🚑 0.00  🔬 0.00  **FUD** XXX  Ⓠ ▣

**AMA:** 2005,Aug,7-8; 2005,Jul,11-12

**85170**  **Clot retraction**
🚑 0.00  🔬 0.00  **FUD** XXX  Ⓠ ▣

**AMA:** 2005,Aug,7-8; 2005,Jul,11-12

**85175**  **Clot lysis time, whole blood dilution**
🚑 0.00  🔬 0.00  **FUD** XXX  Ⓠ ▣

**AMA:** 2005,Aug,7-8; 2005,Jul,11-12

**85210**  **Clotting; factor II, prothrombin, specific**
*EXCLUDES*  Prothrombin time (85610-85611)
Russell viper venom time (85612-85613)
🚑 0.00  🔬 0.00  **FUD** XXX  Ⓠ ▣

**AMA:** 2005,Aug,7-8; 2005,Jul,11-12

**85220**  **factor V (AcG or proaccelerin), labile factor**
🚑 0.00  🔬 0.00  **FUD** XXX  Ⓠ ▣

**AMA:** 2005,Aug,7-8; 2005,Jul,11-12

**85230**  **factor VII (proconvertin, stable factor)**
🚑 0.00  🔬 0.00  **FUD** XXX  Ⓠ ▣

**AMA:** 2005,Aug,7-8; 2005,Jul,11-12

**85240**  **factor VIII (AHG), 1-stage**
🚑 0.00  🔬 0.00  **FUD** XXX  Ⓠ ▣

**AMA:** 2005,Aug,7-8; 2005,Jul,11-12

**85244**  **factor VIII related antigen**
🚑 0.00  🔬 0.00  **FUD** XXX  Ⓠ ▣

**AMA:** 2005,Aug,7-8; 2005,Jul,11-12

**85245**  **factor VIII, VW factor, ristocetin cofactor**
🚑 0.00  🔬 0.00  **FUD** XXX  Ⓠ ▣

**AMA:** 2005,Aug,7-8; 2005,Jul,11-12

**85246**  **factor VIII, VW factor antigen**
🚑 0.00  🔬 0.00  **FUD** XXX  Ⓠ ▣

**AMA:** 2005,Aug,7-8; 2005,Jul,11-12

**85247**  **factor VIII, von Willebrand factor, multimetric analysis**
🚑 0.00  🔬 0.00  **FUD** XXX  Ⓠ ▣

**AMA:** 2005,Aug,7-8; 2005,Jul,11-12

**85250**  factor IX (PTC or Christmas)
 0.00   0.00   **FUD** XXX
AMA: 2005,Aug,7-8; 2005,Jul,11-12

**85260**  factor X (Stuart-Prower)
 0.00   0.00   **FUD** XXX
AMA: 2005,Aug,7-8; 2005,Jul,11-12

**85270**  factor XI (PTA)
 0.00   0.00   **FUD** XXX
AMA: 2005,Aug,7-8; 2005,Jul,11-12

**85280**  factor XII (Hageman)
 0.00   0.00   **FUD** XXX
AMA: 2005,Aug,7-8; 2005,Jul,11-12

**85290**  factor XIII (fibrin stabilizing)
 0.00   0.00   **FUD** XXX
AMA: 2005,Aug,7-8; 2005,Jul,11-12

**85291**  factor XIII (fibrin stabilizing), screen solubility
 0.00   0.00   **FUD** XXX
AMA: 2005,Aug,7-8; 2005,Jul,11-12

**85292**  prekallikrein assay (Fletcher factor assay)
 0.00   0.00   **FUD** XXX
AMA: 2005,Aug,7-8; 2005,Jul,11-12

**85293**  high molecular weight kininogen assay (Fitzgerald factor assay)
 0.00   0.00   **FUD** XXX
AMA: 2005,Aug,7-8; 2005,Jul,11-12

**85300**  Clotting inhibitors or anticoagulants; antithrombin III, activity
 0.00   0.00   **FUD** XXX
AMA: 2005,Aug,7-8; 2005,Jul,11-12

**85301**  antithrombin III, antigen assay
 0.00   0.00   **FUD** XXX
AMA: 2005,Aug,7-8; 2005,Jul,11-12

**85302**  protein C, antigen
 0.00   0.00   **FUD** XXX
AMA: 2005,Aug,7-8; 2005,Jul,11-12

**85303**  protein C, activity
 0.00   0.00   **FUD** XXX
AMA: 2005,Aug,7-8; 2005,Jul,11-12

**85305**  protein S, total
 0.00   0.00   **FUD** XXX
AMA: 2005,Jul,11-12; 2005,Aug,7-8

**85306**  protein S, free
 0.00   0.00   **FUD** XXX
AMA: 2005,Aug,7-8; 2005,Jul,11-12

**85307**  Activated Protein C (APC) resistance assay
 0.00   0.00   **FUD** XXX
AMA: 2005,Aug,7-8; 2005,Jul,11-12

**85335**  Factor inhibitor test
 0.00   0.00   **FUD** XXX
AMA: 2005,Aug,7-8; 2005,Jul,11-12

**85337**  Thrombomodulin
EXCLUDES  Mixing studies for inhibitors (85732)
 0.00   0.00   **FUD** XXX
AMA: 2005,Aug,7-8; 2005,Jul,11-12

**85345**  Coagulation time; Lee and White
 0.00   0.00   **FUD** XXX
AMA: 2005,Aug,7-8; 2005,Jul,11-12

**85347**  activated
 0.00   0.00   **FUD** XXX
AMA: 2005,Aug,7-8; 2005,Jul,11-12

**85348**  other methods
 0.00   0.00   **FUD** XXX
AMA: 2005,Aug,7-8; 2005,Jul,11-12

**85360**  Euglobulin lysis
 0.00   0.00   **FUD** XXX
AMA: 2005,Aug,7-8; 2005,Jul,11-12

**85362**  Fibrin(ogen) degradation (split) products (FDP) (FSP); agglutination slide, semiquantitative
EXCLUDES  Immunoelectrophoresis (86320)
 0.00   0.00   **FUD** XXX
AMA: 2005,Aug,7-8; 2005,Jul,11-12

**85366**  paracoagulation
 0.00   0.00   **FUD** XXX
AMA: 2005,Aug,7-8; 2005,Jul,11-12

**85370**  quantitative
 0.00   0.00   **FUD** XXX
AMA: 2005,Aug,7-8; 2005,Jul,11-12

**85378**  Fibrin degradation products, D-dimer; qualitative or semiquantitative
 0.00   0.00   **FUD** XXX
AMA: 2017,Jan,8; 2016,Jan,13; 2015,Jan,16; 2014,Jan,11

**85379**  quantitative
INCLUDES  Ultrasensitive and standard sensitivity quantitative D-dimer
 0.00   0.00   **FUD** XXX
AMA: 2005,Aug,7-8; 2005,Jul,11-12

**85380**  ultrasensitive (eg, for evaluation for venous thromboembolism), qualitative or semiquantitative
 0.00   0.00   **FUD** XXX
AMA: 2017,Jan,8; 2016,Jan,13; 2015,Jan,16; 2014,Jan,11

**85384**  Fibrinogen; activity
 0.00   0.00   **FUD** XXX
AMA: 2005,Jul,11-12; 2005,Aug,7-8

**85385**  antigen
 0.00   0.00   **FUD** XXX
AMA: 2005,Jul,11-12; 2005,Aug,7-8

**85390**  Fibrinolysins or coagulopathy screen, interpretation and report
 0.00   0.00   **FUD** XXX
AMA: 2005,Jul,11-12; 2005,Aug,7-8

**85396**  Coagulation/fibrinolysis assay, whole blood (eg, viscoelastic clot assessment), including use of any pharmacologic additive(s), as indicated, including interpretation and written report, per day
 0.59   0.59   **FUD** XXX
AMA: 2005,Aug,7-8; 2005,Jul,11-12

**85397**  Coagulation and fibrinolysis, functional activity, not otherwise specified (eg, ADAMTS-13), each analyte
 0.00   0.00   **FUD** XXX

**85400**  Fibrinolytic factors and inhibitors; plasmin
 0.00   0.00   **FUD** XXX
AMA: 2005,Aug,7-8; 2005,Jul,11-12

**85410**  alpha-2 antiplasmin
 0.00   0.00   **FUD** XXX
AMA: 2005,Aug,7-8; 2005,Jul,11-12

**85415**  plasminogen activator
 0.00   0.00   **FUD** XXX
AMA: 2005,Aug,7-8; 2005,Jul,11-12

**85420**  plasminogen, except antigenic assay
 0.00   0.00   **FUD** XXX
AMA: 2005,Aug,7-8; 2005,Jul,11-12

**85421**  plasminogen, antigenic assay
 0.00   0.00   **FUD** XXX
AMA: 2005,Aug,7-8; 2005,Jul,11-12

**85441**  Heinz bodies; direct
 0.00   0.00   **FUD** XXX
AMA: 2005,Aug,7-8; 2005,Jul,11-12

● New Code   ▲ Revised Code   ○ Reinstated   ● New Web Release   ▲ Revised Web Release   Unlisted   Not Covered   # Resequenced
⊘ AMA Mod 51 Exempt   ⑨ Optum Mod 51 Exempt   ⑥ Mod 63 Exempt   ✗ Non-FDA Drug   ★ Telemedicine   Ⓜ Maternity   Ⓐ Age Edit   ✚ Add-on   AMA: CPT Asst
© 2017 Optum360, LLC          CPT © 2017 American Medical Association. All Rights Reserved.

| | | |
|---|---|---|
| **85445** | **induced, acetyl phenylhydrazine** | |
| | 🔶 0.00   ⚗ 0.00   **FUD** XXX | Q ▣ |
| | AMA: 2005,Aug,7-8; 2005,Jul,11-12 | |

| | | |
|---|---|---|
| **85460** | **Hemoglobin or RBCs, fetal, for fetomaternal hemorrhage; differential lysis (Kleihauer-Betke)** | Ⓜ ♀ |
| | EXCLUDES  Hemoglobin F (83030, 83033) | |
| | Hemolysins (86940-86941) | |
| | 🔶 0.00   ⚗ 0.00   **FUD** XXX | Q ▣ |
| | AMA: 2017,Jan,8; 2016,Jan,13; 2015,Jan,16; 2014,Jan,11 | |

| | | |
|---|---|---|
| **85461** | **rosette** | Ⓜ ♀ |
| | 🔶 0.00   ⚗ 0.00   **FUD** XXX | Q ▣ |
| | AMA: 2005,Jul,11-12; 2005,Aug,7-8 | |

| | | |
|---|---|---|
| **85475** | **Hemolysin, acid** | |
| | INCLUDES  Ham test | |
| | EXCLUDES  Hemolysins and agglutinins (86940-86941) | |
| | 🔶 0.00   ⚗ 0.00   **FUD** XXX | Q ▣ |
| | AMA: 2005,Aug,7-8; 2005,Jul,11-12 | |

| | | |
|---|---|---|
| **85520** | **Heparin assay** | |
| | 🔶 0.00   ⚗ 0.00   **FUD** XXX | Q ▣ |
| | AMA: 2005,Aug,7-8; 2005,Jul,11-12 | |

| | | |
|---|---|---|
| **85525** | **Heparin neutralization** | |
| | 🔶 0.00   ⚗ 0.00   **FUD** XXX | Q ▣ |
| | AMA: 2017,Aug,9 | |

| | | |
|---|---|---|
| **85530** | **Heparin-protamine tolerance test** | |
| | 🔶 0.00   ⚗ 0.00   **FUD** XXX | Q ▣ |
| | AMA: 2005,Aug,7-8; 2005,Jul,11-12 | |

| | | |
|---|---|---|
| **85536** | **Iron stain, peripheral blood** | |
| | EXCLUDES  Iron stains on bone marrow or other tissues with physician evaluation (88313) | |
| | 🔶 0.00   ⚗ 0.00   **FUD** XXX | Q ▣ |
| | AMA: 2005,Aug,7-8; 2005,Jul,11-12 | |

| | | |
|---|---|---|
| **85540** | **Leukocyte alkaline phosphatase with count** | |
| | 🔶 0.00   ⚗ 0.00   **FUD** XXX | Q ▣ |
| | AMA: 2005,Aug,7-8; 2005,Jul,11-12 | |

| | | |
|---|---|---|
| **85547** | **Mechanical fragility, RBC** | |
| | 🔶 0.00   ⚗ 0.00   **FUD** XXX | Q ▣ |
| | AMA: 2005,Aug,7-8; 2005,Jul,11-12 | |

| | | |
|---|---|---|
| **85549** | **Muramidase** | |
| | 🔶 0.00   ⚗ 0.00   **FUD** XXX | Q ▣ |
| | AMA: 2005,Aug,7-8; 2005,Jul,11-12 | |

| | | |
|---|---|---|
| **85555** | **Osmotic fragility, RBC; unincubated** | |
| | 🔶 0.00   ⚗ 0.00   **FUD** XXX | Q ▣ |
| | AMA: 2005,Aug,7-8; 2005,Jul,11-12 | |

| | | |
|---|---|---|
| **85557** | **incubated** | |
| | 🔶 0.00   ⚗ 0.00   **FUD** XXX | Q ▣ |
| | AMA: 2005,Aug,7-8; 2005,Jul,11-12 | |

| | | |
|---|---|---|
| **85576** | **Platelet, aggregation (in vitro), each agent** | |
| | EXCLUDES  Thromboxane metabolite(s), including thromboxane, when performed, in urine (84431) | |
| | 🔶 0.00   ⚗ 0.00   **FUD** XXX | ✖ Q ▣ |
| | AMA: 2017,Jan,8; 2016,Jan,13; 2015,Jan,16; 2014,Jan,11; 2012,Jan,15-42 | |

| | | |
|---|---|---|
| **85597** | **Phospholipid neutralization; platelet** | |
| | 🔶 0.00   ⚗ 0.00   **FUD** XXX | Q ▣ |
| | AMA: 2017,Jan,8; 2016,Jan,13; 2015,Jan,16; 2014,Jan,11 | |

| | | |
|---|---|---|
| **85598** | **hexagonal phospholipid** | |
| | 🔶 0.00   ⚗ 0.00   **FUD** XXX | Q ▣ |
| | AMA: 2017,Jan,8; 2016,Jan,13; 2015,Jan,16; 2014,Jan,11 | |

| | | |
|---|---|---|
| **85610** | **Prothrombin time;** | |
| | 🔶 0.00   ⚗ 0.00   **FUD** XXX | ✖ Q ▣ |
| | AMA: 2005,Aug,7-8; 2005,Jul,11-12 | |

| | | |
|---|---|---|
| **85611** | **substitution, plasma fractions, each** | |
| | 🔶 0.00   ⚗ 0.00   **FUD** XXX | Q ▣ |
| | AMA: 2005,Aug,7-8; 2005,Jul,11-12 | |

| | | |
|---|---|---|
| **85612** | **Russell viper venom time (includes venom); undiluted** | |
| | 🔶 0.00   ⚗ 0.00   **FUD** XXX | Q ▣ |
| | AMA: 2005,Aug,7-8; 2005,Jul,11-12 | |

| | | |
|---|---|---|
| **85613** | **diluted** | |
| | 🔶 0.00   ⚗ 0.00   **FUD** XXX | Q ▣ |
| | AMA: 2005,Aug,7-8; 2005,Jul,11-12 | |

| | | |
|---|---|---|
| **85635** | **Reptilase test** | |
| | 🔶 0.00   ⚗ 0.00   **FUD** XXX | Q ▣ |
| | AMA: 2005,Aug,7-8; 2005,Jul,11-12 | |

| | | |
|---|---|---|
| **85651** | **Sedimentation rate, erythrocyte; non-automated** | |
| | 🔶 0.00   ⚗ 0.00   **FUD** XXX | ✖ Q |
| | AMA: 2005,Aug,7-8; 2005,Jul,11-12 | |

| | | |
|---|---|---|
| **85652** | **automated** | |
| | INCLUDES  Westergren test | |
| | 🔶 0.00   ⚗ 0.00   **FUD** XXX | Q ▣ |
| | AMA: 2005,Aug,7-8; 2005,Jul,11-12 | |

| | | |
|---|---|---|
| **85660** | **Sickling of RBC, reduction** | |
| | EXCLUDES  Hemoglobin electrophoresis (83020) | |
| | 🔶 0.00   ⚗ 0.00   **FUD** XXX | Q ▣ |
| | AMA: 2005,Aug,7-8; 2005,Jul,11-12 | |

| | | |
|---|---|---|
| **85670** | **Thrombin time; plasma** | |
| | 🔶 0.00   ⚗ 0.00   **FUD** XXX | Q ▣ |
| | AMA: 2005,Jul,11-12; 2005,Aug,7-8 | |

| | | |
|---|---|---|
| **85675** | **titer** | |
| | 🔶 0.00   ⚗ 0.00   **FUD** XXX | Q ▣ |
| | AMA: 2005,Jul,11-12; 2005,Aug,7-8 | |

| | | |
|---|---|---|
| **85705** | **Thromboplastin inhibition, tissue** | |
| | EXCLUDES  Individual clotting factors (85245-85247) | |
| | 🔶 0.00   ⚗ 0.00   **FUD** XXX | Q ▣ |
| | AMA: 2005,Aug,7-8; 2005,Jul,11-12 | |

## 85730-85732 Partial Thromboplastin Time (PTT)

EXCLUDES  Agglutinins (86000, 86156-86157)
Antiplasmin (85410)
Antithrombin III (85300-85301)
Blood banking procedures (86850-86999)

| | | |
|---|---|---|
| **85730** | **Thromboplastin time, partial (PTT); plasma or whole blood** | |
| | INCLUDES  Hicks-Pitney test | |
| | 🔶 0.00   ⚗ 0.00   **FUD** XXX | Q ▣ |
| | AMA: 2005,Aug,7 8; 2005,Jul,11-12 | |

| | | |
|---|---|---|
| **85732** | **substitution, plasma fractions, each** | |
| | 🔶 0.00   ⚗ 0.00   **FUD** XXX | Q ▣ |
| | AMA: 2017,Jan,8; 2016,Jan,13; 2015,Jan,16; 2014,Jan,11 | |

## 85810-85999 Blood Viscosity and Unlisted Hematology Procedures

| | | |
|---|---|---|
| **85810** | **Viscosity** | |
| | 🔶 0.00   ⚗ 0.00   **FUD** XXX | Q |
| | AMA: 2017,Jan,8; 2016,Jan,13; 2015,Jan,16; 2014,Jan,11; 2012,Jan,15-42 | |

| | | |
|---|---|---|
| **85999** | **Unlisted hematology and coagulation procedure** | |
| | 🔶 0.00   ⚗ 0.00   **FUD** XXX | Q |
| | AMA: 2017,Aug,9; 2017,Jan,8; 2016,Jan,13; 2015,Jan,16; 2014,Jan,11 | |

## 86000-86063 Antibody Testing

| | | |
|---|---|---|
| **86000** | **Agglutinins, febrile (eg, Brucella, Francisella, Murine typhus, Q fever, Rocky Mountain spotted fever, scrub typhus), each antigen** | |
| | EXCLUDES  Infectious agent antibodies (86602-86804) | |
| | 🔶 0.00   ⚗ 0.00   **FUD** XXX | Q |
| | AMA: 2017,Jan,8; 2016,Jan,13; 2015,Jan,16; 2014,Jan,11 | |

| | | |
|---|---|---|
| **86001** | **Allergen specific IgG quantitative or semiquantitative, each allergen** | |
| | 🔶 0.00   ⚗ 0.00   **FUD** XXX | Q ▣ |
| | AMA: 2005,Aug,7-8; 2005,Jul,11-12 | |

▲ **86003** **Allergen specific IgE; quantitative or semiquantitative, crude allergen extract, each**
  *EXCLUDES* *Total quantitative IgE (82785)*
  💶 0.00   ⚖ 0.00   **FUD** XXX     Ⓠ ▱
  **AMA:** 2017,Jan,8; 2016,Jan,13; 2015,Jan,16; 2014,Jan,11

▲ **86005** **qualitative, multiallergen screen (eg, disk, sponge, card)**
  *EXCLUDES* *Total qualitative IgE (83518)*
  💶 0.00   ⚖ 0.00   **FUD** XXX     Ⓠ
  **AMA:** 2017,Jan,8; 2016,Jan,13; 2015,Jan,16; 2014,Jan,11

● **86008** **quantitative or semiquantitative, recombinant or purified component, each**

**86021** **Antibody identification; leukocyte antibodies**
  💶 0.00   ⚖ 0.00   **FUD** XXX     Ⓠ ▱
  **AMA:** 2005,Jul,11-12; 2005,Aug,7-8

**86022** **platelet antibodies**
  💶 0.00   ⚖ 0.00   **FUD** XXX     Ⓠ ▱
  **AMA:** 2005,Jul,11-12; 2005,Aug,7-8

**86023** **platelet associated immunoglobulin assay**
  💶 0.00   ⚖ 0.00   **FUD** XXX     Ⓠ ▱
  **AMA:** 2005,Jul,11-12; 2005,Aug,7-8

**86038** **Antinuclear antibodies (ANA);**
  💶 0.00   ⚖ 0.00   **FUD** XXX     Ⓠ ▱
  **AMA:** 2005,Aug,7-8; 2005,Jul,11-12

**86039** **titer**
  💶 0.00   ⚖ 0.00   **FUD** XXX     Ⓠ ▱
  **AMA:** 2005,Aug,7-8; 2005,Jul,11-12

**86060** **Antistreptolysin 0; titer**
  💶 0.00   ⚖ 0.00   **FUD** XXX     Ⓠ ▱
  **AMA:** 2005,Jul,11-12; 2005,Aug,7-8

**86063** **screen**
  💶 0.00   ⚖ 0.00   **FUD** XXX     Ⓠ
  **AMA:** 2005,Jul,11-12; 2005,Aug,7-8

## 86077-86079 Blood Bank Services

**86077** **Blood bank physician services; difficult cross match and/or evaluation of irregular antibody(s), interpretation and written report**
  💶 1.49   ⚖ 1.60   **FUD** XXX     Ⓠ1 80
  **AMA:** 2005,Aug,7-8; 2005,Jul,11-12

**86078** **investigation of transfusion reaction including suspicion of transmissible disease, interpretation and written report**
  💶 1.48   ⚖ 1.60   **FUD** XXX     Ⓠ1 80
  **AMA:** 2005,Aug,7-8; 2005,Jul,11-12

**86079** **authorization for deviation from standard blood banking procedures (eg, use of outdated blood, transfusion of Rh incompatible units), with written report**
  💶 1.48   ⚖ 1.59   **FUD** XXX     Ⓠ1 80
  **AMA:** 2005,Aug,7-8; 2005,Jul,11-12

## 86140-86344 [86152, 86153] Diagnostic Immunology Testing

**86140** **C-reactive protein;**
  💶 0.00   ⚖ 0.00   **FUD** XXX     Ⓠ
  **AMA:** 2005,Aug,7-8; 2005,Jul,11-12

**86141** **high sensitivity (hsCRP)**
  💶 0.00   ⚖ 0.00   **FUD** XXX     Ⓠ ▱
  **AMA:** 2005,Aug,7-8; 2005,Jul,11-12

**86146** **Beta 2 Glycoprotein I antibody, each**
  💶 0.00   ⚖ 0.00   **FUD** XXX     Ⓠ
  **AMA:** 2005,Aug,7-8; 2005,Jul,11-12

**86147** **Cardiolipin (phospholipid) antibody, each Ig class**
  💶 0.00   ⚖ 0.00   **FUD** XXX     Ⓠ
  **AMA:** 2005,Aug,7-8; 2005,Jul,11-12

\# **86152** **Cell enumeration using immunologic selection and identification in fluid specimen (eg, circulating tumor cells in blood);**
  💶 0.00   ⚖ 0.00   **FUD** XXX     Ⓠ ▱
  *EXCLUDES* *Flow cytometric immunophenotyping (88184-88189)*
  *Flow cytometric quantitation (86355-86357, 86359-86361, 86367)*
  Code also physician interpretation/report when performed ([86153])

\# **86153** **physician interpretation and report, when required**
  💶 0.00   ⚖ 0.00   **FUD** 000     Ⓑ ▱
  *EXCLUDES* *Flow cytometric immunophenotyping (88184-88189)*
  *Flow cytometric quantitation (86355-86357, 86359-86361, 86367)*
  Code first cell enumeration, when performed ([86152])

**86148** **Anti-phosphatidylserine (phospholipid) antibody**
  *EXCLUDES* *Antiprothrombin (phospholipid cofactor) antibody (86849)*
  💶 0.00   ⚖ 0.00   **FUD** XXX     Ⓠ
  **AMA:** 2017,Jan,8; 2016,Jan,13; 2015,Jan,16; 2014,Jan,11

*86152* **Resequenced code. See code following 86147.**

*86153* **Resequenced code. See code before 86148.**

**86155** **Chemotaxis assay, specify method**
  💶 0.00   ⚖ 0.00   **FUD** XXX     Ⓠ
  **AMA:** 2005,Aug,7-8; 2005,Jul,11-12

**86156** **Cold agglutinin; screen**
  💶 0.00   ⚖ 0.00   **FUD** XXX     Ⓠ
  **AMA:** 2005,Aug,7-8; 2005,Jul,11-12

**86157** **titer**
  💶 0.00   ⚖ 0.00   **FUD** XXX     Ⓠ ▱
  **AMA:** 2005,Aug,7-8; 2005,Jul,11-12

**86160** **Complement; antigen, each component**
  💶 0.00   ⚖ 0.00   **FUD** XXX     Ⓠ
  **AMA:** 2005,Aug,7-8; 2005,Jul,11-12

**86161** **functional activity, each component**
  💶 0.00   ⚖ 0.00   **FUD** XXX     Ⓠ
  **AMA:** 2005,Aug,7-8; 2005,Jul,11-12

**86162** **total hemolytic (CH50)**
  💶 0.00   ⚖ 0.00   **FUD** XXX     Ⓠ
  **AMA:** 2005,Aug,7-8; 2005,Jul,11-12

**86171** **Complement fixation tests, each antigen**
  💶 0.00   ⚖ 0.00   **FUD** XXX     Ⓠ
  **AMA:** 2005,Aug,7-8; 2005,Jul,11-12

~~**86185** Counterimmunoelectrophoresis, each antigen~~

**86200** **Cyclic citrullinated peptide (CCP), antibody**
  💶 0.00   ⚖ 0.00   **FUD** XXX     Ⓠ
  **AMA:** 2017,Jan,8; 2016,Jan,13; 2015,Jan,16; 2014,Jan,11

**86215** **Deoxyribonuclease, antibody**
  💶 0.00   ⚖ 0.00   **FUD** XXX     Ⓠ ▱
  **AMA:** 2005,Aug,7-8; 2005,Jul,11-12

**86225** **Deoxyribonucleic acid (DNA) antibody; native or double stranded**
  *EXCLUDES* *HIV antibody tests (86701-86703)*
  💶 0.00   ⚖ 0.00   **FUD** XXX     Ⓠ ▱
  **AMA:** 2005,Aug,7-8; 2005,Jul,11-12

**86226** **single stranded**
  *EXCLUDES* *Anti D.S, DNA, IFA, eg, using C. Lucilae (86255-86256)*
  💶 0.00   ⚖ 0.00   **FUD** XXX     Ⓠ ▱
  **AMA:** 2005,Aug,7-8; 2005,Jul,11-12

**86235** **Extractable nuclear antigen, antibody to, any method (eg, nRNP, SS-A, SS-B, Sm, RNP, Sc170, J01), each antibody**
  💶 0.00   ⚖ 0.00   **FUD** XXX     Ⓠ ▱
  **AMA:** 2005,Aug,7-8; 2005,Jul,11-12

**86243** ~~Fc receptor~~

● New Code   ▲ Revised Code   ○ Reinstated   ● New Web Release   ▲ Revised Web Release   Unlisted   Not Covered   # Resequenced
⊘ AMA Mod 51 Exempt   ⑨ Optum Mod 51 Exempt   ⊛ Mod 63 Exempt   ✗ Non-FDA Drug   ★ Telemedicine   Ⓜ Maternity   ▲ Age Edit   + Add-on   **AMA:** CPT Asst
© 2017 Optum360, LLC     CPT © 2017 American Medical Association. All Rights Reserved.

**86255** **Fluorescent noninfectious agent antibody; screen, each antibody**
🔲 0.00   ⚖ 0.00   **FUD** XXX                    Ⓠ 🖼

AMA: 2005,Aug,9-10; 2005,Aug,7-8

**86256** **titer, each antibody**
> EXCLUDES   *Fluorescent technique for antigen identification in tissue (88346, [88350])*
> *FTA (86780)*
> *Gel (agar) diffusion tests (86331)*
> *Indirect fluorescence (88346, [88350])*

🔲 0.00   ⚖ 0.00   **FUD** XXX                    Ⓠ 🖼

AMA: 2005,Aug,9-10; 2005,Aug,7-8

**86277** **Growth hormone, human (HGH), antibody**
🔲 0.00   ⚖ 0.00   **FUD** XXX                    Ⓠ

AMA: 2005,Aug,7-8; 2005,Jul,11-12

**86280** **Hemagglutination inhibition test (HAI)**
> EXCLUDES   *Antibodies to infectious agents (86602-86804)*
> *Rubella (86762)*

🔲 0.00   ⚖ 0.00   **FUD** XXX                    Ⓠ

AMA: 2005,Aug,7-8; 2005,Jul,11-12

**86294** **Immunoassay for tumor antigen, qualitative or semiquantitative (eg, bladder tumor antigen)**
> EXCLUDES   *Qualitative NMP22 protein (86386)*

🔲 0.00   ⚖ 0.00   **FUD** XXX              ❎ Ⓠ 🖼

AMA: 2005,Aug,7-8; 2005,Jul,11-12

**86300** **Immunoassay for tumor antigen, quantitative; CA 15-3 (27.29)**
🔲 0.00   ⚖ 0.00   **FUD** XXX                    Ⓠ 🖼

AMA: 2005,Aug,7-8; 2005,Jul,11-12

**86301** **CA 19-9**
🔲 0.00   ⚖ 0.00   **FUD** XXX                    Ⓠ 🖼

AMA: 2005,Aug,7-8; 2005,Jul,11-12

**86304** **CA 125**
> EXCLUDES   *Measurement of serum HER-2/neu oncoprotein (83950)*

🔲 0.00   ⚖ 0.00   **FUD** XXX                    Ⓠ 🖼

AMA: 2005,Aug,7-8; 2005,Jul,11-12

**86305** **Human epididymis protein 4 (HE4)**
🔲 0.00   ⚖ 0.00   **FUD** XXX                    Ⓠ

**86308** **Heterophile antibodies; screening**
> EXCLUDES   *Antibodies to infectious agents (86602-86804)*

🔲 0.00   ⚖ 0.00   **FUD** XXX              ❎ Ⓠ

AMA: 2005,Jul,11-12; 2005,Aug,7-8

**86309** **titer**
> EXCLUDES   *Antibodies to infectious agents (86602-86804)*

🔲 0.00   ⚖ 0.00   **FUD** XXX                    Ⓠ

AMA: 2005,Jul,11-12; 2005,Aug,7-8

**86310** **titers after absorption with beef cells and guinea pig kidney**
> EXCLUDES   *Antibodies to infectious agents (86602-86804)*

🔲 0.00   ⚖ 0.00   **FUD** XXX                    Ⓠ

AMA: 2005,Jul,11-12; 2005,Aug,7-8

**86316** **Immunoassay for tumor antigen, other antigen, quantitative (eg, CA 50, 72-4, 549), each**
🔲 0.00   ⚖ 0.00   **FUD** XXX                    Ⓠ 🖼

AMA: 2017,Jan,8; 2016,Jan,13; 2015,Jan,16; 2014,Jan,11; 2012,Jan,15-42

**86317** **Immunoassay for infectious agent antibody, quantitative, not otherwise specified**
> EXCLUDES   *Immunoassay techniques for antigens (83516, 83518-83520, 87301-87450, 87810-87899)*
> *Particle agglutination test (86403)*

🔲 0.00   ⚖ 0.00   **FUD** XXX                    Ⓠ 🖼

AMA: 2005,Jul,11-12; 2005,Aug,7-8

**86318** **Immunoassay for infectious agent antibody, qualitative or semiquantitative, single step method (eg, reagent strip)**
🔲 0.00   ⚖ 0.00   **FUD** XXX              ❎ Ⓠ

AMA: 2017,Jan,8; 2016,Jan,13; 2015,Jan,16; 2014,Jan,11; 2012,Jan,15-42

**86320** **Immunoelectrophoresis; serum**
🔲 0.00   ⚖ 0.00   **FUD** XXX                    Ⓠ 🖼

AMA: 2005,Jul,11-12; 2005,Aug,7-8

**86325** **other fluids (eg, urine, cerebrospinal fluid) with concentration**
🔲 0.00   ⚖ 0.00   **FUD** XXX                    Ⓠ 🖼

AMA: 2005,Jul,11-12; 2005,Aug,7-8

**86327** **crossed (2-dimensional assay)**
🔲 0.00   ⚖ 0.00   **FUD** XXX                    Ⓠ 🖼

AMA: 2005,Jul,11-12; 2005,Aug,7-8

**86329** **Immunodiffusion; not elsewhere specified**
🔲 0.00   ⚖ 0.00   **FUD** XXX                    Ⓠ 🖼

AMA: 2017,Jan,8; 2016,Jan,13; 2015,Jan,16; 2014,Jan,11; 2012,Jan,15-42

**86331** **gel diffusion, qualitative (Ouchterlony), each antigen or antibody**
🔲 0.00   ⚖ 0.00   **FUD** XXX                    Ⓠ 🖼

AMA: 2005,Aug,7-8; 2005,Jul,11-12

**86332** **Immune complex assay**
🔲 0.00   ⚖ 0.00   **FUD** XXX                    Ⓠ

AMA: 2005,Aug,7-8; 2005,Jul,11-12

**86334** **Immunofixation electrophoresis; serum**
🔲 0.00   ⚖ 0.00   **FUD** XXX                    Ⓠ 🖼

AMA: 2005,Jul,11-12; 2005,Aug,7-8

**86335** **other fluids with concentration (eg, urine, CSF)**
🔲 0.00   ⚖ 0.00   **FUD** XXX                    Ⓠ 🖼

AMA: 2005,Aug,7-8; 2005,Jul,11-12

**86336** **Inhibin A**
🔲 0.00   ⚖ 0.00   **FUD** XXX                    Ⓠ

AMA: 2005,Aug,7-8; 2005,Jul,11-12

**86337** **Insulin antibodies**
🔲 0.00   ⚖ 0.00   **FUD** XXX                    Ⓠ

AMA: 2005,Aug,7-8; 2005,Jul,11-12

**86340** **Intrinsic factor antibodies**
🔲 0.00   ⚖ 0.00   **FUD** XXX                    Ⓠ

AMA: 2005,Jul,11-12; 2005,Aug,7-8

**86341** **Islet cell antibody**
🔲 0.00   ⚖ 0.00   **FUD** XXX                    Ⓠ

AMA: 2017,Jan,8; 2016,Jan,13; 2015,Jan,16; 2014,Jan,11

**86343** **Leukocyte histamine release test (LHR)**
🔲 0.00   ⚖ 0.00   **FUD** XXX                    Ⓠ

AMA: 2005,Aug,7-8; 2005,Jul,11-12

**86344** **Leukocyte phagocytosis**
🔲 0.00   ⚖ 0.00   **FUD** XXX                    Ⓠ 🖼

AMA: 2005,Aug,7-8; 2005,Jul,11-12

## 86352 Assay Cellular Function

**86352** **Cellular function assay involving stimulation (eg, mitogen or antigen) and detection of biomarker (eg, ATP)**
🔲 0.00   ⚖ 0.00   **FUD** XXX                    Ⓠ 🖼

## 86353 Lymphocyte Mitogen Response Assay

**CMS:** 100-03,190.8 Lymphocyte Mitogen Response Assays

**86353** **Lymphocyte transformation, mitogen (phytomitogen) or antigen induced blastogenesis**
> EXCLUDES   *Cellular function assay involving stimulation and detection of biomarker (86352)*

🔲 0.00   ⚖ 0.00   **FUD** XXX                    Ⓠ 🖼

AMA: 2005,Aug,7-8; 2005,Jul,11-12

26/TC PC/TC Only   A2-Z3 ASC Payment   50 Bilateral   ♂ Male Only   ♀ Female Only   🔲 Facility RVU   ⚖ Non-Facility RVU   🖼 CCI
FUD Follow-up Days   CMS: IOM (Pub 100)   A-Y OPPSI   80/80 Surg Assist Allowed / w/Doc   📊 Lab Crosswalk   📊 Radiology Crosswalk   ❎ CLIA

CPT © 2017 American Medical Association. All Rights Reserved.          © 2017 Optum360, LLC

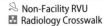

## 86355-86593 Additional Diagnostic Immunology Testing

**86355** **B cells, total count**
EXCLUDES *Flow cytometry interpretation (88187-88189)*
0.00   0.00   **FUD** XXX   Q ⊡
AMA: 2017,Jan,8; 2016,Jan,13; 2015,Jan,16; 2014,Jan,11

**86356** **Mononuclear cell antigen, quantitative (eg, flow cytometry), not otherwise specified, each antigen**
EXCLUDES *Flow cytometry interpretation (88187-88189)*
0.00   0.00   **FUD** XXX   Q ⊡
AMA: 2017,Jan,8; 2016,Jan,13; 2015,Jan,16; 2014,Jan,11

**86357** **Natural killer (NK) cells, total count**
EXCLUDES *Flow cytometry interpretation (88187-88189)*
0.00   0.00   **FUD** XXX   Q ⊡
AMA: 2017,Jan,8; 2016,Jan,13; 2015,Jan,16; 2014,Jan,11

**86359** **T cells; total count**
EXCLUDES *Flow cytometry interpretation (88187-88189)*
0.00   0.00   **FUD** XXX   Q ⊡
AMA: 2017,Jan,8; 2016,Jan,13; 2015,Jan,16; 2014,Jan,11

**86360** **absolute CD4 and CD8 count, including ratio**
EXCLUDES *Flow cytometry interpretation (88187-88189)*
0.00   0.00   **FUD** XXX   Q ⊡
AMA: 2017,Jan,8; 2016,Jan,13; 2015,Jan,16; 2014,Jan,11

**86361** **absolute CD4 count**
EXCLUDES *Flow cytometry interpretation (88187-88189)*
0.00   0.00   **FUD** XXX   Q ⊡
AMA: 2017,Jan,8; 2016,Jan,13; 2015,Jan,16; 2014,Jan,11

**86367** **Stem cells (ie, CD34), total count**
EXCLUDES *Flow cytometry interpretation (88187-88189)*
0.00   0.00   **FUD** XXX   Q ⊡
AMA: 2017,Jan,8; 2016,Jan,13; 2015,Jan,16; 2014,Jan,11; 2013,Oct,3

**86376** **Microsomal antibodies (eg, thyroid or liver-kidney), each**
0.00   0.00   **FUD** XXX   Q ⊡
AMA: 2005,Jul,11-12; 2005,Aug,7-8

~~**86378** **Migration inhibitory factor test (MIF)**~~

**86382** **Neutralization test, viral**
0.00   0.00   **FUD** XXX   Q ⊡
AMA: 2005,Aug,7-8; 2005,Jul,11-12

**86384** **Nitroblue tetrazolium dye test (NTD)**
0.00   0.00   **FUD** XXX   Q ⊡
AMA: 2005,Aug,7-8; 2005,Jul,11-12

**86386** **Nuclear Matrix Protein 22 (NMP22), qualitative**
0.00   0.00   **FUD** XXX   ✗ Q
AMA: 2005,Aug,7-8; 2005,Jul,11-12

**86403** **Particle agglutination; screen, each antibody**
0.00   0.00   **FUD** XXX   Q
AMA: 2005,Jul,11-12; 2005,Aug,7-8

**86406** **titer, each antibody**
0.00   0.00   **FUD** XXX   Q
AMA: 2005,Jul,11-12; 2005,Aug,7-8

**86430** **Rheumatoid factor; qualitative**
0.00   0.00   **FUD** XXX   Q
AMA: 2005,Aug,7-8; 2005,Jul,11-12

**86431** **quantitative**
0.00   0.00   **FUD** XXX   Q
AMA: 2005,Aug,7-8; 2005,Jul,11-12

**86480** **Tuberculosis test, cell mediated immunity antigen response measurement; gamma interferon**
0.00   0.00   **FUD** XXX   Q ⊡
AMA: 2017,Jan,8; 2016,Jan,13; 2015,Jan,16; 2014,Jan,11

**86481** **enumeration of gamma interferon-producing T-cells in cell suspension**
0.00   0.00   **FUD** XXX   Q ⊡
AMA: 2010,Dec,7-10

**86485** **Skin test; candida**
0.00   0.00   **FUD** XXX   01 80 TC
AMA: 2005,Jul,11-12; 2005,Aug,7-8

**86486** **unlisted antigen, each**
0.14   0.14   **FUD** XXX   01 80 TC
AMA: 2008,Apr,5-7

**86490** **coccidioidomycosis**
2.06   2.06   **FUD** XXX   01 80 TC
AMA: 2005,Aug,7-8; 2005,Jul,11-12

**86510** **histoplasmosis**
0.17   0.17   **FUD** XXX   01 80 TC
AMA: 2005,Aug,7-8; 2005,Jul,11-12

**86580** **tuberculosis, intradermal**
INCLUDES   Heaf test
Intradermal Mantoux test
EXCLUDES   *Skin test for allergy (95012-95199)*
*Tuberculosis test, cell mediated immunity measurement of gamma interferon antigen response (86480)*
0.23   0.23   **FUD** XXX   01 80 TC ⊡
AMA: 2005,Aug,7-8; 2005,Jul,11-12

**86590** **Streptokinase, antibody**
EXCLUDES   *Antibodies to infectious agents (86602-86804)*
0.00   0.00   **FUD** XXX   Q
AMA: 2005,Jul,11-12; 2005,Aug,7-8

**86592** **Syphilis test, non-treponemal antibody; qualitative (eg, VDRL, RPR, ART)**
INCLUDES   Wasserman test
EXCLUDES   *Antibodies to infectious agents (86602-86804)*
0.00   0.00   **FUD** XXX   A
AMA: 2005,Jul,11-12; 2005,Aug,7-8

**86593** **quantitative**
EXCLUDES   *Antibodies to infectious agents (86602-86804)*
0.00   0.00   **FUD** XXX   A
AMA: 2005,Jul,11-12; 2005,Aug,7-8

## 86602-86698 Testing for Antibodies to Infectious Agents: Actinomyces- Histoplasma

INCLUDES   Qualitative or semiquantitative immunoassays performed by multiple-step methods for the detection of antibodies to infectious agents
EXCLUDES   *Detection of:*
*Antibodies other than those to infectious agents, see specific antibody or method*
*Infectious agent/antigen (87260-87899 [87623, 87624, 87625, 87806])*
*Immunoassays by single-step method (86318)*

**86602** **Antibody; actinomyces**
0.00   0.00   **FUD** XXX   Q
AMA: 2017,Jan,8; 2016,Jan,13; 2015,Jan,16; 2014,Jan,11

**86603** **adenovirus**
0.00   0.00   **FUD** XXX   Q
AMA: 2005,Jul,11-12; 2005,Aug,7-8

**86606** **Aspergillus**
0.00   0.00   **FUD** XXX   Q
AMA: 2005,Jul,11-12; 2005,Aug,7-8

**86609** **bacterium, not elsewhere specified**
0.00   0.00   **FUD** XXX   Q
AMA: 2005,Jul,11-12; 2005,Aug,7-8

**86611** **Bartonella**
0.00   0.00   **FUD** XXX   Q
AMA: 2005,Jul,11-12; 2005,Aug,7-8

**86612** **Blastomyces**
0.00   0.00   **FUD** XXX   Q
AMA: 2005,Jul,11-12; 2005,Aug,7-8

**86615** **Bordetella**
0.00   0.00   **FUD** XXX   Q
AMA: 2005,Jul,11-12; 2005,Aug,7-8

● New Code   ▲ Revised Code   ○ Reinstated   ● New Web Release   ▲ Revised Web Release   Unlisted   Not Covered   # Resequenced
⊘ AMA Mod 51 Exempt   ⑤ Optum Mod 51 Exempt   ⑥ Mod 63 Exempt   ✗ Non-FDA Drug   ★ Telemedicine   Ⓜ Maternity   Ⓐ Age Edit   ✛ Add-on   AMA: CPT Asst

**86617**    **Borrelia burgdorferi (Lyme disease) confirmatory test (eg, Western Blot or immunoblot)**
🔲 0.00    ⚖ 0.00    **FUD** XXX      Ⓠ
AMA: 2005,Jul,11-12; 2005,Aug,7-8

**86618**    **Borrelia burgdorferi (Lyme disease)**
🔲 0.00    ⚖ 0.00    **FUD** XXX      ✖ Ⓠ
AMA: 2005,Jul,11-12; 2005,Aug,7-8

**86619**    **Borrelia (relapsing fever)**
🔲 0.00    ⚖ 0.00    **FUD** XXX      Ⓠ
AMA: 2005,Jul,11-12; 2005,Aug,7-8

**86622**    **Brucella**
🔲 0.00    ⚖ 0.00    **FUD** XXX      Ⓠ
AMA: 2005,Jul,11-12; 2005,Aug,7-8

**86625**    **Campylobacter**
🔲 0.00    ⚖ 0.00    **FUD** XXX      Ⓠ
AMA: 2005,Jul,11-12; 2005,Aug,7-8

**86628**    **Candida**
EXCLUDES    *Candida skin test (86485)*
🔲 0.00    ⚖ 0.00    **FUD** XXX      Ⓠ
AMA: 2005,Jul,11-12; 2005,Aug,7-8

**86631**    **Chlamydia**
🔲 0.00    ⚖ 0.00    **FUD** XXX      Ⓐ
AMA: 2005,Jul,11-12; 2005,Aug,7-8

**86632**    **Chlamydia, IgM**
EXCLUDES    *Chlamydia antigen (87270, 87320)*
        *Fluorescent antibody technique (86255-86256)*
🔲 0.00    ⚖ 0.00    **FUD** XXX      Ⓐ
AMA: 2005,Jul,11-12; 2005,Aug,7-8

**86635**    **Coccidioides**
🔲 0.00    ⚖ 0.00    **FUD** XXX      Ⓠ
AMA: 2005,Jul,11-12; 2005,Aug,7-8

**86638**    **Coxiella burnetii (Q fever)**
🔲 0.00    ⚖ 0.00    **FUD** XXX      Ⓠ
AMA: 2005,Jul,11-12; 2005,Aug,7-8

**86641**    **Cryptococcus**
🔲 0.00    ⚖ 0.00    **FUD** XXX      Ⓠ
AMA: 2005,Jul,11-12; 2005,Aug,7-8

**86644**    **cytomegalovirus (CMV)**
🔲 0.00    ⚖ 0.00    **FUD** XXX      Ⓠ
AMA: 2005,Jul,11-12; 2005,Aug,7-8

**86645**    **cytomegalovirus (CMV), IgM**
🔲 0.00    ⚖ 0.00    **FUD** XXX      Ⓠ
AMA: 2017,Jan,8; 2016,Jan,13; 2015,Jan,16; 2014,Jan,11

**86648**    **Diphtheria**
🔲 0.00    ⚖ 0.00    **FUD** XXX      Ⓠ
AMA: 2005,Jul,11-12; 2005,Aug,7-8

**86651**    **encephalitis, California (La Crosse)**
🔲 0.00    ⚖ 0.00    **FUD** XXX      Ⓠ
AMA: 2005,Jul,11-12; 2005,Aug,7-8

**86652**    **encephalitis, Eastern equine**
🔲 0.00    ⚖ 0.00    **FUD** XXX      Ⓠ
AMA: 2005,Jul,11-12; 2005,Aug,7-8

**86653**    **encephalitis, St. Louis**
🔲 0.00    ⚖ 0.00    **FUD** XXX      Ⓠ
AMA: 2005,Jul,11-12; 2005,Aug,7-8

**86654**    **encephalitis, Western equine**
🔲 0.00    ⚖ 0.00    **FUD** XXX      Ⓠ
AMA: 2005,Jul,11-12; 2005,Aug,7-8

**86658**    **enterovirus (eg, coxsackie, echo, polio)**
EXCLUDES    *Antibodies to:*
        *Trichinella (86784)*
        *Trypanosoma—see code for specific methodology*
        *Tuberculosis (86580)*
        *Viral—see code for specific methodology*
🔲 0.00    ⚖ 0.00    **FUD** XXX      Ⓠ
AMA: 2005,Jul,11-12; 2005,Aug,7-8

**86663**    **Epstein-Barr (EB) virus, early antigen (EA)**
🔲 0.00    ⚖ 0.00    **FUD** XXX      Ⓠ
AMA: 2005,Jul,11-12; 2005,Aug,7-8

**86664**    **Epstein-Barr (EB) virus, nuclear antigen (EBNA)**
🔲 0.00    ⚖ 0.00    **FUD** XXX      Ⓠ
AMA: 2005,Jul,11-12; 2005,Aug,7-8

**86665**    **Epstein-Barr (EB) virus, viral capsid (VCA)**
🔲 0.00    ⚖ 0.00    **FUD** XXX      Ⓠ
AMA: 2005,Jul,11-12; 2005,Aug,7-8

**86666**    **Ehrlichia**
🔲 0.00    ⚖ 0.00    **FUD** XXX      Ⓠ
AMA: 2005,Jul,11-12; 2005,Aug,7-8

**86668**    **Francisella tularensis**
🔲 0.00    ⚖ 0.00    **FUD** XXX      Ⓠ
AMA: 2005,Jul,11-12; 2005,Aug,7-8

**86671**    **fungus, not elsewhere specified**
🔲 0.00    ⚖ 0.00    **FUD** XXX      Ⓠ
AMA: 2005,Jul,11-12; 2005,Aug,7-8

**86674**    **Giardia lamblia**
🔲 0.00    ⚖ 0.00    **FUD** XXX      Ⓠ
AMA: 2005,Jul,11-12; 2005,Aug,7-8

**86677**    **Helicobacter pylori**
🔲 0.00    ⚖ 0.00    **FUD** XXX      Ⓠ
AMA: 2017,Jan,8; 2016,Jan,13; 2015,Jan,16; 2014,Jan,11

**86682**    **helminth, not elsewhere specified**
🔲 0.00    ⚖ 0.00    **FUD** XXX      Ⓠ
AMA: 2005,Jul,11-12; 2005,Aug,7-8

**86684**    **Haemophilus influenza**
🔲 0.00    ⚖ 0.00    **FUD** XXX      Ⓠ
AMA: 2005,Jul,11-12; 2005,Aug,7-8

**86687**    **HTLV-I**
🔲 0.00    ⚖ 0.00    **FUD** XXX      Ⓠ
AMA: 2005,Jul,11-12; 2005,Aug,7-8

**86688**    **HTLV-II**
🔲 0.00    ⚖ 0.00    **FUD** XXX      Ⓠ
AMA: 2005,Jul,11-12; 2005,Aug,7-8

**86689**    **HTLV or HIV antibody, confirmatory test (eg, Western Blot)**
🔲 0.00    ⚖ 0.00    **FUD** XXX      Ⓠ
AMA: 2017,Jan,8; 2016,Jan,13; 2015,Jan,16; 2014,Jan,11

**86692**    **hepatitis, delta agent**
EXCLUDES    *Hepatitis delta agent, antigen (87380)*
🔲 0.00    ⚖ 0.00    **FUD** XXX      Ⓠ
AMA: 2005,Jul,11-12; 2005,Aug,7-8

**86694**    **herpes simplex, non-specific type test**
🔲 0.00    ⚖ 0.00    **FUD** XXX      Ⓠ
AMA: 2005,Jul,11-12; 2005,Aug,7-8

**86695**    **herpes simplex, type 1**
🔲 0.00    ⚖ 0.00    **FUD** XXX      Ⓠ
AMA: 2017,Jan,8; 2016,Jan,13; 2015,Jan,16; 2014,Jan,11

**86696**    **herpes simplex, type 2**
🔲 0.00    ⚖ 0.00    **FUD** XXX      Ⓠ
AMA: 2005,Jul,11-12; 2005,Aug,7-8

**86698**    **histoplasma**
🔲 0.00    ⚖ 0.00    **FUD** XXX      Ⓠ
AMA: 2005,Jul,11-12; 2005,Aug,7-8

## 86701-86703 Testing for HIV Antibodies

**CMS:** 100-03,190.14 Human Immunodeficiency Virus Testing (Diagnosis); 100-03,190.9 Serologic Testing for Acquired Immunodeficiency Syndrome (AIDS)

INCLUDES Qualitative or semiquantitative immunoassays performed by multiple-step methods for the detection of antibodies to infectious agents

EXCLUDES Confirmatory test for HIV antibody (86689)
HIV-1 antigen (87390)
HIV-1 antigen(s) with HIV 1 and 2 antibodies, single result (87389)
HIV-2 antigen (87391)
Immunoassays by single-step method (86318)
Code also modifier 92 for test performed using a kit or transportable instrument comprising all or part of a single-use, disposable analytical chamber

**86701** **Antibody; HIV-1**
0.00 0.00 **FUD** XXX
**AMA:** 2017,Jan,8; 2016,Jan,13; 2015,Jan,16; 2014,Jan,11

**86702** **HIV-2**
0.00 0.00 **FUD** XXX
**AMA:** 2017,Jan,8; 2016,Jan,13; 2015,Jan,16; 2014,Jan,11

**86703** **HIV-1 and HIV-2, single result**
0.00 0.00 **FUD** XXX
**AMA:** 2017,Jan,8; 2016,Jan,13; 2015,Jan,16; 2014,Jan,11

## 86704-86804 Testing for Infectious Disease Antibodies: Hepatitis—Yersinia

INCLUDES Qualitative or semiquantitative immunoassays performed by multiple-step methods for the detection of antibodies to infectious agents

EXCLUDES Detection of:
Antibodies other than those to infectious agents, see specific antibody or method
Infectious agent/antigen (87260-87899 [87623, 87624, 87625, 87806])
Immunoassays by single-step method (86318)

**86704** **Hepatitis B core antibody (HBcAb); total**
0.00 0.00 **FUD** XXX
**AMA:** 2017,Jan,8; 2016,Jan,13; 2015,Jan,16; 2014,Jan,11

**86705** **IgM antibody**
0.00 0.00 **FUD** XXX
**AMA:** 2017,Jan,8; 2016,Jan,13; 2015,Jan,16; 2014,Jan,11

**86706** **Hepatitis B surface antibody (HBsAb)**
0.00 0.00 **FUD** XXX
**AMA:** 2005,Jul,11-12; 2005,Aug,7-8

**86707** **Hepatitis Be antibody (HBeAb)**
0.00 0.00 **FUD** XXX
**AMA:** 2005,Jul,11-12; 2005,Aug,7-8

**86708** **Hepatitis A antibody (HAAb)**
0.00 0.00 **FUD** XXX
**AMA:** 2017,Jan,8; 2016,Jan,13; 2015,Jan,16; 2014,Jan,11; 2012,Jan,15-42

**86709** **Hepatitis A antibody (HAAb), IgM antibody**
0.00 0.00 **FUD** XXX
**AMA:** 2017,Jan,8; 2016,Jan,13; 2015,Jan,16; 2014,Jan,11; 2012,Jan,15-42

**86710** **Antibody; influenza virus**
0.00 0.00 **FUD** XXX
**AMA:** 2017,Jan,8; 2016,Jan,13; 2015,Jan,16; 2014,Jan,11

**86711** **JC (John Cunningham) virus**
0.00 0.00 **FUD** XXX

**86713** **Legionella**
0.00 0.00 **FUD** XXX
**AMA:** 2005,Jul,11-12; 2005,Aug,7-8

**86717** **Leishmania**
0.00 0.00 **FUD** XXX
**AMA:** 2005,Jul,11-12; 2005,Aug,7-8

**86720** **Leptospira**
0.00 0.00 **FUD** XXX
**AMA:** 2005,Jul,11-12; 2005,Aug,7-8

**86723** **Listeria monocytogenes**
0.00 0.00 **FUD** XXX
**AMA:** 2005,Jul,11-12; 2005,Aug,7-8

**86727** **lymphocytic choriomeningitis**
0.00 0.00 **FUD** XXX
**AMA:** 2005,Jul,11-12; 2005,Aug,7-8

**86729** lymphogranuloma venereum

**86732** **mucormycosis**
0.00 0.00 **FUD** XXX
**AMA:** 2005,Jul,11-12; 2005,Aug,7-8

**86735** **mumps**
0.00 0.00 **FUD** XXX
**AMA:** 2017,Jan,8; 2016,Jan,13; 2015,Jan,16; 2014,Jan,11; 2012,Jan,15-42

**86738** **mycoplasma**
0.00 0.00 **FUD** XXX
**AMA:** 2005,Jul,11-12; 2005,Aug,7-8

**86741** **Neisseria meningitidis**
0.00 0.00 **FUD** XXX
**AMA:** 2005,Jul,11-12; 2005,Aug,7-8

**86744** **Nocardia**
0.00 0.00 **FUD** XXX
**AMA:** 2005,Jul,11-12; 2005,Aug,7-8

**86747** **parvovirus**
0.00 0.00 **FUD** XXX
**AMA:** 2005,Jul,11-12; 2005,Aug,7-8

**86750** **Plasmodium (malaria)**
0.00 0.00 **FUD** XXX
**AMA:** 2005,Jul,11-12; 2005,Aug,7-8

**86753** **protozoa, not elsewhere specified**
0.00 0.00 **FUD** XXX
**AMA:** 2005,Jul,11-12; 2005,Aug,7-8

**86756** **respiratory syncytial virus**
0.00 0.00 **FUD** XXX
**AMA:** 2005,Jul,11-12; 2005,Aug,7-8

**86757** **Rickettsia**
0.00 0.00 **FUD** XXX
**AMA:** 2005,Jul,11-12; 2005,Aug,7-8

**86759** **rotavirus**
0.00 0.00 **FUD** XXX
**AMA:** 2005,Jul,11-12; 2005,Aug,7-8

**86762** **rubella**
0.00 0.00 **FUD** XXX
**AMA:** 2005,Jul,11-12; 2005,Aug,7-8

**86765** **rubeola**
0.00 0.00 **FUD** XXX
**AMA:** 2005,Jul,11-12; 2005,Aug,7-8

**86768** **Salmonella**
0.00 0.00 **FUD** XXX
**AMA:** 2005,Jul,11-12; 2005,Aug,7-8

**86771** **Shigella**
0.00 0.00 **FUD** XXX
**AMA:** 2005,Jul,11-12; 2005,Aug,7-8

**86774** **tetanus**
0.00 0.00 **FUD** XXX
**AMA:** 2005,Jul,11-12; 2005,Aug,7-8

**86777** **Toxoplasma**
0.00 0.00 **FUD** XXX
**AMA:** 2005,Jul,11-12; 2005,Aug,7-8

**86778** **Toxoplasma, IgM**
0.00 0.00 **FUD** XXX
**AMA:** 2005,Jul,11-12; 2005,Aug,7-8

**86780** **Treponema pallidum**
0.00 0.00 **FUD** XXX
EXCLUDES Nontreponemal antibody analysis syphilis testing (86592-86593)

| | 86784 | **Trichinella** |
|---|---|---|
| | | 0.00  0.00  **FUD** XXX |
| | | AMA: 2005,Jul,11-12; 2005,Aug,7-8 |

| | 86787 | **varicella-zoster** |
|---|---|---|
| | | 0.00  0.00  **FUD** XXX |
| | | AMA: 2005,Jul,11-12; 2005,Aug,7-8 |

| | 86788 | **West Nile virus, IgM** |
|---|---|---|
| | | 0.00  0.00  **FUD** XXX |

| | 86789 | **West Nile virus** |
|---|---|---|
| | | 0.00  0.00  **FUD** XXX |

| | 86790 | **virus, not elsewhere specified** |
|---|---|---|
| | | 0.00  0.00  **FUD** XXX |
| | | AMA: 2005,Jul,11-12; 2005,Aug,7-8 |

| | 86793 | **Yersinia** |
|---|---|---|
| | | 0.00  0.00  **FUD** XXX |
| | | AMA: 2005,Jul,11-12; 2005,Aug,7-8 |

● 86794 **Zika virus, IgM**

86800 **Thyroglobulin antibody**
 EXCLUDES *Thyroglobulin (84432)*
 0.00  0.00  **FUD** XXX
 AMA: 2005,Jul,11-12; 2005,Aug,7-8

86803 **Hepatitis C antibody;**
 0.00  0.00  **FUD** XXX
 AMA: 2005,Jul,11-12; 2005,Aug,7-8

86804 **confirmatory test (eg, immunoblot)**
 0.00  0.00  **FUD** XXX
 AMA: 2017,Jan,8; 2016,Jan,13; 2015,Jan,16; 2014,Jan,11

## 86805-86808 Pre-Transplant Antibody Cross Matching

86805 **Lymphocytotoxicity assay, visual crossmatch; with titration**
 0.00  0.00  **FUD** XXX
 AMA: 2017,Jan,8; 2016,Jan,13; 2015,Jan,16; 2014,Jan,11

86806 **without titration**
 0.00  0.00  **FUD** XXX
 AMA: 2005,Aug,7-8; 2005,Jul,11-12

86807 **Serum screening for cytotoxic percent reactive antibody (PRA); standard method**
 0.00  0.00  **FUD** XXX
 AMA: 2017,Jan,8; 2016,Jan,13; 2015,Jan,16; 2014,Jan,11; 2012,Jan,15-42

86808 **quick method**
 0.00  0.00  **FUD** XXX
 AMA: 2017,Jan,8; 2016,Jan,13; 2015,Jan,16; 2014,Jan,11; 2012,Jan,15-42

## 86812-86826 Histocompatibility Testing

**CMS:** 100-03,110.23 Stem Cell Transplantation; 100-03,190.1 Histocompatibility Testing; 100-04,3,90.3 Stem Cell Transplantation; 100-04,3,90.3.1 Allogeneic Stem Cell Transplantation; 100-04,3,90.3.3 Billing for Allogeneic Stem Cell Transplants; 100-04,32,90 Billing for Stem Cell Transplantation; 100-04,4,231.11 Billing for Allogeneic Stem Cell Transplants

 EXCLUDES *HLA typing by molecular pathology techniques (81370-81383)*

86812 **HLA typing; A, B, or C (eg, A10, B7, B27), single antigen**
 0.00  0.00  **FUD** XXX
 AMA: 2017,Jan,8; 2016,Jan,13; 2015,Jan,16; 2014,Jan,11; 2012,May,3-10; 2012,Jan,15-42

86813 **A, B, or C, multiple antigens**
 0.00  0.00  **FUD** XXX
 AMA: 2017,Jan,8; 2016,Jan,13; 2015,Jan,16; 2014,Jan,11; 2012,May,3-10; 2012,Jan,15-42

86816 **DR/DQ, single antigen**
 0.00  0.00  **FUD** XXX
 AMA: 2017,Jan,8; 2016,Jan,13; 2015,Jan,16; 2014,Jan,11; 2012,May,3-10; 2012,Jan,15-42

86817 **DR/DQ, multiple antigens**
 0.00  0.00  **FUD** XXX
 AMA: 2017,Jan,8; 2016,Jan,13; 2015,Jan,16; 2014,Jan,11; 2012,May,3-10; 2012,Jan,15-42

86821 **lymphocyte culture, mixed (MLC)**
 0.00  0.00  **FUD** XXX
 AMA: 2017,Jan,8; 2016,Jan,13; 2015,Jan,16; 2014,Jan,11; 2012,Jan,15-42

~~86822~~ ~~lymphocyte culture, primed (PLC)~~

86825 **Human leukocyte antigen (HLA) crossmatch, non-cytotoxic (eg, using flow cytometry); first serum sample or dilution**
 0.00  0.00  **FUD** XXX
 INCLUDES Autologous HLA crossmatch
 EXCLUDES *B cells (86355)*
 *Flow cytometry (88184-88189)*
 *Lymphocytotoxicity visual crossmatch (86805-86806)*
 *T cells (86359)*

+ 86826 **each additional serum sample or sample dilution (List separately in addition to primary procedure)**
 0.00  0.00  **FUD** XXX
 INCLUDES Autologous HLA crossmatch
 EXCLUDES *B cells (86355)*
 *Flow cytometry (88184-88189)*
 *Lymphocytotoxicity visual crossmatch (86805-86806)*
 *T cells (86359)*
 Code first (86825)

## 86828-86849 HLA Antibodies

86828 **Antibody to human leukocyte antigens (HLA), solid phase assays (eg, microspheres or beads, ELISA, flow cytometry); qualitative assessment of the presence or absence of antibody(ies) to HLA Class I and Class II HLA antigens**
 0.00  0.00  **FUD** XXX
 Code also solid phase testing of untreated and treated specimens of either class of HLA after treatment (86828-86833)

86829 **qualitative assessment of the presence or absence of antibody(ies) to HLA Class I or Class II HLA antigens**
 0.00  0.00  **FUD** XXX
 Code also solid phase testing of untreated and treated specimens of either class of HLA after treatment (86828-86833)

86830 **antibody Identification by qualitative panel using complete HLA phenotypes, HLA Class I**
 0.00  0.00  **FUD** XXX
 Code also solid phase testing of untreated and treated specimens of either class of HLA after treatment (86828-86833)

86831 **antibody identification by qualitative panel using complete HLA phenotypes, HLA Class II**
 0.00  0.00  **FUD** XXX
 Code also solid phase testing of untreated and treated specimens of either class of HLA after treatment (86828-86833)

86832 **high definition qualitative panel for identification of antibody specificities (eg, individual antigen per bead methodology), HLA Class I**
 0.00  0.00  **FUD** XXX
 Code also solid phase testing of untreated and treated specimens of either class of HLA after treatment (86828-86833)

86833 **high definition qualitative panel for identification of antibody specificities (eg, individual antigen per bead methodology), HLA Class II**
 0.00  0.00  **FUD** XXX
 Code also solid phase testing of untreated and treated specimens of either class of HLA after treatment (86828-86833)

86834 **semi-quantitative panel (eg, titer), HLA Class I**
 0.00  0.00  **FUD** XXX

86835 **semi-quantitative panel (eg, titer), HLA Class II**
 0.00  0.00  **FUD** XXX

**26/TC** PC/TC Only   **A2-Z3** ASC Payment   **50** Bilateral   ♂ Male Only   ♀ Female Only   Facility RVU   Non-Facility RVU   CCI
**FUD** Follow-up Days   **CMS:** IOM (Pub 100)   **A-Y** OPPSI   **80/80** Surg Assist Allowed / w/Doc   Lab Crosswalk   Radiology Crosswalk   **X** CLIA

**404**
CPT © 2017 American Medical Association. All Rights Reserved.
© 2017 Optum360, LLC

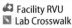

**86849**    **Unlisted immunology procedure**
　🔲 0.00　　🔲 0.00　　**FUD** XXX　　N
　AMA: 2017,Jan,8; 2016,Jan,13; 2015,Jan,16; 2014,Jan,11;
　2012,Jan,15-42

## 86850-86999 Transfusion Services

EXCLUDES　Apheresis (36511-36512)
　　　　　Therapeutic phlebotomy (99195)

**86850**    **Antibody screen, RBC, each serum technique**
　🔲 0.00　　🔲 0.00　　**FUD** XXX　　Q1
　AMA: 2017,Jan,8; 2016,Jan,13; 2015,Jan,16; 2014,Jan,11

**86860**    **Antibody elution (RBC), each elution**
　🔲 0.00　　🔲 0.00　　**FUD** XXX　　Q1
　AMA: 2005,Jul,11-12; 2005,Aug,7-8

**86870**    **Antibody identification, RBC antibodies, each panel for each serum technique**
　🔲 0.00　　🔲 0.00　　**FUD** XXX　　Q2
　AMA: 2017,Jan,8; 2016,Jan,13; 2015,Jan,16; 2014,Jan,11;
　2012,Jan,15-42

**86880**    **Antihuman globulin test (Coombs test); direct, each antiserum**
　🔲 0.00　　🔲 0.00　　**FUD** XXX　　Q1
　AMA: 2005,Aug,7-8; 2005,Jul,11-12

**86885**    **indirect, qualitative, each reagent red cell**
　🔲 0.00　　🔲 0.00　　**FUD** XXX　　Q1
　AMA: 2017,Jan,8; 2016,Jan,13; 2015,Jan,16; 2014,Jan,11

**86886**    **indirect, each antibody titer**
　EXCLUDES　Indirect antihuman globulin (Coombs) test for RBC
　　　　　antibody identification using reagent red cell
　　　　　panels (86870)
　　　　　Indirect antihuman globulin (Coombs) test for RBC
　　　　　antibody screening (86850)
　🔲 0.00　　🔲 0.00　　**FUD** XXX　　Q1
　AMA: 2017,Jan,8; 2016,Jan,13; 2015,Jan,16; 2014,Jan,11

**86890**    **Autologous blood or component, collection processing and storage; predeposited**
　🔲 0.00　　🔲 0.00　　**FUD** XXX　　Q1
　AMA: 2017,Jan,8; 2016,Jan,13; 2015,Jan,16; 2014,Jan,11

**86891**    **intra- or postoperative salvage**
　🔲 0.00　　🔲 0.00　　**FUD** XXX　　Q1
　AMA: 2005,Aug,7-8; 2005,Jul,11-12

**86900**    **Blood typing, serologic; ABO**
　🔲 0.00　　🔲 0.00　　**FUD** XXX　　Q1
　AMA: 2005,Jul,11-12; 2005,Aug,7-8

**86901**    **Rh (D)**
　🔲 0.00　　🔲 0.00　　**FUD** XXX　　Q1
　AMA: 2017,Jan,8; 2016,Jan,13; 2015,Jan,16; 2014,Jan,11

**86902**    **antigen testing of donor blood using reagent serum, each antigen test**
　Code also one time for each antigen for each unit of blood when
　　　multiple units are tested for the same antigen
　🔲 0.00　　🔲 0.00　　**FUD** XXX　　Q1
　AMA: 2010,Dec,7-10

**86904**    **antigen screening for compatible unit using patient serum, per unit screened**
　🔲 0.00　　🔲 0.00　　**FUD** XXX　　Q1
　AMA: 2005,Aug,7-8; 2005,Jul,11-12

**86905**    **RBC antigens, other than ABO or Rh (D), each**
　🔲 0.00　　🔲 0.00　　**FUD** XXX　　Q1
　AMA: 2005,Jul,11-12; 2005,Aug,7-8

**86906**    **Rh phenotyping, complete**
　EXCLUDES　Use of molecular pathology procedures for human
　　　　　erythrocyte antigen typing (81403)
　🔲 0.00　　🔲 0.00　　**FUD** XXX　　Q1
　AMA: 2005,Jul,11-12; 2005,Aug,7-8

**86910**    **Blood typing, for paternity testing, per individual; ABO, Rh and MN**
　🔲 0.00　　🔲 0.00　　**FUD** XXX　　E
　AMA: 2005,Jul,11-12; 2005,Aug,7-8

**86911**    **each additional antigen system**
　🔲 0.00　　🔲 0.00　　**FUD** XXX　　E
　AMA: 2005,Jul,11-12; 2005,Aug,7-8

**86920**    **Compatibility test each unit; immediate spin technique**
　🔲 0.00　　🔲 0.00　　**FUD** XXX　　Q1
　AMA: 2017,Jan,8; 2016,Jan,13; 2015,Jan,16; 2014,Jan,11

**86921**    **incubation technique**
　🔲 0.00　　🔲 0.00　　**FUD** XXX　　Q1
　AMA: 2017,Jan,8; 2016,Jan,13; 2015,Jan,16; 2014,Jan,11

**86922**    **antiglobulin technique**
　🔲 0.00　　🔲 0.00　　**FUD** XXX　　Q1
　AMA: 2017,Jan,8; 2016,Jan,13; 2015,Jan,16; 2014,Jan,11

**86923**    **electronic**
　EXCLUDES　Other compatibility test techniques (86920-86922)
　🔲 0.00　　🔲 0.00　　**FUD** XXX　　Q1
　AMA: 2017,Jan,8; 2016,Jan,13; 2015,Jan,16; 2014,Jan,11

**86927**    **Fresh frozen plasma, thawing, each unit**
　🔲 0.00　　🔲 0.00　　**FUD** XXX　　S
　AMA: 2005,Aug,7-8; 2005,Jul,11-12

**86930**    **Frozen blood, each unit; freezing (includes preparation)**
　🔲 0.00　　🔲 0.00　　**FUD** XXX　　Q1
　AMA: 2017,Jan,8; 2016,Jan,13; 2015,Jan,16; 2014,Jan,11

**86931**    **thawing**
　🔲 0.00　　🔲 0.00　　**FUD** XXX　　Q1
　AMA: 2017,Jan,8; 2016,Jan,13; 2015,Jan,16; 2014,Jan,11

**86932**    **freezing (includes preparation) and thawing**
　🔲 0.00　　🔲 0.00　　**FUD** XXX　　Q1
　AMA: 2017,Jan,8; 2016,Jan,13; 2015,Jan,16; 2014,Jan,11

**86940**    **Hemolysins and agglutinins; auto, screen, each**
　🔲 0.00　　🔲 0.00　　**FUD** XXX　　Q
　AMA: 2005,Aug,7-8; 2005,Jul,11-12

**86941**    **incubated**
　🔲 0.00　　🔲 0.00　　**FUD** XXX　　Q
　AMA: 2005,Jul,11-12; 2005,Aug,7-8

**86945**    **Irradiation of blood product, each unit**
　🔲 0.00　　🔲 0.00　　**FUD** XXX　　Q1
　AMA: 2017,Jan,8; 2016,Jan,13; 2015,Jan,16; 2014,Jan,11;
　2012,Jan,15-42

**86950**    **Leukocyte transfusion**
　EXCLUDES　Infusion allogeneic lymphocytes (38242)
　　　　　Leukapheresis (36511)
　🔲 0.00　　🔲 0.00　　**FUD** XXX　　Q1
　AMA: 2017,Jan,8; 2016,Jan,13; 2015,Jan,16; 2013,Oct,3

**86960**    **Volume reduction of blood or blood product (eg, red blood cells or platelets), each unit**
　🔲 0.00　　🔲 0.00　　**FUD** XXX　　Q1
　AMA: 2017,Jan,8; 2016,Jan,13; 2015,Jan,16; 2014,Jan,11

**86965**    **Pooling of platelets or other blood products**
　EXCLUDES　Autologous WBC injection (0481T)
　　　　　Injection of platelet rich plasma (0232T)
　🔲 0.00　　🔲 0.00　　**FUD** XXX　　Q1
　AMA: 2017,Jan,8; 2016,Jan,13; 2015,Jan,16; 2014,Jan,11

**86970**    **Pretreatment of RBCs for use in RBC antibody detection, identification, and/or compatibility testing; incubation with chemical agents or drugs, each**
　🔲 0.00　　🔲 0.00　　**FUD** XXX　　Q1
　AMA: 2005,Jul,11-12; 2005,Aug,7-8

**86971**    **incubation with enzymes, each**
　🔲 0.00　　🔲 0.00　　**FUD** XXX　　Q1
　AMA: 2005,Jul,11-12; 2005,Aug,7-8

**86972** by density gradient separation
🚑 0.00   ✂ 0.00   **FUD** XXX    [01]
AMA: 2005,Jul,11-12; 2005,Aug,7-8

**86975** Pretreatment of serum for use in RBC antibody identification; incubation with drugs, each
🚑 0.00   ✂ 0.00   **FUD** XXX    [01]
AMA: 2005,Jul,11-12; 2005,Aug,7-8

**86976** by dilution
🚑 0.00   ✂ 0.00   **FUD** XXX    [01]
AMA: 2005,Jul,11-12; 2005,Aug,7-8

**86977** incubation with inhibitors, each
🚑 0.00   ✂ 0.00   **FUD** XXX    [01]
AMA: 2005,Jul,11-12; 2005,Aug,7-8

**86978** by differential red cell absorption using patient RBCs or RBCs of known phenotype, each absorption
🚑 0.00   ✂ 0.00   **FUD** XXX    [01]
AMA: 2005,Jul,11-12; 2005,Aug,7-8

**86985** Splitting of blood or blood products, each unit
🚑 0.00   ✂ 0.00   **FUD** XXX    [01]
AMA: 2017,Jan,8; 2016,Jan,13; 2015,Jan,16; 2014,Jan,11; 2012,May,11-12

**86999** Unlisted transfusion medicine procedure
🚑 0.00   ✂ 0.00   **FUD** XXX    [01]
AMA: 2017,Jan,8; 2016,Jan,13; 2015,Jan,16; 2014,Jan,11; 2012,May,11-12; 2012,Jan,15-42

## 87003-87118 Identification of Microorganisms

INCLUDES   Bacteriology, mycology, parasitology, and virology
EXCLUDES   Additional tests using molecular probes, chromatography, nucleic acid resequencing, or immunologic techniques (87140-87158)
Code also modifier 59 for multiple specimens or sites
Code also modifier 91 for repeat procedures performed on the same day

**87003** Animal inoculation, small animal, with observation and dissection
🚑 0.00   ✂ 0.00   **FUD** XXX    [Q][▢]
AMA: 2005,Aug,7-8; 2005,Jul,11-12

**87015** Concentration (any type), for infectious agents
EXCLUDES   Direct smear for ova and parasites (87177)
🚑 0.00   ✂ 0.00   **FUD** XXX    [Q][▢]
AMA: 2005,Aug,7-8; 2005,Jul,11-12

**87040** Culture, bacterial; blood, aerobic, with isolation and presumptive identification of isolates (includes anaerobic culture, if appropriate)
🚑 0.00   ✂ 0.00   **FUD** XXX    [Q][▢]
AMA: 2017,Jan,8; 2016,Jan,13; 2015,Jan,16; 2014,Jan,11; 2012,Jan,15-42

**87045** stool, aerobic, with isolation and preliminary examination (eg, KIA, LIA), Salmonella and Shigella species
🚑 0.00   ✂ 0.00   **FUD** XXX    [Q][▢]
AMA: 2005,Aug,7-8; 2005,Jul,11-12

**87046** stool, aerobic, additional pathogens, isolation and presumptive identification of isolates, each plate
🚑 0.00   ✂ 0.00   **FUD** XXX    [Q][▢]
AMA: 2017,Jan,8; 2016,Jan,13; 2015,Jan,16; 2014,Jan,11

**87070** any other source except urine, blood or stool, aerobic, with isolation and presumptive identification of isolates
EXCLUDES   Urine (87088)
🚑 0.00   ✂ 0.00   **FUD** XXX    [Q][▢]
AMA: 2017,Jan,8; 2016,Jan,13; 2015,Jan,16; 2014,Jan,11; 2012,Jan,15-42

**87071** quantitative, aerobic with isolation and presumptive identification of isolates, any source except urine, blood or stool
EXCLUDES   Urine (87088)
🚑 0.00   ✂ 0.00   **FUD** XXX    [Q][▢]
AMA: 2017,Jan,8; 2016,Jan,13; 2015,Jan,16; 2014,Jan,11

**87073** quantitative, anaerobic with isolation and presumptive identification of isolates, any source except urine, blood or stool
EXCLUDES   Definitive identification of isolates (87076, 87077)
     Typing of isolates (87140-87158)
🚑 0.00   ✂ 0.00   **FUD** XXX    [Q][▢]
AMA: 2017,Jan,8; 2016,Jan,13; 2015,Jan,16; 2014,Jan,11

**87075** any source, except blood, anaerobic with isolation and presumptive identification of isolates
🚑 0.00   ✂ 0.00   **FUD** XXX    [Q][▢]
AMA: 2005,Aug,7-8; 2005,Jul,11-12

**87076** anaerobic isolate, additional methods required for definitive identification, each isolate
🚑 0.00   ✂ 0.00   **FUD** XXX    [Q][▢]
AMA: 2017,Jan,8; 2016,Jan,13; 2015,Jan,16; 2014,Jan,11

**87077** aerobic isolate, additional methods required for definitive identification, each isolate
🚑 0.00   ✂ 0.00   **FUD** XXX    [✖][Q][▢]
AMA: 2017,Jan,8; 2016,Jan,13; 2015,Jan,16; 2014,Jan,11; 2012,Jan,15-42

**87081** Culture, presumptive, pathogenic organisms, screening only;
🚑 0.00   ✂ 0.00   **FUD** XXX    [Q][▢]
AMA: 2017,Jan,8; 2016,Jan,13; 2015,Jan,16; 2014,Jan,11

**87084** with colony estimation from density chart
🚑 0.00   ✂ 0.00   **FUD** XXX    [Q][▢]
AMA: 2005,Aug,7-8; 2005,Jul,11-12

**87086** Culture, bacterial; quantitative colony count, urine
🚑 0.00   ✂ 0.00   **FUD** XXX    [Q][▢]
AMA: 2017,Jan,8; 2016,Jan,13; 2015,Jan,16; 2014,Jan,11; 2012,Jan,15-42

**87088** with isolation and presumptive identification of each isolate, urine
🚑 0.00   ✂ 0.00   **FUD** XXX    [Q][▢]
AMA: 2017,Jan,8; 2016,Jan,13; 2015,Jan,16; 2014,Jan,11; 2012,Jan,15-42

**87101** Culture, fungi (mold or yeast) isolation, with presumptive identification of isolates; skin, hair, or nail
🚑 0.00   ✂ 0.00   **FUD** XXX    [Q][▢]
AMA: 2017,Jan,8; 2016,Jan,13; 2015,Jan,16; 2014,Jan,11; 2012,Jan,15-42

**87102** other source (except blood)
🚑 0.00   ✂ 0.00   **FUD** XXX    [Q][▢]
AMA: 2005,Aug,7-8; 2005,Jul,11-12

**87103** blood
🚑 0.00   ✂ 0.00   **FUD** XXX    [Q][▢]
AMA: 2005,Aug,7-8; 2005,Jul,11-12

**87106** Culture, fungi, definitive identification, each organism; yeast
🚑 0.00   ✂ 0.00   **FUD** XXX    [Q][▢]
AMA: 2005,Aug,7-8; 2005,Jul,11-12

**87107** mold
🚑 0.00   ✂ 0.00   **FUD** XXX    [Q][▢]
AMA: 2005,Aug,7-8; 2005,Jul,11-12

**87109** Culture, mycoplasma, any source
🚑 0.00   ✂ 0.00   **FUD** XXX    [Q][▢]
AMA: 2005,Aug,7-8; 2005,Jul,11-12

**87110** Culture, chlamydia, any source
EXCLUDES   Immunofluorescence staining of shell vials (87140)
🚑 0.00   ✂ 0.00   **FUD** XXX    [A][▢]
AMA: 2005,Aug,7-8; 2005,Jul,11-12

26/TC PC/TC Only    A2-Z3 ASC Payment    50 Bilateral    ♂ Male Only    ♀ Female Only    🚑 Facility RVU    ✂ Non-Facility RVU    ▢ CCI
**FUD** Follow-up Days    **CMS:** IOM (Pub 100)    A-Y OPPSI    80/80 Surg Assist Allowed / w/Doc    ▢ Lab Crosswalk    ▢ Radiology Crosswalk    ✖ CLIA
CPT © 2017 American Medical Association. All Rights Reserved.

© 2017 Optum360, LLC

**87116** Culture, tubercle or other acid-fast bacilli (eg, TB, AFB, mycobacteria) any source, with isolation and presumptive identification of isolates

> EXCLUDES   Concentration (87015)

🔧 0.00   ✂ 0.00   **FUD** XXX   ⓠ🔲

**AMA:** 2005,Aug,7-8; 2005,Jul,11-12

**87118** Culture, mycobacterial, definitive identification, each isolate

🔧 0.00   ✂ 0.00   **FUD** XXX   ⓠ🔲

**AMA:** 2005,Aug,7-8; 2005,Jul,11-12

## 87140-87158 Additional Culture Typing Techniques

> INCLUDES   Bacteriology, mycology, parasitology, and virology
> EXCLUDES   Use of molecular procedure codes as a substitute for codes in this range (81200-81408 [81161, 81162, 81287, 81288])

Code also definitive identification
Code also modifier 59 for multiple specimens or sites
Code also modifier 91 for repeat procedures performed on the same day

**87140** Culture, typing; immunofluorescent method, each antiserum

🔧 0.00   ✂ 0.00   **FUD** XXX   ⓠ🔲

**AMA:** 2017,Jan,8; 2016,Jan,13; 2015,Jan,16; 2014,Jan,11

**87143** gas liquid chromatography (GLC) or high pressure liquid chromatography (HPLC) method

🔧 0.00   ✂ 0.00   **FUD** XXX   ⓠ🔲

**AMA:** 2005,Aug,7-8; 2005,Jul,11-12

**87147** immunologic method, other than immunofluorescence (eg, agglutination grouping), per antiserum

🔧 0.00   ✂ 0.00   **FUD** XXX   ⓠ🔲

**AMA:** 2017,Jan,8; 2016,Jan,13; 2015,Jan,16; 2014,Jan,11; 2012,Jan,15-42

**87149** identification by nucleic acid (DNA or RNA) probe, direct probe technique, per culture or isolate, each organism probed

🔧 0.00   ✂ 0.00   **FUD** XXX   ⓠ🔲

**AMA:** 2017,Jan,8; 2016,Jan,13; 2015,Jan,16; 2014,Jan,11; 2013,Sep,3-12; 2012,May,3-10

**87150** identification by nucleic acid (DNA or RNA) probe, amplified probe technique, per culture or isolate, each organism probed

🔧 0.00   ✂ 0.00   **FUD** XXX   ⓠ🔲

**AMA:** 2017,Jan,8; 2016,Jan,13; 2015,Jan,16; 2014,Jan,11; 2013,Sep,3-12; 2012,May,3-10

**87152** identification by pulse field gel typing

🔧 0.00   ✂ 0.00   **FUD** XXX   ⓠ🔲

**AMA:** 2017,Jan,8; 2016,Jan,13; 2015,Jan,16; 2014,Jan,11; 2013,Sep,3-12; 2012,May,3-10

**87153** identification by nucleic acid sequencing method, each isolate (eg, sequencing of the 16S rRNA gene)

🔧 0.00   ✂ 0.00   **FUD** XXX   ⓠ🔲

**AMA:** 2017,Jan,8; 2016,Jan,13; 2015,Jan,16; 2013,Sep,3-12; 2012,May,3-10

**87158** other methods

🔧 0.00   ✂ 0.00   **FUD** XXX   ⓠ🔲

**AMA:** 2017,Jan,8; 2016,Jan,13; 2015,Jan,16; 2014,Jan,11

## 87164-87255 Identification of Organism from Primary Source and Sensitivity Studies

> INCLUDES   Bacteriology, mycology, parasitology, and virology
> EXCLUDES   Additional tests using molecular probes, chromatography, or immunologic techniques (87140-87158)

Code also modifier 59 for multiple specimens or sites
Code also modifier 91 for repeat procedures performed on the same day

**87164** Dark field examination, any source (eg, penile, vaginal, oral, skin); includes specimen collection

🔧 0.00   ✂ 0.00   **FUD** XXX   ⓠ🔲

**AMA:** 2005,Jul,11-12; 2005,Aug,7-8

**87166** without collection

🔧 0.00   ✂ 0.00   **FUD** XXX   ⓠ🔲

**AMA:** 2005,Aug,7-8; 2005,Jul,11-12

**87168** Macroscopic examination; arthropod

🔧 0.00   ✂ 0.00   **FUD** XXX   ⓠ🔲

**AMA:** 2005,Aug,7-8; 2005,Jul,11-12

**87169** parasite

🔧 0.00   ✂ 0.00   **FUD** XXX   ⓠ🔲

**AMA:** 2005,Aug,7-8; 2005,Jul,11-12

**87172** Pinworm exam (eg, cellophane tape prep)

🔧 0.00   ✂ 0.00   **FUD** XXX   ⓠ🔲

**AMA:** 2005,Aug,7-8; 2005,Jul,11-12

**87176** Homogenization, tissue, for culture

🔧 0.00   ✂ 0.00   **FUD** XXX   ⓠ🔲

**AMA:** 2005,Aug,7-8; 2005,Jul,11-12

**87177** Ova and parasites, direct smears, concentration and identification

> EXCLUDES   Coccidia or microsporidia exam (87207)
> Complex special stain (trichrome, iron hematoxylin) (87209)
> Concentration for infectious agents (87015)
> Direct smears from primary source (87207)
> Nucleic acid probes in cytologic material (88365)

🔧 0.00   ✂ 0.00   **FUD** XXX   ⓠ🔲

**AMA:** 2017,Jan,8; 2016,Jan,13; 2015,Jan,16; 2014,Jan,11; 2012,Jan,15-42

**87181** Susceptibility studies, antimicrobial agent; agar dilution method, per agent (eg, antibiotic gradient strip)

🔧 0.00   ✂ 0.00   **FUD** XXX   ⓠ🔲

**AMA:** 2017,Jan,8; 2016,Jan,13; 2015,Jan,16; 2014,Jan,11

**87184** disk method, per plate (12 or fewer agents)

🔧 0.00   ✂ 0.00   **FUD** XXX   ⓠ🔲

**AMA:** 2017,Jan,8; 2016,Jan,13; 2015,Jan,16; 2014,Jan,11

**87185** enzyme detection (eg, beta lactamase), per enzyme

🔧 0.00   ✂ 0.00   **FUD** XXX   ⓠ🔲

**AMA:** 2017,Jan,8; 2016,Jan,13; 2015,Jan,16; 2014,Jan,11

**87186** microdilution or agar dilution (minimum inhibitory concentration [MIC] or breakpoint), each multi-antimicrobial, per plate

🔧 0.00   ✂ 0.00   **FUD** XXX   ⓠ🔲

**AMA:** 2017,Jan,8; 2016,Jan,13; 2015,Jan,16; 2014,Jan,11

**+ 87187** microdilution or agar dilution, minimum lethal concentration (MLC), each plate (List separately in addition to code for primary procedure)

Code first (87186, 87188)

🔧 0.00   ✂ 0.00   **FUD** XXX   ⓠ🔲

**AMA:** 2017,Jan,8; 2016,Jan,13; 2015,Jan,16; 2014,Jan,11

**87188** macrobroth dilution method, each agent

🔧 0.00   ✂ 0.00   **FUD** XXX   ⓠ🔲

**AMA:** 2017,Jan,8; 2016,Jan,13; 2015,Jan,16; 2014,Jan,11

**87190** mycobacteria, proportion method, each agent

> EXCLUDES   Other mycobacterial susceptibility studies (87181, 87184, 87186, 87188)

🔧 0.00   ✂ 0.00   **FUD** XXX   ⓠ🔲

**AMA:** 2005,Aug,7-8; 2005,Jul,11-12

**87197** Serum bactericidal titer (Schlichter test)

🔧 0.00   ✂ 0.00   **FUD** XXX   ⓠ🔲

**AMA:** 2005,Aug,7-8; 2005,Jul,11-12

**87205** Smear, primary source with interpretation; Gram or Giemsa stain for bacteria, fungi, or cell types

🔧 0.00   ✂ 0.00   **FUD** XXX   ⓠ🔲

**AMA:** 2017,Jan,8; 2016,Jan,13; 2015,Jan,16; 2014,Jan,11; 2012,Jan,15-42

**87206** fluorescent and/or acid fast stain for bacteria, fungi, parasites, viruses or cell types

🔧 0.00   ✂ 0.00   **FUD** XXX   ⓠ🔲

**AMA:** 2005,Aug,7-8; 2005,Jul,11-12

● New Code   ▲ Revised Code   ○ Reinstated   ● New Web Release   ▲ Revised Web Release   Unlisted   Not Covered   # Resequenced
⊘ AMA Mod 51 Exempt   ⑤ Optum Mod 51 Exempt   ⑥ Mod 63 Exempt   ∦ Non-FDA Drug   ★ Telemedicine   Ⓜ Maternity   Ⓐ Age Edit   + Add-on   **AMA:** CPT Asst
© 2017 Optum360, LLC          CPT © 2017 American Medical Association. All Rights Reserved.          **407**

**87207**    special stain for inclusion bodies or parasites (eg, malaria, coccidia, microsporidia, trypanosomes, herpes viruses)

> EXCLUDES   Direct smears with concentration and identification (87177)
>
> Thick smear preparation (87015)

0.00   0.00   **FUD** XXX

AMA: 2017,Jan,8; 2016,Jan,13; 2015,Jan,16; 2014,Jan,11

**87209**    complex special stain (eg, trichrome, iron hemotoxylin) for ova and parasites

0.00   0.00   **FUD** XXX

AMA: 2017,Jan,8; 2016,Jan,13; 2015,Jan,16; 2014,Jan,11

**87210**    wet mount for infectious agents (eg, saline, India ink, KOH preps)

> EXCLUDES   KOH evaluation of skin, hair, or nails (87220)

0.00   0.00   **FUD** XXX

AMA: 2017,Jan,8; 2016,May,13

**87220**    Tissue examination by KOH slide of samples from skin, hair, or nails for fungi or ectoparasite ova or mites (eg, scabies)

0.00   0.00   **FUD** XXX

AMA: 2005,Aug,7-8; 2005,Jul,11-12

**87230**    Toxin or antitoxin assay, tissue culture (eg, Clostridium difficile toxin)

0.00   0.00   **FUD** XXX

AMA: 2005,Aug,7-8; 2005,Jul,11-12

**87250**    Virus isolation; inoculation of embryonated eggs, or small animal, includes observation and dissection

0.00   0.00   **FUD** XXX

AMA: 2005,Aug,7-8; 2005,Jul,11-12

**87252**    tissue culture inoculation, observation, and presumptive identification by cytopathic effect

0.00   0.00   **FUD** XXX

AMA: 2005,Aug,7-8; 2005,Jul,11-12

**87253**    tissue culture, additional studies or definitive identification (eg, hemabsorption, neutralization, immunofluorescence stain), each isolate

> EXCLUDES   Electron microscopy (88348)
>
> Inclusion bodies in:
>
> Fluids (88106)
>
> Smears (87207-87210)
>
> Tissue sections (88304-88309)

0.00   0.00   **FUD** XXX

AMA: 2005,Aug,7-8; 2005,Jul,11-12

**87254**    centrifuge enhanced (shell vial) technique, includes identification with immunofluorescence stain, each virus

Code also (87252)

0.00   0.00   **FUD** XXX

AMA: 2017,Jan,8; 2016,Jan,13; 2015,Jan,16; 2014,Jan,11

**87255**    including identification by non-immunologic method, other than by cytopathic effect (eg, virus specific enzymatic activity)

0.00   0.00   **FUD** XXX

AMA: 2017,Jan,8; 2016,Jan,13; 2015,Jan,16; 2014,Jan,11

## 87260-87300 Fluorescence Microscopy by Organism

INCLUDES   Primary source only

EXCLUDES   Comparable tests on culture material (87140-87158)

Identification of antibodies (86602-86804)

Nonspecific agent detection (87299, 87449-87450, 87797-87799, 87899)

Code also modifier 59 for different species or strains reported by the same code

**87260**    Infectious agent antigen detection by immunofluorescent technique; adenovirus

0.00   0.00   **FUD** XXX

AMA: 2005,Jul,11-12; 2005,Aug,7-8

**87265**    Bordetella pertussis/parapertussis

0.00   0.00   **FUD** XXX

AMA: 2005,Jul,11-12; 2005,Aug,7-8

**87267**    Enterovirus, direct fluorescent antibody (DFA)

0.00   0.00   **FUD** XXX

AMA: 2017,Jan,8; 2016,Jan,13; 2015,Jan,16; 2014,Jan,11

**87269**    giardia

0.00   0.00   **FUD** XXX

AMA: 2005,Jul,11-12; 2005,Aug,7-8

**87270**    Chlamydia trachomatis

0.00   0.00   **FUD** XXX

AMA: 2005,Jul,11-12; 2005,Aug,7-8

**87271**    Cytomegalovirus, direct fluorescent antibody (DFA)

0.00   0.00   **FUD** XXX

AMA: 2017,Jan,8; 2016,Jan,13; 2015,Jan,16; 2014,Jan,11

**87272**    cryptosporidium

0.00   0.00   **FUD** XXX

AMA: 2005,Jul,11-12; 2005,Aug,7-8

**87273**    Herpes simplex virus type 2

0.00   0.00   **FUD** XXX

AMA: 2005,Jul,11-12; 2005,Aug,7-8

**87274**    Herpes simplex virus type 1

0.00   0.00   **FUD** XXX

AMA: 2005,Jul,11-12; 2005,Aug,7-8

**87275**    influenza B virus

0.00   0.00   **FUD** XXX

AMA: 2017,Jan,8; 2016,Jan,13; 2015,Jan,16; 2014,Jan,11

**87276**    influenza A virus

0.00   0.00   **FUD** XXX

AMA: 2017,Jan,8; 2016,Jan,13; 2015,Jan,16; 2014,Jan,11

**87277**    ~~Legionella micdadei~~

**87278**    Legionella pneumophila

0.00   0.00   **FUD** XXX

AMA: 2005,Jul,11-12; 2005,Aug,7-8

**87279**    Parainfluenza virus, each type

0.00   0.00   **FUD** XXX

AMA: 2005,Jul,11-12; 2005,Aug,7-8

**87280**    respiratory syncytial virus

0.00   0.00   **FUD** XXX

AMA: 2005,Jul,11-12; 2005,Aug,7-8

**87281**    Pneumocystis carinii

0.00   0.00   **FUD** XXX

AMA: 2005,Jul,11-12; 2005,Aug,7-8

**87283**    Rubeola

0.00   0.00   **FUD** XXX

AMA: 2005,Jul,11-12; 2005,Aug,7-8

**87285**    Treponema pallidum

0.00   0.00   **FUD** XXX

AMA: 2005,Jul,11-12; 2005,Aug,7-8

**87290**    Varicella zoster virus

0.00   0.00   **FUD** XXX

AMA: 2005,Jul,11-12; 2005,Aug,7-8

**87299**    not otherwise specified, each organism

0.00   0.00   **FUD** XXX

AMA: 2017,Jan,8; 2016,Jan,13; 2015,Jan,16; 2014,Jan,11

**87300**    Infectious agent antigen detection by immunofluorescent technique, polyvalent for multiple organisms, each polyvalent antiserum

> EXCLUDES   Physician evaluation of infectious disease agents by immunofluorescence (88346)

0.00   0.00   **FUD** XXX

AMA: 2005,Jul,11-12; 2005,Aug,7-8

26/TC PC/TC Only   A2-73 ASC Payment   50 Bilateral   ♂ Male Only   ♀ Female Only   Facility RVU   Non-Facility RVU   CCI

FUD Follow-up Days   CMS: IOM (Pub 100)   A-Y OPPSI   80/80 Surg Assist Allowed / w/Doc   Lab Crosswalk   Radiology Crosswalk   CLIA

408    CPT © 2017 American Medical Association. All Rights Reserved.    © 2017 Optum360, LLC

## 87301-87451 Enzyme Immunoassay Technique by Organism

INCLUDES Primary source only

EXCLUDES *Comparable tests on culture material (87140-87158)*
*Identification of antibodies (86602-86804)*
*Nonspecific agent detection (87449-87450, 87797-87799, 87899)*
Code also modifier 59 for different species or strains reported by the same code

**87301** **Infectious agent antigen detection by immunoassay technique, (eg, enzyme immunoassay [EIA], enzyme-linked immunosorbent assay [ELISA], immunochemiluminometric assay [IMCA]) qualitative or semiquantitative, multiple-step method; adenovirus enteric types 40/41**
0.00    0.00    **FUD** XXX    Q
**AMA:** 2017,Jan,8; 2016,Jan,13; 2015,Jan,16; 2014,Jan,11

**87305** **Aspergillus**
0.00    0.00    **FUD** XXX    Q

**87320** **Chlamydia trachomatis**
0.00    0.00    **FUD** XXX    A ▢
**AMA:** 2005,Jul,11-12; 2005,Aug,7-8

**87324** **Clostridium difficile toxin(s)**
0.00    0.00    **FUD** XXX    Q ▢
**AMA:** 2005,Jul,11-12; 2005,Aug,7-8

**87327** **Cryptococcus neoformans**
EXCLUDES *Cryptococcus latex agglutination (86403)*
0.00    0.00    **FUD** XXX    Q
**AMA:** 2005,Jul,11-12; 2005,Aug,7-8

**87328** **cryptosporidium**
0.00    0.00    **FUD** XXX    Q ▢
**AMA:** 2005,Jul,11-12; 2005,Aug,7-8

**87329** **giardia**
0.00    0.00    **FUD** XXX    Q ▢
**AMA:** 2005,Jul,11-12; 2005,Aug,7-8

**87332** **cytomegalovirus**
0.00    0.00    **FUD** XXX    Q ▢
**AMA:** 2005,Jul,11-12; 2005,Aug,7-8

**87335** **Escherichia coli 0157**
EXCLUDES *Giardia antigen (87329)*
0.00    0.00    **FUD** XXX    Q
**AMA:** 2005,Jul,11-12; 2005,Aug,7-8

**87336** **Entamoeba histolytica dispar group**
0.00    0.00    **FUD** XXX    Q
**AMA:** 2005,Jul,11-12; 2005,Aug,7-8

**87337** **Entamoeba histolytica group**
0.00    0.00    **FUD** XXX    Q
**AMA:** 2005,Jul,11-12; 2005,Aug,7-8

**87338** **Helicobacter pylori, stool**
0.00    0.00    **FUD** XXX    X Q ▢
**AMA:** 2017,Jan,8; 2016,Jan,13; 2015,Jan,16; 2014,Jan,11

**87339** **Helicobacter pylori**
EXCLUDES *H. pylori:*
*Breath and blood by mass spectrometry (83013-83014)*
*Liquid scintillation counter (78267-78268)*
*Stool (87338)*
0.00    0.00    **FUD** XXX    Q ▢
**AMA:** 2005,Jul,11-12; 2005,Aug,7-8

**87340** **hepatitis B surface antigen (HBsAg)**
0.00    0.00    **FUD** XXX    Q
**AMA:** 2017,Jan,8; 2016,Jan,13; 2015,Jan,16; 2014,Jan,11

**87341** **hepatitis B surface antigen (HBsAg) neutralization**
0.00    0.00    **FUD** XXX    A
**AMA:** 2005,Jul,11-12; 2005,Aug,7-8

**87350** **hepatitis Be antigen (HBeAg)**
0.00    0.00    **FUD** XXX    Q ▢
**AMA:** 2005,Jul,11-12; 2005,Aug,7-8

**87380** **hepatitis, delta agent**
0.00    0.00    **FUD** XXX    Q
**AMA:** 2005,Jul,11-12; 2005,Aug,7-8

**87385** **Histoplasma capsulatum**
0.00    0.00    **FUD** XXX    Q
**AMA:** 2005,Jul,11-12; 2005,Aug,7-8

**87389** **HIV-1 antigen(s), with HIV-1 and HIV-2 antibodies, single result**
0.00    0.00    **FUD** XXX    Q ▢
Code also modifier 92 for test performed using a kit or transportable instrument that is all or in part consists of a single-use, disposable analytical chamber

**87390** **HIV-1**
0.00    0.00    **FUD** XXX    Q ▢
**AMA:** 2005,Jul,11-12; 2005,Aug,7-8

**87391** **HIV-2**
0.00    0.00    **FUD** XXX    Q
**AMA:** 2005,Jul,11-12; 2005,Aug,7-8

**87400** **Influenza, A or B, each**
0.00    0.00    **FUD** XXX    Q ▢
**AMA:** 2017,Jan,8; 2016,Jan,13; 2015,Jan,16; 2014,Jan,11; 2012,Jan,15-42

**87420** **respiratory syncytial virus**
0.00    0.00    **FUD** XXX    Q
**AMA:** 2005,Jul,11-12; 2005,Aug,7-8

**87425** **rotavirus**
0.00    0.00    **FUD** XXX    Q ▢
**AMA:** 2005,Jul,11-12; 2005,Aug,7-8

**87427** **Shiga-like toxin**
0.00    0.00    **FUD** XXX    Q
**AMA:** 2005,Jul,11-12; 2005,Aug,7-8

**87430** **Streptococcus, group A**
0.00    0.00    **FUD** XXX    Q ▢
**AMA:** 2017,Jan,8; 2016,Jan,13; 2015,Jan,16; 2012,Jan,15-42

**87449** **Infectious agent antigen detection by immunoassay technique, (eg, enzyme immunoassay [EIA], enzyme-linked immunosorbent assay [ELISA], immunochemiluminometric assay [IMCA]), qualitative or semiquantitative; multiple-step method, not otherwise specified, each organism**
0.00    0.00    **FUD** XXX    X Q ▢
**AMA:** 2017,Jan,8; 2016,Jan,13; 2015,Jan,16; 2014,Jan,11; 2012,Jan,15-42

**87450** **single step method, not otherwise specified, each organism**
0.00    0.00    **FUD** XXX    Q
**AMA:** 2005,Jul,11-12; 2005,Aug,7-8

**87451** **multiple step method, polyvalent for multiple organisms, each polyvalent antiserum**
0.00    0.00    **FUD** XXX    Q
**AMA:** 2005,Jul,11-12; 2005,Aug,7-8

## 87470-87801 [87623, 87624, 87625] Detection Infectious Agent by Probe Techniques

INCLUDES Primary source only

EXCLUDES *Comparable tests on culture material (87140-87158)*
*Identification of antibodies (86602-86804)*
*Nonspecific agent detection (87299, 87449-87450, 87797-87799, 87899)*
*Use of molecular procedure codes as a substitute for codes in this range (81161-81408 [81105, 81106, 81107, 81108, 81109, 81110, 81111, 81112, 81120, 81121, 81161, 81162, 81230, 81231, 81238, 81269, 81283, 81287, 81288, 81334])*
Code also modifier 59 for different species or strains reported by the same code

**87470** ~~Infectious agent detection by nucleic acid (DNA or RNA); Bartonella henselae and Bartonella quintana, direct probe technique~~

● New Code    ▲ Revised Code    ○ Reinstated    ● New Web Release    ▲ Revised Web Release    Unlisted    Not Covered    # Resequenced
⊘ AMA Mod 51 Exempt    ⑤ Optum Mod 51 Exempt    ⑥ Mod 63 Exempt    ✔ Non-FDA Drug    ★ Telemedicine    Ⓜ Maternity    Ⓐ Age Edit    ✛ Add-on    **AMA:** CPT Asst
© 2017 Optum360, LLC    CPT © 2017 American Medical Association. All Rights Reserved.    **409**

**87471** Infectious agent detection by nucleic acid (DNA or RNA); Bartonella henselae and Bartonella quintana, amplified probe technique

🔲 0.00    🔲 0.00    **FUD** XXX    ⊡⊡

**AMA:** 2017,Jan,8; 2016,Jan,13; 2015,Jan,16; 2013,Sep,3-12; 2012,May,3-10

**87472** Bartonella henselae and Bartonella quintana, quantification

🔲 0.00    🔲 0.00    **FUD** XXX    ⊡⊡

**AMA:** 2017,Jan,8; 2016,Jan,13; 2015,Jan,16; 2013,Sep,3-12; 2012,May,3-10

**87475** Borrelia burgdorferi, direct probe technique

🔲 0.00    🔲 0.00    **FUD** XXX    ⊡⊡

**AMA:** 2017,Jan,8; 2016,Jan,13; 2015,Jan,16; 2013,Sep,3-12; 2012,May,3-10

**87476** Borrelia burgdorferi, amplified probe technique

🔲 0.00    🔲 0.00    **FUD** XXX    ⊡⊡

**AMA:** 2017,Jan,8; 2016,Jan,13; 2015,Jan,16; 2013,Sep,3-12; 2012,May,3-10

**87477** ~~Borrelia burgdorferi, quantification~~

**87480** Candida species, direct probe technique

🔲 0.00    🔲 0.00    **FUD** XXX    ⊡⊡

**AMA:** 2017,Jan,8; 2016,Jan,13; 2015,Jan,16; 2013,Sep,3-12; 2012,May,3-10

**87481** Candida species, amplified probe technique

🔲 0.00    🔲 0.00    **FUD** XXX    ⊡⊡

**AMA:** 2017,Jan,8; 2016,Jan,13; 2015,Jan,16; 2013,Sep,3-12; 2012,May,3-10

**87482** Candida species, quantification

🔲 0.00    🔲 0.00    **FUD** XXX    ⊡⊡

**AMA:** 2017,Jan,8; 2016,Jan,13; 2015,Jan,16; 2013,Sep,3-12; 2012,May,3-10

**87483** central nervous system pathogen (eg, Neisseria meningitidis, Streptococcus pneumoniae, Listeria, Haemophilus influenzae, E. coli, Streptococcus agalactiae, enterovirus, human parechovirus, herpes simplex virus type 1 and 2, human herpesvirus 6, cytomegalovirus, varicella zoster virus, Cryptococcus), includes multiplex reverse transcription, when performed, and multiplex amplified probe technique, multiple types or subtypes, 12-25 targets

🔲 0.00    🔲 0.00    **FUD** XXX    ⊡⊡

**87485** Chlamydia pneumoniae, direct probe technique

🔲 0.00    🔲 0.00    **FUD** XXX    ⊡⊡

**AMA:** 2017,Jan,8; 2016,Jan,13; 2015,Jan,16; 2013,Sep,3-12; 2012,May,3-10

**87486** Chlamydia pneumoniae, amplified probe technique

🔲 0.00    🔲 0.00    **FUD** XXX    ⊡⊡

**AMA:** 2017,Jan,8; 2016,Jan,13; 2015,Jan,16; 2013,Sep,3-12; 2012,May,3-10

**87487** Chlamydia pneumoniae, quantification

🔲 0.00    🔲 0.00    **FUD** XXX    ⊡⊡

**AMA:** 2017,Jan,8; 2016,Jan,13; 2015,Jan,16; 2013,Sep,3-12; 2012,May,3-10

**87490** Chlamydia trachomatis, direct probe technique

🔲 0.00    🔲 0.00    **FUD** XXX    Ⓐ⊡

**AMA:** 2017,Jan,8; 2016,Jan,13; 2015,Jan,16; 2013,Sep,3-12; 2012,May,3-10

**87491** Chlamydia trachomatis, amplified probe technique

🔲 0.00    🔲 0.00    **FUD** XXX    Ⓐ⊡

**AMA:** 2017,Jan,8; 2016,Jan,13; 2015,Jan,16; 2013,Jun,13; 2012,May,3-10

**87492** Chlamydia trachomatis, quantification

🔲 0.00    🔲 0.00    **FUD** XXX    ⊡⊡

**AMA:** 2017,Jan,8; 2016,Jan,13; 2015,Jan,16; 2013,Sep,3-12; 2012,May,3-10

**87493** Clostridium difficile, toxin gene(s), amplified probe technique

🔲 0.00    🔲 0.00    **FUD** XXX    ⊡⊡

**AMA:** 2017,Jan,8; 2016,Jan,13; 2015,Jan,16; 2014,Jan,11; 2013,Sep,3-12; 2012,May,3-10

**87495** cytomegalovirus, direct probe technique

🔲 0.00    🔲 0.00    **FUD** XXX    ⊡⊡

**AMA:** 2017,Jan,8; 2016,Jan,13; 2015,Jan,16; 2013,Sep,3-12; 2012,May,3-10

**87496** cytomegalovirus, amplified probe technique

🔲 0.00    🔲 0.00    **FUD** XXX    ⊡⊡

**AMA:** 2017,Jan,8; 2016,Jan,13; 2015,Jan,16; 2013,Sep,3-12; 2012,May,3-10

**87497** cytomegalovirus, quantification

🔲 0.00    🔲 0.00    **FUD** XXX    ⊡⊡

**AMA:** 2017,Jan,8; 2016,Jan,13; 2015,Jan,16; 2013,Sep,3-12; 2012,May,3-10

**87498** enterovirus, amplified probe technique, includes reverse transcription when performed

🔲 0.00    🔲 0.00    **FUD** XXX    ⊡⊡

**AMA:** 2017,Jan,8; 2016,Jan,13; 2015,Jan,16; 2013,Sep,3-12; 2012,May,3-10

**87500** vancomycin resistance (eg, enterococcus species van A, van B), amplified probe technique

🔲 0.00    🔲 0.00    **FUD** XXX    ⊡⊡

**AMA:** 2017,Jan,8; 2016,Jan,13; 2015,Jan,16; 2014,Jan,11; 2013,Sep,3-12; 2012,May,3-10

**87501** influenza virus, includes reverse transcription, when performed, and amplified probe technique, each type or subtype

🔲 0.00    🔲 0.00    **FUD** XXX    ⊡⊡

**AMA:** 2017,Jan,8; 2016,Jan,13; 2015,Jan,16; 2013,Sep,3-12; 2012,May,3-10

**87502** influenza virus, for multiple types or sub-types, includes multiplex reverse transcription, when performed, and multiplex amplified probe technique, first 2 types or sub-types

🔲 0.00    🔲 0.00    **FUD** XXX    ☒⊡⊡

**AMA:** 2017,Jan,8; 2016,Jan,13; 2015,Jan,16; 2013,Sep,3-12; 2012,May,3-10

+ **87503** Influenza virus, for multiple types or sub-types, includes multiplex reverse transcription, when performed, and multiplex amplified probe technique, each additional influenza virus type or sub-type beyond 2 (List separately in addition to code for primary procedure)

Code first (87502)

🔲 0.00    🔲 0.00    **FUD** XXX    ⊡⊡

**AMA:** 2017,Jan,8; 2016,Jan,13; 2015,Jan,16; 2013,Sep,3-12; 2012,May,3-10

**87505** gastrointestinal pathogen (eg, Clostridium difficile, E. coli, Salmonella, Shigella, norovirus, Giardia), includes multiplex reverse transcription, when performed, and multiplex amplified probe technique, multiple types or subtypes, 3-5 targets

🔲 0.00    🔲 0.00    **FUD** XXX    ⊡⊡

**87506** gastrointestinal pathogen (eg, Clostridium difficile, E. coli, Salmonella, Shigella, norovirus, Giardia), includes multiplex reverse transcription, when performed, and multiplex amplified probe technique, multiple types or subtypes, 6-11 targets

🔲 0.00    🔲 0.00    **FUD** XXX    ⊡⊡

**87507** gastrointestinal pathogen (eg, Clostridium difficile, E. coli, Salmonella, Shigella, norovirus, Giardia), includes multiplex reverse transcription, when performed, and multiplex amplified probe technique, multiple types or subtypes, 12-25 targets

🔲 0.00    🔲 0.00    **FUD** XXX    ⊡⊡

87510 **Gardnerella vaginalis, direct probe technique**
🚑 0.00 ⚕ 0.00 **FUD** XXX 🔲🖳
**AMA:** 2017,Jan,8; 2016,Jan,13; 2015,Jan,16; 2013,Sep,3-12; 2012,May,3-10

87511 **Gardnerella vaginalis, amplified probe technique**
🚑 0.00 ⚕ 0.00 **FUD** XXX 🔲🖳
**AMA:** 2017,Jan,8; 2016,Jan,13; 2015,Jan,16; 2013,Sep,3-12; 2012,May,3-10

87512 **Gardnerella vaginalis, quantification**
🚑 0.00 ⚕ 0.00 **FUD** XXX 🔲🖳
**AMA:** 2017,Jan,8; 2016,Jan,13; 2015,Jan,16; 2013,Sep,3-12; 2012,May,3-10

87515 ~~hepatitis B virus, direct probe technique~~

87516 **hepatitis B virus, amplified probe technique**
🚑 0.00 ⚕ 0.00 **FUD** XXX 🔲🖳
**AMA:** 2017,Jan,8; 2016,Jan,13; 2015,Jan,16; 2013,Sep,3-12; 2012,May,3-10

87517 **hepatitis B virus, quantification**
🚑 0.00 ⚕ 0.00 **FUD** XXX 🔲🖳
**AMA:** 2017,Jan,8; 2016,Jan,13; 2015,Jan,16; 2013,Sep,3-12; 2012,May,3-10

87520 **hepatitis C, direct probe technique**
🚑 0.00 ⚕ 0.00 **FUD** XXX 🔲🖳
**AMA:** 2017,Jan,8; 2016,Jan,13; 2015,Jan,16; 2013,Sep,3-12; 2012,May,3-10

87521 **hepatitis C, amplified probe technique, includes reverse transcription when performed**
🚑 0.00 ⚕ 0.00 **FUD** XXX 🔲🖳
**AMA:** 2017,Jan,8; 2016,Jan,13; 2015,Jan,16; 2013,Sep,3-12; 2012,May,3-10

87522 **hepatitis C, quantification, includes reverse transcription when performed**
🚑 0.00 ⚕ 0.00 **FUD** XXX 🔲🖳
**AMA:** 2017,Jan,8; 2016,Jan,13; 2015,Jan,16; 2013,Sep,3-12; 2012,May,3-10

87525 **hepatitis G, direct probe technique**
🚑 0.00 ⚕ 0.00 **FUD** XXX 🔲🖳
**AMA:** 2017,Jan,8; 2016,Jan,13; 2015,Jan,16; 2013,Sep,3-12; 2012,May,3-10

87526 **hepatitis G, amplified probe technique**
🚑 0.00 ⚕ 0.00 **FUD** XXX 🔲🖳
**AMA:** 2017,Jan,8; 2016,Jan,13; 2015,Jan,16; 2013,Sep,3-12; 2012,May,3-10

87527 **hepatitis G, quantification**
🚑 0.00 ⚕ 0.00 **FUD** XXX 🔲🖳
**AMA:** 2017,Jan,8; 2016,Jan,13; 2015,Jan,16; 2013,Sep,3-12; 2012,May,3-10

87528 **Herpes simplex virus, direct probe technique**
🚑 0.00 ⚕ 0.00 **FUD** XXX 🔲🖳
**AMA:** 2017,Jan,8; 2016,Jan,13; 2015,Jan,16; 2013,Sep,3-12; 2012,May,3-10

87529 **Herpes simplex virus, amplified probe technique**
🚑 0.00 ⚕ 0.00 **FUD** XXX 🔲🖳
**AMA:** 2017,Jan,8; 2016,Jan,13; 2015,Jan,16; 2013,Sep,3-12; 2012,May,3-10

87530 **Herpes simplex virus, quantification**
🚑 0.00 ⚕ 0.00 **FUD** XXX 🔲🖳
**AMA:** 2017,Jan,8; 2016,Jan,13; 2015,Jan,16; 2013,Sep,3-12; 2012,May,3-10

87531 **Herpes virus-6, direct probe technique**
🚑 0.00 ⚕ 0.00 **FUD** XXX 🔲🖳
**AMA:** 2017,Jan,8; 2016,Jan,13; 2015,Jan,16; 2013,Sep,3-12; 2012,May,3-10

87532 **Herpes virus-6, amplified probe technique**
🚑 0.00 ⚕ 0.00 **FUD** XXX 🔲🖳
**AMA:** 2017,Jan,8; 2016,Jan,13; 2015,Jan,16; 2013,Sep,3-12; 2012,May,3-10

87533 **Herpes virus-6, quantification**
🚑 0.00 ⚕ 0.00 **FUD** XXX 🔲🖳
**AMA:** 2017,Jan,8; 2016,Jan,13; 2015,Jan,16; 2013,Sep,3-12; 2012,May,3-10

87534 **HIV-1, direct probe technique**
🚑 0.00 ⚕ 0.00 **FUD** XXX 🔲🖳
**AMA:** 2017,Jan,8; 2016,Jan,13; 2015,Jan,16; 2013,Sep,3-12; 2012,May,3-10

87535 **HIV-1, amplified probe technique, includes reverse transcription when performed**
🚑 0.00 ⚕ 0.00 **FUD** XXX 🔲🖳
**AMA:** 2017,Jan,8; 2016,Jan,13; 2015,Jan,16; 2014,Jan,11; 2013,Sep,3-12; 2012,May,3-10

87536 **HIV-1, quantification, includes reverse transcription when performed**
🚑 0.00 ⚕ 0.00 **FUD** XXX 🔲🖳
**AMA:** 2017,Jan,8; 2016,Jan,13; 2015,Jan,16; 2014,Jan,11; 2013,Sep,3-12; 2012,May,3-10; 2012,Jan,15-42

87537 **HIV-2, direct probe technique**
🚑 0.00 ⚕ 0.00 **FUD** XXX 🔲🖳
**AMA:** 2017,Jan,8; 2016,Jan,13; 2015,Jan,16; 2013,Sep,3-12; 2012,May,3-10

87538 **HIV-2, amplified probe technique, includes reverse transcription when performed**
🚑 0.00 ⚕ 0.00 **FUD** XXX 🔲🖳
**AMA:** 2017,Jan,8; 2016,Jan,13; 2015,Jan,16; 2013,Sep,3-12; 2012,May,3-10

87539 **HIV-2, quantification, includes reverse transcription when performed**
🚑 0.00 ⚕ 0.00 **FUD** XXX 🔲🖳
**AMA:** 2017,Jan,8; 2016,Jan,13; 2015,Jan,16; 2013,Sep,3-12; 2012,May,3-10

\# 87623 **Human Papillomavirus (HPV), low-risk types (eg, 6, 11, 42, 43, 44)**
🚑 0.00 ⚕ 0.00 **FUD** XXX 🔲🖳

\# 87624 **Human Papillomavirus (HPV), high-risk types (eg, 16, 18, 31, 33, 35, 39, 45, 51, 52, 56, 58, 59, 68)**
INCLUDES Low- and high-risk types in one assay
🚑 0.00 ⚕ 0.00 **FUD** XXX 🔲🖳
**AMA:** 2017,Jan,8; 2016,Jan,13; 2015,Oct,9

\# 87625 **Human Papillomavirus (HPV), types 16 and 18 only, includes type 45, if performed**
EXCLUDES *HPV detection (genotyping) (0500T)*
🚑 0.00 ⚕ 0.00 **FUD** XXX 🔲🖳
**AMA:** 2017,Jan,8; 2016,Jan,13; 2015,Oct,9; 2015,Jun,10

87540 **Legionella pneumophila, direct probe technique**
🚑 0.00 ⚕ 0.00 **FUD** XXX 🔲🖳
**AMA:** 2017,Jan,8; 2016,Jan,13; 2015,Jan,16; 2013,Sep,3-12; 2012,May,3-10

87541 **Legionella pneumophila, amplified probe technique**
🚑 0.00 ⚕ 0.00 **FUD** XXX 🔲🖳
**AMA:** 2017,Jan,8; 2016,Jan,13; 2015,Jan,16; 2013,Sep,3-12; 2012,May,3-10

87542 **Legionella pneumophila, quantification**
🚑 0.00 ⚕ 0.00 **FUD** XXX 🔲🖳
**AMA:** 2017,Jan,8; 2016,Jan,13; 2015,Jan,16; 2013,Sep,3-12; 2012,May,3-10

87550 **Mycobacteria species, direct probe technique**
🚑 0.00 ⚕ 0.00 **FUD** XXX 🔲🖳
**AMA:** 2017,Jan,8; 2016,Jan,13; 2015,Jan,16; 2013,Sep,3-12; 2012,May,3-10

87551 **Mycobacteria species, amplified probe technique**
🚑 0.00 ⚕ 0.00 **FUD** XXX 🔲🖳
**AMA:** 2017,Jan,8; 2016,Jan,13; 2015,Jan,16; 2013,Sep,3-12; 2012,May,3-10

---

● New Code  ▲ Revised Code  ○ Reinstated  ● New Web Release  ▲ Revised Web Release  Unlisted  Not Covered  # Resequenced
⊘ AMA Mod 51 Exempt  ⑤ Optum Mod 51 Exempt  ⑥ Mod 63 Exempt  ✔ Non-FDA Drug  ★ Telemedicine  Ⓜ Maternity  Ⓐ Age Edit  ✚ Add-on  **AMA:** CPT Asst

**Pathology and Laboratory** *(side tab)*

**87552 — 87652** *(side tab)*

**87552**    **Mycobacteria species, quantification**
     🚑 0.00    🔬 0.00    **FUD** XXX     � symbols
     **AMA:** 2017,Jan,8; 2016,Jan,13; 2015,Jan,16; 2013,Sep,3-12; 2012,May,3-10

**87555**    **Mycobacteria tuberculosis, direct probe technique**
     🚑 0.00    🔬 0.00    **FUD** XXX
     **AMA:** 2017,Jan,8; 2016,Jan,13; 2015,Jan,16; 2013,Sep,3-12; 2012,May,3-10

**87556**    **Mycobacteria tuberculosis, amplified probe technique**
     🚑 0.00    🔬 0.00    **FUD** XXX
     **AMA:** 2017,Jan,8; 2016,Jan,13; 2015,Jan,16; 2013,Sep,3-12; 2012,May,3-10

**87557**    **Mycobacteria tuberculosis, quantification**
     🚑 0.00    🔬 0.00    **FUD** XXX
     **AMA:** 2017,Jan,8; 2016,Jan,13; 2015,Jan,16; 2013,Sep,3-12; 2012,May,3-10

**87560**    **Mycobacteria avium-intracellulare, direct probe technique**
     🚑 0.00    🔬 0.00    **FUD** XXX
     **AMA:** 2017,Jan,8; 2016,Jan,13; 2015,Jan,16; 2013,Sep,3-12; 2012,May,3-10

**87561**    **Mycobacteria avium-intracellulare, amplified probe technique**
     🚑 0.00    🔬 0.00    **FUD** XXX
     **AMA:** 2017,Jan,8; 2016,Jan,13; 2015,Jan,16; 2013,Sep,3-12; 2012,May,3-10

**87562**    **Mycobacteria avium-intracellulare, quantification**
     🚑 0.00    🔬 0.00    **FUD** XXX
     **AMA:** 2017,Jan,8; 2016,Jan,13; 2015,Jan,16; 2013,Sep,3-12; 2012,May,3-10

**87580**    **Mycoplasma pneumoniae, direct probe technique**
     🚑 0.00    🔬 0.00    **FUD** XXX
     **AMA:** 2017,Jan,8; 2016,Jan,13; 2015,Jan,16; 2013,Sep,3-12; 2012,May,3-10

**87581**    **Mycoplasma pneumoniae, amplified probe technique**
     🚑 0.00    🔬 0.00    **FUD** XXX
     **AMA:** 2017,Jan,8; 2016,Jan,13; 2015,Jan,16; 2013,Sep,3-12; 2012,May,3-10

**87582**    **Mycoplasma pneumoniae, quantification**
     🚑 0.00    🔬 0.00    **FUD** XXX
     **AMA:** 2017,Jan,8; 2016,Jan,13; 2015,Jan,16; 2013,Sep,3-12; 2012,May,3-10

**87590**    **Neisseria gonorrhoeae, direct probe technique**
     🚑 0.00    🔬 0.00    **FUD** XXX
     **AMA:** 2017,Jan,8; 2016,Jan,13; 2015,Jan,16; 2013,Sep,3-12; 2012,May,3-10

**87591**    **Neisseria gonorrhoeae, amplified probe technique**
     🚑 0.00    🔬 0.00    **FUD** XXX
     **AMA:** 2017,Jan,8; 2016,Jan,13; 2015,Jan,16; 2013,Sep,3-12; 2013,Jun,13; 2012,May,3-10

**87592**    **Neisseria gonorrhoeae, quantification**
     🚑 0.00    🔬 0.00    **FUD** XXX
     **AMA:** 2017,Jan,8; 2016,Jan,13; 2015,Jan,16; 2013,Sep,3-12; 2012,May,3-10

*87623*    **Resequenced code. See code following 87539.**

*87624*    **Resequenced code. See code following 87539.**

*87625*    **Resequenced code. See code before 87540.**

**87631**    **respiratory virus (eg, adenovirus, influenza virus, coronavirus, metapneumovirus, parainfluenza virus, respiratory syncytial virus, rhinovirus), includes multiplex reverse transcription, when performed, and multiplex amplified probe technique, multiple types or subtypes, 3-5 targets**
     **INCLUDES** Detection of multiple respiratory viruses with one test
     **EXCLUDES** *Assays for typing or subtyping influenza viruses only (87501-87503)*
           *Single test for detection of multiple infectious organisms (87800-87801)*
     🚑 0.00    🔬 0.00    **FUD** XXX
     **AMA:** 2017,Jan,8; 2016,Jan,13; 2015,Jan,16; 2013,Sep,3-12

**87632**    **respiratory virus (eg, adenovirus, influenza virus, coronavirus, metapneumovirus, parainfluenza virus, respiratory syncytial virus, rhinovirus), includes multiplex reverse transcription, when performed, and multiplex amplified probe technique, multiple types or subtypes, 6-11 targets**
     **INCLUDES** Detection of multiple respiratory viruses with one test
     **EXCLUDES** *Assays for typing or subtyping influenza viruses only (87501-87503)*
           *Single test to detect multiple infectious organisms (87800-87801)*
     🚑 0.00    🔬 0.00    **FUD** XXX
     **AMA:** 2017,Jan,8; 2016,Jan,13; 2015,Jan,16; 2013,Sep,3-12

**87633**    **respiratory virus (eg, adenovirus, influenza virus, coronavirus, metapneumovirus, parainfluenza virus, respiratory syncytial virus, rhinovirus), includes multiplex reverse transcription, when performed, and multiplex amplified probe technique, multiple types or subtypes, 12-25 targets**
     **INCLUDES** Detection of multiple respiratory viruses with one test
     **EXCLUDES** *Assays for typing or subtyping influenza viruses only (87501-87503)*
           *Single test to detect multiple infectious organisms (87800-87801)*
     🚑 0.00    🔬 0.00    **FUD** XXX
     **AMA:** 2017,Jan,8; 2016,Jan,13; 2015,Jan,16; 2013,Sep,3-12

● **87634**    **respiratory syncytial virus, amplified probe technique**
     **EXCLUDES** *Assays for RSV with other respiratory viruses (87631-87633)*

**87640**    **Staphylococcus aureus, amplified probe technique**
     🚑 0.00    🔬 0.00    **FUD** XXX
     **AMA:** 2017,Jan,8; 2016,Jan,13; 2015,Jan,16; 2014,Jan,11; 2013,Sep,3-12; 2012,May,3-10

**87641**    **Staphylococcus aureus, methicillin resistant, amplified probe technique**
     **EXCLUDES** *Assays that detect methicillin resistance and identify Staphylococcus aureus using a single nucleic acid sequence (87641)*
     🚑 0.00    🔬 0.00    **FUD** XXX
     **AMA:** 2017,Jan,8; 2016,Jan,13; 2015,Jan,16; 2014,Jan,11; 2013,Sep,3-12; 2012,May,3-10

**87650**    **Streptococcus, group A, direct probe technique**
     🚑 0.00    🔬 0.00    **FUD** XXX
     **AMA:** 2017,Jan,8; 2016,Jan,13; 2015,Jan,16; 2013,Sep,3-12; 2012,May,3-10

**87651**    **Streptococcus, group A, amplified probe technique**
     🚑 0.00    🔬 0.00    **FUD** XXX
     **AMA:** 2017,Jan,8; 2016,Jan,13; 2015,Jan,16; 2013,Sep,3-12; 2012,May,3-10

**87652**    **Streptococcus, group A, quantification**
     🚑 0.00    🔬 0.00    **FUD** XXX
     **AMA:** 2017,Jan,8; 2016,Jan,13; 2015,Jan,16; 2013,Sep,3-12; 2012,May,3-10

| 87653 | **Streptococcus, group B, amplified probe technique** |
|---|---|

 🖐 0.00   ⚕ 0.00   **FUD** XXX   ▢ 🖵

**AMA:** 2017,Jan,8; 2016,Jan,13; 2015,Jan,16; 2014,Jan,11; 2013,Sep,3-12; 2012,May,3-10

| 87660 | **Trichomonas vaginalis, direct probe technique** |
|---|---|

 🖐 0.00   ⚕ 0.00   **FUD** XXX   ▢ 🖵

**AMA:** 2017,Jan,8; 2016,Jan,13; 2015,Jan,16; 2013,Sep,3-12; 2012,May,3-10

| 87661 | **Trichomonas vaginalis, amplified probe technique** |
|---|---|

 🖐 0.00   ⚕ 0.00   **FUD** XXX   ▢ 🖵

● | 87662 | **Zika virus, amplified probe technique** |
|---|---|

| 87797 | **Infectious agent detection by nucleic acid (DNA or RNA), not otherwise specified; direct probe technique, each organism** |
|---|---|

 🖐 0.00   ⚕ 0.00   **FUD** XXX   ▢ 🖵

**AMA:** 2017,Jan,8; 2016,Aug,9; 2016,Jan,13; 2015,Jan,16; 2014,Jan,11; 2013,Sep,3-12; 2012,May,3-10

| 87798 | **amplified probe technique, each organism** |
|---|---|

 🖐 0.00   ⚕ 0.00   **FUD** XXX   ▢ 🖵

**AMA:** 2017,Jan,8; 2016,Jan,13; 2015,Jan,16; 2014,Jan,11; 2013,Sep,3-12; 2012,May,3-10

| 87799 | **quantification, each organism** |
|---|---|

 🖐 0.00   ⚕ 0.00   **FUD** XXX   ▢ 🖵

**AMA:** 2017,Jan,8; 2016,Jan,13; 2015,Jan,16; 2013,Sep,3-12; 2012,May,3-10

| 87800 | **Infectious agent detection by nucleic acid (DNA or RNA), multiple organisms; direct probe(s) technique** |
|---|---|

INCLUDES  Single test to detect multiple infectious organisms

EXCLUDES  *Detection of specific infectious agents not otherwise specified (87797-87799)*

*Each specific organism nucleic acid detection from a primary source (87471-87660 [87623, 87624, 87625])*

 🖐 0.00   ⚕ 0.00   **FUD** XXX   Ⓐ 🖵

**AMA:** 2017,Jan,8; 2016,Aug,9; 2016,Jan,13; 2015,Jan,16; 2013,Sep,3-12; 2012,May,3-10

| 87801 | **amplified probe(s) technique** |
|---|---|

INCLUDES  Single test to detect multiple infectious organisms

EXCLUDES  *Detection of multiple respiratory viruses with one test (87631-87633)*

*Detection of specific infectious agents not otherwise specified (87797-87799)*

*Each specific organism nucleic acid detection from a primary source (87471-87660 [87623, 87624, 87625])*

 🖐 0.00   ⚕ 0.00   **FUD** XXX   ✕ ▢ 🖵

**AMA:** 2017,Jan,8; 2016,Jan,13; 2015,Jan,16; 2014,Jan,11; 2013,Sep,3-12; 2013,Jun,13; 2012,May,3-10

## 87802-87899 [87806] Detection Infectious Agent by Immunoassay with Direct Optical Observation

| 87802 | **Infectious agent antigen detection by immunoassay with direct optical observation; Streptococcus, group B** |
|---|---|

 🖐 0.00   ⚕ 0.00   **FUD** XXX   ▢ 🖵

**AMA:** 2005,Aug,7-8; 2005,Jul,11-12

| 87803 | **Clostridium difficile toxin A** |
|---|---|

 🖐 0.00   ⚕ 0.00   **FUD** XXX   ▢ 🖵

**AMA:** 2005,Aug,7-8; 2005,Jul,11-12

\# | 87806 | **HIV-1 antigen(s), with HIV-1 and HIV-2 antibodies** |
|---|---|

 🖐 0.00   ⚕ 0.00   **FUD** XXX   ▢ 🖵

| 87804 | **Influenza** |
|---|---|

 🖐 0.00   ⚕ 0.00   **FUD** XXX   ✕ ▢ 🖵

**AMA:** 2017,Jan,8; 2016,Jan,13; 2015,Jan,16; 2014,Jan,11; 2012,Jan,15-42

| *87806* | **Resequenced code. See code following 87803.** |
|---|---|

| 87807 | **respiratory syncytial virus** |
|---|---|

 🖐 0.00   ⚕ 0.00   **FUD** XXX   ✕ ▢ 🖵

**AMA:** 2005,Jul,11-12; 2005,Aug,7-8

| 87808 | **Trichomonas vaginalis** |
|---|---|

 🖐 0.00   ⚕ 0.00   **FUD** XXX   ✕ ▢ 🖵

| 87809 | **adenovirus** |
|---|---|

 🖐 0.00   ⚕ 0.00   **FUD** XXX   ✕ ▢ 🖵

**AMA:** 2017,Jan,8; 2016,Jan,13; 2015,Jan,16; 2014,Jan,11

| 87810 | **Chlamydia trachomatis** |
|---|---|

 🖐 0.00   ⚕ 0.00   **FUD** XXX   Ⓐ 🖵

**AMA:** 2017,Jan,8; 2016,Jan,13; 2015,Jan,16; 2014,Jan,11

| 87850 | **Neisseria gonorrhoeae** |
|---|---|

 🖐 0.00   ⚕ 0.00   **FUD** XXX   Ⓐ 🖵

**AMA:** 2017,Jan,8; 2016,Jan,13; 2015,Jan,16; 2014,Jan,11

| 87880 | **Streptococcus, group A** |
|---|---|

 🖐 0.00   ⚕ 0.00   **FUD** XXX   ✕ ▢ 🖵

**AMA:** 2017,Jan,8; 2016,Jan,13; 2015,Jan,16; 2014,Jan,11; 2012,Jan,15-42

| 87899 | **not otherwise specified** |
|---|---|

 🖐 0.00   ⚕ 0.00   **FUD** XXX   ✕ ▢ 🖵

**AMA:** 2017,Jan,8; 2016,Jan,13; 2015,Jan,16; 2014,Jan,11; 2012,Jan,15-42

## 87900-87999 [87906, 87910, 87912] Drug Sensitivity Genotype/Phenotype

| 87900 | **Infectious agent drug susceptibility phenotype prediction using regularly updated genotypic bioinformatics** |
|---|---|

 🖐 0.00   ⚕ 0.00   **FUD** XXX   ▢ 🖵

**AMA:** 2017,Jan,8; 2016,Jan,13; 2015,Dec,18; 2015,Jan,16; 2014,Jan,11; 2013,Sep,3-12; 2012,May,3-10

\# | 87910 | **Infectious agent genotype analysis by nucleic acid (DNA or RNA); cytomegalovirus** |
|---|---|

EXCLUDES  *HPV detection (genotyping) (0500T)*

*HIV-1 infectious agent phenotype prediction (87900)*

 🖐 0.00   ⚕ 0.00   **FUD** XXX   ▢

**AMA:** 2017,Jan,8; 2016,Jan,13; 2015,Jan,16

| 87901 | **HIV-1, reverse transcriptase and protease regions** |
|---|---|

EXCLUDES  *Infectious agent drug susceptibility phenotype prediction for HIV-1 (87900)*

 🖐 0.00   ⚕ 0.00   **FUD** XXX   ▢ 🖵

**AMA:** 2017,Jan,8; 2016,Jan,13; 2015,Jan,16; 2014,Jan,11; 2013,Sep,3-12; 2012,May,3-10

\# | 87906 | **HIV-1, other region (eg, integrase, fusion)** |
|---|---|

 🖐 0.00   ⚕ 0.00   **FUD** XXX   ▢ 🖵

**AMA:** 2017,Jan,8; 2016,Jan,13; 2015,Jan,16

\# | 87912 | **Hepatitis B virus** |
|---|---|

 🖐 0.00   ⚕ 0.00   **FUD** XXX   ▢ 🖵

**AMA:** 2017,Jan,8; 2016,Jan,13; 2015,Jan,16

| 87902 | **Hepatitis C virus** |
|---|---|

 🖐 0.00   ⚕ 0.00   **FUD** XXX   ▢ 🖵

**AMA:** 2017,Jan,8; 2016,Jan,13; 2015,Dec,18; 2015,Nov,10; 2015,Jan,16; 2014,Jan,11; 2013,Sep,3-12; 2012,May,3-10

| 87903 | **Infectious agent phenotype analysis by nucleic acid (DNA or RNA) with drug resistance tissue culture analysis, HIV 1; first through 10 drugs tested** |
|---|---|

 🖐 0.00   ⚕ 0.00   **FUD** XXX   ▢ 🖵

**AMA:** 2017,Jan,8; 2016,Jan,13; 2015,Jan,16; 2014,Jan,11; 2013,Sep,3-12; 2012,May,3-10

+ | 87904 | **each additional drug tested (List separately in addition to code for primary procedure)** |
|---|---|

Code first (87903)

 🖐 0.00   ⚕ 0.00   **FUD** XXX   ▢ 🖵

**AMA:** 2017,Jan,8; 2016,Jan,13; 2015,Jan,16; 2014,Jan,11; 2013,Sep,3-12; 2012,May,3-10; 2012,Jan,15-42

| 87905 | **Infectious agent enzymatic activity other than virus (eg, sialidase activity in vaginal fluid)** |
|---|---|

 🖐 0.00   ⚕ 0.00   **FUD** XXX   ✕ ▢ 🖵

EXCLUDES  *Isolation of a virus identified by a nonimmunologic method, and by noncytopathic effect (87255)*

| *87906* | **Resequenced code. See code following 87901.** |
|---|---|

| 87910 | Resequenced code. See code following 87900. |
|---|---|
| 87912 | Resequenced code. See code before 87902. |

**87999** Unlisted microbiology procedure
🔧 0.00 ⚕ 0.00 **FUD** XXX ⬛N
**AMA:** 2017,Jan,8; 2016,Jan,13; 2015,Jan,16; 2014,Jan,11

## 88000-88099 Autopsy Services

**CMS:** 100-02,15,80.1 Payment for Clinical Laboratory Services
**INCLUDES** Services for physicians only

**88000** Necropsy (autopsy), gross examination only; without CNS
🔧 0.00 ⚕ 0.00 **FUD** XXX ⬛E
**AMA:** 2017,Jan,8; 2016,Jan,13; 2015,Jan,16; 2014,Jan,11

**88005** with brain
🔧 0.00 ⚕ 0.00 **FUD** XXX ⬛E
**AMA:** 2005,Jul,11-12; 2005,Aug,7-8

**88007** with brain and spinal cord
🔧 0.00 ⚕ 0.00 **FUD** XXX ⬛E
**AMA:** 2005,Jul,11-12; 2005,Aug,7-8

**88012** infant with brain ⬛A
🔧 0.00 ⚕ 0.00 **FUD** XXX ⬛E
**AMA:** 2005,Jul,11-12; 2005,Aug,7-8

**88014** stillborn or newborn with brain ⬛A
🔧 0.00 ⚕ 0.00 **FUD** XXX ⬛E
**AMA:** 2005,Jul,11-12; 2005,Aug,7-8

**88016** macerated stillborn ⬛A
🔧 0.00 ⚕ 0.00 **FUD** XXX ⬛E
**AMA:** 2005,Jul,11-12; 2005,Aug,7-8

**88020** Necropsy (autopsy), gross and microscopic; without CNS
🔧 0.00 ⚕ 0.00 **FUD** XXX ⬛E
**AMA:** 2005,Jul,11-12; 2005,Aug,7-8

**88025** with brain
🔧 0.00 ⚕ 0.00 **FUD** XXX ⬛E
**AMA:** 2005,Jul,11-12; 2005,Aug,7-8

**88027** with brain and spinal cord
🔧 0.00 ⚕ 0.00 **FUD** XXX ⬛E
**AMA:** 2005,Jul,11-12; 2005,Aug,7-8

**88028** infant with brain ⬛A
🔧 0.00 ⚕ 0.00 **FUD** XXX ⬛E
**AMA:** 2005,Jul,11-12; 2005,Aug,7-8

**88029** stillborn or newborn with brain ⬛A
🔧 0.00 ⚕ 0.00 **FUD** XXX ⬛E
**AMA:** 2005,Jul,11-12; 2005,Aug,7-8

**88036** Necropsy (autopsy), limited, gross and/or microscopic; regional
🔧 0.00 ⚕ 0.00 **FUD** XXX ⬛E
**AMA:** 2005,Jul,11-12; 2005,Aug,7-8

**88037** single organ
🔧 0.00 ⚕ 0.00 **FUD** XXX ⬛E
**AMA:** 2005,Jul,11-12; 2005,Aug,7-8

**88040** Necropsy (autopsy); forensic examination
🔧 0.00 ⚕ 0.00 **FUD** XXX ⬛E
**AMA:** 2005,Jul,11-12; 2005,Aug,7-8

**88045** coroner's call
🔧 0.00 ⚕ 0.00 **FUD** XXX ⬛E
**AMA:** 2005,Jul,11-12; 2005,Aug,7-8

**88099** Unlisted necropsy (autopsy) procedure
🔧 0.00 ⚕ 0.00 **FUD** XXX ⬛E
**AMA:** 2017,Jan,8; 2016,Jan,13; 2015,Jan,16; 2014,Jan,11

## 88104-88140 Cytopathology: Other Than Cervical/Vaginal

**88104** Cytopathology, fluids, washings or brushings, except cervical or vaginal; smears with interpretation
🔧 2.10 ⚕ 2.10 **FUD** XXX 🔲01 🔲80 🔲
**AMA:** 2017,Jan,8; 2016,Jan,13; 2015,Jan,16; 2014,Jan,11; 2012,Jan,15-42

**88106** simple filter method with interpretation
**EXCLUDES** Cytopathology smears with interpretation (88104)
Selective cellular enhancement (nongynecological) including filter transfer techniques (88112)
🔧 1.81 ⚕ 1.81 **FUD** XXX 🔲01 🔲80
**AMA:** 2017,Jan,8; 2016,Jan,13; 2015,Jan,16; 2014,Jan,11

**88108** Cytopathology, concentration technique, smears and interpretation (eg, Saccomanno technique)
**EXCLUDES** Cervical or vaginal smears (88150-88155)
Gastric intubation with lavage (43754-43755)
🔲 (74340)
🔧 1.77 ⚕ 1.77 **FUD** XXX 🔲01 🔲80 🔲
**AMA:** 2017,Jan,8; 2016,Jan,13; 2015,Jan,16; 2014,Jan,11

**88112** Cytopathology, selective cellular enhancement technique with interpretation (eg, liquid based slide preparation method), except cervical or vaginal
**EXCLUDES** Cytopathology cellular enhancement technique (88108)
🔧 1.92 ⚕ 1.92 **FUD** XXX 🔲01 🔲80 🔲
**AMA:** 2005,Aug,7-8; 2005,Jul,11-12

**88120** Cytopathology, in situ hybridization (eg, FISH), urinary tract specimen with morphometric analysis, 3-5 molecular probes, each specimen; manual
**EXCLUDES** More than five probes (88399)
Morphometric in situ hybridization on specimens other than urinary tract (88367-88368 [88373, 88374])
🔧 17.8 ⚕ 17.8 **FUD** XXX 🔲02 🔲80 🔲
**AMA:** 2010,Dec,7-10

**88121** using computer-assisted technology
**EXCLUDES** More than five probes (88399)
Morphometric in situ hybridization on specimens other than urinary tract (88367-88368 [88373, 88374])
🔧 15.4 ⚕ 15.4 **FUD** XXX 🔲01 🔲80 🔲
**AMA:** 2010,Dec,7-10

**88125** Cytopathology, forensic (eg, sperm)
🔧 0.59 ⚕ 0.59 **FUD** XXX 🔲01 🔲80 🔲
**AMA:** 2005,Aug,7-8; 2005,Jul,11-12

**88130** Sex chromatin identification; Barr bodies
🔧 0.00 ⚕ 0.00 **FUD** XXX 🔲Q 🔲
**AMA:** 2005,Aug,7-8; 2005,Jul,11-12

**88140** peripheral blood smear, polymorphonuclear drumsticks
**EXCLUDES** Guard stain (88313)
🔧 0.00 ⚕ 0.00 **FUD** XXX 🔲Q 🔲
**AMA:** 2017,Jan,8; 2016,Jan,13; 2015,Jan,16; 2014,Jan,11

## 88141-88155 Pap Smears

**CMS:** 100-03,210.2 Screening Pap Smears/Pelvic Examinations for Early Cancer Detection
**EXCLUDES** Non-Bethesda method (88150-88153)

**88141** Cytopathology, cervical or vaginal (any reporting system), requiring interpretation by physician ♀
Code also (88142-88153, 88164-88167, 88174-88175)
🔧 0.92 ⚕ 0.92 **FUD** XXX ⬛N 🔲80 🔲26
**AMA:** 2017,Jan,8; 2016,Jan,13; 2015,Jan,16; 2014,Jan,11; 2012,Jan,15-42

**88142** Cytopathology, cervical or vaginal (any reporting system), collected in preservative fluid, automated thin layer preparation; manual screening under physician supervision ♀
**INCLUDES** Bethesda or non-Bethesda method
🔧 0.00 ⚕ 0.00 **FUD** XXX 🔲Q 🔲
**AMA:** 2017,Jan,8; 2016,Jan,13; 2015,Jan,16; 2014,Jan,11

26/TC PC/TC Only   12-Z3 ASC Payment   50 Bilateral   ♂ Male Only   ♀ Female Only   🔧 Facility RVU   ⚕ Non-Facility RVU   🔲 CCI
**FUD** Follow-up Days   **CMS:** IOM (Pub 100)   A-Y OPPSI   80/80 Surg Assist Allowed / w/Doc   ⬛N Lab Crosswalk   🔲 Radiology Crosswalk   ⊠ CLIA

414
CPT © 2017 American Medical Association. All Rights Reserved.
© 2017 Optum360, LLC

**88143**    with manual screening and rescreening under physician supervision ♀

> **INCLUDES** Bethesda or non-Bethesda method
>
> **EXCLUDES** *Automated screening of automated thin layer preparation (88174-88175)*

📋 0.00    ⚖ 0.00    **FUD** XXX    🔲 🖵

**AMA:** 2017,Jan,8; 2016,Jan,13; 2015,Jan,16; 2014,Jan,11; 2012,Jan,15-42

**88147**    Cytopathology smears, cervical or vaginal; screening by automated system under physician supervision ♀

· 📋 0.00    ⚖ 0.00    **FUD** XXX    🔲 🖵

**AMA:** 2017,Jan,8; 2016,Jan,13; 2015,Jan,16; 2014,Jan,11; 2012,Jan,15-42

**88148**    screening by automated system with manual rescreening under physician supervision ♀

📋 0.00    ⚖ 0.00    **FUD** XXX    🔲 🖵

**AMA:** 2017,Jan,8; 2016,Jan,13; 2015,Jan,16; 2014,Jan,11

**88150**    Cytopathology, slides, cervical or vaginal; manual screening under physician supervision ♀

> **EXCLUDES** *Bethesda method Pap smears (88164-88167)*

📋 0.00    ⚖ 0.00    **FUD** XXX    🔲 🖵

**AMA:** 2017,Jan,8; 2016,Jan,13; 2015,Jan,16; 2014,Jan,11

**88152**    with manual screening and computer-assisted rescreening under physician supervision ♀

> **EXCLUDES** *Bethesda method Pap smears (88164-88167)*

📋 0.00    ⚖ 0.00    **FUD** XXX    🔲 🖵

**AMA:** 2017,Jan,8; 2016,Jan,13; 2015,Jan,16; 2014,Jan,11

**88153**    with manual screening and rescreening under physician supervision ♀

> **EXCLUDES** *Bethesda method Pap smears (88164-88167)*

📋 0.00    ⚖ 0.00    **FUD** XXX    🔲 🖵

**AMA:** 2017,Jan,8; 2016,Jan,13; 2015,Jan,16; 2014,Jan,11; 2012,Jan,15-42

~~**88154**    with manual screening and computer-assisted rescreening using cell selection and review under physician supervision~~

+   **88155**    Cytopathology, slides, cervical or vaginal, definitive hormonal evaluation (eg, maturation index, karyopyknotic index, estrogenic index) (List separately in addition to code[s] for other technical and interpretation services) ♀

> Code first (88142-88153, 88164-88167, 88174-88175)

📋 0.00    ⚖ 0.00    **FUD** XXX    🔲 🖵

**AMA:** 2017,Jan,8; 2016,Jan,13; 2015,Jan,16; 2014,Jan,11; 2012,Jan,15-42

## 88160-88162 Cytopathology Smears (Other Than Pap)

**88160**    Cytopathology, smears, any other source; screening and interpretation

📋 2.05    ⚖ 2.05    **FUD** XXX    🔟 🔟 🖵

**AMA:** 2006,Dec,10-12; 2005,Jul,11-12

**88161**    preparation, screening and interpretation

📋 1.85    ⚖ 1.85    **FUD** XXX    🔟 🔟 🖵

**AMA:** 2017,Jan,8; 2016,Jan,13; 2015,Jan,16; 2014,Jan,11

**88162**    extended study involving over 5 slides and/or multiple stains

> **EXCLUDES** *Aerosol collection of sputum (89220)*
> *Special stains (88312-88314)*

📋 2.82    ⚖ 2.82    **FUD** XXX    🔟 🔟 🖵

**AMA:** 2005,Aug,7-8; 2005,Jul,11-12

## 88164-88167 Pap Smears: Bethesda System

**CMS:** 100-03,210.2 Screening Pap Smears/Pelvic Examinations for Early Cancer Detection

> **EXCLUDES** *Non-Bethesda method (88150-88153)*

**88164**    Cytopathology, slides, cervical or vaginal (the Bethesda System); manual screening under physician supervision ♀

📋 0.00    ⚖ 0.00    **FUD** XXX    🔲 🖵

**AMA:** 2017,Jan,8; 2016,Jan,13; 2015,Jan,16; 2014,Jan,11

**88165**    with manual screening and rescreening under physician supervision ♀

📋 0.00    ⚖ 0.00    **FUD** XXX    🔲 🖵

**AMA:** 2017,Jan,8; 2016,Jan,13; 2015,Jan,16; 2014,Jan,11; 2012,Jan,15-42

**88166**    with manual screening and computer-assisted rescreening under physician supervision ♀

📋 0.00    ⚖ 0.00    **FUD** XXX    🔲 🖵

**AMA:** 2017,Jan,8; 2016,Jan,13; 2015,Jan,16; 2014,Jan,11

**88167**    with manual screening and computer-assisted rescreening using cell selection and review under physician supervision ♀

> **EXCLUDES** *Fine needle aspiration (10021-10022)*

📋 0.00    ⚖ 0.00    **FUD** XXX    🔲 🖵

**AMA:** 2017,Jan,8; 2016,Jan,13; 2015,Jan,16; 2014,Jan,11

## 88172-88173 [88177] Cytopathology of Needle Biopsy

> **EXCLUDES** *Fine needle aspiration (10021-10022)*

**88172**    Cytopathology, evaluation of fine needle aspirate; immediate cytohistologic study to determine adequacy for diagnosis, first evaluation episode, each site

> **INCLUDES** The submission of a complete set of cytologic material for evaluation regardless of the number of needle passes performed or slides prepared from each site
>
> **EXCLUDES** *Cytologic examination during intraoperative pathology consultation (88333-88334)*

📋 1.62    ⚖ 1.62    **FUD** XXX    🔟 🔟 🖵

**AMA:** 2017,Jan,8; 2016,Jan,13; 2016,Jan,11; 2015,Jan,16; 2014,Jan,11; 2012,Jan,15-42

**88173**    interpretation and report

> **INCLUDES** The interpretation and report from each anatomical site no matter how many passes or evaluation episodes are performed during the aspiration
>
> **EXCLUDES** *Cytologic examination during intraoperative pathology consultation (88333-88334)*
> *Fine needle aspiration (10021-10022)*

📋 4.34    ⚖ 4.34    **FUD** XXX    🔟 🔟 🖵

**AMA:** 2017,Jan,8; 2016,Jan,13; 2015,Jan,16; 2014,Jan,11; 2012,Jan,15-42

+  #   **88177**    immediate cytohistologic study to determine adequacy for diagnosis, each separate additional evaluation episode, same site (List separately in addition to code for primary procedure)

> Code also each additional immediate repeat evaluation episode(s) required from the same site (e.g., previous sample is inadequate)
> Code first (88172)

📋 0.86    ⚖ 0.86    **FUD** ZZZ    🅽 🔟

**AMA:** 2017,Jan,8; 2016,Jan,11

## 88174-88177 Pap Smears: Automated Screening

> **EXCLUDES** *Non-Bethesda method (88150-88153)*

**88174**    Cytopathology, cervical or vaginal (any reporting system), collected in preservative fluid, automated thin layer preparation; screening by automated system, under physician supervision ♀

> **INCLUDES** Bethesda or non-Bethesda method

📋 0.00    ⚖ 0.00    **FUD** XXX    🔲 🖵

**AMA:** 2017,Jan,8; 2016,Jan,13; 2015,Jan,16; 2014,Jan,11

**88175**    with screening by automated system and manual rescreening or review, under physician supervision ♀

> **INCLUDES** Bethesda or non-Bethesda method
>
> **EXCLUDES** *Manual screening (88142-88143)*

📋 0.00    ⚖ 0.00    **FUD** XXX    🔲 🖵

**AMA:** 2017,Jan,8; 2016,Jan,13; 2015,Jan,16; 2014,Jan,11; 2012,Jan,15-42

*88177*    Resequenced code. See code following 88173.

● New Code    ▲ Revised Code    ○ Reinstated    ● New Web Release    ▲ Revised Web Release    Unlisted    Not Covered    # Resequenced
⊘ AMA Mod 51 Exempt    ⑨ Optum Mod 51 Exempt    ⑥ Mod 63 Exempt    ∕ Non-FDA Drug    ★ Telemedicine    Ⓜ Maternity    Ⓐ Age Edit    + Add-on    **AMA:** CPT Asst
© 2017 Optum360, LLC                          CPT © 2017 American Medical Association. All Rights Reserved.

## 88182-88199 Cytopathology Using the Fluorescence-Activated Cell Sorter

**88182**   **Flow cytometry, cell cycle or DNA analysis**
*EXCLUDES*   *DNA ploidy analysis by morphometric technique (88358)*
🖐 3.38   ✎ 3.38   **FUD** XXX   [02] [80] ▭
**AMA:** 2017,Jan,8; 2016,Jan,13; 2015,Jan,16; 2013,Oct,3

**88184**   **Flow cytometry, cell surface, cytoplasmic, or nuclear marker, technical component only; first marker**
🖐 1.72   ✎ 1.72   **FUD** XXX   [02] [80] [TC] ▭
**AMA:** 2017,Jan,8; 2016,Jan,13; 2015,Jan,16; 2014,Jan,11; 2013,Oct,3

+ **88185**   **each additional marker (List separately in addition to code for first marker)**
Code first (88184)
🖐 1.05   ✎ 1.05   **FUD** ZZZ   [N] [80] [TC] ▭
**AMA:** 2017,Jan,8; 2016,Jan,13; 2015,Jan,16; 2014,Jan,11; 2013,Oct,3; 2012,Jan,15-42

**88187**   **Flow cytometry, interpretation; 2 to 8 markers**
*EXCLUDES*   *Antibody assessment by flow cytometry (83516-83520, 86000-86849 [86152, 86153])*
*Cell enumeration by immunologic selection and identification ([86152, 86153])*
*Interpretation (86355-86357, 86359-86361, 86367)*
🖐 1.65   ✎ 1.65   **FUD** XXX   [B] [80] [26] ▭
**AMA:** 2017,Jan,8; 2016,Jan,13; 2015,Jan,16; 2014,Jan,11; 2013,Oct,3; 2012,Jan,15-42

**88188**   **9 to 15 markers**
*EXCLUDES*   *Antibody assessment by flow cytometry (83516-83520, 86000-86849 [86152, 86153])*
*Cell enumeration by immunologic selection and identification ([86152, 86153])*
*Interpretation (86355-86357, 86359-86361, 86367)*
🖐 2.10   ✎ 2.10   **FUD** XXX   [B] [80] [26] ▭
**AMA:** 2017,Jan,8; 2016,Jan,13; 2015,Jan,16; 2014,Jan,11; 2013,Oct,3; 2012,Jan,15-42

**88189**   **16 or more markers**
*EXCLUDES*   *Antibody assessment by flow cytometry (83516-83520, 86000-86849 [86152, 86153])*
*Cell enumeration using immunologic selection and identification in fluid sample ([86152, 86153])*
*Interpretation (86355-86357, 86359-86361, 86367)*
🖐 2.58   ✎ 2.58   **FUD** XXX   [B] [80] [26] ▭
**AMA:** 2017,Jan,8; 2016,Jan,13; 2015,Jan,16; 2014,Jan,11; 2013,Oct,3; 2012,Jan,15-42

**88199**   **Unlisted cytopathology procedure**
*EXCLUDES*   *Electron microscopy (88348)*
🖐 0.00   ✎ 0.00   **FUD** XXX   [01] [80]
**AMA:** 2017,Jan,8; 2016,Jan,13; 2015,Jan,16; 2014,Jan,11

## 88230-88299 Cytogenic Studies

**CMS:** 100-03,190.3 Cytogenic Studies
*EXCLUDES*   *Acetylcholinesterase (82013)*
*Alpha-fetoprotein (amniotic fluid or serum) (82105-82106)*
*Microdissection (88380)*
*Molecular pathology codes (81200-81383 [81105, 81106, 81107, 81108, 81109, 81110, 81111, 81112, 81120, 81121, 81161, 81162, 81230, 81231, 81238, 81269, 81283, 81287, 81288, 81334], 81400-81408, [81479], 81410-81471 [81448], 81500-81512, 81599)*

**88230**   **Tissue culture for non-neoplastic disorders; lymphocyte**
🖐 0.00   ✎ 0.00   **FUD** XXX   [Q]
**AMA:** 2017,Jan,8; 2016,Jan,13; 2015,Jan,16; 2014,Jan,11

**88233**   **skin or other solid tissue biopsy**
🖐 0.00   ✎ 0.00   **FUD** XXX   [Q]
**AMA:** 2017,Jan,8; 2016,Jan,13; 2015,Jan,16; 2014,Jan,11

**88235**   **amniotic fluid or chorionic villus cells**   [M]
🖐 0.00   ✎ 0.00   **FUD** XXX   [Q]
**AMA:** 2017,Jan,8; 2016,Jan,13; 2015,Jan,16; 2014,Jan,11

**88237**   **Tissue culture for neoplastic disorders; bone marrow, blood cells**
🖐 0.00   ✎ 0.00   **FUD** XXX   [Q]
**AMA:** 2017,Jan,8; 2016,Jan,13; 2015,Jan,16; 2014,Jan,11

**88239**   **solid tumor**
🖐 0.00   ✎ 0.00   **FUD** XXX   [Q]
**AMA:** 2017,Jan,8; 2016,Jan,13; 2015,Jan,16; 2014,Jan,11

**88240**   **Cryopreservation, freezing and storage of cells, each cell line**
*EXCLUDES*   *Therapeutic cryopreservation and storage (38207)*
🖐 0.00   ✎ 0.00   **FUD** XXX   [Q] ▭
**AMA:** 2017,Jan,8; 2016,Jan,13; 2015,Jan,16; 2014,Jan,11; 2013,Oct,3

**88241**   **Thawing and expansion of frozen cells, each aliquot**
*EXCLUDES*   *Therapeutic thawing of prior harvest (38208)*
🖐 0.00   ✎ 0.00   **FUD** XXX   [Q] ▭
**AMA:** 2017,Jan,8; 2016,Jan,13; 2015,Jan,16; 2014,Jan,11; 2013,Oct,3

**88245**   **Chromosome analysis for breakage syndromes; baseline Sister Chromatid Exchange (SCE), 20-25 cells**
🖐 0.00   ✎ 0.00   **FUD** XXX   [Q] ▭
**AMA:** 2017,Jan,8; 2016,Jan,13; 2015,Jan,16; 2014,Jan,11

**88248**   **baseline breakage, score 50-100 cells, count 20 cells, 2 karyotypes (eg, for ataxia telangiectasia, Fanconi anemia, fragile X)**
🖐 0.00   ✎ 0.00   **FUD** XXX   [Q] ▭
**AMA:** 2017,Jan,8; 2016,Jan,13; 2015,Jan,16; 2014,Jan,11

**88249**   **score 100 cells, clastogen stress (eg, diepoxybutane, mitomycin C, ionizing radiation, UV radiation)**
🖐 0.00   ✎ 0.00   **FUD** XXX   [Q] ▭
**AMA:** 2017,Jan,8; 2016,Jan,13; 2015,Jan,16; 2014,Jan,11

**88261**   **Chromosome analysis; count 5 cells, 1 karyotype, with banding**
🖐 0.00   ✎ 0.00   **FUD** XXX   [Q] ▭
**AMA:** 2017,Jan,8; 2016,Jan,13; 2015,Jan,16; 2014,Jan,11

**88262**   **count 15-20 cells, 2 karyotypes, with banding**
🖐 0.00   ✎ 0.00   **FUD** XXX   [Q] ▭
**AMA:** 2017,Jan,8; 2016,Jan,13; 2015,Jan,16; 2014,Jan,11; 2012,Jan,15-42

**88263**   **count 45 cells for mosaicism, 2 karyotypes, with banding**
🖐 0.00   ✎ 0.00   **FUD** XXX   [Q] ▭
**AMA:** 2017,Jan,8; 2016,Jan,13; 2015,Jan,16; 2014,Jan,11

**88264**   **analyze 20-25 cells**
🖐 0.00   ✎ 0.00   **FUD** XXX   [Q] ▭
**AMA:** 2017,Jan,8; 2016,Jan,13; 2015,Jan,16; 2014,Jan,11

**88267**   **Chromosome analysis, amniotic fluid or chorionic villus, count 15 cells, 1 karyotype, with banding**   [M] ♀
🖐 0.00   ✎ 0.00   **FUD** XXX   [Q] ▭
**AMA:** 2017,Jan,8; 2016,Jan,13; 2015,Jan,16; 2014,Jan,11

**88269**   **Chromosome analysis, in situ for amniotic fluid cells, count cells from 6-12 colonies, 1 karyotype, with banding**   [M] ♀
🖐 0.00   ✎ 0.00   **FUD** XXX   [Q] ▭
**AMA:** 2017,Jan,8; 2016,Jan,13; 2015,Jan,16; 2014,Jan,11

**88271**   **Molecular cytogenetics; DNA probe, each (eg, FISH)**
*EXCLUDES*   *Cytogenomic microarray analysis (81228-81229, 81405-81406, [81479])*
*Fetal chromosome analysis using maternal blood (81420-81422)*
🖐 0.00   ✎ 0.00   **FUD** XXX   [Q] ▭
**AMA:** 2017,Apr,3; 2017,Jan,8; 2016,Jan,13; 2015,Jan,16; 2014,Jan,11; 2013,Sep,3-12; 2012,May,3-10; 2012,Jan,15-42

**88272**   **chromosomal in situ hybridization, analyze 3-5 cells (eg, for derivatives and markers)**
🖐 0.00   ✎ 0.00   **FUD** XXX   [Q] ▭
**AMA:** 2017,Jan,8; 2016,Jan,13; 2015,Jan,16; 2014,Jan,11; 2013,Sep,3-12; 2012,May,3-10; 2012,Jan,15-42

[26]/[TC] PC/TC Only   [A2]-[Z3] ASC Payment   [50] Bilateral   ♂ Male Only   ♀ Female Only   🖐 Facility RVU   ✎ Non-Facility RVU   ▭ CCI
**FUD** Follow-up Days   **CMS:** IOM (Pub 100)   [A]-[Y] OPPSI   [80]/[80] Surg Assist Allowed / w/Doc   ☒ Lab Crosswalk   ☒ Radiology Crosswalk   ☒ CLIA
CPT © 2017 American Medical Association. All Rights Reserved.
416                                                                                    © 2017 Optum360, LLC

88273 **chromosomal in situ hybridization, analyze 10-30 cells (eg, for microdeletions)**
🖩 0.00  ☊ 0.00  **FUD** XXX  🔲🖵
**AMA:** 2017,Jan,8; 2016,Jan,13; 2015,Jan,16; 2014,Jan,11; 2013,Sep,3-12; 2012,May,3-10; 2012,Jan,15-42

88274 **interphase in situ hybridization, analyze 25-99 cells**
🖩 0.00  ☊ 0.00  **FUD** XXX  🔲🖵
**AMA:** 2017,Jan,8; 2016,Jan,13; 2015,Jan,16; 2014,Jan,11; 2013,Sep,3-12; 2012,May,3-10; 2012,Jan,15-42

88275 **interphase in situ hybridization, analyze 100-300 cells**
🖩 0.00  ☊ 0.00  **FUD** XXX  🔲🖵
**AMA:** 2017,Jan,8; 2016,Jan,13; 2015,Jan,16; 2014,Jan,11; 2013,Sep,3-12; 2012,May,3-10; 2012,Jan,15-42

88280 **Chromosome analysis; additional karyotypes, each study**
🖩 0.00  ☊ 0.00  **FUD** XXX  🔲🖵
**AMA:** 2017,Jan,8; 2016,Jan,13; 2015,Jan,16; 2014,Jan,11

88283 **additional specialized banding technique (eg, NOR, C-banding)**
🖩 0.00  ☊ 0.00  **FUD** XXX  🔲🖵
**AMA:** 2017,Jan,8; 2016,Jan,13; 2015,Jan,16; 2014,Jan,11

88285 **additional cells counted, each study**
🖩 0.00  ☊ 0.00  **FUD** XXX  🔲🖵
**AMA:** 2017,Jan,8; 2016,Jan,13; 2015,Jan,16; 2014,Jan,11; 2012,Jan,15-42

88289 **additional high resolution study**
🖩 0.00  ☊ 0.00  **FUD** XXX  🔲🖵
**AMA:** 2017,Jan,8; 2016,Jan,13; 2015,Jan,16; 2014,Jan,11

88291 **Cytogenetics and molecular cytogenetics, interpretation and report**
🖩 0.92  ☊ 0.92  **FUD** XXX  Ⓜ 80 26 🖵
**AMA:** 2017,Jan,8; 2016,Jan,13; 2015,Jan,16; 2014,Jan,11

88299 **Unlisted cytogenetic study**
🖩 0.00  ☊ 0.00  **FUD** XXX  01 80
**AMA:** 2017,Jan,8; 2016,Jan,13; 2015,Jan,16; 2014,Jan,11

# 88300 Evaluation of Surgical Specimen: Gross Anatomy

**CMS:** 100-02,15,80.1 Payment for Clinical Laboratory Services
INCLUDES  Attainment, examination, and reporting
Unit of service is the specimen
EXCLUDES  Additional procedures (88311-88365 [88341, 88350], 88399)
Microscopic exam (88302-88309)

88300 **Level I - Surgical pathology, gross examination only**
🖩 0.46  ☊ 0.46  **FUD** XXX  01 80
**AMA:** 2017,Jan,8; 2016,Jan,13; 2015,Jan,16; 2014,Jan,11; 2012,Jan,15-42

# 88302-88309 Evaluation of Surgical Specimens: Gross and Microscopic Anatomy

**CMS:** 100-02,15,80.1 Payment for Clinical Laboratory Services
INCLUDES  Attainment, examination, and reporting
Unit of service is the specimen
EXCLUDES  Additional procedures (88311-88365 [88341, 88350], 88399)
Mohs surgery (17311-17315)

88302 **Level II - Surgical pathology, gross and microscopic examination**
INCLUDES  Confirming identification and absence of disease:
Appendix, incidental
Fallopian tube, sterilization
Fingers or toes traumatic amputation
Foreskin, newborn
Hernia sac, any site
Hydrocele sac
Nerve
Skin, plastic repair
Sympathetic ganglion
Testis, castration
Vaginal mucosa, incidental
Vas deferens, sterilization
🖩 0.87  ☊ 0.87  **FUD** XXX  01 80 🖵
**AMA:** 2017,Jan,8; 2016,Jan,13; 2015,Jan,16; 2014,Feb,10; 2014,Jan,11; 2012,Jan,15-42

88304 **Level III - Surgical pathology, gross and microscopic examination**
INCLUDES  Abortion, induced
Abscess
Anal tag
Aneurysm-atrial/ventricular
Appendix, other than incidental
Artery, atheromatous plaque
Bartholin's gland cyst
Bone fragment(s), other than pathologic fracture
Bursa/ synovial cyst
Carpal tunnel tissue
Cartilage, shavings
Cholesteatoma
Colon, colostomy stoma
Conjunctiva-biopsy/pterygium
Cornea
Diverticulum-esophagus/small intestine
Dupuytren's contracture tissue
Femoral head, other than fracture
Fissure/fistula
Foreskin, other than newborn
Gallbladder
Ganglion cyst
Hematoma
Hemorrhoids
Hydatid of Morgagni
Intervertebral disc
Joint, loose body
Meniscus
Mucocele, salivary
Neuroma-Morton's/traumatic
Pilonidal cyst/sinus
Polyps, inflammatory-nasal/sinusoidal
Skin-cyst/tag/debridement
Soft tissue, debridement
Soft tissue, lipoma
Spermatocele
Tendon/tendon sheath
Testicular appendage
Thrombus or embolus
Tonsil and/or adenoids
Varicocele
Vas deferens, other than sterilization
Vein, varicosity
🖩 1.16  ☊ 1.16  **FUD** XXX  01 80 🖵
**AMA:** 2017,Jan,8; 2016,Jan,13; 2015,Jan,16; 2014,Feb,10; 2014,Jan,11; 2012,Jan,15-42

## 88305 Level IV - Surgical pathology, gross and microscopic examination

INCLUDES
Abortion, spontaneous/missed
Artery, biopsy
Bone exostosis
Bone marrow, biopsy
Brain/meninges, other than for tumor resection
Breast biopsy without microscopic assessment of surgical margin
Breast reduction mammoplasty
Bronchus, biopsy
Cell block, any source
Cervix, biopsy
Colon, biopsy
Duodenum, biopsy
Endocervix, curettings/biopsy
Endometrium, curettings/biopsy
Esophagus, biopsy
Extremity, amputation, traumatic
Fallopian tube, biopsy
Fallopian tube, ectopic pregnancy
Femoral head, fracture
Finger/toes, amputation, nontraumatic
Gingiva/oral mucosa, biopsy
Heart valve
Joint resection
Kidney biopsy
Larynx biopsy
Leiomyoma(s), uterine myomectomy-without uterus
Lip, biopsy/wedge resection
Lung, transbronchial biopsy
Lymph node, biopsy
Muscle, biopsy
Nasal mucosa, biopsy
Nasopharynx/oropharynx, biopsy
Nerve biopsy
Odontogenic/dental cyst
Omentum, biopsy
Ovary, biopsy/wedge resection
Ovary with or without tube, nonneoplastic
Parathyroid gland
Peritoneum, biopsy
Pituitary tumor
Placenta, other than third trimester
Pleura/pericardium biopsy/tissue
Polyp:
    Cervical/endometrial
    Colorectal
    Stomach/small intestine
Prostate:
    Needle biopsy
    TUR
Salivary gland, biopsy
Sinus, paranasal biopsy
Skin, other than cyst/tag/debridement/plastic repair
Small intestine, biopsy
Soft tissue, other than tumor/mas/lipoma/debridement
Spleen
Stomach biopsy
Synovium
Testis, other than tumor/biopsy, castration
Thyroglossal duct/brachial cleft cyst
Tongue, biopsy
Tonsil, biopsy
Trachea biopsy
Ureter, biopsy
Urethra, biopsy
Urinary bladder, biopsy
Uterus, with or without tubes and ovaries, for prolapse
Vagina biopsy
Vulva/labial biopsy

🖪 1.94    ✎ 1.94    **FUD** XXX      01 80 🖵

**AMA:** 2017,Jan,8; 2016,Jan,13; 2015,Jan,16; 2014,Feb,10; 2014,Jan,11; 2012,Jan,15-42

## 88307 Level V - Surgical pathology, gross and microscopic examination

INCLUDES
Adrenal resection
Bone, biopsy/curettings
Bone fragment(s), pathologic fractures
Brain, biopsy
Brain meninges, tumor resection
Breast, excision of lesion, requiring microscopic evaluation of surgical margins
Breast, mastectomy-partial/simple
Cervix, conization
Colon, segmental resection, other than for tumor
Extremity, amputation, nontraumatic
Eye, enucleation
Kidney, partial/total nephrectomy
Larynx, partial/total resection
Liver
    Biopsy, needle/wedge
    Partial resection
Lung, wedge biopsy
Lymph nodes, regional resection
Mediastinum, mass
Myocardium, biopsy
Odontogenic tumor
Ovary with or without tube, neoplastic
Pancreas, biopsy
Placenta, third trimester
Prostate, except radical resection
Salivary gland
Sentinel lymph node
Small intestine, resection, other than for tumor
Soft tissue mass (except lipoma)-biopsy/simple excision
Stomach-subtotal/total resection, other than for tumor
Testis, biopsy
Thymus, tumor
Thyroid, total/lobe
Ureter, resection
Urinary bladder, TUR
Uterus, with or without tubes and ovaries, other than neoplastic/prolapse

🖪 7.52    ✎ 7.52    **FUD** XXX      02 80 🖵

**AMA:** 2017,Jan,8; 2016,Jan,13; 2015,Jan,16; 2014,Feb,10; 2014,Jan,11; 2012,Jan,15-42

 **26/TC** PC/TC Only   **FUD** Follow-up Days    **A2-Z3** ASC Payment   **CMS:** IOM (Pub 100)    **50** Bilateral   **A-Y** OPPSI    ♂ Male Only   **80/80** Surg Assist Allowed / w/Doc    ♀ Female Only    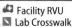 Facility RVU   Lab Crosswalk    ✎ Non-Facility RVU   Radiology Crosswalk    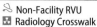 CCI   CLIA

**418**      CPT © 2017 American Medical Association. All Rights Reserved.      © 2017 Optum360, LLC

88309 **Level VI - Surgical pathology, gross and microscopic examination**

INCLUDES Bone resection
Breast, mastectomy-with regional lymph nodes
Colon:
  Segmental resection for tumor
  Total resection
Esophagus, partial/total resection
Extremity, disarticulation
Fetus, with dissection
Larynx, partial/total resection-with regional lymph nodes
Lung-total/lobe/segment resection
Pancreas, total/subtotal resection
Prostate, radical resection
Small intestine, resection for tumor
Soft tissue tumor, extensive resection
Stomach, subtotal/total resection for tumor
Testis, tumor
Tongue/tonsil, resection for tumor
Urinary bladder, partial/total resection
Uterus, with or without tubes and ovaries, neoplastic
Vulva, total/subtotal resection

EXCLUDES *Evaluation of fine needle aspirate (88172-88173)*
*Fine needle aspiration (10021-10022)*

📋 11.5    ✂ 11.5    **FUD** XXX    Q2 80 📋

**AMA:** 2017,Jan,8; 2016,Jan,13; 2015,Jan,16; 2014,Feb,10; 2014,Jan,11; 2012,Jan,15-42

## 88311-88399 [88341, 88350, 88364, 88373, 88374, 88377] Additional Surgical Pathology Services

**CMS:** 100-02,15,80.1 Payment for Clinical Laboratory Services

+ 88311 **Decalcification procedure (List separately in addition to code for surgical pathology examination)**

Code first surgical pathology exam (88302-88309)
📋 0.63    ✂ 0.63    **FUD** XXX    N 80

**AMA:** 2017,Jan,8; 2016,Jan,13; 2015,Jan,16; 2014,Jan,11; 2012,Jan,15-42

88312 **Special stain including interpretation and report; Group I for microorganisms (eg, acid fast, methenamine silver)**

INCLUDES Reporting one unit for each special stain performed on a surgical pathology block, cytologic sample, or hematologic smear

📋 2.78    ✂ 2.78    **FUD** XXX    Q1 80

**AMA:** 2017,Jan,8; 2016,Jan,13; 2015,Jan,16; 2014,Jan,11; 2012,Jan,15-42

88313 **Group II, all other (eg, iron, trichrome), except stain for microorganisms, stains for enzyme constituents, or immunocytochemistry and immunohistochemistry**

INCLUDES Reporting one unit for each special stain performed on a surgical pathology block, cytologic sample, or hematologic smear

EXCLUDES *Immunocytochemistry and immunohistochemistry (88342)*

📋 1.97    ✂ 1.97    **FUD** XXX    Q1 80 📋

**AMA:** 2017,Jan,8; 2016,Jan,13; 2015,Jan,16; 2014,Jan,11; 2012,Jan,15-42

+ 88314 **histochemical stain on frozen tissue block (List separately in addition to code for primary procedure)**

INCLUDES Reporting one unit for each special stain on each frozen surgical pathology block

EXCLUDES *Routine frozen section stain during Mohs surgery (17311-17315)*
*Special stain performed on frozen tissue section specimen to identify enzyme constituents (88319)*

Code also modifier 59 for nonroutine histochemical stain on frozen section during Mohs surgery
Code first (17311-17315, 88302-88309, 88331-88332)
📋 2.21    ✂ 2.21    **FUD** XXX    N 80

**AMA:** 2017,Jan,8; 2016,Jan,13; 2015,Jan,16; 2014,Jan,11

88319 **Group III, for enzyme constituents**

INCLUDES Reporting one unit for each special stain on each frozen surgical pathology block

EXCLUDES *Detection of enzyme constituents by immunohistochemical or immunocytochemical methodology (88342)*

📋 2.51    ✂ 2.51    **FUD** XXX    Q2 80

**AMA:** 2017,Jan,8; 2016,Jan,13; 2015,Jan,16; 2014,Jan,11

88321 **Consultation and report on referred slides prepared elsewhere**

📋 2.46    ✂ 2.92    **FUD** XXX    Q1 80 📋

**AMA:** 2017,Jan,8; 2016,Jan,13; 2015,Jan,16; 2014,Jan,11; 2013,Jun,13; 2012,Jan,15-42

88323 **Consultation and report on referred material requiring preparation of slides**

📋 3.67    ✂ 3.67    **FUD** XXX    Q1 80 📋

**AMA:** 2017,Jan,8; 2016,Jan,13; 2015,Jan,16; 2014,Jan,11; 2013,Jun,13; 2012,Jan,15-42

88325 **Consultation, comprehensive, with review of records and specimens, with report on referred material**

📋 4.41    ✂ 5.33    **FUD** XXX    Q1 80 📋

**AMA:** 2017,Jan,8; 2016,Jan,13; 2015,Jan,16; 2014,Jan,11; 2013,Jun,13; 2012,Jan,15-42

88329 **Pathology consultation during surgery;**

📋 1.06    ✂ 1.48    **FUD** XXX    Q1 80 📋

**AMA:** 2017,Jan,8; 2016,Jan,13; 2015,Jan,16; 2014,Feb,10; 2014,Jan,11; 2012,Jan,15-42

88331 **first tissue block, with frozen section(s), single specimen**

Code also cytologic evaluation performed at same time (88334)
📋 2.75    ✂ 2.75    **FUD** XXX    Q1 80 📋

**AMA:** 2017,Jan,8; 2016,Jan,13; 2015,Jan,16; 2014,Feb,10; 2014,Jan,11

+ 88332 **each additional tissue block with frozen section(s) (List separately in addition to code for primary procedure)**

Code first (88331)
📋 1.49    ✂ 1.49    **FUD** XXX    N 80 📋

**AMA:** 2017,Jan,8; 2016,Jan,13; 2015,Jan,16; 2014,Feb,10; 2014,Jan,11

88333 **cytologic examination (eg, touch prep, squash prep), initial site**

EXCLUDES *Intraprocedural cytologic evaluation of fine needle aspirate (88172)*
*Nonintraoperative cytologic examination (88160-88162)*

📋 2.66    ✂ 2.66    **FUD** XXX    Q2 80 📋

**AMA:** 2017,Jan,8; 2016,Jan,13; 2015,Jan,16; 2014,Feb,10; 2014,Jan,11; 2012,Jan,15-42

+ 88334 **cytologic examination (eg, touch prep, squash prep), each additional site (List separately in addition to code for primary procedure)**

EXCLUDES *Intraprocedural cytologic evaluation of fine needle aspirate (88172)*
*Nonintraoperative cytologic examination (88160-88162)*
*Percutaneous needle biopsy requiring intraprocedural cytologic examination (88333)*

Code first (88331, 88333)
📋 1.68    ✂ 1.68    **FUD** XXX    N 80 📋

**AMA:** 2017,Jan,8; 2016,Jan,13; 2015,Jan,16; 2014,Feb,10; 2014,Jan,11

*88341* **Resequenced code. See code following 88342.**

● New Code    ▲ Revised Code    ○ Reinstated    ● New Web Release    ▲ Revised Web Release    Unlisted    Not Covered    # Resequenced
⊘ AMA Mod 51 Exempt    ⑨ Optum Mod 51 Exempt    ⊚ Mod 63 Exempt    ✗ Non-FDA Drug    ★ Telemedicine    Ⓜ Maternity    Ⓐ Age Edit    + Add-on    **AMA:** CPT Asst
© 2017 Optum360, LLC    CPT © 2017 American Medical Association. All Rights Reserved.    **419**

**88342** Immunohistochemistry or immunocytochemistry, per specimen; initial single antibody stain procedure

EXCLUDES *Morphometric analysis, tumor immunohistochemistry, on same antibody (88360-88361)*
*Use of code more than one time for each specific antibody*

🚑 3.02  Ⓢ 3.02  **FUD** XXX  02 80 ▣

**AMA:** 2017,Jan,8; 2016,Jan,13; 2015,Jun,10; 2015,Jan,16; 2014,Jun,14; 2014,Jan,11; 2012,Jan,15-42

+ # **88341** each additional single antibody stain procedure (List separately in addition to code for primary procedure)

Code first (88342)

EXCLUDES *Morphometric analysis (88360-88361)*
*Use of code more than one time for each specific antibody*

🚑 2.57  Ⓢ 2.57  **FUD** ZZZ  N 80

**AMA:** 2017,Jan,8; 2016,Jan,13; 2015,Jun,10

**88344** each multiplex antibody stain procedure

INCLUDES Staining with multiple antibodies on the same slide

EXCLUDES *Morphometric analysis, tumor immunohistochemistry, on same antibody (88360-88361)*
*Use of code more than one time for each specific antibody*

🚑 4.87  Ⓢ 4.87  **FUD** XXX  01 80 ▣

**AMA:** 2017,Jan,8; 2016,Jan,13; 2015,Jun,10

**88346** Immunofluorescence, per specimen; initial single antibody stain procedure

EXCLUDES *Fluorescent in situ hybridization studies (88364-88369 [88364, 88373, 88374, 88377])*
*Multiple immunofluorescence analysis (88399)*

🚑 2.67  Ⓢ 2.67  **FUD** XXX  02 80 ▣

**AMA:** 2017,Jan,8; 2016,Jan,13; 2015,Jan,16; 2014,Jan,11

+ # **88350** each additional single antibody stain procedure (List separately in addition to code for primary procedure)

🚑 2.07  Ⓢ 2.07  **FUD** ZZZ  N 80

EXCLUDES *Fluorescent in situ hybridization studies (88364-88369 [88364, 88373, 88374, 88377])*
*Multiple immunofluorescence analysis (88399)*

Code first (88346)

**88348** Electron microscopy, diagnostic

🚑 9.79  Ⓢ 9.79  **FUD** XXX  02 80

**AMA:** 2011,Dec,14-18; 2005,Jul,11-12

**88350** Resequenced code. See code following 88346.

**88355** Morphometric analysis; skeletal muscle

🚑 4.03  Ⓢ 4.03  **FUD** XXX  01 80 ▣

**AMA:** 2017,Jan,8; 2016,Jan,13; 2015,Jan,16; 2014,Jan,11

**88356** nerve

🚑 5.91  Ⓢ 5.91  **FUD** XXX  01 80 ▣

**AMA:** 2017,Jan,8; 2016,Jan,13; 2015,Jan,16; 2014,Jun,14; 2014,Jan,11

**88358** tumor (eg, DNA ploidy)

EXCLUDES *Special stain, Group II (88313)*

🚑 2.53  Ⓢ 2.53  **FUD** XXX  02 80 ▣

**AMA:** 2017,Jan,8; 2016,Jan,13; 2015,Jan,16; 2014,Jan,11; 2012,Jan,15-42

**88360** Morphometric analysis, tumor immunohistochemistry (eg, Her-2/neu, estrogen receptor/progesterone receptor), quantitative or semiquantitative, per specimen, each single antibody stain procedure; manual

EXCLUDES *Additional stain procedures unless each test is for different antibody (88341, 88342, 88344)*
*Morphometric analysis using in situ hybridization techniques (88367-88368 [88373, 88374])*

🚑 3.96  Ⓢ 3.96  **FUD** XXX  02 80 ▣

**AMA:** 2017,Jan,8; 2016,Jan,13; 2015,Jun,10; 2015,Jan,16; 2014,Jun,14; 2014,Jan,11

**88361** using computer-assisted technology

EXCLUDES *Additional stain procedures unless each test is for different antibody (88341, 88342, 88344)*
*Morphometric analysis using in situ hybridization techniques (88367-88368 [88373, 88374])*

🚑 4.37  Ⓢ 4.37  **FUD** XXX  02 80 ▣

**AMA:** 2017,Jan,8; 2016,Jan,13; 2015,Jun,10; 2015,Jan,16; 2014,Jun,14; 2014,Jan,11

**88362** Nerve teasing preparations

🚑 6.54  Ⓢ 6.54  **FUD** XXX  02 80 ▣

**AMA:** 2017,Jan,8; 2016,Jan,13; 2015,Jan,16; 2014,Jan,11

**88363** Examination and selection of retrieved archival (ie, previously diagnosed) tissue(s) for molecular analysis (eg, KRAS mutational analysis)

INCLUDES Archival retrieval only

🚑 0.57  Ⓢ 0.67  **FUD** XXX  01 80

**AMA:** 2017,Jan,8; 2016,Jan,13; 2015,Jan,16; 2014,Jan,11

**88364** Resequenced code. See code following 88365.

**88365** In situ hybridization (eg, FISH), per specimen; initial single probe stain procedure

EXCLUDES *Morphometric analysis probe stain procedures with same probe (88367, [88374], 88368, [88377])*

🚑 5.01  Ⓢ 5.01  **FUD** XXX  01 80 ▣

**AMA:** 2017,Jan,8; 2016,Jan,13; 2015,Jan,16; 2014,Jan,11; 2013,Sep,3-12; 2012,May,3-10; 2012,Jan,15-42

+ # **88364** each additional single probe stain procedure (List separately in addition to code for primary procedure)

🚑 3.71  Ⓢ 3.71  **FUD** ZZZ  N 80 ▣

Code first (88365)

**88366** each multiplex probe stain procedure

🚑 7.25  Ⓢ 7.25  **FUD** XXX  01 80 ▣

EXCLUDES *Morphometric analysis probe stain procedures (88367, [88374], 88368, [88377])*

**88367** Morphometric analysis, in situ hybridization (quantitative or semi-quantitative), using computer-assisted technology, per specimen; initial single probe stain procedure

EXCLUDES *In situ hybridization probe stain procedures for same probe (88365, 88366, 88368, [88377])*
*Morphometric in situ hybridization evaluation of urinary tract cytologic specimens (88120-88121)*

🚑 2.99  Ⓢ 2.99  **FUD** XXX  02 80 ▣

**AMA:** 2017,Jan,8; 2016,Jan,13; 2015,Jan,16; 2014,Jan,11; 2013,Sep,3-12; 2012,May,3-10; 2012,Jan,15-42

+ # **88373** each additional single probe stain procedure (List separately in addition to code for primary procedure)

🚑 2.23  Ⓢ 2.23  **FUD** ZZZ  N 80

Code first (88367)

# **88374** each multiplex probe stain procedure

🚑 9.57  Ⓢ 9.57  **FUD** XXX  01 80 ▣

EXCLUDES *In situ hybridization probe stain procedures for same probe (88365, 88366, 88368, [88377])*

**88368** Morphometric analysis, in situ hybridization (quantitative or semi-quantitative), manual, per specimen; initial single probe stain procedure

EXCLUDES *In situ hybridization probe stain procedures for same probe (88365, 88366-88367, [88374])*
*Morphometric in situ hybridization evaluation of urinary tract cytologic specimens (88120-88121)*

🚑 3.30  Ⓢ 3.30  **FUD** XXX  02 80 ▣

**AMA:** 2017,Jan,8; 2016,Jan,13; 2015,Jan,16; 2014,Jan,11; 2013,Sep,3-12; 2012,May,3-10; 2012,Jan,15-42

+ **88369** each additional single probe stain procedure (List separately in addition to code for primary procedure)

🚑 3.02  Ⓢ 3.02  **FUD** ZZZ  N 80 ▣

Code first (88368)

26/TC PC/TC Only   A2-Z3 ASC Payment   50 Bilateral   ♂ Male Only   ♀ Female Only   🚑 Facility RVU   Ⓢ Non-Facility RVU   ▣ CCI
**FUD** Follow-up Days   **CMS:** IOM (Pub 100)   A-Y OPPSI   80/80 Surg Assist Allowed / w/Doc   ◩ Lab Crosswalk   ◧ Radiology Crosswalk   ⊠ CLIA

**420**
CPT © 2017 American Medical Association. All Rights Reserved.
© 2017 Optum360, LLC

# 88377    each multiplex probe stain procedure

⚡ 11.4    ⚖ 11.4    **FUD** XXX    Q1 80

EXCLUDES    *In situ hybridization probe stain procedures for same probe (88365, 88366-88367, [88374])*

88371    **Protein analysis of tissue by Western Blot, with interpretation and report;**

⚡ 0.00    ⚖ 0.00    **FUD** XXX    N 🖵

**AMA:** 2017,Jan,8; 2016,Jan,13; 2015,Dec,18; 2015,Jan,16; 2014,Jan,11

88372    **immunological probe for band identification, each**

⚡ 0.00    ⚖ 0.00    **FUD** XXX    N 🖵

**AMA:** 2017,Jan,8; 2016,Jan,13; 2015,Jan,16; 2014,Jan,11

*88373*    **Resequenced code. See code following 88367.**

*88374*    **Resequenced code. See code following 88367.**

88375    **Optical endomicroscopic image(s), interpretation and report, real-time or referred, each endoscopic session**

EXCLUDES    *Endoscopic procedures that include optical endomicroscopy (43206, 43252, 0397T)*

⚡ 1.31    ⚖ 1.31    **FUD** XXX    B 80 26 🖵

**AMA:** 2017,Jan,8; 2016,Jan,13; 2015,Jan,16; 2013,Aug,5

*88377*    **Resequenced code. See code following 88369.**

88380    **Microdissection (ie, sample preparation of microscopically identified target); laser capture**

EXCLUDES    *Microdissection, manual procedure (88381)*

⚡ 3.86    ⚖ 3.86    **FUD** XXX    N 80 🖵

**AMA:** 2017,Jan,8; 2016,Jan,13; 2015,Jan,16; 2014,Jan,11; 2013,Sep,3-12; 2012,May,3-10

88381    **manual**

EXCLUDES    *Microdissection, laser capture procedure (88380)*

⚡ 3.43    ⚖ 3.43    **FUD** XXX    N 80 🖵

**AMA:** 2017,Jan,8; 2016,Jan,13; 2015,Jan,16; 2014,Jan,11; 2013,Sep,3-12; 2012,May,3-10; 2012,May,14-15

88387    **Macroscopic examination, dissection, and preparation of tissue for non-microscopic analytical studies (eg, nucleic acid-based molecular studies); each tissue preparation (eg, a single lymph node)**

EXCLUDES    *Pathology consultation during surgery (88329-88334, 88388)*
*Tissue preparation for microbiologic cultures or flow cytometric studies*

⚡ 1.08    ⚖ 1.08    **FUD** XXX    N 80 🖵

**AMA:** 2017,Jan,8; 2016,Jan,13; 2015,Jan,16; 2014,Jan,11; 2012,Jan,15-42

+    88388    **in conjunction with a touch imprint, intraoperative consultation, or frozen section, each tissue preparation (eg, a single lymph node) (List separately in addition to code for primary procedure)**

EXCLUDES    *Tissue preparation for microbiologic cultures or flow cytometric studies*

Code first (88329-88334)

⚡ 0.98    ⚖ 0.98    **FUD** XXX    N 80 🖵

**AMA:** 2017,Jan,8; 2016,Jan,13; 2015,Jan,16; 2014,Jan,11; 2012,Jan,15-42

88399    **Unlisted surgical pathology procedure**

⚡ 0.00    ⚖ 0.00    **FUD** XXX    Q1 80

**AMA:** 2017,Jan,8; 2016,Jan,13; 2015,Jan,16; 2014,Jun,14; 2014,Jan,11; 2012,Jan,15-42

## 88720-88749 Transcutaneous Procedures

EXCLUDES    *Transcutaneous oxyhemoglobin measurement (0493T)*
*Wavelength fluorescent spectroscopy of advanced glycation end products (skin) (88749)*

88720    **Bilirubin, total, transcutaneous**

EXCLUDES    *Transdermal oxygen saturation testing (94760-94762)*

⚡ 0.00    ⚖ 0.00    **FUD** XXX    Q 🖵

**AMA:** 2017,Jan,8; 2016,Jan,13; 2015,Jan,16; 2014,Jan,11

88738    **Hemoglobin (Hgb), quantitative, transcutaneous**

EXCLUDES    *In vitro hemoglobin measurement (85018)*

⚡ 0.00    ⚖ 0.00    **FUD** XXX    Q

**AMA:** 2017,Jan,8; 2016,Jan,13; 2015,Jan,16; 2014,Jan,11

88740    **Hemoglobin, quantitative, transcutaneous, per day; carboxyhemoglobin**

EXCLUDES    *In vitro carboxyhemoglobin measurement (82375)*

⚡ 0.00    ⚖ 0.00    **FUD** XXX    Q

**AMA:** 2017,Jan,8; 2016,Jan,13; 2015,Jan,16; 2014,Jan,11

88741    **methemoglobin**

EXCLUDES    *In vitro quantitative methemoglobin measurement (83050)*

⚡ 0.00    ⚖ 0.00    **FUD** XXX    Q 🖵

**AMA:** 2017,Jan,8; 2016,Jan,13; 2015,Jan,16; 2014,Jan,11

88749    **Unlisted in vivo (eg, transcutaneous) laboratory service**

INCLUDES    *All in vivo measurements not specifically listed*

⚡ 0.00    ⚖ 0.00    **FUD** XXX    Q

**AMA:** 2010,Dec,7-10

## 89049-89240 Other Pathology Services

89049    **Caffeine halothane contracture test (CHCT) for malignant hyperthermia susceptibility, including interpretation and report**

⚡ 1.87    ⚖ 7.54    **FUD** XXX    Q1 80

**AMA:** 2017,Jan,8; 2016,Jan,13; 2015,Jan,16; 2014,Jan,11; 2012,Jan,15-42

89050    **Cell count, miscellaneous body fluids (eg, cerebrospinal fluid, joint fluid), except blood;**

⚡ 0.00    ⚖ 0.00    **FUD** XXX    Q 🖵

**AMA:** 2017,Jan,8; 2016,Jan,13; 2015,Jan,16; 2014,Jan,11

89051    **with differential count**

⚡ 0.00    ⚖ 0.00    **FUD** XXX    Q 🖵

**AMA:** 2017,Jan,8; 2016,Jan,13; 2015,Jan,16; 2014,Jan,11

89055    **Leukocyte assessment, fecal, qualitative or semiquantitative**

⚡ 0.00    ⚖ 0.00    **FUD** XXX    Q

**AMA:** 2017,Jan,8; 2016,Jan,13; 2015,Jan,16; 2014,Jan,11

89060    **Crystal identification by light microscopy with or without polarizing lens analysis, tissue or any body fluid (except urine)**

EXCLUDES    *Crystal identification on paraffin embedded tissue*

⚡ 0.00    ⚖ 0.00    **FUD** XXX    Q 🖵

**AMA:** 2017,Jan,8; 2016,Jan,13; 2015,Jan,16; 2014,Jan,11

89125    **Fat stain, feces, urine, or respiratory secretions**

⚡ 0.00    ⚖ 0.00    **FUD** XXX    Q 🖵

**AMA:** 2017,Jan,8; 2016,Jan,13; 2015,Jan,16; 2014,Jan,11

89160    **Meat fibers, feces**

⚡ 0.00    ⚖ 0.00    **FUD** XXX    Q 🖵

**AMA:** 2017,Jan,8; 2016,Jan,13; 2015,Jan,16; 2014,Jan,11

89190    **Nasal smear for eosinophils**

⚡ 0.00    ⚖ 0.00    **FUD** XXX    Q 🖵

**AMA:** 2017,Jan,8; 2016,Jan,13; 2015,Jan,16; 2014,Jan,11; 2012,Jan,15-42

89220    **Sputum, obtaining specimen, aerosol induced technique (separate procedure)**

⚡ 0.46    ⚖ 0.46    **FUD** XXX    Q1 80 TC

**AMA:** 2017,Jan,8; 2016,Jan,13; 2015,Jan,16; 2014,Jan,11

89230    **Sweat collection by iontophoresis**

⚡ 0.12    ⚖ 0.12    **FUD** XXX    Q1 80 TC 🖵

**AMA:** 2017,Jan,8; 2016,Jan,13; 2015,Jan,16; 2014,Jan,11

89240    **Unlisted miscellaneous pathology test**

⚡ 0.00    ⚖ 0.00    **FUD** XXX    Q1 80

**AMA:** 2017,Jan,8; 2016,Jan,13; 2015,Jan,16; 2014,Jan,11; 2012,Jan,15-42

---

● New Code    ▲ Revised Code    ○ Reinstated    ● New Web Release    ▲ Revised Web Release    Unlisted    Not Covered    # Resequenced
⊘ AMA Mod 51 Exempt    ⑤ Optum Mod 51 Exempt    ⑥⑤ Mod 63 Exempt    ✗ Non-FDA Drug    ★ Telemedicine    Ⓜ Maternity    Ⓐ Age Edit    + Add-on    **AMA:** CPT Asst

© 2017 Optum360, LLC    CPT © 2017 American Medical Association. All Rights Reserved.

## 89250-89398 Infertility Treatment Services

**CMS:** 100-02,1,100 Treatment for Infertility

**89250**  **Culture of oocyte(s)/embryo(s), less than 4 days;**
    🖑 0.00   🔬 0.00  **FUD** XXX     01
    **AMA:** 2017,Jan,8; 2016,Jan,13; 2015,Jan,16; 2014,Jan,11; 2012,Jan,15-42

**89251**  **with co-culture of oocyte(s)/embryos**
    EXCLUDES  *Extended culture of oocyte(s)/embryo(s) (89272)*
    🖑 0.00   🔬 0.00  **FUD** XXX     02 🖵
    **AMA:** 2017,Jan,8; 2016,Jan,13; 2015,Jan,16; 2014,Jan,11; 2012,Jan,15-42

**89253**  **Assisted embryo hatching, microtechniques (any method)**
    🖑 0.00   🔬 0.00  **FUD** XXX     01
    **AMA:** 2017,Jan,8; 2016,Jan,13; 2015,Jan,16; 2014,Jan,11; 2012,Jan,15-42

**89254**  **Oocyte identification from follicular fluid**
    🖑 0.00   🔬 0.00  **FUD** XXX     01
    **AMA:** 2017,Jan,8; 2016,Jan,13; 2015,Jan,16; 2014,Jan,11; 2012,Jan,15-42

**89255**  **Preparation of embryo for transfer (any method)**
    🖑 0.00   🔬 0.00  **FUD** XXX     01
    **AMA:** 2017,Jan,8; 2016,Jan,13; 2015,Jan,16; 2014,Jan,11; 2012,Jan,15-42

**89257**  **Sperm identification from aspiration (other than seminal fluid)**
    EXCLUDES  *Semen analysis (89300-89320)*
               *Sperm identification from testis tissue (89264)*
    🖑 0.00   🔬 0.00  **FUD** XXX     01 🖵
    **AMA:** 2017,Jan,8; 2016,Jan,13; 2015,Jan,16; 2014,Jan,11; 2012,Jan,15-42

**89258**  **Cryopreservation; embryo(s)**
    🖑 0.00   🔬 0.00  **FUD** XXX     02
    **AMA:** 2017,Jan,8; 2016,Jan,13; 2015,Jan,16; 2014,Jan,11; 2012,Jan,15-42

**89259**  **sperm**
    EXCLUDES  *Cryopreservation of testicular reproductive tissue (89335)*
    🖑 0.00   🔬 0.00  **FUD** XXX     01
    **AMA:** 2017,Jan,8; 2016,Jan,13; 2015,Jan,16; 2014,Jan,11; 2012,Jan,15-42

**89260**  **Sperm isolation; simple prep (eg, sperm wash and swim-up) for insemination or diagnosis with semen analysis**
    🖑 0.00   🔬 0.00  **FUD** XXX     01 🖵
    **AMA:** 2017,Jan,8; 2016,Jan,13; 2015,Jan,16; 2014,Jan,11; 2012,Jan,15-42

**89261**  **complex prep (eg, Percoll gradient, albumin gradient) for insemination or diagnosis with semen analysis**
    EXCLUDES  *Semen analysis without sperm wash or swim-up (89320)*
    🖑 0.00   🔬 0.00  **FUD** XXX     01 🖵
    **AMA:** 2017,Jan,8; 2016,Jan,13; 2015,Jan,16; 2014,Jan,11; 2012,Jan,15-42

**89264**  **Sperm identification from testis tissue, fresh or cryopreserved** ♂
    EXCLUDES  *Biopsy of testis (54500, 54505)*
               *Semen analysis (89300-89320)*
               *Sperm identification from aspiration (89257)*
    🖑 0.00   🔬 0.00  **FUD** XXX     01 🖵
    **AMA:** 2017,Jan,8; 2016,Jan,13; 2015,Jan,16; 2014,Jan,11; 2012,Jan,15-42

**89268**  **Insemination of oocytes**
    🖑 0.00   🔬 0.00  **FUD** XXX     01
    **AMA:** 2017,Jan,8; 2016,Jan,13; 2015,Jan,16; 2014,Jan,11; 2012,Jan,15-42

**89272**  **Extended culture of oocyte(s)/embryo(s), 4-7 days**
    🖑 0.00   🔬 0.00  **FUD** XXX     02
    **AMA:** 2017,Jan,8; 2016,Jan,13; 2015,Jan,16; 2014,Jan,11; 2012,Jan,15-42

**89280**  **Assisted oocyte fertilization, microtechnique; less than or equal to 10 oocytes**
    🖑 0.00   🔬 0.00  **FUD** XXX     02
    **AMA:** 2017,Jan,8; 2016,Jan,13; 2015,Jan,16; 2014,Jan,11; 2012,Jan,15-42

**89281**  **greater than 10 oocytes**
    🖑 0.00   🔬 0.00  **FUD** XXX     01
    **AMA:** 2017,Jan,8; 2016,Jan,13; 2015,Jan,16; 2014,Jan,11; 2012,Jan,15-42

**89290**  **Biopsy, oocyte polar body or embryo blastomere, microtechnique (for pre-implantation genetic diagnosis); less than or equal to 5 embryos**
    🖑 0.00   🔬 0.00  **FUD** XXX     01
    **AMA:** 2017,Jan,8; 2016,Jan,13; 2015,Jan,16; 2014,Jan,11; 2012,Jan,15-42

**89291**  **greater than 5 embryos**
    🖑 0.00   🔬 0.00  **FUD** XXX     01
    **AMA:** 2017,Jan,8; 2016,Jan,13; 2015,Jan,16; 2014,Jan,11; 2012,Jan,15-42

**89300**  **Semen analysis; presence and/or motility of sperm including Huhner test (post coital)** ♀
    🖑 0.00   🔬 0.00  **FUD** XXX     ✖ 🔲 🖵
    **AMA:** 2017,Jan,8; 2016,Jan,13; 2015,Jan,16; 2014,Jan,11; 2012,Jan,15-42

**89310**  **motility and count (not including Huhner test)** ♂
    🖑 0.00   🔬 0.00  **FUD** XXX     🔲 🖵
    **AMA:** 2017,Jan,8; 2016,Jan,13; 2015,Jan,16; 2014,Jan,11; 2012,Jan,15-42

**89320**  **volume, count, motility, and differential** ♂
    EXCLUDES  *Skin testing (86485-86580, 95012-95199)*
    🖑 0.00   🔬 0.00  **FUD** XXX     🔲 🖵
    **AMA:** 2017,Jan,8; 2016,Jan,13; 2015,Jan,16; 2014,Jan,11; 2012,Jan,15-42

**89321**  **sperm presence and motility of sperm, if performed** ♂
    EXCLUDES  *Hyaluronan binding assay (HBA) (89398)*
    🖑 0.00   🔬 0.00  **FUD** XXX     ✖ 🔲 🖵
    **AMA:** 2017,Jan,8; 2016,Jan,13; 2015,Jan,16; 2014,Jan,11; 2012,Jan,15-42

**89322**  **volume, count, motility, and differential using strict morphologic criteria (eg, Kruger)** ♂
    🖑 0.00   🔬 0.00  **FUD** XXX     🔲 🖵
    **AMA:** 2017,Jan,8; 2016,Jan,13; 2015,Jan,16; 2014,Jan,11; 2012,Jan,15-42

**89325**  **Sperm antibodies** ♂
    EXCLUDES  *Medicolegal identification of sperm (88125)*
    🖑 0.00   🔬 0.00  **FUD** XXX     🔲 🖵
    **AMA:** 2017,Jan,8; 2016,Jan,13; 2015,Jan,16; 2014,Jan,11; 2012,Jan,15-42

**89329**  **Sperm evaluation; hamster penetration test** ♂
    🖑 0.00   🔬 0.00  **FUD** XXX     🔲 🖵
    **AMA:** 2017,Jan,8; 2016,Jan,13; 2015,Jan,16; 2014,Jan,11; 2012,Jan,15-42

**89330**  **cervical mucus penetration test, with or without spinnbarkeit test** ♂
    🖑 0.00   🔬 0.00  **FUD** XXX     🔲 🖵
    **AMA:** 2017,Jan,8; 2016,Jan,13; 2015,Jan,16; 2014,Jan,11; 2012,Jan,15-42

**89331**  **Sperm evaluation, for retrograde ejaculation, urine (sperm concentration, motility, and morphology, as indicated)** ♂
    EXCLUDES  *Detection of sperm in urine (81015)*
    *Code also semen analysis on concurrent sperm specimen (89300-89322)*
    🖑 0.00   🔬 0.00  **FUD** XXX     🔲 🖵
    **AMA:** 2017,Jan,8; 2016,Jan,13; 2015,Jan,16; 2014,Jan,11; 2012,Jan,15-42

| 26/TC PC/TC Only | A2-Z3 ASC Payment | 50 Bilateral | ♂ Male Only | ♀ Female Only | 🖑 Facility RVU | 🔬 Non-Facility RVU | 🖵 CCI |
| FUD Follow-up Days | CMS: IOM (Pub 100) | A-Y OPPSI | 80/80 Surg Assist Allowed / w/Doc | | 🔲 Lab Crosswalk | 🔲 Radiology Crosswalk | ✖ CLIA |

422                CPT © 2017 American Medical Association. All Rights Reserved.           © 2017 Optum360, LLC

89335 **Cryopreservation, reproductive tissue, testicular**

EXCLUDES *Cryopreservation of:*
*Embryo(s) (89258)*
*Oocytes:*
*Immature ([0357T])*
*Mature (89337)*
*Ovarian tissue (0058T)*
*Sperm (89259)*

🔄 0.00 ✂ 0.00 **FUD** XXX 〔Q1〕

**AMA:** 2017,Jan,8; 2016,Jan,13; 2015,Jan,16; 2014,Jan,11; 2012,Jan,15-42

89337 **Cryopreservation, mature oocyte(s)** ♀

EXCLUDES *Cryopreservation of immature oocyte[s] ([0357T])*

🔄 0.00 ✂ 0.00 **FUD** XXX 〔Q1〕▯

**AMA:** 2017,Jan,8; 2016,Jan,13; 2015,Jan,16

89342 **Storage (per year); embryo(s)**

🔄 0.00 ✂ 0.00 **FUD** XXX 〔Q1〕

**AMA:** 2017,Jan,8; 2016,Jan,13; 2015,Jan,16; 2014,Jan,11; 2012,Jan,15-42

89343 **sperm/semen**

🔄 0.00 ✂ 0.00 **FUD** XXX 〔Q1〕

**AMA:** 2017,Jan,8; 2016,Jan,13; 2015,Jan,16; 2014,Jan,11; 2012,Jan,15-42

89344 **reproductive tissue, testicular/ovarian**

🔄 0.00 ✂ 0.00 **FUD** XXX 〔Q1〕

**AMA:** 2017,Jan,8; 2016,Jan,13; 2015,Jan,16; 2014,Jan,11; 2012,Jan,15-42

89346 **oocyte(s)**

🔄 0.00 ✂ 0.00 **FUD** XXX 〔Q2〕

**AMA:** 2017,Jan,8; 2016,Jan,13; 2015,Jan,16; 2014,Jan,11; 2012,Jan,15-42

89352 **Thawing of cryopreserved; embryo(s)**

🔄 0.00 ✂ 0.00 **FUD** XXX 〔Q1〕

**AMA:** 2017,Jan,8; 2016,Jan,13; 2015,Jan,16; 2014,Jan,11; 2012,Jan,15-42

89353 **sperm/semen, each aliquot**

🔄 0.00 ✂ 0.00 **FUD** XXX 〔Q1〕

**AMA:** 2017,Jan,8; 2016,Jan,13; 2015,Jan,16; 2014,Jan,11; 2012,Jan,15-42

89354 **reproductive tissue, testicular/ovarian**

🔄 0.00 ✂ 0.00 **FUD** XXX 〔Q1〕

**AMA:** 2017,Jan,8; 2016,Jan,13; 2015,Jan,16; 2014,Jan,11; 2012,Jan,15-42

89356 **oocytes, each aliquot**

🔄 0.00 ✂ 0.00 **FUD** XXX 〔Q1〕

**AMA:** 2017,Jan,8; 2016,Jan,13; 2015,Jan,16; 2014,Jan,11; 2012,Jan,15-42

89398 **Unlisted reproductive medicine laboratory procedure**

🔄 0.00 ✂ 0.00 **FUD** XXX 〔Q1〕

INCLUDES Hyaluronan binding assay (HBA)

## 0001U-0023U Proprietary Laboratory Analysis (PLA)

In response to the Protecting Access to Medicare Act of 2014 (PAMA), which focuses on payment and coding of clinical laboratory studies paid for under the Medicare Clinical Laboratory Fee Schedule (CLFS), the AMA has developed a new category of CPT codes, known as Proprietary Laboratory Analysis (PLA), which will be released on a quarterly basis. These alphanumeric codes will appear at the end of the Pathology and Laboratory chapter of the CPT book and will include a wide range of tests. Codes 0001U-0003U have an effective date of February 1, 2017. Codes 0004U and 0005U are effective May 1, 2017. Codes 0006U-0017U are effective August 1, 2017. Codes 0018U-0023U are effective October 1, 2017.

INCLUDES All necessary investigative services
PLA codes take priority over other CPT codes

EXCLUDES *Additional procedures necessary before cell lysis (88380-88381)*

● 0001U **Red blood cell antigen typing, DNA, human erythrocyte antigen gene analysis of 35 antigens from 11 blood groups, utilizing whole blood, common RBC alleles reported**

🔄 0.00 ✂ 0.00 **FUD** 000 〔A〕▯

INCLUDES PreciseType® HEA Test, Immucor, Inc.

● 0002U **Oncology (colorectal), quantitative assessment of three urine metabolites (ascorbic acid, succinic acid and carnitine) by liquid chromatography with tandem mass spectrometry (LC-MS/MS) using multiple reaction monitoring acquisition, algorithm reported as likelihood of adenomatous polyps**

🔄 0.00 ✂ 0.00 **FUD** 000 〔Q〕▯

INCLUDES PolypDX™, Atlantic Diagnostic Laboratories, LLC, Metabolomic Technologies, Inc.

● 0003U **Oncology (ovarian) biochemical assays of five proteins (apolipoprotein A-1, CA 125 II, follicle stimulating hormone, human epididymis protein 4, transferrin), utilizing serum, algorithm reported as a likelihood score**

🔄 0.00 ✂ 0.00 **FUD** 000 〔Q〕▯

INCLUDES Overa (OVA1 Next Generation), Aspira Labs, Inc., Vermillion, Inc.

● 0004U **Infectious disease (bacterial), DNA, 27 resistance genes, PCR amplification and probe hybridization in microarray format (molecular detection and identification of AmpC, carbapenemase and ESBL coding genes), bacterial culture colonies, report of genes detected or not detected, per isolate**

🔄 0.00 ✂ 0.00 **FUD** 000 〔A〕

INCLUDES Gram-Negative Bacterial Resistance Gene PCR Panel, Mayo Clinic, Check-Points Health BV, Wageningen, Netherlands

● 0005U **Oncology (prostate) gene expression profile by real-time RT-PCR of 3 genes (ERG, PCA3, and SPDEF), urine, algorithm reported as risk score**

🔄 0.00 ✂ 0.00 **FUD** 000 〔Q〕

INCLUDES ExosomeDx®, Prostate (IntelliScore), Exosome Diagnostics, Inc.

● 0006U **Prescription drug monitoring, 120 or more drugs and substances, definitive tandem mass spectrometry with chromatography, urine, qualitative report of presence (including quantitative levels, when detected) or absence of each drug or substance with description and severity of potential interactions, with identified substances, per date of service**

🔄 0.00 ✂ 0.00 **FUD** 000 〔Q〕

INCLUDES Aegis Drug-Drug Interaction Test, Aegis Sciences Corporation

● 0007U **Drug test(s), presumptive, with definitive confirmation of positive results, any number of drug classes, urine, includes specimen verification including DNA authentication in comparison to buccal DNA, per date of service**

🔄 0.00 ✂ 0.00 **FUD** 000 〔Q〕

INCLUDES ToxProtect, Genotox Laboratories LTD

EXCLUDES *PLA code with the same clinical descriptor (see appendix L for clarification of code) (0020U)*

● 0008U **Helicobacter pylori detection and antibiotic resistance, DNA, 16S and 23S rRNA, gyrA, pbp1, rdxA and rpoB, next generation sequencing, formalin-fixed paraffin embedded or fresh tissue, predictive, reported as positive or negative for resistance to clarithromycin, fluoroquinolones, metronidazole, amoxicillin, tetracycline and rifabutin**

🔄 0.00 ✂ 0.00 **FUD** 000 〔A〕

INCLUDES AmHPR Helicobacter pylori Antibiotic Resistance Next Generation Sequencing Panel, American Molecular Laboratories, Inc.

● 0009U **Oncology (breast cancer), ERBB2 (HER2) copy number by FISH, tumor cells from formalin fixed paraffin embedded tissue isolated using image-based dielectrophoresis (DEP) sorting, reported as ERBB2 gene amplified or non-amplified**

🔄 0.00 ✂ 0.00 **FUD** 000 〔Q〕

INCLUDES DEPArray™ HER2, PacificDx

● New Code ▲ Revised Code ○ Reinstated ● New Web Release ▲ Revised Web Release Unlisted Not Covered # Resequenced
⊘ AMA Mod 51 Exempt ⑤ Optum Mod 51 Exempt ⊚ Mod 63 Exempt ✗ Non-FDA Drug ★ Telemedicine Ⓜ Maternity Ⓐ Age Edit + Add-on **AMA:** CPT Asst
© 2017 Optum360, LLC         CPT © 2017 American Medical Association. All Rights Reserved.         **423**

● 0010U **Infectious disease (bacterial), strain typing by whole genome sequencing, phylogenetic-based report of strain relatedness, per submitted isolate**
    🔹 0.00   🔹 0.00   **FUD** 000                    [A]
    INCLUDES    Bacterial Typing by Whole Genome Sequencing, Mayo Clinic

● 0011U **Prescription drug monitoring, evaluation of drugs present by LC-MS/MS, using oral fluid, reported as a comparison to an estimated steady-state range, per date of service including all drug compounds and metabolites**
    🔹 0.00   🔹 0.00   **FUD** 000                    [Q]
    INCLUDES    Cordant CORE™, Cordant Health Solutions

● 0012U **Germline disorders, gene rearrangement detection by whole genome next-generation sequencing, DNA, whole blood, report of specific gene rearrangement(s)**
    🔹 0.00   🔹 0.00   **FUD** 000                    [A]
    INCLUDES    MatePair Targeted Rearrangements, Congenital, Mayo Clinic

● 0013U **Oncology (solid organ neoplasia), gene rearrangement detection by whole genome next-generation sequencing, DNA, fresh or frozen tissue or cells, report of specific gene rearrangement(s)**
    🔹 0.00   🔹 0.00   **FUD** 000                    [A]
    INCLUDES    MatePair Targeted Rearrangements, Oncology, Mayo Clinic

● 0014U **Hematology (hematolymphoid neoplasia), gene rearrangement detection by whole genome next-generation sequencing, DNA, whole blood or bone marrow, report of specific gene rearrangement(s)**
    🔹 0.00   🔹 0.00   **FUD** 000                    [A]
    INCLUDES    MatePair Targeted Rearrangements, Hematologic, Mayo Clinic

● 0015U **Drug metabolism (adverse drug reactions), DNA, 22 drug metabolism and transporter genes, real-time PCR, blood or buccal swab, genotype and metabolizer status for therapeutic decision support**
    🔹 0.00   🔹 0.00   **FUD** 000                    [Q]
    INCLUDES    OneOme RightMed Pharmacogenomic Test, OneOme, LLC

● 0016U **Oncology (hematolymphoid neoplasia), RNA, BCR/ABL1 major and minor breakpoint fusion transcripts, quantitative PCR amplification, blood or bone marrow, report of fusion not detected or detected with quantitation**
    🔹 0.00   🔹 0.00   **FUD** 000                    [A]
    INCLUDES    BCR-ABL1 major and minor breakpoint fusion transcripts, University of Iowa, Department of Pathology, Asuragen

● 0017U **Oncology (hematolymphoid neoplasia), JAK2 mutation, DNA, PCR amplification of exons 12-14 and sequence analysis, blood or bone marrow, report of JAK2 mutation not detected or detected**
    🔹 0.00   🔹 0.00   **FUD** 000                    [A]
    INCLUDES    JAK2 Mutation, University of Iowa, Department of Pathology

● 0018U **Oncology (thyroid), microRNA profiling by RT-PCR of 10 microRNA sequences, utilizing fine needle aspirate, algorithm reported as a positive or negative result for moderate to high risk of malignancy**
    INCLUDES    ThyraMIR, Interpace Diagnostics

● 0019U **Oncology, RNA, gene expression by whole transcriptome sequencing, formalin-fixed paraffin embedded tissue or fresh frozen tissue, predictive algorithm reported as potential targets for therapeutic agents**
    INCLUDES    OncoTarget/OncoTreat, Columbia University Department of Pathology and Cell Biology, Darwin Health

● 0020U **Drug test(s), presumptive, with definitive confirmation of positive results, any number of drug classes, urine, with specimen verification including DNA authentication in comparison to buccal DNA, per date of service**
    INCLUDES    ToxLok, InSource Diagnostics, Agena Bioscience, Inc.
    EXCLUDES    PLA code with the same clinical descriptor (see appendix L for clarification of code) (0007U)

● 0021U **Oncology (prostate), detection of 8 autoantibodies (ARF 6, NKX3-1, 5'-UTR-BMI1, CEP 164, 3'-UTR-Ropporin, Desmocollin, AURKAIP-1, CSNK2A2), multiplexed immunoassay and flow cytometry serum, algorithm reported as risk score**
    INCLUDES    Apifiny®, Armune BioScience, Inc.

● 0022U **Targeted genomic sequence analysis panel, non-small cell lung neoplasia, DNA and RNA analysis, 23 genes, interrogation for sequence variants and rearrangements, reported as presence/absence of variants and associated therapy(ies) to consider**
    INCLUDES    Oncomine™ Dx Target Test, Thermo Fisher Scientific

● 0023U **Oncology (acute myelogenous leukemia), DNA, genotyping of internal tandem duplication, p.D835, p.I836, using mononuclear cells, reported as detection or non-detection of FLT3 mutation and indication for or against the use of midostaurin**
    INCLUDES    LeukoStrat® CDx FLT3 Mutation Assay, LabPMM LLC, an Invivoscribe Technologies, Inc. company, Invivoscribe Technologies, Inc.

## 90281-90399 Immunoglobulin Products

INCLUDES Immune globulin product only
Anti-infectives
Antitoxins
Isoantibodies
Monoclonal antibodies
Code also (96365-96372, 96374-96375)

**90281** Immune globulin (Ig), human, for intramuscular use

INCLUDES Gamastan

🚑 0.00 👐 0.00 **FUD** XXX ⑤Ⓔ▢

**AMA:** 2017,Jan,8; 2016,Jan,13; 2015,Jan,16; 2014,Jan,11; 2012,Jan,15-42

**90283** Immune globulin (IgIV), human, for intravenous use

🚑 0.00 👐 0.00 **FUD** XXX ⑤Ⓔ▢

**AMA:** 2017,Jan,8; 2016,Jan,13; 2015,Jan,16; 2014,Jan,11; 2012,Jan,15-42

**90284** Immune globulin (SCIg), human, for use in subcutaneous infusions, 100 mg, each

🚑 0.00 👐 0.00 **FUD** XXX ⑤Ⓔ▢

**AMA:** 2017,Jan,8; 2016,Jan,13; 2015,Jan,16; 2012,Jan,15-42

**90287** Botulinum antitoxin, equine, any route

🚑 0.00 👐 0.00 **FUD** XXX ⑤Ⓔ▢

**AMA:** 2017,Jan,8; 2016,Jan,13; 2015,Jan,16; 2014,Jan,11; 2012,Jan,15-42

**90288** Botulism immune globulin, human, for intravenous use

🚑 0.00 👐 0.00 **FUD** XXX ⑤Ⓔ▢

**AMA:** 2017,Jan,8; 2016,Jan,13; 2015,Jan,16; 2014,Jan,11; 2012,Jan,15-42

**90291** Cytomegalovirus immune globulin (CMV-IgIV), human, for intravenous use

INCLUDES Cytogram

🚑 0.00 👐 0.00 **FUD** XXX ⑤Ⓔ▢

**AMA:** 2017,Jan,8; 2016,Jan,13; 2015,Jan,16; 2014,Jan,11; 2012,Jan,15-42

**90296** Diphtheria antitoxin, equine, any route

🚑 0.00 👐 0.00 **FUD** XXX ⑤Ⓔ▢

**AMA:** 2017,Jan,8; 2016,Jan,13; 2015,Jan,16; 2014,Jan,11; 2012,Jan,15-42

**90371** Hepatitis B immune globulin (HBIg), human, for intramuscular use

INCLUDES HBIG

🚑 0.00 👐 0.00 **FUD** XXX ⑤Ⓚ☒▢

**AMA:** 2017,Jan,8; 2016,Jan,13; 2015,Jan,16; 2014,Jan,11; 2012,Jan,15-42

**90375** Rabies immune globulin (RIg), human, for intramuscular and/or subcutaneous use

INCLUDES HyperRAB

🚑 0.00 👐 0.00 **FUD** XXX ⑤Ⓚ☒▢

**AMA:** 2017,Jan,8; 2016,Jan,13; 2015,Jan,16; 2012,Jan,15-42

**90376** Rabies immune globulin, heat-treated (RIg-HT), human, for intramuscular and/or subcutaneous use

🚑 0.00 👐 0.00 **FUD** XXX ⑤Ⓚ☒▢

**AMA:** 2017,Jan,8; 2016,Jan,13; 2015,Jan,16; 2012,Jan,15-42

**90378** Respiratory syncytial virus, monoclonal antibody, recombinant, for intramuscular use, 50 mg, each

INCLUDES Synagis

🚑 0.00 👐 0.00 **FUD** XXX ⑤Ⓚ▢

**AMA:** 2017,Jan,8; 2016,Jan,13; 2015,Jan,16; 2014,Jan,11; 2012,Jan,15-42

**90384** Rho(D) immune globulin (RhIg), human, full-dose, for intramuscular use

🚑 0.00 👐 0.00 **FUD** XXX ⑤Ⓔ▢

**AMA:** 2017,Jan,8; 2016,Jan,13; 2015,Jan,16; 2014,Jan,11; 2012,Jan,15-42

**90385** Rho(D) immune globulin (RhIg), human, mini-dose, for intramuscular use

🚑 0.00 👐 0.00 **FUD** XXX ⑤ⓃⓂ▢

**AMA:** 2017,Jan,8; 2016,Jan,13; 2015,Jan,16; 2014,Jan,11; 2012,Jan,15-42

**90386** Rho(D) immune globulin (RhIgIV), human, for intravenous use

🚑 0.00 👐 0.00 **FUD** XXX ⑤Ⓔ▢

**AMA:** 2017,Jan,8; 2016,Jan,13; 2015,Jan,16; 2014,Jan,11; 2012,Jan,15-42

**90389** Tetanus immune globulin (TIg), human, for intramuscular use

INCLUDES HyperTET S/D (Tetanus Immune Globulin)

🚑 0.00 👐 0.00 **FUD** XXX ⑤Ⓔ▢

**AMA:** 2017,Jan,8; 2016,Jan,13; 2015,Jan,16; 2014,Jan,11; 2012,Jan,15-42

**90393** Vaccinia immune globulin, human, for intramuscular use

🚑 0.00 👐 0.00 **FUD** XXX ⑤Ⓔ▢

**AMA:** 2017,Jan,8; 2016,Jan,13; 2015,Jan,16; 2014,Jan,11; 2012,Jan,15-42

**90396** Varicella-zoster immune globulin, human, for intramuscular use

INCLUDES VariZIG

🚑 0.00 👐 0.00 **FUD** XXX ⑤Ⓚ▢

**AMA:** 2017,Jan,8; 2016,Jan,13; 2015,Jan,16; 2014,Jan,11; 2012,Jan,15-42

**90399** Unlisted immune globulin

🚑 0.00 👐 0.00 **FUD** XXX ⑤Ⓔ▢

**AMA:** 2017,Jan,8; 2016,Jan,13; 2015,Jan,16; 2014,Jan,11; 2012,Jan,15-42

## 90460-90461 Injections Provided with Counseling

INCLUDES All components of influenza vaccine, report X 1 only
Combination vaccines which comprise multiple vaccine components
Components (all antigens) in vaccines to prevent disease due to specific organisms
Counseling by physician or other qualified health care professional
Multi-valent antigens or multiple antigen serotypes against single organisms are considered one component
Patient/family face-to-face counseling by doctor or qualified health care professional for patients 18 years of age and younger

EXCLUDES *Administration of influenza and pneumococcal vaccine for Medicare patients (G0008-G0009)*
*Allergy testing (95004-95028)*
*Bacterial/viral/fungal skin tests (86485-86580)*
*Diagnostic or therapeutic injections (96365-96372, 96374-96375)*
*Vaccines provided without face-to-face counseling from a physician or qualified health care professional or to patients over the age of 18 (90471-90474)*

Code also significant, separately identifiable E&M service when appropriate
Code also toxoid/vaccine (90476-90749 [90620, 90621, 90625, 90630, 90644, 90672, 90673, 90674, 90750, 90756])

**90460** Immunization administration through 18 years of age via any route of administration, with counseling by physician or other qualified health care professional; first or only component of each vaccine or toxoid administered Ⓐ

Code also each additional component in a vaccine (e.g., A 5-year-old receives DtaP-IPV IM administration, and MMR/Varicella vaccines SQ administration. Report initial component X 2, and additional components X 6)

🚑 0.72 👐 0.72 **FUD** XXX Ⓑ⑧⓪

**AMA:** 2017,Jan,8; 2016,Oct,6; 2016,Jan,13; 2015,May,6; 2015,Apr,9; 2015,Apr,10; 2015,Jan,16; 2014,Mar,10; 2014,Jan,11; 2013,Aug,10; 2012,Jul,7; 2012,Jan,43

**+    90461**    **each additional vaccine or toxoid component administered (List separately in addition to code for primary procedure)**    🅐

Code also each additional component in a vaccine (e.g., A 5-year-old receives DtaP-IPV IM administration, and MMR/Varicella vaccines SQ administration. Report initial component X 2, and additional components X 6)

Code first the initial component in each vaccine provided (90460)

🔧 0.36    ✂ 0.36    **FUD** ZZZ    🅑 80 ▭

**AMA:** 2017,Jan,8; 2016,Oct,6; 2016,Jan,13; 2015,May,6; 2015,Apr,10; 2015,Jan,16; 2014,Mar,10; 2014,Jan,11; 2013,Aug,10; 2012,Jul,7; 2012,Jan,43

## 90471-90474 Injections and Other Routes of Administration Without Physician Counseling

**CMS:** 100-04,18,10.4 CWF Edits for Influenza Virus and Pneumococcal Vaccinations

EXCLUDES    Administration of influenza and pneumococcal vaccine for Medicare patients (G0008-G0009)
Administration of vaccine with counseling (90460-90461)
Allergy testing (95004-95028)
Bacterial/viral/fungal skin tests (86485-86580)
Diagnostic or therapeutic injections (96365-96371, 96374)
Patient/family face-to-face counseling

Code also significant separately identifiable E&M service when appropriate
Code also toxoid/vaccine (90476-90749 [90620, 90621, 90625, 90630, 90644, 90672, 90673, 90674, 90750, 90756])

**90471**    **Immunization administration (includes percutaneous, intradermal, subcutaneous, or intramuscular injections); 1 vaccine (single or combination vaccine/toxoid)**

EXCLUDES    Intranasal/oral administration (90473)

🔧 0.72    ✂ 0.72    **FUD** XXX    🆂 80 ▭

**AMA:** 2017,Jan,8; 2016,Oct,6; 2016,Jan,13; 2015,May,6; 2015,Apr,9; 2015,Apr,10; 2015,Jan,16; 2014,Mar,10; 2014,Jan,11; 2013,Aug,10; 2012,Jul,7; 2012,Jan,15-42

**+    90472**    **each additional vaccine (single or combination vaccine/toxoid) (List separately in addition to code for primary procedure)**

EXCLUDES    BCG vaccine, intravesical administration (51720, 90586)
Immune globulin administration (96365-96371, 96374)
Immune globulin product (90281-90399)

Code first initial vaccine (90460, 90471, 90473)

🔧 0.36    ✂ 0.36    **FUD** ZZZ    🅝 80 ▭

**AMA:** 2017,Jan,8; 2016,Oct,6; 2016,Jan,13; 2015,May,6; 2015,Apr,10; 2015,Apr,9; 2015,Jan,16; 2014,Mar,10; 2014,Jan,11; 2013,Aug,10; 2012,Jul,7; 2012,Jan,15-42

**90473**    **Immunization administration by intranasal or oral route; 1 vaccine (single or combination vaccine/toxoid)**

EXCLUDES    Administration by injection (90471)

🔧 0.72    ✂ 0.72    **FUD** XXX    🆂 80 ▭

**AMA:** 2017,Jan,8; 2016,Jan,13; 2015,May,6; 2015,Jan,16; 2014,Mar,10; 2014,Jan,11; 2013,Aug,10; 2012,Jul,7

**+    90474**    **each additional vaccine (single or combination vaccine/toxoid) (List separately in addition to code for primary procedure)**

Code first initial vaccine (90460, 90471, 90473)

🔧 0.36    ✂ 0.36    **FUD** ZZZ    🅝 80 ▭

**AMA:** 2017,Jan,8; 2016,Jan,13; 2015,May,6; 2015,Apr,9; 2015,Jan,16; 2014,Mar,10; 2014,Jan,11; 2013,Aug,10; 2012,Jul,7

## 90476-90756 [90620, 90621, 90625, 90630, 90644, 90672, 90673, 90674, 90750, 90756] Vaccination Products

INCLUDES    Patient's age for coding purposes, not for product license
Vaccine product only

EXCLUDES    Coding of each component of a combination vaccine individually
Immune globulins and administration (90281-90399, 96365-96375)

Code also administration of vaccine (90460-90474)
Code also significant separately identifiable E&M service when appropriate

**90476**    **Adenovirus vaccine, type 4, live, for oral use**

INCLUDES    Adeno-4

🔧 0.00    ✂ 0.00    **FUD** XXX    🆂 🅝 N1 ▭

**AMA:** 2017,Jan,8; 2016,Jan,13; 2015,May,6; 2015,Jan,16; 2014,Jan,11; 2013,Aug,10; 2012,Jan,15-42

**90477**    **Adenovirus vaccine, type 7, live, for oral use**

INCLUDES    Adeno-7

🔧 0.00    ✂ 0.00    **FUD** XXX    🆂 🅜 ▭

**AMA:** 2017,Jan,8; 2016,Jan,13; 2015,May,6; 2015,Jan,16; 2014,Jan,11; 2013,Aug,10; 2012,Jan,15-42

**90581**    **Anthrax vaccine, for subcutaneous or intramuscular use**

INCLUDES    BioThrax

🔧 0.00    ✂ 0.00    **FUD** XXX    🆂 🅔 ▭

**AMA:** 2017,Jan,8; 2016,Jan,13; 2015,May,6; 2015,Jan,16; 2014,Jan,11; 2013,Aug,10; 2012,Jan,15-42

**90585**    **Bacillus Calmette-Guerin vaccine (BCG) for tuberculosis, live, for percutaneous use**

INCLUDES    Mycobax

🔧 0.00    ✂ 0.00    **FUD** XXX    🆂 🅜 ▭

**AMA:** 2017,Jan,8; 2016,Jan,13; 2015,May,6; 2015,Jan,16; 2014,Jan,11; 2013,Aug,10; 2012,Jan,15-42

**90586**    **Bacillus Calmette-Guerin vaccine (BCG) for bladder cancer, live, for intravesical use**

INCLUDES    TheraCys
TICE BCG

🔧 0.00    ✂ 0.00    **FUD** XXX    🆂 🅑 ▭

**AMA:** 2017,Jan,8; 2016,Jan,13; 2015,May,6; 2015,Jan,16; 2014,Jan,11; 2013,Aug,10; 2012,Jan,15-42

●    **90587**    **Dengue vaccine, quadrivalent, live, 3 dose schedule, for subcutaneous use**

🔧 0.00    ✂ 0.00    **FUD** 000    ⚡ 🅔

*90620*    **Resequenced code. See code following 90734.**

*90621*    **Resequenced code. See code following 90734.**

*90625*    **Resequenced code. See code following 90723.**

*90630*    **Resequenced code. See code following 90654.**

**90632**    **Hepatitis A vaccine (HepA), adult dosage, for intramuscular use**    🅐

INCLUDES    Havrix
Vaqta

🔧 0.00    ✂ 0.00    **FUD** XXX    🆂 🅝 N1 ▭

**AMA:** 2017,Jan,8; 2016,Jan,13; 2015,May,6; 2015,Jan,16; 2014,Jan,11; 2013,Aug,10; 2012,Jan,15-42

**90633**    **Hepatitis A vaccine (HepA), pediatric/adolescent dosage-2 dose schedule, for intramuscular use**    🅐

INCLUDES    Havrix
Vaqta

🔧 0.00    ✂ 0.00    **FUD** XXX    🆂 🅝 N1 ▭

**AMA:** 2017,Jan,8; 2016,Jan,13; 2015,May,6; 2015,Jan,16; 2014,Jan,11; 2013,Aug,10; 2012,Jan,15-42

**90634**    **Hepatitis A vaccine (HepA), pediatric/adolescent dosage-3 dose schedule, for intramuscular use**    🅐

INCLUDES    Havrix

🔧 0.00    ✂ 0.00    **FUD** XXX    🆂 🅝 N1 ▭

**AMA:** 2017,Jan,8; 2016,Jan,13; 2015,May,6; 2015,Jan,16; 2014,Jan,11; 2013,Aug,10; 2012,Jan,15-42

**90636**    **Hepatitis A and hepatitis B vaccine (HepA-HepB), adult dosage, for intramuscular use**    🅐

INCLUDES    Twinrix

🔧 0.00    ✂ 0.00    **FUD** XXX    🆂 🅝 N1 ▭

**AMA:** 2017,Jan,8; 2016,Jan,13; 2015,May,6; 2015,Jan,16; 2014,Jan,11; 2013,Aug,10; 2012,Jan,15-42

*90644*    **Resequenced code. See code following 90732.**

**90647**    **Haemophilus influenzae type b vaccine (Hib), PRP-OMP conjugate, 3 dose schedule, for intramuscular use**

INCLUDES    PedvaxHIB

🔧 0.00    ✂ 0.00    **FUD** XXX    🆂 🅝 🅜 ▭

**AMA:** 2017,Jan,8; 2016,Jan,13; 2015,May,6; 2015,Jan,16; 2014,Jan,11; 2013,Aug,10; 2012,Jan,15-42

| 26/TC PC/TC Only | A2-Z3 ASC Payment | 50 Bilateral | ♂ Male Only | ♀ Female Only | 🔧 Facility RVU | ✂ Non-Facility RVU | ▭ CCI |
| FUD Follow-up Days | CMS: IOM (Pub 100) | A-Y OPPSI | 80/80 Surg Assist Allowed / w/Doc | | 🄛 Lab Crosswalk | 🄡 Radiology Crosswalk | ✖ CLIA |

**426**                                        CPT © 2017 American Medical Association. All Rights Reserved.                              © 2017 Optum360, LLC

**90648** Haemophilus influenzae type b vaccine (Hib), PRP-T conjugate, 4 dose schedule, for intramuscular use

INCLUDES ActHIB
Hiberix
OmniHIB

🚲 0.00  👤 0.00  **FUD** XXX  Ⓢ Ⓝ Ⓜ 🖃

**AMA:** 2017,Jan,8; 2016,Jan,13; 2015,May,6; 2015,Jan,16; 2014,Jan,11; 2013,Aug,10; 2012,Jan,15-42

**90649** Human Papillomavirus vaccine, types 6, 11, 16, 18, quadrivalent (4vHPV), 3 dose schedule, for intramuscular use

INCLUDES Gardasil

🚲 0.00  👤 0.00  **FUD** XXX  Ⓢ Ⓜ 🖃

**AMA:** 2017,Jan,8; 2016,Jan,13; 2015,May,6; 2015,Jan,16; 2014,Jan,11; 2013,Aug,10; 2012,Jan,15-42

**90650** Human Papillomavirus vaccine, types 16, 18, bivalent (2vHPV), 3 dose schedule, for intramuscular use

INCLUDES Cervarix

🚲 0.00  👤 0.00  **FUD** XXX  Ⓢ Ⓜ 🖃

**AMA:** 2017,Jan,8; 2016,Jan,13; 2015,May,6; 2015,Jan,16; 2014,Jan,11; 2013,Aug,10; 2012,Jan,15-42

▲ **90651** Human Papillomavirus vaccine types 6, 11, 16, 18, 31, 33, 45, 52, 58, nonavalent (9vHPV), 2 or 3 dose schedule, for intramuscular use

INCLUDES GARDASIL 9

🚲 0.00  👤 0.00  **FUD** XXX  Ⓢ Ⓜ 🖃

**AMA:** 2017,Jan,8; 2016,Jan,13; 2015,May,6; 2015,Jan,16

**90653** Influenza vaccine, inactivated (IIV), subunit, adjuvanted, for intramuscular use

🚲 0.00  👤 0.00  **FUD** XXX  Ⓢ Ⓛ Ⓛ1 🖃

**AMA:** 2017,Jan,8; 2016,Oct,6; 2016,Jan,13; 2015,May,6; 2015,Jan,16; 2014,Jan,11; 2013,Aug,10

**90654** Influenza virus vaccine, trivalent (IIV3), split virus, preservative-free, for intradermal use

INCLUDES Fluzone intradermal

🚲 0.00  👤 0.00  **FUD** XXX  Ⓢ Ⓛ Ⓛ1 🖃

**AMA:** 2017,Jan,8; 2016,Jan,13; 2015,May,6; 2015,Apr,9; 2015,Jan,16; 2014,Jan,11; 2013,Aug,10; 2012,Jan,15-42

\# **90630** Influenza virus vaccine, quadrivalent (IIV4), split virus, preservative free, for intradermal use

INCLUDES Fluzone Intradermal Quadrivalent

🚲 0.00  👤 0.00  **FUD** XXX  Ⓢ Ⓛ Ⓛ1 🖃

**AMA:** 2017,Jan,8; 2016,Jan,13; 2015,May,6; 2015,Jan,16

**90655** Influenza virus vaccine, trivalent (IIV3), split virus, preservative free, 0.25 mL dosage, for intramuscular use

INCLUDES Afluria
Fluzone, no preservative, pediatric dose

🚲 0.00  👤 0.00  **FUD** XXX  Ⓢ Ⓛ Ⓛ1 🖃

**AMA:** 2017,Jan,8; 2016,Oct,6; 2016,May,9; 2016,Jan,13; 2015,May,6; 2015,Jan,16; 2014,Jan,11; 2013,Aug,10; 2012,Jan,15-42

**90656** Influenza virus vaccine, trivalent (IIV3), split virus, preservative free, 0.5 mL dosage, for intramuscular use  Ⓐ

INCLUDES Afluria
Fluvarix
Fluvirin
Fluzone, influenza virus vaccine, no preservative

🚲 0.00  👤 0.00  **FUD** XXX  Ⓢ Ⓛ Ⓛ1 🖃

**AMA:** 2017,Jan,8; 2016,Oct,6; 2016,May,9; 2016,Jan,13; 2015,May,6; 2015,Jan,16; 2014,Jan,11; 2013,Aug,10; 2012,Jan,15-42

**90657** Influenza virus vaccine, trivalent (IIV3), split virus, 0.25 mL dosage, for intramuscular use  Ⓐ

INCLUDES Afluria
Flulaval
Fluvirin
Fluzone (5 ml vial [0.25ml dose])

🚲 0.00  👤 0.00  **FUD** XXX  Ⓢ Ⓛ Ⓛ1 🖃

**AMA:** 2017,Jan,8; 2016,Oct,6; 2016,May,9; 2016,Jan,13; 2015,May,6; 2015,Jan,16; 2014,Jan,11; 2013,Aug,10; 2012,Jan,15-42

**90658** Influenza virus vaccine, trivalent (IIV3), split virus, 0.5 mL dosage, for intramuscular use  Ⓐ

INCLUDES Afluria
Flulaval
Fluvirin
Fluzone

🚲 0.00  👤 0.00  **FUD** XXX  Ⓢ Ⓔ 🖃

**AMA:** 2017,Jan,8; 2016,Oct,6; 2016,May,9; 2016,Jan,13; 2015,May,6; 2015,Jan,16; 2014,Jan,11; 2013,Aug,10; 2012,Jan,15-42

**90660** Influenza virus vaccine, trivalent, live (LAIV3), for intranasal use

INCLUDES FluMist

🚲 0.00  👤 0.00  **FUD** XXX  Ⓢ Ⓛ Ⓛ1 🖃

**AMA:** 2017,Jan,8; 2016,Jan,13; 2015,May,6; 2015,Jan,16; 2014,Jan,11; 2013,Aug,10; 2012,Jan,15-42

\# **90672** Influenza virus vaccine, quadrivalent, live (LAIV4), for intranasal use

🚲 0.00  👤 0.00  **FUD** XXX  Ⓢ Ⓛ Ⓛ1 🖃

**AMA:** 2017,Jan,8; 2016,Jan,13; 2015,May,6; 2015,Jan,16; 2014,Jan,11; 2013,Aug,10

**90661** Influenza virus vaccine (ccIIV3), derived from cell cultures, subunit, preservative and antibiotic free, for intramuscular use

INCLUDES Flucelvax

🚲 0.00  👤 0.00  **FUD** XXX  Ⓢ Ⓛ Ⓛ1 🖃

**AMA:** 2017,Jan,8; 2016,Oct,6; 2016,Jan,13; 2015,May,6; 2015,Jan,16; 2014,Jan,11; 2013,Aug,10; 2012,Jan,15-42

\# **90674** Influenza virus vaccine, quadrivalent (ccIIV4), derived from cell cultures, subunit, preservative and antibiotic free, 0.5 mL dosage, for intramuscular use

🚲 0.00  👤 0.00  **FUD** XXX  Ⓢ Ⓛ Ⓛ1 🖃

**AMA:** 2017,Jan,8; 2016,Oct,6

● \# **90756** Influenza virus vaccine, quadrivalent (ccIIV4), derived from cell cultures, subunit, antibiotic free, 0.5mL dosage, for intramuscular use

🚲 0.00  👤 0.00  **FUD** 000

INCLUDES Flucelvax Quadrivalent

\# **90673** Influenza virus vaccine, trivalent (RIV3), derived from recombinant DNA, hemagglutinin (HA) protein only, preservative and antibiotic free, for intramuscular use

🚲 0.00  👤 0.00  **FUD** XXX  Ⓢ Ⓛ Ⓛ1 🖃

**AMA:** 2017,Jan,8; 2016,Jan,13; 2015,May,6; 2015,Jan,16; 2014,Mar,10; 2014,Jan,11

**90662** Influenza virus vaccine (IIV), split virus, preservative free, enhanced immunogenicity via increased antigen content, for intramuscular use

INCLUDES Fluzone high-dose

🚲 0.00  👤 0.00  **FUD** XXX  Ⓢ Ⓛ Ⓛ1 🖃

**AMA:** 2017,Jan,8; 2016,Jan,13; 2015,May,6; 2015,Jan,16; 2014,Jan,11; 2013,Aug,10; 2012,Jan,15-42

**90664** Influenza virus vaccine, live (LAIV), pandemic formulation, for intranasal use

🚲 0.00  👤 0.00  **FUD** XXX  Ⓢ Ⓔ 🖃

**AMA:** 2017,Jan,8; 2016,Jan,13; 2015,May,6; 2015,Jan,16; 2014,Jan,11; 2013,Aug,10; 2012,Jan,15-42

● New Code  ▲ Revised Code  ○ Reinstated  ● New Web Release  ▲ Revised Web Release  Unlisted  Not Covered  # Resequenced
⊘ AMA Mod 51 Exempt  Ⓢ Optum Mod 51 Exempt  63 Mod 63 Exempt  ✗ Non-FDA Drug  ★ Telemedicine  Ⓜ Maternity  Ⓐ Age Edit  + Add-on  **AMA:** CPT Asst

**90666** Influenza virus vaccine (IIV), pandemic formulation, split virus, preservative free, for intramuscular use

    📷 0.00    ⬚ 0.00    **FUD** XXX    ✎ ⑤ E 🖼

    **AMA:** 2017,Jan,8; 2016,Jan,13; 2015,May,6; 2015,Jan,16; 2014,Jan,11; 2013,Aug,10; 2012,Jan,15-42

**90667** Influenza virus vaccine (IIV), pandemic formulation, split virus, adjuvanted, for intramuscular use

    📷 0.00    ⬚ 0.00    **FUD** XXX    ✎ ⑤ E 🖼

    **AMA:** 2017,Jan,8; 2016,Jan,13; 2015,May,6; 2015,Jan,16; 2014,Jan,11; 2013,Aug,10; 2012,Jan,15-42

**90668** Influenza virus vaccine (IIV), pandemic formulation, split virus, for intramuscular use

    📷 0.00    ⬚ 0.00    **FUD** XXX    ✎ ⑤ E 🖼

    **AMA:** 2017,Jan,8; 2016,Jan,13; 2015,May,6; 2015,Jan,16; 2014,Jan,11; 2013,Aug,10; 2012,Jan,15-42

**90670** Pneumococcal conjugate vaccine, 13 valent (PCV13), for intramuscular use

    INCLUDES    Prevnar 13

    📷 0.00    ⬚ 0.00    **FUD** XXX    ⑤ L L1 🖼

    **AMA:** 2017,Jan,8; 2016,Jan,13; 2015,May,6; 2015,Jan,16; 2014,Jan,11; 2013,Aug,10; 2012,Jan,15-42

*90672* Resequenced code. See code following 90660.

*90673* Resequenced code. See code before 90662.

*90674* Resequenced code. See code following 90661.

**90675** Rabies vaccine, for intramuscular use

    INCLUDES    Imovax

                RabAvert

    📷 0.00    ⬚ 0.00    **FUD** XXX    ⑤ K K2 🖼

    **AMA:** 2017,Jan,8; 2016,Jan,13; 2015,May,6; 2015,Jan,16; 2014,Jan,11; 2013,Aug,10; 2012,Jan,15-42

**90676** Rabies vaccine, for intradermal use

    📷 0.00    ⬚ 0.00    **FUD** XXX    ⑤ K K2 🖼

    **AMA:** 2017,Jan,8; 2016,Jan,13; 2015,May,6; 2015,Jan,16; 2014,Jan,11; 2013,Aug,10; 2012,Jul,7; 2012,Jan,15-42

**90680** Rotavirus vaccine, pentavalent (RV5), 3 dose schedule, live, for oral use

    INCLUDES    RotaTeq

    📷 0.00    ⬚ 0.00    **FUD** XXX    ⑤ N N1 🖼

    **AMA:** 2017,Jan,8; 2016,Jan,13; 2015,May,6; 2015,Jan,16; 2014,Jan,11; 2013,Aug,10; 2012,Jan,15-42

**90681** Rotavirus vaccine, human, attenuated (RV1), 2 dose schedule, live, for oral use

    INCLUDES    Rotarix

    📷 0.00    ⬚ 0.00    **FUD** XXX    ⑤ M 🖼

    **AMA:** 2017,Jan,8; 2016,Jan,13; 2015,May,6; 2015,Jan,16; 2014,Jan,11; 2013,Aug,10; 2012,Jul,7; 2012,Jan,15-42

● **90682** Influenza virus vaccine, quadrivalent (RIV4), derived from recombinant DNA, hemagglutinin (HA) protein only, preservative and antibiotic free, for intramuscular use

    INCLUDES    Flublok

    📷 0.00    ⬚ 0.00    **FUD** XXX    ⑤ L L1 🖼

    **AMA:** 2017,Jan,8

**90685** Influenza virus vaccine, quadrivalent (IIV4), split virus, preservative free, 0.25 mL, for intramuscular use    A

    INCLUDES    Fluzone Quadrivalent

    📷 0.00    ⬚ 0.00    **FUD** XXX    ⑤ L L1 🖼

    **AMA:** 2017,Jan,8; 2016,Oct,6; 2016,May,9; 2016,Jan,13; 2015,May,6; 2015,Jan,16; 2014,Mar,10; 2014,Jan,11; 2013,Aug,10

**90686** Influenza virus vaccine, quadrivalent (IIV4), split virus, preservative free, 0.5 mL dosage, for intramuscular use    A

    INCLUDES    Afluria

                FluLaval Quadrivalent

                Fluarix Quadrivalent

                Fluzone Quadrivalent

    📷 0.00    ⬚ 0.00    **FUD** XXX    ⑤ L L1 🖼

    **AMA:** 2017,Jan,8; 2016,Oct,6; 2016,May,9; 2016,Jan,13; 2015,May,6; 2015,Jan,16; 2014,Mar,10; 2014,Jan,11; 2013,Aug,10

**90687** Influenza virus vaccine, quadrivalent (IIV4), split virus, 0.25 mL dosage, for intramuscular use    A

    INCLUDES    Fluzone Quadrivalent

    📷 0.00    ⬚ 0.00    **FUD** XXX    ⑤ L L1 🖼

    **AMA:** 2017,Jan,8; 2016,Oct,6; 2016,May,9; 2016,Jan,13; 2015,May,6; 2015,Jan,16; 2014,Mar,10; 2014,Jan,11; 2013,Aug,10

**90688** Influenza virus vaccine, quadrivalent (IIV4), split virus, 0.5 mL dosage, for intramuscular use    A

    INCLUDES    FluLaval Quadrivalent

                Fluzone Quadrivalent

    📷 0.00    ⬚ 0.00    **FUD** XXX    ⑤ L L1 🖼

    **AMA:** 2017,Jan,8; 2016,Oct,6; 2016,May,9; 2016,Jan,13; 2015,May,6; 2015,Jan,16; 2014,Mar,10; 2014,Jan,11; 2013,Aug,10

**90690** Typhoid vaccine, live, oral

    INCLUDES    Vivotif

    📷 0.00    ⬚ 0.00    **FUD** XXX    ⑤ N N1 🖼

    **AMA:** 2017,Jan,8; 2016,Jan,13; 2015,May,6; 2015,Jan,16; 2014,Jan,11; 2013,Aug,10; 2012,Jan,15-42

**90691** Typhoid vaccine, Vi capsular polysaccharide (ViCPs), for intramuscular use

    INCLUDES    Typhim Vi

    📷 0.00    ⬚ 0.00    **FUD** XXX    ⑤ N N1 🖼

    **AMA:** 2017,Jan,8; 2016,Jan,13; 2015,May,6; 2015,Jan,16; 2014,Jan,11; 2013,Aug,10; 2012,Jan,15-42

**90696** Diphtheria, tetanus toxoids, acellular pertussis vaccine and inactivated poliovirus vaccine (DTaP-IPV), when administered to children 4 through 6 years of age, for intramuscular use    A

    INCLUDES    KINRIX

                Quadracel

    📷 0.00    ⬚ 0.00    **FUD** XXX    ⑤ N N1 🖼

    **AMA:** 2017,Jan,8; 2016,Jan,13; 2015,May,6; 2015,Jan,16; 2014,Jan,11; 2013,Aug,10; 2012,Jan,15-42

**90697** Diphtheria, tetanus toxoids, acellular pertussis vaccine, inactivated poliovirus vaccine, Haemophilus influenzae type b PRP-OMP conjugate vaccine, and hepatitis B vaccine (DTaP-IPV-Hib-HepB), for intramuscular use

    📷 0.00    ⬚ 0.00    **FUD** XXX    ✎ ⑤ M 🖼

    **AMA:** 2017,Jan,8; 2016,Jan,13; 2015,May,6; 2015,Jan,16

**90698** Diphtheria, tetanus toxoids, acellular pertussis vaccine, Haemophilus influenzae type b, and inactivated poliovirus vaccine, (DTaP-IPV/Hib), for intramuscular use

    INCLUDES    Pentacel

    📷 0.00    ⬚ 0.00    **FUD** XXX    ⑤ N N1 🖼

    **AMA:** 2017,Jan,8; 2016,Jan,13; 2015,May,6; 2015,Jan,16; 2014,Jan,11; 2013,Aug,10; 2012,Jan,15-42

**90700** Diphtheria, tetanus toxoids, and acellular pertussis vaccine (DTaP), when administered to individuals younger than 7 years, for intramuscular use    A

    INCLUDES    Daptacel

                Infanrix

    📷 0.00    ⬚ 0.00    **FUD** XXX    ⑤ N 🖼

    **AMA:** 2017,Jan,8; 2016,Jan,13; 2015,May,6; 2015,Jan,16; 2014,Jan,11; 2013,Aug,10; 2012,Jul,7; 2012,Jan,15-42

**90702** Diphtheria and tetanus toxoids adsorbed (DT) when administered to individuals younger than 7 years, for intramuscular use    A

    INCLUDES    Diphtheria and Tetanus Toxoids Adsorbed USP (For Pediatric Use)

    📷 0.00    ⬚ 0.00    **FUD** XXX    ⑤ N 🖼

    **AMA:** 2017,Jan,8; 2016,Jan,13; 2015,May,6; 2015,Jan,16; 2014,Jan,11; 2013,Aug,10; 2012,Jan,15-42

---

| 26/TC PC/TC Only | A2-Z3 ASC Payment | 50 Bilateral | ♂ Male Only | ♀ Female Only | 📷 Facility RVU | ⬚ Non-Facility RVU | 🖼 CCI |
|---|---|---|---|---|---|---|---|
| **FUD** Follow-up Days | **CMS:** IOM (Pub 100) | A-Y OPPSI | 80/80 Surg Assist Allowed / w/Doc | | 🔬 Lab Crosswalk | ☢ Radiology Crosswalk | ❌ CLIA |

CPT © 2017 American Medical Association. All Rights Reserved.

© 2017 Optum360, LLC

**90707** Measles, mumps and rubella virus vaccine (MMR), live, for subcutaneous use

INCLUDES M-M-R II

🔲 0.00   🔾 0.00   **FUD** XXX   ⑤ Ⓝ 🖵

**AMA:** 2017,Jan,8; 2016,Jan,13; 2015,May,6; 2015,Jan,16; 2014,Jan,11; 2013,Aug,10; 2012,Jul,7; 2012,Jan,15-42

**90710** Measles, mumps, rubella, and varicella vaccine (MMRV), live, for subcutaneous use

INCLUDES ProQuad

🔲 0.00   🔾 0.00   **FUD** XXX   ⑤ Ⓝ 🖵

**AMA:** 2017,Jan,8; 2016,Jan,13; 2015,May,6; 2015,Jan,16; 2014,Jan,11; 2013,Aug,10; 2012,Jan,15-42

**90713** Poliovirus vaccine, inactivated (IPV), for subcutaneous or intramuscular use

INCLUDES IPOL

🔲 0.00   🔾 0.00   **FUD** XXX   ⑤ Ⓝ 🖵

**AMA:** 2017,Jan,8; 2016,Jan,13; 2015,May,6; 2015,Jan,16; 2014,Jan,11; 2013,Aug,10; 2012,Jan,15-42

**90714** Tetanus and diphtheria toxoids adsorbed (Td), preservative free, when administered to individuals 7 years or older, for intramuscular use Ⓐ

INCLUDES Tenivac
Tetanus-diphtheria toxoids adsorbed

🔲 0.00   🔾 0.00   **FUD** XXX   ⑤ Ⓝ 🖵

**AMA:** 2017,Jan,8; 2016,Jan,13; 2015,May,6; 2015,Jan,16; 2014,Jan,11; 2013,Aug,10; 2012,Jan,15-42

**90715** Tetanus, diphtheria toxoids and acellular pertussis vaccine (Tdap), when administered to individuals 7 years or older, for intramuscular use Ⓐ

INCLUDES Adacel
Boostrix

🔲 0.00   🔾 0.00   **FUD** XXX   ⑤ Ⓝ 🖵

**AMA:** 2017,Jan,8; 2016,Jan,13; 2015,May,6; 2015,Jan,16; 2014,Jan,11; 2013,Aug,10; 2012,Jan,15-42

**90716** Varicella virus vaccine (VAR), live, for subcutaneous use

INCLUDES Varivax

🔲 0.00   🔾 0.00   **FUD** XXX   ⑤ Ⓜ 🖵

**AMA:** 2017,Jan,8; 2016,Jan,13; 2015,May,6; 2015,Mar,3; 2015,Jan,16; 2014,Jan,11; 2013,Aug,10; 2012,Jan,15-42

**90717** Yellow fever vaccine, live, for subcutaneous use

INCLUDES YF-VAX

🔲 0.00   🔾 0.00   **FUD** XXX   ⑤ Ⓝ ⑪ 🖵

**AMA:** 2017,Jan,8; 2016,Jan,13; 2015,May,6; 2015,Jan,16; 2014,Jan,11; 2013,Aug,10; 2012,Jan,15-42

**90723** Diphtheria, tetanus toxoids, acellular pertussis vaccine, hepatitis B, and inactivated poliovirus vaccine (DTaP-HepB-IPV), for intramuscular use

INCLUDES PEDIARIX

🔲 0.00   🔾 0.00   **FUD** XXX   ⑤ Ⓜ 🖵

**AMA:** 2017,Jan,8; 2016,Jan,13; 2015,May,6; 2015,Jan,16; 2014,Jan,11; 2013,Aug,10; 2012,Jan,15-42

\# **90625** Cholera vaccine, live, adult dosage, 1 dose schedule, for oral use Ⓐ

🔲 0.00   🔾 0.00   **FUD** XXX   ⑤ Ⓔ 🖵

**AMA:** 2017,Jan,8; 2016,Oct,6; 2016,Jan,13

**90732** Pneumococcal polysaccharide vaccine, 23-valent (PPSV23), adult or immunosuppressed patient dosage, when administered to individuals 2 years or older, for subcutaneous or intramuscular use Ⓐ

INCLUDES Pneumovax 23

🔲 0.00   🔾 0.00   **FUD** XXX   ⑤ Ⓛ ⑪ 🖵

**AMA:** 2017,Jan,8; 2016,Jan,13; 2015,May,6; 2015,Jan,16; 2014,Jan,11; 2013,Aug,10; 2012,Jan,15-42

\# **90644** Meningococcal conjugate vaccine, serogroups C & Y and Haemophilus influenzae type b vaccine (Hib-MenCY), 4 dose schedule, when administered to children 6 weeks-18 months of age, for intramuscular use Ⓐ

INCLUDES MenHibrix

🔲 0.00   🔾 0.00   **FUD** XXX   ⑤ Ⓜ 🖵

**AMA:** 2017,Jan,8; 2016,Jan,13; 2015,May,6; 2015,Jan,16; 2014,Jan,11; 2013,Aug,10; 2012,Jan,15-42

**90733** Meningococcal polysaccharide vaccine, serogroups A, C, Y, W-135, quadrivalent (MPSV4), for subcutaneous use

INCLUDES Menomune-A/C/Y/W-135

🔲 0.00   🔾 0.00   **FUD** XXX   ⑤ Ⓜ 🖵

**AMA:** 2017,Jan,8; 2016,Jan,13; 2015,May,6; 2015,Jan,16; 2014,Jan,11; 2013,Aug,10; 2012,Jan,15-42

**90734** Meningococcal conjugate vaccine, serogroups A, C, Y and W-135, quadrivalent (MCV4 or MenACWY), for intramuscular use

INCLUDES Menactra
Menveo

🔲 0.00   🔾 0.00   **FUD** XXX   ⑤ Ⓜ 🖵

**AMA:** 2017,Jan,8; 2016,Oct,6; 2016,Jan,13; 2015,May,6; 2015,Jan,16; 2014,Jan,11; 2013,Aug,10; 2012,Jan,15-42

▲ \# **90620** Meningococcal recombinant protein and outer membrane vesicle vaccine, serogroup B (MenB-4C), 2 dose schedule, for intramuscular use

INCLUDES Bexsero

🔲 0.00   🔾 0.00   **FUD** XXX   ⑤ Ⓜ 🖵

**AMA:** 2017,Jan,8; 2016,Jan,13; 2015,May,6; 2015,Jan,16

▲ \# **90621** Meningococcal recombinant lipoprotein vaccine, serogroup B (MenB-FHbp), 2 or 3 dose schedule, for intramuscular use

INCLUDES Trumenba

🔲 0.00   🔾 0.00   **FUD** XXX   ⑤ Ⓜ 🖵

**AMA:** 2017,Jan,8; 2016,Jan,13; 2015,May,6; 2015,Jan,16

**90736** Zoster (shingles) vaccine (HZV), live, for subcutaneous injection

INCLUDES Zostavax

🔲 0.00   🔾 0.00   **FUD** XXX   ⑤ Ⓜ 🖵

**AMA:** 2017,Jan,8; 2016,Jan,13; 2015,May,6; 2015,Jan,16; 2014,Jan,11; 2013,Aug,10; 2012,Jan,15-42

● \# **90750** Zoster (shingles) vaccine (HZV), recombinant, sub-unit, adjuvanted, for intramuscular injection

🔲 0.00   🔾 0.00   **FUD** XXX   ✗ ⑤ Ⓔ 🖵

**90738** Japanese encephalitis virus vaccine, inactivated, for intramuscular use

INCLUDES Ixiaro

🔲 0.00   🔾 0.00   **FUD** XXX   ⑤ Ⓜ 🖵

**AMA:** 2017,Jan,8; 2016,Jan,13; 2015,May,6; 2015,Jan,16; 2014,Jan,11; 2013,Aug,10; 2012,Jan,15-42

**90739** Hepatitis B vaccine (HepB), adult dosage, 2 dose schedule, for intramuscular use

🔲 0.00   🔾 0.00   **FUD** XXX   ✗ ⑤ Ⓔ 🖵

**AMA:** 2017,Jan,8; 2016,Jan,13; 2015,May,6; 2015,Jan,16; 2014,Jan,11; 2013,Aug,10

**90740** Hepatitis B vaccine (HepB), dialysis or immunosuppressed patient dosage, 3 dose schedule, for intramuscular use

INCLUDES Recombivax HB

🔲 0.00   🔾 0.00   **FUD** XXX   ⑤ Ⓕ ⑭ 🖵

**AMA:** 2017,Jan,8; 2016,Jan,13; 2015,May,6; 2015,Jan,16; 2014,Jan,11; 2013,Aug,10; 2012,Jan,15-42

**90743** Hepatitis B vaccine (HepB), adolescent, 2 dose schedule, for intramuscular use Ⓐ

INCLUDES Energix-B
Recombivax HB

🔲 0.00   🔾 0.00   **FUD** XXX   ⑤ Ⓕ ⑭ 🖵

**AMA:** 2017,Jan,8; 2016,Jan,13; 2015,May,6; 2015,Jan,16; 2014,Jan,11; 2013,Aug,10; 2012,Jan,15-42

---

● New Code   ▲ Revised Code   ○ Reinstated   ● New Web Release   ▲ Revised Web Release   Unlisted   Not Covered   \# Resequenced
⊘ AMA Mod 51 Exempt   ⑤ Optum Mod 51 Exempt   ⑥⑨ Mod 63 Exempt   ✗ Non-FDA Drug   ★ Telemedicine   Ⓜ Maternity   Ⓐ Age Edit   ＋ Add-on   **AMA:** CPT Asst

© 2017 Optum360, LLC   CPT © 2017 American Medical Association. All Rights Reserved.

**90744** **Hepatitis B vaccine (HepB), pediatric/adolescent dosage, 3 dose schedule, for intramuscular use** Ⓐ

INCLUDES  Energix-B
Flucelvax Quadrivalent
Recombivax HB

🔩 0.00  📏 0.00  **FUD** XXX  ⑤Ⓕ🄵🄴▱

**AMA:** 2017,Jan,8; 2016,Jan,13; 2015,May,6; 2015,Jan,16; 2014,Jan,11; 2013,Aug,10; 2012,Jan,15-42

**90746** **Hepatitis B vaccine (HepB), adult dosage, 3 dose schedule, for intramuscular use**

INCLUDES  Energix-B
Recombivax HB

🔩 0.00  📏 0.00  **FUD** XXX  ⑤Ⓕ🄵🄴▱

**AMA:** 2017,Jan,8; 2016,Jan,13; 2015,May,6; 2015,Jan,16; 2014,Jan,11; 2013,Aug,10; 2012,Jan,15-42

**90747** **Hepatitis B vaccine (HepB), dialysis or immunosuppressed patient dosage, 4 dose schedule, for intramuscular use**

INCLUDES  Energix-B
RECOMBIVAX dialysis

🔩 0.00  📏 0.00  **FUD** XXX  ⑤Ⓕ🄵🄴▱

**AMA:** 2017,Jan,8; 2016,Jan,13; 2015,May,6; 2015,Jan,16; 2014,Jan,11; 2013,Aug,10; 2012,Jan,15-42

**90748** **Hepatitis B and Haemophilus influenzae type b vaccine (Hib-HepB), for intramuscular use**

INCLUDES  COMVAX

🔩 0.00  📏 0.00  **FUD** XXX  ⑤Ⓔ▱

**AMA:** 2017,Jan,8; 2016,Jan,13; 2015,May,6; 2015,Jan,16; 2014,Jan,11; 2013,Aug,10; 2012,Jul,7; 2012,Jan,15-42

**90749** **Unlisted vaccine/toxoid**

🔩 0.00  📏 0.00  **FUD** XXX  ⑤Ⓝ🄽▱

**AMA:** 2017,Jan,8; 2016,Jan,13; 2015,May,6; 2015,Jan,16; 2014,Jan,11; 2012,Jan,15-42

**90750** **Resequenced code. See code following 90736.**

**90756** **Resequenced code. See code following 90661.**

## 90785 Complex Interactive Encounter

**CMS:** 100-02,15,160 Clinical Psychologist Services; 100-02,15,170 Clinical Social Worker (CSW) Services; 100-03,10.3 Inpatient Pain Rehabilitation Programs; 100-03,10.4 Outpatient Hospital Pain Rehabilitation Programs; 100-03,130.1 Inpatient Stays for Alcoholism Treatment; 100-04,12,100 Teaching Physician Services

INCLUDES  At least one of the following activities:
Discussion of a sentinel event demanding third-party involvement (eg, abuse or neglect reported to a state agency)
Interference by the behavior or emotional state of caregiver to understand and assist in the plan of treatment
Managing discordant communication complicating care among participating members (eg, arguing, reactivity)
Use of nonverbal communication methods (eg, toys, other devices, or translator) to eliminate communication barriers
Complicated issues of communication affecting provision of the psychiatric service
Involved communication with:
Emotionally charged or dissonant family members
Patients wanting others present during the visit (e.g., family member, translator)
Patients with impaired or undeveloped verbal skills
Patients with third parties responsible for their care (eg, parents, guardians)
Third-party involvement (eg, schools, probation and parole officers, child protective agencies)

EXCLUDES  *Adaptive behavior treatment (0364T-0367T, 0373T-0374T)*
*Crisis psychotherapy (90839-90840)*

+ **90785** **Interactive complexity (List separately in addition to the code for primary procedure)**

Code first, when performed (99201-99255 [99224, 99225, 99226], 99304-99337, 99341-99350, 90791-90792, 90832-90834, 90836-90838, 90853)

🔩 0.39  📏 0.39  **FUD** ZZZ  Ⓝ▱

**AMA:** 2017,Jan,8; 2016,Dec,11; 2016,Jan,13; 2015,Jan,16; 2013,Jun,3-5; 2013,May,12

## 90791-90792 Psychiatric Evaluations

**CMS:** 100-02,15,170 Clinical Social Worker (CSW) Services; 100-03,10.3 Inpatient Pain Rehabilitation Programs; 100-03,130.1 Inpatient Stays for Alcoholism Treatment; 100-03,130.2 Outpatient Hospital Services for Alcoholism; 100-04,12,100 Teaching Physician Services; 100-04,12,190.3 List of Telehealth Services; 100-04,12,190.6 Payment Methodology for Physician/Practitioner at the Distant Site ; 100-04,12,190.6.1 Submission of Telehealth Claims for Distant Site Practitioners; 100-04,12,190.7 Contractor Editing of Telehealth Claims

INCLUDES  Diagnostic assessment or reassessment without psychotherapy services

EXCLUDES  *Adaptive behavior treatment (0368T-0371T)*
*Crisis psychotherapy (90839-90840)*
*E&M services (99201-99337 [99224, 99225, 99226], 99341-99350, 99366-99368, 99401-99444)*

Code also interactive complexity services when applicable (90785)

**90791** **Psychiatric diagnostic evaluation**

🔩 3.56  📏 3.68  **FUD** XXX  ★🄾🄱▱

**AMA:** 2017,Jan,8; 2016,Jan,13; 2015,Jan,16; 2014,Jun,3; 2014,Jan,11; 2013,Dec,16; 2013,Jun,3-5; 2013,May,12

**90792** **Psychiatric diagnostic evaluation with medical services**

🔩 4.01  📏 4.13  **FUD** XXX  ★🄾🄱▱

**AMA:** 2017,Jan,8; 2016,Jan,13; 2015,Jan,16; 2014,Jun,3; 2014,Jan,11; 2013,Dec,16; 2013,Jun,3-5

## 90832-90838 Psychotherapy Services

**CMS:** 100-02,15,160 Clinical Psychologist Services; 100-02,15,170 Clinical Social Worker (CSW) Services; 100-03,130.1 Inpatient Stays for Alcoholism Treatment; 100-03,130.2 Outpatient Hospital Services for Alcoholism; 100-03,130.3 Chemical Aversion Therapy for Treatment of Alcoholism; 100-04,12,100 Teaching Physician Services; 100-04,12,160 Independent Psychologist Services; 100-04,12,170 Clinical Psychologist Services; 100-04,12,190.3 List of Telehealth Services; 100-04,12,190.6 Payment Methodology for Physician/Practitioner at the Distant Site ; 100-04,12,190.6.1 Submission of Telehealth Claims for Distant Site Practitioners; 100-04,12,190.7 Contractor Editing of Telehealth Claims

INCLUDES  Face-to-face time with patient (family, other informers may also be present)
Pharmacologic management in time allocated to psychotherapy service codes
Psychotherapy only (90832, 90834, 90837)
Psychotherapy with separately identifiable medical E&M services includes add-on codes (90833, 90836, 90838)
Service times of no less than 16 minutes
Services provided in all settings
Therapeutic communication to:
Ameliorate the patient's mental and behavioral symptoms
Modify behavior
Support and encourage personality growth and development
Treatment for:
Behavior disturbances
Mental illness

EXCLUDES  *Adaptive behavior treatment (0364T-0367T, 0373T-0374T)*
*Crisis psychotherapy (90839-90840)*
*Family psychotherapy (90846-90847)*

Code also interactive complexity services with the time the provider spends performing the service reflected in the time for the appropriate psychotherapy code (90785)

**90832** **Psychotherapy, 30 minutes with patient**

🔩 1.77  📏 1.79  **FUD** XXX  ★🄾🄱▱

**AMA:** 2017,Sep,11; 2017,Jan,8; 2016,Dec,11; 2016,Jan,13; 2015,Oct,9; 2015,Jan,16; 2014,Aug,5; 2014,Feb,3; 2013,Aug,13; 2013,Jun,3-5; 2013,May,12; 2013,Jan,3-5

+ **90833** **Psychotherapy, 30 minutes with patient when performed with an evaluation and management service (List separately in addition to the code for primary procedure)**

Code first (99201-99255 [99224, 99225, 99226], 99341-99350)

🔩 1.84  📏 1.86  **FUD** ZZZ  ★Ⓝ▱

**AMA:** 2017,Jan,8; 2016,Dec,11; 2016,Jan,13; 2015,Oct,9; 2015,Jan,16; 2014,Aug,5; 2014,Feb,3; 2013,Aug,13; 2013,Jun,3-5; 2013,May,12; 2013,Jan,3-5

**90834** **Psychotherapy, 45 minutes with patient**

🔩 2.36  📏 2.38  **FUD** XXX  ★🄾🄱▱

**AMA:** 2017,Jan,8; 2016,Dec,11; 2016,Jan,13; 2015,Oct,9; 2015,Jan,16; 2014,Jun,3; 2014,Feb,3; 2013,Aug,13; 2013,Jun,3-5; 2013,May,12; 2013,Jan,3-5

| 26/🄣 PC/TC Only | 🄰2-🅉8 ASC Payment | 50 Bilateral | ♂ Male Only | ♀ Female Only | 🔩 Facility RVU | 📏 Non-Facility RVU | ▱ CCI |
| **FUD** Follow-up Days | **CMS:** IOM (Pub 100) | 🄰-🅈 OPPSI | 80/🄐 Surg Assist Allowed / w/Doc | | 📋 Lab Crosswalk | 🄳 Radiology Crosswalk | ❎ CLIA |

430      CPT © 2017 American Medical Association. All Rights Reserved.      © 2017 Optum360, LLC

**+ 90836** **Psychotherapy, 45 minutes with patient when performed with an evaluation and management service (List separately in addition to the code for primary procedure)**
> Code first (99201-99255 [99224, 99225, 99226], 99304-99337, 99341-99350)
> 🔳 2.33   ⚖ 2.35   **FUD** ZZZ                          ★ Ⓝ 🖵
> **AMA:** 2017,Jan,8; 2016,Dec,11; 2016,Jan,13; 2015,Oct,9; 2015,Jan,16; 2014,Feb,3; 2013,Aug,13; 2013,Jun,3-5; 2013,May,12; 2013,Jan,3-5

**90837** **Psychotherapy, 60 minutes with patient**
> Code also prolonged service for psychotherapy performed without E&M service face-to-face with the patient lasting 90 minutes or longer (99354-99357)
> 🔳 3.55   ⚖ 3.57   **FUD** XXX                          ★ 03 🖵
> **AMA:** 2017,Jan,8; 2016,Dec,11; 2016,Jan,13; 2015,Oct,9; 2015,Oct,3; 2015,Jan,16; 2014,Apr,6; 2014,Feb,3; 2013,Aug,13; 2013,Jun,3-5; 2013,May,12; 2013,Jan,3-5

**+ 90838** **Psychotherapy, 60 minutes with patient when performed with an evaluation and management service (List separately in addition to the code for primary procedure)**
> Code first (99201-99255 [99224, 99225, 99226], 99304-99337, 99341-99350)
> 🔳 3.08   ⚖ 3.10   **FUD** ZZZ                          ★ Ⓝ 🖵
> **AMA:** 2017,Jan,8; 2016,Dec,11; 2016,Jan,13; 2015,Oct,9; 2015,Jan,16; 2014,Apr,6; 2014,Feb,3; 2013,Aug,13; 2013,Jun,3-5; 2013,May,12; 2013,Jan,3-5

## 90839-90840 Services for Patients in Crisis

**CMS:** 100-02,15,170 Clinical Social Worker (CSW) Services; 100-03,130.1 Inpatient Stays for Alcoholism Treatment; 100-03,130.3 Chemical Aversion Therapy for Treatment of Alcoholism; 100-04,12,100 Teaching Physician Services; 100-04,12,160 Independent Psychologist Services; 100-04,12,160.1 Payment of Independent Psychologist Services; 100-04,12,170 Clinical Psychologist Services

> INCLUDES   30 minutes or more of face-to-face time with the patient (for all or part of the service) and/or family providing crisis psychotherapy
> All time spent exclusively with patient (for all or part of the service) and/or family, even if time is not continuous
> Emergent care to a patient in severe distress (eg, life threatening or complex)
> Institute interventions to minimize psychological trauma
> Measures to ease the crisis and reestablish safety
> Psychotherapy
> EXCLUDES   *Adaptive behavior treatment (0364T-0367T, 0373T-0374T)*
> *Other psychiatric services (90785-90899)*

**90839** **Psychotherapy for crisis; first 60 minutes**
> INCLUDES   First 30-74 minutes of crisis psychotherapy per day
> EXCLUDES   *Use of code more than one time per day, even when service is not continuous on that date.*
> 🔳 3.70   ⚖ 3.73   **FUD** XXX                          03 80 🖵
> **AMA:** 2017,Jan,8; 2016,Jan,13; 2015,Oct,9; 2015,Jan,16; 2014,Aug,5; 2013,Jun,3-5

**+ 90840** **each additional 30 minutes (List separately in addition to code for primary service)**
> INCLUDES   Up to 30 minutes of time beyond the initial 74 minutes
> Code first (90839)
> 🔳 1.77   ⚖ 1.78   **FUD** ZZZ                          Ⓝ 80 🖵
> **AMA:** 2017,Jan,8; 2016,Jan,13; 2015,Oct,9; 2015,Jan,16; 2014,Aug,5; 2013,Jun,3-5

## 90845-90863 Additional Psychotherapy Services

**CMS:** 100-02,15,170 Clinical Social Worker (CSW) Services; 100-03,10.3 Inpatient Pain Rehabilitation Programs; 100-03,10.4 Outpatient Hospital Pain Rehabilitation Programs

> EXCLUDES   *Adaptive behavior treatment (0364T-0367T, 0373T-0374T)*
> *Analysis/programming of neurostimulators for vagus nerve stimulation therapy (95970, 95974-95975)*
> *Crisis psychotherapy (90839-90840)*

**90845** **Psychoanalysis**
> 🔳 2.55   ⚖ 2.56   **FUD** XXX                          ★ 03 80 🖵
> **AMA:** 2017,Jan,8; 2016,Jan,13; 2015,Oct,9; 2015,Jan,16; 2014,Jan,11; 2012,Jan,15-42

**90846** **Family psychotherapy (without the patient present), 50 minutes**
> EXCLUDES   *Adaptive behavior treatment (0368T-0371T)*
> *Service times of less than 26 minutes*
> 🔳 2.86   ⚖ 2.88   **FUD** XXX                          ★ 03 80 🖵
> **AMA:** 2017,Mar,10; 2017,Jan,8; 2016,Dec,11; 2016,Jan,13; 2015,Oct,9; 2015,Jan,16; 2014,Jan,11; 2013,Dec,16; 2013,Jun,3-5

**90847** **Family psychotherapy (conjoint psychotherapy) (with patient present), 50 minutes**
> EXCLUDES   *Adaptive behavior treatment (0368T-0371T)*
> *Service times of less than 26 minutes*
> 🔳 2.97   ⚖ 2.99   **FUD** XXX                          ★ 03 80 🖵
> **AMA:** 2017,Jan,8; 2016,Dec,11; 2016,Jan,13; 2015,Oct,9; 2015,Jan,16; 2014,Jan,11; 2013,Dec,16; 2013,Jun,3-5

**90849** **Multiple-family group psychotherapy**
> 🔳 0.88   ⚖ 0.98   **FUD** XXX                          03 80 🖵
> **AMA:** 2017,Jan,8; 2016,Jan,13; 2015,Oct,9; 2015,Jan,16; 2014,Aug,14; 2014,Jan,11

**90853** **Group psychotherapy (other than of a multiple-family group)**
> EXCLUDES   *Adaptive behavior social skills group (0372T)*
> Code also group psychotherapy with interactive complexity (90785)
> 🔳 0.71   ⚖ 0.72   **FUD** XXX                          03 80 🖵
> **AMA:** 2017,Mar,10; 2017,Jan,8; 2016,Jan,13; 2015,Oct,9; 2015,Jan,16; 2014,Aug,14; 2014,Jun,3; 2014,Jan,11; 2013,Jun,3-5

**+ 90863** **Pharmacologic management, including prescription and review of medication, when performed with psychotherapy services (List separately in addition to the code for primary procedure)**
> INCLUDES   Pharmacologic management in time allocated to psychotherapy service codes
> Code first (90832, 90834, 90837)
> 🔳 0.00   ⚖ 0.00   **FUD** XXX                          ★ Ⓔ 🖵
> **AMA:** 2017,Jan,8; 2016,Jan,13; 2015,Jan,16; 2013,Jun,3-5

## 90865-90870 Other Psychiatric Treatment

> EXCLUDES   *Adaptive behavior treatment (0364T-0367T, 0373T-0374T)*
> *Analysis/programming of neurostimulators for vagus nerve stimulation therapy (95970, 95974, 95975)*
> *Crisis psychotherapy (90839-90840)*

**90865** **Narcosynthesis for psychiatric diagnostic and therapeutic purposes (eg, sodium amobarbital (Amytal) interview)**
> 🔳 3.62   ⚖ 4.71   **FUD** XXX                          03 80 🖵
> **AMA:** 2017,Jan,8; 2016,Jan,13; 2015,Jan,16; 2014,Jan,11

**90867** **Therapeutic repetitive transcranial magnetic stimulation (TMS) treatment; initial, including cortical mapping, motor threshold determination, delivery and management**
> 🔳 0.00   ⚖ 0.00   **FUD** 000                          Ⓢ 🖵
> INCLUDES   Evaluation E&M services related directly to:
>           Cortical mapping
>           Delivery and management of TMS services
>           Motor threshold determination
> EXCLUDES   *Electromyography (95860, 95870)*
> *Evoked potential studies (95928-95929)*
> *Medication management*
> *Navigated transcranial magnetic stimulation (nTMS) motor function mapping for treatment planning, upper and lower extremity (64999)*
> *Significant, separately identifiable E&M service*
> *Significant, separately identifiable psychotherapy service*
> *Use of code more than one time for each course of treatment*

---

● New Code   ▲ Revised Code   ○ Reinstated   ● New Web Release   ▲ Revised Web Release   Unlisted   Not Covered   # Resequenced
⊘ AMA Mod 51 Exempt   ⑤¹ Optum Mod 51 Exempt   ⑥³ Mod 63 Exempt   ✗ Non-FDA Drug   ★ Telemedicine   Ⓜ Maternity   Ⓐ Age Edit   + Add-on   **AMA:** CPT Asst
© 2017 Optum360, LLC                      CPT © 2017 American Medical Association. All Rights Reserved.                      **431**

Medicine

90868 — 90935

**90868**    subsequent delivery and management, per session

🚑 0.00    ⚗ 0.00    **FUD** 000     S ▣

INCLUDES   E&M services related directly to:
    Cortical mapping
    Delivery and management of TMS services
    Motor threshold determination

EXCLUDES   *Medication management*
*Navigated transcranial magnetic stimulation (nTMS)*
*    motor function mapping for treatment planning,*
*    upper and lower extremity (64999)*
*Significant, separately identifiable E&M service*
*Significant, separately identifiable psychotherapy*
*    service*

**90869**    subsequent motor threshold re-determination with delivery and management

🚑 0.00    ⚗ 0.00    **FUD** 000     S ▣

INCLUDES   E&M services related directly to:
    Cortical mapping
    Delivery and management of TMS services
    Motor threshold determination

EXCLUDES   *Electromyography (95860, 95870)*
*Evoked potential studies (95928-95929)*
*Medication management*
*Navigated transcranial magnetic stimulation (nTMS)*
*    motor function mapping for treatment planning,*
*    upper and lower extremity (64999)*
*Significant, separately identifiable E&M service*
*Significant, separately identifiable psychotherapy*
*    service*

**90870**    **Electroconvulsive therapy (includes necessary monitoring)**

🚑 3.12    ⚗ 4.98    **FUD** 000     S 80 ▣

**AMA:** 2017,Jan,8; 2016,Jan,13; 2015,Jan,16; 2014,Jan,11

## 90875-90880 Psychiatric Therapy with Biofeedback or Hypnosis

**CMS:** 100-02,15,170 Clinical Social Worker (CSW) Services; 100-04,12,160 Independent Psychologist Services; 100-04,12,160.1 Payment of Independent Psychologist Services; 100-04,12,170 Clinical Psychologist Services

EXCLUDES   *Adaptive behavior treatment (0364T-0367T, 0373T-0374T)*
*Analysis/programming of neurostimulators for vagus nerve stimulation*
*    therapy (95970, 95974, 95975)*
*Crisis psychotherapy (90839-90840)*

**90875**    **Individual psychophysiological therapy incorporating biofeedback training by any modality (face-to-face with the patient), with psychotherapy (eg, insight oriented, behavior modifying or supportive psychotherapy); 30 minutes**

🚑 1.73    ⚗ 1.74    **FUD** XXX     E ▣

**AMA:** 2017,Jan,8; 2016,Jan,13; 2015,Jan,16; 2014,Jan,11; 2012,Jan,15-42

**90876**    **45 minutes**

🚑 2.74    ⚗ 3.05    **FUD** XXX     E ▣

**AMA:** 2017,Jan,8; 2016,Jan,13; 2015,Jan,16; 2014,Jan,11

**90880**    **Hypnotherapy**

🚑 2.62    ⚗ 2.85    **FUD** XXX     Q3 80 ▣

**AMA:** 2017,Jan,8; 2016,Jan,13; 2015,Jan,16; 2014,Jan,11

## 90882-90899 Psychiatric Services without Patient Face-to-Face Contact

**CMS:** 100-04,12,160 Independent Psychologist Services; 100-04,12,160.1 Payment of Independent Psychologist Services

EXCLUDES   *Adaptive behavior treatment (0364T-0367T, 0373T-0374T)*
*Analysis/programming of neurostimulators for vagus nerve stimulation*
*    therapy (95970, 95974, 95975)*
*Crisis psychotherapy (90839-90840)*

**90882**    **Environmental intervention for medical management purposes on a psychiatric patient's behalf with agencies, employers, or institutions**

🚑 0.00    ⚗ 0.00    **FUD** XXX     E ▣

**AMA:** 2017,Jan,8; 2016,Jan,13; 2015,Jan,16; 2014,Jan,11

**90885**    **Psychiatric evaluation of hospital records, other psychiatric reports, psychometric and/or projective tests, and other accumulated data for medical diagnostic purposes**

🚑 1.40    ⚗ 1.40    **FUD** XXX     N ▣

**AMA:** 2017,Jan,8; 2016,Jan,13; 2015,Jan,16; 2014,Jan,11; 2012,Jan,15-42

**90887**    **Interpretation or explanation of results of psychiatric, other medical examinations and procedures, or other accumulated data to family or other responsible persons, or advising them how to assist patient**

EXCLUDES   *Adaptive behavior treatment (0368T-0371T)*

🚑 2.14    ⚗ 2.49    **FUD** XXX     N ▣

**AMA:** 2017,Jan,8; 2016,Jan,13; 2015,Jan,16; 2014,Jan,11; 2012,Jan,15-42

**90889**    **Preparation of report of patient's psychiatric status, history, treatment, or progress (other than for legal or consultative purposes) for other individuals, agencies, or insurance carriers**

🚑 0.00    ⚗ 0.00    **FUD** XXX     N ▣

**AMA:** 2017,Jan,8; 2016,Jan,13; 2015,Jan,16; 2014,Jan,11

**90899**    **Unlisted psychiatric service or procedure**

🚑 0.00    ⚗ 0.00    **FUD** XXX     Q3 80

**AMA:** 2017,Jan,8; 2016,Jan,13; 2015,Jan,16; 2014,Jan,11; 2012,Jan,15-42

## 90901-90911 Biofeedback Therapy

**CMS:** 100-05,5,40.7 Biofeedback Training for Urinary Incontinence

EXCLUDES   *Psychophysiological therapy utilizing biofeedback training (90875-90876)*

**90901**    **Biofeedback training by any modality**

🚑 0.55    ⚗ 1.04    **FUD** 000     A 80 ▣

**AMA:** 2017,Jan,8; 2016,Jan,13; 2015,Jan,16; 2014,Jan,11; 2012,Jan,15-42

**90911**    **Biofeedback training, perineal muscles, anorectal or urethral sphincter, including EMG and/or manometry**

EXCLUDES   *Rectal sensation/tone/compliance testing (91120)*
*Treatment for incontinence, pulsed magnetic*
*    neuromodulation (53899)*

🚑 1.26    ⚗ 2.39    **FUD** 000     S 80 ▣

**AMA:** 2017,Jan,8; 2016,Jan,13; 2015,Jan,16; 2014,Sep,13; 2014,Jan,11; 2012,Jan,15-42

## 90935-90940 Hemodialysis Services: Inpatient ESRD and Outpatient Non-ESRD

**CMS:** 100-02,11,20 Renal Dialysis Items and Services; 100-04,3,100.6 Inpatient Renal Services

EXCLUDES   *Attendance by physician or other qualified health care provider for a prolonged*
*    period of time (99354-99360 [99415, 99416])*
*Blood specimen collection from partial/complete implantable venous access*
*    device (36591)*
*Declotting of cannula (36831, 36833, 36860-36861)*
*Hemodialysis home visit by non-physician health care professional (99512)*
*Therapeutic apheresis procedures (36511-36516)*
*Thrombolytic agent declotting of implanted vascular access device/catheter*
*    (36593)*

Code also significant separately identifiable E&M service not related to dialysis procedure or renal failure with modifier 25 (99201-99215, 99217-99223 [99224, 99225, 99226], 99231-99239, 99241-99245, 99281-99285, 99291-99292, 99304-99318, 99324-99337, 99341-99350, 99466-99467, 99468-99476, 99477-99480)

**90935**    **Hemodialysis procedure with single evaluation by a physician or other qualified health care professional**

INCLUDES   All E&M services related to the patient's renal disease
    rendered on a day dialysis is performed
    Inpatient ESRD and non-ESRD procedures
    Only one evaluation of the patient related to
      hemodialysis procedure
    Outpatient non-ESRD dialysis

🚑 2.04    ⚗ 2.04    **FUD** 000     S 80 ▣

**AMA:** 2017,Jan,8; 2016,Jan,13; 2015,Jan,16; 2014,Jan,11

26/TC PC/TC Only    A2-Z3 ASC Payment    50 Bilateral    ♂ Male Only    ♀ Female Only    🚑 Facility RVU    ⚗ Non-Facility RVU    ▣ CCI
**FUD** Follow-up Days    **CMS:** IOM (Pub 100)    A-Y OPPSI    80/80 Surg Assist Allowed / w/Doc    📋 Lab Crosswalk    ⊞ Radiology Crosswalk    ✖ CLIA

432      CPT © 2017 American Medical Association. All Rights Reserved.      © 2017 Optum360, LLC

## 90937 Hemodialysis procedure requiring repeated evaluation(s) with or without substantial revision of dialysis prescription

INCLUDES  All E&M services related to the patient's renal disease rendered on a day dialysis is performed
Inpatient ESRD and non-ESRD procedures
Outpatient non-ESRD dialysis
Re-evaluation of the patient during hemodialysis procedure

2.94    2.94    **FUD** 000                                          B 80

**AMA:** 2017,Jan,8; 2016,Jan,13; 2015,Jan,16; 2014,Jan,11

## 90940 Hemodialysis access flow study to determine blood flow in grafts and arteriovenous fistulae by an indicator method

EXCLUDES  Hemodialysis access duplex scan (93990)

0.00    0.00    **FUD** XXX                                          N

**AMA:** 2017,Jan,8; 2016,Jan,13; 2015,Jan,16; 2014,Jan,11; 2012,Jan,15-42

# 90945-90947 Dialysis Techniques Other Than Hemodialysis

**CMS:** 100-04,12,40.3 Global Surgery Review; 100-04,3,100.6 Inpatient Renal Services

INCLUDES  All E&M services related to the patient's renal disease rendered on the day dialysis is performed
Procedures other than hemodialysis:
    Continuous renal replacement therapies
    Hemofiltration
    Peritoneal dialysis

EXCLUDES  Attendance by physician or other qualified health care provider for a prolonged period of time (99354-99360 [99415, 99416])
Hemodialysis
Tunneled intraperitoneal catheter insertion
    Open (49421)
    Percutaneous (49418)
Code also significant, separately identifiable E&M service not related to dialysis procedure or renal failure with modifier 25 (99201-99215, 99217-99223 [99224, 99225, 99226], 99231-99239, 99241-99245, 99281-99285, 99291-99292, 99304-99318, 99324-99337, 99341-99350, 99466-99480 [99485, 99486])

## 90945 Dialysis procedure other than hemodialysis (eg, peritoneal dialysis, hemofiltration, or other continuous renal replacement therapies), with single evaluation by a physician or other qualified health care professional

INCLUDES  Only one evaluation of the patient related to the procedure
EXCLUDES  Peritoneal dialysis home infusion (99601, 99602)

2.42    2.42    **FUD** 000                                          V 80

**AMA:** 2017,Jan,8; 2016,Jan,13; 2015,Jan,16; 2014,Jan,11; 2012,Jan,15-42

## 90947 Dialysis procedure other than hemodialysis (eg, peritoneal dialysis, hemofiltration, or other continuous renal replacement therapies) requiring repeated evaluations by a physician or other qualified health care professional, with or without substantial revision of dialysis prescription

EXCLUDES  Re-evaluation during a procedure

3.50    3.50    **FUD** 000                                          B 80

**AMA:** 2017,Jan,8; 2016,Jan,13; 2015,Jan,16; 2014,Jan,11; 2012,Jan,15-42

# 90951-90962 End-stage Renal Disease Monthly Outpatient Services

**CMS:** 100-02,11,20 Renal Dialysis Items and Services ; 100-04,12,190.3 List of Telehealth Services; 100-04,12,190.3.4 ESRD-Related Services as a Telehealth Service; 100-04,8,140.1 ESRD-Related Services Under the Monthly Capitation Payment

INCLUDES  Establishing dialyzing cycle
Management of dialysis visits
Outpatient E&M of dialysis visits
Patient management during dialysis for a month
Telephone calls

EXCLUDES  ESRD/non-ESRD dialysis services performed in an inpatient setting (90935-90937, 90945-90947)
Non-ESRD dialysis services performed in an outpatient setting (90935-90937, 90945-90947)
Non-ESRD related E&M services that cannot be performed during the dialysis session
Services provided during the time transitional care management services are being provided (99495-99496)
Services provided in the same month with chronic care management (99487-99489)

## 90951 End-stage renal disease (ESRD) related services monthly, for patients younger than 2 years of age to include monitoring for the adequacy of nutrition, assessment of growth and development, and counseling of parents; with 4 or more face-to-face visits by a physician or other qualified health care professional per month    A

26.6    26.6    **FUD** XXX                                  ★ M 80

**AMA:** 2017,Jan,8; 2016,Jan,13; 2015,Jan,16; 2014,Oct,3; 2014,Jan,11; 2013,Nov,3; 2013,Apr,3-4

## 90952 with 2-3 face-to-face visits by a physician or other qualified health care professional per month    A

0.00    0.00    **FUD** XXX                                  ★ M 80

**AMA:** 2017,Jan,8; 2016,Jan,13; 2015,Jan,16; 2014,Oct,3; 2014,Jan,11; 2013,Nov,3; 2013,Apr,3-4

## 90953 with 1 face-to-face visit by a physician or other qualified health care professional per month    A

0.00    0.00    **FUD** XXX                                    M 80

**AMA:** 2017,Jan,8; 2016,Jan,13; 2015,Jan,16; 2014,Oct,3; 2014,Jan,11; 2013,Nov,3; 2013,Apr,3-4

## 90954 End-stage renal disease (ESRD) related services monthly, for patients 2-11 years of age to include monitoring for the adequacy of nutrition, assessment of growth and development, and counseling of parents; with 4 or more face-to-face visits by a physician or other qualified health care professional per month    A

23.0    23.0    **FUD** XXX                                  ★ M 80

**AMA:** 2017,Jan,8; 2016,Jan,13; 2015,Jan,16; 2014,Oct,3; 2014,Jan,11; 2013,Nov,3; 2013,Apr,3-4

## 90955 with 2-3 face-to-face visits by a physician or other qualified health care professional per month    A

12.9    12.9    **FUD** XXX                                  ★ M 80

**AMA:** 2017,Jan,8; 2016,Jan,13; 2015,Jan,16; 2014,Oct,3; 2014,Jan,11; 2013,Nov,3; 2013,Apr,3-4

## 90956 with 1 face-to-face visit by a physician or other qualified health care professional per month    A

8.98    8.98    **FUD** XXX                                    M 80

**AMA:** 2017,Jan,8; 2016,Jan,13; 2015,Jan,16; 2014,Oct,3; 2014,Jan,11; 2013,Nov,3; 2013,Apr,3-4

## 90957 End-stage renal disease (ESRD) related services monthly, for patients 12-19 years of age to include monitoring for the adequacy of nutrition, assessment of growth and development, and counseling of parents; with 4 or more face-to-face visits by a physician or other qualified health care professional per month    A

18.1    18.1    **FUD** XXX                                  ★ M 80

**AMA:** 2017,Jan,8; 2016,Jan,13; 2015,Jan,16; 2014,Oct,3; 2014,Jan,11; 2013,Nov,3; 2013,Apr,3-4

● New Code    ▲ Revised Code    ○ Reinstated    ● New Web Release    ▲ Revised Web Release    Unlisted    Not Covered    # Resequenced
Ⓢ AMA Mod 51 Exempt    ⑨ Optum Mod 51 Exempt    ⑨ Mod 63 Exempt    ✗ Non-FDA Drug    ★ Telemedicine    M Maternity    A Age Edit    + Add-on    AMA: CPT Asst
© 2017 Optum360, LLC                              CPT © 2017 American Medical Association. All Rights Reserved.                              433

**90958**    with 2-3 face-to-face visits by a physician or other qualified health care professional per month [A]

📋 12.3    ⚕ 12.3    **FUD** XXX    ★ [M] [80] [▣]

**AMA:** 2017,Jan,8; 2016,Jan,13; 2015,Jan,16; 2014,Oct,3; 2014,Jan,11; 2013,Nov,3; 2013,Apr,3-4

**90959**    with 1 face-to-face visit by a physician or other qualified health care professional per month [A]

📋 8.36    ⚕ 8.36    **FUD** XXX    [M] [80] [▣]

**AMA:** 2017,Jan,8; 2016,Jan,13; 2015,Jan,16; 2014,Oct,3; 2014,Jan,11; 2013,Nov,3; 2013,Apr,3-4

**90960**    End-stage renal disease (ESRD) related services monthly, for patients 20 years of age and older; with 4 or more face-to-face visits by a physician or other qualified health care professional per month [A]

📋 8.00    ⚕ 8.00    **FUD** XXX    ★ [M] [80] [▣]

**AMA:** 2017,Jan,8; 2016,Jan,13; 2015,Jan,16; 2014,Oct,3; 2014,Jan,11; 2013,Nov,3; 2013,Apr,3-4

**90961**    with 2-3 face-to-face visits by a physician or other qualified health care professional per month [A]

📋 6.72    ⚕ 6.72    **FUD** XXX    ★ [M] [80] [▣]

**AMA:** 2017,Jan,8; 2016,Jan,13; 2015,Jan,16; 2014,Oct,3; 2014,Jan,11; 2013,Nov,3; 2013,Apr,3-4

**90962**    with 1 face-to-face visit by a physician or other qualified health care professional per month [A]

📋 5.18    ⚕ 5.18    **FUD** XXX    [M] [80] [▣]

**AMA:** 2017,Jan,8; 2016,Jan,13; 2015,Jan,16; 2014,Oct,3; 2014,Jan,11; 2013,Nov,3; 2013,Apr,3-4

## 90963-90966 End-stage Renal Disease Monthly Home Dialysis Services

**CMS:** 100-02,11,20 Renal Dialysis Items and Services ; 100-04,12,190.3.4 ESRD-Related Services as a Telehealth Service; 100-04,8,140.1 ESRD-Related Services Under the Monthly Capitation Payment; 100-04,8,140.1.1 Payment for Managing Patients on Home Dialysis

[INCLUDES]    ESRD services for home dialysis patients
Services provided for a full month

[EXCLUDES]    *Services provided during the time transitional care management services are being provided (99495-99496)*
*Services provided in the same month with chronic care management (99487-99489)*

**90963**    End-stage renal disease (ESRD) related services for home dialysis per full month, for patients younger than 2 years of age to include monitoring for the adequacy of nutrition, assessment of growth and development, and counseling of parents [A]

📋 15.3    ⚕ 15.3    **FUD** XXX    [M] [80] [▣]

**AMA:** 2017,Jan,8; 2016,Jan,13; 2015,Jan,16; 2014,Oct,3; 2014,Jan,11; 2013,Nov,3; 2013,Apr,3-4

**90964**    End-stage renal disease (ESRD) related services for home dialysis per full month, for patients 2-11 years of age to include monitoring for the adequacy of nutrition, assessment of growth and development, and counseling of parents [A]

📋 13.4    ⚕ 13.4    **FUD** XXX    [M] [80] [▣]

**AMA:** 2017,Jan,8; 2016,Jan,13; 2015,Jan,16; 2014,Oct,3; 2014,Jan,11; 2013,Nov,3; 2013,Apr,3-4

**90965**    End-stage renal disease (ESRD) related services for home dialysis per full month, for patients 12-19 years of age to include monitoring for the adequacy of nutrition, assessment of growth and development, and counseling of parents [A]

📋 12.8    ⚕ 12.8    **FUD** XXX    [M] [80] [▣]

**AMA:** 2017,Jan,8; 2016,Jan,13; 2015,Jan,16; 2014,Oct,3; 2014,Jan,11; 2013,Nov,3; 2013,Apr,3-4

**90966**    End-stage renal disease (ESRD) related services for home dialysis per full month, for patients 20 years of age and older [A]

📋 6.70    ⚕ 6.70    **FUD** XXX    [M] [80] [▣]

**AMA:** 2017,Jan,8; 2016,Jan,13; 2015,Jan,16; 2014,Oct,3; 2014,Jan,11; 2013,Nov,3; 2013,Apr,3-4

## 90967-90970 End-stage Renal Disease Services: Partial Month

**CMS:** 100-02,11,20 Renal Dialysis Items and Services

[INCLUDES]    ESRD services for less than a full month, such as:
A patient who is transient, dies, recovers, or undergoes kidney transplant
Outpatient ESRD-related services initiated prior to completion of assessment
Patient spending part of the month as a hospital inpatient
Services reported on a daily basis, less the days of hospitalization

[EXCLUDES]    *Services provided during the time transitional care management services are being provided (99495-99496)*
*Services provided in the same month with chronic care management (99487-99489)*

**90967**    End-stage renal disease (ESRD) related services for dialysis less than a full month of service, per day; for patients younger than 2 years of age [A]

📋 0.51    ⚕ 0.51    **FUD** XXX    [M] [80] [▣]

**AMA:** 2017,Jan,8; 2016,Jan,13; 2015,Jan,16; 2014,Oct,3; 2014,Jan,11; 2013,Nov,3; 2013,Apr,3-4

**90968**    for patients 2-11 years of age [A]

📋 0.44    ⚕ 0.44    **FUD** XXX    [M] [80] [▣]

**AMA:** 2017,Jan,8; 2016,Jan,13; 2015,Jan,16; 2014,Oct,3; 2014,Jan,11; 2013,Nov,3; 2013,Apr,3-4

**90969**    for patients 12-19 years of age [A]

📋 0.43    ⚕ 0.43    **FUD** XXX    [M] [80] [▣]

**AMA:** 2017,Jan,8; 2016,Jan,13; 2015,Jan,16; 2014,Oct,3; 2014,Jan,11; 2013,Nov,3; 2013,Apr,3-4

**90970**    for patients 20 years of age and older [A]

📋 0.22    ⚕ 0.22    **FUD** XXX    [M] [80] [▣]

**AMA:** 2017,Jan,8; 2016,Jan,13; 2015,Jan,16; 2014,Oct,3; 2014,Jan,11; 2013,Nov,3; 2013,Apr,3-4

## 90989-90993 Dialysis Training Services

**CMS:** 100-04,3,100.6 Inpatient Renal Services

**90989**    Dialysis training, patient, including helper where applicable, any mode, completed course

📋 0.00    ⚕ 0.00    **FUD** XXX    [B] [▣]

**AMA:** 2017,Jan,8; 2016,Jan,13; 2015,Jan,16; 2014,Jan,11; 2012,Jan,15-42

**90993**    Dialysis training, patient, including helper where applicable, any mode, course not completed, per training session

📋 0.00    ⚕ 0.00    **FUD** XXX    [B] [▣]

**AMA:** 2017,Jan,8; 2016,Jan,13; 2015,Jan,16; 2014,Jan,11; 2012,Jan,15-42

## 90997-90999 Hemoperfusion and Unlisted Dialysis Procedures

**CMS:** 100-04,3,100.6 Inpatient Renal Services

**90997**    Hemoperfusion (eg, with activated charcoal or resin)

📋 2.54    ⚕ 2.54    **FUD** 000    [B] [80] [▣]

**AMA:** 1999,Nov,1; 1997,Nov,1

**90999**    Unlisted dialysis procedure, inpatient or outpatient

📋 0.00    ⚕ 0.00    **FUD** XXX    [B] [80]

**AMA:** 1999,Nov,1; 1997,Nov,1

## 91010-91022 Esophageal Manometry

**91010**    Esophageal motility (manometric study of the esophagus and/or gastroesophageal junction) study with interpretation and report;

[EXCLUDES]    *Esophageal motility studies with high-resolution esophageal pressure topography (91299)*
Code also for esophageal motility studies with stimulant or perfusion (91013)

📋 4.97    ⚕ 4.97    **FUD** 000    [S] [80] [▣]

**AMA:** 2005,May,3-6; 1997,Nov,1

[26]/[TC] PC/TC Only    [A2]-[Z3] ASC Payment    [50] Bilateral    ♂ Male Only    ♀ Female Only    📋 Facility RVU    ⚕ Non-Facility RVU    [▣] CCI
**FUD** Follow-up Days    **CMS:** IOM (Pub 100)    [A]-[Y] OPPSI    [80]/[80] Surg Assist Allowed / w/Doc    📊 Lab Crosswalk    ❌ Radiology Crosswalk    ❌ CLIA

CPT © 2017 American Medical Association. All Rights Reserved.    © 2017 Optum360, LLC

+ **91013** **with stimulation or perfusion (eg, stimulant, acid or alkali perfusion) (List separately in addition to code for primary procedure)**

　　　💰 0.66　　⚕ 0.66　　**FUD** ZZZ　　　　　　Ⓝ 80 🖵

　　　*EXCLUDES* *Esophageal motility studies with high-resolution esophageal pressure topography (91299)*
　　　*Use of code more than one time for each session*
　　　Code first (91010)

**91020** **Gastric motility (manometric) studies**

　　　*EXCLUDES* *Gastrointestinal imaging by wireless capsule (91112)*
　　　💰 6.58　　⚕ 6.58　　**FUD** 000　　　　　　Ⓢ 80 🖵

　　　**AMA:** 2017,Jan,8; 2016,Jan,13; 2015,Jan,16; 2013,Sep,13-14

Liver
Stomach

Gastric pertains to the stomach; peptic is a term for ulcers caused by digestive juices in the stomach, duodenum or jejunum; duodenal ulcers are more common in young people, gastric in the elderly

Colon
Small intestine
Esophagus
Mucosal and muscle layers
Fundus
Rugae (folds lining the stomach)
Duodenum
Pyloric sphincter
Inner stomach (area where gastric ulcers occur)

**91022** **Duodenal motility (manometric) study**

　　　*EXCLUDES* *Fluoroscopy (76000)*
　　　*Gastric motility study (91020)*
　　　*Gastrointestinal imaging by wireless capsule (91112)*
　　　💰 4.74　　⚕ 4.74　　**FUD** 000　　　　　　Ⓢ 80 🖵

　　　**AMA:** 2017,Jan,8; 2016,Jan,13; 2015,Jan,16; 2013,Sep,13-14

## 91030-91040 Esophageal Reflux Tests

*EXCLUDES* *Duodenal intubation/aspiration (43756-43757)*
*Esophagoscopy (43180-43233 [43211, 43212, 43213, 43214])*
*Insertion of:*
　*Esophageal tamponade tube (43460)*
　*Miller-Abbott tube (44500)*
*Radiologic services, gastrointestinal (74210-74363)*
*Upper gastrointestinal endoscopy (43235-43259 [43233, 43266, 43270])*

**91030** **Esophagus, acid perfusion (Bernstein) test for esophagitis**

　　　💰 3.79　　⚕ 3.79　　**FUD** 000　　　　　　Ⓢ 80 🖵

**91034** **Esophagus, gastroesophageal reflux test; with nasal catheter pH electrode(s) placement, recording, analysis and interpretation**

　　　💰 5.31　　⚕ 5.31　　**FUD** 000　　　　　　Ⓢ 80 🖵

　　　**AMA:** 2017,Jan,8; 2016,Jan,13; 2015,Jan,16; 2014,Feb,11; 2014,Jan,11

**91035** **with mucosal attached telemetry pH electrode placement, recording, analysis and interpretation**

　　　*INCLUDES* Endoscopy only to place device
　　　💰 13.5　　⚕ 13.5　　**FUD** 000　　　　Ⓢ 🖇 80 🖵

　　　**AMA:** 2017,Jan,8; 2016,Jan,13; 2015,Jan,16; 2014,Feb,11; 2014,Jan,11

**91037** **Esophageal function test, gastroesophageal reflux test with nasal catheter intraluminal impedance electrode(s) placement, recording, analysis and interpretation;**

　　　💰 4.52　　⚕ 4.52　　**FUD** 000　　　　　　Ⓢ 80 🖵

　　　**AMA:** 2005,May,3-6

**91038** **prolonged (greater than 1 hour, up to 24 hours)**

　　　💰 12.6　　⚕ 12.6　　**FUD** 000　　　　　　Ⓢ 80 🖵

　　　**AMA:** 2017,Jan,8; 2016,Jan,13; 2015,Jan,16; 2014,Feb,11

**91040** **Esophageal balloon distension study, diagnostic, with provocation when performed**

　　　*EXCLUDES* *Use of code more than one time for each session*
　　　💰 12.0　　⚕ 12.0　　**FUD** 000　　　　　　Ⓢ 80 🖵

　　　**AMA:** 2017,Jan,6

## 91065 Breath Analysis

**CMS:** 100-03,100.5 Diagnostic Breath Analysis

　　*EXCLUDES* *H. pylori breath test analysis, radioactive (C-14) or nonradioactive (C-13) (78268, 83013)*
　　Code also each challenge administered

**91065** **Breath hydrogen or methane test (eg, for detection of lactase deficiency, fructose intolerance, bacterial overgrowth, or oro-cecal gastrointestinal transit)**

　　　💰 2.11　　⚕ 2.11　　**FUD** 000　　　　　　Ⓢ 80 🖵

　　　**AMA:** 2017,Jan,8; 2016,Jan,13; 2015,Jan,16; 2014,Jan,11

## 91110-91299 Additional Gastrointestinal Diagnostic/Therapeutic Procedures

*EXCLUDES* *Abdominal paracentesis (49082-49084)*
*Abdominal paracentesis with medication administration (96440, 96446)*
*Anoscopy (46600-46615)*
*Colonoscopy (45378-45393 [45388, 45390, 45398])*
*Duodenal intubation/aspiration (43756-43757)*
*Esophagoscopy (43180-43233 [43211, 43212, 43213, 43214])*
*Proctosigmoidoscopy (45300-45327)*
*Radiologic services, gastrointestinal (74210-74363)*
*Sigmoidoscopy (45330-45350 [45346])*
*Small intestine/stomal endoscopy (44360-44408 [44381, 44401])*
*Upper gastrointestinal endoscopy (43235-43259 [43233, 43266, 43270])*

**91110** **Gastrointestinal tract imaging, intraluminal (eg, capsule endoscopy), esophagus through ileum, with interpretation and report**

　　　*EXCLUDES* *Imaging of colon (0355T)*
　　　*Imaging of esophagus through ileum (91111)*
　　　Code also modifier 52 if ileum is not visualized
　　　💰 26.1　　⚕ 26.1　　**FUD** XXX　　　　　　Ⓣ 80 🖵

　　　**AMA:** 2017,Jan,8; 2016,Jan,13; 2015,Jan,16; 2014,Jan,11; 2013,Sep,13-14; 2012,Jan,15-42

**91111** **Gastrointestinal tract imaging, intraluminal (eg, capsule endoscopy), esophagus with interpretation and report**

　　　*EXCLUDES* *Imaging of colon (0355T)*
　　　*Imaging of esophagus through ileum (91111)*
　　　*Use of wireless capsule to measure transit times or pressure in gastrointestinal tract (91112)*
　　　💰 21.0　　⚕ 21.0　　**FUD** XXX　　　　　　Ⓣ 80 🖵

　　　**AMA:** 2017,Jan,8; 2016,Jan,13; 2015,Jan,16; 2013,Sep,13-14

**91112** **Gastrointestinal transit and pressure measurement, stomach through colon, wireless capsule, with interpretation and report**

　　　*EXCLUDES* *Colon motility study (91117)*
　　　*Duodenal motility study (91022)*
　　　*Gastric motility studies (91020)*
　　　*pH of body fluid (83986)*
　　　💰 30.3　　⚕ 30.3　　**FUD** XXX　　　　　　Ⓣ 80 🖵

　　　**AMA:** 2017,Jan,8; 2016,Jan,13; 2015,Jan,16; 2013,Sep,13-14

**91117** **Colon motility (manometric) study, minimum 6 hours continuous recording (including provocation tests, eg, meal, intracolonic balloon distension, pharmacologic agents, if performed), with interpretation and report**

　　　*EXCLUDES* *Anal manometry (91122)*
　　　*Rectal sensation, tone and compliance testing (91120)*
　　　*Use of code more than one time regardless of the number of provocations*
　　　*Use of wireless capsule to measure transit times or pressure in gastrointestinal tract (91112)*
　　　💰 3.99　　⚕ 3.99　　**FUD** 000　　　　　　Ⓣ 80 🖵

　　　**AMA:** 2017,Jan,8; 2016,Jan,13; 2015,Jan,16; 2013,Sep,13-14

---

● New Code　▲ Revised Code　○ Reinstated　● New Web Release　▲ Revised Web Release　Unlisted　Not Covered　# Resequenced
⊘ AMA Mod 51 Exempt　⑤⓪ Optum Mod 51 Exempt　⑥③ Mod 63 Exempt　✐ Non-FDA Drug　★ Telemedicine　Ⓜ Maternity　Ⓐ Age Edit　+ Add-on　**AMA:** CPT Asst

**91120** **Rectal sensation, tone, and compliance test (ie, response to graded balloon distention)**
EXCLUDES *Anorectal manometry (91122)*
*Biofeedback training (90911)*
*Colon motility study (91117)*
🖪 12.0  ⚖ 12.0  **FUD** XXX  ⟦S⟧⟦80⟧⟦▭⟧
**AMA:** 2017,Jan,8; 2016,Jan,13; 2015,Jan,16; 2014,Jan,11; 2013,Sep,13-14

**91122** **Anorectal manometry**
EXCLUDES *Colon motility study (91117)*
🖪 6.47  ⚖ 6.47  **FUD** 000  ⟦T⟧⟦80⟧⟦▭⟧
**AMA:** 2013,Sep,13-14

**91132** **Electrogastrography, diagnostic, transcutaneous;**
🖪 4.16  ⚖ 4.16  **FUD** XXX  ⟦S⟧⟦80⟧⟦▭⟧

**91133** **with provocative testing**
🖪 4.85  ⚖ 4.85  **FUD** XXX  ⟦01⟧⟦80⟧⟦▭⟧

**91200** **Liver elastography, mechanically induced shear wave (eg, vibration), without imaging, with interpretation and report**
🖪 1.09  ⚖ 1.09  **FUD** XXX  ⟦01⟧⟦NN⟧⟦80⟧⟦▭⟧
**AMA:** 2014,Dec,13

**91299** **Unlisted diagnostic gastroenterology procedure**
🖪 0.00  ⚖ 0.00  **FUD** XXX  ⟦S⟧⟦80⟧
**AMA:** 2017,Jan,8; 2016,Jan,13; 2015,Jan,16; 2014,Jan,11

## 92002-92014 Ophthalmic Medical Services

**CMS:** 100-02,15,30.4 Optometrist's Services
INCLUDES Routine ophthalmoscopy
Services provided to established patients who have received professional services from the physician or other qualified health care provider or another physician or other qualified health care professional within the same group practice of the exact same specialty and subspecialty within the past three years
Services provided to new patients who have received no professional services from the physician or other qualified health care provider or another physician or other qualified health care professional within the same group practice of the exact same specialty and subspecialty within the past three years
EXCLUDES *Retinal polarization scan (0469T)*
*Surgical procedures on the eye/ocular adnexa (65091-68899 [67810])*
*Visual screening tests (99173-99174 [99177])*

**92002** **Ophthalmological services: medical examination and evaluation with initiation of diagnostic and treatment program; intermediate, new patient**
INCLUDES Evaluation of new/existing condition complicated by new diagnostic or management problem
Integrated services where medical decision making cannot be separated from examination methods
Other diagnostic procedures:
Biomicroscopy
Mydriasis
Ophthalmoscopy
Tonometry
Problems not related to primary diagnosis
The following for intermediate services:
External ocular/adnexal examination
General medical observation
History
🖪 1.36  ⚖ 2.29  **FUD** XXX  ⟦V⟧⟦80⟧⟦▭⟧
**AMA:** 2017,Sep,14; 2017,Jan,8; 2016,Jan,13; 2015,Jan,16; 2014,Jan,11; 2012,Oct,9-11; 2012,Aug,9; 2012,Jan,15-42

**92004** **comprehensive, new patient, 1 or more visits**
INCLUDES General evaluation of complete visual system
Integrated services where medical decision making cannot be separated from examination methods
Single service that need not be performed at one session
The following for comprehensive services:
Basic sensorimotor examination
Biomicroscopy
Dilation (cycloplegia)
External examinations
General medical observation
Gross visual fields
History
Initiation of diagnostic/treatment programs
Mydriasis
Ophthalmoscopic examinations
Other diagnostic procedures
Prescription of medication
Special diagnostic/treatment services
Tonometry
🖪 2.83  ⚖ 4.20  **FUD** XXX  ⟦V⟧⟦80⟧⟦▭⟧
**AMA:** 2017,Sep,14; 2017,Jan,8; 2016,Nov,9; 2016,Jan,13; 2015,Jan,16; 2014,Jan,11; 2012,Aug,9; 2012,Jan,15-42

**92012** **Ophthalmological services: medical examination and evaluation, with initiation or continuation of diagnostic and treatment program; intermediate, established patient**
INCLUDES Evaluation of new/existing condition complicated by new diagnostic or management problem
Integrated services where medical decision making cannot be separated from examination methods
Problems not related to primary diagnosis
The following for intermediate services:
External ocular/adnexal examination
General medical observation
History
Other diagnostic procedures:
Biomicroscopy
Mydriasis
Ophthalmoscopy
Tonometry
🖪 1.50  ⚖ 2.41  **FUD** XXX  ⟦V⟧⟦80⟧⟦▭⟧
**AMA:** 2017,Sep,14; 2017,Jan,8; 2016,Jan,13; 2015,Jan,16; 2014,Jan,11; 2012,Aug,9

**92014** **comprehensive, established patient, 1 or more visits**
INCLUDES General evaluation of complete visual system
Integrated services where medical decision making cannot be separated from examination methods
Single service that need not be performed at one session
The following for comprehensive services:
Basic sensorimotor examination
Biomicroscopy
Dilation (cycloplegia)
External examinations
General medical observation
Gross visual fields
History
Initiation of diagnostic/treatment programs
Mydriasis
Ophthalmoscopic examinations
Other diagnostic procedures
Prescription of medication
Special diagnostic/treatment services
Tonometry
🖪 2.27  ⚖ 3.49  **FUD** XXX  ⟦V⟧⟦80⟧⟦▭⟧
**AMA:** 2017,Sep,14; 2017,Jan,8; 2016,Nov,9; 2016,Jan,13; 2015,Jan,16; 2014,Jan,11; 2012,Oct,9-11; 2012,Aug,9; 2012,Jan,15-42

## 92015-92145 Ophthalmic Special Services

INCLUDES    Routine ophthalmoscopy
*Surgical procedures on the eye/ocular adnexa (65091-68899 [67810])*
Code also E&M services, when performed
Code also general ophthalmological services, when performed (92002-92014)

**92015**    **Determination of refractive state**

INCLUDES    Lens prescription
Absorptive factor
Axis
Impact resistance
Lens power
Prism
Specification of lens type:
Bifocal
Monofocal

EXCLUDES    *Ocular screening, instrument based (99173-99174 [99177])*

0.55    0.56    **FUD** XXX    E

**AMA:** 2017,Jan,8; 2016,Mar,10; 2016,Jan,13; 2015,Jan,16; 2014,Jan,11; 2013,Mar,6-7; 2012,Jan,15-42

**92018**    **Ophthalmological examination and evaluation, under general anesthesia, with or without manipulation of globe for passive range of motion or other manipulation to facilitate diagnostic examination; complete**

4.12    4.12    **FUD** XXX    J  80

**AMA:** 2017,Jan,8; 2016,Jan,13; 2015,Jan,16; 2014,Jan,11

**92019**    **limited**

2.05    2.05    **FUD** XXX    J  80

**AMA:** 2017,Jan,8; 2016,Jan,13; 2015,Jan,16; 2014,Jan,11

**92020**    **Gonioscopy (separate procedure)**

EXCLUDES    *Gonioscopy under general anesthesia (92018)*

0.60    0.76    **FUD** XXX    01  80

**AMA:** 2017,Jan,8; 2016,Jan,13; 2015,Jan,16; 2014,Jan,11

**92025**    **Computerized corneal topography, unilateral or bilateral, with interpretation and report**

EXCLUDES    *Corneal transplant procedures (65710-65771)*
*Manual keratoscopy*

1.07    1.07    **FUD** XXX    01  80

**AMA:** 2017,Jan,8; 2016,Jan,13; 2015,Jan,16; 2014,Jan,11; 2012,Oct,9-11; 2012,Jan,15-42

**92060**    **Sensorimotor examination with multiple measurements of ocular deviation (eg, restrictive or paretic muscle with diplopia) with interpretation and report (separate procedure)**

1.84    1.84    **FUD** XXX    01  80

**AMA:** 2017,Jan,8; 2016,Jan,13; 2015,Jan,16; 2014,Jan,11

**92065**    **Orthoptic and/or pleoptic training, with continuing medical direction and evaluation**

1.53    1.53    **FUD** XXX    01  80

**AMA:** 2017,Jan,8; 2016,Jan,13; 2015,Jan,16; 2014,Jan,11; 2012,Jan,15-42

**92071**    **Fitting of contact lens for treatment of ocular surface disease**

EXCLUDES    *Contact lens service for keratoconus (92072)*
Code also supply of lens with appropriate supply code or (99070)

0.95    1.07    **FUD** XXX    N  N1  80  50

**AMA:** 2012,Aug,9

**92072**    **Fitting of contact lens for management of keratoconus, initial fitting**

EXCLUDES    *Contact lens service for disease of ocular surface (92071)*
*Subsequent fittings (99211-99215, 92012-92014)*
Code also supply of lens with appropriate supply code or (99070)

2.91    3.79    **FUD** XXX    N  80

**AMA:** 2017,Sep,14; 2017,Jan,8; 2016,Jan,13; 2015,Jan,16; 2014,Jan,11; 2012,Aug,9

**92081**    **Visual field examination, unilateral or bilateral, with interpretation and report; limited examination (eg, tangent screen, Autoplot, arc perimeter, or single stimulus level automated test, such as Octopus 3 or 7 equivalent)**

INCLUDES    Gross visual testing/confrontation testing

0.96    0.96    **FUD** XXX    01  80

**AMA:** 2017,Jan,8; 2016,Jan,13; 2015,Jan,16; 2014,Jan,11; 2012,Oct,9-11; 2012,Jan,15-42

**92082**    **intermediate examination (eg, at least 2 isopters on Goldmann perimeter, or semiquantitative, automated suprathreshold screening program, Humphrey suprathreshold automatic diagnostic test, Octopus program 33)**

INCLUDES    Gross visual testing/confrontation testing

1.37    1.37    **FUD** XXX    01  80

**AMA:** 2017,Jan,8; 2016,Jan,13; 2015,Jan,16; 2014,Jan,11; 2012,Oct,9-11

**92083**    **extended examination (eg, Goldmann visual fields with at least 3 isopters plotted and static determination within the central 30°, or quantitative, automated threshold perimetry, Octopus program G-1, 32 or 42, Humphrey visual field analyzer full threshold programs 30-2, 24-2, or 30/60-2)**

INCLUDES    Gross visual field testing/confrontation testing

EXCLUDES    *Assessment of visual field by transmission of data by patient to a surveillance center (0378T-0379T)*

1.82    1.82    **FUD** XXX    01  60

**AMA:** 2017,Jan,8; 2016,Jan,13; 2015,Jan,16; 2014,Jan,11; 2012,Oct,9-11

**92100**    **Serial tonometry (separate procedure) with multiple measurements of intraocular pressure over an extended time period with interpretation and report, same day (eg, diurnal curve or medical treatment of acute elevation of intraocular pressure)**

EXCLUDES    *Intraocular pressure monitoring for 24 hours or more (0329T)*
*Ocular blood flow measurements (0198T)*
*Single-episode tonometry (99201-99215, 92002-92004)*

0.97    2.26    **FUD** XXX    N  80

**AMA:** 2017,Jan,8; 2016,Jan,13; 2015,Jan,16; 2014,May,5; 2014,Jan,11; 2012,Oct,9-11; 2012,Aug,9; 2012,Jan,15-42

**92132**    **Scanning computerized ophthalmic diagnostic imaging, anterior segment, with interpretation and report, unilateral or bilateral**

EXCLUDES    *Imaging of anterior segment with specular microscopy and endothelial cell analysis (92286)*
*Scanning computerized ophthalmic diagnostic imaging of optic nerve and retina (92133-92134)*
*Tear film imaging (0330T)*

0.88    0.88    **FUD** XXX    01  80

**AMA:** 2017,Jan,8; 2016,Jan,13; 2015,Jan,16; 2014,May,5; 2014,Jan,11; 2013,Apr,7; 2013,Mar,6-7; 2012,Oct,9-11

**92133**    **Scanning computerized ophthalmic diagnostic imaging, posterior segment, with interpretation and report, unilateral or bilateral; optic nerve**

EXCLUDES    *Remote imaging for retinal disease (92227-92228)*
*Scanning computerized ophthalmic imaging of retina at same visit (92134)*

1.06    1.06    **FUD** XXX    01  80

**AMA:** 2017,Jan,8; 2016,Jan,13; 2015,Jan,16; 2014,Nov,10; 2014,Jan,11; 2012,Oct,9-11

**92134**    **retina**

EXCLUDES    *Remote imaging for retinal disease (92227-92228)*
*Scanning computerized ophthalmic imaging of optic nerve at same visit (92133)*

1.16    1.16    **FUD** XXX    01  80

**AMA:** 2017,Jan,8; 2016,Jan,13; 2015,Jan,16; 2014,Nov,10; 2014,Jan,11; 2012,Oct,9-11

● New Code    ▲ Revised Code    ○ Reinstated    ● New Web Release    ▲ Revised Web Release    Unlisted    Not Covered    # Resequenced
⊘ AMA Mod 51 Exempt    ⑨ Optum Mod 51 Exempt    ⑥⑨ Mod 63 Exempt    ✗ Non-FDA Drug    ★ Telemedicine    Ⓜ Maternity    Ⓐ Age Edit    ✛ Add-on    **AMA:** CPT Asst

92136 **Ophthalmic biometry by partial coherence interferometry with intraocular lens power calculation**

> *EXCLUDES* *Tear film imaging (0330T)*
> 2.54  2.54  **FUD** XXX  [01] [80] [□]
> **AMA:** 2017,Jan,8; 2016,Jan,13; 2015,Jan,16; 2014,May,5; 2014,Jan,11; 2012,Jan,15-42

92145 **Corneal hysteresis determination, by air impulse stimulation, unilateral or bilateral, with interpretation and report**

> 0.51  0.51  **FUD** XXX  [01] [80] [□]

## 92225-92287 Other Ophthalmology Services

> *EXCLUDES* *Prescription, fitting, and/or medical supervision of ocular prosthesis adaptation by physician (99201-99215, 99241-99245, 92002-92014)*

92225 **Ophthalmoscopy, extended, with retinal drawing (eg, for retinal detachment, melanoma), with interpretation and report; initial**

> *EXCLUDES* *Ophthalmoscopy under general anesthesia (92018)*
> 0.61  0.76  **FUD** XXX  [01] [80] [□]
> **AMA:** 2017,Jan,8; 2016,Jan,13; 2015,Jan,16; 2014,Jan,11; 2012,Oct,9-11; 2012,Jan,15-42

92226 **subsequent**

> 0.54  0.70  **FUD** XXX  [01] [80] [□]
> **AMA:** 2017,Jan,8; 2016,Jan,13; 2015,Jan,16; 2014,Jan,11

92227 **Remote imaging for detection of retinal disease (eg, retinopathy in a patient with diabetes) with analysis and report under physician supervision, unilateral or bilateral**

> *EXCLUDES* *When services provided with E&M services as part of a single organ system or (92002-92014, 92133-92134, 92228, 92250)*
> 0.41  0.41  **FUD** XXX  ★ [01] [80] [TC] [□]
> **AMA:** 2017,Jan,8; 2016,Jul,8; 2016,Jan,13; 2015,Jan,16; 2014,Jan,11; 2012,Oct,9-11; 2012,Jan,15-42

92228 **Remote imaging for monitoring and management of active retinal disease (eg, diabetic retinopathy) with physician review, interpretation and report, unilateral or bilateral**

> *EXCLUDES* *When services provided with E&M services as part of a single organ system or (92002-92014, 92133-92134, 92227, 92250)*
> 0.98  0.98  **FUD** XXX  ★ [01] [80] [□]
> **AMA:** 2017,Jan,8; 2016,Jan,13; 2015,Jan,16; 2014,Jan,11; 2012,Oct,9-11; 2012,Jan,15-42

92230 **Fluorescein angioscopy with interpretation and report**

> 0.93  1.63  **FUD** XXX  [01] [80] [□]
> **AMA:** 2017,Jan,8; 2016,Jan,13; 2015,Jan,16; 2014,Jan,11

92235 **Fluorescein angiography (includes multiframe imaging) with interpretation and report, unilateral or bilateral**

> *EXCLUDES* *Fluorescein and indocyanine-green angiography (92242)*
> 2.42  2.42  **FUD** XXX  [S] [80] [□]
> **AMA:** 2017,Jun,8; 2017,Jan,8; 2016,Jan,13; 2015,Jan,16; 2014,Jan,11

92240 **Indocyanine-green angiography (includes multiframe imaging) with interpretation and report, unilateral or bilateral**

> *EXCLUDES* *Fluorescein and indocyanine-green angiography (92242)*
> 5.87  5.87  **FUD** XXX  [S] [80] [□]
> **AMA:** 2017,Jun,8; 2017,Jan,8; 2016,Jan,13; 2015,Jan,16; 2014,Jan,11; 2012,Oct,9-11

92242 **Fluorescein angiography and indocyanine-green angiography (includes multiframe imaging) performed at the same patient encounter with interpretation and report, unilateral or bilateral**

> *EXCLUDES* *Fluorescein angiography only (92235)*
> *Indocyanine-green angiography only (92240)*
> 6.40  6.40  **FUD** XXX  [S] [80] [□]
> **AMA:** 2017,Jun,8

92250 **Fundus photography with interpretation and report**

> 1.86  1.86  **FUD** XXX  [01] [80] [CLIA]
> **AMA:** 2017,Jan,8; 2016,Jul,8; 2016,Jan,13; 2015,May,9; 2015,Jan,16; 2014,Dec,16; 2014,Dec,16; 2014,Nov,10; 2014,Jan,11; 2012,Oct,9-11

92260 **Ophthalmodynamometry**

> *EXCLUDES* *Ophthalmoscopy under general anesthesia (92018)*
> 0.31  0.52  **FUD** XXX  [01] [80] [□]
> **AMA:** 2017,Jan,8; 2016,Jan,13; 2015,Jan,16; 2014,Jan,11

92265 **Needle oculoelectromyography, 1 or more extraocular muscles, 1 or both eyes, with interpretation and report**

> 2.41  2.41  **FUD** XXX  [01] [80] [□]
> **AMA:** 2017,Jan,8; 2016,Jan,13; 2015,Jan,16; 2014,Jan,11; 2012,Oct,9-11

92270 **Electro-oculography with interpretation and report**

> *EXCLUDES* *Recording of saccadic eye movements (92700)*
> *Vestibular function testing (92537-92538, 92540-92542, 92544-92548)*
> 2.59  2.59  **FUD** XXX  [01] [80] [□]
> **AMA:** 2017,Jan,8; 2016,Jan,13; 2015,Sep,7; 2015,Jan,16; 2014,Jan,11; 2012,Oct,9-11; 2012,Jan,15-42

92275 **Electroretinography with interpretation and report**

> *EXCLUDES* *Vestibular function tests/electronystagmography (92541-92548)*
> (76511-76529)
> 4.20  4.20  **FUD** XXX  [S] [80] [□]
> **AMA:** 2017,Jan,8; 2016,Jan,13; 2015,Jan,16; 2014,Jan,11; 2012,Oct,9-11

92283 **Color vision examination, extended, eg, anomaloscope or equivalent**

> *EXCLUDES* *Color vision testing with pseudoisochromatic plates (e.g., HRR, Ishihara) (92002-92004, 92012-92014, 99172)*
> 1.58  1.58  **FUD** XXX  [01] [80] [□]
> **AMA:** 2017,Jan,8; 2016,Jan,13; 2015,Jan,16; 2014,Jan,11; 2012,Oct,9-11

92284 **Dark adaptation examination with interpretation and report**

> 1.77  1.77  **FUD** XXX  [01] [80] [□]
> **AMA:** 2017,Jan,8; 2016,Jan,13; 2015,Jan,16; 2014,Jan,11; 2012,Oct,9-11

92285 **External ocular photography with interpretation and report for documentation of medical progress (eg, close-up photography, slit lamp photography, goniophotography, stereo-photography)**

> *EXCLUDES* *Tear film imaging (0330T)*
> 0.59  0.59  **FUD** XXX  [01] [80] [□]
> **AMA:** 2017,Jan,8; 2016,Jan,13; 2015,Jan,16; 2014,May,5; 2014,Jan,11; 2012,Oct,9-11; 2012,Jan,15-42

92286 **Anterior segment imaging with interpretation and report; with specular microscopy and endothelial cell analysis**

> 1.09  1.09  **FUD** XXX  [01] [80] [□]
> **AMA:** 2017,Jan,8; 2016,Jan,13; 2015,Jan,16; 2014,Jan,11; 2013,Mar,6-7; 2012,Oct,9-11

92287 **with fluorescein angiography**

> 3.89  3.89  **FUD** XXX  [01] [80] [□]
> **AMA:** 2017,Jan,8; 2016,Jan,13; 2015,Jan,16; 2014,Jan,11; 2013,Mar,6-7

## 92310-92326 Services Related to Contact Lenses

**CMS:** 100-02,15,30.4 Optometrist's Services

INCLUDES Incidental revision of lens during training period
Patient training/instruction
Specification of optical/physical characteristics:
Curvature
Flexibility
Gas-permeability
Power
Size

EXCLUDES *Extended wear lenses follow up (92012-92014)*
*General ophthalmological services*
*Therapeutic/surgical use of contact lens (68340, 92071-92072)*

**92310** Prescription of optical and physical characteristics of and fitting of contact lens, with medical supervision of adaptation; corneal lens, both eyes, except for aphakia
Code also modifier 52 for one eye
🔲 1.69 ⚖ 2.71 **FUD** XXX 　 E 🖵

**AMA:** 2017,Jan,8; 2016,Jan,13; 2015,Jan,16; 2014,Jan,11; 2012,Oct,9-11

**92311** corneal lens for aphakia, 1 eye
🔲 1.58 ⚖ 2.85 **FUD** XXX 　 01 80 🖵

**AMA:** 2017,Jan,8; 2016,Jan,13; 2015,Jan,16; 2014,Jan,11; 2012,Oct,9-11

**92312** corneal lens for aphakia, both eyes
🔲 1.83 ⚖ 3.32 **FUD** XXX 　 01 80 🖵

**AMA:** 2017,Jan,8; 2016,Jan,13; 2015,Jan,16; 2014,Jan,11; 2012,Oct,9-11

**92313** corneoscleral lens
🔲 1.34 ⚖ 2.72 **FUD** XXX 　 01 80 🖵

**AMA:** 2017,Jan,8; 2016,Jan,13; 2015,Jan,16; 2014,Jan,11; 2012,Oct,9-11

**92314** Prescription of optical and physical characteristics of contact lens, with medical supervision of adaptation and direction of fitting by independent technician; corneal lens, both eyes except for aphakia
Code also modifier 52 for one eye
🔲 1.00 ⚖ 2.25 **FUD** XXX 　 E 🖵

**AMA:** 2017,Jan,8; 2016,Jan,13; 2015,Jan,16; 2014,Jan,11; 2012,Oct,9-11

**92315** corneal lens for aphakia, 1 eye
🔲 0.63 ⚖ 2.09 **FUD** XXX 　 01 80 🖵

**AMA:** 2017,Jan,8; 2016,Jan,13; 2015,Jan,16; 2014,Jan,11; 2012,Oct,9-11

**92316** corneal lens for aphakia, both eyes
🔲 0.94 ⚖ 2.62 **FUD** XXX 　 01 80 🖵

**AMA:** 2017,Jan,8; 2016,Jan,13; 2015,Jan,16; 2014,Jan,11; 2012,Oct,9-11

**92317** corneoscleral lens
🔲 0.65 ⚖ 2.14 **FUD** XXX 　 01 80 🖵

**AMA:** 2017,Jan,8; 2016,Jan,13; 2015,Jan,16; 2014,Jan,11

**92325** Modification of contact lens (separate procedure), with medical supervision of adaptation
🔲 1.19 ⚖ 1.19 **FUD** XXX 　 01 80 🖵

**AMA:** 2017,Jan,8; 2016,Jan,13; 2015,Jan,16; 2014,Jan,11; 2012,Oct,9-11

**92326** Replacement of contact lens
🔲 0.99 ⚖ 0.99 **FUD** XXX 　 01 80 🖵

**AMA:** 2017,Jan,8; 2016,Jan,13; 2015,Jan,16; 2014,Jan,11

## 92340-92499 Services Related to Eyeglasses

**CMS:** 100-02,15,30.4 Optometrist's Services

INCLUDES Anatomical facial characteristics measurement
Final adjustment of spectacles to visual axes/anatomical topography
Written laboratory specifications

EXCLUDES *Supply of materials*

**92340** Fitting of spectacles, except for aphakia; monofocal
🔲 0.53 ⚖ 1.00 **FUD** XXX 　 E 🖵

**AMA:** 2017,Jan,8; 2016,Jan,13; 2015,Jan,16; 2014,Jan,11; 2013,Mar,6-7

**92341** bifocal
🔲 0.68 ⚖ 1.14 **FUD** XXX 　 E 🖵

**AMA:** 2017,Jan,8; 2016,Jan,13; 2015,Jan,16; 2014,Jan,11; 2013,Mar,6-7

**92342** multifocal, other than bifocal
🔲 0.76 ⚖ 1.23 **FUD** XXX 　 E 🖵

**AMA:** 2017,Jan,8; 2016,Jan,13; 2015,Jan,16; 2014,Jan,11; 2013,Mar,6-7

**92352** Fitting of spectacle prosthesis for aphakia; monofocal
🔲 0.53 ⚖ 1.14 **FUD** XXX 　 01 🖵

**AMA:** 2017,Jan,8; 2016,Jan,13; 2015,Jan,16; 2014,Jan,11; 2013,Mar,6-7

**92353** multifocal
🔲 0.72 ⚖ 1.33 **FUD** XXX 　 01 🖵

**AMA:** 2017,Jan,8; 2016,Jan,13; 2015,Jan,16; 2014,Jan,11; 2013,Mar,6-7

**92354** Fitting of spectacle mounted low vision aid; single element system
🔲 0.38 ⚖ 0.38 **FUD** XXX 　 01 🖵

**AMA:** 2017,Jan,8; 2016,Jan,13; 2015,Jan,16; 2014,Jan,11; 2013,Mar,6-7

**92355** telescopic or other compound lens system
🔲 0.59 ⚖ 0.59 **FUD** XXX 　 01 🖵

**AMA:** 2017,Jan,8; 2016,Jan,13; 2015,Jan,16; 2014,Jan,11; 2013,Mar,6-7

**92358** Prosthesis service for aphakia, temporary (disposable or loan, including materials)
🔲 0.32 ⚖ 0.32 **FUD** XXX 　 01 🖵

**AMA:** 2017,Jan,8; 2016,Jan,13; 2015,Jan,16; 2014,Jan,11; 2013,Mar,6-7

**92370** Repair and refitting spectacles; except for aphakia
🔲 0.46 ⚖ 0.87 **FUD** XXX 　 E 🖵

**AMA:** 2017,Jan,8; 2016,Jan,13; 2015,Jan,16; 2014,Jan,11; 2013,Mar,6-7

**92371** spectacle prosthesis for aphakia
🔲 0.33 ⚖ 0.33 **FUD** XXX 　 01 🖵

**AMA:** 2017,Jan,8; 2016,Jan,13; 2015,Jan,16; 2014,Jan,11; 2013,Mar,6-7

**92499** Unlisted ophthalmological service or procedure
🔲 0.00 ⚖ 0.00 **FUD** XXX 　 01 80

**AMA:** 2017,Jan,8; 2016,Jan,13; 2015,Jan,16; 2014,Jan,11

## 92502-92526 Special Procedures of the Ears/Nose/Throat

INCLUDES Anterior rhinoscopy, tuning fork testing, otoscopy, or removal non-impacted cerumen
Diagnostic/treatment services not generally included in an E&M service

EXCLUDES *Laryngoscopy with stroboscopy (31579)*

**92502** Otolaryngologic examination under general anesthesia
🔲 2.74 ⚖ 2.74 **FUD** 000 　 T 80 🖵

**AMA:** 2017,Jan,8; 2016,Sep,6

**92504** Binocular microscopy (separate diagnostic procedure)
🔲 0.27 ⚖ 0.84 **FUD** XXX 　 N 80 🖵

**AMA:** 2017,Jan,8; 2016,Sep,6; 2016,Jan,13; 2015,Jan,16; 2014,Jan,11; 2013,Oct,14; 2012,Jan,15-42

**92507** Treatment of speech, language, voice, communication, and/or auditory processing disorder; individual

EXCLUDES *Adaptive behavior treatment (0364T-0365T, 0368T-0369T)*
*Auditory rehabilitation:*
*Postlingual hearing loss (92633)*
*Prelingual hearing loss (92630)*
*Programming of cochlear implant (92601-92604)*
🔲 2.23 ⚖ 2.23 **FUD** XXX 　 A 80 🖵

**AMA:** 2017,Jan,8; 2016,Sep,6; 2016,Jan,13; 2015,Jan,16; 2014,Jan,11; 2013,Oct,7

● New Code 　▲ Revised Code 　○ Reinstated 　● New Web Release 　▲ Revised Web Release 　Unlisted 　Not Covered 　# Resequenced
⊘ AMA Mod 51 Exempt 　⑨ Optum Mod 51 Exempt 　⑥³ Mod 63 Exempt 　✗ Non-FDA Drug 　★ Telemedicine 　Ⓜ Maternity 　Ⓐ Age Edit 　+ Add-on 　**AMA:** CPT Asst
© 2017 Optum360, LLC 　　CPT © 2017 American Medical Association. All Rights Reserved. 　　**439**

**Medicine** (sidebar)

**92508 — 92542** (sidebar)

**92508**  group, 2 or more individuals
EXCLUDES  *Adaptive behavior treatment (0366T-0367T, 0372T)*
*Auditory rehabilitation:*
*Postlingual hearing loss (92633)*
*Prelingual hearing loss (92630)*
*Programming of cochlear implant (92601-92604)*
0.65   0.65   **FUD** XXX        A 80
**AMA:** 2017,Jan,8; 2016,Sep,6; 2016,Jan,13; 2015,Jan,16; 2014,Jun,3; 2014,Jan,11; 2013,Oct,7

**92511**  Nasopharyngoscopy with endoscope (separate procedure)
EXCLUDES  *Diagnostic flexible laryngoscopy (31575)*
*Transnasal esophagoscopy (43197-43198)*
1.08   3.12   **FUD** 000        T 80
**AMA:** 2017,Jul,7; 2017,Jan,8; 2016,Dec,13; 2016,Sep,6

**92512**  Nasal function studies (eg, rhinomanometry)
0.81   1.71   **FUD** XXX        S 80
**AMA:** 2017,Jan,8; 2016,Sep,6

**92516**  Facial nerve function studies (eg, electroneuronography)
0.65   1.97   **FUD** XXX        S 80
**AMA:** 2017,Jan,8; 2016,Sep,6

**92520**  Laryngeal function studies (ie, aerodynamic testing and acoustic testing)
EXCLUDES  *Other laryngeal function testing (92700)*
*Swallowing/laryngeal sensory testing with flexible fiberoptic endoscope (92611-92617)*
Code also modifier 52 for single test
1.17   2.15   **FUD** XXX        Q1 80
**AMA:** 2017,Jan,8; 2016,Sep,6; 2016,Jan,13; 2015,Jan,16; 2014,Jan,11

**92521**  Evaluation of speech fluency (eg, stuttering, cluttering)
INCLUDES  Ability to execute motor movements needed for speech
Comprehension of written and verbal expression
Determination of patient's ability to create and communicate expressive thought
Evaluation of the ability to produce speech sound
3.14   3.14   **FUD** XXX        A 80
**AMA:** 2017,Jan,8; 2016,Sep,6; 2016,Jan,13; 2015,Jan,16; 2014,Jun,3

**92522**  Evaluation of speech sound production (eg, articulation, phonological process, apraxia, dysarthria);
INCLUDES  Ability to execute motor movements needed for speech
Comprehension of written and verbal expression
Determination of patient's ability to create and communicate expressive thought
Evaluation of the ability to produce speech sound
2.60   2.60   **FUD** XXX        A 80
**AMA:** 2017,Jan,8; 2016,Sep,6; 2016,Jan,13; 2015,Jan,16; 2014,Jun,3

**92523**  with evaluation of language comprehension and expression (eg, receptive and expressive language)
INCLUDES  Ability to execute motor movements needed for speech
Comprehension of written and verbal expression
Determination of patient's ability to create and communicate expressive thought
Evaluation of the ability to produce speech sound
5.55   5.55   **FUD** XXX        A 80
**AMA:** 2017,Jan,8; 2016,Sep,6; 2016,Jan,13; 2015,Jan,16; 2014,Jun,3

**92524**  Behavioral and qualitative analysis of voice and resonance
INCLUDES  Ability to execute motor movements needed for speech
Comprehension of written and verbal expression
Determination of patient's ability to create and communicate expressive thought
Evaluation of the ability to produce speech sound
2.51   2.51   **FUD** XXX        A 80
**AMA:** 2017,Jan,8; 2016,Sep,6; 2016,Jan,13; 2015,Jan,16; 2014,Jun,3

**92526**  Treatment of swallowing dysfunction and/or oral function for feeding
2.43   2.43   **FUD** XXX        A 80
**AMA:** 2017,Jan,8; 2016,Sep,6

## 92531-92548 Vestibular Function Tests

**92531**  Spontaneous nystagmus, including gaze
EXCLUDES  *When performed with E&M services (99201-99215, 99218-99223 [99224, 99225, 99226], 99231-99236, 99241-99245, 99304-99318, 99324-99337)*
0.00   0.00   **FUD** XXX        N
**AMA:** 1997,Nov,1

**92532**  Positional nystagmus test
EXCLUDES  *When performed with E&M services (99201-99215, 99218-99223 [99224, 99225, 99226], 99231-99236, 99241-99245, 99304-99318, 99324-99337)*
0.00   0.00   **FUD** XXX        N
**AMA:** 2002,May,7; 1997,Nov,1

**92533**  Caloric vestibular test, each irrigation (binaural, bithermal stimulation constitutes 4 tests)
INCLUDES  Barany caloric test
0.00   0.00   **FUD** XXX        N
**AMA:** 2017,Jan,8; 2016,Jan,13; 2015,Jan,16; 2014,Jan,11

**92534**  Optokinetic nystagmus test
0.00   0.00   **FUD** XXX        N
**AMA:** 2002,May,7; 1997,Nov,1

**92537**  Caloric vestibular test with recording, bilateral; bithermal (ie, one warm and one cool irrigation in each ear for a total of four irrigations)
EXCLUDES  *Electro-oculography (92270)*
*Monothermal caloric vestibular test (92538)*
Code also modifier 52 when only three irrigations are performed
1.14   1.14   **FUD** XXX        S 80
**AMA:** 2015,Sep,7

**92538**  monothermal (ie, one irrigation in each ear for a total of two irrigations)
EXCLUDES  *Electro-oculography (92270)*
*Monothermal caloric vestibular test (92538)*
Code also modifier 52 if only one irrigation is performed
0.58   0.58   **FUD** XXX        S 80
**AMA:** 2015,Sep,7

**92540**  Basic vestibular evaluation, includes spontaneous nystagmus test with eccentric gaze fixation nystagmus, with recording, positional nystagmus test, minimum of 4 positions, with recording, optokinetic nystagmus test, bidirectional foveal and peripheral stimulation, with recording, and oscillating tracking test, with recording
EXCLUDES  *Vestibular function tests (92270, 92541-92542, 92544-92545)*
2.89   2.89   **FUD** XXX        S 80
**AMA:** 2017,Jan,8; 2016,Jan,13; 2015,Sep,7

**92541**  Spontaneous nystagmus test, including gaze and fixation nystagmus, with recording
EXCLUDES  *Vestibular function tests (92270, 92540, 92542, 92544-92545)*
0.70   0.70   **FUD** XXX        Q1 80
**AMA:** 2017,Jan,8; 2016,Jan,13; 2015,Sep,7; 2015,Jan,16; 2014,Jan,11; 2012,Jan,15-42

**92542**  Positional nystagmus test, minimum of 4 positions, with recording
EXCLUDES  *Vestibular function tests (92270, 92540-92541, 92544-92545)*
0.79   0.79   **FUD** XXX        Q1 80
**AMA:** 2017,Jan,8; 2016,Jan,13; 2015,Sep,7; 2015,Jan,16; 2014,Jan,11; 2012,Jan,15-42

**92544** Optokinetic nystagmus test, bidirectional, foveal or peripheral stimulation, with recording

*EXCLUDES* *Vestibular function tests (92270, 92540-92542, 92545)*
0.48    0.48    **FUD** XXX    S 80 ▢

**AMA:** 2017,Jan,8; 2016,Jan,13; 2015,Sep,7; 2015,Jan,16; 2014,Jan,11

**92545** Oscillating tracking test, with recording

*EXCLUDES* *Vestibular function tests (92270, 92540-92542, 92544)*
0.43    0.43    **FUD** XXX    S 80 ▢

**AMA:** 2017,Jan,8; 2016,Jan,13; 2015,Sep,7; 2015,Jan,16; 2014,Jan,11; 2012,Jan,15-42

**92546** Sinusoidal vertical axis rotational testing

*EXCLUDES* *Electro-oculography (92270)*
2.90    2.90    **FUD** XXX    S 80 ▢

**AMA:** 2017,Jan,8; 2016,Jan,13; 2015,Sep,7; 2015,Jan,16; 2014,Jan,11; 2013,Jun,13; 2012,Jan,15-42

+ **92547** Use of vertical electrodes (List separately in addition to code for primary procedure)

*EXCLUDES* *Electro-oculography (92700)*
Code first (92540-92546)
0.17    0.17    **FUD** ZZZ    N 80 TC ▢

**AMA:** 2017,Jan,8; 2016,Jan,13; 2015,Sep,7; 2015,Jan,16; 2014,Jan,11; 2012,Jan,15-42

**92548** Computerized dynamic posturography

*EXCLUDES* *Electro-oculography (92270)*
2.81    2.81    **FUD** XXX    Q1 80 ▢

**AMA:** 2017,Jan,8; 2016,Jan,13; 2015,Sep,7; 2015,Jan,16; 2014,Jan,11; 2012,Jan,15-42

## 92550-92597 [92558] Hearing and Speech Tests

*INCLUDES* Diagnostic/treatment services not generally included in a comprehensive otorhinolaryngologic evaluation or office visit
Testing of both ears
Tuning fork and whisper tests
Use of calibrated electronic equipment, recording of results, and a report with interpretation
*EXCLUDES* *Evaluation of speech/language/hearing problems using observation/assessment of performance (92521-92524)*
Code also modifier 52 for unilateral testing

**92550** Tympanometry and reflex threshold measurements

*INCLUDES* Tympanometry, acoustic reflex testing individual codes (92567-92568)
0.60    0.60    **FUD** XXX    Q1 80 ▢

**AMA:** 2017,Jan,8; 2016,Jan,13; 2015,Jan,16; 2014,Aug,3

**92551** Screening test, pure tone, air only
0.34    0.34    **FUD** XXX    E ▢

**AMA:** 2017,Jan,8; 2016,Jan,13; 2015,Jan,16; 2014,Aug,3

**92552** Pure tone audiometry (threshold); air only

*EXCLUDES* *Automated test (0208T)*
0.89    0.89    **FUD** XXX    Q1 80 TC ▢

**AMA:** 2017,Jan,8; 2016,Jan,13; 2015,Jan,16; 2014,Aug,3

**92553** air and bone

*EXCLUDES* *Automated test (0209T)*
1.06    1.06    **FUD** XXX    Q1 80 TC ▢

**AMA:** 2017,Jan,8; 2016,Jan,13; 2015,Jan,16; 2014,Aug,3; 2014,Jan,11

**92555** Speech audiometry threshold;

*EXCLUDES* *Automated test (0210T)*
0.66    0.66    **FUD** XXX    Q1 80 TC ▢

**AMA:** 2017,Jan,8; 2016,Jan,13; 2015,Jan,16; 2014,Aug,3

**92556** with speech recognition

*EXCLUDES* *Automated test (0211T)*
1.07    1.07    **FUD** XXX    Q1 80 TC ▢

**AMA:** 2017,Jan,8; 2016,Jan,13; 2015,Jan,16; 2014,Aug,3; 2014,Jan,11

**92557** Comprehensive audiometry threshold evaluation and speech recognition (92553 and 92556 combined)

*EXCLUDES* *Automated test (0208T-0212T)*
*Evaluation/selection of hearing aid (92590-92595)*
0.93    1.07    **FUD** XXX    Q1 80 ▢

**AMA:** 2017,Jan,8; 2016,Jan,13; 2015,Jan,16; 2014,Aug,3; 2014,Jan,11

*92558* **Resequenced code. See code following 92586.**

**92559** Audiometric testing of groups

*INCLUDES* For group testing, indicate tests performed
0.00    0.00    **FUD** XXX    E ▢

**AMA:** 2017,Jan,8; 2016,Jan,13; 2015,Jan,16; 2014,Aug,3

**92560** Bekesy audiometry; screening
0.00    0.00    **FUD** XXX    E ▢

**AMA:** 2017,Jan,8; 2016,Jan,13; 2015,Jan,16; 2014,Aug,3

**92561** diagnostic
1.09    1.09    **FUD** XXX    Q1 80 TC ▢

**AMA:** 2017,Jan,8; 2016,Jan,13; 2015,Jan,16; 2014,Aug,3

**92562** Loudness balance test, alternate binaural or monaural

*INCLUDES* ABLB test
1.31    1.31    **FUD** XXX    Q1 80 TC ▢

**AMA:** 2017,Jan,8; 2016,Jan,13; 2015,Jan,16; 2014,Aug,3

**92563** Tone decay test
0.87    0.87    **FUD** XXX    Q1 80 TC ▢

**AMA:** 2017,Jan,8; 2016,Jan,13; 2015,Jan,16; 2014,Aug,3

**92564** Short increment sensitivity index (SISI)
0.77    0.77    **FUD** XXX    Q1 80 TC ▢

**AMA:** 2017,Jan,8; 2016,Jan,13; 2015,Jan,16; 2014,Aug,3; 2014,Jan,11

**92565** Stenger test, pure tone
0.44    0.44    **FUD** XXX    Q1 80 TC ▢

**AMA:** 2017,Jan,8; 2016,Jan,13; 2015,Jan,16; 2014,Aug,3

**92567** Tympanometry (impedance testing)
0.31    0.41    **FUD** XXX    Q1 80 ▢

**AMA:** 2017,Jan,8; 2016,Jan,13; 2015,Jan,16; 2014,Aug,3; 2014,Jan,11

**92568** Acoustic reflex testing, threshold
0.44    0.45    **FUD** XXX    Q1 80 ▢

**AMA:** 2017,Jan,8; 2016,Jan,13; 2015,Jan,16; 2014,Aug,3; 2014,Jan,11; 2012,Jan,15-42

**92570** Acoustic immittance testing, includes tympanometry (impedance testing), acoustic reflex threshold testing, and acoustic reflex decay testing

*INCLUDES* Tympanometry, acoustic reflex testing individual codes (92567-92568)
0.85    0.91    **FUD** XXX    Q1 80 ▢

**AMA:** 2017,Jan,8; 2016,Jan,13; 2015,Jan,16; 2014,Aug,3

**92571** Filtered speech test
0.77    0.77    **FUD** XXX    Q1 80 TC ▢

**AMA:** 2017,Jan,8; 2016,Jan,13; 2015,Jan,16; 2014,Aug,3; 2014,Jan,11

**92572** Staggered spondaic word test
0.89    0.89    **FUD** XXX    Q1 80 TC ▢

**AMA:** 2017,Jan,8; 2016,Jan,13; 2015,Jan,16; 2014,Aug,3; 2014,Jan,11

**92575** Sensorineural acuity level test
1.65    1.65    **FUD** XXX    Q1 80 TC ▢

**AMA:** 2017,Jan,8; 2016,Jan,13; 2015,Jan,16; 2014,Aug,3

**92576** Synthetic sentence identification test
1.03    1.03    **FUD** XXX    Q1 80 TC ▢

**AMA:** 2017,Jan,8; 2016,Jan,13; 2015,Jan,16; 2014,Aug,3; 2014,Jan,11

**92577** Stenger test, speech
0.43    0.43    **FUD** XXX    Q1 80 TC ▢

**AMA:** 2017,Jan,8; 2016,Jan,13; 2015,Jan,16; 2014,Aug,3

**Medicine**

**92579 — 92606**

92579    **Visual reinforcement audiometry (VRA)**
  1.09   1.29   **FUD** XXX    01 80
  **AMA:** 2017,Jan,8; 2016,Jan,13; 2015,Jan,16; 2014,Aug,3

92582    **Conditioning play audiometry**
  1.89   1.89   **FUD** XXX    01 80 TC
  **AMA:** 2017,Jan,8; 2016,Jan,13; 2015,Jan,16; 2014,Aug,3

92583    **Select picture audiometry**
  1.42   1.42   **FUD** XXX    01 80 TC
  **AMA:** 2017,Jan,8; 2016,Jan,13; 2015,Jan,16; 2014,Aug,3

92584    **Electrocochleography**
  2.08   2.08   **FUD** XXX    S 80 TC
  **AMA:** 2017,Jan,8; 2016,Jan,13; 2015,Jan,16; 2014,Aug,3;
  2014,Jan,11; 2012,Jan,15-42

92585    **Auditory evoked potentials for evoked response audiometry and/or testing of the central nervous system; comprehensive**
  3.83   3.83   **FUD** XXX    S 80
  **AMA:** 2017,Jan,8; 2016,Jan,13; 2015,Jan,16; 2014,Aug,3;
  2013,May,8-10

92586    **limited**
  2.44   2.44   **FUD** XXX    S 80 TC
  **AMA:** 2017,Jan,8; 2016,Jan,13; 2015,Jan,16; 2014,Aug,3

\#  92558    **Evoked otoacoustic emissions, screening (qualitative measurement of distortion product or transient evoked otoacoustic emissions), automated analysis**
  0.00   0.00   **FUD** XXX    E
  **AMA:** 2017,Jan,8; 2016,Jan,13; 2015,Jan,16; 2014,Aug,3

92587    **Distortion product evoked otoacoustic emissions; limited evaluation (to confirm the presence or absence of hearing disorder, 3-6 frequencies) or transient evoked otoacoustic emissions, with interpretation and report**
  0.61   0.61   **FUD** XXX    S 80
  **AMA:** 2017,Jan,8; 2016,Jan,13; 2015,Jan,16; 2014,Aug,3;
  2014,Jan,11

92588    **comprehensive diagnostic evaluation (quantitative analysis of outer hair cell function by cochlear mapping, minimum of 12 frequencies), with interpretation and report**
  EXCLUDES *Evaluation of central auditory function (92620-92621)*
  0.94   0.94   **FUD** XXX    S 80
  **AMA:** 2017,Jan,8; 2016,Jan,13; 2015,Jan,16; 2014,Aug,3

92590    **Hearing aid examination and selection; monaural**
  0.00   0.00   **FUD** XXX    E
  **AMA:** 2017,Jan,8; 2016,Jan,13; 2015,Jan,16; 2014,Aug,3;
  2014,Jul,4

92591    **binaural**
  0.00   0.00   **FUD** XXX    E
  **AMA:** 2017,Jan,8; 2016,Jan,13; 2015,Jan,16; 2014,Aug,3

92592    **Hearing aid check; monaural**
  0.00   0.00   **FUD** XXX    E
  **AMA:** 2017,Jan,8; 2016,Jan,13; 2015,Jan,16; 2014,Aug,3

92593    **binaural**
  0.00   0.00   **FUD** XXX    E
  **AMA:** 2017,Jan,8; 2016,Jan,13; 2015,Jan,16; 2014,Aug,3

92594    **Electroacoustic evaluation for hearing aid; monaural**
  0.00   0.00   **FUD** XXX    E
  **AMA:** 2017,Jan,8; 2016,Jan,13; 2015,Jan,16; 2014,Aug,3

92595    **binaural**
  0.00   0.00   **FUD** XXX    E
  **AMA:** 2017,Jan,8; 2016,Jan,13; 2015,Jan,16; 2014,Aug,3

92596    **Ear protector attenuation measurements**
  1.17   1.17   **FUD** XXX    01 80 TC
  **AMA:** 2017,Jan,8; 2016,Jan,13; 2015,Jan,16; 2014,Aug,3

92597    *Resequenced code. See code following 92604.*

## 92601-92609 [92597, 92618] Services Related to Hearing and Speech Devices

INCLUDES   Diagnostic/treatment services not generally included in a comprehensive otorhinolaryngologic evaluation or office visit

92601    **Diagnostic analysis of cochlear implant, patient younger than 7 years of age; with programming**   A
  INCLUDES   Connection to cochlear implant
   Postoperative analysis/fitting of previously placed external devices
   Stimulator programming
  EXCLUDES   *Cochlear implant placement (69930)*
  3.45   4.19   **FUD** XXX    S 80
  **AMA:** 2017,Jan,8; 2016,Sep,6; 2016,Jan,13; 2015,Jan,16;
  2014,Jul,4; 2014,Jan,11; 2013,Oct,7; 2012,Jan,15-42

92602    **subsequent reprogramming**   A
  INCLUDES   Internal stimulator re-programming
   Subsequent sessions for external transmitter measurements/adjustment
  EXCLUDES   *Analysis with programming (92601)*
   *Aural rehabilitation services after a cochlear implant (92626-92627, 92630-92633)*
   *Cochlear implant placement (69930)*
  1.88   2.34   **FUD** XXX    S 80
  **AMA:** 2017,Jan,8; 2016,Sep,6; 2016,Jan,13; 2015,Jan,16;
  2014,Jul,4; 2014,Jan,11; 2013,Oct,7; 2012,Jan,15-42

92603    **Diagnostic analysis of cochlear implant, age 7 years or older; with programming**   A
  INCLUDES   Connection to cochlear implant
   Post-operative analysis/fitting of previously placed external devices
   Stimulator programming
  EXCLUDES   *Cochlear implant placement (69930)*
  3.47   4.30   **FUD** XXX    S 80
  **AMA:** 2017,Jan,8; 2016,Sep,6; 2016,Jan,13; 2015,Jan,16;
  2014,Jul,4; 2014,Jan,11; 2013,Oct,7; 2012,Jan,15-42

92604    **subsequent reprogramming**   A
  INCLUDES   Internal stimulator re-programming
   Subsequent sessions for external transmitter measurements/adjustment
  EXCLUDES   *Analysis with programming (92603)*
   *Cochlear implant placement (69930)*
  1.93   2.55   **FUD** XXX    S 80
  **AMA:** 2017,Jan,8; 2016,Sep,6; 2016,Jan,13; 2015,Jan,16;
  2014,Jul,4; 2014,Jan,11; 2013,Oct,7; 2012,Jan,15-42

\#  92597    **Evaluation for use and/or fitting of voice prosthetic device to supplement oral speech**
  EXCLUDES   *Augmentative or alternative communication device services (92605, [92618], 92607-92608)*
  2.05   2.05   **FUD** XXX    A 80
  **AMA:** 2017,Jan,8; 2016,Jan,13; 2015,Jan,16; 2014,Jan,11

92605    **Evaluation for prescription of non-speech-generating augmentative and alternative communication device, face-to-face with the patient; first hour**
  EXCLUDES   *Prosthetic voice device fitting or use evaluation (92597)*
  2.52   2.64   **FUD** XXX    A
  **AMA:** 2017,Jan,8; 2016,Jan,13; 2015,Jan,16; 2014,Jan,11;
  2013,Oct,7

+ \#  92618    **each additional 30 minutes (List separately in addition to code for primary procedure)**
  0.94   0.96   **FUD** ZZZ    A
  Code first (92605)

92606    **Therapeutic service(s) for the use of non-speech-generating device, including programming and modification**
  2.02   2.35   **FUD** XXX    A
  **AMA:** 2017,Jan,8; 2016,Jan,13; 2015,Jan,16; 2014,Jan,11

**92607** Evaluation for prescription for speech-generating augmentative and alternative communication device, face-to-face with the patient; first hour

*EXCLUDES* *Evaluation for prescription of non-speech generating device (92605)*

*Evaluation for use/fitting of voice prosthetic (92597)*

🔧 3.61   ⚕ 3.61   **FUD** XXX                    Ⓐ 80 🖥

**AMA:** 2017,Jan,8; 2016,Jan,13; 2015,Jan,16; 2014,Jan,11; 2013,Oct,7

**+  92608** each additional 30 minutes (List separately in addition to code for primary procedure)

Code first initial hour (92607)

🔧 1.50   ⚕ 1.50   **FUD** ZZZ                    Ⓐ 80 🖥

**AMA:** 2017,Jan,8; 2016,Jan,13; 2015,Jan,16; 2014,Jan,11; 2013,Oct,7

**92609** Therapeutic services for the use of speech-generating device, including programming and modification

*EXCLUDES* *Therapeutic services for use of non-speech generating device (92606)*

🔧 3.12   ⚕ 3.12   **FUD** XXX                    Ⓐ 80 🖥

**AMA:** 2017,Jan,8; 2016,Jan,13; 2015,Jan,16; 2014,Jan,11

## 92610-92618 Swallowing Evaluations

**92610** Evaluation of oral and pharyngeal swallowing function

*EXCLUDES* *Evaluation with flexible endoscope (92612-92617)*

*Motion fluoroscopic evaluation of swallowing function (92611)*

🔧 2.07   ⚕ 2.43   **FUD** XXX                    Ⓐ 80 🖥

**AMA:** 2017,Apr,8; 2017,Jan,8; 2016,Jan,13; 2015,Jan,16; 2014,Jan,11

**92611** Motion fluoroscopic evaluation of swallowing function by cine or video recording

*EXCLUDES* *Diagnostic flexible laryngoscopy (31575)*

*Evaluation of oral/pharyngeal swallowing function (92610)*

📷 (74230)

🔧 2.46   ⚕ 2.46   **FUD** XXX                    Ⓐ 80 🖥

**AMA:** 2017,Apr,8; 2017,Jan,8; 2016,Sep,6; 2016,Jan,13; 2015,Jan,16; 2014,Jul,5; 2014,Jan,11

**92612** Flexible endoscopic evaluation of swallowing by cine or video recording;

*EXCLUDES* *Diagnostic flexible fiberoptic laryngoscopy (31575)*

*Flexible endoscopic examination/testing without cine or video recording (92700)*

🔧 1.95   ⚕ 5.31   **FUD** XXX                    Ⓐ 80 🖥

**AMA:** 2017,Jul,7; 2017,Apr,8; 2017,Jan,8; 2016,Dec,13; 2016,Sep,6; 2016,Jan,13; 2015,Jan,16; 2014,Jan,11; 2012,Jan,15-42

**92613** interpretation and report only

*EXCLUDES* *Diagnostic flexible laryngoscopy (31575)*

*Oral/pharyngeal swallowing function examination (92610)*

*Swallowing function motion fluoroscopic examination (92611)*

🔧 1.09   ⚕ 1.09   **FUD** XXX                    Ⓑ 80 🖥

**AMA:** 2017,Jul,7; 2017,Apr,8; 2017,Jan,8; 2016,Dec,13; 2016,Sep,6; 2016,Jan,13; 2015,Jan,16; 2014,Jan,11

**92614** Flexible endoscopic evaluation, laryngeal sensory testing by cine or video recording;

*EXCLUDES* *Diagnostic flexible laryngoscopy (31575)*

*Flexible endoscopic examination/testing without cine or video recording (92700)*

🔧 1.91   ⚕ 4.09   **FUD** XXX                    Ⓐ 80 🖥

**AMA:** 2017,Jul,7; 2017,Apr,8; 2017,Jan,8; 2016,Dec,13; 2016,Sep,6; 2016,Jan,13; 2015,Jan,16; 2014,Jan,11

**92615** interpretation and report only

*EXCLUDES* *Diagnostic flexible laryngoscopy (31575)*

🔧 0.95   ⚕ 0.95   **FUD** XXX                    Ⓔ 80 🖥

**AMA:** 2017,Jul,7; 2017,Apr,8; 2017,Jan,8; 2016,Dec,13; 2016,Sep,6; 2016,Jan,13; 2015,Jan,16; 2014,Jan,11

**92616** Flexible endoscopic evaluation of swallowing and laryngeal sensory testing by cine or video recording;

*EXCLUDES* *Diagnostic flexible fiberoptic laryngoscopy (31575)*

*Flexible endoscopic examination/testing without cine or video recording (92700)*

🔧 2.87   ⚕ 5.86   **FUD** XXX                    Ⓐ 80 🖥

**AMA:** 2017,Jul,7; 2017,Apr,8; 2017,Jan,8; 2016,Dec,13; 2016,Sep,6; 2016,Jan,13; 2015,Jan,16; 2014,Jan,11

**92617** interpretation and report only

*EXCLUDES* *Diagnostic flexible laryngoscopy (31575)*

🔧 1.19   ⚕ 1.19   **FUD** XXX                    Ⓔ 80 🖥

**AMA:** 2017,Jul,7; 2017,Apr,8; 2017,Jan,8; 2016,Dec,13; 2016,Sep,6; 2016,Jan,13; 2015,Jan,16; 2014,Jan,11

*92618* Resequenced code. See code following 92605.

## 92620-92700 Diagnostic Hearing Evaluations and Rehabilitation

*INCLUDES* Diagnostic/treatment services not generally included in a comprehensive otorhinolaryngologic evaluation or office visit

**92620** Evaluation of central auditory function, with report; initial 60 minutes

*EXCLUDES* *Voice analysis (92521-92524)*

🔧 2.35   ⚕ 2.68   **FUD** XXX                    ⑨1 80 🖥

**AMA:** 2017,Jan,8; 2016,Jan,13; 2015,Jan,16; 2014,Aug,3

**+  92621** each additional 15 minutes (List separately in addition to code for primary procedure)

*EXCLUDES* *Voice analysis (92521-92524)*

Code first (92620)

🔧 0.54   ⚕ 0.63   **FUD** ZZZ                    Ⓝ 80 🖥

**AMA:** 2017,Jan,8; 2016,Jan,13; 2015,Jan,16; 2014,Aug,3

**92625** Assessment of tinnitus (includes pitch, loudness matching, and masking)

*EXCLUDES* *Loudness test (92562)*

Code also modifier 52 for unilateral procedure

🔧 1.78   ⚕ 2.00   **FUD** XXX                    ⑨1 80 🖥

**AMA:** 2017,Jan,8; 2016,Jan,13; 2015,Jan,16; 2014,Aug,3

**92626** Evaluation of auditory rehabilitation status; first hour

*INCLUDES* Assessment to determine patient's proficiency in the use of remaining hearing to identify speech

Face-to-face time spent with the patient or family

🔧 2.17   ⚕ 2.55   **FUD** XXX                    ⑨1 80 🖥

**AMA:** 2017,Jan,8; 2016,Sep,6; 2016,Jan,13; 2015,Jan,16; 2014,Jul,4; 2014,May,10; 2014,Jan,11

**+  92627** each additional 15 minutes (List separately in addition to code for primary procedure)

*INCLUDES* Assessment to determine patient's proficiency in the use of remaining hearing to identify speech

Face-to-face time spent with the patient or family

Code first initial hour (92626)

🔧 0.51   ⚕ 0.63   **FUD** ZZZ                    Ⓝ 80 🖥

**AMA:** 2017,Jan,8; 2016,Sep,6; 2016,Jan,13; 2015,Jan,16; 2014,Jul,4; 2014,Jan,11

**92630** Auditory rehabilitation; prelingual hearing loss

🔧 0.00   ⚕ 0.00   **FUD** XXX                    Ⓔ 🖥

**AMA:** 2017,Jan,8; 2016,Sep,6; 2016,Jan,13; 2015,Jan,16; 2014,Jan,11; 2013,Oct,7

**92633** postlingual hearing loss

🔧 0.00   ⚕ 0.00   **FUD** XXX                    Ⓔ 🖥

**AMA:** 2017,Jan,8; 2016,Sep,6; 2016,Jan,13; 2015,Jan,16; 2014,Jan,11; 2013,Oct,7

**92640** Diagnostic analysis with programming of auditory brainstem implant, per hour

🔧 2.72   ⚕ 3.16   **FUD** XXX                    Ⓢ 80 🖥

*EXCLUDES* *Nonprogramming services (cardiac monitoring)*

---

● New Code   ▲ Revised Code   ○ Reinstated   ● New Web Release   ▲ Revised Web Release   Unlisted   Not Covered   # Resequenced
⊘ AMA Mod 51 Exempt   ⑨ Optum Mod 51 Exempt   ⊛ Mod 63 Exempt   ✗ Non-FDA Drug   ★ Telemedicine   Ⓜ Maternity   Ⓐ Age Edit   + Add-on   **AMA:** CPT Asst

© 2017 Optum360, LLC                    CPT © 2017 American Medical Association. All Rights Reserved.

**92700**    Unlisted otorhinolaryngological service or procedure

     INCLUDES    Lombard test

     0.00    0.00    **FUD** XXX      01 80

     **AMA:** 2017,Apr,8; 2017,Jan,8; 2016,Sep,6; 2016,Jan,13; 2015,Sep,7; 2015,Sep,12; 2015,Jan,16; 2014,May,10; 2014,Jan,11; 2012,Jan,15-42

## 92920-92953 Emergency Cardiac Procedures

**92920**    Resequenced code. See code following 92998.

**92921**    Resequenced code. See code following 92998.

**92924**    Resequenced code. See code following 92998.

**92925**    Resequenced code. See code following 92998.

**92928**    Resequenced code. See code following 92998.

**92929**    Resequenced code. See code following 92998.

**92933**    Resequenced code. See code following 92998.

**92934**    Resequenced code. See code following 92998.

**92937**    Resequenced code. See code following 92998.

**92938**    Resequenced code. See code following 92998.

**92941**    Resequenced code. See code following 92998.

**92943**    Resequenced code. See code following 92998.

**92944**    Resequenced code. See code following 92998.

**92950**    Cardiopulmonary resuscitation (eg, in cardiac arrest)

     INCLUDES    Cardiac defibrilllation

     EXCLUDES    *Critical care services (99291-99292)*

     5.35    8.61    **FUD** 000      S 80

     **AMA:** 2017,Jan,8; 2016,Jan,13; 2015,Jan,16; 2014,Jan,11; 2012,Oct,14; 2012,Sep,16; 2012,Jul,12-14; 2012,Jan,15-42

**92953**    Temporary transcutaneous pacing

     EXCLUDES    *Direction of ambulance/rescue personnel by physician or other qualified health care professional (99288)*

     0.03    0.03    **FUD** 000      03 80

     **AMA:** 2017,Jan,8; 2016,Jan,13; 2015,Jan,16; 2014,May,4; 2014,Jan,11

## 92960-92961 Cardioversion

**92960**    Cardioversion, elective, electrical conversion of arrhythmia; external

     3.14    4.49    **FUD** 000      S 80

     **AMA:** 2017,Jan,8; 2016,Jan,13; 2015,Jan,16; 2014,Jan,11; 2012,Jan,15-42; 2012,Jan,13-14

**92961**    internal (separate procedure)

     EXCLUDES    *Device evaluation for implantable defibrillator/multi-lead pacemaker system (93282-93284, 93287, 93289, 93295-93296)*

         *Electrophysiological studies (93618-93624, 93631, 93640-93642)*

         *Intracardiac ablation (93650-93657, 93662)*

     7.23    7.23    **FUD** 000      S

     **AMA:** 2017,Jan,8; 2016,Jan,13; 2015,Feb,3; 2015,Jan,16; 2014,Jan,11

## 92970-92979 Circulatory Assist: External/Internal

     EXCLUDES    *Atrial septostomy, balloon (92992)*

         *Catheter placement for use in circulatory assist devices (intra-aortic balloon pump) (33970)*

**92970**    Cardioassist-method of circulatory assist; internal

     5.36    5.36    **FUD** 000      C 80

     **AMA:** 1997,Nov,1

**92971**    external

     2.93    2.93    **FUD** 000      C 80

     **AMA:** 1997,Nov,1

**92973**    Resequenced code. See code following 92998.

**92974**    Resequenced code. See code following 92998.

**92975**    Resequenced code. See code following 92998.

**92977**    Resequenced code. See code following 92998.

**92978**    Resequenced code. See code following 92998.

**92979**    Resequenced code. See code following 92998.

## 92986-92993 Percutaneous Procedures of Heart Valves and Septum

**92986**    Percutaneous balloon valvuloplasty; aortic valve

     38.3    38.3    **FUD** 090      J 80

     **AMA:** 2017,Jan,8; 2016,Jan,13; 2015,Feb,3; 2015,Jan,16; 2014,Jan,11; 2013,Jan,6-8

**92987**    mitral valve

     39.6    39.6    **FUD** 090      J 80

     **AMA:** 2017,Jan,8; 2016,Jan,13; 2015,Feb,3

**92990**    pulmonary valve

     31.5    31.5    **FUD** 090      J 80

     **AMA:** 2017,Jan,8; 2016,Jan,13; 2015,Jul,10; 2015,Feb,3

**92992**    Atrial septectomy or septostomy; transvenous method, balloon (eg, Rashkind type) (includes cardiac catheterization)

     0.00    0.00    **FUD** 090      C 80

     **AMA:** 2017,Jan,8; 2016,Jul,3; 2016,Jan,13; 2015,Jan,16; 2014,Jan,11; 2012,Jan,15-42

**92993**    blade method (Park septostomy) (includes cardiac catheterization)

     0.00    0.00    **FUD** 090      C 80

     **AMA:** 2017,Jan,8; 2016,Jul,3; 2016,Jan,13; 2015,Jan,16; 2014,Jan,11

## 92997-92998 Percutaneous Angioplasty: Pulmonary Artery

**92997**    Percutaneous transluminal pulmonary artery balloon angioplasty; single vessel

     18.8    18.8    **FUD** 000      J 80

     **AMA:** 2017,Jul,3; 2017,Jan,8; 2016,Mar,5; 2016,Jan,13; 2015,Feb,3

+ **92998**    each additional vessel (List separately in addition to code for primary procedure)

     Code first single vessel (92997)

     9.31    9.31    **FUD** ZZZ      N 80

     **AMA:** 2017,Jul,3; 2017,Jan,8; 2016,Mar,5; 2016,Jan,13; 2015,Feb,3

26/TC PC/TC Only    A2-A3 ASC Payment    50 Bilateral    ♂ Male Only    ♀ Female Only    Facility RVU    Non-Facility RVU    CCI

**FUD** Follow-up Days    **CMS:** IOM (Pub 100)    A-Y OPPSI    80/80 Surg Assist Allowed / w/Doc    Lab Crosswalk    Radiology Crosswalk    CLIA

444       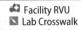 CPT © 2017 American Medical Association. All Rights Reserved.      © 2017 Optum360, LLC

## [92920, 92921, 92924, 92925, 92928, 92929, 92933, 92934, 92937, 92938, 92941, 92943, 92944] Intravascular Coronary Procedures

**INCLUDES**
Accessing the vessel
Additional procedures performed in a third branch of a major coronary artery
All procedures performed in all segments of branches of coronary arteries
  Branches of left anterior descending (diagonals), left circumflex (marginals), and right (posterior descending, posterolaterals)
  Distal, proximal, and mid segments
All procedures performed in all segments of major coronary arteries through the native vessels:
  Distal, proximal, and mid segments
  Left main, left anterior descending, left circumflex, right, and ramus intermedius arteries
All procedures performed in major coronary arteries or recognized coronary artery branches through a coronary artery bypass graft
  A sequential bypass graft with more than a single distal anastomosis as one graft
  Branching bypass grafts (eg, "Y" grafts) include a coronary vessel for the primary graft, with each branch off the primary graft making up an additional coronary vessel
  Each coronary artery bypass graft denotes a single coronary vessel
  Embolic protection devices when used
Arteriotomy closure through the access sheath
Atherectomy (eg, directional, laser, rotational)
Balloon angioplasty (eg, cryoplasty, cutting balloon, wired balloons)
Cardiac catheterization and related procedures when included in the coronary revascularization service (93454-93461, 93563-93564)
Imaging once procedure is complete
Percutaneous coronary interventions (PCI) for disease of coronary vessels, native and bypass grafts
Procedures in branches of the left main and ramus intermedius coronary arteries as they are unrecognized for purposes of individual code assignment
Radiological supervision and interpretation of intervention(s)
Reporting the most comprehensive treatment in a given vessel according to a hierarchy of intensity for the base and add-on codes:
  Add-on codes: 92944 = 92938 > 92934 > 92925 > 92929 > 92921
  Base codes (report only one): 92943 = 92941 = 92933 > 92924 > 92937 = 92928 > 92920
Revascularization achieved with a single procedure when a single lesion continues from one target vessel (major artery, branch, or bypass graft) to ...
Selective vessel catheterization
Stenting (eg, balloon expandable, bare metal, covered, drug eluting, self-expanding)
Traversing of the lesion
**EXCLUDES** *Application of intravascular radioelements (77770-77772)*
*Insertion of device for coronary intravascular brachytherapy (92974)*
*Reduction of septum (eg, alcohol ablation) (93799)*
Code also add-on codes for procedures performed during the same session in additional recognized branches of the target vessel
Code also diagnostic angiography at the time of the interventional procedure when:
  A previous study is available, but documentation states the patient's condition has changed since the previous study or visualization of the anatomy/pathology is inadequate, or a change occurs during the procedure warranting additional evaluation of an area outside the current target area
  No previous catheter-based coronary angiography study is available, and a full diagnostic study is performed, with the decision to perform the intervention based on that study, or
Code also diagnostic angiography performed at a session separate from the interventional procedure
Code also individual base codes for treatment of a segment of a major native coronary artery and another segment of the same artery that requires treatment through a bypass graft when performed at the same time
Code also procedures for both vessels for a bifurcation lesion
Code also procedures performed in second branch of a major coronary artery
Code also treatment of arterial segment requiring access through a bypass graft

---

\# **92920** Percutaneous transluminal coronary angioplasty; single major coronary artery or branch
    🔳 15.4   ⚖ 15.4   **FUD** 000     J 80 ▢
    **AMA:** 2017,Jul,3; 2017,Jan,8; 2016,Jan,13; 2015,Jan,16; 2014,Dec,6; 2013,Jan,3-5

Catheter is advanced to affected portion of coronary artery

A stent is placed

Aorta

Left coronary artery

Plaque

Right coronary artery

Inflated balloon

A balloon may be inflated or other intravascular therapy may accompany the procedure

+ \# **92921** each additional branch of a major coronary artery (List separately in addition to code for primary procedure)
    Code first (92920, 92924, 92928, 92933, 92937, 92941, 92943)
    🔳 0.00   ⚖ 0.00   **FUD** ZZZ     N ▢
    **AMA:** 2017,Jul,3; 2017,Jan,8; 2016,Jan,13; 2015,Jan,16; 2014,Dec,6; 2014,Sep,13; 2013,Jan,3-5

\# **92924** Percutaneous transluminal coronary atherectomy, with coronary angioplasty when performed; single major coronary artery or branch
    🔳 18.4   ⚖ 18.4   **FUD** 000     J 80 ▢
    **AMA:** 2017,Jul,3; 2017,Jan,8; 2016,Jan,13; 2015,Jan,16; 2014,Dec,6; 2013,Jan,3-5

+ \# **92925** each additional branch of a major coronary artery (List separately in addition to code for primary procedure)
    Code first (92924, 92928, 92933, 92937, 92941, 92943)
    🔳 0.00   ⚖ 0.00   **FUD** ZZZ     N ▢
    **AMA:** 2017,Jul,3; 2017,Jan,8; 2016,Jan,13; 2015,Jan,16; 2014,Dec,6; 2014,Sep,13; 2013,Jan,3-5

\# **92928** Percutaneous transcatheter placement of intracoronary stent(s), with coronary angioplasty when performed; single major coronary artery or branch
    🔳 17.2   ⚖ 17.2   **FUD** 000     J 80 ▢
    **AMA:** 2017,Jul,3; 2017,Feb,14; 2017,Jan,8; 2017,Jan,6; 2016,Jan,13; 2015,Jan,16; 2014,Dec,6; 2014,Sep,13; 2014,Mar,13; 2014,Jan,3; 2013,Jan,3-5

+ \# **92929** each additional branch of a major coronary artery (List separately in addition to code for primary procedure)
    Code first (92928, 92933, 92937, 92941, 92943)
    🔳 0.00   ⚖ 0.00   **FUD** ZZZ     N ▢
    **AMA:** 2017,Jul,3; 2017,Jan,8; 2017,Jan,6; 2016,Jan,13; 2015,Jan,16; 2014,Dec,6; 2014,Sep,13; 2013,Jan,3-5

**Medicine**

**92933 — 93005**

# # 92933  Percutaneous transluminal coronary atherectomy, with intracoronary stent, with coronary angioplasty when performed; single major coronary artery or branch

🚑 19.3  ⚕ 19.3  **FUD** 000  [J][80][CCI]

**AMA:** 2017,Jul,3; 2017,Jan,8; 2016,Jan,13; 2015,Jan,16; 2014,Dec,6; 2013,Jan,3-5

+ # 92934  each additional branch of a major coronary artery (List separately in addition to code for primary procedure)

Code first (92933, 92937, 92941, 92943)

🚑 0.00  ⚕ 0.00  **FUD** ZZZ  [N][CCI]

**AMA:** 2017,Jul,3; 2017,Jan,8; 2016,Jan,13; 2015,Jan,16; 2014,Dec,6; 2014,Sep,13; 2013,Jan,3-5

# 92937  Percutaneous transluminal revascularization of or through coronary artery bypass graft (internal mammary, free arterial, venous), any combination of intracoronary stent, atherectomy and angioplasty, including distal protection when performed; single vessel

🚑 17.2  ⚕ 17.2  **FUD** 000  [J][80][CCI]

**AMA:** 2017,Jul,3; 2017,Feb,14; 2017,Jan,8; 2016,Jan,13; 2015,Jan,16; 2014,Dec,6; 2014,Mar,13; 2013,Jan,3-5

+ # 92938  each additional branch subtended by the bypass graft (List separately in addition to code for primary procedure)

Code first (92937)

🚑 0.00  ⚕ 0.00  **FUD** ZZZ  [N][CCI]

**AMA:** 2017,Jul,3; 2017,Jan,8; 2016,Jan,13; 2015,Jan,16; 2014,Dec,6; 2014,Sep,13; 2014,Mar,13; 2013,Jan,3-5

# 92941  Percutaneous transluminal revascularization of acute total/subtotal occlusion during acute myocardial infarction, coronary artery or coronary artery bypass graft, any combination of intracoronary stent, atherectomy and angioplasty, including aspiration thrombectomy when performed, single vessel

INCLUDES  Aspiration thrombectomy, when performed
Embolic protection
Rheolytic thrombectomy

Code also treatment of additional vessels, when appropriate (92920-92938, 92943-92944)

🚑 19.3  ⚕ 19.3  **FUD** 000  [J][80][CCI]

**AMA:** 2017,Jul,3; 2017,Feb,14; 2017,Jan,8; 2016,Jan,13; 2015,Jan,16; 2014,Dec,6; 2014,Mar,13; 2014,Jan,3; 2013,Jan,3-5

# 92943  Percutaneous transluminal revascularization of chronic total occlusion, coronary artery, coronary artery branch, or coronary artery bypass graft, any combination of intracoronary stent, atherectomy and angioplasty; single vessel

INCLUDES  Lack of antegrade flow with angiography and clinical criteria indicative of chronic total occlusion

🚑 19.3  ⚕ 19.3  **FUD** 000  [J][80][CCI]

**AMA:** 2017,Jul,3; 2017,Jan,8; 2016,Jan,13; 2015,Jan,16; 2014,Dec,6; 2013,Jan,3-5

+ # 92944  each additional coronary artery, coronary artery branch, or bypass graft (List separately in addition to code for primary procedure)

EXCLUDES  Application of intravascular radioelements (77770-77772)

Code first (92924, 92928, 92933, 92937, 92941, 92943)

🚑 0.00  ⚕ 0.00  **FUD** ZZZ  [N][CCI]

**AMA:** 2017,Jul,3; 2017,Jan,8; 2016,Jan,13; 2015,Jan,16; 2014,Dec,6; 2014,Sep,13; 2013,Jan,3-5

## [92973, 92974, 92975, 92977, 92978, 92979] Additional Coronary Artery Procedures

+ # 92973  Percutaneous transluminal coronary thrombectomy mechanical (List separately in addition to code for primary procedure)

EXCLUDES  Aspiration thrombectomy

Code first (92920, 92924, 92928, 92933, 92937, 92941, 92943, 92975, 93454-93461, 93563-93564)

🚑 5.15  ⚕ 5.15  **FUD** ZZZ  [N][80][CCI]

**AMA:** 2017,Feb,14; 2017,Jan,8; 2016,Jan,13; 2015,Jan,16; 2014,Dec,6; 2014,Jan,11; 2012,Jan,15-42

+ # 92974  Transcatheter placement of radiation delivery device for subsequent coronary intravascular brachytherapy (List separately in addition to code for primary procedure)

EXCLUDES  Application of intravascular radioelements (77770-77772)

Code first (92920, 92924, 92928, 92933, 92937, 92941, 92943, 93454-93461)

🚑 4.72  ⚕ 4.72  **FUD** ZZZ  [N][80][CCI]

**AMA:** 2017,Feb,14; 2017,Jan,8; 2016,Jan,13; 2015,Jan,16; 2014,Dec,6; 2014,Jan,11

# 92975  Thrombolysis, coronary; by intracoronary infusion, including selective coronary angiography

EXCLUDES  Thrombolysis, cerebral (37195)
Thrombolysis other than coronary ([37211, 37212, 37213, 37214])

🚑 10.9  ⚕ 10.9  **FUD** 000  [C][80][CCI]

**AMA:** 1997,Nov,1; 1991,Win,1

# 92977  by intravenous infusion

EXCLUDES  Thrombolysis, cerebral (37195)
Thrombolysis other than coronary ([37211, 37212, 37213, 37214])

🚑 1.96  ⚕ 1.96  **FUD** XXX  [T][80][CCI]

**AMA:** 1997,Nov,1; 1991,Win,1

+ # 92978  Endoluminal imaging of coronary vessel or graft using intravascular ultrasound (IVUS) or optical coherence tomography (OCT) during diagnostic evaluation and/or therapeutic intervention including imaging supervision, interpretation and report; initial vessel (List separately in addition to code for primary procedure)

Code first primary procedure (92920, 92924, 92928, 92933, 92937, 92941, 92943, 92975, 93454-93461, 93563-93564)

🚑 0.00  ⚕ 0.00  **FUD** ZZZ  [N][80][CCI]

**AMA:** 2017,Jan,8; 2016,Jan,13; 2015,Jan,16; 2014,Dec,6; 2014,Jan,11; 2013,Dec,16; 2012,Jan,15-42

+ # 92979  each additional vessel (List separately in addition to code for primary procedure)

INCLUDES  Transducer manipulations/repositioning in the vessel examined, before and after therapeutic intervention

EXCLUDES  Intravascular spectroscopy (0205T)

Code first initial vessel (92978)

🚑 0.00  ⚕ 0.00  **FUD** ZZZ  [N][80][CCI]

**AMA:** 2017,Jan,8; 2016,Jan,13; 2015,Jan,16; 2014,Dec,6; 2014,Jan,11; 2013,Dec,16

## 93000-93010 Electrocardiographic Services

INCLUDES  Specific order for the service, a separate written and signed report, and documentation of medical necessity

EXCLUDES  Acoustic cardiography (93799)
Echocardiography (93303-93350)
Use of these codes for the review of telemetry monitoring strips

93000  Electrocardiogram, routine ECG with at least 12 leads; with interpretation and report

🚑 0.48  ⚕ 0.48  **FUD** XXX  [M][80][CCI]

**AMA:** 2017,Jan,8; 2016,Jan,13; 2015,Jan,16; 2014,Jan,11

93005  tracing only, without interpretation and report

🚑 0.24  ⚕ 0.24  **FUD** XXX  [Q1][80][TC][CCI]

**AMA:** 2017,Jan,8; 2016,Apr,8; 2016,Jan,13; 2015,Jan,16; 2014,Jan,11

---

93010 **interpretation and report only**
🔲 0.24 ◔ 0.24 **FUD** XXX
⧉ 🅱 80 26 ▭
**AMA:** 2017,Jan,8; 2016,Apr,8; 2016,Jan,13; 2015,Jan,16;
2014,Jan,11

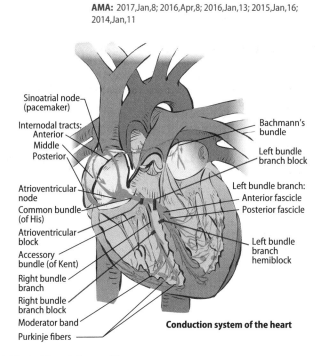

Sinoatrial node
(pacemaker)
Internodal tracts:
Anterior
Middle
Posterior
Atrioventricular
node
Common bundle
(of His)
Atrioventricular
block
Accessory
bundle (of Kent)
Right bundle
branch
Right bundle
branch block
Moderator band
Purkinje fibers
Bachmann's
bundle
Left bundle
branch block
Left bundle branch:
Anterior fascicle
Posterior fascicle
Left bundle
branch
hemiblock

**Conduction system of the heart**

## 93015-93018 Stress Test

93015 **Cardiovascular stress test using maximal or submaximal treadmill or bicycle exercise, continuous electrocardiographic monitoring, and/or pharmacological stress; with supervision, interpretation and report**
🔲 2.16 ◔ 2.16 **FUD** XXX 🅱 80 ▭
**AMA:** 2017,Jan,8; 2016,Jan,13; 2015,Jan,16; 2014,Jan,11;
2012,Jan,15-42

93016 **supervision only, without interpretation and report**
🔲 0.63 ◔ 0.63 **FUD** XXX 🅱 80 26 ▭
**AMA:** 2017,Jan,8; 2016,Jan,13; 2015,Jan,16; 2014,Jan,11;
2012,Jan,15-42

93017 **tracing only, without interpretation and report**
🔲 1.11 ◔ 1.11 **FUD** XXX Q1 80 TC ▭
**AMA:** 2017,Jan,8; 2016,Jan,13; 2015,Jan,16; 2014,Jan,11;
2012,Jan,15-42

93018 **interpretation and report only**
🔲 0.42 ◔ 0.42 **FUD** XXX 🅱 80 26 ▭
**AMA:** 2017,Jan,8; 2016,Jan,13; 2015,Jan,16; 2014,Jan,11;
2012,Jan,15-42

## 93024 Provocation Test for Coronary Vasospasm

93024 **Ergonovine provocation test**
🔲 3.16 ◔ 3.16 **FUD** XXX Q1 80 ▭

## 93025 Microvolt T-Wave Alternans

**CMS:** 100-03,20.30 Microvolt T-Wave Alternans (MTWA); 100-04,32,370 Microvolt T-wave Alternans;
100-04,32,370.1 Coding and Claims Processing for MTWA; 100-04,32,370.2 Messaging for MTWA
INCLUDES Specific order for the service, a separate written and signed report, and
documentation of medical necessity
EXCLUDES *Echocardiography (93303-93350)*
*Use of these codes for the review of telemetry monitoring strips*

93025 **Microvolt T-wave alternans for assessment of ventricular arrhythmias**
🔲 4.60 ◔ 4.60 **FUD** XXX 🆂 80 ▭
**AMA:** 2017,Jan,8; 2016,Jan,13; 2015,Jan,16; 2014,Jan,11

## 93040-93042 Rhythm Strips

INCLUDES Specific order for the service, a separate written and signed report, and
documentation of medical necessity
EXCLUDES *Device evaluation (93261, 93279-93289 [93260], 93291-93296, 93298-93299)*
*Echocardiography (93303-93350)*
*Use of these codes for the review of telemetry monitoring strips*

93040 **Rhythm ECG, 1-3 leads; with interpretation and report**
🔲 0.36 ◔ 0.36 **FUD** XXX 🅱 80 ▭
**AMA:** 2017,Jan,8; 2016,Jan,13; 2015,Jan,16; 2014,Jan,11;
2012,Nov,6-9; 2012,Aug,6-8; 2012,Jan,15-42

93041 **tracing only without interpretation and report**
🔲 0.16 ◔ 0.16 **FUD** XXX Q1 80 TC ▭
**AMA:** 2017,Jan,8; 2016,Jan,13; 2015,Jan,16; 2014,Jan,11;
2012,Aug,6-8; 2012,Jan,15-42

93042 **interpretation and report only**
🔲 0.20 ◔ 0.20 **FUD** XXX 🅱 80 26 ▭
**AMA:** 2017,Jan,8; 2016,Jan,13; 2015,Jan,16; 2014,Jan,11;
2012,Aug,6-8; 2012,Jan,15-42

## 93050 Arterial Waveform Analysis

EXCLUDES *Use of code with any intra-arterial diagnostic or interventional procedure*

93050 **Arterial pressure waveform analysis for assessment of central arterial pressures, includes obtaining waveform(s), digitization and application of nonlinear mathematical transformations to determine central arterial pressures and augmentation index, with interpretation and report, upper extremity artery, non-invasive**
🔲 0.50 ◔ 0.50 **FUD** XXX Q1 80 ▭

## 93224-93227 Holter Monitor

INCLUDES Cardiac monitoring using in-person as well as remote technology for the
assessment of electrocardiographic data
Up to 48 hours of recording on a continuous basis
EXCLUDES *Echocardiography (93303-93355)*
*Implantable patient activated cardiac event recorders (33282, 93285, 93291, 93298)*
*More than 48 hours of monitoring (0295T-0298T)*
Code also modifier 52 when less than 12 hours of continuous recording is provided

93224 **External electrocardiographic recording up to 48 hours by continuous rhythm recording and storage; includes recording, scanning analysis with report, review and interpretation by a physician or other qualified health care professional**
🔲 2.58 ◔ 2.58 **FUD** XXX 🅼 80 ▭
**AMA:** 2017,Jan,8; 2016,Jan,13; 2015,Jan,16; 2014,Jan,11;
2012,Jan,15-42

93225 **recording (includes connection, recording, and disconnection)**
🔲 0.75 ◔ 0.75 **FUD** XXX Q1 80 TC ▭
**AMA:** 2017,Jan,8; 2016,Jan,13; 2015,Jan,16; 2014,Jan,11;
2012,Jan,15-42

93226 **scanning analysis with report**
🔲 1.07 ◔ 1.07 **FUD** XXX Q1 80 TC ▭
**AMA:** 2017,Jan,8; 2016,Jan,13; 2015,Jan,16; 2014,Jan,11;
2012,Jan,15-42

93227 **review and interpretation by a physician or other qualified health care professional**
🔲 0.76 ◔ 0.76 **FUD** XXX 🅼 80 26 ▭
**AMA:** 2017,Jan,8; 2016,Jan,13; 2015,Jan,16; 2014,Jan,11;
2012,Jan,15-42

● New Code ▲ Revised Code ○ Reinstated ● New Web Release ▲ Revised Web Release Unlisted Not Covered # Resequenced
⊘ AMA Mod 51 Exempt ⑤ Optum Mod 51 Exempt ⑥ Mod 63 Exempt ✗ Non-FDA Drug ★ Telemedicine Ⓜ Maternity Ⓐ Age Edit + Add-on **AMA:** CPT Asst
© 2017 Optum360, LLC CPT © 2017 American Medical Association. All Rights Reserved. **447**

Medicine

## 93228-93229 Remote Cardiovascular Telemetry

INCLUDES    Cardiac monitoring using in-person as well as remote technology for the assessment of electrocardiographic data
Mobile telemetry monitors with the capacity to:
Detect arrhythmias
Real-time data analysis for the evaluation quality of the signal
Records ECG rhythm on a continuous basis using external electrodes on the patient
Transmit a tracing at any time
Transmit data to an attended surveillance center where a technician is available to respond to device or rhythm alerts and contact the physician or qualified health care professional if needed
EXCLUDES    Use of code more than one time in a 30-day period

**93228    External mobile cardiovascular telemetry with electrocardiographic recording, concurrent computerized real time data analysis and greater than 24 hours of accessible ECG data storage (retrievable with query) with ECG triggered and patient selected events transmitted to a remote attended surveillance center for up to 30 days; review and interpretation with report by a physician or other qualified health care professional**

EXCLUDES    Cardiovascular monitors that do not perform automatic ECG triggered transmissions to an attended surveillance center (93224-93227, 93268-93272)
📧 0.74    ⅀ 0.74    FUD XXX    ★ M 80 26 🖵
AMA: 2017,Jan,8; 2016,Jan,13; 2015,Jan,16; 2014,Jan,11; 2012,Jan,15-42

**93229    technical support for connection and patient instructions for use, attended surveillance, analysis and transmission of daily and emergent data reports as prescribed by a physician or other qualified health care professional**

EXCLUDES    Cardiovascular monitors that do not perform automatic ECG triggered transmissions to an attended surveillance center (93224-93227, 93268-93272)
📧 20.3    ⅀ 20.3    FUD XXX    ★ S 80 TC 🖵
AMA: 2017,Jan,8; 2016,Jan,13; 2015,Jan,16; 2014,Jan,11; 2012,Jan,15-42

## 93260-93272 Event Monitors

INCLUDES    ECG rhythm derived elements, which differ from physiologic data and include rhythm of the heart, rate, ST analysis, heart rate variability, T-wave alternans, among others
Event monitors that:
Record parts of ECGs in response to patient activation or an automatic detection algorithm (or both)
Require attended surveillance
Transmit data upon request (although not immediately when activated)
EXCLUDES    Monitoring of cardiovascular devices (93279-93289 [93260], 93291-93296, 93298-93299)

**93260    Resequenced code. See code following 93284.**

**93261    Resequenced code. See code following 93289.**

**93268    External patient and, when performed, auto activated electrocardiographic rhythm derived event recording with symptom-related memory loop with remote download capability up to 30 days, 24-hour attended monitoring; includes transmission, review and interpretation by a physician or other qualified health care professional**

EXCLUDES    Implanted patient activated cardiac event recording (33282, 93285, 93291, 93298)
📧 5.76    ⅀ 5.76    FUD XXX    ★ M 80 🖵
AMA: 2017,Jan,8; 2016,Jan,13; 2015,Jan,16; 2014,Jan,11; 2012,Jan,15-42

**93270    recording (includes connection, recording, and disconnection)**
📧 0.26    ⅀ 0.26    FUD XXX    ★ 01 80 TC 🖵
AMA: 2017,Jan,8; 2016,Jan,13; 2015,Jan,16; 2014,Jan,11; 2012,Jan,15-42

**93271    transmission and analysis**
📧 4.78    ⅀ 4.78    FUD XXX    ★ S 80 TC 🖵
AMA: 2017,Jan,8; 2016,Jan,13; 2015,Jan,16; 2014,Jan,11; 2012,Jan,15-42

**93272    review and interpretation by a physician or other qualified health care professional**
📧 0.72    ⅀ 0.72    FUD XXX    ★ M 80 26 🖵
AMA: 2017,Jan,8; 2016,Jan,13; 2015,Jan,16; 2014,Jan,11; 2012,Jan,15-42

## 93278 Signal-averaged Electrocardiography

EXCLUDES    Echocardiography (93303-93355)
Code also modifier 26 for the interpretation and report only

**93278    Signal-averaged electrocardiography (SAECG), with or without ECG**
📧 0.86    ⅀ 0.86    FUD XXX    01 80 🖵
AMA: 2017,Jan,8; 2016,Jan,13; 2015,Jan,16; 2014,Jan,11; 2012,Jan,15-42

## 93279-93299 [93260, 93261] Monitoring of Cardiovascular Devices

INCLUDES    Implantable cardiovascular monitor (ICM) interrogation:
Analysis of at least one recorded physiologic cardiovascular data element from either internal or external sensors
Programmed parameters
Implantable defibrillator interrogation:
Battery
Capture and sensing functions
Leads
Presence or absence of therapy for ventricular tachyarrhythmias
Programmed parameters
Underlying heart rhythm
Implantable loop recorder (ILR) interrogation:
Heart rate and rhythm during recorded episodes from both patient-initiated and device detected events
Programmed parameters
In-person interrogation/device evaluation (93288)
In-person peri-procedural device evaluation/programming of device system parameters (93286)
Interrogation evaluation of device
Pacemaker interrogation:
Battery
Capture and sensing functions
Heart rhythm
Leads
Programmed parameters
Time period established by the initiation of remote monitoring or the 91st day of implantable defibrillator or pacemaker monitoring or the 31st day of ILR monitoring and extending for the succeeding 30- or 90-day period
EXCLUDES    Evaluation of subcutaneous implantable defibrillator device (93260, 93261)
Wearable device monitoring (93224-93272)

**93279    Programming device evaluation (in person) with iterative adjustment of the implantable device to test the function of the device and select optimal permanent programmed values with analysis, review and report by a physician or other qualified health care professional; single lead pacemaker system**

EXCLUDES    External ECG event recording up to 30 days (93268-93272)
Peri-procedural and interrogation device evaluation (93286, 93288)
Rhythm strips (93040-93042)
📧 1.42    ⅀ 1.42    FUD XXX    01 80 🖵
AMA: 2017,Jan,8; 2016,Aug,5; 2016,May,5; 2016,Jan,13; 2015,Jan,16; 2014,Nov,5; 2014,Jul,3; 2014,Jan,11; 2013,Jul,7-9; 2013,Jun,6-8

**93280    dual lead pacemaker system**

EXCLUDES    External ECG event recording up to 30 days (93268-93272)
Peri-procedural and interrogation device evaluation (93286, 93288)
Rhythm strips (93040-93042)
📧 1.65    ⅀ 1.65    FUD XXX    01 80 🖵
AMA: 2017,Jan,8; 2016,Aug,5; 2016,May,5; 2016,Jan,13; 2015,Jan,16; 2014,Nov,5; 2014,Jul,3; 2014,Jan,11; 2013,Jul,7-9; 2013,Jun,6-8

**93281** **multiple lead pacemaker system**

> *EXCLUDES* External ECG event recording up to 30 days
> (93268-93272)
> Peri-procedural and interrogation device evaluation
> (93286, 93288)
> Rhythm strips (93040-93042)

🚑 1.94 ⚕ 1.94 **FUD** XXX  `01` `80` 🖵

**AMA:** 2017,Jan,8; 2016,Aug,5; 2016,May,5; 2016,Jan,13;
2015,Jan,16; 2014,Nov,5; 2014,Jul,3; 2014,Jan,11; 2013,Jul,7-9;
2013,Jun,6-8

**93282** **single lead transvenous implantable defibrillator system**

> *EXCLUDES* Device evaluation subcutaneous lead defibrillator
> system (93260)
> External ECG event recording up to 30 days
> (93268-93272)
> Peri-procedural and interrogation device evaluation
> (93287, 93289)
> Rhythm strips (93040-93042)
> Wearable cardio-defibrillator system services (93745)

🚑 1.79 ⚕ 1.79 **FUD** XXX  `01` `80` 🖵

**AMA:** 2017,Jan,8; 2016,Aug,5; 2016,Jan,13; 2015,Jan,16;
2014,Nov,5; 2014,Jul,3; 2014,Jan,11; 2013,Jul,7-9; 2013,Jun,6-8

**93283** **dual lead transvenous implantable defibrillator system**

> *EXCLUDES* External ECG event recording up to 30 days
> (93268-93272)
> Peri-procedural and interrogation device evaluation
> (93287, 93289)
> Rhythm strips (93040-93042)

🚑 2.31 ⚕ 2.31 **FUD** XXX  `01` `80` 🖵

**AMA:** 2017,Jan,8; 2016,Aug,5; 2016,Jan,13; 2015,Jan,16;
2014,Nov,5; 2014,Jul,3; 2014,Jan,11; 2013,Jul,7-9; 2013,Jun,6-8

**93284** **multiple lead transvenous implantable defibrillator system**

> *EXCLUDES* External ECG event recording up to 30 days
> (93268-93272)
> Peri-procedural and interrogation device evaluation
> (93287, 93289)
> Rhythm strips (93040-93042)

🚑 2.56 ⚕ 2.56 **FUD** XXX  `01` `80` 🖵

**AMA:** 2017,Jan,8; 2016,Aug,5; 2016,Jan,13; 2015,Jan,16;
2014,Nov,5; 2014,Jul,3; 2014,Jan,11; 2013,Jul,7-9; 2013,Jun,6-8

**# 93260** **implantable subcutaneous lead defibrillator system**

> *EXCLUDES* Device evaluation (93261, 93282, 93287)
> External ECG event recording up to 30 days
> (93268-93272)
> Insertion/removal/replacement implantable defibrillator
> (33240, 33241, [33262], [33270, 33271, 33272,
> 33273])
> Rhythm strips (93040-93042)

🚑 1.84 ⚕ 1.84 **FUD** XXX  `01` `80` 🖵

**AMA:** 2017,Jan,8; 2016,Aug,5; 2016,Jan,13; 2015,Jan,16;
2014,Nov,5

**93285** **implantable loop recorder system**

> *EXCLUDES* Device evaluation (93279-93284, 93291)
> External ECG event recording up to 30 days
> (93268-93272)
> Implantation of patient-activated cardiac event recorder
> (33282)
> Rhythm strips (93040-93042)

🚑 1.19 ⚕ 1.19 **FUD** XXX  `01` `80` 🖵

**AMA:** 2017,Jan,8; 2016,Aug,5; 2016,Jan,13; 2015,Jan,16;
2014,Nov,5; 2014,Jul,3; 2014,Jan,11

**93286** **Peri-procedural device evaluation (in person) and programming of device system parameters before or after a surgery, procedure, or test with analysis, review and report by a physician or other qualified health care professional; single, dual, or multiple lead pacemaker system**

> *INCLUDES* One evaluation and programming (if performed once
> before and once after, report as two units)
> *EXCLUDES* Device evaluation (93279-93281, 93288)
> External ECG event recording up to 30 days
> (93268-93272)
> Rhythm strips (93040-93042)
> Services related to cardiac contractility modulation
> systems (0408T-0411T, 0414T-0415T)
> Subcutaneous implantable defibrillator peri-procedural
> device evaluation and programming (93260,
> 93261)

🚑 0.77 ⚕ 0.77 **FUD** XXX  `N` `80` 🖵

**AMA:** 2017,Jan,8; 2016,Aug,5; 2016,May,5; 2016,Jan,13;
2015,Jan,16; 2014,Nov,5; 2014,Jul,3; 2014,Jan,11; 2013,Jul,7-9;
2013,Jun,6-8

**93287** **single, dual, or multiple lead implantable defibrillator system**

> *INCLUDES* One evaluation and programming (if performed once
> before and once after, report as two units)
> *EXCLUDES* Device evaluation (93282-93284, 93289)
> External ECG event recording up to 30 days
> (93268-93272)
> Rhythm strips (93040-93042)
> Services related to cardiac contractility modulation
> systems (0408T-0411T, 0414T-0415T)
> Subcutaneous implantable defibrillator peri-procedural
> device evaluation and programming (93260,
> 93261)

🚑 1.04 ⚕ 1.04 **FUD** XXX  `N` `80` 🖵

**AMA:** 2017,Jan,8; 2016,Aug,5; 2016,May,5; 2016,Jan,13;
2015,Jan,16; 2014,Nov,5; 2014,Jul,3; 2014,Jan,11; 2013,Jul,7-9;
2013,Jun,6-8

**93288** **Interrogation device evaluation (in person) with analysis, review and report by a physician or other qualified health care professional, includes connection, recording and disconnection per patient encounter; single, dual, or multiple lead pacemaker system**

> *EXCLUDES* Device evaluation (93279-93281, 93286, 93294-93295)
> External ECG event recording up to 30 days
> (93268-93272)
> Rhythm strips (93040-93042)

🚑 1.06 ⚕ 1.06 **FUD** XXX  `01` `80` 🖵

**AMA:** 2017,Jan,8; 2016,Aug,5; 2016,May,5; 2016,Jan,13;
2015,Jan,16; 2014,Nov,5; 2014,Jul,3; 2014,Jan,11; 2013,Jul,7-9;
2013,Jun,6-8

**93289** **single, dual, or multiple lead transvenous implantable defibrillator system, including analysis of heart rhythm derived data elements**

> *EXCLUDES* Monitoring physiologic cardiovascular data elements
> derived from an implantable defibrillator (93290)
> *EXCLUDES* Device evaluation (93261, 93282-93284, 93287,
> 93295-93296)
> External ECG event recording up to 30 days
> (93268-93272)
> Rhythm strips (93040-93042)

🚑 1.86 ⚕ 1.86 **FUD** XXX  `01` `80` 🖵

**AMA:** 2017,Jan,8; 2016,Aug,5; 2016,May,5; 2016,Jan,13;
2015,Jan,16; 2014,Nov,5; 2014,Jul,3; 2014,Jan,11; 2013,Jul,7-9;
2013,Jun,6-8

**#** **93261** **implantable subcutaneous lead defibrillator system**

EXCLUDES Device evaluation (93260, 93287, 93289)
External ECG event recording up to 30 days (93268-93272)
Insertion/removal/replacement implantable defibrillator (33240, 33241, [33262], [33270, 33271, 33272, 33273])
Rhythm strips (93040-93042)

🚑 1.69  ⚕ 1.69  **FUD** XXX   01 80 🖥

AMA: 2017,Jan,8; 2016,Aug,5; 2016,Jan,13; 2015,Jan,16; 2014,Nov,5

**93290** **implantable cardiovascular monitor system, including analysis of 1 or more recorded physiologic cardiovascular data elements from all internal and external sensors**

EXCLUDES Device evaluation (93297, 93299)
Heart rhythm derived data (93289)

🚑 0.89  ⚕ 0.89  **FUD** XXX   01 80 🖥

AMA: 2017,Jan,8; 2016,Aug,5; 2016,Jan,13; 2015,Jan,16; 2014,Nov,5; 2014,Jul,3; 2014,Jan,11; 2013,Apr,10-11; 2012,Jan,15-42

**93291** **implantable loop recorder system, including heart rhythm derived data analysis**

EXCLUDES Device evaluation (93288-93290 [93261], 93298-93299)
External ECG event recording up to 30 days (93268-93272)
Implantation of patient-activated cardiac event recorder (33282)
Rhythm strips (93040-93042)

🚑 1.04  ⚕ 1.04  **FUD** XXX   01 80 🖥

AMA: 2017,Jan,8; 2016,Aug,5; 2016,Jan,13; 2015,Jan,16; 2014,Nov,5; 2014,Jul,3; 2014,Jan,11

**93292** **wearable defibrillator system**

EXCLUDES External ECG event recording up to 30 days (93268-93272)
Rhythm strips (93040-93042)
Wearable cardioverter-defibrillator system (93745)

🚑 0.92  ⚕ 0.92  **FUD** XXX   01 80 🖥

AMA: 2017,Jan,8; 2016,Aug,5; 2016,Jan,13; 2015,Jan,16; 2014,Nov,5; 2014,Jul,3; 2014,Jan,11

**93293** **Transtelephonic rhythm strip pacemaker evaluation(s) single, dual, or multiple lead pacemaker system, includes recording with and without magnet application with analysis, review and report(s) by a physician or other qualified health care professional, up to 90 days**

EXCLUDES Device evaluation (93294)
External ECG event recording up to 30 days (93268-93272)
Rhythm strips (93040-93042)
Use of code more than one time in a 90-day period
Use of code when monitoring period is less than 30 days

🚑 1.52  ⚕ 1.52  **FUD** XXX   01 80 🖥

AMA: 2017,Jan,8; 2016,Aug,5; 2016,Jan,13; 2015,Jan,16; 2014,Nov,5; 2014,Jul,3; 2014,Jan,11

**93294** **Interrogation device evaluation(s) (remote), up to 90 days; single, dual, or multiple lead pacemaker system with interim analysis, review(s) and report(s) by a physician or other qualified health care professional**

EXCLUDES Device evaluation (93288, 93293)
External ECG event recording up to 30 days (93268-93272)
Rhythm strips (93040-93042)
Use of code more than one time in a 90-day period
Use of code when monitoring period is less than 30 days

🚑 0.96  ⚕ 0.96  **FUD** XXX   M 80 26 🖥

AMA: 2017,Jan,8; 2016,Aug,5; 2016,Jan,13; 2015,Jan,16; 2014,Nov,5; 2014,Jul,3; 2014,Jan,11; 2012,Jun,3-9

**93295** **single, dual, or multiple lead implantable defibrillator system with interim analysis, review(s) and report(s) by a physician or other qualified health care professional**

EXCLUDES Device evaluation (93289)
External ECG event recording up to 30 days (93268-93272)
Remote monitoring of physiological cardiovascular data (93297)
Rhythm strips (93040-93042)
Use of code more than one time in a 90-day period
Use of code when monitoring period is less than 30 days

🚑 1.92  ⚕ 1.92  **FUD** XXX   M 80 26 🖥

AMA: 2017,Jan,8; 2016,Aug,5; 2016,Jan,13; 2015,Jan,16; 2014,Nov,5; 2014,Jul,3; 2014,Jan,11

**93296** **single, dual, or multiple lead pacemaker system or implantable defibrillator system, remote data acquisition(s), receipt of transmissions and technician review, technical support and distribution of results**

EXCLUDES Device evaluation (93288-93289, 93299)
External ECG event recording up to 30 days (93268-93272)
Rhythm strips (93040-93042)
Use of code more than one time in a 90-day period
Use of code when monitoring period is less than 30 days

🚑 0.74  ⚕ 0.74  **FUD** XXX   01 80 TC 🖥

AMA: 2017,Jan,8; 2016,Aug,5; 2016,Jan,13; 2015,Jan,16; 2014,Nov,5; 2014,Jul,3; 2014,Jan,11

**93297** **Interrogation device evaluation(s), (remote) up to 30 days; implantable cardiovascular monitor system, including analysis of 1 or more recorded physiologic cardiovascular data elements from all internal and external sensors, analysis, review(s) and report(s) by a physician or other qualified health care professional**

EXCLUDES Device evaluation (93290, 93298)
Heart rhythm derived data (93295)
Use of code more than one time in a 30-day period
Use of code when monitoring period is less than 10 days

🚑 0.75  ⚕ 0.75  **FUD** XXX   M 80 26 🖥

AMA: 2017,Jan,8; 2016,Aug,5; 2016,Jan,13; 2015,Jan,16; 2014,Nov,5; 2014,Jul,3; 2014,Jan,11; 2013,Apr,10-11

**93298** **implantable loop recorder system, including analysis of recorded heart rhythm data, analysis, review(s) and report(s) by a physician or other qualified health care professional**

EXCLUDES Device evaluation (93291, 93297)
External ECG event recording up to 30 days (93268-93272)
Implantation of patient-activated cardiac event recorder (33282)
Rhythm strips (93040-93042)
Use of code more than one time in a 30-day period
Use of code when monitoring period is less than 10 days

🚑 0.76  ⚕ 0.76  **FUD** XXX   ★ M 80 26 🖥

AMA: 2017,Jan,8; 2016,Aug,5; 2016,Jan,13; 2015,Jan,16; 2014,Nov,5; 2014,Jul,3; 2014,Jan,11

**93299** **implantable cardiovascular monitor system or implantable loop recorder system, remote data acquisition(s), receipt of transmissions and technician review, technical support and distribution of results**

EXCLUDES Device evaluation (93290-93291, 93296)
External ECG event recording up to 30 days (93268-93272)
Rhythm strips (93040-93042)
Use of code more than one time in a 30-day period
Use of code when monitoring period is less than 10 days

🚑 0.00  ⚕ 0.00  **FUD** XXX   ★ 01 80 TC 🖥

AMA: 2017,Jan,8; 2016,Aug,5; 2016,Jan,13; 2015,Jan,16; 2014,Nov,5; 2014,Jul,3; 2014,Jan,11; 2013,Apr,10-11

26/TC PC/TC Only    A2-Z3 ASC Payment    50 Bilateral    ♂ Male Only    ♀ Female Only    🚑 Facility RVU    ⚕ Non-Facility RVU    🖥 CCI
FUD Follow-up Days    CMS: IOM (Pub 100)    A-Y OPPSI    80/80 Surg Assist Allowed / w/Doc    🔬 Lab Crosswalk    ❖ Radiology Crosswalk    ❌ CLIA

450   CPT © 2017 American Medical Association. All Rights Reserved.   © 2017 Optum360, LLC

## 93303-93355 Echocardiography

INCLUDES Interpretation and report
Obtaining ultrasonic signals from heart/great arteries
Report of study which includes:
Description of recognized abnormalities
Documentation of all clinically relevant findings which includes obtained
quantitative measurements
Interpretation of all information obtained
Two-dimensional image/doppler ultrasonic signal documentation
Ultrasound exam of:
Adjacent great vessels
Cardiac chambers/valves
Pericardium
EXCLUDES Contrast agents and/or drugs used for pharmacological stress
Echocardiography, fetal (76825-76828)
Ultrasound with thorough examination of the organ(s) or anatomic
region/documentation of the image/final written report

**93303** **Transthoracic echocardiography for congenital cardiac anomalies; complete**
6.69   6.69   **FUD** XXX    S 80
AMA: 2017,Jan,8; 2016,Jan,13; 2015,May,10; 2015,Jan,16;
2014,Jan,11; 2013,Dec,14; 2013,Aug,3; 2012,Jan,15-42

**93304** **follow-up or limited study**
4.39   4.39   **FUD** XXX    S 80
AMA: 2017,Jan,8; 2016,Jan,13; 2015,May,10; 2015,Jan,16;
2014,Jan,11; 2013,Dec,14; 2013,Aug,3

**93306** **Echocardiography, transthoracic, real-time with image documentation (2D), includes M-mode recording, when performed, complete, with spectral Doppler echocardiography, and with color flow Doppler echocardiography**
INCLUDES Doppler and color flow
Two-dimensional and M-mode
EXCLUDES Transthoracic without spectral and color doppler
(93307)
6.45   6.45   **FUD** XXX    S 80
AMA: 2017,Jan,8; 2016,Apr,8; 2016,Jan,13; 2015,May,10;
2015,Jan,16; 2013,Aug,3

**93307** **Echocardiography, transthoracic, real-time with image documentation (2D), includes M-mode recording, when performed, complete, without spectral or color Doppler echocardiography**
INCLUDES Additional structures that may be viewed such as
pulmonary vein or artery, pulmonic valve,
inferior vena cava
Obtaining/recording appropriate measurements
Two-dimensional/selected M-mode exam of:
Adjacent portions of the aorta
Aortic/mitral/tricuspid valves
Left/right atria
Left/right ventricles
Pericardium
Using multiple views as required to obtain a complete
functional/anatomic evaluation
EXCLUDES Doppler echocardiography (93320-93321, 93325)
3.67   3.67   **FUD** XXX    S 80
AMA: 2017,Jan,8; 2016,Apr,8; 2016,Jan,13; 2015,May,10;
2015,Jan,16; 2014,Jan,11; 2013,Aug,3; 2012,Jan,15-42

**93308** **Echocardiography, transthoracic, real-time with image documentation (2D), includes M-mode recording, when performed, follow-up or limited study**
INCLUDES An exam that does not evaluate/document the
attempt to evaluate all the structures that
comprise the complete echocardiographic exam
3.53   3.53   **FUD** XXX    S 80
AMA: 2017,Jan,8; 2016,Apr,8; 2016,Jan,13; 2015,May,10;
2015,Jan,16; 2014,Jan,11; 2013,Aug,3; 2012,Mar,9-10;
2012,Jan,15-42

**93312** **Echocardiography, transesophageal, real-time with image documentation (2D) (with or without M-mode recording); including probe placement, image acquisition, interpretation and report**
EXCLUDES Transesophageal echocardiography (93355)
6.96   6.96   **FUD** XXX    S 80
AMA: 2017,Jan,8; 2016,Jan,13; 2015,Jan,16; 2014,Jul,8;
2014,Jan,11; 2013,Aug,3; 2012,Oct,14; 2012,Jan,15-42

**93313** **placement of transesophageal probe only**
EXCLUDES Excludes procedure if performed by same person
performing transesophageal echocardiography
(93355)
0.33   0.33   **FUD** XXX    S 80
AMA: 2017,Jan,8; 2016,Jan,13; 2015,Jan,16; 2014,Jul,8;
2014,Jan,11; 2013,Aug,3

**93314** **image acquisition, interpretation and report only**
EXCLUDES Transesophageal echocardiography (93355)
6.69   6.69   **FUD** XXX    N 80
AMA: 2017,Jan,8; 2016,Jan,13; 2015,Jan,16; 2014,Jul,8;
2014,Jan,11; 2013,Aug,3

**93315** **Transesophageal echocardiography for congenital cardiac anomalies; including probe placement, image acquisition, interpretation and report**
EXCLUDES Transesophageal echocardiography (93355)
0.00   0.00   **FUD** XXX    S 80
AMA: 2017,Jan,8; 2016,Jan,13; 2015,Jan,16; 2014,Jul,8;
2014,Jan,11; 2013,Dec,14; 2013,Aug,3

**93316** **placement of transesophageal probe only**
EXCLUDES Transesophageal echocardiography (93355)
0.77   0.77   **FUD** XXX    S 80
AMA: 2017,Jan,8; 2016,Jan,13; 2015,Jan,16; 2014,Jan,11;
2013,Dec,14; 2013,Aug,3

**93317** **image acquisition, interpretation and report only**
EXCLUDES Transesophageal echocardiography (93355)
0.00   0.00   **FUD** XXX    N 80
AMA: 2017,Jan,8; 2016,Jan,13; 2015,Jan,16; 2014,Jan,11;
2013,Dec,14; 2013,Aug,3

**93318** **Echocardiography, transesophageal (TEE) for monitoring purposes, including probe placement, real time 2-dimensional image acquisition and interpretation leading to ongoing (continuous) assessment of (dynamically changing) cardiac pumping function and to therapeutic measures on an immediate time basis**
EXCLUDES Transesophageal echocardiography (93355)
0.00   0.00   **FUD** XXX    S 80
AMA: 2017,Jan,8; 2016,Jan,13; 2015,Jan,16; 2014,Jan,11;
2013,Aug,3

+ **93320** **Doppler echocardiography, pulsed wave and/or continuous wave with spectral display (List separately in addition to codes for echocardiographic imaging); complete**
EXCLUDES Transesophageal echocardiography (93355)
Code first (93303-93304, 93312, 93314-93315, 93317,
93350-93351)
1.53   1.53   **FUD** ZZZ    N 80
AMA: 2017,Jan,8; 2016,Jan,13; 2015,Jan,16; 2014,Jan,11;
2013,Aug,3

+ **93321** **follow-up or limited study (List separately in addition to codes for echocardiographic imaging)**
EXCLUDES Transesophageal echocardiography (93355)
Code first (93303-93304, 93308, 93312, 93314-93315, 93317,
93350-93351)
0.77   0.77   **FUD** ZZZ    N 80
AMA: 2017,Jan,8; 2016,Jan,13; 2015,Jan,16; 2014,Jan,11;
2013,Aug,3

● New Code   ▲ Revised Code   ○ Reinstated   ● New Web Release   ▲ Revised Web Release   Unlisted   Not Covered   # Resequenced
Ⓢ AMA Mod 51 Exempt   Ⓢ Optum Mod 51 Exempt   ⑥ Mod 63 Exempt   ✏ Non-FDA Drug   ★ Telemedicine   Ⓜ Maternity   Ⓐ Age Edit   + Add-on   AMA: CPT Asst
© 2017 Optum360, LLC     CPT © 2017 American Medical Association. All Rights Reserved.     **451**

**Medicine**

**93325 — 93451**

+ **93325** Doppler echocardiography color flow velocity mapping (List separately in addition to codes for echocardiography)

> *EXCLUDES* *Transesophageal echocardiography (93355)*
> Code first (76825-76828, 93303-93304, 93308, 93312, 93314-93315, 93317, 93350-93351)
> 🔲 0.72  ⚐ 0.72  **FUD** ZZZ    [N] [80] 🔲
> **AMA:** 2017,Jan,8; 2016,Jul,8; 2016,Jan,13; 2015,Jan,16; 2014,Jan,11; 2013,Aug,3

**93350** Echocardiography, transthoracic, real-time with image documentation (2D), includes M-mode recording, when performed, during rest and cardiovascular stress test using treadmill, bicycle exercise and/or pharmacologically induced stress, with interpretation and report;

> *EXCLUDES* *Cardiovascular stress test, complete procedure (93015)*
> Code also exercise stress testing (93016-93018)
> 🔲 6.80  ⚐ 6.80  **FUD** XXX    [S] [80] 🔲
> **AMA:** 2017,Jan,8; 2016,Apr,8; 2016,Jan,13; 2015,Jan,16; 2014,Jul,8; 2014,Jan,11; 2013,Aug,3; 2012,Jan,15-42

**93351** including performance of continuous electrocardiographic monitoring, with supervision by a physician or other qualified health care professional

> *INCLUDES* Stress echocardiogram performed with a complete cardiovascular stress test
> *EXCLUDES* *Cardiovascular stress test (93015-93018)*
> *Echocardiography (93350)*
> *Professional only components of complete stress test and stress echocardiogram performed in a facility by same physician, report with modifier 26*
> *Use of code for professional component (modifier 26 appended) with (93016, 93018, 93350)*
> Code also components of cardiovascular stress test when professional services not performed by same physician performing stress echocardiogram (93016-93018)
> 🔲 7.66  ⚐ 7.66  **FUD** XXX    [S] 🔲
> **AMA:** 2017,Jan,8; 2016,Apr,8; 2016,Jan,13; 2015,Jan,16; 2014,Jul,8; 2014,Jan,11; 2013,Aug,3; 2012,Jan,15-42

+ **93352** Use of echocardiographic contrast agent during stress echocardiography (List separately in addition to code for primary procedure)

> *EXCLUDES* *Use of code more than one time for each stress echocardiogram*
> Code first (93350, 93351)
> 🔲 0.96  ⚐ 0.96  **FUD** ZZZ    [M] [80] 🔲
> **AMA:** 2017,Jan,8; 2016,Jan,13; 2015,Jan,16; 2014,Jan,11; 2013,Aug,3; 2012,Jan,15-42

**93355** Echocardiography, transesophageal (TEE) for guidance of a transcatheter intracardiac or great vessel(s) structural intervention(s) (eg, TAVR, transcatheter pulmonary valve replacement, mitral valve repair, paravalvular regurgitation repair, left atrial appendage occlusion/closure, ventricular septal defect closure) (peri-and intra-procedural), real-time image acquisition and documentation, guidance with quantitative measurements, probe manipulation, interpretation, and report, including diagnostic transesophageal echocardiography and, when performed, administration of ultrasound contrast, Doppler, color flow, and 3D

> 🔲 6.47  ⚐ 6.47  **FUD** XXX    [N] [80] 🔲
> *EXCLUDES* *3D rendering (76376-76377)*
> *Doppler echocardiography (93320-93321, 93325)*
> *Transesophageal echocardiography (93312-93318)*
> *Transesophageal probe positioning by different provider (93313)*

## 93451-93505 Heart Catheterization

> *INCLUDES* Access site imaging and placement of closure device
> Catheter insertion and positioning
> Contrast injection (except as listed below)
> Imaging and insertion of closure device
> Radiology supervision and interpretation
> Roadmapping angiography
> *EXCLUDES* *Congenital cardiac cath procedures (93530-93533)*
> Code also separately identifiable:
> Aortography (93567)
> Noncardiac angiography (see radiology and vascular codes)
> Pulmonary angiography (93568)
> Right ventricular or atrial injection (93566)

**93451** Right heart catheterization including measurement(s) of oxygen saturation and cardiac output, when performed

> *INCLUDES* Cardiac output review
> Insertion catheter into 1+ right cardiac chambers or areas
> Obtaining samples for blood gas
> *EXCLUDES* *Catheterization procedures that include right side of heart (93453, 93456-93457, 93460-93461)*
> *Indicator dilution studies (93561-93562)*
> *Mitral valve repair (0345T)*
> *Percutaneous repair congenital interatrial defect (93580)*
> *Swan-Ganz catheter insertion (93503)*
> Code also administration of medication or exercise to repeat assessment of hemodynamic measurement (93463-93464)
> 🔲 20.5  ⚐ 20.5  **FUD** 000    ⃠ [J] [80] 🔲
> **AMA:** 2017,Jul,3; 2017,Jan,8; 2016,Mar,5; 2016,Jan,13; 2015,Sep,3; 2015,Jan,16; 2014,Jul,3; 2014,Jan,11; 2013,May,12; 2012,Mar,9-10

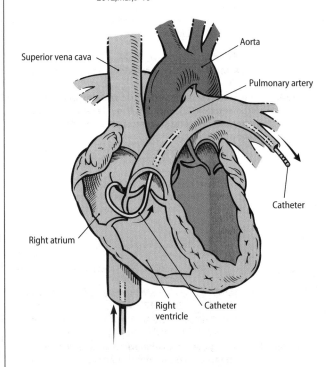

Aorta

Superior vena cava

Pulmonary artery

Catheter

Right atrium

Right ventricle    Catheter

🔲 PC/TC Only    [A2]-[Z3] ASC Payment    [50] Bilateral    ♂ Male Only    ♀ Female Only    🔲 Facility RVU    ⚐ Non-Facility RVU    🔲 CCI
**FUD** Follow-up Days    **CMS:** IOM (Pub 100)    [A]-[Y] OPPSI    [80]/[80] Surg Assist Allowed / w/Doc    🔲 Lab Crosswalk    🔲 Radiology Crosswalk    ⊠ CLIA
CPT © 2017 American Medical Association. All Rights Reserved.    © 2017 Optum360, LLC

**93452** **Left heart catheterization including intraprocedural injection(s) for left ventriculography, imaging supervision and interpretation, when performed**

INCLUDES Insertion of catheter into left cardiac chambers

EXCLUDES *Catheterization procedures that include injections for left ventriculography (93453, 93458-93461)*
*Injection procedures (93561-93565)*
*Percutaneous repair congenital interatrial defect (93580)*
*Services related to cardiac contractility modulation systems (0408T-0411T, 0414T-0415T)*
*Swan-Ganz catheter insertion (93503)*

Code also administration of medication or exercise to repeat assessment of hemodynamic measurement (93463-93464)

Code also transapical or transseptal puncture (93462)

📷 23.3   ⚖ 23.3   **FUD** 000   [J] [80] [📷]

**AMA:** 2017,Jul,3; 2017,Jan,8; 2016,Jan,13; 2015,Jan,16; 2014,Jul,3; 2014,Jan,11; 2013,May,12; 2013,Jan,6-8; 2012,Mar,9-10

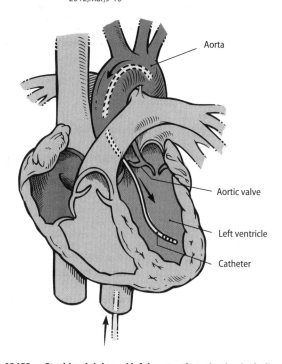

Aorta

Aortic valve

Left ventricle

Catheter

**93453** **Combined right and left heart catheterization including intraprocedural injection(s) for left ventriculography, imaging supervision and interpretation, when performed**

INCLUDES Cardiac output review
Insertion catheter into 1+ right cardiac chambers or areas
Insertion of catheter into left cardiac chambers
Obtaining samples for blood gas

EXCLUDES *Catheterization procedures (93451-93452, 93456-93461)*
*Injection procedures (93561-93565)*
*Mitral valve repair (0345T)*
*Percutaneous repair congenital interatrial defect (93580)*
*Services related to cardiac contractility modulation systems (0408T-0411T, 0414T-0415T)*
*Swan-Ganz catheter insertion (93503)*

Code also administration of medication or exercise to repeat assessment of hemodynamic measurement (93463-93464)

Code also transapical or transseptal puncture (93462)

📷 30.3   ⚖ 30.3   **FUD** 000   [J] [80] [📷]

**AMA:** 2017,Jul,3; 2017,Jan,8; 2016,Mar,5; 2016,Jan,13; 2015,Sep,3; 2015,Jan,16; 2014,Jul,3; 2014,Jan,11; 2013,May,12; 2013,Jan,6-8; 2012,Mar,9-10

**93454** **Catheter placement in coronary artery(s) for coronary angiography, including intraprocedural injection(s) for coronary angiography, imaging supervision and interpretation;**

EXCLUDES *Injection procedures (93561-93565)*
*Mitral valve repair (0345T)*
*Swan-Ganz catheter insertion (93503)*

📷 23.7   ⚖ 23.7   **FUD** 000   [J] [80] [📷]

**AMA:** 2017,Feb,14; 2017,Jan,8; 2016,Mar,5; 2016,Jan,13; 2015,Jan,16; 2014,Dec,6; 2014,Jul,3; 2014,Jan,11; 2013,May,12; 2012,Mar,9-10

**93455** **with catheter placement(s) in bypass graft(s) (internal mammary, free arterial, venous grafts) including intraprocedural injection(s) for bypass graft angiography**

EXCLUDES *Injection procedures (93561-93565)*
*Percutaneous repair congenital interatrial defect (93580)*
*Swan-Ganz catheter insertion (93503)*

📷 27.7   ⚖ 27.7   **FUD** 000   [J] [80] [📷]

**AMA:** 2017,Jan,8; 2016,Mar,5; 2016,Jan,13; 2015,Jan,16; 2014,Dec,6; 2014,Jul,3; 2014,Jan,11; 2013,May,12; 2012,Mar,9-10

**93456** **with right heart catheterization**

INCLUDES Cardiac output review
Insertion catheter into 1+ right cardiac chambers or areas
Obtaining samples for blood gas

EXCLUDES *Injection procedures (93561-93565)*
*Mitral valve repair (0345T)*
*Percutaneous repair congenital interatrial defect (93580)*
*Swan-Ganz catheter insertion (93503)*

Code also administration of medication or exercise to repeat assessment of hemodynamic measurement (93463-93464)

📷 29.9   ⚖ 29.9   **FUD** 000   [⊘] [J] [80] [📷]

**AMA:** 2017,Jul,3; 2017,Jan,8; 2016,Mar,5; 2016,Jan,13; 2015,Sep,3; 2015,Jan,16; 2014,Dec,6; 2014,Jul,3; 2014,Jan,11; 2013,May,12; 2012,Mar,9-10

**93457** **with catheter placement(s) in bypass graft(s) (internal mammary, free arterial, venous grafts) including intraprocedural injection(s) for bypass graft angiography and right heart catheterization**

INCLUDES Cardiac output review
Insertion catheter into 1+ right cardiac chambers or areas
Obtaining samples for blood gas

EXCLUDES *Injection procedures (93561-93565)*
*Percutaneous repair congenital interatrial defect (93580)*
*Swan-Ganz catheter insertion (93503)*

Code also administration of medication or exercise to repeat assessment of hemodynamic measurement (93463-93464)

📷 33.9   ⚖ 33.9   **FUD** 000   [J] [80] [📷]

**AMA:** 2017,Jan,8; 2016,Mar,5; 2016,Jan,13; 2015,Sep,3; 2015,Jan,16; 2014,Dec,6; 2014,Jul,3; 2014,Jan,11; 2013,May,12; 2012,Mar,9-10

**93458** **with left heart catheterization including intraprocedural injection(s) for left ventriculography, when performed**

INCLUDES Insertion of catheter into left cardiac chambers

EXCLUDES *Injection procedures (93561-93565)*
*Percutaneous repair congenital interatrial defect (93580)*
*Services related to cardiac contractility modulation systems (0408T-0411T, 0414T-0415T)*
*Swan-Ganz catheter insertion (93503)*

Code also administration of medication or exercise to repeat assessment of hemodynamic measurement (93463-93464)

Code also transapical or transseptal puncture (93462)

📷 28.5   ⚖ 28.5   **FUD** 000   [J] [80] [📷]

**AMA:** 2017,Jul,3; 2017,Jan,8; 2016,Mar,5; 2016,Jan,13; 2015,Sep,3; 2015,Jan,16; 2014,Dec,6; 2014,Jul,3; 2014,Jan,11; 2013,May,12; 2013,Jan,6-8; 2012,Mar,9-10

93452 — 93458

● New Code   ▲ Revised Code   ○ Reinstated   ● New Web Release   ▲ Revised Web Release   Unlisted   Not Covered   # Resequenced
⊘ AMA Mod 51 Exempt   ⑨ Optum Mod 51 Exempt   ⑨ Mod 63 Exempt   ⁄ Non-FDA Drug   ★ Telemedicine   Ⓜ Maternity   Ⓐ Age Edit   + Add-on   **AMA:** CPT Asst

© 2017 Optum360, LLC   CPT © 2017 American Medical Association. All Rights Reserved.

**93459**    with left heart catheterization including intraprocedural injection(s) for left ventriculography, when performed, catheter placement(s) in bypass graft(s) (internal mammary, free arterial, venous grafts) with bypass graft angiography

INCLUDES    Insertion of catheter into left cardiac chambers

EXCLUDES    Injection procedures (93561-93565)
Percutaneous repair congenital interatrial defect (93580)
Services related to cardiac contractility modulation systems (0408T-0411T, 0414T-0415T)
Swan-Ganz catheter insertion (93503)

Code also administration of medication or exercise to repeat assessment of hemodynamic measurement (93463-93464)
Code also transapical or transseptal puncture (93462)

⚙ 31.6    ⚕ 31.6    **FUD** 000            J 80 ▣

**AMA:** 2017,Jul,3; 2017,Jan,8; 2016,Mar,5; 2016,Jan,13; 2015,Sep,3; 2015,Jan,16; 2014,Dec,6; 2014,Jul,3; 2014,Jan,11; 2013,May,12; 2013,Jan,6-8; 2012,Mar,9-10

**93460**    with right and left heart catheterization including intraprocedural injection(s) for left ventriculography, when performed

INCLUDES    Cardiac output review
Insertion catheter into 1+ right cardiac chambers or areas
Insertion of catheter into left cardiac chambers
Obtaining samples for blood gas

EXCLUDES    Injection procedures (93561-93565)
Percutaneous repair congenital interatrial defect (93580)
Services related to cardiac contractility modulation systems (0408T-0411T, 0414T-0415T)
Swan-Ganz catheter insertion (93503)

Code also administration of medication or exercise to repeat assessment of hemodynamic measurement (93463-93464)
Code also transapical or transseptal puncture (93462)

⚙ 34.1    ⚕ 34.1    **FUD** 000            J 80 ▣

**AMA:** 2017,Jul,3; 2017,Jan,8; 2016,Mar,5; 2016,Jan,13; 2015,Sep,3; 2015,Jan,16; 2014,Dec,6; 2014,Jul,3; 2014,Jan,11; 2013,May,12; 2013,Jan,6-8; 2012,Mar,9-10

**93461**    with right and left heart catheterization including intraprocedural injection(s) for left ventriculography, when performed, catheter placement(s) in bypass graft(s) (internal mammary, free arterial, venous grafts) with bypass graft angiography

INCLUDES    Cardiac output review
Insertion catheter into 1+ right cardiac chambers or areas
Insertion of catheter into left cardiac chambers
Obtaining samples for blood gas

EXCLUDES    Injection procedures (93561-93565)
Mitral valve repair (0345T)
Percutaneous repair congenital interatrial defect (93580)
Services related to cardiac contractility modulation systems (0408T-0411T, 0414T-0415T)
Swan-Ganz catheter insertion (93503)

Code also administration of medication or exercise to repeat assessment of hemodynamic measurement (93463-93464)
Code also transapical or transseptal puncture (93462)

⚙ 39.0    ⚕ 39.0    **FUD** 000            J 80 ▣

**AMA:** 2017,Jul,3; 2017,Jan,8; 2016,Mar,5; 2016,Jan,13; 2015,Sep,3; 2015,Jan,16; 2014,Dec,6; 2014,Jul,3; 2014,Jan,11; 2013,May,12; 2013,Jan,6-8; 2012,Mar,9-10

+ **93462**    Left heart catheterization by transseptal puncture through intact septum or by transapical puncture (List separately in addition to code for primary procedure)

INCLUDES    Insertion of catheter into left cardiac chambers

EXCLUDES    Comprehensive electrophysiologic evaluation (93656)
Transseptal approach for percutaneous closure paravalvular leak (93590)
Mitral valve repair (0345T)

Code also percutaneous closure paravalvular leak when a transapical puncture is performed (93590-93591)
Code first (33477, 93452-93453, 93458-93461, 93582, 93653-93654)

⚙ 6.09    ⚕ 6.09    **FUD** ZZZ            N 80 ▣

**AMA:** 2017,Sep,3; 2017,Jul,3; 2017,Jan,8; 2016,Jan,13; 2015,Sep,3; 2015,Jan,16; 2014,Jul,3; 2014,Jan,11; 2013,Jun,6-8; 2013,May,12; 2012,Mar,9-10

+ **93463**    Pharmacologic agent administration (eg, inhaled nitric oxide, intravenous infusion of nitroprusside, dobutamine, milrinone, or other agent) including assessing hemodynamic measurements before, during, after and repeat pharmacologic agent administration, when performed (List separately in addition to code for primary procedure)

EXCLUDES    Coronary interventional procedures (92920-92944, 92975, 92977)
Use of code more than one time per catheterization

Code first (33477, 93451-93453, 93456-93461, 93530-93533, 93580-93581)

⚙ 2.82    ⚕ 2.82    **FUD** ZZZ            N 80 ▣

**AMA:** 2017,Jan,8; 2016,Jan,13; 2015,Jan,16; 2014,Dec,6; 2014,Jul,3; 2014,Jan,11; 2012,Mar,9-10

+ **93464**    Physiologic exercise study (eg, bicycle or arm ergometry) including assessing hemodynamic measurements before and after (List separately in addition to code for primary procedure)

EXCLUDES    Administration of pharmacologic agent (93463)
Bundle of His recording (93600)
Use of code more than one time per catheterization

Code first (33477, 93451-93453, 93456-93461, 93530-93533)

⚙ 7.22    ⚕ 7.22    **FUD** ZZZ            N 80 ▣

**AMA:** 2017,Jan,8; 2016,Jan,13; 2015,Jan,16; 2014,Jul,3; 2014,Jan,11; 2012,Mar,9-10

**93503**    Insertion and placement of flow directed catheter (eg, Swan-Ganz) for monitoring purposes

EXCLUDES    Diagnostic cardiac catheterization (93451-93461, 93530-93533)
Subsequent monitoring (99356-99357)

⚙ 3.69    ⚕ 3.69    **FUD** 000            ⊘ T 80 ▣

**AMA:** 2017,Jan,8; 2016,Jan,13; 2015,Jan,16; 2014,Jan,11; 2012,Jan,15-42

93505 **Endomyocardial biopsy**

> *EXCLUDES* *Intravascular brachytherapy radionuclide insertion (77770-77772)*
> *Transcatheter insertion of brachytherapy delivery device (92974)*

🔧 19.8   ⚕ 19.8   **FUD** 000   [T] [80] [▭]

**AMA:** 2017,Jan,8; 2016,Jan,13; 2015,Jan,16; 2014,Jan,11; 2012,Jan,15-42

Fluoroscopic guidance may be via brachial, femoral, subclavian, or jugular vein

Brachial vein access

Right atrium and ventricle

Catheter

A biopsy tome is inserted through the catheter and several tiny tissue samples are collected from the walls of the heart

## 93530-93533 Congenital Heart Defect Catheterization

> *INCLUDES* Access site imaging and placement of closure device
> Cardiac output review
> Insertion catheter into 1+ right cardiac chambers or areas
> Obtaining samples for blood gas
> Radiology supervision and interpretation
> Roadmapping angiography
> *EXCLUDES* *Cardiac cath on noncongenital heart (93451-93453, 93456-93461)*
> *Percutaneous repair congenital interatrial defect (93580)*
> *Swan-Ganz catheter insertion (93503)*
> Code also (93563-93568)

93530 **Right heart catheterization, for congenital cardiac anomalies**

🔧 0.00   ⚕ 0.00   **FUD** 000   [J] [80] [▭]

**AMA:** 2017,Jul,3; 2017,Jan,8; 2016,Mar,5; 2016,Jan,13; 2015,Sep,3; 2015,Jan,16; 2014,Jul,3; 2014,Jan,11; 2013,May,12; 2012,Mar,9-10; 2012,Jan,15-42

93531 **Combined right heart catheterization and retrograde left heart catheterization, for congenital cardiac anomalies**

🔧 0.00   ⚕ 0.00   **FUD** 000   [J] [80] [▭]

**AMA:** 2017,Jul,3; 2017,Jan,8; 2016,Mar,5; 2016,Jan,13; 2015,Sep,3; 2015,Jan,16; 2014,Jul,3; 2014,Jan,11; 2012,Mar,9-10

93532 **Combined right heart catheterization and transseptal left heart catheterization through intact septum with or without retrograde left heart catheterization, for congenital cardiac anomalies**

🔧 0.00   ⚕ 0.00   **FUD** 000   [J] [80] [▭]

**AMA:** 2017,Jul,3; 2017,Jan,8; 2016,Mar,5; 2016,Jan,13; 2015,Sep,3; 2015,Jan,16; 2014,Jul,3; 2014,Jan,11; 2012,Mar,9-10; 2012,Jan,15-42

93533 **Combined right heart catheterization and transseptal left heart catheterization through existing septal opening, with or without retrograde left heart catheterization, for congenital cardiac anomalies**

🔧 0.00   ⚕ 0.00   **FUD** 000   [J] [80] [▭]

**AMA:** 2017,Jul,3; 2017,Jan,8; 2016,Mar,5; 2016,Jan,13; 2015,Sep,3; 2015,Jan,16; 2014,Jul,3; 2014,Jan,11; 2012,Mar,9-10

## 93561-93568 Injection Procedures

> *INCLUDES* Catheter repositioning
> Radiology supervision and interpretation
> Using automatic power injector

93561 **Indicator dilution studies such as dye or thermodilution, including arterial and/or venous catheterization; with cardiac output measurement (separate procedure)**

> *EXCLUDES* *Cardiac output, radioisotope method (78472-78473, 78481)*
> *Catheterization procedures (93451-93462)*
> *Percutaneous closure patent ductus arteriosus (93582)*

🔧 0.00   ⚕ 0.00   **FUD** 000   [N] [80] [▭]

**AMA:** 2017,Jan,8; 2016,Jan,13; 2015,Jan,16; 2014,Jul,3; 2014,Jan,11; 2012,Jan,15-42

93562 **subsequent measurement of cardiac output**

> *EXCLUDES* *Cardiac output, radioisotope method (78472-78473, 78481)*
> *Catheterization procedures (93451-93462)*
> *Percutaneous closure patent ductus arteriosus (93582)*

🔧 0.00   ⚕ 0.00   **FUD** 000   [N] [80] [▭]

**AMA:** 2017,Jan,8; 2016,Jan,13; 2015,Jan,16; 2014,Jul,3; 2014,May,4; 2014,Jan,11

+ 93563 **Injection procedure during cardiac catheterization including imaging supervision, interpretation, and report; for selective coronary angiography during congenital heart catheterization (List separately in addition to code for primary procedure)**

> *EXCLUDES* *Catheterization procedures (93452-93461)*
> *Mitral valve repair (0345T)*
> Code first (93530-93533)

🔧 1.70   ⚕ 1.70   **FUD** ZZZ   [N] [80] [▭]

**AMA:** 2017,Jan,8; 2016,Mar,5; 2016,Jan,13; 2015,Jan,16; 2014,Dec,6; 2014,Jan,11; 2013,Jan,6-8

+ 93564 **for selective opacification of aortocoronary venous or arterial bypass graft(s) (eg, aortocoronary saphenous vein, free radial artery, or free mammary artery graft) to one or more coronary arteries and in situ arterial conduits (eg, internal mammary), whether native or used for bypass to one or more coronary arteries during congenital heart catheterization, when performed (List separately in addition to code for primary procedure)**

> *EXCLUDES* *Catheterization procedures (93452-93461)*
> *Mitral valve repair (0345T)*
> *Percutaneous repair congenital interatrial defect (93580)*
> Code first (93530-93533)

🔧 1.79   ⚕ 1.79   **FUD** ZZZ   [N] [80] [▭]

**AMA:** 2017,Jan,8; 2016,Mar,5; 2016,Jan,13; 2015,Jan,16; 2014,Dec,6; 2014,Jan,11; 2013,Jan,6-8

+ 93565 **for selective left ventricular or left atrial angiography (List separately in addition to code for primary procedure)**

> *EXCLUDES* *Catheterization procedures (93452-93461)*
> *Percutaneous repair congenital interatrial defect (93580)*
> Code first (93530-93533)

🔧 1.32   ⚕ 1.32   **FUD** ZZZ   [N] [80] [▭]

**AMA:** 2017,Jan,8; 2016,Jan,13; 2015,Jan,16; 2014,Jan,11; 2013,Jan,6-8

+ 93566 **for selective right ventricular or right atrial angiography (List separately in addition to code for primary procedure)**

> *EXCLUDES* *Percutaneous repair congenital interatrial defect (93580)*
> *Use for right ventriculography when performed during insertion leadless pacemaker (0387T)*
> Code first (93451, 93453, 93456-93457, 93460-93461, 93530-93533)

🔧 1.35   ⚕ 4.58   **FUD** ZZZ   [N] [80] [▭]

**AMA:** 2017,Jan,8; 2016,Aug,5; 2016,May,5; 2016,Mar,5; 2016,Jan,13; 2015,May,3; 2015,Jan,16; 2014,Jan,11; 2013,Jan,6-8

---

● New Code   ▲ Revised Code   ○ Reinstated   ● New Web Release   ▲ Revised Web Release   Unlisted   Not Covered   # Resequenced
⊘ AMA Mod 51 Exempt   ⑤ Optum Mod 51 Exempt   ⑥ Mod 63 Exempt   ✗ Non-FDA Drug   ★ Telemedicine   Ⓜ Maternity   Ⓐ Age Edit   + Add-on   **AMA:** CPT Asst

© 2017 Optum360, LLC   CPT © 2017 American Medical Association. All Rights Reserved.

**+ 93567** **for supravalvular aortography (List separately in addition to code for primary procedure)**

> *EXCLUDES* *Abdominal aortography or non-supravalvular thoracic aortography at same time as cardiac catheterization (36221, 75600-75630)*
>
> Code first (93451-93461, 93530-93533)
>
> ⊞ 1.53   ⅗ 3.87   **FUD** ZZZ   Ⓝ 80 ▭
>
> **AMA:** 2017,Jan,8; 2016,Mar,5; 2016,Jan,13; 2015,Jan,16; 2014,Jan,11; 2013,Jan,6-8

**+ 93568** **for pulmonary angiography (List separately in addition to code for primary procedure)**

> Code first (93451, 93453, 93456-93457, 93460-93461, 93530-93533)
>
> ⊞ 1.38   ⅗ 4.10   **FUD** ZZZ   Ⓝ 80 ▭
>
> **AMA:** 2017,Jan,8; 2016,Mar,5; 2016,Jan,13; 2015,Jan,16; 2014,Jan,11; 2013,Jan,6-8

## 93571-93572 Coronary Artery Doppler Studies

> *INCLUDES* Doppler transducer manipulations/repositioning within the vessel examined, during coronary angiography/therapeutic intervention (angioplasty)

**+ 93571** **Intravascular Doppler velocity and/or pressure derived coronary flow reserve measurement (coronary vessel or graft) during coronary angiography including pharmacologically induced stress; initial vessel (List separately in addition to code for primary procedure)**

> Code first (92920, 92924, 92928, 92933, 92937, 92941, 92943, 92975, 93454-93461, 93563-93564)
>
> ⊞ 0.00   ⅗ 0.00   **FUD** ZZZ   Ⓝ 80 ▭
>
> **AMA:** 2017,Jan,8; 2016,Jan,13; 2015,Dec,18; 2015,May,10; 2015,Jan,16; 2014,Dec,6; 2014,Jan,11

**+ 93572** **each additional vessel (List separately in addition to code for primary procedure)**

> Code first initial vessel (93571)
>
> ⊞ 0.00   ⅗ 0.00   **FUD** ZZZ   Ⓝ 80 ▭
>
> **AMA:** 2017,Jan,8; 2016,Jan,13; 2015,Dec,18; 2015,May,10; 2015,Jan,16; 2014,Dec,6; 2014,Jan,11

## 93580-93583 Percutaneous Repair of Congenital Heart Defects

**93580** **Percutaneous transcatheter closure of congenital interatrial communication (ie, Fontan fenestration, atrial septal defect) with implant**

> *INCLUDES* Injection of contrast for right heart atrial/ventricular angiograms (93564-93566)
> Right heart catheterization (93451, 93453, 93456-93457, 93460-93461, 93530-93533)
>
> *EXCLUDES* *Bypass graft angiography (93455)*
> *Injection of contrast for left heart atrial/ventricular angiograms (93458-93459)*
> *Left heart catheterization (93452, 93458-93459)*
> Code also echocardiography, when performed (93303-93317, 93662)
>
> ⊞ 28.4   ⅗ 28.4   **FUD** 000   Ⓙ 80 ▭
>
> **AMA:** 2017,Jan,8; 2016,Jan,13; 2015,Jan,16; 2014,Jan,11; 2012,Jan,15-42

**93581** **Percutaneous transcatheter closure of a congenital ventricular septal defect with implant**

> *INCLUDES* Injection of contrast for right heart atrial/ventricular angiograms (93564-93566)
> Right heart catheterization (93451, 93453, 93456-93457, 93460-93461, 93530-93533)
>
> *EXCLUDES* *Bypass graft angiography (93455)*
> *Injection of contrast for left heart atrial/ventricular angiograms (93458-93459)*
> *Left heart catheterization (93452, 93458-93459)*
> Code also echocardiography, when performed (93303-93317, 93662)
>
> ⊞ 39.0   ⅗ 39.0   **FUD** 000   Ⓙ 80 ▭
>
> **AMA:** 2017,Jan,8; 2016,Jan,13; 2015,Jan,16; 2014,Jan,11; 2012,Jan,15-42

**93582** **Percutaneous transcatheter closure of patent ductus arteriosus**

> *INCLUDES* Aorta catheter placement (36200)
> Aortography (75600-75605, 93567)
> Heart catheterization (93451-93461, 93530-93533)
>
> *EXCLUDES* *Catheterization pulmonary artery (36013-36014)*
> *Intracardiac echocardiographic services (93662)*
> *Left heart catheterization performed via transapical puncture or transseptal puncture through intact septum (93462)*
> *Ligation repair (33820, 33822, 33824)*
> *Other cardiac angiographic procedures (93563-93566, 93568)*
> *Other echocardiographic services by different provider (93315-93317)*
>
> ⊞ 19.0   ⅗ 19.0   **FUD** 000   Ⓙ 80 ▭
>
> **AMA:** 2017,Jan,8; 2016,Jan,13; 2015,Jan,16; 2014,Jul,3

**93583** **Percutaneous transcatheter septal reduction therapy (eg, alcohol septal ablation) including temporary pacemaker insertion when performed**

> ⊞ 21.6   ⅗ 21.6   **FUD** 000   Ⓒ 80 ▭
>
> *INCLUDES* Alcohol injection (93463)
> Coronary angiography during the procedure to roadmap, guide the intervention, measure the vessel, and complete the angiography (93454-93461, 93531-93533, 93563, 93563, 93565)
> Left heart catheterization (93452-93453, 93458-93461, 93531-93533)
> Temporary pacemaker insertion (33210)
>
> *EXCLUDES* *Intracardiac echocardiographic services when performed (93662)*
> *Myectomy (surgical ventriculomyotomy) to treat idiopathic hypertrophic subaortic stenosis (33416)*
> *Other echocardiographic services rendered by different provider (93312-93317)*
> Code also diagnostic cardiac catheterization procedures if the patient's condition (clinical indication) has changed since the intervention or prior study, there is no available prior catheter-based diagnostic study of the treatment zone, or the prior study is not adequate (93451, 93454-93457, 93530, 93563-93564, 93566-93568)

## 93590-93592 Percutaneous Repair Paravalvular Leak

> *INCLUDES* Access with insertion and positioning of device
> Angiography
> Fluoroscopy (76000)
> Imaging guidance
> Left heart catheterization (93452-93453, 93459-93461, 93531-93533)
> Code also diagnostic right heart catheterization and angiography performed when:
> Code also when there is no previous study and a complete diagnostic study is performed; append modifier 59
> Code also if a previous study is available, but documentation states the patient's condition has changed since the previous study; visualization is insufficient; or a change necessitates reevaluation; append modifier 59

**93590** **Percutaneous transcatheter closure of paravalvular leak; initial occlusion device, mitral valve**

> *INCLUDES* Transseptal puncture (93462)
> Code also for transapical puncture (93462)
>
> ⊞ 34.7   ⅗ 34.7   **FUD** 000   Ⓙ J8 80 ▭
>
> **AMA:** 2017,Sep,3

**93591** **initial occlusion device, aortic valve**

> *EXCLUDES* *Transapical or transseptal puncture (93462)*
>
> ⊞ 28.8   ⅗ 28.8   **FUD** 000   Ⓙ J8 80 ▭
>
> **AMA:** 2017,Sep,3

**+ 93592** **each additional occlusion device (List separately in addition to code for primary procedure)**

> Code first (93590-93591)
>
> ⊞ 12.6   ⅗ 12.6   **FUD** ZZZ   Ⓝ 80 ▭
>
> **AMA:** 2017,Sep,3

## 93600-93603 Recording of Intracardiac Electrograms

INCLUDES Unusual situations where there may be recording/pacing/attempt at arrhythmia induction from only one side of the heart

EXCLUDES *Comprehensive electrophysiological studies (93619-93620, 93653-93654, 93656)*

**93600** **Bundle of His recording**
🔧 0.00 ⚕ 0.00 **FUD** 000 ⊘ J 80 ▭

**AMA:** 2017,Jan,8; 2016,Jan,13; 2015,Jan,16; 2014,Apr,3; 2014,Jan,11; 2013,Jul,7-9; 2013,Jun,6-8; 2012,Jan,15-42

**93602** **Intra-atrial recording**
🔧 0.00 ⚕ 0.00 **FUD** 000 ⊘ J 80 ▭

**AMA:** 2017,Jan,8; 2016,Jan,13; 2015,Jan,16; 2014,Apr,3; 2014,Jan,11; 2013,Jul,7-9; 2013,Jun,6-8; 2012,Jan,15-42

**93603** **Right ventricular recording**
🔧 0.00 ⚕ 0.00 **FUD** 000 ⊘ J 80 ▭

**AMA:** 2017,Jan,8; 2016,Jan,13; 2015,Jan,16; 2014,Apr,3; 2014,Jan,11; 2013,Jul,7-9; 2013,Jun,6-8

## 93609-93613 Intracardiac Mapping and Pacing

**+** **93609** **Intraventricular and/or intra-atrial mapping of tachycardia site(s) with catheter manipulation to record from multiple sites to identify origin of tachycardia (List separately in addition to code for primary procedure)**

EXCLUDES *Intracardiac 3D mapping (93613)*
*Intracardiac ablation with 3D mapping (93654)*
Code first (93620, 93653, 93656)
🔧 0.00 ⚕ 0.00 **FUD** ZZZ N 80 ▭

**AMA:** 2017,Jan,8; 2016,Jan,13; 2015,Jan,16; 2014,Apr,3; 2014,Jan,11; 2013,Jul,7-9; 2013,Jun,6-8

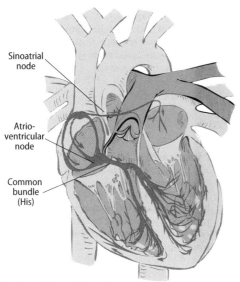

Sinoatrial node

Atrio-ventricular node

Common bundle (His)

**Tachycardia is rapid heartbeat**

**93610** **Intra-atrial pacing**

INCLUDES Unusual situations where there may be recording/pacing/attempt at arrhythmia induction from only one side of the heart

EXCLUDES *Comprehensive electrophysiological studies (93619-93620)*
*Intracardiac ablation (93653-93654, 93656)*
🔧 0.00 ⚕ 0.00 **FUD** 000 ⊘ J 80 ▭

**AMA:** 2017,Jan,8; 2016,Jan,13; 2015,Jan,16; 2014,Apr,3; 2014,Jan,11; 2013,Jul,7-9; 2013,Jun,6-8

**93612** **Intraventricular pacing**

INCLUDES Unusual situations where there may be recording/pacing/attempt at arrhythmia induction from only one side of the heart

EXCLUDES *Comprehensive electrophysiological studies (93619-93622)*
*Intracardiac ablation (93653-93654, 93656)*
🔧 0.00 ⚕ 0.00 **FUD** 000 ⊘ J 80 ▭

**AMA:** 2017,Jan,8; 2016,Jan,13; 2015,Jan,16; 2014,Apr,3; 2014,Jan,11; 2013,Jul,7-9; 2013,Jun,6-8

**+** **93613** **Intracardiac electrophysiologic 3-dimensional mapping (List separately in addition to code for primary procedure)**

EXCLUDES *Intracardiac ablation with 3D mapping (93654)*
*Mapping of tachycardia site (93609)*
Code first (93620, 93653, 93656)
🔧 11.5 ⚕ 11.5 **FUD** ZZZ N 80 ▭

**AMA:** 2017,Jan,8; 2016,Jan,13; 2015,Jan,16; 2014,Apr,3; 2014,Jan,11; 2013,Jul,7-9; 2013,Jun,6-8

## 93615-93616 Recording and Pacing via Esophagus

**93615** **Esophageal recording of atrial electrogram with or without ventricular electrogram(s);**
🔧 0.00 ⚕ 0.00 **FUD** 000 ⊘ J 80 ▭

**AMA:** 2017,Jan,8; 2016,Jan,13; 2015,Jan,16; 2014,Jan,11

**93616** **with pacing**
🔧 0.00 ⚕ 0.00 **FUD** 000 ⊘ J 80 ▭

**AMA:** 2017,Jan,8; 2016,Jan,13; 2015,Jan,16; 2014,Jan,11

## 93618 Pacing to Produce an Arrhythmia

**CMS:** 100-03,20.12 Diagnostic Endocardial Electrical Stimulation (Pacing)

INCLUDES Unusual situations where there may be recording/pacing/attempt at arrhythmia induction from only one side of the heart

EXCLUDES *Comprehensive electrophysiological studies (93619-93622)*
*Intracardiac ablation (93653-93654, 93656)*
*Intracardiac phonocardiogram (93799)*

**93618** **Induction of arrhythmia by electrical pacing**
🔧 0.00 ⚕ 0.00 **FUD** 000 ⊘ J 80 ▭

**AMA:** 2017,Jan,8; 2016,Jan,13; 2015,Jan,16; 2014,Apr,3; 2014,Jan,11; 2013,Jul,7-9; 2013,Jun,6-8; 2012,Jan,15-42

## 93619-93623 Comprehensive Electrophysiological Studies

**CMS:** 100-03,20.12 Diagnostic Endocardial Electrical Stimulation (Pacing)

**93619** **Comprehensive electrophysiologic evaluation with right atrial pacing and recording, right ventricular pacing and recording, His bundle recording, including insertion and repositioning of multiple electrode catheters, without induction or attempted induction of arrhythmia**

INCLUDES Evaluation of sinus node/atrioventricular node/His-Purkinje conduction system without arrhythmia induction

EXCLUDES *Comprehensive electrophysiological studies (93620-93622)*
*Intracardiac ablation (93653-93657)*
*Intracardiac pacing (93610, 93612, 93618)*
*Recording of intracardiac electrograms (93600-93603)*
🔧 0.00 ⚕ 0.00 **FUD** 000 J 80 ▭

**AMA:** 2017,Jan,8; 2016,Jan,13; 2015,Jan,16; 2014,Apr,3; 2014,Jan,11; 2013,Jul,7-9; 2013,Jun,6-8; 2012,Nov,6-9; 2012,Jan,15-42

**93620** Comprehensive electrophysiologic evaluation including insertion and repositioning of multiple electrode catheters with induction or attempted induction of arrhythmia; with right atrial pacing and recording, right ventricular pacing and recording, His bundle recording

> INCLUDES Recording/pacing/attempted arrhythmia induction from one or more site(s) in the heart
> EXCLUDES *Comprehensive electrophysiological study without induction/attempted induction arrhythmia (93619)*
> *Intracardiac ablation (93653-93657)*
> *Intracardiac pacing (93610, 93612, 93618)*
> *Recording of intracardiac electrograms (93600-93603)*
> 🚑 0.00    ⚕ 0.00    **FUD** 000    J 80 ▢
> **AMA:** 2017,Jan,8; 2016,Jan,13; 2015,Jan,16; 2014,Apr,3; 2014,Jan,11; 2013,Jul,7-9; 2013,Jun,6-8; 2012,Nov,6-9; 2012,Jan,15-42

+ **93621** with left atrial pacing and recording from coronary sinus or left atrium (List separately in addition to code for primary procedure)

> INCLUDES Recording/pacing/attempted arrhythmia induction from one or more site(s) in the heart
> EXCLUDES *Intracardiac ablation (93656)*
> Code first (93620, 93653-93654)
> 🚑 0.00    ⚕ 0.00    **FUD** ZZZ    N 80 ▢
> **AMA:** 2017,Jan,8; 2016,Jan,13; 2015,Jan,16; 2014,Apr,3; 2014,Jan,11; 2013,Jul,7-9; 2013,Jun,6-8; 2012,Nov,6-9; 2012,Jan,15-42

+ **93622** with left ventricular pacing and recording (List separately in addition to code for primary procedure)

> EXCLUDES *Intracardiac ablation (93654)*
> Code first (93620, 93653, 93656)
> 🚑 0.00    ⚕ 0.00    **FUD** ZZZ    N 80 ▢
> **AMA:** 2017,Jan,8; 2016,Jan,13; 2015,Jan,16; 2014,Apr,3; 2014,Jan,11; 2013,Jul,7-9; 2013,Jun,6-8; 2012,Nov,6-9; 2012,Jan,15-42

+ **93623** Programmed stimulation and pacing after intravenous drug infusion (List separately in addition to code for primary procedure)

> INCLUDES Recording/pacing/attempted arrhythmia induction from one or more site(s) in the heart
> Code first comprehensive electrophysiologic evaluation (93610, 93612, 93619-93620, 93653-93654, 93656)
> 🚑 0.00    ⚕ 0.00    **FUD** ZZZ    N 80 ▢
> **AMA:** 2017,Jan,8; 2016,Jan,13; 2015,Jan,16; 2014,Apr,3; 2014,Jan,11; 2013,Jul,7-9; 2012,Jan,15-42

## 93624-93631 Followup and Intraoperative Electrophysiologic Studies

**CMS:** 100-03,20.12 Diagnostic Endocardial Electrical Stimulation (Pacing)

**93624** Electrophysiologic follow-up study with pacing and recording to test effectiveness of therapy, including induction or attempted induction of arrhythmia

> INCLUDES Recording/pacing/attempted arrhythmia induction from one or more site(s) in the heart
> 🚑 0.00    ⚕ 0.00    **FUD** 000    J 80 ▢
> **AMA:** 2017,Jan,8; 2016,Jan,13; 2015,Jan,16; 2014,Jan,11

**93631** Intra-operative epicardial and endocardial pacing and mapping to localize the site of tachycardia or zone of slow conduction for surgical correction

> EXCLUDES *Operative ablation of an arrhythmogenic focus or pathway by a separate provider (33250-33261)*
> 🚑 0.00    ⚕ 0.00    **FUD** 000    🚫 N 80 ▢
> **AMA:** 2017,Jan,8; 2016,Jan,13; 2015,Jan,16; 2014,Jan,11

## 93640-93644 Electrophysiologic Studies of Cardioverter-Defibrillators

> INCLUDES Recording/pacing/attempted arrhythmia induction from one or more site(s) in the heart

**93640** Electrophysiologic evaluation of single or dual chamber pacing cardioverter-defibrillator leads including defibrillation threshold evaluation (induction of arrhythmia, evaluation of sensing and pacing for arrhythmia termination) at time of initial implantation or replacement;

> 🚑 0.00    ⚕ 0.00    **FUD** 000    N 80 ▢
> **AMA:** 2017,Jan,8; 2016,Jan,13; 2015,Jan,16; 2014,Jan,11; 2012,Jun,3-9

**93641** with testing of single or dual chamber pacing cardioverter-defibrillator pulse generator

> EXCLUDES *Single/dual chamber pacing cardioverter-defibrillators reprogramming/electronic analysis, subsequent/periodic (93282-93283, 93289, 93292, 93295, 93642)*
> 🚑 0.00    ⚕ 0.00    **FUD** 000    N 80 ▢
> **AMA:** 2017,Jan,8; 2016,Jan,13; 2015,Jan,16; 2014,Apr,3; 2014,Jan,11; 2012,Jun,3-9

**93642** Electrophysiologic evaluation of single or dual chamber transvenous pacing cardioverter-defibrillator (includes defibrillation threshold evaluation, induction of arrhythmia, evaluation of sensing and pacing for arrhythmia termination, and programming or reprogramming of sensing or therapeutic parameters)

> 🚑 9.79    ⚕ 9.79    **FUD** 000    J 80 ▢
> **AMA:** 2017,Jan,8; 2016,Jan,13; 2015,Jan,16; 2014,Apr,3; 2014,Jan,11; 2013,Jul,7-9; 2013,Jun,6-8

**93644** Electrophysiologic evaluation of subcutaneous implantable defibrillator (includes defibrillation threshold evaluation, induction of arrhythmia, evaluation of sensing for arrhythmia termination, and programming or reprogramming of sensing or therapeutic parameters)

> 🚑 6.18    ⚕ 6.18    **FUD** 000    N 80 ▢
> EXCLUDES *Insertion/replacement subcutaneous implantable defibrillator ([33270])*
> *Subcutaneous cardioverter-defibrillator electrophysiologic evaluation, subsequent/periodic (93260-93261)*

## 93650-93657 Intracardiac Ablation

> INCLUDES Ablation services include selective delivery of cryo-energy or radiofrequency to targeted tissue
> Electrophysiologic studies performed in the same session with ablation

**93650** Intracardiac catheter ablation of atrioventricular node function, atrioventricular conduction for creation of complete heart block, with or without temporary pacemaker placement

> 🚑 17.2    ⚕ 17.2    **FUD** 000    J 80 ▢
> **AMA:** 2017,Jan,8; 2016,Jan,13; 2015,Jan,16; 2014,Jan,11; 2012,May,14-15; 2012,Apr,17-18

26/TC PC/TC Only    A2-Z3 ASC Payment    50 Bilateral    ♂ Male Only    ♀ Female Only    🚑 Facility RVU    ⚕ Non-Facility RVU    ▢ CCI
FUD Follow-up Days    CMS: IOM (Pub 100)    A-Y OPPSI    80/80 Surg Assist Allowed / w/Doc    ◼ Lab Crosswalk    ◼ Radiology Crosswalk    ✖ CLIA
458    CPT © 2017 American Medical Association. All Rights Reserved.    © 2017 Optum360, LLC

**93653** Comprehensive electrophysiologic evaluation including insertion and repositioning of multiple electrode catheters with induction or attempted induction of an arrhythmia with right atrial pacing and recording, right ventricular pacing and recording (when necessary), and His bundle recording (when necessary) with intracardiac catheter ablation of arrhythmogenic focus; with treatment of supraventricular tachycardia by ablation of fast or slow atrioventricular pathway, accessory atrioventricular connection, cavo-tricuspid isthmus or other single atrial focus or source of atrial re-entry

> EXCLUDES  *Comprehensive electrophysiological studies (93619-93620)*
> *Electrophysiologic evaluation pacing cardioverter defibrillator (93642)*
> *Intracardiac ablation with transseptal catheterization (93656)*
> *Intracardiac ablation with treatment ventricular arrhythmia (93654)*
> *Intracardiac pacing (93610, 93612, 93618)*
> *Recording of intracardiac electrograms (93600-93603)*

24.3   24.3   **FUD** 000   J 80 ▭

**AMA:** 2017,Jan,8; 2016,Jan,13; 2015,Jan,16; 2014,Apr,3; 2013,Jul,7-9; 2013,Jun,6-8

**93654** with treatment of ventricular tachycardia or focus of ventricular ectopy including intracardiac electrophysiologic 3D mapping, when performed, and left ventricular pacing and recording, when performed

> EXCLUDES  *Comprehensive electrophysiological studies (93619-93620, 93622)*
> *Device evaluation (93279-93284, 93286-93289)*
> *Electrophysiologic evaluation pacing cardioverter defibrillator (93642)*
> *Intracardiac ablation with transseptal catheterization (93656)*
> *Intracardiac ablation with treatment supraventricular tachycardia (93653)*
> *Intracardiac pacing (93609-93613, 93618)*
> *Recording of intracardiac electrograms (93600-93603)*

32.6   32.6   **FUD** 000   J 80 ▭

**AMA:** 2017,Jan,8; 2016,Jan,13; 2015,Jan,16; 2014,Apr,3; 2013,Jul,7-9; 2013,Jun,6-8

**+ 93655** Intracardiac catheter ablation of a discrete mechanism of arrhythmia which is distinct from the primary ablated mechanism, including repeat diagnostic maneuvers, to treat a spontaneous or induced arrhythmia (List separately in addition to code for primary procedure)

Code first (93653-93654, 93656)

12.4   12.4   **FUD** ZZZ   N 80 ▭

**AMA:** 2017,Jan,8; 2016,Jan,13; 2015,Jan,16; 2014,Apr,3; 2013,Jul,7-9; 2013,Jun,6-8

**93656** Comprehensive electrophysiologic evaluation including transseptal catheterizations, insertion and repositioning of multiple electrode catheters with induction or attempted induction of an arrhythmia including left or right atrial pacing/recording when necessary, right ventricular pacing/recording when necessary, and His bundle recording when necessary with intracardiac catheter ablation of atrial fibrillation by pulmonary vein isolation

> INCLUDES  His bundle recording when indicated
> Left atrial pacing/recording
> Right ventricular pacing/recording

> EXCLUDES  *Comprehensive electrophysiological studies (93619-93621)*
> *Device evaluation (93279-93284, 93286-93289)*
> *Electrophysiologic evaluation with treatment ventricular tachycardia (93654)*
> *Left heart catheterization by transseptal puncture (93462)*
> *Intracardiac ablation with treatment supraventricular tachycardia (93653)*
> *Intracardiac pacing (93610, 93612, 93618)*
> *Recording of intracardiac electrograms (93600-93603)*

32.7   32.7   **FUD** 000   J 80 ▭

**AMA:** 2017,Jan,8; 2016,Jan,13; 2015,Jan,16; 2014,Apr,3; 2013,Jul,7-9; 2013,Jun,6-8

**+ 93657** Additional linear or focal intracardiac catheter ablation of the left or right atrium for treatment of atrial fibrillation remaining after completion of pulmonary vein isolation (List separately in addition to code for primary procedure)

Code first (93656)

12.3   12.3   **FUD** ZZZ   N 80 ▭

**AMA:** 2017,Jan,8; 2016,Jan,13; 2015,Jan,16; 2014,Apr,3; 2013,Jul,7-9; 2013,Jun,6-8

## 93660-93662 Other Tests for Cardiac Function

**93660** Evaluation of cardiovascular function with tilt table evaluation, with continuous ECG monitoring and intermittent blood pressure monitoring, with or without pharmacological intervention

> EXCLUDES  *Autonomic nervous system function testing (95921, 95924, [95943])*

4.48   4.48   **FUD** 000   S 80 ▭

**AMA:** 2017,Jan,8; 2016,Jan,13; 2015,Jan,16; 2014,Jan,11; 2012,Nov,6-9

**+ 93662** Intracardiac echocardiography during therapeutic/diagnostic intervention, including imaging supervision and interpretation (List separately in addition to code for primary procedure)

> EXCLUDES  *Internal cardioversion (92961)*

Code first (as appropriate) (92987, 93453, 93460-93462, 93532, 93580-93581, 93620-93622, 93653-93654, 93656)

0.00   0.00   **FUD** ZZZ   N 80 ▭

**AMA:** 2017,Jan,8; 2016,Jan,13; 2015,Jan,16; 2014,Jan,11; 2012,Jan,15-42

## 93668 Rehabilitation Services: Peripheral Arterial Disease

> INCLUDES  Monitoring:
> Other cardiovascular limitations for adjustment of workload
> Patient's claudication threshold
> Motorized treadmill or track
> Sessions lasting 45-60 minutes
> Supervision by exercise physiologist/nurse
> Code also appropriate E&M service, when performed

**93668** Peripheral arterial disease (PAD) rehabilitation, per session

0.00   0.00   **FUD** XXX   S ▭

**AMA:** 2008,Mar,4-5

● New Code   ▲ Revised Code   ○ Reinstated   ● New Web Release   ▲ Revised Web Release   Unlisted   Not Covered   # Resequenced
⊘ AMA Mod 51 Exempt   Ⓢ Optum Mod 51 Exempt   Ⓢ Mod 63 Exempt   ✒ Non-FDA Drug   ★ Telemedicine   Ⓜ Maternity   Ⓐ Age Edit   + Add-on   AMA: CPT Asst
© 2017 Optum360, LLC   CPT © 2017 American Medical Association. All Rights Reserved.

**Medicine**

## 93701-93702 Thoracic Electrical Bioimpedance

EXCLUDES *Bioelectrical impedance analysis whole body (0358T)*
*Indirect measurement of left ventricular filling pressure by computerized calibration of the arterial waveform response to Valsalva (93799)*

**93701** **Bioimpedance-derived physiologic cardiovascular analysis**
🔹 0.69 🔸 0.69 **FUD** XXX  [01][80][TC][▯]
**AMA:** 2017,Jan,8; 2016,Jan,13; 2015,Jan,16; 2014,Jan,11

**93702** **Bioimpedance spectroscopy (BIS), extracellular fluid analysis for lymphedema assessment(s)**
🔹 3.49 🔸 3.49 **FUD** XXX  [S][80][TC][▯]

## 93724 Electronic Analysis of Pacemaker Function

**93724** **Electronic analysis of antitachycardia pacemaker system (includes electrocardiographic recording, programming of device, induction and termination of tachycardia via implanted pacemaker, and interpretation of recordings)**
🔹 7.69 🔸 7.69 **FUD** 000  [S][80][▯]
**AMA:** 2017,Jan,8; 2016,Jan,13; 2015,Jan,16; 2014,Jan,11

## 93740 Temperature Gradient Assessment

**93740** **Temperature gradient studies**
🔹 0.23 🔸 0.23 **FUD** XXX  [01][▯]

## 93745 Wearable Cardioverter-Defibrillator System Services

EXCLUDES *Device evaluation (93282, 93292)*

**93745** **Initial set-up and programming by a physician or other qualified health care professional of wearable cardioverter-defibrillator includes initial programming of system, establishing baseline electronic ECG, transmission of data to data repository, patient instruction in wearing system and patient reporting of problems or events**
🔹 0.00 🔸 0.00 **FUD** XXX  [S][80][▯]
**AMA:** 2009,Mar,5-7; 2009,Feb,3-12

## 93750 Ventricular Assist Device (VAD) Interrogation

**CMS:** 100-03,20.9 Artificial Hearts and Related Devices; 100-03,20.9.1 Ventricular Assist Devices; 100-04,32,320.1 Artificial Hearts Prior to May 1, 2008; 100-04,32,320.2 Coding for Artificial Hearts After May 1, 2008; 100-04,32,320.3 Ventricular Assist Devices; 100-04,32,320.3.1 Post-cardiotomy; 100-04,32,320.3.2 Bridge- to -Transplantation

EXCLUDES *Insertion of ventricular assist device (33975-33976, 33979)*
*Removal/replacement ventricular assist device (33981-33983)*

**93750** **Interrogation of ventricular assist device (VAD), in person, with physician or other qualified health care professional analysis of device parameters (eg, drivelines, alarms, power surges), review of device function (eg, flow and volume status, septum status, recovery), with programming, if performed, and report**
🔹 1.32 🔸 1.58 **FUD** XXX  [S][80][▯]
**AMA:** 2017,Jan,8; 2016,Jan,13; 2015,Jan,16; 2014,Jan,11

## 93770 Peripheral Venous Blood Pressure Assessment

**CMS:** 100-03,20.19 Ambulatory Blood Pressure Monitoring (20.19)
EXCLUDES *Cannulization, central venous (36500, 36555-36556)*

**93770** **Determination of venous pressure**
🔹 0.23 🔸 0.23 **FUD** XXX  [N][▯]

## 93784-93790 Ambulatory Blood Pressure Monitoring

**CMS:** 100-03,20.19 Ambulatory Blood Pressure Monitoring (20.19); 100-04,32,10.1 Ambulatory Blood Pressure Monitoring Billing Requirements

**93784** **Ambulatory blood pressure monitoring, utilizing a system such as magnetic tape and/or computer disk, for 24 hours or longer; including recording, scanning analysis, interpretation and report**
🔹 1.52 🔸 1.52 **FUD** XXX  [B][80][▯]
**AMA:** 1991,Win,1

**93786** **recording only**
🔹 0.84 🔸 0.84 **FUD** XXX  [01][80][TC][▯]

**93788** **scanning analysis with report**
🔹 0.15 🔸 0.15 **FUD** XXX  [01][80][TC][▯]

**93790** **review with interpretation and report**
🔹 0.53 🔸 0.53 **FUD** XXX  [M][80][26][▯]

## 93792-93793 INR Monitoring

**CMS:** 100-03,190.11 Home PT/INR Monitoring for Anticoagulation Management; 100-04,32,60.4.1 Anticoagulation Management: Covered Diagnosis Codes

EXCLUDES *Chronic care management ([99490], 99487, 99489)*
*Online evaluation and management services by a physician or other qualified health care professional (99444, 98969)*
*Telephone assessment and management service by nonphysician healthcare professional (98966-98968)*
*Telephone evaluation and management service by physician or other qualified healthcare professional (99441-99443)*
*Transitional care management (99495-99496)*

● **93792** **Patient/caregiver training for initiation of home international normalized ratio (INR) monitoring under the direction of a physician or other qualified health care professional, face-to-face, including use and care of the INR monitor, obtaining blood sample, instructions for reporting home INR test results, and documentation of patient's/caregiver's ability to perform testing and report results**
Code also INR home monitoring equipment with appropriate supply code or (99070)
Code also significantly separately identifiable E&M service on same date of service using modifier 25

● **93793** **Anticoagulant management for a patient taking warfarin, must include review and interpretation of a new home, office, or lab international normalized ratio (INR) test result, patient instructions, dosage adjustment (as needed), and scheduling of additional test(s), when performed**
EXCLUDES *E&M services on same date of service (99201-99215, 99241-99245)*
*Use of code more than one time per day*

## 93797-93799 Cardiac Rehabilitation

**CMS:** 100-02,15,232 Cardiac Rehabilitation and Intensive Cardiac Rehabilitation; 100-04,32,140.2 Cardiac Rehabilitation On or After January 1, 2010; 100-04,32,140.2.1 Coding Cardiac Rehabilitation Services On or After January 1, 2010; 100-04,32,140.2.2.2 Institutional Claims for CR and ICR Services; 100-04,32,140.2.2.4 CR Services Exceeding 36 Sessions; 100-04,32,140.3 Intensive Cardiac Rehabilitation On or After January 1, 2010; 100-08,15,4.2.8 Cardiac Rehabilitation (CR) and Intensive Cardiac Rehabilitation (ICR)

**93797** **Physician or other qualified health care professional services for outpatient cardiac rehabilitation; without continuous ECG monitoring (per session)**
🔹 0.25 🔸 0.46 **FUD** 000  [S][80][▯]

**93798** **with continuous ECG monitoring (per session)**
🔹 0.40 🔸 0.71 **FUD** 000  [S][80][▯]
**AMA:** 2005,Nov,1-9

**93799** **Unlisted cardiovascular service or procedure**
🔹 0.00 🔸 0.00 **FUD** XXX  [S][80]
**AMA:** 2017,Jan,8; 2016,May,5; 2016,Jan,13; 2015,Jan,16; 2014,Jan,11; 2013,Dec,16; 2012,Jan,15-42

## 93880-93895 Noninvasive Tests Extracranial/Intracranial Arteries

INCLUDES Patient care required to perform/supervise studies and interpret results
EXCLUDES *Hand-held dopplers that do not provide a hard copy or vascular flow bidirectional analysis (See E&M codes)*

**93880** **Duplex scan of extracranial arteries; complete bilateral study**
EXCLUDES *Common carotid intima-media thickness (IMT) studies (93895, 0126T)*
🔹 5.73 🔸 5.73 **FUD** XXX  [S][80][▯]
**AMA:** 2017,Jan,8; 2016,Jan,13; 2015,Jan,16; 2014,Jan,11

**93882** **unilateral or limited study**
EXCLUDES *Common carotid intima-media thickness (IMT) studies (93895, 0126T)*
🔹 3.65 🔸 3.65 **FUD** XXX  [S][80][▯]
**AMA:** 2017,Jan,8; 2016,Jan,13; 2015,Jan,16; 2014,Jan,11

[26/TC] PC/TC Only | [M2-Z3] ASC Payment | [50] Bilateral | ♂ Male Only | ♀ Female Only | 🔹 Facility RVU | 🔸 Non-Facility RVU | ▯ CCI
**FUD** Follow-up Days | **CMS:** IOM (Pub 100) | [A-Y] OPPSI | [80/80] Surg Assist Allowed / w/Doc | 🔳 Lab Crosswalk | 🔳 Radiology Crosswalk | 🔳 CLIA

**460** CPT © 2017 American Medical Association. All Rights Reserved. © 2017 Optum360, LLC

93701 — 93882

**93886** **Transcranial Doppler study of the intracranial arteries; complete study**

INCLUDES Complete transcranial doppler (TCD) study
Ultrasound evaluation of right/left anterior circulation territories and posterior circulation territory

🔧 7.81   ⚕ 7.81   **FUD** XXX                    S 80 🖵

**AMA:** 2017,Jan,8; 2016,Jan,13; 2015,Jan,16; 2014,Jan,11

**93888** **limited study**

INCLUDES Limited TCD study
Ultrasound examination of two or fewer of these territories (right/left anterior circulation, posterior circulation)

🔧 4.25   ⚕ 4.25   **FUD** XXX                    S 80 🖵

**AMA:** 2017,Jan,8; 2016,Jan,13; 2015,Jan,16; 2014,Jan,11

**93890** **vasoreactivity study**

EXCLUDES Limited TCD study (93888)

🔧 8.05   ⚕ 8.05   **FUD** XXX                    Q1 80 🖵

**AMA:** 2017,Jan,8; 2016,Jan,13; 2015,Jan,16; 2014,Jan,11

**93892** **emboli detection without intravenous microbubble injection**

EXCLUDES Limited TCD study (93888)

🔧 9.31   ⚕ 9.31   **FUD** XXX                    Q1 80 🖵

**AMA:** 2017,Jan,8; 2016,Jan,13; 2015,Jan,16; 2014,Jan,11

**93893** **emboli detection with intravenous microbubble injection**

EXCLUDES Limited TCD study (93888)

🔧 9.80   ⚕ 9.80   **FUD** XXX                    Q1 80 🖵

**AMA:** 2017,Jan,8; 2016,Jan,13; 2015,Jan,16; 2014,Jan,11

**93895** **Quantitative carotid intima media thickness and carotid atheroma evaluation, bilateral**

🔧 0.00   ⚕ 0.00   **FUD** XXX                    E 80 🖵

EXCLUDES Common carotid intima-media thickness (IMT) study (0126T)
Complete and limited duplex studiies (93880, 93882)

## 93922-93971 Noninvasive Vascular Studies: Extremities

**CMS:** 100-04,8,180 Noninvasive Studies for ESRD Patients

INCLUDES Patient care required to perform/supervise studies and interpret results

EXCLUDES Hand-held dopplers that do not provide a hard copy or provided vascular flow bidirectional analysis (see E&M codes)

**93922** **Limited bilateral noninvasive physiologic studies of upper or lower extremity arteries, (eg, for lower extremity: ankle/brachial indices at distal posterior tibial and anterior tibial/dorsalis pedis arteries plus bidirectional, Doppler waveform recording and analysis at 1-2 levels, or ankle/brachial indices at distal posterior tibial and anterior tibial/dorsalis pedis arteries plus volume plethysmography at 1-2 levels, or ankle/brachial indices at distal posterior tibial and anterior tibial/dorsalis pedis arteries with, transcutaneous oxygen tension measurement at 1-2 levels)**

INCLUDES Evaluation of:
Doppler analysis of bidirectional blood flow
Nonimaging physiologic recordings of pressure
Oxygen tension measurements and/or plethysmography
Lower extremity (potential levels include high thigh, low thigh, calf, ankle, metatarsal and toes) limited study includes either:
Ankle/brachial indices at distal posterior tibial and anterior tibial/dorsalis pedis arteries plus bidirectional Doppler waveform recording and analysis as 1-2 levels; OR
Ankle/brachial indices at distal posterior tibial and anterior tibial/dorsalis pedis arteries plus volume plethysmography at 1-2 levels; OR
Ankle/brachial indices at distal posterior tibial and anterior tibial/dorsalis pedis arteries with transcutaneous oxygen tension measurements at 1-2 levels
Unilateral provocative functional measurement
Unilateral study of 3 or move levels
Upper extremity (potential levels include arm, forearm, wrist, and digits) limited study includes:
Doppler-determined systolic pressures and bidirectional waveform recording with analysis at 1-2 levels; OR
Doppler-determined systolic pressures and transcutaneous oxygen tension measurements at 1-2 levels; OR
Doppler-determined systolic pressures and volume plethysmography at 1-2 levels

EXCLUDES Endothelial function assessment (0337T)
Transcutaneous oxyhemoglobin measurement (0493T)
Use of code more than one time for the lower extremity(s)
Use of code more than one time for the upper extremity(s)
Code also modifier 52 for unilateral study of 1-2 levels
Code also twice with modifier 59 for upper and lower extremity study

🔧 2.51   ⚕ 2.51   **FUD** XXX                    Q1 80 🖵

**AMA:** 2017,Jan,8; 2016,Jan,13; 2015,Jan,16; 2014,Jan,9; 2014,Jan,11; 2013,Jun,13; 2012,Jun,15-16

---

**93923** Complete bilateral noninvasive physiologic studies of upper or lower extremity arteries, 3 or more levels (eg, for lower extremity: ankle/brachial indices at distal posterior tibial and anterior tibial/dorsalis pedis arteries plus segmental blood pressure measurements with bidirectional Doppler waveform recording and analysis, at 3 or more levels, or ankle/brachial indices at distal posterior tibial and anterior tibial/dorsalis pedis arteries plus segmental volume plethysmography at 3 or more levels, or ankle/brachial indices at distal posterior tibial and anterior tibial/dorsalis pedis arteries plus segmental transcutaneous oxygen tension measurements at 3 or more levels), or single level study with provocative functional maneuvers (eg, measurements with postural provocative tests, or measurements with reactive hyperemia)

INCLUDES Evaluation of:
Doppler analysis of bidirectional blood flow
Nonimaging physiologic recordings of pressures
Oxygen tension measurements
Lower extremity:
Ankle/brachial indices at distal posterior tibial and anterior tibial/dorsalis pedis arteries plus bidirectional Doppler waveform recording and analysis at 3 or more levels; OR
Ankle/brachial indices at distal posterior tibial and anterior tibial/dorsalis pedis arteries with transcutaneous oxygen tension measurements at 3 or more levels; OR
Ankle/brachial indices at distal posterior tibial and anterior tibial/dorsalis pedis arteries plus volume plethysmography at 3 or more levels; OR
Provocative functional maneuvers and measurement at a single level
Upper extremity complete study:
Doppler-determined systolic pressures and bidirectional waveform recording with analysis at 3 or more levels; OR
Doppler-determined systolic pressures and transcutaneous oxygen tension measurements at 3 or more levels; OR
Doppler-determined systolic pressures and volume plethysmography at 3 or more levels; OR
Provocative functional maneuvers and measurement at a single level

EXCLUDES Endothelial function assessment (0337T)
Unilateral study at 3 or more levels (93922)
Use of code more than one time for the lower extremity(s)
Use of code more than one time for the upper extremity(s)
Code also twice with modifier 59 for upper and lower extremity study

3.90 3.90 FUD XXX S 80

AMA: 2017,Jan,8; 2016,Jan,13; 2015,Jan,16; 2014,Jan,9; 2014,Jan,11; 2012,Jun,15-16; 2012,Jan,15-42

**93924** Noninvasive physiologic studies of lower extremity arteries, at rest and following treadmill stress testing, (ie, bidirectional Doppler waveform or volume plethysmography recording and analysis at rest with ankle/brachial indices immediately after and at timed intervals following performance of a standardized protocol on a motorized treadmill plus recording of time of onset of claudication or other symptoms, maximal walking time, and time to recovery) complete bilateral study

INCLUDES Evaluation of:
Doppler analysis of bidirectional blood flow
Non-imaging physiologic recordings of pressures
Oxygen tension measurements
Plethysmography

EXCLUDES Noninvasive vascular studies of extremities (93922-93923)
Other types of exercise

4.86 4.86 FUD XXX S 80

AMA: 2017,Jan,8; 2016,Jan,13; 2015,Jan,16; 2014,Jan,9; 2014,Jan,11; 2012,Jun,15-16

**93925** Duplex scan of lower extremity arteries or arterial bypass grafts; complete bilateral study

7.33 7.33 FUD XXX S 80

AMA: 2017,Jan,8; 2016,Sep,9; 2016,Jan,13; 2015,Jan,16; 2014,Jan,11

**93926** unilateral or limited study

4.30 4.30 FUD XXX S 80

AMA: 2017,Jan,8; 2016,Sep,9; 2016,Jan,13; 2015,Jan,16; 2014,Jan,11

**93930** Duplex scan of upper extremity arteries or arterial bypass grafts; complete bilateral study

5.89 5.89 FUD XXX S 80

AMA: 2017,Jan,8; 2016,Sep,9; 2016,Jan,13; 2015,Jan,16; 2014,Jan,11

**93931** unilateral or limited study

3.64 3.64 FUD XXX S 80

AMA: 2017,Jan,8; 2016,Sep,9; 2016,Jan,13; 2015,Jan,16; 2014,Jan,11

**93970** Duplex scan of extremity veins including responses to compression and other maneuvers; complete bilateral study

EXCLUDES Endovenous ablation (36475-36476, 36478-36479)

5.58 5.58 FUD XXX S 80

AMA: 2017,Jan,8; 2016,Nov,3; 2016,Sep,9; 2016,Jan,13; 2015,Jan,16; 2014,Oct,6; 2014,Jan,11; 2012,Feb,11; 2012,Jan,13-14

**93971** unilateral or limited study

EXCLUDES Endovenous ablation (36475-36476, 36478-36479)

3.40 3.40 FUD XXX S 80

AMA: 2017,Jan,8; 2016,Nov,3; 2016,Sep,9; 2016,Jan,13; 2015,Aug,8; 2015,Jan,16; 2014,Oct,6; 2014,Jan,11; 2012,Feb,11; 2012,Jan,15-42; 2012,Jan,13-14

## 93975-93982 Noninvasive Vascular Studies: Abdomen/Chest/Pelvis

**93975** Duplex scan of arterial inflow and venous outflow of abdominal, pelvic, scrotal contents and/or retroperitoneal organs; complete study

7.98 7.98 FUD XXX S 80

AMA: 2017,Jan,8; 2016,Aug,9; 2016,Jan,13; 2015,Mar,9; 2015,Jan,16; 2014,Jun,14; 2014,Jan,11; 2012,Jan,15-42

**93976** limited study

4.63 4.63 FUD XXX S 80

AMA: 2017,Jan,8; 2016,Aug,9; 2016,Jan,13; 2015,Mar,9; 2015,Jan,16; 2014,Jan,11; 2012,Jan,15-42

**93978** Duplex scan of aorta, inferior vena cava, iliac vasculature, or bypass grafts; complete study

EXCLUDES Ultrasound screening for abdominal aortic aneurysm (76706)

5.40 5.40 FUD XXX S 80

AMA: 2017,Jan,8; 2016,Jan,13; 2015,Jan,16; 2014,Jan,11

**93979** unilateral or limited study

EXCLUDES Ultrasound screening for abdominal aortic aneurysm (76706)

3.39 3.39 FUD XXX Q 80

AMA: 2017,Jan,8; 2016,Jan,13; 2015,Jan,16; 2014,Jun,14; 2014,Jan,11

**93980** Duplex scan of arterial inflow and venous outflow of penile vessels; complete study

3.44 3.44 FUD XXX S 80

AMA: 2017,Jan,8; 2016,Jan,13; 2015,Jan,16; 2014,Jan,11

**93981** follow-up or limited study

2.09 2.09 FUD XXX S 80

AMA: 2017,Jan,8; 2016,Jan,13; 2015,Jan,16; 2014,Jan,11

**93982** ~~Noninvasive physiologic study of implanted wireless pressure sensor in aneurysmal sac following endovascular repair, complete study including recording, analysis of pressure and waveform tracings, interpretation and report~~

## 93990-93998 Noninvasive Vascular Studies: Hemodialysis Access

**93990** Duplex scan of hemodialysis access (including arterial inflow, body of access and venous outflow)

> **EXCLUDES** *Hemodialysis access flow measurement by indicator method (90940)*
> 🚑 4.51   ⚕ 4.51   **FUD** XXX    [01] [80] 🖵
> **AMA:** 2017,Jan,8; 2016,Jan,13; 2015,Jan,16; 2014,Jan,11

**93998** Unlisted noninvasive vascular diagnostic study

> 🚑 0.00   ⚕ 0.00   **FUD** XXX    [01] [80] 🖵
> **AMA:** 2017,Jan,8; 2016,Jan,13; 2015,Jan,16; 2014,Jan,9; 2012,Oct,13; 2012,Sep,9

## 94002-94005 Ventilator Management Services

**94002** Ventilation assist and management, initiation of pressure or volume preset ventilators for assisted or controlled breathing; hospital inpatient/observation, initial day

> **EXCLUDES** *E&M services*
> 🚑 2.63   ⚕ 2.63   **FUD** XXX    [03] [80] 🖵
> **AMA:** 2017,Jan,8; 2016,Jan,13; 2015,Jan,16; 2014,Oct,8; 2014,May,4; 2014,Jan,11; 2012,Jan,15-42

**94003** hospital inpatient/observation, each subsequent day

> **EXCLUDES** *E&M services*
> 🚑 1.90   ⚕ 1.90   **FUD** XXX    [03] [80] 🖵
> **AMA:** 2017,Jan,8; 2016,Jan,13; 2015,Jan,16; 2014,Oct,8; 2014,May,4; 2014,Jan,11

**94004** nursing facility, per day

> **EXCLUDES** *E&M services*
> 🚑 1.40   ⚕ 1.40   **FUD** XXX    [B] [80] 🖵
> **AMA:** 2017,Jan,8; 2016,Jan,13; 2015,Jan,16; 2014,Oct,8; 2014,Jan,11

**94005** Home ventilator management care plan oversight of a patient (patient not present) in home, domiciliary or rest home (eg, assisted living) requiring review of status, review of laboratories and other studies and revision of orders and respiratory care plan (as appropriate), within a calendar month, 30 minutes or more

> Code also when a different provider reports care plan oversight in the same 30 days (99339-99340, 99374-99378)
> 🚑 2.63   ⚕ 2.63   **FUD** XXX    [M] 🖵
> **AMA:** 2017,Jan,8; 2016,Jan,13; 2015,Jan,16; 2014,Oct,8; 2014,Jan,11; 2012,Jan,15-42

## 94010-94799 Respiratory Services: Diagnostic and Therapeutic

> **INCLUDES** Laboratory procedure(s)
> Test results interpretation
> **EXCLUDES** *Separately identifiable E&M service*

**94010** Spirometry, including graphic record, total and timed vital capacity, expiratory flow rate measurement(s), with or without maximal voluntary ventilation

> **INCLUDES** Measurement of expiratory airflow and volumes
> **EXCLUDES** *Diffusing capacity (94729)*
> *Other respiratory function services (94150, 94200, 94375, 94728)*
> 🚑 1.01   ⚕ 1.01   **FUD** XXX    [01] [80] 🖵
> **AMA:** 2017,Jan,8; 2016,Jan,13; 2015,Sep,9; 2015,Jan,16; 2014,Mar,11; 2014,Jan,11; 2013,Dec,12; 2012,Nov,13-14; 2012,Nov,11-12; 2012,Aug,6-8; 2012,Jan,15-42

**94011** Measurement of spirometric forced expiratory flows in an infant or child through 2 years of age

> 🚑 2.61   ⚕ 2.61   **FUD** XXX    [01] [80] 🖵
> **AMA:** 2017,Jan,8; 2016,Jan,13; 2015,Jan,16; 2014,Jan,11; 2013,Dec,12; 2012,Aug,6-8

**94012** Measurement of spirometric forced expiratory flows, before and after bronchodilator, in an infant or child through 2 years of age

> 🚑 4.20   ⚕ 4.20   **FUD** XXX    [01] [80] 🖵
> **AMA:** 2017,Jan,8; 2016,Jan,13; 2015,Jan,16; 2014,Jan,11; 2013,Dec,12; 2012,Aug,6-8

**94013** Measurement of lung volumes (ie, functional residual capacity [FRC], forced vital capacity [FVC], and expiratory reserve volume [ERV]) in an infant or child through 2 years of age

> 🚑 0.57   ⚕ 0.57   **FUD** XXX    [S] [80] 🖵
> **AMA:** 2017,Jan,8; 2016,Jan,13; 2015,Jan,16; 2014,Jan,11; 2013,Dec,12; 2012,Aug,6-8

**94014** Patient-initiated spirometric recording per 30-day period of time; includes reinforced education, transmission of spirometric tracing, data capture, analysis of transmitted data, periodic recalibration and review and interpretation by a physician or other qualified health care professional

> 🚑 1.60   ⚕ 1.60   **FUD** XXX    [01] [80] 🖵
> **AMA:** 2017,Jan,8; 2016,Jan,13; 2015,Jan,16; 2014,Jan,11; 2013,Dec,12; 2012,Aug,6-8

**94015** recording (includes hook-up, reinforced education, data transmission, data capture, trend analysis, and periodic recalibration)

> 🚑 0.88   ⚕ 0.88   **FUD** XXX    [01] [80] [TC] 🖵
> **AMA:** 2017,Jan,8; 2016,Jan,13; 2015,Jan,16; 2014,Jan,11; 2013,Dec,12; 2012,Aug,6-8

**94016** review and interpretation only by a physician or other qualified health care professional

> 🚑 0.72   ⚕ 0.72   **FUD** XXX    [A] [80] [26] 🖵
> **AMA:** 2017,Jan,8; 2016,Jan,13; 2015,Jan,16; 2014,Jan,11; 2013,Dec,12; 2012,Aug,6-8

**94060** Bronchodilation responsiveness, spirometry as in 94010, pre- and post-bronchodilator administration

> **INCLUDES** Spirometry performed prior to and after a bronchodilator has been administered
> **EXCLUDES** *Bronchospasm prolonged exercise test with pre- and post-spirometry (94617)*
> *Diffusing capacity (94729)*
> *Other respiratory function services (94150, 94200, 94375, 94640, 94728)*
> Code also bronchodilator supply with appropriate supply code or (99070)
> 🚑 1.72   ⚕ 1.72   **FUD** XXX    [S] [80] 🖵
> **AMA:** 2017,Jan,8; 2016,Jan,13; 2015,Sep,9; 2015,Jan,16; 2014,Mar,11; 2014,Jan,11; 2013,Dec,12; 2012,Aug,6-8; 2012,Jan,15-42

**94070** Bronchospasm provocation evaluation, multiple spirometric determinations as in 94010, with administered agents (eg, antigen[s], cold air, methacholine)

> **EXCLUDES** *Diffusing capacity (94729)*
> *Inhalation treatment (diagnostic or therapeutic) (94640)*
> Code also antigen(s) administration with appropriate supply code or (99070)
> 🚑 1.70   ⚕ 1.70   **FUD** XXX    [S] [80] 🖵
> **AMA:** 2017,Jan,8; 2016,Jan,13; 2015,Sep,9; 2015,Jan,16; 2014,Jan,11; 2013,Dec,12; 2012,Nov,11-12; 2012,Aug,6-8

**94150** Vital capacity, total (separate procedure)

> **EXCLUDES** *Other respiratory function services (94010, 94060, 94728)*
> *Thoracic gas volumes (94726-94727)*
> 🚑 0.71   ⚕ 0.71   **FUD** XXX    [01] 🖵
> **AMA:** 2017,Jan,8; 2016,Jan,13; 2015,Jan,16; 2014,Mar,11; 2014,Jan,11; 2013,Dec,12; 2012,Aug,6-8; 2012,Jan,15-42

**94200** Maximum breathing capacity, maximal voluntary ventilation

> **EXCLUDES** *Other respiratory function services (94010, 94060)*
> 🚑 0.73   ⚕ 0.73   **FUD** XXX    [01] [80] 🖵
> **AMA:** 2017,Jan,8; 2016,Jan,13; 2015,Jan,16; 2014,Mar,11; 2014,Jan,11; 2013,Dec,12; 2012,Aug,6-8; 2012,Jan,15-42

Medicine

94250 — 94667

**94250** **Expired gas collection, quantitative, single procedure (separate procedure)**
> EXCLUDES *Complex pulmonary stress test (94621)*
> ✈ 0.75 ⚕ 0.75 **FUD** XXX [01][80][⌨]
>
> **AMA:** 2017,Jan,8; 2016,Jan,13; 2015,Dec,16; 2015,Jan,16; 2014,Jan,11; 2013,Dec,12; 2012,Aug,6-8

**94375** **Respiratory flow volume loop**
> INCLUDES Identification of obstruction patterns in central or peripheral airways (inspiratory and/or expiratory)
> EXCLUDES *Diffusing capacity (94729)*
> *Other respiratory function services (94010, 94060, 94728)*
> ✈ 1.12 ⚕ 1.12 **FUD** XXX [01][80][⌨]
>
> **AMA:** 2017,Jan,8; 2016,Jan,13; 2015,Jan,16; 2014,Mar,11; 2014,Jan,11; 2013,Dec,12; 2012,Aug,6-8

**94400** **Breathing response to CO2 (CO2 response curve)**
> EXCLUDES *Inhalation treatment (diagnostic or therapeutic) (94640)*
> ✈ 1.61 ⚕ 1.61 **FUD** XXX [01][80][⌨]
>
> **AMA:** 2017,Jan,8; 2016,Jan,13; 2015,Sep,9; 2015,Jan,16; 2014,Mar,11; 2014,Jan,11; 2013,Dec,12; 2012,Aug,6-8; 2012,Jan,15-42

**94450** **Breathing response to hypoxia (hypoxia response curve)**
> EXCLUDES *HAST - high altitude simulation test (94452, 94453)*
> ✈ 1.96 ⚕ 1.96 **FUD** XXX [01][80][⌨]
>
> **AMA:** 2017,Jan,8; 2016,Jan,13; 2015,Jan,16; 2014,Jan,11; 2013,Dec,12; 2012,Aug,6-8

**94452** **High altitude simulation test (HAST), with interpretation and report by a physician or other qualified health care professional;**
> EXCLUDES *HAST test with supplemental oxygen titration (94453)*
> *Noninvasive pulse oximetry (94760-94761)*
> *Obtaining arterial blood gases (36600)*
> ✈ 1.63 ⚕ 1.63 **FUD** XXX [01][80][⌨]
>
> **AMA:** 2017,Jan,8; 2016,Jan,13; 2015,Jan,16; 2014,Jan,11; 2013,Dec,12; 2012,Aug,6-8

**94453** **with supplemental oxygen titration**
> EXCLUDES *HAST test without supplemental oxygen titration (94452)*
> *Noninvasive pulse oximetry (94760-94761)*
> *Obtaining arterial blood gases (36600)*
> ✈ 2.26 ⚕ 2.26 **FUD** XXX [01][80][⌨]
>
> **AMA:** 2017,Jan,8; 2016,Jan,13; 2015,Jan,16; 2014,Jan,11; 2013,Dec,12; 2012,Aug,6-8

**94610** **Intrapulmonary surfactant administration by a physician or other qualified health care professional through endotracheal tube**
> INCLUDES Reporting once per dosing episode
> EXCLUDES *Intubation, endotracheal (31500)*
> *Neonatal critical care (99468-99472)*
> ✈ 1.59 ⚕ 1.59 **FUD** XXX [⊘][01][80][⌨]
>
> **AMA:** 2017,Jan,8; 2016,Jan,13; 2015,Jan,16; 2014,Jan,11; 2013,Dec,12; 2012,Aug,6-8; 2012,Jan,15-42

● **94617** **Exercise test for bronchospasm, including pre- and post-spirometry, electrocardiographic recording(s), and pulse oximetry**
> EXCLUDES *Cardiovascular stress test (93015-93018)*
> *ECG monitoring (93000-93010, 93040-93042)*
> *Pulse oximetry (94760-94761)*

● **94618** **Pulmonary stress testing (eg, 6-minute walk test), including measurement of heart rate, oximetry, and oxygen titration, when performed**
> EXCLUDES *Pulse oximetry (94760-94761)*

**94620** ~~Pulmonary stress testing; simple (eg, 6-minute walk test, prolonged exercise test for bronchospasm with pre- and post-spirometry and oximetry)~~
> To report, see 94618

▲ **94621** **Cardiopulmonary exercise testing, including measurements of minute ventilation, CO2 production, O2 uptake, and electrocardiographic recordings**
> EXCLUDES *Cardiovascular stress test (93015-93018)*
> *ECG monitoring (93000-93010, 93040-93042)*
> *Expired gas collection (94250)*
> *Oxygen uptake expired gas analysis (94680-94690)*
> *Pulse oximetry (94760-94761)*
> ✈ 4.60 ⚕ 4.60 **FUD** XXX [S][80][⌨]
>
> **AMA:** 2017,Jan,8; 2016,Jan,13; 2015,Jan,16; 2014,Jan,11; 2013,Dec,12; 2012,Nov,13-14; 2012,Aug,6-8; 2012,Jan,15-42

**94640** **Pressurized or nonpressurized inhalation treatment for acute airway obstruction for therapeutic purposes and/or for diagnostic purposes such as sputum induction with an aerosol generator, nebulizer, metered dose inhaler or intermittent positive pressure breathing (IPPB) device**
> EXCLUDES *1 hour or more of continuous inhalation treatment (94644, 94645)*
> *Other respiratory function services (94060, 94070, 94400)*
> Code also modifier 76 when more than 1 inhalation treatment is performed on the same date
> ✈ 0.52 ⚕ 0.52 **FUD** XXX [01][80][⌨]
>
> **AMA:** 2017,Jan,8; 2016,Jan,13; 2015,Sep,9; 2015,Jan,16; 2014,Mar,11; 2014,Jan,11; 2013,Dec,12; 2012,Aug,6-8; 2012,Jan,15-42

**94642** **Aerosol inhalation of pentamidine for pneumocystis carinii pneumonia treatment or prophylaxis**
> ✈ 0.00 ⚕ 0.00 **FUD** XXX [01][80][⌨]
>
> **AMA:** 2017,Jan,8; 2016,Jan,13; 2015,Jan,16; 2014,Jan,11; 2013,Dec,12; 2012,Aug,6-8

**94644** **Continuous inhalation treatment with aerosol medication for acute airway obstruction; first hour**
> EXCLUDES *Services that are less than 1 hour (94640)*
> ✈ 1.25 ⚕ 1.25 **FUD** XXX [01][80][⌨]
>
> **AMA:** 2017,Jan,8; 2016,Jan,13; 2015,Sep,9; 2015,Jan,16; 2014,Mar,11; 2014,Jan,11; 2013,Dec,12; 2012,Aug,6-8

+ **94645** **each additional hour (List separately in addition to code for primary procedure)**
> Code first initial hour (94644)
> ✈ 0.41 ⚕ 0.41 **FUD** XXX [N][80][⌨]
>
> **AMA:** 2017,Jan,8; 2016,Jan,13; 2015,Sep,9; 2015,Jan,16; 2014,Mar,11; 2014,Jan,11; 2013,Dec,12; 2012,Aug,6-8

**94660** **Continuous positive airway pressure ventilation (CPAP), initiation and management**
> ✈ 1.09 ⚕ 1.80 **FUD** XXX [01][80][⌨]
>
> **AMA:** 2017,Jan,8; 2016,Jan,13; 2015,Jan,16; 2014,Oct,8; 2014,May,4; 2014,Jan,11; 2013,Dec,12; 2012,Aug,6-8; 2012,Jan,15-42

**94662** **Continuous negative pressure ventilation (CNP), initiation and management**
> ✈ 1.00 ⚕ 1.00 **FUD** XXX [03][80][⌨]
>
> **AMA:** 2017,Jan,8; 2016,Jan,13; 2015,Jan,16; 2014,May,4; 2014,Jan,11; 2013,Dec,12; 2012,Aug,6-8; 2012,Jan,15-42

**94664** **Demonstration and/or evaluation of patient utilization of an aerosol generator, nebulizer, metered dose inhaler or IPPB device**
> INCLUDES Reporting only one time per day of service
> ✈ 0.49 ⚕ 0.49 **FUD** XXX [01][80][⌨]
>
> **AMA:** 2017,Jan,8; 2016,Jan,13; 2015,Jan,16; 2014,Jan,11; 2013,Dec,12; 2012,Aug,6-8; 2012,Jan,15-42

**94667** **Manipulation chest wall, such as cupping, percussing, and vibration to facilitate lung function; initial demonstration and/or evaluation**
> ✈ 0.75 ⚕ 0.75 **FUD** XXX [01][80][⌨]
>
> **AMA:** 2017,Jan,8; 2016,Jan,13; 2015,Sep,9; 2015,Jan,16; 2014,Mar,11; 2014,Jan,11; 2013,Dec,12; 2012,Aug,6-8; 2012,Jan,15-42

26/TC PC/TC Only | A2-Z3 ASC Payment | 50 Bilateral | ♂ Male Only | ♀ Female Only | ✈ Facility RVU | ⚕ Non-Facility RVU | ⌨ CCI
FUD Follow-up Days | CMS: IOM (Pub 100) | A-Y OPPSI | 80/80 Surg Assist Allowed / w/Doc | ▨ Lab Crosswalk | ▦ Radiology Crosswalk | ☒ CLIA

464
CPT © 2017 American Medical Association. All Rights Reserved.
© 2017 Optum360, LLC

**94668** **subsequent**

🖩 0.83 ⚖ 0.83 **FUD** XXX 〔Q1〕〔80〕🖵

**AMA:** 2017,Jan,8; 2016,Jan,13; 2015,Sep,9; 2015,Jan,16; 2014,Mar,11; 2014,Jan,11; 2013,Dec,12; 2012,Aug,6-8; 2012,Jan,15-42

**94669** **Mechanical chest wall oscillation to facilitate lung function, per session**

INCLUDES Application of an external wrap or vest to provide mechanical oscillation

🖩 0.93 ⚖ 0.93 **FUD** XXX 〔Q1〕〔80〕🖵

**AMA:** 2017,Jan,8; 2016,Jan,13; 2015,Jan,16; 2014,Jan,11; 2013,Dec,12

**94680** **Oxygen uptake, expired gas analysis; rest and exercise, direct, simple**

EXCLUDES Cardiopulmonary stress testing (94621)

🖩 1.61 ⚖ 1.61 **FUD** XXX 〔Q1〕〔80〕🖵

**AMA:** 2017,Jan,8; 2016,Jan,13; 2015,Jan,16; 2014,Jan,11; 2013,Dec,12; 2012,Aug,6-8

**94681** **including CO2 output, percentage oxygen extracted**

EXCLUDES Cardiopulmonary stress testing (94621)

🖩 1.53 ⚖ 1.53 **FUD** XXX 〔Q1〕〔80〕🖵

**AMA:** 2017,Jan,8; 2016,Jan,13; 2015,Jan,16; 2014,Jan,11; 2013,Dec,12; 2012,Aug,6-8

**94690** **rest, indirect (separate procedure)**

EXCLUDES Arterial puncture (36600)
Cardiopulmonary stress testing (94621)

🖩 1.45 ⚖ 1.45 **FUD** XXX 〔Q1〕〔80〕🖵

**AMA:** 2017,Jan,8; 2016,Jan,13; 2015,Jan,16; 2014,Jan,11; 2013,Dec,12; 2012,Aug,6-8

**94726** **Plethysmography for determination of lung volumes and, when performed, airway resistance**

INCLUDES Airway resistance
Determination of:
Functional residual capacity
Residual volume
Total lung capacity

EXCLUDES Airway resistance (94728)
Bronchial provocation (94070)
Diffusing capacity (94729)
Gas dilution or washout (94727)
Spirometry (94010, 94060)

🖩 1.49 ⚖ 1.49 **FUD** XXX 〔Q1〕〔80〕🖵

**AMA:** 2017,Jan,8; 2016,Jan,13; 2015,Jan,16; 2014,Jan,11; 2013,Dec,12; 2013,May,11; 2012,Aug,6-8; 2012,Jan,3-5

**94727** **Gas dilution or washout for determination of lung volumes and, when performed, distribution of ventilation and closing volumes**

EXCLUDES Bronchial provocation (94070)
Diffusing capacity (94729)
Plethysmography for lung volume/airway resistance (94726)
Spirometry (94010, 94060)

🖩 1.19 ⚖ 1.19 **FUD** XXX 〔Q1〕〔80〕🖵

**AMA:** 2017,Jan,8; 2016,Jan,13; 2015,Jan,16; 2014,Jan,11; 2013,Dec,12; 2013,May,11; 2012,Aug,6-8; 2012,Jan,3-5

**94728** **Airway resistance by impulse oscillometry**

EXCLUDES Diffusing capacity (94729)
Gas dilution techniques
Other respiratory function services (94010, 94060, 94070, 94375, 94726)

🖩 1.12 ⚖ 1.12 **FUD** XXX 〔Q1〕〔80〕🖵

**AMA:** 2017,Jan,8; 2016,Jan,13; 2015,Jan,16; 2014,Mar,11; 2014,Jan,11; 2013,Dec,12; 2013,May,11; 2012,Aug,6-8; 2012,Jan,3-5

**+ 94729** **Diffusing capacity (eg, carbon monoxide, membrane) (List separately in addition to code for primary procedure)**

Code first (94010, 94060, 94070, 94375, 94726-94728)

🖩 1.54 ⚖ 1.54 **FUD** ZZZ 〔N〕〔80〕🖵

**AMA:** 2017,Jan,8; 2016,Jan,13; 2015,Jan,16; 2014,Jan,11; 2013,Dec,12; 2012,Aug,6-8; 2012,Jan,3-5

**94750** **Pulmonary compliance study (eg, plethysmography, volume and pressure measurements)**

🖩 2.23 ⚖ 2.23 **FUD** XXX 〔Q1〕〔80〕🖵

**AMA:** 2017,Jan,8; 2016,Jan,13; 2015,Jan,16; 2014,Jan,11; 2013,Dec,12; 2012,Aug,6-8

**94760** **Noninvasive ear or pulse oximetry for oxygen saturation; single determination**

EXCLUDES Blood gases (82803-82810)
Cardiopulmonary stress testing (94621)
Exercise test for bronchospasm (94617)
Pulmonary stress testing (94618)

🖩 0.09 ⚖ 0.09 **FUD** XXX 〔N〕〔80〕〔TC〕🖵

**AMA:** 2017,Jan,8; 2016,Jan,13; 2015,Jan,16; 2014,May,4; 2014,Jan,11; 2013,Dec,12; 2012,Aug,6-8; 2012,Jan,15-42

**94761** **multiple determinations (eg, during exercise)**

EXCLUDES Cardiopulmonary stress testing (94621)
Exercise test for bronchospasm (94617)
Pulmonary stress testing (94618)

🖩 0.13 ⚖ 0.13 **FUD** XXX 〔N〕〔80〕〔TC〕🖵

**AMA:** 2017,Jan,8; 2016,Jan,13; 2015,Jan,16; 2014,May,4; 2014,Jan,11; 2013,Dec,12; 2012,Aug,6-8; 2012,Jan,15-42

**94762** **by continuous overnight monitoring (separate procedure)**

🖩 0.69 ⚖ 0.69 **FUD** XXX 〔Q3〕〔80〕〔TC〕🖵

**AMA:** 2017,Jan,8; 2016,Jan,13; 2015,Jan,16; 2014,May,4; 2014,Jan,11; 2013,Dec,12; 2012,Aug,6-8

**94770** **Carbon dioxide, expired gas determination by infrared analyzer**

EXCLUDES Arterial catheterization/cannulation (36620)
Arterial puncture (36600)
Bronchoscopy (31622-31654 [31651])
Flow directed catheter placement (93503)
Needle biopsy of the lung (32405)
Orotracheal/nasotracheal intubation (31500)
Placement of central venous catheter (36555-36556)
Therapeutic phlebotomy (99195)
Thoracentesis (32554-32555)
Venipuncture (36410)

🖩 0.21 ⚖ 0.21 **FUD** XXX 〔S〕〔80〕🖵

**AMA:** 2017,Jan,8; 2016,Jan,13; 2015,Jan,16; 2014,Mar,11; 2014,Jan,11; 2013,Dec,12; 2012,Aug,6-8

**94772** **Circadian respiratory pattern recording (pediatric pneumogram), 12-24 hour continuous recording, infant** 🅰

EXCLUDES Electromyograms/EEG/ECG/respiration recordings

🖩 0.00 ⚖ 0.00 **FUD** XXX 〔S〕〔80〕🖵

**AMA:** 2017,Jan,8; 2016,Jan,13; 2015,Jan,16; 2014,Jan,11; 2013,Dec,12; 2012,Aug,6-8

**94774** **Pediatric home apnea monitoring event recording including respiratory rate, pattern and heart rate per 30-day period of time; includes monitor attachment, download of data, review, interpretation, and preparation of a report by a physician or other qualified health care professional** 🅰

INCLUDES Oxygen saturation monitoring
EXCLUDES Event monitors (93268-93272)
Holter monitor (93224-93227)
Pediatric home apnea services (94775-94777)
Remote cardiovascular telemetry (93228-93229)
Sleep testing (95805-95811 [95800, 95801])

🖩 0.00 ⚖ 0.00 **FUD** YYY 〔B〕〔80〕🖵

**AMA:** 2017,Jan,8; 2016,Jan,13; 2015,Jan,16; 2014,Jan,11; 2013,Dec,12; 2012,Aug,6-8

● New Code ▲ Revised Code ○ Reinstated ● New Web Release ▲ Revised Web Release Unlisted Not Covered # Resequenced
⊘ AMA Mod 51 Exempt ⑤ Optum Mod 51 Exempt ⊚ Mod 63 Exempt ⩘ Non-FDA Drug ★ Telemedicine Ⓜ Maternity 🅰 Age Edit + Add-on **AMA:** CPT Asst

**94775** monitor attachment only (includes hook-up, initiation of recording and disconnection) [A]

> INCLUDES Oxygen saturation monitoring
> EXCLUDES *Event monitors (93268-93272)*
> *Holter monitor (93224-93227)*
> *Remote cardiovascular telemetry (93228-93229)*
> *Sleep testing (95805-95811 [95800, 95801])*

🖫 0.00  ⅍ 0.00  **FUD** YYY  [S] [80] [TC] [▭]

**AMA:** 2017,Jan,8; 2016,Jan,13; 2015,Jan,16; 2014,Jan,11; 2013,Dec,12; 2012,Aug,6-8

**94776** monitoring, download of information, receipt of transmission(s) and analyses by computer only [A]

> INCLUDES Oxygen saturation monitoring
> EXCLUDES *Event monitors (93268-93272)*
> *Holter monitor (93224-93227)*
> *Remote cardiovascular telemetry (93228-93229)*
> *Sleep testing (95805-95811 [95800, 95801])*

🖫 0.00  ⅍ 0.00  **FUD** YYY  [S] [80] [TC] [▭]

**AMA:** 2017,Jan,8; 2016,Jan,13; 2015,Jan,16; 2014,Jan,11; 2013,Dec,12; 2012,Aug,6-8

**94777** review, interpretation and preparation of report only by a physician or other qualified health care professional [A]

> INCLUDES Oxygen saturation monitoring
> EXCLUDES *Event monitors (93268-93272)*
> *Holter monitor (93224-93227)*
> *Remote cardiovascular telemetry (93228-93229)*
> *Sleep testing (95805-95811 [95800, 95801])*

🖫 0.00  ⅍ 0.00  **FUD** YYY  [B] [80] [26] [▭]

**AMA:** 2017,Jan,8; 2016,Jan,13; 2015,Jan,16; 2014,Jan,11; 2013,Dec,12; 2012,Aug,6-8

**94780** Car seat/bed testing for airway integrity, neonate, with continual nursing observation and continuous recording of pulse oximetry, heart rate and respiratory rate, with interpretation and report; 60 minutes [A]

> EXCLUDES *Pediatric and neonatal critical care services (99468-99476, 99477-99480)*
> *Pulse oximetry (94760-94761)*
> *Rhythm strips (93040-93042)*
> *Use of code for less than 60 minutes of service*

🖫 0.70  ⅍ 1.68  **FUD** XXX  [01] [▭]

**AMA:** 2017,Jan,8; 2016,Jan,13; 2015,May,10; 2015,Jan,16; 2014,Jan,11; 2013,Dec,12; 2012,Aug,6-8

+ **94781** each additional full 30 minutes (List separately in addition to code for primary procedure) [A]

Code first (94780)

🖫 0.25  ⅍ 0.65  **FUD** ZZZ  [N] [▭]

**AMA:** 2017,Jan,8; 2016,Jan,13; 2015,May,10; 2015,Jan,16; 2014,Jan,11; 2013,Dec,12; 2012,Aug,6-8

**94799** Unlisted pulmonary service or procedure

🖫 0.00  ⅍ 0.00  **FUD** XXX  [01] [80]

**AMA:** 2017,Jan,8; 2016,Jan,13; 2015,Dec,16; 2015,May,10; 2015,Jan,16; 2014,Jan,11; 2013,Dec,12; 2012,Nov,13-14; 2012,Aug,6-8; 2012,Jan,15-42

## 95004-95071 Allergy Tests

> EXCLUDES *Drugs administered for intractable/severe allergic reaction (eg, antihistamines, epinephrine, steroids) (96372)*
> *E&M services when reporting test interpretation/report*
> *Laboratory tests for allergies (86000-86999 [86152, 86153])*

Code also medical conferences regarding use of equipment (eg, air filters, humidifiers, dehumidifiers), climate therapy, physical, occupational, and recreation therapy using appropriate E&M codes

Code also significant, separately identifiable E&M services using modifier 25, when performed (99201-99215, 99217-99223 [99224, 99225, 99226], 99231-99233, 99241-99255, 99281-99285, 99304-99318, 99324-99337, 99341-99350, 99381-99429)

**95004** Percutaneous tests (scratch, puncture, prick) with allergenic extracts, immediate type reaction, including test interpretation and report, specify number of tests

🖫 0.19  ⅍ 0.19  **FUD** XXX  [01] [80] [▭]

**AMA:** 2017,Jan,8; 2016,Jan,13; 2015,Jan,16; 2014,Jan,11; 2013,Jan,9-10; 2012,Jan,15-42

**95012** Nitric oxide expired gas determination

🖫 0.54  ⅍ 0.54  **FUD** XXX  [01] [80]

**AMA:** 2017,Jan,8; 2016,Jan,13; 2015,Jan,16; 2014,Mar,11; 2014,Jan,11; 2013,Jan,9-10; 2012,Jan,15-42

**95017** Allergy testing, any combination of percutaneous (scratch, puncture, prick) and intracutaneous (intradermal), sequential and incremental, with venoms, immediate type reaction, including test interpretation and report, specify number of tests

🖫 0.10  ⅍ 0.22  **FUD** XXX  [01] [80] [▭]

**AMA:** 2017,Jan,8; 2016,Jan,13; 2015,Jul,9; 2015,Jan,16; 2013,Jan,9-10

**95018** Allergy testing, any combination of percutaneous (scratch, puncture, prick) and intracutaneous (intradermal), sequential and incremental, with drugs or biologicals, immediate type reaction, including test interpretation and report, specify number of tests

🖫 0.20  ⅍ 0.58  **FUD** XXX  [01] [80] [▭]

**AMA:** 2017,Jan,8; 2016,Jan,13; 2015,Jul,9; 2015,Jan,16; 2013,Jan,9-10

**95024** Intracutaneous (intradermal) tests with allergenic extracts, immediate type reaction, including test interpretation and report, specify number of tests

🖫 0.03  ⅍ 0.22  **FUD** XXX  [01] [80] [▭]

**AMA:** 2017,Jan,8; 2016,Jan,13; 2015,Jan,16; 2014,Jan,11; 2013,Jan,9-10; 2012,Jan,15-42

**95027** Intracutaneous (intradermal) tests, sequential and incremental, with allergenic extracts for airborne allergens, immediate type reaction, including test interpretation and report, specify number of tests

🖫 0.13  ⅍ 0.13  **FUD** XXX  [01] [80] [▭]

**AMA:** 2017,Jan,8; 2016,Jan,13; 2015,Jan,16; 2014,Jan,11; 2013,Jan,9-10; 2012,Jan,15-42

**95028** Intracutaneous (intradermal) tests with allergenic extracts, delayed type reaction, including reading, specify number of tests

🖫 0.38  ⅍ 0.38  **FUD** XXX  [01] [80] [TC] [▭]

**AMA:** 2017,Jan,8; 2016,Jan,13; 2015,Jan,16; 2014,Jan,11; 2013,Jan,9-10

**95044** Patch or application test(s) (specify number of tests)

🖫 0.16  ⅍ 0.16  **FUD** XXX  [01] [80] [▭]

**AMA:** 2017,Jan,8; 2016,Jan,13; 2015,Jan,16; 2014,Jan,11; 2013,Jan,9-10

**95052** Photo patch test(s) (specify number of tests)

🖫 0.19  ⅍ 0.19  **FUD** XXX  [01] [80] [▭]

**AMA:** 2017,Jan,8; 2016,Jan,13; 2015,Jan,16; 2014,Jan,11; 2013,Jan,9-10

**95056** Photo tests

🖫 1.25  ⅍ 1.25  **FUD** XXX  [01] [80] [▭]

**AMA:** 2017,Jan,8; 2016,Jan,13; 2015,Jan,16; 2014,Jan,11; 2013,Jan,9-10

| [26]/[TC] PC/TC Only | [A2]-[Z3] ASC Payment | [50] Bilateral | ♂ Male Only | 🖫 Facility RVU | ⅍ Non-Facility RVU | [▭] CCI |
|---|---|---|---|---|---|---|
| **FUD** Follow-up Days | **CMS:** IOM (Pub 100) | [A]-[Y] OPPSI | [80]/[80] Surg Assist Allowed / w/Doc | [▨] Lab Crosswalk | [▨] Radiology Crosswalk | [X] CLIA |

466

CPT © 2017 American Medical Association. All Rights Reserved.  © 2017 Optum360, LLC

**95060** **Ophthalmic mucous membrane tests**
🔧 1.00   ⚖ 1.00   **FUD** XXX    Q1 80 TC 🔲
**AMA:** 2017,Jan,8; 2016,Jan,13; 2015,Jan,16; 2014,Jan,11; 2013,Jan,9-10

**95065** **Direct nasal mucous membrane test**
🔧 0.71   ⚖ 0.71   **FUD** XXX    Q1 80 TC 🔲
**AMA:** 2017,Jan,8; 2016,Jan,13; 2015,Jan,16; 2014,Jan,11; 2013,Jan,9-10

**95070** **Inhalation bronchial challenge testing (not including necessary pulmonary function tests); with histamine, methacholine, or similar compounds**
EXCLUDES   *Pulmonary function tests (94060, 94070)*
🔧 0.87   ⚖ 0.87   **FUD** XXX    S 80 TC 🔲
**AMA:** 2017,Jan,8; 2016,Jan,13; 2015,Jan,16; 2014,Jan,11; 2013,Jan,9-10; 2012,Nov,11-12

**95071** **with antigens or gases, specify**
EXCLUDES   *Pulmonary function tests (94060, 94070)*
🔧 1.03   ⚖ 1.03   **FUD** XXX    Q1 80 TC 🔲
**AMA:** 2017,Jan,8; 2016,Jan,13; 2015,Jan,16; 2014,Jan,11; 2013,Jan,9-10; 2012,Nov,11-12

## 95076-95079 Challenge Ingestion Testing

**CMS:** 100-03,110.12 Challenge Ingestion Food Testing
INCLUDES   Assessment and monitoring for allergic reactions (eg, blood pressure, peak flow meter)
  Testing time until the test ends or to the point an E&M service is needed
EXCLUDES   *Use of code to report testing time less than 61 minutes, such as a positive challenge resulting in ending the test (use E&M codes as appropriate)*
Code also interventions when appropriate (eg, injection of epinephrine or steroid)

**95076** **Ingestion challenge test (sequential and incremental ingestion of test items, eg, food, drug or other substance); initial 120 minutes of testing**
INCLUDES   First 120 minutes of testing time (not face-to-face time with physician)
🔧 2.08   ⚖ 3.28   **FUD** XXX    S 80 🔲
**AMA:** 2017,Jan,8; 2016,Jan,13; 2015,Jan,16; 2013,Jan,9-10

**+** **95079** **each additional 60 minutes of testing (List separately in addition to code for primary procedure)**
INCLUDES   Includes each 60 minutes of additional testing time (not face-to-face time with physician)
  Code first (95076)
🔧 1.90   ⚖ 2.34   **FUD** ZZZ    N 80 🔲
**AMA:** 2017,Jan,8; 2016,Jan,13; 2015,Jan,16; 2013,Jan,9-10

## 95115-95199 Allergy Immunotherapy

**CMS:** 100-03,110.9 Antigens Prepared for Sublingual Administration
INCLUDES   Allergen immunotherapy professional services
EXCLUDES   *Bacterial/viral/fungal extracts skin testing (86485-86580, 95028)*
  *Special reports for allergy patients (99080)*
  *The following procedures for testing: (See Pathology/Immunology section or code:) (95199)*
  *Leukocyte histamine release (LHR)*
  *Lymphocytic transformation test (LTT)*
  *Mast cell degranulation test (MCDT)*
  *Migration inhibitory factor test (MIF)*
  *Nitroblue tetrazolium dye test (NTD)*
  *Radioallergosorbent testing (RAST)*
  *Rat mast cell technique (RMCT)*
  *Transfer factor test (TFT)*
Code also significant separately identifiable E&M services, when performed

**95115** **Professional services for allergen immunotherapy not including provision of allergenic extracts; single injection**
🔧 0.25   ⚖ 0.25   **FUD** XXX    S 80 🔲
**AMA:** 2017,Jan,8; 2016,Jan,13; 2015,Jan,16; 2014,Jan,11; 2013,Jan,9-10

**95117** **2 or more injections**
🔧 0.29   ⚖ 0.29   **FUD** XXX    S 80 🔲
**AMA:** 2017,Jan,8; 2016,Jan,13; 2015,Jan,16; 2014,Jan,11; 2013,Jan,9-10; 2012,Jan,15-42

**95120** **Professional services for allergen immunotherapy in the office or institution of the prescribing physician or other qualified health care professional, including provision of allergenic extract; single injection**
🔧 0.00   ⚖ 0.00   **FUD** XXX    E 🔲
**AMA:** 2017,Jan,8; 2016,Jan,13; 2015,Jan,16; 2014,Jan,11; 2013,Jan,9-10

**95125** **2 or more injections**
🔧 0.00   ⚖ 0.00   **FUD** XXX    E 🔲
**AMA:** 2017,Jan,8; 2016,Jan,13; 2015,Jan,16; 2014,Jan,11; 2013,Jan,9-10; 2012,Jan,15-42

**95130** **single stinging insect venom**
🔧 0.00   ⚖ 0.00   **FUD** XXX    E 🔲
**AMA:** 2017,Jan,8; 2016,Jan,13; 2015,Jan,16; 2014,Jan,11; 2013,Jan,9-10; 2012,Jan,15-42

**95131** **2 stinging insect venoms**
🔧 0.00   ⚖ 0.00   **FUD** XXX    E 🔲
**AMA:** 2017,Jan,8; 2016,Jan,13; 2015,Jan,16; 2014,Jan,11; 2013,Jan,9-10; 2012,Jan,15-42

**95132** **3 stinging insect venoms**
🔧 0.00   ⚖ 0.00   **FUD** XXX    E 🔲
**AMA:** 2017,Jan,8; 2016,Jan,13; 2015,Jan,16; 2014,Jan,11; 2013,Jan,9-10; 2012,Jan,15-42

**95133** **4 stinging insect venoms**
🔧 0.00   ⚖ 0.00   **FUD** XXX    E 🔲
**AMA:** 2017,Jan,8; 2016,Jan,13; 2015,Jan,16; 2014,Jan,11; 2013,Jan,9-10; 2012,Jan,15-42

**95134** **5 stinging insect venoms**
🔧 0.00   ⚖ 0.00   **FUD** XXX    E 🔲
**AMA:** 2017,Jan,8; 2016,Jan,13; 2015,Jan,16; 2014,Jan,11; 2013,Jan,9-10; 2012,Jan,15-42

**95144** **Professional services for the supervision of preparation and provision of antigens for allergen immunotherapy, single dose vial(s) (specify number of vials)**
INCLUDES   Single dose vial/single dose of antigen administered in one injection
🔧 0.09   ⚖ 0.37   **FUD** XXX    S 80 🔲
**AMA:** 2017,Jan,8; 2016,Jan,13; 2015,Jan,16; 2014,Jan,11; 2013,Jan,9-10; 2012,Jan,15-42

**95145** **Professional services for the supervision of preparation and provision of antigens for allergen immunotherapy (specify number of doses); single stinging insect venom**
🔧 0.09   ⚖ 0.71   **FUD** XXX    S 80 🔲
**AMA:** 2017,Jan,8; 2016,Jan,13; 2015,Jan,16; 2014,Jan,11; 2013,Jan,9-10; 2012,Jan,15-42

**95146** **2 single stinging insect venoms**
🔧 0.09   ⚖ 1.30   **FUD** XXX    S 80 🔲
**AMA:** 2017,Jan,8; 2016,Jan,13; 2015,Jan,16; 2014,Jan,11; 2013,Jan,9-10

**95147** **3 single stinging insect venoms**
🔧 0.09   ⚖ 1.38   **FUD** XXX    S 80 🔲
**AMA:** 2017,Jan,8; 2016,Jan,13; 2015,Jan,16; 2014,Jan,11; 2013,Jan,9-10

**95148** **4 single stinging insect venoms**
🔧 0.09   ⚖ 1.95   **FUD** XXX    S 80 🔲
**AMA:** 2017,Jan,8; 2016,Jan,13; 2015,Jan,16; 2014,Jan,11; 2013,Jan,9-10

**95149** **5 single stinging insect venoms**
🔧 0.09   ⚖ 2.58   **FUD** XXX    S 80 🔲
**AMA:** 2017,Jan,8; 2016,Jan,13; 2015,Jan,16; 2014,Jan,11; 2013,Jan,9-10

**95165** **Professional services for the supervision of preparation and provision of antigens for allergen immunotherapy; single or multiple antigens (specify number of doses)**
🔧 0.09   ⚖ 0.37   **FUD** XXX    S 80 🔲
**AMA:** 2017,Jan,8; 2016,Jan,13; 2015,Jan,16; 2014,Jan,11; 2013,Jan,9-10; 2012,Jan,15-42

© 2017 Optum360, LLC   CPT © 2017 American Medical Association. All Rights Reserved.

95170 **whole body extract of biting insect or other arthropod (specify number of doses)**

> INCLUDES  A dose which is the amount of antigen(s) administered in a single injection from a multiple dose vial

> 0.09  0.27  **FUD** XXX  S 80 ▭

> **AMA:** 2017,Jan,8; 2016,Jan,13; 2015,Jan,16; 2014,Jan,11; 2013,Jan,9-10; 2012,Jan,15-42

95180 **Rapid desensitization procedure, each hour (eg, insulin, penicillin, equine serum)**

> 2.87  3.77  **FUD** XXX  Q1 80 ▭

> **AMA:** 2017,Jan,8; 2016,Jan,13; 2015,Jan,16; 2014,Jan,11; 2013,Jan,9-10

95199 **Unlisted allergy/clinical immunologic service or procedure**

> 0.00  0.00  **FUD** XXX  Q1 80

> **AMA:** 2017,Jan,8; 2016,Jan,13; 2015,Jan,16; 2014,Jan,11; 2013,Jan,9-10

## 95249-95251 [95249] Glucose Monitoring By Subcutaneous Device

> EXCLUDES  *Physiologic data collection/interpretation (99091)*
> *Use of code more than one time per month*
> Code also when data receiver owned by patient for placement of sensor, hook-up, monitor calibration, training, and printout (95999)

95249 *Resequenced code. See code following 95250.*

▲ 95250 **Ambulatory continuous glucose monitoring of interstitial tissue fluid via a subcutaneous sensor for a minimum of 72 hours; physician or other qualified health care professional (office) provided equipment, sensor placement, hook-up, calibration of monitor, patient training, removal of sensor, and printout of recording**

> EXCLUDES  *Subcutaneous pocket with insertion interstitial glucose monitor (0446T)*

> 4.45  4.45  **FUD** XXX  V 80 TC ▭

> **AMA:** 2017,Jan,8; 2016,Jan,13; 2015,Jan,16; 2014,Jan,11

● # 95249 **patient-provided equipment, sensor placement, hook-up, calibration of monitor, patient training, and printout of recording**

> 0.00  0.00  **FUD** 000

> INCLUDES  Performing complete collection of initial data in the provider's office

> EXCLUDES  *Subcutaneous pocket with insertion interstitial glucose monitor (0446T)*
> *Use of code more than one time during the period the patient owns the data receiver*

▲ 95251 **analysis, interpretation and report**

> 1.24  1.24  **FUD** XXX  B 80 26 ▭

> **AMA:** 2017,Jan,8; 2016,Jan,13; 2015,Jan,16; 2014,Jan,11

## 95782-95811 [95782, 95783, 95800, 95801] Sleep Studies

> INCLUDES  Assessment of sleep disorders in adults and children
> Continuous and simultaneous monitoring and recording of physiological sleep parameters of 6 hours or more
> Evaluation of patient's response to therapies
> Physician:
> Interpretation
> Recording
> Report
> Recording sessions may be:
> Attended studies that include the presence of a technologist or qualified health care professional to respond to the needs of the patient or technical issues at the bedside
> Remote without the presence of a technologist or a qualified health professional
> Unattended without the presence of a technologist or qualified health care professional
> Testing parameters include:
> Actigraphy: Use of a noninvasive portable device to record gross motor movements to approximate periods of sleep and wakefulness
> Electrooculogram (EOG): Records electrical activity associated with eye movements
> Maintenance of wakefulness test (MWT): An attended study used to determine the patient's ability to stay awake
> Multiple sleep latency test (MSLT): Attended study to determine the tendency of the patient to fall asleep
> Peripheral arterial tonometry (PAT): Pulsatile volume changes in a digit are measured to determine activity in the sympathetic nervous system for respiratory analysis
> Polysomnography: An attended continuous, simultaneous recording of physiological parameters of sleep for at least 6 hours in a sleep laboratory setting that also includes four or more of the following:
> 1. Airflow-oral and/or nasal
> 2. Bilateral anterior tibialis EMG
> 3. Electrocardiogram (ECG)
> 4. Oxyhemoglobin saturation, SpO2
> 5. Respiratory effort
> Positive airway pressure (PAP): Noninvasive devices used to treat sleep-related disorders
> Respiratory airflow (ventilation): Assessment of air movement during inhalation and exhalation as measured by nasal pressure sensors and thermistor
> Respiratory analysis: Assessment of components of respiration obtained by other methods such as airflow or peripheral arterial tone
> Respiratory effort: Use of the diaphragm and/or intercostal muscle for airflow is measured using transducers to estimate thoracic and abdominal motion
> Respiratory movement: Measures the movement of the chest and abdomen during respiration
> Sleep latency: Pertains to the time it takes to get to sleep
> Sleep staging: Determination of the separate levels of sleep according to physiological measurements
> Total sleep time: Determined by the use of actigraphy and other methods
> Use of portable and in-laboratory technology

> EXCLUDES  *E&M services*

95782 **Resequenced code. See code following 95811.**

95783 **Resequenced code. See code following 95811.**

95800 **Resequenced code. See code following 95806.**

95801 **Resequenced code. See code following 95806.**

95803 **Actigraphy testing, recording, analysis, interpretation, and report (minimum of 72 hours to 14 consecutive days of recording)**

> EXCLUDES  *Sleep studies (95806-95811 [95800, 95801])*
> *Use of code more than one time in a 14-day period*

> 3.98  3.98  **FUD** XXX  Q1 80 ▭

> **AMA:** 2017,Jan,8; 2016,Jan,13; 2015,Jan,16; 2014,Jan,11

| 26/TC PC/TC Only | A2-Z3 ASC Payment | 50 Bilateral | ♂ Male Only | ♀ Female Only | Facility RVU | Non-Facility RVU | CCI |
| FUD Follow-up Days | CMS: IOM (Pub 100) | A-Y OPPSI | 80/80 Surg Assist Allowed / w/Doc | | Lab Crosswalk | Radiology Crosswalk | CLIA |

468

CPT © 2017 American Medical Association. All Rights Reserved.  © 2017 Optum360, LLC

95805    **Multiple sleep latency or maintenance of wakefulness testing, recording, analysis and interpretation of physiological measurements of sleep during multiple trials to assess sleepiness**

> INCLUDES    Physiological sleep parameters as measured by:
> Frontal, central, and occipital EEG leads (3 leads)
> Left and right EOG
> Submental EMG lead
>
> EXCLUDES    *Polysomnography (95808-95811)*
> *Sleep study, not attended (95806)*
>
> Code also modifier 52 when less than four nap opportunities are recorded
>
> 📋 12.0    ⚖ 12.0    **FUD** XXX          S 80 ▣
>
> **AMA:** 2017,Jan,8; 2016,Jan,13; 2015,Jan,16; 2014,Jan,11; 2013,Feb,14-15

95806    **Sleep study, unattended, simultaneous recording of, heart rate, oxygen saturation, respiratory airflow, and respiratory effort (eg, thoracoabdominal movement)**

> EXCLUDES    *Arterial waveform analysis (93050)*
> *Event monitors (93268-93272)*
> *Holter monitor (93224-93227)*
> *Remote cardiovascular telemetry (93228-93229)*
> *Rhythm strips (93041-93042)*
> *Unattended sleep study with measurement of a minimum heart rate, oxygen saturation, and respiratory analysis (95801)*
> *Unattended sleep study with measurement of heart rate, oxygen saturation, respiratory analysis, and sleep time (95800)*
>
> Code also modifier 52 for fewer than 6 hours of recording
>
> 📋 4.79    ⚖ 4.79    **FUD** XXX          S 80 ▣
>
> **AMA:** 2017,Jan,8; 2016,Jan,13; 2015,Jan,16; 2014,Jan,11; 2013,Jul,11-12; 2013,Feb,14-15; 2012,Jan,15-42

\#  95800    **Sleep study, unattended, simultaneous recording; heart rate, oxygen saturation, respiratory analysis (eg, by airflow or peripheral arterial tone), and sleep time**

> 📋 5.04    ⚖ 5.04    **FUD** XXX          S 80 ▣
>
> **AMA:** 2017,Jan,8; 2016,Jan,13; 2015,Jan,16; 2014,Jan,11; 2013,Feb,14-15

\#  95801    **minimum of heart rate, oxygen saturation, and respiratory analysis (eg, by airflow or peripheral arterial tone)**

> 📋 2.57    ⚖ 2.57    **FUD** XXX          Q1 80 ▣
>
> **AMA:** 2017,Jan,8; 2016,Jan,13; 2015,Jan,16; 2014,Jan,11; 2013,Feb,14-15

95807    **Sleep study, simultaneous recording of ventilation, respiratory effort, ECG or heart rate, and oxygen saturation, attended by a technologist**

> EXCLUDES    *Polysomnography (95808-95811)*
> *Sleep study, not attended (95806)*
>
> Code also modifier 52 for fewer than 6 hours of recording
>
> 📋 13.1    ⚖ 13.1    **FUD** XXX          S 80 ▣
>
> **AMA:** 2017,Jan,8; 2016,Jan,13; 2015,Jan,16; 2014,Jan,11; 2013,Feb,14-15

95808    **Polysomnography; any age, sleep staging with 1-3 additional parameters of sleep, attended by a technologist**

> EXCLUDES    *Sleep study, not attended (95806)*
>
> 📋 18.0    ⚖ 18.0    **FUD** XXX          S 80 ▣
>
> **AMA:** 2017,Jan,8; 2016,Jan,13; 2015,Jan,16; 2014,Jan,11; 2013,Feb,14-15; 2012,Jan,15-42

95810    **age 6 years or older, sleep staging with 4 or more additional parameters of sleep, attended by a technologist**    Ⓐ

> EXCLUDES    *Sleep study, not attended (95806)*
>
> Code also modifier 52 for fewer than 6 hours of recording
>
> 📋 17.5    ⚖ 17.5    **FUD** XXX          S 80 ▣
>
> **AMA:** 2017,Jan,8; 2016,Jan,13; 2015,Jan,16; 2014,Jan,11; 2013,Feb,14-15

95811    **age 6 years or older, sleep staging with 4 or more additional parameters of sleep, with initiation of continuous positive airway pressure therapy or bilevel ventilation, attended by a technologist**    Ⓐ

> EXCLUDES    *Sleep study, not attended (95806)*
>
> Code also modifier 52 for fewer than 6 hours of recording
>
> 📋 18.4    ⚖ 18.4    **FUD** XXX          S 80 ▣
>
> **AMA:** 2017,Jan,8; 2016,Jan,13; 2015,Jan,16; 2014,Oct,8; 2014,Jan,11; 2013,Feb,14-15

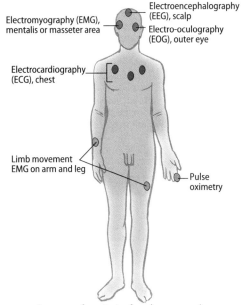

Electromyography (EMG), mentalis or masseter area

Electroencephalography (EEG), scalp

Electro-oculography (EOG), outer eye

Electrocardiography (ECG), chest

Limb movement EMG on arm and leg

Pulse oximetry

Core areas of monitoring for polysomnography

\#  95782    **younger than 6 years, sleep staging with 4 or more additional parameters of sleep, attended by a technologist**    Ⓐ

> 📋 28.8    ⚖ 28.8    **FUD** XXX          S 80 ▣
>
> **AMA:** 2017,Jan,8; 2016,Jan,13; 2015,Jan,16; 2014,Jan,11; 2013,Feb,14-15

\#  95783    **younger than 6 years, sleep staging with 4 or more additional parameters of sleep, with initiation of continuous positive airway pressure therapy or bi-level ventilation, attended by a technologist**    Ⓐ

> Code also modifier 52 for fewer than 7 hours of recording
>
> 📋 32.7    ⚖ 32.7    **FUD** XXX          S 80 ▣
>
> **AMA:** 2017,Jan,8; 2016,Jan,13; 2015,Jan,16; 2014,Oct,8; 2014,Jan,11; 2013,Feb,14-15

● New Code    ▲ Revised Code    ○ Reinstated    ● New Web Release    ▲ Revised Web Release    Unlisted    Not Covered    # Resequenced
⊘ AMA Mod 51 Exempt    ⑤ Optum Mod 51 Exempt    ⑥³ Mod 63 Exempt    ✗ Non-FDA Drug    ★ Telemedicine    Ⓜ Maternity    Ⓐ Age Edit    + Add-on    **AMA:** CPT Asst
© 2017 Optum360, LLC                              CPT © 2017 American Medical Association. All Rights Reserved.                              **469**

## 95812-95830 Evaluation of Brain Activity by Electroencephalogram

**INCLUDES** Only time when time is being recorded and data are being collected and does not include set-up and take-down

**EXCLUDES** E&M services

**95812** **Electroencephalogram (EEG) extended monitoring; 41-60 minutes**

**INCLUDES** Hyperventilation

Only time when recording is taking place and data are being collected and does not include set-up and take-down

Photic stimulation

Physician interpretation

Recording of 41-60 minutes

Report

**EXCLUDES** EEG digital analysis (95957)

EEG during nonintracranial surgery (95955)

EEG monitoring, 24-hour (95950-95953, 95956)

Wada test (95958)

Code also modifier 26 for physician interpretation only

🖩 9.15     9.15   **FUD** XXX                    S 80 ▢

**AMA:** 2017,Jan,8; 2016,Jan,13; 2015,Jan,16; 2014,Jan,11; 2012,Jan,15-42

**95813** **greater than 1 hour**

**INCLUDES** Hyperventilation

Only time when recording is taking place and data are being collected and does not include set-up and take-down

Photic stimulation

Physician interpretation

Recording of 61 minutes or more

Report

**EXCLUDES** EEG digital analysis (95957)

EEG during nonintracranial surgery (95955)

EEG monitoring, 24-hour (95950-95953, 95956)

Wada test (95958)

Code also modifier 26 for physician interpretation only

🖩 11.5     11.5   **FUD** XXX                  S 80 ▢

**AMA:** 2017,Jan,8; 2016,Jan,13; 2015,Jan,16; 2014,Jan,11; 2012,Jan,15-42

**95816** **Electroencephalogram (EEG); including recording awake and drowsy**

**INCLUDES** Photic stimulation

Physician interpretation

Recording of 20-40 minutes

Report

**EXCLUDES** EEG digital analysis (95957)

EEG during nonintracranial surgery (95955)

EEG monitoring, 24-hour (95950-95953, 95956)

Wada test (95958)

Code also modifier 26 for physician interpretation only

🖩 10.2     10.2   **FUD** XXX                  S 80 ▢

**AMA:** 2017,Jan,8; 2016,Jan,13; 2015,Dec,16; 2015,Jan,16; 2014,Jan,11; 2012,Jan,15-42

**95819** **including recording awake and asleep**

**INCLUDES** Hyperventilation

Photic stimulation

Physician interpretation

Recording of 20-40 minutes

Report

**EXCLUDES** EEG digital analysis (95957)

EEG during nonintracranial surgery (95955)

EEG monitoring, 24-hour (95950-95953, 95956)

Wada test (95958)

Code also modifier 26 for interpretation only

🖩 11.7     11.7   **FUD** XXX                  S 80 ▢

**AMA:** 2017,Jan,8; 2016,Jan,13; 2015,Dec,16; 2015,Jan,16; 2014,Jan,11

**95822** **recording in coma or sleep only**

**INCLUDES** Hyperventilation

Photic stimulation

Physician interpretation

Recording of 20-40 minutes

Report

**EXCLUDES** EEG digital analysis (95957)

EEG during nonintracranial surgery (95955)

EEG monitoring, 24-hour (95950-95953, 95956)

Wada test (95958)

Code also modifier 26 for interpretation only

🖩 10.6     10.6   **FUD** XXX                  S 80 ▢

**AMA:** 2017,Jan,8; 2016,Jan,13; 2015,Jan,16; 2014,Dec,18; 2014,Jan,11; 2013,May,8-10

**95824** **cerebral death evaluation only**

**INCLUDES** Physician interpretation

Recording

Report

**EXCLUDES** EEG digital analysis (95957)

EEG during nonintracranial surgery (95955)

EEG monitoring, 24-hour (95950-95953, 95956)

Wada test (95958)

Code also modifier 26 for physician interpretation only

🖩 0.00     0.00   **FUD** XXX                  S 80 ▢

**AMA:** 2003,Dec,4; 2001,Nov,4

**95827** **all night recording**

**INCLUDES** Physician interpretation

Recording

Report

**EXCLUDES** EEG digital analysis (95957)

EEG during nonintracranial surgery (95955)

EEG monitoring, 24-hour (95950-95953, 95956)

Wada test (95958)

Code also modifier 26 for interpretation only

🖩 18.7     18.7   **FUD** XXX                  S 80 ▢

**AMA:** 2003,Dec,4; 2001,Nov,4

**95829** **Electrocorticogram at surgery (separate procedure)**

**INCLUDES** Physician interpretation

Recording

Report

Code also modifier 26 for interpretation only

🖩 54.1     54.1   **FUD** XXX                  N 80 ▢

**AMA:** 2003,Dec,4; 2001,Nov,4

**95830** **Insertion by physician or other qualified health care professional of sphenoidal electrodes for electroencephalographic (EEG) recording**

🖩 2.61     6.20   **FUD** XXX                  B 80 ▢

**AMA:** 2003,Dec,4; 2001,Nov,4

## 95831-95857 Evaluation of Muscles and Range of Motion

**CMS:** 100-02,15,230.4 Services By a Physical/Occupational Therapist in Private Practice

**EXCLUDES** E&M services

**95831** **Muscle testing, manual (separate procedure) with report; extremity (excluding hand) or trunk**

🖩 0.45     0.89   **FUD** XXX                  A 80 ▢

**AMA:** 2017,Jan,8; 2016,Dec,16; 2016,Jan,13; 2015,Jan,16; 2014,Jan,11; 2013,Aug,7; 2012,Jan,15-42

**95832** **hand, with or without comparison with normal side**

🖩 0.48     0.88   **FUD** XXX                  A 80 ▢

**AMA:** 2017,Jan,8; 2016,Dec,16; 2016,Jan,13; 2015,Jan,16; 2014,Jan,11; 2013,Aug,7; 2012,Jan,15-42

**95833** **total evaluation of body, excluding hands**

🖩 0.61     1.05   **FUD** XXX                  A 80 ▢

**AMA:** 2017,Jan,8; 2016,Dec,16; 2016,Jan,13; 2015,Jan,16; 2014,Jan,11; 2013,Aug,7; 2012,Oct,14; 2012,Sep,16

**95834** **total evaluation of body, including hands**

🖩 0.89     1.48   **FUD** XXX                  A 80 ▢

**AMA:** 2017,Jan,8; 2016,Jan,13; 2015,Jan,16; 2014,Jan,11; 2013,Aug,7

| 26/TC PC/TC Only | 12-Z3 ASC Payment | 50 Bilateral | ♂ Male Only | ♀ Female Only | 🖩 Facility RVU | & Non-Facility RVU | ▢ CCI |
|---|---|---|---|---|---|---|---|
| FUD Follow-up Days | CMS: IOM (Pub 100) | A-Y OPPSI | 80/80 Surg Assist Allowed / w/Doc | | 🖩 Lab Crosswalk | 🖩 Radiology Crosswalk | ✕ CLIA |

470                                   CPT © 2017 American Medical Association. All Rights Reserved.                          © 2017 Optum360, LLC

| 95851 | Range of motion measurements and report (separate procedure); each extremity (excluding hand) or each trunk section (spine) |
|---|---|

📖 0.22   ⅋ 0.51   **FUD** XXX                    [A] [80] 🖵

**AMA:** 2017,Jan,8; 2016,Dec,16; 2016,Jan,13; 2015,Jan,16; 2014,Jan,11; 2013,Aug,7; 2012,Jan,15-42

**95852**   **hand, with or without comparison with normal side**

📖 0.16   ⅋ 0.44   **FUD** XXX                    [A] [80] 🖵

**AMA:** 2017,Jan,8; 2016,Jan,13; 2015,Jan,16; 2014,Jan,11; 2013,Aug,7

**95857**   **Cholinesterase inhibitor challenge test for myasthenia gravis**

📖 0.85   ⅋ 1.53   **FUD** XXX                    [S] [80] 🖵

**AMA:** 2017,Jan,8; 2016,Jan,13; 2015,Jan,16; 2014,Jan,11

# 95860-95887 [95885, 95886, 95887] Evaluation of Nerve and Muscle Function: EMGs with/without Nerve Conduction Studies

INCLUDES   Physician interpretation
Recording
Report
EXCLUDES   E&M services

**95860**   **Needle electromyography; 1 extremity with or without related paraspinal areas**

INCLUDES   Testing of five or more muscles per extremity
EXCLUDES   Dynamic electromyography during motion analysis studies (96002-96003)
Guidance for chemodenervation (95873-95874)

📖 3.46   ⅋ 3.46   **FUD** XXX                    [Q1] [80] 🖵

**AMA:** 2017,Jan,8; 2016,Jan,13; 2015,Mar,6; 2015,Jan,16; 2014,Jan,11; 2013,May,8-10; 2013,Mar,3-5; 2012,Feb,8; 2012,Jan,15-42

**95861**   **2 extremities with or without related paraspinal areas**

INCLUDES   Testing of five or more muscles per extremity
EXCLUDES   Dynamic electromyography during motion analysis studies (96002-96003)
Guidance for chemodenervation (95873-95874)

📖 4.92   ⅋ 4.92   **FUD** XXX                    [Q1] [80] 🖵

**AMA:** 2017,Jan,8; 2016,Jan,13; 2015,Mar,6; 2015,Jan,16; 2014,Jan,11; 2013,May,8-10; 2013,Mar,3-5; 2012,Feb,8; 2012,Jan,15-42

**95863**   **3 extremities with or without related paraspinal areas**

INCLUDES   Testing of five or more muscles per extremity
EXCLUDES   Dynamic electromyography during motion analysis studies (96002-96003)
Guidance for chemodenervation (95873-95874)

📖 6.18   ⅋ 6.18   **FUD** XXX                    [S] [80] 🖵

**AMA:** 2017,Jan,8; 2016,Jan,13; 2015,Mar,6; 2015,Jan,16; 2014,Jan,11; 2013,May,8-10; 2013,Mar,3-5; 2012,Feb,8; 2012,Jan,15-42

**95864**   **4 extremities with or without related paraspinal areas**

INCLUDES   Testing of five or more muscles per extremity
EXCLUDES   Dynamic electromyography during motion analysis studies (96002-96003)
Guidance for chemodenervation (95873-95874)

📖 6.95   ⅋ 6.95   **FUD** XXX                    [S] [80] 🖵

**AMA:** 2017,Jan,8; 2016,Jan,13; 2015,Mar,6; 2015,Jan,16; 2014,Jan,11; 2013,May,8-10; 2013,Mar,3-5; 2012,Feb,8; 2012,Jan,15-42

**95865**   **larynx**

EXCLUDES   Dynamic electromyography during motion analysis studies (96002-96003)
Guidance for chemodenervation (95873-95874)
Code also modifier 52 for unilateral procedure

📖 4.15   ⅋ 4.15   **FUD** XXX                    [Q1] [80] 🖵

**AMA:** 2017,Jan,8; 2016,Jan,13; 2015,Mar,6; 2015,Jan,16; 2014,Jan,6; 2014,Jan,11; 2013,May,8-10; 2012,Jan,15-42

**95866**   **hemidiaphragm**

EXCLUDES   Dynamic electromyography during motion analysis studies (96002-96003)
Guidance for chemodenervation (95873-95874)

📖 3.84   ⅋ 3.84   **FUD** XXX                    [Q1] [80] 🖵

**AMA:** 2017,Jan,8; 2016,Jan,13; 2015,Mar,6; 2015,Jan,16; 2014,Jan,11; 2013,May,8-10; 2012,Jan,15-42

**95867**   **cranial nerve supplied muscle(s), unilateral**

EXCLUDES   Guidance for chemodenervation (95873-95874)

📖 2.74   ⅋ 2.74   **FUD** XXX                    [S] [80] 🖵

**AMA:** 2017,Jan,8; 2016,Jan,13; 2015,Mar,6; 2015,Jan,16; 2014,Jan,11; 2013,May,8-10; 2013,Mar,3-5; 2012,Feb,8; 2012,Jan,15-42

**95868**   **cranial nerve supplied muscles, bilateral**

EXCLUDES   Guidance for chemodenervation (95873-95874)

📖 3.81   ⅋ 3.81   **FUD** XXX                    [S] [80] 🖵

**AMA:** 2017,Jan,8; 2016,Jan,13; 2015,Mar,6; 2015,Jan,16; 2014,Jan,11; 2013,May,8-10; 2013,Mar,3-5; 2012,Feb,8; 2012,Jan,15-42

**95869**   **thoracic paraspinal muscles (excluding T1 or T12)**

EXCLUDES   Dynamic electromyography during motion analysis studies (96002-96003)
Guidance for chemodenervation (95873-95874)

📖 2.59   ⅋ 2.59   **FUD** XXX                    [Q1] [80] 🖵

**AMA:** 2017,Jan,8; 2016,Jan,13; 2015,Mar,6; 2015,Jan,16; 2014,Jan,11; 2013,May,8-10; 2013,Mar,3-5; 2012,Feb,8; 2012,Jan,15-42

**95870**   **limited study of muscles in 1 extremity or non-limb (axial) muscles (unilateral or bilateral), other than thoracic paraspinal, cranial nerve supplied muscles, or sphincters**

INCLUDES   Adson test
Testing of four or less muscles per extremity
EXCLUDES   Anal/urethral sphincter/detrusor/urethra/perineum musculature (51785-51792)
Complete study of extremities (95860-95864)
Dynamic electromyography during motion analysis studies (96002-96003)
Eye muscles (92265)
Guidance for chemodenervation (95873-95874)

📖 2.62   ⅋ 2.62   **FUD** XXX                    [Q1] [80] 🖵

**AMA:** 2017,Jan,8; 2016,Jan,13; 2015,Mar,6; 2015,Jan,16; 2014,Jan,11; 2013,May,8-10; 2013,Mar,3-5; 2012,Feb,8; 2012,Jan,15-42

**95872**   **Needle electromyography using single fiber electrode, with quantitative measurement of jitter, blocking and/or fiber density, any/all sites of each muscle studied**

EXCLUDES   Dynamic electromyography during motion analysis studies (96002-96003)

📖 5.58   ⅋ 5.58   **FUD** XXX                    [S] [80] 🖵

**AMA:** 2017,Jan,8; 2016,Jan,13; 2015,Mar,6; 2015,Jan,16; 2014,Jan,11; 2012,Jan,15-42

+ # **95885**   **Needle electromyography, each extremity, with related paraspinal areas, when performed, done with nerve conduction, amplitude and latency/velocity study; limited (List separately in addition to code for primary procedure)**

📖 1.66   ⅋ 1.66   **FUD** ZZZ                    [N] [80] 🖵

**AMA:** 2017,Jul,10; 2017,Jan,8; 2016,Jan,13; 2015,Mar,6; 2015,Jan,16; 2014,Jan,11; 2013,Sep,17; 2013,May,8-10; 2013,Mar,3-5; 2012,Feb,8; 2012,Jan,15-42

+ # **95886**   **complete, five or more muscles studied, innervated by three or more nerves or four or more spinal levels (List separately in addition to code for primary procedure)**

📖 2.58   ⅋ 2.58   **FUD** ZZZ                    [N] [80] 🖵

**AMA:** 2017,Jul,10; 2017,Jan,8; 2016,Jan,13; 2015,Mar,6; 2015,Jan,16; 2014,Jan,11; 2013,Sep,17; 2013,May,8-10; 2013,Mar,3-5; 2012,Feb,8; 2012,Jan,15-42

---

● New Code   ▲ Revised Code   ○ Reinstated   ● New Web Release   ▲ Revised Web Release   Unlisted   Not Covered   # Resequenced
⊘ AMA Mod 51 Exempt   ⑤ Optum Mod 51 Exempt   ⑥³ Mod 63 Exempt   ✗ Non-FDA Drug   ★ Telemedicine   Ⓜ Maternity   Ⓐ Age Edit   + Add-on   **AMA:** CPT Asst

**Medicine**

**+ #  95887  Needle electromyography, non-extremity (cranial nerve supplied or axial) muscle(s) done with nerve conduction, amplitude and latency/velocity study (List separately in addition to code for primary procedure)**

🚑 2.28   ⚖ 2.28   **FUD** ZZZ   N 80 ▣

**AMA:** 2017,Jul,10; 2017,Jan,8; 2016,Jan,13; 2015,Mar,6; 2015,Jan,16; 2014,Jan,11; 2014,Jan,8; 2013,Mar,3-5; 2012,Jul,12-14; 2012,Feb,8; 2012,Jan,15-42

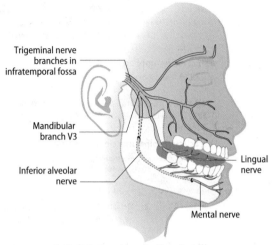

Trigeminal nerve branches in infratemporal fossa

Mandibular branch V3

Inferior alveolar nerve

Lingual nerve

Mental nerve

Cranial nerves: trigeminal branches of lower face and select facial nerves

Needle EMG is performed to determine conduction, amplitude, and latency/velocity

**+  95873  Electrical stimulation for guidance in conjunction with chemodenervation (List separately in addition to code for primary procedure)**

EXCLUDES  *Chemodenervation larynx (64617)*
*Needle electromyography (95860-95870)*
*Needle electromyography guidance for chemodenervation (95874)*
*Use of more than one guidance code for each code for chemodenervation*
Code first chemodenervation (64612, 64615-64616, 64642-64647)

🚑 2.07   ⚖ 2.07   **FUD** ZZZ   N 80 ▣

**AMA:** 2017,Jan,8; 2016,Jan,13; 2015,Mar,6; 2015,Jan,16; 2014,Jan,6; 2014,Jan,11; 2013,Apr,5-6; 2012,Jan,15-42

**+  95874  Needle electromyography for guidance in conjunction with chemodenervation (List separately in addition to code for primary procedure)**

EXCLUDES  *Chemodenervation larynx (64617)*
*Needle electromyography (95860-95870)*
*Needle electromyography guidance for chemodenervation (95873)*
*Use of more than one guidance code for each code for chemodenervation*
Code first chemodenervation (64612, 64615-64616, 64642-64647)

🚑 2.09   ⚖ 2.09   **FUD** ZZZ   N 80 ▣

**AMA:** 2017,Jan,8; 2016,Jan,13; 2015,Mar,6; 2015,Jan,16; 2014,Oct,14; 2014,Jan,6; 2014,Jan,11; 2013,Apr,5-6; 2012,Jan,15-42

**95875  Ischemic limb exercise test with serial specimen(s) acquisition for muscle(s) metabolite(s)**

🚑 3.32   ⚖ 3.32   **FUD** XXX   S 80 ▣

**AMA:** 2017,Jan,8; 2016,Jan,13; 2015,Mar,6; 2015,Jan,16; 2014,Jan,11; 2012,Jan,15-42

**95885**  Resequenced code. See code following 95872.

**95886**  Resequenced code. See code following 95872.

**95887**  Resequenced code. See code before 95873.

## 95905-95913 Evaluation of Nerve Function: Nerve Conduction Studies

INCLUDES  Conduction studies of motor and sensory nerves
Reports from on-site examiner including the work product of the interpretation of results using established methodologies, calculations, comparisons to normal studies, and interpretation by physician or other qualified health care professional
Single conduction study comprising a sensory and motor conduction test with/without F or H wave testing, and all orthodromic and antidromic impulses
Total number of tests performed indicate which code is appropriate

EXCLUDES  *Use of code for more than one study when multiple sites on the same nerve are tested*

Code also electromyography performed with nerve conduction studies, as appropriate ([95885, 95886, 95887])

**95905  Motor and/or sensory nerve conduction, using preconfigured electrode array(s), amplitude and latency/velocity study, each limb, includes F-wave study when performed, with interpretation and report**

INCLUDES  Study with preconfigured electrodes that are customized to a specific body location

EXCLUDES  *Needle electromyography ([95885, 95886])*
*Nerve conduction studies (95907-95913)*
*Use of this code more than one time for each limb studied*

🚑 2.02   ⚖ 2.02   **FUD** XXX   🚫 01 80 ▣

**AMA:** 2017,Jan,8; 2016,Jan,13; 2015,Jan,16; 2014,Jan,11; 2013,Mar,3-5; 2012,Feb,8

**95907  Nerve conduction studies; 1-2 studies**

🚑 2.76   ⚖ 2.76   **FUD** XXX   S 80 ▣

**AMA:** 2017,Jan,8; 2016,Jan,13; 2015,Jan,16; 2014,Jan,11; 2013,Sep,17; 2013,May,8-10; 2013,Mar,3-5

**95908  3-4 studies**

🚑 3.55   ⚖ 3.55   **FUD** XXX   S 80 ▣

**AMA:** 2017,Jan,8; 2016,Jan,13; 2015,Mar,6; 2015,Jan,16; 2014,Jan,11; 2013,Sep,17; 2013,May,8-10; 2013,Mar,3-5

**95909  5-6 studies**

🚑 4.23   ⚖ 4.23   **FUD** XXX   S 80 ▣

**AMA:** 2017,Jan,8; 2016,Jan,13; 2015,Jan,16; 2014,Jan,11; 2013,Sep,17; 2013,May,8-10; 2013,Mar,3-5

**95910  7-8 studies**

🚑 5.59   ⚖ 5.59   **FUD** XXX   S 80 ▣

**AMA:** 2017,Jan,8; 2016,Jan,13; 2015,Jan,16; 2014,Jan,11; 2013,Sep,17; 2013,May,8-10; 2013,Mar,3-5

**95911  9-10 studies**

🚑 6.66   ⚖ 6.66   **FUD** XXX   S 80 ▣

**AMA:** 2017,Jan,8; 2016,Jan,13; 2015,Jan,16; 2014,Jan,11; 2013,Sep,17; 2013,May,8-10; 2013,Mar,3-5

**95912  11-12 studies**

🚑 7.35   ⚖ 7.35   **FUD** XXX   S 80 ▣

**AMA:** 2017,Jan,8; 2016,Jan,13; 2015,Jan,16; 2014,Jan,11; 2013,Sep,17; 2013,May,8-10; 2013,Mar,3-5

**95913  13 or more studies**

🚑 8.44   ⚖ 8.44   **FUD** XXX   S 80 ▣

**AMA:** 2017,Jan,8; 2016,Jan,13; 2015,Jan,16; 2014,Jan,11; 2013,Sep,17; 2013,May,8-10; 2013,Mar,3-5

## [95940, 95941] Intraoperative Neurophysiological Monitoring

**INCLUDES** Monitoring, testing, and data evaluation during surgical procedures by a monitoring professional dedicated only to performing the necessary testing and monitoring

Monitoring services provided by the anesthesiologist or surgeon separately

**EXCLUDES** *Baseline neurophysiologic monitoring*
*EEG during nonintracranial surgery (95955)*
*Electrocorticography (95829)*
*Intraoperative cortical and subcortical mapping (95961-95962)*
*Neurostimulator programming/analysis (95970-95975)*
*Time required for set-up, recording, interpretation, and removal of electrodes*

Code also baseline studies (eg, EMGs, NCVs), no more than one time per operative session

Code also services provided after midnight using the date when monitoring started and the total monitoring time

Code also standby time prior to procedure (99360)

Code first (92585, 95822, 95860-95870, 95907-95913, 95925-95937 [95938, 95939])

**+ # 95940** **Continuous intraoperative neurophysiology monitoring in the operating room, one on one monitoring requiring personal attendance, each 15 minutes (List separately in addition to code for primary procedure)**

**INCLUDES** 15 minute increments of monitoring service

A total of all monitoring time for procedures overlapping midnight

Based on time spent monitoring, regardless of number of tests or parameters monitored

Continuous intraoperative neurophysiologic monitoring by a dedicated monitoring professional in the operating room providing one-on-one patient care

Monitoring time may begin prior to the incision

Monitoring time that is distinct from baseline neurophysiologic study/s time or other services (eg, mapping)

**EXCLUDES** *Time spent in executing or interpreting the baseline neurophysiologic study or studies*

Code also monitoring from outside of the operating room, when applicable ([95941])

🔧 0.93    ⚒ 0.93    **FUD** XXX    N N1 80 ▣

**AMA:** 2017,Aug,8; 2017,Jan,8; 2016,Jan,13; 2015,Jan,16; 2014,Apr,10; 2014,Apr,5; 2013,May,8-10

**+ # 95941** **Continuous intraoperative neurophysiology monitoring, from outside the operating room (remote or nearby) or for monitoring of more than one case while in the operating room, per hour (List separately in addition to code for primary procedure)**

**INCLUDES** Based on time spent monitoring, regardless of number of tests or parameters monitored

Monitoring time that is distinct from baseline neurophysiologic study/s time or other services (eg, mapping)

One hour increments of monitoring service

🔧 0.00    ⚒ 0.00    **FUD** XXX    N N1 ▣

**AMA:** 2017,Aug,8; 2017,Jan,8; 2016,Jan,13; 2015,Jan,16; 2014,Dec,18; 2014,Apr,10; 2014,Apr,5; 2014,Jan,11; 2013,May,8-10; 2013,Feb,16-17

## 95921-95924 [95943] Evaluation of Autonomic Nervous System

**INCLUDES** Physician interpretation
Recording
Report
Testing for autonomic dysfunction including site and autonomic subsystems

**95921** **Testing of autonomic nervous system function; cardiovagal innervation (parasympathetic function), including 2 or more of the following: heart rate response to deep breathing with recorded R-R interval, Valsalva ratio, and 30:15 ratio**

**INCLUDES** Display on a monitor

Minimum of two of the following elements are performed:

Cardiovascular function as indicated by a 30:15 ration (R/R interval at beat 30)/(R-R interval at beat 15)

Heart rate response to deep breathing obtained by visual quantitative analysis of recordings with patient taking 5-6 breaths per minute

Valsalva ratio (at least 2) obtained by dividing the highest heart rate by the lowest

Monitoring of heart rate by electrocardiography of rate obtained from time between two successive R waves (R-R interval)

Storage of data for waveform analysis

Testing most usually in prone position

Tilt table testing, when performed

**EXCLUDES** *Autonomic nervous system testing with sympathetic adrenergic function testing (95922, 95924)*

*Simultaneous measures of parasympathetic and sympathetic function ([95943])*

🔧 2.41    ⚒ 2.41    **FUD** XXX    S 80 ▣

**AMA:** 2017,Jan,8; 2016,Jan,13; 2015,Jan,16; 2014,Jan,11; 2012,Nov,6-9; 2012,Jan,15-42

**95922** **vasomotor adrenergic innervation (sympathetic adrenergic function), including beat-to-beat blood pressure and R-R interval changes during Valsalva maneuver and at least 5 minutes of passive tilt**

**EXCLUDES** *Autonomic nervous system testing with parasympathetic function (95921, 95924)*

*Simultaneous measures of parasympathetic and sympathetic function ([95943])*

🔧 2.83    ⚒ 2.83    **FUD** XXX    Q1 80 ▣

**AMA:** 2017,Jan,8; 2016,Jan,13; 2015,Jan,16; 2014,Jan,11; 2012,Nov,6-9; 2012,Jan,15-42

**95923** **sudomotor, including 1 or more of the following: quantitative sudomotor axon reflex test (QSART), silastic sweat imprint, thermoregulatory sweat test, and changes in sympathetic skin potential**

🔧 3.99    ⚒ 3.99    **FUD** XXX    Q1 80 ▣

**AMA:** 2017,Jan,8; 2016,Jan,13; 2015,Jan,16; 2014,Jan,11; 2012,Nov,6-9; 2012,Jan,15-42

**95924** **combined parasympathetic and sympathetic adrenergic function testing with at least 5 minutes of passive tilt**

**INCLUDES** Tilt table testing of adrenergic and parasympathetic function

**EXCLUDES** *Autonomic nervous system testing with parasympathetic function (95921-95922)*

*Simultaneous measures of parasympathetic and sympathetic function ([95943])*

🔧 4.32    ⚒ 4.32    **FUD** XXX    S 80 ▣

**AMA:** 2017,Jan,8; 2016,Jan,13; 2015,Jan,16; 2012,Nov,6-9

**Medicine** (left side tab)

**95943 — 95951** (left side tab)

\# **95943** Simultaneous, independent, quantitative measures of both parasympathetic function and sympathetic function, based on time-frequency analysis of heart rate variability concurrent with time-frequency analysis of continuous respiratory activity, with mean heart rate and blood pressure measures, during rest, paced (deep) breathing, Valsalva maneuvers, and head-up postural change

EXCLUDES *Autonomic nervous system testing (95921-95922, 95924)*

*Rhythm ECG (93040)*

⚕ 0.00 ✂ 0.00 **FUD** XXX  [S] [80] [▭]

**AMA:** 2017,Jan,8; 2016,Jan,13; 2015,Jan,16; 2012,Nov,6-9

## 95925-95943 [95938, 95939] Neurotransmission Studies

**95925** Short-latency somatosensory evoked potential study, stimulation of any/all peripheral nerves or skin sites, recording from the central nervous system; in upper limbs

EXCLUDES *Auditory evoked potentials (92585)*

*Evoked potential study in both upper and lower limbs ([95938])*

*Evoked potential study in lower limbs (95926)*

⚕ 3.92 ✂ 3.92 **FUD** XXX  [S] [80] [▭]

**AMA:** 2017,Jan,8; 2016,Jan,13; 2015,Jan,16; 2014,Jan,11; 2013,May,8-10; 2012,Apr,17-18

**95926** in lower limbs

EXCLUDES *Auditory evoked potentials (92585)*

*Evoked potential study in both upper and lower limbs ([95938])*

*Evoked potential study in upper limbs (95925)*

⚕ 3.80 ✂ 3.80 **FUD** XXX  [S] [80] [▭]

**AMA:** 2017,Jan,8; 2016,Jan,13; 2015,Jan,16; 2014,Jan,11; 2013,May,8-10; 2012,Apr,17-18; 2012,Jan,15-42

\# **95938** in upper and lower limbs

⚕ 9.69 ✂ 9.69 **FUD** XXX  [S] [80] [▭]

**AMA:** 2017,Jan,8; 2016,Jan,13; 2015,Jan,16; 2014,Jan,11; 2013,May,8-10; 2013,Feb,16-17; 2012,Apr,17-18

**95927** in the trunk or head

EXCLUDES *Auditory evoked potentials (92585)*

Code also modifier 52 for unilateral test

⚕ 3.90 ✂ 3.90 **FUD** XXX  [S] [80] [▭]

**AMA:** 2017,Jan,8; 2016,Jan,13; 2015,Jan,16; 2014,Jan,11; 2013,May,8-10

**95928** Central motor evoked potential study (transcranial motor stimulation); upper limbs

EXCLUDES *Central motor evoked potential study lower limbs (95929)*

⚕ 6.04 ✂ 6.04 **FUD** XXX  [S] [80] [▭]

**AMA:** 2017,Jan,8; 2016,Jan,13; 2015,Jan,16; 2013,May,8-10

**95929** lower limbs

EXCLUDES *Central motor evoked potential study upper limbs (95928)*

⚕ 6.22 ✂ 6.22 **FUD** XXX  [S] [80] [▭]

**AMA:** 2017,Jan,8; 2016,Jan,13; 2015,Jan,16; 2014,Dec,6; 2013,May,8-10

\# **95939** in upper and lower limbs

EXCLUDES *Central motor evoked potential study of either lower or upper limbs (95928-95929)*

⚕ 14.2 ✂ 14.2 **FUD** XXX  [S] [80] [▭]

**AMA:** 2017,Jan,8; 2016,Jan,13; 2015,Jan,16; 2014,Jan,11; 2013,May,8-10; 2012,Apr,17-18

▲ **95930** Visual evoked potential (VEP) checkerboard or flash testing, central nervous system except glaucoma, with interpretation and report

EXCLUDES *Visual acuity screening using automated visual evoked potential devices (0333T)*

*Visual evoked glaucoma testing ([0464T])*

⚕ 3.66 ✂ 3.66 **FUD** XXX  [S] [80] [▭]

**AMA:** 2017,Jan,8; 2016,Jan,13; 2015,Jan,16; 2014,Aug,8; 2013,May,8-10

**95933** Orbicularis oculi (blink) reflex, by electrodiagnostic testing

⚕ 2.17 ✂ 2.17 **FUD** XXX  [QT] [80] [▭]

**AMA:** 2017,Jul,10; 2017,Jan,8; 2016,Jan,13; 2015,Jan,16; 2013,May,8-10

**95937** Neuromuscular junction testing (repetitive stimulation, paired stimuli), each nerve, any 1 method

⚕ 2.32 ✂ 2.32 **FUD** XXX  [S] [80] [▭]

**AMA:** 2017,Jan,8; 2016,Feb,13; 2016,Jan,13; 2015,Jan,16; 2014,Jan,11; 2013,May,8-10; 2013,Mar,3-5

Nerve

Muscle

Nerve fascicles

Model of normal neuromuscular junction

Acetylcholine reaction

A selected neuromusular junction is repeatedly stimulated. The test is useful to demonstrate reduced muscle action potential from fatigue

**95938** Resequenced code. See code following 95926.

**95939** Resequenced code. See code following 95929.

**95940** Resequenced code. See code following 95913.

**95941** Resequenced code. See code following 95913.

**95943** Resequenced code. See code following 95924.

## 95950-95962 Electroencephalography For Seizure Monitoring/Intraoperative Use

EXCLUDES *E&M services*

**95950** Monitoring for identification and lateralization of cerebral seizure focus, electroencephalographic (eg, 8 channel EEG) recording and interpretation, each 24 hours

INCLUDES Only time when recording is taking place and data are being collected and does not include set-up and take-down

Recording for more than 12 hours up to 24 hours

EXCLUDES *Use of code more than one time per 24-hour period*

Code also modifier 52 only when recording is 12 hours or less

⚕ 9.43 ✂ 9.43 **FUD** XXX  [S] [80] [▭]

**AMA:** 2017,Jan,8; 2016,Jan,13; 2015,Jan,16; 2014,Jan,11

**95951** Monitoring for localization of cerebral seizure focus by cable or radio, 16 or more channel telemetry, combined electroencephalographic (EEG) and video recording and interpretation (eg, for presurgical localization), each 24 hours

INCLUDES Interpretations during recording with changes to care of patient

Only time when recording is taking place and data are being collected and does not include set-up and take-down

Recording for more than 12 hours up to 24 hours

EXCLUDES *Use of code more than one time per 24-hour period*

Code also modifier 52 only when recording is 12 hours or less

⚕ 0.00 ✂ 0.00 **FUD** XXX  [S] [80] [▭]

**AMA:** 2017,Jan,8; 2016,Jan,13; 2015,Jan,16; 2014,Dec,16; 2014,Dec,16; 2014,Jan,11; 2013,Aug,13; 2012,Jan,15-42

**95953** Monitoring for localization of cerebral seizure focus by computerized portable 16 or more channel EEG, electroencephalographic (EEG) recording and interpretation, each 24 hours, unattended

INCLUDES Only time when recording is taking place and data are being collected and does not include set-up and take-down
Recording for more than 12 hours up to 24 hours
EXCLUDES *Use of code more than one time per 24-hour period*
Code also modifier 52 only when recording is 12 hours or less
⚙ 12.0  ⚖ 12.0  **FUD** XXX  S 80 ▣
**AMA:** 2017,Jan,8; 2016,Jan,13; 2015,Jan,16; 2014,Dec,16; 2014,Dec,16; 2014,Jan,11

**95954** Pharmacological or physical activation requiring physician or other qualified health care professional attendance during EEG recording of activation phase (eg, thiopental activation test)
⚙ 12.8  ⚖ 12.8  **FUD** XXX  S 80 ▣
**AMA:** 2017,Jan,8; 2016,Jan,13; 2015,Jan,16; 2014,Jan,11

**95955** Electroencephalogram (EEG) during nonintracranial surgery (eg, carotid surgery)
⚙ 6.05  ⚖ 6.05  **FUD** XXX  N 80 ▣
**AMA:** 2017,Jan,8; 2016,Jan,13; 2015,Jan,16; 2014,Dec,18

**95956** Monitoring for localization of cerebral seizure focus by cable or radio, 16 or more channel telemetry, electroencephalographic (EEG) recording and interpretation, each 24 hours, attended by a technologist or nurse

INCLUDES Only time when recording is taking place and data are being collected and does not include set-up and take-down
Recording for more than 12 hours up to 24 hours
EXCLUDES *Use of code more than one time per 24-hour period*
Code also modifier 52 only when recording is 12 hours or less
⚙ 46.0  ⚖ 46.0  **FUD** XXX  S 80 ▣
**AMA:** 2017,Jan,8; 2016,Jan,13; 2015,Jan,16; 2014,Jan,11

**95957** Digital analysis of electroencephalogram (EEG) (eg, for epileptic spike analysis)
⚙ 8.64  ⚖ 8.64  **FUD** XXX  N 80 ▣
**AMA:** 2017,Jan,8; 2016,Jan,13; 2015,Jan,16; 2014,Jan,11

**95958** Wada activation test for hemispheric function, including electroencephalographic (EEG) monitoring
⚙ 16.4  ⚖ 16.4  **FUD** XXX  S 80 ▣
**AMA:** 2000,Jul,1; 1998,Nov,1

**95961** Functional cortical and subcortical mapping by stimulation and/or recording of electrodes on brain surface, or of depth electrodes, to provoke seizures or identify vital brain structures; initial hour of attendance by a physician or other qualified health care professional

INCLUDES One hour of attendance by physician or other qualified health care professional
Code also each additional hour of attendance by physician or other qualified health care professional, when appropriate (95962)
Code also modifier 52 for 30 minutes or less of attendance by physician or other qualified health care professional
⚙ 8.68  ⚖ 8.68  **FUD** XXX  S 80 ▣
**AMA:** 2017,Jan,8; 2016,Jan,13; 2015,Jan,16; 2014,Jan,11; 2012,Jan,15-42

**+ 95962** each additional hour of attendance by a physician or other qualified health care professional (List separately in addition to code for primary procedure)

INCLUDES One hour of attendance by physician or other qualified health care professional
Code first initial hour (95961)
⚙ 7.43  ⚖ 7.43  **FUD** ZZZ  N 80 ▣
**AMA:** 2017,Jan,8; 2016,Jan,13; 2015,Jan,16; 2014,Jan,11; 2012,Jan,15-42

## 95965-95967 Magnetoencephalography

INCLUDES Physician interpretation
Recording
Report
EXCLUDES *CT provided along with magnetoencephalography (70450-70470, 70496)*
*Electroencephalography provided along with magnetoencephalography (95812-95827)*
*E&M services*
*MRI provided along with magnetoencephalography (70551-70553)*
*Somatosensory evoked potentials/auditory evoked potentials/visual evoked potentials provided along with magnetic evoked field responses (92585, 95925, 95926, 95930)*

**95965** Magnetoencephalography (MEG), recording and analysis; for spontaneous brain magnetic activity (eg, epileptic cerebral cortex localization)
⚙ 0.00  ⚖ 0.00  **FUD** XXX  S 80 ▣
**AMA:** 1997,Nov,1

**95966** for evoked magnetic fields, single modality (eg, sensory, motor, language, or visual cortex localization)
⚙ 0.00  ⚖ 0.00  **FUD** XXX  S 80 ▣
**AMA:** 1997,Nov,1

**+ 95967** for evoked magnetic fields, each additional modality (eg, sensory, motor, language, or visual cortex localization) (List separately in addition to code for primary procedure)
Code first single modality (95966)
⚙ 0.00  ⚖ 0.00  **FUD** ZZZ  N 80 ▣
**AMA:** 1997,Nov,1

## 95970-95982 Evaluation of Implanted Neurostimulator

INCLUDES Simple intraoperative or subsequent programming of neurostimulator (three or less of the following); or complex neurostimulator (three or more of the following):
8 or more electrode contacts
Alternating electrode polarities
Cycling
Dose time
More than 1 clinical feature
Number of channels
Number of programs
Pulse amplitude
Pulse duration
Pulse frequency
Rate
Stimulation train duration
Train spacing
EXCLUDES *E&M services*
*Neurostimulator electrodes:*
*Implantation (43647, 43881, 61850-61870, 63650-63655, 64553-64580)*
*Revision/removal (43648, 43882, 61880, 63661-63664, 64585)*
*Neurostimulator pulse generator/receiver:*
*Insertion (61885, 63685, 64590)*
*Revision/removal (61888, 63688, 64595)*

**95970** Electronic analysis of implanted neurostimulator pulse generator system (eg, rate, pulse amplitude, pulse duration, configuration of wave form, battery status, electrode selectability, output modulation, cycling, impedance and patient compliance measurements); simple or complex brain, spinal cord, or peripheral (ie, cranial nerve, peripheral nerve, sacral nerve, neuromuscular) neurostimulator pulse generator/transmitter, without reprogramming
⚙ 0.69  ⚖ 1.93  **FUD** XXX  Q1 80 ▣
**AMA:** 2017,Jan,8; 2016,Jul,7; 2016,Jan,13; 2015,Jan,16; 2014,Jan,11; 2012,Jan,15-42

**95971** simple spinal cord, or peripheral (ie, peripheral nerve, sacral nerve, neuromuscular) neurostimulator pulse generator/transmitter, with intraoperative or subsequent programming
⚙ 1.16  ⚖ 1.43  **FUD** XXX  S 80 ▣
**AMA:** 2017,Jan,8; 2016,Jul,7; 2016,Jan,13; 2015,Jan,16; 2014,Jan,11; 2012,Oct,14; 2012,Jan,15-42

**95972** complex spinal cord, or peripheral (ie, peripheral nerve, sacral nerve, neuromuscular) (except cranial nerve) neurostimulator pulse generator/transmitter, with intraoperative or subsequent programming

🔌 1.19    1.65  **FUD** XXX    S 80 ▣

**AMA:** 2017,Jan,8; 2016,Jul,7; 2016,Jan,13; 2015,Jan,16; 2014,Aug,5; 2014,Jan,11

**95974** complex cranial nerve neurostimulator pulse generator/transmitter, with intraoperative or subsequent programming, with or without nerve interface testing, first hour

Code also modifier 52 for service less than 31 minutes

🔌 4.69    5.90  **FUD** XXX    S 80 ▣

**AMA:** 2017,Jan,8; 2016,Jul,7; 2016,Jan,13; 2015,Jan,16; 2014,Aug,5; 2014,Jan,11; 2012,Jan,15-42

+ **95975** complex cranial nerve neurostimulator pulse generator/transmitter, with intraoperative or subsequent programming, each additional 30 minutes after first hour (List separately in addition to code for primary procedure)

Code first initial hour (95974)

🔌 2.65    3.17  **FUD** ZZZ    N 80 ▣

**AMA:** 2017,Jan,8; 2016,Jul,7; 2016,Jan,13; 2015,Jan,16; 2014,Jan,11; 2012,Jan,15-42

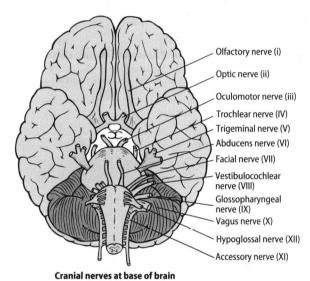

Olfactory nerve (i)
Optic nerve (ii)
Oculomotor nerve (iii)
Trochlear nerve (IV)
Trigeminal nerve (V)
Abducens nerve (VI)
Facial nerve (VII)
Vestibulocochlear nerve (VIII)
Glossopharyngeal nerve (IX)
Vagus nerve (X)
Hypoglossal nerve (XII)
Accessory nerve (XI)

**Cranial nerves at base of brain**

**95978** Electronic analysis of implanted neurostimulator pulse generator system (eg, rate, pulse amplitude and duration, battery status, electrode selectability and polarity, impedance and patient compliance measurements), complex deep brain neurostimulator pulse generator/transmitter, with initial or subsequent programming; first hour

Code also modifier 52 for service less than 31 minutes

🔌 5.49    7.08  **FUD** XXX    S 80 ▣

**AMA:** 2017,Jan,8; 2016,Jul,7; 2016,Jan,13; 2015,Jan,16; 2014,Aug,5; 2014,Jan,11

+ **95979** each additional 30 minutes after first hour (List separately in addition to code for primary procedure)

Code first initial hour (95978)

🔌 2.56    3.07  **FUD** ZZZ    N 80 ▣

**AMA:** 2017,Jan,8; 2016,Jul,7; 2016,Jan,13; 2015,Jan,16; 2014,Jan,11

**95980** Electronic analysis of implanted neurostimulator pulse generator system (eg, rate, pulse amplitude and duration, configuration of wave form, battery status, electrode selectability, output modulation, cycling, impedance and patient measurements) gastric neurostimulator pulse generator/transmitter; intraoperative, with programming

INCLUDES  Gastric neurostimulator of lesser curvature

EXCLUDES  *Analysis, with programming when performed, of vagus nerve trunk stimulator for morbid obesity (0312T, 0317T)*

🔌 1.32    1.32  **FUD** XXX    N 80 ▣

**AMA:** 2017,Jan,8; 2016,Jul,7; 2016,Jan,13; 2015,Jan,16; 2014,Jan,11; 2012,Jan,15-42

**95981** subsequent, without reprogramming

EXCLUDES  *Analysis, with programming when performed, of vagus nerve trunk stimulator for morbid obesity (0312T, 0317T)*

🔌 0.51    0.91  **FUD** XXX    Q1 80 ▣

**AMA:** 2017,Jan,8; 2016,Jul,7; 2016,Jan,13; 2015,Jan,16; 2014,Jan,11

**95982** subsequent, with reprogramming

EXCLUDES  *Analysis, with programming when performed, of vagus nerve trunk stimulator for morbid obesity (0312T, 0317T)*

🔌 1.04    1.50  **FUD** XXX    Q1 80 ▣

**AMA:** 2017,Jan,8; 2016,Jul,7; 2016,Jan,13; 2015,Jan,16; 2014,Jan,11

## 95990-95991 Refill/Upkeep of Implanted Drug Delivery Pump to Central Nervous System

EXCLUDES  *Analysis/reprogramming of implanted pump for infusion (62367-62370)*
*E&M services*

**95990** Refilling and maintenance of implantable pump or reservoir for drug delivery, spinal (intrathecal, epidural) or brain (intraventricular), includes electronic analysis of pump, when performed;

🔌 2.56    2.56  **FUD** XXX    S 80 ▣

**AMA:** 2017,Jan,8; 2016,Jan,13; 2015,Jan,16; 2014,Jan,11; 2012,Aug,10-12; 2012,Jul,3-6; 2012,Jan,15-42

**95991** requiring skill of a physician or other qualified health care professional

🔌 1.13    3.37  **FUD** XXX    T 80 ▣

**AMA:** 2017,Jan,8; 2016,Jan,13; 2015,Jan,16; 2014,Jan,11; 2012,Aug,10-12; 2012,Jul,3-6

## 95992-95999 Other and Unlisted Neurological Procedures

**95992** Canalith repositioning procedure(s) (eg, Epley maneuver, Semont maneuver), per day

EXCLUDES  *Nystagmus testing (92531-92532)*

🔌 1.06    1.22  **FUD** XXX    ⊘ A 80 ▣

**AMA:** 2017,Jan,8; 2016,Jan,13; 2015,Jan,16; 2014,Jan,11

**95999** Unlisted neurological or neuromuscular diagnostic procedure

🔌 0.00    0.00  **FUD** XXX    Q1 80

**AMA:** 2017,Jan,8; 2016,Jan,13; 2015,Aug,8; 2015,Jan,16; 2014,Jan,11; 2012,Jan,15-42

## 96000-96004 Motion Analysis Studies

**CMS:** 100-02,15,230.4 Services By a Physical/Occupational Therapist in Private Practice

INCLUDES  Services provided as part of major therapeutic/diagnostic decision making
Services provided in a dedicated motion analysis department capable of:
3-D kinetics/dynamic electromyography
Computerized 3-D kinematics
Videotaping from the front/back/both sides

EXCLUDES  *E&M services*
*Gait training (97116)*
*Needle electromyography (95860-95872 [95885, 95886, 95887])*

**96000** Comprehensive computer-based motion analysis by video-taping and 3D kinematics;

🔌 2.71    2.71  **FUD** XXX    S 80 ▣

**AMA:** 2017,Jan,8; 2016,Jan,13; 2015,Jan,16; 2014,Jan,11

| 26/TC PC/TC Only | A2-Z3 ASC Payment | 50 Bilateral | ♂ Male Only | ♀ Female Only | 🔌 Facility RVU | ⚖ Non-Facility RVU | ▣ CCI |
| **FUD** Follow-up Days | **CMS:** IOM (Pub 100) | A-Y OPPSI | 80/80 Surg Assist Allowed / w/Doc | | ▮ Lab Crosswalk | ▦ Radiology Crosswalk | ✖ CLIA |

**476**  CPT © 2017 American Medical Association. All Rights Reserved.  © 2017 Optum360, LLC

**96001** **with dynamic plantar pressure measurements during walking**

    🚑 3.47    ⚕ 3.47    **FUD** XXX      S 80 🖥

    **AMA:** 2017,Jan,8; 2016,Jan,13; 2015,Jan,16; 2014,Jan,11

**96002** **Dynamic surface electromyography, during walking or other functional activities, 1-12 muscles**

    🚑 0.62    ⚕ 0.62    **FUD** XXX      S 80 🖥

    **AMA:** 2017,Jan,8; 2016,Jan,13; 2015,Aug,8; 2015,Jan,16; 2014,Jan,11

**96003** **Dynamic fine wire electromyography, during walking or other functional activities, 1 muscle**

    🚑 0.47    ⚕ 0.47    **FUD** XXX      Q1 80 🖥

    **AMA:** 2017,Jan,8; 2016,Jan,13; 2015,Jan,16; 2014,Jan,11

**96004** **Review and interpretation by physician or other qualified health care professional of comprehensive computer-based motion analysis, dynamic plantar pressure measurements, dynamic surface electromyography during walking or other functional activities, and dynamic fine wire electromyography, with written report**

    🚑 3.33    ⚕ 3.33    **FUD** XXX      B 80 26 🖥

    **AMA:** 2017,Jan,8; 2016,Jan,13; 2015,Aug,8; 2015,Jan,16; 2014,Jan,11

## 96020 Neurofunctional Brain Testing

INCLUDES    Selection/administration of testing of:
       Cognition
       Determination of validity of neurofunctional testing relative to separately interpreted functional magnetic resonance images
       Functional neuroimaging
       Language
       Memory
       Monitoring performance of testing
       Movement
       Other neurological functions
       Sensation

EXCLUDES    *Clinical depression treatment by repetitive transcranial magnetic stimulation (90867-90868)*
     *E&M services on the same date*
     *MRI of the brain (70554-70555)*
     *Neuropsychological testing on the same date (96116-96120)*
     *Psychological testing on the same date (96101-96103)*

**96020** **Neurofunctional testing selection and administration during noninvasive imaging functional brain mapping, with test administered entirely by a physician or other qualified health care professional (ie, psychologist), with review of test results and report**

    🚑 0.00    ⚕ 0.00    **FUD** XXX      N 80 🖥

    **AMA:** 2017,Jan,8; 2016,Jan,13; 2015,Jan,16; 2014,Jan,11

## 96040 Genetic Counseling Services

INCLUDES    Analysis for genetic risk assessment
       Counseling of patient/family
       Counseling services
       Face-to-face interviews
       Obtaining structured family genetic history
       Pedigree construction
       Review of medical data/family information
       Services provided by trained genetic counselor
       Services provided during one or more sessions
       Thirty minutes of face-to-face time and is reported one time for each 16-30 minutes of the service

EXCLUDES    *Education/genetic counseling by a physician or other qualified health care provider to a group (99078)*
     *Education/genetic counseling by a physician or other qualified health care provider to an individual; use appropriate E&M code*
     *Education regarding genetic risks by a nonphysician to a group (98961, 98962)*
     *Genetic counseling and/or risk factor reduction intervention from a physician or other qualified health care provider provided to patients without symptoms/diagnosis (99401-99412)*
     *Use of code when 15 minutes or less of face-to-face time is provided*

**96040** **Medical genetics and genetic counseling services, each 30 minutes face-to-face with patient/family**

    🚑 1.33    ⚕ 1.33    **FUD** XXX      ★ B 🖥

    **AMA:** 2017,Jan,8; 2016,Jan,13; 2015,Jan,16; 2014,Jan,11

## 96101-96127 Cognitive Capability Assessments

**CMS:** 100-02,15,80.2 Psychological and Neuropsychological Tests

INCLUDES    Cognitive function testing of the central nervous system

EXCLUDES    *Cognitive skills development (97127, 97533)*
     *Physician conducted mini-mental status examination; use appropriate E&M code*

**96101** **Psychological testing (includes psychodiagnostic assessment of emotionality, intellectual abilities, personality and psychopathology, eg, MMPI, Rorschach, WAIS), per hour of the psychologist's or physician's time, both face-to-face time administering tests to the patient and time interpreting these test results and preparing the report**

    INCLUDES    Situations when more time is needed to assimilate other clinical data sources including tests administered by a technician or computer and previously reported
         Time spent face to face, interpretation, and preparing report

    EXCLUDES    *Adaptive behavior services (0364T-0367T, 0373T-0374T)*
         *Use of code for less than 31 minutes of time*

    🚑 2.23    ⚕ 2.25    **FUD** XXX      Q3 80 🖥

    **AMA:** 2017,Jul,10; 2017,Jan,8; 2016,Sep,9; 2016,Jan,13; 2015,Aug,5; 2015,Jan,16; 2014,Jun,3; 2014,Jan,11; 2012,Jan,15-42

**96102** **Psychological testing (includes psychodiagnostic assessment of emotionality, intellectual abilities, personality and psychopathology, eg, MMPI and WAIS), with qualified health care professional interpretation and report, administered by technician, per hour of technician time, face-to-face**

    EXCLUDES    *Adaptive behavior services (0364T-0367T, 0373T-0374T)*
         *Use of code for less than 31 minutes of time*

    🚑 0.67    ⚕ 1.75    **FUD** XXX      Q3 80 🖥

    **AMA:** 2017,Jan,8; 2016,Sep,9; 2016,Jan,13; 2015,Aug,5; 2015,Jan,16; 2014,Jan,11

**96103** **Psychological testing (includes psychodiagnostic assessment of emotionality, intellectual abilities, personality and psychopathology, eg, MMPI), administered by a computer, with qualified health care professional interpretation and report**

    EXCLUDES    *Adaptive behavior services (0364T-0367T, 0373T-0374T)*

    🚑 0.75    ⚕ 0.78    **FUD** XXX      Q1 80 🖥

    **AMA:** 2017,Jan,8; 2016,Sep,9; 2016,Jan,13; 2015,Aug,5; 2015,Jan,16; 2014,Jan,11; 2012,Jan,15-42

**96105** **Assessment of aphasia (includes assessment of expressive and receptive speech and language function, language comprehension, speech production ability, reading, spelling, writing, eg, by Boston Diagnostic Aphasia Examination) with interpretation and report, per hour**

    EXCLUDES    *Adaptive behavior services (0364T-0367T, 0373T-0374T)*
         *Use of code for less than 31 minutes of time*

    🚑 3.04    ⚕ 3.04    **FUD** XXX      A 80 🖥

    **AMA:** 2017,Jan,8; 2016,Jan,13; 2015,Aug,5; 2015,Jan,16; 2014,Jan,11

**96110** **Developmental screening (eg, developmental milestone survey, speech and language delay screen), with scoring and documentation, per standardized instrument**

    EXCLUDES    *Adaptive behavior services (0364T-0367T, 0373T-0374T)*

    🚑 0.27    ⚕ 0.27    **FUD** XXX      E 🖥

    **AMA:** 2017,Feb,14; 2017,Jan,8; 2016,Jan,13; 2015,Aug,5; 2015,Jan,16; 2014,Jun,3; 2014,Jan,11

**96111** **Developmental testing, (includes assessment of motor, language, social, adaptive, and/or cognitive functioning by standardized developmental instruments) with interpretation and report**

    EXCLUDES    *Adaptive behavior services (0364T-0367T, 0373T-0374T)*

    🚑 3.54    ⚕ 3.71    **FUD** XXX      Q3 80 🖥

    **AMA:** 2017,Jan,8; 2016,Jan,13; 2015,Aug,5; 2015,Jan,16; 2014,Jan,11

---

● New Code    ▲ Revised Code    ○ Reinstated    ● New Web Release    ▲ Revised Web Release    Unlisted    Not Covered    # Resequenced
⊘ AMA Mod 51 Exempt    ⑤ Optum Mod 51 Exempt    ⑥ Mod 63 Exempt    ✗ Non-FDA Drug    ★ Telemedicine    Ⓜ Maternity    Ⓐ Age Edit    + Add-on    **AMA:** CPT Asst
© 2017 Optum360, LLC        CPT © 2017 American Medical Association. All Rights Reserved.

**96116** Neurobehavioral status exam (clinical assessment of thinking, reasoning and judgment, eg, acquired knowledge, attention, language, memory, planning and problem solving, and visual spatial abilities), per hour of the psychologist's or physician's time, both face-to-face time with the patient and time interpreting test results and preparing the report

> INCLUDES Time spent face to face, interpretation, and preparing report

> EXCLUDES *Adaptive behavior services (0364T-0367T, 0373T-0374T)*
> *Use of code for less than 31 minutes of time*

> 🔲 2.44 🔲 2.60 **FUD** XXX ★ 🔲 🔲 🔲

> **AMA:** 2017,Jan,8; 2016,Jan,13; 2015,Aug,5; 2015,Jan,16; 2014,Jun,3; 2014,Jan,11; 2012,Jan,15-42

**96118** Neuropsychological testing (eg, Halstead-Reitan Neuropsychological Battery, Wechsler Memory Scales and Wisconsin Card Sorting Test), per hour of the psychologist's or physician's time, both face-to-face time administering tests to the patient and time interpreting these test results and preparing the report

> INCLUDES Situations when more time is needed to assimilate other clinical data sources including tests administered by a technician or computer and previously reported
> Time spent face to face, interpretation, and preparing report

> EXCLUDES *Adaptive behavior services (0364T-0367T, 0373T-0374T)*
> *Use of code for less than 31 minutes of time*

> 🔲 2.22 🔲 2.75 **FUD** XXX 🔲 🔲 🔲

> **AMA:** 2017,Jan,8; 2016,Jan,13; 2015,Aug,5; 2015,Jan,16; 2014,Jun,3; 2014,Jan,11; 2012,Jan,15-42

**96119** Neuropsychological testing (eg, Halstead-Reitan Neuropsychological Battery, Wechsler Memory Scales and Wisconsin Card Sorting Test), with qualified health care professional interpretation and report, administered by technician, per hour of technician time, face-to-face

> EXCLUDES *Adaptive behavior services (0364T-0367T, 0373T-0374T)*
> *Use of code for less than 31 minutes of time*

> 🔲 0.67 🔲 2.24 **FUD** XXX 🔲 🔲 🔲

> **AMA:** 2017,Jan,8; 2016,Jan,13; 2015,Aug,5; 2015,Jan,16; 2014,Jan,11

**96120** Neuropsychological testing (eg, Wisconsin Card Sorting Test), administered by a computer, with qualified health care professional interpretation and report

> EXCLUDES *Adaptive behavior services (0364T-0367T, 0373T-0374T)*
> *Use of code for less than 31 minutes of time*

> 🔲 0.74 🔲 1.36 **FUD** XXX 🔲 🔲 🔲

> **AMA:** 2017,Jan,8; 2016,Jan,13; 2015,Aug,5; 2015,Jan,16; 2014,Jan,11; 2012,Jan,15-42

**96125** Standardized cognitive performance testing (eg, Ross Information Processing Assessment) per hour of a qualified health care professional's time, both face-to-face time administering tests to the patient and time interpreting these test results and preparing the report

> INCLUDES Time spent face to face, interpretation, and preparing report

> EXCLUDES *Adaptive behavior services (0364T-0367T, 0373T-0374T)*
> *Neuropsychological testing (96118-96120)*
> *Psychological testing (96101-96103)*
> *Use of code for less than 31 minutes of time*

> 🔲 3.28 🔲 3.28 **FUD** XXX 🔲 🔲 🔲

> **AMA:** 2017,Jan,8; 2016,Jan,13; 2015,Aug,5; 2015,Jan,16; 2014,Jan,11; 2012,Jan,15-42

**96127** Brief emotional/behavioral assessment (eg, depression inventory, attention-deficit/hyperactivity disorder [ADHD] scale), with scoring and documentation, per standardized instrument

> 🔲 0.16 🔲 0.16 **FUD** XXX 🔲 🔲 🔲 🔲

> **AMA:** 2017,Feb,14; 2017,Jan,8; 2016,Jan,13; 2015,Aug,5

## 96150-96155 Biopsychosocial Assessment/Intervention

> INCLUDES Services for patients that have primary physical illnesses/diagnoses/symptoms who may benefit from assessments/interventions that focus on the biopsychosocial factors related to the patient's health status
> Services used to identify the following factors which are important to the prevention/treatment/management of physical health problems:
> Behavioral
> Cognitive
> Emotional
> Psychological
> Social

> EXCLUDES *Adaptive behavior services (0364T-0367T, 0373T-0374T)*
> *E&M services on the same date*
> *Preventive medicine counseling services (99401-99412)*
> *Psychotherapy services (90785-90899)*

**96150** Health and behavior assessment (eg, health-focused clinical interview, behavioral observations, psychophysiological monitoring, health-oriented questionnaires), each 15 minutes face-to-face with the patient; initial assessment

> 🔲 0.60 🔲 0.61 **FUD** XXX ★ 🔲 🔲 🔲

> **AMA:** 2017,Jan,8; 2016,Jan,13; 2015,Jan,16; 2014,Sep,13; 2014,Jun,3; 2014,Jan,11; 2013,May,12; 2012,Jan,15-42

**96151** re-assessment

> 🔲 0.58 🔲 0.59 **FUD** XXX ★ 🔲 🔲 🔲

> **AMA:** 2017,Jan,8; 2016,Jan,13; 2015,Jan,16; 2014,Sep,13; 2014,Jun,3; 2014,Jan,11; 2013,May,12; 2012,Jan,15-42

**96152** Health and behavior intervention, each 15 minutes, face-to-face; individual

> 🔲 0.55 🔲 0.56 **FUD** XXX ★ 🔲 🔲 🔲

> **AMA:** 2017,Jan,8; 2016,Jan,13; 2015,Jan,16; 2014,Sep,13; 2014,Jun,3; 2014,Jan,11; 2013,May,12; 2012,Jan,15-42

**96153** group (2 or more patients)

> 🔲 0.12 🔲 0.13 **FUD** XXX ★ 🔲 🔲 🔲

> **AMA:** 2017,Jan,8; 2016,Jan,13; 2015,Jan,16; 2014,Sep,13; 2014,Jun,3; 2014,Jan,11; 2013,May,12; 2012,Jan,15-42

**96154** family (with the patient present)

> 🔲 0.54 🔲 0.55 **FUD** XXX ★ 🔲 🔲 🔲

> **AMA:** 2017,Jan,8; 2016,Jan,13; 2015,Jan,16; 2014,Sep,13; 2014,Jun,3; 2014,Jan,11; 2013,May,12; 2012,Jan,15-42

**96155** family (without the patient present)

> 🔲 0.64 🔲 0.64 **FUD** XXX 🔲 🔲

> **AMA:** 2017,Jan,8; 2016,Jan,13; 2015,Jan,16; 2014,Sep,13; 2014,Jun,3; 2014,Jan,11; 2013,May,12; 2012,Jan,15-42

## 96160-96161 Health Risk Assessments

**96160** Administration of patient-focused health risk assessment instrument (eg, health hazard appraisal) with scoring and documentation, per standardized instrument

> 🔲 0.13 🔲 0.13 **FUD** ZZZ 🔲 🔲

> **AMA:** 2017,Feb,14; 2017,Jan,8; 2016,Nov,5

**96161** Administration of caregiver-focused health risk assessment instrument (eg, depression inventory) for the benefit of the patient, with scoring and documentation, per standardized instrument

> 🔲 0.13 🔲 0.13 **FUD** ZZZ 🔲 🔲

> **AMA:** 2017,Feb,14; 2017,Jan,8; 2016,Nov,5

🔲/🔲 PC/TC Only    🔲-🔲 ASC Payment    🔲 Bilateral    ♂ Male Only    ♀ Female Only    🔲 Facility RVU    🔲 Non-Facility RVU    🔲 CCI
**FUD** Follow-up Days    **CMS:** IOM (Pub 100)    🔲-🔲 OPPSI    🔲/🔲 Surg Assist Allowed / w/Doc    🔲 Lab Crosswalk    🔲 Radiology Crosswalk    🔲 CLIA
CPT © 2017 American Medical Association. All Rights Reserved.

478     © 2017 Optum360, LLC

## 96360-96361 Intravenous Fluid Infusion for Hydration (Nonchemotherapy)

**CMS:** 100-04,4,230.2 OPPS Drug Administration

INCLUDES Administration of prepackaged fluids and electrolytes
Coding hierarchy rules for facility reporting only:
　Chemotherapy services are primary to diagnostic, prophylactic, and therapeutic services
　Diagnostic, prophylactic, and therapeutic services are primary to hydration services
　Infusions are primary to pushes
　Pushes are primary to injections
　　Constant observance/attendance of person administering the drug or substance
　　Infusion of 15 minutes or less
Direct supervision by physician or other qualified health care provider:
　Direction of personnel
Minimal supervision for:
　Consent
　Safety oversight
　Supervision of personnel
Report the initial code for the primary reason for the visit regardless of the order in which the infusions or injections are given
The following if done to facilitate the injection/infusion:
　Flush at the end of infusion
　Indwelling IV, subcutaneous catheter/port access
　Local anesthesia
　Start of IV
　Supplies/tubing/syringes
　Treatment plan verification

EXCLUDES *Catheter/port declotting (36593)*
*Drugs/other substances*
*Minimal infusion to keep the vein open or during other therapeutic infusions*
*Services provided by physicians or other qualified health care providers in facility settings*
*Significant separately identifiable E&M service if performed*
*Use of a code for a second initial service on the same date for accessing a multi-lumen catheter, restarting an IV, or when two IV lines are needed to meet an infusion rate*
*Use of code for infusion for hydration that is 31 minutes or less*

**96360** **Intravenous infusion, hydration; initial, 31 minutes to 1 hour**

EXCLUDES *Use of code if service is performed as a concurrent infusion*

🚑 1.63　⚖ 1.63　**FUD** XXX　　　S 80 ▣

**AMA:** 2017,Jan,8; 2016,Jan,13; 2015,Jan,16; 2014,May,10; 2014,Jan,11; 2013,Oct,3

**+ 96361** **each additional hour (List separately in addition to code for primary procedure)**

INCLUDES Hydration infusion of more than 30 minutes beyond 1 hour
Hydration provided as a secondary or subsequent service after a different initial service via the same IV access site
Code first (96360)

🚑 0.43　⚖ 0.43　**FUD** ZZZ　　　S 80 ▣

**AMA:** 2017,Jan,8; 2016,Jan,13; 2015,Jan,16; 2014,May,10; 2014,Jan,11; 2013,Oct,3

## 96365-96371 Infusions: Diagnostic/Preventive/Therapeutic

**CMS:** 100-04,4,230.2 OPPS Drug Administration

INCLUDES Administration of fluid
Administration of substances/drugs
An infusion of 16 minutes or more
Coding hierarchy rules for facility reporting:
　Chemotherapy services are primary to diagnostic, prophylactic, and therapeutic services
　Diagnostic, prophylactic, and therapeutic services are primary to hydration services
　Infusions are primary to pushes
　Pushes are primary to injections
Constant presence of health care professional administering the substance/drug
Direct supervision of physician or other qualified health care provider:
　Consent
　Direction of personnel
　Patient assessment
　Safety oversight
　Supervision of personnel
The following if done to facilitate the injection/infusion:
　Flush at the end of infusion
　Indwelling IV, subcutaneous catheter/port access
　Local anesthesia
　Start of IV
　Supplies/tubing/syringes
Training to assess patient and monitor vital signs
Training to prepare/dose/dispose
Treatment plan verification

EXCLUDES *Catheter/port declotting (36593)*
*Services provided by physicians or other qualified health care providers in facility settings*
*Significant separately identifiable E&M service, when performed*
*Use of a code for a second initial service on the same date for accessing a multi-lumen catheter, restarting an IV, or when two IV lines are needed to meet an infusion rate*
*Use of code with other procedures for which IV push or infusion is an integral part of the procedure*
Code also drugs/materials

**96365** **Intravenous infusion, for therapy, prophylaxis, or diagnosis (specify substance or drug); initial, up to 1 hour**

Code also second initial service with modifier 59 when patient's condition or drug protocol mandates the use of two IV lines

🚑 1.95　⚖ 1.95　**FUD** XXX　　　S 80 ▣

**AMA:** 2017,Jan,8; 2016,Jan,13; 2015,Jan,16; 2014,Jan,11; 2012,Jan,15-42

**+ 96366** **each additional hour (List separately in addition to code for primary procedure)**

INCLUDES Additional hours of sequential infusion
Infusion intervals of more than 30 minutes beyond one hour
Second and subsequent infusions of the same drug or substance
Code also additional infusion, when appropriate (96367)
Code first (96365)

🚑 0.53　⚖ 0.53　**FUD** ZZZ　　　S 80 ▣

**AMA:** 2017,Jan,8; 2016,Jan,13; 2015,Jan,16; 2014,Jan,11; 2012,Jan,15-42

**+ 96367** **additional sequential infusion of a new drug/substance, up to 1 hour (List separately in addition to code for primary procedure)**

INCLUDES A secondary or subsequent service with a new drug or substance after a different initial service via the same IV access

EXCLUDES *Use of code more than one time per sequential infusion of the same mix*

Code first (96365, 96374, 96409, 96413)

🚑 0.87　⚖ 0.87　**FUD** ZZZ　　　S 80 ▣

**AMA:** 2017,Jan,8; 2016,Jan,13; 2015,Jan,16; 2014,Jan,11; 2012,Jan,15-42

**+ 96368** **concurrent infusion (List separately in addition to code for primary procedure)**

EXCLUDES *Use of code more than one time per date of service*

Code first (96365, 96366, 96413, 96415, 96416)

🚑 0.58　⚖ 0.58　**FUD** ZZZ　　　N 80 ▣

**AMA:** 2017,Jan,8; 2016,Jan,13; 2015,Jan,16; 2014,Jan,11

---

● New Code　▲ Revised Code　○ Reinstated　● New Web Release　▲ Revised Web Release　Unlisted　Not Covered　# Resequenced
⊘ AMA Mod 51 Exempt　⑤⓪ Optum Mod 51 Exempt　⑥③ Mod 63 Exempt　✗ Non-FDA Drug　★ Telemedicine　Ⓜ Maternity　Ⓐ Age Edit　+ Add-on　**AMA:** CPT Asst

© 2017 Optum360, LLC　CPT © 2017 American Medical Association. All Rights Reserved.

**96369**    **Subcutaneous infusion for therapy or prophylaxis (specify substance or drug); initial, up to 1 hour, including pump set-up and establishment of subcutaneous infusion site(s)**

> EXCLUDES   *Infusions of 15 minutes or less (96372)*
>
> *Use of code more than one time per encounter*

🚑 5.03    ⚕ 5.03    **FUD** XXX      [S] [80] [▣]

**AMA:** 2017,Jan,8; 2016,Jan,13; 2015,Jan,16; 2014,Jan,11

+ **96370**    **each additional hour (List separately in addition to code for primary procedure)**

> INCLUDES   Infusions of more than 30 minutes beyond one hour

Code first (96369)

🚑 0.43    ⚕ 0.43    **FUD** ZZZ      [S] [80] [▣]

**AMA:** 2017,Jan,8; 2016,Jan,13; 2015,Jan,16; 2014,Jan,11

+ **96371**    **additional pump set-up with establishment of new subcutaneous infusion site(s) (List separately in addition to code for primary procedure)**

> EXCLUDES   *Use of code more than one time per encounter*

Code first (96369)

🚑 1.93    ⚕ 1.93    **FUD** ZZZ      [S] [80] [▣]

**AMA:** 2017,Jan,8; 2016,Jan,13; 2015,Jan,16; 2014,Jan,11

## 96372-96379 Injections: Diagnostic/Preventive/Therapeutic

**CMS:** 100-04,4,230.2 OPPS Drug Administration

> INCLUDES   Administration of fluid
> Administration of substances/drugs
> Coding hierarchy rules for facility reporting:
> > Chemotherapy services are primary to diagnostic, prophylactic, and therapeutic services
> > Infusions are primary to pushes
> > Pushes are primary to injections
>
> Constant presence of health care professional administering the substance/drug
> Direct supervision by physician or other qualified health care provider:
> > Consent
> > Direction of personnel
> > Patient assessment
> > Safety oversight
> > Supervision of personnel
>
> Infusion of 15 minutes or less
> The following if done to facilitate the injection/infusion:
> > Flush at the end of infusion
> > Indwelling IV, subcutaneous catheter/port access
> > Local anesthesia
> > Start of IV
> > Supplies/tubing/syringes
>
> Training to assess patient and monitor vital signs
> Training to prepare/dose/dispose
> Treatment plan verification

> EXCLUDES   *Catheter/port declotting (36593)*
> *Services provided by physicians or other qualified health care providers in facility settings*
> *Significant separately identifiable E&M service, when performed*
> *Use of a code for a second initial service on the same date for accessing a multi-lumen catheter, restarting an IV, or when two IV lines are needed to meet an infusion rate*
> *Use of code with other procedures for which IV push or infusion is an integral part of the procedure*

Code also drugs/materials

**96372**    **Therapeutic, prophylactic, or diagnostic injection (specify substance or drug); subcutaneous or intramuscular**

> INCLUDES   Direct supervision by physician or other qualified health care provider when reported by the physician/other qualified health care provider. When reported by a hospital, physician/other qualified health care provider need not be present.
> Hormonal therapy injections (non-antineoplastic) (96372)

> EXCLUDES   *Administration of vaccines/toxoids (90460-90474)*
> *Allergen immunotherapy injections (95115-95117)*
> *Antineoplastic hormonal injections (96402)*
> *Antineoplastic nonhormonal injections (96401)*
> *Injections administered without direct supervision by physician or other qualified health care provider (99211)*

🚑 0.72    ⚕ 0.72    **FUD** XXX      [S] [80] [▣]

**AMA:** 2017,Jan,8; 2016,Oct,9; 2016,Jan,13; 2015,Jan,16; 2014,Jan,9; 2014,Jan,11; 2013,Jan,9-10; 2012,Jan,15-42

**96373**    **intra-arterial**

🚑 0.54    ⚕ 0.54    **FUD** XXX      [S] [80] [▣]

**AMA:** 2017,Jan,8; 2016,Jan,13; 2015,Jan,16; 2014,Jan,11

**96374**    **intravenous push, single or initial substance/drug**

> Code also second initial service with modifier 59 when patient's condition or drug protocol mandates the use of two IV lines

🚑 1.62    ⚕ 1.62    **FUD** XXX      [S] [80] [▣]

**AMA:** 2017,Jan,8; 2016,Jan,13; 2015,Nov,3; 2015,Jan,16; 2014,Jan,11; 2013,Jun,9-11; 2013,Feb,3-6

+ **96375**    **each additional sequential intravenous push of a new substance/drug (List separately in addition to code for primary procedure)**

> INCLUDES   IV push of a new substance/drug provided as a secondary or subsequent service after a different initial service via same IV access site

Code first (96365, 96374, 96409, 96413)

🚑 0.63    ⚕ 0.63    **FUD** ZZZ      [S] [80] [▣]

**AMA:** 2017,Jan,8; 2016,Jan,13; 2015,Nov,3; 2015,Jan,16; 2014,Jan,11; 2013,Feb,3-6

26/TC PC/TC Only    A2-Z3 ASC Payment    50 Bilateral    ♂ Male Only    ♀ Female Only    🚑 Facility RVU    ⚕ Non-Facility RVU    ▣ CCI

FUD Follow-up Days    CMS: IOM (Pub 100)    A-Y OPPSI    80/80 Surg Assist Allowed / w/Doc    ▣ Lab Crosswalk    ▣ Radiology Crosswalk    ☒ CLIA

CPT © 2017 American Medical Association. All Rights Reserved.

© 2017 Optum360, LLC

**+ 96376** each additional sequential intravenous push of the same substance/drug provided in a facility (List separately in addition to code for primary procedure)

> **INCLUDES** Facilities only
>
> **EXCLUDES** *IV push performed within 30 minutes of a reported push of the same substance or drug*
>
> *Services performed by any nonfacilty provider*
>
> Code first (96365, 96374, 96409, 96413)
>
> 🚑 0.00 ✂ 0.00 **FUD** ZZZ ☒☐
>
> **AMA:** 2017,Jan,8; 2016,Jan,13; 2015,Jan,16; 2014,Nov,14; 2014,Jan,11

**96377** Application of on-body injector (includes cannula insertion) for timed subcutaneous injection

> 🚑 0.00 ✂ 0.00 **FUD** XXX ☒☐
>
> **AMA:** 2017,Jan,8; 2016,Oct,9

**96379** Unlisted therapeutic, prophylactic, or diagnostic intravenous or intra-arterial injection or infusion

> 🚑 0.00 ✂ 0.00 **FUD** XXX ☒☒
>
> **AMA:** 2017,Jan,8; 2016,Jan,13; 2015,Jan,16; 2014,Jan,11

# 96401-96411 Chemotherapy and Other Complex Drugs, Biologicals: Injection and IV Push

**CMS:** 100-03,110.2 Certain Drugs Distributed by the National Cancer Institute; 100-03,110.6 Scalp Hypothermia During Chemotherapy, to Prevent Hair Loss; 100-04,4,230.2 OPPS Drug Administration

> **INCLUDES** Highly complex services that require direct supervision for:
> Consent
> Patient assessment
> Safety oversight
> Supervision
> More intense work and monitoring of clinical staff by physician or other qualified health care provider due to greater risk of severe patient reactions
> Parenteral administration of:
> Anti-neoplastic agents for noncancer diagnoses
> Monoclonal antibody agents
> Nonradionuclide antineoplastic drugs
> Other biologic response modifiers
>
> **EXCLUDES** *Use of a code for a second initial service on the same date for accessing a multi-lumen catheter, restarting an IV, or when two IV lines are needed to meet an infusion rate*

**96401** Chemotherapy administration, subcutaneous or intramuscular; non-hormonal anti-neoplastic

> **EXCLUDES** *Services performed by physicians or other qualified health care providers in facility settings*
>
> 🚑 2.10 ✂ 2.10 **FUD** XXX ☒☒☐
>
> **AMA:** 2017,Jan,8; 2016,Jan,13; 2015,Jan,16; 2014,Jan,11; 2012,Jan,15-42

**96402** hormonal anti-neoplastic

> **EXCLUDES** *Services performed by physicians or other qualified health care providers in facility settings*
>
> 🚑 0.92 ✂ 0.92 **FUD** XXX ☒☒☐
>
> **AMA:** 2017,Jan,8; 2016,Jan,13; 2015,Jan,16; 2014,Jan,11; 2012,Jan,15-42

**96405** Chemotherapy administration; intralesional, up to and including 7 lesions

> 🚑 0.86 ✂ 2.31 **FUD** 000 ☒☐
>
> **AMA:** 2017,Jan,8; 2016,Jan,13; 2015,Jan,16; 2014,Jan,11; 2012,Jan,15-42

**96406** intralesional, more than 7 lesions

> 🚑 1.32 ✂ 3.38 **FUD** 000 ☒☐
>
> **AMA:** 2017,Jan,8; 2016,Jan,13; 2015,Jan,16; 2014,Jan,11; 2012,Jan,15-42

**96409** intravenous, push technique, single or initial substance/drug

> **INCLUDES** Push technique includes:
> Administration of injection directly into vessel or access line by health care professional; or
> Infusion less than or equal to 15 minutes
>
> **EXCLUDES** *Insertion of arterial and venous cannula(s) for extracorporeal circulation (36823)*
>
> *Services performed by physicians or other qualified health care providers in facility settings*
>
> Code also second initial service with modifier 59 when patient's condition or drug protocol mandates the use of two IV lines
>
> 🚑 3.13 ✂ 3.13 **FUD** XXX ☒☒☐
>
> **AMA:** 2017,Jan,8; 2016,Jan,13; 2015,Jan,16; 2014,Jan,11; 2012,Jan,15-42

**+ 96411** intravenous, push technique, each additional substance/drug (List separately in addition to code for primary procedure)

> **INCLUDES** Push technique includes:
> Administration of injection directly into vessel or access line by health care professional; or
> Infusion less than or equal to 15 minutes
>
> **EXCLUDES** *Insertion of arterial and venous cannula(s) for extracorporeal circulation (36823)*
>
> *Services performed by physicians or other qualified health care providers in facility settings*
>
> Code first initial substance/drug (96409, 96413)
>
> 🚑 1.76 ✂ 1.76 **FUD** ZZZ ☒☒☐
>
> **AMA:** 2017,Jan,8; 2016,Jan,13; 2015,Jan,16; 2014,Jan,11; 2012,Jan,15-42

● New Code  ▲ Revised Code  ○ Reinstated  ● New Web Release  ▲ Revised Web Release  Unlisted  Not Covered  # Resequenced
⊘ AMA Mod 51 Exempt  ⑤ Optum Mod 51 Exempt  ⑥ Mod 63 Exempt  ✗ Non-FDA Drug  ★ Telemedicine  Ⓜ Maternity  Ⓐ Age Edit  + Add-on  **AMA:** CPT Asst

© 2017 Optum360, LLC  CPT © 2017 American Medical Association. All Rights Reserved.  **481**

Medicine

## 96413-96417 Chemotherapy and Complex Drugs, Biologicals: Intravenous Infusion

**CMS:** 100-03,110.2 Certain Drugs Distributed by the National Cancer Institute; 100-03,110.6 Scalp Hypothermia During Chemotherapy, to Prevent Hair Loss; 100-04,230.2 OPPS Drug Administration

INCLUDES Highly complex services that require direct supervision for:
Consent
Patient assessment
Safety oversight
Supervision
More intense work and monitoring of clinical staff by physician or other qualified health care provider due to greater risk of severe patient reactions
Parenteral administration of:
Anti-neoplastic agents for noncancer diagnoses
Monoclonal antibody agents
Nonradionuclide antineoplastic drugs
Other biologic response modifiers
The following in the administration:
Access to IV/catheter/port
Drug preparation
Flushing at the completion of the infusion
Hydration fluid
Routine tubing/syringe/supplies
Starting the IV
Use of local anesthesia

EXCLUDES *Administration of nonchemotherapy agents such as antibiotics/steroids/analgesics*
*Declotting of catheter/port (36593)*
*Home infusion (99601-99602)*
*Insertion of arterial and venous cannula(s) for extracorporeal circulation (36823)*
*Services provided by physicians or other qualified health care providers in facility settings*
*Use of a code for a second initial service on the same date for accessing a multi-lumen catheter, restarting an IV, or when two IV lines are needed to meet an infusion rate*

Code also drug or substance
Code also significant separately identifiable E&M service, when performed

### 96413 Chemotherapy administration, intravenous infusion technique; up to 1 hour, single or initial substance/drug

INCLUDES Push technique includes:
Administration of injection directly into vessel or access line by health care professional; or
Infusion less than or equal to 15 minutes

EXCLUDES *Hydration administered as secondary or subsequent service via same IV access site (96361)*
*Therapeutic/prophylactic/diagnostic drug infusion/injection through the same intravenous access (96366, 96367, 96375)*

Code also second initial service with modifier 59 when patient's condition or drug protocol mandates the use of two IV lines

🖩 3.89   ⚖ 3.89   **FUD** XXX                                   S 80 ▢

**AMA:** 2017,Jan,8; 2016,Jan,13; 2015,Jan,16; 2014,Jan,11; 2012,Jan,15-42

### + 96415 each additional hour (List separately in addition to code for primary procedure)

INCLUDES Infusion intervals of more than 30 minutes past 1-hour increments
Code first initial hour (96413)

🖩 0.80   ⚖ 0.80   **FUD** ZZZ                                   S 80 ▢

**AMA:** 2017,Jan,8; 2016,Jan,13; 2015,Jan,16; 2014,Jan,11; 2012,Jan,15-42

### 96416 initiation of prolonged chemotherapy infusion (more than 8 hours), requiring use of a portable or implantable pump

EXCLUDES *Portable or implantable infusion pump/reservoir refilling/maintenance for drug delivery (96521-96523)*

🖩 3.93   ⚖ 3.93   **FUD** XXX                                   S 80 ▢

**AMA:** 2017,Jan,8; 2016,Jan,13; 2015,Jan,16; 2014,Jan,11; 2012,Jan,15-42

### + 96417 each additional sequential infusion (different substance/drug), up to 1 hour (List separately in addition to code for primary procedure)

INCLUDES Push technique includes:
Administration of injection directly into vessel or access line by health care professional; or
Infusion less than or equal to 15 minutes

EXCLUDES *Additional hour(s) of sequential infusion (96415)*
*Use of code more than one time per sequential infusion*

Code first initial substance/drug (96413)

🖩 1.84   ⚖ 1.84   **FUD** ZZZ                                   S 80 ▢

**AMA:** 2017,Jan,8; 2016,Jan,13; 2015,Jan,16; 2014,Jan,11; 2012,Jan,15-42

## 96420-96425 Chemotherapy and Complex Drugs, Biologicals: Intra-arterial

**CMS:** 100-03,110.2 Certain Drugs Distributed by the National Cancer Institute; 100-03,110.6 Scalp Hypothermia During Chemotherapy, to Prevent Hair Loss; 100-04,4,230.2 OPPS Drug Administration

INCLUDES Highly complex services that require direct supervision for:
Consent
Patient assessment
Safety oversight
Supervision
More intense work and monitoring of clinical staff by physician or other qualified health care provider due to greater risk of severe patient reactions
Parenteral administration of:
Anti-neoplastic agents for noncancer diagnoses
Monoclonal antibody agents
Non-radionuclide antineoplastic drugs
Other biologic response modifiers
The following in the administration:
Access to IV/catheter/port
Drug preparation
Flushing at the completion of the infusion
Hydration fluid
Routine tubing/syringe/supplies
Starting the IV
Use of local anesthesia

EXCLUDES *Administration of non-chemotherapy agents such as antibiotics/steroids/analgesics*
*Declotting of catheter/port (36593)*
*Home infusion (99601-99602)*
*Services provided by physicians or other qualified health care providers in facility settings*
*Use of a code for a second initial service on the same date for accessing a multi-lumen catheter, restarting an IV, or when two IV lines are needed*

Code also drug or substance
Code also significant separately identifiable E&M service, when performed

### 96420 Chemotherapy administration, intra-arterial; push technique

INCLUDES Push technique includes:
Administration of injection directly into vessel or access line by health care professional; or
Infusion less than or equal to 15 minutes
Regional chemotherapy perfusion

EXCLUDES *Insertion of arterial and venous cannula(s) for extracorporeal circulation (36823)*
*Placement of intra-arterial catheter*

🖩 3.00   ⚖ 3.00   **FUD** XXX                                   S 80 ▢

**AMA:** 2017,Jan,8; 2016,Mar,3; 2016,Jan,13; 2015,Nov,3; 2015,Jan,16; 2014,Jan,11; 2013,Nov,6; 2012,Jan,15-42

### 96422 infusion technique, up to 1 hour

INCLUDES Push technique includes:
Administration of injection directly into vessel or access line by health care professional; or
Infusion less than or equal to 15 minutes
Regional chemotherapy perfusion

EXCLUDES *Insertion of arterial and venous cannula(s) for extracorporeal circulation (36823)*
*Placement of intra-arterial catheter*

🖩 5.22   ⚖ 5.22   **FUD** XXX                                   S 80 ▢

**AMA:** 2017,Jan,8; 2016,Mar,3; 2016,Jan,13; 2015,Nov,3; 2015,Jan,16; 2014,Jan,11; 2012,Jan,15-42

+ 96423 **infusion technique, each additional hour (List separately in addition to code for primary procedure)**

INCLUDES Infusion intervals of more than 30 minutes past 1-hour increments
Regional chemotherapy perfusion

EXCLUDES Insertion of arterial and venous cannula(s) for extracorporeal circulation (36823)
Placement of intra-arterial catheter

Code first initial hour (96422)

🚑 2.12  ✂ 2.12  **FUD** ZZZ  [S] [80] [📠]

**AMA:** 2017,Jan,8; 2016,Mar,3; 2016,Jan,13; 2015,Nov,3; 2015,Jan,16; 2014,Jan,11; 2012,Jan,15-42

96425 **infusion technique, initiation of prolonged infusion (more than 8 hours), requiring the use of a portable or implantable pump**

INCLUDES Regional chemotherapy perfusion

EXCLUDES Insertion of arterial and venous cannula(s) for extracorporeal circulation (36823)
Placement of intra-arterial catheter
Portable or implantable infusion pump/reservoir refilling/maintenance for drug delivery (96521-96523)

🚑 5.17  ✂ 5.17  **FUD** XXX  [S] [80] [📠]

**AMA:** 2017,Jan,8; 2016,Mar,3; 2016,Jan,13; 2015,Nov,3; 2015,Jan,16; 2014,Jan,11; 2012,Jan,15-42

## 96440-96450 Chemotherapy Administration: Intrathecal/Peritoneal Cavity/Pleural Cavity

**CMS:** 100-03,110.2 Certain Drugs Distributed by the National Cancer Institute; 100-04,4,230.2 OPPS Drug Administration

96440 **Chemotherapy administration into pleural cavity, requiring and including thoracentesis**

🚑 3.59  ✂ 22.0  **FUD** 000  [S] [80] [📠]

**AMA:** 2017,Jan,8; 2016,Jan,13; 2015,Jan,16; 2014,Jan,11; 2012,Jan,15-42

96446 **Chemotherapy administration into the peritoneal cavity via indwelling port or catheter**

🚑 0.82  ✂ 5.73  **FUD** XXX  [S] [80] [📠]

**AMA:** 2017,Jan,8; 2016,Jan,13; 2015,Jan,16; 2014,Jan,11; 2012,Jan,15-42

96450 **Chemotherapy administration, into CNS (eg, intrathecal), requiring and including spinal puncture**

EXCLUDES Chemotherapy administration, intravesical/bladder (51720)
Fluoroscopy (77003)
Insertion of catheter/reservoir:
Intraventricular (61210, 61215)
Subarachnoid (62350-62351, 62360-62362)

🚑 2.30  ✂ 5.13  **FUD** 000  [S] [80] [📠]

**AMA:** 2017,Jan,8; 2016,Jan,13; 2015,Jan,16; 2014,Jan,11; 2012,Jan,15-42

## 96521-96523 Refill/Upkeep of Drug Delivery Device

**CMS:** 100-04,4,230.2 OPPS Drug Administration

INCLUDES Highly complex services that require direct supervision for:
Consent
Patient assessment
Safety oversight
Supervision
Parenteral administration of:
Anti-neoplastic agents for noncancer diagnoses
Monoclonal antibody agents
Non-radionuclide antineoplastic drugs
Other biologic response modifiers
The following in the administration:
Access to IV/catheter/port
Drug preparation
Flushing at the completion of the infusion
Hydration fluid
Routine tubing/syringe/supplies
Starting the IV
Use of local anesthesia
Therapeutic drugs other than chemotherapy

EXCLUDES Administration of non-chemotherapy agents such as antibiotics/steroids/analgesics
Blood specimen collection from completely implantable venous access device (36591)
Declotting of catheter/port (36593)
Home infusion (99601-99602)
Services provided by physicians or other qualified health care providers in facility settings

Code also drug or substance
Code also significant separately identifiable E&M service, when performed

96521 **Refilling and maintenance of portable pump**

🚑 3.95  ✂ 3.95  **FUD** XXX  [S] [80] [📠]

**AMA:** 2017,Jan,8; 2016,Jan,13; 2015,Jan,16; 2014,Jan,11

96522 **Refilling and maintenance of implantable pump or reservoir for drug delivery, systemic (eg, intravenous, intra-arterial)**

EXCLUDES Implantable infusion pump refilling/maintenance for spinal/brain drug delivery (95990-95991)

🚑 3.22  ✂ 3.22  **FUD** XXX  [S] [80] [📠]

**AMA:** 2017,Jan,8; 2016,Jan,13; 2015,Jan,16; 2014,Jan,11; 2012,Aug,10-12

96523 **Irrigation of implanted venous access device for drug delivery systems**

EXCLUDES Direct supervision by physician or other qualified health care provider in facility settings
Use of code with any other services on the same date of service

🚑 0.70  ✂ 0.70  **FUD** XXX  [Q1] [80] [📠]

**AMA:** 2017,Jan,8; 2016,Jan,13; 2015,Jan,16; 2014,Jan,11; 2012,Jan,15-42

**Medicine** *(side tab)*
**96542 — 96904** *(side tab)*

## 96542-96549 Chemotherapy Injection Into Brain

**CMS:** 100-04,4,230.2 OPPS Drug Administration

**INCLUDES**    Highly complex services that require direct supervision for:
- Consent
- Patient assessment
- Safety oversight
- Supervision

Parenteral administration of:
- Anti-neoplastic agents for noncancer diagnoses
- Monoclonal antibody agents
- Non-radionuclide antineoplastic drugs
- Other biologic response modifiers

The following in the administration:
- Access to IV/catheter/port
- Drug preparation
- Flushing at the completion of the infusion
- Hydration fluid
- Routine tubing/syringe/supplies
- Starting the IV
- Use of local anesthesia

**EXCLUDES** *Administration of non-chemotherapy agents such as antibiotics/steroids/analgesics*
*Blood specimen collection from completely implantable venous access device (36591)*
*Declotting of catheter/port (36593)*
*Home infusion (99601-99602)*

Code also drug or substance
Code also significant separately identifiable E&M service, when performed

**96542**    **Chemotherapy injection, subarachnoid or intraventricular via subcutaneous reservoir, single or multiple agents**

       **EXCLUDES** *Oral radioactive isotope therapy (79005)*

       📋 1.20    ⚕ 3.51    **FUD** XXX      S 80 🖵

       **AMA:** 2017,Jan,8; 2016,Jan,13; 2015,Jan,16; 2014,Jan,11

**96549**    **Unlisted chemotherapy procedure**

       📋 0.00    ⚕ 0.00    **FUD** XXX      S 80

       **AMA:** 2017,Jan,8; 2016,Jan,13; 2015,Jan,16; 2014,Jan,11; 2012,Jan,15-42

## 96567-96574 Destruction of Lesions: Photodynamic Therapy

**EXCLUDES** *Ocular photodynamic therapy (67221)*

▲ **96567**    **Photodynamic therapy by external application of light to destroy premalignant lesions of the skin and adjacent mucosa with application and illumination/activation of photosensitive drug(s), per day**

       **INCLUDES**   Services provided without direct participation by physician or other qualified healthcare professional

       📋 3.82    ⚕ 3.82    **FUD** XXX      01 80 🖵

       **AMA:** 2017,Jan,8; 2016,Jan,13; 2015,Jan,16; 2014,Jan,11; 2012,Jan,15-42

+ **96570**    **Photodynamic therapy by endoscopic application of light to ablate abnormal tissue via activation of photosensitive drug(s); first 30 minutes (List separately in addition to code for endoscopy or bronchoscopy procedures of lung and gastrointestinal tract)**

       Code also for 38-52 minutes (96571)
       Code also modifier 52 when services with report are less than 23 minutes
       Code first (31641, 43229)

       📋 1.63    ⚕ 1.63    **FUD** ZZZ      N 🖵

       **AMA:** 2017,Jan,8; 2016,Jan,13; 2015,Jan,16; 2014,Jan,11; 2013,Apr,8-9

+ **96571**    **each additional 15 minutes (List separately in addition to code for endoscopy or bronchoscopy procedures of lung and gastrointestinal tract)**

       **EXCLUDES** *23-37 minutes of service (96570)*
       Code first (96570)
       Code first when appropriate (31641, 43229)

       📋 0.75    ⚕ 0.75    **FUD** ZZZ      N 🖵

       **AMA:** 2017,Jan,8; 2016,Jan,13; 2015,Jan,16; 2014,Jan,11; 2013,Apr,8-9

● **96573**    **Photodynamic therapy by external application of light to destroy premalignant lesions of the skin and adjacent mucosa with application and illumination/activation of photosensitizing drug(s) provided by a physician or other qualified health care professional, per day**

       **INCLUDES**   Application of photosensitizer to lesions at an anatomical site
       Debridement, when performed
       Use of light to activate photosensitizer for destruction of premalignant lesions

       **EXCLUDES** *Debridement lesion with photodynamic therapy provided by physician or other qualified healthcare professional (96574)*
       *Photodynamic therapy by external application of light to same anatomical site (96567)*
       *Services provided to same area on same date of services as photodynamic therapy:*
       *Biopsy (11100-11101)*
       *Debridement (11000-11001, 11004-11005)*
       *Excision of lesion (11400-11471)*
       *Shaving of lesion (11300-11313)*

● **96574**    **Debridement of premalignant hyperkeratotic lesion(s) (ie, targeted curettage, abrasion) followed with photodynamic therapy by external application of light to destroy premalignant lesions of the skin and adjacent mucosa with application and illumination/activation of photosensitizing drug(s) provided by a physician or other qualified health care professional, per day**

       **INCLUDES**   Application of photosensitizer to lesions at an anatomical site
       Debridement, when performed
       Use of light to activate photosensitizer for destruction of premalignant lesions

       **EXCLUDES** *Photodynamic therapy by external application of light for destruction of premalignant lesions (96573)*
       *Photodynamic therapy by external application of light to same anatomical site (96567)*
       *Services provided to same area on same date of services as photodynamic therapy:*
       *Biopsy (11100-11101)*
       *Debridement (11000-11001, 11004-11005)*
       *Excision of lesion (11400-11471)*
       *Shaving of lesion (11300-11313)*

## 96900-96999 Diagnostic/Therapeutic Skin Procedures

**EXCLUDES** *E&M services*
*Injection, intralesional (11900-11901)*

**96900**    **Actinotherapy (ultraviolet light)**

       **EXCLUDES** *Rhinophototherapy (30999)*
       🔬 (88160-88161)

       📋 0.59    ⚕ 0.59    **FUD** XXX      01 80 🖵

       **AMA:** 2017,Jan,8; 2016,Nov,9; 2016,Sep,3; 2016,Jan,13; 2015,Jan,16; 2014,Jan,11; 2012,Jul,9; 2012,Jan,15-42

**96902**    **Microscopic examination of hairs plucked or clipped by the examiner (excluding hair collected by the patient) to determine telogen and anagen counts, or structural hair shaft abnormality**

       🔬 (88160-88161)

       📋 0.59    ⚕ 0.61    **FUD** XXX      N 🖵

       **AMA:** 1997,Nov,1

**96904**    **Whole body integumentary photography, for monitoring of high risk patients with dysplastic nevus syndrome or a history of dysplastic nevi, or patients with a personal or familial history of melanoma**

       🔬 (88160-88161)

       📋 1.77    ⚕ 1.77    **FUD** XXX      N 80 🖵

       **AMA:** 2006,Dec,10-12

---

**96910** Photochemotherapy; tar and ultraviolet B (Goeckerman treatment) or petrolatum and ultraviolet B
📷 (88160-88161)
🚑 2.01 ⚕ 2.01 **FUD** XXX    01 80 📠
**AMA:** 2017,Jan,8; 2016,Sep,3; 2016,Jan,13; 2015,Jan,16; 2014,Jan,11; 2012,Jul,9

**96912** psoralens and ultraviolet A (PUVA)
📷 (88160-88161)
🚑 2.58 ⚕ 2.58 **FUD** XXX    01 80 📠
**AMA:** 2017,Jan,8; 2016,Sep,3; 2016,Jan,13; 2015,Jan,16; 2014,Jan,11; 2012,Jul,9

**96913** Photochemotherapy (Goeckerman and/or PUVA) for severe photoresponsive dermatoses requiring at least 4-8 hours of care under direct supervision of the physician (includes application of medication and dressings)
📷 (88160-88161)
🚑 3.66 ⚕ 3.66 **FUD** XXX    T 80 📠
**AMA:** 2017,Jan,8; 2016,Sep,3

**96920** Laser treatment for inflammatory skin disease (psoriasis); total area less than 250 sq cm
EXCLUDES *Destruction by laser of:*
*Benign lesions (17110-17111)*
*Cutaneous vascular proliferative lesions (17106-17108)*
*Malignant lesions (17260-17286)*
*Premalignant lesions (17000-17004)*
📷 (88160-88161)
🚑 1.92 ⚕ 4.41 **FUD** 000    01 📠
**AMA:** 2017,Jan,8; 2016,Sep,3; 2016,Jan,13; 2015,Jan,16; 2014,Jan,11; 2013,May,12; 2012,Jul,9; 2012,Jan,15-42

**96921** 250 sq cm to 500 sq cm
EXCLUDES *Destruction by laser of:*
*Benign lesions (17110-17111)*
*Cutaneous vascular proliferative lesions (17106-17108)*
*Malignant lesions (17260-17286)*
*Premalignant lesions (17000-17004)*
📷 (88160-88161)
🚑 2.17 ⚕ 4.86 **FUD** 000    01 📠
**AMA:** 2017,Jan,8; 2016,Sep,3; 2016,Jan,13; 2015,Jan,16; 2014,Jan,11; 2013,May,12; 2012,Jul,9; 2012,Jan,15-42

**96922** over 500 sq cm
EXCLUDES *Destruction by laser of:*
*Benign lesions (17110-17111)*
*Cutaneous vascular proliferative lesions (17106-17108)*
*Malignant lesions (17260-17286)*
*Premalignant lesions (17000-17004)*
📷 (88160-88161)
🚑 3.48 ⚕ 6.71 **FUD** 000    01 📠
**AMA:** 2017,Jan,8; 2016,Sep,3; 2016,Jan,13; 2015,Jan,16; 2014,Jan,11; 2013,May,12; 2012,Jul,9; 2012,Jan,15-42

**96931** Reflectance confocal microscopy (RCM) for cellular and sub-cellular imaging of skin; image acquisition and interpretation and report, first lesion
EXCLUDES *Optical coherence tomography for skin imaging (0470T-0471T)*
*Reflectance confocal microscopy examination without generated mosaic images (96999)*
🚑 4.51 ⚕ 4.51 **FUD** XXX    M 80 📠
**AMA:** 2017,Sep,9

**96932** image acquisition only, first lesion
EXCLUDES *Optical coherence tomography for skin imaging (0470T-0471T)*
*Reflectance confocal microscopy examination without generated mosaic images (96999)*
🚑 2.92 ⚕ 2.92 **FUD** XXX    01 80 TC 📠
**AMA:** 2017,Sep,9

**96933** interpretation and report only, first lesion
EXCLUDES *Optical coherence tomography for skin imaging (0470T-0471T)*
*Reflectance confocal microscopy examination without generated mosaic images (96999)*
🚑 1.28 ⚕ 1.28 **FUD** XXX    B 80 26 📠
**AMA:** 2017,Sep,9

+ **96934** image acquisition and interpretation and report, each additional lesion (List separately in addition to code for primary procedure)
EXCLUDES *Optical coherence tomography for skin imaging (0470T-0471T)*
*Reflectance confocal microscopy examination without generated mosaic images (96999)*
Code first (96931)
🚑 2.32 ⚕ 2.32 **FUD** ZZZ    N 80 📠
**AMA:** 2017,Sep,9

+ **96935** image acquisition only, each additional lesion (List separately in addition to code for primary procedure)
EXCLUDES *Optical coherence tomography for skin imaging (0470T-0471T)*
*Reflectance confocal microscopy examination without generated mosaic images (96999)*
Code first (96932)
🚑 0.98 ⚕ 0.98 **FUD** ZZZ    N 80 TC 📠
**AMA:** 2017,Sep,9

+ **96936** interpretation and report only, each additional lesion (List separately in addition to code for primary procedure)
EXCLUDES *Optical coherence tomography for skin imaging (0470T-0471T)*
*Reflectance confocal microscopy examination without generated mosaic images (96999)*
Code first (96933)
🚑 1.22 ⚕ 1.22 **FUD** ZZZ    N 80 26 📠
**AMA:** 2017,Sep,9

**96999** Unlisted special dermatological service or procedure
🚑 0.00 ⚕ 0.00 **FUD** XXX    01 80
**AMA:** 2017,Sep,9; 2017,Jan,8; 2016,Sep,3; 2016,Jan,13; 2015,Jan,16; 2014,Jan,11; 2013,May,12; 2012,Jul,9

# [97161, 97162, 97163, 97164] Assessment: Physical Therapy

**CMS:** 100-02,15,230.4 Services By a Physical/Occupational Therapist in Private Practice; 100-04,5,10.3.2 Therapy Cap Exceptions; 100-04,5,10.6 Functional Reporting; 100-04,5,20.2 Reporting Units of Service

INCLUDES Creation of care plan
Evaluation of body systems as defined in the 1997 E&M documentation guidelines:
Cardiovascular system: Vital signs, edema of extremities
Integumentary system: Inspection for abnormalities of skin
Mental status: Orientation, judgment, thought processes
Musculoskeletal system: Evaluation of gait and station, range of motion, muscle strength, height and weight
Neuromuscular evaluation: Balance, abnormal movements

\# **97161** Physical therapy evaluation: low complexity, requiring these components: A history with no personal factors and/or comorbidities that impact the plan of care; An examination of body system(s) using standardized tests and measures addressing 1-2 elements from any of the following: body structures and functions, activity limitations, and/or participation restrictions; A clinical presentation with stable and/or uncomplicated characteristics; and Clinical decision making of low complexity using standardized patient assessment instrument and/or measurable assessment of functional outcome. Typically, 20 minutes are spent face-to-face with the patient and/or family.
🚑 2.30 ⚕ 2.30 **FUD** XXX    A 80 📠
**AMA:** 2017,Aug,3; 2017,Jun,6; 2017,Jan,8

● New Code ▲ Revised Code ○ Reinstated ● New Web Release ▲ Revised Web Release Unlisted Not Covered # Resequenced
⊘ AMA Mod 51 Exempt ⑤ Optum Mod 51 Exempt ⑥ Mod 63 Exempt ⁄ Non-FDA Drug ★ Telemedicine M Maternity A Age Edit + Add-on **AMA:** CPT Asst
© 2017 Optum360, LLC     CPT © 2017 American Medical Association. All Rights Reserved.     **485**

\# **97162** Physical therapy evaluation: moderate complexity, requiring these components: A history of present problem with 1-2 personal factors and/or comorbidities that impact the plan of care; An examination of body systems using standardized tests and measures in addressing a total of 3 or more elements from any of the following: body structures and functions, activity limitations, and/or participation restrictions; An evolving clinical presentation with changing characteristics; and Clinical decision making of moderate complexity using standardized patient assessment instrument and/or measurable assessment of functional outcome. Typically, 30 minutes are spent face-to-face with the patient and/or family.

🚑 2.30 ⚕ 2.30 **FUD** XXX 　　 A 80 ▭

**AMA:** 2017,Aug,3; 2017,Jun,6; 2017,Jan,8

\# **97163** Physical therapy evaluation: high complexity, requiring these components: A history of present problem with 3 or more personal factors and/or comorbidities that impact the plan of care; An examination of body systems using standardized tests and measures addressing a total of 4 or more elements from any of the following: body structures and functions, activity limitations, and/or participation restrictions; A clinical presentation with unstable and unpredictable characteristics; and Clinical decision making of high complexity using standardized patient assessment instrument and/or measurable assessment of functional outcome. Typically, 45 minutes are spent face-to-face with the patient and/or family.

🚑 2.30 ⚕ 2.30 **FUD** XXX 　　 A 80 ▭

**AMA:** 2017,Aug,3; 2017,Jun,6; 2017,Jan,8

\# **97164** Re-evaluation of physical therapy established plan of care, requiring these components: An examination including a review of history and use of standardized tests and measures is required; and Revised plan of care using a standardized patient assessment instrument and/or measurable assessment of functional outcome Typically, 20 minutes are spent face-to-face with the patient and/or family.

🚑 1.55 ⚕ 1.55 **FUD** XXX 　　 A 80 ▭

**AMA:** 2017,Aug,3; 2017,Jun,6; 2017,Jan,8

## [97165, 97166, 97167, 97168] Assessment: Occupational Therapy

**CMS:** 100-02,15,230.4 Services By a Physical/Occupational Therapist in Private Practice; 100-04,5,10.3.2 Therapy Cap Exceptions; 100-04,5,10.6 Functional Reporting; 100-04,5,20.2 Reporting Units of Service

INCLUDES Creation of care plan
Evaluations as appropriate
Medical history
Occupational status
Past history of therapy

\# **97165** Occupational therapy evaluation, low complexity, requiring these components: An occupational profile and medical and therapy history, which includes a brief history including review of medical and/or therapy records relating to the presenting problem; An assessment(s) that identifies 1-3 performance deficits (ie, relating to physical, cognitive, or psychosocial skills) that result in activity limitations and/or participation restrictions; and Clinical decision making of low complexity, which includes an analysis of the occupational profile, analysis of data from problem-focused assessment(s), and consideration of a limited number of treatment options. Patient presents with no comorbidities that affect occupational performance. Modification of tasks or assistance (eg, physical or verbal) with assessment(s) is not necessary to enable completion of evaluation component. Typically, 30 minutes are spent face-to-face with the patient and/or family.

🚑 2.62 ⚕ 2.62 **FUD** XXX 　　 A 80 ▭

**AMA:** 2017,Jun,6; 2017,Feb,3; 2017,Jan,8

\# **97166** Occupational therapy evaluation, moderate complexity, requiring these components: An occupational profile and medical and therapy history, which includes an expanded review of medical and/or therapy records and additional review of physical, cognitive, or psychosocial history related to current functional performance; An assessment(s) that identifies 3-5 performance deficits (ie, relating to physical, cognitive, or psychosocial skills) that result in activity limitations and/or participation restrictions; and Clinical decision making of moderate analytic complexity, which includes an analysis of the occupational profile, analysis of data from detailed assessment(s), and consideration of several treatment options. Patient may present with comorbidities that affect occupational performance. Minimal to moderate modification of tasks or assistance (eg, physical or verbal) with assessment(s) is necessary to enable patient to complete evaluation component. Typically, 45 minutes are spent face-to-face with the patient and/or family.

🚑 2.62 ⚕ 2.62 **FUD** XXX 　　 A 80 ▭

**AMA:** 2017,Jun,6; 2017,Feb,3; 2017,Jan,8

\# **97167** Occupational therapy evaluation, high complexity, requiring these components: An occupational profile and medical and therapy history, which includes review of medical and/or therapy records and extensive additional review of physical, cognitive, or psychosocial history related to current functional performance; An assessment(s) that identifies 5 or more performance deficits (ie, relating to physical, cognitive, or psychosocial skills) that result in activity limitations and/or participation restrictions; and Clinical decision making of high analytic complexity, which includes an analysis of the patient profile, analysis of data from comprehensive assessment(s), and consideration of multiple treatment options. Patient presents with comorbidities that affect occupational performance. Significant modification of tasks or assistance (eg, physical or verbal) with assessment(s) is necessary to enable patient to complete evaluation component. Typically, 60 minutes are spent face-to-face with the patient and/or family.

🚑 2.62 ⚕ 2.62 **FUD** XXX 　　 A 80 ▭

**AMA:** 2017,Jun,6; 2017,Feb,3; 2017,Jan,8

\# **97168** Re-evaluation of occupational therapy established plan of care, requiring these components: An assessment of changes in patient functional or medical status with revised plan of care; An update to the initial occupational profile to reflect changes in condition or environment that affect future interventions and/or goals; and A revised plan of care. A formal reevaluation is performed when there is a documented change in functional status or a significant change to the plan of care is required. Typically, 30 minutes are spent face-to-face with the patient and/or family.

🚑 1.74 ⚕ 1.74 **FUD** XXX 　　 A 80 ▭

**AMA:** 2017,Jun,6; 2017,Feb,3; 2017,Jan,8

---

26/TC PC/TC Only 　 A2-Z3 ASC Payment 　 50 Bilateral 　 ♂ Male Only 　 ♀ Female Only 　 🚑 Facility RVU 　 ⚕ Non-Facility RVU 　 ▭ CCI
**FUD** Follow-up Days 　 **CMS:** IOM (Pub 100) 　 A-Y OPPSI 　 80/80 Surg Assist Allowed / w/Doc 　 ▣ Lab Crosswalk 　 ▣ Radiology Crosswalk 　 ✖ CLIA

486 　　　　　　　　　　　　　　　　　　 CPT © 2017 American Medical Association. All Rights Reserved. 　　　　　　　　　　　 © 2017 Optum360, LLC

## [97169, 97170, 97171, 97172] Assessment: Athletic Training

INCLUDES Creation of care plan
Evaluation of body systems as defined in the 1997 E&M documentation guidelines:
Cardiovascular system: Vital signs, edema of extremities
Integumentary system: Inspection for abnormalities of skin
Musculoskeletal system: Evaluation of gait and station, range of motion, muscle strength, height and weight
Neuromuscular evaluation: Balance, abnormal movements

\# **97169** **Athletic training evaluation, low complexity, requiring these components: A history and physical activity profile with no comorbidities that affect physical activity; An examination of affected body area and other symptomatic or related systems addressing 1-2 elements from any of the following: body structures, physical activity, and/or participation deficiencies; and Clinical decision making of low complexity using standardized patient assessment instrument and/or measurable assessment of functional outcome. Typically, 15 minutes are spent face-to-face with the patient and/or family.**
🔧 0.00   ⚕ 0.00   **FUD** XXX                                    E 🖼
**AMA:** 2017,Jun,6; 2017,Jan,8

\# **97170** **Athletic training evaluation, moderate complexity, requiring these components: A medical history and physical activity profile with 1-2 comorbidities that affect physical activity; An examination of affected body area and other symptomatic or related systems addressing a total of 3 or more elements from any of the following: body structures, physical activity, and/or participation deficiencies; and Clinical decision making of moderate complexity using standardized patient assessment instrument and/or measurable assessment of functional outcome. Typically, 30 minutes are spent face-to-face with the patient and/or family.**
🔧 0.00   ⚕ 0.00   **FUD** XXX                                    E 🖼
**AMA:** 2017,Jun,6; 2017,Jan,8

\# **97171** **Athletic training evaluation, high complexity, requiring these components: A medical history and physical activity profile, with 3 or more comorbidities that affect physical activity; A comprehensive examination of body systems using standardized tests and measures addressing a total of 4 or more elements from any of the following: body structures, physical activity, and/or participation deficiencies; Clinical presentation with unstable and unpredictable characteristics; and Clinical decision making of high complexity using standardized patient assessment instrument and/or measurable assessment of functional outcome. Typically, 45 minutes are spent face-to-face with the patient and/or family.**
🔧 0.00   ⚕ 0.00   **FUD** XXX                                    E 🖼
**AMA:** 2017,Jun,6; 2017,Jan,8

\# **97172** **Re-evaluation of athletic training established plan of care requiring these components: An assessment of patient's current functional status when there is a documented change; and A revised plan of care using a standardized patient assessment instrument and/or measurable assessment of functional outcome with an update in management options, goals, and interventions. Typically, 20 minutes are spent face-to-face with the patient and/or family.**
🔧 0.00   ⚕ 0.00   **FUD** XXX                                    E 🖼
**AMA:** 2017,Jun,6; 2017,Jan,8

## 97010-97028 Physical Therapy Treatment Modalities: Supervised

**CMS:** 100-02,15,230 Practice of Physical Therapy, Occupational Therapy, and Speech-Language Pathology; 100-02,15,230.1 Practice of Physical Therapy; 100-02,15,230.2 Practice of Occupational Therapy; 100-02,15,230.4 Services By a Physical/Occupational Therapist in Private Practice; 100-03,10.3 Inpatient Pain Rehabilitation Programs; 100-03,10.4 Outpatient Hospital Pain Rehabilitation Programs; 100-03,160.17 Payment for L-Dopa /Associated Inpatient Hospital Services; 100-04,5,10 Part B Outpatient Rehabilitation and Comprehensive Outpatient Rehabilitation Facility (CORF) Services - General; 100-04,5,10.2 Financial Limitation for Outpatient Rehabilitation Services; 100-04,5,20.2 Reporting Units of Service

INCLUDES Adding incremental intervals of treatment time for the same visit to calculate the total service time
EXCLUDES Direct patient contact by the provider
Electromyography (95860-95872 [95885, 95886, 95887])
EMG biofeedback training (90901)
Muscle and range of motion tests (95831-95857)
Nerve conduction studies (95905-95913)
Transcutaneous nerve stimulation (TNS) (64550)

**97010** **Application of a modality to 1 or more areas; hot or cold packs**
🔧 0.17   ⚕ 0.17   **FUD** XXX                          ⑤ A 🖼
**AMA:** 2017,Jan,8; 2016,Jun,8; 2016,Jan,13; 2015,Jan,16; 2014,Jan,11; 2012,Jan,15-42

**97012** **traction, mechanical**
🔧 0.46   ⚕ 0.46   **FUD** XXX                          ⑤ A 80 🖼
**AMA:** 2017,Jan,8; 2016,Jun,8; 2016,Jan,13; 2015,Jan,16; 2014,Jan,11; 2012,Jan,15-42

**97014** **electrical stimulation (unattended)**
EXCLUDES Acupuncture with electrical stimulation (97813, 97814)
🔧 0.45   ⚕ 0.45   **FUD** XXX                          ⑤ E 🖼
**AMA:** 2017,Jan,8; 2016,Jan,13; 2015,Jan,16; 2014,Jan,11; 2012,Jan,15-42

**97016** **vasopneumatic devices**
🔧 0.55   ⚕ 0.55   **FUD** XXX                          ⑤ A 80 🖼
**AMA:** 2017,Jan,8; 2016,Jan,13; 2015,Jan,16; 2014,Jan,11; 2012,Jan,15-42

**97018** **paraffin bath**
🔧 0.31   ⚕ 0.31   **FUD** XXX                          ⑤ A 80 🖼
**AMA:** 2017,Jan,8; 2016,Jan,13; 2015,Jan,16; 2014,Jan,11; 2012,Jan,15-42

**97022** **whirlpool**
🔧 0.67   ⚕ 0.67   **FUD** XXX                          ⑤ A 80 🖼
**AMA:** 2017,Jan,8; 2016,Jan,13; 2015,Jan,16; 2014,Jan,11; 2012,Jan,15-42

**97024** **diathermy (eg, microwave)**
🔧 0.19   ⚕ 0.19   **FUD** XXX                          ⑤ A 80 🖼
**AMA:** 2017,Jan,8; 2016,Jan,13; 2015,Jan,16; 2014,Jan,11; 2012,Jan,15-42

**97026** **infrared**
🔧 0.17   ⚕ 0.17   **FUD** XXX                          ⑤ A 80 🖼
**AMA:** 2017,Jan,8; 2016,Jan,13; 2015,Jan,16; 2014,Jan,11; 2012,Jan,15-42

**97028** **ultraviolet**
🔧 0.21   ⚕ 0.21   **FUD** XXX                          ⑤ A 80 🖼
**AMA:** 2017,Jan,8; 2016,Jan,13; 2015,Jan,16; 2014,Jan,11; 2012,Jan,15-42

## 97032-97039 Physical Therapy Treatment Modalities: Constant Attendance

**CMS:** 100-02,15,230 Practice of Physical Therapy, Occupational Therapy, and Speech-Language Pathology; 100-02,15,230.1 Practice of Physical Therapy; 100-02,15,230.2 Practice of Occupational Therapy; 100-02,15,230.4 Services By a Physical/Occupational Therapist in Private Practice; 100-03,10.3 Inpatient Pain Rehabilitation Programs; 100-03,10.4 Outpatient Hospital Pain Rehabilitation Programs; 100-03,160.17 Payment for L-Dopa /Associated Inpatient Hospital Services; 100-04,5,10 Part B Outpatient Rehabilitation and Comprehensive Outpatient Rehabilitation Facility (CORF) Services - General; 100-04,5,20.2 Reporting Units of Service

INCLUDES — Adding incremental intervals of treatment time for the same visit to calculate the total service time
Direct patient contact by the provider

EXCLUDES — *Electromyography (95860-95872 [95885, 95886, 95887])*
*EMG biofeedback training (90901)*
*Muscle and range of motion tests (95831-95857)*
*Nerve conduction studies (95905-95913)*
*Transcutaneous nerve stimulation (TNS) (64550)*

**97032** **Application of a modality to 1 or more areas; electrical stimulation (manual), each 15 minutes**

EXCLUDES — *Transcutaneous electrical modulation pain reprocessing (TEMPR) (scrambler therapy) (0278T)*

📑 0.54 ⚖ 0.54 **FUD** XXX (S) A 80 CCI

**AMA:** 2017,Jan,8; 2016,Jan,13; 2015,Jan,16; 2014,Jan,11; 2012,Jan,15-42

**97033** **iontophoresis, each 15 minutes**

📑 0.62 ⚖ 0.62 **FUD** XXX (S) A 80 CCI

**AMA:** 2017,Jan,8; 2016,Jan,13; 2015,Jan,16; 2014,Jan,11

**97034** **contrast baths, each 15 minutes**

📑 0.51 ⚖ 0.51 **FUD** XXX (S) A 80 CCI

**AMA:** 2017,Jan,8; 2016,Jan,13; 2015,Jan,16; 2014,Jan,11

**97035** **ultrasound, each 15 minutes**

📑 0.36 ⚖ 0.36 **FUD** XXX (S) A 80 CCI

**AMA:** 2017,Jan,8; 2016,Jan,13; 2015,Jan,16; 2014,Jan,11; 2012,Jan,15-42

**97036** **Hubbard tank, each 15 minutes**

📑 0.93 ⚖ 0.93 **FUD** XXX (S) A 80 CCI

**AMA:** 2017,Jan,8; 2016,Jan,13; 2015,Jan,16; 2014,Jan,11

**97039** **Unlisted modality (specify type and time if constant attendance)**

📑 0.00 ⚖ 0.00 **FUD** XXX A 80 CCI

**AMA:** 2017,Jan,8; 2016,Nov,9; 2016,Jun,8; 2016,Jan,13; 2015,Jan,16; 2014,Jan,11; 2012,Jan,15-42

## 97110-97546 Other Therapeutic Techniques With Direct Patient Contact

**CMS:** 100-02,15,230 Practice of Physical Therapy, Occupational Therapy, and Speech-Language Pathology; 100-02,15,230.1 Practice of Physical Therapy; 100-02,15,230.2 Practice of Occupational Therapy; 100-02,15,230.4 Services By a Physical/Occupational Therapist in Private Practice; 100-03,10.3 Inpatient Pain Rehabilitation Programs; 100-03,10.4 Outpatient Hospital Pain Rehabilitation Programs; 100-04,5,10 Part B Outpatient Rehabilitation and Comprehensive Outpatient Rehabilitation Facility (CORF) Services - General; 100-04,5,10.2 Financial Limitation for Outpatient Rehabilitation Services; 100-04,5,20.2 Reporting Units of Service

INCLUDES — Application of clinical skills/services to improve function
Direct patient contact by the provider

EXCLUDES — *Electromyography (95860-95872 [95885, 95886, 95887])*
*EMG biofeedback training (90901)*
*Muscle and range of motion tests (95831-95857)*
*Nerve conduction studies (95905-95913)*
*Transcutaneous nerve stimulation (TNS) (64550)*

**97110** **Therapeutic procedure, 1 or more areas, each 15 minutes; therapeutic exercises to develop strength and endurance, range of motion and flexibility**

📑 0.92 ⚖ 0.92 **FUD** XXX (S) A 80 CCI

**AMA:** 2017,Jan,8; 2016,Jun,8; 2016,Jan,13; 2015,Jan,16; 2014,Aug,5; 2014,Mar,13; 2014,Jan,11; 2012,Mar,9-10; 2012,Jan,15-42

**97112** **neuromuscular reeducation of movement, balance, coordination, kinesthetic sense, posture, and/or proprioception for sitting and/or standing activities**

📑 0.96 ⚖ 0.96 **FUD** XXX (S) A 80 CCI

**AMA:** 2017,Jan,8; 2016,Jan,13; 2015,Jan,16; 2014,Mar,13; 2014,Jan,11; 2012,Mar,9-10; 2012,Jan,15-42

**97113** **aquatic therapy with therapeutic exercises**

📑 1.22 ⚖ 1.22 **FUD** XXX (S) A 80 CCI

**AMA:** 2017,Jan,8; 2016,Jan,13; 2015,Jan,16; 2014,Mar,13; 2014,Jan,11; 2012,Jan,15-42

**97116** **gait training (includes stair climbing)**

EXCLUDES — *Comprehensive gait/motion analysis (96000-96003)*

📑 0.80 ⚖ 0.80 **FUD** XXX (S) A 80 CCI

**AMA:** 2017,Jan,8; 2016,Jan,13; 2015,Jan,16; 2014,Mar,13; 2014,Jan,11; 2012,Jan,15-42

**97124** **massage, including effleurage, petrissage and/or tapotement (stroking, compression, percussion)**

EXCLUDES — *Myofascial release (97140)*

📑 0.74 ⚖ 0.74 **FUD** XXX (S) A 80 CCI

**AMA:** 2017,Jan,8; 2016,Jun,8; 2016,Jan,13; 2015,Jan,16; 2014,Mar,13; 2014,Jan,11; 2012,Jan,15-42

● **97127** **Therapeutic interventions that focus on cognitive function (eg, attention, memory, reasoning, executive function, problem solving, and/or pragmatic functioning) and compensatory strategies to manage the performance of an activity (eg, managing time or schedules, initiating, organizing and sequencing tasks), direct (one-on-one) patient contact**

EXCLUDES — *Adaptive behavior treatment (0364T-0365T, 0368T-0369T)*
*Use of code more than one time per day*

**97139** **Unlisted therapeutic procedure (specify)**

📑 0.00 ⚖ 0.00 **FUD** XXX A 80 CCI

**AMA:** 2017,Jan,8; 2016,Jan,13; 2015,Jan,16; 2014,Mar,13; 2014,Jan,11; 2012,Jan,15-42

**97140** **Manual therapy techniques (eg, mobilization/ manipulation, manual lymphatic drainage, manual traction), 1 or more regions, each 15 minutes**

📑 0.85 ⚖ 0.85 **FUD** XXX (S) A 80 CCI

**AMA:** 2017,Jan,8; 2016,Nov,9; 2016,Sep,9; 2016,Aug,3; 2016,Jan,13; 2015,Mar,9; 2015,Jan,16; 2014,Mar,13; 2014,Jan,11; 2012,Jan,15-42

**97150** **Therapeutic procedure(s), group (2 or more individuals)**

INCLUDES — Constant attendance by the physician/therapist
Reporting this procedure for each member of group

EXCLUDES — *Adaptive behavior services (0366T-0367T, 0372T)*
*Osteopathic manipulative treatment (98925-98929)*

📑 0.49 ⚖ 0.49 **FUD** XXX (S) A 80 CCI

**AMA:** 2017,Jan,8; 2016,Jan,13; 2015,Jan,16; 2014,Mar,13; 2014,Jan,11; 2012,Jan,15-42

**97161** **Resequenced code. See code before 97010.**

**97162** **Resequenced code. See code before 97010.**

**97163** **Resequenced code. See code before 97010.**

**97164** **Resequenced code. See code before 97010.**

**97165** **Resequenced code. See code before 97010.**

**97166** **Resequenced code. See code before 97010.**

**97167** **Resequenced code. See code before 97010.**

**97168** **Resequenced code. See code before 97010.**

**97169** **Resequenced code. See code before 97010.**

**97170** **Resequenced code. See code before 97010.**

**97171** **Resequenced code. See code before 97010.**

**97172** **Resequenced code. See code before 97010.**

**97530** **Therapeutic activities, direct (one-on-one) patient contact (use of dynamic activities to improve functional performance), each 15 minutes**

📑 0.99 ⚖ 0.99 **FUD** XXX (S) A 80 CCI

**AMA:** 2017,Jan,8; 2016,Jan,13; 2015,Jan,16; 2014,Mar,13; 2014,Jan,11; 2012,Jan,15-42

| 26/TC PC/TC Only | A2-Z3 ASC Payment | 50 Bilateral | ♂ Male Only | ♀ Female Only | 📑 Facility RVU | ⚖ Non-Facility RVU | CCI |
| FUD Follow-up Days | CMS: IOM (Pub 100) | A-Y OPPSI | 80/80 Surg Assist Allowed / w/Doc | | Lab Crosswalk | Radiology Crosswalk | CLIA |

488

CPT © 2017 American Medical Association. All Rights Reserved.

© 2017 Optum360, LLC

97532 ~~Development of cognitive skills to improve attention, memory, problem solving (includes compensatory training), direct (one-on-one) patient contact, each 15 minutes~~

To report, see 97127

97533 **Sensory integrative techniques to enhance sensory processing and promote adaptive responses to environmental demands, direct (one-on-one) patient contact, each 15 minutes**

🚑 0.83 ⚗ 0.83 **FUD** XXX (51) A 80 🖵

**AMA:** 2017,Jan,8; 2016,Jan,13; 2015,Jan,16; 2014,Mar,13; 2014,Jan,11

97535 **Self-care/home management training (eg, activities of daily living (ADL) and compensatory training, meal preparation, safety procedures, and instructions in use of assistive technology devices/adaptive equipment) direct one-on-one contact, each 15 minutes**

🚑 0.99 ⚗ 0.99 **FUD** XXX (51) A 80 🖵

**AMA:** 2017,Jan,8; 2016,Aug,3; 2016,Jan,13; 2015,Jun,10; 2015,Mar,9; 2015,Jan,16; 2014,Mar,13; 2014,Jan,11; 2012,Jan,15-42

97537 **Community/work reintegration training (eg, shopping, transportation, money management, avocational activities and/or work environment/modification analysis, work task analysis, use of assistive technology device/adaptive equipment), direct one-on-one contact, each 15 minutes**

*EXCLUDES* *Wheelchair management/propulsion training (97542)*

🚑 0.86 ⚗ 0.86 **FUD** XXX (51) A 80 🖵

**AMA:** 2017,Jan,8; 2016,Jan,13; 2015,Jan,16; 2014,Mar,13; 2014,Jan,11

97542 **Wheelchair management (eg, assessment, fitting, training), each 15 minutes**

🚑 0.87 ⚗ 0.87 **FUD** XXX (51) A 80 🖵

**AMA:** 2017,Jan,8; 2016,Jan,13; 2015,Jun,10; 2015,Jan,16; 2014,Mar,13; 2014,Jan,11

97545 **Work hardening/conditioning; initial 2 hours**

🚑 0.00 ⚗ 0.00 **FUD** XXX (51) A 80 🖵

**AMA:** 2017,Jan,8; 2016,Jan,13; 2015,Jan,16; 2014,Mar,13; 2014,Jan,11; 2012,Jan,15-42

+ 97546 **each additional hour (List separately in addition to code for primary procedure)**

Code first initial 2 hours (97545)

🚑 0.00 ⚗ 0.00 **FUD** ZZZ (51) A 80 🖵

**AMA:** 2017,Jan,8; 2016,Jan,13; 2015,Jan,16; 2014,Mar,13; 2014,Jan,11; 2012,Jan,15-42

## 97597-97610 Treatment of Wounds

**CMS:** 100-02,15,230.4 Services By a Physical/Occupational Therapist in Private Practice; 100-03,270.3 Blood-derived Products for Chronic Nonhealing Wounds; 100-04,4,200.9 Billing for "Sometimes Therapy" Services that May be Paid as Non-Therapy Services; 100-04,5,10 Part B Outpatient Rehabilitation and Comprehensive Outpatient Rehabilitation Facility (CORF) Services - General

*INCLUDES* Direct patient contact
Removing devitalized/necrotic tissue and promoting healing

*EXCLUDES* *Burn wound debridement (16020-16030)*

97597 **Debridement (eg, high pressure waterjet with/without suction, sharp selective debridement with scissors, scalpel and forceps), open wound, (eg, fibrin, devitalized epidermis and/or dermis, exudate, debris, biofilm), including topical application(s), wound assessment, use of a whirlpool, when performed and instruction(s) for ongoing care, per session, total wound(s) surface area; first 20 sq cm or less**

*INCLUDES* Chemical cauterization (17250)

🚑 0.66 ⚗ 2.13 **FUD** 000 (51) T 80 🖵

**AMA:** 2017,Jan,8; 2016,Oct,3; 2016,Aug,9; 2016,Jan,13; 2015,Jan,16; 2014,Jun,11; 2014,Jan,11; 2012,Oct,3-8; 2012,Mar,3; 2012,Jan,6-10; 2012,Jan,15-42

Wound may be washed, addressed with scissors, and/or tweezers and scalpel

+ 97598 **each additional 20 sq cm, or part thereof (List separately in addition to code for primary procedure)**

*INCLUDES* Chemical cauterization (17250)

Code first (97597)

🚑 0.31 ⚗ 0.70 **FUD** ZZZ (51) N 80 🖵

**AMA:** 2017,Jan,8; 2016,Oct,3; 2016,Aug,9; 2016,Jan,13; 2015,Jan,16; 2014,Jun,11; 2014,Jan,11; 2012,Mar,3; 2012,Jan,15-42; 2012,Jan,6-10

97602 **Removal of devitalized tissue from wound(s), non-selective debridement, without anesthesia (eg, wet-to-moist dressings, enzymatic, abrasion, larval therapy), including topical application(s), wound assessment, and instruction(s) for ongoing care, per session**

*INCLUDES* Chemical cauterization (17250)

🚑 0.00 ⚗ 0.00 **FUD** XXX (51) 01 🖵

**AMA:** 2017,Jan,8; 2016,Oct,3; 2016,Jan,13; 2015,Jan,16; 2014,Jun,11; 2014,Jan,11; 2012,Dec,12; 2012,Mar,3; 2012,Jan,15-42; 2012,Jan,6-10

● New Code  ▲ Revised Code  ○ Reinstated  ● New Web Release  ▲ Revised Web Release  Unlisted  Not Covered  # Resequenced
⊘ AMA Mod 51 Exempt  (51) Optum Mod 51 Exempt  (63) Mod 63 Exempt  ✗ Non-FDA Drug  ★ Telemedicine  M Maternity  A Age Edit  + Add-on  **AMA:** CPT Asst
© 2017 Optum360, LLC                    CPT © 2017 American Medical Association. All Rights Reserved.                    **489**

**97605** Negative pressure wound therapy (eg, vacuum assisted drainage collection), utilizing durable medical equipment (DME), including topical application(s), wound assessment, and instruction(s) for ongoing care, per session; total wound(s) surface area less than or equal to 50 square centimeters

> EXCLUDES   Negative pressure wound therapy using disposable medical equipment (97607-97608)

🚑 0.71   ✂ 1.17   **FUD** XXX      ⑤ 01 80 💻

**AMA:** 2017,Jan,8; 2016,Feb,13; 2016,Jan,13; 2015,Jan,16; 2014,Nov,8; 2014,Jan,11; 2012,Jan,15-42

**97606** total wound(s) surface area greater than 50 square centimeters

> EXCLUDES   Negative pressure wound therapy using disposable medical equipment (97607-97608)

🚑 0.77   ✂ 1.38   **FUD** XXX      ⑤ 01 80 💻

**AMA:** 2017,Jan,8; 2016,Feb,13; 2016,Jan,13; 2015,Jan,16; 2014,Nov,8; 2014,Jan,11; 2012,Jan,15-42

**97607** Negative pressure wound therapy, (eg, vacuum assisted drainage collection), utilizing disposable, non-durable medical equipment including provision of exudate management collection system, topical application(s), wound assessment, and instructions for ongoing care, per session; total wound(s) surface area less than or equal to 50 square centimeters

> EXCLUDES   Negative pressure wound therapy using durable medical equipment (97605-97606)

🚑 0.00   ✂ 0.00   **FUD** XXX      ⑤ T 80 💻

**AMA:** 2017,Jan,8; 2016,Jan,13; 2015,Jan,16; 2014,Nov,8

**97608** total wound(s) surface area greater than 50 square centimeters

> EXCLUDES   Negative pressure wound therapy using durable medical equipment (97605-97606)

🚑 0.00   ✂ 0.00   **FUD** XXX      ⑤ T 80 💻

**AMA:** 2017,Jan,8; 2016,Jan,13; 2015,Jan,16; 2014,Nov,8

**97610** Low frequency, non-contact, non-thermal ultrasound, including topical application(s), when performed, wound assessment, and instruction(s) for ongoing care, per day

🚑 0.45   ✂ 3.39   **FUD** XXX      ⑤ 01 80 💻

**AMA:** 2017,Jan,8; 2016,Jan,13; 2015,Jan,16; 2014,Jun,11

## 97750-97799 Assessments and Training

**CMS:** 100-02,15,230.1 Practice of Physical Therapy; 100-02,15,230.2 Practice of Occupational Therapy; 100-02,15,230.4 Services By a Physical/Occupational Therapist in Private Practice; 100-04,5,10 Part B Outpatient Rehabilitation and Comprehensive Outpatient Rehabilitation Facility (CORF) Services - General

**97750** Physical performance test or measurement (eg, musculoskeletal, functional capacity), with written report, each 15 minutes

> INCLUDES   Direct patient contact
> EXCLUDES   Muscle/range of motion testing and electromyography/nerve velocity determination (95831-95857, 95860-95872, [95885, 95886, 95887], 95907-95913)

🚑 0.93   ✂ 0.93   **FUD** XXX      ⑤ A 80 💻

**AMA:** 2017,Jan,8; 2016,Jan,13; 2015,Jan,16; 2014,Jan,11; 2013,Aug,7; 2012,Jan,15-42

**97755** Assistive technology assessment (eg, to restore, augment or compensate for existing function, optimize functional tasks and/or maximize environmental accessibility), direct one-on-one contact, with written report, each 15 minutes

> INCLUDES   Direct patient contact
> EXCLUDES   Augmentative/alternative communication device (92605, 92607)
> Muscle/range of motion testing and electromyography/nerve velocity determination (95831-95857, 95860-95872, [95885, 95886, 95887], 95907-95913)

🚑 1.01   ✂ 1.01   **FUD** XXX      ⑤ A 80 💻

**AMA:** 1996,Sep,7; 1995,Sum,5

▲ **97760** Orthotic(s) management and training (including assessment and fitting when not otherwise reported), upper extremity(ies), lower extremity(ies) and/or trunk, initial orthotic(s) encounter, each 15 minutes

> EXCLUDES   Gait training, if performed on the same extremity (97116)

🚑 1.08   ✂ 1.08   **FUD** XXX      ⑤ A 80 💻

**AMA:** 2017,Jan,8; 2016,Jan,13; 2015,Jan,16; 2014,Jan,11

▲ **97761** Prosthetic(s) training, upper and/or lower extremity(ies), initial prosthetic(s) encounter, each 15 minutes

🚑 0.94   ✂ 0.94   **FUD** XXX      ⑤ A 80 💻

**AMA:** 2017,Jan,8; 2016,Jan,13; 2015,Jan,16; 2014,Jan,11; 2012,Jan,15-42

**97762** ~~Checkout for orthotic/prosthetic use, established patient, each 15 minutes~~

> To report, see 97763

● **97763** Orthotic(s)/prosthetic(s) management and/or training, upper extremity(ies), lower extremity(ies), and/or trunk, subsequent orthotic(s)/prosthetic(s) encounter, each 15 minutes    ⑤

> EXCLUDES   Initial encounter for orthotics and prosthetics management and training (97760-97761)

**97799** Unlisted physical medicine/rehabilitation service or procedure

🚑 0.00   ✂ 0.00   **FUD** XXX      A 80

**AMA:** 2017,Jan,8; 2016,Nov,9; 2016,Jan,13; 2015,Jan,16; 2014,Jan,11

## 97802-97804 Medical Nutrition Therapy Services

**CMS:** 100-03,180.1 Medical Nutrition Therapy; 100-04,12,190.3 List of Telehealth Services; 100-04,12,190.6 Payment Methodology for Physician/Practitioner at the Distant Site ; 100-04,12,190.6.1 Submission of Telehealth Claims for Distant Site Practitioners; 100-04,12,190.7 Contractor Editing of Telehealth Claims; 100-04,4,300 Medical Nutrition Therapy Services; 100-04,4,300.6 CWF Edits for MNT/DSMT

> EXCLUDES   Medical nutrition therapy assessment/intervention provided by physician or other qualified health care provider; use appropriate E&M codes

**97802** Medical nutrition therapy; initial assessment and intervention, individual, face-to-face with the patient, each 15 minutes

🚑 0.92   ✂ 0.98   **FUD** XXX      ★ A 80 💻

**AMA:** 2017,Jan,8; 2016,Jan,13; 2015,Jan,16; 2014,Jan,11

**97803** re-assessment and intervention, individual, face-to-face with the patient, each 15 minutes

🚑 0.78   ✂ 0.85   **FUD** XXX      ★ A 80 💻

**AMA:** 2017,Jan,8; 2016,Jan,13; 2015,Jan,16; 2014,Jan,11

**97804** group (2 or more individual(s)), each 30 minutes

🚑 0.43   ✂ 0.45   **FUD** XXX      ★ A 80 💻

**AMA:** 2017,Jan,8; 2016,Jan,13; 2015,Jan,16; 2014,Jan,11

## 97810-97814 Acupuncture

**CMS:** 100-03,10.3 Inpatient Pain Rehabilitation Programs; 100-03,10.4 Outpatient Hospital Pain Rehabilitation Programs; 100-03,30.3 Acupuncture; 100-03,30.3.1 Acupuncture for Fibromyalgia; 100-03,30.3.2 Acupuncture for Osteoarthritis

> INCLUDES   15 minute increments of face-to-face contact with the patient
> Reporting only one code for each 15 minute increment

Code also significant separately identifiable E&M service using modifier 25, when performed

**97810** Acupuncture, 1 or more needles; without electrical stimulation, initial 15 minutes of personal one-on-one contact with the patient

> EXCLUDES   Treatment with electrical stimulation (97813-97814)

🚑 0.87   ✂ 1.03   **FUD** XXX      E 💻

**AMA:** 2017,Jan,8; 2016,Jan,13; 2015,Jan,16; 2014,Jan,11; 2012,Jan,15-42

+ **97811** without electrical stimulation, each additional 15 minutes of personal one-on-one contact with the patient, with re-insertion of needle(s) (List separately in addition to code for primary procedure)

> EXCLUDES   Treatment with electrical stimulation (97813-97814)
> Code first initial 15 minutes (97810)

🚑 0.72   ✂ 0.77   **FUD** ZZZ      E 💻

**AMA:** 2017,Jan,8; 2016,Jan,13; 2015,Jan,16; 2014,Jan,11

**97813**    with electrical stimulation, initial 15 minutes of personal one-on-one contact with the patient

> EXCLUDES *Treatment without electrical stimulation (97813-97814)*
> 🚑 0.94   ✂ 1.10   **FUD** XXX      E 🖳
> **AMA:** 2017,Jan,8; 2016,Jan,13; 2015,Jan,16; 2014,Jan,11

**+**   **97814**    with electrical stimulation, each additional 15 minutes of personal one-on-one contact with the patient, with re-insertion of needle(s) (List separately in addition to code for primary procedure)

> EXCLUDES *Treatment without electrical stimulation (97813-97814)*
> Code first initial 15 minutes (97813)
> 🚑 0.79   ✂ 0.87   **FUD** ZZZ      E 🖳
> **AMA:** 2017,Jan,8; 2016,Jan,13; 2015,Jan,16; 2014,Jan,11

## 98925-98929 Osteopathic Manipulation

**CMS:** 100-03,150.1 Manipulation

> INCLUDES Physician applied manual treatment done to eliminate/alleviate somatic dysfunction and related disorders using a variety of techniques
> The following body regions:
>    Abdomen/visceral region
>    Cervical region
>    Head region
>    Lower extremities
>    Lumbar region
>    Pelvic region
>    Rib cage region
>    Sacral region
>    Thoracic region
>    Upper extremities
> Code also significant separately identifiable E&M service using modifier 25, when performed

**98925**    Osteopathic manipulative treatment (OMT); 1-2 body regions involved

> 🚑 0.68   ✂ 0.89   **FUD** 000      Q1 80 🖳
> **AMA:** 2017,Jan,8; 2016,Jan,13; 2015,Jan,16; 2014,Jan,11; 2012,Jan,15-42

**98926**    3-4 body regions involved

> 🚑 1.02   ✂ 1.29   **FUD** 000      Q1 80 🖳
> **AMA:** 2017,Jan,8; 2016,Jan,13; 2015,Jan,16; 2014,Jan,11; 2012,Jan,15-42

**98927**    5-6 body regions involved

> 🚑 1.35   ✂ 1.69   **FUD** 000      Q1 80 🖳
> **AMA:** 2017,Jan,8; 2016,Jan,13; 2015,Jan,16; 2014,Jan,11; 2012,Jan,15-42

**98928**    7-8 body regions involved

> 🚑 1.69   ✂ 2.06   **FUD** 000      Q1 80 🖳
> **AMA:** 2017,Jan,8; 2016,Jan,13; 2015,Jan,16; 2014,Jan,11; 2012,May,14-15; 2012,Jan,15-42

**98929**    9-10 body regions involved

> 🚑 2.05   ✂ 2.46   **FUD** 000      Q1 80 🖳
> **AMA:** 2017,Jan,8; 2016,Jan,13; 2015,Jan,16; 2014,Jan,11; 2012,Jan,15-42

## 98940-98943 Chiropractic Manipulation

**CMS:** 100-01,5,70.6 Chiropractors; 100-02,15,240 Chiropractic Services - General; 100-02,15,240.1.3 Necessity for Treatment; 100-02,15,30.5 Chiropractor's Services; 100-03,150.1 Manipulation

> INCLUDES Form of manual treatment performed to influence joint/neurophysical function
> The following five extraspinal regions:
>    Abdomen
>    Head, including temporomandibular joint, excluding atlanto-occipital region
>    Lower extremities
>    Rib cage, not including costotransverse/costovertebral joints
>    Upper extremities
> The following five spinal regions:
>    Cervical region (atlanto-occipital joint)
>    Lumbar region
>    Pelvic region (sacro-iliac joint)
>    Sacral region
>    Thoracic region (costovertebral/costotransverse joints)
> Code also significant separately identifiable E&M service using modifier 25 when performed

**98940**    Chiropractic manipulative treatment (CMT); spinal, 1-2 regions

> 🚑 0.64   ✂ 0.80   **FUD** 000      Q1 80 🖳
> **AMA:** 2017,Jan,8; 2016,Jan,13; 2015,Jan,16; 2014,Jan,11; 2013,Dec,14; 2012,Jan,15-42

**98941**    spinal, 3-4 regions

> 🚑 0.98   ✂ 1.15   **FUD** 000      Q1 80 🖳
> **AMA:** 2017,Jan,8; 2016,Jan,13; 2015,Jan,16; 2014,Jan,11; 2013,Dec,14; 2012,Jan,15-42

**98942**    spinal, 5 regions

> 🚑 1.33   ✂ 1.50   **FUD** 000      Q1 80 🖳
> **AMA:** 2017,Jan,8; 2016,Jan,13; 2015,Jan,16; 2014,Jan,11; 2013,Dec,14; 2012,Jan,15-42

**98943**    extraspinal, 1 or more regions

> 🚑 0.67   ✂ 0.77   **FUD** XXX      E 🖳
> **AMA:** 2017,Jan,8; 2016,Jan,13; 2015,Jan,16; 2014,Jan,11; 2013,Dec,14; 2012,Jan,15-42

## 98960-98962 Self-Management Training

> INCLUDES Education/training services:
>    Prescribed by a physician or other qualified health care professional
>    Provided by a qualified nonphysician health care provider
>    Standardized curriculum that may be modified as necessary for:
>      Clinical needs
>      Cultural norms
>      Health literacy
>    Teaching the patient how to manage the illness/delay the comorbidity(s)
> EXCLUDES *Genetic counseling education services (96040, 98961-98962)*
> *Health/behavior assessment (96150-96155)*
> *Medical nutrition therapy (97802-97804)*
> *The following services:*
> *Counseling/education to a group (99078)*
> *Counseling/education to individuals (99201-99215, 99217-99223 [99224, 99225, 99226], 99231-99233, 99241-99255, 99281-99285, 99304-99318, 99324-99337, 99341-99350, 99401-99429)*
> *Counseling/risk factor reduction without symptoms/established disease (99401-99412)*

**98960**    Education and training for patient self-management by a qualified, nonphysician health care professional using a standardized curriculum, face-to-face with the patient (could include caregiver/family) each 30 minutes; individual patient

> 🚑 0.79   ✂ 0.79   **FUD** XXX      ★ E 🖳
> **AMA:** 2017,Jan,8; 2016,Jan,13; 2015,Jan,16; 2014,Oct,3; 2014,Jan,11; 2013,Nov,3; 2013,Apr,3-4

**98961**    2-4 patients

> INCLUDES Group education regarding genetic risks
> 🚑 0.38   ✂ 0.38   **FUD** XXX      ★ E 🖳
> **AMA:** 2017,Jan,8; 2016,Jan,13; 2015,Jan,16; 2014,Oct,3; 2014,Jan,11; 2013,Nov,3; 2013,Apr,3-4

**98962**  **5-8 patients**

INCLUDES  Group education regarding genetic risks

📋 0.28  ⚕ 0.28  **FUD** XXX  ★ E 🖳

AMA: 2017,Jan,8; 2016,Jan,13; 2015,Jan,16; 2014,Oct,3; 2014,Jan,11; 2013,Nov,3; 2013,Apr,3-4

## 98966-98968 Nonphysician Telephone Services

INCLUDES  Assessment and management services provided by telephone by a qualified health care professional
Episode of care initiated by an established patient or his/her guardian
EXCLUDES  *Call initiated by the qualified health care professional*
*Calls during the postoperative period of a procedure*
*Decision to see the patient at the next available urgent care appointment*
*Decision to see the patient within 24 hours of the call*
*Monitoring of INR*
*Patient management services during same time frame as (99487-99489, 99495-99496)*
*Telephone services provided by a physician (99441-99443)*
*Telephone services that are considered a part of a previous or subsequent service*
*Use of codes if same codes billed within the past seven days*

**98966**  Telephone assessment and management service provided by a qualified nonphysician health care professional to an established patient, parent, or guardian not originating from a related assessment and management service provided within the previous 7 days nor leading to an assessment and management service or procedure within the next 24 hours or soonest available appointment; 5-10 minutes of medical discussion

📋 0.36  ⚕ 0.39  **FUD** XXX  E 🖳

AMA: 2017,Jan,8; 2016,Jan,13; 2015,Jan,16; 2014,Oct,3; 2014,Jan,11; 2013,Oct,11; 2013,Nov,3; 2013,Apr,3-4

**98967**  **11-20 minutes of medical discussion**

📋 0.72  ⚕ 0.76  **FUD** XXX  E 🖳

AMA: 2017,Jan,8; 2016,Jan,13; 2015,Jan,16; 2014,Oct,3; 2014,Jan,11; 2013,Oct,11; 2013,Nov,3; 2013,Apr,3-4

**98968**  **21-30 minutes of medical discussion**

📋 1.08  ⚕ 1.12  **FUD** XXX  E 🖳

AMA: 2017,Jan,8; 2016,Jan,13; 2015,Jan,16; 2014,Oct,3; 2014,Jan,11; 2013,Oct,11; 2013,Nov,3; 2013,Apr,3-4

## 98969 Nonphysician Online Service

INCLUDES  On-line assessment and management service provided by a qualified health care professional
Timely reply to the patient as well as:
Ordering laboratory services
Permanent record of the service; either hard copy or electronic
Providing a prescription
Related telephone calls
EXCLUDES  *Monitoring of INR (93792-93793)*
*On-line evaluation service:*
*Provided during the postoperative period of a procedure*
*Provided more than once in a seven day period*
*Related to a service provided in the previous seven days*
*Patient management services during same time frame as (99487-99489, 99495-99496)*

**98969**  Online assessment and management service provided by a qualified nonphysician health care professional to an established patient or guardian, not originating from a related assessment and management service provided within the previous 7 days, using the Internet or similar electronic communications network

📋 0.00  ⚕ 0.00  **FUD** XXX  E 🖳

AMA: 2017,Jan,8; 2016,Jan,13; 2015,Jan,16; 2014,Oct,3; 2014,Jan,11; 2013,Oct,11; 2013,Nov,3; 2013,Apr,3-4

## 99000-99091 Supplemental Services and Supplies

INCLUDES  Supplemental reporting for services adjunct to the basic service provided

**99000**  Handling and/or conveyance of specimen for transfer from the office to a laboratory

📋 0.00  ⚕ 0.00  **FUD** XXX  E 🖳

AMA: 2017,Jan,8; 2016,Jan,13; 2015,Jan,16; 2014,Jan,11; 2012,Jan,15-42

**99001**  Handling and/or conveyance of specimen for transfer from the patient in other than an office to a laboratory (distance may be indicated)

📋 0.00  ⚕ 0.00  **FUD** XXX  E 🖳

AMA: 2017,Jan,8; 2016,Jan,13; 2015,Jan,16; 2014,Jan,11; 2012,Jan,15-42

**99002**  Handling, conveyance, and/or any other service in connection with the implementation of an order involving devices (eg, designing, fitting, packaging, handling, delivery or mailing) when devices such as orthotics, protectives, prosthetics are fabricated by an outside laboratory or shop but which items have been designed, and are to be fitted and adjusted by the attending physician or other qualified health care professional

EXCLUDES  *Venous blood routine collection (36415)*

📋 0.00  ⚕ 0.00  **FUD** XXX  B 🖳

AMA: 2017,Jan,8; 2016,Jan,13; 2015,Jan,16; 2014,Jan,11; 2012,Jan,15-42

**99024**  Postoperative follow-up visit, normally included in the surgical package, to indicate that an evaluation and management service was performed during a postoperative period for a reason(s) related to the original procedure

📋 0.00  ⚕ 0.00  **FUD** XXX  B 🖳

AMA: 2017,Jul,9; 2017,Jan,3; 2017,Jan,8; 2016,Jan,13; 2015,Mar,3; 2015,Jan,16; 2014,Jan,11; 2012,Jan,15-42

**99026**  Hospital mandated on call service; in-hospital, each hour

EXCLUDES  *Physician stand-by services with prolonged physician attendance (99360)*
*Time spent providing procedures or services that may be separately reported*

📋 0.00  ⚕ 0.00  **FUD** XXX  E 🖳

AMA: 2017,Jan,8; 2016,Jan,13; 2015,Jan,16; 2014,Jan,11; 2012,Jan,15-42

**99027**  **out-of-hospital, each hour**

EXCLUDES  *Physician stand-by services with prolonged physician attendance (99360)*
*Time spent providing procedures or services that may be separately reported*

📋 0.00  ⚕ 0.00  **FUD** XXX  E 🖳

AMA: 2017,Jan,8; 2016,Jan,13; 2015,Jan,16; 2014,Jan,11; 2012,Jan,15-42

**99050**  Services provided in the office at times other than regularly scheduled office hours, or days when the office is normally closed (eg, holidays, Saturday or Sunday), in addition to basic service

Code also more than one adjunct code per encounter when appropriate
Code first basic service provided

📋 0.00  ⚕ 0.00  **FUD** XXX  SI B 🖳

AMA: 2017,Jan,8; 2016,Jan,13; 2015,Jan,16; 2014,Jan,11; 2012,Jan,15-42

**99051**  Service(s) provided in the office during regularly scheduled evening, weekend, or holiday office hours, in addition to basic service

Code also more than one adjunct code per encounter when appropriate
Code first basic service provided

📋 0.00  ⚕ 0.00  **FUD** XXX  SI B 🖳

AMA: 2017,Jan,8; 2016,Jan,13; 2015,Jan,16; 2014,Jan,11; 2012,Jan,15-42

**99053**  Service(s) provided between 10:00 PM and 8:00 AM at 24-hour facility, in addition to basic service

Code also more than one adjunct code per encounter when appropriate
Code first basic service provided

📋 0.00  ⚕ 0.00  **FUD** XXX  SI B 🖳

AMA: 2017,Jan,8; 2016,Jan,13; 2015,Jan,16; 2014,Jan,11; 2012,Jan,15-42

26/TC PC/TC Only  A2-A3 ASC Payment  50 Bilateral  ♂ Male Only  ♀ Female Only  📋 Facility RVU  ⚕ Non-Facility RVU  🖳 CCI
FUD Follow-up Days  CMS: IOM (Pub 100)  A-Y OPPSI  80/80 Surg Assist Allowed / w/Doc  🅽 Lab Crosswalk  🅡 Radiology Crosswalk  ❌ CLIA
CPT © 2017 American Medical Association. All Rights Reserved.
© 2017 Optum360, LLC

**99056** **Service(s) typically provided in the office, provided out of the office at request of patient, in addition to basic service**

Code also more than one adjunct code per encounter when appropriate

Code first basic service provided

🚑 0.00 ⚕ 0.00 **FUD** XXX ⑤ Ⓑ ▭

**AMA:** 2017,Jan,8; 2016,Jan,13; 2015,Jan,16; 2014,Jan,11; 2012,Jan,15-42

**99058** **Service(s) provided on an emergency basis in the office, which disrupts other scheduled office services, in addition to basic service**

Code also more than one adjunct code per encounter when appropriate

Code first basic service provided

🚑 0.00 ⚕ 0.00 **FUD** XXX ⑤ Ⓑ ▭

**AMA:** 2017,Jan,8; 2016,Jan,13; 2015,Jan,16; 2014,Jan,11; 2012,Jan,15-42

**99060** **Service(s) provided on an emergency basis, out of the office, which disrupts other scheduled office services, in addition to basic service**

Code also more than one adjunct code per encounter when appropriate

Code first basic service provided

🚑 0.00 ⚕ 0.00 **FUD** XXX ⑤ Ⓑ ▭

**AMA:** 2017,Jan,8; 2016,Jan,13; 2015,Jan,16; 2014,Jan,11; 2012,Jan,15-42

**99070** **Supplies and materials (except spectacles), provided by the physician or other qualified health care professional over and above those usually included with the office visit or other services rendered (list drugs, trays, supplies, or materials provided)**

EXCLUDES Spectacles supply

🚑 0.00 ⚕ 0.00 **FUD** XXX Ⓑ ▭

**AMA:** 2017,Sep,14; 2017,Jan,6; 2017,Jan,8; 2016,Jan,13; 2015,Jan,16; 2014,Mar,11; 2014,Jan,11; 2013,Dec,12; 2013,Mar,6-7; 2012,Nov,11-12; 2012,Aug,9; 2012,Apr,10; 2012,Jan,15-42

**99071** **Educational supplies, such as books, tapes, and pamphlets, for the patient's education at cost to physician or other qualified health care professional**

🚑 0.00 ⚕ 0.00 **FUD** XXX Ⓑ ▭

**AMA:** 2017,Jan,8; 2016,Jan,13; 2015,Jan,16; 2014,Oct,3; 2014,Jan,11; 2013,Nov,3; 2013,Apr,3-4; 2012,Jan,15-42

**99075** **Medical testimony**

🚑 0.00 ⚕ 0.00 **FUD** XXX Ⓔ ▭

**AMA:** 2017,Jan,8; 2016,Jan,13; 2015,Jan,16; 2014,Jan,11; 2012,Jan,15-42

**99078** **Physician or other qualified health care professional qualified by education, training, licensure/regulation (when applicable) educational services rendered to patients in a group setting (eg, prenatal, obesity, or diabetic instructions)**

🚑 0.00 ⚕ 0.00 **FUD** XXX Ⓝ ▭

**AMA:** 2017,Jan,8; 2016,Jan,13; 2015,Jan,16; 2014,Oct,3; 2014,Jan,11; 2013,Nov,3; 2013,Apr,3-4; 2012,Jan,15-42

**99080** **Special reports such as insurance forms, more than the information conveyed in the usual medical communications or standard reporting form**

EXCLUDES Completion of workmen's compensation forms (99455-99456)

🚑 0.00 ⚕ 0.00 **FUD** XXX Ⓑ ▭

**AMA:** 2017,Jan,8; 2016,Jan,13; 2015,Jan,16; 2014,Oct,3; 2014,Jan,11; 2013,Nov,3; 2013,Apr,3-4; 2012,Jan,15-42

**99082** **Unusual travel (eg, transportation and escort of patient)**

🚑 0.00 ⚕ 0.00 **FUD** XXX Ⓑ 80 ▭

**AMA:** 2017,Jan,8; 2016,Jan,13; 2015,Jan,16; 2014,Jan,11; 2012,Jan,15-42

**99090** **Analysis of clinical data stored in computers (eg, ECGs, blood pressures, hematologic data)**

EXCLUDES Collection/interpretation by health care professional/physician of physiologic data stored/transmitted by patient or caregiver (99091)

Use of this code when a more specific CPT code exists for cardiographic services, glucose monitoring, or musculoskeletal function testing (93227, 93272, 95250, 97750, 0206T)

🚑 0.00 ⚕ 0.00 **FUD** XXX Ⓑ ▭

**AMA:** 2017,Jan,8; 2016,Jan,13; 2015,Jan,16; 2014,Oct,3; 2014,May,4; 2014,Jan,11; 2013,Nov,3; 2013,Apr,3-4; 2012,Jan,15-42

**99091** **Collection and interpretation of physiologic data (eg, ECG, blood pressure, glucose monitoring) digitally stored and/or transmitted by the patient and/or caregiver to the physician or other qualified health care professional, qualified by education, training, licensure/regulation (when applicable) requiring a minimum of 30 minutes of time**

🚑 1.59 ⚕ 1.59 **FUD** XXX Ⓝ ▭

**AMA:** 2017,Jan,8; 2016,Jan,13; 2015,Jan,16; 2014,Oct,3; 2014,Jan,11; 2013,Nov,3; 2013,Apr,3-4; 2012,Jan,15-42

## 99100-99140 Modifying Factors for Anesthesia Services

**CMS:** 100-04,12,140.3 Payment for Qualified Nonphysician Anesthetists; 100-04,12,140.3.3 Billing Modifiers; 100-04,12,140.3.4 General Billing Instructions; 100-04,12,140.4.1 Anesthesiologist/Qualified Nonphysican Anesthetist; 100-04,12,140.4.2 Anesthetist and Anesthesiologist in a Single Procedure; 100-04,12,140.4.4 Conversion Factors for Anesthesia Services; 100-04,4,250.3.2 Anesthesia in a Hospital Outpatient Setting

Code first primary anesthesia procedure

+ **99100** **Anesthesia for patient of extreme age, younger than 1 year and older than 70 (List separately in addition to code for primary anesthesia procedure)** Ⓐ

EXCLUDES Anesthesia services for infants one year old or less at the time of surgery (00326, 00561, 00834, 00836)

🚑 0.00 ⚕ 0.00 **FUD** ZZZ Ⓑ ▭

**AMA:** 2017,Jan,8; 2016,Jan,13; 2015,Jan,16; 2014,Jan,11

+ **99116** **Anesthesia complicated by utilization of total body hypothermia (List separately in addition to code for primary anesthesia procedure)**

EXCLUDES Anesthesia for procedures on heart/pericardial sac/great vessels of chest with pump oxygenator (00561)

🚑 0.00 ⚕ 0.00 **FUD** ZZZ Ⓑ ▭

**AMA:** 2017,Jan,8; 2016,Jan,13; 2015,Jan,16; 2014,Jan,11

+ **99135** **Anesthesia complicated by utilization of controlled hypotension (List separately in addition to code for primary anesthesia procedure)**

EXCLUDES Anesthesia for procedures on heart/pericardial sac/great vessels of chest with pump oxygenator (00561)

🚑 0.00 ⚕ 0.00 **FUD** ZZZ Ⓑ ▭

**AMA:** 2017,Jan,8; 2016,Jan,13; 2015,Jan,16; 2014,Jan,11

+ **99140** **Anesthesia complicated by emergency conditions (specify) (List separately in addition to code for primary anesthesia procedure)**

INCLUDES Conditions where postponement of treatment could be dangerous to life or health

🚑 0.00 ⚕ 0.00 **FUD** ZZZ Ⓑ ▭

**AMA:** 2017,Jan,8; 2016,Jan,13; 2015,Jan,16; 2014,Jan,11; 2012,Jan,15-42

● New Code ▲ Revised Code ○ Reinstated ● New Web Release ▲ Revised Web Release Unlisted Not Covered # Resequenced
⊘ AMA Mod 51 Exempt ⑤ Optum Mod 51 Exempt ⑥ Mod 63 Exempt ✗ Non-FDA Drug ★ Telemedicine Ⓜ Maternity Ⓐ Age Edit + Add-on **AMA:** CPT Asst
© 2017 Optum360, LLC CPT © 2017 American Medical Association. All Rights Reserved.

## 99151-99157 Moderate Sedation Services

**INCLUDES**    Intraservice work that begins with administration of the sedation drugs and ends when the procedure is over
Monitoring of:
   Patient response to the drugs
   Vital signs
Ordering and providing the drug to the patient (first and subsequent)
Pre- and postservice procedures

**99151**    **Moderate sedation services provided by the same physician or other qualified health care professional performing the diagnostic or therapeutic service that the sedation supports, requiring the presence of an independent trained observer to assist in the monitoring of the patient's level of consciousness and physiological status; initial 15 minutes of intraservice time, patient younger than 5 years of age**

> **INCLUDES**    First 15 minutes of intraservice time for patients under age 5
> Services provided to patients by same provider of the service for which moderate sedation is necessary with monitoring by a trained observer

   0.67    2.18    **FUD** XXX        ⊘ N ▣

**AMA:** 2017,Sep,11; 2017,Jun,3; 2017,Jan,3

**99152**    **initial 15 minutes of intraservice time, patient age 5 years or older**

> **INCLUDES**    First 15 minutes of intraservice time for patients age 5 and over
> Services provided to patients by same provider of the service for which moderate sedation is necessary with monitoring by a trained observer

   0.35    1.45    **FUD** XXX        ⊘ N ▣

**AMA:** 2017,Sep,11; 2017,Jun,3; 2017,Jan,3

+ **99153**    **each additional 15 minutes intraservice time (List separately in addition to code for primary service)**

> **INCLUDES**    Services provided to patients by same provider of the service for which moderate sedation is necessary with monitoring by a trained observer (99155-99157)
>
> **EXCLUDES**    Services provided to patients by a physician/other qualified health care professional other than the provider rendering the service

Code first (99151-99152)

   0.31    0.31    **FUD** ZZZ        N TC ▣

**AMA:** 2017,Sep,11; 2017,Jun,3; 2017,Jan,3

**99155**    **Moderate sedation services provided by a physician or other qualified health care professional other than the physician or other qualified health care professional performing the diagnostic or therapeutic service that the sedation supports; initial 15 minutes of intraservice time, patient younger than 5 years of age**

> **INCLUDES**    First 15 minutes of intraservice time for patients under age 5
> Services provided to patients by a physician/other qualified health care professional other than the provider rendering the service for which moderate sedation is necessary

   2.63    2.63    **FUD** XXX        N ▣

**AMA:** 2017,Sep,11; 2017,Jun,3; 2017,Jan,3

**99156**    **initial 15 minutes of intraservice time, patient age 5 years or older**

> **INCLUDES**    First 15 minutes of intraservice time for patients age 5 and over
> Services provided to patients by a physician/other qualified health care professional other than the provider rendering the service for which moderate sedation is necessary

   2.15    2.15    **FUD** XXX        N ▣

**AMA:** 2017,Sep,11; 2017,Jun,3; 2017,Jan,3

+ **99157**    **each additional 15 minutes intraservice time (List separately in addition to code for primary service)**

> **INCLUDES**    Each subsequent 15 minutes of services
> Services provided to patients by a physician/other qualified health care professional other than the provider rendering the service for which moderate sedation is necessary (99151-99152)
>
> **EXCLUDES**    Services provided to patients by same provider of the service for which moderate sedation is necessary with monitoring by a trained observer (99151-99152)

Code first (99155-99156)

   1.63    1.63    **FUD** ZZZ        N ▣

**AMA:** 2017,Sep,11; 2017,Jun,3; 2017,Jan,3

## 99170 Specialized Examination of Child

**EXCLUDES**    Moderate sedation (99151-99157)

**99170**    **Anogenital examination, magnified, in childhood for suspected trauma, including image recording when performed**        A

   2.50    4.67    **FUD** 000        T ▣

**AMA:** 2017,Jan,8; 2016,Jan,13; 2015,Jan,16; 2014,Sep,7; 2014,Jan,11

## 99172-99173 Visual Acuity Screening Tests

**INCLUDES**    Graduated visual acuity stimuli that allow a quantitative determination/estimation of visual acuity

**EXCLUDES**    General ophthalmological or E&M services

**99172**    **Visual function screening, automated or semi-automated bilateral quantitative determination of visual acuity, ocular alignment, color vision by pseudoisochromatic plates, and field of vision (may include all or some screening of the determination[s] for contrast sensitivity, vision under glare)**

> **EXCLUDES**    Screening for visual acuity, amblyogenic factors, retinal polarization scan (99173, 99174 [99177], 0469T)

   0.00    0.00    **FUD** XXX        E ▣

**AMA:** 2017,Jan,8; 2016,Jan,13; 2015,Jan,16; 2014,Jan,11; 2012,Jan,15-42

**99173**    **Screening test of visual acuity, quantitative, bilateral**

> **EXCLUDES**    Screening for visual function, amblyogenic factors (99172, 99174, [99177])

   0.09    0.09    **FUD** XXX        E ▣

**AMA:** 2017,Jan,8; 2016,Jan,13; 2015,Jan,16; 2014,Jan,11

## 99174 [99177] Screening For Amblyogenic Factors

**EXCLUDES**    General ophthalmological services (92002-92014)
Screening for visual acuity (99172-99173, [99177])

**99174**    **Instrument-based ocular screening (eg, photoscreening, automated-refraction), bilateral; with remote analysis and report**

> **EXCLUDES**    Ocular screening on-site analysis ([99177])

   0.00    0.00    **FUD** XXX        E ▣

**AMA:** 2017,Jan,8; 2016,Mar,10; 2016,Jan,13; 2015,Jan,16; 2014,Jan,11; 2013,Mar,6-7

\# **99177**    **with on-site analysis**

> **EXCLUDES**    Remote ocular screening (99174)
> Retinal polarization scan (0469T)

   0.00    0.00    **FUD** XXX        E ▣

**AMA:** 2017,Jan,8; 2016,Mar,10

## 99175-99177 Drug Administration to Induce Vomiting

**EXCLUDES**    Diagnostic gastric lavage (43754-43755)
Diagnostic gastric intubation (43754-43755)

**99175**    **Ipecac or similar administration for individual emesis and continued observation until stomach adequately emptied of poison**

   0.45    0.45    **FUD** XXX        N 80 ▣

**AMA:** 1997,Nov,1

*99177*    **Resequenced code. See code following 99174.**

26/TC PC/TC Only    A2-Z3 ASC Payment    50 Bilateral    ♂ Male Only    ♀ Female Only    Facility RVU    Non-Facility RVU    ▣ CCI
**FUD** Follow-up Days    **CMS:** IOM (Pub 100)    A-Y OPPSI    80/80 Surg Assist Allowed / w/Doc    Lab Crosswalk    Radiology Crosswalk    ✖ CLIA

494                 CPT © 2017 American Medical Association. All Rights Reserved.               © 2017 Optum360, LLC

## 99183-99184 Hyperbaric Oxygen Therapy

**CMS:** 100-03,20.29 Hyperbaric Oxygen Therapy; 100-04,32,30.1 HBO Therapy for Lower Extremity Diabetic Wounds

*EXCLUDES* *E&M services, when performed*
*Other procedures such as wound debridement, when performed*

**99183** **Physician or other qualified health care professional attendance and supervision of hyperbaric oxygen therapy, per session**

🔧 3.14 ⚕ 3.14 **FUD** XXX B 80 26 ▭

**AMA:** 2017,Jan,8; 2016,Jan,13; 2015,Jan,16; 2014,Jan,11; 2012,Jan,15-42

**99184** **Initiation of selective head or total body hypothermia in the critically ill neonate, includes appropriate patient selection by review of clinical, imaging and laboratory data, confirmation of esophageal temperature probe location, evaluation of amplitude EEG, supervision of controlled hypothermia, and assessment of patient tolerance of cooling** A

*EXCLUDES* *Use of code more than one time per hospitalization*

🔧 6.04 ⚕ 6.04 **FUD** XXX C 80 ▭

**AMA:** 2017,Jan,8; 2016,Jan,13; 2015,Oct,8

## 99188 Topical Fluoride Application

**99188** **Application of topical fluoride varnish by a physician or other qualified health care professional**

🔧 0.00 ⚕ 0.00 **FUD** XXX E 80 ▭

## 99190-99192 Assemble and Manage Pump with Oxygenator/Heat Exchange

**99190** **Assembly and operation of pump with oxygenator or heat exchanger (with or without ECG and/or pressure monitoring); each hour**

🔧 0.00 ⚕ 0.00 **FUD** XXX C ▭

**AMA:** 1997,Nov,1

**99191** **45 minutes**

🔧 0.00 ⚕ 0.00 **FUD** XXX C ▭

**AMA:** 1997,Nov,1

**99192** **30 minutes**

🔧 0.00 ⚕ 0.00 **FUD** XXX C ▭

**AMA:** 1997,Nov,1

## 99195-99199 Therapeutic Phlebotomy and Unlisted Procedures

**99195** **Phlebotomy, therapeutic (separate procedure)**

🔧 2.83 ⚕ 2.83 **FUD** XXX Q1 80 ▭

**AMA:** 2017,Jan,8; 2016,Jan,13; 2015,Jan,16; 2014,Jan,11; 2012,Jan,15-42

**99199** **Unlisted special service, procedure or report**

🔧 0.00 ⚕ 0.00 **FUD** XXX B 80

**AMA:** 2017,Jan,8; 2016,Jan,13; 2015,Jan,16; 2014,Jan,11; 2012,Oct,13; 2012,Sep,9; 2012,Jun,15-16

## 99500-99602 Home Visit By Non-Physician Professionals

*INCLUDES* Services performed by non-physician providers
Services provided in patient's:
Assisted living apartment
Custodial care facility
Group home
Non-traditional private home
Residence
School

*EXCLUDES* *Home visits performed by physicians (99341-99350)*
*Other services/procedures provided by physicians to patients at home*

Code also home visit E&M codes if health care provider is authorized to use (99341-99350)
Code also significant separately identifiable E&M service, when performed

**99500** **Home visit for prenatal monitoring and assessment to include fetal heart rate, non-stress test, uterine monitoring, and gestational diabetes monitoring** M ♀

🔧 0.00 ⚕ 0.00 **FUD** XXX E ▭

**AMA:** 2017,Jan,8; 2016,Jan,13; 2015,Jan,16; 2014,Jan,11; 2012,Jan,15-42

**99501** **Home visit for postnatal assessment and follow-up care** M ♀

🔧 0.00 ⚕ 0.00 **FUD** XXX E ▭

**AMA:** 2017,Jan,8; 2016,Jan,13; 2015,Jan,16; 2014,Jan,11

**99502** **Home visit for newborn care and assessment** A

🔧 0.00 ⚕ 0.00 **FUD** XXX E ▭

**AMA:** 2017,Jan,8; 2016,Jan,13; 2015,Jan,16; 2014,Jan,11

**99503** **Home visit for respiratory therapy care (eg, bronchodilator, oxygen therapy, respiratory assessment, apnea evaluation)**

🔧 0.00 ⚕ 0.00 **FUD** XXX E ▭

**AMA:** 2017,Jan,8; 2016,Jan,13; 2015,Jan,16; 2014,Jan,11

**99504** **Home visit for mechanical ventilation care**

🔧 0.00 ⚕ 0.00 **FUD** XXX E ▭

**AMA:** 2017,Jan,8; 2016,Jan,13; 2015,Jan,16; 2014,Jan,11

**99505** **Home visit for stoma care and maintenance including colostomy and cystostomy**

🔧 0.00 ⚕ 0.00 **FUD** XXX E ▭

**AMA:** 2017,Jan,8; 2016,Jan,13; 2015,Jan,16; 2014,Jan,11

**99506** **Home visit for intramuscular injections**

🔧 0.00 ⚕ 0.00 **FUD** XXX E ▭

**AMA:** 2017,Jan,8; 2016,Jan,13; 2015,Jan,16; 2014,Jan,11

**99507** **Home visit for care and maintenance of catheter(s) (eg, urinary, drainage, and enteral)**

🔧 0.00 ⚕ 0.00 **FUD** XXX E ▭

**AMA:** 2017,Jan,8; 2016,Jan,13; 2015,Jan,16; 2014,Jan,11

**99509** **Home visit for assistance with activities of daily living and personal care**

*EXCLUDES* *Medical nutrition therapy/assessment home services (97802-97804)*
*Self-care/home management training (97535)*
*Speech therapy home services (92507-92508)*

🔧 0.00 ⚕ 0.00 **FUD** XXX E ▭

**AMA:** 2017,Jan,8; 2016,Jan,13; 2015,Jan,16; 2014,Jan,11

**99510** **Home visit for individual, family, or marriage counseling**

🔧 0.00 ⚕ 0.00 **FUD** XXX E ▭

**AMA:** 2017,Jan,8; 2016,Jan,13; 2015,Jan,16; 2014,Jan,11

**99511** **Home visit for fecal impaction management and enema administration**

🔧 0.00 ⚕ 0.00 **FUD** XXX E ▭

**AMA:** 2017,Jan,8; 2016,Jan,13; 2015,Jan,16; 2014,Jan,11

**99512** **Home visit for hemodialysis**

*EXCLUDES* *Peritoneal dialysis home infusion (99601-99602)*

🔧 0.00 ⚕ 0.00 **FUD** XXX E ▭

**AMA:** 2017,Jan,8; 2016,Jan,13; 2015,Jan,16; 2014,Jan,11

---

**99600** **Unlisted home visit service or procedure**
    📤 0.00    ✂ 0.00    **FUD** XXX    E ▣
    **AMA:** 2017,Jan,8; 2016,Jan,13; 2015,Jan,16; 2014,Jan,11;
    2012,Jan,15-42

**99601** **Home infusion/specialty drug administration, per visit (up to 2 hours);**
    📤 0.00    ✂ 0.00    **FUD** XXX    E ▣
    **AMA:** 2005,Nov,1-9; 2003,Oct,7

+ **99602** **each additional hour (List separately in addition to code for primary procedure)**
    Code first (99601)
    📤 0.00    ✂ 0.00    **FUD** XXX    E ▣
    **AMA:** 2005,Nov,1-9; 2003,Oct,7

## 99605-99607 Medication Management By Pharmacist

INCLUDES  Direct (face-to-face) assessment and intervention by a pharmacist for the
    purpose of:
    Managing medication complications and/or interactions
    Maximizing the patient's response to drug therapy
  Documenting the following required elements:
    Advice given regarding improvement of treatment compliance and
      outcomes
    Profile of medications (prescription and nonprescription)
    Review of applicable patient history

EXCLUDES  *Routine tasks associated with dispensing and related activities (e.g., providing*
    *product information)*

**99605** **Medication therapy management service(s) provided by a pharmacist, individual, face-to-face with patient, with assessment and intervention if provided; initial 15 minutes, new patient**
    📤 0.00    ✂ 0.00    **FUD** XXX    E ▣
    **AMA:** 2017,Jan,8; 2016,Jan,13; 2015,Jan,16; 2014,Oct,3;
    2014,Jan,11; 2013,Nov,3; 2013,Apr,3-4; 2012,Jan,15-42

**99606** **initial 15 minutes, established patient**
    📤 0.00    ✂ 0.00    **FUD** XXX    E ▣
    **AMA:** 2017,Jan,8; 2016,Jan,13; 2015,Jan,16; 2014,Oct,3;
    2014,Jan,11; 2013,Nov,3; 2013,Apr,3-4; 2012,Jan,15-42

+ **99607** **each additional 15 minutes (List separately in addition to code for primary service)**
    Code first (99605, 99606)
    📤 0.00    ✂ 0.00    **FUD** XXX    E ▣
    **AMA:** 2017,Jan,8; 2016,Jan,13; 2015,Jan,16; 2014,Oct,3;
    2014,Jan,11; 2013,Nov,3; 2013,Apr,3-4; 2012,Jan,15-42

26/TC PC/TC Only    A2-Z3 ASC Payment    50 Bilateral    ♂ Male Only    ♀ Female Only    📤 Facility RVU    ✂ Non-Facility RVU    ▣ CCI
FUD Follow-up Days    CMS: IOM (Pub 100)    A-Y OPPSI    80/80 Surg Assist Allowed / w/Doc    Lab Crosswalk    Radiology Crosswalk    CLIA

496    CPT © 2017 American Medical Association. All Rights Reserved.    © 2017 Optum360, LLC

# Evaluation and Management (E/M) Services Guidelines

Information unique to this section is defined or identified below.

For additional information about evaluation and management services, see Appendix C: Evaluation and Management Extended Guidelines. This appendix includes comprehensive explanations and instructions for the correct selection of an E&M service code based on federal documentation standards.

## Classification of Evaluation and Management (E/M) Services

The E/M section is divided into broad categories such as office visits, hospital visits, and consultations. Most of the categories are further divided into two or more subcategories of E/M services. For example, there are two subcategories of office visits (new patient and established patient) and there are two subcategories of hospital visits (initial and subsequent). The subcategories of E/M services are further classified into levels of E/M services that are identified by specific codes. This classification is important because the nature of work varies by type of service, place of service, and the patient's status.

The basic format of the levels of E/M services is the same for most categories. First, a unique code number is listed. Second, the place and/or type of service is specified, eg, office consultation. Third, the content of the service is defined, eg, comprehensive history and comprehensive examination. (See "Levels of E/M Services," for details on the content of E/M services.) Fourth, the nature of the presenting problem(s) usually associated with a given level is described. Fifth, the time typically required to provide the service is specified. (A detailed discussion of time is provided separately.)

## Definitions of Commonly Used Terms

Certain key words and phrases are used throughout the E/M section. The following definitions are intended to reduce the potential for differing interpretations and to increase the consistency of reporting by physicians in differing specialties. E/M services may also be reported by other qualified health care professionals who are authorized to perform such services within the scope of their practice.

### New and Established Patient

Solely for the purposes of distinguishing between new and established patients, professional services are those face-to-face services rendered by physicians and other qualified health care professionals who may report E/M services with a specific CPT® code or codes. A new patient is one who has not received any professional services from the physician/qualified health care professional or another physician/qualified health care professional of the exact same specialty and subspecialty who belongs to the same group practice, within the past three years.

An established patient is one who has received professional services from the physician/qualified health care professional or another physician/qualified health care professional of the exact same specialty and subspecialty who belongs to the same group practice, within the past three years. See the decision tree at right.

When a physician/qualified health care professional is on call or covering for another physician/qualified health care professional, the patient's encounter is classified as it would have been by the physician/qualified health care professional who is not available. When advanced practice nurses and physician assistants are working with physicians, they are considered as working in the exact same specialty and exact same subspecialties as the physician.

No distinction is made between new and established patients in the emergency department. E/M services in the emergency department category may be reported for any new or established patient who presents for treatment in the emergency department.

The decision tree in the next column is provided to aid in determining whether to report the E/M service provided as a new or an established patient encounter.

## Chief Complaint

A chief complaint is a concise statement describing the symptom, problem, condition, diagnosis, or other factor that is the reason for the encounter, usually stated in the patient's words.

## Concurrent Care and Transfer of Care

Concurrent care is the provision of similar services (e.g., hospital visits) to the same patient by more than one physician or other qualified health care professional on the same day. When concurrent care is provided, no special reporting is required. Transfer of care is the process whereby a physician or other qualified health care professional who is managing some or all of a patient's problems relinquishes this responsibility to another physician or other qualified health care professional who explicitly agrees to accept this responsibility and who, from the initial encounter, is not providing consultative services. The physician or other qualified health care professional transferring care is then no longer providing care for these problems though he or she may continue providing care for other conditions when appropriate. Consultation codes should not be reported by the physician or other qualified health care professional who has agreed to accept transfer of care before an initial evaluation, but they are appropriate to report if the decision to accept transfer of care cannot be made until after the initial consultation evaluation, regardless of site of service.

## Decision Tree for New vs Established Patients

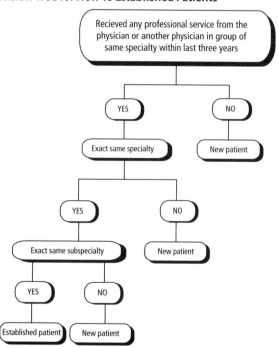

## Counseling

Counseling is a discussion with a patient and/or family concerning one or more of the following areas:

- Diagnostic results, impressions, and/or recommended diagnostic studies

- Prognosis

- Risks and benefits of management (treatment) options

- Instructions for management (treatment) and/or follow-up

- Importance of compliance with chosen management (treatment) options

- Risk factor reduction

- Patient and family education
  (For psychotherapy, see 90832–90834, 90836–90840)

## Family History

A review of medical events in the patient's family that includes significant information about:

- The health status or cause of death of parents, siblings, and children
- Specific diseases related to problems identified in the Chief Complaint or History of the Present Illness, and/or System Review
- Diseases of family members that may be hereditary or place the patient at risk

## History of Present Illness

A chronological description of the development of the patient's present illness from the first sign and/or symptom to the present. This includes a description of location, quality, severity, timing, context, modifying factors, and associated signs and symptoms significantly related to the presenting problem(s).

## Levels of E/M Services

Within each category or subcategory of E/M service, there are three to five levels of E/M services available for reporting purposes. Levels of E/M services are not interchangeable among the different categories or subcategories of service. For example, the first level of E/M services in the subcategory of office visit, new patient, does not have the same definition as the first level of E/M services in the subcategory of office visit, established patient.

The levels of E/M services include examinations, evaluations, treatments, conferences with or concerning patients, preventive pediatric and adult health supervision, and similar medical services, such as the determination of the need and/or location for appropriate care. Medical screening includes the history, examination, and medical decision-making required to determine the need and/or location for appropriate care and treatment of the patient (eg, office and other outpatient setting, emergency department, nursing facility). The levels of E/M services encompass the wide variations in skill, effort, time, responsibility, and medical knowledge required for the prevention or diagnosis and treatment of illness or injury and the promotion of optimal health. Each level of E/M services may be used by all physicians or other qualified health care professionals.

The descriptors for the levels of E/M services recognize seven components, six of which are used in defining the levels of E/M services. These components are:

- History
- Examination
- Medical decision making
- Counseling
- Coordination of care
- Nature of presenting problem
- Time

The first three of these components (history, examination, and medical decision making) are considered the key components in selecting a level of E/M services. (See "Determine the Extent of History Obtained.")

The next three components (counseling, coordination of care, and the nature of the presenting problem) are considered contributory factors in the majority of encounters. Although the first two of these contributory factors are important E/M services, it is not required that these services be provided at every patient encounter.

Coordination of care with other physicians, other qualified health care professionals, or agencies without a patient encounter on that day is reported using the case management codes.

The final component, time, is discussed in detail below.

Any specifically identifiable procedure (ie, identified with a specific CPT code) performed on or subsequent to the date of initial or subsequent E/M services should be reported separately.

The actual performance and/or interpretation of diagnostic tests/studies ordered during a patient encounter are not included in the levels of E/M services. Physician performance of diagnostic tests/studies for which specific CPT codes are available may be reported separately, in addition to the appropriate E/M code. The physician's interpretation of the results of diagnostic tests/studies (ie, professional component) with preparation of a separate distinctly identifiable signed written report may also be reported separately, using the appropriate CPT code with modifier 26 appended.

The physician or other health care professional may need to indicate that on the day a procedure or service identified by a CPT code was performed, the patient's condition required a significant separately identifiable E/M service above and beyond other services provided or beyond the usual preservice and postservice care associated with the procedure that was performed. The E/M service may be caused or prompted by the symptoms or condition for which the procedure and/or service was provided. This circumstance may be reported by adding modifier 25 to the appropriate level of E/M service. As such, different diagnoses are not required for reporting of the procedure and the E/M services on the same date.

## Nature of Presenting Problem

A presenting problem is a disease, condition, illness, injury, symptom, sign, finding, complaint, or other reason for encounter, with or without a diagnosis being established at the time of the encounter. The E/M codes recognize five types of presenting problems that are defined as follows:

**Minimal:** A problem that may not require the presence of the physician or other qualified health care professional, but service is provided under the physician's or other qualified health care professional's supervision.

**Self-limited or minor:** A problem that runs a definite and prescribed course, is transient in nature, and is not likely to permanently alter health status OR has a good prognosis with management/compliance.

**Low severity:** A problem where the risk of morbidity without treatment is low; there is little to no risk of mortality without treatment; full recovery without functional impairment is expected.

**Moderate severity:** A problem where the risk of morbidity without treatment is moderate; there is moderate risk of mortality without treatment; uncertain prognosis OR increased probability of prolonged functional impairment.

**High severity:** A problem where the risk of morbidity without treatment is high to extreme; there is a moderate to high risk of mortality without treatment OR high probability of severe, prolonged functional impairment.

## Past History

A review of the patient's past experiences with illnesses, injuries, and treatments that includes significant information about:

- Prior major illnesses and injuries
- Prior operations
- Prior hospitalizations
- Current medications
- Allergies (eg, drug, food)
- Age appropriate immunization status
- Age appropriate feeding/dietary status

## Social History

An age appropriate review of past and current activities that includes significant information about:

- Marital status and/or living arrangements
- Current employment
- Occupational history
- Military history
- Use of drugs, alcohol, and tobacco
- Level of education
- Sexual history
- Other relevant social factors

CPT © 2017 American Medical Association. All Rights Reserved.

© 2017 Optum360, LLC

## System Review (Review of Systems)
An inventory of body systems obtained through a series of questions seeking to identify signs and/or symptoms that the patient may be experiencing or has experienced. For the purposes of the CPT codebook the following elements of a system review have been identified:

- Constitutional symptoms (fever, weight loss, etc)
- Eyes
- Ears, nose, mouth, throat
- Cardiovascular
- Respiratory
- Gastrointestinal
- Genitourinary
- Musculoskeletal
- Integumentary (skin and/or breast)
- Neurological
- Psychiatric
- Endocrine
- Hematologic/lymphatic
- Allergic/immunologic

The review of systems helps define the problem, clarify the differential diagnosis, identify needed testing, or serves as baseline data on other systems that might be affected by any possible management options.

## Time
The inclusion of time in the definitions of levels of E/M services has been implicit in prior editions of the CPT codebook. The inclusion of time as an explicit factor beginning in *CPT 1992* is done to assist in selecting the most appropriate level of E/M services. It should be recognized that the specific times expressed in the visit code descriptors are averages and, therefore, represent a range of times that may be higher or lower depending on actual clinical circumstances.

Time is not a descriptive component for the emergency department levels of E/M services because emergency department services are typically provided on a variable intensity basis, often involving multiple encounters with several patients over an extended period of time. Therefore, it is often difficult to provide accurate estimates of the time spent face-to-face with the patient.

Studies to establish levels of E/M services employed surveys of practicing physicians to obtain data on the amount of time and work associated with typical E/M services. Since "work" is not easily quantifiable, the codes must rely on other objective, verifiable measures that correlate with physicians' estimates of their "work." It has been demonstrated that estimations of intraservice time, both within and across specialties, is a variable that is predictive of the "work" of E/M services. This same research has shown there is a strong relationship between intraservice time and total time for E/M services. Intraservice time, rather than total time, was chosen for inclusion with the codes because of its relative ease of measurement and because of its direct correlation with measurements of the total amount of time and work associated with typical E/M services.

Intraservice times are defined as face-to-face time for office and other outpatient visits and as unit/floor time for hospital and other inpatient visits. This distinction is necessary because most of the work of typical office visits takes place during the face-to-face time with the patient, while most of the work of typical hospital visits takes place during the time spent on the patient's floor or unit. When prolonged time occurs in either the office or the inpatient areas, the appropriate add-on code should be reported.

**Face-to-face time (office and other outpatient visits and office consultations):** For coding purposes, face-to-face time for these services is defined as only that time spent face-to-face with the patient and/or family. This includes the time spent performing such tasks as obtaining a history, performing an examination, and counseling the patient.

Time is also spent doing work before or after the face-to-face time with the patient, performing such tasks as reviewing records and tests, arranging for

further services, and communicating further with other professionals and the patient through written reports and telephone contact.

This non-face-to-face time for office services—also called pre- and postencounter time—is not included in the time component described in the E/M codes. However, the pre- and post-non-face-to-face work associated with an encounter was included in calculating the total work of typical services in physician surveys.

Thus, the face-to-face time associated with the services described by any E/M code is a valid proxy for the total work done before, during, and after the visit.

**Unit/floor time (hospital observation services, inpatient hospital care, initial inpatient hospital consultations, nursing facility):** For reporting purposes, intraservice time for these services is defined as unit/floor time, which includes the time present on the patient's hospital unit and at the bedside rendering services for that patient. This includes the time to establish and/or review the patient's chart, examine the patient, write notes, and communicate with other professionals and the patient's family.

In the hospital, pre- and post-time includes time spent off the patient's floor performing such tasks as reviewing pathology and radiology findings in another part of the hospital.

This pre- and postvisit time is not included in the time component described in these codes. However, the pre- and postwork performed during the time spent off the floor or unit was included in calculating the total work of typical services in physician surveys.

Thus, the unit/floor time associated with the services described by any code is a valid proxy for the total work done before, during, and after the visit.

## Unlisted Service
An E/M service may be provided that is not listed in this section of the CPT codebook. When reporting such a service, the appropriate unlisted code may be used to indicate the service, identifying it by "Special Report," as discussed in the following paragraph. The "Unlisted Services" and accompanying codes for the E/M section are as follows:

| 99429 | Unlisted preventive medicine service |
| 99499 | Unlisted evaluation and management service |

## Special Report
An unlisted service or one that is unusual, variable, or new may require a special report demonstrating the medical appropriateness of the service. Pertinent information should include an adequate definition or description of the nature, extent, and need for the procedure and the time, effort, and equipment necessary to provide the service. Additional items that may be included are complexity of symptoms, final diagnosis, pertinent physical findings, diagnostic and therapeutic procedures, concurrent problems, and follow-up care.

## Instructions for Selecting a Level of E/M Service

### Review the Reporting Instructions for the Selected Category or Subcategory
Most of the categories and many of the subcategories of service have special guidelines or instructions unique to that category or subcategory. Where these are indicated, eg, "Inpatient Hospital Care," special instructions will be presented preceding the levels of E/M services.

### Review the Level of E/M Service Descriptors and Examples in the Selected Category or Subcategory
The descriptors for the levels of E/M services recognize seven components, six of which are used in defining the levels of E/M services. These components are:

- History
- Examination
- Medical decision making

- Counseling
- Coordination of care
- Nature of presenting problem
- Time

The first three of these components (ie, history, examination, and medical decision making) should be considered the key components in selecting the level of E/M services. An exception to this rule is in the case of visits that consist predominantly of counseling or coordination of care.

The nature of the presenting problem and time are provided in some levels to assist the physician in determining the appropriate level of E/M service.

## Determine the Extent of History Obtained

The extent of the history is dependent upon clinical judgment and on the nature of the presenting problem(s). The levels of E/M services recognize four types of history that are defined as follows:

**Problem focused:** Chief complaint; brief history of present illness or problem.

**Expanded problem focused:** Chief complaint; brief history of present illness; problem pertinent system review.

**Detailed:** Chief complaint; extended history of present illness; problem pertinent system review extended to include a review of a limited number of additional systems; pertinent past, family, and/or social history directly related to the patient's problems.

**Comprehensive:** Chief complaint; extended history of present illness; review of systems that is directly related to the problem(s) identified in the history of the present illness plus a review of all additional body systems; complete past, family, and social history.

The comprehensive history obtained as part of the preventive medicine E/M service is not problem-oriented and does not involve a chief complaint or present illness. It does, however, include a comprehensive system review and comprehensive or interval past, family, and social history as well as a comprehensive assessment/history of pertinent risk factors.

## Determine the Extent of Examination Performed

The extent of the examination performed is dependent on clinical judgment and on the nature of the presenting problem(s). The levels of E/M services recognize four types of examination that are defined as follows:

**Problem focused:** A limited examination of the affected body area or organ system.

**Expanded problem focused:** A limited examination of the affected body area or organ system and other symptomatic or related organ system(s).

**Detailed:** An extended examination of the affected body area(s) and other symptomatic or related organ system(s).

**Comprehensive:** A general multisystem examination or a complete examination of a single organ system. Note: The comprehensive examination performed as part of the preventive medicine E/M service is multisystem, but its extent is based on age and risk factors identified.

For the purposes of these CPT definitions, the following body areas are recognized:

- Head, including the face
- Neck
- Chest, including breasts and axilla
- Abdomen
- Genitalia, groin, buttocks
- Back
- Each extremity

For the purposes of these CPT definitions, the following organ systems are recognized:

- Eyes
- Ears, nose, mouth, and throat
- Cardiovascular
- Respiratory
- Gastrointestinal
- Genitourinary
- Musculoskeletal
- Skin
- Neurologic
- Psychiatric
- Hematologic/lymphatic/immunologic

## Determine the Complexity of Medical Decision Making

Medical decision making refers to the complexity of establishing a diagnosis and/or selecting a management option as measured by:

- The number of possible diagnoses and/or the number of management options that must be considered
- The amount and/or complexity of medical records, diagnostic tests, and/or other information that must be obtained, reviewed, and analyzed
- The risk of significant complications, morbidity, and/or mortality, as well as comorbidities associated with the patient's presenting problem(s), the diagnostic procedure(s), and/or the possible management options

Four types of medical decision making are recognized: straightforward, low complexity, moderate complexity, and high complexity. To qualify for a given type of decision making, two of the three elements in Table 1 must be met or exceeded.

Comorbidities and underlying diseases, in and of themselves, are not considered in selecting a level of E/M services unless their presence significantly increases the complexity of the medical decision making.

## Select the Appropriate Level of E/M Services Based on the Following

For the following categories/subcategories, all of the key components, ie, history, examination, and medical decision making, must meet or exceed the stated requirements to qualify for a particular level of E/M service: office, new patient; hospital observation services; initial hospital care; office consultations; initial inpatient consultations; emergency department services; initial nursing facility care; domiciliary care, new patient; and home, new patient.

For the following categories/subcategories, two of the three key components (ie, history, examination, and medical decision making) must meet or exceed the stated requirements to qualify for a particular level of E/M services: office, established patient; subsequent hospital care; subsequent nursing facility care; domiciliary care, established patient; and home, established patient.

When counseling and/or coordination of care dominates (more than 50 percent) the encounter with the patient and/or family (face-to-face time in the office or other outpatient setting or floor/unit time in the hospital or nursing facility), then time shall be considered the key or controlling factor to qualify for a particular level of E/M services. This includes time spent with parties who have assumed responsibility for the care of the patient or decision making whether or not they are family members (e.g., foster parents, person acting in loco parentis, legal guardian). The extent of counseling and/or coordination of care must be documented in the medical record.

## CONSULTATION CODES AND MEDICARE REIMBURSEMENT

The Centers for Medicare and Medicaid Services (CMS) no longer provides benefits for CPT consultation codes. CMS has, however, redistributed the value of the consultation codes across the other E/M codes for services which are covered by Medicare. CMS has retained codes 99241 - 99251 in the Medicare Physician Fee Schedule for those private payers that use this data for reimbursement. Note that private payers may choose to follow CMS or CPT guidelines, and the use of consultation codes should be verified with individual payers.

## Table 1

### Complexity of Medical Decision Making

| Number of Diagnoses or Management Options | Amount and/or Complexity of Data to Be Reviewed | Risk of Complications and/or Morbidity or Mortality | Type of Decision Making |
|---|---|---|---|
| minimal | minimal or none | minimal | straightforward |
| limited | limited | low | low complexity |
| multiple | moderate | moderate | moderate complexity |
| extensive | extensive | high | high complexity |

**Evaluation and Management**

## 99201-99215 Outpatient and Other Visits

**CMS:** 100-04,11,40.1.3 Independent Attending Physician Services; 100-04,12,100.1.1 Teaching Physicians E/M Services; 100-04,12,190.3 List of Telehealth Services; 100-04,12,190.6 Payment Methodology for Physician/Practitioner at the Distant Site ; 100-04,12,190.6.1 Submission of Telehealth Claims for Distant Site Practitioners; 100-04,12,190.7 Contractor Editing of Telehealth Claims; 100-04,12,230 Primary Care Incentive Payment Program; 100-04,12,230.1 Definition of Primary Care Practitioners and Services; 100-04,12,230.2 Coordination with Other Payments; 100-04,12,230.3 Claims Processing and Payment; 100-04,12,30.6.10 Consultation Services; 100-04,12,30.6.15.1 Prolonged Services With Direct Face-to-Face Patient Contact Service (Codes 99354 - 99357); 100-04,12,30.6.4 Services Furnished Incident to Physician's Service; 100-04,12,30.6.7 Payment for Office or Other Outpatient E&M Visits; 100-04,12,40.3 Global Surgery Review; 100-04,18,80.2 Contractor BIlling Requirements; 100-04,32,130.1 Billing and Payment of External counterpulsation (ECP)

**INCLUDES**     Established patients: received prior professional services from the physician or qualified health care professional or another physician or qualified health care professional in the practice of the exact same specialty and subspecialty in the previous three years (99211-99215)

New patients: have not received professional services from the physician or qualified health care professional or any other physician or qualified health care professional in the same practice in the exact same specialty and subspecialty in the previous three years (99201-99205)

Office visits

Outpatient services (including services prior to a formal admission to a facility)

**EXCLUDES**     Services provided in:

Emergency department (99281-99285)

Hospital observation (99217-99220 [99224, 99225, 99226])

Hospital observation or inpatient with same day admission and discharge (99234-99236)

**99201**     Office or other outpatient visit for the evaluation and management of a new patient, which requires these 3 key components: A problem focused history; A problem focused examination; Straightforward medical decision making. Counseling and/or coordination of care with other physicians, other qualified health care professionals, or agencies are provided consistent with the nature of the problem(s) and the patient's and/or family's needs. Usually, the presenting problem(s) are self limited or minor. Typically, 10 minutes are spent face-to-face with the patient and/or family.

      📁 0.76    ⚗ 1.24    **FUD** XXX          ★ B 80 🖥

      **AMA:** 2017,Aug,3; 2017,Jun,6; 2017,Jan,8; 2016,Dec,11; 2016,Sep,6; 2016,Mar,10; 2016,Jan,7; 2016,Jan,13; 2015,Dec,3; 2015,Oct,3; 2015,Jan,16; 2015,Jan,12; 2014,Nov,14; 2014,Oct,8; 2014,Oct,3; 2014,Aug,3; 2014,Jan,11; 2013,Aug,13; 2013,Jun,3-5; 2013,Jan,9-10; 2012,Aug,3-5; 2012,Apr,10; 2012,Jan,15-42; 2012,Jan,3-5

**99202**     Office or other outpatient visit for the evaluation and management of a new patient, which requires these 3 key components: An expanded problem focused history; An expanded problem focused examination; Straightforward medical decision making. Counseling and/or coordination of care with other physicians, other qualified health care professionals, or agencies are provided consistent with the nature of the problem(s) and the patient's and/or family's needs. Usually, the presenting problem(s) are of low to moderate severity. Typically, 20 minutes are spent face-to-face with the patient and/or family.

      📁 1.43    ⚗ 2.11    **FUD** XXX          ★ B 80 🖥

      **AMA:** 2017,Aug,3; 2017,Jun,6; 2017,Jan,8; 2016,Dec,11; 2016,Sep,6; 2016,Mar,10; 2016,Jan,13; 2016,Jan,7; 2015,Dec,3; 2015,Oct,3; 2015,Jan,12; 2015,Jan,16; 2014,Nov,14; 2014,Oct,8; 2014,Oct,3; 2014,Aug,3; 2014,Jan,11; 2013,Aug,13; 2013,Jun,3-5; 2013,Jan,9-10; 2012,Aug,3-5; 2012,Apr,10; 2012,Jan,3-5; 2012,Jan,15-42

**99203**     Office or other outpatient visit for the evaluation and management of a new patient, which requires these 3 key components: A detailed history; A detailed examination; Medical decision making of low complexity. Counseling and/or coordination of care with other physicians, other qualified health care professionals, or agencies are provided consistent with the nature of the problem(s) and the patient's and/or family's needs. Usually, the presenting problem(s) are of moderate severity. Typically, 30 minutes are spent face-to-face with the patient and/or family.

      📁 2.17    ⚗ 3.05    **FUD** XXX          ★ B 80 🖥

      **AMA:** 2017,Aug,3; 2017,Jun,6; 2017,Jan,8; 2016,Dec,11; 2016,Sep,6; 2016,Mar,10; 2016,Jan,7; 2016,Jan,13; 2015,Dec,3; 2015,Oct,3; 2015,Jan,16; 2015,Jan,12; 2014,Nov,14; 2014,Oct,3; 2014,Oct,8; 2014,Aug,3; 2014,Jan,11; 2013,Aug,13; 2013,Jun,3-5; 2013,Jan,9-10; 2012,Aug,3-5; 2012,Apr,10; 2012,Jan,15-42; 2012,Jan,3-5

**99204**     Office or other outpatient visit for the evaluation and management of a new patient, which requires these 3 key components: A comprehensive history; A comprehensive examination; Medical decision making of moderate complexity. Counseling and/or coordination of care with other physicians, other qualified health care professionals, or agencies are provided consistent with the nature of the problem(s) and the patient's and/or family's needs. Usually, the presenting problem(s) are of moderate to high severity. Typically, 45 minutes are spent face-to-face with the patient and/or family.

      📁 3.67    ⚗ 4.63    **FUD** XXX          ★ B 80 🖥

      **AMA:** 2017,Aug,3; 2017,Jun,6; 2017,Jan,8; 2016,Dec,11; 2016,Sep,6; 2016,Mar,10; 2016,Jan,13; 2016,Jan,7; 2015,Dec,3; 2015,Oct,3; 2015,Jan,12; 2015,Jan,16; 2014,Nov,14; 2014,Oct,8; 2014,Oct,3; 2014,Aug,3; 2014,Jan,11; 2013,Aug,13; 2013,Jun,3-5; 2013,Jan,9-10; 2012,Aug,3-5; 2012,Apr,10; 2012,Jan,3-5; 2012,Jan,15-42

**99205**     Office or other outpatient visit for the evaluation and management of a new patient, which requires these 3 key components: A comprehensive history; A comprehensive examination; Medical decision making of high complexity. Counseling and/or coordination of care with other physicians, other qualified health care professionals, or agencies are provided consistent with the nature of the problem(s) and the patient's and/or family's needs. Usually, the presenting problem(s) are of moderate to high severity. Typically, 60 minutes are spent face-to-face with the patient and/or family.

      📁 4.78    ⚗ 5.83    **FUD** XXX          ★ B 80 🖥

      **AMA:** 2017,Aug,3; 2017,Jun,6; 2017,Jan,8; 2016,Dec,11; 2016,Sep,6; 2016,Mar,10; 2016,Jan,13; 2016,Jan,7; 2015,Dec,3; 2015,Oct,3; 2015,Jan,12; 2015,Jan,16; 2014,Nov,14; 2014,Oct,8; 2014,Oct,3; 2014,Aug,3; 2014,Jan,11; 2013,Aug,13; 2013,Jun,3-5; 2013,Jan,9-10; 2012,Aug,3-5; 2012,Apr,10; 2012,Jan,3-5; 2012,Jan,15-42

**99211**     Office or other outpatient visit for the evaluation and management of an established patient, that may not require the presence of a physician or other qualified health care professional. Usually, the presenting problem(s) are minimal. Typically, 5 minutes are spent performing or supervising these services.

      📁 0.26    ⚗ 0.57    **FUD** XXX          B 80 🖥

      **AMA:** 2017,Aug,3; 2017,Jun,6; 2017,Mar,10; 2017,Jan,8; 2016,Dec,11; 2016,Sep,6; 2016,Mar,10; 2016,Jan,13; 2016,Jan,7; 2015,Dec,3; 2015,Oct,3; 2015,Jan,12; 2015,Jan,16; 2014,Nov,14; 2014,Oct,8; 2014,Oct,3; 2014,Aug,3; 2014,Mar,13; 2014,Jan,11; 2013,Nov,3; 2013,Aug,13; 2013,Jun,3-5; 2013,Mar,13; 2013,Jan,9-10; 2012,Aug,3-5; 2012,Apr,10; 2012,Jan,3-5; 2012,Jan,15-42

**26/TC** PC/TC Only    **A2-Z3** ASC Payment    **50** Bilateral    ♂ Male Only    ♀ Female Only    📁 Facility RVU    ⚗ Non-Facility RVU    🖥 CCI

**FUD** Follow-up Days    **CMS:** IOM (Pub 100)    **A-Y** OPPSI    **80/80** Surg Assist Allowed / w/Doc    🔲 Lab Crosswalk    🔲 Radiology Crosswalk    ✖ CLIA

502                                         CPT © 2017 American Medical Association. All Rights Reserved.                © 2017 Optum360, LLC

**99212** Office or other outpatient visit for the evaluation and management of an established patient, which requires at least 2 of these 3 key components: A problem focused history; A problem focused examination; Straightforward medical decision making. Counseling and/or coordination of care with other physicians, other qualified health care professionals, or agencies are provided consistent with the nature of the problem(s) and the patient's and/or family's needs. Usually, the presenting problem(s) are self limited or minor. Typically, 10 minutes are spent face-to-face with the patient and/or family.

    🚑 0.72   ⚕ 1.23  **FUD** XXX   ★ B 80 🖵

    **AMA:** 2017,Aug,3; 2017,Jun,6; 2017,Jan,8; 2016,Dec,11; 2016,Sep,6; 2016,Mar,10; 2016,Jan,13; 2016,Jan,7; 2015,Dec,3; 2015,Oct,3; 2015,Jan,12; 2015,Jan,16; 2014,Nov,14; 2014,Oct,3; 2014,Oct,8; 2014,Aug,3; 2014,Jan,11; 2013,Nov,3; 2013,Aug,13; 2013,Jun,3-5; 2013,Mar,13; 2013,Jan,9-10; 2012,Aug,3-5; 2012,Mar,4-7; 2012,Apr,10; 2012,Jan,15-42; 2012,Jan,3-5

**99213** Office or other outpatient visit for the evaluation and management of an established patient, which requires at least 2 of these 3 key components: An expanded problem focused history; An expanded problem focused examination; Medical decision making of low complexity. Counseling and coordination of care with other physicians, other qualified health care professionals, or agencies are provided consistent with the nature of the problem(s) and the patient's and/or family's needs. Usually, the presenting problem(s) are of low to moderate severity. Typically, 15 minutes are spent face-to-face with the patient and/or family.

    🚑 1.44   ⚕ 2.06  **FUD** XXX   ★ B 80 🖵

    **AMA:** 2017,Aug,3; 2017,Jun,6; 2017,Jan,8; 2016,Dec,11; 2016,Sep,6; 2016,Mar,10; 2016,Jan,13; 2016,Jan,7; 2015,Dec,3; 2015,Oct,3; 2015,Jan,12; 2015,Jan,16; 2014,Nov,14; 2014,Oct,8; 2014,Oct,3; 2014,Aug,3; 2014,Jan,11; 2013,Nov,3; 2013,Aug,13; 2013,Jun,3-5; 2013,Mar,13; 2013,Jan,9-10; 2012,Aug,3-5; 2012,Apr,10; 2012,Mar,4-7; 2012,Jan,15-42; 2012,Jan,3-5

**99214** Office or other outpatient visit for the evaluation and management of an established patient, which requires at least 2 of these 3 key components: A detailed history; A detailed examination; Medical decision making of moderate complexity. Counseling and/or coordination of care with other physicians, other qualified health care professionals, or agencies are provided consistent with the nature of the problem(s) and the patient's and/or family's needs. Usually, the presenting problem(s) are of moderate to high severity. Typically, 25 minutes are spent face-to-face with the patient and/or family.

    🚑 2.22   ⚕ 3.03  **FUD** XXX   ★ B 80 🖵

    **AMA:** 2017,Aug,3; 2017,Jun,6; 2017,Jan,8; 2016,Dec,11; 2016,Sep,6; 2016,Mar,10; 2016,Jan,13; 2016,Jan,7; 2015,Dec,3; 2015,Oct,3; 2015,Jan,12; 2015,Jan,16; 2014,Nov,14; 2014,Oct,3; 2014,Oct,8; 2014,Aug,3; 2014,Jan,11; 2013,Nov,3; 2013,Aug,13; 2013,Jun,3-5; 2013,Mar,13; 2013,Jan,9-10; 2012,Aug,3-5; 2012,Apr,10; 2012,Mar,4-7; 2012,Jan,15-42; 2012,Jan,3-5

**99215** Office or other outpatient visit for the evaluation and management of an established patient, which requires at least 2 of these 3 key components: A comprehensive history; A comprehensive examination; Medical decision making of high complexity. Counseling and/or coordination of care with other physicians, other qualified health care professionals, or agencies are provided consistent with the nature of the problem(s) and the patient's and/or family's needs. Usually, the presenting problem(s) are of moderate to high severity. Typically, 40 minutes are spent face-to-face with the patient and/or family.

    🚑 3.14   ⚕ 4.08  **FUD** XXX   ★ B 80 🖵

    **AMA:** 2017,Aug,3; 2017,Jun,6; 2017,Jan,8; 2016,Dec,11; 2016,Sep,6; 2016,Mar,10; 2016,Jan,7; 2016,Jan,13; 2015,Dec,3; 2015,Oct,3; 2015,Jan,16; 2015,Jan,12; 2014,Nov,14; 2014,Oct,3; 2014,Oct,8; 2014,Aug,3; 2014,Jan,11; 2013,Nov,3; 2013,Aug,13; 2013,Jun,3-5; 2013,Mar,13; 2013,Jan,9-10; 2012,Aug,3-5; 2012,Apr,10; 2012,Jan,15-42; 2012,Jan,3-5

## 99217-99220 Facility Observation Visits: Initial and Discharge

**CMS:** 100-04,11,40.1.3 Independent Attending Physician Services; 100-04,12,100.1.1 Teaching Physicians E/M Services; 100-04,12,30.6.4 Services Furnished Incident to Physician's Service; 100-04,12,30.6.8 Payment for Hospital Observation Services; 100-04,12,40.3 Global Surgery Review; 100-04,32,130.1 Billing and Payment of External counterpulsation (ECP)

    **INCLUDES** Services provided on the same date in other settings or departments associated with the observation status admission (99201-99215, 99281-99285, 99304-99318, 99324-99337, 99341-99350, 99381-99429)

    Services provided to new and established patients admitted to a hospital specifically for observation (not required to be a designated area of the hospital)

    **EXCLUDES** *Services provided by physicians or another qualified health care professional other than the admitting physician ([99224, 99225, 99226], 99241-99245)*

    *Services provided to a patient admitted and discharged from observation status on the same date (99234-99236)*

    *Services provided to a patient admitted to the hospital following observation status (99221-99223)*

    *Services provided to a patient discharged from inpatient care (99238-99239)*

▲ **99217** Observation care discharge day management (This code is to be utilized to report all services provided to a patient on discharge from outpatient hospital "observation status" if the discharge is on other than the initial date of "observation status." To report services to a patient designated as "observation status" or "inpatient status" and discharged on the same date, use the codes for Observation or Inpatient Care Services [including Admission and Discharge Services, 99234-99236 as appropriate.])

    **INCLUDES** Discussing the observation admission with the patient

    Final patient evaluation:

      Discharge instructions

      Sign off on discharge medical records

    🚑 2.06   ⚕ 2.06  **FUD** XXX   B 80 🖵

    **AMA:** 2017,Aug,3; 2017,Jun,6; 2017,Jan,8; 2016,Dec,11; 2016,Jan,13; 2016,Jan,7; 2015,Dec,3; 2015,Jan,16; 2014,Nov,14; 2014,Oct,8; 2014,Jan,11; 2013,Jun,3-5; 2013,Jan,9-10; 2012,Jul,10-11

● New Code  ▲ Revised Code  ○ Reinstated  ● New Web Release  ▲ Revised Web Release  Unlisted  Not Covered  # Resequenced

⊘ AMA Mod 51 Exempt  ⑤ Optum Mod 51 Exempt  ㊿ Mod 63 Exempt  ⚡ Non-FDA Drug  ★ Telemedicine  Ⓜ Maternity  🄰 Age Edit  + Add-on  **AMA:** CPT Asst

**Evaluation and Management**

**99218 — 99226**

▲ 99218 Initial observation care, per day, for the evaluation and management of a patient which requires these 3 key components: A detailed or comprehensive history; A detailed or comprehensive examination; and Medical decision making that is straightforward or of low complexity. Counseling and/or coordination of care with other physicians, other qualified health care professionals, or agencies are provided consistent with the nature of the problem(s) and the patient's and/or family's needs. Usually, the problem(s) requiring admission to outpatient hospital "observation status" are of low severity. Typically, 30 minutes are spent at the bedside and on the patient's hospital floor or unit.

🚑 2.82   ⚕ 2.82   **FUD** XXX                    B 80 🖵

**AMA:** 2017,Aug,3; 2017,Jun,6; 2017,Jan,8; 2016,Dec,11; 2016,Jan,13; 2016,Jan,7; 2015,Dec,3; 2015,Jul,3; 2015,Mar,3; 2015,Jan,16; 2014,Nov,14; 2014,Oct,8; 2014,Jan,11; 2013,Aug,13; 2013,Jun,3-5; 2013,Jan,9-10; 2012,Aug,3-5; 2012,Jul,10-11; 2012,Jan,15-42

▲ 99219 Initial observation care, per day, for the evaluation and management of a patient, which requires these 3 key components: A comprehensive history; A comprehensive examination; and Medical decision making of moderate complexity. Counseling and/or coordination of care with other physicians, other qualified health care professionals, or agencies are provided consistent with the nature of the problem(s) and the patient's and/or family's needs. Usually, the problem(s) requiring admission to outpatient hospital "observation status" are of moderate severity. Typically, 50 minutes are spent at the bedside and on the patient's hospital floor or unit.

🚑 3.84   ⚕ 3.84   **FUD** XXX                    B 80 🖵

**AMA:** 2017,Aug,3; 2017,Jun,6; 2017,Jan,8; 2016,Dec,11; 2016,Jan,13; 2016,Jan,7; 2015,Dec,3; 2015,Jul,3; 2015,Jan,16; 2014,Nov,14; 2014,Oct,8; 2014,Jan,11; 2013,Aug,13; 2013,Jun,3-5; 2013,Jan,9-10; 2012,Aug,3-5; 2012,Jul,10-11; 2012,Jan,15-42

▲ 99220 Initial observation care, per day, for the evaluation and management of a patient, which requires these 3 key components: A comprehensive history; A comprehensive examination; and Medical decision making of high complexity. Counseling and/or coordination of care with other physicians, other qualified health care professionals, or agencies are provided consistent with the nature of the problem(s) and the patient's and/or family's needs. Usually, the problem(s) requiring admission to outpatient hospital "observation status" are of high severity. Typically, 70 minutes are spent at the bedside and on the patient's hospital floor or unit.

🚑 5.25   ⚕ 5.25   **FUD** XXX                    B 80 🖵

**AMA:** 2017,Aug,3; 2017,Jun,6; 2017,Jan,8; 2016,Dec,11; 2016,Jan,13; 2016,Jan,7; 2015,Dec,3; 2015,Jul,3; 2015,Jan,16; 2014,Nov,14; 2014,Oct,8; 2014,Jan,11; 2013,Aug,13; 2013,Jun,3-5; 2013,Jan,9-10; 2012,Aug,3-5; 2012,Jul,10-11; 2012,Jan,15-42

## [99224, 99225, 99226] Facility Observation Visits: Subsequent

**CMS:** 100-04,11,40.1.3 Independent Attending Physician Services; 100-04,12,100.1.1 Teaching Physicians E/M Services; 100-04,12,30.6.4 Services Furnished Incident to Physician's Service; 100-04,12,30.6.8 Payment for Hospital Observation Services; 100-04,12,30.6.9.1 Initial Hospital Care and Observation or Inpatient Care Services

INCLUDES   Changes in patient's status (e.g., physical condition, history; response to medical management)
Medical record review
Review of diagnostic test results
Services provided on the same date in other settings or departments associated with the observation status admission (99201-99215, 99281-99285, 99304-99318, 99324-99337, 99341-99350, 99381-99429)

EXCLUDES   *Observation admission and discharge on the same day (99234-99236)*

\# 99224 Subsequent observation care, per day, for the evaluation and management of a patient, which requires at least 2 of these 3 key components: Problem focused interval history; Problem focused examination; Medical decision making that is straightforward or of low complexity. Counseling and/or coordination of care with other physicians, other qualified health care professionals, or agencies are provided consistent with the nature of the problem(s) and the patient's and/or family's needs. Usually, the patient is stable, recovering, or improving. Typically, 15 minutes are spent at the bedside and on the patient's hospital floor or unit.

🚑 1.13   ⚕ 1.13   **FUD** XXX                    B 80 🖵

**AMA:** 2017,Aug,3; 2017,Jun,6; 2017,Jan,8; 2016,Dec,11; 2016,Jan,13; 2016,Jan,7; 2015,Dec,3; 2015,Jan,16; 2014,Nov,14; 2014,Oct,8; 2014,Jan,11; 2013,Aug,13; 2013,Jun,3-5; 2013,Jan,9-10; 2012,Aug,3-5; 2012,Jul,10-11

\# 99225 Subsequent observation care, per day, for the evaluation and management of a patient, which requires at least 2 of these 3 key components: An expanded problem focused interval history; An expanded problem focused examination; Medical decision making of moderate complexity. Counseling and/or coordination of care with other physicians, other qualified health care professionals, or agencies are provided consistent with the nature of the problem(s) and the patient's and/or family's needs. Usually, the patient is responding inadequately to therapy or has developed a minor complication. Typically, 25 minutes are spent at the bedside and on the patient's hospital floor or unit.

🚑 2.06   ⚕ 2.06   **FUD** XXX                    B 80 🖵

**AMA:** 2017,Aug,3; 2017,Jun,6; 2017,Jan,8; 2016,Dec,11; 2016,Jan,13; 2016,Jan,7; 2015,Dec,3; 2015,Jan,16; 2014,Nov,14; 2014,Oct,8; 2014,Jan,11; 2013,Aug,13; 2013,Jun,3-5; 2013,Jan,9-10; 2012,Aug,3-5; 2012,Jul,10-11

\# 99226 Subsequent observation care, per day, for the evaluation and management of a patient, which requires at least 2 of these 3 key components: A detailed interval history; A detailed examination; Medical decision making of high complexity. Counseling and/or coordination of care with other physicians, other qualified health care professionals, or agencies are provided consistent with the nature of the problem(s) and the patient's and/or family's needs. Usually, the patient is unstable or has developed a significant complication or a significant new problem. Typically, 35 minutes are spent at the bedside and on the patient's hospital floor or unit.

🚑 2.97   ⚕ 2.97   **FUD** XXX                    B 80 🖵

**AMA:** 2017,Aug,3; 2017,Jun,6; 2017,Jan,8; 2016,Dec,11; 2016,Jan,13; 2016,Jan,7; 2015,Dec,3; 2015,Jan,16; 2014,Nov,14; 2014,Oct,8; 2014,Jan,11; 2013,Aug,13; 2013,Jun,3-5; 2013,Jan,9-10; 2012,Aug,3-5; 2012,Jul,10-11

## 99221-99233 Inpatient Hospital Visits: Initial and Subsequent

**CMS:** 100-04,11,40.1.3 Independent Attending Physician Services; 100-04,12,100.1.1 Teaching Physicians E/M Services; 100-04,12,30.6.10 Consultation Services; 100-04,12,30.6.15.1 Prolonged Services With Direct Face-to-Face Patient Contact Service (Codes 99354 - 99357); 100-04,12,30.6.4 Services Furnished Incident to Physician's Service; 100-04,12,30.6.9 Payment for Inpatient Hospital Visits - General

INCLUDES Initial physician services provided to the patient in the hospital or "partial" hospital settings (99221-99223)

   Services provided on the date of admission in other settings or departments associated with an observation status admission (99201-99215, 99281-99285, 99304-99318, 99324-99337, 99341-99350, 99381-99397)

   Services provided to a new or established patient

EXCLUDES *Inpatient admission and discharge on the same date (99234-99236)*

   *Inpatient E&M services provided by other than the admitting physician*

**99221** Initial hospital care, per day, for the evaluation and management of a patient, which requires these 3 key components: A detailed or comprehensive history; A detailed or comprehensive examination; and Medical decision making that is straightforward or of low complexity. Counseling and/or coordination of care with other physicians, other qualified health care professionals, or agencies are provided consistent with the nature of the problem(s) and the patient's and/or family's needs. Usually, the problem(s) requiring admission are of low severity. Typically, 30 minutes are spent at the bedside and on the patient's hospital floor or unit.

  🚑 2.87 ⚕ 2.87 **FUD** XXX B 80 🖵

  **AMA:** 2017,Aug,3; 2017,Jun,6; 2017,Jan,8; 2016,Dec,11; 2016,Mar,10; 2016,Jan,13; 2016,Jan,7; 2015,Dec,18; 2015,Dec,3; 2015,Jul,3; 2015,Jan,16; 2014,Nov,14; 2014,Oct,8; 2014,Jan,11; 2013,Aug,13; 2013,Jun,3-5; 2013,Jan,9-10; 2012,Aug,3-5; 2012,Jul,10-11; 2012,Jul,12-14; 2012,Jan,15-42

**99222** Initial hospital care, per day, for the evaluation and management of a patient, which requires these 3 key components: A comprehensive history; A comprehensive examination; and Medical decision making of moderate complexity. Counseling and/or coordination of care with other physicians, other qualified health care professionals, or agencies are provided consistent with the nature of the problem(s) and the patient's and/or family's needs. Usually, the problem(s) requiring admission are of moderate severity. Typically, 50 minutes are spent at the bedside and on the patient's hospital floor or unit.

  🚑 3.87 ⚕ 3.87 **FUD** XXX B 80 🖵

  **AMA:** 2017,Aug,3; 2017,Jun,6; 2017,Jan,8; 2016,Dec,11; 2016,Mar,10; 2016,Jan,13; 2016,Jan,7; 2015,Dec,18; 2015,Dec,3; 2015,Jul,3; 2015,Mar,3; 2015,Jan,16; 2014,Nov,14; 2014,Oct,8; 2014,Jan,11; 2013,Aug,13; 2013,Jun,3-5; 2013,Jan,9-10; 2012,Aug,3-5; 2012,Jul,12-14; 2012,Jul,10-11; 2012,Jan,15-42

**99223** Initial hospital care, per day, for the evaluation and management of a patient, which requires these 3 key components: A comprehensive history; A comprehensive examination; and Medical decision making of high complexity. Counseling and/or coordination of care with other physicians, other qualified health care professionals, or agencies are provided consistent with the nature of the problem(s) and the patient's and/or family's needs. Usually, the problem(s) requiring admission are of high severity. Typically, 70 minutes are spent at the bedside and on the patient's hospital floor or unit.

  🚑 5.73 ⚕ 5.73 **FUD** XXX B 80 🖵

  **AMA:** 2017,Aug,3; 2017,Jun,6; 2017,Jan,8; 2016,Dec,11; 2016,Mar,10; 2016,Jan,13; 2016,Jan,7; 2015,Dec,18; 2015,Dec,3; 2015,Jul,3; 2015,Jan,16; 2014,Nov,14; 2014,Oct,8; 2014,Jan,11; 2013,Aug,13; 2013,Jun,3-5; 2013,Jan,9-10; 2012,Aug,3-5; 2012,Jul,12-14; 2012,Jul,10-11; 2012,Jan,15-42

*99224* **Resequenced code. See code following 99220.**

*99225* **Resequenced code. See code following 99220.**

*99226* **Resequenced code. See code before 99221.**

**99231** Subsequent hospital care, per day, for the evaluation and management of a patient, which requires at least 2 of these 3 key components: A problem focused interval history; A problem focused examination; Medical decision making that is straightforward or of low complexity. Counseling and/or coordination of care with other physicians, other qualified health care professionals, or agencies are provided consistent with the nature of the problem(s) and the patient's and/or family's needs. Usually, the patient is stable, recovering or improving. Typically, 15 minutes are spent at the bedside and on the patient's hospital floor or unit.

  🚑 1.11 ⚕ 1.11 **FUD** XXX ★ B 80 🖵

  **AMA:** 2017,Aug,3; 2017,Jun,6; 2017,Jan,8; 2016,Dec,11; 2016,Jan,13; 2016,Jan,7; 2015,Dec,3; 2015,Jul,3; 2015,Jan,16; 2014,Nov,14; 2014,Oct,8; 2014,May,4; 2014,Jan,11; 2013,Sep,17; 2013,Aug,13; 2013,Jun,3-5; 2013,Jan,9-10; 2012,Aug,3-5; 2012,Jul,12-14; 2012,Jan,15-42

**99232** Subsequent hospital care, per day, for the evaluation and management of a patient, which requires at least 2 of these 3 key components: An expanded problem focused interval history; An expanded problem focused examination; Medical decision making of moderate complexity. Counseling and/or coordination of care with other physicians, other qualified health care professionals, or agencies are provided consistent with the nature of the problem(s) and the patient's and/or family's needs. Usually, the patient is responding inadequately to therapy or has developed a minor complication. Typically, 25 minutes are spent at the bedside and on the patient's hospital floor or unit.

  🚑 2.04 ⚕ 2.04 **FUD** XXX ★ B 80 🖵

  **AMA:** 2017,Aug,3; 2017,Jun,6; 2017,Jan,8; 2016,Dec,11; 2016,Oct,8; 2016,Jan,13; 2016,Jan,7; 2015,Dec,3; 2015,Jul,3; 2015,Jan,16; 2014,Nov,14; 2014,Oct,8; 2014,Jan,11; 2013,Aug,13; 2013,Jun,3-5; 2013,Jan,9-10; 2012,Aug,3-5; 2012,Jul,12-14; 2012,Jan,15-42

**99233** Subsequent hospital care, per day, for the evaluation and management of a patient, which requires at least 2 of these 3 key components: A detailed interval history; A detailed examination; Medical decision making of high complexity. Counseling and/or coordination of care with other physicians, other qualified health care professionals, or agencies are provided consistent with the nature of the problem(s) and the patient's and/or family's needs. Usually, the patient is unstable or has developed a significant complication or a significant new problem. Typically, 35 minutes are spent at the bedside and on the patient's hospital floor or unit.

  🚑 2.95 ⚕ 2.95 **FUD** XXX ★ B 80 🖵

  **AMA:** 2017,Aug,3; 2017,Jun,6; 2017,Jan,8; 2016,Dec,11; 2016,Oct,8; 2016,Jan,13; 2016,Jan,7; 2015,Dec,3; 2015,Jul,3; 2015,Jan,16; 2014,Nov,14; 2014,Oct,8; 2014,May,4; 2014,Jan,11; 2013,Aug,13; 2013,Jun,3-5; 2013,Jan,9-10; 2012,Aug,3-5; 2012,Jul,12-14; 2012,Jan,15-42

● New Code ▲ Revised Code ○ Reinstated ● New Web Release ▲ Revised Web Release Unlisted Not Covered # Resequenced
⊘ AMA Mod 51 Exempt ⑨ Optum Mod 51 Exempt ⑥ Mod 63 Exempt ✗ Non-FDA Drug ★ Telemedicine Ⓜ Maternity Ⓐ Age Edit + Add-on **AMA:** CPT Asst
© 2017 Optum360, LLC CPT © 2017 American Medical Association. All Rights Reserved.

Evaluation and Management

99234 — 99239

## 99234-99236 Observation/Inpatient Visits: Admitted/Discharged on Same Date

**CMS:** 100-04,11,40.1.3 Independent Attending Physician Services; 100-04,12,100.1.1 Teaching Physicians E/M Services; 100-04,12,30.6.4 Services Furnished Incident to Physician's Service; 100-04,12,30.6.8 Payment for Hospital Observation Services; 100-04,12,30.6.9 Swing Bed Visits; 100-04,12,30.6.9.1 Initial Hospital Care and Observation or Inpatient Care Services; 100-04,12,30.6.9.2 Hospital Discharge Management; 100-04,12,40.3 Global Surgery Review

**INCLUDES** Admission and discharge services on the same date in an observation or inpatient setting
All services provided by admitting physician or other qualified health care professional on same date of service, even when initiated in another setting (e.g., emergency department, nursing facility, office)

**EXCLUDES** *Services provided to patients admitted to observation and discharged on a different date (99217-99220, [99224, 99225, 99226])*

**99234** Observation or inpatient hospital care, for the evaluation and management of a patient including admission and discharge on the same date, which requires these 3 key components: A detailed or comprehensive history; A detailed or comprehensive examination; and Medical decision making that is straightforward or of low complexity. Counseling and/or coordination of care with other physicians, other qualified health care professionals, or agencies are provided consistent with the nature of the problem(s) and the patient's and/or family's needs. Usually the presenting problem(s) requiring admission are of low severity. Typically, 40 minutes are spent at the bedside and on the patient's hospital floor or unit.

    🖫 3.77    ⚕ 3.77    **FUD** XXX    B 80 ▭

    **AMA:** 2017,Aug,3; 2017,Jun,6; 2017,Jan,8; 2016,Dec,11; 2016,Jan,13; 2015,Jul,3; 2015,Jan,16; 2014,Oct,8; 2014,Jan,11; 2013,Jun,3-5; 2012,Jul,10-11; 2012,Jan,15-42

**99235** Observation or inpatient hospital care, for the evaluation and management of a patient including admission and discharge on the same date, which requires these 3 key components: A comprehensive history; A comprehensive examination; and Medical decision making of moderate complexity. Counseling and/or coordination of care with other physicians, other qualified health care professionals, or agencies are provided consistent with the nature of the problem(s) and the patient's and/or family's needs. Usually the presenting problem(s) requiring admission are of moderate severity. Typically, 50 minutes are spent at the bedside and on the patient's hospital floor or unit.

    🖫 4.78    ⚕ 4.78    **FUD** XXX    B 80 ▭

    **AMA:** 2017,Aug,3; 2017,Jun,6; 2017,Jan,8; 2016,Dec,11; 2016,Jan,13; 2015,Jul,3; 2015,Jan,16; 2014,Oct,8; 2014,Jan,11; 2013,Jun,3-5; 2012,Jul,10-11; 2012,Jan,15-42

**99236** Observation or inpatient hospital care, for the evaluation and management of a patient including admission and discharge on the same date, which requires these 3 key components: A comprehensive history; A comprehensive examination; and Medical decision making of high complexity. Counseling and/or coordination of care with other physicians, other qualified health care professionals, or agencies are provided consistent with the nature of the problem(s) and the patient's and/or family's needs. Usually the presenting problem(s) requiring admission are of high severity. Typically, 55 minutes are spent at the bedside and on the patient's hospital floor or unit.

    🖫 6.16    ⚕ 6.16    **FUD** XXX    B 80 ▭

    **AMA:** 2017,Aug,3; 2017,Jun,6; 2017,Jan,8; 2016,Dec,11; 2016,Jan,13; 2015,Jul,3; 2015,Jan,16; 2014,Oct,8; 2014,Jan,11; 2013,Jun,3-5; 2012,Jul,10-11; 2012,Jan,15-42

## 99238-99239 Inpatient Hospital Discharge Services

**CMS:** 100-04,11,40.1.3 Independent Attending Physician Services; 100-04,12,100.1.1 Teaching Physicians E/M Services; 100-04,12,30.6.4 Services Furnished Incident to Physician's Service; 100-04,12,30.6.9 Payment for Inpatient Hospital Visits - General; 100-04,12,30.6.9.1 Initial Hospital Care and Observation or Inpatient Care Services; 100-04,12,30.6.9.2 Subsequent Hospital Visit and Discharge Management; 100-04,12,40.3 Global Surgery Review

**INCLUDES** All services on discharge day when discharge and admission are not the same day
Discharge instructions
Final patient evaluation
Final preparation of the patient's medical records
Provision of prescriptions/referrals, as needed
Review of the inpatient admission

**EXCLUDES** *Admission/discharge on same date (99234-99236)*
*Discharge from observation (99217)*
*Discharge from nursing facility (99315-99316)*
*Healthy newborn evaluated and discharged on same date (99463)*
*Services provided by other than attending physician or other qualified health care professional on date of discharge (99231-99233)*

**99238** Hospital discharge day management; 30 minutes or less

    🖫 2.05    ⚕ 2.05    **FUD** XXX    B 80 ▭

    **AMA:** 2017,Aug,3; 2017,Jun,6; 2017,Jan,8; 2016,Dec,11; 2016,Jan,13; 2015,Jan,16; 2014,Oct,8; 2014,Jan,11; 2013,Aug,13; 2013,Jun,3-5; 2012,Jul,10-11; 2012,Jul,12-14; 2012,Jan,15-42

**99239** more than 30 minutes

    🖫 3.04    ⚕ 3.04    **FUD** XXX    B 80 ▭

    **AMA:** 2017,Aug,3; 2017,Jun,6; 2017,Jan,8; 2016,Dec,11; 2016,Jan,13; 2015,Jan,16; 2014,Oct,8; 2014,Jan,11; 2013,Aug,13; 2013,Jun,3-5; 2012,Jul,12-14; 2012,Jan,15-42

## 99241-99245 Consultations: Office and Outpatient

**CMS:** 100-04,11,40.1.3 Independent Attending Physician Services; 100-04,12,190.6 Payment Methodology for Physician/Practitioner at the Distant Site ; 100-04,12,190.6.1 Submission of Telehealth Claims for Distant Site Practitioners; 100-04,12,190.7 Contractor Editing of Telehealth Claims; 100-04,12,30.6.10 Consultation Services; 100-04,12,30.6.15.1 Prolonged Services With Direct Face-to-Face Patient Contact Service (Codes 99354 - 99357); 100-04,12,30.6.4 Services Furnished Incident to Physician's Service; 100-04,12,30.6.9.1 Initial Hospital Care and Observation or Inpatient Care Services; 100-04,12,40.3 Global Surgery Review; 100-04,32,130.1 Billing and Payment of External counterpulsation (ECP); 100-04,4,160 Clinic and Emergency Visits Under OPPS

**INCLUDES**  A third-party mandated consultation
All outpatient consultations provided in the office, outpatient or other ambulatory facility, domiciliary/rest home, emergency department, patient's home, and hospital observation
Documentation of a request for a consultation from an appropriate source
Documentation of the need for consultation in the patient's medical record
One consultation per consultant
Provision by a physician or qualified nonphysician practitioner whose advice, opinion, recommendation, suggestion, direction, or counsel, etc., is requested for evaluating/treating a patient since that individual's expertise in a specific medical area is beyond the scope of knowledge of the requesting physician
Provision of a written report of findings/recommendations from the consultant to the referring physician

**EXCLUDES**  *Another appropriately requested and documented consultation pertaining to the same/new problem; repeat use of consultation codes*
*Any distinctly recognizable procedure/service provided on or following the consultation*
*Assumption of care (all or partial); report subsequent codes as appropriate for the place of service (99211-99215, 99334-99337, 99347-99350)*
*Consultation prompted by the patient/family; report codes for office, domiciliary/rest home, or home visits instead (99201-99215, 99324-99337, 99341-99350)*
*Services provided to Medicare patients; E&M code as appropriate for the place of service or HCPCS code (99201-99215, 99221-99223, 99231-99233, G0406-G0408, G0425-G0427)*

**99241** Office consultation for a new or established patient, which requires these 3 key components: A problem focused history; A problem focused examination; and Straightforward medical decision making. Counseling and/or coordination of care with other physicians, other qualified health care professionals, or agencies are provided consistent with the nature of the problem(s) and the patient's and/or family's needs. Usually, the presenting problem(s) are self limited or minor. Typically, 15 minutes are spent face-to-face with the patient and/or family.

 0.92  1.34  **FUD** XXX  ★E

**AMA:** 2017,Aug,3; 2017,Jun,6; 2017,Jan,8; 2016,Dec,11; 2016,Sep,6; 2016,Jan,13; 2016,Jan,7; 2015,Jan,12; 2015,Jan,16; 2014,Nov,14; 2014,Oct,8; 2014,Sep,13; 2014,Aug,3; 2014,Jan,11; 2013,Jun,3-5; 2013,Jan,9-10; 2012,Aug,3-5; 2012,Apr,10; 2012,Jan,15-42

**99242** Office consultation for a new or established patient, which requires these 3 key components: An expanded problem focused history; An expanded problem focused examination; and Straightforward medical decision making. Counseling and/or coordination of care with other physicians, other qualified health care professionals, or agencies are provided consistent with the nature of the problem(s) and the patient's and/or family's needs. Usually, the presenting problem(s) are of low severity. Typically, 30 minutes are spent face-to-face with the patient and/or family.

 1.93  2.52  **FUD** XXX  ★E

**AMA:** 2017,Aug,3; 2017,Jun,8; 2017,Jun,6; 2017,Jan,8; 2016,Dec,11; 2016,Sep,6; 2016,Jan,13; 2016,Jan,7; 2015,Jan,16; 2015,Jan,12; 2014,Nov,14; 2014,Oct,8; 2014,Sep,13; 2014,Aug,3; 2014,Jan,11; 2013,Jun,3-5; 2013,Jan,9-10; 2012,Aug,3-5; 2012,Apr,10; 2012,Jan,15-42

**99243** Office consultation for a new or established patient, which requires these 3 key components: A detailed history; A detailed examination; and Medical decision making of low complexity. Counseling and/or coordination of care with other physicians, other qualified health care professionals, or agencies are provided consistent with the nature of the problem(s) and the patient's and/or family's needs. Usually, the presenting problem(s) are of moderate severity. Typically, 40 minutes are spent face-to-face with the patient and/or family.

 2.70  3.45  **FUD** XXX  ★E

**AMA:** 2017,Aug,3; 2017,Jun,6; 2017,Jan,8; 2016,Dec,11; 2016,Sep,6; 2016,Jan,7; 2016,Jan,13; 2015,Jan,16; 2015,Jan,12; 2014,Nov,14; 2014,Oct,8; 2014,Sep,13; 2014,Aug,3; 2014,Jan,11; 2013,Jun,3-5; 2013,Jan,9-10; 2012,Aug,3-5; 2012,Apr,10; 2012,Jan,15-42

**99244** Office consultation for a new or established patient, which requires these 3 key components: A comprehensive history; A comprehensive examination; and Medical decision making of moderate complexity. Counseling and/or coordination of care with other physicians, other qualified health care professionals, or agencies are provided consistent with the nature of the problem(s) and the patient's and/or family's needs. Usually, the presenting problem(s) are of moderate to high severity. Typically, 60 minutes are spent face-to-face with the patient and/or family.

 4.34  5.16  **FUD** XXX  ★E

**AMA:** 2017,Aug,3; 2017,Jun,6; 2017,Jan,8; 2016,Dec,11; 2016,Sep,6; 2016,Jan,13; 2016,Jan,7; 2015,Jan,12; 2015,Jan,16; 2014,Nov,14; 2014,Oct,8; 2014,Sep,13; 2014,Aug,3; 2014,Jan,11; 2013,Aug,12; 2013,Jun,3-5; 2013,Jan,9-10; 2012,Aug,3-5; 2012,Apr,10; 2012,Jan,15-42

**99245** Office consultation for a new or established patient, which requires these 3 key components: A comprehensive history; A comprehensive examination; and Medical decision making of high complexity. Counseling and/or coordination of care with other physicians, other qualified health care professionals, or agencies are provided consistent with the nature of the problem(s) and the patient's and/or family's needs. Usually, the presenting problem(s) are of moderate to high severity. Typically, 80 minutes are spent face-to-face with the patient and/or family.

 5.37  6.29  **FUD** XXX  ★E

**AMA:** 2017,Aug,3; 2017,Jun,6; 2017,Jan,8; 2016,Dec,11; 2016,Sep,6; 2016,Jan,13; 2016,Jan,7; 2015,Jan,12; 2015,Jan,16; 2014,Nov,14; 2014,Oct,8; 2014,Sep,13; 2014,Aug,3; 2014,Jan,11; 2013,Jun,3-5; 2013,Jan,9-10; 2012,Aug,3-5; 2012,Apr,10; 2012,Jan,15-42

● New Code   ▲ Revised Code   ○ Reinstated   ● New Web Release   ▲ Revised Web Release   Unlisted   Not Covered   # Resequenced
Ⓢ AMA Mod 51 Exempt   ⑤ Optum Mod 51 Exempt   ⑤ Mod 63 Exempt   ✗ Non-FDA Drug   ★ Telemedicine   Ⓜ Maternity   Ⓐ Age Edit   ✛ Add-on   **AMA:** CPT Asst
© 2017 Optum360, LLC          CPT © 2017 American Medical Association. All Rights Reserved.

## 99251-99255 Consultations: Inpatient

**CMS:** 100-04,11,40.1.3 Independent Attending Physician Services; 100-04,12,190.6 Payment Methodology for Physician/Practitioner at the Distant Site ; 100-04,12,190.6.1 Submission of Telehealth Claims for Distant Site Practitioners; 100-04,12,190.7 Contractor Editing of Telehealth Claims; 100-04,12,30.6.10 Consultation Services; 100-04,12,30.6.15.1 Prolonged Services With Direct Face-to-Face Patient Contact Service (Codes 99354 - 99357); 100-04,12,30.6.4 Services Furnished Incident to Physician's Service; 100-04,12,30.6.9.1 Initial Hospital Care and Observation or Inpatient Care Services; 100-04,12,40.3 Global Surgery Review

**INCLUDES** A third-party mandated consultation

All inpatient consultations include services provided in the hospital inpatient or partial hospital settings and nursing facilities

Consultation services provided outpatient for the same inpatient hospitalization (99241-99245)

Documentation of a request for a consultation from an appropriate source

Documentation of the need for consultation in the patient's medical record

One consultation by consultant per admission

Provision by a physician or qualified nonphysician practitioner whose advice, opinion, recommendation, suggestion, direction, or counsel, etc. is requested for evaluating/treating a patient since that individual's expertise in a specific medical area is beyond the scope of knowledge of the requesting physician

Provision of a written report of findings/recommendations from the consultant to the referring physician

**EXCLUDES** *Another appropriately requested and documented consultation pertaining to the same/new problem: repeat use of consultation codes*

*Any distinctly recognizable procedure/service provided on or following the consultation*

*Assumption of care (all or partial): report subsequent codes as appropriate for the place of service (99231-99233, 99307-99310)*

*Consultation prompted by the patient/family: report codes for office, domiciliary/rest home, or home visits instead (99201-99215, 99324-99337, 99341-99350)*

*Services provided to Medicare patients; E&M code as appropriate for the place of service or HCPCS code (99201-99215, 99221-99223, 99231-99233, G0406-G0408, G0425-G0427)*

**99251** Inpatient consultation for a new or established patient, which requires these 3 key components: A problem focused history; A problem focused examination; and Straightforward medical decision making. Counseling and/or coordination of care with other physicians, other qualified health care professionals, or agencies are provided consistent with the nature of the problem(s) and the patient's and/or family's needs. Usually, the presenting problem(s) are self limited or minor. Typically, 20 minutes are spent at the bedside and on the patient's hospital floor or unit.

    📁 1.38    🔍 1.38    **FUD** XXX        ★ E ▭

**AMA:** 2017,Aug,3; 2017,Jun,6; 2017,Jan,8; 2016,Dec,11; 2016,Jan,13; 2016,Jan,7; 2015,Jan,16; 2014,Nov,14; 2014,Oct,8; 2014,Jan,11; 2013,Jun,3-5; 2013,Jan,9-10; 2012,Aug,3-5; 2012,Jan,15-42

**99252** Inpatient consultation for a new or established patient, which requires these 3 key components: An expanded problem focused history; An expanded problem focused examination; and Straightforward medical decision making. Counseling and/or coordination of care with other physicians, other qualified health care professionals, or agencies are provided consistent with the nature of the problem(s) and the patient's and/or family's needs. Usually, the presenting problem(s) are of low severity. Typically, 40 minutes are spent at the bedside and on the patient's hospital floor or unit.

    📁 2.11    🔍 2.11    **FUD** XXX        ★ E ▭

**AMA:** 2017,Aug,3; 2017,Jun,6; 2017,Jan,8; 2016,Dec,11; 2016,Jan,7; 2016,Jan,13; 2015,Jan,16; 2014,Nov,14; 2014,Oct,8; 2014,Jan,11; 2013,Jun,3-5; 2013,Jan,9-10; 2012,Aug,3-5; 2012,Jan,15-42

**99253** Inpatient consultation for a new or established patient, which requires these 3 key components: A detailed history; A detailed examination; and Medical decision making of low complexity. Counseling and/or coordination of care with other physicians, other qualified health care professionals, or agencies are provided consistent with the nature of the problem(s) and the patient's and/or family's needs. Usually, the presenting problem(s) are of moderate severity. Typically, 55 minutes are spent at the bedside and on the patient's hospital floor or unit.

    📁 3.24    🔍 3.24    **FUD** XXX        ★ E ▭

**AMA:** 2017,Aug,3; 2017,Jun,6; 2017,Jan,8; 2016,Dec,11; 2016,Jan,13; 2016,Jan,7; 2015,Jan,16; 2014,Nov,14; 2014,Oct,8; 2014,Jan,11; 2013,Jun,3-5; 2013,Jan,9-10; 2012,Aug,3-5; 2012,Jan,15-42

**99254** Inpatient consultation for a new or established patient, which requires these 3 key components: A comprehensive history; A comprehensive examination; and Medical decision making of moderate complexity. Counseling and/or coordination of care with other physicians, other qualified health care professionals, or agencies are provided consistent with the nature of the problem(s) and the patient's and/or family's needs. Usually, the presenting problem(s) are of moderate to high severity. Typically, 80 minutes are spent at the bedside and on the patient's hospital floor or unit.

    📁 4.71    🔍 4.71    **FUD** XXX        ★ E ▭

**AMA:** 2017,Aug,3; 2017,Jun,6; 2017,Jan,8; 2016,Dec,11; 2016,Jan,7; 2016,Jan,13; 2015,Jan,16; 2014,Nov,14; 2014,Oct,8; 2014,Jan,11; 2013,Jun,3-5; 2013,Jan,9-10; 2012,Aug,3-5; 2012,Jan,15-42

**99255** Inpatient consultation for a new or established patient, which requires these 3 key components: A comprehensive history; A comprehensive examination; and Medical decision making of high complexity. Counseling and/or coordination of care with other physicians, other qualified health care professionals, or agencies are provided consistent with the nature of the problem(s) and the patient's and/or family's needs. Usually, the presenting problem(s) are of moderate to high severity. Typically, 110 minutes are spent at the bedside and on the patient's hospital floor or unit.

    📁 5.68    🔍 5.68    **FUD** XXX        ★ E ▭

**AMA:** 2017,Aug,3; 2017,Jun,6; 2017,Jan,8; 2016,Dec,11; 2016,Jan,7; 2016,Jan,13; 2015,Jan,16; 2014,Nov,14; 2014,Oct,8; 2014,Jan,11; 2013,Jun,3-5; 2013,Jan,9-10; 2012,Aug,3-5; 2012,Jan,15-42

## 99281-99288 Emergency Department Visits

**CMS:** 100-04,11,40.1.3 Independent Attending Physician Services; 100-04,12,30.6.11 Emergency Department Visits; 100-04,4,160 Clinic and Emergency Visits Under OPPS

**INCLUDES** Any amount of time spent with the patient, which usually involves a series of encounters while the patient is in the emergency department

Care provided to new and established patients

**EXCLUDES** *Critical care services (99291-99292)*

*Observation services (99217-99220, 99234-99236)*

**99281** Emergency department visit for the evaluation and management of a patient, which requires these 3 key components: A problem focused history; A problem focused examination; and Straightforward medical decision making. Counseling and/or coordination of care with other physicians, other qualified health care professionals, or agencies are provided consistent with the nature of the problem(s) and the patient's and/or family's needs. Usually, the presenting problem(s) are self limited or minor.

    📁 0.60    🔍 0.60    **FUD** XXX        J 80 ▭

**AMA:** 2017,Aug,3; 2017,Jun,6; 2017,Jan,8; 2016,Jan,13; 2016,Jan,7; 2015,Jan,16; 2015,Jan,12; 2014,Nov,14; 2014,Oct,8; 2014,Jan,11; 2013,Jun,3-5; 2013,Jan,9-10; 2012,Jan,15-42

| 26/TC PC/TC Only | A2-Z3 ASC Payment | 50 Bilateral | ♂ Male Only | ♀ Female Only | 📁 Facility RVU | 🔍 Non-Facility RVU | ▭ CCI |
|---|---|---|---|---|---|---|---|
| **FUD** Follow-up Days | **CMS:** IOM (Pub 100) | A-Y OPPSI | 80/80 Surg Assist Allowed / w/Doc | | ▥ Lab Crosswalk | ▣ Radiology Crosswalk | ✖ CLIA |

508        CPT © 2017 American Medical Association. All Rights Reserved.        © 2017 Optum360, LLC

**99282** Emergency department visit for the evaluation and management of a patient, which requires these 3 key components: An expanded problem focused history; An expanded problem focused examination; and Medical decision making of low complexity. Counseling and/or coordination of care with other physicians, other qualified health care professionals, or agencies are provided consistent with the nature of the problem(s) and the patient's and/or family's needs. Usually, the presenting problem(s) are of low to moderate severity.

📁 1.17    ⚖ 1.17    **FUD** XXX    [J] [80] [🖥]

**AMA:** 2017,Aug,3; 2017,Jun,6; 2017,Jan,8; 2016,Jan,7; 2016,Jan,13; 2015,Jan,16; 2015,Jan,12; 2014,Nov,14; 2014,Oct,8; 2014,Jan,11; 2013,Jun,3-5; 2013,Jan,9-10; 2012,Jan,15-42

**99283** Emergency department visit for the evaluation and management of a patient, which requires these 3 key components: An expanded problem focused history; An expanded problem focused examination; and Medical decision making of moderate complexity. Counseling and/or coordination of care with other physicians, other qualified health care professionals, or agencies are provided consistent with the nature of the problem(s) and the patient's and/or family's needs. Usually, the presenting problem(s) are of moderate severity.

📁 1.75    ⚖ 1.75    **FUD** XXX    [J] [80] [🖥]

**AMA:** 2017,Aug,3; 2017,Jun,6; 2017,Jan,8; 2016,Jan,13; 2016,Jan,7; 2015,Jan,12; 2015,Jan,16; 2014,Nov,14; 2014,Oct,8; 2014,Jan,11; 2013,Jun,3-5; 2013,Jan,9-10; 2012,Jan,15-42

**99284** Emergency department visit for the evaluation and management of a patient, which requires these 3 key components: A detailed history; A detailed examination; and Medical decision making of moderate complexity. Counseling and/or coordination of care with other physicians, other qualified health care professionals, or agencies are provided consistent with the nature of the problem(s) and the patient's and/or family's needs. Usually, the presenting problem(s) are of high severity, and require urgent evaluation by the physician, or other qualified health care professionals but do not pose an immediate significant threat to life or physiologic function.

📁 3.32    ⚖ 3.32    **FUD** XXX    [J] [80] [🖥]

**AMA:** 2017,Aug,3; 2017,Jun,6; 2017,Jan,8; 2016,Jan,13; 2016,Jan,7; 2015,Jan,16; 2015,Jan,12; 2014,Nov,14; 2014,Oct,8; 2014,Jan,11; 2013,Jun,3-5; 2013,Jan,9-10; 2012,Jan,15-42

**99285** Emergency department visit for the evaluation and management of a patient, which requires these 3 key components within the constraints imposed by the urgency of the patient's clinical condition and/or mental status: A comprehensive history; A comprehensive examination; and Medical decision making of high complexity. Counseling and/or coordination of care with other physicians, other qualified health care professionals, or agencies are provided consistent with the nature of the problem(s) and the patient's and/or family's needs. Usually, the presenting problem(s) are of high severity and pose an immediate significant threat to life or physiologic function.

📁 4.90    ⚖ 4.90    **FUD** XXX    [J] [80] [🖥]

**AMA:** 2017,Aug,3; 2017,Jun,6; 2017,Jan,8; 2016,Jan,7; 2016,Jan,13; 2015,Jan,16; 2015,Jan,12; 2014,Nov,14; 2014,Oct,8; 2014,Jan,11; 2013,Jun,3-5; 2013,Jan,9-10; 2012,Jan,15-42

**99288** Physician or other qualified health care professional direction of emergency medical systems (EMS) emergency care, advanced life support

[INCLUDES]    Management provided by an emergency/intensive care based physician or other qualified health care professional via voice contact to ambulance/rescue staff for services such as heart monitoring and drug administration

📁 0.00    ⚖ 0.00    **FUD** XXX    [B] [🖥]

**AMA:** 2017,Aug,3; 2017,Jun,6; 2017,Jan,8; 2016,Jan,13; 2015,Jan,16; 2014,Oct,8; 2014,Jan,11; 2013,May,6-7

## 99291-99292 Critical Care Visits: Patients 72 Months of Age and Older

**CMS:** 100-04,11,40.1.3 Independent Attending Physician Services; 100-04,12,30.6.4 Services Furnished Incident to Physician's Service; 100-04,12,30.6.9 Swing Bed Visits; 100-04,12,40.3 Global Surgery Review; 100-04,4,160 Clinic and Emergency Visits Under OPPS; 100-04,4,160.1 Critical Care Services

[INCLUDES]    30 minutes or more of direct care provided by the physician or other qualified health care professional to a critically ill or injured patient, regardless of the location
All activities performed outside of the unit or off the floor
All time spent exclusively with patient/family/caregivers on the nursing unit or elsewhere
Outpatient critical care provided to neonates and pediatric patients up through 71 months of age
Physician or other qualified health care professional presence during interfacility transfer for critically ill/injured patients over 24 months of age
Professional services for interpretation of:
    Blood gases
    Chest films (71045-71046)
    Measurement of cardiac output (93561-93562)
    Other computer stored information (99090)
    Pulse oximetry (94760-94762)
Professional services for:
    Gastric intubation (43752-43753)
    Transcutaneous pacing, temporary (92953)
    Venous access, arterial puncture (36000, 36410, 36415, 36591, 36600)
    Ventilation assistance and management, includes CPAP, CNP (94002-94004, 94660, 94662)

[EXCLUDES]    All services that are less than 30 minutes; report appropriate E&M code
Critical care services provided via remote real-time interactive videoconferencing (0188T, 0189T)
Inpatient critical care services provided to child 2 through 5 years of age (99475-99476)
Inpatient critical care services provided to infants 29 days through 24 months of age (99471-99472)
Inpatient critical care services provided to neonates that are age 28 days or less (99468-99469)
Other procedures not listed as included performed by the physician or other qualified health care professional rendering critical care
Patients who are not critically ill but in the critical care department (report appropriate E&M code)
Physician or other qualified health care professional presence during interfacility transfer for critically ill/injured patients under 24 months of age (99466-99467)
Supervisory services of control physician during interfacility transfer for critically ill/injured patients under 24 months of age ([99485, 99486])

**99291** Critical care, evaluation and management of the critically ill or critically injured patient; first 30-74 minutes

📁 6.32    ⚖ 7.75    **FUD** XXX    [J] [80] [🖥]

**AMA:** 2017,Aug,3; 2017,Jun,6; 2017,Jan,8; 2016,Oct,8; 2016,Aug,9; 2016,May,3; 2016,Jan,13; 2015,Jul,3; 2015,Feb,10; 2015,Jan,16; 2014,Oct,8; 2014,Oct,14; 2014,Aug,5; 2014,May,4; 2014,Jan,11; 2013,May,6-7; 2013,Feb,16-17; 2012,Oct,14; 2012,Sep,16; 2012,Jul,12-14; 2012,Jan,15-42

**+ 99292** each additional 30 minutes (List separately in addition to code for primary service)

Code first (99291)

📁 3.17    ⚖ 3.47    **FUD** ZZZ    [N] [80] [🖥]

**AMA:** 2017,Aug,3; 2017,Jun,6; 2017,Jan,8; 2016,Aug,9; 2016,May,3; 2016,Jan,13; 2015,Jul,3; 2015,Feb,10; 2015,Jan,16; 2014,Oct,14; 2014,Oct,8; 2014,Aug,5; 2014,May,4; 2014,Jan,11; 2013,May,6-7; 2013,Feb,16-17; 2012,Jan,15-42

---

● New Code    ▲ Revised Code    ○ Reinstated    ● New Web Release    ▲ Revised Web Release    Unlisted    Not Covered    # Resequenced
⊘ AMA Mod 51 Exempt    ⑤ Optum Mod 51 Exempt    ⑥³ Mod 63 Exempt    ✗ Non-FDA Drug    ★ Telemedicine    [M] Maternity    [A] Age Edit    + Add-on    **AMA:** CPT Asst

© 2017 Optum360, LLC                    CPT © 2017 American Medical Association. All Rights Reserved.

## 99304-99310 Nursing Facility Visits

**CMS:** 100-04,11,40.1.3 Independent Attending Physician Services; 100-04,12,230 Primary Care Incentive Payment Program; 100-04,12,230.1 Definition of Primary Care Practitioners and Services; 100-04,12,230.2 Coordination with Other Payments; 100-04,12,230.3 Claims Processing and Payment; 100-04,12,30.6.10 Consultation Services; 100-04,12,30.6.13 Nursing Facility Visits; 100-04,12,30.6.15.1 Prolonged Services With Direct Face-to-Face Patient Contact Service (Codes 99354 - 99357); 100-04,12,30.6.4 Services Furnished Incident to Physician's Service; 100-04,12,30.6.9 Swing Bed Visits

**INCLUDES** All E&M services provided by the admitting physician on the date of nursing facility admission in other locations (e.g., office, emergency department)
Initial care, subsequent care, discharge, and yearly assessments
Initial services include patient assessment and physician participation in developing a plan of care (99304-99306)
Services provided in a psychiatric residential treatment center
Services provided to new and established patients in a nursing facility (skilled, intermediate, and long-term care facilities)
Subsequent services include physician review of medical records, reassessment, and review of test results (99307-99310)

**EXCLUDES** Care plan oversight services (99379-99380)
Code also hospital discharge services on the same date of admission or readmission to the nursing home (99217, 99234-99236, 99238-99239)

**99304** Initial nursing facility care, per day, for the evaluation and management of a patient, which requires these 3 key components: A detailed or comprehensive history; A detailed or comprehensive examination; and Medical decision making that is straightforward or of low complexity. Counseling and/or coordination of care with other physicians, other qualified health care professionals, or agencies are provided consistent with the nature of the problem(s) and the patient's and/or family's needs. Usually, the problem(s) requiring admission are of low severity. Typically, 25 minutes are spent at the bedside and on the patient's facility floor or unit.
🔧 2.58   🔧 2.58   **FUD** XXX   B 80 📷
**AMA:** 2017,Aug,3; 2017,Jun,6; 2017,Jan,8; 2016,Dec,11; 2016,Jan,13; 2016,Jan,7; 2015,Jan,16; 2014,Nov,14; 2014,Oct,8; 2014,Jan,11; 2013,Jun,3-5; 2013,Jan,9-10; 2012,Aug,3-5; 2012,Jul,12-14; 2012,Jan,3-5

**99305** Initial nursing facility care, per day, for the evaluation and management of a patient, which requires these 3 key components: A comprehensive history; A comprehensive examination; and Medical decision making of moderate complexity. Counseling and/or coordination of care with other physicians, other qualified health care professionals, or agencies are provided consistent with the nature of the problem(s) and the patient's and/or family's needs. Usually, the problem(s) requiring admission are of moderate severity. Typically, 35 minutes are spent at the bedside and on the patient's facility floor or unit.
🔧 3.68   🔧 3.68   **FUD** XXX   B 80 📷
**AMA:** 2017,Aug,3; 2017,Jun,6; 2017,Jan,8; 2016,Dec,11; 2016,Jan,13; 2016,Jan,7; 2015,Jan,16; 2014,Nov,14; 2014,Oct,8; 2014,Jan,11; 2013,Jun,3-5; 2013,Jan,9-10; 2012,Aug,3-5; 2012,Jul,12-14; 2012,Jan,3-5

**99306** Initial nursing facility care, per day, for the evaluation and management of a patient, which requires these 3 key components: A comprehensive history; A comprehensive examination; and Medical decision making of high complexity. Counseling and/or coordination of care with other physicians, other qualified health care professionals, or agencies are provided consistent with the nature of the problem(s) and the patient's and/or family's needs. Usually, the problem(s) requiring admission are of high severity. Typically, 45 minutes are spent at the bedside and on the patient's facility floor or unit.
🔧 4.71   🔧 4.71   **FUD** XXX   B 80 📷
**AMA:** 2017,Aug,3; 2017,Jun,6; 2017,Jan,8; 2016,Dec,11; 2016,Jan,13; 2016,Jan,7; 2015,Jan,16; 2014,Nov,14; 2014,Oct,8; 2014,Jan,11; 2013,Jun,3-5; 2013,Jan,9-10; 2012,Aug,3-5; 2012,Jul,12-14; 2012,Jan,3-5

**99307** Subsequent nursing facility care, per day, for the evaluation and management of a patient, which requires at least 2 of these 3 key components: A problem focused interval history; A problem focused examination; Straightforward medical decision making. Counseling and/or coordination of care with other physicians, other qualified health care professionals, or agencies are provided consistent with the nature of the problem(s) and the patient's and/or family's needs. Usually, the patient is stable, recovering, or improving. Typically, 10 minutes are spent at the bedside and on the patient's facility floor or unit.
🔧 1.26   🔧 1.26   **FUD** XXX   ★ B 80 📷
**AMA:** 2017,Aug,3; 2017,Jun,6; 2017,Jan,8; 2016,Dec,11; 2016,Jan,13; 2016,Jan,7; 2015,Jan,16; 2014,Nov,14; 2014,Oct,8; 2014,Jan,11; 2013,Jun,3-5; 2013,Jan,9-10; 2012,Aug,3-5; 2012,Jul,12-14; 2012,Jan,15-42; 2012,Jan,3-5

**99308** Subsequent nursing facility care, per day, for the evaluation and management of a patient, which requires at least 2 of these 3 key components: An expanded problem focused interval history; An expanded problem focused examination; Medical decision making of low complexity. Counseling and/or coordination of care with other physicians, other qualified health care professionals, or agencies are provided consistent with the nature of the problem(s) and the patient's and/or family's needs. Usually, the patient is responding inadequately to therapy or has developed a minor complication. Typically, 15 minutes are spent at the bedside and on the patient's facility floor or unit.
🔧 1.95   🔧 1.95   **FUD** XXX   ★ B 80 📷
**AMA:** 2017,Aug,3; 2017,Jun,6; 2017,Jan,8; 2016,Dec,11; 2016,Jan,13; 2016,Jan,7; 2015,Jan,16; 2014,Nov,14; 2014,Oct,8; 2014,Jan,11; 2013,Jun,3-5; 2013,Jan,9-10; 2012,Aug,3-5; 2012,Jul,12-14; 2012,Jan,3-5

**99309** Subsequent nursing facility care, per day, for the evaluation and management of a patient, which requires at least 2 of these 3 key components: A detailed interval history; A detailed examination; Medical decision making of moderate complexity. Counseling and/or coordination of care with other physicians, other qualified health care professionals, or agencies are provided consistent with the nature of the problem(s) and the patient's and/or family's needs. Usually, the patient has developed a significant complication or a significant new problem. Typically, 25 minutes are spent at the bedside and on the patient's facility floor or unit.
🔧 2.58   🔧 2.58   **FUD** XXX   ★ B 80 📷
**AMA:** 2017,Aug,3; 2017,Jun,6; 2017,Jan,8; 2016,Dec,11; 2016,Jan,13; 2016,Jan,7; 2015,Jan,16; 2014,Nov,14; 2014,Oct,8; 2014,Jan,11; 2013,Jun,3-5; 2013,Jan,9-10; 2012,Aug,3-5; 2012,Jul,12-14; 2012,Jan,3-5

**99310** Subsequent nursing facility care, per day, for the evaluation and management of a patient, which requires at least 2 of these 3 key components: A comprehensive interval history; A comprehensive examination; Medical decision making of high complexity. Counseling and/or coordination of care with other physicians, other qualified health care professionals, or agencies are provided consistent with the nature of the problem(s) and the patient's and/or family's needs. The patient may be unstable or may have developed a significant new problem requiring immediate physician attention. Typically, 35 minutes are spent at the bedside and on the patient's facility floor or unit.
🔧 3.84   🔧 3.84   **FUD** XXX   ★ B 80 📷
**AMA:** 2017,Aug,3; 2017,Jun,6; 2017,Jan,8; 2016,Dec,11; 2016,Jan,13; 2016,Jan,7; 2015,Jan,16; 2014,Nov,14; 2014,Oct,8; 2014,Jan,11; 2013,Jun,3-5; 2013,Jan,9-10; 2012,Aug,3-5; 2012,Jan,15-42; 2012,Jan,3-5

26/TC PC/TC Only   A2-Z3 ASC Payment   50 Bilateral   ♂ Male Only   ♀ Female Only   🔧 Facility RVU   🔧 Non-Facility RVU   📷 CCI
**FUD** Follow-up Days   **CMS:** IOM (Pub 100)   A-Y OPPSI   80/80 Surg Assist Allowed / w/Doc   🔧 Lab Crosswalk   🔧 Radiology Crosswalk   ❌ CLIA

CPT © 2017 American Medical Association. All Rights Reserved.

© 2017 Optum360, LLC

## 99315-99316 Nursing Home Discharge

**CMS:** 100-04,11,40.1.3 Independent Attending Physician Services; 100-04,12,230 Primary Care Incentive Payment Program; 100-04,12,230.1 Definition of Primary Care Practitioners and Services; 100-04,12,230.2 Coordination with Other Payments; 100-04,12,230.3 Claims Processing and Payment; 100-04,12,30.6.13 Nursing Facility Visits; 100-04,12,30.6.4 Services Furnished Incident to Physician's Service; 100-04,12,40.3 Global Surgery Review

INCLUDES Discharge services include all time spent by the physician or other qualified health care professional for:
Completion of discharge records
Discharge instructions for patient and caregivers
Discussion regarding the stay in the facility
Final patient examination
Provide prescriptions and referrals as appropriate

**99315** **Nursing facility discharge day management; 30 minutes or less**

🚑 2.07 ⚕ 2.07 **FUD** XXX B 80 ▣

**AMA:** 2017,Aug,3; 2017,Jun,6; 2017,Jan,8; 2016,Dec,11; 2016,Jan,13; 2016,Jan,7; 2015,Jan,16; 2014,Nov,14; 2014,Oct,8; 2014,Jan,11; 2013,Jun,3-5; 2013,Jan,9-10; 2012,Jul,12-14; 2012,Jan,15-42; 2012,Jan,3-5

**99316** **more than 30 minutes**

🚑 2.99 ⚕ 2.99 **FUD** XXX B 80 ▣

**AMA:** 2017,Aug,3; 2017,Jun,6; 2017,Jan,8; 2016,Dec,11; 2016,Jan,13; 2016,Jan,7; 2015,Jan,16; 2014,Nov,14; 2014,Oct,8; 2014,Jan,11; 2013,Jun,3-5; 2013,Jan,9-10; 2012,Jul,12-14; 2012,Jan,15-42; 2012,Jan,3-5

## 99318 Annual Nursing Home Assessment

**CMS:** 100-04,12,230 Primary Care Incentive Payment Program; 100-04,12,230.1 Definition of Primary Care Practitioners and Services; 100-04,12,230.2 Coordination with Other Payments; 100-04,12,230.3 Claims Processing and Payment; 100-04,12,30.6.13 Nursing Facility Visits; 100-04,12,30.6.15.1 Prolonged Services With Direct Face-to-Face Patient Contact Service (Codes 99354 - 99357); 100-04,12,30.6.4 Services Furnished Incident to Physician's Service; 100-04,12,30.6.9 Swing Bed Visits

INCLUDES Includes nursing facility visits on same date of service as (99304-99316)

**99318** **Evaluation and management of a patient involving an annual nursing facility assessment, which requires these 3 key components: A detailed interval history; A comprehensive examination; and Medical decision making that is of low to moderate complexity. Counseling and/or coordination of care with other physicians, other qualified health care professionals, or agencies are provided consistent with the nature of the problem(s) and the patient's and/or family's needs. Usually, the patient is stable, recovering, or improving. Typically, 30 minutes are spent at the bedside and on the patient's facility floor or unit.**

🚑 2.72 ⚕ 2.72 **FUD** XXX B 80 ▣

**AMA:** 2017,Aug,3; 2017,Jun,6; 2017,Jan,8; 2016,Dec,11; 2016,Jan,13; 2016,Jan,7; 2015,Jan,16; 2014,Nov,14; 2014,Oct,8; 2014,Jan,11; 2013,Jun,3-5; 2013,Jan,9-10; 2012,Jan,3-5

## 99324-99337 Domiciliary Care, Rest Home, Assisted Living Visits

**CMS:** 100-04,11,40.1.3 Independent Attending Physician Services; 100-04,12,230 Primary Care Incentive Payment Program; 100-04,12,230.1 Definition of Primary Care Practitioners and Services; 100-04,12,230.2 Coordination with Other Payments; 100-04,12,230.3 Claims Processing and Payment; 100-04,12,30.6.14 Domiciliary Care, Rest Home, Assisted Living Visits; 100-04,12,30.6.15.1 Prolonged Services With Direct Face-to-Face Patient Contact Service (Codes 99354 - 99357); 100-04,12,30.6.4 Services Furnished Incident to Physician's Service

INCLUDES E&M services for patients residing in assisted living, domiciliary care, and rest homes where medical care is not included
Services provided to new patients or established patients (99324-99328, 99334-99337)

EXCLUDES *Care plan oversight services provided to a patient in a rest home under the care of a home health agency (99374-99375)*
*Care plan oversight services provided to a patient under the care of a hospice agency (99377-99378)*

**99324** **Domiciliary or rest home visit for the evaluation and management of a new patient, which requires these 3 key components: A problem focused history; A problem focused examination; and Straightforward medical decision making. Counseling and/or coordination of care with other physicians, other qualified health care professionals, or agencies are provided consistent with the nature of the problem(s) and the patient's and/or family's needs. Usually, the presenting problem(s) are of low severity. Typically, 20 minutes are spent with the patient and/or family or caregiver.**

🚑 1.56 ⚕ 1.56 **FUD** XXX B 80 ▣

**AMA:** 2017,Aug,3; 2017,Jun,6; 2017,Jan,8; 2016,Dec,11; 2016,Jan,13; 2016,Jan,7; 2015,Jan,16; 2014,Nov,14; 2014,Oct,8; 2014,Oct,3; 2014,Jan,11; 2013,Jun,3-5; 2013,Jan,9-10; 2012,Aug,3-5; 2012,Apr,10; 2012,Jan,3-5

**99325** **Domiciliary or rest home visit for the evaluation and management of a new patient, which requires these 3 key components: An expanded problem focused history; An expanded problem focused examination; and Medical decision making of low complexity. Counseling and/or coordination of care with other physicians, other qualified health care professionals, or agencies are provided consistent with the nature of the problem(s) and the patient's and/or family's needs. Usually, the presenting problem(s) are of moderate severity. Typically, 30 minutes are spent with the patient and/or family or caregiver.**

🚑 2.27 ⚕ 2.27 **FUD** XXX B 80 ▣

**AMA:** 2017,Aug,3; 2017,Jun,6; 2017,Jan,8; 2016,Dec,11; 2016,Jan,13; 2016,Jan,7; 2015,Jan,16; 2014,Nov,14; 2014,Oct,8; 2014,Oct,3; 2014,Jan,11; 2013,Jun,3-5; 2013,Jan,9-10; 2012,Aug,3-5; 2012,Apr,10; 2012,Jan,3-5

**99326** **Domiciliary or rest home visit for the evaluation and management of a new patient, which requires these 3 key components: A detailed history; A detailed examination; and Medical decision making of moderate complexity. Counseling and/or coordination of care with other physicians, other qualified health care professionals, or agencies are provided consistent with the nature of the problem(s) and the patient's and/or family's needs. Usually, the presenting problem(s) are of moderate to high severity. Typically, 45 minutes are spent with the patient and/or family or caregiver.**

🚑 3.94 ⚕ 3.94 **FUD** XXX B 80 ▣

**AMA:** 2017,Aug,3; 2017,Jun,6; 2017,Jan,8; 2016,Dec,11; 2016,Jan,13; 2016,Jan,7; 2015,Jan,16; 2014,Nov,14; 2014,Oct,8; 2014,Oct,3; 2014,Jan,11; 2013,Jun,3-5; 2013,Jan,9-10; 2012,Aug,3-5; 2012,Apr,10; 2012,Jan,3-5

**99327** Domiciliary or rest home visit for the evaluation and management of a new patient, which requires these 3 key components: A comprehensive history; A comprehensive examination; and Medical decision making of moderate complexity. Counseling and/or coordination of care with other physicians, other qualified health care professionals, or agencies are provided consistent with the nature of the problem(s) and the patient's and/or family's needs. Usually, the presenting problem(s) are of high severity. Typically, 60 minutes are spent with the patient and/or family or caregiver.

    📠 5.25   ⚕ 5.25   **FUD** XXX    B 80 ▢

    **AMA:** 2017,Aug,3; 2017,Jun,6; 2017,Jan,8; 2016,Dec,11; 2016,Jan,13; 2016,Jan,7; 2015,Jan,16; 2014,Nov,14; 2014,Oct,8; 2014,Oct,3; 2014,Jan,11; 2013,Jun,3-5; 2013,Jan,9-10; 2012,Aug,3-5; 2012,Apr,10; 2012,Jan,3-5

**99328** Domiciliary or rest home visit for the evaluation and management of a new patient, which requires these 3 key components: A comprehensive history; A comprehensive examination; and Medical decision making of high complexity. Counseling and/or coordination of care with other physicians, other qualified health care professionals, or agencies are provided consistent with the nature of the problem(s) and the patient's and/or family's needs. Usually, the patient is unstable or has developed a significant new problem requiring immediate physician attention. Typically, 75 minutes are spent with the patient and/or family or caregiver.

    📠 6.15   ⚕ 6.15   **FUD** XXX    B 80 ▢

    **AMA:** 2017,Aug,3; 2017,Jun,6; 2017,Jan,8; 2016,Dec,11; 2016,Jan,13; 2016,Jan,7; 2015,Jan,16; 2014,Nov,14; 2014,Oct,8; 2014,Oct,3; 2014,Jan,11; 2013,Jun,3-5; 2013,Jan,9-10; 2012,Aug,3-5; 2012,Apr,10; 2012,Jan,3-5

**99334** Domiciliary or rest home visit for the evaluation and management of an established patient, which requires at least 2 of these 3 key components: A problem focused interval history; A problem focused examination; Straightforward medical decision making. Counseling and/or coordination of care with other physicians, other qualified health care professionals, or agencies are provided consistent with the nature of the problem(s) and the patient's and/or family's needs. Usually, the presenting problem(s) are self-limited or minor. Typically, 15 minutes are spent with the patient and/or family or caregiver.

    📠 1.70   ⚕ 1.70   **FUD** XXX    B 80 ▢

    **AMA:** 2017,Aug,3; 2017,Jun,6; 2017,Jan,8; 2016,Dec,11; 2016,Jan,13; 2016,Jan,7; 2015,Jan,16; 2014,Nov,14; 2014,Oct,8; 2014,Oct,3; 2014,Jan,11; 2013,Nov,3; 2013,Jun,3-5; 2013,Jan,9-10; 2012,Aug,3-5; 2012,Apr,10; 2012,Jan,3-5

**99335** Domiciliary or rest home visit for the evaluation and management of an established patient, which requires at least 2 of these 3 key components: An expanded problem focused interval history; An expanded problem focused examination; Medical decision making of low complexity. Counseling and/or coordination of care with other physicians, other qualified health care professionals, or agencies are provided consistent with the nature of the problem(s) and the patient's and/or family's needs. Usually, the presenting problem(s) are of low to moderate severity. Typically, 25 minutes are spent with the patient and/or family or caregiver.

    📠 2.68   ⚕ 2.68   **FUD** XXX    B 80 ▢

    **AMA:** 2017,Aug,3; 2017,Jun,6; 2017,Jan,8; 2016,Dec,11; 2016,Jan,13; 2016,Jan,7; 2015,Jan,16; 2014,Nov,14; 2014,Oct,8; 2014,Oct,3; 2014,Jan,11; 2013,Nov,3; 2013,Jun,3-5; 2013,Jan,9-10; 2012,Aug,3-5; 2012,Apr,10; 2012,Jan,3-5

**99336** Domiciliary or rest home visit for the evaluation and management of an established patient, which requires at least 2 of these 3 key components: A detailed interval history; A detailed examination; Medical decision making of moderate complexity. Counseling and/or coordination of care with other physicians, other qualified health care professionals, or agencies are provided consistent with the nature of the problem(s) and the patient's and/or family's needs. Usually, the presenting problem(s) are of moderate to high severity. Typically, 40 minutes are spent with the patient and/or family or caregiver.

    📠 3.81   ⚕ 3.81   **FUD** XXX    B 80 ▢

    **AMA:** 2017,Aug,3; 2017,Jun,6; 2017,Jan,8; 2016,Dec,11; 2016,Jan,13; 2016,Jan,7; 2015,Jan,16; 2014,Nov,14; 2014,Oct,8; 2014,Oct,3; 2014,Jan,11; 2013,Nov,3; 2013,Jun,3-5; 2013,Jan,9-10; 2012,Aug,3-5; 2012,Apr,10; 2012,Jan,3-5

**99337** Domiciliary or rest home visit for the evaluation and management of an established patient, which requires at least 2 of these 3 key components: A comprehensive interval history; A comprehensive examination; Medical decision making of moderate to high complexity. Counseling and/or coordination of care with other physicians, other qualified health care professionals, or agencies are provided consistent with the nature of the problem(s) and the patient's and/or family's needs. Usually, the presenting problem(s) are of moderate to high severity. The patient may be unstable or may have developed a significant new problem requiring immediate physician attention. Typically, 60 minutes are spent with the patient and/or family or caregiver.

    📠 5.45   ⚕ 5.45   **FUD** XXX    B 80 ▢

    **AMA:** 2017,Aug,3; 2017,Jun,6; 2017,Jan,8; 2016,Dec,11; 2016,Jan,13; 2016,Jan,7; 2015,Jan,16; 2014,Nov,14; 2014,Oct,8; 2014,Oct,3; 2014,Jan,11; 2013,Nov,3; 2013,Jun,3-5; 2013,Jan,9-10; 2012,Aug,3-5; 2012,Apr,10; 2012,Jan,3-5

## 99339-99340 Care Plan Oversight: Rest Home, Domiciliary Care, Assisted Living, and Home

**CMS:** 100-04,12,180 Payment of Care Plan Oversight (CPO); 100-04,12,180.1 Billing for Care Plan Oversight (CPO); 100-04,12,230 Primary Care Incentive Payment Program; 100-04,12,230.1 Definition of Primary Care Practitioners and Services; 100-04,12,230.2 Coordination with Other Payments; 100-04,12,230.3 Claims Processing and Payment; 100-04,12,30.6.14 Domiciliary Care, Rest Home, Assisted Living Visits; 100-04,12,30.6.4 Services Furnished Incident to Physician's Service

INCLUDES   Care plan oversight for patients residing in assisted living, domiciliary care, private residences, and rest homes
    Patient management services during same time frame as (99441-99444, 99487-99489, 99495-99496, 98966-98969)

EXCLUDES   *Care plan oversight services furnished under a home health agency, nursing facility, or hospice (99374-99380)*

**99339** Individual physician supervision of a patient (patient not present) in home, domiciliary or rest home (eg, assisted living facility) requiring complex and multidisciplinary care modalities involving regular physician development and/or revision of care plans, review of subsequent reports of patient status, review of related laboratory and other studies, communication (including telephone calls) for purposes of assessment or care decisions with health care professional(s), family member(s), surrogate decision maker(s) (eg, legal guardian) and/or key caregiver(s) involved in patient's care, integration of new information into the medical treatment plan and/or adjustment of medical therapy, within a calendar month; 15-29 minutes

    📠 2.18   ⚕ 2.18   **FUD** XXX    B ▢

    **AMA:** 2017,Aug,3; 2017,Jun,6; 2017,Jan,8; 2016,Jan,13; 2015,Jan,16; 2014,Oct,8; 2014,Oct,3; 2014,Jan,11; 2013,Nov,3; 2013,Sep,15-16; 2013,Jun,3-5; 2013,Apr,3-4; 2012,Jan,15-42; 2012,Jan,3-5

26/TC PC/TC Only    A2-Z3 ASC Payment    50 Bilateral    ♂ Male Only    ♀ Female Only    📠 Facility RVU    ⚕ Non-Facility RVU    ▢ CCI
**FUD** Follow-up Days    **CMS:** IOM (Pub 100)    A-Y OPPSI    80/80 Surg Assist Allowed / w/Doc    🔲 Lab Crosswalk    📊 Radiology Crosswalk    ❌ CLIA

**512**         CPT © 2017 American Medical Association. All Rights Reserved.         © 2017 Optum360, LLC

**99340** **30 minutes or more**
🚑 3.06 ⚒ 3.06 **FUD** XXX B 📠
**AMA:** 2017,Aug,3; 2017,Jun,6; 2017,Jan,8; 2016,Jan,13; 2015,Jan,16; 2014,Oct,8; 2014,Oct,3; 2014,Jan,11; 2013,Nov,3; 2013,Sep,15-16; 2013,Jun,3-5; 2013,Apr,3-4; 2012,Jan,15-42; 2012,Jan,3-5

## 99341-99350 Home Visits

**CMS:** 100-04,11,40.1.3 Independent Attending Physician Services; 100-04,12,230 Primary Care Incentive Payment Program; 100-04,12,230.1 Definition of Primary Care Practitioners and Services; 100-04,12,230.2 Coordination with Other Payments; 100-04,12,230.3 Claims Processing and Payment; 100-04,12,30.6.14 Domiciliary Care, Rest Home, Assisted Living Visits; 100-04,12,30.6.14.1 Home Visits; 100-04,12,30.6.15.1 Prolonged Services With Direct Face-to-Face Patient Contact Service (Codes 99354 - 99357); 100-04,12,30.6.4 Services Furnished Incident to Physician's Service; 100-04,12,40.3 Global Surgery Review

INCLUDES Services for a new patient or an established patient (99341-99345, 99347-99350)
Services provided to a patient in a private home
EXCLUDES *Services provided to patients under home health agency or hospice care (99374-99378)*

**99341** Home visit for the evaluation and management of a new patient, which requires these 3 key components: A problem focused history; A problem focused examination; and Straightforward medical decision making. Counseling and/or coordination of care with other physicians, other qualified health care professionals, or agencies are provided consistent with the nature of the problem(s) and the patient's and/or family's needs. Usually, the presenting problem(s) are of low severity. Typically, 20 minutes are spent face-to-face with the patient and/or family.
🚑 1.55 ⚒ 1.55 **FUD** XXX B 80 📠
**AMA:** 2017,Aug,3; 2017,Jun,6; 2017,Jan,8; 2016,Dec,11; 2016,Jan,13; 2016,Jan,7; 2015,Jan,16; 2014,Nov,14; 2014,Oct,8; 2014,Oct,3; 2014,Jan,11; 2013,Jun,3-5; 2013,Jan,9-10; 2012,Aug,3-5; 2012,Apr,10; 2012,Jan,3-5

**99342** Home visit for the evaluation and management of a new patient, which requires these 3 key components: An expanded problem focused history; An expanded problem focused examination; and Medical decision making of low complexity. Counseling and/or coordination of care with other physicians, other qualified health care professionals, or agencies are provided consistent with the nature of the problem(s) and the patient's and/or family's needs. Usually, the presenting problem(s) are of moderate severity. Typically, 30 minutes are spent face-to-face with the patient and/or family.
🚑 2.24 ⚒ 2.24 **FUD** XXX B 80 📠
**AMA:** 2017,Aug,3; 2017,Jun,6; 2017,Jan,8; 2016,Dec,11; 2016,Jan,7; 2016,Jan,13; 2015,Jan,16; 2014,Nov,14; 2014,Oct,8; 2014,Oct,3; 2014,Jan,11; 2013,Jun,3-5; 2013,Jan,9-10; 2012,Aug,3-5; 2012,Apr,10; 2012,Jan,3-5

**99343** Home visit for the evaluation and management of a new patient, which requires these 3 key components: A detailed history; A detailed examination; and Medical decision making of moderate complexity. Counseling and/or coordination of care with other physicians, other qualified health care professionals, or agencies are provided consistent with the nature of the problem(s) and the patient's and/or family's needs. Usually, the presenting problem(s) are of moderate to high severity. Typically, 45 minutes are spent face-to-face with the patient and/or family.
🚑 3.68 ⚒ 3.68 **FUD** XXX B 80 📠
**AMA:** 2017,Aug,3; 2017,Jun,6; 2017,Jan,8; 2016,Dec,11; 2016,Jan,13; 2016,Jan,7; 2015,Jan,16; 2014,Nov,14; 2014,Oct,8; 2014,Oct,3; 2014,Jan,11; 2013,Jun,3-5; 2013,Jan,9-10; 2012,Aug,3-5; 2012,Apr,10; 2012,Jan,3-5

**99344** Home visit for the evaluation and management of a new patient, which requires these 3 key components: A comprehensive history; A comprehensive examination; and Medical decision making of moderate complexity. Counseling and/or coordination of care with other physicians, other qualified health care professionals, or agencies are provided consistent with the nature of the problem(s) and the patient's and/or family's needs. Usually, the presenting problem(s) are of high severity. Typically, 60 minutes are spent face-to-face with the patient and/or family.
🚑 5.16 ⚒ 5.16 **FUD** XXX B 80 📠
**AMA:** 2017,Aug,3; 2017,Jun,6; 2017,Jan,8; 2016,Dec,11; 2016,Jan,13; 2016,Jan,7; 2015,Jan,16; 2014,Nov,14; 2014,Oct,8; 2014,Oct,3; 2014,Jan,11; 2013,Jun,3-5; 2013,Jan,9-10; 2012,Aug,3-5; 2012,Apr,10; 2012,Jan,3-5

**99345** Home visit for the evaluation and management of a new patient, which requires these 3 key components: A comprehensive history; A comprehensive examination; and Medical decision making of high complexity. Counseling and/or coordination of care with other physicians, other qualified health care professionals, or agencies are provided consistent with the nature of the problem(s) and the patient's and/or family's needs. Usually, the patient is unstable or has developed a significant new problem requiring immediate physician attention. Typically, 75 minutes are spent face-to-face with the patient and/or family.
🚑 6.25 ⚒ 6.25 **FUD** XXX B 80 📠
**AMA:** 2017,Aug,3; 2017,Jun,6; 2017,Jan,8; 2016,Dec,11; 2016,Jan,13; 2016,Jan,7; 2015,Jan,16; 2014,Nov,14; 2014,Oct,8; 2014,Oct,3; 2014,Jan,11; 2013,Jun,3-5; 2013,Jan,9-10; 2012,Aug,3-5; 2012,Apr,10; 2012,Jan,3-5

**99347** Home visit for the evaluation and management of an established patient, which requires at least 2 of these 3 key components: A problem focused interval history; A problem focused examination; Straightforward medical decision making. Counseling and/or coordination of care with other physicians, other qualified health care professionals, or agencies are provided consistent with the nature of the problem(s) and the patient's and/or family's needs. Usually, the presenting problem(s) are self limited or minor. Typically, 15 minutes are spent face-to-face with the patient and/or family.
🚑 1.56 ⚒ 1.56 **FUD** XXX B 80 📠
**AMA:** 2017,Aug,3; 2017,Jun,6; 2017,Jan,8; 2016,Dec,11; 2016,Jan,13; 2016,Jan,7; 2015,Jan,16; 2014,Nov,14; 2014,Oct,8; 2014,Oct,3; 2014,Jan,11; 2013,Nov,3; 2013,Jun,3-5; 2013,Jan,9-10; 2012,Aug,3-5; 2012,Apr,10; 2012,Jan,3-5

**99348** Home visit for the evaluation and management of an established patient, which requires at least 2 of these 3 key components: An expanded problem focused interval history; An expanded problem focused examination; Medical decision making of low complexity. Counseling and/or coordination of care with other physicians, other qualified health care professionals, or agencies are provided consistent with the nature of the problem(s) and the patient's and/or family's needs. Usually, the presenting problem(s) are of low to moderate severity. Typically, 25 minutes are spent face-to-face with the patient and/or family.
🚑 2.38 ⚒ 2.38 **FUD** XXX B 80 📠
**AMA:** 2017,Aug,3; 2017,Jun,6; 2017,Jan,8; 2016,Dec,11; 2016,Jan,13; 2016,Jan,7; 2015,Jan,16; 2014,Nov,14; 2014,Oct,8; 2014,Oct,3; 2014,Jan,11; 2013,Nov,3; 2013,Jun,3-5; 2013,Jan,9-10; 2012,Aug,3-5; 2012,Apr,10; 2012,Jan,3-5

● New Code ▲ Revised Code ○ Reinstated ● New Web Release ▲ Revised Web Release Unlisted Not Covered # Resequenced
⊘ AMA Mod 51 Exempt ⑤⓪ Optum Mod 51 Exempt ⑥③ Mod 63 Exempt ✗ Non-FDA Drug ★ Telemedicine Ⓜ Maternity Ⓐ Age Edit + Add-on **AMA:** CPT Asst
© 2017 Optum360, LLC CPT © 2017 American Medical Association. All Rights Reserved.

**Evaluation and Management**

**99349**    **Home visit for the evaluation and management of an established patient, which requires at least 2 of these 3 key components: A detailed interval history; A detailed examination; Medical decision making of moderate complexity. Counseling and/or coordination of care with other physicians, other qualified health care professionals, or agencies are provided consistent with the nature of the problem(s) and the patient's and/or family's needs. Usually, the presenting problem(s) are moderate to high severity. Typically, 40 minutes are spent face-to-face with the patient and/or family.**

   3.63    3.63    **FUD** XXX      B 80

**AMA:** 2017,Aug,3; 2017,Jun,6; 2017,Jan,8; 2016,Dec,11; 2016,Jan,13; 2016,Jan,7; 2015,Jan,16; 2014,Nov,14; 2014,Oct,8; 2014,Oct,3; 2014,Jan,11; 2013,Nov,3; 2013,Jun,3-5; 2013,Jan,9-10; 2012,Aug,3-5; 2012,Apr,10; 2012,Jan,3-5

**99350**    **Home visit for the evaluation and management of an established patient, which requires at least 2 of these 3 key components: A comprehensive interval history; A comprehensive examination; Medical decision making of moderate to high complexity. Counseling and/or coordination of care with other physicians, other qualified health care professionals, or agencies are provided consistent with the nature of the problem(s) and the patient's and/or family's needs. Usually, the presenting problem(s) are of moderate to high severity. The patient may be unstable or may have developed a significant new problem requiring immediate physician attention. Typically, 60 minutes are spent face-to-face with the patient and/or family.**

   5.03    5.03    **FUD** XXX      B 80

**AMA:** 2017,Aug,3; 2017,Jun,6; 2017,Jan,8; 2016,Dec,11; 2016,Jan,13; 2016,Jan,7; 2015,Jan,16; 2014,Nov,14; 2014,Oct,8; 2014,Oct,3; 2014,Jan,11; 2013,Nov,3; 2013,Jun,3-5; 2013,Jan,9-10; 2012,Aug,3-5; 2012,Apr,10; 2012,Jan,3-5

## 99354-99357 Prolonged Services Direct Contact

**CMS:** 100-04,11,40.1.3 Independent Attending Physician Services; 100-04,12,30.6.15.1 Prolonged Services With Direct Face-to-Face Patient Contact Service (Codes 99354 - 99357); 100-04,12,30.6.4 Services Furnished Incident to Physician's Service

INCLUDES    Personal contact with the patient by the physician or other qualified health professional

Services extending beyond the customary service provided in the inpatient or outpatient setting

Time spent providing additional indirect contact services on the floor or unit of the hospital or nursing facility during the same session as the direct contact

Time spent providing prolonged services on a date of service, even when the time is not continuous

EXCLUDES    *Services less than 30 minutes, less than 15 minutes after the first hour, or after the final 30 minutes*

*Services provided independent of the date of personal contact with the patient (99358-99359)*

Code first E&M service code, as appropriate

**+**    **99354**    **Prolonged evaluation and management or psychotherapy service(s) (beyond the typical service time of the primary procedure) in the office or other outpatient setting requiring direct patient contact beyond the usual service; first hour (List separately in addition to code for office or other outpatient Evaluation and Management or psychotherapy service)**

EXCLUDES    *Prolonged service provided by clinical staff under supervision ([99415, 99416])*

*Use of code more than one time per date of service*

Code first (99201-99215, 99241-99245, 99324-99337, 99341-99350, 90837, 90847)

   3.45    3.66    **FUD** ZZZ     ★ N 80

**AMA:** 2017,Jan,8; 2016,Dec,11; 2016,Jan,13; 2015,Oct,9; 2015,Oct,3; 2015,Jan,16; 2014,Oct,8; 2014,Jun,14; 2014,Apr,6; 2014,Jan,11; 2013,Oct,11; 2013,Jun,3-5; 2013,May,12; 2012,Aug,3-5; 2012,Apr,10

**+**    **99355**    **each additional 30 minutes (List separately in addition to code for prolonged service)**

EXCLUDES    *Prolonged service provided by clinical staff under supervision ([99415, 99416])*

Code first (99354)

   2.56    2.76    **FUD** ZZZ     ★ N 80

**AMA:** 2017,Jan,8; 2016,Dec,11; 2016,Jan,13; 2015,Oct,9; 2015,Oct,3; 2015,Jan,16; 2014,Oct,8; 2014,Jun,14; 2014,Apr,6; 2014,Jan,11; 2013,Oct,11; 2013,Jun,3-5; 2013,May,12; 2012,Aug,3-5; 2012,Apr,10

**+**    **99356**    **Prolonged service in the inpatient or observation setting, requiring unit/floor time beyond the usual service; first hour (List separately in addition to code for inpatient Evaluation and Management service)**

EXCLUDES    *Use of code more than one time per date of service*

Code first (99218-99223 [99224, 99225, 99226], 99231-99236, 99251-99255, 99304-99310, 90837)

   2.60    2.60    **FUD** ZZZ     C 80

**AMA:** 2017,Jan,8; 2016,Dec,11; 2016,Jan,13; 2015,Oct,9; 2015,Oct,3; 2015,Jan,16; 2014,Oct,8; 2014,Jun,14; 2014,Apr,6; 2014,Jan,11; 2013,Oct,11; 2013,Jun,3-5; 2013,May,12; 2012,Aug,3-5; 2012,Jul,10-11

**+**    **99357**    **each additional 30 minutes (List separately in addition to code for prolonged service)**

Code first (99356)

   2.60    2.60    **FUD** ZZZ     C 80

**AMA:** 2017,Jan,8; 2016,Dec,11; 2016,Jan,13; 2015,Oct,9; 2015,Oct,3; 2015,Jan,16; 2014,Oct,8; 2014,Jun,14; 2014,Apr,6; 2014,Jan,11; 2013,Oct,11; 2013,Jun,3-5; 2013,May,12; 2012,Aug,3-5; 2012,Jul,10-11

## 99358-99359 Prolonged Services Indirect Contact

**CMS:** 100-04,11,40.1.3 Independent Attending Physician Services; 100-04,12,30.6.15.2 Prolonged Services Without Face to Face Service; 100-04,12,30.6.4 Services Furnished Incident to Physician's Service

INCLUDES    Services extending beyond the customary service

Time spent providing indirect contact services by the physician or other qualified health care professional in relation to patient management where face-to-face services have or will occur on a different date

Time spent providing prolonged services performed on a date of service (which may be other than the date of the primary service) that are not continuous

EXCLUDES    *Any additional unit or floor time in the hospital or nursing facility during the same evaluation and management session*

*Behavioral health integration care management services (99484)*

*Care plan oversight (99339-99340, 99374-99380)*

*Chronic care management services provided during the same month ([99490])*

*INR monitoring services (93792-93793)*

*Online medical services (99444)*

*Patient management services during same time frame as (99487-99489, 99495-99496)*

*Psychiatric collaborative care management services during the same month (99492-99494)*

*Services less than 30 minutes, less than 15 minutes after the first hour, or after the final 30 minutes*

*Time spent in medical team conference (99366-99368)*

*Use of code more than one time per date of service*

Code also E&M or other services provided

**99358**    **Prolonged evaluation and management service before and/or after direct patient care; first hour**

EXCLUDES    *Use of code more than one time per date of service*

   3.16    3.16    **FUD** XXX     N 80

**AMA:** 2017,Jan,8; 2016,Jan,13; 2015,Jan,16; 2014,Oct,3; 2014,Oct,8; 2014,Jan,11; 2013,Oct,11; 2013,Nov,3; 2013,Apr,3-4; 2012,Aug,3-5

**+**    **99359**    **each additional 30 minutes (List separately in addition to code for prolonged service)**

Code first (99358)

   1.52    1.52    **FUD** ZZZ     N 80

**AMA:** 2017,Jan,8; 2016,Jan,13; 2015,Jan,16; 2014,Oct,3; 2014,Oct,8; 2014,Jan,11; 2013,Oct,11; 2013,Nov,3; 2013,Apr,3-4; 2012,Aug,3-5

26/TC PC/TC Only    A2-Z3 ASC Payment    50 Bilateral    ♂ Male Only    ♀ Female Only    Facility RVU    Non-Facility RVU    CCI

**FUD** Follow-up Days    **CMS:** IOM (Pub 100)    A-Y OPPSI    80/80 Surg Assist Allowed / w/Doc    Lab Crosswalk    Radiology Crosswalk    CLIA

**514**      CPT © 2017 American Medical Association. All Rights Reserved.      © 2017 Optum360, LLC

## [99415, 99416] Prolonged Clinical Staff Services Under Supervision

INCLUDES  Time spent by clinical staff providing prolonged face-to-face services extending beyond the customary service under the supervision of a physician or other qualified health professional

Time spent by clinical staff providing prolonged services on a date of service, even when the time is not continuous

EXCLUDES  *Prolonged service provided by physician or other qualified health care professional (99354-99357)*

*Services less than 45 minutes*

*Services provided to more than two patients at the same time*

Code also E&M or other services provided

**+ # 99415  Prolonged clinical staff service (the service beyond the typical service time) during an evaluation and management service in the office or outpatient setting, direct patient contact with physician supervision; first hour (List separately in addition to code for outpatient Evaluation and Management service)**

EXCLUDES  *Use of code more than one time per date of service*

Code first (99201-99215)

🚑 0.25  ⚖ 0.25  **FUD** ZZZ  N 80 TC 🖵

**AMA:** 2017,Jan,8; 2016,Mar,8; 2016,Feb,13; 2016,Jan,13; 2015,Oct,3

**+ # 99416  each additional 30 minutes (List separately in addition to code for prolonged service)**

EXCLUDES  *Services less than 30 minutes, less than 15 minutes after the first hour, or after the final 30 minutes*

Code first ([99415])

🚑 0.13  ⚖ 0.13  **FUD** ZZZ  N 80 TC 🖵

**AMA:** 2017,Jan,8; 2016,Mar,8; 2016,Feb,13; 2016,Jan,13; 2015,Oct,3

## 99360 Standby Services

**CMS:** 100-04,12,30.6.15.3 Standby Services; 100-04,12,30.6.4 Services Furnished Incident to Physician's Service

INCLUDES  Services requested by physician or qualified health care professional that involve no direct patient contact

Total standby time for the day

EXCLUDES  *Delivery attendance (99464)*

*Less than 30 minutes of standby time*

*On-call services mandated by the hospital (99026-99027)*

Code also as appropriate (99460, 99465)

**99360  Standby service, requiring prolonged attendance, each 30 minutes (eg, operative standby, standby for frozen section, for cesarean/high risk delivery, for monitoring EEG)**

🚑 1.73  ⚖ 1.73  **FUD** XXX  B 🖵

**AMA:** 2017,Jan,8; 2016,Jan,13; 2015,Jan,16; 2014,Oct,8; 2014,Apr,5; 2014,Jan,11; 2013,May,8-10; 2012,Jan,15-42

## 99363-99364 Supervision of Warfarin Therapy

**99363  ~~Anticoagulant management for an outpatient taking warfarin, physician review and interpretation of International Normalized Ratio (INR) testing, patient instructions, dosage adjustment (as needed), and ordering of additional tests; initial 90 days of therapy (must include a minimum of 8 INR measurements)~~**

To report, see 93792-93793

**99364  ~~each subsequent 90 days of therapy (must include a minimum of 3 INR measurements)~~**

To report, see 93792-93793

## 99366-99368 Interdisciplinary Conferences

**CMS:** 100-04,11,40.1.3 Independent Attending Physician Services

INCLUDES  Documentation of participation, contribution, and recommendations of the conference

Face-to-face participation by minimum of three qualified people from different specialties or disciplines

Only participants who have performed face-to-face evaluations or direct treatment to the patient within the previous 60 days

Start of the review of an individual patient and ends at conclusion of review

EXCLUDES  *Conferences of less than 30 minutes (not reportable)*

*More than one individual from the same specialty at the same encounter*

*Patient management services during same time frame as (99487-99489, 99495-99496)*

*Time spent record keeping or writing a report*

**99366  Medical team conference with interdisciplinary team of health care professionals, face-to-face with patient and/or family, 30 minutes or more, participation by nonphysician qualified health care professional**

INCLUDES  Team conferences of 30 minutes or more

EXCLUDES  *Team conferences by a physician with patient or family present, see appropriate evaluation and management service code*

🚑 1.19  ⚖ 1.21  **FUD** XXX  N 🖵

**AMA:** 2017,Jan,8; 2016,Jan,13; 2015,Jan,16; 2014,Oct,8; 2014,Oct,3; 2014,Jun,3; 2014,Jan,11; 2013,Nov,3; 2013,Apr,3-4; 2012,Jan,15-42

**99367  Medical team conference with interdisciplinary team of health care professionals, patient and/or family not present, 30 minutes or more; participation by physician**

INCLUDES  Team conferences of 30 minutes or more

🚑 1.59  ⚖ 1.59  **FUD** XXX  N 🖵

**AMA:** 2017,Jan,8; 2016,Jan,13; 2015,Jan,16; 2014,Oct,8; 2014,Jun,3; 2014,Jan,11; 2013,Nov,3; 2013,Apr,3-4

**99368  participation by nonphysician qualified health care professional**

INCLUDES  Team conferences of 30 minutes or more

🚑 1.04  ⚖ 1.04  **FUD** XXX  N 🖵

**AMA:** 2017,Jan,8; 2016,Jan,13; 2015,Jan,16; 2014,Oct,8; 2014,Oct,3; 2014,Jun,3; 2014,Jan,11; 2013,Nov,3; 2013,Apr,3-4; 2012,Jan,15-42

● New Code  ▲ Revised Code  ○ Reinstated  ● New Web Release  ▲ Revised Web Release  Unlisted  Not Covered  # Resequenced

⊘ AMA Mod 51 Exempt  ⑤ Optum Mod 51 Exempt  ⑥ Mod 63 Exempt  ✗ Non-FDA Drug  ★ Telemedicine  Ⓜ Maternity  Ⓐ Age Edit  + Add-on  **AMA:** CPT Asst

© 2017 Optum360, LLC    CPT © 2017 American Medical Association. All Rights Reserved.    **515**

## 99374-99380 Care Plan Oversight: Patient Under Care of HHA, Hospice, or Nursing Facility

**CMS:** 100-04,11,40.1.3 Independent Attending Physician Services; 100-04,12,180 Payment of Care Plan Oversight (CPO); 100-04,12,180.1 Billing for Care Plan Oversight (CPO); 100-04,12,30.6.4 Services Furnished Incident to Physician's Service

**INCLUDES**   Analysis of reports, diagnostic tests, treatment plans

Discussions with other health care providers, outside of the practice, involved in the patient's care

Establishment of and revisions to care plans within a 30-day period

Payment to one physician per month for covered care plan oversight services (must be the same one who signed the plan of care)

**EXCLUDES**   *Care plan oversight services provided in a hospice agency (99377-99378)*

*Care plan oversight services provided in assisted living, domiciliary care, or private residence, not under care of a home health agency or hospice (99339-99340)*

*Patient management services during same time frame as (99441-99444, 99487-99498, 99495-99496, 98966-98969)*

*Routine postoperative care provided during a global surgery period*

*Time discussing treatment with patient and/or caregivers*

Code also office/outpatient visits, hospital, home, nursing facility, domiciliary, or non-face-to-face services

**99374**   **Supervision of a patient under care of home health agency (patient not present) in home, domiciliary or equivalent environment (eg, Alzheimer's facility) requiring complex and multidisciplinary care modalities involving regular development and/or revision of care plans by that individual, review of subsequent reports of patient status, review of related laboratory and other studies, communication (including telephone calls) for purposes of assessment or care decisions with health care professional(s), family member(s), surrogate decision maker(s) (eg, legal guardian) and/or key caregiver(s) involved in patient's care, integration of new information into the medical treatment plan and/or adjustment of medical therapy, within a calendar month; 15-29 minutes**

      1.59    1.98   **FUD** XXX       B ▣

      **AMA:** 2017,Jan,8; 2016,Jan,13; 2015,Jan,16; 2014,Oct,8; 2014,Oct,3; 2014,Jan,11; 2013,Nov,3; 2013,Sep,15-16; 2013,Jul,11-12; 2013,Apr,3-4

**99375**   **30 minutes or more**

      2.49    2.95   **FUD** XXX       E ▣

      **AMA:** 2017,Jan,8; 2016,Jan,13; 2015,Jan,16; 2014,Oct,8; 2014,Oct,3; 2014,Jan,11; 2013,Nov,3; 2013,Sep,15-16; 2013,Jul,11-12; 2013,Apr,3-4

**99377**   **Supervision of a hospice patient (patient not present) requiring complex and multidisciplinary care modalities involving regular development and/or revision of care plans by that individual, review of subsequent reports of patient status, review of related laboratory and other studies, communication (including telephone calls) for purposes of assessment or care decisions with health care professional(s), family member(s), surrogate decision maker(s) (eg, legal guardian) and/or key caregiver(s) involved in patient's care, integration of new information into the medical treatment plan and/or adjustment of medical therapy, within a calendar month; 15-29 minutes**

      1.59    1.98   **FUD** XXX       B ▣

      **AMA:** 2017,Jan,8; 2016,Jan,13; 2015,Jan,16; 2014,Oct,8; 2014,Oct,3; 2014,Jan,11; 2013,Nov,3; 2013,Sep,15-16; 2013,Jul,11-12; 2013,Apr,3-4

**99378**   **30 minutes or more**

      2.49    2.95   **FUD** XXX       E ▣

      **AMA:** 2017,Jan,8; 2016,Jan,13; 2015,Jan,16; 2014,Oct,8; 2014,Oct,3; 2014,Jan,11; 2013,Nov,3; 2013,Sep,15-16; 2013,Jul,11-12; 2013,Apr,3-4

**99379**   **Supervision of a nursing facility patient (patient not present) requiring complex and multidisciplinary care modalities involving regular development and/or revision of care plans by that individual, review of subsequent reports of patient status, review of related laboratory and other studies, communication (including telephone calls) for purposes of assessment or care decisions with health care professional(s), family member(s), surrogate decision maker(s) (eg, legal guardian) and/or key caregiver(s) involved in patient's care, integration of new information into the medical treatment plan and/or adjustment of medical therapy, within a calendar month; 15-29 minutes**

      1.59    1.98   **FUD** XXX       B ▣

      **AMA:** 2017,Jan,8; 2016,Jan,13; 2015,Jan,16; 2014,Oct,8; 2014,Oct,3; 2014,Jan,11; 2013,Nov,3; 2013,Sep,15-16; 2013,Jul,11-12; 2013,Apr,3-4

**99380**   **30 minutes or more**

      2.49    2.95   **FUD** XXX       B ▣

      **AMA:** 2017,Jan,8; 2016,Jan,13; 2015,Jan,16; 2014,Oct,8; 2014,Oct,3; 2014,Jan,11; 2013,Nov,3; 2013,Sep,15-16; 2013,Jul,11-12; 2013,Apr,3-4

## 99381-99397 Preventive Medicine Visits

**CMS:** 100-04,11,40.1.3 Independent Attending Physician Services; 100-04,12,30.6.2 Medically Necessary and Preventive Medicine Service on Same Date; 100-04,12,30.6.4 Services Furnished Incident to Physician's Service

**INCLUDES**   Care of a small problem or preexisting condition that requires no extra work

New patients or established patients (99381-99387, 99391-99397)

Regular preventive care (e.g., well-child exams) for all age groups

**EXCLUDES**   *Behavioral change interventions (99406-99409)*

*Counseling/risk factor reduction interventions not provided with a preventive medical examination (99401-99412)*

*Diagnostic tests and other procedures*

Code also immunization counseling, administration, and product (90460-90461, 90471-90474, 90476-90749 [90620, 90621, 90625, 90630, 90644, 90672, 90673, 90674, 90750, 90756])

Code also significant, separately identifiable E&M service on the same date for substantial problems requiring additional work using modifier 25 and (99201-99215)

**99381**   **Initial comprehensive preventive medicine evaluation and management of an individual including an age and gender appropriate history, examination, counseling/anticipatory guidance/risk factor reduction interventions, and the ordering of laboratory/diagnostic procedures, new patient; infant (age younger than 1 year)**   A

      2.17    3.11   **FUD** XXX       E ▣

      **AMA:** 2017,Jan,8; 2016,Mar,8; 2016,Jan,13; 2015,Jan,16; 2014,Oct,8; 2014,Jan,11; 2013,Jan,9-10; 2012,Jan,15-42

**99382**   **early childhood (age 1 through 4 years)**   A

      2.30    3.25   **FUD** XXX       E ▣

      **AMA:** 2017,Jan,8; 2016,Mar,8; 2016,Jan,13; 2015,Jan,16; 2014,Oct,8; 2014,Jan,11; 2013,Jan,9-10

**99383**   **late childhood (age 5 through 11 years)**   A

      2.45    3.39   **FUD** XXX       E ▣

      **AMA:** 2017,Jan,8; 2016,Mar,8; 2016,Jan,13; 2015,Jan,16; 2014,Oct,8; 2014,Jan,11; 2013,Jan,9-10

**99384**   **adolescent (age 12 through 17 years)**   A

      2.89    3.81   **FUD** XXX       E ▣

      **AMA:** 2017,Jan,8; 2016,Mar,8; 2016,Jan,13; 2015,Jan,16; 2015,Jan,12; 2014,Oct,8; 2014,Jan,11; 2013,Jan,9-10

**99385**   **18-39 years**   A

      2.77    3.69   **FUD** XXX       E ▣

      **AMA:** 2017,Jan,8; 2016,Mar,8; 2016,Jan,13; 2015,Jan,16; 2015,Jan,12; 2014,Oct,8; 2014,Jan,11; 2013,Jan,9-10

**99386**   **40-64 years**   A

      3.37    4.29   **FUD** XXX       E ▣

      **AMA:** 2017,Jan,8; 2016,Mar,8; 2016,Jan,13; 2015,Jan,16; 2015,Jan,12; 2014,Oct,8; 2014,Jan,11; 2013,Jan,9-10

**26/TC** PC/TC Only   **A2-A3** ASC Payment   **50** Bilateral   ♂ Male Only   ♀ Female Only   ⚡ Facility RVU   ✂ Non-Facility RVU   ▢ CCI

**FUD** Follow-up Days   **CMS:** IOM (Pub 100)   **A-Y** OPPSI   **80/81** Surg Assist Allowed / w/Doc   ▣ Lab Crosswalk   ▣ Radiology Crosswalk   ✖ CLIA

CPT © 2017 American Medical Association. All Rights Reserved.       © 2017 Optum360, LLC

**99387** **65 years and older**
3.61  4.65  **FUD** XXX
AMA: 2017,Jan,8; 2016,Mar,8; 2016,Jan,13; 2015,Jan,16; 2014,Oct,8; 2014,Jan,11; 2013,Jan,9-10

**99391** **Periodic comprehensive preventive medicine reevaluation and management of an individual including an age and gender appropriate history, examination, counseling/anticipatory guidance/risk factor reduction interventions, and the ordering of laboratory/diagnostic procedures, established patient; infant (age younger than 1 year)**
1.98  2.79  **FUD** XXX
AMA: 2017,Jan,8; 2016,Mar,8; 2016,Jan,13; 2015,Jan,16; 2014,Oct,8; 2014,Jan,11; 2013,Jan,9-10

**99392** **early childhood (age 1 through 4 years)**
2.17  2.98  **FUD** XXX
AMA: 2017,Jan,8; 2016,Mar,8; 2016,Jan,13; 2015,Jan,16; 2014,Oct,8; 2014,Jan,11; 2013,Jan,9-10

**99393** **late childhood (age 5 through 11 years)**
2.17  2.97  **FUD** XXX
AMA: 2017,Jan,8; 2016,Mar,8; 2016,Jan,13; 2015,Jan,16; 2014,Oct,8; 2014,Jan,11; 2013,Jan,9-10

**99394** **adolescent (age 12 through 17 years)**
2.45  3.26  **FUD** XXX
AMA: 2017,Jan,8; 2016,Mar,8; 2016,Jan,13; 2015,Jan,16; 2015,Jan,12; 2014,Oct,8; 2014,Jan,11; 2013,Jan,9-10

**99395** **18-39 years**
2.52  3.33  **FUD** XXX
AMA: 2017,Jan,8; 2016,Mar,8; 2016,Jan,13; 2015,Jan,16; 2015,Jan,12; 2014,Oct,8; 2014,Jan,11; 2013,Jan,9-10

**99396** **40-64 years**
2.74  3.55  **FUD** XXX
AMA: 2017,Sep,11; 2017,Jan,8; 2016,Mar,8; 2016,Jan,13; 2015,Jan,16; 2015,Jan,12; 2014,Oct,8; 2014,Jan,11; 2013,Jan,9-10; 2012,Mar,4-7

**99397** **65 years and older**
2.89  3.82  **FUD** XXX
AMA: 2017,Jan,8; 2016,Mar,8; 2016,Jan,13; 2015,Jan,16; 2014,Oct,8; 2014,Jan,11; 2013,Jan,9-10; 2012,Jan,15-42

# 99401-99416 Counseling Services: Risk Factor and Behavioral Change Modification

INCLUDES   Face-to-face services for new and established patients based on time increments of 15 to 60 minutes
Health and behavioral services provided on the same day (96150-96155)
Issues such as a healthy diet, exercise, alcohol and drug abuse
Services provided by a physician or other qualified healthcare professional for the purpose of promoting health and reducing illness and injury

EXCLUDES   *Counseling and risk factor reduction interventions included in preventive medicine services (99381-99397)*
*Counseling services provided to patient groups with existing symptoms or illness (99078)*
Code also significant, separately identifiable E&M services when performed and append modifier 25 to that service

**99401** **Preventive medicine counseling and/or risk factor reduction intervention(s) provided to an individual (separate procedure); approximately 15 minutes**
0.69  1.02  **FUD** XXX
AMA: 2017,Jan,8; 2016,Mar,8; 2016,Jan,13; 2015,Jan,16; 2014,Oct,8; 2014,Aug,5; 2014,Jan,11; 2013,Jan,9-10

**99402** **approximately 30 minutes**
1.42  1.74  **FUD** XXX
AMA: 2017,Jan,8; 2016,Mar,8; 2016,Jan,13; 2015,Jan,16; 2014,Oct,8; 2014,Aug,5; 2014,Jan,11; 2013,Jan,9-10

**99403** **approximately 45 minutes**
2.11  2.44  **FUD** XXX
AMA: 2017,Jan,8; 2016,Mar,8; 2016,Jan,13; 2015,Jan,16; 2014,Oct,8; 2014,Aug,5; 2014,Jan,11; 2013,Jan,9-10

**99404** **approximately 60 minutes**
2.82  3.14  **FUD** XXX
AMA: 2017,Jan,8; 2016,Mar,8; 2016,Jan,13; 2015,Jan,16; 2014,Oct,8; 2014,Aug,5; 2014,Jan,11; 2013,Jan,9-10

**99406** **Smoking and tobacco use cessation counseling visit; intermediate, greater than 3 minutes up to 10 minutes**
0.35  0.41  **FUD** XXX   ★ S 80
AMA: 2017,Jan,8; 2016,Mar,8; 2016,Jan,13; 2015,Jan,16; 2014,Oct,8; 2014,Jan,11; 2013,Jan,9-10; 2012,Jan,15-42

**99407** **intensive, greater than 10 minutes**
INCLUDES   Time duration of (99406)
0.73  0.79  **FUD** XXX   ★ S 80
AMA: 2017,Jan,8; 2016,Mar,8; 2016,Jan,13; 2015,Jan,16; 2014,Oct,8; 2014,Jan,11; 2013,Jan,9-10; 2012,Jan,15-42

**99408** **Alcohol and/or substance (other than tobacco) abuse structured screening (eg, AUDIT, DAST), and brief intervention (SBI) services; 15 to 30 minutes**
INCLUDES   Health risk assessment (96160-96161)
Only initial screening and brief intervention
Services of 15 minutes or more
0.94  0.99  **FUD** XXX   ★ E
AMA: 2017,Jan,8; 2016,Nov,5; 2016,Mar,8; 2016,Jan,13; 2015,Jan,16; 2014,Oct,8; 2014,Jan,11; 2013,Jan,9-10

**99409** **greater than 30 minutes**
INCLUDES   Health risk assessment (96160-96161)
Only initial screening and brief intervention
Time duration of (99408)
1.88  1.93  **FUD** XXX   ★ E
AMA: 2017,Jan,8; 2016,Nov,5; 2016,Mar,8; 2016,Jan,13; 2015,Jan,16; 2014,Oct,8; 2014,Jan,11; 2013,Jan,9-10

**99411** **Preventive medicine counseling and/or risk factor reduction intervention(s) provided to individuals in a group setting (separate procedure); approximately 30 minutes**
0.22  0.46  **FUD** XXX
AMA: 2017,Jan,8; 2016,Mar,8; 2016,Jan,13; 2015,Jan,16; 2014,Oct,8; 2014,Jan,11; 2013,Jan,9-10

**99412** **approximately 60 minutes**
0.36  0.60  **FUD** XXX
AMA: 2017,Jan,8; 2016,Mar,8; 2016,Jan,13; 2015,Jan,16; 2014,Oct,8; 2014,Jan,11; 2013,Jan,9-10

**99415** *Resequenced code. See code following 99359.*

**99416** *Resequenced code. See code following 99359.*

# 99429 Other Preventive Medicine

**99429** **Unlisted preventive medicine service**
0.00  0.00  **FUD** XXX
AMA: 2017,Jan,8; 2016,Mar,8; 2016,Jan,13; 2015,Jan,16; 2014,Oct,8; 2014,Jan,11; 2013,Jan,9-10

● New Code   ▲ Revised Code   ○ Reinstated   ● New Web Release   ▲ Revised Web Release   Unlisted   Not Covered   # Resequenced
⊘ AMA Mod 51 Exempt   ⑪ Optum Mod 51 Exempt   ⑥ Mod 63 Exempt   ✗ Non-FDA Drug   ★ Telemedicine   Ⓜ Maternity   Ⓐ Age Edit   + Add-on   AMA: CPT Asst
© 2017 Optum360, LLC          CPT © 2017 American Medical Association. All Rights Reserved.          **517**

## 99441-99443 Telephone Calls for Patient Management

**CMS:** 100-04,11,40.1.3 Independent Attending Physician Services

**INCLUDES**
Episodes of care initiated by an established patient or the patient or guardian of an established patient
Non-face-to-face E&M services provided by a physician or other health care provider qualified to report E&M services
Related E&M services provided within:
Postoperative period of a completed procedure
Seven days prior to the service

**EXCLUDES**
*Patient management services during same time frame as (99339-99340, 99374-99380, 99487-99489, 99495-99496, 93792-93793)*
*Services provided by a qualified nonphysician health care professional unable to report E&M codes (98966-98968)*
*Use of codes more than one time for telephone and online services when reported within a seven day period of time by the same provider*

**99441** **Telephone evaluation and management service by a physician or other qualified health care professional who may report evaluation and management services provided to an established patient, parent, or guardian not originating from a related E/M service provided within the previous 7 days nor leading to an E/M service or procedure within the next 24 hours or soonest available appointment; 5-10 minutes of medical discussion**
0.36   0.39   **FUD** XXX   E
**AMA:** 2017,Jan,8; 2016,Jan,13; 2015,Jan,16; 2014,Oct,8; 2014,Oct,3; 2014,Jan,11; 2013,Oct,11; 2013,Nov,3; 2013,Apr,3-4

**99442** **11-20 minutes of medical discussion**
0.72   0.76   **FUD** XXX   E
**AMA:** 2017,Jan,8; 2016,Jan,13; 2015,Jan,16; 2014,Oct,8; 2014,Oct,3; 2014,Jan,11; 2013,Oct,11; 2013,Nov,3; 2013,Apr,3-4

**99443** **21-30 minutes of medical discussion**
1.08   1.12   **FUD** XXX   E
**AMA:** 2017,Jan,8; 2016,Jan,13; 2015,Jan,16; 2014,Oct,8; 2014,Oct,3; 2014,Jan,11; 2013,Oct,11; 2013,Nov,3; 2013,Apr,3-4

## 99444 Online Patient Management Services

**CMS:** 100-04,11,40.1.3 Independent Attending Physician Services

**INCLUDES**
All related communications such as related phone calls, prescription and lab orders
Permanent electronic or hardcopy storage
Physician evaluation and management services provided via the internet in response to a patient's on-line inquiry
Physician's personal timely response
Related E&M services provided within:
Postoperative period of a completed procedure
Seven days prior to the service

**EXCLUDES**
*Online medical evaluation by a qualified nonphysician health care professional (98969)*
*Patient management services during same time frame as (99339-99340, 99374-99380, 99487-99489, 99495-99496, 93792-93793)*

**99444** **Online evaluation and management service provided by a physician or other qualified health care professional who may report evaluation and management services provided to an established patient or guardian, not originating from a related E/M service provided within the previous 7 days, using the Internet or similar electronic communications network**
0.00   0.00   **FUD** XXX   E
**AMA:** 2017,Jan,8; 2016,Jan,13; 2015,Jan,16; 2014,Oct,8; 2014,Oct,3; 2014,Jan,11; 2013,Oct,11; 2013,Nov,3; 2013,Apr,3-4; 2012,Nov,13-14

## 99446-99449 Online and Telephone Consultative Services

**CMS:** 100-04,11,40.1.3 Independent Attending Physician Services

**INCLUDES**
Multiple telephone and/or internet contact needed to complete the consultation (e.g., test result(s) follow-up)
New or established patient with new problem or exacerbation of existing problem and not seen within the last 14 days
Review of pertinent lab, imaging and/or pathology studies, medical records, medications reported only once within a 7 day period

**EXCLUDES**
*Any service less than 5 minutes*
*Communication with family with or without the patient present (99441-99444, 98966-98969)*
*Online services*
*Physician to patient (99444)*
*Qualified health care professional to patient (98969)*
*Requesting physician's time 30 minutes over the typical E&M service and patient is not on-site (99358-99359)*
*Requesting physician's time 30 minutes over the typical E&M service and patient is on-site (99354-99357)*
*Telephone services*
*Physician to patient (99441-99443)*
*Qualified health care professional to patient (98966-98968)*
*Transfer of care only*

**99446** **Interprofessional telephone/Internet assessment and management service provided by a consultative physician including a verbal and written report to the patient's treating/requesting physician or other qualified health care professional; 5-10 minutes of medical consultative discussion and review**
0.00   0.00   **FUD** XXX   E
**AMA:** 2017,Jan,8; 2016,Jan,13; 2015,Jan,16; 2014,Oct,8; 2014,Jun,14; 2013,Oct,11

**99447** **11-20 minutes of medical consultative discussion and review**
0.00   0.00   **FUD** XXX   E
**AMA:** 2017,Jan,8; 2016,Jan,13; 2015,Jan,16; 2014,Oct,8; 2014,Jun,14; 2013,Oct,11

**99448** **21-30 minutes of medical consultative discussion and review**
0.00   0.00   **FUD** XXX   E
**AMA:** 2017,Jan,8; 2016,Jan,13; 2015,Jan,16; 2014,Oct,8; 2014,Jun,14; 2013,Oct,11

**99449** **31 minutes or more of medical consultative discussion and review**
0.00   0.00   **FUD** XXX   E
**AMA:** 2017,Jan,8; 2016,Jan,13; 2015,Jan,16; 2014,Oct,8; 2014,Jun,14; 2013,Oct,11

## 99450-99456 Life/Disability Insurance Eligibility Visits

**CMS:** 100-04,12,30.6.4 Services Furnished Incident to Physician's Service

**INCLUDES**
Assessment services for insurance eligibility and work-related disability without medical management of the patient's illness/injury
Services provided to new/established patients at any site of service

**EXCLUDES**
*Any additional E&M services or procedures performed on the same date of service: report with appropriate code*

**99450** **Basic life and/or disability examination that includes: Measurement of height, weight, and blood pressure; Completion of a medical history following a life insurance pro forma; Collection of blood sample and/or urinalysis complying with "chain of custody" protocols; and Completion of necessary documentation/certificates.**
0.00   0.00   **FUD** XXX   E
**AMA:** 2017,Jan,8; 2016,Jan,13; 2015,Jan,16; 2014,Oct,8; 2014,Jan,11

CPT © 2017 American Medical Association. All Rights Reserved.          © 2017 Optum360, LLC

**99455** Work related or medical disability examination by the treating physician that includes: Completion of a medical history commensurate with the patient's condition; Performance of an examination commensurate with the patient's condition; Formulation of a diagnosis, assessment of capabilities and stability, and calculation of impairment; Development of future medical treatment plan; and Completion of necessary documentation/certificates and report.

INCLUDES    Special reports (99080)

🔹 0.00    ⚕ 0.00    **FUD** XXX                    B 80 💻

**AMA:** 2017,Jan,8; 2016,Jan,13; 2015,Jan,16; 2014,Oct,8; 2014,Jan,11; 2013,Aug,13

**99456** Work related or medical disability examination by other than the treating physician that includes: Completion of a medical history commensurate with the patient's condition; Performance of an examination commensurate with the patient's condition; Formulation of a diagnosis, assessment of capabilities and stability, and calculation of impairment; Development of future medical treatment plan; and Completion of necessary documentation/certificates and report.

INCLUDES    Special reports (99080)

🔹 0.00    ⚕ 0.00    **FUD** XXX                    B 80 💻

**AMA:** 2017,Jan,8; 2016,Jan,13; 2015,Jan,16; 2014,Oct,8; 2014,Jan,11; 2013,Aug,13

## 99460-99463 Evaluation and Management Services for Age 28 Days or Less

**CMS:** 100-04,12,30.6.4 Services Furnished Incident to Physician's Service

INCLUDES    Family consultation
Healthy newborn history and physical
Medical record documentation
Ordering of diagnostic test and treatments
Services provided to healthy newborns age 28 days or less

EXCLUDES    Neonatal intensive and critical care services (99466-99469 [99485, 99486], 99477-99480)
Newborn follow up services in an office or outpatient setting (99201-99215, 99381, 99391)
Newborn hospital discharge services if provided on a date subsequent to the admission date (99238-99239)
Nonroutine neonatal inpatient evaluation and management services (99221-99233)

Code also circumcision (54150)
Code also attendance at delivery (99464)
Code also emergency resuscitation services (99465)

**99460** Initial hospital or birthing center care, per day, for evaluation and management of normal newborn infant    A

🔹 2.83    ⚕ 2.83    **FUD** XXX                    V 80 💻

**AMA:** 2017,Jan,8; 2016,Jan,13; 2015,Jan,16; 2014,Oct,8; 2014,Jan,11

**99461** Initial care, per day, for evaluation and management of normal newborn infant seen in other than hospital or birthing center    A

🔹 1.79    ⚕ 2.63    **FUD** XXX                    M 80 💻

**AMA:** 2017,Jan,8; 2016,Jan,13; 2015,Jan,16; 2014,Oct,8; 2014,Jan,11

**99462** Subsequent hospital care, per day, for evaluation and management of normal newborn    A

🔹 1.26    ⚕ 1.26    **FUD** XXX                    C 80 💻

**AMA:** 2017,Jan,8; 2016,Jan,13; 2015,Jan,16; 2014,Oct,8; 2014,Jan,11

**99463** Initial hospital or birthing center care, per day, for evaluation and management of normal newborn infant admitted and discharged on the same date    A

🔹 3.38    ⚕ 3.38    **FUD** XXX                    V 80 💻

**AMA:** 2017,Jan,8; 2016,Jan,13; 2015,Jan,16; 2014,Oct,8; 2014,Jan,11

## 99464-99465 Newborn Delivery Attendance/Resuscitation

**CMS:** 100-04,12,30.6.4 Services Furnished Incident to Physician's Service

**99464** Attendance at delivery (when requested by the delivering physician or other qualified health care professional) and initial stabilization of newborn    A

EXCLUDES    Resuscitation at delivery (99465)

🔹 2.18    ⚕ 2.18    **FUD** XXX                    N 80 💻

**AMA:** 2017,Jan,8; 2016,Jan,13; 2015,Jan,16; 2014,Oct,8; 2014,Jan,11

**99465** Delivery/birthing room resuscitation, provision of positive pressure ventilation and/or chest compressions in the presence of acute inadequate ventilation and/or cardiac output    A

EXCLUDES    Attendance at delivery (99464)
Code also any necessary procedures performed as part of the resuscitation

🔹 4.32    ⚕ 4.32    **FUD** XXX                    S 80 💻

**AMA:** 2017,Jan,8; 2016,Jan,13; 2015,Jan,16; 2014,Oct,8; 2014,Jan,11

## 99466-99467 Critical Care Transport Age 24 Months or Younger

**CMS:** 100-04,12,30.6.4 Services Furnished Incident to Physician's Service

INCLUDES    Face-to-face care starting when the physician assumes responsibility of the patient at the referring facility until the receiving facility accepts the patient
Physician presence during interfacility transfer of critically ill/injured patient 24 months of age or less
Services provided by the physician during transport:
Blood gases
Chest x-rays (71045-71046)
Data stored in computers (e.g., ECGs, blood pressures, hematologic data) (99090)
Gastric intubation (43752-43753)
Interpretation of cardiac output measurements (93562)
Pulse oximetry (94760-94762)
Routine monitoring:
Heart rate
Respiratory rate
Temporary transcutaneous pacing (92953)
Vascular access procedures (36000, 36400, 36405-36406, 36415, 36591, 36600)
Ventilatory management (94002-94003, 94660, 94662)

EXCLUDES    Neonatal hypothermia (99184)
Patient critical care transport services with personal contact with patient of less than 30 minutes
Physician directed emergency care via two-way voice communication with transporting staff (99288, [99485, 99486])
Services less than 30 minutes in duration (see E&M codes)
Services of the physician directing transport (control physician) ([99485, 99486])

Code also any services not designated as included in the critical care transport service

**99466** Critical care face-to-face services, during an interfacility transport of critically ill or critically injured pediatric patient, 24 months of age or younger; first 30-74 minutes of hands-on care during transport    A

🔹 6.89    ⚕ 6.89    **FUD** XXX                    N 80 💻

**AMA:** 2017,Jan,8; 2016,Jan,13; 2015,Jan,16; 2014,Oct,8; 2014,Jan,11; 2013,May,6-7

**+ 99467** each additional 30 minutes (List separately in addition to code for primary service)    A

Code first (99466)

🔹 3.46    ⚕ 3.46    **FUD** ZZZ                    N 80 💻

**AMA:** 2017,Jan,8; 2016,Jan,13; 2015,Jan,16; 2014,Oct,8; 2014,Jan,11; 2013,May,6-7

● New Code    ▲ Revised Code    ○ Reinstated    ● New Web Release    ▲ Revised Web Release    Unlisted    Not Covered    # Resequenced
⊘ AMA Mod 51 Exempt    ⑨ Optum Mod 51 Exempt    ⑥③ Mod 63 Exempt    ✂ Non-FDA Drug    ★ Telemedicine    Ⓜ Maternity    Ⓐ Age Edit    + Add-on    AMA: CPT Asst
© 2017 Optum360, LLC                    CPT © 2017 American Medical Association. All Rights Reserved.

## [99485, 99486] Critical Care Transport Supervision Age 24 Months or Younger

**INCLUDES** Advice for treatment to the transport team from the control physician
Non face-to-face care starts with first contact by the control physician with the transport team and ends when patient responsibility is assumed by the receiving facility

**EXCLUDES** *Emergency systems physician direction for pediatric patient older than 24 months (99288)*
*Services provided by transport team*
*Services less than 15 minutes*
*Services performed by control physician for the same time period*
*Services performed by same physician providing critical care transport (99466-99467)*

\#    **99485**    **Supervision by a control physician of interfacility transport care of the critically ill or critically injured pediatric patient, 24 months of age or younger, includes two-way communication with transport team before transport, at the referring facility and during the transport, including data interpretation and report; first 30 minutes** Ⓐ

🚑 2.17    ⚗ 2.17    **FUD** XXX    Ⓑ 🏳

**AMA:** 2017,Jan,8; 2016,Jan,13; 2015,Jan,16; 2014,Oct,8; 2013,May,6-7

\+ \#    **99486**    **each additional 30 minutes (List separately in addition to code for primary procedure)** Ⓐ

Code first ([99485])

🚑 1.88    ⚗ 1.88    **FUD** XXX    Ⓑ 🏳

**AMA:** 2017,Jan,8; 2016,Jan,13; 2015,Jan,16; 2014,Oct,8; 2013,May,6-7

## 99468-99476 Critical Care Age 5 Years or Younger

**CMS:** 100-04,12,30.6.4 Services Furnished Incident to Physician's Service

**INCLUDES** All services included in codes 99291-99292 as well as the following which may be reported by facilities only:
Administration of blood/blood components (36430, 36440)
Administration of intravenous fluids (96360-96361)
Administration of surfactant (94610)
Bladder aspiration, suprapubic (51100)
Bladder catheterization (51701, 51702)
Car seat evaluation (94780-94781)
Catheterization umbilical artery (36660)
Catheterization umbilical vein (36510)
Central venous catheter, centrally inserted (36555)
Endotracheal intubation (31500)
Lumbar puncture (62270)
Oral or nasogastric tube placement (43752)
Pulmonary function testing, performed at the bedside (94375)
Pulse or ear oximetry (94760-94762)
Vascular access, arteries (36140, 36620)
Vascular access, venous (36400-36406, 36420, 36600)
Ventilatory management (94002-94004, 94660)
Initial and subsequent care provided to a critically ill infant or child
Other hospital care or intensive care services by same group or individual done on same day that patient was transferred to initial neonatal/pediatric critical care
Readmission to critical unit on same day or during the same stay (subsequent care)

**EXCLUDES** *Critical care services for patients 6 years of age or older (99291-99292)*
*Critical care services provided by a second physician or physician of a different specialty (99291-99292)*
*Interfacility transport services by same or different individual of same or different specialty or group on same date of service (99466-99467, [99485, 99486])*
*Neonatal hypothermia (99184)*
*Remote critical care (0188T-0189T)*
*Services performed by individual in another group receiving a patient transferred to a lower level of care (99231-99233, 99478-99480)*
*Services performed by individual transferring a patient to a lower level of care (99231-99233, 99291-99292)*
*Services performed by same or different individual in same group on same day (99291-99292)*
*Services performed by transferring individual prior to transfer of patient to an individual in a different group (99221-99233, 99291-99292, 99460-99462, 99477-99480)*

Code also normal newborn care if done on same day by same group or individual that provides critical care. Report modifier 25 with initial critical care code (99460-99462)

**99468**    **Initial inpatient neonatal critical care, per day, for the evaluation and management of a critically ill neonate, 28 days of age or younger** Ⓐ

🚑 28.1    ⚗ 28.1    **FUD** XXX    Ⓒ 80 🏳

**AMA:** 2017,Jan,8; 2016,May,3; 2016,Jan,13; 2015,Oct,8; 2015,Jul,3; 2015,Feb,10; 2015,Jan,16; 2014,Oct,8; 2014,May,4; 2014,Jan,11; 2012,Aug,6-8

**99469**    **Subsequent inpatient neonatal critical care, per day, for the evaluation and management of a critically ill neonate, 28 days of age or younger** Ⓐ

🚑 11.3    ⚗ 11.3    **FUD** XXX    Ⓒ 80 🏳

**AMA:** 2017,Jan,8; 2016,May,3; 2016,Jan,13; 2015,Oct,8; 2015,Jul,3; 2015,Feb,10; 2015,Jan,16; 2014,Oct,8; 2014,May,4; 2014,Jan,11; 2012,Aug,6-8

**99471**    **Initial inpatient pediatric critical care, per day, for the evaluation and management of a critically ill infant or young child, 29 days through 24 months of age** Ⓐ

🚑 24.4    ⚗ 24.4    **FUD** XXX    Ⓒ 80 🏳

**AMA:** 2017,Jan,8; 2016,May,3; 2016,Jan,13; 2015,Jul,3; 2015,Feb,10; 2015,Jan,16; 2014,Oct,8; 2014,Jan,11; 2012,Aug,6-8

**99472**    **Subsequent inpatient pediatric critical care, per day, for the evaluation and management of a critically ill infant or young child, 29 days through 24 months of age** Ⓐ

🚑 11.6    ⚗ 11.6    **FUD** XXX    Ⓒ 80 🏳

**AMA:** 2017,Jan,8; 2016,May,3; 2016,Jan,13; 2015,Jul,3; 2015,Feb,10; 2015,Jan,16; 2014,Oct,8; 2014,Jan,11; 2012,Aug,6-8

26/TC PC/TC Only    A2-Z3 ASC Payment    50 Bilateral    ♂ Male Only    🚑 Facility RVU    ⚗ Non-Facility RVU    □ CCI
**FUD** Follow-up Days    **CMS:** IOM (Pub 100)    A-Y OPPSI    80/80 Surg Assist Allowed / w/Doc    ▪ Lab Crosswalk    ▪ Radiology Crosswalk    ✖ CLIA
**520**                                                  ♀ Female Only
CPT © 2017 American Medical Association. All Rights Reserved.                                          © 2017 Optum360, LLC

**99475** Initial inpatient pediatric critical care, per day, for the evaluation and management of a critically ill infant or young child, 2 through 5 years of age   🅰
    🔁 16.3    ⚖ 16.3    **FUD** XXX     Ⓒ 80 🖵
    **AMA:** 2017,Jan,8; 2016,May,3; 2016,Jan,13; 2015,Jul,3; 2015,Feb,10; 2015,Jan,16; 2014,Oct,8; 2014,Jan,11

**99476** Subsequent inpatient pediatric critical care, per day, for the evaluation and management of a critically ill infant or young child, 2 through 5 years of age   🅰
    🔁 9.74    ⚖ 9.74    **FUD** XXX     Ⓒ 80 🖵
    **AMA:** 2017,Jan,8; 2016,May,3; 2016,Jan,13; 2015,Jul,3; 2015,Feb,10; 2015,Jan,16; 2014,Oct,8; 2014,Jan,11

## 99477-99480 Initial Inpatient Neonatal Intensive Care and Other Services

**CMS:** 100-04,12,30.6.4 Services Furnished Incident to Physician's Service

INCLUDES     All services included in codes 99291-99292 as well as the following that may be reported by facilities only:
    Adjustments to enteral and/or parenteral nutrition
    Airway and ventilator management (31500, 94002-94004, 94375, 94610, 94660)
    Bladder catheterization (51701-51702)
    Blood transfusion (36430, 36440)
    Car seat evaluation (94780-94781)
    Constant and/or frequent monitoring of vital signs
    Continuous observation by the healthcare team
    Heat maintenance
    Intensive cardiac or respiratory monitoring
    Oral or nasogastric tube insertion (43752)
    Oxygen saturation (94760-94762)
    Spinal puncture (62270)
    Suprapubic catheterization (51100)
    Vascular access procedures (36000, 36140, 36400, 36405-36406, 36420, 36510, 36555, 36600, 36620, 36660)

EXCLUDES    *Critical care services for patient transferred after initial or subsequent intensive care is provided (99291-99292)*
    *Initial day intensive care provided by transferring individual same day neonate/infant transferred to a lower level of care (99477)*
    *Inpatient neonatal/pediatric critical care services received on same day (99468-99476)*
    *Necessary resuscitation services done as part of delivery care prior to admission*
    *Neonatal hypothermia (99184)*
    *Services provided by receiving individual when patient is transferred for critical care (99468-99476)*
    *Services for receiving provider when patient improves after the initial day and is transferred to a lower level of care (99231-99233, 99478-99480)*
    *Subsequent care of a sick neonate, under 28 days of age, more than 5000 grams, not requiring critical or intensive care services (99231-99233)*
Code also care provided by receiving individual when patient is transferred to an individual in different group (99231-99233, 99462)
Code also initial neonatal intensive care service when physician or other qualified health care professional is present for delivery and/or neonate requires resuscitation (99464-99465); append modifier 25 to (99477)

**99477** Initial hospital care, per day, for the evaluation and management of the neonate, 28 days of age or younger, who requires intensive observation, frequent interventions, and other intensive care services   🅰
     EXCLUDES   *Initiation of care of a critically ill neonate (99468)*
       *Initiation of inpatient care of a normal newborn (99460)*
    🔁 10.0    ⚖ 10.0    **FUD** XXX     Ⓒ 80 🖵
    **AMA:** 2017,Jan,8; 2016,Jan,13; 2015,Jul,3; 2015,Jan,16; 2014,Oct,8; 2014,Jan,11; 2012,Aug,6-8

**99478** Subsequent intensive care, per day, for the evaluation and management of the recovering very low birth weight infant (present body weight less than 1500 grams)   🅰
    🔁 3.97    ⚖ 3.97    **FUD** XXX     Ⓒ 80 🖵
    **AMA:** 2017,Jan,8; 2016,Jan,13; 2015,Jul,3; 2015,Jan,16; 2014,Oct,8; 2014,Jan,11; 2012,Aug,6-8

**99479** Subsequent intensive care, per day, for the evaluation and management of the recovering low birth weight infant (present body weight of 1500-2500 grams)   🅰
    🔁 3.53    ⚖ 3.53    **FUD** XXX     Ⓒ 80 🖵
    **AMA:** 2017,Jan,8; 2016,Jan,13; 2015,Jul,3; 2015,Jan,16; 2014,Oct,8; 2014,Jan,11; 2012,Aug,6-8

**99480** Subsequent intensive care, per day, for the evaluation and management of the recovering infant (present body weight of 2501-5000 grams)   🅰
    🔁 3.41    ⚖ 3.41    **FUD** XXX     Ⓒ 80 🖵
    **AMA:** 2017,Jan,8; 2016,Jan,13; 2015,Jul,3; 2015,Jan,16; 2014,Oct,8; 2014,Jan,11; 2012,Aug,6-8

## 99483-99486 Cognitive Impairment Services

INCLUDES    Evaluation and care plans for new or existing patients with symptoms of cognitive impairment
    Assessment and care plan services during the same time frame as:
     E&M services (99201-99215, 99241-99245, 99324-99337, 99341-99350, 99355-99368 [99415, 99416], 99497-99498)
     Medication management (99605-99607)
     Need for services evaluation (e.g., legal, financial, meals, personal care)
     Patient and caregiver focused risk assessment (96160-96161)
     Psychiatric and psychological services (90785, 90791-90792, 96103, 96127)
    Consideration of other conditions that may cause cognitive impairment (e.g., infection, hydrocephalus, stroke, medications)

EXCLUDES    *Use of code more than one time per 180 day period*

● **99483** Assessment of and care planning for a patient with cognitive impairment, requiring an independent historian, in the office or other outpatient, home or domiciliary or rest home, with all of the following required elements: Cognition-focused evaluation including a pertinent history and examination; Medical decision making of moderate or high complexity; Functional assessment (eg, basic and instrumental activities of daily living), including decision-making capacity; Use of standardized instruments for staging of dementia (eg, functional assessment staging test [FAST], clinical dementia rating [CDR]); Medication reconciliation and review for high-risk medications; Evaluation for neuropsychiatric and behavioral symptoms, including depression, including use of standardized screening instrument(s); Evaluation of safety (eg, home), including motor vehicle operation; Identification of caregiver(s), caregiver knowledge, caregiver needs, social supports, and the willingness of caregiver to take on caregiving tasks; Development, updating or revision, or review of an Advance Care Plan; Creation of a written care plan, including initial plans to address any neuropsychiatric symptoms, neuro-cognitive symptoms, functional limitations, and referral to community resources as needed (eg, rehabilitation services, adult day programs, support groups) shared with the patient and/or caregiver with initial education and support. Typically, 50 minutes are spent face-to-face with the patient and/or family or caregiver.

*99484* Resequenced code. See code following 99498.

*99485* Resequenced code. See code following 99467.

*99486* Resequenced code. See code following 99467.

---

● New Code    ▲ Revised Code    ○ Reinstated    ● New Web Release    ▲ Revised Web Release    Unlisted    Not Covered    # Resequenced
Ⓢ AMA Mod 51 Exempt    Ⓢ Optum Mod 51 Exempt    ⑥³ Mod 63 Exempt    ✗ Non-FDA Drug    ★ Telemedicine    Ⓜ Maternity    🅰 Age Edit    + Add-on    **AMA:** CPT Asst
© 2017 Optum360, LLC      CPT © 2017 American Medical Association. All Rights Reserved.      **521**

**Evaluation and Management**

**99490 — 99493**

## [99490] Coordination of Services for Chronic Care

**CMS:** 100-02,13,110.5 Chronic Care Management (CCM) Services

INCLUDES  Case management services provided to patients that:
Have two or more conditions anticipated to endure more than 12 months or until the patient's death
Require at least 20 minutes of staff time monthly
Risk is high that conditions will result in decompensation, deterioration, or death
Patient management services during same time frame as (99339-99340, 99358-99359, 99366-99368, 99374-99380, 99441-99444, [99490], 99487, 99489, 99495-99496, 90951-90970, 93792-93793, 93792-93793, 98960-98962, 98969, 99071, 99078, 99080, 99090-99091, 99605-99607)
Services performed during a postoperative surgical period

EXCLUDES  Psychiatric collaborative care management (99484, 99492-99494)

\# **99490** **Chronic care management services, at least 20 minutes of clinical staff time directed by a physician or other qualified health care professional, per calendar month, with the following required elements: multiple (two or more) chronic conditions expected to last at least 12 months, or until the death of the patient; chronic conditions place the patient at significant risk of death, acute exacerbation/decompensation, or functional decline; comprehensive care plan established, implemented, revised, or monitored.**

⚕ 0.91   ⚖ 1.19   **FUD** XXX   S ▢

**AMA:** 2017,Jan,8; 2016,Jan,13; 2015,Feb,3; 2015,Jan,16; 2014,Oct,3

## 99487-99490 Coordination of Complex Services for Chronic Care

INCLUDES  All clinical non-face-to-face time with patient, family, and caregivers
Only services given by physician or other qualified health caregiver who has the role of care coordination for the patient for the month
Patient management services during same time frame as (99339-99340, 99358-99359, 99366-99368, 99374-99380, 99441-99444, 99495-99496, 90951-90970, 93792-93793, 98960-98962, 98966-98969, 99071, 99078, 99080, 99090-99091, 99605-99607)
Services provided to patients in a rest home, domiciliary, assisted living facility, or at home that include:
Caregiver education to family or patient, addressing independent living and self-management
Communication with patient and all caregivers and professionals regarding care
Determining which community and health resources would benefit the patient
Developing and maintaining a care plan
Facilitation of services and care
Health outcomes data and registry documentation
Providing communication with home health and other patient utilized services
Support for treatment and medication adherence
Services that address activities of daily living, psychosocial, and medical needs

EXCLUDES  E&M services by same/different individual during time frame of care management services
Psychiatric collaborative care management (99484, 99492-99494)

**99487** **Complex chronic care management services, with the following required elements: multiple (two or more) chronic conditions expected to last at least 12 months, or until the death of the patient, chronic conditions place the patient at significant risk of death, acute exacerbation/decompensation, or functional decline, establishment or substantial revision of a comprehensive care plan, moderate or high complexity medical decision making; 60 minutes of clinical staff time directed by a physician or other qualified health care professional, per calendar month**

INCLUDES  Clinical services, 60 to 74 minutes, during a calendar month

⚕ 1.47   ⚖ 2.61   **FUD** XXX   S 80 ▢

**AMA:** 2017,Apr,9; 2017,Jan,8; 2016,Jan,13; 2015,Jan,16; 2014,Oct,8; 2014,Oct,3; 2014,Jun,3; 2014,Feb,3; 2014,Jan,11; 2013,Nov,3; 2013,Sep,15-16; 2013,Apr,3-4; 2013,Jan,3-5

+ **99489** **each additional 30 minutes of clinical staff time directed by a physician or other qualified health care professional, per calendar month (List separately in addition to code for primary procedure)**

EXCLUDES  Clinical services less than 30 minutes beyond the initial 60 minutes of care, per calendar month
Code first (99487)

⚕ 0.74   ⚖ 1.31   **FUD** ZZZ   N 80 ▢

**AMA:** 2017,Apr,9; 2017,Jan,8; 2016,Jan,13; 2015,Jan,16; 2014,Oct,8; 2014,Oct,3; 2014,Jun,3; 2014,Jan,11; 2013,Nov,3; 2013,Sep,15-16; 2013,Apr,3-4; 2013,Jan,3-5

**99490** Resequenced code. See code before 99487.

## 99492-99494 Psychiatric Collaborative Care

INCLUDES  Services provided during a calendar month by a physician or other qualified healthcare profession for patients with a psychiatric diagnosis
Assessment of behavioral health status
Creation of and updating a care plan
Treatment provided during an episode of care during which goals may be met, not achieved, or there is a lack of services during a period of six months

EXCLUDES  Additional services provided by a behavioral health care manager during the same calendar month period (do not count as time for 99492-99494):
Psychiatric evaluation (90791-90792)
Psychotherapy (99406-99407, 99408-99409, 90832-90834, 90836-90838, 90839-90840, 90846-90847, 90849, 90853)
Services provided by a psychiatric consultant (do not count as time for 99492-99494): (E&M services) and psychiatric evaluation (90791-90792)

● **99492** **Initial psychiatric collaborative care management, first 70 minutes in the first calendar month of behavioral health care manager activities, in consultation with a psychiatric consultant, and directed by the treating physician or other qualified health care professional, with the following required elements: outreach to and engagement in treatment of a patient directed by the treating physician or other qualified health care professional; initial assessment of the patient, including administration of validated rating scales, with the development of an individualized treatment plan; review by the psychiatric consultant with modifications of the plan if recommended; entering patient in a registry and tracking patient follow-up and progress using the registry, with appropriate documentation, and participation in weekly caseload consultation with the psychiatric consultant; and provision of brief interventions using evidence-based techniques such as behavioral activation, motivational interviewing, and other focused treatment strategies.**

EXCLUDES  Services of less than 36 minutes
Subsequent collaborative care managment in same calendar month (99493)

● **99493** **Subsequent psychiatric collaborative care management, first 60 minutes in a subsequent month of behavioral health care manager activities, in consultation with a psychiatric consultant, and directed by the treating physician or other qualified health care professional, with the following required elements: tracking patient follow-up and progress using the registry, with appropriate documentation; participation in weekly caseload consultation with the psychiatric consultant; ongoing collaboration with and coordination of the patient's mental health care with the treating physician or other qualified health care professional and any other treating mental health providers; additional review of progress and recommendations for changes in treatment, as indicated, including medications, based on recommendations provided by the psychiatric consultant; provision of brief interventions using evidence-based techniques such as behavioral activation, motivational interviewing, and other focused treatment strategies; monitoring of patient outcomes using validated rating scales; and relapse prevention planning with patients as they achieve remission of symptoms and/or other treatment goals and are prepared for discharge from active treatment.**

EXCLUDES  Initial collaborative care managment in same calendar month (99492)

| 26/TC PC/TC Only | A2-Z3 ASC Payment | 50 Bilateral | ♂ Male Only | ♀ Female Only | ⚕ Facility RVU | ⚖ Non-Facility RVU | ▢ CCI |
| FUD Follow-up Days | CMS: IOM (Pub 100) | A-Y OPPSI | 80/80 Surg Assist Allowed / w/Doc | | ▨ Lab Crosswalk | ▨ Radiology Crosswalk | ✕ CLIA |

CPT © 2017 American Medical Association. All Rights Reserved.

© 2017 Optum360, LLC

● + **99494** Initial or subsequent psychiatric collaborative care management, each additional 30 minutes in a calendar month of behavioral health care manager activities, in consultation with a psychiatric consultant, and directed by the treating physician or other qualified health care professional (List separately in addition to code for primary procedure)

    🔟 0.00   🔗 0.00  **FUD** 000

    INCLUDES  Coordination of care with emergency department staff
    Code first (99492, 99493)

## 99495-99496 Management of Transitional Care Services

**CMS:** 100-02,13,110.4 Transitional Care Management (TCM) Services; 100-04,12,190.3 List of Telehealth Services

INCLUDES  First interaction (face-to-face, by telephone, or electronic) with patient or his/her caregiver and must be done within 2 working days of discharge
Initial face-to-face; must be done within code time frame and include medication management
New or established patient with moderate to high complexity medical decision making needs during care transitions
Patient management services during same time frame as (99339-99340, 99358-99359, 99366-99368, 99374-99380, 99441-99444, 99487-99489, 90951-90970, 93792-93793, 98960-98962, 98966-98969, 99071, 99078, 99080, 99090-99091, 99605-99607)
Services from discharge day up to 29 days post discharge
Subsequent discharge within 30 days
Without face-to-face patient care given by physician or other qualified health care professional includes:
  Arrangement of follow-up and referrals with community resources and providers
  Contacting qualified health care professionals for specific problems of patient
  Discharge information review
  Need for follow-up care review based on tests and treatments
  Patient, family, and caregiver education
Without face-to-face patient care given by staff under the guidance of physician or other qualified health care professional includes:
  Caregiver education to family or patient, addressing independent living and self-management
  Communication with patient and all caregivers and professionals regarding care
  Determining which community and health resources would benefit the patient
  Providing communication with home health and other patient utilized services
  Support for treatment and medication adherence
  The facilitation of services and care
EXCLUDES  E&M services after the first face-to-face visit

**99495** Transitional Care Management Services with the following required elements: Communication (direct contact, telephone, electronic) with the patient and/or caregiver within 2 business days of discharge Medical decision making of at least moderate complexity during the service period Face-to-face visit, within 14 calendar days of discharge

    🔟 3.12   🔗 4.61  **FUD** XXX    ★ V 80 ▣

    **AMA:** 2017,Jan,8; 2016,Jan,13; 2015,Jan,16; 2014,Oct,8; 2014,Oct,3; 2014,Mar,13; 2014,Jan,11; 2013,Nov,3; 2013,Dec,11; 2013,Sep,15-16; 2013,Aug,13; 2013,Jul,11-12; 2013,Apr,3-4; 2013,Jan,3-5

**99496** Transitional Care Management Services with the following required elements: Communication (direct contact, telephone, electronic) with the patient and/or caregiver within 2 business days of discharge Medical decision making of high complexity during the service period Face-to-face visit, within 7 calendar days of discharge

    🔟 4.52   🔗 6.52  **FUD** XXX    ★ V 80 ▣

    **AMA:** 2017,Jan,8; 2016,Jan,13; 2015,Jan,16; 2014,Oct,8; 2014,Oct,3; 2014,Mar,13; 2014,Jan,11; 2013,Nov,3; 2013,Sep,15-16; 2013,Aug,13; 2013,Jul,11-12; 2013,Apr,3-4; 2013,Jan,3-5

## 99497-99498 Advance Directive Guidance

**CMS:** 100-02,15,280.5.1 Advance Care Planning with an Annual Wellness Visit; 100-04,18,140.8 Advance Care Planning with an Annual Wellness Visit (AWV); 100-04,4,200.11 Advance Care Planning as an Optional Element of an Annual Wellness Visit

EXCLUDES  Critical care services (99291-99292, 99468-99469, 99471-99472, 99475-99476, 99477-99480, 99483)
    Services for cognitive care (99483)
    Treatment/management for an active problem (see appropriate E&M service)

**99497** Advance care planning including the explanation and discussion of advance directives such as standard forms (with completion of such forms, when performed), by the physician or other qualified health care professional; first 30 minutes, face-to-face with the patient, family member(s), and/or surrogate

    🔟 2.17   🔗 2.31  **FUD** XXX    01 80 ▣

    **AMA:** 2017,Jan,8; 2016,Feb,7; 2016,Jan,13; 2015,Jan,16; 2014,Dec,11

+ **99498** each additional 30 minutes (List separately in addition to code for primary procedure)

    🔟 2.02   🔗 2.02  **FUD** ZZZ    N 80 ▣

    **AMA:** 2017,Jan,8; 2016,Feb,7; 2016,Jan,13; 2015,Jan,16; 2014,Dec,11

## [99484] Behavioral Health Integration Care

INCLUDES  Care management services requiring 20 minutes or more per calendar month
Coordination of care with emergency department staff
Face to face services when necessary
Provided as an outpatient service
Provision of services by clinical staff and reported by supervising physician or other qualified healthcare professional
Provision of services to patients with whom there is an ongoing relationship
Treatment plan and specific service components
EXCLUDES  Other services for which the time or activities associated with that service aren't used to meet requirements for 99484:
    Chronic care management ([99490], 99487-99489)
    Psychiatric collaborative care in same calendar month (99492-99494)
    Psychotherapy services (90785-90899)

● # **99484** Care management services for behavioral health conditions, at least 20 minutes of clinical staff time, directed by a physician or other qualified health care professional, per calendar month, with the following required elements: initial assessment or follow-up monitoring, including the use of applicable validated rating scales; behavioral health care planning in relation to behavioral/psychiatric health problems, including revision for patients who are not progressing or whose status changes; facilitating and coordinating treatment such as psychotherapy, pharmacotherapy, counseling and/or psychiatric consultation; and continuity of care with a designated member of the care team.

    🔟 0.00   🔗 0.00  **FUD** 000

## 99499 Unlisted Evaluation and Management Services

**CMS:** 100-04,12,30.6.10 Consultation Services; 100-04,12,30.6.4 Services Furnished Incident to Physician's Service; 100-04,12,30.6.9.1 Initial Hospital Care and Observation or Inpatient Care Services

**99499** Unlisted evaluation and management service

    🔟 0.00   🔗 0.00  **FUD** XXX    B 80

    **AMA:** 2017,Jan,8; 2016,Jan,13; 2015,Jan,16; 2014,Oct,8; 2014,Jan,11; 2012,Nov,13-14; 2012,Jul,10-11; 2012,Apr,10; 2012,Jan,15-42

## 0001F-0015F Quality Measures with Multiple Components

INCLUDES    Several measures grouped within a single code descriptor to make possible reporting for clinical conditions when all of the components have been met

**0001F**    Heart failure assessed (includes assessment of all the following components) (CAD): Blood pressure measured (2000F) Level of activity assessed (1003F) Clinical symptoms of volume overload (excess) assessed (1004F) Weight, recorded (2001F) Clinical signs of volume overload (excess) assessed (2002F)

INCLUDES    Blood pressure measured (2000F)
Clinical signs of volume overload (excess) assessed (2002F)
Clinical symptoms of volume overload (excess) assessed (1004F)
Level of activity assessed (1003F)
Weight recorded (2001F)

🚑 0.00    ⚕ 0.00    **FUD** XXX              E

**AMA:** 2017,Jan,8; 2016,Jan,13; 2015,Jan,16; 2014,Jan,11

**0005F**    Osteoarthritis assessed (OA) Includes assessment of all the following components: Osteoarthritis symptoms and functional status assessed (1006F) Use of anti-inflammatory or over-the-counter (OTC) analgesic medications assessed (1007F) Initial examination of the involved joint(s) (includes visual inspection, palpation, range of motion) (2004F)

INCLUDES    Initial examination of the involved joint(s) (includes visual inspection/palpation/range of motion) (2004F)
Osteoarthritis symptoms and functional status assessed (1006F)
Use of anti-inflammatory or over-the-counter (OTC) analgesic medications assessed (1007F)

🚑 0.00    ⚕ 0.00    **FUD** XXX              E

**AMA:** 2005,Oct,1-5

**0012F**    Community-acquired bacterial pneumonia assessment (includes all of the following components) (CAP): Co-morbid conditions assessed (1026F) Vital signs recorded (2010F) Mental status assessed (2014F) Hydration status assessed (2018F)

🚑 0.00    ⚕ 0.00    **FUD** XXX              E

INCLUDES    Co-morbid conditions assessed (1026F)
Hydration status assessed (2018F)
Mental status assessed (2014F)
Vital signs recorded (2010F)

**0014F**    Comprehensive preoperative assessment performed for cataract surgery with intraocular lens (IOL) placement (includes assessment of all of the following components) (EC): Dilated fundus evaluation performed within 12 months prior to cataract surgery (2020F) Pre-surgical (cataract) axial length, corneal power measurement and method of intraocular lens power calculation documented (must be performed within 12 months prior to surgery) (3073F) Preoperative assessment of functional or medical indication(s) for surgery prior to the cataract surgery with intraocular lens placement (must be performed within 12 months prior to cataract surgery) (3325F)

INCLUDES    Evaluation of dilated fundus done within 12 months prior to surgery (2020F)
Preoperative assessment of functional or medical indications done within 12 months prior to surgery (3325F)
Presurgical measurement of axial length, corneal power, and IOL power calculation performed within 12 months prior to surgery (3073F)

🚑 0.00    ⚕ 0.00    **FUD** XXX              E

**AMA:** 2008,Mar,8-12

**0015F**    Melanoma follow up completed (includes assessment of all of the following components) (ML): History obtained regarding new or changing moles (1050F) Complete physical skin exam performed (2029F) Patient counseled to perform a monthly self skin examination (5005F)

INCLUDES    Complete physical skin exam (2029F)
Counseling to perform monthly skin self-examination (5005F)
History obtained of new or changing moles (1050F)

🚑 0.00    ⚕ 0.00    **FUD** XXX              E

**AMA:** 2008,Mar,8-12

## 0500F-0584F Care Provided According to Prevailing Guidelines

INCLUDES    Measures of utilization or patient care provided for certain clinical purposes

**0500F**    Initial prenatal care visit (report at first prenatal encounter with health care professional providing obstetrical care. Report also date of visit and, in a separate field, the date of the last menstrual period [LMP]) (Prenatal)    M ♀

🚑 0.00    ⚕ 0.00    **FUD** XXX              E

**AMA:** 2017,Jan,8; 2016,Jan,13; 2015,Jan,16; 2014,Jan,11

**0501F**    Prenatal flow sheet documented in medical record by first prenatal visit (documentation includes at minimum blood pressure, weight, urine protein, uterine size, fetal heart tones, and estimated date of delivery). Report also: date of visit and, in a separate field, the date of the last menstrual period [LMP] (Note: If reporting 0501F Prenatal flow sheet, it is not necessary to report 0500F Initial prenatal care visit) (Prenatal)    M ♀

🚑 0.00    ⚕ 0.00    **FUD** XXX              E

**AMA:** 2004,Nov,1

**0502F**    Subsequent prenatal care visit (Prenatal) [Excludes: patients who are seen for a condition unrelated to pregnancy or prenatal care (eg, an upper respiratory infection; patients seen for consultation only, not for continuing care)]    M ♀

EXCLUDES    Patients seen for an unrelated pregnancy/prenatal care condition (e.g., upper respiratory infection; patients seen for consultation only, not for continuing care)

🚑 0.00    ⚕ 0.00    **FUD** XXX              E

**AMA:** 2004,Nov,1

**0503F**    Postpartum care visit (Prenatal)    M ♀

🚑 0.00    ⚕ 0.00    **FUD** XXX              E

**AMA:** 2004,Nov,1

**0505F**    Hemodialysis plan of care documented (ESRD, P-ESRD)

🚑 0.00    ⚕ 0.00    **FUD** XXX              E

**AMA:** 2008,Mar,8-12

**0507F**    Peritoneal dialysis plan of care documented (ESRD)

🚑 0.00    ⚕ 0.00    **FUD** XXX              E

**AMA:** 2008,Mar,8-12

**0509F**    Urinary incontinence plan of care documented (GER)

🚑 0.00    ⚕ 0.00    **FUD** XXX              M

**0513F**    Elevated blood pressure plan of care documented (CKD)

🚑 0.00    ⚕ 0.00    **FUD** XXX              M

**AMA:** 2008,Mar,8-12

**0514F**    Plan of care for elevated hemoglobin level documented for patient receiving Erythropoiesis-Stimulating Agent therapy (ESA) (CKD)

🚑 0.00    ⚕ 0.00    **FUD** XXX              E

**AMA:** 2008,Mar,8-12

**0516F**    Anemia plan of care documented (ESRD)

🚑 0.00    ⚕ 0.00    **FUD** XXX              E

**AMA:** 2008,Mar,8-12

**0517F**    Glaucoma plan of care documented (EC)

🚑 0.00    ⚕ 0.00    **FUD** XXX              M

**AMA:** 2008,Mar,8-12

**0518F**   Falls plan of care documented (GER)
🚑 0.00   ⚘ 0.00   **FUD** XXX   M
AMA: 2008,Mar,8-12

**0519F**   Planned chemotherapy regimen, including at a minimum: drug(s) prescribed, dose, and duration, documented prior to initiation of a new treatment regimen (ONC)
🚑 0.00   ⚘ 0.00   **FUD** XXX   E
AMA: 2008,Mar,8-12

**0520F**   Radiation dose limits to normal tissues established prior to the initiation of a course of 3D conformal radiation for a minimum of 2 tissue/organ (ONC)
🚑 0.00   ⚘ 0.00   **FUD** XXX   M
AMA: 2008,Mar,8-12

**0521F**   Plan of care to address pain documented (COA) (ONC)
🚑 0.00   ⚘ 0.00   **FUD** XXX   M
AMA: 2008,Mar,8-12

**0525F**   Initial visit for episode (BkP)
🚑 0.00   ⚘ 0.00   **FUD** XXX   E
AMA: 2008,Mar,8-12

**0526F**   Subsequent visit for episode (BkP)
🚑 0.00   ⚘ 0.00   **FUD** XXX   M
AMA: 2008,Mar,8-12

**0528F**   Recommended follow-up interval for repeat colonoscopy of at least 10 years documented in colonoscopy report (End/Polyp)
🚑 0.00   ⚘ 0.00   **FUD** XXX   M

**0529F**   Interval of 3 or more years since patient's last colonoscopy, documented (End/Polyp)
🚑 0.00   ⚘ 0.00   **FUD** XXX   M

**0535F**   Dyspnea management plan of care, documented (Pall Cr)
🚑 0.00   ⚘ 0.00   **FUD** XXX   E

**0540F**   Glucorticoid Management Plan Documented (RA)
🚑 0.00   ⚘ 0.00   **FUD** XXX   M

**0545F**   Plan for follow-up care for major depressive disorder, documented (MDD ADOL)
🚑 0.00   ⚘ 0.00   **FUD** XXX   E

**0550F**   Cytopathology report on routine nongynecologic specimen finalized within two working days of accession date (PATH)
🚑 0.00   ⚘ 0.00   **FUD** XXX   E

**0551F**   Cytopathology report on nongynecologic specimen with documentation that the specimen was non-routine (PATH)
🚑 0.00   ⚘ 0.00   **FUD** XXX   E

**0555F**   Symptom management plan of care documented (HF)
🚑 0.00   ⚘ 0.00   **FUD** XXX   E

**0556F**   Plan of care to achieve lipid control documented (CAD)
🚑 0.00   ⚘ 0.00   **FUD** XXX   E

**0557F**   Plan of care to manage anginal symptoms documented (CAD)
🚑 0.00   ⚘ 0.00   **FUD** XXX   E

**0575F**   HIV RNA control plan of care, documented (HIV)
🚑 0.00   ⚘ 0.00   **FUD** XXX   E

**0580F**   Multidisciplinary care plan developed or updated (ALS)
🚑 0.00   ⚘ 0.00   **FUD** XXX   E

**0581F**   Patient transferred directly from anesthetizing location to critical care unit (Peri2)
🚑 0.00   ⚘ 0.00   **FUD** XXX   M

**0582F**   Patient not transferred directly from anesthetizing location to critical care unit (Peri2)
🚑 0.00   ⚘ 0.00   **FUD** XXX   E

**0583F**   Transfer of care checklist used (Peri2)
🚑 0.00   ⚘ 0.00   **FUD** XXX   M

**0584F**   Transfer of care checklist not used (Peri2)
🚑 0.00   ⚘ 0.00   **FUD** XXX   E

## 1000F-1505F Elements of History/Review of Systems

INCLUDES   Measures for specific aspects of patient history or review of systems

**1000F**   Tobacco use assessed (CAD, CAP, COPD, PV) (DM)
🚑 0.00   ⚘ 0.00   **FUD** XXX   E
AMA: 2017,Jan,8; 2016,Jan,13; 2015,Jan,16; 2014,Jan,11

**1002F**   Anginal symptoms and level of activity assessed (NMA-No Measure Associated)
🚑 0.00   ⚘ 0.00   **FUD** XXX   E
AMA: 2004,Nov,1

**1003F**   Level of activity assessed (NMA-No Measure Associated)
🚑 0.00   ⚘ 0.00   **FUD** XXX   E
AMA: 2006,Dec,10-12

**1004F**   Clinical symptoms of volume overload (excess) assessed (NMA-No Measure Associated)
🚑 0.00   ⚘ 0.00   **FUD** XXX   E
AMA: 2006,Dec,10-12

**1005F**   Asthma symptoms evaluated (includes documentation of numeric frequency of symptoms or patient completion of an asthma assessment tool/survey/questionnaire) (NMA-No Measure Associated)
🚑 0.00   ⚘ 0.00   **FUD** XXX   E

**1006F**   Osteoarthritis symptoms and functional status assessed (may include the use of a standardized scale or the completion of an assessment questionnaire, such as the SF-36, AAOS Hip & Knee Questionnaire) (OA) [Instructions: Report when osteoarthritis is addressed during the patient encounter]
🚑 0.00   ⚘ 0.00   **FUD** XXX   M

INCLUDES   Osteoarthritis when it is addressed during the patient encounter

**1007F**   Use of anti-inflammatory or analgesic over-the-counter (OTC) medications for symptom relief assessed (OA)
🚑 0.00   ⚘ 0.00   **FUD** XXX   E

**1008F**   Gastrointestinal and renal risk factors assessed for patients on prescribed or OTC non-steroidal anti-inflammatory drug (NSAID) (OA)
🚑 0.00   ⚘ 0.00   **FUD** XXX   E

**1010F**   Severity of angina assessed by level of activity (CAD)
🚑 0.00   ⚘ 0.00   **FUD** XXX   E

**1011F**   Angina present (CAD)
🚑 0.00   ⚘ 0.00   **FUD** XXX   E

**1012F**   Angina absent (CAD)
🚑 0.00   ⚘ 0.00   **FUD** XXX   E

**1015F**   Chronic obstructive pulmonary disease (COPD) symptoms assessed (Includes assessment of at least 1 of the following: dyspnea, cough/sputum, wheezing), or respiratory symptom assessment tool completed (COPD)
🚑 0.00   ⚘ 0.00   **FUD** XXX   E

**1018F**   Dyspnea assessed, not present (COPD)
🚑 0.00   ⚘ 0.00   **FUD** XXX   E

**1019F**   Dyspnea assessed, present (COPD)
🚑 0.00   ⚘ 0.00   **FUD** XXX   E

**1022F**   Pneumococcus immunization status assessed (CAP, COPD)
🚑 0.00   ⚘ 0.00   **FUD** XXX   E
AMA: 2010,Jul,3-5; 2008,Mar,8-12

**1026F**   Co-morbid conditions assessed (eg, includes assessment for presence or absence of: malignancy, liver disease, congestive heart failure, cerebrovascular disease, renal disease, chronic obstructive pulmonary disease, asthma, diabetes, other co-morbid conditions) (CAP)
🚑 0.00   ⚘ 0.00   **FUD** XXX   E

**1030F**   Influenza immunization status assessed (CAP)
🚑 0.00   ⚘ 0.00   **FUD** XXX   E
AMA: 2008,Mar,8-12

**1031F** Smoking status and exposure to second hand smoke in the home assessed (Asthma)
📇 0.00 ⅋ 0.00 **FUD** XXX E

**1032F** Current tobacco smoker or currently exposed to secondhand smoke (Asthma)
📇 0.00 ⅋ 0.00 **FUD** XXX E

**1033F** Current tobacco non-smoker and not currently exposed to secondhand smoke (Asthma)
📇 0.00 ⅋ 0.00 **FUD** XXX E

**1034F** Current tobacco smoker (CAD, CAP, COPD, PV) (DM)
📇 0.00 ⅋ 0.00 **FUD** XXX E
**AMA:** 2008,Mar,8-12

**1035F** Current smokeless tobacco user (eg, chew, snuff) (PV)
📇 0.00 ⅋ 0.00 **FUD** XXX E
**AMA:** 2008,Mar,8-12

**1036F** Current tobacco non-user (CAD, CAP, COPD, PV) (DM) (IBD)
📇 0.00 ⅋ 0.00 **FUD** XXX M
**AMA:** 2008,Mar,8-12

**1038F** Persistent asthma (mild, moderate or severe) (Asthma)
📇 0.00 ⅋ 0.00 **FUD** XXX M
**AMA:** 2017,Jan,8; 2016,Jan,13; 2015,Jan,16; 2014,Jan,11

**1039F** Intermittent asthma (Asthma)
📇 0.00 ⅋ 0.00 **FUD** XXX M
**AMA:** 2017,Jan,8; 2016,Jan,13; 2015,Jan,16; 2014,Jan,11

**1040F** DSM-5 criteria for major depressive disorder documented at the initial evaluation (MDD, MDD ADOL)
📇 0.00 ⅋ 0.00 **FUD** XXX E
**AMA:** 2008,Mar,8-12

**1050F** History obtained regarding new or changing moles (ML)
📇 0.00 ⅋ 0.00 **FUD** XXX E
**AMA:** 2008,Mar,8-12

**1052F** Type, anatomic location, and activity all assessed (IBD)
📇 0.00 ⅋ 0.00 **FUD** XXX E

**1055F** Visual functional status assessed (EC)
📇 0.00 ⅋ 0.00 **FUD** XXX E

**1060F** Documentation of permanent or persistent or paroxysmal atrial fibrillation (STR)
📇 0.00 ⅋ 0.00 **FUD** XXX E

**1061F** Documentation of absence of permanent and persistent and paroxysmal atrial fibrillation (STR)
📇 0.00 ⅋ 0.00 **FUD** XXX E

**1065F** Ischemic stroke symptom onset of less than 3 hours prior to arrival (STR)
📇 0.00 ⅋ 0.00 **FUD** XXX E

**1066F** Ischemic stroke symptom onset greater than or equal to 3 hours prior to arrival (STR)
📇 0.00 ⅋ 0.00 **FUD** XXX E

**1070F** Alarm symptoms (involuntary weight loss, dysphagia, or gastrointestinal bleeding) assessed; none present (GERD)
📇 0.00 ⅋ 0.00 **FUD** XXX E

**1071F** 1 or more present (GERD)
📇 0.00 ⅋ 0.00 **FUD** XXX E

**1090F** Presence or absence of urinary incontinence assessed (GER)
📇 0.00 ⅋ 0.00 **FUD** XXX M

**1091F** Urinary incontinence characterized (eg, frequency, volume, timing, type of symptoms, how bothersome) (GER)
📇 0.00 ⅋ 0.00 **FUD** XXX E

**1100F** Patient screened for future fall risk; documentation of 2 or more falls in the past year or any fall with injury in the past year (GER)
📇 0.00 ⅋ 0.00 **FUD** XXX M
**AMA:** 2008,Mar,8-12

**1101F** documentation of no falls in the past year or only 1 fall without injury in the past year (GER)
📇 0.00 ⅋ 0.00 **FUD** XXX M
**AMA:** 2008,Mar,8-12

**1110F** Patient discharged from an inpatient facility (eg, hospital, skilled nursing facility, or rehabilitation facility) within the last 60 days (GER)
📇 0.00 ⅋ 0.00 **FUD** XXX E

**1111F** Discharge medications reconciled with the current medication list in outpatient medical record (COA) (GER)
📇 0.00 ⅋ 0.00 **FUD** XXX M

**1116F** Auricular or periauricular pain assessed (AOE)
📇 0.00 ⅋ 0.00 **FUD** XXX E
**AMA:** 2008,Mar,8-12

**1118F** GERD symptoms assessed after 12 months of therapy (GERD)
📇 0.00 ⅋ 0.00 **FUD** XXX E
**AMA:** 2008,Mar,8-12

**1119F** Initial evaluation for condition (HEP C)(EPI, DSP)
📇 0.00 ⅋ 0.00 **FUD** XXX E
**AMA:** 2008,Mar,8-12

**1121F** Subsequent evaluation for condition (HEP C)(EPI)
📇 0.00 ⅋ 0.00 **FUD** XXX E
**AMA:** 2008,Mar,8-12

**1123F** Advance Care Planning discussed and documented advance care plan or surrogate decision maker documented in the medical record (DEM) (GER, Pall Cr)
📇 0.00 ⅋ 0.00 **FUD** XXX M
**AMA:** 2008,Mar,8-12

**1124F** Advance Care Planning discussed and documented in the medical record, patient did not wish or was not able to name a surrogate decision maker or provide an advance care plan (DEM) (GER, Pall Cr)
📇 0.00 ⅋ 0.00 **FUD** XXX M
**AMA:** 2008,Mar,8-12

**1125F** Pain severity quantified; pain present (COA) (ONC)
📇 0.00 ⅋ 0.00 **FUD** XXX M
**AMA:** 2008,Mar,8-12

**1126F** no pain present (COA) (ONC)
📇 0.00 ⅋ 0.00 **FUD** XXX M
**AMA:** 2008,Mar,8-12

**1127F** New episode for condition (NMA-No Measure Associated)
📇 0.00 ⅋ 0.00 **FUD** XXX E
**AMA:** 2008,Mar,8-12

**1128F** Subsequent episode for condition (NMA-No Measure Associated)
📇 0.00 ⅋ 0.00 **FUD** XXX E
**AMA:** 2008,Mar,8-12

**1130F** Back pain and function assessed, including all of the following: Pain assessment and functional status and patient history, including notation of presence or absence of "red flags" (warning signs) and assessment of prior treatment and response, and employment status (BkP)
📇 0.00 ⅋ 0.00 **FUD** XXX E
**AMA:** 2008,Mar,8-12

**1134F** Episode of back pain lasting 6 weeks or less (BkP)
📇 0.00 ⅋ 0.00 **FUD** XXX E
**AMA:** 2008,Mar,8-12

**1135F** Episode of back pain lasting longer than 6 weeks (BkP)
📇 0.00 ⅋ 0.00 **FUD** XXX E
**AMA:** 2008,Mar,8-12

**1136F** Episode of back pain lasting 12 weeks or less (BkP)
📇 0.00 ⅋ 0.00 **FUD** XXX E
**AMA:** 2008,Mar,8-12

---

● New Code ▲ Revised Code ○ Reinstated ● New Web Release ▲ Revised Web Release Unlisted Not Covered # Resequenced
⊘ AMA Mod 51 Exempt ⑤ Optum Mod 51 Exempt ⑥ Mod 63 Exempt ✗ Non-FDA Drug ★ Telemedicine Ⓜ Maternity Ⓐ Age Edit + Add-on **AMA:** CPT Asst

© 2017 Optum360, LLC CPT © 2017 American Medical Association. All Rights Reserved.

**Category II Codes**

**1137F — 2019F**

**1137F** Episode of back pain lasting longer than 12 weeks (BkP)
🚑 0.00   ⅗ 0.00   **FUD** XXX    E
**AMA:** 2008,Mar,8-12

**1150F** Documentation that a patient has a substantial risk of death within 1 year (Pall Cr)
🚑 0.00   ⅗ 0.00   **FUD** XXX    E

**1151F** Documentation that a patient does not have a substantial risk of death within one year (Pall Cr)
🚑 0.00   ⅗ 0.00   **FUD** XXX    E

**1152F** Documentation of advanced disease diagnosis, goals of care prioritize comfort (Pall Cr)
🚑 0.00   ⅗ 0.00   **FUD** XXX    E

**1153F** Documentation of advanced disease diagnosis, goals of care do not prioritize comfort (Pall Cr)
🚑 0.00   ⅗ 0.00   **FUD** XXX    E

**1157F** Advance care plan or similar legal document present in the medical record (COA)
🚑 0.00   ⅗ 0.00   **FUD** XXX    E

**1158F** Advance care planning discussion documented in the medical record (COA)
🚑 0.00   ⅗ 0.00   **FUD** XXX    M

**1159F** Medication list documented in medical record (COA)
🚑 0.00   ⅗ 0.00   **FUD** XXX    E

**1160F** Review of all medications by a prescribing practitioner or clinical pharmacist (such as, prescriptions, OTCs, herbal therapies and supplements) documented in the medical record (COA)
🚑 0.00   ⅗ 0.00   **FUD** XXX    E

**1170F** Functional status assessed (COA) (RA)
🚑 0.00   ⅗ 0.00   **FUD** XXX    M

**1175F** Functional status for dementia assessed and results reviewed (DEM)
🚑 0.00   ⅗ 0.00   **FUD** XXX    M

**1180F** All specified thromboembolic risk factors assessed (AFIB)
🚑 0.00   ⅗ 0.00   **FUD** XXX    E

**1181F** Neuropsychiatric symptoms assessed and results reviewed (DEM)
🚑 0.00   ⅗ 0.00   **FUD** XXX    M

**1182F** Neuropsychiatric symptoms, one or more present (DEM)
🚑 0.00   ⅗ 0.00   **FUD** XXX    E

**1183F** Neuropsychiatric symptoms, absent (DEM)
🚑 0.00   ⅗ 0.00   **FUD** XXX    E

**1200F** Seizure type(s) and current seizure frequency(ies) documented (EPI)
🚑 0.00   ⅗ 0.00   **FUD** XXX    E

**1205F** Etiology of epilepsy or epilepsy syndrome(s) reviewed and documented (EPI)
🚑 0.00   ⅗ 0.00   **FUD** XXX    E

**1220F** Patient screened for depression (SUD)
🚑 0.00   ⅗ 0.00   **FUD** XXX    E

**1400F** Parkinson's disease diagnosis reviewed (Prkns)
🚑 0.00   ⅗ 0.00   **FUD** XXX    E

**1450F** Symptoms improved or remained consistent with treatment goals since last assessment (HF)
🚑 0.00   ⅗ 0.00   **FUD** XXX    E

**1451F** Symptoms demonstrated clinically important deterioration since last assessment (HF)
🚑 0.00   ⅗ 0.00   **FUD** XXX    E

**1460F** Qualifying cardiac event/diagnosis in previous 12 months (CAD)
🚑 0.00   ⅗ 0.00   **FUD** XXX    M

**1461F** No qualifying cardiac event/diagnosis in previous 12 months (CAD)
🚑 0.00   ⅗ 0.00   **FUD** XXX    M

**1490F** Dementia severity classified, mild (DEM)
🚑 0.00   ⅗ 0.00   **FUD** XXX    E

**1491F** Dementia severity classified, moderate (DEM)
🚑 0.00   ⅗ 0.00   **FUD** XXX    E

**1493F** Dementia severity classified, severe (DEM)
🚑 0.00   ⅗ 0.00   **FUD** XXX    E

**1494F** Cognition assessed and reviewed (DEM)
🚑 0.00   ⅗ 0.00   **FUD** XXX    E

**1500F** Symptoms and signs of distal symmetric polyneuropathy reviewed and documented (DSP)
🚑 0.00   ⅗ 0.00   **FUD** XXX    E

**1501F** Not initial evaluation for condition (DSP)
🚑 0.00   ⅗ 0.00   **FUD** XXX    E

**1502F** Patient queried about pain and pain interference with function using a valid and reliable instrument (DSP)
🚑 0.00   ⅗ 0.00   **FUD** XXX    E

**1503F** Patient queried about symptoms of respiratory insufficiency (ALS)
🚑 0.00   ⅗ 0.00   **FUD** XXX    E

**1504F** Patient has respiratory insufficiency (ALS)
🚑 0.00   ⅗ 0.00   **FUD** XXX    E

**1505F** Patient does not have respiratory insufficiency (ALS)
🚑 0.00   ⅗ 0.00   **FUD** XXX    E

## 2000F-2060F Elements of Examination

INCLUDES   Components of clinical assessment or physical exam

**2000F** Blood pressure measured (CKD)(DM)
🚑 0.00   ⅗ 0.00   **FUD** XXX    M
**AMA:** 2017,Jan,8; 2016,Jan,13; 2015,Jan,16; 2014,Jan,11

**2001F** Weight recorded (PAG)
🚑 0.00   ⅗ 0.00   **FUD** XXX    E
**AMA:** 2006,Dec,10-12

**2002F** Clinical signs of volume overload (excess) assessed (NMA-No Measure Associated)
🚑 0.00   ⅗ 0.00   **FUD** XXX    E
**AMA:** 2006,Dec,10-12

**2004F** Initial examination of the involved joint(s) (includes visual inspection, palpation, range of motion) (OA) [Instructions: Report only for initial osteoarthritis visit or for visits for new joint involvement]
INCLUDES   Visits for initial osteoarthritis examination or new joint involvement
🚑 0.00   ⅗ 0.00   **FUD** XXX    E
**AMA:** 2004,Feb,3; 2003,Aug,1

**2010F** Vital signs (temperature, pulse, respiratory rate, and blood pressure) documented and reviewed (CAP) (EM)
🚑 0.00   ⅗ 0.00   **FUD** XXX    E

**2014F** Mental status assessed (CAP) (EM)
🚑 0.00   ⅗ 0.00   **FUD** XXX    E

**2015F** Asthma impairment assessed (Asthma)
🚑 0.00   ⅗ 0.00   **FUD** XXX    E

**2016F** Asthma risk assessed (Asthma)
🚑 0.00   ⅗ 0.00   **FUD** XXX    E

**2018F** Hydration status assessed (normal/mildly dehydrated/severely dehydrated) (CAP)
🚑 0.00   ⅗ 0.00   **FUD** XXX    E

**2019F** Dilated macular exam performed, including documentation of the presence or absence of macular thickening or hemorrhage and the level of macular degeneration severity (EC)
🚑 0.00   ⅗ 0.00   **FUD** XXX    M

2020F    Dilated fundus evaluation performed within 12 months prior to cataract surgery (EC)
🚑 0.00   ⚕ 0.00   **FUD** XXX                     E
**AMA:** 2008,Mar,8-12

2021F    Dilated macular or fundus exam performed, including documentation of the presence or absence of macular edema and level of severity of retinopathy (EC)
🚑 0.00   ⚕ 0.00   **FUD** XXX                     E

2022F    Dilated retinal eye exam with interpretation by an ophthalmologist or optometrist documented and reviewed (DM)
🚑 0.00   ⚕ 0.00   **FUD** XXX                     M
**AMA:** 2008,Mar,8-12

2024F    7 standard field stereoscopic photos with interpretation by an ophthalmologist or optometrist documented and reviewed (DM)
🚑 0.00   ⚕ 0.00   **FUD** XXX                     M
**AMA:** 2008,Mar,8-12

2026F    Eye imaging validated to match diagnosis from 7 standard field stereoscopic photos results documented and reviewed (DM)
🚑 0.00   ⚕ 0.00   **FUD** XXX                     M
**AMA:** 2008,Mar,8-12

2027F    Optic nerve head evaluation performed (EC)
🚑 0.00   ⚕ 0.00   **FUD** XXX                     M

2028F    Foot examination performed (includes examination through visual inspection, sensory exam with monofilament, and pulse exam - report when any of the 3 components are completed) (DM)
🚑 0.00   ⚕ 0.00   **FUD** XXX                     E

2029F    Complete physical skin exam performed (ML)
🚑 0.00   ⚕ 0.00   **FUD** XXX                     E
**AMA:** 2008,Mar,8-12

2030F    Hydration status documented, normally hydrated (PAG)
🚑 0.00   ⚕ 0.00   **FUD** XXX                     E

2031F    Hydration status documented, dehydrated (PAG)
🚑 0.00   ⚕ 0.00   **FUD** XXX                     E

2035F    Tympanic membrane mobility assessed with pneumatic otoscopy or tympanometry (OME)
🚑 0.00   ⚕ 0.00   **FUD** XXX                     E
**AMA:** 2008,Mar,8-12

2040F    Physical examination on the date of the initial visit for low back pain performed, in accordance with specifications (BkP)
🚑 0.00   ⚕ 0.00   **FUD** XXX                     E
**AMA:** 2008,Mar,8-12

2044F    Documentation of mental health assessment prior to intervention (back surgery or epidural steroid injection) or for back pain episode lasting longer than 6 weeks (BkP)
🚑 0.00   ⚕ 0.00   **FUD** XXX                     E
**AMA:** 2008,Mar,8-12

2050F    Wound characteristics including size and nature of wound base tissue and amount of drainage prior to debridement documented (CWC)
🚑 0.00   ⚕ 0.00   **FUD** XXX                     E

2060F    Patient interviewed directly on or before date of diagnosis of major depressive disorder (MDD ADOL)
🚑 0.00   ⚕ 0.00   **FUD** XXX                     E

## 3006F-3776F Findings from Diagnostic or Screening Tests

INCLUDES   Results and medical decision making with regards to ordered tests:
Clinical laboratory tests
Other examination procedures
Radiological examinations

3006F    Chest X-ray results documented and reviewed (CAP)
🚑 0.00   ⚕ 0.00   **FUD** XXX                     E
**AMA:** 2017,Jan,8; 2016,Jan,13; 2015,Jan,16; 2014,Jan,11

3008F    Body Mass Index (BMI), documented (PV)
🚑 0.00   ⚕ 0.00   **FUD** XXX                     E

3011F    Lipid panel results documented and reviewed (must include total cholesterol, HDL-C, triglycerides and calculated LDL-C) (CAD)
🚑 0.00   ⚕ 0.00   **FUD** XXX                     E

3014F    Screening mammography results documented and reviewed (PV)
🚑 0.00   ⚕ 0.00   **FUD** XXX                     M
**AMA:** 2008,Mar,8-12

3015F    Cervical cancer screening results documented and reviewed (PV)                                                ♀
🚑 0.00   ⚕ 0.00   **FUD** XXX                     E

3016F    Patient screened for unhealthy alcohol use using a systematic screening method (PV) (DSP)
🚑 0.00   ⚕ 0.00   **FUD** XXX                     E

3017F    Colorectal cancer screening results documented and reviewed (PV)
🚑 0.00   ⚕ 0.00   **FUD** XXX                     M
**AMA:** 2008,Mar,8-12

3018F    Pre-procedure risk assessment and depth of insertion and quality of the bowel prep and complete description of polyp(s) found, including location of each polyp, size, number and gross morphology and recommendations for follow-up in final colonoscopy report documented (End/Polyp)
🚑 0.00   ⚕ 0.00   **FUD** XXX                     E

3019F    Left ventricular ejection fraction (LVEF) assessment planned post discharge (HF)
🚑 0.00   ⚕ 0.00   **FUD** XXX                     E

3020F    Left ventricular function (LVF) assessment (eg, echocardiography, nuclear test, or ventriculography) documented in the medical record (Includes quantitative or qualitative assessment results) (NMA-No Measure Associated)
🚑 0.00   ⚕ 0.00   **FUD** XXX                     E
**AMA:** 2006,Dec,10-12

3021F    Left ventricular ejection fraction (LVEF) less than 40% or documentation of moderately or severely depressed left ventricular systolic function (CAD, HF)
🚑 0.00   ⚕ 0.00   **FUD** XXX                     M

3022F    Left ventricular ejection fraction (LVEF) greater than or equal to 40% or documentation as normal or mildly depressed left ventricular systolic function (CAD, HF)
🚑 0.00   ⚕ 0.00   **FUD** XXX                     M

3023F    Spirometry results documented and reviewed (COPD)
🚑 0.00   ⚕ 0.00   **FUD** XXX                     M

3025F    Spirometry test results demonstrate FEV1/FVC less than 70% with COPD symptoms (eg, dyspnea, cough/sputum, wheezing) (CAP, COPD)
🚑 0.00   ⚕ 0.00   **FUD** XXX                     E

3027F    Spirometry test results demonstrate FEV1/FVC greater than or equal to 70% or patient does not have COPD symptoms (COPD)
🚑 0.00   ⚕ 0.00   **FUD** XXX                     E

**3028F** Oxygen saturation results documented and reviewed (includes assessment through pulse oximetry or arterial blood gas measurement) (CAP, COPD) (EM)
🛏 0.00    ⚕ 0.00    **FUD** XXX                                          E

**3035F** Oxygen saturation less than or equal to 88% or a PaO2 less than or equal to 55 mm Hg (COPD)
🛏 0.00    ⚕ 0.00    **FUD** XXX                                          E

**3037F** Oxygen saturation greater than 88% or PaO2 greater than 55 mm Hg (COPD)
🛏 0.00    ⚕ 0.00    **FUD** XXX                                          E

**3038F** Pulmonary function test performed within 12 months prior to surgery (Lung/Esop Cx)
🛏 0.00    ⚕ 0.00    **FUD** XXX                                          E

**3040F** Functional expiratory volume (FEV1) less than 40% of predicted value (COPD)
🛏 0.00    ⚕ 0.00    **FUD** XXX                                          E

**3042F** Functional expiratory volume (FEV1) greater than or equal to 40% of predicted value (COPD)
🛏 0.00    ⚕ 0.00    **FUD** XXX                                          E

**3044F** Most recent hemoglobin A1c (HbA1c) level less than 7.0% (DM)
🛏 0.00    ⚕ 0.00    **FUD** XXX                                          M

**3045F** Most recent hemoglobin A1c (HbA1c) level 7.0-9.0% (DM)
🛏 0.00    ⚕ 0.00    **FUD** XXX                                          M

**3046F** Most recent hemoglobin A1c level greater than 9.0% (DM)
🛏 0.00    ⚕ 0.00    **FUD** XXX                                          M
**EXCLUDES** *Levels of hemoglobin A1c less than or equal to 9.0% (3044F-3045F)*

**3048F** Most recent LDL-C less than 100 mg/dL (CAD) (DM)
🛏 0.00    ⚕ 0.00    **FUD** XXX                                          E

**3049F** Most recent LDL-C 100-129 mg/dL (CAD) (DM)
🛏 0.00    ⚕ 0.00    **FUD** XXX                                          E

**3050F** Most recent LDL-C greater than or equal to 130 mg/dL (CAD) (DM)
🛏 0.00    ⚕ 0.00    **FUD** XXX                                          E

**3055F** Left ventricular ejection fraction (LVEF) less than or equal to 35% (HF)
🛏 0.00    ⚕ 0.00    **FUD** XXX                                          E

**3056F** Left ventricular ejection fraction (LVEF) greater than 35% or no LVEF result available (HF)
🛏 0.00    ⚕ 0.00    **FUD** XXX                                          E

**3060F** Positive microalbuminuria test result documented and reviewed (DM)
🛏 0.00    ⚕ 0.00    **FUD** XXX                                          M

**3061F** Negative microalbuminuria test result documented and reviewed (DM)
🛏 0.00    ⚕ 0.00    **FUD** XXX                                          M

**3062F** Positive macroalbuminuria test result documented and reviewed (DM)
🛏 0.00    ⚕ 0.00    **FUD** XXX                                          M

**3066F** Documentation of treatment for nephropathy (eg, patient receiving dialysis, patient being treated for ESRD, CRF, ARF, or renal insufficiency, any visit to a nephrologist) (DM)
🛏 0.00    ⚕ 0.00    **FUD** XXX                                          M

**3072F** Low risk for retinopathy (no evidence of retinopathy in the prior year) (DM)
🛏 0.00    ⚕ 0.00    **FUD** XXX                                          M
**AMA:** 2008,Mar,8-12

**3073F** Pre-surgical (cataract) axial length, corneal power measurement and method of intraocular lens power calculation documented within 12 months prior to surgery (EC)
🛏 0.00    ⚕ 0.00    **FUD** XXX                                          E
**AMA:** 2008,Mar,8-12

**3074F** Most recent systolic blood pressure less than 130 mm Hg (DM), (HTN, CKD, CAD)
🛏 0.00    ⚕ 0.00    **FUD** XXX                                          E
**AMA:** 2008,Mar,8-12

**3075F** Most recent systolic blood pressure 130-139 mm Hg (DM) (HTN, CKD, CAD)
🛏 0.00    ⚕ 0.00    **FUD** XXX                                          E
**AMA:** 2008,Mar,8-12

**3077F** Most recent systolic blood pressure greater than or equal to 140 mm Hg (HTN, CKD, CAD) (DM)
🛏 0.00    ⚕ 0.00    **FUD** XXX                                          E
**AMA:** 2008,Mar,8-12

**3078F** Most recent diastolic blood pressure less than 80 mm Hg (HTN, CKD, CAD) (DM)
🛏 0.00    ⚕ 0.00    **FUD** XXX                                          E
**AMA:** 2008,Mar,8-12

**3079F** Most recent diastolic blood pressure 80-89 mm Hg (HTN, CKD, CAD) (DM)
🛏 0.00    ⚕ 0.00    **FUD** XXX                                          E
**AMA:** 2008,Mar,8-12

**3080F** Most recent diastolic blood pressure greater than or equal to 90 mm Hg (HTN, CKD, CAD) (DM)
🛏 0.00    ⚕ 0.00    **FUD** XXX                                          E
**AMA:** 2008,Mar,8-12

**3082F** Kt/V less than 1.2 (Clearance of urea [Kt]/volume [V]) (ESRD, P-ESRD)
🛏 0.00    ⚕ 0.00    **FUD** XXX                                          E
**AMA:** 2008,Mar,8-12

**3083F** Kt/V equal to or greater than 1.2 and less than 1.7 (Clearance of urea [Kt]/volume [V]) (ESRD, P-ESRD)
🛏 0.00    ⚕ 0.00    **FUD** XXX                                          E
**AMA:** 2008,Mar,8-12

**3084F** Kt/V greater than or equal to 1.7 (Clearance of urea [Kt]/volume [V]) (ESRD, P-ESRD)
🛏 0.00    ⚕ 0.00    **FUD** XXX                                          E
**AMA:** 2008,Mar,8-12

**3085F** Suicide risk assessed (MDD, MDD ADOL)
🛏 0.00    ⚕ 0.00    **FUD** XXX                                          E

**3088F** Major depressive disorder, mild (MDD)
🛏 0.00    ⚕ 0.00    **FUD** XXX                                          E

**3089F** Major depressive disorder, moderate (MDD)
🛏 0.00    ⚕ 0.00    **FUD** XXX                                          E

**3090F** Major depressive disorder, severe without psychotic features (MDD)
🛏 0.00    ⚕ 0.00    **FUD** XXX                                          E

**3091F** Major depressive disorder, severe with psychotic features (MDD)
🛏 0.00    ⚕ 0.00    **FUD** XXX                                          E

**3092F** Major depressive disorder, in remission (MDD)
🛏 0.00    ⚕ 0.00    **FUD** XXX                                          E

**3093F** Documentation of new diagnosis of initial or recurrent episode of major depressive disorder (MDD)
🛏 0.00    ⚕ 0.00    **FUD** XXX                                          E
**AMA:** 2008,Mar,8-12

**3095F** Central dual-energy X-ray absorptiometry (DXA) results documented (OP)(IBD)
🛏 0.00    ⚕ 0.00    **FUD** XXX                                          M

**3096F** Central dual-energy X-ray absorptiometry (DXA) ordered (OP)(IBD)
🛏 0.00    ⚕ 0.00    **FUD** XXX                                          E

**3100F** Carotid imaging study report (includes direct or indirect reference to measurements of distal internal carotid diameter as the denominator for stenosis measurement) (STR, RAD)
🛏 0.00    ⚕ 0.00    **FUD** XXX                                          M
**AMA:** 2008,Mar,8-12

26/TC PC/TC Only          42-Z3 ASC Payment          50 Bilateral          ♂ Male Only          ♀ Female Only          🛏 Facility RVU          ⚕ Non-Facility RVU          ▣ CCI
FUD Follow-up Days     CMS: IOM (Pub 100)     A-Y OPPSI          80/80 Surg Assist Allowed / w/Doc          ▣ Lab Crosswalk          ▣ Radiology Crosswalk          ☒ CLIA

CPT © 2017 American Medical Association. All Rights Reserved.          © 2017 Optum360, LLC

**3110F** Documentation in final CT or MRI report of presence or absence of hemorrhage and mass lesion and acute infarction (STR)
 🖤 0.00  ⚕ 0.00  **FUD** XXX  Ⓔ

**3111F** CT or MRI of the brain performed in the hospital within 24 hours of arrival or performed in an outpatient imaging center, to confirm initial diagnosis of stroke, TIA or intracranial hemorrhage (STR)
 🖤 0.00  ⚕ 0.00  **FUD** XXX  Ⓔ

**3112F** CT or MRI of the brain performed greater than 24 hours after arrival to the hospital or performed in an outpatient imaging center for purpose other than confirmation of initial diagnosis of stroke, TIA, or intracranial hemorrhage (STR)
 🖤 0.00  ⚕ 0.00  **FUD** XXX  Ⓔ

**3115F** Quantitative results of an evaluation of current level of activity and clinical symptoms (HF)
 🖤 0.00  ⚕ 0.00  **FUD** XXX  Ⓔ

**3117F** Heart failure disease specific structured assessment tool completed (HF)
 🖤 0.00  ⚕ 0.00  **FUD** XXX  Ⓔ

**3118F** New York Heart Association (NYHA) Class documented (HF)
 🖤 0.00  ⚕ 0.00  **FUD** XXX  Ⓔ

**3119F** No evaluation of level of activity or clinical symptoms (HF)
 🖤 0.00  ⚕ 0.00  **FUD** XXX  Ⓔ

**3120F** 12-Lead ECG Performed (EM)
 🖤 0.00  ⚕ 0.00  **FUD** XXX  Ⓔ

**3126F** Esophageal biopsy report with a statement about dysplasia (present, absent, or indefinite, and if present, contains appropriate grading) (PATH)
 🖤 0.00  ⚕ 0.00  **FUD** XXX  Ⓜ

**3130F** Upper gastrointestinal endoscopy performed (GERD)
 🖤 0.00  ⚕ 0.00  **FUD** XXX  Ⓔ

**3132F** Documentation of referral for upper gastrointestinal endoscopy (GERD)
 🖤 0.00  ⚕ 0.00  **FUD** XXX  Ⓔ

**3140F** Upper gastrointestinal endoscopy report indicates suspicion of Barrett's esophagus (GERD)
 🖤 0.00  ⚕ 0.00  **FUD** XXX  Ⓔ

**3141F** Upper gastrointestinal endoscopy report indicates no suspicion of Barrett's esophagus (GERD)
 🖤 0.00  ⚕ 0.00  **FUD** XXX  Ⓔ

**3142F** Barium swallow test ordered (GERD)
 🖤 0.00  ⚕ 0.00  **FUD** XXX  Ⓔ
 INCLUDES Documentation of barium swallow test

**3150F** Forceps esophageal biopsy performed (GERD)
 🖤 0.00  ⚕ 0.00  **FUD** XXX  Ⓔ

**3155F** Cytogenetic testing performed on bone marrow at time of diagnosis or prior to initiating treatment (HEM)
 🖤 0.00  ⚕ 0.00  **FUD** XXX  Ⓜ
 **AMA:** 2008,Mar,8-12

**3160F** Documentation of iron stores prior to initiating erythropoietin therapy (HEM)
 🖤 0.00  ⚕ 0.00  **FUD** XXX  Ⓜ
 **AMA:** 2008,Mar,8-12

**3170F** Flow cytometry studies performed at time of diagnosis or prior to initiating treatment (HEM)
 🖤 0.00  ⚕ 0.00  **FUD** XXX  Ⓜ
 **AMA:** 2008,Mar,8-12

**3200F** Barium swallow test not ordered (GERD)
 🖤 0.00  ⚕ 0.00  **FUD** XXX  Ⓔ

**3210F** Group A Strep Test Performed (PHAR)
 🖤 0.00  ⚕ 0.00  **FUD** XXX  Ⓜ
 **AMA:** 2008,Mar,8-12

**3215F** Patient has documented immunity to Hepatitis A (HEP-C)
 🖤 0.00  ⚕ 0.00  **FUD** XXX  Ⓔ
 **AMA:** 2008,Mar,8-12

**3216F** Patient has documented immunity to Hepatitis B (HEP-C)(IBD)
 🖤 0.00  ⚕ 0.00  **FUD** XXX  Ⓔ
 **AMA:** 2008,Mar,8-12

**3218F** RNA testing for Hepatitis C documented as performed within 6 months prior to initiation of antiviral treatment for Hepatitis C (HEP-C)
 🖤 0.00  ⚕ 0.00  **FUD** XXX  Ⓔ
 **AMA:** 2008,Mar,8-12

**3220F** Hepatitis C quantitative RNA testing documented as performed at 12 weeks from initiation of antiviral treatment (HEP-C)
 🖤 0.00  ⚕ 0.00  **FUD** XXX  Ⓔ
 **AMA:** 2008,Mar,8-12

**3230F** Documentation that hearing test was performed within 6 months prior to tympanostomy tube insertion (OME)
 🖤 0.00  ⚕ 0.00  **FUD** XXX  Ⓔ
 **AMA:** 2008,Mar,8-12

**3250F** Specimen site other than anatomic location of primary tumor (PATH)
 🖤 0.00  ⚕ 0.00  **FUD** XXX  Ⓜ

**3260F** pT category (primary tumor), pN category (regional lymph nodes), and histologic grade documented in pathology report (PATH)
 🖤 0.00  ⚕ 0.00  **FUD** XXX  Ⓜ
 **AMA:** 2008,Mar,8-12

**3265F** Ribonucleic acid (RNA) testing for Hepatitis C viremia ordered or results documented (HEP C)
 🖤 0.00  ⚕ 0.00  **FUD** XXX  Ⓔ
 **AMA:** 2008,Mar,8-12

**3266F** Hepatitis C genotype testing documented as performed prior to initiation of antiviral treatment for Hepatitis C (HEP C)
 🖤 0.00  ⚕ 0.00  **FUD** XXX  Ⓔ
 **AMA:** 2008,Mar,8-12

**3267F** Pathology report includes pT category, pN category, Gleason score, and statement about margin status (PATH)
 🖤 0.00  ⚕ 0.00  **FUD** XXX  Ⓜ

**3268F** Prostate-specific antigen (PSA), and primary tumor (T) stage, and Gleason score documented prior to initiation of treatment (PRCA)
 🖤 0.00  ⚕ 0.00  **FUD** XXX  Ⓔ
 **AMA:** 2008,Mar,8-12

**3269F** Bone scan performed prior to initiation of treatment or at any time since diagnosis of prostate cancer (PRCA)
 🖤 0.00  ⚕ 0.00  **FUD** XXX  Ⓜ
 **AMA:** 2008,Mar,8-12

**3270F** Bone scan not performed prior to initiation of treatment nor at any time since diagnosis of prostate cancer (PRCA)
 🖤 0.00  ⚕ 0.00  **FUD** XXX  Ⓜ
 **AMA:** 2008,Mar,8-12

**3271F** Low risk of recurrence, prostate cancer (PRCA)
 🖤 0.00  ⚕ 0.00  **FUD** XXX  Ⓔ
 **AMA:** 2008,Mar,8-12

**3272F** Intermediate risk of recurrence, prostate cancer (PRCA)
 🖤 0.00  ⚕ 0.00  **FUD** XXX  Ⓔ
 **AMA:** 2008,Mar,8-12

**3273F** High risk of recurrence, prostate cancer (PRCA)
 🖤 0.00  ⚕ 0.00  **FUD** XXX  Ⓔ
 **AMA:** 2008,Mar,8-12

**3274F** Prostate cancer risk of recurrence not determined or neither low, intermediate nor high (PRCA)
📋 0.00 ⚖ 0.00 **FUD** XXX      E
AMA: 2008,Mar,8-12

**3278F** Serum levels of calcium, phosphorus, intact Parathyroid Hormone (PTH) and lipid profile ordered (CKD)
📋 0.00 ⚖ 0.00 **FUD** XXX      E
AMA: 2008,Mar,8-12

**3279F** Hemoglobin level greater than or equal to 13 g/dL (CKD, ESRD)
📋 0.00 ⚖ 0.00 **FUD** XXX      E
AMA: 2008,Mar,8-12

**3280F** Hemoglobin level 11 g/dL to 12.9 g/dL (CKD, ESRD)
📋 0.00 ⚖ 0.00 **FUD** XXX      E
AMA: 2008,Mar,8-12

**3281F** Hemoglobin level less than 11 g/dL (CKD, ESRD)
📋 0.00 ⚖ 0.00 **FUD** XXX      E
AMA: 2008,Mar,8-12

**3284F** Intraocular pressure (IOP) reduced by a value of greater than or equal to 15% from the pre-intervention level (EC)
📋 0.00 ⚖ 0.00 **FUD** XXX      M
AMA: 2008,Mar,8-12

**3285F** Intraocular pressure (IOP) reduced by a value less than 15% from the pre-intervention level (EC)
📋 0.00 ⚖ 0.00 **FUD** XXX      M
AMA: 2008,Mar,8-12

**3288F** Falls risk assessment documented (GER)
📋 0.00 ⚖ 0.00 **FUD** XXX      M
AMA: 2008,Mar,8-12

**3290F** Patient is D (Rh) negative and unsensitized (Pre-Cr)
📋 0.00 ⚖ 0.00 **FUD** XXX      E
AMA: 2008,Mar,8-12

**3291F** Patient is D (Rh) positive or sensitized (Pre-Cr)
📋 0.00 ⚖ 0.00 **FUD** XXX      E
AMA: 2008,Mar,8-12

**3292F** HIV testing ordered or documented and reviewed during the first or second prenatal visit (Pre-Cr)
📋 0.00 ⚖ 0.00 **FUD** XXX      E

**3293F** ABO and Rh blood typing documented as performed (Pre-Cr)
📋 0.00 ⚖ 0.00 **FUD** XXX      E

**3294F** Group B Streptococcus (GBS) screening documented as performed during week 35-37 gestation (Pre-Cr)
📋 0.00 ⚖ 0.00 **FUD** XXX      E

**3300F** American Joint Committee on Cancer (AJCC) stage documented and reviewed (ONC)
📋 0.00 ⚖ 0.00 **FUD** XXX      M
AMA: 2008,Mar,8-12

**3301F** Cancer stage documented in medical record as metastatic and reviewed (ONC)
EXCLUDES *Cancer staging measures (3321F-3390F)*
📋 0.00 ⚖ 0.00 **FUD** XXX      M
AMA: 2008,Mar,8-12

**3315F** Estrogen receptor (ER) or progesterone receptor (PR) positive breast cancer (ONC)
📋 0.00 ⚖ 0.00 **FUD** XXX      E
AMA: 2008,Mar,8-12

**3316F** Estrogen receptor (ER) and progesterone receptor (PR) negative breast cancer (ONC)
📋 0.00 ⚖ 0.00 **FUD** XXX      E
AMA: 2008,Mar,8-12

**3317F** Pathology report confirming malignancy documented in the medical record and reviewed prior to the initiation of chemotherapy (ONC)
📋 0.00 ⚖ 0.00 **FUD** XXX      E
AMA: 2008,Mar,8-12

**3318F** Pathology report confirming malignancy documented in the medical record and reviewed prior to the initiation of radiation therapy (ONC)
📋 0.00 ⚖ 0.00 **FUD** XXX      E
AMA: 2008,Mar,8-12

**3319F** 1 of the following diagnostic imaging studies ordered: chest x-ray, CT, Ultrasound, MRI, PET, or nuclear medicine scans (ML)
📋 0.00 ⚖ 0.00 **FUD** XXX      M
AMA: 2008,Mar,8-12

**3320F** None of the following diagnostic imaging studies ordered: chest X-ray, CT, Ultrasound, MRI, PET, or nuclear medicine scans (ML)
📋 0.00 ⚖ 0.00 **FUD** XXX      M
AMA: 2008,Mar,8-12

**3321F** AJCC Cancer Stage 0 or IA Melanoma, documented (ML)
📋 0.00 ⚖ 0.00 **FUD** XXX      M

**3322F** Melanoma greater than AJCC Stage 0 or IA (ML)
📋 0.00 ⚖ 0.00 **FUD** XXX      M

**3323F** Clinical tumor, node and metastases (TNM) staging documented and reviewed prior to surgery (Lung/Esop Cx)
📋 0.00 ⚖ 0.00 **FUD** XXX      E

**3324F** MRI or CT scan ordered, reviewed or requested (EPI)
📋 0.00 ⚖ 0.00 **FUD** XXX      E

**3325F** Preoperative assessment of functional or medical indication(s) for surgery prior to the cataract surgery with intraocular lens placement (must be performed within 12 months prior to cataract surgery) (EC)
📋 0.00 ⚖ 0.00 **FUD** XXX      E
AMA: 2008,Mar,8-12

**3328F** Performance status documented and reviewed within 2 weeks prior to surgery (Lung/Esop Cx)
📋 0.00 ⚖ 0.00 **FUD** XXX      E

**3330F** Imaging study ordered (BkP)
📋 0.00 ⚖ 0.00 **FUD** XXX      E
AMA: 2008,Mar,8-12

**3331F** Imaging study not ordered (BkP)
📋 0.00 ⚖ 0.00 **FUD** XXX      E
AMA: 2008,Mar,8-12

**3340F** Mammogram assessment category of "incomplete: need additional imaging evaluation" documented (RAD)
📋 0.00 ⚖ 0.00 **FUD** XXX      M
AMA: 2008,Mar,8-12

**3341F** Mammogram assessment category of "negative," documented (RAD)
📋 0.00 ⚖ 0.00 **FUD** XXX      M
AMA: 2008,Mar,8-12

**3342F** Mammogram assessment category of "benign," documented (RAD)
📋 0.00 ⚖ 0.00 **FUD** XXX      M
AMA: 2008,Mar,8-12

**3343F** Mammogram assessment category of "probably benign," documented (RAD)
📋 0.00 ⚖ 0.00 **FUD** XXX      M
AMA: 2008,Mar,8-12

**3344F** Mammogram assessment category of "suspicious," documented (RAD)
📋 0.00 ⚖ 0.00 **FUD** XXX      M
AMA: 2008,Mar,8-12

**3345F** Mammogram assessment category of "highly suggestive of malignancy," documented (RAD)
📞 0.00  🔊 0.00  **FUD** XXX  Ⓜ
**AMA:** 2008,Mar,8-12

**3350F** Mammogram assessment category of "known biopsy proven malignancy," documented (RAD)
📞 0.00  🔊 0.00  **FUD** XXX  Ⓜ
**AMA:** 2008,Mar,8-12

**3351F** Negative screen for depressive symptoms as categorized by using a standardized depression screening/assessment tool (MDD)
📞 0.00  🔊 0.00  **FUD** XXX  Ⓔ

**3352F** No significant depressive symptoms as categorized by using a standardized depression assessment tool (MDD)
📞 0.00  🔊 0.00  **FUD** XXX  Ⓔ

**3353F** Mild to moderate depressive symptoms as categorized by using a standardized depression screening/assessment tool (MDD)
📞 0.00  🔊 0.00  **FUD** XXX  Ⓔ

**3354F** Clinically significant depressive symptoms as categorized by using a standardized depression screening/assessment tool (MDD)
📞 0.00  🔊 0.00  **FUD** XXX  Ⓔ

**3370F** AJCC Breast Cancer Stage 0 documented (ONC)
📞 0.00  🔊 0.00  **FUD** XXX  Ⓔ

**3372F** AJCC Breast Cancer Stage I: T1mic, T1a or T1b (tumor size ≤ 1 cm) documented (ONC)
📞 0.00  🔊 0.00  **FUD** XXX  Ⓔ

**3374F** AJCC Breast Cancer Stage I: T1c (tumor size > 1 cm to 2 cm) documented (ONC)
📞 0.00  🔊 0.00  **FUD** XXX  Ⓔ

**3376F** AJCC Breast Cancer Stage II documented (ONC)
📞 0.00  🔊 0.00  **FUD** XXX  Ⓔ

**3378F** AJCC Breast Cancer Stage III documented (ONC)
📞 0.00  🔊 0.00  **FUD** XXX  Ⓔ

**3380F** AJCC Breast Cancer Stage IV documented (ONC)
📞 0.00  🔊 0.00  **FUD** XXX  Ⓔ

**3382F** AJCC colon cancer, Stage 0 documented (ONC)
📞 0.00  🔊 0.00  **FUD** XXX  Ⓔ

**3384F** AJCC colon cancer, Stage I documented (ONC)
📞 0.00  🔊 0.00  **FUD** XXX  Ⓔ

**3386F** AJCC colon cancer, Stage II documented (ONC)
📞 0.00  🔊 0.00  **FUD** XXX  Ⓔ

**3388F** AJCC colon cancer, Stage III documented (ONC)
📞 0.00  🔊 0.00  **FUD** XXX  Ⓔ

**3390F** AJCC colon cancer, Stage IV documented (ONC)
📞 0.00  🔊 0.00  **FUD** XXX  Ⓔ

**3394F** Quantitative HER2 immunohistochemistry (IHC) evaluation of breast cancer consistent with the scoring system defined in the ASCO/CAP guidelines (PATH)
📞 0.00  🔊 0.00  **FUD** XXX  Ⓜ

**3395F** Quantitative non-HER2 immunohistochemistry (IHC) evaluation of breast cancer (eg, testing for estrogen or progesterone receptors [ER/PR]) performed (PATH)
📞 0.00  🔊 0.00  **FUD** XXX  Ⓜ

**3450F** Dyspnea screened, no dyspnea or mild dyspnea (Pall Cr)
📞 0.00  🔊 0.00  **FUD** XXX  Ⓔ

**3451F** Dyspnea screened, moderate or severe dyspnea (Pall Cr)
📞 0.00  🔊 0.00  **FUD** XXX  Ⓔ

**3452F** Dyspnea not screened (Pall Cr)
📞 0.00  🔊 0.00  **FUD** XXX  Ⓔ

**3455F** TB screening performed and results interpreted within six months prior to initiation of first-time biologic disease modifying anti-rheumatic drug therapy for RA (RA)
📞 0.00  🔊 0.00  **FUD** XXX  Ⓜ

**3470F** Rheumatoid arthritis (RA) disease activity, low (RA)
📞 0.00  🔊 0.00  **FUD** XXX  Ⓜ

**3471F** Rheumatoid arthritis (RA) disease activity, moderate (RA)
📞 0.00  🔊 0.00  **FUD** XXX  Ⓜ

**3472F** Rheumatoid arthritis (RA) disease activity, high (RA)
📞 0.00  🔊 0.00  **FUD** XXX  Ⓜ

**3475F** Disease prognosis for rheumatoid arthritis assessed, poor prognosis documented (RA)
📞 0.00  🔊 0.00  **FUD** XXX  Ⓜ

**3476F** Disease prognosis for rheumatoid arthritis assessed, good prognosis documented (RA)
📞 0.00  🔊 0.00  **FUD** XXX  Ⓜ

**3490F** History of AIDS-defining condition (HIV)
📞 0.00  🔊 0.00  **FUD** XXX  Ⓔ

**3491F** HIV indeterminate (infants of undetermined HIV status born of HIV-infected mothers) (HIV)
📞 0.00  🔊 0.00  **FUD** XXX  Ⓔ

**3492F** History of nadir CD4+ cell count <350 cells/mm3 (HIV)
📞 0.00  🔊 0.00  **FUD** XXX  Ⓔ

**3493F** No history of nadir CD4+ cell count <350 cells/mm3 and no history of AIDS-defining condition (HIV)
📞 0.00  🔊 0.00  **FUD** XXX  Ⓔ

**3494F** CD4+ cell count <200 cells/mm3 (HIV)
📞 0.00  🔊 0.00  **FUD** XXX  Ⓔ

**3495F** CD4+ cell count 200 - 499 cells/mm3 (HIV)
📞 0.00  🔊 0.00  **FUD** XXX  Ⓔ

**3496F** CD4+ cell count ≥ 500 cells/mm3 (HIV)
📞 0.00  🔊 0.00  **FUD** XXX  Ⓔ

**3497F** CD4+ cell percentage <15% (HIV)
📞 0.00  🔊 0.00  **FUD** XXX  Ⓔ

**3498F** CD4+ cell percentage ≥ 15% (HIV)
📞 0.00  🔊 0.00  **FUD** XXX  Ⓔ

**3500F** CD4+ cell count or CD4+ cell percentage documented as performed (HIV)
📞 0.00  🔊 0.00  **FUD** XXX  Ⓔ

**3502F** HIV RNA viral load below limits of quantification (HIV)
📞 0.00  🔊 0.00  **FUD** XXX  Ⓔ

**3503F** HIV RNA viral load not below limits of quantification (HIV)
📞 0.00  🔊 0.00  **FUD** XXX  Ⓔ

**3510F** Documentation that tuberculosis (TB) screening test performed and results interpreted (HIV) (IBD)
📞 0.00  🔊 0.00  **FUD** XXX  Ⓔ

**3511F** Chlamydia and gonorrhea screenings documented as performed (HIV)
📞 0.00  🔊 0.00  **FUD** XXX  Ⓔ

**3512F** Syphilis screening documented as performed (HIV)
📞 0.00  🔊 0.00  **FUD** XXX  Ⓔ

**3513F** Hepatitis B screening documented as performed (HIV)
📞 0.00  🔊 0.00  **FUD** XXX  Ⓔ

**3514F** Hepatitis C screening documented as performed (HIV)
📞 0.00  🔊 0.00  **FUD** XXX  Ⓔ

**3515F** Patient has documented immunity to Hepatitis C (HIV)
📞 0.00  🔊 0.00  **FUD** XXX  Ⓔ

**3517F** Hepatitis B Virus (HBV) status assessed and results interpreted within one year prior to receiving a first course of anti-TNF (tumor necrosis factor) therapy (IBD)
📞 0.00  🔊 0.00  **FUD** XXX  Ⓜ

● New Code   ▲ Revised Code   ○ Reinstated   ● New Web Release   ▲ Revised Web Release   Unlisted   Not Covered   # Resequenced
🚫 AMA Mod 51 Exempt   ⑤ Optum Mod 51 Exempt   ⑥ Mod 63 Exempt   ✓ Non-FDA Drug   ★ Telemedicine   Ⓜ Maternity   Ⓐ Age Edit   + Add-on   **AMA:** CPT Asst
© 2017 Optum360, LLC                    CPT © 2017 American Medical Association. All Rights Reserved.                    **533**

| 3520F | Clostridium difficile testing performed (IBD) |
|---|---|

🏥 0.00   🔬 0.00   **FUD** XXX   E

| 3550F | Low risk for thromboembolism (AFIB) |
|---|---|

| 3551F | Intermediate risk for thromboembolism (AFIB) |
|---|---|

🏥 0.00   🔬 0.00   **FUD** XXX   E

| 3552F | High risk for thromboembolism (AFIB) |
|---|---|

🏥 0.00   🔬 0.00   **FUD** XXX   E

| 3555F | Patient had International Normalized Ratio (INR) measurement performed (AFIB) |
|---|---|

🏥 0.00   🔬 0.00   **FUD** XXX   E

**AMA:** 2010,Jul,3-5

| 3570F | Final report for bone scintigraphy study includes correlation with existing relevant imaging studies (eg, X-ray, MRI, CT) corresponding to the same anatomical region in question (NUC_MED) |
|---|---|

🏥 0.00   🔬 0.00   **FUD** XXX   M

| 3572F | Patient considered to be potentially at risk for fracture in a weight-bearing site (NUC_MED) |
|---|---|

🏥 0.00   🔬 0.00   **FUD** XXX   E

| 3573F | Patient not considered to be potentially at risk for fracture in a weight-bearing site (NUC_MED) |
|---|---|

🏥 0.00   🔬 0.00   **FUD** XXX   E

| 3650F | Electroencephalogram (EEG) ordered, reviewed or requested (EPI) |
|---|---|

🏥 0.00   🔬 0.00   **FUD** XXX   E

| 3700F | Psychiatric disorders or disturbances assessed (Prkns) |
|---|---|

🏥 0.00   🔬 0.00   **FUD** XXX   E

| 3720F | Cognitive impairment or dysfunction assessed (Prkns) |
|---|---|

🏥 0.00   🔬 0.00   **FUD** XXX   M

| 3725F | Screening for depression performed (DEM) |
|---|---|

🏥 0.00   🔬 0.00   **FUD** XXX   M

| 3750F | Patient not receiving dose of corticosteroids greater than or equal to 10mg/day for 60 or greater consecutive days (IBD) |
|---|---|

🏥 0.00   🔬 0.00   **FUD** XXX   E

| 3751F | Electrodiagnostic studies for distal symmetric polyneuropathy conducted (or requested), documented, and reviewed within 6 months of initial evaluation for condition (DSP) |
|---|---|

🏥 0.00   🔬 0.00   **FUD** XXX   E

| 3752F | Electrodiagnostic studies for distal symmetric polyneuropathy not conducted (or requested), documented, or reviewed within 6 months of initial evaluation for condition (DSP) |
|---|---|

🏥 0.00   🔬 0.00   **FUD** XXX   E

| 3753F | Patient has clear clinical symptoms and signs that are highly suggestive of neuropathy AND cannot be attributed to another condition, AND has an obvious cause for the neuropathy (DSP) |
|---|---|

🏥 0.00   🔬 0.00   **FUD** XXX   E

| 3754F | Screening tests for diabetes mellitus reviewed, requested, or ordered (DSP) |
|---|---|

🏥 0.00   🔬 0.00   **FUD** XXX   E

| 3755F | Cognitive and behavioral impairment screening performed (ALS) |
|---|---|

🏥 0.00   🔬 0.00   **FUD** XXX   E

| 3756F | Patient has pseudobulbar affect, sialorrhea, or ALS-related symptoms (ALS) |
|---|---|

🏥 0.00   🔬 0.00   **FUD** XXX   E

| 3757F | Patient does not have pseudobulbar affect, sialorrhea, or ALS-related symptoms (ALS) |
|---|---|

🏥 0.00   🔬 0.00   **FUD** XXX   E

| 3758F | Patient referred for pulmonary function testing or peak cough expiratory flow (ALS) |
|---|---|

🏥 0.00   🔬 0.00   **FUD** XXX   E

| 3759F | Patient screened for dysphagia, weight loss, and impaired nutrition, and results documented (ALS) |
|---|---|

🏥 0.00   🔬 0.00   **FUD** XXX   E

| 3760F | Patient exhibits dysphagia, weight loss, or impaired nutrition (ALS) |
|---|---|

🏥 0.00   🔬 0.00   **FUD** XXX   E

| 3761F | Patient does not exhibit dysphagia, weight loss, or impaired nutrition (ALS) |
|---|---|

🏥 0.00   🔬 0.00   **FUD** XXX   E

| 3762F | Patient is dysarthric (ALS) |
|---|---|

🏥 0.00   🔬 0.00   **FUD** XXX   E

| 3763F | Patient is not dysarthric (ALS) |
|---|---|

🏥 0.00   🔬 0.00   **FUD** XXX   E

| 3775F | Adenoma(s) or other neoplasm detected during screening colonoscopy (SCADR) |
|---|---|

🏥 0.00   🔬 0.00   **FUD** XXX   M

| 3776F | Adenoma(s) or other neoplasm not detected during screening colonoscopy (SCADR) |
|---|---|

🏥 0.00   🔬 0.00   **FUD** XXX   M

## 4000F-4563F Therapies Provided (Includes Preventive Services)

INCLUDES   Behavioral/pharmacologic/procedural therapies
Preventive services including patient education/counseling

| 4000F | Tobacco use cessation intervention, counseling (COPD, CAP, CAD, Asthma) (DM) (PV) |
|---|---|

🏥 0.00   🔬 0.00   **FUD** XXX   E

**AMA:** 2017,Jan,8; 2016,Jan,13; 2015,Jan,16; 2014,Jan,11

| 4001F | Tobacco use cessation intervention, pharmacologic therapy (COPD, CAD, CAP, PV, Asthma) (DM) (PV) |
|---|---|

🏥 0.00   🔬 0.00   **FUD** XXX   E

**AMA:** 2008,Mar,8-12; 2004,Nov,1

| 4003F | Patient education, written/oral, appropriate for patients with heart failure, performed (NMA-No Measure Associated) |
|---|---|

🏥 0.00   🔬 0.00   **FUD** XXX   E

**AMA:** 2004,Nov,1

| 4004F | Patient screened for tobacco use and received tobacco cessation intervention (counseling, pharmacotherapy, or both), if identified as a tobacco user (PV, CAD) |
|---|---|

🏥 0.00   🔬 0.00   **FUD** XXX   M

| 4005F | Pharmacologic therapy (other than minerals/vitamins) for osteoporosis prescribed (OP) (IBD) |
|---|---|

🏥 0.00   🔬 0.00   **FUD** XXX   E

| 4008F | Beta-blocker therapy prescribed or currently being taken (CAD,HF) |
|---|---|

🏥 0.00   🔬 0.00   **FUD** XXX   M

| 4010F | Angiotensin Converting Enzyme (ACE) Inhibitor or Angiotensin Receptor Blocker (ARB) therapy prescribed or currently being taken (CAD, CKD, HF) (DM) |
|---|---|

🏥 0.00   🔬 0.00   **FUD** XXX   M

| 4011F | Oral antiplatelet therapy prescribed (CAD) |
|---|---|

🏥 0.00   🔬 0.00   **FUD** XXX   E

**AMA:** 2004,Nov,1

| 4012F | Warfarin therapy prescribed (NMA-No Measure Associated) |
|---|---|

🏥 0.00   🔬 0.00   **FUD** XXX   E

| 4013F | Statin therapy prescribed or currently being taken (CAD) |
|---|---|

🏥 0.00   🔬 0.00   **FUD** XXX   E

| 4014F | Written discharge instructions provided to heart failure patients discharged home (Instructions include all of the following components: activity level, diet, discharge medications, follow-up appointment, weight monitoring, what to do if symptoms worsen) (NMA-No Measure Associated) |
|---|---|

🏥 0.00   🔬 0.00   **FUD** XXX   E

26/TC PC/TC Only   A2-A8 ASC Payment   50 Bilateral   ♂ Male Only   ♀ Female Only   🏥 Facility RVU   🔬 Non-Facility RVU   ☐ CCI
**FUD** Follow-up Days   **CMS:** IOM (Pub 100)   A-Y OPPSI   80/80 Surg Assist Allowed / w/Doc   🔬 Lab Crosswalk   ☢ Radiology Crosswalk   ✖ CLIA

534   CPT © 2017 American Medical Association. All Rights Reserved.   © 2017 Optum360, LLC

**4015F** Persistent asthma, preferred long term control medication or an acceptable alternative treatment, prescribed (NMA-No Measure Associated)

🔧 0.00　✂ 0.00　**FUD** XXX　　　E

EXCLUDES　*Use of code with modifier 1P*

Code also modifier 2P for patient reasons for not prescribing

**4016F** Anti-inflammatory/analgesic agent prescribed (OA) (Use for prescribed or continued medication[s], including over-the-counter medication[s])

🔧 0.00　✂ 0.00　**FUD** XXX　　　E

INCLUDES　Over-the-counter medication(s)

Prescribed/continued medication(s)

**4017F** Gastrointestinal prophylaxis for NSAID use prescribed (OA)

🔧 0.00　✂ 0.00　**FUD** XXX　　　E

**4018F** Therapeutic exercise for the involved joint(s) instructed or physical or occupational therapy prescribed (OA)

🔧 0.00　✂ 0.00　**FUD** XXX　　　E

**4019F** Documentation of receipt of counseling on exercise and either both calcium and vitamin D use or counseling regarding both calcium and vitamin D use (OP)

🔧 0.00　✂ 0.00　**FUD** XXX　　　E

**4025F** Inhaled bronchodilator prescribed (COPD)

🔧 0.00　✂ 0.00　**FUD** XXX　　　E

**4030F** Long-term oxygen therapy prescribed (more than 15 hours per day) (COPD)

🔧 0.00　✂ 0.00　**FUD** XXX　　　E

**4033F** Pulmonary rehabilitation exercise training recommended (COPD)

🔧 0.00　✂ 0.00　**FUD** XXX　　　E

Code also dyspnea assessed, present (1019F)

**4035F** Influenza immunization recommended (COPD) (IBD)

🔧 0.00　✂ 0.00　**FUD** XXX　　　E

AMA: 2008,Mar,8-12

**4037F** Influenza immunization ordered or administered (COPD, PV, CKD, ESRD)(IBD)

🔧 0.00　✂ 0.00　**FUD** XXX　　　E

AMA: 2008,Mar,8-12

**4040F** Pneumococcal vaccine administered or previously received (COPD) (PV), (IBD)

🔧 0.00　✂ 0.00　**FUD** XXX　　　M

AMA: 2008,Mar,8-12

**4041F** Documentation of order for cefazolin OR cefuroxime for antimicrobial prophylaxis (PERI 2)

🔧 0.00　✂ 0.00　**FUD** XXX　　　E

**4042F** Documentation that prophylactic antibiotics were neither given within 4 hours prior to surgical incision nor given intraoperatively (PERI 2)

🔧 0.00　✂ 0.00　**FUD** XXX　　　E

**4043F** Documentation that an order was given to discontinue prophylactic antibiotics within 48 hours of surgical end time, cardiac procedures (PERI 2)

🔧 0.00　✂ 0.00　**FUD** XXX　　　E

**4044F** Documentation that an order was given for venous thromboembolism (VTE) prophylaxis to be given within 24 hours prior to incision time or 24 hours after surgery end time (PERI 2)

🔧 0.00　✂ 0.00　**FUD** XXX　　　M

**4045F** Appropriate empiric antibiotic prescribed (CAP), (EM)

🔧 0.00　✂ 0.00　**FUD** XXX　　　E

**4046F** Documentation that prophylactic antibiotics were given within 4 hours prior to surgical incision or given intraoperatively (PERI 2)

🔧 0.00　✂ 0.00　**FUD** XXX　　　E

**4047F** Documentation of order for prophylactic parenteral antibiotics to be given within 1 hour (if fluoroquinolone or vancomycin, 2 hours) prior to surgical incision (or start of procedure when no incision is required) (PERI 2)

🔧 0.00　✂ 0.00　**FUD** XXX　　　E

**4048F** Documentation that administration of prophylactic parenteral antibiotic was initiated within 1 hour (if fluoroquinolone or vancomycin, 2 hours) prior to surgical incision (or start of procedure when no incision is required) as ordered (PERI 2)

🔧 0.00　✂ 0.00　**FUD** XXX　　　E

**4049F** Documentation that order was given to discontinue prophylactic antibiotics within 24 hours of surgical end time, non-cardiac procedure (PERI 2)

🔧 0.00　✂ 0.00　**FUD** XXX　　　E

**4050F** Hypertension plan of care documented as appropriate (NMA-No Measure Associated)

🔧 0.00　✂ 0.00　**FUD** XXX　　　E

**4051F** Referred for an arteriovenous (AV) fistula (ESRD, CKD)

🔧 0.00　✂ 0.00　**FUD** XXX　　　E

AMA: 2008,Mar,8-12

**4052F** Hemodialysis via functioning arteriovenous (AV) fistula (ESRD)

🔧 0.00　✂ 0.00　**FUD** XXX　　　E

AMA: 2008,Mar,8-12

**4053F** Hemodialysis via functioning arteriovenous (AV) graft (ESRD)

🔧 0.00　✂ 0.00　**FUD** XXX　　　E

AMA: 2008,Mar,8-12

**4054F** Hemodialysis via catheter (ESRD)

🔧 0.00　✂ 0.00　**FUD** XXX　　　E

AMA: 2008,Mar,8-12

**4055F** Patient receiving peritoneal dialysis (ESRD)

🔧 0.00　✂ 0.00　**FUD** XXX　　　E

AMA: 2008,Mar,8-12

**4056F** Appropriate oral rehydration solution recommended (PAG)

🔧 0.00　✂ 0.00　**FUD** XXX　　　E

**4058F** Pediatric gastroenteritis education provided to caregiver (PAG)

🔧 0.00　✂ 0.00　**FUD** XXX　　　E

**4060F** Psychotherapy services provided (MDD, MDD ADOL)

🔧 0.00　✂ 0.00　**FUD** XXX　　　E

**4062F** Patient referral for psychotherapy documented (MDD, MDD ADOL)

🔧 0.00　✂ 0.00　**FUD** XXX　　　E

**4063F** Antidepressant pharmacotherapy considered and not prescribed (MDD ADOL)

🔧 0.00　✂ 0.00　**FUD** XXX　　　E

**4064F** Antidepressant pharmacotherapy prescribed (MDD, MDD ADOL)

🔧 0.00　✂ 0.00　**FUD** XXX　　　E

**4065F** Antipsychotic pharmacotherapy prescribed (MDD)

🔧 0.00　✂ 0.00　**FUD** XXX　　　E

**4066F** Electroconvulsive therapy (ECT) provided (MDD)

🔧 0.00　✂ 0.00　**FUD** XXX　　　E

**4067F** Patient referral for electroconvulsive therapy (ECT) documented (MDD)

🔧 0.00　✂ 0.00　**FUD** XXX　　　E

**4069F** Venous thromboembolism (VTE) prophylaxis received (IBD)

🔧 0.00　✂ 0.00　**FUD** XXX　　　E

---

● New Code　▲ Revised Code　○ Reinstated　● New Web Release　▲ Revised Web Release　Unlisted　Not Covered　# Resequenced
Ⓢ AMA Mod 51 Exempt　Ⓢ Optum Mod 51 Exempt　Ⓢ Mod 63 Exempt　✕ Non-FDA Drug　★ Telemedicine　Ⓜ Maternity　Ⓐ Age Edit　✚ Add-on　**AMA:** CPT Asst

© 2017 Optum360, LLC　　CPT © 2017 American Medical Association. All Rights Reserved.

**4070F** Deep vein thrombosis (DVT) prophylaxis received by end of hospital day 2 (STR)
 0.00  0.00  **FUD** XXX  E

**4073F** Oral antiplatelet therapy prescribed at discharge (STR)
 0.00  0.00  **FUD** XXX  E

**4075F** Anticoagulant therapy prescribed at discharge (STR)
 0.00  0.00  **FUD** XXX  E

**4077F** Documentation that tissue plasminogen activator (t-PA) administration was considered (STR)
 0.00  0.00  **FUD** XXX  E

**4079F** Documentation that rehabilitation services were considered (STR)
 0.00  0.00  **FUD** XXX  E

**4084F** Aspirin received within 24 hours before emergency department arrival or during emergency department stay (EM)
 0.00  0.00  **FUD** XXX  E

**4086F** Aspirin or clopidogrel prescribed or currently being taken (CAD)
 0.00  0.00  **FUD** XXX  M

**4090F** Patient receiving erythropoietin therapy (HEM)
 0.00  0.00  **FUD** XXX  M
**AMA:** 2008,Mar,8-12

**4095F** Patient not receiving erythropoietin therapy (HEM)
 0.00  0.00  **FUD** XXX  E
**AMA:** 2008,Mar,8-12

**4100F** Bisphosphonate therapy, intravenous, ordered or received (HEM)
 0.00  0.00  **FUD** XXX  M
**AMA:** 2008,Mar,8-12

**4110F** Internal mammary artery graft performed for primary, isolated coronary artery bypass graft procedure (CABG)
 0.00  0.00  **FUD** XXX  M

**4115F** Beta blocker administered within 24 hours prior to surgical incision (CABG)
 0.00  0.00  **FUD** XXX  M

**4120F** Antibiotic prescribed or dispensed (URI, PHAR), (A-BRONCH)
 0.00  0.00  **FUD** XXX  M
**AMA:** 2008,Mar,8-12

**4124F** Antibiotic neither prescribed nor dispensed (URI, PHAR), (A-BRONCH)
 0.00  0.00  **FUD** XXX  M
**AMA:** 2008,Mar,8-12

**4130F** Topical preparations (including OTC) prescribed for acute otitis externa (AOE)
 0.00  0.00  **FUD** XXX  M
**AMA:** 2010,Jan,6-7; 2008,Mar,8-12

**4131F** Systemic antimicrobial therapy prescribed (AOE)
 0.00  0.00  **FUD** XXX  M
**AMA:** 2008,Mar,8-12

**4132F** Systemic antimicrobial therapy not prescribed (AOE)
 0.00  0.00  **FUD** XXX  M
**AMA:** 2008,Mar,8-12

**4133F** Antihistamines or decongestants prescribed or recommended (OME)
 0.00  0.00  **FUD** XXX  E
**AMA:** 2008,Mar,8-12

**4134F** Antihistamines or decongestants neither prescribed nor recommended (OME)
 0.00  0.00  **FUD** XXX  E
**AMA:** 2008,Mar,8-12

**4135F** Systemic corticosteroids prescribed (OME)
 0.00  0.00  **FUD** XXX  E
**AMA:** 2008,Mar,8-12

**4136F** Systemic corticosteroids not prescribed (OME)
 0.00  0.00  **FUD** XXX  E
**AMA:** 2008,Mar,8-12

**4140F** Inhaled corticosteroids prescribed (Asthma)
 0.00  0.00  **FUD** XXX  E

**4142F** Corticosteroid sparing therapy prescribed (IBD)
 0.00  0.00  **FUD** XXX  E

**4144F** Alternative long-term control medication prescribed (Asthma)
 0.00  0.00  **FUD** XXX  E

**4145F** Two or more anti-hypertensive agents prescribed or currently being taken (CAD, HTN)
 0.00  0.00  **FUD** XXX  E

**4148F** Hepatitis A vaccine injection administered or previously received (HEP-C)
 0.00  0.00  **FUD** XXX  E

**4149F** Hepatitis B vaccine injection administered or previously received (HEP-C, HIV) (IBD)
 0.00  0.00  **FUD** XXX  E

**4150F** Patient receiving antiviral treatment for Hepatitis C (HEP-C)
 0.00  0.00  **FUD** XXX  E
**AMA:** 2008,Mar,8-12

**4151F** Patient did not start or is not receiving antiviral treatment for Hepatitis C during the measurement period (HEP-C)
 0.00  0.00  **FUD** XXX  E
**AMA:** 2008,Mar,8-12

**4153F** Combination peginterferon and ribavirin therapy prescribed (HEP-C)
 0.00  0.00  **FUD** XXX  E
**AMA:** 2008,Mar,8-12

**4155F** Hepatitis A vaccine series previously received (HEP-C)
 0.00  0.00  **FUD** XXX  E
**AMA:** 2008,Mar,8-12

**4157F** Hepatitis B vaccine series previously received (HEP-C)
 0.00  0.00  **FUD** XXX  E
**AMA:** 2008,Mar,8-12

**4158F** Patient counseled about risks of alcohol use (HEP-C)
 0.00  0.00  **FUD** XXX  E
**AMA:** 2008,Mar,8-12

**4159F** Counseling regarding contraception received prior to initiation of antiviral treatment (HEP-C)
 0.00  0.00  **FUD** XXX  E
**AMA:** 2008,Mar,8-12

**4163F** Patient counseling at a minimum on all of the following treatment options for clinically localized prostate cancer: active surveillance, and interstitial prostate brachytherapy, and external beam radiotherapy, and radical prostatectomy, provided prior to initiation of treatment (PRCA)
 0.00  0.00  **FUD** XXX  E
**AMA:** 2008,Mar,8-12

**4164F** Adjuvant (ie, in combination with external beam radiotherapy to the prostate for prostate cancer) hormonal therapy (gonadotropin-releasing hormone [GnRH] agonist or antagonist) prescribed/administered (PRCA)
 0.00  0.00  **FUD** XXX  M
**AMA:** 2008,Mar,8-12

**4165F** 3-dimensional conformal radiotherapy (3D-CRT) or intensity modulated radiation therapy (IMRT) received (PRCA)
 0.00  0.00  **FUD** XXX  E
**AMA:** 2008,Mar,8-12

26/TC PC/TC Only  A2-Z3 ASC Payment  50 Bilateral  ♂ Male Only  ♀ Female Only   Facility RVU   Non-Facility RVU   CCI
FUD Follow-up Days  CMS: IOM (Pub 100)  A-Y OPPSI  80/80 Surg Assist Allowed / w/Doc   Lab Crosswalk   Radiology Crosswalk  CLIA

536
CPT © 2017 American Medical Association. All Rights Reserved.
© 2017 Optum360, LLC

**4167F** Head of bed elevation (30-45 degrees) on first ventilator day ordered (CRIT)

🚑 0.00   ⚕ 0.00   **FUD** XXX   E

AMA: 2008,Mar,8-12

**4168F** Patient receiving care in the intensive care unit (ICU) and receiving mechanical ventilation, 24 hours or less (CRIT)

🚑 0.00   ⚕ 0.00   **FUD** XXX   E

AMA: 2008,Mar,8-12

**4169F** Patient either not receiving care in the intensive care unit (ICU) OR not receiving mechanical ventilation OR receiving mechanical ventilation greater than 24 hours (CRIT)

🚑 0.00   ⚕ 0.00   **FUD** XXX   E

AMA: 2008,Mar,8-12

**4171F** Patient receiving erythropoiesis-stimulating agents (ESA) therapy (CKD)

🚑 0.00   ⚕ 0.00   **FUD** XXX   E

AMA: 2008,Mar,8-12

**4172F** Patient not receiving erythropoiesis-stimulating agents (ESA) therapy (CKD)

🚑 0.00   ⚕ 0.00   **FUD** XXX   E

AMA: 2008,Mar,8-12

**4174F** Counseling about the potential impact of glaucoma on visual functioning and quality of life, and importance of treatment adherence provided to patient and/or caregiver(s) (EC)

🚑 0.00   ⚕ 0.00   **FUD** XXX   E

AMA: 2008,Mar,8-12

**4175F** Best-corrected visual acuity of 20/40 or better (distance or near) achieved within the 90 days following cataract surgery (EC)

🚑 0.00   ⚕ 0.00   **FUD** XXX   M

AMA: 2008,Mar,8-12

**4176F** Counseling about value of protection from UV light and lack of proven efficacy of nutritional supplements in prevention or progression of cataract development provided to patient and/or caregiver(s) (NMA-No Measure Associated)

🚑 0.00   ⚕ 0.00   **FUD** XXX   E

**4177F** Counseling about the benefits and/or risks of the Age-Related Eye Disease Study (AREDS) formulation for preventing progression of age-related macular degeneration (AMD) provided to patient and/or caregiver(s) (EC)

🚑 0.00   ⚕ 0.00   **FUD** XXX   M

AMA: 2008,Mar,8-12

**4178F** Anti-D immune globulin received between 26 and 30 weeks gestation (Pre-Cr)   M

🚑 0.00   ⚕ 0.00   **FUD** XXX   E

AMA: 2008,Mar,8-12

**4179F** Tamoxifen or aromatase inhibitor (AI) prescribed (ONC)

🚑 0.00   ⚕ 0.00   **FUD** XXX   E

AMA: 2008,Mar,8-12

**4180F** Adjuvant chemotherapy referred, prescribed, or previously received for Stage III colon cancer (ONC)

🚑 0.00   ⚕ 0.00   **FUD** XXX   E

AMA: 2008,Mar,8-12

**4181F** Conformal radiation therapy received (NMA-No Measure Associated)

🚑 0.00   ⚕ 0.00   **FUD** XXX   E

**4182F** Conformal radiation therapy not received (NMA-No Measure Associated)

🚑 0.00   ⚕ 0.00   **FUD** XXX   E

**4185F** Continuous (12-months) therapy with proton pump inhibitor (PPI) or histamine H2 receptor antagonist (H2RA) received (GERD)

🚑 0.00   ⚕ 0.00   **FUD** XXX   E

AMA: 2008,Mar,8-12

**4186F** No continuous (12-months) therapy with either proton pump inhibitor (PPI) or histamine H2 receptor antagonist (H2RA) received (GERD)

🚑 0.00   ⚕ 0.00   **FUD** XXX   E

AMA: 2008,Mar,8-12

**4187F** Disease modifying anti-rheumatic drug therapy prescribed or dispensed (RA)

🚑 0.00   ⚕ 0.00   **FUD** XXX   E

**4188F** Appropriate angiotensin converting enzyme (ACE)/angiotensin receptor blockers (ARB) therapeutic monitoring test ordered or performed (AM)

🚑 0.00   ⚕ 0.00   **FUD** XXX   E

AMA: 2008,Mar,8-12

**4189F** Appropriate digoxin therapeutic monitoring test ordered or performed (AM)

🚑 0.00   ⚕ 0.00   **FUD** XXX   E

AMA: 2008,Mar,8-12

**4190F** Appropriate diuretic therapeutic monitoring test ordered or performed (AM)

🚑 0.00   ⚕ 0.00   **FUD** XXX   E

AMA: 2008,Mar,8-12

**4191F** Appropriate anticonvulsant therapeutic monitoring test ordered or performed (AM)

🚑 0.00   ⚕ 0.00   **FUD** XXX   E

AMA: 2008,Mar,8-12

**4192F** Patient not receiving glucocorticoid therapy (RA)

🚑 0.00   ⚕ 0.00   **FUD** XXX   M

**4193F** Patient receiving <10 mg daily prednisone (or equivalent), or RA activity is worsening, or glucocorticoid use is for less than 6 months (RA)

🚑 0.00   ⚕ 0.00   **FUD** XXX   M

**4194F** Patient receiving ≥10 mg daily prednisone (or equivalent) for longer than 6 months, and improvement or no change in disease activity (RA)

🚑 0.00   ⚕ 0.00   **FUD** XXX   M

**4195F** Patient receiving first-time biologic disease modifying anti-rheumatic drug therapy for rheumatoid arthritis (RA)

🚑 0.00   ⚕ 0.00   **FUD** XXX   M

**4196F** Patient not receiving first-time biologic disease modifying anti-rheumatic drug therapy for rheumatoid arthritis (RA)

🚑 0.00   ⚕ 0.00   **FUD** XXX   M

**4200F** External beam radiotherapy as primary therapy to prostate with or without nodal irradiation (PRCA)

🚑 0.00   ⚕ 0.00   **FUD** XXX   E

AMA: 2008,Mar,8-12

**4201F** External beam radiotherapy with or without nodal irradiation as adjuvant or salvage therapy for prostate cancer patient (PRCA)

🚑 0.00   ⚕ 0.00   **FUD** XXX   E

AMA: 2008,Mar,8-12

**4210F** Angiotensin converting enzyme (ACE) or angiotensin receptor blockers (ARB) medication therapy for 6 months or more (MM)

🚑 0.00   ⚕ 0.00   **FUD** XXX   E

AMA: 2008,Mar,8-12

**4220F** Digoxin medication therapy for 6 months or more (MM)

🚑 0.00   ⚕ 0.00   **FUD** XXX   E

AMA: 2008,Mar,8-12

**4221F** Diuretic medication therapy for 6 months or more (MM)

🚑 0.00   ⚕ 0.00   **FUD** XXX   E

AMA: 2008,Mar,8-12

**4230F** Anticonvulsant medication therapy for 6 months or more (MM)

🚑 0.00   ⚕ 0.00   **FUD** XXX   E

AMA: 2008,Mar,8-12

---

● New Code   ▲ Revised Code   ○ Reinstated   ● New Web Release   ▲ Revised Web Release   Unlisted   Not Covered   # Resequenced
⊘ AMA Mod 51 Exempt   Ⓢ Optum Mod 51 Exempt   ⓒ Mod 63 Exempt   ✎ Non-FDA Drug   ★ Telemedicine   M Maternity   A Age Edit   + Add-on   **AMA:** CPT Asst
© 2017 Optum360, LLC          CPT © 2017 American Medical Association. All Rights Reserved.

Category II Codes · 4240F — 4470F

**4240F** Instruction in therapeutic exercise with follow-up provided to patients during episode of back pain lasting longer than 12 weeks (BkP)

🖫 0.00 ◿ 0.00 **FUD** XXX E

AMA: 2008,Mar,8-12

**4242F** Counseling for supervised exercise program provided to patients during episode of back pain lasting longer than 12 weeks (BkP)

🖫 0.00 ◿ 0.00 **FUD** XXX E

AMA: 2008,Mar,8-12

**4245F** Patient counseled during the initial visit to maintain or resume normal activities (BkP)

🖫 0.00 ◿ 0.00 **FUD** XXX E

AMA: 2008,Mar,8-12

**4248F** Patient counseled during the initial visit for an episode of back pain against bed rest lasting 4 days or longer (BkP)

🖫 0.00 ◿ 0.00 **FUD** XXX E

AMA: 2008,Mar,8-12

**4250F** Active warming used intraoperatively for the purpose of maintaining normothermia, or at least 1 body temperature equal to or greater than 36 degrees Centigrade (or 96.8 degrees Fahrenheit) recorded within the 30 minutes immediately before or the 15 minutes immediately after anesthesia end time (CRIT)

🖫 0.00 ◿ 0.00 **FUD** XXX E

AMA: 2008,Mar,8-12

**4255F** Duration of general or neuraxial anesthesia 60 minutes or longer, as documented in the anesthesia record (CRIT) (Peri2)

🖫 0.00 ◿ 0.00 **FUD** XXX M

**4256F** Duration of general or neuraxial anesthesia less than 60 minutes, as documented in the anesthesia record (CRIT) (Peri2)

🖫 0.00 ◿ 0.00 **FUD** XXX E

**4260F** Wound surface culture technique used (CWC)

🖫 0.00 ◿ 0.00 **FUD** XXX E

**4261F** Technique other than surface culture of the wound exudate used (eg, Levine/deep swab technique, semi-quantitative or quantitative swab technique) or wound surface culture technique not used (CWC)

🖫 0.00 ◿ 0.00 **FUD** XXX E

**4265F** Use of wet to dry dressings prescribed or recommended (CWC)

🖫 0.00 ◿ 0.00 **FUD** XXX E

**4266F** Use of wet to dry dressings neither prescribed nor recommended (CWC)

🖫 0.00 ◿ 0.00 **FUD** XXX E

**4267F** Compression therapy prescribed (CWC)

🖫 0.00 ◿ 0.00 **FUD** XXX E

**4268F** Patient education regarding the need for long term compression therapy including interval replacement of compression stockings received (CWC)

🖫 0.00 ◿ 0.00 **FUD** XXX E

**4269F** Appropriate method of offloading (pressure relief) prescribed (CWC)

🖫 0.00 ◿ 0.00 **FUD** XXX E

**4270F** Patient receiving potent antiretroviral therapy for 6 months or longer (HIV)

🖫 0.00 ◿ 0.00 **FUD** XXX E

**4271F** Patient receiving potent antiretroviral therapy for less than 6 months or not receiving potent antiretroviral therapy (HIV)

🖫 0.00 ◿ 0.00 **FUD** XXX E

**4274F** Influenza immunization administered or previously received (HIV) (P-ESRD)

🖫 0.00 ◿ 0.00 **FUD** XXX E

**4276F** Potent antiretroviral therapy prescribed (HIV)

🖫 0.00 ◿ 0.00 **FUD** XXX E

**4279F** Pneumocystis jiroveci pneumonia prophylaxis prescribed (HIV)

🖫 0.00 ◿ 0.00 **FUD** XXX E

**4280F** Pneumocystis jiroveci pneumonia prophylaxis prescribed within 3 months of low CD4+ cell count or percentage (HIV)

🖫 0.00 ◿ 0.00 **FUD** XXX E

**4290F** Patient screened for injection drug use (HIV)

🖫 0.00 ◿ 0.00 **FUD** XXX E

**4293F** Patient screened for high-risk sexual behavior (HIV)

🖫 0.00 ◿ 0.00 **FUD** XXX E

**4300F** Patient receiving warfarin therapy for nonvalvular atrial fibrillation or atrial flutter (AFIB)

🖫 0.00 ◿ 0.00 **FUD** XXX E

**4301F** Patient not receiving warfarin therapy for nonvalvular atrial fibrillation or atrial flutter (AFIB)

🖫 0.00 ◿ 0.00 **FUD** XXX E

**4305F** Patient education regarding appropriate foot care and daily inspection of the feet received (CWC)

🖫 0.00 ◿ 0.00 **FUD** XXX E

**4306F** Patient counseled regarding psychosocial and pharmacologic treatment options for opioid addiction (SUD)

🖫 0.00 ◿ 0.00 **FUD** XXX E

**4320F** Patient counseled regarding psychosocial and pharmacologic treatment options for alcohol dependence (SUD)

🖫 0.00 ◿ 0.00 **FUD** XXX E

**4322F** Caregiver provided with education and referred to additional resources for support (DEM)

🖫 0.00 ◿ 0.00 **FUD** XXX M

**4324F** Patient (or caregiver) queried about Parkinson's disease medication related motor complications (Prkns)

🖫 0.00 ◿ 0.00 **FUD** XXX E

**4325F** Medical and surgical treatment options reviewed with patient (or caregiver) (Prkns)

🖫 0.00 ◿ 0.00 **FUD** XXX M

**4326F** Patient (or caregiver) queried about symptoms of autonomic dysfunction (Prkns)

🖫 0.00 ◿ 0.00 **FUD** XXX E

**4328F** Patient (or caregiver) queried about sleep disturbances (Prkns)

🖫 0.00 ◿ 0.00 **FUD** XXX E

**4330F** Counseling about epilepsy specific safety issues provided to patient (or caregiver(s)) (EPI)

🖫 0.00 ◿ 0.00 **FUD** XXX E

**4340F** Counseling for women of childbearing potential with epilepsy (EPI)

🖫 0.00 ◿ 0.00 **FUD** XXX M

**4350F** Counseling provided on symptom management, end of life decisions, and palliation (DEM)

🖫 0.00 ◿ 0.00 **FUD** XXX E

**4400F** Rehabilitative therapy options discussed with patient (or caregiver) (Prkns)

🖫 0.00 ◿ 0.00 **FUD** XXX M

**4450F** Self-care education provided to patient (HF)

🖫 0.00 ◿ 0.00 **FUD** XXX E

**4470F** Implantable cardioverter-defibrillator (ICD) counseling provided (HF)

🖫 0.00 ◿ 0.00 **FUD** XXX E

26/TC PC/TC Only    A2-Z3 ASC Payment    50 Bilateral    ♂ Male Only    ♀ Female Only    🖫 Facility RVU    ◿ Non-Facility RVU    ▢ CCI

**FUD** Follow-up Days    **CMS:** IOM (Pub 100)    A-Y OPPSI    80/80 Surg Assist Allowed / w/Doc    ▤ Lab Crosswalk    ▦ Radiology Crosswalk    ✖ CLIA

538          CPT © 2017 American Medical Association. All Rights Reserved.        © 2017 Optum360, LLC

**4480F** Patient receiving ACE inhibitor/ARB therapy and beta-blocker therapy for 3 months or longer (HF)
📋 0.00   ✂ 0.00   **FUD** XXX                    E

**4481F** Patient receiving ACE inhibitor/ARB therapy and beta-blocker therapy for less than 3 months or patient not receiving ACE inhibitor/ARB therapy and beta-blocker therapy (HF)
📋 0.00   ✂ 0.00   **FUD** XXX                    E

**4500F** Referred to an outpatient cardiac rehabilitation program (CAD)
📋 0.00   ✂ 0.00   **FUD** XXX                    M

**4510F** Previous cardiac rehabilitation for qualifying cardiac event completed (CAD)
📋 0.00   ✂ 0.00   **FUD** XXX                    M

**4525F** Neuropsychiatric intervention ordered (DEM)
📋 0.00   ✂ 0.00   **FUD** XXX                    M

**4526F** Neuropsychiatric intervention received (DEM)
📋 0.00   ✂ 0.00   **FUD** XXX                    M

**4540F** Disease modifying pharmacotherapy discussed (ALS)
📋 0.00   ✂ 0.00   **FUD** XXX                    E

**4541F** Patient offered treatment for pseudobulbar affect, sialorrhea, or ALS-related symptoms (ALS)
📋 0.00   ✂ 0.00   **FUD** XXX                    E

**4550F** Options for noninvasive respiratory support discussed with patient (ALS)
📋 0.00   ✂ 0.00   **FUD** XXX                    E

**4551F** Nutritional support offered (ALS)
📋 0.00   ✂ 0.00   **FUD** XXX                    E

**4552F** Patient offered referral to a speech language pathologist (ALS)
📋 0.00   ✂ 0.00   **FUD** XXX                    E

**4553F** Patient offered assistance in planning for end of life issues (ALS)
📋 0.00   ✂ 0.00   **FUD** XXX                    E

**4554F** Patient received inhalational anesthetic agent (Peri2)
📋 0.00   ✂ 0.00   **FUD** XXX                    M

**4555F** Patient did not receive inhalational anesthetic agent (Peri2)
📋 0.00   ✂ 0.00   **FUD** XXX                    E

**4556F** Patient exhibits 3 or more risk factors for post-operative nausea and vomiting (Peri2)
📋 0.00   ✂ 0.00   **FUD** XXX                    M

**4557F** Patient does not exhibit 3 or more risk factors for post-operative nausea and vomiting (Peri2)
📋 0.00   ✂ 0.00   **FUD** XXX                    E

**4558F** Patient received at least 2 prophylactic pharmacologic anti-emetic agents of different classes preoperatively and intraoperatively (Peri2)
📋 0.00   ✂ 0.00   **FUD** XXX                    E

**4559F** At least 1 body temperature measurement equal to or greater than 35.5 degrees Celsius (or 95.9 degrees Fahrenheit) recorded within the 30 minutes immediately before or the 15 minutes immediately after anesthesia end time (Peri2)
📋 0.00   ✂ 0.00   **FUD** XXX                    E

**4560F** Anesthesia technique did not involve general or neuraxial anesthesia (Peri2)
📋 0.00   ✂ 0.00   **FUD** XXX                    E

**4561F** Patient has a coronary artery stent (Peri2)
📋 0.00   ✂ 0.00   **FUD** XXX                    E

**4562F** Patient does not have a coronary artery stent (Peri2)
📋 0.00   ✂ 0.00   **FUD** XXX                    E

**4563F** Patient received aspirin within 24 hours prior to anesthesia start time (Peri2)
📋 0.00   ✂ 0.00   **FUD** XXX                    E

## 5005F-5250F Results Conveyed and Documented

INCLUDES   Patient's:
    Functional status
    Morbidity/mortality
    Satisfaction/experience with care
    Review/communication of test results to patients

**5005F** Patient counseled on self-examination for new or changing moles (ML)
📋 0.00   ✂ 0.00   **FUD** XXX                    E
**AMA:** 2008,Mar,8-12

**5010F** Findings of dilated macular or fundus exam communicated to the physician or other qualified health care professional managing the diabetes care (EC)
📋 0.00   ✂ 0.00   **FUD** XXX                    M

**5015F** Documentation of communication that a fracture occurred and that the patient was or should be tested or treated for osteoporosis (OP)
📋 0.00   ✂ 0.00   **FUD** XXX                    M

**5020F** Treatment summary report communicated to physician(s) or other qualified health care professional(s) managing continuing care and to the patient within 1 month of completing treatment (ONC)
📋 0.00   ✂ 0.00   **FUD** XXX                    E
**AMA:** 2008,Mar,8-12

**5050F** Treatment plan communicated to provider(s) managing continuing care within 1 month of diagnosis (ML)
📋 0.00   ✂ 0.00   **FUD** XXX                    M
**AMA:** 2008,Mar,8-12

**5060F** Findings from diagnostic mammogram communicated to practice managing patient's on-going care within 3 business days of exam interpretation (RAD)
📋 0.00   ✂ 0.00   **FUD** XXX                    E
**AMA:** 2008,Mar,8-12

**5062F** Findings from diagnostic mammogram communicated to the patient within 5 days of exam interpretation (RAD)
📋 0.00   ✂ 0.00   **FUD** XXX                    E
**AMA:** 2008,Mar,8-12

**5100F** Potential risk for fracture communicated to the referring physician or other qualified health care professional within 24 hours of completion of the imaging study (NUC_MED)
📋 0.00   ✂ 0.00   **FUD** XXX                    E

**5200F** Consideration of referral for a neurological evaluation of appropriateness for surgical therapy for intractable epilepsy within the past 3 years (EPI)
📋 0.00   ✂ 0.00   **FUD** XXX                    E

**5250F** Asthma discharge plan provided to patient (Asthma)
📋 0.00   ✂ 0.00   **FUD** XXX                    E

## 6005F-6150F Elements Related to Patient Safety Processes

INCLUDES   Patient safety practices

**6005F** Rationale (eg, severity of illness and safety) for level of care (eg, home, hospital) documented (CAP)
📋 0.00   ✂ 0.00   **FUD** XXX                    E
**AMA:** 2017,Jan,8; 2016,Jan,13; 2015,Jan,16; 2014,Jan,11

**6010F** Dysphagia screening conducted prior to order for or receipt of any foods, fluids, or medication by mouth (STR)
📋 0.00   ✂ 0.00   **FUD** XXX                    E

**6015F** Patient receiving or eligible to receive foods, fluids, or medication by mouth (STR)
📋 0.00   ✂ 0.00   **FUD** XXX                    E

**6020F** NPO (nothing by mouth) ordered (STR)
📋 0.00   ✂ 0.00   **FUD** XXX                    E

● New Code    ▲ Revised Code    ○ Reinstated    ● New Web Release    ▲ Revised Web Release    Unlisted    Not Covered    # Resequenced
⊘ AMA Mod 51 Exempt    ⑤ Optum Mod 51 Exempt    ⑥³ Mod 63 Exempt    ✗ Non-FDA Drug    ★ Telemedicine    M Maternity    A Age Edit    + Add-on    **AMA:** CPT Asst

**6030F** All elements of maximal sterile barrier technique, hand hygiene, skin preparation and, if ultrasound is used, sterile ultrasound techniques followed (CRIT)
📷 0.00  ✂ 0.00  **FUD** XXX                    M
**AMA:** 2008,Mar,8-12

**6040F** Use of appropriate radiation dose reduction devices OR manual techniques for appropriate moderation of exposure, documented (RAD)
📷 0.00  ✂ 0.00  **FUD** XXX                    E

**6045F** Radiation exposure or exposure time in final report for procedure using fluoroscopy, documented (RAD)
📷 0.00  ✂ 0.00  **FUD** XXX                    E
**AMA:** 2008,Mar,8-12

**6070F** Patient queried and counseled about anti-epileptic drug (AED) side effects (EPI)
📷 0.00  ✂ 0.00  **FUD** XXX                    E

**6080F** Patient (or caregiver) queried about falls (Prkns, DSP)
📷 0.00  ✂ 0.00  **FUD** XXX                    E

**6090F** Patient (or caregiver) counseled about safety issues appropriate to patient's stage of disease (Prkns)
📷 0.00  ✂ 0.00  **FUD** XXX                    E

**6100F** Timeout to verify correct patient, correct site, and correct procedure, documented (PATH)
📷 0.00  ✂ 0.00  **FUD** XXX                    E

**6101F** Safety counseling for dementia provided (DEM)
📷 0.00  ✂ 0.00  **FUD** XXX                    M

**6102F** Safety counseling for dementia ordered (DEM)
📷 0.00  ✂ 0.00  **FUD** XXX                    M

**6110F** Counseling provided regarding risks of driving and the alternatives to driving (DEM)
📷 0.00  ✂ 0.00  **FUD** XXX                    E

**6150F** Patient not receiving a first course of anti-TNF (tumor necrosis factor) therapy (IBD)
📷 0.00  ✂ 0.00  **FUD** XXX                    E

## 7010F-7025F Recall/Reminder System in Place

INCLUDES   Capabilities of the provider
Measures that address the setting or system of care provided

**7010F** Patient information entered into a recall system that includes: target date for the next exam specified and a process to follow up with patients regarding missed or unscheduled appointments (ML)
📷 0.00  ✂ 0.00  **FUD** XXX                    M
**AMA:** 2008,Mar,8-12

**7020F** Mammogram assessment category (eg, Mammography Quality Standards Act [MQSA], Breast Imaging Reporting and Data System [BI-RADS], or FDA approved equivalent categories) entered into an internal database to allow for analysis of abnormal interpretation (recall) rate (RAD)
📷 0.00  ✂ 0.00  **FUD** XXX                    E
**AMA:** 2008,Mar,8-12

**7025F** Patient information entered into a reminder system with a target due date for the next mammogram (RAD)
📷 0.00  ✂ 0.00  **FUD** XXX                    M
**AMA:** 2008,Mar,8-12

## 9001F-9007F No Measure Associated

INCLUDES   Aspects of care not associated with measures at the current time

**9001F** Aortic aneurysm less than 5.0 cm maximum diameter on centerline formatted CT or minor diameter on axial formatted CT (NMA-No Measure Associated)
📷 0.00  ✂ 0.00  **FUD** XXX                    E

**9002F** Aortic aneurysm 5.0 - 5.4 cm maximum diameter on centerline formatted CT or minor diameter on axial formatted CT (NMA-No Measure Associated)
📷 0.00  ✂ 0.00  **FUD** XXX                    E

**9003F** Aortic aneurysm 5.5 - 5.9 cm maximum diameter on centerline formatted CT or minor diameter on axial formatted CT (NMA-No Measure Associated)
📷 0.00  ✂ 0.00  **FUD** XXX                    M

**9004F** Aortic aneurysm 6.0 cm or greater maximum diameter on centerline formatted CT or minor diameter on axial formatted CT (NMA-No Measure Associated)
📷 0.00  ✂ 0.00  **FUD** XXX                    M

**9005F** Asymptomatic carotid stenosis: No history of any transient ischemic attack or stroke in any carotid or vertebrobasilar territory (NMA-No Measure Associated)
📷 0.00  ✂ 0.00  **FUD** XXX                    E

**9006F** Symptomatic carotid stenosis: Ipsilateral carotid territory TIA or stroke less than 120 days prior to procedure (NMA-No Measure Associated)
📷 0.00  ✂ 0.00  **FUD** XXX                    M

**9007F** Other carotid stenosis: Ipsilateral TIA or stroke 120 days or greater prior to procedure or any prior contralateral carotid territory or vertebrobasilar TIA or stroke (NMA-No Measure Associated)
📷 0.00  ✂ 0.00  **FUD** XXX                    M

## 0042T

**0042T** Cerebral perfusion analysis using computed tomography with contrast administration, including post-processing of parametric maps with determination of cerebral blood flow, cerebral blood volume, and mean transit time

⚕ 0.00  ⚕ 0.00  **FUD** XXX  N N1 80 🖵

**AMA:** 2003,Nov,5

## 0051T-0053T

~~**0051T** Implantation of a total replacement heart system (artificial heart) with recipient cardiectomy~~

To report, see ~33927-33929

~~**0052T** Replacement or repair of thoracic unit of a total replacement heart system (artificial heart)~~

To report. see ~33927-33929

~~**0053T** Replacement or repair of implantable component or components of total replacement heart system (artificial heart), excluding thoracic unit~~

To report. see ~33927-33929

## 0054T-0055T

+ **0054T** Computer-assisted musculoskeletal surgical navigational orthopedic procedure, with image-guidance based on fluoroscopic images (List separately in addition to code for primary procedure)

Code first primary procedure

⚕ 0.00  ⚕ 0.00  **FUD** XXX  N N1 80 🖵

**AMA:** 2017,Jan,8; 2016,Jan,13; 2015,Jan,16; 2014,Jan,11; 2012,Jan,15-42

+ **0055T** Computer-assisted musculoskeletal surgical navigational orthopedic procedure, with image-guidance based on CT/MRI images (List separately in addition to code for primary procedure)

INCLUDES Performance of both CT and MRI in same session (1 unit)

Code first primary procedure

⚕ 0.00  ⚕ 0.00  **FUD** XXX  N N1 80 🖵

**AMA:** 2017,Jan,8; 2016,Jan,13; 2015,Jan,16; 2014,Jan,11; 2012,Jan,15-42

## 0058T [0357T]

EXCLUDES Cryopreservation of:
Embryos (89258)
Oocyte(s), mature (89337)
Sperm (89259)
Testicular reproductive tissue (89335)

**0058T** Cryopreservation; reproductive tissue, ovarian

⚕ 0.00  ⚕ 0.00  **FUD** XXX  Q1 80 🖵

**AMA:** 2004,Apr,1; 2004,Jun,7

\# **0357T** immature oocyte(s)  ♀

⚕ 0.00  ⚕ 0.00  **FUD** XXX  Q1 N1 80 🖵

## 0071T-0072T

EXCLUDES Insertion bladder catheter (51702)
MRI guidance for parenchymal tissue ablation (77022)

**0071T** Focused ultrasound ablation of uterine leiomyomata, including MR guidance; total leiomyomata volume less than 200 cc of tissue  ♀

⚕ 0.00  ⚕ 0.00  **FUD** XXX  J 80 🖵

**AMA:** 2005,Mar,1-6; 2005,Dec,3-6

**0072T** total leiomyomata volume greater or equal to 200 cc of tissue  ♀

⚕ 0.00  ⚕ 0.00  **FUD** XXX  J 80 🖵

**AMA:** 2005,Mar,1-6; 2005,Dec,3-6

## 0075T-0076T

**0075T** Transcatheter placement of extracranial vertebral artery stent(s), including radiologic supervision and interpretation, open or percutaneous; initial vessel

INCLUDES All diagnostic services for stenting
Ipsilateral extracranial vertebral selective catheterization when confirming the need for stenting

EXCLUDES Selective catheterization and imaging when stenting is not required (report only selective catheterization codes)

⚕ 0.00  ⚕ 0.00  **FUD** XXX  C 80 🖵

**AMA:** 2017,Jan,8; 2016,Jan,13; 2015,Jan,16; 2014,Mar,8

+ **0076T** each additional vessel (List separately in addition to code for primary procedure)

Code first (0075T)

⚕ 0.00  ⚕ 0.00  **FUD** XXX  C 80 🖵

**AMA:** 2017,Jan,8; 2016,Jan,13; 2015,Jan,16; 2014,Mar,8

## 0085T

**0085T** Breath test for heart transplant rejection

⚕ 0.00  ⚕ 0.00  **FUD** XXX  E 🖵

**AMA:** 2005,May,7-12

## 0095T-0098T

INCLUDES Fluoroscopy

+ **0095T** Removal of total disc arthroplasty (artificial disc), anterior approach, each additional interspace, cervical (List separately in addition to code for primary procedure)

EXCLUDES Lumbar disc (0164T)
Revision of total disc arthroplasty, cervical (22861)
Revision of total disc arthroplasty, lumbar (22862)

Code first (22864)

⚕ 0.00  ⚕ 0.00  **FUD** XXX  C 80 🖵

**AMA:** 2006,Feb,1-6; 2005,Jun,6-8

+ **0098T** Revision including replacement of total disc arthroplasty (artificial disc), anterior approach, each additional interspace, cervical (List separately in addition to code for primary procedure)

EXCLUDES Application of intervertebral biomechanical device(s) at the same level (22853-22854, [22859])
Removal of total disc arthroplasty (0095T)
Spinal cord decompression (63001-63048)

Code first (22861)

⚕ 0.00  ⚕ 0.00  **FUD** XXX  C 80 🖵

**AMA:** 2006,Feb,1-6; 2005,Jun,6-8

## 0100T-0159T

**0100T** Placement of a subconjunctival retinal prosthesis receiver and pulse generator, and implantation of intra-ocular retinal electrode array, with vitrectomy

EXCLUDES Evaluation and initial programming of implantable retinal electrode array device (0472T)

⚕ 0.00  ⚕ 0.00  **FUD** XXX  T J8 80 🖵

**AMA:** 2017,Jan,8; 2016,Jan,13; 2015,Jan,16; 2014,Jan,11; 2012,Jan,15-42

**0101T** Extracorporeal shock wave involving musculoskeletal system, not otherwise specified, high energy

EXCLUDES Extracorporeal shock wave therapy for healing of integumentary system wounds (28899)

⚕ 0.00  ⚕ 0.00  **FUD** XXX  J J8 80 🖵

**AMA:** 2017,Jan,8; 2016,Jan,13; 2015,Jan,16; 2014,Jan,11; 2012,Jan,15-42

**0102T** Extracorporeal shock wave, high energy, performed by a physician, requiring anesthesia other than local, involving lateral humeral epicondyle

⚕ 0.00  ⚕ 0.00  **FUD** XXX  J G2 80 🖵

**AMA:** 2017,Jan,8; 2016,Jan,13; 2015,Jan,16; 2014,Jan,11; 2012,Jan,15-42

---

**0106T** Quantitative sensory testing (QST), testing and interpretation per extremity; using touch pressure stimuli to assess large diameter sensation

⚕ 0.00　✂ 0.00　**FUD** XXX　　[Q1] [80] ▢

**AMA:** 2017,Jan,8; 2016,Jan,13; 2015,Jan,16; 2014,Jan,11; 2012,Jan,15-42

**0107T** using vibration stimuli to assess large diameter fiber sensation

⚕ 0.00　✂ 0.00　**FUD** XXX　　[Q1] [80] ▢

**AMA:** 2017,Jan,8; 2016,Jan,13; 2015,Jan,16; 2014,Jan,11

**0108T** using cooling stimuli to assess small nerve fiber sensation and hyperalgesia

⚕ 0.00　✂ 0.00　**FUD** XXX　　[Q1] [80] ▢

**AMA:** 2017,Jan,8; 2016,Jan,13; 2015,Jan,16; 2014,Jan,11

**0109T** using heat-pain stimuli to assess small nerve fiber sensation and hyperalgesia

⚕ 0.00　✂ 0.00　**FUD** XXX　　[Q1] [80] ▢

**AMA:** 2017,Jan,8; 2016,Jan,13; 2015,Jan,16; 2014,Jan,11

**0110T** using other stimuli to assess sensation

⚕ 0.00　✂ 0.00　**FUD** XXX　　[Q1] [80] ▢

**AMA:** 2017,Jan,8; 2016,Jan,13; 2015,Jan,16; 2014,Jan,11

**0111T** Long-chain (C20-22) omega-3 fatty acids in red blood cell (RBC) membranes

EXCLUDES　Very long chain fatty acids (82726)

⚕ 0.00　✂ 0.00　**FUD** XXX　　[A] ▢

**AMA:** 2017,Jan,8; 2016,Jan,13; 2015,Jan,16; 2014,Jan,11

**0126T** Common carotid intima-media thickness (IMT) study for evaluation of atherosclerotic burden or coronary heart disease risk factor assessment

EXCLUDES　Duplex scan extracranial arteries (93880-93882)
　　　　　Evaluation carotid intima media and atheroma (93895)

⚕ 0.00　**FUD** XXX　　[Q1] [N1] [80] ▢

**AMA:** 2017,Jan,8; 2016,Jan,13; 2015,Jan,16; 2014,Jan,11

+ **0159T** Computer-aided detection, including computer algorithm analysis of MRI image data for lesion detection/characterization, pharmacokinetic analysis, with further physician review for interpretation, breast MRI (List separately in addition to code for primary procedure)

EXCLUDES　3D rendering (76376-76377)

Code first (77058-77059)

⚕ 0.00　✂ 0.00　**FUD** ZZZ　　[N] [N1] [80] ▢

**AMA:** 2017,Jan,8; 2016,Jan,13; 2015,Jan,16; 2014,Jan,11

## 0163T-0165T

**CMS:** 100-03,150.10 Lumbar Artificial Disc Replacement (LADR)

INCLUDES　Fluoroscopy

EXCLUDES　Application of intervertebral biomechanical device(s) at the same level (22853-22854, [22859])
　　　　　Cervical disc procedures (22856)
　　　　　Decompression (63001-63048)
　　　　　Exploration retroperitoneal area at same level (49010)

+ **0163T** Total disc arthroplasty (artificial disc), anterior approach, including discectomy to prepare interspace (other than for decompression), each additional interspace, lumbar (List separately in addition to code for primary procedure)

Code first (22857)

⚕ 0.00　✂ 0.00　**FUD** YYY　　[C] [80] ▢

**AMA:** 2017,Jan,8; 2016,Jan,13; 2015,Jan,16; 2014,Jan,11

+ **0164T** Removal of total disc arthroplasty, (artificial disc), anterior approach, each additional interspace, lumbar (List separately in addition to code for primary procedure)

Code first (22865)

⚕ 0.00　✂ 0.00　**FUD** YYY　　[C] [80] ▢

**AMA:** 2017,Jan,8; 2016,Jan,13; 2015,Jan,16; 2014,Jan,11

+ **0165T** Revision including replacement of total disc arthroplasty (artificial disc), anterior approach, each additional interspace, lumbar (List separately in addition to code for primary procedure)

Code first (22862)

⚕ 0.00　✂ 0.00　**FUD** YYY　　[C] [80] ▢

**AMA:** 2017,Jan,8; 2016,Jan,13; 2015,Jan,16; 2014,Jan,11

## 0174T-0175T

+ **0174T** Computer-aided detection (CAD) (computer algorithm analysis of digital image data for lesion detection) with further physician review for interpretation and report, with or without digitization of film radiographic images, chest radiograph(s), performed concurrent with primary interpretation (List separately in addition to code for primary procedure)

Code first (71045-71048)

⚕ 0.00　✂ 0.00　**FUD** XXX　　[N] [N1] [80] ▢

**AMA:** 2007,Jul,6-10; 2007,Mar,7-8

**0175T** Computer-aided detection (CAD) (computer algorithm analysis of digital image data for lesion detection) with further physician review for interpretation and report, with or without digitization of film radiographic images, chest radiograph(s), performed remote from primary interpretation

INCLUDES　Chest x-rays (71045-71048)

⚕ 0.00　✂ 0.00　**FUD** XXX　　[N] [N1] [80] ▢

**AMA:** 2007,Jul,6-10; 2007,Mar,7-8

## 0178T-0180T

~~**0178T** Electrocardiogram, 64 leads or greater, with graphic presentation and analysis; with interpretation and report~~

To report, see ~93799

~~**0179T** tracing and graphics only, without interpretation and report~~

To report, see ~93799

~~**0180T** interpretation and report only~~

To report, see ~93799

## 0184T

**0184T** Excision of rectal tumor, transanal endoscopic microsurgical approach (ie, TEMS), including muscularis propria (ie, full thickness)

INCLUDES　Operating microscope (66990)
　　　　　Proctosigmoidoscopy (45300, 45308-45309, 45315, 45317, 45320)

EXCLUDES　Nonendoscopic excision of rectal tumor (45160, 45171-45172)

⚕ 0.00　✂ 0.00　**FUD** XXX　　[J] [80] ▢

**AMA:** 2017,Jan,8; 2016,Feb,12; 2016,Jan,13; 2015,Jan,16; 2014,Jan,11

---

| [26]/[TC] PC/TC Only | [A2]-[Z3] ASC Payment | [50] Bilateral | ♂ Male Only | ♀ Female Only | ⚕ Facility RVU | ✂ Non-Facility RVU | ▢ CCI |
| **FUD** Follow-up Days | **CMS:** IOM (Pub 100) | [A]-[Y] OPPSI | [80]/[80] Surg Assist Allowed / w/Doc | | ▣ Lab Crosswalk | ▣ Radiology Crosswalk | ☒ CLIA |

542

CPT © 2017 American Medical Association. All Rights Reserved.　　　© 2017 Optum360, LLC

## 0188T-0189T

INCLUDES 30 minutes or more of direct medical care by a physician(s) or other qualified health care professional(s) to a critically ill or critically injured patient from an off-site location
Additional on-site critical care services when a critically ill or injured patient requires critical care resources not available on-site
Other critical care services provided during the same time period by provider or other individual (99291-99292, 99468-99476)
Real time ability to:
Document the remote care services in the medical record
Enter orders electronically
Evaluate patients with high fidelity audio/video capabilities
Observe patient monitors, infusion pumps, ventilators
Talk to patients and family members
Videoconference with the health care team on-site in the patient's room
Real-time access to the patient's:
Clinical laboratory test results
Diagnostic test results
Medical records
Radiographic images
Review and/or interpretation of all diagnostic information
Time spent with the patient, family, or surrogate decision makers to obtain a medical history, review the patient's condition/prognosis, or discuss treatment options from the remote site
EXCLUDES *Time spent away from the remote site without real-time capabilities*
*Time spent for services that do not directly contribute to patient treatment*

**0188T** **Remote real-time interactive video-conferenced critical care, evaluation and management of the critically ill or critically injured patient; first 30-74 minutes**
INCLUDES First 30 to 74 minutes of remote critical care each day
Remote critical care less than 30 minutes total duration
🔄 0.00   ⚖ 0.00   **FUD** XXX                        ★ M 🖵
**AMA:** 2017,Jan,8; 2016,May,3; 2016,Jan,13; 2015,Jan,16; 2014,Jan,11; 2012,Jan,15-42

+ **0189T** **each additional 30 minutes (List separately in addition to code for primary service)**
INCLUDES Up to 30 minutes each beyond the first 74 minutes
Code first (0188T)
🔄 0.00   ⚖ 0.00   **FUD** XXX                        ★ M 🖵
**AMA:** 2017,Jan,8; 2016,May,3; 2016,Jan,13; 2015,Jan,16; 2014,Jan,11; 2012,Jan,15-42

## 0190T-0191T [0253T, 0376T]

+ **0190T** **Placement of intraocular radiation source applicator (List separately in addition to primary procedure)**
EXCLUDES *Insertion of brachytherapy source by radiation oncologist (see Clinical Brachytherapy Section)*
Code also brachytherapy source
Code first (67036)
🔄 0.00   ⚖ 0.00   **FUD** XXX                        N N1 80 🖵
**AMA:** 2008,Jan,6-7

**0191T** **Insertion of anterior segment aqueous drainage device, without extraocular reservoir, internal approach, into the trabecular meshwork; initial insertion**
🔄 0.00   ⚖ 0.00   **FUD** XXX                        J J8 80 🖵
**AMA:** 2017,Jan,8; 2016,Jan,13; 2015,Jan,16; 2014,Jan,11; 2012,Dec,12

+ # **0376T** **each additional device insertion (List separately in addition to code for primary procedure)**
🔄 0.00   ⚖ 0.00   **FUD** XXX                        N N1 80 🖵
Code first (0191T)

# **0253T** **Insertion of anterior segment aqueous drainage device, without extraocular reservoir, internal approach, into the suprachoroidal space**
🔄 0.00   ⚖ 0.00   **FUD** YYY                        J J8 80 🖵
EXCLUDES *Insertion aqueous drainage device, external approach (66183)*

## 0195T-0196T

INCLUDES Application of intervertebral biomechanical device(s) at the same level (22853-22854, [22859])
Computed tomography (76380, 76497, 77011-77012)
Epidurography (72275)
Fluoroscopy (76000, 76496, 77002-77003)
Grafts (20930-20938)
Instrumentation (22840, 22845)
Lumbar arthrodesis (22558)
Pelvic fixation (22848)

**0195T** **Arthrodesis, pre-sacral interbody technique, disc space preparation, discectomy, without instrumentation, with image guidance, includes bone graft when performed; L5-S1 interspace**
🔄 0.00   ⚖ 0.00   **FUD** XXX                        C 80 🖵
**AMA:** 2017,Jan,8; 2016,Jan,13; 2015,Jan,16; 2013,Jul,3-5; 2012,Apr,14-16

+ **0196T** **L4-L5 interspace (List separately in addition to code for primary procedure)**
Code first (0195T)
🔄 0.00   ⚖ 0.00   **FUD** XXX                        C 80 🖵
**AMA:** 2017,Jan,8; 2016,Jan,13; 2015,Jan,16; 2013,Jul,3-5; 2012,Apr,14-16

## 0198T

**0198T** **Measurement of ocular blood flow by repetitive intraocular pressure sampling, with interpretation and report**
🔄 0.00   ⚖ 0.00   **FUD** XXX                        Q1 80 🖵
**AMA:** 2017,Jan,8; 2016,Jan,13; 2015,Jan,16; 2014,Jan,11; 2012,Aug,9; 2012,Jan,15-42

## 0200T-0201T

INCLUDES Deep bone biopsy (20225)

**0200T** **Percutaneous sacral augmentation (sacroplasty), unilateral injection(s), including the use of a balloon or mechanical device, when used, 1 or more needles, includes imaging guidance and bone biopsy, when performed**
🔄 0.00   ⚖ 0.00   **FUD** XXX              J 02 80 50 🖵
**AMA:** 2017,Jan,8; 2016,Jan,13; 2015,Dec,18; 2015,Apr,8; 2015,Jan,8

**0201T** **Percutaneous sacral augmentation (sacroplasty), bilateral injections, including the use of a balloon or mechanical device, when used, 2 or more needles, includes imaging guidance and bone biopsy, when performed**
🔄 0.00   ⚖ 0.00   **FUD** XXX                   J 02 80 🖵
**AMA:** 2017,Jan,8; 2016,Jan,13; 2015,Dec,18; 2015,Apr,8; 2015,Jan,8

## 0202T-0207T

**0202T** **Posterior vertebral joint(s) arthroplasty (eg, facet joint[s] replacement), including facetectomy, laminectomy, foraminotomy, and vertebral column fixation, injection of bone cement, when performed, including fluoroscopy, single level, lumbar spine**
🔄 0.00   ⚖ 0.00   **FUD** XXX                        C 80 🖵
INCLUDES Instrumentation (22840, 22853-22854, [22859])
Laminectomy (63005, 63012, 63017, 63047)
Laminotomy (63030, 63042)
Lumbar arthroplasty (22857)
Percutaneous lumbar vertebral augmentation (22514)
Percutaneous vertebroplasty (22511)
Spinal cord decompression (63056)

+ **0205T** **Intravascular catheter-based coronary vessel or graft spectroscopy (eg, infrared) during diagnostic evaluation and/or therapeutic intervention including imaging supervision, interpretation, and report, each vessel (List separately in addition to code for primary procedure)**
🔄 0.00   ⚖ 0.00   **FUD** ZZZ                        N N1 80 🖵
Code first (92920, 92924, 92928, 92933, 92937, 92941, 92943, 92975, 93454-93461, 93563-93564)

---

**0206T** Computerized database analysis of multiple cycles of digitized cardiac electrical data from two or more ECG leads, including transmission to a remote center, application of multiple nonlinear mathematical transformations, with coronary artery obstruction severity assessment

🔧 0.00   ⚖ 0.00   **FUD** XXX   01 N1 80 TC ▭

Code also 12-lead ECG when performed (93000-93010)

**0207T** Evacuation of meibomian glands, automated, using heat and intermittent pressure, unilateral

🔧 0.00   ⚖ 0.00   **FUD** XXX   01 80 ▭

**AMA:** 2017,Jan,8; 2016,Jan,13; 2015,Jan,16; 2014,May,5

## 0208T-0212T

EXCLUDES   *Manual audiometric testing by a qualified health care professional, using audiometers (92551-92557)*

**0208T** Pure tone audiometry (threshold), automated; air only

🔧 0.00   ⚖ 0.00   **FUD** XXX   01 80 TC ▭

**AMA:** 2017,Jan,8; 2016,Jan,13; 2015,Jan,16; 2014,Aug,3

**0209T** air and bone

🔧 0.00   ⚖ 0.00   **FUD** XXX   01 80 TC ▭

**AMA:** 2017,Jan,8; 2016,Jan,13; 2015,Jan,16; 2014,Aug,3; 2014,Jan,11

**0210T** Speech audiometry threshold, automated;

🔧 0.00   ⚖ 0.00   **FUD** XXX   01 80 TC ▭

**AMA:** 2014,Aug,3

**0211T** with speech recognition

🔧 0.00   ⚖ 0.00   **FUD** XXX   01 80 TC ▭

**AMA:** 2017,Jan,8; 2016,Jan,13; 2015,Jan,16; 2014,Aug,3; 2014,Jan,11

**0212T** Comprehensive audiometry threshold evaluation and speech recognition (0209T, 0211T combined), automated

🔧 0.00   ⚖ 0.00   **FUD** XXX   01 80 TC ▭

**AMA:** 2017,Jan,8; 2016,Jan,13; 2015,Jan,16; 2014,Aug,3; 2014,Jan,11

## 0213T-0215T

**0213T** Injection(s), diagnostic or therapeutic agent, paravertebral facet (zygapophyseal) joint (or nerves innervating that joint) with ultrasound guidance, cervical or thoracic; single level

🔧 0.00   ⚖ 0.00   **FUD** XXX   T R2 80 50 ▭

**AMA:** 2017,Jan,8; 2016,Jan,13; 2015,Jan,16; 2014,Jan,11

+ **0214T** second level (List separately in addition to code for primary procedure)

Code first (0213T)

🔧 0.00   ⚖ 0.00   **FUD** ZZZ   N N1 80 50 ▭

**AMA:** 2017,Jan,8; 2016,Jan,13; 2015,Jan,16; 2014,Jan,11

+ **0215T** third and any additional level(s) (List separately in addition to code for primary procedure)

EXCLUDES   *Use of code more than one time per date of service*

Code first (0213T-0214T)

🔧 0.00   ⚖ 0.00   **FUD** ZZZ   N N1 80 50 ▭

**AMA:** 2017,Jan,8; 2016,Jan,13; 2015,Jan,16; 2014,Jan,11

## 0216T-0218T

EXCLUDES   *Injection with CT or fluoroscopic guidance (64490-64495)*

**0216T** Injection(s), diagnostic or therapeutic agent, paravertebral facet (zygapophyseal) joint (or nerves innervating that joint) with ultrasound guidance, lumbar or sacral; single level

🔧 0.00   ⚖ 0.00   **FUD** XXX   T R2 80 50 ▭

**AMA:** 2017,Jan,8; 2016,Jan,13; 2015,Jan,16; 2014,Jan,11

+ **0217T** second level (List separately in addition to code for primary procedure)

Code first (0216T)

🔧 0.00   ⚖ 0.00   **FUD** ZZZ   N N1 80 50 ▭

**AMA:** 2017,Jan,8; 2016,Jan,13; 2015,Jan,16; 2014,Jan,11

+ **0218T** third and any additional level(s) (List separately in addition to code for primary procedure)

EXCLUDES   *Use of code more than one time per date of service*

Code first (0216T-0217T)

🔧 0.00   ⚖ 0.00   **FUD** ZZZ   N N1 80 50 ▭

**AMA:** 2017,Jan,8; 2016,Jan,13; 2015,Jan,16; 2014,Jan,11

## 0219T-0222T

INCLUDES   Allografts at same level (20930-20931)
Application of intervertebral biomechanical device(s) at the same level (22853-22854, [22859])
Arthrodesis at same level (22600-22614)
Instrumentation at same level (22840)
Radiologic services

**0219T** Placement of a posterior intrafacet implant(s), unilateral or bilateral, including imaging and placement of bone graft(s) or synthetic device(s), single level; cervical

🔧 0.00   ⚖ 0.00   **FUD** XXX   C 80 ▭

**AMA:** 2017,Jan,8; 2016,Jan,13; 2015,Jan,16; 2014,Jan,11; 2012,Jun,10-11; 2012,Jan,15-42

**0220T** thoracic

🔧 0.00   ⚖ 0.00   **FUD** XXX   C 80 ▭

**AMA:** 2017,Jan,8; 2016,Jan,13; 2015,Jan,16; 2014,Jan,11; 2012,Jun,10-11; 2012,Jan,15-42

**0221T** lumbar

🔧 0.00   ⚖ 0.00   **FUD** XXX   J 80 ▭

**AMA:** 2017,Jan,8; 2016,Jan,13; 2015,Jan,16; 2014,Jan,11; 2012,Jun,10-11; 2012,Jan,15-42

+ **0222T** each additional vertebral segment (List separately in addition to code for primary procedure)

Code first (0219T-0221T)

🔧 0.00   ⚖ 0.00   **FUD** ZZZ   N 80 ▭

**AMA:** 2017,Jan,8; 2016,Jan,13; 2015,Jan,16; 2014,Jan,11; 2012,Jun,10-11; 2012,Jan,15-42

## 0228T-0232T

**0228T** Injection(s), anesthetic agent and/or steroid, transforaminal epidural, with ultrasound guidance, cervical or thoracic; single level

🔧 0.00   ⚖ 0.00   **FUD** XXX   T 02 50 ▭

**AMA:** 2017,Jan,8; 2016,Jan,13; 2015,Jan,16; 2014,Jan,11; 2012,Jan,15-42

+ **0229T** each additional level (List separately in addition to code for primary procedure)

Code first (0228T)

🔧 0.00   ⚖ 0.00   **FUD** XXX   N N1 50 ▭

**AMA:** 2017,Jan,8; 2016,Jan,13; 2015,Jan,16; 2014,Jan,11; 2012,Jan,15-42

**0230T** Injection(s), anesthetic agent and/or steroid, transforaminal epidural, with ultrasound guidance, lumbar or sacral; single level

🔧 0.00   ⚖ 0.00   **FUD** XXX   T 02 50 ▭

**AMA:** 2017,Jan,8; 2016,Jan,13; 2015,Jan,16; 2014,Jan,11; 2012,Jan,15-42

+ **0231T** each additional level (List separately in addition to code for primary procedure)

INCLUDES   Ultrasound guidance (76942, 76998-76999)

EXCLUDES   *Injection performed with CT of fluoroscopic guidance (64479-64484)*

Code first (0230T)

🔧 0.00   ⚖ 0.00   **FUD** XXX   N N1 50 ▭

**AMA:** 2017,Jan,8; 2016,Jan,13; 2015,Jan,16; 2014,Jan,11; 2012,Jan,15-42

0232T **Injection(s), platelet rich plasma, any site, including image guidance, harvesting and preparation when performed**

> INCLUDES   Arthrocentesis (20600-20610)
> Blood collection (36415, 36592)
> Imaging guidance (76942, 77002, 77012, 77021)
> Injections (20550-20551)
> Platelet/blood product pooling (86965)
> Tissue grafts (20926)
>
> EXCLUDES   *Aspiration of bone marrow for grafting, biopsy, harvesting for transplant (38220-38221, 38230)*
> *Injections white cell concentrate (0481T)*
>
> 🔧 0.00   ✂ 0.00   **FUD** XXX   01 N1 🖥
>
> **AMA:** 2017,Jan,8; 2016,Jan,13; 2015,Jan,16; 2014,Jan,11; 2012,Oct,14; 2012,May,11-12

## 0234T-0238T

> INCLUDES   Atherectomy by any technique in arteries above the inguinal ligaments
> Radiology supervision and interpretation
> EXCLUDES   *Accessing and catheterization of the vessel*
> *Atherectomy performed below the inguinal ligaments (37225, 37227, 37229, 37231, 37233, 37235)*
> *Closure of the arteriotomy by any technique*
> *Negotiating the lesion*
> *Other interventions to the same or different vessels*
> *Protection from embolism*

0234T **Transluminal peripheral atherectomy, open or percutaneous, including radiological supervision and interpretation; renal artery**

> 🔧 0.00   ✂ 0.00   **FUD** YYY   J 80 🖥
>
> **AMA:** 2017,Jan,8; 2016,Jan,13; 2015,Jan,16; 2014,Jan,11

0235T **visceral artery (except renal), each vessel**

> 🔧 0.00   ✂ 0.00   **FUD** YYY   C 80 🖥
>
> **AMA:** 2017,Jan,8; 2016,Jan,13; 2015,Jan,16; 2014,Jan,11

0236T **abdominal aorta**

> 🔧 0.00   ✂ 0.00   **FUD** YYY   J 80 🖥
>
> **AMA:** 2017,Jan,8; 2016,Jan,13; 2015,Jan,16; 2014,Jan,11

0237T **brachiocephalic trunk and branches, each vessel**

> 🔧 0.00   ✂ 0.00   **FUD** YYY   J 80 🖥
>
> **AMA:** 2017,Jan,8; 2016,Jan,13; 2015,Jan,16; 2014,Jan,11

0238T **iliac artery, each vessel**

> 🔧 0.00   ✂ 0.00   **FUD** YYY   J J6 80 🖥
>
> **AMA:** 2017,Jan,8; 2016,Jan,13; 2015,Jan,16; 2014,Jan,11

## 0249T-0255T

0249T **Ligation, hemorrhoidal vascular bundle(s), including ultrasound guidance**

> INCLUDES   Ultrasound guidance (76872, 76942, 76998)
> EXCLUDES   *Anoscopy (46600)*
> *Hemorrhoidectomy (46221, [46945, 46946], 46250-46262)*
> *Placement seton (46020)*
>
> 🔧 0.00   ✂ 0.00   **FUD** YYY   J G2 80 🖥
>
> **AMA:** 2017,Jan,8; 2016,Jan,13; 2015,Mar,9

*0253T* **Resequenced code. See code before 0195T.**

▲ 0254T **Endovascular repair of iliac artery bifurcation (eg, aneurysm, pseudoaneurysm, arteriovenous malformation, trauma, dissection) using bifurcated endograft from the common iliac artery into both the external and internal iliac artery, including all selective and/or nonselective catheterization(s) required for device placement and all associated radiological supervision and interpretation, unilateral**

> 🔧 0.00   ✂ 0.00   **FUD** YYY   C 80 🖥
>
> **AMA:** 2017,Jan,8; 2016,Jan,13; 2015,Jan,16; 2014,Jan,11; 2013,Dec,8

~~0255T~~ ~~radiological supervision and interpretation~~

> To report, see 0254T

## 0263T-0265T

> EXCLUDES   *Bone marrow and stem cell services (38204-38242 [38243])*

0263T **Intramuscular autologous bone marrow cell therapy, with preparation of harvested cells, multiple injections, one leg, including ultrasound guidance, if performed; complete procedure including unilateral or bilateral bone marrow harvest**

> 🔧 0.00   ✂ 0.00   **FUD** XXX   S G2 80 🖥
>
> INCLUDES   Duplex scan (93925-93926)
> Ultrasound guidance (76942)

0264T **complete procedure excluding bone marrow harvest**

> 🔧 0.00   ✂ 0.00   **FUD** XXX   S G2 80 🖥
>
> INCLUDES   Bone marrow harvest only (0265T)
> Duplex scan (93925-93926)
> Ultrasound guidance (76942)

0265T **unilateral or bilateral bone marrow harvest only for intramuscular autologous bone marrow cell therapy**

> 🔧 0.00   ✂ 0.00   **FUD** XXX   S G2 80 🖥
>
> EXCLUDES   *Complete procedure (0263T-0264T)*

## 0266T-0273T

0266T **Implantation or replacement of carotid sinus baroreflex activation device; total system (includes generator placement, unilateral or bilateral lead placement, intra-operative interrogation, programming, and repositioning, when performed)**

> 🔧 0.00   ✂ 0.00   **FUD** YYY   C 80 🖥
>
> INCLUDES   Components of complete procedure (0267T-0268T)

0267T **lead only, unilateral (includes intra-operative interrogation, programming, and repositioning, when performed)**

> 🔧 0.00   ✂ 0.00   **FUD** YYY   T 80 🖥
>
> EXCLUDES   *Complete procedure (0266T)*
> *Device interrogation (0272T-0273T)*
> *Removal/revision device or components (0269T-0271T)*

0268T **pulse generator only (includes intra-operative interrogation, programming, and repositioning, when performed)**

> 🔧 0.00   ✂ 0.00   **FUD** YYY   J 80 🖥
>
> EXCLUDES   *Complete procedure (0266T)*
> *Device interrogation (0272T-0273T)*
> *Removal/revision device or components (0269T-0271T)*

0269T **Revision or removal of carotid sinus baroreflex activation device; total system (includes generator placement, unilateral or bilateral lead placement, intra-operative interrogation, programming, and repositioning, when performed)**

> 🔧 0.00   ✂ 0.00   **FUD** XXX   Q2 G2 80 🖥
>
> EXCLUDES   *Device interrogation (0272T-0273T)*
> *Implantation/replacement device and/or components (0266T-0268T)*
> *Removal/revision device or components (0269T-0271T)*

0270T **lead only, unilateral (includes intra-operative interrogation, programming, and repositioning, when performed)**

> 🔧 0.00   ✂ 0.00   **FUD** XXX   Q2 G2 80 🖥
>
> EXCLUDES   *Device interrogation (0272T-0273T)*
> *Implantation/replacement device and/or components (0266T-0268T)*
> *Removal/revision device or components (0269T-0271T)*

0271T **pulse generator only (includes intra-operative interrogation, programming, and repositioning, when performed)**

> 🔧 0.00   ✂ 0.00   **FUD** XXX   Q2 G2 80 🖥
>
> EXCLUDES   *Device interrogation (0272T-0273T)*
> *Implantation/replacement device and/or components (0266T-0268T)*
> *Removal/revision device or components (0269T-0271T)*

---

● New Code   ▲ Revised Code   ○ Reinstated   ⬤ New Web Release   ▲ Revised Web Release   Unlisted   Not Covered   # Resequenced
⊘ AMA Mod 51 Exempt   ⑤⓪ Optum Mod 51 Exempt   ⑥③ Mod 63 Exempt   ✏ Non-FDA Drug   ★ Telemedicine   M Maternity   A Age Edit   + Add-on   **AMA:** CPT Asst

Category III Codes

0272T — 0298T

**0272T** Interrogation device evaluation (in person), carotid sinus baroreflex activation system, including telemetric iterative communication with the implantable device to monitor device diagnostics and programmed therapy values, with interpretation and report (eg, battery status, lead impedance, pulse amplitude, pulse width, therapy frequency, pathway mode, burst mode, therapy start/stop times each day);

    📓 0.00　 ✂ 0.00　**FUD** XXX　　　　S 80 ▭

　　　*EXCLUDES* Device interrogation (0273T)
　　　Implantation/replacement device and/or components (0266T-0268T)
　　　Removal/revision device or components (0269T-0271T)

**0273T** with programming

    📓 0.00　 ✂ 0.00　**FUD** XXX　　　　S 80 ▭

　　　*EXCLUDES* Device interrogation (0272T)
　　　Implantation/replacement device and/or components (0266T-0268T)
　　　Removal/revision device or components (0269T-0271T)

### 0274T-0275T

*EXCLUDES* Laminotomy/hemilaminectomy by open and endoscopically assisted approach (63020-63035)
Percutaneous decompression of nucleus pulposus of intervertebral disc by needle-based technique (62287)

**0274T** Percutaneous laminotomy/laminectomy (interlaminar approach) for decompression of neural elements, (with or without ligamentous resection, discectomy, facetectomy and/or foraminotomy), any method, under indirect image guidance (eg, fluoroscopic, CT), single or multiple levels, unilateral or bilateral; cervical or thoracic

    📓 0.00　 ✂ 0.00　**FUD** YYY　　　　J 62 80 ▭

**AMA:** 2017,Feb,12; 2017,Jan,8; 2016,Jan,13; 2015,Jan,16; 2014,Jan,11; 2012,Jul,3-6; 2012,Jan,13-14

**0275T** lumbar

    📓 0.00　 ✂ 0.00　**FUD** XXX　　　　J 62 ▭

**AMA:** 2017,Feb,12; 2017,Jan,8; 2016,Jan,13; 2015,Jan,16; 2014,Jan,11; 2012,Jul,3-6; 2012,Jan,13-14

### 0278T

**0278T** Transcutaneous electrical modulation pain reprocessing (eg, scrambler therapy), each treatment session (includes placement of electrodes)

    📓 0.00　 ✂ 0.00　**FUD** XXX　　　　01 N1 80 ▭

### 0290T

Code first (65710, 65730, 65750, 65755)

**+　0290T** Corneal incisions in the recipient cornea created using a laser, in preparation for penetrating or lamellar keratoplasty (List separately in addition to code for primary procedure)

    📓 0.00　 ✂ 0.00　**FUD** ZZZ　　　　N N1 80 ▭

**AMA:** 2017,Jan,8; 2016,Jan,13; 2015,Jan,16; 2014,Jan,11; 2012,Aug,9

### 0293T-0294T

**0293T** ~~Insertion of left atrial hemodynamic monitor; complete system, includes implanted communication module and pressure sensor lead in left atrium including transseptal access, radiological supervision and interpretation, and associated injection procedures, when performed~~

**0294T** ~~pressure sensor lead at time of insertion of pacing cardioverter-defibrillator pulse generator including radiological supervision and interpretation and associated injection procedures, when performed (List separately in addition to code for primary procedure)~~

### 0295T-0298T

*EXCLUDES* External echocardiograph monitoring up to 48 hours (93224-93227)
External electrocardiographic monitoring (93260-93272)
Mobile cardiovascular telemetry with echocardiograph recording (93228-93229)

**0295T** External electrocardiographic recording for more than 48 hours up to 21 days by continuous rhythm recording and storage; includes recording, scanning analysis with report, review and interpretation

    📓 0.00　 ✂ 0.00　**FUD** XXX　　　　M 80 ▭

**AMA:** 2017,Jan,8; 2016,Jan,13; 2015,Jan,16; 2014,Jan,11; 2013,Feb,16-17

**0296T** recording (includes connection and initial recording)

    📓 0.00　 ✂ 0.00　**FUD** XXX　　　　01 80 ▭

**AMA:** 2017,Jan,8; 2016,Jan,13; 2015,Jan,16; 2014,Jan,11; 2013,Feb,16-17

**0297T** scanning analysis with report

    📓 0.00　 ✂ 0.00　**FUD** XXX　　　　01 80 ▭

**AMA:** 2017,Jan,8; 2016,Jan,13; 2015,Jan,16; 2014,Jan,11; 2013,Feb,16-17

**0298T** review and interpretation

    📓 0.00　 ✂ 0.00　**FUD** XXX　　　　M 80 ▭

**AMA:** 2017,Jan,8; 2016,Jan,13; 2015,Jan,16; 2014,Jan,11; 2013,Feb,16-17

### 0299T-0300T

**0299T** ~~Extracorporeal shock wave for integumentary wound healing, high energy, including topical application and dressing care; initial wound~~

　　　To report, see ~28899

**0300T** ~~each additional wound (List separately in addition to code for primary procedure)~~

　　　To report, see ~28899

### 0301T

**0301T** ~~Destruction/reduction of malignant breast tumor with externally applied focused microwave, including interstitial placement of disposable catheter with combined temperature monitoring probe and microwave focusing sensocatheter under ultrasound thermotherapy guidance~~

　　　To report, see ~19499

### 0302T-0304T

**0302T** ~~Insertion or removal and replacement of intracardiac ischemia monitoring system including imaging supervision and interpretation when performed and intra-operative interrogation and programming when performed; complete system (includes device and electrode)~~

**0303T** ~~electrode only~~

**0304T** ~~device only~~

### 0305T-0307T

**0305T** ~~Programming device evaluation (in person) of intracardiac ischemia monitoring system with iterative adjustment of programmed values, with analysis, review, and report~~

**0306T** ~~Interrogation device evaluation (in person) of intracardiac ischemia monitoring system with analysis, review, and report~~

**0307T** ~~Removal of intracardiac ischemia monitoring device~~

26/TC PC/TC Only　　A2-Z3 ASC Payment　　50 Bilateral　　♂ Male Only　　♀ Female Only　　📓 Facility RVU　　✂ Non-Facility RVU　　▭ CCI
**FUD** Follow-up Days　　**CMS:** IOM (Pub 100)　　A-Y OPPSI　　80/I80 Surg Assist Allowed / w/Doc　　⬛ Lab Crosswalk　　⬛ Radiology Crosswalk　　✖ CLIA
CPT © 2017 American Medical Association. All Rights Reserved.　　　© 2017 Optum360, LLC

## 0308T-0310T

**0308T** Insertion of ocular telescope prosthesis including removal of crystalline lens or intraocular lens prosthesis

> INCLUDES Injection procedures (66020, 66030)
> Iridectomy when performed (66600-66635, 66761)
> Operating microscope (69990)
> Repositioning of intraocular lens (66825)
>
> EXCLUDES Cataract extraction (66982-66986)

> 🚑 0.00   ✂ 0.00   **FUD** YYY          J J8 50 ▣
>
> **AMA:** 2017,Jan,8; 2016,Jan,13; 2015,Jan,16; 2014,Jan,11; 2013,Mar,6-7

**0309T** ~~Arthrodesis, pre-sacral interbody technique, including disc space preparation, discectomy, with posterior instrumentation, with image guidance, includes bone graft, when performed, lumbar, L4-L5 interspace (List separately in addition to code for primary procedure)~~

> To report, see ~22899

**0310T** ~~Motor function mapping using non-invasive navigated transcranial magnetic stimulation (nTMS) for therapeutic treatment planning, upper and lower extremity~~

> To report, see ~64999

## 0312T-0317T

> EXCLUDES Analysis and/or programming (or reprogramming) of vagus nerve stimulator (95970, 95974-95975)
> Implantation, replacement, removal, and/or revision of vagus nerve neurostimulator (electrode array and/or pulse generator) for stimulation of vagus nerve other than at the esophagogastric junction (64568-64570)

**0312T** Vagus nerve blocking therapy (morbid obesity); laparoscopic implantation of neurostimulator electrode array, anterior and posterior vagal trunks adjacent to esophagogastric junction (EGJ), with implantation of pulse generator, includes programming

> 🚑 0.00   ✂ 0.00   **FUD** XXX          J 80 ▣
>
> **AMA:** 2017,Jan,8; 2016,Jan,13; 2015,Jan,16; 2013,Jan,11-12

**0313T** laparoscopic revision or replacement of vagal trunk neurostimulator electrode array, including connection to existing pulse generator

> 🚑 0.00   ✂ 0.00   **FUD** XXX          T G2 80 ▣
>
> **AMA:** 2017,Jan,8; 2016,Jan,13; 2015,Jan,16; 2013,Jan,11-12

**0314T** laparoscopic removal of vagal trunk neurostimulator electrode array and pulse generator

> 🚑 0.00   ✂ 0.00   **FUD** YYY          02 G2 80 ▣
>
> **AMA:** 2017,Jan,8; 2016,Jan,13; 2015,Jan,16; 2013,Jan,11-12

**0315T** removal of pulse generator

> EXCLUDES Removal with replacement pulse generator (0316T)
>
> 🚑 0.00   ✂ 0.00   **FUD** XXX          02 G2 80 ▣
>
> **AMA:** 2017,Jan,8; 2016,Jan,13; 2015,Jan,16; 2013,Jan,11-12

**0316T** replacement of pulse generator

> EXCLUDES Removal without replacement pulse generator (0315T)
>
> 🚑 0.00   ✂ 0.00   **FUD** XXX          J J8 80 ▣
>
> **AMA:** 2017,Jan,8; 2016,Jan,13; 2015,Jan,16; 2013,Jan,11-12

**0317T** neurostimulator pulse generator electronic analysis, includes reprogramming when performed

> 🚑 0.00   ✂ 0.00   **FUD** XXX          01 80 ▣
>
> **AMA:** 2017,Jan,8; 2016,Jan,13; 2015,Jan,16; 2013,Jan,11-12

## 0329T-0330T

**0329T** Monitoring of intraocular pressure for 24 hours or longer, unilateral or bilateral, with interpretation and report

> 🚑 0.00   ✂ 0.00   **FUD** YYY          E ▣
>
> **AMA:** 2017,Jan,8; 2016,Jan,13; 2015,Jan,16; 2014,May,5

**0330T** Tear film imaging, unilateral or bilateral, with interpretation and report

> 🚑 0.00   ✂ 0.00   **FUD** YYY          01 N1 ▣
>
> **AMA:** 2017,Jan,8; 2016,Jan,13; 2015,Jan,16; 2014,May,5

## 0331T-0332T

> EXCLUDES Myocardial infarction avid imaging (78466, 78468, 78469)

**0331T** Myocardial sympathetic innervation imaging, planar qualitative and quantitative assessment;

> 🚑 0.00   ✂ 0.00   **FUD** YYY          S Z2 ▣
>
> **AMA:** 2017,Jan,8; 2016,Jan,13; 2015,Jan,16; 2014,Jun,14

**0332T** with tomographic SPECT

> 🚑 0.00   ✂ 0.00   **FUD** YYY          S Z2 ▣
>
> **AMA:** 2017,Jan,8; 2016,Jan,13; 2015,Jan,16; 2014,Jun,14

## 0333T [0464T]

▲ **0333T** Visual evoked potential, screening of visual acuity, automated, with report

> EXCLUDES Visual evoked potential testing for glaucoma (0464T)
>
> 🚑 0.00   ✂ 0.00   **FUD** YYY          E ▣
>
> **AMA:** 2017,Jan,8; 2016,Jan,13; 2015,Jan,16; 2014,Aug,8

● # **0464T** Visual evoked potential, testing for glaucoma, with interpretation and report

> 🚑 0.00   ✂ 0.00   **FUD** YYY          S ▣
>
> EXCLUDES Visual evoked potential for visual acuity (0333T)

## 0335T-0337T

**0335T** Extra-osseous subtalar joint implant for talotarsal stabilization

> 🚑 0.00   ✂ 0.00   **FUD** YYY          J J8 ▣

**0337T** Endothelial function assessment, using peripheral vascular response to reactive hyperemia, non-invasive (eg, brachial artery ultrasound, peripheral artery tonometry), unilateral or bilateral

> 🚑 0.00   ✂ 0.00   **FUD** YYY          01 ▣
>
> EXCLUDES Noninvasive vascular studies extremities (93922-93923)

## 0338T-0339T

> INCLUDES Selective catheter placement renal arteries (36251-36254)

**0338T** Transcatheter renal sympathetic denervation, percutaneous approach including arterial puncture, selective catheter placement(s) renal artery(ies), fluoroscopy, contrast injection(s), intraprocedural roadmapping and radiological supervision and interpretation, including pressure gradient measurements, flush aortogram and diagnostic renal angiography when performed; unilateral

> 🚑 0.00   ✂ 0.00   **FUD** YYY          J G2 ▣

**0339T** bilateral

> 🚑 0.00   ✂ 0.00   **FUD** YYY          J G2 ▣

## 0340T-0342T

**0340T** ~~Ablation, pulmonary tumor(s), including pleura or chest wall when involved by tumor extension, percutaneous, cryoablation, unilateral, includes imaging guidance~~

> To report. see 32994

**0341T** Quantitative pupillometry with interpretation and report, unilateral or bilateral

> 🚑 0.00   ✂ 0.00   **FUD** YYY          N M1 ▣

**0342T** Therapeutic apheresis with selective HDL delipidation and plasma reinfusion

> 🚑 0.00   ✂ 0.00   **FUD** YYY          S G2 ▣

## 0345T-0347T

**0345T** Transcatheter mitral valve repair percutaneous approach via the coronary sinus

> EXCLUDES Cardiac catheterization procedures integral to valve procedure (93451-93454, 93456-93461, 93563-93564)
> Repair of mitral valve including transseptal puncture (33418-33419)
> Transcatheter implantation/replacement mitral valve (TMVI) (0483T-0484T)
>
> 🚑 0.00   ✂ 0.00   **FUD** YYY          C ▣
>
> **AMA:** 2017,Jan,8; 2016,Jan,13; 2015,Sep,3

---

● New Code   ▲ Revised Code   ○ Reinstated   ● New Web Release   ▲ Revised Web Release   Unlisted   Not Covered   # Resequenced
Ⓢ AMA Mod 51 Exempt   ⑩ Optum Mod 51 Exempt   ⊛ Mod 63 Exempt   ✔ Non-FDA Drug   ★ Telemedicine   M Maternity   A Age Edit   + Add-on   **AMA:** CPT Asst

Category III Codes

0346T — 0363T

**+ 0346T** Ultrasound, elastography (List separately in addition to code for primary procedure)

 0.00  0.00 **FUD** YYY  N N1 CCI

 Code first (76536, 76604, 76641-76642, 76700, 76705, 76770, 76775, 76830, 76856-76857, 76870, 76872, 76881-76882)

**0347T** Placement of interstitial device(s) in bone for radiostereometric analysis (RSA)

 0.00  0.00 **FUD** YYY  01 N1 CCI

 **AMA:** 2017,Jan,8; 2016,Jan,13; 2015,Jun,8

## 0348T-0350T

**0348T** Radiologic examination, radiostereometric analysis (RSA); spine, (includes cervical, thoracic and lumbosacral, when performed)

 0.00  0.00 **FUD** YYY  01 N1 CCI

 **AMA:** 2017,Jan,8; 2016,Jan,13; 2015,Jun,8

**0349T** upper extremity(ies), (includes shoulder, elbow, and wrist, when performed)

 0.00  0.00 **FUD** YYY  01 N1 CCI

 **AMA:** 2017,Jan,8; 2016,Jan,13; 2015,Jun,8

**0350T** lower extremity(ies), (includes hip, proximal femur, knee, and ankle, when performed)

 0.00  0.00 **FUD** YYY  01 N1 CCI

 **AMA:** 2017,Jan,8; 2016,Jan,13; 2015,Jun,8

## 0351T-0354T

**0351T** Optical coherence tomography of breast or axillary lymph node, excised tissue, each specimen; real-time intraoperative

 INCLUDES  Interpretation and report (0352T)

 0.00  0.00 **FUD** YYY  N N1 CCI

 **AMA:** 2017,Jan,8; 2016,Jan,13; 2015,Apr,6

**0352T** interpretation and report, real-time or referred

 INCLUDES  Interpretation and report (0351T)

 0.00  0.00 **FUD** YYY  B CCI

 **AMA:** 2017,Jan,8; 2016,Jan,13; 2015,Apr,6

**0353T** Optical coherence tomography of breast, surgical cavity; real-time intraoperative

 INCLUDES  Interpretation and report (0354T)

 EXCLUDES  Use of code more than one time per session

 0.00  0.00 **FUD** YYY  N N1 CCI

 **AMA:** 2017,Jan,8; 2016,Jan,13; 2015,Apr,6

**0354T** interpretation and report, real time or referred

 0.00  0.00 **FUD** YYY  B CCI

 **AMA:** 2017,Jan,8; 2016,Jan,13; 2015,Apr,6

## 0355T-0358T

**0355T** Gastrointestinal tract imaging, intraluminal (eg, capsule endoscopy), colon, with interpretation and report

 0.00  0.00 **FUD** YYY  J CCI

 INCLUDES  Distal ileum imaging when performed

 EXCLUDES  Capsule endoscopy esophagus only (91111)
 Capsule endoscopy esophagus through ileum (91110)

**0356T** Insertion of drug-eluting implant (including punctal dilation and implant removal when performed) into lacrimal canaliculus, each

 EXCLUDES  Drug-eluting ocular insert (0444T-0445T)

 0.00  0.00 **FUD** YYY  01 N1 CCI

 **AMA:** 2017,Aug,7

*0357T* **Resequenced code. See code following 0058T.**

**0358T** Bioelectrical impedance analysis whole body composition assessment, with interpretation and report

 0.00  0.00 **FUD** YYY  01 CCI

## 0359T

 INCLUDES  Adaptive behavior evaluation by physician/other qualified health care professional with assistance of technician(s)

 EXCLUDES  Evaluation for occupational therapy ([97165, 97166, 97167, 97168])
 The following services when provided on the same date of service:
 Assessment/evaluation/testing of cognitive function (96101-96125)
 Behavior/health assessment (96150-96155)
 Psychiatric services (90785-90899)

**0359T** Behavior identification assessment, by the physician or other qualified health care professional, face-to-face with patient and caregiver(s), includes administration of standardized and non-standardized tests, detailed behavioral history, patient observation and caregiver interview, interpretation of test results, discussion of findings and recommendations with the primary guardian(s)/caregiver(s), and preparation of report

 0.00  0.00 **FUD** YYY  S CCI

 **AMA:** 2017,Jan,8; 2016,Jan,13; 2015,Jan,16; 2014,Jun,3

## 0360T-0363T

 INCLUDES  Follow-up assessments
 Provided to patients with destructive behaviors
 Only the time of one technician when more than one is in attendance
 Time reported during one day only

 EXCLUDES  The following services when provided on the same date of service:
 Assessment/evaluation/testing of cognitive function (96101-96125)
 Behavior/health assessment (96150-96155)
 Psychiatric services (90785-90899)

**0360T** Observational behavioral follow-up assessment, includes physician or other qualified health care professional direction with interpretation and report, administered by one technician; first 30 minutes of technician time, face-to-face with the patient

 INCLUDES  Time based on face-to-face time provided by one technician and not the collective time of several technicians

 EXCLUDES  Less than 16 minutes of face-to-face technician time

 0.00  0.00 **FUD** YYY  S CCI

 **AMA:** 2017,Jan,8; 2016,Jan,13; 2015,Jan,16; 2014,Jun,3

**+ 0361T** each additional 30 minutes of technician time, face-to-face with the patient (List separately in addition to code for primary service)

 Code first (0360T)

 0.00  0.00 **FUD** ZZZ  N CCI

 **AMA:** 2017,Jan,8; 2016,Jan,13; 2015,Jan,16; 2014,Jun,3

**0362T** Exposure behavioral follow-up assessment, includes physician or other qualified health care professional direction with interpretation and report, administered by physician or other qualified health care professional with the assistance of one or more technicians; first 30 minutes of technician(s) time, face-to-face with the patient

 INCLUDES  Time based on face-to-face time provided by one technician and not the collective time of several technicians

 0.00  0.00 **FUD** YYY  S CCI

 **AMA:** 2017,Jan,8; 2016,Jan,13; 2015,Jan,16; 2014,Jun,3

**+ 0363T** each additional 30 minutes of technician(s) time, face-to-face with the patient (List separately in addition to code for primary procedure)

 0.00  0.00 **FUD** ZZZ  N CCI

 **AMA:** 2017,Jan,8; 2016,Jan,13; 2015,Jan,16; 2014,Jun,3

26/TC PC/TC Only
FUD Follow-up Days
A2-Z3 ASC Payment
CMS: IOM (Pub 100)
50 Bilateral
A-Y OPPSI
♂ Male Only
80/80 Surg Assist Allowed / w/Doc
♀ Female Only
 Facility RVU
 Lab Crosswalk
 Non-Facility RVU
 Radiology Crosswalk
 CCI
 CLIA
CPT © 2017 American Medical Association. All Rights Reserved.
© 2017 Optum360, LLC

## 0364T-0372T

**0364T** Adaptive behavior treatment by protocol, administered by technician, face-to-face with one patient; first 30 minutes of technician time

> *EXCLUDES* *Assessment/evaluation/testing of cognitive function (96101-96155)*
> *Cognitive function interventions (97127)*
> *Psychiatric services (90785-90899)*
> *Treatment of speech language disorder, individual (92507)*

📋 0.00   ✂ 0.00   **FUD** YYY                    S 🖥

**AMA:** 2017,Jan,8; 2016,Sep,6; 2016,Jan,13; 2015,Jan,16; 2014,Jun,3

**+  0365T** each additional 30 minutes of technician time (List separately in addition to code for primary procedure)

> *EXCLUDES* *Assessment/evaluation/testing of cognitive function (96101-96155)*
> *Cognitive function interventions (97127)*
> *Psychiatric services (90785-90899)*
> *Treatment of speech language disorder, individual (92507)*

Code first (0364T)

📋 0.00   ✂ 0.00   **FUD** ZZZ                    N 🖥

**AMA:** 2017,Jan,8; 2016,Sep,6; 2016,Jan,13; 2015,Jan,16; 2014,Jun,3

**0366T** Group adaptive behavior treatment by protocol, administered by technician, face-to-face with two or more patients; first 30 minutes of technician time

> *EXCLUDES* *Assessment/evaluation/testing of cognitive function (96101-96155)*
> *Cognitive function interventions (97127)*
> *Groups comprising more than eight patients*
> *Psychiatric services (90785-90899)*
> *Therapeutic procedures (97150)*
> *Treatment of speech language disorder, group (92508)*

📋 0.00   ✂ 0.00   **FUD** YYY                    S 🖥

**AMA:** 2017,Jan,8; 2016,Sep,6; 2016,Jan,13; 2015,Jan,16; 2014,Jun,3

**+  0367T** each additional 30 minutes of technician time (List separately in addition to code for primary procedure)

> *EXCLUDES* *Assessment/evaluation/testing of cognitive function (96101-96125)*
> *Cognitive function interventions (97127)*
> *Groups comprising more than eight patients*
> *Psychiatric services (90785-90899)*
> *Therapeutic procedures (97150)*
> *Treatment of speech language disorder, individual (92507)*

Code first (0366T)

📋 0.00   ✂ 0.00   **FUD** ZZZ                    N 🖥

**AMA:** 2017,Jan,8; 2016,Sep,6; 2016,Jan,13; 2015,Jan,16; 2014,Jun,3

**0368T** Adaptive behavior treatment with protocol modification administered by physician or other qualified health care professional with one patient; first 30 minutes of patient face-to-face time

> *EXCLUDES* *Cognitive function interventions (97127)*
> *Explanation/interpretation psychiatric and other services (90887)*
> *Family psychotherapy (90846-90847)*
> *Psychiatric diagnostic evaluation (90791-90792)*
> *Treatment of speech language disorder, individual (92507)*

📋 0.00   ✂ 0.00   **FUD** YYY                    S 🖥

**AMA:** 2017,Jan,8; 2016,Sep,6; 2016,Jan,13; 2015,Jan,16; 2014,Jun,3

**+  0369T** each additional 30 minutes of patient face-to-face time (List separately in addition to code for primary procedure)

> *EXCLUDES* *Cognitive function interventions (97127)*
> *Explanation/interpretation psychiatric and other services (90887)*
> *Family psychotherapy (90846-90847)*
> *Psychiatric diagnostic evaluation (90791-90792)*
> *Treatment of speech language disorder, individual (92507)*

Code first (0368T)

📋 0.00   ✂ 0.00   **FUD** ZZZ                    N 🖥

**AMA:** 2017,Jan,8; 2016,Sep,6; 2016,Jan,13; 2015,Jan,16; 2014,Jun,3

**0370T** Family adaptive behavior treatment guidance, administered by physician or other qualified health care professional (without the patient present)

> *EXCLUDES* *Cognitive function interventions (97127)*
> *Explanation/interpretation psychiatric and other services (90887)*
> *Family psychotherapy (90846-90847)*
> *Psychiatric diagnostic evaluation (90791-90792)*

📋 0.00   ✂ 0.00   **FUD** YYY                    S 🖥

**AMA:** 2017,Jan,8; 2016,Jan,13; 2015,Jan,16; 2014,Jun,3

**0371T** Multiple-family group adaptive behavior treatment guidance, administered by physician or other qualified health care professional (without the patient present)

> *EXCLUDES* *Explanation/interpretation psychiatric and other services (90887)*
> *Family psychotherapy (90846-90847)*
> *Groups comprising more than eight patients*
> *Psychiatric diagnostic evaluation (90791-90792)*

📋 0.00   ✂ 0.00   **FUD** YYY                    S 🖥

**AMA:** 2017,Jan,8; 2016,Jan,13; 2015,Jan,16; 2014,Jun,3

**0372T** Adaptive behavior treatment social skills group, administered by physician or other qualified health care professional face-to-face with multiple patients

> *EXCLUDES* *Group psychotherapy (90853)*
> *Groups comprising more than eight patients*
> *Therapeutic procedures (97150)*
> *Treatment of speech language disorder, group (92508)*

📋 0.00   ✂ 0.00   **FUD** YYY                    S 🖥

**AMA:** 2017,Jan,8; 2016,Sep,6; 2016,Jan,13; 2015,Jan,16; 2014,Jun,3

## 0373T-0374T

> *EXCLUDES* *Assessment/evaluation/testing of cognitive function (96101-96155)*
> *Psychiatric services (90785-90899)*

**0373T** Exposure adaptive behavior treatment with protocol modification requiring two or more technicians for severe maladaptive behavior(s); first 60 minutes of technicians' time, face-to-face with patient

📋 0.00   ✂ 0.00   **FUD** YYY                    S 🖥

**AMA:** 2017,Jan,8; 2016,Jan,13; 2015,Jan,16; 2014,Jun,3

**+  0374T** each additional 30 minutes of technicians' time face-to-face with patient (List separately in addition to code for primary procedure)

Code first (0373T)

📋 0.00   ✂ 0.00   **FUD** ZZZ                    N 🖥

**AMA:** 2014,Jun,3

## 0375T

**0375T** Total disc arthroplasty (artificial disc), anterior approach, including discectomy with end plate preparation (includes osteophytectomy for nerve root or spinal cord decompression and microdissection), cervical, three or more levels

> *EXCLUDES* *Procedures performed at same level with (22853-22854, [22859], 22856, [22858])*

📋 0.00   ✂ 0.00   **FUD** XXX                    C 80 🖥

**AMA:** 2017,Jan,8; 2016,Jan,13; 2015,Apr,7

● New Code   ▲ Revised Code   ○ Reinstated   ● New Web Release   ▲ Revised Web Release   Unlisted   Not Covered   # Resequenced
⊘ AMA Mod 51 Exempt   Ⓢ Optum Mod 51 Exempt   ⊚ Mod 63 Exempt   ✗ Non-FDA Drug   ★ Telemedicine   M Maternity   A Age Edit   + Add-on   **AMA:** CPT Asst
© 2017 Optum360, LLC                        CPT © 2017 American Medical Association. All Rights Reserved.                        549

## 0376T-0377T

*0376T*   Resequenced code. See code following 0191T.

**0377T**   **Anoscopy with directed submucosal injection of bulking agent for fecal incontinence**

    🔧 0.00     ⚕ 0.00     **FUD** XXX       J R2 80 ▢

    *INCLUDES*   Diagnostic anoscopy (46600)

## 0378T-0380T

**0378T**   **Visual field assessment, with concurrent real time data analysis and accessible data storage with patient initiated data transmitted to a remote surveillance center for up to 30 days; review and interpretation with report by a physician or other qualified health care professional**

    🔧 0.00     ⚕ 0.00     **FUD** XXX       B 80 ▢

    **AMA:** 2017,Jan,8; 2016,Jan,13; 2015,Jan,10

**0379T**   **technical support and patient instructions, surveillance, analysis and transmission of daily and emergent data reports as prescribed by a physician or other qualified health care professional**

    🔧 0.00     ⚕ 0.00     **FUD** XXX       Q1 N1 80 ▢

    **AMA:** 2017,Jan,8; 2016,Jan,13; 2015,Jan,10

**0380T**   **Computer-aided animation and analysis of time series retinal images for the monitoring of disease progression, unilateral or bilateral, with interpretation and report**

    🔧 0.00     ⚕ 0.00     **FUD** XXX       Q1 N1 80 ▢

    **AMA:** 2016,Feb,12

## 0381T-0386T

**0381T**   **External heart rate and 3-axis accelerometer data recording up to 14 days to assess changes in heart rate and to monitor motion analysis for the purposes of diagnosing nocturnal epilepsy seizure events; includes report, scanning analysis with report, review and interpretation by a physician or other qualified health care professional**

    🔧 0.00     ⚕ 0.00     **FUD** XXX       M 80 ▢

    *EXCLUDES*   *External heart rate and data recording for 15 days or more (0383T-0386T)*

**0382T**   **review and interpretation only**

    🔧 0.00     ⚕ 0.00     **FUD** XXX       M 80 ▢

    *EXCLUDES*   *External heart rate and data recording for 15 days or more (0383T-0386T)*

**0383T**   **External heart rate and 3-axis accelerometer data recording from 15 to 30 days to assess changes in heart rate and to monitor motion analysis for the purposes of diagnosing nocturnal epilepsy seizure events; includes report, scanning analysis with report, review and interpretation by a physician or other qualified health care professional**

    🔧 0.00     ⚕ 0.00     **FUD** XXX       M 80 ▢

    *EXCLUDES*   *External heart rate and data recording for 14 days or less (0381T-0382T)*

            *External heart rate and data recording for 30 days or more (0385T-0386T)*

**0384T**   **review and interpretation only**

    🔧 0.00     ⚕ 0.00     **FUD** XXX       M 80 ▢

    *EXCLUDES*   *External heart rate and data recording for 14 days or less (0381T-0382T)*

            *External heart rate and data recording for 30 days or more (0385T-0386T)*

**0385T**   **External heart rate and 3-axis accelerometer data recording more than 30 days to assess changes in heart rate and to monitor motion analysis for the purposes of diagnosing nocturnal epilepsy seizure events; includes report, scanning analysis with report, review and interpretation by a physician or other qualified health care professional**

    🔧 0.00     ⚕ 0.00     **FUD** XXX       M 80 ▢

    *EXCLUDES*   *External heart rate and data recording for 30 days or less (0381T-0384T)*

**0386T**   **review and interpretation only**

    🔧 0.00     ⚕ 0.00     **FUD** XXX       M 80 ▢

    *EXCLUDES*   *External heart rate and data recording for 30 days or less (0381T-0384T)*

## 0387T-0391T

**0387T**   **Transcatheter insertion or replacement of permanent leadless pacemaker, ventricular**

    *INCLUDES*   Device evaluation (0389T-0391T)

            Fluoroscopy (76000)

            Lead removal when replacement performed (0388T)

            Right ventriculography (93566)

            Venography, femoral (75820)

    *EXCLUDES*   *Procedures related to pacemaker systems with leads (33202-33203, 33206-33222 [33221], 33224-33226)*

    🔧 0.00     ⚕ 0.00     **FUD** XXX       J J8 80 ▢

    **AMA:** 2017,Jan,8; 2016,Aug,5; 2016,May,5; 2016,Jan,13; 2015,May,3; 2015,Jan,16; 2014,Dec,16; 2014,Dec,16

**0388T**   **Transcatheter removal of permanent leadless pacemaker, ventricular**

    *INCLUDES*   Fluoroscopy (76000)

            Right ventriculography (93566)

            Venography, femoral (75820)

    *EXCLUDES*   *Insertion or replacement of device (0387T)*

            *Procedures related to pacemaker systems with leads (33233-33238 [33227, 33228, 33229])*

    🔧 0.00     ⚕ 0.00     **FUD** XXX       T R2 80 ▢

    **AMA:** 2017,Jan,8; 2016,Aug,5; 2016,May,5; 2016,Jan,13; 2015,May,3; 2015,Jan,16; 2014,Dec,16; 2014,Dec,16

**0389T**   **Programming device evaluation (in person) with iterative adjustment of the implantable device to test the function of the device and select optimal permanent programmed values with analysis, review and report, leadless pacemaker system**

    *EXCLUDES*   *Device evaluation (0390T-0391T)*

            *Insertion or replacement of device (0387T)*

            *Procedures to program pacemaker systems with leads (93279-93281)*

    🔧 0.00     ⚕ 0.00     **FUD** XXX       Q1 80 ▢

    **AMA:** 2017,Jan,8; 2016,Aug,5; 2016,May,5; 2016,Jan,13; 2015,May,3; 2015,Jan,16; 2014,Dec,16; 2014,Dec,16

**0390T**   **Peri-procedural device evaluation (in person) and programming of device system parameters before or after a surgery, procedure or test with analysis, review and report, leadless pacemaker system**

    *EXCLUDES*   *Device evaluation (0389T, 0391T)*

            *Insertion or replacement of device (0387T)*

            *Procedures for peri-procedural evaluation and programming of pacemaker systems with leads (93286-93287)*

    🔧 0.00     ⚕ 0.00     **FUD** XXX       N N1 80 ▢

    **AMA:** 2017,Jan,8; 2016,Aug,5; 2016,May,5; 2016,Jan,13; 2015,May,3; 2015,Jan,16; 2014,Dec,16; 2014,Dec,16

**0391T**   **Interrogation device evaluation (in person) with analysis, review and report, includes connection, recording and disconnection per patient encounter, leadless pacemaker system**

    *EXCLUDES*   *Device evaluation (0389T-0390T)*

            *Insertion or replacement of device (0387T)*

            *Procedures for interrogation device evaluaiton of pacemaker systems with leads (93288-93289)*

    🔧 0.00     ⚕ 0.00     **FUD** XXX       Q1 80 ▢

    **AMA:** 2017,Jan,8; 2016,Aug,5; 2016,May,5; 2016,Jan,13; 2015,May,3

---

26/TC PC/TC Only    A2-Z3 ASC Payment    50 Bilateral    ♂ Male Only    ♀ Female Only    🔧 Facility RVU    ⚕ Non-Facility RVU    ▢ CCI

**FUD** Follow-up Days    **CMS:** IOM (Pub 100)    A-Y OPPSI    80/80 Surg Assist Allowed / w/Doc    🔬 Lab Crosswalk    ☢ Radiology Crosswalk    ✖ CLIA

550      CPT © 2017 American Medical Association. All Rights Reserved.      © 2017 Optum360, LLC

## 0394T-0395T

EXCLUDES Radiation oncology procedures (77261-77263, 77300, 77306-77307, 77316-77318, 77332-77334, 77336, 77427-77499, 77761-77772, 77778, 77789)

**0394T** **High dose rate electronic brachytherapy, skin surface application, per fraction, includes basic dosimetry, when performed**

🔲 0.00    ⚖ 0.00    **FUD** XXX    S Z2 80 ▢

EXCLUDES Superficial non-brachytherapy radiation (77401)

**0395T** **High dose rate electronic brachytherapy, interstitial or intracavitary treatment, per fraction, includes basic dosimetry, when performed**

🔲 0.00    ⚖ 0.00    **FUD** XXX    S Z2 80 ▢

EXCLUDES High dose rate skin surface application (0394T)

## 0396T-0399T

+ **0396T** **Intra-operative use of kinetic balance sensor for implant stability during knee replacement arthroplasty (List separately in addition to code for primary procedure)**

🔲 0.00    ⚖ 0.00    **FUD** XXX    N N1 80 ▢

Code first (27445-27447, 27486-27488)

+ **0397T** **Endoscopic retrograde cholangiopancreatography (ERCP), with optical endomicroscopy (List separately in addition to code for primary procedure)**

🔲 0.00    ⚖ 0.00    **FUD** XXX    N N1 80 ▢

INCLUDES Optical endomicroscopic image(s) (88375)

EXCLUDES Use of code more than one time per operative session

Code first (43260-43265, [43274], [43275], [43276], [43277], [43278])

**0398T** **Magnetic resonance image guided high intensity focused ultrasound (MRgFUS), stereotactic ablation lesion, intracranial for movement disorder including stereotactic navigation and frame placement when performed**

🔲 0.00    ⚖ 0.00    **FUD** XXX    S 80 ▢

INCLUDES Application stereotactic headframe (61800)
Stereotactic computer-assisted navigation (61781)

+ **0399T** **Myocardial strain imaging (quantitative assessment of myocardial mechanics using image-based analysis of local myocardial dynamics) (List separately in addition to code for primary procedure)**

🔲 0.00    ⚖ 0.00    **FUD** XXX    N N1 80

EXCLUDES Use of code more than one time per operative session

Code first (93303-93312, 93314-93315, 93317, 93350-93351, 93355)

## 0400T-0401T

**0400T** **Multi-spectral digital skin lesion analysis of clinically atypical cutaneous pigmented lesions for detection of melanomas and high risk melanocytic atypia; one to five lesions**

🔲 0.00    ⚖ 0.00    **FUD** XXX    N N1 80

**0401T** **six or more lesions**

🔲 0.00    ⚖ 0.00    **FUD** XXX    N N1 80 ▢

INCLUDES Treatment of one to five lesions (0400T)

## 0402T

**0402T** **Collagen cross-linking of cornea (including removal of the corneal epithelium and intraoperative pachymetry when performed)**

INCLUDES Corneal epithelium removal (65435)
Corneal pachymetry (76514)
Operating microscope (69990)

🔲 0.00    ⚖ 0.00    **FUD** XXX    T R2 80 ▢

**AMA:** 2017,Jan,8; 2016,Feb,12

## 0403T [0488T]

INCLUDES Intensive behavioral counseling by trained lifestyle coach
Standardized course with an emphasis on weight, exercise, stress management, and nutrition

**0403T** **Preventive behavior change, intensive program of prevention of diabetes using a standardized diabetes prevention program curriculum, provided to individuals in a group setting, minimum 60 minutes, per day**

EXCLUDES Online/electronic diabetes prevention program ([0488T])
Self-management training and education by nonphysician health care professional (98960-98962)

🔲 0.00    ⚖ 0.00    **FUD** XXX    E 80

**AMA:** 2015,Aug,4

● # **0488T** **Preventive behavior change, online/electronic structured intensive program for prevention of diabetes using a standardized diabetes prevention program curriculum, provided to an individual, per 30 days**

🔲 0.00    ⚖ 0.00    **FUD** 000

INCLUDES In person elements when appropriate

EXCLUDES Group diabetes prevention program (0403T)
Self-management training and education by nonphysician health care professional (98960-98962)

## 0404T-0405T

**0404T** **Transcervical uterine fibroid(s) ablation with ultrasound guidance, radiofrequency** ♀

🔲 0.00    ⚖ 0.00    **FUD** XXX    J 80 ▢

**0405T** **Oversight of the care of an extracorporeal liver assist system patient requiring review of status, review of laboratories and other studies, and revision of orders and liver assist care plan (as appropriate), within a calendar month, 30 minutes or more of non-face-to-face time**

🔲 0.00    ⚖ 0.00    **FUD** XXX    B 80 ▢

## 0406T-0407T

INCLUDES Sinus procedures when performed on the same side (31200-31205, 31231, 31237, 31240, 31254-31255, 31288, 31290)

**0406T** **Nasal endoscopy, surgical, ethmoid sinus, placement of drug eluting implant;**

🔲 0.00    ⚖ 0.00    **FUD** XXX    Q2 N1 80 ▢

**AMA:** 2017,Jan,8; 2016,Feb,10

**0407T** **with biopsy, polypectomy or debridement**

EXCLUDES Endoscopy of sinus when performed on the same side (0406T)

🔲 0.00    ⚖ 0.00    **FUD** XXX    Q2 N1 80 ▢

**AMA:** 2017,Jan,8; 2016,Feb,10

## 0408T-0418T

**0408T** **Insertion or replacement of permanent cardiac contractility modulation system, including contractility evaluation when performed, and programming of sensing and therapeutic parameters; pulse generator with transvenous electrodes**

🔲 0.00    ⚖ 0.00    **FUD** XXX    J J8 80 ▢

INCLUDES Device evaluation (93286-93287, 0415T, 0417T-0418T)
Insertion or replacement of entire system

EXCLUDES Cardiac catheterization (93452-93453, 93458-93461)

Code also removal of each electrode when pulse generator and electrodes are removed and replaced (0410T-0411T)

**0409T** **pulse generator only**

🔲 0.00    ⚖ 0.00    **FUD** XXX    J J8 80 ▢

INCLUDES Device evaluation (93286-93287, 0415T, 0417T-0418T)

EXCLUDES Cardiac catheterization (93452-93453, 93458-93461)

**0410T** **atrial electrode only**

🔲 0.00    ⚖ 0.00    **FUD** XXX    J J8 80 ▢

INCLUDES Device evaluation (93286-93287, 0415T, 0417T-0418T)
Each atrial electrode inserted or replaced

EXCLUDES Cardiac catheterization (93452-93453, 93458-93461)

---

**0411T**    ventricular electrode only

     📠 0.00    🔪 0.00    **FUD** XXX      J J8 80 🖵

     INCLUDES    Device evaluation (93286-93287, 0415T, 0417T-0418T)
          Each ventricular electrode inserted or replaced
     EXCLUDES    Cardiac catheterization (93452-93453, 93458-93461)
          Insertion or replacement of complete CCM system
            (0408T)

**0412T**    **Removal of permanent cardiac contractility modulation system; pulse generator only**

     📠 0.00    🔪 0.00    **FUD** XXX      Q2 G2 80 🖵

     EXCLUDES    Device evaluation (0417T-0418T)
          Insertion or replacement of complete CCM system
            (0408T)

**0413T**    transvenous electrode (atrial or ventricular)

     📠 0.00    🔪 0.00    **FUD** XXX      Q2 G2 80 🖵

     INCLUDES    Each electrode removed
     EXCLUDES    Device evaluation (0417T-0418T)
          Insertion or replacement of complete CCM system
            (0408T)
     Code also removal and replacement of electrode(s), as
          appropriate (0410T-0411T)
     Code also removal of pulse generator when leads also removed
          (0412T)

**0414T**    **Removal and replacement of permanent cardiac contractility modulation system pulse generator only**

     📠 0.00    🔪 0.00    **FUD** XXX      J J8 80 🖵

     EXCLUDES    Cardiac catheterization (93452-93453, 93458-93461)
          Device evaluation (93286-93287, 0417T-0418T)
     Code also replacement of pulse generator when leads also
          removed and replaced (0408T, 0412T-0413T)

**0415T**    **Repositioning of previously implanted cardiac contractility modulation transvenous electrode, (atrial or ventricular lead)**

     📠 0.00    🔪 0.00    **FUD** XXX      T G2 80 🖵

     EXCLUDES    Cardiac catheterization (93452-93453, 93458-93461)
          Device evaluation (93286-93287, 0417T-0418T)
          Insertion or replacement of entire system or components
            (0408T-0411T)

**0416T**    **Relocation of skin pocket for implanted cardiac contractility modulation pulse generator**

     📠 0.00    🔪 0.00    **FUD** XXX      T G2 80 🖵

**0417T**    **Programming device evaluation (in person) with iterative adjustment of the implantable device to test the function of the device and select optimal permanent programmed values with analysis, including review and report, implantable cardiac contractility modulation system**

     📠 0.00    🔪 0.00    **FUD** XXX      Q1 80 🖵

     EXCLUDES    Insertion/replacement/removal/repositioning of device
          or components (0408T-0415T, 0418T)

**0418T**    **Interrogation device evaluation (in person) with analysis, review and report, includes connection, recording and disconnection per patient encounter, implantable cardiac contractility modulation system**

     📠 0.00    🔪 0.00    **FUD** XXX      Q1 80 🖵

     EXCLUDES    Insertion/replacement/removal/repositioning of device
          or components (0408T-0415T, 0417T)

## 0419T-0420T

     EXCLUDES    Neurofibroma excision (64792)
          Use of code more than one time per session

**0419T**    **Destruction of neurofibroma, extensive (cutaneous, dermal extending into subcutaneous); face, head and neck, greater than 50 neurofibromas**

     📠 0.00    🔪 0.00    **FUD** XXX      T R2 80 🖵

     **AMA:** 2017,Jan,8; 2016,Apr,3

**0420T**    **trunk and extremities, extensive, greater than 100 neurofibromas**

     📠 0.00    🔪 0.00    **FUD** XXX      T R2 80 🖵

     **AMA:** 2017,Jan,8; 2016,Apr,3

## 0421T-0423T

**0421T**    **Transurethral waterjet ablation of prostate, including control of post-operative bleeding, including ultrasound guidance, complete (vasectomy, meatotomy, cystourethroscopy, urethral calibration and/or dilation, and internal urethrotomy are included when performed)**    ♂

     📠 0.00    🔪 0.00    **FUD** XXX      E 80 🖵

     EXCLUDES    Transrectal ultrasound (76872)
          Transurethral prostate resection (52500, 52630)

**0422T**    **Tactile breast imaging by computer-aided tactile sensors, unilateral or bilateral**

     📠 0.00    🔪 0.00    **FUD** XXX      Q1 Z2 80 🖵

**0423T**    **Secretory type II phospholipase A2 (sPLA2-IIA)**

     📠 0.00    🔪 0.00    **FUD** XXX      A

     EXCLUDES    Lipoprotein-associated phospholipase A2 [LpPLA2]
          (83698)

## 0424T-0436T

     INCLUDES    Phrenic nerve stimulation system includes:
          Pulse generator
          Sensing lead (placed in azygos vein)
          Stimulation lead (placed into right brachiocephalic vein or left
            periocardiophrenic vein)

**0424T**    **Insertion or replacement of neurostimulator system for treatment of central sleep apnea; complete system (transvenous placement of right or left stimulation lead, sensing lead, implantable pulse generator)**

     📠 0.00    🔪 0.00    **FUD** XXX      J G2 80 🖵

     INCLUDES    Device evaluation (0434T-0436T)
          Insertion or replacement system components
            (0424T-0427T)
          Repositioning of leads (0432T-0433T)
     Code also when pulse generator and all leads are removed and
          replaced (0428T-0430T)

**0425T**    sensing lead only

     📠 0.00    🔪 0.00    **FUD** XXX      J G2 80 🖵

     EXCLUDES    Device evaluation (0434T-0436T)
          Insertion/replacement complete system (0424T)
          Repositioning of leads (0432T-0433T)

**0426T**    stimulation lead only

     📠 0.00    🔪 0.00    **FUD** XXX      J G2 80 🖵

     EXCLUDES    Device evaluation (0434T-0436T)
          Insertion/replacement complete system (0424T)
          Repositioning of leads (0432T-0433T)

**0427T**    pulse generator only

     📠 0.00    🔪 0.00    **FUD** XXX      J G2 80 🖵

     EXCLUDES    Device evaluation (0434T-0436T)
          Insertion/replacement complete system (0424T)
          Repositioning of leads (0432T-0433T)

**0428T**    **Removal of neurostimulator system for treatment of central sleep apnea; pulse generator only**

     📠 0.00    🔪 0.00    **FUD** XXX      Q2 G2 80 🖵

     EXCLUDES    Device evaluation (0434T-0436T)
          Removal with replacement of pulse generator and all
            leads (0424T, 0429T-0430T)
          Repositioning of leads (0432T-0433T)
     Code also when a lead is removed (0429T-0430T)

**0429T**    sensing lead only

     📠 0.00    🔪 0.00    **FUD** XXX      Q2 G2 80 🖵

     INCLUDES    Removal of one sensing lead
     EXCLUDES    Device evaluation (0434T-0436T)

**0430T**    stimulation lead only

     INCLUDES    Removal of one stimulation lead
     EXCLUDES    Device evaluation (0434T-0436T)

     📠 0.00    🔪 0.00    **FUD** XXX      Q2 G2 80 🖵

     **AMA:** 2015,Aug,4

**0431T** Removal and replacement of neurostimulator system for treatment of central sleep apnea, pulse generator only

0.00   0.00   **FUD** XXX   J 62 80

EXCLUDES  Device evaluation (0434T-0436T)
Replacement or removal of generator and all three leads (0424T, 0428T-0430T)

**0432T** Repositioning of neurostimulator system for treatment of central sleep apnea; stimulation lead only

0.00   0.00   **FUD** XXX   T 62 80

EXCLUDES  Device evaluation (0434T-0436T)
Insertion/replacement complete system or components (0424T-0427T)

**0433T** sensing lead only

0.00   0.00   **FUD** XXX   T 62 80

EXCLUDES  Device evaluation (0434T-0436T)
Insertion/replacement complete system or components (0424T-0427T)

**0434T** Interrogation device evaluation implanted neurostimulator pulse generator system for central sleep apnea

0.00   0.00   **FUD** XXX   S 62 80

EXCLUDES  Insertion/replacement complete system or components (0424T-0427T)
Removal of system or components (0428T-0431T)
Repositioning leads (0432T-0433T)

**0435T** Programming device evaluation of implanted neurostimulator pulse generator system for central sleep apnea; single session

0.00   0.00   **FUD** XXX   S 80

EXCLUDES  Device evaluation (0436T)
Insertion/replacement complete system or components (0424T-0427T)
Removal of system or components (0428T-0431T)
Repositioning leads (0432T-0433T)

**0436T** during sleep study

0.00   0.00   **FUD** XXX   S 80

EXCLUDES  Device evaluation (0435T)
Insertion/replacement complete system or components (0424T-0427T)
Removal of system or components (0428T-0431T)
Repositioning leads (0432T-0433T)
Use of code more than one time for each sleep study

## 0437T-0439T

+ **0437T** Implantation of non-biologic or synthetic implant (eg, polypropylene) for fascial reinforcement of the abdominal wall (List separately in addition to code for primary procedure)

0.00   0.00   **FUD** ZZZ   N N1 80

EXCLUDES  Implantation mesh, other material for repair incisional or ventral hernia (49560-49561, 49565-49566, 49568)
Insertion mesh, other material for closure of wound caused by necrotizing soft tissue infection (11004-11006, 49568)

+ ~~**0438T**~~ ~~Transperineal placement of biodegradable material, peri-prostatic (via needle), single or multiple, includes image guidance~~

To report, see 55874

+ **0439T** Myocardial contrast perfusion echocardiography, at rest or with stress, for assessment of myocardial ischemia or viability (List separately in addition to code for primary procedure)

Code first (93306-93308, 93350-93351)

0.00   0.00   **FUD** ZZZ   N N1 80

AMA: 2017,Jan,8; 2016,Apr,8

## 0440T-0442T

EXCLUDES  Insertion/removal drug-eluting stent into canaliculus

**0440T** Ablation, percutaneous, cryoablation, includes imaging guidance; upper extremity distal/peripheral nerve

0.00   0.00   **FUD** YYY   J 62 80

**0441T** lower extremity distal/peripheral nerve

0.00   0.00   **FUD** YYY   J 62 80

**0442T** nerve plexus or other truncal nerve (eg, brachial plexus, pudendal nerve)

0.00   0.00   **FUD** YYY   J 62 80

## 0443T

+ **0443T** Real-time spectral analysis of prostate tissue by fluorescence spectroscopy, including imaging guidance (List separately in addition to code for primary procedure)   ♂

0.00   0.00   **FUD** ZZZ   N N1 80

EXCLUDES  Use of code more than one time for each session
Code also (55700)

## 0444T-0445T

EXCLUDES  Insertion/removal drug-eluting stent into canaliculus (0356T)

**0444T** Initial placement of a drug-eluting ocular insert under one or more eyelids, including fitting, training, and insertion, unilateral or bilateral

0.00   0.00   **FUD** YYY   N N1 80

AMA: 2017,Aug,7

**0445T** Subsequent placement of a drug-eluting ocular insert under one or more eyelids, including re-training, and removal of existing insert, unilateral or bilateral

0.00   0.00   **FUD** YYY   N N1 80

AMA: 2017,Aug,7

## 0446T-0448T

EXCLUDES  Placement non-implantable interstitial glucose sensor without pocket (95250)

**0446T** Creation of subcutaneous pocket with insertion of implantable interstitial glucose sensor, including system activation and patient training

0.00   0.00   **FUD** YYY   T J8

EXCLUDES  Interpretation/report of ambulatory glucose monitoring of interstitial tissue (95251)
Removal interstitial glucose sensor (0447T-0448T)

**0447T** Removal of implantable interstitial glucose sensor from subcutaneous pocket via incision

0.00   0.00   **FUD** YYY   02 62

**0448T** Removal of implantable interstitial glucose sensor with creation of subcutaneous pocket at different anatomic site and insertion of new implantable sensor, including system activation

0.00   0.00   **FUD** YYY   T 62

EXCLUDES  Initial insertion of sensor (0446T)
Removal of sensor (0447T)

## 0449T-0450T

EXCLUDES  Removal by internal approach of aqueous drainage device without extraocular reservoir in subconjunctival space (92499)

**0449T** Insertion of aqueous drainage device, without extraocular reservoir, internal approach, into the subconjunctival space; initial device

0.00   0.00   **FUD** YYY   J J8

+ **0450T** each additional device (List separately in addition to code for primary procedure)

0.00   0.00   **FUD** YYY   N N1

Code first (0449T)

---

## 0451T-0463T

**INCLUDES** Access procedures (36000-36010)
Catheterization of vessel (36200-36228)
Diagnostic angiography (75600-75774)
Imaging guidance (76000-76001, 76936-76937, 77001-77002, 77011-77012, 77021)
Injection procedures (93561-93572)
Radiological supervision and interpretation

**EXCLUDES** Cardiac catheterization (93451-93533)

**0451T** Insertion or replacement of a permanently implantable aortic counterpulsation ventricular assist system, endovascular approach, and programming of sensing and therapeutic parameters; complete system (counterpulsation device, vascular graft, implantable vascular hemostatic seal, mechano-electrical skin interface and subcutaneous electrodes)

🔧 0.00   ✂ 0.00   **FUD** YYY                      C ▭

**EXCLUDES** Aortic counterpulsation ventricular assist system procedures (0452T-0458T)
Insertion intra-aortic balloon assist device (33967, 33970, 33973)
Insertion/replacement extracorporeal ventricular assist device (33975-33976, 33981)
Insertion/replacement intracorporeal ventricular assist device (33979, 33982-33983)
Insertion ventricular assist device (33990-33991)

**0452T** aortic counterpulsation device and vascular hemostatic seal

🔧 0.00   ✂ 0.00   **FUD** YYY                      C ▭

**EXCLUDES** Insertion intra-aortic balloon assist device (33973)
Insertion intracorporeal ventricular assist device (33979, 33982-33983)
Insertion/replacement counterpulsation ventricular assist system procedures (0451T)
Insertion ventricular assist device (33990-33991)
Removal counterpulsation ventricular assist system (0455T-0456T)

**0453T** mechano-electrical skin interface

🔧 0.00   ✂ 0.00   **FUD** YYY                      J ▭

**EXCLUDES** Insertion intra-aortic balloon assist device (33973)
Insertion intracorporeal ventricular assist device (33979, 33982-33983)
Insertion/replacement counterpulsation ventricular assist system procedures (0451T)
Insertion ventricular assist device (33990-33991)
Removal counterpulsation ventricular assist system (0455T, 0457T)

**0454T** subcutaneous electrode

🔧 0.00   ✂ 0.00   **FUD** YYY                      J ▭

**INCLUDES** Each electrode inserted or replaced

**EXCLUDES** Insertion intra-aortic balloon assist device (33973, 33982-33983)
Insertion/replacement counterpulsation ventricular assist system (0451T)
Insertion/replacement intracorporeal ventricular assist device (33979, 33982-33983)
Insertion ventricular assist device (33990-33991)
Removal device or component (0455T, 0458T)

**0455T** Removal of permanently implantable aortic counterpulsation ventricular assist system; complete system (aortic counterpulsation device, vascular hemostatic seal, mechano-electrical skin interface and electrodes)

🔧 0.00   ✂ 0.00   **FUD** YYY                      C ▭

**EXCLUDES** Insertion/replacement system or component (0451T-0454T)
Removal:
Extracorporeal ventricular assist device (33977-33978)
Intra-aortic balloon assist device (33968, 33971, 33974)
Intracorporeal ventricular assist device (33980)
Percutaneous ventricular assist device (33992)
System or component (0456T-0458T)

**0456T** aortic counterpulsation device and vascular hemostatic seal

🔧 0.00   ✂ 0.00   **FUD** YYY                      C ▭

**EXCLUDES** Insertion/replacement system or component (0451T-0454T)
Removal:
Aortic counterpulsation ventricular assist system (0455T)
Intra-aortic balloon assist device (33974)
Intracorporeal ventricular assist device (33980)
Percutaneous ventricular assist device (33992)

**0457T** mechano-electrical skin interface

🔧 0.00   ✂ 0.00   **FUD** YYY                      Q2 ▭

**EXCLUDES** Insertion/replacement system or component (0451T, 0453T)
Removal:
Aortic counterpulsation ventricular assist system (0455T)
Intra-aortic balloon assist device (33974)
Intracorporeal ventricular assist device (33980)
Percutaneous ventricular assist device (33992)

**0458T** subcutaneous electrode

🔧 0.00   ✂ 0.00   **FUD** YYY                      Q2 ▭

**INCLUDES** Each electrode removed

**EXCLUDES** Insertion/replacement system or component (0451T, 0454T)
Removal:
Aortic counterpulsation ventricular assist system (0455T)
Intra-aortic balloon assist device (33974)
Intracorporeal ventricular assist device (33980)
Percutaneous ventricular assist device (33992)

**0459T** Relocation of skin pocket with replacement of implanted aortic counterpulsation ventricular assist device, mechano-electrical skin interface and electrodes

🔧 0.00   ✂ 0.00   **FUD** YYY                      C ▭

**EXCLUDES** Repositioning percutaneous ventricular assist device (33993)

**0460T** Repositioning of previously implanted aortic counterpulsation ventricular assist device; subcutaneous electrode

🔧 0.00   ✂ 0.00   **FUD** YYY                      T ▭

**INCLUDES** Reporting for repositioning of each electrode

**EXCLUDES** Insertion/replacement system or component (0451T, 0454T)
Repositioning of percutaneous ventricular assist device (33993)

**0461T** aortic counterpulsation device

🔧 0.00   ✂ 0.00   **FUD** YYY                      C ▭

**EXCLUDES** Repositioning percutaneous ventricular assist device (33993)

**0462T** Programming device evaluation (in person) with iterative adjustment of the implantable mechano-electrical skin interface and/or external driver to test the function of the device and select optimal permanent programmed values with analysis, including review and report, implantable aortic counterpulsation ventricular assist system, per day

🔧 0.00   ✂ 0.00   **FUD** YYY                      S ▭

**EXCLUDES** Device evaluation (0463T)
Insertion/replacement system or component (0451T-0454T)
Relocation of pocket (0459T)
Removal system or component (0455T-0458T)
Repositioning device (0460T-0461T)

**0463T** Interrogation device evaluation (in person) with analysis, review and report, includes connection, recording and disconnection per patient encounter, implantable aortic counterpulsation ventricular assist system, per day

🚗 0.00 ⚕ 0.00 **FUD** YYY [S] 🖃

EXCLUDES Device evaluation (0462T)
Insertion/replacement system or component (0451T-0454T)
Relocation of pocket (0459T)
Removal system or component (0455T-0458T)
Repositioning device (0460T-0461T)

## 0464T

*0464T* Resequenced code. See code following 0333T.

## 0465T-0469T

EXCLUDES Replacement/revision cranial nerve neurostimulator electrode array (64569)

● **0465T** Suprachoroidal injection of a pharmacologic agent (does not include supply of medication)

🚗 0.00 ⚕ 0.00 **FUD** YYY [T] [G2] 🖃

EXCLUDES Intravitreal implantation or injection (67025-67028)

● + **0466T** Insertion of chest wall respiratory sensor electrode or electrode array, including connection to pulse generator (List separately in addition to code for primary procedure)

EXCLUDES Revision/removal chest wall respiratory sensor electrode or array (0467T-0468T)

Code first (64568)

🚗 0.00 ⚕ 0.00 **FUD** YYY [N] [N1] 🖃

AMA: 2017,Jan,8; 2016,Nov,6

● **0467T** Revision or replacement of chest wall respiratory sensor electrode or electrode array, including connection to existing pulse generator

EXCLUDES Insertion/removal chest wall respiratory sensor electrode or array (0466T, 0468T)
Replacement/revision cranial nerve neurostimulator electrode array (64569)

🚗 0.00 ⚕ 0.00 **FUD** YYY [Q2] [N1] 🖃

AMA: 2017,Jan,8; 2016,Nov,6

● **0468T** Removal of chest wall respiratory sensor electrode or electrode array

EXCLUDES Insertion/removal chest wall respiratory sensor electrode or array (0466T-0467T)
Removal cranial neurostimulator electrode array (64570)

🚗 0.00 ⚕ 0.00 **FUD** YYY [Q2] [N1] 🖃

AMA: 2017,Jan,8; 2016,Nov,6

● **0469T** Retinal polarization scan, ocular screening with on-site automated results, bilateral

🚗 0.00 ⚕ 0.00 **FUD** XXX [E] 🖃

INCLUDES Ophthalmic medical services (92002-92014)
EXCLUDES Ocular screening (99174, [99177])

## 0470T-0471T

EXCLUDES Optical coherence tomography of coronary vessel or graft (92978-92979)
Reflectance confocal microscopy (RCM) for cellular and subcellular skin imaging (96931-96936)

● **0470T** Optical coherence tomography (OCT) for microstructural and morphological imaging of skin, image acquisition, interpretation, and report; first lesion

🚗 0.00 ⚕ 0.00 **FUD** XXX [M] 🖃

● + **0471T** each additional lesion (List separately in addition to code for primary procedure)

🚗 0.00 ⚕ 0.00 **FUD** XXX [N] 🖃

Code first (0470T)

## 0472T-0474T

● **0472T** Device evaluation, interrogation, and initial programming of intraocular retinal electrode array (eg, retinal prosthesis), in person, with iterative adjustment of the implantable device to test functionality, select optimal permanent programmed values with analysis, including visual training, with review and report by a qualified health care professional

🚗 0.00 ⚕ 0.00 **FUD** XXX [Q1] 🖃

● **0473T** Device evaluation and interrogation of intraocular retinal electrode array (eg, retinal prosthesis), in person, including reprogramming and visual training, when performed, with review and report by a qualified health care professional

🚗 0.00 ⚕ 0.00 **FUD** XXX [Q1]

INCLUDES Reprogramming of device (0473T)
EXCLUDES Placement of intra-ocular retinal electrode display (0100T)

● **0474T** Insertion of anterior segment aqueous drainage device, with creation of intraocular reservoir, internal approach, into the supraciliary space

🚗 0.00 ⚕ 0.00 **FUD** XXX [J] [J8] 🖃

## 0475T-0478T

● **0475T** Recording of fetal magnetic cardiac signal using at least 3 channels; patient recording and storage, data scanning with signal extraction, technical analysis and result, as well as supervision, review, and interpretation of report by a physician or other qualified health care professional

🚗 0.00 ⚕ 0.00 **FUD** XXX [M] 🖃

● **0476T** patient recording, data scanning, with raw electronic signal transfer of data and storage

🚗 0.00 ⚕ 0.00 **FUD** XXX [Q1] 🖃

● **0477T** signal extraction, technical analysis, and result

🚗 0.00 ⚕ 0.00 **FUD** XXX [Q1]

● **0478T** review, interpretation, report by physician or other qualified health care professional

🚗 0.00 ⚕ 0.00 **FUD** XXX [M]

## 0479T-0480T

EXCLUDES Ablative laser treatment for additional square cm for open wound (0492T)
Cicatricial lesion excision
Use of code more than one time per day

● **0479T** Fractional ablative laser fenestration of burn and traumatic scars for functional improvement; first 100 cm2 or part thereof, or 1% of body surface area of infants and children

● + **0480T** each additional 100 cm2, or each additional 1% of body surface area of infants and children, or part thereof (List separately in addition to code for primary procedure)

🚗 0.00 ⚕ 0.00 **FUD** 000

Code first (0479T)

## 0481T-0482T

● **0481T** Injection(s), autologous white blood cell concentrate (autologous protein solution), any site, including image guidance, harvesting and preparation, when performed

EXCLUDES Autologous WBC injection (0481T)
Blood collection (36415, 36592)
Bone marrow procedures (38220-38222, 38230)
Imaging guidance (76942, 77002, 77012, 77021)
Injection of platelet rich plasma (0232T)
Injections to tendon, ligament, or fascia (20550-20551)
Joint aspiration or injection (20600-20611)
Other tissue grafts (20926)
Pooling of platelets (86965)

---

● **+ 0482T** Absolute quantitation of myocardial blood flow, positron emission tomography (PET), rest and stress (List separately in addition to code for primary procedure)

  🔧 0.00  ✂ 0.00  **FUD** 000

  *EXCLUDES* *Metabolic evaluation of heart (78459)*
  *PET perfusion study of heart (78491-78492)*
  Code first (78491-78492)

## 0483T-0484T

  *INCLUDES* Access and closure
  Angiography
  Balloon valvuloplasty
  Contrast injections
  Fluoroscopy
  Radiological supervision and interpretation
  Valve deployment and repositioning
  Ventriculography

  *EXCLUDES* *Diagnostic heart catheterization (93451-93453, 93456-93461, 93530-93533)*
  Code also cardiopulmonary bypass when provided (33367-33369)
  Code also diagnostic cardiac catheterization procedures if there is no previous study available and append modifier 59
   The condition of the patient has changed
   The previous study is inadequate

● **0483T** Transcatheter mitral valve implantation/replacement (TMVI) with prosthetic valve; percutaneous approach, including transseptal puncture, when performed

● **0484T** transthoracic exposure (eg, thoracotomy, transapical)

## 0485T-0486T

● **0485T** Optical coherence tomography (OCT) of middle ear, with interpretation and report; unilateral

● **0486T** bilateral

## 0487T-0488T

● **0487T** Biomechanical mapping, transvaginal, with report

  *0488T* Resequenced code. See code following 0403T.

## 0489T-0490T

  *EXCLUDES* *Joint injection/aspiration (20600, 20604)*
  *Liposuction procedures (15876-15879)*
  *Tissue grafts (20926)*

● **0489T** Autologous adipose-derived regenerative cell therapy for scleroderma in the hands; adipose tissue harvesting, isolation and preparation of harvested cells including incubation with cell dissociation enzymes, removal of non-viable cells and debris, determination of concentration and dilution of regenerative cells

● **0490T** multiple injections in one or both hands

  *EXCLUDES* *Single injections*

## 0491T-0493T

● **0491T** Ablative laser treatment, non-contact, full field and fractional ablation, open wound, per day, total treatment surface area; first 20 sq cm or less

● **+ 0492T** each additional 20 sq cm, or part thereof (List separately in addition to code for primary procedure)

  🔧 0.00  ✂ 0.00  **FUD** 000

  *EXCLUDES* *Laser fenestration for scars (0479T-0480T)*
  Code first (0491T)

● **0493T** Near-infrared spectroscopy studies of lower extremity wounds (eg, for oxyhemoglobin measurement)

## 0494T-0496T

● **0494T** Surgical preparation and cannulation of marginal (extended) cadaver donor lung(s) to ex vivo organ perfusion system, including decannulation, separation from the perfusion system, and cold preservation of the allograft prior to implantation, when performed

● **0495T** Initiation and monitoring marginal (extended) cadaver donor lung(s) organ perfusion system by physician or qualified health care professional, including physiological and laboratory assessment (eg, pulmonary artery flow, pulmonary artery pressure, left atrial pressure, pulmonary vascular resistance, mean/peak and plateau airway pressure, dynamic compliance and perfusate gas analysis), including bronchoscopy and X ray when performed; first two hours in sterile field

● **+ 0496T** each additional hour (List separately in addition to code for primary procedure)

  🔧 0.00  ✂ 0.00  **FUD** 000

  Code first (0495T)

## 0497T-0498T

  *EXCLUDES* *ECG event monitoring (93268, 93271-93272)*
  *ECG rhythm strips (93040-93042)*
  *External ECG monitoring for more than 48 hours and less than 21 days (0295T-0298T)*
  *Remote telemetry (93228-93229)*

● **0497T** External patient-activated, physician- or other qualified health care professional-prescribed, electrocardiographic rhythm derived event recorder without 24 hour attended monitoring; in-office connection

● **0498T** review and interpretation by a physician or other qualified health care professional per 30 days with at least one patient-generated triggered event

## 0499T-0500T

● **0499T** Cystourethroscopy, with mechanical dilation and urethral therapeutic drug delivery for urethral stricture or stenosis, including fluoroscopy, when performed

  *EXCLUDES* *Cystourethroscopy for stricture (52281, 52283)*

● **0500T** Infectious agent detection by nucleic acid (DNA or RNA), human papillomavirus (HPV) for five or more separately reported high-risk HPV types (eg, 16, 18, 31, 33, 35, 39, 45, 51, 52, 56, 58, 59, 68) (ie, genotyping)

  *EXCLUDES* *Less than five high-risk HPV types ([87624, 87625])*

## 0501T-0504T

  *EXCLUDES* *Use of code more than one time for each CT angiogram*

● **0501T** Noninvasive estimated coronary fractional flow reserve (FFR) derived from coronary computed tomography angiography data using computation fluid dynamics physiologic simulation software analysis of functional data to assess the severity of coronary artery disease; data preparation and transmission, analysis of fluid dynamics and simulated maximal coronary hyperemia, generation of estimated FFR model, with anatomical data review in comparison with estimated FFR model to reconcile discordant data, interpretation and report

  *INCLUDES* All components of complete test (0501T-0504T)

● **0502T** data preparation and transmission

● **0503T** analysis of fluid dynamics and simulated maximal coronary hyperemia, and generation of estimated FFR model

● **0504T** anatomical data review in comparison with estimated FFR model to reconcile discordant data, interpretation and report

---

26/TC PC/TC Only  A2-Z3 ASC Payment  50 Bilateral  ♂ Male Only  ♀ Female Only  🔧 Facility RVU  ✂ Non-Facility RVU  ▭ CCI
FUD Follow-up Days  CMS: IOM (Pub 100)  A-Y OPPSI  80/80 Surg Assist Allowed / w/Doc  📟 Lab Crosswalk  📟 Radiology Crosswalk  ✖ CLIA

556  CPT © 2017 American Medical Association. All Rights Reserved.  © 2017 Optum360, LLC

# Appendix A — Modifiers

## CPT Modifiers

A modifier is a two-position alpha or numeric code appended to a CPT® code to clarify the services being billed. Modifiers provide a means by which a service can be altered without changing the procedure code. They add more information, such as the anatomical site, to the code. In addition, they help to eliminate the appearance of duplicate billing and unbundling. Modifiers are used to increase accuracy in reimbursement, coding consistency, editing, and to capture payment data.

**22**  **Increased Procedural Services:** When the work required to provide a service is substantially greater than typically required, it may be identified by adding modifier 22 to the usual procedure code. Documentation must support the substantial additional work and the reason for the additional work (ie, increased intensity, time, technical difficulty of procedure, severity of patient's condition, physical and mental effort required).
**Note:** This modifier should not be appended to an E/M service.

**23**  **Unusual Anesthesia:** Occasionally, a procedure, which usually requires either no anesthesia or local anesthesia, because of unusual circumstances must be done under general anesthesia. This circumstance may be reported by adding modifier 23 to the procedure code of the basic service.

**24**  **Unrelated Evaluation and Management Service by the Same Physician or Other Qualified Health Care Professional During a Postoperative Period:** The physician or other qualified health care professional may need to indicate that an evaluation and management service was performed during a postoperative period for a reason(s) unrelated to the original procedure. This circumstance may be reported by adding modifier 24 to the appropriate level of E/M service.

**25**  **Significant, Separately Identifiable Evaluation and Management Service by the Same Physician or Other Qualified Health Care Professional on the Same Day of the Procedure or Other Service:** It may be necessary to indicate that on the day a procedure or service identified by a CPT code was performed, the patient's condition required a significant, separately identifiable E/M service above and beyond the other service provided or beyond the usual preoperative and postoperative care associated with the procedure that was performed. A significant, separately identifiable E/M service is defined or substantiated by documentation that satisfies the relevant criteria for the respective E/M service to be reported (see Evaluation and Management Services Guidelines for instructions on determining level of E/M service). The E/M service may be prompted by the symptom or condition for which the procedure and/or service was provided. As such, different diagnoses are not required for reporting of the E/M services on the same date. This circumstance may be reported by adding modifier 25 to the appropriate level of E/M service.
**Note:** This modifier is not used to report an E/M service that resulted in a decision to perform surgery. See modifier 57. For significant, separately identifiable non-E/M services, see modifier 59.

**26**  **Professional Component:** Certain procedures are a combination of a physician or other qualified health care professional component and a technical component. When the physician or other qualified health care professional component is reported separately, the service may be identified by adding modifier 26 to the usual procedure number.

**32**  **Mandated Services:** Services related to mandated consultation and/or related services (eg, third-party payer, governmental, legislative or regulatory requirement) may be identified by adding modifier 32 to the basic procedure.

**33**  **Preventive Services:** When the primary purpose of the service is the delivery of an evidence-based service in accordance with a U.S. Preventive Services Task Force A or B rating in effect and other preventive services identified in preventive services mandates (legislative or regulatory), the service may be identified by adding 33 to the procedure. For separately reported services specifically identified as preventive, the modifier should not be used.

**47**  **Anesthesia by Surgeon:** Regional or general anesthesia provided by the surgeon may be reported by adding modifier 47 to the basic service. (This does not include local anesthesia.)
**Note:** Modifier 47 would not be used as a modifier for the anesthesia procedures 00100-01999.

**50**  **Bilateral Procedure:** Unless otherwise identified in the listings, bilateral procedures that are performed at the same session should be identified by adding modifier 50 to the appropriate 5-digit code.

**51**  **Multiple Procedures:** When multiple procedures, other than E/M services, Physical Medicine and Rehabilitation services or provision of supplies (e.g., vaccines), are performed at the same session by the same individual, the primary procedure or service may be reported as listed. The additional procedure(s) or service(s) may be identified by appending modifier 51 to the additional procedure or service code(s).
**Note:** This modifier should not be appended to designated "add-on" codes.

**52**  **Reduced Services:** Under certain circumstances a service or procedure is partially reduced or eliminated at the discretion of the physician or other qualified health care professional. Under these circumstances the service provided can be identified by its usual procedure number and the addition of modifier 52, signifying that the service is reduced. This provides a means of reporting reduced services without disturbing the identification of the basic service.
**Note:** For hospital outpatient reporting of a previously scheduled procedure/service that is partially reduced or cancelled as a result of extenuating circumstances or those that threaten the well-being of the patient prior to or after administration of anesthesia, see modifiers 73 and 74 (see modifiers approved for ASC hospital outpatient use).

**53**  **Discontinued Procedure:** Under certain circumstances, the physician or other qualified health care professional may elect to terminate a surgical or diagnostic procedure. Due to extenuating circumstances or those that threaten the well being of the patient, it may be necessary to indicate that a surgical or diagnostic procedure was started but discontinued. This circumstance may be reported by adding modifier 53 to the code reported by the physician for the discontinued procedure.
**Note:** This modifier is not used to report the elective cancellation of a procedure prior to the patient's anesthesia induction and/or surgical preparation in the operating suite. For outpatient hospital/ambulatory surgery center (ASC) reporting of a previously scheduled procedure/service that is partially reduced or cancelled as a result of extenuating circumstances or those that threaten the well being of the patient prior to or after administration of anesthesia, see modifiers 73 and 74 (see modifiers approved for ASC hospital outpatient use).

**54**  **Surgical Care Only:** When 1 physician or other qualified health care professional performs a surgical procedure and another provides preoperative and/or postoperative management, surgical services may be identified by adding modifier 54 to the usual procedure number.

**55**  **Postoperative Management Only:** When 1 physician or other qualified health care professional performed the postoperative management and another performed the surgical procedure, the postoperative component may be identified by adding modifier 55 to the usual procedure number.

**56**  **Preoperative Management Only:** When 1 physician or other qualified health care professional performed the preoperative care and evaluation and another performed the surgical procedure, the preoperative component may be identified by adding modifier 56 to the usual procedure number.

**57**  **Decision for Surgery:** An evaluation and management service that resulted in the initial decision to perform the surgery may be identified by adding modifier 57 to the appropriate level of E/M service.

**58** **Staged or Related Procedure or Service by the Same Physician or Other Qualified Health Care Professional During the Postoperative Period:** It may be necessary to indicate that the performance of a procedure or service during the postoperative period was (a) planned or anticipated (staged); (b) more extensive than the original procedure; or (c) for therapy following a surgical procedure. This circumstance may be reported by adding modifier 58 to the staged or related procedure. **Note:** For treatment of a problem that requires a return to the operating or procedure room (eg, unanticipated clinical condition), see modifier 78.

**59** **Distinct Procedural Service:** Under certain circumstances, it may be necessary to indicate that a procedure or service was distinct or independent from other non-E/M services performed on the same day. Modifier 59 is used to identify procedures/services, other than E/M services, that are not normally reported together but are appropriate under the circumstances. Documentation must support a different session, different procedure or surgery, different site or organ system, separate incision/excision, separate lesion, or separate injury (or area of injury in extensive injuries) not ordinarily encountered or performed on the same day by the same individual. However, when another already established modifier is appropriate it should be used rather than modifier 59. Only if no more descriptive modifier is available and the use of modifier 59 best explains the circumstances, should modifier 59 be used. **Note:** Modifier 59 should not be appended to an E/M service. To report a separate and distinct E/M service with a non-E/M service performed on the same date, see modifier 25. See also "Level II (HCPCS/National) Modifiers."

**62** **Two Surgeons:** When 2 surgeons work together as primary surgeons performing distinct part(s) of a procedure, each surgeon should report his/her distinct operative work by adding modifier 62 to the procedure code and any associated add-on code(s) for that procedure as long as both surgeons continue to work together as primary surgeons. Each surgeon should report the cosurgery once using the same procedure code. If additional procedure(s) (including add-on procedure[s]) are performed during the same surgical session, separate code(s) may also be reported with modifier 62 added. **Note:** If a cosurgeon acts as an assistant in the performance of additional procedure(s), other than those reported with the modifier 62, during the same surgical session, those services may be reported using separate procedure code(s) with modifier 80 or modifier 82 added, as appropriate.

**63** **Procedure Performed on Infants less than 4 kg:** Procedures performed on neonates and infants up to a present body weight of 4 kg may involve significantly increased complexity and physician or other qualified health care professional work commonly associated with these patients. This circumstance may be reported by adding modifier 63 to the procedure number. **Note:** Unless otherwise designated, this modifier may only be appended to procedures/services listed in the 20005-69990 code series. Modifier 63 should not be appended to any CPT codes listed in the Evaluation and Management Services, Anesthesia, Radiology, Pathology/Laboratory, or Medicine sections.

**66** **Surgical Team:** Under some circumstances, highly complex procedures (requiring the concomitant services of several physicians or other qualified health care professionals, often of different specialties, plus other highly skilled, specially trained personnel, various types of complex equipment) are carried out under the "surgical team" concept. Such circumstances may be identified by each participating individual with the addition of modifier 66 to the basic procedure number used for reporting services.

**76** **Repeat Procedure or Service by Same Physician or Other Qualified Health Care Professional:** It may be necessary to indicate that a procedure or service was repeated by the same physician or other qualified health care professional subsequent to the original procedure or service. This circumstance may be reported by adding modifier 76 to the repeated procedure or service. **Note:** This modifier should not be appended to an E/M service.

**77** **Repeat Procedure by Another Physician or Other Qualified Health Care Professional:** It may be necessary to indicate that a basic procedure or service was repeated by another physician or other qualified health care professional subsequent to the original procedure or service. This circumstance may be reported by adding modifier 77 to the repeated procedure or service. **Note:** This modifier should not be appended to an E/M service.

**78** **Unplanned Return to the Operating/Procedure Room by the Same Physician or Other Qualified Health Care Professional Following Initial Procedure for a Related Procedure During the Postoperative Period:** It may be necessary to indicate that another procedure was performed during the postoperative period of the initial procedure (unplanned procedure following initial procedure). When this procedure is related to the first, and requires the use of an operating/procedure room, it may be reported by adding modifier 78 to the related procedure. (For repeat procedures, see modifier 76.)

**79** **Unrelated Procedure or Service by the Same Physician or Other Qualified Health Care Professional During the Postoperative Period:** The individual may need to indicate that the performance of a procedure or service during the postoperative period was unrelated to the original procedure. This circumstance may be reported by using modifier 79. (For repeat procedures on the same day, see modifier 76.)

**80** **Assistant Surgeon:** Surgical assistant services may be identified by adding modifier 80 to the usual procedure number(s).

**81** **Minimum Assistant Surgeon:** Minimum surgical assistant services are identified by adding modifier 81 to the usual procedure number.

**82** **Assistant Surgeon (when qualified resident surgeon not available):** The unavailability of a qualified resident surgeon is a prerequisite for use of modifier 82 appended to the usual procedure code number(s).

**90** **Reference (Outside) Laboratory:** When laboratory procedures are performed by a party other than the treating or reporting physician or other qualified health care professional, the procedure may be identified by adding modifier 90 to the usual procedure number.

**91** **Repeat Clinical Diagnostic Laboratory Test:** In the course of treatment of the patient, it may be necessary to repeat the same laboratory test on the same day to obtain subsequent (multiple) test results. Under these circumstances, the laboratory test performed can be identified by its usual procedure number and the addition of modifier 91. **Note:** This modifier may not be used when tests are rerun to confirm initial results; due to testing problems with specimens or equipment; or for any other reason when a normal, one-time, reportable result is all that is required. This modifier may not be used when another code(s) describes a series of test results (eg, glucose tolerance tests, evocative/suppression testing). This modifier may only be used for a laboratory test(s) performed more than once on the same day on the same patient.

**92** **Alternative Laboratory Platform Testing:** When laboratory testing is being performed using a kit or transportable instrument that wholly or in part consists of a single use, disposable analytical chamber, the service may be identified by adding modifier 92 to the usual laboratory procedure code (HIV testing 86701-86703, and 87389). The test does not require permanent dedicated space, hence by its design may be hand carried or transported to the vicinity of the patient for immediate testing at that site, although location of the testing is not in itself determinative of the use of this modifier.

CPT © 2017 American Medical Association. All Rights Reserved.

© 2017 Optum360, LLC

Appendix A — Modifiers

**95 Synchronous Telemedicine Service Rendered Via a Real-Time Interactive Audio and Video Telecommunications System:** Synchronous telemedicine service is defined as a **real-time** interaction between a physician or other qualified health care professional and a patient who is located at a distant site from the physician or other qualified health care professional. The totality of the communication of information exchanged between the physician or other qualified health care professional and patient during the course of the synchronous telemedicine service must be of an amount and nature that would be sufficient to meet the key components and/or requirements of the same service when rendered via a face-to-face interaction. Modifier 95 may only be appended to the services listed in Appendix F. Appendix F is the list of CPT codes for services that are typically performed face-to-face, but may be rendered via real-time (synchronous) interactive audio and video telecommunications system.

**96 Habilitative Services:** When a service or procedure that may be either habilitative or rehabilitative in nature is provided for habilitative purposes, the physician or other qualified health care professional may add modifier 96 to the service or procedure code to indicate that the service or procedure provided was a habilitative service. Habilitative services help an individual learn skills and functioning for daily living that the individual has not yet developed, and then keep and/or improve those learned skills. Habilitative services also help an individual keep, learn, or improve skills and functioning for daily living.

**97 Rehabilitative Services:** When a service or procedure that may be either habilitative or rehabilitative in nature is provided for rehabilitative purposes, the physician or other qualified health care professional may add modifier 97 to the service or procedure code to indicate that the service or procedure provided was a rehabilitative service. Rehabilitative services help an individual keep, get back, or improve skills and functioning for daily living that have been lost or impaired because the individual was sick, hurt, or disabled.

**99 Multiple Modifiers:** Under certain circumstances 2 or more modifiers may be necessary to completely delineate a service. In such situations, modifier 99 should be added to the basic procedure and other applicable modifiers may be listed as part of the description of the service.

## Anesthesia Physical Status Modifiers

All anesthesia services are reported by use of the five-digit anesthesia procedure code with the appropriate physical status modifier appended.

Under certain circumstances, when other modifier(s) are appropriate, they should be reported in addition to the physical status modifier.

**P1** A normal healthy patient

**P2** A patient with mild systemic disease

**P3** A patient with severe systemic disease

**P4** A patient with severe systemic disease that is a constant threat to life

**P5** A moribund patient who is not expected to survive without the operation

**P6** A declared brain-dead patient whose organs are being removed for donor purposes

## Modifiers Approved for Ambulatory Surgery Center (ASC) Hospital Outpatient Use

### CPT Level I Modifiers

**25 Significant, Separately Identifiable Evaluation and Management Service by the Same Physician or Other Qualified Health Care Professional on the Same Day of the Procedure or Other Service:** It may be necessary to indicate that on the day a procedure or service identified by a CPT code was performed, the patient's condition required a significant, separately identifiable E/M service above and beyond the other service provided or beyond the usual preoperative and

postoperative care associated with the procedure that was performed. A significant, separately identifiable E/M service is defined or substantiated by documentation that satisfies the relevant criteria for the respective E/M service to be reported (see Evaluation and Management Services Guidelines for instructions on determining level of E/M service). The E/M service may be prompted by the symptom or condition for which the procedure and/or service was provided. As such, different diagnoses are not required for reporting of the E/M services on the same date. This circumstance may be reported by adding modifier 25 to the appropriate level of E/M service.
**Note:** This modifier is not used to report an E/M service that resulted in a decision to perform surgery. See modifier 57. For significant, separately identifiable non-E/M services, see modifier 59.

**27 Multiple Outpatient Hospital E/M Encounters on the Same Date:** For hospital outpatient reporting purposes, utilization of hospital resources related to separate and distinct E/M encounters performed in multiple outpatient hospital settings on the same date may be reported by adding modifier 27 to each appropriate level outpatient and/or emergency department E/M code(s). This modifier provides a means of reporting circumstances involving evaluation and management services provided by a physician(s) in more than one (multiple) outpatient hospital setting(s) (eg, hospital emergency department, clinic).
**Note:** This modifier is not to be used for physician reporting of multiple E/M services performed by the same physician on the same date. For physician reporting of all outpatient evaluation and management services provided by the same physician on the same date and performed in multiple outpatient settings (eg, hospital emergency department, clinic), see Evaluation and Management, Emergency Department, or Preventive Medicine Services codes.

**50 Bilateral Procedure:** Unless otherwise identified in the listings, bilateral procedures that are performed at the same session should be identified by adding modifier 50 to the appropriate 5-digit code.

**52 Reduced Services:** Under certain circumstances a service or procedure is partially reduced or eliminated at the discretion of the physician or other qualified health care professional. Under these circumstances the service provided can be identified by its usual procedure number and the addition of modifier 52, signifying that the service is reduced. This provides a means of reporting reduced services without disturbing the identification of the basic service.
**Note:** For hospital outpatient reporting of a previously scheduled procedure/service that is partially reduced or cancelled as a result of extenuating circumstances or those that threaten the well-being of the patient prior to or after administration of anesthesia, see modifiers 73 and 74 (see modifiers approved for ASC hospital outpatient use).

**58 Staged or Related Procedure or Service by the Same Physician or Other Qualified Health Care Professional During the Postoperative Period:** It may be necessary to indicate that the performance of a procedure or service during the postoperative period was (a) planned or anticipated (staged); (b) more extensive than the original procedure; or (c) for therapy following a surgical procedure. This circumstance may be reported by adding modifier 58 to the staged or related procedure.
**Note:** For treatment of a problem that requires a return to the operating or procedure room (eg, unanticipated clinical condition), see modifier 78.

**59 Distinct Procedural Service:** Under certain circumstances, it may be necessary to indicate that a procedure or service was distinct or independent from other non-E/M services performed on the same day. Modifier 59 is used to identify procedures/services, other than E/M services, that are not normally reported together but are appropriate under the circumstances. Documentation must support a different session, different procedure or surgery, different site or organ system, separate incision/excision, separate lesion, or separate injury (or area of injury in extensive injuries) not ordinarily encountered or performed on the same day by the same individual. However, when another already established modifier is appropriate it should be used rather than modifier 59. Only if no more descriptive modifier is available and the use of modifier 59 best explains the circumstances, should modifier 59 be used.
**Note:** Modifier 59 should not be appended to an E/M service. To report a separate and distinct E/M service with a non-E/M service

performed on the same date, see modifier 25. See also "Level II (HCPCS/National) Modifiers."

**73  Discontinued Out-Patient Hospital/Ambulatory Surgery Center (ASC) Procedure Prior to the Administration of Anesthesia:** Due to extenuating circumstances or those that threaten the well being of the patient, the physician may cancel a surgical or diagnostic procedure subsequent to the patient's surgical preparation (including sedation when provided, and being taken to the room where the procedure is to be performed), but prior to the administration of anesthesia (local, regional block(s), or general). Under these circumstances, the intended service that is prepared for but cancelled can be reported by its usual procedure number and the addition of modifier 73.
**Note:** The elective cancellation of a service prior to the administration of anesthesia and/or surgical preparation of the patient should not be reported. For physician reporting of a discontinued procedure, see modifier 53.

**74  Discontinued Out-Patient Hospital/Ambulatory Surgery Center (ASC) Procedure After Administration of Anesthesia:** Due to extenuating circumstances or those that threaten the well being of the patient, the physician may terminate a surgical or diagnostic procedure after the administration of anesthesia (local, regional block(s), general) or after the procedure was started (incision made, intubation started, scope inserted, etc.). Under these circumstances, the procedure started but terminated can be reported by its usual procedure number and the addition of modifier 74.
**Note:** The elective cancellation of a service prior to the administration of anesthesia and/or surgical preparation of the patient should not be reported. For physician reporting of a discontinued procedure, see modifier 53.

**76  Repeat Procedure or Service by Same Physician or Other Qualified Health Care Professional:** It may be necessary to indicate that a procedure or service was repeated by the same physician or other qualified health care professional subsequent to the original procedure or service. This circumstance may be reported by adding modifier 76 to the repeated procedure or service.
**Note:** This modifier should not be appended to an E/M service.

**77  Repeat Procedure by Another Physician or Other Qualified Health Care Professional:** It may be necessary to indicate that a basic procedure or service was repeated by another physician or other qualified health care professional subsequent to the original procedure or service. This circumstance may be reported by adding modifier 77 to the repeated procedure or service.
**Note:** This modifier should not be appended to an E/M service.

**78  Unplanned Return to the Operating/Procedure Room by the Same Physician or Other Qualified Health Care Professional Following Initial Procedure for a Related Procedure During the Postoperative Period:** It may be necessary to indicate that another procedure was performed during the postoperative period of the initial procedure (unplanned procedure following initial procedure). When this procedure is related to the first, and requires the use of an operating/procedure room, it may be reported by adding modifier 78 to the related procedure. (For repeat procedures, see modifier 76.)

**79  Unrelated Procedure or Service by the Same Physician During the Postoperative Period:** The individual may need to indicate that the performance of a procedure or service during the postoperative period was unrelated to the original procedure. This circumstance may be reported by using modifier 79. (For repeat procedures on the same day, see modifier 76.)

**91  Repeat Clinical Diagnostic Laboratory Test:** In the course of treatment of the patient, it may be necessary to repeat the same laboratory test on the same day to obtain subsequent (multiple) test results. Under these circumstances, the laboratory test performed can be identified by its usual procedure number and the addition of modifier 91.
**Note:** This modifier may not be used when tests are rerun to confirm initial results; due to testing problems with specimens or equipment; or for any other reason when a normal, one-time, reportable result is all that is required. This modifier may not be used when another code(s) describe a series of test results (eg, glucose tolerance tests, evocative/suppression testing). This modifier may only be used for a laboratory test(s) performed more than once on the same day on the same patient.

## Level II (HCPCS/National) Modifiers
The HCPCS Level II modifiers included here are those most commonly used when coding procedures. See your 2018 HCPCS Level II book for a complete listing

### Anatomical Modifiers
| | |
|---|---|
| **E1** | Upper left, eyelid |
| **E2** | Lower left, eyelid |
| **E3** | Upper right, eyelid |
| **E4** | Lower right, eyelid |
| **F1** | Left hand, second digit |
| **F2** | Left hand, third digit |
| **F3** | Left hand, fourth digit |
| **F4** | Left hand, fifth digit |
| **F5** | Right hand, thumb |
| **F6** | Right hand, second digit |
| **F7** | Right hand, third digit |
| **F8** | Right hand, fourth digit |
| **F9** | Right hand, fifth digit |
| **FA** | Left hand, thumb |
| **LT** | Left side (used to identify procedures performed on the left side of the body) |
| **RT** | Right side (used to identify procedures performed on the right side of the body) |
| **T1** | Left foot, second digit |
| **T2** | Left foot, third digit |
| **T3** | Left foot, fourth digit |
| **T4** | Left foot, fifth digit |
| **T5** | Right foot, great toe |
| **T6** | Right foot, second digit |
| **T7** | Right foot, third digit |
| **T8** | Right foot, fourth digit |
| **T9** | Right foot, fifth digit |
| **TA** | Left foot, great toe |

## Anesthesia Modifiers
| | |
|---|---|
| **AA** | Anesthesia services performed personally by anesthesiologist |
| **AD** | Medical supervision by a physician: more than four concurrent anesthesia procedures |
| **G8** | Monitored anesthesia care (MAC) for deep complex, complicated, or markedly invasive surgical procedure |
| **G9** | Monitored anesthesia care for patient who has history of severe cardiopulmonary condition |
| **QK** | Medical direction of two, three, or four concurrent anesthesia procedures involving qualified individuals |
| **QS** | Monitored anesthesia care service |
| **QX** | CRNA service: with medical direction by a physician |
| **QY** | Medical direction of one certified registered nurse anesthetist (CRNA) by an anesthesiologist |
| **QZ** | CRNA service: without medical direction by a physician |

## Coronary Artery Modifiers
| | |
|---|---|
| **LC** | Left circumflex coronary artery |
| **LD** | Left anterior descending coronary artery |
| **LM** | Left main coronary artery |
| **RC** | Right coronary artery |
| **RI** | Ramus intermedius coronary artery |

CPT © 2017 American Medical Association. All Rights Reserved.

© 2017 Optum360, LLC

## Other Modifiers

**CT** Computed tomography services furnished using equipment that does not meet each of the attributes of the national electrical manufacturers association (NEMA) xr-29-2013 standard

**EA** Erythropoetic stimulating agent (ESA) administered to treat anemia due to anticancer chemotherapy

**EB** Erythropoetic stimulating agent (ESA) administered to treat anemia due to anticancer radiotherapy

**EC** Erythropoetic stimulating agent (ESA) administered to treat anemia not due to anticancer radiotherapy or anticancer chemotherapy

**FP** Service provided as part of family planning program

**FX** X-ray taken using film

**G7** Pregnancy resulted from rape or incest or pregnancy certified by physician as life threatening

**GA** Waiver of liability statement issued as required by payer policy, individual case

**GQ** Via asynchronous telecommunications system

**GT** Via interactive audio and video telecommunication systems

**GU** Waiver of liability statement issued as required by payer policy, routine notice

**GX** Notice of liability issued, voluntary under payer policy

**GY** Item or service statutorily excluded, does not meet the definition of any Medicare benefit or for non-Medicare insurers, is not a contract benefit

**GZ** Item or service expected to be denied as not reasonable and necessary

**PI** Positron emission tomography (PET) or PET/computed tomography (CT) to inform the initial treatment strategy of tumors that are biopsy proven or strongly suspected of being cancerous based on other diagnostic testing

**PS** Positron emission tomography (PET) or PET/computed tomography (CT) to inform the subsequent treatment strategy of cancerous tumor when the beneficiary's treating physician determines that the PET study is needed to inform subsequent anti-tumor strategy

**PT** Colorectal cancer screening test; converted to diagnostic test or other procedure

**Q7** One Class A finding

**Q8** Two Class B findings

**Q9** One Class B and 2 Class C findings

**QC** Single channel monitoring

**QW** CLIA waived test

**TC** Technical component. Under certain circumstances, a charge may be made for the technical component alone. Under those circumstances the technical component charge is identified by adding modifier 'TC' to the usual procedure number. Technical component charges are institutional charges and not billed separately by physicians. However, portable x-ray suppliers only bill for technical component and should utilize modifier TC. The charge data from portable x-ray suppliers will then be used to build customary and prevailing profiles.

**\* XE** Separate encounter, a service that Is distinct because it occurred during a separate encounter

**\* XP** Separate practitioner, a service that is distinct because it was performed by a different practitioner

**\* XS** Separate structure, a service that is distinct because it was performed on a separate organ/structure

**\* XU** Unusual non-overlapping service, the use of a service that is distinct because it does not overlap usual components of the main service

\* CMS instituted additional HCPCS modifiers to define explicit subsets of modifier 59 Distinct Procedural Service.

## Category II Modifiers

**1P** Performance measure exclusion modifier due to medical reasons
Includes:
- Not indicated (absence of organ/limb, already received/performed, other)
- Contraindicated (patient allergic history, potential adverse drug interaction, other)
- Other medical reasons

**2P** Performance measure exclusion modifier due to patient reasons
Includes:
- Patient declined
- Economic, social, or religious reasons
- Other patient reasons

**3P** Performance measure exclusion modifier due to system reasons
Includes:
- Resources to perform the services not available (eg, equipment, supplies)
- Insurance coverage or payer-related limitations
- Other reasons attributable to health care delivery system

**8P** Performance measure reporting modifier - action not performed, reason not otherwise specified

# Appendix B — New, Changed and Deleted Codes

## New Codes

**00731** Anesthesia for upper gastrointestinal endoscopic procedures, endoscope introduced proximal to duodenum; not otherwise specified

**00732**      endoscopic retrograde cholangiopancreatography (ERCP)

**00811** Anesthesia for lower intestinal endoscopic procedures, endoscope introduced distal to duodenum; not otherwise specified

**00812**      screening colonoscopy

**00813** Anesthesia for combined upper and lower gastrointestinal endoscopic procedures, endoscope introduced both proximal to and distal to the duodenum

**15730** Midface flap (ie, zygomaticofacial flap) with preservation of vascular pedicle(s)

**15733** Muscle, myocutaneous, or fasciocutaneous flap; head and neck with named vascular pedicle (ie, buccinators, genioglossus, temporalis, masseter, sternocleidomastoid, levator scapulae)

**19294** Preparation of tumor cavity, with placement of a radiation therapy applicator for intraoperative radiation therapy (IORT) concurrent with partial mastectomy (List separately in addition to code for primary procedure)

**20939** Bone marrow aspiration for bone grafting, spine surgery only, through separate skin or fascial incision (List separately in addition to code for primary procedure)

**31241** Nasal/sinus endoscopy, surgical; with ligation of sphenopalatine artery

**31253** Nasal/sinus endoscopy, surgical with ethmoidectomy; total (anterior and posterior), including frontal sinus exploration, with removal of tissue from frontal sinus, when performed

**31257** Nasal/sinus endoscopy, surgical with ethmoidectomy; total (anterior and posterior), including sphenoidotomy

**31259** Nasal/sinus endoscopy, surgical with ethmoidectomy; total (anterior and posterior), including sphenoidotomy, with removal of tissue from the sphenoid sinus

**31298** Nasal/sinus endoscopy, surgical; with dilation of frontal and sphenoid sinus ostia (eg, balloon dilation)

**32994** Ablation therapy for reduction or eradication of 1 or more pulmonary tumor(s) including pleura or chest wall when involved by tumor extension, percutaneous, including imaging guidance when performed, unilateral; cryoablation

**33927** Implantation of a total replacement heart system (artificial heart) with recipient cardiectomy

**33928** Removal and replacement of total replacement heart system (artificial heart)

**33929** Removal of a total replacement heart system (artificial heart) for heart transplantation (List separately in addition to code for primary procedure)

**34701** Endovascular repair of infrarenal aorta by deployment of an aorto-aortic tube endograft including pre-procedure sizing and device selection, all nonselective catheterization(s), all associated radiological supervision and interpretation, all endograft extension(s) placed in the aorta from the level of the renal arteries to the aortic bifurcation, and all angioplasty/stenting performed from the level of the renal arteries to the aortic bifurcation; for other than rupture (eg, for aneurysm, pseudoaneurysm, dissection, penetrating ulcer)

**34702**      for rupture including temporary aortic and/or iliac balloon occlusion, when performed (eg, for aneurysm, pseudoaneurysm, dissection, penetrating ulcer, traumatic disruption)

**34703** Endovascular repair of infrarenal aorta and/or iliac artery(ies) by deployment of an aorto-uni-iliac endograft including pre-procedure sizing and device selection, all nonselective catheterization(s), all associated radiological supervision and interpretation, all endograft extension(s) placed in the aorta from the level of the renal arteries to the iliac bifurcation, and all angioplasty/stenting performed from the level of the renal arteries to the iliac bifurcation; for other than rupture (eg, for aneurysm, pseudoaneurysm, dissection, penetrating ulcer)

**34704**      for rupture including temporary aortic and/or iliac balloon occlusion, when performed (eg, for aneurysm, pseudoaneurysm, dissection, penetrating ulcer, traumatic disruption)

**34705** Endovascular repair of infrarenal aorta and/or iliac artery(ies) by deployment of an aorto-bi-iliac endograft including pre-procedure sizing and device selection, all nonselective catheterization(s), all associated radiological supervision and interpretation, all endograft extension(s) placed in the aorta from the level of the renal arteries to the iliac bifurcation, and all angioplasty/stenting performed from the level of the renal arteries to the iliac bifurcation; for other than rupture (eg, for aneurysm, pseudoaneurysm, dissection, penetrating ulcer)

**34706**      for rupture including temporary aortic and/or iliac balloon occlusion, when performed (eg, for aneurysm, pseudoaneurysm, dissection, penetrating ulcer, traumatic disruption)

**34707** Endovascular repair of iliac artery by deployment of an ilio-iliac tube endograft including pre-procedure sizing and device selection, all nonselective catheterization(s), all associated radiological supervision and interpretation, and all endograft extension(s) proximally to the aortic bifurcation and distally to the iliac bifurcation, and treatment zone angioplasty/stenting, when performed, unilateral; for other than rupture (eg, for aneurysm, pseudoaneurysm, dissection, arteriovenous malformation)

**34708**      for rupture including temporary aortic and/or iliac balloon occlusion, when performed (eg, for aneurysm, pseudoaneurysm, dissection, arteriovenous malformation, traumatic disruption)

**34709** Placement of extension prosthesis(es) distal to the common iliac artery(ies) or proximal to the renal artery(ies) for endovascular repair of infrarenal abdominal aortic or iliac aneurysm, false aneurysm, dissection, penetrating ulcer, including pre-procedure sizing and device selection, all nonselective catheterization(s), all associated radiological supervision and interpretation, and treatment zone angioplasty/stenting, when performed, per vessel treated (List separately in addition to code for primary procedure)

**34710** Delayed placement of distal or proximal extension prosthesis for endovascular repair of infrarenal abdominal aortic or iliac aneurysm, false aneurysm, dissection, endoleak, or endograft migration, including pre-procedure sizing and device selection, all nonselective catheterization(s), all associated radiological supervision and interpretation, and treatment zone angioplasty/stenting, when performed; initial vessel treated

**34711**      each additional vessel treated (List separately in addition to code for primary procedure)

**34712** Transcatheter delivery of enhanced fixation device(s) to the endograft (eg, anchor, screw, tack) and all associated radiological supervision and interpretation

**34713** Percutaneous access and closure of femoral artery for delivery of endograft through a large sheath (12 French or larger), including ultrasound guidance, when performed, unilateral (List separately in addition to code for primary procedure)

| | |
|---|---|
| 34714 | Open femoral artery exposure with creation of conduit for delivery of endovascular prosthesis or for establishment of cardiopulmonary bypass, by groin incision, unilateral (List separately in addition to code for primary procedure) |
| 34715 | Open axillary/subclavian artery exposure for delivery of endovascular prosthesis by infraclavicular or supraclavicular incision, unilateral (List separately in addition to code for primary procedure) |
| 34716 | Open axillary/subclavian artery exposure with creation of conduit for delivery of endovascular prosthesis or for establishment of cardiopulmonary bypass, by infraclavicular or supraclavicular incision, unilateral (List separately in addition to code for primary procedure) |
| 36465 | Injection of non-compounded foam sclerosant with ultrasound compression maneuvers to guide dispersion of the injectate, inclusive of all imaging guidance and monitoring; single incompetent extremity truncal vein (eg, great saphenous vein, accessory saphenous vein) |
| 36466 | multiple incompetent truncal veins (eg, great saphenous vein, accessory saphenous vein), same leg |
| 36482 | Endovenous ablation therapy of incompetent vein, extremity, by transcatheter delivery of a chemical adhesive (eg, cyanoacrylate) remote from the access site, inclusive of all imaging guidance and monitoring, percutaneous; first vein treated |
| 36483 | subsequent vein(s) treated in a single extremity, each through separate access sites (List separately in addition to code for primary procedure) |
| 38222 | Diagnostic bone marrow; biopsy(ies) and aspiration(s) |
| 38573 | Laparoscopy, surgical with bilateral total pelvic lymphadenectomy and peri-aortic lymph node sampling, peritoneal washings, peritoneal biopsy(ies), omentectomy, and diaphragmatic washings, including diaphragmatic and other serosal biopsy(ies), when performed |
| 43286 | Esophagectomy, total or near total, with laparoscopic mobilization of the abdominal and mediastinal esophagus and proximal gastrectomy, with laparoscopic pyloric drainage procedure if performed, with open cervical pharyngogastrostomy or esophagogastrostomy (ie, laparoscopic transhiatal esophagectomy) |
| 43287 | Esophagectomy, distal two-thirds, with laparoscopic mobilization of the abdominal and lower mediastinal esophagus and proximal gastrectomy, with laparoscopic pyloric drainage procedure if performed, with separate thoracoscopic mobilization of the middle and upper mediastinal esophagus and thoracic esophagogastrostomy (ie, laparoscopic thoracoscopic esophagectomy, Ivor Lewis esophagectomy) |
| 43288 | Esophagectomy, total or near total, with thoracoscopic mobilization of the upper, middle, and lower mediastinal esophagus, with separate laparoscopic proximal gastrectomy, with laparoscopic pyloric drainage procedure if performed, with open cervical pharyngogastrostomy or esophagogastrostomy (ie, thoracoscopic, laparoscopic and cervical incision esophagectomy, McKeown esophagectomy, tri-incisional esophagectomy) |
| 55874 | Transperineal placement of biodegradable material, peri-prostatic, single or multiple injection(s), including image guidance, when performed |
| 58575 | Laparoscopy, surgical, total hysterectomy for resection of malignancy (tumor debulking), with omentectomy including salpingo-oophorectomy, unilateral or bilateral, when performed |
| 64912 | Nerve repair; with nerve allograft, each nerve, first strand (cable) |
| 64913 | Nerve repair; with nerve allograft, each additional strand (List separately in addition to code for primary procedure) |
| 71045 | Radiologic examination, chest; single view |
| 71046 | 2 views |
| 71047 | 3 views |
| 71048 | 4 or more views |
| 74018 | Radiologic examination, abdomen; 1 view |
| 74019 | 2 views |
| 74021 | 3 or more views |

| | |
|---|---|
| 81175 | ASXL1 (additional sex combs like 1, transcriptional regulator) (eg, myelodysplastic syndrome, myeloproliferative neoplasms, chronic myelomonocytic leukemia), gene analysis; full gene sequence |
| 81176 | targeted sequence analysis (eg, exon 12) |
| 81230 | CYP3A4 (cytochrome P450 family 3 subfamily A member 4) (eg, drug metabolism), gene analysis, common variant(s) (eg, *2, *22) |
| 81231 | CYP3A5 (cytochrome P450 family 3 subfamily A member 5) (eg, drug metabolism), gene analysis, common variants (eg, *2, *3, *4, *5, *6, *7) |
| 81232 | DPYD (dihydropyrimidine dehydrogenase) (eg, 5-fluorouracil/5-FU and capecitabine drug metabolism), gene analysis, common variant(s) (eg, *2A, *4, *5, *6) |
| 81238 | F9 (coagulation factor IX) (eg, hemophilia B), full gene sequence |
| 81247 | G6PD (glucose-6-phosphate dehydrogenase) (eg, hemolytic anemia, jaundice), gene analysis; common variant(s) (eg, A, A-) |
| 81248 | known familial variant(s) |
| 81249 | full gene sequence |
| 81258 | HBA1/HBA2 (alpha globin 1 and alpha globin 2) (eg, alpha thalassemia, Hb Bart hydrops fetalis syndrome, HbH disease), gene analysis; known familial variant |
| 81259 | full gene sequence |
| 81269 | duplication/deletion variants |
| 81105 | Human Platelet Antigen 1 genotyping (HPA-1), ITGB3 (integrin, beta 3 [platelet glycoprotein IIIa], antigen CD61 [GPIIIa]) (eg, neonatal alloimmune thrombocytopenia [NAIT], post-transfusion purpura), gene analysis, common variant, HPA-1a/b (L33P) |
| 81106 | Human Platelet Antigen 2 genotyping (HPA-2), GP1BA (glycoprotein Ib [platelet], alpha polypeptide [GPIba]) (eg, neonatal alloimmune thrombocytopenia [NAIT], post-transfusion purpura), gene analysis, common variant, HPA-2a/b (T145M) |
| 81107 | Human Platelet Antigen 3 genotyping (HPA-3), ITGA2B (integrin, alpha 2b [platelet glycoprotein IIb of IIb/IIIa complex], antigen CD41 [GPIIb]) (eg, neonatal alloimmune thrombocytopenia [NAIT], post-transfusion purpura), gene analysis, common variant, HPA-3a/b (I843S) |
| 81108 | Human Platelet Antigen 4 genotyping (HPA-4), ITGB3 (integrin, beta 3 [platelet glycoprotein IIIa], antigen CD61 [GPIIIa]) (eg, neonatal alloimmune thrombocytopenia [NAIT], post-transfusion purpura), gene analysis, common variant, HPA-4a/b (R143Q) |
| 81109 | Human Platelet Antigen 5 genotyping (HPA-5), ITGA2 (integrin, alpha 2 [CD49B, alpha 2 subunit of VLA-2 receptor] [GPIa]) (eg, neonatal alloimmune thrombocytopenia [NAIT], post-transfusion purpura), gene analysis, common variant (eg, HPA-5a/b (K505E)) |
| 81110 | Human Platelet Antigen 6 genotyping (HPA-6w), ITGB3 (integrin, beta 3 [platelet glycoprotein IIIa, antigen CD61] [GPIIIa]) (eg, neonatal alloimmune thrombocytopenia [NAIT], post-transfusion purpura), gene analysis, common variant, HPA-6a/b (R489Q) |
| 81111 | Human Platelet Antigen 9 genotyping (HPA-9w), ITGA2B (integrin, alpha 2b [platelet glycoprotein IIb of IIb/IIIa complex, antigen CD41] [GPIIb]) (eg, neonatal alloimmune thrombocytopenia [NAIT], post-transfusion purpura), gene analysis, common variant, HPA-9a/b (V837M) |
| 81112 | Human Platelet Antigen 15 genotyping (HPA-15), CD109 (CD109 molecule) (eg, neonatal alloimmune thrombocytopenia [NAIT], post-transfusion purpura), gene analysis, common variant, HPA-15a/b (S682Y) |
| 81120 | IDH1 (isocitrate dehydrogenase 1 [NADP+], soluble) (eg, glioma), common variants (eg, R132H, R132C) |
| 81121 | IDH2 (isocitrate dehydrogenase 2 [NADP+], mitochondrial) (eg, glioma), common variants (eg, R140W, R172M) |
| 81283 | IFNL3 (interferon, lambda 3) (eg, drug response), gene analysis, rs12979860 variant |
| 81334 | RUNX1 (runt related transcription factor 1) (eg, acute myeloid leukemia, familial platelet disorder with associated myeloid malignancy), gene analysis, targeted sequence analysis (eg, exons 3-8) |
| 81328 | SLCO1B1 (solute carrier organic anion transporter family, member 1B1) (eg, adverse drug reaction), gene analysis, common variant(s) (eg, *5) |

CPT © 2017 American Medical Association. All Rights Reserved.

© 2017 Optum360, LLC

81335 TPMT (thiopurine S-methyltransferase) (eg, drug metabolism), gene analysis, common variants (eg, *2, *3)

81346 TYMS (thymidylate synthetase) (eg, 5-fluorouracil/5-FU drug metabolism), gene analysis, common variant(s) (eg, tandem repeat variant)

81361 HBB (hemoglobin, subunit beta) (eg, sickle cell anemia, beta thalassemia, hemoglobinopathy); common variant(s) (eg, HbS, HbC, HbE)

81362     known familial variant(s)

81363     duplication/deletion variant(s)

81364     full gene sequence

81448 Hereditary peripheral neuropathies (eg, Charcot-Marie-Tooth, spastic paraplegia), genomic sequence analysis panel, must include sequencing of at least 5 peripheral neuropathy-related genes (eg, BSCL2, GJB1, MFN2, MPZ, REEP1, SPAST, SPG11, SPTLC1)

81520 Oncology (breast), mRNA gene expression profiling by hybrid capture of 58 genes (50 content and 8 housekeeping), utilizing formalin-fixed paraffin-embedded tissue, algorithm reported as a recurrence risk score

81521 Oncology (breast), mRNA, microarray gene expression profiling of 70 content genes and 465 housekeeping genes, utilizing fresh frozen or formalin-fixed paraffin-embedded tissue, algorithm reported as index related to risk of distant metastasis

81541 Oncology (prostate), mRNA gene expression profiling by real-time RT-PCR of 46 genes (31 content and 15 housekeeping), utilizing formalin-fixed paraffin-embedded tissue, algorithm reported as a disease-specific mortality risk score

81551 Oncology (prostate), promoter methylation profiling by real-time PCR of 3 genes (GSTP1, APC, RASSF1), utilizing formalin-fixed paraffin-embedded tissue, algorithm reported as a likelihood of prostate cancer detection on repeat biopsy

86008 Allergen specific IgE; quantitative or semiquantitative, recombinant or purified component, each

86794 Antibody; Zika virus, IgM

87634 Infectious agent detection by nucleic acid (DNA or RNA); respiratory syncytial virus, amplified probe technique

87662 Infectious agent detection by nucleic acid (DNA or RNA); Zika virus, amplified probe technique

0001U Red blood cell antigen typing, DNA, human erythrocyte antigen gene analysis of 35 antigens from 11 blood groups, utilizing whole blood, common RBC alleles reported

0002U Oncology (colorectal), quantitative assessment of three urine metabolites (ascorbic acid, succinic acid and carnitine) by liquid chromatography with tandem mass spectrometry (LC-MS/MS) using multiple reaction monitoring acquisition, algorithm reported as likelihood of adenomatous polyps

0003U Oncology (ovarian) biochemical assays of five proteins (apolipoprotein A-1, CA 125 II, follicle stimulating hormone, human epididymis protein 4, transferrin), utilizing serum, algorithm reported as a likelihood score

0004U Infectious disease (bacterial), DNA, 27 resistance genes, PCR amplification and probe hybridization in microarray format (molecular detection and identification of AmpC, carbapenemase and ESBL coding genes), bacterial culture colonies, report of genes detected or not detected, per isolate

0005U Oncology (prostate) gene expression profile by real-time RT-PCR of 3 genes (ERG, PCA3, and SPDEF), urine, algorithm reported as risk score

0006U Prescription drug monitoring, 120 or more drugs and substances, definitive tandem mass spectrometry with chromatography, urine, qualitative report of presence (including quantitative levels, when detected) or absence of each drug or substance with description and severity of potential interactions, with identified substances, per date of service

0007U Drug test(s), presumptive, with definitive confirmation of positive results, any number of drug classes, urine, includes specimen verification including DNA authentication in comparison to buccal DNA, per date of service

0008U Helicobacter pylori detection and antibiotic resistance, DNA, 16S and 23S rRNA, gyrA, pbp1, rdxA and rpoB, next generation sequencing, formalin-fixed paraffin-embedded or fresh tissue, predictive, reported as positive or negative for resistance to clarithromycin, fluoroquinolones, metronidazole, amoxicillin, tetracycline and rifabutin

0009U Oncology (breast cancer), ERBB2 (HER2) copy number by FISH, tumor cells from formalin-fixed paraffin-embedded tissue isolated using image-based dielectrophoresis (DEP) sorting, reported as ERBB2 gene amplified or non-amplified

0010U Infectious disease (bacterial), strain typing by whole genome sequencing, phylogenetic-based report of strain relatedness, per submitted isolate

0011U Prescription drug monitoring, evaluation of drugs present by LC-MS/MS, using oral fluid, reported as a comparison to an estimated steady-state range, per date of service including all drug compounds and metabolites

0012U Germline disorders, gene rearrangement detection by whole genome next-generation sequencing, DNA, whole blood, report of specific gene rearrangement(s)

0013U Oncology (solid organ neoplasia), gene rearrangement detection by whole genome next-generation sequencing, DNA, fresh or frozen tissue or cells, report of specific gene rearrangement(s)

0014U Hematology (hematolymphoid neoplasia), gene rearrangement detection by whole genome next-generation sequencing, DNA, whole blood or bone marrow, report of specific gene rearrangement(s)

0015U Drug metabolism (adverse drug reactions), DNA, 22 drug metabolism and transporter genes, real-time PCR, blood or buccal swab, genotype and metabolizer status for therapeutic decision support

0016U Oncology (hematolymphoid neoplasia), RNA, BCR/ABL1 major and minor breakpoint fusion transcripts, quantitative PCR amplification, blood or bone marrow, report of fusion not detected or detected with quantitation

0017U Oncology (hematolymphoid neoplasia), JAK2 mutation, DNA, PCR amplification of exons 12-14 and sequence analysis, blood or bone marrow, report of JAK2 mutation not detected or detected

90587 Dengue vaccine, quadrivalent, live, 3 dose schedule, for subcutaneous use

90756 Influenza virus vaccine, quadrivalent (ccIIV4), derived from cell cultures, subunit, antibiotic free, 0.5 mL dosage, for intramuscular use

93792 Patient/caregiver training for initiation of home international normalized ratio (INR) monitoring under the direction of a physician or other qualified health care professional, face-to-face, including use and care of the INR monitor, obtaining blood sample, instructions for reporting home INR test results, and documentation of patient's/caregiver's ability to perform testing and report results

93793 Anticoagulant management for a patient taking warfarin, must include review and interpretation of a new home, office, or lab international normalized ratio (INR) test result, patient instructions, dosage adjustment (as needed), and scheduling of additional test(s), when performed

94617 Exercise test for bronchospasm, including pre- and post-spirometry, electrocardiographic recording(s), and pulse oximetry

94618 Pulmonary stress testing (eg, 6-minute walk test), including measurement of heart rate, oximetry, and oxygen titration, when performed

95249 Ambulatory continuous glucose monitoring of interstitial tissue fluid via a subcutaneous sensor for a minimum of 72 hours; patient-provided equipment, sensor placement, hook-up, calibration of monitor, patient training, and printout of recording

96573 Photodynamic therapy by external application of light to destroy premalignant lesions of the skin and adjacent mucosa with application and illumination/activation of photosensitizing drug(s) provided by a physician or other qualified health care professional, per day

96574 Debridement of premalignant hyperkeratotic lesion(s) (ie, targeted curettage, abrasion) followed with photodynamic therapy by external application of light to destroy premalignant lesions of the skin and adjacent mucosa with application and illumination/activation of photosensitizing drug(s) provided by a physician or other qualified health care professional, per day

97127 Therapeutic interventions that focus on cognitive function (eg, attention, memory, reasoning, executive function, problem solving, and/or pragmatic functioning) and compensatory strategies to manage the performance of an activity (eg, managing time or schedules, initiating, organizing and sequencing tasks), direct (one-on-one) patient contact

97763 Orthotic(s)/prosthetic(s) management and/or training, upper extremity(ies), lower extremity(ies), and/or trunk, subsequent orthotic(s)/prosthetic(s) encounter, each 15 minutes

99483 Assessment of and care planning for a patient with cognitive impairment, requiring an independent historian, in the office or other outpatient, home or domiciliary or rest home, with all of the following required elements:

- Cognition-focused evaluation including a pertinent history and examination;
- Medical decision making of moderate or high complexity;
- Functional assessment (eg, basic and instrumental activities of daily living), including decision-making capacity;
- Use of standardized instruments for staging of dementia (eg, functional assessment staging test [FAST], clinical dementia rating [CDR]);
- Medication reconciliation and review for high-risk medications;
- Evaluation for neuropsychiatric and behavioral symptoms, including depression, including use of standardized screening instrument(s);
- Evaluation of safety (eg, home), including motor vehicle operation;
- Identification of caregiver(s), caregiver knowledge, caregiver needs, social supports, and the willingness of caregiver to take on caregiving tasks;
- Development, updating or revision, or review of an Advance Care Plan;
- Creation of a written care plan, including initial plans to address any neuropsychiatric symptoms, neuro-cognitive symptoms, functional limitations, and referral to community resources as needed (eg, rehabilitation services, adult day programs, support groups) shared with the patient and/or caregiver with initial education and support.
- Typically, 50 minutes are spent face-to-face with the patient and/or family or caregiver.

99484 Care management services for behavioral health conditions, at least 20 minutes of clinical staff time, directed by a physician or other qualified health care professional, per calendar month, with the following required elements:

- initial assessment or follow-up monitoring, including the use of applicable validated rating scales;
- behavioral health care planning in relation to behavioral/psychiatric health problems, including revision for patients who are not progressing or whose status changes;
- facilitating and coordinating treatment such as psychotherapy, pharmacotherapy, counseling and/or psychiatric consultation; and
- continuity of care with a designated member of the care team.

98492 Initial psychiatric collaborative care management, first 70 minutes in the first calendar month of behavioral health care manager activities, in consultation with a psychiatric consultant, and directed by the treating physician or other qualified health care professional, with the following required elements:

- outreach to and engagement in treatment of a patient directed by the treating physician or other qualified health care professional;
- initial assessment of the patient, including administration of validated rating scales, with the development of an individualized treatment plan;
- review by the psychiatric consultant with modifications of the plan if recommended;
- entering patient in a registry and tracking patient follow-up and progress using the registry, with appropriate documentation, and participation in weekly caseload consultation with the psychiatric consultant; and

- provision of brief interventions using evidence-based techniques such as behavioral activation, motivational interviewing, and other focused treatment strategies.

99493 Subsequent psychiatric collaborative care management, first 60 minutes in a subsequent month of behavioral health care manager activities, in consultation with a psychiatric consultant, and directed by the treating physician or other qualified health care professional, with the following required elements:

- tracking patient follow-up and progress using the registry, with appropriate documentation;
- participation in weekly caseload consultation with the psychiatric consultant;
- ongoing collaboration with and coordination of the patient's mental health care with the treating physician or other qualified health care professional and any other treating mental health providers;
- additional review of progress and recommendations for changes in treatment, as indicated, including medications, based on recommendations provided by the psychiatric consultant;
- provision of brief interventions using evidence-based techniques such as behavioral activation, motivational interviewing, and other focused treatment strategies;
- monitoring of patient outcomes using validated rating scales; and
- relapse prevention planning with patients as they achieve remission of symptoms and/or other treatment goals and are prepared for discharge from active treatment.

99494 Initial or subsequent psychiatric collaborative care management, each additional 30 minutes in a calendar month of behavioral health care manager activities, in consultation with a psychiatric consultant, and directed by the treating physician or other qualified health care professional (List separately in addition to code for primary procedure)

0488T Preventive behavior change, online/electronic structured intensive program for prevention of diabetes using a standardized diabetes prevention program curriculum, provided to an individual, per 30 days

0468T Removal of chest wall respiratory sensor electrode or electrode array

0469T Retinal polarization scan, ocular screening with on-site automated results, bilateral

0470T Optical coherence tomography (OCT) for microstructural and morphological imaging of skin, image acquisition, interpretation, and report; first lesion

0471T each additional lesion (List separately in addition to code for primary procedure)

0472T Device evaluation, interrogation, and initial programming of intraocular retinal electrode array (eg, retinal prosthesis), in person, with iterative adjustment of the implantable device to test functionality, select optimal permanent programmed values with analysis, including visual training, with review and report by a qualified health care professional

0473T Device evaluation and interrogation of intraocular retinal electrode array (eg, retinal prosthesis), in person, including reprogramming and visual training, when performed, with review and report by a qualified health care professional

0474T Insertion of anterior segment aqueous drainage device, with creation of intraocular reservoir, internal approach, into the supraciliary space

0475T Recording of fetal magnetic cardiac signal using at least 3 channels; patient recording and storage, data scanning with signal extraction, technical analysis and result, as well as supervision, review, and interpretation of report by a physician or other qualified health care professional

0476T patient recording, data scanning, with raw electronic signal transfer of data and storage

0477T signal extraction, technical analysis, and result

0478T review, interpretation, report by physician or other qualified health care professional

0479T Fractional ablative laser fenestration of burn and traumatic scars for functional improvement; first 100 cm2 or part thereof, or 1% of body surface area of infants and children

CPT © 2017 American Medical Association. All Rights Reserved.

© 2017 Optum360, LLC

**0480T** each additional 100 cm2, or each additional 1% of body surface area of infants and children, or part thereof (List separately in addition to code for primary procedure)

**0481T** Injection(s), autologous white blood cell concentrate (autologous protein solution), any site, including image guidance, harvesting and preparation, when performed

**0482T** Absolute quantitation of myocardial blood flow, positron emission tomography (PET), rest and stress (List separately in addition to code for primary procedure)

**0483T** Transcatheter mitral valve implantation/replacement (TMVI) with prosthetic valve; percutaneous approach, including transseptal puncture, when performed

**0484T** transthoracic exposure (eg, thoracotomy, transapical)

**0485T** Optical coherence tomography (OCT) of middle ear, with interpretation and report; unilateral

**0486T** bilateral

**0487T** Biomechanical mapping, transvaginal, with report

**0489T** Autologous adipose-derived regenerative cell therapy for scleroderma in the hands; adipose tissue harvesting, isolation and preparation of harvested cells including incubation with cell dissociation enzymes, removal of non-viable cells and debris, determination of concentration and dilution of regenerative cells

**0490T** multiple injections in one or both hands

**0491T** Ablative laser treatment, non-contact, full field and fractional ablation, open wound, per day, total treatment surface area; first 20 sq cm or less

**0492T** each additional 20 sq cm, or part thereof (List separately in addition to code for primary procedure)

**0493T** Near-infrared spectroscopy studies of lower extremity wounds (eg, for oxyhemoglobin measurement)

**0494T** Surgical preparation and cannulation of marginal (extended) cadaver donor lung(s) to ex vivo organ perfusion system, including decannulation, separation from the perfusion system, and cold preservation of the allograft prior to implantation, when performed

**0495T** Initiation and monitoring marginal (extended) cadaver donor lung(s) organ perfusion system by physician or qualified health care professional, including physiological and laboratory assessment (eg, pulmonary artery flow, pulmonary artery pressure, left atrial pressure, pulmonary vascular resistance, mean/peak and plateau airway pressure, dynamic compliance and perfusate gas analysis), including bronchoscopy and X ray when performed; first two hours in sterile field

**0496T** each additional hour (List separately in addition to code for primary procedure)

**0497T** External patient-activated, physician- or other qualified health care professional-prescribed, electrocardiographic rhythm derived event recorder without 24 hour attended monitoring; in-office connection

**0498T** review and interpretation by a physician or other qualified health care professional per 30 days with at least one patient-generated triggered event

**0499T** Cystourethroscopy, with mechanical dilation and urethral therapeutic drug delivery for urethral stricture or stenosis, including fluoroscopy, when performed

**0500T** Infectious agent detection by nucleic acid (DNA or RNA), Human Papillomavirus (HPV) for five or more separately reported high-risk HPV types (eg, 16, 18, 31, 33, 35, 39, 45, 51, 52, 56, 58, 59, 68) (ie, genotyping)

**0501T** Noninvasive estimated coronary fractional flow reserve (FFR) derived from coronary computed tomography angiography data using computation fluid dynamics physiologic simulation software analysis of functional data to assess the severity of coronary artery disease; data preparation and transmission, analysis of fluid dynamics and simulated maximal coronary hyperemia, generation of estimated FFR model, with anatomical data review in comparison with estimated FFR model to reconcile discordant data, interpretation and report

**0502T** data preparation and transmission

**0503T** analysis of fluid dynamics and simulated maximal coronary hyperemia, and generation of estimated FFR model

**0504T** anatomical data review in comparison with estimated FFR model to reconcile discordant data, interpretation and report

# Changed Codes

**17250** Chemical cauterization of granulation tissue (ie, proud flesh, sinus or fistula)

**31254** Nasal/sinus endoscopy, surgical with ethmoidectomy; with ethmoidectomy, partial (anterior)

**31255** with ethmoidectomy, total (anterior and posterior)

**31276** Nasal/sinus endoscopy, surgical, with frontal sinus exploration, with or without including removal of tissue from frontal sinus, when performed

**31645** Bronchoscopy, rigid or flexible, including fluoroscopic guidance, when performed; with therapeutic aspiration of tracheobronchial tree, initial (eg, drainage of lung abscess)

**31646** Bronchoscopy, rigid or flexible, including fluoroscopic guidance, when performed; with therapeutic aspiration of tracheobronchial tree, subsequent, same hospital stay

**32998** Ablation therapy for reduction or eradication of 1 or more pulmonary tumor(s) including pleura or chest wall when involved by tumor extension, percutaneous, radiofrequency including imaging guidance when performed, unilateral, radiofrequency

**34812** Open femoral artery exposure for delivery of endovascular prosthesis, by groin incision, unilateral (List separately in addition to code for primary procedure)

**34820** Open iliac artery exposure for delivery of endovascular prosthesis or iliac occlusion during endovascular therapy, by abdominal or retroperitoneal incision, unilateral (List separately in addition to code for primary procedure)

**34833** Open iliac artery exposure with creation of conduit for delivery of aortic or iliac endovascular prosthesis or for establishment of cardiopulmonary bypass, by abdominal or retroperitoneal incision, unilateral (List separately in addition to code for primary procedure)

**34834** Open brachial artery exposure to assist in the deployment of aortic or iliac endovascular prosthesis by arm incision, unilateral for delivery of endovascular prosthesis, unilateral (List separately in addition to code for primary procedure)

**36140** Introduction of needle or intracatheter, upper or lower extremity artery extremity artery

**36468** Single or multiple injections Injection(s) of sclerosing solutions, sclerosant for spider veins (telangiectasia), limb or trunk

**36470** Injection of sclerosing solution sclerosant; single incompetent vein (other than telangiectasia)

**36471** multiple incompetent veins (other than telangiectasia), same leg

**36516** Therapeutic apheresis; with extracorporeal immunoadsorption, selective adsorption or selective filtration and plasma reinfusion

**36908** Transcatheter placement of intravascular stent(s), central dialysis segment, performed through dialysis circuit, including all imaging and radiological supervision and interpretation required to perform the stenting, and all angioplasty in the central dialysis segment (List separately in addition to code for primary procedure)

**38220** Bone Diagnostic bone marrow; aspiration only(s)

**38221** biopsy, needle or trocar(ies)

**43112** Total or near total esophagectomy, with thoracotomy; with pharyngogastrostomy or cervical esophagogastrostomy, with or without pyloroplasty (ie, McKeown esophagectomy or tri-incisional esophagectomy)

**57240** Anterior colporrhaphy, repair of cystocele with or without repair of urethrocele, including cystourethroscopy, when performed

**57260** Combined anteroposterior colporrhaphy, including cystourethroscopy, when performed;

**57265** with enterocele repair

64550   Application of surface (transcutaneous) neurostimulator (eg, TENS unit)

76000   Fluoroscopy (separate procedure), up to 1 hour physician or other qualified health care professional time, ~~other than 71023 or 71034 (eg, cardiac fluoroscopy)~~

76881   Ultrasound, ~~extremity, nonvascular, complete~~ joint (ie, joint space and peri-articular soft tissue structures) real-time with image documentation~~; complete~~

76882   Ultrasound, limited, ~~anatomic specific~~ joint or other nonvascular extremity structure(s) (eg, joint space, peri-articular tendon[s], muscle[s], nerve[s], other soft tissue structure[s], or soft tissue mass[es]), real-time with image documentation

80305   Drug test(s), presumptive, any number of drug classes, any number of devices or procedures (eg, immunoassay); capable of being read by direct optical observation only (eg, dipsticks utilizing immunoassay [eg, dipsticks, cups, cards, or cartridges]), includes sample validation when performed, per date of service

80306         read by instrument assisted direct optical observation (eg, ~~dipsticks~~ utilizing immunoassay [eg, dipsticks, cups, cards, or cartridges]), includes sample validation when performed, per date of service

80307         by instrument chemistry analyzers (eg, utilizing immunoassay [eg, EIA, ELISA, EMIT, FPIA, IA, KIMS, RIA]), chromatography (eg, GC, HPLC), and mass spectrometry either with or without chromatography, (eg, DART, DESI, GC-MS, GC-MS/MS, LC-MS, LC-MS/MS, LDTD, MALDI, TOF) includes sample validation when performed, per date of service

81257   HBA1/HBA2 (alpha globin 1 and alpha globin 2) (eg, alpha thalassemia, Hb Bart hydrops fetalis syndrome, HbH disease), gene analysis;, ~~for~~ common deletions or variant (eg, Southeast Asian, Thai, Filipino, Mediterranean, alpha3.7, alpha4.2, alpha20.5, Constant Spring)

81400   Molecular pathology procedure, Level 1 (eg, identification of single germline variant [eg, SNP] by techniques such as restriction enzyme digestion or melt curve analysis)

~~DPYD (dihydropyrimidine dehydrogenase) (eg, 5-fluorouracil/5-FU and capecitabine drug metabolism), IVS14+1G>A variant~~

~~Human Platelet Antigen 1 genotyping (HPA-1), ITGB3 (integrin, beta 3 [platelet glycoprotein IIIa], antigen CD61 [GPIIIa]) (eg, neonatal alloimmune thrombocytopenia [NAIT], post-transfusion purpura), HPA-1a/b (L33P)~~

~~Human Platelet Antigen 2 genotyping (HPA-2), GP1BA (glycoprotein Ib [platelet], alpha polypeptide [GPIbα]) (eg, neonatal alloimmune thrombocytopenia [NAIT], post-transfusion purpura), HPA-2a/b (T145M)~~

~~Human Platelet Antigen 3 genotyping (HPA-3), ITGA2B (integrin, alpha 2b [platelet glycoprotein IIb of IIb/IIIa complex], antigen CD41 [GPIIb]) (eg, neonatal alloimmune thrombocytopenia [NAIT], post-transfusion purpura), HPA-3a/b (I843S)~~

~~Human Platelet Antigen 4 genotyping (HPA-4), ITGB3 (integrin, beta 3 [platelet glycoprotein IIIa], antigen CD61 [GPIIIa]) (eg, neonatal alloimmune thrombocytopenia [NAIT], post-transfusion purpura), HPA-4a/b (R143Q)~~

~~Human Platelet Antigen 5 genotyping (HPA-5), ITGA2 (integrin, alpha 2 [CD49B, alpha 2 subunit of VLA-2 receptor] [GPIa]) (eg, neonatal alloimmune thrombocytopenia [NAIT], post-transfusion purpura), HPA-5a/b (K505E)~~

~~Human Platelet Antigen 6 genotyping (HPA-6w), ITGB3 (integrin, beta 3 [platelet glycoprotein IIIa, antigen CD61] [GPIIIa]) (eg, neonatal alloimmune thrombocytopenia [NAIT], post-transfusion purpura), HPA-6a/b (R489Q)~~

~~Human Platelet Antigen 9 genotyping (HPA-9w), ITGA2B (integrin, alpha 2b [platelet glycoprotein IIb of IIb/IIIa complex, antigen CD41] [GPIIb]) (eg, neonatal alloimmune thrombocytopenia [NAIT], post-transfusion purpura), HPA-9a/b (V837M)~~

~~Human Platelet Antigen 15 genotyping (HPA-15), CD109 (CD109 molecule) (eg, neonatal alloimmune thrombocytopenia [NAIT], post-transfusion purpura), HPA-15a/b (S682Y)~~

~~IL28B (interleukin 28B [interferon, lambda 3]) (eg, drug response), rs12979860 variant~~

~~SLCO1B1 (solute carrier organic anion transporter family, member 1B1) (eg, adverse drug reaction), V174A variant~~

81401   Molecular pathology procedure, Level 2 (eg, 2-10 SNPs, 1 methylated variant, or 1 somatic variant [typically using nonsequencing target variant analysis], or detection of a dynamic mutation disorder/triplet repeat)

~~CYP3A4 (cytochrome P450, family 3, subfamily A, polypeptide 4) (eg, drug metabolism), common variants (eg, *2, *3, *4, *5, *6)~~

~~CYP3A5 (cytochrome P450, family 3, subfamily A, polypeptide 5) (eg, drug metabolism), common variants (eg, *2, *3, *4, *5, *6)~~

~~HBB (hemoglobin, beta) (eg, sickle cell anemia, hemoglobin C, hemoglobin E), common variants (eg, HbS, HbC, HbE)~~

LINC00518 (long intergenic non-protein coding RNA 518) (eg, melanoma), expression analysis

PRAME (preferentially expressed antigen in melanoma) (eg, melanoma), expression analysis

~~TPMT (thiopurine S-methyltransferase) (eg, drug metabolism), common variants (eg, *2, *3)~~

~~TYMS (thymidylate synthetase) (eg, 5-fluorouracil/5-FU drug metabolism), tandem repeat variant~~

81403   Molecular pathology procedure, Level 4 (eg, analysis of single exon by DNA sequence analysis, analysis of >10 amplicons using multiplex PCR in 2 or more independent reactions, mutation scanning or duplication/deletion variants of 2-5 exons)

~~HBB (hemoglobin, beta, beta-globin) (eg, beta thalassemia), duplication/deletion analysis~~

~~IDH1 (isocitrate dehydrogenase 1 [NADP], soluble) (eg, glioma), common exon 4 variants (eg, R132H, R132C)IDH2 (isocitrate dehydrogenase 2 [NADP], mitochondrial) (eg, glioma), common exon 4 variants (eg, R140W, R172M)~~

~~IDH2 (isocitrate dehydrogenase 2 [NADP], mitochondrial) (eg, glioma), common exon 4 variants (eg, R140W, R172M)~~

81404   Molecular pathology procedure, Level 5 (eg, analysis of 2-5 exons by DNA sequence analysis, mutation scanning or duplication/deletion variants of 6-10 exons, or characterization of a dynamic mutation disorder/triplet repeat by Southern blot analysis)

~~HBA1/HBA2 (alpha globin 1 and alpha globin 2) (eg, alpha thalassemia), duplication/deletion analysis~~

~~HBB (hemoglobin, beta, Beta-Globin) (eg, thalassemia), full gene sequence~~

81405   Molecular pathology procedure, Level 6 (eg, analysis of 6-10 exons by DNA sequence analysis, mutation scanning or duplication/deletion variants of 11-25 exons, regionally targeted cytogenomic array analysis)

CPOX (coproporphyrinogen oxidase) (eg, hereditary coproporphyria), full gene sequence

CTRC (chymotrypsin C) (eg, hereditary pancreatitis), full gene sequence

~~F9 (coagulation factor IX) (eg, hemophilia B), full gene sequence~~

~~HBA1/HBA2 (alpha globin 1 and alpha globin 2) (eg, thalassemia), full gene sequence~~

PKLR (pyruvate kinase, liver and RBC) (eg, pyruvate kinase deficiency), full gene sequence

81406   Molecular pathology procedure, Level 7 (eg, analysis of 11-25 exons by DNA sequence analysis, mutation scanning or duplication/deletion variants of 26-50 exons, cytogenomic array analysis for neoplasia)

ANOS1 (anosmin-1) (eg, Kallmann syndrome 1), full gene sequence

HMBS (hydroxymethylbilane synthase) (eg, acute intermittent porphyria), full gene sequence

~~KAL1 (Kallmann syndrome 1 sequence) (eg, Kallmann syndrome), full gene sequence~~

PPOX (protoporphyrinogen oxidase) (eg, variegate porphyria), full gene sequence

81432  Hereditary breast cancer-related disorders (eg, hereditary breast cancer, hereditary ovarian cancer, hereditary endometrial cancer); genomic sequence analysis panel, must include sequencing of at least ~~14~~10 genes, always including ~~ATM~~, BRCA1, BRCA2, ~~BRIP1~~, CDH1, MLH1, MSH2, MSH6, ~~NBN~~, PALB2, PTEN, ~~RAD51C~~, STK11, and TP53

81439  ~~Inherited~~ Hereditary cardiomyopathy (eg, hypertrophic cardiomyopathy, dilated cardiomyopathy, arrhythmogenic right ventricular cardiomyopathy), genomic sequence analysis panel, must include sequencing of at least 5 cardiomyopathy-related genes ~~including~~ (eg, DSG2, MYBPC3, MYH7, PKP2, TTN)

82042  Albumin; ~~urine or~~ other source, quantitative, each specimen

82043  Albumin; urine (eg, microalbumin), quantitative

82044  Albumin; urine (eg, microalbumin), semiquantitative (eg, reagent strip assay)

86003  Allergen specific IgE; quantitative or semiquantitative, ~~each~~ crude allergen extract, each

86005          qualitative, multiallergen screen (~~dipstick~~ eg, ~~paddle~~ disk, ~~or disk~~ sponge, card)

90651  Human Papillomavirus vaccine types 6, 11, 16, 18, 31, 33, 45, 52, 58, nonavalent (9vHPV), 2 or 3 dose schedule, for intramuscular use

90620  Meningococcal recombinant protein and outer membrane vesicle vaccine, serogroup B ~~(MenB)~~ (MenB-4C), 2 dose schedule, for intramuscular use

90621  Meningococcal recombinant lipoprotein vaccine, serogroup B ~~(MenB)~~ (MenB-FHbp), 2 or 3 dose schedule, for intramuscular use

94621  ~~Pulmonary stress~~Cardiopulmonary exercise testing~~;~~, including measurements of minute ventilation, CO2 production, O2 uptake, and electrocardiographic recordings ~~complex (including measurements of CO2 production, O2 uptake, and electrocardiographic recordings)~~

95250  Ambulatory continuous glucose monitoring of interstitial tissue fluid via a subcutaneous sensor for a minimum of 72 hours; physician or other qualified health care professional (office) provided equipment, sensor placement, hook-up, calibration of monitor, patient training, removal of sensor, and printout of recording

95251          analysis, interpretation and report

95930  Visual evoked potential (VEP) checkerboard or flash testing, central nervous system except glaucoma, ~~checkerboard or flash~~with interpretation and report

96567  Photodynamic therapy by external application of light to destroy premalignant ~~and/or malignant lesions~~ of the skin and adjacent mucosa with application and (~~eg, lip) by~~ illumination/activation of photosensitive drug(s), ~~each phototherapy exposure session~~ per day

97760  Orthotic(s) management and training (including assessment and fitting when not otherwise reported), upper extremity~~(s)~~(ies), lower extremity(s)(ies) and/or trunk, initial orthotic(s) encounter, each 15 minutes

97761  Prosthetic(s) training, upper and/or lower extremity(ies), initial prosthetic(s) encounter, each 15 minutes

99217  **Observation care discharge** day management (This code is to be utilized to report all services provided to a patient on discharge from outpatient hospital "observation status" if the discharge is on other than the initial date of "observation status." To report services to a patient designated as "observation status" or "inpatient status" and discharged on the same date, use the codes for Observation or Inpatient Care Services [including Admission and Discharge Services, 99234-99236 as appropriate.])

99218  **Initial observation care,** per day, for the evaluation and management of a patient which requires these 3 key components:
- **A detailed or comprehensive history;**
- **A detailed or comprehensive examination; and**
- **Medical decision making that is straightforward or of low complexity.**

Counseling and/or coordination of care with other physicians, other qualified health care professionals, or agencies are provided consistent with the nature of the problem(s) and the patient's and/or family's needs.

Usually, the problem(s) requiring admission to outpatient hospital "observation status" are of low severity. Typically, 30 minutes are spent at the bedside and on the patient's hospital floor or unit.

99219  **Initial observation care,** per day, for the evaluation and management of a patient, which requires these 3 key components:
- **A comprehensive history;**
- **A comprehensive examination; and**
- **Medical decision making of moderate complexity.**

Counseling and/or coordination of care with other physicians, other qualified health care professionals, or agencies are provided consistent with the nature of the problem(s) and the patient's and/or family's needs.

Usually, the problem(s) requiring admission to outpatient hospital "observation status" are of moderate severity. Typically, 50 minutes are spent at the bedside and on the patient's hospital floor or unit.

99220  **Initial observation care,** per day, for the evaluation and management of a patient, which requires these 3 key components:
- **A comprehensive history;**
- **A comprehensive examination; and**
- **Medical decision making of high complexity.**

Counseling and/or coordination of care with other physicians, other qualified health care professionals, or agencies are provided consistent with the nature of the problem(s) and the patient's and/or family's needs.

Usually, the problem(s) requiring admission to outpatient hospital "observation status" are of high severity. Typically, 70 minutes are spent at the bedside and on the patient's hospital floor or unit.

0254T  Endovascular repair of iliac artery bifurcation (eg, aneurysm, pseudoaneurysm, arteriovenous malformation, trauma, dissection) using bifurcated ~~endoprosthesis~~ endograft from the common iliac artery into both the external and internal iliac artery, including all selective and/or nonselective catheterization(s) required for device placement and all associated radiological supervision and interpretation, unilateral

## Deleted Codes

| | | | | | | |
|---|---|---|---|---|---|---|
| 0051T | 0052T | 0053T | 00740 | 00810 | 01180 | 01190 |
| 01682 | 0178T | 0179T | 0180T | 0255T | 0293T | 0294T |
| 0299T | 0300T | 0301T | 0302T | 0303T | 0304T | 0305T |
| 0306T | 0307T | 0309T | 0310T | 0340T | 0438T | 15732 |
| 29582 | 29583 | 31320 | 34800 | 34802 | 34803 | 34804 |
| 34805 | 34806 | 34825 | 34826 | 34900 | 36120 | 36515 |
| 71021 | 71022 | 71023 | 71030 | 71034 | 71035 | 74000 |
| 74010 | 74020 | 75658 | 75952 | 75953 | 75954 | 77422 |
| 78190 | 83499 | 84061 | 86185 | 86243 | 86378 | 86729 |
| 86822 | 87277 | 87470 | 87477 | 87515 | 88154 | 93982 |
| 94620 | 97532 | 97762 | 99363 | 99364 | | |

Note: In the row starting 55450: 55450, 64565, 69820, 69840, 71010, 71015, 71020

## Web Release New and Changed Codes

Codes indicated as "Web Release" codes indicate CPT codes that are in *Current Procedural Coding Expert* for the current year, but will not be in the AMA CPT book until the following year. This can also include those codes designated by the AMA as new or revised for 2018 but that actually appeared in the 2017 Optum360 book. These codes will have the appropriate new or changed icon appended to match the CPT code book, however. See the complete list below:

### New codes and changes to codes in the 2018 *Current Procedural Coding Expert* that will not appear in the CPT code book until 2019 are indicated with the following icons: ● ▲ These icons will be green in the body of the book.

0018U  Oncology (thyroid), microRNA profiling by RT-PCR of 10 microRNA sequences, utilizing fine needle aspirate, algorithm reported as a positive or negative result for moderate to high risk of malignancy

0019U   Oncology, RNA, gene expression by whole transcriptome sequencing, formalin-fixed paraffin embedded tissue or fresh frozen tissue, predictive algorithm reported as potential targets for therapeutic agents

0020U   Drug test(s), presumptive, with definitive confirmation of positive results, any number of drug classes, urine, with specimen verification including DNA authentication in comparison to buccal DNA, per date of service

0021U   Oncology (prostate), detection of 8 autoantibodies (ARF 6, NKX3-1, 5'-UTR-BMI1, CEP 164, 3'-UTR-Ropporin, Desmocollin, AURKAIP-1, CSNK2A2), multiplexed immunoassay and flow cytometry serum, algorithm reported as risk score

0022U   Targeted genomic sequence analysis panel, non-small cell lung neoplasia, DNA and RNA analysis, 23 genes, interrogation for sequence variants and rearrangements, reported as presence/absence of variants and associated therapy(ies) to consider

0023U   Oncology (acute myelogenous leukemia), DNA, genotyping of internal tandem duplication, p.D835, p.I836, using mononuclear cells, reported as detection or non-detection of FLT3 mutation and indication for or against the use of midostaurin

## Codes and changes that were new to *Current Procedural Coding Expert* for 2017 and are now in the 2018 CPT code book include:

0333T   Visual evoked potential, screening of visual acuity, automated, with report

0464T   Visual evoked potential, testing for glaucoma, with interpretation and report

0465T   Suprachoroidal injection of a pharmacologic agent (does not include supply of medication)

0466T   Insertion of chest wall respiratory sensor electrode or electrode array, including connection to pulse generator (List separately in addition to code for primary procedure)

0467T   Revision or replacement of chest wall respiratory sensor electrode or electrode array, including connection to existing pulse generator

90682   Influenza virus vaccine, quadrivalent (RIV4), derived from recombinant DNA, hemagglutinin (HA) protein only, preservative and antibiotic free, for intramuscular use

90750   Zoster (shingles) vaccine (HZV), recombinant, sub-unit, adjuvanted, for intramuscular use

CPT © 2017 American Medical Association. All Rights Reserved.                                    © 2017 Optum360, LLC

# Appendix C — Evaluation and Management Extended Guidelines

This appendix provides an overview of evaluation and management (E/M) services, tables that identify the documentation elements associated with each code, and the federal documentation guidelines with emphasis on the 1997 exam guidelines. This set of guidelines represent the most complete discussion of the elements of the currently accepted versions. The 1997 version identifies both general multi-system physical examinations and single-system examinations, but providers may also use the original 1995 version of the E/M guidelines; both are currently supported by the Centers for Medicare and Medicaid Services (CMS) for audit purposes.

The levels of E/M services define the wide variations in skill, effort, and time and are required for preventing and/or diagnosing and treating illness or injury, and promoting optimal health. These codes are intended to represent physician work, and because much of this work involves the amount of training, experience, expertise, and knowledge that a provider may employ when treating a given patient, the true indications of the level of this work may be difficult to recognize without some explanation.

At first glance, selecting an E/M code may appear to be difficult, but the system of coding clinical visits may be mastered once the requirements for code selection are learned and used.

## Providers

The AMA advises coders that while a particular service or procedure may be assigned to a specific section, the service or procedure itself is not limited to use only by that specialty group (see paragraphs 2 and 3 under "Instructions for Use of the CPT® Codebook" on page xii of the AMA CPT Book). Additionally, the procedures and services listed throughout the book are for use by any qualified physician or other qualified health care professional or entity (e.g., hospitals, laboratories, or home health agencies).

The use of the phrase "physician or other qualified health care professional" (OQHCP) was adopted to identify a health care provider other than a physician. This type of provider is further described in CPT as an individual "qualified by education, training, licensure/regulation (when applicable), and facility privileging (when applicable)." State licensure guidelines determine the scope of practice and a qualified health care professional must practice within these guidelines, even if more restrictive than the CPT guidelines. The qualified health care professional may report services independently or under incident-to guidelines. The professionals within this definition are separate from "clinical staff" and are able to practice independently. CPT defines clinical staff as "a person who works under the supervision of a physician or other qualified health care professional and who is allowed, by law, regulation, and facility policy to perform or assist in the performance of a specified professional service, but who does not individually report that professional service." Keep in mind that there may be other policies or guidance that can affect who may report a specific service.

## Types of E/M Services

When approaching E/M, the first choice that a provider must make is what type of code to use. The following tables outline the E/M codes for different levels of care for:

- Office or other outpatient services—new patient
- Office or other outpatient services—established patient
- Hospital observation services—initial care, subsequent, and discharge
- Hospital inpatient services—initial care, subsequent, and discharge
- Observation or inpatient care (including admission and discharge services)
- Consultations—office or other outpatient
- Consultations—inpatient
- Emergency department services
- Critical care
- Nursing facility—initial services
- Nursing facility—subsequent services

- Nursing facility—discharge and annual assessment
- Domiciliary, rest home, or custodial care—new patient
- Domiciliary, rest home, or custodial care—established patient
- Home services—new patient
- Home services—established patient
- Newborn care services
- Neonatal and pediatric interfacility transport
- Neonatal and pediatric critical care—inpatient
- Neonate and infant intensive care services—initial and continuing

The specifics of the code components that determine code selection are listed in the table and discussed in the next section. Before a level of service is decided upon, the correct type of service is identified.

A new patient is a patient who has not received any face-to-face professional services from the physician or other qualified health care provider within the past three years. An established patient is a patient who has received face-to-face professional services from the physician or other qualified health care provider within the past three years. In the case of group practices, if a physician or other qualified health care provider of the exact same specialty or subspecialty has seen the patient within three years, the patient is considered established.

If a physician or other qualified health care provider is on call or covering for another physician or other qualified health care provider, the patient's encounter is classified as it would have been by the physician or other qualified health care provider who is not available. Thus, a locum tenens physician or other qualified health care provider who sees a patient on behalf of the patient's attending physician or other qualified health care provider may not bill a new patient code unless the attending physician or other qualified health care provider has not seen the patient for any problem within three years.

Office or other outpatient services are E/M services provided in the physician or other qualified health care provider's office, the outpatient area, or other ambulatory facility. Until the patient is admitted to a health care facility, he/she is considered to be an outpatient. Hospital observation services are E/M services provided to patients who are designated or admitted as "observation status" in a hospital.

Codes 99218-99220 are used to indicate initial observation care. These codes include the initiation of the observation status, supervision of patient care including writing orders, and the performance of periodic reassessments. These codes are used only by the provider "admitting" the patient for observation.

Codes 99234-99236 are used to indicate evaluation and management services to a patient who is admitted to and discharged from observation status or hospital inpatient on the same day. If the patient is admitted as an inpatient from observation on the same day, use the appropriate level of Initial Hospital Care (99221-99223).

Code 99217 indicates discharge from observation status. It includes the final physical examination of the patient, instructions, and preparation of the discharge records. It should not be used when admission and discharge are on the same date of service. As mentioned above, report codes 99234-99236 to appropriately describe same day observation services.

If a patient is in observation longer than one day, subsequent observation care codes 99224-99226 should be reported. If the patient is discharged on the second day, observation discharge code 99217 should be reported. If the patient status is changed to inpatient on a subsequent date, the appropriate inpatient code, 99221-99233, should be reported.

Initial hospital care is defined as E/M services provided during the first hospital inpatient encounter with the patient by the admitting provider. (If a physician other than the admitting physician performs the initial inpatient encounter, refer to consultations or subsequent hospital care in the CPT book.) Subsequent hospital care includes all follow-up encounters with the patient by all physicians or other qualified health care providers.

As there may only be one admitting physician, HCPCS Level II modifier AI Principal physician of record, should be appended to the initial hospital care code by the attending physician or other qualified health care provider.

A consultation is the provision of a physician or other qualified health care provider's opinion or advice about a patient for a specific problem at the request of another physician or other appropriate source. CPT also states that a consultation may be performed when a physician or other qualified health care provider is determining whether to accept the transfer of patient care at the request of another physician or appropriate source. An office or other outpatient consultation is a consultation provided in the consultant's office, in the emergency department, or in an outpatient or other ambulatory facility including hospital observation services, home services, domiciliary, rest home, or custodial care. An inpatient consultation is a consultation provided in the hospital or partial hospital nursing facility setting. Report only one inpatient consultation by a consultant for each admission to the hospital or nursing facility.

If a consultant participates in the patient's management after the opinion or advice is provided, use codes for subsequent hospital or observation care or for office or other outpatient services (established patient), as appropriate.

Under CMS guidelines, the inpatient and office/outpatient consultation codes contained in the CPT manual are not covered services.

All outpatient consultation services will be reported for Medicare using the appropriate new or established evaluation and management (E/M) codes.

Inpatient consultation services for the initial encounter should be reported by the physician providing the service using initial hospital care codes 99221–99223, and subsequent inpatient care codes 99231–99233.

Codes 99487, 99489, and 99490 are used to report evaluation and management services for chronic care management. These codes represent management and support services provided by clinical staff, under the direction of a physician or other qualified health care professional, to patients residing at home or in a domiciliary, rest home, or assisted living facility. The qualified provider oversees the management and/or coordination of services for all medical conditions, psychosocial needs, and activities of daily living. These codes are reported only once per calendar month and have specific time-based thresholds.

Codes 99497-99498 are used to report the discussion and explanation of advanced directives by a physician or other qualified health care professional. These codes represent a face-to-face service between the provider and a patient, family member, or surrogate. These codes are time-based codes and, since no active management of the problem(s) is undertaken during this time, may be reported on the same day as another E/M service.

Beginning in 2017, certain codes that CPT considers appropriate telehealth services are identified with the ★ icon and reported with modifier 95 Synchronous telemedicine service rendered via a real-time interactive audio and video telecommunications system. Medicare recognizes certain CPT and HCPCS Level II G codes as telehealth services reported with modifier GT. Check with individual payers for telehealth modifier guidance.

## Office or Other Outpatient Services—New Patient

| E/M Code | History[1] | Exam[1] | Medical Decision Making[1] | Problem Severity | Coordination of Care; Counseling | Time Spent Face-to-Face (avg.) |
|---|---|---|---|---|---|---|
| 99201 | Problem-focused | Problem-focused | Straight-forward | Minor or self-limited | Consistent with problem(s) and patient's needs | 10 min. |
| 99202 | Expanded problem-focused | Expanded problem-focused | Straight-forward | Low to moderate | Consistent with problem(s) and patient's needs | 20 min. |
| 99203 | Detailed | Detailed | Low complexity | Moderate | Consistent with problem(s) and patient's needs | 30 min. |
| 99204 | Comprehensive | Comprehensive | Moderate complexity | Moderate to high | Consistent with problem(s) and patient's needs | 45 min. |
| 99205 | Comprehensive | Comprehensive | High complexity | Moderate to high | Consistent with problem(s) and patient's needs | 60 min. |

1 Key component. For new patients, all three components (history, exam, and medical decision making) are crucial for selecting the correct code.

 CPT © 2017 American Medical Association. All Rights Reserved. © 2017 Optum360, LLC

## Office or Other Outpatient Services—Established Patient[1]

| E/M Code | History[2] | Exam[2] | Medical Decision Making[2] | Problem Severity | Coordination of Care; Counseling | Time Spent Face-to-Face (avg.) |
|---|---|---|---|---|---|---|
| 99211 | — | — | Physician supervision, but presence not required | Minimal | Consistent with problem(s) and patient's needs | 5 min. |
| 99212 | Problem-focused | Problem-focused | Straight-forward | Minor or self-limited | Consistent with problem(s) and patient's needs | 10 min. |
| 99213 | Expanded problem-focused | Expanded problem-focused | Low complexity | Low to moderate | Consistent with problem(s) and patient's needs | 15 min. |
| 99214 | Detailed | Detailed | Moderate complexity | Moderate to high | Consistent with problem(s) and patient's needs | 25 min. |
| 99215 | Comprehensive | Comprehensive | High complexity | Moderate to high | Consistent with problem(s) and patient's needs | 40 min. |

1  Includes follow-up, periodic reevaluation, and evaluation and management of new problems.
2  Key component. For established patients, at least two of the three components (history, exam, and medical decision making) are needed to select the correct code.

## Hospital Observation Services

| E/M Code | History[1] | Exam[1] | Medical Decision Making[1] | Problem Severity | Coordination of Care; Counseling | Time Spent Bedside and on Unit/Floor (avg.) |
|---|---|---|---|---|---|---|
| 99217 | Observation care discharge day management | | | | | |
| 99218 | Detailed or comprehensive | Detailed or comprehensive | Straight-forward or low complexity | Low | Consistent with problem(s) and patient's needs | 30 min. |
| 99219 | Comprehensive | Comprehensive | Moderate complexity | Moderate | Consistent with problem(s) and patient's needs | 50 min. |
| 99220 | Comprehensive | Comprehensive | High complexity | High | Consistent with problem(s) and patient's needs | 70 min. |

1  Key component. All three components (history, exam, and medical decision making) are crucial for selecting the correct code.

## Subsequent Hospital Observation Services[1]

| E/M Code[2] | History[3] | Exam[3] | Medical Decision Making[3] | Problem Severity | Coordination of Care; Counseling | Time Spent Bedside and on Unit/Floor (avg.) |
|---|---|---|---|---|---|---|
| 99224 | Problem-focused interval | Problem-focused | Straight-forward or low complexity | Stable, recovering, or improving | Consistent with problem(s) and patient's needs | 15 min. |
| 99225 | Expanded problem-focused interval | Expanded problem-focused | Moderate complexity | Inadequate response to treatment; minor complications | Consistent with problem(s) and patient's needs | 25 min. |
| 99226 | Detailed interval | Detailed | High complexity | Unstable; significant new problem or significant complication | Consistent with problem(s) and patient's needs | 35 min. |

1  All subsequent levels of service include reviewing the medical record, diagnostic studies, and changes in the patient's status, such as history, physical condition, and response to treatment since the last assessment.
2  These codes are resequenced in CPT and are printed following codes 99217-99220.
3  Key component. For subsequent care, at least two of the three components (history, exam, and medical decision making) are needed to select the correct code.

## Hospital Inpatient Services—Initial Care[1]

| E/M Code | History[2] | Exam[2] | Medical Decision Making[2] | Problem Severity | Coordination of Care; Counseling | Time Spent Bedside and on Unit/Floor (avg.) |
|---|---|---|---|---|---|---|
| 99221 | Detailed or comprehensive | Detailed or comprehensive | Straight-forward or low complexity | Low | Consistent with problem(s) and patient's needs | 30 min. |
| 99222 | Comprehensive | Comprehensive | Moderate complexity | Moderate | Consistent with problem(s) and patient's needs | 50 min. |
| 99223 | Comprehensive | Comprehensive | High complexity | High | Consistent with problem(s) and patient's needs | 70 min. |

1　The admitting physician should append modifier AI, Principal physician of record, for Medicare patients

2　Key component. For initial care, all three components (history, exam, and medical decision making) are crucial for selecting the correct code.

## Hospital Inpatient Services—Subsequent Care[1]

| E/M Code | History[2] | Exam[2] | Medical Decision Making[2] | Problem Severity | Coordination of Care; Counseling | Time Spent Bedside and on Unit/Floor (avg.) |
|---|---|---|---|---|---|---|
| 99231 | Problem-focused interval | Problem-focused | Straight-forward or low complexity | Stable, recovering or Improving | Consistent with problem(s) and patient's needs | 15 min. |
| 99232 | Expanded problem-focused interval | Expanded problem-focused | Moderate complexity | Inadequate response to treatment; minor complications | Consistent with problem(s) and patient's needs | 25 min. |
| 99233 | Detailed interval | Detailed | High complexity | Unstable; significant new problem or significant complication | Consistent with problem(s) and patient's needs | 35 min. |
| 99238 | Hospital discharge day management | | | | | 30 min. or less |
| 99239 | Hospital discharge day management | | | | | > 30 min. |

1　All subsequent levels of service include reviewing the medical record, diagnostic studies, and changes in the patient's status, such as history, physical condition, and response to treatment since the last assessment.

2　Key component. For subsequent care, at least two of the three components (history, exam, and medical decision making) are needed to select the correct code.

## Observation or Inpatient Care Services (Including Admission and Discharge Services)

| E/M Code | History[1] | Exam[1] | Medical Decision Making[1] | Problem Severity | Coordination of Care; Counseling | Time |
|---|---|---|---|---|---|---|
| 99234 | Detailed or comprehensive | Detailed or comprehensive | Straight-forward or low complexity | Low | Consistent with problem(s) and patient's needs | 40 min. |
| 99235 | Comprehensive | Comprehensive | Moderate | Moderate | Consistent with problem(s) and patient's needs | 50 min. |
| 99236 | Comprehensive | Comprehensive | High | High | Consistent with problem(s) and patient's needs | 55 min. |

1　Key component. All three components (history, exam, and medical decision making) are crucial for selecting the correct code.

## Consultations—Office or Other Outpatient

| E/M Code | History[1] | Exam[1] | Medical Decision Making[1] | Problem Severity | Coordination of Care; Counseling | Time Spent Face-to-Face (avg.) |
|---|---|---|---|---|---|---|
| 99241 | Problem-focused | Problem-focused | Straight-forward | Minor or self-limited | Consistent with problem(s) and patient's needs | 15 min. |
| 99242 | Expanded problem-focused | Expanded problem-focused | Straight-forward | Low | Consistent with problem(s) and patient's needs | 30 min. |
| 99243 | Detailed | Detailed | Low complexity | Moderate | Consistent with problem(s) and patient's needs | 40 min. |
| 99244 | Comprehensive | Comprehensive | Moderate complexity | Moderate to high | Consistent with problem(s) and patient's needs | 60 min. |
| 99245 | Comprehensive | Comprehensive | High complexity | Moderate to high | Consistent with problem(s) and patient's needs | 80 min. |

1  Key component. For office or other outpatient consultations, all three components (history, exam, and medical decision making) are crucial for selecting the correct code.

## Consultations—Inpatient[1]

| E/M Code | History[2] | Exam[2] | Medical Decision Making[2] | Problem Severity | Coordination of Care; Counseling | Time Spent Bedside and on Unit/Floor (avg.) |
|---|---|---|---|---|---|---|
| 99251 | Problem-focused | Problem-focused | Straight-forward | Minor or self-limited | Consistent with problem(s) and patient's needs | 20 min. |
| 99252 | Expanded problem-focused | Expanded problem-focused | Straight-forward | Low | Consistent with problem(s) and patient's needs | 40 min. |
| 99253 | Detailed | Detailed | Low complexity | Moderate | Consistent with problem(s) and patient's needs | 55 min. |
| 99254 | Comprehensive | Comprehensive | Moderate complexity | Moderate to high | Consistent with problem(s) and patient's needs | 80 min. |
| 99255 | Comprehensive | Comprehensive | High complexity | Moderate to high | Consistent with problem(s) and patient's needs | 110 min. |

1  These codes are used for hospital inpatients, residents of nursing facilities or patients in a partial hospital setting.

2  Key component. For initial inpatient consultations, all three components (history, exam, and medical decision making) are crucial for selecting the correct code.

## Emergency Department Services, New or Established Patient

| E/M Code | History[1] | Exam[1] | Medical Decision Making[1] | Problem Severity[3] | Coordination of Care; Counseling | Time Spent[2] Face-to-Face (avg.) |
|---|---|---|---|---|---|---|
| 99281 | Problem-focused | Problem-focused | Straight-forward | Minor or self-limited | Consistent with problem(s) and patient's needs | N/A |
| 99282 | Expanded problem-focused | Expanded problem-focused | Low complexity | Low to moderate | Consistent with problem(s) and patient's needs | N/A |
| 99283 | Expanded problem-focused | Expanded problem-focused | Moderate complexity | Moderate | Consistent with problem(s) and patient's needs | N/A |
| 99284 | Detailed | Detailed | Moderate complexity | High; requires urgent evaluation | Consistent with problem(s) and patient's needs | N/A |
| 99285 | Comprehensive | Comprehensive | High complexity | High; poses immediate/ significant threat to life or physiologic function | Consistent with problem(s) and patient's needs | N/A |
| 99288[4] | | | High complexity | | | N/A |

1 Key component. For emergency department services, all three components (history, exam, and medical decision making) are crucial for selecting the correct code and must be adequately documented in the medical record to substantiate the level of service reported.

2 Typical times have not been established for this category of services.

3 NOTE: The severity of the patient's problem, while taken into consideration when evaluating and treating the patient, does not automatically determine the level of E/M service unless the medical record documentation reflects the severity of the patient's illness, injury, or condition in the details of the history, physical examination, and medical decision making process. Federal auditors will "downcode" the level of E/M service despite the nature of the patient's problem when the documentation does not support the E/M code reported.

4 Code 99288 is used to report two-way communication with emergency medical services personnel in the field.

## Critical Care

| E/M Code | Patient Status | Physician Attendance | Time[1] |
|---|---|---|---|
| 99291 | Critically ill or critically injured | Constant | First 30–74 minutes |
| 99292 | Critically ill or critically injured | Constant | Each additional 30 minutes beyond the first 74 minutes |

1 Per the guidelines for time in *CPT 2016 page xv*, "A unit of time is attained when the mid-point is passed. For example, an hour is attained when 31 minutes have elapsed (more than midway between zero and 60 minutes)."

## Nursing Facility Services—Initial Nursing Facility Care[1]

| E/M Code | History[1] | Exam[1] | Medical Decision Making[1] | Problem Severity | Coordination of Care; Counseling |
|---|---|---|---|---|---|
| 99304 | Detailed or comprehensive | Detailed or comprehensive | Straight-forward or low complexity | Low | 25 min. |
| 99305 | Comprehensive | Comprehensive | Moderate complexity | Moderate | 35 min. |
| 99306 | Comprehensive | Comprehensive | High complexity | High | 45 min. |

1 These services must be performed by the physician. See CPT Corrections Document – CPT 2013 page 3 or guidelines CPT 2016 page 26.

2 Key component. For new patients, all three components (history, exam, and medical decision making) are crucial for selecting the correct code.

CPT © 2017 American Medical Association. All Rights Reserved.

© 2017 Optum360, LLC

## Nursing Facility Services—Subsequent Nursing Facility Care

| E/M Code | History[1] | Exam[1] | Medical Decision Making[2] | Problem Severity | Coordination of Care; Counseling |
|---|---|---|---|---|---|
| 99307 | Problem-focused interval | Problem-focused | Straight-forward | Stable, recovering or improving | 10 min. |
| 99308 | Expanded problem-focused interval | Expanded problem-focused | Low complexity | Responding inadequately or has developed a minor complication | 15 min. |
| 99309 | Detailed interval | Detailed | Moderate complexity | Significant complication or a significant new problem | 25 min. |
| 99310 | Comprehensive interval | Comprehensive | High complexity | Developed a significant new problem requiring immediate attention | 35 min. |

1 Key component. For established patients, at least two of the three components (history, exam, and medical decision making) are needed for selecting the correct code.

## Nursing Facility Discharge and Annual Assessment

| E/M Code | History[1] | Exam[1] | Medical Decision Making[1] | Problem Severity | Time Spent Bedside and on Unit/Floor (avg.) |
|---|---|---|---|---|---|
| 99315 | Nursing facility discharge day management | | | | 30 min. or less |
| 99316 | Nursing facility discharge day management | | | | more than 30 min. |
| 99318 | Detailed interval | Comprehensive | Low to moderate complexity | Stable, recovering or improving | 30 min. |

1 Key component. For annual nursing facility assessment, all three components (history, exam, and medical decision making) are crucial for selecting the correct code.

## Domiciliary, Rest Home (e.g., Boarding Home) or Custodial Care Services—New Patient

| E/M Code | History[1] | Exam[1] | Medical Decision Making[1] | Problem Severity | Coordination of Care; Counseling | Time Spent Face-to-Face (avg.) |
|---|---|---|---|---|---|---|
| 99324 | Problem-focused | Problem-focused | Straight-forward | Low | Consistent with problem(s) and patient's needs | 20 min. |
| 99325 | Expanded problem-focused | Expanded problem-focused | Low complexity | Moderate | Consistent with problem(s) and patient's needs | 30 min. |
| 99326 | Detailed | Detailed | Moderate complexity | Moderate to high | Consistent with problem(s) and patient's needs | 45 min. |
| 99327 | Comprehensive | Comprehensive | Moderate complexity | High | Consistent with problem(s) and patient's needs | 60 min. |
| 99328 | Comprehensive | Comprehensive | High complexity | Unstable or developed a new problem requiring immediate physician attention | Consistent with problem(s) and patient's needs | 75 min. |

1 Key component. For new patients, all three components (history, exam, and medical decision making) are crucial for selecting the correct code and must be adequately documented in the medical record to substantiate the level of service reported.

## Domiciliary, Rest Home (e.g., Boarding Home) or Custodial Care Services— Established Patient

| E/M Code | History[1] | Exam[1] | Medical Decision Making[1] | Problem Severity | Coordination of Care; Counseling | Time Spent Face-to-Face (avg.) |
|---|---|---|---|---|---|---|
| 99334 | Problem-focused interval | Problem-focused | Straight-forward | Minor or self-limited | Consistent with problem(s) and patient's needs | 15 min. |
| 99335 | Expanded problem-focused interval | Expanded problem-focused | Low complexity | Low to moderate | Consistent with problem(s) and patient's needs | 25 min. |
| 99336 | Detailed interval | Detailed | Moderate complexity | Moderate to high | Consistent with problem(s) and patient's needs | 40 min. |
| 99337 | Comprehensive interval | Comprehensive | Moderate to high complexity | Moderate to high | Consistent with problem(s) and patient's needs | 60 min. |

1 Key component. For established patients, at least two of the three components (history, exam, and medical decision making) are needed for selecting the correct code.

## Domiciliary, Rest Home (e.g., Assisted Living Facility), or Home Care Plan Oversight Services

| E/M Code | Intent of Service | Presence of Patient | Time |
|---|---|---|---|
| 99339 | Individual physician supervision of a patient (patient not present) in home, domiciliary or rest home (e.g., assisted living facility) requiring complex and multidisciplinary care modalities involving regular physician development and/or revision of care plans, review of subsequent reports of patient status, review of related laboratory and other studies, communication (including telephone calls) for purposes of assessment or care decisions with health care professional(s), family member(s), surrogate decision maker(s) (e.g., legal guardian) and/or key caregiver(s) involved in patient's care, integration of new information into the medical treatment plan and/or adjustment of medical therapy, within a calendar month | Patient not present | 15–29 min. |
| 99340 | Same as 99339 | Patient not present | 30 min. or more |

## Home Services—New Patient

| E/M Code | History[1] | Exam[1] | Medical Decision Making[1] | Problem Severity | Coordination of Care; Counseling | Time Spent Face-to-Face (avg.) |
|---|---|---|---|---|---|---|
| 99341 | Problem-focused | Problem-focused | Straight-forward complexity | Low | Consistent with problem(s) and patient's needs | 20 min. |
| 99342 | Expanded problem-focused | Expanded problem-focused | Low complexity | Moderate | Consistent with problem(s) and patient's needs | 30 min. |
| 99343 | Detailed | Detailed | Moderate complexity | Moderate to high | Consistent with problem(s) and patient's needs | 45 min. |
| 99344 | Comprehensive | Comprehensive | Moderate complexity | High | Consistent with problem(s) and patient's needs | 60 min. |
| 99345 | Comprehensive | Comprehensive | High complexity | Usually the patient has developed a significant new problem requiring immediate physician attention | Consistent with problem(s) and patient's needs | 75 min. |

1 Key component. For new patients, all three components (history, exam, and medical decision making) are crucial for selecting the correct code and must be adequately documented in the medical record to substantiate the level of service reported.

CPT © 2017 American Medical Association. All Rights Reserved.

## Home Services—Established Patient

| E/M Code | History[1] | Exam[1] | Medical Decision Making[1] | Problem Severity | Coordination of Care; Counseling | Time Spent Face-to-Face (avg.) |
|---|---|---|---|---|---|---|
| 99347 | Problem-focused interval | Problem-focused | Straight-forward | Minor or self-limited | Consistent with problem(s) and patient's needs | 15 min. |
| 99348 | Expanded problem-focused interval | Expanded problem-focused | Low complexity | Low to moderate | Consistent with problem(s) and patient's needs | 25 min. |
| 99349 | Detailed interval | Detailed | Moderate complexity | Moderate to high | Consistent with problem(s) and patient's needs | 40 min. |
| 99350 | Comprehensive interval | Comprehensive | Moderate to high complexity | Moderate to high Usually the patient has developed a significant new problem requiring immediate physician attention | Consistent with problem(s) and patient's needs | 60 min. |

1 Key component. For established patients, at least two of the three components (history, exam, and medical decision making) are needed for selecting the correct code.

## Newborn Care Services

| E/M Code | Patient Status | Type of Visit |
|---|---|---|
| 99460 | Normal newborn | Inpatient initial inpatient hospital or birthing center per day |
| 99461 | Normal newborn | Inpatient initial treatment not in hospital or birthing center per day |
| 99462 | Normal newborn | Inpatient subsequent per day |
| 99463 | Normal newborn | Inpatient initial inpatient and discharge in hospital or birthing center per day |
| 99464 | Unstable newborn | Attendance at delivery |
| 99465 | High-risk newborn at delivery | Resuscitation, ventilation, and cardiac treatment |

## Neonatal and Pediatric Interfacility Transportation

| E/M Code | Patient Status | Type of Visit |
|---|---|---|
| 99466 | Critically ill or injured infant or young child, to 24 months | Face-to-face transportation from one facility to another, initial 30-74 minutes |
| 99467 | Critically ill or injured infant or young child, to 24 months | Face-to-face transportation from one facility to another, each additional 30 minutes |
| 99485[1] | Critically ill or injured infant or young child, to 24 months | Supervision of patient transport from one facility to another, initial 30 minutes |
| 99486[1] | Critically ill or injured infant or young child, to 24 months | Supervision of patient transport from one facility to another, each additional 30 minutes |

1 These codes are resequenced in CPT and are printed following codes 99466-99467.

## Inpatient Neonatal and Pediatric Critical Care

| E/M Code | Patient Status | Type of Visit |
|---|---|---|
| 99468[1] | Critically ill neonate, aged 28 days or less | Inpatient initial per day |
| 99469[2] | Critically ill neonate, aged 28 days or less | Inpatient subsequent per day |
| 99471 | Critically ill infant or young child, aged 29 days to 24 months | Inpatient initial per day |
| 99472 | Critically ill infant or young child, aged 29 days to 24 months | Inpatient subsequent per day |
| 99475 | Critically ill infant or young child, 2 to 5 years[3] | Inpatient initial per day |
| 99476 | Critically ill infant or young child, 2 to 5 years | Inpatient subsequent per day |

1 Codes 99468, 99471, and 99475 may be reported only once per admission.
2 Codes 99469, 99472, and 99476 may be reported only once per day and by only one provider.
3 See 99291-99292 for patients 6 years of age and older.

## Neonate and Infant Initial and Continuing Intensive Care Services

| E/M Code | Patient Status | Type of Visit |
|---|---|---|
| 99477 | Neonate, aged 28 days or less | Inpatient initial per day |
| 99478 | Infant with present body weight of less than 1500 grams, no longer critically ill | Inpatient subsequent per day |
| 99479 | Infant with present body weight of 1500-2500 grams, no longer critically ill | Inpatient subsequent per day |
| 99480 | Infant with present body weight of 2501-5000 grams, no longer critically ill | Inpatient subsequent per day |

## Levels of E/M Services

Confusion may be experienced when first approaching E/M due to the way that each description of a code component or element seems to have another layer of description beneath. The three key components—history, exam, and decision making—are each comprised of elements that combine to create varying levels of that component.

For example, an expanded problem-focused history includes the chief complaint, a brief history of the present illness, and a system review focusing on the patient's problems. The level of exam is not made up of different elements but rather distinguished by the extent of exam across body areas or organ systems.

The single largest source of confusion are the "labels" or names applied to the varying degrees of history, exam, and decision-making. Terms such as expanded problem-focused, detailed, and comprehensive are somewhat meaningless unless they are defined. The lack of definition in CPT guidelines relative to these terms is precisely what caused the first set of federal guidelines to be developed in 1995 and again in 1997.

## Documentation Guidelines for Evaluation and Management Services

Both versions of the federal guidelines go well beyond CPT guidelines in defining specific code requirements. The current version of the CPT guidelines does not explain the number of history of present illness (HPI) elements or the specific number of organ systems or body areas to be examined as they are in the federal guidelines. Adherence to some version of the guidelines is required when billing E/M to federal payers, but at this time, the CPT guidelines do not incorporate this level of detail into the code definitions. Although that could be interpreted to mean that non-governmental payers have a lesser documentation standard, it is best to adopt one set of the federal versions for all payer types for both consistency and ease of use.

The 1997 guidelines supply a great amount of detail relative to history and exam and will give the provider clear direction to follow when documenting elements. With that stated, the 1995 guidelines are equally valid and place a lesser documentation burden on the provider in regards to the physical exam.

The 1995 guidelines ask only for a notation of "normal" on systems with normal findings. The only narrative required is for abnormal findings. The 1997 version calls for much greater detail, or an "elemental" or "bullet-point" approach to organ systems, although a notation of normal is sufficient when addressing the elements within a system. The 1997 version works well in a template or electronic health record (EHR) format for recording E/M services.

The 1997 version did produce the single system specialty exam guidelines. When reviewing the complete guidelines listed below, note the differences between exam requirements in the 1995 and 1997 versions.

### A Comparison of 1995 and 1997 Exam Guidelines

There are four types of exams indicated in the levels of E/M codes. Although the descriptors or labels are the same under 1995 and 1997 guidelines, the degree of detail required is different. The remaining content on this topic references the 1997 general multi-system speciality examination, at the end of this chapter.

The levels under each set of guidelines are:

**1995 Exam Guidelines:**

| | |
|---|---|
| Problem focused: | One body area or system |
| Expanded problem focused: | Two to seven body areas or organ systems |
| Detailed: | Two to seven body areas or organ systems |
| Comprehensive: | Eight or more organ systems or a complete single-system examination |

**1997 Exam Guidelines:**

| | |
|---|---|
| Problem-focused: | Perform and document examination of one to five bullet point elements in one or more organ systems/body areas from the general multi-system examination |
| OR | |
| | Perform or document examination of one to five bullet point elements from one of the 10 single-organ-system examinations, shaded or unshaded boxes |
| Expanded problem-focused: | Perform and document examination of at least six bullet point elements in one or more organ systems from the general multi-system examination |
| OR | |
| | Perform and document examination of at least six bullet point elements from one of the 10 single-organ-system examinations, shaded or unshaded boxes |
| Detailed: | Perform and document examination of at least six organ systems or body areas, including at least two bullet point elements for each organ system or body area from the general multi-system examination |
| OR | |
| | Perform and document examination of at least 12 bullet point elements in two or more organ systems or body areas from the general multisystem examination |
| OR | |
| | Perform and document examination of at least 12 bullet elements from one of the single-organ-system examinations, shaded or unshaded boxes |
| Comprehensive: | Perform and document examination of at least nine organ systems or body areas, with all bullet elements for each organ system or body area (unless specific instructions are expected to limit examination content with at least two bullet elements for each organ system or body area) from the general multi-system examination |
| OR | |

CPT © 2017 American Medical Association. All Rights Reserved.

© 2017 Optum360, LLC

Perform and document examination of all bullet point elements from one of the 10 single-organ system examinations with documentation of every element in shaded boxes and at least one element in each unshaded box from the single-organ-system examination.

# The Documentation Guidelines

The following guidelines were developed jointly by the American Medical Association (AMA) and the Centers for Medicare and Medicaid Services (CMS). Their mutual goal was to provide physicians and claims reviewers with advice about preparing or reviewing documentation for Evaluation and Management (E/M) services.

## I.    Introduction

### What is Documentation and Why Is It Important?
Medical record documentation is required to record pertinent facts, findings, and observations about an individual's health history, including past and present illnesses, examinations, tests, treatments, and outcomes. The medical record chronologically documents the care of the patient and is an important element contributing to high quality care. The medical record facilitates:

- The ability of the physician and other health care professionals to evaluate and plan the patient's immediate treatment and to monitor his/her health care over time
- Communication and continuity of care among physicians and other health care professionals involved in the patient's care
- Accurate and timely claims review and payment
- Appropriate utilization review and quality of care evaluations
- Collection of data that may be useful for research and education

An appropriately documented medical record can reduce many of the problems associated with claims processing and may serve as a legal document to verify the care provided, if necessary.

### What Do Payers Want and Why?
Because payers have a contractual obligation to enrollees, they may require reasonable documentation that services are consistent with the insurance coverage provided. They may request information to validate:

- The site of service
- The medical necessity and appropriateness of the diagnostic and/or therapeutic services provided
- Services provided have been accurately reported

## II.   General Principles of Medical Record Documentation
The principles of documentation listed below are applicable to all types of medical and surgical services in all settings. For Evaluation and Management (E/M) services, the nature and amount of physician work and documentation varies by type of service, place of service, and the patient's status. The general principles listed below may be modified to account for these variable circumstances in providing E/M services.

- The medical record should be complete and legible
- The documentation of each patient encounter should include:
  - A reason for the encounter and relevant history, physical examination findings, and prior diagnostic test results
  - Assessment, clinical impression, or diagnosis
  - Plan for care
  - Date and legible identity of the practitioner
- If not documented, the rationale for ordering diagnostic and other ancillary services should be easily inferred
- Past and present diagnoses should be accessible to the treating and/or consulting physician
- Appropriate health risk factors should be identified
- The patient's progress, response to, and changes in treatment and revision of diagnosis should be documented
- The CPT and ICD-9-CM codes reported on the health insurance claim form or billing statement should be supported by the documentation in the medical record

## III.  Documentation of E/M Services 1995 and 1997
The following information provides definitions and documentation guidelines for the three key components of E/M services and for visits that consist predominately of counseling or coordination of care. The three key components—history, examination, and medical decision making—appear in the descriptors for office and other outpatient services, hospital observation services, hospital inpatient services, consultations, emergency department services, nursing facility services, domiciliary care services, and home services. While some of the text of the CPT guidelines has been repeated in this document, the reader should refer to CMS or CPT for the complete descriptors for E/M services and instructions for selecting a level of service. Documentation guidelines are identified by the symbol DG.

The descriptors for the levels of E/M services recognize seven components that are used in defining the levels of E/M services. These components are:

- History
- Examination
- Medical decision making
- Counseling
- Coordination of care
- Nature of presenting problem
- Time

The first three of these components (i.e., history, examination, and medical decision making) are the key components in selecting the level of E/M services. In the case of visits that consist predominately of counseling or coordination of care, time is the key or controlling factor to qualify for a particular level of E/M service.

Because the level of E/M service is dependent on two or three key components, performance and documentation of one component (e.g., examination) at the highest level does not necessarily mean that the encounter in its entirety qualifies for the highest level of E/M service.

These Documentation Guidelines for E/M services reflect the needs of the typical adult population. For certain groups of patients, the recorded information may vary slightly from that described here. Specifically, the medical records of infants, children, adolescents, and pregnant women may have additional or modified information, as appropriate, recorded in each history and examination area.

As an example, newborn records may include under history of the present illness (HPI) the details of the mother's pregnancy and the infant's status at birth; social history will focus on family structure; and family history will focus on congenital anomalies and hereditary disorders in the family. In addition, the content of a pediatric examination will vary with the age and development of the child. Although not specifically defined in these documentation guidelines, these patient group variations on history and examination are appropriate.

### A.    Documentation of History
The levels of E/M services are based on four types of history (Problem Focused, Expanded Problem Focused, Detailed, and Comprehensive). Each type of history includes some or all of the following elements:

- Chief complaint (CC)
- History of present illness (HPI)
- Review of systems (ROS)
- Past, family, and/or social history (PFSH)

The extent of history of present illness, review of systems, and past, family, and/or social history that is obtained and documented is dependent upon clinical judgment and the nature of the presenting problem.

The chart below shows the progression of the elements required for each type of history. To qualify for a given type of history all three elements in the table must be met. (A chief complaint is indicated at all levels.)

- DG:    The CC, ROS, and PFSH may be listed as separate elements of history or they may be included in the description of the history of present illness

- DG:    A ROS and/or a PFSH obtained during an earlier encounter does not need to be re-recorded if there is evidence that the physician reviewed and updated the previous information. This may occur when a physician updates his/her own record or in an institutional setting or group practice where many physicians use a common record. The review and update may be documented by:

    – Describing any new ROS and/or PFSH information or noting there has been no change in the information

    – Noting the date and location of the earlier ROS and/or PFSH

- DG:    The ROS and/or PFSH may be recorded by ancillary staff or on a form completed by the patient. To document that the physician reviewed the information, there must be a notation supplementing or confirming the information recorded by others

- DG:    If the physician is unable to obtain a history from the patient or other source, the record should describe the patient's condition or other circumstance that precludes obtaining a history

Definitions and specific documentation guidelines for each of the elements of history are listed below.

## Chief Complaint (CC)

The CC is a concise statement describing the symptom, problem, condition, diagnosis, physician recommended return, or other factor that is the reason for the encounter, usually stated in the patient's words.

- DG:    The medical record should clearly reflect the chief complaint

## History of Present Illness (HPI)

The HPI is a chronological description of the development of the patient's present illness from the first sign and/or symptom or from the previous encounter to the present. It includes the following elements:

- Location
- Quality
- Severity
- Duration
- Timing
- Context
- Modifying factors
- Associated signs and symptoms

Brief and extended HPIs are distinguished by the amount of detail needed to accurately characterize the clinical problem.

A brief HPI consists of one to three elements of the HPI.

- DG:    The medical record should describe one to three elements of the present illness (HPI)

An extended HPI consists of at least four elements of the HPI or the status of at least three chronic or inactive conditions.

- DG:    The medical record should describe at least four elements of the present illness (HPI) or the status of at least three chronic or inactive conditions

Beginning with services performed on or after September 10, 2013, CMS has stated that physicians and other qualified health care professionals will be able to use the 1997 guidelines for an extended history of present illness (HPI) in combination with other elements from the 1995 documentation guidelines to document a particular level of evaluation and management service.

| History of Present Illness | Review of systems (ROS) | PFSH | Type of History |
|---|---|---|---|
| Brief | N/A | N/A | Problem-focused |
| Brief | Problem Pertinent | N/A | Expanded Problem-Focused |
| Extended | Extended | Pertinent | Detailed |
| Extended | Complete | Complete | Comprehensive |

## Review of Systems (ROS)

A ROS is an inventory of body systems obtained through a series of questions seeking to identify signs and/or symptoms that the patient may be experiencing or has experienced. For purposes of ROS, the following systems are recognized:

- Constitutional symptoms (e.g., fever, weight loss)
- Eyes
- Ears, nose, mouth, throat
- Cardiovascular
- Respiratory
- Gastrointestinal
- Genitourinary
- Musculoskeletal
- Integumentary (skin and/or breast)
- Neurological
- Psychiatric
- Endocrine
- Hematologic/lymphatic
- Allergic/immunologic

A problem pertinent ROS inquires about the system directly related to the problem identified in the HPI.

- DG:    The patient's positive responses and pertinent negatives for the system related to the problem should be documented

An extended ROS inquires about the system directly related to the problem identified in the HPI and a limited number of additional systems.

- DG:    The patient's positive responses and pertinent negatives for two to nine systems should be documented

A complete ROS inquires about the system directly related to the problem identified in the HPI plus all additional body systems.

- DG:    At least 10 organ systems must be reviewed. Those systems with positive or pertinent negative responses must be individually documented. For the remaining systems, a notation indicating all other systems are negative is permissible. In the absence of such a notation, at least 10 systems must be individually documented

## Past, Family, and/or Social History (PFSH)

The PFSH consists of a review of three areas:

- Past history (the patient's past experiences with illnesses, operations, injuries, and treatment)
- Family history (a review of medical events in the patient's family, including diseases that may be hereditary or place the patient at risk)
- Social history (an age appropriate review of past and current activities)

For certain categories of E/M services that include only an interval history, it is not necessary to record information about the PFSH. Those categories are subsequent hospital care, follow-up inpatient consultations, and subsequent nursing facility care.

A pertinent PFSH is a review of the history area directly related to the problem identified in the HPI.

- DG:    At least one specific item from any of the three history areas must be documented for a pertinent PFSH

A complete PFSH is a review of two or all three of the PFSH history areas, depending on the category of the E/M service. A review of all three history areas is required for services that by their nature include a comprehensive assessment or reassessment of the patient. A review of two of the three history areas is sufficient for other services.

- DG: A least one specific item from two of the three history areas must be documented for a complete PFSH for the following categories of E/M services: office or other outpatient services, established patient; emergency department; domiciliary care, established patient; and home care, established patient

- DG: At least one specific item from each of the three history areas must be documented for a complete PFSH for the following categories of E/M services: office or other outpatient services, new patient; hospital observation services; hospital inpatient services, initial care; consultations; comprehensive nursing facility assessments; domiciliary care, new patient; and home care, new patient

## B. Documentation of Examination 1997 Guidelines

The levels of E/M services are based on four types of examination:

- Problem Focused: A limited examination of the affected body area or organ system
- Expanded Problem Focused: A limited examination of the affected body area or organ system and any other symptomatic or related body area or organ system
- Detailed: An extended examination of the affected body area or organ system and any other symptomatic or related body area or organ system
- Comprehensive: A general multi-system examination or complete examination of a single organ system and other symptomatic or related body area or organ system

These types of examinations have been defined for general multi-system and the following single organ systems:

- Cardiovascular
- Ears, nose, mouth, and throat
- Eyes
- Genitourinary (Female)
- Genitourinary (Male)
- Hematologic/lymphatic/immunologic
- Musculoskeletal
- Neurological
- Psychiatric
- Respiratory
- Skin

Any physician regardless of specialty may perform a general multi-system examination or any of the single organ system examinations. The type (general multi-system or single organ system) and content of examination are selected by the examining physician and are based upon clinical judgment, the patient's history, and the nature of the presenting problem.

The content and documentation requirements for each type and level of examination are summarized below and described in detail in a table found later on in this document. In the table, organ systems and body areas recognized by CPT for purposes of describing examinations are shown in the left column. The content, or individual elements, of the examination pertaining to that body area or organ system are identified by bullets (•) in the right column.

Parenthetical examples "(e.g., ...)," have been used for clarification and to provide guidance regarding documentation. Documentation for each

element must satisfy any numeric requirements (such as "Measurement of any three of the following seven...") included in the description of the element. Elements with multiple components but with no specific numeric requirement (such as "Examination of liver and spleen") require documentation of at least one component. It is possible for a given examination to be expanded beyond what is defined here. When that occurs, findings related to the additional systems and/or areas should be documented.

- DG: Specific abnormal and relevant negative findings from the examination of the affected or symptomatic body area or organ system should be documented. A notation of "abnormal" without elaboration is insufficient

- DG: Abnormal or unexpected findings from the examination of any asymptomatic body area or organ system should be described

- DG: A brief statement or notation indicating "negative" or "normal" is sufficient to document normal findings related to an unaffected areas or asymptomatic organ system

### General Multi-System Examinations

General multi-system examinations are described in detail later in this document. To qualify for a given level of multi-system examination, the following content and documentation requirements should be met:

- Problem Focused Examination: It should include performance and documentation of one to five elements identified by a bullet (•) in one or more organ systems or body areas
- Expanded Problem Focused Examination: It should include performance and documentation of at least six elements identified by a bullet (•) in one or more organ systems or body areas
- Detailed Examination: It should include at least six organ systems or body areas. For each system/area selected, performance and documentation of at least two elements identified by a bullet (•) is expected. Alternatively, a detailed examination may include performance and documentation of at least 12 elements identified by a bullet (•) in two or more organ systems or body areas
- Comprehensive Examination: It should include at least nine organ systems or body areas. For each system/area selected, all elements of the examination identified by a bullet (•) should be performed, unless specific directions limit the content of the examination. For each area/system, documentation of at least two elements identified by a bullet (•) is expected

### Single Organ System Examinations

The single organ system examinations recognized by CMS include eyes; ears, nose, mouth, and throat; cardiovascular; respiratory; genitourinary (male and female); musculoskeletal; neurologic; hematologic, lymphatic, and immunologic; skin; and psychiatric. Note that for each specific single organ examination type, the performance and documentation of the stated number of elements, identified by a bullet (•) should be included, whether in a box with a shaded or unshaded border. The following content and documentation requirements must be met to qualify for a given level:

- Problem Focused Examination: one to five elements
- Expanded Problem Focused Examination: at least six elements
- Detailed Examination: at least 12 elements (other than eye and psychiatric examinations)
- Comprehensive Examination: all elements (Documentation of every element in a box with a shaded border and at least one element in a box with an unshaded border is expected)

# Content and Documentation Requirements

## *General Multisystem Examination 1997*

| System/Body Area | Elements of Examination |
|---|---|
| Constitutional | • Measurement of any three of the following seven vital signs: 1) sitting or standing blood pressure, 2) supine blood pressure, 3) pulse rate and regularity, 4) respiration, 5) temperature, 6) height, 7) weight (May be measured and recorded by ancillary staff).<br>• General appearance of patient (e.g., development, nutrition, body habitus, deformities attention to grooming) |
| Eyes | • Inspection of conjunctivae and lids<br>• Examination of pupils and irises (e.g., reaction to light and accommodation, size and symmetry)<br>• Ophthalmoscopic examination of optic discs (e.g., size, C/D ratio, appearance) and posterior segments (e.g., vessel changes, exudates, hemorrhages) |
| Ears, nose, mouth, and throat | • External inspection of ears and nose (e.g., overall appearance, scars, lesions, masses)<br>• Otoscopic examination of external auditory canals and tympanic membranes<br>• Assessment of hearing (e.g., whispered voice, finger rub, tuning fork)<br>• Inspection of nasal mucosa, septum and turbinates<br>• Inspection of lips, teeth and gums<br>• Examination of oropharynx: oral mucosa, salivary glands, hard and soft palates, tongue, tonsils and posterior pharynx |
| Neck | • Examination of neck (e.g., masses, overall appearance, symmetry, tracheal position, crepitus)<br>• Examination of thyroid (e.g., enlargement, tenderness, mass) |
| Respiratory | • Assessment of respiratory effort (e.g., intercostal retractions, use of accessory muscles, diaphragmatic movement)<br>• Percussion of chest (e.g., dullness, flatness, hyperresonance)<br>• Palpation of chest (e.g., tactile fremitus)<br>• Auscultation of lungs (e.g., breath sounds, adventitious sounds, rubs) |
| Cardiovascular | • Palpation of heart (e.g., location, size, thrills)<br>• Auscultation of heart with notation of abnormal sounds and murmurs<br>• Examination of:<br>  — carotid arteries (e.g., pulse amplitude, bruits)<br>  — abdominal aorta (e.g., size, bruits)<br>  — femoral arteries (e.g., pulse amplitude, bruits)<br>  — pedal pulses (e.g., pulse amplitude)<br>  — extremities for edema and/or varicosities |
| Chest (Breasts) | • Inspection of breasts (e.g., symmetry, nipple discharge)<br>• Palpation of breasts and axillae (e.g., masses or lumps, tenderness) |
| Gastrointestinal (Abdomen) | • Examination of abdomen with notation of presence of masses or tenderness<br>• Examination of liver and spleen<br>• Examination for presence or absence of hernia<br>• Examination (when indicated) of anus, perineum and rectum, including sphincter tone, presence of hemorrhoids, rectal masses<br>• Obtain stool sample for occult blood test when indicated |
| Genitourinary | **Male:**<br>• Examination of the scrotal contents (e.g., hydrocele, spermatocele, tenderness of cord, testicular mass)<br>• Examination of the penis<br>• Digital rectal examination of prostate gland (e.g., size, symmetry, nodularity tenderness)<br>**Female:**<br>• Pelvic examination (with or without specimen collection for smears and cultures), including:<br>  — examination of external genitalia (e.g., general appearance, hair distribution, lesions) and vagina (e.g., general appearance, estrogen effect, discharge, lesions, pelvic support, cystocele, rectocele)<br>  — examination of urethra (e.g., masses, tenderness, scarring)<br>  — examination of bladder (e.g., fullness, masses, tenderness)<br>• Cervix (e.g., general appearance, lesions, discharge)<br>• Uterus (e.g., size, contour, position, mobility, tenderness, consistency, descent or support)<br>• Adnexa/parametria (e.g., masses, tenderness) |
| Lymphatic | Palpation of lymph nodes in **two or more** areas:<br>• Neck<br>• Groin<br>• Axillae<br>• Other |

CPT © 2017 American Medical Association. All Rights Reserved.

© 2017 Optum360, LLC

| System/Body Area | Elements of Examination |
|---|---|
| Musculoskeletal | • Examination of gait and station *(if circled, add to total at bottom of column to the left)<br>• Inspection and/or palpation of digits and nails (e.g., clubbing, cyanosis, inflammatory conditions, petechiae, ischemia, infections, nodes) *(if circled, add to total at bottom of column to the left)<br>Examination of joints, bones and muscles of **one or more of the following six** areas: 1) head and neck; 2) spine, ribs, and pelvis; 3) right upper extremity; 4) left upper extremity; 5) right lower extremity; and 6) left lower extremity. The examination of a given area includes:<br>• Inspection and/or palpation with notation of presence of any misalignment, asymmetry, crepitation, defects, tenderness, masses, effusions<br>• Assessment of range of motion with notation of any pain, crepitation or contracture<br>• Assessment of stability with notation of any dislocation (luxation), subluxation, or laxity<br>• Assessment of muscle strength and tone (e.g., flaccid, cog wheel, spastic) with notation of any atrophy or abnormal movements |
| Skin | • Inspection of skin and subcutaneous tissue (e.g., rashes, lesions, ulcers)<br>• Palpation of skin and subcutaneous tissue (e.g., induration, subcutaneous nodules, tightening) |
| Neurologic | • Test cranial nerves with notation of any deficits<br>• Examination of deep tendon reflexes with notation of pathological reflexes (e.g., Babinski)<br>• Examination of sensation (e.g., by touch, pin, vibration, proprioception) |
| Psychiatric | • Description of patient's judgment and insight<br>• Brief assessment of mental status including:<br>— Orientation to time, place and person<br>— Recent and remote memory<br>— Mood and affect (e.g., depression, anxiety, agitation) |

### Content and Documentation Requirements

| Level of exam | Perform and document |
|---|---|
| Problem focused | **One to five** elements identified by a bullet. |
| Expanded problem focused | **At least six** elements identified by a bullet. |
| Detailed | **At least 12** elements identified by a bullet, whether in a box with a shaded or unshaded border |
| Comprehensive | Performance of **all** elements identified by a bullet; whether in a box or with a shaded or unshaded box. Documentation of every element in each with a shaded border and at least one element in a box with un shaded border is expected |

| Number of Diagnoses or Management Options | Amount and/or Complexity of Data to be Reviewed | Risk of Complications and/or Morbidity or Mortality | Type of Decision Making |
|---|---|---|---|
| Minimal | Minimal or None | Minimal | Straightforward |
| Limited | Limited | Low | Low Complexity |
| Multiple | Moderate | Moderate | Moderate Complexity |
| Extensive | Extensive | High | High Complexity |

### C. Documentation of the Complexity of Medical Decision Making 1995 and 1997

The levels of E/M services recognize four types of medical decision-making (straightforward, low complexity, moderate complexity, and high complexity). Medical decision-making refers to the complexity of establishing a diagnosis and/or selecting a management option as measured by:

• The number of possible diagnoses and/or the number of management options that must be considered

• The amount and/or complexity of medical records, diagnostic tests, and/or other information that must be obtained, reviewed, and analyzed

• The risk of significant complications, morbidity, and/or mortality, as well as comorbidities, associated with the patient's presenting problem, the diagnostic procedure, and/or the possible management options

The following chart shows the progression of the elements required for each level of medical decision-making. To qualify for a given type of decision-making, two of the three elements in the table must be either met or exceeded.

Each of the elements of medical decision-making is described below.

**Number of Diagnoses or Management Options**

The number of possible diagnoses and/or the number of management options that must be considered is based on the number and types of problems addressed during the encounter, the complexity of establishing a diagnosis, and the management decisions that are made by the physician.

Generally, decision making with respect to a diagnosed problem is easier than that for an identified but undiagnosed problem. The number and type of diagnostic tests employed may be an indicator of the number of possible diagnoses. Problems that are improving or resolving are less complex than those that are worsening or failing to change as expected. The need to seek advice from others is another indicator of complexity of diagnostic or management problems.

• DG: For each encounter, an assessment, clinical impression, or diagnosis should be documented. It may be explicitly stated or implied in documented decisions regarding management plans and/or further evaluation

— For a presenting problem with an established diagnosis, the record should reflect whether the problem is: a) improved, well controlled, resolving, or resolved; or b) inadequately controlled, worsening, or failing to change as expected

— For a presenting problem without an established diagnosis, the assessment or clinical impression may be stated in the form of a differential diagnosis or as a "possible," "probable," or "rule-out" (R/O) diagnosis

- DG: The initiation of, or changes in, treatment should be documented. Treatment includes a wide range of management options including patient instructions, nursing instructions, therapies, and medications

- DG: If referrals are made, consultations requested, or advice sought, the record should indicate to whom or where the referral or consultation is made or from whom the advice is requested

## Amount and/or Complexity of Data to be Reviewed

The amount and complexity of data to be reviewed is based on the types of diagnostic testing ordered or reviewed. A decision to obtain and review old medical records and/or obtain history from sources other than the patient increases the amount and complexity of data to be reviewed.

Discussion of contradictory or unexpected test results with the physician who performed or interpreted the test is an indication of the complexity of data being reviewed. On occasion, the physician who ordered a test may personally review the image, tracing, or specimen to supplement information from the physician who prepared the test report or interpretation; this is another indication of the complexity of data being reviewed.

- DG: If a diagnostic service (test or procedure) is ordered, planned, scheduled, or performed at the time of the E/M encounter, the type of service (e.g., lab or x-ray) should be documented

- DG: The review of lab, radiology, and/or other diagnostic tests should be documented. A simple notation such as WBC elevated" or "chest x-ray unremarkable" is acceptable. Alternatively, the review may be documented by initialing and dating the report containing the test results

- DG: A decision to obtain old records or a decision to obtain additional history from the family, caretaker, or other source to supplement that obtained from the patient should be documented

- DG: Relevant findings from the review of old records and/or the receipt of additional history from the family, caretaker, or other source to supplement that obtained from the patient should be documented. If there is no relevant information beyond that already obtained, that fact should be documented. A notation of "old records reviewed" or "additional history obtained from family" without elaboration is insufficient

- DG: The results of discussion of laboratory, radiology, or other diagnostic tests with the physician who performed or interpreted the study should be documented

- DG: The direct visualization and independent interpretation of an image, tracing, or specimen previously or subsequently interpreted by another physician should be documented

## Risk of Significant Complications, Morbidity, and/or Mortality

The risk of significant complications, morbidity, and/or mortality is based on the risks associated with the presenting problem, the diagnostic procedure, and the possible management options.

- DG: Comorbidities/underlying disease or other factors that increase the complexity of medical decision making by increasing the risk of complications, morbidity, and/or mortality should be documented

- DG: If a surgical or invasive diagnostic procedure is ordered, planned, or scheduled at the time of the E/M encounter, the type of procedure (e.g., laparoscopy) should be documented

- DG: If a surgical or invasive diagnostic procedure is performed at the time of the E/M encounter, the specific procedure should be documented

- DG: The referral for or decision to perform a surgical or invasive diagnostic procedure on an urgent basis should be documented or implied

The following Table of Risk may be used to help determine whether the risk of significant complications, morbidity, and/or mortality is minimal, low, moderate, or high. Because the determination of risk is complex and not readily quantifiable, the table includes common clinical examples rather than absolute measures of risk. The assessment of risk of the presenting problem is based on the risk related to the disease process anticipated between the present encounter and the next one. The assessment of risk of selecting diagnostic procedures and management options is based on the risk during and immediately following any procedures or treatment. The highest level of risk in any one category (presenting problem, diagnostic procedure, or management options) determines the overall risk.

CPT © 2017 American Medical Association. All Rights Reserved.  © 2017 Optum360, LLC

## Table of Risk

| Level of Risk | Presenting Problem(s) | Diagnostic Procedure(s) Ordered | Management Options Selected |
|---|---|---|---|
| Minimal | One self-limited or minor problem (e.g., cold, insect bite, tinea corporis) | Laboratory test requiring veinpuncture<br>Chest x-rays<br>EKG/EEG<br>Urinalysis<br>Ultrasound (e.g., echocardiography)<br>KOH prep | Rest<br>Gargles<br>Elastic bandages<br>Superficial dressings |
| Low | Two or more self-limited or minor problems<br>One stable chronic illness (e.g., well controlled hypertension, non-insulin dependent diabetes, cataract, BPH)<br>Acute, uncomplicated illness or injury (e.g., cystitis, allergic rhinitis, simple sprain) | Physiologic tests not under stress (e.g., pulmonary function tests)<br>Non-cardiovascular imaging studies with contrast (e.g., barium enema)<br>Superficial needle biopsies<br>Clinical laboratory tests requiring arterial puncture<br>Skin biopsies | Over-the-counter drugs<br>Minor surgery with no identified risk factors<br>Physical therapy<br>Occupational therapy<br>IV fluids without additives |
| Moderate | One or more chronic illnesses with mild exacerbation, progression or side effects of treatment<br>Two or more stable chronic illnesses<br>Undiagnosed new problem with uncertain prognosis (e.g., lump in breast)<br>Acute illness with systemic symptoms (e.g., pyelonephritis, pneumonitis, colitis)<br>Acute complicated injury (e.g., head injury with brief loss of consciousness) | Physiologic tests not under stress (e.g., cardiac stress test, fetal contraction stress test)<br>Diagnostic endoscopies with no identified risk factors<br>Deep needle or incisional biopsy<br>Cardiovascular imaging studies with contrast and no identified risk factors (e.g., arteriogram, cardiac catheterization)<br>Obtain fluid from body cavity (e.g., lumbar puncture, thoracentesis, culdocentesis) | Minor surgery with identified risk factors<br>Effective major surgery (open, percutaneous or endoscopic) with no identified risk factors<br>Prescription drug management<br>Therapeutic nuclear medicine<br>IV fluids with additives<br>Closed treatment of fracture or dislocation without manipulation |
| High | One or more chronic illnesses with severe exacerbation, progression or side effects of treatment<br>Acute/chronic illnesses that may pose a threat to life or bodily function (e.g., multiple trauma, acute MI, pulmonary embolus, severe respiratory distress, progressive severe rheumatoid arthritis, psychiatric illness with potential threat to self or others, peritonitis, acute renal failure<br>An abrupt change in neurologic status (e.g., seizure, TIA, weakness or sensory loss) | Cardiovascular imaging studies with contrast with identified risk factors<br>Cardiac electrophysiological tests<br>Diagnostic endoscopies with identified risk factors<br>Discography | Elective major surgery (open, percutaneous or endoscopic) with identified risk factors<br>Emergency major surgery (open, percutaneous or endoscopic)<br>Parenteral controlled substances<br>Drug therapy requiring intensive monitoring for toxicity<br>Decision not to resuscitate or to de-escalate care because of poor prognosis |

### D. Documentation of an Encounter Dominated by Counseling or Coordination of Care

In the case where counseling and/or coordination of care dominates (more than 50 percent) the physician/patient and/or family encounter (face-to-face time in the office or other outpatient setting or floor-unit time in the hospital or nursing facility), time is considered the key or controlling factor to qualify for a particular level of E/M service.

- DG: If the physician elects to report the level of service based on counseling and/or coordination of care, the total length of time of the encounter (face-to-face or floor time, as appropriate) should be documented and the record should describe the counseling and/or activities to coordinate care

# Appendix D — Crosswalk of Deleted Codes

The deleted code crosswalk is meant to be used as a reference tool to find active codes that could be used in place of the deleted code. This will not always be an exact match. Please review the code descriptions and guidelines before selecting a code.

| Code | Cross reference |
|------|-----------------|
| 00740 | To report, see 00731-00732 |
| 00810 | To report, see 00811-00813 |
| 15732 | To report, see 15733 |
| 34800 | To report, see 34701-34708 |
| 34802 | To report, see 34701-34708 |
| 34803 | To report, see 34701-34708 |
| 34804 | To report, see 34701-34708 |
| 34805 | To report, see 34701-34708 |
| 34806 | To report, see 34701-34708 |
| 34825 | To report, see 34709-34711 |
| 34826 | To report, see 34709-34711 |
| 34900 | To report, see 34707-34708 |
| 36515 | To report, see 36516 |
| 55450 | To report, see 55250 |
| 71010 | To report, see 71045 |
| 71015 | To report, see 71045 |
| 71020 | To report, see 71046 |
| 71021 | To report, see 71047 |

| Code | Cross reference |
|------|-----------------|
| 71022 | To report, see 71047-71048 |
| 71023 | To report, see 71046, 76000-76001 |
| 71030 | To report, see 71048 |
| 71034 | To report, see 71048, 76000-76001 |
| 71035 | To report, see 71046-71048 |
| 74000 | To report, see 74018 |
| 74010 | To report, see 74019, 74021 |
| 74020 | To report, see 74019, 74021 |
| 75658 | To report, see 75710 |
| 75952 | To report, see 34701, 34711, 0254T |
| 75953 | To report, see 34701-34711, 0254T |
| 75954 | To report, see 34701-34711, 0254T |
| 94620 | To report, see 94618 |
| 97532 | To report, see 97127 |
| 97762 | To report, see 97763 |
| 99363 | To report, see 93792-93793 |
| 99364 | To report, see 93792-93793 |
| 0051T | To report, see 33927-33929 |

| Code | Cross reference |
|------|-----------------|
| 0052T | To report, see 33927-33929 |
| 0053T | To report, see 33927-33929 |
| 0178T | To report, see 93799 |
| 0179T | To report, see 93799 |
| 0180T | To report, see 93799 |
| 0255T | To report, see 0254T |
| 0299T | To report, see 28899 |
| 0300T | To report, see 28899 |
| 0301T | To report, see 19499 |
| 0309T | To report, see 22899 |
| 0310T | To report, see 64999 |
| 0340T | To report, see 32994 |
| 0438T | To report, see 55874 |

# Appendix E — Resequenced Codes

| Code | Reference |
|------|-----------|
| 11045 | See code following 11042. |
| 11046 | See code following 11043. |
| 21552 | See code following 21555. |
| 21554 | See code following 21556. |
| 22858 | See code following 22856. |
| 22859 | See code following 22854. |
| 23071 | See code following 23075. |
| 23073 | See code following 23076. |
| 24071 | See code following 24075 |
| 24073 | See code following 24076. |
| 25071 | See code following 25075. |
| 25073 | See code following 25076. |
| 26111 | See code following 26115. |
| 26113 | See code following 26116. |
| 27043 | See code following 27047. |
| 27045 | See code following 27048. |
| 27059 | See code following 27049. |
| 27329 | See code following 27360. |
| 27337 | See code following 27327. |
| 27339 | See code following 27328. |
| 27632 | See code following 27618. |
| 27634 | See code following 27619. |
| 28039 | See code following 28043. |
| 28041 | See code following 28045. |
| 28295 | See code following 28296. |
| 29914 | See code following 29863. |
| 29915 | See code following 29863. |
| 29916 | See code before 29866. |
| 31253 | See code following 31255. |
| 31257 | See code following 31255. |
| 31259 | See code following 31255. |
| 31551 | See code following 31580. |
| 31552 | See code following 31580. |
| 31553 | See code following 31580. |
| 31554 | See code following 31580. |
| 31572 | See code following 31578. |
| 31573 | See code following 31578. |
| 31574 | See code following 31578. |
| 31651 | See code following 31647. |
| 32994 | See code following 31255. |
| 33221 | See code following 33213. |
| 33227 | See code following 33233. |
| 33228 | See code following 33233. |
| 33229 | See code before 33234. |
| 33230 | See code following 33240. |
| 33231 | See code before 33241. |
| 33262 | See code following 33241. |
| 33263 | See code following 33241. |
| 33264 | See code before 33243. |
| 33270 | See code following 33249. |
| 33271 | See code following 33249. |
| 33272 | See code following 33249. |
| 33273 | See code following 33249. |
| 33962 | See code following 33959. |
| 33963 | See code following 33959. |

| Code | Reference |
|------|-----------|
| 33964 | See code following 33959. |
| 33965 | See code following 33959. |
| 33966 | See code following 33959. |
| 33969 | See code following 33959. |
| 33984 | See code following 33959. |
| 33985 | See code following 33959. |
| 33986 | See code following 33959. |
| 33987 | See code following 33959. |
| 33988 | See code following 33959. |
| 33989 | See code following 33959. |
| 34812 | See code following 34713. |
| 34820 | See code following 34714. |
| 34833 | See code following 34714. |
| 34834 | See code following 34714. |
| 36465 | See code following 36471. |
| 36466 | See code following 36471. |
| 36482 | See code following 36479. |
| 36483 | See code following 36479. |
| 37211 | See code following 37200. |
| 37212 | See code following 37200. |
| 37213 | See code following 37200. |
| 37214 | See code following 37200. |
| 37246 | See code following 37235. |
| 37247 | See code following 37235. |
| 37248 | See code following 37235. |
| 37249 | See code following 37235. |
| 38243 | See code following 38241. |
| 42310 | See code following 43259. |
| 43211 | See code following 43217. |
| 43212 | See code following 43217. |
| 43213 | See code following 43220. |
| 43214 | See code following 43220. |
| 43233 | Resequenced 43249. |
| 43266 | Resequenced 43255. |
| 43270 | See code following 43257. |
| 43274 | See code following 43265. |
| 43275 | See code following 43265. |
| 43276 | See code following 43265. |
| 43277 | See code before 43273. |
| 43278 | See code before 43273. |
| 44381 | See code following 44382. |
| 44401 | See code following 44392. |
| 45346 | See code following 45338. |
| 45388 | See code following 45382. |
| 45390 | See code following 45392. |
| 45398 | See code following 45393. |
| 45399 | See code before 45990. |
| 46220 | See code before 46230. |
| 46320 | See code following 46230. |
| 46945 | See code following 46221. |
| 46946 | See code following 46221. |
| 46947 | See code following 46762. |
| 50430 | See code following 43259 |
| 50431 | See code following 43259. |
| 50432 | See code following 43259. |

| Code | Reference |
|------|-----------|
| 50433 | See code following 43259. |
| 50434 | See code following 43259. |
| 50435 | See code following 43259. |
| 51797 | See code following 51729. |
| 52356 | See code following 52353. |
| 58674 | See code before 58541. |
| 64461 | See code following 64484. |
| 64462 | See code following 64484. |
| 64463 | See code following 64484. |
| 64633 | See code following 64620. |
| 64634 | See code following 64620. |
| 64635 | See code following 64620. |
| 64636 | See code before 64630. |
| 67810 | See code following 67715. |
| 77085 | See code following 77081. |
| 77086 | See code before 77084. |
| 77295 | See code before 77300. |
| 77385 | See code following 77417. |
| 77386 | See code following 77417. |
| 77387 | See code following 77417. |
| 77424 | See code before 77422. |
| 77425 | See code before 77422. |
| 80081 | See code following 80055. |
| 80164 | See code following 80201. |
| 80165 | See code following 80201. |
| 80171 | See code following 80169. |
| 80305 | See code before 80150. |
| 80306 | See code before 80150. |
| 80307 | See code before 80150. |
| 80320 | See code before 80150. |
| 80321 | See code before 80150. |
| 80322 | See code before 80150. |
| 80323 | See code before 80150. |
| 80324 | See code before 80150. |
| 80325 | See code before 80150. |
| 80326 | See code before 80150. |
| 80327 | See code before 80150. |
| 80328 | See code before 80150. |
| 80329 | See code before 80150. |
| 80330 | See code before 80150. |
| 80331 | See code before 80150. |
| 80332 | See code before 80150. |
| 80333 | See code before 80150. |
| 80334 | See code before 80150. |
| 80335 | See code before 80150. |
| 80336 | See code before 80150. |
| 80337 | See code before 80150. |
| 80338 | See code before 80150. |
| 80339 | See code before 80150. |
| 80340 | See code before 80150. |
| 80341 | See code before 80150. |
| 80342 | See code before 80150. |
| 80343 | See code before 80150. |
| 80344 | See code before 80150. |
| 80345 | See code before 80150. |

| Code | Reference | Code | Reference | Code | Reference |
|------|-----------|------|-----------|------|-----------|
| 80346 | See code before 80150. | 81287 | See code following 81290. | 92944 | See code following 92998. |
| 80347 | See code before 80150. | 81288 | See code following 81292. | 92973 | See code following 92998. |
| 80348 | See code before 80150. | 81334 | See code following 81326. | 92974 | See code following 92998. |
| 80349 | See code before 80150. | 81448 | See code following 81438. | 92975 | See code following 92998. |
| 80350 | See code before 80150. | 81479 | See code following 81408. | 92977 | See code following 92998. |
| 80351 | See code before 80150. | 82042 | See code following 82045. | 92978 | See code following 92998. |
| 80352 | See code before 80150. | 82652 | See code following 82306. | 92979 | See code following 92998. |
| 80353 | See code before 80150. | 83992 | See code following 80365. | 93260 | See code following 93284. |
| 80354 | See code before 80150. | 86152 | See code following 86147. | 93261 | See code following 93289. |
| 80355 | See code before 80150. | 86153 | See code before 86148. | 95249 | See code following 95250. |
| 80356 | See code before 80150. | 87623 | See code following 87539. | 95782 | See code following 95811. |
| 80357 | See code before 80150. | 87624 | See code following 87539. | 95783 | See code following 95811. |
| 80358 | See code before 80150. | 87625 | See code before 87540. | 95800 | See code following 95806. |
| 80359 | See code before 80150. | 87806 | See code following 87803. | 95801 | See code following 95806. |
| 80360 | See code before 80150. | 87906 | See code following 87901. | 95885 | See code following 95872. |
| 80361 | See code before 80150. | 87910 | See code following 87900. | 95886 | See code following 95872. |
| 80362 | See code before 80150. | 87912 | See code before 87902. | 95887 | See code before 95873. |
| 80363 | See code before 80150. | 88177 | See code following 88173. | 95938 | See code following 95926. |
| 80364 | See code before 80150. | 88341 | See code following 88342. | 95939 | See code following 95929. |
| 80365 | See code following 80364. | 88350 | See code following 88346. | 95940 | See code following 95913. |
| 80366 | See code following 83992. | 88364 | See code following 88365. | 95941 | See code following 95913. |
| 80367 | See code following 80366. | 88373 | See code following 88367. | 95943 | See code following 95924. |
| 80368 | See code following 80367. | 88374 | See code following 88367. | 97161 | See code before 97010. |
| 80369 | See code following 80368. | 88377 | See code following 88369. | 97162 | See code before 97010. |
| 80370 | See code following 80369. | 90620 | See code following 90734. | 97163 | See code before 97010. |
| 80371 | See code following 80370. | 90621 | See code following 90734. | 97164 | See code before 97010. |
| 80372 | See code following 80371. | 90625 | See code following 90723. | 97165 | See code before 97010. |
| 80373 | See code following 80372. | 90630 | See code following 90654. | 97166 | See code before 97010. |
| 80374 | See code following 80373. | 90644 | See code following 90732. | 97167 | See code before 97010. |
| 80375 | See code following 80374. | 90672 | See code following 90660. | 97168 | See code before 97010. |
| 80376 | See code following 80375. | 90673 | See code following 90662. | 97169 | See code before 97010. |
| 80377 | See code following 80376. | 90674 | See code following 90661. | 97170 | See code before 97010. |
| 81105 | See code following 81269. | 90750 | See code following 90736 | 97171 | See code before 97010. |
| 81106 | See code following 81269. | 90756 | See code following 90661. | 97172 | See code before 97010. |
| 81107 | See code following 81269. | 92558 | See code following 92586. | 99177 | See code following 99174. |
| 81108 | See code following 81269. | 92597 | See code following 92604. | 99224 | See code following 99220. |
| 81109 | See code following 81269. | 92618 | See code following 92605. | 99225 | See code following 99220. |
| 81110 | See code following 81269. | 92920 | See code following 92998. | 99226 | See code before 99221. |
| 81111 | See code following 81269. | 92921 | See code following 92998. | 99415 | See code following 99359. |
| 81112 | See code following 81269. | 92924 | See code following 92998. | 99416 | See code following 99359. |
| 81120 | See code following 81269. | 92925 | See code following 92998. | 99484 | See code following 99498. |
| 81121 | See code following 81269. | 92928 | See code following 92998. | 99485 | See code following 99467. |
| 81161 | See code before 81232. | 92929 | See code following 92998. | 99486 | See code following 99467. |
| 81162 | See code following 81211. | 92933 | See code following 92998. | 99490 | See code before 99487. |
| 81230 | See code following 81227. | 92934 | See code following 92998. | 0253T | See code following 0195T. |
| 81231 | See code following 81227. | 92937 | See code following 92998. | 0357T | See code following 0058T. |
| 81238 | See code following 81241. | 92938 | See code following 92998. | 0376T | See code following 0191T. |
| 81269 | See code following 81259. | 92941 | See code following 92998. | 0464T | See code following 0333T. |
| 81283 | See code following 81269. | 92943 | See code following 92998. | 0488T | See code following 0403T. |

CPT © 2017 American Medical Association. All Rights Reserved.

© 2017 Optum360, LLC

# Appendix F — Add-on Codes, Modifier 51 Exempt, Optum Modifier 51 Exempt, Modifier 63 Exempt, and Modifier 95 Telemedicine Services

Codes specified as add-on, exempt from modifier 51 and 63, and modifier 95 (telemedicine services) are listed. The lists are designed to be read left to right rather than vertically.

## Add-on Codes

| | | | | | | |
|---|---|---|---|---|---|---|
| 0054T | 0055T | 0076T | 0095T | 0098T | 0159T | 0163T |
| 0164T | 0165T | 0174T | 0189T | 0190T | 01953 | 01968 |
| 01969 | 0196T | 0205T | 0214T | 0215T | 0217T | 0218T |
| 0222T | 0229T | 0231T | 0290T | 0346T | 0361T | 0363T |
| 0365T | 0367T | 0369T | 0374T | 0376T | 0396T | 0397T |
| 0399T | 0437T | 0439T | 0443T | 0450T | 0466T | 0471T |
| 0480T | 0482T | 0492T | 0496T | 10036 | 11001 | 11008 |
| 11045 | 11046 | 11047 | 11101 | 11201 | 11732 | 11922 |
| 13102 | 13122 | 13133 | 13153 | 14302 | 15003 | 15005 |
| 15101 | 15111 | 15116 | 15121 | 15131 | 15136 | 15151 |
| 15152 | 15156 | 15157 | 15201 | 15221 | 15241 | 15261 |
| 15272 | 15274 | 15276 | 15278 | 15777 | 15787 | 15847 |
| 16036 | 17003 | 17312 | 17314 | 17315 | 19001 | 19082 |
| 19084 | 19086 | 19126 | 19282 | 19284 | 19286 | 19288 |
| 19294 | 19297 | 20929 | 20930 | 20931 | 20936 | 20937 |
| 20938 | 20939 | 20985 | 22103 | 22116 | 22208 | 22216 |
| 22226 | 22328 | 22512 | 22515 | 22527 | 22534 | 22552 |
| 22585 | 22614 | 22632 | 22634 | 22840 | 22841 | 22842 |
| 22843 | 22844 | 22845 | 22846 | 22847 | 22848 | 22853 |
| 22854 | 22858 | 22859 | 22868 | 22870 | 26125 | 26861 |
| 26863 | 27358 | 27692 | 29826 | 31627 | 31632 | 31633 |
| 31637 | 31649 | 31651 | 31654 | 32501 | 32506 | 32507 |
| 32667 | 32668 | 32674 | 33141 | 33225 | 33257 | 33258 |
| 33259 | 33367 | 33368 | 33369 | 33419 | 33508 | 33517 |
| 33518 | 33519 | 33521 | 33522 | 33523 | 33530 | 33572 |
| 33768 | 33884 | 33924 | 33929 | 33987 | 34709 | 34711 |
| 34713 | 34714 | 34715 | 34716 | 34808 | 34812 | 34813 |
| 34820 | 34833 | 34834 | 35306 | 35390 | 35400 | 35500 |
| 35572 | 35600 | 35681 | 35682 | 35683 | 35685 | 35686 |
| 35697 | 35700 | 36218 | 36227 | 36228 | 36248 | 36474 |
| 36476 | 36479 | 36483 | 36907 | 36908 | 36909 | 37185 |
| 37186 | 37222 | 37223 | 37232 | 37233 | 37234 | 37235 |
| 37237 | 37239 | 37247 | 37249 | 37252 | 37253 | 38102 |
| 38746 | 38747 | 38900 | 43273 | 43283 | 43338 | 43635 |
| 44015 | 44121 | 44128 | 44139 | 44203 | 44213 | 44701 |
| 44955 | 47001 | 47542 | 47543 | 47544 | 47550 | 48400 |
| 49326 | 49327 | 49412 | 49435 | 49568 | 49905 | 50606 |
| 50705 | 50706 | 51797 | 52442 | 56606 | 57267 | 58110 |
| 58611 | 59525 | 60512 | 61316 | 61517 | 61610 | 61611 |
| 61612 | 61641 | 61642 | 61651 | 61781 | 61782 | 61783 |
| 61797 | 61799 | 61800 | 61864 | 61868 | 62148 | 62160 |
| 63035 | 63043 | 63044 | 63048 | 63057 | 63066 | 63076 |
| 63078 | 63082 | 63086 | 63088 | 63091 | 63103 | 63295 |
| 63308 | 63621 | 64462 | 64480 | 64484 | 64491 | 64492 |
| 64494 | 64495 | 64634 | 64636 | 64643 | 64645 | 64727 |
| 64778 | 64783 | 64787 | 64832 | 64837 | 64859 | 64872 |
| 64874 | 64876 | 64901 | 64902 | 64913 | 65757 | 66990 |
| 67225 | 67320 | 67331 | 67332 | 67334 | 67335 | 67340 |
| 69990 | 74301 | 74713 | 75565 | 75774 | 76125 | 76802 |
| 76810 | 76812 | 76814 | 76937 | 77001 | 77002 | 77003 |
| 77063 | 77293 | 78020 | 78496 | 78730 | 81266 | 81416 |
| 81426 | 81536 | 82952 | 86826 | 87187 | 87503 | 87904 |
| 88155 | 88177 | 88185 | 88311 | 88314 | 88332 | 88334 |
| 88341 | 88350 | 88364 | 88369 | 88373 | 88388 | 90461 |
| 90472 | 90474 | 90785 | 90833 | 90836 | 90838 | 90840 |
| 90863 | 91013 | 92547 | 92608 | 92618 | 92621 | 92627 |
| 92921 | 92925 | 92929 | 92934 | 92938 | 92944 | 92973 |
| 92974 | 92978 | 92979 | 92998 | 93320 | 93321 | 93325 |
| 93352 | 93462 | 93463 | 93464 | 93563 | 93564 | 93565 |
| 93566 | 93567 | 93568 | 93571 | 93572 | 93592 | 93609 |
| 93613 | 93621 | 93622 | 93623 | 93655 | 93657 | 93662 |
| 94645 | 94729 | 94781 | 95079 | 95873 | 95874 | 95885 |
| 95886 | 95887 | 95940 | 95941 | 95962 | 95967 | 95975 |
| 95979 | 96361 | 96366 | 96367 | 96368 | 96370 | 96371 |
| 96375 | 96376 | 96411 | 96415 | 96417 | 96423 | 96570 |
| 96571 | 96934 | 96935 | 96936 | 97546 | 97598 | 97811 |
| 97814 | 99100 | 99116 | 99135 | 99140 | 99153 | 99157 |
| 99292 | 99354 | 99355 | 99356 | 99357 | 99359 | 99415 |
| 99416 | 99467 | 99486 | 99489 | 99494 | 99498 | 99602 |
| 99607 | | | | | | |

## AMA Modifer 51 Exempt Codes

| | | | | | | |
|---|---|---|---|---|---|---|
| 17004 | 20697 | 20974 | 20975 | 31500 | 36620 | 44500 |
| 61107 | 93451 | 93456 | 93503 | 93600 | 93602 | 93603 |
| 93610 | 93612 | 93615 | 93616 | 93618 | 93631 | 94610 |
| 95905 | 95992 | 99151 | 99152 | | | |

## Modifier 63 Exempt Codes

| | | | | | | |
|---|---|---|---|---|---|---|
| 30540 | 30545 | 31520 | 33470 | 33502 | 33503 | 33505 |
| 33506 | 33610 | 33611 | 33619 | 33647 | 33670 | 33690 |
| 33694 | 33730 | 33732 | 33735 | 33736 | 33750 | 33755 |
| 33762 | 33778 | 33786 | 33922 | 33946 | 33947 | 33948 |
| 33949 | 36415 | 36420 | 36450 | 36456 | 36460 | 36510 |
| 36660 | 39503 | 43313 | 43314 | 43520 | 43831 | 44055 |
| 44126 | 44127 | 44128 | 46070 | 46705 | 46715 | 46716 |
| 46730 | 46735 | 46740 | 46742 | 46744 | 47700 | 47701 |
| 49215 | 49491 | 49492 | 49495 | 49496 | 49600 | 49605 |
| 49606 | 49610 | 49611 | 53025 | 54000 | 54150 | 54160 |
| 63700 | 63702 | 63704 | 63706 | 65820 | | |

## Optum Modifier 51 Exempt Codes

| | | | | | | |
|---|---|---|---|---|---|---|
| 90281 | 90283 | 90284 | 90287 | 90288 | 90291 | 90296 |
| 90371 | 90375 | 90376 | 90378 | 90384 | 90385 | 90386 |
| 90389 | 90393 | 90396 | 90399 | 90476 | 90477 | 90581 |
| 90585 | 90586 | 90620 | 90621 | 90625 | 90630 | 90632 |
| 90633 | 90634 | 90636 | 90644 | 90647 | 90648 | 90649 |
| 90650 | 90651 | 90653 | 90654 | 90655 | 90656 | 90657 |
| 90658 | 90660 | 90661 | 90662 | 90664 | 90666 | 90667 |
| 90668 | 90670 | 90672 | 90673 | 90674 | 90675 | 90676 |
| 90680 | 90681 | 90685 | 90686 | 90687 | 90688 | 90690 |
| 90691 | 90696 | 90697 | 90698 | 90700 | 90702 | 90707 |
| 90710 | 90713 | 90714 | 90715 | 90716 | 90717 | 90723 |
| 90732 | 90733 | 90734 | 90736 | 90738 | 90739 | 90740 |
| 90743 | 90744 | 90746 | 90747 | 90748 | 90749 | 90750 |
| 97010 | 97012 | 97014 | 97016 | 97018 | 97022 | 97024 |
| 97026 | 97028 | 97032 | 97033 | 97034 | 97035 | 97036 |
| 97110 | 97112 | 97113 | 97116 | 97124 | 97140 | 97150 |
| 97530 | 97532 | 97533 | 97535 | 97537 | 97542 | 97545 |
| 97546 | 97597 | 97598 | 97602 | 97605 | 97606 | 97607 |
| 97608 | 97610 | 97750 | 97755 | 97760 | 97761 | 97762 |
| 97763 | 99050 | 99051 | 99053 | 99056 | 99058 | 99060 |

## Telemedicine Services Codes

The codes on the following list may be used to report telemedicine services when modifier 95 Synchronous Telemedicine Service Rendered via a Real-Time Interactive Audio and Visual Telecommunications System, is appended.

| | | | | | | |
|---|---|---|---|---|---|---|
| 0188T | 0189T | 90791 | 90792 | 90832 | 90833 | 90834 |
| 90836 | 90837 | 90838 | 90845 | 90846 | 90847 | 90863 |
| 90951 | 90952 | 90954 | 90955 | 90957 | 90958 | 90960 |
| 90961 | 92227 | 92228 | 93228 | 93229 | 93268 | 93270 |
| 93271 | 93272 | 93298 | 93299 | 96040 | 96116 | 96150 |
| 96151 | 96152 | 96153 | 96154 | 97802 | 97803 | 97804 |
| 98960 | 98961 | 98962 | 99201 | 99202 | 99203 | 99204 |
| 99205 | 99212 | 99213 | 99214 | 99215 | 99231 | 99232 |
| 99233 | *99241 | *99242 | *99243 | *99244 | *99245 | *99251 |
| *99252 | *99253 | *99254 | *99255 | 99307 | 99308 | 99309 |
| 99310 | 99354 | 99355 | 99406 | 99407 | 99408 | 99409 |
| 99495 | 99496 | | | | | |

* Consultations are noncovered by Medicare

# Appendix G — Medicare Internet-only Manuals (IOMs)

The Centers for Medicare and Medicaid Services restructured its paper-based manual system as a web-based system on October 1, 2003. Called the online CMS manual system, it combines all of the various program instructions into internet-only manuals (IOMs), which are used by all CMS programs and contractors. In many instances, the references from the online manuals in appendix G contain a mention of the old paper manuals from which the current information was obtained when the manuals were converted. This information is shown in the header of the text, in the following format, when applicable, as A3-3101, HO-210, and B3-2049. Complete versions of all of the manuals can be found at https://www.cms.gov/Regulations-and-Guidance/Guidance/Manuals/Internet-Only-Manuals-IOMs.html.

Effective with implementation of the IOMs, the former method of publishing program memoranda (PMs) to communicate program instructions was replaced by the following four templates:

- One-time notification
- Manual revisions
- Business requirements
- Confidential requirements

The web-based system has been organized by functional area (e.g., eligibility, entitlement, claims processing, benefit policy, program integrity) in an effort to eliminate redundancy within the manuals, simplify updating, and make CMS program instructions available more quickly. The web-based system contains the functional areas included below:

| Pub. 100 | Introduction |
| --- | --- |
| Pub. 100-01 | Medicare General Information, Eligibility, and Entitlement Manual |
| Pub. 100-02 | Medicare Benefit Policy Manual |
| Pub. 100-03 | Medicare National Coverage Determinations (NCD) Manual |
| Pub. 100-04 | Medicare Claims Processing Manual |
| Pub. 100-05 | Medicare Secondary Payer Manual |
| Pub. 100-06 | Medicare Financial Management Manual |
| Pub. 100-07 | State Operations Manual |
| Pub. 100-08 | Medicare Program Integrity Manual |
| Pub. 100-09 | Medicare Contractor Beneficiary and Provider Communications Manual |
| Pub. 100-10 | Quality Improvement Organization Manual |
| Pub. 100-11 | Programs of All-Inclusive Care for the Elderly (PACE) Manual |
| Pub. 100-12 | State Medicaid Manual (under development) |
| Pub. 100-13 | Medicaid State Children's Health Insurance Program (under development) |
| Pub. 100-14 | Medicare ESRD Network Organizations Manual |
| Pub. 100-15 | Medicaid Integrity Program (MIP) |
| Pub. 100-16 | Medicare Managed Care Manual |
| Pub. 100-17 | CMS/Business Partners Systems Security Manual |
| Pub. 100-18 | Medicare Prescription Drug Benefit Manual |
| Pub. 100-19 | Demonstrations |
| Pub. 100-20 | One-Time Notification |
| Pub. 100-21 | Recurring Update Notification |
| Pub. 100-22 | Medicare Quality Reporting Incentive Programs Manual |
| Pub. 100-24 | State Buy-In Manual |
| Pub. 100-25 | Information Security Acceptable Risk Safeguards Manual |

A brief description of the Medicare manuals primarily used for *CPC Expert* follows:

The *National Coverage Determinations Manual* (NCD), is organized according to categories such as diagnostic services, supplies, and medical procedures. The table of contents lists each category and subject within that category. Revision transmittals identify any new or background material, recap the changes, and provide an effective date for the change.

When complete, the manual will contain two chapters. Chapter 1 currently includes a description of CMS's national coverage determinations. When available, chapter 2 will contain a list of HCPCS codes related to each coverage determination. The manual is organized in accordance with CPT category sequences.

The *Medicare Benefit Policy Manual* contains Medicare general coverage instructions that are not national coverage determinations. As a general rule, in the past these instructions have been found in chapter II of the *Medicare Carriers Manual,* the *Medicare Intermediary Manual*, other provider manuals, and program memoranda.

The *Medicare Claims Processing Manual* contains instructions for processing claims for contractors and providers.

The *Medicare Program Integrity Manual* communicates the priorities and standards for the Medicare integrity programs.

## Medicare IOM references

### 100-01, 3, 20.5

**Blood Deductibles (Part A and Part B)**

Program payment may not be made for the first 3 pints of whole blood or equivalent units of packed red cells received under Part A and Part B combined in a calendar year. However, blood processing (e.g., administration, storage) is not subject to the deductible.

The blood deductibles are in addition to any other applicable deductible and coinsurance amounts for which the patient is responsible.

The deductible applies only to the first 3 pints of blood furnished in a calendar year, even if more than one provider furnished blood.

### 100-01, 5, 70.6

**Chiropractors**

**A. General**

A licensed chiropractor who meets uniform minimum standards (see subsection C) is a physician for specified services. Coverage extends only to treatment by means of manual manipulation of the spine to correct a subluxation demonstrated by X-ray, provided such treatment is legal in the State where performed. All other services furnished or ordered by chiropractors are not covered. An X-ray obtained by a chiropractor for his or her own diagnostic purposes before commencing treatment may suffice for claims documentation purposes. This means that if a chiropractor orders, takes, or interprets an X-ray to demonstrate a subluxation of the spine, the X-ray can be used for claims processing purposes. However, there is no coverage or payment for these services or for any other diagnostic or therapeutic service ordered or furnished by the chiropractor. In addition, in performing manual manipulation of the spine, some chiropractors use manual devices that are hand-held with the thrust of the force of the device being controlled manually. While such manual manipulation may be covered, there is no separate payment permitted for use of this device.

**B. Licensure and Authorization to Practice**

A chiropractor must be licensed or legally authorized to furnish chiropractic services by the State or jurisdiction in which the services are furnished.

**C. Uniform Minimum Standards**

I. Prior to July 1, 1974, Chiropractors licensed or authorized to practice prior to July 1, 1974, and those individuals who commenced their studies in a chiropractic college before that date must meet all of the following minimum standards to render payable services under the program:

  a. Preliminary education equal to the requirements for graduation from an accredited high school or other secondary school;

  b. Graduation from a college of chiropractic approved by the State's chiropractic examiners that included the completion of a course of study covering a period of not less than 3 school years of 6 months each year in actual continuous attendance covering adequate course of study in the subjects of anatomy, physiology, symptomatology and diagnosis, hygiene and sanitation, chemistry, histology, pathology, and principles and practice of chiropractic, including clinical instruction in vertebral palpation, nerve tracing and adjusting; and

c. Passage of an examination prescribed by the State's chiropractic examiners covering the subjects listed in subsection b.

2. After June 30, 1974 - Individuals commencing their studies in a chiropractic college after June 30, 1974, must meet all of the following additional requirements:

a. Satisfactory completion of 2 years of pre-chiropractic study at the college level;

b. Satisfactory completion of a 4-year course of 8 months each year (instead of a 3-year course of 6 months each year) at a college or school of chiropractic that includes not less than 4,000 hours in the scientific and chiropractic courses specified in subsection1.b, plus courses in the use and effect of X-ray and chiropractic analysis; and

c. The practitioner must be over 21 years of age.

## 100-02, 1, 90
### Termination of Pregnancy
B3-4276.1,.2

Effective for services furnished on or after October 1, 1998, Medicare will cover abortions procedures in the following situations:

1. If the pregnancy is the result of an act or rape or incest; or

2. In the case where a woman suffers from a physical disorder, physical injury, or physical illness, including a life-endangering physical condition caused by the pregnancy itself that would, as certified by a physician, place the woman in danger of death unless an abortion is performed.

NOTE: The "G7" modifier must be used with the following CPT codes in order for these services to be covered when the pregnancy resulted from rape or incest, or the pregnancy is certified by a physician as life threatening to the mother:

59840, 59841, 59850, 59851, 59852, 59855, 59856, 59857, 59866

## 100-02, 1, 100
### Treatment for Infertility
A3-3101.13

Effective for services rendered on or after January 15, 1980, reasonable and necessary services associated with treatment for infertility are covered under Medicare. Like pregnancy (see Sec. 80 above), infertility is a condition sufficiently at variance with the usual state of health to make it appropriate for a person who normally would be expected to be fertile to seek medical consultation and treatment. Contractors should coordinate with QIOs to see that utilization guidelines are established for this treatment if inappropriate utilization or abuse is suspected.

## 100-02, 11, 20
### Renal Dialysis Items and Services
Medicare provides payment under the ESRD PPS for all renal dialysis services for outpatient maintenance dialysis when they are furnished to Medicare ESRD patients for the treatment of ESRD by a Medicare certified ESRD facility or a special purpose dialysis facility. Renal dialysis services are the items and services included under the composite rate and the ESRD-related items and services that were separately paid as of December 31, 2010 that were used for the treatment of ESRD.

Renal dialysis services are furnished in various settings including hospital outpatient ESRD facilities, independent ESRD facilities, or in the patient's home. Renal dialysis items and services furnished at ESRD facilities differ according to the types of patients being treated, the types of equipment and supplies used, the preferences of the treating physician, and the capability and makeup of the staff. Although not all facilities provide an identical range of services, the most common elements of dialysis treatment include:

- Laboratory Tests;

- Drugs and Biologicals;

- Equipment and supplies - dialysis machine use and maintenance;

- Personnel services;

- Administrative services;

- Overhead costs;

- Monitoring access and related declotting or referring the patient, and

- Direct nursing services include registered nurses, licensed practical nurses, technicians, social workers, and dietitians.

## 100-02, 11, 20.2
### Laboratory Services
All laboratory services furnished to individuals for the treatment of ESRD are included in the ESRD PPS as Part B services and are not paid separately as of January 1, 2011. The laboratory services include but are not limited to:

- Laboratory tests included under the composite rate as of December 31, 2010 (discussed below); and

- Former separately billable Part B laboratory tests that were billed by ESRD facilities and independent laboratories for ESRD patients.

Composite rate laboratory tests are listed in §20.2.E of this chapter. More information regarding composite rate laboratory tests can be found in Pub. 100-4, Medicare Claims Processing Manual, chapter 8, §50.1, §60.1, and §80. As discussed below, composite rate laboratory services should not be reported on claims.

The distinction of what is considered to be a renal dialysis laboratory test is a clinical decision determined by the ESRD patient's ordering practitioner. If a laboratory test is ordered for the treatment of ESRD, then the laboratory test is not paid separately.

Payment for all renal dialysis laboratory tests furnished under the ESRD PPS is made directly to the ESRD facility responsible for the patient's care. The ESRD facility must furnish the laboratory tests directly or under arrangement and report renal dialysis laboratory tests on the ESRD facility claim (with the exception of composite rate laboratory services).

An ESRD facility must report renal dialysis laboratory services on its claims in order for the laboratory tests to be included in the outlier payment calculation. Renal dialysis laboratory services that were or would have been paid separately under Medicare Part B prior to January 1, 2011, are priced for the outlier payment calculation using the Clinical Laboratory Fee Schedule. Further information regarding the outlier policy can be found in §60.D of this chapter.

Certain laboratory services will be subject to Part B consolidated billing requirements and will no longer be separately payable when provided to ESRD beneficiaries by providers other than the renal dialysis facility. The list below includes the renal dialysis laboratory tests that are routinely performed for the treatment of ESRD. Payment for the laboratory tests identified on this list is included in the ESRD PPS. The laboratory tests listed in the table are used to enforce consolidated billing edits to ensure that payment is not made for renal dialysis laboratory tests outside of the ESRD PPS. The list of renal dialysis laboratory tests is not an all-inclusive list. If any laboratory test is ordered for the treatment of ESRD, then the laboratory test is considered to be included in the ESRD PPS and is the responsibility of the ESRD facility. Additional renal dialysis laboratory tests may be added through administrative issuances in the future.

LABS SUBJECT TO ESRD CONSOLIDATED BILLING

| CPT/ HCPCS | Short Description |
|---|---|
| 80047 | Basic Metabolic Panel (Calcium, ionized) |
| 80048 | Basic Metabolic Panel (Calcium, total) |
| 80051 | Electrolyte Panel |
| 80053 | Comprehensive Metabolic Panel |
| 80061 | Lipid Panel |
| 80069 | Renal Function Panel |
| 80076 | Hepatic Function Panel |
| 82040 | Assay of serum albumin |
| 82108 | Assay of aluminum |
| 82306 | Vitamin d, 25 hydroxy |
| 82310 | Assay of calcium |
| 82330 | Assay of calcium, Ionized |
| 82374 | Assay, blood carbon dioxide |
| 82379 | Assay of carnitine |
| 82435 | Assay of blood chloride |
| 82565 | Assay of creatinine |
| 82570 | Assay of urine creatinine |
| 82575 | Creatinine clearance test |
| 82607 | Vitamin B-12 |
| 82652 | Vit d 1, 25-dihydroxy |
| 82668 | Assay of erythropoietin |
| 82728 | Assay of ferritin |
| 82746 | Blood folic acid serum |
| 83540 | Assay of iron |
| 83550 | Iron binding test |
| 83735 | Assay of magnesium |
| 83970 | Assay of parathormone |
| 84075 | Assay alkaline phosphatase |
| 84100 | Assay of phosphorus |
| 84132 | Assay of serum potassium |
| 84134 | Assay of prealbumin |

CPT © 2017 American Medical Association. All Rights Reserved.

© 2017 Optum360, LLC

| CPT/ HCPCS | Short Description |
|---|---|
| 84155 | Assay of protein, serum |
| 84157 | Assay of protein by other source |
| 84295 | Assay of serum sodium |
| 84466 | Assay of transferrin |
| 84520 | Assay of urea nitrogen |
| 84540 | Assay of urine/urea-n |
| 84545 | Urea-N clearance test |
| 85014 | Hematocrit |
| 85018 | Hemoglobin |
| 85025 | Complete (cbc), automated (HgB, Hct, RBC, WBC, and Platelet count) and automated differential WBC count. |
| 85027 | Complete (cbc), automated (HgB, Hct, RBC, WBC, and Platelet count) |
| 85041 | Automated rbc count |
| 85044 | Manual reticulocyte count |
| 85045 | Automated reticulocyte count |
| 85046 | Reticyte/hgb concentrate |
| 85048 | Automated leukocyte count |
| 86704 | Hep b core antibody, total |
| 86705 | Hep b core antibody, igm |
| 86706 | Hep b surface antibody |
| 87040 | Blood culture for bacteria |
| 87070 | Culture, bacteria, other |
| 87071 | Culture bacteri aerobic othr |
| 87073 | Culture bacteria anaerobic |
| 87075 | Cultr bacteria, except blood |
| 87076 | Culture anaerobe ident, each |
| 87077 | Culture aerobic identify |
| 87081 | Culture screen only |
| 87340 | Hepatitis b surface ag, eia |
| G0306 | CBC/diff wbc w/o platelet |
| G0307 | CBC without platelet |

### A. Automated Multi-Channel Chemistry (AMCC) Tests

During the ESRD PPS transition period (see §70 of this chapter) ESRD facilities are required to report the renal dialysis AMCC tests with the appropriate modifiers (CD, CE, or CF) on their claims for purposes of applying the 50/50 rule under the composite rate portion of the blended payment. Refer to §70.B of this chapter for additional information regarding the composite rate portion of the blended payment during the transition.

The 50/50 rule is necessary for those ESRD facilities that chose to go through the transition period. If the 50/50 rule allows for separate payment, then the laboratory tests are priced using the clinical laboratory fee schedule. Information regarding the 50/50 rule can be found in §20.2.E of this chapter and in Pub. 100-4, Medicare Claims Processing Manual, chapter 16, §40.6.

NOTE: An ESRD facility billing a renal dialysis AMCC test must use the CF modifier when the AMCC is not in the composite rate but is a renal dialysis service. AMCC tests that are furnished to individuals for reasons other than for the treatment of ESRD should be billed with the AY modifier to Medicare directly by the entity furnishing the service with the AY modifier.

### B. Laboratory Services Furnished for Reasons Other Than for the Treatment of ESRD

#### 1. Independent Laboratory

A patient's physician or practitioner may order a laboratory test that is included on the list of items and services subject to consolidated billing edits for reasons other than for the treatment of ESRD. When this occurs, the patient's physician or practitioner should notify the independent laboratory or the ESRD facility (with the appropriate clinical laboratory certification in accordance with the Clinical Laboratory Improvement Act) that furnished the laboratory service that the test is not a renal dialysis service and that entity may bill Medicare separately using the AY modifier. The AY modifier serves as an attestation that the item or service is medically necessary for the patient but is not being used for the treatment of ESRD.

#### 2. Hospital-Based Laboratory

Hospital outpatient clinical laboratories furnishing renal dialysis laboratory tests to ESRD patients for reasons other than for the treatment of ESRD may submit a claim for separate payment using the AY modifier. The AY modifier serves as an attestation that the item or service is medically necessary for the patient but is not being used for the treatment of ESRD.

### C. Laboratory Services Performed in Emergency Rooms or Emergency Departments

In an emergency room or emergency department, the ordering physician or practitioner may not know at the time the laboratory test is being ordered, if it is being ordered as a renal dialysis service. Consequently, emergency rooms or

emergency departments are not required to append an AY modifier to these laboratory tests when submitting claims with dates of service on or after January 1, 2012.

When a renal dialysis laboratory service is furnished to an ESRD patient in an emergency room or emergency department on a different date of service, hospitals can append an ET modifier to the laboratory tests furnished to ESRD patients to indicate that the laboratory test was furnished in conjunction with the emergency visit. Appending the ET modifier indicates that the laboratory service being furnished on a day other than the emergency visit is related to the emergency visit and at the time the ordering physician was unable to determine if the test was ordered for reasons of treating the patient's ESRD.

Allowing laboratory testing to bypass consolidated billing edits in the emergency room or department does not mean that ESRD facilities should send patients to other settings for routine laboratory testing for the purpose of not assuming financial responsibility of renal dialysis items and services. For additional information regarding laboratory services furnished in a variety of settings, see Pub. 100-4, Medicare Claims Processing Manual, chapter 16, §30.3 and §40.6.

### D. Hepatitis B Laboratory Services for Transient Patients

Laboratory testing for hepatitis B is a renal dialysis service. Effective January 1, 2011, hepatitis B testing is included in the ESRD PPS and therefore cannot be billed separately to Medicare.

The Conditions for Coverage for ESRD facilities require routine hepatitis B testing (42 CFR §494.30(a)(1)). The ESRD facility is responsible for the payment of the laboratory test, regardless of frequency. If an ESRD patient wishes to travel, the patient's home ESRD facility should have systems in place for communicating hepatitis B test results to the destination ESRD facility.

### E. Laboratory Services Included Under Composite Rate

Prior to the implementation of the ESRD PPS, the costs of certain ESRD laboratory services furnished for outpatient maintenance dialysis by either the ESRD facility's staff or an independent laboratory, were included in the composite rate calculations. Therefore, payment for all of these laboratory tests was included in the ESRD facility's composite rate and the tests could not have been billed separately to the Medicare program.

All laboratory services that were included under the composite rate are included under the ESRD PPS unless otherwise specified. Payments for these laboratory tests are included in the ESRD PPS and are not paid separately under the composite rate portion of the blended payment and are not eligible for outlier payments. Therefore, composite rate laboratory services should not be reported on the claim. Laboratory tests included in the composite payment rate are identified below.

#### 1. Routinely Covered Tests Paid Under Composite Rate

The tests listed below are usually performed for dialysis patients and were routinely covered at the frequency specified in the absence of indications to the contrary, (i.e., no documentation of medical necessity was required other than knowledge of the patient's status as an ESRD beneficiary). When any of these tests were performed at a frequency greater than that specified, the additional tests were separately billable and were covered only if they were medically justified by accompanying documentation. A diagnosis of ESRD alone was not sufficient medical evidence to warrant coverage of the additional tests. The nature of the illness or injury (diagnosis, complaint, or symptom) requiring the performance of the test(s) must have been present, along with ICD diagnosis coding, on the claim for payment.

   a. Hemodialysis, IPD, CCPD, and Hemofiltration

   - Per Treatment - All hematocrit, hemoglobin, and clotting time tests furnished incident to dialysis treatments;

   - Weekly - Prothrombin time for patients on anticoagulant therapy and Serum Creatinine;

   - Weekly or Thirteen Per Quarter - BUN;

   - Monthly - Serum Calcium, Serum Potassium, Serum Chloride, CBC, Serum Bicarbonate, Serum Phosphorous, Total Protein, Serum Albumin, Alkaline Phosphatase, aspartate amino transferase (AST) (SGOT) and LDH; and

   - Automated Multi-Channel Chemistry (AMCC) - If an automated battery of tests, such as the SMA-12, is performed and contains most of the tests listed in one of the weekly or monthly categories, it is not necessary to separately identify any tests in the battery that are not listed. Further information concerning automated tests and the "50 percent rule" can be found below and in Pub. 100-4, Medicare Claims Processing Manual, chapter 16, §40.6.1.

   b. CAPD

   - Monthly – BUN, Creatinine, Sodium, Potassium, CO2, Calcium, Magnesium, Phosphate, Total Protein, Albumin, Alkaline Phosphatase, LDH, AST, SGOT, HCT, Hbg, and Dialysate Protein.

Under the ESRD PPS, frequency requirements do not apply for the purpose of payment. However, laboratory tests should be ordered as necessary and should not be restricted because of financial reasons.

#### 2. Separately Billable Tests Under the Composite Rate

The following list identifies certain separately billable laboratory tests that were covered routinely and without documentation of medical necessity other than knowledge of the patient's status as an ESRD beneficiary, when furnished at specified frequencies. If they were performed at a frequency greater than that specified, they were covered only if accompanied by medical documentation. A diagnosis of ESRD alone was not sufficient documentation. The medical necessity of the test(s), the nature of the illness or injury (diagnosis, complaint or symptom) requiring the performance of the test(s) must have been furnished on claims using the ICD diagnosis coding system.

— Separately Billable Tests for Hemodialysis, IPD, CCPD, and Hemofiltration

Serum Aluminum - one every 3 months

Serum Ferritin - one every 3 months

— Separately Billable Tests for CAPD

WBC, RBC, and Platelet count – One every 3 months

Residual renal function and 24 hour urine volume – One every 6 months

Under the ESRD PPS frequency requirements do not apply for the purpose of payment. However, laboratory tests should be ordered as necessary and should not be restricted because of financial reasons.

**3. Automated Multi-Channel Chemistry (AMCC) Tests Under the Composite Rate**

Clinical diagnostic laboratory tests that comprise the AMCC (listed in Appendix A and B) could be considered to be composite rate and non-composite rate laboratory services. Composite rate payment was paid by the A/B MAC (A). To determine if separate payment was allowed for non-composite rate tests for a particular date of service, 50 percent or more of the covered tests must be non-composite rate tests. This policy also applies to the composite rate portion of the blended payment during the transition. Beginning January 1, 2014, the 50 percent rule will no longer apply and no separate payment will be made under the composite rate portion of the blended payment.

Medicare applied the following to AMCC tests for ESRD beneficiaries:

— Payment was the lowest rate for services performed by the same provider, for the same beneficiary, for the same date of service.

— The A/B MAC identified, for a particular date of service, the AMCC tests ordered that were included in the composite rate and those that were not included. The composite rate tests were defined for Hemodialysis, IPD, CCPD, and Hemofiltration (see Appendix A) and for CAPD (see Appendix B).

— If 50 percent or more of the covered tests were included under the composite rate payment, then all submitted tests were included within the composite payment. In this case, no separate payment in addition to the composite rate was made for any of the separately billable tests.

— If less than 50 percent of the covered tests were composite rate tests, all AMCC tests submitted for that Date of Service (DOS) were separately payable.

— A non-composite rate test was defined as any test separately payable outside of the composite rate or beyond the normal frequency covered under the composite rate that was reasonable and necessary.

Three pricing modifiers identify the different payment situations for ESRD AMCC tests. The physician who ordered the tests was responsible for identifying the appropriate modifier when ordering the tests.

— CD - AMCC test had been ordered by an ESRD facility or Medicare capitation payment (MCP) physician that was part of the composite rate and was not separately billable

— CE - AMCC test had been ordered by an ESRD facility or MCP physician that was a composite rate test but was beyond the normal frequency covered under the rate and was separately reimbursable based on medical necessity

— CF - AMCC test had been ordered by an ESRD facility or MCP physician that was not part of the composite rate and was separately billable

The ESRD clinical diagnostic laboratory tests identified with modifiers "CD", "CE" or "CF" may not have been billed as organ or disease panels. Effective October 1, 2003, all ESRD clinical diagnostic laboratory tests must be billed individually. See Pub. 100-4, Medicare Claims Processing Manual, chapter 16, §40.6.1, for additional billing and payment instructions as well as examples of the 50/50 rule.

For ESRD dialysis patients, CPT code 82330 Calcium; ionized shall be included in the calculation for the 50/50 rule (Pub. 100-4, Medicare Claims Processing Manual, chapter 16, §40.6.1). When CPT code 82330 is billed as a substitute for CPT code 82310, Calcium; total, it shall be billed with modifier CD or CE. When CPT code 82330 is billed in addition to CPT 82310, it shall be billed with CF modifier.

## 100-2, 13, 220

### Preventive Health Services

(Rev. 230, Issued: 12-09-16, Effective: 03-09-17, Implementation: 03-09-17)

RHCs and FQHCs are paid for the professional component of allowable preventive services when all of the program requirements are met and frequency limits (where applicable) have not been exceeded. The beneficiary copayment and deductible (where applicable) is waived by the Affordable Care Act for the IPPE and AWV, and for Medicare-covered preventive services recommended by the USPSTF with a grade or A or B.

## 100-2, 13, 220.1

### Preventive Health Services in RHCs

(Rev. 230, Issued: 12-09-16, Effective: 03-09-17, Implementation: 03-09-17)

Influenza (G0008) and Pneumococcal Vaccines (G0009)

Influenza and pneumococcal vaccines and their administration are paid at 100 percent of reasonable cost through the cost report. No visit is billed, and these costs should not be included on the claim. The beneficiary coinsurance and deductible are waived.

Hepatitis B Vaccine (G0010)

Hepatitis B vaccine and its administration is included in the RHC visit and is not separately billable. The cost of the vaccine and its administration can be included in the line item for the otherwise qualifying visit. A visit cannot be billed if vaccine administration is the only service the RHC provides. The beneficiary coinsurance and deductible are waived.

Initial Preventive Physical Exam (G0402)

The IPPE is a one-time exam that must occur within the first 12 months following the beneficiary's enrollment. The IPPE can be billed as a stand-alone visit if it is the only medical service provided on that day with a RHC practitioner. If an IPPE visit is furnished on the same day as another billable visit, two visits may be billed. The beneficiary coinsurance and deductible are waived.

Annual Wellness Visit (G0438 and G0439)

The AWV is a personalized prevention plan for beneficiaries who are not within the first 12 months of their first Part B coverage period and have not received an IPPE or AWV within the past 12 months. The AWV can be billed as a stand-alone visit if it is the only medical service provided on that day with a RHC practitioner. If the AWV is furnished on the same day as another medical visit, it is not a separately billable visit. The beneficiary coinsurance and deductible are waived.

Diabetes Self-Management Training (G0108) and Medical Nutrition Therapy (97802 and 97803)

Diabetes self-management training or medical nutrition therapy provided by a registered dietician or nutritional professional at a RHC may be considered incident to a visit with a RHC practitioner provided all applicable conditions are met. DSMT and MNT are not billable visits in a RHC, although the cost may be allowable on the cost report. RHCs cannot bill a visit for services furnished by registered dieticians or nutritional professionals. However, RHCs are permitted to become certified providers of DSMT services and report the cost of such services on their cost report for inclusion in the computation of their AIR. The beneficiary coinsurance and deductible apply.

Screening Pelvic and Clinical Breast Examination (G0101)

Screening pelvic and clinical breast examination can be billed as a stand-alone visit if it is the only medical service provided on that day with a RHC practitioner. If it is furnished on the same day as another medical visit, it is not a separately billable visit. The beneficiary coinsurance and deductible are waived.

Screening Papanicolaou Smear (Q0091)

Screening Papanicolaou smear can be billed as a stand-alone visit if it is the only medical service provided on that day with a RHC practitioner. If it is furnished on the same day as another medical visit, it is not a separately billable visit. The beneficiary coinsurance and deductible are waived.

Prostate Cancer Screening (G0102)

Prostate cancer screening can be billed as a stand-alone visit if it is the only medical service provided on that day with a RHC practitioner. If it is furnished on the same day as another medical visit, it is not a separately billable visit. The beneficiary coinsurance and deductible apply.

Glaucoma Screening (G0117 and G0118)

Glaucoma screening for high risk patients can be billed as a stand-alone visit if it is the only medical service provided on that day with a RHC practitioner. If it is furnished on the same day as another medical visit, it is not a separately billable visit. The beneficiary coinsurance and deductible apply.

Lung Cancer Screening Using Low Dose Computed Tomography (LDCT) (G0296)

LDCT can be billed as a stand-alone visit if it is the only medical service provided on that day with a RHC practitioner. If it is furnished on the same day as another medical visit, it is not a separately billable visit. The beneficiary coinsurance and deductible are waived.

**NOTE:** Hepatitis C Screening (G0472) is a technical service only and therefore it is not paid as part of the RHC visit.

## 100-2, 13, 220.3

### Preventive Health Services in FQHCs

(Rev. 230, Issued: 12-09-16, Effective: 03-09-17, Implementation: 03-09-17)

FQHCs must provide preventive health services on site or by arrangement with another provider. These services must be furnished by or under the direct supervision of a physician, NP, PA, CNM, CP, or CSW. Section 330(b)(1)(A)(i)(III) of the Public Health Service (PHS) Act required preventive health services can be found at http://bphc.hrsa.gov/policiesregulations/legislation/index.html, and include:

• prenatal and perinatal services;

• appropriate cancer screening;

- well-child services;

- immunizations against vaccine-preventable diseases;

- screenings for elevated blood lead levels, communicable diseases, and cholesterol;

- pediatric eye, ear, and dental screenings to determine the need for vision and hearing correction and dental care;

- voluntary family planning services; and

- preventive dental services.

**NOTE:** The cost of providing these services may be included in the FQHC cost report but they do not necessarily qualify as FQHC billable visits or for the waiver of the beneficiary coinsurance.

Influenza (G0008) and Pneumococcal Vaccines (G0009)

Influenza and pneumococcal vaccines and their administration are paid at 100 percent of reasonable cost through the cost report. The cost is included in the cost report and no visit is billed. FQHCs must include these charges on the claim if furnished as part of an encounter. The beneficiary coinsurance is waived.

Hepatitis B Vaccine (G0010)

Hepatitis B vaccine and its administration is included in the FQHC visit and is not separately billable. The cost of the vaccine and its administration can be included in the line item for the otherwise qualifying visit. A visit cannot be billed if vaccine administration is the only service the FQHC provides. The beneficiary coinsurance is waived.

Initial Preventive Physical Exam (G0402)

The IPPE is a one-time exam that must occur within the first 12 months following the beneficiary's enrollment. The IPPE can be billed as a stand-alone visit if it is the only medical service provided on that day with a FQHC practitioner. If an IPPE visit is furnished on the same day as another billable visit, FQHCs may not bill for a separate visit. These FQHCs will have an adjustment of 1.3416 to their PPS rate. The beneficiary coinsurance is waived.

Annual Wellness Visit (G0438 and G0439)

The AWV is a personalized prevention plan for beneficiaries who are not within the first 12 months of their first Part B coverage period and have not received an IPPE or AWV within the past12 months. The AWV can be billed as a stand-alone visit if it is the only medical service provided on that day with a FQHC practitioner. If the AWV is furnished on the same day as another medical visit, it is not a separately billable visit. FQHCs that are authorized to bill under the FQHC PPS will have an adjustment of 1.3416 to their PPS rate. The beneficiary coinsurance is waived.

Diabetes Self-Management Training (G0108) and Medical Nutrition Therapy (97802 and 97803)

DSMT and MNT furnished by certified DSMT and MNT providers are billable visits in FQHCs when they are provided in a one-on-one, face-to-face encounter and all program requirements are met. Other diabetes counseling or medical nutrition services provided by a registered dietician at the FQHC may be considered incident to a visit with a FQHC provider. The beneficiary coinsurance is waived for MNT services and is applicable for DSMT.

DSMT must be furnished by a certified DSMT practitioner, and MNT must be furnished by a registered dietitian or nutrition professional. Program requirements for DSMT services are set forth in 42 CFR 410 Subpart H for DSMT and in Part 410, Subpart G for MNT services, and additional guidance can be found at Pub. 100-02, chapter 15, section 300.

Screening Pelvic and Clinical Breast Examination (G0101)

Screening pelvic and clinical breast examination can be billed as a stand-alone visit if it is the only medical service provided on that day with a FQHC practitioner. If it is furnished on the same day as another medical visit, it is not a separately billable visit. The beneficiary coinsurance is waived.

Screening Papanicolaou Smear (Q0091)

Screening Papanicolaou smear can be billed as a stand-alone visit if it is the only medical service provided on that day with a FQHC practitioner. If it is furnished on the same day as another medical visit, it is not a separately billable visit. The beneficiary coinsurance is waived.

Prostate Cancer Screening (G0102)

Prostate cancer screening can be billed as a stand-alone visit if it is the only medical service provided on that day with a FQHC practitioner. If it is furnished on the same day as another medical visit, it is not a separately billable visit. The beneficiary coinsurance applies.

Glaucoma Screening (G0117 and G0118)

Glaucoma screening for high risk patients can be billed as a stand-alone visit if it is the only medical service provided on that day with a FQHC practitioner. If it is furnished on the same day as another medical visit, it is not a separately billable visit. The beneficiary coinsurance applies.

Lung Cancer Screening Using Low Dose Computed Tomography (LDCT) (G0296)

LDCT can be billed as a stand-alone visit if it is the only medical service provided on that day with a FQHC practitioner. If it is furnished on the same day as another medical visit, it is not a separately billable visit. The beneficiary coinsurance is waived.

**NOTE:** Hepatitis C Screening (G0472) is a technical service only and therefore not paid as part of the FQHC visit.

## 100-02, 15, 20.1

### *Physician Expense for Surgery, Childbirth, and Treatment for Infertility*
B3-2005.l

**A. Surgery and Childbirth**

Skilled medical management is covered throughout the events of pregnancy, beginning with diagnosis, continuing through delivery and ending after the necessary postnatal care. Similarly, in the event of termination of pregnancy, regardless of whether terminated spontaneously or for therapeutic reasons (i.e., where the life of the mother would be endangered if the fetus were brought to term), the need for skilled medical management and/or medical services is equally important as in those cases carried to full term. After the infant is delivered and is a separate individual, items and services furnished to the infant are not covered on the basis of the mother's eligibility.

Most surgeons and obstetricians bill patients an all-inclusive package charge intended to cover all services associated with the surgical procedure or delivery of the child. All expenses for surgical and obstetrical care, including preoperative/prenatal examinations and tests and post-operative/postnatal services, are considered incurred on the date of surgery or delivery, as appropriate. This policy applies whether the physician bills on a package charge basis, or itemizes the bill separately for these items.

Occasionally, a physician's bill may include charges for additional services not directly related to the surgical procedure or the delivery. Such charges are considered incurred on the date the additional services are furnished.

The above policy applies only where the charges are imposed by one physician or by a clinic on behalf of a group of physicians. Where more than one physician imposes charges for surgical or obstetrical services, all preoperative/prenatal and post-operative/postnatal services performed by the physician who performed the surgery or delivery are considered incurred on the date of the surgery or delivery. Expenses for services rendered by other physicians are considered incurred on the date they were performed.

**B. Treatment for Infertility**

Reasonable and necessary services associated with treatment for infertility are covered under Medicare. Infertility is a condition sufficiently at variance with the usual state of health to make it appropriate for a person who normally is expected to be fertile to seek medical consultation and treatment.

## 100-02, 15, 30.4

### *Optometrist's Services*
B3-2020.25

Effective April 1, 1987, a doctor of optometry is considered a physician with respect to all services the optometrist is authorized to perform under State law or regulation. To be covered under Medicare, the services must be medically reasonable and necessary for the diagnosis or treatment of illness or injury, and must meet all applicable coverage requirements. See the Medicare Benefit Policy Manual, Chapter 16, "General Exclusions from Coverage," for exclusions from coverage that apply to vision care services, and the Medicare Claims Processing Manual, Chapter 12, "Physician/Practitioner Billing," for information dealing with payment for items and services furnished by optometrists.

**A. FDA Monitored Studies of Intraocular Lenses**

Special coverage rules apply to situations in which an ophthalmologist is involved in a Food and Drug Administration (FDA) monitored study of the safety and efficacy of an investigational Intraocular Lens (IOL). The investigation process for IOLs is unique in that there is a core period and an adjunct period. The core study is a traditional, well-controlled clinical investigation with full record keeping and reporting requirements. The adjunct study is essentially an extended distribution phase for lenses in which only limited safety data are compiled. Depending on the lens being evaluated, the adjunct study may be an extension of the core study or may be the only type of investigation to which the lens may be subject.

All eye care services related to the investigation of the IOL must be provided by the investigator (i.e., the implanting ophthalmologist) or another practitioner (including a doctor of optometry) who provides services at the direction or under the supervision of the investigator and who has an agreement with the investigator that information on the patient is given to the investigator so that he or she may report on the patient to the IOL manufacturer. Eye care services furnished by anyone other than the investigator (or a practitioner who assists the investigator, as described in the preceding paragraph) are not covered during the period the IOL is being investigated, unless the services are not related to the investigation.

**B. Concurrent Care**

Where more than one practitioner furnishes concurrent care, services furnished to a beneficiary by both an ophthalmologist and another physician (including an optometrist) may be recognized for payment if it is determined that each practitioner's services were reasonable and necessary. (See Sec.30.E.)

## 100-02, 15, 30.5

### *Chiropractor's Services*

B3-2020.26

A chiropractor must be licensed or legally authorized to furnish chiropractic services by the State or jurisdiction in which the services are furnished. In addition, a licensed chiropractor must meet the following uniform minimum standards to be considered a physician for Medicare coverage. Coverage extends only to treatment by means of manual manipulation of the spine to correct a subluxation provided such treatment is legal in the State where performed. All other services furnished or ordered by chiropractors are not covered. If a chiropractor orders, takes, or interprets an x-ray or other diagnostic procedure to demonstrate a subluxation of the spine, the x-ray can be used for documentation. However, there is no coverage or payment for these services or for any other diagnostic or therapeutic service ordered or furnished by the chiropractor. For detailed information on using x-rays to determine subluxation, see Sec.240.1.2. In addition, in performing manual manipulation of the spine, some chiropractors use manual devices that are hand-held with the thrust of the force of the device being controlled manually. While such manual manipulation may be covered, there is no separate payment permitted for use of this device.

### A. Uniform Minimum Standards

**Prior to July 1, 1974**

Chiropractors licensed or authorized to practice prior to July 1, 1974, and those individuals who commenced their studies in a chiropractic college before that date must meet all of the following three minimum standards to render payable services under the program:

- Preliminary education equal to the requirements for graduation from an accredited high school or other secondary school;

- Graduation from a college of chiropractic approved by the State's chiropractic examiners that included the completion of a course of study covering a period of not less than 3 school years of 6 months each year in actual continuous attendance covering adequate course of study in the subjects of anatomy, physiology, symptomatology and diagnosis, hygiene and sanitation, chemistry, histology, pathology, and principles and practice of chiropractic, including clinical instruction in vertebral palpation, nerve tracing, and adjusting; and

- Passage of an examination prescribed by the State's chiropractic examiners covering the subjects listed above.

**After June 30, 1974**

Individuals commencing their studies in a chiropractic college after June 30, 1974, must meet all of the above three standards and all of the following additional requirements:

- Satisfactory completion of 2 years of pre-chiropractic study at the college level;

- Satisfactory completion of a 4-year course of 8 months each year (instead of a 3-year course of 6 months each year) at a college or school of chiropractic that includes not less than 4,000 hours in the scientific and chiropractic courses specified in the second bullet under "Prior to July 1, 1974" above, plus courses in the use and effect of x-ray and chiropractic analysis; and

- The practitioner must be over 21 years of age.

### B. Maintenance Therapy

Under the Medicare program, Chiropractic maintenance therapy is not considered to be medically reasonable or necessary, and is therefore not payable. Maintenance therapy is defined as a treatment plan that seeks to prevent disease, promote health, and prolong and enhance the quality of life; or therapy that is performed to maintain or prevent deterioration of a chronic condition. When further clinical improvement cannot reasonably be expected from continuous ongoing care, and the chiropractic treatment becomes supportive rather than corrective in nature, the treatment is then considered maintenance therapy. For information on how to indicate on a claim a treatment is or is not maintenance, see Sec.240.1.3.

## 100-02, 15, 50.4.4.2

### *Immunizations*

Vaccinations or inoculations are excluded as immunizations unless they are directly related to the treatment of an injury or direct exposure to a disease or condition, such as anti-rabies treatment, tetanus antitoxin or booster vaccine, botulin antitoxin, antivenin sera, or immune globulin. In the absence of injury or direct exposure, preventive immunization (vaccination or inoculation) against such diseases as smallpox, polio, diphtheria, etc., is not covered. However, pneumococcal, hepatitis B, and influenza virus vaccines are exceptions to this rule. (See items A, B, and C below.) In cases where a vaccination or inoculation is excluded from coverage, related charges are also not covered.

### A. Pneumococcal Pneumonia Vaccinations

1. Background and History of Coverage:

   Section 1861(s)(10)(A) of the Social Security Act and regulations at 42 CFR 410.57 authorize Medicare coverage under Part B for pneumococcal vaccine and its administration.

   For services furnished on or after May 1, 1981 through September 18, 2014, the Medicare Part B program covered pneumococcal pneumonia vaccine and its administration when furnished in compliance with any applicable State law by any provider of services or any entity or individual with a supplier number. Coverage included an initial vaccine administered only to persons at high risk of serious pneumococcal disease (including all people 65 and older; immunocompetent adults at increased risk of pneumococcal disease or its complications because of chronic illness; and individuals with compromised immune systems), with revaccination administered only to persons at highest risk of serious pneumococcal infection and those likely to have a rapid decline in pneumococcal antibody levels, provided that at least 5 years had passed since the previous dose of pneumococcal vaccine.

   Those administering the vaccine did not require the patient to present an immunization record prior to administering the pneumococcal vaccine, nor were they compelled to review the patient's complete medical record if it was not available, relying on the patient's verbal history to determine prior vaccination status.

   Effective July 1, 2000, Medicare no longer required for coverage purposes that a doctor of medicine or osteopathy order the vaccine. Therefore, a beneficiary could receive the vaccine upon request without a physician's order and without physician supervision.

2. Coverage Requirements:

   Effective for claims with dates of service on and after September 19, 2014, an initial pneumococcal vaccine may be administered to all Medicare beneficiaries who have never received a pneumococcal vaccination under Medicare Part B. A different, second pneumococcal vaccine may be administered 1 year after the first vaccine was administered (i.e., 11 full months have passed following the month in which the last pneumococcal vaccine was administered).

   Those administering the vaccine should not require the patient to present an immunization record prior to administering the pneumococcal vaccine, nor should they feel compelled to review the patient's complete medical record if it is not available. Instead, provided that the patient is competent, it is acceptable to rely on the patient's verbal history to determine prior vaccination status.

   Medicare does not require for coverage purposes that a doctor of medicine or osteopathy order the vaccine. Therefore, the beneficiary may receive the vaccine upon request without a physician's order and without physician supervision.

### B. Hepatitis B Vaccine

Effective for services furnished on or after September 1, 1984, P.L. 98-369 provides coverage under Part B for hepatitis B vaccine and its administration, furnished to a Medicare beneficiary who is at high or intermediate risk of contracting hepatitis B. High-risk groups currently identified include (see exception below):

- ESRD patients;

- Hemophiliacs who receive Factor VIII or IX concentrates;

- Clients of institutions for the mentally retarded;

- Persons who live in the same household as a Hepatitis B Virus (HBV) carrier;

- Homosexual men;

- Illicit injectable drug abusers; and

- Persons diagnosed with diabetes mellitus.

Intermediate risk groups currently identified include:

- Staff in institutions for the mentally retarded; and

- Workers in health care professions who have frequent contact with blood or blood-derived body fluids during routine work.

EXCEPTION: Persons in both of the above-listed groups in paragraph B, would not be considered at high or intermediate risk of contracting hepatitis B, however, if there were laboratory evidence positive for antibodies to hepatitis B. (ESRD patients are routinely tested for hepatitis B antibodies as part of their continuing monitoring and therapy.)

For Medicare program purposes, the vaccine may be administered upon the order of a doctor of medicine or osteopathy, by a doctor of medicine or osteopathy, or by home health agencies, skilled nursing facilities, ESRD facilities, hospital outpatient departments, and persons recognized under the incident to physicians' services provision of law.

A charge separate from the ESRD composite rate will be recognized and paid for administration of the vaccine to ESRD patients.

### C. Influenza Virus Vaccine

Effective for services furnished on or after May 1, 1993, the Medicare Part B program covers influenza virus vaccine and its administration when furnished in compliance with any applicable State law by any provider of services or any entity or individual with a supplier number. Typically, these vaccines are administered once a flu season. Medicare does not require, for coverage purposes, that a doctor of medicine or osteopathy order the vaccine. Therefore, the beneficiary may receive the vaccine upon request without a physician's order and without physician supervision.

## 100-02, 15, 80.1

### *Clinical Laboratory Services*

Section 1833 and 1861 of the Act provides for payment of clinical laboratory services under Medicare Part B. Clinical laboratory services involve the biological, microbiological, serological, chemical, immunohematological, hematological, biophysical, cytological, pathological, or other examination of materials derived from the human body for the diagnosis, prevention, or treatment of a disease or assessment of a medical condition. Laboratory services must meet all applicable requirements of the Clinical Laboratory Improvement Amendments of 1988 (CLIA), as set forth at 42 CFR part 493. Section 1862(a)(1)(A) of the Act provides that Medicare payment may not be made for services that are not reasonable and necessary. Clinical laboratory services must be ordered and used promptly by the physician who is treating the beneficiary as described in 42 CFR 410.32(a), or by a qualified nonphysician practitioner, as described in 42 CFR 410.32(a)(3).

See section 80.6 of this manual for related physician ordering instructions.

See the Medicare Claims Processing Manual Chapter 16 for related claims processing instructions.

## 100-02, 15, 80.2

### Psychological Tests and Neuropsychological Tests

Medicare Part B coverage of psychological tests and neuropsychological tests is authorized under section 1861(s)(3) of the Social Security Act. Payment for psychological and neuropsychological tests is authorized under section 1842(b)(2)(A) of the Social Security Act. The payment amounts for the new psychological and neuropsychological tests (CPT codes 96102, 96103, 96119 and 96120) that are effective January 1, 2006, and are billed for tests administered by a technician or a computer reflect a site of service payment differential for the facility and non-facility settings.

Additionally, there is no authorization for payment for diagnostic tests when performed on an "incident to" basis.

Under the diagnostic tests provision, all diagnostic tests are assigned a certain level of supervision. Generally, regulations governing the diagnostic tests provision require that only physicians can provide the assigned level of supervision for diagnostic tests.

However, there is a regulatory exception to the supervision requirement for diagnostic psychological and neuropsychological tests in terms of who can provide the supervision.

That is, regulations allow a clinical psychologist (CP) or a physician to perform the general supervision assigned to diagnostic psychological and neuropsychological tests.

In addition, nonphysician practitioners such as nurse practitioners (NPs), clinical nurse specialists (CNSs) and physician assistants (PAs) who personally perform diagnostic psychological and neuropsychological tests are excluded from having to perform these tests under the general supervision of a physician or a CP. Rather, NPs and CNSs must perform such tests under the requirements of their respective benefit instead of the requirements for diagnostic psychological and neuropsychological tests. Accordingly, NPs and CNSs must perform tests in collaboration (as defined under Medicare law at section 1861(aa)(6) of the Act) with a physician. PAs perform tests under the general supervision of a physician as required for services furnished under the PA benefit.

Furthermore, physical therapists (PTs), occupational therapists (OTs) and speech language pathologists (SLPs) are authorized to bill three test codes as "sometimes therapy" codes. Specifically, CPT codes 96105, 96110 and 96111 may be performed by these therapists. However, when PTs, OTs and SLPs perform these three tests, they must be performed under the general supervision of a physician or a CP.

#### Who May Bill for Diagnostic Psychological and Neuropsychological Tests CPs - see qualifications under chapter 15, section 160 of the Benefits Policy Manual, Pub. 100-2.

- NPs -to the extent authorized under State scope of practice. See qualifications under chapter 15, section 200 of the Benefits Policy Manual, Pub. 100-2.
- CNSs -to the extent authorized under State scope of practice. See qualifications under chapter 15, section 210 of the Benefits Policy Manual, Pub. 100-2.
- PAs - to the extent authorized under State scope of practice. See qualifications under chapter 15, section 190 of the Benefits Policy Manual, Pub. 100-2.
- Independently Practicing Psychologists (IPPs) PTs, OTs and SLPs - see qualifications under chapter 15, sections 220-230.6 of the Benefits Policy Manual, Pub. 100-2.

Psychological and neuropsychological tests performed by a psychologist (who is not a CP) practicing independently of an institution, agency, or physician's office are covered when a physician orders such tests. An IPP is any psychologist who is licensed or certified to practice psychology in the State or jurisdiction where furnishing services or, if the jurisdiction does not issue licenses, if provided by any practicing psychologist. (It is CMS' understanding that all States, the District of Columbia, and Puerto Rico license psychologists, but that some trust territories do not. Examples of psychologists, other than CPs, whose psychological and neuropsychological tests are covered under the diagnostic tests provision include, but are not limited to, educational psychologists and counseling psychologists.)

The carrier must secure from the appropriate State agency a current listing of psychologists holding the required credentials to determine whether the tests of a particular IPP are covered under Part B in States that have statutory licensure or certification. In States or territories that lack statutory licensing or certification, the carrier checks individual qualifications before provider numbers are issued. Possible reference sources are the national directory of membership of the American Psychological Association, which provides data about the educational background of individuals and indicates which members are board-certified, the records and directories of the State or territorial psychological association, and the National Register of Health Service Providers. If qualification is dependent on a doctoral degree from a currently accredited program, the carrier verifies the date of accreditation of the school involved, since such accreditation is not retroactive. If the

listed reference sources do not provide enough information (e.g., the psychologist is not a member of one of these sources), the carrier contacts the psychologist personally for the required information. Generally, carriers maintain a continuing list of psychologists whose qualifications have been verified.

NOTE: When diagnostic psychological tests are performed by a psychologist who is not practicing independently, but is on the staff of an institution, agency, or clinic, that entity bills for the psychological tests.

The carrier considers psychologists as practicing independently when:

- They render services on their own responsibility, free of the administrative and professional control of an employer such as a physician, institution or agency;
- The persons they treat are their own patients; and
- They have the right to bill directly, collect and retain the fee for their services.

A psychologist practicing in an office located in an institution may be considered an independently practicing psychologist when both of the following conditions exist:

- The office is confined to a separately-identified part of the facility which is used solely as the psychologist's office and cannot be construed as extending throughout the entire institution; and
- The psychologist conducts a private practice, i.e., services are rendered to patients from outside the institution as well as to institutional patients.

#### Payment for Diagnostic Psychological and Neuropsychological Tests

Expenses for diagnostic psychological and neuropsychological tests are not subject to the outpatient mental health treatment limitation, that is, the payment limitation on treatment services for mental, psychoneurotic and personality disorders as authorized under Section 1833(c) of the Act. The payment amount for the new psychological and neuropsychological tests (CPT codes 96102, 96103, 96119 and 96120) that are billed for tests performed by a technician or a computer reflect a site of service payment differential for the facility and non-facility settings. CPs, NPs, CNSs and PAs are required by law to accept assigned payment for psychological and neuropsychological tests. However, while IPPs are not required by law to accept assigned payment for these tests, they must report the name and address of the physician who ordered the test on the claim form when billing for tests.

#### CPT Codes for Diagnostic Psychological and Neuropsychological Tests

The range of CPT codes used to report psychological and neuropsychological tests is 96101-96120. CPT codes 96101, 96102, 96103, 96105, 96110, and 96111 are appropriate for use when billing for psychological tests. CPT codes 96116, 96118, 96119 and 96120 are appropriate for use when billing for neuropsychological tests.

All of the tests under this CPT code range 96101-96120 are indicated as active codes under the physician fee schedule database and are covered if medically necessary.

#### Payment and Billing Guidelines for Psychological and Neuropsychological Tests

The technician and computer CPT codes for psychological and neuropsychological tests include practice expense, malpractice expense and professional work relative value units.

Accordingly, CPT psychological test code 96101 should not be paid when billed for the same tests or services performed under psychological test codes 96102 or 96103. CPT neuropsychological test code 96118 should not be paid when billed for the same tests or services performed under neuropsychological test codes 96119 or 96120. However, CPT codes 96101 and 96118 can be paid separately on the rare occasion when billed on the same date of service for different and separate tests from 96102, 96103, 96119 and 96120.

Under the physician fee schedule, there is no payment for services performed by students or trainees. Accordingly, Medicare does not pay for services represented by CPT codes 96102 and 96119 when performed by a student or a trainee. However, the presence of a student or a trainee while the test is being administered does not prevent a physician, CP, IPP, NP, CNS or PA from performing and being paid for the psychological test under 96102 or the neuropsychological test under 96119.

## 100-02, 15, 80.5.5

### Frequency Standards

Medicare pays for a screening BMM once every 2 years (at least 23 months have passed since the month the last covered BMM was performed).

When medically necessary, Medicare may pay for more frequent BMMs. Examples include, but are not limited to, the following medical circumstances:

- Monitoring beneficiaries on long-term glucocorticoid (steroid) therapy of more than 3 months.
- Confirming baseline BMMs to permit monitoring of beneficiaries in the future.

## 100-02, 15, 150.1

### Treatment of Temporomandibular Joint (TMJ) Syndrome

There are a wide variety of conditions that can be characterized as TMJ, and an equally wide variety of methods for treating these conditions. Many of the procedures fall within the Medicare program's statutory exclusion that prohibits payment for items and services that have not been demonstrated to be reasonable and necessary for the diagnosis and treatment of illness or injury (§1862(a)(1) of the Act). Other services and appliances used to treat TMJ fall within the Medicare program's statutory exclusion at 1862(a)(12), which prohibits payment "for services in connection with the care, treatment, filling, removal, or replacement of teeth or structures directly supporting teeth...." For these reasons, a diagnosis of TMJ on a claim is insufficient. The actual condition or symptom must be determined.

## 100-02, 15, 160

### Clinical Psychologist Services

#### A. Clinical Psychologist (CP) Defined

To qualify as a clinical psychologist (CP), a practitioner must meet the following requirements: Hold a doctoral degree in psychology; Be licensed or certified, on the basis of the doctoral degree in psychology, by the State in which he or she practices, at the independent practice level of psychology to furnish diagnostic, assessment, preventive, and therapeutic services directly to individuals.

#### B. Qualified Clinical Psychologist Services Defined

Effective July 1, 1990, the diagnostic and therapeutic services of CPs and services and supplies furnished incident to such services are covered as the services furnished by a physician or as incident to physician's services are covered. However, the CP must be legally authorized to perform the services under applicable licensure laws of the State in which they are furnished.

#### C. Types of Clinical Psychologist Services

That May Be Covered Diagnostic and therapeutic services that the CP is legally authorized to perform in accordance with State law and/or regulation. Carriers pay all qualified CPs based on the physician fee schedule for the diagnostic and therapeutic services. (Psychological tests by practitioners who do not meet the requirements for a CP may be covered under the provisions for diagnostic tests as described in Sec. 80.2.

Services and supplies furnished incident to a CP's services are covered if the requirements that apply to services incident to a physician's services, as described in Sec.60 are met. These services must be:

- Mental health services that are commonly furnished in CPs' offices;
- An integral, although incidental, part of professional services performed by the CP;
- Performed under the direct personal supervision of the CP; i.e., the CP must be physically present and immediately available;
- Furnished without charge or included in the CP's bill; and
- Performed by an employee of the CP (or an employee of the legal entity that employs the supervising CP) under the common law control test of the Act, as set forth in 20 CFR 404.1007 and Sec.RS 2101.020 of the Retirement and Survivors Insurance part of the Social Security Program Operations Manual System.
- Diagnostic psychological testing services when furnished under the general supervision of a CP.

Carriers are required to familiarize themselves with appropriate State laws and/or regulations governing a CP's scope of practice.

#### D. Noncovered Services

The services of CPs are not covered if the service is otherwise excluded from Medicare coverage even though a clinical psychologist is authorized by State law to perform them.

For example, Sec.1862(a)(1)(A) of the Act excludes from coverage services that are not "reasonable and necessary for the diagnosis or treatment of an illness or injury or to improve the functioning of a malformed body member." Therefore, even though the services are authorized by State law, the services of a CP that are determined to be not reasonable and necessary are not covered. Additionally, any therapeutic services that are billed by CPs under CPT psychotherapy codes that include medical evaluation and management services are not covered.

#### E. Requirement for Consultation

When applying for a Medicare provider number, a CP must submit to the carrier a signed Medicare provider/supplier enrollment form that indicates an agreement to the effect that, contingent upon the patient's consent, the CP will attempt to consult with the patient's attending or primary care physician in accordance with accepted professional ethical norms, taking into consideration patient confidentiality.

If the patient assents to the consultation, the CP must attempt to consult with the patient's physician within a reasonable time after receiving the consent. If the CP's attempts to consult directly with the physician are not successful, the CP must notify the physician within a reasonable time that he or she is furnishing services to the patient. Additionally, the CP must document, in the patient's medical record, the date the patient consented or declined consent to consultations, the date of consultation, or, if attempts to consult did not succeed, that date and manner of notification to the physician.

The only exception to the consultation requirement for CPs is in cases where the patient's primary care or attending physician refers the patient to the CP. Also, neither a CP nor a primary care nor attending physician may bill Medicare or the patient for this required consultation.

#### F. Outpatient Mental Health Services Limitation

All covered therapeutic services furnished by qualified CPs are subject to the outpatient mental health services limitation in Pub 100-1, Medicare General Information, Eligibility, and Entitlement Manual, Chapter 3, "Deductibles, Coinsurance Amounts, and Payment Limitations," Sec.30, (i.e., only 62 1/2 percent of

expenses for these services are considered incurred expenses for Medicare purposes). The limitation does not apply to diagnostic services.

G. Assignment Requirement Assignment iSec. required.

## 100-02, 15, 170

### Clinical Social Worker (CSW) Services
B3-2152

See the Medicare Claims Processing Manual Chapter 12, Physician/Nonphysician Practitioners, §150, "Clinical Social Worker Services," for payment requirements.

#### A. Clinical Social Worker Defined

Section 1861(hh) of the Act defines a "clinical social worker" as an individual who:

- Possesses a master's or doctor's degree in social work;
- Has performed at least two years of supervised clinical social work; and
- Is licensed or certified as a clinical social worker by the State in which the services are performed; or
- In the case of an individual in a State that does not provide for licensure or certification, has completed at least 2 years or 3,000 hours of post master's degree supervised clinical social work practice under the supervision of a master's level social worker in an appropriate setting such as a hospital, SNF, or clinic.

#### B. Clinical Social Worker Services Defined

Section 1861(hh)(2) of the Act defines "clinical social worker services" as those services that the CSW is legally authorized to perform under State law (or the State regulatory mechanism provided by State law) of the State in which such services are performed for the diagnosis and treatment of mental illnesses. Services furnished to an inpatient of a hospital or an inpatient of a SNF that the SNF is required to provide as a requirement for participation are not included. The services that are covered are those that are otherwise covered if furnished by a physician or as incident to a physician's professional service.

#### C. Covered Services

Coverage is limited to the services a CSW is legally authorized to perform in accordance with State law (or State regulatory mechanism established by State law). The services of a CSW may be covered under Part B if they are:

- The type of services that are otherwise covered if furnished by a physician, or as incident to a physician's service. (See §30 for a description of physicians' services and §70 of Pub 100-1, the Medicare General Information, Eligibility, and Entitlement Manual, Chapter 5, for the definition of a physician.);
- Performed by a person who meets the definition of a CSW (See subsection A.); and
- Not otherwise excluded from coverage. Carriers should become familiar with the State law or regulatory mechanism governing a CSW's scope of practice in their service area.

#### D. Noncovered Services

Services of a CSW are not covered when furnished to inpatients of a hospital or to inpatients of a SNF if the services furnished in the SNF are those that the SNF is required to furnish as a condition of participation in Medicare. In addition, CSW services are not covered if they are otherwise excluded from Medicare coverage even though a CSW is authorized by State law to perform them. For example, the Medicare law excludes from coverage services that are not "reasonable and necessary for the diagnosis or treatment of an illness or injury or to improve the functioning of a malformed body member."

#### E. Outpatient Mental Health Services Limitation

All covered therapeutic services furnished by qualified CSWs are subject to the outpatient psychiatric services limitation in Pub 100-1, Medicare General Information, Eligibility, and Entitlement Manual, Chapter 3, "Deductibles, Coinsurance Amounts, and Payment Limitations," §30, (i.e., only 62 1/2 percent of expenses for these services are considered incurred expenses for Medicare purposes). The limitation does not apply to diagnostic services.

#### F. Assignment Requirement
Assignment is required.

## 100-02, 15, 180

### Nurse-Midwife (CNM) Services
B3-2154

#### A. General

Effective on or after July 1, 1988, the services provided by a certified nurse-midwife or incident to the certified nurse-midwife's services are covered. Payment is made under assignment only. See the Medicare Claims Processing Manual, Chapter 12, "Physician and Nonphysician Practitioners," §130, for payment methodology for nurse midwife services.

#### B. Certified Nurse-Midwife Defined

A certified nurse-midwife is a registered nurse who has successfully completed a program of study and clinical experience in nurse-midwifery, meeting guidelines prescribed by the Secretary, or who has been certified by an organization recognized by the Secretary. The Secretary has recognized certification by the American College of Nurse-Midwives and State qualifying requirements in those States that specify a

*Appendix G — Medicare Internet-only Manuals (IOMs)*

program of education and clinical experience for nurse-midwives for these purposes. A nurse-midwife must:

- Be currently licensed to practice in the State as a registered professional nurse; and

- Meet one of the following requirements:

  1. Be legally authorized under State law or regulations to practice as a nurse-midwife and have completed a program of study and clinical experience for nurse-midwives, as specified by the State; or

  2. If the State does not specify a program of study and clinical experience that nurse-midwives must complete to practice in that State, the nurse-midwife must:

     a. Be currently certified as a nurse-midwife by the American College of Nurse-Midwives;

     b. Have satisfactorily completed a formal education program (of at least one academic year) that, upon completion, qualifies the nurse to take the certification examination offered by the American College of Nurse-Midwives; or

     c. Have successfully completed a formal education program for preparing registered nurses to furnish gynecological and obstetrical care to women during pregnancy, delivery, and the postpartum period, and care to normal newborns, and have practiced as a nurse-midwife for a total of 12 months during any 18-month period from August 8, 1976, to July 16, 1982.

### C. Covered Services
1. General - Effective January 1, 1988, through December 31, 1993, the coverage of nurse-midwife services was restricted to the maternity cycle. The maternity cycle is a period that includes pregnancy, labor, and the immediate postpartum period.

   Beginning with services furnished on or after January 1, 1994, coverage is no longer limited to the maternity cycle. Coverage is available for services furnished by a nurse-midwife that he or she is legally authorized to perform in the State in which the services are furnished and that would otherwise be covered if furnished by a physician, including obstetrical and gynecological services.

2. Incident To- Services and supplies furnished incident to a nurse midwife's service are covered if they would have been covered when furnished incident to the services of a doctor of medicine or osteopathy, as described in §60.

### D. Noncovered Services
The services of nurse-midwives are not covered if they are otherwise excluded from Medicare coverage even though a nurse-midwife is authorized by State law to perform them. For example, the Medicare program excludes from coverage routine physical checkups and services that are not reasonable and necessary for the diagnosis or treatment of an illness or injury or to improve the functioning of a malformed body member. Coverage of service to the newborn continues only to the point that the newborn is or would normally be treated medically as a separate individual. Items and services furnished the newborn from that point are not covered on the basis of the mother's eligibility.

### E. Relationship With Physician
Most States have licensure and other requirements applicable to nurse-midwives. For example, some require that the nurse-midwife have an arrangement with a physician for the referral of the patient in the event a problem develops that requires medical attention. Others may require that the nurse-midwife function under the general supervision of a physician. Although these and similar State requirements must be met in order for the nurse-midwife to provide Medicare covered care, they have no effect on the nurse-midwife's right to personally bill for and receive direct Medicare payment. That is, billing does not have to flow through a physician or facility. See §60.2 for coverage of services performed by nurse-midwives incident to the service of physicians.

### F. Place of Service
There is no restriction on place of service. Therefore, nurse-midwife services are covered if provided in the nurse-midwife's office, in the patient's home, or in a hospital or other facility, such as a clinic or birthing center owned or operated by a nurse-midwife.

### G. Assignment Requirement
Assignment is required.

## 100-02, 15, 220

### *Coverage of Outpatient Rehabilitation Therapy Services (Physical Therapy, Occupational Therapy, and Speech-Language Pathology Services) Under Medical Insurance*
A comprehensive knowledge of the policies that apply to therapy services cannot be obtained through manuals alone. The most definitive policies are Local Coverage Determinations found at the Medicare Coverage Database www.cms.hhs.gov/mcd. A list of Medicare contractors is found at the CMS Web site. Specific questions about all Medicare policies should be addressed to the contractors through the contact information supplied on their Web sites. General Medicare questions may be addressed to the Medicare regional offices http://www.cms.hhs.gov/RegionalOffices/.

### A. Definitions
The following defines terms used in this section and §230:

ACTIVE PARTICIPATION of the clinician in treatment means that the clinician personally furnishes in its entirety at least 1 billable service on at least 1 day of treatment.

ASSESSMENT is separate from evaluation, and is included in services or procedures, (it is not separately payable). The term assessment as used in Medicare manuals related to therapy services is distinguished from language in Current Procedural Terminology (CPT) codes that specify assessment, e.g., 97755, Assistive Technology Assessment, which may be payable). Assessments shall be provided only by clinicians, because assessment requires professional skill to gather data by observation and patient inquiry and may include limited objective testing and measurement to make clinical judgments regarding the patient's condition(s). Assessment determines, e.g., changes in the patient's status since the last visit/treatment day and whether the planned procedure or service should be modified. Based on these assessment data, the professional may make judgments about progress toward goals and/or determine that a more complete evaluation or re-evaluation (see definitions below) is indicated. Routine weekly assessments of expected progression in accordance with the plan are not payable as re-evaluations.

CERTIFICATION is the physician's/nonphysician practitioner's (NPP) approval of the plan of care. Certification requires a dated signature on the plan of care or some other document that indicates approval of the plan of care.

The CLINICIAN is a term used in this manual and in Pub 100-4, chapter 5, section 10 or section 20, to refer to only a physician, nonphysician practitioner or a therapist (but not to an assistant, aide or any other personnel) providing a service within their scope of practice and consistent with state and local law. Clinicians make clinical judgments and are responsible for all services they are permitted to supervise. Services that require the skills of a therapist, may be appropriately furnished by clinicians, that is, by or under the supervision of qualified physicians/NPPs when their scope of practice, state and local laws allow it and their personal professional training is judged by Medicare contractors as sufficient to provide to the beneficiary skills equivalent to a therapist for that service.

COMPLEXITIES are complicating factors that may influence treatment, e.g., they may influence the type, frequency, intensity and/or duration of treatment. Complexities may be represented by diagnoses (ICD codes), by patient factors such as age, severity, acuity, multiple conditions, and motivation, or by the patient's social circumstances such as the support of a significant other or the availability of transportation to therapy.

A DATE may be in any form (written, stamped or electronic). The date may be added to the record in any manner and at any time, as long as the dates are accurate. If they are different, refer to both the date a service was performed and the date the entry to the record was made. For example, if a physician certifies a plan and fails to date it, staff may add "Received Date" in writing or with a stamp. The received date is valid for certification/re-certification purposes. Also, if the physician faxes the referral, certification, or re-certification and forgets to date it, the date that prints out on the fax is valid. If services provided on one date are documented on another date, both dates should be documented.

The EPISODE of Outpatient Therapy – For the purposes of therapy policy, an outpatient therapy episode is defined as the period of time, in calendar days, from the first day the patient is under the care of the clinician (e.g., for evaluation or treatment) for the current condition(s) being treated by one therapy discipline (PT, or OT, or SLP) until the last date of service for that discipline in that setting.

During the episode, the beneficiary may be treated for more than one condition; including conditions with an onset after the episode has begun. For example, a beneficiary receiving PT for a hip fracture who, after the initial treatment session, develops low back pain would also be treated under a PT plan of care for rehabilitation of low back pain. That plan may be modified from the initial plan, or it may be a separate plan specific to the low back pain, but treatment for both conditions concurrently would be considered the same episode of PT treatment. If that same patient developed a swallowing problem during intubation for the hip surgery, the first day of treatment by the SLP would be a new episode of SLP care.

EVALUATION is a separately payable comprehensive service provided by a clinician, as defined above, that requires professional skills to make clinical judgments about conditions for which services are indicated based on objective measurements and subjective evaluations of patient performance and functional abilities. Evaluation is warranted e.g., for a new diagnosis or when a condition is treated in a new setting. These evaluative judgments are essential to development of the plan of care, including goals and the selection of interventions.

FUNCTIONAL REPORTING, which is required on claims for all outpatient therapy services pursuant to 42CFR410.59, 410.60, and 410.62, uses nonpayable G-codes and related modifiers to convey information about the patient's functional status at specified points during therapy. (See Pub 100-4, chapter 5, section 10.6)

RE-EVALUATION provides additional objective information not included in other documentation. Re-evaluation is separately payable and is periodically indicated during an episode of care when the professional assessment of a clinician indicates a significant improvement, or decline, or change in the patient's condition or functional status that was not anticipated in the plan of care.

Although some state regulations and state practice acts require re-evaluation at specific times, for Medicare payment, reevaluations must also meet Medicare coverage guidelines. The decision to provide a reevaluation shall be made by a clinician.

INTERVAL of certified treatment (certification interval) consists of 90 calendar days or less, based on an individual's needs. A physician/NPP may certify a plan of care for an interval length that is less than 90 days. There may be more than one certification interval in an episode of care. The certification interval is not the same as a Progress Report period.

MAINTENANCE PROGRAM (MP) means a program established by a therapist that consists of activities and/or mechanisms that will assist a beneficiary in maximizing or maintaining the progress he or she has made during therapy or to prevent or slow further deterioration due to a disease or illness.

NONPHYSICIAN PRACTITIONERS (NPP) means physician assistants, clinical nurse specialists, and nurse practitioners, who may, if state and local laws permit it, and when appropriate rules are followed, provide, certify or supervise therapy services.

PHYSICIAN with respect to outpatient rehabilitation therapy services means a doctor of medicine, osteopathy (including an osteopathic practitioner), podiatric medicine, or optometry (for low vision rehabilitation only). Chiropractors and doctors of dental surgery or dental medicine are not considered physicians for therapy services and may neither refer patients for rehabilitation therapy services nor establish therapy plans of care.

PATIENT, client, resident, and beneficiary are terms used interchangeably to indicate enrolled recipients of Medicare covered services.

PROVIDERS of services are defined in §1861(u) of the Act, 42CFR400.202 and 42CFR485 Subpart H as participating hospitals, critical access hospitals (CAH), skilled nursing facilities (SNF), comprehensive outpatient rehabilitation facilities (CORF), home health agencies (HHA), hospices, participating clinics, rehabilitation agencies or outpatient rehabilitation facilities (ORF). Providers are also defined as public health agencies with agreements only to furnish outpatient therapy services, or community mental health centers with agreements only to furnish partial hospitalization services. To qualify as providers of services, these providers must meet certain conditions enumerated in the law and enter into an agreement with the Secretary in which they agree not to charge any beneficiary for covered services for which the program will pay and to refund any erroneous collections made. Note that the word PROVIDER in sections 220 and 230 is not used to mean a person who provides a service, but is used as in the statute to mean a facility or agency such as rehabilitation agency or home health agency.

QUALIFIED PROFESSIONAL means a physical therapist, occupational therapist, speech-language pathologist, physician, nurse practitioner, clinical nurse specialist, or physician's assistant, who is licensed or certified by the state to furnish therapy services, and who also may appropriately furnish therapy services under Medicare policies. Qualified professional may also include a physical therapist assistant (PTA) or an occupational therapy assistant (OTA) when furnishing services under the supervision of a qualified therapist, who is working within the state scope of practice in the state in which the services are furnished. Assistants are limited in the services they may furnish (see section 230.1 and 230.2) and may not supervise other therapy caregivers.

QUALIFIED PERSONNEL means staff (auxiliary personnel) who have been educated and trained as therapists and qualify to furnish therapy services only under direct supervision incident to a physician or NPP. See §230.5 of this chapter. Qualified personnel may or may not be licensed as therapists but meet all of the requirements for therapists with the exception of licensure.

SIGNATURE means a legible identifier of any type acceptable according to policies in Pub. 100-08, Medicare Program Integrity Manual, chapter 3, §3.3.2.4 concerning signatures.

SUPERVISION LEVELS for outpatient rehabilitation therapy services are the same as those for diagnostic tests defined in 42CFR410.32. Depending on the setting, the levels include personal supervision (in the room), direct supervision (in the office suite), and general supervision (physician/NPP is available but not necessarily on the premises).

SUPPLIERS of therapy services include individual practitioners such as physicians, NPPs, physical therapists and occupational therapists who have Medicare provider numbers. Regulatory references on physical therapists in private practice (PTPPs) and occupational therapists in private practice (OTPPs) are at 42CFR410.60 (C)(1), 485.701-729, and 486.150-163.

THERAPIST refers only to qualified physical therapists, occupational therapists and speech-language pathologists, as defined in §230. Qualifications that define therapists are in §§230.1, 230.2, and 230.3. Skills of a therapist are defined by the scope of practice for therapists in the state).

THERAPY (or outpatient rehabilitation services) includes only outpatient physical therapy (PT), occupational therapy (OT) and speech-language pathology (SLP) services paid using the Medicare Physician Fee Schedule or the same services when provided in hospitals that are exempt from the hospital Outpatient Prospective Payment System and paid on a reasonable cost basis, including critical access hospitals.

Therapy services referred to in this chapter are those skilled services furnished according to the standards and conditions in CMS manuals, (e.g., in this chapter

and in Pub. 100-4, Medicare Claims Processing Manual, chapter 5), within their scope of practice by qualified professionals or qualified personnel, as defined in this section, represented by procedures found in the American Medical Association's "Current Procedural Terminology (CPT)." A list of CPT (HCPCS) codes is provided in Pub. 100-4, chapter 5, §20, and in Local Coverage Determinations developed by contractors.

TREATMENT DAY means a single calendar day on which treatment, evaluation and/or reevaluation is provided. There could be multiple visits, treatment sessions/encounters on a treatment day.

VISITS OR TREATMENT SESSIONS begin at the time the patient enters the treatment area (of a building, office, or clinic) and continue until all services (e.g., activities, procedures, services) have been completed for that session and the patient leaves that area to participate in a non-therapy activity. It is likely that not all minutes in the visits/treatment sessions are billable (e.g., rest periods). There may be two treatment sessions in a day, for example, in the morning and afternoon. When there are two visits/ treatment sessions in a day, plans of care indicate treatment amount of twice a day.

## B. References

Paper Manuals. The following manuals, now outdated, were resources for the Internet Only Manuals:

- Part A Medicare Intermediary Manual, (Pub. 13)
- Part B Medicare Carrier Manual, (Pub. 14)
- Hospital Manual, (Pub. 10)
- Outpatient Physical Therapy/CORF Manual, (Pub. 9)

Regulation and Statute. The information in this section is based in part on the following current references:

- 42CFR refers to Title 42, Code of Federal Regulation (CFR).
- The Act refers to the Social Security Act.

Internet Only Manuals. Current Policies that concern providers and suppliers of therapy services are located in many places throughout CMS Manuals. Sites that may be of interest include:

- Pub.100-1 GENERAL INFORMATION, ELIGIBILITY, AND ENTITLEMENT
  - Chapter 1- General Overview
    - 10.1 - Hospital Insurance (Part A) for Inpatient Hospital, Hospice, Home Health and SNF Services - A Brief Description
    - 10.2 - Home Health Services
    - 10.3 - Supplementary Medical Insurance (Part B) - A Brief Description
    - 20.2 - Discrimination Prohibited
- Pub. 100-2, MEDICARE BENEFIT POLICY MANUAL
  - Ch 6 - Hospital Services Covered Under Part B
    - 10 - Medical and Other Health Services Furnished to Inpatients of Participating Hospitals
    - 20 - Outpatient Hospital Services
    - 20.2 - Outpatient Defined
    - 20.4.1 - Diagnostic Services Defined
    - 70 - Outpatient Hospital Psychiatric Services
  - Ch 8 - Coverage of Extended Care (SNF) Services Under Hospital Insurance
    - 30.4. - Direct Skilled Rehabilitation Services to Patients
    - 40 - Physician Certification and Recertification for Extended Care Services
    - 50.3 - Physical Therapy, Speech-Language Pathology, and Occupational Therapy Furnished by the Skilled Nursing Facility or by Others Under Arrangements with the Facility and Under Its Supervision
    - 70.3 - Inpatient Physical Therapy, Occupational Therapy, and Speech Pathology Services
  - Ch 12 - Comprehensive Outpatient Rehabilitation Facility (CORF) Coverage
    - 10 - Comprehensive Outpatient Rehabilitation Facility (CORF) Services Provided by Medicare
    - 20 - Required and Optional CORF Services
    - 20.1 - Required Services
    - 20.2 - Optional CORF Services
    - 30 - Rules for Provision of Services
    - 30.1 - Rules for Payment of CORF Services
    - 40 - Specific CORF Services
    - 40.1 - Physicians' Services
    - 40.2 - Physical Therapy Services
    - 40.3 - Occupational Therapy Services
    - 40.4 - Speech Language Pathology Services
- Pub. 100-3 MEDICARE NATIONAL COVERAGE DETERMINATIONS MANUAL
  - Part 1

CPT © 2017 American Medical Association. All Rights Reserved.                     © 2017 Optum360, LLC

Specific policies may differ by setting. Other policies concerning therapy services are found in other manuals. When a therapy service policy is specific to a setting, it takes precedence over these general outpatient policies. For special rules on:

- CORFs - See chapter 12 of this manual and also Pub. 100-4, chapter 5;
- SNF - See chapter 8 of this manual and also Pub. 100-4, chapter 6, for SNF claims/billing;
- HHA - See chapter 7 of this manual, and Pub. 100-4, chapter 10;
- GROUP THERAPY AND STUDENTS - See Pub. 100-2, chapter 15, §230;
- ARRANGEMENTS - Pub. 100-1, chapter 5, §10.3;
- COVERAGE is described in the Medicare Program Integrity Manual, Pub. 100-08, chapter 13, §13.5.1; and
- THERAPY CAPS - See Pub. 100-4, chapter 5, §10.2, for a complete description of this financial limitation.

### C. General
Therapy services are a covered benefit in §§1861(g), 1861(p), and 1861(ll) of the Act. Therapy services may also be provided incident to the services of a physician/NPP under §§1861(s)(2) and 1862(a)(20) of the Act.

Covered therapy services are furnished by providers, by others under arrangements with and under the supervision of providers, or furnished by suppliers (e.g., physicians, NPP, enrolled therapists), who meet the requirements in Medicare manuals for therapy services.

Where a prospective payment system (PPS) applies, therapy services are paid when services conform to the requirements of that PPS. Reimbursement for therapy provided to Part A inpatients of hospitals or residents of SNFs in covered stays is included in the respective PPS rates.

Payment for therapy provided by an HHA under a plan of treatment is included in the home health PPS rate. Therapy may be billed by an HHA on bill type 34x if there are no home health services billed under a home health plan of care at the same time (e.g., the patient is not homebound), and there is a valid therapy plan of treatment.

In addition to the requirements described in this chapter, the services must be furnished in accordance with health and safety requirements set forth in regulations at 42CFR484, and 42CFR485.

When therapy services may be furnished appropriately in a community pool by a clinician in a physical therapist or occupational therapist private practice, physician office, outpatient hospital, or outpatient SNF, the practice/office or provider shall rent or lease the pool, or a specific portion of the pool. The use of that part of the pool during specified times shall be restricted to the patients of that practice or provider.

The written agreement to rent or lease the pool shall be available for review on request. When part of the pool is rented or leased, the agreement shall describe the part of the pool that is used exclusively by the patients of that practice/office or provider and the times that exclusive use applies. Other providers, including rehabilitation agencies (previously referred to as OPTs and ORFs) and CORFs, are subject to the requirements outlined in the respective State Operations Manual regarding rented or leased community pools.

## 100-02, 15, 230
### *Practice of Physical Therapy, Occupational Therapy, and Speech-Language Pathology*

#### A. Group Therapy Services.
Contractors pay for outpatient physical therapy services (which includes outpatient speech-language pathology services) and outpatient occupational therapy services provided simultaneously to two or more individuals by a practitioner as group therapy services (97150). The individuals can be, but need not be performing the same activity. The physician or therapist involved in group therapy services must be in constant attendance, but one-on-one patient contact is not required.

#### B. Therapy Students
1. General

   Only the services of the therapist can be billed and paid under Medicare Part B. The services performed by a student are not reimbursed even if provided under "line of sight" supervision of the therapist; however, the presence of the student "in the room" does not make the service unbillable. Pay for the direct (one-to-one) patient contact services of the physician or therapist provided to Medicare Part B patients. Group therapy services performed by a therapist or physician may be billed when a student is also present "in the room".

   EXAMPLES:

   Therapists may bill and be paid for the provision of services in the following scenarios:

   - The qualified practitioner is present and in the room for the entire session. The student participates in the delivery of services when the qualified practitioner is directing the service, making the skilled judgment, and is responsible for the assessment and treatment.

   - The qualified practitioner is present in the room guiding the student in service delivery when the therapy student and the therapy assistant student are participating in the provision of services, and the practitioner is not engaged in treating another patient or doing other tasks at the same time.

   - The qualified practitioner is responsible for the services and as such, signs all documentation. (A student may, of course, also sign but it is not necessary since the Part B payment is for the clinician's service, not for the student's services).

2. Therapy Assistants as Clinical Instructors

   Physical therapist assistants and occupational therapy assistants are not precluded from serving as clinical instructors for therapy students, while providing services within their scope of work and performed under the direction and supervision of a licensed physical or occupational therapist to a Medicare beneficiary.

3. Services Provided Under Part A and Part B

   The payment methodologies for Part A and B therapy services rendered by a student are different. Under the MPFS (Medicare Part B), Medicare pays for services provided by physicians and practitioners that are specifically authorized by statute. Students do not meet the definition of practitioners under Medicare Part B. Under SNF PPS, payments are based upon the case mix or Resource Utilization Group (RUG) category that describes the patient. In the rehabilitation groups, the number of therapy minutes delivered to the patient determines the RUG category. Payment levels for each category are based upon the costs of caring for patients in each group rather than providing pecific payment for each therapy service as is done in Medicare Part B.

## 100-02, 15, 230.1
### *Practice of Physical Therapy*

#### A. General
Physical therapy services are those services provided within the scope of practice of physical therapists and necessary for the diagnosis and treatment of impairments, functional limitations, disabilities or changes in physical function and health status. (See Pub. 100-3, the Medicare National Coverage Determinations Manual, for specific conditions or services.) For descriptions of aquatic therapy in a community center pool see section 220C of this chapter.

#### B. Qualified Physical Therapist Defined
Reference: 42CFR484.4

The new personnel qualifications for physical therapists were discussed in the 2008 Physician Fee Schedule. See the Federal Register of November 27, 2007, for the full text. See also the correction notice for this rule, published in the Federal Register on January 15, 2008.

The regulation provides that a qualified physical therapist (PT) is a person who is licensed, if applicable, as a PT by the state in which he or she is practicing unless licensure does not apply, has graduated from an accredited PT education program and passed a national examination approved by the state in which PT services are provided.

The phrase, "by the state in which practicing" includes any authorization to practice provided by the same state in which the service is provided, including temporary licensure, regardless of the location of the entity billing the services. The curriculum accreditation is provided by the Commission on Accreditation in Physical Therapy Education (CAPTE) or, for those who graduated before CAPTE, curriculum approval was provided by the American Physical Therapy Association (APTA). For internationally educated PTs, curricula are approved by a credentials evaluation organization either approved by the APTA or identified in 8 CFR 212.15(e) as it relates to PTs. For example, in 2007, 8 CFR 212.15(e) approved the credentials evaluation provided by the Federation of State Boards of Physical Therapy (FSBPT) and the Foreign Credentialing Commission on Physical Therapy (FCCPT). The requirements above apply to all PTs effective January 1, 2010, if they have not met any of the following requirements prior to January 1, 2010.

Physical therapists whose current license was obtained on or prior to December 31, 2009, qualify to provide PT services to Medicare beneficiaries if they:

- graduated from a CAPTE approved program in PT on or before December 31, 2009 (examination is not required); or,

- graduated on or before December 31, 2009, from a PT program outside the U.S. that is determined to be substantially equivalent to a U.S. program by a credentials evaluating organization approved by either the APTA or identified in 8 CFR 212.15(e) and also passed an examination for PTs approved by the state in which practicing.

Or, PTs whose current license was obtained before January 1, 2008, may meet the requirements in place on that date (i.e., graduation from a curriculum approved by either the APTA, the Committee on Allied Health Education and Accreditation of the American Medical Association, or both).

Or, PTs meet the requirements who are currently licensed and were licensed or qualified as a PT on or before December 31, 1977, and had 2 years appropriate experience as a PT, and passed a proficiency examination conducted, approved, or sponsored by the U.S. Public Health Service.

Or, PTs meet the requirements if they are currently licensed and before January 1, 1966, they were:

- admitted to membership by the APTA; or

- admitted to registration by the American Registry of Physical Therapists; or

- graduated from a 4-year PT curriculum approved by a State Department of Education; or

- licensed or registered and prior to January 1, 1970, they had 15 years of fulltime experience in PT under the order and direction of attending and referring doctors of medicine or osteopathy.

Or, PTs meet requirements if they are currently licensed and they were trained outside the U.S. before January 1, 2008, and after 1928 graduated from a PT curriculum approved in the country in which the curriculum was located, if that country had an organization that was a member of the World Confederation for Physical Therapy, and that PT qualified as a member of the organization.

For outpatient PT services that are provided incident to the services of physicians/NPPs, the requirement for PT licensure does not apply; all other personnel qualifications do apply. The qualified personnel providing PT services incident to the services of a physician/NPP must be trained in an accredited PT curriculum. For example, a person who, on or before December 31, 2009, graduated from a PT curriculum accredited by CAPTE, but who has not passed the national examination or obtained a license, could provide Medicare outpatient PT therapy services incident to the services of a physician/NPP if the physician assumes responsibility for the services according to the incident to policies. On or after January 1, 2010, although licensure does not apply, both education and examination requirements that are effective January 1, 2010, apply to qualified personnel who provide PT services incident to the services of a physician/NPP.

### C. Services of Physical Therapy Support Personnel
Reference: 42CFR 484.4

Personnel Qualifications. The new personnel qualifications for physical therapist assistants (PTA) were discussed in the 2008 Physician Fee Schedule. See the Federal Register of November 27, 2007, for the full text. See also the correction notice for this rule, published in the Federal Register on January 15, 2008.

The regulation provides that a qualified PTA is a person who is licensed as a PTA unless licensure does not apply, is registered or certified, if applicable, as a PTA by the state in which practicing, and graduated from an approved curriculum for PTAs, and passed a national examination for PTAs. The phrase, "by the state in which practicing" includes any authorization to practice provided by the same state in which the service is provided, including temporary licensure, regardless of the location or the entity billing for the services. Approval for the curriculum is provided by CAPTE or, if internationally or military trained PTAs apply, approval will be through a credentialing body for the curriculum for PTAs identified by either the American Physical Therapy Association or identified in 8 CFR 212.15(e). A national examination for PTAs is, for example the one furnished by the Federation of State Boards of Physical Therapy. These requirements above apply to all PTAs effective January 1, 2010, if they have not met any of the following requirements prior to January 1, 2010.

Those PTAs also qualify who, on or before December 31, 2009, are licensed, registered or certified as a PTA and met one of the two following requirements:

1. Is licensed or otherwise regulated in the state in which practicing; or

2. In states that have no licensure or other regulations, or where licensure does not apply, PTAs have:

   — graduated on or before December 31, 2009, from a 2-year college-level program approved by the APTA or CAPTE; and

   — effective January 1, 2010, those PTAs must have both graduated from a CAPTE approved curriculum and passed a national examination for PTAs; or

   — PTAs may also qualify if they are licensed, registered or certified as a PTA, if applicable and meet requirements in effect before January 1, 2008, that is,

     – they have graduated before January 1, 2008, from a 2 year college level program approved by the APTA; or

     – on or before December 31, 1977, they were licensed or qualified as a PTA and passed a proficiency examination conducted, approved, or sponsored by the U.S. Public Health Service.

Services. The services of PTAs used when providing covered therapy benefits are included as part of the covered service. These services are billed by the supervising physical therapist. PTAs may not provide evaluation services, make clinical judgments or decisions or take responsibility for the service. They act at the direction and under the supervision of the treating physical therapist and in accordance with state laws.

A physical therapist must supervise PTAs. The level and frequency of supervision differs by setting (and by state or local law). General supervision is required for PTAs in all settings except private practice (which requires direct supervision) unless state practice requirements are more stringent, in which case state or local requirements must be followed. See specific settings for details. For example, in clinics, rehabilitation services, either on or off the organization's premises, those services are supervised by a qualified physical therapist who makes an onsite supervisory visit at least once every 30 days or more frequently if required by state or local laws or regulation.

The services of a PTA shall not be billed as services incident to a physician/NPP's service, because they do not meet the qualifications of a therapist.

The cost of supplies (e.g., theraband, hand putty, electrodes) used in furnishing covered therapy care is included in the payment for the HCPCS codes billed by the physical therapist, and are, therefore, not separately billable. Separate coverage and billing provisions apply to items that meet the definition of brace in Sec.130.

Services provided by aides, even if under the supervision of a therapist, are not therapy services and are not covered by Medicare. Although an aide may help the therapist by providing unskilled services, those services that are unskilled are not covered by Medicare and shall be denied as not reasonable and necessary if they are billed as therapy services.

### D. Application of Medicare Guidelines to PT Services
This subsection will be used in the future to illustrate the application of the above guidelines to some of the physical therapy modalities and procedures utilized in the treatment of patients.

## 100-02, 15, 230.2

### *Practice of Occupational Therapy*

230.2 - Practice of Occupational Therapy (Rev. 88, Issued: 05-07-08, Effective: 01-01-08, Implementation: 06-09-08)

#### A. General
Occupational therapy services are those services provided within the scope of practice of occupational therapists and necessary for the diagnosis and treatment of impairments, functional disabilities or changes in physical function and health status. (See Pub. 100- 03, the Medicare National Coverage Determinations Manual, for specific conditions or services.)

Occupational therapy is medically prescribed treatment concerned with improving or restoring functions which have been impaired by illness or injury or, where function has been permanently lost or reduced by illness or injury, to improve the individual's ability to perform those tasks required for independent functioning. Such therapy may involve:

- The evaluation, and reevaluation as required, of a patient's level of function by administering diagnostic and prognostic tests;

- The selection and teaching of task-oriented therapeutic activities designed to restore physical function; e.g., use of woodworking activities on an inclined table to restore shoulder, elbow, and wrist range of motion lost as a result of burns;

- The planning, implementing, and supervising of individualized therapeutic activity programs as part of an overall "active treatment" program for a patient with a diagnosed psychiatric illness; e.g., the use of sewing activities which require following a pattern to reduce confusion and restore reality orientation in a schizophrenic patient;

- The planning and implementing of therapeutic tasks and activities to restore sensoryintegrative function; e.g., providing motor and tactile activities to increase sensory input and improve response for a stroke patient with functional loss resulting in a distorted body image;

- The teaching of compensatory technique to improve the level of independence in the activities of daily living, for example:

— Teaching a patient who has lost the use of an arm how to pare potatoes and chop vegetables with one hand;

— Teaching an upper extremity amputee how to functionally utilize a prosthesis;

— Teaching a stroke patient new techniques to enable the patient to perform feeding, dressing, and other activities as independently as possible; or

— Teaching a patient with a hip fracture/hip replacement techniques of standing tolerance and balance to enable the patient to perform such functional activities as dressing and homemaking tasks.

The designing, fabricating, and fitting of orthotics and self-help devices; e.g., making a hand splint for a patient with rheumatoid arthritis to maintain the hand in a functional position or constructing a device which would enable an individual to hold a utensil and feed independently; or Vocational and prevocational assessment and training, subject to the limitations specified in item B below.

Only a qualified occupational therapist has the knowledge, training, and experience required to evaluate and, as necessary, reevaluate a patient's level of function, determine whether an occupational therapy program could reasonably be expected to improve, restore, or compensate for lost function and, where appropriate, recommend to the physician/NPP a plan of treatment.

### B. Qualified Occupational Therapist Defined
Reference: 42CFR484.4 The new personnel qualifications for occupational therapists (OT) were discussed in the 2008 Physician Fee Schedule. See the Federal Register of November 27, 2007, for the full text. See also the correction notice for this rule, published in the Federal Register on January 15, 2008.

The regulation provides that a qualified OT is an individual who is licensed, if licensure applies, or otherwise regulated, if applicable, as an OT by the state in which practicing, and graduated from an accredited education program for OTs, and is eligible to take or has passed the examination for OTs administered by the National Board for Certification in Occupational Therapy, Inc. (NBCOT). The phrase, "by the state in which practicing" includes any authorization to practice provided by the same state in which the service is provided, including temporary licensure, regardless of the location of the entity billing the services. The education program for U.S. trained OTs is accredited by the Accreditation Council for Occupational Therapy Education (ACOTE). The requirements above apply to all OTs effective January 1, 2010, if they have not met any of the following requirements prior to January 1, 2010.

The OTs may also qualify if on or before December 31, 2009:

- they are licensed or otherwise regulated as an OT in the state in which practicing (regardless of the qualifications they met to obtain that licensure or regulation); or

- when licensure or other regulation does not apply, OTs have graduated from an OT education program accredited by ACOTE and are eligible to take, or have successfully completed the NBCOT examination for OTs.

Also, those OTs who met the Medicare requirements for OTs that were in 42CFR484.4 prior to January 1, 2008, qualify to provide OT services for Medicare beneficiaries if:

- on or before January 1, 2008, they graduated an OT program approved jointly by the American Medical Association and the AOTA, or

- they are eligible for the National Registration Examination of AOTA or the National Board for Certification in OT.

Also, they qualify who on or before December 31, 1977, had 2 years of appropriate experience as an occupational therapist, and had achieved a satisfactory grade on a proficiency examination conducted, approved, or sponsored by the U.S. Public Health Service.

Those educated outside the U.S. may meet the same qualifications for domestic trained OTs. For example, they qualify if they were licensed or otherwise regulated by the state in which practicing on or before December 31, 2009. Or they are qualified if they:

- graduated from an OT education program accredited as substantially equivalent to a U.S. OT education program by ACOTE, the World Federation of Occupational Therapists, or a credentialing body approved by AOTA; and

- passed the NBCOT examination for OT; and

- Effective January 1, 2010, are licensed or otherwise regulated, if applicable as an OT by the state in which practicing.

For outpatient OT services that are provided incident to the services of physicians/NPPs, the requirement for OT licensure does not apply; all other personnel qualifications do apply. The qualified personnel providing OT services incident to the services of a physician/NPP must be trained in an accredited OT curriculum. For example, a person who, on or before December 31, 2009, graduated from an OT curriculum accredited by ACOTE and is eligible to take or has successfully completed the entry-level certification examination for OTs developed and administered by NBCOT, could provide Medicare outpatient OT services incident to the services of a physician/NPP if the physician assumes responsibility for the services according to the incident to policies. On or after January 1, 2010, although licensure does not apply, both education and examination requirements that are effective January 1, 2010, apply to qualified personnel who provide OT services incident to the services of a physician/NPP.

### C. Services of Occupational Therapy Support Personnel
Reference: 42CFR 484.4

The new personnel qualifications for occupational therapy assistants were discussed in the 2008 Physician Fee Schedule. See the Federal Register of November 27, 2007, for the full text. See also the correction notice for this rule, published in the Federal Register on January 15, 2008.

The regulation provides that an occupational therapy assistant is a person who is licensed, unless licensure does not apply, or otherwise regulated, if applicable, as an OTA by the state in which practicing, and graduated from an OTA education program accredited by ACOTE and is eligible to take or has successfully completed the NBCOT examination for OTAs. The phrase, "by the state in which practicing" includes any authorization to practice provided by the same state in which the service is provided, including temporary licensure, regardless of the location of the entity billing the services.

If the requirements above are not met, an OTA may qualify if, on or before December 31, 2009, the OTA is licensed or otherwise regulated as an OTA, if applicable, by the state in which practicing, or meets any qualifications defined by the state in which practicing.

Or, where licensure or other state regulation does not apply, OTAs may qualify if they have, on or before December 31, 2009:

- completed certification requirements to practice as an OTA established by a credentialing organization approved by AOTA; and

- after January 1, 2010, they have also completed an education program accredited by ACOTE and passed the NBCOT examination for OTAs.

OTAs who qualified under the policies in effect prior to January 1, 2008, continue to qualify to provide OT directed and supervised OTA services to Medicare beneficiaries.

Therefore, OTAs qualify who after December 31, 1977, and on or before December 31, 2007:

- completed certification requirements to practice as an OTA established by a credentialing organization approved by AOTA; or

- completed the requirements to practice as an OTA applicable in the state in which practicing.

Those OTAs who were educated outside the U.S. may meet the same requirements as domestically trained OTAs. Or, if educated outside the U.S. on or after January 1, 2008, they must have graduated from an OTA program accredited as substantially equivalent to OTA entry level education in the U.S. by ACOTE, its successor organization, or the World Federation of Occupational Therapists or a credentialing body approved by AOTA. In addition, they must have passed an exam for OTAs administered by NBCOT.

Services. The services of OTAs used when providing covered therapy benefits are included as part of the covered service. These services are billed by the supervising occupational therapist. OTAs may not provide evaluation services, make clinical judgments or decisions or take responsibility for the service. They act at the direction and under the supervision of the treating occupational therapist and in accordance with state laws.

An occupational therapist must supervise OTAs. The level and frequency of supervision differs by setting (and by state or local law). General supervision is required for OTAs in all settings except private practice (which requires direct supervision) unless state practice requirements are more stringent, in which case state or local requirements must be followed. See specific settings for details. For example, in clinics, rehabilitation agencies, and public health agencies, 42CFR485.713 indicates that when an OTA provides services, either on or off the organization's premises, those services are supervised by a qualified occupational therapist who makes an onsite supervisory visit at least once every 30 days or more frequently if required by state or local laws or regulation.

The services of an OTA shall not be billed as services incident to a physician/NPP's service, because they do not meet the qualifications of a therapist.

The cost of supplies (e.g., looms, ceramic tiles, or leather) used in furnishing covered therapy care is included in the payment for the HCPCS codes billed by the occupational therapist and are, therefore, not separately billable. Separate coverage and billing provisions apply to items that meet the definition of brace in Sec.130 of this manual.

Services provided by aides, even if under the supervision of a therapist, are not therapy services in the outpatient setting and are not covered by Medicare. Although an aide may help the therapist by providing unskilled services, those services that are unskilled are not covered by Medicare and shall be denied as not reasonable and necessary if they are billed as therapy services.

### D. Application of Medicare Guidelines to Occupational Therapy Services
Occupational therapy may be required for a patient with a specific diagnosed psychiatric illness. If such services are required, they are covered assuming the coverage criteria are met. However, where an individual's motivational needs are not related to a specific diagnosed psychiatric illness, the meeting of such needs does not usually require an individualized therapeutic program. Such needs can be met through general activity programs or the efforts of other professional personnel involved in the care of the patient. Patient motivation is an appropriate and inherent function of all health disciplines, which is interwoven with other functions performed by such personnel for the patient. Accordingly, since the special skills of an occupational therapist are not required, an occupational therapy program for individuals who do not have a specific diagnosed psychiatric illness is not to be considered reasonable and necessary for the treatment of an illness or injury. Services furnished under such a program are not covered.

Occupational therapy may include vocational and prevocational assessment and training. When services provided by an occupational therapist are related solely to specific employment opportunities, work skills, or work settings, they are not reasonable or necessary for the diagnosis or treatment of an illness or injury and are not covered. However, carriers and intermediaries exercise care in applying this exclusion, because the assessment of level of function and the teaching of compensatory techniques to improve the level of function, especially in activities of daily living, are services which occupational therapists provide for both vocational and nonvocational purposes. For example, an assessment of sitting and standing tolerance might be nonvocational for a mother of young children or a retired individual living alone, but could also be a vocational test for a sales clerk. Training an amputee in the use of prosthesis for telephoning is necessary for everyday activities as well as for employment purposes. Major changes in life style may be mandatory for an individual with a substantial disability. The techniques of adjustment cannot be considered exclusively vocational or nonvocational.

## 100-02, 15, 230.4

### Services Furnished by a Therapist in Private Practice

#### A. General

See section 220 of this chapter for definitions. Therapist refers only to a qualified physical therapist, occupational therapist or speech-language pathologist. TPP refers to therapists in private practice (qualified physical therapists, occupational therapists and speech-language pathologists).

In order to qualify to bill Medicare directly as a therapist, each individual must be enrolled as a private practitioner and employed in one of the following practice types: an unincorporated solo practice, unincorporated partnership, unincorporated group practice, physician/NPP group or groups that are not professional corporations, if allowed by state and local law. Physician/NPP group practices may employ TPP if state and local law permits this employee relationship.

For purposes of this provision, a physician/NPP group practice is defined as one or more physicians/NPPs enrolled with Medicare who may bill as one entity. For further details on issues concerning enrollment, see the provider enrollment Web site at www.cms.hhs.gov/MedicareProviderSupEnroll and Pub. 100-08, Medicare Program Integrity Manual, chapter15, section 15.4.4.9.

Private practice also includes therapists who are practicing therapy as employees of another supplier, of a professional corporation or other incorporated therapy practice. Private practice does not include individuals when they are working as employees of an institutional provider.

Services should be furnished in the therapist's or group's office or in the patient's home. The office is defined as the location(s) where the practice is operated, in the state(s) where the therapist (and practice, if applicable) is legally authorized to furnish services, during the hours that the therapist engages in the practice at that location. If services are furnished in a private practice office space, that space shall be owned, leased, or rented by the practice and used for the exclusive purpose of operating the practice. For descriptions of aquatic therapy in a community center pool see section 220C of this chapter.

Therapists in private practice must be approved as meeting certain requirements, but do not execute a formal provider agreement with the Secretary.

If therapists who have their own Medicare National Provider Identifier (NPI) are employed by therapist groups, physician/NPP groups, or groups that are not professional organizations, the requirement that therapy space be owned, leased, or rented may be satisfied by the group that employs the therapist. Each therapist employed by a group should enroll as a TPP.

When therapists with a Medicare NPI provide services in the physician's/NPP's office in which they are employed, and bill using their NPI for each therapy service, then the direct supervision requirement for enrolled staff apply.

When the therapist who has a Medicare NPI is employed in a physician's/NPP's office the services are ordinarily billed as services of the therapist, with the therapist identified on the claim as the supplier of services. However, services of the therapist who has a Medicare NPI may also be billed by the physician/NPP as services incident to the physician's/NPP's service. (See §230.5 for rules related to therapy services incident to a physician.) In that case, the physician/NPP is the supplier of service, the NPI of the supervising physician/NPP is reported on the claim with the service and all the rules for both therapy services and incident to services (§230.5) must be followed.

#### B. Private Practice Defined

Reference: Federal Register November, 1998, pages 58863-58869; 42CFR 410.38(b), 42CFR410.59, 42CFR410.60, 42CFR410.62

The contractor considers a therapist to be in private practice if the therapist maintains office space at his or her own expense and furnishes services only in that space or the patient's home. Or, a therapist is employed by another supplier and furnishes services in facilities established at the expense of that supplier.

The therapist need not be in full-time private practice but must be engaged in private practice on a regular basis; i.e., the therapist is recognized as a private practitioner and for that purpose has access to the necessary equipment to provide an adequate program of therapy.

The therapy services must be provided either by or under the direct supervision of the TPP. Each TPP should be enrolled as a Medicare provider. If a therapist is not enrolled, the services of that therapist must be directly supervised by an enrolled therapist. Direct supervision requires that the supervising private practice therapist be present in the office suite at the time the service is performed. These direct

supervision requirements apply only in the private practice setting and only for therapists and their assistants. In other outpatient settings, supervision rules differ. The services of support personnel must be included in the therapist's bill. The supporting personnel, including other therapists, must be W-2 or 1099 employees of the TPP or other qualified employer.

Coverage of outpatient therapy under Part B includes the services of a qualified TPP when furnished in the therapist's office or the beneficiary's home. For this purpose, "home" includes an institution that is used as a home, but not a hospital, CAH or SNF, (Federal Register Nov. 2, 1998, pg 58869).

#### C. Assignment

Reference: Nov. 2, 1998 Federal Register, pg. 58863

See also Pub. 100-4 chapter 1, §30.2.

When physicians, NPPs, or TPPs obtain provider numbers, they have the option of accepting assignment (participating) or not accepting assignment (nonparticipating). In contrast, providers, such as outpatient hospitals, SNFs, rehabilitation agencies, and CORFs, do not have the option. For these providers, assignment is mandatory.

If physicians/NPPs, or TPPs accept assignment (are participating), they must accept the Medicare Physician Fee Schedule amount as payment. Medicare pays 80% and the patient is responsible for 20%. In contrast, if they do not accept assignment, Medicare will only pay 95% of the fee schedule amount. However, when these services are not furnished on an assignment-related basis, the limiting charge applies. (See §1848(g)(2)(c) of the Act.)

NOTE: Services furnished by a therapist in the therapist's office under arrangements with hospitals in rural communities and public health agencies (or services provided in the beneficiary's home under arrangements with a provider of outpatient physical or occupational therapy services) are not covered under this provision. See section 230.6.

## 100-02, 15, 232

### Cardiac Rehabilitation (CR) and Intensive Cardiac Rehabilitation (ICR) Services Furnished On or After January 1, 2010

Cardiac rehabilitation (CR) services mean a physician-supervised program that furnishes physician prescribed exercise, cardiac risk factor modification, including education, counseling, and behavioral intervention; psychosocial assessment, outcomes assessment, and other items/services as determined by the Secretary under certain conditions. Intensive cardiac rehabilitation (ICR) services mean a physician-supervised program that furnishes the same items/services under the same conditions as a CR program but must also demonstrate, as shown in peer-reviewed published research, that it improves patients' cardiovascular disease through specific outcome measurements described in 42 CFR 410.49(c). Effective January 1, 2010, Medicare Part B pays for CR/ICR programs and related items/services if specific criteria is met by the Medicare beneficiary, the CR/ICR program itself, the setting in which is it administered, and the physician administering the program, as outlined below:

#### CR/ICR Program Beneficiary Requirements:

Medicare covers CR/ICR program services for beneficiaries who have experienced one or more of the following:

- Acute myocardial infarction within the preceding 12 months;
- Coronary artery bypass surgery;
- Current stable angina pectoris;
- Heart valve repair or replacement;
- Percutaneous transluminal coronary angioplasty (PTCA) or coronary stenting;
- Heart or heart-lung transplant.

For cardiac rehabilitation only: Stable, chronic heart failure defined as patients with left ventricular ejection fraction of 35% or less and New York Heart Association (NYHA) class II to IV symptoms despite being on optimal heart failure therapy for at least 6 weeks. (Effective February 18, 2014.)

#### CR/ICR Program Component Requirements:

- Physician-prescribed exercise. This physical activity includes aerobic exercise combined with other types of exercise (i.e., strengthening, stretching) as determined to be appropriate for individual patients by a physician each day CR/ICR items/services are furnished.
- Cardiac risk factor modification. This includes education, counseling, and behavioral intervention, tailored to the patients' individual needs.
- Psychosocial assessment. This assessment means an evaluation of an individual's mental and emotional functioning as it relates to the individual's rehabilitation. It should include: (1) an assessment of those aspects of the individual's family and home situation that affects the individual's rehabilitation treatment, and, (2) a psychosocial evaluation of the individual's response to, and rate of progress under, the treatment plan.
- Outcomes assessment. These should include: (i) minimally, assessments from the commencement and conclusion of CR/ICR, based on patient-centered outcomes which must be measured by the physician immediately at the beginning and end of the program, and, (ii) objective clinical measures of the effectiveness of the CR/ICR program for the individual patient, including exercise performance and self-reported measures of exertion and behavior.

- Individualized treatment plan. This plan should be written and tailored to each individual patient and include (i) a description of the individual's diagnosis; (ii) the type, amount, frequency, and duration of the CR/ICR items/services furnished; and (iii) the goals set for the individual under the plan. The individualized treatment plan must be established, reviewed, and signed by a physician every 30 days.

As specified at 42 CFR 410.49(f)(1), CR sessions are limited to a maximum of 2 1-hour sessions per day for up to 36 sessions over up to 36 weeks with the option for an additional 36 sessions over an extended period of time if approved by the contractor under section 1862(a)(1)(A) of the Act. ICR sessions are limited to 72 1-hour sessions (as defined in section 1848(b)(5) of the Act), up to 6 sessions per day, over a period of up to 18 weeks.

### CR/ICR Program Setting Requirements:
CR/ICR services must be furnished in a physician's office or a hospital outpatient setting (for ICR, the hospital outpatient setting must provide ICR using an approved ICR program). All settings must have a physician immediately available and accessible for medical consultations and emergencies at all times when items/services are being furnished under the program. This provision is satisfied if the physician meets the requirements for direct supervision of physician office services as specified at 42 CFR 410.26, and for hospital outpatient services as specified at 42 CFR 410.27.

### ICR Program Approval Requirements:
All prospective ICR programs must be approved through the national coverage determination (NCD) process. To be approved as an ICR program, it must demonstrate through peer-reviewed, published research that it has accomplished one or more of the following for its patients: (i) positively affected the progression of coronary heart disease, (ii) reduced the need for coronary bypass surgery, or, (iii) reduced the need for percutaneous coronary interventions.

An ICR program must also demonstrate through peer-reviewed, published research that it accomplished a statistically significant reduction in five or more of the following measures for patients from their levels before CR services to after CR services: (i) low density lipoprotein, (ii) triglycerides, (iii) body mass index, (iv) systolic blood pressure, (v) diastolic blood pressure, and (vi) the need for cholesterol, blood pressure, and diabetes medications.

A list of approved ICR programs, identified through the NCD process, will be posted to the CMS Web site and listed in the Federal Register.

Once an ICR program is approved through the NCD process, all prospective ICR sites wishing to furnish ICR items/services via an approved ICR program may enroll with their local contractor to become an ICR program supplier using the designated forms as specified at 42 CFR 424.510, and report specialty code 31 to be identified as an enrolled ICR supplier. For purposes of appealing an adverse determination concerning site approval, an ICR site is considered a supplier (or prospective supplier) as defined in 42 CFR 498.2.

### CR/ICR Program Physician Requirements:
Physicians responsible for CR/ICR programs are identified as medical directors who oversee or supervise the CR/ICR program at a particular site. The medical director, in consultation with staff, is involved in directing the progress of individuals in the program. The medical director, as well as physicians acting as the supervising physician, must possess all of the following: (1) expertise in the management of individuals with cardiac pathophysiology, (2) cardiopulmonary training in basic life support or advanced cardiac life support, and (3) licensed to practice medicine in the state in which the CR/ICR program is offered. Direct physician supervision may be provided by a supervising physician or the medical director.

(See Pub. 100-3, Medicare National Coverage Determinations Manual, Chapter 1, Part 1, section 20.10.1, Pub. 100-4, Medicare Claims Processing Manual, Chapter 32, section 140, Pub. 100-08, Medicare Program Integrity Manual, Chapter 15, section 15.4.2.8, for specific claims processing, coding, and billing requirements for CR/ICR program services.)

## 100-02, 15, 240

### Chiropractic Services - General
B3-2250, B3-4118

The term "physician" under Part B includes a chiropractor who meets the specified qualifying requirements set forth in Sec.30.5 but only for treatment by means of manual manipulation of the spine to correct a subluxation.

Effective for claims with dates of services on or after January 1, 2000, an x-ray is not required to demonstrate the subluxation.

Implementation of the chiropractic benefit requires an appreciation of the differences between chiropractic theory and experience and traditional medicine due to fundamental differences regarding etiology and theories of the pathogenesis of disease. Judgments about the reasonableness of chiropractic treatment must be based on the application of chiropractic principles. So that Medicare beneficiaries receive equitable adjudication of claims based on such principles and are not deprived of the benefits intended by the law, carriers may use chiropractic consultation in carrier review of Medicare chiropractic claims.

Payment is based on the physician fee schedule and made to the beneficiary or, on assignment, to the chiropractor.

### A. Verification of Chiropractor's Qualifications
Carriers must establish a reference file of chiropractors eligible for payment as physicians under the criteria in Sec.30.1. They pay only chiropractors on file. Information needed to establish such files is furnished by the CMS RO.

The RO is notified by the appropriate State agency which chiropractors are licensed and whether each meets the national uniform standards.

## 100-02, 15, 240.1.3

### Necessity for Treatment
The patient must have a significant health problem in the form of a neuromusculoskeletal condition necessitating treatment, and the manipulative services rendered must have a direct therapeutic relationship to the patient's condition and provide reasonable expectation of recovery or improvement of function. The patient must have a subluxation of the spine as demonstrated by x-ray or physical exam, as described above.

Most spinal joint problems fall into the following categories:

- Acute subluxation-A patient's condition is considered acute when the patient is being treated for a new injury, identified by x-ray or physical exam as specified above. The result of chiropractic manipulation is expected to be an improvement in, or arrest of progression, of the patient's condition.

- Chronic subluxation-A patient's condition is considered chronic when it is not expected to significantly improve or be resolved with further treatment (as is the case with an acute condition), but where the continued therapy can be expected to result in some functional improvement. Once the clinical status has remained stable for a given condition, without expectation of additional objective clinical improvements, further manipulative treatment is considered maintenance therapy and is not covered.

For Medicare purposes, a chiropractor must place an AT modifier on a claim when providing active/corrective treatment to treat acute or chronic subluxation. However the presence of the AT modifier may not in all instances indicate that the service is reasonable and necessary. As always, contractors may deny if appropriate after medical review.

### A. Maintenance Therapy
Maintenance therapy includes services that seek to prevent disease, promote health and prolong and enhance the quality of life, or maintain or prevent deterioration of a chronic condition. When further clinical improvement cannot reasonably be expected from continuous ongoing care, and the chiropractic treatment becomes supportive rather than corrective in nature, the treatment is then considered maintenance therapy. The AT modifier must not be placed on the claim when maintenance therapy has been provided. Claims without the AT modifier will be considered as maintenance therapy and denied. Chiropractors who give or receive from beneficiaries an ABN shall follow the instructions in Pub. 100-4, Medicare Claims Processing Manual, chapter 23, section 20.9.1.1 and include a GA (or in rare instances a GZ) modifier on the claim.

### B. Contraindications
Dynamic thrust is the therapeutic force or maneuver delivered by the physician during manipulation in the anatomic region of involvement. A relative contraindication is a condition that adds significant risk of injury to the patient from dynamic thrust, but does not rule out the use of dynamic thrust. The doctor should discuss this risk with the patient and record this in the chart. The following are relative contraindications to dynamic thrust:

- Articular hyper mobility and circumstances where the stability of the joint is uncertain;

- Severe demineralization of bone;

- Benign bone tumors (spine);

- Bleeding disorders and anticoagulant therapy; and

- Radiculopathy with progressive neurological signs.

- Dynamic thrust is absolutely contraindicated near the site of demonstrated subluxation and proposed manipulation in the following:

- Acute arthropathies characterized by acute inflammation and ligamentous laxity and anatomic subluxation or dislocation; including acute rheumatoid arthritis and ankylosing spondylitis;

- Acute fractures and dislocations or healed fractures and dislocations with signs of instability;

- An unstable os odontoideum;

- Malignancies that involve the vertebral column;

- Infection of bones or joints of the vertebral column;

- Signs and symptoms of myelopathy or cauda equina syndrome;

- For cervical spinal manipulations, vertebrobasilar insufficiency syndrome; and

- A significant major artery aneurysm near the proposed manipulation.

## 100-02, 15, 280.5.1

### Advance Care Planning (ACP) Furnished as an Optional Element with an Annual Wellness Visit (AWV) Upon Agreement with the Patient

(Rev. 216 Issued: 12-22-15, Effective: 01-01-16, Implementation: 01-04-16)

Beginning in CY 2016, CMS will treat an AWV and voluntary ACP that are furnished on the same day and by the same provider as a preventive service. Voluntary ACP services, upon agreement with the patient, will be an optional element of the AWV. (See section 1861(hhh)(2)(G) of the Act.) When ACP services are furnished as a part of an AWV, according to sections 1833(a)(1) and 1833(b)(10) of the Act, the coinsurance and deductible are waived.

Voluntary advance care planning means the face-to-face service between a physician (or other qualified health care professional) and the patient discussing advance directives, with or without completing relevant legal forms. An advance directive is a document appointing an agent and/or recording the wishes of a patient pertaining to his/her medical treatment at a future time should he/she lack decisional capacity at that time.

See Pub. 100-04, *Medicare Claims Processing Manual*, chapter 18, section 140.8 for claims processing and billing instructions.

## 100-02, 15, 290

### Foot Care

#### A. Treatment of Subluxation of Foot

Subluxations of the foot are defined as partial dislocations or displacements of joint surfaces, tendons ligaments, or muscles of the foot. Surgical or nonsurgical treatments undertaken for the sole purpose of correcting a subluxated structure in the foot as an isolated entity are not covered.

However, medical or surgical treatment of subluxation of the ankle joint (talo-crural joint) is covered. In addition, reasonable and necessary medical or surgical services, diagnosis, or treatment for medical conditions that have resulted from or are associated with partial displacement of structures is covered. For example, if a patient has osteoarthritis that has resulted in a partial displacement of joints in the foot, and the primary treatment is for the osteoarthritis, coverage is provided.

#### B. Exclusions from Coverage

The following foot care services are generally excluded from coverage under both Part A and Part B. (See Sec. 290.F and Sec. 290.G for instructions on applying foot care exclusions.)

1. Treatment of Flat Foot

    The term "flat foot" is defined as a condition in which one or more arches of the foot have flattened out. Services or devices directed toward the care or correction of such conditions, including the prescription of supportive devices, are not covered.

2. Routine Foot Care

    Except as provided above, routine foot care Is excluded from coverage. Services that normally are considered routine and not covered by Medicare include the following:

    — The cutting or removal of corns and calluses;

    — The trimming, cutting, clipping, or debriding of nails; and

    — Other hygienic and preventive maintenance care, such as cleaning and soaking the feet, the use of skin creams to maintain skin tone of either ambulatory or bedfast patients, and any other service performed in the absence of localized illness, injury, or symptoms involving the foot.

3. Supportive Devices for Feet Orthopedic shoes and other supportive devices for the feet generally are not covered.

    However, this exclusion does not apply to such a shoe if it is an integral part of a leg brace, and its expense is included as part of the cost of the brace. Also, this exclusion does not apply to therapeutic shoes furnished to diabetics.

#### C. Exceptions to Routine Foot Care Exclusion

1. Necessary and Integral Part of Otherwise Covered Services

    In certain circumstances, services ordinarily considered to be routine may be covered if they are performed as a necessary and integral part of otherwise covered services, such as diagnosis and treatment of ulcers, wounds, or infections.

2. Treatment of Warts on Foot

    The treatment of warts (including plantar warts) on the foot is covered to the same extent as services provided for the treatment of warts located elsewhere on the body.

3. Presence of Systemic Condition

    The presence of a systemic condition such as metabolic, neurologic, or peripheral vascular disease may require scrupulous foot care by a professional that in the absence of such condition(s) would be considered routine (and, therefore, excluded from coverage). Accordingly, foot care that would otherwise be considered routine may be covered when systemic condition(s) result in severe circulatory embarrassment or areas of diminished sensation in the individual's legs or feet. (See subsection A.)

In these instances, certain foot care procedures that otherwise are considered routine (e.g., cutting or removing corns and calluses, or trimming, cutting, clipping, or debriding nails) may pose a hazard when performed by a nonprofessional person on patients with such systemic conditions. (See Sec.290.G for procedural instructions.)

4. Mycotic Nails

    In the absence of a systemic condition, treatment of mycotic nails may be covered.

    The treatment of mycotic nails for an ambulatory patient is covered only when the physician attending the patient's mycotic condition documents that (1) there is clinical evidence of mycosis of the toenail, and (2) the patient has marked limitation of ambulation, pain, or secondary infection resulting from the thickening and dystrophy of the infected toenail plate.

    The treatment of mycotic nails for a nonambulatory patient is covered only when the physician attending the patient's mycotic condition documents that (1) there is clinical evidence of mycosis of the toenail, and (2) the patient suffers from pain or secondary infection resulting from the thickening and dystrophy of the infected toenail plate.

    For the purpose of these requirements, documentation means any written information that is required by the carrier in order for services to be covered. Thus, the information submitted with claims must be substantiated by information found in the patient's medical record. Any information, including that contained in a form letter, used for documentation purposes is subject to carrier verification in order to ensure that the information adequately justifies coverage of the treatment of mycotic nails.

#### D. Systemic Conditions That Might Justify Coverage

Although not intended as a comprehensive list, the following metabolic, neurologic, and peripheral vascular diseases (with synonyms in parentheses) most commonly represent the underlying conditions that might justify coverage for routine foot care.

Diabetes mellitus *

Arteriosclerosis obliterans (A.S.O., arteriosclerosis of the extremities, occlusive peripheral arteriosclerosis)

Buerger's disease (thromboangiitis obliterans)

Chronic thrombophlebitis *

Peripheral neuropathies involving the feet -

— Associated with malnutrition and vitamin deficiency *

    – Malnutrition (general, pellagra)

    – Alcoholism

    – Malabsorption (celiac disease, tropical sprue)

    – Pernicious anemia Associated with carcinoma *

— Associated with diabetes mellitus *

— Associated with drugs and toxins *

— Associated with multiple sclerosis *

— Associated with uremia (chronic renal disease) *

— Associated with traumatic injury

— Associated with leprosy or neurosyphilis

— Associated with hereditary disorders

    – Hereditary sensory radicular neuropathy

    – Angiokeratoma corporis diffusum (Fabry's)

    – Amyloid neuropathy

When the patient's condition is one of those designated by an asterisk (*), routine procedures are covered only if the patient is under the active care of a doctor of medicine or osteopathy who documents the condition.

#### E. Supportive Devices for Feet Orthopedic shoes and other supportive devices for the feet generally are not covered.

However, this exclusion does not apply to such a shoe if it is an integral part of a leg brace, and its expense is included as part of the cost of the brace. Also, this exclusion does not apply to therapeutic shoes furnished to diabetics.

#### F. Presumption of Coverage

In evaluating whether the routine services can be reimbursed, a presumption of coverage may be made where the evidence available discloses certain physical and/or clinical findings consistent with the diagnosis and indicative of severe peripheral involvement.

For purposes of applying this presumption the following findings are pertinent:

**Class A Findings**

Nontraumatic amputation of foot or integral skeletal portion thereof.

**Class B Findings**

Absent posterior tibial pulse;

Advanced trophic changes as: hair growth (decrease or absence) nail changes (thickening) pigmentary changes (discoloration) skin texture (thin, shiny) skin color (rubor or redness) (Three required); and

Absent dorsalis pedis pulse.

    CPT © 2017 American Medical Association. All Rights Reserved.    © 2017 Optum360, LLC

**Class C Findings**

Claudication;

Temperature changes (e.g., cold feet);

Edema;

Paresthesias (abnormal spontaneous sensations in the feet); and

Burning.

The presumption of coverage may be applied when the physician rendering the routine foot care has identified:

1. A Class A finding;
2. Two of the Class B findings; or
3. One Class B and two Class C findings.

Cases evidencing findings falling short of these alternatives may involve podiatric treatment that may constitute covered care and should be reviewed by the intermediary's medical staff and developed as necessary.

For purposes of applying the coverage presumption where the routine services have been rendered by a podiatrist, the contractor may deem the active care requirement met if the claim or other evidence available discloses that the patient has seen an M.D. or D.O. for treatment and/or evaluation of the complicating disease process during the 6-month period prior to the rendition of the routine-type services. The intermediary may also accept the podiatrist's statement that the diagnosing and treating M.D. or D.O. also concurs with the podiatrist's findings as to the severity of the peripheral involvement indicated.

Services ordinarily considered routine might also be covered if they are performed as a necessary and integral part of otherwise covered services, such as diagnosis and treatment of diabetic ulcers, wounds, and infections.

**G. Application of Foot Care Exclusions to Physician's Services**

The exclusion of foot care is determined by the nature of the service. Thus, payment for an excluded service should be denied whether performed by a podiatrist, osteopath, or a doctor of medicine, and without regard to the difficulty or complexity of the procedure.

When an itemized bill shows both covered services and noncovered services not integrally related to the covered service, the portion of charges attributable to the noncovered services should be denied. (For example, if an itemized bill shows surgery for an ingrown toenail and also removal of calluses not necessary for the performance of toe surgery, any additional charge attributable to removal of the calluses should be denied.) In reviewing claims involving foot care, the carrier should be alert to the following exceptional situations:

1. Payment may be made for incidental noncovered services performed as a necessary and integral part of, and secondary to, a covered procedure. For example, if trimming of toenails is required for application of a cast to a fractured foot, the carrier need not allocate and deny a portion of the charge for the trimming of the nails. However, a separately itemized charge for such excluded service should be disallowed. When the primary procedure is covered the administration of anesthesia necessary for the performance of such procedure is also covered.

2. Payment may be made for initial diagnostic services performed in connection with a specific symptom or complaint if it seems likely that its treatment would be covered even though the resulting diagnosis may be one requiring only noncovered care.

The name of the M.D. or D.O. who diagnosed the complicating condition must be submitted with the claim. In those cases, where active care is required, the approximate date the beneficiary was last seen by such physician must also be indicated.

NOTE: Section 939 of P.L. 96-499 removed "warts" from the routine foot care exclusion effective July 1, 1981.

Relatively few claims for routine-type care are anticipated considering the severity of conditions contemplated as the basis for this exception. Claims for this type of foot care should not be paid in the absence of convincing evidence that nonprofessional performance of the service would have been hazardous for the beneficiary because of an underlying systemic disease. The mere statement of a diagnosis such as those mentioned in Sec.D above does not of itself indicate the severity of the condition. Where development is indicated to verify diagnosis and/or severity the carrier should follow existing claims processing practices, which may include review of carrier's history and medical consultation as well as physician contacts.

The rules in Sec.290.F concerning presumption of coverage also apply.

Codes and policies for routine foot care and supportive devices for the feet are not exclusively for the use of podiatrists. These codes must be used to report foot care services regardless of the specialty of the physician who furnishes the services. Carriers must instruct physicians to use the most appropriate code available when billing for routine foot care.

## 100-02, 16, 10

### *General Exclusions From Coverage*

A3-3150, HO-260, HHA-232, B3-2300

No payment can be made under either the hospital insurance or supplementary medicalinsurance program for certain items and services, when the following conditions exist:

- Not reasonable and necessary (§20);
- No legal obligation to pay for or provide (§40);
- Paid for by a governmental entity (§50);
- Not provided within United States (§60);
- Resulting from war (§70);
- Personal comfort (§80);
- Routine services and appliances (§90);
- Custodial care (§110);
- Cosmetic surgery (§120);
- Charges by immediate relatives or members of household (§130);
- Dental services (§140);
- Paid or expected to be paid under workers' compensation (§150);
- Nonphysician services provided to a hospital inpatient that were not provided directly or arranged for by the hospital (§170);
- Services Related to and Required as a Result of Services Which are not Covered Under Medicare (§180);
- Excluded foot care services and supportive devices for feet (§30); or
- Excluded investigational devices (See Chapter 14, §30).

## 100-02, 16, 100

### *Hearing Aids and Auditory Implants*

Section 1862(a)(7) of the Social Security Act states that no payment may be made under part A or part B for any expenses incurred for items or services "where such expenses are for . . . hearing aids or examinations therefore. . . ." This policy is further reiterated at 42 CFR 411.15(d) which specifically states that "hearing aids or examination for the purpose of prescribing, fitting, or changing hearing aids" are excluded from coverage.

Hearing aids are amplifying devices that compensate for impaired hearing. Hearing aids include air conduction devices that provide acoustic energy to the cochlea via stimulation of the tympanic membrane with amplified sound. They also include bone conduction devices that provide mechanical energy to the cochlea via stimulation of the scalp with amplified mechanical vibration or by direct contact with the tympanic membrane or middle ear ossicles.

Certain devices that produce perception of sound by replacing the function of the middle ear, cochlea or auditory nerve are payable by Medicare as prosthetic devices. These devices are indicated only when hearing aids are medically inappropriate or cannot be utilized due to congenital malformations, chronic disease, severe sensorineural hearing loss or surgery. The following are prosthetic devices:

- Cochlear implants and auditory brainstem implants, i.e., devices that replace the function of cochlear structures or auditory nerve and provide electrical energy to auditory nerve fibers and other neural tissue via implanted electrode arrays.

- Osseointegrated implants, i.e., devices implanted in the skull that replace the function of the middle ear and provide mechanical energy to the cochlea via a mechanical transducer.

Medicare contractors deny payment for an item or service that is associated with any hearing aid as defined above. See Sec.180 for policy for the medically necessary treatment of complications of implantable hearing aids, such as medically necessary removals of implantable hearing aids due to infection.

## 100-02, 16, 120

### *Cosmetic Surgery*

A3-3160, HO-260.11, B3-2329

Cosmetic surgery or expenses incurred in connection with such surgery is not covered. Cosmetic surgery includes any surgical procedure directed at improving appearance, except when required for the prompt (i.e., as soon as medically feasible) repair of accidental injury or for the improvement of the functioning of a malformed body member. For example, this exclusion does not apply to surgery in connection with treatment of severe burns or repair of the face following a serious automobile accident, or to surgery for therapeutic purposes which coincidentally also serves some cosmetic purpose.

## 100-02, 16, 180

### *Services Related to and Required as a Result of Services Which Are Not Covered Under Medicare*

B3-2300.1, A3-3101.14, HO-210.12

Medical and hospital services are sometimes required to treat a condition that arises as a result of services that are not covered because they are determined to be not reasonable and necessary or because they are excluded from coverage for other reasons. Services "related to" noncovered services (e.g., cosmetic surgery, noncovered organ transplants, noncovered artificial organ implants, etc.), including

**Appendix G — Medicare Internet-only Manuals (IOMs)**

services related to follow-up care and complications of noncovered services which require treatment during a hospital stay in which the noncovered service was performed, are not covered services under Medicare. Services "not related to" noncovered services are covered under Medicare. Following are examples of services "related to" and "not related to" noncovered services while the beneficiary is an inpatient:

- A beneficiary was hospitalized for a noncovered service and broke a leg while in the hospital. Services related to care of the broken leg during this stay is a clear example of "not related to" services and are covered under Medicare.

- A beneficiary was admitted to the hospital for covered services, but during the course of hospitalization became a candidate for a noncovered transplant or implant and actually received the transplant or implant during that hospital stay. When the original admission was entirely unrelated to the diagnosis that led to a recommendation for a noncovered transplant or implant, the services related to the admitting condition would be covered.

- A beneficiary was admitted to the hospital for covered services related to a condition which ultimately led to identification of a need for transplant and receipt of a transplant during the same hospital stay. If, on the basis of the nature of the services and a comparison of the date they are received with the date on which the beneficiary is identified as a transplant candidate, the services could reasonably be attributed to preparation for the noncovered transplant, the services would be "related to" noncovered services and would also be noncovered.

Following is an example of services received subsequent to a noncovered inpatient stay:

- After a beneficiary has been discharged from the hospital stay in which the beneficiary received noncovered services, medical and hospital services required to treat a condition or complication that arises as a result of the prior noncovered services may be covered when they are reasonable and necessary in all other respects. Thus, coverage could be provided for subsequent inpatient stays or outpatient treatment ordinarily covered by Medicare, even if the need for treatment arose because of a previous noncovered procedure. Some examples of services that may be found to be covered under this policy are the reversal of intestinal bypass surgery for obesity, repair of complications from transsexual surgery or from cosmetic surgery, removal of a noncovered bladder stimulator, or treatment of any infection at the surgical site of a noncovered transplant that occurred following discharge from the hospital.

However, any subsequent services that could be expected to have been incorporated into a global fee are considered to have been paid in the global fee, and may not be paid again. Thus, where a patient undergoes cosmetic surgery and the treatment regimen calls for a series of postoperative visits to the surgeon for evaluating the patient's progress, these visits are not paid.

## 100-03, 10.2

### NCD for Transcutaneous Electrical Nerve Stimulation (TENS) for Acute Post-Operative Pain (10.2)

**Indications and Limitations of Coverage**

The use of Transcutaneous Electrical Nerve Stimulation (TENS) for the relief of acute post-operative pain is covered under Medicare. TENS may be covered whether used as an adjunct to the use of drugs, or as an alternative to drugs, in the treatment of acute pain resulting from surgery.

TENS devices, whether durable or disposable, may be used in furnishing this service. When used for the purpose of treating acute post-operative pain, TENS devices are considered supplies. As such they may be hospital supplies furnished inpatients covered under Part A, or supplies incident to a physician's service when furnished in connection with surgery done on an outpatient basis, and covered under Part B.

It is expected that TENS, when used for acute post-operative pain, will be necessary for relatively short periods of time, usually 30 days or less. In cases when TENS is used for longer periods, Medicare Administrative Contractors should attempt to ascertain whether TENS is no longer being used for acute pain but rather for chronic pain, in which case the TENS device may be covered as durable medical equipment as described in §160.27.

Cross-references:

Medicare Benefit Policy Manual, Chapter 1, "Inpatient Hospital Services," §40;

Medicare Benefit Policy Manual, Chapter 2, "Hospital Services Covered Under Part B," §§20, 20.4, and 80; Medicare Benefit Policy Manual, Chapter 15, "Covered Medical and other Health Services, §110."

## 100-03, 10.3

### NCD for Inpatient Hospital Pain Rehabilitation Programs (10.3)

Since pain rehabilitation programs of a lesser scope than that described above would raise a question as to whether the program could be provided in a less intensive setting than on an inpatient hospital basis, carefully evaluate such programs to determine whether the program does, in fact, necessitate a hospital level of care. Some pain rehabilitation programs may utilize services and devices which are excluded from coverage, e.g., acupuncture (see 35-8), biofeedback (see 35-27), dorsal column stimulator (see 65-8), and family counseling services (see 35-l4). In determining whether the scope of a pain program does necessitate inpatient

hospital care, evaluate only those services and devices which are covered. Although diagnostic tests may be an appropriate part of pain rehabilitation programs, such tests would be covered in an individual case only where they can be reasonably related to a patient's illness, complaint, symptom, or injury and where they do not represent an unnecessary duplication of tests previously performed.

An inpatient program of 4 weeks' duration is generally required to modify pain behavior. After this period it would be expected that any additional rehabilitation services which might be required could be effectively provided on an outpatient basis under an outpatient pain rehabilitation program (see 10.4 of the NCD Manual) or other outpatient program. The first 7-I0 days of such an inpatient program constitute, in effect, an evaluation period. If a patient is unable to adjust to the program within this period, it is generally concluded that it is unlikely that the program will be effective and the patient is discharged from the program. On occasions a program longer than 4 weeks may be required in a particular case. In such a case there should be documentation to substantiate that inpatient care beyond a 4-week period was reasonable and necessary. Similarly, where it appears that a patient participating in a program is being granted frequent outside passes, a question would exist as to whether an inpatient program is reasonable and necessary for the treatment of the patient's condition.

An inpatient hospital stay for the purpose of participating in a pain rehabilitation program would be covered as reasonable and necessary to the treatment of a patient's condition where the pain is attributable to a physical cause, the usual methods of treatment have not been successful in alleviating it, and a significant loss of ability to function independently has resulted from the pain. Chronic pain patients often have psychological problems which accompany or stem from the physical pain and it is appropriate to include psychological treatment in the multidisciplinary approach. However, patients whose pain symptoms result from a mental condition, rather than from any physical cause, generally cannot be succesfully treated in a pain rehabilitation program.

## 100-03, 10.4

### NCD for Outpatient Hospital Pain Rehabilitation Programs (10.4)

Coverage of services furnished under outpatient hospital pain rehabilitation programs, including services furnished in group settings under individualized plans of treatment, is available if the patient's pain is attributable to a physical cause, the usual methods of treatment have not been successful in alleviating it, and a significant loss of ability by the patient to function independently has resulted from the pain. If a patient meets these conditions and the program provides services of the types discussed in §10.3, the services provided under the program may be covered. Non-covered services (e.g., vocational counseling, meals for outpatients, or acupuncture) continue to be excluded from coverage, and A/B Medicare Administrative Contractors would not be precluded from finding, in the case of particular patients, that the pain rehabilitation program is not reasonable and necessary under §1862(a)(1) of the Social Security Act for the treatment of their conditions.

## 100-03, 10.5

### NCD for Autogenous Epidural Blood Graft (10.5)

Autogenous epidural blood grafts are considered a safe and effective remedy for severe headaches that may occur after performance of spinal anesthesia, spinal taps or myelograms, and are covered.

## 100-03, 10.6

### NCD for Anesthesia in Cardiac Pacemaker Surgery (10.6)

The use of general or monitored anesthesia during transvenous cardiac pacemaker surgery may be reasonable and necessary and therefore covered under Medicare only if adequate documentation of medical necessity is provided on a case-by-case basis. The Medicare Adminstrative Contractor obtains advice from its medical consultants or from appropriate specialty physicians or groups in its locality regarding the adequacy of documentation before deciding whether a particular claim should be covered.

A second type of pacemaker surgery that is sometimes performed involves the use of the thoracic method of implantation which requires open surgery. Where the thoracic method is employed, general anesthesia is always used and should not require special medical documentation.

## 100-03, 20.2

### NCD for Extracranial-Intracranial (EC-IC) Arterial Bypass Surgery (20.2)

Extracranial-Intracranial (EC-IC) arterial bypass surgery is not a covered procedure when it is performed as a treatment for ischemic cerebrovascular disease of the carotid or middle cerebral arteries which includes the treatment or prevention of strokes. The premise that this procedure which bypasses narrowed arterial segments, improves the blood supply to the brain and reduces the risk of having a stroke has not been demonstrated to be any more effective than no surgical intervention. Accordingly, EC-IC arterial bypass surgery is not considered reasonable and necessary within the meaning of §1862(a)(1) of the Act when it is performed as a treatment for ischemic cerebrovascular disease of the carotid or middle cerebral arteries.

## 100-03, 20.8.4

### Leadless Pacemakers

(Rev. 201, Issued: 07-28-17, Effective: 01-18-18, Implementation: 08-29-17- for MAC local edits; January 2, 2018 - for MCS shared edits)

**A. General**

The leadless pacemaker eliminates the need for a device pocket and insertion of a pacing lead which are integral elements of traditional pacing systems. The removal of these elements eliminate an important source of complications associated with traditional pacing systems while providing similar benefits. Leadless pacemakers are delivered via catheter to the heart, and function similarly to other transvenous single-chamber ventricular pacemakers.

**B. Nationally Covered Indications**

Effective January 18, 2017, the Centers for Medicare & Medicaid Services (CMS) covers leadless pacemakers through Coverage with Evidence Development (CED). CMS covers leadless pacemakers when procedures are performed in Food and Drug Administration (FDA) approved studies. CMS also covers, in prospective longitudinal studies, leadless

pacemakers that are used in accordance with the FDA approved label for devices that have either:

- an associated ongoing FDA approved post-approval study; or

- completed an FDA post-approval study.

Each study must be approved by CMS and as a fully-described, written part of its protocol, must address the following research questions:

- What are the peri-procedural and post-procedural complications of leadless pacemakers?

- What are the long term outcomes of leadless pacemakers?

- What are the effects of patient characteristics (age, gender, comorbidities) on the use and health effects of leadless pacemakers?

CMS will review studies to determine if they meet the 13 criteria listed below. If CMS determines that they meet these criteria, the study will be posted on CMS' CED website (https://www.cms.gov/Medicare/Coverage/Coverage-with-Evidence-Development/index.html).

a. The principal purpose of the study is to test whether the item or service meaningfully improves health outcomes of affected beneficiaries who are represented by the enrolled subjects.

b. The rationale for the study is well supported by available scientific and medical evidence.

c. The study results are not anticipated to unjustifiably duplicate existing knowledge.

d. The study design is methodologically appropriate and the anticipated number of enrolled subjects is sufficient to answer the research question(s) being asked in the National Coverage Determination.

e. The study is sponsored by an organization or individual capable of completing it successfully.

f. The research study is in compliance with all applicable Federal regulations concerning the protection of human subjects found in the Code of Federal Regulations (CFR) at 45 CFR Part 46. If a study is regulated by the Food and Drug Administration (FDA), it is also in compliance with 21 CFR Parts 50 and 56. In addition, to further enhance the protection of human subjects in studies conducted under CED, the study must provide and obtain meaningful informed consent from patients regarding the risks associated with the study items and/or services, and the use and eventual disposition of the collected data.

g. All aspects of the study are conducted according to appropriate standards of scientific integrity.

h. The study has a written protocol that clearly demonstrates adherence to the standards listed here as Medicare requirements.

i. The study is not designed to exclusively test toxicity or disease pathophysiology in healthy individuals. Such studies may meet this requirement only if the disease or condition being studied is life threatening as defined in 21 CFR §312.81(a) and the patient has no other viable treatment options.

j. The clinical research studies and registries are registered on the www.ClinicalTrials.gov website by the principal sponsor/investigator prior to the enrollment of the first study subject. Registries are also registered in the Agency for Healthcare Research and Quality (AHRQ) Registry of Patient Registries (RoPR).

k. The research study protocol specifies the method and timing of public release of all prespecified outcomes to be measured including release of outcomes if outcomes are negative or study is terminated early. The results must be made public within 12 months of the study's primary completion date, which is the date the final subject had final data collection for the primary endpoint, even if the trial does not achieve its primary aim. The results must include number started/completed, summary results for primary and secondary outcome measures, statistical analyses, and adverse events. Final results must be reported in a publicly accessibly manner; either in a peer-reviewed scientific journal (in print or on-line), in an on-line publicly accessible registry dedicated to the dissemination of clinical trial information such as ClinicalTrials.gov, or in journals

willing to publish in abbreviated format (e.g., for studies with negative or incomplete results).

l. The study protocol must explicitly discuss beneficiary subpopulations affected by the item or service under investigation, particularly traditionally underrepresented groups in clinical studies, how the inclusion and exclusion criteria effect enrollment of these populations, and a plan for the retention and reporting of said populations in the trial. If the inclusion and exclusion criteria are expected to have a negative effect on the recruitment or retention of underrepresented populations, the protocol must discuss why these criteria are necessary.

m. The study protocol explicitly discusses how the results are or are not expected to be generalizable to affected beneficiary subpopulations. Separate discussions in the protocol may be necessary for populations eligible for Medicare due to age, disability or Medicaid eligibility.

Consistent with section 1142 of the Act, the Agency for Healthcare Research and Quality (AHRQ) supports clinical research studies that CMS determines meet the above-listed standards and address the above-listed research questions.

All clinical research study protocols must be reviewed and approved by CMS. The principal investigator must submit the complete study protocol, identify the relevant CMS research question(s) that will be addressed and cite the location of the detailed analysis plan for those questions in the protocol, plus provide a statement addressing how the study satisfies each of the standards of scientific integrity (a. through m. listed above), as well as the investigator's contact information, to the address below. The information will be reviewed, and approved studies will be identified on the CMS website.

Director, Coverage and Analysis Group
Re: Leadless Pacemakers CED
Centers for Medicare & Medicaid Services (CMS)
7500 Security Blvd., Mail Stop S3-02-01
Baltimore, MD 21244-1850

Email address for protocol submissions: clinicalstudynotification@cms.hhs.gov

Email subject line: "CED [NCD topic (i.e. Leadless Pacemakers)] [name of sponsor/primary investigator]"

**C. Nationally Non-Covered Indications**

Leadless pacemakers are non-covered when furnished outside of a CMS approved CED study.

**D. Other**

NA

## 100-03, 20.9

### Artificial Hearts and Related Devices (Various Effective Dates Below)

**A. General**

An artificial heart is a biventricular replacement device which requires removal of a substantial part of the native heart, including both ventricles. Removal of this device is not compatible with life, unless the patient has a heart transplant.

**B. Nationally Covered Indications**

1. Bridge-to-transplant (BTT) (effective for services performed on or after May 1, 2008)

   An artificial heart for bridge-to-transplantation (BTT) is covered when performed under coverage with evidence development (CED) when a clinical study meets all of the criteria listed below. The clinical study must address at least one of the following questions:

   — Were there unique circumstances such as expertise available in a particular facility or an unusual combination of conditions in particular patients that affected their outcomes?

   — What will be the average time to device failure when the device is made available to larger numbers of patients?

   — Do results adequately give a reasonable indication of the full range of outcomes (both positive and negative) that might be expected from more widespread use?

   The clinical study must meet all of the criteria stated in Section D of this policy. The above information should be mailed to: Director, Coverage and Analysis Group, Centers for Medicare & Medicaid Services (CMS), Re: Artificial Heart, Mailstop S3-02-01, 7500 Security Blvd, Baltimore, MD 21244-1850.

   Clinical studies that are determined by CMS to meet the above requirements will be listed on the CMS Web site at: http://www.cms.gov/Medicare/Coverage/Coverage-with-Evidence-Development/Artificial-Hearts.html.

2. Destination therapy (DT) (effective for services performed on or after May 1, 2008)

   An artificial heart for destination therapy (DT) is covered when performed under CED when a clinical study meets all of the criteria listed below. The clinical study must address at least one of the following questions:

   — Were there unique circumstances such as expertise available in a particular facility or an unusual combination of conditions in particular patients that affected their outcomes?

— What will be the average time to device failure when the device is made available to larger numbers of patients?

— Do results adequately give a reasonable indication of the full range of outcomes (both positive and negative) that might be expected from more widespread use?

The clinical study must meet all of the criteria stated in Section D of this policy. The above information should be mailed to: Director, Coverage and Analysis Group, Centers for Medicare & Medicaid Services, Re: Artificial Heart, Mailstop S3-02-01, 7500 Security Blvd, Baltimore, MD 21244-1850.

Clinical studies that are determined by CMS to meet the above requirements will be listed on the CMS Web site at: http://www.cms.gov/Medicare/Coverage/Coverage-with-Evidence-Development/Artificial-Hearts.html.

### C. Nationally Non-Covered Indications

All other indications for the use of artificial hearts not otherwise listed remain non-covered, except in the context of Category B investigational device exemption clinical trials (42 CFR 405) or as a routine cost in clinical trials defined under section 310.1 of the National Coverage Determinations (NCD) Manual.

### D. Other

Clinical study criteria:

- The study must be reviewed and approved by the Food and Drug Administration (FDA).
- The principal purpose of the research study is to test whether a particular intervention potentially improves the participants' health outcomes.
- The research study is well supported by available scientific and medical information, or it is intended to clarify or establish the health outcomes of interventions already in common clinical use.
- The research study does not unjustifiably duplicate existing studies.
- The research study design is appropriate to answer the research question being asked in the study.
- The research study is sponsored by an organization or individual capable of executing the proposed study successfully.
- The research study is in compliance with all applicable Federal regulations concerning the protection of human subjects found at 45 CFR Part 46. If a study is FDA-regulated it also must be in compliance with 21 CFR Parts 50 and 56.
- All aspects of the research study are conducted according to appropriate standards of scientific integrity (see http://www.icmje.org).
- The research study has a written protocol that clearly addresses, or incorporates by reference, the standards listed here as Medicare requirements for CED.
- The clinical research study is not designed to exclusively test toxicity or disease pathophysiology in healthy individuals. Trials of all medical technologies measuring therapeutic outcomes as one of the objectives meet this standard only if the disease or condition being studied is life threatening as defined in 21 CFR §312.81(a) and the patient has no other viable treatment options.
- The clinical research study is registered on the www.ClinicalTrials.gov Web site by the principal sponsor/investigator as demonstrated by having a Clinicaltrials.gov Identifier.
- The research study protocol specifies the method and timing of public release of all pre-specified outcomes to be measured including release of outcomes if outcomes are negative or study is terminated early. The results must be made public within 24 months of the end of data collection. If a report is planned to be published in a peer-reviewed journal, then that initial release may be an abstract that meets the requirements of the International Committee of Medical Journal Editors (ICMJE) (http://www.icmje.org). However a full report of the outcomes must be made public no later than three (3) years after the end of data collection.
- The research study protocol must explicitly discuss subpopulations affected by the treatment under investigation, particularly traditionally under-represented groups in clinical studies, how the inclusion and exclusion criteria effect enrollment of these populations, and a plan for the retention and reporting of said populations in the trial. If the inclusion and exclusion criteria are expected to have a negative effect on the recruitment or retention of under-represented populations, the protocol must discuss why these criteria are necessary.
- The research study protocol explicitly discusses how the results are or are not expected to be generalizable to the Medicare population to infer whether Medicare patients may benefit from the intervention. Separate discussions in the protocol may be necessary for populations eligible for Medicare due to age, disability, or Medicaid eligibility.

Consistent with section 1142 of the Social Security Act (the Act), the Agency for Healthcare Research and Quality (AHRQ) supports clinical research studies that CMS determines meet the above-listed standards and address the above-listed research questions.

The principal investigator of an artificial heart clinical study seeking Medicare payment should submit the following documentation to CMS and should expect to be notified when the CMS review is complete:

- Complete study protocol (must be dated or identified with a version number);
- Protocol summary;

- Statement that the submitted protocol version has been agreed upon by the FDA;
- Statement that the above study standards are met;
- Statement that the study addresses at least one of the above questions related to artificial hearts;
- Complete contact information (phone number, email address, and mailing address); and,
- Clinicaltrials.gov Identifier.

## 100-03, 20.9.1

### Ventricular Assist Devices (Various Effective Dates Below)

#### A. General

A ventricular assist device (VAD) is surgically attached to one or both intact ventricles and is used to assist or augment the ability of a damaged or weakened native heart to pump blood. Improvement in the performance of the native heart may allow the device to be removed.

#### B. Nationally Covered Indications

1. Post-cardiotomy (effective for services performed on or after October 18, 1993) Post-cardiotomy is the period following open-heart surgery. VADs used for support of blood circulation post-cardiotomy are covered only if they have received approval from the Food and Drug Administration (FDA) for that purpose, and the VADs are used according to the FDA-approved labeling instructions.

2. Bridge-to-Transplant (effective for services performed on or after January 22, 1996)

   The VADs used for bridge to transplant are covered only if they have received approval from the FDA for that purpose, and the VADs are used according to FDA-approved labeling instructions. All of the following criteria must be fulfilled in order for Medicare coverage to be provided for a VAD used as a bridge to transplant:

   — The patient is approved for heart transplantation by a Medicare-approved heart transplant center and is active on the Organ Procurement and Transplantation Network (OPTN) heart transplant waitlist.

   — The implanting site, if different than the Medicare-approved transplant center, must receive written permission from the Medicare-approved transplant center under which the patient is listed prior to implantation of the VAD.

3. Destination Therapy (DT) (effective for services performed on or after October 1, 2003)

   Destination therapy (DT) is for patients that require mechanical cardiac support. The VADs used for DT are covered only if they have received approval from the FDA for that purpose.

   Patient Selection (effective November 9, 2010):

   The VADs are covered for patients who have chronic end-stage heart failure (New York Heart Association Class IV end-stage left ventricular failure) who are not candidates for heart transplantation at the time of VAD implant, and meet the following conditions:Have failed to respond to optimal medical management (including beta-blockers and ACE inhibitors if tolerated) for 45 of the last 60 days, or have been balloon pump-dependent for 7 days, or IV inotrope-dependent for 14 days; and,

   — Have a left ventricular ejection fraction (LVEF) <25%; and,

   — Have demonstrated functional limitation with a peak oxygen consumption of =14 ml/kg/min unless balloon pump- or inotrope-dependent or physically unable to perform the test. Facility Criteria (effective October 30, 2013):

   Facilities currently credentialed by the Joint Commission for placement of VADs as DT may continue as Medicare-approved facilities until October 30, 2014. At the conclusion of this transition period, these facilities must be in compliance with the following criteria as determined by a credentialing organization. As of the effective date, new facilities must meet the following criteria as a condition of coverage of this procedure as DT under section 1862(a)(1)(A) of the Social Security Act (the Act):

   Beneficiaries receiving VADs for DT must be managed by an explicitly identified cohesive, multidisciplinary team of medical professionals with the appropriate qualifications, training, and experience. The team embodies collaboration and dedication across medical specialties to offer optimal patient-centered care. Collectively, the team must ensure that patients and caregivers have the knowledge and support necessary to participate in shared decision making and to provide appropriate informed consent. The team members must be based at the facility and must include individuals with experience working with patients before and after placement of a VAD.

   The team must include, at a minimum:

   – At least one physician with cardiothoracic surgery privileges and individual experience implanting at least 10 durable, intracorporeal, left VADs as BTT or DT over the course of the previous 36 months with activity in the last year.

   – At least one cardiologist trained in advanced heart failure with clinical competence in medical and device-based management including VADs, and clinical competence in the management of patients before and after heart transplant.

– A VAD program coordinator.

– A social worker.

– A palliative care specialist. Facilities must be credentialed by an organization approved by the Centers for Medicare & Medicaid Services.

### C. Nationally Non-Covered Indications

All other indications for the use of VADs not otherwise listed remain non-covered, except in the context of Category B investigational device exemption clinical trials (42 CFR 405) or as a routine cost in clinical trials defined under section 310.1 of the National Coverage Determinations (NCD) Manual.

### D. Other

This policy does not address coverage of VADs for right ventricular support, biventricular support, use in beneficiaries under the age of 18, use in beneficiaries with complex congenital heart disease, or use in beneficiaries with acute heart failure without a history of chronic heart failure. Coverage under section 1862(a)(1)(A) of the Act for VADs in these situations will be made by local Medicare Administrative Contractors within their respective jurisdictions.

## 100-03, 20.12

### NCD for Diagnostic Endocardial Electrical Stimulation (Pacing) (20.12)

Diagnostic endocardial electrical stimulation (EES), also called programmed electrical stimulation of the heart, is covered under Medicare when used for patients with severe cardiac arrhythmias.

## 100-03, 20.19

### NCD for Ambulatory Blood Pressure Monitoring (20.19)

ABPM must be performed for at least 24 hours to meet coverage criteria.

ABPM is only covered for those patients with suspected white coat hypertension. Suspected white coat hypertension is defined as

1) office blood pressure > 140/90 mm Hg on at least three separate clinic/office visits with two separate measurements made at each visit;

2) at least two documented blood pressure measurements taken outside the office which are < 140/90 mm Hg; and

3) no evidence of end-organ damage.

The information obtained by ABPM is necessary in order to determine the appropriate management of the patient. ABPM is not covered for any other uses. In the rare circumstance that ABPM needs to be performed more than once in a patient, the qualifying criteria described above must be met for each subsequent ABPM test.

For those patients that undergo ABPM and have an ambulatory blood pressure of < 135/85 with no evidence of end-organ damage, it is likely that their cardiovascular risk is similar to that of normotensives. They should be followed over time. Patients for which ABPM demonstrates a blood pressure of > 135/85 may be at increased cardiovascular risk, and a physician may wish to consider antihypertensive therapy.

## 100-03, 20.26

### NCD for Partial Ventriculectomy (20.26)

Since the mortality rate is high and there are no published scientific articles or clinical studies regarding partial ventriculectomy, this procedure cannot be considered reasonable and necessary within the meaning of Sec.1862(a)(1) of the Act. Therefore, partial ventriculectomy is not covered by Medicare.

## 100-03, 20.28

### NCD for Therapeutic Embolization (20.28)

Therapeutic embolization is covered when done for hemorrhage, and for other conditions amenable to treatment by the procedure, when reasonable and necessary for the individual patient. Renal embolization for the treatment of renal adenocarcinoma continues to be covered, effective December 15, 1978, as one type of therapeutic embolization, to:

• Reduce tumor vascularity preoperatively;

• Reduce tumor bulk in inoperable cases; or

• Palliate specific symptoms.

## 100-03, 20.29

### NCD for Hyperbaric Oxygen Therapy (20.29)

#### A. Covered Conditions

Program reimbursement for HBO therapy will be limited to that which is administered in a chamber (including the one man unit) and is limited to the following conditions:

1. Acute carbon monoxide intoxication,

2. Decompression illness,

3. Gas embolism,

4. Gas gangrene,

5. Acute traumatic peripheral ischemia. HBO therapy is a valuable adjunctive treatment to be used in combination with accepted standard therapeutic measures when loss of function, limb, or life is threatened.

6. Crush injuries and suturing of severed limbs. As in the previous conditions, HBO therapy would be an adjunctive treatment when loss of function, limb, or life is threatened.

7. Progressive necrotizing infections (necrotizing fasciitis),

8. Acute peripheral arterial insufficiency,

9. Preparation and preservation of compromised skin grafts (not for primary management of wounds),

10. Chronic refractory osteomyelitis, unresponsive to conventional medical and surgical management,

11. Osteoradionecrosis as an adjunct to conventional treatment,

12. Soft tissue radionecrosis as an adjunct to conventional treatment,

13. Cyanide poisoning,

14. Actinomycosis, only as an adjunct to conventional therapy when the disease process is refractory to antibiotics and surgical treatment,

14. Diabetic wounds of the lower extremities in patients who meet the following three criteria:

    a. Patient has type I or type II diabetes and has a lower extremity wound that is due to diabetes;

    b. Patient has a wound classified as Wagner grade III or higher; and

    c. Patient has failed an adequate course of standard wound therapy.

The use of HBO therapy is covered as adjunctive therapy only after there are no measurable signs of healing for at least 30 -days of treatment with standard wound therapy and must be used in addition to standard wound care. Standard wound care in patients with diabetic wounds includes: assessment of a patient's vascular status and correction of any vascular problems in the affected limb if possible, optimization of nutritional status, optimization of glucose control, debridement by any means to remove devitalized tissue, maintenance of a clean, moist bed of granulation tissue with appropriate moist dressings, appropriate off-loading, and necessary treatment to resolve any infection that might be present. Failure to respond to standard wound care occurs when there are no measurable signs of healing for at least 30 consecutive days. Wounds must be evaluated at least every 30 days during administration of HBO therapy. Continued treatment with HBO therapy is not covered if measurable signs of healing have not been demonstrated within any 30-day period of treatment.

#### B. Noncovered Conditions

All other indications not specified under Sec.270.4(A) are not covered under the Medicare program. No program payment may be made for any conditions other than those listed in Sec. 270.4(A).

No program payment may be made for HBO in the treatment of the following conditions:

1. Cutaneous, decubitus, and stasis ulcers.

2. Chronic peripheral vascular insufficiency.

3. Anaerobic septicemia and infection other than clostridial.

4. Skin burns (thermal).

5. Senility.

6. Myocardial infarction.

7. Cardiogenic shock.

8. Sickle cell anemia.

9. Acute thermal and chemical pulmonary damage, i.e., smoke inhalation with pulmonary insufficiency.

10. Acute or chronic cerebral vascular insufficiency.

11. Hepatic necrosis.

12. Aerobic septicemia.

13. Nonvascular causes of chronic brain syndrome (Pick's disease, Alzheimer's disease, Korsakoff's disease).

14. Tetanus.

15. Systemic aerobic infection.

16. Organ transplantation.

17. Organ storage.

18. Pulmonary emphysema.

19. Exceptional blood loss anemia.

20. Multiple Sclerosis.

21. Arthritic Diseases.

22. Acute cerebral edema.

## C. Topical Application of Oxygen

This method of administering oxygen does not meet the definition of HBO therapy as stated above. Also, its clinical efficacy has not been established. Therefore, no Medicare reimbursement may be made for the topical application of oxygen.

## 100-03, 20.30

### NCD for Microvolt T-Wave Alternans (MTWA) (20.30)

#### B. Nationally Covered Indications

Microvolt T-wave Alternans diagnostic testing is covered for the evaluation of patients at risk for SCD, only when the spectral analysis method is used.

#### C. Nationally Non-Covered Indications

Microvolt T-wave Alternans diagnostic test is non-covered for the evaluation of patients at risk for SCD if measurement is not performed employing the spectral analysis.

#### D. Other

N/A

## 100-03, 20.32

### Transcatheter Aortic Valve Replacement (TAVR)

#### A. General

Transcatheter aortic valve replacement (TAVR - also known as TAVI or transcatheter aortic valve implantation) is used in the treatment of aortic stenosis. A bioprosthetic valve is inserted percutaneously using a catheter and implanted in the orifice of the aortic valve.

#### B. Nationally Covered Indications

The Centers for Medicare & Medicaid Services (CMS) covers transcatheter aortic valve replacement (TAVR) under Coverage with Evidence Development (CED) with the following conditions:

A. TAVR is covered for the treatment of symptomatic aortic valve stenosis when furnished according to a Food and Drug Administration (FDA)-approved indication and when all of the following conditions are met:

1. The procedure is furnished with a complete aortic valve and implantation system that has received FDA premarket approval (PMA) for that system's FDA approved indication.

2. Two cardiac surgeons have independently examined the patient face-to-face and evaluated the patient's suitability for open aortic valve replacement (AVR) surgery; and both surgeons have documented the rationale for their clinical judgment and the rationale is available to the heart team.

3. The patient (preoperatively and postoperatively) is under the care of a heart team: a cohesive, multi-disciplinary, team of medical professionals. The heart team concept embodies collaboration and dedication across medical specialties to offer optimal patient-centered care.

   TAVR must be furnished in a hospital with the appropriate infrastructure that includes but is not limited to:

   a. On-site heart valve surgery program,

   b. Cardiac catheterization lab or hybrid operating room/catheterization lab equipped with a fixed radiographic imaging system with flat-panel fluoroscopy, offering quality imaging,

   c. Non-invasive imaging such as echocardiography, vascular ultrasound, computed tomography (CT) and magnetic resonance (MR),

   d. Sufficient space, in a sterile environment, to accommodate necessary equipment for cases with and without complications,

   e. Post-procedure intensive care facility with personnel experienced in managing patients who have undergone open-heart valve procedures,

   f. Appropriate volume requirements per the applicable qualifications below.

   There are two sets of qualifications; the first set outlined below is for hospital programs and heart teams without previous TAVR experience and the second set is for those with TAVR experience.

   Qualifications to begin a TAVR program for hospitals without TAVR experience:

   The hospital program must have the following:

   a. $\geq$ 50 total AVRs in the previous year prior to TAVR, including = 10 high-risk patients, and;

   b. $\geq$ 2 physicians with cardiac surgery privileges, and;

   c. $\geq$ 1000 catheterizations per year, including = 400 percutaneous coronary interventions (PCIs) per year.

   Qualifications to begin a TAVR program for heart teams without TAVR experience:

   The heart team must include:

   a. Cardiovascular surgeon with:

      i. $\geq$ 100 career AVRs including 10 high-risk patients; or,

      ii. $\geq$ 25 AVRs in one year; or,

      iii. $\geq$ 50 AVRs in 2 years; and which include at least 20 AVRs in the last year prior to TAVR initiation; and,

   b. Interventional cardiologist with:

      i. Professional experience with 100 structural heart disease procedures lifetime; or,

      ii. 30 left-sided structural procedures per year of which 60% should be balloon aortic valvuloplasty (BAV). Atrial septal defect and patent foramen ovale closure are not considered left-sided procedures; and,

   c. Additional members of the heart team such as echocardiographers, imaging specialists, heart failure specialists, cardiac anesthesiologists, intensivists, nurses, and social workers; and,

   d. Device-specific training as required by the manufacturer.

   Qualifications for hospital programs with TAVR experience:

   The hospital program must maintain the following:

   a. $\geq$ 20 AVRs per year or = 40 AVRs every 2 years; and,

   b. $\geq$ 2 physicians with cardiac surgery privileges; and,

   c. $\geq$ 1000 catheterizations per year, including = 400 percutaneous coronary interventions (PCIs) per year.

   Qualifications for heart teams with TAVR experience:

   The heart team must include:

   a. cardiovascular surgeon and an interventional cardiologist whose combined experience maintains the following:

      i. $\geq$ 20 TAVR procedures in the prior year, or,

      ii. $\geq$ 40 TAVR procedures in the prior 2 years; and,

   b. Additional members of the heart team such as echocardiographers, imaging specialists, heart failure specialists, cardiac anesthesiologists, intensivists, nurses, and social workers.

4. The heart team's interventional cardiologist(s) and cardiac surgeon(s) must jointly participate in the intra-operative technical aspects of TAVR.

5. The heart team and hospital are participating in a prospective, national, audited registry that: 1) consecutively enrolls TAVR patients; 2) accepts all manufactured devices; 3) follows the patient for at least one year; and, 4) complies with relevant regulations relating to protecting human research subjects, including 45 CFR Part 46 and 21 CFR Parts 50 & 56. The following outcomes must be tracked by the registry; and the registry must be designed to permit identification and analysis of patient, practitioner and facility level variables that predict each of these outcomes:

   i. Stroke;

   ii. All cause mortality;

   iii. Transient Ischemic Attacks (TIAs);

   iv. Major vascular events;

   v. Acute kidney injury;

   vi. Repeat aortic valve procedures;

   vii. Quality of Life (QoL).

   The registry should collect all data necessary and have a written executable analysis plan in place to address the following questions (to appropriately address some questions, Medicare claims or other outside data may be necessary):

   – When performed outside a controlled clinical study, how do outcomes and adverse events compare to the pivotal clinical studies?

   – How do outcomes and adverse events in subpopulations compare to patients in the pivotal clinical studies?

   – What is the long term ($\geq$ 5 year) durability of the device?

   – What are the long term ($\geq$ 5 year) outcomes and adverse events?

   – How do the demographics of registry patients compare to the pivotal studies?

   Consistent with section 1142 of the Act, the Agency for Healthcare Research and Quality (AHRQ) supports clinical research studies that CMS determines meet the above-listed standards and address the above-listed research questions.

B. TAVR is covered for uses that are not expressly listed as an FDA-approved indication when performed within a clinical study that fulfills all of the following.

1. The heart team's interventional cardiologist(s) and cardiac surgeon(s) must jointly participate in the intra-operative technical aspects of TAVR.

2. As a fully-described, written part of its protocol, the clinical research study must critically evaluate not only each patient's quality of life pre- and post-TAVR (minimum of 1 year), but must also address at least one of the following questions: § What is the incidence of stroke?

   – What is the rate of all cause mortality?

   – What is the incidence of transient ischemic attacks (TIAs)?

CPT © 2017 American Medical Association. All Rights Reserved.

© 2017 Optum360, LLC

– What is the incidence of major vascular events?

– What is the incidence of acute kidney injury?

– What is the incidence of repeat aortic valve procedures?

3. The clinical study must adhere to the following standards of scientific integrity and relevance to the Medicare population:

a. The principal purpose of the research study is to test whether a particular intervention potentially improves the participants' health outcomes.

b. The research study is well supported by available scientific and medical information or it is intended to clarify or establish the health outcomes of interventions already in common clinical use.

c. The research study does not unjustifiably duplicate existing studies.

d. The research study design is appropriate to answer the research question being asked in the study.

e. The research study is sponsored by an organization or individual capable of executing the proposed study successfully.

f. The research study is in compliance with all applicable Federal regulations concerning the protection of human subjects found in the Code of Federal Regulations (CFR) at 45 CFR Part 46. If a study is regulated by the Food and Drug Administration (FDA), it also must be in compliance with 21 CFR Parts 50 and 56. In particular, the informed consent includes a straightforward explanation of the reported increased risks of stroke and vascular complications that have been published for TAVR.

g. All aspects of the research study are conducted according to appropriate standards of scientific integrity (see http://www.icmje.org).

h. The research study has a written protocol that clearly addresses, or incorporates by reference, the standards listed as Medicare coverage requirements.

i. The clinical research study is not designed to exclusively test toxicity or disease pathophysiology in healthy individuals. Trials of all medical technologies measuring therapeutic outcomes as one of the objectives meet this standard only if the disease or condition being studied is life threatening as defined in 21 CFR §312.81(a) and the patient has no other viable treatment options.

j. The clinical research study is registered on the www.ClinicalTrials.gov website by the principal sponsor/investigator prior to the enrollment of the first study subject.

k. The research study protocol specifies the method and timing of public release of all pre-specified outcomes to be measured including release of outcomes if outcomes are negative or study is terminated early. The results must be made public within 24 months of the end of data collection. If a report is planned to be published in a peer reviewed journal, then that initial release may be an abstract that meets the requirements of the International Committee of Medical Journal Editors (http://www.icmje.org). However a full report of the outcomes must be made public no later than three (3) years after the end of data collection.

l. The research study protocol must explicitly discuss subpopulations affected by the treatment under investigation, particularly traditionally underrepresented groups in clinical studies, how the inclusion and exclusion criteria affect enrollment of these populations, and a plan for the retention and reporting of said populations on the trial. If the inclusion and exclusion criteria are expected to have a negative effect on the recruitment or retention of underrepresented populations, the protocol must discuss why these criteria are necessary.

m. The research study protocol explicitly discusses how the results are or are not expected to be generalizable to the Medicare population to infer whether Medicare patients may benefit from the intervention. Separate discussions in the protocol may be necessary for populations eligible for Medicare due to age, disability or Medicaid eligibility. Consistent with section 1142 of the Act, AHRQ supports clinical research studies that CMS determines meet the above-listed standards and address the above-listed research questions.

4. The principal investigator must submit the complete study protocol, identify the relevant CMS research question(s) that will be addressed, and cite the location of the detailed analysis plan for those questions in the protocol, plus provide a statement addressing how the study satisfies each of the standards of scientific integrity (a. through m. listed above), as well as the investigator's contact information, to the address below. The information will be reviewed, and approved studies will be identified on the CMS Website.

> Director, Coverage and Analysis Group
> Re: TAVR CED
> Centers for Medicare & Medicaid Services (CMS)
> 7500 Security Blvd., Mail Stop S3-02-01
> Baltimore, MD 21244-1850

**C. Nationally Non-Covered Indications**

TAVR is not covered for patients in whom existing co-morbidities would preclude the expected benefit from correction of the aortic stenosis.

**D.**

NA

(This NCD last reviewed May 2012.)

## 100-03, 20.34

### *Percutaneous Left Atrial Appendage Closure (LAAC)*

(Rev. 192, Issued: 05-06-16, Effective: 02-08-16, Implementation: 10-03-16)

**A. General**

Patients with atrial fibrillation (AF), an irregular heartbeat, are at an increased risk of stroke. The left atrial appendage (LAA) is a tubular structure that opens into the left atrium and has been shown to be one potential source for blood clots that can cause strokes. While thinning the blood with anticoagulant medications has been proven to prevent strokes, percutaneous LAA closure (LAAC) has been studied as a non-pharmacologic alternative for patients with AF.

**B. Nationally Covered Indications**

The Centers for Medicare & Medicaid Services (CMS) covers percutaneous LAAC for non-valvular atrial fibrillation (NVAF) through Coverage with Evidence Development (CED) with the following conditions:

a. LAAC devices are covered when the device has received Food and Drug Administration (FDA) Premarket Approval (PMA) for that device's FDA-approved indication and meet all of the conditions specified below:

The patient must have:

- A CHADS2 score ≥ 2 (Congestive heart failure, Hypertension, Age >75, Diabetes, Stroke/transient ischemia attack/thromboembolism) or CHA2DS2-VASc score ≥ 3 (Congestive heart failure, Hypertension, Age ≥ 65, Diabetes, Stroke/transient ischemia attack/thromboembolism, Vascular disease, Sex category)

- A formal shared decision making interaction with an independent non-interventional physician using an evidence-based decision tool on oral anticoagulation in patients with NVAF prior to LAAC. Additionally, the shared decision making interaction must be documented in the medical record.

- A suitability for short-term warfarin but deemed unable to take long-term oral anticoagulation following the conclusion of shared decision making, as LAAC is only covered as a second line therapy to oral anticoagulants. The patient (preoperatively and postoperatively) is under the care of a cohesive, multidisciplinary team (MDT) of medical professionals. The procedure must be furnished in a hospital with an established structural heart disease (SHD) and/or electrophysiology (EP) program.

The procedure must be performed by an interventional cardiologist(s), electrophysiologist(s), or cardiovascular surgeon (s) that meet the following criteria:

- Has received training prescribed by the manufacturer on the safe and effective use of the device prior to performing LAAC; and,

- Has performed ≥ 25 interventional cardiac procedures that involve transseptal puncture through an intact septum; and,

- Continues to perform ≥ 25 interventional cardiac procedures that involve transseptal puncture through an intact septum, of which at least 12 are LAAC, over a 2-year period.

The patient is enrolled in, and the MDT and hospital must participate in, a prospective, national, audited registry that: 1) consecutively enrolls LAAC patients, and, 2) tracks the following annual outcomes for each patient for a period of at least 4 years from the time of the LAAC:

- Operator-specific complications

- Device-specific complications including device thrombosis

- Stroke, adjudicated, by type

- Transient Ischemic Attack (TIA)

- Systemic embolism

- Death

- Major bleeding, by site and severity

The registry must be designed to permit identification and analysis of patient, practitioner, and facility level factors that predict patient risk for these outcomes. The registry must collect all data necessary to conduct analyses adjusted for relevant confounders, and have a written executable analysis plan in place to address the following questions:

- How do the outcomes listed above compare to outcomes in the pivotal clinical trials in the short term (≤12 months) and in the long term (≥ 4 years)?

- What is the long term (≥ 4 year) durability of the device?

- What are the short term (≤12 months) and the long term (≥4 years) device-specific complications including device thromboses?

To appropriately address some of these questions, Medicare claims or other outside data may be necessary.

Registries must be reviewed and approved by CMS. Potential registry sponsors must submit all registry documentation to CMS for approval, including the written executable analysis plan and auditing plan. CMS will review the qualifications of candidate registries to ensure that the approved registry follows standard data collection practices, and collects data necessary to evaluate the patient outcomes specified above. The registry's national clinical trial number must be recorded on the claim.

Consistent with section 1142 of the Social Security Act (the Act), the Agency for Healthcare Research and Quality (AHRQ) supports clinical research studies that CMS determines address the above-listed research questions and the a-m criteria listed in Section c. of this decision.

All approved registries will be posted on the CED website located at: https://www.cms.gov/Medicare/Coverage/Coverage-with-Evidence-Development/index.html.

b.  LAAC is covered for NVAF patients not included in Section a. of this decision when performed within an FDA-approved randomized controlled trial (RCT) if such trials meet the criteria established below:

As a fully-described written part of its protocol, the RCT must critically answer, in comparison to optimal medical therapy, the following questions:

•  As a primary endpoint, what is the true incidence of ischemic stroke and systemic embolism?

•  As a secondary endpoint, what is cardiovascular mortality and all-cause mortality?

FDA-approved RCTs must be reviewed and approved by CMS. Consistent with section 1142 of the Act, AHRQ supports clinical research studies that CMS determines address the above-listed research questions and the a-m criteria listed in section c. of this decision.

The principal investigator must submit the complete study protocol, identify the relevant CMS research question(s) that will be addressed, and cite the location of the detailed analysis plan for those questions in the protocol, plus provide a statement addressing how the study satisfies each of the standards of scientific integrity a. through m. listed in section c. of this decision, as well as the investigator's contact information, to the address below.

Director, Coverage and Analysis Group Re: LAAC CED Centers for Medicare & Medicaid Services 7500 Security Blvd., Mail Stop S3-02-01 Baltimore, MD 21244-1850

c.  All clinical studies, RCTs and registries submitted for review must adhere to the following standards of scientific integrity and relevance to the Medicare population:

a.  The principal purpose of the study is to test whether the item or service meaningfully improves health outcomes of affected beneficiaries who are represented by the enrolled subjects.

b.  The rationale for the study is well supported by available scientific and medical evidence.

c.  The study results are not anticipated to unjustifiably duplicate existing knowledge.

d.  The study design is methodologically appropriate and the anticipated number of enrolled subjects is sufficient to answer the research question(s) being asked in the National Coverage Determination.

e.  The study is sponsored by an organization or individual capable of completing it successfully.

f.  The research study is in compliance with all applicable Federal regulations concerning the protection of human subjects found in the Code of Federal Regulations (CFR) at 45 CFR Part 46. If a study is regulated by the FDA, it is also in compliance with 21 CFR Parts 50 and 56. In addition, to further enhance the protection of human subjects in studies conducted under CED, the study must provide and obtain meaningful informed consent from patients regarding the risks associated with the study items and/or services, and the use and eventual disposition of the collected data.

g.  All aspects of the study are conducted according to appropriate standards of scientific integrity.

h.  The study has a written protocol that clearly demonstrates adherence to the standards listed here as Medicare requirements.

i.  The study is not designed to exclusively test toxicity or disease pathophysiology in healthy individuals. Such studies may meet this requirement only if the disease or condition being studied is life threatening as defined in 21 CFR §312.81(a) and the patient has no other viable treatment options.

j.  The clinical research studies and registries are registered on the www.ClinicalTrials.gov website by the principal sponsor/investigator prior to the enrollment of the first study subject. Registries are also registered in the AHRQ Registry of Patient Registries (RoPR).

k.  The research study protocol specifies the method and timing of public release of all prespecified outcomes to be measured including release of outcomes if outcomes are negative or study is terminated early. The results must be made public within 12 months of the study's primary completion date, which is the date the final subject had final data collection for the primary endpoint, even if the trial does not achieve its primary aim. The results must include number started/completed, summary results for primary and secondary outcome measures, statistical analyses, and adverse events. Final results must be reported in a publicly accessibly manner; either in a peer-reviewed scientific journal (in print or on-line), in an on-line publicly accessible registry dedicated

to the dissemination of clinical trial information such as ClinicalTrials.gov, or in journals willing to publish in abbreviated format (e.g., for studies with negative or incomplete results).

l.  The study protocol must explicitly discuss beneficiary subpopulations affected by the item or service under investigation, particularly traditionally underrepresented groups in clinical studies, how the inclusion and exclusion criteria effect enrollment of these populations, and a plan for the retention and reporting of said populations in the trial. If the inclusion and exclusion criteria are expected to have a negative effect on the recruitment or retention of underrepresented populations, the protocol must discuss why these criteria are necessary.

m.  The study protocol explicitly discusses how the results are or are not expected to be generalizable to affected beneficiary subpopulations. Separate discussions in the protocol may be necessary for populations eligible for Medicare due to age, disability, or Medicaid eligibility.

**C.  Nationally Non-Covered Indications**

LAAC is non-covered for the treatment of NVAF when not furnished under CED according to the above-noted criteria.

(This NCD last reviewed February 2016.)

## 100-03, 30.3

### NCD for Acupuncture (30.3)

Although acupuncture has been used for thousands of years in China and for decades in parts of Europe, it is a new agent of unknown use and efficacy in the United States. Even in those areas of the world where it has been widely used, its mechanism is not known. Three units of the National Institutes of Health, the National Institute of General Medical Sciences, National Institute of Neurological Diseases and Stroke, and Fogarty International Center have been designed to assess and identify specific opportunities and needs for research attending the use of acupuncture for surgical anesthesia and relief of chronic pain. Until the pending scientific assessment of the technique has been completed and its efficacy has been established, Medicare reimbursement for acupuncture, as an anesthetic or as an analgesic or for other therapeutic purposes, may not be made. Accordingly, acupuncture is not considered reasonable and necessary within the meaning of §1862(a)(1) of the Act.

## 100-03, 30.3.1

### NCD for Acupuncture for Fibromyalgia (30.3.1)

**General**

Although acupuncture has been used for thousands of years in China and for decades in parts of Europe, it is still a relatively new agent of unknown use and efficacy in the United States. Even in those areas of the world where it has been widely used, its mechanism is not known. Three units of the National Institutes of Health, the National Institute of General Medical Sciences, National Institute of Neurological Diseases and Stroke, and Fogarty International Center were designated to assess and identify specific opportunities and needs for research attending the use of acupuncture for surgical anesthesia and relief of chronic pain. Following thorough review, and pending completion of the scientific assessment and efficacy of the technique, CMS initially issued a national noncoverage determination for acupuncture in May 1980.

**Nationally Covered Indications**

Not applicable.

**Nationally Noncovered Indications**

After careful reconsideration of its initial noncoverage determination for acupuncture, CMS concludes that there is no convincing evidence for the use of acupuncture for pain relief in patients with fibromyalgia. Study design flaws presently prohibit assessing acupuncture's utility for improving health outcomes. Accordingly, CMS determines that acupuncture is not considered reasonable and necessary for the treatment of fibromyalgia within the meaning of §1862(a)(1) of the Social Security Act, and the national noncoverage determination for acupuncture continues.

(This NCD last reviewed April 2004.)

## 100-03, 30.3.2

### NCD for Acupuncture for Osteoarthritis (30.3.2)

**General**

Although acupuncture has been used for thousands of years in China and for decades in parts of Europe, it is still a relatively new agent of unknown use and efficacy in the United States. Even in those areas of the world where it has been widely used, its mechanism is not known. Three units of the National Institutes of Health, the National Institute of General Medical Sciences, National Institute of Neurological Diseases and Stroke, and Fogarty International Center were designated to assess and identify specific opportunities and needs for research attending the use of acupuncture for surgical anesthesia and relief of chronic pain. Following thorough review, and pending completion of the scientific assessment and efficacy of the technique, CMS initially issued a national noncoverage determination for acupuncture in May 1980.

CPT © 2017 American Medical Association. All Rights Reserved.

© 2017 Optum360, LLC

**Nationally Covered Indications**

Not applicable.

**Nationally Noncovered Indications**

After careful reconsideration of its initial noncoverage determination for acupuncture, CMS concludes that there is no convincing evidence for the use of acupuncture for pain relief in patients with osteoarthritis. Study design flaws presently prohibit assessing acupuncture's utility for improving health outcomes. Accordingly, CMS determines that acupuncture is not considered reasonable and necessary for the treatment of osteoarthritis within the meaning of §1862(a)(1) of the Social Security Act, and the national noncoverage determination for acupuncture continues.

(This NCD last reviewed April 2004.)

## 100-03, 80.7

### NCD for Refractive Keratoplasty (80.7)

The correction of common refractive errors by eyeglasses, contact lenses or other prosthetic devices is specifically excluded from coverage. The use of radial keratotomy and/or keratoplasty for the purpose of refractive error compensation is considered a substitute or alternative to eye glasses or contact lenses, which are specifically excluded by Sec.1862(a)(7) of the Act (except in certain cases in connection with cataract surgery). In addition, many in the medical community consider such procedures cosmetic surgery, which is excluded by section Sec.1862(a)(10) of the Act. Therefore, radial keratotomy and keratoplasty to treat refractive defects are not covered.

Keratoplasty that treats specific lesions of the cornea, such as phototherapeutic keratectomy that removes scar tissue from the visual field, deals with an abnormality of the eye and is not cosmetic surgery. Such cases may be covered under Sec.1862(a)(1)(A) of the Act.

The use of lasers to treat ophthalmic disease constitutes opthalmalogic surgery. Coverage is restricted to practitioners who have completed an approved training program in ophthalmologic surgery.

## 100-03, 80.10

### NCD for Phaco-Emulsification procedure - cataract extraction (80.10)

In view of recommendations of authoritative sources in the field of ophthalmology, the subject technique is viewed as an accepted procedure for removal of cataracts. Accordingly, program reimbursement may be made for necessary services furnished in connection with cataract extraction utilizing the phaco-emulsification procedure.

## 100-03, 80.12

### NCD for Intraocular Lenses (IOLs) (80.12)

Intraocular lens implantation services, as well as the lens itself, may be covered if reasonable and necessary for the individual. Implantation services may include hospital, surgical, and other medical services, including pre-implantation ultrasound (A-scan) eye measurement of one or both eyes.

## 100-03, 100.1

### 100.1 - Bariatric Surgery for Treatment of Co-Morbid Conditions Related to Morbid Obesity

Please note, sections 40.5, 100.8, 100.11, and 100.14 have been removed from the National Coverage Determination (NCD) Manual and incorporated into NCD 100.1.

#### A. General

Obesity may be caused by medical conditions such as hypothyroidism, Cushing's disease, and hypothalamic lesions, or can aggravate a number of cardiac and respiratory diseases as well as diabetes and hypertension. Non-surgical services in connection with the treatment of obesity are covered when such services are an integral and necessary part of a course of treatment for one of these medical conditions.

In addition, supplemented fasting is a type of very low calorie weight reduction regimen used to achieve rapid weight loss. The reduced calorie intake is supplemented by a mixture of protein, carbohydrates, vitamins, and minerals. Serious questions exist about the safety of prolonged adherence for 2 months or more to a very low calorie weight reduction regimen as a general treatment for obesity, because of instances of cardiopathology and sudden death, as well as possible loss of body protein.

Bariatric surgery procedures are performed to treat comorbid conditions associated with morbid obesity. Two types of surgical procedures are employed. Malabsorptive procedures divert food from the stomach to a lower part of the digestive tract where the normal mixing of digestive fluids and absorption of nutrients cannot occur. Restrictive procedures restrict the size of the stomach and decrease intake. Surgery can combine both types of procedures.

The following are descriptions of bariatric surgery procedures:

1. Roux-en-Y Gastric Bypass (RYGBP)

   The RYGBP achieves weight loss by gastric restriction and malabsorption. Reduction of the stomach to a small gastric pouch (30 cc) results in feelings of satiety following even small meals. This small pouch is connected to a segment of the jejunum, bypassing the duodenum and very proximal small intestine, thereby reducing absorption. RYGBP procedures can be open or laparoscopic.

2. Biliopancreatic Diversion with Duodenal Switch (BPD/DS) or Gastric Reduction Duodenal Switch (BPD/GRDS)

   The BPD achieves weight loss by gastric restriction and malabsorption. The stomach is partially resected, but the remaining capacity is generous compared to that achieved with RYGBP. As such, patients eat relatively normal-sized meals and do not need to restrict intake radically, since the most proximal areas of the small intestine (i.e., the duodenum and jejunum) are bypassed, and substantial malabsorption occurs. The partial BPD/DS or BPD/GRDS is a variant of the BPD procedure. It involves resection of the greater curvature of the stomach, preservation of the pyloric sphincter, and transection of the duodenum above the ampulla of Vater with a duodeno-ileal anastomosis and a lower ileo-ileal anastomosis. BPD/DS or BPD/GRDS procedures can be open or laparoscopic.

3. Adjustable Gastric Banding (AGB)

   The AGB achieves weight loss by gastric restriction only. A band creating a gastric pouch with a capacity of approximately 15 to 30 cc's encircles the uppermost portion of the stomach. The band is an inflatable doughnut-shaped balloon, the diameter of which can be adjusted in the clinic by adding or removing saline via a port that is positioned beneath the skin. The bands are adjustable, allowing the size of the gastric outlet to be modified as needed, depending on the rate of a patient's weight loss. AGB procedures are laparoscopic only.

4. Sleeve Gastrectomy

   Sleeve gastrectomy is a 70%-80% greater curvature gastrectomy (sleeve resection of the stomach) with continuity of the gastric lesser curve being maintained while simultaneously reducing stomach volume. In the past, sleeve gastrectomy was the first step in a two-stage procedure when performing RYGBP, but more recently has been offered as a stand-alone surgery. Sleeve gastrectomy procedures can be open or laparoscopic.

5. Vertical Gastric Banding (VGB)

   The VGB achieves weight loss by gastric restriction only. The upper part of the stomach is stapled, creating a narrow gastric inlet or pouch that remains connected with the remainder of the stomach. In addition, a non-adjustable band is placed around this new inlet in an attempt to prevent future enlargement of the stoma (opening). As a result, patients experience a sense of fullness after eating small meals. Weight loss from this procedure results entirely from eating less. VGB procedures are essentially no longer performed.

#### B. Nationally Covered Indications

Effective for services performed on and after February 21, 2006, Open and laparoscopic Roux-en-Y gastric bypass (RYGBP), open and laparoscopic Biliopancreatic Diversion with Duodenal Switch (BPD/DS) or Gastric Reduction Duodenal Switch (BPD/GRDS), and laparoscopic adjustable gastric banding (LAGB) are covered for Medicare beneficiaries who have a body-mass index = 35, have at least one co-morbidity related to obesity, and have been previously unsuccessful with medical treatment for obesity.

Effective for dates of service on and after February 21, 2006, these procedures are only covered when performed at facilities that are: (1) certified by the American College of Surgeons as a Level 1 Bariatric Surgery Center (program standards and requirements in effect on February 15, 2006); or (2) certified by the American Society for Bariatric Surgery as a Bariatric Surgery Center of Excellence (program standards and requirements in effect on February 15, 2006). Effective for dates of service on and after September 24, 2013, facilities are no longer required to be certified.

Effective for services performed on and after February 12, 2009, the Centers for Medicare & Medicaid Services (CMS) determines that Type 2 diabetes mellitus is a co-morbidity for purposes of this NCD.

A list of approved facilities and their approval dates are listed and maintained on the CMS Coverage Web site at http://www.cms.gov/Medicare/Medicare-General-Information/MedicareApprovedFacilitie/Bariatric-Surgery.html , and published in the Federal Register for services provided up to and including date of service September 23, 2013.

#### C. Nationally Non-Covered Indications

Treatments for obesity alone remain non-covered.

Supplemented fasting is not covered under the Medicare program as a general treatment for obesity (see section D. below for discretionary local coverage).

The following bariatric surgery procedures are non-covered for all Medicare beneficiaries:

- Open adjustable gastric banding;
- Open sleeve gastrectomy;
- Laparoscopic sleeve gastrectomy (prior to June 27, 2012);
- Open and laparoscopic vertical banded gastroplasty;
- Intestinal bypass surgery; and,
- Gastric balloon for treatment of obesity.

#### D. Other

Effective for services performed on and after June 27, 2012, Medicare Administrative Contractors (MACs) acting within their respective jurisdictions may determine coverage of stand-alone laparoscopic sleeve gastrectomy (LSG) for the treatment of co-morbid conditions related to obesity in Medicare beneficiaries only when all of the following conditions a.-c. are satisfied.

a.  The beneficiary has a body-mass index (BMI) = 35 kg/m2,

b.  The beneficiary has at least one co-morbidity related to obesity, and,

c.  The beneficiary has been previously unsuccessful with medical treatment for obesity.

The determination of coverage for any bariatric surgery procedures that are not specifically identified in an NCD as covered or non-covered, for Medicare beneficiaries who have a body-mass index = 35, have at least one co-morbidity related to obesity, and have been previously unsuccessful with medical treatment for obesity, is left to the local MACs.

Where weight loss is necessary before surgery in order to ameliorate the complications posed by obesity when it coexists with pathological conditions such as cardiac and respiratory diseases, diabetes, or hypertension (and other more conservative techniques to achieve this end are not regarded as appropriate), supplemented fasting with adequate monitoring of the patient is eligible for coverage on a case-by-case basis or pursuant to a local coverage determination. The risks associated with the achievement of rapid weight loss must be carefully balanced against the risk posed by the condition requiring surgical treatment.

## 100-03, 100.5

### NCD for Diagnostic Breath Analyses (100.5)

The Following Breath Test is Covered:

*   Lactose breath hydrogen to detect lactose malabsorption.

The Following Breath Tests are Excluded from Coverage;

*   Lactulose breath hydrogen for diagnosing small bowel bacterial overgrowth and measuring small bowel transit time.

*   $CO_2$ for diagnosing bile acid malabsorption.

*   $CO_2$ for diagnosing fat malabsorption.

## 100-03, 100.13

### NCD for Laparoscopic Cholecystectomy (100.13)

Laparoscopic cholecystectomy is a covered surgical procedure in which a diseased gall bladder is removed through the use of instruments introduced via cannulae, with vision of the operative field maintained by use of a high-resolution television camera-monitor system (video laparoscope). For inpatient claims, use ICD-9-CM code 51.23, Laparoscopic cholecystectomy. For all other claims, use CPT codes 49310 for laparoscopy, surgical; cholecystectomy (any method), and 49311 for laparoscopy, surgical: cholecystectomy with cholangiography.

## 100-03, 110.1

### NCD for Hyperthermia for Treatment of Cancer (110.1)

Local hyperthermia is covered under Medicare when used in connection with radiation therapy for the treatment of primary or metastatic cutaneous or subcutaneous superficial malignancies. It is not covered when used alone or in connection with chemotherapy.

## 100-03, 110.2

### NCD for Certain Drugs Distributed by the National Cancer Institute (110.2)

Under its Cancer Therapy Evaluation, the Division of Cancer Treatment of the National Cancer Institute (NCI), in cooperation with the Food and Drug Administration, approves and distributes certain drugs for use in treating terminally ill cancer patients. One group of these drugs, designated as Group C drugs, unlike other drugs distributed by the NCI, is not limited to use in clinical trials for the purpose of testing their efficacy. Drugs are classified as Group C drugs only if there is sufficient evidence demonstrating their efficacy within a tumor type and that they can be safely administered.

A physician is eligible to receive Group C drugs from the Divison of Cancer Treatment only if the following requirements are met:

*   A physician must be registered with the NCI as an investigator by having completed an FD-Form 1573;

*   A written request for the drug, indicating the disease to be treated, must be submitted to the NCI;

*   The use of the drug must be limited to indications outlined in the NCI's guidelines; and

*   All adverse reactions must be reported to the Investigational Drug Branch of the Division of Cancer Treatment.

In view of these NCI controls on distribution and use of Group C drugs, A/B Medicare Adminstrative Contractors (MACs) may assume, in the absence of evidence to the contrary, that a Group C drug and the related hospital stay are covered if all other applicable coverage requirements are satisfied.

If there is reason to question coverage in a particular case, the matter should be resolved with the assistance of the Quality Improvement Organization (QIO), or if there is none, the assistance of the MAC's medical consultants.

Information regarding those drugs which are classified as Group C drugs may be obtained from:

Chief, Investigational Drug Branch
Cancer Therapy Evaluation Program
Executive Plaza North, Suite 7134
National Cancer Institute
Rockville, Maryland 20852-7426

## 100-03, 110.4

### Extracorporeal Photopheresis

#### A. General

Extracorporeal photopheresis is a medical procedure in which a patient's white blood cells are exposed first to a drug called 8-methoxypsoralen (8-MOP) and then to ultraviolet A (UVA) light. The procedure starts with the removal of the patient's blood, which is centrifuged to isolate the white blood cells. The drug is typically administered directly to the white blood cells after they have been removed from the patient (referred to as ex vivo administration) but the drug can alternatively be administered directly to the patient before the white blood cells are withdrawn. After UVA light exposure, the treated white blood cells are then re-infused into the patient.

#### B. Nationally Covered Indications

The Centers for Medicare & Medicaid Services (CMS) has determined that extracorporeal photopheresis is reasonable and necessary under §1862(a)(1)(A) of the Social Security Act (the Act) under the following circumstances:

1.  Effective April 8, 1988, Medicare provides coverage for:

    Palliative treatment of skin manifestations of cutaneous T-cell lymphoma that has not responded to other therapy.

2.  Effective December 19, 2006, Medicare also provides coverage for:

    Patients with acute cardiac allograft rejection whose disease is refractory to standard immunosuppressive drug treatment; and,

    Patients with chronic graft versus host disease whose disease is refractory to standard immunosuppressive drug treatment.

3.  Effective April 30, 2012, Medicare also provides coverage for:

    Extracorporeal photopheresis for the treatment of bronchiolitis obliterans syndrome (BOS) following lung allograft transplantation only when extracorporeal photopheresis is provided under a clinical research study that meets the following conditions:

    The clinical research study meets the requirements specified below to assess the effect of extracorporeal photopheresis for the treatment of BOS following lung allograft transplantation. The clinical study must address one or more aspects of the following question:

    Prospectively, do Medicare beneficiaries who have received lung allografts, developed BOS refractory to standard immunosuppressive therapy, and received extracorporeal photopheresis , experience improved patient-centered health outcomes as indicated by:

    a.  improved forced expiratory volume in one second (FEV1);

    b.  improved survival after transplant; and/or,

    c.  improved quality of life?

        The required clinical study must adhere to the following standards of scientific integrity and relevance to the Medicare population:

    a.  The principal purpose of the research study is to test whether extracorporeal photopheresis potentially improves the participants' health outcomes.

    b.  The research study is well supported by available scientific and medical information or it is intended to clarify or establish the health outcomes of interventions already in common clinical use.

    c.  The research study does not unjustifiably duplicate existing studies.

    d.  The research study design is appropriate to answer the research question being asked in the study.

    e.  The research study is sponsored by an organization or individual capable of successfully executing the proposed study.

    f.  The research study is in compliance with all applicable Federal regulations concerning the protection of human subjects found at 45 CFR Part 46. If a study is regulated by the Food and Drug Administration (FDA), it must also be in compliance with 21 CFR parts 50 and 56.

    g.  All aspects of the research study are conducted according to appropriate standards of scientific integrity (see http://www.icmje.org).

    h.  The research study has a written protocol that clearly addresses, or incorporates by reference, the standards listed here as Medicare requirements for coverage with evidence development.

    i.  The clinical research study is not designed to exclusively test toxicity or disease pathophysiology in healthy individuals. Trials of all medical technologies measuring therapeutic outcomes as one of the objectives meet this standard only if the disease or condition being studied is life threatening as defined in 21 CFR § 312.81(a) and the patient has no other viable treatment options.

j. The clinical research study is registered on the ClinicalTrials.gov website by the principal sponsor/investigator prior to the enrollment of the first study subject.

k. The research study protocol specifies the method and timing of public release of all prespecified outcomes to be measured including release of outcomes if outcomes are negative or study is terminated early. The results must be made public within 24 months of the end of data collection. If a report is planned to be published in a peer-reviewed journal, then that initial release may be an abstract that meets the requirements of the International Committee of Medical Journal Editors (http://www.icmje.org).

l. The research study protocol must explicitly discuss subpopulations affected by the treatment under investigation, particularly traditionally underrepresented groups in clinical studies, how the inclusion and exclusion criteria effect enrollment of these populations, and a plan for the retention and reporting of said populations on the trial. If the inclusion and exclusion criteria are expected to have a negative effect on the recruitment or retention of underrepresented populations, the protocol must discuss why these criteria are necessary.

m. The research study protocol explicitly discusses how the results are or are not expected to be generalizable to the Medicare population to infer whether Medicare patients may benefit from the intervention. Separate discussions in the protocol may be necessary for populations eligible for Medicare due to age, disability or Medicaid eligibility.

Consistent with section 1142 of the Act, the Agency for Healthcare Research and Quality supports clinical research studies that CMS determines meet the above-listed standards and address the above-listed research questions.

Any clinical study under which there is coverage of extracorporeal photopheresis for this indication pursuant to this national coverage determination (NCD) must be approved by April 30, 2014. If there are no approved clinical studies on this date, this NCD will expire and coverage of extracorporeal photopheresis for BOS will revert to the coverage policy in effect prior to the issuance of the final decision memorandum for this NCD.

#### C. Nationally Non-Covered Indications

All other indications for extracorporeal photopheresis not otherwise indicated above as covered remain non-covered.

#### D. Other

Claims processing instructions can be found in chapter 32, section 190 of the Medicare Claims Processing Manual.

(This NCD last reviewed April 2012.)

## 100-03, 110.6

### NCD for Scalp Hypothermia During Chemotherapy, to Prevent Hair Loss (110.6)

While ice-filled bags or bandages or other devices used for scalp hypothermia during chemotherapy may be covered as supplies of the kind commonly furnished without a separate charge, no separate charge for them would be recognized.

## 100-03, 110.7

### NCD for Blood Transfusions (110.7)

#### B. Policy Governing Transfusions

For Medicare coverage purposes, it is important to distinguish between a transfusion itself and preoperative blood services; e.g., collection, processing, storage. Medically necessary transfusion of blood, regardless of the type, may generally be a covered service under both Part A and Part B of Medicare. Coverage does not make a distinction between the transfusion of homologous, autologous, or donor-directed blood. With respect to the coverage of the services associated with the preoperative collection, processing, and storage of autologous and donor-directed blood, the following policies apply.

1. Hospital Part A and B Coverage and Payment

   Under Sec.1862(a)(14) of the Act, non-physician services furnished to hospital patients are covered and paid for as hospital services. As provided in Sec.1886 of the Act, under the prospective [payment system (PPS), the diagnosis related group (DRG) payment to the hospital includes all covered blood and blood processing expenses, whether or not the blood is eventually used.

   Under its provider agreement, a hospital is required to furnish or arrange for all covered services furnished to hospital patients. medicare payment is made to the hospital, under PPS or cost reimbursement, for covered inpatient services, and it is intended to reflect payment for all costs of furnishing those services.

2. Nonhospital Part B Coverage

   Under Part B, to be eligible for separate coverage, a service must fit the definition of one of the services authorized by Sec.1832 of the Act. These services are defined in 42 CFR 410.10 and do not include a separate category for a supplier's services associated with blood donation services, either autologous or

donor-directed. That is, the collection, processing, and storage of blood for later transfusion into the beneficiary is not recognized as a separate service under Part B. Therefore, there is no avenue through which a blood supplier can receive direct payment under Part B for blood donation services.

#### C. Perioperative Blood Salvage

When the perioperative blood salvage process is used in surgery on a hospital patient, payment made to the hospital (under PPS or through cost reimbursement) for the procedure in which that process is used is intended to encompass payment for all costs relating to that process.

## 100-03, 110.8

### NCD for Blood Platelet Transfusions (110.8)

Blood platelet transplants are safe and effective for the correction of thrombocytopenia and other blood defects. It is covered under Medicare when treatment is reasonable and necessary for the individual patient.

## 100-03, 110.8.1

### NCD for Stem Cell Transplantation (110.8.1)

#### Indications and Limitations of Coverage

1. Allogeneic Hematopoietic Stem Cell Transplantation (HSCT)

   Allogeneic hematopoietic stem cell transplantation (HSCT) is a procedure in which a portion of a healthy donor's stem cell or bone marrow is obtained and prepared for intravenous infusion.

   a. Nationally Covered Indications

      The following uses of allogeneic HSCT are covered under Medicare:

      i. Effective for services performed on or after August 1, 1978, for the treatment of leukemia, leukemia in remission, or aplastic anemia when it is reasonable and necessary,

      ii. Effective for services performed on or after June 3, 1985, for the treatment of severe combined immunodeficiency disease (SCID) and for the treatment of Wiskott-Aldrich syndrome.

      iii. Effective for services performed on or after August 4, 2010, for the treatment of Myelodysplastic Syndromes (MDS) pursuant to Coverage with Evidence Development (CED) in the context of a Medicare-approved, prospective clinical study.

   The MDS refers to a group of diverse blood disorders in which the bone marrow does not produce enough healthy, functioning blood cells. These disorders are varied with regard to clinical characteristics, cytologic and pathologic features, and cytogenetics. The abnormal production of blood cells in the bone marrow leads to low blood cell counts, referred to as cytopenias, which are a hallmark feature of MDS along with a dysplastic and hypercellular-appearing bone marrow.

   Medicare payment for these beneficiaries will be restricted to patients enrolled in an approved clinical study. In accordance with the Stem Cell Therapeutic and Research Act of 2005 (US Public Law 109-129) a standard dataset is collected for all allogeneic transplant patients in the United States by the Center for International Blood and Marrow Transplant Research. The elements in this dataset, comprised of two mandatory forms plus one additional form, encompass the information we require for a study under CED.

   A prospective clinical study seeking Medicare payment for treating a beneficiary with allogeneic HSCT for MDS pursuant to CED must meet one or more aspects of the following questions:

   — Prospectively, compared to Medicare beneficiaries with MDS who do not receive HSCT, do Medicare beneficiaries with MDS who receive HSCT have improved outcomes as indicated by:

      – Relapse-free mortality,

      – progression free survival,

      – relapse, and

      – overall survival?

   — Prospectively, in Medicare beneficiaries with MDS who receive HSCT, how do International Prognostic Scoring System (IPSS) score, patient age, cytopenias and comorbidities predict the following outcomes:

      – Relapse-free mortality,

      – progression free survival,

      – relapse, and

      – overall survival?

   — Prospectively, in Medicare beneficiaries with MDS who receive HSCT, what treatment facility characteristics predict meaningful clinical improvement in the following outcomes:

      – Relapse-free mortality,

      – progression free survival,

      – relapse, and

      – overall survival?

In addition, the clinical study must adhere to the following standards of scientific integrity and relevance to the Medicare population:

a. The principal purpose of the research study is to test whether a particular intervention potentially improves the participants' health outcomes.

b. The research study is well supported by available scientific and medical information or it is intended to clarify or establish the health outcomes of interventions already in common clinical use.

c. The research study does not unjustifiably duplicate existing studies.

d. The research study design is appropriate to answer the research question being asked in the study.

e. The research study is sponsored by an organization or individual capable of executing the proposed study successfully.

f. The research study is in compliance with all applicable Federal regulations concerning the protection of human subjects found at 45 CFR Part 46.

g. All aspects of the research study are conducted according to appropriate standards of scientific integrity (see http://www.icmje.org).

h. The research study has a written protocol that clearly addresses, or incorporates by reference, the standards listed here as Medicare requirements for CED coverage.

i. The clinical research study is not designed to exclusively test toxicity or disease pathophysiology in healthy individuals. Trials of all medical technologies measuring therapeutic outcomes as one of the objectives meet this standard only if the disease or condition being studied is life threatening as defined in 21 CFR §312.81(a) and the patient has no other viable treatment options.

j. The clinical research study is registered on the ClinicalTrials.gov Web site by the principal sponsor/investigator prior to the enrollment of the first study subject.

k. The research study protocol specifies the method and timing of public release of all pre-specified outcomes to be measured including release of outcomes if outcomes are negative or study is terminated early. The results must be made public within 24 months of the end of data collection. If a report is planned to be published in a peer-reviewed journal, then that initial release may be an abstract that meets the requirements of the International Committee of Medical Journal Editors (http://www.icmje.org). However a full report of the outcomes must be made public no later than 3 years after the end of data collection.

l. The research study protocol must explicitly discuss subpopulations affected by the treatment under investigation, particularly traditionally underrepresented groups in clinical studies, how the inclusion and exclusion criteria effect enrollment of these populations, and a plan for the retention and reporting of said populations on the trial. If the inclusion and exclusion criteria are expected to have a negative effect on the recruitment or retention of underrepresented populations, the protocol must discuss why these criteria are necessary.

m. The research study protocol explicitly discusses how the results are or are not expected to be generalizable to the Medicare population to infer whether Medicare patients may benefit from the intervention. Separate discussions in the protocol may be necessary for populations eligible for Medicare due to age, disability or Medicaid eligibility.

Consistent with section 1142 of the Social Security Act, the Agency for Health Research and Quality (AHRQ) supports clinical research studies that CMS determines meet the above-listed standards and address the above-listed research questions.

The clinical research study should also have the following features:

— It should be a prospective, longitudinal study with clinical information from the period before HSCT and short- and long-term follow-up information.

— Outcomes should be measured and compared among pre-specified subgroups within the cohort.

— The study should be powered to make inferences in subgroup analyses.

— Risk stratification methods should be used to control for selection bias. Data elements to be used in risk stratification models should include:

Patient selection:

— Patient Age at diagnosis of MDS and at transplantation

— Date of onset of MDS

— Disease classification (specific MDS subtype at diagnosis prior to preparative/conditioning regimen using World Health Organization (WHO) classifications). Include presence/absence of refractory cytopenias

— Comorbid conditions

— IPSS score (and WHO-adapted Prognostic Scoring System (WPSS) score, if applicable) at diagnosis and prior to transplantation

— Score immediately prior to transplantation and one year post-transplantation

— Disease assessment at diagnosis at start of preparative regimen and last assessment prior to preparative regimen Subtype of MDS (refractory anemia with or without blasts, degree of blasts, etc.)

— Type of preparative/conditioning regimen administered (myeloabalative, non-myeloablative, reduced–intensity conditioning)

— Donor type

— Cell Source

— IPSS Score at diagnosis

Facilities must submit the required transplant essential data to the Stem Cell Therapeutics Outcomes Database.

b. Nationally Non-Covered Indications

Effective for services performed on or after May 24, 1996, allogeneic HSCT is not covered as treatment for multiple myeloma.

2. Autologous Stem Cell Transplantation (AuSCT)

Autologous stem cell transplantation (AuSCT) is a technique for restoring stem cells using the patient's own previously stored cells.

a. Nationally Covered Indications

i. Effective for services performed on or after April 28, 1989, AuSCT is considered reasonable and necessary under §l862(a)(1)(A) of the Social Security Act (the Act) for the following conditions and is covered under Medicare for patients with:

• Acute leukemia in remission who have a high probability of relapse and who have no human leucocyte antigens (HLA)-matched;

• Resistant non-Hodgkin's lymphomas or those presenting with poor prognostic features following an initial response;

• Recurrent or refractory neuroblastoma; or

• Advanced Hodgkin's disease who have failed conventional therapy and have no HLA-matched donor.

ii. Effective October 1, 2000, single AuSCT is only covered for Durie-Salmon Stage II or III patients that fit the following requirements:

• Newly diagnosed or responsive multiple myeloma. This includes those patients with previously untreated disease, those with at least a partial response to prior chemotherapy (defined as a 50% decrease either in measurable paraprotein [serum and/or urine] or in bone marrow infiltration, sustained for at least 1 month), and those in responsive relapse; and,

• Adequate cardiac, renal, pulmonary, and hepatic function.

iii. Effective for services performed on or after March 15, 2005, when recognized clinical risk factors are employed to select patients for transplantation, high dose melphalan (HDM) together with AuSCT is reasonable and necessary for Medicare beneficiaries of any age group with primary amyloid light chain (AL) amyloidosis who meet the following criteria:

• Amyloid deposition in 2 or fewer organs; and,

• Cardiac left ventricular ejection fraction (EF) greater than 45%.

b. Nationally Non-Covered Indications

Insufficient data exist to establish definite conclusions regarding the efficacy of AuSCT for the following conditions:

– Acute leukemia not in remission;

– Chronic granulocytic leukemia;

– Solid tumors (other than neuroblastoma);

– Up to October 1, 2000, multiple myeloma;

– Tandem transplantation (multiple rounds of AuSCT) for patients with multiple myeloma;

– Effective October 1, 2000, non primary AL amyloidosis; and,

– Effective October 1, 2000, thru March 14, 2005, primary AL amyloidosis for Medicare beneficiaries age 64 or older.

In these cases, AuSCT is not considered reasonable and necessary within the meaning of §l862(a)(1)(A) of the Act and is not covered under Medicare.

**B. Other**

All other indications for stem cell transplantation not otherwise noted above as covered or non-covered nationally remain at Medicare Administrative Contractor discretion.

## 100-03, 110.9

### NCD for Antigens Prepared for Sublingual Administration (110.9)

For antigens provided to patients on or after November 17, 1996, Medicare does not cover such antigens if they are to be administered sublingually, i.e., by placing drops under the patient's tongue. This kind of allergy therapy has not been proven to be safe and effective. Antigens are covered only if they are administered by injection.

CPT © 2017 American Medical Association. All Rights Reserved.

© 2017 Optum360, LLC

## 100-03, 110.12

### NCD for Challenge Ingestion Food Testing (110.12)

This procedure is covered when it is used on an outpatient basis if it is reasonable and necessary for the individual patient.

Challenge ingestion food testing has not been proven to be effective in the diagnosis of rheumatoid arthritis, depression, or respiratory disorders. Accordingly, its use in the diagnosis of these conditions is not reasonable and necessary within the meaning of section 1862(a)(1) of the Medicare law, and no program payment is made for this procedure when it is so used.

## 100-03, 110.14

### NCD for Apheresis (Therapeutic Pheresis) (110.14)

#### B. Indications

Apheresis is covered for the following indications:

- Plasma exchange for acquired myasthenia gravis;
- Leukapheresis in the treatment of leukemekia
- Plasmapheresis in the treatment of primary macroglobulinemia (Waldenstrom);
- Treatment of hyperglobulinemias, including (but not limited to) multiple myelomas, cryoglobulinemia and hyperviscosity syndromes;
- Plasmapheresis or plasma exchange as a last resort treatment of thrombobotic thrombocytopenic purpura (TTP);
- Plasmapheresis or plasma exchange in the last resort treatment of life threatening rheumatoid vasculitis;
- Plasma perfusion of charcoal filters for treatment of pruritis of cholestatic liver disease;
- Plasma exchange in the treatment of Goodpasture's Syndrome;
- Plasma exchange in the treatment of glomerulonephritis associated with antiglomerular basement membrane antibodies and advancing renal failure or pulmonary hemorrhage;
- Treatment of chronic relapsing polyneuropathy for patients with severe or life threatening symptoms who have failed to respond to conventional therapy;
- Treatment of life threatening scleroderma and polymyositis when the patient is unresponsive to conventional therapy;
- Treatment of Guillain-Barre Syndrome; and
- Treatment of last resort for life threatening systemic lupus erythematosus (SLE) when conventional therapy has failed to prevent clinical deterioration.

#### C. Settings

Apheresis is covered only when performed in a hospital setting (either inpatient or outpatient). or in a nonhospital setting. e.g. physician directed clinic when the following conditions are met:

- A physician (or a number of physicians) is present to perform medical services and to respond to medical emergencies at all times during patient care hours;
- Each patient is under the care of a physician; and
- All nonphysician services are furnished under the direct, personal supervision of a physician.

## 100-03, 110.16

### NCD for Nonselective (Random) Transfusions and Living Related Donor Specific Transfusions (DST) in Kidney Transplantation (110.16)

These pretransplant transfusions are covered under Medicare without a specific limitation on the number of transfusions, subject to the normal Medicare blood deductible provisions. Where blood is given directly to the transplant patient; e.g., in the case of donor specific transfusions, the blood is considered replaced for purposes of the blood deductible provisions.

## 100-03, 110.23

### Stem Cell Transplantation (Formerly 110.8.1) (Various Effective Dates Below)

(Rev. 193, Issued; 07-01-16, Effective: 01-27-16, Implementation: 10-03-16)

#### A. General

Stem cell transplantation is a process in which stem cells are harvested from either a patient's (autologous) or donor's (allogeneic) bone marrow or peripheral blood for intravenous infusion. Autologous stem cell transplantation (AuSCT) is a technique for restoring stem cells using the patient's own previously stored cells. AuSCT must be used to effect hematopoietic reconstitution following severely myelotoxic doses of chemotherapy (HDCT) and/or radiotherapy used to treat various malignancies. Allogeneic hematopoietic stem cell transplantation (HSCT) is a procedure in which a portion of a healthy donor's stem cell or bone marrow is obtained and prepared for intravenous infusion. Allogeneic HSCT may be used to restore function in recipients having an inherited or acquired deficiency or defect. Hematopoietic stem cells are multi-potent stem cells that give rise to all the blood cell types; these stem cells form

blood and immune cells. A hematopoietic stem cell is a cell isolated from blood or bone marrow that can renew itself, differentiate to a variety of specialized cells, can mobilize out of the bone marrow into circulating blood, and can undergo programmed cell death, called apoptosis - a process by which cells that are unneeded or detrimental will self-destruct.

The Centers for Medicare & Medicaid Services (CMS) is clarifying that bone marrow and peripheral blood stem cell transplantation is a process which includes mobilization, harvesting, and transplant of bone marrow or peripheral blood stem cells and the administration of high dose chemotherapy or radiotherapy prior to the actual transplant. When bone marrow or peripheral blood stem cell transplantation is covered, all necessary steps are included in coverage. When bone marrow or peripheral blood stem cell transplantation is non-covered, none of the steps are covered.

#### B. Nationally Covered Indications

I. Allogeneic Hematopoietic Stem Cell Transplantation (HSCT)

a) Effective for services performed on or after August 1, 1978, for the treatment of leukemia, leukemia in remission, or aplastic anemia when it is reasonable and necessary,

b) Effective for services performed on or after June 3, 1985, for the treatment of severe combined immunodeficiency disease (SCID) and for the treatment of Wiskott-Aldrich syndrome.

c) Effective for services performed on or after August 4, 2010, for the treatment of Myelodysplastic Syndromes (MDS) pursuant to Coverage with Evidence Development (CED) in the context of a Medicare-approved, prospective clinical study.

MDS refers to a group of diverse blood disorders in which the bone marrow does not produce enough healthy, functioning blood cells. These disorders are varied with regard to clinical characteristics, cytologic and pathologic features, and cytogenetics. The abnormal production of blood cells in the bone marrow leads to low blood cell counts, referred to as cytopenias, which are a hallmark feature of MDS along with a dysplastic and hypercellular-appearing bone marrow

Medicare payment for these beneficiaries will be restricted to patients enrolled in an approved clinical study. In accordance with the Stem Cell Therapeutic and Research Act of 2005 (US Public Law 109-129) a standard dataset is collected for all allogeneic transplant patients in the United States by the Center for International Blood and Marrow Transplant Research. The elements in this dataset, comprised of two mandatory forms plus one additional form, encompass the information we require for a study under CED.

A prospective clinical study seeking Medicare payment for treating a beneficiary with allogeneic HSCT for MDS pursuant to CED must meet one or more aspects of the following questions:

1. Prospectively, compared to Medicare beneficiaries with MDS who do not receive HSCT, do Medicare beneficiaries with MDS who receive HSCT have improved outcomes as indicated by:

- Relapse-free mortality,
- progression free survival,
- relapse, and
- overall survival?

2. Prospectively, in Medicare beneficiaries with MDS who receive HSCT, how do International Prognostic Scoring System (IPSS) scores, patient age, cytopenias, and comorbidities predict the following outcomes:

- Relapse-free mortality,
- progression free survival,
- relapse, and
- overall survival?

3. Prospectively, in Medicare beneficiaries with MDS who receive HSCT, what treatment facility characteristics predict meaningful clinical improvement in the following outcomes:

- Relapse-free mortality,
- progression free survival,
- relapse, and
- overall survival?

In addition, the clinical study must adhere to the following standards of scientific integrity and relevance to the Medicare population:

a. The principal purpose of the research study is to test whether a particular intervention potentially improves the participants' health outcomes.

b. The research study is well supported by available scientific and medical information or it is intended to clarify or establish the health outcomes of interventions already in common clinical use.

c. The research study does not unjustifiably duplicate existing studies.

d. The research study design is appropriate to answer the research question being asked in the study.

e. The research study is sponsored by an organization or individual capable of executing the proposed study successfully.

CPT © 2017 American Medical Association. All Rights Reserved.

f. The research study is in compliance with all applicable Federal regulations concerning the protection of human subjects found at 45 CFR Part 46. If a study is regulated by the Food and Drug Administration (FDA), it must be in compliance with 21 CFR parts 50 and 56.

g. All aspects of the research study are conducted according to appropriate standards of scientific integrity (see http://www.icmje.org).

h. The research study has a written protocol that clearly addresses, or incorporates by reference, the standards listed here as Medicare requirements for CED coverage.

i. The clinical research study is not designed to exclusively test toxicity or disease pathophysiology in healthy individuals. Trials of all medical technologies measuring therapeutic outcomes as one of the objectives meet this standard only if the disease or condition being studied is life threatening as defined in 21 CFR §312.81(a) and the patient has no other viable treatment options.

j. The clinical research study is registered on the ClinicalTrials.gov Web site by the principal sponsor/investigator prior to the enrollment of the first study subject.

k. The research study protocol specifies the method and timing of public release of all pre-specified outcomes to be measured including release of outcomes if outcomes are negative or study is terminated early. The results must be made public within 24 months of the end of data collection. If a report is planned to be published in a peer-reviewed journal, then that initial release may be an abstract that meets the requirements of the International Committee of Medical Journal Editors (http://www.icmje.org). However a full report of the outcomes must be made public no later than 3 years after the end of data collection.

l. The research study protocol must explicitly discuss subpopulations affected by the treatment under investigation, particularly traditionally underrepresented groups in clinical studies, how the inclusion and exclusion criteria effect enrollment of these populations, and a plan for the retention and reporting of said populations on the trial. If the inclusion and exclusion criteria are expected to have a negative effect on the recruitment or retention of underrepresented populations, the protocol must discuss why these criteria are necessary.

m. The research study protocol explicitly discusses how the results are or are not expected to be generalizable to the Medicare population to infer whether Medicare patients may benefit from the intervention. Separate discussions in the protocol may be necessary for populations eligible for Medicare due to age, disability or Medicaid eligibility.

Consistent with section 1142 of the Social Security Act, the Agency for Health Research and Quality (AHRQ) supports clinical research studies that CMS determines meet the above-listed standards and address the above-listed research questions.

The clinical research study should also have the following features:

- It should be a prospective, longitudinal study with clinical information from the period before HSCT and short- and long-term follow-up information.

- Outcomes should be measured and compared among pre-specified subgroups within the cohort.

- The study should be powered to make inferences in subgroup analyses.

- Risk stratification methods should be used to control for selection bias. Data elements to be used in risk stratification models should include:

Patient selection:

– Patient Age at diagnosis of MDS and at transplantation

– Date of onset of MDS

– Disease classification (specific MDS subtype at diagnosis prior to preparative/conditioning regimen using World Health Organization (WHO) classifications). Include presence/absence of refractory cytopenias

– Comorbid conditions

– IPSS score (and WHO-adapted Prognostic Scoring System (WPSS) score, if applicable) at diagnosis and prior to transplantation

– Score immediately prior to transplantation and one year post-transplantation

– Disease assessment at diagnosis at start of preparative regimen and last assessment prior to preparative regimen Subtype of MDS (refractory anemia with or without blasts, degree of blasts, etc.)

– Type of preparative/conditioning regimen administered (myeloablative, non-myeloablative, reduced–intensity conditioning)

– Donor type

– Cell Source

Facilities must submit the required transplant essential data to the Stem Cell Therapeutics Outcomes Database.

d) Effective for claims with dates of service on or after January 27, 2016, allogeneic HSCT for multiple myeloma is covered by Medicare only for beneficiaries with Durie-Salmon Stage II or III multiple myeloma, or

International Staging System (ISS) Stage II or Stage III multiple myeloma, and participating in an approved prospective clinical study that meets the criteria below. There must be appropriate statistical techniques to control for selection bias and confounding by age, duration of diagnosis, disease classification, International Myeloma Working Group (IMWG) classification, ISS stage, comorbid conditions, type of preparative/conditioning regimen, graft vs. host disease (GVHD) prophylaxis, donor type and cell source.

A prospective clinical study seeking Medicare coverage for allogeneic HSCT for multiple myeloma pursuant to CED must address the following question:

Compared to patients who do not receive allogeneic HSCT, do Medicare beneficiaries with multiple myeloma who receive allogeneic HSCT have improved outcomes as indicated by:

– Graft vs. host disease (acute and chronic);

– Other transplant-related adverse events;

– Overall survival; and

– (optional) Quality of life?

All CMS-approved clinical studies and registries must adhere to the below listed standards of scientific integrity and relevance to the Medicare population as listed in section g.

e) Effective for claims with dates of service on or after January 27, 2016, allogeneic HSCT for myelofibrosis (MF) is covered by Medicare only for beneficiaries with Dynamic International Prognostic Scoring System (DIPSSplus) intermediate-2 or High primary or secondary MF and participating in an approved prospective clinical study. All Medicare approved studies must use appropriate statistical techniques in the analysis to control for selection bias and potential confounding by age, duration of diagnosis, disease classification, DIPSSplus score, comorbid conditions, type of preparative/conditioning regimen, graft vs. host disease (GVHD) prophylaxis, donor type and cell source.

A prospective clinical study seeking Medicare coverage for allogeneic HSCT for myelofibrosis pursuant to Coverage with Evidence Development (CED) must address the following question:

Compared to patients who do not receive allogeneic HSCT, do Medicare beneficiaries with MF who receive allogeneic HSCT transplantation have improved outcomes as indicated by:

– Graft vs. host disease (acute and chronic);

– Other transplant-related adverse events;

– Overall survival; and

– (optional) Quality of life?

All CMS-approved clinical studies and registries must adhere to the below listed standards of scientific integrity and relevance to the Medicare population as listed in section g.

f) Effective for claims with dates of service on or after January 27, 2016, allogeneic HSCT for sickle cell disease (SCD) is covered by Medicare only for beneficiaries with severe, symptomatic SCD who participate in an approved prospective clinical study.

A prospective clinical study seeking Medicare coverage for allogeneic HSCT for sickle cell disease pursuant to Coverage with Evidence Development (CED) must address the following question:

Compared to patients who do not receive allogeneic HSCT, do Medicare beneficiaries with SCD who receive allogeneic HSCT have improved outcomes as indicated by:

– Graft vs. host disease (acute and chronic),

– Other transplant-related adverse events;

– Overall survival; and

– (optional) Quality of life?

All CMS-approved clinical studies and registries must adhere to the below listed standards of scientific integrity and relevance to the Medicare population listed in section g:

g) All CMS-approved clinical studies and registries in sections d, e and f must adhere to the below listed standards of scientific integrity and relevance to the Medicare population:

a. The principal purpose of the study is to test whether the item or service meaningfully improves health outcomes of affected beneficiaries who are represented by the enrolled subjects.

b. The rationale for the study is well supported by available scientific and medical evidence.

c. The study results are not anticipated to unjustifiably duplicate existing knowledge.

d. The study design is methodologically appropriate and the anticipated number of enrolled subjects is sufficient to answer the research question(s) being asked in the National Coverage Determination.

e. The study is sponsored by an organization or individual capable of completing it successfully.

CPT © 2017 American Medical Association. All Rights Reserved.

© 2017 Optum360, LLC

f. The research study is in compliance with all applicable Federal regulations concerning the protection of human subjects found in the Code of Federal Regulations (CFR) at 45 CFR Part 46. If a study is regulated by the Food and Drug Administration (FDA), it is also in compliance with 21 CFR Parts 50 and 56. In addition, to further enhance the protection of human subjects in studies conducted under CED, the study must provide and obtain meaningful informed consent from patients regarding the risks associated with the study items and/or services, and the use and eventual disposition of the collected data.

g. All aspects of the study are conducted according to appropriate standards of scientific integrity.

h. The study has a written protocol that clearly demonstrates adherence to the standards listed here as Medicare requirements.

i. The study is not designed to exclusively test toxicity or disease pathophysiology in healthy individuals. Such studies may meet this requirement only if the disease or condition being studied is life threatening as defined in 21 CFR §312.81(a) and the patient has no other viable treatment options.

j. The clinical research studies and registries are registered on the www.ClinicalTrials.gov website by the principal sponsor/investigator prior to the enrollment of the first study subject. Registries are also registered in the Agency for Healthcare Quality (AHRQ) Registry of Patient Registries (RoPR).

k. The research study protocol specifies the method and timing of public release of all prespecified outcomes to be measured including release of outcomes if outcomes are negative or study is terminated early. The results must be made public within 12 months of the study's primary completion date, which is the date the final subject had final data collection for the primary endpoint, even if the trial does not achieve its primary aim. The results must include number started/completed, summary results for primary and secondary outcome measures, statistical analyses, and adverse events. Final results must be reported in a publicly accessibly manner; either in a peer-reviewed scientific journal (in print or on-line), in an on-line publicly accessible registry dedicated to the dissemination of clinical trial information such as ClinicalTrials.gov, or in journals willing to publish in abbreviated format (e.g., for studies with negative or incomplete results).

l. The study protocol must explicitly discuss beneficiary subpopulations affected by the item or service under investigation, particularly traditionally underrepresented groups in clinical studies, how the inclusion and exclusion criteria effect enrollment of these populations, and a plan for the retention and reporting of said populations in the trial. If the inclusion and exclusion criteria are expected to have a negative effect on the recruitment or retention of underrepresented populations, the protocol must discuss why these criteria are necessary.

m. The study protocol explicitly discusses how the results are or are not expected to be generalizable to affected beneficiary subpopulations. Separate discussions in the protocol may be necessary for populations eligible for Medicare due to age, disability or Medicaid eligibility.

Consistent with section 1142 of the Act, the Agency for Healthcare Research and Quality (AHRQ) supports clinical research studies that CMS determines meet the above-listed standards and address the above-listed research questions.

II. Autologous Stem Cell Transplantation (AuSCT)

a) Effective for services performed on or after April 28, 1989, AuSCT is considered reasonable and necessary under §1862(a)(1)(A) of the Act for the following conditions and is covered under Medicare for patients with:

1. Acute leukemia in remission who have a high probability of relapse and who have no human leucocyte antigens (HLA)-matched;

2. Resistant non-Hodgkin's lymphomas or those presenting with poor prognostic features following an initial response;

3. Recurrent or refractory neuroblastoma; or,

4. Advanced Hodgkin's disease who have failed conventional therapy and have no HLA-matched donor.

b) Effective October 1, 2000, single AuSCT is only covered for Durie-Salmon Stage II or III patients that fit the following requirements:

– Newly diagnosed or responsive multiple myeloma. This includes those patients with previously untreated disease, those with at least a partial response to prior chemotherapy (defined as a 50% decrease either in measurable paraprotein [serum and/or urine] or in bone marrow infiltration, sustained for at least 1 month), and those in responsive relapse; and

– Adequate cardiac, renal, pulmonary, and hepatic function.

c) Effective for services performed on or after March 15, 2005, when recognized clinical risk factors are employed to select patients for transplantation, high dose melphalan (HDM) together with AuSCT is reasonable and necessary for Medicare beneficiaries of any age group with primary amyloid light chain (AL) amyloidosis who meet the following criteria:

– Amyloid deposition in 2 or fewer organs; and,

– Cardiac left ventricular ejection fraction (EF) greater than 45%.

**C. Nationally Non-Covered Indications**

I. Allogeneic Hematopoietic Stem Cell Transplantation (HSCT)

Effective for claims with dates of service on or after May 24, 1996, through January 26, 2016, allogeneic HSCT is not covered as treatment for multiple myeloma.

II. Autologous Stem Cell Transplantation (AuSCT)

Insufficient data exist to establish definite conclusions regarding the efficacy of AuSCT for the following conditions:

a) Acute leukemia not in remission;

b) Chronic granulocytic leukemia;

c) Solid tumors (other than neuroblastoma);

d) Up to October 1, 2000, multiple myeloma;

e) Tandem transplantation (multiple rounds of AuSCT) for patients with multiple myeloma;

f) Effective October 1, 2000, non primary AL amyloidosis; and,

g) Effective October 1, 2000, through March 14, 2005, primary AL amyloidosis for Medicare beneficiaries age 64 or older.

In these cases, AuSCT is not considered reasonable and necessary within the meaning of §l862(a)(1)(A) of the Act and is not covered under Medicare.

**D. Other**

All other indications for stem cell transplantation not otherwise noted above as covered or non-covered remain at local Medicare Administrative Contractor discretion.

(This NCD last reviewed January 2016.)

## 100-03, 130.1

### NCD for Inpatient Hospital Stays for Treatment of Alcoholism (130.1)

**A. Inpatient Hospital Stay for Alcohol Detoxification**

Many hospitals provide detoxification services during the more acute stages of alcoholism or alcohol withdrawal. When the high probability or occurrence of medical complications (e.g., delirium, confusion, trauma, or unconsciousness) during detoxification for acute alcoholism or alcohol withdrawal necessitates the constant availability of physicians and/or complex medical equipment found only in the hospital setting, inpatient hospital care during this period is considered reasonable and necessary and is therefore covered under the program. Generally, detoxification can be accomplished within two to three days with an occasional need for up to five days where the patient's condition dictates. This limit (five days) may be extended in an individual case where there is a need for a longer period for detoxification for a particular patient.

In such cases, however, there should be documentation by a physician which substantiates that a longer period of detoxification was reasonable and necessary. When the detoxification needs of an individual no longer require an inpatient hospital setting, coverage should be denied on the basis that inpatient hospital care is not reasonable and necessary as required by §1862(a)(l) of the Social Security Act (the Act). Following detoxification a patient may be transferred to an inpatient rehabilitation unit or discharged to a residential treatment program or outpatient treatment setting.

**B. Inpatient Hospital Stay for Alcohol Rehabilitation**

Hospitals may also provide structured inpatient alcohol rehabilitation programs to the chronic alcoholic. These programs are composed primarily of coordinated educational and psychotherapeutic services provided on a group basis. Depending on the subject matter, a series of lectures, discussions, films, and group therapy sessions are led by either physicians, psychologists, or alcoholism counselors from the hospital or various outside organizations. In addition, individual psychotherapy and family counseling (see §70.1) may be provided in selected cases. These programs are conducted under the supervision and direction of a physician. Patients may directly enter an inpatient hospital rehabilitation program after having undergone detoxification in the same hospital or in another hospital or may enter an inpatient hospital rehabilitation program without prior hospitalization for detoxification.

Alcohol rehabilitation can be provided in a variety of settings other than the hospital setting. In order for an inpatient hospital stay for alcohol rehabilitation to be covered under Medicare it must be medically necessary for the care to be provided in the inpatient hospital setting rather than in a less costly facility or on an outpatient basis. Inpatient hospital care for receipt of an alcohol rehabilitation program would generally be medically necessary where either (l) there is documentation by the physician that recent alcohol rehabilitation services in a less intensive setting or on an outpatient basis have proven unsuccessful and, as a consequence, the patient requires the supervision and intensity of services which can only be found in the controlled environment of the hospital, or (2) only the hospital environment can assure the medical management or control of the patient's concomitant conditions during the course of alcohol rehabilitation. (However, a patient's concomitant condition may make the use of certain alcohol treatment modalities medically inappropriate.)

In addition, the "active treatment" criteria (see the Medicare Benefit Policy Manual, Chapter 2, "Inpatient Psychiatric Hospital Services," §20) should be applied to psychiatric care in the general hospital as well as to psychiatric care in a psychiatric hospital. Since alcoholism is classifiable as a psychiatric condition the "active treatment" criteria must also be met in order for alcohol rehabilitation services to be covered under Medicare. (Thus, it is the combined need for "active treatment" and for covered care which can only be provided in the inpatient hospital setting, rather than the fact that rehabilitation immediately follows a period of detoxification which provides the basis for coverage of inpatient hospital alcohol rehabilitation programs.)

Generally 16-19 days of rehabilitation services are sufficient to bring a patient to a point where care could be continued in other than an inpatient hospital setting. An inpatient hospital stay for alcohol rehabilitation may be extended beyond this limit in an individual case where a longer period of alcohol rehabilitation is medically necessary. In such cases, however, there should be documentation by a physician which substantiates the need for such care. Where the rehabilitation needs of an individual no longer require an inpatient hospital setting, coverage should be denied on the basis that inpatient hospital care is not reasonable and necessary as required by §1862 (a)(I) of the Act.

Subsequent admissions to the inpatient hospital setting for alcohol rehabilitation follow-up, reinforcement, or "recap" treatments are considered to be readmissions (rather than an extension of the original stay) and must meet the requirements of this section for coverage under Medicare. Prior admissions to the inpatient hospital setting - either in the same hospital or in a different hospital - may be an indication that the "active treatment" requirements are not met (i.e., there is no reasonable expectation of improvement) and the stay should not be covered. Accordingly, there should be documentation to establish that "readmission" to the hospital setting for alcohol rehabilitation services can reasonably be expected to result in improvement of the patient's condition. For example, the documentation should indicate what changes in the patient's medical condition, social or emotional status, or treatment plan make improvement likely, or why the patient's initial hospital treatment was not sufficient.

### C. Combined Alcohol Detoxification/Rehabilitation Programs

Medicare Administrative Contractors (MACs) should apply the guidelines in A. and B. above to both phases of a combined inpatient hospital alcohol detoxification/rehabilitation program. Not all patients who require the inpatient hospital setting for detoxification also need the inpatient hospital setting for rehabilitation. (See §130.1 for coverage of outpatient hospital alcohol rehabilitation services.) Where the inpatient hospital setting is medically necessary for both alcohol detoxification and rehabilitation, generally a 3-week period is reasonable and necessary to bring the patient to the point where care can be continued in other than an inpatient hospital setting.

Decisions regarding reasonableness and necessity of treatment, the need for an inpatient hospital level of care, and length of treatment should be made by A/B MAC (A) based on accepted medical practice with the advice of their medical consultant. (In hospitals under PSRO review, PSRO determinations of medical necessity of services and appropriateness of the level of care at which services are provided are binding on A/B MAC (A) for purposes of adjudicating claims for payment.)

## 100-03, 130.2

### NCD for Outpatient Hospital Services for Treatment of Alcoholism (130.2)

Coverage is available for both diagnostic and therapeutic services furnished for the treatment of alcoholism by the hospital to outpatients subject to the same rules applicable to outpatient hospital services in general. While there is no coverage for day hospitalization programs, per se, individual services which meet the requirements in the Medicare Benefit Policy Manual, Chapter 6, Sec.20 may be covered. (Meals, transportation and recreational and social activities do not fall within the scope of covered outpatient hospital services under Medicare.)

All services must be reasonable and necessary for diagnosis or treatment of the patient's condition (see the Medicare Benefit Policy Manual, chapter 16 Sec.20). Thus, educational services and family counseling would only be covered where they are directly related to treatment of the patient's condition. The frequency of treatment and period of time over which it occurs must also be reasonable and necessary.

## 100-03, 130.3

### NCD for Chemical AversionTherapy for Treatment of Alcoholism (130.3)

Chemical aversion therapy is a behavior modification technique that is used in the treatment of alcoholism. Chemical aversion therapy facilitates alcohol abstinence through the development of conditioned aversions to the taste, smell, and sight of alcohol beverages. This is accomplished by repeatedly pairing alcohol with unpleasant symptoms (e.g., nausea) which have been induced by one of several chemical agents. While a number of drugs have been employed in chemical aversion therapy, the three most commonly used are emetine, apomorphine, and lithium. None of the drugs being used, however, have yet been approved by the Food and Drug Administration specifically for use in chemical aversion therapy for alcoholism. Accordingly, when these drugs are being employed in conjunction with this therapy, patients undergoing this treatment need to be kept under medical observation.

Available evidence indicates that chemical aversion therapy may be an effective component of certain alcoholism treatment programs, particularly as part of multi-modality treatment programs which include other behavioral techniques and therapies, such as psychotherapy. Based on this evidence, the Centers for Medicare & Medicaid Services' medical consultants have recommended that chemical aversion therapy be covered under Medicare. However, since chemical aversion therapy is a

demanding therapy which may not be appropriate for all Medicare beneficiaries needing treatment for alcoholism, a physician should certify to the appropriateness of chemical aversion therapy in the individual case. Therefore, if chemical aversion therapy for treatment of alcoholism is determined to be reasonable and necessary for an individual patient, it is covered under Medicare.

When it is medically necessary for a patient to receive chemical aversion therapy as a hospital inpatient, coverage for care in that setting is available. (See §130.1 regarding coverage of multi-modality treatment programs.) Follow-up treatments for chemical aversion therapy can generally be provided on an outpatient basis. Thus, where a patient is admitted as an inpatient for receipt of chemical aversion therapy, there must be documentation by the physician of the need in the individual case for the inpatient hospital admission.

Decisions regarding reasonableness and necessity of treatment and the need for an inpatient hospital level of care should be made by the A/B MAC (A) based on accepted medical practice with the advice of their medical consultant. (In hospitals under Quality Improvement Organization (QIO) review, QIO determinations of medical necessity of services and appropriateness of the level of care at which services are provided are binding on the A/B MAC (A) for purposes of adjudicating claims for payment.)

## 100-03, 140.1

### NCD for Abortion (140.1)

Abortions are not covered Medicare procedures except:

1. If the pregnancy is the result of an act of rape or incest; or

2. In the case where a woman suffers from a physical disorder, physical injury, or physical illness, including a life-endangering physical condition caused by or arising from the pregnancy itself, that would, as certified by a physician, place the woman in danger of death unless an abortion is performed.

## 100-03, 140.2

### NCD for Breast Reconstruction Following Mastectomy (140.2)

Reconstruction of the affected and the contralateral unaffected breast following a medically necessary mastectomy is considered a relatively safe and effective noncosmetic procedure. Accordingly, program payment may be made for breast reconstruction surgery following removal of a breast for any medical reason.

Program payment may not be made for breast reconstruction for cosmetic reasons. (Cosmetic surgery is excluded from coverage under Sec.I862(a)(I0) of the Social Security Act.)

## 100-03, 140.5

### NCD for Laser Procedures (140.5)

Medicare recognizes the use of lasers for many medical indications. Procedures performed with lasers are sometimes used in place of more conventional techniques. In the absence of a specific noncoverage instruction, and where a laser has been approved for marketing by the Food and Drug Administration, Medicare Administrative Contractor discretion may be used to determine whether a procedure performed with a laser is reasonable and necessary and, therefore, covered.

The determination of coverage for a procedure performed using a laser is made on the basis that the use of lasers to alter, revise, or destroy tissue is a surgical procedure. Therefore, coverage of laser procedures is restricted to practitioners with training in the surgical management of the disease or condition being treated.

## 100-03, 150.1

### NCD for Manipulation (150.1)

Manipulation of the Rib Cage.--Manual manipulation of the rib cage contributes to the treatment of respiratory conditions such as bronchitis, emphysema, and asthma as part of a regimen which includes other elements of therapy, and is covered only under such circumstances.

Manipulation of the Head.--Manipulation of the occipitocervical or temporomandibular regions of the head when indicated for conditions affecting those portions of the head and neck is a covered service.

## 100-03, 150.2

### NCD for Osteogenic Stimulators (150.2)

**Electrical Osteogenic Stimulators**

**B. Nationally Covered Indications**
1. Noninvasive Stimulator.

   The noninvasive stimulator device is covered only for the following indications:

   — Nonunion of long bone fractures;

   — Failed fusion, where a minimum of nine months has elapsed since the last surgery;

   — Congenital pseudarthroses; and

   — Effective July 1, 1996, as an adjunct to spinal fusion surgery for patients at high risk of pseudarthrosis due to previously failed spinal fusion at the same site or for those undergoing multiple level fusion. A multiple level fusion involves 3 or more vertebrae (e.g., L3-L5, L4-S1, etc.).

— Effective September 15, 1980, nonunion of long bone fractures is considered to exist only after 6 or more months have elapsed without healing of the fracture.

— Effective April 1, 2000, nonunion of long bone fractures is considered to exist only when serial radiographs have confirmed that fracture healing has ceased for 3 or more months prior to starting treatment with the electrical osteogenic stimulator. Serial radiographs must include a minimum of 2 sets of radiographs, each including multiple views of the fracture site, separated by a minimum of 90 days.

2. Invasive (Implantable) Stimulator.

The invasive stimulator device is covered only for the following indications:

— Nonunion of long bone fractures

— Effective July 1, 1996, as an adjunct to spinal fusion surgery for patients at high risk of pseudarthrosis due to previously failed spinal fusion at the same site or for those undergoing multiple level fusion. A multiple level fusion involves 3 or more vertebrae (e.g., L3-5, L4-S1, etc.)

— Effective September 15, 1980, nonunion of long bone fractures is considered to exist only after 6 or more months have elapsed without healing of the fracture.

— Effective April 1, 2000, non union of long bone fractures is considered to exist only when serial radiographs have confirmed that fracture healing has ceased for 3 or more months prior to starting treatment with the electrical osteogenic stimulator. Serial radiographs must include a minimum of 2 sets of radiographs, each including multiple views of the fracture site, separated by a minimum of 90 days.

— Effective for services performed on or after January 1, 2001, ultrasonic osteogenic stimulators are covered as medically reasonable and necessary for the treatment of non-union fractures. In demonstrating nonunion of fractures, we would expect:

  – A minimum of two sets of radiographs obtained prior to starting treatment with the osteogenic stimulator, separated by a minimum of 90 days. Each radiograph must include multiple views of the fracture site accompanied with a written interpretation by a physician stating that there has been no clinically significant evidence of fracture healing between the two sets of radiographs.

  – Indications that the patient failed at least one surgical intervention for the treatment of the fracture.

— Effective April 27, 2005, upon the recommendation of the ultrasound stimulation for nonunion fracture healing, CMS determins that the evidence is adequate to condlude that noninvasive ultrasound stimulation for the treatment of nonunion bone fractures prior to surfical intervention is reasonable and necessary. In demonstrating non-union fracturs, CMS expects:

  – A minimum of 2 sets of radiographs, obtained prior to starting treating with the osteogenic stimulator, separated by a minimum of 90 days. Each radiograph set must include multiple views of the fracture site accompanied with a written interpretation by a physician stating that there has been no clinically significant evidence of fracture healing between the 2 sets of radiographs.

### C. Nationally Non-Covered Indications

Nonunion fractures of the skull, vertebrae and those that are tumor-related are excluded from coverage.

Ultrasonic osteogenic stimulators may not be used concurrently with other non-invasive osteogenic devices.

Ultrasonic osteogenic stimulators for fresh fractures and delayed unions remain non-covered.

(This NCD last reviewed June 2005)

## 100-03, 150.7

### NCD for Prolotherapy, Joint Sclerotherapy, and Ligamentous Injections with Sclerosing Agents (150.7)

The medical effectiveness of the above therapies has not been verified by scientifically controlled studies. Accordingly, reimbursement for these modalities should be denied on the ground that they are not reasonable and necessary as required by Sec.1862(a)(1) of the Act.

## 100-03, 150.10

### NCD for Lumbar Artificial Disc Replacement (LADR) (150.10)

#### A. General

The lumbar artificial disc replacement (LADR) is a surgical procedure on the lumbar spine that involves complete removal of the damaged or diseased lumbar intervertebral disc and implantation of an artificial disc. The procedure may be done as an alternative to lumbar spinal fusion and is intended to reduce pain, increase movement at the site of surgery and restore intervertebral disc height. The Food and

Drug Administration has approved the use of LADR for spine arthroplasty in skeletally mature patients with degenerative or discogenic disc disease at one level for L3 to S1.

#### B. Nationally Covered Indications
N/A

#### C. Nationally Non-Covered Indications
Effective for services performed from May 16, 2006 through August 13, 2007, the Centers for Medicare and Medicaid Services (CMS) has found that LADR with the ChariteTM lumbar artificial disc is not reasonable and necessary for the Medicare population over 60 years of age; therefore, LADR with the ChariteTM lumbar artificial disc is non-covered for Medicare beneficiaries over 60 years of age.

Effective for services performed on or after August 14, 2007, CMS has found that LADR is not reasonable and necessary for the Medicare population over 60 years of age; therefore, LADR is non-covered for Medicare beneficiaries over 60 years of age.

#### D. Other
For Medicare beneficiaries 60 years of age and younger, there is no national coverage determination for LADR, leaving such determinations to continue to be made by the local Medicare Administrative Contractors.

For dates of service May 16, 2006 through August 13, 2007, Medicare coverage under the investigational device exemption (IDE) for LADR with a disc other than the ChariteTM lumbar disc in eligible clinical trials is not impacted.

## 100-03, 160.8

### NCD for Electroencephalographic (EEG) Monitoring During Surgical Procedures Involving the Cerebral Vasculature (160.8)
CIM 35-57

Electroencephalographic (EEG) monitoring is a safe and reliable technique for the assessment of gross cerebral blood flow during general anesthesia and is covered under Medicare. Very characteristic changes in the EEG occur when cerebral perfusion is inadequate for cerebral function. EEG monitoring as an indirect measure of cerebral perfusion requires the expertise of an electroencephalographer, a neurologist trained in EEG, or an advanced EEG technician for its proper interpretation.

The EEG monitoring may be covered routinely in carotid endarterectomies and in other neurological procedures where cerebral perfusion could be reduced. Such other procedures might include aneurysm surgery where hypotensive anesthesia is used or other cerebral vascular procedures where cerebral blood flow may be interrupted.

## 100-03, 160.17

### NCD for L-DOPA (160.17)

#### A. Part A Payment for L-Dopa and Associated Inpatient Hospital Services
A hospital stay and related ancillary services for the administration of L-Dopa are covered if medically required for this purpose. Whether a drug represents an allowable inpatient hospital cost during such stay depends on whether it meets the definition of a drug in Sec.1861(t) of the Act; i.e., on its inclusion in the compendia named in the Act or approval by the hospital's pharmacy and drug therapeutics (P&DT) or equivalent committee. (Levodopa (L-Dopa) has been favorably evaluated for the treatment of Parkinsonism by A.M.A. Drug Evaluations, First Edition 1971, the replacement compendia for "New Drugs.")

Inpatient hospital services are frequently not required in many cases when L-Dopa therapy is initiated. Therefore, determine the medical need for inpatient hospital services on the basis of medical facts in the individual case. It is not necessary to hospitalize the typical, well-functioning, ambulatory Parkinsonian patient who has no concurrent disease at the start of L-Dopa treatment. It is reasonable to provide inpatient hospital services for Parkinsonian patients with concurrent diseases, particularly of the cardiovascular, gastrointestinal, and neuropsychiatric systems. Although many patients require hospitalization for a period of under 2 weeks, a 4-week period of inpatient care is not unreasonable.

Laboratory tests in connection with the administration of L-Dopa - The tests medically warranted in connection with the achievement of optimal dosage and the control of the side effects of L-Dopa include a complete blood count, liver function tests such as SGOT, SGPT, and/or alkaline phosphatase, BUN or creatinine and urinalysis, blood sugar, and electrocardiogram.

Whether or not the patient is hospitalized, laboratory tests in certain cases are reasonable at weekly intervals although some physicians prefer to perform the tests much less frequently.

Physical therapy furnished in connection with administration of L-Dopa - Where, following administration of the drug, the patient experiences a reduction of rigidity which permits the reestablishment of a restorative goal for him/her, physical therapy services required to enable him/her to achieve this goal are payable provided they require the skills of a qualified physical therapist and are furnished by or under the supervision of such a therapist. However, once the individual's restoration potential has been achieved, the services required to maintain him/her at this level do not generally require the skills of a qualified physical therapist. In such situations, the role of the therapist is to evaluate the patient's needs in consultation with his/her physician and design a program of exercise appropriate to the capacity and tolerance of the patient and treatment objectives of the physician, leaving to others the actual carrying out of the program. While the evaluative services rendered by a qualified physical therapist are payable as physical therapy, services furnished by others in connection with the carrying out of the maintenance program established by the therapist are not.

#### B. Part A Reimbursement for L-Dopa Therapy in SNFs

Initiation of L-Dopa therapy can be appropriately carried out in the SNF setting, applying the same guidelines used for initiation of L-Dopa therapy in the hospital, including the types of patients who should be covered for inpatient services, the role of physical therapy, and the use of laboratory tests. (See subsection A.) Where inpatient care is required and L-Dopa therapy is initiated in the SNF, limit the stay to a maximum of 4 weeks; but in many cases the need may be no longer than 1 or 2 weeks, depending upon the patient's condition. However, where L-Dopa therapy is begun in the hospital and the patient is transferred to an SNF for continuation of the therapy, a combined length of stay in hospital and SNF of no longer than 4 weeks is reasonable (i.e., 1 week hospital stay followed by 3 weeks SNF stay; or 2 weeks hospital stay followed by 2 weeks SNF stay; etc.). Medical need must be demonstrated in cases where the combined length of stay in hospital and SNF is longer than 4 weeks. The choice of hospital or SNF, and the decision regarding the relative length of time spent in each, should be left to the medical judgment of the treating physician.

#### C. L-Dopa Coverage Under Part B

Part B reimbursement may not be made for the drug L-Dopa since it is a self-administrable drug. However, physician services rendered in connection with its administration and control of its side effects are covered if determined to be reasonable and necessary. Initiation of L-Dopa therapy on an outpatient basis is possible in most cases. Visit frequency ranging from every week to every 2 or 3 months is acceptable. However, after half a year of therapy, visits more frequent than every month would usually not be reasonable.

### 100-03, 180.1

#### NCD for Medical Nutrition Therapy (180.1)

Effective October 1, 2002, basic coverage of MNT for the first year a beneficiary receives MNT with either a diagnosis of renal disease or diabetes as defined at 42 CFR Sec.410.130 is 3 hours. Also effective October 1, 2002, basic coverage in subsequent years for renal disease or diabetes is 2 hours. The dietitian/nutritionist may choose how many units are performed per day as long as all of the other requirements in this NCD and 42 CFR Secs.410.130-410.134 are met. Pursuant to the exception at 42 CFR Sec.410.132(b)(5), additional hours are considered to be medically necessary and covered if the treating physician determines that there is a change in medical condition, diagnosis, or treatment regimen that requires a change in MNT and orders additional hours during that episode of care.

Effective October 1, 2002, if the treating physician determines that receipt of both MNT and DSMT is medically necessary in the same episode of care, Medicare will cover both DSMT and MNT initial and subsequent years without decreasing either benefit as long as DSMT and MNT are not provided on the same date of service. The dietitian/nutritionist may choose how many units are performed per day as long as all of the other requirements in the NCD and 42 CFR Secs.410.130-410.134 are met. Pursuant to the exception at 42 CFR 410.132(b)(5), additional hours are considered to be medically necessary and covered if the treating physician determines that there is a change in medical condition, diagnosis, or treatment regimen that requires a change in MNT and orders additional hours during that episode of care.

### 100-03, 190.1

#### NCD for Histocompatibility Testing (190.1)

This testing is safe and effective when it is performed on patients:

- In preparation for a kidney transplant;
- In preparation for bone marrow transplantation;
- In preparation for blood platelet transfusions (particularly where multiple infusions are involved); or
- Who are suspected of having ankylosing spondylitis.

This testing is covered under Medicare when used for any of the indications listed in A, B, and C and if it is reasonable and necessary for the patient.

It is covered for ankylosing spondylitis in cases where other methods of diagnosis would not be appropriate or have yielded inconclusive results. Request documentation supporting the medical necessity of the test from the physician in all cases where ankylosing spondylitis is indicated as the reason for the test.

### 100-03, 190.8

#### NCD for Lymphocyte Mitogen Response Assays (190.8)

It is a covered test under Medicare when it is medically necessary to assess lymphocytic function in diagnosed immunodeficiency diseases and to monitor immunotherapy.

It is not covered when it is used to monitor the treatment of cancer, because its use for that purpose is experimental.

### 100-03, 190.9

#### NCD for Serologic Testing for Acquired Immunodeficiency Syndrome (AIDS) (190.9)

These tests may be covered when performed to help determine a diagnosis for symptomatic patients. They are not covered when furnished as part of a screening program for asymptomatic persons.

Note: Two enzyme-linked immunosorbent assay (ELISA) tests that were conducted on the same specimen must both be positive before Medicare will cover the Western blot test.

### 100-03, 190.11

#### NCD for Home Prothrombin Time International Normalized Ratio (INR) Monitoring for Anticoagulation Management (190.11)

#### A. General

Use of the International Normalized Ratio (INR) or prothrombin time (PT) - standard measurement for reporting the blood's clotting time) - allows physicians to determine the level of anticoagulation in a patient independent of the laboratory reagents used. The INR is the ratio of the patient's PT (extrinsic or tissue-factor dependent coagulation pathway) compared to the mean PT for a group of normal individuals. Maintaining patients within his/her prescribed therapeutic range minimizes adverse events associated with inadequate or excessive anticoagulation such as serious bleeding or thromboembolic events. Patient self-testing and self-management through the use of a home INR monitor may be used to improve the time in therapeutic rate (TTR) for select groups of patients. Increased TTR leads to improved clinical outcomes and reductions in thromboembolic and hemorrhagic events.

Warfarin (also prescribed under other trade names, e.g., Coumadin(R)) is a self-administered, oral anticoagulant (blood thinner) medication that affects the vitamin K- dependent clotting factors II, VII, IX and X. It is widely used for various medical conditions, and has a narrow therapeutic index, meaning it is a drug with less than a 2-fold difference between median lethal dose and median effective dose. For this reason, since October 4, 2006, it falls under the category of a Food and Drug dministration (FDA) "black-box" drug whose dosage must be closely monitored to avoid serious complications. A PT/INR monitoring system is a portable testing device that includes a finger-stick and an FDA-cleared meter that measures the time it takes for a person's blood plasma to clot.

#### B. Nationally Covered Indications

For services furnished on or after March 19, 2008, Medicare will cover the use of home PT/INR monitoring for chronic, oral anticoagulation management for patients with mechanical heart valves, chronic atrial fibrillation, or venous thromboembolism (inclusive of deep venous thrombosis and pulmonary embolism) on warfarin. The monitor and the home testing must be prescribed by a treating physician as provided at 42 CFR 410.32(a), and all of the following requirements must be met:

1. The patient must have been anticoagulated for at least 3 months prior to use of the home INR device; and,

2. The patient must undergo a face-to-face educational program on anticoagulation anagement and must have demonstrated the correct use of the device prior to its use in the home; and,

3. The patient continues to correctly use the device in the context of the management of the anticoagulation therapy following the initiation of home monitoring; and,

4. Self-testing with the device should not occur more frequently than once a week.

#### C. Nationally Non-Covered Indications
N/A

#### D. Other

1. All other indications for home PT/INR monitoring not indicated as nationally covered above remain at local Medicare contractor discretion.

2. This national coverage determination (NCD) is distinct from, and makes no changes to, the PT clinical laboratory NCD at section 190.17 of Publication 100-3 of the NCD Manual.

### 100-03, 190.14

#### NCD for Human Immunodeficiency Virus (HIV) Testing (Diagnosis) (190.14)

#### Indications and Limitations of Coverage

#### Indications

Diagnostic testing to establish HIV infection may be indicated when there is a strong clinical suspicion supported by one or more of the following clinical findings:

- The patient has a documented, otherwise unexplained, AIDS-defining or AIDS-associated opportunistic infection.

- The patient has another documented sexually transmitted disease which identifies significant risk of exposure to HIV and the potential for an early or subclinical infection.

- The patient has documented acute or chronic hepatitis B or C infection that identifies a significant risk of exposure to HIV and the potential for an early or subclinical infection.

- The patient has a documented AIDS-defining or AIDS-associated neoplasm.

- The patient has a documented AIDS-associated neurologic disorder or otherwise unexplained dementia.

- The patient has another documented AIDS-defining clinical condition, or a history of other severe, recurrent, or persistent conditions which suggest an underlying immune deficiency (for example, cutaneous or mucosal disorders).

- The patient has otherwise unexplained generalized signs and symptoms suggestive of a chronic process with an underlying immune deficiency (for example, fever, weight loss, malaise, fatigue, chronic diarrhea, failure to thrive, chronic cough, hemoptysis, shortness of breath, or lymphadenopathy).

- The patient has otherwise unexplained laboratory evidence of a chronic disease process with an underlying immune deficiency (for example, anemia, leukopenia, pancytopenia, lymphopenia, or low CD4+ lymphocyte count).

- The patient has signs and symptoms of acute retroviral syndrome with fever, malaise, lymphadenopathy, and skin rash.

- The patient has documented exposure to blood or body fluids known to be capable of transmitting HIV (for example, needlesticks and other significant blood exposures) and antiviral therapy is initiated or anticipated to be initiated.

- The patient is undergoing treatment for rape. (HIV testing is a part of the rape treatment protocol.)

**Limitations**

HIV antibody testing in the United States is usually performed using HIV-1 or HIV-½ combination tests. HIV-2 testing is indicated if clinical circumstances suggest HIV-2 is likely (that is, compatible clinical findings and HIV-1 test negative). HIV-2 testing may also be indicated in areas of the country where there is greater prevalence of HIV-2 infections.

The Western Blot test should be performed only after documentation that the initial EIA tests are repeatedly positive or equivocal on a single sample.

- The HIV antigen tests currently have no defined diagnostic usage.

- Direct viral RNA detection may be performed in those situations where serologic testing does not establish a diagnosis but strong clinical suspicion persists (for example, acute retroviral syndrome, nonspecific serologic evidence of HIV, or perinatal HIV infection).

- If initial serologic tests confirm an HIV infection, repeat testing is not indicated.

- If initial serologic tests are HIV EIA negative and there is no indication for confirmation of infection by viral RNA detection, the interval prior to retesting is 3-6 months.

- Testing for evidence of HIV infection using serologic methods may be medically appropriate in situations where there is a risk of exposure to HIV. However, in the absence of a documented AIDS defining or HIV- associated disease, an HIV associated sign or symptom, or documented exposure to a known HIV-infected source, the testing is considered by Medicare to be screening and thus is not covered by Medicare (for example, history of multiple blood component transfusions, exposure to blood or body fluids not resulting in consideration of therapy, history of transplant, history of illicit drug use, multiple sexual partners, same-sex encounters, prostitution, or contact with prostitutes).

- The CPT Editorial Panel has issued a number of codes for infectious agent detection by direct antigen or nucleic acid probe techniques that have not yet been developed or are only being used on an investigational basis. Laboratory providers are advised to remain current on FDA-approval status for these tests.

## 100-03, 190.15

### NCD for Blood Counts (190.15)

**Indications**

Indications for a CBC or hemogram include red cell, platelet, and white cell disorders. Examples of these indications are enumerated individually below.

1. Indications for a CBC generally include the evaluation of bone marrow dysfunction as a result of neoplasms, therapeutic agents, exposure to toxic substances, or pregnancy. The CBC is also useful in assessing peripheral destruction of blood cells, suspected bone marrow failure or bone marrow infiltrate, suspected myeloproliferative, myelodysplastic, or lymphoproliferative processes, and immune disorders.

2. Indications for hemogram or CBC related to red cell (RBC) parameters of the hemogram include signs, symptoms, test results, illness, or disease that can be associated with anemia or other red blood cell disorder (e.g., pallor, weakness, fatigue, weight loss, bleeding, acute injury associated with blood loss or suspected blood loss, abnormal menstrual bleeding, hematuria, hematemesis, hematochezia, positive fecal occult blood test, malnutrition, vitamin deficiency, malabsorption, neuropathy, known malignancy, presence of acute or chronic disease that may have associated anemia, coagulation or hemostatic disorders, postural dizziness, syncope, abdominal pain, change in bowel habits, chronic marrow hypoplasia or decreased RBC production, tachycardia, systolic heart murmur, congestive heart failure, dyspnea, angina, nailbed deformities, growth retardation, jaundice, hepatomegaly, splenomegaly, lymphadenopathy, ulcers on the lower extremities).

3. Indications for hemogram or CBC related to red cell (RBC) parameters of the hemogram include signs, symptoms, test results, illness, or disease that can be associated with polycythemia (for example, fever, chills, ruddy skin, conjunctival redness, cough, wheezing, cyanosis, clubbing of the fingers, orthopnea, heart murmur, headache, vague cognitive changes including memory changes, sleep apnea, weakness, pruritus, dizziness, excessive sweating, visual symptoms, weight loss, massive obesity, gastrointestinal bleeding, paresthesias, dyspnea, joint symptoms, epigastric distress, pain and erythema of the fingers or toes, venous or arterial thrombosis, thromboembolism, myocardial infarction, stroke, transient ischemic attacks, congenital heart disease, chronic obstructive pulmonary disease, increased erythropoietin production associated with neoplastic, renal or hepatic disorders, androgen or diuretic use, splenomegaly, hepatomegaly, diastolic hypertension.)

4. Specific indications for CBC with differential count related to the WBC include signs, symptoms, test results, illness, or disease associated with leukemia, infections or inflammatory processes, suspected bone marrow failure or bone marrow infiltrate, suspected myeloproliferative, myelodysplastic or lymphoproliferative disorder, use of drugs that may cause leukopenia, and immune disorders (e.g., fever, chills, sweats, shock, fatigue, malaise, tachycardia, tachypnea, heart murmur, seizures, alterations of consciousness, meningismus, pain such as headache, abdominal pain, arthralgia, odynophagia, or dysuria, redness or swelling of skin, soft tissue bone, or joint, ulcers of the skin or mucous membranes, gangrene, mucous membrane discharge, bleeding, thrombosis, respiratory failure, pulmonary infiltrate, jaundice, diarrhea, vomiting, hepatomegaly, splenomegaly, lymphadenopathy, opportunistic infection such as oral candidiasis.)

5. Specific indications for CBC related to the platelet count include signs, symptoms, test results, illness, or disease associated with increased or decreased platelet production and destruction, or platelet dysfunction (e.g., gastrointestinal bleeding, genitourinary tract bleeding, bilateral epistaxis, thrombosis, ecchymosis, purpura, jaundice, petechiae, fever, heparin therapy, suspected DIC, shock, pre-eclampsia, neonate with maternal ITP, massive transfusion, recent platelet transfusion, cardiopulmonary bypass, hemolytic uremic syndrome, renal diseases, lymphadenopathy, hepatomegaly, splenomegaly, hypersplenism, neurologic abnormalities, viral or other infection, myeloproliferative, myelodysplastic, or lymphoproliferative disorder, thrombosis, exposure to toxic agents, excessive alcohol ingestion, autoimmune disorders (SLE, RA and other).

6. Indications for hemogram or CBC related to red cell (RBC) parameters of the hemogram include, in addition to those already listed, thalassemia, suspected hemoglobinopathy, lead poisoning, arsenic poisoning, and spherocytosis.

7. Specific indications for CBC with differential count related to the WBC include, in addition to those already listed, storage diseases; mucopolysaccharidoses, and use of drugs that cause leukocytosis such as G-CSF or GM-CSF.

8. Specific indications for CBC related to platelet count include, in addition to those already listed, May-Hegglin syndrome and Wiskott-Aldrich syndrome.

**Limitations**

1. Testing of patients who are asymptomatic, or who do not have a condition that could be expected to result in a hematological abnormality, is screening and is not a covered service.

2. In some circumstances it may be appropriate to perform only a hemoglobin or hematocrit to assess the oxygen carrying capacity of the blood. When the ordering provider requests only a hemoglobin or hematocrit, the remaining components of the CBC are not covered.

3. When a blood count is performed for an end-stage renal disease (ESRD) patient, and is billed outside the ESRD rate, documentation of the medical necessity for the blood count must be submitted with the claim.

4. In some patients presenting with certain signs, symptoms or diseases, a single CBC may be appropriate. Repeat testing may not be indicated unless abnormal results are found, or unless there is a change in clinical condition. If repeat testing is performed, a more descriptive diagnosis code (e.g., anemia) should be reported to support medical necessity. However, repeat testing may be indicated where results are normal in patients with conditions where there is a continued risk for the development of hematologic abnormality.

## 100-03, 190.18

### Serum Iron Studies

**Indications:**

1. Ferritin (82728), iron (83540) and either iron binding capacity (83550) or transferrin (84466) are useful in the differential diagnosis of iron deficiency, anemia, and for iron overload conditions.

   a. The following presentations are examples that may support the use of these studies for evaluating iron deficiency:

   - Certain abnormal blood count values (i.e., decreased mean corpuscular volume (MCV), decreased hemoglobin/hematocrit when the MCV is low or normal, or increased red cell distribution width (RDW) and low or normal MCV);

   - Abnormal appetite (pica);

Appendix G — Medicare Internet-only Manuals (IOMs)

– Acute or chronic gastrointestinal blood loss;

– Hematuria;

– Menorrhagia;

– Malabsorption;

– Status post-gastrectomy;

– Status post-gastrojejunostomy;

– Malnutrition;

– Preoperative autologous blood collection(s);

– Malignant, chronic inflammatory and infectious conditions associated with anemia which may present in a similar manner to iron deficiency anemia;

– Following a significant surgical procedure where blood loss had occurred and had not been repaired with adequate iron replacement.

b. The following presentations are examples that may support the use of these studies for evaluating iron overload:

– Chronic Hepatitis;

– Diabetes;

– Hyperpigmentation of skin;

– Arthropathy;

– Cirrhosis;

– Hypogonadism;

– Hypopituitarism;

– Impaired porphyrin metabolism;

– Heart failure;

– Multiple transfusions;

– Sideroblastic anemia;

– Thalassemia major;

– Cardiomyopathy, cardiac dysrhythmias and conduction disturbances.

2. Follow-up testing may be appropriate to monitor response to therapy, e.g., oral or parenteral iron, ascorbic acid, and erythropoietin.

3. Iron studies may be appropriate in patients after treatment for other nutritional deficiency anemias, such as folate and vitamin B12, because iron deficiency may not be revealed until such a nutritional deficiency is treated.

4. Serum ferritin may be appropriate for monitoring iron status in patients with chronic renal disease with or without dialysis.

5. Serum iron may also be indicated for evaluation of toxic effects of iron and other metals (e.g., nickel, cadmium, aluminum, lead) whether due to accidental, intentional exposure or metabolic causes.

**Limitations:**

1. Iron studies should be used to diagnose and manage iron deficiency or iron overload states. These tests are not to be used solely to assess acute phase reactants where disease management will be unchanged. For example, infections and malignancies are associated with elevations in acute phase reactants such as ferritin, and decreases in serum iron concentration, but iron studies would only be medically necessary if results of iron studies might alter the management of the primary diagnosis or might warrant direct treatment of an iron disorder or condition.

2. If a normal serum ferritin level is documented, repeat testing would not ordinarily be medically necessary unless there is a change in the patient's condition, and ferritin assessment is needed for the ongoing management of the patient. For example, a patient presents with new onset insulin-dependent diabetes mellitus and has a serum ferritin level performed for the suspicion of hemochromatosis. If the ferritin level is normal, the repeat ferritin for diabetes mellitus would not be medically necessary.

3. When an End Stage Renal Disease (ESRD) patient is tested for ferritin, testing more frequently than every three months (the frequency authorized by 3167.3, Fiscal Intermediary manual) requires documentation of medical necessity [e.g., other than "Chronic Renal Failure" (ICD-9-CM 585) or "Renal Failure, Unspecified" (ICD-9-CM 586)].

4. It is ordinarily not necessary to measure both transferrin and TIBC at the same time because TIBC is an indirect measure of transferrin. When transferrin is ordered as part of the nutritional assessment for evaluating malnutrition, it is not necessary to order other iron studies unless iron deficiency or iron overload is suspected as well.

5. It is not ordinarily necessary to measure both iron/TIBC (or transferrin) and ferritin in initial patient testing. If clinically indicated after evaluation of the initial iron studies, it may be appropriate to perform additional iron studies either on the initial specimen or on a subsequently obtained specimen. After a diagnosis of iron deficiency or iron overload is established, either iron/TIBC (or transferrin) or ferritin may be medically necessary for monitoring, but not both.

6. It would not ordinarily be considered medically necessary to do a ferritin as a preoperative test except in the presence of anemia or recent autologous blood collections prior to the surgery.

## 100-03, 190.19

### Collagen Crosslinks, Any Method

**Indications:**

Generally speaking, collagen crosslink testing is useful mostly in "fast losers" of bone. The age when these bone markers can help direct therapy is often pre-Medicare. By the time a fast loser of bone reaches age 65, she will most likely have been stabilized by appropriate therapy or have lost so much bone mass that further testing is useless. Coverage for bone marker assays may be established, however, for younger Medicare beneficiaries and for those men and women who might become fast losers because of some other therapy such as glucocorticoids. Safeguards should be incorporated to prevent excessive use of tests in patients for whom they have no clinical relevance.

Collagen crosslinks testing is used to:

• Identify individuals with elevated bone resorption, who have osteoporosis in whom response to treatment is being monitored;

• Predict response (as assessed by bone mass measurements) to FDA approved antiresorptive therapy in postmenopausal women; and

• Assess response to treatment of patients with osteoporosis, Paget's disease of the bone, or risk for osteoporosis where treatment may include FDA approved antiresorptive agents, anti-estrogens or selective estrogen receptor moderators.

**Limitations:**

Because of significant specimen to specimen collagen crosslink physiologic variability (15-20%), current recommendations for appropriate utilization include: one or two base-line assays from specified urine collections on separate days; followed by a repeat assay about three months after starting anti-resorptive therapy; followed by a repeat assay in 12 months after the three-month assay; and thereafter not more than annually, unless there is a change in therapy in which circumstance an additional test may be indicated three months after the initiation of new therapy.

Some collagen crosslink assays may not be appropriate for use in some disorders, according to FDA labeling restrictions.

Note: Scroll down for links to the quarterly Covered Code Lists (including narrative).

## 100-03, 190.20

### NCD for Blood Glucose Testing (190.20)

**Indications:**

Blood glucose values are often necessary for the management of patients with diabetes mellitus, where hyperglycemia and hypoglycemia are often present. They are also critical in the determination of control of blood glucose levels in the patient with impaired fasting glucose (FPG 110-125 mg/dL), the patient with insulin resistance syndrome and/or carbohydrate intolerance (excessive rise in glucose following ingestion of glucose or glucose sources of food), in the patient with a hypoglycemic disorder such as nesidioblastosis or insulinoma, and in patients with a catabolic or malnutrition state. In addition to those conditions already listed, glucose testing may be medically necessary in patients with tuberculosis, unexplained chronic or recurrent infections, alcoholism, coronary artery disease (especially in women), or unexplained skin conditions (including pruritis, local skin infections, ulceration and gangrene without an established cause).

Many medical conditions may be a consequence of a sustained elevated or depressed glucose level. These include comas, seizures or epilepsy, confusion, abnormal hunger, abnormal weight loss or gain, and loss of sensation. Evaluation of glucose may also be indicated in patients on medications known to affect carbohydrate metabolism.

Effective January 1, 2005, the Medicare law expanded coverage to diabetic screening services. Some forms of blood glucode testing covered under this national coverage determination may be covered for screening purposes subject to specified frequencies. See 42 CFR 410.18 and section 90, chapter 18 of the Claims Processing Manual, for a full description of this screening benefit.

**Limitations:**

Frequent home blood glucose testing by diabetic patients should be encouraged. In stable, non-hospitalized patients who are unable or unwilling to do home monitoring, it may be reasonable and necessary to measure quantitative blood glucose up to four times annually.

Depending upon the age of the patient, type of diabetes, degree of control, complications of diabetes, and other co-morbid conditions, more frequent testing than four times annually may be reasonable and necessary.

In some patients presenting with nonspecific signs, symptoms, or diseases not normally associated with disturbances in glucose metabolism, a single blood glucose test may be medically necessary. Repeat testing may not be indicated unless abnormal results are found or unless there is a change in clinical condition. If repeat testing is performed, a specific diagnosis code (e.g., diabetes) should be reported to support medical necessity. However, repeat testing may be indicated where results are normal in patients with conditions where there is a confirmed continuing risk of glucose metabolism abnormality (e.g., monitoring glucocorticoid therapy).

CPT © 2017 American Medical Association. All Rights Reserved.　　　　　　　© 2017 Optum360, LLC

## 100-03, 190.22

### NCD for Thyroid Testing (190.22)

#### Indications

Thyroid function tests are used to define hyper function, euthyroidism, or hypofunction of thyroid disease. Thyroid testing may be reasonable and necessary to:

- Distinguish between primary and secondary hypothyroidism;

- Confirm or rule out primary hypothyroidism;

- Monitor thyroid hormone levels (for example, patients with goiter, thyroid nodules, or thyroid cancer);

- Monitor drug therapy in patients with primary hypothyroidism;

- Confirm or rule out primary hyperthyroidism; and

- Monitor therapy in patients with hyperthyroidism.

Thyroid function testing may be medically necessary in patients with disease or neoplasm of the thyroid and other endocrine glands. Thyroid function testing may also be medically necessary in patients with metabolic disorders; malnutrition; hyperlipidemia; certain types of anemia; psychosis and non-psychotic personality disorders; unexplained depression; ophthalmologic disorders; various cardiac arrhythmias; disorders of menstruation; skin conditions; myalgias; and a wide array of signs and symptoms, including alterations in consciousness; malaise; hypothermia; symptoms of the nervous and musculoskeletal system; skin and integumentary system; nutrition and metabolism; cardiovascular; and gastrointestinal system.

It may be medically necessary to do follow-up thyroid testing in patients with a personal history of malignant neoplasm of the endocrine system and in patients on long-term thyroid drug therapy.

#### Limitations

Testing may be covered up to two times a year in clinically stable patients; more frequent testing may be reasonable and necessary for patients whose thyroid therapy has been altered or in whom symptoms or signs of hyperthyroidism or hypothyroidism are noted.

## 100-03, 190.23

### NCD for Lipid Testing (190.23)

#### Indications and Limitations of Coverage

#### Indications

The medical community recognizes lipid testing as appropriate for evaluating atherosclerotic cardiovascular disease. Conditions in which lipid testing may be indicated include:

- Assessment of patients with atherosclerotic cardiovascular disease.

- Evaluation of primary dyslipidemia.

- Any form of atherosclerotic disease, or any disease leading to the formation of atherosclerotic disease.

- Diagnostic evaluation of diseases associated with altered lipid metabolism, such as: nephrotic syndrome, pancreatitis, hepatic disease, and hypo and hyperthyroidism.

- Secondary dyslipidemia, including diabetes mellitus, disorders of gastrointestinal absorption, chronic renal failure.

- Signs or symptoms of dyslipidemias, such as skin lesions.

- As follow-up to the initial screen for coronary heart disease (total cholesterol + HDL cholesterol) when total cholesterol is determined to be high (>240 mg/dL), or borderline-high (200-240 mg/dL) plus two or more coronary heart disease risk factors, or an HDL cholesterol, <35 mg/dl.

To monitor the progress of patients on anti-lipid dietary management and pharmacologic therapy for the treatment of elevated blood lipid disorders, total cholesterol, HDL cholesterol and LDL cholesterol may be used. Triglycerides may be obtained if this lipid fraction is also elevated or if the patient is put on drugs (for example, thiazide diuretics, beta blockers, estrogens, glucocorticoids, and tamoxifen) which may raise the triglyceride level.

When monitoring long term anti-lipid dietary or pharmacologic therapy and when following patients with borderline high total or LDL cholesterol levels, it may be reasonable to perform the lipid panel annually. A lipid panel at a yearly interval will usually be adequate while measurement of the serum total cholesterol or a measured LDL should suffice for interim visits if the patient does not have hypertriglyceridemia.

Any one component of the panel or a measured LDL may be reasonable and necessary up to six times the first year for monitoring dietary or pharmacologic therapy. More frequent total cholesterol HDL cholesterol, LDL cholesterol and triglyceride testing may be indicated for marked elevations or for changes to anti-lipid therapy due to inadequate initial patient response to dietary or pharmacologic therapy. The LDL cholesterol or total cholesterol may be measured three times yearly after treatment goals have been achieved.

Electrophoretic or other quantitation of lipoproteins may be indicated if the patient has a primary disorder of lipoid metabolism.

Effective January 1, 2005, the Medicare law expanded coverage to cardiovascular screening services. Several of the procedures included in this NCD may be covered for screening purposes subject to specified frequencies. See 42 CFR 410.17 and section 100, chapter 18, of the Claims Processing Manual, for a full description of this benefit.

#### Limitations

Lipid panel and hepatic panel testing may be used for patients with severe psoriasis which has not responded to conventional therapy and for which the retinoid etretinate has been prescribed and who have developed hyperlipidemia or hepatic toxicity. Specific examples include erythroderma and generalized pustular type and psoriasis associated with arthritis.

Routine screening and prophylactic testing for lipid disorder are not covered by Medicare. While lipid screening may be medically appropriate, Medicare by statute does not pay for it. Lipid testing in asymptomatic individuals is considered to be screening regardless of the presence of other risk factors such as family history, tobacco use, etc.

Once a diagnosis is established, one or several specific tests are usually adequate for monitoring the course of the disease. Less specific diagnoses (for example, other chest pain) alone do not support medical necessity of these tests.

When monitoring long term anti-lipid dietary or pharmacologic therapy and when following patients with borderline high total or LDL cholesterol levels, it is reasonable to perform the lipid panel annually. A lipid panel at a yearly interval will usually be adequate while measurement of the serum total cholesterol or a measured LDL should suffice for interim visits if the patient does not have hypertriglyceridemia.

Any one component of the panel or a measured LDL may be medically necessary up to six times the first year for monitoring dietary or pharmacologic therapy. More frequent total cholesterol HDL cholesterol, LDL cholesterol and triglyceride testing may be indicated for marked elevations or for changes to anti-lipid therapy due to inadequate initial patient response to dietary or pharmacologic therapy. The LDL cholesterol or total cholesterol may be measured three times yearly after treatment goals have been achieved.

If no dietary or pharmacological therapy is advised, monitoring is not necessary.

When evaluating non-specific chronic abnormalities of the liver (for example, elevations of transaminase, alkaline phosphatase, abnormal imaging studies, etc.), a lipid panel would generally not be indicated more than twice per year.

## 100-03, 190.26

### NCD for Carcinoembryonic Antigen (CEA)

Carcinoembryonic antigen (CEA) is a protein polysaccharide found in some carcinomas. It is effective as a biochemical marker for monitoring the response of certain malignancies to therapy.

#### Indications

CEA may be medically necessary for follow-up of patients with colorectal carcinoma. It would however only be medically necessary at treatment decision-making points. In some clinical situations (e.g. adenocarcinoma of the lung, small cell carcinoma of the lung, and some gastrointestinal carcinomas) when a more specific marker is not expressed by the tumor, CEA may be a medically necessary alternative marker for monitoring. Preoperative CEA may also be helpful in determining the post-operative adequacy of surgical resection and subsequent medical management. In general, a single tumor marker will suffice in following patients with colorectal carcinoma or other malignancies that express such tumor markers.

In following patients who have had treatment for colorectal carcinoma, ASCO guideline suggests that if resection of liver metastasis would be indicated, it is recommended that post-operative CEA testing be performed every two to three months in patients with initial stage II or stage III disease for at least two years after diagnosis.

For patients with metastatic solid tumors which express CEA, CEA may be measured at the start of the treatment and with subsequent treatment cycles to assess the tumor's response to therapy.

#### Limitations:

Serum CEA determinations are generally not indicated more frequently than once per chemotherapy treatment cycle for patients with metastatic solid tumors which express CEA or every two months post-surgical treatment for patients who have had colorectal carcinoma. However, it may be proper to order the test more frequently in certain situations, for example, when there has been a significant change from prior CEA level or a significant change in patient status which could reflect disease progression or recurrence.

Testing with a diagnosis of an in situ carcinoma is not reasonably done more frequently than once, unless the result is abnormal, in which case the test may be repeated once.

## 100-03, 190.3

### NCD for Cytogenetic Studies (190.3)

Medicare covers these tests when they are reasonable and necessary for the diagnosis or treatment of the following conditions:

- Genetic disorders (e.g., mongolism) in a fetus (See Medicare Benefit Policy Manual, Chapter 15, "Covered medical and Other health Services," Sec. 20.1)

- Failure of sexual development;

- Chronic myelogenous leukemia;

- Acute leukemias lymphoid (FAB L1-L3), myeloid (FAB M0-M7), and unclassified; or

- Mylodysplasia

## 100-03, 190.31

### NCD for Prostate Specific Antigen (PSA) (190.31)

**Indications:**

PSA is of proven value in differentiating benign from malignant disease in men with lower urinary tract signs and symptoms (e.g., hematuria, slow urine stream, hesitancy, urgency, frequency, nocturia and incontinence) as well as with patients with palpably abnormal prostate glands on physician exam, and in patients with other laboratory or imaging studies that suggest the possibility of a malignant prostate disorder. PSA is also a marker used to follow the progress of prostate cancer once a diagnosis has been established, such as in detecting metastatic or persistent disease in patients who may require additional treatment. PSA testing may also be useful in the differential diagnosis of men presenting with as yet undiagnosed disseminated metastatic disease.

**Limitations:**

Generally, for patients with lower urinary tract signs or symptoms, the test is performed only once per year unless there is a change in the patient's medical condition.

Testing with a diagnosis of in situ carcinoma is not reasonably done more frequently than once, unless the result is abnormal, in which case the test may be repeated once.

## 100-03, 210.1

### NCD for Prostate Cancer Screening Tests (210.1)

**Indications and Limitations of Coverage**

CIM 50-55

Covered

#### A. General

Section 4103 of the Balanced Budget Act of 1997 provides for coverage of certain prostate cancer screening tests subject to certain coverage, frequency, and payment limitations. Medicare will cover prostate cancer screening tests/procedures for the early detection of prostate cancer. Coverage of prostate cancer screening tests includes the following procedures furnished to an individual for the early detection of prostate cancer:

- Screening digital rectal examination; and
- Screening prostate specific antigen blood test

#### B. Screening Digital Rectal Examinations

Screening digital rectal examinations are covered at a frequency of once every 12 months for men who have attained age 50 (at least 11 months have passed following the month in which the last Medicare-covered screening digital rectal examination was performed). Screening digital rectal examination means a clinical examination of an individual's prostate for nodules or other abnormalities of the prostate. This screening must be performed by a doctor of medicine or osteopathy (as defined in §1861(r)(1) of the Act), or by a physician assistant, nurse practitioner, clinical nurse specialist, or certified nurse midwife (as defined in §1861(aa) and §1861(gg) of the Act) who is authorized under State law to perform the examination, fully knowledgeable about the beneficiary's medical condition, and would be responsible for using the results of any examination performed in the overall management of the beneficiary's specific medical problem.

#### C. Screening Prostate Specific Antigen Tests

Screening prostate specific antigen tests are covered at a frequency of once every 12 months for men who have attained age 50 (at least 11 months have passed following the month in which the last Medicare-covered screening prostate specific antigen test was performed). Screening prostate specific antigen tests (PSA) means a test to detect the marker for adenocarcinoma of prostate. PSA is a reliable immunocytochemical marker for primary and metastatic adenocarcinoma of prostate. This screening must be ordered by the beneficiary's physician or by the beneficiary's physician assistant, nurse practitioner, clinical nurse specialist, or certified nurse midwife (the term "attending physician"; is defined in §1861(r)(1) of the Act to mean a doctor of medicine or osteopathy and the terms ";physician assistant, nurse practitioner, clinical nurse specialist, or certified nurse midwife"; are defined in §1861(aa) and §1861(gg) of the Act) who is fully knowledgeable about the beneficiary's medical condition, and who would be responsible for using the results of any examination (test) performed in the overall management of the beneficiary's specific medical problem.

## 100-03, 210.2

### NCD for Screening Pap Smears and Pelvic Examinations for Early Detection of Cervical or Vaginal Cancer (210.2)

#### Screening Pap Smear

A screening pap smear and related medically necessary services provided to a woman for the early detection of cervical cancer (including collection of the sample of cells and a physician's interpretation of the test results) and pelvic examination (including clinical breast examination) are covered under Medicare Part B when ordered by a physician (or authorized practitioner) under one of the following conditions:

- She has not had such a test during the preceding two years or is a woman of childbearing age (Â§1861(nn) of the Social Security Act (the Act).
- There is evidence (on the basis of her medical history or other findings) that she is at high risk of developing cervical cancer and her physician (or authorized practitioner) recommends that she have the test performed more frequently than every two years.

High risk factors for cervical and vaginal cancer are:

- Early onset of sexual activity (under 16 years of age)
- Multiple sexual partners (five or more in a lifetime)
- History of sexually transmitted disease (including HIV infection)
- Fewer than three negative or any pap smears within the previous seven years; and
- DES (diethylstilbestrol) - exposed daughters of women who took DES during pregnancy.

NOTE: Claims for pap smears must indicate the beneficiary's low or high risk status by including the appropriate diagnosis code on the line item (Item 24E of the Form CMS-1500).

#### Definitions

A woman as described in Â§1861(nn) of the Act is a woman who is of childbearing age and has had a pap smear test during any of the preceding 3 years that indicated the presence of cervical or vaginal cancer or other abnormality, or is at high risk of developing cervical or vaginal cancer.

A woman of childbearing age is one who is premenopausal and has been determined by a physician or other qualified practitioner to be of childbearing age, based upon the medical history or other findings.

Other qualified practitioner, as defined in 42 CFR 410.56(a) includes a certified nurse midwife (as defined in Â§1861(gg) of the Act), or a physician assistant, nurse practitioner, or clinical nurse specialist (as defined in Â§1861(aa) of the Act) who is authorized under State law to perform the examination.

#### Screening Pelvic Examination

Section 4102 of the Balanced Budget Act of 1997 provides for coverage of screening pelvic examinations (including a clinical breast examination) for all female beneficiaries, subject to certain frequency and other limitations. A screening pelvic examination (including a clinical breast examination) should include at least seven of the following eleven elements:

- Inspection and palpation of breasts for masses or lumps, tenderness, symmetry, or nipple discharge.
- Digital rectal examination including sphincter tone, presence of hemorrhoids, and rectal masses. Pelvic examination (with or without specimen collection for smears and cultures) including:
- External genitalia (for example, general appearance, hair distribution, or lesions).
- Urethral meatus (for example, size, location, lesions, or prolapse).
- Urethra (for example, masses, tenderness, or scarring).
- Bladder (for example, fullness, masses, or tenderness).
- Vagina (for example, general appearance, estrogen effect, discharge lesions, pelvic support, cystocele, or rectocele).
- Cervix (for example, general appearance, lesions, or discharge).
- Uterus (for example, size, contour, position, mobility, tenderness, consistency, descent, or support).
- Adnexa/parametria (for example, masses, tenderness, organomegaly, or nodularity).
- Anus and perineum.

This description is from Documentation Guidelines for Evaluation and Management Services, published in May 1997 and was developed by the Centers for Medicare & Medicaid Services and the American Medical Association.

## 100-03, 210.2.1

### Screening for Cervical Cancer with Human Papillomavirus (HPV) Testing (Effective July 9, 2015)

(Rev. 189, Issued: 02-05-16, Effective: 07-05-16; Implementation: 03-07-16 - for non-shared MAC edits; 07-05-16 - CWF analysis and design; 10-03-16 - CWF Coding, Testing and Implementation, MCS, and FISS Implementation; 01-03-17 - Requirement BR9434.04.8.2)

#### A. General

Medicare covers a screening pelvic examination and Pap test for all female beneficiaries at 12 or 24 month intervals, based on specific risk factors. See 42 C.F.R. §410.56; Medicare National Coverage Determinations Manual, §210.2.1 Current Medicare coverage does not include the HPV testing. Pursuant to §1861(ddd) of the Social Security Act, the Secretary may add coverage of "additional preventive services" if certain statutory requirements are met.

#### B. Nationally Covered Indications

Effective for services performed on or after July 9, 2015, CMS has determined that the evidence is sufficient to add Human Papillomavirus (HPV) testing once every five years as an additional preventive service benefit under the Medicare program for asymptomatic beneficiaries aged 30 to 65 years in conjunction with the Pap smear test. CMS will cover screening for cervical cancer with the appropriate U.S. Food and Drug Administration (FDA) approved/cleared laboratory tests, used consistent with FDA approved labeling and in compliance with the Clinical Laboratory Improvement Act (CLIA) regulations.

### C. Nationally Non-Covered Indications

Unless specifically covered in this NCD, any other NCD, by statute or regulation, preventive services are non-covered by Medicare.

### D. Other

(This NCD last reviewed July 2015.)

## 100-03, 220.6.9

### NCD for PET (FDG) for Refractory Seizures (220.6.9)

Beginning July 1, 2001, Medicare covers FDG PET for pre-surgical evaluation for the purpose of localization of a focus of refractory seizure activity.

Limitations: Covered only for pre-surgical evaluation.

Documentation that these conditions are met should be maintained by the referring physician in the beneficiary's medical record, as is normal business practice.

(This NCD last reviewed June 2001.)

## 100-03, 220.6.17

### NCD for Positron Emission Tomography (FDG) for Oncologic Conditions (220.6.17)

### A. General

FDG (2-[F18] fluoro-2-deoxy-D-glucose) Positron Emission Tomography (PET) is a minimally-invasive diagnostic imaging procedure used to evaluate glucose metabolism in normal tissue as well as in diseased tissues in conditions such as cancer, ischemic heart disease, and some neurologic disorders. FDG is an injected radionuclide (or radiopharmaceutical) that emits sub-atomic particles, known as positrons, as it decays. FDG PET uses a positron camera (tomograph) to measure the decay of FDG. The rate of FDG decay provides biochemical information on glucose metabolism in the tissue being studied. As malignancies can cause abnormalities of metabolism and blood flow, FDG PET evaluation may indicate the probable presence or absence of a malignancy based upon observed differences in biologic activity compared to adjacent tissues.

The Centers for Medicare and Medicaid Services (CMS) was asked by the National Oncologic PET Registry (NOPR) to reconsider section 220.6 of the National Coverage Determinations (NCD) Manual to end the prospective data collection requirements under Coverage with Evidence Development (CED) across all oncologic indications of FDG PET imaging. The CMS received public input indicating that the current coverage framework of prospective data collection under CED be ended for all oncologic uses of FDG PET imaging.

1. Framework

   Effective for claims with dates of service on and after June 11, 2013, CMS is adopting a coverage framework that ends the prospective data collection requirements by NOPR under CED for all oncologic uses of FDG PET imaging. CMS is making this change for all NCDs that address coverage of FDG PET for oncologic uses addressed in this decision. This decision does not change coverage for any use of PET imaging using radiopharmaceuticals NaF-18 (fluorine-18 labeled sodium fluoride), ammonia N-13, or rubidium-82 (Rb-82).

2. Initial Anti-Tumor Treatment Strategy

   CMS continues to believe that the evidence is adequate to determine that the results of FDG PET imaging are useful in determining the appropriate initial anti-tumor treatment strategy for beneficiaries with suspected cancer and improve health outcomes and thus are reasonable and necessary under §1862(a)(1)(A) of the Social Security Act (the Act).

   Therefore, CMS continues to nationally cover one FDG PET study for beneficiaries who have cancers that are biopsy proven or strongly suspected based on other diagnostic testing when the beneficiary's treating physician determines that the FDG PET study is needed to determine the location and/or extent of the tumor for the following therapeutic purposes related to the initial anti-tumor treatment strategy:

   — To determine whether or not the beneficiary is an appropriate candidate for an invasive diagnostic or therapeutic procedure; or

   — To determine the optimal anatomic location for an invasive procedure; or

   — To determine the anatomic extent of tumor when the recommended antitumor treatment reasonably depends on the extent of the tumor.

   See the table at the end of this section for a synopsis of all nationally covered and noncovered oncologic uses of FDG PET imaging.

   #### B.1. Initial Anti-Tumor Treatment Strategy Nationally Covered Indications

   a. CMS continues to nationally cover FDG PET imaging for the initial anti-tumor treatment strategy for male and female breast cancer only when used in staging distant metastasis.

   b. CMS continues to nationally cover FDG PET to determine initial anti-tumor treatment strategy for melanoma other than for the evaluation of regional lymph nodes.

   c. CMS continues to nationally cover FDG PET imaging for the detection of pre-treatment metastasis (i.e., staging) in newly diagnosed cervical cancers following conventional imaging.

   #### C.1. Initial Anti-Tumor Treatment Strategy Nationally Non-Covered Indications

   a. CMS continues to nationally non-cover initial anti-tumor treatment strategy in Medicare beneficiaries who have adenocarcinoma of the prostate.

   b. CMS continues to nationally non-cover FDG PET imaging for diagnosis of breast cancer and initial staging of axillary nodes.

   c. CMS continues to nationally non-cover FDG PET imaging for initial anti-tumor treatment strategy for the evaluation of regional lymph nodes in melanoma.

   d. CMS continues to nationally non-cover FDG PET imaging for the diagnosis of cervical cancer related to initial anti-tumor treatment strategy.

3. Subsequent Anti-Tumor Treatment Strategy

   #### B.2. Subsequent Anti-Tumor Treatment Strategy Nationally Covered Indications

   Three FDG PET scans are nationally covered when used to guide subsequent management of anti-tumor treatment strategy after completion of initial anti-cancer therapy. Coverage of more than three FDG PET scans to guide subsequent management of anti-tumor treatment strategy after completion of initial anti-cancer therapy shall be determined by the local Medicare Administrative Contractors.

4. Synopsis of Coverage of FDG PET for Oncologic Conditions

   Effective for claims with dates of service on and after June 11, 2013, the chart below summarizes national FDG PET coverage for oncologic conditions:

| FDG PET for Cancers Tumor Type | Initial Treatment Strategy (formerly "diagnosis" & "staging") | Subsequent Treatment Strategy (formerly "restaging" & "monitoring response to treatment") |
|---|---|---|
| Colorectal | Cover | Cover |
| Esophagus | Cover | Cover |
| Head & Neck (not Thyroid, CNS) | Cover | Cover |
| Lymphoma | Cover | Cover |
| Non-Small Cell Lung | Cover | Cover |
| Ovary | Cover | Cover |
| Brain | Cover | Cover |
| Cervix | Cover w/exception* | Cover |
| Small Cell Lung | Cover | Cover |
| Soft Tissue Sarcoma | Cover | Cover |
| Pancreas | Cover | Cover |
| Testes | Cover | Cover |
| Prostate | Non-cover | Cover |
| Thyroid | Cover | Cover |
| Breast (male and female) | Cover w/exception* | Cover |
| Melanoma | Cover w/exception* | Cover |
| All Other Solid Tumors | Cover | Cover |
| Myeloma | Cover | Cover |
| All other cancers not listed | Cover | Cover |

\* Cervix: Nationally non-covered for the initial diagnosis of cervical cancer related to initial anti-tumor treatment strategy. All other indications for initial anti-tumor treatment strategy for cervical cancer are nationally covered.

\* Breast: Nationally non-covered for initial diagnosis and/or staging of axillary lymph nodes. Nationally covered for initial staging of metastatic disease. All other indications for initial anti-tumor treatment strategy for breast cancer are nationally covered.

\* Melanoma: Nationally non-covered for initial staging of regional lymph nodes. All other indications for initial anti-tumor treatment strategy for melanoma are nationally covered.

### D. Other
N/A

## 100-03, 220.6.19

### Positron Emission Tomography NaF-18 (NaF-18 PET) to Identify Bone Metastasis of Cancer (Effective February 26, 2010)

### A. General

Positron Emission Tomography (PET) is a non-invasive, diagnostic imaging procedure that assesses the level of metabolic activity and perfusion in various organ systems of the body. A positron camera (tomograph) is used to produce cross-sectional tomographic images, which are obtained from positron-emitting radioactive tracer substances (radiopharmaceuticals) such as F-18 sodium fluoride. NaF-18 PET has been recognized as an excellent technique for imaging areas of altered osteogenic activity in bone. The clinical value of detecting and assessing the initial extent of metastatic cancer in bone is attested by a number of professional guidelines for oncology. Imaging to detect bone metastases is also recommended when a patient, following completion of initial treatment, is symptomatic with bone pain suspicious for metastases from a known primary tumor.

### B. Nationally Covered Indications

Effective February 26, 2010, the Centers for Medicare & Medicaid Services (CMS) will cover NaF-18 PET imaging when the beneficiary's treating physician determines that the NaF-18 PET study is needed to inform to inform the initial antitumor treatment strategy or to guide subsequent antitumor treatment strategy after the completion of initial treatment, and when the beneficiary is enrolled in, and the NaF-18 PET provider is participating in, the following type of prospective clinical study:

A NaF-18 PET clinical study that is designed to collect additional information at the time of the scan to assist in initial antitumor treatment planning or to guide subsequent treatment strategy by the identification, location and quantification of bone metastases in beneficiaries in whom bone metastases are strongly suspected based on clinical symptoms or the results of other diagnostic studies. Qualifying clinical studies must ensure that specific hypotheses are addressed; appropriate data elements are collected; hospitals and providers are qualified to provide the PET scan and interpret the results; participating hospitals and providers accurately report data on all enrolled patients not included in other qualifying trials through adequate auditing mechanisms; and all patient confidentiality, privacy, and other Federal laws must be followed.

The clinical studies for which Medicare will provide coverage must answer one or more of the following questions:

Prospectively, in Medicare beneficiaries whose treating physician determines that the NaF-18 PET study results are needed to inform the initial antitumor treatment strategy or to guide subsequent antitumor treatment strategy after the completion of initial treatment, does the addition of NaF-18 PET imaging lead to:

- A change in patient management to more appropriate palliative care; or
- A change in patient management to more appropriate curative care; or
- Improved quality of life; or Improved survival?

The study must adhere to the following standards of scientific integrity and relevance to the Medicare population:

a. The principal purpose of the research study is to test whether a particular intervention potentially improves the participants' health outcomes.

b. The research study is well-supported by available scientific and medical information or it is intended to clarify or establish the health outcomes of interventions already in common clinical use.

c. The research study does not unjustifiably duplicate existing studies.

d. The research study design is appropriate to answer the research question being asked in the study.

e. The research study is sponsored by an organization or individual capable of executing the proposed study successfully.

f. The research study is in compliance with all applicable Federal regulations concerning the protection of human subjects found in the Code of Federal Regulations (CFR) at 45 CFR Part 46. If a study is regulated by the Food and Drug Administration (FDA), it also must be in compliance with 21 CFR Parts 50 and 56.

g. All aspects of the research study are conducted according to the appropriate standards of scientific integrity.

h. The research study has a written protocol that clearly addresses, or incorporates by reference, the Medicare standards.

i. The clinical research study is not designed to exclusively test toxicity or disease pathophysiology in healthy individuals. Trials of all medical technologies measuring therapeutic outcomes as one of the objectives meet this standard only if the disease or condition being studied is life-threatening as defined in 21 CFR Sec.312.81(a) and the patient has no other viable treatment options.

j. The clinical research study is registered on the www.ClinicalTrials.gov Web site by the principal sponsor/investigator prior to the enrollment of the first study subject.

k. The research study protocol specifies the method and timing of public release of all pre-specified outcomes to be measured including release of outcomes if outcomes are negative or study is terminated early. The results must be made public within 24 months of the end of data collection. If a report is planned to be published in a peer-reviewed journal, then that initial release may be an abstract that meets the requirements of the International Committee of Medical Journal Editors. However, a full report of the outcomes must be made public no later than three (3) years after the end of data collection.

l. The research study protocol must explicitly discuss subpopulations affected by the treatment under investigation, particularly traditionally underrepresented groups in clinical studies, how the inclusion and exclusion criteria affect enrollment of these populations, and a plan for the retention and reporting of said populations on the trial. If the inclusion and exclusion criteria are expected to

have a negative effect on the recruitment or retention of underrepresented populations, the protocol must discuss why these criteria are necessary.

m. The research study protocol explicitly discusses how the results are or are not expected to be generalizable to the Medicare population to infer whether Medicare patients may benefit from the intervention. Separate discussions in the protocol may be necessary for populations eligible for Medicare due to age, disability or Medicaid eligibility.

Consistent with section 1142 of the Social Security Act (the Act), the Agency for Healthcare Research and Quality (AHRQ) supports clinical research studies that the Centers for Medicare and Medicaid Services (CMS) determines meet the above-listed standards and address the above-listed research questions.

### C. Nationally Non-Covered Indications

Effective February 26, 2010, CMS determines that the evidence is not sufficient to determine that the results of NaF-18 PET imaging to identify bone metastases improve health outcomes of beneficiaries with cancer and is not reasonable and necessary under Sec.1862(a)(1)(A) of the Act unless it is to inform initial antitumor treatment strategy or to guide subsequent antitumor treatment strategy after completion of initial treatment, and then only under CED. All other uses and clinical indications of NaF-18 PET are nationally non-covered.

### D. Other

The only radiopharmaceutical diagnostic imaging agents covered by Medicare for PET cancer imaging are 2-[F-18] Fluoro-D-Glucose (FDG) and NaF-18 (sodium fluoride-18). All other PET radiopharmaceutical diagnostic imaging agents are non-covered for this indication.

(This NCD was last reviewed in February 2010.)

## 100-03, 220.13

### NCD for Percutaneous Image-Guided Breast Biopsy (220.13)

Percutaneous image-guided breast biopsy is a method of obtaining a breast biopsy through a percutaneous incision by employing image guidance systems. Image guidance systems may be either ultrasound or stereotactic.

The Breast Imaging Reporting and Data System (or BIRADS system) employed by the American College of Radiology provides a standardized lexicon with which radiologists may report their interpretation of a mammogram. The BIRADS grading of mammograms is as follows: Grade I-Negative, Grade II-Benign finding, Grade III-Probably benign, Grade IV-Suspicious abnormality, and Grade V-Highly suggestive of malignant neoplasm.

### A. Non-Palpable Breast Lesions

Effective January 1, 2003, Medicare covers percutaneous image-guided breast biopsy using stereotactic or ultrasound imaging for a radiographic abnormality that is non-palpable and is graded as a BIRADS III, IV, or V.

### B. Palpable Breast Lesions

Effective January 1, 2003, Medicare covers percutaneous image guided breast biopsy using stereotactic or ultrasound imaging for palpable lesions that are difficult to biopsy using palpation alone. Medicare Administrative Contractors have the discretion to decide what types of palpable lesions are difficult to biopsy using palpation.

## 100-03, 230.1

### NCD for Treatment of Kidney Stones (230.1)

In addition to the traditional surgical/endoscopic techniques for the treatment of kidney stones, the following lithotripsy techniques are also covered for services rendered on or after March 15, 1985.

Extracorporeal Shock Wave Lithotripsy.--Extracorporeal Shock Wave Lithotripsy (ESWL) is a non-invasive method of treating kidney stones using a device called a lithotriptor. The lithotriptor uses shock waves generated outside of the body to break up upper urinary tract stones. It focuses the shock waves specifically on stones under X-ray visualization, pulverizing them by repeated shocks. ESWL is covered under Medicare for use in the treatment of upper urinary tract kidney stones.

Percutaneous Lithotripsy.--Percutaneous lithotripsy (or nephrolithotomy) is an invasive method of treating kidney stones by using ultrasound, electrohydraulic or mechanical lithotripsy. A probe is inserted through an incision in the skin directly over the kidney and applied to the stone. A form of lithotripsy is then used to fragment the stone. Mechanical or electrohydraulic lithotripsy may be used as an alternative or adjunct to ultrasonic lithotripsy. Percutaneous lithotripsy of kidney stones by ultrasound or by the related techniques of electrohydraulic or mechanical lithotripsy is covered under Medicare.

The following is covered for services rendered on or after January 16, 1988.

Transurethral Ureteroscopic Lithotripsy.--Transurethral ureteroscopic lithotripsy is a method of fragmenting and removing ureteral and renal stones through a cystoscope. The cystoscope is inserted through the urethra into the bladder. Catheters are passed through the scope into the opening where the ureters enter the bladder. Instruments passed through this opening into the ureters are used to manipulate and ultimately disintegrate stones, using either mechanical crushing, transcystoscopic electrohydraulic shock waves, ultrasound or laser. Transurethral ureteroscopic lithotripsy for the treatment of urinary tract stones of the kidney or ureter is covered under Medicare.

## 100-03, 230.3

### NCD for Sterilization (230.3)

#### A. Nationally Covered Conditions
Payment may be made only where sterilization is a necessary part of the treatment of an illness or injury, e.g., removal of a uterus because of a tumor, removal of diseased ovaries.

Sterilization of a mentally challenged beneficiary is covered if it is a necessary part of the treatment of an illness or injury (bilateral oophorectomy or bilateral orchidectomy in a case of cancer of the prostate). The Medicare Administrative Contractor denies claims when the pathological evidence of the necessity to perform any such procedures to treat an illness or injury is absent; and

Monitor such surgeries closely and obtain the information needed to determine whether in fact the surgery was performed as a means of treating an illness or injury or only to achieve sterilization.

#### B. Nationally Non-Covered Conditions
- Elective hysterectomy, tubal ligation, and vasectomy, if the primary indication for these procedures is sterilization;
- A sterilization that is performed because a physician believes another pregnancy would endanger the overall general health of the woman is not considered to be reasonable and necessary for the diagnosis or treatment of illness or injury within the meaning of §1862(a)(1) of the Social Security Act. The same conclusion would apply where the sterilization is performed only as a measure to prevent the possible development of, or effect on, a mental condition should the individual become pregnant; and sterilization of a mentally retarded person where the purpose is to prevent conception, rather than the treatment of an illness or injury.

## 100-03, 230.4

### NCD for Diagnosis and Treatment of Impotence (230.4)

Program payment may be made for diagnosis and treatment of sexual impotence. Impotence is a failure of a body part for which the diagnosis, and frequently the treatment, require medical expertise. Depending on the cause of the condition, treatment may be surgical; e.g., implantation of a penile prosthesis, or nonsurgical; e.g., medical or psychotherapeutic treatment. Since causes and, therefore, appropriate treatment vary, if abuse is suspected it may be necessary to request documentation of appropriateness in individual cases. If treatment is furnished to patients (other than hospital inpatients) in connection with a mental condition, apply the psychiatric service limitation described in the Medicare General Information, Eligibility, and Entitlement Manual, Chapter 3.

## 100-03, 230.10

### NCD for Incontinence Control Devices (230.10)

#### A - Mechanical/Hydraulic Incontinence Control Devices
Mechanical/hydraulic incontinence control devices are accepted as safe and effective in the management of urinary incontinence in patients with permanent anatomic and neurologic dysfunctions of the bladder. This class of devices achieves control of urination by compression of the urethra. The materials used and the success rate may vary somewhat from device to device. Such a device is covered when its use is reasonable and necessary for the individual patient.

#### B - Collagen Implant
A collagen implant, which is injected into the submucosal tissues of the urethra and/or the bladder neck and into tissues adjacent to the urethra, is a prosthetic device used in the treatment of stress urinary incontinence resulting from intrinsic sphincter deficiency (ISD). ISD is a cause of stress urinary incontinence in which the urethral sphincter is unable to contract and generate sufficient resistance in the bladder, especially during stress maneuvers.

Prior to collagen implant therapy, a skin test for collagen sensitivity must be administered and evaluated over a 4 week period.

In male patients, the evaluation must include a complete history and physical examination and a simple cystometrogram to determine that the bladder fills and stores properly. The patient then is asked to stand upright with a full bladder and to cough or otherwise exert abdominal pressure on his bladder. If the patient leaks, the diagnosis of ISD is established.

In female patients, the evaluation must include a complete history and physical examination (including a pelvic exam) and a simple cystometrogram to rule out abnormalities of bladder compliance and abnormalities of urethral support. Following that determination, an abdominal leak point pressure (ALLP) test is performed. Leak point pressure, stated in cm H2O, is defined as the intra-abdominal pressure at which leakage occurs from the bladder (around a catheter) when the bladder has been filled with a minimum of 150 cc fluid. If the patient has an ALLP of less than 100 cm H$_2$O, the diagnosis of ISD is established.

To use a collagen implant, physicians must have urology training in the use of a cystoscope and must complete a collagen implant training program.

Coverage of a collagen implant, and the procedure to inject it, is limited to the following types of patients with stress urinary incontinence due to ISD:
- Male or female patients with congenital sphincter weakness secondary to conditions such as myelomeningocele or epispadias;
- Male or female patients with acquired sphincter weakness secondary to spinal cord lesions;
- Male patients following trauma, including prostatectomy and/or radiation; and
- Female patients without urethral hypermobility and with abdominal leak point pressures of 100 cm H2O or less.

Patients whose incontinence does not improve with 5 injection procedures (5 separate treatment sessions) are considered treatment failures, and no further treatment of urinary incontinence by collagen implant is covered. Patients who have a reoccurrence of incontinence following successful treatment with collagen implants in the past (e.g., 6-12 months previously) may benefit from additional treatment sessions. Coverage of additional sessions may be allowed but must be supported by medical justification.

## 100-03, 260.1

### Adult Liver Transplantation

#### A. General
Liver transplantation, which is in situ replacement of a patient's liver with a donor liver, in certain circumstances, may be an accepted treatment for patients with end-stage liver disease due to a variety of causes. The procedure is used in selected patients as a treatment for malignancies, including primary liver tumors and certain metastatic tumors, which are typically rare but lethal with very limited treatment options. It has also been used in the treatment of patients with extrahepatic perihilar malignancies. Examples of malignancies include extrahepatic unresectable cholangiocarcinoma (CCA), liver metastases due to a neuroendocrine tumor (NET), and, hemangioendothelioma (HAE). Despite potential short- and long-term complications, transplantation may offer the only chance of cure for selected patients while providing meaningful palliation for some others.

#### B. Nationally Covered Indications
Effective July 15, 1996, adult liver transplantation when performed on beneficiaries with end- stage liver disease other than hepatitis B or malignancies is covered under Medicare when performed in a facility which is approved by the Centers for Medicare & Medicaid Services (CMS) as meeting institutional coverage criteria.

Effective December 10, 1999, adult liver transplantation when performed on beneficiaries with end-stage liver disease other than malignancies is covered under Medicare when performed in a facility which is approved by CMS as meeting institutional coverage criteria.

Effective September 1, 2001, Medicare covers adult liver transplantation for hepatocellular carcinoma when the following conditions are met:
- The patient is not a candidate for subtotal liver resection;
- The patient's tumor(s) is less than or equal to 5 cm in diameter;
- There is no macrovascular involvement;
- There is no identifiable extrahepatic spread of tumor to surrounding lymph nodes, lungs, abdominal organs or bone; and,
- The transplant is furnished in a facility that is approved by CMS as meeting institutional coverage criteria for liver transplants (see 65 FR 15006).

Effective June 21, 2012, Medicare Adminstrative Contractors acting within their respective jurisdictions may determine coverage of adult liver transplantation for the following malignancies: (1) extrahepatic unresectable cholangiocarcinoma (CCA); (2) liver metastases due to a neuroendocrine tumor (NET); and, (3) hemangioendothelioma (HAE).

1. Follow-Up Care

   Follow-up care or re-transplantation required as a result of a covered liver transplant is covered, provided such services are otherwise reasonable and necessary. Follow-up care is also covered for patients who have been discharged from a hospital after receiving non-covered liver transplant. Coverage for follow-up care is for items and services that are reasonable and necessary as determined by Medicare guidelines.

2. Immunosuppressive Drugs

   See the Medicare Benefit Policy Manual, Chapter 15, "Covered Medical and Other Health Services," §50.5.1 and the Medicare Claims Processing Manual, Chapter 17, "Drugs and Biologicals," §80.3.

#### C. Nationally Non-Covered Indications
Adult liver transplantation for other malignancies remains excluded from coverage.

#### D. Other
Coverage of adult liver transplantation is effective as of the date of the facility's approval, but for applications received before July 13, 1991, can be effective as early as March 8, 1990. (See 56 FR 15006 dated April 12, 1991.)

(This NCD last reviewed June 2012.)

## 100-03, 260.2

### NCD for Pediatric Liver Transplantation (260.2)
Liver transplantation is covered for children (under age 18) with extrahepatic biliary atresia or any other form of end stage liver disease, except that coverage is not provided for children with a malignancy extending beyond the margins of the liver or those with persistent viremia.

Liver transplantation is covered for Medicare beneficiaries when performed in a pediatric hospital that performs pediatric liver transplants if the hospital submits an application which CMS approves documenting that:

- The hospital's pediatric liver transplant program is operated jointly by the hospital and another facility that has been found by CMS to meet the institutional coverage criteria in the "Federal Register" notice of April 12, 1991;

- The unified program shares the same transplant surgeons and quality assurance program (including oversight committee, patient protocol, and patient selection criteria); and

- The hospital is able to provide the specialized facilities, services, and personnel that are required by pediatric liver transplant patients.

## 100-03, 260.3

### NCD for Pancreas Transplants (260.3)

#### B. Nationally Covered Indications

Effective for services performed on or after July 1, 1999, whole organ pancreas transplantation is nationally covered by Medicare when performed simultaneous with or after a kidney transplant. If the pancreas transplant occurs after the kidney transplant, immunosuppressive therapy begins with the date of discharge from the inpatient stay for the pancreas transplant.

Effective for services performed on or after April 26, 2006, pancreas transplants alone (PA) are reasonable and necessary for Medicare beneficiaries in the following limited circumstances:

1. PA will be limited to those facilities that are Medicare-approved for kidney transplantation. (Approved centers can be found at http://www.cms.hhs.gov/ESRDGeneralInformation/02_Data.asp#TopOfPage

2. Patients must have a diagnosis of type I diabetes:

   — Patient with diabetes must be beta cell autoantibody positive; or

   — Patient must demonstrate insulinopenia defined as a fasting C-peptide level that is less than or equal to 110% of the lower limit of normal of the laboratory's measurement method. Fasting C-peptide levels will only be considered valid with a concurrently obtained fasting glucose <225 mg/dL;

3. Patients must have a history of medically-uncontrollable labile (brittle) insulin-dependent diabetes mellitus with documented recurrent, severe, acutely life-threatening metabolic complications that require hospitalization. Aforementioned complications include frequent hypoglycemia unawareness or recurring severe ketoacidosis, or recurring severe hypoglycemic attacks;

4. Patients must have been optimally and intensively managed by an endocrinologist for at least 12 months with the most medically-recognized advanced insulin formulations and delivery systems;

5. Patients must have the emotional and mental capacity to understand the significant risks associated with surgery and to effectively manage the lifelong need for immunosuppression; and,

6. Patients must otherwise be a suitable candidate for transplantation.

#### C. Nationally Non-Covered Indications

The following procedure is not considered reasonable and necessary within the meaning of section 1862(a)(1)(A) of the Social Security Act:

1. Transplantation of partial pancreatic tissue or islet cells (except in the context of a clinical trial (see section 260.3.1 of the National Coverage Determinations Manual).

#### D. Other

Not applicable.

(This NCD last reviewed April 2006.)

## 100-03, 260.5

### NCD for Intestinal and Multi-Visceral Transplantation (260.5)

#### A. General

Medicare covers intestinal and multi-visceral transplantation for the purpose of restoring intestinal function in patients with irreversible intestinal failure. Intestinal failure is defined as the loss of absorptive capacity of the small bowel secondary to severe primary gastrointestinal disease or surgically induced short bowel syndrome. It may be associated with both mortality and profound morbidity. Multi-visceral transplantation includes organs in the digestive system (stomach, duodenum, pancreas, liver and intestine).

The evidence supports the fact that aged patients generally do not survive as well as younger patients receiving intestinal transplantation. Nonetheless, some older patients who are free from other contraindications have received the procedure and are progressing well, as evidenced by the United Network for Organ Sharing (UNOS) data. Thus, it is not appropriate to include specific exclusions from coverage, such as an age limitation, in the national coverage policy.

#### B. Nationally Covered Indications

Effective for services performed on or after April 1, 2001, this procedure is covered only when performed for patients who have failed total parenteral nutrition (TPN) and only when performed in centers that meet approval criteria.

1. Failed TPN

   The TPN delivers nutrients intravenously, avoiding the need for absorption through the small bowel. TPN failure includes the following:

   — Impending or overt liver failure due to TPN induced liver injury. The clinical manifestations include elevated serum bilirubin and/or liver enzymes, splenomegaly, thrombocytopenia, gastroesophageal varices, coagulopathy, stomal bleeding or hepatic fibrosis/cirrhosis.

   — Thrombosis of the major central venous channels; jugular, subclavian, and femoral veins. Thrombosis of two or more of these vessels is considered a life threatening complication and failure of TPN therapy. The sequelae of central venous thrombosis are lack of access for TPN infusion, fatal sepsis due to infected thrombi, pulmonary embolism, Superior Vena Cava syndrome, or chronic venous insufficiency.

   — Frequent line infection and sepsis. The development of two or more episodes of systemic sepsis secondary to line infection per year that requires hospitalization indicates failure of TPN therapy. A single episode of line related fungemia, septic shock and/or Acute Respiratory Distress Syndrome are considered indicators of TPN failure.

   — Frequent episodes of severe dehydration despite intravenous fluid supplement in addition to TPN. Under certain medical conditions such as secretory diarrhea and non-constructable gastrointestinal tract, the loss of the gastrointestinal and pancreatobiliary secretions exceeds the maximum intravenous infusion rates that can be tolerated by the cardiopulmonary system. Frequent episodes of dehydration are deleterious to all body organs particularly kidneys and the central nervous system with the development of multiple kidney stones, renal failure, and permanent brain damage.

2. Approved Transplant Facilities

   Intestinal transplantation is covered by Medicare if performed in an approved facility. The criteria for approval of centers will be based on a volume of 10 intestinal transplants per year with a 1-year actuarial survival of 65 percent using the Kaplan-Meier technique.

#### C. Nationally Non-covered Indications

All other indications remain non-covered.

#### D. Other

NA.

(This NCD last reviewed May 2006.)

## 100-03, 260.9

### NCD for Heart Transplants (260.9)

#### A. General

Cardiac transplantation is covered under Medicare when performed in a facility which is approved by Medicare as meeting institutional coverage criteria. (See CMS Ruling 87-1.)

#### B. Exceptions

In certain limited cases, exceptions to the criteria may be warranted if there is justification and if the facility ensures our objectives of safety and efficacy. Under no circumstances will exceptions be made for facilities whose transplant programs have been in existence for less than two years, and applications from consortia will not be approved.

Although consortium arrangements will not be approved for payment of Medicare heart transplants, consideration will be given to applications from heart transplant facilities that consist of more than one hospital where all of the following conditions exist:

- The hospitals are under the common control or have a formal affiliation arrangement with each other under the auspices of an organization such as a university or a legally-constituted medical research institute; and

- The hospitals share resources by routinely using the same personnel or services in their transplant programs. The sharing of resources must be supported by the submission of operative notes or other information that documents the routine use of the same personnel and services in all of the individual hospitals. At a minimum, shared resources means:

- The individual members of the transplant team, consisting of the cardiac transplant surgeons, cardiologists and pathologists, must practice in all the hospitals and it can be documented that they otherwise function as members of the transplant team;

- The same organ procurement organization, immunology, and tissue-typing services must be used by all the hospitals;

- The hospitals submit, in the manner required (Kaplan-Meier method) their individual and pooled experience and survival data; and

- The hospitals otherwise meet the remaining Medicare criteria for heart transplant facilities; that is, the criteria regarding patient selection, patient management, program commitment, etc.

#### C. Pediatric Hospitals

Cardiac transplantation is covered for Medicare beneficiaries when performed in a pediatric hospital that performs pediatric heart transplants if the hospital submits an application which CMS approves as documenting that:

- The hospital's pediatric heart transplant program is operated jointly by the hospital and another facility that has been found by CMS to meet the institutional coverage criteria in CMS Ruling 87-1;

- The unified program shares the same transplant surgeons and quality assurance program (including oversight committee, patient protocol, and patient selection criteria); and

- The hospital is able to provide the specialized facilities, services, and personnel that are required by pediatric heart transplant patients.

### D. Follow-Up Care

Follow-up care required as a result of a covered heart transplant is covered, provided such services are otherwise reasonable and necessary. Follow-up care is also covered for patients who have been discharged from a hospital after receiving a noncovered heart transplant. Coverage for follow-up care would be for items and services that are reasonable and necessary, as determined by Medicare guidelines. (See the Medicare Benefit Policy Manual, Chapter 16, "General Exclusions from Coverage," Sec.180.)

### E. Immunosuppressive Drugs

See the Medicare Claims Processing Manual, Chapter 17, "Drugs and Biologicals," Sec.80.3.1, and Chapter 8, "Outpatient ESRD Hospital, Independent Facility, and Physician/Supplier Claims," Sec.120.1.

### F. Artificial Hearts

Medicare does not cover the use of artificial hearts as a permanent replacement for a human heart or as a temporary life-support system until a human heart becomes available for transplant (often referred to as a "bridge to transplant"). Medicare does cover a ventricular assist device (VAD) when used in conjunction with specific criteria listed in Sec.20.9 of the NCD Manual.

## 100-03, 270.3

### NCD for Blood-Derived Products for Chronic Non-Healing Wounds (270.3)

#### A. General

Wound healing is a dynamic, interactive process that involves multiple cells and proteins. There are three progressive stages of normal wound healing, and the typical wound healing duration is about 4 weeks. While cutaneous wounds are a disruption of the normal, anatomic structure and function of the skin, subcutaneous wounds involve tissue below the skin's surface. Wounds are categorized as either acute, in where the normal wound healing stages are not yet completed but it is presumed they will be, resulting in orderly and timely wound repair, or chronic, in where a wound has failed to progress through the normal wound healing stages and repair itself within a sufficient time period.

Platelet-rich plasma (PRP) is produced in an autologous or homologous manner. Autologous PRP is comprised of blood from the patient who will ultimately receive the PRP. Alternatively, homologous PRP is derived from blood from multiple donors.

Blood is donated by the patient and centrifuged to produce an autologous gel for treatment of chronic, non-healing cutaneous wounds that persists for 30 days or longer and fail to properly complete the healing process. Autologous blood derived products for chronic, non-healing wounds includes both: (1) platelet derived growth factor (PDGF) products (such as Procuren), and (2) PRP (such as AutoloGel).

The PRP is different from previous products in that it contains whole cells including white cells, red cells, plasma, platelets, fibrinogen, stem cells, macrophages, and fibroblasts.

The PRP is used by physicians in clinical settings in treating chronic, non-healing wounds, open, cutaneous wounds, soft tissue, and bone. Alternatively, PDGF does not contain cells and was previously marketed as a product to be used by patients at home.

#### B. Nationally Covered Indications

Effective August 2, 2012, upon reconsideration, The Centers for Medicare and Medicaid Services (CMS) has determined that platelet-rich plasma (PRP) – an autologous blood-derived product, will be covered only for the treatment of chronic non-healing diabetic, venous and/or pressure wounds and only when the following conditions are met:

The patient is enrolled in a clinical trial that addresses the following questions using validated and reliable methods of evaluation. Clinical study applications for coverage pursuant to this National coverage Determination (NCD) must be received by August 2, 2014.

The clinical research study must meet the requirements specified below to assess the effect of PRP for the treatment of chronic non-healing diabetic, venous and/or pressure wounds. The clinical study must address:

Prospectively, do Medicare beneficiaries that have chronic non-healing diabetic, venous and/or pressure wounds who receive well-defined optimal usual care along with PRP therapy, experience clinically significant health outcomes compared to patients who receive well-defined optimal usual care for chronic non-healing diabetic, venous and/or pressure wounds as indicated by addressing at least one of the following:

a. Complete wound healing?

b. Ability to return to previous function and resumption of normal activities?

c. Reduction of wound size or healing trajectory which results in the patient's ability to return to previous function and resumption of normal activities?

The required clinical trial of PRP must adhere to the following standards of scientific integrity and relevance to the Medicare population:

a. The principal purpose of the CLINICAL STUDY is to test whether PRP improves the participants' health outcomes.

b. The CLINICAL STUDY is well supported by available scientific and medical information or it is intended to clarify or establish the health outcomes of interventions already in common clinical use.

c. The CLINICAL STUDY does not unjustifiably duplicate existing studies.

d. The CLINICAL STUDY design is appropriate to answer the research question being asked in the study.

e. The CLINICAL STUDY is sponsored by an organization or individual capable of executing the proposed study successfully.

f. The CLINICAL STUDY is in compliance with all applicable Federal regulations concerning the protection of human subjects found at 45 CFR Part 46.

g. All aspects of the CLINICAL STUDY are conducted according to appropriate standards of scientific integrity set by the International Committee of Medical Journal Editors (http://www.icmje.org).

h. The CLINICAL STUDY has a written protocol that clearly addresses, or incorporates by reference, the standards listed here as Medicare requirements for coverage with evidence development (CED).

i. The CLINICAL STUDY is not designed to exclusively test toxicity or disease pathophysiology in healthy individuals. Trials of all medical technologies measuring therapeutic outcomes as one of the objectives meet this standard only if the disease or condition being studied is life threatening as defined in 21 CFR §312.81(a) and the patient has no other viable treatment options.

j. The CLINICAL STUDY is registered on the ClinicalTrials.gov website by the principal sponsor/investigator prior to the enrollment of the first study subject.

k. The CLINICAL STUDY protocol specifies the method and timing of public release of all pre-specified outcomes to be measured including release of outcomes if outcomes are negative or study is terminated early. The results must be made public within 24 months of the end of data collection. If a report is planned to be published in a peer reviewed journal, then that initial release may be an abstract that meets the requirements of the International Committee of Medical Journal Editors (http://www.icmje.org). However a full report of the outcomes must be made public no later than three (3) years after the end of data collection.

l. The CLINICAL STUDY protocol must explicitly discuss subpopulations affected by the treatment under investigation, particularly traditionally underrepresented groups in clinical studies, how the inclusion and exclusion criteria effect enrollment of these populations, and a plan for the retention and reporting of said populations on the trial. If the inclusion and exclusion criteria are expected to have a negative effect on the recruitment or retention of underrepresented populations, the protocol must discuss why these criteria are necessary.

m. The CLINICAL STUDY protocol explicitly discusses how the results are or are not expected to be generalizable to the Medicare population to infer whether Medicare patients may benefit from the intervention. Separate discussions in the protocol may be necessary for populations eligible for Medicare due to age, disability or Medicaid eligibility. Consistent with §1142 of the Social Security Act (the Act), the Agency for Healthcare Research and Quality (AHRQ) supports clinical research studies that CMS determines meet the above-listed standards and address the above-listed research questions.

Any clinical study undertaken pursuant to this NCD must be approved no later than August 2, 2014. If there are no approved clinical studies on or before August 2, 2014, this CED will expire. Any clinical study approved will adhere to the timeframe designated in the approved clinical study protocol.

#### C. Nationally Non-Covered Indications

1. Effective December 28, 1992, the Centers for Medicare & Medicaid Services (CMS) issued a national non-coverage determination for platelet-derived wound-healing formulas intended to treat patients with chronic, non-healing wounds. This decision was based on a lack of sufficient published data to determine safety and efficacy, and a public health service technology assessment.

## 100-04, 3, 90.1

### Kidney Transplant - General

A3-3612, HO-E414

A major treatment for patients with ESRD is kidney transplantation. This involves removing a kidney, usually from a living relative of the patient or from an unrelated person who has died, and surgically placing the kidney into the patient. After the beneficiary receives a kidney transplant, Medicare pays the transplant hospital for the transplant and appropriate standard acquisition charges. Special provisions apply to payment. For the list of approved Medicare certified transplant facilities, refer to the following Web site:

http://www.cms.hhs.gov/CertificationandComplianc/20_Transplant.asp#TopOfPage

A transplant hospital may acquire cadaver kidneys by:

- Excising kidneys from cadavers in its own hospital; and
- Arrangements with a freestanding organ procurement organization (OPO) that provides cadaver kidneys to any transplant hospital or by a hospital based OPO.

A transplant hospital that is also a certified organ procurement organization may acquire cadaver kidneys by:

- Having its organ procurement team excise kidneys from cadavers in other hospitals;
- Arrangements with participating community hospitals, whether they excise kidneys on a regular or irregular basis; and
- Arrangements with an organ procurement organization that services the transplant hospital as a member of a network.

When the transplant hospital also excises the cadaver kidney, the cost of the procedure is included in its kidney acquisition costs and is considered in arriving at its standard cadaver kidney acquisition charge. When the transplant hospital excises a kidney to provide another hospital, it may use its standard cadaver kidney acquisition charge or its standard detailed departmental charges to bill that hospital.

When the excising hospital is not a transplant hospital, it bills its customary charges for services used in excising the cadaver kidney to the transplant hospital or organ procurement agency.

If the transplanting hospital's organ procurement team excises the cadaver kidney at another hospital, the cost of operating such a team is included in the transplanting hospital's kidney acquisition costs, along with the reasonable charges billed by the other hospital of its services.

## 100-04, 3, 90.1.1

### The Standard Kidney Acquisition Charge

There are two basic standard charges that must be developed by transplant hospitals from costs expected to be incurred in the acquisition of kidneys:

- The standard charge for acquiring a live donor kidney; and
- The standard charge for acquiring a cadaver kidney.

The standard charge is not a charge representing the acquisition cost of a specific kidney; rather, it is a charge that reflects the average cost associated with each type of kidney acquisition.

When the transplant hospital bills the program for the transplant, it shows its standard kidney acquisition charge on revenue code 081X. Kidney acquisition charges are not considered for the IPPS outlier calculation.

Acquisition services are billed from the excising hospital to the transplant hospital. A billing form is not submitted from the excising hospital to the FI. The transplant hospital keeps an itemized statement that identifies the services furnished, the charges, the person receiving the service (donor/recipient), and whether this is a potential transplant donor or recipient. These charges are reflected in the transplant hospital's kidney acquisition costcenter and are used in determining the hospital's standard charge for acquiring a live donor's kidney or a cadaver's kidney. The standard charge is not a charge representing the acquisition cost of a specific kidney. Rather, it is a charge that reflects the average cost associated with each type of kidney acquisition. Also, it is an all-inclusive charge for all services required in acquisition of a kidney, i.e., tissue typing, post-operative evaluation.

### A. Billing For Blood And Tissue Typing of the Transplant Recipient Whether or Not Medicare Entitlement Is Established

Tissue typing and pre-transplant evaluation can be reflected only through the kidney acquisition charge of the hospital where the transplant will take place. The transplant hospital includes in its kidney acquisition cost center the reasonable charges it pays to the independent laboratory or other hospital which typed the potential transplant recipient, either before or after his entitlement. It also includes reasonable charges paid for physician tissue typing services, applicable to live donors and recipients (during the preentitlement period and after entitlement, but prior to hospital admission for transplantation).

### B. Billing for Blood and Tissue Typing and Other Pre-Transplant Evaluation of Live Donors

The entitlement date of the beneficiary who will receive the transplant is not a consideration in reimbursing for the services to donors, since no bill is submitted directly to Medicare. All charges for services to donors prior to admission into the hospital for excision are "billed" indirectly to Medicare through the live donor acquisition charge of transplanting hospitals.

### C. Billing Donor And Recipient Pre-Transplant Services (Performed by Transplant Hospitals or Other Providers) to the Kidney Acquisition Cost Center

The transplant hospital prepares an itemized statement of the services rendered for submittal to its cost accounting department. Regular Medicare billing forms are not necessary for this purpose, since no bills are submitted to the A/B MAC (A) at this point.

The itemized statement should contain information that identifies the person receiving the service (donor/recipient), the health care insurance number, the service rendered and the charge for the service, as well as a statement as to whether this is a potential transplant donor or recipient. If it is a potential donor, the provider must identify the prospective recipient.

EXAMPLE:

Mary Jones
Health care insurance number
200 Adams St.
Anywhere, MS

Transplant donor evaluation services for recipient:

John Jones
Health care insurance number
200 Adams St.
Anywhere, MS

Services performed in a hospital other than the potential transplant hospital or by an independent laboratory are billed by that facility to the potential transplant hospital. This holds true regardless of where in the United States the service is performed. For example, if the donor services are performed in a Florida hospital and the transplant is to take place in a California hospital, the Florida hospital bills the California hospital (as described in above). The Florida hospital is paid by the California hospital, which recoups the monies through the kidney acquisition cost center.

### D. Billing for Cadaveric Donor Services

Normally, various tests are performed to determine the type and suitability of a cadaver kidney. Such tests may be performed by the excising hospital (which may also be a transplant hospital) or an independent laboratory. When the excising-only hospital performs the tests, it includes the related charges on its bill to the transplant hospital or to the organ procurement agency. When the tests are performed by the transplant hospital, it uses the related costs in establishing the standard charge for acquiring the cadaver kidney. The transplant hospital includes the costs and charges in the appropriate departments for final cost settlement purposes. When the tests are performed by an independent laboratory for the excising-only hospital or the transplant hospital, the laboratory bills the hospital that engages its services or the organ procurement agency. The excising-only hospital includes such charges in its charges to the transplant hospital, which then includes the charges in developing its standard charge for acquiring the cadaver kidney. It is the transplant hospitals' responsibility to assure that the independent laboratory does not bill both hospitals. The cost of these services cannot be billed directly to the program, since such tests and other procedures performed on a cadaver are not identifiable to a specific patient.

### E. Billing For Physicians' Services Prior to Transplantation

Physicians' services applicable to kidney excisions involving live donors and recipients (during the pre-entitlement period and after entitlement, but prior to entrance into the hospital for transplantation) as well as all physicians' services applicable to cadavers are considered Part A hospital services (kidney acquisition costs).

### F. Billing for Physicians' Services After Transplantation

All physicians' services rendered to the living donor and all physicians' services rendered to the transplant recipient are billed to the Medicare program in the same manner as all Medicare Part B services are billed. All donor physicians' services must be billed to the account of the recipient (i.e., the recipient's Medicare number).

### G. Billing For Physicians' Renal Transplantation Services

To ensure proper payment when submitting a Part B bill for the renal surgeon's services to the recipient, the appropriate HCPCS codes must be submitted, including HCPCS codes for concurrent surgery, as applicable.

The bill must include all living donor physicians' services, e.g., Revenue Center code 081X.

## 100-04, 3, 90.1.2

### Billing for Kidney Transplant and Acquisition Services

Applicable standard kidney acquisition charges are identified separately by revenue code 0811 (Living Donor Kidney Acquisition) or 0812 (Cadaver Donor Kidney Acquisition). Where interim bills are submitted, the standard acquisition charge appears on the billing form for the period during which the transplant took place. This charge is in addition to the hospital's charges for services rendered directly to the Medicare recipient.

The contractor deducts kidney acquisition charges for PPS hospitals for processing through Pricer. These costs, incurred by approved kidney transplant hospitals, are not included in the kidney transplant prospective payment. They are paid on a reasonable cost basis. Interim payment is paid as a "pass through" item. (See the Provider Reimbursement Manual, Part 1, §2802 B.8.) The contractor includes kidney acquisition charges under the appropriate revenue code in CWF.

### Bill Review Procedures

The Medicare Code Editor (MCE) creates a Limited Coverage edit for kidney transplant procedure codes. Where these procedure codes are identified by MCE, the contractor checks the provider number to determine if the provider is an approved transplant center, and checks the effective approval date. The contractor shall also determine if the facility is certified for adults and/or pediatric transplants dependent upon the patient's age. If payment is appropriate (i.e., the center is approved and the service is on or after the approval date) it overrides the limited coverage edit.

## 100-04, 3, 90.2

### Heart Transplants

Cardiac transplantation is covered under Medicare when performed in a facility which is approved by Medicare as meeting institutional coverage criteria. On April 6, 1987, CMS Ruling 87-1, "Criteria for Medicare Coverage of Heart Transplants" was published in the "Federal Register." For Medicare coverage purposes, heart transplants are medically reasonable and necessary when performed in facilities that meet these criteria. If a hospital wishes to bill Medicare for heart transplants, it must submit an application and documentation, showing its ongoing compliance with each criterion.

If a contractor has any questions concerning the effective or approval dates of its hospitals, it should contact its RO.

For a complete list of approved transplant centers, visit:

http://www.cms.hhs.gov/CertificationandComplianc/20_Transplant.asp#TopOfPage

#### A. Effective Dates

The effective date of coverage for heart transplants performed at facilities applying after July 6, 1987, is the date the facility receives approval as a heart transplant facility. Coverage is effective for discharges October 17, 1986 for facilities that would have qualified and that applied by July 6, 1987. All transplant hospitals will be recertified under the final rule, Federal Register / Vol. 72, No. 61 / Friday, March 30, 2007, / Rules and Regulations.

The CMS informs each hospital of its effective date in an approval letter.

#### B. Drugs

Medicare Part B covers immunosuppressive drugs following a covered transplant in an approved facility.

#### C. Noncovered Transplants

Medicare will not cover transplants or re-transplants in facilities that have not been approved as meeting the facility criteria. If a beneficiary is admitted for and receives a heart transplant from a hospital that is not approved, physicians' services, and inpatient services associated with the transplantation procedure are not covered.

If a beneficiary received a heart transplant from a hospital while it was not an approved facility and later requires services as a result of the noncovered transplant, the services are covered when they are reasonable and necessary in all other respects.

#### D. Charges for Heart Acquisition Services

The excising hospital bills the OPO, who in turn bills the transplant (implant) hospital for applicable services. It should not submit a bill to its contractor. The transplant hospital must keep an itemized statement that identifies the services rendered, the charges, the person receiving the service (donor/recipient), and whether this person is a potential transplant donor or recipient. These charges are reflected in the transplant hospital's heart acquisition cost center and are used in determining its standard charge for acquiring a donor's heart. The standard charge is not a charge representing the acquisition cost of a specific heart; rather, it reflects the average cost associated with each type of heart acquisition. Also, it is an all inclusive charge for all services required in acquisition of a heart, i.e., tissue typing, post-operative evaluation, etc.

#### E. Bill Review Procedures

The contractor takes the following actions to process heart transplant bills. It may accomplish them manually or modify its MCE and Grouper interface programs to handle the processing.

1. MCE Interface

   The MCE creates a Limited Coverage edit for heart transplant procedure codes. Where these procedure codes are identified by MCE, the contractor checks the provider number to determine if the provider is an approved transplant center, and checks the effective approval date. The contractor shall also determine if the facility is certified for adults and/or pediatric transplants dependent upon the patient's age. If payment is appropriate (i.e., the center is approved and the service is on or after the approval date) it overrides the limited coverage edit.

2. Handling Heart Transplant Billings From Nonapproved Hospitals

   Where a heart transplant and covered services are provided by a nonapproved hospital, the bill data processed through Grouper and Pricer must exclude transplant procedure codes and related charges.

## 100-04, 3, 90.3

### Stem Cell Transplantation

(Rev. 3556, Issued: 07-01-16; Effective: 1-27-16; Implementation: 10-3-16)

#### A. General

Stem cell transplantation is a process in which stem cells are harvested from either a patient's (autologous) or donor's (allogeneic) bone marrow or peripheral blood for intravenous infusion. Autologous stem cell transplantation (AuSCT) is a technique for restoring stem cells using the patient's own previously stored cells. AuSCTmust be used to effect hematopoietic reconstitution following severely myelotoxic doses of chemotherapy (HDCT) and/or radiotherapy used to treat various malignancies. Allogeneic hematopoietic stem cell transplantation (HSCT) is a procedure in which a portion of a healthy donor's stem cell or bone marrow is obtained and prepared for intravenous infusion. Allogeneic HSCTmay be used to restore function in recipients having an inherited or acquired deficiency or defect. Hematopoietic stem cells are

multi-potent stem cells that give rise to all the blood cell types; these stem cells form blood and immune cells. A hematopoietic stem cell is a cell isolated from blood or bone marrow that can renew itself, differentiate to a variety of specialized cells, can mobilize out of the bone marrow into circulating blood, and can undergo programmed cell death, called apoptosis - a process by which cells that are unneeded or detrimental will self-destruct.

The Centers for Medicare & Medicaid Services (CMS) is clarifying that bone marrow and peripheral blood stem cell transplantation is a process which includes mobilization, harvesting, and transplant of bone marrow or peripheral blood stem cells and the administration of high dose chemotherapy or radiotherapy prior to the actual transplant. When bone marrow or peripheral blood stem cell transplantation is covered, all necessary steps are included in coverage. When bone marrow or peripheral blood stem cell transplantation is non-covered, none of the steps are covered.

Allogeneic and autologous stem cell transplants are covered under Medicare for specific diagnoses. Effective October 1, 1990, these cases were assigned to MS-DRG 009, Bone Marrow Transplant.

The A/B MAC (A)'s Medicare Code Editor (MCE) will edit stem cell transplant procedure codes against diagnosis codes to determine which cases meet specified coverage criteria. Cases with a diagnosis code for a covered condition will pass (as covered) the MCE noncovered procedure edit. When a stem cell transplant case is selected for review based on the random selection of beneficiaries, the QIO will review the case on a post-payment basis to assure proper coverage decisions.

Bone marrow transplant codes that are reported with an ICD-9-CM that is "not otherwise specified" are returned to the hospital for a more specific procedure code. ICD-10-PCS codes are more precise and clearly identify autologous and nonautologous stem cells.

The A/B MAC (A) may choose to review if data analysis deems it a priority.

#### B. Nationally Covered Indications

I. Allogeneic Hematopoietic Stem Cell Transplantation (HSCT)

   a. General

   Allogeneic stem cell transplantation (ICD-9-CM Procedure Codes 41.02, 41.03, 41.05, and 41.08,; ICD-10-PCS codes 30230G1, 30230Y1, 30233G1, 30233Y1, 30240G1, 30240Y1, 30243G1, 30243Y1, 30250G1, 30250Y1, 30253G1, 30253Y1, 30260G1, 30260Y1, 30263G1, and 30263Y1) is a procedure in which a portion of a healthy donor's stem cells are obtained and prepared for intravenous infusion to restore normal hematopoietic function in recipients having an inherited or acquired hematopoietic deficiency or defect. See Pub. 100-03, National Coverage Determinations (NCD) Manual, chapter 1, section 110.23, for further information about this policy, and Pub. 100-04, CPM, chapter 32, section 90, for information on coding.

   Expenses incurred by a donor are a covered benefit to the recipient/beneficiary but, except for physician services, are not paid separately. Services to the donor include physician services, hospital care in connection with screening the stem cell, and ordinary follow-up care.

   b. Covered Conditions

      i. Effective for services performed on or after August 1, 1978: For the treatment of leukemia, leukemia in remission, or aplastic anemia when it is reasonable and necessary;

      ii. Effective for services performed on or after June 3, 1985: For the treatment of severe combined immunodeficiency disease (SCID), and for the treatment of Wiskott-Aldrich syndrome;

      iii. Effective for services performed on or after August 4, 2010: For the treatment of Myelodysplastic Syndromes (MDS) pursuant to Coverage with Evidence Development (CED) in the context of a Medicare-approved, prospective clinical study.

      iv. Effective for claims with dates of service on or after January 27, 2016:

   1. Allogeneic HSCT for multiple myeloma is covered by Medicare only for beneficiaries with Durie-Salmon Stage II or III multiple myeloma, or International Staging System (ISS) Stage II or Stage III multiple myeloma, and participating in an approved prospective clinical study.

   2. Allogeneic HSCT for myelofibrosis (MF) is covered by Medicare only for beneficiaries with Dynamic International Prognostic Scoring System (DIPSSplus) intermediate-2 or High primary or secondary MF and participating in an approved prospective clinical study.

   3. Allogeneic HSCT for sickle cell disease (SCD) is covered by Medicare only for beneficiaries with severe, symptomatic SCD who participate in an approved prospective clinical study.

II. Autologous Stem Cell Transplantation (AuSCT)

   a. General

   Autologous stem cell transplantation (ICD-9-CM Procedure Codes 41.01, 41.04, 41.07, and 41.09; ICD-10-PCS codes 30230AZ, 30230G0, 30230Y0, 30233G0, 30233Y0, 30240G0, 30240Y0, 30243G0, 30243Y0, 30250G0, 30250Y0, 30253G0, 30253Y0, 30260G0, 30260Y0, 30263G0, and 30263Y0) is a technique for restoring stem cells using the patient's own previously stored cells. AuSCT must be used to effect hematopoietic reconstitution following severely myelotoxic doses of chemotherapy (high dose chemotherapy (HDCT)) and/or radiotherapy used to treat various malignancies. Refer to Pub. 100-03, NCD Manual, chapter 1, section

© 2017 Optum360, LLC     CPT © 2017 American Medical Association. All Rights Reserved.

110.23, for further information about this policy, and Pub. 100-04, CPM, chapter 32, section 90, for information on coding.

b. Covered Conditions

1. Effective for services performed on or after April 28, 1989: Acute leukemia in remission who have a high probability of relapse and who have no human leucocyte antigens (HLA)-matched; Resistant non-Hodgkin's lymphomas or those presenting with poor prognostic features following an initial response; Recurrent or refractory neuroblastoma; or, Advanced Hodgkin's disease who have failed conventional therapy and have no HLA-matched donor.

2. Effective for services performed on or after October 1, 2000: Single AuSCT is only covered for Durie-Salmon Stage II or III patients that fit the following requirements:

    • Newly diagnosed or responsive multiple myeloma. This includes those patients with previously untreated disease, those with at least a partial response to prior chemotherapy (defined as a 50% decrease either in measurable paraprotein [serum and/or urine] or in bone marrow infiltration, sustained for at least 1 month), and those in responsive relapse; and

    • Adequate cardiac, renal, pulmonary, and hepatic function.

3. Effective for services performed on or after March 15, 2005: When recognized clinical risk factors are employed to select patients for transplantation, high dose melphalan (HDM) together with AuSCT is reasonable and necessary for Medicare beneficiaries of any age group with primary amyloid light chain (AL) amyloidosis who meet the following criteria:

    • Amyloid deposition in 2 or fewer organs; and,

    • Cardiac left ventricular ejection fraction (EF) greater than 45%.

**C. Nationally Non-Covered Indications**

I. Allogeneic Hematopoietic Stem Cell Transplantation (HSCT)

Effective for claims with dates of service on or after May 24, 1996, through January 26, 2016, allogeneic HSCT is not covered as treatment for multiple myeloma. Refer to Pub. 100-03, NCD Manual, chapter 1, section 110.23, for further information about this policy, and Pub. 100-04, CPM, chapter 32, section 90, for information on coding.

II. Autologous Stem Cell Transplantation (AuSCT)

Insufficient data exist to establish definite conclusions regarding the efficacy of AuSCT for the following conditions:

    a) Acute leukemia not in remission;

    b) Chronic granulocytic leukemia;

    c) Solid tumors (other than neuroblastoma); Up to October 1, 2000, multiple myeloma;

    e) Tandem transplantation (multiple rounds of AuSCT) for patients with multiple myeloma;

    f) Effective October 1, 2000, non primary AL amyloidosis; and,

    g) Effective October 1, 2000, through March 14, 2005, primary AL amyloidosis for Medicare beneficiaries age 64 or older. In these cases, AuSCT is not considered reasonable and necessary within the meaning of §l862(a)(1)(A) of the Act and is not covered under Medicare. Refer to Pub. 100-03, NCD Manual, chapter 1, section 110.23, for further information about this policy, and Pub. 100-04, CPM, chapter 32, section 90, for information on coding.

**D. Other**

All other indications for stem cell transplantation not otherwise noted above as covered or non-covered remain at local Medicare Administrative Contractor discretion.

## 100-4, 3, 90.3.1

### *Billing for Stem Cell Transplantation*

(Rev. 3571, Issued: 07-29-16; Effective: 01-01-17; Implementation; 01-03-17)

**A. Billing for Allogeneic Stem Cell Transplants**

**1. Definition of Acquisition Charges for Allogeneic Stem Cell Transplants**

Acquisition charges for allogeneic stem cell transplants include, but are not limited to, charges for the costs of the following services:

• National Marrow Donor Program fees, if applicable, for stem cells from an unrelated donor;

• Tissue typing of donor and recipient;

• Donor evaluation;

• Physician pre-admission/pre-procedure donor evaluation services;

• Costs associated with harvesting procedure (e.g., general routine and special care services, procedure/operating room and other ancillary services, apheresis services, etc.);

• Post-operative/post-procedure evaluation of donor; and

• Preparation and processing of stem cells.

Payment for these acquisition services is included in the MS-DRG payment for the allogeneic stem cell transplant when the transplant occurs in the inpatient setting, and in the OPPS APC payment for the allogeneic stem cell transplant when the transplant occurs in the outpatient setting. The Medicare contractor does not make separate payment for these acquisition services, because hospitals may bill and receive payment only for services provided to the Medicare beneficiary who is the recipient of the stem cell transplant and whose illness is being treated with the stem cell transplant. Unlike the acquisition costs of solid organs for transplant (e.g., hearts and kidneys), which are paid on a reasonable cost basis, acquisition costs for allogeneic stem cells are included in prospective payment.

Acquisition charges for stem cell transplants apply only to allogeneic transplants, for which stem cells are obtained from a donor (other than the recipient himself or herself). Acquisition charges do not apply to autologous transplants (transplanted stem cells are obtained from the recipient himself or herself), because autologous transplants involve services provided to the beneficiary only (and not to a donor), for which the hospital may bill and receive payment (see Pub. 100-04, chapter 4, §231.10 and paragraph B of this section for information regarding billing for autologous stem cell transplants).

**2. Billing for Acquisition Services**

The hospital bills and shows acquisition charges for allogeneic stem cell transplants based on the status of the patient (i.e., inpatient or outpatient) when the transplant is furnished. See Pub. 100-04, chapter 4, §231.11 for instructions regarding billing for acquisition services for allogeneic stem cell transplants that are performed in the outpatient setting.

When the allogeneic stem cell transplant occurs in the inpatient setting, the hospital identifies stem cell acquisition charges for allogeneic bone marrow/stem cell transplants separately by using revenue code 0815 (Stem Cell Acquisition). Revenue code 0815 charges should include all services required to acquire stem cells from a donor, as defined above.

On the recipient's transplant bill, the hospital reports the acquisition charges, cost report days, and utilization days for the donor's hospital stay (if applicable) and/or charges for other encounters in which the stem cells were obtained from the donor. The donor is covered for medically necessary inpatient hospital days of care or outpatient care provided in connection with the allogeneic stem cell transplant under Part A. Expenses incurred for complications are paid only if they are directly and immediately attributable to the stem cell donation procedure. The hospital reports the acquisition charges on the billing form for the recipient, as described in the first paragraph of this section. It does not charge the donor's days of care against the recipient's utilization record. For cost reporting purposes, it includes the covered donor days and charges as Medicare days and charges.

The transplant hospital keeps an itemized statement that identifies the services furnished, the charges, the person receiving the service (donor/recipient), and whether this is a potential transplant donor or recipient. These charges will be reflected in the transplant hospital's stem cell/bone marrow acquisition cost center. For allogeneic stem cell acquisition services in cases that do not result in transplant, due to death of the intended recipient or other causes, hospitals include the costs associated with the acquisition services on the Medicare cost report.

The hospital shows charges for the transplant itself in revenue center code 0362 or another appropriate cost center. Selection of the cost center is up to the hospital.

**B. Billing for Autologous Stem Cell Transplants**

The hospital bills and shows all charges for autologous stem cell harvesting, processing, and transplant procedures based on the status of the patient (i.e., inpatient or outpatient) when the services are furnished. It shows charges for the actual transplant, in revenue center code 0362 or another appropriate cost center. ICD-9-CM or ICD-10-PCS codes are used to identify inpatient procedures.

The HCPCS codes describing autologous stem cell harvesting procedures may be billed and are separately payable under the OPPS when provided in the hospital outpatient setting of care. Autologous harvesting procedures are distinct from the acquisition services described in Pub. 100-04, chapter 4, §231.11 and section A. above for allogeneic stem cell transplants, which include services provided when stem cells are obtained from a donor and not from the patient undergoing the stem cell transplant. The HCPCS codes describing autologous stem cell processing procedures also may be billed and are separately payable under the OPPS when provided to hospital outpatients.

Payment for autologous stem cell harvesting procedures performed in the hospital inpatient setting of care, with transplant also occurring in the inpatient setting of care, is included in the MS-DRG payment for the autologous stem cell transplant.

## 100-04, 3, 90.3.2

### *Autologous Stem Cell Transplantation (AuSCT)*

Autologous Stem Cell Transplantation (AuSCT)

**A. General**

Autologous stem cell transplantation (AuSCT) (ICD-9-CM procedure code 41.01, 41.04, 41.07, and 41.09 and CPT-4 code 38241) is a technique for restoring stem cells using the patient's own previously stored cells. AuSCT must be used to effect hematopoietic reconstitution following severely myelotoxic doses of chemotherapy (high dose chemotherapy (HDCT)) and/or radiotherapy used to treat various malignancies.

**Appendix G — Medicare Internet-only Manuals (IOMs)**

**If ICD-9-CM is applicable, use the following Procedure Codes and Descriptions**

| ICD-9-CM Code | Description |
| --- | --- |
| 41.01 | Autologous bone marrow transplant without purging |
| 41.04 | Autologous hematopoietic stem cell transplant without purging |
| 41.07 | Autologous hematopoietic stem cell transplant with purging |
| 41.09 | Autologous bone marrow transplant with purging |

**If ICD-10-PCS is applicable, use the following Procedure Codes and Descriptions**

| ICD-10-PCS Code | Description |
| --- | --- |
| 30230AZ | Transfusion of Embryonic Stem Cells into Peripheral Vein, Open Approach |
| 30230G0 | Transfusion of Autologous Bone Marrow into Peripheral Vein, Open Approach |
| 30230Y0 | Transfusion of Autologous Hematopoietic Stem Cells into Peripheral Vein, Open Approach |
| 30233G0 | Transfusion of Autologous Bone Marrow into Peripheral Vein, Percutaneous Approach |
| 30233Y0 | Transfusion of Autologous Hematopoietic Stem Cells into Peripheral Vein, Percutaneous Approach |
| 30240G0 | Transfusion of Autologous Bone Marrow into Central Vein, Open Approach |
| 30240Y0 | Transfusion of Autologous Bone Marrow into Central Vein, Open Approach |
| 30243G0 | Transfusion of Autologous Bone Marrow into Central Vein, Percutaneous Approach |
| 30243Y0 | Transfusion of Autologous Hematopoietic Stem Cells into Central Vein, Percutaneous Approach |
| 30250G0 | Transfusion of Autologous Bone Marrow into Peripheral Artery, Open Approach |
| 30250Y0 | Transfusion of Autologous Hematopoietic Stem Cells into Peripheral Artery, Open Approach |
| 30253G0 | Transfusion of Autologous Bone Marrow into Peripheral Artery, Percutaneous Approach |
| 30253Y0 | Transfusion of Autologous Hematopoietic Stem Cells into Peripheral Artery, Percutaneous Approach |
| 30260G0 | Transfusion of Autologous Bone Marrow into Central Artery, Open Approach |
| 30260Y0 | Transfusion of Autologous Hematopoietic Stem Cells into Central Artery, Open Approach |
| 30263G0 | Transfusion of Autologous Bone Marrow into Central Artery, Percutaneous Approach |
| 30263Y0 | Transfusion of Autologous Hematopoietic Stem Cells into Central Artery, Percutaneous Approach |

**B. Covered Conditions**
1. Effective for services performed on or after April 28, 1989:

For acute leukemia in remission for patients who have a high probability of relapse and who have no human leucocyte antigens (HLA)-matched the following diagnosis codes are reported:

**If ICD-9-CM is applicable, use the following Diagnosis Codes and Descriptions**

| Diagnosis Code | Description |
| --- | --- |
| 204.01 | Lymphoid leukemia, acute, in remission |
| 205.01 | Myeloid leukemia, acute, in remission |
| 206.01 | Monocytic leukemia, acute, in remission |
| 207.01 | Acute erythremia and erythroleukemia, in remission |
| 208.01 | Leukemia of unspecified cell type, acute, in remission |

**If ICD-10-CM is applicable, use the following Diagnosis Codes and Descriptions**

| Diagnosis Code | Description |
| --- | --- |
| C91.01 | Acute lymphoblastic leukemia, in remission |
| C92.01 | Acute myeloblastic leukemia, in remission |
| C92.41 | Acute promyelocytic leukemia, in remission |
| C92.51 | Acute myelomonocytic leukemia, in remission |
| C92.61 | Acute myeloid leukemia with 11q23-abnormality in remission |
| C92.A1 | Acute myeloid leukemia with multilineage dysplasia, in remission |
| C93.01 | Acute monoblastic/monocytic leukemia, in remission |
| C94.01 | Acute erythroid leukemia, in remission |
| C94.21 | Acute megakaryoblastic leukemia, in remission |
| C94.41 | Acute parmyelosis with myelofibrosis, in remission |

| Diagnosis Code | Description |
| --- | --- |
| C95.01 | Acute leukemia of unspecified cell type, in remission |

For resistant non-Hodgkin's lymphomas (or those presenting with poor prognostic features following an initial response the following diagnosis codes are reported:

**If ICD-9-CM is applicable, use the following code ranges:**
200.00 - 200.08,

200.10 - 00.18,

200.20 - 200.28,

200.80 - 200.88,

202.00 - 202.08,

202.80 - 202.88, and

202.90 - 202.98.

**If ICD-10-CM is applicable use the following code ranges:**
C82.00 - C85.29,

C85.80 - C86.6,

C96.4, and

C96.Z - C96.9.

For recurrent or refractory neuroblastoma (see ICD-9-CM Neoplasm by site, malignant for the appropriate diagnosis code)

If ICD-10-CM is applicable the following ranges are reported:

C00 - C96, and

D00 - D09 Resistant non-Hodgkin's lymphomas

For advanced Hodgkin's disease patients who have failed conventional therapy and have no HLA-matched donor the following diagnosis codes are reported:

If ICD-9-CM is applicable, 201.00-201.98.

If ICD-10-CM is applicable, C81.00 – C81.99.

2. Effective for services performed on or after October 1, 2000:

Durie-Salmon Stage II or III that fit the following requirement are covered: Newly diagnosed or responsive multiple myeloma (if ICD-9-CM is applicable, diagnosis codes 203.00 and 238.6, and, if ICD-10-CM is applicable, diagnosis codes C90.00 and D47.Z9). This includes those patients with previously untreated disease, those with at least a partial response to prior chemotherapy (defined as a 50% decrease either in measurable paraprotein [serum and/or urine] or in bone marrow infiltration, sustained for at least 1 month), and those in responsive relapse, and adequate cardiac, renal, pulmonary, and hepatic function.

3. Effective for Services On or After March 15, 2005

Effective for services performed on or after March 15, 2005 when recognized clinical risk factors are employed to select patients for transplantation, high-dose melphalan (HDM), together with AuSCT, in treating Medicare beneficiaries of any age group with primary amyloid light-chain (AL) amyloidosis who meet the following criteria:

Amyloid deposition in 2 or fewer organs; and,

Cardiac left ventricular ejection fraction (EF) of 45% or greater.

**C. Noncovered Conditions**
Insufficient data exist to establish definite conclusions regarding the efficacy of autologous stem cell transplantation for the following conditions:

- Acute leukemia not in remission:
  - If ICD-9-CM is applicable, diagnosis codes 204.00, 205.00, 206.00, 207.00 and 208.00 are noncovered;
  - If ICD-10-CM is applicable, diagnosis codes C91.00, C92.00, C92.40, C92.50, C92.60, C92.A0, C93.00, C94.00, and C95.00 are noncovered.
- Chronic granulocytic leukemia:
  - If ICD-9-CM is applicable, diagnosis codes 205.10 and 205.11;
  - If ICD-10-CM is applicable, diagnosis codes C92.10 and C92.11.
- Solid tumors (other than neuroblastoma):
  - If ICD-9-CM is applicable, diagnosis codes 140.0-199.1;
  - If ICD-10-CM is applicable, diagnosis codes C00.0 - C80.2 and D00.0 - D09.9. Multiple myeloma (ICD-9-CM codes 203.00 and 238.6), through September 30, 2000.
- Tandem transplantation (multiple rounds of autologous stem cell transplantation) for patients with multiple myeloma
  - If ICD-9-CM is applicable, diagnosis codes 203.00 and 238.6 and,
  - If ICD-10-CM is applicable, diagnosis codes C90.00 and D47.Z9)
- Non-primary (AL) amyloidosis,
  - If ICD-9-CM is applicable, diagnosis code 277.3. Effective October 1, 2000; ICD-9-CM code 277.3 was expanded to codes 277.30, 277.31, and 277.39 effective October 1, 2006.
  - If ICD-10-CM is applicable, diagnosis codes are E85.0 – E85.9. or

- Primary (AL) amyloidosis
  - If ICD-9-CM is applicable, diagnosis codes 277.30, 277.31, and 277.39 and for Medicare beneficiaries age 64 or older, effective October 1, 2000, through March 14, 2005.
  - If ICD-10-CM is applicable, diagnosis codes are E85.Ø - E85.9.

NOTE: Coverage for conditions other than these specifically designated as covered or non-covered is left to the discretion of the A/B MAC (A).

## 100-04, 3, 90.3.3

### Billing for Stem Cell Transplantation

#### A. Billing for Allogeneic Stem Cell Transplants

1. Definition of Acquisition Charges for Allogeneic Stem Cell Transplants

   Acquisition charges for allogeneic stem cell transplants include, but are not limited to, charges for the costs of the following services:

   - National Marrow Donor Program fees, if applicable, for stem cells from an unrelated donor;
   - Tissue typing of donor and recipient;
   - Donor evaluation;
   - Physician pre-admission/pre-procedure donor evaluation services;
   - Costs associated with harvesting procedure (e.g., general routine and special care services, procedure/operating room and other ancillary services, apheresis services, etc.);
   - Post-operative/post-procedure evaluation of donor; and
   - Preparation and processing of stem cells.

   Payment for these acquisition services is included in the MS-DRG payment for the allogeneic stem cell transplant when the transplant occurs in the inpatient setting, and in the OPPS APC payment for the allogeneic stem cell transplant when the transplant occurs in the outpatient setting. The Medicare contractor does not make separate payment for these acquisition services, because hospitals may bill and receive payment only for services provided to the Medicare beneficiary who is the recipient of the stem cell transplant and whose illness is being treated with the stem cell transplant. Unlike the acquisition costs of solid organs for transplant (e.g., hearts and kidneys), which are paid on a reasonable cost basis, acquisition costs for allogeneic stem cells are included in prospective payment.

   Acquisition charges for stem cell transplants apply only to allogeneic transplants, for which stem cells are obtained from a donor (other than the recipient himself or herself). Acquisition charges do not apply to autologous transplants (transplanted stem cells are obtained from the recipient himself or herself), because autologous transplants involve services provided to the beneficiary only (and not to a donor), for which the hospital may bill and receive payment (see Pub. 100-4, chapter 4, §231.10 and paragraph B of this section for information regarding billing for autologous stem cell transplants).

2. Billing for Acquisition Services

   The hospital bills and shows acquisition charges for allogeneic stem cell transplants based on the status of the patient (i.e., inpatient or outpatient) when the transplant is furnished. See Pub. 100-4, chapter 4, §231.11 for instructions regarding billing for acquisition services for allogeneic stem cell transplants that are performed in the outpatient setting.

   When the allogeneic stem cell transplant occurs in the inpatient setting, the hospital identifies stem cell acquisition charges for allogeneic bone marrow/stem cell transplants separately in FL 42 of Form CMS-1450 (or electronic equivalent) by using revenue code 0819 (Other Organ Acquisition). Revenue code 0819 charges should include all services required to acquire stem cells from a donor, as defined above.

   On the recipient's transplant bill, the hospital reports the acquisition charges, cost report days, and utilization days for the donor's hospital stay (if applicable) and/or charges for other encounters in which the stem cells were obtained from the donor. The donor is covered for medically necessary inpatient hospital days of care or outpatient care provided in connection with the allogeneic stem cell transplant under Part A. Expenses incurred for complications are paid only if they are directly and immediately attributable to the stem cell donation procedure. The hospital reports the acquisition charges on the billing form for the recipient, as described in the first paragraph of this section. It does not charge the donor's days of care against the recipient's utilization record. For cost reporting purposes, it includes the covered donor days and charges as Medicare days and charges.

   The transplant hospital keeps an itemized statement that identifies the services furnished, the charges, the person receiving the service (donor/recipient), and whether this is a potential transplant donor or recipient. These charges will be reflected in the transplant hospital's stem cell/bone marrow acquisition cost center. For allogeneic stem cell acquisition services in cases that do not result in transplant, due to death of the intended recipient or other causes, hospitals include the costs associated with the acquisition services on the Medicare cost report.

   The hospital shows charges for the transplant itself in revenue center code 0362 or another appropriate cost center. Selection of the cost center is up to the hospital.

#### B. Billing for Autologous Stem Cell Transplants

The hospital bills and shows all charges for autologous stem cell harvesting, processing, and transplant procedures based on the status of the patient (i.e., inpatient or outpatient) when the services are furnished. It shows charges for the actual transplant, described by the appropriate ICD-9-CM procedure or CPT codes, in revenue center code 0362 or another appropriate cost center. ICD-9-CM or ICD-10-PCS codes are used to identify inpatient procedures.

The CPT codes describing autologous stem cell harvesting procedures may be billed and are separately payable under the OPPS when provided in the hospital outpatient setting of care. Autologous harvesting procedures are distinct from the acquisition services described in Pub. 100-4, chapter 4, §231.11 and section A. above for allogeneic stem cell transplants, which include services provided when stem cells are obtained from a donor and not from the patient undergoing the stem cell transplant. The CPT codes describing autologous stem cell processing procedures also may be billed and are separately payable under the OPPS when provided to hospital outpatients.

Payment for autologous stem cell harvesting procedures performed in the hospital inpatient setting of care, with transplant also occurring in the inpatient setting of care, is included in the MS-DRG payment for the autologous stem cell transplant.

## 100-04, 3, 90.4

### Liver Transplants

#### A. Background

For Medicare coverage purposes, liver transplants are considered medically reasonable and necessary for specified conditions when performed in facilities that meet specific criteria. Coverage guidelines may be found in Publication 100-3, Section 260.1.

Effective for claims with dates of service June 21, 2012 and later, contractors may, at their discretion cover adult liver transplantation for patients with extrahepatic unresectable cholangiocarcinoma (CCA), (2) liver metastases due to a neuroendocrine tumor (NET) or (3) hemangioendothelimo (HAE) when furnished in an approved Liver Transplant Center (below). All other nationally non-covered malignancies continue to remain nationally non-covered.

To review the current list of approved Liver Transplant Centers, see http://www.cms.hhs.gov/CertificationandComplianc/20_Transplant.asp#TopOfPage

## 100-04, 3, 90.4.1

### Standard Liver Acquisition Charge
A3-3615.1, A3-3615.3

Each transplant facility must develop a standard charge for acquiring a cadaver liver from costs it expects to incur in the acquisition of livers.

This standard charge is not a charge that represents the acquisition cost of a specific liver. Rather, it is a charge that reflects the average cost associated with a liver acquisition.

Services associated with liver acquisition are billed from the organ procurement organization or, in some cases, the excising hospital to the transplant hospital. The excising hospital does not submit a billing form to the FI. The transplant hospital keeps an itemized statement that identifies the services furnished, the charges, the person receiving the service (donor/recipient), and the potential transplant donor. These charges are reflected in the transplant hospital's liver acquisition cost center and are used in determining the hospital's standard charge for acquiring a cadaver's liver. The standard charge is not a charge representing the acquisition cost of a specific liver. Rather, it is a charge that reflects the average cost associated with liver acquisition. Also, it is an all inclusive charge for all services required in acquisition of a liver, e.g., tissue typing, transportation of organ, and surgeons' retrieval fees.

## 100-04, 3, 90.4.2

### Billing for Liver Transplant and Acquisition Services

The inpatient claim is completed in accordance with instructions in chapter 25 for the beneficiary who receives a covered liver transplant. Applicable standard liver acquisition charges are identified separately in FL 42 by revenue code 0817 (Donor-Liver). Where interim bills are submitted, the standard acquisition charge appears on the billing form for the period during which the transplant took place. This charge is in addition to the hospital's charge for services furnished directly to the Medicare recipient.

The contractor deducts liver acquisition charges for IPPS hospitals prior to processing through Pricer. Costs of liver acquisition incurred by approved liver transplant facilities are not included in prospective payment DRG 480 (Liver Transplant). They are paid on a reasonable cost basis. This item is a "pass-through" cost for which interim payments are made. (See the Provider Reimbursement Manual, Part 1, §2802 B.8.) The contractor includes liver acquisition charges under revenue code 0817 in the HUIP record that it sends to CWF and the QIO.

## A. Bill Review Procedures

The contractor takes the following actions to process liver transplant bills.

1. Operative Report

   The contractor requires the operative report with all claims for liver transplants, or sends a development request to the hospital for each liver transplant with a diagnosis code for a covered condition.

2. MCE Interface

   The MCE contains a limited coverage edit for liver transplant procedures using ICD-9-CM code 50.59 if ICD-9 is applicable, and, if ICD-10 is applicable, using ICD-10-PCS codes 0FY00Z0, 0FY00Z1, and 0FY00Z2.

   Where a liver transplant procedure code is identified by the MCE, the contractor shall check the provider number and effective date to determine if the provider is an approved liver transplant facility at the time of the transplant, and the contractor shall also determine if the facility is certified for adults and/or pediatric transplants dependent upon the patient's age. If yes, the claim is suspended for review of the operative report to determine whether the beneficiary has at least one of the covered conditions when the diagnosis code is for a covered condition. If payment is appropriate (i.e., the facility is approved, the service is furnished on or after the approval date, and the beneficiary has a covered condition), the contractor sends the claim to Grouper and Pricer.

   If none of the diagnoses codes are for a covered condition, or if the provider is not an approved liver transplant facility, the contractor denies the claim.

   NOTE: Some noncovered conditions are included in the covered diagnostic codes. (The diagnostic codes are broader than the covered conditions. Do not pay for noncovered conditions.)

3. Grouper

   If the bill shows a discharge date before March 8, 1990, the liver transplant procedure is not covered. If the discharge date is March 8, 1990 or later, the contractor processes the bill through Grouper and Pricer. If the discharge date is after March 7, 1990, and before October 1, 1990, Grouper assigned CMS DRG 191 or 192. The contractor sent the bill to Pricer with review code 08. Pricer would then overlay CMS DRG 191 or 192 with CMS DRG 480 and the weights and thresholds for CMS DRG 480 to price the bill. If the discharge date is after September 30, 1990, Grouper assigns CMS DRG 480 and Pricer is able to price without using review code 08. If the discharge date is after September 30, 2007, Grouper assigns MS-DRG 005 or 006 (Liver transplant with MCC or Intestinal Transplant or Liver transplant without MCC, respectively) and Pricer is able to price without using review code 08.

4. Liver Transplant Billing From Non-approved Hospitals

   Where a liver transplant and covered services are provided by a non-approved hospital, the bill data processed through Grouper and Pricer must exclude transplant procedure codes and related charges.

   When CMS approves a hospital to furnish liver transplant services, it informs the hospital of the effective date in the approval letter. The contractor will receive a copy of the letter.

## 100-04, 3, 90.5

### Pancreas Transplants Kidney Transplants

(Rev. 3481, Issued: 03-18-16. Effective: 06-20-16, Implementation: 06-20-16)

### A. Background

Effective July 1, 1999, Medicare covered pancreas transplantation when performed simultaneously with or following a kidney transplant if ICD-9 is applicable, ICD-9-CM procedure code 55.69. If ICD-10 is applicable, the following ICD-10-PCS codes will be used:

   0TY00Z0,

   0TY00Z1,

   0TY00Z2,

   0TY10Z0.

   0TY10Z1, and

   0TY10Z2.

Pancreas transplantation is performed to induce an insulin independent, euglycemic state in diabetic patients. The procedure is generally limited to those patients with severe secondary complications of diabetes including kidney failure. However, pancreas transplantation is sometimes performed on patients with labile diabetes and hypoglycemic unawareness.

Medicare has had a policy of not covering pancreas transplantation. The Office of Health Technology Assessment performed an assessment on pancreas-kidney transplantation in 1994. They found reasonable graft survival outcomes for patients receiving either simultaneous pancreas-kidney (SPK) transplantation or pancreas after kidney (PAK) transplantation. For a list of facilities approved to perform SPK or PAK, refer to the following Web site: https://www.cms.gov/Medicare/Provider-Enrollment-and-Certification/CertificationandComplianc/downloads/ApprovedTransplantPrograms.pdf

## B. Billing for Pancreas Transplants

There are no special provisions related to managed care participants. Managed care plans are required to provide all Medicare covered services. Medicare does not restrict which hospitals or physicians may perform pancreas transplantation.

The transplant procedure and revenue code 0360 for the operating room are paid under these codes. Procedures must be reported using the current ICD-9-CM procedure codes for pancreas and kidney transplants. Providers must place at least one of the following transplant procedure codes on the claim:

### If ICD-9 Is Applicable

   52.80    Transplant of pancreas

   52.82    Homotransplant of pancreas

The Medicare Code Editor (MCE) has been updated to include 52.80 and 52.82 as limited coverage procedures. The contractor must determine if the facility is approved for the transplant and certified for either pediatric or adult transplants dependent upon the age of the patient.

Effective October 1, 2000, ICD-9-CM code 52.83 was moved in the MCE to non-covered. The contractor must override any deny edit on claims that came in with 52.82 prior to October 1, 2000 and adjust, as 52.82 is the correct code.

If the discharge date is July 1, 1999, or later: the contractor processes the bill through Grouper and Pricer.

### If ICD-10 is applicable, the following procedure codes (ICD-10-PCS) are:

   0FYG0Z0 Transplantation of Pancreas, Allogeneic, Open Approach

   0FYG0Z1 Transplantation of Pancreas, Syngeneic, Open Approach

Pancreas transplantation is reasonable and necessary for the following diagnosis codes. However, since this is not an all-inclusive list, the contractor is permitted to determine if any additional diagnosis codes will be covered for this procedure.

If ICD-9-CM is applicable, Diabetes Diagnosis Codes and Descriptions

| ICD-9-CM Code | Description |
|---|---|
| 250.00 | Diabetes mellitus without mention of complication, type II (non-insulin dependent) (NIDDM) (adult onset) or unspecified type, not stated as uncontrolled. |
| 250.01 | Diabetes mellitus without mention of complication, type I (insulin dependent) (IDDM) (juvenile), not stated as uncontrolled. |
| 250.02 | Diabetes mellitus without mention of complication, type II (non-insulin dependent) (NIDDM) (adult onset) or unspecified type, uncontrolled. |
| 250.03 | Diabetes mellitus without mention of complication, type I (insulin dependent) (IDDM) (juvenile), uncontrolled. |
| 250.1X | Diabetes with ketoacidosis |
| 250.2X | Diabetes with hyperosmolarity |
| 250.3X | Diabetes with coma |
| 250.4X | Diabetes with renal manifestations |
| 250.5X | Diabetes with ophthalmic manifestations |
| 250.6X | Diabetes with neurological manifestations |
| 250.7X | Diabetes with peripheral circulatory disorders |
| 250.8X | Diabetes with other specified manifestations |
| 250.9X | Diabetes with unspecified complication |

NOTE: X=0-3

If ICD-10-CM is applicable, the diagnosis codes are: E10.10 - E10.9

Hypertensive Renal Diagnosis Codes and Descriptions if ICD-9-CM is applicable :

| ICD-9-CM Code | Description |
|---|---|
| 403.01 | Malignant hypertensive renal disease, with renal failure |
| 403.11 | Benign hypertensive renal disease, with renal failure |
| 403.91 | Unspecified hypertensive renal disease, with renal failure |
| 404.02 | Malignant hypertensive heart and renal disease, with renal failure |
| 404.03 | Malignant hypertensive heart and renal disease, with congestive heart failure or renal failure |
| 404.12 | Benign hypertensive heart and renal disease, with renal failure |
| 404.13 | Benign hypertensive heart and renal disease, with congestive heart failure or renal failure |
| 404.92 | Unspecified hypertensive heart and renal disease, with renal failure |
| 404.93 | Unspecified hypertensive heart and renal disease, with congestive heart failure or renal failure |
| 585.1–585.6, 585.9 | Chronic Renal Failure Code |

If ICD-10-CM is applicable, diagnosis codes and descriptions are:

| ICD-10-CM code | Description |
|---|---|
| I12.0 | Hypertensive chronic kidney disease with stage 5 chronic kidney disease or end stage renal disease |
| I13.11 | Hypertensive heart and chronic kidney disease without heart failure, with stage 5 chronic kidney disease, or end stage renal disease |
| I13.2 | Hypertensive heart and chronic kidney disease with heart failure and with stage 5 chronic kidney disease, or end stage renal disease |
| N18.1 | Chronic kidney disease, stage 1 |
| N18.2 | Chronic kidney disease, stage 2 (mild) |
| N18.3 | Chronic kidney disease, stage 3 (moderate) |
| N18.4 | Chronic kidney disease, stage 4 (severe) |
| N18.5 | Chronic kidney disease, stage 5 |
| N18.6 | End stage renal disease |
| N18.9 | Chronic kidney disease, unspecified |

**NOTE:** If a patient had a kidney transplant that was successful, the patient no longer has chronic kidney failure, therefore it would be inappropriate for the provider to bill ICD-9-CM codes 585.1 - 585.6, 585.9 or, if ICD-10-CM is applicable, the diagnosis codes N18.1 - N18.9 on such a patient. In these cases one of the following codes should be present on the claim or in the beneficiary's history.

The provider uses the following ICD-9-CM status codes only when a kidney transplant was performed before the pancreas transplant and ICD-9 is applicable:

| ICD-9-CM code | Description |
|---|---|
| V42.0 | Organ or tissue replaced by transplant kidney |
| V43.89 | Organ tissue replaced by other means, kidney or pancreas |

If ICD-10-CM is applicable, the following ICD-10-CM status codes will be used:

| ICD-10-CM code | Description |
|---|---|
| Z48.22 | Encounter for aftercare following kidney transplant |
| Z94.0 | Kidney transplant status |

**NOTE:** If a kidney and pancreas transplants are performed simultaneously, the claim should contain a diabetes diagnosis code and a renal failure code or one of the hypertensive renal failure diagnosis codes. The claim should also contain two transplant procedure codes. If the claim is for a pancreas transplant only, the claim should contain a diabetes diagnosis code and a status code to indicate a previous kidney transplant. If the status code is not on the claim for the pancreas transplant, the contractor will search the beneficiary's claim history for a status code indicating a prior kidney transplant.

### C. Drugs
If the pancreas transplant occurs after the kidney transplant, immunosuppressive therapy will begin with the date of discharge from the inpatient stay for the pancreas transplant.

### D. Charges for Pancreas Acquisition Services
A separate organ acquisition cost center has been established for pancreas transplantation. The Medicare cost report will include a separate line to account for pancreas transplantation costs. The 42 CFR 412.2(e)(4) was changed to include pancreas in the list of organ acquisition costs that are paid on a reasonable cost basis.

Acquisition costs for pancreas transplantation as well as kidney transplants will occur in Revenue Center 081X. The contractor overrides any claims that suspend due to repetition of revenue code 081X on the same claim if the patient had a simultaneous kidney/pancreas transplant. It pays for acquisition costs for both kidney and pancreas organs if transplants are performed simultaneously. It will not pay for more than two organ acquisitions on the same claim.

### E. Medicare Summary Notices (MSN) and Remittance Advice Messages
If the provider submits a claim for simultaneous pancreas kidney transplantation or pancreas transplantation following a kidney transplant, and omits one of the appropriate diagnosis/procedure codes, the contractor shall reject the claim.

The following reflects the remittance advice messages and associated codes that will appear when rejecting/denying claims under this policy. This CARC/RARC combination is compliant with CAQH CORE Business Scenario 3.

Group Code: CO

CARC: B15

RARC: N/A

MSN: 16.32

If no evidence of a prior kidney transplant is presented, then the contractor shall deny the claim.

The following reflects the remittance advice messages and associated codes that will appear when rejecting/denying claims under this policy. This CARC/RARC combination is compliant with CAQH CORE Business Scenario 3.

Group Code: CO

CARC: 50

RARC: MA126

MSN: 15.4

## 100-04, 3, 90.5.1

### Pancreas Transplants Alone (PA)
Rev.3481, Issued: 03-18-16. Effective: 06-20-16, Implementation: 06-20-16

### A. General
Pancreas transplantation is performed to induce an insulin-independent, euglycemic state in diabetic patients. The procedure is generally limited to those patients with severe secondary complications of diabetes, including kidney failure. However, pancreas transplantation is sometimes performed on patients

with labile diabetes and hypoglycemic unawareness. Medicare has had a long-standing policy of not covering pancreas transplantation, as the safety and effectiveness of the procedure had not been demonstrated. The Office of Health Technology Assessment performed an assessment of pancreas-kidney transplantation in 1994. It found reasonable graft survival outcomes for patients receiving either simultaneous pancreas-kidney transplantation or pancreas-after-kidney transplantation.

### B. Nationally Covered Indications
CMS determines that whole organ pancreas transplantation will be nationally covered by Medicare when performed simultaneous with or after a kidney transplant. If the pancreas transplant occurs after the kidney transplant, immunosuppressive therapy will begin with the date of discharge from the inpatient stay for the pancreas transplant.

### C. Billing and Claims Processing
Contractors shall pay for Pancreas Transplantation Alone (PA) effective for services on or after April 26, 2006 when performed in those facilities that are Medicare-approved for kidney transplantation. Approved facilities are located at the following address: https://www.cms.gov/Medicare/Provider-Enrollment-and-Certification/Certification andComplianc/downloads/ApprovedTransplantPrograms.pdf

Contractors who receive claims for PA services that were performed in an unapproved facility, should reject such claims. The following reflects the remittance advice messages and associated codes that will appear when rejecting/denying claims under this policy. This CARC/RARC combination is compliant with CAQH CORE Business Scenario 3.

Group Code: CO

CARC: 58

RARC: N/A

MSN: 16.2.

Payment will be made for a PA service performed in an approved facility, and which meets the coverage guidelines mentioned above for beneficiaries with type I diabetes.

All-Inclusive List of Covered Diagnosis Codes for PA if ICD-9-CM is applicable

(NOTE: "X" = 1 and 3 only)

| ICD-9-CM code | Description |
|---|---|
| 250.0X | Diabetes mellitus without mention of complication, type I (insulin dependent) (IDDM) (juvenile), not stated as uncontrolled. |
| 250.1X | Diabetes with ketoacidosis |
| 250.2X | Diabetes with hyperosmolarity |
| 250.3X | Diabetes with coma |
| 250.4X | Diabetes with renal manifestations |
| 250.5X | Diabetes with ophthalmic manifestations |
| 250.6X | Diabetes with neurological manifestations |
| 250.7X | Diabetes with peripheral circulatory disorders |
| 250.8X | Diabetes with other specified manifestations |
| 250.9X | Diabetes with unspecified complication |

**If ICD-10-CM is applicable, the provider uses the following range of ICD-10-CM codes:**
E10.10 – E10.9.

**Procedure Codes**

**If ICD-9 CM is applicable**
52.80 - Transplant of pancreas

52.82 - Homotransplant of pancreas

**If ICD-10 is applicable, the provider uses the following ICD-10-PCS codes:**
0FYG0Z0 Transplantation of Pancreas, Allogeneic, Open Approach

0FYG0Z1 Transplantation of Pancreas, Syngeneic, Open Approach

CPT © 2017 American Medical Association. All Rights Reserved.

© 2017 Optum360, LLC

Contractors who receive claims for PA that are not billed using the covered diagnosis/procedure codes listed above shall reject such claims. The MCE edits to ensure that the transplant is covered based on the diagnosis. The MCE also considers ICD-9-CM codes 52.80 and 52.82 and ICD-10-PCS codes ØFYGØZØ and ØFYGØZ1 as limited coverage dependent upon whether the facility is approved to perform the transplant and is certified for the age of the patient.

The following reflects the remittance advice messages and associated codes that will appear when rejecting/denying claims under this policy. This CARC/RARC combination is compliant with CAQH CORE Business Scenario 3.

> Group Code: CO
>
> CARC: 50
>
> RARC: N/A
>
> MSN: 15.4

Contractors shall hold the provider liable for denied\rejected claims unless the hospital issues a Hospital Issued Notice of Non-coverage (HINN) or a physician issues an Advanced Beneficiary Notice (ABN) for Part-B for physician services.

### D. Charges for Pancreas Alone Acquisition Services

A separate organ acquisition cost center has been established for pancreas transplantation. The Medicare cost report will include a separate line to account for pancreas transplantation costs. The 42 CFR 412.2(e)(4) was changed to include PA in the list of organ acquisition costs that are paid on a reasonable cost basis.

Acquisition costs for PA transplantation are billed in Revenue Code 081X. The contractor removes acquisition charges prior to sending the claims to Pricer so such charges are not included in the outlier calculation.

## 100-04, 3, 90.6

### Intestinal and Multi-Visceral Transplants

(Rev. 3481, Issued: 03-18-16. Effective: 06-20-16, Implementation: 06-20-16)

### A. Background

Effective for services on or after April 1, 2001, Medicare covers intestinal and multi-visceral transplantation for the purpose of restoring intestinal function in patients with irreversible intestinal failure. Intestinal failure is defined as the loss of absorptive capacity of the small bowel secondary to severe primary gastrointestinal disease or surgically induced short bowel syndrome. Intestinal failure prevents oral nutrition and may be associated with both mortality and profound morbidity. Multi-Visceral transplantation includes organs in the digestive system (stomach, duodenum, liver, and intestine). See §260.5 of the National Coverage Determinations Manual for further information.

### B. Approved Transplant Facilities

Medicare will cover intestinal transplantation if performed in an approved facility. The approved facilities are located at: https://www.cms.gov/Medicare/Provider-Enrollment-and-Certification/Certification andComplianc/downloads/ApprovedTransplantPrograms.pdf

### C. Billing

If ICD-9-CM is applicable, ICD-9-CM procedure code 46.97 is effective for discharges on or after April 1, 2001. If ICD-10 is applicable, the ICD-10-PCS procedure codes are ØDY8ØZØ, ØDY8ØZ1, ØDY8ØZ2, ØDYEØZØ, ØDYEØZ1, and ØDYEØZ2. The Medicare Code Editor (MCE) lists these codes as limited coverage procedures. The contractor shall override the MCE when this procedure code is listed and the coverage criteria are met in an approved transplant facility, and also determine if the facility is certified for adults and/or pediatric transplants dependent upon the patient's age.

For these procedures where the provider is approved as transplant facility and certified for the adult and/or pediatric population, and the service is performed on or after the transplant approval date, the contractor must suspend the claim for clerical review of the operative report to determine whether the beneficiary has at least one of the covered conditions listed when the diagnosis code is for a covered condition.

This review is not part of the contractor's medical review workload. Instead, the contractor should complete this review as part of its claims processing workload.

If ICD-9-CM is applicable, charges for ICD-9-CM procedure code 46.97, and, if ICD-10 is applicable, the ICD-10-PCS procedure codes ØDY8ØZØ, ØDY8ØZ1, ØDY8ØZ2, ØDYEØZØ, ØDYEØZ1, or ØDYEØZ2 should be billed under revenue code 0360, Operating Room Services.

For discharge dates on or after October 1, 2001, acquisition charges are billed under revenue code 081X, Organ Acquisition. For discharge dates between April 1, 2001, and September 30, 2001, hospitals were to report the acquisition charges on the claim, but there was no interim pass-through payment made for these costs.

Bill the procedure used to obtain the donor's organ on the same claim, using appropriate ICD procedure codes.

The 11X bill type should be used when billing for intestinal transplants.

Immunosuppressive therapy for intestinal transplantation is covered and should be billed consistent with other organ transplants under the current rules.

If ICD-9-CM is applicable, there is no specific ICD-9-CM diagnosis code for intestinal failure. Diagnosis codes exist to capture the causes of intestinal failure. Some examples of intestinal failure include but are not limited to the following conditions and their associated ICD-9-CM codes:

- Volvulus 560.2,

- Volvulus gastroschisis 756.79, other [congenital] anomalies of abdominal wall,
- Volvulus gastroschisis 569.89, other specified disorders of intestine,
- Necrotizing enterocolitis 777.5, necrotizing enterocolitis in fetus or newborn,
- Necrotizing enterocolitis 014.8, other tuberculosis of intestines, peritoneum, and mesenteric,
- Necrotizing enterocolitis and splanchnic vascular thrombosis 557.0, acute vascular insufficiency of intestine,
- Inflammatory bowel disease 569.9, unspecified disorder of intestine,
- Radiation enteritis 777.5, necrotizing enterocolitis in fetus or newborn, and
- Radiation enteritis 558.1.

If ICD-10-CM is applicable, some diagnosis codes that may be used for intestinal failure are:

- Volvulus K56.2,
- Enteroptosis K63.4,
- Other specified diseases of intestine K63.89,
- Other specified diseases of the digestive system K92.89,
- Postsurgical malabsorption, not elsewhere classified K91.2,
- Other congenital malformations of abdominal wall Q79.59,
- Necrotizing enterocolitis in newborn, unspecified P77.9,
- Stage 1 necrotizing enterocolitis in newborn P77.1,
- Stage 2 necrotizing enterocolitis in newborn P77.2, and
- Stage 3 necrotizing enterocolitis in newborn P77.3

### D. Acquisition Costs

A separate organ acquisition cost center was established for acquisition costs incurred on or after October 1, 2001. The Medicare Cost Report will include a separate line to account for these transplantation costs.

For intestinal and multi-visceral transplants performed between April 1, 2001, and October 1, 2001, the DRG payment was payment in full for all hospital services related to this procedure.

### E. Medicare Summary Notices (MSN), Remittance Advice Messages, and Notice of Utilization Notices (NOU)

If an intestinal transplant is billed by an unapproved facility after April 1, 2001, the contractor shall deny the claim.

The following reflects the remittance advice messages and associated codes that will appear when rejecting/denying claims under this policy. This CARC/RARC combination is compliant with CAQH CORE Business Scenario 3.

> Group Code: CO
>
> CARC: 171
>
> RARC: N/A

MSN: 21.6 or 21.18 or 16.2

## 100-04, 3, 100.1

### Billing for Abortion Services

(Rev. 3481, Issued: 03-18-16. Effective: 06-20-16, Implementation: 06-20-16)

Effective October 1, 1998, abortions are not covered under the Medicare program except for instances where the pregnancy is a result of an act of rape or incest; or the woman suffers from a physical disorder, physical injury, or physical illness, including a life endangering physical condition caused by the pregnancy itself that would, as certified by a physician, place the woman in danger of death unless an abortion is performed.

### A. "G" Modifier

The "G7" modifier is defined as "the pregnancy resulted from rape or incest, or pregnancy certified by physician as life threatening."

Beginning July 1, 1999, providers should bill for abortion services using the new Modifier G7. This modifier can be used on claims with dates of services October 1, 1998, and after. CWF will be able to recognize the modifier beginning July 1, 1999.

### B. A/B MAC (A) Billing Instructions

1. Hospital Inpatient Billing

   Hospitals use bill type 11X. Medicare will pay only when one of the following condition codes is reported:

| Condition Code | Description |
| --- | --- |
| AA | Abortion Performed due to Rape |
| AB | Abortion Performed due to Incest |
| AD | Abortion Performed due to life endangering physical condition |

With one of the following:

**If ICD-9-CM Is Applicable:**
- an appropriate ICD principal diagnosis code that will group to DRG 770 (Abortion W D&C, Aspiration Curettage Or Hysterotomy) or

© 2017 Optum360, LLC

CPT © 2017 American Medical Association. All Rights Reserved.

- an appropriate ICD principal diagnosis code and one of the following ICD-9-CM operating room procedure that will group to DRG 779 (Abortion W/O D&C):69.01, 69.02, 69.51, 74.91.

If ICD-10-CM is applicable, one of the following ICD-10-PCS codes are used:

| ICD-10-PCS code | Description |
| --- | --- |
| 10A07ZZ | Abortion of Products of Conception, Via Natural or Artificial Opening |
| 10A08ZZ | Abortion of Products of Conception, Via Natural or Artificial Opening Endoscopic |
| 10D17ZZ | Extraction of Products of Conception, Retained, Via Natural or Artificial Opening |
| 10D18ZZ | Extraction of Products of Conception, Retained, Via Natural or Artificial Opening Endoscopic |
| 10A07ZZ | Abortion of Products of Conception, Via Natural or Artificial Opening |
| 10A08ZZ | Abortion of Products of Conception, Via Natural or Artificial Opening Endoscopic |
| 10A00ZZ | Abortion of Products of Conception, Open Approach |
| 10A03ZZ | Abortion of Products of Conception, Percutaneous Approach |
| 10A04ZZ | Abortion of Products of Conception, Percutaneous Endoscopic Approach |

Providers must use ICD-9-CM codes 69.01 and 69.02 if ICD-9-CM is applicable, or, if ICD-10-CM is applicable, the related 1CD-10-PCS codes to describe exactly the procedure or service performed.

The A/B MAC (A) must manually review claims with the above ICD-9-CM/ICD-10-PCS procedure codes to verify that all of the above conditions are met.

2. Outpatient Billing

Hospitals will use bill type 13X and 85X. Medicare will pay only if one of the following CPT codes is used with the "G7" modifier.

| | | | | |
| --- | --- | --- | --- | --- |
| 59840 | 59851 | 59856 | 59841 | 59852 |
| 59857 | 59850 | 59855 | 59866 | |

### C. Common Working File (CWF) Edits

For hospital outpatient claims, CWF will bypass its edits for a managed care beneficiary who is having an abortion outside their plan and the claim is submitted with the "G7" modifier and one of the above CPT codes.

For hospital inpatient claims, CWF will bypass its edits for a managed care beneficiary who is having an abortion outside their plan and the claim is submitted with one of the above inpatient procedure codes.

### D. Medicare Summary Notices (MSN)/Explanation of Your Medicare Benefits Remittance Advice Message

If a claim is submitted with one of the above CPT procedure codes but no "G7" modifier, the claim is denied.

The following reflects the remittance advice messages and associated codes that will appear when rejecting/denying claims under this policy. This CARC/RARC combination is compliant with CAQH CORE Business Scenario 3.

Group Code: CO

CARC: 272

RARC: N/A

MSN: 21.21

## 100-04, 3, 100.6

### Inpatient Renal Services

HO-E400

Section 405.103l of Subpart J of Regulation 5 stipulates that only approved hospitals may bill for ESRD services. Hence, to allow hospitals to bill and be reimbursed for inpatient dialysis services furnished under arrangements, both facilities participating in the arrangement must meet the conditions of 405.2120 and 405.2160 of Subpart U of Regulation 5. In order for renal dialysis facilities to have a written arrangement with each other to provide inpatient dialysis care both facilities must meet the minimum utilization rate requirement, i.e., two dialysis stations with a performance capacity of at least four dialysis treatments per week.

Dialysis may be billed by an SNF as a service if: (a) it is provided by a hospital with which the facility has a transfer agreement in effect, and that hospital is approved to provide staff-assisted dialysis for the Medicare program; or (b) it is furnished directly by an SNF meeting all nonhospital maintenance dialysis facility requirements, including minimum utilization requirements. (See 1861(h)(6), 1861(h)(7), title XVIII.)

## 100-04, 4, 20.6.12

### Use of HCPCS Modifier – CT

(Rev. 3425, Issued: 12-18-15, Effective: 01-01-16, Implementation: 01-04-16)

Effective January 1, 2016, the definition of modifier – CT is "Computed tomography services furnished using equipment that does not meet each of the attributes of the National Electrical Manufacturers Association (NEMA) XR-29-2013 standard." This modifier is required to be reported on claims for computed tomography (CT) scans described by applicable HCPCS codes that are furnished on non-NEMA Standard XR-29-2013-compliant equipment. The applicable CT services are identified by HCPCS codes 70450 through 70498; 71250 through 71275; 72125 through 72133; 72191 through 72194; 73200 through 73206; 73700 through 73706; 74150 through 74178; 74261 through 74263; and 75571 through 75574 (and any succeeding codes).

This modifier should not be reported with codes that describe CT scans not listed above.

## 100-04, 4, 160

### Clinic and Emergency Visits

CMS has acknowledged from the beginning of the OPPS that CMS believes that CPT Evaluation and Management (E/M) codes were designed to reflect the activities of physicians and do not describe well the range and mix of services provided by hospitals during visits of clinic and emergency department patients. While awaiting the development of a national set of facility-specific codes and guidelines, providers should continue to apply their current internal guidelines to the existing CPT codes. Each hospital's internal guidelines should follow the intent of the CPT code descriptors, in that the guidelines should be designed to reasonably relate the intensity of hospital resources to the different levels of effort represented by the codes. Hospitals should ensure that their guidelines accurately reflect resource distinctions between the five levels of codes.

Effective January 1, 2007, CMS is distinguishing between two types of emergency departments: Type A emergency departments and Type B emergency departments.

A Type A emergency department is defined as an emergency department that is available 24 hours a day, 7 days a week and is either licensed by the State in which it is located under applicable State law as an emergency room or emergency department or it is held out to the public (by name, posted signs, advertising, or other means) as a place that provides for emergency medical conditions on an urgent basis without requiring a previously scheduled appointment.

A Type B emergency department is defined as an emergency department that meets the definition of a "dedicated emergency department" as defined in 42 CFR 489.24 under the EMTALA regulations. It must meet at least one of the following requirements: (1) It is licensed by the State in which it is located under applicable State law as an emergency room or emergency department; (2) It is held out to the public (by name, posted signs, advertising, or other means) as a place that provides care for emergency medical conditions on an urgent basis without requiring a previously scheduled appointment; or (3) During the calendar year immediately preceding the calendar year in which a determination under 42 CFR 489.24 is being made, based on a representative sample of patient visits that occurred during that calendar year, it provides at least one-third of all of its outpatient visits for the treatment of emergency medical conditions on an urgent basis without requiring a previously scheduled appointment.

Hospitals must bill for visits provided in Type A emergency departments using CPT emergency department E/M codes. Hospitals must bill for visits provided in Type B emergency departments using the G-codes that describe visits provided in Type B emergency departments.

Hospitals that will be billing the new Type B ED visit codes may need to update their internal guidelines to report these codes.

Emergency department and clinic visits are paid in some cases separately and in other cases as part of a composite APC payment. See section 10.2.1 of this chapter for further details.

## 100-4, 4, 200.1

### Billing for Corneal Tissue

(Rev. 3425, Issued: 12-18-15, Effective: 01-01-16, Implementation: 01-04-16)

Corneal tissue will be paid on a cost basis, not under OPPS, only when it is used in a corneal transplant procedure described by one of the following CPT codes: 65710, 65730, 65750, 65755, 65756, 65765, 65767, and any successor code or new code describing a new type of corneal transplant procedure that uses eye banked corneal tissue. In all other procedures cornea tissue is packaged. To receive cost based reimbursement hospitals must bill charges for corneal tissue using HCPCS code V2785.

## 100-4, 4, 200.3.1

### Billing Instructions for IMRT Planning and Delivery

(Rev. 3685, Issued: 12-22-16, Effective: 01-01-17, Implementation: 01-03-17)

Payment for the services identified by CPT codes 77014, 77280, 77285, 77290, 77295, 77306 through 77321, 77331, and 77370 are included in the APC payment for CPT code 77301 (IMRT planning). These codes should not be reported in addition to CPT code 77301 when provided prior to or as part of the development of the IMRT plan. In addition, CPT codes 77280-77290 (simulation-aided field settings) should not be reported for verification of the treatment field during a course of IMRT.

## 100-4, 4, 200.3.2

### Billing for Multi-Source Photon (Cobalt 60-Based) Stereotactic Radiosurgery (SRS) Planning and Delivery

(Rev. 3685, Issued: 12-22-16, Effective: 01-01-17, Implementation: 01-03-17)

Effective for services furnished on or after January 1, 2014, hospitals must report SRS planning and delivery services using only the CPT codes that accurately describe the service furnished. For the delivery services, hospitals must report CPT code 77371, 77372, or 77373.

| CPT Code | Long Descriptor |
|---|---|
| 77371 | Radiation treatment delivery, stereotactic radiosurgery (srs), complete course of treatment of cranial lesion(s) consisting of 1 session; multi- source cobalt 60 based |
| 77372 | Radiation treatment delivery, stereotactic radiosurgery (srs), complete course of treatment of cranial lesion(s) consisting of 1 session; linear accelerator based |
| 77373 | Stereotactic body radiation therapy, treatment delivery, per fraction to 1 or more lesions, including image guidance, entire course not to exceed 5 fractions |

As instructed in the CY 2014 OPPS/ASC final rule, CPT code 77371 is to be used only for single session cranial SRS cases performed with a Cobalt-60 device, and CPT code 77372 is to be used only for single session cranial SRS cases performed with a linac-based device. The term "cranial" means that the pathological lesion(s) that are the target of the radiation is located in the patient's cranium or head. The term "single session" means that the entire intracranial lesion(s) that comprise the patient's diagnosis are treated during a single treatment session on a single day. CPT code 77372 is never to be used for the first fraction or any other fraction of a fractionated SRS treatment. CPT code 77372 is to be used only for single session cranial linac-based SRS treatment. Fractionated SRS treatment is any SRS delivery service requiring more thana single session of SRS treatment for a cranial lesion, up to a total of no more than five fractions, and one to five sessions (but no more than five) for non-cranial lesions. CPT code 77373 is to be used for any fraction (including the first fraction) in any series of fractionated treatments, regardless of the anatomical location of the lesion or lesions being radiated. Fractionated cranial SRS is any cranial SRS that exceeds one treatment session and fractionated non-cranial SRS is any non-cranial SRS, regardless of the number of fractions but never more than five. Therefore, CPT code 77373 is the exclusive code (and the use of no other SRS treatment delivery code is permitted) for any and all fractionated SRS treatment services delivered anywhere in the body, including, but not limited to, the cranium or head. 77372 is not to be used for the first fraction of a fractionated cranial SRS treatment series and must only be used in cranial SRS when there is a single treatment session to treat the patient's entire condition.

In addition, for the planning services, hospitals must report the specific CPT code that accurately describes the service provided. The planning services may include but are not limited to CPT code 77290, 77295, 77300, 77334, or 77370.

| CPT Code | Long Descriptor |
|---|---|
| 77290 | Therapeutic radiology simulation-aided field setting; complex |
| 77295 | Therapeutic radiology simulation-aided field setting; 3-dimensional |
| 77300 | Basic radiation dosimetry calculation, central axis depth dose calculation, tdf, nsd, gap calculation, off axis factor, tissue inhomogeneity factors, calculation of non-ionizing radiation surface and depth dose, as required during course of treatment, only when prescribed by the treating physician |
| 77334 | Treatment devices, design and construction; complex (irregular blocks, special shields, compensators, wedges, molds or casts) |
| 77370 | Special medical radiation physics consultation |

Effective for cranial single session stereotactic radiosurgery procedures (CPT code 77371 or 77372) furnished on or after January 1, 2016 until December 31, 2017, costs for certain adjunctive services (e.g., planning and preparation) are not factored into the APC payment rate for APC 5627 (Level 7 Radiation Therapy). Rather, the ten planning and preparation codes listed in table below, will be paid according to their assigned status indicator when furnished 30 days prior or 30 days post SRS treatment delivery.

In addition, hospitals must report modifier "CP" (Adjunctive service related to a procedure assigned to a comprehensive ambulatory payment classification [C-APC] procedure) on TOB 13X claims for any other services (excluding the ten codes in table below) that are adjunctive or related to SRS treatment but billed on a different claim and within either 30 days prior or 30 days after the date of service for either CPT code 77371 (Radiation treatment delivery, stereotactic radiosurgery, complete course of treatment cranial lesion(s) consisting of 1 session; multi-source Cobalt 60-based) or CPT code 77372 (Linear accelerator based). The "CP" modifier need not be reported with the ten planning and preparation CPT codes table below. Adjunctive/related services include but are not necessarily limited to imaging, clinical treatment planning/preparation, and consultations. Any service related to the SRS delivery should have the CP modifier appended. We would not expect the "CP" modifier to be

reported with services such as chemotherapy administration as this is considered to be a distinct service that is not directly adjunctive, integral, or dependent on delivery of SRS treatment.

Excluded Planning and Preparation CPT Codes

| CPT Code | CY 2017 Short Descriptor | CY 2017 Opps Status Indicator |
|---|---|---|
| 70551 | Mri brain stem w/o dye | Q3 |
| 70552 | Mri brain stem w/dye | Q3 |
| 70553 | Mri brain stem w/o & w/dye | Q3 |
| 77011 | Ct scan for localization | N |
| 77014 | Ct scan for therapy guide | N |
| 77280 | Set radiation therapy field | S |
| 77285 | Set radiation therapy field | S |
| 77290 | Set radiation therapy field | S |
| 77295 | 3-d radiotherapy plan | S |
| 77336 | Radiation physics consult | S |

## 100-04, 4, 200.11

### Billing Advance Care Planning (ACP) as an Optional Element of an Annual Wellness Visit (AWV)

(Rev. 3739, Issued: 03-17-17, Effective: 01-01-16, Implementation: 06-19-17)

Effective January 1, 2016 payment for the service described by CPT code 99497 (Advance care planning including the explanation and discussion of advance directives such as standard forms (with completion of such forms, when performed), by the physician or other qualified health care professional; first 30 minutes, face-to-face with the patient, family member(s), and/or surrogate) is conditionally packaged under the OPPS and is consequently assigned to a conditionally packaged payment status indicator of "Q1." When this service is furnished with another service paid under the OPPS, payment is packaged; when it is the only service furnished, payment is made separately. CPT code 99498 (Advance care planning including the explanation and discussion of advance directives such as standard forms (with completion of such forms, when performed), by the physician or other qualified health care professional; each additional 30 minutes (List separately in addition to code for primary procedure)) is an add-on code and therefore payment for the service described by this code is unconditionally packaged (assigned status indicator "N") in the OPPS in accordance with 42 CFR 419.2(b)(18).

In addition, for services furnished on or after January 1, 2016, Advance Care Planning (ACP) is treated as a preventive service when furnished with an AWV. The Medicare coinsurance and Part B deductible are waived for ACP when furnished as an optional element of an AWV.

The codes for the optional ACP services furnished as part of an AWV are 99497 (Advance care planning including the explanation and discussion of advance directives such as standard forms (with completion of such forms, when performed), by the physician or other qualified health professional; first 30 minutes, face-to-face with the patient, family member(s) and/or surrogate;) and an add-on code 99498 (each additional 30 minutes (List separately in addition to code for primary procedure)). When ACP services are provided as a part of an AWV, practitioners would report CPT code 99497

(and add-on CPT code 99498 when applicable) for the ACP services in addition to either of the AWV codes (G0438 or G0439).

The deductible and coinsurance for ACP will only be waived when billed on the same day and on the same claim as an AWV (code G0438 or G0439), and must also be furnished by the same provider. Waiver of the deductible and coinsurance for ACP is limited to once per year. Payment for an AWV is limited to once per year. If the AWV billed with ACP is denied for exceeding the once per year limit, the deductible and coinsurance will be applied to the ACP.

Also see Pub. 100-02, Medicare Benefit Policy Manual, chapter 15, section 280.5.1 for more information.

## 100-04, 4, 231.10

### Billing for Autologous Stem Cell Transplants

(Rev.3556, Issued: 07-01-2016; Effective: 1-27-16; Implementation: 10-3-16)

The hospital bills and shows all charges for autologous stem cell harvesting, processing, and transplant procedures based on the status of the patient (i.e., inpatient or outpatient) when the services are furnished. It shows charges for the actual transplant, described by the appropriate ICD procedure or CPT codes in Revenue Center 0362 (Operating Room Services; Organ Transplant, Other than Kidney) or another appropriate cost center.

The CPT codes describing autologous stem cell harvesting procedures may be billed and are separately payable under the Outpatient Prospective Payment System (OPPS) when provided in the hospital outpatient setting of care. Autologous harvesting procedures are distinct from the acquisition services described in Pub. 100-04, Chapter 3, §90.3.1 and §231.11 of this chapter for allogeneic stem cell transplants, which include services provided when stem cells are obtained from a donor and not from the patient undergoing the stem cell transplant.

The CPT codes describing autologous stem cell processing procedures also may be billed and are separately payable under the OPPS when provided to hospital outpatients.

## 100-4, 4, 231.11

### Billing for Allogeneic Stem Cell Transplants

(Rev. 3571, Issued: 07-29-16, Effective: 01-01-17, Implementation: 01-03-17)

#### 1. Definition of Acquisition Charges for Allogeneic Stem Cell Transplants

Acquisition charges for allogeneic stem cell transplants include, but are not limited to, charges for the costs of the following services:

- National Marrow Donor Program fees, if applicable, for stem cells from an unrelated donor;
- Tissue typing of donor and recipient;
- Donor evaluation;
- Physician pre-procedure donor evaluation services;
- Costs associated with harvesting procedure (e.g., general routine and special care services, procedure/operating room and other ancillary services, apheresis services,etc.);
- Post-operative/post-procedure evaluation of donor; and
- Preparation and processing of stem cells.

Payment for these acquisition services is included in the OPPS C-APC payment for the allogeneic stem cell transplant when the transplant occurs in the hospital outpatient setting, and in the MS-DRG payment for the allogeneic stem cell transplant when the transplant occurs in the inpatient setting. The Medicare contractor does not make separate payment for these acquisition services, because hospitals may bill and receive payment only for services provided to the Medicare beneficiary who is the recipient of the stem cell transplant and whose illness is being treated with the stem cell transplant. Unlike the acquisition costs of solid organs for transplant (e.g., hearts and kidneys), which are paid on a reasonable cost basis, acquisition costs for allogeneic stem cells are included in prospective payment. Recurring update notifications describing changes to and billing instructions for various payment policies implemented in the OPPS are issued annually.

Acquisition charges for stem cell transplants apply only to allogeneic transplants, for which stem cells are obtained from a donor (other than the recipient himself or herself). Acquisition charges do not apply to autologous transplants (transplanted stem cells are obtained from the recipient himself or herself), because autologous transplants involve services provided to the beneficiary only (and not to a donor), for which the hospital may bill and receive payment (see Pub. 100-04, chapter 3, §90.3.1 and §231.10 of this chapter for information regarding billing for autologous stem cell transplants).

#### 2. Billing for Acquisition Services

The hospital bills and shows acquisition charges for allogeneic stem cell transplants based on the status of the patient (i.e., inpatient or outpatient) when the transplant is furnished. See Pub. 100-04, chapter 3, §90.3.1 for instructions regarding billing for acquisition services for allogeneic stem cell transplants that are performed in the inpatient setting.

Effective January 1, 2017, when the allogeneic stem cell transplant occurs in the outpatient setting, the hospital identifies stem cell acquisition charges for allogeneic bone marrow/stem cell transplants separately in FL 42 of Form CMS-1450 (or electronic equivalent) by using revenue code 0815 (Other Organ Acquisition). Revenue code 0815 charges should include all services required to acquire stem cells from a donor, as defined above, and should be reported on the same date of service as the transplant procedure in order to be appropriately packaged for payment purposes.

The transplant hospital keeps an itemized statement that identifies the services furnished, the charges, the person receiving the service (donor/recipient), and whether this is a potential transplant donor or recipient. These charges will be reflected in the transplant hospital's stem cell/bone marrow acquisition cost center. For allogeneic stem cell acquisition services in cases that do not result in transplant, due to death of the intended recipient or other causes, hospitals include the costs associated with the acquisition services on the Medicare cost report.

In the case of an allogeneic transplant in the hospital outpatient setting, the hospital reports the transplant itself with the appropriate CPT code, and a charge under revenue

center code 0362 or another appropriate cost center. Selection of the cost center is up to the hospital.

## 100-04, 4, 250.16

### Multiple Procedure Payment Reduction (MPPR) on Certain Diagnostic Imaging Procedures Rendered by Physicians

(Rev. 3578, Issued: 08-05 Effective: 01-01-17, Implementation: 01-03-17)

Diagnostic imaging procedures rendered by a physician that has reassigned their billing rights to a Method II CAH are payable by Medicare when the procedures are eligible and billed on type of bill 85x with revenue code (RC) 096x, 097x and/or 098x.

The MPPR on diagnostic imaging applies when multiple services are furnished by the same physician to the same patient in the same session on the same day. Full payment is made for each service with the highest payment under the MPFS. Effective for dates of services on or after January 1, 2012, payment is made at 75 percent for each subsequent service; and effective for dates of services on or after January 1, 2017, payment is made at 95 percent for each subsequent service.

## 100-04, 4, 290.5.3

### Billing and Payment for Observation Services Furnished Beginning January 1, 2016

(Rev. 3425, Issued: 12-18-15, Effective: 01-01-16, Implementation: 01-04-16)

Observation services are reported using HCPCS code G0378 (Hospital observation service, per hour). Beginning January 1, 2008, HCPCS code G0378 for hourly observation services is assigned status indicator N, signifying that its payment is always packaged. No separate payment is made for observation services reported with HCPCS code G0378, and APC 0339 is deleted as of January 1, 2008. In most circumstances, observation services are supportive and ancillary to the other services provided to a patient. Beginning January 1, 2016, in certain circumstances when observation services are billed in conjunction with a clinic visit, Type A emergency department visit (Level 1 through 5), Type B emergency department visit (Level 1 through 5), critical care services, or a direct referral as an integral part of a patient's extended encounter of care, comprehensive payment may be made for all services on the claim including, the entire extended care encounter through comprehensive APC 8011 (Comprehensive Observation Services) when certain criteria are met. For information about comprehensive APCs, see §10.2.3 (Comprehensive APCs) of this chapter.

There is no limitation on diagnosis for payment of APC 8011; however, comprehensive APC payment will not be made when observation services are reported in association with a surgical procedure (T status procedure) or the hours of observation care reported are less than 8. The I/OCE evaluates every claim received to determine if payment through a comprehensive APC is appropriate. If payment through a comprehensive APC is inappropriate, the I/OCE, in conjunction with the Pricer, determines the appropriate status indicator, APC, and payment for every code on a claim.

All of the following requirements must be met in order for a hospital to receive a comprehensive APC payment through the Comprehensive Observation Services APC (APC 8011):

1. Observation Time

a. Observation time must be documented in the medical record.

b. Hospital billing for observation services begins at the clock time documented in the patient's medical record, which coincides with the time that observation services are initiated in accordance with a physician's order for observation services.

c. A beneficiary's time receiving observation services (and hospital billing) ends when all clinical or medical interventions have been completed, including follow-up care furnished by hospital staff and physicians that may take place after a physician has ordered the patient be released or admitted as an inpatient.

d. The number of units reported with HCPCS code G0378 must equal or exceed 8 hours.

2. Additional Hospital Services

a. The claim for observation services must include one of the following services in addition to the reported observation services. The additional services listed below must have a line item date of service on the same day or the day before the date reported for observation:

- A Type A or B emergency department visit (CPT codes 99281 through 99285 or HCPCS codes G0380 through G0384); or

- A clinic visit (HCPCS code G0463); or

- Critical care (CPT code 99291); or

- Direct referral for observation care reported with HCPCS code G0379 (APC 5013) must be reported on the same date of service as the date reported for observation services.

b. No procedure with a T status indicator or a J1 status indicator can be reported on the claim.

3. Physician Evaluation

a. The beneficiary must be in the care of a physician during the period of observation, as documented in the medical record by outpatient registration, discharge, and other appropriate progress notes that are timed, written, and signed by the physician.

b. The medical record must include documentation that the physician explicitly assessed patient risk to determine that the beneficiary would benefit from observation care.

Criteria 1 and 3 related to observation care beginning and ending time and physician evaluation apply regardless of whether the hospital believes that the criteria will be met for payment of the extended encounter through the Comprehensive Observation Services APC (APC 8011).

CPT © 2017 American Medical Association. All Rights Reserved.

© 2017 Optum360, LLC

Only visits, critical care and observation services that are billed on a 13X bill type may be considered for a comprehensive APC payment through the Comprehensive Observation Services APC (APC 8011).

Non-repetitive services provided on the same day as either direct referral for observation care or observation services must be reported on the same claim because the OCE claim-by-claim logic cannot function properly unless all services related to the episode of observation care, including hospital clinic visits, emergency department visits, critical care services, and T status procedures, are reported on the same claim. Additional guidance can be found in chapter 1, section 50.2.2 of this manual.

If a claim for services provided during an extended assessment and management encounter including observation care does not meet all of the requirements listed above, then the usual APC logic will apply to separately payable items and services on the claim; the special logic for direct admission will apply, and payment for the observation care will be packaged into payments for other separately payable services provided to the beneficiary in the same encounter.

## 100-04, 5, 10

### Part B Outpatient Rehabilitation and Comprehensive Outpatient Rehabilitation Facility (CORF) Services - General

(Rev. 3454, Issued: 02-04-16, Effective: 07-01-16, Implementation: 07-05-16)

Language in this section is defined or described in Pub. 100-02, chapter 15, sections 220 and 230.

Section §1834(k)(5) to the Social Security Act (the Act), requires that all claims for outpatient rehabilitation services and comprehensive outpatient rehabilitation facility (CORF) services, be reported using a uniform coding system. The CMS chose HCPCS (Healthcare Common Procedure Coding System) as the coding system to be used for the reporting of these services. This coding requirement is effective for all claims for outpatient rehabilitation services and CORF services submitted on or after April 1, 1998.

The Act also requires payment under a prospective payment system for outpatient rehabilitation services including CORF services. Effective for claims with dates of service on or after January 1, 1999, the Medicare Physician Fee Schedule (MPFS) became the method of payment for outpatient therapy services furnished by:

- Comprehensive outpatient rehabilitation facilities (CORFs);
- Outpatient physical therapy providers (OPTs), also known as rehabilitation agencies;
- Hospitals (to outpatients and inpatients who are not in a covered Part A stay);
- Skilled nursing facilities (SNFs) (to residents not in a covered Part A stay and to nonresidents who receive outpatient rehabilitation services from the SNF); and
- Home health agencies (HHAs) (to individuals who are not homebound or otherwise are not receiving services under a home health plan of care (POC)).

**NOTE:** No provider or supplier other than the SNF will be paid for therapy services during the time the beneficiary is in a covered SNF Part A stay. For information regarding SNF consolidated billing see chapter 6, section 10 of this manual.

Similarly, under the HH prospective payment system, HHAs are responsible to provide, either directly or under arrangements, all outpatient rehabilitation therapy services to beneficiaries receiving services under a home health POC. No other provider or supplier will be paid for these services during the time the beneficiary is in a covered Part A stay. For information regarding HH consolidated billing see chapter10, section 20 of this manual.

Section 143 of the Medicare Improvements for Patients and Provider's Act of 2008 (MIPPA) authorizes the Centers for Medicare & Medicaid Services (CMS) to enroll speech-language pathologists (SLP) as suppliers of Medicare services and for SLPs to begin billing Medicare for outpatient speech-language pathology services furnished in private practice beginning July 1, 2009. Enrollment will allow SLPs in private practice to bill Medicare and receive direct payment for their services. Previously, the Medicare program could only pay SLP services if an institution, physician or nonphysician practitioner billed them.

In Chapter 23, as part of the CY 2009 Medicare Physician Fee Schedule Database, the descriptor for PC/TC indicator "7", as applied to certain HCPCS/CPT codes, is described as specific to the services of privately practicing therapists. Payment may not be made if the service is provided to either a hospital outpatient or a hospital inpatient by a physical therapist, occupational therapist, or speech-language pathologist in private practice.

The MPFS is used as a method of payment for outpatient rehabilitation services furnished under arrangement with any of these providers.

In addition, the MPFS is used as the payment system for CORF services identified by the HCPCS codes in §20. Assignment is mandatory.

Services that are paid subject to the MPFS are adjusted based on the applicable payment locality. Rehabilitation agencies and CORFs with service locations in different payment localities shall follow the instructions for multiple service locations in chapter 1, section 170.1.1.

The Medicare allowed charge for the services is the lower of the actual charge or the MPFS amount. The Medicare payment for the services is 80 percent of the allowed charge after the Part B deductible is met. Coinsurance is made at 20 percent of the lower of the actual charge or the MPFS amount. The general coinsurance rule (20

percent of the actual charges) does not apply when making payment under the MPFS. This is a final payment.

The MPFS does not apply to outpatient rehabilitation services furnished by critical access hospitals (CAHs) or hospitals in Maryland. CAHs are to be paid on a reasonable cost basis. Maryland hospitals are paid under the Maryland All-Payer Model.

Contractors process outpatient rehabilitation claims from hospitals, including CAHs, SNFs, HHAs, CORFs, outpatient rehabilitation agencies, and outpatient physical therapy providers for which they have received a tie in notice from the Regional Office (RO). These provider types submit their claims to the contractors using the ASC X12 837 institutional claim format or the CMS-1450 paper form when permissible. Contractors also process claims from physicians, certain nonphysician practitioners (NPPs), therapists in private practices (TPPs), (which are limited to physical and occupational therapists, and speech-language pathologists in private practices), and physician-directed clinics that bill for services furnished incident to a physician's service (see Pub. 100-02, Medicare Benefit Policy Manual, chapter 15, for a definition of "incident to"). These provider types submit their claims to the contractor using the ASC X 12 837 professional claim format or the CMS-1500 paper form when permissible.

There are different fee rates for nonfacility and facility services. Chapter 23 describes the differences in these two rates. (See fields 28 and 29 of the record therein described). Facility rates apply to professional services performed in a facility other than the professional's office. Nonfacility rates apply when the service is performed in the professional's office. The nonfacility rate (that is paid when the provider performs the services in its own facility) accommodates overhead and indirect expenses the provider incurs by operating its own facility. Thus it is somewhat higher than the facility rate.

Contractors pay the nonfacility rate on institutional claims for services performed in the provider's facility. Contractors may pay professional claims using the facility or nonfacility rate depending upon where the service is performed (place of service on the claim), and the provider specialty.

Contractors pay the codes in §20 under the MPFS on professional claims regardless of whether they may be considered rehabilitation services. However, contractors must use this list for institutional claims to determine whether to pay under outpatient rehabilitation rules or whether payment rules for other types of service may apply, e.g., OPPS for hospitals, reasonable costs for CAHs.

Note that because a service is considered an outpatient rehabilitation service does not automatically imply payment for that service. Additional criteria, including coverage, plan of care and physician certification must also be met. These criteria are described in Pub. 100-02, Medicare Benefit Policy Manual, chapters 1 and 15.

Payment for rehabilitation services provided to Part A inpatients of hospitals or SNFs is included in the respective PPS rate. Also, for SNFs (but not hospitals), if the beneficiary has Part B, but not Part A coverage (e.g., Part A benefits are exhausted), the SNF must bill for any rehabilitation service.

Payment for rehabilitation therapy services provided by home health agencies under a home health plan of care is included in the home health PPS rate. HHAs may submit bill type 34X and be paid under the MPFS if there are no home health services billed under a home health plan of care at the same time, and there is a valid rehabilitation POC (e.g., the patient is not homebound).

An institutional employer (other than a SNF) of the TPPs, or physician performing outpatient services, (e.g., hospital, CORF, etc.), or a clinic billing on behalf of the physician or therapist may bill the contractor on a professional claim.

The MPFS is the basis of payment for outpatient rehabilitation services furnished by TPPs, physicians, and certain nonphysician practitioners or for diagnostic tests provided incident to the services of such physicians or nonphysician practitioners. (See Pub. 100-02, Medicare Benefit Policy Manual, Chapter 15, for a definition of "incident to, therapist, therapy and related instructions.") Such services are billed to the contractor on the professional claim format. Assignment is mandatory.

The following table identifies the provider and supplier types, and identifies which claim format they may use to submit claims for outpatient therapy services to the contractor.

| "Provider/Supplier Service" Type | Format | Bill Type | Comment |
|---|---|---|---|
| Inpatient SNF Part A | Institutional | 21X | Included in PPS |
| Inpatient hospital Part B | Institutional | 12X | Hospital may obtain services under arrangements and bill, or rendering provider may bill. |
| Inpatient SNF Part B (audiology tests are not included) | Institutional | 22X | SNF must provide and bill, or obtain under arrangements and bill. |
| Outpatient hospital | Institutional | 13X | Hospital may provide and bill or obtain under arrangements and bill. |
| Outpatient SNF | Institutional | 23X | SNF must provide and bill or obtain under arrangements and bill. |

| "Provider/Supplier Service" Type | Format | Bill Type | Comment |
|---|---|---|---|
| HHA billing for services not rendered under a Part A or Part B home health plan of care, but rendered under a therapy plan of care. | Institutional | 34X | Service not under home health plan of care. |
| Outpatient physical therapy providers (OPTs), also known as rehabilitation agencies | Institutional | 74X | Paid MPFS for outpatient rehabilitation services. |
| Comprehensive Outpatient Rehabilitation Facility (CORF) | Institutional | 75X | Paid MPFS for outpatient rehabilitation services and all other services except drugs. Drugs are paid 95% of the AWP. |
| Physician, NPPs, TPPs, (therapy services in hospital or SNF) | Professional | See Chapter 26 for place of service coding. | Payment may not be made for therapy services to Part A inpatients of hospitals or SNFs, or for Part B SNF residents. **NOTE:** Payment may be made to physicians and NPPs for their professional services defined as "sometimes therapy" (not part of a therapy plan) in certain situations; for example, when furnished to a beneficiary registered as an outpatient of a hospital. |
| Physician/NPP/TPPs office, or patient's home | Professional | See Chapter 26 for place of service coding. | Paid via MPFS. |
| Critical Access Hospital - inpatient Part B | Institutional | 12X | Rehabilitation services are paid at cost. |
| Critical Access Hospital – outpatient Part B | Institutional | 85X | Rehabilitation services are paid at cost. |

For a list of the outpatient rehabilitation HCPCS codes see §20.

If a contractor receives an institutional claim for one of these HCPCS codes with dates of service on or after July 1, 2003, that does not appear on the supplemental file it currently uses to pay the therapy claims, it contacts its professional claims area to obtain the non-facility price in order to pay the claim.

**NOTE:** The list of codes in §20 contains commonly utilized codes for outpatient rehabilitation services. Contractors may consider other codes on institutional claims for payment under the MPFS as outpatient rehabilitation services to the extent that such codes are determined to be medically reasonable and necessary and could be performed within the scope of practice of the therapist providing the service.

## 100-4, 5, 10.3.2

### Exceptions Process

(Rev. 3670, Issued: 12-01-16, Effective: 01-01-17, Implementation: 01-03-17)

An exception may be made when the patient's condition is justified by documentation indicating that the beneficiary requires continued skilled therapy, i.e., therapy beyond the amount payable under the therapy cap, to achieve their prior functional status or maximum expected functional status within a reasonable amount of time.

No special documentation is submitted to the contractor for exceptions. The clinician is responsible for consulting guidance in the Medicare manuals and in the professional literature to determine if the beneficiary may qualify for the exception because documentation justifies medically necessary services above the caps. The clinician's opinion is not binding on the Medicare contractor who makes the final determination concerning whether the claim is payable.

Documentation justifying the services shall be submitted in response to any Additional Documentation Request (ADR) for claims that are selected for medical review. Follow the documentation requirements in Pub. 100-02, chapter 15, section 220.3. If medical records are requested for review, clinicians may include, at their discretion, a summary that specifically addresses the justification for therapy cap exception.

In making a decision about whether to utilize the exception, clinicians shall consider, for example, whether services are appropriate to--

The patient's condition, including the diagnosis, complexities, and severity;

The services provided, including their type, frequency, and duration;

The interaction of current active conditions and complexities that directly and significantly influence the treatment such that it causes services to exceed caps.

In addition, the following should be considered before using the exception process:

**1. Exceptions for Evaluation Services**

Evaluation. The CMS will accept therapy evaluations from caps after the therapy caps are reached when evaluation is necessary, e.g., to determine if the current status of the beneficiary requires therapy services. For example, the following CPT codes for evaluation procedures may be appropriate:

> 92521, 92522, 92523, 92524, 92597, 92607, 92608, 92610, 92611, 92612, 92614, 92616, 96105, 96125. 97161, 97162, 97163, 97164, 97165, 97166, 97167, and 97168.

These codes will continue to be reported as outpatient therapy procedures as listed in the Annual Therapy Update for the current year at: http://www.cms.gov/TherapyServices/05_Annual_Therapy_Update.asp#TopOfPage.

They are not diagnostic tests. Definitions of evaluations and documentation are found in Pub. 100-02, chapter 15, sections 220 and 230.

Other Services. There are a number of sources that suggest the amount of certain services that may be typical, either per service, per episode, per condition, or per discipline. For example, see the CSC - Therapy Cap Report, 3/21/2008, and CSC – Therapy Edits Tables 4/14/2008 at www.cms.hhs.gov/TherapyServices (Studies and Reports), or more recent utilization reports. Professional literature and guidelines from professional associations also provide a basis on which to estimate whether the type, frequency, and intensity of services are appropriate to an individual. Clinicians and contractors should utilize available evidence related to the patient's condition to justify provision of medically necessary services to individual beneficiaries, especially when they exceed caps. Contractors shall not limit medically necessary services that are justified by scientific research applicable to the beneficiary. Neither contractors nor clinicians shall utilize professional literature and scientific reports to justify payment for continued services after an individual's goals have been met earlier than is typical. Conversely, professional literature and scientific reports shall not be used as justification to deny payment to patients whose needs are greater than is typical or when the patient's condition is not represented by the literature.

**2. Exceptions for Medically Necessary Services**

Clinicians may utilize the process for exception for any diagnosis or condition for which they can justify services exceeding the cap. Regardless of the diagnosis or condition, the patient must also meet other requirements for coverage.

Bill the most relevant diagnosis. As always, when billing for therapy services, the diagnosis code that best relates to the reason for the treatment shall be on the claim, unless there is a compelling reason to report another diagnosis code. For example, when a patient with diabetes is being treated with therapy for gait training due to amputation, the preferred diagnosis is abnormality of gait (which characterizes the treatment). Where it is possible in accordance with State and local laws and the contractors' local coverage determinations, avoid using vague or general diagnoses. When a claim includes several types of services, or where the physician/NPP must supply the diagnosis, it may not be possible to use the most relevant therapy diagnosis code in the primary position. In that case, the relevant diagnosis code should, if possible, be on the claim in another position.

Codes representing the medical condition that caused the treatment are used when there is no code representing the treatment. Complicating conditions are preferably used in non-primary positions on the claim and are billed in the primary position only in the rare circumstance that there is no more relevant code.

The condition or complexity that caused treatment to exceed caps must be related to the therapy goals and must either be the condition that is being treated or a complexity that directly and significantly impacts the rate of recovery of the condition being treated such that it is appropriate to exceed the caps. Documentation for an exception should indicate how the complexity (or combination of complexities) directly and significantly affects treatment for a therapy condition.

If the contractor has determined that certain codes do not characterize patients who require medically necessary services, providers/suppliers may not use those codes, but must utilize a billable diagnosis code allowed by their contractor to describe the patient's condition. Contractors shall not apply therapy caps to services based on the patient's condition, but only on the medical necessity of the service for the condition. If a service would be payable before the cap is reached and is still medically necessary after the cap is reached, that service is excepted.

Contact your contractor for interpretation if you are not sure that a service is applicable for exception.

It is very important to recognize that most conditions would not ordinarily result in services exceeding the cap. Use the KX modifier only in cases where the condition of the individual patient is such that services are APPROPRIATELY provided in an episode that exceeds the cap. Routine use of the KX modifier for all patients with these conditions will likely show up on data analysis as aberrant and invite inquiry. Be sure that documentation is sufficiently detailed to support the use of the modifier.

In justifying exceptions for therapy caps, clinicians and contractors should not only consider the medical diagnoses and medical complications that might directly and significantly influence the amount of treatment required. Other variables (such as the availability of a caregiver at home) that affect appropriate treatment shall also be considered. Factors that influence the need for treatment should be supportable by published research, clinical guidelines from professional sources, and/or clinical or common sense. See Pub. 100-02, chapter 15, section 220.3 for information related to documentation of the evaluation, and section 220.2 on medical necessity for some factors that complicate treatment.

**NOTE:** The patient's lack of access to outpatient hospital therapy services alone, when outpatient hospital therapy services are excluded from the limitation, does not justify excepted services. Residents of skilled nursing facilities prevented by consolidated billing from accessing hospital services, debilitated patients for whom transportation to the hospital is a physical hardship, or lack of therapy services at hospitals in the beneficiary's county may or may not qualify as justification for continued services above the caps. The patient's condition and complexities might justify extended services, but their location does not. For dates of service on or after October 1, 2012, therapy services furnished in an outpatient hospital are not excluded from the limitation.

## 100-04, 5, 10.6

### Functional Reporting

(Rev. 3670, Issued: 12-01-16, Effective: 01-01-17, Implementation: 01-03-17)

**A. General**

Section 3005(g) of the Middle Class Tax Relief and Jobs Creation Act (MCTRJCA) amended Section 1833(g) of the Act to require a claims-based data collection system for outpatient therapy services, including physical therapy (PT), occupational therapy (OT) and speech-language pathology (SLP) services. 42 CFR 410.59, 410.60, 410.61, 410.62 and 410.105 implement this requirement. The system will collect data on beneficiary function during the course of therapy services in order to better understand beneficiary conditions, outcomes, and expenditures.

Beneficiary unction information is reported using 42 nonpayable functional G-codes and seven severity/complexity modifiers on claims for PT, OT, and SLP services. Functional reporting on one functional limitation at a time is required periodically throughout an entire PT, OT, or SLP therapy episode of care.

The nonpayable G-codes and severity modifiers provide information about the beneficiary's functional status at the outset of the therapy episode of care, including projected goal status, at specified points during treatment, and at the time of discharge. These G-codes, along with the associated modifiers, are required at specified intervals on all claims for outpatient therapy services – not just those over the cap.

**B. Application of New Coding Requirements**

This functional data reporting and collection system is effective for therapy services with dates of service on and after January 1, 2013. A testing period will be in effect from January 1, 2013, until July 1, 2013, to allow providers and practitioners to use the new coding requirements to assure that systems work. Claims for therapy services furnished on and after July 1, 2013, that do not contain the required functional G-code/modifier information will be returned or rejected, as applicable.

**C. Services Affected**

These requirements apply to all claims for services furnished under the Medicare Part B outpatient therapy benefit and the PT, OT, and SLP services furnished under the CORF benefit. They also apply to the therapy services furnished personally by and incident to the service of a physician or a nonphysician practitioner (NPP), including a nurse practitioner (NP), a certified nurse specialist (CNS), or a physician assistant (PA), as applicable.

**D. Providers and Practitioners Affected.**

The functional reporting requirements apply to the therapy services furnished by the following providers: hospitals, CAHs, SNFs, CORFs, rehabilitation agencies, and HHAs (when the beneficiary is not under a home health plan of care). It applies to the following practitioners: physical therapists, occupational therapists, and speech-language pathologists in private practice (TPPs), physicians, and NPPs as noted above. The term "clinician" is applied to these practitioners throughout this manual section. (See definition section of Pub. 100-02, chapter 15, section 220.)

**E. Function-related G-codes**

There are 42 functional G-codes, 14 sets of three codes each. Six of the G-code sets are generally for PT and OT functional limitations and eight sets of G-codes are for SLP functional limitations.

The following G-codes are for functional limitations typically seen in beneficiaries receiving PT or OT services. The first four of these sets describe categories of functional limitations and the final two sets describe "other" functional limitations, which are to be used for functional limitations not described by one of the four categories.

**NONPAYABLE G-CODES FOR FUNCTIONAL LIMITATIONS**

| | Long Descriptor | Short Descriptor |
|---|---|---|
| **Mobility G-code Set** | | |
| G8978 | Mobility: walking & moving around functional limitation, current status, at therapy episode outset and at reporting intervals | Mobility current status |
| G8979 | Mobility: walking & moving around functional limitation, projected goal status, at therapy episode outset, at reporting intervals, and at discharge or to end reporting | Mobility goal status |
| G8980 | Mobility: walking & moving around functional limitation, discharge status, at discharge from therapy or to end reporting | Mobility D/C status |
| **Changing & Maintaining Body Position G-code Set** | | |
| G8981 | Changing & maintaining body position functional limitation, current status, at therapy episode outset and at reporting intervals | Body pos current status |
| G8982 | Changing & maintaining body position functional limitation, projected goal status, at therapy episode outset, at reporting intervals, and at discharge or to end reporting | Body pos goal status |
| G8983 | Changing & maintaining body position functional limitation, discharge status, at discharge from therapy or to end reporting | Body pos D/C status |
| **Carrying, Moving & Handling Objects G-code Set** | | |
| G8984 | Carrying, moving & handling objects functional limitation, current status, at therapy episode outset and at reporting intervals | Carry current status |
| G8985 | Carrying, moving & handling objects functional limitation, projected goal status, at therapy episode outset, at reporting intervals, and at discharge or to end reporting | Carry goal status |
| G8986 | Carrying, moving & handling objects functional limitation, discharge status, at discharge from therapy or to end reporting | Carry D/C status |
| **Self Care G-code Set** | | |
| G8987 | Self care functional limitation, current status, at therapy episode outset and at reporting intervals | Self care current status |
| G8988 | Self care functional limitation, projected goal status, at therapy episode outset, at reporting intervals, and at discharge or to end reporting | Self care goal status |
| G8989 | Self care functional limitation, discharge status, at discharge from therapy or to end reporting | Self care D/C status |

- The following "other PT/OT" functional G-codes are used to report:
- a beneficiary's functional limitation that is not defined by one of the above four categories;
- a beneficiary whose therapy services are not intended to treat a functional limitation;
- or a beneficiary's functional limitation when an overall, composite or other score from a functional assessment too is used and it does not clearly represent a functional limitation defined by one of the above four code sets.

| | Long Descriptor | Short Descriptor |
|---|---|---|
| **Other PT/OT Primary G-code Set** | | |
| G8990 | Other physical or occupational therapy primary functional limitation, current status, at therapy episode outset and at reporting intervals | Other PT/OT current status |
| G8991 | Other physical or occupational therapy primary functional limitation, projected goal status, at therapy episode outset, at reporting intervals, and at discharge or to end reporting | Other PT/OT goal status |
| G8992 | Other physical or occupational therapy primary functional limitation, discharge status, at discharge from therapy or to end reporting | Other PT/OT D/C status |
| **Other PT/OT Subsequent G-code Set** | | |
| G8993 | Other physical or occupational therapy subsequent functional limitation, current status, at therapy episode outset and at reporting intervals | Sub PT/OT current status |
| G8994 | Other physical or occupational therapy subsequent functional limitation, projected goal status, at therapy episode outset, at reporting intervals, and at discharge or to end reporting | Sub PT/OT goal status |

| | Long Descriptor | Short Descriptor |
|---|---|---|
| G8995 | Other physical or occupational subsequent functional limitation, discharge from therapy or end reporting. | Sub PT/OT D/C status |

The following G-codes are for functional limitations typically seen in beneficiaries receiving SLP services. Seven are for specific functional communication measures, which are modeled after the National Outcomes Measurement System (NOMS), and one is for any "other" measure not described by one of the other seven.

| | Long Descriptor | Short Descriptor |
|---|---|---|
| **Swallowing G-code Set** | | |
| G8996 | Swallowing functional limitation, current status, at therapy episode outset and at reporting intervals | Swallow current status |
| G8997 | Swallowing functional limitation, projected goal status, at therapy episode outset, at reporting intervals, and at discharge or to end reporting | Swallow goal status |
| G8998 | Swallowing functional limitation, discharge status, at discharge from therapy or to end reporting | Swallow D/C status |
| **Motor Speech G-code Set (Note: These codes are not sequentially numbered)** | | |
| G8999 | Motor speech functional limitation, current status, at therapy episode outset and at reporting intervals | Motor speech current status |
| G9186 | Motor speech functional limitation, projected goal status at therapy episode outset, at reporting intervals, and at discharge or to end reporting | Motor speech goal status |
| G9158 | Motor speech functional limitation, discharge status, at discharge from therapy or to end reporting | Motor speech D/C status |
| **Spoken Language Comprehension G-code Set** | | |
| G9159 | Spoken language comprehension functional limitation, current status, at therapy episode outset and at reporting intervals | Lang comp current status |
| G9160 | Spoken language comprehension functional limitation, projected goal status, at therapy episode outset, at reporting intervals, and at discharge or to end reporting | Lang comp goal status |
| G9161 | Spoken language comprehension functional limitation, discharge status, at discharge from therapy or to end reporting | Lang comp D/C status |
| **Spoken Language Expressive G-code Set** | | |
| G9162 | Spoken language expression functional limitation, current status, at therapy episode outset and at reporting intervals | Lang express current status |
| G9163 | Spoken language expression functional limitation, projected goal status, at therapy episode outset, at reporting intervals, and at discharge or to end reporting | Lang press goal status |
| G9164 | Spoken language expression functional limitation, discharge status, at discharge from therapy or to end reporting | Lang express D/C status |
| **Attention G-code Set** | | |
| G9165 | Attention functional limitation, current status, at therapy episode outset and at reporting intervals | Atten current status |
| G9166 | Attention functional limitation, projected goal status, at therapy episode outset, at reporting intervals, and at discharge or to end reporting | Atten goal status |
| G9167 | Attention functional limitation, discharge status, at discharge from therapy or to end reporting | Atten D/C status |
| **Memory G-code Set** | | |
| G9168 | Memory functional limitation, current status, at therapy episode outset and at reporting intervals | Memory current status |
| G9169 | Memory functional limitation, projected goal status, at therapy episode outset, at reporting intervals, and at discharge or to end reporting | Memory goal status |
| G9170 | Memory functional limitation, discharge status, at discharge from therapy or to end reporting | Memory D/C status |
| **Voice G-code Set** | | |
| G9171 | Voice functional limitation, current status, at therapy episode outset and at reporting intervals | Voice current status |

| | Long Descriptor | Short Descriptor |
|---|---|---|
| G9172 | Voice functional limitation, projected goal status, at therapy episode outset, at reporting intervals, and at discharge or to end reporting | Voice goal status |
| G9173 | Voice functional limitation, discharge status, at discharge from therapy or to end reporting | Voice D/C status |

The following "other SLP" G-code set is used to report:

- on one of the other eight NOMS-defined functional measures not described by the above code sets; or
- to report an overall, composite or other score from assessment tool that does not clearly represent one of the above seven categorical SLP functional measures.

| | Long Descriptor | Short Descriptor |
|---|---|---|
| **Other Speech Language Pathology G-code Set** | | |
| G9174 | Other speech language pathology functional limitation, current status, at therapy episode outset and at reporting intervals | Speech lang current status |
| G9175 | Other speech language pathology functional limitation, projected goal status, at therapy episode outset, at reporting intervals, and at discharge or to end reporting | Speech lang goal status |
| G9176 | Other speech language pathology functional limitation, discharge status, at discharge from therapy or to end reporting | Speech lang D/C status |

**F. Severity/Complexity Modifiers**

For each nonpayable functional G-code, one of the modifiers listed below must be used to report the severity/complexity for that functional limitation.

| Modifier | Impairment Limitation Restriction |
|---|---|
| CH | 0 percent impaired, limited or restricted |
| CI | At least 1 percent but less than 20 percent impaired, limited or restricted |
| CJ | At least 20 percent but less than 40 percent impaired, limited or restricted |
| CK | At least 40 percent but less than 60 percent impaired, limited or restricted |
| CL | At least 60 percent but less than 80 percent impaired, limited or restricted |
| CM | At least 80 percent but less than 100 percent impaired, limited or restricted |
| CN | 100 percent impaired, limited or restricted |

The severity modifiers reflect the beneficiary's percentage of functional impairment as determined by the clinician furnishing the therapy services.

**G. Required Reporting of Functional G-codes and Severity Modifiers**

The functional G-codes and severity modifiers listed above are used in the required reporting on therapy claims at certain specified points during therapy episodes of care. Claims containing these functional G-codes must also contain another billable and separately payable (non-bundled) service. Only one functional limitation shall be reported at a given time for each related therapy plan of care (POC).

Functional reporting using the G-codes and corresponding severity modifiers is required reporting on specified therapy claims. Specifically, they are required on claims:

- At the outset of a therapy episode of care (i.e., on the claim for the date of service (DOS) of the initial therapy service);
- At least once every 10 treatment days, which corresponds with the progress reporting period;
- When an evaluative procedure, including a re-evaluative one, (HCPCS/CPT codes 92521, 92522, 92523, 92524, 92597, 92607, 92608, 92610, 92611, 92612, 92614, 92616, 96105, 96125, 97161, 97162, 97163, 97164, 97165, 97166, 97167, 97168) is furnished and billed;
- At the time of discharge from the therapy episode of care–(i.e., on the date services related to the discharge [progress] report are furnished); and
- At the time reporting of a particular functional limitation is ended in cases where the need for further therapy is necessary.
- At the time reporting is begun for a new or different functional limitation within the same episode of care (i.e., after the reporting of the prior functional limitation is ended)

Functional reporting is required on claims throughout the entire episode of care. When the beneficiary has reached his or her goal or progress has been maximized on the initially selected functional limitation, but the need for treatment continues, reporting is required for a second functional limitation using another set of G-codes. In these situations two or more functional limitations will be reported for a

CPT © 2017 American Medical Association. All Rights Reserved.

© 2017 Optum360, LLC

beneficiary during the therapy episode of care. Thus, reporting on more than one functional limitation may be required for some beneficiaries but not simultaneously.

When the beneficiary stops coming to therapy prior to discharge, the clinician should report the functional information on the last claim. If the clinician is unaware that the beneficiary is not returning for therapy until after the last claim is submitted, the clinician cannot report the discharge status.

When functional reporting is required on a claim for therapy services, two G-codes will generally be required.

Two exceptions exist:

1. Therapy services under more than one therapy POC. Claims may contain more than two nonpayable functional G-codes when in cases where a beneficiary receives therapy services under multiple POCs (PT, OT, and/or SLP) from the same therapy provider.

2. One-Time Therapy Visit. When a beneficiary is seen and future therapy services are either not medically indicated or are going to be furnished by another provider, the clinician reports on the claim for the DOS of the visit, all three G-codes in the appropriate code set (current status, goal status and discharge status), along with corresponding severity modifiers. Each reported functional G-code must also contain the following line of service information:

- Functional severity modifier

- Therapy modifier indicating the related discipline/POC -- GP, GO or GN -- for PT, OT, and SLP services, respectively

- Date of the related therapy service

- Nominal charge, e.g., a penny, for institutional claims submitted to the FIs and A/MACs. For professional claims, a zero charge is acceptable for the service line. If provider billing software requires an amount for professional claims, a nominal charge, e.g., a penny, may be included. Note: The KX modifier is not required on the claim line for nonpayable G-codes, but would be required with the procedure code for medically necessary therapy services furnished once the beneficiary's annual cap has been reached.

The following example demonstrates how the G-codes and modifiers are used. In this example, the clinician determines that the beneficiary's mobility restriction is the most clinically relevant functional limitation and selects the Mobility G-code set (G8978 – G8980) to represent the beneficiary's functional limitation. The clinician also determines the severity/complexity of the beneficiary's functional limitation and selects the appropriate modifier. In this example, the clinician determines that the beneficiary has a 75 percent mobility restriction for which the CL modifier is applicable. The clinician expects that at the end of therapy the beneficiaries will have only a 15 percent mobility restriction for which the CI modifier is applicable. When the beneficiary attains the mobility goal, therapy continues to be medically necessary to addresss a functional limitation for which there is no categorical G-code. The clinician reports this using (G8990 – G8992).

At the outset of therapy. On the DOS for which the initial evaluative procedure is furnished or the initial treatment day of a therapy POC, the claim for the service will also include two G-codes as shown below.

- G8978-CL to report the functional limitation (Mobility with current mobility limitation of "at least 60 percent but less than 80 percent impaired, limited or restricted")

- G8979-CI to report the projected goal for a mobility restriction of "at least 1 percent but less than 20 percent impaired, limited or restricted."

At the end of each progress reporting period. On the claim for the DOS when the services related to the progress report (which must be done at least once each 10 treatment days) are furnished, the clinician will report the same two G-codes but the modifier for the current status may be different.

- G8978 with the appropriate modifier are reported to show the beneficiary's current status as of this DOS. So if thebeneficiary has made no progress, this claim will include G8978-CL. If the beneficiary made progress and now has a mobility restriction of 65 percent CL would still be the appropriate modifier for 65 percent, and G8978-CL would be reported in this case. If the beneficiary now has a mobility restriction of 45 percent, G8978-CK would be reported.

- G8979-CI would be reported to show the projected goal. This severity modifier would not change unless the clinician adjusts the beneficiary's goal. This step is repeated as necessary and clinically appropriate, adjusting the current status modifier used as the beneficiary progresses through therapy.

- At the time the beneficiary is discharged from the therapy episode. The final claim for therapy episode will include two G-codes.

- G8979-CI would be reported to show the projected goal. G8980-CI would be reported if the beneficiary attained the 15 percent mobility goal. Alternatively, if the beneficiary's mobility restriction only reached 25 percent; G8980-CJ would be reported. To end reporting of one functional limitation. As noted above, functional reporting is required to continue throughout the entire episode of care. Accordingly, when further therapy is medically necessary after the beneficiary attains the goal for the first reported functional limitation, the clinician would end reporting of the first functional limitation by using the same G-codes and modifiers that would be used at the time of discharge. Using the mobility example, to end reporting of the mobility functional limitation, G8979-CI and G8980-CI would be reported on the same DOS that coincides with end of that progress reporting period.

To begin reporting of a second functional limitation. At the time reporting is begun for a new and different functional limitation, within the same episode of care (i.e., after the reporting of the prior functional limitation is ended). Reporting on the second functional limitation, however, is not begun until the DOS of the next treatment day -- which is day one of the new progress reporting period. When the next functional limitation to be reported is NOT defined by one of the other three PT/OT categorical codes, the G-code set (G8990 - G8992) for the "other PT/OT primary" functional limitation is used, rather than the G-code set for the "other PT/OT subsequent" because it is the first reported "other PT/OT" functional limitation. This reporting begins on the DOS of the first treatment day following the mobility "discharge" reporting, which is counted as the initial service for the "other PT/OT primary" functional limitation and the first treatment day of the new progress reporting period. In this case, G8990 and G8991, along with the corresponding modifiers, are reported on the claim for therapy services.

The table below illustrates when reporting is required using this example and what G-codes would be used.

Example of Required Reporting

| Key: Reporting Period (RP) | Begin RP #1 for Mobility at Episode Outset | End RP#1for Mobility at Progress Report | Mobility RP #2 Begins Next Treatment Day | End RP#2 for Mobility at Progress Report | Mobility RP #3 Begins Next Treatment Day | D/C or End Reporting for \Mobility | Begin RP #1 for Other PT/OT Primary |
|---|---|---|---|---|---|---|---|
| Mobility: Walking & Moving Around | | | | | | | |
| G8978 – Current Status | X | X | | X | | | |
| G 8979– Goal Status | X | X | | X | | X | |
| G8980 – Discharge Status | | | | | | X | |
| Other PT/OT Primary | | | | | | | |
| G8990 – Current Status | | | | | | | X |
| G8991 – Goal Status | | | | | | | X |
| G8992 – Discharge Status | | | | | | | |
| No Functional Reporting Req'd | | | X | | X | | |

### H. Required Tracking and Documentation of Functional G-codes and Severity Modifiers

The clinician who furnishes the services must not only report the functional information on the therapy claim, but, he/she must track and document the G-codes and severity modifiers used for this reporting in the beneficiary's medical record of therapy services.

For details related to the documentation requirements, refer to Pub. 100-02, Medicare Benefit Policy Manual, chapter 15, section 220.4, - MCTRJCA-required Functional Reporting. For coverage rules related to MCTRJCA and therapy goals, refer to Pub. 100-02: a) for outpatient therapy services, see chapter 15, section 220.1.2 B and b) for instructions specific to PT, OT, and SLP services in the CORF, see chapter 12, section 10.

## 100-4, 5, 20.2

### Reporting of Service Units With HCPCS

(Rev. 3670, Issued: 12-01-16, Effective: 01-01-17, Implementation: 01-03-17)

#### A. General

Effective with claims submitted on or after April 1, 1998, providers billing on the ASC X12 837 institutional claim format or Form CMS-1450 were required to report the number of units for outpatient rehabilitation services based on the procedure or service, e.g., based on the HCPCS code reported instead of the revenue code. This was already in

effect for billing on the Form CMS-1500, and CORFs were required to report their full range of CORF services on the institutional claim. These unit-reporting requirements continue with the standards required for electronically submitting health care claims under the Health Insurance Portability and Accountability Act of 1996 (HIPAA) - the currently adopted version of the ASC X12 837 transaction standards and implementation guides. The Administrative Simplification Compliance Act mandates that claims that are sent to Medicare electronically unless certain exceptions are met.

#### B. Timed and Untimed Codes

When reporting service units for HCPCS codes where the procedure is not defined by a specific timeframe ("untimed" HCPCS), the provider enters "1" in the field labeled units. For timed codes, units are reported based on the number of times the procedure is performed, as described in the HCPCS code definition.

EXAMPLE: A beneficiary received a speech-language pathology evaluation represented by HCPCS "untimed" code 92521. Regardless of the number of minutes spent providing this service only one unit of service is appropriately billed on the same day.

Several CPT codes used for therapy modalities, procedures, and tests and measurements specify that the direct (one on one) time spent in patient contact is 15 minutes. Providers report these "timed" procedure codes for services delivered on any single calendar day using CPT codes and the appropriate number of 15 minute units of service.

**EXAMPLE:** A beneficiary received a total of 60 minutes of occupational therapy, e.g., HCPCS "timed" code 97530 which is defined in 15 minute units, on a given date of service. The provider would then report 4 units of 97530.

### C. Counting Minutes for Timed Codes in 15 Minute Units

When only one service is provided in a day, providers should not bill for services performed for less than 8 minutes. For any single timed CPT code in the same day measured in 15 minute units, providers bill a single 15-minute unit for treatment greater than or equal to 8 minutes through and including 22 minutes. If the duration of a single modality or procedure in a day is greater than or equal to 23 minutes, through and including 37 minutes, then 2 units should be billed. Time intervals for 1 through 8 units are as follows:

**Units Number of Minutes**

1 unit: ≥ 8 minutes through 22 minutes

2 units:≥ 23 minutes through 37 minutes

3 units:≥ 38 minutes through 52 minutes

4 units:≥ 53 minutes through 67 minutes

5 units:≥ 68 minutes through 82 minutes

6 units:≥ 83 minutes through 97 minutes

7 units:≥ 98 minutes through 112 minutes

8 units:≥ 113 minutes through 127 minutes

The pattern remains the same for treatment times in excess of 2 hours.

If a service represented by a 15 minute timed code is performed in a single day for at least 15 minutes, that service shall be billed for at least one unit. If the service is performed for at least 30 minutes, that service shall be billed for at least two units, etc. It is not appropriate to count all minutes of treatment in a day toward the units for one code if other services were performed for more than 15 minutes. See examples 2 and 3 below.

When more than one service represented by 15 minute timed codes is performed in a single day, the total number of minutes of service (as noted on the chart above) determines the number of timed units billed. See example 1 below.

If any 15 minute timed service that is performed for 7 minutes or less than 7 minutes on the same day as another 15 minute timed service that was also performed for 7 minutes or less and the total time of the two is 8 minutes or greater than 8 minutes, then bill one unit for the service performed for the most minutes. This is correct because the total time is greater than the minimum time for one unit. The same logic is applied when three or more different services are provided for 7 minutes or less than 7 minutes. See example 5 below.

The expectation (based on the work values for these codes) is that a provider's direct patient contact time for each unit will average 15 minutes in length. If a provider has a consistent practice of billing less than 15 minutes for a unit, these situations should be highlighted for review.

If more than one 15 minute timed CPT code is billed during a single calendar day, then the total number of timed units that can be billed is constrained by the total treatment minutes for that day. See all examples below.

Pub. 100-02, Medicare Benefit Policy Manual, Chapter 15, Section 220.3B, Documentation Requirements for Therapy Services, indicates that the amount of time for each specific intervention/modality provided to the patient is not required to be documented in the Treatment Note. However, the total number of timed minutes must be documented. These examples indicate how to count the appropriate number of units for the total therapy minutes provided.

Example 1 –

24 minutes of neuromuscular reeducation, code 97112,

23 minutes of therapeutic exercise, code 97110,

Total timed code treatment time was 47 minutes.

See the chart above. The 47 minutes falls within the range for 3 units = 38 to 52 minutes.

Appropriate billing for 47 minutes is only 3 timed units. Each of the codes is performed for more than 15 minutes, so each shall be billed for at least 1 unit. The correct coding is 2 units of code 97112 and one unit of code 97110, assigning more timed units to the service that took the most time.

Example 2 –

20 minutes of neuromuscular reeducation (97112)

20 minutes therapeutic exercise (97110),

40 Total timed code minutes.

Appropriate billing for 40 minutes is 3 units. Each service was done at least 15 minutes and should be billed for at least one unit, but the total allows 3 units. Since the time for each service is the same, choose either code for 2 units and bill the other for 1 unit. Do not bill 3 units for either one of the codes.

Example 3 –

33 minutes of therapeutic exercise (97110),

7 minutes of manual therapy (97140),

40 Total timed minutes

Appropriate billing for 40 minutes is for 3 units. Bill 2 units of 97110 and 1 unit of 97140. Count the first 30 minutes of 97110 as two full units. Compare the remaining time for 97110 (33-30 = 3 minutes) to the time spent on 97140 (7 minutes) and bill the larger, which is 97140.

Example 4 –

18 minutes of therapeutic exercise (97110),

13 minutes of manual therapy (97140),

10 minutes of gait training (97116),

8 minutes of ultrasound (97035),

49 Total timed minutes

Appropriate billing is for 3 units. Bill the procedures you spent the most time providing. Bill 1 unit each of 97110, 97116, and 97140. You are unable to bill for the ultrasound because the total time of timed units that can be billed is constrained by the total timed code treatment minutes (i.e., you may not bill 4 units for less than 53 minutes regardless of how many services were performed). You would still document the ultrasound in the treatment notes.

Example 5 –

7 minutes of neuromuscular reeducation (97112)

7 minutes therapeutic exercise (97110)

7 minutes manual therapy (97140)

21 Total timed minutes

Appropriate billing is for one unit. The qualified professional (See definition in Pub. 100-02, chapter 15, section 220) shall select one appropriate CPT code (97112, 97110, 97140) to bill since each unit was performed for the same amount of time and only one unit is allowed.

**NOTE:** The above schedule of times is intended to provide assistance in rounding time into 15-minute increments. It does not imply that any minute until the eighth should be excluded from the total count. The total minutes of active treatment counted for all 15 minute timed codes includes all direct treatment time for the timed codes. Total treatment minutes - including minutes spent providing services represented by untimed codes - are also documented. For documentation in the medical record of the services provided see Pub. 100-02, chapter 15, section 220.3.

### D. Specific Limits for HCPCS

The Deficit Reduction Act of 2005, section 5107 requires the implementation of clinically appropriate code edits to eliminate improper payments for outpatient therapy services. The following codes may be billed, when covered, only at or below the number of units indicated on the chart per treatment day. When higher amounts of units are billed than those indicated in the table below, the units on the claim line that exceed the limit shall be denied as medically unnecessary (according to 1862(a)(1)(A)). Denied claims may be appealed and an ABN is appropriate to notify the beneficiary of liability.

This chart does not include all of the codes identified as therapy codes; refer to section 20 of this chapter for further detail on these and other therapy codes. For example, therapy codes called "always therapy" must always be accompanied by therapy modifiers identifying the type of therapy plan of care under which the service is provided.

Use the chart in the following manner:

The codes that are allowed one unit for "Allowed Units" in the chart below may be billed no more than once per provider, per discipline, per date of service, per patient.

The codes allowed 0 units in the column for "Allowed Units", may not be billed under a plan of care indicated by the discipline in that column. Some codes may be billed by one discipline (e.g., PT) and not by others (e.g., OT or SLP).

When physicians/NPPs bill "always therapy" codes they must follow the policies of the type of therapy they are providing e.g., utilize a plan of care, bill with the appropriate

therapy modifier (GP, GO, GN), bill the allowed units on the chart below for PT, OT or SLP depending on the plan. A physician/NPP shall not bill an "always therapy" code unless the service is provided under a therapy plan of care. Therefore, NA stands for "Not Applicable" in the chart below.

When a "sometimes therapy" code is billed by a physician/NPP, but as a medical service, and not under a therapy plan of care, the therapy modifier shall not be used, but the number of units billed must not exceed the number of units indicated in the chart below per patient, per provider/supplier, per day.

**NOTE:** As of April 1, 2017, the chart below uses the CPT Consumer Friendly Code Descriptions which are intended only to assist the reader in identifying the service related to the CPT/HCPCS code. The reader is reminded that these descriptions cannot be used in place of the CPT long descriptions which officially define each of the services. The table below no longer contains a column noting whether a code is "timed" or "untimed" as this notation is not relevant to the number of units allowed

CPT © 2017 American Medical Association. All Rights Reserved.

© 2017 Optum360, LLC

per code on claims for the listed therapy services. We note that the official long descriptors for the CPT codes can be found in the latest CPT code book.

| CPT/ HCPCS Code | CPT Consumer Friendly Code Descriptions and Claim Line Outlier/Edit Details | PT Allowed Units | OT Allowed Units | SLP Allowed Units | Physician /NPP Not Under Therapy POC |
|---|---|---|---|---|---|
| 92521 | Evaluation of speech fluency | 0 | 0 | 1 | NA |
| 92522 | Evaluation of speech sound production | 0 | 0 | 1 | NA |
| 92523 | Evaluation of speech sound production with evaluation of language comprehension and expression | 0 | 0 | 1 | NA |
| 92524 | Behavioral and qualitative analysis of voice and resonance | 0 | 0 | 1 | NA |
| 92597 | Evaluation for use and/or fitting of voice prosthetic device to supplement oral speech | 0 | 0 | 1 | NA |
| 92607 | Evaluation of patient with prescription of speech-generating and alternative communication device | 0 | 0 | 1 | NA |
| 92611 | Fluoroscopic and video recorded motion evaluation of swallowing function | 0 | 1 | 1 | 1 |
| 92612 | Evaluation and recording of swallowing using an endoscope Evaluation and recording of swallowing using an endoscope | 0 | 1 | 1 | 1 |
| 92614 | Evaluation and recording of voice box sensory function using an endoscope | 0 | 1 | 1 | 1 |
| 92616 | Evaluation and recording of swallowing and voice box sensory function using an endoscope | 0 | 1 | 1 | 1 |
| 95833 | Manual muscle testing of whole body | 1 | 1 | 0 | 1 |
| 95834 | Manual muscle testing of whole body including hands | 1 | 1 | 0 | 1 |
| 96110 | Developmental screening | 1 | 1 | 1 | 1 |
| 96111 | Developmental testing | 1 | 1 | 1 | 1 |
| 97161 | Evaluation of physical therapy, typically 20 minutes | 1 | 0 | 0 | NA |
| 97162 | Evaluation of physical therapy, typically 30 minutes | 1 | 0 | 0 | NA |
| 97163 | Evaluation of physical therapy, typically 45 minutes | 1 | 0 | 0 | NA |
| 97164 | Re-evaluation of physical therapy, typically 20 minutes | 1 | 0 | 0 | NA |
| 97165 | Evaluation of occupational therapy, typically 30 minutes | 0 | 1 | 0 | NA |
| 97166 | Evaluation of occupational therapy, typically 45 minutes | 0 | 1 | 0 | NA |
| 97167 | Evaluation of occupational therapy, typically 60 minutes | 0 | 1 | 0 | NA |
| 97168 | Re-evaluation of occupational therapy established plan of care, typically 30 minutes | 0 | 1 | 0 | NA |

## 100-04, 8, 140.1

### Payment for ESRD-Related Services Under the Monthly Capitation Payment (Center Based Patients)

Physicians and practitioners managing center based patients on dialysis are paid a monthly rate for most outpatient dialysis-related physician services furnished to a Medicare ESRD beneficiary. The payment amount varies based on the number of visits provided within each month and the age of the ESRD beneficiary. Under this methodology, separate codes are billed for providing one visit per month, two to three visits per month and four or more visits per month. The lowest payment amount applies when a physician provides one visit per month; a higher payment is provided for two to three visits per month. To receive the highest payment amount, a physician or practitioner would have to provide at least four ESRD-related visits per

month. The MCP is reported once per month for services performed in an outpatient setting that are related to the patients' ESRD.

The physician or practitioner who provides the complete assessment, establishes the patient's plan of care, and provides the ongoing management is the physician or practitioner who submits the bill for the monthly service.

a. Month defined.

For purposes of billing for physician and practitioner ESRD related services, the term 'month' means a calendar month. The first month the beneficiary begins dialysis treatments is the date the dialysis treatments begin through the end of the calendar month. Thereafter, the term 'month' refers to a calendar month.

b. Determination of the age of beneficiary.

The beneficiary's age at the end of the month is the age of the patient for determining the appropriate age related ESRD-related services code.

c. Qualifying Visits Under the MCP

- General policy.

Visits must be furnished face-to-face by a physician, clinical nurse specialist, nurse practitioner, or physician's assistant.

- Visits furnished by another physician or practitioner (who is not the MCP physician or practitioner).

The MCP physician or practitioner may use other physicians or qualified nonphysician practitioners to provide some of the visits during the month. The MCP physician or practitioner does not have to be present when these other physicians or practitioners provide visits. In this instance, the rules are consistent with the requirements for hospital split/shared evaluation and management visits. The non-MCP physician or practitioner must be a partner, an employee of the same group practice, or an employee of the MCP physician or practitioner. For example, the physician or practitioner furnishing visits under the MCP may be either a W-2 employee or 1099 independent contractor.

When another physician is used to furnish some of the visits during the month, the physician who provides the complete assessment, establishes the patient's plan of care, and provides the ongoing management should bill for the MCP service.

If the nonphysician practitioner is the practitioner who performs the complete assessment and establishes the plan of care, then the MCP service should be billed under the PIN of the clinical nurse specialist, nurse practitioner, or physician assistant.

- Residents, interns and fellows.

Patient visits by residents, interns and fellows enrolled in an approved Medicare graduate medical education (GME) program may be counted towards the MCP visits if the teaching MCP physician is present during the visit.

- Patients designated/admitted as hospital observation status.

ESRD-related visits furnished to patients in hospital observation status that occur on or after January 1, 2005, should be counted for purposes of billing the MCP codes. Visits furnished to patients in hospital observation status are included when submitting MCP claims for ESRD-related services.

- ESRD-related visits furnished to beneficiaries residing in a SNF.

ESRD-related visits furnished to beneficiaries residing in a SNF should be counted for purposes of billing the MCP codes.

- SNF residents admitted as an inpatient.

Inpatient visits are not counted for purposes of the MCP service. If the beneficiary residing in a SNF is admitted to the hospital as an inpatient, the appropriate inpatient visit code should be billed.

- ESRD Related Visits as a Telehealth Service

ESRD-related services with 2 or 3 visits per month and ESRD-related services with 4 or more visits per month may be furnished as a telehealth service. However, at least one visit per month is required in person to examine the vascular access site. A clinical examination of the vascular access site must be furnished face-to-face (not as a telehealth service) by a physician, nurse practitioner or physician's assistant. For more information on how ESRD-related visits may be furnished as a Medicare telehealth service and for general Medicare telehealth policy see Pub. 100-2, Medicare Benefit Policy manual, chapter 15, section 270. For claims processing instructions see Pub. 100-4, Medicare Claims Processing manual chapter 12, section 190.

## 100-04, 8, 140.1.1

### Payment for Managing Patients on Home Dialysis

Physicians and practitioners managing ESRD patients who dialyze at home are paid a single monthly rate based on the age of the beneficiary. The MCP physician (or practitioner) must furnish at least one face-to-face patient visit per month for the home dialysis MCP service. Documentation by the MCP physician (or practitioner) should support at least one face-to-face encounter per month with the home dialysis patient. Medicare contractors may waive the requirement for a monthly face-to-face visit for the home dialysis MCP service on a case by case basis, for example, when the nephrologist's notes indicate that the physician actively and adequately managed

© 2017 Optum360, LLC

CPT © 2017 American Medical Association. All Rights Reserved.

the care of the home dialysis patient throughout the month. The management of home dialysis patients who remain a home dialysis patient the entire month should be coded using the ESRD-related services for home dialysis patients HCPCS codes.

When another physician is used to furnish some of the visits during the month, the physician who provides the complete assessment, establishes the patient's plan of care, and provides the ongoing management should bill for the MCP service.

If the nonphysician practitioner is the practitioner who performs the complete assessment and establishes the plan of care, then the MCP service should be billed under the PIN of the clinical nurse specialist, nurse practitioner, or physician assistant.

Residents, interns and fellows. Patient visits by residents, interns and fellows enrolled in an approved Medicare graduate medical education (GME) program may be counted towards the MCP visits if the teaching MCP physician is present during the visit.

a. Month defined.

For purposes of billing for physician and practitioner ESRD related services, the term 'month' means a calendar month. The first month the beneficiary begins dialysis treatments is the date the dialysis treatments begin through the end of the calendar month. Thereafter, the term 'month' refers to a calendar month.

b. Qualifying Visits under the MCP

- General policy.

Visits must be furnished face-to-face by a physician, clinical nurse specialist, nurse practitioner, or physician's assistant.

- Visits furnished by another physician or practitioner (who is not the MCP physician or practitioner).

The MCP physician or practitioner may use other physicians or qualified nonphysician practitioners to provide the visit(s) during the month. The MCP physician or practitioner does not have to be present when these other physicians or practitioners provide visit(s). The non-MCP physician or practitioner must be a partner, an employee of the same group practice, or an employee of the MCP physician or practitioner. For example, the physician or practitioner furnishing visits under the MCP may be either a W-2 employee or 1099 independent contractor.

When another physician is used to furnish some of the visits during the month, the physician who provides the complete assessment, establishes the patient's plan of care, and provides the ongoing management should bill for the MCP service.

If the nonphysician practitioner is the practitioner who performs the complete assessment and establishes the plan of care, then the MCP service should be billed under the PIN of the clinical nurse specialist, nurse practitioner, or physician assistant.

- Residents, interns and fellows.

Patient visits by residents, interns and fellows enrolled in an approved Medicare graduate medical education (GME) program may be counted towards the MCP visits if the teaching MCP physician is present during the visit.

## 100-4, 8, 180

### Noninvasive Studies for ESRD Patients - Facility and Physician Services

(Rev. 3650, Issued: 11-10-16, Effective: 02-10-17, Implementation: 02-10-17)

For Medicare coverage of noninvasive vascular studies, see the Medicare Benefit Policy Manual, Chapter 11.

For dialysis to take place there must be a means of access so that the exchange of waste products may occur. As part of the dialysis treatment, ESRD facilities are responsible for monitoring access, and when occlusions occur, either declot the access or refer the patient for appropriate treatment. Procedures associated with monitoring access involve taking venous pressure, aspirating thrombus, observing elevated recirculation time, reduced urea reduction ratios, or collapsed shunt, etc. All such procedures are covered under the composite rate.

ESRD facilities may not monitor access through noninvasive vascular studies such as duplex and Doppler flow scans and bill separately for these procedures. Noninvasive vascular studies are not covered as a separately billable service if used to monitor a patient's vascular access site.

Medicare pays for the technical component of the procedure in the composite payment rate.

Where there are signs and symptoms of vascular access problems, Doppler flow studies may be used as a means to obtain diagnostic information to permit medical intervention to address the problem. Doppler flow studies may be considered medically necessary in the presence of signs or symptoms of possible failure of the ESRD patient's vascular access site, and when the results are used in determining the clinical course of the treatment for the patient.

The only Current Procedural Terminology (CPT) billing code for noninvasive vascular testing of a hemodialysis access site is 93990. A/B MACs (B) must deny separate billing of the technical component of this code if it is performed on any patient for whom the ESRD composite rate for dialysis is being paid, unless there is appropriate medical indication of the need for a Doppler flow study.

When a dialysis patient exhibits signs and symptoms of compromise to the vascular access site, Doppler flow studies may provide diagnostic information that will determine the appropriate medical intervention. Medicare considers a Doppler flow study medically necessary when the beneficiary's dialysis access site manifests signs or symptoms associated with vascular compromise, and when the results of this test are necessary to determine the clinical course of treatment.

Examples supporting the medical necessity for Doppler flow studies include:

a. Elevated dynamic venous pressure >200mm HG when measured during dialysis with the blood pump set on a 200cc/min.,

b. Access recirculation of 12 percent or greater,

c. An otherwise unexplained urea reduction ration <60 oercebtm abd

d. An access with a palpable "water hammer" pulse on examination, (which implies venous outflow obstruction).

Unless the documentation is provided supporting the necessity of more than one study, Medicare will limit payment to either a Doppler flow study or an arteriogram (fistulogram, venogram), but not both.

An example of when both studies may be clinically necessary is when a Doppler flow study demonstrates reduced flow (blood flow rate less than 800cc/min or a decreased flow of 25 percent or greater from previous study) and the physician requires an arteriogram to further define the extent of the problem. The patient's medical record(s) must provide documentation supporting the need for more than one imaging study.

This policy is applicable to claims from ESRD facilities and all other sources, such as independent diagnostic testing facilities, and hospital outpatient departments.

A/B MACs (B) shall develop LMRP for Doppler flow studies if this service meets the criteria listed in the Medicare Program Integrity Manual, Chapter 1. This provides guidance to contractors on the scope, purpose, and meaning of LMRP.

The professional component of the procedure is included in the monthly capitation payment (MCP) (See §140 above.) The professional component should be denied for code 93990 if billed by the MCP physician. Medically necessary services that are included or bundled into the MCP (e.g., test interpretations) are separately payable when furnished by physicians other than the MCP physician.

The contractor shall use the following remittance advice messages and associated codes when rejecting/denying claims under this policy. This CARC/RARC combination is compliant with CAQH CORE Business Scenario Four.

Group Code: CO
CARC: 24
RARC: N/A
MSN:16.32

Billing for monitoring of hemodialysis access using CPT codes for noninvasive vascular studies other than 93990 is considered a misrepresentation of the service actually

provided and contractors will consider this action for fraud investigation. They will conduct data analysis on a periodic basis for noninvasive diagnostic studies of the extremities (including CPT codes 93922, 93923, 93924, 93925, 93926, 93930, 93931, 93965, 93970, 93971). Contractors should handle aberrant findings under normal program safeguard processes by taking whatever corrective action is deemed necessary.

## 100-04, 9, 182

### Medical Nutrition Therapy (MNT) Services

#### A - FQHCs

Previously, MNT type services were considered incident to services under the FQHC benefit, if all relevant program requirements were met. Therefore, separate all-inclusive encounter rate payment could not be made for the provision of MNT services. With passage of DRA, effective January 1, 2006, FQHCs are eligible for a separate payment under Part B for these services provided they meet all program requirements. Payment is made at the all-inclusive encounter rate to the FQHC. This payment can be in addition to payment for any other qualifying visit on the same date of service as the beneficiary received qualifying MNT services.

For FQHCs to qualify for a separate visit payment for MNT services, the services must be a one-on-one face-to-face encounter. Group sessions don't constitute a billable visit for any FQHC services. Rather, the cost of group sessions is included in the calculation of the all-inclusive FQHC visit rate. To receive payment for MNT services, the MNT services must be billed on TOB 73X with the appropriate individual MNT HCPCS code (codes 97802, 97803, or G0270) and with the appropriate site of service revenue code in the 052X revenue code series. This payment can be in addition to payment for any other qualifying visit on the same date of service as the beneficiary received qualifying MNT services as long as the claim for MNT services contain the appropriate coding specified above.

**NOTE:** MNT is not a qualifying visit on the same day that DSMT is provided.

Additional information on MNT can be found in Chapter 4, section 300 of this manual.

Group services (HCPCS 97804 or G0271) do not meet the criteria for a separate qualifying encounter. All line items billed on TOB 73x with HCPCS code 97804 or G0271 will be denied.

### B - RHCs

Separate payment to RHCs for these practitioners/services continues to be precluded as these services are not within the scope of Medicare-covered RHC benefits. All line items billed on TOB 71x with HCPCS codes for MNT services will be denied.

## 100-04, 11, 40.1.3

### Independent Attending Physician Services

When hospice coverage is elected, the beneficiary waives all rights to Medicare Part B payments for professional services that are related to the treatment and management of his/her terminal illness during any period his/her hospice benefit election is in force, except for professional services of an independent attending physician, who is not an employee of the designated hospice nor receives compensation from the hospice for those services. For purposes of administering the hospice benefit provisions, an "attending physician" means an individual who:

- Is a doctor of medicine or osteopathy or

- A nurse practitioner (for professional services related to the terminal illness that are furnished on or after December 8, 2003); and

- Is identified by the individual, at the time he/she elects hospice coverage, as having the most significant role in the determination and delivery of their medical care.

Hospices should reiterate with patients that they must not see independent physicians for care related to their terminal illness other than their independent attending physician unless the hospice arranges it.

Even though a beneficiary elects hospice coverage, he/she may designate and use an independent attending physician, who is not employed by nor receives compensation from the hospice for professional services furnished, in addition to the services of hospice-employed physicians. The professional services of an independent attending physician, who may be a nurse practitioner as defined in Chapter 9, that are reasonable and necessary for the treatment and management of a hospice patient's terminal illness are not considered Medicare Part A hospice services.

Where the service is related to the hospice patient's terminal illness but was furnished by someone other than the designated "attending physician" [or a physician substituting for the attending physician]) the physician or other provider must look to the hospice for payment.

Professional services related to the hospice patient's terminal condition that were furnished by an independent attending physician, who may be a nurse practitioner, are billed to the Medicare contractor through Medicare Part B. When the independent attending physician furnishes a terminal illness related service that includes both a professional and technical component (e.g., x-rays), he/she bills the professional component of such services to the Medicare contractor on a professional claim and looks to the hospice for payment for the technical component. Likewise, the independent attending physician, who may be a nurse practitioner, would look to the hospice for payment for terminal illness related services furnished that have no professional component (e.g., clinical lab tests). The remainder of this section explains this in greater detail.

When a Medicare beneficiary elects hospice coverage he/she may designate an attending physician, who may be a nurse practitioner, not employed by the hospice, in addition to receiving care from hospice-employed physicians. The professional services of a non-hospice affiliated attending physician for the treatment and management of a hospice patient's terminal illness are not considered Medicare Part A "hospice services." These independent attending physician services are billed through Medicare Part B to the Medicare contractor, provided they were not furnished under a payment arrangement with the hospice. The independent attending physician codes services with the GV modifier "Attending physician not employed or paid under agreement by the patient's hospice provider" when billing his/her professional services furnished for the treatment and management of a hospice patient's terminal condition. The Medicare contractor makes payment to the independent attending physician or beneficiary, as appropriate, based on the payment and deductible rules applicable to each covered service.

Payments for the services of an independent attending physician are not counted in determining whether the hospice cap amount has been exceeded because Part B services provided by an independent attending physician are not part of the hospice's care.

Services provided by an independent attending physician who may be a nurse practitioner must be coordinated with any direct care services provided by hospice physicians.

Only the direct professional services of an independent attending physician, who may be a nurse practitioner, to a patient may be billed; the costs for services such as lab or x-rays are not to be included in the bill.

If another physician covers for a hospice patient's designated attending physician, the services of the substituting physician are billed by the designated attending physician under the reciprocal or locum tenens billing instructions. In such instances, the attending physician bills using the GV modifier in conjunction with either the Q5 or Q6 modifier.

When services related to a hospice patient's terminal condition are furnished under a payment arrangement with the hospice by the designated attending physician who may be a nurse practitioner (i.e., by a non-independent physician/nurse practitioner), the physician must look to the hospice for payment. In this situation the physicians'

services are Part A hospice services and are billed by the hospice to its Medicare contractor.

Medicare contractors must process and pay for covered, medically necessary Part B services that physicians furnish to patients after their hospice benefits are revoked even if the patient remains under the care of the hospice. Such services are billed without the GV or GW modifiers. Make payment based on applicable Medicare payment and deductible rules for each covered service even if the beneficiary continues to be treated by the hospice after hospice benefits are revoked.

The CWF response contains the periods of hospice entitlement. This information is a permanent part of the notice and is furnished on all CWF replies and automatic notices. Medicare contractor use the CWF reply for validating dates of hospice coverage and to research, examine and adjudicate services coded with the GV or GW modifiers.

## 100-04, 12, 20.4.7

### Services That Do Not Meet the National Electrical Manufacturers Association (NEMA) Standard XR-29-2013

(Rev. 3402, Issued: 11-06-15, Effective: 01-01-16, Implementation: 01-04-16)

Section 218(a) of the Protecting Access to Medicare Act of 2014 (PAMA) is titled "Quality Incentives To Promote Patient Safety and Public Health in Computed Tomography Diagnostic Imaging." It amends the Social Security Act (SSA) by reducing payment for the technical component (and the technical component of the global fee) of the Physician Fee Schedule service (5 percent in 2016 and 15 percent in 2017 and subsequent years) for computed tomography (CT) services identified by CPT codes 70450-70498, 71250-71275, 72125-72133, 72191-72194, 73200-73206, 73700-73706,

74150-74178, 74261-74263, and 75571-75574 furnished using equipment that does not meet each of the attributes of the National Electrical Manufacturers Association (NEMA) Standard XR-29-2013, entitled "Standard Attributes on CT Equipment Related to Dose Optimization and Management."

The statutory provision requires that information be provided and attested to by a supplier and a hospital outpatient department that indicates whether an applicable CT service was furnished that was not consistent with the NEMA CT equipment standard, and that such information may be included on a claim and may be a modifier. The statutory provision also provides that such information shall be verified, as appropriate, as part of the periodic accreditation of suppliers under SSA section 1834(e) and hospitals under SSA section 1865(a). Any reduced expenditures resulting from this provision are not budget neutral. To implement this provision, CMS created modifier "CT" (Computed tomography services furnished using equipment that does not meet each of the attributes of the National Electrical Manufacturers Association (NEMA) XR-29-2013 standard).

Beginning in 2016, claims for CT scans described by above-listed CPT codes (and any successor codes) that are furnished on non-NEMA Standard XR-29-2013-compliant CT scans must include modifier "CT" that will result in the applicable payment reduction.

A list of codes subject to the CT modifier will be maintained in the web supporting files for the annual rule.

Beginning January 1, 2016, a payment reduction of 5 percent applies to the technical component (and the technical component of the global fee) for Computed Tomography (CT) services furnished using equipment that is inconsistent with the CT equipment standard and for which payment is made under the physician fee schedule. This payment reduction becomes 15 percent beginning January 1, 2017, and after.

## 100-04, 12, 30.1

### Digestive System

B3-15100

#### A. Upper Gastrointestinal Endoscopy Including Endoscopic Ultrasound (EUS) (Code 43259)

If the person performing the original diagnostic endoscopy has access to the EUS and the clinical situation requires an EUS, the EUS may be done at the same time. The procedure, diagnostic and EUS, is reported under the same code, CPT 43259. This code conforms to CPT guidelines for the indented codes. The service represented by the indented code, in this case code 43259 for EUS, includes the service represented by the unintended code preceding the list of indented codes. Therefore, when a diagnostic examination of the upper gastrointestinal tract "including esophagus, stomach, and either the duodenum or jejunum as appropriate," includes the use of endoscopic ultrasonography, the service is reported by a single code, namely 43259.

Interpretation, whether by a radiologist or endoscopist, is reported under CPT code 76975-26. These codes may both be reported on the same day.

#### B. Incomplete Colonoscopies (Codes 45330 and 45378)

An incomplete colonoscopy, e.g., the inability to extend beyond the splenic flexure, is billed and paid using colonoscopy code 45378 with modifier "-53." The Medicare physician fee schedule database has specific values for code 45378-53. These values are the same as for code 45330, sigmoidoscopy, as failure to extend beyond the splenic flexure means that a sigmoidoscopy rather than a colonoscopy has been performed.

However, code 45378-53 should be used when an incomplete colonoscopy has been done because other MPFSDB indicators are different for codes 45378 and 45330.

## 100-04, 12, 30.6.2

### Billing for Medically Necessary Visit on Same Occasion as Preventive Medicine Service

See Chapter 18 for payment for covered preventive services.

When a physician furnishes a Medicare beneficiary a covered visit at the same place and on the same occasion as a noncovered preventive medicine service (CPT codes 99381- 99397), consider the covered visit to be provided in lieu of a part of the preventive medicine service of equal value to the visit. A preventive medicine service (CPT codes 99381-99397) is a noncovered service. The physician may charge the beneficiary, as a charge for the noncovered remainder of the service, the amount by which the physician's current established charge for the preventive medicine service exceeds his/her current established charge for the covered visit. Pay for the covered visit based on the lesser of the fee schedule amount or the physician's actual charge for the visit. The physician is not required to give the beneficiary written advance notice of noncoverage of the part of the visit that constitutes a routine preventive visit. However, the physician is responsible for notifying the patient in advance of his/her liability for the charges for services that are not medically necessary to treat the illness or injury.

There could be covered and noncovered procedures performed during this encounter (e.g., screening x-ray, EKG, lab tests.). These are considered individually. Those procedures which are for screening for asymptomatic conditions are considered noncovered and, therefore, no payment is made. Those procedures ordered to diagnose or monitor a symptom, medical condition, or treatment are evaluated for medical necessity and, if covered, are paid.

## 100-04, 12, 30.6.4

### Evaluation and Management (E/M) Services Furnished Incident to Physician's Service by Nonphysician Practitioners

When evaluation and management services are furnished incident to a physician's service by a nonphysician practitioner, the physician may bill the CPT code that describes the evaluation and management service furnished.

When evaluation and management services are furnished incident to a physician's service by a nonphysician employee of the physician, not as part of a physician service, the physician bills code 99211 for the service.

A physician is not precluded from billing under the "incident to" provision for services provided by employees whose services cannot be paid for directly under the Medicare program. Employees of the physician may provide services incident to the physician's service, but the physician alone is permitted to bill Medicare.

Services provided by employees as "incident to" are covered when they meet all the requirements for incident to and are medically necessary for the individual needs of the patient.

## 100-04, 12, 30.6.7

### Payment for Office or Other Outpatient Evaluation and Management (E/M) Visits

#### A. Definition of New Patient for Selection of E/M Visit Code

Interpret the phrase "new patient" to mean a patient who has not received any professional services, i.e., E/M service or other face-to-face service (e.g., surgical procedure) from the physician or physician group practice (same physician specialty) within the previous 3 years. For example, if a professional component of a previous procedure is billed in a 3 year time period, e.g., a lab interpretation is billed and no E/M service or other face-to-face service with the patient is performed, then this patient remains a new patient for the initial visit. An interpretation of a diagnostic test, reading an x-ray or EKG etc., in the absence of an E/M service or other face-to-face service with the patient does not affect the designation of a new patient.

#### B. Office/Outpatient E/M Visits Provided on Same Day for Unrelated Problems

As for all other E/M services except where specifically noted, carriers may not pay two E/M office visits billed by a physician (or physician of the same specialty from the same group practice) for the same beneficiary on the same day unless the physician documents that the visits were for unrelated problems in the office or outpatient setting which could not be provided during the same encounter (e.g., office visit for blood pressure medication evaluation, followed five hours later by a visit for evaluation of leg pain following an accident).

#### C. Office/Outpatient or Emergency Department E/M Visit on Day of Admission to Nursing Facility

Carriers may not pay a physician for an emergency department visit or an office visit and a comprehensive nursing facility assessment on the same day. Bundle E/M visits on the same date provided in sites other than the nursing facility into the initial nursing facility care code when performed on the same date as the nursing facility admission by the same physician.

#### D. Drug Administration Services and E/M Visits Billed on Same Day of Service

Carriers must advise physicians that CPT code 99211 cannot be paid if it is billed with a drug administration service such as a chemotherapy or nonchemotherapy drug infusion code (effective January 1, 2004). This drug administration policy was

expanded in the Physician Fee Schedule Final Rule, November 15, 2004, to also include a therapeutic or diagnostic injection code (effective January 1, 2005). Therefore, when a medically necessary, significant and separately identifiable E/M service (which meets a higher complexity level than CPT code 99211) is performed, in addition to one of these drug administration services, the appropriate E/M CPT code should be reported with modifier -25. Documentation should support the level of E/M service billed. For an E/M service provided on the same day, a different diagnosis is not required.

## 100-04, 12, 30.6.8

### Payment for Hospital Observation Services and Observation or Inpatient Care Services (Including Admission and Discharge Services)

#### A. Who May Bill Observation Care Codes

Observation care is a well-defined set of specific, clinically appropriate services, which include ongoing short term treatment, assessment, and reassessment, that are furnished while a decision is being made regarding whether patients will require further treatment as hospital inpatients or if they are able to be discharged from the hospital. Observation services are commonly ordered for patients who present to the emergency department and who then require a significant period of treatment or monitoring in order to make a decision concerning their admission or discharge.

In only rare and exceptional cases do reasonable and necessary outpatient observation services span more than 48 hours. In the majority of cases, the decision whether to discharge a patient from the hospital following resolution of the reason for the observation care or to admit the patient as an inpatient can be made in less than 48 hours, usually in less than 24 hours.

Contractors pay for initial observation care billed by only the physician who ordered hospital outpatient observation services and was responsible for the patient during his/her observation care. A physician who does not have inpatient admitting privileges but who is authorized to furnish hospital outpatient observation services may bill these codes.

For a physician to bill observation care codes, there must be a medical observation record for the patient which contains dated and timed physician's orders regarding the observation services the patient is to receive, nursing notes, and progress notes prepared by the physician while the patient received observation services. This record must be in addition to any record prepared as a result of an emergency department or outpatient clinic encounter.

Payment for an initial observation care code is for all the care rendered by the ordering physician on the date the patient's observation services began. All other physicians who furnish consultations or additional evaluations or services while the patient is receiving hospital outpatient observation services must bill the appropriate outpatient service codes.

For example, if an internist orders observation services and asks another physician to additionally evaluate the patient, only the internist may bill the initial and subsequent observation care codes. The other physician who evaluates the patient must bill the new or established office or other outpatient visit codes as appropriate.

For information regarding hospital billing of observation services, see Chapter 4, §290.

#### B. Physician Billing for Observation Care Following Initiation of Observation Services

Similar to initial observation codes, payment for a subsequent observation care code is for all the care rendered by the treating physician on the day(s) other than the initial or discharge date. All other physicians who furnish consultations or additional evaluations or services while the patient is receiving hospital outpatient observation services must bill the appropriate outpatient service codes.

When a patient receives observation care for less than 8 hours on the same calendar date, the Initial Observation Care, from CPT code range 99218 – 99220, shall be reported by the physician. The Observation Care Discharge Service, CPT code 99217, shall not be reported for this scenario.

When a patient is admitted for observation care and then is discharged on a different calendar date, the physician shall report Initial Observation Care, from CPT code range 99218 – 99220, and CPT observation care discharge CPT code 99217. On the rare occasion when a patient remains in observation care for 3 days, the physician shall report an initial observation care code (99218-99220) for the first day of observation care, a subsequent observation care code (99224-99226) for the second day of observation care, and an observation care discharge CPT code 99217 for the observation care on the discharge date. When observation care continues beyond 3 days, the physician shall report a subsequent observation care code (99224-99226) for each day between the first day of observation care and the discharge date.

When a patient receives observation care for a minimum of 8 hours, but less than 24 hours, and is discharged on the same calendar date, Observation or Inpatient Care Services (Including Admission and Discharge Services) from CPT code range 99234 – 99236 shall be reported. The observation discharge, CPT code 99217, cannot also be reported for this scenario.

#### C. Documentation Requirements for Billing Observation or Inpatient Care Services (Including Admission and Discharge Services)

The physician shall satisfy the E/M documentation guidelines for furnishing observation care or inpatient hospital care. In addition to meeting the

CPT © 2017 American Medical Association. All Rights Reserved.

© 2017 Optum360, LLC

documentation requirements for history, examination, and medical decision making, documentation in the medical record shall include:

- Documentation stating the stay for observation care or inpatient hospital care involves 8 hours, but less than 24 hours;
- Documentation identifying the billing physician was present and personally performed the services; and
- Documentation identifying the order for observation services, progress notes, and discharge notes were written by the billing physician.

In the rare circumstance when a patient receives observation services for more than 2 calendar dates, the physician shall bill observation services furnished on day(s) other than the initial or discharge date using subsequent observation care codes. The physician may not use the subsequent hospital care codes since the patient is not an inpatient of the hospital.

### D. Admission to Inpatient Status Following Observation Care
If the same physician who ordered hospital outpatient observation services also admits the patient to inpatient status before the end of the date on which the patient began receiving hospital outpatient observation services, pay only an initial hospital visit for the evaluation and management services provided on that date. Medicare payment for the initial hospital visit includes all services provided to the patient on the date of admission by that physician, regardless of the site of service. The physician may not bill an initial or subsequent observation care code for services on the date that he or she admits the patient to inpatient status. If the patient is admitted to inpatient status from hospital outpatient observation care subsequent to the date of initiation of observation services, the physician must bill an initial hospital visit for the services provided on that date. The physician may not bill the hospital observation discharge management code (code 99217) or an outpatient/office visit for the care provided while the patient received hospital outpatient observation services on the date of admission to inpatient status.

### E. Hospital Observation Services During Global Surgical Period
The global surgical fee includes payment for hospital observation (codes 99217, 99218, 99219, 99220, 99224, 99225, 99226, 99234, 99235, and 99236) services unless the criteria for use of CPT modifiers "-24," "-25," or "-57" are met. Contractors must pay for these services in addition to the global surgical fee only if both of the following requirements are met:

- The hospital observation service meets the criteria needed to justify billing it with CPT modifiers "-24," "-25," or "-57" (decision for major surgery); and
- The hospital observation service furnished by the surgeon meets all of the criteria for the hospital observation code billed.

Examples of the decision for surgery during a hospital observation period are:

- An emergency department physician orders hospital outpatient observation services for a patient with a head injury. A neurosurgeon is called in to evaluate the need for surgery while the patient is receiving observation services and decides that the patient requires surgery. The surgeon would bill a new or established office or other outpatient visit code as appropriate with the "-57" modifier to indicate that the decision for surgery was made during the evaluation. The surgeon must bill the office or other outpatient visit code because the patient receiving hospital outpatient observation services is not an inpatient of the hospital. Only the physician who ordered hospital outpatient observation services may bill for observation care.

- A neurosurgeon orders hospital outpatient observation services for a patient with a head injury. During the observation period, the surgeon makes the decision for surgery. The surgeon would bill the appropriate level of hospital observation code with the "-57" modifier to indicate that the decision for surgery was made while the surgeon was providing hospital observation care.

Examples of hospital observation services during the postoperative period of a surgery are:

- A surgeon orders hospital outpatient observation services for a patient with abdominal pain from a kidney stone on the 80th day following a TURP (performed by that surgeon). The surgeon decides that the patient does not require surgery. The surgeon would bill the observation code with CPT modifier "-24" and documentation to support that the observation services are unrelated to the surgery.

- A surgeon orders hospital outpatient observation services for a patient with abdominal pain on the 80th day following a TURP (performed by that surgeon). While the patient is receiving hospital outpatient observation services, the surgeon decides that the patient requires kidney surgery. The surgeon would bill the observation code with HCPCS modifier "-57" to indicate that the decision for surgery was made while the patient was receiving hospital outpatient observation services. The subsequent surgical procedure would be reported with modifier "-79."

- A surgeon orders hospital outpatient observation services for a patient with abdominal pain on the 20th day following a resection of the colon (performed by that surgeon). The surgeon determines that the patient requires no further colon surgery and discharges the patient. The surgeon may not bill for the observation services furnished during the global period because they were related to the previous surgery.

An example of a billable hospital observation service on the same day as a procedure is when a physician repairs a laceration of the scalp in the emergency department for a patient with a head injury and then subsequently orders hospital outpatient

observation services for that patient. The physician would bill the observation code with a CPT modifier 25 and the procedure code.

## 100-04, 12, 30.6.9
### Payment for Inpatient Hospital Visits - General

#### A. Hospital Visit and Critical Care on Same Day
When a hospital inpatient or office/outpatient evaluation and management service (E/M) are furnished on a calendar date at which time the patient does not require critical care and the patient subsequently requires critical care both the critical Care Services (CPT codes 99291 and 99292) and the previous E/M service may be paid on the same date of service. Hospital emergency department services are not paid for the same date as critical care services when provided by the same physician to the same patient.

During critical care management of a patient those services that do not meet the level of critical care shall be reported using an inpatient hospital care service with CPT Subsequent Hospital Care using a code from CPT code range 99231 – 99233.

Both Initial Hospital Care (CPT codes 99221 – 99223) and Subsequent Hospital Care codes are "per diem" services and may be reported only once per day by the same physician or physicians of the same specialty from the same group practice.

Physicians and qualified nonphysician practitioners (NPPs) are advised to retain documentation for discretionary contractor review should claims be questioned for both hospital care and critical care claims. The retained documentation shall support claims for critical care when the same physician or physicians of the same specialty in a group practice report critical care services for the same patient on the same calendar date as other E/M services.

#### B. Two Hospital Visits Same Day
Contractors pay a physician for only one hospital visit per day for the same patient, whether the problems seen during the encounters are related or not. The inpatient hospital visit descriptors contain the phrase "per day" which means that the code and the payment established for the code represent all services provided on that date. The physician should select a code that reflects all services provided during the date of the service.

#### C. Hospital Visits Same Day But by Different Physicians
In a hospital inpatient situation involving one physician covering for another, if physician A sees the patient in the morning and physician B, who is covering for A, sees the same patient in the evening, contractors do not pay physician B for the second visit. The hospital visit descriptors include the phrase "per day" meaning care for the day.

If the physicians are each responsible for a different aspect of the patient's care, pay both visits if the physicians are in different specialties and the visits are billed with different diagnoses. There are circumstances where concurrent care may be billed by physicians of the same specialty.

#### D. Visits to Patients in Swing Beds
If the inpatient care is being billed by the hospital as inpatient hospital care, the hospital care codes apply. If the inpatient care is being billed by the hospital as nursing facility care, then the nursing facility codes apply.

## 100-04, 12, 30.6.9.1
### Payment for Initial Hospital Care Services and Observation or Inpatient Care Services (Including Admission and Discharge Services)

#### A. Initial Hospital Care From Emergency Room
Contractors pay for an initial hospital care service if a physician sees a patient in the emergency room and decides to admit the person to the hospital. They do not pay for both E/M services. Also, they do not pay for an emergency department visit by the same physician on the same date of service. When the patient is admitted to the hospital via another site of service (e.g., hospital emergency department, physician's office, nursing facility), all services provided by the physician in conjunction with that admission are considered part of the initial hospital care when performed on the same date as the admission.

#### B. Initial Hospital Care on Day Following Visit
Contractors pay both visits if a patient is seen in the office on one date and admitted to the hospital on the next date, even if fewer than 24 hours has elapsed between the visit and the admission.

#### C. Initial Hospital Care and Discharge on Same Day
When the patient is admitted to inpatient hospital care for less than 8 hours on the same date, then Initial Hospital Care, from CPT code range 99221 – 99223, shall be reported by the physician. The Hospital Discharge Day Management service, CPT codes 99238 or 99239, shall not be reported for this scenario.

When a patient is admitted to inpatient initial hospital care and then discharged on a different calendar date, the physician shall report an Initial Hospital Care from CPT code range 99221 – 99223 and a Hospital Discharge Day Management service, CPT code 99238 or 99239.

When a patient has been admitted to inpatient hospital care for a minimum of 8 hours but less than 24 hours and discharged on the same calendar date, Observation or Inpatient Hospital Care Services (Including Admission and Discharge Services), from CPT code range 99234 – 99236, shall be reported.

**D. Documentation Requirements for Billing Observation or Inpatient Care Services (Including Admission and Discharge Services)**

The physician shall satisfy the E/M documentation guidelines for admission to and discharge from inpatient observation or hospital care. In addition to meeting the documentation requirements for history, examination and medical decision making documentation in the medical record shall include:

- Documentation stating the stay for hospital treatment or observation care status involves 8 hours but less than 24 hours;

- Documentation identifying the billing physician was present and personally performed the services; and

- Documentation identifying the admission and discharge notes were written by the billing physician.

**E. Physician Services Involving Transfer From One Hospital to Another; Transfer Within Facility to Prospective Payment System (PPS) Exempt Unit of Hospital; Transfer From One Facility to Another Separate Entity Under Same Ownership and/or Part of Same Complex; or Transfer From One Department to Another Within Single Facility**

Physicians may bill both the hospital discharge management code and an initial hospital care code when the discharge and admission do not occur on the same day if the transfer is between:

- Different hospitals;

- Different facilities under common ownership which do not have merged records; or

- Between the acute care hospital and a PPS exempt unit within the same hospital when there are no merged records.

In all other transfer circumstances, the physician should bill only the appropriate level of subsequent hospital care for the date of transfer.

**F. Initial Hospital Care Service History and Physical That Is Less Than Comprehensive**

When a physician performs a visit that meets the definition of a Level 5 office visit several days prior to an admission and on the day of admission performs less than a comprehensive history and physical, he or she should report the office visit that reflects the services furnished and also report the lowest level initial hospital care code (i.e., code 99221) for the initial hospital admission. Contractors pay the office visit as billed and the Level 1 initial hospital care code.

Physicians who provide an initial visit to a patient during inpatient hospital care that meets the minimum key component work and/or medical necessity requirements shall report an initial hospital care code (99221-99223). The principal physician of record shall append modifier "-AI" (Principal Physician of Record) to the claim for the initial hospital care code. This modifier will identify the physician who oversees the patient's care from all other physicians who may be furnishing specialty care.

Physicians may bill initial hospital care service codes (99221-99223), for services that were reported with CPT consultation codes (99241 – 99255) prior to January 1, 2010, when the furnished service and documentation meet the minimum key component work and/or medical necessity requirements. Physicians must meet all the requirements of the initial hospital care codes, including "a detailed or comprehensive history" and "a detailed or comprehensive examination" to report CPT code 99221, which are greater than the requirements for consultation codes 99251 and 99252.

Subsequent hospital care CPT codes 99231 and 99232, respectively, require "a problem focused interval history" and "an expanded problem focused interval history." An E/M service that could be described by CPT consultation code 99251 or 99252 could potentially meet the component work and medical necessity requirements to report 99231 or 99232. Physicians may report a subsequent hospital care CPT code for services that were reported as CPT consultation codes (99241 – 99255) prior to January 1, 2010, where the medical record appropriately demonstrates that the work and medical necessity requirements are met for reporting a subsequent hospital care code (under the level selected), even though the reported code is for the provider's first E/M service to the inpatient during the hospital stay.

Reporting CPT code 99499 (Unlisted evaluation and management service) should be limited to cases where there is no other specific E/M code payable by Medicare that describes that service.

Reporting CPT code 99499 requires submission of medical records and contractor manual medical review of the service prior to payment. Contractors shall expect reporting under these circumstances to be unusual.

**G. Initial Hospital Care Visits by Two Different M.D.s or D.O.s When They Are Involved in Same Admission**

In the inpatient hospital setting all physicians (and qualified nonphysician practitioners where permitted) who perform an initial evaluation may bill the initial hospital care codes (99221 – 99223) or nursing facility care codes (99304 – 99306). Contractors consider only one M.D. or D.O. to be the principal physician of record (sometimes referred to as the admitting physician.) The principal physician of record is identified in Medicare as the physician who oversees the patient's care from other physicians who may be furnishing specialty care. Only the principal physician of record shall append modifier "-AI" (Principal Physician of Record) in addition to the E/M code. Follow-up visits in the facility setting shall be billed as subsequent hospital care visits and subsequent nursing facility care visits.

## 100-04, 12, 30.6.9.2

### Subsequent Hospital Visit and Hospital Discharge Day Management

**A. Subsequent Hospital Visits During the Global Surgery Period**

(Refer to Secs.40-40.4 on global surgery) The Medicare physician fee schedule payment amount for surgical procedures includes all services (e.g., evaluation and management visits) that are part of the global surgery payment; therefore, contractors shall not pay more than that amount when a bill is fragmented for staged procedures.

**B. Hospital Discharge Day Management Service Hospital Discharge Day**

Management Services, CPT code 99238 or 99239 is a face-to-face evaluation and management (E/M) service between the attending physician and the patient. The E/M discharge day management visit shall be reported for the date of the actual visit by the physician or qualified nonphysician practitioner even if the patient is discharged from the facility on a different calendar date. Only one hospital discharge day management service is payable per patient per hospital stay.

Only the attending physician of record reports the discharge day management service. Physicians or qualified nonphysician practitioners, other than the attending physician, who have been managing concurrent health care problems not primarily managed by the attending physician, and who are not acting on behalf of the attending physician, shall use Subsequent Hospital Care (CPT code range 99231 - 99233) for a final visit.

Medicare pays for the paperwork of patient discharge day management through the pre- and post- service work of an E/M service.

**C. Subsequent Hospital Visit and Discharge Management on Same Day**

Pay only the hospital discharge management code on the day of discharge (unless it is also the day of admission, in which case, refer to Sec.30.6.9.1 C for the policy on Observation or Inpatient Care Services (Including Admission and Discharge Services CPT Codes 99234 - 99236). Contractors do not pay both a subsequent hospital visit in addition to hospital discharge day management service on the same day by the same physician. Instruct physicians that they may not bill for both a hospital visit and hospital discharge management for the same date of service.

**D. Hospital Discharge Management (CPT Codes 99238 and 99239) and Nursing Facility Admission Code When Patient Is Discharged From Hospital and Admitted to Nursing Facility on Same Day**

Contractors pay the hospital discharge code (codes 99238 or 99239) in addition to a nursing facility admission code when they are billed by the same physician with the same date of service.

If a surgeon is admitting the patient to the nursing facility due to a condition that is not as a result of the surgery during the postoperative period of a service with the global surgical period, he/she bills for the nursing facility admission and care with a modifier "-24" and provides documentation that the service is unrelated to the surgery (e.g., return of an elderly patient to the nursing facility in which he/she has resided for five years following discharge from the hospital for cholecystectomy).

Contractors do not pay for a nursing facility admission by a surgeon in the postoperative period of a procedure with a global surgical period if the patient's admission to the nursing facility is to receive post operative care related to the surgery (e.g., admission to a nursing facility to receive physical therapy following a hip replacement). Payment for the nursing facility admission and subsequent nursing facility services are included in the global fee and cannot be paid separately.

**E. Hospital Discharge Management and Death Pronouncement**

Only the physician who personally performs the pronouncement of death shall bill for the face-to-face Hospital Discharge Day Management Service, CPT code 99238 or 99239. The date of the pronouncement shall reflect the calendar date of service on the day it was performed even if the paperwork is delayed to a subsequent date.

## 100-04, 12, 30.6.10

### Consultation Services

Consultation Services versus Other Evaluation and Management (E/M) Visits

Effective January 1, 2010, the consultation codes are no longer recognized for Medicare Part B payment. Physicians shall code patient evaluation and management visits with E/M codes that represent where the visit occurs and that identify the complexity of the visit performed.

In the inpatient hospital setting and the nursing facility setting, physicians (and qualified nonphysician practitioners where permitted) may bill the most appropriate initial hospital care code (99221-99223), subsequent hospital care code (99231 and 99232), initial nursing facility care code (99304-99306), or subsequent nursing facility care code (99307-99310) that reflects the services the physician or practitioner furnished. Subsequent hospital care codes could potentially meet the component work and medical necessity requirements to be reported for an E/M service that could be described by CPT consultation code 99251 or 99252. Contractors shall not find fault in cases where the medical record appropriately demonstrates that the work and medical necessity requirements are met for reporting a subsequent hospital care code (under the level selected), even though the reported code is for the provider's first E/M service to the inpatient during the hospital stay. Unlisted evaluation and management service (code 99499) shall only be reported for consultation services when an E/M service that could be described by codes 99251 or 99252 is furnished, and there is no other specific E/M code payable by Medicare that describes that service. Reporting code 99499 requires submission of medical records and contractor manual medical review of the service prior to payment. CMS expects

CPT © 2017 American Medical Association. All Rights Reserved.                                    © 2017 Optum360, LLC

reporting under these circumstances to be unusual. T he principal physician of record is identified in Medicare as the physician who oversees the patient's care from other physicians who may be furnishing specialty care. The principal physician of record shall append modifier "-AI" (Principal Physician of Record), in addition to the E/M code. Follow-up visits in the facility setting shall be billed as subsequent hospital care visits and subsequent nursing facility care visits.

In the CAH setting, those CAHs that use method II shall bill the appropriate new or established visit code for those physician and non-physician practitioners who have reassigned their billing rights, depending on the relationship status between the physician and patient.

In the office or other outpatient setting where an evaluation is performed, physicians and qualified nonphysician practitioners shall use the CPT codes (99201 – 99215) depending on the complexity of the visit and whether the patient is a new or established patient to that physician. All physicians and qualified nonphysician practitioners shall follow the E/M documentation guidelines for all E/M services. These rules are applicable for Medicare secondary payer claims as well as for claims in which Medicare is the primary payer.

## 100-04, 12, 30.6.11
### *Emergency Department Visits*

#### A. Use of Emergency Department Codes by Physicians Not Assigned to Emergency Department
Any physician seeing a patient registered in the emergency department may use emergency department visit codes (for services matching the code description). It is not required that the physician be assigned to the emergency department.

#### B. Use of Emergency Department Codes In Office
Emergency department coding is not appropriate if the site of service is an office or outpatient setting or any sight of service other than an emergency department. The emergency department codes should only be used if the patient is seen in the emergency department and the services described by the HCPCS code definition are provided. The emergency department is defined as an organized hospital-based facility for the provision of unscheduled or episodic services to patients who present for immediate medical attention.

#### C. Use of Emergency Department Codes to Bill Nonemergency Services
Services in the emergency department may not be emergencies. However the codes (99281 - 99288) are payable if the described services are provided.

However, if the physician asks the patient to meet him or her in the emergency department as an alternative to the physician's office and the patient is not registered as a patient in the emergency department, the physician should bill the appropriate office/outpatient visit codes. Normally a lower level emergency department code would be reported for a nonemergency condition.

#### D. Emergency Department or Office/Outpatient Visits on Same Day As Nursing Facility Admission
Emergency department visit provided on the same day as a comprehensive nursing facility assessment are not paid. Payment for evaluation and management services on the same date provided in sites other than the nursing facility are included in the payment for initial nursing facility care when performed on the same date as the nursing facility admission.

#### E. Physician Billing for Emergency Department Services Provided to Patient by Both Patient's Personal Physician and Emergency Department Physician
If a physician advises his/her own patient to go to an emergency department (ED) of a hospital for care and the physician subsequently is asked by the ED physician to come to the hospital to evaluate the patient and to advise the ED physician as to whether the patient should be admitted to the hospital or be sent home, the physicians should bill as follows:

If the patient is admitted to the hospital by the patient's personal physician, then the patient's regular physician should bill only the appropriate level of the initial hospital care (codes 99221 - 99223) because all evaluation and management services provided by that physician in conjunction with that admission are considered part of the initial hospital care when performed on the same date as the admission. The ED physician who saw the patient in the emergency department should bill the appropriate level of the ED codes.

If the ED physician, based on the advice of the patient's personal physician who came to the emergency department to see the patient, sends the patient home, then the ED physician should bill the appropriate level of emergency department service. The patient's personal physician should also bill the level of emergency department code that describes the service he or she provided in the emergency department. If the patient's personal physician does not come to the hospital to see the patient, but only advises the emergency department physician by telephone, then the patient's personal physician may not bill.

#### F. Emergency Department Physician Requests Another Physician to See the Patient in Emergency Department or Office/Outpatient Setting
If the emergency department physician requests that another physician evaluate a given patient, the other physician should bill an emergency department visit code. If the patient is admitted to the hospital by the second physician performing the evaluation, he or she should bill an initial hospital care code and not an emergency department visit code.

## 100-04, 12, 30.6.13
### *Nursing Facility Services*

#### A. Visits to Perform the Initial Comprehensive Assessment and Annual Assessments
The distinction made between the delegation of physician visits and tasks in a skilled nursing facility (SNF) and in a nursing facility (NF) is based on the Medicare Statute. Section 1819 (b) (6) (A) of the Social Security Act (the Act) governs SNFs while section 1919 (b) (6) (A) of the Act governs NFs. For further information refer to Medlearn Matters article number SE0418 at www.cms.hhs.gov/medlearn/matters.

The federally mandated visits in a SNF and NF must be performed by the physician except as otherwise permitted (42 CFR 483.40 (c) (4) and (f)). The principal physician of record must append the modifier "-AI", (Principal Physician of Record), to the initial nursing facility care code. This modifier will identify the physician who oversees the patient's care from other physicians who may be furnishing specialty care. All other physicians or qualified NPPs who perform an initial evaluation in the NF or SNF may bill the initial nursing facility care code. The initial federally mandated visit is defined in S&C-04-08 (see www.cms.hhs.gov/medlearn/matters) as the initial comprehensive visit during which the physician completes a thorough assessment, develops a plan of care, and writes or verifies admitting orders for the nursing facility resident. For Survey and Certification requirements, a visit must occur no later than 30 days after admission.

Further, per the Long Term Care regulations at 42 CFR 483.40 (c) (4) and (e) (2), in a SNF the physician may not delegate a task that the physician must personally perform. Therefore, as stated in S&C-04-08 the physician may not delegate the initial federally mandated comprehensive visit in a SNF.

The only exception, as to who performs the initial visit, relates to the NF setting. In the NF setting, a qualified NPP (i.e., a nurse practitioner (NP), physician assistant (PA), or a clinical nurse specialist (CNS)), who is not employed by the facility, may perform the initial visit when the State law permits. The evaluation and management (E/M) visit shall be within the State scope of practice and licensure requirements where the E/M visit is performed and the requirements for physician collaboration and physician supervision shall be met.

Under Medicare Part B payment policy, other medically necessary E/M visits may be performed and reported prior to and after the initial visit, if the medical needs of the patient require an E/M visit. A qualified NPP may perform medically necessary E/M visits prior to and after the initial visit if all the requirements for collaboration, general physician supervision, licensure, and billing are met.

The CPT Nursing Facility Services codes shall be used with place of service (POS) 31 (SNF) if the patient is in a Part A SNF stay. They shall be used with POS 32 (nursing facility) if the patient does not have Part A SNF benefits or if the patient is in a NF or in a non-covered SNF stay (e.g., there was no preceding 3-day hospital stay). The CPT Nursing Facility code definition also includes POS 54 (Intermediate Care Facility/Mentally Retarded) and POS 56 (Psychiatric Residential Treatment Center). For further guidance on POS codes and associated CPT codes refer to §30.6.14.

Effective January 1, 2006, the Initial Nursing Facility Care codes 99301– 99303 are deleted.

Beginning January 1, 2006, the new CPT codes, Initial Nursing Facility Care, per day, (99304 – 99306) shall be used to report the initial federally mandated visit. Only a physician may report these codes for an initial federally mandated visit performed in a SNF or NF (with the exception of the qualified NPP in the NF setting who is not employed by the facility and when State law permits, as explained above).

A readmission to a SNF or NF shall have the same payment policy requirements as an initial admission in both the SNF and NF settings.

A physician who is employed by the SNF/NF may perform the E/M visits and bill independently to Medicare Part B for payment. An NPP who is employed by the SNF or NF may perform and bill Medicare Part B directly for those services where it is permitted as discussed above. The employer of the PA shall always report the visits performed by the PA. A physician, NP or CNS has the option to bill Medicare directly or to reassign payment for his/her professional service to the facility.

As with all E/M visits for Medicare Part B payment policy, the E/M documentation guidelines apply.

*Medically Necessary Visits*
Qualified NPPs may perform medically necessary E/M visits prior to and after the physician's initial federally mandated visit in both the SNF and NF. Medically necessary E/M visits for the diagnosis or treatment of an illness or injury or to improve the functioning of a malformed body member are payable under the physician fee schedule under Medicare Part B. A physician or NPP may bill the most appropriate initial nursing facility care code (CPT codes 99304-99306) or subsequent nursing facility care code (CPT codes 99307-99310), even if the E/M service is provided prior to the initial federally mandated visit.

*SNF Setting--Place of Service Code 31*
Following the initial federally mandated visit by the physician, the physician may delegate alternate federally mandated physician visits to a qualified NPP who meets collaboration and physician supervision requirements and is licensed as such by the State and performing within the scope of practice in that State.

*NF Setting--Place of Service Code 32*
Per the regulations at 42 CFR 483.40 (f), a qualified NPP, who meets the collaboration and physician supervision requirements, the State scope of practice and licensure requirements, and who is not employed by the NF, may at the option of the State,

perform the initial federally mandated visit in a NF, and may perform any other federally mandated physician visit in a NF in addition to performing other medically necessary E/M visits.

Questions pertaining to writing orders or certification and recertification issues in the SNF and NF settings shall be addressed to the appropriate State Survey and Certification Agency departments for clarification.

### B. Visits to Comply With Federal Regulations (42 CFR 483.40 (c) (1)) in the SNF and NF

Payment is made under the physician fee schedule by Medicare Part B for federally mandated visits. Following the initial federally mandated visit by the physician or qualified NPP where permitted, payment shall be made for federally mandated visits that monitor and evaluate residents at least once every 30 days for the first 90 days after admission and at least once every 60 days thereafter.

Effective January 1, 2006, the Subsequent Nursing Facility Care, per day, codes 99311– 99313 are deleted.

Beginning January 1, 2006, the new CPT codes, Subsequent Nursing Facility Care, per day, (99307 – 99310) shall be used to report federally mandated physician E/M visits and medically necessary E/M visits.

Carriers shall not pay for more than one E/M visit performed by the physician or qualified NPP for the same patient on the same date of service. The Nursing Facility Services codes represent a "per day" service.

The federally mandated E/M visit may serve also as a medically necessary E/M visit if the situation arises (i.e., the patient has health problems that need attention on the day the scheduled mandated physician E/M visit occurs). The physician/qualified NPP shall bill only one E/M visit.

Beginning January 1, 2006, the new CPT code, Other Nursing Facility Service (99318), may be used to report an annual nursing facility assessment visit on the required schedule of visits on an annual basis. For Medicare Part B payment policy, an annual nursing facility assessment visit code may substitute as meeting one of the federally mandated physician visits if the code requirements for CPT code 99318 are fully met and in lieu of reporting a Subsequent Nursing Facility Care, per day, service (codes 99307 – 99310). It shall not be performed in addition to the required number of federally mandated physician visits. The new CPT annual assessment code does not represent a new benefit service for Medicare Part B physician services.

Qualified NPPs, whether employed or not by the SNF, may perform alternating federally mandated physician visits, at the option of the physician, after the initial federally mandated visit by the physician in a SNF.

Qualified NPPs in the NF setting, who are not employed by the NF and who are working in collaboration with a physician, may perform federally mandated physician visits, at the option of the State.

Medicare Part B payment policy does not pay for additional E/M visits that may be required by State law for a facility admission or for other additional visits to satisfy facility or other administrative purposes. E/M visits, prior to and after the initial federally mandated physician visit, that are reasonable and medically necessary to meet the medical needs of the individual patient (unrelated to any State requirement or administrative purpose) are payable under Medicare Part B.

### C. Visits by Qualified Nonphysician Practitioners

All E/M visits shall be within the State scope of practice and licensure requirements where the visit is performed and all the requirements for physician collaboration and physician supervision shall be met when performed and reported by qualified NPPs. General physician supervision and employer billing requirements shall be met for PA services in addition to the PA meeting the State scope of practice and licensure requirements where the E/M visit is performed.

*Medically Necessary Visits*

Qualified NPPs may perform medically necessary E/M visits prior to and after the physician's initial visit in both the SNF and NF. Medically necessary E/M visits for the diagnosis or treatment of an illness or injury or to improve the functioning of a malformed body member are payable under the physician fee schedule under Medicare Part B. A physician or NPP may bill the most appropriate initial nursing facility care code (CPT codes 99304-99306) or subsequent nursing facility care code (CPT codes 99307-99310), even if the E/M service is provided prior to the initial federally mandated visit.

*SNF Setting--Place of Service Code 31*

Following the initial federally mandated visit by the physician, the physician may delegate alternate federally mandated physician visits to a qualified NPP who meets collaboration and physician supervision requirements and is licensed as such by the State and performing within the scope of practice in that State.

*NF Setting--Place of Service Code 32*

Per the regulations at 42 CFR 483.40 (f), a qualified NPP, who meets the collaboration and physician supervision requirements, the State scope of practice and licensure requirements, and who is not employed by the NF, may at the option of the State, perform the initial federally mandated visit in a NF, and may perform any other federally mandated physician visit in a NF in addition to performing other medically necessary E/M visits.

Questions pertaining to writing orders or certification and recertification issues in the SNF and NF settings shall be addressed to the appropriate State Survey and Certification Agency departments for clarification.

### D. Medically Complex Care

Payment is made for E/M visits to patients in a SNF who are receiving services for medically complex care upon discharge from an acute care facility when the visits are reasonable and medically necessary and documented in the medical record. Physicians and qualified NPPs shall report initial nursing facility care codes for their first visit with the patient. The principal physician of record must append the modifier "-AI" (Principal Physician of Record), to the initial nursing facility care code when billed to identify the physician who oversees the patient's care from other physicians who may be furnishing specialty care. Follow-up visits shall be billed as subsequent nursing facility care visits.

### E. Incident to Services

Where a physician establishes an office in a SNF/NF, the "incident to" services and requirements are confined to this discrete part of the facility designated as his/her office. "Incident to" E/M visits, provided in a facility setting, are not payable under the Physician Fee Schedule for Medicare Part B. Thus, visits performed outside the designated "office" area in the SNF/NF would be subject to the coverage and payment rules applicable to the SNF/NF setting and shall not be reported using the CPT codes for office or other outpatient visits or use place of service code 11.

### F. Use of the Prolonged Services Codes and Other Time-Related Services

Beginning January 1, 2008, typical/average time units for E/M visits in the SNF/NF settings are reestablished. Medically necessary prolonged services for E/M visits (codes 99356 and 99357) in a SNF or NF may be billed with the Nursing Facility Services in the code ranges (99304 – 99306, 99307 – 99310 and 99318).

*Counseling and Coordination of Care Visits*

With the reestablishment of typical/average time units, medically necessary E/M visits for counseling and coordination of care, for Nursing Facility Services in the code ranges (99304 – 99306, 99307 – 99310 and 99318) that are time-based services, may be billed with the appropriate prolonged services codes (99356 and 99357).

### G. Multiple Visits

The complexity level of an E/M visit and the CPT code billed must be a covered and medically necessary visit for each patient (refer to §§1862 (a)(1)(A) of the Act). Claims for an unreasonable number of daily E/M visits by the same physician to multiple patients at a facility within a 24-hour period may result in medical review to determine medical necessity for the visits. The E/M visit (Nursing Facility Services) represents a "per day" service per patient as defined by the CPT code. The medical record must be personally documented by the physician or qualified NPP who performed the E/M visit and the documentation shall support the specific level of E/M visit to each individual patient.

### H. Split/Shared E/M Visit

A split/shared E/M visit cannot be reported in the SNF/NF setting. A split/shared E/M visit is defined by Medicare Part B payment policy as a medically necessary encounter with a patient where the physician and a qualified NPP each personally perform a substantive portion of an E/M visit face-to-face with the same patient on the same date of service. A substantive portion of an E/M visit involves all or some portion of the history, exam or medical decision making key components of an E/M service. The physician and the qualified NPP must be in the same group practice or be employed by the same employer. The split/shared E/M visit applies only to selected E/M visits and settings (i.e., hospital inpatient, hospital outpatient, hospital observation, emergency department, hospital discharge, office and non facility clinic visits, and prolonged visits associated with these E/M visit codes). The split/shared E/M policy does not apply to critical care services or procedures.

### I. SNF/NF Discharge Day Management Service

Medicare Part B payment policy requires a face-to-face visit with the patient provided by the physician or the qualified NPP to meet the SNF/NF discharge day management service as defined by the CPT code. The E/M discharge day management visit shall be reported for the date of the actual visit by the physician or qualified NPP even if the patient is discharged from the facility on a different calendar date. The CPT codes 99315 – 99316 shall be reported for this visit. The Discharge Day Management Service may be reported using CPT code 99315 or 99316, depending on the code requirement, for a patient who has expired, but only if the physician or qualified NPP personally performed the death pronouncement.

## 100-04, 12, 30.6.14

### *Home Care and Domiciliary Care Visits*

#### Physician Visits to Patients Residing in Various Places of Service

The American Medical Association's Current Procedural Terminology (CPT) 2006 new patient codes 99324 - 99328 and established patient codes 99334 - 99337(new codes beginning January 2006), for Domiciliary, Rest Home (e.g., Boarding Home), or Custodial Care Services, are used to report evaluation and management (E/M) services to residents residing in a facility which provides room, board, and other personal assistance services, generally on a long-term basis. These CPT codes are used to report E/M services in facilities assigned places of service (POS) codes 13 (Assisted Living Facility), 14 (Group Home), 33 (Custodial Care Facility) and 55 (Residential Substance Abuse Facility). Assisted living facilities may also be known as adult living facilities.

Physicians and qualified nonphysician practitioners (NPPs) furnishing E/M services to residents in a living arrangement described by one of the POS listed above must use the level of service code in the CPT code range 99324 - 99337 to report the service they provide. The CPT codes 99321 - 99333 for Domiciliary, Rest Home (e.g., Boarding Home), or Custodial Care Services are deleted beginning January, 2006.

Beginning in 2006, reasonable and medically necessary, face-to-face, prolonged services, represented by CPT codes 99354 - 99355, may be reported with the appropriate companion E/M codes when a physician or qualified NPP, provides a prolonged service involving direct (face-to-face) patient contact that is beyond the usual E/M visit service for a Domiciliary, Rest Home (e.g., Boarding Home) or Custodial Care Service. All the requirements for prolonged services at Sec.30.6.15.1 must be met.

The CPT codes 99341 through 99350, Home Services codes, are used to report E/M services furnished to a patient residing in his or her own private residence (e.g., private home, apartment, town home) and not residing in any type of congregate/shared facility living arrangement including assisted living facilities and group homes. The Home Services codes apply only to the specific 2-digit POS 12 (Home). Home Services codes may not be used for billing E/M services provided in settings other than in the private residence of an individual as described above.

Beginning in 2006, E/M services provided to patients residing in a Skilled Nursing Facility (SNF) or a Nursing Facility (NF) must be reported using the appropriate CPT level of service code within the range identified for Initial Nursing Facility Care (new CPT codes 99304 - 99306) and Subsequent Nursing Facility Care (new CPT codes 99307 - 99310). Use the CPT code, Other Nursing Facility Services (new CPT code 99318), for an annual nursing facility assessment. Use CPT codes 99315 - 99316 for SNF/NF discharge services. The CPT codes 99301 - 99303 and 99311 - 99313 are deleted beginning January, 2006. The Home Services codes should not be used for these places of service.

The CPT SNF/NF code definition includes intermediate care facilities (ICFs) and long term care facilities (LTCFs). These codes are limited to the specific 2-digit POS 31 (SNF), 32 (Nursing Facility), 54 (Intermediate Care Facility/Mentally Retarded) and 56 (Psychiatric Residential Treatment Center).

The CPT nursing facility codes should be used with POS 31 (SNF) if the patient is in a Part A SNF stay and POS 32 (nursing facility) if the patient does not have Part A SNF benefits. There is no longer a different payment amount for a Part A or Part B benefit period in these POS settings.

## 100-04, 12, 30.6.14.1

### Home Services
B3-15515, B3-15066

#### A. Requirement for Physician Presence
Home services codes 99341-99350 are paid when they are billed to report evaluation and management services provided in a private residence. A home visit cannot be billed by a physician unless the physician was actually present in the beneficiary's home.

#### B. Homebound Status
Under the home health benefit the beneficiary must be confined to the home for services to be covered. For home services provided by a physician using these codes, the beneficiary does not need to be confined to the home. The medical record must document the medical necessity of the home visit made in lieu of an office or outpatient visit.

#### C. Fee Schedule Payment for Services to Homebound
Patients under General Supervision Payment may be made in some medically underserved areas where there is a lack of medical personnel and home health services for injections, EKGs, and venipunctures that are performed for homebound patients under general physician supervision by nurses and paramedical employees of physicians or physician-directed clinics. Section 10 provides additional information on the provision of services to homebound Medicare patients.

## 100-04, 12, 30.6.15.1

### Prolonged Services With Direct Face-to-Face Patient Contact Service

#### A. Definition
Prolonged physician services (CPT code 99354) in the office or other outpatient setting with direct face-to-face patient contact which require 1 hour beyond the usual service are payable when billed on the same day by the same physician or qualified nonphysician practitioner (NPP) as the companion evaluation and management codes. The time for usual service refers to the typical/average time units associated with the companion evaluation and management service as noted in the CPT code. Each additional 30 minutes of direct face-to-face patient contact following the first hour of prolonged services may be reported by CPT code 99355.

Prolonged physician services (code 99356) in the inpatient setting, with direct face-to-face patient contact which require 1 hour beyond the usual service are payable when they are billed on the same day by the same physician or qualified NPP as the companion evaluation and management codes. Each additional 30 minutes of direct face-to-face patient contact following the first hour of prolonged services may be reported by CPT code 99357.

Prolonged service of less than 30 minutes total duration on a given date is not separately reported because the work involved is included in the total work of the evaluation and management codes.

Code 99355 or 99357 may be used to report each additional 30 minutes beyond the first hour of prolonged services, based on the place of service. These codes may be used to report the final 15 – 30 minutes of prolonged service on a given date, if not otherwise billed. Prolonged service of less than 15 minutes beyond the first hour or less than 15 minutes beyond the final 30 minutes is not reported separately.

#### B. Required Companion Codes
- The companion evaluation and management codes for 99354 are the Office or Other Outpatient visit codes (99201 - 99205, 99212 – 99215), the Domiciliary, Rest Home, or Custodial Care Services codes (99324 – 99328, 99334 – 99337), the Home Services codes (99341 - 99345, 99347 – 99350);
- The companion codes for 99355 are 99354 and one of the evaluation and management codes required for 99354 to be used;
- The companion evaluation and management codes for 99356 are the Initial Hospital Care codes and Subsequent Hospital Care codes (99221 - 99223, 99231 – 99233); Nursing Facility Services codes (99304 -99318); or
- The companion codes for 99357 are 99356 and one of the evaluation and management codes required for 99356 to be used.

Prolonged services codes 99354 – 99357 are not paid unless they are accompanied by the companion codes as indicated.

#### C. Requirement for Physician Presence
Physicians may count only the duration of direct face-to-face contact between the physician and the patient (whether the service was continuous or not) beyond the typical/average time of the visit code billed to determine whether prolonged services can be billed and to determine the prolonged services codes that are allowable. In the case of prolonged office services, time spent by office staff with the patient, or time the patient remains unaccompanied in the office cannot be billed. In the case of prolonged hospital services, time spent reviewing charts or discussion of a patient with house medical staff and not with direct face-to-face contact with the patient, or waiting for test results, for changes in the patient's condition, for end of a therapy, or for use of facilities cannot be billed as prolonged services.

#### D. Documentation
Documentation is not required to accompany the bill for prolonged services unless the physician has been selected for medical review. Documentation is required in the medical record about the duration and content of the medically necessary evaluation and management service and prolonged services billed. The medical record must be appropriately and sufficiently documented by the physician or qualified NPP to show that the physician or qualified NPP personally furnished the direct face-to-face time with the patient specified in the CPT code definitions. The start and end times of the visit shall be documented in the medical record along with the date of service.

#### E. Use of the Codes
Prolonged services codes can be billed only if the total duration of the physician or qualified NPP direct face-to-face service (including the visit) equals or exceeds the threshold time for the evaluation and management service the physician or qualified NPP provided (typical/average time associated with the CPT E/M code plus 30 minutes). If the total duration of direct face-to-face time does not equal or exceed the threshold time for the level of evaluation and management service the physician or qualified NPP provided, the physician or qualified NPP may not bill for prolonged services.

#### F. Threshold Times for Codes 99354 and 99355 (Office or Other Outpatient Setting)
If the total direct face-to-face time equals or exceeds the threshold time for code 99354, but is less than the threshold time for code 99355, the physician should bill the evaluation and management visit code and code 99354. No more than one unit of 99354 is acceptable. If the total direct face-to-face time equals or exceeds the threshold time for code 99355 by no more than 29 minutes, the physician should bill the visit code 99354 and one unit of code 99355. One additional unit of code 99355 is billed for each additional increment of 30 minutes extended duration. Contractors use the following threshold times to determine if the prolonged services codes 99354 and/or 99355 can be billed with the office or other outpatient settings including domiciliary, rest home, or custodial care services and home services codes.

Threshold Time for Prolonged Visit Codes 99354 and/or 99355 Billed with Office/Outpatient Code

| Code | Typical Time for Code | Threshold Time to Bill Code 99354 | Threshold Time to Bill Codes 99354 and 99355 |
|------|----------------------|-----------------------------------|----------------------------------------------|
| 99201 | 10 | 40 | 85 |
| 99202 | 20 | 50 | 95 |
| 99203 | 30 | 60 | 105 |
| 99204 | 45 | 75 | 120 |
| 99205 | 60 | 90 | 135 |
| 99212 | 10 | 40 | 85 |
| 99213 | 15 | 45 | 90 |
| 99214 | 25 | 55 | 100 |
| 99215 | 40 | 70 | 115 |
| 99324 | 20 | 50 | 95 |
| 99325 | 30 | 60 | 105 |
| 99326 | 45 | 75 | 120 |
| 99327 | 60 | 90 | 135 |
| 99328 | 75 | 105 | 150 |
| 99334 | 15 | 45 | 90 |
| 99335 | 25 | 55 | 100 |
| 99336 | 40 | 70 | 115 |

| Code | Typical Time for Code | Threshold Time to Bill Code 99354 | Threshold Time to Bill Codes 99354 and 99355 |
|------|------|------|------|
| 99337 | 60 | 90 | 135 |
| 99341 | 20 | 50 | 95 |
| 99342 | 30 | 60 | 105 |
| 99343 | 45 | 75 | 120 |
| 99344 | 60 | 90 | 135 |
| 99345 | 75 | 105 | 150 |
| 99347 | 15 | 45 | 90 |
| 99348 | 25 | 55 | 100 |
| 99349 | 40 | 70 | 115 |
| 99350 | 60 | 90 | 135 |

### G. Threshold Times for Codes 99356 and 99357

(Inpatient Setting) If the total direct face-to-face time equals or exceeds the threshold time for code 99356, but is less than the threshold time for code 99357, the physician should bill the visit and code 99356. Contractors do not accept more than one unit of code 99356. If the total direct face-to-face time equals or exceeds the threshold time for code 99356 by no more than 29 minutes, the physician bills the visit code 99356 and one unit of code 99357. One additional unit of code 99357 is billed for each additional increment of 30 minutes extended duration. Contractors use the following threshold times to determine if the prolonged services codes 99356 and/or 99357 can be billed with the inpatient setting codes.

Threshold Time for Prolonged Visit Codes 99356 and/or 99357 Billed with Inpatient Setting Codes Code

| Code | Typical Time for Code | Threshold Time to Bill Code 99356 | Threshold Time to Bill Codes 99356 and 99357 |
|------|------|------|------|
| 99221 | 30 | 60 | 105 |
| 99222 | 50 | 80 | 125 |
| 99223 | 70 | 100 | 145 |
| 99231 | 15 | 45 | 90 |
| 99232 | 25 | 55 | 100 |
| 99233 | 35 | 65 | 110 |
| 99304 | 25 | 55 | 100 |
| 99305 | 35 | 65 | 110 |
| 99306 | 45 | 75 | 120 |
| 99307 | 10 | 40 | 85 |
| 99308 | 15 | 45 | 90 |
| 99309 | 25 | 55 | 100 |
| 99310 | 35 | 65 | 110 |
| 99318 | 30 | 60 | 10 |

Add 30 minutes to the threshold time for billing codes 99356 and 99357 to get the threshold time for billing code 99356 and two units of 99357.

### H. Prolonged Services Associated With Evaluation and Management Services Based on Counseling and/or Coordination of Care (Time-Based)

When an evaluation and management service is dominated by counseling and/or coordination of care (the counseling and/or coordination of care represents more than 50% of the total time with the patient) in a face-to-face encounter between the physician or qualified NPP and the patient in the office/clinic or the floor time (in the scenario of an inpatient service), then the evaluation and management code is selected based on the typical/average time associated with the code levels. The time approximation must meet or exceed the specific CPT code billed (determined by the typical/average time associated with the evaluation and management code) and should not be "rounded" to the next higher level.

In those evaluation and management services in which the code level is selected based on time, prolonged services may only be reported with the highest code level in that family of codes as the companion code.

### I. Examples of Billable Prolonged Services

*EXAMPLE 1*

A physician performed a visit that met the definition of an office visit code 99213 and the total duration of the direct face-to-face services (including the visit) was 65 minutes. The physician bills code 99213 and one unit of code 99354.

*EXAMPLE 2*

A physician performed a visit that met the definition of a domiciliary, rest home care visit code 99327 and the total duration of the direct face-to-face contact (including the visit) was 140 minutes. The physician bills codes 99327, 99354, and one unit of code 99355.

*EXAMPLE 3*

A physician performed an office visit to an established patient that was predominantly counseling, spending 75 minutes (direct face-to-face) with the patient. The physician should report CPT code 99215 and one unit of code 99354.

### J. Examples of Nonbillable Prolonged Services

*EXAMPLE 1*

A physician performed a visit that met the definition of visit code 99212 and the total duration of the direct face-to-face contact (including the visit) was 35 minutes. The physician cannot bill prolonged services because the total duration of direct face-to-face service did not meet the threshold time for billing prolonged services.

*EXAMPLE 2*

A physician performed a visit that met the definition of code 99213 and, while the patient was in the office receiving treatment for 4 hours, the total duration of the direct face-to-face service of the physician was 40 minutes. The physician cannot bill prolonged services because the total duration of direct face-to-face service did not meet the threshold time for billing prolonged services.

*EXAMPLE 3*

A physician provided a subsequent office visit that was predominantly counseling, spending 60 minutes (face-to-face) with the patient. The physician cannot code 99214, which has a typical time of 25 minutes, and one unit of code 99354. The physician must bill the highest level code in the code family (99215 which has 40 minutes typical/average time units associated with it). The additional time spent beyond this code is 20 minutes and does not meet the threshold time for billing prolonged services.

## 100-4, 12, 30.6.15.2

### Prolonged Services Without Direct Face-to-Face Patient Contact Service (Codes 99358 - 99359)

(Rev. 3678, Issued: 12-16-16, Effective: 01-01-17, Implementation: 01-03-17)

Until CY 2017, CPT codes 99358 and 99359 were not separately payable and were bundled (included for payment) under the related face-to-face E/M service code. Practitioners were not permitted to bill the patient for services described by CPT codes 99358 and 99359 since they are Medicare covered services and payment was included in the payment for other billable services.

Beginning in CY 2017, CPT codes 99358 and 99359 are separately payable under the physician fee schedule. The CPT prefatory language and reporting rules for these codes apply for Medicare billing. For example, CPT codes 99358 and 99359 cannot be reported during the same service period as complex chronic care management (CCM) services or transitional care management services. They are not reported for time spent in non-face-to-face care described by more specific codes having no upper time limit in the CPT code set. We have posted a file that notes the times assumed to be typical for purposes of PFS rate-setting. That file is available on our website under downloads for our annual regulation at http://www.cms.gov/Medicare/Medicare-Fee-for-Service-Payment/PhysicianFeeSched/PFS-Federal-Regulation-Notices.html. We note that while these typical times are not required to bill the displayed codes, we would expect that only time spent in excess of these times should be reported under CPT codes 99358 and 99359. We note that CPT codes 99358 and 99359 can only be used to report extended qualifying time of the billing physician or other practitioner (not clinical staff). Prolonged services cannot be reported in association with a companion E/M code that also qualifies as the initiating visit for CCM services. Practitioners should instead report the add-on code for CCM initiation, if applicable.

## 100-04, 12, 30.6.15.3

### Physician Standby Service

Standby services are not payable to physicians. Physicians may not bill Medicare or beneficiaries for standby services. Payment for standby services is included in the Part A payment to the facility. Such services are a part of hospital costs to provide quality care.

If hospitals pay physicians for standby services, such services are part of hospital costs to provide quality care.

## 100-04, 12, 40.3

### Claims Review for Global Surgeries

#### A. Relationship to Correct Coding Initiative (CCI)

The CCI policy and computer edits allow A/B MACs (B) to detect instances of fragmented billing for certain intra-operative services and other services furnished on the same day as the surgery that are considered to be components of the surgical procedure and, therefore, included in the global surgical fee. When both correct coding and global surgery edits apply to the same claim, A/B MACs (B) first apply the correct coding edits, then, apply the global surgery edits to the correctly coded services.

#### B. Prepayment Edits to Detect Separate Billing of Services Included in the Global Package

In addition to the correct coding edits, A/B MACs (B) must be capable of detecting certain other services included in the payment for a major or minor surgery or for an endoscopy. On a prepayment basis, A/B MACs (B) identify the services that meet the following conditions:

- Preoperative services that are submitted on the same claim or on a subsequent claim as a surgical procedure; or

- Same day or postoperative services that are submitted on the same claim or on a subsequent claim as a surgical procedure or endoscopy;

  and -

CPT © 2017 American Medical Association. All Rights Reserved.

© 2017 Optum360, LLC

- Services that were furnished within the prescribed global period of the surgical procedure;
- Services that are billed without modifier "-78," "-79," "-24," "25," or "-57" or are billed with modifier "-24" but without the required documentation; and
- Services that are billed with the same provider or group number as the surgical procedure or endoscopy. Also, edit for any visits billed separately during the postoperative period without modifier "-24" by a physician who billed for the postoperative care only with modifier "-55."

A/B MACs (B) use the following evaluation and management codes in establishing edits for visits included in the global package. CPT codes 99241, 99242, 99243, 99244, 99245, 99251, 99252, 99253, 99254, 99255, 99271, 99272, 99273, 99274, and 99275 have been transferred from the excluded category and are now included in the global surgery edits.

**Evaluation and Management Codes for A/B MAC (B) Edits**

| 92012 | 92014 | 99211 | 99212 | 99213 | 99214 | 99215 |
|-------|-------|-------|-------|-------|-------|-------|
| 99217 | 99218 | 99219 | 99220 | 99221 | 99222 | 99223 |
| 99231 | 99232 | 99233 | 99234 | 99235 | 99236 | 99238 |
| 99239 | 99241 | 99242 | 99243 | 99244 | 99245 | 99251 |
| 99252 | 99253 | 99254 | 99255 | 99261 | 99262 | 99263 |
| 99271 | 99272 | 99273 | 99274 | 99275 | 99291 | 99292 |
| 99301 | 99302 | 99303 | 99311 | 99312 | 99313 | 99315 |
| 99316 | 99331 | 99332 | 99333 | 99347 | 99348 | 99349 |
| 99350 | 99374 | 99375 | 99377 | 99378 |       |       |

NOTE: In order for codes 99291 or 99292 to be paid for services furnished during the preoperative or postoperative period, modifier "-25" or "-24," respectively, must be used to indicate that the critical care was unrelated to the specific anatomic injury or general surgical procedure performed.

If a surgeon is admitting a patient to a nursing facility for a condition not related to the global surgical procedure, the physician should bill for the nursing facility admission and care with a "-24" modifier and appropriate documentation. If a surgeon is admitting a patient to a nursing facility and the patient's admission to that facility relates to the global surgical procedure, the nursing facility admission and any services related to the global surgical procedure are included in the global surgery fee.

**C. Exclusions from Prepayment Edits**
A/B MACs (B) exclude the following services from the prepayment audit process and allow separate payment if all usual requirements are met:

- Services listed in §40.1.B; and
- Services billed with the modifier "-25," "-57," "-58," "-78," or "-79."

Exceptions

See §§40.2.A.8, 40.2.A.9, and 40.4.A for instances where prepayment review is required for modifier "-25." In addition, prepayment review is necessary for CPT codes 90935, 90937, 90945, and 90947 when a visit and modifier "-25" are billed with these services.

Exclude the following codes from the prepayment edits required in §40.3.B.

| 92002 | 92004 | 99201 | 99202 | 99203 | 99204 | 99205 |
|-------|-------|-------|-------|-------|-------|-------|
| 99281 | 99282 | 99283 | 99284 | 99285 | 99321 | 99322 |
| 99323 | 99341 | 99342 | 99343 | 99344 | 99345 |       |

## 100-04, 12, 40.7

### *Claims for Bilateral Surgeries*
B3-4827, B3-15040

**A. General**
Bilateral surgeries are procedures performed on both sides of the body during the same operative session or on the same day.

The terminology for some procedure codes includes the terms "bilateral" (e.g., code 27395; Lengthening of the hamstring tendon; multiple, bilateral.) or "unilateral or bilateral" (e.g., code 52290; cystourethroscopy; with ureteral meatotomy, unilateral or bilateral). The payment adjustment rules for bilateral surgeries do not apply to procedures identified by CPT as "bilateral" or "unilateral or bilateral" since the fee schedule reflects any additional work required for bilateral surgeries.

Field 22 of the MFSDB indicates whether the payment adjustment rules apply to a surgical procedure.

**B. Billing Instructions for Bilateral Surgeries**
If a procedure is not identified by its terminology as a bilateral procedure (or unilateral or bilateral), physicians must report the procedure with modifier "-50." They report such procedures as a single line item. (NOTE: This differs from the CPT coding guidelines which indicate that bilateral procedures should be billed as two line items.)

If a procedure is identified by the terminology as bilateral (or unilateral or bilateral), as in codes 27395 and 52290, physicians do not report the procedure with modifier "-50."

**C. Claims Processing System Requirements**
Carriers must be able to:

1. Identify bilateral surgeries by the presence on the claim form or electronic submission of the "-50" modifier or of the same code on separate lines reported once with modifier "-LT" and once with modifier "-RT";
2. Access Field 34 or 35 of the MFSDB to determine the Medicare payment amount;
3. Access Field 22 of the MFSDB:
   — If Field 22 contains an indicator of "0," "2," or "3," the payment adjustment rules for bilateral surgeries do not apply. Base payment on the lower of the billed amount or 100 percent of the fee schedule amount (Field 34 or 35) unless other payment adjustment rules apply.

   NOTE: Some codes which have a bilateral indicator of "0" in the MFSDB may be performed more than once on a given day. These are services that would never be considered bilateral and thus should not be billed with modifier "-50." Where such a code is billed on multiple line tems or with more than 1 in the units field and carriers have determined that the code may be reported more than once, bypass the "0" bilateral indicator and refer to the multiple surgery field for pricing;

   — If Field 22 contains an indicator of "1," the standard adjustment rules apply. Base payment on the lower of the billed amount or 150 percent of the fee schedule amount (Field 34 or 35). (Multiply the payment amount in Field 34 or 35 for the surgery by 150 percent and round to the nearest cent.)
4. Apply the requirements 40 - 40.4 on global surgeries to bilateral surgeries; and
5. Retain the "-50" modifier in history for any bilateral surgeries paid at the adjusted amount.

   (NOTE: The "-50" modifier is not retained for surgeries which are bilateral by definition such as code 27395.)

## 100-04, 12, 40.8

### *Claims for Co-Surgeons and Team Surgeons*
B3-4828, B3-15046

**A. General**
Under some circumstances, the individual skills of two or more surgeons are required to perform surgery on the same patient during the same operative session. This may be required because of the complex nature of the procedure(s) and/or the patient's condition.

In these cases, the additional physicians are not acting as assistants-at-surgery.

**B. Billing Instructions**
The following billing procedures apply when billing for a surgical procedure or procedures that required the use of two surgeons or a team of surgeons:

- If two surgeons (each in a different specialty) are required to perform a specific procedure, each surgeon bills for the procedure with a modifier "-62. " Co-surgery also refers to surgical procedures involving two surgeons performing the parts of the procedure simultaneously, i.e., heart transplant or bilateral knee replacements. Documentation of the medical necessity for two surgeons is required for certain services identified in the MFSDB. (See 40.8.C.5.);
- If a team of surgeons (more than 2 surgeons of different specialties) is required to perform a specific procedure, each surgeon bills for the procedure with a modifier "-66." Field 25 of the MFSDB identifies certain services submitted with a "-66" modifier which must be sufficiently documented to establish that a team was medically necessary. All claims for team surgeons must contain sufficient information to allow pricing "by report."
- If surgeons of different specialties are each performing a different procedure (with specific CPT codes), neither co-surgery nor multiple surgery rules apply (even if the procedures are performed through the same incision). If one of the surgeons performs multiple procedures, the multiple procedure rules apply to that surgeon's services. (See 40.6 for multiple surgery payment rules.)

For co-surgeons (modifier 62), the fee schedule amount applicable to the payment for each co-surgeon is 62.5 percent of the global surgery fee schedule amount. Team surgery (modifier 66) is paid for on a "By Report" basis.

**C. Claims Processing System Requirements**
Carriers must be able to:

1. Identify a surgical procedure performed by two surgeons or a team of surgeons by the presence on the claim form or electronic submission of the "-62" or "-66" modifier;
2. Access Field 34 or 35 of the MFSDB to determine the fee schedule payment amount for the surgery;
3. Access Field 24 or 25, as appropriate, of the MFSDB. These fields provide guidance on whether two or team surgeons are generally required for the surgical procedure;
4. If the surgery is billed with a "-62" or "-66" modifier and Field 24 or 25 contains an indicator of "0," payment adjustment rules for two or team surgeons do not apply:
   — Carriers pay the first bill submitted, and base payment on the lower of the billed amount or 100 percent of the fee schedule amount (Field 34 or 35) unless other payment adjustment rules apply;

— Carriers deny bills received subsequently from other physicians and use the appropriate MSN message in 40.8.D. As these are medical necessity denials, the instructions in the Program Integrity Manual regarding denial of unassigned claims for medical necessity are applied;

5. If the surgery is billed with a "-62" modifier and Field 24 contains an indicator of "1," suspend the claim for manual review of any documentation submitted with the claim. If the documentation supports the need for co-surgeons, base payment for each physician on the lower of the billed amount or 62.5 percent of the fee schedule amount (Field 34 or 35);

6. If the surgery is billed with a "-62" modifier and Field 24 contains an indicator of "2," payment rules for two surgeons apply. Carriers base payment for each physician on the lower of the billed amount or 62.5 percent of the fee schedule amount (Field 34 or 35);

7. If the surgery is billed with a "-66" modifier and Field 25 contains an indicator of "1," carriers suspend the claim for manual review. If carriers determine that team surgeons were medically necessary, each physician is paid on a "by report" basis;

8. If the surgery is billed with a "-66" modifier and Field 25 contains an indicator of "2," carriers pay "by report";

NOTE: A Medicare fee may have been established for some surgical procedures that are billed with the "-66" modifier. In these cases, all physicians on the team must agree on the percentage of the Medicare payment amount each is to receive.

If carriers receive a bill with a "-66" modifier after carriers have paid one surgeon the full Medicare payment amount (on a bill without the modifier), deny the subsequent claim.

9. Apply the rules global surgical packages to each of the physicians participating in a co- or team surgery; and

10. Retain the "-62" and "-66" modifiers in history for any co- or team surgeries.

### D. Beneficiary Liability on Denied Claims for Assistant, Co- surgeon and Team Surgeons

MSN message 23.10 which states "Medicare does not pay for a surgical assistant for this kind of surgery," was established for denial of claims for assistant surgeons. Where such payment is denied because the procedure is subject to the statutory restriction against payment for assistants-at-surgery. Carriers include the following statement in the MSN:

"You cannot be charged for this service." (Unnumbered add-on message.)

Carriers use Group Code CO on the remittance advice to the physician to signify that the beneficiary may not be billed for the denied service and that the physician could be subject to penalties if a bill is issued to the beneficiary.

If Field 23 of the MFSDB contains an indicator of "0" or "1" (assistant-at-surgery may not be paid) for procedures CMS has determined that an assistant surgeon is not generally medically necessary.

For those procedures with an indicator of "0," the limitation on liability provisions described in Chapter 30 apply to assigned claims. Therefore, carriers include the appropriate limitation of liability language from Chapter 21. For unassigned claims, apply the rules in the Program Integrity Manual concerning denial for medical necessity.

Where payment may not be made for a co- or team surgeon, use the following MSN message (MSN message number 15.13):

Medicare does not pay for team surgeons for this procedure.

Where payment may not be made for a two surgeons, use the following MSN message (MSN message number 15.12):

Medicare does not pay for two surgeons for this procedure.

Also see limitation of liability remittance notice REF remark codes M25, M26, and M27.

Use the following message on the remittance notice:

Multiple physicians/assistants are not covered in this case. (Reason code 54.)

## 100-4, 12, 50

### Payment for Anesthesiology Services
(Rev. 3747; Issued: 04-14-17; Effective: 01-01-17; Implementation: 05-15-17)

#### A. General Payment Rule
The fee schedule amount for physician anesthesia services furnished is, with the exceptions noted, based on allowable base and time units multiplied by an anesthesia conversion factor specific to that locality. The base unit for each anesthesia procedure is communicated to the A/B MACs by means of the HCPCS file released annually. CMS releases the conversion factor annually. The base units and conversion factor are available on the CMS website at: https://www.cms.gov/Center/Provider-Type/Anesthesiologists-Center.html.

#### B. Payment at Personally Performed Rate
The A/B MAC must determine the fee schedule payment, recognizing the base unit for the anesthesia code and one time unit per 15 minutes of anesthesia time if:

• The physician personally performed the entire anesthesia service alone;

• The physician is involved with one anesthesia case with a resident, the physician is a teaching physician as defined in §100;

• The physician is involved in the training of physician residents in a single anesthesia case, two concurrent anesthesia cases involving residents or a single anesthesia case involving a resident that is concurrent to another case that meets the requirements for payment at the medically directed rate. The physician meets the teaching physician criteria in §100.1.4;

• The physician is continuously involved in a single case involving a student nurse anesthetist;

• If the physician is involved with a single case with a qualified nonphysician anesthetist (a certified registered nurse anesthetist (CRNA) or an anesthesiologist's assistant)), A/B MACs may pay the physician service and the qualified nonphysician anesthetist service in accordance with the requirements for payment at the medically directed rate;

Or

• The physician and the CRNA (or anesthesiologist's assistant) are involved in one anesthesia case and the services of each are found to be medically necessary. Documentation must be submitted by both the CRNA and the physician to support payment of the full fee for each of the two providers. The physician reports the AA modifier and the CRNA reports the QZ modifier.

#### C. Payment at the Medically Directed Rate
The A/B MAC determines payment at the medically directed rate for the physician on the basis of 50 percent of the allowance for the service performed by the physician alone. Payment will be made at the medically directed rate if the physician medically directs qualified individuals (all of whom could be CRNAs, anesthesiologists' assistants, interns, residents, or combinations of these individuals) in two, three, or four concurrent cases and the physician performs the followingactivities.

• Performs a pre-anesthetic examination and evaluation;

• Prescribes the anesthesia plan;

• Personally participates in the most demanding procedures in the anesthesia plan, including, if applicable, induction and emergence;

• Ensures that any procedures in the anesthesia plan that he or she does not perform are performed by a qualified individual;

• Monitors the course of anesthesia administration at frequent intervals;

• Remains physically present and available for immediate diagnosis and treatment of emergencies; and

• Provides indicated post-anesthesia care.

The physician must document in the medical record that he or she performed the pre-anesthetic examination and evaluation. Physicians must also document that they provided indicated post-anesthesia care, were present during some portion of the anesthesia monitoring, and were present during the most demanding procedures in the anesthesia plan, including induction and emergence, where indicated.

NOTE: Concurrency refers to to the maximum number of procedures that the physician is medically directing within the context of a single procedure andwhether these other procedures overlap each other. Concurrency is not dependent on each of the cases involving a Medicare patient. For example, if an anesthesiologist medically directs three concurrent procedures, two of which involve non-Medicare patients and the remaining a Medicare patient, this represents three concurrent cases.

The requirements for payment at the medically directed rate also apply to cases involving student nurse anesthetists if the physician medically directs two concurrent cases, with each of the two cases involving a student nurse anesthetist, or the physician directs one case involving a student nurse anesthetist and another involving a qualified individual (for example: CRNA, anesthesiologist's assistant, intern or resident).

The requirements for payment at the medically directed rate do not apply to a single resident case that is concurrent to another anesthesia case paid at the medically directed rate or to two concurrent anesthesia cases involving residents.

If anesthesiologists are in a group practice, one physician member may provide the pre- anesthesia examination and evaluation while another fulfills the other criteria. Similarly, one physician member of the group may provide post-anesthesia care while another member of the group furnishes the other component parts of the anesthesia service. However, the medical record must indicate that the services were furnished by physicians and identify the physicians who furnished them.

A physician who is concurrently furnishing services that meet the requirements for payment at the medically directed rate cannot ordinarily be involved in furnishing additional services to other patients. However, addressing an emergency of short duration in the immediate area, administering an epidural or caudal anesthetic to ease labor pain, periodic (rather than continuous) monitoring of an obstetrical patient, receiving patients entering the operating suite for the next surgery, checking or discharging patients in the recovery room, or handling scheduling matters, do not substantially diminish the scope of control exercised by the physician and do not constitute a separate service for the purpose of determining whether the requirements for payment at the medically directed rate are met.

However, if the physician leaves the immediate area of the operating suite for other than short durations or devotes extensive time to an emergency case or is otherwise not available to respond to the immediate needs of the surgical patients, the physician's services to the surgical patients would not meet the requirements for payment at the medically directed rate. A/B MACs may not make payment under the feeschedule.

CPT © 2017 American Medical Association. All Rights Reserved.                    © 2017 Optum360, LLC

#### D. Payment at Medically Supervised Rate

The A/B MAC may allow only three base units per procedure when the anesthesiologist is involved in furnishing more than four procedures concurrently or is performing other services while directing the concurrent procedures. An additional time unit may be recognized if the physician can document he or she was present atinduction.

#### E. Billing and Payment for Multiple Anesthesia Procedures

Physicians bill for the anesthesia services associated with multiple bilateral surgeries by reporting the anesthesia procedure with the highest base unit value with the multiple procedure modifier -51. They report the total time for all procedures in the line item with the highest base unit value.

If the same anesthesia CPT code applies to two or more of the surgical procedures, billers enter the anesthesia code with the -51 modifier and the number of surgeries to which the modified CPT code applies.

Payment can be made under the fee schedule for anesthesia services associated with multiple surgical procedures or multiple bilateral procedures. Payment is determined based on the base unit of the anesthesia procedure with the highest base unit value and time units based on the actual anesthesia time of the multiple procedures. See §§40.6-40.7 for billing and claims processing instructions for multiple and bilateral surgeries.

#### F. Payment for Medical and Surgical Services Furnished in Addition to Anesthesia Procedure

Payment may be made under the fee schedule for specific medical and surgical services furnished by the anesthesiologist as long as these services are reasonable and medically necessary or provided that other rebundling provisions (see §30 and Chapter 23) do not preclude separate payment. These services may be furnished in conjunction with the anesthesia procedure to the patient or may be furnished as single services, e.g., during the day of or the day before the anesthesia service. These services include the insertion of a Swan Ganz catheter, the insertion of central venous pressure lines, emergency intubation, and critical care visits.

#### G. Anesthesia Time and Calculation of Anesthesia TimeUnits

Anesthesia time is defined as the period during which an anesthesia practitioner is present with the patient. It starts when the anesthesia practitioner begins to prepare the patient for anesthesia services in the operating room or an equivalent area and ends when the anesthesia practitioner is no longer furnishing anesthesia services to the patient, that is, when the patient may be placed safely under postoperative care. Anesthesia time is a continuous time period from the start of anesthesia to the end of an anesthesia service. In counting anesthesia time for services furnished, the anesthesia practitioner can add blocks of time around an interruption in anesthesia time as long as the anesthesia practitioner is furnishing continuous anesthesia care within the time periods around the interruption.

Actual anesthesia time in minutes is reported on the claim. For anesthesia services furnished, the A/B MAC computes time units by dividing reported anesthesia time by 15 minutes. Round the time unit to one decimal place. The A/B MAC does not recognize time units for CPT code 01996 (daily hospital management of epidural or subarachnoid continuous drug administration).

For purposes of this section, anesthesia practitioner means:

- a physician who performs the anesthesia service alone,
- a CRNA who is furnishing services that do not meet the requirements for payment at the medically directed rate,
- a qualified nonphysician anesthetist who is furnishing services that meet the requirements for payment at the medically directed rate.

The physician who medically directs the qualified nonphysician anesthetist would ordinarily report the same time as the qualified nonphysician anesthetist reports for the service.

#### H. Monitored Anesthesia Care

Monitored anesthesia care involves the intra-operative monitoring by a physician or qualified individual under the medical direction of a physician or of the patient's vital physiological signs in anticipation of the need for administration of general anesthesia or of the development of adverse physiological patient reaction to the surgical procedure. It also includes the performance of a pre-anesthetic examination and evaluation, prescription of the anesthesia care required, administration of any necessary oral or parenteral medications (e.g., atropine, demerol, valium) and provision of indicated postoperative anesthesia care.

The A/B MAC pays for reasonable and medically necessary monitored anesthesia care services on the same basis as other anesthesia services. If the physician personally performs the monitored anesthesia care case, payment is made under the fee schedule using the payment rules for payment at the personally performed rate. If the physician medically directs four or fewer concurrent cases and monitored anesthesia care represents one or more of these concurrentcases, payment is made under the fee schedule using the payment rules for payment at the medically directed rate. Anesthesiologists use the QS modifier to report monitored anesthesia care cases, in addition to reporting the actual anesthesia time and one of the payment modifiers on the claim.

#### I. Anesthesia Claims Modifiers

Physicians report the appropriate modifier to denote whether the service meets the requirements for payment at the personally performed rate, medically directed rate, or medically supervised rate.

    AA - Anesthesia Services performed personally by the anesthesiologist

    AD - Medical Supervision by a physician; more than 4 concurrent anesthesia procedures

    G8 - Monitored anesthesia care (MAC) for deep complex, complicated, or markedly invasive surgical procedures

    G9 - Monitored anesthesia care for patient who has a history of severe cardio-pulmonary condition

    QK - Medical direction of two, three or four concurrent anesthesia procedures involving qualified individuals

    QS - Monitored anesthesia care service

**NOTE:** The QS modifier can be used by a physician or a qualified nonphysician anesthetist and is for informational purposes. Providers must report actual anesthesia time and one of the payment modifiers on the claim.

    QY - Medical direction of one qualified nonphysician anesthetist by an anesthesiologist

    GC - These services have been performed by a resident under the direction of a teaching physician.

**NOTE:** The GC modifier is reported by the teaching physician to indicate he/she rendered the service in compliance with the teaching physician requirements in §100 of this chapter. One of the payment modifiers must be used in conjunction with the GC modifier.

The A/B MAC must determine payment for anesthesia in accordance with these instructions. They must be able to determine the uniform base unit that is assigned to the anesthesia code and apply the appropriate reduction where the anesthesia procedure meets the requirements for payment at the medically directed rate. They must also be able to determine the number of anesthesia time units from actual anesthesia time reported on the claim. The A/B MAC must multiply allowable units by the anesthesia-specific conversion factor used to determine fee schedule payment for the payment area.

#### J. Moderate Sedation Services Furnished in Conjunction with and in Support of Procedural Services

Anesthesia services range in complexity. The continuum of anesthesia services, from least intense to most intense in complexity is as follows: local or topical anesthesia, moderate (conscious) sedation, regional anesthesia and general anesthesia. Moderate sedation is a drug induced depression of consciousness during which the patient responds purposefully to verbal commands, either alone or accompanied by light tactile stimulation. Moderate sedation does not include minimal sedation, deep sedation or monitored anesthesia care.

Practitioners will report the appropriate CPT and/or HCPCS code that describes the moderate sedation services furnished during a patient encounter, which are furnished in conjunction with and in support of a procedural service, consistent with CPT guidance.

Refer to §50 and §140 of this chapter for information regarding reporting of anesthesia services furnished in conjunction with and in support of procedural services.

#### K. Anesthesia for Diagnostic or Therapeutic Nerve Blocks and Services Lower in Intensity than Moderate Sedation

If the anesthesiologist or CRNA provides anesthesia for diagnostic or therapeutic nerve blocks or injections and a different provider performs the block or injection, then the anesthesiologist or CRNA may report the anesthesia service using the appropriate CPT code consistent with CPT guidance. The service must meet the criteria for monitored anesthesia care as described in this section. If the anesthesiologist or CRNA provides both the anesthesia service and the block or injection, then the anesthesiologist or CRNA may report the anesthesia service and the injection or block. However, the anesthesia service must meet the requirements for moderate sedation and if a lower level complexity anesthesia service is provided, then the moderate sedation code should not be reported.

If the physician performing the medical or surgical procedure also provides a level of anesthesia lower in intensity than moderate sedation, such as a local or topical anesthesia, then the moderate sedation code should not be reported and no separate payment should be allowed by the A/B MAC.

## 100-04, 12, 100

### *Teaching Physician Services*

#### Definitions

For purposes of this section, the following definitions apply.

Resident -An individual who participates in an approved graduate medical education (GME) program or a physician who is not in an approved GME program but who is authorized to practice only in a hospital setting. The term includes interns and fellows in GME programs recognized as approved for purposes of direct GME payments made by the FI. Receiving a staff or faculty appointment or participating in a fellowship does not by itself alter the status of "resident". Additionally, this status remains unaffected regardless of whether a hospital includes the physician in its full time equivalency count of residents.

Student- An individual who participates in an accredited educational program (e.g., a medical school) that is not an approved GME program. A student is never considered to be an intern or a resident. Medicare does not pay for any service furnished by a student. See 100.1.1B for a discussion concerning E/M service documentation performed by students.

**Teaching Physician** -A physician (other than another resident) who involves residents in the care of his or her patients.

**Direct Medical and Surgical Services** -Services to individual beneficiaries that are either personally furnished by a physician or furnished by a resident under the supervision of a physician in a teaching hospital making the reasonable cost election for physician services furnished in teaching hospitals. All payments for such services are made by the FI for the hospital.

**Teaching Hospital** -A hospital engaged in an approved GME residency program in medicine, osteopathy, dentistry, or podiatry.

**Teaching Setting** -Any provider, hospital-based provider, or nonprovider setting in which Medicare payment for the services of residents is made by the FI under the direct graduate medical education payment methodology or freestanding SNF or HHA in which such payments are made on a reasonable cost basis.

**Critical or Key Portion**- That part (or parts) of a service that the teaching physician determines is (are) a critical or key portion(s). For purposes of this section, these terms are interchangeable.

**Documentation**- Notes recorded in the patient's medical records by a resident, and/or teaching physician or others as outlined in the specific situations below regarding the service furnished. Documentation may be dictated and typed or hand-written, or computer-generated and typed or handwritten. Documentation must be dated and include a legible signature or identity. Pursuant to 42 CFR 415.172 (b), documentation must identify, at a minimum, the service furnished, the participation of the teaching physician in providing the service, and whether the teaching physician was physically present. In the context of an electronic medical record, the term 'macro' means a command in a computer or dictation application that automatically generates predetermined text that is not edited by the user.

When using an electronic medical record, it is acceptable for the teaching physician to use a macro as the required personal documentation if the teaching physician adds it personally in a secured (password protected) system. In addition to the teaching physician's macro, either the resident or the teaching physician must provide customized information that is sufficient to support a medical necessity determination. The note in the electronic medical record must sufficiently describe the specific services furnished to the specific patient on the specific date. It is insufficient documentation if both the resident and the teaching physician use macros only.

**Physically Present**- The teaching physician is located in the same room (or partitioned or curtained area, if the room is subdivided to accommodate multiple patients) as the patient and/or performs a face-to-face service.

## 100-04, 12, 100.1.1

### Evaluation and Management (E/M) Services

#### A. General Documentation Instructions and Common Scenarios

Evaluation and Management (E/M) Services -- For a given encounter, the selection of the appropriate level of E/M service should be determined according to the code definitions in the American Medical Association's Current Procedural Terminology (CPT) and any applicable documentation guidelines.

For purposes of payment, E/M services billed by teaching physicians require that they personally document at least the following:

- That they performed the service or were physically present during the key or critical portions of the service when performed by the resident; and

- The participation of the teaching physician in the management of the patient.

When assigning codes to services billed by teaching physicians, reviewers will combine the documentation of both the resident and the teaching physician.

Documentation by the resident of the presence and participation of the teaching physician is not sufficient to establish the presence and participation of the teaching physician.

On medical review, the combined entries into the medical record by the teaching physician and the resident constitute the documentation for the service and together must support the medical necessity of the service.

Following are four common scenarios for teaching physicians providing E/M services:

Scenario 1:

The teaching physician personally performs all the required elements of an E/M service without a resident. In this scenario the resident may or may not have performed the E/M service independently.

In the absence of a note by a resident, the teaching physician must document as he/she would document an E/M service in a nonteaching setting.

Where a resident has written notes, the teaching physician's note may reference the resident's note. The teaching physician must document that he/she performed the critical or key portion(s) of the service, and that he/she was directly involved in the management of the patient. For payment, the composite of the teaching physician's entry and the resident's entry together must support the medical necessity of the billed service and the level of the service billed by the teaching physician.

Scenario 2:

The resident performs the elements required for an E/M service in the presence of, or jointly with, the teaching physician and the resident documents the service. In this case, the teaching physician must document that he/she was present during the performance of the critical or key portion(s) of the service and that he/she was directly involved in the management of the patient. The teaching physician's note should reference the resident's note. For payment, the composite of the teaching physician's entry and the resident's entry together must support the medical necessity and the level of the service billed by the teaching physician.

Scenario 3:

The resident performs some or all of the required elements of the service in the absence of the teaching physician and documents his/her service. The teaching physician independently performs the critical or key portion(s) of the service with or without the resident present and, as appropriate, discusses the case with the resident. In this instance, the teaching physician must document that he/she personally saw the patient, personally performed critical or key portions of the service, and participated in the management of the patient. The teaching physician's note should reference the resident's note. For payment, the composite of the teaching physician's entry and the resident's entry together must support the medical necessity of the billed service and the level of the service billed by the teaching physician.

Scenario 4:

When a medical resident admits a patient to a hospital late at night and the teaching physician does not see the patient until later, including the next calendar day:

- The teaching physician must document that he/she personally saw the patient and participated in the management of the patient. The teaching physician may reference the resident's note in lieu of re-documenting the history of present illness, exam, medical decision-making, review of systems and/or past family/social history provided that the patient's condition has not changed, and the teaching physician agrees with the resident's note.

- The teaching physician's note must reflect changes in the patient's condition and clinical course that require that the resident's note be amended with further information to address the patient's condition and course at the time the patient is seen personally by the teaching physician.

- The teaching physician's bill must reflect the date of service he/she saw the patient and his/her personal work of obtaining a history, performing a physical, and participating in medical decision-making regardless of whether the combination of the teaching physician's and resident's documentation satisfies criteria for a higher level of service. For payment, the composite of the teaching physician's entry and the resident's entry together must support the medical necessity of the billed service and the level of the service billed by the teaching physician.

Following are examples of minimally acceptable documentation for each of these scenarios:

Scenario 1:

Admitting Note: "I performed a history and physical examination of the patient and discussed his management with the resident. I reviewed the resident's note and agree with the documented findings and plan of care."

Follow-up Visit: "Hospital Day #3. I saw and evaluated the patient. I agree with the findings and the plan of care as documented in the resident's note."

Follow-up Visit: "Hospital Day #5. I saw and examined the patient. I agree with the resident's note except the heart murmur is louder, so I will obtain an echo to evaluate."

(NOTE: In this scenario if there are no resident notes, the teaching physician must document as he/she would document an E/M service in a non-teaching setting.)

Scenario 2:

Initial or Follow-up Visit: "I was present with the resident during the history and exam. I discussed the case with the resident and agree with the findings and plan as documented in the resident's note."

Follow-up Visit: "I saw the patient with the resident and agree with the resident's findings and plan."

Scenarios 3 and 4:

Initial Visit: "I saw and evaluated the patient. I reviewed the resident's note and agree, except that picture is more consistent with pericarditis than myocardial ischemia. Will begin NSAIDs."

Initial or Follow-up Visit: "I saw and evaluated the patient. Discussed with resident and agree with resident's findings and plan as documented in the resident's note."

Follow-up Visit: "See resident's note for details. I saw and evaluated the patient and agree with the resident's finding and plans as written."

Follow-up Visit: "I saw and evaluated the patient. Agree with resident's note but lower extremities are weaker, now 3/5; MRI of L/S Spine today."

Following are examples of unacceptable documentation:

- "Agree with above." followed by legible countersignature or identity;

- "Rounded, Reviewed, Agree." followed by legible countersignature or identity;

- "Discussed with resident. Agree." followed by legible countersignature or identity;

- "Seen and agree." followed by legible countersignature or identity;
- "Patient seen and evaluated." followed by legible countersignature or identity; and
- A legible countersignature or identity alone.

Such documentation is not acceptable, because the documentation does not make it possible to determine whether the teaching physician was present, evaluated the patient, and/or had any involvement with the plan of care.

### B. E/M Service Documentation Provided By Students

Any contribution and participation of a student to the performance of a billable service (other than the review of systems and/or past family/social history which are not separately billable, but are taken as part of an E/M service) must be performed in the physical presence of a teaching physician or physical presence of a resident in a service meeting the requirements set forth in this section for teaching physician billing.

Students may document services in the medical record. However, the documentation of an E/M service by a student that may be referred to by the teaching physician is limited to documentation related to the review of systems and/or past family/social history. The teaching physician may not refer to a student's documentation of physical exam findings or medical decision making in his or her personal note. If the medical student documents E/M services, the teaching physician must verify and redocument the history of present illness as well as perform and redocument the physical exam and medical decision making activities of the service.

### C. Exception for E/M Services Furnished in Certain Primary Care Centers

Teaching physicians providing E/M services with a GME program granted a primary care exception may bill Medicare for lower and mid-level E/M services provided by residents. For the E/M codes listed below, teaching physicians may submit claims for services furnished by residents in the absence of a teaching physician:

| New Patient | Established Patient |
|---|---|
| 99201 | 99211 |
| 99202 | 99212 |
| 99203 | 99213 |

Effective January 1, 2005, the following code is included under the primary care exception: HCPCS code G0402 (Initial preventive physical examination; face-to-face visit services limited to new beneficiary during the first 12 months of Medicare enrollment).

Effective January 1, 2011, the following codes are included under the primary care exception: HCPCS codes G0438 (Annual wellness visit, including personal preventive plan service, first visit) and G0439 (Annual wellness visit, including personal preventive plan service, subsequent visit).

If a service other than those listed above needs to be furnished, then the general teaching physician policy set forth in §100.1 applies. For this exception to apply, a center must attest in writing that all the following conditions are met for a particular residency program. Prior approval is not necessary, but centers exercising the primary care exception must maintain records demonstrating that they qualify for the exception.

The services must be furnished in a center located in the outpatient department of a hospital or another ambulatory care entity in which the time spent by residents in patient care activities is included in determining direct GME payments to a teaching hospital by the hospital's FI. This requirement is not met when the resident is assigned to a physician's office away from the center or makes home visits. In the case of a nonhospital entity, verify with the FI that the entity meets the requirements of a written agreement between the hospital and the entity set forth at 42 CFR 413.78(e)(3)(ii).

Under this exception, residents providing the billable patient care service without the physical presence of a teaching physician must have completed at least 6 months of a GME approved residency program. Centers must maintain information under the provisions at 42 CFR 413.79(a)(6).

Teaching physicians submitting claims under this exception may not supervise more than four residents at any given time and must direct the care from such proximity as to constitute immediate availability. Teaching physicians may include residents with less than 6 months in a GME approved residency program in the mix of four residents under the teaching physician's supervision. However, the teaching physician must be physically present for the critical or key portions of services furnished by the residents with less than 6 months in a GME approved residency program. That is, the primary care exception does not apply in the case of residents with less than 6 months in a GME approved residency program.

Teaching physicians submitting claims under this exception must:

- Not have other responsibilities (including the supervision of other personnel) at the time the service was provided by the resident;
- Have the primary medical responsibility for patients cared for by the residents;
- Ensure that the care provided was reasonable and necessary;
- Review the care provided by the resident during or immediately after each visit. This must include a review of the patient's medical history, the resident's findings on physical examination, the patient's diagnosis, and treatment plan (i.e., record of tests and therapies); and
- Document the extent of his/her own participation in the review and direction of the services furnished to each patient.

Patients under this exception should consider the center to be their primary location for health care services. The residents must be expected to generally provide care to the same group of established patients during their residency training. The types of services furnished by residents under this exception include:

- Acute care for undifferentiated problems or chronic care for ongoing conditions including chronic mental illness;
- Coordination of care furnished by other physicians and providers; and,
- Comprehensive care not limited by organ system or diagnosis.

Residency programs most likely qualifying for this exception include family practice, general internal medicine, geriatric medicine, pediatrics, and obstetrics/gynecology.

Certain GME programs in psychiatry may qualify in special situations such as when the program furnishes comprehensive care for chronically mentally ill patients. These would be centers in which the range of services the residents are trained to furnish, and actually do furnish, include comprehensive medical care as well as psychiatric care. For example, antibiotics are being prescribed as well as psychotropic drugs.

## 100-4, 12, 140.1

### Qualified NonphysicianAnesthetists

(Rev. 3747; Issued: 04-14-17; Effective: 01-01-17; Implementation: 05-15-17)

For payment purposes, the term "qualified nonphysician anesthetist" is used to refer to both certified registered nurse anesthetists (CRNAs) and anesthesiologists' assistants unless otherwise separately discussed.

An anesthesiologist's assistant means a person who:

- Works under the direction of an anesthesiologist;
- Is in compliance with all applicable requirements of State law, including any licensure requirements the state imposes on nonphysician anesthetists; and
- Is a graduate of a medical school based anesthesiologist assistant educational program that –
  - Is accredited by the Committee on Allied Health Education and Accreditation;

And

  - Includes approximately two years of specialized basic science and clinical education in anesthesia at a level that builds on a premedical undergraduate science background.

A CRNA is a registered nurse who:

- is licensed as a registered professional nurse by the State in which the nurse practices;
- Meets any licensure requirements the State imposes with respect to nonphysician anesthetists;
- Has graduated from a nurse anesthesia educational program that meets the standards of the Council on Accreditation of Nurse Anesthesia Programs; and
- Meets the following criteria:
  - Has passed a certification examination of the Council on Certification of Nurse Anesthetists or the Council on Recertification of Nurse Anesthetists;

Or

  - Is a graduate of a nurse anesthesia educational program that meets the standards of the Council of Accreditation of Nurse Anesthesia Educational Programs, and within 24 months of graduation, has passed a certification examination of the Council on Certification of Nurse Anesthetists or the Council on Recertification of Nurse Anesthetists.

## 100-4, 12, 140.2

### Entity or Individual to Whom Fee Schedule is Payable for Qualified NonphysicianAnesthetists

(Rev. 3747; Issued: 04-14-17; Effective: 01-01-17; Implementation: 05-15-17)

Payment for the services of a qualified nonphysician anesthetist may be made directly to the qualified nonphysician anesthetist who furnished the anesthesia services or to a hospital, physician, group practice, or ASC with which the qualified nonphysician anesthetist has an employment or contractual relationship.

## 100-4, 12, 140.3

### Anesthesia Fee Schedule Payment for Qualified NonphysicianAnesthetists

(Rev. 3747; Issued: 04-14-17; Effective: 01-01-17; Implementation: 05-15-17)

Payment for the services furnished by qualified nonphysician anesthetists are subject to the usual Part B coinsurance and deductible, and are made only on an assignment basis. The assignment agreed to by the qualified nonphysician anesthetist is binding upon any other person or entity claiming payment for the service. Except for deductible and coinsurance amounts, any person who knowingly and willfully presents or causes to be presented to a Medicare beneficiary a bill or request for payment for services of a qualified nonphysician anesthetist for which payment may be made on an assignment-related basis is subject to civil monetary penalties.

The fee schedule for anesthesia services furnished by qualified nonphysician anesthetists is the least of 80 percent of:

- The actual charge;
- The applicable locality anesthesia conversion factor multiplied by the sum of allowable base and time units.

## 100-4, 12, 140.3.1

### Conversion Factors Used for Qualified Nonphysician Anesthetists

(Rev. 3747; Issued: 04-14-17; Effective: 01-01-17; Implementation: 05-15-17)

The conversion factors applicable to anesthesia services are increased by the update factor used to update physicians' services under the physician fee schedule. They are generally published in November of the year preceding the year in which they apply.

## 100-4, 12, 140.3.2

### Anesthesia Time and Calculation of Anesthesia TimeUnits

(Rev. 3747; Issued: 04-14-17; Effective: 01-01-17; Implementation: 05-15-17)

Anesthesia time means the time during which a qualified nonphysician anesthetist is present with the patient. It starts when the qualified nonphysician anesthetist begins to prepare the patient for anesthesia services in the operating room or an equivalent area and ends when the qualified nonphysician anesthetist is no longer furnishing anesthesia services to the patient, that is, when the patient may be placed safely under postoperative care. Anesthesia time is a continuous time period from the start of anesthesia to the end of an anesthesia service. In counting anesthesia time, the qualified nonphysician anesthetist can add blocks of time around an interruption in anesthesia time as long as the qualified nonphysician anesthetist is furnishing continuous anesthesia care within the time periods around the interruption.

## 100-4, 12, 140.3.3

### Billing Modifiers

(Rev. 3747; Issued: 04-14-17; Effective: 01-01-17; Implementation: 05-15-17)

The following modifiers are used by qualified nonphysician anesthetists when billing for anesthesia services:

- QX – Qualified nonphysician anesthetist service: With medical direction by a physician.
- QZ – CRNA service: Without medical direction by a physician.
- QS – Monitored anesthesia care services
  - **NOTE:** The QS modifier can be used by a physician or a qualified nonphysician anesthetist and is for informational purposes. Providers must report actual anesthesia time and one of the payment modifiers on the claim.

## 100-4, 12, 140.3.4

### General Billing Instructions

(Rev. 3747; Issued: 04-14-17; Effective: 01-01-17; Implementation: 05-15-17)

Claims for reimbursement for qualified nonphysician anesthetist services should be completed in accordance with existing billing instructions for anesthesiologists with the following additions.

- If an employer-physician furnishes concurrent medical direction for a procedure involving CRNAs and the medical direction service is unassigned, the physician should bill on an assigned basis on a separate claim for the qualified nonphysician anesthetist service. If the physician is participating or takes assignment, both services should be billed on one claim but as separate line items.
- All claims forms must have the provider billing number of the qualified nonphysician anesthetist and/or the employer of the qualified nonphysician anesthetist performing the service in either block 24.H of the Form CMS-1500 and/or block 31 as applicable. Verify that the billing number is valid before making payment.

Payments should be calculated in accordance with Medicare payment rules in §140.3. The A/B MAC must institute all necessary payment edits to assure that duplicate payments are not made to physicians for qualified nonphysician anesthetist services or to a qualified nonphysician anesthetist directly for bills submitted on their behalf by qualified billers.

A CRNA is identified on the provider file by specialty code 43. An anesthesiologist's assistant is identified on the provider file by specialty code 32.

## 100-4, 12, 140.4.1

### An Anesthesiologist and Qualified Nonphysician Anesthetist Work Together

(Rev. 3747; Issued: 04-14-17; Effective: 01-01-17; Implementation: 05-15-17)

A/B MACs will distribute educational releases and use other established means to ensure that anesthesiologists understand the requirements for medical direction of qualified nonphysician anesthetists.

A/B MACs will perform reviews of payments for anesthesiology services to identify situations in which an excessive number of concurrent anesthesiology services may have been performed. They will use peer practice and their experience in developing review criteria. They will also periodically review a sample of claims for medical direction of four or fewer concurrent anesthesia procedures. During this process physicians may be requested to submit documentation of the names of procedures performed and the names of the anesthetists medically directed.

Physicians who cannot supply the necessary documentation for the sample claims must submit documentation with all subsequent claims before payment will be made.

## 100-4, 12, 140.4.2

### Qualified Nonphysician Anesthetist and an Anesthesiologist in a Single Anesthesia Procedure

(Rev. 3747; Issued: 04-14-17; Effective: 01-01-17; Implementation: 05-15-17)

Where a single anesthesia procedure involves both a physician medical direction service and the service of the medically directed qualified nonphysician anesthetist, the payment amount for the service of each is 50 percent of the allowance otherwise recognized had the service been furnished by the anesthesiologist alone. For the single medically directed service, the physician will use the QY modifier and the qualified nonphysician anesthetist will use the QX modifier.

In unusual circumstances when it is medically necessary for both the CRNA and the anesthesiologist to be completely and fully involved during a procedure, full payment for the services of each provider is allowed. The physician would report using the AA modifier and the CRNA would report using the QZ modifier. Documentation must be submitted by each provider to support payment of the full fee.

## 100-04, 12, 140.4.3

### Payment for Medical or Surgical Services Furnished by CRNAs

Payment shall be made for reasonable and necessary medical or surgical services furnished by CRNAs if they are legally authorized to perform these services in the state in which services are furnished. Payment is determined under the physician fee schedule on the basis of the national physician fee schedule conversion factor, the geographic adjustment factor, and the resource-based relative value units for the medical or surgical service.

## 100-04, 12, 140.4.4

### Conversion Factors for Anesthesia Services of Qualified Nonphysician Anesthetists Furnished on or After January 1, 1992

Conversion factors used to determine fee schedule payments for anesthesia services furnished by qualified nonphysician anesthetists on or after January 1, 1992, are determined based on a statutory methodology.

For example, for anesthesia services furnished by a medically directed qualified nonphysician anesthetist in 1994, the medically directed allowance is 60 percent of the allowance that would be recognized for the anesthesia service if the physician personally performed the service without an assistant, i.e., alone. For subsequent years, the medically directed allowance is the following percent of the personally performed allowance.

| | |
|---|---|
| Services furnished in 1995 | 57.5 percent |
| Services furnished in 1996 | 55.0 percent |
| Services furnished in 1997 | 52.5 percent |
| Services furnished in 1998 and after | 50.0 percent |

## 100-4, 12, 140.5

### Payment for Anesthesia Services Furnished by a Teaching CRNA

(Rev. 3747; Issued: 04-14-17; Effective: 01-01-17; Implementation: 05-15-17)

Payment can be made under Part B to a teaching CRNA who supervises a single case involving a student nurse anesthetist where the CRNA is continuously present. The CRNA reports the service using the QZ modifier. No payment is made under Part B for the service provided by a student nurse anesthetist.

The A/B MAC may allow payment, as follows, if a teaching CRNA is involved in cases with two student nurse anesthetists:

- Recognize the full base units (assigned to the anesthesia code) where the teaching CRNA is present with the student nurse anesthetist throughout pre and post anesthesia care;and
- Recognize the actual time the teaching CRNA is personally present with the student nurse anesthetist. Anesthesia time may be discontinuous. For example, a teaching CRNA is involved in two concurrent cases with student nurse anesthetists. Case 1 runs from 9:00 a.m. to 11:00 a.m. and case 2 runs from 9:45a.m. to 11:30 a.m. The teaching CRNA is present in case 1 from 9:00 a.m. to 9:30 a.m. and from 10:15 a.m. to 10:30 a.m. From 9:45 a.m. to 10:14 a.m. and from 10:31 a.m. to 11:30 a.m., the CRNA is present in case 2. The CRNA may report 45 minutes of anesthesia time for case 1 (i.e., 3 time units) and 88 minutes (i.e., 5.9 units) of anesthesia time for case 2.

The teaching CRNA must document his/her involvement in cases with student nurse anesthetists. The documentation must be sufficient to support the payment of the fee and available for review upon request.

The teaching CRNA (not under the medical direction of a physician), can be paid for his or her involvement in each of two concurrent cases with student nurse anesthetists; allow payment at the regular fee schedule rate. The teaching CRNA reports the anesthesia service using the QZmodifier.

To bill the anesthesia base units, the teaching CRNA must be present with the student nurse anesthetist during pre and post anesthesia care for each of the two cases. To bill anesthesia time for each case, the teaching CRNA must continue to devote his or her time to the two concurrent cases and not be involved in other activities. The teaching CRNA can decide how to allocate his or her time to optimize patient care in the two cases based on the complexity of the anesthesia cases, the experience and skills of the student nurse anesthetists, and the patients' health status and other factors. The teaching CRNA must document his or her involvement in the cases with the student nurse anesthetists.

## 100-04, 12, 160

### Independent Psychologist Services
B3-2150, B3-2070.2 See the Medicare Benefit Policy Manual, Chapter 15, for coverage requirements.

There are a number of types of psychologists. Educational psychologists engage in identifying and treating education-related issues. In contrast, counseling psychologists provide services that include a broader realm including phobias, familial issues, etc.

Psychometrists are psychologists who have been trained to administer and interpret tests.

However, clinical psychologists are defined as a provider of diagnostic and therapeutic services. Because of the differences in services provided, services provided by psychologists who do not provide clinical services are subject to different billing guidelines. One service often provided by nonclinical psychologist is diagnostic testing.

NOTE: Diagnostic psychological testing services performed by persons who meet these requirements are covered as other diagnostic tests. When, however, the psychologist is not practicing independently, but is on the staff of an institution, agency, or clinic, that entity bills for the diagnostic services.

Expenses for such testing are not subject to the payment limitation on treatment for mental, psychoneurotic, and personality disorders. Independent psychologists are not required by law to accept assignment when performing psychological tests. However, regardless of whether the psychologist accepts assignment, he or she must report on the claim form the name and address of the physician who ordered the test.

## 100-04, 12, 160.1

### Payment
Diagnostic testing services are not subject to the outpatient mental health limitation. Refer to §210, below, for a discussion of the outpatient mental health limitation. The diagnostic testing services performed by a psychologist (who is not a clinical psychologist) practicing independently of an institution, agency, or physician's office are covered as other diagnostic tests if a physician orders such testing. Medicare covers this type of testing as an outpatient service if furnished by any psychologist who is licensed or certified to practice psychology in the State or jurisdiction where he or she is furnishing services or, if the jurisdiction does not issue licenses, if provided by any practicing psychologist. (It is CMS' understanding that all States, the District of Columbia, and Puerto Ricolicense psychologists, but that some trust territories do not. Examples of psychologists, other than clinical psychologists, whose services are covered under this provision include, but are not limited to, educational psychologists and counseling psychologists.)

To determine whether the diagnostic psychological testing services of a particular independent psychologist are covered under Part B in States which have statutory licensure or certification, carriers must secure from the appropriate State agency a current listing of psychologists holding the required credentials. In States or territories which lack statutory licensing and certification, carriers must check individual qualifications as claims are submitted. Possible reference sources are the national directory of membership of the American Psychological Association, which provides data about the educational background of individuals and indicates which members are board-certified, and records and directories of the State or territorial psychological association. If qualification is dependent on a doctoral degree from a currently accredited program, carriers must verify the date of accreditation of the school involved, since such accreditation is not retroactive. If the reference sources listed above do not provide enough information (e.g., the psychologist is not a member of the association), carriers must contact the psychologist personally for the required information. Carriers may wish to maintain a continuing list of psychologists whose qualifications have been verified.

Medicare excludes expenses for diagnostic testing from the payment limitation on treatment for mental/psychoneurotic/personality disorders.

Carriers must identify the independent psychologist's choice whether or not to accept assignment when performing psychological tests.

Carriers must accept an independent psychologist claim only if the psychologist reports the name/UPIN of the physician who ordered a test.

Carriers pay nonparticipating independent psychologists at 95 percent of the physician fee schedule allowed amount.

Carriers pay participating independent psychologists at 100 percent of the physician fee schedule allowed amount. Independent psychologists are identified on the provider file by specialty code 62 and provider type 35.

## 100-04, 12, 170

### Clinical Psychologist Services
B3-2150 See Medicare Benefit Policy Manual, Chapter 15, for general coverage requirements.

Direct payment may be made under Part B for professional services. However, services furnished incident to the professional services of CPs to hospital patients remain bundled.

Therefore, payment must continue to be made to the hospital (by the FI) for such "incident to" services.

## 100-04, 12, 180

### Care Plan Oversight Services
The Medicare Benefit Policy Manual, Chapter 15, contains requirements for coverage for medical and other health services including those of physicians and non-physician practitioners.

Care plan oversight (CPO) is the physician supervision of a patient receiving complex and/or multidisciplinary care as part of Medicare-covered services provided by a participating home health agency or Medicare approved hospice.

CPO services require complex or multidisciplinary care modalities involving:

- Regular physician development and/or revision of care plans;
- Review of subsequent reports of patient status;
- Review of related laboratory and other studies;
- Communication with other health professionals not employed in the same practice who are involved in the patient's care;
- Integration of new information into the medical treatment plan; and/or
- Adjustment of medical therapy.

The CPO services require recurrent physician supervision of a patient involving 30 or more minutes of the physician's time per month. Services not countable toward the 30 minutes threshold that must be provided in order to bill for CPO include, but are not limited to:

- Time associated with discussions with the patient, his or her family or friends to adjust medication or treatment;
- Time spent by staff getting or filing charts;
- Travel time; and/or Physician's time spent telephoning prescriptions into the pharmacist unless the telephone conversation involves discussions of pharmaceutical therapies.

Implicit in the concept of CPO is the expectation that the physician has coordinated an aspect of the patient's care with the home health agency or hospice during the month for which CPO services were billed. The physician who bills for CPO must be the same physician who signs the plan of care.

Nurse practitioners, physician assistants, and clinical nurse specialists, practicing within the scope of State law, may bill for care plan oversight. These non-physician practitioners must have been providing ongoing care for the beneficiary through evaluation and management services. These non-physician practitioners may not bill for CPO if they have been involved only with the delivery of the Medicare-covered home health or hospice service.

**A. Home Health CPO**
Non-physician practitioners can perform CPO only if the physician signing the plan of care provides regular ongoing care under the same plan of care as does the NPP billing for CPO and either:

- The physician and NPP are part of the same group practice; or
- If the NPP is a nurse practitioner or clinical nurse specialist, the physician signing the plan of care also has a collaborative agreement with the NPP; or
- If the NPP is a physician assistant, the physician signing the plan of care is also the physician who provides general supervision of physician assistant services for the practice.

Billing may be made for care plan oversight services furnished by an NPP when:

- The NPP providing the care plan oversight has seen and examined the patient;
- The NPP providing care plan oversight is not functioning as a consultant whose participation is limited to a single medical condition rather than multidisciplinary coordination of care; and
- The NPP providing care plan oversight integrates his or her care with that of the physician who signed the plan of care.

NPPs may not certify the beneficiary for home health care.

**B. Hospice CPO**
The attending physician or nurse practitioner (who has been designated as the attending physician) may bill for hospice CPO when they are acting as an "attending physician".

An "attending physician" is one who has been identified by the individual, at the time he/she elects hospice coverage, as having the most significant role in the determination and delivery of their medical care. They are not employed nor paid by the hospice. The care plan oversight services are billed using Form CMS-1500 or electronic equivalent.

For additional information on hospice CPO, see Chapter 11, 40.1.3.1 of this manual.

## 100-04, 12, 180.1

### Care Plan Oversight Billing Requirements

#### A. Codes for Which Separate Payment May Be Made

Effective January 1, 1995, separate payment may be made for CPO oversight services for 30 minutes or more if the requirements specified in the Medicare Benefits Policy Manual, Chapter 15 are met.

Providers billing for CPO must submit the claim with no other services billed on that claim and may bill only after the end of the month in which the CPO services were rendered. CPO services may not be billed across calendar months and should be submitted (and paid) only for one unit of service.

Physicians may bill and be paid separately for CPO services only if all the criteria in the Medicare Benefit Policy Manual, Chapter 15 are met.

#### B. Physician Certification and Recertification of Home Health Plans of Care

Effective 2001, two new HCPCS codes for the certification and recertification and development of plans of care for Medicare-covered home health services were created.

See the Medicare General Information, Eligibility, and Entitlement Manual, Pub. 100-1, Chapter 4, "Physician Certification and Recertification of Services," 10-60, and the Medicare Benefit Policy Manual, Pub. 100-2, Chapter 7, "Home Health Services", 30.

The home health agency certification code can be billed only when the patient has not received Medicare-covered home health services for at least 60 days. The home health agency recertification code is used after a patient has received services for at least 60 days (or one certification period) when the physician signs the certification after the initial certification period. The home health agency recertification code will be reported only once every 60 days, except in the rare situation when the patient starts a new episode before 60 days elapses and requires a new plan of care to start a new episode.

#### C. Provider Number of Home Health Agency (HHA) or Hospice

For claims for CPO submitted on or after January 1, 1997, physicians must enter on the Medicare claim form the 6-character Medicare provider number of the HHA or hospice providing Medicare-covered services to the beneficiary for the period during which CPO services was furnished and for which the physician signed the plan of care. Physicians are responsible for obtaining the HHA or hospice Medicare provider numbers.

Additionally, physicians should provide their UPIN to the HHA or hospice furnishing services to their patient.

NOTE: There is currently no place on the HIPAA standard ASC X12N 837 professional format to specifically include the HHA or hospice provider number required for a care plan oversight claim. For this reason, the requirement to include the HHA or hospice provider number on a care plan oversight claim is temporarily waived until a new version of this electronic standard format is adopted under HIPAA and includes a place to provide the HHA and hospice provider numbers for care plan oversight claims.

## 100-04, 12, 190.3

### List of Medicare Telehealth Services

(Rev. 3476, Issued: 03-11-16, Effective: 01-01-15, Effective: 04-11-16)

The use of a telecommunications system may substitute for an in-person encounter for professional consultations, office visits, office psychiatry services, and a limited number of other physician fee schedule (PFS) services. The various services and corresponding current procedure terminology (CPT) or Healthcare Common Procedure Coding System (HCPCS) codes are listed on the CMS website at www.cms.gov/Medicare/Medicare-General-Information/Telehealth/.

NOTE: Beginning January 1, 2010, CMS eliminated the use of all consultation codes, except for inpatient telehealth consultation G-codes. CMS no longer recognizes office/outpatient or inpatient consultation CPT codes for payment of office/outpatient or inpatient visits. Instead, physicians and practitioners are instructed to bill a new or established patient office/outpatient visit CPT code or appropriate hospital or nursing facility care code, as appropriate to the particular patient, for all office/outpatient or inpatient visits.

## 100-04, 12, 190.3.4

### Payment for ESRD-Related Services as a Telehealth Service

(Rev. 3476, Issued: 03-11-16, Effective: 01-01-15, Effective: 04-11-16)

The ESRD-related services included in the monthly capitation payment (MCP) with 2 or 3 visits per month and ESRD-related services with 4 or more visits per month may be paid as Medicare telehealth services. However, at least 1 visit must be furnished face-to-face "hands on" to examine the vascular access site by a physician, clinical nurse specialist, nurse practitioner, or physician assistant. An interactive audio and

video telecommunications system may be used for providing additional visits required under the 2-to-3 visit MCP and the 4-or-more visit MCP. The medical record must indicate that at least one of the visits was furnished face-to-face "hands on" by a physician, clinical nurse specialist, nurse practitioner, or physician assistant.

The MCP physician, for example, the physician or practitioner who is responsible for the complete monthly assessment of the patient and establishes the patient's plan of care, may use other physicians and practitioners to furnish ESRD-related visits through an interactive audio and video telecommunications system. The non-MCP physician or practitioner must have a relationship with the billing physician or practitioner such as a partner, employees of the same group practice or an employee of the MCP physician, for example, the non MCP physician or practitioner is either a W-2 employee or 1099 independent contractor. However, the physician or practitioner who is responsible for the complete monthly assessment and establishes the ESRD beneficiary's plan of care should bill for the MCP in any given month.

#### Clinical Criteria

The visit, including a clinical examination of the vascular access site, must be conducted face-to-face "hands on" by a physician, clinical nurse specialist, nurse practitioner or physician's assistant. For additional visits, the physician or practitioner at the distant site is required, at a minimum, to use an interactive audio and video telecommunications system that allows the physician or practitioner to provide medical management services for a maintenance dialysis beneficiary. For example, an ESRD-related visit conducted via telecommunications system must permit the physician or practitioner at the distant site to perform an assessment of whether the dialysis is working effectively and whether the patient is tolerating the procedure well (physiologically and psychologically). During this assessment, the physician or practitioner at the distant site must be able to determine whether alteration in any aspect of the beneficiary's prescription is indicated, due to such changes as the estimate of the patient's dry weight.

## 100-04, 12, 190.3.5

### Payment for Subsequent Hospital Care Services and Subsequent Nursing Facility Care Services as Telehealth Services

(Rev. 3476, Issued: 03-11-16, Effective: 01-01-15, Effective: 04-11-16)

Subsequent hospital care services are limited to one telehealth visit every 3 days. The frequency limit of the benefit is not intended to apply to consulting physicians or practitioners, who should continue to report initial or follow-up inpatient telehealth consultations using the applicable HCPCS G-codes.

Similarly, subsequent nursing facility care services are limited to one telehealth visit every 30 days. Furthermore, subsequent nursing facility care services reported for a Federally-mandated periodic visit under 42 CFR 483.40(c) may not be furnished through telehealth. The frequency limit of the benefit is not intended to apply to consulting physicians or practitioners, who should continue to report initial or follow-up inpatient telehealth consultations using the applicable HCPCS G-codes.

Inpatient telehealth consultations are furnished to beneficiaries in hospitals or skilled nursing facilities via telehealth at the request of the physician of record, the attending physician, or another appropriate source. The physician or practitioner who furnishes the initial inpatient consultation via telehealth cannot be the physician or practitioner of record or the attending physician or practitioner, and the initial inpatient telehealth consultation would be distinct from the care provided by the physician or practitioner of record or the attending physician or practitioner. Counseling and coordination of care with other providers or agencies is included as well, consistent with the nature of the problem(s) and the patient's needs. Initial and follow-up inpatient telehealth consultations are subject to the criteria for inpatient telehealth consultation services, as described in section 190.3 of this chapter.

## 100-04, 12, 190.3.6

### Payment for Diabetes Self-Management Training (DSMT) as a Telehealth Service

(Rev. 3476, Issued: 03-11-16, Effective: 01-01-15, Effective: 04-11-16)

Individual and group DSMT services may be paid as a Medicare telehealth service; however, at least 1 hour of the 10 hour benefit in the year following the initial DSMT service must be furnished in-person to allow for effective injection training. The injection training may be furnished through either individual or group DSMT services. By reporting the –GT or –GQ modifier with HCPCS code G0108 (Diabetes outpatient self-management training services, individual, per 30 minutes) or G0109 (Diabetes outpatient self-management training services, group session (2 or more), per 30 minutes), the distant site practitioner certifies that the beneficiary has received or will receive 1 hour of in-person DSMT services for purposes of injection training during the year following the initial DSMT service.

As specified in 42 CFR 410.141(e) and stated in Pub. 100-02, Medicare Benefit Policy Manual, chapter 15, section 300.2, individual DSMT services may be furnished by a physician, individual, or entity that furnishes other services for which direct Medicare payment may be made and that submits necessary documentation to, and is accredited by, an accreditation organization approved by CMS. However, consistent with the statutory requirements of section 1834(m)(1) of the Act, as provided in 42 CFR 410.78(b)(1) and (b)(2) and stated in section 190.6 of this chapter, Medicare telehealth services, including individual DSMT services furnished as a telehealth service, could only be furnished by a licensed PA, NP, CNS, CNM, clinical psychologist, clinical social worker, or registered dietitian or nutrition professional.

## 100-04, 12, 190.5

### *Originating Site Facility Fee Payment Methodology*
(Rev. 3476, Issued: 03-11-16, Effective: 01-01-15, Effective: 04-11-16)

1. Originating site defined

The term originating site means the location of an eligible Medicare beneficiary at the time the service being furnished via a telecommunications system occurs. For asynchronous, store and forward telecommunications technologies, an originating site is only a Federal telemedicine demonstration program conducted in Alaska or Hawaii.

2. Facility fee for originating site

The originating site facility fee is a separately billable Part B payment. The contractor pays it outside of other payment methodologies. This fee is subject to post payment verification.

For telehealth services furnished from October 1, 2001, through December 31, 2002, the originating site facility fee was the lesser of $20 or the actual charge. For services furnished on or after January 1 of each subsequent year, the originating site facility fee is updated by the Medicare Economic Index. The updated fee is included in the Medicare Physician Fee Schedule (MPFS) Final Rule, which is published by November 1 prior to the start of the calendar year for which it is effective. The updated fee for each calendar year is also issued annually in a Recurring Update Notification instruction for January of each year.

3. Payment amount:

The originating site facility fee is a separately billable Part B payment. The payment amount to the originating site is the lesser of 80 percent of the actual charge or 80 percent of the originating site facility fee, except CAHs. The beneficiary is responsible for any unmet deductible amount and Medicare coinsurance.

The originating site facility fee payment methodology for each type of facility is clarified below.

Hospital outpatient department. When the originating site is a hospital outpatient department, payment for the originating site facility fee must be made as described above and not under the OPPS. Payment is not based on the OPPS payment methodology.

Hospital inpatient. For hospital inpatients, payment for the originating site facility fee must be made outside the diagnostic related group (DRG) payment, since this is a Part B benefit, similar to other services paid separately from the DRG payment, (e.g., hemophilia blood clotting factor).

Critical access hospitals. When the originating site is a critical access hospital, make payment separately from the cost-based reimbursement methodology. For CAH's, the payment amount is 80 percent of the originating site facility fee.

Federally qualified health centers (FQHCs) and rural health clinics (RHCs). The originating site facility fee for telehealth services is not an FQHC or RHC service. When an FQHC or RHC serves as the originating site, the originating site facility fee must be paid separately from the center or clinic all-inclusive rate.

Physicians' and practitioners' offices. When the originating site is a physician's or practitioner's office, the payment amount, in accordance with the law, is the lesser of 80 percent of the actual charge or 80 percent of the originating site facility fee, regardless of geographic location. The A/B MAC (B) shall not apply the geographic practice cost index (GPCI) to the originating site facility fee. This fee is statutorily set and is not subject to the geographic payment adjustments authorized under the MPFS.

Hospital-based or critical access-hospital based renal dialysis center (or their satellites). When a hospital-based or critical access hospital-based renal dialysis center (or their satellites) serves as the originating site, the originating site facility fee is covered in addition to any composite rate or MCP amount.

Skilled nursing facility (SNF). The originating site facility fee is outside the SNF prospective payment system bundle and, as such, is not subject to SNF consolidated billing. The originating site facility fee is a separately billable Part B payment.

Community Mental Health Center (CMHC). The originating site facility fee is not a partial hospitalization service. The originating site facility fee does not count towards the number of services used to determine payment for partial hospitalization services. The originating site facility fee is not bundled in the per diem payment for partial hospitalization. The originating site facility fee is a separately billable Part B payment.

To receive the originating facility site fee, the provider submits claims with HCPCS code "Q3014, telehealth originating site facility fee"; short description "telehealth facility fee." The type of service for the telehealth originating site facility fee is "9, other items and services." For A/B MAC (B) processed claims, the "office" place of service (code 11) is the only payable setting for code Q3014. There is no participation payment differential for code Q3014. Deductible and coinsurance rules apply to Q3014. By submitting Q3014 HCPCS code, the originating site authenticates they are located in either a rural HPSA or non-MSA county.

This benefit may be billed on bill types 12X, 13X, 22X, 23X, 71X, 72X, 73X, 76X, and 85X. Unless otherwise applicable, report the originating site facility fee under revenue code 078X and include HCPCS code "Q3014, telehealth originating site facility fee."

Hospitals and critical access hospitals bill their A/B/MAC (A) for the originating site facility fee. Telehealth bills originating in inpatient hospitals must be submitted on a 12X TOB using the date of discharge as the line item date of service.

Independent and provider-based RHCs and FQHCs bill the appropriate A/B/MAC (A) using the RHC or FQHC bill type and billing number. HCPCS code Q3014 is the only non-RHC/FQHC service that is billed using the clinic/center bill type and provider number. All RHCs and FQHCs must use revenue code 078X when billing for the originating site facility fee. For all other non-RHC/FQHC services, provider based RHCs and FQHCs must bill using the base provider's bill type and billing number. Independent RHCs and FQHCs must bill the A/B MAC (B) for all other non-RHC/FQHC services. If an RHC/FQHC visit occurs on the same day as a telehealth service, the RHC/FQHC serving as an originating site must bill for HCPCS code Q3014 telehealth originating site facility fee on a separate revenue line from the RHC/FQHC visit using revenue code 078X.

Hospital-based or CAH-based renal dialysis centers (including satellites) bill their A/B/MAC (A) for the originating site facility fee. Telehealth bills originating in renal dialysis centers must be submitted on a 72X TOB. All hospital-based or CAH-based renal dialysis centers (including satellites) must use revenue code 078X when billing for the originating site facility fee. The renal dialysis center serving as an originating site must bill for HCPCS code Q3014, telehealth originating site facility fee, on a separate revenue line from any other services provided to the beneficiary.

Skilled nursing facilities (SNFs) bill their A/B/MAC (A) for the originating site facility fee. Telehealth bills originating in SNFs must be submitted on TOB 22X or 23X. For SNF inpatients in a covered Part A stay, the originating site facility fee must be submitted on a 22X TOB. All SNFs must use revenue code 078X when billing for the originating site facility fee. The SNF serving as an originating site must bill for HCPCS code Q3014, telehealth originating site facility fee, on a separate revenue line from any other services provided to the beneficiary.

Community mental health centers (CMHCs) bill their A/B/MAC (A) for the originating site facility fee. Telehealth bills originating in CMHCs must be submitted on a 76X TOB. All CMHCs must use revenue code 078X when billing for the originating site facility fee. The CMHC serving as an originating site must bill for HCPCS code Q3014, telehealth originating site facility fee, on a separate revenue line from any other services provided to the beneficiary. Note that Q3014 does not count towards the number of services used to determine per diem payments for partial hospitalization services.

The beneficiary is responsible for any unmet deductible amount and Medicare coinsurance.

## 100-04, 12, 190.6

### *Payment Methodology for Physician/Practitioner at the Distant Site*
(Rev. 3586, Issued: 08-12-16, Effective: 01-01-17, Effective: 01-03-17)

1. Distant Site Defined

The term "distant site" means the site where the physician or practitioner, providing the professional service, is located at the time the service is provided via a telecommunications system.

2. Payment Amount (professional fee)

The payment amount for the professional service provided via a telecommunications system by the physician or practitioner at the distant site is equal to the current fee schedule amount for the service provided at the facility rate. Payment for an office visit, consultation, individual psychotherapy or pharmacologic management via a telecommunications system should be made at the same facility amount as when these services are furnished without the use of a telecommunications system. For Medicare payment to occur, the service must be within a practitioner's scope of practice under State law. The beneficiary is responsible for any unmet deductible amount and applicable coinsurance.

3. Medicare Practitioners Who May Receive Payment at the Distant Site (i.e., at a site other than where beneficiary is)

As a condition of Medicare Part B payment for telehealth services, the physician or practitioner at the distant site must be licensed to provide the service under state law. When the physician or practitioner at the distant site is licensed under state law to provide a covered telehealth service (i.e., professional consultation, office and other outpatient visits, individual psychotherapy, and pharmacologic management) then he or she may bill for and receive payment for this service when delivered via a telecommunications system.

If the physician or practitioner at the distant site is located in a CAH that has elected Method II, and the physician or practitioner has reassigned his/her benefits to the CAH, the CAH bills its regular A/B/MAC (A) for the professional services provided at the distant site via a telecommunications system, in any of the revenue codes 096x, 097x or 098x. All requirements for billing distant site telehealth services apply.

4. Medicare Practitioners Who May Bill for Covered Telehealth Services are Listed Below (subject to State law)

> Physician
> Nurse practitioner
> Physician assistant
> Nurse-midwife
> Clinical nurse specialist
> Clinical psychologist*
> Clinical social worker*
> Registered dietitian or nutrition professional
> Certified registered nurse anesthetist

*Clinical psychologists and clinical social workers cannot bill for psychotherapy services that include medical evaluation and management services under Medicare. These practitioners may not bill or receive payment for the following CPT codes: 90805, 90807, and 90809.

## 100-4, 12, 190.6.1
### Submission of Telehealth Claims for Distant Site Practitioners
(Rev. 3586, Issued: 08-12-16, Effective: 01-01-17, Implementation: 01-03-17)

Claims for telehealth services are submitted to the contractors that process claims for the performing physician/practitioner's service area. Physicians/practitioners submit the appropriate HCPCS procedure code for covered professional telehealth services with place of service code 02 (Telehealth) along with the "GT" modifier ("via interactive audio and video telecommunications system"). By coding and billing the "GT" modifier with a covered telehealth procedure code, the distant site physician/practitioner certifies that the beneficiary was present at an eligible originating site when the telehealth service was furnished. By coding and billing the "GT" modifier with a covered ESRD-related service telehealth code, the distant site physician/practitioner certifies that 1 visit per month was furnished face-to-face "hands on" to examine the vascular access site. Refer to section 190.3.4 of this chapter for the conditions of telehealth payment for ESRD-related services.

In situations where a CAH has elected payment Method II for CAH outpatients, and the practitioner has reassigned his/her benefits to the CAH, A/B/MACs (A) should make payment for telehealth services provided by the physician or practitioner at 80 percent of the MPFS facility amount for the distant site service. In all other cases, except for MNT services as discussed in Section 190.7- A/B MAC (B) Editing of Telehealth Claims, telehealth services provided by the physician or practitioner at the distant site are billed to the A/B/MAC (B).

Physicians and practitioners at the distant site bill their A/B/MAC (B) for covered telehealth services, for example, "99245 GT." Physicians' and practitioners' offices serving as a telehealth originating site bill their A/B/MAC (B) for the originating site facility fee.

## 100-4, 12, 190.7
### A/B MAC (B) Editing of Telehealth Claims
(Rev. 3721, Issued: 02-24-17, Effective: 05-25-17, Implementation: 05-25-17)

Medicare telehealth services (as listed in section 190.3) are billed with either the "GT" or "GQ" modifier. The contractor shall approve covered telehealth services if the physician or practitioner is licensed under State law to provide the service. Contractors must familiarize themselves with licensure provisions of States for which they process claims and disallow telehealth services furnished by physicians or practitioners who are not authorized to furnish the applicable telehealth service under State law. For example, if a nurse practitioner is not licensed to provide individual psychotherapy under State law, he or she would not be permitted to receive payment for individual psychotherapy under Medicare. The contractor shall install edits to ensure that only properly licensed physicians and practitioners are paid for covered telehealth services.

If a contractor receives claims for professional telehealth services coded with the "GQ" modifier (representing "via asynchronous telecommunications system"), it shall approve/pay for these services only if the physician or practitioner is affiliated with a Federal telemedicine demonstration conducted in Alaska or Hawaii. The contractor may require the physician or practitioner at the distant site to document his or her participation in a Federal telemedicine demonstration program conducted in Alaska or Hawaii prior to paying for telehealth services provided via asynchronous, store and forward technologies.

Contractors shall deny telehealth services if the physician or practitioner is not eligible to bill for them.

The following reflects the remittance advice messages and associated codes that will appear when rejecting/denying claims under this policy. This CARC/RARC combination is compliant with CAQH CORE Business Scenario 3.

> Group Code: CO
> CARC: 185
> RARC: N/A
> MSN: 21.18

If a service is billed with one of the telehealth modifiers and the procedure code is not designated as a covered telehealth service, the contractor denies the service.

The following reflects the remittance advice messages and associated codes that will appear when rejecting/denying claims under this policy. This CARC/RARC combination is compliant with CAQH CORE Business Scenario 3.

> Group Code: CO
> CARC: 96
> RARC: N776
> MSN: 9.4

The only claims from institutional facilities that FIs shall pay for telehealth services at the distant site, except for MNT services, are for physician or practitioner services when the distant site is located in a CAH that has elected Method II, and the physician or practitioner has reassigned his/her benefits to the CAH. The CAH bills its regular FI for the professional services provided at the distant site via a telecommunications system, in any of the revenue codes 096x, 097x or 098x. All requirements for billing distant site telehealth services apply.

Claims from hospitals or CAHs for MNT services are submitted to the hospital's or CAH's regular FI. Payment is based on the non-facility amount on the Medicare Physician Fee Schedule for the particular HCPCS codes.

## 100-04, 12, 230
### Primary Care Incentive Payment Program (PCIP)

Section 5501(a) of the Affordable Care Act revises Section 1833 of the Social Security Act (the Act) by adding a new paragraph, (x), "Incentive Payments for Primary Care Services." Section 1833(x) of the Act states that in the case of primary care services furnished on or after January 1, 2011, and before January 1, 2016, there shall be a 10 percent incentive payment for such services under Part B when furnished by a primary care practitioner.

Information regarding Primary Care Incentive Payment Program (PCIP) payments made to critical access hospitals (CAHs) paid under the optional method can be found in Pub. 100-4, Chapter 4, §250.12 of this manual.

## 100-04, 12, 230.1
### Definition of Primary Care Practitioners and Primary Care Services
Primary care practitioners are defined as:

1. A physician who has a primary specialty designation of family medicine, internal medicine, geriatric medicine, or pediatric medicine for whom primary care services accounted for at least 60 percent of the allowed charges under Part B for the practitioner in a prior period as determined appropriate by the Secretary; or

2. A nurse practitioner, clinical nurse specialist, or physician assistant for whom primary care services accounted for at least 60 percent of the allowed charges under Part B for the practitioner in a prior period as determined appropriate by the Secretary.

Primary care services are defined as HCPCS Codes:

1. 99201 through 99215 for new and established patient office or outpatient evaluation and management (E/M) visits;

2. 99304 through 99340 for initial, subsequent, discharge, and other nursing facility E/M services; new and established patient domiciliary, rest home or custodial care E/M services; and domiciliary, rest home or home care plan oversight services; and

3. 99341 through 99350 for new and established patient home E/M visits.

**Practitioner Identification**
Eligible practitioners will be identified on claims by the National Provider Identifier (NPI) number of the rendering practitioner. If the claim is submitted by a practitioner's group practice, the rendering practitioner's NPI must be included on the line-item for the primary care service and reflect an eligible HCPCS as identified. In order to be eligible for the PCIP, physician assistants, clinical nurse specialists, and nurse practitioners must be billing for their services under their own NPI and not furnishing services incident to physicians' services. Regardless of the specialty area in which they may be practicing, the specific nonphysician practitioners are eligible for the PCIP based on their profession and historical percentage of allowed charges as primary care services that equals or exceeds the 60 percent threshold.

Beginning in calendar year (CY) 2011, primary care practitioners will be identified based on their primary specialty of enrollment in Medicare and percentage of allowed charges for primary care services that equals or exceeds the 60 percent threshold from Medicare claims data 2 years prior to the bonus payment year.

Eligible practitioners for PCIP payments in a given calendar year (CY) will be listed by eligible NPI in the Primary Care Incentive Payment Program Eligibility File, available after January 31, of the payment year on their Medicare contractor's website. Practitioners should contact their contractor with any questions regarding their eligibility for the PCIP.

## 100-04, 12, 230.2
### Coordination with Other Payments

Section 5501(a)(3) of the Affordable Care Act provides payment under the PCIP as an additional payment amount for specified primary care services without regard to any additional payment for the service under Section 1833(m) of the Act. Therefore, an eligible primary care physician furnishing a primary care service in a health professional shortage area (HPSA) may receive both a HPSA physician bonus payment (as described in the Medicare Claims Processing Manual, Pub. 100-4, Chapter 12, §90.4) under the HPSA physician bonus program and a PCIP incentive payment under the new program beginning in CY 2011.

## 100-04, 12, 230.3
### Claims Processing and Payment

**A. General Overview**
Incentive payments will be made on a quarterly basis and shall be equal to 10 percent of the amount paid for such services under the Medicare Physician Fee Schedule (PFS) for those services furnished during the bonus payment year. For information on PCIP payments to CAHs paid under the optional method, see the Medicare Claims Processing Manual, Pub. 100-4, Chapter 4, §250.12.

On an annual basis Medicare contractors shall receive a Primary Care Incentive Payment Program Eligibility File that they shall post to their website. The file will list the NPIs of all practitioners who are eligible to receive PCIP payments for the upcoming CY.

**B. Method of Payment**

- Calculate and pay qualifying primary care practitioners an additional 10 percent incentive payment;

- Calculate the payment based on the amount actually paid for the services, not the Medicare approved amounts;

- Combine the PCIP incentive payments, when appropriate, with other incentive payments, including the HPSA physician bonus payment, and the HPSA Surgical Incentive Payment Program (HSIP) payment;

- Provide a special remittance form that is forwarded with the incentive payment so that physicians and practitioners can identify which type of incentive payment (HPSA physician and/or PCIP) was paid for which services.

- Practitioners should contact their contractor with any questions regarding PCIP payments.

**C. Changes for Contractor Systems**

The Medicare Carrier System, (MCS), Common Working File (CWF) and the National Claims History (NCH) shall be modified to accept a new PCIP indicator on the claim line. Once the type of incentive payment has been identified by the shared systems, the shared system shall modify their systems to set the indicator on the claim line as follows:

   1 = HPSA;

   2 = PSA;

   3 = HPSA and PSA;

   4 = HSIP;

   5 = HPSA and HSIP;

   6 = PCIP;

   7 = HPSA and PCIP; and

   Space = Not Applicable.

The contractor shared system shall send the HIGLAS 810 invoice for incentive payment invoices, including the new PCIP payment. The contractor shall also combine the provider's HPSA physician bonus, physician scarcity (PSA) bonus (if it should become available at a later date), HSIP payment and/or PCIP payment invoice per provider. The contractor shall receive the HIGLAS 835 payment file from HIGLAS showing a single incentive payment per provider

## 100-04, 13, 30.1.3.1

### A/B MAC (A) Payment for Low Osmolar Contrast Material (LOCM) (Radiology)

The LOCM is paid on a reasonable cost basis when rendered by a SNF to its Part B patients (in addition to payment for the radiology procedure) when it is used in one of the situations listed below.

The following HCPCS are used when billing for LOCM.

| HCPCS Code | Description (January 1. 1994, and later) |
|---|---|
| A4644 | Supply of low osmolar contrast material (100-199 mgs of iodine); |
| A4645 | Supply of low osmolar contrast material (200-299 mgs of iodine); or |
| A4646 | Supply of low osmolar contrast material (300-399 mgs of iodine). |

When billing for LOCM, SNFs use revenue code 0636. If the SNF charge for the radiology procedure includes a charge for contrast material, the SNF must adjust the charge for the radiology procedure to exclude any amount for the contrast material.

NOTE: LOCM is never billed with revenue code 0255 or as part of the radiology procedure.

The A/B MAC (A) will edit for the intrathecal procedure codes and the following codes to determine if payment for LOCM is to be made. If an intrathecal procedure code is not present, or one of the ICD codes is not present to indicate that a required medical condition is met, the A/B MAC (A) will deny payment for LOCM. In these instances, LOCM is not covered and should not be billed to Medicare.

When LOCM Is Separately Billable and Related Coding Requirements

- In all intrathecal injections. HCPCS codes that indicate intrathecal injections are:

   70010, 70015, 72240, 72255, 72265, 72270, 72285, 72295

   One of these must be included on the claim; or

- In intravenous and intra-arterial injections only when certain medical conditions are present in an outpatient. The SNF must verify the existence of at least one of the following medical conditions, and report the applicable diagnosis code(s) either as a principal diagnosis code or other diagnosis codes on the claim:

   — A history of previous adverse reaction to contrast material. The applicable ICD-9-CM codes are V14.8 and V14.9. The applicable ICD-10-CM codes are Z88.8 and Z88.9. The conditions which should not be considered adverse reactions are a sensation of heat, flushing, or a single episode of nausea or vomiting. If the adverse reaction occurs on that visit with the induction of contrast material, codes describing hives, urticaria, etc. should also be present, as well as a code describing the external cause of injury and poisoning, ICD-9-CM code E947.8. The applicable ICD-10 CM codes are:

T50.8X5A Adverse effect of diagnostic agents, initial encounter, T50.8X5S Adverse effect of diagnostic agents, sequela , T50.995A Adverse effect of other drugs, medicaments and biological substances, initial encounter, or T50.995S Adverse effect of other drugs, medicaments and biological substances, sequela;

— A history or condition of asthma or allergy. The applicable ICD-9-CM codes are V07.1, V14.0 through V14.9, V15.0, 493.00, 493.01, 493.10, 493.11, 493.20, 493.21, 493.90, 493.91, 495.0, 495.1, 495.2, 495.3, 495.4, 495.5, 495.6, 495.7, 495.8, 495.9, 995.0, 995.1, 995.2, and 995.3. The applicable ICD-10-CM codes are in the table below:

ICD-10-CM Codes

| J44.0 | J44.9 | J45.20 | J45.22 | J45.30 | J45.32 | J45.40 |
|---|---|---|---|---|---|---|
| J45.42 | J45.50 | J45.52 | J45.902 | J45.909 | J45.998 | J67.0 |
| J67.1 | JJ67.2 | J67.3 | J67.4 | J67.5 | J67.6 | J67.7 |
| J67.8 | J67.9 | J96.00 | J96.01 | J96.02 | J96.90 | J96.91 |
| J96.92 | T36.0X5A | T36.1X5A | T36.2X5A | T36.3X5A | T36.4X5A | T36.5X5A |
| T36.6X5A | T36.7X5A | T36.8X5A | T36.95XA | T37.0X5A | T37.1X5A | T37.2X5A |
| T37.3X5A | T37.8X5A | T37.95XA | T38.0X5A | T38.1X5A | T38.2X5A | T38.3X5A |
| T38.4X5A | T38.6X5A | T38.7X5A | T38.805A | T38.815A | T38.895A | T38.905A |
| T38.995A | T39.015A | T39.095A | T39.1X5A | T39.2X5A | T39.2X5A | T39.315A |
| T39.395A | T39.4X5A | T39.8X5A | T39.95XA | T40.0X5A | T40.1X5A | T40.2X5A |
| T40.3X5A | T40.4X5A | T40.5X5A | T40.605A | T40.695A | T40.7X5A | T40.8X5A |
| T40.905A | T40.995A | T41.0X5A | T41.1X5A | T41.205A | T41.295A | T41.3X5A |
| T41.4X5A | T41.X5A | T41.5X5A | T42.0X5A | T42.1X5A | T42.2X5A | T42.3X5A |
| T42.4X5A | T42.5X5A | T42.6X5A | 427.5XA | 428.X5A | T43.015A | T43.025A |
| T43.1X5A | T43.205A | T43.215A | T43.225A | T43.295A | T43.3X5A | T43.4X5A |
| T43.505A | T43.595A | T43.605A | T43.615A | T43.625A | T43.635A | T43.695A |
| T43.8X5A | T43.95XA | T44.0X5A | T44.1X5A | T44.2X5A | T44.3X5A | T44.6X5A |
| T44.7X5A | T44.8X5A | T44.905A | T44.995A | T45.0X5A | T45.1X5A | T45.2X5A |
| T45.3X5A | T45.4X5A | T45.515A | T45.525A | T45.605A | T45.615A | T45.625A |
| T45.695A | T45.7X5A | T45.8X5A | T45.95XA | T46.0X5A | T46.1X5A | T46.2X5A |
| T46.3X5A | T46.4X5A | T46.5X5A | T46.6X5A | T46.7X5A | T46.8X5A | T46.905A |
| T46.995A | T47.0X5A | T47.1X5A | T47.2X5A | T47.3X5A | T47.4X5A | T47.5X5A |
| T47.6X5A | T47.7X5A | T47.8X5A | T47.95XA | T48.0X5A | T48.1X5A | T48.205A |
| T48.295A | T48.3X5A | T48.4X5A | T48.5X5A | T48.6X5A | T48.905A | T48.995A |
| T49.0X5A | T49.1X5A | T49.2X5A | T49.3X5A | T49.4X5A | T49.5X5A | T49.6X5A |
| T49.6X5A | T47.X5A9 | T49.8X5A | T49.95XA | T50.0X5A | T50.1X5A | T50.2X5A |
| T50.3X5A | T50.4X5A | T50.5X5A | T50.6X5A | T50.7X5A | T50.8X5A | T50.905a |
| T50.995A | T50.A15A | T50.A25A | T50.A95A | T50.B15A | T50.B95A | T50.Z15A |
| T50.Z95A | T78.2XXA | T78.3XXA | T78.40XA | T78.41XA | T88.52XA | T88.59XA |
| T88.6XXA | Z51.89 | Z88.0 | Z88.1 | Z88.2 | Z88.3 | Z88.4 |
| Z88.5 | Z88.6 | Z88.7 | Z88.8 | Z88.9 | Z91.010 | |

— Significant cardiac dysfunction including recent or imminent cardiac decompensation, severe arrhythmia, unstable angina pectoris, recent myocardial infarction, and pulmonary hypertension. The applicable ICD-9-CM codes are:

ICD-9-CM

| 402.00 | 402.01 | 402.10 | 402.11 | 402.90 | 402.91 | 404.00 |
|---|---|---|---|---|---|---|
| 404.01 | 404.02 | 404.03 | 404.10 | 404.11 | 404.12 | 404.13 |
| 404.90 | 404.91 | 404.92 | 404.93 | 410.00 | 410.01 | 410.02 |
| 410.10 | 410.11 | 410.12 | 410.20 | 410.21 | 410.22 | 410.30 |
| 410.31 | 410.32 | 410.40 | 410.41 | 410.42 | 410.50 | 410.51 |
| 410.52 | 410.60 | 410.61 | 410.62 | 410.70 | 410.71 | 410.72 |
| 410.80 | 410.81 | 410.82 | 410.90 | 410.91 | 410.92 | 411.1 |
| 415.0 | 416.0 | 416.1 | 416.8 | 416.9 | 420.0 | 420.90 |
| 420.91 | 420.99 | 424.90 | 424.91 | 424.99 | 427.0 | 427.1 |
| 427.2 | 427.31 | 427.32 | 427.41 | 427.42 | 427.5 | 427.60 |
| 427.61 | 427.69 | 427.81 | 427.89 | 427.9 | 428.0 | 428.1 |
| 428.9 | 429.0 | 429.1 | 429.2 | 429.3 | 429.4 | 429.5 |
| 429.6 | 429.71 | 429.79 | 429.81 | 429.82 | 429.89 | 429.9 |
| 785.50 | 785.51 | 785.59 | | | | |

— The applicable ICD-10-CM codes are in the table below:

ICD-10-CM Codes

| A18.84 | I11.0 | I11.9 | I13.0 | I13.10 | I13.11 | I13.2 |
|---|---|---|---|---|---|---|
| I20.0 | I21.01 | I21.02 | I21.09 | I21.11 | I21.19 | I21.21 |
| I21.29 | I21.3 | I21.4 | I22.1 | I22.2 | I22.8 | I23.0 |
| I23.1 | I23.2 | I23.3 | I23.4 | I23.5 | I23.6 | I23.7 |
| I23.8 | I25.10 | I25.110 | I25.700 | I25.710 | I25.720 | I25.730 |
| I25.750 | I25.760 | I25.790 | I26.01 | I26.02 | I26.09 | I27.0 |
| I27.1 | I27.2 | I27.81 | I27.89 | I27.9 | I30.0 | I30.1 |
| I30.8 | I30.9 | I32 | I38 | I39 | I46.2 | I46.8 |
| I46.9 | I47.0 | I471 | I472 | I47.9 | I48.0 | I48.1 |
| I48.1 | I48.2 | I48.3 | I48.4 | I48.91 | I48.92 | I49.01 |
| I49.02 | I49.1 | I49.2 | I49.3 | I49.40 | I49.49 | I49.5 |
| I49.8 | I49.9 | I50.1 | I50.20 | I50.21 | I50.22 | I50.23 |
| I50.30 | I50.31 | I50.32 | I50.33 | I50.40 | I50.41 | I50.42 |
| I50.43 | I50.9 | I51 | I51.0 | I51.1 | I51.2 | I51.3 |
| I51.4 | I51.5 | I51.7 | I51.89 | I51.9 | I52 | I97.0 |
| I97.110 | I97.111 | I97.120 | I97.121 | I97.130 | I97.131 | I97.190 |
| I97.191 | M32.11 | M32.12 | R00.1 | R57.0 | R57.8 | R57.9 |

— Generalized severe debilitation. The applicable ICD-9-CM codes are: 203.00, 203.01, all codes for diabetes mellitus, 518.81, 585, 586, 799.3, 799.4, and V46.1. The applicable ICD-10-CM codes are: J96.850, J96.00 through J96.02, J96.90 through J96.91, N18.1 through N19, R53.81, R64, and Z99.11 through Z99.12. Or

— Sickle Cell disease. The applicable ICD-9-CM codes are 282.4, 282.60, 282.61, 282.62, 282.63, and 282.69. The applicable ICD-10-CM codes are D56.0 through D56.3, D56.5 through D56.9, D57.00 through D57.1, D57.20, D57.411 through D57.419, and D57.811 through D57.819.

## 100-04, 13, 40.1.1

### Magnetic Resonance Angiography (MRA) Coverage Summary

Section 1861(s)(2)(C) of the Social Security Act provides for coverage of diagnostic testing. Coverage of magnetic resonance angiography (MRA) of the head and neck, and MRA of the peripheral vessels of the lower extremities is limited as described in Publication (Pub.) 100-3, the Medicare National Coverage Determinations (NCD) Manual. This instruction has been revised as of July 1, 2003, based on a determination that coverage is reasonable and necessary in additional circumstances. Under that instruction, MRA is generally covered only to the extent that it is used as a substitute for contrast angiography, except to the extent that there are documented circumstances consistent with that instruction that demonstrates the medical necessity of both tests. Prior to June 3, 2010, there was no coverage of MRA outside of the indications and circumstances described in that instruction.

Effective for claims with dates of service on or after June 3, 2010, contractors have the discretion to cover or not cover all indications of MRA (and magnetic resonance imaging (MRI)) that are not specifically nationally covered or nationally non-covered as stated in section 220.2 of the NCD Manual.

Because the status codes for HCPCS codes 71555, 71555-TC, 71555-26, 74185, 74185-TC, and 74185-26 were changed in the Medicare Physician Fee Schedule Database from 'N' to 'R' on April 1, 1998, any MRA claims with those HCPCS codes with dates of service between April 1, 1998, and June 30, 1999, are to be processed according to the contractor's discretionary authority to determine payment in the absence of national policy.

Effective for claims with dates of service on or after February 24, 2011, Medicare will provide coverage for MRIs for beneficiaries with implanted cardiac pacemakers or implantable cardioverter defibrillators if the beneficiary is enrolled in an approved clinical study under the Coverage with Study Participation form of Coverage with Evidence Development that meets specific criteria per Pub. 100-3, the NCD Manual, chapter 1, section 220.2.C.1

## 100-04, 13, 40.1.2

### HCPCS Coding Requirements

Providers must report HCPCS codes when submitting claims for MRA of the chest, abdomen, head, neck or peripheral vessels of lower extremities. The following HCPCS codes should be used to report these services:

| MRA of head | 70544, 70544-26, 70544-TC |
|---|---|
| MRA of head | 70545, 70545-26, 70545-TC |
| MRA of head | 70546, 70546-26, 70546-TC |
| MRA of neck | 70547, 70547-26, 70547-TC |
| MRA of neck | 70548, 70548-26, 70548-TC |
| MRA of neck | 70549, 70549-26, 70549-TC |

| MRA of chest | 71555, 71555-26, 71555-TC |
|---|---|
| MRA of pelvis | 72198, 72198-26, 72198-TC |
| MRA of abdomen (dates of service on or after July 1, 2003) – see below. | 74185, 74185-26, 74185-TC |
| MRA of peripheral vessels of lower extremities | 73725, 73725-26, 73725-TC |

## 100-04, 13, 60

### Positron Emission Tomography (PET) Scans - General Information

Positron emission tomography (PET) is a noninvasive imaging procedure that assesses perfusion and the level of metabolic activity in various organ systems of the human body. A positron camera (tomograph) is used to produce cross-sectional tomographic images which are obtained by detecting radioactivity from a radioactive tracer substance (radiopharmaceutical) that emits a radioactive tracer substance (radiopharmaceutical FDG) such as 2 -[F-18] flouro-D-glucose FDG, that is administered intravenously to the patient.

The Medicare National Coverage Determinations (NCD) Manual, Chapter 1, Sec.220.6, contains additional coverage instructions to indicate the conditions under which a PET scan is performed.

**A. Definitions**

For all uses of PET, excluding Rubidium 82 for perfusion of the heart, myocardial viability and refractory seizures, the following definitions apply:

- **Diagnosis:** PET is covered only in clinical situations in which the PET results may assist in avoiding an invasive diagnostic procedure, or in which the PET results may assist in determining the optimal anatomical location to perform an invasive diagnostic procedure. In general, for most solid tumors, a tissue diagnosis is made prior to the performance of PET scanning. PET scans following a tissue diagnosis are generally performed for the purpose of staging, rather than diagnosis. Therefore, the use of PET in the diagnosis of lymphoma, esophageal and colorectal cancers, as well as in melanoma, should be rare. PET is not covered for other diagnostic uses, and is not covered for screening (testing of patients without specific signs and symptoms of disease).

- **Staging:** PET is covered in clinical situations in which (1) (a) the stage of the cancer remains in doubt after completion of a standard diagnostic workup, including conventional imaging (computed tomography, magnetic resonance imaging, or ultrasound) or, (b) the use of PET would also be considered reasonable and necessary if it could potentially replace one or more conventional imaging studies when it is expected that conventional study information is insufficient for the clinical management of the patient and, (2) clinical management of the patient would differ depending on the stage of the cancer identified.

  NOTE: Effective for services on or after April 3, 2009, the terms "diagnosis" and "staging" will be replaced with "Initial Treatment Strategy." For further information on this new term, refer to Pub. 100-3, NCD Manual, section 220.6.17.

- **Restaging:** PET will be covered for restaging: (1) after the completion of treatment for the purpose of detecting residual disease, (2) for detecting suspected recurrence, or metastasis, (3) to determine the extent of a known recurrence, or (4) if it could potentially replace one or more conventional imaging studies when it is expected that conventional study information is to determine the extent of a known recurrence, or if study information is insufficient for the clinical management of the patient. Restaging applies to testing after a course of treatment is completed and is covered subject to the conditions above.

- **Monitoring:** Use of PET to monitor tumor response to treatment during the planned course of therapy (i.e., when a change in therapy is anticipated).

  NOTE: Effective for services on or after April 3, 2009, the terms "restaging" and "monitoring" will be replaced with "Subsequent Treatment Strategy." For further information on this new term, refer to Pub. 100-3, NCD Manual, section 220.6.17.

**B. Limitations**

For staging and restaging: PET is covered in either/or both of the following circumstances:

- The stage of the cancer remains in doubt after completion of a standard diagnostic workup, including conventional imaging (computed tomography, magnetic resonance imaging, or ultrasound); and/or

- The clinical management of the patient would differ depending on the stage of the cancer identified. PET will be covered for restaging after the completion of treatment for the purpose of detecting residual disease, for detecting suspected recurrence, or to determine the extent of a known recurrence. Use of PET would also be considered reasonable and necessary if it could potentially replace one or more conventional imaging studies when it is expected that conventional study information is insufficient for the clinical management of the patient.

The PET is not covered for other diagnostic uses, and is not covered for screening (testing of patients without specific symptoms). Use of PET to monitor tumor response during the planned course of therapy (i.e. when no change in therapy is being contemplated) is not covered.

CPT © 2017 American Medical Association. All Rights Reserved.

© 2017 Optum360, LLC

## 100-04, 13, 60.2

### Use of Gamma Cameras and Full Ring and Partial Ring PET Scanners for PET Scans

See the Medicare NCD Manual, Section 220.6, concerning 2-[F-18] Fluoro-D-Glucose (FDG) PET scanners and details about coverage.

On July 1, 2001, HCPCS codes G0210 - G0230 were added to allow billing for all currently covered indications for FDG PET. Although the codes do not indicate the type of PET scanner, these codes were used until January 1, 2002, by providers to bill for services in a manner consistent with the coverage policy.

Effective January 1, 2002, HCPCS codes G0210 - G0230 were updated with new descriptors to properly reflect the type of PET scanner used. In addition, four new HCPCS codes became effective for dates of service on and after January 1, 2002, (G0231, G0232, G0233, G0234) for covered conditions that may be billed if a gamma camera is used for the PET scan. For services performed from January 1, 2002, through January 27, 2005, providers should bill using the revised HCPCS codes G0210 - G0234.

Beginning January 28, 2005 providers should bill using the appropriate CPT code.

## 100-04, 13, 60.3

### PET Scan Qualifying Conditions and HCPCS Code Chart

Below is a summary of all covered PET scan conditions, with effective dates.

NOTE: The G codes below except those a # can be used to bill for PET Scan services through January 27, 2005. Effective for dates of service on or after January 28, 2005, providers must bill for PET Scan services using the appropriate CPT codes. See section 60.3.1. The G codes with a # can continue to be used for billing after January 28, 2005 and these remain non-covered by Medicare. (NOTE: PET Scanners must be FDA-approved.)

| Conditions | Coverage Effective Date | **** HCPCS/CPT |
|---|---|---|
| *Myocardial perfusion imaging (following previous PET G0030-G0047) single study, rest or stress (exercise and/or pharmacologic) | 3/14/95 | G0030 |
| *Myocardial perfusion imaging (following previous PET G0030-G0047) multiple studies, rest or stress (exercise and/or pharmacologic) | 3/14/95 | G0031 |
| *Myocardial perfusion imaging (following rest SPECT, 78464); single study, rest or stress (exercise and/or pharmacologic) | 3/14/95 | G0032 |
| *Myocardial perfusion imaging (following rest SPECT 78464); multiple studies, rest or stress (exercise and/or pharmacologic) | 3/14/95 | G0033 |
| *Myocardial perfusion (following stress SPECT 78465); single study, rest or stress (exercise and/or pharmacologic) | 3/14/95 | G0034 |
| *Myocardial Perfusion Imaging (following stress SPECT 78465); multiple studies, rest or stress (exercise and/or pharmacologic) | 3/14/95 | G0035 |
| *Myocardial Perfusion Imaging (following coronary angiography 93510-93529); single study, rest or stress (exercise and/or pharmacologic) | 3/14/95 | G0036 |
| *Myocardial Perfusion Imaging, (following coronary angiography), 93510-93529); multiple studies, rest or stress (exercise and/or pharmacologic) | 3/14/95 | G0037 |
| *Myocardial Perfusion Imaging (following stress planar myocardial perfusion, 78460); single study, rest or stress (exercise and/or pharmacologic) | 3/14/95 | G0038 |
| *Myocardial Perfusion Imaging (following stress planar myocardial perfusion, 78460); multiple studies, rest or stress (exercise and/or pharmacologic) | 3/14/95 | G0039 |
| *Myocardial Perfusion Imaging (following stress echocardiogram 93350); single study, rest or stress (exercise and/or pharmacologic) | 3/14/95 | G0040 |
| *Myocardial Perfusion Imaging (following stress echocardiogram, 93350); multiple studies, rest or stress (exercise and/or pharmacologic) | 3/14/95 | G0041 |
| *Myocardial Perfusion Imaging (following stress nuclear ventriculogram 78481 or 78483); single study, rest or stress (exercise and/or pharmacologic) | 3/14/95 | G0042 |
| *Myocardial Perfusion Imaging (following stress nuclear ventriculogram 78481 or 78483); multiple studies, rest or stress (exercise and/or pharmacologic) | 3/14/95 | G0043 |

| Conditions | Coverage Effective Date | **** HCPCS/CPT |
|---|---|---|
| *Myocardial Perfusion Imaging (following stress ECG, 93000); single study, rest or stress (exercise and/or pharmacologic) | 3/14/95 | G0044 |
| *Myocardial perfusion (following stress ECG, 93000), multiple studies; rest or stress (exercise and/or pharmacologic) | 3/14/95 | 0045 |
| *Myocardial perfusion (following stress ECG, 93015), single study; rest or stress (exercise and/or pharmacologic) | 3/14/95 | G0046 |
| *Myocardial perfusion (following stress ECG, 93015); multiple studies, rest or stress (exercise and/or pharmacologic) | 3/14/95 | G0047 |
| PET imaging regional or whole body; single pulmonary nodule | 1/1/98 | G0125 |
| Lung cancer, non-small cell (PET imaging whole body) Diagnosis, Initial Staging, Restaging | 7/1/01 | G0210 G0211 G0212 |
| Colorectal cancer (PET imaging whole body) Diagnosis, Initial Staging, Restaging | 7/1/01 | G0213 G0214 G0215 |
| Melanoma (PET imaging whole body) Diagnosis, Initial Staging, Restaging | 7/1/01 | G0216 G0217 G0218 |
| Melanoma for non-covered indications | 7/1/01 | #G0219 |
| Lymphoma (PET imaging whole body) Diagnosis, Initial Staging, Restaging | 7/1/01 | G0220 G0221 G0222 |
| Head and neck cancer; excluding thyroid and CNS cancers (PET imaging whole body or regional) Diagnosis, Initial Staging, Restaging | 7/1/01 | G0223 G0224 G0225 |
| Esophageal cancer (PET imaging whole body) Diagnosis, Initial Staging, Restaging | 7/1/01 | G0226 G0227 G0228 |
| Metabolic brain imaging for pre-surgical evaluation of refractory seizures | 7/1/01 | G0229 |
| Metabolic assessment for myocardial viability following inconclusive SPECT study | 7/1/01 | G0230 |
| Recurrence of colorectal or colorectal metastatic cancer (PET whole body, gamma cameras only) | 1/1/02 | G0231 |
| Staging and characterization of lymphoma (PET whole body, gamma cameras only) | 1/1/02 | G0232 |
| Recurrence of melanoma or melanoma metastatic cancer (PET whole body, gamma cameras only) | 1/1/02 | G0233 |
| Regional or whole body, for solitary pulmonary nodule following CT, or for initial staging of nonsmall cell lung cancer (gamma cameras only) | 1/1/02 | G0234 |
| Non-Covered Service PET imaging, any site not otherwise specified | 1/28/05 | #G0235 |
| Non-Covered Service Initial diagnosis of breast cancer and/or surgical planning for breast cancer (e.g., initial staging of axillary lymph nodes), not covered (full- and partialring PET scanners only) | 10/1/02 | #G0252 |
| Breast cancer, staging/restaging of local regional recurrence or distant metastases, i.e., staging/restaging after or prior to course of treatment (full- and partial-ring PET scanners only) | 10/1/02 | G0253 |
| Breast cancer, evaluation of responses to treatment, performed during course of treatment (full- and partial-ring PET scanners only) | 10/1/02 | G0254 |
| Myocardial imaging, positron emission tomography (PET), metabolic evaluation | 10/1/02 | 78459 |
| Restaging or previously treated thyroid cancer of follicular cell origin following negative I-131 whole body scan (full- and partial-ring PET scanner only) | 10/1/03 | G0296 |
| Tracer Rubidium**82 (Supply of Radiopharmaceutical Diagnostic Imaging Agent) (This is only billed through Outpatient Perspective Payment System, OPPS.) (Carriers must use HCPCS Code A4641). | 10/1/03 | Q3000 |

| Conditions | Coverage Effective Date | **** HCPCS/CPT |
|---|---|---|
| ***Supply of Radiopharmaceutical Diagnostic Imaging Agent, Ammonia N-13*** | 01/1/04 | A9526 |
| PET imaging, brain imaging for the differential diagnosis of Alzheimer's disease with aberrant features vs. fronto-temporal dementia | 09/15/04 | Appropriate CPT Code from section 60.3.1 |
| PET Cervical Cancer Staging as adjunct to conventional imaging, other staging, diagnosis, restaging, monitoring | 1/28/05 | Appropriate CPT Code from section 60.3.1 |

\* NOTE: Carriers must report A4641 for the tracer Rubidium 82 when used with PET scan codes G0030 through G0047 for services performed on or before January 27, 2005

\*\* NOTE: Not FDG PET

\*\*\* NOTE: For dates of service October 1, 2003, through December 31, 2003, use temporary code Q4078 for billing this radiopharmaceutical.

## 100-04, 13, 60.3.1

### Appropriate CPT Codes Effective for PET Scans for Services Performed on or After January 28, 2005

NOTE: All PET scan services require the use of a radiopharmaceutical diagnostic imaging agent (tracer). The applicable tracer code should be billed when billing for a PET scan service. See section 60.3.2 below for applicable tracer codes.

| CPT Code | Description |
|---|---|
| 78459 | Myocardial imaging, positron emission tomography (PET), metabolic evaluation |
| 78491 | Myocardial imaging, positron emission tomography (PET), perfusion, single study at rest or stress |
| 78492 | Myocardial imaging, positron emission tomography (PET), perfusion, multiple studies at rest and/or stress |
| 78608 | Brain imaging, positron emission tomography (PET); metabolic evaluation |
| 78811 | Tumor imaging, positron emission tomography (PET); limited area (eg, chest, head/neck) |
| 78812 | Tumor imaging, positron emission tomography (PET); skull base to mid-thigh |
| 78813 | Tumor imaging, positron emission tomography (PET); whole body |
| 78814 | Tumor imaging, positron emission tomography (PET) with concurrently acquired computed tomography (CT) for attenuation correction and anatomical localization; limited area (eg, chest, head/neck) |
| 78815 | Tumor imaging, positron emission tomography (PET) with concurrently acquired computed tomography (CT) for attenuation correction and anatomical localization; skull base to mid-thigh |
| 78816 | Tumor imaging, positron emission tomography (PET) with concurrently acquired computed tomography (CT) for attenuation correction and anatomical localization; whole body |

## 100-04, 13, 60.3.2

### Tracer Codes Required for PET Scans

**The following tracer codes are applicable only to CPT 78491 and 78492. They can not be reported with any other code.**

**Institutional providers billing the fiscal intermediary**

| HCPCS | Description |
|---|---|
| *A9555 | Rubidium Rb-82, Diagnostic, Per study dose, Up To 60 Millicuries |
| * Q3000 (Deleted effective 12/31/05) | Supply of Radiopharmaceutical Diagnostic Imaging Agent, Rubidium Rb-82, per dose |
| A9526 | Nitrogen N-13 Ammonia, Diagnostic, Per study dose, Up To 40 Millicuries |

\* NOTE: For claims with dates of service prior to 1/01/06, providers report Q3000 for supply of radiopharmaceutical diagnostic imaging agent, Rubidium Rb-82. For claims with dates of service 1/01/06 and later, providers report A9555 for radiopharmaceutical diagnostic imaging agent, Rubidium Rb-82 in place of Q3000.

**Physicians / practitioners billing the carrier:**

| *A4641 | Supply of Radiopharmaceutical Diagnostic Imaging Agent, Not Otherwise Classified |
|---|---|
| A9526 | Nitrogen N-13 Ammonia, Diagnostic, Per study dose, Up To 40 Millicuries |
| A9555 | Rubidium Rb-82, Diagnostic, Per study dose, Up To 60 Millicuries |

\* NOTE: Effective January 1, 2008, tracer code A4641 is not applicable for PET Scans.

**The following tracer codes are applicable only to CPT 78459, 78608, 78811-78816. They can not be reported with any other code:**

**Institutional providers billing the fiscal intermediary:**

| * A9552 | Fluorodeoxyglucose F18, FDG, Diagnostic, Per study dose, Up to 45 Millicuries |
|---|---|
| * C1775 (Deleted effective 12/31/05) | Supply of Radiopharmaceutical Diagnostic Imaging Agent, Fluorodeoxyglucose F18, (2-Deoxy-2-18F Fluoro-D-Glucose), Per dose (4-40 Mci/Ml) |
| **A4641 | Supply of Radiopharmaceutical Diagnostic Imaging Agent, Not Otherwise Classified |
| A9580 | Sodium Fluoride F-18, Diagnostic, per study dose, up to 30 Millicuries |

\* NOTE: For claims with dates of service prior to 1/01/06, OPPS hospitals report C1775 for supply of radiopharmaceutical diagnostic imaging agent, Fluorodeoxyglucose F18. For claims with dates of service January 1, 2006 and later, providers report A9552 for radiopharmaceutical diagnostic imaging agent, Fluorodeoxyglucose F18 in place of C1775.

\*\* NOTE: Effective January 1, 2008, tracer code A4641 is not applicable for PET Scans.

\*\*\* NOTE: Effective for claims with dates of service February 26, 2010 and later, tracer code A9580 is applicable for PET Scans.

**Physicians / practitioners billing the carrier:**

| A9552 | Fluorodeoxyglucose F18, FDG, Diagnostic, Per study dose, Up to 45 Millicuries |
|---|---|
| *A4641 | Supply of Radiopharmaceutical Diagnostic Imaging Agent, Not Otherwise Classified |
| A9580 | Sodium Fluoride F-18, Diagnostic, per study dose, up to 30 Millicuries |

\* NOTE: Effective January 1, 2008, tracer code A4641 is not applicable for PET Scans.

\*\*\* NOTE: Effective for claims with dates of service February 26, 2010 and later, tracer code A9580 is applicable for PET Scans.

**Positron Emission Tomography Reference Table**

| CPT | Short Descriptor | Tracer/Code | or | Tracer/Code | Comment |
|---|---|---|---|---|---|
| 78459 | Myocardial imaging, positron emission tomography (PET), metabolic imaging | FDG A9552 | -- | -- | N/A |
| 78491 | Myocardial imaging, positron emission tomography (PET), perfusion; single study at rest or stress | N-13 A9526 | or | Rb-82 A9555 | N/A |
| 78492 | Myocardial imaging, positron emission tomography (PET), perfusion; multiple studies at rest and/or stress | N-13 A9526 | or | Rb-82 A9555 | N/A |
| 78608 | Brain imaging, positron emission tomography (PET); metabolic evaluation | FDG A9552 | -- | -- | Covered indications: Alzheimer's disease/dementias, intractable seizures. Note: This code is also covered for dedicated PET brain tumor imaging. |
| 78609 | Brain imaging, positron emission tomography (PET); perfusion evaluation | -- | -- | -- | Nationally noncovered |

CPT © 2017 American Medical Association. All Rights Reserved.

© 2017 Optum360, LLC

| CPT | Short Descriptor | Tracer/Code | or | Tracer/Code | Comment |
|---|---|---|---|---|---|
| 78811 | Positron emission tomography (PET) imaging; limited area (e.g, chest, head/neck) | FDG A9552 | or | NaF-18 A9580 | NaF-18 PET is covered only to identify bone metastasis of cancer. |
| 78812 | Positron emission tomography (PET) imaging, skull base to mid-thigh | FDG A9552 | or | NaF-18 A9580 | NaF-18 PET is covered only to identify bone metastasis of cancer. |
| 78813 | Positron emission tomography (PET) imaging, whole body | FDG A9552 | or | NaF-18 A9580 | NaF-18 PET is covered only to identify bone metastasis of cancer. |
| 78814 | PET/CT imaging, limited area (e.g., chest, head/neck) | FDG A9552 | or | NaF-18 A9580 | NaF-18 PET is covered only to identify bone metastasis of cancer. |
| 78815 | PET/CT imaging skull base to mid-thigh | FDG A9552 | or | NaF-18 A9580 | NaF-18 PET is covered only to identify bone metastasis of cancer. |
| 78816 | PET/CT imaging, whole body | FDG A9552 | or | NaF-18 A9580 | NaF-18 PET is covered only to identify bone metastasis of cancer. |

## 100-4, 13, 60.12

### Coverage for PET Scans for Dementia and Neurodegenerative Diseases

(Rev. 3650, Issued: 11-10-16, Effective: 02-10-17, Implementation: 02-10-17)

Effective for dates of service on or after September 15, 2004, Medicare will cover FDG PET scans for a differential diagnosis of fronto-temporal dementia (FTD) and Alzheimer's disease OR; its use in a CMS-approved practical clinical trial focused on the utility of FDG-PET in the diagnosis or treatment of dementing neurodegenerative diseases. Refer to Pub. 100-03, NCD Manual, section 220.6.13, for complete coverage conditions and clinical trial requirements and section 60.15 of this manual for claims processing information.

### A. A/B MAC (A and B) Billing Requirements for PET Scan Claims for FDG-PET for the Differential Diagnosis of Fronto-temporal Dementia and Alzheimer's Disease:

CPT Code for PET Scans for Dementia and Neurodegenerative Diseases

Contractors shall advise providers to use the appropriate CPT code from section 60.3.1 for dementia and neurodegenerative diseases for services performed on or after January 28, 2005.

Diagnosis Codes for PET Scans for Dementia and Neurodegenerative Diseases

The contractor shall ensure one of the following appropriate diagnosis codes is present on claims for PET Scans for AD:

- If ICD-9-CM is applicable, ICD-9 codes are: 290.0, 290.10 - 290.13, 290.20 - 290, 21, 290.3, 331.0, 331.11, 331.19, 331.2, 331.9, 780.93
- If ICD-10-CM is applicable, ICD-10 codes are: F03.90, F03.90 plus F05, G30.9, G31.01, G31.9, R41.2 or R41.3

Medicare contractors shall deny claims when submitted with an appropriate CPT code from section 60.3.1 and with a diagnosis code other than the range of codes listed above.

Medicare contractors shall instruct providers to issue an Advanced Beneficiary Notice to beneficiaries advising them of potential financial liability prior to delivering the service if one of the appropriate diagnosis codes will not be present on the claim.

The contractor shall use the following remittance advice messages and associated codes when rejecting/denying claims under this policy. This CARC/RARC combination is compliant with CAQH CORE Business Scenario Three.

Group Code: PR (if claim is received with a GA modifier) otherwise CO

CARC: 11

RARC: N/A

MSN: 16.48

Provider Documentation Required with the PET Scan Claim

Medicare contractors shall inform providers to ensure the conditions mentioned in the NCD Manual, section 220.6.13, have been met. The information must also be maintained in the beneficiary's medical record:

- Date of onset of symptoms;
- Diagnosis of clinical syndrome (normal aging, mild cognitive impairment or MCI: mild, moderate, or severe dementia);
- Mini mental status exam (MMSE) or similar test score;
- Presumptive cause (possible, probably, uncertain AD);
- Any neuropsychological testing performed;

- Results of any structural imaging (MRI, CT) performed;
- Relevant laboratory tests (B12, thyroid hormone); and,
- Number and name of prescribed medications.

### B. Billing Requirements for Beta Amyloid Positron Emission Tomography (PET) in Dementia and Neurodegenerative Disease:

Effective for claims with dates of service on and after September 27, 2013, Medicare will only allow coverage with evidence development (CED) for Positron Emission Tomography (PET) beta amyloid (also referred to as amyloid-beta (Aβ)) imaging (HCPCS A9586)or (HCPCS A9599) (one PET Aβ scan per patient).

**NOTE:** Please note that effective January 1, 2014 the following code A9599 will be updated in the IOCE and HCPCS update. This code will be contractor priced.

Medicare Summary Notices, Remittance Advice Remark Codes, and Claim Adjustment Reason Codes

Effective for dates of service on or after September 27, 2013, contractors shall return as unprocessable/return to provider claims for PET Aβ imaging, through CED during a clinical trial, not containing the following:

- Condition code 30, (A/B MAC (A) only)
- Modifier Q0 and/or modifier Q1 as appropriate
- ICD-9 dx code V70.7/ICD-10 dx code Z00.6 (on either the primary/secondary position)
- A PET HCPCS code (78811 or 78814)
- At least, one Dx code from the table below,

| ICD-9 Codes | Corresponding ICD-10 Codes |
|---|---|
| 290.0 Senile dementia, uncomplicated | F03.90 Unspecified dementia without behavioral disturbance |
| 290.10 Presenile dementia, uncomplicated | F03.90 Unspecified dementia without behavioral disturbance |
| 290.11 Presenile dementia with delirium | F03.90 Unspecified dementia without behavioral disturbance |
| 290.12 Presenile dementia with delusional features | F03.90 Unspecified dementia without behavioral disturbance |
| 290.13 Presenile dementia with depressive features | F03.90 Unspecified dementia without behavioral disturbance |
| 290.20 Senile dementia with delusional features | F03.90 Unspecified dementia without behavioral disturbance |
| 290.21 Senile dementia with depressive features | F03.90 Unspecified dementia without behavioral disturbance |
| 290.3 Senile dementia with delirium | F03.90 Unspecified dementia without behavioral disturbance |
| 290.40 Vascular dementia, uncomplicated | F01.50 Vascular dementia without behavioral disturbance |
| 290.41 Vascular dementia with delirium | F01.51 Vascular dementia with behavioral disturbance |
| 290.42 Vascular dementia with delusions | F01.51 Vascular dementia with behavioral disturbance |
| 290.43 Vascular dementia with depressed mood | F01.51 Vascular dementia with behavioral disturbance |
| 294.10 Dementia in conditions classified elsewhere without behavioral disturbance | F02.80 Dementia in other diseases classified elsewhere without behavioral disturbance |
| 294.11 Dementia in conditions classified elsewhere with behavioral disturbance | F02.81 Dementia in other diseases classified elsewhere with behavioral disturbance |
| 294.20 Dementia, unspecified, without behavioral disturbance | F03.90 Unspecified dementia without behavioral disturbance |
| 294.21 Dementia, unspecified, with behavioral disturbance | F03.91 Unspecified dementia with behavioral disturbance |
| 331.11 Pick's Disease | G31.01 Pick's disease |
| 331.19 Other Frontotemporal dementia | G31.09 Other frontotemporal dementia |
| 331.6 Corticobasal degeneration | G31.85 Corticobasal degeneration |
| 331.82 Dementia with Lewy Bodies | G31.83 Dementia with Lewy bodies |
| 331.83 Mild cognitive impairment, so stated | G31.84 Mild cognitive impairment, so stated |
| 780.93 Memory LossR41.1 Anterograde amnesia | R41.2 Retrograde amnesia<br><br>R41.3 Other amnesia (Amnesia NOS, Memory loss NOS) |
| V70.7 Examination for normal comparison or control in clinical | Z00.6 Encounter for examination for normal comparison and control in clinical research program |

and

- Aβ HCPCS code A9586 or A9599

The contractor shall use the following remittance advice messages and associated codes when returning claims under this policy. This CARC/RARC combination is compliant with CAQH CORE Business Scenario Two.

Group Code: CO
CARC: 4
RARC: N517, N519
MSN: N/A

Contractors shall line-item deny claims for PET Aβ, HCPCS code A9586 or A9599, where a previous PET Aβ, HCPCS code A9586 or A9599 is paid in history.

The contractor shall use the following remittance advice messages and associated codes when rejecting/denying claims under this policy. This CARC/RARC combination is compliant with CAQH CORE Business Scenario Three.

Group Code: PR (if claim is received with a GA modifier) otherwise CO
CARC: 149
RARC: N587
MSN: 20.12

## 100-04, 13, 60.13

### Billing Requirements for PET Scans for Specific Indications of Cervical Cancer for Services Performed on or After January 28, 2005

Contractors shall accept claims for these services with the appropriate CPT code listed in section 60.3.1. Refer to Pub. 100-3, section 220.6.17, for complete coverage guidelines for this new PET oncology indication. The implementation date for these CPT codes will be April 18, 2005. Also see section 60.17, of this chapter for further claims processing instructions for cervical cancer indications.

## 100-04, 13, 60.15

### Billing Requirements for CMS - Approved Clinical Trials and Coverage With Evidence Development Claims for PET Scans for Neurodegenerative Diseases, Previously Specified Cancer Indications, and All Other Cancer Indications Not Previously Specified

#### A/B MACs (A and B)

Effective for services on or after January 28, 2005, contractors shall accept and pay for claims for Positron Emission Tomography (PET) scans for lung cancer, esophageal cancer, colorectal cancer, lymphoma, melanoma, head & neck cancer, breast cancer, thyroid cancer, soft tissue sarcoma, brain cancer, ovarian cancer, pancreatic cancer, small cell lung cancer, and testicular cancer, as well as for neurodegenerative diseases and all other cancer indications not previously mentioned in this chapter, if these scans were performed as part of a Centers for Medicare & Medicaid (CMS)-approved clinical trial. (See Pub. 100-3, National Coverage Determinations (NCD) Manual, sections 220.6.13 and 220.6.17.)

Contractors shall also be aware that PET scans for all cancers not previously specified at Pub. 100-3, NCD Manual, section 220.6.17, remain nationally non-covered unless performed in conjunction with a CMS-approved clinical trial.

Effective for dates of service on or after June 11, 2013, Medicare has ended the coverage with evidence development (CED) requirement for FDG (2-[F18] fluoro-2-deoxy-D-glucose) PET and PET/computed tomography (CT) and PET/magnetic resonance imaging (MRI) for all oncologic indications contained in section 220.6.17 of the NCD Manual. Modifier -Q0 (Investigational clinical service provided in a clinical research study that is in an approved clinical research study) or -Q1 (routine clinical service

provided in a clinical research study that is in an approved clinical research study) is no longer mandatory for these services when performed on or after June 11, 2013.

#### A/B MACs (B) Only

A/B MACs (B) shall pay claims for PET scans for beneficiaries participating in a CMS-approved clinical trial submitted with an appropriate current procedural terminology (CPT) code from section 60.3.1 of this chapter and modifier Q0/Q1 for services performed on or after January 1, 2008, through June 10, 2013. (NOTE: Modifier QR (Item or service provided in a Medicare specified study) and QA (FDA investigational device exemption) were replaced by modifier Q0 effective January 1, 2008.) Modifier QV (item or service provided as routine care in a Medicare qualifying clinical trial) was replaced by modifier Q1 effective January 1, 2008.) Beginning with services performed on or after June 11, 2013, modifier Q0/Q1 is no longer required for PET FDG services.

#### A/B MACs (A) Only

In order to pay claims for PET scans on behalf of beneficiaries participating in a CMS-approved clinical trial, A/B MACs (A) require providers to submit claims with, if ICD-9-CM is applicable, ICD-9 code V70.7; if ICD-10-CM is applicable, ICD-10 code Z00.6 in the primary/secondary diagnosis position using the ASC X12 837 institutional claim format or on Form CMS-1450, with the appropriate principal diagnosis code and an appropriate CPT code from section 60.3.1. Effective for PET scan claims for dates of service on or after January 28, 2005, through December 31, 2007, A/B MACs (A) shall accept claims with the QR, QV, or QA modifier on other than

inpatient claims. Effective for services on or after January 1, 2008, through June 10, 2013, modifier Q0 replaced the-QR and QA modifier, modifier Q1 replaced the QV modifier. Modifier Q0/Q1 is no longer required for services performed on or after June 11, 2013.

## 100-4, 13, 60.16

### Billing and Coverage Changes for PET Scans Effective for Services on or After April 3, 2009

(Rev. 3650, Issued: 11-10-16, Effective: 02-10-17, Implementation: 02-10-17)

#### A. Summary of Changes

Effective for services on or after April 3, 2009, Medicare will not cover the use of FDG PET imaging to determine initial treatment strategy in patients with adenocarcinoma of the prostate.

Medicare will also not cover FDG PET imaging for subsequent treatment strategy for tumor types other than breast, cervical, colorectal, esophagus, head and neck (non-CNS/thyroid), lymphoma, melanoma, myeloma, non-small cell lung, and ovarian, unless

the FDG PET is provided under the coverage with evidence development (CED) paradigm (billed with modifier -Q0/-Q1, see section 60.15 of this chapter).

Medicare will cover FDG PET imaging for initial treatment strategy for myeloma.

Effective for services performed on or after June 11, 2013, Medicare has ended the CED requirement for FDG PET and PET/CT and PET/MRI for all oncologic indications contained in section 220.6.17 of the NCD Manual. Effective for services on or after June 11, 2013, the Q0/Q1 modifier is no longer required.

Beginning with services performed on or after June 11, 2013, contractors shall pay for up to three (3) FDG PET scans when used to guide subsequent management of anti-tumor treatment strategy (modifier PS) after completion of initial anti-cancer therapy (modifier PI) for the exact same cancer diagnosis.

Coverage of any additional FDG PET scans (that is, beyond 3) used to guide subsequent management of anti-tumor treatment strategy after completion of initial anti-tumor therapy for the same cancer diagnosis will be determined by the A/B MACs (A or B). Claims will include the KX modifier indicating the coverage criteria is met for coverage of four or more FDG PET scans for subsequent treatment strategy for the same cancer diagnosis under this NCD.

A different cancer diagnosis whether submitted with a PI or a PS modifier will begin the count of one initial and three subsequent FDG PET scans not requiring the KX modifier and four or more FDG PET scans for subsequent treatment strategy for the same cancer diagnosis requiring the KX modifier.

**NOTE:** The presence or absence of an initial treatment strategy claim in a beneficiary's record does not impact the frequency criteria for subsequent treatment strategy claims for the same cancer diagnosis.

**NOTE:** Providers please refer to the following link for a list of appropriate diagnosis codes, http://cms.gov/medicare/coverage/determinationprocess/downloads/petforsolidtumorsoncologicdxcodesattachment_NCD220_6_17.pdf

For further information regarding the changes in coverage, refer to Pub.100-03, NCD Manual, section 220.6.17.

#### B. Modifiers for PET Scans

Effective for claims with dates of service on or after April 3, 2009, the following modifiers have been created for use to inform for the initial treatment strategy of biopsy-proven or strongly suspected tumors or subsequent treatment strategy of cancerous tumors:

PI Positron Emission Tomography (PET) or PET/Computed Tomography (CT) to inform the initial treatment strategy of tumors that are biopsy proven or strongly suspected of being cancerous based on other diagnostic testing.

Short descriptor: PET tumor init tx strat

PS Positron Emission Tomography (PET) or PET/Computed Tomography (CT) to inform the subsequent treatment strategy of cancerous tumors when the beneficiary's treatment physician determines that the PET study is needed to inform subsequent anti-tumor strategy.

Short descriptor: PS - PET tumor subsq tx strategy

#### C. Billing for A/B MACs (A and B)

Effective for claims with dates of service on or after April 3, 2009, contractors shall accept FDG PET claims billed to inform initial treatment strategy with the following CPT codes AND modifier PI: 78608, 78811, 78812, 78813, 78814, 78815, 78816.

Effective for claims with dates of service on or after April 3, 2009, contractors shall accept FDG PET claims with modifier PS for the subsequent treatment strategy for solid tumors using a CPT code above AND a cancer diagnosis code.

Contractors shall also accept FDG PET claims billed to inform initial treatment strategy or subsequent treatment strategy when performed under CED with one of the PET or PET/CT CPT codes above AND modifier PI OR modifier PS AND a cancer diagnosis code AND modifier Q0/Q1. Effective for services performed on or after June 11, 2013, the CED requirement has ended and modifier Q0/Q1, along with condition code 30 (institutional claims only), or ICD-9 code V70.7, (both institutional and practitioner claims) are no longer required.

CPT © 2017 American Medical Association. All Rights Reserved.                    © 2017 Optum360, LLC

**D. Medicare Summary Notices, Remittance Advice Remark Codes, and Claim Adjustment Reason Codes**

Effective for dates of service on or after April 3, 2009, contractors shall return as unprocessable/return to provider claims that do not include the PI modifier with one of the PET/PET/CT CPT codes listed in subsection C. above when billing for the initial treatment strategy for solid tumors in accordance with Pub.100-03, NCD Manual, section 220.6.17.

In addition, contractors shall return as unprocessable/return to provider claims that do not include the PS modifier with one of the CPT codes listed in subsection C. above when billing for the subsequent treatment strategy for solid tumors in accordance with Pub.100-03, NCD Manual, section 220.6.17.

The contractor shall use the following remittance advice messages and associated codes when returning claims under this policy. This CARC/RARC combination is compliant with CAQH CORE Business Scenario Two.

Group Code: CO
CARC: 4
RARC: MA130
MSN: N/A

Effective for claims with dates of service on or after April 3, 2009, through June 10, 2013, contractors shall return as unprocessable/return to provider FDG PET claims billed to inform initial treatment strategy or subsequent treatment strategy when performed under CED without one of the PET/PET/CT CPT codes listed in subsection C. above AND modifier PI OR modifier PS AND a cancer diagnosis code AND modifier Q0/Q1.

The contractor shall use the following remittance advice messages and associated codes when returning claims under this policy. This CARC/RARC combination is compliant with CAQH CORE Business Scenario Two.

Group Code: CO
CARC: 4
RARC: MA130
MSN: N/A

Effective April 3, 2009, contractors shall deny claims with ICD-9/ICD-10 diagnosis code 185/C61 for FDG PET imaging for the initial treatment strategy of patients with adenocarcinoma of the prostate.

For dates of service prior to June 11, 2013, contractors shall also deny claims for FDG PET imaging for subsequent treatment strategy for tumor types other than breast, cervical, colorectal, esophagus, head and neck (non-CNS/thyroid), lymphoma, melanoma, myeloma, non-small cell lung, and ovarian, unless the FDG PET is provided under CED (submitted with the Q0/Q1 modifier) and use the following messages:

The contractor shall use the following remittance advice messages and associated codes when rejecting/denying claims under this policy. This CARC/RARC combination is compliant with CAQH CORE Business Scenario Three.

Group Code: PR (if claim is received with a GA modifier) otherwise CO
CARC: 50
RARC: N/A
MSN: 15.4

Effective for dates of service on or after June 11, 2013, contractors shall use the following messages when denying claims in excess of three for PET FDG scans for subsequent treatment strategy when the KX modifier is not included, identified by CPT codes 78608, 78811, 78812, 78813, 78814, 78815, or 78816, modifier PS, HCPCS A9552, and the same cancer diagnosis code.

The contractor shall use the following remittance advice messages and associated codes when rejecting/denying claims under this policy. This CARC/RARC combination is compliant with CAQH CORE Business Scenario Three.

Group Code: PR (if claim is received with a GA modifier) otherwise CO
CARC: 96
RARC: N435
MSN: 23.17

## 100-4, 13, 60.17

### Billing and Coverage Changes for PET Scans for Cervical Cancer Effective for Services on or After November 10, 2009

(Rev. 3650, Issued: 11-10-16, Effective: 02-10-17, Implementation: 02-10-17)

**A. Billing Changes for A/B MACs (A and B)**

Effective for claims with dates of service on or after November 10, 2009, contractors shall accept FDG PET oncologic claims billed to inform initial treatment strategy; specifically for staging in beneficiaries who have biopsy-proven cervical cancer when the beneficiary's treating physician determines the FDG PET study is needed to determine the location and/or extent of the tumor as specified in Pub. 100-03, section 220.6.17.

EXCEPTION: CMS continues to non-cover FDG PET for initial diagnosis of cervical cancer related to initial treatment strategy.

**NOTE:** Effective for claims with dates of service on and after November 10, 2009, the –Q0 modifier is no longer necessary for FDG PET for cervical cancer.

**B. Medicare Summary Notices, Remittance Advice Remark Codes, and Claim Adjustment Reason Codes**

Additionally, contractors shall return as unprocessable /return to provider for FDG PET for cervical cancer for initial treatment strategy billed without the following: one of the PET/PET/ CT CPT codes listed in 60.16 C above AND modifier PI AND a cervical cancer diagnosis code.

The contractor shall use the following remittance advice messages and associated codes when returning claims under this policy. This CARC/RARC combination is compliant with CAQH CORE Business Scenario Two.

Group Code: CO
CARC: 4
RARC: MA130
MSN: N/A

## 100-4, 13, 60.18

### Billing and Coverage Changes for PET (NaF-18) Scans to Identify Bone Metastasis of Cancer Effective for Claims With Dates of Services on or After February 26, 2010

(Rev. 3650, Issued: 11-10-16, Effective: 02-10-17, Implementation: 02-10-17)

**A. Billing Changes for A/B MACs (A and B)**

Effective for claims with dates of service on and after February 26, 2010, contractors shall pay for NaF-18 PET oncologic claims to inform initial treatment strategy (PI) or subsequent treatment strategy (PS) for suspected or biopsy proven bone metastasis ONLY in the context of a clinical study and as specified in Pub. 100-03, section 220.6. All other claims for NaF-18 PET oncology claims remain non-covered.

**B. Medicare Summary Notices, Remittance Advice Remark Codes, and Claim Adjustment Reason Codes**

Effective for claims with dates of service on or after February 26, 2010, contractors shall return as unprocessable NaF-18 PET oncologic claims billed with modifier TC or globally (for A/B MACs (A) modifier TC or globally does not apply) and HCPCS A9580 to inform the initial treatment strategy or subsequent treatment strategy for bone metastasis that do not include ALL of the following:

- PI or PS modifier AND
- PET or PET/CT CPT code (78811, 78812, 78813, 78814, 78815, 78816) AND
- Cancer diagnosis code AND
- Q0 modifier - Investigational clinical service provided in a clinical research study, are present on the claim.

**NOTE:** For institutional claims, continue to include ICD-9 diagnosis code V70.7 or ICD-10 diagnosis code Z00.6 and condition code 30 to denote a clinical study.

The contractor shall use the following remittance advice messages and associated codes when returning claims under this policy. This CARC/RARC combination is compliant with CAQH CORE Business Scenario Two

Group Code: CO
CARC: 4
RARC: MA130
MSN: N/A

Effective for claims with dates of service on or after February 26, 2010, contractors shall accept PET oncologic claims billed with modifier 26 and modifier KX to inform the initial treatment strategy or subsequent treatment strategy for bone metastasis that include the following:

- PI or PS modifier AND
- PET or PET/CT CPT code (78811, 78812, 78813, 78814, 78815, 78816) AND
- Cancer diagnosis code AND
- Q0 modifier - Investigational clinical service provided in a clinical research study, are present on the claim.

**NOTE:** If modifier KX is present on the professional component service, Contractors shall process the service as PET NaF-18 rather than PET with FDG.

Contractors shall also return as unprocessable NaF-18 PET oncologic professional component claims (i.e., claims billed with modifiers 26 and KX) to inform the initial treatment strategy or subsequent treatment strategy for bone metastasis billed with HCPCS A9580.

The contractor shall use the following remittance advice messages and associated codes when returning claims under this policy. This CARC/RARC combination is compliant with CAQH CORE Business Scenario Two.

Group Code: CO
CARC: 4
RARC: MA130
MSN: N/A

Claim Adjustment Reason Code 97 – The benefit for this service is included in the payment/allowance for another service/procedure that has already been adjudicated.

NOTE: Refer to the 835 Healthcare Policy identification Segment (loop 2110 Service Payment Information REF), if present.

## 100-04, 13, 70.3

### Radiation Treatment Delivery (CPT 77401 - 77417)

Carriers pay for these TC services on a daily basis under CPT codes 77401-77416 for radiation treatment delivery. They do not use local codes and RVUs in paying for the TC of radiation oncology services. Multiple treatment sessions on the same day are payable as long as there has been a distinct break in therapy services, and the individual sessions are of the character usually furnished on different days. Carriers pay for CPT code 77417 (Therapeutic radiology port film(s)) on a weekly (five fractions) basis.

## 100-04, 13, 70.4

### Clinical Brachytherapy (CPT Codes 77750 - 77799)

Carriers must apply the bundled services policy to procedures in this family of codes other than CPT code 77776. For procedures furnished in settings in which TC payments are made, carriers must pay separately for the expendable source associated with these procedures under CPT code 79900 except in the case of remote after-loading high intensity brachytherapy procedures (CPT codes 77781-77784). In the four codes cited, the expendable source is included in the RVUs for the TC of the procedures.

## 100-04, 13, 70.5

### Radiation Physics Services (CPT Codes 77300 - 77399)

Carriers pay for the PC and TC of CPT codes 77300-77334 and 77399 on the same basis as they pay for radiologic services generally. For professional component billings in all settings, carriers presume that the radiologist participated in the provision of the service, e.g., reviewed/validated the physicist's calculation. CPT codes 77336 and 77370 are technical services only codes that are payable by carriers in settings in which only technical component is are payable.

## 100-04, 13, 80.1

### Physician Presence

Radiologic supervision and interpretation (S&I) codes are used to describe the personal supervision of the performance of the radiologic portion of a procedure by one or more physicians and the interpretation of the findings. In order to bill for the supervision aspect of the procedure, the physician must be present during its performance. This kind of personal supervision of the performance of the procedure is a service to an individual beneficiary and differs from the type of general supervision of the radiologic procedures performed in a hospital for which FIs pay the costs as physician services to the hospital. The interpretation of the procedure may be performed later by another physician. In situations in which a cardiologist, for example, bills for the supervision (the "S") of the S&I code, and a radiologist bills for the interpretation (the "I") of the code, both physicians should use a "-52" modifier indicating a reduced service, e.g., only one of supervision and/or interpretation. Payment for the fragmented S&I code is no more than if a single physician furnished both aspects of the procedure.

## 100-04, 13, 80.2

### Multiple Procedure Reduction

Carriers make no multiple procedure reductions in the S&I or primary non-radiologic codes in these types of procedures, or in any procedure codes for which the descriptor and RVUs reflect a multiple service reduction. For additional procedure codes that do not reflect such a reduction, carriers apply the multiple procedure reductions.

## 100-04, 16, 40.6.1

### Automated Multi-Channel Chemistry (AMCC) Tests for ESRD Beneficiaries

Instructions for Services Provided on and After January 1, 2011

Section 153b of the MIPPA requires that all ESRD-related laboratory tests must be reported by the ESRD facility whether provided directly or under arrangements with an independent laboratory. When laboratory services are billed by providers other than the ESRD facility and the laboratory test furnished is designated as a laboratory test that is included in the ESRD PPS (ESRD-related), the claim will be rejected or denied. In the event that an ESRD-related laboratory test was furnished to an ESRD beneficiary for reasons other than for the treatment of ESRD, the provider may submit a claim for separate payment using modifier AY. The AY modifier serves as an attestation that the item or service is medically necessary for the dialysis patient but is not being used for the treatment of ESRD. The items and services subject to consolidated billing located on the CMS website includes the list of ESRD-related laboratory tests that are routinely performed for the treatment of ESRD.

For services provided on or after January 1, 2011, the 50/50 rule no longer applies to independent laboratory claims for AMCC tests furnished to ESRD beneficiaries. The 50/50 rule modifiers (CD, CE, and CF) are no longer required for independent laboratories effective for dates of service on and after January 1, 2011. However, for services provided between January 1, 2011 and March 31, 2015, the 50/50 rule modifiers are still required for use by ESRD facilities that are receiving the transitional blended payment amount (the transition ends in CY 2014). For services provided on

or after April 1, 2015, the 50/50 rule modifiers are no longer required for use by ESRD facilities.

Effective for dates of service on and after January 1, 2012, contractors shall allow organ disease panel codes (i.e., HCPCS codes 80047, 80048, 80051, 80053, 80061, 80069, and 80076) to be billed by independent laboratories for AMCC panel tests furnished to ESRD eligible beneficiaries if:

- The beneficiary is not receiving dialysis treatment for any reason (e.g., post-transplant beneficiaries), or
- The test is not related to the treatment of ESRD, in which case the supplier would append modifier "AY".

Contractors shall make payment for organ disease panels according to the Clinical Laboratory Fee Schedule and shall apply the normal ESRD PPS editing rules for independent laboratory claims. The aforementioned organ disease panel codes were added to the list of bundled ESRD PPS laboratory tests in January 2012.

Effective for dates of service on and after April 1, 2015, contractors shall allow organ disease panel codes (i.e., HCPCS codes 80047, 80048, 80051, 80053, 80061, 80069, and 80076) to be billed by ESRD facilities for AMCC panel tests furnished to ESRD eligible beneficiaries if:

- These codes best describe the laboratory services provided to the beneficiary, which are paid under the ESRD PPS, or
- The test is not related to the treatment of ESRD, in which case the ESRD facility would append modifier "AY" and the service may be paid separately from the ESRD PPS.

**Instructions for Services Provided Prior to January 1, 2011**

For claims with dates of service prior to January 1, 2011, Medicare will apply the following rules to Automated Multi-Channel Chemistry (AMCC) tests for ESRD beneficiaries:

- Payment is at the lowest rate for tests performed by the same provider, for the same beneficiary, for the same date of service.
- The facility/laboratory must identify, for a particular date of service, the AMCC tests ordered that are included in the composite rate and those that are not included. See Publication 100-2, Chapter 11, Section 30.2.2 for the chart detailing the composite rate tests for Hemodialysis, Intermittent Peritoneal Dialysis (IPD), Continuous Cycling Peritoneal Dialysis (CCPD), and Hemofiltration as well as a second chart detailing the composite rate tests for Continuous Ambulatory Peritoneal Dialysis (CAPD).
- If 50 percent or more of the covered tests are included under the composite rate payment, then all submitted tests are included within the composite payment. In this case, no separate payment in addition to the composite rate is made for any of the separately billable tests.
- If less than 50 percent of the covered tests are composite rate tests, all AMCC tests submitted for that Date of Service (DOS) for that beneficiary are separately payable.
- A noncomposite rate test is defined as any test separately payable outside of the composite rate or beyond the normal frequency covered under the composite rate that is reasonable and necessary.
- For carrier processed claims, all chemistries ordered for beneficiaries with chronic dialysis for ESRD must be billed individually and must be rejected when billed as a panel.

(See §100.6UH for details regarding pricing modifiers.)

Implementation of this Policy:

ESRD facilities when ordering an ESRD-related AMCC must specify for each test within the AMCC whether the test:

a. Is part of the composite rate and not separately payable;

b. Is a composite rate test but is, on the date of the order, beyond the frequency covered under the composite rate and thus separately payable; or

c. Is not part of the ESRD composite rate and thus separately payable.

Laboratories must:

a. Identify which tests, if any, are not included within the ESRD facility composite rate payment

b. Identify which tests ordered for chronic dialysis for ESRD as follows:

　1) Modifier CD: AMCC Test has been ordered by an ESRD facility or MCP physician that is part of the composite rate and is not separately billable.

　2) Modifier CE: AMCC Test has been ordered by an ESRD facility or MCP physician that is a composite rate test but is beyond the normal frequency covered under the rate and is separately reimbursable based on medical necessity.

　3) Modifier CF: AMCC Test has been ordered by an ESRD facility or MCP physician that is not part of the composite rate and is separately billable.

c. Bill all tests ordered for a chronic dialysis ESRD beneficiary individually and not as a panel.

The shared system must calculate the number of AMCC tests provided for any given date of service. Sum all AMCC tests with a CD modifier and divide the sum of all tests with a CD, CE, and CF modifier for the same beneficiary and provider for any given date of service.

 CPT © 2017 American Medical Association. All Rights Reserved. © 2017 Optum360, LLC

If the result of the calculation for a date of service is 50 percent or greater, do not pay for the tests.

If the result of the calculation for a date of service is less than 50 percent, pay for all of the tests.

For FI processed claims, all tests for a date of service must be billed on the monthly ESRD bill. Providers that submit claims to a FI must send in an adjustment if they identify additional tests that have not been billed.

Carrier standard systems shall adjust the previous claim when the incoming claim for a date of service is compared to a claim on history and the action is adjust payment. Carrier standard systems shall spread the payment amount over each line item on both claims (the claim on history and the incoming claim).

The organ and disease oriented panels (80048, 80051, 80053, and 80076) are subject to the 50 percent rule. However, clinical diagnostic laboratories shall not bill these services as panels, they must be billed individually. Laboratory tests that are not covered under the composite rate and that are furnished to CAPD end stage renal disease (ESRD) patients dialyzing at home are billed in the same way as any other test furnished home patients.

FI Business Requirements for ESRD Reimbursement of AMCC Tests:

| Requirement # | Requirements | Responsibility |
|---|---|---|
| 1.1 | The FI shared system must RTP a claim for AMCC tests when a claim for that date of service has already been submitted. | Shared system |
| 1.2 | Based upon the presence of the CD, CE and CF payment modifiers, identify the AMCC tests ordered that are included and not included in the composite rate payment. | Shared System |
| 1.3 | Based upon the determination of requirement 1.2, if 50 percent or more of the covered tests are included under the composite rate, no separate payment is made. | Shared System |
| 1.4 | Based upon the determination of requirement 1.2, if less than 50 percent are covered tests included under the composite rate, all AMCC tests for that date of service are payable. | Shared System |
| 1.5 | Effective for claims with dates of service on or after January 1, 2006, include any line items with a modifier 91 used in conjunction with the "CD," "CE," or "CF" modifier in the calculation of the 50/50 rule. | Shared System |
| 1.6 | FIs must return any claims for additional tests for any date of service within the billing period when the provider has already submitted a claim. Instruct the provider to adjust the first claim. | FI or Shared System |
| 1.7 | After the calculation of the 50/50 rule, services used to determine the payment amount may never exceed 22. Effective for claims with dates of service on or after January 1, 2006, accept all valid line items submitted for the date of service and pay a maximum of the ATP 22 rate. | Shared System |

Carrier Business Requirements for ESRD Reimbursement of AMCC Tests:

| Requirement # | Requirements | Responsibility |
|---|---|---|
| 1 | The standard systems shall calculate payment at the lowest rate for these automated tests even if reported on separate claims for services performed by the same provider, for the same beneficiary, for the same date of service. | Standard Systems |
| 2 | Standard Systems shall identify the AMCC tests ordered that are included and are not included in the composite rate payment based upon the presence of the "CD," "CE" and "CF" modifiers. | Standard Systems |
| 3 | Based upon the determination of requirement 2 if 50 percent or more of the covered services are included under the composite rate payment, Standard Systems shall indicate that no separate payment is provided for the services submitted for that date of service. | Standard Systems |

| Requirement # | Requirements | Responsibility |
|---|---|---|
| 4 | Based upon the determination of requirement 2 if less than 50 percent are covered services included under the composite rate, Standard Systems shall indicate that all AMCC tests for that date of service are payable under the 50/50 rule. | Standard Systems |
| 5 | Effective for claims with dates of service on or after January 1, 2006, include any line items with a modifier 91 used in conjunction with the "CD," "CE," or "CF" modifier in the calculation of the 50/50 rule. | Standard Systems |
| 6 | Standard Systems shall adjust the previous claim when the incoming claim is compared to the claim on history and the action is to deny the previous claim. Spread the payment amount over each line item on both claims (the adjusted claim and the incoming claim). | Standard Systems |
| 7 | Standard Systems shall spread the adjustment across the incoming claim unless the adjusted amount would exceed the submitted amount of the services on the claim. | Standard System |
| 8 | After the calculation of the 50/50 rule, services used to determine the payment amount may never exceed 22. Accept all valid line items for the date of service and pay a maximum of the ATP 22 rate. | Standard Systems |

### Examples of the Application of the 50/50 Rule

The following examples are to illustrate how claims should be paid. The percentages in the action section represent the number of composite rate tests over the total tests. If this percentage is 50 percent or greater, no payment should be made for the claim.

**Example 1:**
**Provider Name: Jones Hospital**
**DOS 2/1/02**

| Claim/Services | |
|---|---|
| | 82040 Mod CD |
| | 82310 Mod CD |
| | 82374 Mod CD |
| | 82435 Mod CD |
| | 82947 Mod CF |
| | 84295 Mod CF |
| | 82040 Mod CD (Returned as duplicate) |
| | 84075 Mod CE |
| | 82310 Mod CE |
| | 84155 Mod CE |

ACTION: 9 services total, 2 non-composite rate tests, 3 composite rate tests beyond the frequency, 4 composite rate tests; 4/9 = 44.4%<50% pay at ATP 09

**Example 2:**
**Provider Name: Bon Secours Renal Facility**
**DOS 2/15/02**

| Claim/Services | |
|---|---|
| | 82040 Mod CE and Mod 91 |
| | 84450 Mod CE |
| | 82310 Mod CE |
| | 82247 Mod CF |
| | 82465 No modifier present |
| | 82565 Mod CE |
| | 84550 Mod CF |
| | 82040 Mod CD |
| | 84075 Mod CE |
| | 82435 Mod CE |
| | 82550 Mod CF |
| | 82947 Mod CF |
| | 82977 Mod CF |

ACTION: 12 services total, 5 non-composite rate tests, 6 composite rate tests beyond the frequency, 1 composite rate test; 1/12 = 8.3%<50% pay at ATP 12

**Example 3:**
**Provider Name: Sinai Hospital Renal Facility**
**DOS 4/02/02**

| Claim/Services | |
|---|---|
| | 82565 Mod CD |
| | 83615 Mod CD |
| | 82247 Mod CF |
| | 82248 Mod CF |
| | 82040 Mod CD |
| | 84450 Mod CD |
| | 82565 Mod CE |

## 100-04, 16, 70.8

### Certificate of Waiver

Effective September 1, 1992, all laboratory testing sites (except as provided in 42 CFR 493.3(b)) must have either a CLIA certificate of waiver, certificate for provider-performed microscopy procedures, certificate of registration, certificate of compliance, or certificate of accreditation to legally perform clinical laboratory testing on specimens from individuals in the United States.

The Food and Drug Administration approves CLIA waived tests on a flow basis. The CMS identifies CLIA waived tests by providing an updated list of waived tests to the Medicare contractors on a quarterly basis via a Recurring Update Notification. To be recognized as a waived test, some CLIA waived tests have unique HCPCS procedure codes and some must have a QW modifier included with the HCPCS code.

For a list of specific HCPCS codes subject to CLIA see

http://www.cms.hhs.gov/CLIA/downloads/waivetbl.pdf

## 100-4, 16, 90.2

### Organ or Disease Oriented Panels

(Rev. 3619, Issued: 10-07-16, Effective: 01-10-17 Implementation: 01-10-17)

Organ or disease panels must be paid at the lower of the billed charge, the fee amount for the panel, or the sum of the fee amounts for all components. When panels contain one or more automated tests, the A/B MAC (A) or (B) determines the correct price for the panel by comparing the price for the automated profile laboratory tests with the sum of the fee amounts for individual tests. Payment for the total panel may not exceed the sum total of the fee amounts for individual covered tests. All Medicare coverage rules apply.

The Medicare shared systems must calculate the correct payment amount. The CMS furnishes fee prices for each code but the A/B MAC (A) or (B) system must compare individual codes billed with codes and prices for related individual tests. (With each HCPCS update, HCPCS codes are reviewed and the system is updated). Once the codes are identified, A/B MACs (A) and (B) publish panel codes to providers.

The only acceptable Medicare definition for the component tests included in the CPT codes for organ or disease oriented panels is the American Medical Association (AMA) definition of component tests. The CMS will not pay for the panel code unless all of the tests in the definition are performed. If the laboratory has a custom panel that includes other tests, in addition to those in the defined CPT or HCPCS panels, the additional tests, whether on the list of automated tests or not, are billed separately in addition to the CPT or HCPCS panel code.

**NOTE:** If a laboratory chooses, it can bill each of the component tests of these panels individually, but payment will be based upon the above rules.

## TABLE OF CHEMISTRY PANELS

| Chemistry | CPT | Hepatic Function Panel 80076 | Basic Metabolic Panel (Calcium, ionized) 80047 | Basic Metabolic Panel (Calcium, total) 80048 | Comprehensive Metabolic Panel 80053 | Renal Function Panel 80069 | Lipid[1] Panel 80061 | Electrolyte Panel 80051 |
|---|---|---|---|---|---|---|---|---|
| Albumin | 82040 | X | | | X | X | | |
| Alkaline phosphatase | 84075 | X | | | X | | | |
| ALT (SGPT) | 84460 | X | | | X | | | |
| AST (SGOT) | 84450 | X | | | X | | | |
| Bilirubin, total | 82247 | X | | | X | | | |
| Bilirubin, direct | 82248 | X | | | | | | |
| Calcium | 82310 | | | X | X | X | | |
| Calcium ionized | 82330 | | X | | | | | |
| Chloride | 82435 | | X | X | X | X | | X |
| Cholesterol | 82465 | | | | | | X | |
| CK, CPK | 82550 | | | | | | | |
| CO2 (bicarbonate) | 82374 | | X | X | X | X | | X |
| Creatinine | 82565 | | X | X | X | X | | |
| GGT | 82977 | | | | | | | |
| Glucose | 82947 | | X | X | X | X | | |
| LDH | 83615 | | | | | | | |
| Phosphorus | 84100 | | | | | X | | |
| Potassium | 84132 | | X | X | X | X | | X |
| Protein | 84155 | X | | | X | | | |
| Sodium | 84295 | | X | X | X | X | | X |
| Triglycerides | 84478 | | | | | | X | |
| Urea nitrogen (BUN) | 84520 | | X | X | X | X | | |
| Uric Acid | 84550 | | | | | | | |

1　CPT code 83718 is billed with Organ/Disease Panel 80061 but is not included in the AMCC bundling.

## 100-4, 18, 1.2

### Table of Preventive and Screening Services

(Rev. 3827, Issued: 08-01-17; Effective: 07-01-17; Implementation: 01-02-18)

| Service | CPT/ HCPCS Code | Long Descriptor | USPSTF Rating | Coins./ Deductible |
|---|---|---|---|---|
| Initial Preventive Physical Examination, IPPE | G0402 | Initial preventive physical examination; face to face visits, services limited to new beneficiary during the first 12 months of Medicare enrollment | *Not Rated | WAIVED |
| | G0403 | Electrocardiogram, routine ECG with 12 leads; performed as a screening for the initial preventive physical examination with interpretation and report | | Not Waived |
| | G0404 | Electrocardiogram, routine ECG with 12 leads; tracing only, without interpretation and report, performed as a screening for the initial preventive physical examination | | Not Waived |
| | G0405 | Electrocardiogram, routine ECG with 12 leads; interpretation and report only, performed as a screening for the initial preventive physical examination | | Not Waived |

| Service | CPT/ HCPCS Code | Long Descriptor | USPSTF Rating | Coins./ Deductible |
|---------|-----------------|-----------------|---------------|--------------------|
| Ultrasound Screening for Abdominal Aortic Aneurysm (AAA) furnished prior to January 1, 2017 | 76706 | Ultrasound, abdominal aorta, real time with image documentation, screening study for abdominal aortic aneurysm (AAA) | B | WAIVED |
| Cardio-vascular Disease Screening | 80061 | Lipid panel | A | WAIVED |
| | 82465 | Cholesterol, serum or whole blood, total | | WAIVED |
| | 83718 | Lipoprotein, direct measurement; high density cholesterol (hdl cholesterol) | | WAIVED |
| | 84478 | Triglycerides | | WAIVED |
| Diabetes Screening Tests | 82947 | Glucose; quantitative, blood (except reagent strip) | B | WAIVED |
| | 82950 | Glucose; post glucose dose (includes glucose) | | WAIVED |
| | 82951 | Glucose; tolerance test (gtt), three specimens (includes glucose) | *Not Rated | WAIVED |
| Diabetes Self-Management Training Services (DSMT) | G0108 | Diabetes outpatient self-management training services, individual, per 30 minutes | *Not Rated | Not Waived |
| | G0109 | Diabetes outpatient self-management training services, group session (2 or more), per 30 minutes | | Not Waived |
| Ultrasound Screening for Abdominal Aortic Aneurysm (AAA) furnished prior to January 1, 2017 | G0389 | Ultrasound, B-scan and /or real time with image documentation; for abdominal aortic aneurysm (AAA) ultrasound screening | B | WAIVED |
| Medical Nutrition Therapy (MNT) Services | 97802 | Medical nutrition therapy; initial assessment and intervention, individual, face-to-face with the patient, each 15 minutes | B | WAIVED |
| | 97803 | Medical nutrition therapy; re-assessment and intervention, individual, face-to-face with the patient, each 15 minutes | | WAIVED |
| | 97804 | Medical nutrition therapy; group (2 or more individual(s)), each 30 minutes | | WAIVED |
| | G0270 | Medical nutrition therapy; reassessment and subsequent intervention(s) following second referral in same year for change in diagnosis, medical condition or treatment regimen (including additional hours needed for renal disease), individual, face to face with the patient, each 15 minutes | B | WAIVED |
| | G0271 | Medical nutrition therapy, reassessment and subsequent intervention(s) following second referral in same year for change in diagnosis, medical condition, or treatment regimen (including additional hours needed for renal disease), group (2 or more individuals), each 30 minutes | | WAIVED |

| Service | CPT/ HCPCS Code | Long Descriptor | USPSTF Rating | Coins./ Deductible |
|---------|-----------------|-----------------|---------------|--------------------|
| Screening Pap Test | G0123 | Screening cytopathology, cervical or vaginal (any reporting system), collected in preservative fluid, automated thin layer preparation, screening by cytotechnologist under physician supervision | A | WAIVED |
| | G0124 | Screening cytopathology, cervical or vaginal (any reporting system), collected in preservative fluid, automated thin layer preparation, requiring interpretation by physician | | WAIVED |
| | G0141 | Screening cytopathology smears, cervical or vaginal, performed by automated system, with manual rescreening, requiring interpretation by physician | A | WAIVED |
| | G0143 | Screening cytopathology, cervical or vaginal (any reporting system), collected in preservative fluid, automated thin layer preparation, with manual screening and rescreening by cytotechnologist under physician supervision | A | WAIVED |
| | G0144 | Screening cytopathology, cervical or vaginal (any reporting system), collected in preservative fluid, automated thin layer preparation, with screening by automated system, under physician supervision | A | WAIVED |
| | G0145 | Screening cytopathology, cervical or vaginal (any reporting system), collected in preservative fluid, automated thin layer preparation, with screening by automated system and manual rescreening under physician supervision | A | WAIVED |
| | G0147 | Screening cytopathology smears, cervical or vaginal, performed by automated system under physician supervision | A | WAIVED |
| | G0148 | Screening cytopathology smears, cervical or vaginal, performed by automated system with manual rescreening | A | WAIVED |
| | P3000 | Screening papanicolaou smear, cervical or vaginal, up to three smears, by technician under physician supervision | | WAIVED |
| | P3001 | Screening papanicolaou smear, cervical or vaginal, up to three smears, requiring interpretation by physician | | WAIVED |
| | Q0091 | Screening papanicolaou smear; obtaining, preparing and conveyance of cervical or vaginal smear to laboratory | | WAIVED |
| Screening Pelvic Exam | G0101 | Cervical or vaginal cancer screening; pelvic and clinical breast examination | A | WAIVED |

© 2017 Optum360, LLC   CPT © 2017 American Medical Association. All Rights Reserved.

**Appendix G — Medicare Internet-only Manuals (IOMs)**

| Service | CPT/HCPCS Code | Long Descriptor | USPSTF Rating | Coins./Deductible |
|---|---|---|---|---|
| Screening Mammography | 77052 | Computer-aided detection (computer algorithm analysis of digital image data for lesion detection) with further physician review for interpretation, with or without digitization of film radiographic images; screening mammography (list separately in addition to code for primary procedure) | B | WAIVED |
| | 77057 | Screening mammography, bilateral (2-view film study of each breast) | | WAIVED |
| | 77063 | Screening digital breast tomosynthesis, bilateral | B | WAIVED |
| | G0202 | Screening mammography, producing direct 2-D digital image, bilateral, all views | | WAIVED |
| Bone Mass Measurement | G0130 | Single energy x-ray absorptiometry (sexa) bone density study, one or more sites; appendicular skeleton (peripheral) (e.g., radius, wrist, heel) | | WAIVED |
| | 77078 | Computed tomography, bone mineral density study, 1 or more sites; axial skeleton (e.g., hips, pelvis, spine) | B | WAIVED |
| | 77079 | Computed tomography, bone mineral density study, 1 or more sites; appendicular skeleton (peripheral) (e.g., radius, wrist, heel) | | WAIVED |
| | 77080 | Dual-energy x-ray absorptiometry (dxa), bone density study, 1 or more sites; axial skeleton (e.g., hips, pelvis, spine) | | WAIVED |
| | 77081 | Dual-energy x-ray absorptiometry (dxa), bone density study, 1 or more sites; appendicular skeleton (peripheral) (e.g., radius, wrist, heel) | | WAIVED |
| | 77083 | Radiographic absorptiometry (e.g., photo densitometry, radiogrammetry), 1 or more sites | | WAIVED |
| | 76977 | Ultrasound bone density measurement and interpretation, peripheral site(s), any method | | WAIVED |

**NOTE:** For Colorectal Cancer Screening, effective January 1, 2015, when anesthesia service 00810 is performed in conjunction with screening colonoscopy services G0105 or G0121, coinsurance and deductible will be waived for anesthesia service 00810 when modifier 33 is entered on the anesthesia claim.

When a screening colonoscopy becomes a diagnostic colonoscopy, anesthesia code 00810 should be submitted with only the PT modifier and only the deductible will be waived.

| Service | CPT/HCPCS Code | Long Descriptor | USPSTF Rating | Coins./Deductible |
|---|---|---|---|---|
| Colorectal Cancer Screening | G0104 | Colorectal cancer screening; flexible sigmoidoscopy | A | WAIVED |
| | G0105 | Colorectal cancer screening; colonoscopy on individual at high risk | | WAIVED |
| | G0106 | Colorectal cancer screening; alternative to G0104, screening sigmoidoscopy, barium enema | *Not Rated | Coins. Applies & Ded. is waived |
| | G0120 | Colorectal cancer screening; alternative to G0105, screening colonoscopy, barium enema. | | Coins. Applies & Ded. is waived |
| | G0121 | Colorectal cancer screening; colonoscopy on individual not meeting criteria for high risk | | WAIVED |
| | 82270 | Blood, occult, by peroxidase activity (e.g., guaiac), qualitative; feces, consecutive | A | WAIVED |
| | G0328 | Colorectal cancer screening; fecal occult blood test, immunoassay, 1-3 simultaneous | | WAIVED |

| Service | CPT/HCPCS Code | Long Descriptor | USPSTF Rating | Coins./Deductible |
|---|---|---|---|---|
| Prostate Cancer Screening | G0102 | Prostate cancer screening; digital rectal examination | D | Not Waived |
| | G0103 | Prostate cancer screening; prostate specific antigen test (PSA) | | WAIVED |
| Glaucoma Screening | G0117 | Glaucoma screening for high risk patients furnished by an optometrist or ophthalmologist | I | Not Waived |
| | G0118 | Glaucoma screening for high risk patient furnished under the direct supervision of an optometrist or ophthalmologist | | Not Waived |
| Influenza Virus Vaccine | 90630 | Influenza virus vaccine, quadrivalent (IIV4), split virus, preservative free, for intradermal use | B | WAIVED |
| | 90653 | Influenza virus vaccine, inactivated, subunit, adjuvanted, for intramuscular use | | WAIVED |
| | 90654 | Influenza virus vaccine, split virus, preservative free, for intradermal use, for adults ages 18-64 | | WAIVED |
| | 90655 | Influenza virus vaccine, split virus, preservative free, when administered to children 6-35 months of age, for intramuscular use | | WAIVED |
| | 90656 | Influenza virus vaccine, split virus, preservative free, when administered to individuals 3 years and older, for intramuscular use | | WAIVED |
| | 90657 | Influenza virus vaccine, split virus, when administered to children 6-35 months of age, for intramuscular use | | WAIVED |
| | 90658 | Influenza virus vaccine, trivalent (IIV3), split virus, 0.5 mL dosage, for intramuscular use | | WAIVED |
| | 90660 | Influenza virus vaccine, live, for intranasal use | | WAIVED |
| | 90661 | Influenza virus vaccine, derived from cell cultures, subunit, preservative and antibiotic free, for intramuscular use | | WAIVED |
| | 90662 | Influenza virus vaccine, split virus, preservative free, enhanced immunogenicity via increased antigen content, for intramuscular use | | WAIVED |

| Service | CPT/ HCPCS Code | Long Descriptor | USPSTF Rating | Coins./ Deductible |
|---|---|---|---|---|
| | 90672 | Influenza virus vaccine, live, quadrivalent, for intranasal use | | WAIVED |
| | 90673 | Influenza virus vaccine, trivalent, derived from recombinant DNA (RIV3), hemagglutinin (HA) protein only, preservative and antibiotic free, for intramuscular use | | WAIVED |
| | 90674 | Influenza virus vaccine, quadrivalent (ccIIV4), derived from cell cultures, subunit, preservative and antibiotic free, 0.5 mL dosage, for intramuscular use | | WAIVED |
| | 90682 | Influenza virus vaccine, quadrivalent (RIV4), derived from recombinant DNA, hemagglutinin (HA) protein only, preservative and antibiotic free, for intramuscular use | | WAIVED |
| | 90685 | Influenza virus vaccine, quadrivalent, split virus, preservative free, when administered to children 6- 35 months of age, for intramuscular use | | WAIVED |
| | 90686 | Influenza virus vaccine, quadrivalent, split virus, preservative free, when administered to individuals 3 years of age and older, for intramuscular use | | WAIVED |
| | 90687 | Influenza virus vaccine, quadrivalent, split virus, when administered to children 6-35 months of age, for intramuscular use | | WAIVED |
| | 90688 | Influenza virus vaccine, quadrivalent, split virus, when administered to individuals 3 years of age and older, for intramuscular use | | WAIVED |
| | 90756 | Influenza virus vaccine, quadrivalent (ccIIV4), derived from cell cultures, subunit, antibiotic free, 0.5mL dosage, for intramuscular use | | WAIVED |
| | G0008 | Administration of influenza virus vaccine | | WAIVED |
| Pneumo-coccal Vaccine | 90669 | Pneumococcal conjugate vaccine, polyvalent, when administered to children younger than 5 years, for intramuscular use | B | WAIVED |
| | 90670 | Pneumococcal conjugate vaccine, 13 valent, for intramuscular use | | WAIVED |
| | 90732 | Pneumococcal polysaccharide vaccine, 23-valent, adult or immunosuppressed patient dosage, when administered to individuals 2 years or older, for subcutaneous or intramuscular use | | WAIVED |
| | G0009 | Administration of pneumococcal vaccine | | WAIVED |
| Hepatitis B Vaccine | 90739 | Hepatitis B vaccine, adult dosage (2 dose schedule), for intramuscular use | A | WAIVED |
| | 90740 | Hepatitis B vaccine, dialysis or immunosuppressed patient dosage (3 dose schedule), for intramuscular use | | WAIVED |
| | 90743 | Hepatitis B vaccine, adolescent (2 dose schedule), for intramuscular use | | WAIVED |
| | 90744 | Hepatitis B vaccine, pediatric/adolescent dosage (3 dose schedule), for intramuscular use | | WAIVED |

| Service | CPT/ HCPCS Code | Long Descriptor | USPSTF Rating | Coins./ Deductible |
|---|---|---|---|---|
| | 90746 | Hepatitis B vaccine, adult dosage, for intramuscular use | | WAIVED |
| | 90747 | Hepatitis B vaccine, dialysis or immunosuppressed patient dosage (4 dose schedule), for intramuscular use | | WAIVED |
| | G0010 | Administration of Hepatitis B vaccine | A | WAIVED |
| Hepatitis C Virus Screening | G0472 | Screening for Hepatitis C antibody | B | WAIVED |
| HIV Screening | G0432 | Infectious agent antigen detection by enzyme immunoassay (EIA) technique, qualitative or semi-qualitative, multiple- step method, HIV-1 or HIV-2, screening | A | WAIVED |
| | G0433 | Infectious agent antigen detection by enzyme- linked immunosorbent assay (ELISA) technique, antibody, HIV-1 or HIV-2, screening | | WAIVED |
| | G0435 | Infectious agent antigen detection by rapid antibody test of oral mucosa transudate, HIV-1 or HIV- 2 , screening | | WAIVED |
| Smoking Cessation for services furnished prior to October 1, 2016 | G0436 | Smoking and tobacco cessation counseling visit for the asymptomatic patient; intermediate, greater than 3 minutes, up to 10 minutes | A | WAIVED |
| | G0437 | Smoking and tobacco cessation counseling visit for the asymptomatic patient intensive, greater than 10 minutes | | WAIVED |
| Smoking Cessation for services furnished on or after October 1, 2016 | 99406 | Smoking and tobacco cessation counseling visit for the asymptomatic patient; intermediate, greater than 3 minutes, up to 10 minutes | A | WAIVED |
| | 99407 | Smoking and tobacco cessation counseling visit for the asymptomatic patient intensive, greater than 10 minutes | | |
| Annual Wellness Visit | G0438 | Annual wellness visit, including PPPS, first visit | *Not Rated | WAIVED |
| | G0439 | Annual wellness visit, including PPPS, subsequent visit | | WAIVED |
| Intensive Behavioral Therapy for Obesity | G0447 | Face-to-Face Behavioral Counseling for Obesity, 15 minutes | B | WAIVED |
| | G0473 | Face-to-face behavioral counseling for obesity, group (2-10), 30 minute(s) | | |
| Lung Cancer Screening | G0296 | Counseling visit to discuss need for lung cancer screening (LDCT) using low dose CT scan (service is for eligibility determination and shared decision making) | B | WAIVED |
| | G0297 | Low dose CT scan (LDCT) for lung cancer screening | | |

## 100-4, 18, 10.2.1

### *Healthcare Common Procedure Coding System (HCPCS) and Diagnosis Codes*

(Rev. 3827, Issued: 08-04-17; Effective: 08-01-17; Implementation: 07-03-17)

Vaccines and their administration are reported using separate codes. The following codes are for reporting the vaccines only.

| HCPCS | Definition |
|---|---|
| 90630 | Influenza virus vaccine, quadrivalent (IIV4), split virus, preservative free, for intradermal use |
| 90653 | Influenza virus vaccine, inactivated, subunit, adjuvanted, for intramuscular use |
| 90654 | Influenza virus vaccine, split virus, preservative-free, for intradermal use, for adults ages 18 – 64; |

| HCPCS | Definition |
|-------|------------|
| 90655 | Influenza virus vaccine, split virus, preservative free, for children 6-35 months of age, for intramuscular use; |
| 90656 | Influenza virus vaccine, split virus, preservative free, for use in individuals 3 years and above, for intramuscular use; |
| 90657 | Influenza virus vaccine, split virus, for children 6-35 months of age, for intramuscular use; |
| 90658 | Influenza virus vaccine, trivalent (IIV3), split virus, 0.5 mL dosage, for intramuscular use |
| 90660 | Influenza virus vaccine, live, for intranasal use; |
| 90661 | Influenza virus vaccine, derived from cell cultures, subunit, preservative and antibiotic free, for intramuscular use |
| 90662 | Influenza virus vaccine, split virus, preservative free, enhanced immunogenicity via increased antigen content, for intramuscular use |
| 90669 | Pneumococcal conjugate vaccine, polyvalent, for children under 5 years, for intramuscular use |
| 90670 | Pneumococcal conjugate vaccine, 13 valent, for intramuscular use |
| 90672 | Influenza virus vaccine, live, quadrivalent, for intranasal use; |
| 90673 | Influenza virus vaccine, trivalent, derived from recombinant DNA (RIV3), hemagglutinin (HA) protein only, preservative and antibiotic free, for intramuscular use |
| 90674 | Influenza virus vaccine, quadrivalent (ccIIV4), derived from cell cultures, subunit, preservative and antibiotic free, 0.5 mL dosage, for intramuscular use |
| 90682 | Influenza virus vaccine, quadrivalent (RIV4), derived from recombinant DNA, hemagglutinin (HA) protein only, preservative and antibiotic free, for intramuscular use |
| 90685 | Influenza virus vaccine, quadrivalent, split virus, preservative free, when administered to children 6-35 months of age, for intramuscular use |
| 90686 | Influenza virus vaccine, quadrivalent, split virus, preservative free, when administered to individuals 3 years of age and older, for intramuscular use |
| 90687 | Influenza virus vaccine, quadrivalent, split virus, when administered to children 6-35 months of age, for intramuscular use |
| 90688 | Influenza virus vaccine, quadrivalent, split virus, when administered to individuals 3 years of age and older, for intramuscular use |
| 90732 | Pneumococcal polysaccharide vaccine, 23-valent, adult or immunosuppressed patient dosage, for use in individuals 2 years or older, for subcutaneous or intramuscular use; |
| 90739 | Hepatitis B vaccine, adult dosage (2 dose schedule), for intramuscular use |
| 90740 | Hepatitis B vaccine, dialysis or immunosuppressed patient dosage (3 dose schedule), for intramuscular use; |
| 90743 | Hepatitis B vaccine, adolescent (2 dose schedule), for intramuscular use; |
| 90744 | Hepatitis B vaccine, pediatric/adolescent dosage (3 dose schedule), for intramuscular use; |
| 90746 | Hepatitis B vaccine, adult dosage, for intramuscular use; and |
| 90747 | Hepatitis B vaccine, dialysis or immunosuppressed patient dosage (4 dose schedule), for intramuscular use. |
| 90756 | Influenza virus vaccine, quadrivalent (ccIIV4), derived from cell cultures, subunit, antibiotic free, 0.5mL dosage, for intramuscular use |

The following codes are for reporting administration of the vaccines only. The administration of the vaccines is billed using:

| HCPCS | Definition |
|-------|------------|
| G0008 | Administration of influenza virus vaccine; |
| G0009 | Administration of pneumococcal vaccine; and |
| *G0010 | Administration of hepatitis B vaccine. |
| *90471 | Immunization administration. (For OPPS hospitals billing for the hepatitis B vaccine administration) |
| *90472 | Each additional vaccine. (For OPPS hospitals billing for the hepatitis B vaccine administration) |

**\* NOTE:** For claims with dates of service prior to January 1, 2006, OPPS and non-OPPS hospitals report G0010 for hepatitis B vaccine administration. For claims with dates of service January 1, 2006 until December 31, 2010, OPPS hospitals report 90471 or 90472 for hepatitis B vaccine administration as appropriate in place of G0010. Beginning January 1, 2011, providers should report G0010 for billing under the OPPS rather than 90471 or 90472 to ensure correct waiver of coinsurance and deductible for the administration of hepatitis B vaccine.

One of the following diagnosis codes must be reported as appropriate. If the sole purpose for the visit is to receive a vaccine or if a vaccine is the only service billed on a claim, the applicable following diagnosis code may be used.

| ICD-9-CM Diagnosis Code | Description |
|-------------------------|-------------|
| V03.82 | Pneumococcus |
| V04.81** | Influenza |
| V06.6*** | Pneumococcus and Influenza |
| V05.3 | Hepatitis B |

**\*\*Effective for influenza virus claims with dates of service October 1, 2003 and later.

**\*\*\*Effective October 1, 2006, providers may report ICD-9-CM diagnosis code V06.6 on claims for pneumococcus and/or influenza virus vaccines when the purpose of the visit was to receive both vaccines.

NOTE: ICD-10-CM diagnosis code Z23 may be used for an encounter for immunizations effective October 1, 2015, when ICD-10 was implemented.

If a diagnosis code for pneumococcus, hepatitis B, or influenza virus vaccination is not reported on a claim, contractors may not enter the diagnosis on the claim. Contractors must follow current resolution processes for claims with missing diagnosis codes.

If the diagnosis code and the narrative description are correct, but the HCPCS code is incorrect, the A/B MAC (A or B) may correct the HCPCS code and pay the claim. For example, if the reported diagnosis code is V04.81 and the narrative description (if annotated on the claim) says "flu shot" but the HCPCS code is incorrect, contractors may change the HCPCS code and pay for the flu vaccine. Effective October 1, 2006, A/B MACs (B) should follow the instructions in Pub. 100-04, Chapter 1, Section 80.3.2.1.1 (A/B MAC (B) Data Element Requirements) for claims submitted without a HCPCScode.

Claims for hepatitis B vaccinations must report the I.D. Number of the referring physician. In addition, if a doctor of medicine or osteopathy does not order the influenza virus vaccine, the A/B MACs (A) claims require:

- UPIN code SLF000 to be reported on claims submitted prior to May 23, 2008, when Medicare began accepting NPIs, only

- The provider's own NPI to be reported in the NPI field for the attending physician on claims submitted on or after May 23, 2008, when NPI requirements were implemented.

## 100-04, 18, 10.2.2.1

### Payment for Pneumococcal Pneumonia Virus, Influenza Virus, and Hepatitis B Virus Vaccines and Their Administration on Institutional Claims

(Rev. 3754, Issued: 04-21-17; Effective: 07-01-17; Implementation: 07-03-17)

Payment for Vaccines

Payment for these vaccines is as follows:

| Facility | Type of Bill | Payment |
|----------|--------------|---------|
| Hospitals, other than Indian Health Service (IHS) Hospitals and Critical Access Hospitals (CAHs) | 012x, 013x | Reasonable cost |
| IHS Hospitals | 012x, 013x, 083x | 95% of AWP |
| IHS CAHs | 085x | 95% of AWP |
| CAHs Method I and Method II | 085x | Reasonable cost |
| Skilled Nursing Facilities | 022x, 023x | Reasonable cost |
| Home Health Agencies | 034x | Reasonable cost |
| Hospice | 081x, 082x | 95% of the AWP |
| Comprehensive Outpatient Rehabilitation Facilities | 075x | 95% of the AWP |
| Independent Renal Dialysis Facilities | 072x | 95% of the AWP |
| Hospital-based Renal Dialysis Facilities | 072x | Reasonable cost |

**Payment for Vaccine Administration**

Payment for the administration of Influenza Virus and PPV vaccines is as follows:

| Facility | Type of Bill | Payment |
|----------|--------------|---------|
| Hospitals, other than IHS Hospitals and CAHs | 012x, 013x | Outpatient Prospective Payment System (OPPS) for hospitals subject to OPPS<br><br>Reasonable cost for hospitals not subject to OPPS |
| IHS Hospitals | 012x, 013x, 083x | MPFS as indicated in guidelines below. |

| Facility | Type of Bill | Payment |
|---|---|---|
| IHS CAHs | 085x | MPFS as indicated in guidelines below. |
| CAHs Method I and II | 085x | Reasonable cost |
| Skilled Nursing Facilities | 022x, 023x | MPFS |
| Home Health Agencies | 034x | OPPS |
| Hospices | 081x, 082x | MPFS |
| Comprehensive Outpatient Rehabilitation Facilities | 075x | MPFS |
| Independent RDFs | 072x | MPFS |
| Hospital-based RDFs | 072x | Reasonable cost |

Payment for the administration of Hepatitis B vaccine is as follows:

| Facility | Type of Bill | Payment |
|---|---|---|
| Hospitals other than IHS hospitals and CAHs | 012x, 013x | Outpatient Prospective Payment System (OPPS) for hospitals subject to OPPS |
| | | Reasonable cost for hospitals not subject to OPPS |
| IHS Hospitals | 012x, 013x, 083x | MPFS |
| CAHs | 085x | Reasonable cost |
| Method I and II | | |
| IHS CAHs | 085x | MPFS |
| Skilled Nursing Facilities | 022x, 023x | MPFS |
| Home Health Agencies | 034x | OPPS |
| Hospices | 081x, 082x | MPFS |
| Comprehensive Outpatient Rehabilitation Facilities | 075x | MPFS |
| Independent RDFs | 072x | MPFS |
| Hospital-based RDFs | 072x | Reasonable cost |

## 100-04, 18, 10.4.1

### CWF Edits on A/B MAC (A) Claims

(Rev. 3827; Issued: 08-04-17; Effective: 08-01-17; Implementation: 01-02-18)

In order to prevent duplicate payment by the same A/B MAC (A), CWF edits by line item on the A/B MAC (A) number, the beneficiary Health Insurance Claim (HIC) number, and the date of service, the influenza virus procedure codes 90630, 90653, 90654, 90655, 90656, 90657, 90658, 90660, 90661, 90662, 90672, 90673, 90674, 90682, 90685, 90686, 90687, 90688, or 90756 and the pneumococcal procedure codes 90669, 90670, or 90732, and the administration codes G0008 or G0009.

If CWF receives a claim with either HCPCS codes 90630, 90653, 90654, 90655, 90656, 90657, 90658, 90658, 90660, 90661, 90662, 90672, 90673, 90674, 90682, 90685, 90686, 90687, 90688, or 90756 and it already has on record a claim with the same HIC number, same A/B MAC (A) number, same date of service, and any one of those HCPCS codes, the second claim submitted to CWF rejects.

If CWF receives a claim with HCPCS codes 90669, 90670, or 90732 and it already has

on record a claim with the same HIC number, same A/B MAC (A) number, same date of service, and the same HCPCS code, the second claim submitted to CWF rejects when all four items match.

If CWF receives a claim with HCPCS administration codes G0008 or G0009 and it already has on record a claim with the same HIC number, same A/B MAC (A) number, same date of service, and same procedure code, CWF rejects the second claim submitted when all four items match.

CWF returns to the A/B MAC (A) a reject code "7262" for this edit. A/B MACs (A) must deny the second claim and use the same messages they currently use for the denial of duplicate claims.

## 100-04, 18, 10.4.2

### CWF Edits on A/B MAC (B) Claims

(Rev. 3827, Issued: 08-04-17; Effective: 07-01-17; Implementation: 01-02-18)

In order to prevent duplicate payment by the same A/B MAC (B), CWF will edit by line item on the A/B MAC (B) number, the HIC number, the date of service, the influenza virus procedure codes 90630, 90653, 90654, 90655, 90656, 90657, 90658, 90660, 90661, 90662, 90672, 90673, 90674, 90682, 90685, 90686, 90687, 90688, or 90756; the pneumococcal procedure codes 90669, 90670, or 90732; and the administration code G0008 or G0009.

If CWF receives a claim with either HCPCS codes 90630, 90653, 90654, 90655, 90656, 90657, 90658, 90660, 90661, 90662, 90672, 90673, 90674, 90682, 90685, 90686, 90687, 90688, or 90756 and it already has on record a claim with the same HIC number, same A/B MAC (B) number, same date of service, and any one of those HCPCS codes, the second claim submitted to CWF will reject.

If CWF receives a claim with HCPCS codes 90669, 90670, or 90732 and it already has on record a claim with the same HIC number, same A/B MAC (B) number, same date of service, and the same HCPCS code, the second claim submitted to CWF will reject when all four items match.

If CWF receives a claim with HCPCS administration codes G0008 or G0009 and it already has on record a claim with the same HIC number, same A/B MAC (B) number, same date of service, and same procedure code, CWF will reject the second claim submitted.

CWF will return to the A/B MAC (B) a specific reject code for this edit. A/B MACs (B) must deny the second claim and use the same messages they currently use for the denial of duplicate claims.

In order to prevent duplicate payment by the centralized billing contractor and local A/B MAC (B), CWF will edit by line item for A/B MAC (B) number, same HIC number, same date of service, the influenza virus procedure codes 90630, 90653, 90654, 90655, 90656, 90657, 90658, 90660, 90661, 90662, 90672, 90673, 90674, 90682, 90685, 90686, 90687, 90688, or 90756; the pneumococcal procedure codes 90669, 90670, or 90732; and the administration code G0008 or G0009.

If CWF receives a claim with either HCPCS codes 90630, 90653, 90654, 90655, 90656, 90657, 90658, 90660, 90661, 90662, 90672, 90673, 90674, 90682, 90685, 90686, 90687, 90688, or 90756 and it already has on record a claim with a different A/B MAC (B) number, but same HIC number, same date of service, and any one of those same HCPCS codes, the second claim submitted to CWF will reject.

If CWF receives a claim with HCPCS codes 90669, 90670, or 90732 and it already has on record a claim with the same HIC number, different A/B MAC (B) number, same date of service, and the same HCPCS code, the second claim submitted to CWF will reject.

If CWF receives a claim with HCPCS administration codes G0008 or G0009 and it already has on record a claim with a different A/B MAC (B) number, but the same HIC number, same date of service, and same procedure code, CWF will reject the second claim submitted.

CWF will return a specific reject code for this edit. A/B MACs (B) must deny the second claim. For the second edit, the reject code should automatically trigger the following Medicare Summary Notice (MSN) and Remittance Advice (RA) messages.

MSN: 7.2 – "This is a duplicate of a claim processed by another contractor. You should receive a Medicare Summary Notice from them."

Claim Adjustment Reason Code 18 – Exact duplicate claim/service

## 100-04, 18, 10.4.3

### CWF Crossover Edits A/B MAC (B) Claims

(Rev. 5827, Issued: 08-04-17; Effective: 08-01-17; Implementation: 01-02-18)

When CWF receives a claim from the A/B MAC (B), it will review Part B outpatient claims history to verify that a duplicate claim has not already been posted.

CWF will edit on the beneficiary HIC number; the date of service; the influenza virus procedure codes 90630, 90653, 90654, 90655, 90656, 90657, 90658, 90660, 90661, 90662, 90672, 90673, 90674, 90682, 90685, 90686, 90687, 90688, or 90756; the pneumococcal procedure codes 90669, 90670, or 90732; and the administration code G0008 or G0009.

CWF will return a specific reject code for this edit. A/B MACs (B) must deny the second claim and use the same messages they currently use for the denial of duplicate claims.

## 100-04, 18, 60

### Colorectal Cancer Screening

(Rev. 3436, Issued: 12-30-15, Effective: 10-09-14, Implementation: 09-08-15 for non-shared MAC edits; 01-04-16 - For all shared system changes.)

See the Medicare Benefit Policy Manual, Chapter 15, and the Medicare National Coverage Determinations (NCD) Manual, Chapter 1, Section 210.3 for Medicare Part B coverage requirements and effective dates of colorectal cancer screening services.

Effective for services furnished on or after January 1, 1998, payment may be made for colorectal cancer screening for the early detection of cancer. For screening colonoscopy services (one of the types of services included in this benefit) prior to July 2001, coverage was limited to high-risk individuals. For services July 1, 2001, and later screening colonoscopies are covered for individuals not at high risk.

The following services are considered colorectal cancer screening services:

- Fecal-occult blood test (FOBT),1-3 simultaneous determinations (guaiac-based);
- Flexible sigmoidoscopy;
- Colonoscopy; and,
- Barium enema

Effective for services on or after January 1, 2004, payment may be made for the following colorectal cancer screening service as an alternative for the guaiac-based FOBT, 1-3 simultaneous determinations:

- Fecal-occult blood test, immunoassay, 1-3 simultaneous determinations

Effective for claims with dates of service on or after October 9, 2014, payment may be made for colorectal cancer screening using the Cologuard™ multitarget stool DNA (sDNA) test:

G0464 (Colorectal cancer screening; stool-based DNA and fecal occult hemoglobin (e.g., KRAS, NDRG4 and BMP3).

## 100-04, 18, 80.2

### A/B Medicare Administrative Contractor (MAC) (B) Billing Requirements

Effective for dates of service on and after January 1, 2005, through December 31, 2008, contractors shall recognize the HCPCS codes G0344, G0366, G0367, and G0368 shown above in §80.1 for an IPPE. The type of service (TOS) for each of these codes is as follows:

G0344: TOS = 1

G0366: TOS = 5

G0367: TOS = 5

G0368: TOS = 5

Contractors shall pay physicians or qualified nonphysician practitioners for only one IPPE performed not later than 6 months after the date the individual's first coverage begins under Medicare Part B, but only if that coverage period begins on or after January 1, 2005.

Effective for dates of service on and after January 1, 2009, contractors shall recognize the HCPCS codes G0402, G0403, G0404, and G0405 shown above in §80.1 for an IPPE. The TOS for each of these codes is as follows:

G0402: TOS = 1

G0403: TOS = 5

G0404: TOS = 5

G0405: TOS = 5

Under the MIPPA of 2008, contractors shall pay physicians or qualified nonphysician practitioners for only one IPPE performed not later than 12 months after the date the individual's first coverage begins under Medicare Part B only if that coverage period begins on or after January 1, 2009.

Contractors shall allow payment for a medically necessary Evaluation and Management (E/M) service at the same visit as the IPPE when it is clinically appropriate. Physicians and qualified nonphysician practitioners shall use CPT codes 99201-99215 to report an E/M with CPT modifier 25 to indicate that the E/M is a significant, separately identifiable service from the IPPE code reported (G0344 or G0402, whichever applies based on the date the IPPE is performed). Refer to chapter 12, § 30.6.1.1, of this manual for the physician/practitioner billing correct coding and payment policy regarding E/M services.

If the EKG performed as a component of the IPPE is not performed by the primary physician or qualified NPP during the IPPE visit, another physician or entity may perform and/or interpret the EKG. The referring physician or qualified NPP needs to make sure that the performing physician or entity bills the appropriate G code for the screening EKG, and not a CPT code in the 93000 series. **Both the IPPE and the EKG should be billed in order for the beneficiary to receive the complete IPPE service.** Effective for dates of service on and after January 1, 2009, the screening EKG is optional and is no longer a mandated service of an IPPE if performed as a result of a referral from an IPPE.

Should the same physician or NPP need to perform an additional medically necessary EKG in the 93000 series on the same day as the IPPE, report the appropriate EKG CPT code(s) with modifier 59, indicating that the EKG is a distinct procedural service.

Physicians or qualified nonphysician practitioners shall bill the contractor the appropriate HCPCS codes for IPPE on the Form CMS-1500 claim or an approved electronic format. The HCPCS codes for an IPPE and screening EKG are paid under the Medicare Physician Fee Schedule (MPFS).

See §1.3 of this chapter for waiver of cost sharing requirements of coinsurance, copayment and deductible for furnished preventive services available in Medicare.

## 100-04, 18, 140.8

### Advance Care Planning (ACP) as an Optional Element of an Annual Wellness Visit (AWV)

(Rev. 3428 Issued: 12-22-15, Effective: 01-01-16, Implementation: 01-04-16)

For services furnished on or after January 1, 2016, Advance Care Planning (ACP) is treated as a preventive service when furnished with an AWV. The Medicare coinsurance and Part B deductible are waived for ACP when furnished as an optional element of an AWV.

The codes for the optional ACP services furnished as part of an AWV are 99497 (Advance care planning including the explanation and discussion of advance directives such as standard forms (with completion of such forms, when performed), by the physician or other qualified health professional; first 30 minutes, face-to-face with the patient, family member(s) and/or surrogate;) and an add-on code 99498 (each additional 30 minutes (List separately in addition to code for primary procedure)). When ACP services are provided as a part of an AWV, practitioners would report CPT code 99497 (and add-on CPT code 99498 when applicable) for the ACP services in addition to either of the AWV codes (G0438 or G0439).

The deductible and coinsurance for ACP will only be waived when billed with modifier 33 on the same day and on the same claim as an AWV (code G0438 or G0439), and must also be furnished by the same provider. Waiver of the deductible

and coinsurance for ACP is limited to once per year. Payment for an AWV is limited to once per year. If the AWV billed with ACP is denied for exceeding the once per year limit, the deductible and coinsurance will be applied to the ACP.

Also see Pub. 100-02, *Medicare Benefit Policy Manual*, chapter 15, section 280.5.1 for more information.

## 100-04, 32, 10.1

### Ambulatory Blood Pressure Monitoring (ABPM) Billing Requirements

#### A. Coding Applicable to A/B MACs (A and B)

Effective April 1, 2002, a National Coverage Decision was made to allow for Medicare coverage of ABPM for those beneficiaries with suspected "white coat hypertension" (WCH). ABPM involves the use of a non-invasive device, which is used to measure blood pressure in 24-hour cycles. These 24-hour measurements are stored in the device and are later interpreted by a physician. Suspected "WCH" is defined as: (1) Clinic/office blood pressure >140/90 mm Hg on at least three separate clinic/office visits with two separate measurements made at each visit; (2) At least two documented separate blood pressure measurements taken outside the clinic/office which are < 140/90 mm Hg; and (3) No evidence of end-organ damage. ABPM is not covered for any other uses. Coverage policy can be found in Medicare National Coverage Determinations Manual, Chapter 1, Part 1, §20.19. (http://www.cms.hhs.gov/manuals/103_cov_determ/ncd103index.asp).

The ABPM must be performed for at least 24 hours to meet coverage criteria. Payment is not allowed for institutionalized beneficiaries, such as those receiving Medicare covered skilled nursing in a facility. In the rare circumstance that ABPM needs to be performed more than once for a beneficiary, the qualifying criteria described above must be met for each subsequent ABPM test.

Effective dates for applicable Common Procedure Coding System (HCPCS) codes for ABPM for suspected WCH and their covered effective dates are as follows:

| HCPCS | Definition | Effective Date |
|---|---|---|
| 93784 | ABPM, utilizing a system such as magnetic tape and/or computer disk, for 24 hours or longer; including recording, scanning analysis, interpretation and report. | 04/01/2002 |
| 93786 | ABPM, utilizing a system such as magnetic tape and/or computer disk, for 24 hours or longer; recording only. | 04/01/2002 |
| 93788 | ABPM, utilizing a system such as magnetic tape and/or computer disk, for 24 hours or longer; scanning analysis with report. | 01/01/2004 |
| 93790 | ABPM, utilizing a system such as magnetic tape and/or computer disk, for 24 hours or longer; physician review with interpretation and report. | 04/01/2002 |

In addition, one of the following diagnosis codes must be present:

| | Diagnosis Code | Description |
|---|---|---|
| If ICD-9-CM is applicable | 796.2 | Elevated blood pressure reading without diagnosis of hypertension. |
| If ICD-10-CM is applicable | R03.0 | Elevated blood pressure reading without diagnosis of hypertension |

#### B. A/B MAC (A) Billing Instructions

The applicable types of bills acceptable when billing for ABPM services are 13X, 23X, 71X, 73X, 75X, and 85X. Chapter 25 of this manual provides general billing instructions that must be followed for bills submitted to A/B MACs (A). The A/B MACs (A) pay for hospital outpatient ABPM services billed on a 13X type of bill with HCPCS 93786 and/or 93788 as follows: (1) Outpatient Prospective Payment System (OPPS) hospitals pay based on the Ambulatory Payment Classification (APC); (2) non-OPPS hospitals (Indian Health Services Hospitals, Hospitals that provide Part B services only, and hospitals located in American Samoa, Guam, Saipan and the Virgin Islands) pay based on reasonable cost, except for Maryland Hospitals which are paid based on a percentage of cost. Effective 4/1/06, type of bill 14X is for non-patient laboratory specimens and is no longer applicable for ABPM.

The A/B MACs (A) pay for comprehensive outpatient rehabilitation facility (CORF) ABPM services billed on a 75x type of bill with HCPCS code 93786 and/or 93788 based on the Medicare Physician Fee Schedule (MPFS) amount for that HCPCS code.

The A/B MACs (A) pay for ABPM services for critical access hospitals (CAHs) billed on a 85x type of bill as follows: (1) for CAHs that elected the Standard Method and billed HCPCS code 93786 and/or 93788, pay based on reasonable cost for that HCPCS code; and (2) for CAHs that elected the Optional Method and billed any combination of HCPCS codes 93786, 93788 and 93790 pay based on reasonable cost for HCPCS 93786 and 93788 and pay 115% of the MPFS amount for HCPCS code 93790.

The A/B MACs (A) pay for ABPM services for skilled nursing facility (SNF) outpatients billed on a 23x type of bill with HCPCS code 93786 and/or 93788, based on the MPFS.

The A/B MACs (A) accept independent and provider-based rural health clinic (RHC) bills for visits under the all-inclusive rate when the RHC bills on a 71x type of bill with revenue code 052x for providing the professional component of ABPM services. The A/B MACs (A) should not make a separate payment to a RHC for the professional component of ABPM services in addition to the all-inclusive rate. RHCs are not required to use ABPM HCPCS codes for professional services covered under the all-inclusive rate.

The A/B MACs (A) accept free-standing and provider-based federally qualified health center (FQHC) bills for visits under the all-inclusive rate when the FQHC bills on a 73x type of bill with revenue code 052x for providing the professional component of ABPM services.

The A/B MACs (A) should not make a separate payment to a FQHC for the professional component of ABPM services in addition to the all-inclusive rate. FQHCs are not required to use ABPM HCPCS codes for professional services covered under the all-inclusive rate.

The A/B MACs (A) pay provider-based RHCs/FQHCs for the technical component of ABPM services when billed under the base provider's number using the above requirements for that particular base provider type, i.e., a OPPS hospital based RHC would be paid for the ABPM technical component services under the OPPS using the APC for code 93786 and/or 93788 when billed on a 13x type of bill.

Independent and free-standing RHC/FQHC practitioners are only paid for providing the technical component of ABPM services when billed to the A/B MAC (B) following the MAC's instructions.

### C. A/B MAC (B) Claims
A/B MACs (B) pay for ABPM services billed with ICD-9-CM diagnosis code 796.2 (if ICD-9 is applicable) or, if ICD-10 is applicable, ICD-10-CM diagnosis code R03.0 and HCPCS codes 93784 or for any combination of 93786, 93788 and 93790, based on the MPFS for the specific HCPCS code billed.

### D. Coinsurance and Deductible
The A/B MACs (A and B) shall apply coinsurance and deductible to payments for ABPM services except for services billed to the A/B MAC (A) by FQHCs. For FQHCs only co-insurance applies.

## 100-04, 32, 30.1

### Billing Requirements for HBO Therapy for the Treatment of Diabetic Wounds of the Lower Extremities
Hyperbaric Oxygen Therapy is a modality in which the entire body is exposed to oxygen under increased atmospheric pressure. Effective April 1, 2003, a National Coverage Decision expanded the use of HBO therapy to include coverage for the treatment of diabetic wounds of the lower extremities. For specific coverage criteria for HBO Therapy, refer to the National Coverage Determinations Manual, Chapter 1, section 20.29.

NOTE: Topical application of oxygen does not meet the definition of HBO therapy as stated above. Also, its clinical efficacy has not been established. Therefore, no Medicare reimbursement may be made for the topical application of oxygen.

I. Billing Requirements for A/B MACs (A)

Claims for HBO therapy should be submitted using the ASC X12 837 institutional claim format or, in rare cases, on Form CMS-1450.

a. Applicable Bill Types

The applicable hospital bill types are 11X, 13X and 85X.

b. Procedural Coding

99183– Physician attendance and supervision of hyperbaric oxygen therapy, per session.

C1300 – Hyperbaric oxygen under pressure, full body chamber, per 30-minute interval.

NOTE: Code C1300 is not available for use other than in a hospital outpatient department. In skilled nursing facilities (SNFs), HBO therapy is part of the SNF PPS payment for beneficiaries in covered Part A stays.

For hospital inpatients and critical access hospitals (CAHs) not electing Method I, HBO therapy is reported under revenue code 940 without any HCPCS code. For inpatient services, if ICD-9-is applicable, show ICD-9-CM procedure code 93.59. If ICD-10 is applicable, show ICD-10-PCS code 5A05121.

For CAHs electing Method I, HBO therapy is reported under revenue code 940 along with HCPCS code 99183.

c. Payment Requirements for A/B MACs (A)

Payment is as follows:

A/B MAC (A) payment is allowed for HBO therapy for diabetic wounds of the lower extremities when performed as a physician service in a hospital outpatient setting and for inpatients. Payment is allowed for claims with valid diagnosis codes as shown above with dates of service on or after April 1, 2003. Those claims with invalid codes should be denied as not medically necessary.

For hospitals, payment will be based upon the Ambulatory Payment Classification (APC) or the inpatient Diagnosis Related Group (DRG). Deductible and coinsurance apply.

Payment to Critical Access Hospitals (electing Method I) is made under cost reimbursement. For Critical Access Hospitals electing Method II, the technical component is paid under cost reimbursement and the professional component is paid under the Physician Fee Schedule.

II. A/B MAC (B) Billing Requirements

Claims for this service should be submitted using the ASC X12 837 professional claim format or Form CMS-1500.

The following HCPCS code applies:

99183 – Physician attendance and supervision of hyperbaric oxygen therapy, per session.

a. Payment Requirements for A/B MACs (B)

Payment and pricing information will occur through updates to the Medicare Physician Fee Schedule Database (MPFSDB). Pay for this service on the basis of the MPFSDB. Deductible and coinsurance apply. Claims from physicians or other practitioners where assignment was not taken, are subject to the Medicare limiting charge.

III. Medicare Summary Notices (MSNs)

Use the following MSN Messages where appropriate:

In situations where the claim is being denied on the basis that the condition does not meet our coverage requirements, use one of the following MSN Messages:

"Medicare does not pay for this item or service for this condition." (MSN Message 16.48)

The Spanish version of the MSN message should read:

"Medicare no paga por este articulo o servicio para esta afeccion."

In situations where, based on the above utilization policy, medical review of the claim results in a determination that the service is not medically necessary, use the following MSN message:

"The information provided does not support the need for this service or item." (MSN Message 15.4)

The Spanish version of the MSN message should read:

"La informacion proporcionada no confirma la necesidad para este servicio o articulo."

### IV. Remittance Advice Notices
Use appropriate existing remittance advice remark codes and claim adjustment reason codes at the line level to express the specific reason if you deny payment for HBO therapy for the treatment of diabetic wounds of lower extremities.

## 100-04, 32, 60.4.1

### Allowable Covered Diagnosis Codes
Allowable Covered Diagnosis Codes

For services furnished on or after July 1, 2002, the applicable ICD-9-CM diagnosis code for this benefit is V43.3, organ or tissue replaced by other means; heart valve.

For services furnished on or after March 19, 2008, the applicable ICD-9-CM diagnosis codes for this benefit are:

- V43.3 (organ or tissue replaced by other means; heart valve),
- 289.81 (primary hypercoagulable state),
- 451.0-451.9 (includes 451.11, 451.19, 451.2, 451.80-451.84, 451.89) (phlebitis & thrombophlebitis),
- 453.0-453.3 (other venous embolism & thrombosis),
- 453.40-453.49 (includes 453.40-453.42, 453.8-453.9) (venous embolism and thrombosis of the deep vessels of the lower extremity, and other specified veins/unspecified sites)
- 415.11-415.12, 415.19 (pulmonary embolism & infarction) or,
- 427.31 (atrial fibrillation (established) (paroxysmal)).

For services furnished on or after the implementation of ICD-10 the applicable ICD-10-CM diagnosis codes for this benefit are:

**Heart Valve Replacement**

- Z95.2 - Presence of prosthetic heart valve

**Primary Hypercoagulable State**

| ICD-10-CM | Code Description |
| --- | --- |
| D68.51 | Activated protein C resistance |
| D68.52 | Prothrombin gene mutation |
| D68.59 | Other primary thrombophilia |
| D68.61 | Antiphospholipid syndrome |
| D68.62 | Lupus anticoagulant syndrome |

**Phlebitis & Thrombophlebitis**

| ICD-10-CM | Code Description |
| --- | --- |
| I80.00 | Phlebitis and thrombophlebitis of superficial vessels of unspecified lower extremity |
| I80.01 | Phlebitis and thrombophlebitis of superficial vessels of right lower extremity |

| ICD-10-CM | Code Description |
|-----------|-----------------|
| I80.02 | Phlebitis and thrombophlebitis of superficial vessels of left lower extremity |
| I80.03 | Phlebitis and thrombophlebitis of superficial vessels of lower extremities, bilateral |
| I80.10 | Phlebitis and thrombophlebitis of unspecified femoral vein |
| I80.11 | Phlebitis and thrombophlebitis of right femoral vein |
| I80.12 | Phlebitis and thrombophlebitis of left femoral vein |
| I80.13 | Phlebitis and thrombophlebitis of femoral vein, bilateral |
| I80.201 | Phlebitis and thrombophlebitis of unspecified deep vessels of right lower extremity |
| I80.202 | Phlebitis and thrombophlebitis of unspecified deep vessels of left lower extremity |
| I80.203 | Phlebitis and thrombophlebitis of unspecified deep vessels of lower extremities, bilateral |
| I80.209 | Phlebitis and thrombophlebitis of unspecified deep vessels of unspecified lower extremity |
| I80.221 | Phlebitis and thrombophlebitis of right popliteal vein |
| I80.222 | Phlebitis and thrombophlebitis of left popliteal vein |
| I80.223 | Phlebitis and thrombophlebitis of popliteal vein, bilateral |
| I80.229 | Phlebitis and thrombophlebitis of unspecified popliteal vein |
| I80.231 | Phlebitis and thrombophlebitis of right tibial vein |
| I80.232 | Phlebitis and thrombophlebitis of left tibial vein |
| I80.233 | Phlebitis and thrombophlebitis of tibial vein, bilateral |
| I80.239 | Phlebitis and thrombophlebitis of unspecified tibial vein |
| I80.291 | Phlebitis and thrombophlebitis of other deep vessels of right lower extremity |
| I80.292 | Phlebitis and thrombophlebitis of other deep vessels of left lower extremity |
| I80.293 | Phlebitis and thrombophlebitis of other deep vessels of lower extremity, bilateral |
| I80.299 | Phlebitis and thrombophlebitis of other deep vessels of unspecified lower extremity |
| I80.3 | Phlebitis and thrombophlebitis of lower extremities, unspecified |
| I80.211 | Phlebitis and thrombophlebitis of right iliac vein |
| I80.212 | Phlebitis and thrombophlebitis of left iliac vein |
| I80.213 | Phlebitis and thrombophlebitis of iliac vein, bilateral |
| I80.219 | Phlebitis and thrombophlebitis of unspecified iliac vein |
| I80.8 | Phlebitis and thrombophlebitis of other sites |
| I80.9 | Phlebitis and thrombophlebitis of unspecified site |

**Other Venous Embolism & Thrombosis**

| ICD-10-CM | Code Description |
|-----------|-----------------|
| I82.0 | Budd- Chiari syndrome |
| I82.1 | Thrombophlebitis migrans |
| I82.211 | Chronic embolism and thrombosis of superior vena cava |
| I82.220 | Acute embolism and thrombosis of inferior vena cava |
| I82.221 | Chronic embolism and thrombosis of inferior vena cava |
| I82.291 | Chronic embolism and thrombosis of other thoracic veins |
| I82.3 | Embolism and thrombosis of renal vein |

**Venous Embolism and thrombosis of the deep vessels of the lower extremity, and other specified veins/unspecified sites**

| ICD-10-CM | Code Description |
|-----------|-----------------|
| I82.401 | Acute embolism and thrombosis of unspecified deep veins of right lower extremity |
| I82.402 | Acute embolism and thrombosis of unspecified deep veins of left lower extremity |
| I82.403 | Acute embolism and thrombosis of unspecified deep veins of lower extremity, bilateral |
| I82.409 | Acute embolism and thrombosis of unspecified deep veins of unspecified lower extremity |
| I82.411 | Acute embolism and thrombosis of right femoral vein |
| I82.412 | Acute embolism and thrombosis of left femoral vein |
| I82.413 | Acute embolism and thrombosis of femoral vein, bilateral |
| I82.419 | Acute embolism and thrombosis of unspecified femoral vein |
| I82.421 | Acute embolism and thrombosis of right iliac vein |
| I82.422 | Acute embolism and thrombosis of left iliac vein |
| I82.423 | Acute embolism and thrombosis of iliac vein, bilateral |
| I82.429 | Acute embolism and thrombosis of unspecified iliac vein |

| ICD-10-CM | Code Description |
|-----------|-----------------|
| I82.431 | Acute embolism and thrombosis of right popliteal vein |
| I82.432 | Acute embolism and thrombosis of left popliteal vein |
| I82.433 | Acute embolism and thrombosis of popliteal vein, bilateral |
| I82.439 | Acute embolism and thrombosis of unspecified popliteal vein |
| I82.4Y1 | Acute embolism and thrombosis of unspecified deep veins of right proximal lower extremity |
| I82.4Y2 | Acute embolism and thrombosis of unspecified deep veins of left proximal lower extremity |
| I82.4Y3 | Acute embolism and thrombosis of unspecified deep veins of proximal lower extremity, bilateral |
| I82.4Y9 | Acute embolism and thrombosis of unspecified deep veins of unspecified proximal lower extremity |
| I82.441 | Acute embolism and thrombosis of right tibial vein |
| I82.442 | Acute embolism and thrombosis of left tibial vein |
| I82.443 | Acute embolism and thrombosis of tibial vein, bilateral |
| I82.449 | Acute embolism and thrombosis of unspecified tibial vein |
| I82.491 | Acute embolism and thrombosis of other specified deep vein of right lower extremity |
| I82.492 | Acute embolism and thrombosis of other specified deep vein of left lower extremity |
| I82.493 | Acute embolism and thrombosis of other specified deep vein of lower extremity, bilateral |
| I82.499 | Acute embolism and thrombosis of other specified deep vein of unspecified lower extremity |
| I82.4Z1 | Acute embolism and thrombosis of unspecified deep veins of right distal lower extremity |
| I82.4Z2 | Acute embolism and thrombosis of unspecified deep veins of left distal lower extremity |
| I82.4Z3 | Acute embolism and thrombosis of unspecified deep veins of distal lower extremity, bilateral |
| I82.4Z9 | Acute embolism and thrombosis of unspecified deep veins of unspecified distal lower extremity |
| I82.501 | Chronic embolism and thrombosis of unspecified deep veins of right lower extremity |
| I82.502 | Chronic embolism and thrombosis of unspecified deep veins of left lower extremity |
| I82.503 | Chronic embolism and thrombosis of unspecified deep veins of lower extremity, bilateral |
| I82.509 | Chronic embolism and thrombosis of unspecified deep veins of unspecified lower extremity |
| I82.591 | Chronic embolism and thrombosis of other specified deep vein of right lower extremity |
| I82.592 | Chronic embolism and thrombosis of other specified deep vein of left lower extremity |
| I82.593 | Chronic embolism and thrombosis of other specified deep vein of lower extremity, bilateral |
| I82.599 | Chronic embolism and thrombosis of other specified deep vein of unspecified lower extremity |
| I82.511 | Chronic embolism and thrombosis of right femoral vein |
| I82.512 | Chronic embolism and thrombosis of left femoral vein |
| I82.513 | Chronic embolism and thrombosis of femoral vein, bilateral |
| I82.519 | Chronic embolism and thrombosis of unspecified femoral vein |
| I82.521 | Chronic embolism and thrombosis of right iliac vein |
| I82.522 | Chronic embolism and thrombosis of left iliac vein |
| I82.523 | Chronic embolism and thrombosis of iliac vein, bilateral |
| I82.529 | Chronic embolism and thrombosis of unspecified iliac vein |
| I82.531 | Chronic embolism and thrombosis of right popliteal vein |
| I82.532 | Chronic embolism and thrombosis of left popliteal vein |
| I82.533 | Chronic embolism and thrombosis of popliteal vein, bilateral |
| I82.539 | Chronic embolism and thrombosis of unspecified popliteal vein |
| I82.5Y1 | Chronic embolism and thrombosis of unspecified deep veins of right proximal lower extremity |
| I82.5Y2 | Chronic embolism and thrombosis of unspecified deep veins of left proximal lower extremity |
| I82.5Y3 | Chronic embolism and thrombosis of unspecified deep veins of proximal lower extremity, bilateral |
| I82.5Y9 | Chronic embolism and thrombosis of unspecified deep veins of unspecified proximal lower extremity |
| I82.541 | Chronic embolism and thrombosis of right tibial vein |
| I82.542 | Chronic embolism and thrombosis of left tibial vein |

CPT © 2017 American Medical Association. All Rights Reserved.

© 2017 Optum360, LLC

| ICD-10-CM | Code Description |
|-----------|------------------|
| I82.543 | Chronic embolism and thrombosis of tibial vein, bilateral |
| I82.549 | Chronic embolism and thrombosis of unspecified tibial vein |
| I82.5Z1 | Chronic embolism and thrombosis of unspecified deep veins of right distal lower extremity |
| I82.5Z2 | Chronic embolism and thrombosis of unspecified deep veins of left distal lower extremity |
| I82.5Z3 | Chronic embolism and thrombosis of unspecified deep veins of distal lower extremity, bilateral |
| I82.5Z9 | Chronic embolism and thrombosis of unspecified deep veins of unspecified distal lower extremity |
| I82.611 | Acute embolism and thrombosis of superficial veins of right upper extremity |
| I82.612 | Acute embolism and thrombosis of superficial veins of left upper extremity |
| I82.613 | Acute embolism and thrombosis of superficial veins of upper extremity, bilateral |
| I82.619 | Acute embolism and thrombosis of superficial veins of unspecified upper extremity |
| I82.621 | Acute embolism and thrombosis of deep veins of right upper extremity |
| I82.622 | Acute embolism and thrombosis of deep veins of left upper extremity |
| I82.623 | Acute embolism and thrombosis of deep veins of upper extremity, bilateral |
| I82.629 | Acute embolism and thrombosis of deep veins of unspecified upper extremity |
| I82.601 | Acute embolism and thrombosis of unspecified veins of right upper extremity |
| I82.602 | Acute embolism and thrombosis of unspecified veins of left upper extremity |
| I82.603 | Acute embolism and thrombosis of unspecified veins of upper extremity, bilateral |
| I82.609 | Acute embolism and thrombosis of unspecified veins of unspecified upper extremity |
| I82.A11 | Acute embolism and thrombosis of right axillary vein |
| I82.A12 | Acute embolism and thrombosis of left axillary vein |
| I82.A13 | Acute embolism and thrombosis of axillary vein, bilateral |
| I82.A19 | Acute embolism and thrombosis of unspecified axillary vein |
| I82.A21 | Chronic embolism and thrombosis of right axillary vein |
| I82.A22 | Chronic embolism and thrombosis of left axillary vein |
| I82.A23 | Chronic embolism and thrombosis of axillary vein, bilateral |
| I82.A29 | Chronic embolism and thrombosis of unspecified axillary vein |
| I82.B11 | Acute embolism and thrombosis of right subclavian vein |
| I82.B12 | Acute embolism and thrombosis of left subclavian vein |
| I82.B13 | Acute embolism and thrombosis of subclavian vein, bilateral |
| I82.B19 | Acute embolism and thrombosis of unspecified subclavian vein |
| I82.B21 | Chronic embolism and thrombosis of right subclavian vein |
| I82.B22 | Chronic embolism and thrombosis of left subclavian vein |
| I82.B23 | Chronic embolism and thrombosis of subclavian vein, bilateral |
| I82.B29 | Chronic embolism and thrombosis of unspecified subclavian vein |
| I82.C11 | Acute embolism and thrombosis of right internal jugular vein |
| I82.C12 | Acute embolism and thrombosis of left internal jugular vein |
| I82.C13 | Acute embolism and thrombosis of internal jugular vein, bilateral |
| I82.C19 | Acute embolism and thrombosis of unspecified internal jugular vein |
| I82.C21 | Chronic embolism and thrombosis of right internal jugular vein |
| I82.C22 | Chronic embolism and thrombosis of left internal jugular vein |
| I82.C23 | Chronic embolism and thrombosis of internal jugular vein, bilateral |
| I82.C29 | Chronic embolism and thrombosis of unspecified internal jugular vein |
| I82.210 | Acute embolism and thrombosis of superior vena cava |
| I82.290 | Acute embolism and thrombosis of other thoracic veins |
| I82.701 | Chronic embolism and thrombosis of unspecified veins of right upper extremity |
| I82.702 | Chronic embolism and thrombosis of unspecified veins of left upper extremity |
| I82.703 | Chronic embolism and thrombosis of unspecified veins of upper extremity, bilateral |
| I82.709 | Chronic embolism and thrombosis of unspecified veins of unspecified upper extremity |
| I82.711 | Chronic embolism and thrombosis of superficial veins of right upper extremity |

| ICD-10-CM | Code Description |
|-----------|------------------|
| I82.712 | Chronic embolism and thrombosis of superficial veins of left upper extremity |
| I82.713 | Chronic embolism and thrombosis of superficial veins of upper extremity, bilateral |
| I82.719 | Chronic embolism and thrombosis of superficial veins of unspecified upper extremity |
| I82.721 | Chronic embolism and thrombosis of deep veins of right upper extremity |
| I82.722 | Chronic embolism and thrombosis of deep veins of left upper extremity |
| I82.723 | Chronic embolism and thrombosis of deep veins of upper extremity, bilateral |
| I82.729 | Chronic embolism and thrombosis of deep veins of unspecified upper extremity |
| I82.811 | Embolism and thrombosis of superficial veins of right lower extremities |
| I82.812 | Embolism and thrombosis of superficial veins of left lower extremities |
| I82.813 | Embolism and thrombosis of superficial veins of lower extremities, bilateral |
| I82.819 | Embolism and thrombosis of superficial veins of unspecified lower extremities |
| I82.890 | Acute embolism and thrombosis of other specified veins |
| I82.891 | Chronic embolism and thrombosis of other specified veins |
| I82.90 | Acute embolism and thrombosis of unspecified vein |
| I82.91 | Chronic embolism and thrombosis of unspecified vein |

**Pulmonary Embolism & Infarction**

| ICD-10-CM | Code Description |
|-----------|------------------|
| I26.90 | Septic pulmonary embolism without acute cor pulmonale |
| I26.99 | Other pulmonary embolism without acute cor pulmonale |
| I26.01 | Septic pulmonary embolism with acute cor pulmonale |
| I26.90 | Septic pulmonary embolism without acute cor pulmonale |
| I26.09 | Other pulmonary embolism with acute cor pulmonale |
| I26.99 | Other pulmonary embolism without acute cor pulmonale |

**Atrial Fibrillation**

| ICD-10-CM | Code Description |
|-----------|------------------|
| I48.0 | Paroxysmal atrial fibrillation |
| I48.2 | Chronic atrial fibrillation |
| I48 | -91 Unspecified atrial fibrillation Other |
| I23.6 | Thrombosis of atrium, auricular appendage, and ventricle as current complications following acute myocardial infarction |
| I27.82 | Chronic pulmonary embolism |
| I67.6 | Nonpyogenic thrombosis of intracranial venous system |
| O22.50 | Cerebral venous thrombosis in pregnancy, unspecified trimester |
| O22.51 | Cerebral venous thrombosis in pregnancy, first trimester |
| O22.52 | Cerebral venous thrombosis in pregnancy, second trimester |
| O22.53 | Cerebral venous thrombosis in pregnancy, third trimester |
| O87.3 | Cerebral venous thrombosis in the puerperium |
| Z79.01 | Long term (current) use of anticoagulants |

Coverage policy can be found in Pub. 100-3, Medicare National Coverage Determinations Manual, Chapter 1, section 190.11 PT/INR. (http://www.cms.hhs.gov/manuals/103_cov_determ/ncd103index.asp

## 100-04, 32, 60.5.2

### *Applicable Diagnosis Codes for A/B Macs*

For services furnished on or after July 1, 2002, the applicable ICD-9-CM diagnosis code for this benefit is V43.3, organ or tissue replaced by other means; heart valve.

For services furnished on or after March 19, 2008, the applicable ICD-9-CM diagnosis codes for this benefit are:

- V43.3 (organ or tissue replaced by other means; heart valve),
- 289.81 (primary hypercoagulable state),
- 451.0-451.9 (includes 451.11, 451.19, 451.2, 451.80-451.84, 451.89) (phlebitis & thrombophlebitis),
- 453.0-453.3 (other venous embolism & thrombosis),
- 453.40-453.49 (includes 453.40-453.42, 453.8-453.9) (venous embolism and thrombosis of the deep vessels of the lower extremity, and other specified veins/unspecified sites)

- 415.11-415.12, 415.19 (pulmonary embolism & infarction) or,
- 427.31 (atrial fibrillation (established) (paroxysmal)).

For services furnished on or after implementation of ICD-10 the applicable ICD-10-CM diagnosis codes for this benefit are:

### Heart Valve Replacement
- Z95.2 - Presence of prosthetic heart valve

### Primary Hypercoagulable State

| ICD-10-CM | Code Description |
|---|---|
| D68.51 | Activated protein C resistance |
| D68.52 | Prothrombin gene mutation |
| D68.59 | Other primary thrombophilia |
| D68.61 | Antiphospholipid syndrome |
| D68.62 | Lupus anticoagulant syndrome |

### Phlebitis & Thrombophlebitis

| ICD-10-CM | Code Description |
|---|---|
| I80.00 | Phlebitis and thrombophlebitis of superficial vessels of unspecified lower extremity |
| I80.01 | Phlebitis and thrombophlebitis of superficial vessels of right lower extremity |
| I80.02 | Phlebitis and thrombophlebitis of superficial vessels of left lower extremity |
| I80.03 | Phlebitis and thrombophlebitis of superficial vessels of lower extremities, bilateral |
| I80.10 | Phlebitis and thrombophlebitis of unspecified femoral vein |
| I80.11 | Phlebitis and thrombophlebitis of right femoral vein |
| I80.12 | Phlebitis and thrombophlebitis of left femoral vein |
| I80.13 | Phlebitis and thrombophlebitis of femoral vein, bilateral |
| I80.201 | Phlebitis and thrombophlebitis of unspecified deep vessels of right lower extremity |
| I80.202 | Phlebitis and thrombophlebitis of unspecified deep vessels of left lower extremity |
| I80.203 | Phlebitis and thrombophlebitis of unspecified deep vessels of lower extremities, bilateral |
| I80.209 | Phlebitis and thrombophlebitis of unspecified deep vessels of unspecified lower extremity |
| I80.221 | Phlebitis and thrombophlebitis of right popliteal vein |
| I80.222 | Phlebitis and thrombophlebitis of left popliteal vein |
| I80.223 | Phlebitis and thrombophlebitis of popliteal vein, bilateral |
| I80.229 | Phlebitis and thrombophlebitis of unspecified popliteal vein |
| I80.231 | Phlebitis and thrombophlebitis of right tibial vein |
| I80.232 | Phlebitis and thrombophlebitis of left tibial vein |
| I80.233 | Phlebitis and thrombophlebitis of tibial vein, bilateral |
| I80.239 | Phlebitis and thrombophlebitis of unspecified tibial vein |
| I80.291 | Phlebitis and thrombophlebitis of other deep vessels of right lower extremity |
| I80.292 | Phlebitis and thrombophlebitis of other deep vessels of left lower extremity |
| I80.293 | Phlebitis and thrombophlebitis of other deep vessels of lower extremity, bilateral |
| I80.299 | Phlebitis and thrombophlebitis of other deep vessels of unspecified lower extremity |
| I80.3 | Phlebitis and thrombophlebitis of lower extremities, unspecified |
| I80.211 | Phlebitis and thrombophlebitis of right iliac vein |
| I80.212 | Phlebitis and thrombophlebitis of left iliac vein |
| I80.213 | Phlebitis and thrombophlebitis of iliac vein, bilateral |
| I80.219 | Phlebitis and thrombophlebitis of unspecified iliac vein |
| I80.8 | Phlebitis and thrombophlebitis of other sites |
| I80.9 | Phlebitis and thrombophlebitis of unspecified site |

### Other Venous Embolism & Thrombosis

| ICD-10-CM | Code Description |
|---|---|
| I82.0 | Budd- Chiari syndrome |
| I82.1 | Thrombophlebitis migrans |
| I82.211 | Chronic embolism and thrombosis of superior vena cava |
| I82220 | Acute embolism and thrombosis of inferior vena cava |
| I82.221 | Chronic embolism and thrombosis of inferior vena cava |
| I82.291 | Chronic embolism and thrombosis of other thoracic veins |
| I82.3 | Embolism and thrombosis of renal vein |

### Venous Embolism and thrombosis of the deep vessels of the lower extremity, and other specified veins/unspecified sites

| ICD-10-CM | Code Description |
|---|---|
| I82.401 | Acute embolism and thrombosis of unspecified deep veins of right lower extremity |
| I82.402 | Acute embolism and thrombosis of unspecified deep veins of left lower extremity |
| I82.403 | Acute embolism and thrombosis of unspecified deep veins of lower extremity, bilateral |
| I82.409 | Acute embolism and thrombosis of unspecified deep veins of unspecified lower extremity |
| I82.411 | Acute embolism and thrombosis of right femoral vein |
| I82.412 | Acute embolism and thrombosis of left femoral vein |
| I82.413 | Acute embolism and thrombosis of femoral vein, bilateral |
| I82.419 | Acute embolism and thrombosis of unspecified femoral vein |
| I82.421 | Acute embolism and thrombosis of right iliac vein |
| I82.422 | Acute embolism and thrombosis of left iliac vein |
| I82.423 | Acute embolism and thrombosis of iliac vein, bilateral |
| I82.429 | Acute embolism and thrombosis of unspecified iliac vein |
| I82.431 | Acute embolism and thrombosis of right popliteal vein |
| I82.432 | Acute embolism and thrombosis of left popliteal vein |
| I82.433 | Acute embolism and thrombosis of popliteal vein, bilateral |
| I82.439 | Acute embolism and thrombosis of unspecified popliteal vein |
| I82.4Y1 | Acute embolism and thrombosis of unspecified deep veins of right proximal lower extremity |
| I82.4Y2 | Acute embolism and thrombosis of unspecified deep veins of left proximal lower extremity |
| I82.4Y3 | Acute embolism and thrombosis of unspecified deep veins of proximal lower extremity, bilateral |
| I82.4Y9 | Acute embolism and thrombosis of unspecified deep veins of unspecified proximal lower extremity |
| I82.441 | Acute embolism and thrombosis of right tibial vein |
| I82.442 | Acute embolism and thrombosis of left tibial vein |
| I82.443 | Acute embolism and thrombosis of tibial vein, bilateral |
| I82.449 | Acute embolism and thrombosis of unspecified tibial vein |
| I82.491 | Acute embolism and thrombosis of other specified deep vein of right lower extremity |
| I82.492 | Acute embolism and thrombosis of other specified deep vein of left lower extremity |
| I82.493 | Acute embolism and thrombosis of other specified deep vein of lower extremity, bilateral |
| I82.499 | Acute embolism and thrombosis of other specified deep vein of unspecified lower extremity |
| I82.4Z1 | Acute embolism and thrombosis of unspecified deep veins of right distal lower extremity |
| I82.4Z2 | Acute embolism and thrombosis of unspecified deep veins of left distal lower extremity |
| I82.4Z3 | Acute embolism and thrombosis of unspecified deep veins of distal lower extremity, bilateral |
| I82.4Z9 | Acute embolism and thrombosis of unspecified deep veins of unspecified distal lower extremity |
| I82.501 | Chronic embolism and thrombosis of unspecified deep veins of right lower extremity |
| I82.502 | Chronic embolism and thrombosis of unspecified deep veins of left lower extremity |
| I82.503 | Chronic embolism and thrombosis of unspecified deep veins of lower extremity, bilateral |
| I82.509 | Chronic embolism and thrombosis of unspecified deep veins of unspecified lower extremity |
| I82.591 | Chronic embolism and thrombosis of other specified deep vein of right lower extremity |
| I82.592 | Chronic embolism and thrombosis of other specified deep vein of left lower extremity |
| I82.593 | Chronic embolism and thrombosis of other specified deep vein of lower extremity, bilateral |
| I82.599 | Chronic embolism and thrombosis of other specified deep vein of unspecified lower extremity |
| I82.511 | Chronic embolism and thrombosis of right femoral vein |
| I82.512 | Chronic embolism and thrombosis of left femoral vein |
| I82.513 | Chronic embolism and thrombosis of femoral vein, bilateral |
| I82.519 | Chronic embolism and thrombosis of unspecified femoral vein |
| I82.521 | Chronic embolism and thrombosis of right iliac vein |

CPT © 2017 American Medical Association. All Rights Reserved.
© 2017 Optum360, LLC

| ICD-10-CM | Code Description |
|---|---|
| I82.522 | Chronic embolism and thrombosis of left iliac vein |
| I82.523 | Chronic embolism and thrombosis of iliac vein, bilateral |
| I82.529 | Chronic embolism and thrombosis of unspecified iliac vein |
| I82.531 | Chronic embolism and thrombosis of right popliteal vein |
| I82.532 | Chronic embolism and thrombosis of left popliteal vein |
| I82.533 | Chronic embolism and thrombosis of popliteal vein, bilateral |
| I82.539 | Chronic embolism and thrombosis of unspecified popliteal vein |
| I82.5Y1 | Chronic embolism and thrombosis of unspecified deep veins of right proximal lower extremity |
| I82.5Y2 | Chronic embolism and thrombosis of unspecified deep veins of left proximal lower extremity |
| I82.5Y3 | Chronic embolism and thrombosis of unspecified deep veins of proximal lower extremity, bilateral |
| I82.5Y9 | Chronic embolism and thrombosis of unspecified deep veins of unspecified proximal lower extremity |
| I82.541 | Chronic embolism and thrombosis of right tibial vein |
| I82.42 | Chronic embolism and thrombosis of left tibial vein |
| I82.543 | Chronic embolism and thrombosis of tibial vein, bilateral |
| I82.549 | Chronic embolism and thrombosis of unspecified tibial vein |
| I82.5Z1 | Chronic embolism and thrombosis of unspecified deep veins of right distal lower extremity |
| I82.5Z2 | Chronic embolism and thrombosis of unspecified deep veins of left distal lower extremity |
| I82.5Z3 | Chronic embolism and thrombosis of unspecified deep veins of distal lower extremity, bilateral |
| I82.5Z9 | Chronic embolism and thrombosis of unspecified deep veins of unspecified distal lower extremity |
| I82.611 | Acute embolism and thrombosis of superficial veins of right upper extremity |
| I82.612 | Acute embolism and thrombosis of superficial veins of left upper extremity |
| I82.613 | Acute embolism and thrombosis of superficial veins of upper extremity, bilateral |
| I82.619 | Acute embolism and thrombosis of superficial veins of unspecified upper extremity |
| I82.621 | Acute embolism and thrombosis of deep veins of right upper extremity |
| I82.622 | Acute embolism and thrombosis of deep veins of left upper extremity |
| I82.623 | Acute embolism and thrombosis of deep veins of upper extremity, bilateral |
| I82.629 | Acute embolism and thrombosis of deep veins of unspecified upper extremity |
| I82.601 | Acute embolism and thrombosis of unspecified veins of right upper extremity |
| I82.602 | Acute embolism and thrombosis of unspecified veins of left upper extremity |
| I82.603 | Acute embolism and thrombosis of unspecified veins of upper extremity, bilateral |
| I82.609 | Acute embolism and thrombosis of unspecified veins of unspecified upper extremity |
| I82.A11 | Acute embolism and thrombosis of right axillary vein |
| I82.A12 | Acute embolism and thrombosis of left axillary vein |
| I82.A13 | Acute embolism and thrombosis of axillary vein, bilateral |
| I82.A19 | Acute embolism and thrombosis of unspecified axillary vein |
| I82.A21 | Chronic embolism and thrombosis of right axillary vein |
| I82.A22 | Chronic embolism and thrombosis of left axillary vein |
| I82.A23 | Chronic embolism and thrombosis of axillary vein, bilateral |
| I82.A29 | Chronic embolism and thrombosis of unspecified axillary vein |
| I82.B11 | Acute embolism and thrombosis of right subclavian vein |
| I82.B12 | Acute embolism and thrombosis of left subclavian vein |
| I82.B13 | Acute embolism and thrombosis of subclavian vein, bilateral |
| I82.B19 | Acute embolism and thrombosis of unspecified subclavian vein |
| I82.B21 | Chronic embolism and thrombosis of right subclavian vein |
| I82.B22 | Chronic embolism and thrombosis of left subclavian vein |
| I82.B23 | Chronic embolism and thrombosis of subclavian vein, bilateral |
| I82.B29 | Chronic embolism and thrombosis of unspecified subclavian vein |
| I82.C11 | Acute embolism and thrombosis of right internal jugular vein |
| I82.C12 | Acute embolism and thrombosis of left internal jugular vein |
| I82.C13 | Acute embolism and thrombosis of internal jugular vein, bilateral |

| ICD-10-CM | Code Description |
|---|---|
| I82.C19 | Acute embolism and thrombosis of unspecified internal jugular vein |
| I82.C21 | Chronic embolism and thrombosis of right internal jugular vein |
| I82.C22 | Chronic embolism and thrombosis of left internal jugular vein |
| I82.C23 | Chronic embolism and thrombosis of internal jugular vein, bilateral |
| I82.C29 | Chronic embolism and thrombosis of unspecified internal jugular vein |
| I82.210 | Acute embolism and thrombosis of superior vena cava |
| I82.290 | Acute embolism and thrombosis of other thoracic veins |
| I82.701 | Chronic embolism and thrombosis of unspecified veins of right upper extremity |
| I82.702 | Chronic embolism and thrombosis of unspecified veins of left upper extremity |
| I82.703 | Chronic embolism and thrombosis of unspecified veins of upper extremity, bilateral |
| I82.709 | Chronic embolism and thrombosis of unspecified veins of unspecified upper extremity |
| I82.711 | Chronic embolism and thrombosis of superficial veins of right upper extremity |
| I82.712 | Chronic embolism and thrombosis of superficial veins of left upper extremity |
| I82.713 | Chronic embolism and thrombosis of superficial veins of upper extremity, bilateral |
| I82.719 | Chronic embolism and thrombosis of superficial veins of unspecified upper extremity |
| I82.721 | Chronic embolism and thrombosis of deep veins of right upper extremity |
| I82.722 | Chronic embolism and thrombosis of deep veins of left upper extremity |
| I82.723 | Chronic embolism and thrombosis of deep veins of upper extremity, bilateral |
| I82.729 | Chronic embolism and thrombosis of deep veins of unspecified upper extremity |
| I82.811 | Embolism and thrombosis of superficial veins of right lower extremities |
| I82.812 | Embolism and thrombosis of superficial veins of left lower extremities |
| I82.813 | Embolism and thrombosis of superficial veins of lower extremities, bilateral |
| I82.819 | Embolism and thrombosis of superficial veins of unspecified lower extremities |
| I82.890 | Acute embolism and thrombosis of other specified veins |
| I82.891 | Chronic embolism and thrombosis of other specified veins |
| I82.90 | Acute embolism and thrombosis of unspecified vein |
| I82.91 | Chronic embolism and thrombosis of unspecified vein |

**Pulmonary Embolism & Infarction**

| ICD-10-CM | Code Description |
|---|---|
| I26.01 | Septic pulmonary embolism with acute cor pulmonale |
| I26.90 | Septic pulmonary embolism without acute cor pulmonale |
| I26.09 | Other pulmonary embolism with acute cor pulmonale |
| I26.99 | Other pulmonary embolism without acute cor pulmonale |

**Atrial Fibrillation**

| ICD-10-CM | Code Description |
|---|---|
| I48.0 | Paroxysmal atrial fibrillation |
| I48.2 | Chronic atrial fibrillation |
| I48. | -91 Unspecified atrial fibrillation Other |
| I23.6 | Thrombosis of atrium, auricular appendage, and ventricle as current complications following acute myocardial infarction |
| I27.82 | Chronic pulmonary embolism |
| I67.6 | Nonpyogenic thrombosis of intracranial venous system |
| O22.50 | Cerebral venous thrombosis in pregnancy, unspecified trimester |
| O22.51 | Cerebral venous thrombosis in pregnancy, first trimester |
| O22.52 | Cerebral venous thrombosis in pregnancy, second trimester |
| O22.53 | Cerebral venous thrombosis in pregnancy, third trimester |
| O87.3 | Cerebral venous thrombosis in the puerperium |
| Z79.01 | Long term (current) use of anticoagulants |
| Z86.718 | Personal history of other venous thrombosis and embolism |
| Z95.4 | Presence of other heart |

Coverage policy can be found in Pub. 100-3, Medicare National Coverage Determinations Manual, Chapter 1, section 190.11 PT/INR. (http://www.cms.hhs.gov/manuals/103_cov_determ/ncd103index.asp)

© 2017 Optum360, LLC

CPT © 2017 American Medical Association. All Rights Reserved.

## 100-04, 32, 80.8

### CWF Utilization Edits

#### Edit 1

Should CWF receive a claim from an FI for G0245 or G0246 and a second claim from a contractor for either G0245 or G0246 (or vice versa) and they are different dates of service and less than 6 months apart, the second claim will reject. CWF will edit to allow G0245 or G0246 to be paid no more than every 6 months for a particular beneficiary, regardless of who furnished the service. If G0245 has been paid, regardless of whether it was posted as a facility or professional claim, it must be 6 months before G0245 can be paid again or G0246 can be paid. If G0246 has been paid, regardless of whether it was posted as a facility or professional claim, it must be 6 months before G0246 can be paid again or G0245 can be paid. CWF will not impose limits on how many times each code can be paid for a beneficiary as long as there has been 6 months between each service.

The CWF will return a specific reject code for this edit to the contractors and FIs that will be identified in the CWF documentation. Based on the CWF reject code, the contractors and FIs must deny the claims and return the following messages:

MSN 18.4 -- This service is being denied because it has not been __ months since your last examination of this kind (NOTE: Insert 6 as the appropriate number of months.)

RA claim adjustment reason code 96 - Non-covered charges, along with remark code M86 - Service denied because payment already made for same/similar procedure within set time frame.

#### Edit 2

The CWF will edit to allow G0247 to pay only if either G0245 or G0246 has been submitted and accepted as payable on the same date of service. CWF will return a specific reject code for this edit to the contractors and FIs that will be identified in the CWF documentation. Based on this reject code, contractors and FIs will deny the claims and return the following messages:

MSN 21.21 - This service was denied because Medicare only covers this service under certain circumstances.

RA claim adjustment reason code 107 - The related or qualifying claim/service was not identified on this claim.

#### Edit 3

Once a beneficiary's condition has progressed to the point where routine foot care becomes a covered service, payment will no longer be made for LOPS evaluation and management services. Those services would be considered to be included in the regular exams and treatments afforded to the beneficiary on a routine basis. The physician or provider must then just bill the routine foot care codes, per Pub 100-2, Chapter 15, Sec. 290.

The CWF will edit to reject LOPS codes G0245, G0246, and/or G0247 when on the beneficiary's record it shows that one of the following routine foot care codes were billed and paid within the prior 6 months: 11055, 11056, 11057, 11719, 11720, and/or 11721.

The CWF will return a specific reject code for this edit to the contractors and FIs that will be identified in the CWF documentation. Based on the CWF reject code, the contractors and FIs must deny the claims and return the following messages:

MSN 21.21 - This service was denied because Medicare only covers this service under certain circumstances.

The RA claim adjustment reason code 96 - Non-covered charges, along with remark code M86 - Service denied because payment already made for same/similar procedure within set time frame.

## 100-04, 32, 90

### Stem Cell Transplantation

Rev.3556, Issued: 07-01-2016; Effective: 1-27-16; Implementation: 10-3-16

#### A. General

Stem cell transplantation is a process in which stem cells are harvested from either a patient's (autologous) or donor's (allogeneic) bone marrow or peripheral blood for intravenous infusion.

Allogeneic and autologous stem cell transplants are covered under Medicare for specific diagnoses. See Pub. 100-03, National Coverage Determinations Manual, section 110.23, for a complete description of covered and noncovered conditions. For Part A hospital inpatient claims processing instructions, refer to Pub. 100-04, Chapter 3, section 90. The following sections contain claims processing instructions for all other claims.

#### B. Nationally Covered Indications

I. Allogeneic Hematopoietic Stem Cell Transplantation (HSCT)

HCPCS Code 38240

ICD-9-CM Procedure Codes 41.02, 41.03, 41.05, and 41.08

ICD-10-PCS Procedure Codes 30230G1, 30230Y1, 30233G1, 30233Y1, 30240G1, 30240Y1, 30243G1, 30243Y1, 30250G1, 30250Y1, 30253G1, 30253Y1, 30260G1, 30260Y1, 30263G1, and 30263Y1

a. Effective for services performed on or after August 1, 1978:

i. For the treatment of leukemia, leukemia in remission (ICD-9-CM codes 204.00 through 208.91; see table below for ICD-10-CM codes)

| ICD-10 | Description |
|---|---|
| C91.01 | Acute lymphoblastic leukemia, in remission |
| C91.11 | Chronic lymphocytic leukemia of B-cell type in remission |
| C91.31 | Prolymphocytic leukemia of B-cell type, in remission |
| C91.51 | Adult T-cell lymphoma/leukemia (HTLV-1-associated), in remission |
| C91.61 | Prolymphocytic leukemia of T-cell type, in remission |
| C91.91 | Lymphoid leukemia, unspecified, in remission |
| C91.A1 | Mature B-cell leukemia Burkitt-type, in remission |
| C91.Z1 | Other lymphoid leukemia, in remission |
| C92.01 | Acute myeloblastic leukemia, in remission |
| C92.11 | Chronic myeloid leukemia, BCR/ABL-positive, in remission |
| C92.21 | Atypical chronic myeloid leukemia, BCR/ABL-negative, in remission |
| C92.31 | Myeloid sarcoma, in remission |
| C92.41 | Acute promyelocytic leukemia, in remission |
| C92.51 | Acute myelomonocytic leukemia, in remission |
| C92.61 | Acute myeloid leukemia with 11q23-abnormality in remission |
| C92.91 | Myeloid leukemia, unspecified in remission |
| C92.A1 | Acute myeloid leukemia with multilineage dysplasia, in remission |
| C92.Z1 | Other myeloid leukemia, in remission |
| C93.01 | Acute monoblastic/monocytic leukemia, in remission |
| C93.11 | Chronic myelomonocytic leukemia, in remission |
| C93.31 | Juvenile myelomonocytic leukemia, in remission |
| C93.91 | Monocytic leukemia, unspecified in remission |
| C93.Z1 | Other monocytic leukemia, in remission |
| C94.01 | Acute erythroid leukemia, in remission |
| C94.21 | Acute megakaryoblastic leukemia, in remission |
| C94.31 | Mast cell leukemia, in remission |
| C94.81 | Other specified leukemias, in remission |
| C95.01 | Acute leukemia of unspecified cell type, in remission |
| C95.11 | Chronic leukemia of unspecified cell type, in remission |
| C95.91 | Leukemia, unspecified, in remission |
| D45 | Polycythemia vera |

ii. For the treatment of aplastic anemia (ICD-9-CM codes 284.0 through 284.9; see table below for ICD-10-CM codes)

| ICD-10 | Description |
|---|---|
| D60.0 | Chronic acquired pure red cell aplasia |
| D60.1 | Transient acquired pure red cell aplasia |
| D60.8 | Other acquired pure red cell aplasias |
| D60.9 | Acquired pure red cell aplasia, unspecified |
| D61.01 | Constitutional (pure) red blood cell aplasia |
| D61.09 | Other constitutional aplastic anemia |
| D61.1 | Drug-induced aplastic anemia |
| D61.2 | Aplastic anemia due to other external agents |
| D61.3 | Idiopathic aplastic anemia |
| D61.810 | Antineoplastic chemotherapy induced pancytopenia |
| D61.811 | Other drug-induced pancytopenia |
| D61.818 | Other pancytopenia |
| D61.82 | Myelophthisis |
| D61.89 | Other specified aplastic anemias and other bone marrow failure syndromes |
| D61.9 | Aplastic anemia, unspecified |

b. Effective for services performed on or after June 3, 1985:

i. For the treatment of severe combined immunodeficiency disease (SCID) (ICD-9-CM code 279.2; ICD-10-CM codes D81.0, D81.1, D81.2, D81.6, D81.7, D81.89, and D81.9). ii. For the treatment of Wiskott-Aldrich syndrome (ICD-9-CM code 279.12; ICD-10-CM code D82.0)

c. Effective for services performed on or after August 4, 2010: For the treatment of Myelodysplastic Syndromes (MDS) (ICD-9-CM codes 238.72, 238.73, 238.74, 238.75 and ICD-10-CM codes D46.A, D46.B, D46.C, D46.0, D46.1, D46.20, D46.21, D46.22, D46.4, D46.9, D46.Z) pursuant to Coverage with Evidence Development (CED) in the context of a Medicare-approved, prospective clinical study. Refer to Pub. 100-03, NCD Manual, chapter 1, section 110.23, for further information about this policy. See section F below for billing instructions.

d. Effective for services performed on or after January 27, 2016:

   i. Allogeneic HSCT for multiple myeloma (ICD-10-CM codes C90.00, C90.01, and C90.02) is covered by Medicare only for beneficiaries with Durie-Salmon Stage II or III multiple myeloma, or International Staging System (ISS) Stage II or Stage III multiple myeloma, and participating in an approved prospective clinical study. Refer to Pub. 100-03, NCD Manual, chapter 1, section 110.23, for further information about this policy. See section F below for billing instructions.

   ii. Allogeneic HSCT for myelofibrosis (MF) (ICD-10-CM codes C94.40, C94.41, C94.42, D47.4, and D75.81) is covered by Medicare only for beneficiaries with Dynamic International Prognostic Scoring System (DIPSSplus) intermediate-2 or High primary or secondary MF and participating in an approved prospective clinical study. Refer to Pub. 100-03, NCD Manual, chapter 1, section 110.23, for further information about this policy. See section F below for billing instructions.

   iii. Allogeneic HSCT for sickle cell disease (SCD) (ICD-10-CM codes D57.00, D57.01, D57.02, D57.1, D57.20, D57.211, D57.212, D57.219, D57.40, D57.411, D57.412, D57.419, D57.80, D57.811, D57.812, and D57.819) is covered by Medicare only for beneficiaries with severe, symptomatic SCD who participate in an approved prospective clinical study. Refer to Pub. 100-03, NCD Manual, chapter 1, section 110.23, for further information about this policy. See section F below for billing instructions.

II. Autologous Stem Cell Transplantation (AuSCT)

HCPCS Code 38241

ICD-9-CM Procedure Codes 41.01, 41.04, 41.07, and 41.09;

ICD-10-PCS Procedure Codes 30230AZ, 30230G0, 30230Y0, 30233G0, 30233Y0, 30240G0, 30240Y0, 30243G0, 30243Y0, 30250G0, 30250Y0, 30253G0, 30253Y0, 30260G0, 30260Y0, 30263G0, and 30263Y0

a. Effective for services performed on or after April 28, 1989: Acute leukemia in remission who have a high probability of relapse and who have no human leucocyte antigens (HLA)-matched (ICD-9-CM codes 204.01, 205.01, 206.01, 207.01, 208.01; ICD-10-CM diagnosis codes C91.01, C92.01, C92,41, C92.51, C92.61, C92.A1, C93.01, C94.01, C94.21, C94.41, C95.01); Resistant non-Hodgkin's lymphomas or those presenting with poor prognostic features following an initial response (ICD-9-CM codes 200.00 - 200.08, 200.10-200.18, 200.20-200.28, 200.80-200.88, 202.00-202.08, 202.80-202.88 or 202.90-202.98; ICD-10-CM diagnosis codes C82.00-C85.29, C85.80-C86.6, C96.4, and C96.Z-C96.9); Recurrent or refractory neuroblastoma (see ICD-9-CM codes Neoplasm by site, malignant for the appropriate diagnosis code; if ICD-10-CM is applicable the following ranges are reported: C00 - C96, and D00 - D09 Resistant non-Hodgkin's lymphomas); or, Advanced Hodgkin's disease who have failed conventional therapy and have no HLA-matched donor (ICD-9-CM codes 201.00 - 201.98; ICD-10-CM codes C81.00 - C81.99).

b. Effective for services performed on or after October 1, 2000: Single AuSCT is only covered for Durie-Salmon Stage II or III multiple myeloma patients (ICD-9-CM codes 203.00 or 238.6; ICD-10-CM codes C90.00, C90.01, C90.02 and D47.Z9) that fit the following requirements:

   • Newly diagnosed or responsive multiple myeloma. This includes those patients with previously untreated disease, those with at least a partial response to prior chemotherapy (defined as a 50% decrease either in measurable paraprotein [serum and/or urine] or in bone marrow infiltration, sustained for at least 1 month), and those in responsive relapse; and • Adequate cardiac, renal, pulmonary, and hepatic function.

c. Effective for services performed on or after March 15, 2005: When recognized clinical risk factors are employed to select patients for transplantation, high dose melphalan (HDM) together with AuSCT is reasonable and necessary for Medicare beneficiaries of any age group with primary amyloid light chain (AL) amyloidosis (ICD-9-CM code 277.3 or 277.39) who meet the following criteria:

   • Amyloid deposition in 2 or fewer organs; and,

   • Cardiac left ventricular ejection fraction (EF) greater than 45%.

| ICD-9-CM code | Description | ICD-10-CM code | Description |
|---|---|---|---|
| 277.30 | Amyloidosis, unspecified | E85.9 | Amyloidosis, unspecified |
| 277.39 | Other amyloidosis | E85.8 | Other amyloidosis |
| | | E85.4 | Organ-limited amyloidosis |

As the ICD-9-CM codes 277.3, and 277.39 for amyloidosis do not differentiate between primary and non-primary, A/B MACs (B) should perform prepay reviews on all claims with a diagnosis of ICD-9-CM code 277.3 to determine whether payment is appropriate.

If ICD-10-CM is applicable, as the applicable ICD-10 CM codes E85.4, E85.8, and E85.9 for amyloidosis do not differentiate between primary and non-primary, A/B MACs (B) should perform prepay reviews on all claims with a diagnosis of ICD-10-CM code E85.4, E85.8, and E85.9 to determine whether payment is appropriate.

**C. Nationally Non-Covered Indications**

I. Allogeneic Hematopoietic Stem Cell Transplantation (HSCT)

Effective for claims with dates of service on or after May 24, 1996, through January 27, 2016, allogeneic HSCT is not covered as treatment for multiple myeloma (if ICD-9-CM is applicable, ICD-9-CM code 203.00 and 203.01; or if ICD-10-CM is applicable, ICD-10-CMcodes C90.00, C90.01, C90.02 and D47.Z9).

II. Autologous Stem Cell Transplantation (AuSCT)

AuSCT is not considered reasonable and necessary within the meaning of §I862(a)(1)(A) of the Act and is not covered under Medicare for the following conditions:

   a) Acute leukemia not in remission (if ICD-9-CM is applicable, ICD-9-CM codes 204.00, 205.00, 206.00, 207.00 and 208.00; or if ICD-10-CM is applicable, ICD-10-CM codes C91.00, C92.00, C93.00, C94.00, andC95.00)

   b) Chronic granulocytic leukemia (if ICD-9-CM is applicable, ICD-9-CM codes 205.10 and 205.11; or if ICD-10-CM is applicable, ICD-10-CM codes C92.10 andC92.11);

   c) Solid tumors (other than neuroblastoma) (if ICD-9-CM is applicable, ICD-9-CM codes 140.0 through 199.1; or if ICD-10-CM is applicable, ICD-10-CM codesC00.0 – C80.2 and D00.0 – D09.9);

   d) Up to October 1, 2000, multiple myeloma (if ICD-9-CM is applicable, ICD-9-CM code 203.00 and 203.01; or if ICD-10-CM is applicable, ICD-10-CM codes C90.00, C90.01, C90.02 and D47.Z9);

   e) Tandem transplantation (multiple rounds of AuSCT) for patients with multiple myeloma (if ICD-9-CM is applicable, ICD-9-CM code 203.00 and 203.01; or if ICD-10-CM is applicable, ICD-10-CM codes C90.00, C90.01, C90.02 and D47.Z9);

   f) Effective October 1, 2000, non-primary AL amyloidosis (see table below for applicable ICD codes); and,

   g) Effective October 1, 2000, through March 14, 2005, primary AL amyloidosis for Medicare beneficiaries age 64 or older (see table below for applicable ICD codes).

| ICD-9-CM codes | Description | ICD-10-CM codes | Description |
|---|---|---|---|
| 277.30 | Amyloidosis, unspecified | E85.9 | Amyloidosis, unspecified |
| 277.31 | Familial Mediterranean fever | E85.0 | Non-neuropathic heredofamilial amyloidosis |
| 277.39 | Other amyloidosis | E85.8 | Other amyloidosis |
| | | E85.1 | Neuropathic heredofamilial amyloidosis |
| | | E85.2 | Heredofamilial amyloidosis, unspecified |
| | | E85.3 | Secondary systemic amyloidosis |
| | | E85.4 | Organ-limited amyloidosis |

As the ICD-9-CM code 277.3 and 277.39 for amyloidosis do not differentiate between primary and non-primary, A/B MACs (B) should perform prepay reviews on all claims with a diagnosis of ICD-9-CM code 277.3 and 277.39 to determine whether payment is appropriate.

If ICD-10-CM is applicable, as the applicable ICD-10 CM codes E85.4, E85.8, and E85.9 for amyloidosis do not differentiate between primary and non-primary, A/B MACs (B) should perform prepay reviews on all claims with a diagnosis of ICD-10-CM code E85.4, E85.8, and E85.9 to determine whether payment is appropriate.

**D. Other**

All other indications for stem cell transplantation not otherwise noted above as covered or non-covered remain at local Medicare Administrative Contractor discretion.

**E. Suggested MSN and RA Messages**

The contractor shall use an appropriate MSN and RA message such as the following:

MSN - 15.4, The information provided does not support the need for this service or item;

RA - 150, Payment adjusted because the payer deems the information submitted does not support this level of service.

**F. Clinical Trials for Allogeneic Hematopoietic Stem Cell Transplantation (HSCT) for Myelodysplastic Syndrome (MDS), Multiple Myeloma, Myelofibrosis (MF), and for Sickle Cell Disease (SCD)**

I. Background

Effective for services performed on or after August 4, 2010, contractors shall pay for claims for allogeneic HSCT for the treatment of Myelodysplastic Syndromes (MDS) pursuant to Coverage with Evidence Development (CED) in the context of a Medicare-approved, prospective clinical study.

Effective for services performed on or after January 27, 2016, contractors shall pay for claims for allogeneic HSCT for the treatment of multiple myeloma, myelofibrosis

(MF), and for sickle cell disease (SCD) pursuant to CED, in the context of a Medicare-approved, prospective clinical study.

Refer to Pub.100-03, National Coverage Determinations Manual, Chapter 1, section 110.23, for more information about this policy, and Pub. 100-04, Medicare Claims Processing Manual, Chapter 3, section 90.3, for information on inpatient billing of this CED.

II.  Adjudication Requirements Payable Conditions. For claims with dates of service on and after August 4, 2010, contractors shall pay for claims for allogeneic HSCT for MDS when the service was provided pursuant to a Medicare-approved clinical study under CED; these services are paid only in the inpatient setting (Type of Bill (TOB) 11X), as outpatient Part B (TOB 13X), and in Method II critical access hospitals (TOB 85X).

Contractors shall require the following coding in order to pay for these claims:

- Existing Medicare-approved clinical trial coding conventions, as required in Pub. 100-04, Medicare Claims Processing Manual, Chapter 32, section 69, and inpatient billing requirements regarding acquisition of stem cells in Pub. 100-04, Medicare Claims Processing Manual, Chapter 3, section 90.3.1.

- If ICD-9-CM is applicable, for Inpatient Hospital Claims: ICD-9-CM procedure codes 41.02, 41.03, 41.05, and 41.08 or,

- If ICD-10-CM is applicable, ICD-10-PCS, procedure codes 30230G1, 30230Y1, 30233G1, 30233Y1, 30240G1, 30240Y1, 30243G1, 30243Y1, 30250G1,30250Y1, 30253G1, 30253Y1, 30260G1, 30260Y1, 30263G1, and 30263Y1

- If Outpatient Hospital or Professional Claims: HCPCS procedure code 38240

- If ICD-9-CM is applicable, ICD-9-CM diagnosis codes 238.72, 238.73, 238.74, 238.75 or,

- If ICD-10-CM is applicable, ICD-10-CM codes D46.A, D46.B, D46.C, D46.0, D46.1, D46.20, D46.21, D46.22, D46.4, D46.9, D46.Z,

- Professional claims only: place of service codes 19, 21, or 22.

Payable Conditions. For claims with dates of service on and after January 27, 2016, contractors shall pay for claims for allogeneic HSCT for multiple myeloma, myelofibrosis (MF), and for sickle cell disease (SCD) when the service was provided pursuant to a Medicare-approved clinical study under CED; these services are paid only in the inpatient setting (Type of Bill (TOB) 11X), as outpatient Part B (TOB 13X), and in Method II critical access hospitals (TOB 85X).

Contractors shall require the following coding in order to pay for these claims:

- Existing Medicare-approved clinical trial coding conventions, as required in Pub. 100-04, Medicare Claims Processing Manual, Chapter 32, section 69, and inpatient billing requirements regarding acquisition of stem cells in Pub. 100-04, Medicare Claims Processing Manual, Chapter 3, section 90.3.1.

- ICD-10-PCS codes 30230G1, 30230Y1, 30233G1, 30233Y1, 30240G1, 30240Y1, 30243G1, 30243Y1, 30250G1, 30250Y1, 30253G1, 30253Y1, 30260G1, 30260Y1, 30263G1, and 30263Y1

- If Outpatient Hospital or Professional Claims: HCPCS procedure code 38240

- ICD-10-CM diagnosis codes C90.00, C90.01, C90.02, C94.40, C94.41, C94.42, D47.4, D75.81, D57.00, D57.01, D57.02, D57.1, D57.20, D57.211, D57.212, D57.219, D57.40, D57.411, D57.412, D57.419, D57.80, D57.811, D57.812, and D57.819

- Professional claims only: place of service codes 19, 21, or 22.

Denials. Contractors shall deny claims failing to meet any of the above criteria. In addition, contractors shall apply the following requirements:

- Providers shall issue a hospital issued notice of non-coverage (HINN) or advance beneficiary notice (ABN) to the beneficiary if the services performed are not provided in accordance with CED.

- Contractors shall deny claims that do not meet the criteria for coverage with the following messages:

CARC 50 - These are non-covered services because this is not deemed a 'medical necessity' by the payer.

**NOTE:** Refer to the 835 Healthcare Policy Identification Segment (loop 2110 Service Payment Information REF), if present.

RARC N386 - This decision was based on a National Coverage Determination (NCD). An NCD provides a coverage determination as to whether a particular item or service is covered. A copy of this policy is available at http:www.cms.hhs.gov/mcd/search.asp. If you do not have web access, you may contact the contractor to request a copy of the NCD.

Group Code – Patient Responsibility (PR) if HINN/ABN issued, otherwise Contractual Obligation (CO)

MSN 16.77 – This service/item was not covered because it was not provided as part of a qualifying trial/study. (Este servicio/artículo no fue cubierto porque no estaba incluido como parte de un ensayo clínico/estudio calificado.)

MSN 15.20 – The following policies [NCD 110.23] were used when we made this decision. (Las siguientes políticas [NCD 110.23] fueron utilizadas cuando se tomó esta decisión.)

## 100-04, 32, 90.2

### HCPCS and Diagnosis Coding

**Allogeneic Stem Cell Transplantation**

- Effective for services performed on or after August 1, 1978:

  - For the treatment of leukemia or leukemia in remission, providers shall use ICD-9-CM codes 204.00 through 208.91 and HCPCS code 38240.

  - For the treatment of aplastic anemia, providers shall use ICD-9-CM codes 284.0 through 284.9 and HCPCS code 38240.

- Effective for services performed on or after June 3, 1985:

  - For the treatment of severe combined immunodeficiency disease, providers shall use ICD-9-CM code 279.2 and HCPCS code 38240.

  - For the treatment of Wiskott-Aldrich syndrome, providers shall use ICD-9-CM code 279.12 and HCPCS code 38240.

- Effective for services performed on or after May 24, 1996:

  - Allogeneic stem cell transplantation, HCPCS code 38240 is not covered as treatment for the diagnosis of multiple myeloma ICD-9-CM codes 203.00 or 203.01.

Autologous Stem Cell Transplantation.--Is covered under the following circumstances effective for services performed on or after April 28, 1989:

- For the treatment of patients with acute leukemia in remission who have a high probability of relapse and who have no human leucocyte antigens (HLA) matched, providers shall use ICD-9-CM code 204.01 lymphoid; ICD-9-CM code 205.01 myeloid; ICD-9-CM code 206.01 monocytic; or ICD-9-CM code 207.01 acute erythremia and erythroleukemia; or ICD-9-CM code 208.01 unspecified cell type and HCPCS code 38241.

- For the treatment of resistant non-Hodgkin's lymphomas for those patients presenting with poor prognostic features following an initial response, providers shall use ICD-9-CM codes 200.00 - 200.08, 200.10-200.18, 200.20-200.28, 200.80-200.88, 202.00-202.08, 202.80-202.88 or 202.90-202.98 and HCPCS code 38241.

- For the treatment of recurrent or refractory neuroblastoma, providers shall use ICD-9-CM codes Neoplasm by site, malignant, the appropriate HCPCS code and HCPCS code 38241.

- For the treatment of advanced Hodgkin's disease for patients who have failed conventional therapy and have no HLA-matched donor, providers shall use ICD-9-CM codes 201.00 - 201.98 and HCPCS code 38241.

Autologous Stem Cell Transplantation.--Is covered under the following circumstances effective for services furnished on or after October 1, 2000:

- For the treatment of multiple myeloma (only for beneficiaries who are less than age 78, have Durie-Salmon stage II or III newly diagnosed or responsive multiple myeloma, and have adequate cardiac, renal, pulmonary and hepatic functioning), providers shall use ICD- 9-CM code 203.00 or 238.6 and HCPCS code 38241.

- For the treatment of recurrent or refractory neuroblastoma, providers shall use appropriate code (see ICD-9-CM neoplasm by site, malignant) and HCPCS code 38241.

- Effective for services performed on or after March 15, 2005, when recognized clinical risk factors are employed to select patients for transplantation, high-dose melphalan (HDM) together with autologous stem cell transplantation (HDM/AuSCT) is reasonable and necessary for Medicare beneficiaries of any age group for the treatment of primary amyloid light chain (AL) amyloidosis, ICD-9-CM code 277.3 who meet the following criteria:

- Amyloid deposition in 2 or fewer organs; and,

- Cardiac left ventricular ejection fraction (EF) greater than 45%.

## 100-04, 32, 90.2.1

### HCPCS and Diagnosis Coding for Stem Cell Transplantation - ICD-10-CM Applicable

ICD-10 is applicable to services on and after the implementation of ICD-.

For services provided use the appropriate code from the ICD-10 CM codes in the table below. See §90.2 for a list of covered conditions.

| ICD-10 | Description |
|--------|-------------|
| C91.01 | Acute lymphoblastic leukemia, in remission |
| C91.11 | Chronic lymphocytic leukemia of B-cell type in remission |
| C91.31 | Prolymphocytic leukemia of B-cell type, in remission |
| C91.51 | Adult T-cell lymphoma/leukemia (HTLV-1-associated), in remission |
| C91.61 | Prolymphocytic leukemia of T-cell type, in remission |
| C91.91 | Lymphoid leukemia, unspecified, in remission |
| C91.A1 | Mature B-cell leukemia Burkitt-type, in remission |

CPT © 2017 American Medical Association. All Rights Reserved.                    © 2017 Optum360, LLC

| ICD-10 | Description |
|---|---|
| C91.Z1 | Other lymphoid leukemia, in remission |
| C92.01 | Acute myeloblastic leukemia, in remission |
| C92.11 | Chronic myeloid leukemia, BCR/ABL-positive, in remission |
| C92.21 | Atypical chronic myeloid leukemia, BCR/ABL-negative, in remission |
| C92.31 | Myeloid sarcoma, in remission |
| C92.41 | Acute promyelocytic leukemia, in remission |
| C92.51 | Acute myelomonocytic leukemia, in remission |
| C92.61 | Acute myeloid leukemia with 11q23-abnormality in remission |
| C92.91 | Myeloid leukemia, unspecified in remission |
| C92.A1 | Acute myeloid leukemia with multilineage dysplasia, in remission |
| C92.Z1 | Other myeloid leukemia, in remission |
| C93.01 | Acute monoblastic/monocytic leukemia, in remission |
| C93.11 | Chronic myelomonocytic leukemia, in remission |
| C93.31 | Juvenile myelomonocytic leukemia, in remission |
| C93.91 | Monocytic leukemia, unspecified in remission |
| C93.91 | Monocytic leukemia, unspecified in remission |
| C93.Z1 | Other monocytic leukemia, in remission |
| C94.01 | Acute erythroid leukemia, in remission |
| C94.21 | Acute megakaryoblastic leukemia, in remission |
| C94.31 | Mast cell leukemia, in remission |
| C94.81 | Other specified leukemias, in remission |
| C95.01 | Acute leukemia of unspecified cell type, in remission |
| C95.11 | Chronic leukemia of unspecified cell type, in remission |
| C95.91 | Leukemia, unspecified, in remission |
| D45 | Polycythemia vera |
| D61.01 | Constitutional (pure) red blood cell aplasia |
| D61.09 | Other constitutional aplastic anemia |
| D82.0 | Wiskott-Aldrich syndrome |
| D81.0 | Severe combined immunodeficiency [SCID] with reticular dysgenesis |
| D81.1 | Severe combined immunodeficiency [SCID] with low T- and B-cell numbers |
| D81.2 | Severe combined immunodeficiency [SCID] with low or normal B-cell numbers |
| D81.6 | Major histocompatibility complex class I deficiency |
| D81.7 | Major histocompatibility complex class II deficiency |
| D81.89 | Other combined immunodeficiencies |
| D81.9 | Combined immunodeficiency, unspecified |
| D81.2 | Severe combined immunodeficiency [SCID] with low or normal B-cell numbers |
| D81.6 | Major histocompatibility complex class I deficiency |
| D60.0 | Chronic acquired pure red cell aplasia |
| D60.1 | Transient acquired pure red cell aplasia |
| D60.8 | Other acquired pure red cell aplasias |
| D60.9 | Acquired pure red cell aplasia, unspecified |
| D61.01 | Constitutional (pure) red blood cell aplasia |
| D61.09 | Other constitutional aplastic anemia |
| D61.1 | Drug-induced aplastic anemia |
| D61.2 | Aplastic anemia due to other external agents |
| D61.3 | Idiopathic aplastic anemia |
| D61.810 | Antineoplastic chemotherapy induced pancytopenia |
| D61.811 | Other drug-induced pancytopenia |
| D61.818 | Other pancytopenia |
| D61.82 | Myelophthisis |
| D61.89 | Other specified aplastic anemias and other bone marrow failure syndromes |
| D61.9 | Aplastic anemia, unspecified |

- If ICD-10-CM is applicable, the following ranges of ICD-10-CM codes are also covered for AuSCT: Resistant non-Hodgkin's lymphomas, ICD-10-CM diagnosis codes C82.00-C85.29, C85.80-C86.6, C96.4, and C96.Z-C96.9.
- Tandem transplantation (multiple rounds of autologous stem cell transplantation) for patients with multiple myeloma, ICD-10-CM codes C90.00 and D47.Z9

**NOTE:** The following conditions are not covered:

- Acute leukemia not in remission
- Chronic granulocytic leukemia
- Solid tumors (other than neuroblastoma)

- Multiple myeloma
- For Medicare beneficiaries age 64 or older, all forms of amyloidosis, primary and non-primary
- Non-primary amyloidosis

Also coverage for conditions other than those specifically designated as covered in §90.2 or specifically designated as non-covered in this section or in §90.3 will be at the discretion of the individual contractor.

## 100-04, 32, 90.3

### Non-Covered Conditions

Autologous stem cell transplantation is not covered for the following conditions:

- Acute leukemia not in remission (If ICD-9-CM is applicable, ICD-9-CM codes 204.00, 205.00, 206.00, 207.00 and 208.00) or (If ICD-10-CM is applicable, ICD-10-CM codes C91.00, C92.00, C93.00, C94.00, and C95.00)
- Chronic granulocytic leukemia (ICD-9-CM codes 205.10 and 205.11 if ICD-9-CM is applicable) or (if ICD-10-CM is applicable, ICD-10-CM codes C92.10 and C92.11);
- Solid tumors (other than neuroblastoma) (ICD-9-CM codes 140.0 through 199.1 if ICD-9-CM is applicable or if ICD-10-CM is applicable, ICD-10-CM codes C00.0 – C80.2 and D00.0 – D09.9.)
- Effective for services rendered on or after May 24, 1996 through September 30, 2000, multiple myeloma (ICD-9-CM code 203.00 and 203.01 if ICD-9-CM is applicable or if ICD-10-CM is applicable, ICD-10-CM codes C90.00 and D47.Z9);
- Effective for services on or after October 1, 2000, through March 14, 2005, for Medicare beneficiaries age 64 or older, all forms of amyloidosis, primary and non-primary
- Effective for services on or after 10/01/00, for all Medicare beneficiaries, non-primary amyloidosis

| ICD-9-CM | Description | ICD-10-CM | Description |
|---|---|---|---|
| 277.30 | Amyloidosis, unspecified | E85.9 | Amyloidosis, unspecified |
| 277.31 | Familial Mediterranean fever | E85.0 | Non-neuropathic heredofamilial amyloidosis |
| 277.39 | Other amyloidosis | E85.1 | Neuropathic heredofamilial amyloidosis |
| 277.39 | Other amyloidosis | E85.2 | Heredofamilial amyloidosis, unspecified |
| 277.39 | Other amyloidosis | E85.3 | Secondary systemic amyloidosis |
| 277.39 | Other amyloidosis | E85.4 | Organ-limited amyloidosis |
| 277.39 | Other amyloidosis | E85.8 | Other amyloidosis |

**NOTE:** Coverage for conditions other than those specifically designated as covered in 90.2 or 90.2.1 or specifically designated as non-covered in this section will be at the discretion of the individual A/B MAC (B).

## 100-04, 32, 90.4

### Edits

NOTE: Coverage for conditions other than those specifically designated as covered in 80.2 or specifically designated as non-covered in this section will be at the discretion of the individual A/B MAC (B).

Appropriate diagnosis to procedure code edits should be implemented for the non-covered conditions and services in 90.2 90.2.1, and 90.3 as applicable.

As the ICD-9-CM code 277.3 for amyloidosis does not differentiate between primary and non-primary, A/B MACs (B) should perform prepay reviews on all claims with a diagnosis of ICD-9-CM code 277.3 and a HCPCS procedure code of 38241 to determine whether payment is appropriate.

If ICD-10-CM is applicable, the applicable ICD-10 CM codes are: E85.0, E85.1, E85.2, E85.3, E85.4, E85.8, and E85.9.

## 100-04, 32, 90.6

### Clinical Trials for Allogeneic Hematopoietic Stem Cell Transplantation (HSCT) for Myelodysplastic Syndrome (MDS)

#### A. Background

Myelodysplastic Syndrome (MDS) refers to a group of diverse blood disorders in which the bone marrow does not produce enough healthy, functioning blood cells. These disorders are varied with regard to clinical characteristics, cytologic and pathologic features, and cytogenetics.

On August 4, 2010, the Centers for Medicare & Medicaid Services (CMS) issued a national coverage determination (NCD) stating that CMS believes that the evidence does not demonstrate that the use of allogeneic hematopoietic stem cell transplantation (HSCT) improves health outcomes in Medicare beneficiaries with MDS. Therefore, allogeneic HSCT for MDS is not reasonable and necessary under §1862(a)(1)(A) of the Social Security Act (the Act). However, allogeneic HSCT for MDS is reasonable and necessary under §1862(a)(1)(E) of the Act and therefore covered by Medicare ONLY if provided pursuant to a Medicare-approved clinical study under

Coverage with Evidence Development (CED). Refer to Pub.100-3, NCD Manual, Chapter 1, section 110.8.1, for more information about this policy, and Pub. 100-4, MCP Manual, Chapter 3, section 90.3.1, for information on CED.

**B. Adjudication Requirements**

Payable Conditions. For claims with dates of service on and after August 4, 2010, contractors shall pay for claims for HSCT for MDS when the service was provided pursuant to a Medicare-approved clinical study under CED; these services are paid only in the inpatient setting (Type of Bill (TOB) 11X), as outpatient Part B (TOB 13X), and in Method II critical access hospitals (TOB 85X). Contractors shall require the following coding in order to pay for these claims:

- Existing Medicare-approved clinical trial coding conventions, as required in Pub. 100-4, MCP Manual, Chapter 32, section 69, and inpatient billing requirements regarding acquisition of stem cells in Pub. 100-4, MCP Manual, Chapter 3, section 90.3.3.

- If ICD-9-CM is applicable, for Inpatient Hospital Claims: ICD-9-CM procedure codes 41.02, 41.03, 41.05, and 41.08 or,

- If ICD-10-CM is applicable, ICD-10-PCS, procedure codes 30230G1, 30230Y1, 30233G1, 30233Y1, 30240G1, 30240Y1, 30243G1, 30243Y1, 30250G1,30250Y1, 30253G1, 30253Y1, 30260G1, 30260Y1, 30263G1, and 30263Y1

- If Outpatient Hospital or Professional Claims: HCPCS procedure code 38240

- If ICD-9-CM is applicable, ICD-9-CM diagnosis code 238.75 or If ICD-10-CM is applicable, ICD-10-CM diagnosis codes D46.9, D46.Z, or Z00.6 Professional claims only: place of service codes 21 or 22.

Denials. Contractors shall deny claims failing to meet any of the above criteria. In addition, contractors shall apply the following requirements:

- Providers shall issue a hospital issued notice of non-coverage (HINN) or advance beneficiary notice (ABN) to the beneficiary if the services performed are not provided in accordance with CED.

- Contractors shall deny claims that do not meet the criteria for coverage with the following messages:

  CARC 50 - These are non-covered services because this is not deemed a 'medical necessity' by the payer.

  NOTE: Refer to the 835 Healthcare Policy Identification Segment (loop 2110 Service Payment Information REF), if present.

  RARC N386 - This decision was based on a National Coverage Determination (NCD). An NCD provides a coverage determination as to whether a particular item or service is covered. A copy of this policy is available at http://www.cms.hhs.gov/mcd/search.asp. If you do not have web access, you may contact the contractor to request a copy of the NCD.

  Group Code – Patient Responsibility (PR) if HINN/ABN issued, otherwise Contractual Obligation (CO)

  MSN 16.77 – This service/item was not covered because it was not provided as part of a qualifying trial/study. (Este servicio/artículo no fue cubierto porque no estaba incluido como parte de un ensayo clínico/estudio calificado.)

## 100-04, 32, 120.2

### Coding and General Billing Requirements

Physicians and hospitals must report one of the following Current Procedural Terminology (CPT) codes on the claim:

66982   Extracapsular cataract removal with insertion of intraocular lens prosthesis (one stage procedure), manual or mechanical technique (e.g., irrigation and aspiration or phacoemulsification), complex requiring devices or techniques not generally used in routine cataract surgery (e.g., iris expansion device, suture support for intraocular lens, or primary posterior capsulorrhexis) or performed on patients in the amblyogenic development stage.

66983   Intracapsular cataract with insertion of intraocular lens prosthesis (one stage procedure)

66984   Extracapsular cataract removal with insertion of intraocular lens prosthesis (one stage procedure), manual or mechanical technique (e.g., irrigation and aspiration or phacoemulsification)

66985   Insertion of intraocular lens prosthesis (secondary implant), not associated with concurrent cataract extraction

66986   Exchange of intraocular lens

In addition, physicians inserting a P-C IOL or A-C IOL in an office setting may bill code V2632 (posterior chamber intraocular lens) for the IOL. Medicare will make payment for the lens based on reasonable cost for a conventional IOL. Place of Service (POS) = 11.

Effective for dates of service on and after January 1, 2006, physician, hospitals and ASCs may also bill the non-covered charges related to the P-C function of the IOL using HCPCS code V2788. Effective for dates of service on and after January 22, 2007 through January 1, 2008, non-covered charges related to A-C function of the IOL can be billed using HCPCS code V2788. The type of service indicator for the non-covered billed charges is Q. (The type of service is applied by the Medicare carrier and not the provider). Effective for A-C IOL insertion services on or after January 1, 2008,

physicians, hospitals and ASCs should use V2787 rather than V2788 to report any additional charges that accrue.

When denying the non-payable charges submitted with V2787 or V2788, contractors shall use an appropriate Medical Summary Notice (MSN) such as 16.10 (Medicare does not pay for this item or service) and an appropriate claim adjustment reason code such as 96 (non-covered charges) for claims submitted with the non-payable charges.

Hospitals and physicians may use the proper CPT code(s) to bill Medicare for evaluation and management services usually associated with services following cataract extraction surgery, if appropriate.

**A - Applicable Bill Types**

The hospital applicable bill types are 12X, 13X, 83X and 85X.

**B - Other Special Requirements for Hospitals**

Hospitals shall continue to pay CAHs method 2 claims under current payment methodologies for conditional IOLs.

## 100-04, 32, 130.1

### Billing and Payment Requirements

Effective for dates of service on or after January 1, 2000, use HCPCS code G0166 (External counterpulsation, per session) to report ECP services. The codes for external cardiac assist (92971), ECG rhythm strip and report (93040 or 93041), pulse oximetry (94760 or 94761) and plethysmography (93922 or 93923) or other monitoring tests for examining the effects of this treatment are not clinically necessary with this service and should not be paid on the same day, unless they occur in a clinical setting not connected with the delivery of the ECP. Daily evaluation and management service, e.g., 99201-99205, 99211-99215, 99217-99220, 99241-99245, cannot be billed with the ECP treatments. Any evaluation and management service must be justified with adequate documentation of the medical necessity of the visit. Deductible and coinsurance apply.

## 100-04, 32, 140.2

### Cardiac Rehabilitation Program Services Furnished On or After January 1, 2010

As specified at 42 CFR 410.49, Medicare covers cardiac rehabilitation items and services for patients who have experienced one or more of the following:

- An acute myocardial infarction within the preceding 12 months; or

- A coronary artery bypass surgery; or

- Current stable angina pectoris; or

- Heart valve repair or replacement; or

- Percutaneous transluminal coronary angioplasty (PTCA) or coronary stenting; or

- A heart or heart-lung transplant or;

- Stable, chronic heart failure defined as patients with left ventricular ejection fraction of 35% or less and New York Heart Association (NYHA) class II to IV symptoms despite being on optimal heart failure therapy for at least 6 weeks (effective February 18, 2014).

Cardiac rehabilitation programs must include the following components:

- Physician-prescribed exercise each day cardiac rehabilitation items and services are furnished;

- Cardiac risk factor modification, including education, counseling, and behavioral intervention at least once during the program, tailored to patients' individual needs;

- Psychosocial assessment;

- Outcomes assessment; and

- An individualized treatment plan detailing how components are utilized for each patient.

Cardiac rehabilitation items and services must be furnished in a physician's office or a hospital outpatient setting. All settings must have a physician immediately available and accessible for medical consultations and emergencies at all times items and services are being furnished under the program. This provision is satisfied if the physician meets the requirements for the direct supervision of physician's office services as specified at 42 CFR 410.26 and for hospital outpatient therapeutic services as specified at 42 CFR 410.27.

As specified at 42 CFR 410.49(f)(1), cardiac rehabilitation program sessions are limited to a maximum of 2 1-hour sessions per day for up to 36 sessions over up to 36 weeks, with the option for an additional 36 sessions over an extended period of time if approved by the Medicare contractor.

## 100-04, 32, 140.2.1

### Coding Requirements for Cardiac Rehabilitation Services Furnished On or After January 1, 2010

The following are the applicable CPT codes for cardiac rehabilitation services: 93797 - Physician services for outpatient cardiac rehabilitation; without continuous ECG monitoring (per session) and 93798 - Physician services for outpatient cardiac rehabilitation; with continuous ECG monitoring (per session) Effective for dates of service on or after January 1, 2010, hospitals and practitioners may report a maximum of 2 1-hour sessions per day. In order to report one session of cardiac rehabilitation services in a day, the duration of treatment must be at least 31 minutes. Two sessions of cardiac rehabilitation services may only be reported in the same day if the duration of treatment is at least 91 minutes. In other words, the first session would account for 60 minutes and the second session would account for at least 31 minutes if two sessions are reported. If several shorter periods of cardiac rehabilitation services are furnished on a given day, the minutes of service during those periods must be added together for reporting in 1-hour session increments.

Example: If the patient receives 20 minutes of cardiac rehabilitation services in the day, no cardiac rehabilitation session may be reported because less than 31 minutes of services were furnished.

Example: If the patient receives 20 minutes of cardiac rehabilitation services in the morning and 35 minutes of cardiac rehabilitation services in the afternoon of a single day, the hospital or practitioner would report 1 session of cardiac rehabilitation services under 1 unit of the appropriate CPT code for the total duration of 55 minutes of cardiac rehabilitation services on that day.

Example: If the patient receives 70 minutes of cardiac rehabilitation services in the morning and 25 minutes of cardiac rehabilitation services in the afternoon of a single day, the hospital or practitioner would report two sessions of cardiac rehabilitation services under the appropriate CPT code(s) because the total duration of cardiac rehabilitation services on that day of 95 minutes exceeds 90 minutes.

Example: If the patient receives 70 minutes of cardiac rehabilitation services in the morning and 85 minutes of cardiac rehabilitation services in the afternoon of a single day, the hospital or practitioner would report two sessions of cardiac rehabilitation services under the appropriate CPT code(s) for the total duration of cardiac rehabilitation services of 155 minutes. A maximum of two sessions per day may be reported, regardless of the total duration of cardiac rehabilitation services.

## 100-04, 32, 140.2.2.2

### Requirements for CR and ICR Services on Institutional Claims

Effective for claims with dates of service on and after January 1, 2010, contractors shall pay for CR and ICR services when submitted on Types of Bill (TOBs) 13X and 85X only. All other TOBs shall be denied.

The following messages shall be used when contractors deny CR and ICR claims for TOBs 13X and 85X:

Claim Adjustment Reason Code (CARC) 171 – Payment is denied when performed/billed by this type of provider in this type of facility.

Remittance Advice Remark Code (RARC) N428 - Service/procedure not covered when performed in this place of service.

Medicare Summary Notice (MSN) 21.25 - This service was denied because Medicare only covers this service in certain settings.

Group Code PR (Patient Responsibility) – Where a claim is received with the GA modifier indicating that a signed ABN is on file.

Group Code CO (Contractor Responsibility) – Where a claim is received with the GZ modifier indicating that no signed ABN is on file.

## 100-04, 32, 140.2.2.4

### Edits for CR Services Exceeding 36 Sessions

Effective for claims with dates of service on or after January 1, 2010, contractors shall deny all claims with HCPCS 93797 and 93798 (both professional and institutional claims) that exceed 36 CR sessions when a KX modifier is not included on the claim line.

The following messages shall be used when contractors deny CR claims that exceed 36 sessions, when a KX modifier is not included on the claim line:

Claim Adjustment Reason Code (CARC) 119 – Benefit maximum for this period or occurrence has been reached.

RARC N435 - Exceeds number/frequency approved/allowed within time period without support documentation.

MSN 23.17- Medicare won't cover these services because they are not considered medically necessary.

Spanish Version - Medicare no cubrirá estos servicios porque no son considerados necesarios por razones médicas.

Group Code PR (Patient Responsibility) – Where a claim is received with the GA modifier indicating that a signed ABN is on file.

Group Code CO (Contractor Responsibility) – Where a claim is received with the GZ modifier indicating that no signed ABN is on file.

Contractors shall not research and adjust CR claims paid for more than 36 sessions processed prior to the implementation of CWF edits. However, contractors may adjust claims brought to their attention.

## 100-04, 32, 140.3

### Intensive Cardiac Rehabilitation Program Services Furnished On or After January 1, 2010

As specified at 42 CFR 410.49, Medicare covers intensive cardiac rehabilitation items and services for patients who have experienced one or more of the following:

- An acute myocardial infarction within the preceding 12 months; or
- A coronary artery bypass surgery; or
- Current stable angina pectoris; or
- Heart valve repair or replacement; or
- Percutaneous transluminal coronary angioplasty (PTCA) or coronary stenting; or
- A heart or heart-lung transplant or;
- A stable, chronic heart failure defined as patients with left ventricular ejection fraction of 35% or less and New York Heart Association (NYHA) class II to IV symptoms despite being on optimal heart failure therapy for at least 6 weeks (effective February 18, 2014).

Intensive cardiac rehabilitation programs must include the following components:

- Physician-prescribed exercise each day cardiac rehabilitation items and services are furnished;
- Cardiac risk factor modification, including education, counseling, and behavioral intervention at least once during the program, tailored to patients' individual needs;
- Psychosocial assessment;
- Outcomes assessment; and
- An individualized treatment plan detailing how components are utilized for each patient.

Intensive cardiac rehabilitation programs must be approved by Medicare. In order to be approved, a program must demonstrate through peer-reviewed published research that it has accomplished one or more of the following for its patients:

- Positively affected the progression of coronary heart disease;
- Reduced the need for coronary bypass surgery; and
- Reduced the need for percutaneous coronary interventions.

An intensive cardiac rehabilitation program must also demonstrate through peer-reviewed published research that it accomplished a statistically significant reduction in 5 or more of the following measures for patients from their levels before cardiac rehabilitation services to after cardiac rehabilitation services:

- Low density lipoprotein;
- Triglycerides;
- Body mass index;
- Systolic blood pressure;
- Diastolic blood pressure; and
- The need for cholesterol, blood pressure, and diabetes medications.

Intensive cardiac rehabilitation items and services must be furnished in a physician's office or a hospital outpatient setting. All settings must have a physician immediately available and accessible for medical consultations and emergencies at all times items and services are being furnished under the program. This provision is satisfied if the physician meets the requirements for direct supervision of physician office services as specified at 42 CFR 410.26 and for hospital outpatient therapeutic services as specified at 42 CFR 410.27.

As specified at 42 CFR 410.49(f)(2), intensive cardiac rehabilitation program sessions are limited to 72 1-hour sessions, up to 6 sessions per day, over a period of up to 18 weeks.

## 100-04, 32, 150.1

### Bariatric Surgery for Treatment of Co-Morbid Conditions Related to Morbid Obesity

Effective for services on or after February 21, 2006, Medicare has determined that the following bariatric surgery procedures are reasonable and necessary under certain conditions for the treatment of morbid obesity. The patient must have a body-mass index (BMI) =35, have at least one co-morbidity related to obesity, and have been previously unsuccessful with medical treatment for obesity. This medical information must be documented in the patient's medical record. In addition, the procedure must be performed at an approved facility. A list of approved facilities may be found at http://www.cms.gov/Medicare/Medicare-General-Information/MedicareApprovedFa cilitie/Bariatric-Surgery.html

Effective for services performed on and after February 12, 2009, Medicare has determined that Type 2 diabetes mellitus is a co-morbidity for purposes of processing bariatric surgery claims.

Effective for dates of service on and after September 24, 2013, the Centers for Medicare & Medicaid Services (CMS) has removed the certified facility requirements for Bariatric Surgery for Treatment of Co-Morbid Conditions Related to Morbid Obesity.

© 2017 Optum360, LLC

Please note the additional national coverage determinations related to bariatric surgery will be consolidated and subsumed into Publication 100-3, Chapter 1, section 100.1. These include sections 40.5, 100.8, 100.11 and 100.14.

- Open Roux-en-Y gastric bypass (RYGBP)
- Laparoscopic Roux-en-Y gastric bypass (RYGBP)
- Laparoscopic adjustable gastric banding (LAGB)
- Open biliopancreatic diversion with duodenal switch (BPD/DS) or gastric reduction duodenal switch (BPD/GRDS)
- Laparoscopic biliopancreatic diversion with duodenal switch (BPD/DS) or gastric reduction duodenal switch (BPD/GRDS)
- Laparoscopic sleeve gastrectomy (LSG) (Effective June 27, 2012, covered at Medicare Administrative Contractor (MAC) discretion.

## 100-04, 32, 150.2

### HCPCS Procedure Codes for Bariatric Surgery

#### A. Covered HCPCS Procedure Codes

For services on or after February 21, 2006, the following HCPCS procedure codes are covered for bariatric surgery:

43770 Laparoscopy, surgical, gastric restrictive procedure; placement of adjustable gastric band (gastric band and subcutaneous port components).

43644 Laparoscopy, surgical, gastric restrictive procedure; with gastric bypass and Roux-en-Y gastroenterostomy (roux limb 150 cm or less).

43645 Laparoscopy with gastric bypass and small intestine reconstruction to limit absorption. (Do not report 43645 in conjunction with 49320, 43847.)

43845 Gastric restrictive procedure with partial gastrectomy, pylorus-preserving duodenoileostomy and ileoieostomy (50 to 100 cm common channel) to limit absorption (biliopancreatic diversion with duodenal switch).

43846 Gastric restrictive procedure, with gastric bypass for morbid obesity; with short limb (150 cm or less Roux-en-Y gastroenterostomy. (For greater than 150 cm, use 43847.) (For laparoscopic procedure, use 43644.)

43847 With small intestine reconstruction to limit absorption.

43775 Laparoscopy, surgical, gastric restrictive procedure; longitudinal gastrectomy (i.e., sleeve gastrectomy) (Effective June 27, 2012, covered at contractor's discretion.)

#### B. Noncovered HCPCS Procedure Codes

For services on or after February 21, 2006, the following HCPCS procedure codes are non-covered for bariatric surgery:

43842 Gastric restrictive procedure, without gastric bypass, for morbid obesity; vertical banded gastroplasty.

NOC code 43999 used to bill for:

Laparoscopic vertical banded gastroplasty

Open sleeve gastrectomy

Laparoscopic sleeve gastrectomy (for contractor non-covered instances)

Open adjustable gastric banding

## 100-04, 32, 150.5

### ICD Diagnosis Codes for BMI Greater Than or Equal to 35

The following ICD-9 diagnosis codes identify BMI >=35 :

V85.35 - Body Mass Index 35.0-35.9, adult

V85.36 - Body Mass Index 36.0-36.9, adult

V85.37 - Body Mass Index 37.0-37.9, adult

V85.38 - Body Mass Index 38.0-38.9, adult

V85.39 - Body Mass Index 39.0-39.9, adult

V85.41 - Body Mass Index 40.0-44.9, adult

V85.42 - Body Mass Index 45.0-49.9, adult

V85.43 - Body Mass Index 50.0-59.9, adult

V85.44 - Body Mass Index 60.0-69.9, adult

V85.45 - Body Mass Index 70.0 and over, adult

The following ICD-10 diagnosis codes identify BMI >=35:

Z6835 - Body Mass Index 35.0-35.9, adult

Z6836 - Body Mass Index 36.0-36.9, adult.

Z6837 - Body Mass Index 37.0-37.9, adult

Z6838 - Body Mass Index 38.0-38.9, adult

Z6839 - Body Mass Index 39.0-39.9, adult

Z6841 - Body Mass Index 40.0-44.9, adult

Z6842 - Body Mass Index 45.0-49.9, adult

Z6843 - Body Mass Index 50.0-59.9, adult

Z6844 - Body Mass Index 60.0-69.9, adult

Z6845 - Body Mass Index 70.0 and over, adult

## 100-04, 32, 150.6

### Claims Guidance for Payment

Covered Bariatric Surgery Procedures for Treatment of Co-Morbid Conditions Related to Morbid Obesity

Contractors shall process covered bariatric surgery claims as follows:

1. Identify bariatric surgery claims.

   Contractors identify inpatient bariatric surgery claims by the presence of ICD-9/ICD-10 diagnosis code 278.01/E66.01as the primary diagnosis (for morbid obesity) and one of the covered ICD-9/ICD-10 procedure codes listed in §150.3.

   Contractors identify practitioner bariatric surgery claims by the presence of ICD-9/ICD-10 diagnosis code 278.01/E66.01 as the primary diagnosis (for morbid obesity) and one of the covered HCPCS procedure codes listed in §150.2.

2. Perform facility certification validation for all bariatric surgery claims on a pre-pay basis up to and including date of service September 23, 2013.

   A list of approved facilities are found at the link noted in section 150.1, section A, above.

3. Review bariatric surgery claims data and determine whether a pre- or post-pay sample of bariatric surgery claims need further review to assure that the beneficiary has a BMI =35 (V85.35-V85.45/Z68.35-Z68.45) (see ICD-10 equivalents above in section 150.5), and at least one co-morbidity related to obesity

   The A/B MAC medical director may define the appropriate method for addressing the obesity-related co-morbid requirement.

   Effective for dates of service on and after September 24, 2013, CMS has removed the certified facility requirements for Bariatric Surgery for Treatment of Co-Morbid Conditions Related to Morbid Obesity.

NOTE: If ICD-9/ICD-10 diagnosis code 278.01/E66.01 is present, but a covered procedure code (listed in §150.2 or §150.3) is/are not present, the claim is not for bariatric surgery and should be processed under normal procedures.

## 100-04, 32, 161

### Intracranial Percutaneous Transluminal Angioplasty (PTA) With Stenting

#### A. Background

In the past, PTA to treat obstructive lesions of the cerebral arteries was non-covered by Medicare because the safety and efficacy of the procedure had not been established. This national coverage determination (NCD) meant that the procedure was also non-covered for beneficiaries participating in Food and Drug Administration (FDA)-approved investigational device exemption (IDE) clinical trials.

#### B. Policy

On February 9, 2006, a request for reconsideration of this NCD initiated a national coverage analysis. CMS reviewed the evidence and determined that intracranial PTA with stenting is reasonable and necessary under §1862(a)(1)(A) of the Social Security Act for the treatment of cerebral vessels (as specified in The National Coverage Determinations Manual, Chapter 1, part 1, section 20.7) only when furnished in accordance with FDA-approved protocols governing Category B IDE clinical trials. All other indications for intracranial PTA with stenting remain non-covered.

#### C. Billing

Providers of covered intracranial PTA with stenting shall use Category B IDE billing requirements, as listed above in section 68.4. In addition to these requirements, providers must bill the appropriate procedure and diagnosis codes for the date of service to receive payment. That is, under Part A, providers must bill intracranial PTA using ICD-9-CM procedure codes 00.62 and 00.65, if ICD-9-CM is applicable, or, if ICD-10-PCS is applicable, ICD-10-PCS procedure codes 037G34Z, 037G3DZ, 037G3ZZ, 037G44Z, 037G4DZ, 037G4ZZ, 03CG3ZZ, 057L3DZ, 057L4DZ and 05CL3ZZ. ICD-9-CM diagnosis code 437.0 or ICD-10-CM diagnosis code 167.2applies, depending on the date of service.

Under Part B, providers must bill HCPCS procedure code 37799. If ICD-9-CM is applicable ICD-9-CM diagnosis code 437.0 or if ICD-10-CM is applicable,ICD-10-CM diagnosis code 167.2 applies.

NOTE: ICD- codes are subject to modification. Providers must always ensure they are using the latest and most appropriate codes.

## 100-04, 32, 190

### Billing Requirements for Extracorporeal Photopheresis

Effective for dates of services on and after December 19, 2006, Medicare has expanded coverage for extracorporeal photopheresis for patients with acute cardiac allograft rejection whose disease is refractory to standard immunosuppresive drug treatment and patients with chronic graft versus host disease whose disease is refractory to standard immunosuppresive drug treatment. (See Pub. 100-3, chapter 1, section 110.4, for complete coverage guidelines).

Effective for claims with dates of service on or after April 30, 2012, CMS has expanded coverage for extracorporeal photopheresis for the treatment of BOS following lung allograft transplantation only when extracorporeal photopheresis is provided under a clinical research study that meets specific requirements to assess the effect of extracorporeal photopheresis for the treatment of BOS following lung allograft transplantation. Further coverage criteria is outlined in Publication 100-3, Section 110.4 of the NCD.

## 100-04, 32, 190.2

### Healthcare Common Procedural Coding System (HCPCS), Applicable Diagnosis Codes and Procedure Code

The following HCPCS procedure code is used for billing extracorporeal photopheresis:

- 36522 - Photopheresis, extracorporeal

The following are the applicable ICD-9-CM diagnosis codes for the new expanded coverage:

- 996.83 - Complications of transplanted heart, or,
- 996.85 - Complications of transplanted bone marrow, or,
- 996.88 – Complications of transplanted organ, stem cell

Effective for services for BOS following lung allograft transplantation the following is a list of applicable ICD-9-CM diagnosis codes:

- 996.84 – Complications of transplanted lung
- 491.9 - Unspecified chronic bronchitis
- 491.20 – Obstructive chronic bronchitis without exacerbation
- 491.21 – Obstructive chronic bronchitis with (acute) exacerbation
- 496 – Chronic airway obstruction, not elsewhere classified

The following is the applicable ICD-9-CM procedure code for the new expanded coverage:

- 99.88 - Therapeutic photopheresis

NOTE: Contractors shall edit for an appropriate oncological and autoimmune disorder diagnosis for payment of extracorporeal photopheresis according to the NCD.

Effective for claims with dates of service on or after April 30, 2012, in addition to HCPCS 36522, the following ICD-9-CM codes are applicable for extracorporeal photopheresis for the treatment of BOS following lung allograft transplantation only when extracorporeal photopheresis is provided under a clinical research study as outlined in Section 190 above:

A reference listing of ICD-9 CM and ICD-10-CM coding and descriptions is listed V70.7 below:

| ICD9 | Long Description | ICD10 | ICD10 Description |
|------|------------------|-------|-------------------|
| 491.20 | Obstructive chronic | J44.9 | Chronic obstructive bronchitis without exacerbation pulmonary disease, unspecified |
| 491.21 | Obstructive chronic bronchitis with (acute) exacerbation | J44.1 | Chronic obstructive pulmonary disease with (acute) exacerbation |
| 491.9 | Unspecified chronic bronchitis | J42 | Unspecified chronic bronchitis |
| 496 | Chronic airway obstruction, not elsewhere classified | J44.9 | Chronic obstructive pulmonary disease, unspecified |
| 996.84 | Complications of transplanted lung | T86.810 | Lung transplant rejection |
| 996.84 | Complications of transplanted lung | T86.811 | Lung transplant failure |
| 996.84 | Complications of transplanted lung | T86.812 | Lung transplant infection (not recommended for extracorporeal photopheresis coverage) |
| 996.84 | Complications of transplanted lung | T86.818 | Other complications of lung transplant |
| 996.84 | Complications of transplanted lung | T86.819 | Unspecified complication of lung transplant |
| 996.88 | Complications of Transplanted organ, Stem cell | T86.5 | Complications of Stem Cell Transplant |
| V70.7 | Examination of participant in clinical trial | Z00.6 | Encounter for examination for normal comparison and control in clinical research program (needed for CED) |

Contractors must also report modifier Q0 - (investigational clinical service provided in a clinical research study that is in an approved research study) or Q1 (routine clinical service provided in a clinical research study that is in an approved clinical research study) as appropriate on these claims. Contractors must use diagnosis code V70.7/Z00.6 and condition code 30 (A/B MAC (A) only), along with value code D4 and the 8-digit clinical identifier number (A/MACs only) for these claims.

## 100-04, 32, 190.3

### Medicare Summary Notices (MSNs), Remittance Advice Remark Codes (RAs) and Claim Adjustment Reason Code

Contractors shall continue to use the appropriate existing messages that they have in place when denying claims submitted that do not meet the Medicare coverage criteria for extracorporeal photopheresis.

Contractors shall deny claims when the service is not rendered to an inpatient or outpatient of a hospital, including critical access hospitals (CAHs) using the following codes:

- Claim Adjustment Reason code: 58 – "Claim/service denied/reduced because treatment was deemed by payer to have been rendered in an inappropriate or invalid place of service."
- MSN 16.2 - "This service cannot be paid when provided in this location/facility." Spanish translation: "Este servicio no se puede pagar cuando es suministrado en esta sitio/facilidad." (Include either MSN 36.1 or 36.2 dependant on liablity.)
- RA MA 30 - "Missing/incomplete/invalid type of bill." (FIs and A/MACs only)
- Group Code - CO (Contractual Obligations) or PR (Patient Responsibility) dependant on liability. Contractors shall return to provider/ return as unprocessable claims for BOS containing HCPCS procedure code 36522 along with one of the following ICD-9-CM diagnosis codes: 996.84, 491.9, 491.20, 491.21, and 496 but is missing Diagnosis code V70.7 (as secondary diagnosis, Institutional only), Condition code 30 Institutional claims only), Clinical trial modifier Q0. Use the following messages:
  — CARC 4 – The procedure code is inconsistent with the modifier used or a required modifier is missing. Note: Refer to the 835 Healthcare Policy Identification Segment (loop 2110 Service Payment Information REF), if present.
  — RARC MA 130 – Your claim contains incomplete and/or invalid information, and no appeal rights are afforded because the claim is unprocessable. Please submit a new claim with the complete/correct information.
  — RARC M16 – Alert: Please see our web site, mailings, or bulletins for more details concerning this policy/procedure/decision.

## 100-04, 32, 220.1

### 220.1 - General

Effective for services on or after September 29, 2008, the Center for Medicare & Medicaid Services (CMS) made the decision that Thermal Intradiscal Procedures (TIPS) are not reasonable and necessary for the treatment of low back pain. Therefore, TIPs are non-covered. Refer to Pub.100-3, Medicare National Coverage Determination (NCD) Manual Chapter 1, Part 2, Section 150.11, for further information on the NCD.

## 100-04, 32, 290.1.1

### Coding Requirements for TAVR Services Furnished on or After January 1, 2013

Beginning January 1, 2013, the following are the applicable Current Procedural Terminology (CPT) codes for TAVR:

- 33361 Transcatheter aortic valve replacement (TAVR/TAVI) with prosthetic valve; percutaneous femoral artery approach
- 33362 Transcatheter aortic valve replacement (TAVR/TAVI) with prosthetic valve; open femoral approach
- 33363 Transcatheter aortic valve replacement (TAVR/TAVI) with prosthetic valve; open axillary artery approach
- 33364 Transcatheter aortic valve replacement (TAVR/TAVI) with prosthetic valve; open iliac artery approach
- 3336 Transcatheter aortic valve replacement (TAVR/TAVI) with prosthetic valve; transaortic approach (e.g., median sternotomy, mediastinotomy)
- 0318T Transcatheter aortic valve replacement (TAVR/TAVI) with prosthetic valve; transapical approach (e.g., left thoracotomy)

Beginning January 1, 2014, temporary CPT code 0318T above is retired. TAVR claims with dates of service on and after January 1, 2014 shall instead use permanent CPT code:

- 33366 Transcatheter aortic valve replacement (TAVR/TAVI) with prosthetic valve; transapical exposure (e.g., left thoracotomy)

## 100-04, 32, 290.2

### Claims Processing Requirements for TAVR Services on Professional Claims

#### Place of Service (POS) Professional Claims

Effective for claims with dates of service on and after May 1, 2012, place of service (POS) code 21 shall be used for TAVR services. All other POS codes shall be denied.

The following messages shall be used when Medicare contractors deny TAVR claims for POS:

Claim Adjustment Reason Code (CARC) 58: "Treatment was deemed by the payer to have been rendered in an inappropriate or invalid place of service. NOTE: Refer to the 835 Healthcare Policy Identification Segment (loop 2110 Service Payment Information REF), if present."

Remittance advice remark code (RARC) N428: "Not covered when performed in this place of service."

Medicare Summary Notice (MSN) 21.25: "This service was denied because Medicare only covers this service in certain settings."

Spanish Version: "El servicio fue denegado porque Medicare solamente lo cubre en ciertas situaciones."

#### Professional Claims Modifier -62

For TAVR claims processed on or after July 1, 2013, contractors shall pay claim lines with 0256T, 0257T, 0258T, 0259T, 33361, 33362, 33363, 33364, 33365 & 0318T only when billed with modifier -62. Claim lines billed without modifier -62 shall be returned as unprocessable.

Beginning January 1, 2014, temporary CPT code 0318T above is retired. TAVR claims with dates of service on and after January 1, 2014 shall instead use permanent CPT code 33366.

The following messages shall be used when Medicare contractors return TAVR claims billed without modifier -62 as unprocessable:

CARC 4: "The procedure code is inconsistent with the modifier used or a required modifier is missing. Note: Refer to the 835 Healthcare Policy Identification Segment (loop 2110 Service Payment Information REF), if present."

RARC N29: "Missing documentation/orders/notes/summary/report/chart."

RARC MA130: "Your claim contains incomplete and/or invalid information, and no appeal rights are afforded because the claim is unprocessable. Please submit a new claim with the complete/correct information."

#### Professional Claims Modifier -Q0

For claims processed on or after July 1, 2013, contractors shall pay TAVR claim lines for 0256T, 0257T, 0258T, 0259T, 33361, 33362, 33363, 33364, 33365 & 0318T when billed with modifier -Q0. Claim lines billed without modifier -Q0 shall be returned as unprocessable.

Beginning January 1, 2014, temporary CPT code 0318T above is retired. TAVR claims with dates of service on and after January 1, 2014 shall instead use permanent CPT code 33366.

The following messages shall be used when Medicare contractors return TAVR claims billed without modifier -Q0 as unprocessable:

CARC 4: "The procedure code is inconsistent with the modifier used or a required modifier is missing. Note: Refer to the 835 Healthcare Policy Identification Segment (loop 2110 Service Payment Information REF), if present."

RARC N29: "Missing documentation/orders/notes/summary/report/chart."

RARC MA130: "Your claim contains incomplete and/or invalid information, and no appeal rights are afforded because the claim is unprocessable. Please submit a new claim with the complete/correct information."

For claims processed on or after July 1, 2013, contractors shall pay TAVR claim lines for 0256T, 0257T, 0258T, 0259T, 33361, 33362, 33363, 33364, 33365 & 0318T when billed with diagnosis code V70.7 (ICD-10=Z00.6). Claim lines billed without diagnosis code V70.7 (ICD-10=Z00.6) shall be returned as unprocessable.

Beginning January 1, 2014, temporary CPT code 0318T above is retired. TAVR claims with dates of service on and after January 1, 2014 shall instead use permanent CPT code 33366.

The following messages shall be used when Medicare contractors return TAVR claims billed without diagnosis code V70.7 (ICD-10=Z00.6) as unprocessable:

CARC 16: "Claim/service lacks information which is needed for adjudication. At least one Remark Code must be provided (may be comprised of either the NCPDP Reject Reason Code, or Remittance Advice Remark Code that is not an ALERT)."

RARC M76: "Missing/incomplete/invalid diagnosis or condition"

RARC MA130: "Your claim contains incomplete and/or invalid information, and no appeal rights are afforded because the claim is unprocessable. Please submit a new claim with the complete/correct information."

#### Professional Claims 8-digit ClinicalTrials.gov Identifier Number

For claims processed on or after July 1, 2013, contractors shall pay TAVR claim lines for 0256T, 0257T, 0258T, 0259T, 33361, 33362, 33363, 33364, 33365 & 0318T when billed with the numeric, 8-digit clinicaltrials.gov identifier number preceded by the two alpha characters "CT" when placed in Field 19 of paper Form CMS-1500, or when entered without the "CT" prefix in the electronic 837P in Loop 2300REF02(REF01=P4).

Claim lines billed without an 8-digit clinicaltrials.gov identifier number shall be returned as unprocessable.

Beginning January 1, 2014, temporary CPT code 0318T above is retired. TAVR claims with dates of service on and after January 1, 2014 shall instead use permanent CPT code 33366.

The following messages shall be used when Medicare contractors return TAVR claims billed without an 8-digit clinicaltrials.gov identifier number as unprocessable:

CARC 16: "Claim/service lacks information which is needed for adjudication. At least one Remark Code must be provided (may be comprised of either NCPDP Reject Reason Code, or Remittance Advice Remark Code that is not an ALERT)."

RARC MA50: "Missing/incomplete/invalid Investigational Device Exemption number for FDA-approved clinical trial services."

RARC MA130: "Your claim contains incomplete and/or invalid information, and no appeal rights are afforded because the claim is unprocessable. Please submit a new claim with the complete/correct information."

NOTE: Clinicaltrials.gov identifier numbers for TAVR are listed on our website:

(http://www.cms.gov/Medicare/Coverage/Coverage-with-Evidence-Development/Transcatheter-Aortic-Valve-Replacement-TAVR-.html)

290.3 - Claims Processing Requirements for TAVR Services on Inpatient Hospital Claims

(Rev.2827. Issued: 11-29-13, Effective: 01-01-14, Implementation: 01-06-14)

Inpatient hospitals shall bill for TAVR on an 11X TOB effective for discharges on or after May 1, 2012. Refer to Section 69 of this chapter for further guidance on billing under CED.

Inpatient hospital discharges for TAVR shall be covered when billed with:

- V70.7 and Condition Code 30.

- An 8-digit clinicaltrials.gov identifier number listed on the CMS website (effective July 1, 2013)

Inpatient hospital discharges for TAVR shall be rejected when billed without:

- V70.7 and Condition Code 30.

- An 8-digit clinicaltrials.gov identifier number listed on the CMS website (effective July 1, 2013)

Claims billed by hospitals not participating in the trial/registry shall be rejected with the following messages:

CARC: 50 -These are non-covered services because this is not deemed a "medical necessity" by the payer.

RARC N386 - This decision was based on a National Coverage Determination (NCD). An NCD provides a coverage determination as to whether a particular item or service is covered. A copy of this policy is available at http://www.cms.hhs.gov/mcd/search.asp. If you do not have web access, you may contact the contractor to request a copy of the NCD.

#### Group Code –Contractual Obligation (CO)

MSN 16.77 – This service/item was not covered because it was not provided as part of a qualifying trial/study. (Este servicio/artículo no fue cubierto porque no estaba incluido como parte de un ensayo clínico/estudio calificado.)

## 100-04, 32, 290.3

### Claims Processing Requirements for TAVR Services on Inpatient Hospital Claims

Inpatient hospitals shall bill for TAVR on an 11X TOB effective for discharges on or after May 1, 2012. Refer to Section 69 of this chapter for further guidance on billing under CED.

Inpatient hospital discharges for TAVR shall be covered when billed with:

- V70.7 and Condition Code 30.

- An 8-digit clinicaltrials.gov identifier number listed on the CMS website (effective July 1, 2013)

Inpatient hospital discharges for TAVR shall be rejected when billed without:

- V70.7 and Condition Code 30.

- An 8-digit clinicaltrials.gov identifier number listed on the CMS website (effective July 1, 2013)

Claims billed by hospitals not participating in the trial/registry shall be rejected with the following messages:

CARC: 50 -These are non-covered services because this is not deemed a "medical necessity" by the payer.

RARC N386 - This decision was based on a National Coverage Determination (NCD). An NCD provides a coverage determination as to whether a particular item or service is covered. A copy of this policy is available at http://www.cms.hhs.gov/mcd/search.asp. If you do not have web access, you may contact the contractor to request a copy of the NCD.

Group Code –Contractual Obligation (CO)

MSN 16.77 – This service/item was not covered because it was not provided as part of a qualifying trial/study. (Este servicio/artículo no fue cubierto porque no estaba incluido como parte de un ensayo clínico/estudio calificado.)

## 100-04, 32, 290.4

### Claims Processing Requirements for TAVR Services for Medicare Advantage (MA) Plan Participants

MA plans are responsible for payment of TAVR services for MA plan participants. Medicare coverage for TAVR is included under section 310.1 of the NCD Manual (Routine Costs in Clinical Trials).

## 100-04, 32, 320.1

### Coding Requirements for Artificial Hearts Furnished Before May 1, 2008

Effective for discharges before May 1, 2008, Medicare does not cover the use of artificial hearts, either as a permanent replacement for a human heart or as a temporary life-support system until a human heart becomes available for transplant (often referred to a "bridge to transplant").

## 100-04, 32, 320.2

### Coding Requirements for Artificial Hearts Furnished On or After May 1, 2008

Effective for discharges on or after May 1, 2008, the use of artificial hearts will be covered by Medicare under Coverage with Evidence Development (CED) when beneficiaries are enrolled in a clinical study that meets all of the criteria listed in IOM Pub. 100-3, Medicare NCD Manual, section 20.9.

#### Claims Coding

For claims with dates of service on or after May 1, 2008, artificial hearts in the context of an approved clinical study for a Category A IDE, refer to section 69 in this manual for more detail on CED billing. Appropriate ICD-10 diagnosis and procedure codes are included below:

| ICD-10 Diagnosis Code | Definition | Discharges Effective |
|---|---|---|
| I09.81 | Rheumatic heart failure | On or After ICD-10 Implementation |
| I11.0 | Hypertensive heart disease with heart failure | |
| I13.0 | Hypertensive heart and chronic kidney disease with heart failure and stage 1 through stage 4 chronic kidney disease, or unspecified chronic kidney disease | |
| I13.2 | Hypertensive heart and chronic kidney disease with heart failure and with stage 5 chronic kidney disease, or end stage renal disease | |
| I20.0 | Unstable angina | |
| I21.01 | ST elevation (STEMI) myocardial infarction involving left main coronary artery | |
| I21.02 | ST elevation (STEMI) myocardial infarction involving left anterior descending coronary artery | |
| I21.09 | ST elevation (STEMI) myocardial infarction involving other coronary artery of anterior wall | |
| I21.11 | ST elevation (STEMI) myocardial infarction involving right coronary artery | |
| I21.19 | ST elevation (STEMI) myocardial infarction involving other coronary artery of inferior wall | |
| I21.21 | ST elevation (STEMI) myocardial infarction involving left circumflex coronary artery | |
| I21.29 | ST elevation (STEMI) myocardial infarction involving other sites | |
| I21.3 | ST elevation (STEMI) myocardial infarction of unspecified site | |
| I21.4 | Non-ST elevation (NSTEMI) myocardial infarction | |
| I22.0 | Subsequent ST elevation (STEMI) myocardial infarction of anterior wall | |
| I22.1 | Subsequent ST elevation (STEMI) myocardial infarction of inferior wall | |
| I22.2 | Subsequent non-ST elevation (NSTEMI) myocardial infarction | |
| I22.8 | Subsequent ST elevation (STEMI) myocardial infarction of other sites | |
| I22.9 | Subsequent ST elevation (STEMI) myocardial infarction of unspecified site | |
| I24.0 | Acute coronary thrombosis not resulting in myocardial infarction | |

| ICD-10 Diagnosis Code | Definition | Discharges Effective |
|---|---|---|
| I24.1 | Dressler's syndrome | On or After ICD-10 Implementation |
| I24.8 | Other forms of acute ischemic heart disease | |
| I24.9 | Acute ischemic heart disease, unspecified | |
| I25.10 | Atherosclerotic heart disease of native coronary artery without angina pectoris | |
| I25.110 | Atherosclerotic heart disease of native coronary artery with unstable angina pectoris | |
| I25.111 | Atherosclerotic heart disease of native coronary artery with angina pectoris with documented spasm | |
| I25.118 | Atherosclerotic heart disease of native coronary artery with other forms of angina pectoris | |
| I25.119 | Atherosclerotic heart disease of native coronary artery with unspecified angina pectoris | |
| I25.5 | Ischemic cardiomyopathy | |
| I25.6 | Silent myocardial ischemia | |
| I25.700 | Atherosclerosis of coronary artery bypass graft(s), unspecified, with unstable angina pectoris | |
| I25.701 | Atherosclerosis of coronary artery bypass graft(s), unspecified, with angina pectoris with documented spasm | |
| I25.708 | Atherosclerosis of coronary artery bypass graft(s), unspecified, with other forms of angina pectoris | |
| I25.709 | Atherosclerosis of coronary artery bypass graft(s), unspecified, with unspecified angina pectoris | |
| I25.710 | Atherosclerosis of autologous vein coronary artery bypass graft(s) with unstable angina pectoris | |
| I25.711 | Atherosclerosis of autologous vein coronary artery bypass graft(s) with angina pectoris with documented spasm | |
| I25.718 | Atherosclerosis of autologous vein coronary artery bypass graft(s) with other forms of angina pectoris | |
| I25.719 | Atherosclerosis of autologous vein coronary artery bypass graft(s) with unspecified angina pectoris | |
| I25.720 | Atherosclerosis of autologous artery coronary artery bypass graft(s) with unstable angina pectoris | |
| I25.721 | Atherosclerosis of autologous artery coronary artery bypass graft(s) with angina pectoris with documented spasm | |
| I25.728 | Atherosclerosis of autologous artery coronary artery bypass graft(s) with other forms of angina pectoris | |
| I25.729 | Atherosclerosis of autologous artery coronary artery bypass graft(s) with unspecified angina pectoris | |
| I25.730 | Atherosclerosis of nonautologous biological coronary artery bypass graft(s) with unstable angina pectoris | |
| I25.731 | Atherosclerosis of nonautologous biological coronary artery bypass graft(s) with angina pectoris with documented spasm | |
| I25.738 | Atherosclerosis of nonautologous biological coronary artery bypass graft(s) with other forms of angina pectoris | |
| I25.739 | Atherosclerosis of nonautologous biological coronary artery bypass graft(s) with unspecified angina pectoris | |
| I25.750 | Atherosclerosis of native coronary artery of transplanted heart with unstable angina | |
| I25.751 | Atherosclerosis of native coronary artery of transplanted heart with angina pectoris with documented spasm | |
| I25.758 | Atherosclerosis of native coronary artery of transplanted heart with other forms of angina pectoris | |

| ICD-10 Diagnosis Code | Definition | Discharges Effective |
|---|---|---|
| I25.759 | Atherosclerosis of native coronary artery of transplanted heart with unspecified angina pectoris | On or After ICD-10 Implementation |
| I25.760 | Atherosclerosis of bypass graft of coronary artery of transplanted heart with unstable angina | |
| I25.761 | Atherosclerosis of bypass graft of coronary artery of transplanted heart with angina pectoris with documented spasm | |
| I25.768 | Atherosclerosis of bypass graft of coronary artery of transplanted heart with other forms of angina pectoris | |
| I25.769 | Atherosclerosis of bypass graft of coronary artery of transplanted heart with unspecified angina pectoris | |
| I25.790 | Atherosclerosis of other coronary artery bypass graft(s) with unstable angina pectoris | |
| I25.791 | Atherosclerosis of other coronary artery bypass graft(s) with angina pectoris with documented spasm | |
| I25.798 | Atherosclerosis of other coronary artery bypass graft(s) with other forms of angina pectoris | |
| I25.799 | Atherosclerosis of other coronary artery bypass graft(s) with unspecified angina pectoris | |
| I25.810 | Atherosclerosis of coronary artery bypass graft(s) without angina pectoris | |
| I25.811 | Atherosclerosis of native coronary artery of transplanted heart without angina pectoris | |
| I25.812 | Atherosclerosis of bypass graft of coronary artery of transplanted heart without angina pectoris | |
| I25.89 | Other forms of chronic ischemic heart disease | |
| I25.9 | Chronic ischemic heart disease, unspecified | |
| I34.0 | Nonrheumatic mitral (valve) insufficiency | |
| I34.1 | Nonrheumatic mitral (valve) prolapse | |
| I34.2 | Nonrheumatic mitral (valve) stenosis | |
| I34.8 | Other nonrheumatic mitral valve disorders | |
| I34.9 | Nonrheumatic mitral valve disorder, unspecified | |
| I35.0 | Nonrheumatic aortic (valve) stenosis | |
| I35.1 | Nonrheumatic aortic (valve) insufficiency | |
| I35.2 | Nonrheumatic aortic (valve) stenosis with insufficiency | |
| I35.8 | Other nonrheumatic aortic valve disorders | |
| I35.9 | Nonrheumatic aortic valve disorder, unspecified | |
| I36.0 | Nonrheumatic tricuspid (valve) stenosis | |
| I36.1 | Nonrheumatic tricuspid (valve) insufficiency | |
| I36.2 | Nonrheumatic tricuspid (valve) stenosis with insufficiency | |
| I36.8 | Other nonrheumatic tricuspid valve disorders | |
| I36.9 | Nonrheumatic tricuspid valve disorder, unspecified | |
| I37.0 | Nonrheumatic pulmonary valve stenosis | |
| I37.1 | Nonrheumatic pulmonary valve insufficiency | |
| I37.2 | Nonrheumatic pulmonary valve stenosis with insufficiency | |
| I37.8 | Other nonrheumatic pulmonary valve disorders | |
| I37.9 | Nonrheumatic pulmonary valve disorder, unspecified | |
| I38 | Endocarditis, valve unspecified | |
| I39 | Endocarditis and heart valve disorders in diseases classified elsewhere | |
| I42.0 | Dilated cardiomyopathy | |
| I42.2 | Other hypertrophic cardiomyopathy | |
| I42.3 | Endomyocardial (eosinophilic) disease | |
| I42.4 | Endocardial fibroelastosis | |
| I42.5 | Other restrictive cardiomyopathy | |
| I42.6 | Alcoholic cardiomyopathy | |
| I42.7 | Cardiomyopathy due to drug and external agent | |

| ICD-10 Diagnosis Code | Definition | Discharges Effective |
|---|---|---|
| I42.8 | Other cardiomyopathies | On or After ICD-10 Implementation |
| I42.9 | Cardiomyopathy, unspecified | |
| I43 | Cardiomyopathy in diseases classified elsewhere | |
| I46.2 | Cardiac arrest due to underlying cardiac condition | |
| I46.8 | Cardiac arrest due to other underlying condition | |
| I46.9 | Cardiac arrest, cause unspecified | |
| I47.0 | Re-entry ventricular arrhythmia | |
| I47.1 | Supraventricular tachycardia | |
| I47.2 | Ventricular tachycardia | |
| I47.9 | Paroxysmal tachycardia, unspecified | |
| I48.0 | Atrial fibrillation | |
| I48.1 | Atrial flutter | |
| I49.01 | Ventricular fibrillation | |
| I49.02 | Ventricular flutter | |
| I49.1 | Atrial premature depolarization | |
| I49.2 | Junctional premature depolarization | |
| I49.3 | Ventricular premature depolarization | |
| I49.40 | Unspecified premature depolarization | |
| I49.49 | Other premature depolarization | |
| I49.5 | Sick sinus syndrome | |
| I49.8 | Other specified cardiac arrhythmias | |
| I49.9 | Cardiac arrhythmia, unspecified | |
| I50.1 | Left ventricular failure | |
| I50.20 | Unspecified systolic (congestive) heart failure | |
| I50.21 | Acute systolic (congestive) heart failure | |
| I50.22 | Chronic systolic (congestive) heart failure | |
| I50.23 | Acute on chronic systolic (congestive) heart failure | |
| I50.30 | Unspecified diastolic (congestive) heart failure | |
| I50.31 | Acute diastolic (congestive) heart failure | |
| I50.32 | Chronic diastolic (congestive) heart failure | |
| I50.33 | Acute on chronic diastolic (congestive) heart failure | |
| I50.40 | Unspecified combined systolic (congestive) and diastolic (congestive) heart failure | |
| I50.41 | Acute combined systolic (congestive) and diastolic (congestive) heart failure | |
| I50.42 | Chronic combined systolic (congestive) and diastolic (congestive) heart failure | |
| I50.43 | Acute on chronic combined systolic (congestive) and diastolic (congestive) heart failure | |
| I50.9 | Heart failure, unspecified | |
| I51.4 | Myocarditis, unspecified | |
| I51.9 | Heart disease, unspecified | |
| I52 | Other heart disorders in diseases classified elsewhere | |
| I97.0 | Postcardiotomy syndrome | |
| I97.110 | Postprocedural cardiac insufficiency following cardiac surgery | |
| I97.111 | Postprocedural cardiac insufficiency following other surgery | |
| I97.120 | Postprocedural cardiac arrest following cardiac surgery | |
| I97.121 | Postprocedural cardiac arrest following other surgery | |
| I97.130 | Postprocedural heart failure following cardiac surgery | |
| I97.131 | Postprocedural heart failure following other surgery | |
| I97.190 | Other postprocedural cardiac functional disturbances following cardiac surgery | |
| I97.191 | Other postprocedural cardiac functional disturbances following other surgery | |
| I97.710 | Intraoperative cardiac arrest during cardiac surgery | |

CPT © 2017 American Medical Association. All Rights Reserved.

© 2017 Optum360, LLC

| ICD-10 Diagnosis Code | Definition | Discharges Effective |
|---|---|---|
| I97.711 | Intraoperative cardiac arrest during other surgery | On or After ICD-10 Implementation |
| I97.790 | Other intraoperative cardiac functional disturbances during cardiac surgery | |
| I97.791 | Other intraoperative cardiac functional disturbances during other surgery | |
| I97.88 | Other intraoperative complications of the circulatory system, not elsewhere classified | |
| I97.89 | Other postprocedural complications and disorders of the circulatory system, not elsewhere classified | |
| M32.11 | Endocarditis in systemic lupus erythematosus | |
| O90.89 | Other complications of the puerperium, not elsewhere classified | |
| Q20.0 | Common arterial trunk | |
| Q20.1 | Double outlet right ventricle | |
| Q20.2 | Double outlet left ventricle | |
| Q20.3 | Discordant ventriculoarterial connection | |
| Q20.4 | Double inlet ventricle | |
| Q20.5 | Discordant atrioventricular connection | |
| Q20.6 | Isomerism of atrial appendages | |
| Q20.8 | Other congenital malformations of cardiac chambers and connections | |
| Q20.9 | Congenital malformation of cardiac chambers and connections, unspecified | |
| Q21.0 | Ventricular septal defect | |
| Q21.1 | Atrial septal defect | |
| Q21.2 | Atrioventricular septal defect | |
| Q21.3 | Tetralogy of Fallot | |
| Q21.4 | Aortopulmonary septal defect | |
| Q21.8 | Other congenital malformations of cardiac septa | |
| Q21.9 | Congenital malformation of cardiac septum, unspecified | |
| Q22.0 | Pulmonary valve atresia | |
| Q22.1 | Congenital pulmonary valve stenosis | |
| Q22.2 | Congenital pulmonary valve insufficiency | |
| Q22.3 | Other congenital malformations of pulmonary valve | |
| Q22.4 | Congenital tricuspid stenosis | |
| Q22.5 | Ebstein's anomaly | |
| Q22.6 | Hypoplastic right heart syndrome | |
| Q22.8 | Other congenital malformations of tricuspid valve | |
| Q22.9 | Congenital malformation of tricuspid valve, unspecified | |
| Q23.0 | Congenital stenosis of aortic valve | |
| Q23.1 | Congenital insufficiency of aortic valve | |
| Q23.2 | Congenital mitral stenosis | |
| Q23.3 | Congenital mitral insufficiency | |
| Q23.4 | Hypoplastic left heart syndrome | |
| Q23.8 | Other congenital malformations of aortic and mitral valves | |
| Q23.9 | Congenital malformation of aortic and mitral valves, unspecified | |
| Q24.0 | Dextrocardia | |
| Q24.1 | Levocardia | |
| Q24.2 | Cor triatriatum | |
| Q24.3 | Pulmonary infundibular stenosis | |
| Q24.4 | Congenital subaortic stenosis | |
| Q24.5 | Malformation of coronary vessels | |
| Q24.6 | Congenital heart block | |
| Q24.8 | Other specified congenital malformations of heart | |
| Q24.9 | Congenital malformation of heart, unspecified | |
| R00.1 | Bradycardia, unspecified | |
| R57.0 | Cardiogenic shock | |

| ICD-10 Diagnosis Code | Definition | Discharges Effective |
|---|---|---|
| T82.221A | Breakdown (mechanical) of biological heart valve graft, initial encounter | On or After ICD-10 Implementation |
| T82.222A | Displacement of biological heart valve graft, initial encounter | |
| T82.223A | Leakage of biological heart valve graft, initial encounter | |
| T82.228A | Other mechanical complication of biological heart valve graft, initial encounter | |
| T82.512A | Breakdown (mechanical) of artificial heart, initial encounter | |
| T82.514A | Breakdown (mechanical) of infusion catheter, initial encounter | |
| T82.518A | Breakdown (mechanical) of other cardiac and vascular devices and implants, initial encounter | |
| T82.519A | Breakdown (mechanical) of unspecified cardiac and vascular devices and implants, initial encounter | |
| T82.522A | Displacement of artificial heart, initial encounter | |
| T82.524A | Displacement of infusion catheter, initial encounter | |
| T82.528A | Displacement of other cardiac and vascular devices and implants, initial encounter | |
| T82.529A | Displacement of unspecified cardiac and vascular devices and implants, initial encounter | |
| T82.532A | Leakage of artificial heart, initial encounter | |
| T82.534A | Leakage of infusion catheter, initial encounter | |
| T82.538A | Leakage of other cardiac and vascular devices and implants, initial encounter | |
| T82.539A | Leakage of unspecified cardiac and vascular devices and implants, initial encounter | |
| T82.592A | Other mechanical complication of artificial heart, initial encounter | |
| T82.594A | Other mechanical complication of infusion catheter, initial encounter | |
| T82.598A | Other mechanical complication of other cardiac and vascular devices and implants, initial encounter | |
| T82.599A | Other mechanical complication of unspecified cardiac and vascular devices and implants, initial encounter | |
| T86.20 | Unspecified complication of heart transplant | |
| T86.21 | Heart transplant rejection | |
| T86.22 | Heart transplant failure | |
| T86.23 | Heart transplant infection | |
| T86.290 | Cardiac allograft vasculopathy | |
| T86.298 | Other complications of heart transplant | |
| T86.30 | Unspecified complication of heart-lung transplant | |
| T86.31 | Heart-lung transplant rejection | |
| T86.32 | Heart-lung transplant failure | |
| T86.33 | Heart-lung transplant infection | |
| T86.39 | Other complications of heart-lung transplant | |
| Z48.21 | Encounter for aftercare following heart transplant | |
| Z48.280 | Encounter for aftercare following heart-lung transplant | |
| Z94.1 | Heart transplant status | |
| Z94.3 | Heart and lungs transplant status | |
| Z95.9 | Presence of cardiac and vascular implant and graft, unspecified | |
| Q24.0 | Dextrocardia | |
| Q24.1 | Levocardia | |
| Q24.2 | Cor triatriatum | |
| Q24.3 | Pulmonary infundibular stenosis | |
| Q24.4 | Congenital subaortic stenosis | |
| Q24.5 | Malformation of coronary vessels | |
| Q24.6 | Congenital heart block | |
| Q24.8 | Other specified congenital malformations of heart | |

Appendix G — Medicare Internet-only Manuals (IOMs)

| ICD-10 Diagnosis Code | Definition | Discharges Effective |
|---|---|---|
| Q24.9 | Congenital malformation of heart, unspecified | On or After ICD-10 Implementation |
| R00.1 | Bradycardia, unspecified | |
| R57.0 | Cardiogenic shock | |
| T82.221A | Breakdown (mechanical) of biological heart valve graft, initial encounter | |
| T82.222A | Displacement of biological heart valve graft, initial encounter | |
| T82.223A | Leakage of biological heart valve graft, initial encounter | |
| T82.228A | Other mechanical complication of biological heart valve graft, initial encounter | |
| T82.512A | Breakdown (mechanical) of artificial heart, initial encounter | |
| T82.514A | Breakdown (mechanical) of infusion catheter, initial encounter | |
| T82.518A | Breakdown (mechanical) of other cardiac and vascular devices and implants, initial encounter | |
| T82.519A | Breakdown (mechanical) of unspecified cardiac and vascular devices and implants, initial encounter | |
| T82.522A | Displacement of artificial heart, initial encounter | |
| T82.524A | Displacement of infusion catheter, initial encounter | |
| T82.528A | Displacement of other cardiac and vascular devices and implants, initial encounter | |
| T82.529A | Displacement of unspecified cardiac and vascular devices and implants, initial encounter | |
| T82.532A | Leakage of artificial heart, initial encounter | |
| T82.534A | Leakage of infusion catheter, initial encounter | |
| T82.538A | Leakage of other cardiac and vascular devices and implants, initial encounter | |
| T82.539A | Leakage of unspecified cardiac and vascular devices and implants, initial encounter | |
| T82.592A | Other mechanical complication of artificial heart, initial encounter | |
| T82.594A | Other mechanical complication of infusion catheter, initial encounter | |
| T82.598A | Other mechanical complication of other cardiac and vascular devices and implants, initial encounter | |
| T82.599A | Other mechanical complication of unspecified cardiac and vascular devices and implants, initial encounter | |
| T86.20 | Unspecified complication of heart transplant | |
| T86.21 | Heart transplant rejection | |
| T86.22 | Heart transplant failure | |
| T86.23 | Heart transplant infection | |
| T86.290 | Cardiac allograft vasculopathy | |
| T86.298 | Other complications of heart transplant | |
| T86.30 | Unspecified complication of heart-lung transplant | |
| T86.31 | Heart-lung transplant rejection | |
| T86.32 | Heart-lung transplant failure | |
| T86.33 | Heart-lung transplant infection | |
| T86.39 | Other complications of heart-lung transplant | |
| Z48.21 | Encounter for aftercare following heart transplant | |
| Z48.280 | Encounter for aftercare following heart-lung transplant | |
| Z94.1 | Heart transplant status | |
| Z94.3 | Heart and lungs transplant status | |
| Z95.9 | Presence of cardiac and vascular implant and graft, unspecified | |
| 02RK0JZ | Replacement of Right Ventricle with Synthetic Substitute, Open Approach | |
| 02RL0JZ | Revision of Synthetic Substitute in Heart, Open Approach | |
| 02WA0JZ | Revision of Synthetic Substitute in Heart, Open Approach | |

**NOTE:** Total artificial heart is reported with a "cluster" of 2 codes for open replacement with synthetic substitute of the right and left ventricles- 02RK0JZ + 02RL0JZ

## 100-04, 32, 320.3

### Ventricular Assist Devices

Medicare may cover a Ventricular Assist Device (VAD). A VAD is used to assist a damaged or weakened heart in pumping blood. VADs are used as a bridge to a heart transplant, for support of blood circulation post-cardiotomy or destination therapy. Refer to the IOM Pub. 100-3, NCD Manual, section 20.9.1 for coverage criteria.

## 100-04, 32, 320.3.1

### Post-cardiotomy

Post-cardiotomy is the period following open-heart surgery. VADs used for support of blood circulation post-cardiotomy are covered only if they have received approval from the Food and Drug Administration (FDA) for that purpose, and the VADs are used according to the FDA-approved labeling instructions

## 100-04, 32, 320.3.2

### Bridge- to -Transplantation (BTT)

Coverage for BTT is restricted to patients listed for heart transplantation. The Centers for Medicare & Medicaid Services (CMS) has clearly identified that the patient must be active on the waitlist maintained by the Organ Procurement and Transplantation Network. CMS has also removed the general time requirement that patients receive a transplant as soon as medically reasonable.

## 100-04, 32, 370

### Microvolt T-wave Alternans (MTWA)

On March 21, 2006, the Centers for Medicare & Medicaid Services (CMS) began national coverage of microvolt T-wave Alternans (MTWA) diagnostic testing when it was performed using only the spectral analysis (SA) method for the evaluation of patients at risk for sudden cardiac death (SCD) from ventricular arrhythmias and patients who may be candidates for Medicare coverage of the placement of an implantable cardiac defibrillator (ICD).

Effective for claims with dates of service on and after January 13, 2015, Medicare Administrative Contractors (MACs) may determine coverage of MTWA diagnostic testing when it is performed using methods of analysis other than SA for the evaluation of patients at risk for SCD from ventricular arrhythmias. Further information can be found at Publication 100-3, section 20.30, of the National Coverage Determinations Manual.

## 100-04, 32, 370.1

### Coding and Claims Processing for MTWA

Effective for claims with dates of service on and after March 21, 2006, MACs shall accept CPT 93025 (MTWA for assessment of ventricular arrhythmias) for MTWA diagnostic testing for the evaluation of patients at risk for SCD with the SA method of analysis only. All other methods of analysis for MTWA are non-covered.

Effective for claims with dates of service on and after January 13, 2015, MACs shall at their discretion determine coverage for CPT 93025 for MTWA diagnostic testing for the evaluation of patients at risk for SCD with methods of analysis other than SA. The –KX modifier shall be used as an attestation by the practitioner and/or provider of the service that documentation is on file verifying the MTWA was performed using a method of analysis other than SA for the evaluation of patients at risk for SCD from ventricular arrhythmias and that all other NCD criteria was met.

NOTE: The –KX modifier is NOT required on MTWA claims for the evaluation of patients at risk for SCD if the SA analysis method is used.

NOTE: This diagnosis code list/translation was approved by CMS/Coverage. It may or may not be a complete list of covered indications/diagnosis codes that are covered but should serve as a finite starting point.

As this policy indicates, individual A/B MACs within their respective jurisdictions have the discretion to make coverage determinations they deem reasonable and necessary under section 1862(a)1)(A) of the Social Security Act. Therefore, A/B MACs may have additional covered diagnosis codes in their individual policies where contractor discretion is appropriate.

**ICD-9 Codes**

| 410.11 | Acute myocardial infarction of other anterior wall, initial episode of care |
|---|---|
| 410.11 | Acute myocardial infarction of other anterior wall, initial episode of care |
| 410.01 | Acute myocardial infarction of anterolateral wall, initial episode of care |
| 410.11 | Acute myocardial infarction of other anterior wall, initial episode of care |
| 410.31 | Acute myocardial infarction of inferoposterior wall, initial episode of care |
| 410.21 | Acute myocardial infarction of inferolateral wall, initial episode of care |
| 410.41 | Acute myocardial infarction of other inferior wall, initial episode of care |
| 410.81 | Acute myocardial infarction of other specified sites, initial episode of care |

CPT © 2017 American Medical Association. All Rights Reserved.

© 2017 Optum360, LLC

| 410.51 | Acute myocardial infarction of other lateral wall, initial episode of care |
| 410.61 | True posterior wall infarction, initial episode of care |
| 410.81 | Acute myocardial infarction of other specified sites, initial episode of care |
| 410.91 | Acute myocardial infarction of unspecified site, initial episode of care |
| 410.71 | Subendocardial infarction, initial episode of care |
| 410.01 | Acute myocardial infarction of anterolateral wall, initial episode of care |
| 410.11 | Acute myocardial infarction of other anterior wall, initial episode of care |
| 410.21 | Acute myocardial infarction of inferolateral wall, initial episode of care |
| 410.31 | Acute myocardial infarction of inferoposterior wall, initial episode of care |
| 410.41 | Acute myocardial infarction of other inferior wall, initial episode of care |
| 410.71 | Subendocardial infarction, initial episode of care |
| 410.51 | Acute myocardial infarction of other lateral wall, initial episode of care |
| 410.61 | True posterior wall infarction, initial episode of care |
| 410.81 | Acute myocardial infarction of other specified sites, initial episode of care |
| 410.91 | Acute myocardial infarction of unspecified site, initial episode of care |
| 411.89 | Other acute and subacute forms of ischemic heart disease, other |
| 411.89 | Other acute and subacute forms of ischemic heart disease, other |
| 427.1 | Paroxysmal ventricular tachycardia |
| 427.1 | Paroxysmal ventricular tachycardia |
| 427.41 | Ventricular fibrillation |
| 427.42 | Ventricular flutter |
| 780.2 | Syncope and collapse |
| V45.89 | Other postprocedural status |

### ICD-10 Codes

| I21.01 | ST elevation (STEMI) myocardial infarction involving left main coronary artery |
| I21.02 | ST elevation (STEMI) myocardial infarction involving left anterior descending coron |
| I21.09 | ST elevation (STEMI) myocardial infarction involving other coronary artery of anteri |
| I21.09 | ST elevation (STEMI) myocardial infarction involving other coronary artery of anteri |
| I21.11 | ST elevation (STEMI) myocardial infarction involving right coronary artery |
| I21.19 | ST elevation (STEMI) myocardial infarction involving other coronary artery of inferi |
| I21.19 | ST elevation (STEMI) myocardial infarction involving other coronary artery of inferi |
| I21.21 | ST elevation (STEMI) myocardial infarction involving left circumflex coronary artery |
| I21.29 | ST elevation (STEMI) myocardial infarction involving other sites |
| I21.29 | ST elevation (STEMI) myocardial infarction involving other sites |
| I21.29 | ST elevation (STEMI) myocardial infarction involving other sites |
| I21.3 | ST elevation (STEMI) myocardial infarction of unspecified site |
| I21.4 | Non-ST elevation (NSTEMI) myocardial infarction |
| I22.0 | Subsequent ST elevation (STEMI) myocardial infarction of anterior wall |
| I22.0 | Subsequent ST elevation (STEMI) myocardial infarction of anterior wall |
| I22.1 | Subsequent ST elevation (STEMI) myocardial infarction of inferior wall |
| I22.1 | Subsequent ST elevation (STEMI) myocardial infarction of inferior wall |
| I22.1 | Subsequent ST elevation (STEMI) myocardial infarction of inferior wall |
| I22.2 | Subsequent non-ST elevation (NSTEMI) myocardial infarction |
| I22.8 | Subsequent ST elevation (STEMI) myocardial infarction of other sites |
| I22.8 | Subsequent ST elevation (STEMI) myocardial infarction of other sites |
| I22.8 | Subsequent ST elevation (STEMI) myocardial infarction of other sites |
| I22.9 | Subsequent ST elevation (STEMI) myocardial infarction of unspecified site |
| I24.8 | Other forms of acute ischemic heart disease |
| I24.9 | Acute ischemic heart disease, unspecified |
| I47.0 | Re-entry ventricular arrhythmia |
| I47.2 | Ventricular tachycardia |
| I49.01 | Ventricular fibrillation |
| I49.02 | Ventricular flutter |
| R55 | Syncope and collapse |
| Z98.89 | Other specified postprocedural states |

## 100-04, 32, 370.2

### Messaging for MTWA

Effective for claims with dates of service on and after January 13, 2015, MACs shall deny claims for MTWA CPT 93025 with methods of analysis other than SA without modifier -KX using the following messages:

CARC 4: "The procedure code is inconsistent with the modifier used or a required modifier is missing. Note: Refer to the 835 Healthcare Policy Identification Segment (loop 2110 Service Payment Information REF), if present."

RARC N657 – This should be billed with the appropriate code for these services.

Group Code: CO (Contractual Obligation) assigning financial liability to the provider

MSN 15.20 - The following policies [NCD 20.30] were used when we made this decision

Spanish Equivalent - 15.20 - Las siguientes políticas [NCD 20.30] fueron utilizadas cuando se tomó esta decisión.

## 100-04, 32, 380

### Leadless Pacemakers

(Rev. 3815, Issued: 07-28-17, Effective: 01-18-18, Implementation: 08-29-17 - for MAC local edits; January 2, 2018 - for MCS shared edits)

Effective for dates of service on or after January 18, 2017, contractors shall cover leadless pacemakers through Coverage with Evidence Development (CED) when procedures are performed in CMS-approved CED studies. Please refer to the National Coverage Determinations Manual (Publication 100-03, Section 20.8.4) for more information.

## 100-04, 32, 380.1

### Leadless Pacemaker Coding and Billing Requirements for Professional Claims

(Rev. 3815, Issued: 07-28-17, Effective: 01-18-18, Implementation: 08-29-17 - for MAC local edits; January 2, 2018 - for MCS shared edits)

Effective for dates of service on or after January 18, 2017, contractors shall allow the following procedure codes on claims for leadless pacemakers:

0387T Transcatheter insertion or replacement of permanent leadless pacemaker, ventricular

0389T Programming device evaluation (in person) with iterative adjustment of the implantable device to test the function of the device and select optimal permanent programmed values with analysis, review and report, leadless pacemaker system.

0390T Peri-procedural device evaluation (in person) and programming of device system parameters before or after surgery, procedure or test with analysis, review and report, leadless pacemaker system.

0391T Interrogation device evaluation (in person) with analysis, review and report, includes connection, recording and disconnection per patient encounter, leadless pacemaker system.

Effective for dates of service on or after January 18, 2017, contractors shall allow the following ICD-10 diagnosis codes on claims for leadless pacemakers:

Z00.6 – Encounter for examination for normal comparison and control in clinical research program.

## 100-04, 32, 380.1.1

### Leadless Pacemaker Place of Service Restrictions

(Rev. 3815, Issued: 07-28-17, Effective: 01-18-18, Implementation: 08-29-17 - for MAC local edits; January 2, 2018 - for MCS shared edits)

Effective for dates of service on or after January 18, 2017, contractors shall only pay claims for leadless pacemakers when services are provided in one of the following places of service (POS):

POS 06 – Indian Health Service Provider Based Facility

POS 21 – Inpatient Hospital

POS 22 - On Campus-Outpatient Hospital

POS 26 – Military Treatment Facility

## 100-04, 32, 380.1.2

### Leadless Pacemaker Modifier

(Rev. 3815, Issued: 07-28-17, Effective: 01-18-18, Implementation: 08-29-17 - for MAC local edits; January 2, 2018 - for MCS shared edits)

Effective for claims with dates of service on or after January 18, 2017, modifier Q0 – Investigational clinical service provided in a clinical research study that is an approved clinical research study, must also be included.

© 2017 Optum360, LLC

## 100-05, 10.3.2

### Exceptions Process

(Rev. 3367 Issued: 10-07-2015, Effective: 01-01-2016, Implementation: 01-04-2016)

An exception may be made when the patient's condition is justified by documentation indicating that the beneficiary requires continued skilled therapy, i.e., therapy beyond the amount payable under the therapy cap, to achieve their prior functional status or maximum expected functional status within a reasonable amount of time.

No special documentation is submitted to the contractor for exceptions. The clinician is responsible for consulting guidance in the Medicare manuals and in the professional literature to determine if the beneficiary may qualify for the exception because documentation justifies medically necessary services above the caps. The clinician's opinion is not binding on the Medicare contractor who makes the final determination concerning whether the claim is payable.

Documentation justifying the services shall be submitted in response to any Additional Documentation Request (ADR) for claims that are selected for medical review. Follow the documentation requirements in Pub. 100-02, chapter 15, section 220.3. If medical records are requested for review, clinicians may include, at their discretion, a summary that specifically addresses the justification for therapy cap exception.

In making a decision about whether to utilize the exception, clinicians shall consider, for example, whether services are appropriate to--

The patient's condition, including the diagnosis, complexities, and severity;

The services provided, including their type, frequency, and duration;

The interaction of current active conditions and complexities that directly and significantly influence the treatment such that it causes services to exceed caps.

In addition, the following should be considered before using the exception process:

1. Exceptions for Evaluation Services

Evaluation. The CMS will except therapy evaluations from caps after the therapy caps are reached when evaluation is necessary, e.g., to determine if the current status of the beneficiary requires therapy services. For example, the following CPT codes for evaluation procedures may be appropriate:

92521, 92522, 92523, 92524, 92597, 92607, 92608, 92610, 92611, 92612, 92614, 92616, 96105, 96125, 97001, 97002, 97003, 97004.

These codes will continue to be reported as outpatient therapy procedures as listed in the Annual Therapy Update for the current year at: http://www.cms.gov/TherapyServices/05_Annual_Therapy_Update.asp#TopOfPage.

They are not diagnostic tests. Definitions of evaluations and documentation are found in Pub. 100-02, chapter 15, sections 220 and 230.

Other Services. There are a number of sources that suggest the amount of certain services that may be typical, either per service, per episode, per condition, or per discipline. For example, see the CSC - Therapy Cap Report, 3/21/2008, and CSC – Therapy Edits Tables 4/14/2008 at www.cms.hhs.gov/TherapyServices (Studies and Reports), or more recent utilization reports. Professional literature and guidelines from professional associations also provide a basis on which to estimate whether the type, frequency, and intensity of services are appropriate to an individual. Clinicians and contractors should utilize available evidence related to the patient's condition to justify provision of medically necessary services to individual beneficiaries, especially when they exceed caps. Contractors shall not limit medically necessary services that are justified by scientific research applicable to the beneficiary. Neither contractors nor clinicians shall utilize professional literature and scientific reports to justify payment for continued services after an individual's goals have been met earlier than is typical. Conversely, professional literature and scientific reports shall not be used as justification to deny payment to patients whose needs are greater than is typical or when the patient's condition is not represented by the literature.

2. Exceptions for Medically Necessary Services

Clinicians may utilize the process for exception for any diagnosis or condition for which they can justify services exceeding the cap. Regardless of the diagnosis or condition, the patient must also meet other requirements for coverage.

Bill the most relevant diagnosis. As always, when billing for therapy services, the diagnosis code that best relates to the reason for the treatment shall be on the claim, unless there is a compelling reason to report another diagnosis code. For example, when a patient with diabetes is being treated with therapy for gait training due to amputation, the preferred diagnosis is abnormality of gait (which characterizes the treatment). Where it is possible in accordance with State and local laws and the contractors' local coverage determinations, avoid using vague or general diagnoses. When a claim includes several types of services, or where the physician/NPP must supply the diagnosis, it may not be possible to use the most relevant therapy diagnosis code in the primary position. In that case, the relevant diagnosis code should, if possible, be on the claim in another position.

Codes representing the medical condition that caused the treatment are used when there is no code representing the treatment. Complicating conditions are preferably used in non-primary positions on the claim and are billed in the primary position only in the rare circumstance that there is no more relevant code.

The condition or complexity that caused treatment to exceed caps must be related to the therapy goals and must either be the condition that is being treated or a complexity that directly and significantly impacts the rate of recovery of the condition being treated such that it is appropriate to exceed the caps. Documentation for an exception should indicate how the complexity (or combination of complexities) directly and significantly affects treatment for a therapy condition.

If the contractor has determined that certain codes do not characterize patients who require medically necessary services, providers/suppliers may not use those codes, but must utilize a billable diagnosis code allowed by their contractor to describe the patient's condition. Contractors shall not apply therapy caps to services based on the patient's condition, but only on the medical necessity of the service for the condition. If a service would be payable before the cap is reached and is still medically necessary after the cap is reached, that service is excepted.

Contact your contractor for interpretation if you are not sure that a service is applicable for exception.

It is very important to recognize that most conditions would not ordinarily result in services exceeding the cap. Use the KX modifier only in cases where the condition of the individual patient is such that services are APPROPRIATELY provided in an episode that exceeds the cap. Routine use of the KX modifier for all patients with these conditions will likely show up on data analysis as aberrant and invite inquiry. Be sure that documentation is sufficiently detailed to support the use of the modifier.

In justifying exceptions for therapy caps, clinicians and contractors should not only consider the medical diagnoses and medical complications that might directly and significantly influence the amount of treatment required. Other variables (such as the availability of a caregiver at home) that affect appropriate treatment shall also be considered. Factors that influence the need for treatment should be supportable by published research, clinical guidelines from professional sources, and/or clinical or common sense. See Pub. 100-02, chapter 15, section 220.3 for information related to documentation of the evaluation, and section 220.2 on medical necessity for some factors that complicate treatment.

**NOTE:** The patient's lack of access to outpatient hospital therapy services alone, when outpatient hospital therapy services are excluded from the limitation, does not justify excepted services. Residents of skilled nursing facilities prevented by consolidated billing from accessing hospital services, debilitated patients for whom transportation to the hospital is a physical hardship, or lack of therapy services at hospitals in the beneficiary's county may or may not qualify as justification for continued services above the caps. The patient's condition and complexities might justify extended services, but their location does not. For dates of service on or after October 1, 2012, therapy services furnished in an outpatient hospital are not excluded from the limitation.

CPT © 2017 American Medical Association. All Rights Reserved.                    © 2017 Optum360, LLC

In 2015, Congress passed the Medicare Access and CHIP Reauthorization Act (MACRA), which included sweeping changes for practitioners who provide services reimbursed under the Medicare physician fee schedule (MPFS). The act focused on repealing the faulty Medicare sustainable growth rate, focusing on quality of patient outcomes, and controlling Medicare spending.

A MACRA final rule in October 2016 established the Quality Payment Program (QPP) that was effective January 1, 2017.

The QPP has two tracks:

- The merit-based incentive payment system (MIPS)
- Alternative payment models (APMs).

MIPS uses the existing quality and value reporting systems—Physician Quality Reporting System (PQRS) (which ends January 1, 2019), Medicare meaningful use (MU), and value-based modifier (VBM) programs—to define certain performance categories that determine an overall score. Eligible clinicians (ECs) can obtain a composite performance score (CPS) of up to 100 points from these weighted performance categories. This performance score then defines the payment adjustments in the second calendar year after the year the score is obtained. For instance, the score obtained for the 2017 performance year is linked to payment for Medicare Part B services in 2019.

The performance categories, along with the weights used to determine the overall score, are:

- Quality (60 percent for 2017)
- Advancing care information (previously called meaningful use) (25 percent for 2017)
- Clinical practice improvement activities (CPIA) (15 percent for 2017)
- Resource use (0 percent for 2017)

ECs may also choose to participate in APMs. These payment models, created in conjunction with the clinician community, provide additional incentives to those clinicians in the APM who provide high-quality care as cost-efficiently as possible. APMs can be created around specific clinical conditions, a care episode, or a patient population type. An APM can also be described as a new way of paying the healthcare provider for the care rendered to Medicare patients.

Advanced APMs are a subset of APMs; practices participating in an advanced APM can earn even more incentives because the ECs take on risk related to their patients' outcomes. For calendar years 2019 through 2024, clinicians participating in advanced APMs have the potential to earn an additional 5 percent incentive payment; furthermore, they are exempt from having to participate in MIPS as long as they have sufficiently participated in the advanced APM.

Under MACRA, advanced APMs must meet the basic definition of an APM while also meeting additional criteria such as in the following list.

- All participants must use certified electronic health record technology (CEHRT).
- Participants must employ quality measures that are equivalent to those in the MIPS quality performance category.
- APM entities must bear more than nominal financial risk for monetary losses.
- Entities must be "medical home models," which were expanded under the authority of the Center for Medicare and Medicaid Innovation (section 1115A[c] of the act).

Calendar year 2017 is the transition year of the QPP that allows clinicians to choose a preferred pathway of participation as well as their pace of participation. Eligible clinicians have three flexible options for submitting data to the MIPS and a fourth option to join advanced APMs. Under the QPP, providers can receive increased payment by providing high-quality care and by controlling costs. ECs who successfully report determined criteria—defined by the pathway chosen—receive a larger payment depending on how successful they are at meeting performance thresholds. Those who do not participate or who do not fulfill the defined requirements receive a negative penalty; failure to participate in a track in 2017 results in a 4 percent payment reduction in 2019.

ECs can receive incentives under the QPP. Once the performance threshold is established, ALL ECs who score above that threshold are eligible to receive a positive payment adjustment. Keep in mind that the key requirement is that an EC **submit data** to avoid the negative payment adjustment and receive the incentives. CMS has redesigned the scoring so that clinicians are able to know how well they are doing in the program, as benchmarks are known in advance of participating.

The first year of the QPP took effect on January 1, 2017. As the years progress, the QPP will expand: more quality measures will be developed; the number of accountable care organizations will increase, allowing more practitioners to participate in the advanced APMs; and the impact to Medicare reimbursement will be greater. Other refinements will be made as eligible professionals and the Centers for Medicare and Medicaid Services (CMS) navigate these changes.

## Proposed 2018 Changes

Proposed changes to MIPS effective 2018 include, but are not limited to, the following:

- The performance period requirements would be increased; specifically, a full year of data would be required for both the quality and cost performance categories without factoring cost scores into final scores (maintaining cost impact at 0 percent):
  - increase improvement activities (IA) and advanced care information (ACI) categories to report a minimum of 90 days of data
  - allow scoring of performance category measures submitted through multiple mechanisms in 2018 versus reporting via only one reporting mechanism per performance category (i.e., three quality measures reported through a registry and three through CEHRT)
- Virtual groups would be offered as an additional participation option. CMS is soliciting feedback on the definition of a virtual group as well as the composition, election process, agreements, and reporting requirements.
- So that more small practices and ECs in rural or health professional shortage areas (HPSA) could be excluded from MIPS participation, the low-volume threshold would be raised to ECs or groups with less than $90,000 in Medicare Part B billings or those who provide care to fewer than 200 Part B beneficiaries. CMS is seeking comments regarding adding an opt-in option that would take effect in 2019.
- ECs may be able to earn a minimum of 15 out of 100 points to avoid a negative payment adjustment; this represents an increase from the current three-point threshold. For example, ECs could earn the total 15 points in 2018 by fully participating in the IA performance category.
  - Clinicians earning more than 15 points would become eligible for a slight bonus; if they accumulate 70 or more points, they could earn an additional bonus (0.5 to 10 percent).
- ECs could continue to use the 2014 edition of CEHRT for 2018 while being encouraged to use the 2015 edition.
- Bonus points may be awarded in the scoring process for:
  - exclusive use of the 2015 edition of CEHRT
  - care provided to complex patients using hierarchical condition categories (HCC) or dual-eligible method (this will equate to an additional one to three points to the EC depending on the medical complexity associated with the patient)
  - ECs in small practices contingent upon the ECs submitting data in a minimum of one performance category (5 points)
- MIPS performance improvement would be added in to the score for the quality performance category.

- A new option to use facility-based scoring for facility-based clinicians would be added:
  - 75 percent of the services ECs and groups perform must be in the emergency department or the inpatient setting.
  - Implementation would be limited for quality and cost performance categories.
  - Voluntary facility-based scoring would have to align with the Hospital Valued Based Purchasing (Hospital VBP) Program to limit burdens on clinicians; the measurement option would convert hospital total performance score to a MIPS quality and cost performance category score.
  - All measures adopted for the 2019 Hospital VBP Program would be included on the MIPS list of quality and cost measures during the 2020 MIPS payment year.
  - ECs could opt in or opt out of facility-based scoring.
- A new hardship exemption would be added in the ACI performance category for small practices.
- Three points would continue to be granted to small practices for incomplete quality performance category measures data; for all others, one point would be granted for incompleteness versus the current three points.
- Additional activities would be considered for the IA performance category.

CMS is looking for input and feedback on broadening the definition of physician-focused payment models (PFPM) to include payment arrangements that involve both Medicaid and the Children's Health Insurance Program (CHIP) as qualifying federal payers versus only CMS. Additionally, CMS is considering viewing PFPMs as advanced APMs though the agency will not make any guarantees.

Beginning in the 2019 performance period, participation in Medicaid, Medicare Advantage, and private payer arrangements that meet certain criteria ("Other Payer Advanced APMs") may be included when determining whether eligible clinicians earn the 5 percent incentive payment and are exempt from MIPS. Under the all-payer combination option, eligible clinicians must first be in advanced APMs under Medicare for payment arrangements to be considered with non-Medicare payers, including Medicaid.

Other changes CMS has proposed include:

- Providing additional information regarding how the quality performance category will be scored under the APM scoring standard for non-ACO models previously weighted at zero
- Adding a fourth "snapshot" date of December 31 for full tax identification number APMs for determining eligibility for participating in a MIPS APM for purposes of the scoring standard—this would permit participants who join certain APMs between September 1 and December 31 to benefit from that scoring standard. CMS recognizes how significantly this program changes how clinicians are paid under the Medicare program. CMS uses stakeholder feedback to continue to look for ways to promote flexibility and encourage participation as the agency eases clinicians into "full participation."

Because of the complexity and newness of the QPP, the program is likely to be revised and further clarified in the future. It is important that providers keep apprised of these changes and review internal policies and processes to guarantee that they earn the highest possible positive adjustment in payment.

For additional information, go to the CMS website at https://www.cms.gov/Medicare/Quality-Initiatives-Patient-Assessment-Instruments/Value-Based-Programs/MACRA-MIPS-and-APMs/MACRA-MIPS-and-APMs.html.

Optum360's new *MACRA Quality Payment Program Guide* contains detailed information about the QPP—it explains the program and provides the pertinent information key to deciding on the measures most applicable to specific practice and reporting options. To order, go to optum360coding.com.

     CPT © 2017 American Medical Association. All Rights Reserved.                    © 2017 Optum360, LLC

# Appendix I — Medically Unlikely Edits (MUEs)

The Centers for Medicare & Medicaid Services (CMS) began to publish many of the edits used in the medically unlikely edits (MUE) program for the first time effective October 2008. What follows below is a list of the published CPT codes that have MUEs assigned to them and the number of units allowed with each code. CMS publishes the updates on a quarterly basis. Not all MUEs will be published, however. MUEs intended to detect and discourage any questionable payments will not be published as the agency feels the efficacy of these edits would be compromised. CMS added another component to the MUEs—the MUE Adjudication Indicator (MAI). The appropriate MAI can be found in parentheses following the MUE in this table and specify the maximum units of service (UOS) for a CPT/HCPCS code for the service. The MAI designates whether the UOS edit is applied to the line or claim.

The three MAIs are defined as follows:

**MAI 1 (Line Edit)** This MAI will continue to be adjudicated as the line edit on the claim and is auto-adjudicated by the contractor.

**MAI 2 (Date of Service Edit, Policy)** This MAI is considered to be the "absolute date of service edit" and is based on policy. The total unit of services (UOS) for that CPT code and that date of service (DOS) are combined for this edit. Medicare contractors are required to review all claims for the same patient, same date of service, and same provider.

**MAI 3 (Date of Service Edit: Clinical)** This MAI is also a date-of-service edit but is based upon clinical standards. The review takes current and previously submitted claims for the same patient, same date of service, and same provider into account. When medical necessity is clearly documented, the edit may be bypassed or the claim resubmitted.

The quarterly updates are published on the CMS website at http://www.cms.gov/NationalCorrectCodInitEd/MUE.html.

## Professional

| CPT | MUE | CPT | MUE | CPT | MUE | CPT | MUE | CPT | MUE | CPT | MUE | CPT | MUE | CPT | MUE |
|-----|-----|-----|-----|-----|-----|-----|-----|-----|-----|-----|-----|-----|-----|-----|-----|
| 0001M | 1 | 0180T | 1 | 0255T | 2 | 0331T | 1 | 0377T | 1 | 0421T | 1 | 0463T | 1 | 11044 | 1 |
| 0001U | 1 | 0184T | 1 | 0263T | 1 | 0332T | 1 | 0378T | 1 | 0422T | 1 | 0464T | 1 | 11045 | 12 |
| 0002M | 1 | 0190T | 2 | 0264T | 1 | 0333T | 1 | 0379T | 1 | 0423T | 1 | 0465T | 1 | 11046 | 10 |
| 0002U | 1 | 0191T | 2 | 0265T | 1 | 0335T | 2 | 0380T | 1 | 0424T | 1 | 0466T | 1 | 11047 | 10 |
| 0003M | 1 | 0195T | 1 | 0266T | 1 | 0337T | 1 | 0381T | 1 | 0425T | 1 | 0467T | 1 | 11055 | 1 |
| 0003U | 1 | 0196T | 1 | 0267T | 1 | 0338T | 1 | 0382T | 1 | 0426T | 1 | 0468T | 1 | 11056 | 1 |
| 0004M | 1 | 0198T | 2 | 0268T | 1 | 0339T | 1 | 0383T | 1 | 0427T | 1 | 0469T | 1 | 11057 | 1 |
| 0006M | 1 | 0200T | 1 | 0269T | 1 | 0340T | 2 | 0384T | 1 | 0428T | 1 | 0470T | 1 | 11100 | 1 |
| 0007M | 1 | 0201T | 1 | 0270T | 1 | 0341T | 1 | 0385T | 1 | 0429T | 1 | 0471T | 2 | 11101 | 6 |
| 0008M | 1 | 0202T | 1 | 0271T | 1 | 0342T | 1 | 0386T | 1 | 0430T | 1 | 0472T | 1 | 11200 | 1 |
| 0009M | 1 | 0205T | 3 | 0272T | 1 | 0345T | 1 | 0387T | 1 | 0431T | 1 | 0473T | 1 | 11201 | 0 |
| 0042T | 1 | 0206T | 1 | 0273T | 1 | 0346T | 1 | 0388T | 1 | 0432T | 1 | 0474T | 2 | 11300 | 5 |
| 0051T | 1 | 0207T | 2 | 0274T | 1 | 0347T | 1 | 0389T | 1 | 0433T | 1 | 0475T | 1 | 11301 | 6 |
| 0052T | 1 | 0208T | 1 | 0275T | 1 | 0348T | 1 | 0390T | 1 | 0434T | 1 | 0476T | 1 | 11302 | 4 |
| 0053T | 1 | 0209T | 1 | 0278T | 1 | 0349T | 1 | 0391T | 1 | 0435T | 1 | 0477T | 1 | 11303 | 3 |
| 0054T | 1 | 0210T | 1 | 0290T | 1 | 0350T | 1 | 0394T | 2 | 0436T | 1 | 0478T | 1 | 11305 | 4 |
| 0055T | 1 | 0211T | 1 | 0293T | 1 | 0351T | 5 | 0395T | 2 | 0437T | 1 | 10021 | 4 | 11306 | 4 |
| 0058T | 1 | 0212T | 1 | 0294T | 1 | 0352T | 5 | 0396T | 2 | 0438T | 1 | 10022 | 4 | 11307 | 3 |
| 0071T | 1 | 0213T | 1 | 0295T | 1 | 0353T | 2 | 0397T | 1 | 0439T | 1 | 10030 | 2 | 11308 | 4 |
| 0072T | 1 | 0214T | 1 | 0296T | 1 | 0354T | 2 | 0398T | 1 | 0440T | 3 | 10035 | 1 | 11310 | 4 |
| 0075T | 1 | 0215T | 1 | 0297T | 1 | 0355T | 1 | 0399T | 1 | 0441T | 3 | 10036 | 2 | 11311 | 4 |
| 0076T | 1 | 0216T | 1 | 0298T | 1 | 0356T | 4 | 0400T | 1 | 0442T | 3 | 10040 | 1 | 11312 | 3 |
| 0095T | 1 | 0217T | 1 | 0299T | 1 | 0357T | 1 | 0401T | 1 | 0443T | 1 | 10060 | 1 | 11313 | 3 |
| 0098T | 2 | 0218T | 1 | 0300T | 1 | 0358T | 1 | 0402T | 2 | 0444T | 1 | 10061 | 1 | 11400 | 3 |
| 0100T | 1 | 0219T | 1 | 0301T | 1 | 0359T | 1 | 0403T | 1 | 0445T | 1 | 10080 | 1 | 11401 | 3 |
| 0101T | 1 | 0220T | 1 | 0302T | 1 | 0360T | 1 | 0404T | 1 | 0446T | 1 | 10081 | 1 | 11402 | 2 |
| 0102T | 2 | 0221T | 1 | 0303T | 1 | 0361T | 3 | 0405T | 1 | 0447T | 1 | 10120 | 3 | 11403 | 2 |
| 0106T | 4 | 0222T | 1 | 0304T | 1 | 0362T | 1 | 0406T | 2 | 0448T | 1 | 10121 | 2 | 11404 | 2 |
| 0107T | 4 | 0228T | 1 | 0305T | 1 | 0363T | 3 | 0407T | 2 | 0449T | 1 | 10140 | 2 | 11406 | 2 |
| 0108T | 4 | 0229T | 2 | 0306T | 1 | 0364T | 1 | 0408T | 1 | 0450T | 2 | 10160 | 3 | 11420 | 3 |
| 0109T | 4 | 0230T | 1 | 0307T | 1 | 0365T | 15 | 0409T | 1 | 0451T | 1 | 10180 | 2 | 11421 | 3 |
| 0110T | 4 | 0231T | 2 | 0308T | 1 | 0366T | 1 | 0410T | 1 | 0452T | 1 | 11000 | 1 | 11422 | 3 |
| 0111T | 1 | 0232T | 1 | 0309T | 1 | 0367T | 5 | 0411T | 1 | 0453T | 1 | 11001 | 1 | 11423 | 2 |
| 0126T | 1 | 0234T | 2 | 0310T | 1 | 0368T | 1 | 0412T | 1 | 0454T | 3 | 11004 | 1 | 11424 | 2 |
| 0159T | 2 | 0235T | 2 | 0312T | 1 | 0369T | 11 | 0413T | 1 | 0455T | 1 | 11005 | 1 | 11426 | 2 |
| 0163T | 1 | 0236T | 1 | 0313T | 1 | 0370T | 2 | 0414T | 1 | 0456T | 1 | 11006 | 1 | 11440 | 4 |
| 0164T | 4 | 0237T | 2 | 0314T | 1 | 0371T | 2 | 0415T | 1 | 0457T | 1 | 11008 | 1 | 11441 | 3 |
| 0165T | 4 | 0238T | 2 | 0315T | 1 | 0372T | 2 | 0416T | 1 | 0458T | 3 | 11010 | 2 | 11442 | 3 |
| 0174T | 1 | 0249T | 1 | 0316T | 1 | 0373T | 1 | 0417T | 1 | 0459T | 1 | 11011 | 2 | 11443 | 2 |
| 0175T | 1 | 0253T | 1 | 0317T | 1 | 0374T | 10 | 0418T | 1 | 0460T | 3 | 11012 | 2 | 11444 | 2 |
| 0178T | 1 | 0254T | 2 | 0329T | 1 | 0375T | 1 | 0419T | 1 | 0461T | 1 | 11042 | 1 | 11446 | 2 |
| 0179T | 1 | | | 0330T | 1 | 0376T | 2 | 0420T | 1 | 0462T | 1 | 11043 | 1 | 11450 | 1 |

**Appendix I — Medically Unlikely Edits (MUEs) — Professional**

| CPT | MUE | CPT | MUE | CPT | MUE | CPT | MUE | CPT | MUE | CPT | MUE | CPT | MUE | CPT | MUE |
|---|---|---|---|---|---|---|---|---|---|---|---|---|---|---|---|
| 11451 | 1 | 12017 | 1 | 15150 | 1 | 15829 | 1 | 17273 | 4 | 19350 | 1 | 20816 | 3 | 21086 | 1 |
| 11462 | 1 | 12018 | 1 | 15151 | 1 | 15830 | 1 | 17274 | 4 | 19355 | 1 | 20822 | 3 | 21087 | 1 |
| 11463 | 1 | 12020 | 2 | 15152 | 5 | 15832 | 1 | 17276 | 3 | 19357 | 1 | 20824 | 1 | 21088 | 1 |
| 11470 | 3 | 12021 | 3 | 15155 | 1 | 15833 | 1 | 17280 | 6 | 19361 | 1 | 20827 | 1 | 21100 | 1 |
| 11471 | 2 | 12031 | 1 | 15156 | 1 | 15834 | 1 | 17281 | 6 | 19364 | 1 | 20838 | 1 | 21110 | 2 |
| 11600 | 2 | 12032 | 1 | 15157 | 1 | 15835 | 1 | 17282 | 5 | 19366 | 1 | 20900 | 2 | 21116 | 1 |
| 11601 | 2 | 12034 | 1 | 15200 | 1 | 15836 | 1 | 17283 | 4 | 19367 | 1 | 20902 | 2 | 21120 | 1 |
| 11602 | 3 | 12035 | 1 | 15201 | 9 | 15837 | 2 | 17284 | 3 | 19368 | 1 | 20910 | 1 | 21121 | 1 |
| 11603 | 2 | 12036 | 1 | 15220 | 1 | 15838 | 1 | 17286 | 3 | 19369 | 1 | 20912 | 1 | 21122 | 1 |
| 11604 | 2 | 12037 | 1 | 15221 | 9 | 15839 | 2 | 17311 | 4 | 19370 | 1 | 20920 | 1 | 21123 | 1 |
| 11606 | 2 | 12041 | 1 | 15240 | 1 | 15840 | 1 | 17312 | 6 | 19371 | 1 | 20922 | 1 | 21125 | 2 |
| 11620 | 2 | 12042 | 1 | 15241 | 9 | 15841 | 2 | 17313 | 3 | 19380 | 1 | 20924 | 2 | 21127 | 2 |
| 11621 | 2 | 12044 | 1 | 15260 | 1 | 15842 | 2 | 17314 | 4 | 19396 | 1 | 20926 | 2 | 21137 | 1 |
| 11622 | 2 | 12045 | 1 | 15261 | 6 | 15845 | 2 | 17315 | 15 | 20005 | 4 | 20931 | 1 | 21138 | 1 |
| 11623 | 2 | 12046 | 1 | 15271 | 1 | 15847 | 1 | 17340 | 1 | 20100 | 2 | 20937 | 1 | 21139 | 1 |
| 11624 | 2 | 12047 | 1 | 15272 | 3 | 15851 | 1 | 17360 | 1 | 20101 | 2 | 20938 | 1 | 21141 | 1 |
| 11626 | 2 | 12051 | 1 | 15273 | 1 | 15852 | 1 | 17380 | 1 | 20102 | 3 | 20950 | 2 | 21142 | 1 |
| 11640 | 2 | 12052 | 1 | 15274 | 60 | 15860 | 1 | 19000 | 2 | 20103 | 4 | 20955 | 1 | 21143 | 1 |
| 11641 | 2 | 12053 | 1 | 15275 | 1 | 15876 | 1 | 19001 | 5 | 20150 | 2 | 20956 | 1 | 21145 | 1 |
| 11642 | 3 | 12054 | 1 | 15276 | 3 | 15877 | 1 | 19020 | 2 | 20200 | 2 | 20957 | 1 | 21146 | 1 |
| 11643 | 2 | 12055 | 1 | 15277 | 1 | 15878 | 1 | 19030 | 1 | 20205 | 4 | 20962 | 1 | 21147 | 1 |
| 11644 | 2 | 12056 | 1 | 15278 | 15 | 15879 | 1 | 19081 | 1 | 20206 | 3 | 20969 | 2 | 21150 | 1 |
| 11646 | 2 | 12057 | 1 | 15570 | 2 | 15920 | 1 | 19082 | 2 | 20220 | 4 | 20970 | 1 | 21151 | 1 |
| 11719 | 1 | 13100 | 1 | 15572 | 2 | 15922 | 1 | 19083 | 1 | 20225 | 4 | 20972 | 2 | 21154 | 1 |
| 11720 | 1 | 13101 | 1 | 15574 | 2 | 15931 | 1 | 19084 | 2 | 20240 | 4 | 20973 | 1 | 21155 | 1 |
| 11721 | 1 | 13102 | 9 | 15576 | 2 | 15933 | 1 | 19085 | 1 | 20245 | 4 | 20974 | 1 | 21159 | 1 |
| 11730 | 1 | 13120 | 1 | 15600 | 2 | 15934 | 1 | 19086 | 2 | 20250 | 3 | 20975 | 1 | 21160 | 1 |
| 11732 | 9 | 13121 | 1 | 15610 | 2 | 15935 | 1 | 19100 | 4 | 20251 | 3 | 20979 | 1 | 21172 | 1 |
| 11740 | 3 | 13122 | 9 | 15620 | 2 | 15936 | 1 | 19101 | 3 | 20500 | 2 | 20982 | 1 | 21175 | 1 |
| 11750 | 6 | 13131 | 1 | 15630 | 2 | 15937 | 1 | 19105 | 2 | 20501 | 2 | 20983 | 1 | 21179 | 1 |
| 11755 | 4 | 13132 | 1 | 15650 | 1 | 15940 | 2 | 19110 | 1 | 20520 | 4 | 20985 | 2 | 21180 | 1 |
| 11760 | 4 | 13133 | 7 | 15731 | 1 | 15941 | 2 | 19112 | 2 | 20525 | 4 | 21010 | 1 | 21181 | 1 |
| 11762 | 2 | 13151 | 1 | 15732 | 3 | 15944 | 2 | 19120 | 1 | 20526 | 1 | 21011 | 4 | 21182 | 1 |
| 11765 | 4 | 13152 | 1 | 15734 | 4 | 15945 | 2 | 19125 | 1 | 20527 | 2 | 21012 | 3 | 21183 | 1 |
| 11770 | 1 | 13153 | 2 | 15736 | 2 | 15946 | 2 | 19126 | 3 | 20550 | 5 | 21013 | 4 | 21184 | 1 |
| 11771 | 1 | 13160 | 2 | 15738 | 4 | 15950 | 2 | 19260 | 2 | 20551 | 5 | 21014 | 3 | 21188 | 1 |
| 11772 | 1 | 14000 | 2 | 15740 | 3 | 15951 | 2 | 19271 | 1 | 20552 | 1 | 21015 | 1 | 21193 | 1 |
| 11900 | 1 | 14001 | 2 | 15750 | 2 | 15952 | 2 | 19272 | 1 | 20553 | 1 | 21016 | 2 | 21194 | 1 |
| 11901 | 1 | 14020 | 4 | 15756 | 2 | 15953 | 2 | 19281 | 1 | 20555 | 1 | 21025 | 2 | 21195 | 1 |
| 11920 | 1 | 14021 | 3 | 15757 | 2 | 15956 | 2 | 19282 | 2 | 20600 | 6 | 21026 | 2 | 21196 | 1 |
| 11921 | 1 | 14040 | 4 | 15758 | 2 | 15958 | 2 | 19283 | 1 | 20604 | 4 | 21029 | 1 | 21198 | 1 |
| 11922 | 1 | 14041 | 3 | 15760 | 2 | 16000 | 1 | 19284 | 2 | 20605 | 2 | 21030 | 1 | 21199 | 1 |
| 11950 | 1 | 14060 | 4 | 15770 | 2 | 16020 | 1 | 19285 | 1 | 20606 | 2 | 21031 | 2 | 21206 | 1 |
| 11951 | 1 | 14061 | 2 | 15775 | 1 | 16025 | 1 | 19286 | 2 | 20610 | 2 | 21032 | 1 | 21208 | 1 |
| 11952 | 1 | 14301 | 2 | 15776 | 1 | 16030 | 1 | 19287 | 1 | 20611 | 2 | 21034 | 1 | 21209 | 1 |
| 11954 | 1 | 14302 | 8 | 15777 | 1 | 16035 | 1 | 19288 | 2 | 20612 | 2 | 21040 | 2 | 21210 | 2 |
| 11960 | 2 | 14350 | 2 | 15780 | 1 | 16036 | 8 | 19296 | 1 | 20615 | 1 | 21044 | 1 | 21215 | 2 |
| 11970 | 2 | 15002 | 1 | 15781 | 1 | 17000 | 1 | 19297 | 2 | 20650 | 4 | 21045 | 1 | 21230 | 2 |
| 11971 | 2 | 15003 | 60 | 15782 | 1 | 17003 | 13 | 19298 | 1 | 20660 | 1 | 21046 | 2 | 21235 | 2 |
| 11976 | 1 | 15004 | 1 | 15783 | 1 | 17004 | 1 | 19300 | 1 | 20661 | 1 | 21047 | 2 | 21240 | 1 |
| 11980 | 1 | 15005 | 19 | 15786 | 1 | 17106 | 1 | 19301 | 1 | 20662 | 1 | 21048 | 2 | 21242 | 1 |
| 11981 | 1 | 15040 | 1 | 15787 | 2 | 17107 | 1 | 19302 | 1 | 20663 | 1 | 21049 | 1 | 21243 | 1 |
| 11982 | 1 | 15050 | 1 | 15788 | 1 | 17108 | 1 | 19303 | 1 | 20664 | 1 | 21050 | 1 | 21244 | 1 |
| 11983 | 1 | 15100 | 1 | 15789 | 1 | 17110 | 1 | 19304 | 1 | 20665 | 1 | 21060 | 1 | 21245 | 2 |
| 12001 | 1 | 15101 | 40 | 15792 | 1 | 17111 | 1 | 19305 | 1 | 20670 | 3 | 21070 | 1 | 21246 | 2 |
| 12002 | 1 | 15110 | 1 | 15793 | 1 | 17250 | 4 | 19306 | 1 | 20680 | 3 | 21073 | 1 | 21247 | 1 |
| 12004 | 1 | 15111 | 5 | 15819 | 1 | 17260 | 7 | 19307 | 1 | 20690 | 2 | 21076 | 1 | 21248 | 2 |
| 12005 | 1 | 15115 | 1 | 15820 | 1 | 17261 | 7 | 19316 | 1 | 20692 | 2 | 21077 | 1 | 21249 | 2 |
| 12006 | 1 | 15116 | 2 | 15821 | 1 | 17262 | 6 | 19318 | 1 | 20693 | 2 | 21079 | 1 | 21255 | 1 |
| 12007 | 1 | 15120 | 1 | 15822 | 1 | 17263 | 5 | 19324 | 1 | 20694 | 2 | 21080 | 1 | 21256 | 1 |
| 12011 | 1 | 15121 | 8 | 15823 | 1 | 17264 | 3 | 19325 | 1 | 20696 | 2 | 21081 | 1 | 21260 | 1 |
| 12013 | 1 | 15130 | 1 | 15824 | 1 | 17266 | 2 | 19328 | 1 | 20697 | 4 | 21082 | 1 | 21261 | 1 |
| 12014 | 1 | 15131 | 2 | 15825 | 1 | 17270 | 6 | 19330 | 1 | 20802 | 1 | 21083 | 1 | 21263 | 1 |
| 12015 | 1 | 15135 | 1 | 15826 | 1 | 17271 | 4 | 19340 | 1 | 20805 | 1 | 21084 | 1 | 21267 | 1 |
| 12016 | 1 | 15136 | 1 | 15828 | 1 | 17272 | 5 | 19342 | 1 | 20808 | 1 | 21085 | 1 | 21268 | 1 |

CPT © 2017 American Medical Association. All Rights Reserved.                    © 2017 Optum360, LLC

| CPT | MUE | CPT | MUE | CPT | MUE | CPT | MUE | CPT | MUE | CPT | MUE | CPT | MUE | CPT | MUE |
|---|---|---|---|---|---|---|---|---|---|---|---|---|---|---|---|
| 21270 | 1 | 21552 | 4 | 22505 | 1 | 22902 | 4 | 23466 | 1 | 24126 | 1 | 24577 | 1 | 25150 | 1 |
| 21275 | 1 | 21554 | 2 | 22510 | 1 | 22903 | 3 | 23470 | 1 | 24130 | 1 | 24579 | 1 | 25151 | 1 |
| 21280 | 1 | 21555 | 4 | 22511 | 1 | 22904 | 1 | 23472 | 1 | 24134 | 1 | 24582 | 1 | 25170 | 1 |
| 21282 | 1 | 21556 | 3 | 22512 | 3 | 22905 | 1 | 23473 | 1 | 24136 | 1 | 24586 | 1 | 25210 | 2 |
| 21295 | 1 | 21557 | 1 | 22513 | 1 | 23000 | 1 | 23474 | 1 | 24138 | 1 | 24587 | 1 | 25215 | 1 |
| 21296 | 1 | 21558 | 1 | 22514 | 1 | 23020 | 1 | 23480 | 1 | 24140 | 1 | 24600 | 1 | 25230 | 1 |
| 21310 | 1 | 21600 | 5 | 22515 | 4 | 23030 | 2 | 23485 | 1 | 24145 | 1 | 24605 | 1 | 25240 | 1 |
| 21315 | 1 | 21610 | 1 | 22532 | 1 | 23031 | 1 | 23490 | 1 | 24147 | 1 | 24615 | 1 | 25246 | 1 |
| 21320 | 1 | 21615 | 1 | 22533 | 1 | 23035 | 1 | 23491 | 1 | 24149 | 1 | 24620 | 1 | 25248 | 3 |
| 21325 | 1 | 21616 | 1 | 22534 | 3 | 23040 | 1 | 23500 | 1 | 24150 | 1 | 24635 | 1 | 25250 | 1 |
| 21330 | 1 | 21620 | 1 | 22548 | 1 | 23044 | 1 | 23505 | 1 | 24152 | 1 | 24640 | 1 | 25251 | 1 |
| 21335 | 1 | 21627 | 1 | 22551 | 1 | 23065 | 2 | 23515 | 1 | 24155 | 1 | 24650 | 1 | 25259 | 1 |
| 21336 | 1 | 21630 | 1 | 22552 | 5 | 23066 | 2 | 23520 | 1 | 24160 | 1 | 24655 | 1 | 25260 | 9 |
| 21337 | 1 | 21632 | 1 | 22554 | 1 | 23071 | 2 | 23525 | 1 | 24164 | 1 | 24665 | 1 | 25263 | 4 |
| 21338 | 1 | 21685 | 1 | 22556 | 1 | 23073 | 2 | 23530 | 1 | 24200 | 3 | 24666 | 1 | 25265 | 4 |
| 21339 | 1 | 21700 | 1 | 22558 | 1 | 23075 | 3 | 23532 | 1 | 24201 | 3 | 24670 | 1 | 25270 | 8 |
| 21340 | 1 | 21705 | 1 | 22585 | 7 | 23076 | 2 | 23540 | 1 | 24220 | 1 | 24675 | 1 | 25272 | 4 |
| 21343 | 1 | 21720 | 1 | 22586 | 1 | 23077 | 1 | 23545 | 1 | 24300 | 1 | 24685 | 1 | 25274 | 4 |
| 21344 | 1 | 21725 | 1 | 22590 | 1 | 23078 | 1 | 23550 | 1 | 24301 | 2 | 24800 | 1 | 25275 | 2 |
| 21345 | 1 | 21740 | 1 | 22595 | 1 | 23100 | 1 | 23552 | 1 | 24305 | 4 | 24802 | 1 | 25280 | 9 |
| 21346 | 1 | 21742 | 1 | 22600 | 1 | 23101 | 2 | 23570 | 1 | 24310 | 3 | 24900 | 1 | 25290 | 12 |
| 21347 | 1 | 21743 | 1 | 22610 | 1 | 23105 | 1 | 23575 | 1 | 24320 | 2 | 24920 | 1 | 25295 | 9 |
| 21348 | 1 | 21750 | 1 | 22612 | 1 | 23106 | 1 | 23585 | 1 | 24330 | 1 | 24925 | 1 | 25300 | 1 |
| 21355 | 1 | 21811 | 1 | 22614 | 13 | 23107 | 1 | 23600 | 1 | 24331 | 1 | 24930 | 1 | 25301 | 1 |
| 21356 | 1 | 21812 | 1 | 22630 | 1 | 23120 | 1 | 23605 | 1 | 24332 | 1 | 24931 | 1 | 25310 | 5 |
| 21360 | 1 | 21813 | 1 | 22632 | 4 | 23125 | 1 | 23615 | 1 | 24340 | 1 | 24935 | 1 | 25312 | 5 |
| 21365 | 1 | 21820 | 1 | 22633 | 1 | 23130 | 1 | 23616 | 1 | 24341 | 2 | 24940 | 1 | 25315 | 1 |
| 21366 | 1 | 21825 | 1 | 22634 | 4 | 23140 | 1 | 23620 | 1 | 24342 | 2 | 25000 | 2 | 25316 | 1 |
| 21385 | 1 | 21920 | 3 | 22800 | 1 | 23145 | 1 | 23625 | 1 | 24343 | 1 | 25001 | 1 | 25320 | 1 |
| 21386 | 1 | 21925 | 3 | 22802 | 1 | 23146 | 1 | 23630 | 1 | 24344 | 1 | 25020 | 1 | 25332 | 1 |
| 21387 | 1 | 21930 | 5 | 22804 | 1 | 23150 | 1 | 23650 | 1 | 24345 | 1 | 25023 | 1 | 25335 | 1 |
| 21390 | 1 | 21931 | 3 | 22808 | 1 | 23155 | 1 | 23655 | 1 | 24346 | 1 | 25024 | 1 | 25337 | 1 |
| 21395 | 1 | 21932 | 4 | 22810 | 1 | 23156 | 1 | 23660 | 1 | 24357 | 2 | 25025 | 1 | 25350 | 1 |
| 21400 | 1 | 21933 | 3 | 22812 | 1 | 23170 | 1 | 23665 | 1 | 24358 | 2 | 25028 | 4 | 25355 | 1 |
| 21401 | 1 | 21935 | 1 | 22818 | 1 | 23172 | 1 | 23670 | 1 | 24359 | 2 | 25031 | 2 | 25360 | 1 |
| 21406 | 1 | 21936 | 1 | 22819 | 1 | 23174 | 1 | 23675 | 1 | 24360 | 1 | 25035 | 2 | 25365 | 1 |
| 21407 | 1 | 22010 | 2 | 22830 | 1 | 23180 | 1 | 23680 | 1 | 24361 | 1 | 25040 | 1 | 25370 | 1 |
| 21408 | 1 | 22015 | 2 | 22840 | 1 | 23182 | 1 | 23700 | 1 | 24362 | 1 | 25065 | 3 | 25375 | 1 |
| 21421 | 1 | 22100 | 1 | 22842 | 1 | 23184 | 1 | 23800 | 1 | 24363 | 1 | 25066 | 2 | 25390 | 1 |
| 21422 | 1 | 22101 | 1 | 22843 | 1 | 23190 | 1 | 23802 | 1 | 24365 | 1 | 25071 | 3 | 25391 | 1 |
| 21423 | 1 | 22102 | 1 | 22844 | 1 | 23195 | 1 | 23900 | 1 | 24366 | 1 | 25073 | 3 | 25392 | 1 |
| 21431 | 1 | 22103 | 3 | 22845 | 1 | 23200 | 1 | 23920 | 1 | 24370 | 1 | 25075 | 6 | 25393 | 1 |
| 21432 | 1 | 22110 | 1 | 22846 | 1 | 23210 | 1 | 23921 | 1 | 24371 | 1 | 25076 | 5 | 25394 | 1 |
| 21433 | 1 | 22112 | 1 | 22847 | 1 | 23220 | 1 | 23930 | 2 | 24400 | 1 | 25077 | 1 | 25400 | 1 |
| 21435 | 1 | 22114 | 1 | 22848 | 1 | 23330 | 2 | 23931 | 2 | 24410 | 1 | 25078 | 1 | 25405 | 1 |
| 21436 | 1 | 22116 | 3 | 22849 | 1 | 23333 | 1 | 23935 | 2 | 24420 | 1 | 25085 | 1 | 25415 | 1 |
| 21440 | 2 | 22206 | 1 | 22850 | 1 | 23334 | 1 | 24000 | 1 | 24430 | 1 | 25100 | 1 | 25420 | 1 |
| 21445 | 2 | 22207 | 1 | 22852 | 1 | 23335 | 1 | 24006 | 1 | 24435 | 1 | 25101 | 1 | 25425 | 1 |
| 21450 | 1 | 22208 | 6 | 22853 | 5 | 23350 | 1 | 24065 | 2 | 24470 | 1 | 25105 | 1 | 25426 | 1 |
| 21451 | 1 | 22210 | 1 | 22854 | 5 | 23395 | 1 | 24066 | 2 | 24495 | 1 | 25107 | 1 | 25430 | 1 |
| 21452 | 1 | 22212 | 1 | 22855 | 1 | 23397 | 1 | 24071 | 3 | 24498 | 1 | 25109 | 4 | 25431 | 1 |
| 21453 | 1 | 22214 | 1 | 22856 | 1 | 23400 | 1 | 24073 | 3 | 24500 | 1 | 25110 | 3 | 25440 | 1 |
| 21454 | 1 | 22216 | 6 | 22857 | 1 | 23405 | 2 | 24075 | 5 | 24505 | 1 | 25111 | 1 | 25441 | 1 |
| 21461 | 1 | 22220 | 1 | 22858 | 1 | 23406 | 1 | 24076 | 4 | 24515 | 1 | 25112 | 1 | 25442 | 1 |
| 21462 | 1 | 22222 | 1 | 22859 | 5 | 23410 | 1 | 24077 | 1 | 24516 | 1 | 25115 | 1 | 25443 | 1 |
| 21465 | 1 | 22224 | 1 | 22861 | 1 | 23412 | 1 | 24079 | 1 | 24530 | 1 | 25116 | 1 | 25444 | 1 |
| 21470 | 1 | 22226 | 4 | 22862 | 1 | 23415 | 1 | 24100 | 1 | 24535 | 1 | 25118 | 5 | 25445 | 1 |
| 21480 | 1 | 22310 | 1 | 22864 | 1 | 23420 | 1 | 24101 | 1 | 24538 | 1 | 25119 | 1 | 25446 | 1 |
| 21485 | 1 | 22315 | 1 | 22865 | 1 | 23430 | 1 | 24102 | 1 | 24545 | 1 | 25120 | 1 | 25447 | 4 |
| 21490 | 1 | 22318 | 1 | 22867 | 1 | 23440 | 1 | 24105 | 1 | 24546 | 1 | 25125 | 1 | 25449 | 1 |
| 21497 | 1 | 22319 | 1 | 22868 | 1 | 23450 | 1 | 24110 | 1 | 24560 | 1 | 25126 | 1 | 25450 | 1 |
| 21501 | 3 | 22325 | 1 | 22869 | 1 | 23455 | 1 | 24115 | 1 | 24565 | 1 | 25130 | 1 | 25455 | 1 |
| 21502 | 1 | 22326 | 1 | 22870 | 1 | 23460 | 1 | 24116 | 1 | 24566 | 1 | 25135 | 1 | 25490 | 1 |
| 21510 | 1 | 22327 | 1 | 22900 | 3 | 23462 | 1 | 24120 | 1 | 24575 | 1 | 25136 | 1 | 25491 | 1 |
| 21550 | 3 | 22328 | 6 | 22901 | 2 | 23465 | 1 | 24125 | 1 | 24576 | 1 | 25145 | 1 | 25492 | 1 |

| CPT | MUE | CPT | MUE | CPT | MUE | CPT | MUE | CPT | MUE | CPT | MUE | CPT | MUE | CPT | MUE |
|---|---|---|---|---|---|---|---|---|---|---|---|---|---|---|---|
| 25500 | 1 | 26060 | 5 | 26460 | 4 | 26675 | 1 | 27065 | 1 | 27246 | 1 | 27394 | 1 | 27516 | 1 |
| 25505 | 1 | 26070 | 2 | 26471 | 4 | 26676 | 3 | 27066 | 1 | 27248 | 1 | 27395 | 1 | 27517 | 1 |
| 25515 | 1 | 26075 | 4 | 26474 | 4 | 26685 | 3 | 27067 | 1 | 27250 | 1 | 27396 | 1 | 27519 | 1 |
| 25520 | 1 | 26080 | 4 | 26476 | 4 | 26686 | 3 | 27070 | 1 | 27252 | 1 | 27397 | 1 | 27520 | 1 |
| 25525 | 1 | 26100 | 1 | 26477 | 4 | 26700 | 3 | 27071 | 1 | 27253 | 1 | 27400 | 1 | 27524 | 1 |
| 25526 | 1 | 26105 | 2 | 26478 | 6 | 26705 | 3 | 27075 | 1 | 27254 | 1 | 27403 | 1 | 27530 | 1 |
| 25530 | 1 | 26110 | 3 | 26479 | 4 | 26706 | 4 | 27076 | 1 | 27256 | 1 | 27405 | 2 | 27532 | 1 |
| 25535 | 1 | 26111 | 4 | 26480 | 4 | 26715 | 4 | 27077 | 1 | 27257 | 1 | 27407 | 2 | 27535 | 1 |
| 25545 | 1 | 26113 | 4 | 26483 | 4 | 26720 | 4 | 27078 | 1 | 27258 | 1 | 27409 | 1 | 27536 | 1 |
| 25560 | 1 | 26115 | 4 | 26485 | 4 | 26725 | 4 | 27080 | 1 | 27259 | 1 | 27412 | 1 | 27538 | 1 |
| 25565 | 1 | 26116 | 2 | 26489 | 3 | 26727 | 4 | 27086 | 1 | 27265 | 1 | 27415 | 1 | 27540 | 1 |
| 25574 | 1 | 26117 | 2 | 26490 | 3 | 26735 | 4 | 27087 | 1 | 27266 | 1 | 27416 | 1 | 27550 | 1 |
| 25575 | 1 | 26118 | 1 | 26492 | 2 | 26740 | 3 | 27090 | 1 | 27267 | 1 | 27418 | 1 | 27552 | 1 |
| 25600 | 1 | 26121 | 1 | 26494 | 1 | 26742 | 3 | 27091 | 1 | 27268 | 1 | 27420 | 1 | 27556 | 1 |
| 25605 | 1 | 26123 | 1 | 26496 | 1 | 26746 | 3 | 27093 | 1 | 27269 | 1 | 27422 | 1 | 27557 | 1 |
| 25606 | 1 | 26125 | 4 | 26497 | 2 | 26750 | 3 | 27095 | 1 | 27275 | 2 | 27424 | 1 | 27558 | 1 |
| 25607 | 1 | 26130 | 1 | 26498 | 1 | 26755 | 3 | 27096 | 1 | 27279 | 1 | 27425 | 1 | 27560 | 1 |
| 25608 | 1 | 26135 | 4 | 26499 | 2 | 26756 | 3 | 27097 | 1 | 27280 | 1 | 27427 | 1 | 27562 | 1 |
| 25609 | 1 | 26140 | 3 | 26500 | 4 | 26765 | 5 | 27098 | 1 | 27282 | 1 | 27428 | 1 | 27566 | 1 |
| 25622 | 1 | 26145 | 6 | 26502 | 3 | 26770 | 3 | 27100 | 1 | 27284 | 1 | 27429 | 1 | 27570 | 1 |
| 25624 | 1 | 26160 | 5 | 26508 | 1 | 26775 | 4 | 27105 | 1 | 27286 | 1 | 27430 | 1 | 27580 | 1 |
| 25628 | 1 | 26170 | 5 | 26510 | 4 | 26776 | 4 | 27110 | 1 | 27290 | 1 | 27435 | 1 | 27590 | 1 |
| 25630 | 1 | 26180 | 4 | 26516 | 1 | 26785 | 3 | 27111 | 1 | 27295 | 1 | 27437 | 1 | 27591 | 1 |
| 25635 | 1 | 26185 | 1 | 26517 | 1 | 26820 | 1 | 27120 | 1 | 27301 | 3 | 27438 | 1 | 27592 | 1 |
| 25645 | 1 | 26200 | 2 | 26518 | 1 | 26841 | 1 | 27122 | 1 | 27303 | 2 | 27440 | 1 | 27594 | 1 |
| 25650 | 1 | 26205 | 1 | 26520 | 4 | 26842 | 1 | 27125 | 1 | 27305 | 1 | 27441 | 1 | 27596 | 1 |
| 25651 | 1 | 26210 | 2 | 26525 | 4 | 26843 | 2 | 27130 | 1 | 27306 | 1 | 27442 | 1 | 27598 | 1 |
| 25652 | 1 | 26215 | 2 | 26530 | 4 | 26844 | 2 | 27132 | 1 | 27307 | 1 | 27443 | 1 | 27600 | 1 |
| 25660 | 1 | 26230 | 2 | 26531 | 4 | 26850 | 5 | 27134 | 1 | 27310 | 1 | 27445 | 1 | 27601 | 1 |
| 25670 | 1 | 26235 | 2 | 26535 | 4 | 26852 | 2 | 27137 | 1 | 27323 | 2 | 27446 | 1 | 27602 | 1 |
| 25671 | 1 | 26236 | 2 | 26536 | 4 | 26860 | 1 | 27138 | 1 | 27324 | 3 | 27447 | 1 | 27603 | 2 |
| 25675 | 1 | 26250 | 2 | 26540 | 4 | 26861 | 4 | 27140 | 1 | 27325 | 1 | 27448 | 1 | 27604 | 2 |
| 25676 | 1 | 26260 | 1 | 26541 | 4 | 26862 | 1 | 27146 | 1 | 27326 | 1 | 27450 | 1 | 27605 | 1 |
| 25680 | 1 | 26262 | 1 | 26542 | 4 | 26863 | 3 | 27147 | 1 | 27327 | 5 | 27454 | 1 | 27606 | 1 |
| 25685 | 1 | 26320 | 4 | 26545 | 4 | 26910 | 4 | 27151 | 1 | 27328 | 4 | 27455 | 1 | 27607 | 2 |
| 25690 | 1 | 26340 | 4 | 26546 | 2 | 26951 | 8 | 27156 | 1 | 27329 | 1 | 27457 | 1 | 27610 | 1 |
| 25695 | 1 | 26341 | 2 | 26548 | 3 | 26952 | 5 | 27158 | 1 | 27330 | 1 | 27465 | 1 | 27612 | 1 |
| 25800 | 1 | 26350 | 6 | 26550 | 1 | 26990 | 2 | 27161 | 1 | 27331 | 1 | 27466 | 1 | 27613 | 4 |
| 25805 | 1 | 26352 | 2 | 26551 | 1 | 26991 | 1 | 27165 | 1 | 27332 | 1 | 27468 | 1 | 27614 | 3 |
| 25810 | 1 | 26356 | 4 | 26553 | 1 | 26992 | 2 | 27170 | 1 | 27333 | 1 | 27470 | 1 | 27615 | 1 |
| 25820 | 1 | 26357 | 2 | 26554 | 1 | 27000 | 1 | 27175 | 1 | 27334 | 1 | 27472 | 1 | 27616 | 1 |
| 25825 | 1 | 26358 | 2 | 26555 | 2 | 27001 | 1 | 27176 | 1 | 27335 | 1 | 27475 | 1 | 27618 | 4 |
| 25830 | 1 | 26370 | 3 | 26556 | 2 | 27003 | 1 | 27177 | 1 | 27337 | 4 | 27477 | 1 | 27619 | 4 |
| 25900 | 1 | 26372 | 1 | 26560 | 2 | 27005 | 1 | 27178 | 1 | 27339 | 4 | 27479 | 1 | 27620 | 1 |
| 25905 | 1 | 26373 | 2 | 26561 | 2 | 27006 | 1 | 27179 | 1 | 27340 | 1 | 27485 | 1 | 27625 | 1 |
| 25907 | 1 | 26390 | 2 | 26562 | 2 | 27025 | 1 | 27181 | 1 | 27345 | 1 | 27486 | 1 | 27626 | 1 |
| 25909 | 1 | 26392 | 2 | 26565 | 3 | 27027 | 1 | 27185 | 1 | 27347 | 1 | 27487 | 1 | 27630 | 2 |
| 25915 | 1 | 26410 | 4 | 26567 | 3 | 27030 | 1 | 27187 | 1 | 27350 | 1 | 27488 | 1 | 27632 | 4 |
| 25920 | 1 | 26412 | 3 | 26568 | 2 | 27033 | 1 | 27197 | 1 | 27355 | 1 | 27495 | 1 | 27634 | 2 |
| 25922 | 1 | 26415 | 2 | 26580 | 1 | 27035 | 1 | 27198 | 1 | 27356 | 1 | 27496 | 1 | 27635 | 1 |
| 25924 | 1 | 26416 | 2 | 26587 | 2 | 27036 | 1 | 27200 | 1 | 27357 | 1 | 27497 | 1 | 27637 | 1 |
| 25927 | 1 | 26418 | 4 | 26590 | 2 | 27040 | 2 | 27202 | 1 | 27358 | 1 | 27498 | 1 | 27638 | 1 |
| 25929 | 1 | 26420 | 4 | 26591 | 4 | 27041 | 3 | 27220 | 1 | 27360 | 2 | 27499 | 1 | 27640 | 1 |
| 25931 | 1 | 26426 | 4 | 26593 | 9 | 27043 | 3 | 27222 | 1 | 27364 | 1 | 27500 | 1 | 27641 | 1 |
| 26010 | 2 | 26428 | 2 | 26596 | 1 | 27045 | 3 | 27226 | 1 | 27365 | 1 | 27501 | 1 | 27645 | 1 |
| 26011 | 3 | 26432 | 2 | 26600 | 2 | 27047 | 4 | 27227 | 1 | 27370 | 1 | 27502 | 1 | 27646 | 1 |
| 26020 | 4 | 26433 | 2 | 26605 | 3 | 27048 | 2 | 27228 | 1 | 27372 | 2 | 27503 | 1 | 27647 | 1 |
| 26025 | 1 | 26434 | 2 | 26607 | 2 | 27049 | 1 | 27230 | 1 | 27380 | 2 | 27506 | 1 | 27648 | 1 |
| 26030 | 1 | 26437 | 4 | 26608 | 5 | 27050 | 1 | 27232 | 1 | 27381 | 2 | 27507 | 1 | 27650 | 1 |
| 26034 | 2 | 26440 | 6 | 26615 | 4 | 27052 | 1 | 27235 | 1 | 27385 | 2 | 27508 | 1 | 27652 | 1 |
| 26035 | 1 | 26442 | 5 | 26641 | 1 | 27054 | 1 | 27236 | 1 | 27386 | 2 | 27509 | 1 | 27654 | 1 |
| 26037 | 1 | 26445 | 5 | 26645 | 1 | 27057 | 1 | 27238 | 1 | 27390 | 1 | 27510 | 1 | 27656 | 1 |
| 26040 | 1 | 26449 | 5 | 26650 | 1 | 27059 | 1 | 27240 | 1 | 27391 | 1 | 27511 | 1 | 27658 | 2 |
| 26045 | 1 | 26450 | 6 | 26665 | 1 | 27060 | 1 | 27244 | 1 | 27392 | 1 | 27513 | 1 | 27659 | 2 |
| 26055 | 5 | 26455 | 6 | 26670 | 2 | 27062 | 1 | 27245 | 1 | 27393 | 1 | 27514 | 1 | 27664 | 2 |

CPT © 2017 American Medical Association. All Rights Reserved.

© 2017 Optum360, LLC

| CPT | MUE | CPT | MUE | CPT | MUE | CPT | MUE | CPT | MUE | CPT | MUE | CPT | MUE | CPT | MUE |
|---|---|---|---|---|---|---|---|---|---|---|---|---|---|---|---|
| 27665 | 2 | 27830 | 1 | 28120 | 2 | 28360 | 1 | 29010 | 1 | 29827 | 1 | 30110 | 1 | 31231 | 1 |
| 27675 | 1 | 27831 | 1 | 28122 | 4 | 28400 | 1 | 29015 | 1 | 29828 | 1 | 30115 | 1 | 31233 | 1 |
| 27676 | 1 | 27832 | 1 | 28124 | 4 | 28405 | 1 | 29035 | 1 | 29830 | 1 | 30117 | 2 | 31235 | 1 |
| 27680 | 3 | 27840 | 1 | 28126 | 4 | 28406 | 1 | 29040 | 1 | 29834 | 1 | 30118 | 1 | 31237 | 1 |
| 27681 | 1 | 27842 | 1 | 28130 | 1 | 28415 | 1 | 29044 | 1 | 29835 | 1 | 30120 | 1 | 31238 | 1 |
| 27685 | 2 | 27846 | 1 | 28140 | 4 | 28420 | 1 | 29046 | 1 | 29836 | 1 | 30124 | 2 | 31239 | 1 |
| 27686 | 3 | 27848 | 1 | 28150 | 4 | 28430 | 1 | 29049 | 1 | 29837 | 1 | 30125 | 1 | 31240 | 1 |
| 27687 | 1 | 27860 | 1 | 28153 | 6 | 28435 | 1 | 29055 | 1 | 29838 | 1 | 30130 | 1 | 31254 | 1 |
| 27690 | 2 | 27870 | 1 | 28160 | 5 | 28436 | 1 | 29058 | 1 | 29840 | 1 | 30140 | 1 | 31255 | 1 |
| 27691 | 2 | 27871 | 1 | 28171 | 1 | 28445 | 1 | 29065 | 1 | 29843 | 1 | 30150 | 1 | 31256 | 1 |
| 27692 | 4 | 27880 | 1 | 28173 | 2 | 28446 | 1 | 29075 | 1 | 29844 | 1 | 30160 | 1 | 31267 | 1 |
| 27695 | 1 | 27881 | 1 | 28175 | 2 | 28450 | 2 | 29085 | 1 | 29845 | 1 | 30200 | 1 | 31276 | 1 |
| 27696 | 1 | 27882 | 1 | 28190 | 3 | 28455 | 3 | 29086 | 2 | 29846 | 1 | 30210 | 1 | 31287 | 1 |
| 27698 | 2 | 27884 | 1 | 28192 | 2 | 28456 | 2 | 29105 | 1 | 29847 | 1 | 30220 | 1 | 31288 | 1 |
| 27700 | 1 | 27886 | 1 | 28193 | 2 | 28465 | 3 | 29125 | 1 | 29848 | 1 | 30300 | 1 | 31290 | 1 |
| 27702 | 1 | 27888 | 1 | 28200 | 4 | 28470 | 2 | 29126 | 1 | 29850 | 1 | 30310 | 1 | 31291 | 1 |
| 27703 | 1 | 27889 | 1 | 28202 | 2 | 28475 | 5 | 29130 | 3 | 29851 | 1 | 30320 | 1 | 31292 | 1 |
| 27704 | 1 | 27892 | 1 | 28208 | 4 | 28476 | 4 | 29131 | 2 | 29855 | 1 | 30400 | 1 | 31293 | 1 |
| 27705 | 1 | 27893 | 1 | 28210 | 2 | 28485 | 5 | 29200 | 1 | 29856 | 1 | 30410 | 1 | 31294 | 1 |
| 27707 | 1 | 27894 | 1 | 28220 | 1 | 28490 | 1 | 29240 | 1 | 29860 | 1 | 30420 | 1 | 31295 | 1 |
| 27709 | 1 | 28001 | 2 | 28222 | 1 | 28495 | 1 | 29260 | 1 | 29861 | 1 | 30430 | 1 | 31296 | 1 |
| 27712 | 1 | 28002 | 3 | 28225 | 1 | 28496 | 1 | 29280 | 2 | 29862 | 1 | 30435 | 1 | 31297 | 1 |
| 27715 | 1 | 28003 | 2 | 28226 | 1 | 28505 | 1 | 29305 | 1 | 29863 | 1 | 30450 | 1 | 31300 | 1 |
| 27720 | 1 | 28005 | 3 | 28230 | 1 | 28510 | 4 | 29325 | 1 | 29866 | 1 | 30460 | 1 | 31320 | 1 |
| 27722 | 1 | 28008 | 2 | 28232 | 6 | 28515 | 4 | 29345 | 1 | 29867 | 1 | 30462 | 1 | 31360 | 1 |
| 27724 | 1 | 28010 | 4 | 28234 | 6 | 28525 | 4 | 29355 | 1 | 29868 | 1 | 30465 | 1 | 31365 | 1 |
| 27725 | 1 | 28011 | 4 | 28238 | 1 | 28530 | 1 | 29358 | 1 | 29870 | 1 | 30520 | 1 | 31367 | 1 |
| 27726 | 1 | 28020 | 2 | 28240 | 1 | 28531 | 1 | 29365 | 1 | 29871 | 1 | 30540 | 1 | 31368 | 1 |
| 27727 | 1 | 28022 | 4 | 28250 | 1 | 28540 | 1 | 29405 | 1 | 29873 | 1 | 30545 | 1 | 31370 | 1 |
| 27730 | 1 | 28024 | 4 | 28260 | 1 | 28545 | 1 | 29425 | 1 | 29874 | 1 | 30560 | 1 | 31375 | 1 |
| 27732 | 1 | 28035 | 1 | 28261 | 1 | 28546 | 1 | 29435 | 1 | 29875 | 1 | 30580 | 2 | 31380 | 1 |
| 27734 | 1 | 28039 | 3 | 28262 | 1 | 28555 | 1 | 29440 | 1 | 29876 | 1 | 30600 | 1 | 31382 | 1 |
| 27740 | 1 | 28041 | 3 | 28264 | 1 | 28570 | 1 | 29445 | 1 | 29877 | 1 | 30620 | 1 | 31390 | 1 |
| 27742 | 1 | 28043 | 4 | 28270 | 6 | 28575 | 1 | 29450 | 1 | 29879 | 1 | 30630 | 1 | 31395 | 1 |
| 27745 | 1 | 28045 | 4 | 28272 | 6 | 28576 | 1 | 29505 | 1 | 29880 | 1 | 30801 | 1 | 31400 | 1 |
| 27750 | 1 | 28046 | 1 | 28280 | 1 | 28585 | 1 | 29515 | 1 | 29881 | 1 | 30802 | 1 | 31420 | 1 |
| 27752 | 1 | 28047 | 1 | 28285 | 4 | 28600 | 2 | 29520 | 1 | 29882 | 1 | 30901 | 1 | 31500 | 2 |
| 27756 | 1 | 28050 | 2 | 28286 | 1 | 28605 | 2 | 29530 | 1 | 29883 | 1 | 30903 | 1 | 31502 | 1 |
| 27758 | 1 | 28052 | 2 | 28288 | 5 | 28606 | 3 | 29540 | 1 | 29884 | 1 | 30905 | 1 | 31505 | 1 |
| 27759 | 1 | 28054 | 2 | 28289 | 1 | 28615 | 5 | 29550 | 1 | 29885 | 1 | 30906 | 1 | 31510 | 1 |
| 27760 | 1 | 28055 | 1 | 28291 | 1 | 28630 | 2 | 29580 | 1 | 29886 | 1 | 30915 | 1 | 31511 | 1 |
| 27762 | 1 | 28060 | 1 | 28292 | 1 | 28635 | 2 | 29581 | 1 | 29887 | 1 | 30920 | 1 | 31512 | 1 |
| 27766 | 1 | 28062 | 1 | 28295 | 1 | 28636 | 4 | 29582 | 1 | 29888 | 1 | 30930 | 1 | 31513 | 1 |
| 27767 | 1 | 28070 | 2 | 28296 | 1 | 28645 | 4 | 29583 | 1 | 29889 | 1 | 31000 | 1 | 31515 | 1 |
| 27768 | 1 | 28072 | 4 | 28297 | 1 | 28660 | 4 | 29584 | 1 | 29891 | 1 | 31002 | 1 | 31520 | 1 |
| 27769 | 1 | 28080 | 4 | 28298 | 1 | 28665 | 4 | 29700 | 2 | 29892 | 1 | 31020 | 1 | 31525 | 1 |
| 27780 | 1 | 28086 | 2 | 28299 | 1 | 28666 | 4 | 29705 | 1 | 29893 | 1 | 31030 | 1 | 31526 | 1 |
| 27781 | 1 | 28088 | 2 | 28300 | 1 | 28675 | 4 | 29710 | 1 | 29894 | 1 | 31032 | 1 | 31527 | 1 |
| 27784 | 1 | 28090 | 2 | 28302 | 1 | 28705 | 1 | 29720 | 1 | 29895 | 1 | 31040 | 1 | 31528 | 1 |
| 27786 | 1 | 28092 | 2 | 28304 | 1 | 28715 | 1 | 29730 | 1 | 29897 | 1 | 31050 | 1 | 31529 | 1 |
| 27788 | 1 | 28100 | 1 | 28305 | 1 | 28725 | 1 | 29740 | 1 | 29898 | 1 | 31051 | 1 | 31530 | 1 |
| 27792 | 1 | 28102 | 1 | 28306 | 1 | 28730 | 1 | 29750 | 1 | 29899 | 1 | 31070 | 1 | 31531 | 1 |
| 27808 | 1 | 28103 | 1 | 28307 | 1 | 28735 | 1 | 29800 | 1 | 29900 | 2 | 31075 | 1 | 31535 | 1 |
| 27810 | 1 | 28104 | 2 | 28308 | 4 | 28737 | 1 | 29804 | 1 | 29901 | 2 | 31080 | 1 | 31536 | 1 |
| 27814 | 1 | 28106 | 1 | 28309 | 1 | 28740 | 5 | 29805 | 1 | 29902 | 2 | 31081 | 1 | 31540 | 1 |
| 27816 | 1 | 28107 | 1 | 28310 | 1 | 28750 | 1 | 29806 | 1 | 29904 | 1 | 31084 | 1 | 31541 | 1 |
| 27818 | 1 | 28108 | 2 | 28312 | 4 | 28755 | 1 | 29807 | 1 | 29905 | 1 | 31085 | 1 | 31545 | 1 |
| 27822 | 1 | 28110 | 1 | 28313 | 4 | 28760 | 1 | 29819 | 1 | 29906 | 1 | 31086 | 1 | 31546 | 1 |
| 27823 | 1 | 28111 | 1 | 28315 | 1 | 28800 | 1 | 29820 | 1 | 29907 | 1 | 31087 | 1 | 31551 | 1 |
| 27824 | 1 | 28112 | 4 | 28320 | 1 | 28805 | 1 | 29821 | 1 | 29914 | 1 | 31090 | 1 | 31552 | 1 |
| 27825 | 1 | 28113 | 1 | 28322 | 2 | 28810 | 6 | 29822 | 1 | 29915 | 1 | 31200 | 1 | 31553 | 1 |
| 27826 | 1 | 28114 | 1 | 28340 | 2 | 28820 | 6 | 29823 | 1 | 29916 | 1 | 31201 | 1 | 31554 | 1 |
| 27827 | 1 | 28116 | 1 | 28341 | 2 | 28825 | 10 | 29824 | 1 | 30000 | 1 | 31205 | 1 | 31560 | 1 |
| 27828 | 1 | 28118 | 1 | 28344 | 1 | 28890 | 1 | 29825 | 1 | 30020 | 1 | 31225 | 1 | 31561 | 1 |
| 27829 | 1 | 28119 | 1 | 28345 | 2 | 29000 | 1 | 29826 | 1 | 30100 | 2 | 31230 | 1 | 31570 | 1 |

| CPT | MUE | CPT | MUE | CPT | MUE | CPT | MUE | CPT | MUE | CPT | MUE | CPT | MUE | CPT | MUE |
|---|---|---|---|---|---|---|---|---|---|---|---|---|---|---|---|
| 31571 | 1 | 31770 | 2 | 32609 | 1 | 33215 | 2 | 33369 | 1 | 33600 | 1 | 33814 | 1 | 33978 | 1 |
| 31572 | 1 | 31775 | 1 | 32650 | 1 | 33216 | 1 | 33390 | 1 | 33602 | 1 | 33820 | 1 | 33979 | 1 |
| 31573 | 1 | 31780 | 1 | 32651 | 1 | 33217 | 1 | 33391 | 1 | 33606 | 1 | 33822 | 1 | 33980 | 1 |
| 31574 | 1 | 31781 | 1 | 32652 | 1 | 33218 | 1 | 33404 | 1 | 33608 | 1 | 33824 | 1 | 33981 | 1 |
| 31575 | 1 | 31785 | 1 | 32653 | 1 | 33220 | 1 | 33405 | 1 | 33610 | 1 | 33840 | 1 | 33982 | 1 |
| 31576 | 1 | 31786 | 1 | 32654 | 1 | 33221 | 1 | 33406 | 1 | 33611 | 1 | 33845 | 1 | 33983 | 1 |
| 31577 | 1 | 31800 | 1 | 32655 | 1 | 33222 | 1 | 33410 | 1 | 33612 | 1 | 33851 | 1 | 33984 | 1 |
| 31578 | 1 | 31805 | 1 | 32656 | 1 | 33223 | 1 | 33411 | 1 | 33615 | 1 | 33852 | 1 | 33985 | 1 |
| 31579 | 1 | 31820 | 1 | 32658 | 1 | 33224 | 1 | 33412 | 1 | 33617 | 1 | 33853 | 1 | 33986 | 1 |
| 31580 | 1 | 31825 | 1 | 32659 | 1 | 33225 | 1 | 33413 | 1 | 33619 | 1 | 33860 | 1 | 33987 | 1 |
| 31584 | 1 | 31830 | 1 | 32661 | 1 | 33226 | 1 | 33414 | 1 | 33620 | 1 | 33863 | 1 | 33988 | 1 |
| 31587 | 1 | 32035 | 1 | 32662 | 1 | 33227 | 1 | 33415 | 1 | 33621 | 1 | 33864 | 1 | 33989 | 1 |
| 31590 | 1 | 32036 | 1 | 32663 | 1 | 33228 | 1 | 33416 | 1 | 33622 | 1 | 33870 | 1 | 33990 | 1 |
| 31591 | 1 | 32096 | 1 | 32664 | 1 | 33229 | 1 | 33417 | 1 | 33641 | 1 | 33875 | 1 | 33991 | 1 |
| 31592 | 1 | 32097 | 1 | 32665 | 1 | 33230 | 1 | 33418 | 1 | 33645 | 1 | 33877 | 1 | 33992 | 1 |
| 31595 | 1 | 32098 | 1 | 32666 | 1 | 33231 | 1 | 33419 | 1 | 33647 | 1 | 33880 | 1 | 33993 | 1 |
| 31600 | 1 | 32100 | 1 | 32667 | 3 | 33233 | 1 | 33420 | 1 | 33660 | 1 | 33881 | 1 | 34001 | 1 |
| 31601 | 1 | 32110 | 1 | 32668 | 2 | 33234 | 1 | 33422 | 1 | 33665 | 1 | 33883 | 1 | 34051 | 1 |
| 31603 | 1 | 32120 | 1 | 32669 | 2 | 33235 | 1 | 33425 | 1 | 33670 | 1 | 33884 | 2 | 34101 | 1 |
| 31605 | 1 | 32124 | 1 | 32670 | 1 | 33236 | 1 | 33426 | 1 | 33675 | 1 | 33886 | 1 | 34111 | 2 |
| 31610 | 1 | 32140 | 1 | 32671 | 1 | 33237 | 1 | 33427 | 1 | 33676 | 1 | 33889 | 1 | 34151 | 2 |
| 31611 | 1 | 32141 | 1 | 32672 | 1 | 33238 | 1 | 33430 | 1 | 33677 | 1 | 33891 | 1 | 34201 | 1 |
| 31612 | 1 | 32150 | 1 | 32673 | 1 | 33240 | 1 | 33460 | 1 | 33681 | 1 | 33910 | 1 | 34203 | 1 |
| 31613 | 1 | 32151 | 1 | 32674 | 1 | 33241 | 1 | 33463 | 1 | 33684 | 1 | 33915 | 1 | 34401 | 1 |
| 31614 | 1 | 32160 | 1 | 32701 | 1 | 33243 | 1 | 33464 | 1 | 33688 | 1 | 33916 | 1 | 34421 | 1 |
| 31615 | 1 | 32200 | 2 | 32800 | 1 | 33244 | 1 | 33465 | 1 | 33690 | 1 | 33917 | 1 | 34451 | 1 |
| 31622 | 1 | 32215 | 1 | 32810 | 1 | 33249 | 1 | 33468 | 1 | 33692 | 1 | 33920 | 1 | 34471 | 1 |
| 31623 | 1 | 32220 | 1 | 32815 | 1 | 33250 | 1 | 33470 | 1 | 33694 | 1 | 33922 | 1 | 34490 | 1 |
| 31624 | 1 | 32225 | 1 | 32820 | 1 | 33251 | 1 | 33471 | 1 | 33697 | 1 | 33924 | 1 | 34501 | 1 |
| 31625 | 1 | 32310 | 1 | 32850 | 1 | 33254 | 1 | 33474 | 1 | 33702 | 1 | 33925 | 1 | 34502 | 1 |
| 31626 | 1 | 32320 | 1 | 32851 | 1 | 33255 | 1 | 33475 | 1 | 33710 | 1 | 33926 | 1 | 34510 | 2 |
| 31627 | 1 | 32400 | 2 | 32852 | 1 | 33256 | 1 | 33476 | 1 | 33720 | 1 | 33930 | 1 | 34520 | 1 |
| 31628 | 1 | 32405 | 2 | 32853 | 1 | 33257 | 1 | 33477 | 1 | 33722 | 1 | 33933 | 1 | 34530 | 1 |
| 31629 | 1 | 32440 | 1 | 32854 | 1 | 33258 | 1 | 33478 | 1 | 33724 | 1 | 33935 | 1 | 34800 | 1 |
| 31630 | 1 | 32442 | 1 | 32855 | 1 | 33259 | 1 | 33496 | 1 | 33726 | 1 | 33940 | 1 | 34802 | 1 |
| 31631 | 1 | 32445 | 1 | 32856 | 1 | 33261 | 1 | 33500 | 1 | 33730 | 1 | 33944 | 1 | 34803 | 1 |
| 31632 | 2 | 32480 | 1 | 32900 | 1 | 33262 | 1 | 33501 | 1 | 33732 | 1 | 33945 | 1 | 34804 | 1 |
| 31633 | 2 | 32482 | 1 | 32905 | 1 | 33263 | 1 | 33502 | 1 | 33735 | 1 | 33946 | 1 | 34805 | 1 |
| 31634 | 1 | 32484 | 2 | 32906 | 1 | 33264 | 1 | 33503 | 1 | 33736 | 1 | 33947 | 1 | 34806 | 1 |
| 31635 | 1 | 32486 | 1 | 32940 | 1 | 33265 | 1 | 33504 | 1 | 33737 | 1 | 33948 | 1 | 34808 | 1 |
| 31636 | 1 | 32488 | 1 | 32960 | 1 | 33266 | 1 | 33505 | 1 | 33750 | 1 | 33949 | 1 | 34812 | 1 |
| 31637 | 2 | 32491 | 1 | 32997 | 1 | 33270 | 1 | 33506 | 1 | 33755 | 1 | 33951 | 1 | 34813 | 1 |
| 31638 | 1 | 32501 | 1 | 32998 | 1 | 33271 | 1 | 33507 | 1 | 33762 | 1 | 33952 | 1 | 34820 | 1 |
| 31640 | 1 | 32503 | 1 | 33010 | 1 | 33272 | 1 | 33508 | 1 | 33764 | 1 | 33953 | 1 | 34825 | 1 |
| 31641 | 1 | 32504 | 1 | 33011 | 1 | 33273 | 1 | 33510 | 1 | 33766 | 1 | 33954 | 1 | 34826 | 4 |
| 31643 | 1 | 32505 | 1 | 33015 | 1 | 33282 | 1 | 33511 | 1 | 33767 | 1 | 33955 | 1 | 34830 | 1 |
| 31645 | 1 | 32506 | 3 | 33020 | 1 | 33284 | 1 | 33512 | 1 | 33768 | 1 | 33956 | 1 | 34831 | 1 |
| 31646 | 2 | 32507 | 2 | 33025 | 1 | 33300 | 1 | 33513 | 1 | 33770 | 1 | 33957 | 1 | 34832 | 1 |
| 31647 | 1 | 32540 | 1 | 33030 | 1 | 33305 | 1 | 33514 | 1 | 33771 | 1 | 33958 | 1 | 34833 | 1 |
| 31648 | 1 | 32550 | 2 | 33031 | 1 | 33310 | 1 | 33516 | 1 | 33774 | 1 | 33959 | 1 | 34834 | 1 |
| 31649 | 2 | 32551 | 2 | 33050 | 1 | 33315 | 1 | 33517 | 1 | 33775 | 1 | 33962 | 1 | 34839 | 1 |
| 31651 | 3 | 32552 | 2 | 33120 | 1 | 33320 | 1 | 33518 | 1 | 33776 | 1 | 33963 | 1 | 34841 | 1 |
| 31652 | 1 | 32553 | 1 | 33130 | 1 | 33321 | 1 | 33519 | 1 | 33777 | 1 | 33964 | 1 | 34842 | 1 |
| 31653 | 1 | 32554 | 2 | 33140 | 1 | 33322 | 1 | 33521 | 1 | 33778 | 1 | 33965 | 1 | 34843 | 1 |
| 31654 | 1 | 32555 | 2 | 33141 | 1 | 33330 | 1 | 33522 | 1 | 33779 | 1 | 33966 | 1 | 34844 | 1 |
| 31660 | 1 | 32556 | 2 | 33202 | 1 | 33335 | 1 | 33523 | 1 | 33780 | 1 | 33967 | 1 | 34845 | 1 |
| 31661 | 1 | 32557 | 2 | 33203 | 1 | 33340 | 1 | 33530 | 1 | 33781 | 1 | 33968 | 1 | 34846 | 1 |
| 31717 | 1 | 32560 | 1 | 33206 | 1 | 33361 | 1 | 33533 | 1 | 33782 | 1 | 33969 | 1 | 34847 | 1 |
| 31720 | 1 | 32561 | 1 | 33207 | 1 | 33362 | 1 | 33534 | 1 | 33783 | 1 | 33970 | 1 | 34848 | 1 |
| 31725 | 1 | 32562 | 1 | 33208 | 1 | 33363 | 1 | 33535 | 1 | 33786 | 1 | 33971 | 1 | 34900 | 1 |
| 31730 | 1 | 32601 | 1 | 33210 | 1 | 33364 | 1 | 33536 | 1 | 33788 | 1 | 33973 | 1 | 35001 | 1 |
| 31750 | 1 | 32604 | 1 | 33211 | 1 | 33365 | 1 | 33542 | 1 | 33800 | 1 | 33974 | 1 | 35002 | 1 |
| 31755 | 1 | 32606 | 1 | 33212 | 1 | 33366 | 1 | 33545 | 1 | 33802 | 1 | 33975 | 1 | 35005 | 1 |
| 31760 | 1 | 32607 | 1 | 33213 | 1 | 33367 | 1 | 33548 | 1 | 33803 | 1 | 33976 | 1 | 35011 | 1 |
| 31766 | 1 | 32608 | 1 | 33214 | 1 | 33368 | 1 | 33572 | 3 | 33813 | 1 | 33977 | 1 | 35013 | 1 |

CPT © 2017 American Medical Association. All Rights Reserved.

© 2017 Optum360, LLC

| CPT | MUE | CPT | MUE | CPT | MUE | CPT | MUE | CPT | MUE | CPT | MUE | CPT | MUE | CPT | MUE |
|---|---|---|---|---|---|---|---|---|---|---|---|---|---|---|---|
| 35021 | 1 | 35508 | 1 | 35691 | 1 | 36410 | 3 | 36680 | 1 | 37233 | 2 | 38242 | 1 | 40800 | 2 |
| 35022 | 1 | 35509 | 1 | 35693 | 1 | 36415 | 2 | 36800 | 1 | 37234 | 2 | 38243 | 1 | 40801 | 2 |
| 35045 | 2 | 35510 | 1 | 35694 | 1 | 36420 | 2 | 36810 | 1 | 37235 | 2 | 38300 | 1 | 40804 | 2 |
| 35081 | 1 | 35511 | 1 | 35695 | 1 | 36425 | 2 | 36815 | 1 | 37236 | 1 | 38305 | 1 | 40805 | 2 |
| 35082 | 1 | 35512 | 1 | 35697 | 2 | 36430 | 1 | 36818 | 1 | 37237 | 2 | 38308 | 1 | 40806 | 2 |
| 35091 | 1 | 35515 | 1 | 35700 | 2 | 36440 | 1 | 36819 | 1 | 37238 | 1 | 38380 | 1 | 40808 | 4 |
| 35092 | 1 | 35516 | 1 | 35701 | 1 | 36450 | 1 | 36820 | 1 | 37239 | 2 | 38381 | 1 | 40810 | 4 |
| 35102 | 1 | 35518 | 1 | 35721 | 1 | 36455 | 1 | 36821 | 2 | 37241 | 2 | 38382 | 1 | 40812 | 4 |
| 35103 | 1 | 35521 | 1 | 35741 | 1 | 36456 | 1 | 36823 | 1 | 37242 | 2 | 38500 | 2 | 40814 | 4 |
| 35111 | 1 | 35522 | 1 | 35761 | 2 | 36460 | 2 | 36825 | 1 | 37243 | 1 | 38505 | 3 | 40816 | 2 |
| 35112 | 1 | 35523 | 1 | 35800 | 2 | 36468 | 1 | 36830 | 2 | 37244 | 2 | 38510 | 1 | 40818 | 2 |
| 35121 | 1 | 35525 | 1 | 35820 | 2 | 36470 | 1 | 36831 | 1 | 37246 | 1 | 38520 | 1 | 40819 | 2 |
| 35122 | 1 | 35526 | 1 | 35840 | 2 | 36471 | 2 | 36832 | 2 | 37247 | 2 | 38525 | 1 | 40820 | 5 |
| 35131 | 1 | 35531 | 2 | 35860 | 2 | 36473 | 1 | 36833 | 1 | 37248 | 1 | 38530 | 1 | 40830 | 2 |
| 35132 | 1 | 35533 | 1 | 35870 | 1 | 36474 | 2 | 36835 | 1 | 37249 | 2 | 38542 | 1 | 40831 | 2 |
| 35141 | 1 | 35535 | 1 | 35875 | 2 | 36475 | 1 | 36838 | 1 | 37252 | 1 | 38550 | 1 | 40840 | 1 |
| 35142 | 1 | 35536 | 1 | 35876 | 2 | 36476 | 2 | 36860 | 2 | 37253 | 5 | 38555 | 1 | 40842 | 1 |
| 35151 | 1 | 35537 | 1 | 35879 | 2 | 36478 | 1 | 36861 | 2 | 37500 | 1 | 38562 | 1 | 40843 | 1 |
| 35152 | 1 | 35538 | 1 | 35881 | 2 | 36479 | 2 | 36901 | 1 | 37565 | 1 | 38564 | 1 | 40844 | 1 |
| 35180 | 2 | 35539 | 1 | 35883 | 1 | 36481 | 1 | 36902 | 1 | 37600 | 1 | 38570 | 1 | 40845 | 1 |
| 35182 | 2 | 35540 | 1 | 35884 | 1 | 36500 | 4 | 36903 | 1 | 37605 | 1 | 38571 | 1 | 41000 | 2 |
| 35184 | 2 | 35556 | 1 | 35901 | 1 | 36510 | 1 | 36904 | 1 | 37606 | 1 | 38572 | 1 | 41005 | 2 |
| 35188 | 2 | 35558 | 1 | 35903 | 2 | 36511 | 1 | 36905 | 1 | 37607 | 1 | 38700 | 1 | 41006 | 2 |
| 35189 | 1 | 35560 | 1 | 35905 | 1 | 36512 | 1 | 36906 | 1 | 37609 | 1 | 38720 | 1 | 41007 | 2 |
| 35190 | 2 | 35563 | 1 | 35907 | 1 | 36513 | 1 | 36907 | 1 | 37615 | 2 | 38724 | 1 | 41008 | 2 |
| 35201 | 2 | 35565 | 1 | 36000 | 4 | 36514 | 1 | 36908 | 1 | 37616 | 1 | 38740 | 1 | 41009 | 2 |
| 35206 | 2 | 35566 | 1 | 36002 | 2 | 36515 | 1 | 36909 | 1 | 37617 | 3 | 38745 | 1 | 41010 | 1 |
| 35207 | 3 | 35570 | 1 | 36005 | 2 | 36516 | 1 | 37140 | 1 | 37618 | 2 | 38746 | 1 | 41015 | 2 |
| 35211 | 3 | 35571 | 2 | 36010 | 2 | 36522 | 1 | 37145 | 1 | 37619 | 1 | 38747 | 1 | 41016 | 2 |
| 35216 | 2 | 35572 | 2 | 36011 | 4 | 36555 | 2 | 37160 | 1 | 37650 | 1 | 38760 | 1 | 41017 | 2 |
| 35221 | 3 | 35583 | 1 | 36012 | 4 | 36556 | 2 | 37180 | 1 | 37660 | 1 | 38765 | 1 | 41018 | 2 |
| 35226 | 3 | 35585 | 2 | 36013 | 2 | 36557 | 2 | 37181 | 1 | 37700 | 1 | 38770 | 1 | 41019 | 1 |
| 35231 | 2 | 35587 | 2 | 36014 | 2 | 36558 | 2 | 37182 | 1 | 37718 | 1 | 38780 | 1 | 41100 | 3 |
| 35236 | 2 | 35600 | 2 | 36015 | 4 | 36560 | 2 | 37183 | 1 | 37722 | 1 | 38790 | 1 | 41105 | 3 |
| 35241 | 2 | 35601 | 1 | 36100 | 2 | 36561 | 2 | 37184 | 1 | 37735 | 1 | 38792 | 1 | 41108 | 2 |
| 35246 | 2 | 35606 | 1 | 36120 | 2 | 36563 | 1 | 37185 | 2 | 37760 | 1 | 38794 | 1 | 41110 | 2 |
| 35251 | 2 | 35612 | 1 | 36140 | 3 | 36565 | 1 | 37186 | 2 | 37761 | 1 | 38900 | 1 | 41112 | 2 |
| 35256 | 2 | 35616 | 1 | 36160 | 2 | 36566 | 1 | 37187 | 1 | 37765 | 1 | 39000 | 1 | 41113 | 2 |
| 35261 | 1 | 35621 | 1 | 36200 | 2 | 36568 | 2 | 37188 | 1 | 37766 | 1 | 39010 | 1 | 41114 | 2 |
| 35266 | 2 | 35623 | 1 | 36215 | 6 | 36569 | 2 | 37191 | 1 | 37780 | 1 | 39200 | 1 | 41115 | 1 |
| 35271 | 2 | 35626 | 3 | 36216 | 4 | 36570 | 2 | 37192 | 1 | 37785 | 1 | 39220 | 1 | 41116 | 2 |
| 35276 | 2 | 35631 | 4 | 36217 | 2 | 36571 | 2 | 37193 | 1 | 37788 | 2 | 39401 | 1 | 41120 | 1 |
| 35281 | 2 | 35632 | 1 | 36218 | 6 | 36575 | 2 | 37195 | 1 | 37790 | 1 | 39402 | 1 | 41130 | 1 |
| 35286 | 2 | 35633 | 1 | 36221 | 1 | 36576 | 2 | 37197 | 2 | 38100 | 1 | 39501 | 1 | 41135 | 1 |
| 35301 | 2 | 35634 | 1 | 36222 | 1 | 36578 | 2 | 37200 | 2 | 38101 | 1 | 39503 | 1 | 41140 | 1 |
| 35302 | 1 | 35636 | 1 | 36223 | 1 | 36580 | 2 | 37211 | 1 | 38102 | 1 | 39540 | 1 | 41145 | 1 |
| 35303 | 1 | 35637 | 1 | 36224 | 1 | 36581 | 2 | 37212 | 1 | 38115 | 1 | 39541 | 1 | 41150 | 1 |
| 35304 | 1 | 35638 | 1 | 36225 | 1 | 36582 | 2 | 37213 | 1 | 38120 | 1 | 39545 | 1 | 41153 | 1 |
| 35305 | 1 | 35642 | 1 | 36226 | 1 | 36583 | 2 | 37214 | 1 | 38200 | 1 | 39560 | 1 | 41155 | 1 |
| 35306 | 2 | 35645 | 1 | 36227 | 1 | 36584 | 2 | 37215 | 1 | 38205 | 1 | 39561 | 1 | 41250 | 2 |
| 35311 | 1 | 35646 | 1 | 36228 | 4 | 36585 | 2 | 37217 | 1 | 38206 | 1 | 40490 | 3 | 41251 | 2 |
| 35321 | 1 | 35647 | 1 | 36245 | 6 | 36589 | 2 | 37218 | 1 | 38208 | 0 | 40500 | 2 | 41252 | 2 |
| 35331 | 1 | 35650 | 1 | 36246 | 4 | 36590 | 2 | 37220 | 2 | 38209 | 0 | 40510 | 2 | 41500 | 1 |
| 35341 | 3 | 35654 | 1 | 36247 | 3 | 36591 | 2 | 37221 | 2 | 38210 | 0 | 40520 | 2 | 41510 | 1 |
| 35351 | 1 | 35656 | 1 | 36248 | 6 | 36592 | 1 | 37222 | 2 | 38211 | 0 | 40525 | 2 | 41512 | 1 |
| 35355 | 1 | 35661 | 1 | 36251 | 1 | 36593 | 2 | 37223 | 2 | 38212 | 0 | 40527 | 2 | 41520 | 1 |
| 35361 | 1 | 35663 | 1 | 36252 | 1 | 36595 | 2 | 37224 | 2 | 38213 | 0 | 40530 | 2 | 41530 | 1 |
| 35363 | 1 | 35665 | 1 | 36253 | 1 | 36596 | 2 | 37225 | 2 | 38214 | 0 | 40650 | 2 | 41800 | 2 |
| 35371 | 1 | 35666 | 2 | 36254 | 1 | 36597 | 2 | 37226 | 2 | 38215 | 0 | 40652 | 2 | 41805 | 3 |
| 35372 | 1 | 35671 | 2 | 36260 | 1 | 36598 | 2 | 37227 | 2 | 38220 | 1 | 40654 | 2 | 41806 | 3 |
| 35390 | 1 | 35681 | 1 | 36261 | 1 | 36600 | 4 | 37228 | 2 | 38221 | 1 | 40700 | 1 | 41820 | 4 |
| 35400 | 1 | 35682 | 1 | 36262 | 1 | 36620 | 3 | 37229 | 2 | 38230 | 1 | 40701 | 1 | 41821 | 2 |
| 35500 | 2 | 35683 | 1 | 36400 | 1 | 36625 | 2 | 37230 | 2 | 38232 | 1 | 40702 | 1 | 41822 | 1 |
| 35501 | 1 | 35685 | 2 | 36405 | 1 | 36640 | 1 | 37231 | 2 | 38240 | 1 | 40720 | 1 | 41823 | 1 |
| 35506 | 1 | 35686 | 1 | 36406 | 1 | 36660 | 1 | 37232 | 2 | 38241 | 1 | 40761 | 1 | 41825 | 2 |

**Appendix I — Medically Unlikely Edits (MUEs) — Professional**

| CPT | MUE | CPT | MUE | CPT | MUE | CPT | MUE | CPT | MUE | CPT | MUE | CPT | MUE | CPT | MUE |
|-----|-----|-----|-----|-----|-----|-----|-----|-----|-----|-----|-----|-----|-----|-----|-----|
| 41826 | 2 | 42808 | 2 | 43212 | 1 | 43327 | 1 | 43774 | 1 | 44186 | 1 | 44620 | 2 | 45340 | 1 |
| 41827 | 2 | 42809 | 1 | 43213 | 1 | 43328 | 1 | 43775 | 1 | 44187 | 1 | 44625 | 1 | 45341 | 1 |
| 41828 | 4 | 42810 | 1 | 43214 | 1 | 43330 | 1 | 43800 | 1 | 44188 | 1 | 44626 | 1 | 45342 | 1 |
| 41830 | 2 | 42815 | 1 | 43215 | 1 | 43331 | 1 | 43810 | 1 | 44202 | 1 | 44640 | 2 | 45346 | 1 |
| 41850 | 2 | 42820 | 1 | 43216 | 1 | 43332 | 1 | 43820 | 1 | 44203 | 2 | 44650 | 2 | 45347 | 1 |
| 41870 | 2 | 42821 | 1 | 43217 | 1 | 43333 | 1 | 43825 | 1 | 44204 | 2 | 44660 | 1 | 45349 | 1 |
| 41872 | 4 | 42825 | 1 | 43220 | 1 | 43334 | 1 | 43830 | 1 | 44205 | 1 | 44661 | 1 | 45350 | 1 |
| 41874 | 4 | 42826 | 1 | 43226 | 1 | 43335 | 1 | 43831 | 1 | 44206 | 1 | 44680 | 1 | 45378 | 1 |
| 42000 | 1 | 42830 | 1 | 43227 | 1 | 43336 | 1 | 43832 | 1 | 44207 | 1 | 44700 | 1 | 45379 | 1 |
| 42100 | 3 | 42831 | 1 | 43229 | 1 | 43337 | 1 | 43840 | 2 | 44208 | 1 | 44701 | 1 | 45380 | 1 |
| 42104 | 3 | 42835 | 1 | 43231 | 1 | 43338 | 1 | 43843 | 1 | 44210 | 1 | 44705 | 1 | 45381 | 1 |
| 42106 | 2 | 42836 | 1 | 43232 | 1 | 43340 | 1 | 43845 | 1 | 44211 | 1 | 44715 | 1 | 45382 | 1 |
| 42107 | 2 | 42842 | 1 | 43233 | 1 | 43341 | 1 | 43846 | 1 | 44212 | 1 | 44720 | 2 | 45384 | 1 |
| 42120 | 1 | 42844 | 1 | 43235 | 1 | 43351 | 1 | 43847 | 1 | 44213 | 1 | 44721 | 2 | 45385 | 1 |
| 42140 | 1 | 42845 | 1 | 43236 | 1 | 43352 | 1 | 43848 | 1 | 44227 | 1 | 44800 | 1 | 45386 | 1 |
| 42145 | 1 | 42860 | 1 | 43237 | 1 | 43360 | 1 | 43850 | 1 | 44300 | 1 | 44820 | 1 | 45388 | 1 |
| 42160 | 2 | 42870 | 1 | 43238 | 1 | 43361 | 1 | 43855 | 1 | 44310 | 2 | 44850 | 1 | 45389 | 1 |
| 42180 | 1 | 42890 | 1 | 43239 | 1 | 43400 | 1 | 43860 | 1 | 44312 | 1 | 44900 | 1 | 45390 | 1 |
| 42182 | 1 | 42892 | 1 | 43240 | 1 | 43401 | 1 | 43865 | 1 | 44314 | 1 | 44950 | 1 | 45391 | 1 |
| 42200 | 1 | 42894 | 1 | 43241 | 1 | 43405 | 1 | 43870 | 1 | 44316 | 1 | 44955 | 1 | 45392 | 1 |
| 42205 | 1 | 42900 | 1 | 43242 | 1 | 43410 | 1 | 43880 | 1 | 44320 | 1 | 44960 | 1 | 45393 | 1 |
| 42210 | 1 | 42950 | 1 | 43243 | 1 | 43415 | 1 | 43881 | 1 | 44322 | 1 | 44970 | 1 | 45395 | 1 |
| 42215 | 1 | 42953 | 1 | 43244 | 1 | 43420 | 1 | 43882 | 1 | 44340 | 1 | 45000 | 1 | 45397 | 1 |
| 42220 | 1 | 42955 | 1 | 43245 | 1 | 43425 | 1 | 43886 | 1 | 44345 | 1 | 45005 | 1 | 45398 | 1 |
| 42225 | 1 | 42960 | 1 | 43246 | 1 | 43450 | 1 | 43887 | 1 | 44346 | 1 | 45020 | 1 | 45400 | 1 |
| 42226 | 1 | 42961 | 1 | 43247 | 1 | 43453 | 1 | 43888 | 1 | 44360 | 1 | 45100 | 2 | 45402 | 1 |
| 42227 | 1 | 42962 | 1 | 43248 | 1 | 43460 | 1 | 44005 | 1 | 44361 | 1 | 45108 | 1 | 45500 | 1 |
| 42235 | 1 | 42970 | 1 | 43249 | 1 | 43496 | 1 | 44010 | 1 | 44363 | 1 | 45110 | 1 | 45505 | 1 |
| 42260 | 1 | 42971 | 1 | 43250 | 1 | 43500 | 1 | 44015 | 1 | 44364 | 1 | 45111 | 1 | 45520 | 1 |
| 42280 | 1 | 42972 | 1 | 43251 | 1 | 43501 | 1 | 44020 | 2 | 44365 | 1 | 45112 | 1 | 45540 | 1 |
| 42281 | 1 | 43020 | 1 | 43252 | 1 | 43502 | 1 | 44021 | 1 | 44366 | 1 | 45113 | 1 | 45541 | 1 |
| 42300 | 2 | 43030 | 1 | 43253 | 1 | 43510 | 1 | 44025 | 1 | 44369 | 1 | 45114 | 1 | 45550 | 1 |
| 42305 | 2 | 43045 | 1 | 43254 | 1 | 43520 | 1 | 44050 | 1 | 44370 | 1 | 45116 | 1 | 45560 | 1 |
| 42310 | 2 | 43100 | 1 | 43255 | 2 | 43605 | 1 | 44055 | 1 | 44372 | 1 | 45119 | 1 | 45562 | 1 |
| 42320 | 2 | 43101 | 1 | 43257 | 1 | 43610 | 2 | 44100 | 1 | 44373 | 1 | 45120 | 1 | 45563 | 1 |
| 42330 | 2 | 43107 | 1 | 43259 | 1 | 43611 | 2 | 44110 | 1 | 44376 | 1 | 45121 | 1 | 45800 | 1 |
| 42335 | 2 | 43108 | 1 | 43260 | 1 | 43620 | 1 | 44111 | 1 | 44377 | 1 | 45123 | 1 | 45805 | 1 |
| 42340 | 1 | 43112 | 1 | 43261 | 1 | 43621 | 1 | 44120 | 1 | 44378 | 1 | 45126 | 1 | 45820 | 1 |
| 42400 | 2 | 43113 | 1 | 43262 | 2 | 43622 | 1 | 44121 | 4 | 44379 | 1 | 45130 | 1 | 45825 | 1 |
| 42405 | 2 | 43116 | 1 | 43263 | 1 | 43631 | 1 | 44125 | 1 | 44380 | 1 | 45135 | 1 | 45900 | 1 |
| 42408 | 1 | 43117 | 1 | 43264 | 1 | 43632 | 1 | 44126 | 1 | 44381 | 1 | 45136 | 1 | 45905 | 1 |
| 42409 | 1 | 43118 | 1 | 43265 | 1 | 43633 | 1 | 44127 | 1 | 44382 | 1 | 45150 | 1 | 45910 | 1 |
| 42410 | 1 | 43121 | 1 | 43266 | 1 | 43634 | 1 | 44128 | 2 | 44384 | 1 | 45160 | 1 | 45915 | 1 |
| 42415 | 1 | 43122 | 1 | 43270 | 1 | 43635 | 1 | 44130 | 3 | 44385 | 1 | 45171 | 2 | 45990 | 1 |
| 42420 | 1 | 43123 | 1 | 43273 | 1 | 43640 | 1 | 44132 | 1 | 44386 | 1 | 45172 | 2 | 46020 | 2 |
| 42425 | 1 | 43124 | 1 | 43274 | 2 | 43641 | 1 | 44133 | 1 | 44388 | 1 | 45190 | 1 | 46030 | 1 |
| 42426 | 1 | 43130 | 1 | 43275 | 1 | 43644 | 1 | 44135 | 1 | 44389 | 1 | 45300 | 1 | 46040 | 2 |
| 42440 | 1 | 43135 | 1 | 43276 | 2 | 43645 | 1 | 44136 | 1 | 44390 | 1 | 45303 | 1 | 46045 | 2 |
| 42450 | 2 | 43180 | 1 | 43277 | 3 | 43647 | 1 | 44137 | 1 | 44391 | 1 | 45305 | 1 | 46050 | 2 |
| 42500 | 2 | 43191 | 1 | 43278 | 1 | 43648 | 1 | 44139 | 1 | 44392 | 1 | 45307 | 1 | 46060 | 2 |
| 42505 | 2 | 43192 | 1 | 43279 | 1 | 43651 | 1 | 44140 | 2 | 44394 | 1 | 45308 | 1 | 46070 | 1 |
| 42507 | 1 | 43193 | 1 | 43280 | 1 | 43652 | 1 | 44141 | 1 | 44401 | 1 | 45309 | 1 | 46080 | 1 |
| 42509 | 1 | 43194 | 1 | 43281 | 1 | 43653 | 1 | 44143 | 1 | 44402 | 1 | 45315 | 1 | 46083 | 2 |
| 42510 | 1 | 43195 | 1 | 43282 | 1 | 43752 | 2 | 44144 | 1 | 44403 | 1 | 45317 | 1 | 46200 | 1 |
| 42550 | 2 | 43196 | 1 | 43283 | 1 | 43753 | 1 | 44145 | 1 | 44404 | 1 | 45320 | 1 | 46220 | 1 |
| 42600 | 2 | 43197 | 1 | 43284 | 1 | 43754 | 1 | 44146 | 1 | 44405 | 1 | 45321 | 1 | 46221 | 1 |
| 42650 | 2 | 43198 | 1 | 43285 | 1 | 43755 | 1 | 44147 | 1 | 44406 | 1 | 45327 | 1 | 46230 | 1 |
| 42660 | 2 | 43200 | 1 | 43300 | 1 | 43756 | 1 | 44150 | 1 | 44407 | 1 | 45330 | 1 | 46250 | 1 |
| 42665 | 2 | 43201 | 1 | 43305 | 1 | 43757 | 1 | 44151 | 1 | 44408 | 1 | 45331 | 1 | 46255 | 1 |
| 42700 | 2 | 43202 | 1 | 43310 | 1 | 43760 | 2 | 44155 | 1 | 44500 | 1 | 45332 | 1 | 46257 | 1 |
| 42720 | 1 | 43204 | 1 | 43312 | 1 | 43761 | 2 | 44156 | 1 | 44602 | 1 | 45333 | 1 | 46258 | 1 |
| 42725 | 1 | 43205 | 1 | 43313 | 1 | 43770 | 1 | 44157 | 1 | 44603 | 1 | 45334 | 1 | 46260 | 1 |
| 42800 | 3 | 43206 | 1 | 43314 | 1 | 43771 | 1 | 44158 | 1 | 44604 | 1 | 45335 | 1 | 46261 | 1 |
| 42804 | 3 | 43210 | 1 | 43320 | 1 | 43772 | 1 | 44160 | 1 | 44605 | 1 | 45337 | 1 | 46262 | 1 |
| 42806 | 1 | 43211 | 1 | 43325 | 1 | 43773 | 1 | 44180 | 1 | 44615 | 4 | 45338 | 1 | 46270 | 1 |

CPT © 2017 American Medical Association. All Rights Reserved.

© 2017 Optum360, LLC

| CPT | MUE | CPT | MUE | CPT | MUE | CPT | MUE | CPT | MUE | CPT | MUE | CPT | MUE | CPT | MUE |
|-----|-----|-----|-----|-----|-----|-----|-----|-----|-----|-----|-----|-----|-----|-----|-----|
| 46275 | 1 | 47142 | 1 | 47800 | 1 | 49411 | 1 | 49900 | 1 | 50541 | 1 | 50930 | 2 | 51800 | 1 |
| 46280 | 1 | 47143 | 1 | 47801 | 1 | 49412 | 1 | 49904 | 1 | 50542 | 1 | 50940 | 1 | 51820 | 1 |
| 46285 | 1 | 47144 | 1 | 47802 | 1 | 49418 | 1 | 49905 | 1 | 50543 | 1 | 50945 | 1 | 51840 | 1 |
| 46288 | 1 | 47145 | 1 | 47900 | 1 | 49419 | 1 | 49906 | 1 | 50544 | 1 | 50947 | 1 | 51841 | 1 |
| 46320 | 2 | 47146 | 3 | 48000 | 1 | 49421 | 1 | 50010 | 1 | 50545 | 1 | 50948 | 1 | 51845 | 1 |
| 46500 | 1 | 47147 | 2 | 48001 | 1 | 49422 | 1 | 50020 | 1 | 50546 | 1 | 50951 | 1 | 51860 | 1 |
| 46505 | 1 | 47300 | 2 | 48020 | 1 | 49423 | 2 | 50040 | 1 | 50547 | 1 | 50953 | 1 | 51865 | 1 |
| 46600 | 1 | 47350 | 1 | 48100 | 1 | 49424 | 3 | 50045 | 1 | 50548 | 1 | 50955 | 1 | 51880 | 1 |
| 46601 | 1 | 47360 | 1 | 48102 | 1 | 49425 | 1 | 50060 | 1 | 50551 | 1 | 50957 | 1 | 51900 | 1 |
| 46604 | 1 | 47361 | 1 | 48105 | 1 | 49426 | 1 | 50065 | 1 | 50553 | 1 | 50961 | 1 | 51920 | 1 |
| 46606 | 1 | 47362 | 1 | 48120 | 1 | 49427 | 1 | 50070 | 1 | 50555 | 1 | 50970 | 1 | 51925 | 1 |
| 46607 | 1 | 47370 | 1 | 48140 | 1 | 49428 | 1 | 50075 | 1 | 50557 | 1 | 50972 | 1 | 51940 | 1 |
| 46608 | 1 | 47371 | 1 | 48145 | 1 | 49429 | 1 | 50080 | 1 | 50561 | 1 | 50974 | 1 | 51960 | 1 |
| 46610 | 1 | 47380 | 1 | 48146 | 1 | 49435 | 1 | 50081 | 1 | 50562 | 1 | 50976 | 1 | 51980 | 1 |
| 46611 | 1 | 47381 | 1 | 48148 | 1 | 49436 | 1 | 50100 | 1 | 50570 | 1 | 50980 | 1 | 51990 | 1 |
| 46612 | 1 | 47382 | 1 | 48150 | 1 | 49440 | 1 | 50120 | 1 | 50572 | 1 | 51020 | 1 | 51992 | 1 |
| 46614 | 1 | 47383 | 1 | 48152 | 1 | 49441 | 1 | 50125 | 1 | 50574 | 1 | 51030 | 1 | 52000 | 1 |
| 46615 | 1 | 47400 | 1 | 48153 | 1 | 49442 | 1 | 50130 | 1 | 50575 | 1 | 51040 | 1 | 52001 | 1 |
| 46700 | 1 | 47420 | 1 | 48154 | 1 | 49446 | 1 | 50135 | 1 | 50576 | 1 | 51045 | 2 | 52005 | 2 |
| 46705 | 1 | 47425 | 1 | 48155 | 1 | 49450 | 1 | 50200 | 1 | 50580 | 1 | 51050 | 1 | 52007 | 1 |
| 46706 | 1 | 47460 | 1 | 48400 | 1 | 49451 | 1 | 50205 | 1 | 50590 | 1 | 51060 | 1 | 52010 | 1 |
| 46707 | 1 | 47480 | 1 | 48500 | 1 | 49452 | 1 | 50220 | 1 | 50592 | 1 | 51065 | 1 | 52204 | 1 |
| 46710 | 1 | 47490 | 1 | 48510 | 1 | 49460 | 1 | 50225 | 1 | 50593 | 1 | 51080 | 1 | 52214 | 1 |
| 46712 | 1 | 47531 | 2 | 48520 | 1 | 49465 | 1 | 50230 | 1 | 50600 | 1 | 51100 | 1 | 52224 | 1 |
| 46715 | 1 | 47532 | 1 | 48540 | 1 | 49491 | 1 | 50234 | 1 | 50605 | 1 | 51101 | 1 | 52234 | 1 |
| 46716 | 1 | 47533 | 1 | 48545 | 1 | 49492 | 1 | 50236 | 1 | 50606 | 1 | 51102 | 1 | 52235 | 1 |
| 46730 | 1 | 47534 | 2 | 48547 | 1 | 49495 | 1 | 50240 | 1 | 50610 | 1 | 51500 | 1 | 52240 | 1 |
| 46735 | 1 | 47535 | 1 | 48548 | 1 | 49496 | 1 | 50250 | 1 | 50620 | 1 | 51520 | 1 | 52250 | 1 |
| 46740 | 1 | 47536 | 2 | 48550 | 1 | 49500 | 1 | 50280 | 1 | 50630 | 1 | 51525 | 1 | 52260 | 1 |
| 46742 | 1 | 47537 | 1 | 48551 | 1 | 49501 | 1 | 50290 | 1 | 50650 | 1 | 51530 | 1 | 52265 | 1 |
| 46744 | 1 | 47538 | 2 | 48552 | 2 | 49505 | 1 | 50300 | 1 | 50660 | 1 | 51535 | 1 | 52270 | 1 |
| 46746 | 1 | 47539 | 2 | 48554 | 1 | 49507 | 1 | 50320 | 1 | 50684 | 1 | 51550 | 1 | 52275 | 1 |
| 46748 | 1 | 47540 | 2 | 48556 | 1 | 49520 | 1 | 50323 | 1 | 50686 | 2 | 51555 | 1 | 52276 | 1 |
| 46750 | 1 | 47541 | 1 | 49000 | 1 | 49521 | 1 | 50325 | 1 | 50688 | 2 | 51565 | 1 | 52277 | 1 |
| 46751 | 1 | 47542 | 2 | 49002 | 1 | 49525 | 1 | 50327 | 1 | 50690 | 2 | 51570 | 1 | 52281 | 1 |
| 46753 | 1 | 47543 | 1 | 49010 | 1 | 49540 | 1 | 50328 | 1 | 50693 | 2 | 51575 | 1 | 52282 | 1 |
| 46754 | 1 | 47544 | 1 | 49020 | 2 | 49550 | 1 | 50329 | 1 | 50694 | 2 | 51580 | 1 | 52283 | 1 |
| 46760 | 1 | 47550 | 1 | 49040 | 2 | 49553 | 1 | 50340 | 1 | 50695 | 2 | 51585 | 1 | 52285 | 1 |
| 46761 | 1 | 47552 | 1 | 49060 | 2 | 49555 | 1 | 50360 | 1 | 50700 | 1 | 51590 | 1 | 52287 | 1 |
| 46762 | 1 | 47553 | 1 | 49062 | 1 | 49557 | 1 | 50365 | 1 | 50705 | 2 | 51595 | 1 | 52290 | 1 |
| 46900 | 1 | 47554 | 1 | 49082 | 1 | 49560 | 2 | 50370 | 1 | 50706 | 2 | 51596 | 1 | 52300 | 1 |
| 46910 | 1 | 47555 | 1 | 49083 | 2 | 49561 | 2 | 50380 | 1 | 50715 | 1 | 51597 | 1 | 52301 | 1 |
| 46916 | 1 | 47556 | 1 | 49084 | 1 | 49565 | 2 | 50382 | 1 | 50722 | 1 | 51600 | 1 | 52305 | 1 |
| 46917 | 1 | 47562 | 1 | 49180 | 2 | 49566 | 2 | 50384 | 1 | 50725 | 1 | 51605 | 1 | 52310 | 1 |
| 46922 | 1 | 47563 | 1 | 49185 | 2 | 49568 | 2 | 50385 | 1 | 50727 | 1 | 51610 | 1 | 52315 | 2 |
| 46924 | 1 | 47564 | 1 | 49203 | 1 | 49570 | 1 | 50386 | 1 | 50728 | 1 | 51700 | 1 | 52317 | 1 |
| 46930 | 1 | 47570 | 1 | 49204 | 1 | 49572 | 1 | 50387 | 1 | 50740 | 1 | 51701 | 2 | 52318 | 1 |
| 46940 | 1 | 47600 | 1 | 49205 | 1 | 49580 | 1 | 50389 | 1 | 50750 | 1 | 51702 | 2 | 52320 | 1 |
| 46942 | 1 | 47605 | 1 | 49215 | 1 | 49582 | 1 | 50390 | 2 | 50760 | 1 | 51703 | 2 | 52325 | 1 |
| 46945 | 1 | 47610 | 1 | 49220 | 1 | 49585 | 1 | 50391 | 1 | 50770 | 1 | 51705 | 1 | 52327 | 1 |
| 46946 | 1 | 47612 | 1 | 49250 | 1 | 49587 | 1 | 50395 | 1 | 50780 | 1 | 51710 | 1 | 52330 | 1 |
| 46947 | 1 | 47620 | 1 | 49255 | 1 | 49590 | 1 | 50396 | 1 | 50782 | 1 | 51715 | 1 | 52332 | 1 |
| 47000 | 3 | 47700 | 1 | 49320 | 1 | 49600 | 1 | 50400 | 1 | 50783 | 1 | 51720 | 1 | 52334 | 1 |
| 47001 | 3 | 47701 | 1 | 49321 | 1 | 49605 | 1 | 50405 | 1 | 50785 | 1 | 51725 | 1 | 52341 | 1 |
| 47010 | 3 | 47711 | 1 | 49322 | 1 | 49606 | 1 | 50430 | 2 | 50800 | 1 | 51726 | 1 | 52342 | 1 |
| 47015 | 1 | 47712 | 1 | 49323 | 1 | 49610 | 1 | 50431 | 2 | 50810 | 1 | 51727 | 1 | 52343 | 1 |
| 47100 | 3 | 47715 | 1 | 49324 | 1 | 49611 | 1 | 50432 | 2 | 50815 | 1 | 51728 | 1 | 52344 | 1 |
| 47120 | 2 | 47720 | 1 | 49325 | 1 | 49650 | 1 | 50433 | 2 | 50820 | 1 | 51729 | 1 | 52345 | 1 |
| 47122 | 1 | 47721 | 1 | 49326 | 1 | 49651 | 1 | 50434 | 2 | 50825 | 1 | 51736 | 1 | 52346 | 1 |
| 47125 | 1 | 47740 | 1 | 49327 | 1 | 49652 | 2 | 50435 | 2 | 50830 | 1 | 51741 | 1 | 52351 | 1 |
| 47130 | 1 | 47741 | 1 | 49400 | 1 | 49653 | 2 | 50500 | 1 | 50840 | 1 | 51784 | 1 | 52352 | 1 |
| 47133 | 1 | 47760 | 1 | 49402 | 1 | 49654 | 2 | 50520 | 1 | 50845 | 1 | 51785 | 1 | 52353 | 1 |
| 47135 | 1 | 47765 | 1 | 49405 | 2 | 49655 | 2 | 50525 | 1 | 50860 | 1 | 51792 | 1 | 52354 | 1 |
| 47140 | 1 | 47780 | 1 | 49406 | 2 | 49656 | 2 | 50526 | 1 | 50900 | 1 | 51797 | 1 | 52355 | 1 |
| 47141 | 1 | 47785 | 1 | 49407 | 1 | 49657 | 2 | 50540 | 1 | 50920 | 2 | 51798 | 1 | 52356 | 1 |

| CPT | MUE | CPT | MUE | CPT | MUE | CPT | MUE | CPT | MUE | CPT | MUE | CPT | MUE | CPT | MUE |
|---|---|---|---|---|---|---|---|---|---|---|---|---|---|---|---|
| 52400 | 1 | 53850 | 1 | 54416 | 1 | 55725 | 1 | 57160 | 1 | 57720 | 1 | 58605 | 1 | 59320 | 1 |
| 52402 | 1 | 53852 | 1 | 54417 | 1 | 55801 | 1 | 57170 | 1 | 57800 | 1 | 58611 | 1 | 59325 | 1 |
| 52441 | 1 | 53855 | 1 | 54420 | 1 | 55810 | 1 | 57180 | 1 | 58100 | 1 | 58615 | 1 | 59350 | 1 |
| 52442 | 6 | 53860 | 1 | 54430 | 1 | 55812 | 1 | 57200 | 1 | 58110 | 1 | 58660 | 1 | 59400 | 1 |
| 52450 | 1 | 54000 | 1 | 54435 | 1 | 55815 | 1 | 57210 | 1 | 58120 | 1 | 58661 | 1 | 59409 | 2 |
| 52500 | 1 | 54001 | 1 | 54437 | 1 | 55821 | 1 | 57220 | 1 | 58140 | 1 | 58662 | 1 | 59410 | 1 |
| 52601 | 1 | 54015 | 1 | 54438 | 1 | 55831 | 1 | 57230 | 1 | 58145 | 1 | 58670 | 1 | 59412 | 1 |
| 52630 | 1 | 54050 | 1 | 54440 | 1 | 55840 | 1 | 57240 | 1 | 58146 | 1 | 58671 | 1 | 59414 | 1 |
| 52640 | 1 | 54055 | 1 | 54450 | 1 | 55842 | 1 | 57250 | 1 | 58150 | 1 | 58672 | 1 | 59425 | 1 |
| 52647 | 1 | 54056 | 1 | 54500 | 1 | 55845 | 1 | 57260 | 1 | 58152 | 1 | 58673 | 1 | 59426 | 1 |
| 52648 | 1 | 54057 | 1 | 54505 | 1 | 55860 | 1 | 57265 | 1 | 58180 | 1 | 58674 | 1 | 59430 | 1 |
| 52649 | 1 | 54060 | 1 | 54512 | 1 | 55862 | 1 | 57267 | 2 | 58200 | 1 | 58700 | 1 | 59510 | 1 |
| 52700 | 1 | 54065 | 1 | 54520 | 1 | 55865 | 1 | 57268 | 1 | 58210 | 1 | 58720 | 1 | 59514 | 1 |
| 53000 | 1 | 54100 | 2 | 54522 | 1 | 55866 | 1 | 57270 | 1 | 58240 | 1 | 58740 | 1 | 59515 | 1 |
| 53010 | 1 | 54105 | 2 | 54530 | 1 | 55870 | 1 | 57280 | 1 | 58260 | 1 | 58750 | 1 | 59525 | 1 |
| 53020 | 1 | 54110 | 1 | 54535 | 1 | 55873 | 1 | 57282 | 1 | 58262 | 1 | 58752 | 1 | 59610 | 1 |
| 53025 | 1 | 54111 | 1 | 54550 | 1 | 55875 | 1 | 57283 | 1 | 58263 | 1 | 58760 | 1 | 59612 | 2 |
| 53040 | 1 | 54112 | 1 | 54560 | 1 | 55876 | 1 | 57284 | 1 | 58267 | 1 | 58770 | 1 | 59614 | 1 |
| 53060 | 1 | 54115 | 1 | 54600 | 1 | 55920 | 1 | 57285 | 1 | 58270 | 1 | 58800 | 1 | 59618 | 1 |
| 53080 | 1 | 54120 | 1 | 54620 | 1 | 56405 | 2 | 57287 | 1 | 58275 | 1 | 58805 | 1 | 59620 | 1 |
| 53085 | 1 | 54125 | 1 | 54640 | 1 | 56420 | 1 | 57288 | 1 | 58280 | 1 | 58820 | 1 | 59622 | 1 |
| 53200 | 1 | 54130 | 1 | 54650 | 1 | 56440 | 1 | 57289 | 1 | 58285 | 1 | 58822 | 1 | 59812 | 1 |
| 53210 | 1 | 54135 | 1 | 54660 | 1 | 56441 | 1 | 57291 | 1 | 58290 | 1 | 58825 | 1 | 59820 | 1 |
| 53215 | 1 | 54150 | 1 | 54670 | 1 | 56442 | 1 | 57292 | 1 | 58291 | 1 | 58900 | 1 | 59821 | 1 |
| 53220 | 1 | 54160 | 1 | 54680 | 1 | 56501 | 1 | 57295 | 1 | 58292 | 1 | 58920 | 1 | 59830 | 1 |
| 53230 | 1 | 54161 | 1 | 54690 | 1 | 56515 | 1 | 57296 | 1 | 58293 | 1 | 58925 | 1 | 59840 | 1 |
| 53235 | 1 | 54162 | 1 | 54692 | 1 | 56605 | 1 | 57300 | 1 | 58294 | 1 | 58940 | 1 | 59841 | 1 |
| 53240 | 1 | 54163 | 1 | 54700 | 1 | 56606 | 6 | 57305 | 1 | 58301 | 1 | 58943 | 1 | 59850 | 1 |
| 53250 | 1 | 54164 | 1 | 54800 | 1 | 56620 | 1 | 57307 | 1 | 58321 | 1 | 58950 | 1 | 59851 | 1 |
| 53260 | 1 | 54200 | 1 | 54830 | 1 | 56625 | 1 | 57308 | 1 | 58322 | 1 | 58951 | 1 | 59852 | 1 |
| 53265 | 1 | 54205 | 1 | 54840 | 1 | 56630 | 1 | 57310 | 1 | 58323 | 1 | 58952 | 1 | 59855 | 1 |
| 53270 | 1 | 54220 | 1 | 54860 | 1 | 56631 | 1 | 57311 | 1 | 58340 | 1 | 58953 | 1 | 59856 | 1 |
| 53275 | 1 | 54230 | 1 | 54861 | 1 | 56632 | 1 | 57320 | 1 | 58345 | 1 | 58954 | 1 | 59857 | 1 |
| 53400 | 1 | 54231 | 1 | 54865 | 1 | 56633 | 1 | 57330 | 1 | 58346 | 1 | 58956 | 1 | 59866 | 1 |
| 53405 | 1 | 54235 | 1 | 54900 | 1 | 56634 | 1 | 57335 | 1 | 58350 | 1 | 58957 | 1 | 59870 | 1 |
| 53410 | 1 | 54240 | 1 | 54901 | 1 | 56637 | 1 | 57400 | 1 | 58353 | 1 | 58958 | 1 | 59871 | 1 |
| 53415 | 1 | 54250 | 1 | 55000 | 1 | 56640 | 1 | 57410 | 1 | 58356 | 1 | 58960 | 1 | 60000 | 1 |
| 53420 | 1 | 54300 | 1 | 55040 | 1 | 56700 | 1 | 57415 | 1 | 58400 | 1 | 58970 | 1 | 60100 | 3 |
| 53425 | 1 | 54304 | 1 | 55041 | 1 | 56740 | 1 | 57420 | 1 | 58410 | 1 | 58974 | 1 | 60200 | 2 |
| 53430 | 1 | 54308 | 1 | 55060 | 1 | 56800 | 1 | 57421 | 1 | 58520 | 1 | 58976 | 2 | 60210 | 1 |
| 53431 | 1 | 54312 | 1 | 55100 | 2 | 56805 | 1 | 57423 | 1 | 58540 | 1 | 59000 | 2 | 60212 | 1 |
| 53440 | 1 | 54316 | 1 | 55110 | 1 | 56810 | 1 | 57425 | 1 | 58541 | 1 | 59001 | 2 | 60220 | 1 |
| 53442 | 1 | 54318 | 1 | 55120 | 1 | 56820 | 1 | 57426 | 1 | 58542 | 1 | 59012 | 2 | 60225 | 1 |
| 53444 | 1 | 54322 | 1 | 55150 | 1 | 56821 | 1 | 57452 | 1 | 58543 | 1 | 59015 | 2 | 60240 | 1 |
| 53445 | 1 | 54324 | 1 | 55175 | 1 | 57000 | 1 | 57454 | 1 | 58544 | 1 | 59020 | 2 | 60252 | 1 |
| 53446 | 1 | 54326 | 1 | 55180 | 1 | 57010 | 1 | 57455 | 1 | 58545 | 1 | 59025 | 2 | 60254 | 1 |
| 53447 | 1 | 54328 | 1 | 55200 | 1 | 57020 | 1 | 57456 | 1 | 58546 | 1 | 59030 | 2 | 60260 | 1 |
| 53448 | 1 | 54332 | 1 | 55250 | 1 | 57022 | 1 | 57460 | 1 | 58548 | 1 | 59050 | 2 | 60270 | 1 |
| 53449 | 1 | 54336 | 1 | 55300 | 1 | 57023 | 1 | 57461 | 1 | 58550 | 1 | 59051 | 2 | 60271 | 1 |
| 53450 | 1 | 54340 | 1 | 55400 | 1 | 57061 | 1 | 57500 | 1 | 58552 | 1 | 59070 | 2 | 60280 | 1 |
| 53460 | 1 | 54344 | 1 | 55450 | 1 | 57065 | 1 | 57505 | 1 | 58553 | 1 | 59072 | 2 | 60281 | 1 |
| 53500 | 1 | 54348 | 1 | 55500 | 1 | 57100 | 3 | 57510 | 1 | 58554 | 1 | 59074 | 2 | 60300 | 2 |
| 53502 | 1 | 54352 | 1 | 55520 | 1 | 57105 | 2 | 57511 | 1 | 58555 | 1 | 59076 | 2 | 60500 | 1 |
| 53505 | 1 | 54360 | 1 | 55530 | 1 | 57106 | 1 | 57513 | 1 | 58558 | 1 | 59100 | 1 | 60502 | 1 |
| 53510 | 1 | 54380 | 1 | 55535 | 1 | 57107 | 1 | 57520 | 1 | 58559 | 1 | 59120 | 1 | 60505 | 1 |
| 53515 | 1 | 54385 | 1 | 55540 | 1 | 57109 | 1 | 57522 | 1 | 58560 | 1 | 59121 | 1 | 60512 | 1 |
| 53520 | 1 | 54390 | 1 | 55550 | 1 | 57110 | 1 | 57530 | 1 | 58561 | 1 | 59130 | 1 | 60520 | 1 |
| 53600 | 1 | 54400 | 1 | 55600 | 1 | 57111 | 1 | 57531 | 1 | 58562 | 1 | 59135 | 1 | 60521 | 1 |
| 53601 | 1 | 54401 | 1 | 55605 | 1 | 57112 | 1 | 57540 | 1 | 58563 | 1 | 59136 | 1 | 60522 | 1 |
| 53605 | 1 | 54405 | 1 | 55650 | 1 | 57120 | 1 | 57545 | 1 | 58565 | 1 | 59140 | 1 | 60540 | 1 |
| 53620 | 1 | 54406 | 1 | 55680 | 1 | 57130 | 1 | 57550 | 1 | 58570 | 1 | 59150 | 1 | 60545 | 1 |
| 53621 | 1 | 54408 | 1 | 55700 | 1 | 57135 | 2 | 57555 | 1 | 58571 | 1 | 59151 | 1 | 60600 | 1 |
| 53660 | 1 | 54410 | 1 | 55705 | 1 | 57150 | 1 | 57556 | 1 | 58572 | 1 | 59160 | 1 | 60605 | 1 |
| 53661 | 1 | 54411 | 1 | 55706 | 1 | 57155 | 1 | 57558 | 1 | 58573 | 1 | 59200 | 1 | 60650 | 1 |
| 53665 | 1 | 54415 | 1 | 55720 | 1 | 57156 | 1 | 57700 | 1 | 58600 | 1 | 59300 | 1 | 61000 | 1 |

CPT © 2017 American Medical Association. All Rights Reserved.

© 2017 Optum360, LLC

| CPT | MUE | CPT | MUE | CPT | MUE | CPT | MUE | CPT | MUE | CPT | MUE | CPT | MUE | CPT | MUE |
|---|---|---|---|---|---|---|---|---|---|---|---|---|---|---|---|
| 61001 | 1 | 61543 | 1 | 61703 | 1 | 62256 | 1 | 63056 | 1 | 63307 | 1 | 64505 | 1 | 64742 | 1 |
| 61020 | 2 | 61544 | 1 | 61705 | 1 | 62258 | 1 | 63057 | 3 | 63308 | 3 | 64508 | 1 | 64744 | 1 |
| 61026 | 2 | 61545 | 1 | 61708 | 1 | 62263 | 1 | 63064 | 1 | 63600 | 2 | 64510 | 1 | 64746 | 1 |
| 61050 | 1 | 61546 | 1 | 61710 | 1 | 62264 | 1 | 63066 | 1 | 63610 | 1 | 64517 | 1 | 64755 | 1 |
| 61055 | 1 | 61548 | 1 | 61711 | 1 | 62267 | 2 | 63075 | 1 | 63615 | 1 | 64520 | 1 | 64760 | 1 |
| 61070 | 2 | 61550 | 1 | 61720 | 1 | 62268 | 1 | 63076 | 3 | 63620 | 1 | 64530 | 1 | 64763 | 1 |
| 61105 | 1 | 61552 | 1 | 61735 | 1 | 62269 | 2 | 63077 | 1 | 63621 | 2 | 64550 | 1 | 64766 | 1 |
| 61107 | 1 | 61556 | 1 | 61750 | 2 | 62270 | 2 | 63078 | 3 | 63650 | 2 | 64553 | 1 | 64771 | 2 |
| 61108 | 1 | 61557 | 1 | 61751 | 2 | 62272 | 1 | 63081 | 1 | 63655 | 1 | 64555 | 2 | 64772 | 2 |
| 61120 | 1 | 61558 | 1 | 61760 | 1 | 62273 | 2 | 63082 | 6 | 63661 | 1 | 64561 | 1 | 64774 | 2 |
| 61140 | 1 | 61559 | 1 | 61770 | 1 | 62280 | 1 | 63085 | 1 | 63662 | 1 | 64565 | 2 | 64776 | 1 |
| 61150 | 1 | 61563 | 2 | 61781 | 1 | 62281 | 1 | 63086 | 2 | 63663 | 1 | 64566 | 1 | 64778 | 1 |
| 61151 | 1 | 61564 | 1 | 61782 | 1 | 62282 | 1 | 63087 | 1 | 63664 | 1 | 64568 | 1 | 64782 | 2 |
| 61154 | 1 | 61566 | 1 | 61783 | 1 | 62284 | 1 | 63088 | 4 | 63685 | 1 | 64569 | 1 | 64783 | 2 |
| 61156 | 1 | 61567 | 1 | 61790 | 1 | 62287 | 1 | 63090 | 1 | 63688 | 1 | 64570 | 1 | 64784 | 3 |
| 61210 | 1 | 61570 | 1 | 61791 | 1 | 62290 | 5 | 63091 | 3 | 63700 | 1 | 64575 | 2 | 64786 | 1 |
| 61215 | 1 | 61571 | 1 | 61796 | 1 | 62291 | 4 | 63101 | 1 | 63702 | 1 | 64580 | 2 | 64787 | 4 |
| 61250 | 1 | 61575 | 1 | 61797 | 4 | 62292 | 1 | 63102 | 1 | 63704 | 1 | 64581 | 2 | 64788 | 5 |
| 61253 | 1 | 61576 | 1 | 61798 | 1 | 62294 | 1 | 63103 | 3 | 63706 | 1 | 64585 | 2 | 64790 | 1 |
| 61304 | 1 | 61580 | 1 | 61799 | 4 | 62302 | 1 | 63170 | 1 | 63707 | 1 | 64590 | 1 | 64792 | 2 |
| 61305 | 1 | 61581 | 1 | 61800 | 1 | 62303 | 1 | 63172 | 1 | 63709 | 1 | 64595 | 1 | 64795 | 2 |
| 61312 | 2 | 61582 | 1 | 61850 | 1 | 62304 | 1 | 63173 | 1 | 63710 | 1 | 64600 | 2 | 64802 | 1 |
| 61313 | 2 | 61583 | 1 | 61860 | 1 | 62305 | 1 | 63180 | 1 | 63740 | 1 | 64605 | 1 | 64804 | 1 |
| 61314 | 2 | 61584 | 1 | 61863 | 1 | 62320 | 1 | 63182 | 1 | 63741 | 1 | 64610 | 1 | 64809 | 1 |
| 61315 | 1 | 61585 | 1 | 61864 | 1 | 62321 | 1 | 63185 | 1 | 63744 | 1 | 64611 | 1 | 64818 | 1 |
| 61316 | 1 | 61586 | 1 | 61867 | 1 | 62322 | 1 | 63190 | 1 | 63746 | 1 | 64612 | 1 | 64820 | 4 |
| 61320 | 2 | 61590 | 1 | 61868 | 2 | 62323 | 1 | 63191 | 1 | 64400 | 4 | 64615 | 1 | 64821 | 1 |
| 61321 | 1 | 61591 | 1 | 61870 | 1 | 62324 | 1 | 63194 | 1 | 64402 | 1 | 64616 | 1 | 64822 | 1 |
| 61322 | 1 | 61592 | 1 | 61880 | 1 | 62325 | 1 | 63195 | 1 | 64405 | 1 | 64617 | 1 | 64823 | 1 |
| 61323 | 1 | 61595 | 1 | 61885 | 2 | 62326 | 1 | 63196 | 1 | 64408 | 1 | 64620 | 5 | 64831 | 1 |
| 61330 | 1 | 61596 | 1 | 61886 | 1 | 62327 | 1 | 63197 | 1 | 64410 | 1 | 64630 | 1 | 64832 | 3 |
| 61332 | 1 | 61597 | 1 | 61888 | 1 | 62350 | 1 | 63198 | 1 | 64413 | 1 | 64632 | 1 | 64834 | 1 |
| 61333 | 1 | 61598 | 1 | 62000 | 1 | 62351 | 1 | 63199 | 1 | 64415 | 1 | 64633 | 1 | 64835 | 1 |
| 61340 | 1 | 61600 | 1 | 62005 | 1 | 62355 | 1 | 63200 | 1 | 64416 | 1 | 64634 | 4 | 64836 | 1 |
| 61343 | 1 | 61601 | 1 | 62010 | 1 | 62360 | 1 | 63250 | 1 | 64417 | 1 | 64635 | 1 | 64837 | 2 |
| 61345 | 1 | 61605 | 1 | 62100 | 1 | 62361 | 1 | 63251 | 1 | 64418 | 1 | 64636 | 4 | 64840 | 1 |
| 61450 | 1 | 61606 | 1 | 62115 | 1 | 62362 | 1 | 63252 | 1 | 64420 | 3 | 64640 | 5 | 64856 | 2 |
| 61458 | 1 | 61607 | 1 | 62117 | 1 | 62365 | 1 | 63265 | 1 | 64421 | 3 | 64642 | 1 | 64857 | 2 |
| 61460 | 1 | 61608 | 1 | 62120 | 1 | 62367 | 1 | 63266 | 1 | 64425 | 1 | 64643 | 3 | 64858 | 1 |
| 61480 | 1 | 61610 | 1 | 62121 | 1 | 62368 | 1 | 63267 | 1 | 64430 | 1 | 64644 | 1 | 64859 | 2 |
| 61500 | 1 | 61611 | 1 | 62140 | 1 | 62369 | 1 | 63268 | 1 | 64435 | 1 | 64645 | 3 | 64861 | 1 |
| 61501 | 1 | 61612 | 1 | 62141 | 1 | 62370 | 1 | 63270 | 1 | 64445 | 1 | 64646 | 1 | 64862 | 1 |
| 61510 | 1 | 61613 | 1 | 62142 | 2 | 62380 | 1 | 63271 | 1 | 64446 | 1 | 64647 | 1 | 64864 | 2 |
| 61512 | 1 | 61615 | 1 | 62143 | 2 | 63001 | 1 | 63272 | 1 | 64447 | 1 | 64650 | 1 | 64865 | 1 |
| 61514 | 2 | 61616 | 1 | 62145 | 2 | 63003 | 1 | 63273 | 1 | 64448 | 1 | 64653 | 1 | 64866 | 1 |
| 61516 | 1 | 61618 | 2 | 62146 | 2 | 63005 | 1 | 63275 | 1 | 64449 | 1 | 64680 | 1 | 64868 | 1 |
| 61517 | 1 | 61619 | 2 | 62147 | 1 | 63011 | 1 | 63276 | 1 | 64450 | 10 | 64681 | 1 | 64872 | 1 |
| 61518 | 1 | 61623 | 2 | 62148 | 1 | 63012 | 1 | 63277 | 1 | 64455 | 1 | 64702 | 2 | 64874 | 1 |
| 61519 | 1 | 61624 | 2 | 62160 | 1 | 63015 | 1 | 63278 | 1 | 64461 | 1 | 64704 | 4 | 64876 | 1 |
| 61520 | 1 | 61626 | 2 | 62161 | 1 | 63016 | 1 | 63280 | 1 | 64462 | 1 | 64708 | 3 | 64885 | 1 |
| 61521 | 1 | 61630 | 1 | 62162 | 1 | 63017 | 1 | 63281 | 1 | 64463 | 1 | 64712 | 1 | 64886 | 1 |
| 61522 | 1 | 61635 | 2 | 62163 | 1 | 63020 | 1 | 63282 | 1 | 64479 | 1 | 64713 | 1 | 64890 | 2 |
| 61524 | 2 | 61645 | 3 | 62164 | 1 | 63030 | 1 | 63283 | 1 | 64480 | 4 | 64714 | 1 | 64891 | 2 |
| 61526 | 1 | 61650 | 1 | 62165 | 1 | 63035 | 4 | 63285 | 1 | 64483 | 1 | 64716 | 2 | 64892 | 2 |
| 61530 | 1 | 61651 | 2 | 62180 | 1 | 63040 | 1 | 63286 | 1 | 64484 | 4 | 64718 | 1 | 64893 | 2 |
| 61531 | 1 | 61680 | 1 | 62190 | 1 | 63042 | 1 | 63287 | 1 | 64486 | 1 | 64719 | 1 | 64895 | 2 |
| 61533 | 2 | 61682 | 1 | 62192 | 1 | 63043 | 4 | 63290 | 1 | 64487 | 1 | 64721 | 1 | 64896 | 2 |
| 61534 | 1 | 61684 | 1 | 62194 | 1 | 63044 | 4 | 63295 | 1 | 64488 | 1 | 64722 | 4 | 64897 | 2 |
| 61535 | 2 | 61686 | 1 | 62200 | 1 | 63045 | 1 | 63300 | 1 | 64489 | 1 | 64726 | 2 | 64898 | 2 |
| 61536 | 1 | 61690 | 1 | 62201 | 1 | 63046 | 1 | 63301 | 1 | 64490 | 1 | 64727 | 2 | 64901 | 2 |
| 61537 | 1 | 61692 | 1 | 62220 | 1 | 63047 | 1 | 63302 | 1 | 64491 | 1 | 64732 | 1 | 64902 | 1 |
| 61538 | 1 | 61697 | 2 | 62223 | 1 | 63048 | 5 | 63303 | 1 | 64492 | 1 | 64734 | 1 | 64905 | 1 |
| 61539 | 1 | 61698 | 1 | 62225 | 2 | 63050 | 1 | 63304 | 1 | 64493 | 1 | 64736 | 1 | 64907 | 1 |
| 61540 | 1 | 61700 | 2 | 62230 | 2 | 63051 | 1 | 63305 | 1 | 64494 | 1 | 64738 | 1 | 64910 | 3 |
| 61541 | 1 | 61702 | 1 | 62252 | 2 | 63055 | 1 | 63306 | 1 | 64495 | 1 | 64740 | 1 | 64911 | 2 |

**Appendix I — Medically Unlikely Edits (MUEs) — Professional**

| CPT | MUE | CPT | MUE | CPT | MUE | CPT | MUE | CPT | MUE | CPT | MUE | CPT | MUE |
|---|---|---|---|---|---|---|---|---|---|---|---|---|---|
| 65091 | 1 | 65900 | 1 | 67041 | 1 | 67825 | 1 | 68700 | 1 | 69641 | 1 | 70355 | 1 | 72072 | 1 |
| 65093 | 1 | 65920 | 1 | 67042 | 1 | 67830 | 1 | 68705 | 2 | 69642 | 1 | 70360 | 2 | 72074 | 1 |
| 65101 | 1 | 65930 | 1 | 67043 | 1 | 67835 | 1 | 68720 | 1 | 69643 | 1 | 70370 | 1 | 72080 | 1 |
| 65103 | 1 | 66020 | 1 | 67101 | 1 | 67840 | 4 | 68745 | 1 | 69644 | 1 | 70371 | 1 | 72081 | 1 |
| 65105 | 1 | 66030 | 1 | 67105 | 1 | 67850 | 3 | 68750 | 1 | 69645 | 1 | 70380 | 2 | 72082 | 1 |
| 65110 | 1 | 66130 | 1 | 67107 | 1 | 67875 | 1 | 68760 | 4 | 69646 | 1 | 70390 | 2 | 72083 | 1 |
| 65112 | 1 | 66150 | 1 | 67108 | 1 | 67880 | 1 | 68761 | 4 | 69650 | 1 | 70450 | 3 | 72084 | 1 |
| 65114 | 1 | 66155 | 1 | 67110 | 1 | 67882 | 1 | 68770 | 1 | 69660 | 1 | 70460 | 1 | 72100 | 2 |
| 65125 | 1 | 66160 | 1 | 67113 | 1 | 67900 | 1 | 68801 | 4 | 69661 | 1 | 70470 | 2 | 72110 | 1 |
| 65130 | 1 | 66170 | 1 | 67115 | 1 | 67901 | 1 | 68810 | 1 | 69662 | 1 | 70480 | 1 | 72114 | 1 |
| 65135 | 1 | 66172 | 1 | 67120 | 1 | 67902 | 1 | 68811 | 1 | 69666 | 1 | 70481 | 1 | 72120 | 1 |
| 65140 | 1 | 66174 | 1 | 67121 | 1 | 67903 | 1 | 68815 | 1 | 69667 | 1 | 70482 | 1 | 72125 | 1 |
| 65150 | 1 | 66175 | 1 | 67141 | 1 | 67904 | 1 | 68816 | 1 | 69670 | 1 | 70486 | 1 | 72126 | 1 |
| 65155 | 1 | 66179 | 1 | 67145 | 1 | 67906 | 1 | 68840 | 1 | 69676 | 1 | 70487 | 1 | 72127 | 1 |
| 65175 | 1 | 66180 | 1 | 67208 | 1 | 67908 | 1 | 68850 | 1 | 69700 | 1 | 70488 | 1 | 72128 | 1 |
| 65205 | 1 | 66183 | 1 | 67210 | 1 | 67909 | 1 | 69000 | 1 | 69711 | 1 | 70490 | 1 | 72129 | 1 |
| 65210 | 1 | 66184 | 1 | 67218 | 1 | 67911 | 4 | 69005 | 1 | 69714 | 1 | 70491 | 1 | 72130 | 1 |
| 65220 | 1 | 66185 | 1 | 67220 | 1 | 67912 | 1 | 69020 | 1 | 69715 | 1 | 70492 | 1 | 72131 | 1 |
| 65222 | 1 | 66220 | 1 | 67221 | 1 | 67914 | 2 | 69100 | 3 | 69717 | 1 | 70496 | 2 | 72132 | 1 |
| 65235 | 1 | 66225 | 1 | 67225 | 1 | 67915 | 2 | 69105 | 1 | 69718 | 1 | 70498 | 2 | 72133 | 1 |
| 65260 | 1 | 66250 | 1 | 67227 | 1 | 67916 | 2 | 69110 | 1 | 69720 | 1 | 70540 | 1 | 72141 | 1 |
| 65265 | 1 | 66500 | 1 | 67228 | 1 | 67917 | 2 | 69120 | 1 | 69725 | 1 | 70542 | 1 | 72142 | 1 |
| 65270 | 1 | 66505 | 1 | 67229 | 1 | 67921 | 2 | 69140 | 1 | 69740 | 1 | 70543 | 1 | 72146 | 1 |
| 65272 | 1 | 66600 | 1 | 67250 | 1 | 67922 | 2 | 69145 | 1 | 69745 | 1 | 70544 | 2 | 72147 | 1 |
| 65273 | 1 | 66605 | 1 | 67255 | 1 | 67923 | 2 | 69150 | 1 | 69801 | 1 | 70545 | 1 | 72148 | 1 |
| 65275 | 1 | 66625 | 1 | 67311 | 1 | 67924 | 2 | 69155 | 1 | 69805 | 1 | 70546 | 1 | 72149 | 1 |
| 65280 | 1 | 66630 | 1 | 67312 | 1 | 67930 | 2 | 69200 | 1 | 69806 | 1 | 70547 | 1 | 72156 | 1 |
| 65285 | 1 | 66635 | 1 | 67314 | 1 | 67935 | 2 | 69205 | 1 | 69820 | 1 | 70548 | 1 | 72157 | 1 |
| 65286 | 1 | 66680 | 1 | 67316 | 1 | 67938 | 2 | 69209 | 1 | 69840 | 1 | 70549 | 1 | 72158 | 1 |
| 65290 | 1 | 66682 | 1 | 67318 | 1 | 67950 | 2 | 69210 | 1 | 69905 | 1 | 70551 | 2 | 72170 | 2 |
| 65400 | 1 | 66700 | 1 | 67320 | 2 | 67961 | 4 | 69220 | 1 | 69910 | 1 | 70552 | 2 | 72190 | 1 |
| 65410 | 1 | 66710 | 1 | 67331 | 1 | 67966 | 4 | 69222 | 1 | 69915 | 1 | 70553 | 2 | 72191 | 1 |
| 65420 | 1 | 66711 | 1 | 67332 | 1 | 67971 | 1 | 69300 | 1 | 69930 | 1 | 70554 | 1 | 72192 | 1 |
| 65426 | 1 | 66720 | 1 | 67334 | 1 | 67973 | 1 | 69310 | 1 | 69950 | 1 | 70555 | 1 | 72193 | 1 |
| 65430 | 1 | 66740 | 1 | 67335 | 1 | 67974 | 1 | 69320 | 1 | 69955 | 1 | 70557 | 1 | 72194 | 1 |
| 65435 | 1 | 66761 | 1 | 67340 | 2 | 67975 | 1 | 69420 | 1 | 69960 | 1 | 70558 | 1 | 72195 | 1 |
| 65436 | 1 | 66762 | 1 | 67343 | 1 | 68020 | 1 | 69421 | 1 | 69970 | 1 | 70559 | 1 | 72196 | 1 |
| 65450 | 1 | 66770 | 1 | 67345 | 1 | 68040 | 1 | 69424 | 1 | 69990 | 1 | 71010 | 6 | 72197 | 1 |
| 65600 | 1 | 66820 | 1 | 67346 | 1 | 68100 | 1 | 69433 | 1 | 70010 | 1 | 71015 | 2 | 72198 | 1 |
| 65710 | 1 | 66821 | 1 | 67400 | 1 | 68110 | 1 | 69436 | 1 | 70015 | 1 | 71020 | 4 | 72200 | 2 |
| 65730 | 1 | 66825 | 1 | 67405 | 1 | 68115 | 1 | 69440 | 1 | 70030 | 2 | 71021 | 1 | 72202 | 1 |
| 65750 | 1 | 66830 | 1 | 67412 | 1 | 68130 | 1 | 69450 | 1 | 70100 | 2 | 71022 | 1 | 72220 | 1 |
| 65755 | 1 | 66840 | 1 | 67413 | 1 | 68135 | 1 | 69501 | 1 | 70110 | 2 | 71023 | 1 | 72240 | 1 |
| 65756 | 1 | 66850 | 1 | 67414 | 1 | 68200 | 1 | 69502 | 1 | 70120 | 1 | 71030 | 1 | 72255 | 1 |
| 65757 | 1 | 66852 | 1 | 67415 | 1 | 68320 | 1 | 69505 | 1 | 70130 | 1 | 71034 | 1 | 72265 | 1 |
| 65770 | 1 | 66920 | 1 | 67420 | 1 | 68325 | 1 | 69511 | 1 | 70134 | 1 | 71035 | 3 | 72270 | 1 |
| 65772 | 1 | 66930 | 1 | 67430 | 1 | 68326 | 2 | 69530 | 1 | 70140 | 2 | 71100 | 2 | 72275 | 3 |
| 65775 | 1 | 66940 | 1 | 67440 | 1 | 68328 | 2 | 69535 | 1 | 70150 | 1 | 71101 | 2 | 72285 | 4 |
| 65778 | 1 | 66982 | 1 | 67445 | 1 | 68330 | 1 | 69540 | 1 | 70160 | 1 | 71110 | 1 | 72295 | 5 |
| 65779 | 1 | 66983 | 1 | 67450 | 1 | 68335 | 1 | 69550 | 1 | 70170 | 2 | 71111 | 1 | 73000 | 2 |
| 65780 | 1 | 66984 | 1 | 67500 | 1 | 68340 | 1 | 69552 | 1 | 70190 | 1 | 71120 | 1 | 73010 | 2 |
| 65781 | 1 | 66985 | 1 | 67505 | 1 | 68360 | 1 | 69554 | 1 | 70200 | 2 | 71130 | 1 | 73020 | 2 |
| 65782 | 1 | 66986 | 1 | 67515 | 1 | 68362 | 1 | 69601 | 1 | 70210 | 1 | 71250 | 2 | 73030 | 4 |
| 65785 | 1 | 66990 | 1 | 67550 | 1 | 68371 | 1 | 69602 | 1 | 70220 | 1 | 71260 | 2 | 73040 | 2 |
| 65800 | 1 | 67005 | 1 | 67560 | 1 | 68400 | 1 | 69603 | 1 | 70240 | 1 | 71270 | 1 | 73050 | 1 |
| 65810 | 1 | 67010 | 1 | 67570 | 1 | 68420 | 2 | 69604 | 1 | 70250 | 2 | 71275 | 1 | 73060 | 2 |
| 65815 | 1 | 67015 | 1 | 67700 | 2 | 68500 | 1 | 69605 | 1 | 70260 | 1 | 71550 | 1 | 73070 | 2 |
| 65820 | 1 | 67025 | 1 | 67710 | 1 | 68505 | 1 | 69610 | 1 | 70300 | 1 | 71551 | 1 | 73080 | 2 |
| 65850 | 1 | 67027 | 1 | 67715 | 1 | 68510 | 1 | 69620 | 1 | 70310 | 1 | 71552 | 1 | 73085 | 2 |
| 65855 | 1 | 67028 | 1 | 67800 | 1 | 68520 | 1 | 69631 | 1 | 70320 | 1 | 71555 | 1 | 73090 | 2 |
| 65860 | 1 | 67030 | 1 | 67801 | 1 | 68525 | 1 | 69632 | 1 | 70328 | 1 | 72020 | 4 | 73092 | 2 |
| 65865 | 1 | 67031 | 1 | 67805 | 1 | 68530 | 1 | 69633 | 1 | 70330 | 1 | 72040 | 3 | 73100 | 2 |
| 65870 | 1 | 67036 | 1 | 67808 | 1 | 68540 | 1 | 69635 | 1 | 70332 | 2 | 72050 | 1 | 73110 | 3 |
| 65875 | 1 | 67039 | 1 | 67810 | 2 | 68550 | 1 | 69636 | 1 | 70336 | 1 | 72052 | 1 | 73115 | 2 |
| 65880 | 1 | 67040 | 1 | 67820 | 1 | | | 69637 | 1 | 70350 | 1 | 72070 | 1 | 73120 | 3 |

CPT © 2017 American Medical Association. All Rights Reserved.

© 2017 Optum360, LLC

| CPT | MUE | CPT | MUE | CPT | MUE | CPT | MUE | CPT | MUE | CPT | MUE | CPT | MUE | CPT | MUE |
|---|---|---|---|---|---|---|---|---|---|---|---|---|---|---|---|
| 73130 | 3 | 74230 | 1 | 75736 | 2 | 76536 | 1 | 77053 | 2 | 77525 | 1 | 78272 | 1 | 78805 | 1 |
| 73140 | 3 | 74235 | 1 | 75741 | 1 | 76604 | 1 | 77054 | 2 | 77600 | 1 | 78278 | 2 | 78806 | 1 |
| 73200 | 2 | 74240 | 2 | 75743 | 1 | 76641 | 2 | 77058 | 1 | 77605 | 1 | 78282 | 1 | 78807 | 1 |
| 73201 | 2 | 74241 | 1 | 75746 | 1 | 76642 | 2 | 77059 | 1 | 77610 | 1 | 78290 | 1 | 78808 | 1 |
| 73202 | 2 | 74245 | 1 | 75756 | 2 | 76700 | 1 | 77063 | 1 | 77615 | 1 | 78291 | 1 | 78811 | 1 |
| 73206 | 2 | 74246 | 1 | 75774 | 7 | 76705 | 2 | 77065 | 1 | 77620 | 1 | 78300 | 1 | 78812 | 1 |
| 73218 | 2 | 74247 | 1 | 75801 | 1 | 76706 | 1 | 77066 | 1 | 77750 | 1 | 78305 | 1 | 78813 | 1 |
| 73219 | 2 | 74249 | 1 | 75803 | 1 | 76770 | 1 | 77067 | 1 | 77761 | 1 | 78306 | 1 | 78814 | 1 |
| 73220 | 2 | 74250 | 1 | 75805 | 1 | 76775 | 2 | 77071 | 1 | 77762 | 1 | 78315 | 1 | 78815 | 1 |
| 73221 | 2 | 74251 | 1 | 75807 | 1 | 76776 | 2 | 77072 | 1 | 77763 | 1 | 78320 | 1 | 78816 | 1 |
| 73222 | 2 | 74260 | 1 | 75809 | 1 | 76800 | 1 | 77073 | 1 | 77767 | 2 | 78414 | 1 | 79005 | 1 |
| 73223 | 2 | 74261 | 1 | 75810 | 1 | 76801 | 1 | 77074 | 1 | 77768 | 2 | 78428 | 1 | 79101 | 1 |
| 73501 | 2 | 74262 | 1 | 75820 | 2 | 76802 | 2 | 77075 | 1 | 77770 | 2 | 78445 | 1 | 79200 | 1 |
| 73502 | 2 | 74270 | 1 | 75822 | 1 | 76805 | 1 | 77076 | 1 | 77771 | 2 | 78451 | 1 | 79300 | 1 |
| 73503 | 2 | 74280 | 1 | 75825 | 1 | 76810 | 2 | 77077 | 1 | 77772 | 2 | 78452 | 1 | 79403 | 1 |
| 73521 | 2 | 74283 | 1 | 75827 | 1 | 76811 | 1 | 77078 | 1 | 77778 | 1 | 78453 | 1 | 79440 | 1 |
| 73522 | 2 | 74290 | 1 | 75831 | 1 | 76812 | 2 | 77080 | 1 | 77789 | 2 | 78454 | 1 | 79445 | 1 |
| 73523 | 2 | 74300 | 1 | 75833 | 1 | 76813 | 1 | 77081 | 1 | 77790 | 1 | 78456 | 1 | 80047 | 2 |
| 73525 | 2 | 74301 | 1 | 75840 | 1 | 76814 | 2 | 77084 | 1 | 78012 | 1 | 78457 | 1 | 80048 | 2 |
| 73551 | 2 | 74328 | 1 | 75842 | 1 | 76815 | 1 | 77085 | 1 | 78013 | 1 | 78458 | 1 | 80051 | 2 |
| 73552 | 2 | 74329 | 1 | 75860 | 2 | 76816 | 3 | 77086 | 1 | 78014 | 1 | 78459 | 1 | 80053 | 1 |
| 73560 | 4 | 74330 | 1 | 75870 | 1 | 76817 | 1 | 77261 | 1 | 78015 | 1 | 78466 | 1 | 80061 | 1 |
| 73562 | 4 | 74340 | 1 | 75872 | 1 | 76818 | 3 | 77262 | 1 | 78016 | 1 | 78468 | 1 | 80069 | 1 |
| 73564 | 4 | 74355 | 1 | 75880 | 1 | 76819 | 3 | 77263 | 1 | 78018 | 1 | 78469 | 1 | 80074 | 1 |
| 73565 | 1 | 74360 | 1 | 75885 | 1 | 76820 | 3 | 77280 | 2 | 78020 | 1 | 78472 | 1 | 80076 | 1 |
| 73580 | 2 | 74363 | 2 | 75887 | 1 | 76821 | 3 | 77285 | 1 | 78070 | 1 | 78473 | 1 | 80081 | 1 |
| 73590 | 3 | 74400 | 1 | 75889 | 1 | 76825 | 3 | 77290 | 1 | 78071 | 1 | 78481 | 1 | 80150 | 2 |
| 73592 | 2 | 74410 | 1 | 75891 | 1 | 76826 | 3 | 77293 | 1 | 78072 | 1 | 78483 | 1 | 80155 | 1 |
| 73600 | 3 | 74415 | 1 | 75893 | 2 | 76827 | 3 | 77295 | 1 | 78075 | 1 | 78491 | 1 | 80156 | 2 |
| 73610 | 3 | 74420 | 2 | 75894 | 2 | 76828 | 3 | 77300 | 10 | 78102 | 1 | 78492 | 1 | 80157 | 2 |
| 73615 | 2 | 74425 | 2 | 75898 | 2 | 76830 | 1 | 77301 | 1 | 78103 | 1 | 78494 | 1 | 80158 | 2 |
| 73620 | 3 | 74430 | 1 | 75901 | 1 | 76831 | 1 | 77306 | 1 | 78104 | 1 | 78496 | 1 | 80159 | 2 |
| 73630 | 3 | 74440 | 1 | 75902 | 2 | 76856 | 1 | 77307 | 1 | 78110 | 1 | 78579 | 1 | 80162 | 2 |
| 73650 | 2 | 74445 | 1 | 75952 | 1 | 76857 | 1 | 77316 | 1 | 78111 | 1 | 78580 | 1 | 80163 | 1 |
| 73660 | 2 | 74450 | 1 | 75953 | 4 | 76870 | 1 | 77317 | 1 | 78120 | 1 | 78582 | 1 | 80164 | 2 |
| 73700 | 2 | 74455 | 1 | 75954 | 2 | 76872 | 1 | 77318 | 1 | 78121 | 1 | 78597 | 1 | 80165 | 1 |
| 73701 | 2 | 74470 | 2 | 75956 | 1 | 76873 | 1 | 77321 | 1 | 78122 | 1 | 78598 | 1 | 80168 | 2 |
| 73702 | 2 | 74485 | 2 | 75957 | 1 | 76881 | 2 | 77331 | 3 | 78130 | 1 | 78600 | 1 | 80169 | 1 |
| 73706 | 2 | 74710 | 1 | 75958 | 2 | 76882 | 2 | 77332 | 4 | 78135 | 1 | 78601 | 1 | 80170 | 2 |
| 73718 | 2 | 74712 | 1 | 75959 | 1 | 76885 | 1 | 77333 | 2 | 78140 | 1 | 78605 | 1 | 80171 | 1 |
| 73719 | 2 | 74713 | 2 | 75970 | 1 | 76886 | 1 | 77334 | 10 | 78185 | 1 | 78606 | 1 | 80173 | 2 |
| 73720 | 2 | 74740 | 1 | 75984 | 2 | 76930 | 1 | 77336 | 1 | 78190 | 1 | 78607 | 1 | 80175 | 1 |
| 73721 | 3 | 74742 | 2 | 75989 | 2 | 76932 | 1 | 77338 | 1 | 78191 | 1 | 78608 | 1 | 80176 | 1 |
| 73722 | 2 | 74775 | 1 | 76000 | 3 | 76936 | 1 | 77370 | 1 | 78195 | 1 | 78610 | 1 | 80177 | 1 |
| 73723 | 2 | 75557 | 1 | 76001 | 1 | 76937 | 2 | 77371 | 1 | 78201 | 1 | 78630 | 1 | 80178 | 2 |
| 73725 | 2 | 75559 | 1 | 76010 | 2 | 76940 | 1 | 77372 | 1 | 78202 | 1 | 78635 | 1 | 80180 | 1 |
| 74000 | 4 | 75561 | 1 | 76080 | 3 | 76941 | 3 | 77373 | 1 | 78205 | 1 | 78645 | 1 | 80183 | 1 |
| 74010 | 2 | 75563 | 1 | 76098 | 3 | 76942 | 1 | 77401 | 1 | 78206 | 1 | 78647 | 1 | 80184 | 2 |
| 74020 | 2 | 75565 | 1 | 76100 | 2 | 76945 | 2 | 77402 | 2 | 78215 | 1 | 78650 | 1 | 80185 | 2 |
| 74022 | 2 | 75571 | 1 | 76101 | 1 | 76946 | 1 | 77407 | 2 | 78216 | 1 | 78660 | 1 | 80186 | 2 |
| 74150 | 1 | 75572 | 1 | 76102 | 1 | 76948 | 1 | 77412 | 2 | 78226 | 1 | 78700 | 1 | 80188 | 2 |
| 74160 | 1 | 75573 | 1 | 76120 | 1 | 76965 | 2 | 77417 | 1 | 78227 | 1 | 78701 | 1 | 80190 | 2 |
| 74170 | 1 | 75574 | 1 | 76125 | 1 | 76970 | 2 | 77422 | 1 | 78230 | 1 | 78707 | 1 | 80192 | 2 |
| 74174 | 1 | 75600 | 1 | 76376 | 2 | 76975 | 1 | 77423 | 1 | 78231 | 1 | 78708 | 1 | 80194 | 2 |
| 74175 | 1 | 75605 | 1 | 76377 | 2 | 76977 | 1 | 77424 | 1 | 78232 | 1 | 78709 | 1 | 80195 | 2 |
| 74176 | 2 | 75625 | 1 | 76380 | 2 | 76998 | 1 | 77425 | 1 | 78258 | 1 | 78710 | 1 | 80197 | 2 |
| 74177 | 2 | 75630 | 1 | 76506 | 1 | 77001 | 2 | 77427 | 1 | 78261 | 1 | 78725 | 1 | 80198 | 2 |
| 74178 | 1 | 75635 | 1 | 76510 | 2 | 77002 | 1 | 77431 | 1 | 78262 | 1 | 78730 | 1 | 80199 | 1 |
| 74181 | 1 | 75658 | 1 | 76511 | 2 | 77003 | 1 | 77432 | 1 | 78264 | 1 | 78740 | 1 | 80200 | 2 |
| 74182 | 1 | 75705 | 20 | 76512 | 2 | 77011 | 1 | 77435 | 1 | 78265 | 1 | 78761 | 1 | 80201 | 2 |
| 74183 | 1 | 75710 | 2 | 76513 | 2 | 77012 | 1 | 77469 | 1 | 78266 | 1 | 78800 | 1 | 80202 | 2 |
| 74185 | 1 | 75716 | 1 | 76514 | 1 | 77013 | 1 | 77470 | 1 | 78267 | 1 | 78801 | 1 | 80203 | 1 |
| 74190 | 1 | 75726 | 3 | 76516 | 1 | 77014 | 2 | 77520 | 1 | 78268 | 1 | 78802 | 1 | 80299 | 3 |
| 74210 | 1 | 75731 | 1 | 76519 | 2 | 77021 | 1 | 77522 | 1 | 78270 | 1 | 78803 | 1 | 80305 | 1 |
| 74220 | 1 | 75733 | 1 | 76529 | 2 | 77022 | 1 | 77523 | 1 | 78271 | 1 | 78804 | 1 | 80306 | 1 |

| CPT | MUE | CPT | MUE | CPT | MUE | CPT | MUE | CPT | MUE | CPT | MUE | CPT | MUE | CPT | MUE |
|---|---|---|---|---|---|---|---|---|---|---|---|---|---|---|---|
| 80307 | 1 | 81227 | 1 | 81327 | 1 | 81493 | 1 | 82248 | 2 | 82627 | 1 | 83013 | 1 | 83735 | 4 |
| 80400 | 1 | 81228 | 1 | 81330 | 1 | 81500 | 1 | 82252 | 1 | 82633 | 1 | 83014 | 1 | 83775 | 1 |
| 80402 | 1 | 81229 | 1 | 81331 | 1 | 81503 | 1 | 82261 | 1 | 82634 | 1 | 83015 | 1 | 83785 | 1 |
| 80406 | 1 | 81235 | 1 | 81332 | 1 | 81504 | 1 | 82270 | 1 | 82638 | 1 | 83018 | 4 | 83789 | 4 |
| 80408 | 1 | 81240 | 1 | 81340 | 1 | 81506 | 1 | 82271 | 1 | 82652 | 1 | 83020 | 2 | 83825 | 2 |
| 80410 | 1 | 81241 | 1 | 81341 | 1 | 81507 | 1 | 82272 | 1 | 82656 | 1 | 83021 | 2 | 83835 | 2 |
| 80412 | 1 | 81242 | 1 | 81342 | 1 | 81508 | 1 | 82274 | 1 | 82657 | 3 | 83026 | 1 | 83857 | 1 |
| 80414 | 1 | 81243 | 1 | 81350 | 1 | 81509 | 1 | 82286 | 1 | 82658 | 2 | 83030 | 1 | 83861 | 2 |
| 80415 | 1 | 81244 | 1 | 81355 | 1 | 81510 | 1 | 82300 | 1 | 82664 | 2 | 83033 | 1 | 83864 | 1 |
| 80416 | 1 | 81245 | 1 | 81370 | 1 | 81511 | 1 | 82306 | 1 | 82668 | 1 | 83036 | 1 | 83872 | 2 |
| 80417 | 1 | 81246 | 1 | 81371 | 1 | 81512 | 1 | 82308 | 1 | 82670 | 2 | 83037 | 1 | 83873 | 1 |
| 80418 | 1 | 81250 | 1 | 81372 | 1 | 81519 | 1 | 82310 | 2 | 82671 | 1 | 83045 | 1 | 83874 | 2 |
| 80420 | 1 | 81251 | 1 | 81373 | 2 | 81525 | 1 | 82330 | 2 | 82672 | 1 | 83050 | 1 | 83876 | 1 |
| 80422 | 1 | 81252 | 1 | 81374 | 1 | 81528 | 1 | 82331 | 1 | 82677 | 1 | 83051 | 1 | 83880 | 1 |
| 80424 | 1 | 81253 | 1 | 81375 | 1 | 81535 | 1 | 82340 | 1 | 82679 | 1 | 83060 | 1 | 83883 | 6 |
| 80426 | 1 | 81254 | 1 | 81376 | 5 | 81536 | 11 | 82355 | 2 | 82693 | 2 | 83065 | 1 | 83885 | 2 |
| 80428 | 1 | 81255 | 1 | 81377 | 2 | 81538 | 1 | 82360 | 2 | 82696 | 1 | 83068 | 1 | 83915 | 1 |
| 80430 | 1 | 81256 | 1 | 81378 | 1 | 81539 | 1 | 82365 | 2 | 82705 | 1 | 83069 | 1 | 83916 | 2 |
| 80432 | 1 | 81257 | 1 | 81379 | 1 | 81540 | 1 | 82370 | 2 | 82710 | 1 | 83070 | 1 | 83918 | 1 |
| 80434 | 1 | 81260 | 1 | 81380 | 2 | 81545 | 1 | 82373 | 1 | 82715 | 3 | 83080 | 2 | 83919 | 1 |
| 80435 | 1 | 81261 | 1 | 81381 | 3 | 81595 | 1 | 82374 | 2 | 82725 | 1 | 83088 | 1 | 83921 | 2 |
| 80436 | 1 | 81262 | 1 | 81382 | 6 | 82009 | 1 | 82375 | 1 | 82726 | 1 | 83090 | 2 | 83930 | 2 |
| 80438 | 1 | 81263 | 1 | 81383 | 2 | 82010 | 1 | 82376 | 1 | 82728 | 1 | 83150 | 1 | 83935 | 2 |
| 80439 | 1 | 81264 | 1 | 81400 | 2 | 82013 | 1 | 82378 | 1 | 82731 | 1 | 83491 | 1 | 83937 | 1 |
| 80500 | 1 | 81265 | 1 | 81401 | 2 | 82016 | 1 | 82379 | 1 | 82735 | 1 | 83497 | 1 | 83945 | 2 |
| 80502 | 1 | 81266 | 2 | 81402 | 1 | 82017 | 1 | 82380 | 1 | 82746 | 1 | 83498 | 2 | 83950 | 1 |
| 81000 | 2 | 81267 | 1 | 81403 | 4 | 82024 | 4 | 82382 | 1 | 82747 | 1 | 83499 | 1 | 83951 | 1 |
| 81001 | 2 | 81268 | 4 | 81404 | 5 | 82030 | 1 | 82383 | 1 | 82757 | 1 | 83500 | 1 | 83970 | 2 |
| 81002 | 2 | 81270 | 1 | 81405 | 2 | 82040 | 1 | 82384 | 2 | 82759 | 1 | 83505 | 1 | 83986 | 2 |
| 81003 | 2 | 81272 | 1 | 81406 | 2 | 82042 | 2 | 82387 | 1 | 82760 | 1 | 83516 | 4 | 83987 | 1 |
| 81005 | 2 | 81273 | 1 | 81407 | 1 | 82043 | 1 | 82390 | 1 | 82775 | 1 | 83518 | 1 | 83992 | 2 |
| 81007 | 1 | 81275 | 1 | 81408 | 2 | 82044 | 1 | 82397 | 3 | 82776 | 1 | 83519 | 5 | 83993 | 1 |
| 81015 | 2 | 81276 | 1 | 81410 | 1 | 82045 | 1 | 82415 | 1 | 82777 | 1 | 83520 | 8 | 84030 | 1 |
| 81020 | 1 | 81287 | 1 | 81411 | 1 | 82075 | 2 | 82435 | 2 | 82784 | 6 | 83525 | 4 | 84035 | 1 |
| 81025 | 1 | 81288 | 1 | 81412 | 1 | 82085 | 1 | 82436 | 1 | 82785 | 1 | 83527 | 1 | 84060 | 1 |
| 81050 | 2 | 81290 | 1 | 81413 | 1 | 82088 | 2 | 82438 | 1 | 82787 | 4 | 83528 | 1 | 84061 | 1 |
| 81161 | 1 | 81291 | 1 | 81414 | 1 | 82103 | 1 | 82441 | 1 | 82800 | 1 | 83540 | 2 | 84066 | 1 |
| 81162 | 1 | 81292 | 1 | 81415 | 1 | 82104 | 1 | 82465 | 1 | 82805 | 2 | 83550 | 1 | 84075 | 2 |
| 81170 | 1 | 81293 | 1 | 81416 | 2 | 82105 | 1 | 82480 | 1 | 82810 | 2 | 83570 | 1 | 84078 | 1 |
| 81200 | 1 | 81294 | 1 | 81417 | 1 | 82106 | 2 | 82482 | 1 | 82820 | 1 | 83582 | 1 | 84080 | 1 |
| 81201 | 1 | 81295 | 1 | 81420 | 1 | 82107 | 1 | 82485 | 1 | 82930 | 1 | 83586 | 1 | 84081 | 1 |
| 81202 | 1 | 81296 | 1 | 81422 | 1 | 82108 | 1 | 82495 | 1 | 82938 | 1 | 83593 | 1 | 84085 | 1 |
| 81203 | 1 | 81297 | 1 | 81425 | 1 | 82120 | 1 | 82507 | 1 | 82941 | 1 | 83605 | 3 | 84087 | 1 |
| 81205 | 1 | 81298 | 1 | 81426 | 2 | 82127 | 1 | 82523 | 1 | 82943 | 1 | 83615 | 2 | 84100 | 2 |
| 81206 | 1 | 81299 | 1 | 81427 | 1 | 82128 | 2 | 82525 | 2 | 82945 | 4 | 83625 | 2 | 84105 | 1 |
| 81207 | 1 | 81300 | 1 | 81430 | 1 | 82131 | 2 | 82528 | 1 | 82946 | 1 | 83630 | 1 | 84106 | 1 |
| 81208 | 1 | 81301 | 1 | 81431 | 1 | 82135 | 1 | 82530 | 4 | 82947 | 5 | 83631 | 1 | 84110 | 1 |
| 81209 | 1 | 81302 | 1 | 81432 | 1 | 82136 | 2 | 82533 | 5 | 82950 | 3 | 83632 | 1 | 84112 | 1 |
| 81210 | 1 | 81303 | 1 | 81433 | 1 | 82139 | 2 | 82540 | 1 | 82951 | 2 | 83633 | 1 | 84119 | 1 |
| 81211 | 1 | 81304 | 1 | 81434 | 1 | 82140 | 2 | 82542 | 6 | 82952 | 3 | 83655 | 2 | 84120 | 1 |
| 81212 | 1 | 81310 | 1 | 81435 | 1 | 82143 | 2 | 82550 | 3 | 82955 | 1 | 83661 | 3 | 84126 | 1 |
| 81213 | 1 | 81311 | 1 | 81436 | 1 | 82150 | 2 | 82552 | 3 | 82960 | 1 | 83662 | 4 | 84132 | 2 |
| 81214 | 1 | 81313 | 1 | 81437 | 1 | 82154 | 1 | 82553 | 3 | 82963 | 1 | 83663 | 3 | 84133 | 2 |
| 81215 | 1 | 81314 | 1 | 81438 | 1 | 82157 | 1 | 82554 | 1 | 82965 | 1 | 83664 | 3 | 84134 | 1 |
| 81216 | 1 | 81315 | 1 | 81439 | 1 | 82160 | 1 | 82565 | 2 | 82977 | 1 | 83670 | 1 | 84135 | 1 |
| 81217 | 1 | 81316 | 1 | 81440 | 1 | 82163 | 1 | 82570 | 3 | 82978 | 1 | 83690 | 2 | 84138 | 1 |
| 81218 | 1 | 81317 | 1 | 81442 | 1 | 82164 | 1 | 82575 | 1 | 82979 | 1 | 83695 | 1 | 84140 | 1 |
| 81219 | 1 | 81318 | 1 | 81445 | 1 | 82172 | 3 | 82585 | 1 | 82985 | 1 | 83698 | 1 | 84143 | 2 |
| 81220 | 1 | 81319 | 1 | 81450 | 1 | 82175 | 2 | 82595 | 1 | 83001 | 1 | 83700 | 1 | 84144 | 1 |
| 81221 | 1 | 81321 | 1 | 81455 | 1 | 82180 | 1 | 82600 | 1 | 83002 | 1 | 83701 | 1 | 84145 | 1 |
| 81222 | 1 | 81322 | 1 | 81460 | 1 | 82190 | 2 | 82607 | 1 | 83003 | 5 | 83704 | 1 | 84146 | 3 |
| 81223 | 1 | 81323 | 1 | 81465 | 1 | 82232 | 2 | 82608 | 1 | 83006 | 1 | 83718 | 1 | 84150 | 2 |
| 81224 | 1 | 81324 | 1 | 81470 | 1 | 82239 | 1 | 82610 | 1 | 83009 | 1 | 83719 | 1 | 84152 | 1 |
| 81225 | 1 | 81325 | 1 | 81471 | 1 | 82240 | 1 | 82615 | 1 | 83010 | 1 | 83721 | 1 | 84153 | 1 |
| 81226 | 1 | 81326 | 1 | 81490 | 1 | 82247 | 2 | 82626 | 1 | 83012 | 1 | 83727 | 1 | 84154 | 1 |

CPT © 2017 American Medical Association. All Rights Reserved.
© 2017 Optum360, LLC

Appendix I — Medically Unlikely Edits (MUEs) — Professional

| CPT | MUE | CPT | MUE | CPT | MUE | CPT | MUE | CPT | MUE | CPT | MUE | CPT | MUE | CPT | MUE |
|---|---|---|---|---|---|---|---|---|---|---|---|---|---|---|---|
| 84155 | 1 | 84488 | 1 | 85292 | 1 | 86021 | 1 | 86359 | 1 | 86701 | 1 | 86860 | 2 | 87158 | 1 |
| 84156 | 1 | 84490 | 1 | 85293 | 1 | 86022 | 1 | 86360 | 1 | 86702 | 2 | 86870 | 2 | 87164 | 2 |
| 84157 | 2 | 84510 | 1 | 85300 | 2 | 86023 | 3 | 86361 | 1 | 86703 | 1 | 86880 | 4 | 87166 | 2 |
| 84160 | 2 | 84512 | 1 | 85301 | 1 | 86038 | 1 | 86367 | 1 | 86704 | 1 | 86885 | 1 | 87168 | 2 |
| 84163 | 1 | 84520 | 4 | 85302 | 1 | 86039 | 1 | 86376 | 2 | 86705 | 1 | 86886 | 3 | 87169 | 2 |
| 84165 | 1 | 84525 | 1 | 85303 | 2 | 86060 | 1 | 86378 | 1 | 86706 | 2 | 86890 | 1 | 87172 | 1 |
| 84166 | 2 | 84540 | 2 | 85305 | 2 | 86063 | 1 | 86382 | 3 | 86707 | 1 | 86891 | 1 | 87176 | 2 |
| 84181 | 3 | 84545 | 1 | 85306 | 2 | 86077 | 1 | 86384 | 1 | 86708 | 1 | 86900 | 1 | 87177 | 3 |
| 84182 | 6 | 84550 | 1 | 85307 | 2 | 86078 | 1 | 86386 | 1 | 86709 | 1 | 86901 | 1 | 87181 | 12 |
| 84202 | 1 | 84560 | 2 | 85335 | 2 | 86079 | 1 | 86406 | 2 | 86710 | 4 | 86902 | 6 | 87184 | 8 |
| 84203 | 1 | 84577 | 1 | 85337 | 1 | 86140 | 1 | 86430 | 2 | 86711 | 2 | 86904 | 2 | 87185 | 4 |
| 84206 | 1 | 84578 | 1 | 85345 | 1 | 86141 | 1 | 86431 | 2 | 86713 | 3 | 86905 | 8 | 87186 | 12 |
| 84207 | 1 | 84580 | 1 | 85347 | 5 | 86146 | 3 | 86480 | 1 | 86717 | 8 | 86906 | 1 | 87187 | 3 |
| 84210 | 1 | 84583 | 1 | 85348 | 1 | 86147 | 4 | 86481 | 1 | 86720 | 2 | 86920 | 9 | 87188 | 6 |
| 84220 | 1 | 84585 | 1 | 85360 | 1 | 86148 | 3 | 86485 | 1 | 86723 | 2 | 86921 | 2 | 87190 | 9 |
| 84228 | 1 | 84586 | 1 | 85362 | 2 | 86152 | 1 | 86486 | 2 | 86727 | 2 | 86922 | 5 | 87197 | 1 |
| 84233 | 1 | 84588 | 1 | 85366 | 1 | 86153 | 1 | 86490 | 1 | 86729 | 0 | 86923 | 10 | 87205 | 3 |
| 84234 | 1 | 84590 | 1 | 85370 | 1 | 86155 | 1 | 86510 | 1 | 86732 | 2 | 86927 | 2 | 87206 | 6 |
| 84235 | 1 | 84591 | 1 | 85378 | 1 | 86156 | 1 | 86580 | 1 | 86735 | 2 | 86930 | 0 | 87207 | 3 |
| 84238 | 3 | 84597 | 1 | 85379 | 2 | 86157 | 1 | 86590 | 1 | 86738 | 2 | 86931 | 1 | 87209 | 4 |
| 84244 | 2 | 84600 | 2 | 85380 | 1 | 86160 | 4 | 86592 | 2 | 86741 | 2 | 86932 | 2 | 87210 | 4 |
| 84252 | 1 | 84620 | 1 | 85384 | 2 | 86161 | 2 | 86593 | 2 | 86744 | 2 | 86940 | 1 | 87220 | 3 |
| 84255 | 2 | 84630 | 2 | 85385 | 1 | 86162 | 1 | 86602 | 3 | 86747 | 2 | 86941 | 1 | 87230 | 3 |
| 84260 | 1 | 84681 | 1 | 85390 | 3 | 86171 | 2 | 86603 | 2 | 86750 | 4 | 86945 | 2 | 87250 | 1 |
| 84270 | 1 | 84702 | 2 | 85396 | 1 | 86185 | 1 | 86609 | 14 | 86753 | 3 | 86950 | 1 | 87252 | 2 |
| 84275 | 1 | 84703 | 1 | 85397 | 3 | 86200 | 1 | 86611 | 4 | 86756 | 2 | 86960 | 1 | 87253 | 2 |
| 84285 | 1 | 84704 | 1 | 85400 | 1 | 86215 | 1 | 86612 | 2 | 86757 | 6 | 86965 | 1 | 87254 | 7 |
| 84295 | 3 | 84830 | 1 | 85410 | 1 | 86225 | 1 | 86615 | 6 | 86759 | 2 | 86970 | 1 | 87255 | 2 |
| 84300 | 2 | 85002 | 1 | 85415 | 2 | 86226 | 1 | 86617 | 2 | 86762 | 2 | 86971 | 1 | 87260 | 1 |
| 84302 | 1 | 85004 | 1 | 85420 | 2 | 86235 | 10 | 86618 | 2 | 86765 | 2 | 86972 | 1 | 87265 | 1 |
| 84305 | 1 | 85007 | 1 | 85421 | 1 | 86243 | 1 | 86619 | 2 | 86768 | 5 | 86975 | 1 | 87267 | 1 |
| 84307 | 1 | 85008 | 1 | 85441 | 1 | 86255 | 5 | 86622 | 2 | 86771 | 2 | 86976 | 1 | 87269 | 1 |
| 84311 | 2 | 85009 | 1 | 85445 | 1 | 86256 | 9 | 86625 | 1 | 86774 | 2 | 86977 | 1 | 87270 | 1 |
| 84315 | 1 | 85013 | 1 | 85460 | 1 | 86277 | 1 | 86628 | 3 | 86777 | 2 | 86978 | 1 | 87271 | 1 |
| 84375 | 1 | 85014 | 2 | 85461 | 1 | 86280 | 1 | 86631 | 6 | 86778 | 2 | 86985 | 1 | 87272 | 1 |
| 84376 | 1 | 85018 | 2 | 85475 | 1 | 86294 | 1 | 86632 | 3 | 86780 | 2 | 87003 | 1 | 87273 | 1 |
| 84377 | 1 | 85025 | 2 | 85520 | 1 | 86300 | 2 | 86635 | 4 | 86784 | 1 | 87015 | 4 | 87274 | 1 |
| 84378 | 2 | 85027 | 2 | 85525 | 2 | 86301 | 1 | 86638 | 6 | 86787 | 2 | 87040 | 2 | 87275 | 1 |
| 84379 | 1 | 85032 | 1 | 85530 | 1 | 86304 | 1 | 86641 | 2 | 86788 | 1 | 87045 | 3 | 87276 | 1 |
| 84392 | 1 | 85041 | 1 | 85536 | 1 | 86305 | 1 | 86644 | 2 | 86789 | 2 | 87046 | 6 | 87277 | 1 |
| 84402 | 1 | 85044 | 1 | 85540 | 1 | 86308 | 1 | 86645 | 1 | 86790 | 4 | 87070 | 3 | 87278 | 1 |
| 84403 | 2 | 85045 | 1 | 85547 | 1 | 86309 | 1 | 86648 | 2 | 86793 | 2 | 87071 | 4 | 87279 | 1 |
| 84410 | 1 | 85046 | 2 | 85549 | 1 | 86310 | 1 | 86651 | 2 | 86800 | 1 | 87073 | 3 | 87280 | 1 |
| 84425 | 1 | 85048 | 2 | 85555 | 1 | 86316 | 2 | 86652 | 2 | 86803 | 1 | 87075 | 6 | 87281 | 1 |
| 84430 | 1 | 85049 | 2 | 85557 | 1 | 86317 | 6 | 86653 | 2 | 86804 | 1 | 87076 | 6 | 87283 | 1 |
| 84431 | 1 | 85055 | 1 | 85576 | 7 | 86318 | 2 | 86654 | 2 | 86805 | 2 | 87077 | 10 | 87285 | 1 |
| 84432 | 1 | 85060 | 1 | 85597 | 1 | 86320 | 1 | 86658 | 12 | 86807 | 2 | 87081 | 6 | 87290 | 1 |
| 84436 | 1 | 85097 | 1 | 85598 | 1 | 86325 | 2 | 86663 | 2 | 86808 | 1 | 87084 | 1 | 87299 | 1 |
| 84437 | 1 | 85130 | 1 | 85610 | 4 | 86327 | 1 | 86664 | 2 | 86812 | 1 | 87086 | 3 | 87300 | 2 |
| 84439 | 1 | 85170 | 1 | 85611 | 2 | 86329 | 3 | 86665 | 2 | 86813 | 1 | 87088 | 6 | 87301 | 1 |
| 84442 | 1 | 85175 | 1 | 85612 | 1 | 86331 | 12 | 86666 | 4 | 86816 | 1 | 87101 | 4 | 87305 | 1 |
| 84443 | 4 | 85210 | 2 | 85613 | 3 | 86332 | 1 | 86668 | 2 | 86817 | 1 | 87102 | 4 | 87320 | 1 |
| 84445 | 1 | 85220 | 2 | 85635 | 1 | 86334 | 2 | 86671 | 3 | 86821 | 1 | 87103 | 2 | 87324 | 2 |
| 84446 | 1 | 85230 | 2 | 85651 | 1 | 86335 | 2 | 86674 | 3 | 86822 | 1 | 87106 | 4 | 87327 | 1 |
| 84449 | 1 | 85240 | 2 | 85652 | 1 | 86336 | 1 | 86677 | 3 | 86825 | 1 | 87107 | 4 | 87328 | 2 |
| 84450 | 1 | 85244 | 1 | 85660 | 1 | 86337 | 1 | 86682 | 2 | 86826 | 2 | 87109 | 2 | 87329 | 2 |
| 84460 | 1 | 85245 | 2 | 85670 | 2 | 86340 | 1 | 86684 | 2 | 86828 | 1 | 87110 | 2 | 87332 | 1 |
| 84466 | 1 | 85246 | 2 | 85675 | 1 | 86341 | 1 | 86687 | 1 | 86829 | 1 | 87116 | 2 | 87335 | 1 |
| 84478 | 1 | 85247 | 2 | 85705 | 1 | 86343 | 1 | 86688 | 1 | 86830 | 2 | 87118 | 3 | 87336 | 1 |
| 84479 | 1 | 85250 | 2 | 85730 | 4 | 86344 | 1 | 86689 | 2 | 86831 | 2 | 87140 | 3 | 87337 | 1 |
| 84480 | 1 | 85260 | 2 | 85732 | 4 | 86352 | 1 | 86692 | 2 | 86832 | 2 | 87143 | 2 | 87338 | 1 |
| 84481 | 1 | 85270 | 2 | 85810 | 2 | 86353 | 7 | 86694 | 2 | 86833 | 1 | 87149 | 4 | 87339 | 1 |
| 84482 | 1 | 85280 | 2 | 86000 | 6 | 86355 | 7 | 86695 | 2 | 86834 | 1 | 87150 | 12 | 87340 | 1 |
| 84484 | 2 | 85290 | 2 | 86001 | 20 | 86356 | 7 | 86696 | 2 | 86835 | 1 | 87152 | 1 | 87341 | 1 |
| 84485 | 1 | 85291 | 1 | 86005 | 2 | 86357 | 1 | 86698 | 3 | 86850 | 3 | 87153 | 3 | 87350 | 1 |

| CPT | MUE | CPT | MUE | CPT | MUE | CPT | MUE | CPT | MUE | CPT | MUE | CPT | MUE | CPT | MUE |
|---|---|---|---|---|---|---|---|---|---|---|---|---|---|---|---|
| 87380 | 1 | 87540 | 1 | 88140 | 1 | 88321 | 1 | 89281 | 1 | 90662 | 1 | 90870 | 2 | 92071 | 2 |
| 87385 | 2 | 87541 | 1 | 88141 | 1 | 88323 | 1 | 89290 | 1 | 90664 | 1 | 90880 | 1 | 92072 | 1 |
| 87389 | 1 | 87542 | 1 | 88142 | 1 | 88325 | 1 | 89291 | 1 | 90666 | 1 | 90885 | 0 | 92081 | 1 |
| 87390 | 1 | 87550 | 1 | 88143 | 1 | 88329 | 2 | 89300 | 1 | 90667 | 1 | 90887 | 0 | 92082 | 1 |
| 87391 | 1 | 87551 | 2 | 88147 | 1 | 88331 | 11 | 89310 | 1 | 90668 | 1 | 90889 | 0 | 92083 | 1 |
| 87400 | 2 | 87552 | 1 | 88148 | 1 | 88332 | 13 | 89320 | 1 | 90670 | 1 | 90901 | 1 | 92100 | 1 |
| 87420 | 1 | 87555 | 1 | 88150 | 1 | 88333 | 4 | 89321 | 1 | 90672 | 1 | 90911 | 1 | 92132 | 1 |
| 87425 | 1 | 87556 | 1 | 88152 | 1 | 88334 | 5 | 89322 | 1 | 90673 | 1 | 90935 | 1 | 92133 | 1 |
| 87427 | 2 | 87557 | 1 | 88153 | 1 | 88341 | 9 | 89325 | 1 | 90674 | 1 | 90937 | 1 | 92134 | 1 |
| 87430 | 1 | 87560 | 1 | 88154 | 1 | 88342 | 3 | 89329 | 1 | 90675 | 1 | 90940 | 1 | 92136 | 2 |
| 87449 | 3 | 87561 | 1 | 88155 | 1 | 88344 | 1 | 89330 | 1 | 90676 | 1 | 90945 | 1 | 92145 | 1 |
| 87450 | 2 | 87562 | 1 | 88160 | 4 | 88346 | 2 | 89331 | 1 | 90680 | 1 | 90947 | 1 | 92225 | 2 |
| 87451 | 2 | 87580 | 1 | 88161 | 4 | 88348 | 1 | 89335 | 1 | 90681 | 1 | 90951 | 1 | 92226 | 2 |
| 87470 | 1 | 87581 | 1 | 88162 | 3 | 88350 | 8 | 89337 | 1 | 90682 | 1 | 90952 | 1 | 92227 | 1 |
| 87471 | 1 | 87582 | 1 | 88164 | 1 | 88355 | 1 | 89342 | 1 | 90685 | 1 | 90953 | 1 | 92228 | 1 |
| 87472 | 1 | 87590 | 1 | 88165 | 1 | 88356 | 1 | 89343 | 1 | 90686 | 1 | 90954 | 1 | 92230 | 2 |
| 87475 | 1 | 87591 | 3 | 88166 | 1 | 88358 | 2 | 89344 | 1 | 90687 | 1 | 90955 | 1 | 92235 | 1 |
| 87476 | 1 | 87592 | 1 | 88167 | 1 | 88360 | 6 | 89346 | 1 | 90688 | 1 | 90956 | 1 | 92240 | 1 |
| 87477 | 1 | 87623 | 1 | 88172 | 5 | 88361 | 6 | 89352 | 1 | 90690 | 1 | 90957 | 1 | 92242 | 1 |
| 87480 | 1 | 87624 | 1 | 88173 | 5 | 88362 | 1 | 89353 | 1 | 90691 | 1 | 90958 | 1 | 92250 | 1 |
| 87481 | 1 | 87625 | 1 | 88174 | 1 | 88363 | 2 | 89354 | 1 | 90696 | 1 | 90959 | 1 | 92260 | 1 |
| 87482 | 1 | 87631 | 1 | 88175 | 1 | 88364 | 3 | 89356 | 2 | 90697 | 1 | 90960 | 1 | 92265 | 1 |
| 87483 | 1 | 87632 | 1 | 88177 | 6 | 88365 | 4 | 90284 | 0 | 90698 | 1 | 90961 | 1 | 92270 | 1 |
| 87485 | 1 | 87633 | 1 | 88182 | 2 | 88366 | 2 | 90296 | 1 | 90700 | 1 | 90962 | 1 | 92275 | 1 |
| 87486 | 1 | 87640 | 1 | 88184 | 2 | 88367 | 3 | 90371 | 10 | 90702 | 1 | 90963 | 1 | 92283 | 1 |
| 87487 | 1 | 87641 | 1 | 88187 | 2 | 88368 | 3 | 90375 | 20 | 90707 | 1 | 90964 | 1 | 92284 | 1 |
| 87490 | 1 | 87650 | 1 | 88188 | 2 | 88369 | 3 | 90376 | 20 | 90710 | 1 | 90965 | 1 | 92285 | 1 |
| 87491 | 3 | 87651 | 1 | 88189 | 2 | 88371 | 1 | 90378 | 4 | 90713 | 1 | 90966 | 1 | 92286 | 1 |
| 87492 | 1 | 87652 | 1 | 88230 | 2 | 88372 | 1 | 90385 | 1 | 90714 | 1 | 90967 | 1 | 92287 | 1 |
| 87493 | 2 | 87653 | 1 | 88233 | 2 | 88373 | 3 | 90393 | 1 | 90715 | 1 | 90968 | 1 | 92311 | 1 |
| 87495 | 1 | 87660 | 1 | 88235 | 2 | 88374 | 5 | 90396 | 1 | 90716 | 1 | 90969 | 1 | 92312 | 1 |
| 87496 | 1 | 87661 | 1 | 88237 | 4 | 88375 | 1 | 90460 | 9 | 90717 | 1 | 90970 | 1 | 92313 | 1 |
| 87497 | 2 | 87797 | 3 | 88239 | 3 | 88377 | 5 | 90461 | 8 | 90732 | 1 | 90989 | 1 | 92315 | 1 |
| 87498 | 1 | 87798 | 13 | 88240 | 1 | 88380 | 1 | 90471 | 1 | 90733 | 1 | 90993 | 1 | 92316 | 1 |
| 87500 | 1 | 87799 | 3 | 88241 | 3 | 88381 | 1 | 90472 | 4 | 90734 | 1 | 90997 | 1 | 92317 | 1 |
| 87501 | 1 | 87800 | 2 | 88245 | 1 | 88387 | 2 | 90473 | 1 | 90736 | 1 | 91010 | 1 | 92325 | 1 |
| 87502 | 1 | 87801 | 3 | 88248 | 1 | 88388 | 1 | 90474 | 1 | 90738 | 1 | 91013 | 1 | 92326 | 2 |
| 87503 | 1 | 87802 | 2 | 88249 | 1 | 88720 | 1 | 90476 | 1 | 90739 | 1 | 91020 | 1 | 92352 | 0 |
| 87505 | 1 | 87803 | 3 | 88261 | 2 | 88738 | 1 | 90477 | 1 | 90740 | 1 | 91022 | 1 | 92353 | 0 |
| 87506 | 1 | 87804 | 3 | 88262 | 2 | 88740 | 1 | 90581 | 1 | 90743 | 1 | 91030 | 1 | 92354 | 0 |
| 87507 | 1 | 87806 | 1 | 88263 | 1 | 88741 | 1 | 90585 | 1 | 90744 | 1 | 91034 | 1 | 92355 | 0 |
| 87510 | 1 | 87807 | 2 | 88264 | 1 | 89049 | 1 | 90586 | 1 | 90746 | 1 | 91035 | 1 | 92358 | 0 |
| 87511 | 1 | 87808 | 1 | 88267 | 2 | 89050 | 2 | 90587 | 1 | 90747 | 1 | 91037 | 1 | 92371 | 0 |
| 87512 | 1 | 87809 | 2 | 88269 | 2 | 89051 | 2 | 90620 | 1 | 90750 | 1 | 91038 | 1 | 92502 | 1 |
| 87515 | 1 | 87810 | 2 | 88271 | 16 | 89055 | 2 | 90621 | 1 | 90785 | 3 | 91040 | 1 | 92504 | 1 |
| 87516 | 1 | 87850 | 1 | 88272 | 12 | 89060 | 2 | 90625 | 1 | 90791 | 1 | 91065 | 2 | 92507 | 1 |
| 87517 | 1 | 87880 | 2 | 88273 | 3 | 89125 | 2 | 90630 | 1 | 90792 | 1 | 91110 | 1 | 92508 | 1 |
| 87520 | 1 | 87899 | 4 | 88274 | 5 | 89160 | 1 | 90632 | 1 | 90832 | 2 | 91111 | 1 | 92511 | 1 |
| 87521 | 1 | 87900 | 1 | 88275 | 12 | 89190 | 1 | 90633 | 1 | 90833 | 2 | 91112 | 1 | 92512 | 1 |
| 87522 | 1 | 87901 | 1 | 88280 | 1 | 89220 | 1 | 90634 | 1 | 90834 | 2 | 91117 | 1 | 92516 | 1 |
| 87525 | 1 | 87902 | 1 | 88283 | 5 | 89230 | 1 | 90636 | 1 | 90836 | 2 | 91120 | 1 | 92520 | 1 |
| 87526 | 1 | 87903 | 1 | 88285 | 10 | 89250 | 1 | 90644 | 1 | 90837 | 2 | 91122 | 1 | 92521 | 1 |
| 87527 | 1 | 87904 | 14 | 88289 | 1 | 89251 | 1 | 90647 | 1 | 90838 | 2 | 91132 | 1 | 92522 | 1 |
| 87528 | 1 | 87905 | 2 | 88291 | 1 | 89253 | 1 | 90648 | 1 | 90839 | 1 | 91133 | 1 | 92523 | 1 |
| 87529 | 2 | 87906 | 2 | 88300 | 4 | 89254 | 1 | 90649 | 1 | 90840 | 3 | 91200 | 1 | 92524 | 1 |
| 87530 | 2 | 87910 | 1 | 88302 | 4 | 89255 | 1 | 90650 | 1 | 90845 | 1 | 92002 | 1 | 92526 | 1 |
| 87531 | 1 | 87912 | 1 | 88304 | 5 | 89257 | 1 | 90651 | 1 | 90846 | 1 | 92004 | 1 | 92531 | 0 |
| 87532 | 1 | 88104 | 5 | 88305 | 16 | 89258 | 1 | 90653 | 1 | 90847 | 1 | 92012 | 1 | 92532 | 0 |
| 87533 | 1 | 88106 | 5 | 88307 | 8 | 89259 | 1 | 90654 | 1 | 90849 | 1 | 92014 | 1 | 92534 | 0 |
| 87534 | 1 | 88108 | 6 | 88309 | 3 | 89260 | 1 | 90655 | 1 | 90853 | 1 | 92018 | 1 | 92537 | 1 |
| 87535 | 1 | 88112 | 6 | 88311 | 4 | 89261 | 1 | 90656 | 1 | 90863 | 1 | 92019 | 1 | 92538 | 1 |
| 87536 | 1 | 88120 | 2 | 88312 | 9 | 89264 | 1 | 90657 | 1 | 90865 | 1 | 92020 | 1 | 92540 | 1 |
| 87537 | 1 | 88121 | 2 | 88313 | 8 | 89268 | 1 | 90658 | 1 | 90867 | 1 | 92025 | 1 | 92541 | 1 |
| 87538 | 1 | 88125 | 1 | 88314 | 6 | 89272 | 1 | 90660 | 1 | 90868 | 1 | 92060 | 1 | 92542 | 1 |
| 87539 | 1 | 88130 | 1 | 88319 | 11 | 89280 | 1 | 90661 | 1 | 90869 | 1 | 92065 | 1 | 92544 | 1 |

CPT © 2017 American Medical Association. All Rights Reserved.

© 2017 Optum360, LLC

| CPT | MUE | CPT | MUE | CPT | MUE | CPT | MUE | CPT | MUE | CPT | MUE | CPT | MUE | CPT | MUE |
|---|---|---|---|---|---|---|---|---|---|---|---|---|---|---|---|
| 92545 | 1 | 92937 | 2 | 93294 | 1 | 93609 | 1 | 94004 | 1 | 95079 | 2 | 95905 | 2 | 96119 | 6 |
| 92546 | 1 | 92938 | 6 | 93295 | 1 | 93610 | 1 | 94010 | 1 | 95115 | 1 | 95907 | 1 | 96120 | 1 |
| 92547 | 1 | 92941 | 1 | 93296 | 1 | 93612 | 1 | 94011 | 1 | 95117 | 1 | 95908 | 1 | 96125 | 2 |
| 92548 | 1 | 92943 | 2 | 93297 | 1 | 93613 | 1 | 94012 | 1 | 95120 | 0 | 95909 | 1 | 96127 | 2 |
| 92550 | 1 | 92944 | 3 | 93298 | 1 | 93615 | 1 | 94013 | 1 | 95125 | 0 | 95910 | 1 | 96150 | 8 |
| 92552 | 1 | 92950 | 2 | 93299 | 1 | 93616 | 1 | 94014 | 1 | 95130 | 0 | 95911 | 1 | 96151 | 6 |
| 92553 | 1 | 92953 | 2 | 93303 | 1 | 93618 | 1 | 94015 | 1 | 95131 | 0 | 95912 | 1 | 96152 | 6 |
| 92555 | 1 | 92960 | 2 | 93304 | 1 | 93619 | 1 | 94016 | 1 | 95132 | 0 | 95913 | 1 | 96153 | 8 |
| 92556 | 1 | 92961 | 1 | 93306 | 1 | 93620 | 1 | 94060 | 1 | 95133 | 0 | 95921 | 1 | 96154 | 8 |
| 92557 | 1 | 92970 | 1 | 93307 | 1 | 93621 | 1 | 94070 | 1 | 95134 | 0 | 95922 | 1 | 96160 | 1 |
| 92558 | 0 | 92971 | 1 | 93308 | 1 | 93622 | 1 | 94150 | 0 | 95144 | 30 | 95923 | 1 | 96161 | 1 |
| 92561 | 1 | 92973 | 2 | 93312 | 1 | 93623 | 1 | 94200 | 1 | 95145 | 10 | 95924 | 1 | 96360 | 1 |
| 92562 | 1 | 92974 | 1 | 93313 | 1 | 93624 | 1 | 94250 | 1 | 95146 | 10 | 95925 | 1 | 96361 | 8 |
| 92563 | 1 | 92975 | 1 | 93314 | 1 | 93631 | 1 | 94375 | 1 | 95147 | 10 | 95926 | 1 | 96365 | 1 |
| 92564 | 1 | 92977 | 1 | 93315 | 1 | 93640 | 1 | 94400 | 1 | 95148 | 10 | 95927 | 1 | 96366 | 8 |
| 92565 | 1 | 92978 | 1 | 93316 | 1 | 93641 | 1 | 94450 | 1 | 95149 | 10 | 95928 | 1 | 96367 | 4 |
| 92567 | 1 | 92979 | 2 | 93317 | 1 | 93642 | 1 | 94452 | 1 | 95165 | 30 | 95929 | 1 | 96368 | 1 |
| 92568 | 1 | 92986 | 1 | 93318 | 1 | 93644 | 1 | 94453 | 1 | 95170 | 10 | 95930 | 1 | 96369 | 1 |
| 92570 | 1 | 92987 | 1 | 93320 | 1 | 93650 | 1 | 94610 | 2 | 95180 | 6 | 95933 | 1 | 96370 | 3 |
| 92571 | 1 | 92990 | 1 | 93321 | 1 | 93653 | 1 | 94620 | 1 | 95250 | 1 | 95937 | 4 | 96371 | 1 |
| 92572 | 1 | 92992 | 1 | 93325 | 1 | 93654 | 1 | 94621 | 1 | 95251 | 1 | 95938 | 1 | 96372 | 4 |
| 92575 | 1 | 92993 | 1 | 93350 | 1 | 93655 | 2 | 94640 | 4 | 95782 | 1 | 95939 | 1 | 96373 | 2 |
| 92576 | 1 | 92997 | 1 | 93351 | 1 | 93656 | 1 | 94642 | 1 | 95783 | 1 | 95940 | 32 | 96374 | 1 |
| 92577 | 1 | 92998 | 2 | 93352 | 1 | 93657 | 1 | 94644 | 1 | 95800 | 1 | 95943 | 1 | 96375 | 6 |
| 92579 | 1 | 93000 | 3 | 93355 | 1 | 93660 | 1 | 94645 | 2 | 95801 | 1 | 95950 | 1 | 96376 | 0 |
| 92582 | 1 | 93005 | 3 | 93451 | 1 | 93662 | 1 | 94660 | 1 | 95803 | 1 | 95951 | 1 | 96377 | 1 |
| 92583 | 1 | 93010 | 5 | 93452 | 1 | 93701 | 1 | 94662 | 1 | 95805 | 1 | 95953 | 1 | 96401 | 3 |
| 92584 | 1 | 93015 | 1 | 93453 | 1 | 93702 | 1 | 94664 | 1 | 95806 | 1 | 95954 | 1 | 96402 | 2 |
| 92585 | 1 | 93016 | 1 | 93454 | 1 | 93724 | 1 | 94667 | 1 | 95807 | 1 | 95955 | 1 | 96405 | 1 |
| 92586 | 1 | 93017 | 1 | 93455 | 1 | 93740 | 0 | 94668 | 2 | 95808 | 1 | 95956 | 1 | 96406 | 1 |
| 92587 | 1 | 93018 | 1 | 93456 | 1 | 93745 | 1 | 94669 | 4 | 95810 | 1 | 95957 | 1 | 96409 | 1 |
| 92588 | 1 | 93024 | 1 | 93457 | 1 | 93750 | 4 | 94680 | 1 | 95811 | 1 | 95958 | 1 | 96411 | 3 |
| 92596 | 1 | 93025 | 1 | 93458 | 1 | 93770 | 0 | 94681 | 1 | 95812 | 1 | 95961 | 1 | 96413 | 1 |
| 92597 | 1 | 93040 | 3 | 93459 | 1 | 93784 | 1 | 94690 | 1 | 95813 | 1 | 95962 | 5 | 96415 | 8 |
| 92601 | 1 | 93041 | 2 | 93460 | 1 | 93786 | 1 | 94726 | 1 | 95816 | 1 | 95965 | 1 | 96416 | 1 |
| 92602 | 1 | 93042 | 3 | 93461 | 1 | 93788 | 1 | 94727 | 1 | 95819 | 1 | 95966 | 1 | 96417 | 3 |
| 92603 | 1 | 93050 | 1 | 93462 | 1 | 93790 | 1 | 94728 | 1 | 95822 | 1 | 95967 | 3 | 96420 | 1 |
| 92604 | 1 | 93224 | 1 | 93463 | 1 | 93797 | 2 | 94729 | 1 | 95824 | 1 | 95970 | 1 | 96422 | 2 |
| 92605 | 0 | 93225 | 1 | 93464 | 1 | 93798 | 2 | 94750 | 1 | 95827 | 1 | 95971 | 1 | 96423 | 1 |
| 92607 | 1 | 93226 | 1 | 93503 | 2 | 93880 | 1 | 94760 | 1 | 95829 | 1 | 95972 | 1 | 96425 | 1 |
| 92608 | 4 | 93227 | 1 | 93505 | 1 | 93882 | 1 | 94761 | 1 | 95830 | 1 | 95974 | 1 | 96440 | 1 |
| 92609 | 1 | 93228 | 1 | 93530 | 1 | 93886 | 1 | 94762 | 1 | 95831 | 5 | 95975 | 2 | 96446 | 1 |
| 92610 | 1 | 93229 | 1 | 93531 | 1 | 93888 | 1 | 94770 | 1 | 95832 | 1 | 95978 | 1 | 96450 | 1 |
| 92611 | 1 | 93260 | 1 | 93532 | 1 | 93890 | 1 | 94772 | 1 | 95833 | 1 | 95979 | 6 | 96521 | 2 |
| 92612 | 1 | 93261 | 1 | 93533 | 1 | 93892 | 1 | 94774 | 1 | 95834 | 1 | 95980 | 1 | 96522 | 1 |
| 92613 | 1 | 93268 | 1 | 93561 | 1 | 93893 | 1 | 94775 | 1 | 95851 | 3 | 95981 | 1 | 96523 | 1 |
| 92614 | 1 | 93270 | 1 | 93562 | 1 | 93922 | 1 | 94776 | 1 | 95852 | 1 | 95982 | 1 | 96542 | 1 |
| 92615 | 1 | 93271 | 1 | 93563 | 1 | 93923 | 1 | 94777 | 1 | 95857 | 1 | 95990 | 1 | 96567 | 1 |
| 92616 | 1 | 93272 | 1 | 93564 | 1 | 93924 | 1 | 94780 | 1 | 95860 | 1 | 95991 | 1 | 96570 | 1 |
| 92617 | 1 | 93278 | 1 | 93565 | 1 | 93925 | 1 | 94781 | 2 | 95861 | 1 | 95992 | 1 | 96571 | 2 |
| 92618 | 1 | 93279 | 1 | 93566 | 1 | 93926 | 1 | 95004 | 80 | 95863 | 1 | 96000 | 1 | 96900 | 1 |
| 92620 | 1 | 93280 | 1 | 93567 | 1 | 93930 | 1 | 95012 | 2 | 95864 | 1 | 96001 | 1 | 96902 | 0 |
| 92621 | 4 | 93281 | 1 | 93568 | 1 | 93931 | 1 | 95017 | 27 | 95865 | 1 | 96002 | 1 | 96904 | 1 |
| 92625 | 1 | 93282 | 1 | 93571 | 1 | 93970 | 1 | 95018 | 19 | 95866 | 1 | 96003 | 1 | 96910 | 1 |
| 92626 | 1 | 93283 | 1 | 93572 | 2 | 93971 | 1 | 95024 | 40 | 95867 | 1 | 96004 | 1 | 96912 | 1 |
| 92627 | 6 | 93284 | 1 | 93580 | 1 | 93975 | 1 | 95027 | 90 | 95868 | 1 | 96020 | 1 | 96913 | 1 |
| 92640 | 1 | 93285 | 1 | 93581 | 1 | 93976 | 1 | 95028 | 30 | 95869 | 1 | 96040 | 4 | 96920 | 1 |
| 92920 | 3 | 93286 | 2 | 93582 | 1 | 93978 | 1 | 95044 | 80 | 95870 | 4 | 96101 | 8 | 96921 | 1 |
| 92921 | 6 | 93287 | 2 | 93583 | 1 | 93979 | 1 | 95052 | 20 | 95872 | 4 | 96102 | 4 | 96922 | 1 |
| 92924 | 2 | 93288 | 1 | 93590 | 1 | 93980 | 1 | 95056 | 1 | 95873 | 1 | 96103 | 1 | 96931 | 1 |
| 92925 | 6 | 93289 | 1 | 93591 | 1 | 93981 | 1 | 95060 | 1 | 95874 | 1 | 96105 | 3 | 96932 | 1 |
| 92928 | 3 | 93290 | 1 | 93592 | 2 | 93982 | 1 | 95065 | 1 | 95875 | 2 | 96110 | 3 | 96933 | 1 |
| 92929 | 6 | 93291 | 1 | 93600 | 1 | 93990 | 2 | 95070 | 1 | 95885 | 4 | 96111 | 1 | 96934 | 2 |
| 92933 | 2 | 93292 | 1 | 93602 | 1 | 94002 | 1 | 95071 | 1 | 95886 | 4 | 96116 | 4 | 96935 | 2 |
| 92934 | 6 | 93293 | 1 | 93603 | 1 | 94003 | 1 | 95076 | 1 | 95887 | 1 | 96118 | 8 | 96936 | 2 |

CPT © 2017 American Medical Association. All Rights Reserved.

| CPT | MUE | CPT | MUE | CPT | MUE | CPT | MUE | CPT | MUE | CPT | MUE | CPT | MUE | CPT | MUE |
|---|---|---|---|---|---|---|---|---|---|---|---|---|---|---|---|
| 97010 | 0 | 99002 | 0 | 99285 | 1 | 99477 | 1 | A4250 | 0 | A4385 | 2 | A4663 | 0 | A5102 | 0 |
| 97012 | 1 | 99024 | 0 | 99288 | 0 | 99478 | 1 | A4252 | 0 | A4389 | 2 | A4670 | 0 | A5105 | 0 |
| 97014 | 0 | 99050 | 0 | 99291 | 1 | 99479 | 1 | A4253 | 0 | A4392 | 2 | A4671 | 0 | A5112 | 0 |
| 97016 | 1 | 99051 | 0 | 99292 | 8 | 99480 | 1 | A4255 | 0 | A4397 | 0 | A4672 | 0 | A5113 | 0 |
| 97018 | 1 | 99053 | 0 | 99304 | 1 | 99485 | 1 | A4256 | 0 | A4398 | 0 | A4673 | 0 | A5114 | 0 |
| 97022 | 1 | 99056 | 0 | 99305 | 1 | 99486 | 4 | A4257 | 0 | A4399 | 0 | A4674 | 0 | A5120 | 150 |
| 97024 | 1 | 99058 | 0 | 99306 | 1 | 99487 | 1 | A4258 | 0 | A4400 | 0 | A4680 | 0 | A5121 | 0 |
| 97026 | 1 | 99060 | 0 | 99307 | 1 | 99490 | 1 | A4259 | 0 | A4402 | 0 | A4690 | 0 | A5122 | 0 |
| 97028 | 1 | 99070 | 0 | 99308 | 1 | 99495 | 1 | A4261 | 0 | A4404 | 0 | A4706 | 0 | A5126 | 0 |
| 97032 | 4 | 99071 | 0 | 99309 | 1 | 99496 | 1 | A4262 | 0 | A4407 | 2 | A4707 | 0 | A5131 | 0 |
| 97033 | 4 | 99078 | 0 | 99310 | 1 | 99497 | 1 | A4263 | 0 | A4410 | 2 | A4708 | 0 | A5500 | 0 |
| 97034 | 2 | 99080 | 0 | 99315 | 1 | 99498 | 3 | A4264 | 0 | A4413 | 2 | A4709 | 0 | A5501 | 0 |
| 97035 | 2 | 99082 | 1 | 99316 | 1 | 99605 | 0 | A4265 | 0 | A4416 | 2 | A4714 | 0 | A5503 | 0 |
| 97036 | 3 | 99090 | 0 | 99318 | 1 | 99606 | 0 | A4266 | 0 | A4419 | 2 | A4719 | 0 | A5504 | 0 |
| 97110 | 6 | 99091 | 0 | 99324 | 1 | 99607 | 0 | A4267 | 0 | A4423 | 2 | A4720 | 0 | A5505 | 0 |
| 97112 | 4 | 99100 | 1 | 99325 | 1 | A0021 | 0 | A4268 | 0 | A4426 | 2 | A4721 | 0 | A5506 | 0 |
| 97113 | 6 | 99116 | 0 | 99326 | 1 | A0080 | 0 | A4269 | 0 | A4429 | 2 | A4722 | 0 | A5507 | 0 |
| 97116 | 4 | 99135 | 0 | 99327 | 1 | A0090 | 0 | A4270 | 0 | A4432 | 2 | A4723 | 0 | A5508 | 0 |
| 97124 | 4 | 99140 | 0 | 99328 | 1 | A0100 | 0 | A4300 | 0 | A4435 | 2 | A4724 | 0 | A5510 | 0 |
| 97140 | 6 | 99151 | 2 | 99334 | 1 | A0110 | 0 | A4301 | 1 | A4455 | 0 | A4725 | 0 | A5512 | 0 |
| 97150 | 1 | 99152 | 2 | 99335 | 1 | A0120 | 0 | A4305 | 0 | A4459 | 0 | A4726 | 0 | A5513 | 0 |
| 97161 | 1 | 99153 | 9 | 99336 | 1 | A0130 | 0 | A4306 | 0 | A4461 | 2 | A4728 | 0 | A6000 | 0 |
| 97162 | 1 | 99155 | 2 | 99337 | 1 | A0140 | 0 | A4310 | 0 | A4465 | 0 | A4730 | 0 | A6022 | 0 |
| 97163 | 1 | 99156 | 2 | 99341 | 1 | A0160 | 0 | A4311 | 0 | A4467 | 0 | A4736 | 0 | A6154 | 0 |
| 97164 | 1 | 99157 | 6 | 99342 | 1 | A0170 | 0 | A4312 | 0 | A4470 | 0 | A4737 | 0 | A6196 | 0 |
| 97165 | 1 | 99170 | 1 | 99343 | 1 | A0180 | 0 | A4313 | 0 | A4480 | 0 | A4740 | 0 | A6197 | 0 |
| 97166 | 1 | 99175 | 1 | 99344 | 1 | A0190 | 0 | A4314 | 0 | A4490 | 0 | A4750 | 0 | A6198 | 0 |
| 97167 | 1 | 99177 | 1 | 99345 | 1 | A0200 | 0 | A4315 | 0 | A4495 | 0 | A4755 | 0 | A6199 | 0 |
| 97168 | 1 | 99183 | 1 | 99347 | 1 | A0210 | 0 | A4316 | 0 | A4500 | 0 | A4760 | 0 | A6203 | 0 |
| 97169 | 1 | 99184 | 1 | 99348 | 1 | A0225 | 0 | A4320 | 0 | A4510 | 0 | A4765 | 0 | A6204 | 0 |
| 97170 | 1 | 99191 | 1 | 99349 | 1 | A0380 | 0 | A4322 | 0 | A4520 | 0 | A4766 | 0 | A6205 | 0 |
| 97171 | 1 | 99192 | 1 | 99350 | 1 | A0382 | 0 | A4326 | 0 | A4550 | 0 | A4770 | 0 | A6206 | 0 |
| 97172 | 1 | 99195 | 2 | 99354 | 1 | A0384 | 0 | A4327 | 0 | A4553 | 0 | A4771 | 0 | A6207 | 0 |
| 97530 | 6 | 99201 | 1 | 99355 | 4 | A0390 | 0 | A4328 | 0 | A4554 | 0 | A4772 | 0 | A6208 | 0 |
| 97532 | 8 | 99202 | 1 | 99356 | 1 | A0392 | 0 | A4330 | 0 | A4555 | 0 | A4773 | 0 | A6209 | 0 |
| 97533 | 4 | 99203 | 1 | 99357 | 4 | A0394 | 0 | A4332 | 2 | A4556 | 0 | A4774 | 0 | A6210 | 0 |
| 97535 | 8 | 99204 | 1 | 99358 | 1 | A0396 | 0 | A4335 | 0 | A4557 | 0 | A4802 | 0 | A6211 | 0 |
| 97537 | 8 | 99205 | 1 | 99359 | 2 | A0398 | 0 | A4337 | 0 | A4558 | 0 | A4860 | 0 | A6212 | 0 |
| 97542 | 8 | 99211 | 1 | 99366 | 0 | A0420 | 0 | A4338 | 0 | A4561 | 1 | A4870 | 0 | A6213 | 0 |
| 97545 | 1 | 99212 | 2 | 99367 | 0 | A0422 | 0 | A4340 | 0 | A4562 | 1 | A4890 | 0 | A6214 | 0 |
| 97546 | 2 | 99213 | 2 | 99368 | 0 | A0424 | 0 | A4344 | 0 | A4565 | 2 | A4911 | 0 | A6215 | 0 |
| 97597 | 1 | 99214 | 2 | 99406 | 1 | A0425 | 250 | A4346 | 0 | A4566 | 0 | A4913 | 0 | A6216 | 0 |
| 97598 | 8 | 99215 | 1 | 99407 | 1 | A0426 | 2 | A4351 | 0 | A4570 | 0 | A4918 | 0 | A6217 | 0 |
| 97602 | 0 | 99217 | 1 | 99415 | 1 | A0427 | 2 | A4352 | 0 | A4575 | 0 | A4927 | 0 | A6218 | 0 |
| 97605 | 1 | 99218 | 1 | 99416 | 4 | A0428 | 4 | A4354 | 0 | A4580 | 0 | A4928 | 0 | A6219 | 0 |
| 97606 | 1 | 99219 | 1 | 99446 | 1 | A0429 | 2 | A4355 | 0 | A4590 | 0 | A4929 | 0 | A6220 | 0 |
| 97607 | 1 | 99220 | 1 | 99447 | 1 | A0430 | 1 | A4356 | 0 | A4595 | 0 | A4930 | 0 | A6222 | 0 |
| 97608 | 1 | 99221 | 1 | 99448 | 1 | A0431 | 1 | A4357 | 0 | A4602 | 0 | A4931 | 0 | A6223 | 0 |
| 97610 | 1 | 99222 | 1 | 99449 | 1 | A0432 | 1 | A4358 | 0 | A4606 | 0 | A4932 | 0 | A6224 | 0 |
| 97750 | 8 | 99223 | 1 | 99455 | 1 | A0433 | 1 | A4361 | 0 | A4611 | 0 | A5051 | 0 | A6228 | 0 |
| 97755 | 8 | 99224 | 1 | 99456 | 1 | A0434 | 2 | A4362 | 0 | A4614 | 0 | A5052 | 0 | A6229 | 0 |
| 97760 | 6 | 99225 | 1 | 99460 | 1 | A0435 | 999 | A4363 | 1 | A4618 | 1 | A5053 | 0 | A6230 | 0 |
| 97761 | 6 | 99226 | 1 | 99461 | 1 | A0436 | 300 | A4364 | 0 | A4625 | 30 | A5054 | 0 | A6231 | 0 |
| 97762 | 4 | 99231 | 1 | 99462 | 1 | A0888 | 0 | A4367 | 0 | A4627 | 0 | A5055 | 0 | A6234 | 0 |
| 97802 | 8 | 99232 | 1 | 99463 | 1 | A0998 | 0 | A4368 | 1 | A4633 | 0 | A5056 | 90 | A6235 | 0 |
| 97803 | 8 | 99233 | 1 | 99464 | 1 | A4210 | 0 | A4375 | 2 | A4635 | 0 | A5057 | 90 | A6236 | 0 |
| 97804 | 6 | 99234 | 1 | 99465 | 1 | A4211 | 0 | A4376 | 2 | A4638 | 0 | A5061 | 0 | A6237 | 0 |
| 98925 | 1 | 99235 | 1 | 99466 | 1 | A4212 | 0 | A4377 | 2 | A4640 | 0 | A5062 | 0 | A6238 | 0 |
| 98926 | 1 | 99236 | 1 | 99467 | 4 | A4220 | 1 | A4378 | 2 | A4642 | 1 | A5063 | 0 | A6239 | 0 |
| 98927 | 1 | 99238 | 1 | 99468 | 1 | A4221 | 0 | A4379 | 2 | A4648 | 5 | A5071 | 0 | A6240 | 0 |
| 98928 | 1 | 99239 | 1 | 99469 | 1 | A4222 | 0 | A4380 | 2 | A4649 | 1 | A5072 | 0 | A6241 | 0 |
| 98929 | 1 | 99281 | 1 | 99471 | 1 | A4224 | 0 | A4381 | 2 | A4650 | 3 | A5073 | 0 | A6242 | 0 |
| 98940 | 1 | 99282 | 1 | 99472 | 1 | A4225 | 0 | A4382 | 2 | A4653 | 0 | A5081 | 0 | A6243 | 0 |
| 98941 | 1 | 99283 | 1 | 99475 | 1 | A4232 | 0 | A4383 | 2 | A4657 | 0 | A5082 | 0 | A6244 | 0 |
| 98942 | 1 | 99284 | 1 | 99476 | 1 | A4235 | 0 | A4384 | 2 | A4660 | 0 | A5093 | 0 | A6245 | 0 |

CPT © 2017 American Medical Association. All Rights Reserved.                    © 2017 Optum360, LLC

| CPT | MUE | CPT | MUE | CPT | MUE | CPT | MUE | CPT | MUE | CPT | MUE | CPT | MUE | CPT | MUE |
|---|---|---|---|---|---|---|---|---|---|---|---|---|---|---|---|
| A6246 | 0 | A7036 | 0 | A9542 | 1 | B5200 | 0 | C8901 | 1 | C9606 | 1 | E0200 | 0 | E0370 | 0 |
| A6247 | 0 | A7037 | 0 | A9543 | 1 | C1716 | 4 | C8902 | 1 | C9607 | 1 | E0202 | 0 | E0371 | 0 |
| A6248 | 0 | A7039 | 0 | A9546 | 1 | C1717 | 10 | C8903 | 1 | C9608 | 2 | E0203 | 0 | E0372 | 0 |
| A6250 | 0 | A7040 | 2 | A9547 | 2 | C1719 | 99 | C8904 | 1 | C9725 | 1 | E0205 | 0 | E0373 | 0 |
| A6251 | 0 | A7041 | 2 | A9548 | 2 | C1721 | 1 | C8905 | 1 | C9727 | 1 | E0210 | 0 | E0424 | 0 |
| A6252 | 0 | A7044 | 0 | A9550 | 1 | C1722 | 1 | C8906 | 1 | C9728 | 1 | E0215 | 0 | E0425 | 0 |
| A6253 | 0 | A7047 | 0 | A9551 | 1 | C1730 | 0 | C8907 | 1 | C9733 | 1 | E0217 | 0 | E0430 | 0 |
| A6254 | 0 | A7048 | 2 | A9552 | 1 | C1731 | 0 | C8908 | 1 | C9734 | 1 | E0218 | 0 | E0431 | 0 |
| A6255 | 0 | A7501 | 0 | A9553 | 1 | C1732 | 0 | C8909 | 1 | C9739 | 1 | E0221 | 0 | E0434 | 0 |
| A6256 | 0 | A7504 | 0 | A9554 | 1 | C1733 | 0 | C8910 | 1 | C9740 | 1 | E0225 | 0 | E0435 | 0 |
| A6257 | 0 | A7507 | 0 | A9555 | 2 | C1749 | 1 | C8911 | 1 | C9741 | 1 | E0231 | 0 | E0439 | 0 |
| A6258 | 0 | A7520 | 0 | A9556 | 10 | C1764 | 1 | C8912 | 1 | C9744 | 1 | E0232 | 0 | E0440 | 0 |
| A6259 | 0 | A7524 | 0 | A9557 | 2 | C1767 | 2 | C8913 | 1 | E0100 | 0 | E0235 | 0 | E0441 | 0 |
| A6260 | 0 | A7527 | 0 | A9558 | 7 | C1771 | 1 | C8914 | 1 | E0105 | 0 | E0236 | 0 | E0442 | 0 |
| A6261 | 0 | A9152 | 0 | A9559 | 1 | C1772 | 1 | C8918 | 1 | E0110 | 0 | E0239 | 0 | E0443 | 0 |
| A6262 | 0 | A9153 | 0 | A9560 | 2 | C1776 | 10 | C8919 | 1 | E0111 | 0 | E0240 | 0 | E0444 | 0 |
| A6266 | 0 | A9155 | 1 | A9561 | 1 | C1778 | 4 | C8920 | 1 | E0112 | 0 | E0241 | 0 | E0445 | 0 |
| A6402 | 0 | A9180 | 0 | A9562 | 2 | C1782 | 1 | C8921 | 1 | E0113 | 0 | E0242 | 0 | E0446 | 0 |
| A6403 | 0 | A9270 | 0 | A9563 | 10 | C1785 | 1 | C8922 | 1 | E0114 | 0 | E0243 | 0 | E0455 | 0 |
| A6404 | 0 | A9272 | 0 | A9564 | 20 | C1786 | 1 | C8923 | 1 | E0116 | 0 | E0244 | 0 | E0457 | 0 |
| A6410 | 2 | A9273 | 0 | A9566 | 1 | C1813 | 1 | C8924 | 1 | E0117 | 0 | E0245 | 0 | E0459 | 0 |
| A6413 | 0 | A9274 | 0 | A9567 | 2 | C1815 | 1 | C8925 | 1 | E0118 | 0 | E0246 | 0 | E0462 | 0 |
| A6501 | 0 | A9275 | 0 | A9568 | 0 | C1817 | 1 | C8926 | 1 | E0130 | 0 | E0247 | 0 | E0465 | 0 |
| A6502 | 0 | A9276 | 0 | A9569 | 1 | C1820 | 2 | C8927 | 1 | E0135 | 0 | E0248 | 0 | E0466 | 0 |
| A6503 | 0 | A9277 | 0 | A9570 | 1 | C1822 | 1 | C8928 | 1 | E0140 | 0 | E0249 | 0 | E0470 | 0 |
| A6504 | 0 | A9278 | 0 | A9571 | 1 | C1830 | 2 | C8929 | 1 | E0141 | 0 | E0250 | 0 | E0471 | 0 |
| A6505 | 0 | A9279 | 0 | A9572 | 1 | C1840 | 1 | C8930 | 1 | E0143 | 0 | E0251 | 0 | E0472 | 0 |
| A6506 | 0 | A9280 | 0 | A9575 | 200 | C1841 | 1 | C8931 | 1 | E0144 | 0 | E0255 | 0 | E0480 | 0 |
| A6507 | 0 | A9281 | 0 | A9576 | 40 | C1842 | 1 | C8932 | 1 | E0147 | 0 | E0256 | 0 | E0481 | 0 |
| A6508 | 0 | A9282 | 0 | A9577 | 50 | C1882 | 1 | C8933 | 1 | E0148 | 0 | E0260 | 0 | E0482 | 0 |
| A6509 | 0 | A9283 | 0 | A9578 | 50 | C1886 | 1 | C8957 | 2 | E0149 | 0 | E0261 | 0 | E0483 | 0 |
| A6510 | 0 | A9284 | 0 | A9579 | 100 | C1891 | 1 | C9113 | 0 | E0153 | 0 | E0265 | 0 | E0484 | 0 |
| A6511 | 0 | A9285 | 0 | A9580 | 1 | C1900 | 1 | C9132 | 5500 | E0154 | 0 | E0266 | 0 | E0485 | 0 |
| A6513 | 0 | A9286 | 0 | A9581 | 20 | C2613 | 2 | C9140 | 22000 | E0155 | 0 | E0270 | 0 | E0486 | 0 |
| A6530 | 0 | A9300 | 0 | A9582 | 1 | C2616 | 1 | C9248 | 0 | E0156 | 0 | E0271 | 0 | E0487 | 0 |
| A6531 | 0 | A9500 | 3 | A9583 | 18 | C2619 | 1 | C9250 | 1 | E0157 | 0 | E0272 | 0 | E0500 | 0 |
| A6532 | 0 | A9501 | 1 | A9584 | 1 | C2620 | 1 | C9254 | 0 | E0158 | 0 | E0273 | 0 | E0550 | 0 |
| A6533 | 0 | A9502 | 3 | A9585 | 300 | C2621 | 1 | C9257 | 5 | E0159 | 2 | E0274 | 0 | E0555 | 0 |
| A6534 | 0 | A9503 | 1 | A9586 | 1 | C2622 | 1 | C9275 | 1 | E0160 | 0 | E0275 | 0 | E0560 | 0 |
| A6535 | 0 | A9504 | 1 | A9587 | 54 | C2623 | 2 | C9285 | 2 | E0161 | 0 | E0276 | 0 | E0561 | 0 |
| A6536 | 0 | A9505 | 4 | A9588 | 10 | C2624 | 1 | C9290 | 266 | E0162 | 0 | E0277 | 0 | E0562 | 0 |
| A6537 | 0 | A9507 | 1 | A9599 | 1 | C2626 | 1 | C9293 | 700 | E0163 | 0 | E0280 | 0 | E0565 | 0 |
| A6538 | 0 | A9508 | 2 | A9600 | 7 | C2630 | 0 | C9352 | 3 | E0165 | 0 | E0290 | 0 | E0570 | 0 |
| A6539 | 0 | A9509 | 5 | A9604 | 1 | C2631 | 1 | C9353 | 4 | E0167 | 0 | E0291 | 0 | E0572 | 0 |
| A6540 | 0 | A9510 | 1 | A9606 | 203 | C2634 | 24 | C9354 | 300 | E0168 | 0 | E0292 | 0 | E0574 | 0 |
| A6541 | 0 | A9512 | 30 | A9700 | 2 | C2635 | 124 | C9355 | 3 | E0170 | 0 | E0293 | 0 | E0575 | 0 |
| A6544 | 0 | A9515 | 1 | B4081 | 0 | C2636 | 690 | C9356 | 125 | E0171 | 0 | E0294 | 0 | E0580 | 0 |
| A6545 | 0 | A9516 | 4 | B4082 | 0 | C2637 | 0 | C9358 | 800 | E0172 | 0 | E0295 | 0 | E0585 | 0 |
| A6549 | 0 | A9517 | 200 | B4083 | 0 | C2638 | 150 | C9359 | 30 | E0175 | 0 | E0296 | 0 | E0600 | 0 |
| A7000 | 0 | A9520 | 1 | B4087 | 0 | C2639 | 150 | C9360 | 300 | E0181 | 0 | E0297 | 0 | E0601 | 0 |
| A7003 | 0 | A9521 | 2 | B4088 | 0 | C2640 | 150 | C9361 | 10 | E0182 | 0 | E0300 | 0 | E0602 | 0 |
| A7005 | 0 | A9524 | 10 | B4149 | 0 | C2641 | 150 | C9362 | 60 | E0184 | 0 | E0301 | 0 | E0603 | 0 |
| A7006 | 0 | A9526 | 2 | B4153 | 0 | C2642 | 120 | C9363 | 500 | E0185 | 0 | E0302 | 0 | E0604 | 0 |
| A7013 | 0 | A9527 | 195 | B4157 | 0 | C2643 | 120 | C9364 | 600 | E0186 | 0 | E0303 | 0 | E0605 | 0 |
| A7014 | 0 | A9528 | 10 | B4160 | 0 | C2644 | 500 | C9447 | 1 | E0187 | 0 | E0304 | 0 | E0606 | 0 |
| A7016 | 0 | A9529 | 10 | B4164 | 0 | C2645 | 4608 | C9460 | 1 | E0188 | 0 | E0305 | 0 | E0607 | 0 |
| A7017 | 0 | A9530 | 200 | B4168 | 0 | C5271 | 1 | C9482 | 150 | E0189 | 0 | E0310 | 0 | E0610 | 0 |
| A7020 | 0 | A9531 | 100 | B4172 | 0 | C5272 | 3 | C9483 | 120 | E0190 | 0 | E0315 | 0 | E0615 | 0 |
| A7025 | 0 | A9532 | 10 | B4176 | 0 | C5273 | 1 | C9497 | 1 | E0191 | 0 | E0316 | 0 | E0616 | 1 |
| A7026 | 0 | A9536 | 1 | B4178 | 0 | C5274 | 35 | C9600 | 3 | E0193 | 0 | E0325 | 0 | E0617 | 0 |
| A7027 | 0 | A9537 | 1 | B4180 | 0 | C5275 | 1 | C9601 | 2 | E0194 | 0 | E0326 | 0 | E0618 | 0 |
| A7028 | 0 | A9538 | 1 | B4189 | 0 | C5276 | 3 | C9602 | 2 | E0196 | 0 | E0328 | 0 | E0619 | 0 |
| A7029 | 0 | A9539 | 2 | B4199 | 0 | C5277 | 1 | C9603 | 2 | E0197 | 0 | E0329 | 0 | E0620 | 0 |
| A7032 | 0 | A9540 | 2 | B5000 | 0 | C5278 | 15 | C9604 | 2 | E0198 | 0 | E0350 | 0 | E0621 | 0 |
| A7035 | 0 | A9541 | 1 | B5100 | 0 | C8900 | 1 | C9605 | 2 | E0199 | 0 | E0352 | 0 | E0625 | 0 |

© 2017 Optum360, LLC

CPT © 2017 American Medical Association. All Rights Reserved.

**Appendix I — Medically Unlikely Edits (MUEs) — Professional**

| CPT | MUE | CPT | MUE | CPT | MUE | CPT | MUE | CPT | MUE | CPT | MUE | CPT | MUE | CPT | MUE |
|---|---|---|---|---|---|---|---|---|---|---|---|---|---|---|---|
| E0627 | 0 | E0830 | 0 | E1012 | 0 | E1285 | 0 | E2000 | 0 | E2366 | 0 | E2631 | 0 | G0293 | 1 |
| E0629 | 0 | E0840 | 0 | E1014 | 0 | E1290 | 0 | E2100 | 0 | E2367 | 0 | E2632 | 0 | G0294 | 1 |
| E0630 | 0 | E0849 | 0 | E1015 | 0 | E1295 | 0 | E2101 | 0 | E2368 | 0 | E2633 | 0 | G0296 | 1 |
| E0635 | 0 | E0850 | 0 | E1016 | 0 | E1300 | 0 | E2120 | 0 | E2369 | 0 | G0008 | 1 | G0297 | 1 |
| E0636 | 0 | E0855 | 0 | E1017 | 0 | E1310 | 0 | E2201 | 0 | E2370 | 0 | G0009 | 1 | G0302 | 1 |
| E0637 | 0 | E0856 | 0 | E1018 | 0 | E1352 | 0 | E2202 | 0 | E2371 | 0 | G0010 | 1 | G0303 | 1 |
| E0638 | 0 | E0860 | 0 | E1020 | 0 | E1353 | 0 | E2203 | 0 | E2373 | 0 | G0027 | 1 | G0304 | 1 |
| E0639 | 0 | E0870 | 0 | E1028 | 0 | E1354 | 0 | E2204 | 0 | E2374 | 0 | G0101 | 1 | G0305 | 1 |
| E0640 | 0 | E0880 | 0 | E1029 | 0 | E1355 | 0 | E2205 | 0 | E2375 | 0 | G0102 | 1 | G0306 | 1 |
| E0641 | 0 | E0890 | 0 | E1030 | 0 | E1356 | 0 | E2206 | 0 | E2376 | 0 | G0103 | 1 | G0307 | 1 |
| E0642 | 0 | E0900 | 0 | E1031 | 0 | E1357 | 0 | E2207 | 0 | E2377 | 0 | G0104 | 1 | G0328 | 1 |
| E0650 | 0 | E0910 | 0 | E1035 | 0 | E1358 | 0 | E2208 | 0 | E2378 | 0 | G0105 | 1 | G0329 | 1 |
| E0651 | 0 | E0911 | 0 | E1037 | 0 | E1372 | 0 | E2209 | 0 | E2381 | 0 | G0106 | 1 | G0333 | 0 |
| E0652 | 0 | E0912 | 0 | E1038 | 0 | E1390 | 0 | E2210 | 0 | E2382 | 0 | G0108 | 6 | G0337 | 1 |
| E0655 | 0 | E0920 | 0 | E1039 | 0 | E1391 | 0 | E2211 | 0 | E2383 | 0 | G0109 | 12 | G0339 | 1 |
| E0656 | 0 | E0930 | 0 | E1050 | 0 | E1392 | 0 | E2212 | 0 | E2384 | 0 | G0117 | 1 | G0340 | 2 |
| E0657 | 0 | E0935 | 0 | E1060 | 0 | E1405 | 0 | E2213 | 0 | E2385 | 0 | G0118 | 1 | G0341 | 1 |
| E0660 | 0 | E0936 | 0 | E1070 | 0 | E1406 | 0 | E2214 | 0 | E2386 | 0 | G0120 | 1 | G0342 | 1 |
| E0665 | 0 | E0940 | 0 | E1083 | 0 | E1500 | 0 | E2215 | 0 | E2387 | 0 | G0121 | 1 | G0343 | 1 |
| E0666 | 0 | E0941 | 0 | E1084 | 0 | E1510 | 0 | E2216 | 0 | E2388 | 0 | G0123 | 1 | G0364 | 2 |
| E0667 | 0 | E0942 | 0 | E1085 | 0 | E1520 | 0 | E2217 | 0 | E2389 | 0 | G0124 | 1 | G0365 | 2 |
| E0668 | 0 | E0944 | 0 | E1086 | 0 | E1530 | 0 | E2218 | 0 | E2390 | 0 | G0127 | 1 | G0372 | 1 |
| E0669 | 0 | E0945 | 0 | E1087 | 0 | E1540 | 0 | E2219 | 0 | E2391 | 0 | G0128 | 1 | G0379 | 0 |
| E0670 | 0 | E0946 | 0 | E1088 | 0 | E1550 | 0 | E2220 | 0 | E2392 | 0 | G0130 | 1 | G0396 | 1 |
| E0671 | 0 | E0947 | 0 | E1089 | 0 | E1560 | 0 | E2221 | 0 | E2394 | 0 | G0141 | 1 | G0397 | 1 |
| E0672 | 0 | E0948 | 0 | E1090 | 0 | E1570 | 0 | E2222 | 0 | E2395 | 0 | G0143 | 1 | G0398 | 1 |
| E0673 | 0 | E0950 | 0 | E1092 | 0 | E1575 | 0 | E2224 | 0 | E2396 | 0 | G0144 | 1 | G0399 | 1 |
| E0675 | 0 | E0951 | 0 | E1093 | 0 | E1580 | 0 | E2225 | 0 | E2397 | 0 | G0145 | 1 | G0400 | 1 |
| E0676 | 1 | E0952 | 0 | E1100 | 0 | E1590 | 0 | E2226 | 0 | E2402 | 0 | G0147 | 1 | G0402 | 1 |
| E0691 | 0 | E0955 | 0 | E1110 | 0 | E1592 | 0 | E2227 | 0 | E2500 | 0 | G0148 | 1 | G0403 | 1 |
| E0692 | 0 | E0956 | 0 | E1130 | 0 | E1594 | 0 | E2228 | 0 | E2502 | 0 | G0166 | 2 | G0404 | 1 |
| E0693 | 0 | E0957 | 0 | E1140 | 0 | E1600 | 0 | E2230 | 0 | E2504 | 0 | G0168 | 2 | G0405 | 1 |
| E0694 | 0 | E0958 | 0 | E1150 | 0 | E1610 | 0 | E2231 | 0 | E2506 | 0 | G0175 | 1 | G0406 | 1 |
| E0700 | 0 | E0959 | 0 | E1160 | 0 | E1615 | 0 | E2291 | 1 | E2508 | 0 | G0177 | 0 | G0407 | 1 |
| E0705 | 0 | E0960 | 0 | E1161 | 0 | E1620 | 0 | E2292 | 1 | E2510 | 0 | G0179 | 1 | G0408 | 1 |
| E0710 | 0 | E0961 | 0 | E1170 | 0 | E1625 | 0 | E2293 | 1 | E2511 | 0 | G0180 | 1 | G0410 | 4 |
| E0720 | 0 | E0966 | 0 | E1171 | 0 | E1630 | 0 | E2294 | 1 | E2512 | 0 | G0181 | 1 | G0411 | 4 |
| E0730 | 0 | E0967 | 0 | E1172 | 0 | E1632 | 0 | E2295 | 0 | E2601 | 0 | G0182 | 1 | G0412 | 1 |
| E0731 | 0 | E0968 | 0 | E1180 | 0 | E1634 | 0 | E2300 | 0 | E2602 | 0 | G0186 | 1 | G0413 | 1 |
| E0740 | 0 | E0970 | 0 | E1190 | 0 | E1635 | 0 | E2301 | 0 | E2603 | 0 | G0202 | 1 | G0414 | 1 |
| E0744 | 0 | E0971 | 0 | E1195 | 0 | E1636 | 0 | E2310 | 0 | E2604 | 0 | G0204 | 2 | G0415 | 1 |
| E0745 | 0 | E0973 | 0 | E1200 | 0 | E1637 | 0 | E2311 | 0 | E2605 | 0 | G0206 | 2 | G0416 | 1 |
| E0746 | 1 | E0974 | 0 | E1220 | 0 | E1639 | 0 | E2312 | 0 | E2606 | 0 | G0235 | 1 | G0420 | 2 |
| E0747 | 0 | E0978 | 0 | E1221 | 0 | E1700 | 0 | E2313 | 0 | E2607 | 0 | G0237 | 8 | G0421 | 4 |
| E0748 | 0 | E0981 | 0 | E1222 | 0 | E1701 | 0 | E2321 | 0 | E2608 | 0 | G0238 | 8 | G0422 | 6 |
| E0749 | 1 | E0982 | 0 | E1223 | 0 | E1702 | 0 | E2322 | 0 | E2609 | 0 | G0239 | 1 | G0423 | 6 |
| E0755 | 0 | E0983 | 0 | E1224 | 0 | E1800 | 0 | E2323 | 0 | E2611 | 0 | G0245 | 1 | G0424 | 2 |
| E0760 | 0 | E0984 | 0 | E1225 | 0 | E1801 | 0 | E2324 | 0 | E2612 | 0 | G0246 | 1 | G0425 | 1 |
| E0761 | 0 | E0985 | 0 | E1226 | 0 | E1802 | 0 | E2325 | 0 | E2613 | 0 | G0247 | 1 | G0426 | 1 |
| E0762 | 0 | E0986 | 0 | E1228 | 0 | E1805 | 0 | E2326 | 0 | E2614 | 0 | G0248 | 1 | G0427 | 1 |
| E0764 | 0 | E0988 | 0 | E1229 | 0 | E1806 | 0 | E2327 | 0 | E2615 | 0 | G0249 | 3 | G0429 | 1 |
| E0765 | 0 | E0990 | 0 | E1230 | 0 | E1810 | 0 | E2328 | 0 | E2616 | 0 | G0250 | 1 | G0432 | 1 |
| E0766 | 0 | E0992 | 0 | E1231 | 0 | E1811 | 0 | E2329 | 0 | E2617 | 0 | G0257 | 0 | G0433 | 1 |
| E0769 | 0 | E0994 | 0 | E1232 | 0 | E1812 | 0 | E2330 | 0 | E2619 | 0 | G0259 | 2 | G0435 | 1 |
| E0770 | 1 | E0995 | 0 | E1233 | 0 | E1815 | 0 | E2331 | 0 | E2620 | 0 | G0260 | 2 | G0438 | 1 |
| E0776 | 0 | E1002 | 0 | E1234 | 0 | E1816 | 0 | E2340 | 0 | E2621 | 0 | G0268 | 1 | G0439 | 1 |
| E0779 | 0 | E1003 | 0 | E1235 | 0 | E1818 | 0 | E2341 | 0 | E2622 | 0 | G0270 | 8 | G0442 | 1 |
| E0780 | 0 | E1004 | 0 | E1236 | 0 | E1820 | 0 | E2342 | 0 | E2623 | 0 | G0271 | 4 | G0443 | 1 |
| E0781 | 1 | E1005 | 0 | E1237 | 0 | E1821 | 0 | E2343 | 0 | E2624 | 0 | G0276 | 1 | G0444 | 1 |
| E0782 | 1 | E1006 | 0 | E1238 | 0 | E1825 | 0 | E2351 | 0 | E2625 | 0 | G0277 | 5 | G0445 | 1 |
| E0783 | 1 | E1007 | 0 | E1240 | 0 | E1830 | 0 | E2358 | 0 | E2626 | 0 | G0278 | 1 | G0446 | 1 |
| E0784 | 0 | E1008 | 0 | E1250 | 0 | E1831 | 0 | E2359 | 0 | E2627 | 0 | G0281 | 1 | G0447 | 2 |
| E0785 | 1 | E1009 | 0 | E1260 | 0 | E1840 | 0 | E2361 | 0 | E2628 | 0 | G0283 | 1 | G0448 | 1 |
| E0786 | 1 | E1010 | 0 | E1270 | 0 | E1841 | 0 | E2363 | 0 | E2629 | 0 | G0288 | 1 | G0451 | 1 |
| E0791 | 0 | E1011 | 0 | E1280 | 0 | E1902 | 0 | E2365 | 0 | E2630 | 0 | G0289 | 1 | G0452 | 6 |

CPT © 2017 American Medical Association. All Rights Reserved.

© 2017 Optum360, LLC

| CPT | MUE | CPT | MUE | CPT | MUE | CPT | MUE | CPT | MUE | CPT | MUE | CPT | MUE | CPT | MUE |
|---|---|---|---|---|---|---|---|---|---|---|---|---|---|---|---|
| G0453 | 40 | J0153 | 180 | J0596 | 840 | J1094 | 0 | J1580 | 9 | J2182 | 100 | J2760 | 2 | J3357 | 520 |
| G0454 | 1 | J0171 | 20 | J0597 | 250 | J1100 | 120 | J1595 | 1 | J2185 | 30 | J2765 | 10 | J3360 | 6 |
| G0455 | 1 | J0178 | 4 | J0598 | 100 | J1110 | 3 | J1599 | 300 | J2210 | 1 | J2770 | 6 | J3364 | 0 |
| G0458 | 1 | J0180 | 150 | J0600 | 3 | J1120 | 2 | J1600 | 2 | J2212 | 240 | J2778 | 10 | J3365 | 0 |
| G0459 | 1 | J0190 | 0 | J0610 | 15 | J1130 | 300 | J1602 | 300 | J2248 | 150 | J2780 | 16 | J3370 | 12 |
| G0460 | 1 | J0200 | 0 | J0620 | 1 | J1160 | 2 | J1610 | 2 | J2250 | 22 | J2783 | 60 | J3380 | 300 |
| G0463 | 0 | J0202 | 12 | J0630 | 1 | J1162 | 1 | J1620 | 0 | J2260 | 4 | J2785 | 4 | J3385 | 92 |
| G0466 | 1 | J0205 | 0 | J0636 | 100 | J1165 | 50 | J1626 | 30 | J2265 | 400 | J2786 | 500 | J3396 | 150 |
| G0467 | 1 | J0207 | 4 | J0637 | 20 | J1170 | 350 | J1630 | 5 | J2270 | 9 | J2788 | 1 | J3400 | 0 |
| G0468 | 1 | J0210 | 4 | J0638 | 180 | J1180 | 2 | J1631 | 9 | J2274 | 250 | J2790 | 1 | J3410 | 8 |
| G0469 | 1 | J0215 | 30 | J0640 | 24 | J1190 | 8 | J1640 | 626 | J2278 | 999 | J2791 | 50 | J3411 | 4 |
| G0470 | 1 | J0220 | 1 | J0641 | 1200 | J1200 | 8 | J1642 | 100 | J2280 | 4 | J2792 | 400 | J3415 | 6 |
| G0471 | 2 | J0221 | 300 | J0670 | 12 | J1205 | 4 | J1644 | 40 | J2300 | 4 | J2793 | 320 | J3420 | 1 |
| G0472 | 1 | J0256 | 3500 | J0690 | 12 | J1212 | 1 | J1645 | 10 | J2310 | 4 | J2794 | 100 | J3430 | 25 |
| G0473 | 1 | J0257 | 1400 | J0692 | 12 | J1230 | 6 | J1650 | 30 | J2315 | 380 | J2795 | 200 | J3465 | 40 |
| G0475 | 1 | J0270 | 32 | J0694 | 8 | J1240 | 6 | J1652 | 20 | J2320 | 4 | J2796 | 150 | J3470 | 3 |
| G0476 | 1 | J0275 | 1 | J0695 | 60 | J1245 | 6 | J1655 | 0 | J2323 | 300 | J2800 | 3 | J3471 | 999 |
| G0480 | 1 | J0278 | 15 | J0696 | 16 | J1250 | 2 | J1670 | 1 | J2325 | 0 | J2805 | 3 | J3472 | 2 |
| G0481 | 1 | J0280 | 7 | J0697 | 4 | J1260 | 2 | J1675 | 0 | J2353 | 60 | J2810 | 5 | J3473 | 450 |
| G0482 | 1 | J0282 | 5 | J0698 | 10 | J1265 | 20 | J1700 | 0 | J2354 | 60 | J2820 | 15 | J3475 | 20 |
| G0483 | 1 | J0285 | 5 | J0702 | 18 | J1267 | 150 | J1710 | 0 | J2355 | 2 | J2840 | 460 | J3480 | 40 |
| G0491 | 1 | J0287 | 20 | J0706 | 1 | J1270 | 8 | J1720 | 10 | J2357 | 90 | J2850 | 16 | J3485 | 160 |
| G0492 | 1 | J0288 | 0 | J0710 | 0 | J1290 | 30 | J1725 | 0 | J2358 | 405 | J2860 | 170 | J3486 | 4 |
| G0498 | 1 | J0289 | 50 | J0712 | 120 | J1300 | 120 | J1730 | 0 | J2360 | 2 | J2910 | 0 | J3489 | 5 |
| G0499 | 1 | J0290 | 24 | J0713 | 12 | J1320 | 0 | J1740 | 3 | J2370 | 2 | J2916 | 20 | J3520 | 0 |
| G0500 | 1 | J0295 | 12 | J0714 | 4 | J1322 | 220 | J1741 | 8 | J2400 | 4 | J2920 | 25 | J3530 | 0 |
| G0502 | 1 | J0300 | 8 | J0715 | 0 | J1324 | 108 | J1742 | 2 | J2405 | 64 | J2930 | 25 | J7030 | 5 |
| G0503 | 1 | J0330 | 10 | J0716 | 4 | J1325 | 1 | J1743 | 66 | J2407 | 120 | J2940 | 0 | J7040 | 6 |
| G0504 | 2 | J0348 | 200 | J0717 | 400 | J1327 | 1 | J1744 | 30 | J2410 | 2 | J2941 | 8 | J7042 | 6 |
| G0505 | 1 | J0350 | 0 | J0720 | 15 | J1330 | 1 | J1745 | 150 | J2425 | 125 | J2950 | 0 | J7050 | 10 |
| G0506 | 1 | J0360 | 2 | J0725 | 10 | J1335 | 2 | J1750 | 45 | J2426 | 819 | J2993 | 2 | J7060 | 10 |
| G0507 | 1 | J0364 | 6 | J0735 | 50 | J1364 | 2 | J1756 | 500 | J2430 | 3 | J2995 | 0 | J7070 | 4 |
| G0508 | 1 | J0365 | 0 | J0740 | 2 | J1380 | 4 | J1786 | 900 | J2440 | 4 | J2997 | 8 | J7100 | 2 |
| G0509 | 1 | J0380 | 1 | J0743 | 16 | J1410 | 4 | J1790 | 2 | J2460 | 0 | J3000 | 2 | J7110 | 2 |
| G0659 | 1 | J0390 | 0 | J0744 | 6 | J1430 | 10 | J1800 | 6 | J2469 | 10 | J3010 | 100 | J7120 | 4 |
| G6001 | 2 | J0395 | 0 | J0745 | 2 | J1435 | 1 | J1810 | 0 | J2501 | 2 | J3030 | 1 | J7121 | 4 |
| G6002 | 2 | J0400 | 39 | J0770 | 5 | J1436 | 0 | J1815 | 8 | J2502 | 60 | J3060 | 900 | J7131 | 500 |
| G6003 | 2 | J0401 | 400 | J0775 | 180 | J1438 | 2 | J1817 | 0 | J2503 | 2 | J3070 | 3 | J7175 | 9000 |
| G6004 | 2 | J0456 | 4 | J0780 | 4 | J1439 | 750 | J1830 | 1 | J2504 | 15 | J3090 | 200 | J7178 | 7700 |
| G6005 | 2 | J0461 | 200 | J0795 | 100 | J1442 | 3360 | J1833 | 372 | J2505 | 1 | J3095 | 150 | J7179 | 30000 |
| G6006 | 2 | J0470 | 2 | J0800 | 3 | J1443 | 272 | J1835 | 0 | J2507 | 8 | J3101 | 50 | J7180 | 6000 |
| G6007 | 2 | J0475 | 8 | J0833 | 3 | J1447 | 960 | J1840 | 3 | J2510 | 4 | J3105 | 2 | J7181 | 3850 |
| G6008 | 2 | J0476 | 2 | J0834 | 3 | J1450 | 4 | J1850 | 4 | J2513 | 1 | J3110 | 2 | J7182 | 22000 |
| G6009 | 2 | J0480 | 1 | J0840 | 6 | J1451 | 1 | J1885 | 8 | J2515 | 1 | J3121 | 400 | J7183 | 15000 |
| G6010 | 2 | J0485 | 1500 | J0850 | 9 | J1452 | 0 | J1890 | 0 | J2540 | 75 | J3145 | 750 | J7185 | 4000 |
| G6011 | 2 | J0490 | 160 | J0875 | 300 | J1453 | 150 | J1930 | 120 | J2543 | 16 | J3230 | 2 | J7186 | 8000 |
| G6012 | 2 | J0500 | 4 | J0878 | 1500 | J1455 | 18 | J1931 | 760 | J2545 | 1 | J3240 | 1 | J7187 | 7500 |
| G6013 | 2 | J0515 | 3 | J0881 | 500 | J1457 | 0 | J1940 | 6 | J2547 | 600 | J3243 | 150 | J7188 | 22000 |
| G6014 | 2 | J0520 | 0 | J0882 | 300 | J1458 | 100 | J1942 | 882 | J2550 | 3 | J3246 | 1 | J7189 | 13000 |
| G6015 | 2 | J0558 | 24 | J0883 | 1125 | J1459 | 300 | J1945 | 0 | J2560 | 1 | J3250 | 2 | J7190 | 30000 |
| G6016 | 2 | J0561 | 24 | J0884 | 1125 | J1460 | 10 | J1950 | 12 | J2562 | 48 | J3260 | 8 | J7191 | 0 |
| G6017 | 2 | J0570 | 4 | J0885 | 60 | J1556 | 300 | J1953 | 300 | J2590 | 3 | J3262 | 800 | J7192 | 22000 |
| G9143 | 1 | J0571 | 0 | J0887 | 360 | J1557 | 300 | J1955 | 11 | J2597 | 45 | J3265 | 0 | J7193 | 4000 |
| G9156 | 1 | J0572 | 0 | J0888 | 360 | J1559 | 375 | J1956 | 4 | J2650 | 0 | J3280 | 0 | J7194 | 9000 |
| G9157 | 1 | J0573 | 0 | J0890 | 0 | J1560 | 1 | J1960 | 0 | J2670 | 0 | J3285 | 1 | J7195 | 6000 |
| G9187 | 1 | J0574 | 0 | J0894 | 100 | J1561 | 300 | J1980 | 2 | J2675 | 1 | J3300 | 160 | J7196 | 175 |
| G9480 | 1 | J0575 | 0 | J0895 | 12 | J1562 | 375 | J1990 | 0 | J2680 | 4 | J3301 | 16 | J7197 | 6300 |
| G9678 | 1 | J0583 | 250 | J0897 | 120 | J1566 | 300 | J2001 | 60 | J2690 | 4 | J3302 | 0 | J7198 | 6000 |
| J0120 | 1 | J0585 | 600 | J0945 | 4 | J1568 | 300 | J2010 | 10 | J2700 | 48 | J3303 | 24 | J7200 | 20000 |
| J0129 | 100 | J0586 | 300 | J1000 | 1 | J1569 | 300 | J2020 | 6 | J2704 | 80 | J3305 | 0 | J7201 | 9000 |
| J0130 | 6 | J0587 | 300 | J1020 | 8 | J1570 | 4 | J2060 | 4 | J2710 | 2 | J3310 | 0 | J7202 | 11550 |
| J0131 | 400 | J0588 | 600 | J1030 | 8 | J1571 | 20 | J2150 | 8 | J2720 | 5 | J3315 | 6 | J7205 | 9750 |
| J0132 | 12 | J0592 | 6 | J1040 | 4 | J1572 | 300 | J2170 | 8 | J2724 | 4000 | J3320 | 0 | J7207 | 7500 |
| J0133 | 1200 | J0594 | 320 | J1050 | 1000 | J1573 | 130 | J2175 | 4 | J2725 | 0 | J3350 | 0 | J7209 | 7500 |
| J0135 | 8 | J0595 | 8 | J1071 | 400 | J1575 | 650 | J2180 | 0 | J2730 | 2 | J3355 | 1 | J7297 | 0 |

© 2017 Optum360, LLC

Appendix I — Medically Unlikely Edits (MUEs) — Professional

| CPT | MUE | CPT | MUE | CPT | MUE | CPT | MUE | CPT | MUE | CPT | MUE | CPT | MUE | CPT | MUE |
|---|---|---|---|---|---|---|---|---|---|---|---|---|---|---|---|
| J7298 | 0 | J7634 | 0 | J9043 | 60 | J9303 | 100 | K0605 | 0 | K0870 | 0 | L0635 | 0 | L1660 | 0 |
| J7301 | 0 | J7635 | 0 | J9045 | 22 | J9305 | 150 | K0606 | 0 | K0871 | 0 | L0636 | 0 | L1680 | 0 |
| J7308 | 3 | J7636 | 0 | J9047 | 120 | J9306 | 840 | K0607 | 0 | K0877 | 0 | L0637 | 0 | L1685 | 0 |
| J7309 | 1 | J7637 | 0 | J9050 | 6 | J9307 | 80 | K0608 | 0 | K0878 | 0 | L0638 | 0 | L1686 | 0 |
| J7310 | 2 | J7638 | 0 | J9055 | 120 | J9308 | 280 | K0609 | 0 | K0879 | 0 | L0639 | 0 | L1690 | 0 |
| J7311 | 1 | J7639 | 3 | J9060 | 24 | J9310 | 12 | K0672 | 0 | K0880 | 0 | L0640 | 0 | L1700 | 0 |
| J7312 | 14 | J7640 | 0 | J9065 | 20 | J9315 | 40 | K0730 | 0 | K0884 | 0 | L0641 | 0 | L1710 | 0 |
| J7313 | 38 | J7641 | 0 | J9070 | 55 | J9320 | 4 | K0733 | 0 | K0885 | 0 | L0642 | 0 | L1720 | 0 |
| J7315 | 2 | J7642 | 0 | J9098 | 5 | J9325 | 400 | K0738 | 0 | K0886 | 0 | L0643 | 0 | L1730 | 0 |
| J7316 | 4 | J7643 | 0 | J9100 | 120 | J9328 | 400 | K0740 | 0 | K0890 | 0 | L0648 | 0 | L1755 | 0 |
| J7320 | 50 | J7644 | 3 | J9120 | 5 | J9330 | 50 | K0743 | 0 | K0891 | 0 | L0649 | 0 | L1810 | 0 |
| J7321 | 2 | J7645 | 0 | J9130 | 24 | J9340 | 4 | K0744 | 0 | K0898 | 1 | L0650 | 0 | L1812 | 0 |
| J7322 | 48 | J7647 | 0 | J9145 | 240 | J9351 | 120 | K0745 | 0 | K0900 | 0 | L0651 | 0 | L1820 | 0 |
| J7323 | 2 | J7648 | 0 | J9150 | 12 | J9352 | 50 | K0746 | 0 | L0112 | 0 | L0700 | 0 | L1830 | 0 |
| J7324 | 2 | J7649 | 0 | J9151 | 10 | J9354 | 600 | K0800 | 0 | L0113 | 0 | L0710 | 0 | L1831 | 0 |
| J7325 | 96 | J7650 | 0 | J9155 | 240 | J9355 | 100 | K0801 | 0 | L0120 | 0 | L0810 | 0 | L1832 | 0 |
| J7326 | 2 | J7657 | 0 | J9160 | 7 | J9357 | 4 | K0802 | 0 | L0130 | 0 | L0820 | 0 | L1833 | 0 |
| J7327 | 2 | J7658 | 0 | J9165 | 0 | J9360 | 45 | K0806 | 0 | L0140 | 0 | L0830 | 0 | L1834 | 0 |
| J7328 | 336 | J7659 | 0 | J9171 | 240 | J9370 | 4 | K0807 | 0 | L0150 | 0 | L0859 | 0 | L1836 | 0 |
| J7330 | 1 | J7660 | 0 | J9175 | 10 | J9371 | 5 | K0808 | 0 | L0160 | 0 | L0861 | 0 | L1840 | 0 |
| J7336 | 1120 | J7665 | 127 | J9176 | 1500 | J9390 | 36 | K0812 | 0 | L0170 | 0 | L0970 | 0 | L1843 | 0 |
| J7340 | 1 | J7667 | 0 | J9178 | 150 | J9395 | 20 | K0813 | 0 | L0172 | 0 | L0972 | 0 | L1844 | 0 |
| J7342 | 10 | J7668 | 0 | J9179 | 50 | J9400 | 600 | K0814 | 0 | L0174 | 0 | L0974 | 0 | L1845 | 0 |
| J7500 | 0 | J7669 | 0 | J9181 | 100 | J9600 | 4 | K0815 | 0 | L0180 | 0 | L0976 | 0 | L1846 | 0 |
| J7501 | 1 | J7670 | 0 | J9185 | 2 | K0001 | 0 | K0816 | 0 | L0190 | 0 | L0978 | 0 | L1847 | 0 |
| J7502 | 0 | J7674 | 100 | J9190 | 20 | K0002 | 0 | K0820 | 0 | L0200 | 0 | L0980 | 0 | L1848 | 0 |
| J7503 | 0 | J7676 | 0 | J9200 | 5 | K0003 | 0 | K0821 | 0 | L0220 | 0 | L0982 | 0 | L1850 | 0 |
| J7504 | 15 | J7680 | 0 | J9201 | 20 | K0004 | 0 | K0822 | 0 | L0450 | 0 | L0984 | 0 | L1851 | 0 |
| J7505 | 1 | J7681 | 0 | J9202 | 3 | K0005 | 0 | K0823 | 0 | L0452 | 0 | L1000 | 0 | L1852 | 0 |
| J7507 | 0 | J7682 | 2 | J9205 | 215 | K0006 | 0 | K0824 | 0 | L0454 | 0 | L1001 | 0 | L1860 | 0 |
| J7508 | 0 | J7683 | 0 | J9206 | 42 | K0007 | 0 | K0825 | 0 | L0455 | 0 | L1005 | 0 | L1900 | 0 |
| J7509 | 0 | J7684 | 0 | J9207 | 90 | K0009 | 0 | K0826 | 0 | L0456 | 0 | L1010 | 0 | L1902 | 0 |
| J7510 | 0 | J7685 | 0 | J9208 | 15 | K0015 | 0 | K0827 | 0 | L0457 | 0 | L1020 | 0 | L1904 | 0 |
| J7511 | 9 | J7686 | 1 | J9209 | 55 | K0017 | 0 | K0828 | 0 | L0458 | 0 | L1025 | 0 | L1906 | 0 |
| J7512 | 0 | J8501 | 0 | J9211 | 6 | K0018 | 0 | K0829 | 0 | L0460 | 0 | L1030 | 0 | L1907 | 0 |
| J7513 | 6 | J8510 | 0 | J9212 | 0 | K0019 | 0 | K0830 | 0 | L0462 | 0 | L1040 | 0 | L1910 | 0 |
| J7515 | 0 | J8520 | 0 | J9213 | 12 | K0020 | 0 | K0831 | 0 | L0464 | 0 | L1050 | 0 | L1920 | 0 |
| J7516 | 1 | J8521 | 0 | J9214 | 100 | K0037 | 0 | K0835 | 0 | L0466 | 0 | L1060 | 0 | L1930 | 0 |
| J7517 | 0 | J8530 | 0 | J9215 | 0 | K0038 | 0 | K0836 | 0 | L0467 | 0 | L1070 | 0 | L1932 | 0 |
| J7518 | 0 | J8540 | 0 | J9216 | 2 | K0039 | 0 | K0837 | 0 | L0468 | 0 | L1080 | 0 | L1940 | 0 |
| J7520 | 0 | J8560 | 0 | J9217 | 6 | K0040 | 0 | K0838 | 0 | L0469 | 0 | L1085 | 0 | L1945 | 0 |
| J7525 | 2 | J8562 | 0 | J9218 | 1 | K0041 | 0 | K0839 | 0 | L0470 | 0 | L1090 | 0 | L1950 | 0 |
| J7527 | 0 | J8600 | 0 | J9219 | 1 | K0042 | 0 | K0840 | 0 | L0472 | 0 | L1100 | 0 | L1951 | 0 |
| J7604 | 0 | J8610 | 0 | J9225 | 1 | K0043 | 0 | K0841 | 0 | L0480 | 0 | L1110 | 0 | L1960 | 0 |
| J7605 | 2 | J8650 | 0 | J9226 | 1 | K0044 | 0 | K0842 | 0 | L0482 | 0 | L1120 | 0 | L1970 | 0 |
| J7606 | 2 | J8655 | 1 | J9228 | 1100 | K0045 | 0 | K0843 | 0 | L0484 | 0 | L1200 | 0 | L1971 | 0 |
| J7607 | 0 | J8670 | 180 | J9230 | 5 | K0046 | 0 | K0848 | 0 | L0486 | 0 | L1210 | 0 | L1980 | 0 |
| J7608 | 3 | J8700 | 0 | J9245 | 9 | K0047 | 0 | K0849 | 0 | L0488 | 0 | L1220 | 0 | L1990 | 0 |
| J7609 | 0 | J8705 | 0 | J9250 | 25 | K0050 | 0 | K0850 | 0 | L0490 | 0 | L1230 | 0 | L2000 | 0 |
| J7610 | 0 | J9000 | 20 | J9260 | 20 | K0051 | 0 | K0851 | 0 | L0491 | 0 | L1240 | 0 | L2005 | 0 |
| J7611 | 10 | J9015 | 1 | J9261 | 80 | K0052 | 0 | K0852 | 0 | L0492 | 0 | L1250 | 0 | L2010 | 0 |
| J7612 | 10 | J9017 | 30 | J9262 | 700 | K0053 | 0 | K0853 | 0 | L0621 | 0 | L1260 | 0 | L2020 | 0 |
| J7613 | 10 | J9019 | 60 | J9263 | 700 | K0056 | 0 | K0854 | 0 | L0622 | 0 | L1270 | 0 | L2030 | 0 |
| J7614 | 10 | J9020 | 0 | J9266 | 2 | K0065 | 0 | K0855 | 0 | L0623 | 0 | L1280 | 0 | L2034 | 0 |
| J7615 | 0 | J9025 | 300 | J9267 | 750 | K0069 | 0 | K0856 | 0 | L0624 | 0 | L1290 | 0 | L2035 | 0 |
| J7620 | 6 | J9027 | 100 | J9268 | 1 | K0070 | 0 | K0857 | 0 | L0625 | 0 | L1300 | 0 | L2036 | 0 |
| J7622 | 0 | J9031 | 1 | J9270 | 0 | K0071 | 0 | K0858 | 0 | L0626 | 0 | L1310 | 0 | L2037 | 0 |
| J7624 | 0 | J9032 | 300 | J9271 | 300 | K0072 | 0 | K0859 | 0 | L0627 | 0 | L1499 | 1 | L2038 | 0 |
| J7626 | 2 | J9033 | 300 | J9280 | 12 | K0073 | 0 | K0860 | 0 | L0628 | 0 | L1600 | 0 | L2040 | 0 |
| J7627 | 0 | J9034 | 360 | J9293 | 8 | K0077 | 0 | K0861 | 0 | L0629 | 0 | L1610 | 0 | L2050 | 0 |
| J7628 | 0 | J9035 | 180 | J9295 | 800 | K0105 | 0 | K0862 | 0 | L0630 | 0 | L1620 | 0 | L2060 | 0 |
| J7629 | 0 | J9039 | 210 | J9299 | 440 | K0195 | 0 | K0863 | 0 | L0631 | 0 | L1630 | 0 | L2070 | 0 |
| J7631 | 4 | J9040 | 4 | J9300 | 0 | K0455 | 0 | K0864 | 0 | L0632 | 0 | L1640 | 0 | L2080 | 0 |
| J7632 | 0 | J9041 | 35 | J9301 | 100 | K0462 | 0 | K0868 | 0 | L0633 | 0 | L1650 | 0 | L2090 | 0 |
| J7633 | 0 | J9042 | 200 | J9302 | 200 | K0602 | 0 | K0869 | 0 | L0634 | 0 | L1652 | 0 | L2106 | 0 |

CPT © 2017 American Medical Association. All Rights Reserved.

© 2017 Optum360, LLC

| CPT | MUE | CPT | MUE | CPT | MUE | CPT | MUE | CPT | MUE | CPT | MUE | CPT | MUE | CPT | MUE |
|---|---|---|---|---|---|---|---|---|---|---|---|---|---|---|---|
| L2108 | 0 | L2628 | 0 | L3400 | 0 | L3921 | 0 | L5200 | 0 | L5653 | 0 | L5826 | 0 | L6388 | 0 |
| L2112 | 0 | L2630 | 0 | L3410 | 0 | L3923 | 0 | L5210 | 0 | L5654 | 0 | L5828 | 0 | L6400 | 0 |
| L2114 | 0 | L2640 | 0 | L3420 | 0 | L3924 | 0 | L5220 | 0 | L5655 | 0 | L5830 | 0 | L6450 | 0 |
| L2116 | 0 | L2650 | 0 | L3430 | 0 | L3925 | 0 | L5230 | 0 | L5656 | 0 | L5840 | 0 | L6500 | 0 |
| L2126 | 0 | L2660 | 0 | L3440 | 0 | L3927 | 0 | L5250 | 0 | L5658 | 0 | L5845 | 0 | L6550 | 0 |
| L2128 | 0 | L2670 | 0 | L3450 | 0 | L3929 | 0 | L5270 | 0 | L5661 | 0 | L5848 | 0 | L6570 | 0 |
| L2132 | 0 | L2680 | 0 | L3455 | 0 | L3930 | 0 | L5280 | 0 | L5665 | 0 | L5850 | 0 | L6580 | 0 |
| L2134 | 0 | L2750 | 0 | L3460 | 0 | L3931 | 0 | L5301 | 0 | L5666 | 0 | L5855 | 0 | L6582 | 0 |
| L2136 | 0 | L2755 | 0 | L3465 | 0 | L3933 | 0 | L5312 | 0 | L5668 | 0 | L5856 | 0 | L6584 | 0 |
| L2180 | 0 | L2760 | 0 | L3470 | 0 | L3935 | 0 | L5321 | 0 | L5670 | 0 | L5857 | 0 | L6586 | 0 |
| L2182 | 0 | L2768 | 0 | L3480 | 0 | L3956 | 0 | L5331 | 0 | L5671 | 0 | L5858 | 0 | L6588 | 0 |
| L2184 | 0 | L2780 | 0 | L3485 | 0 | L3960 | 0 | L5341 | 0 | L5672 | 0 | L5859 | 0 | L6590 | 0 |
| L2186 | 0 | L2785 | 0 | L3500 | 0 | L3961 | 0 | L5400 | 0 | L5673 | 0 | L5910 | 0 | L6600 | 0 |
| L2188 | 0 | L2795 | 0 | L3510 | 0 | L3962 | 0 | L5410 | 0 | L5676 | 0 | L5920 | 0 | L6605 | 0 |
| L2190 | 0 | L2800 | 0 | L3520 | 0 | L3967 | 0 | L5420 | 0 | L5677 | 0 | L5925 | 0 | L6610 | 0 |
| L2192 | 0 | L2810 | 0 | L3530 | 0 | L3971 | 0 | L5430 | 0 | L5678 | 0 | L5930 | 0 | L6611 | 0 |
| L2200 | 0 | L2820 | 0 | L3540 | 0 | L3973 | 0 | L5450 | 0 | L5679 | 0 | L5940 | 0 | L6615 | 0 |
| L2210 | 0 | L2830 | 0 | L3550 | 0 | L3975 | 0 | L5460 | 0 | L5680 | 0 | L5950 | 0 | L6616 | 0 |
| L2220 | 0 | L2840 | 0 | L3560 | 0 | L3976 | 0 | L5500 | 0 | L5681 | 0 | L5960 | 0 | L6620 | 0 |
| L2230 | 0 | L2850 | 0 | L3570 | 0 | L3977 | 0 | L5505 | 0 | L5682 | 0 | L5961 | 0 | L6621 | 0 |
| L2232 | 0 | L2861 | 0 | L3580 | 0 | L3978 | 0 | L5510 | 0 | L5683 | 0 | L5962 | 0 | L6623 | 0 |
| L2240 | 0 | L3000 | 0 | L3590 | 0 | L3980 | 0 | L5520 | 0 | L5684 | 0 | L5964 | 0 | L6624 | 0 |
| L2250 | 0 | L3001 | 0 | L3595 | 0 | L3981 | 0 | L5530 | 0 | L5685 | 0 | L5966 | 0 | L6625 | 0 |
| L2260 | 0 | L3002 | 0 | L3600 | 0 | L3982 | 0 | L5535 | 0 | L5686 | 0 | L5968 | 0 | L6628 | 0 |
| L2265 | 0 | L3003 | 0 | L3610 | 0 | L3984 | 0 | L5540 | 0 | L5688 | 0 | L5969 | 0 | L6629 | 0 |
| L2270 | 0 | L3010 | 0 | L3620 | 0 | L3995 | 0 | L5560 | 0 | L5690 | 0 | L5970 | 0 | L6630 | 0 |
| L2275 | 0 | L3020 | 0 | L3630 | 0 | L4000 | 0 | L5570 | 0 | L5692 | 0 | L5971 | 0 | L6632 | 0 |
| L2280 | 0 | L3030 | 0 | L3640 | 0 | L4002 | 0 | L5580 | 0 | L5694 | 0 | L5972 | 0 | L6635 | 0 |
| L2300 | 0 | L3031 | 0 | L3650 | 0 | L4010 | 0 | L5585 | 0 | L5695 | 0 | L5974 | 0 | L6637 | 0 |
| L2310 | 0 | L3040 | 0 | L3660 | 0 | L4020 | 0 | L5590 | 0 | L5696 | 0 | L5975 | 0 | L6638 | 0 |
| L2320 | 0 | L3050 | 0 | L3670 | 0 | L4030 | 0 | L5595 | 0 | L5697 | 0 | L5976 | 0 | L6640 | 0 |
| L2330 | 0 | L3060 | 0 | L3671 | 0 | L4040 | 0 | L5600 | 0 | L5698 | 0 | L5978 | 0 | L6641 | 0 |
| L2335 | 0 | L3070 | 0 | L3674 | 0 | L4045 | 0 | L5610 | 0 | L5699 | 0 | L5979 | 0 | L6642 | 0 |
| L2340 | 0 | L3080 | 0 | L3675 | 0 | L4050 | 0 | L5611 | 0 | L5700 | 0 | L5980 | 0 | L6645 | 0 |
| L2350 | 0 | L3090 | 0 | L3677 | 0 | L4055 | 0 | L5613 | 0 | L5701 | 0 | L5981 | 0 | L6646 | 0 |
| L2360 | 0 | L3100 | 0 | L3678 | 0 | L4060 | 0 | L5614 | 0 | L5702 | 0 | L5982 | 0 | L6647 | 0 |
| L2370 | 0 | L3140 | 0 | L3702 | 0 | L4070 | 0 | L5616 | 0 | L5703 | 0 | L5984 | 0 | L6648 | 0 |
| L2375 | 0 | L3150 | 0 | L3710 | 0 | L4080 | 0 | L5617 | 0 | L5704 | 0 | L5985 | 0 | L6650 | 0 |
| L2380 | 0 | L3160 | 0 | L3720 | 0 | L4090 | 0 | L5618 | 0 | L5705 | 0 | L5986 | 0 | L6655 | 0 |
| L2385 | 0 | L3170 | 0 | L3730 | 0 | L4100 | 0 | L5620 | 0 | L5706 | 0 | L5987 | 0 | L6660 | 0 |
| L2387 | 0 | L3215 | 0 | L3740 | 0 | L4110 | 0 | L5622 | 0 | L5707 | 0 | L5988 | 0 | L6665 | 0 |
| L2390 | 0 | L3216 | 0 | L3760 | 0 | L4130 | 0 | L5624 | 0 | L5710 | 0 | L5990 | 0 | L6670 | 0 |
| L2395 | 0 | L3217 | 0 | L3762 | 0 | L4205 | 0 | L5626 | 0 | L5711 | 0 | L6000 | 0 | L6672 | 0 |
| L2397 | 0 | L3219 | 0 | L3763 | 0 | L4210 | 0 | L5628 | 0 | L5712 | 0 | L6010 | 0 | L6675 | 0 |
| L2405 | 0 | L3221 | 0 | L3764 | 0 | L4350 | 0 | L5629 | 0 | L5714 | 0 | L6020 | 0 | L6676 | 0 |
| L2415 | 0 | L3222 | 0 | L3765 | 0 | L4360 | 0 | L5630 | 0 | L5716 | 0 | L6026 | 0 | L6677 | 0 |
| L2425 | 0 | L3224 | 0 | L3766 | 0 | L4361 | 0 | L5631 | 0 | L5718 | 0 | L6050 | 0 | L6680 | 0 |
| L2430 | 0 | L3225 | 0 | L3806 | 0 | L4370 | 0 | L5632 | 0 | L5722 | 0 | L6055 | 0 | L6682 | 0 |
| L2492 | 0 | L3230 | 0 | L3807 | 0 | L4386 | 0 | L5634 | 0 | L5724 | 0 | L6100 | 0 | L6684 | 0 |
| L2500 | 0 | L3250 | 0 | L3808 | 0 | L4387 | 0 | L5636 | 0 | L5726 | 0 | L6110 | 0 | L6686 | 0 |
| L2510 | 0 | L3251 | 0 | L3809 | 0 | L4392 | 0 | L5637 | 0 | L5728 | 0 | L6120 | 0 | L6687 | 0 |
| L2520 | 0 | L3252 | 0 | L3891 | 0 | L4394 | 0 | L5638 | 0 | L5780 | 0 | L6130 | 0 | L6688 | 0 |
| L2525 | 0 | L3253 | 0 | L3900 | 0 | L4396 | 0 | L5639 | 0 | L5781 | 0 | L6200 | 0 | L6689 | 0 |
| L2526 | 0 | L3300 | 0 | L3901 | 0 | L4397 | 0 | L5640 | 0 | L5782 | 0 | L6205 | 0 | L6690 | 0 |
| L2530 | 0 | L3310 | 0 | L3904 | 0 | L4398 | 0 | L5642 | 0 | L5785 | 0 | L6250 | 0 | L6691 | 0 |
| L2540 | 0 | L3320 | 0 | L3905 | 0 | L4631 | 0 | L5643 | 0 | L5790 | 0 | L6300 | 0 | L6692 | 0 |
| L2550 | 0 | L3330 | 0 | L3906 | 0 | L5000 | 0 | L5644 | 0 | L5795 | 0 | L6310 | 0 | L6693 | 0 |
| L2570 | 0 | L3332 | 0 | L3908 | 0 | L5010 | 0 | L5645 | 0 | L5810 | 0 | L6320 | 0 | L6694 | 0 |
| L2580 | 0 | L3334 | 0 | L3912 | 0 | L5020 | 0 | L5646 | 0 | L5811 | 0 | L6350 | 0 | L6695 | 0 |
| L2600 | 0 | L3340 | 0 | L3913 | 0 | L5050 | 0 | L5647 | 0 | L5812 | 0 | L6360 | 0 | L6696 | 0 |
| L2610 | 0 | L3350 | 0 | L3915 | 0 | L5060 | 0 | L5648 | 0 | L5814 | 0 | L6370 | 0 | L6697 | 0 |
| L2620 | 0 | L3360 | 0 | L3916 | 0 | L5100 | 0 | L5649 | 0 | L5816 | 0 | L6380 | 0 | L6698 | 0 |
| L2622 | 0 | L3370 | 0 | L3917 | 0 | L5105 | 0 | L5650 | 0 | L5818 | 0 | L6382 | 0 | L6703 | 0 |
| L2624 | 0 | L3380 | 0 | L3918 | 0 | L5150 | 0 | L5651 | 0 | L5822 | 0 | L6384 | 0 | L6704 | 0 |
| L2627 | 0 | L3390 | 0 | L3919 | 0 | L5160 | 0 | L5652 | 0 | L5824 | 0 | L6386 | 0 | L6706 | 0 |

**Appendix I — Medically Unlikely Edits (MUEs) — Professional**

| CPT | MUE | CPT | MUE | CPT | MUE | CPT | MUE | CPT | MUE | CPT | MUE | CPT | MUE | CPT | MUE |
|-----|-----|-----|-----|-----|-----|-----|-----|-----|-----|-----|-----|-----|-----|-----|-----|
| L6707 | 0 | L8001 | 0 | L8641 | 4 | P9070 | 2 | Q1005 | 2 | Q4140 | 32 | V2104 | 0 | V2511 | 0 |
| L6708 | 0 | L8002 | 0 | L8642 | 2 | P9071 | 2 | Q2004 | 1 | Q4141 | 25 | V2105 | 0 | V2512 | 0 |
| L6709 | 0 | L8015 | 0 | L8658 | 4 | P9072 | 2 | Q2009 | 100 | Q4142 | 600 | V2106 | 0 | V2513 | 0 |
| L6711 | 0 | L8020 | 0 | L8659 | 4 | P9603 | 300 | Q2017 | 12 | Q4143 | 96 | V2107 | 0 | V2520 | 2 |
| L6712 | 0 | L8030 | 0 | L8670 | 4 | P9604 | 2 | Q2026 | 45 | Q4145 | 160 | V2108 | 0 | V2521 | 2 |
| L6713 | 0 | L8031 | 0 | L8679 | 3 | P9612 | 1 | Q2028 | 1470 | Q4146 | 50 | V2109 | 0 | V2522 | 2 |
| L6714 | 0 | L8032 | 0 | L8681 | 1 | P9615 | 1 | Q2034 | 1 | Q4147 | 150 | V2110 | 0 | V2523 | 2 |
| L6715 | 0 | L8035 | 0 | L8682 | 2 | Q0035 | 1 | Q2035 | 1 | Q4148 | 24 | V2111 | 0 | V2530 | 0 |
| L6721 | 0 | L8039 | 0 | L8683 | 1 | Q0091 | 1 | Q2036 | 1 | Q4149 | 10 | V2112 | 0 | V2531 | 0 |
| L6722 | 0 | L8040 | 0 | L8684 | 1 | Q0111 | 2 | Q2037 | 1 | Q4150 | 32 | V2113 | 0 | V2599 | 2 |
| L6805 | 0 | L8041 | 0 | L8685 | 1 | Q0112 | 3 | Q2038 | 1 | Q4151 | 24 | V2114 | 0 | V2600 | 0 |
| L6810 | 0 | L8042 | 0 | L8686 | 2 | Q0113 | 2 | Q2039 | 1 | Q4152 | 24 | V2115 | 0 | V2610 | 0 |
| L6880 | 0 | L8043 | 0 | L8687 | 1 | Q0114 | 1 | Q2043 | 1 | Q4153 | 6 | V2118 | 0 | V2615 | 0 |
| L6881 | 0 | L8044 | 0 | L8688 | 1 | Q0115 | 1 | Q2049 | 14 | Q4154 | 36 | V2121 | 0 | V2623 | 0 |
| L6882 | 0 | L8045 | 0 | L8689 | 1 | Q0138 | 510 | Q2050 | 14 | Q4155 | 100 | V2199 | 2 | V2624 | 0 |
| L6883 | 0 | L8046 | 0 | L8690 | 2 | Q0139 | 510 | Q2052 | 1 | Q4156 | 49 | V2200 | 0 | V2625 | 0 |
| L6884 | 0 | L8047 | 0 | L8691 | 1 | Q0144 | 0 | Q3014 | 1 | Q4157 | 24 | V2201 | 0 | V2626 | 0 |
| L6885 | 0 | L8048 | 1 | L8692 | 0 | Q0161 | 0 | Q3027 | 30 | Q4158 | 70 | V2202 | 0 | V2627 | 0 |
| L6890 | 0 | L8049 | 0 | L8693 | 1 | Q0162 | 0 | Q3028 | 0 | Q4159 | 28 | V2203 | 0 | V2628 | 0 |
| L6895 | 0 | L8300 | 0 | L8695 | 1 | Q0163 | 0 | Q3031 | 1 | Q4160 | 36 | V2204 | 0 | V2629 | 0 |
| L6900 | 0 | L8310 | 0 | L8696 | 1 | Q0164 | 0 | Q4001 | 1 | Q4161 | 42 | V2205 | 0 | V2630 | 2 |
| L6905 | 0 | L8320 | 0 | P2028 | 1 | Q0166 | 0 | Q4002 | 1 | Q4162 | 4 | V2206 | 0 | V2631 | 2 |
| L6910 | 0 | L8330 | 0 | P2029 | 1 | Q0167 | 0 | Q4003 | 2 | Q4163 | 32 | V2207 | 0 | V2632 | 2 |
| L6915 | 0 | L8400 | 0 | P2033 | 1 | Q0169 | 0 | Q4004 | 2 | Q4164 | 400 | V2208 | 0 | V2700 | 0 |
| L6920 | 0 | L8410 | 0 | P2038 | 1 | Q0173 | 0 | Q4025 | 1 | Q4165 | 100 | V2209 | 0 | V2702 | 0 |
| L6925 | 0 | L8415 | 0 | P3000 | 1 | Q0174 | 0 | Q4026 | 1 | Q4166 | 100 | V2210 | 0 | V2710 | 0 |
| L6930 | 0 | L8417 | 0 | P3001 | 1 | Q0175 | 0 | Q4027 | 1 | Q4167 | 32 | V2211 | 0 | V2715 | 0 |
| L6935 | 0 | L8420 | 0 | P9010 | 2 | Q0177 | 0 | Q4028 | 1 | Q4168 | 160 | V2212 | 0 | V2718 | 0 |
| L6940 | 0 | L8430 | 0 | P9011 | 2 | Q0180 | 0 | Q4074 | 3 | Q4169 | 32 | V2213 | 0 | V2730 | 0 |
| L6945 | 0 | L8435 | 0 | P9012 | 8 | Q0478 | 1 | Q4081 | 100 | Q4170 | 120 | V2214 | 0 | V2744 | 0 |
| L6950 | 0 | L8440 | 0 | P9016 | 3 | Q0479 | 1 | Q4101 | 88 | Q4171 | 100 | V2215 | 0 | V2745 | 0 |
| L6955 | 0 | L8460 | 0 | P9017 | 2 | Q0480 | 1 | Q4102 | 21 | Q4172 | 54 | V2218 | 0 | V2750 | 0 |
| L6960 | 0 | L8465 | 0 | P9019 | 2 | Q0481 | 1 | Q4103 | 0 | Q4173 | 64 | V2219 | 0 | V2755 | 0 |
| L6965 | 0 | L8470 | 0 | P9020 | 2 | Q0482 | 1 | Q4104 | 50 | Q4174 | 8 | V2220 | 0 | V2756 | 0 |
| L6970 | 0 | L8480 | 0 | P9021 | 3 | Q0483 | 1 | Q4105 | 250 | Q4175 | 120 | V2221 | 0 | V2760 | 0 |
| L6975 | 0 | L8485 | 0 | P9022 | 2 | Q0484 | 1 | Q4106 | 76 | Q5101 | 3360 | V2299 | 0 | V2761 | 0 |
| L7007 | 0 | L8500 | 0 | P9023 | 2 | Q0485 | 1 | Q4107 | 50 | Q5102 | 150 | V2300 | 0 | V2762 | 0 |
| L7008 | 0 | L8501 | 0 | P9031 | 12 | Q0486 | 1 | Q4108 | 250 | Q9950 | 5 | V2301 | 0 | V2770 | 0 |
| L7009 | 0 | L8507 | 0 | P9032 | 12 | Q0487 | 1 | Q4110 | 250 | Q9951 | 0 | V2302 | 0 | V2780 | 0 |
| L7040 | 0 | L8509 | 1 | P9033 | 12 | Q0488 | 1 | Q4111 | 56 | Q9953 | 10 | V2303 | 0 | V2781 | 0 |
| L7045 | 0 | L8510 | 0 | P9034 | 2 | Q0489 | 1 | Q4112 | 2 | Q9954 | 18 | V2304 | 0 | V2782 | 0 |
| L7170 | 0 | L8511 | 1 | P9035 | 2 | Q0490 | 1 | Q4113 | 4 | Q9955 | 10 | V2305 | 0 | V2783 | 0 |
| L7180 | 0 | L8514 | 1 | P9036 | 2 | Q0491 | 1 | Q4114 | 6 | Q9956 | 9 | V2306 | 0 | V2784 | 0 |
| L7181 | 0 | L8515 | 1 | P9037 | 2 | Q0492 | 1 | Q4115 | 240 | Q9957 | 3 | V2307 | 0 | V2785 | 2 |
| L7185 | 0 | L8600 | 2 | P9038 | 2 | Q0493 | 1 | Q4116 | 192 | Q9958 | 300 | V2308 | 0 | V2786 | 0 |
| L7186 | 0 | L8604 | 3 | P9039 | 2 | Q0494 | 1 | Q4117 | 200 | Q9959 | 0 | V2309 | 0 | V2790 | 1 |
| L7190 | 0 | L8605 | 4 | P9040 | 3 | Q0495 | 1 | Q4118 | 1000 | Q9960 | 250 | V2310 | 0 | V2797 | 0 |
| L7191 | 0 | L8606 | 5 | P9041 | 5 | Q0497 | 2 | Q4121 | 78 | Q9961 | 200 | V2311 | 0 | V5008 | 0 |
| L7259 | 0 | L8607 | 20 | P9043 | 5 | Q0498 | 1 | Q4122 | 96 | Q9962 | 150 | V2312 | 0 | V5010 | 0 |
| L7360 | 0 | L8609 | 1 | P9044 | 10 | Q0499 | 1 | Q4123 | 160 | Q9963 | 240 | V2313 | 0 | V5011 | 0 |
| L7362 | 0 | L8610 | 2 | P9045 | 20 | Q0501 | 1 | Q4124 | 140 | Q9964 | 0 | V2314 | 0 | V5274 | 0 |
| L7364 | 0 | L8612 | 2 | P9046 | 25 | Q0502 | 1 | Q4125 | 28 | Q9966 | 250 | V2315 | 0 | V5281 | 0 |
| L7366 | 0 | L8613 | 2 | P9047 | 20 | Q0503 | 3 | Q4126 | 32 | Q9967 | 300 | V2318 | 0 | V5282 | 0 |
| L7367 | 0 | L8614 | 2 | P9048 | 1 | Q0504 | 1 | Q4127 | 100 | Q9969 | 3 | V2319 | 0 | V5283 | 0 |
| L7368 | 0 | L8615 | 2 | P9050 | 1 | Q0506 | 8 | Q4128 | 128 | Q9982 | 1 | V2320 | 0 | V5284 | 0 |
| L7400 | 0 | L8616 | 2 | P9051 | 2 | Q0507 | 1 | Q4130 | 100 | Q9983 | 1 | V2321 | 0 | V5285 | 0 |
| L7401 | 0 | L8617 | 2 | P9052 | 2 | Q0508 | 1 | Q4131 | 60 | R0070 | 2 | V2399 | 0 | V5286 | 0 |
| L7402 | 0 | L8618 | 2 | P9053 | 2 | Q0509 | 1 | Q4132 | 50 | R0075 | 2 | V2410 | 0 | V5287 | 0 |
| L7403 | 0 | L8619 | 2 | P9054 | 2 | Q0510 | 0 | Q4133 | 113 | R0076 | 1 | V2430 | 0 | V5288 | 0 |
| L7404 | 0 | L8621 | 600 | P9055 | 2 | Q0511 | 0 | Q4134 | 160 | V2020 | 0 | V2499 | 2 | V5289 | 0 |
| L7405 | 0 | L8622 | 2 | P9056 | 2 | Q0512 | 0 | Q4135 | 900 | V2025 | 0 | V2500 | 0 | V5290 | 0 |
| L7510 | 4 | L8627 | 2 | P9057 | 2 | Q0513 | 0 | Q4136 | 900 | V2100 | 0 | V2501 | 0 | | |
| L7900 | 0 | L8628 | 2 | P9058 | 2 | Q0514 | 0 | Q4137 | 32 | V2101 | 0 | V2502 | 0 | | |
| L7902 | 0 | L8629 | 2 | P9059 | 2 | Q0515 | 0 | Q4138 | 32 | V2102 | 0 | V2503 | 0 | | |
| L8000 | 0 | L8631 | 4 | P9060 | 2 | Q1004 | 2 | Q4139 | 2 | V2103 | 0 | V2510 | 0 | | |

## OPPS

| CPT | MUE | CPT | MUE | CPT | MUE | CPT | MUE | CPT | MUE | CPT | MUE | CPT | MUE | CPT | MUE |
|---|---|---|---|---|---|---|---|---|---|---|---|---|---|---|---|
| 0001M | 1 | 0216T | 1 | 0333T | 1 | 0403T | 0 | 0467T | 1 | 11403 | 2 | 11971 | 2 | 15002 | 1 |
| 0001U | 1 | 0217T | 1 | 0335T | 2 | 0404T | 1 | 0468T | 1 | 11404 | 2 | 11976 | 1 | 15003 | 9 |
| 0002M | 1 | 0218T | 1 | 0337T | 1 | 0405T | 1 | 0469T | 1 | 11406 | 2 | 11980 | 1 | 15004 | 1 |
| 0002U | 1 | 0219T | 1 | 0338T | 1 | 0406T | 2 | 0470T | 1 | 11420 | 3 | 11981 | 1 | 15005 | 2 |
| 0003M | 1 | 0220T | 1 | 0339T | 1 | 0407T | 2 | 0471T | 2 | 11421 | 3 | 11982 | 1 | 15040 | 1 |
| 0003U | 1 | 0221T | 1 | 0340T | 2 | 0408T | 1 | 0472T | 1 | 11422 | 3 | 11983 | 1 | 15050 | 1 |
| 0004M | 1 | 0222T | 1 | 0341T | 1 | 0409T | 1 | 0473T | 1 | 11423 | 2 | 12001 | 1 | 15100 | 1 |
| 0006M | 1 | 0228T | 1 | 0342T | 1 | 0410T | 1 | 0474T | 2 | 11424 | 2 | 12002 | 1 | 15101 | 9 |
| 0007M | 1 | 0229T | 2 | 0345T | 1 | 0411T | 1 | 0475T | 1 | 11426 | 2 | 12004 | 1 | 15110 | 1 |
| 0008M | 1 | 0230T | 1 | 0346T | 1 | 0412T | 1 | 0476T | 1 | 11440 | 4 | 12005 | 1 | 15111 | 2 |
| 0009M | 1 | 0231T | 2 | 0347T | 1 | 0413T | 1 | 0477T | 1 | 11441 | 3 | 12006 | 1 | 15115 | 1 |
| 0042T | 1 | 0232T | 1 | 0348T | 1 | 0414T | 1 | 0478T | 1 | 11442 | 3 | 12007 | 1 | 15116 | 2 |
| 0051T | 1 | 0234T | 2 | 0349T | 1 | 0415T | 1 | 10021 | 4 | 11443 | 2 | 12011 | 1 | 15120 | 1 |
| 0052T | 1 | 0235T | 2 | 0350T | 1 | 0416T | 1 | 10022 | 4 | 11444 | 2 | 12013 | 1 | 15121 | 5 |
| 0053T | 1 | 0236T | 1 | 0351T | 5 | 0417T | 1 | 10030 | 2 | 11446 | 2 | 12014 | 1 | 15130 | 1 |
| 0054T | 1 | 0237T | 2 | 0352T | 5 | 0418T | 1 | 10035 | 1 | 11450 | 1 | 12015 | 1 | 15131 | 2 |
| 0055T | 1 | 0238T | 2 | 0353T | 2 | 0419T | 1 | 10036 | 3 | 11451 | 1 | 12016 | 1 | 15135 | 1 |
| 0058T | 1 | 0249T | 1 | 0354T | 2 | 0420T | 1 | 10040 | 1 | 11462 | 1 | 12017 | 1 | 15136 | 1 |
| 0071T | 1 | 0253T | 1 | 0355T | 1 | 0421T | 1 | 10060 | 1 | 11463 | 1 | 12018 | 1 | 15150 | 1 |
| 0072T | 1 | 0254T | 2 | 0356T | 4 | 0422T | 1 | 10061 | 1 | 11470 | 3 | 12020 | 2 | 15151 | 1 |
| 0075T | 1 | 0255T | 2 | 0357T | 1 | 0423T | 1 | 10080 | 1 | 11471 | 2 | 12021 | 3 | 15152 | 2 |
| 0076T | 1 | 0263T | 1 | 0358T | 1 | 0424T | 1 | 10081 | 1 | 11600 | 2 | 12031 | 1 | 15155 | 1 |
| 0095T | 1 | 0264T | 1 | 0359T | 1 | 0425T | 1 | 10120 | 3 | 11601 | 2 | 12032 | 1 | 15156 | 1 |
| 0098T | 2 | 0265T | 1 | 0360T | 1 | 0426T | 1 | 10121 | 2 | 11602 | 3 | 12034 | 1 | 15157 | 1 |
| 0100T | 1 | 0266T | 1 | 0361T | 3 | 0427T | 1 | 10140 | 2 | 11603 | 2 | 12035 | 1 | 15200 | 1 |
| 0101T | 1 | 0267T | 1 | 0362T | 1 | 0428T | 1 | 10160 | 3 | 11604 | 2 | 12036 | 1 | 15201 | 9 |
| 0102T | 2 | 0268T | 1 | 0363T | 3 | 0429T | 1 | 10180 | 2 | 11606 | 2 | 12037 | 1 | 15220 | 1 |
| 0106T | 4 | 0269T | 1 | 0364T | 1 | 0430T | 1 | 11000 | 1 | 11620 | 2 | 12041 | 1 | 15221 | 9 |
| 0107T | 4 | 0270T | 1 | 0365T | 15 | 0431T | 1 | 11001 | 1 | 11621 | 2 | 12042 | 1 | 15240 | 1 |
| 0108T | 4 | 0271T | 1 | 0366T | 1 | 0432T | 1 | 11004 | 1 | 11622 | 2 | 12044 | 1 | 15241 | 9 |
| 0109T | 4 | 0272T | 1 | 0367T | 5 | 0433T | 1 | 11005 | 1 | 11623 | 2 | 12045 | 1 | 15260 | 1 |
| 0110T | 4 | 0273T | 1 | 0368T | 1 | 0434T | 1 | 11006 | 1 | 11624 | 2 | 12046 | 1 | 15261 | 6 |
| 0111T | 1 | 0274T | 1 | 0369T | 11 | 0435T | 1 | 11008 | 1 | 11626 | 2 | 12047 | 1 | 15271 | 1 |
| 0126T | 1 | 0275T | 1 | 0370T | 2 | 0436T | 1 | 11010 | 2 | 11640 | 2 | 12051 | 1 | 15272 | 3 |
| 0159T | 2 | 0278T | 1 | 0371T | 2 | 0437T | 1 | 11011 | 2 | 11641 | 2 | 12052 | 1 | 15273 | 1 |
| 0163T | 1 | 0290T | 1 | 0372T | 2 | 0438T | 1 | 11012 | 2 | 11642 | 3 | 12053 | 1 | 15274 | 6 |
| 0164T | 4 | 0293T | 1 | 0373T | 1 | 0439T | 1 | 11042 | 1 | 11643 | 2 | 12054 | 1 | 15275 | 1 |
| 0165T | 4 | 0294T | 1 | 0374T | 10 | 0440T | 3 | 11043 | 1 | 11644 | 2 | 12055 | 1 | 15276 | 3 |
| 0174T | 1 | 0295T | 1 | 0375T | 1 | 0441T | 3 | 11044 | 1 | 11646 | 2 | 12056 | 1 | 15277 | 1 |
| 0175T | 1 | 0296T | 1 | 0376T | 2 | 0442T | 3 | 11045 | 12 | 11719 | 1 | 12057 | 1 | 15278 | 3 |
| 0178T | 1 | 0297T | 1 | 0377T | 1 | 0443T | 1 | 11046 | 4 | 11720 | 1 | 13100 | 1 | 15570 | 2 |
| 0179T | 1 | 0298T | 1 | 0378T | 1 | 0444T | 1 | 11047 | 4 | 11721 | 1 | 13101 | 1 | 15572 | 2 |
| 0180T | 1 | 0299T | 1 | 0379T | 1 | 0445T | 1 | 11055 | 1 | 11730 | 1 | 13102 | 9 | 15574 | 2 |
| 0184T | 1 | 0300T | 1 | 0380T | 1 | 0446T | 1 | 11056 | 1 | 11732 | 9 | 13120 | 1 | 15576 | 2 |
| 0190T | 2 | 0301T | 1 | 0381T | 1 | 0447T | 1 | 11057 | 1 | 11740 | 3 | 13121 | 1 | 15600 | 2 |
| 0191T | 2 | 0302T | 1 | 0382T | 1 | 0448T | 1 | 11100 | 1 | 11750 | 6 | 13122 | 9 | 15610 | 2 |
| 0195T | 1 | 0303T | 1 | 0383T | 1 | 0449T | 1 | 11101 | 6 | 11755 | 4 | 13131 | 1 | 15620 | 2 |
| 0196T | 1 | 0304T | 1 | 0384T | 1 | 0450T | 2 | 11200 | 1 | 11760 | 4 | 13132 | 1 | 15630 | 2 |
| 0198T | 2 | 0305T | 1 | 0385T | 1 | 0451T | 1 | 11201 | 0 | 11762 | 2 | 13133 | 7 | 15650 | 1 |
| 0200T | 1 | 0306T | 1 | 0386T | 1 | 0452T | 1 | 11300 | 5 | 11765 | 4 | 13151 | 1 | 15731 | 1 |
| 0201T | 1 | 0307T | 1 | 0387T | 1 | 0453T | 1 | 11301 | 6 | 11770 | 1 | 13152 | 1 | 15732 | 3 |
| 0202T | 1 | 0308T | 1 | 0388T | 1 | 0454T | 3 | 11302 | 4 | 11771 | 1 | 13153 | 2 | 15734 | 4 |
| 0205T | 3 | 0309T | 1 | 0389T | 1 | 0455T | 1 | 11303 | 3 | 11772 | 1 | 13160 | 2 | 15736 | 2 |
| 0206T | 1 | 0310T | 1 | 0390T | 1 | 0456T | 1 | 11305 | 4 | 11900 | 1 | 14000 | 2 | 15738 | 4 |
| 0207T | 2 | 0312T | 1 | 0391T | 1 | 0457T | 1 | 11306 | 4 | 11901 | 1 | 14001 | 2 | 15740 | 3 |
| 0208T | 1 | 0313T | 1 | 0394T | 2 | 0458T | 3 | 11307 | 3 | 11920 | 1 | 14020 | 4 | 15750 | 2 |
| 0209T | 1 | 0314T | 1 | 0395T | 2 | 0459T | 1 | 11308 | 4 | 11921 | 1 | 14021 | 3 | 15756 | 2 |
| 0210T | 1 | 0315T | 1 | 0396T | 2 | 0460T | 3 | 11310 | 4 | 11922 | 1 | 14040 | 4 | 15757 | 2 |
| 0211T | 1 | 0316T | 1 | 0397T | 1 | 0461T | 1 | 11311 | 4 | 11950 | 1 | 14041 | 3 | 15758 | 2 |
| 0212T | 1 | 0317T | 1 | 0398T | 1 | 0462T | 1 | 11312 | 3 | 11951 | 1 | 14060 | 4 | 15760 | 2 |
| 0213T | 1 | 0329T | 1 | 0399T | 1 | 0463T | 1 | 11313 | 3 | 11952 | 1 | 14061 | 2 | 15770 | 2 |
| 0214T | 1 | 0330T | 1 | 0400T | 1 | 0464T | 1 | 11400 | 3 | 11954 | 1 | 14301 | 1 | 15775 | 1 |
| 0215T | 1 | 0331T | 1 | 0401T | 1 | 0465T | 1 | 11401 | 3 | 11960 | 2 | 14302 | 8 | 15776 | 1 |
| | | 0332T | 1 | 0402T | 2 | 0466T | 1 | 11402 | 3 | 11970 | 2 | 14350 | 2 | 15777 | 1 |

© 2017 Optum360, LLC

CPT © 2017 American Medical Association. All Rights Reserved.

| CPT | MUE | CPT | MUE | CPT | MUE | CPT | MUE | CPT | MUE | CPT | MUE | CPT | MUE | CPT | MUE |
|---|---|---|---|---|---|---|---|---|---|---|---|---|---|---|---|
| 15780 | 1 | 16035 | 1 | 19288 | 2 | 20612 | 2 | 21040 | 2 | 21215 | 2 | 21440 | 2 | 22206 | 1 |
| 15781 | 1 | 16036 | 2 | 19296 | 1 | 20615 | 1 | 21044 | 1 | 21230 | 2 | 21445 | 2 | 22207 | 1 |
| 15782 | 1 | 17000 | 1 | 19297 | 2 | 20650 | 4 | 21045 | 1 | 21235 | 2 | 21450 | 1 | 22208 | 6 |
| 15783 | 1 | 17003 | 13 | 19298 | 1 | 20660 | 1 | 21046 | 2 | 21240 | 1 | 21451 | 1 | 22210 | 1 |
| 15786 | 1 | 17004 | 1 | 19300 | 1 | 20661 | 1 | 21047 | 2 | 21242 | 1 | 21452 | 1 | 22212 | 1 |
| 15787 | 2 | 17106 | 1 | 19301 | 1 | 20662 | 1 | 21048 | 2 | 21243 | 1 | 21453 | 1 | 22214 | 1 |
| 15788 | 1 | 17107 | 1 | 19302 | 1 | 20663 | 1 | 21049 | 1 | 21244 | 1 | 21454 | 1 | 22216 | 6 |
| 15789 | 1 | 17108 | 1 | 19303 | 1 | 20664 | 1 | 21050 | 1 | 21245 | 2 | 21461 | 1 | 22220 | 1 |
| 15792 | 1 | 17110 | 1 | 19304 | 1 | 20665 | 1 | 21060 | 1 | 21246 | 2 | 21462 | 1 | 22222 | 1 |
| 15793 | 1 | 17111 | 1 | 19305 | 1 | 20670 | 3 | 21070 | 1 | 21247 | 1 | 21465 | 1 | 22224 | 1 |
| 15819 | 1 | 17250 | 4 | 19306 | 1 | 20680 | 3 | 21073 | 1 | 21248 | 2 | 21470 | 1 | 22226 | 4 |
| 15820 | 1 | 17260 | 7 | 19307 | 1 | 20690 | 2 | 21076 | 1 | 21249 | 2 | 21480 | 1 | 22310 | 1 |
| 15821 | 1 | 17261 | 7 | 19316 | 1 | 20692 | 2 | 21077 | 1 | 21255 | 1 | 21485 | 1 | 22315 | 1 |
| 15822 | 1 | 17262 | 6 | 19318 | 1 | 20693 | 2 | 21079 | 1 | 21256 | 1 | 21490 | 1 | 22318 | 1 |
| 15823 | 1 | 17263 | 5 | 19324 | 1 | 20694 | 2 | 21080 | 1 | 21260 | 1 | 21497 | 1 | 22319 | 1 |
| 15824 | 1 | 17264 | 3 | 19325 | 1 | 20696 | 2 | 21081 | 1 | 21261 | 1 | 21501 | 3 | 22325 | 1 |
| 15825 | 1 | 17266 | 2 | 19328 | 1 | 20697 | 4 | 21082 | 1 | 21263 | 1 | 21502 | 1 | 22326 | 1 |
| 15826 | 1 | 17270 | 6 | 19330 | 1 | 20802 | 1 | 21083 | 1 | 21267 | 1 | 21510 | 1 | 22327 | 1 |
| 15828 | 1 | 17271 | 4 | 19340 | 1 | 20805 | 1 | 21084 | 1 | 21268 | 1 | 21550 | 3 | 22328 | 6 |
| 15829 | 1 | 17272 | 5 | 19342 | 1 | 20808 | 1 | 21085 | 1 | 21270 | 1 | 21552 | 4 | 22505 | 1 |
| 15830 | 1 | 17273 | 4 | 19350 | 1 | 20816 | 3 | 21086 | 1 | 21275 | 1 | 21554 | 2 | 22510 | 1 |
| 15832 | 1 | 17274 | 4 | 19355 | 1 | 20822 | 3 | 21087 | 1 | 21280 | 1 | 21555 | 4 | 22511 | 1 |
| 15833 | 1 | 17276 | 3 | 19357 | 1 | 20824 | 1 | 21088 | 1 | 21282 | 1 | 21556 | 3 | 22512 | 3 |
| 15834 | 1 | 17280 | 6 | 19361 | 1 | 20827 | 1 | 21100 | 1 | 21295 | 1 | 21557 | 1 | 22513 | 1 |
| 15835 | 1 | 17281 | 6 | 19364 | 1 | 20838 | 1 | 21110 | 2 | 21296 | 1 | 21558 | 1 | 22514 | 1 |
| 15836 | 1 | 17282 | 5 | 19366 | 1 | 20900 | 2 | 21116 | 1 | 21310 | 1 | 21600 | 5 | 22515 | 4 |
| 15837 | 2 | 17283 | 4 | 19367 | 1 | 20902 | 2 | 21120 | 1 | 21315 | 1 | 21610 | 1 | 22532 | 1 |
| 15838 | 1 | 17284 | 3 | 19368 | 1 | 20910 | 1 | 21121 | 1 | 21320 | 1 | 21615 | 1 | 22533 | 1 |
| 15839 | 2 | 17286 | 3 | 19369 | 1 | 20912 | 1 | 21122 | 1 | 21325 | 1 | 21616 | 1 | 22534 | 3 |
| 15840 | 1 | 17311 | 4 | 19370 | 1 | 20920 | 1 | 21123 | 1 | 21330 | 1 | 21620 | 1 | 22548 | 1 |
| 15841 | 2 | 17312 | 6 | 19371 | 1 | 20922 | 1 | 21125 | 2 | 21335 | 1 | 21627 | 1 | 22551 | 1 |
| 15842 | 2 | 17313 | 3 | 19380 | 1 | 20924 | 2 | 21127 | 2 | 21336 | 1 | 21630 | 1 | 22552 | 5 |
| 15845 | 2 | 17314 | 4 | 19396 | 1 | 20926 | 2 | 21137 | 1 | 21337 | 1 | 21632 | 1 | 22554 | 1 |
| 15847 | 1 | 17315 | 15 | 20005 | 4 | 20931 | 1 | 21138 | 1 | 21338 | 1 | 21685 | 1 | 22556 | 1 |
| 15850 | 1 | 17340 | 1 | 20100 | 2 | 20937 | 1 | 21139 | 1 | 21339 | 1 | 21700 | 1 | 22558 | 1 |
| 15851 | 1 | 17360 | 1 | 20101 | 2 | 20938 | 1 | 21141 | 1 | 21340 | 1 | 21705 | 1 | 22585 | 7 |
| 15852 | 1 | 17380 | 1 | 20102 | 3 | 20950 | 2 | 21142 | 1 | 21343 | 1 | 21720 | 1 | 22586 | 1 |
| 15860 | 1 | 19000 | 2 | 20103 | 4 | 20955 | 1 | 21143 | 1 | 21344 | 1 | 21725 | 1 | 22590 | 1 |
| 15876 | 1 | 19001 | 5 | 20150 | 2 | 20956 | 1 | 21145 | 1 | 21345 | 1 | 21740 | 1 | 22595 | 1 |
| 15877 | 1 | 19020 | 2 | 20200 | 2 | 20957 | 1 | 21146 | 1 | 21346 | 1 | 21742 | 1 | 22600 | 1 |
| 15878 | 1 | 19030 | 1 | 20205 | 4 | 20962 | 1 | 21147 | 1 | 21347 | 1 | 21743 | 1 | 22610 | 1 |
| 15879 | 1 | 19081 | 1 | 20206 | 3 | 20969 | 2 | 21150 | 1 | 21348 | 1 | 21750 | 1 | 22612 | 1 |
| 15920 | 1 | 19082 | 2 | 20220 | 4 | 20970 | 1 | 21151 | 1 | 21355 | 1 | 21811 | 1 | 22614 | 13 |
| 15922 | 1 | 19083 | 1 | 20225 | 4 | 20972 | 2 | 21154 | 1 | 21356 | 1 | 21812 | 1 | 22630 | 1 |
| 15931 | 1 | 19084 | 2 | 20240 | 4 | 20973 | 1 | 21155 | 1 | 21360 | 1 | 21813 | 1 | 22632 | 4 |
| 15933 | 1 | 19085 | 1 | 20245 | 4 | 20974 | 1 | 21159 | 1 | 21365 | 1 | 21820 | 1 | 22633 | 1 |
| 15934 | 1 | 19086 | 2 | 20250 | 3 | 20975 | 1 | 21160 | 1 | 21366 | 1 | 21825 | 1 | 22634 | 4 |
| 15935 | 1 | 19100 | 4 | 20251 | 3 | 20979 | 1 | 21175 | 1 | 21385 | 1 | 21920 | 3 | 22800 | 1 |
| 15936 | 1 | 19101 | 3 | 20500 | 2 | 20982 | 1 | 21179 | 1 | 21386 | 1 | 21925 | 3 | 22802 | 1 |
| 15937 | 1 | 19105 | 2 | 20501 | 2 | 20983 | 1 | 21180 | 1 | 21387 | 1 | 21930 | 5 | 22804 | 1 |
| 15940 | 2 | 19110 | 1 | 20520 | 4 | 20985 | 2 | 21181 | 1 | 21390 | 1 | 21931 | 3 | 22808 | 1 |
| 15941 | 2 | 19112 | 2 | 20525 | 4 | 21010 | 1 | 21182 | 1 | 21395 | 1 | 21932 | 4 | 22810 | 1 |
| 15944 | 2 | 19120 | 1 | 20526 | 1 | 21011 | 4 | 21183 | 1 | 21400 | 1 | 21933 | 3 | 22812 | 1 |
| 15945 | 2 | 19125 | 1 | 20527 | 2 | 21012 | 3 | 21184 | 1 | 21401 | 1 | 21935 | 1 | 22818 | 1 |
| 15946 | 2 | 19126 | 3 | 20550 | 5 | 21013 | 4 | 21188 | 1 | 21406 | 1 | 21936 | 1 | 22819 | 1 |
| 15950 | 2 | 19260 | 2 | 20551 | 5 | 21014 | 3 | 21193 | 1 | 21407 | 1 | 22010 | 2 | 22830 | 1 |
| 15951 | 2 | 19271 | 1 | 20552 | 1 | 21015 | 1 | 21194 | 1 | 21408 | 1 | 22015 | 2 | 22840 | 1 |
| 15952 | 2 | 19272 | 1 | 20553 | 1 | 21016 | 2 | 21195 | 1 | 21421 | 1 | 22100 | 1 | 22842 | 1 |
| 15953 | 2 | 19281 | 1 | 20555 | 1 | 21025 | 2 | 21196 | 1 | 21422 | 1 | 22101 | 1 | 22843 | 1 |
| 15956 | 2 | 19282 | 2 | 20600 | 6 | 21026 | 2 | 21198 | 1 | 21423 | 1 | 22102 | 1 | 22844 | 1 |
| 15958 | 2 | 19283 | 1 | 20604 | 4 | 21029 | 1 | 21199 | 1 | 21431 | 1 | 22103 | 3 | 22845 | 1 |
| 16000 | 1 | 19284 | 2 | 20605 | 2 | 21030 | 1 | 21206 | 1 | 21432 | 1 | 22110 | 1 | 22846 | 1 |
| 16020 | 1 | 19285 | 1 | 20606 | 2 | 21031 | 2 | 21208 | 1 | 21433 | 1 | 22112 | 1 | 22847 | 1 |
| 16025 | 1 | 19286 | 2 | 20610 | 2 | 21032 | 1 | 21209 | 1 | 21435 | 1 | 22114 | 1 | 22848 | 1 |
| 16030 | 1 | 19287 | 1 | 20611 | 2 | 21034 | 1 | 21210 | 2 | 21436 | 1 | 22116 | 3 | 22849 | 1 |

CPT © 2017 American Medical Association. All Rights Reserved.      © 2017 Optum360, LLC

| CPT | MUE | CPT | MUE | CPT | MUE | CPT | MUE | CPT | MUE | CPT | MUE | CPT | MUE | CPT | MUE |
|---|---|---|---|---|---|---|---|---|---|---|---|---|---|---|---|
| 22850 | 1 | 23334 | 1 | 24000 | 1 | 24430 | 1 | 25100 | 1 | 25420 | 1 | 25909 | 1 | 26392 | 2 |
| 22852 | 1 | 23335 | 1 | 24006 | 1 | 24435 | 1 | 25101 | 1 | 25425 | 1 | 25915 | 1 | 26410 | 4 |
| 22853 | 5 | 23350 | 1 | 24065 | 2 | 24470 | 1 | 25105 | 1 | 25426 | 1 | 25920 | 1 | 26412 | 3 |
| 22854 | 5 | 23395 | 1 | 24066 | 2 | 24495 | 1 | 25107 | 1 | 25430 | 1 | 25922 | 1 | 26415 | 2 |
| 22855 | 1 | 23397 | 1 | 24071 | 3 | 24498 | 1 | 25109 | 4 | 25431 | 1 | 25924 | 1 | 26416 | 2 |
| 22856 | 1 | 23400 | 1 | 24073 | 3 | 24500 | 1 | 25110 | 3 | 25440 | 1 | 25927 | 1 | 26418 | 4 |
| 22857 | 1 | 23405 | 2 | 24075 | 5 | 24505 | 1 | 25111 | 1 | 25441 | 1 | 25929 | 1 | 26420 | 4 |
| 22858 | 1 | 23406 | 1 | 24076 | 4 | 24515 | 1 | 25112 | 1 | 25442 | 1 | 25931 | 1 | 26426 | 4 |
| 22859 | 5 | 23410 | 1 | 24077 | 1 | 24516 | 1 | 25115 | 1 | 25443 | 1 | 26010 | 2 | 26428 | 4 |
| 22861 | 1 | 23412 | 1 | 24079 | 1 | 24530 | 1 | 25116 | 1 | 25444 | 1 | 26011 | 3 | 26432 | 2 |
| 22862 | 1 | 23415 | 1 | 24100 | 1 | 24535 | 1 | 25118 | 5 | 25445 | 1 | 26020 | 4 | 26433 | 2 |
| 22864 | 1 | 23420 | 1 | 24101 | 1 | 24538 | 1 | 25119 | 1 | 25446 | 1 | 26025 | 1 | 26434 | 2 |
| 22865 | 1 | 23430 | 1 | 24102 | 1 | 24545 | 1 | 25120 | 1 | 25447 | 4 | 26030 | 1 | 26437 | 4 |
| 22867 | 1 | 23440 | 1 | 24105 | 1 | 24546 | 1 | 25125 | 1 | 25449 | 1 | 26034 | 2 | 26440 | 6 |
| 22868 | 1 | 23450 | 1 | 24110 | 1 | 24560 | 1 | 25126 | 1 | 25450 | 1 | 26035 | 1 | 26442 | 5 |
| 22869 | 1 | 23455 | 1 | 24115 | 1 | 24565 | 1 | 25130 | 1 | 25455 | 1 | 26037 | 1 | 26445 | 5 |
| 22870 | 1 | 23460 | 1 | 24116 | 1 | 24566 | 1 | 25135 | 1 | 25490 | 1 | 26040 | 1 | 26449 | 5 |
| 22900 | 3 | 23462 | 1 | 24120 | 1 | 24575 | 1 | 25136 | 1 | 25491 | 1 | 26045 | 1 | 26450 | 6 |
| 22901 | 2 | 23465 | 1 | 24125 | 1 | 24576 | 1 | 25145 | 1 | 25492 | 1 | 26055 | 5 | 26455 | 6 |
| 22902 | 4 | 23466 | 1 | 24126 | 1 | 24577 | 1 | 25150 | 1 | 25500 | 1 | 26060 | 5 | 26460 | 4 |
| 22903 | 3 | 23470 | 1 | 24130 | 1 | 24579 | 1 | 25151 | 1 | 25505 | 1 | 26070 | 2 | 26471 | 4 |
| 22904 | 1 | 23472 | 1 | 24134 | 1 | 24582 | 1 | 25170 | 1 | 25515 | 1 | 26075 | 4 | 26474 | 4 |
| 22905 | 1 | 23473 | 1 | 24136 | 1 | 24586 | 1 | 25210 | 2 | 25520 | 1 | 26080 | 4 | 26476 | 4 |
| 23000 | 1 | 23474 | 1 | 24138 | 1 | 24587 | 1 | 25215 | 1 | 25525 | 1 | 26100 | 1 | 26477 | 4 |
| 23020 | 1 | 23480 | 1 | 24140 | 1 | 24600 | 1 | 25230 | 1 | 25526 | 1 | 26105 | 2 | 26478 | 6 |
| 23030 | 2 | 23485 | 1 | 24145 | 1 | 24605 | 1 | 25240 | 1 | 25530 | 1 | 26110 | 3 | 26479 | 4 |
| 23031 | 1 | 23490 | 1 | 24147 | 1 | 24615 | 1 | 25246 | 1 | 25535 | 1 | 26111 | 4 | 26480 | 4 |
| 23035 | 1 | 23491 | 1 | 24149 | 1 | 24620 | 1 | 25248 | 3 | 25545 | 1 | 26113 | 4 | 26483 | 4 |
| 23040 | 1 | 23500 | 1 | 24150 | 1 | 24635 | 1 | 25250 | 1 | 25560 | 1 | 26115 | 4 | 26485 | 4 |
| 23044 | 1 | 23505 | 1 | 24152 | 1 | 24640 | 1 | 25251 | 1 | 25565 | 1 | 26116 | 2 | 26489 | 3 |
| 23065 | 2 | 23515 | 1 | 24155 | 1 | 24650 | 1 | 25259 | 1 | 25574 | 1 | 26117 | 2 | 26490 | 3 |
| 23066 | 2 | 23520 | 1 | 24160 | 1 | 24655 | 1 | 25260 | 7 | 25575 | 1 | 26118 | 1 | 26492 | 2 |
| 23071 | 2 | 23525 | 1 | 24164 | 1 | 24665 | 1 | 25263 | 4 | 25600 | 1 | 26121 | 1 | 26494 | 1 |
| 23073 | 2 | 23530 | 1 | 24200 | 3 | 24666 | 1 | 25265 | 4 | 25605 | 1 | 26123 | 1 | 26496 | 1 |
| 23075 | 3 | 23532 | 1 | 24201 | 3 | 24670 | 1 | 25270 | 8 | 25606 | 1 | 26125 | 4 | 26497 | 2 |
| 23076 | 2 | 23540 | 1 | 24220 | 1 | 24675 | 1 | 25272 | 4 | 25607 | 1 | 26130 | 1 | 26498 | 1 |
| 23077 | 1 | 23545 | 1 | 24300 | 1 | 24685 | 1 | 25274 | 4 | 25608 | 1 | 26135 | 4 | 26499 | 2 |
| 23078 | 1 | 23550 | 1 | 24301 | 2 | 24800 | 1 | 25275 | 2 | 25609 | 1 | 26140 | 3 | 26500 | 4 |
| 23100 | 1 | 23552 | 1 | 24305 | 4 | 24802 | 1 | 25280 | 9 | 25622 | 1 | 26145 | 6 | 26502 | 3 |
| 23101 | 2 | 23570 | 1 | 24310 | 3 | 24900 | 1 | 25290 | 12 | 25624 | 1 | 26160 | 5 | 26508 | 1 |
| 23105 | 1 | 23575 | 1 | 24320 | 2 | 24920 | 1 | 25295 | 9 | 25628 | 1 | 26170 | 5 | 26510 | 4 |
| 23106 | 1 | 23585 | 1 | 24330 | 1 | 24925 | 1 | 25300 | 1 | 25630 | 1 | 26180 | 4 | 26516 | 1 |
| 23107 | 1 | 23600 | 1 | 24331 | 1 | 24930 | 1 | 25301 | 1 | 25635 | 1 | 26185 | 1 | 26517 | 1 |
| 23120 | 1 | 23605 | 1 | 24332 | 1 | 24931 | 1 | 25310 | 5 | 25645 | 1 | 26200 | 2 | 26518 | 1 |
| 23125 | 1 | 23615 | 1 | 24340 | 1 | 24935 | 1 | 25312 | 5 | 25650 | 1 | 26205 | 1 | 26520 | 4 |
| 23130 | 1 | 23616 | 1 | 24341 | 2 | 24940 | 1 | 25315 | 1 | 25651 | 1 | 26210 | 2 | 26525 | 4 |
| 23140 | 1 | 23620 | 1 | 24342 | 2 | 25000 | 2 | 25316 | 1 | 25652 | 1 | 26215 | 2 | 26530 | 4 |
| 23145 | 1 | 23625 | 1 | 24343 | 1 | 25001 | 1 | 25320 | 1 | 25660 | 1 | 26230 | 2 | 26531 | 4 |
| 23146 | 1 | 23630 | 1 | 24344 | 1 | 25020 | 1 | 25332 | 1 | 25670 | 1 | 26235 | 2 | 26535 | 4 |
| 23150 | 1 | 23650 | 1 | 24345 | 1 | 25023 | 1 | 25335 | 1 | 25671 | 1 | 26236 | 2 | 26536 | 4 |
| 23155 | 1 | 23655 | 1 | 24346 | 1 | 25024 | 1 | 25337 | 1 | 25675 | 1 | 26250 | 2 | 26540 | 4 |
| 23156 | 1 | 23660 | 1 | 24357 | 2 | 25025 | 1 | 25350 | 1 | 25676 | 1 | 26260 | 1 | 26541 | 4 |
| 23170 | 1 | 23665 | 1 | 24358 | 2 | 25028 | 4 | 25355 | 1 | 25680 | 1 | 26262 | 1 | 26542 | 4 |
| 23172 | 1 | 23670 | 1 | 24359 | 2 | 25031 | 2 | 25360 | 1 | 25685 | 1 | 26320 | 4 | 26545 | 4 |
| 23174 | 1 | 23675 | 1 | 24360 | 1 | 25035 | 2 | 25365 | 1 | 25690 | 1 | 26340 | 4 | 26546 | 2 |
| 23180 | 1 | 23680 | 1 | 24361 | 1 | 25040 | 1 | 25370 | 1 | 25695 | 1 | 26341 | 2 | 26548 | 3 |
| 23182 | 1 | 23700 | 1 | 24362 | 1 | 25065 | 3 | 25375 | 1 | 25800 | 1 | 26350 | 6 | 26550 | 1 |
| 23184 | 1 | 23800 | 1 | 24363 | 1 | 25066 | 2 | 25390 | 1 | 25805 | 1 | 26352 | 2 | 26551 | 1 |
| 23190 | 1 | 23802 | 1 | 24365 | 1 | 25071 | 3 | 25391 | 1 | 25810 | 1 | 26356 | 4 | 26553 | 1 |
| 23195 | 1 | 23900 | 1 | 24366 | 1 | 25073 | 3 | 25392 | 1 | 25820 | 1 | 26357 | 2 | 26554 | 1 |
| 23200 | 1 | 23920 | 1 | 24370 | 1 | 25075 | 6 | 25393 | 1 | 25825 | 1 | 26358 | 2 | 26555 | 2 |
| 23210 | 1 | 23921 | 1 | 24371 | 1 | 25076 | 5 | 25394 | 1 | 25830 | 1 | 26370 | 3 | 26556 | 2 |
| 23220 | 1 | 23930 | 2 | 24400 | 1 | 25077 | 1 | 25400 | 1 | 25900 | 1 | 26372 | 1 | 26560 | 2 |
| 23330 | 2 | 23931 | 2 | 24410 | 1 | 25078 | 1 | 25405 | 1 | 25905 | 1 | 26373 | 2 | 26561 | 2 |
| 23333 | 1 | 23935 | 2 | 24420 | 1 | 25085 | 1 | 25415 | 1 | 25907 | 1 | 26390 | 2 | 26562 | 2 |

CPT © 2017 American Medical Association. All Rights Reserved.

| CPT | MUE | CPT | MUE | CPT | MUE | CPT | MUE | CPT | MUE | CPT | MUE | CPT | MUE | CPT | MUE |
|---|---|---|---|---|---|---|---|---|---|---|---|---|---|---|---|
| 26565 | 3 | 27027 | 1 | 27185 | 1 | 27347 | 1 | 27487 | 1 | 27630 | 2 | 27780 | 1 | 28086 | 2 |
| 26567 | 3 | 27030 | 1 | 27187 | 1 | 27350 | 1 | 27488 | 1 | 27632 | 4 | 27781 | 1 | 28088 | 2 |
| 26568 | 2 | 27033 | 1 | 27197 | 1 | 27355 | 1 | 27495 | 1 | 27634 | 2 | 27784 | 1 | 28090 | 2 |
| 26580 | 1 | 27035 | 1 | 27198 | 1 | 27356 | 1 | 27496 | 1 | 27635 | 1 | 27786 | 1 | 28092 | 2 |
| 26587 | 2 | 27036 | 1 | 27200 | 1 | 27357 | 1 | 27497 | 1 | 27637 | 1 | 27788 | 1 | 28100 | 1 |
| 26590 | 2 | 27040 | 2 | 27202 | 1 | 27358 | 1 | 27498 | 1 | 27638 | 1 | 27792 | 1 | 28102 | 1 |
| 26591 | 4 | 27041 | 3 | 27220 | 1 | 27360 | 2 | 27499 | 1 | 27640 | 1 | 27808 | 1 | 28103 | 1 |
| 26593 | 9 | 27043 | 3 | 27222 | 1 | 27364 | 1 | 27500 | 1 | 27641 | 1 | 27810 | 1 | 28104 | 2 |
| 26596 | 1 | 27045 | 3 | 27226 | 1 | 27365 | 1 | 27501 | 1 | 27645 | 1 | 27814 | 1 | 28106 | 1 |
| 26600 | 2 | 27047 | 4 | 27227 | 1 | 27370 | 1 | 27502 | 1 | 27646 | 1 | 27816 | 1 | 28107 | 1 |
| 26605 | 3 | 27048 | 2 | 27228 | 1 | 27372 | 2 | 27503 | 1 | 27647 | 1 | 27818 | 1 | 28108 | 2 |
| 26607 | 2 | 27049 | 1 | 27230 | 1 | 27380 | 2 | 27506 | 1 | 27648 | 1 | 27822 | 1 | 28110 | 1 |
| 26608 | 5 | 27050 | 1 | 27232 | 1 | 27381 | 2 | 27507 | 1 | 27650 | 1 | 27823 | 1 | 28111 | 1 |
| 26615 | 4 | 27052 | 1 | 27235 | 1 | 27385 | 2 | 27508 | 1 | 27652 | 1 | 27824 | 1 | 28112 | 4 |
| 26641 | 1 | 27054 | 1 | 27236 | 1 | 27386 | 2 | 27509 | 1 | 27654 | 1 | 27825 | 1 | 28113 | 1 |
| 26645 | 1 | 27057 | 1 | 27238 | 1 | 27390 | 1 | 27510 | 1 | 27656 | 1 | 27826 | 1 | 28114 | 1 |
| 26650 | 1 | 27059 | 1 | 27240 | 1 | 27391 | 1 | 27511 | 1 | 27658 | 2 | 27827 | 1 | 28116 | 1 |
| 26665 | 1 | 27060 | 1 | 27244 | 1 | 27392 | 1 | 27513 | 1 | 27659 | 2 | 27828 | 1 | 28118 | 1 |
| 26670 | 2 | 27062 | 1 | 27245 | 1 | 27393 | 1 | 27514 | 1 | 27664 | 2 | 27829 | 1 | 28119 | 1 |
| 26675 | 1 | 27065 | 1 | 27246 | 1 | 27394 | 1 | 27516 | 1 | 27665 | 2 | 27830 | 1 | 28120 | 2 |
| 26676 | 3 | 27066 | 1 | 27248 | 1 | 27395 | 1 | 27517 | 1 | 27675 | 1 | 27831 | 1 | 28122 | 4 |
| 26685 | 3 | 27067 | 1 | 27250 | 1 | 27396 | 1 | 27519 | 1 | 27676 | 1 | 27832 | 1 | 28124 | 4 |
| 26686 | 3 | 27070 | 1 | 27252 | 1 | 27397 | 1 | 27520 | 1 | 27680 | 3 | 27840 | 1 | 28126 | 4 |
| 26700 | 3 | 27071 | 1 | 27253 | 1 | 27400 | 1 | 27524 | 1 | 27681 | 1 | 27842 | 1 | 28130 | 1 |
| 26705 | 3 | 27075 | 1 | 27254 | 1 | 27403 | 1 | 27530 | 1 | 27685 | 2 | 27846 | 1 | 28140 | 4 |
| 26706 | 4 | 27076 | 1 | 27256 | 1 | 27405 | 2 | 27532 | 1 | 27686 | 3 | 27848 | 1 | 28150 | 4 |
| 26715 | 4 | 27077 | 1 | 27257 | 1 | 27407 | 2 | 27535 | 1 | 27687 | 1 | 27860 | 1 | 28153 | 6 |
| 26720 | 4 | 27078 | 1 | 27258 | 1 | 27409 | 1 | 27536 | 1 | 27690 | 2 | 27870 | 1 | 28160 | 5 |
| 26725 | 4 | 27080 | 1 | 27259 | 1 | 27412 | 1 | 27538 | 1 | 27691 | 2 | 27871 | 1 | 28171 | 1 |
| 26727 | 4 | 27086 | 1 | 27265 | 1 | 27415 | 1 | 27540 | 1 | 27692 | 4 | 27880 | 1 | 28173 | 2 |
| 26735 | 4 | 27087 | 1 | 27266 | 1 | 27416 | 1 | 27550 | 1 | 27695 | 1 | 27881 | 1 | 28175 | 2 |
| 26740 | 3 | 27090 | 1 | 27267 | 1 | 27418 | 1 | 27552 | 1 | 27696 | 1 | 27882 | 1 | 28190 | 3 |
| 26742 | 3 | 27091 | 1 | 27268 | 1 | 27420 | 1 | 27556 | 1 | 27698 | 2 | 27884 | 1 | 28192 | 2 |
| 26746 | 3 | 27093 | 1 | 27269 | 1 | 27422 | 1 | 27557 | 1 | 27700 | 1 | 27886 | 1 | 28193 | 2 |
| 26750 | 3 | 27095 | 1 | 27275 | 2 | 27424 | 1 | 27558 | 1 | 27702 | 1 | 27888 | 1 | 28200 | 4 |
| 26755 | 3 | 27096 | 1 | 27279 | 1 | 27425 | 1 | 27560 | 1 | 27703 | 1 | 27889 | 1 | 28202 | 2 |
| 26756 | 3 | 27097 | 1 | 27280 | 1 | 27427 | 1 | 27562 | 1 | 27704 | 1 | 27892 | 1 | 28208 | 4 |
| 26765 | 5 | 27098 | 1 | 27282 | 1 | 27428 | 1 | 27566 | 1 | 27705 | 1 | 27893 | 1 | 28210 | 2 |
| 26770 | 3 | 27100 | 1 | 27284 | 1 | 27429 | 1 | 27570 | 1 | 27707 | 1 | 27894 | 1 | 28220 | 1 |
| 26775 | 4 | 27105 | 1 | 27286 | 1 | 27430 | 1 | 27580 | 1 | 27709 | 1 | 28001 | 2 | 28222 | 1 |
| 26776 | 4 | 27110 | 1 | 27290 | 1 | 27435 | 1 | 27590 | 1 | 27712 | 1 | 28002 | 3 | 28225 | 1 |
| 26785 | 3 | 27111 | 1 | 27295 | 1 | 27437 | 1 | 27591 | 1 | 27715 | 1 | 28003 | 2 | 28226 | 1 |
| 26820 | 1 | 27120 | 1 | 27301 | 3 | 27438 | 1 | 27592 | 1 | 27720 | 1 | 28005 | 3 | 28230 | 1 |
| 26841 | 1 | 27122 | 1 | 27303 | 2 | 27440 | 1 | 27594 | 1 | 27722 | 1 | 28008 | 2 | 28232 | 6 |
| 26842 | 1 | 27125 | 1 | 27305 | 1 | 27441 | 1 | 27596 | 1 | 27724 | 1 | 28010 | 4 | 28234 | 6 |
| 26843 | 2 | 27130 | 1 | 27306 | 1 | 27442 | 1 | 27598 | 1 | 27725 | 1 | 28011 | 4 | 28238 | 1 |
| 26844 | 2 | 27132 | 1 | 27307 | 1 | 27443 | 1 | 27600 | 1 | 27726 | 1 | 28020 | 2 | 28240 | 1 |
| 26850 | 5 | 27134 | 1 | 27310 | 1 | 27445 | 1 | 27601 | 1 | 27727 | 1 | 28022 | 4 | 28250 | 1 |
| 26852 | 2 | 27137 | 1 | 27323 | 2 | 27446 | 1 | 27602 | 1 | 27730 | 1 | 28024 | 4 | 28260 | 1 |
| 26860 | 1 | 27138 | 1 | 27324 | 3 | 27447 | 1 | 27603 | 2 | 27732 | 1 | 28035 | 1 | 28261 | 1 |
| 26861 | 4 | 27140 | 1 | 27325 | 1 | 27448 | 1 | 27604 | 2 | 27734 | 1 | 28039 | 3 | 28262 | 1 |
| 26862 | 1 | 27146 | 1 | 27326 | 1 | 27450 | 1 | 27605 | 1 | 27740 | 1 | 28041 | 3 | 28264 | 1 |
| 26863 | 3 | 27147 | 1 | 27327 | 5 | 27454 | 1 | 27606 | 1 | 27742 | 1 | 28043 | 4 | 28270 | 6 |
| 26910 | 4 | 27151 | 1 | 27328 | 4 | 27455 | 1 | 27607 | 2 | 27745 | 1 | 28045 | 4 | 28272 | 6 |
| 26951 | 8 | 27156 | 1 | 27329 | 1 | 27457 | 1 | 27610 | 1 | 27750 | 1 | 28046 | 1 | 28280 | 1 |
| 26952 | 5 | 27158 | 1 | 27330 | 1 | 27465 | 1 | 27612 | 1 | 27752 | 1 | 28047 | 1 | 28285 | 4 |
| 26990 | 2 | 27161 | 1 | 27331 | 1 | 27466 | 1 | 27613 | 4 | 27756 | 1 | 28050 | 2 | 28286 | 1 |
| 26991 | 1 | 27165 | 1 | 27332 | 1 | 27468 | 1 | 27614 | 3 | 27758 | 1 | 28052 | 2 | 28288 | 5 |
| 26992 | 2 | 27170 | 1 | 27333 | 1 | 27470 | 1 | 27615 | 1 | 27759 | 1 | 28054 | 2 | 28289 | 1 |
| 27000 | 1 | 27175 | 1 | 27334 | 1 | 27472 | 1 | 27616 | 1 | 27760 | 1 | 28055 | 1 | 28291 | 1 |
| 27001 | 1 | 27176 | 1 | 27335 | 1 | 27475 | 1 | 27618 | 4 | 27762 | 1 | 28060 | 1 | 28292 | 1 |
| 27003 | 1 | 27177 | 1 | 27337 | 4 | 27477 | 1 | 27619 | 4 | 27766 | 1 | 28062 | 1 | 28295 | 1 |
| 27005 | 1 | 27178 | 1 | 27339 | 4 | 27479 | 1 | 27620 | 1 | 27767 | 1 | 28070 | 2 | 28296 | 1 |
| 27006 | 1 | 27179 | 1 | 27340 | 1 | 27485 | 1 | 27625 | 1 | 27768 | 1 | 28072 | 2 | 28297 | 1 |
| 27025 | 1 | 27181 | 1 | 27345 | 1 | 27486 | 1 | 27626 | 1 | 27769 | 1 | 28080 | 4 | 28298 | 1 |

CPT © 2017 American Medical Association. All Rights Reserved.

© 2017 Optum360, LLC

| CPT | MUE | CPT | MUE | CPT | MUE | CPT | MUE | CPT | MUE | CPT | MUE | CPT | MUE | CPT | MUE |
|---|---|---|---|---|---|---|---|---|---|---|---|---|---|---|---|
| 28299 | 1 | 28666 | 4 | 29705 | 1 | 29893 | 1 | 31030 | 1 | 31526 | 1 | 31645 | 1 | 32506 | 3 |
| 28300 | 1 | 28675 | 4 | 29710 | 1 | 29894 | 1 | 31032 | 1 | 31527 | 1 | 31646 | 2 | 32507 | 2 |
| 28302 | 1 | 28705 | 1 | 29720 | 1 | 29895 | 1 | 31040 | 1 | 31528 | 1 | 31647 | 1 | 32540 | 1 |
| 28304 | 1 | 28715 | 1 | 29730 | 1 | 29897 | 1 | 31050 | 1 | 31529 | 1 | 31648 | 1 | 32550 | 2 |
| 28305 | 1 | 28725 | 1 | 29740 | 1 | 29898 | 1 | 31051 | 1 | 31530 | 1 | 31649 | 2 | 32551 | 2 |
| 28306 | 1 | 28730 | 1 | 29750 | 1 | 29899 | 1 | 31070 | 1 | 31531 | 1 | 31651 | 3 | 32552 | 2 |
| 28307 | 1 | 28735 | 1 | 29800 | 1 | 29900 | 2 | 31075 | 1 | 31535 | 1 | 31652 | 1 | 32553 | 1 |
| 28308 | 4 | 28737 | 1 | 29804 | 1 | 29901 | 2 | 31080 | 1 | 31536 | 1 | 31653 | 1 | 32554 | 2 |
| 28309 | 1 | 28740 | 5 | 29805 | 1 | 29902 | 2 | 31081 | 1 | 31540 | 1 | 31654 | 1 | 32555 | 2 |
| 28310 | 1 | 28750 | 1 | 29806 | 1 | 29904 | 1 | 31084 | 1 | 31541 | 1 | 31660 | 1 | 32556 | 2 |
| 28312 | 4 | 28755 | 1 | 29807 | 1 | 29905 | 1 | 31085 | 1 | 31545 | 1 | 31661 | 1 | 32557 | 2 |
| 28313 | 4 | 28760 | 1 | 29819 | 1 | 29906 | 1 | 31086 | 1 | 31546 | 1 | 31717 | 1 | 32560 | 1 |
| 28315 | 1 | 28800 | 1 | 29820 | 1 | 29907 | 1 | 31087 | 1 | 31551 | 1 | 31720 | 3 | 32561 | 1 |
| 28320 | 1 | 28805 | 1 | 29821 | 1 | 29914 | 1 | 31090 | 1 | 31552 | 1 | 31725 | 1 | 32562 | 1 |
| 28322 | 2 | 28810 | 6 | 29822 | 1 | 29915 | 1 | 31200 | 1 | 31553 | 1 | 31730 | 1 | 32601 | 1 |
| 28340 | 2 | 28820 | 6 | 29823 | 1 | 29916 | 1 | 31201 | 1 | 31554 | 1 | 31750 | 1 | 32604 | 1 |
| 28341 | 2 | 28825 | 10 | 29824 | 1 | 30000 | 1 | 31205 | 1 | 31560 | 1 | 31755 | 1 | 32606 | 1 |
| 28344 | 1 | 28890 | 1 | 29825 | 1 | 30020 | 1 | 31225 | 1 | 31561 | 1 | 31760 | 1 | 32607 | 1 |
| 28345 | 2 | 29000 | 1 | 29826 | 1 | 30100 | 2 | 31230 | 1 | 31570 | 1 | 31766 | 1 | 32608 | 1 |
| 28360 | 1 | 29010 | 1 | 29827 | 1 | 30110 | 1 | 31231 | 1 | 31571 | 1 | 31770 | 2 | 32609 | 1 |
| 28400 | 1 | 29015 | 1 | 29828 | 1 | 30115 | 1 | 31233 | 1 | 31572 | 1 | 31775 | 1 | 32650 | 1 |
| 28405 | 1 | 29035 | 1 | 29830 | 1 | 30117 | 2 | 31235 | 1 | 31573 | 1 | 31780 | 1 | 32651 | 1 |
| 28406 | 1 | 29040 | 1 | 29834 | 1 | 30118 | 1 | 31237 | 1 | 31574 | 1 | 31781 | 1 | 32652 | 1 |
| 28415 | 1 | 29044 | 1 | 29835 | 1 | 30120 | 1 | 31238 | 1 | 31575 | 1 | 31785 | 1 | 32653 | 1 |
| 28420 | 1 | 29046 | 1 | 29836 | 1 | 30124 | 2 | 31239 | 1 | 31576 | 1 | 31786 | 1 | 32654 | 1 |
| 28430 | 1 | 29049 | 1 | 29837 | 1 | 30125 | 1 | 31240 | 1 | 31577 | 1 | 31800 | 1 | 32655 | 1 |
| 28435 | 1 | 29055 | 1 | 29838 | 1 | 30130 | 1 | 31254 | 1 | 31578 | 1 | 31805 | 1 | 32656 | 1 |
| 28436 | 1 | 29058 | 1 | 29840 | 1 | 30140 | 1 | 31255 | 1 | 31579 | 1 | 31820 | 1 | 32658 | 1 |
| 28445 | 1 | 29065 | 1 | 29843 | 1 | 30150 | 1 | 31256 | 1 | 31580 | 1 | 31825 | 1 | 32659 | 1 |
| 28446 | 1 | 29075 | 1 | 29844 | 1 | 30160 | 1 | 31267 | 1 | 31584 | 1 | 31830 | 1 | 32661 | 1 |
| 28450 | 2 | 29085 | 1 | 29845 | 1 | 30200 | 1 | 31276 | 1 | 31587 | 1 | 32035 | 1 | 32662 | 1 |
| 28455 | 3 | 29086 | 2 | 29846 | 1 | 30210 | 1 | 31287 | 1 | 31590 | 1 | 32036 | 1 | 32663 | 1 |
| 28456 | 2 | 29105 | 1 | 29847 | 1 | 30220 | 1 | 31288 | 1 | 31591 | 1 | 32096 | 1 | 32664 | 1 |
| 28465 | 3 | 29125 | 1 | 29848 | 1 | 30300 | 1 | 31290 | 1 | 31592 | 1 | 32097 | 1 | 32665 | 1 |
| 28470 | 2 | 29126 | 1 | 29850 | 1 | 30310 | 1 | 31291 | 1 | 31595 | 1 | 32098 | 1 | 32666 | 1 |
| 28475 | 5 | 29130 | 3 | 29851 | 1 | 30320 | 1 | 31292 | 1 | 31600 | 1 | 32100 | 1 | 32667 | 3 |
| 28476 | 4 | 29131 | 2 | 29855 | 1 | 30400 | 1 | 31293 | 1 | 31601 | 1 | 32110 | 1 | 32668 | 2 |
| 28485 | 5 | 29200 | 1 | 29856 | 1 | 30410 | 1 | 31294 | 1 | 31603 | 1 | 32120 | 1 | 32669 | 2 |
| 28490 | 1 | 29240 | 1 | 29860 | 1 | 30420 | 1 | 31295 | 1 | 31605 | 1 | 32124 | 1 | 32670 | 1 |
| 28495 | 1 | 29260 | 1 | 29861 | 1 | 30430 | 1 | 31296 | 1 | 31610 | 1 | 32140 | 1 | 32671 | 1 |
| 28496 | 1 | 29280 | 2 | 29862 | 1 | 30435 | 1 | 31297 | 1 | 31611 | 1 | 32141 | 1 | 32672 | 1 |
| 28505 | 1 | 29305 | 1 | 29863 | 1 | 30450 | 1 | 31300 | 1 | 31612 | 1 | 32150 | 1 | 32673 | 1 |
| 28510 | 4 | 29325 | 1 | 29866 | 1 | 30460 | 1 | 31320 | 1 | 31613 | 1 | 32151 | 1 | 32674 | 1 |
| 28515 | 4 | 29345 | 1 | 29867 | 1 | 30462 | 1 | 31360 | 1 | 31614 | 1 | 32160 | 1 | 32701 | 1 |
| 28525 | 4 | 29355 | 1 | 29868 | 1 | 30465 | 1 | 31365 | 1 | 31615 | 1 | 32200 | 2 | 32800 | 1 |
| 28530 | 1 | 29358 | 1 | 29870 | 1 | 30520 | 1 | 31367 | 1 | 31622 | 1 | 32215 | 1 | 32810 | 1 |
| 28531 | 1 | 29365 | 1 | 29871 | 1 | 30540 | 1 | 31368 | 1 | 31623 | 1 | 32220 | 1 | 32815 | 1 |
| 28540 | 1 | 29405 | 1 | 29873 | 1 | 30545 | 1 | 31370 | 1 | 31624 | 1 | 32225 | 1 | 32820 | 1 |
| 28545 | 1 | 29425 | 1 | 29874 | 1 | 30560 | 1 | 31375 | 1 | 31625 | 1 | 32310 | 1 | 32850 | 1 |
| 28546 | 1 | 29435 | 1 | 29875 | 1 | 30580 | 2 | 31380 | 1 | 31626 | 1 | 32320 | 1 | 32851 | 1 |
| 28555 | 1 | 29440 | 1 | 29876 | 1 | 30600 | 1 | 31382 | 1 | 31627 | 1 | 32400 | 2 | 32852 | 1 |
| 28570 | 1 | 29445 | 1 | 29877 | 1 | 30620 | 1 | 31390 | 1 | 31628 | 1 | 32405 | 2 | 32853 | 1 |
| 28575 | 1 | 29450 | 1 | 29879 | 1 | 30630 | 1 | 31395 | 1 | 31629 | 1 | 32440 | 1 | 32854 | 1 |
| 28576 | 1 | 29505 | 1 | 29880 | 1 | 30801 | 1 | 31400 | 1 | 31630 | 1 | 32442 | 1 | 32855 | 1 |
| 28585 | 1 | 29515 | 1 | 29881 | 1 | 30802 | 1 | 31420 | 1 | 31631 | 1 | 32445 | 1 | 32856 | 1 |
| 28600 | 2 | 29520 | 1 | 29882 | 1 | 30901 | 1 | 31500 | 2 | 31632 | 2 | 32480 | 1 | 32900 | 1 |
| 28605 | 2 | 29530 | 1 | 29883 | 1 | 30903 | 1 | 31502 | 1 | 31633 | 2 | 32482 | 1 | 32905 | 1 |
| 28606 | 3 | 29540 | 1 | 29884 | 1 | 30905 | 1 | 31505 | 1 | 31634 | 1 | 32484 | 2 | 32906 | 1 |
| 28615 | 5 | 29550 | 1 | 29885 | 1 | 30906 | 1 | 31510 | 1 | 31635 | 1 | 32486 | 1 | 32940 | 1 |
| 28630 | 2 | 29580 | 1 | 29886 | 1 | 30915 | 1 | 31511 | 1 | 31636 | 1 | 32488 | 1 | 32960 | 1 |
| 28635 | 2 | 29581 | 1 | 29887 | 1 | 30920 | 1 | 31512 | 1 | 31637 | 2 | 32491 | 1 | 32997 | 1 |
| 28636 | 4 | 29582 | 1 | 29888 | 1 | 30930 | 1 | 31513 | 1 | 31638 | 1 | 32501 | 1 | 32998 | 1 |
| 28645 | 4 | 29583 | 1 | 29889 | 1 | 31000 | 1 | 31515 | 1 | 31640 | 1 | 32503 | 1 | 33010 | 1 |
| 28660 | 4 | 29584 | 1 | 29891 | 1 | 31002 | 1 | 31520 | 1 | 31641 | 1 | 32504 | 1 | 33011 | 1 |
| 28665 | 4 | 29700 | 2 | 29892 | 1 | 31020 | 1 | 31525 | 1 | 31643 | 1 | 32505 | 1 | 33015 | 1 |

© 2017 Optum360, LLC

**Appendix I — Medically Unlikely Edits (MUEs) — OPPS**

| CPT | MUE | CPT | MUE | CPT | MUE | CPT | MUE | CPT | MUE | CPT | MUE | CPT | MUE | CPT | MUE |
|---|---|---|---|---|---|---|---|---|---|---|---|---|---|---|---|
| 33020 | 1 | 33284 | 1 | 33512 | 1 | 33768 | 1 | 33956 | 1 | 34831 | 1 | 35303 | 1 | 35637 | 1 |
| 33025 | 1 | 33300 | 1 | 33513 | 1 | 33770 | 1 | 33957 | 1 | 34832 | 1 | 35304 | 1 | 35638 | 1 |
| 33030 | 1 | 33305 | 1 | 33514 | 1 | 33771 | 1 | 33958 | 1 | 34833 | 1 | 35305 | 1 | 35642 | 1 |
| 33031 | 1 | 33310 | 1 | 33516 | 1 | 33774 | 1 | 33959 | 1 | 34834 | 1 | 35306 | 2 | 35645 | 1 |
| 33050 | 1 | 33315 | 1 | 33517 | 1 | 33775 | 1 | 33962 | 1 | 34839 | 1 | 35311 | 1 | 35646 | 1 |
| 33120 | 1 | 33320 | 1 | 33518 | 1 | 33776 | 1 | 33963 | 1 | 34841 | 1 | 35321 | 1 | 35647 | 1 |
| 33130 | 1 | 33321 | 1 | 33519 | 1 | 33777 | 1 | 33964 | 1 | 34842 | 1 | 35331 | 1 | 35650 | 1 |
| 33140 | 1 | 33322 | 1 | 33521 | 1 | 33778 | 1 | 33965 | 1 | 34843 | 1 | 35341 | 3 | 35654 | 1 |
| 33141 | 1 | 33330 | 1 | 33522 | 1 | 33779 | 1 | 33966 | 1 | 34844 | 1 | 35351 | 1 | 35656 | 1 |
| 33202 | 1 | 33335 | 1 | 33523 | 1 | 33780 | 1 | 33967 | 1 | 34845 | 1 | 35361 | 1 | 35661 | 1 |
| 33203 | 1 | 33340 | 1 | 33530 | 1 | 33781 | 1 | 33968 | 1 | 34846 | 1 | 35363 | 1 | 35663 | 1 |
| 33206 | 1 | 33361 | 1 | 33533 | 1 | 33782 | 1 | 33969 | 1 | 34847 | 1 | 35371 | 1 | 35665 | 1 |
| 33207 | 1 | 33362 | 1 | 33534 | 1 | 33783 | 1 | 33970 | 1 | 34848 | 1 | 35372 | 1 | 35666 | 2 |
| 33208 | 1 | 33363 | 1 | 33535 | 1 | 33786 | 1 | 33971 | 1 | 34900 | 1 | 35390 | 1 | 35671 | 2 |
| 33210 | 1 | 33364 | 1 | 33536 | 1 | 33788 | 1 | 33973 | 1 | 35001 | 1 | 35400 | 1 | 35681 | 1 |
| 33211 | 1 | 33365 | 1 | 33542 | 1 | 33800 | 1 | 33974 | 1 | 35002 | 1 | 35500 | 2 | 35682 | 1 |
| 33212 | 1 | 33366 | 1 | 33545 | 1 | 33802 | 1 | 33975 | 1 | 35005 | 1 | 35501 | 1 | 35683 | 1 |
| 33213 | 1 | 33367 | 1 | 33548 | 1 | 33803 | 1 | 33976 | 1 | 35011 | 1 | 35506 | 1 | 35685 | 2 |
| 33214 | 1 | 33368 | 1 | 33572 | 3 | 33813 | 1 | 33977 | 1 | 35013 | 1 | 35508 | 1 | 35686 | 1 |
| 33215 | 2 | 33369 | 1 | 33600 | 1 | 33814 | 1 | 33978 | 1 | 35021 | 1 | 35509 | 1 | 35691 | 1 |
| 33216 | 1 | 33390 | 1 | 33602 | 1 | 33820 | 1 | 33979 | 1 | 35022 | 1 | 35510 | 1 | 35693 | 1 |
| 33217 | 1 | 33391 | 1 | 33606 | 1 | 33822 | 1 | 33980 | 1 | 35045 | 2 | 35511 | 1 | 35694 | 1 |
| 33218 | 1 | 33404 | 1 | 33608 | 1 | 33824 | 1 | 33981 | 1 | 35081 | 1 | 35512 | 1 | 35695 | 1 |
| 33220 | 1 | 33405 | 1 | 33610 | 1 | 33840 | 1 | 33982 | 1 | 35082 | 1 | 35515 | 1 | 35697 | 2 |
| 33221 | 1 | 33406 | 1 | 33611 | 1 | 33845 | 1 | 33983 | 1 | 35091 | 1 | 35516 | 1 | 35700 | 2 |
| 33222 | 1 | 33410 | 1 | 33612 | 1 | 33851 | 1 | 33984 | 1 | 35092 | 1 | 35518 | 1 | 35701 | 1 |
| 33223 | 1 | 33411 | 1 | 33615 | 1 | 33852 | 1 | 33985 | 1 | 35102 | 1 | 35521 | 1 | 35721 | 1 |
| 33224 | 1 | 33412 | 1 | 33617 | 1 | 33853 | 1 | 33986 | 1 | 35103 | 1 | 35522 | 1 | 35741 | 1 |
| 33225 | 1 | 33413 | 1 | 33619 | 1 | 33860 | 1 | 33987 | 1 | 35111 | 1 | 35523 | 1 | 35761 | 2 |
| 33226 | 1 | 33414 | 1 | 33620 | 1 | 33863 | 1 | 33988 | 1 | 35112 | 1 | 35525 | 1 | 35800 | 2 |
| 33227 | 1 | 33415 | 1 | 33621 | 1 | 33864 | 1 | 33989 | 1 | 35121 | 1 | 35526 | 1 | 35820 | 2 |
| 33228 | 1 | 33416 | 1 | 33622 | 1 | 33870 | 1 | 33990 | 1 | 35122 | 1 | 35531 | 2 | 35840 | 2 |
| 33229 | 1 | 33417 | 1 | 33641 | 1 | 33875 | 1 | 33991 | 1 | 35131 | 1 | 35533 | 1 | 35860 | 2 |
| 33230 | 1 | 33418 | 1 | 33645 | 1 | 33877 | 1 | 33992 | 1 | 35132 | 1 | 35535 | 1 | 35870 | 1 |
| 33231 | 1 | 33419 | 1 | 33647 | 1 | 33880 | 1 | 33993 | 1 | 35141 | 1 | 35536 | 1 | 35875 | 2 |
| 33233 | 1 | 33420 | 1 | 33660 | 1 | 33881 | 1 | 34001 | 1 | 35142 | 1 | 35537 | 1 | 35876 | 2 |
| 33234 | 1 | 33422 | 1 | 33665 | 1 | 33883 | 1 | 34051 | 1 | 35151 | 1 | 35538 | 1 | 35879 | 2 |
| 33235 | 1 | 33425 | 1 | 33670 | 1 | 33884 | 2 | 34101 | 1 | 35152 | 1 | 35539 | 1 | 35881 | 2 |
| 33236 | 1 | 33426 | 1 | 33675 | 1 | 33886 | 1 | 34111 | 2 | 35180 | 2 | 35540 | 1 | 35883 | 1 |
| 33237 | 1 | 33427 | 1 | 33676 | 1 | 33889 | 1 | 34151 | 2 | 35182 | 2 | 35556 | 1 | 35884 | 1 |
| 33238 | 1 | 33430 | 1 | 33677 | 1 | 33891 | 1 | 34201 | 1 | 35184 | 2 | 35558 | 1 | 35901 | 1 |
| 33240 | 1 | 33460 | 1 | 33681 | 1 | 33910 | 1 | 34203 | 1 | 35188 | 2 | 35560 | 1 | 35903 | 2 |
| 33241 | 1 | 33463 | 1 | 33684 | 1 | 33915 | 1 | 34401 | 1 | 35189 | 1 | 35563 | 1 | 35905 | 1 |
| 33243 | 1 | 33464 | 1 | 33688 | 1 | 33916 | 1 | 34421 | 1 | 35190 | 2 | 35565 | 1 | 35907 | 1 |
| 33244 | 1 | 33465 | 1 | 33690 | 1 | 33917 | 1 | 34451 | 1 | 35201 | 2 | 35566 | 1 | 36000 | 4 |
| 33249 | 1 | 33468 | 1 | 33692 | 1 | 33920 | 1 | 34471 | 1 | 35206 | 2 | 35570 | 1 | 36002 | 2 |
| 33250 | 1 | 33470 | 1 | 33694 | 1 | 33922 | 1 | 34490 | 1 | 35207 | 3 | 35571 | 2 | 36005 | 2 |
| 33251 | 1 | 33471 | 1 | 33697 | 1 | 33924 | 1 | 34501 | 1 | 35211 | 3 | 35572 | 2 | 36010 | 2 |
| 33254 | 1 | 33474 | 1 | 33702 | 1 | 33925 | 1 | 34502 | 1 | 35216 | 2 | 35583 | 1 | 36011 | 4 |
| 33255 | 1 | 33475 | 1 | 33710 | 1 | 33926 | 1 | 34510 | 2 | 35221 | 3 | 35585 | 2 | 36012 | 4 |
| 33256 | 1 | 33476 | 1 | 33720 | 1 | 33930 | 1 | 34520 | 1 | 35226 | 3 | 35587 | 2 | 36013 | 2 |
| 33257 | 1 | 33477 | 1 | 33722 | 1 | 33933 | 1 | 34530 | 1 | 35231 | 2 | 35600 | 2 | 36014 | 2 |
| 33258 | 1 | 33478 | 1 | 33724 | 1 | 33935 | 1 | 34800 | 1 | 35236 | 2 | 35601 | 1 | 36015 | 4 |
| 33259 | 1 | 33496 | 1 | 33726 | 1 | 33940 | 1 | 34802 | 1 | 35241 | 2 | 35606 | 1 | 36100 | 2 |
| 33261 | 1 | 33500 | 1 | 33730 | 1 | 33944 | 1 | 34803 | 1 | 35246 | 2 | 35612 | 1 | 36120 | 2 |
| 33262 | 1 | 33501 | 1 | 33732 | 1 | 33945 | 1 | 34804 | 1 | 35251 | 2 | 35616 | 1 | 36140 | 3 |
| 33263 | 1 | 33502 | 1 | 33735 | 1 | 33946 | 1 | 34805 | 1 | 35256 | 2 | 35621 | 1 | 36160 | 2 |
| 33264 | 1 | 33503 | 1 | 33736 | 1 | 33947 | 1 | 34806 | 1 | 35261 | 1 | 35623 | 1 | 36200 | 2 |
| 33265 | 1 | 33504 | 1 | 33737 | 1 | 33948 | 1 | 34808 | 1 | 35266 | 2 | 35626 | 3 | 36215 | 2 |
| 33266 | 1 | 33505 | 1 | 33750 | 1 | 33949 | 1 | 34812 | 1 | 35271 | 2 | 35631 | 4 | 36216 | 2 |
| 33270 | 1 | 33506 | 1 | 33755 | 1 | 33951 | 1 | 34813 | 1 | 35276 | 2 | 35632 | 1 | 36217 | 2 |
| 33271 | 1 | 33507 | 1 | 33762 | 1 | 33952 | 1 | 34820 | 1 | 35281 | 2 | 35633 | 1 | 36218 | 2 |
| 33272 | 1 | 33508 | 1 | 33764 | 1 | 33953 | 1 | 34825 | 1 | 35286 | 2 | 35634 | 1 | 36221 | 1 |
| 33273 | 1 | 33510 | 1 | 33766 | 1 | 33954 | 1 | 34826 | 4 | 35301 | 2 | 35636 | 1 | 36222 | 1 |
| 33282 | 1 | 33511 | 1 | 33767 | 1 | 33955 | 1 | 34830 | 1 | 35302 | 1 | | | 36223 | 1 |

CPT © 2017 American Medical Association. All Rights Reserved.
© 2017 Optum360, LLC

| CPT | MUE | CPT | MUE | CPT | MUE | CPT | MUE | CPT | MUE | CPT | MUE | CPT | MUE | CPT | MUE |
|---|---|---|---|---|---|---|---|---|---|---|---|---|---|---|---|
| 36224 | 1 | 36580 | 2 | 37211 | 1 | 38102 | 1 | 39501 | 1 | 41135 | 1 | 42415 | 1 | 43122 | 1 |
| 36225 | 1 | 36581 | 2 | 37212 | 1 | 38115 | 1 | 39503 | 1 | 41140 | 1 | 42420 | 1 | 43123 | 1 |
| 36226 | 1 | 36582 | 2 | 37213 | 1 | 38120 | 1 | 39540 | 1 | 41145 | 1 | 42425 | 1 | 43124 | 1 |
| 36227 | 1 | 36583 | 2 | 37214 | 1 | 38200 | 1 | 39541 | 1 | 41150 | 1 | 42426 | 1 | 43130 | 1 |
| 36228 | 2 | 36584 | 2 | 37215 | 1 | 38204 | 1 | 39545 | 1 | 41153 | 1 | 42440 | 1 | 43135 | 1 |
| 36245 | 3 | 36585 | 2 | 37217 | 1 | 38205 | 1 | 39560 | 1 | 41155 | 1 | 42450 | 2 | 43180 | 1 |
| 36246 | 4 | 36589 | 2 | 37218 | 1 | 38206 | 1 | 39561 | 1 | 41250 | 2 | 42500 | 2 | 43191 | 1 |
| 36247 | 2 | 36590 | 2 | 37220 | 2 | 38207 | 1 | 40490 | 3 | 41251 | 2 | 42505 | 2 | 43192 | 1 |
| 36248 | 2 | 36591 | 2 | 37221 | 2 | 38208 | 1 | 40500 | 2 | 41252 | 2 | 42507 | 1 | 43193 | 1 |
| 36251 | 1 | 36592 | 1 | 37222 | 2 | 38209 | 1 | 40510 | 2 | 41500 | 1 | 42509 | 1 | 43194 | 1 |
| 36252 | 1 | 36593 | 2 | 37223 | 2 | 38210 | 1 | 40520 | 2 | 41510 | 1 | 42510 | 1 | 43195 | 1 |
| 36253 | 1 | 36595 | 2 | 37224 | 2 | 38211 | 1 | 40525 | 2 | 41512 | 1 | 42550 | 2 | 43196 | 1 |
| 36254 | 1 | 36596 | 2 | 37225 | 2 | 38212 | 1 | 40527 | 2 | 41520 | 1 | 42600 | 2 | 43197 | 1 |
| 36260 | 1 | 36597 | 2 | 37226 | 2 | 38213 | 1 | 40530 | 2 | 41530 | 1 | 42650 | 2 | 43198 | 1 |
| 36261 | 1 | 36598 | 2 | 37227 | 2 | 38214 | 1 | 40650 | 2 | 41800 | 2 | 42660 | 2 | 43200 | 1 |
| 36262 | 1 | 36600 | 4 | 37228 | 2 | 38215 | 1 | 40652 | 2 | 41805 | 3 | 42665 | 2 | 43201 | 1 |
| 36400 | 1 | 36620 | 3 | 37229 | 2 | 38220 | 1 | 40654 | 2 | 41806 | 3 | 42700 | 2 | 43202 | 1 |
| 36405 | 1 | 36625 | 2 | 37230 | 2 | 38221 | 1 | 40700 | 1 | 41820 | 4 | 42720 | 1 | 43204 | 1 |
| 36406 | 1 | 36640 | 1 | 37231 | 2 | 38230 | 1 | 40701 | 1 | 41821 | 2 | 42725 | 1 | 43205 | 1 |
| 36410 | 3 | 36660 | 1 | 37232 | 2 | 38232 | 1 | 40702 | 1 | 41822 | 1 | 42800 | 3 | 43206 | 1 |
| 36415 | 2 | 36680 | 1 | 37233 | 2 | 38240 | 1 | 40720 | 1 | 41823 | 1 | 42804 | 3 | 43210 | 1 |
| 36416 | 6 | 36800 | 1 | 37234 | 2 | 38241 | 1 | 40761 | 1 | 41825 | 2 | 42806 | 1 | 43211 | 1 |
| 36420 | 2 | 36810 | 1 | 37235 | 2 | 38242 | 1 | 40800 | 2 | 41826 | 2 | 42808 | 2 | 43212 | 1 |
| 36425 | 2 | 36815 | 1 | 37236 | 1 | 38243 | 1 | 40801 | 2 | 41827 | 2 | 42809 | 1 | 43213 | 1 |
| 36430 | 1 | 36818 | 1 | 37237 | 2 | 38300 | 1 | 40804 | 2 | 41828 | 4 | 42810 | 1 | 43214 | 1 |
| 36440 | 1 | 36819 | 1 | 37238 | 1 | 38305 | 1 | 40805 | 2 | 41830 | 2 | 42815 | 1 | 43215 | 1 |
| 36450 | 1 | 36820 | 1 | 37239 | 2 | 38308 | 1 | 40806 | 2 | 41850 | 2 | 42820 | 1 | 43216 | 1 |
| 36455 | 1 | 36821 | 2 | 37241 | 2 | 38380 | 1 | 40808 | 4 | 41870 | 2 | 42821 | 1 | 43217 | 1 |
| 36456 | 1 | 36823 | 1 | 37242 | 2 | 38381 | 1 | 40810 | 4 | 41872 | 4 | 42825 | 1 | 43220 | 1 |
| 36460 | 2 | 36825 | 1 | 37243 | 1 | 38382 | 1 | 40812 | 4 | 41874 | 4 | 42826 | 1 | 43226 | 1 |
| 36468 | 1 | 36830 | 2 | 37244 | 2 | 38500 | 2 | 40814 | 4 | 42000 | 1 | 42830 | 1 | 43227 | 1 |
| 36470 | 1 | 36831 | 1 | 37246 | 1 | 38505 | 3 | 40816 | 2 | 42100 | 3 | 42831 | 1 | 43229 | 1 |
| 36471 | 1 | 36832 | 2 | 37247 | 2 | 38510 | 1 | 40818 | 2 | 42104 | 3 | 42835 | 1 | 43231 | 1 |
| 36473 | 1 | 36833 | 1 | 37248 | 1 | 38520 | 1 | 40819 | 2 | 42106 | 2 | 42836 | 1 | 43232 | 1 |
| 36474 | 2 | 36835 | 1 | 37249 | 2 | 38525 | 1 | 40820 | 5 | 42107 | 2 | 42842 | 1 | 43233 | 1 |
| 36475 | 1 | 36838 | 1 | 37252 | 1 | 38530 | 1 | 40830 | 2 | 42120 | 1 | 42844 | 1 | 43235 | 1 |
| 36476 | 2 | 36860 | 2 | 37253 | 5 | 38542 | 1 | 40831 | 2 | 42140 | 1 | 42845 | 1 | 43236 | 1 |
| 36478 | 1 | 36861 | 2 | 37500 | 1 | 38550 | 1 | 40840 | 1 | 42145 | 1 | 42860 | 1 | 43237 | 1 |
| 36479 | 2 | 36901 | 1 | 37565 | 1 | 38555 | 1 | 40842 | 1 | 42160 | 2 | 42870 | 1 | 43238 | 1 |
| 36481 | 1 | 36902 | 1 | 37600 | 1 | 38562 | 1 | 40843 | 1 | 42180 | 1 | 42890 | 1 | 43239 | 1 |
| 36500 | 4 | 36903 | 1 | 37605 | 1 | 38564 | 1 | 40844 | 1 | 42182 | 1 | 42892 | 1 | 43240 | 1 |
| 36510 | 1 | 36904 | 1 | 37606 | 1 | 38570 | 1 | 40845 | 1 | 42200 | 1 | 42894 | 1 | 43241 | 1 |
| 36511 | 1 | 36905 | 1 | 37607 | 1 | 38571 | 1 | 41000 | 2 | 42205 | 1 | 42900 | 1 | 43242 | 1 |
| 36512 | 1 | 36906 | 1 | 37609 | 1 | 38572 | 1 | 41005 | 2 | 42210 | 1 | 42950 | 1 | 43243 | 1 |
| 36513 | 1 | 36907 | 1 | 37615 | 2 | 38700 | 1 | 41006 | 2 | 42215 | 1 | 42953 | 1 | 43244 | 1 |
| 36514 | 1 | 36908 | 1 | 37616 | 1 | 38720 | 1 | 41007 | 2 | 42220 | 1 | 42955 | 1 | 43245 | 1 |
| 36515 | 1 | 36909 | 1 | 37617 | 3 | 38724 | 1 | 41008 | 2 | 42225 | 1 | 42960 | 1 | 43246 | 1 |
| 36516 | 1 | 37140 | 1 | 37618 | 2 | 38740 | 1 | 41009 | 2 | 42226 | 1 | 42961 | 1 | 43247 | 1 |
| 36522 | 1 | 37145 | 1 | 37619 | 1 | 38745 | 1 | 41010 | 1 | 42227 | 1 | 42962 | 1 | 43248 | 1 |
| 36555 | 2 | 37160 | 1 | 37650 | 1 | 38746 | 1 | 41015 | 2 | 42235 | 1 | 42970 | 1 | 43249 | 1 |
| 36556 | 2 | 37180 | 1 | 37660 | 1 | 38747 | 1 | 41016 | 2 | 42260 | 1 | 42971 | 1 | 43250 | 1 |
| 36557 | 2 | 37181 | 1 | 37700 | 1 | 38760 | 1 | 41017 | 2 | 42280 | 1 | 42972 | 1 | 43251 | 1 |
| 36558 | 2 | 37182 | 1 | 37718 | 1 | 38765 | 1 | 41018 | 2 | 42281 | 1 | 43020 | 1 | 43252 | 1 |
| 36560 | 2 | 37183 | 1 | 37722 | 1 | 38770 | 1 | 41019 | 1 | 42300 | 2 | 43030 | 1 | 43253 | 1 |
| 36561 | 2 | 37184 | 1 | 37735 | 1 | 38780 | 1 | 41100 | 3 | 42305 | 2 | 43045 | 1 | 43254 | 1 |
| 36563 | 1 | 37185 | 2 | 37760 | 1 | 38790 | 1 | 41105 | 3 | 42310 | 2 | 43100 | 1 | 43255 | 2 |
| 36565 | 1 | 37186 | 2 | 37761 | 1 | 38792 | 1 | 41108 | 2 | 42320 | 2 | 43101 | 1 | 43257 | 1 |
| 36566 | 1 | 37187 | 1 | 37765 | 1 | 38794 | 1 | 41110 | 2 | 42330 | 2 | 43107 | 1 | 43259 | 1 |
| 36568 | 2 | 37188 | 1 | 37766 | 1 | 38900 | 1 | 41112 | 2 | 42335 | 2 | 43108 | 1 | 43260 | 1 |
| 36569 | 2 | 37191 | 1 | 37780 | 1 | 39000 | 1 | 41113 | 2 | 42340 | 1 | 43112 | 1 | 43261 | 1 |
| 36570 | 2 | 37192 | 1 | 37785 | 1 | 39010 | 1 | 41114 | 2 | 42400 | 2 | 43113 | 1 | 43262 | 2 |
| 36571 | 2 | 37193 | 1 | 37788 | 1 | 39200 | 1 | 41115 | 1 | 42405 | 2 | 43116 | 1 | 43263 | 1 |
| 36575 | 2 | 37195 | 1 | 37790 | 1 | 39220 | 1 | 41116 | 2 | 42408 | 1 | 43117 | 1 | 43264 | 1 |
| 36576 | 2 | 37197 | 2 | 38100 | 1 | 39401 | 1 | 41120 | 1 | 42409 | 1 | 43118 | 1 | 43265 | 1 |
| 36578 | 2 | 37200 | 2 | 38101 | 1 | 39402 | 1 | 41130 | 1 | 42410 | 1 | 43121 | 1 | 43266 | 1 |

**Appendix I — Medically Unlikely Edits (MUEs) — OPPS**

| CPT | MUE | CPT | MUE | CPT | MUE | CPT | MUE | CPT | MUE | CPT | MUE | CPT | MUE | CPT | MUE |
|---|---|---|---|---|---|---|---|---|---|---|---|---|---|---|---|
| 43270 | 1 | 43640 | 1 | 44132 | 1 | 44386 | 1 | 45172 | 2 | 46020 | 2 | 46922 | 1 | 47563 | 1 |
| 43273 | 1 | 43641 | 1 | 44133 | 1 | 44388 | 1 | 45190 | 1 | 46030 | 1 | 46924 | 1 | 47564 | 1 |
| 43274 | 2 | 43644 | 1 | 44135 | 1 | 44389 | 1 | 45300 | 1 | 46040 | 2 | 46930 | 1 | 47570 | 1 |
| 43275 | 1 | 43645 | 1 | 44136 | 1 | 44390 | 1 | 45303 | 1 | 46045 | 2 | 46940 | 1 | 47600 | 1 |
| 43276 | 2 | 43647 | 1 | 44137 | 1 | 44391 | 1 | 45305 | 1 | 46050 | 2 | 46942 | 1 | 47605 | 1 |
| 43277 | 3 | 43648 | 1 | 44139 | 1 | 44392 | 1 | 45307 | 1 | 46060 | 2 | 46945 | 1 | 47610 | 1 |
| 43278 | 1 | 43651 | 1 | 44140 | 2 | 44394 | 1 | 45308 | 1 | 46070 | 1 | 46946 | 1 | 47612 | 1 |
| 43279 | 1 | 43652 | 1 | 44141 | 1 | 44401 | 1 | 45309 | 1 | 46080 | 1 | 46947 | 1 | 47620 | 1 |
| 43280 | 1 | 43653 | 1 | 44143 | 1 | 44402 | 1 | 45315 | 1 | 46083 | 2 | 47000 | 3 | 47700 | 1 |
| 43282 | 1 | 43752 | 2 | 44144 | 1 | 44403 | 1 | 45317 | 1 | 46200 | 1 | 47001 | 3 | 47701 | 1 |
| 43283 | 1 | 43753 | 1 | 44145 | 1 | 44404 | 1 | 45320 | 1 | 46220 | 1 | 47010 | 3 | 47711 | 1 |
| 43284 | 1 | 43754 | 1 | 44146 | 1 | 44405 | 1 | 45321 | 1 | 46221 | 1 | 47015 | 1 | 47712 | 1 |
| 43285 | 1 | 43755 | 1 | 44147 | 1 | 44406 | 1 | 45327 | 1 | 46230 | 1 | 47100 | 3 | 47715 | 1 |
| 43300 | 1 | 43756 | 1 | 44150 | 1 | 44407 | 1 | 45330 | 1 | 46250 | 1 | 47120 | 2 | 47720 | 1 |
| 43305 | 1 | 43757 | 1 | 44151 | 1 | 44408 | 1 | 45331 | 1 | 46255 | 1 | 47122 | 1 | 47721 | 1 |
| 43310 | 1 | 43760 | 2 | 44155 | 1 | 44500 | 1 | 45332 | 1 | 46257 | 1 | 47125 | 1 | 47740 | 1 |
| 43312 | 1 | 43761 | 2 | 44156 | 1 | 44602 | 1 | 45333 | 1 | 46258 | 1 | 47130 | 1 | 47741 | 1 |
| 43313 | 1 | 43770 | 1 | 44157 | 1 | 44603 | 1 | 45334 | 1 | 46260 | 1 | 47133 | 1 | 47760 | 1 |
| 43314 | 1 | 43771 | 1 | 44158 | 1 | 44604 | 1 | 45335 | 1 | 46261 | 1 | 47135 | 1 | 47765 | 1 |
| 43320 | 1 | 43772 | 1 | 44160 | 1 | 44605 | 1 | 45337 | 1 | 46262 | 1 | 47140 | 1 | 47780 | 1 |
| 43325 | 1 | 43773 | 1 | 44180 | 1 | 44615 | 4 | 45338 | 1 | 46270 | 1 | 47141 | 1 | 47785 | 1 |
| 43327 | 1 | 43774 | 1 | 44186 | 1 | 44620 | 2 | 45340 | 1 | 46275 | 1 | 47142 | 1 | 47800 | 1 |
| 43328 | 1 | 43775 | 1 | 44187 | 1 | 44625 | 1 | 45341 | 1 | 46280 | 1 | 47143 | 1 | 47801 | 1 |
| 43330 | 1 | 43800 | 1 | 44188 | 1 | 44626 | 1 | 45342 | 1 | 46285 | 1 | 47144 | 1 | 47802 | 1 |
| 43331 | 1 | 43810 | 1 | 44202 | 1 | 44640 | 2 | 45346 | 1 | 46288 | 1 | 47145 | 1 | 47900 | 1 |
| 43332 | 1 | 43820 | 1 | 44203 | 2 | 44650 | 2 | 45347 | 1 | 46320 | 2 | 47146 | 3 | 48000 | 1 |
| 43333 | 1 | 43825 | 1 | 44204 | 2 | 44660 | 1 | 45349 | 1 | 46500 | 1 | 47147 | 2 | 48001 | 1 |
| 43334 | 1 | 43830 | 1 | 44205 | 1 | 44661 | 1 | 45350 | 1 | 46505 | 1 | 47300 | 2 | 48020 | 1 |
| 43335 | 1 | 43831 | 1 | 44206 | 1 | 44680 | 1 | 45378 | 1 | 46600 | 1 | 47350 | 1 | 48100 | 1 |
| 43336 | 1 | 43832 | 1 | 44207 | 1 | 44700 | 1 | 45379 | 1 | 46601 | 1 | 47360 | 1 | 48102 | 1 |
| 43337 | 1 | 43840 | 2 | 44208 | 1 | 44701 | 1 | 45380 | 1 | 46604 | 1 | 47361 | 1 | 48105 | 1 |
| 43338 | 1 | 43843 | 1 | 44210 | 1 | 44705 | 1 | 45381 | 1 | 46606 | 1 | 47362 | 1 | 48120 | 1 |
| 43340 | 1 | 43845 | 1 | 44211 | 1 | 44715 | 1 | 45382 | 1 | 46607 | 1 | 47370 | 1 | 48140 | 1 |
| 43341 | 1 | 43846 | 1 | 44212 | 1 | 44720 | 2 | 45384 | 1 | 46608 | 1 | 47371 | 1 | 48145 | 1 |
| 43351 | 1 | 43847 | 1 | 44213 | 1 | 44721 | 2 | 45385 | 1 | 46610 | 1 | 47380 | 1 | 48146 | 1 |
| 43352 | 1 | 43848 | 1 | 44227 | 1 | 44800 | 1 | 45386 | 1 | 46611 | 1 | 47381 | 1 | 48148 | 1 |
| 43360 | 1 | 43850 | 1 | 44300 | 1 | 44820 | 1 | 45388 | 1 | 46612 | 1 | 47382 | 1 | 48150 | 1 |
| 43361 | 1 | 43855 | 1 | 44310 | 2 | 44850 | 1 | 45389 | 1 | 46614 | 1 | 47383 | 1 | 48152 | 1 |
| 43400 | 1 | 43860 | 1 | 44312 | 1 | 44900 | 1 | 45390 | 1 | 46615 | 1 | 47400 | 1 | 48153 | 1 |
| 43401 | 1 | 43865 | 1 | 44314 | 1 | 44950 | 1 | 45391 | 1 | 46700 | 1 | 47420 | 1 | 48154 | 1 |
| 43405 | 1 | 43870 | 1 | 44316 | 1 | 44955 | 1 | 45392 | 1 | 46705 | 1 | 47425 | 1 | 48155 | 1 |
| 43410 | 1 | 43880 | 1 | 44320 | 1 | 44960 | 1 | 45393 | 1 | 46706 | 1 | 47460 | 1 | 48400 | 1 |
| 43415 | 1 | 43881 | 1 | 44322 | 1 | 44970 | 1 | 45395 | 1 | 46707 | 1 | 47480 | 1 | 48500 | 1 |
| 43420 | 1 | 43882 | 1 | 44340 | 1 | 45000 | 1 | 45397 | 1 | 46710 | 1 | 47490 | 1 | 48510 | 1 |
| 43425 | 1 | 43886 | 1 | 44345 | 1 | 45005 | 1 | 45398 | 1 | 46712 | 1 | 47531 | 2 | 48520 | 1 |
| 43450 | 1 | 43887 | 1 | 44346 | 1 | 45020 | 1 | 45400 | 1 | 46715 | 1 | 47532 | 1 | 48540 | 1 |
| 43453 | 1 | 43888 | 1 | 44360 | 1 | 45100 | 2 | 45402 | 1 | 46716 | 1 | 47533 | 1 | 48545 | 1 |
| 43460 | 1 | 44005 | 1 | 44361 | 1 | 45108 | 1 | 45500 | 1 | 46730 | 1 | 47534 | 2 | 48547 | 1 |
| 43496 | 1 | 44010 | 1 | 44363 | 1 | 45110 | 1 | 45505 | 1 | 46735 | 1 | 47535 | 1 | 48548 | 1 |
| 43500 | 1 | 44015 | 1 | 44364 | 1 | 45111 | 1 | 45520 | 1 | 46740 | 1 | 47536 | 2 | 48550 | 1 |
| 43501 | 1 | 44020 | 2 | 44365 | 1 | 45112 | 1 | 45540 | 1 | 46742 | 1 | 47537 | 1 | 48551 | 1 |
| 43502 | 1 | 44021 | 1 | 44366 | 1 | 45113 | 1 | 45541 | 1 | 46744 | 1 | 47538 | 2 | 48552 | 2 |
| 43510 | 1 | 44025 | 1 | 44369 | 1 | 45114 | 1 | 45550 | 1 | 46746 | 1 | 47539 | 2 | 48554 | 1 |
| 43520 | 1 | 44050 | 1 | 44370 | 1 | 45116 | 1 | 45560 | 1 | 46748 | 1 | 47540 | 2 | 48556 | 1 |
| 43605 | 1 | 44055 | 1 | 44372 | 1 | 45119 | 1 | 45562 | 1 | 46750 | 1 | 47541 | 1 | 49000 | 1 |
| 43610 | 2 | 44100 | 1 | 44373 | 1 | 45120 | 1 | 45563 | 1 | 46751 | 1 | 47542 | 2 | 49002 | 1 |
| 43611 | 2 | 44110 | 1 | 44376 | 1 | 45121 | 1 | 45800 | 1 | 46753 | 1 | 47543 | 1 | 49010 | 1 |
| 43620 | 1 | 44111 | 1 | 44377 | 1 | 45123 | 1 | 45805 | 1 | 46754 | 1 | 47544 | 1 | 49020 | 2 |
| 43621 | 1 | 44120 | 1 | 44378 | 1 | 45126 | 1 | 45820 | 1 | 46760 | 1 | 47550 | 1 | 49040 | 2 |
| 43622 | 1 | 44121 | 4 | 44379 | 1 | 45130 | 1 | 45825 | 1 | 46761 | 1 | 47552 | 1 | 49060 | 2 |
| 43631 | 1 | 44125 | 1 | 44380 | 1 | 45135 | 1 | 45900 | 1 | 46762 | 1 | 47553 | 1 | 49062 | 1 |
| 43632 | 1 | 44126 | 1 | 44381 | 1 | 45136 | 1 | 45905 | 1 | 46900 | 1 | 47554 | 1 | 49082 | 1 |
| 43633 | 1 | 44127 | 1 | 44382 | 1 | 45150 | 1 | 45910 | 1 | 46910 | 1 | 47555 | 1 | 49083 | 2 |
| 43634 | 1 | 44128 | 2 | 44384 | 1 | 45160 | 1 | 45915 | 1 | 46916 | 1 | 47556 | 1 | 49084 | 1 |
| 43635 | 1 | 44130 | 3 | 44385 | 1 | 45171 | 2 | 45990 | 1 | 46917 | 1 | 47562 | 1 | 49180 | 2 |

CPT © 2017 American Medical Association. All Rights Reserved.     © 2017 Optum360, LLC

Appendix I — Medically Unlikely Edits (MUEs) — OPPS

| CPT | MUE | CPT | MUE | CPT | MUE | CPT | MUE | CPT | MUE | CPT | MUE | CPT | MUE | CPT | MUE |
|---|---|---|---|---|---|---|---|---|---|---|---|---|---|---|---|
| 49185 | 2 | 49568 | 2 | 50385 | 1 | 50727 | 1 | 51700 | 1 | 52317 | 1 | 53446 | 1 | 54326 | 1 |
| 49203 | 1 | 49570 | 1 | 50386 | 1 | 50728 | 1 | 51701 | 2 | 52318 | 1 | 53447 | 1 | 54328 | 1 |
| 49204 | 1 | 49572 | 1 | 50387 | 1 | 50740 | 1 | 51702 | 2 | 52320 | 1 | 53448 | 1 | 54332 | 1 |
| 49205 | 1 | 49580 | 1 | 50389 | 1 | 50750 | 1 | 51703 | 2 | 52325 | 1 | 53449 | 1 | 54336 | 1 |
| 49215 | 1 | 49582 | 1 | 50390 | 2 | 50760 | 1 | 51705 | 2 | 52327 | 1 | 53450 | 1 | 54340 | 1 |
| 49220 | 1 | 49585 | 1 | 50391 | 1 | 50770 | 1 | 51710 | 1 | 52330 | 1 | 53460 | 1 | 54344 | 1 |
| 49250 | 1 | 49587 | 1 | 50395 | 1 | 50780 | 1 | 51715 | 1 | 52332 | 1 | 53500 | 1 | 54348 | 1 |
| 49255 | 1 | 49590 | 1 | 50396 | 1 | 50782 | 1 | 51720 | 1 | 52334 | 1 | 53502 | 1 | 54352 | 1 |
| 49320 | 1 | 49600 | 1 | 50400 | 1 | 50783 | 1 | 51725 | 1 | 52341 | 1 | 53505 | 1 | 54360 | 1 |
| 49321 | 1 | 49605 | 1 | 50405 | 1 | 50785 | 1 | 51726 | 1 | 52342 | 1 | 53510 | 1 | 54380 | 1 |
| 49322 | 1 | 49606 | 1 | 50430 | 2 | 50810 | 1 | 51727 | 1 | 52343 | 1 | 53515 | 1 | 54385 | 1 |
| 49323 | 1 | 49610 | 1 | 50431 | 2 | 50815 | 1 | 51728 | 1 | 52344 | 1 | 53520 | 1 | 54390 | 1 |
| 49324 | 1 | 49611 | 1 | 50432 | 2 | 50820 | 1 | 51729 | 1 | 52345 | 1 | 53600 | 1 | 54400 | 1 |
| 49325 | 1 | 49650 | 1 | 50433 | 2 | 50825 | 1 | 51736 | 1 | 52346 | 1 | 53601 | 1 | 54401 | 1 |
| 49326 | 1 | 49651 | 1 | 50434 | 2 | 50830 | 1 | 51741 | 1 | 52351 | 1 | 53605 | 1 | 54405 | 1 |
| 49327 | 1 | 49652 | 2 | 50435 | 2 | 50840 | 1 | 51784 | 1 | 52352 | 1 | 53620 | 1 | 54406 | 1 |
| 49400 | 1 | 49653 | 2 | 50500 | 1 | 50845 | 1 | 51785 | 1 | 52353 | 1 | 53621 | 1 | 54408 | 1 |
| 49402 | 1 | 49654 | 2 | 50520 | 1 | 50860 | 1 | 51792 | 1 | 52354 | 1 | 53660 | 1 | 54410 | 1 |
| 49405 | 2 | 49655 | 2 | 50525 | 1 | 50900 | 1 | 51797 | 1 | 52355 | 1 | 53661 | 1 | 54411 | 1 |
| 49406 | 2 | 49656 | 2 | 50526 | 1 | 50920 | 2 | 51798 | 1 | 52356 | 1 | 53665 | 1 | 54415 | 1 |
| 49407 | 1 | 49657 | 2 | 50540 | 1 | 50930 | 2 | 51800 | 1 | 52400 | 1 | 53850 | 1 | 54416 | 1 |
| 49411 | 1 | 49900 | 1 | 50541 | 1 | 50940 | 1 | 51820 | 1 | 52402 | 1 | 53852 | 1 | 54417 | 1 |
| 49412 | 1 | 49904 | 1 | 50542 | 1 | 50945 | 1 | 51840 | 1 | 52441 | 1 | 53855 | 1 | 54420 | 1 |
| 49418 | 1 | 49905 | 1 | 50543 | 1 | 50947 | 1 | 51841 | 1 | 52442 | 6 | 53860 | 1 | 54430 | 1 |
| 49419 | 1 | 49906 | 1 | 50544 | 1 | 50948 | 1 | 51845 | 1 | 52450 | 1 | 54000 | 1 | 54435 | 1 |
| 49421 | 1 | 50010 | 1 | 50545 | 1 | 50951 | 1 | 51860 | 1 | 52500 | 1 | 54001 | 1 | 54437 | 1 |
| 49422 | 1 | 50020 | 1 | 50546 | 1 | 50953 | 1 | 51865 | 1 | 52601 | 1 | 54015 | 1 | 54438 | 1 |
| 49423 | 2 | 50040 | 1 | 50547 | 1 | 50955 | 1 | 51880 | 1 | 52630 | 1 | 54050 | 1 | 54440 | 1 |
| 49424 | 3 | 50045 | 1 | 50548 | 1 | 50957 | 1 | 51900 | 1 | 52640 | 1 | 54055 | 1 | 54450 | 1 |
| 49425 | 1 | 50060 | 1 | 50551 | 1 | 50961 | 1 | 51920 | 1 | 52647 | 1 | 54056 | 1 | 54500 | 1 |
| 49426 | 1 | 50065 | 1 | 50553 | 1 | 50970 | 1 | 51925 | 1 | 52648 | 1 | 54057 | 1 | 54505 | 1 |
| 49427 | 1 | 50070 | 1 | 50555 | 1 | 50972 | 1 | 51940 | 1 | 52649 | 1 | 54060 | 1 | 54512 | 1 |
| 49428 | 1 | 50075 | 1 | 50557 | 1 | 50974 | 1 | 51960 | 1 | 52700 | 1 | 54065 | 1 | 54520 | 1 |
| 49429 | 1 | 50080 | 1 | 50561 | 1 | 50976 | 1 | 51980 | 1 | 53000 | 1 | 54100 | 2 | 54522 | 1 |
| 49435 | 1 | 50081 | 1 | 50562 | 1 | 50980 | 1 | 51990 | 1 | 53010 | 1 | 54105 | 2 | 54530 | 1 |
| 49436 | 1 | 50100 | 1 | 50570 | 1 | 51020 | 1 | 51992 | 1 | 53020 | 1 | 54110 | 1 | 54535 | 1 |
| 49440 | 1 | 50120 | 1 | 50572 | 1 | 51030 | 1 | 52000 | 1 | 53025 | 1 | 54111 | 1 | 54550 | 1 |
| 49441 | 1 | 50125 | 1 | 50574 | 1 | 51040 | 1 | 52001 | 1 | 53040 | 1 | 54112 | 1 | 54560 | 1 |
| 49442 | 1 | 50130 | 1 | 50575 | 1 | 51045 | 2 | 52005 | 2 | 53060 | 1 | 54115 | 1 | 54600 | 1 |
| 49446 | 1 | 50135 | 1 | 50576 | 1 | 51050 | 1 | 52007 | 1 | 53080 | 1 | 54120 | 1 | 54620 | 1 |
| 49450 | 1 | 50200 | 1 | 50580 | 1 | 51060 | 1 | 52010 | 1 | 53085 | 1 | 54125 | 1 | 54640 | 1 |
| 49451 | 1 | 50205 | 1 | 50590 | 1 | 51065 | 1 | 52204 | 1 | 53200 | 1 | 54130 | 1 | 54650 | 1 |
| 49452 | 1 | 50220 | 1 | 50592 | 1 | 51080 | 1 | 52214 | 1 | 53210 | 1 | 54135 | 1 | 54660 | 1 |
| 49460 | 1 | 50225 | 1 | 50593 | 1 | 51100 | 1 | 52224 | 1 | 53215 | 1 | 54150 | 1 | 54670 | 1 |
| 49465 | 1 | 50230 | 1 | 50600 | 1 | 51101 | 1 | 52234 | 1 | 53220 | 1 | 54160 | 1 | 54680 | 1 |
| 49491 | 1 | 50234 | 1 | 50605 | 1 | 51102 | 1 | 52235 | 1 | 53230 | 1 | 54161 | 1 | 54690 | 1 |
| 49492 | 1 | 50236 | 1 | 50606 | 1 | 51500 | 1 | 52240 | 1 | 53235 | 1 | 54162 | 1 | 54692 | 1 |
| 49495 | 1 | 50240 | 1 | 50610 | 1 | 51520 | 1 | 52250 | 1 | 53240 | 1 | 54163 | 1 | 54700 | 1 |
| 49496 | 1 | 50250 | 1 | 50620 | 1 | 51525 | 1 | 52260 | 1 | 53250 | 1 | 54164 | 1 | 54800 | 1 |
| 49500 | 1 | 50280 | 1 | 50630 | 1 | 51530 | 1 | 52265 | 1 | 53260 | 1 | 54200 | 1 | 54830 | 1 |
| 49501 | 1 | 50290 | 1 | 50650 | 1 | 51535 | 1 | 52270 | 1 | 53265 | 1 | 54205 | 1 | 54840 | 1 |
| 49505 | 1 | 50300 | 1 | 50660 | 1 | 51550 | 1 | 52275 | 1 | 53270 | 1 | 54220 | 1 | 54860 | 1 |
| 49507 | 1 | 50320 | 1 | 50684 | 1 | 51555 | 1 | 52276 | 1 | 53275 | 1 | 54230 | 1 | 54861 | 1 |
| 49520 | 1 | 50323 | 1 | 50686 | 2 | 51565 | 1 | 52277 | 1 | 53400 | 1 | 54231 | 1 | 54865 | 1 |
| 49521 | 1 | 50325 | 1 | 50688 | 2 | 51570 | 1 | 52281 | 1 | 53405 | 1 | 54235 | 1 | 54900 | 1 |
| 49525 | 1 | 50327 | 1 | 50690 | 2 | 51575 | 1 | 52282 | 1 | 53410 | 1 | 54240 | 1 | 54901 | 1 |
| 49540 | 1 | 50328 | 1 | 50693 | 2 | 51580 | 1 | 52283 | 1 | 53415 | 1 | 54250 | 1 | 55000 | 1 |
| 49550 | 1 | 50329 | 1 | 50694 | 2 | 51585 | 1 | 52285 | 1 | 53420 | 1 | 54300 | 1 | 55040 | 1 |
| 49553 | 1 | 50340 | 1 | 50695 | 2 | 51590 | 1 | 52287 | 1 | 53425 | 1 | 54304 | 1 | 55041 | 1 |
| 49555 | 1 | 50360 | 1 | 50700 | 1 | 51595 | 1 | 52290 | 1 | 53430 | 1 | 54308 | 1 | 55060 | 1 |
| 49557 | 1 | 50365 | 1 | 50705 | 2 | 51596 | 1 | 52300 | 1 | 53431 | 1 | 54312 | 1 | 55100 | 2 |
| 49560 | 2 | 50370 | 1 | 50706 | 2 | 51597 | 1 | 52301 | 1 | 53440 | 1 | 54316 | 1 | 55110 | 1 |
| 49561 | 2 | 50380 | 1 | 50715 | 1 | 51600 | 1 | 52305 | 1 | 53442 | 1 | 54318 | 1 | 55120 | 1 |
| 49565 | 2 | 50382 | 1 | 50722 | 1 | 51605 | 1 | 52310 | 1 | 53444 | 1 | 54322 | 1 | 55150 | 1 |
| 49566 | 2 | 50384 | 1 | 50725 | 1 | 51610 | 1 | 52315 | 2 | 53445 | 1 | 54324 | 1 | 55175 | 1 |

© 2017 Optum360, LLC

**Appendix I — Medically Unlikely Edits (MUEs) — OPPS**

| CPT | MUE | CPT | MUE | CPT | MUE | CPT | MUE | CPT | MUE | CPT | MUE | CPT | MUE | CPT | MUE |
|---|---|---|---|---|---|---|---|---|---|---|---|---|---|---|---|
| 55180 | 1 | 57010 | 1 | 57455 | 1 | 58545 | 1 | 59025 | 2 | 60254 | 1 | 61516 | 1 | 61618 | 2 |
| 55200 | 1 | 57020 | 1 | 57456 | 1 | 58546 | 1 | 59030 | 2 | 60260 | 1 | 61517 | 1 | 61619 | 2 |
| 55250 | 1 | 57022 | 1 | 57460 | 1 | 58548 | 1 | 59050 | 2 | 60270 | 1 | 61518 | 1 | 61623 | 2 |
| 55300 | 1 | 57023 | 1 | 57461 | 1 | 58550 | 1 | 59051 | 2 | 60271 | 1 | 61519 | 1 | 61624 | 2 |
| 55400 | 1 | 57061 | 1 | 57500 | 1 | 58552 | 1 | 59070 | 2 | 60280 | 1 | 61520 | 1 | 61626 | 2 |
| 55450 | 1 | 57065 | 1 | 57505 | 1 | 58553 | 1 | 59072 | 2 | 60281 | 1 | 61521 | 1 | 61630 | 1 |
| 55500 | 1 | 57100 | 3 | 57510 | 1 | 58554 | 1 | 59074 | 2 | 60300 | 2 | 61522 | 1 | 61635 | 2 |
| 55520 | 1 | 57105 | 2 | 57511 | 1 | 58555 | 1 | 59076 | 2 | 60500 | 1 | 61524 | 2 | 61645 | 3 |
| 55530 | 1 | 57106 | 1 | 57513 | 1 | 58558 | 1 | 59100 | 1 | 60502 | 1 | 61526 | 1 | 61650 | 1 |
| 55535 | 1 | 57107 | 1 | 57520 | 1 | 58559 | 1 | 59120 | 1 | 60505 | 1 | 61530 | 1 | 61651 | 2 |
| 55540 | 1 | 57109 | 1 | 57522 | 1 | 58560 | 1 | 59121 | 1 | 60512 | 1 | 61531 | 1 | 61680 | 1 |
| 55550 | 1 | 57110 | 1 | 57530 | 1 | 58561 | 1 | 59130 | 1 | 60520 | 1 | 61533 | 2 | 61682 | 1 |
| 55600 | 1 | 57111 | 1 | 57531 | 1 | 58562 | 1 | 59135 | 1 | 60521 | 1 | 61534 | 1 | 61684 | 1 |
| 55605 | 1 | 57112 | 1 | 57540 | 1 | 58563 | 1 | 59136 | 1 | 60522 | 1 | 61535 | 2 | 61686 | 1 |
| 55650 | 1 | 57120 | 1 | 57545 | 1 | 58565 | 1 | 59140 | 1 | 60540 | 1 | 61536 | 1 | 61690 | 1 |
| 55680 | 1 | 57130 | 1 | 57550 | 1 | 58570 | 1 | 59150 | 1 | 60545 | 1 | 61537 | 1 | 61692 | 1 |
| 55700 | 1 | 57135 | 2 | 57555 | 1 | 58571 | 1 | 59151 | 1 | 60600 | 1 | 61538 | 1 | 61697 | 2 |
| 55705 | 1 | 57150 | 1 | 57556 | 1 | 58572 | 1 | 59160 | 1 | 60605 | 1 | 61539 | 1 | 61698 | 1 |
| 55706 | 1 | 57155 | 1 | 57558 | 1 | 58573 | 1 | 59200 | 1 | 60650 | 1 | 61540 | 1 | 61700 | 2 |
| 55720 | 1 | 57156 | 1 | 57700 | 1 | 58600 | 1 | 59300 | 1 | 61000 | 1 | 61541 | 1 | 61702 | 1 |
| 55725 | 1 | 57160 | 1 | 57720 | 1 | 58605 | 1 | 59320 | 1 | 61001 | 1 | 61543 | 1 | 61703 | 1 |
| 55801 | 1 | 57170 | 1 | 57800 | 1 | 58611 | 1 | 59325 | 1 | 61020 | 2 | 61544 | 1 | 61705 | 1 |
| 55810 | 1 | 57180 | 1 | 58100 | 1 | 58615 | 1 | 59350 | 1 | 61026 | 2 | 61545 | 1 | 61708 | 1 |
| 55812 | 1 | 57200 | 1 | 58110 | 1 | 58660 | 1 | 59400 | 1 | 61050 | 1 | 61546 | 1 | 61710 | 1 |
| 55815 | 1 | 57210 | 1 | 58120 | 1 | 58661 | 1 | 59409 | 2 | 61055 | 1 | 61548 | 1 | 61711 | 1 |
| 55821 | 1 | 57220 | 1 | 58140 | 1 | 58662 | 1 | 59410 | 1 | 61070 | 2 | 61550 | 1 | 61720 | 1 |
| 55831 | 1 | 57230 | 1 | 58145 | 1 | 58670 | 1 | 59412 | 1 | 61105 | 1 | 61552 | 1 | 61735 | 1 |
| 55840 | 1 | 57240 | 1 | 58146 | 1 | 58671 | 1 | 59414 | 1 | 61107 | 1 | 61556 | 1 | 61750 | 2 |
| 55842 | 1 | 57250 | 1 | 58150 | 1 | 58672 | 1 | 59425 | 1 | 61108 | 1 | 61557 | 1 | 61751 | 2 |
| 55845 | 1 | 57260 | 1 | 58152 | 1 | 58673 | 1 | 59426 | 1 | 61120 | 1 | 61558 | 1 | 61760 | 1 |
| 55860 | 1 | 57265 | 1 | 58180 | 1 | 58674 | 1 | 59430 | 1 | 61140 | 1 | 61559 | 1 | 61770 | 1 |
| 55862 | 1 | 57267 | 2 | 58200 | 1 | 58700 | 1 | 59510 | 1 | 61150 | 1 | 61563 | 2 | 61781 | 1 |
| 55865 | 1 | 57268 | 1 | 58210 | 1 | 58720 | 1 | 59514 | 1 | 61151 | 1 | 61564 | 1 | 61782 | 1 |
| 55866 | 1 | 57270 | 1 | 58240 | 1 | 58740 | 1 | 59515 | 1 | 61154 | 1 | 61566 | 1 | 61783 | 1 |
| 55870 | 1 | 57280 | 1 | 58260 | 1 | 58750 | 1 | 59525 | 1 | 61156 | 1 | 61567 | 1 | 61790 | 1 |
| 55873 | 1 | 57282 | 1 | 58262 | 1 | 58752 | 1 | 59610 | 1 | 61210 | 1 | 61570 | 1 | 61791 | 1 |
| 55875 | 1 | 57283 | 1 | 58263 | 1 | 58760 | 1 | 59612 | 2 | 61215 | 1 | 61571 | 1 | 61796 | 1 |
| 55876 | 1 | 57284 | 1 | 58267 | 1 | 58770 | 1 | 59614 | 1 | 61250 | 1 | 61575 | 1 | 61797 | 4 |
| 55920 | 1 | 57285 | 1 | 58270 | 1 | 58800 | 1 | 59618 | 1 | 61253 | 1 | 61576 | 1 | 61798 | 1 |
| 56405 | 2 | 57287 | 1 | 58275 | 1 | 58805 | 1 | 59620 | 1 | 61304 | 1 | 61580 | 1 | 61799 | 4 |
| 56420 | 1 | 57288 | 1 | 58280 | 1 | 58820 | 1 | 59622 | 1 | 61305 | 1 | 61581 | 1 | 61800 | 1 |
| 56440 | 1 | 57289 | 1 | 58285 | 1 | 58822 | 1 | 59812 | 1 | 61312 | 2 | 61582 | 1 | 61850 | 1 |
| 56441 | 1 | 57291 | 1 | 58290 | 1 | 58825 | 1 | 59820 | 1 | 61313 | 2 | 61583 | 1 | 61860 | 1 |
| 56442 | 1 | 57292 | 1 | 58291 | 1 | 58900 | 1 | 59821 | 1 | 61314 | 2 | 61584 | 1 | 61863 | 1 |
| 56501 | 1 | 57295 | 1 | 58292 | 1 | 58920 | 1 | 59830 | 1 | 61315 | 1 | 61585 | 1 | 61864 | 1 |
| 56515 | 1 | 57296 | 1 | 58293 | 1 | 58925 | 1 | 59840 | 1 | 61316 | 1 | 61586 | 1 | 61867 | 1 |
| 56605 | 1 | 57300 | 1 | 58294 | 1 | 58940 | 1 | 59841 | 1 | 61320 | 2 | 61590 | 1 | 61868 | 2 |
| 56606 | 6 | 57305 | 1 | 58301 | 1 | 58943 | 1 | 59850 | 1 | 61321 | 1 | 61591 | 1 | 61870 | 1 |
| 56620 | 1 | 57307 | 1 | 58321 | 1 | 58950 | 1 | 59851 | 1 | 61322 | 1 | 61592 | 1 | 61880 | 1 |
| 56625 | 1 | 57308 | 1 | 58322 | 1 | 58951 | 1 | 59852 | 1 | 61323 | 1 | 61595 | 1 | 61885 | 2 |
| 56630 | 1 | 57310 | 1 | 58323 | 1 | 58952 | 1 | 59855 | 1 | 61330 | 1 | 61596 | 1 | 61886 | 1 |
| 56631 | 1 | 57311 | 1 | 58340 | 1 | 58953 | 1 | 59856 | 1 | 61332 | 1 | 61597 | 1 | 61888 | 1 |
| 56632 | 1 | 57320 | 1 | 58345 | 1 | 58954 | 1 | 59857 | 1 | 61333 | 1 | 61598 | 1 | 62000 | 1 |
| 56633 | 1 | 57330 | 1 | 58346 | 1 | 58956 | 1 | 59866 | 1 | 61340 | 1 | 61600 | 1 | 62005 | 1 |
| 56634 | 1 | 57335 | 1 | 58350 | 1 | 58957 | 1 | 59870 | 1 | 61343 | 1 | 61601 | 1 | 62010 | 1 |
| 56637 | 1 | 57400 | 1 | 58353 | 1 | 58958 | 1 | 59871 | 1 | 61345 | 1 | 61605 | 1 | 62100 | 1 |
| 56640 | 1 | 57410 | 1 | 58356 | 1 | 58960 | 1 | 60000 | 1 | 61450 | 1 | 61606 | 1 | 62115 | 1 |
| 56700 | 1 | 57415 | 1 | 58400 | 1 | 58970 | 1 | 60100 | 3 | 61458 | 1 | 61607 | 1 | 62117 | 1 |
| 56740 | 1 | 57420 | 1 | 58410 | 1 | 58974 | 1 | 60200 | 2 | 61460 | 1 | 61608 | 1 | 62120 | 1 |
| 56800 | 1 | 57421 | 1 | 58520 | 1 | 58976 | 2 | 60210 | 1 | 61480 | 1 | 61610 | 1 | 62121 | 1 |
| 56805 | 1 | 57423 | 1 | 58540 | 1 | 59000 | 2 | 60212 | 1 | 61500 | 1 | 61611 | 1 | 62140 | 1 |
| 56810 | 1 | 57425 | 1 | 58541 | 1 | 59001 | 2 | 60220 | 1 | 61501 | 1 | 61612 | 1 | 62141 | 1 |
| 56820 | 1 | 57426 | 1 | 58542 | 1 | 59012 | 2 | 60225 | 1 | 61510 | 1 | 61613 | 1 | 62142 | 2 |
| 56821 | 1 | 57452 | 1 | 58543 | 1 | 59015 | 2 | 60240 | 1 | 61512 | 1 | 61615 | 1 | 62143 | 2 |
| 57000 | 1 | 57454 | 1 | 58544 | 1 | 59020 | 2 | 60252 | 1 | 61514 | 2 | 61616 | 1 | 62145 | 2 |

CPT © 2017 American Medical Association. All Rights Reserved.     © 2017 Optum360, LLC

| CPT | MUE | CPT | MUE | CPT | MUE | CPT | MUE | CPT | MUE | CPT | MUE | CPT | MUE | CPT | MUE |
|---|---|---|---|---|---|---|---|---|---|---|---|---|---|---|---|
| 62146 | 2 | 63005 | 1 | 63275 | 1 | 64449 | 1 | 64680 | 1 | 64868 | 1 | 65770 | 1 | 66920 | 1 |
| 62147 | 1 | 63011 | 1 | 63276 | 1 | 64450 | 10 | 64681 | 1 | 64872 | 1 | 65772 | 1 | 66930 | 1 |
| 62148 | 1 | 63012 | 1 | 63277 | 1 | 64455 | 1 | 64702 | 2 | 64874 | 1 | 65775 | 1 | 66940 | 1 |
| 62160 | 1 | 63015 | 1 | 63278 | 1 | 64461 | 1 | 64704 | 4 | 64876 | 1 | 65778 | 1 | 66982 | 1 |
| 62161 | 1 | 63016 | 1 | 63280 | 1 | 64462 | 1 | 64708 | 3 | 64885 | 1 | 65779 | 1 | 66983 | 1 |
| 62162 | 1 | 63017 | 1 | 63281 | 1 | 64463 | 1 | 64712 | 1 | 64886 | 1 | 65780 | 1 | 66984 | 1 |
| 62163 | 1 | 63020 | 1 | 63282 | 1 | 64479 | 1 | 64713 | 1 | 64890 | 2 | 65781 | 1 | 66985 | 1 |
| 62164 | 1 | 63030 | 1 | 63283 | 1 | 64480 | 4 | 64714 | 1 | 64891 | 2 | 65782 | 1 | 66986 | 1 |
| 62165 | 1 | 63035 | 4 | 63285 | 1 | 64483 | 1 | 64716 | 2 | 64892 | 2 | 65785 | 1 | 66990 | 1 |
| 62180 | 1 | 63040 | 1 | 63286 | 1 | 64484 | 4 | 64718 | 1 | 64893 | 2 | 65800 | 1 | 67005 | 1 |
| 62190 | 1 | 63042 | 1 | 63287 | 1 | 64486 | 1 | 64719 | 1 | 64895 | 2 | 65810 | 1 | 67010 | 1 |
| 62192 | 1 | 63043 | 4 | 63290 | 1 | 64487 | 1 | 64721 | 1 | 64896 | 2 | 65815 | 1 | 67015 | 1 |
| 62194 | 1 | 63044 | 4 | 63295 | 1 | 64488 | 1 | 64722 | 4 | 64897 | 2 | 65820 | 1 | 67025 | 1 |
| 62200 | 1 | 63045 | 1 | 63300 | 1 | 64489 | 1 | 64726 | 2 | 64898 | 2 | 65850 | 1 | 67027 | 1 |
| 62201 | 1 | 63046 | 1 | 63301 | 1 | 64490 | 1 | 64727 | 2 | 64901 | 2 | 65855 | 1 | 67028 | 1 |
| 62220 | 1 | 63047 | 1 | 63302 | 1 | 64491 | 1 | 64732 | 1 | 64902 | 1 | 65860 | 1 | 67030 | 1 |
| 62223 | 1 | 63048 | 5 | 63303 | 1 | 64492 | 1 | 64734 | 1 | 64905 | 1 | 65865 | 1 | 67031 | 1 |
| 62225 | 2 | 63050 | 1 | 63304 | 1 | 64493 | 1 | 64736 | 1 | 64907 | 1 | 65870 | 1 | 67036 | 1 |
| 62230 | 2 | 63051 | 1 | 63305 | 1 | 64494 | 1 | 64738 | 1 | 64910 | 3 | 65875 | 1 | 67039 | 1 |
| 62252 | 2 | 63055 | 1 | 63306 | 1 | 64495 | 1 | 64740 | 1 | 64911 | 2 | 65880 | 1 | 67040 | 1 |
| 62256 | 1 | 63056 | 1 | 63307 | 1 | 64505 | 1 | 64742 | 1 | 65091 | 1 | 65900 | 1 | 67041 | 1 |
| 62258 | 1 | 63057 | 3 | 63308 | 3 | 64508 | 1 | 64744 | 1 | 65093 | 1 | 65920 | 1 | 67042 | 1 |
| 62263 | 1 | 63064 | 1 | 63600 | 2 | 64510 | 1 | 64746 | 1 | 65101 | 1 | 65930 | 1 | 67043 | 1 |
| 62264 | 1 | 63066 | 1 | 63610 | 1 | 64517 | 1 | 64755 | 1 | 65103 | 1 | 66020 | 1 | 67101 | 1 |
| 62267 | 2 | 63075 | 1 | 63615 | 1 | 64520 | 1 | 64760 | 1 | 65105 | 1 | 66030 | 1 | 67105 | 1 |
| 62268 | 1 | 63076 | 3 | 63620 | 1 | 64530 | 1 | 64763 | 1 | 65110 | 1 | 66130 | 1 | 67107 | 1 |
| 62269 | 2 | 63077 | 1 | 63621 | 2 | 64550 | 1 | 64766 | 1 | 65112 | 1 | 66150 | 1 | 67108 | 1 |
| 62270 | 2 | 63078 | 3 | 63650 | 2 | 64553 | 1 | 64771 | 2 | 65114 | 1 | 66155 | 1 | 67110 | 1 |
| 62272 | 2 | 63081 | 1 | 63655 | 1 | 64555 | 2 | 64772 | 2 | 65125 | 1 | 66160 | 1 | 67113 | 1 |
| 62273 | 2 | 63082 | 6 | 63661 | 1 | 64561 | 1 | 64774 | 2 | 65130 | 1 | 66170 | 1 | 67115 | 1 |
| 62280 | 1 | 63085 | 1 | 63662 | 1 | 64565 | 2 | 64776 | 1 | 65135 | 1 | 66172 | 1 | 67120 | 1 |
| 62281 | 1 | 63086 | 2 | 63663 | 1 | 64566 | 1 | 64778 | 1 | 65140 | 1 | 66174 | 1 | 67121 | 1 |
| 62282 | 1 | 63087 | 1 | 63664 | 1 | 64568 | 1 | 64782 | 2 | 65150 | 1 | 66175 | 1 | 67141 | 1 |
| 62284 | 1 | 63088 | 4 | 63685 | 1 | 64569 | 1 | 64783 | 2 | 65155 | 1 | 66179 | 1 | 67145 | 1 |
| 62287 | 1 | 63090 | 1 | 63688 | 1 | 64570 | 1 | 64784 | 3 | 65175 | 1 | 66180 | 1 | 67208 | 1 |
| 62290 | 5 | 63091 | 3 | 63700 | 1 | 64575 | 2 | 64786 | 1 | 65205 | 1 | 66183 | 1 | 67210 | 1 |
| 62291 | 4 | 63101 | 1 | 63702 | 1 | 64580 | 2 | 64787 | 4 | 65210 | 1 | 66184 | 1 | 67218 | 1 |
| 62292 | 1 | 63102 | 1 | 63704 | 1 | 64581 | 2 | 64788 | 5 | 65220 | 1 | 66185 | 1 | 67220 | 1 |
| 62294 | 1 | 63103 | 3 | 63706 | 1 | 64585 | 2 | 64790 | 1 | 65222 | 1 | 66220 | 1 | 67221 | 1 |
| 62302 | 1 | 63170 | 1 | 63707 | 1 | 64590 | 1 | 64792 | 2 | 65235 | 1 | 66225 | 1 | 67225 | 1 |
| 62303 | 1 | 63172 | 1 | 63709 | 1 | 64595 | 1 | 64795 | 2 | 65260 | 1 | 66250 | 1 | 67227 | 1 |
| 62304 | 1 | 63173 | 1 | 63710 | 1 | 64600 | 2 | 64802 | 1 | 65265 | 1 | 66500 | 1 | 67228 | 1 |
| 62305 | 1 | 63180 | 1 | 63740 | 1 | 64605 | 1 | 64804 | 1 | 65270 | 1 | 66505 | 1 | 67229 | 1 |
| 62320 | 1 | 63182 | 1 | 63741 | 1 | 64610 | 1 | 64809 | 1 | 65272 | 1 | 66600 | 1 | 67250 | 1 |
| 62321 | 1 | 63185 | 1 | 63744 | 1 | 64611 | 1 | 64818 | 1 | 65273 | 1 | 66605 | 1 | 67255 | 1 |
| 62322 | 1 | 63190 | 1 | 63746 | 1 | 64612 | 1 | 64820 | 4 | 65275 | 1 | 66625 | 1 | 67311 | 1 |
| 62323 | 1 | 63191 | 1 | 64400 | 4 | 64615 | 1 | 64821 | 1 | 65280 | 1 | 66630 | 1 | 67312 | 1 |
| 62324 | 1 | 63194 | 1 | 64402 | 1 | 64616 | 1 | 64822 | 1 | 65285 | 1 | 66635 | 1 | 67314 | 1 |
| 62325 | 1 | 63195 | 1 | 64405 | 1 | 64617 | 1 | 64823 | 1 | 65286 | 1 | 66680 | 1 | 67316 | 1 |
| 62326 | 1 | 63196 | 1 | 64408 | 1 | 64620 | 5 | 64831 | 1 | 65290 | 1 | 66682 | 1 | 67318 | 1 |
| 62327 | 1 | 63197 | 1 | 64410 | 1 | 64630 | 1 | 64832 | 3 | 65400 | 1 | 66700 | 1 | 67320 | 2 |
| 62350 | 1 | 63198 | 1 | 64413 | 1 | 64632 | 1 | 64834 | 1 | 65410 | 1 | 66710 | 1 | 67331 | 1 |
| 62351 | 1 | 63199 | 1 | 64415 | 1 | 64633 | 1 | 64835 | 1 | 65420 | 1 | 66711 | 1 | 67332 | 1 |
| 62355 | 1 | 63200 | 1 | 64416 | 1 | 64634 | 4 | 64836 | 1 | 65426 | 1 | 66720 | 1 | 67334 | 1 |
| 62360 | 1 | 63250 | 1 | 64417 | 1 | 64635 | 1 | 64837 | 2 | 65430 | 1 | 66740 | 1 | 67335 | 1 |
| 62361 | 1 | 63251 | 1 | 64418 | 1 | 64636 | 4 | 64840 | 1 | 65435 | 1 | 66761 | 1 | 67340 | 2 |
| 62362 | 1 | 63252 | 1 | 64420 | 3 | 64640 | 5 | 64856 | 2 | 65436 | 1 | 66762 | 1 | 67343 | 1 |
| 62365 | 1 | 63265 | 1 | 64421 | 3 | 64642 | 1 | 64857 | 2 | 65450 | 1 | 66770 | 1 | 67345 | 1 |
| 62367 | 1 | 63266 | 1 | 64425 | 1 | 64643 | 3 | 64858 | 1 | 65600 | 1 | 66820 | 1 | 67346 | 1 |
| 62368 | 1 | 63267 | 1 | 64430 | 1 | 64644 | 1 | 64859 | 2 | 65710 | 1 | 66821 | 1 | 67400 | 1 |
| 62369 | 1 | 63268 | 1 | 64435 | 1 | 64645 | 3 | 64861 | 1 | 65730 | 1 | 66825 | 1 | 67405 | 1 |
| 62370 | 1 | 63270 | 1 | 64445 | 1 | 64646 | 1 | 64862 | 1 | 65750 | 1 | 66830 | 1 | 67412 | 1 |
| 62380 | 1 | 63271 | 1 | 64446 | 1 | 64647 | 1 | 64864 | 2 | 65755 | 1 | 66840 | 1 | 67413 | 1 |
| 63001 | 1 | 63272 | 1 | 64447 | 1 | 64650 | 1 | 64865 | 1 | 65756 | 1 | 66850 | 1 | 67414 | 1 |
| 63003 | 1 | 63273 | 1 | 64448 | 1 | 64653 | 1 | 64866 | 1 | 65757 | 1 | 66852 | 1 | 67415 | 1 |

© 2017 Optum360, LLC

**Appendix I — Medically Unlikely Edits (MUEs) — OPPS**

| CPT | MUE | CPT | MUE | CPT | MUE | CPT | MUE | CPT | MUE | CPT | MUE | CPT | MUE | CPT | MUE |
|---|---|---|---|---|---|---|---|---|---|---|---|---|---|---|---|
| 67420 | 1 | 68325 | 1 | 69511 | 1 | 70134 | 1 | 71035 | 3 | 72270 | 1 | 73725 | 2 | 75559 | 1 |
| 67430 | 1 | 68326 | 2 | 69530 | 1 | 70140 | 2 | 71100 | 2 | 72275 | 3 | 74000 | 4 | 75561 | 1 |
| 67440 | 1 | 68328 | 2 | 69535 | 1 | 70150 | 1 | 71101 | 2 | 72285 | 4 | 74010 | 2 | 75563 | 1 |
| 67445 | 1 | 68330 | 1 | 69540 | 1 | 70160 | 1 | 71110 | 1 | 72295 | 5 | 74020 | 2 | 75565 | 1 |
| 67450 | 1 | 68335 | 1 | 69550 | 1 | 70170 | 2 | 71111 | 1 | 73000 | 2 | 74022 | 2 | 75571 | 1 |
| 67500 | 1 | 68340 | 1 | 69552 | 1 | 70190 | 1 | 71120 | 1 | 73010 | 2 | 74150 | 1 | 75572 | 1 |
| 67505 | 1 | 68360 | 1 | 69554 | 1 | 70200 | 2 | 71130 | 1 | 73020 | 2 | 74160 | 1 | 75573 | 1 |
| 67515 | 1 | 68362 | 1 | 69601 | 1 | 70210 | 1 | 71250 | 2 | 73030 | 4 | 74170 | 1 | 75574 | 1 |
| 67550 | 1 | 68371 | 1 | 69602 | 1 | 70220 | 1 | 71260 | 2 | 73040 | 2 | 74174 | 1 | 75600 | 1 |
| 67560 | 1 | 68400 | 1 | 69603 | 1 | 70240 | 1 | 71270 | 1 | 73050 | 1 | 74175 | 1 | 75605 | 1 |
| 67570 | 1 | 68420 | 1 | 69604 | 1 | 70250 | 2 | 71275 | 1 | 73060 | 2 | 74176 | 2 | 75625 | 1 |
| 67700 | 2 | 68440 | 2 | 69605 | 1 | 70260 | 1 | 71550 | 1 | 73070 | 2 | 74177 | 2 | 75630 | 1 |
| 67710 | 1 | 68500 | 1 | 69610 | 1 | 70300 | 1 | 71551 | 1 | 73080 | 2 | 74178 | 1 | 75635 | 1 |
| 67715 | 1 | 68505 | 1 | 69620 | 1 | 70310 | 1 | 71552 | 1 | 73085 | 2 | 74181 | 1 | 75658 | 1 |
| 67800 | 1 | 68510 | 1 | 69631 | 1 | 70320 | 1 | 71555 | 1 | 73090 | 2 | 74182 | 1 | 75705 | 20 |
| 67801 | 1 | 68520 | 1 | 69632 | 1 | 70328 | 1 | 72020 | 4 | 73092 | 2 | 74183 | 1 | 75710 | 2 |
| 67805 | 1 | 68525 | 1 | 69633 | 1 | 70330 | 1 | 72040 | 3 | 73100 | 2 | 74185 | 1 | 75716 | 1 |
| 67808 | 1 | 68530 | 1 | 69635 | 1 | 70332 | 2 | 72050 | 1 | 73110 | 3 | 74190 | 1 | 75726 | 3 |
| 67810 | 2 | 68540 | 1 | 69636 | 1 | 70336 | 1 | 72052 | 1 | 73115 | 2 | 74210 | 1 | 75731 | 1 |
| 67820 | 1 | 68550 | 1 | 69637 | 1 | 70350 | 1 | 72070 | 1 | 73120 | 3 | 74220 | 1 | 75733 | 1 |
| 67825 | 1 | 68700 | 1 | 69641 | 1 | 70355 | 1 | 72072 | 1 | 73130 | 3 | 74230 | 1 | 75736 | 2 |
| 67830 | 1 | 68705 | 2 | 69642 | 1 | 70360 | 2 | 72074 | 1 | 73140 | 3 | 74235 | 1 | 75741 | 1 |
| 67835 | 1 | 68720 | 1 | 69643 | 1 | 70370 | 1 | 72080 | 1 | 73200 | 2 | 74240 | 2 | 75743 | 1 |
| 67840 | 4 | 68745 | 1 | 69644 | 1 | 70371 | 1 | 72081 | 1 | 73201 | 2 | 74241 | 1 | 75746 | 1 |
| 67850 | 3 | 68750 | 1 | 69645 | 1 | 70380 | 2 | 72082 | 1 | 73202 | 2 | 74245 | 1 | 75756 | 2 |
| 67875 | 1 | 68760 | 4 | 69646 | 1 | 70390 | 2 | 72083 | 1 | 73206 | 2 | 74246 | 1 | 75774 | 7 |
| 67880 | 1 | 68761 | 4 | 69650 | 1 | 70450 | 3 | 72084 | 1 | 73218 | 2 | 74247 | 1 | 75801 | 1 |
| 67882 | 1 | 68770 | 1 | 69660 | 1 | 70460 | 1 | 72100 | 2 | 73219 | 2 | 74249 | 1 | 75803 | 1 |
| 67900 | 1 | 68801 | 4 | 69661 | 1 | 70470 | 2 | 72110 | 1 | 73220 | 2 | 74250 | 1 | 75805 | 1 |
| 67901 | 1 | 68810 | 1 | 69662 | 1 | 70480 | 1 | 72114 | 1 | 73221 | 2 | 74251 | 1 | 75807 | 1 |
| 67902 | 1 | 68811 | 1 | 69666 | 1 | 70481 | 1 | 72120 | 1 | 73222 | 2 | 74260 | 1 | 75809 | 1 |
| 67903 | 1 | 68815 | 1 | 69667 | 1 | 70482 | 1 | 72125 | 1 | 73223 | 2 | 74261 | 1 | 75810 | 1 |
| 67904 | 1 | 68816 | 1 | 69670 | 1 | 70486 | 1 | 72126 | 1 | 73501 | 2 | 74262 | 1 | 75820 | 2 |
| 67906 | 1 | 68840 | 1 | 69676 | 1 | 70487 | 1 | 72127 | 1 | 73502 | 2 | 74270 | 1 | 75822 | 1 |
| 67908 | 1 | 68850 | 1 | 69700 | 1 | 70488 | 1 | 72128 | 1 | 73503 | 2 | 74280 | 1 | 75825 | 1 |
| 67909 | 1 | 69000 | 1 | 69711 | 1 | 70490 | 1 | 72129 | 1 | 73521 | 2 | 74283 | 1 | 75827 | 1 |
| 67911 | 4 | 69005 | 1 | 69714 | 1 | 70491 | 1 | 72130 | 1 | 73522 | 2 | 74290 | 1 | 75831 | 1 |
| 67912 | 1 | 69020 | 1 | 69715 | 1 | 70492 | 1 | 72131 | 1 | 73523 | 2 | 74300 | 1 | 75833 | 1 |
| 67914 | 2 | 69100 | 3 | 69717 | 1 | 70496 | 2 | 72132 | 1 | 73525 | 2 | 74301 | 1 | 75840 | 1 |
| 67915 | 2 | 69105 | 1 | 69718 | 1 | 70498 | 2 | 72133 | 1 | 73551 | 2 | 74328 | 1 | 75842 | 1 |
| 67916 | 2 | 69110 | 1 | 69720 | 1 | 70540 | 1 | 72141 | 1 | 73552 | 2 | 74329 | 1 | 75860 | 2 |
| 67917 | 2 | 69120 | 1 | 69725 | 1 | 70542 | 1 | 72142 | 1 | 73560 | 4 | 74330 | 1 | 75870 | 1 |
| 67921 | 2 | 69140 | 1 | 69740 | 1 | 70543 | 1 | 72146 | 1 | 73562 | 4 | 74340 | 1 | 75872 | 1 |
| 67922 | 2 | 69145 | 1 | 69745 | 1 | 70544 | 2 | 72147 | 1 | 73564 | 4 | 74355 | 1 | 75880 | 1 |
| 67923 | 2 | 69150 | 1 | 69801 | 1 | 70545 | 1 | 72148 | 1 | 73565 | 1 | 74360 | 1 | 75885 | 1 |
| 67924 | 2 | 69155 | 1 | 69805 | 1 | 70546 | 1 | 72149 | 1 | 73580 | 2 | 74363 | 2 | 75887 | 1 |
| 67930 | 2 | 69200 | 1 | 69806 | 1 | 70547 | 1 | 72156 | 1 | 73590 | 3 | 74400 | 1 | 75889 | 1 |
| 67935 | 2 | 69205 | 1 | 69820 | 1 | 70548 | 1 | 72157 | 1 | 73592 | 2 | 74410 | 1 | 75891 | 1 |
| 67938 | 2 | 69209 | 1 | 69840 | 1 | 70549 | 1 | 72158 | 1 | 73600 | 3 | 74415 | 1 | 75893 | 2 |
| 67950 | 2 | 69210 | 1 | 69905 | 1 | 70551 | 2 | 72170 | 2 | 73610 | 3 | 74420 | 2 | 75894 | 2 |
| 67961 | 4 | 69220 | 1 | 69910 | 1 | 70552 | 2 | 72190 | 1 | 73615 | 2 | 74425 | 2 | 75898 | 2 |
| 67966 | 4 | 69222 | 1 | 69915 | 1 | 70553 | 2 | 72191 | 1 | 73620 | 3 | 74430 | 1 | 75901 | 1 |
| 67971 | 1 | 69300 | 1 | 69930 | 1 | 70554 | 1 | 72192 | 1 | 73630 | 3 | 74440 | 1 | 75902 | 2 |
| 67973 | 1 | 69310 | 1 | 69950 | 1 | 70555 | 1 | 72193 | 1 | 73650 | 2 | 74445 | 1 | 75952 | 1 |
| 67974 | 1 | 69320 | 1 | 69955 | 1 | 70557 | 1 | 72194 | 1 | 73660 | 2 | 74450 | 1 | 75953 | 4 |
| 67975 | 1 | 69420 | 1 | 69960 | 1 | 70558 | 1 | 72195 | 1 | 73700 | 2 | 74455 | 1 | 75954 | 1 |
| 68020 | 1 | 69421 | 1 | 69970 | 1 | 70559 | 1 | 72196 | 1 | 73701 | 2 | 74470 | 2 | 75956 | 1 |
| 68040 | 1 | 69424 | 1 | 69990 | 1 | 71010 | 6 | 72197 | 1 | 73702 | 2 | 74485 | 2 | 75957 | 1 |
| 68100 | 1 | 69433 | 1 | 70010 | 1 | 71015 | 2 | 72198 | 1 | 73706 | 2 | 74710 | 1 | 75958 | 2 |
| 68110 | 1 | 69436 | 1 | 70015 | 1 | 71020 | 4 | 72200 | 2 | 73718 | 2 | 74712 | 1 | 75959 | 1 |
| 68115 | 1 | 69440 | 1 | 70030 | 2 | 71021 | 1 | 72202 | 1 | 73719 | 2 | 74713 | 2 | 75970 | 1 |
| 68130 | 1 | 69450 | 1 | 70100 | 2 | 71022 | 1 | 72220 | 1 | 73720 | 2 | 74740 | 1 | 75984 | 2 |
| 68135 | 1 | 69501 | 1 | 70110 | 2 | 71023 | 1 | 72240 | 1 | 73721 | 3 | 74742 | 2 | 75989 | 2 |
| 68200 | 1 | 69502 | 1 | 70120 | 1 | 71030 | 1 | 72255 | 1 | 73722 | 2 | 74775 | 1 | 76000 | 3 |
| 68320 | 1 | 69505 | 1 | 70130 | 1 | 71034 | 1 | 72265 | 1 | 73723 | 2 | 75557 | 1 | 76001 | 1 |

CPT © 2017 American Medical Association. All Rights Reserved.    © 2017 Optum360, LLC

| CPT | MUE | CPT | MUE | CPT | MUE | CPT | MUE | CPT | MUE | CPT | MUE | CPT | MUE | CPT | MUE |
|---|---|---|---|---|---|---|---|---|---|---|---|---|---|---|---|
| 76010 | 2 | 76940 | 1 | 77370 | 1 | 78185 | 1 | 78606 | 1 | 80173 | 2 | 81201 | 1 | 81295 | 1 |
| 76080 | 3 | 76941 | 3 | 77371 | 1 | 78190 | 1 | 78607 | 1 | 80175 | 1 | 81202 | 1 | 81296 | 1 |
| 76098 | 3 | 76942 | 1 | 77372 | 1 | 78191 | 1 | 78608 | 1 | 80176 | 1 | 81203 | 1 | 81297 | 1 |
| 76100 | 2 | 76945 | 1 | 77373 | 1 | 78195 | 1 | 78610 | 1 | 80177 | 1 | 81205 | 1 | 81298 | 1 |
| 76101 | 1 | 76946 | 1 | 77385 | 2 | 78201 | 1 | 78630 | 1 | 80178 | 2 | 81206 | 1 | 81299 | 1 |
| 76102 | 1 | 76948 | 1 | 77386 | 2 | 78202 | 1 | 78635 | 1 | 80180 | 1 | 81207 | 1 | 81300 | 1 |
| 76120 | 1 | 76965 | 2 | 77387 | 2 | 78205 | 1 | 78645 | 1 | 80183 | 1 | 81208 | 1 | 81301 | 1 |
| 76125 | 1 | 76970 | 2 | 77401 | 1 | 78206 | 1 | 78647 | 1 | 80184 | 2 | 81209 | 1 | 81302 | 1 |
| 76376 | 2 | 76975 | 1 | 77402 | 2 | 78215 | 1 | 78650 | 1 | 80185 | 2 | 81210 | 1 | 81303 | 1 |
| 76377 | 1 | 76977 | 1 | 77407 | 2 | 78216 | 1 | 78660 | 1 | 80186 | 2 | 81211 | 1 | 81304 | 1 |
| 76380 | 2 | 76998 | 1 | 77412 | 2 | 78226 | 1 | 78700 | 1 | 80188 | 2 | 81212 | 1 | 81310 | 1 |
| 76506 | 1 | 77001 | 2 | 77417 | 1 | 78227 | 1 | 78701 | 1 | 80190 | 2 | 81213 | 1 | 81311 | 1 |
| 76510 | 1 | 77002 | 1 | 77422 | 1 | 78230 | 1 | 78707 | 1 | 80192 | 2 | 81214 | 1 | 81313 | 1 |
| 76511 | 2 | 77003 | 1 | 77423 | 1 | 78231 | 1 | 78708 | 1 | 80194 | 2 | 81215 | 1 | 81314 | 1 |
| 76512 | 2 | 77011 | 1 | 77424 | 1 | 78232 | 1 | 78709 | 1 | 80195 | 2 | 81216 | 1 | 81315 | 1 |
| 76513 | 2 | 77012 | 1 | 77425 | 1 | 78258 | 1 | 78710 | 1 | 80197 | 2 | 81217 | 1 | 81316 | 1 |
| 76514 | 1 | 77013 | 1 | 77427 | 1 | 78261 | 1 | 78725 | 1 | 80198 | 2 | 81218 | 1 | 81317 | 1 |
| 76516 | 1 | 77014 | 2 | 77431 | 1 | 78262 | 1 | 78730 | 1 | 80199 | 1 | 81219 | 1 | 81318 | 1 |
| 76519 | 1 | 77021 | 1 | 77432 | 1 | 78264 | 1 | 78740 | 1 | 80200 | 2 | 81220 | 1 | 81319 | 1 |
| 76529 | 2 | 77022 | 1 | 77435 | 1 | 78265 | 1 | 78761 | 1 | 80201 | 2 | 81221 | 1 | 81321 | 1 |
| 76536 | 1 | 77053 | 2 | 77469 | 1 | 78266 | 1 | 78800 | 1 | 80202 | 2 | 81222 | 1 | 81322 | 1 |
| 76604 | 1 | 77054 | 2 | 77470 | 1 | 78267 | 1 | 78801 | 1 | 80203 | 1 | 81223 | 1 | 81323 | 1 |
| 76641 | 2 | 77058 | 1 | 77520 | 1 | 78268 | 1 | 78802 | 1 | 80299 | 3 | 81224 | 1 | 81324 | 1 |
| 76642 | 2 | 77059 | 1 | 77522 | 1 | 78270 | 1 | 78803 | 1 | 80305 | 1 | 81225 | 1 | 81325 | 1 |
| 76700 | 1 | 77061 | 1 | 77523 | 1 | 78271 | 1 | 78804 | 1 | 80306 | 1 | 81226 | 1 | 81326 | 1 |
| 76705 | 2 | 77062 | 1 | 77525 | 1 | 78272 | 1 | 78805 | 1 | 80307 | 1 | 81227 | 1 | 81327 | 1 |
| 76706 | 1 | 77063 | 1 | 77600 | 1 | 78278 | 2 | 78806 | 1 | 80400 | 1 | 81228 | 1 | 81330 | 1 |
| 76770 | 1 | 77065 | 1 | 77605 | 1 | 78282 | 1 | 78807 | 1 | 80402 | 1 | 81229 | 1 | 81331 | 1 |
| 76775 | 2 | 77066 | 1 | 77610 | 1 | 78290 | 1 | 78808 | 1 | 80406 | 1 | 81235 | 1 | 81332 | 1 |
| 76776 | 2 | 77067 | 1 | 77615 | 1 | 78291 | 1 | 78811 | 1 | 80408 | 1 | 81240 | 1 | 81340 | 1 |
| 76800 | 1 | 77071 | 1 | 77620 | 1 | 78300 | 1 | 78812 | 1 | 80410 | 1 | 81241 | 1 | 81341 | 1 |
| 76801 | 1 | 77072 | 1 | 77750 | 1 | 78305 | 1 | 78813 | 1 | 80412 | 1 | 81242 | 1 | 81342 | 1 |
| 76802 | 2 | 77073 | 1 | 77761 | 1 | 78306 | 1 | 78814 | 1 | 80414 | 1 | 81243 | 1 | 81350 | 1 |
| 76805 | 1 | 77074 | 1 | 77762 | 1 | 78315 | 1 | 78815 | 1 | 80415 | 1 | 81244 | 1 | 81355 | 1 |
| 76810 | 2 | 77075 | 1 | 77763 | 1 | 78320 | 1 | 78816 | 1 | 80416 | 1 | 81245 | 1 | 81370 | 1 |
| 76811 | 1 | 77076 | 1 | 77767 | 2 | 78414 | 1 | 79005 | 1 | 80417 | 1 | 81246 | 1 | 81371 | 1 |
| 76812 | 2 | 77077 | 1 | 77768 | 2 | 78428 | 1 | 79101 | 1 | 80418 | 1 | 81250 | 1 | 81372 | 1 |
| 76813 | 1 | 77078 | 1 | 77770 | 2 | 78445 | 1 | 79200 | 1 | 80420 | 1 | 81251 | 1 | 81373 | 2 |
| 76814 | 2 | 77080 | 1 | 77771 | 2 | 78451 | 1 | 79300 | 1 | 80422 | 1 | 81252 | 1 | 81374 | 1 |
| 76815 | 1 | 77081 | 1 | 77772 | 2 | 78452 | 1 | 79403 | 1 | 80424 | 1 | 81253 | 1 | 81375 | 1 |
| 76816 | 3 | 77084 | 1 | 77778 | 1 | 78453 | 1 | 79440 | 1 | 80426 | 1 | 81254 | 1 | 81376 | 5 |
| 76817 | 1 | 77085 | 1 | 77789 | 2 | 78454 | 1 | 79445 | 1 | 80428 | 1 | 81255 | 1 | 81377 | 2 |
| 76818 | 3 | 77086 | 1 | 77790 | 1 | 78456 | 1 | 80047 | 2 | 80430 | 1 | 81256 | 1 | 81378 | 1 |
| 76819 | 3 | 77261 | 1 | 78012 | 1 | 78457 | 1 | 80048 | 2 | 80432 | 1 | 81257 | 1 | 81379 | 1 |
| 76820 | 3 | 77262 | 1 | 78013 | 1 | 78458 | 1 | 80051 | 4 | 80434 | 1 | 81260 | 1 | 81380 | 2 |
| 76821 | 3 | 77263 | 1 | 78014 | 1 | 78459 | 1 | 80053 | 1 | 80435 | 1 | 81261 | 1 | 81381 | 3 |
| 76825 | 3 | 77280 | 2 | 78015 | 1 | 78466 | 1 | 80061 | 1 | 80436 | 1 | 81262 | 1 | 81382 | 6 |
| 76826 | 3 | 77285 | 1 | 78016 | 1 | 78468 | 1 | 80069 | 1 | 80438 | 1 | 81263 | 1 | 81383 | 2 |
| 76827 | 3 | 77290 | 1 | 78018 | 1 | 78469 | 1 | 80074 | 1 | 80439 | 1 | 81264 | 1 | 81400 | 2 |
| 76828 | 3 | 77293 | 1 | 78020 | 1 | 78472 | 1 | 80076 | 1 | 80500 | 1 | 81265 | 1 | 81401 | 3 |
| 76830 | 1 | 77295 | 1 | 78070 | 1 | 78473 | 1 | 80081 | 1 | 80502 | 1 | 81266 | 2 | 81402 | 1 |
| 76831 | 1 | 77300 | 10 | 78071 | 1 | 78481 | 1 | 80150 | 2 | 81000 | 2 | 81267 | 1 | 81403 | 3 |
| 76856 | 1 | 77301 | 1 | 78072 | 1 | 78483 | 1 | 80155 | 1 | 81001 | 2 | 81268 | 4 | 81404 | 3 |
| 76857 | 1 | 77306 | 1 | 78075 | 1 | 78491 | 1 | 80156 | 2 | 81002 | 2 | 81270 | 1 | 81405 | 2 |
| 76870 | 1 | 77307 | 1 | 78102 | 1 | 78492 | 1 | 80157 | 2 | 81003 | 2 | 81272 | 1 | 81406 | 3 |
| 76872 | 1 | 77316 | 1 | 78103 | 1 | 78494 | 1 | 80158 | 3 | 81005 | 2 | 81273 | 1 | 81407 | 1 |
| 76873 | 1 | 77317 | 1 | 78104 | 1 | 78496 | 1 | 80159 | 2 | 81007 | 1 | 81275 | 1 | 81408 | 1 |
| 76881 | 2 | 77318 | 1 | 78110 | 1 | 78579 | 1 | 80162 | 2 | 81015 | 2 | 81276 | 1 | 81410 | 1 |
| 76882 | 2 | 77321 | 1 | 78111 | 1 | 78580 | 1 | 80163 | 1 | 81020 | 1 | 81287 | 1 | 81411 | 1 |
| 76885 | 1 | 77331 | 3 | 78120 | 1 | 78582 | 1 | 80164 | 2 | 81025 | 1 | 81288 | 1 | 81412 | 1 |
| 76886 | 1 | 77332 | 4 | 78121 | 1 | 78597 | 1 | 80165 | 1 | 81050 | 2 | 81290 | 1 | 81413 | 1 |
| 76930 | 1 | 77333 | 2 | 78122 | 1 | 78598 | 1 | 80168 | 2 | 81161 | 1 | 81291 | 1 | 81414 | 1 |
| 76932 | 1 | 77334 | 10 | 78130 | 1 | 78600 | 1 | 80169 | 2 | 81162 | 1 | 81292 | 1 | 81415 | 1 |
| 76936 | 1 | 77336 | 1 | 78135 | 1 | 78601 | 1 | 80170 | 2 | 81170 | 1 | 81293 | 1 | 81416 | 2 |
| 76937 | 2 | 77338 | 1 | 78140 | 1 | 78605 | 1 | 80171 | 1 | 81200 | 1 | 81294 | 1 | 81417 | 1 |

© 2017 Optum360, LLC

CPT © 2017 American Medical Association. All Rights Reserved.

Appendix I — Medically Unlikely Edits (MUEs) — OPPS

| CPT | MUE | CPT | MUE | CPT | MUE | CPT | MUE | CPT | MUE | CPT | MUE | CPT | MUE | CPT | MUE |
|---|---|---|---|---|---|---|---|---|---|---|---|---|---|---|---|
| 81420 | 1 | 82107 | 1 | 82485 | 1 | 82938 | 1 | 83593 | 1 | 84085 | 1 | 84403 | 2 | 85045 | 1 |
| 81422 | 1 | 82108 | 1 | 82495 | 1 | 82941 | 1 | 83605 | 3 | 84087 | 1 | 84410 | 1 | 85046 | 1 |
| 81425 | 1 | 82120 | 1 | 82507 | 1 | 82943 | 1 | 83615 | 3 | 84100 | 2 | 84425 | 1 | 85048 | 2 |
| 81426 | 2 | 82127 | 1 | 82523 | 1 | 82945 | 4 | 83625 | 1 | 84105 | 1 | 84430 | 1 | 85049 | 2 |
| 81427 | 1 | 82128 | 2 | 82525 | 2 | 82946 | 1 | 83630 | 1 | 84106 | 1 | 84431 | 1 | 85055 | 1 |
| 81430 | 1 | 82131 | 2 | 82528 | 1 | 82947 | 5 | 83631 | 1 | 84110 | 1 | 84432 | 1 | 85060 | 1 |
| 81431 | 1 | 82135 | 1 | 82530 | 4 | 82950 | 3 | 83632 | 1 | 84112 | 1 | 84436 | 1 | 85097 | 2 |
| 81432 | 1 | 82136 | 2 | 82533 | 5 | 82951 | 1 | 83633 | 1 | 84119 | 1 | 84437 | 1 | 85130 | 1 |
| 81433 | 1 | 82139 | 2 | 82540 | 1 | 82952 | 3 | 83655 | 2 | 84120 | 1 | 84439 | 1 | 85170 | 1 |
| 81434 | 1 | 82140 | 2 | 82542 | 6 | 82955 | 1 | 83661 | 3 | 84126 | 1 | 84442 | 1 | 85175 | 1 |
| 81435 | 1 | 82143 | 2 | 82550 | 3 | 82960 | 1 | 83662 | 4 | 84132 | 3 | 84443 | 4 | 85210 | 2 |
| 81436 | 1 | 82150 | 4 | 82552 | 3 | 82963 | 1 | 83663 | 3 | 84133 | 2 | 84445 | 1 | 85220 | 2 |
| 81437 | 1 | 82154 | 1 | 82553 | 3 | 82965 | 1 | 83664 | 3 | 84134 | 1 | 84446 | 1 | 85230 | 2 |
| 81438 | 1 | 82157 | 1 | 82554 | 2 | 82977 | 1 | 83670 | 1 | 84135 | 1 | 84449 | 1 | 85240 | 2 |
| 81439 | 1 | 82160 | 1 | 82565 | 3 | 82978 | 1 | 83690 | 2 | 84138 | 1 | 84450 | 1 | 85244 | 1 |
| 81440 | 1 | 82163 | 1 | 82570 | 3 | 82979 | 1 | 83695 | 1 | 84140 | 1 | 84460 | 1 | 85245 | 2 |
| 81442 | 1 | 82164 | 1 | 82575 | 1 | 82985 | 1 | 83698 | 1 | 84143 | 2 | 84466 | 1 | 85246 | 2 |
| 81445 | 1 | 82172 | 3 | 82585 | 1 | 83001 | 1 | 83700 | 1 | 84144 | 1 | 84478 | 1 | 85247 | 2 |
| 81450 | 1 | 82175 | 2 | 82595 | 1 | 83002 | 1 | 83701 | 1 | 84145 | 1 | 84479 | 1 | 85250 | 2 |
| 81455 | 1 | 82180 | 1 | 82600 | 1 | 83003 | 5 | 83704 | 1 | 84146 | 3 | 84480 | 1 | 85260 | 2 |
| 81460 | 1 | 82190 | 2 | 82607 | 1 | 83006 | 1 | 83718 | 1 | 84150 | 2 | 84481 | 1 | 85270 | 2 |
| 81465 | 1 | 82232 | 2 | 82608 | 1 | 83009 | 1 | 83719 | 1 | 84152 | 1 | 84482 | 1 | 85280 | 2 |
| 81470 | 1 | 82239 | 1 | 82610 | 1 | 83010 | 1 | 83721 | 1 | 84153 | 1 | 84484 | 4 | 85290 | 2 |
| 81471 | 1 | 82240 | 1 | 82615 | 1 | 83012 | 1 | 83727 | 1 | 84154 | 1 | 84485 | 1 | 85291 | 1 |
| 81490 | 1 | 82247 | 2 | 82626 | 1 | 83013 | 1 | 83735 | 4 | 84155 | 1 | 84488 | 1 | 85292 | 1 |
| 81493 | 1 | 82248 | 2 | 82627 | 1 | 83014 | 1 | 83775 | 1 | 84156 | 1 | 84490 | 1 | 85293 | 1 |
| 81500 | 1 | 82252 | 1 | 82633 | 1 | 83015 | 1 | 83785 | 1 | 84157 | 2 | 84510 | 1 | 85300 | 2 |
| 81503 | 1 | 82261 | 1 | 82634 | 1 | 83018 | 4 | 83789 | 4 | 84160 | 2 | 84512 | 3 | 85301 | 1 |
| 81504 | 1 | 82270 | 1 | 82638 | 1 | 83020 | 2 | 83825 | 2 | 84163 | 1 | 84520 | 4 | 85302 | 1 |
| 81506 | 1 | 82271 | 3 | 82652 | 1 | 83021 | 2 | 83835 | 2 | 84165 | 1 | 84525 | 1 | 85303 | 2 |
| 81507 | 1 | 82272 | 1 | 82656 | 1 | 83026 | 1 | 83857 | 1 | 84166 | 2 | 84540 | 2 | 85305 | 2 |
| 81508 | 1 | 82274 | 1 | 82657 | 3 | 83030 | 1 | 83861 | 2 | 84181 | 3 | 84545 | 1 | 85306 | 2 |
| 81509 | 1 | 82286 | 1 | 82658 | 2 | 83033 | 1 | 83864 | 1 | 84182 | 6 | 84550 | 1 | 85307 | 2 |
| 81510 | 1 | 82300 | 1 | 82664 | 2 | 83036 | 1 | 83872 | 2 | 84202 | 1 | 84560 | 2 | 85335 | 2 |
| 81511 | 1 | 82306 | 1 | 82668 | 1 | 83037 | 1 | 83873 | 1 | 84203 | 1 | 84577 | 1 | 85337 | 1 |
| 81512 | 1 | 82308 | 1 | 82670 | 2 | 83045 | 1 | 83874 | 4 | 84206 | 1 | 84578 | 1 | 85345 | 1 |
| 81519 | 1 | 82310 | 4 | 82671 | 1 | 83050 | 2 | 83876 | 1 | 84207 | 1 | 84580 | 1 | 85347 | 9 |
| 81525 | 1 | 82330 | 4 | 82672 | 1 | 83051 | 1 | 83880 | 1 | 84210 | 1 | 84583 | 1 | 85348 | 4 |
| 81528 | 1 | 82331 | 1 | 82677 | 1 | 83060 | 1 | 83883 | 6 | 84220 | 1 | 84585 | 1 | 85360 | 1 |
| 81535 | 1 | 82340 | 1 | 82679 | 1 | 83065 | 1 | 83885 | 2 | 84228 | 1 | 84586 | 1 | 85362 | 2 |
| 81536 | 11 | 82355 | 2 | 82693 | 2 | 83068 | 1 | 83915 | 1 | 84233 | 1 | 84588 | 1 | 85366 | 1 |
| 81538 | 1 | 82360 | 2 | 82696 | 1 | 83069 | 1 | 83916 | 2 | 84234 | 1 | 84590 | 1 | 85370 | 1 |
| 81539 | 1 | 82365 | 2 | 82705 | 1 | 83070 | 1 | 83918 | 2 | 84235 | 1 | 84591 | 1 | 85378 | 2 |
| 81540 | 1 | 82370 | 2 | 82710 | 1 | 83080 | 2 | 83919 | 1 | 84238 | 3 | 84597 | 1 | 85379 | 2 |
| 81545 | 1 | 82373 | 1 | 82715 | 3 | 83088 | 1 | 83921 | 2 | 84244 | 2 | 84600 | 2 | 85380 | 2 |
| 81595 | 1 | 82374 | 3 | 82725 | 1 | 83090 | 2 | 83930 | 2 | 84252 | 1 | 84620 | 1 | 85384 | 2 |
| 82009 | 3 | 82375 | 4 | 82726 | 1 | 83150 | 1 | 83935 | 2 | 84255 | 2 | 84630 | 2 | 85385 | 1 |
| 82010 | 3 | 82376 | 2 | 82728 | 1 | 83491 | 1 | 83937 | 1 | 84260 | 1 | 84681 | 1 | 85390 | 3 |
| 82013 | 1 | 82378 | 1 | 82731 | 1 | 83497 | 1 | 83945 | 2 | 84270 | 1 | 84702 | 2 | 85396 | 1 |
| 82016 | 1 | 82379 | 1 | 82735 | 1 | 83498 | 2 | 83950 | 1 | 84275 | 1 | 84703 | 1 | 85397 | 3 |
| 82017 | 1 | 82380 | 1 | 82746 | 1 | 83499 | 1 | 83951 | 1 | 84285 | 1 | 84704 | 1 | 85400 | 1 |
| 82024 | 4 | 82382 | 1 | 82747 | 1 | 83500 | 1 | 83970 | 4 | 84295 | 4 | 84830 | 1 | 85410 | 1 |
| 82030 | 1 | 82383 | 1 | 82757 | 1 | 83505 | 1 | 83986 | 2 | 84300 | 2 | 85002 | 1 | 85415 | 2 |
| 82040 | 1 | 82384 | 2 | 82759 | 1 | 83516 | 5 | 83987 | 1 | 84302 | 3 | 85004 | 2 | 85420 | 2 |
| 82042 | 2 | 82387 | 1 | 82760 | 1 | 83518 | 1 | 83992 | 2 | 84305 | 1 | 85007 | 1 | 85421 | 1 |
| 82043 | 1 | 82390 | 1 | 82775 | 1 | 83519 | 5 | 83993 | 1 | 84307 | 1 | 85008 | 1 | 85441 | 1 |
| 82044 | 1 | 82397 | 4 | 82776 | 1 | 83520 | 8 | 84030 | 1 | 84311 | 2 | 85009 | 1 | 85445 | 1 |
| 82045 | 1 | 82415 | 1 | 82777 | 1 | 83525 | 4 | 84035 | 1 | 84315 | 1 | 85013 | 1 | 85460 | 1 |
| 82075 | 2 | 82435 | 3 | 82784 | 6 | 83527 | 1 | 84060 | 1 | 84375 | 1 | 85014 | 4 | 85461 | 1 |
| 82085 | 1 | 82436 | 1 | 82785 | 1 | 83528 | 1 | 84061 | 1 | 84376 | 1 | 85018 | 4 | 85475 | 1 |
| 82088 | 2 | 82438 | 1 | 82787 | 4 | 83540 | 2 | 84066 | 1 | 84377 | 1 | 85025 | 4 | 85520 | 3 |
| 82103 | 1 | 82441 | 1 | 82800 | 2 | 83550 | 1 | 84075 | 2 | 84378 | 2 | 85027 | 4 | 85525 | 2 |
| 82104 | 1 | 82465 | 1 | 82810 | 4 | 83570 | 1 | 84078 | 1 | 84379 | 1 | 85032 | 2 | 85530 | 1 |
| 82105 | 1 | 82480 | 2 | 82820 | 1 | 83582 | 1 | 84080 | 1 | 84392 | 1 | 85041 | 1 | 85536 | 1 |
| 82106 | 2 | 82482 | 1 | 82930 | 1 | 83586 | 1 | 84081 | 1 | 84402 | 1 | 85044 | 1 | 85540 | 1 |

CPT © 2017 American Medical Association. All Rights Reserved.

© 2017 Optum360, LLC

| CPT | MUE | CPT | MUE | CPT | MUE | CPT | MUE | CPT | MUE | CPT | MUE | CPT | MUE | CPT | MUE |
|---|---|---|---|---|---|---|---|---|---|---|---|---|---|---|---|
| 85547 | 1 | 86309 | 1 | 86648 | 2 | 86793 | 2 | 87101 | 4 | 87327 | 1 | 87528 | 1 | 87905 | 2 |
| 85549 | 1 | 86310 | 1 | 86651 | 2 | 86800 | 1 | 87102 | 4 | 87328 | 2 | 87529 | 2 | 87906 | 2 |
| 85555 | 1 | 86316 | 2 | 86652 | 2 | 86803 | 1 | 87103 | 2 | 87329 | 2 | 87530 | 2 | 87910 | 1 |
| 85557 | 1 | 86317 | 6 | 86653 | 2 | 86804 | 1 | 87106 | 4 | 87332 | 1 | 87531 | 1 | 87912 | 1 |
| 85576 | 7 | 86318 | 2 | 86654 | 2 | 86805 | 12 | 87107 | 4 | 87335 | 1 | 87532 | 1 | 88104 | 5 |
| 85597 | 1 | 86320 | 1 | 86658 | 12 | 86807 | 2 | 87109 | 2 | 87336 | 1 | 87533 | 1 | 88106 | 5 |
| 85598 | 1 | 86325 | 2 | 86663 | 2 | 86808 | 1 | 87110 | 2 | 87337 | 1 | 87534 | 1 | 88108 | 6 |
| 85610 | 4 | 86327 | 1 | 86664 | 2 | 86812 | 1 | 87118 | 3 | 87338 | 1 | 87535 | 1 | 88112 | 6 |
| 85611 | 2 | 86329 | 3 | 86665 | 2 | 86813 | 1 | 87140 | 3 | 87339 | 1 | 87536 | 1 | 88120 | 2 |
| 85612 | 1 | 86331 | 12 | 86666 | 4 | 86816 | 1 | 87143 | 2 | 87340 | 1 | 87537 | 1 | 88121 | 2 |
| 85613 | 3 | 86332 | 1 | 86668 | 2 | 86817 | 1 | 87149 | 11 | 87341 | 1 | 87538 | 1 | 88125 | 1 |
| 85635 | 1 | 86334 | 2 | 86671 | 3 | 86821 | 1 | 87150 | 12 | 87350 | 1 | 87539 | 1 | 88130 | 1 |
| 85651 | 1 | 86335 | 2 | 86674 | 3 | 86822 | 1 | 87152 | 1 | 87380 | 1 | 87540 | 1 | 88140 | 1 |
| 85652 | 1 | 86336 | 1 | 86677 | 3 | 86825 | 1 | 87153 | 3 | 87385 | 2 | 87541 | 1 | 88141 | 1 |
| 85660 | 1 | 86337 | 1 | 86682 | 2 | 86826 | 8 | 87164 | 2 | 87389 | 1 | 87542 | 1 | 88142 | 1 |
| 85670 | 2 | 86340 | 1 | 86684 | 2 | 86828 | 2 | 87166 | 2 | 87390 | 1 | 87550 | 1 | 88143 | 1 |
| 85675 | 1 | 86341 | 1 | 86687 | 1 | 86829 | 2 | 87168 | 2 | 87391 | 1 | 87551 | 2 | 88147 | 1 |
| 85705 | 1 | 86343 | 1 | 86688 | 1 | 86830 | 2 | 87169 | 2 | 87400 | 2 | 87552 | 1 | 88148 | 1 |
| 85730 | 4 | 86344 | 1 | 86689 | 2 | 86831 | 2 | 87172 | 1 | 87420 | 1 | 87555 | 1 | 88150 | 1 |
| 85732 | 4 | 86352 | 1 | 86692 | 2 | 86832 | 2 | 87176 | 3 | 87425 | 1 | 87556 | 1 | 88152 | 1 |
| 85810 | 2 | 86353 | 7 | 86694 | 2 | 86833 | 1 | 87177 | 3 | 87427 | 2 | 87557 | 1 | 88153 | 1 |
| 86000 | 6 | 86355 | 1 | 86695 | 2 | 86834 | 1 | 87181 | 12 | 87430 | 1 | 87560 | 1 | 88154 | 1 |
| 86001 | 20 | 86356 | 7 | 86696 | 2 | 86835 | 1 | 87184 | 8 | 87449 | 3 | 87561 | 1 | 88155 | 1 |
| 86005 | 6 | 86357 | 1 | 86698 | 3 | 86850 | 3 | 87185 | 4 | 87450 | 2 | 87562 | 1 | 88160 | 4 |
| 86021 | 1 | 86359 | 1 | 86701 | 1 | 86860 | 2 | 87186 | 12 | 87451 | 2 | 87580 | 1 | 88161 | 4 |
| 86022 | 1 | 86360 | 1 | 86702 | 2 | 86870 | 6 | 87187 | 3 | 87470 | 1 | 87581 | 1 | 88162 | 3 |
| 86023 | 3 | 86361 | 1 | 86703 | 1 | 86880 | 4 | 87188 | 14 | 87471 | 1 | 87582 | 1 | 88164 | 1 |
| 86038 | 1 | 86367 | 2 | 86704 | 1 | 86885 | 3 | 87190 | 10 | 87472 | 1 | 87590 | 1 | 88165 | 1 |
| 86039 | 1 | 86376 | 2 | 86705 | 1 | 86886 | 3 | 87197 | 1 | 87475 | 1 | 87591 | 3 | 88166 | 1 |
| 86060 | 1 | 86378 | 1 | 86706 | 2 | 86890 | 2 | 87206 | 6 | 87476 | 1 | 87592 | 1 | 88167 | 1 |
| 86063 | 1 | 86382 | 3 | 86707 | 1 | 86891 | 2 | 87207 | 3 | 87477 | 1 | 87623 | 1 | 88172 | 7 |
| 86077 | 1 | 86384 | 1 | 86708 | 1 | 86900 | 3 | 87209 | 4 | 87480 | 1 | 87624 | 1 | 88173 | 7 |
| 86078 | 1 | 86386 | 1 | 86709 | 1 | 86901 | 3 | 87210 | 4 | 87481 | 1 | 87625 | 1 | 88174 | 1 |
| 86079 | 1 | 86406 | 2 | 86710 | 4 | 86902 | 40 | 87220 | 3 | 87482 | 1 | 87631 | 1 | 88175 | 1 |
| 86140 | 1 | 86430 | 2 | 86711 | 2 | 86905 | 28 | 87230 | 3 | 87483 | 1 | 87632 | 1 | 88177 | 6 |
| 86141 | 1 | 86431 | 2 | 86713 | 3 | 86906 | 1 | 87250 | 1 | 87485 | 1 | 87633 | 1 | 88182 | 2 |
| 86146 | 3 | 86480 | 1 | 86717 | 8 | 86920 | 19 | 87252 | 4 | 87486 | 1 | 87640 | 1 | 88184 | 2 |
| 86147 | 4 | 86481 | 1 | 86720 | 2 | 86922 | 10 | 87253 | 3 | 87487 | 1 | 87641 | 1 | 88187 | 2 |
| 86148 | 3 | 86485 | 1 | 86723 | 2 | 86923 | 10 | 87254 | 10 | 87490 | 1 | 87650 | 1 | 88188 | 2 |
| 86152 | 1 | 86486 | 2 | 86727 | 2 | 86930 | 3 | 87255 | 2 | 87491 | 3 | 87651 | 1 | 88189 | 2 |
| 86153 | 1 | 86490 | 1 | 86729 | 0 | 86931 | 4 | 87260 | 1 | 87492 | 1 | 87652 | 1 | 88230 | 2 |
| 86155 | 1 | 86510 | 1 | 86732 | 2 | 86940 | 3 | 87265 | 1 | 87493 | 2 | 87653 | 1 | 88233 | 2 |
| 86156 | 1 | 86580 | 1 | 86735 | 2 | 86941 | 3 | 87267 | 1 | 87495 | 1 | 87660 | 1 | 88235 | 2 |
| 86157 | 1 | 86590 | 1 | 86738 | 2 | 86945 | 5 | 87269 | 1 | 87496 | 1 | 87661 | 1 | 88237 | 4 |
| 86160 | 4 | 86592 | 2 | 86741 | 2 | 86950 | 1 | 87270 | 1 | 87497 | 2 | 87797 | 3 | 88239 | 3 |
| 86161 | 2 | 86593 | 2 | 86744 | 2 | 86960 | 3 | 87271 | 1 | 87498 | 1 | 87798 | 21 | 88240 | 3 |
| 86162 | 1 | 86602 | 3 | 86747 | 2 | 86965 | 4 | 87272 | 1 | 87500 | 1 | 87799 | 3 | 88241 | 3 |
| 86171 | 2 | 86603 | 2 | 86750 | 4 | 86971 | 6 | 87273 | 1 | 87501 | 1 | 87800 | 2 | 88245 | 1 |
| 86185 | 1 | 86609 | 14 | 86753 | 3 | 86972 | 2 | 87274 | 1 | 87502 | 1 | 87801 | 3 | 88248 | 1 |
| 86200 | 1 | 86611 | 4 | 86756 | 2 | 86975 | 2 | 87275 | 1 | 87503 | 1 | 87802 | 2 | 88249 | 1 |
| 86215 | 1 | 86612 | 2 | 86757 | 6 | 86976 | 2 | 87276 | 1 | 87505 | 1 | 87803 | 3 | 88261 | 2 |
| 86225 | 1 | 86615 | 6 | 86759 | 2 | 86977 | 2 | 87277 | 1 | 87506 | 1 | 87804 | 3 | 88262 | 2 |
| 86226 | 1 | 86617 | 2 | 86762 | 2 | 87003 | 1 | 87278 | 1 | 87507 | 1 | 87806 | 1 | 88263 | 1 |
| 86235 | 10 | 86618 | 2 | 86765 | 2 | 87015 | 6 | 87279 | 1 | 87510 | 1 | 87807 | 2 | 88264 | 1 |
| 86243 | 1 | 86619 | 2 | 86768 | 5 | 87045 | 3 | 87280 | 1 | 87511 | 1 | 87808 | 1 | 88267 | 2 |
| 86255 | 5 | 86622 | 2 | 86771 | 2 | 87046 | 6 | 87281 | 1 | 87512 | 1 | 87809 | 2 | 88269 | 1 |
| 86256 | 9 | 86625 | 1 | 86774 | 2 | 87071 | 4 | 87283 | 1 | 87515 | 1 | 87810 | 2 | 88271 | 16 |
| 86277 | 1 | 86628 | 2 | 86777 | 2 | 87073 | 3 | 87285 | 1 | 87516 | 1 | 87850 | 1 | 88272 | 12 |
| 86280 | 1 | 86631 | 6 | 86778 | 2 | 87075 | 6 | 87290 | 1 | 87517 | 1 | 87880 | 2 | 88273 | 3 |
| 86294 | 1 | 86632 | 3 | 86780 | 2 | 87076 | 6 | 87299 | 1 | 87520 | 1 | 87899 | 6 | 88274 | 5 |
| 86300 | 2 | 86635 | 4 | 86784 | 1 | 87077 | 10 | 87300 | 2 | 87521 | 1 | 87900 | 1 | 88275 | 12 |
| 86301 | 1 | 86638 | 6 | 86787 | 2 | 87081 | 6 | 87301 | 1 | 87522 | 1 | 87901 | 1 | 88280 | 1 |
| 86304 | 1 | 86641 | 2 | 86788 | 2 | 87084 | 1 | 87305 | 1 | 87525 | 1 | 87902 | 1 | 88283 | 5 |
| 86305 | 1 | 86644 | 2 | 86789 | 2 | 87086 | 3 | 87320 | 1 | 87526 | 1 | 87903 | 1 | 88285 | 10 |
| 86308 | 1 | 86645 | 1 | 86790 | 4 | 87088 | 6 | 87324 | 2 | 87527 | 1 | 87904 | 14 | 88289 | 1 |

| CPT | MUE | CPT | MUE | CPT | MUE | CPT | MUE | CPT | MUE | CPT | MUE | CPT | MUE |
|-----|-----|-----|-----|-----|-----|-----|-----|-----|-----|-----|-----|-----|-----|
| 88291 | 1 | 89251 | 1 | 90647 | 1 | 90838 | 3 | 91132 | 1 | 92522 | 1 | 92618 | 1 | 93279 | 1 |
| 88300 | 4 | 89253 | 1 | 90648 | 1 | 90839 | 1 | 91133 | 1 | 92523 | 1 | 92620 | 1 | 93280 | 1 |
| 88302 | 4 | 89254 | 1 | 90649 | 1 | 90840 | 4 | 91200 | 1 | 92524 | 1 | 92621 | 4 | 93281 | 1 |
| 88304 | 5 | 89255 | 1 | 90650 | 1 | 90845 | 1 | 92002 | 1 | 92526 | 1 | 92625 | 1 | 93282 | 1 |
| 88305 | 16 | 89257 | 1 | 90651 | 1 | 90846 | 2 | 92004 | 1 | 92531 | 1 | 92626 | 1 | 93283 | 1 |
| 88307 | 8 | 89258 | 1 | 90653 | 1 | 90847 | 2 | 92012 | 1 | 92532 | 1 | 92627 | 6 | 93284 | 1 |
| 88309 | 3 | 89259 | 1 | 90654 | 1 | 90849 | 2 | 92014 | 1 | 92533 | 4 | 92640 | 1 | 93285 | 1 |
| 88311 | 4 | 89260 | 1 | 90655 | 1 | 90853 | 5 | 92018 | 1 | 92534 | 1 | 92920 | 3 | 93286 | 2 |
| 88312 | 9 | 89261 | 1 | 90656 | 1 | 90863 | 1 | 92019 | 1 | 92537 | 1 | 92921 | 6 | 93287 | 2 |
| 88313 | 8 | 89264 | 1 | 90657 | 1 | 90865 | 1 | 92020 | 1 | 92538 | 1 | 92924 | 2 | 93288 | 1 |
| 88314 | 6 | 89268 | 1 | 90658 | 1 | 90867 | 1 | 92025 | 1 | 92540 | 1 | 92925 | 6 | 93289 | 1 |
| 88319 | 11 | 89272 | 1 | 90660 | 1 | 90868 | 1 | 92060 | 1 | 92541 | 1 | 92928 | 3 | 93290 | 1 |
| 88321 | 1 | 89280 | 1 | 90661 | 1 | 90869 | 1 | 92065 | 1 | 92542 | 1 | 92929 | 6 | 93291 | 1 |
| 88323 | 1 | 89281 | 1 | 90662 | 1 | 90870 | 2 | 92071 | 2 | 92544 | 1 | 92933 | 2 | 93292 | 1 |
| 88325 | 1 | 89290 | 1 | 90664 | 1 | 90880 | 1 | 92072 | 1 | 92545 | 1 | 92934 | 6 | 93293 | 1 |
| 88329 | 2 | 89291 | 1 | 90666 | 1 | 90885 | 1 | 92081 | 1 | 92546 | 1 | 92937 | 2 | 93294 | 1 |
| 88331 | 11 | 89300 | 1 | 90667 | 1 | 90887 | 1 | 92082 | 1 | 92547 | 1 | 92938 | 6 | 93295 | 1 |
| 88332 | 13 | 89310 | 1 | 90668 | 1 | 90889 | 1 | 92083 | 1 | 92548 | 1 | 92941 | 1 | 93296 | 1 |
| 88333 | 4 | 89320 | 1 | 90670 | 1 | 90901 | 1 | 92100 | 1 | 92550 | 1 | 92943 | 2 | 93297 | 1 |
| 88334 | 5 | 89321 | 1 | 90672 | 1 | 90911 | 1 | 92132 | 1 | 92552 | 1 | 92944 | 3 | 93298 | 1 |
| 88341 | 9 | 89322 | 1 | 90673 | 1 | 90935 | 1 | 92133 | 1 | 92553 | 1 | 92950 | 2 | 93299 | 1 |
| 88342 | 3 | 89325 | 1 | 90674 | 1 | 90937 | 1 | 92134 | 1 | 92555 | 1 | 92953 | 2 | 93303 | 1 |
| 88344 | 1 | 89329 | 1 | 90675 | 1 | 90940 | 1 | 92136 | 1 | 92556 | 1 | 92960 | 2 | 93304 | 1 |
| 88346 | 2 | 89330 | 1 | 90676 | 1 | 90945 | 1 | 92145 | 1 | 92557 | 1 | 92961 | 1 | 93306 | 1 |
| 88348 | 1 | 89331 | 1 | 90680 | 1 | 90947 | 1 | 92225 | 2 | 92558 | 0 | 92970 | 1 | 93307 | 1 |
| 88350 | 8 | 89335 | 1 | 90681 | 1 | 90951 | 3 | 92226 | 2 | 92561 | 1 | 92971 | 1 | 93308 | 1 |
| 88355 | 1 | 89337 | 1 | 90682 | 1 | 90952 | 1 | 92227 | 1 | 92562 | 1 | 92973 | 2 | 93312 | 1 |
| 88356 | 1 | 89342 | 1 | 90685 | 1 | 90953 | 1 | 92228 | 1 | 92563 | 1 | 92974 | 1 | 93313 | 1 |
| 88358 | 2 | 89343 | 1 | 90686 | 1 | 90954 | 1 | 92230 | 2 | 92564 | 1 | 92975 | 1 | 93314 | 1 |
| 88360 | 6 | 89344 | 1 | 90687 | 1 | 90955 | 1 | 92235 | 1 | 92565 | 1 | 92977 | 1 | 93315 | 1 |
| 88361 | 6 | 89346 | 1 | 90688 | 1 | 90956 | 1 | 92240 | 1 | 92567 | 1 | 92978 | 1 | 93316 | 1 |
| 88362 | 1 | 89352 | 1 | 90690 | 1 | 90957 | 1 | 92242 | 1 | 92568 | 1 | 92979 | 2 | 93317 | 1 |
| 88363 | 2 | 89353 | 1 | 90691 | 1 | 90958 | 1 | 92250 | 1 | 92570 | 1 | 92986 | 1 | 93318 | 1 |
| 88364 | 3 | 89354 | 1 | 90696 | 1 | 90959 | 1 | 92260 | 1 | 92571 | 1 | 92987 | 1 | 93320 | 1 |
| 88365 | 4 | 89356 | 2 | 90697 | 1 | 90960 | 1 | 92265 | 1 | 92572 | 1 | 92990 | 1 | 93321 | 1 |
| 88366 | 2 | 90284 | 0 | 90698 | 1 | 90961 | 1 | 92270 | 1 | 92575 | 1 | 92992 | 1 | 93325 | 1 |
| 88367 | 3 | 90296 | 1 | 90700 | 1 | 90962 | 1 | 92275 | 1 | 92576 | 1 | 92993 | 1 | 93350 | 1 |
| 88368 | 3 | 90371 | 10 | 90702 | 1 | 90963 | 1 | 92283 | 1 | 92577 | 1 | 92997 | 1 | 93351 | 1 |
| 88369 | 3 | 90375 | 20 | 90707 | 1 | 90964 | 1 | 92284 | 1 | 92579 | 1 | 92998 | 2 | 93352 | 1 |
| 88371 | 1 | 90376 | 20 | 90710 | 1 | 90965 | 1 | 92285 | 1 | 92582 | 1 | 93000 | 3 | 93355 | 1 |
| 88372 | 1 | 90378 | 4 | 90713 | 1 | 90966 | 1 | 92286 | 1 | 92583 | 1 | 93005 | 5 | 93451 | 1 |
| 88373 | 3 | 90385 | 1 | 90714 | 1 | 90967 | 1 | 92287 | 1 | 92584 | 1 | 93010 | 5 | 93452 | 1 |
| 88374 | 5 | 90393 | 1 | 90715 | 1 | 90968 | 1 | 92311 | 1 | 92585 | 1 | 93015 | 1 | 93453 | 1 |
| 88375 | 1 | 90396 | 1 | 90716 | 1 | 90969 | 1 | 92312 | 1 | 92586 | 1 | 93016 | 1 | 93454 | 1 |
| 88377 | 5 | 90460 | 9 | 90717 | 1 | 90970 | 1 | 92313 | 1 | 92587 | 1 | 93017 | 1 | 93455 | 1 |
| 88380 | 1 | 90461 | 8 | 90732 | 1 | 90989 | 1 | 92315 | 1 | 92588 | 1 | 93018 | 1 | 93456 | 1 |
| 88381 | 1 | 90471 | 1 | 90733 | 1 | 90993 | 1 | 92316 | 1 | 92596 | 1 | 93024 | 1 | 93457 | 1 |
| 88387 | 2 | 90472 | 4 | 90734 | 1 | 90997 | 1 | 92317 | 1 | 92597 | 1 | 93025 | 1 | 93458 | 1 |
| 88388 | 1 | 90473 | 1 | 90736 | 1 | 91010 | 1 | 92325 | 1 | 92601 | 1 | 93040 | 3 | 93459 | 1 |
| 88720 | 1 | 90474 | 1 | 90738 | 1 | 91013 | 1 | 92326 | 2 | 92602 | 1 | 93041 | 3 | 93460 | 1 |
| 88738 | 1 | 90476 | 1 | 90739 | 1 | 91020 | 1 | 92352 | 1 | 92603 | 1 | 93042 | 3 | 93461 | 1 |
| 88740 | 1 | 90477 | 1 | 90740 | 1 | 91022 | 1 | 92353 | 1 | 92604 | 1 | 93050 | 1 | 93462 | 1 |
| 88741 | 1 | 90581 | 1 | 90743 | 1 | 91030 | 1 | 92354 | 1 | 92605 | 1 | 93224 | 1 | 93463 | 1 |
| 89049 | 1 | 90585 | 1 | 90744 | 1 | 91034 | 1 | 92355 | 1 | 92606 | 1 | 93225 | 1 | 93464 | 1 |
| 89050 | 2 | 90586 | 1 | 90746 | 1 | 91035 | 1 | 92358 | 1 | 92607 | 1 | 93226 | 1 | 93503 | 2 |
| 89051 | 2 | 90587 | 1 | 90747 | 1 | 91037 | 1 | 92371 | 1 | 92608 | 4 | 93227 | 1 | 93505 | 1 |
| 89055 | 2 | 90620 | 1 | 90750 | 1 | 91038 | 1 | 92502 | 1 | 92609 | 1 | 93228 | 1 | 93530 | 1 |
| 89060 | 2 | 90621 | 1 | 90785 | 3 | 91040 | 1 | 92504 | 1 | 92610 | 1 | 93229 | 1 | 93531 | 1 |
| 89125 | 2 | 90625 | 1 | 90791 | 1 | 91065 | 2 | 92507 | 1 | 92611 | 1 | 93260 | 1 | 93532 | 1 |
| 89160 | 1 | 90630 | 1 | 90792 | 2 | 91110 | 1 | 92508 | 1 | 92612 | 1 | 93261 | 1 | 93533 | 1 |
| 89190 | 1 | 90632 | 1 | 90832 | 3 | 91111 | 1 | 92511 | 1 | 92613 | 1 | 93268 | 1 | 93561 | 1 |
| 89220 | 2 | 90633 | 1 | 90833 | 3 | 91112 | 1 | 92512 | 1 | 92614 | 1 | 93270 | 1 | 93562 | 1 |
| 89230 | 1 | 90634 | 1 | 90834 | 3 | 91117 | 1 | 92516 | 1 | 92615 | 1 | 93271 | 1 | 93563 | 1 |
| 89240 | 1 | 90636 | 1 | 90836 | 3 | 91120 | 1 | 92520 | 1 | 92616 | 1 | 93272 | 1 | 93564 | 1 |
| 89250 | 1 | 90644 | 1 | 90837 | 3 | 91122 | 1 | 92521 | 1 | 92617 | 1 | 93278 | 1 | 93565 | 1 |

CPT © 2017 American Medical Association. All Rights Reserved.

© 2017 Optum360, LLC

| CPT | MUE | CPT | MUE | CPT | MUE | CPT | MUE | CPT | MUE | CPT | MUE | CPT | MUE | CPT | MUE |
|---|---|---|---|---|---|---|---|---|---|---|---|---|---|---|---|
| 93566 | 1 | 93925 | 1 | 94781 | 2 | 95861 | 1 | 95992 | 1 | 96571 | 2 | 97750 | 8 | 99222 | 0 |
| 93567 | 1 | 93926 | 1 | 95004 | 80 | 95863 | 1 | 96000 | 1 | 96900 | 1 | 97755 | 8 | 99223 | 0 |
| 93568 | 1 | 93930 | 1 | 95012 | 2 | 95864 | 1 | 96001 | 1 | 96902 | 1 | 97760 | 6 | 99224 | 1 |
| 93571 | 1 | 93931 | 1 | 95017 | 27 | 95865 | 1 | 96002 | 1 | 96904 | 1 | 97761 | 6 | 99225 | 1 |
| 93572 | 2 | 93970 | 1 | 95018 | 19 | 95866 | 1 | 96003 | 1 | 96910 | 1 | 97762 | 4 | 99226 | 1 |
| 93580 | 1 | 93971 | 1 | 95024 | 40 | 95867 | 1 | 96004 | 1 | 96912 | 1 | 97802 | 8 | 99231 | 0 |
| 93581 | 1 | 93975 | 1 | 95027 | 90 | 95868 | 1 | 96020 | 1 | 96913 | 1 | 97803 | 8 | 99232 | 0 |
| 93582 | 1 | 93976 | 1 | 95028 | 30 | 95869 | 1 | 96040 | 4 | 96920 | 1 | 97804 | 6 | 99233 | 0 |
| 93583 | 1 | 93978 | 1 | 95044 | 80 | 95870 | 4 | 96101 | 8 | 96921 | 1 | 98925 | 1 | 99234 | 1 |
| 93590 | 1 | 93979 | 1 | 95052 | 20 | 95872 | 4 | 96102 | 4 | 96922 | 1 | 98926 | 1 | 99235 | 1 |
| 93591 | 1 | 93980 | 1 | 95056 | 1 | 95873 | 1 | 96103 | 1 | 96931 | 1 | 98927 | 1 | 99236 | 1 |
| 93592 | 2 | 93981 | 1 | 95060 | 1 | 95874 | 1 | 96105 | 3 | 96932 | 1 | 98928 | 1 | 99238 | 0 |
| 93600 | 1 | 93982 | 1 | 95065 | 1 | 95875 | 2 | 96110 | 3 | 96933 | 1 | 98929 | 1 | 99239 | 0 |
| 93602 | 1 | 93990 | 2 | 95070 | 1 | 95885 | 4 | 96111 | 1 | 96934 | 2 | 98940 | 1 | 99281 | 2 |
| 93603 | 1 | 94002 | 1 | 95071 | 1 | 95886 | 4 | 96116 | 4 | 96935 | 2 | 98941 | 1 | 99282 | 2 |
| 93609 | 1 | 94003 | 1 | 95076 | 1 | 95887 | 1 | 96118 | 8 | 96936 | 2 | 98942 | 1 | 99283 | 2 |
| 93610 | 1 | 94004 | 1 | 95079 | 2 | 95905 | 2 | 96119 | 6 | 97010 | 1 | 99002 | 1 | 99284 | 2 |
| 93612 | 1 | 94010 | 1 | 95115 | 1 | 95907 | 1 | 96120 | 1 | 97012 | 1 | 99024 | 1 | 99285 | 2 |
| 93613 | 1 | 94011 | 1 | 95117 | 1 | 95908 | 1 | 96125 | 2 | 97014 | 0 | 99050 | 1 | 99288 | 1 |
| 93615 | 1 | 94012 | 1 | 95120 | 0 | 95909 | 1 | 96127 | 2 | 97016 | 1 | 99051 | 1 | 99291 | 1 |
| 93616 | 1 | 94013 | 1 | 95125 | 0 | 95910 | 1 | 96150 | 8 | 97018 | 1 | 99053 | 1 | 99292 | 8 |
| 93618 | 1 | 94014 | 1 | 95130 | 0 | 95911 | 1 | 96151 | 6 | 97022 | 1 | 99056 | 1 | 99304 | 1 |
| 93619 | 1 | 94015 | 1 | 95131 | 0 | 95912 | 1 | 96152 | 6 | 97024 | 1 | 99058 | 1 | 99305 | 1 |
| 93620 | 1 | 94016 | 1 | 95132 | 0 | 95913 | 1 | 96153 | 12 | 97026 | 1 | 99060 | 1 | 99306 | 1 |
| 93621 | 1 | 94060 | 1 | 95133 | 0 | 95921 | 1 | 96154 | 8 | 97028 | 1 | 99070 | 1 | 99307 | 1 |
| 93622 | 1 | 94070 | 1 | 95134 | 0 | 95922 | 1 | 96160 | 1 | 97032 | 4 | 99071 | 1 | 99308 | 1 |
| 93623 | 1 | 94150 | 2 | 95144 | 30 | 95923 | 1 | 96161 | 1 | 97033 | 4 | 99078 | 3 | 99309 | 1 |
| 93624 | 1 | 94200 | 1 | 95145 | 10 | 95924 | 1 | 96360 | 1 | 97034 | 2 | 99080 | 1 | 99310 | 1 |
| 93631 | 1 | 94250 | 1 | 95146 | 10 | 95925 | 1 | 96361 | 24 | 97035 | 2 | 99082 | 1 | 99315 | 1 |
| 93640 | 1 | 94375 | 1 | 95147 | 10 | 95926 | 1 | 96365 | 1 | 97036 | 3 | 99090 | 1 | 99316 | 1 |
| 93641 | 1 | 94400 | 1 | 95148 | 10 | 95927 | 1 | 96366 | 24 | 97110 | 8 | 99091 | 1 | 99318 | 1 |
| 93642 | 1 | 94450 | 1 | 95149 | 10 | 95928 | 1 | 96367 | 4 | 97112 | 6 | 99100 | 1 | 99324 | 1 |
| 93644 | 1 | 94452 | 1 | 95165 | 30 | 95929 | 1 | 96368 | 1 | 97113 | 6 | 99116 | 1 | 99325 | 1 |
| 93650 | 1 | 94453 | 1 | 95170 | 10 | 95930 | 1 | 96369 | 1 | 97116 | 4 | 99135 | 1 | 99326 | 1 |
| 93653 | 1 | 94610 | 2 | 95180 | 8 | 95933 | 1 | 96370 | 3 | 97124 | 4 | 99140 | 2 | 99327 | 1 |
| 93654 | 1 | 94620 | 1 | 95250 | 1 | 95937 | 4 | 96371 | 1 | 97140 | 6 | 99151 | 2 | 99328 | 1 |
| 93655 | 2 | 94621 | 1 | 95251 | 1 | 95938 | 1 | 96372 | 5 | 97150 | 2 | 99152 | 2 | 99334 | 1 |
| 93656 | 1 | 94640 | 2 | 95782 | 1 | 95939 | 1 | 96373 | 3 | 97161 | 1 | 99153 | 12 | 99335 | 1 |
| 93657 | 1 | 94642 | 1 | 95783 | 1 | 95940 | 20 | 96374 | 1 | 97162 | 1 | 99155 | 2 | 99336 | 1 |
| 93660 | 1 | 94644 | 1 | 95800 | 1 | 95943 | 1 | 96375 | 6 | 97163 | 1 | 99156 | 2 | 99337 | 1 |
| 93662 | 1 | 94645 | 4 | 95801 | 1 | 95950 | 1 | 96376 | 10 | 97164 | 1 | 99157 | 6 | 99339 | 1 |
| 93701 | 1 | 94660 | 1 | 95803 | 1 | 95951 | 1 | 96377 | 1 | 97165 | 1 | 99170 | 1 | 99340 | 1 |
| 93702 | 1 | 94662 | 1 | 95805 | 1 | 95953 | 1 | 96401 | 4 | 97166 | 1 | 99175 | 1 | 99341 | 1 |
| 93724 | 1 | 94664 | 1 | 95806 | 1 | 95954 | 1 | 96402 | 2 | 97167 | 1 | 99177 | 1 | 99342 | 1 |
| 93740 | 1 | 94667 | 1 | 95807 | 1 | 95955 | 1 | 96405 | 1 | 97168 | 1 | 99183 | 1 | 99343 | 1 |
| 93745 | 1 | 94668 | 5 | 95808 | 1 | 95956 | 1 | 96406 | 1 | 97169 | 1 | 99184 | 1 | 99344 | 1 |
| 93750 | 1 | 94669 | 4 | 95810 | 1 | 95957 | 1 | 96409 | 1 | 97170 | 1 | 99188 | 1 | 99345 | 1 |
| 93770 | 1 | 94680 | 1 | 95811 | 1 | 95958 | 1 | 96411 | 3 | 97171 | 1 | 99191 | 1 | 99347 | 1 |
| 93784 | 1 | 94681 | 1 | 95812 | 1 | 95961 | 1 | 96413 | 1 | 97172 | 1 | 99192 | 1 | 99348 | 1 |
| 93786 | 1 | 94690 | 1 | 95813 | 1 | 95962 | 3 | 96415 | 8 | 97530 | 6 | 99195 | 2 | 99349 | 1 |
| 93788 | 1 | 94726 | 1 | 95816 | 1 | 95965 | 1 | 96416 | 1 | 97532 | 8 | 99201 | 1 | 99350 | 1 |
| 93790 | 1 | 94727 | 1 | 95819 | 1 | 95966 | 1 | 96417 | 3 | 97533 | 4 | 99202 | 1 | 99354 | 1 |
| 93797 | 2 | 94728 | 1 | 95822 | 1 | 95967 | 3 | 96420 | 2 | 97535 | 8 | 99203 | 1 | 99355 | 4 |
| 93798 | 2 | 94729 | 1 | 95824 | 1 | 95970 | 1 | 96422 | 2 | 97537 | 8 | 99204 | 1 | 99356 | 1 |
| 93880 | 1 | 94750 | 1 | 95827 | 1 | 95971 | 1 | 96423 | 2 | 97542 | 8 | 99205 | 1 | 99357 | 1 |
| 93882 | 1 | 94760 | 1 | 95829 | 1 | 95972 | 1 | 96425 | 1 | 97545 | 1 | 99211 | 2 | 99358 | 1 |
| 93886 | 1 | 94761 | 1 | 95830 | 1 | 95974 | 1 | 96440 | 1 | 97546 | 2 | 99212 | 2 | 99359 | 1 |
| 93888 | 1 | 94762 | 1 | 95831 | 5 | 95975 | 2 | 96446 | 1 | 97597 | 1 | 99213 | 2 | 99363 | 1 |
| 93890 | 1 | 94770 | 1 | 95832 | 1 | 95978 | 1 | 96450 | 1 | 97598 | 8 | 99214 | 2 | 99364 | 1 |
| 93892 | 1 | 94772 | 1 | 95833 | 1 | 95979 | 6 | 96521 | 2 | 97602 | 1 | 99215 | 2 | 99366 | 3 |
| 93893 | 1 | 94774 | 1 | 95834 | 1 | 95980 | 1 | 96522 | 1 | 97605 | 1 | 99217 | 1 | 99367 | 1 |
| 93895 | 1 | 94775 | 1 | 95851 | 3 | 95981 | 1 | 96523 | 2 | 97606 | 1 | 99218 | 1 | 99368 | 3 |
| 93922 | 1 | 94776 | 1 | 95852 | 1 | 95982 | 1 | 96542 | 1 | 97607 | 1 | 99219 | 1 | 99374 | 1 |
| 93923 | 1 | 94777 | 1 | 95857 | 1 | 95990 | 1 | 96567 | 1 | 97608 | 1 | 99220 | 1 | 99377 | 1 |
| 93924 | 1 | 94780 | 1 | 95860 | 1 | 95991 | 1 | 96570 | 1 | 97610 | 1 | 99221 | 0 | 99379 | 1 |

**Appendix I — Medically Unlikely Edits (MUEs) — OPPS**

| CPT | MUE | CPT | MUE | CPT | MUE | CPT | MUE | CPT | MUE | CPT | MUE | CPT | MUE | CPT | MUE |
|---|---|---|---|---|---|---|---|---|---|---|---|---|---|---|---|
| 99380 | 1 | A0424 | 0 | A4332 | 2 | A4426 | 2 | A4657 | 0 | A5083 | 5 | A6537 | 0 | A9153 | 0 |
| 99406 | 1 | A0425 | 250 | A4335 | 1 | A4427 | 1 | A4660 | 0 | A5093 | 2 | A6538 | 0 | A9155 | 1 |
| 99407 | 1 | A0426 | 2 | A4337 | 2 | A4428 | 1 | A4663 | 0 | A5102 | 1 | A6539 | 0 | A9180 | 0 |
| 99415 | 1 | A0427 | 2 | A4338 | 3 | A4429 | 2 | A4670 | 0 | A5105 | 1 | A6540 | 0 | A9270 | 0 |
| 99416 | 4 | A0428 | 4 | A4340 | 2 | A4430 | 1 | A4671 | 0 | A5112 | 2 | A6541 | 0 | A9272 | 0 |
| 99446 | 1 | A0429 | 2 | A4344 | 2 | A4431 | 1 | A4672 | 0 | A5113 | 0 | A6544 | 0 | A9273 | 0 |
| 99447 | 1 | A0430 | 1 | A4346 | 2 | A4432 | 2 | A4673 | 0 | A5114 | 0 | A6545 | 2 | A9274 | 0 |
| 99448 | 1 | A0431 | 1 | A4351 | 2 | A4433 | 1 | A4674 | 0 | A5120 | 150 | A6549 | 0 | A9275 | 0 |
| 99449 | 1 | A0432 | 1 | A4352 | 2 | A4434 | 1 | A4680 | 0 | A5121 | 1 | A6550 | 1 | A9276 | 0 |
| 99455 | 1 | A0433 | 1 | A4353 | 3 | A4435 | 2 | A4690 | 0 | A5122 | 1 | A7000 | 0 | A9277 | 0 |
| 99456 | 1 | A0434 | 2 | A4354 | 2 | A4455 | 1 | A4706 | 0 | A5126 | 2 | A7001 | 0 | A9278 | 0 |
| 99460 | 1 | A0435 | 999 | A4355 | 2 | A4459 | 1 | A4707 | 0 | A5131 | 1 | A7002 | 0 | A9279 | 0 |
| 99461 | 1 | A0436 | 300 | A4356 | 2 | A4461 | 2 | A4708 | 0 | A5200 | 2 | A7003 | 0 | A9280 | 0 |
| 99462 | 1 | A0888 | 0 | A4357 | 2 | A4463 | 2 | A4709 | 0 | A5500 | 0 | A7004 | 0 | A9281 | 0 |
| 99463 | 1 | A0998 | 0 | A4361 | 1 | A4465 | 1 | A4714 | 0 | A5501 | 0 | A7005 | 0 | A9282 | 0 |
| 99464 | 1 | A4210 | 0 | A4362 | 2 | A4467 | 0 | A4719 | 0 | A5503 | 0 | A7006 | 0 | A9283 | 0 |
| 99465 | 1 | A4211 | 1 | A4363 | 0 | A4470 | 1 | A4720 | 0 | A5504 | 0 | A7007 | 0 | A9284 | 0 |
| 99466 | 1 | A4212 | 2 | A4364 | 2 | A4480 | 1 | A4721 | 0 | A5505 | 0 | A7010 | 0 | A9285 | 0 |
| 99467 | 4 | A4220 | 1 | A4366 | 1 | A4481 | 2 | A4722 | 0 | A5506 | 0 | A7012 | 0 | A9286 | 0 |
| 99468 | 1 | A4221 | 0 | A4367 | 1 | A4490 | 0 | A4723 | 0 | A5507 | 0 | A7013 | 0 | A9300 | 0 |
| 99469 | 1 | A4222 | 2 | A4368 | 1 | A4495 | 0 | A4724 | 0 | A5508 | 0 | A7014 | 0 | A9500 | 3 |
| 99471 | 1 | A4224 | 1 | A4372 | 1 | A4500 | 0 | A4725 | 0 | A5510 | 0 | A7015 | 0 | A9501 | 1 |
| 99472 | 1 | A4225 | 1 | A4373 | 1 | A4510 | 0 | A4726 | 0 | A5512 | 0 | A7016 | 0 | A9502 | 3 |
| 99475 | 1 | A4232 | 0 | A4375 | 2 | A4520 | 0 | A4728 | 0 | A5513 | 0 | A7017 | 0 | A9503 | 1 |
| 99476 | 1 | A4233 | 0 | A4376 | 2 | A4550 | 3 | A4730 | 0 | A6000 | 0 | A7018 | 0 | A9504 | 1 |
| 99477 | 1 | A4234 | 0 | A4377 | 2 | A4553 | 0 | A4736 | 0 | A6154 | 1 | A7020 | 0 | A9505 | 4 |
| 99478 | 1 | A4235 | 1 | A4378 | 2 | A4554 | 0 | A4737 | 0 | A6205 | 1 | A7025 | 0 | A9507 | 1 |
| 99479 | 1 | A4236 | 0 | A4379 | 2 | A4555 | 0 | A4740 | 0 | A6228 | 2 | A7026 | 0 | A9508 | 2 |
| 99480 | 1 | A4250 | 0 | A4380 | 2 | A4556 | 2 | A4750 | 0 | A6230 | 1 | A7027 | 0 | A9509 | 5 |
| 99485 | 1 | A4252 | 0 | A4381 | 2 | A4557 | 2 | A4755 | 0 | A6236 | 1 | A7028 | 0 | A9510 | 1 |
| 99486 | 4 | A4253 | 0 | A4382 | 2 | A4558 | 1 | A4760 | 0 | A6238 | 3 | A7029 | 0 | A9512 | 30 |
| 99487 | 1 | A4255 | 0 | A4383 | 2 | A4561 | 1 | A4765 | 0 | A6239 | 1 | A7030 | 0 | A9515 | 1 |
| 99490 | 1 | A4256 | 1 | A4384 | 2 | A4562 | 1 | A4766 | 0 | A6240 | 2 | A7031 | 0 | A9516 | 4 |
| 99495 | 1 | A4257 | 0 | A4385 | 2 | A4565 | 2 | A4770 | 0 | A6241 | 1 | A7032 | 0 | A9517 | 200 |
| 99496 | 1 | A4258 | 0 | A4387 | 1 | A4566 | 0 | A4771 | 0 | A6244 | 1 | A7033 | 0 | A9520 | 1 |
| 99497 | 1 | A4259 | 0 | A4388 | 1 | A4570 | 0 | A4772 | 0 | A6246 | 3 | A7034 | 0 | A9521 | 2 |
| 99498 | 3 | A4261 | 0 | A4389 | 1 | A4575 | 0 | A4773 | 0 | A6247 | 2 | A7035 | 0 | A9524 | 10 |
| 99605 | 0 | A4262 | 4 | A4390 | 1 | A4580 | 0 | A4774 | 0 | A6250 | 1 | A7036 | 0 | A9526 | 2 |
| 99606 | 0 | A4263 | 4 | A4391 | 1 | A4590 | 0 | A4802 | 0 | A6256 | 3 | A7037 | 0 | A9527 | 195 |
| 99607 | 0 | A4264 | 0 | A4392 | 2 | A4595 | 2 | A4860 | 0 | A6259 | 3 | A7038 | 0 | A9528 | 10 |
| A0021 | 0 | A4265 | 1 | A4393 | 1 | A4602 | 1 | A4870 | 0 | A6261 | 3 | A7039 | 0 | A9529 | 10 |
| A0080 | 0 | A4266 | 0 | A4396 | 1 | A4604 | 1 | A4890 | 0 | A6262 | 3 | A7040 | 2 | A9530 | 200 |
| A0090 | 0 | A4267 | 0 | A4397 | 1 | A4605 | 1 | A4911 | 0 | A6404 | 2 | A7041 | 2 | A9531 | 100 |
| A0100 | 0 | A4268 | 0 | A4398 | 2 | A4606 | 1 | A4913 | 0 | A6410 | 2 | A7044 | 0 | A9532 | 10 |
| A0110 | 0 | A4269 | 0 | A4399 | 1 | A4611 | 0 | A4918 | 0 | A6411 | 2 | A7045 | 0 | A9536 | 1 |
| A0120 | 0 | A4270 | 3 | A4400 | 1 | A4612 | 0 | A4927 | 0 | A6413 | 0 | A7046 | 0 | A9537 | 1 |
| A0130 | 0 | A4280 | 1 | A4402 | 1 | A4613 | 0 | A4928 | 0 | A6501 | 1 | A7047 | 0 | A9538 | 1 |
| A0140 | 0 | A4300 | 4 | A4404 | 1 | A4614 | 1 | A4929 | 0 | A6502 | 1 | A7048 | 2 | A9539 | 2 |
| A0160 | 0 | A4301 | 1 | A4407 | 2 | A4618 | 1 | A4930 | 0 | A6503 | 1 | A7501 | 1 | A9540 | 2 |
| A0170 | 0 | A4305 | 2 | A4408 | 1 | A4623 | 10 | A4931 | 0 | A6504 | 2 | A7502 | 0 | A9541 | 1 |
| A0180 | 0 | A4306 | 2 | A4409 | 1 | A4624 | 2 | A4932 | 0 | A6505 | 2 | A7503 | 0 | A9542 | 1 |
| A0190 | 0 | A4310 | 2 | A4410 | 2 | A4625 | 30 | A5051 | 1 | A6506 | 2 | A7504 | 180 | A9543 | 1 |
| A0200 | 0 | A4311 | 2 | A4411 | 1 | A4627 | 0 | A5052 | 1 | A6507 | 2 | A7505 | 0 | A9546 | 1 |
| A0210 | 0 | A4312 | 1 | A4412 | 1 | A4628 | 1 | A5053 | 2 | A6508 | 2 | A7506 | 0 | A9547 | 2 |
| A0225 | 0 | A4313 | 1 | A4413 | 2 | A4629 | 1 | A5055 | 1 | A6509 | 1 | A7507 | 200 | A9548 | 2 |
| A0380 | 0 | A4314 | 2 | A4414 | 1 | A4633 | 0 | A5056 | 90 | A6510 | 1 | A7508 | 0 | A9550 | 1 |
| A0382 | 0 | A4315 | 2 | A4415 | 1 | A4635 | 0 | A5057 | 90 | A6511 | 1 | A7509 | 0 | A9551 | 1 |
| A0384 | 0 | A4316 | 1 | A4416 | 2 | A4636 | 0 | A5061 | 2 | A6513 | 1 | A7520 | 4 | A9552 | 1 |
| A0390 | 0 | A4320 | 2 | A4417 | 2 | A4637 | 0 | A5062 | 1 | A6530 | 0 | A7521 | 0 | A9553 | 1 |
| A0392 | 0 | A4322 | 2 | A4418 | 2 | A4638 | 0 | A5063 | 1 | A6531 | 2 | A7522 | 0 | A9554 | 1 |
| A0394 | 0 | A4326 | 1 | A4419 | 2 | A4640 | 0 | A5071 | 2 | A6532 | 2 | A7524 | 2 | A9555 | 2 |
| A0396 | 0 | A4327 | 2 | A4420 | 1 | A4642 | 1 | A5072 | 1 | A6533 | 0 | A7525 | 0 | A9556 | 10 |
| A0398 | 0 | A4328 | 1 | A4423 | 2 | A4648 | 3 | A5073 | 1 | A6534 | 0 | A7526 | 0 | A9557 | 2 |
| A0420 | 0 | A4330 | 1 | A4424 | 1 | A4650 | 3 | A5081 | 2 | A6535 | 0 | A7527 | 2 | A9558 | 7 |
| A0422 | 0 | A4331 | 3 | A4425 | 1 | A4653 | 0 | A5082 | 1 | A6536 | 0 | A9152 | 0 | A9559 | 1 |

CPT © 2017 American Medical Association. All Rights Reserved.     © 2017 Optum360, LLC

| CPT | MUE | CPT | MUE | CPT | MUE | CPT | MUE | CPT | MUE | CPT | MUE | CPT | MUE | CPT | MUE |
|---|---|---|---|---|---|---|---|---|---|---|---|---|---|---|---|
| A9560 | 2 | B5000 | 0 | C1816 | 2 | C2645 | 4608 | C9363 | 500 | E0182 | 0 | E0300 | 0 | E0601 | 0 |
| A9561 | 1 | B5100 | 0 | C1817 | 1 | C5271 | 1 | C9364 | 600 | E0184 | 0 | E0301 | 0 | E0602 | 0 |
| A9562 | 2 | B5200 | 0 | C1818 | 2 | C5272 | 3 | C9447 | 1 | E0185 | 0 | E0302 | 0 | E0603 | 0 |
| A9563 | 10 | B9002 | 0 | C1819 | 4 | C5273 | 1 | C9460 | 100 | E0186 | 0 | E0303 | 0 | E0604 | 0 |
| A9564 | 20 | B9004 | 0 | C1820 | 2 | C5274 | 35 | C9482 | 600 | E0187 | 0 | E0304 | 0 | E0605 | 0 |
| A9566 | 1 | B9006 | 0 | C1821 | 4 | C5275 | 1 | C9483 | 120 | E0188 | 0 | E0305 | 0 | E0606 | 0 |
| A9567 | 2 | C1713 | 20 | C1822 | 1 | C5276 | 3 | C9497 | 1 | E0189 | 0 | E0310 | 0 | E0607 | 0 |
| A9568 | 0 | C1714 | 4 | C1830 | 2 | C5277 | 1 | C9600 | 3 | E0190 | 0 | E0315 | 0 | E0610 | 0 |
| A9569 | 1 | C1715 | 45 | C1840 | 1 | C5278 | 15 | C9601 | 2 | E0191 | 0 | E0316 | 0 | E0615 | 0 |
| A9570 | 1 | C1716 | 4 | C1841 | 0 | C8900 | 1 | C9602 | 2 | E0193 | 0 | E0325 | 0 | E0616 | 1 |
| A9571 | 1 | C1717 | 10 | C1842 | 0 | C8901 | 1 | C9603 | 2 | E0194 | 0 | E0326 | 0 | E0617 | 0 |
| A9572 | 1 | C1719 | 99 | C1874 | 5 | C8902 | 1 | C9604 | 2 | E0196 | 0 | E0328 | 0 | E0618 | 0 |
| A9575 | 200 | C1721 | 1 | C1875 | 4 | C8903 | 1 | C9605 | 2 | E0197 | 0 | E0329 | 0 | E0619 | 0 |
| A9576 | 100 | C1722 | 1 | C1876 | 5 | C8904 | 1 | C9606 | 1 | E0198 | 0 | E0350 | 0 | E0620 | 0 |
| A9577 | 50 | C1724 | 5 | C1877 | 5 | C8905 | 1 | C9607 | 1 | E0199 | 0 | E0352 | 0 | E0621 | 0 |
| A9578 | 50 | C1725 | 9 | C1878 | 2 | C8906 | 1 | C9608 | 2 | E0200 | 0 | E0370 | 0 | E0625 | 0 |
| A9579 | 100 | C1726 | 5 | C1880 | 2 | C8907 | 1 | C9725 | 1 | E0202 | 0 | E0371 | 0 | E0627 | 0 |
| A9580 | 1 | C1727 | 4 | C1881 | 2 | C8908 | 1 | C9726 | 2 | E0203 | 0 | E0372 | 0 | E0629 | 0 |
| A9581 | 20 | C1728 | 5 | C1882 | 1 | C8909 | 1 | C9727 | 1 | E0205 | 0 | E0373 | 0 | E0630 | 0 |
| A9582 | 1 | C1729 | 6 | C1883 | 4 | C8910 | 1 | C9728 | 1 | E0210 | 0 | E0424 | 0 | E0635 | 0 |
| A9583 | 18 | C1730 | 4 | C1884 | 4 | C8911 | 1 | C9733 | 1 | E0215 | 0 | E0425 | 0 | E0636 | 0 |
| A9584 | 1 | C1731 | 2 | C1885 | 2 | C8912 | 1 | C9734 | 1 | E0217 | 0 | E0430 | 0 | E0637 | 0 |
| A9585 | 300 | C1732 | 3 | C1886 | 1 | C8913 | 1 | C9739 | 1 | E0218 | 0 | E0431 | 0 | E0638 | 0 |
| A9586 | 1 | C1733 | 3 | C1887 | 7 | C8914 | 1 | C9740 | 1 | E0221 | 0 | E0433 | 0 | E0639 | 0 |
| A9587 | 54 | C1749 | 1 | C1888 | 2 | C8918 | 1 | C9741 | 1 | E0225 | 0 | E0434 | 0 | E0640 | 0 |
| A9588 | 10 | C1750 | 2 | C1891 | 1 | C8919 | 1 | C9744 | 1 | E0231 | 0 | E0435 | 0 | E0641 | 0 |
| A9599 | 1 | C1751 | 3 | C1892 | 6 | C8920 | 1 | C9898 | 1 | E0232 | 0 | E0439 | 0 | E0642 | 0 |
| A9600 | 7 | C1752 | 2 | C1893 | 6 | C8921 | 1 | E0100 | 0 | E0235 | 0 | E0440 | 0 | E0650 | 0 |
| A9604 | 1 | C1753 | 2 | C1894 | 6 | C8922 | 1 | E0105 | 0 | E0236 | 0 | E0441 | 0 | E0651 | 0 |
| A9606 | 203 | C1754 | 2 | C1895 | 2 | C8923 | 1 | E0110 | 0 | E0239 | 0 | E0442 | 0 | E0652 | 0 |
| A9700 | 2 | C1755 | 2 | C1896 | 2 | C8924 | 1 | E0111 | 0 | E0240 | 0 | E0443 | 0 | E0655 | 0 |
| B4034 | 0 | C1756 | 2 | C1897 | 2 | C8925 | 1 | E0112 | 0 | E0241 | 0 | E0444 | 0 | E0656 | 0 |
| B4035 | 0 | C1757 | 6 | C1898 | 2 | C8926 | 1 | E0113 | 0 | E0242 | 0 | E0445 | 0 | E0657 | 0 |
| B4036 | 0 | C1758 | 2 | C1899 | 2 | C8927 | 1 | E0114 | 0 | E0243 | 0 | E0446 | 0 | E0660 | 0 |
| B4081 | 0 | C1759 | 2 | C1900 | 1 | C8928 | 1 | E0116 | 0 | E0244 | 0 | E0455 | 0 | E0665 | 0 |
| B4082 | 0 | C1760 | 4 | C2613 | 2 | C8929 | 1 | E0117 | 0 | E0245 | 0 | E0457 | 0 | E0666 | 0 |
| B4083 | 0 | C1762 | 4 | C2614 | 3 | C8930 | 1 | E0118 | 0 | E0246 | 0 | E0459 | 0 | E0667 | 0 |
| B4087 | 1 | C1763 | 4 | C2615 | 2 | C8931 | 1 | E0130 | 0 | E0247 | 0 | E0462 | 0 | E0668 | 0 |
| B4088 | 1 | C1764 | 1 | C2616 | 1 | C8932 | 1 | E0135 | 0 | E0248 | 0 | E0465 | 0 | E0669 | 0 |
| B4149 | 0 | C1765 | 4 | C2617 | 4 | C8933 | 1 | E0140 | 0 | E0249 | 0 | E0466 | 0 | E0670 | 0 |
| B4150 | 0 | C1766 | 4 | C2618 | 4 | C8934 | 2 | E0141 | 0 | E0250 | 0 | E0470 | 0 | E0671 | 0 |
| B4152 | 0 | C1767 | 2 | C2619 | 1 | C8935 | 2 | E0143 | 0 | E0251 | 0 | E0471 | 0 | E0672 | 0 |
| B4153 | 0 | C1768 | 3 | C2620 | 1 | C8936 | 2 | E0144 | 0 | E0255 | 0 | E0472 | 0 | E0673 | 0 |
| B4154 | 0 | C1769 | 9 | C2621 | 1 | C8957 | 2 | E0147 | 0 | E0256 | 0 | E0480 | 0 | E0675 | 0 |
| B4155 | 0 | C1770 | 3 | C2622 | 1 | C9113 | 10 | E0148 | 0 | E0260 | 0 | E0481 | 0 | E0676 | 1 |
| B4157 | 0 | C1771 | 1 | C2623 | 4 | C9132 | 5500 | E0149 | 0 | E0261 | 0 | E0482 | 0 | E0691 | 0 |
| B4158 | 0 | C1772 | 1 | C2624 | 1 | C9140 | 22000 | E0153 | 0 | E0265 | 0 | E0483 | 0 | E0692 | 0 |
| B4159 | 0 | C1773 | 3 | C2625 | 4 | C9248 | 25 | E0154 | 0 | E0266 | 0 | E0484 | 0 | E0693 | 0 |
| B4160 | 0 | C1776 | 10 | C2626 | 1 | C9250 | 5 | E0155 | 0 | E0270 | 0 | E0485 | 0 | E0694 | 0 |
| B4161 | 0 | C1777 | 2 | C2627 | 2 | C9254 | 400 | E0156 | 0 | E0271 | 0 | E0486 | 0 | E0700 | 0 |
| B4162 | 0 | C1778 | 4 | C2628 | 4 | C9257 | 8000 | E0157 | 0 | E0272 | 0 | E0487 | 0 | E0705 | 1 |
| B4164 | 0 | C1779 | 2 | C2629 | 4 | C9275 | 1 | E0158 | 0 | E0273 | 0 | E0500 | 0 | E0710 | 0 |
| B4168 | 0 | C1780 | 2 | C2630 | 4 | C9285 | 2 | E0159 | 0 | E0274 | 0 | E0550 | 0 | E0720 | 0 |
| B4172 | 0 | C1781 | 4 | C2631 | 1 | C9290 | 266 | E0160 | 0 | E0275 | 0 | E0555 | 0 | E0730 | 0 |
| B4176 | 0 | C1782 | 1 | C2634 | 24 | C9293 | 700 | E0161 | 0 | E0276 | 0 | E0560 | 0 | E0731 | 0 |
| B4178 | 0 | C1783 | 2 | C2635 | 124 | C9352 | 3 | E0162 | 0 | E0277 | 0 | E0561 | 0 | E0740 | 0 |
| B4180 | 0 | C1784 | 2 | C2636 | 690 | C9353 | 4 | E0163 | 0 | E0280 | 0 | E0562 | 0 | E0744 | 0 |
| B4189 | 0 | C1785 | 1 | C2637 | 0 | C9354 | 300 | E0165 | 0 | E0290 | 0 | E0565 | 0 | E0745 | 0 |
| B4193 | 0 | C1786 | 1 | C2638 | 150 | C9355 | 3 | E0167 | 0 | E0291 | 0 | E0570 | 0 | E0746 | 1 |
| B4197 | 0 | C1787 | 2 | C2639 | 150 | C9356 | 125 | E0168 | 0 | E0292 | 0 | E0572 | 0 | E0747 | 0 |
| B4199 | 0 | C1788 | 2 | C2640 | 150 | C9358 | 800 | E0170 | 0 | E0293 | 0 | E0574 | 0 | E0748 | 0 |
| B4216 | 0 | C1789 | 2 | C2641 | 150 | C9359 | 30 | E0171 | 0 | E0294 | 0 | E0575 | 0 | E0749 | 1 |
| B4220 | 0 | C1813 | 1 | C2642 | 120 | C9360 | 300 | E0172 | 0 | E0295 | 0 | E0580 | 0 | E0755 | 0 |
| B4222 | 0 | C1814 | 2 | C2643 | 120 | C9361 | 10 | E0175 | 0 | E0296 | 0 | E0585 | 0 | E0760 | 0 |
| B4224 | 0 | C1815 | 1 | C2644 | 500 | C9362 | 60 | E0181 | 0 | E0297 | 0 | E0600 | 0 | E0761 | 0 |

| CPT | MUE | CPT | MUE | CPT | MUE | CPT | MUE | CPT | MUE | CPT | MUE | CPT | MUE |
|---|---|---|---|---|---|---|---|---|---|---|---|---|---|
| E0762 | 1 | E0986 | 0 | E1226 | 1 | E1801 | 0 | E2324 | 0 | E2612 | 0 | G0239 | 2 | G0412 | 1 |
| E0764 | 0 | E0988 | 0 | E1228 | 0 | E1802 | 0 | E2325 | 0 | E2613 | 0 | G0245 | 1 | G0413 | 1 |
| E0765 | 0 | E0990 | 2 | E1229 | 0 | E1805 | 0 | E2326 | 0 | E2614 | 0 | G0246 | 1 | G0414 | 1 |
| E0766 | 0 | E0992 | 1 | E1230 | 0 | E1806 | 0 | E2327 | 0 | E2615 | 0 | G0247 | 1 | G0415 | 1 |
| E0769 | 0 | E0994 | 0 | E1231 | 0 | E1810 | 0 | E2328 | 0 | E2616 | 0 | G0248 | 1 | G0416 | 1 |
| E0770 | 1 | E0995 | 2 | E1232 | 0 | E1811 | 0 | E2329 | 0 | E2617 | 0 | G0249 | 3 | G0420 | 2 |
| E0776 | 0 | E1002 | 0 | E1233 | 0 | E1812 | 0 | E2330 | 0 | E2619 | 0 | G0250 | 1 | G0421 | 4 |
| E0779 | 0 | E1003 | 0 | E1234 | 0 | E1815 | 0 | E2331 | 0 | E2620 | 0 | G0257 | 1 | G0422 | 6 |
| E0780 | 0 | E1004 | 0 | E1235 | 0 | E1816 | 0 | E2340 | 0 | E2621 | 0 | G0259 | 2 | G0423 | 6 |
| E0781 | 0 | E1005 | 0 | E1236 | 0 | E1818 | 0 | E2341 | 0 | E2622 | 0 | G0260 | 2 | G0424 | 2 |
| E0782 | 1 | E1006 | 0 | E1237 | 0 | E1820 | 0 | E2342 | 0 | E2623 | 0 | G0268 | 1 | G0425 | 1 |
| E0783 | 1 | E1007 | 0 | E1238 | 0 | E1821 | 0 | E2343 | 0 | E2624 | 0 | G0269 | 2 | G0426 | 1 |
| E0784 | 0 | E1008 | 0 | E1239 | 0 | E1825 | 0 | E2351 | 0 | E2625 | 0 | G0270 | 8 | G0427 | 1 |
| E0785 | 1 | E1009 | 0 | E1240 | 0 | E1830 | 0 | E2358 | 0 | E2626 | 0 | G0271 | 4 | G0429 | 1 |
| E0786 | 1 | E1010 | 0 | E1250 | 0 | E1831 | 0 | E2359 | 0 | E2627 | 0 | G0276 | 1 | G0432 | 1 |
| E0791 | 0 | E1011 | 0 | E1260 | 0 | E1840 | 0 | E2361 | 0 | E2628 | 0 | G0277 | 5 | G0433 | 1 |
| E0830 | 0 | E1012 | 0 | E1270 | 0 | E1841 | 0 | E2363 | 0 | E2629 | 0 | G0278 | 1 | G0435 | 1 |
| E0840 | 0 | E1014 | 0 | E1280 | 0 | E1902 | 0 | E2365 | 0 | E2630 | 0 | G0281 | 1 | G0438 | 1 |
| E0849 | 0 | E1015 | 0 | E1285 | 0 | E2000 | 0 | E2366 | 0 | E2631 | 0 | G0283 | 1 | G0439 | 1 |
| E0850 | 0 | E1016 | 0 | E1290 | 0 | E2100 | 0 | E2367 | 0 | E2632 | 0 | G0288 | 1 | G0442 | 1 |
| E0855 | 0 | E1017 | 0 | E1295 | 0 | E2101 | 0 | E2368 | 0 | E2633 | 0 | G0289 | 1 | G0443 | 1 |
| E0856 | 0 | E1018 | 0 | E1300 | 0 | E2120 | 0 | E2369 | 0 | G0008 | 1 | G0293 | 1 | G0444 | 1 |
| E0860 | 0 | E1020 | 0 | E1310 | 0 | E2201 | 0 | E2370 | 0 | G0009 | 1 | G0294 | 1 | G0445 | 1 |
| E0870 | 0 | E1028 | 0 | E1352 | 0 | E2202 | 0 | E2371 | 0 | G0010 | 1 | G0296 | 1 | G0446 | 1 |
| E0880 | 0 | E1029 | 0 | E1353 | 0 | E2203 | 0 | E2373 | 0 | G0027 | 1 | G0297 | 1 | G0447 | 2 |
| E0890 | 0 | E1030 | 0 | E1354 | 0 | E2204 | 0 | E2374 | 0 | G0101 | 1 | G0302 | 1 | G0448 | 1 |
| E0900 | 0 | E1031 | 0 | E1355 | 0 | E2205 | 0 | E2375 | 0 | G0102 | 1 | G0303 | 1 | G0451 | 1 |
| E0910 | 0 | E1035 | 0 | E1356 | 0 | E2206 | 0 | E2376 | 0 | G0103 | 1 | G0304 | 1 | G0452 | 1 |
| E0911 | 0 | E1036 | 0 | E1357 | 0 | E2207 | 0 | E2377 | 0 | G0104 | 1 | G0305 | 1 | G0453 | 10 |
| E0912 | 0 | E1037 | 0 | E1358 | 0 | E2208 | 0 | E2378 | 0 | G0105 | 1 | G0306 | 4 | G0454 | 1 |
| E0920 | 0 | E1038 | 0 | E1372 | 0 | E2209 | 0 | E2381 | 0 | G0106 | 1 | G0307 | 4 | G0455 | 1 |
| E0930 | 0 | E1039 | 0 | E1390 | 0 | E2210 | 0 | E2382 | 0 | G0108 | 8 | G0328 | 1 | G0458 | 1 |
| E0935 | 0 | E1050 | 0 | E1391 | 0 | E2211 | 0 | E2383 | 0 | G0109 | 12 | G0329 | 1 | G0459 | 1 |
| E0936 | 0 | E1060 | 0 | E1392 | 0 | E2212 | 0 | E2384 | 0 | G0117 | 1 | G0333 | 0 | G0460 | 1 |
| E0940 | 0 | E1070 | 0 | E1405 | 0 | E2213 | 0 | E2385 | 0 | G0118 | 1 | G0337 | 1 | G0463 | 6 |
| E0941 | 0 | E1083 | 0 | E1406 | 0 | E2214 | 0 | E2386 | 0 | G0120 | 1 | G0339 | 1 | G0466 | 1 |
| E0942 | 0 | E1084 | 0 | E1500 | 0 | E2215 | 0 | E2387 | 0 | G0121 | 1 | G0340 | 2 | G0467 | 1 |
| C0944 | 0 | E1085 | 0 | E1510 | 0 | E2216 | 0 | E2388 | 0 | G0123 | 1 | G0341 | 1 | G0468 | 1 |
| E0945 | 0 | E1086 | 0 | E1520 | 0 | E2217 | 0 | E2389 | 0 | G0124 | 1 | G0342 | 1 | G0469 | 1 |
| E0946 | 0 | E1087 | 0 | E1530 | 0 | E2218 | 0 | E2390 | 0 | G0127 | 1 | G0343 | 1 | G0470 | 1 |
| E0947 | 0 | E1088 | 0 | E1540 | 0 | E2219 | 0 | E2391 | 0 | G0128 | 1 | G0364 | 2 | G0471 | 2 |
| E0948 | 0 | E1089 | 0 | E1550 | 0 | E2220 | 0 | E2392 | 0 | G0129 | 6 | G0365 | 2 | G0472 | 1 |
| E0950 | 0 | E1090 | 0 | E1560 | 0 | E2221 | 0 | E2394 | 0 | G0130 | 1 | G0372 | 1 | G0473 | 1 |
| E0951 | 0 | E1092 | 0 | E1570 | 0 | E2222 | 0 | E2395 | 0 | G0141 | 1 | G0378 | 72 | G0475 | 1 |
| E0952 | 0 | E1093 | 0 | E1575 | 0 | E2224 | 0 | E2396 | 0 | G0143 | 1 | G0379 | 1 | G0476 | 1 |
| E0955 | 0 | E1100 | 0 | E1580 | 0 | E2225 | 0 | E2397 | 0 | G0144 | 1 | G0380 | 2 | G0480 | 1 |
| E0956 | 0 | E1110 | 0 | E1590 | 0 | E2226 | 0 | E2402 | 0 | G0145 | 1 | G0381 | 2 | G0481 | 1 |
| E0957 | 0 | E1130 | 0 | E1592 | 0 | E2227 | 0 | E2500 | 0 | G0147 | 1 | G0382 | 2 | G0482 | 1 |
| E0958 | 0 | E1140 | 0 | E1594 | 0 | E2228 | 0 | E2502 | 0 | G0148 | 1 | G0383 | 2 | G0483 | 1 |
| E0959 | 2 | E1150 | 0 | E1600 | 0 | E2230 | 0 | E2504 | 0 | G0166 | 2 | G0384 | 2 | G0491 | 1 |
| E0960 | 0 | E1160 | 0 | E1610 | 0 | E2231 | 0 | E2506 | 0 | G0168 | 2 | G0390 | 1 | G0492 | 1 |
| E0961 | 2 | E1161 | 0 | E1615 | 0 | E2291 | 1 | E2508 | 0 | G0175 | 1 | G0396 | 1 | G0498 | 1 |
| E0966 | 1 | E1170 | 0 | E1620 | 0 | E2292 | 1 | E2510 | 0 | G0176 | 5 | G0397 | 1 | G0499 | 1 |
| E0967 | 0 | E1171 | 0 | E1625 | 0 | E2293 | 1 | E2511 | 0 | G0177 | 5 | G0398 | 1 | G0500 | 1 |
| E0968 | 0 | E1172 | 0 | E1630 | 0 | E2294 | 1 | E2512 | 0 | G0179 | 1 | G0399 | 1 | G0502 | 1 |
| E0970 | 0 | E1180 | 0 | E1632 | 0 | E2295 | 0 | E2601 | 0 | G0180 | 1 | G0400 | 1 | G0503 | 1 |
| E0971 | 2 | E1190 | 0 | E1634 | 0 | E2300 | 0 | E2602 | 0 | G0181 | 1 | G0402 | 1 | G0504 | 2 |
| E0973 | 2 | E1195 | 0 | E1635 | 0 | E2301 | 0 | E2603 | 0 | G0182 | 1 | G0403 | 1 | G0505 | 1 |
| E0974 | 2 | E1200 | 0 | E1636 | 0 | E2310 | 0 | E2604 | 0 | G0186 | 1 | G0404 | 1 | G0506 | 1 |
| E0978 | 1 | E1220 | 0 | E1637 | 0 | E2311 | 0 | E2605 | 0 | G0202 | 1 | G0405 | 1 | G0507 | 1 |
| E0981 | 0 | E1221 | 0 | E1639 | 0 | E2312 | 0 | E2606 | 0 | G0204 | 2 | G0406 | 1 | G0508 | 1 |
| E0982 | 0 | E1222 | 0 | E1700 | 0 | E2313 | 0 | E2607 | 0 | G0206 | 2 | G0407 | 1 | G0509 | 1 |
| E0983 | 0 | E1223 | 0 | E1701 | 0 | E2321 | 0 | E2608 | 0 | G0235 | 1 | G0408 | 1 | G0659 | 1 |
| E0984 | 0 | E1224 | 0 | E1702 | 0 | E2322 | 0 | E2609 | 0 | G0237 | 8 | G0410 | 6 | G6001 | 2 |
| E0985 | 0 | E1225 | 0 | E1800 | 0 | E2323 | 0 | E2611 | 0 | G0238 | 8 | G0411 | 6 | G6002 | 2 |

CPT © 2017 American Medical Association. All Rights Reserved.     © 2017 Optum360, LLC

| CPT | MUE | CPT | MUE | CPT | MUE | CPT | MUE | CPT | MUE | CPT | MUE | CPT | MUE | CPT | MUE |
|---|---|---|---|---|---|---|---|---|---|---|---|---|---|---|---|
| G6003 | 2 | J0401 | 400 | J0775 | 180 | J1438 | 2 | J1817 | 0 | J2503 | 2 | J3070 | 3 | J7175 | 9000 |
| G6004 | 2 | J0456 | 4 | J0780 | 10 | J1439 | 750 | J1830 | 1 | J2504 | 15 | J3090 | 200 | J7178 | 7700 |
| G6005 | 2 | J0461 | 800 | J0795 | 100 | J1442 | 3360 | J1833 | 1116 | J2505 | 1 | J3095 | 150 | J7179 | 30000 |
| G6006 | 2 | J0470 | 2 | J0800 | 3 | J1443 | 272 | J1835 | 0 | J2507 | 8 | J3101 | 50 | J7180 | 6000 |
| G6007 | 2 | J0475 | 8 | J0833 | 3 | J1447 | 960 | J1840 | 3 | J2510 | 4 | J3105 | 4 | J7181 | 3850 |
| G6008 | 2 | J0476 | 2 | J0834 | 3 | J1450 | 4 | J1850 | 14 | J2513 | 1 | J3110 | 2 | J7182 | 22000 |
| G6009 | 2 | J0480 | 1 | J0840 | 18 | J1451 | 200 | J1885 | 8 | J2515 | 8 | J3121 | 400 | J7183 | 15000 |
| G6010 | 2 | J0485 | 1500 | J0850 | 9 | J1452 | 0 | J1890 | 0 | J2540 | 75 | J3145 | 750 | J7185 | 4000 |
| G6011 | 2 | J0490 | 160 | J0875 | 300 | J1453 | 150 | J1930 | 120 | J2543 | 20 | J3230 | 6 | J7186 | 13200 |
| G6012 | 2 | J0500 | 4 | J0878 | 1500 | J1455 | 18 | J1931 | 760 | J2545 | 1 | J3240 | 1 | J7187 | 9600 |
| G6013 | 2 | J0515 | 6 | J0881 | 500 | J1457 | 0 | J1940 | 10 | J2547 | 600 | J3243 | 200 | J7188 | 22000 |
| G6014 | 2 | J0520 | 0 | J0882 | 300 | J1458 | 100 | J1942 | 882 | J2550 | 3 | J3246 | 100 | J7189 | 26000 |
| G6015 | 2 | J0558 | 24 | J0883 | 1250 | J1459 | 300 | J1945 | 0 | J2560 | 16 | J3250 | 4 | J7190 | 30000 |
| G6016 | 2 | J0561 | 24 | J0884 | 1250 | J1460 | 10 | J1950 | 12 | J2562 | 48 | J3260 | 12 | J7191 | 0 |
| G6017 | 2 | J0570 | 4 | J0885 | 60 | J1556 | 300 | J1953 | 300 | J2590 | 15 | J3262 | 800 | J7192 | 22000 |
| G9143 | 1 | J0571 | 0 | J0887 | 360 | J1557 | 300 | J1955 | 11 | J2597 | 45 | J3265 | 0 | J7193 | 20000 |
| G9156 | 1 | J0572 | 0 | J0888 | 360 | J1559 | 375 | J1956 | 4 | J2650 | 0 | J3280 | 0 | J7194 | 9000 |
| G9157 | 1 | J0573 | 0 | J0890 | 0 | J1560 | 1 | J1960 | 0 | J2670 | 0 | J3285 | 9 | J7195 | 20000 |
| G9187 | 0 | J0574 | 0 | J0894 | 100 | J1561 | 300 | J1980 | 8 | J2675 | 1 | J3300 | 160 | J7196 | 175 |
| G9480 | 1 | J0575 | 0 | J0895 | 12 | J1562 | 375 | J1990 | 0 | J2680 | 4 | J3301 | 16 | J7197 | 6300 |
| G9678 | 1 | J0583 | 1250 | J0897 | 120 | J1566 | 300 | J2001 | 400 | J2690 | 4 | J3302 | 0 | J7198 | 30000 |
| J0120 | 1 | J0585 | 600 | J0945 | 4 | J1568 | 300 | J2010 | 10 | J2700 | 48 | J3303 | 24 | J7200 | 20000 |
| J0129 | 100 | J0586 | 300 | J1000 | 1 | J1569 | 300 | J2020 | 6 | J2704 | 400 | J3305 | 0 | J7201 | 9000 |
| J0130 | 6 | J0587 | 300 | J1020 | 8 | J1570 | 4 | J2060 | 10 | J2710 | 10 | J3310 | 0 | J7202 | 11550 |
| J0131 | 400 | J0588 | 600 | J1030 | 8 | J1571 | 20 | J2150 | 8 | J2720 | 10 | J3315 | 6 | J7205 | 9750 |
| J0132 | 300 | J0592 | 12 | J1040 | 4 | J1572 | 300 | J2170 | 8 | J2724 | 4000 | J3320 | 0 | J7207 | 7500 |
| J0133 | 1200 | J0594 | 320 | J1050 | 1000 | J1573 | 130 | J2175 | 6 | J2725 | 0 | J3350 | 0 | J7209 | 7500 |
| J0135 | 8 | J0595 | 12 | J1071 | 400 | J1575 | 650 | J2180 | 0 | J2730 | 2 | J3355 | 1 | J7297 | 0 |
| J0153 | 180 | J0596 | 840 | J1094 | 0 | J1580 | 9 | J2182 | 100 | J2760 | 2 | J3357 | 520 | J7298 | 0 |
| J0171 | 120 | J0597 | 250 | J1100 | 120 | J1595 | 2 | J2185 | 60 | J2765 | 18 | J3360 | 6 | J7301 | 0 |
| J0178 | 4 | J0598 | 100 | J1110 | 3 | J1599 | 300 | J2210 | 5 | J2770 | 7 | J3364 | 0 | J7308 | 3 |
| J0180 | 150 | J0600 | 3 | J1120 | 2 | J1600 | 2 | J2212 | 240 | J2778 | 10 | J3365 | 0 | J7309 | 1 |
| J0190 | 0 | J0610 | 15 | J1130 | 300 | J1602 | 300 | J2248 | 300 | J2780 | 16 | J3370 | 12 | J7310 | 2 |
| J0200 | 0 | J0620 | 1 | J1160 | 3 | J1610 | 3 | J2250 | 30 | J2783 | 60 | J3380 | 300 | J7311 | 1 |
| J0202 | 12 | J0630 | 8 | J1162 | 10 | J1620 | 0 | J2260 | 16 | J2785 | 4 | J3385 | 92 | J7312 | 14 |
| J0205 | 0 | J0636 | 100 | J1165 | 50 | J1626 | 30 | J2265 | 400 | J2786 | 500 | J3396 | 150 | J7313 | 38 |
| J0207 | 4 | J0637 | 20 | J1170 | 50 | J1630 | 7 | J2270 | 15 | J2788 | 1 | J3400 | 0 | J7315 | 2 |
| J0210 | 16 | J0638 | 180 | J1180 | 0 | J1631 | 9 | J2274 | 100 | J2790 | 3 | J3410 | 16 | J7316 | 4 |
| J0215 | 30 | J0640 | 24 | J1190 | 8 | J1640 | 626 | J2278 | 999 | J2791 | 275 | J3411 | 8 | J7320 | 50 |
| J0220 | 20 | J0641 | 1200 | J1200 | 8 | J1642 | 150 | J2280 | 8 | J2792 | 400 | J3415 | 6 | J7321 | 2 |
| J0221 | 300 | J0670 | 10 | J1205 | 4 | J1644 | 50 | J2300 | 10 | J2793 | 320 | J3420 | 1 | J7322 | 48 |
| J0256 | 3500 | J0690 | 16 | J1212 | 1 | J1645 | 10 | J2310 | 10 | J2794 | 100 | J3430 | 50 | J7323 | 2 |
| J0257 | 1400 | J0692 | 12 | J1230 | 5 | J1650 | 30 | J2315 | 380 | J2795 | 2400 | J3465 | 120 | J7324 | 2 |
| J0270 | 32 | J0694 | 12 | J1240 | 6 | J1652 | 20 | J2320 | 4 | J2796 | 150 | J3470 | 3 | J7325 | 96 |
| J0275 | 1 | J0695 | 60 | J1245 | 6 | J1655 | 0 | J2323 | 300 | J2800 | 3 | J3471 | 999 | J7326 | 2 |
| J0278 | 15 | J0696 | 16 | J1250 | 4 | J1670 | 2 | J2325 | 34 | J2805 | 3 | J3472 | 2 | J7327 | 2 |
| J0280 | 10 | J0697 | 12 | J1260 | 2 | J1675 | 0 | J2353 | 60 | J2810 | 20 | J3473 | 450 | J7328 | 336 |
| J0282 | 70 | J0698 | 12 | J1265 | 100 | J1700 | 0 | J2354 | 60 | J2820 | 10 | J3475 | 80 | J7330 | 1 |
| J0285 | 6 | J0702 | 20 | J1267 | 150 | J1710 | 0 | J2355 | 2 | J2840 | 460 | J3480 | 200 | J7336 | 1120 |
| J0287 | 60 | J0706 | 16 | J1270 | 16 | J1720 | 10 | J2357 | 90 | J2850 | 48 | J3485 | 160 | J7340 | 1 |
| J0288 | 0 | J0710 | 0 | J1290 | 60 | J1725 | 0 | J2358 | 405 | J2860 | 170 | J3486 | 4 | J7342 | 10 |
| J0289 | 115 | J0712 | 180 | J1300 | 120 | J1730 | 0 | J2360 | 3 | J2910 | 0 | J3489 | 5 | J7500 | 15 |
| J0290 | 24 | J0713 | 12 | J1320 | 0 | J1740 | 3 | J2370 | 30 | J2916 | 20 | J3520 | 0 | J7501 | 8 |
| J0295 | 12 | J0714 | 12 | J1322 | 220 | J1741 | 32 | J2400 | 4 | J2920 | 25 | J3530 | 0 | J7502 | 60 |
| J0300 | 8 | J0715 | 0 | J1324 | 108 | J1742 | 4 | J2405 | 64 | J2930 | 25 | J7030 | 20 | J7503 | 120 |
| J0330 | 50 | J0716 | 4 | J1325 | 18 | J1743 | 66 | J2407 | 120 | J2940 | 0 | J7040 | 12 | J7504 | 15 |
| J0348 | 200 | J0717 | 400 | J1327 | 99 | J1744 | 90 | J2410 | 2 | J2941 | 8 | J7042 | 12 | J7505 | 1 |
| J0350 | 0 | J0720 | 15 | J1330 | 1 | J1745 | 150 | J2425 | 125 | J2950 | 0 | J7050 | 20 | J7507 | 40 |
| J0360 | 6 | J0725 | 10 | J1335 | 2 | J1750 | 45 | J2426 | 819 | J2993 | 2 | J7060 | 10 | J7508 | 300 |
| J0364 | 6 | J0735 | 50 | J1364 | 8 | J1756 | 500 | J2430 | 3 | J2995 | 0 | J7070 | 7 | J7509 | 60 |
| J0365 | 0 | J0740 | 2 | J1380 | 4 | J1786 | 900 | J2440 | 4 | J2997 | 100 | J7100 | 2 | J7510 | 60 |
| J0380 | 1 | J0743 | 16 | J1410 | 4 | J1790 | 2 | J2460 | 0 | J3000 | 2 | J7110 | 3 | J7511 | 9 |
| J0390 | 0 | J0744 | 8 | J1430 | 10 | J1800 | 12 | J2469 | 10 | J3010 | 100 | J7120 | 20 | J7512 | 300 |
| J0395 | 0 | J0745 | 8 | J1435 | 1 | J1810 | 0 | J2501 | 25 | J3030 | 2 | J7121 | 0 | J7513 | 6 |
| J0400 | 120 | J0770 | 5 | J1436 | 0 | J1815 | 200 | J2502 | 60 | J3060 | 900 | J7131 | 500 | J7515 | 90 |

**Appendix I — Medically Unlikely Edits (MUEs) — OPPS**

| CPT | MUE | CPT | MUE | CPT | MUE | CPT | MUE | CPT | MUE | CPT | MUE | CPT | MUE | CPT | MUE |
|---|---|---|---|---|---|---|---|---|---|---|---|---|---|---|---|
| J7516 | 4 | J8521 | 15 | J9214 | 100 | K0019 | 0 | K0830 | 0 | L0462 | 1 | L1040 | 1 | L1910 | 2 |
| J7517 | 16 | J8530 | 60 | J9215 | 0 | K0020 | 0 | K0831 | 0 | L0464 | 1 | L1050 | 1 | L1920 | 2 |
| J7518 | 12 | J8540 | 48 | J9216 | 2 | K0037 | 0 | K0835 | 0 | L0466 | 1 | L1060 | 1 | L1930 | 2 |
| J7520 | 40 | J8560 | 6 | J9217 | 6 | K0038 | 0 | K0836 | 0 | L0467 | 1 | L1070 | 2 | L1932 | 2 |
| J7525 | 2 | J8562 | 12 | J9218 | 1 | K0039 | 0 | K0837 | 0 | L0468 | 1 | L1080 | 2 | L1940 | 2 |
| J7527 | 20 | J8600 | 40 | J9219 | 1 | K0040 | 0 | K0838 | 0 | L0469 | 1 | L1085 | 1 | L1945 | 2 |
| J7604 | 0 | J8610 | 20 | J9225 | 1 | K0041 | 0 | K0839 | 0 | L0470 | 1 | L1090 | 1 | L1950 | 2 |
| J7605 | 0 | J8650 | 6 | J9226 | 1 | K0042 | 0 | K0840 | 0 | L0472 | 1 | L1100 | 2 | L1951 | 2 |
| J7606 | 0 | J8655 | 1 | J9228 | 1100 | K0043 | 0 | K0841 | 0 | L0480 | 1 | L1110 | 2 | L1960 | 2 |
| J7607 | 0 | J8670 | 180 | J9230 | 5 | K0044 | 0 | K0842 | 0 | L0482 | 1 | L1120 | 3 | L1970 | 2 |
| J7608 | 0 | J8700 | 120 | J9245 | 11 | K0045 | 0 | K0843 | 0 | L0484 | 1 | L1200 | 1 | L1971 | 2 |
| J7609 | 0 | J8705 | 22 | J9250 | 50 | K0046 | 0 | K0848 | 0 | L0486 | 1 | L1210 | 2 | L1980 | 2 |
| J7610 | 0 | J9000 | 20 | J9260 | 20 | K0047 | 0 | K0849 | 0 | L0488 | 1 | L1220 | 1 | L1990 | 2 |
| J7611 | 0 | J9015 | 1 | J9261 | 80 | K0050 | 0 | K0850 | 0 | L0490 | 1 | L1230 | 1 | L2000 | 2 |
| J7612 | 0 | J9017 | 30 | J9262 | 700 | K0051 | 0 | K0851 | 0 | L0491 | 1 | L1240 | 1 | L2005 | 2 |
| J7613 | 0 | J9019 | 60 | J9263 | 700 | K0052 | 0 | K0852 | 0 | L0492 | 1 | L1250 | 2 | L2010 | 2 |
| J7614 | 0 | J9020 | 0 | J9266 | 2 | K0053 | 0 | K0853 | 0 | L0621 | 1 | L1260 | 1 | L2020 | 2 |
| J7615 | 0 | J9025 | 300 | J9267 | 750 | K0056 | 0 | K0854 | 0 | L0622 | 1 | L1270 | 3 | L2030 | 2 |
| J7620 | 0 | J9027 | 100 | J9268 | 1 | K0065 | 0 | K0855 | 0 | L0623 | 1 | L1280 | 2 | L2034 | 2 |
| J7622 | 0 | J9031 | 1 | J9270 | 0 | K0069 | 0 | K0856 | 0 | L0624 | 1 | L1290 | 2 | L2035 | 2 |
| J7624 | 0 | J9032 | 300 | J9271 | 300 | K0070 | 0 | K0857 | 0 | L0625 | 1 | L1300 | 1 | L2036 | 2 |
| J7626 | 0 | J9033 | 300 | J9280 | 12 | K0071 | 0 | K0858 | 0 | L0626 | 1 | L1310 | 1 | L2037 | 2 |
| J7627 | 0 | J9034 | 360 | J9293 | 8 | K0072 | 0 | K0859 | 0 | L0627 | 1 | L1499 | 1 | L2038 | 2 |
| J7628 | 0 | J9035 | 180 | J9295 | 800 | K0073 | 0 | K0860 | 0 | L0628 | 1 | L1600 | 1 | L2040 | 1 |
| J7629 | 0 | J9039 | 210 | J9299 | 440 | K0077 | 0 | K0861 | 0 | L0629 | 1 | L1610 | 1 | L2050 | 1 |
| J7631 | 0 | J9040 | 4 | J9300 | 0 | K0105 | 0 | K0862 | 0 | L0630 | 1 | L1620 | 1 | L2060 | 1 |
| J7632 | 0 | J9041 | 35 | J9301 | 100 | K0195 | 0 | K0863 | 0 | L0631 | 1 | L1630 | 1 | L2070 | 1 |
| J7633 | 0 | J9042 | 200 | J9302 | 200 | K0455 | 0 | K0864 | 0 | L0632 | 1 | L1640 | 1 | L2080 | 1 |
| J7634 | 0 | J9043 | 60 | J9303 | 100 | K0462 | 0 | K0868 | 0 | L0633 | 1 | L1650 | 1 | L2090 | 1 |
| J7635 | 0 | J9045 | 22 | J9305 | 150 | K0552 | 0 | K0869 | 0 | L0634 | 1 | L1652 | 1 | L2106 | 2 |
| J7636 | 0 | J9047 | 120 | J9306 | 840 | K0601 | 0 | K0870 | 0 | L0635 | 1 | L1660 | 1 | L2108 | 2 |
| J7637 | 0 | J9050 | 6 | J9307 | 80 | K0602 | 0 | K0871 | 0 | L0636 | 1 | L1680 | 1 | L2112 | 2 |
| J7638 | 0 | J9055 | 120 | J9308 | 280 | K0603 | 0 | K0877 | 0 | L0637 | 1 | L1685 | 1 | L2114 | 2 |
| J7639 | 0 | J9060 | 24 | J9310 | 12 | K0604 | 0 | K0878 | 0 | L0638 | 1 | L1686 | 1 | L2116 | 2 |
| J7640 | 0 | J9065 | 20 | J9315 | 40 | K0605 | 0 | K0879 | 0 | L0639 | 1 | L1690 | 1 | L2126 | 2 |
| J7641 | 0 | J9070 | 55 | J9320 | 4 | K0606 | 0 | K0880 | 0 | L0640 | 1 | L1700 | 1 | L2128 | 2 |
| J7642 | 0 | J9098 | 5 | J9325 | 400 | K0607 | 0 | K0884 | 0 | L0641 | 1 | L1710 | 1 | L2132 | 2 |
| J7643 | 0 | J9100 | 120 | J9328 | 400 | K0608 | 0 | K0885 | 0 | L0642 | 1 | L1720 | 2 | L2134 | 2 |
| J7644 | 0 | J9120 | 5 | J9330 | 50 | K0609 | 0 | K0886 | 0 | L0643 | 1 | L1730 | 1 | L2136 | 2 |
| J7645 | 0 | J9130 | 24 | J9340 | 4 | K0730 | 0 | K0890 | 0 | L0648 | 1 | L1755 | 2 | L2180 | 2 |
| J7647 | 0 | J9145 | 240 | J9351 | 120 | K0733 | 0 | K0891 | 0 | L0649 | 1 | L1810 | 2 | L2182 | 4 |
| J7648 | 0 | J9150 | 12 | J9352 | 50 | K0738 | 0 | K0898 | 1 | L0650 | 1 | L1812 | 2 | L2184 | 4 |
| J7649 | 0 | J9151 | 10 | J9354 | 600 | K0740 | 0 | K0900 | 0 | L0651 | 1 | L1820 | 2 | L2186 | 4 |
| J7650 | 0 | J9155 | 240 | J9355 | 100 | K0743 | 0 | L0112 | 1 | L0700 | 1 | L1830 | 2 | L2188 | 2 |
| J7657 | 0 | J9160 | 0 | J9357 | 4 | K0800 | 0 | L0113 | 1 | L0710 | 1 | L1831 | 2 | L2190 | 2 |
| J7658 | 0 | J9165 | 0 | J9360 | 45 | K0801 | 0 | L0120 | 1 | L0810 | 1 | L1832 | 2 | L2192 | 2 |
| J7659 | 0 | J9171 | 240 | J9370 | 4 | K0802 | 0 | L0130 | 1 | L0820 | 1 | L1833 | 2 | L2200 | 4 |
| J7660 | 0 | J9175 | 10 | J9371 | 5 | K0806 | 0 | L0140 | 1 | L0830 | 1 | L1834 | 2 | L2210 | 4 |
| J7665 | 127 | J9176 | 1500 | J9390 | 36 | K0807 | 0 | L0150 | 1 | L0859 | 1 | L1836 | 2 | L2220 | 4 |
| J7667 | 0 | J9178 | 150 | J9395 | 20 | K0808 | 0 | L0160 | 1 | L0861 | 1 | L1840 | 2 | L2230 | 2 |
| J7668 | 0 | J9179 | 50 | J9400 | 600 | K0812 | 0 | L0170 | 1 | L0970 | 1 | L1843 | 2 | L2232 | 2 |
| J7669 | 0 | J9181 | 100 | J9600 | 4 | K0813 | 0 | L0172 | 1 | L0972 | 1 | L1844 | 2 | L2240 | 2 |
| J7670 | 0 | J9185 | 2 | K0001 | 0 | K0814 | 0 | L0174 | 1 | L0974 | 1 | L1845 | 2 | L2250 | 2 |
| J7674 | 100 | J9190 | 20 | K0002 | 0 | K0815 | 0 | L0180 | 1 | L0976 | 1 | L1846 | 2 | L2260 | 2 |
| J7676 | 0 | J9200 | 20 | K0003 | 0 | K0816 | 0 | L0190 | 1 | L0978 | 2 | L1847 | 2 | L2265 | 2 |
| J7680 | 0 | J9201 | 20 | K0004 | 0 | K0820 | 0 | L0200 | 1 | L0980 | 1 | L1848 | 2 | L2270 | 2 |
| J7681 | 0 | J9202 | 3 | K0005 | 0 | K0821 | 0 | L0220 | 1 | L0982 | 1 | L1850 | 2 | L2275 | 2 |
| J7682 | 0 | J9205 | 215 | K0006 | 0 | K0822 | 0 | L0450 | 1 | L0984 | 3 | L1851 | 2 | L2280 | 2 |
| J7683 | 0 | J9206 | 42 | K0007 | 0 | K0823 | 0 | L0452 | 1 | L1000 | 1 | L1852 | 2 | L2300 | 1 |
| J7684 | 0 | J9207 | 90 | K0008 | 0 | K0824 | 0 | L0454 | 1 | L1001 | 1 | L1860 | 2 | L2310 | 1 |
| J7685 | 0 | J9208 | 15 | K0009 | 0 | K0825 | 0 | L0455 | 1 | L1005 | 1 | L1900 | 2 | L2320 | 2 |
| J7686 | 0 | J9209 | 55 | K0013 | 0 | K0826 | 0 | L0456 | 1 | L1010 | 2 | L1902 | 2 | L2330 | 2 |
| J8501 | 57 | J9211 | 6 | K0015 | 0 | K0827 | 0 | L0457 | 1 | L1020 | 2 | L1904 | 2 | L2335 | 2 |
| J8510 | 5 | J9212 | 0 | K0017 | 0 | K0828 | 0 | L0458 | 1 | L1025 | 1 | L1906 | 2 | L2340 | 2 |
| J8520 | 50 | J9213 | 12 | K0018 | 0 | K0829 | 0 | L0460 | 1 | L1030 | 1 | L1907 | 2 | L2350 | 2 |

CPT © 2017 American Medical Association. All Rights Reserved.          © 2017 Optum360, LLC

| CPT | MUE | CPT | MUE | CPT | MUE | CPT | MUE | CPT | MUE | CPT | MUE | CPT | MUE | CPT | MUE |
|---|---|---|---|---|---|---|---|---|---|---|---|---|---|---|---|
| L2360 | 2 | L3332 | 2 | L3912 | 2 | L5160 | 2 | L5658 | 2 | L5855 | 2 | L6580 | 2 | L6883 | 2 |
| L2370 | 2 | L3340 | 2 | L3913 | 2 | L5200 | 2 | L5661 | 2 | L5856 | 2 | L6582 | 2 | L6884 | 2 |
| L2375 | 2 | L3350 | 2 | L3915 | 2 | L5210 | 2 | L5665 | 2 | L5857 | 2 | L6584 | 2 | L6885 | 2 |
| L2380 | 2 | L3360 | 2 | L3916 | 2 | L5220 | 2 | L5666 | 2 | L5858 | 2 | L6586 | 2 | L6890 | 2 |
| L2500 | 2 | L3370 | 2 | L3917 | 2 | L5230 | 2 | L5668 | 2 | L5859 | 2 | L6588 | 2 | L6895 | 2 |
| L2510 | 2 | L3380 | 2 | L3918 | 2 | L5250 | 2 | L5670 | 2 | L5910 | 2 | L6590 | 2 | L6900 | 2 |
| L2520 | 2 | L3390 | 2 | L3919 | 2 | L5270 | 2 | L5671 | 2 | L5920 | 2 | L6600 | 2 | L6905 | 2 |
| L2525 | 2 | L3400 | 2 | L3921 | 2 | L5280 | 2 | L5672 | 2 | L5925 | 2 | L6605 | 2 | L6910 | 2 |
| L2526 | 2 | L3410 | 2 | L3923 | 2 | L5301 | 2 | L5676 | 2 | L5930 | 2 | L6610 | 2 | L6915 | 2 |
| L2530 | 2 | L3420 | 2 | L3924 | 2 | L5312 | 2 | L5677 | 2 | L5940 | 2 | L6611 | 2 | L6920 | 2 |
| L2540 | 2 | L3430 | 2 | L3925 | 4 | L5321 | 2 | L5678 | 2 | L5950 | 2 | L6615 | 2 | L6925 | 2 |
| L2550 | 2 | L3440 | 2 | L3927 | 4 | L5331 | 2 | L5680 | 2 | L5960 | 2 | L6616 | 2 | L6930 | 2 |
| L2570 | 2 | L3450 | 2 | L3929 | 2 | L5341 | 2 | L5681 | 2 | L5961 | 1 | L6620 | 2 | L6935 | 2 |
| L2580 | 2 | L3455 | 2 | L3930 | 2 | L5400 | 2 | L5682 | 2 | L5962 | 2 | L6621 | 2 | L6940 | 2 |
| L2600 | 2 | L3460 | 2 | L3931 | 2 | L5410 | 2 | L5683 | 2 | L5964 | 2 | L6623 | 2 | L6945 | 2 |
| L2610 | 2 | L3465 | 2 | L3933 | 3 | L5420 | 2 | L5684 | 2 | L5966 | 2 | L6624 | 2 | L6950 | 2 |
| L2620 | 2 | L3470 | 2 | L3935 | 3 | L5430 | 2 | L5686 | 2 | L5968 | 2 | L6625 | 2 | L6955 | 2 |
| L2622 | 2 | L3480 | 2 | L3960 | 1 | L5450 | 2 | L5688 | 2 | L5969 | 0 | L6628 | 2 | L6960 | 2 |
| L2624 | 2 | L3485 | 2 | L3961 | 1 | L5460 | 2 | L5690 | 2 | L5970 | 2 | L6629 | 2 | L6965 | 2 |
| L2627 | 1 | L3500 | 2 | L3962 | 1 | L5500 | 2 | L5692 | 2 | L5971 | 2 | L6630 | 2 | L6970 | 2 |
| L2628 | 1 | L3510 | 2 | L3967 | 1 | L5505 | 2 | L5694 | 2 | L5972 | 2 | L6635 | 2 | L6975 | 2 |
| L2630 | 1 | L3520 | 2 | L3971 | 1 | L5510 | 2 | L5695 | 2 | L5973 | 2 | L6637 | 2 | L7007 | 2 |
| L2640 | 1 | L3530 | 2 | L3973 | 1 | L5520 | 2 | L5696 | 2 | L5974 | 2 | L6638 | 2 | L7008 | 2 |
| L2650 | 2 | L3540 | 2 | L3975 | 1 | L5530 | 2 | L5697 | 2 | L5975 | 2 | L6640 | 2 | L7009 | 2 |
| L2660 | 1 | L3550 | 2 | L3976 | 1 | L5535 | 2 | L5698 | 2 | L5976 | 2 | L6641 | 2 | L7040 | 2 |
| L2670 | 2 | L3560 | 2 | L3977 | 1 | L5540 | 2 | L5699 | 2 | L5978 | 2 | L6642 | 2 | L7045 | 2 |
| L2680 | 2 | L3570 | 2 | L3978 | 1 | L5560 | 2 | L5700 | 2 | L5979 | 2 | L6645 | 2 | L7170 | 2 |
| L2795 | 2 | L3580 | 2 | L3980 | 2 | L5570 | 2 | L5701 | 2 | L5980 | 2 | L6646 | 2 | L7180 | 2 |
| L2800 | 2 | L3590 | 2 | L3981 | 2 | L5580 | 2 | L5702 | 2 | L5981 | 2 | L6647 | 2 | L7181 | 2 |
| L2820 | 2 | L3595 | 2 | L3982 | 2 | L5585 | 2 | L5703 | 2 | L5982 | 2 | L6648 | 2 | L7185 | 2 |
| L2830 | 2 | L3600 | 2 | L3984 | 2 | L5590 | 2 | L5704 | 2 | L5984 | 2 | L6650 | 2 | L7186 | 2 |
| L2861 | 0 | L3610 | 2 | L4000 | 1 | L5595 | 2 | L5705 | 2 | L5985 | 2 | L6670 | 2 | L7190 | 2 |
| L3000 | 2 | L3620 | 2 | L4010 | 2 | L5600 | 2 | L5706 | 2 | L5986 | 2 | L6672 | 2 | L7191 | 2 |
| L3001 | 2 | L3630 | 2 | L4020 | 2 | L5610 | 2 | L5707 | 2 | L5987 | 2 | L6675 | 2 | L7259 | 2 |
| L3002 | 2 | L3640 | 1 | L4030 | 2 | L5611 | 2 | L5710 | 2 | L5988 | 2 | L6676 | 2 | L7362 | 1 |
| L3003 | 2 | L3650 | 1 | L4040 | 2 | L5613 | 2 | L5711 | 2 | L5990 | 2 | L6677 | 2 | L7366 | 1 |
| L3010 | 2 | L3660 | 1 | L4045 | 2 | L5614 | 2 | L5712 | 2 | L6000 | 2 | L6686 | 2 | L7368 | 1 |
| L3020 | 2 | L3670 | 1 | L4050 | 2 | L5616 | 2 | L5714 | 2 | L6010 | 2 | L6687 | 2 | L7400 | 2 |
| L3030 | 2 | L3671 | 1 | L4055 | 2 | L5617 | 2 | L5716 | 2 | L6020 | 2 | L6688 | 2 | L7401 | 2 |
| L3031 | 2 | L3674 | 1 | L4060 | 2 | L5628 | 2 | L5718 | 2 | L6026 | 2 | L6689 | 2 | L7402 | 2 |
| L3040 | 2 | L3675 | 1 | L4070 | 2 | L5629 | 2 | L5722 | 2 | L6050 | 2 | L6690 | 2 | L7403 | 2 |
| L3050 | 2 | L3677 | 1 | L4080 | 2 | L5630 | 2 | L5724 | 2 | L6055 | 2 | L6693 | 2 | L7404 | 2 |
| L3060 | 2 | L3678 | 1 | L4100 | 2 | L5631 | 2 | L5726 | 2 | L6100 | 2 | L6694 | 2 | L7405 | 2 |
| L3070 | 2 | L3702 | 2 | L4130 | 2 | L5632 | 2 | L5728 | 2 | L6110 | 2 | L6695 | 2 | L7510 | 4 |
| L3080 | 2 | L3710 | 2 | L4210 | 4 | L5634 | 2 | L5780 | 2 | L6120 | 2 | L6696 | 2 | L7900 | 0 |
| L3090 | 2 | L3720 | 2 | L4350 | 2 | L5636 | 2 | L5781 | 2 | L6130 | 2 | L6697 | 2 | L7902 | 0 |
| L3100 | 2 | L3730 | 2 | L4360 | 2 | L5637 | 2 | L5782 | 2 | L6200 | 2 | L6698 | 2 | L8030 | 2 |
| L3140 | 1 | L3740 | 2 | L4361 | 2 | L5638 | 2 | L5785 | 2 | L6205 | 2 | L6703 | 2 | L8031 | 2 |
| L3150 | 1 | L3760 | 2 | L4370 | 2 | L5639 | 2 | L5790 | 2 | L6250 | 2 | L6704 | 2 | L8032 | 2 |
| L3160 | 2 | L3762 | 2 | L4386 | 2 | L5640 | 2 | L5795 | 2 | L6300 | 2 | L6706 | 2 | L8035 | 2 |
| L3170 | 2 | L3763 | 2 | L4387 | 2 | L5642 | 2 | L5810 | 2 | L6310 | 2 | L6707 | 2 | L8039 | 2 |
| L3215 | 0 | L3764 | 2 | L4392 | 2 | L5643 | 2 | L5811 | 2 | L6320 | 2 | L6708 | 2 | L8040 | 1 |
| L3216 | 0 | L3765 | 2 | L4394 | 2 | L5644 | 2 | L5812 | 2 | L6350 | 2 | L6709 | 2 | L8041 | 1 |
| L3217 | 0 | L3766 | 2 | L4396 | 2 | L5645 | 2 | L5814 | 2 | L6360 | 2 | L6711 | 2 | L8042 | 2 |
| L3219 | 0 | L3806 | 2 | L4397 | 2 | L5646 | 2 | L5816 | 2 | L6370 | 2 | L6712 | 2 | L8043 | 1 |
| L3221 | 0 | L3807 | 2 | L4398 | 2 | L5647 | 2 | L5818 | 2 | L6380 | 2 | L6713 | 2 | L8044 | 1 |
| L3222 | 0 | L3808 | 2 | L4631 | 2 | L5648 | 2 | L5822 | 2 | L6382 | 2 | L6714 | 2 | L8045 | 2 |
| L3224 | 2 | L3809 | 2 | L5000 | 2 | L5649 | 2 | L5824 | 2 | L6384 | 2 | L6715 | 5 | L8046 | 1 |
| L3225 | 2 | L3891 | 0 | L5010 | 2 | L5650 | 2 | L5826 | 2 | L6386 | 2 | L6721 | 2 | L8047 | 2 |
| L3230 | 2 | L3900 | 2 | L5020 | 2 | L5651 | 2 | L5828 | 2 | L6388 | 2 | L6722 | 2 | L8048 | 2 |
| L3250 | 2 | L3901 | 2 | L5050 | 2 | L5652 | 2 | L5830 | 2 | L6400 | 2 | L6805 | 2 | L8300 | 1 |
| L3251 | 2 | L3904 | 2 | L5060 | 2 | L5653 | 2 | L5840 | 2 | L6450 | 2 | L6810 | 2 | L8310 | 1 |
| L3252 | 2 | L3905 | 2 | L5100 | 2 | L5654 | 2 | L5845 | 2 | L6500 | 2 | L6880 | 2 | L8320 | 2 |
| L3253 | 2 | L3906 | 2 | L5105 | 2 | L5655 | 2 | L5848 | 2 | L6550 | 2 | L6881 | 2 | L8330 | 2 |
| L3330 | 2 | L3908 | 2 | L5150 | 2 | L5656 | 2 | L5850 | 2 | L6570 | 2 | L6882 | 2 | L8500 | 1 |

**Appendix I — Medically Unlikely Edits (MUEs) — OPPS**

| CPT | MUE | CPT | MUE | CPT | MUE | CPT | MUE | CPT | MUE | CPT | MUE | CPT | MUE | CPT | MUE |
|---|---|---|---|---|---|---|---|---|---|---|---|---|---|---|---|
| L8501 | 2 | P2038 | 1 | Q0091 | 1 | Q0513 | 1 | Q4123 | 160 | Q9950 | 5 | V2210 | 2 | V2623 | 2 |
| L8507 | 3 | P3000 | 1 | Q0111 | 2 | Q0514 | 1 | Q4124 | 280 | Q9951 | 0 | V2211 | 2 | V2624 | 2 |
| L8509 | 1 | P3001 | 1 | Q0112 | 3 | Q0515 | 0 | Q4125 | 28 | Q9953 | 10 | V2212 | 2 | V2625 | 2 |
| L8510 | 1 | P9010 | 4 | Q0113 | 2 | Q1004 | 2 | Q4126 | 0 | Q9954 | 18 | V2213 | 2 | V2626 | 2 |
| L8511 | 1 | P9011 | 4 | Q0114 | 1 | Q1005 | 2 | Q4127 | 100 | Q9955 | 10 | V2214 | 2 | V2627 | 2 |
| L8514 | 1 | P9012 | 12 | Q0115 | 1 | Q2004 | 1 | Q4128 | 128 | Q9956 | 9 | V2215 | 2 | V2628 | 2 |
| L8515 | 1 | P9016 | 12 | Q0138 | 510 | Q2009 | 100 | Q4130 | 160 | Q9957 | 3 | V2218 | 2 | V2629 | 2 |
| L8600 | 2 | P9017 | 24 | Q0139 | 510 | Q2017 | 12 | Q4131 | 98 | Q9958 | 600 | V2219 | 2 | V2630 | 2 |
| L8604 | 3 | P9019 | 12 | Q0144 | 0 | Q2026 | 45 | Q4132 | 50 | Q9959 | 0 | V2220 | 2 | V2631 | 2 |
| L8605 | 4 | P9020 | 5 | Q0161 | 30 | Q2028 | 1470 | Q4133 | 113 | Q9960 | 250 | V2221 | 2 | V2632 | 2 |
| L8606 | 5 | P9021 | 8 | Q0162 | 24 | Q2034 | 1 | Q4134 | 160 | Q9961 | 200 | V2299 | 2 | V2700 | 2 |
| L8607 | 20 | P9022 | 12 | Q0163 | 6 | Q2035 | 1 | Q4135 | 900 | Q9962 | 200 | V2300 | 2 | V2702 | 0 |
| L8609 | 1 | P9023 | 15 | Q0164 | 8 | Q2036 | 1 | Q4136 | 900 | Q9963 | 240 | V2301 | 2 | V2710 | 2 |
| L8610 | 2 | P9031 | 12 | Q0166 | 2 | Q2037 | 1 | Q4137 | 32 | Q9964 | 0 | V2302 | 2 | V2715 | 4 |
| L8612 | 2 | P9032 | 12 | Q0167 | 108 | Q2038 | 1 | Q4138 | 32 | Q9966 | 250 | V2303 | 2 | V2718 | 2 |
| L8613 | 2 | P9033 | 12 | Q0169 | 12 | Q2039 | 1 | Q4139 | 2 | Q9967 | 300 | V2304 | 2 | V2730 | 2 |
| L8614 | 2 | P9034 | 4 | Q0173 | 5 | Q2043 | 1 | Q4140 | 32 | Q9969 | 3 | V2305 | 2 | V2744 | 2 |
| L8615 | 2 | P9035 | 4 | Q0174 | 0 | Q2049 | 20 | Q4141 | 25 | Q9982 | 1 | V2306 | 2 | V2745 | 2 |
| L8616 | 2 | P9036 | 4 | Q0175 | 6 | Q2050 | 20 | Q4142 | 600 | Q9983 | 1 | V2307 | 2 | V2750 | 2 |
| L8617 | 2 | P9037 | 4 | Q0177 | 16 | Q2052 | 0 | Q4143 | 96 | R0070 | 2 | V2308 | 2 | V2755 | 2 |
| L8618 | 2 | P9038 | 4 | Q0180 | 1 | Q3014 | 2 | Q4145 | 160 | R0075 | 2 | V2309 | 2 | V2756 | 0 |
| L8619 | 2 | P9039 | 2 | Q0478 | 1 | Q3027 | 30 | Q4146 | 50 | R0076 | 1 | V2310 | 2 | V2760 | 0 |
| L8621 | 600 | P9040 | 8 | Q0479 | 1 | Q3028 | 0 | Q4147 | 150 | V2020 | 1 | V2311 | 2 | V2761 | 2 |
| L8622 | 2 | P9041 | 100 | Q0480 | 1 | Q3031 | 1 | Q4148 | 24 | V2025 | 0 | V2312 | 2 | V2762 | 0 |
| L8627 | 2 | P9043 | 10 | Q0481 | 1 | Q4001 | 1 | Q4149 | 10 | V2100 | 2 | V2313 | 2 | V2770 | 2 |
| L8628 | 2 | P9044 | 20 | Q0482 | 1 | Q4002 | 1 | Q4150 | 32 | V2101 | 2 | V2314 | 2 | V2780 | 2 |
| L8629 | 2 | P9045 | 20 | Q0483 | 1 | Q4003 | 2 | Q4151 | 24 | V2102 | 2 | V2315 | 2 | V2781 | 2 |
| L8631 | 4 | P9046 | 40 | Q0484 | 1 | Q4004 | 2 | Q4152 | 24 | V2103 | 2 | V2318 | 2 | V2782 | 2 |
| L8641 | 4 | P9047 | 20 | Q0485 | 1 | Q4025 | 1 | Q4153 | 6 | V2104 | 2 | V2319 | 2 | V2783 | 2 |
| L8642 | 2 | P9048 | 2 | Q0486 | 1 | Q4026 | 1 | Q4154 | 36 | V2105 | 2 | V2320 | 2 | V2784 | 2 |
| L8658 | 4 | P9050 | 1 | Q0487 | 1 | Q4027 | 1 | Q4155 | 100 | V2106 | 2 | V2321 | 2 | V2785 | 2 |
| L8659 | 4 | P9051 | 4 | Q0488 | 1 | Q4028 | 1 | Q4156 | 49 | V2107 | 2 | V2399 | 2 | V2786 | 0 |
| L8670 | 4 | P9052 | 3 | Q0489 | 1 | Q4074 | 0 | Q4157 | 24 | V2108 | 2 | V2410 | 2 | V2790 | 1 |
| L8679 | 3 | P9053 | 3 | Q0490 | 1 | Q4081 | 400 | Q4158 | 70 | V2109 | 2 | V2430 | 2 | V2797 | 0 |
| L8680 | 0 | P9054 | 2 | Q0491 | 1 | Q4101 | 176 | Q4159 | 14 | V2110 | 2 | V2499 | 2 | V5008 | 0 |
| L8681 | 1 | P9055 | 2 | Q0492 | 1 | Q4102 | 140 | Q4160 | 72 | V2111 | 2 | V2500 | 2 | V5010 | 0 |
| L8682 | 2 | P9056 | 3 | Q0493 | 1 | Q4103 | 0 | Q4161 | 42 | V2112 | 2 | V2501 | 2 | V5011 | 0 |
| L8683 | 1 | P9057 | 4 | Q0494 | 1 | Q4104 | 250 | Q4162 | 4 | V2113 | 2 | V2502 | 2 | V5274 | 0 |
| L8684 | 1 | P9058 | 4 | Q0495 | 1 | Q4105 | 250 | Q4163 | 32 | V2114 | 2 | V2503 | 2 | V5281 | 0 |
| L8685 | 1 | P9059 | 15 | Q0497 | 2 | Q4106 | 152 | Q4164 | 400 | V2115 | 2 | V2510 | 2 | V5282 | 0 |
| L8686 | 2 | P9060 | 4 | Q0498 | 1 | Q4107 | 128 | Q4165 | 100 | V2118 | 2 | V2511 | 2 | V5283 | 0 |
| L8687 | 1 | P9070 | 15 | Q0499 | 1 | Q4108 | 250 | Q4166 | 300 | V2121 | 2 | V2512 | 2 | V5284 | 0 |
| L8688 | 1 | P9071 | 15 | Q0501 | 1 | Q4110 | 250 | Q4167 | 32 | V2199 | 2 | V2513 | 2 | V5285 | 0 |
| L8689 | 1 | P9072 | 2 | Q0502 | 1 | Q4111 | 112 | Q4168 | 160 | V2200 | 2 | V2520 | 2 | V5286 | 0 |
| L8690 | 2 | P9603 | 100 | Q0503 | 3 | Q4112 | 2 | Q4169 | 32 | V2201 | 2 | V2521 | 2 | V5287 | 0 |
| L8691 | 1 | P9604 | 2 | Q0504 | 1 | Q4113 | 4 | Q4170 | 120 | V2202 | 2 | V2522 | 2 | V5288 | 0 |
| L8692 | 0 | P9612 | 1 | Q0506 | 8 | Q4114 | 6 | Q4171 | 100 | V2203 | 2 | V2523 | 2 | V5289 | 0 |
| L8693 | 1 | P9615 | 1 | Q0507 | 1 | Q4115 | 240 | Q4172 | 128 | V2204 | 2 | V2530 | 2 | V5290 | 0 |
| L8695 | 1 | Q0035 | 1 | Q0508 | 24 | Q4116 | 320 | Q4173 | 64 | V2205 | 2 | V2531 | 2 | | |
| L8696 | 1 | Q0081 | 2 | Q0509 | 1 | Q4117 | 200 | Q4174 | 8 | V2206 | 2 | V2599 | 2 | | |
| P2028 | 1 | Q0083 | 2 | Q0510 | 1 | Q4118 | 1000 | Q4175 | 120 | V2207 | 2 | V2600 | 1 | | |
| P2029 | 1 | Q0084 | 2 | Q0511 | 1 | Q4121 | 156 | Q5101 | 3360 | V2208 | 2 | V2610 | 1 | | |
| P2033 | 1 | Q0085 | 2 | Q0512 | 4 | Q4122 | 96 | Q5102 | 150 | V2209 | 2 | V2615 | 2 | | |

CPT © 2017 American Medical Association. All Rights Reserved.                    © 2017 Optum360, LLC

# Appendix J — Inpatient Only Procedures

**Inpatient Only Procedures**—This appendix identifies services with the status indicator C. Medicare will not pay an OPPS hospital or ASC when they are performed on a Medicare patient as an outpatient. Physicians should refer to this list when scheduling Medicare patients for surgical procedures. CMS updates this list quarterly.

| | | |
|---|---|---|
| 00176 Anesth pharyngeal surgery | 01404 Anesth amputation at knee | 19369 Breast reconstruction |
| 00192 Anesth facial bone surgery | 01442 Anesth knee artery surg | 20661 Application of head brace |
| 00211 Anesth cran surg hematoma | 01444 Anesth knee artery repair | 20664 Application of halo |
| 00214 Anesth skull drainage | 01486 Anesth ankle replacement | 20802 Replantation arm complete |
| 00215 Anesth skull repair/fract | 01502 Anesth lwr leg embolectomy | 20805 Replant forearm complete |
| 00474 Anesth surgery of rib | 01634 Anesth shoulder joint amput | 20808 Replantation hand complete |
| 0051T Implant total heart system | 01636 Anesth forequarter amput | 20816 Replantation digit complete |
| 00524 Anesth chest drainage | 01638 Anesth shoulder replacement | 20824 Replantation thumb complete |
| 0052T Replace thrc unit hrt syst | 0163T Lumb artif diskectomy addl | 20827 Replantation thumb complete |
| 0053T Replace implantable hrt syst | 0164T Remove lumb artif disc addl | 20838 Replantation foot complete |
| 00540 Anesth chest surgery | 01652 Anesth shoulder vessel surg | 20955 Fibula bone graft microvasc |
| 00542 Anesthesia removal pleura | 01654 Anesth shoulder vessel surg | 20956 Iliac bone graft microvasc |
| 00546 Anesth lung chest wall surg | 01656 Anesth arm-leg vessel surg | 20957 Mt bone graft microvasc |
| 00560 Anesth heart surg w/o pump | 0165T Revise lumb artif disc addl | 20962 Other bone graft microvasc |
| 00561 Anesth heart surg <1 yr | 01756 Anesth radical humerus surg | 20969 Bone/skin graft microvasc |
| 00562 Anesth hrt surg w/pmp age 1+ | 0195T Prescrl fuse w/o instr l5/s1 | 20970 Bone/skin graft iliac crest |
| 00567 Anesth CABG w/pump | 0196T Prescrl fuse w/o instr l4/l5 | 21045 Extensive jaw surgery |
| 00580 Anesth heart/lung transplnt | 01990 Support for organ donor | 21141 Lefort i-1 piece w/o graft |
| 00604 Anesth sitting procedure | 0202T Post vert arthrplst 1 lumbar | 21142 Lefort i-2 piece w/o graft |
| 00632 Anesth removal of nerves | 0219T Plmt post facet implt cerv | 21143 Lefort i-3/> piece w/o graft |
| 00670 Anesth spine cord surgery | 0220T Plmt post facet implt thor | 21145 Lefort i-1 piece w/ graft |
| 0075T Perq stent/chest vert art | 0235T Trluml perip athrc visceral | 21146 Lefort i-2 piece w/ graft |
| 0076T S&i stent/chest vert art | 0254T Evasc rpr iliac art bifur | 21147 Lefort i-3/> piece w/ graft |
| 00792 Anesth hemorr/excise liver | 0255T Evasc rpr iliac art bifr s&i | 21151 Lefort ii w/bone grafts |
| 00794 Anesth pancreas removal | 0266T Implt/rpl crtd sns dev total | 21154 Lefort iii w/o lefort i |
| 00796 Anesth for liver transplant | 0293T Ins lt atrl press monitor | 21155 Lefort iii w/ lefort i |
| 00802 Anesth fat layer removal | 0294T Ins lt atrl mont pres lead | 21159 Lefort iii w/fhdw/o lefort i |
| 00844 Anesth pelvis surgery | 0309T Prescrl fuse w/ instr l4/l5 | 21160 Lefort iii w/fhd w/ lefort i |
| 00846 Anesth hysterectomy | 0345T Transcath mtral vlve repair | 21179 Reconstruct entire forehead |
| 00848 Anesth pelvic organ surg | 0375T Total disc arthrp ant appr | 21180 Reconstruct entire forehead |
| 00864 Anesth removal of bladder | 0451T Insj/rplcmt aortic ventr sys | 21182 Reconstruct cranial bone |
| 00865 Anesth removal of prostate | 0452T Insj/rplcmt dev vasc seal | 21183 Reconstruct cranial bone |
| 00866 Anesth removal of adrenal | 0455T Remvl aortic ventr cmpl sys | 21184 Reconstruct cranial bone |
| 00868 Anesth kidney transplant | 0456T Remvl aortic dev vasc seal | 21188 Reconstruction of midface |
| 00882 Anesth major vein ligation | 0459T Relocaj rplcmt aortic ventr | 21194 Reconst lwr jaw w/graft |
| 00904 Anesth perineal surgery | 0461T Repos aortic contrpulsj dev | 21196 Reconst lwr jaw w/fixation |
| 00908 Anesth removal of prostate | 11004 Debride genitalia & perineum | 21247 Reconstruct lower jaw bone |
| 00932 Anesth amputation of penis | 11005 Debride abdom wall | 21255 Reconstruct lower jaw bone |
| 00934 Anesth penis nodes removal | 11006 Debride genit/per/abdom wall | 21268 Revise eye sockets |
| 00936 Anesth penis nodes removal | 11008 Remove mesh from abd wall | 21343 Open tx dprsd front sinus fx |
| 00944 Anesth vaginal hysterectomy | 15756 Free myo/skin flap microvasc | 21344 Open tx compl front sinus fx |
| 0095T Rmvl artific disc addl crvcl | 15757 Free skin flap microvasc | 21347 Opn tx nasomax fx multple |
| 0098T Rev artific disc addl | 15758 Free fascial flap microvasc | 21348 Opn tx nasomax fx w/graft |
| 01140 Anesth amputation at pelvis | 16036 Escharotomy addl incision | 21366 Opn tx complx malar w/grft |
| 01150 Anesth pelvic tumor surgery | 19271 Revision of chest wall | 21422 Treat mouth roof fracture |
| 01212 Anesth hip disarticulation | 19272 Extensive chest wall surgery | 21423 Treat mouth roof fracture |
| 01214 Anesth hip arthroplasty | 19305 Mast radical | 21431 Treat craniofacial fracture |
| 01232 Anesth amputation of femur | 19306 Mast rad urban type | 21432 Treat craniofacial fracture |
| 01234 Anesth radical femur surg | 19361 Breast reconstr w/lat flap | 21433 Treat craniofacial fracture |
| 01272 Anesth femoral artery surg | 19364 Breast reconstruction | 21435 Treat craniofacial fracture |
| 01274 Anesth femoral embolectomy | 19367 Breast reconstruction | 21436 Treat craniofacial fracture |
| 01402 Anesth knee arthroplasty | 19368 Breast reconstruction | 21510 Drainage of bone lesion |

| | | |
|---|---|---|
| 21615 Removal of rib | 22843 Insert spine fixation device | 27138 Revise hip joint replacement |
| 21616 Removal of rib and nerves | 22844 Insert spine fixation device | 27140 Transplant femur ridge |
| 21620 Partial removal of sternum | 22846 Insert spine fixation device | 27146 Incision of hip bone |
| 21627 Sternal debridement | 22847 Insert spine fixation device | 27147 Revision of hip bone |
| 21630 Extensive sternum surgery | 22848 Insert pelv fixation device | 27151 Incision of hip bones |
| 21632 Extensive sternum surgery | 22849 Reinsert spinal fixation | 27156 Revision of hip bones |
| 21705 Revision of neck muscle/rib | 22850 Remove spine fixation device | 27158 Revision of pelvis |
| 21740 Reconstruction of sternum | 22852 Remove spine fixation device | 27161 Incision of neck of femur |
| 21750 Repair of sternum separation | 22855 Remove spine fixation device | 27165 Incision/fixation of femur |
| 21825 Treat sternum fracture | 22857 Lumbar artif diskectomy | 27170 Repair/graft femur head/neck |
| 22010 I&d p-spine c/t/cerv-thor | 22861 Revise cerv artific disc | 27175 Treat slipped epiphysis |
| 22015 I&d abscess p-spine l/s/ls | 22862 Revise lumbar artif disc | 27176 Treat slipped epiphysis |
| 22110 Remove part of neck vertebra | 22864 Remove cerv artif disc | 27177 Treat slipped epiphysis |
| 22112 Remove part thorax vertebra | 22865 Remove lumb artif disc | 27178 Treat slipped epiphysis |
| 22114 Remove part lumbar vertebra | 23200 Resect clavicle tumor | 27181 Treat slipped epiphysis |
| 22116 Remove extra spine segment | 23210 Resect scapula tumor | 27185 Revision of femur epiphysis |
| 22206 Incis spine 3 column thorac | 23220 Resect prox humerus tumor | 27187 Reinforce hip bones |
| 22207 Incis spine 3 column lumbar | 23335 Shoulder prosthesis removal | 27222 Treat hip socket fracture |
| 22208 Incis spine 3 column adl seg | 23472 Reconstruct shoulder joint | 27226 Treat hip wall fracture |
| 22210 Incis 1 vertebral seg cerv | 23474 Revis reconst shoulder joint | 27227 Treat hip fracture(s) |
| 22212 Incis 1 vertebral seg thorac | 23900 Amputation of arm & girdle | 27228 Treat hip fracture(s) |
| 22214 Incis 1 vertebral seg lumbar | 23920 Amputation at shoulder joint | 27232 Treat thigh fracture |
| 22216 Incis addl spine segment | 24900 Amputation of upper arm | 27236 Treat thigh fracture |
| 22220 Incis w/discectomy cervical | 24920 Amputation of upper arm | 27240 Treat thigh fracture |
| 22222 Incis w/discectomy thoracic | 24930 Amputation follow-up surgery | 27244 Treat thigh fracture |
| 22224 Incis w/discectomy lumbar | 24931 Amputate upper arm & implant | 27245 Treat thigh fracture |
| 22226 Revise extra spine segment | 24940 Revision of upper arm | 27248 Treat thigh fracture |
| 22318 Treat odontoid fx w/o graft | 25900 Amputation of forearm | 27253 Treat hip dislocation |
| 22319 Treat odontoid fx w/graft | 25905 Amputation of forearm | 27254 Treat hip dislocation |
| 22325 Treat spine fracture | 25915 Amputation of forearm | 27258 Treat hip dislocation |
| 22326 Treat neck spine fracture | 25920 Amputate hand at wrist | 27259 Treat hip dislocation |
| 22327 Treat thorax spine fracture | 25924 Amputation follow-up surgery | 27268 Cltx thigh fx w/mnpj |
| 22328 Treat each add spine fx | 25927 Amputation of hand | 27269 Optx thigh fx |
| 22532 Lat thorax spine fusion | 26551 Great toe-hand transfer | 27280 Fusion of sacroiliac joint |
| 22533 Lat lumbar spine fusion | 26553 Single transfer toe-hand | 27282 Fusion of pubic bones |
| 22534 Lat thor/lumb addl seg | 26554 Double transfer toe-hand | 27284 Fusion of hip joint |
| 22548 Neck spine fusion | 26556 Toe joint transfer | 27286 Fusion of hip joint |
| 22556 Thorax spine fusion | 26992 Drainage of bone lesion | 27290 Amputation of leg at hip |
| 22558 Lumbar spine fusion | 27005 Incision of hip tendon | 27295 Amputation of leg at hip |
| 22586 Prescrl fuse w/ instr l5-s1 | 27025 Incision of hip/thigh fascia | 27303 Drainage of bone lesion |
| 22590 Spine & skull spinal fusion | 27030 Drainage of hip joint | 27365 Resect femur/knee tumor |
| 22595 Neck spinal fusion | 27036 Excision of hip joint/muscle | 27445 Revision of knee joint |
| 22600 Neck spine fusion | 27054 Removal of hip joint lining | 27448 Incision of thigh |
| 22610 Thorax spine fusion | 27070 Part remove hip bone super | 27450 Incision of thigh |
| 22630 Lumbar spine fusion | 27071 Part removal hip bone deep | 27454 Realignment of thigh bone |
| 22632 Spine fusion extra segment | 27075 Resect hip tumor | 27455 Realignment of knee |
| 22633 Lumbar spine fusion combined | 27076 Resect hip tum incl acetabul | 27457 Realignment of knee |
| 22634 Spine fusion extra segment | 27077 Resect hip tum w/innom bone | 27465 Shortening of thigh bone |
| 22800 Post fusion </6 vert seg | 27078 Rsect hip tum incl femur | 27466 Lengthening of thigh bone |
| 22802 Post fusion 7-12 vert seg | 27090 Removal of hip prosthesis | 27468 Shorten/lengthen thighs |
| 22804 Post fusion 13/> vert seg | 27091 Removal of hip prosthesis | 27470 Repair of thigh |
| 22808 Ant fusion 2-3 vert seg | 27120 Reconstruction of hip socket | 27472 Repair/graft of thigh |
| 22810 Ant fusion 4-7 vert seg | 27122 Reconstruction of hip socket | 27486 Revise/replace knee joint |
| 22812 Ant fusion 8/> vert seg | 27125 Partial hip replacement | 27487 Revise/replace knee joint |
| 22818 Kyphectomy 1-2 segments | 27130 Total hip arthroplasty | 27488 Removal of knee prosthesis |
| 22819 Kyphectomy 3 or more | 27132 Total hip arthroplasty | 27495 Reinforce thigh |
| 22830 Exploration of spinal fusion | 27134 Revise hip joint replacement | 27506 Treatment of thigh fracture |
| 22841 Insert spine fixation device | 27137 Revise hip joint replacement | 27507 Treatment of thigh fracture |

CPT © 2017 American Medical Association. All Rights Reserved.     © 2017 Optum360, LLC

| | | | | | |
|---|---|---|---|---|---|
| 27511 | Treatment of thigh fracture | 32097 | Open wedge/bx lung nodule | 32815 | Close bronchial fistula |
| 27513 | Treatment of thigh fracture | 32098 | Open biopsy of lung pleura | 32820 | Reconstruct injured chest |
| 27514 | Treatment of thigh fracture | 32100 | Exploration of chest | 32850 | Donor pneumonectomy |
| 27519 | Treat thigh fx growth plate | 32110 | Explore/repair chest | 32851 | Lung transplant single |
| 27535 | Treat knee fracture | 32120 | Re-exploration of chest | 32852 | Lung transplant with bypass |
| 27536 | Treat knee fracture | 32124 | Explore chest free adhesions | 32853 | Lung transplant double |
| 27540 | Treat knee fracture | 32140 | Removal of lung lesion(s) | 32854 | Lung transplant with bypass |
| 27556 | Treat knee dislocation | 32141 | Remove/treat lung lesions | 32855 | Prepare donor lung single |
| 27557 | Treat knee dislocation | 32150 | Removal of lung lesion(s) | 32856 | Prepare donor lung double |
| 27558 | Treat knee dislocation | 32151 | Remove lung foreign body | 32900 | Removal of rib(s) |
| 27580 | Fusion of knee | 32160 | Open chest heart massage | 32905 | Revise & repair chest wall |
| 27590 | Amputate leg at thigh | 32200 | Drain open lung lesion | 32906 | Revise & repair chest wall |
| 27591 | Amputate leg at thigh | 32215 | Treat chest lining | 32940 | Revision of lung |
| 27592 | Amputate leg at thigh | 32220 | Release of lung | 32997 | Total lung lavage |
| 27596 | Amputation follow-up surgery | 32225 | Partial release of lung | 33015 | Incision of heart sac |
| 27598 | Amputate lower leg at knee | 32310 | Removal of chest lining | 33020 | Incision of heart sac |
| 27645 | Resect tibia tumor | 32320 | Free/remove chest lining | 33025 | Incision of heart sac |
| 27646 | Resect fibula tumor | 32440 | Remove lung pneumonectomy | 33030 | Partial removal of heart sac |
| 27702 | Reconstruct ankle joint | 32442 | Sleeve pneumonectomy | 33031 | Partial removal of heart sac |
| 27703 | Reconstruction ankle joint | 32445 | Removal of lung extrapleural | 33050 | Resect heart sac lesion |
| 27712 | Realignment of lower leg | 32480 | Partial removal of lung | 33120 | Removal of heart lesion |
| 27715 | Revision of lower leg | 32482 | Bilobectomy | 33130 | Removal of heart lesion |
| 27724 | Repair/graft of tibia | 32484 | Segmentectomy | 33140 | Heart revascularize (tmr) |
| 27725 | Repair of lower leg | 32486 | Sleeve lobectomy | 33141 | Heart tmr w/other procedure |
| 27727 | Repair of lower leg | 32488 | Completion pneumonectomy | 33202 | Insert epicard eltrd open |
| 27880 | Amputation of lower leg | 32491 | Lung volume reduction | 33203 | Insert epicard eltrd endo |
| 27881 | Amputation of lower leg | 32501 | Repair bronchus add-on | 33236 | Remove electrode/thoracotomy |
| 27882 | Amputation of lower leg | 32503 | Resect apical lung tumor | 33237 | Remove electrode/thoracotomy |
| 27886 | Amputation follow-up surgery | 32504 | Resect apical lung tum/chest | 33238 | Remove electrode/thoracotomy |
| 27888 | Amputation of foot at ankle | 32505 | Wedge resect of lung initial | 33243 | Remove eltrd/thoracotomy |
| 28800 | Amputation of midfoot | 32506 | Wedge resect of lung add-on | 33250 | Ablate heart dysrhythm focus |
| 31225 | Removal of upper jaw | 32507 | Wedge resect of lung diag | 33251 | Ablate heart dysrhythm focus |
| 31230 | Removal of upper jaw | 32540 | Removal of lung lesion | 33254 | Ablate atria lmtd |
| 31290 | Nasal/sinus endoscopy surg | 32650 | Thoracoscopy w/pleurodesis | 33255 | Ablate atria w/o bypass ext |
| 31291 | Nasal/sinus endoscopy surg | 32651 | Thoracoscopy remove cortex | 33256 | Ablate atria w/bypass exten |
| 31360 | Removal of larynx | 32652 | Thoracoscopy rem totl cortex | 33257 | Ablate atria lmtd add-on |
| 31365 | Removal of larynx | 32653 | Thoracoscopy remov fb/fibrin | 33258 | Ablate atria x10sv add-on |
| 31367 | Partial removal of larynx | 32654 | Thoracoscopy contrl bleeding | 33259 | Ablate atria w/bypass add-on |
| 31368 | Partial removal of larynx | 32655 | Thoracoscopy resect bullae | 33261 | Ablate heart dysrhythm focus |
| 31370 | Partial removal of larynx | 32656 | Thoracoscopy w/pleurectomy | 33265 | Ablate atria lmtd endo |
| 31375 | Partial removal of larynx | 32658 | Thoracoscopy w/sac fb remove | 33266 | Ablate atria x10sv endo |
| 31380 | Partial removal of larynx | 32659 | Thoracoscopy w/sac drainage | 33300 | Repair of heart wound |
| 31382 | Partial removal of larynx | 32661 | Thoracoscopy w/pericard exc | 33305 | Repair of heart wound |
| 31390 | Removal of larynx & pharynx | 32662 | Thoracoscopy w/mediast exc | 33310 | Exploratory heart surgery |
| 31395 | Reconstruct larynx & pharynx | 32663 | Thoracoscopy w/lobectomy | 33315 | Exploratory heart surgery |
| 31725 | Clearance of airways | 32664 | Thoracoscopy w/ th nrv exc | 33320 | Repair major blood vessel(s) |
| 31760 | Repair of windpipe | 32665 | Thoracoscop w/esoph musc exc | 33321 | Repair major vessel |
| 31766 | Reconstruction of windpipe | 32666 | Thoracoscopy w/wedge resect | 33322 | Repair major blood vessel(s) |
| 31770 | Repair/graft of bronchus | 32667 | Thoracoscopy w/w resect addl | 33330 | Insert major vessel graft |
| 31775 | Reconstruct bronchus | 32668 | Thoracoscopy w/w resect diag | 33335 | Insert major vessel graft |
| 31780 | Reconstruct windpipe | 32669 | Thoracoscopy remove segment | 33340 | Perq clsr tcat l atr apndge |
| 31781 | Reconstruct windpipe | 32670 | Thoracoscopy bilobectomy | 33361 | Replace aortic valve perq |
| 31786 | Remove windpipe lesion | 32671 | Thoracoscopy pneumonectomy | 33362 | Replace aortic valve open |
| 31800 | Repair of windpipe injury | 32672 | Thoracoscopy for lvrs | 33363 | Replace aortic valve open |
| 31805 | Repair of windpipe injury | 32673 | Thoracoscopy w/thymus resect | 33364 | Replace aortic valve open |
| 32035 | Thoracostomy w/rib resection | 32674 | Thoracoscopy lymph node exc | 33365 | Replace aortic valve open |
| 32036 | Thoracostomy w/flap drainage | 32800 | Repair lung hernia | 33366 | Trcath replace aortic valve |
| 32096 | Open wedge/bx lung infiltr | 32810 | Close chest after drainage | 33367 | Replace aortic valve w/byp |

Appendix J — Inpatient Only Procedures

| | | | | | |
|---|---|---|---|---|---|
| 33368 | Replace aortic valve w/byp | 33535 | Cabg arterial three | 33777 | Repair great vessels defect |
| 33369 | Replace aortic valve w/byp | 33536 | Cabg arterial four or more | 33778 | Repair great vessels defect |
| 33390 | Valvuloplasty aortic valve | 33542 | Removal of heart lesion | 33779 | Repair great vessels defect |
| 33391 | Valvuloplasty aortic valve | 33545 | Repair of heart damage | 33780 | Repair great vessels defect |
| 33404 | Prepare heart-aorta conduit | 33548 | Restore/remodel ventricle | 33781 | Repair great vessels defect |
| 33405 | Replacement of aortic valve | 33572 | Open coronary endarterectomy | 33782 | Nikaidoh proc |
| 33406 | Replacement of aortic valve | 33600 | Closure of valve | 33783 | Nikaidoh proc w/ostia implt |
| 33410 | Replacement of aortic valve | 33602 | Closure of valve | 33786 | Repair arterial trunk |
| 33411 | Replacement of aortic valve | 33606 | Anastomosis/artery-aorta | 33788 | Revision of pulmonary artery |
| 33412 | Replacement of aortic valve | 33608 | Repair anomaly w/conduit | 33800 | Aortic suspension |
| 33413 | Replacement of aortic valve | 33610 | Repair by enlargement | 33802 | Repair vessel defect |
| 33414 | Repair of aortic valve | 33611 | Repair double ventricle | 33803 | Repair vessel defect |
| 33415 | Revision subvalvular tissue | 33612 | Repair double ventricle | 33813 | Repair septal defect |
| 33416 | Revise ventricle muscle | 33615 | Repair modified fontan | 33814 | Repair septal defect |
| 33417 | Repair of aortic valve | 33617 | Repair single ventricle | 33820 | Revise major vessel |
| 33418 | Repair tcat mitral valve | 33619 | Repair single ventricle | 33822 | Revise major vessel |
| 33420 | Revision of mitral valve | 33620 | Apply r&l pulm art bands | 33824 | Revise major vessel |
| 33422 | Revision of mitral valve | 33621 | Transthor cath for stent | 33840 | Remove aorta constriction |
| 33425 | Repair of mitral valve | 33622 | Redo compl cardiac anomaly | 33845 | Remove aorta constriction |
| 33426 | Repair of mitral valve | 33641 | Repair heart septum defect | 33851 | Remove aorta constriction |
| 33427 | Repair of mitral valve | 33645 | Revision of heart veins | 33852 | Repair septal defect |
| 33430 | Replacement of mitral valve | 33647 | Repair heart septum defects | 33853 | Repair septal defect |
| 33460 | Revision of tricuspid valve | 33660 | Repair of heart defects | 33860 | Ascending aortic graft |
| 33463 | Valvuloplasty tricuspid | 33665 | Repair of heart defects | 33863 | Ascending aortic graft |
| 33464 | Valvuloplasty tricuspid | 33670 | Repair of heart chambers | 33864 | Ascending aortic graft |
| 33465 | Replace tricuspid valve | 33675 | Close mult vsd | 33870 | Transverse aortic arch graft |
| 33468 | Revision of tricuspid valve | 33676 | Close mult vsd w/resection | 33875 | Thoracic aortic graft |
| 33470 | Revision of pulmonary valve | 33677 | Cl mult vsd w/rem pul band | 33877 | Thoracoabdominal graft |
| 33471 | Valvotomy pulmonary valve | 33681 | Repair heart septum defect | 33880 | Endovasc taa repr incl subcl |
| 33474 | Revision of pulmonary valve | 33684 | Repair heart septum defect | 33881 | Endovasc taa repr w/o subcl |
| 33475 | Replacement pulmonary valve | 33688 | Repair heart septum defect | 33883 | Insert endovasc prosth taa |
| 33476 | Revision of heart chamber | 33690 | Reinforce pulmonary artery | 33884 | Endovasc prosth taa add-on |
| 33477 | Implant tcat pulm vlv perq | 33692 | Repair of heart defects | 33886 | Endovasc prosth delayed |
| 33478 | Revision of heart chamber | 33694 | Repair of heart defects | 33889 | Artery transpose/endovas taa |
| 33496 | Repair prosth valve clot | 33697 | Repair of heart defects | 33891 | Car-car bp grft/endovas taa |
| 33500 | Repair heart vessel fistula | 33702 | Repair of heart defects | 33910 | Remove lung artery emboli |
| 33501 | Repair heart vessel fistula | 33710 | Repair of heart defects | 33915 | Remove lung artery emboli |
| 33502 | Coronary artery correction | 33720 | Repair of heart defect | 33916 | Surgery of great vessel |
| 33503 | Coronary artery graft | 33722 | Repair of heart defect | 33917 | Repair pulmonary artery |
| 33504 | Coronary artery graft | 33724 | Repair venous anomaly | 33920 | Repair pulmonary atresia |
| 33505 | Repair artery w/tunnel | 33726 | Repair pul venous stenosis | 33922 | Transect pulmonary artery |
| 33506 | Repair artery translocation | 33730 | Repair heart-vein defect(s) | 33924 | Remove pulmonary shunt |
| 33507 | Repair art intramural | 33732 | Repair heart-vein defect | 33925 | Rpr pul art unifocal w/o cpb |
| 33510 | Cabg vein single | 33735 | Revision of heart chamber | 33926 | Repr pul art unifocal w/cpb |
| 33511 | Cabg vein two | 33736 | Revision of heart chamber | 33930 | Removal of donor heart/lung |
| 33512 | Cabg vein three | 33737 | Revision of heart chamber | 33933 | Prepare donor heart/lung |
| 33513 | Cabg vein four | 33750 | Major vessel shunt | 33935 | Transplantation heart/lung |
| 33514 | Cabg vein five | 33755 | Major vessel shunt | 33940 | Removal of donor heart |
| 33516 | Cabg vein six or more | 33762 | Major vessel shunt | 33944 | Prepare donor heart |
| 33517 | Cabg artery-vein single | 33764 | Major vessel shunt & graft | 33945 | Transplantation of heart |
| 33518 | Cabg artery-vein two | 33766 | Major vessel shunt | 33946 | Ecmo/ecls initiation venous |
| 33519 | Cabg artery-vein three | 33767 | Major vessel shunt | 33947 | Ecmo/ecls initiation artery |
| 33521 | Cabg artery-vein four | 33768 | Cavopulmonary shunting | 33948 | Ecmo/ecls daily mgmt-venous |
| 33522 | Cabg artery-vein five | 33770 | Repair great vessels defect | 33949 | Ecmo/ecls daily mgmt artery |
| 33523 | Cabg art-vein six or more | 33771 | Repair great vessels defect | 33951 | Ecmo/ecls insj prph cannula |
| 33530 | Coronary artery bypass/reop | 33774 | Repair great vessels defect | 33952 | Ecmo/ecls insj prph cannula |
| 33533 | Cabg arterial single | 33775 | Repair great vessels defect | 33953 | Ecmo/ecls insj prph cannula |
| 33534 | Cabg arterial two | 33776 | Repair great vessels defect | 33954 | Ecmo/ecls insj prph cannula |

CPT © 2017 American Medical Association. All Rights Reserved.

© 2017 Optum360, LLC

| Code | Description | Code | Description | Code | Description |
|---|---|---|---|---|---|
| 33955 | Ecmo/ecls insj ctr cannula | 34848 | Visc & infraren abd 4+ prost | 35515 | Art byp grft subclav-vertbrl |
| 33956 | Ecmo/ecls insj ctr cannula | 35001 | Repair defect of artery | 35516 | Art byp grft subclav-axilary |
| 33957 | Ecmo/ecls repos perph cnula | 35002 | Repair artery rupture neck | 35518 | Art byp grft axillary-axilry |
| 33958 | Ecmo/ecls repos perph cnula | 35005 | Repair defect of artery | 35521 | Art byp grft axill-femoral |
| 33959 | Ecmo/ecls repos perph cnula | 35013 | Repair artery rupture arm | 35522 | Art byp grft axill-brachial |
| 33962 | Ecmo/ecls repos perph cnula | 35021 | Repair defect of artery | 35523 | Art byp grft brchl-ulnr-rdl |
| 33963 | Ecmo/ecls repos perph cnula | 35022 | Repair artery rupture chest | 35525 | Art byp grft brachial-brchl |
| 33964 | Ecmo/ecls repos perph cnula | 35081 | Repair defect of artery | 35526 | Art byp grft aor/carot/innom |
| 33965 | Ecmo/ecls rmvl perph cannula | 35082 | Repair artery rupture aorta | 35531 | Art byp grft aorcel/aormesen |
| 33966 | Ecmo/ecls rmvl prph cannula | 35091 | Repair defect of artery | 35533 | Art byp grft axill/fem/fem |
| 33967 | Insert i-aort percut device | 35092 | Repair artery rupture aorta | 35535 | Art byp grft hepatorenal |
| 33968 | Remove aortic assist device | 35102 | Repair defect of artery | 35536 | Art byp grft splenorenal |
| 33969 | Ecmo/ecls rmvl perph cannula | 35103 | Repair artery rupture aorta | 35537 | Art byp grft aortoiliac |
| 33970 | Aortic circulation assist | 35111 | Repair defect of artery | 35538 | Art byp grft aortobi-iliac |
| 33971 | Aortic circulation assist | 35112 | Repair artery rupture spleen | 35539 | Art byp grft aortofemoral |
| 33973 | Insert balloon device | 35121 | Repair defect of artery | 35540 | Art byp grft aortbifemoral |
| 33974 | Remove intra-aortic balloon | 35122 | Repair artery rupture belly | 35556 | Art byp grft fem-popliteal |
| 33975 | Implant ventricular device | 35131 | Repair defect of artery | 35558 | Art byp grft fem-femoral |
| 33976 | Implant ventricular device | 35132 | Repair artery rupture groin | 35560 | Art byp grft aortorenal |
| 33977 | Remove ventricular device | 35141 | Repair defect of artery | 35563 | Art byp grft ilioiliac |
| 33978 | Remove ventricular device | 35142 | Repair artery rupture thigh | 35565 | Art byp grft iliofemoral |
| 33979 | Insert intracorporeal device | 35151 | Repair defect of artery | 35566 | Art byp fem-ant-post tib/prl |
| 33980 | Remove intracorporeal device | 35152 | Repair ruptd popliteal art | 35570 | Art byp tibial-tib/peroneal |
| 33981 | Replace vad pump ext | 35182 | Repair blood vessel lesion | 35571 | Art byp pop-tibl-prl-other |
| 33982 | Replace vad intra w/o bp | 35189 | Repair blood vessel lesion | 35583 | Vein byp grft fem-popliteal |
| 33983 | Replace vad intra w/bp | 35211 | Repair blood vessel lesion | 35585 | Vein byp fem-tibial peroneal |
| 33984 | Ecmo/ecls rmvl prph cannula | 35216 | Repair blood vessel lesion | 35587 | Vein byp pop-tibl peroneal |
| 33985 | Ecmo/ecls rmvl ctr cannula | 35221 | Repair blood vessel lesion | 35600 | Harvest art for cabg add-on |
| 33986 | Ecmo/ecls rmvl ctr cannula | 35241 | Repair blood vessel lesion | 35601 | Art byp common ipsi carotid |
| 33987 | Artery expos/graft artery | 35246 | Repair blood vessel lesion | 35606 | Art byp carotid-subclavian |
| 33988 | Insertion of left heart vent | 35251 | Repair blood vessel lesion | 35612 | Art byp subclav-subclavian |
| 33989 | Removal of left heart vent | 35271 | Repair blood vessel lesion | 35616 | Art byp subclav-axillary |
| 33990 | Insert vad artery access | 35276 | Repair blood vessel lesion | 35621 | Art byp axillary-femoral |
| 33991 | Insert vad art&vein access | 35281 | Repair blood vessel lesion | 35623 | Art byp axillary-pop-tibial |
| 33992 | Remove vad different session | 35301 | Rechanneling of artery | 35626 | Art byp aorsubcl/carot/innom |
| 33993 | Reposition vad diff session | 35302 | Rechanneling of artery | 35631 | Art byp aor-celiac-msn-renal |
| 34001 | Removal of artery clot | 35303 | Rechanneling of artery | 35632 | Art byp ilio-celiac |
| 34051 | Removal of artery clot | 35304 | Rechanneling of artery | 35633 | Art byp ilio-mesenteric |
| 34151 | Removal of artery clot | 35305 | Rechanneling of artery | 35634 | Art byp iliorenal |
| 34401 | Removal of vein clot | 35306 | Rechanneling of artery | 35636 | Art byp spenorenal |
| 34451 | Removal of vein clot | 35311 | Rechanneling of artery | 35637 | Art byp aortoiliac |
| 34502 | Reconstruct vena cava | 35331 | Rechanneling of artery | 35638 | Art byp aortobi-iliac |
| 34808 | Endovas iliac a device addon | 35341 | Rechanneling of artery | 35642 | Art byp carotid-vertebral |
| 34812 | Xpose for endoprosth femorl | 35351 | Rechanneling of artery | 35645 | Art byp subclav-vertebrl |
| 34813 | Femoral endovas graft add-on | 35355 | Rechanneling of artery | 35646 | Art byp aortobifemoral |
| 34820 | Xpose for endoprosth iliac | 35361 | Rechanneling of artery | 35647 | Art byp aortofemoral |
| 34830 | Open aortic tube prosth repr | 35363 | Rechanneling of artery | 35650 | Art byp axillary-axillary |
| 34831 | Open aortoiliac prosth repr | 35371 | Rechanneling of artery | 35654 | Art byp axill-fem-femoral |
| 34832 | Open aortofemor prosth repr | 35372 | Rechanneling of artery | 35656 | Art byp femoral-popliteal |
| 34833 | Xpose for endoprosth iliac | 35390 | Reoperation carotid add-on | 35661 | Art byp femoral-femoral |
| 34834 | Xpose endoprosth brachial | 35400 | Angioscopy | 35663 | Art byp ilioiliac |
| 34841 | Endovasc visc aorta 1 graft | 35501 | Art byp grft ipsilat carotid | 35665 | Art byp iliofemoral |
| 34842 | Endovasc visc aorta 2 graft | 35506 | Art byp grft subclav-carotid | 35666 | Art byp fem-ant-post tib/prl |
| 34843 | Endovasc visc aorta 3 graft | 35508 | Art byp grft carotid-vertbrl | 35671 | Art byp pop-tibl-prl-other |
| 34844 | Endovasc visc aorta 4 graft | 35509 | Art byp grft contral carotid | 35681 | Composite byp grft pros&vein |
| 34845 | Visc & infraren abd 1 prosth | 35510 | Art byp grft carotid-brchial | 35682 | Composite byp grft 2 veins |
| 34846 | Visc & infraren abd 2 prosth | 35511 | Art byp grft subclav-subclav | 35683 | Composite byp grft 3/> segmt |
| 34847 | Visc & infraren abd 3 prosth | 35512 | Art byp grft subclav-brchial | 35691 | Art trnsposj vertbrl carotid |

| | | |
|---|---|---|
| 35693 Art trnsposj subclavian | 39599 Diaphragm surgery procedure | 43405 Ligate/staple esophagus |
| 35694 Art trnsposj subclav carotid | 41130 Partial removal of tongue | 43410 Repair esophagus wound |
| 35695 Art trnsposj carotid subclav | 41135 Tongue and neck surgery | 43415 Repair esophagus wound |
| 35697 Reimplant artery each | 41140 Removal of tongue | 43425 Repair esophagus opening |
| 35700 Reoperation bypass graft | 41145 Tongue removal neck surgery | 43460 Pressure treatment esophagus |
| 35701 Exploration carotid artery | 41150 Tongue mouth jaw surgery | 43496 Free jejunum flap microvasc |
| 35721 Exploration femoral artery | 41153 Tongue mouth neck surgery | 43500 Surgical opening of stomach |
| 35741 Exploration popliteal artery | 41155 Tongue jaw & neck surgery | 43501 Surgical repair of stomach |
| 35800 Explore neck vessels | 42426 Excise parotid gland/lesion | 43502 Surgical repair of stomach |
| 35820 Explore chest vessels | 42845 Extensive surgery of throat | 43520 Incision of pyloric muscle |
| 35840 Explore abdominal vessels | 42894 Revision of pharyngeal walls | 43605 Biopsy of stomach |
| 35870 Repair vessel graft defect | 42953 Repair throat esophagus | 43610 Excision of stomach lesion |
| 35901 Excision graft neck | 42961 Control throat bleeding | 43611 Excision of stomach lesion |
| 35905 Excision graft thorax | 42971 Control nose/throat bleeding | 43620 Removal of stomach |
| 35907 Excision graft abdomen | 43045 Incision of esophagus | 43621 Removal of stomach |
| 36660 Insertion catheter artery | 43100 Excision of esophagus lesion | 43622 Removal of stomach |
| 36823 Insertion of cannula(s) | 43101 Excision of esophagus lesion | 43631 Removal of stomach partial |
| 37140 Revision of circulation | 43107 Removal of esophagus | 43632 Removal of stomach partial |
| 37145 Revision of circulation | 43108 Removal of esophagus | 43633 Removal of stomach partial |
| 37160 Revision of circulation | 43112 Removal of esophagus | 43634 Removal of stomach partial |
| 37180 Revision of circulation | 43113 Removal of esophagus | 43635 Removal of stomach partial |
| 37181 Splice spleen/kidney veins | 43116 Partial removal of esophagus | 43640 Vagotomy & pylorus repair |
| 37182 Insert hepatic shunt (tips) | 43117 Partial removal of esophagus | 43641 Vagotomy & pylorus repair |
| 37215 Transcath stent cca w/eps | 43118 Partial removal of esophagus | 43644 Lap gastric bypass/roux-en-y |
| 37217 Stent placemt retro carotid | 43121 Partial removal of esophagus | 43645 Lap gastr bypass incl smll i |
| 37218 Stent placemt ante carotid | 43122 Partial removal of esophagus | 43771 Lap revise gastr adj device |
| 37616 Ligation of chest artery | 43123 Partial removal of esophagus | 43775 Lap sleeve gastrectomy |
| 37617 Ligation of abdomen artery | 43124 Removal of esophagus | 43800 Reconstruction of pylorus |
| 37618 Ligation of extremity artery | 43135 Removal of esophagus pouch | 43810 Fusion of stomach and bowel |
| 37660 Revision of major vein | 43279 Lap myotomy heller | 43820 Fusion of stomach and bowel |
| 37788 Revascularization penis | 43283 Lap esoph lengthening | 43825 Fusion of stomach and bowel |
| 38100 Removal of spleen total | 43300 Repair of esophagus | 43832 Place gastrostomy tube |
| 38101 Removal of spleen partial | 43305 Repair esophagus and fistula | 43840 Repair of stomach lesion |
| 38102 Removal of spleen total | 43310 Repair of esophagus | 43843 Gastroplasty w/o v-band |
| 38115 Repair of ruptured spleen | 43312 Repair esophagus and fistula | 43845 Gastroplasty duodenal switch |
| 38380 Thoracic duct procedure | 43313 Esophagoplasty congenital | 43846 Gastric bypass for obesity |
| 38381 Thoracic duct procedure | 43314 Tracheo-esophagoplasty cong | 43847 Gastric bypass incl small i |
| 38382 Thoracic duct procedure | 43320 Fuse esophagus & stomach | 43848 Revision gastroplasty |
| 38562 Removal pelvic lymph nodes | 43325 Revise esophagus & stomach | 43850 Revise stomach-bowel fusion |
| 38564 Removal abdomen lymph nodes | 43327 Esoph fundoplasty lap | 43855 Revise stomach-bowel fusion |
| 38724 Removal of lymph nodes neck | 43328 Esoph fundoplasty thor | 43860 Revise stomach-bowel fusion |
| 38746 Remove thoracic lymph nodes | 43330 Esophagomyotomy abdominal | 43865 Revise stomach-bowel fusion |
| 38747 Remove abdominal lymph nodes | 43331 Esophagomyotomy thoracic | 43880 Repair stomach-bowel fistula |
| 38765 Remove groin lymph nodes | 43332 Transab esoph hiat hern rpr | 43881 Impl/redo electrd antrum |
| 38770 Remove pelvis lymph nodes | 43333 Transab esoph hiat hern rpr | 43882 Revise/remove electrd antrum |
| 38780 Remove abdomen lymph nodes | 43334 Transthor diaphrag hern rpr | 44005 Freeing of bowel adhesion |
| 39000 Exploration of chest | 43335 Transthor diaphrag hern rpr | 44010 Incision of small bowel |
| 39010 Exploration of chest | 43336 Thorabd diaphr hern repair | 44015 Insert needle cath bowel |
| 39200 Resect mediastinal cyst | 43337 Thorabd diaphr hern repair | 44020 Explore small intestine |
| 39220 Resect mediastinal tumor | 43338 Esoph lengthening | 44021 Decompress small bowel |
| 39499 Chest procedure | 43340 Fuse esophagus & intestine | 44025 Incision of large bowel |
| 39501 Repair diaphragm laceration | 43341 Fuse esophagus & intestine | 44050 Reduce bowel obstruction |
| 39503 Repair of diaphragm hernia | 43351 Surgical opening esophagus | 44055 Correct malrotation of bowel |
| 39540 Repair of diaphragm hernia | 43352 Surgical opening esophagus | 44110 Excise intestine lesion(s) |
| 39541 Repair of diaphragm hernia | 43360 Gastrointestinal repair | 44111 Excision of bowel lesion(s) |
| 39545 Revision of diaphragm | 43361 Gastrointestinal repair | 44120 Removal of small intestine |
| 39560 Resect diaphragm simple | 43400 Ligate esophagus veins | 44121 Removal of small intestine |
| 39561 Resect diaphragm complex | 43401 Esophagus surgery for veins | 44125 Removal of small intestine |

CPT © 2017 American Medical Association. All Rights Reserved.
© 2017 Optum360, LLC

Appendix J — Inpatient Only Procedures

| | | |
|---|---|---|
| 44126 | Enterectomy w/o taper cong | 44680 | Surgical revision intestine | 47135 | Transplantation of liver |
| 44127 | Enterectomy w/taper cong | 44700 | Suspend bowel w/prosthesis | 47140 | Partial removal donor liver |
| 44128 | Enterectomy cong add-on | 44715 | Prepare donor intestine | 47141 | Partial removal donor liver |
| 44130 | Bowel to bowel fusion | 44720 | Prep donor intestine/venous | 47142 | Partial removal donor liver |
| 44132 | Enterectomy cadaver donor | 44721 | Prep donor intestine/artery | 47143 | Prep donor liver whole |
| 44133 | Enterectomy live donor | 44800 | Excision of bowel pouch | 47144 | Prep donor liver 3-segment |
| 44135 | Intestine transplnt cadaver | 44820 | Excision of mesentery lesion | 47145 | Prep donor liver lobe split |
| 44136 | Intestine transplant live | 44850 | Repair of mesentery | 47146 | Prep donor liver/venous |
| 44137 | Remove intestinal allograft | 44899 | Bowel surgery procedure | 47147 | Prep donor liver/arterial |
| 44139 | Mobilization of colon | 44900 | Drain appendix abscess open | 47300 | Surgery for liver lesion |
| 44140 | Partial removal of colon | 44960 | Appendectomy | 47350 | Repair liver wound |
| 44141 | Partial removal of colon | 45110 | Removal of rectum | 47360 | Repair liver wound |
| 44143 | Partial removal of colon | 45111 | Partial removal of rectum | 47361 | Repair liver wound |
| 44144 | Partial removal of colon | 45112 | Removal of rectum | 47362 | Repair liver wound |
| 44145 | Partial removal of colon | 45113 | Partial proctectomy | 47380 | Open ablate liver tumor rf |
| 44146 | Partial removal of colon | 45114 | Partial removal of rectum | 47381 | Open ablate liver tumor cryo |
| 44147 | Partial removal of colon | 45116 | Partial removal of rectum | 47400 | Incision of liver duct |
| 44150 | Removal of colon | 45119 | Remove rectum w/reservoir | 47420 | Incision of bile duct |
| 44151 | Removal of colon/ileostomy | 45120 | Removal of rectum | 47425 | Incision of bile duct |
| 44155 | Removal of colon/ileostomy | 45121 | Removal of rectum and colon | 47460 | Incise bile duct sphincter |
| 44156 | Removal of colon/ileostomy | 45123 | Partial proctectomy | 47480 | Incision of gallbladder |
| 44157 | Colectomy w/ileoanal anast | 45126 | Pelvic exenteration | 47550 | Bile duct endoscopy add-on |
| 44158 | Colectomy w/neo-rectum pouch | 45130 | Excision of rectal prolapse | 47570 | Laparo cholecystoenterostomy |
| 44160 | Removal of colon | 45135 | Excision of rectal prolapse | 47600 | Removal of gallbladder |
| 44187 | Lap ileo/jejuno-stomy | 45136 | Excise ileoanal reservoir | 47605 | Removal of gallbladder |
| 44188 | Lap colostomy | 45395 | Lap removal of rectum | 47610 | Removal of gallbladder |
| 44202 | Lap enterectomy | 45397 | Lap remove rectum w/pouch | 47612 | Removal of gallbladder |
| 44203 | Lap resect s/intestine addl | 45400 | Laparoscopic proc | 47620 | Removal of gallbladder |
| 44204 | Laparo partial colectomy | 45402 | Lap proctopexy w/sig resect | 47700 | Exploration of bile ducts |
| 44205 | Lap colectomy part w/ileum | 45540 | Correct rectal prolapse | 47701 | Bile duct revision |
| 44206 | Lap part colectomy w/stoma | 45550 | Repair rectum/remove sigmoid | 47711 | Excision of bile duct tumor |
| 44207 | L colectomy/coloproctostomy | 45562 | Exploration/repair of rectum | 47712 | Excision of bile duct tumor |
| 44208 | L colectomy/coloproctostomy | 45563 | Exploration/repair of rectum | 47715 | Excision of bile duct cyst |
| 44210 | Laparo total proctocolectomy | 45800 | Repair rect/bladder fistula | 47720 | Fuse gallbladder & bowel |
| 44211 | Lap colectomy w/proctectomy | 45805 | Repair fistula w/colostomy | 47721 | Fuse upper gi structures |
| 44212 | Laparo total proctocolectomy | 45820 | Repair rectourethral fistula | 47740 | Fuse gallbladder & bowel |
| 44213 | Lap mobil splenic fl add-on | 45825 | Repair fistula w/colostomy | 47741 | Fuse gallbladder & bowel |
| 44227 | Lap close enterostomy | 46705 | Repair of anal stricture | 47760 | Fuse bile ducts and bowel |
| 44300 | Open bowel to skin | 46710 | Repr per/vag pouch sngl proc | 47765 | Fuse liver ducts & bowel |
| 44310 | Ileostomy/jejunostomy | 46712 | Repr per/vag pouch dbl proc | 47780 | Fuse bile ducts and bowel |
| 44314 | Revision of ileostomy | 46715 | Rep perf anoper fistu | 47785 | Fuse bile ducts and bowel |
| 44316 | Devise bowel pouch | 46716 | Rep perf anoper/vestib fistu | 47800 | Reconstruction of bile ducts |
| 44320 | Colostomy | 46730 | Construction of absent anus | 47801 | Placement bile duct support |
| 44322 | Colostomy with biopsies | 46735 | Construction of absent anus | 47802 | Fuse liver duct & intestine |
| 44345 | Revision of colostomy | 46740 | Construction of absent anus | 47900 | Suture bile duct injury |
| 44346 | Revision of colostomy | 46742 | Repair of imperforated anus | 48000 | Drainage of abdomen |
| 44602 | Suture small intestine | 46744 | Repair of cloacal anomaly | 48001 | Placement of drain pancreas |
| 44603 | Suture small intestine | 46746 | Repair of cloacal anomaly | 48020 | Removal of pancreatic stone |
| 44604 | Suture large intestine | 46748 | Repair of cloacal anomaly | 48100 | Biopsy of pancreas open |
| 44605 | Repair of bowel lesion | 46751 | Repair of anal sphincter | 48105 | Resect/debride pancreas |
| 44615 | Intestinal stricturoplasty | 47010 | Open drainage liver lesion | 48120 | Removal of pancreas lesion |
| 44620 | Repair bowel opening | 47015 | Inject/aspirate liver cyst | 48140 | Partial removal of pancreas |
| 44625 | Repair bowel opening | 47100 | Wedge biopsy of liver | 48145 | Partial removal of pancreas |
| 44626 | Repair bowel opening | 47120 | Partial removal of liver | 48146 | Pancreatectomy |
| 44640 | Repair bowel-skin fistula | 47122 | Extensive removal of liver | 48148 | Removal of pancreatic duct |
| 44650 | Repair bowel fistula | 47125 | Partial removal of liver | 48150 | Partial removal of pancreas |
| 44660 | Repair bowel-bladder fistula | 47130 | Partial removal of liver | 48152 | Pancreatectomy |
| 44661 | Repair bowel-bladder fistula | 47133 | Removal of donor liver | 48153 | Pancreatectomy |

| | | |
|---|---|---|
| 48154 Pancreatectomy | 50280 Removal of kidney lesion | 51525 Removal of bladder lesion |
| 48155 Removal of pancreas | 50290 Removal of kidney lesion | 51530 Removal of bladder lesion |
| 48400 Injection intraop add-on | 50300 Remove cadaver donor kidney | 51550 Partial removal of bladder |
| 48500 Surgery of pancreatic cyst | 50320 Remove kidney living donor | 51555 Partial removal of bladder |
| 48510 Drain pancreatic pseudocyst | 50323 Prep cadaver renal allograft | 51565 Revise bladder & ureter(s) |
| 48520 Fuse pancreas cyst and bowel | 50325 Prep donor renal graft | 51570 Removal of bladder |
| 48540 Fuse pancreas cyst and bowel | 50327 Prep renal graft/venous | 51575 Removal of bladder & nodes |
| 48545 Pancreatorrhaphy | 50328 Prep renal graft/arterial | 51580 Remove bladder/revise tract |
| 48547 Duodenal exclusion | 50329 Prep renal graft/ureteral | 51585 Removal of bladder & nodes |
| 48548 Fuse pancreas and bowel | 50340 Removal of kidney | 51590 Remove bladder/revise tract |
| 48551 Prep donor pancreas | 50360 Transplantation of kidney | 51595 Remove bladder/revise tract |
| 48552 Prep donor pancreas/venous | 50365 Transplantation of kidney | 51596 Remove bladder/create pouch |
| 48554 Transpl allograft pancreas | 50370 Remove transplanted kidney | 51597 Removal of pelvic structures |
| 48556 Removal allograft pancreas | 50380 Reimplantation of kidney | 51800 Revision of bladder/urethra |
| 49000 Exploration of abdomen | 50400 Revision of kidney/ureter | 51820 Revision of urinary tract |
| 49002 Reopening of abdomen | 50405 Revision of kidney/ureter | 51840 Attach bladder/urethra |
| 49010 Exploration behind abdomen | 50500 Repair of kidney wound | 51841 Attach bladder/urethra |
| 49020 Drainage abdom abscess open | 50520 Close kidney-skin fistula | 51865 Repair of bladder wound |
| 49040 Drain open abdom abscess | 50525 Close nephrovisceral fistula | 51900 Repair bladder/vagina lesion |
| 49060 Drain open retroperi abscess | 50526 Close nephrovisceral fistula | 51920 Close bladder-uterus fistula |
| 49062 Drain to peritoneal cavity | 50540 Revision of horseshoe kidney | 51925 Hysterectomy/bladder repair |
| 49203 Exc abd tum 5 cm or less | 50545 Laparo radical nephrectomy | 51940 Correction of bladder defect |
| 49204 Exc abd tum over 5 cm | 50546 Laparoscopic nephrectomy | 51960 Revision of bladder & bowel |
| 49205 Exc abd tum over 10 cm | 50547 Laparo removal donor kidney | 51980 Construct bladder opening |
| 49215 Excise sacral spine tumor | 50548 Laparo remove w/ureter | 53415 Reconstruction of urethra |
| 49220 Multiple surgery abdomen | 50600 Exploration of ureter | 53448 Remov/replc ur sphinctr comp |
| 49255 Removal of omentum | 50605 Insert ureteral support | 54125 Removal of penis |
| 49412 Ins device for rt guide open | 50610 Removal of ureter stone | 54130 Remove penis & nodes |
| 49425 Insert abdomen-venous drain | 50620 Removal of ureter stone | 54135 Remove penis & nodes |
| 49428 Ligation of shunt | 50630 Removal of ureter stone | 54390 Repair penis and bladder |
| 49605 Repair umbilical lesion | 50650 Removal of ureter | 54430 Revision of penis |
| 49606 Repair umbilical lesion | 50660 Removal of ureter | 54438 Replantation of penis |
| 49610 Repair umbilical lesion | 50700 Revision of ureter | 55605 Incise sperm duct pouch |
| 49611 Repair umbilical lesion | 50715 Release of ureter | 55650 Remove sperm duct pouch |
| 49900 Repair of abdominal wall | 50722 Release of ureter | 55801 Removal of prostate |
| 49904 Omental flap extra-abdom | 50725 Release/revise ureter | 55810 Extensive prostate surgery |
| 49905 Omental flap intra-abdom | 50728 Revise ureter | 55812 Extensive prostate surgery |
| 49906 Free omental flap microvasc | 50740 Fusion of ureter & kidney | 55815 Extensive prostate surgery |
| 50010 Exploration of kidney | 50750 Fusion of ureter & kidney | 55821 Removal of prostate |
| 50040 Drainage of kidney | 50760 Fusion of ureters | 55831 Removal of prostate |
| 50045 Exploration of kidney | 50770 Splicing of ureters | 55840 Extensive prostate surgery |
| 50060 Removal of kidney stone | 50780 Reimplant ureter in bladder | 55842 Extensive prostate surgery |
| 50065 Incision of kidney | 50782 Reimplant ureter in bladder | 55845 Extensive prostate surgery |
| 50070 Incision of kidney | 50783 Reimplant ureter in bladder | 55862 Extensive prostate surgery |
| 50075 Removal of kidney stone | 50785 Reimplant ureter in bladder | 55865 Extensive prostate surgery |
| 50100 Revise kidney blood vessels | 50800 Implant ureter in bowel | 56630 Extensive vulva surgery |
| 50120 Exploration of kidney | 50810 Fusion of ureter & bowel | 56631 Extensive vulva surgery |
| 50125 Explore and drain kidney | 50815 Urine shunt to intestine | 56632 Extensive vulva surgery |
| 50130 Removal of kidney stone | 50820 Construct bowel bladder | 56633 Extensive vulva surgery |
| 50135 Exploration of kidney | 50825 Construct bowel bladder | 56634 Extensive vulva surgery |
| 50205 Renal biopsy open | 50830 Revise urine flow | 56637 Extensive vulva surgery |
| 50220 Remove kidney open | 50840 Replace ureter by bowel | 56640 Extensive vulva surgery |
| 50225 Removal kidney open complex | 50845 Appendico-vesicostomy | 57110 Remove vagina wall complete |
| 50230 Removal kidney open radical | 50860 Transplant ureter to skin | 57111 Remove vagina tissue compl |
| 50234 Removal of kidney & ureter | 50900 Repair of ureter | 57112 Vaginectomy w/nodes compl |
| 50236 Removal of kidney & ureter | 50920 Closure ureter/skin fistula | 57270 Repair of bowel pouch |
| 50240 Partial removal of kidney | 50930 Closure ureter/bowel fistula | 57280 Suspension of vagina |
| 50250 Cryoablate renal mass open | 50940 Release of ureter | 57296 Revise vag graft open abd |

 CPT © 2017 American Medical Association. All Rights Reserved. © 2017 Optum360, LLC

Appendix J — Inpatient Only Procedures

| | | |
|---|---|---|
| 57305 Repair rectum-vagina fistula | 59850 Abortion | 61521 Removal of brain lesion |
| 57307 Fistula repair & colostomy | 59851 Abortion | 61522 Removal of brain abscess |
| 57308 Fistula repair transperine | 59852 Abortion | 61524 Removal of brain lesion |
| 57311 Repair urethrovaginal lesion | 59855 Abortion | 61526 Removal of brain lesion |
| 57531 Removal of cervix radical | 59856 Abortion | 61530 Removal of brain lesion |
| 57540 Removal of residual cervix | 59857 Abortion | 61531 Implant brain electrodes |
| 57545 Remove cervix/repair pelvis | 60254 Extensive thyroid surgery | 61533 Implant brain electrodes |
| 58140 Myomectomy abdom method | 60270 Removal of thyroid | 61534 Removal of brain lesion |
| 58146 Myomectomy abdom complex | 60505 Explore parathyroid glands | 61535 Remove brain electrodes |
| 58150 Total hysterectomy | 60521 Removal of thymus gland | 61536 Removal of brain lesion |
| 58152 Total hysterectomy | 60522 Removal of thymus gland | 61537 Removal of brain tissue |
| 58180 Partial hysterectomy | 60540 Explore adrenal gland | 61538 Removal of brain tissue |
| 58200 Extensive hysterectomy | 60545 Explore adrenal gland | 61539 Removal of brain tissue |
| 58210 Extensive hysterectomy | 60600 Remove carotid body lesion | 61540 Removal of brain tissue |
| 58240 Removal of pelvis contents | 60605 Remove carotid body lesion | 61541 Incision of brain tissue |
| 58267 Vag hyst w/urinary repair | 60650 Laparoscopy adrenalectomy | 61543 Removal of brain tissue |
| 58275 Hysterectomy/revise vagina | 61105 Twist drill hole | 61544 Remove & treat brain lesion |
| 58280 Hysterectomy/revise vagina | 61107 Drill skull for implantation | 61545 Excision of brain tumor |
| 58285 Extensive hysterectomy | 61108 Drill skull for drainage | 61546 Removal of pituitary gland |
| 58293 Vag hyst w/uro repair compl | 61120 Burr hole for puncture | 61548 Removal of pituitary gland |
| 58400 Suspension of uterus | 61140 Pierce skull for biopsy | 61550 Release of skull seams |
| 58410 Suspension of uterus | 61150 Pierce skull for drainage | 61552 Release of skull seams |
| 58520 Repair of ruptured uterus | 61151 Pierce skull for drainage | 61556 Incise skull/sutures |
| 58540 Revision of uterus | 61154 Pierce skull & remove clot | 61557 Incise skull/sutures |
| 58548 Lap radical hyst | 61156 Pierce skull for drainage | 61558 Excision of skull/sutures |
| 58605 Division of fallopian tube | 61210 Pierce skull implant device | 61559 Excision of skull/sutures |
| 58611 Ligate oviduct(s) add-on | 61250 Pierce skull & explore | 61563 Excision of skull tumor |
| 58700 Removal of fallopian tube | 61253 Pierce skull & explore | 61564 Excision of skull tumor |
| 58720 Removal of ovary/tube(s) | 61304 Open skull for exploration | 61566 Removal of brain tissue |
| 58740 Adhesiolysis tube ovary | 61305 Open skull for exploration | 61567 Incision of brain tissue |
| 58750 Repair oviduct | 61312 Open skull for drainage | 61570 Remove foreign body brain |
| 58752 Revise ovarian tube(s) | 61313 Open skull for drainage | 61571 Incise skull for brain wound |
| 58760 Fimbrioplasty | 61314 Open skull for drainage | 61575 Skull base/brainstem surgery |
| 58822 Drain ovary abscess percut | 61315 Open skull for drainage | 61576 Skull base/brainstem surgery |
| 58825 Transposition ovary(s) | 61316 Implt cran bone flap to abdo | 61580 Craniofacial approach skull |
| 58940 Removal of ovary(s) | 61320 Open skull for drainage | 61581 Craniofacial approach skull |
| 58943 Removal of ovary(s) | 61321 Open skull for drainage | 61582 Craniofacial approach skull |
| 58950 Resect ovarian malignancy | 61322 Decompressive craniotomy | 61583 Craniofacial approach skull |
| 58951 Resect ovarian malignancy | 61323 Decompressive lobectomy | 61584 Orbitocranial approach/skull |
| 58952 Resect ovarian malignancy | 61332 Explore/biopsy eye socket | 61585 Orbitocranial approach/skull |
| 58953 Tah rad dissect for debulk | 61333 Explore orbit/remove lesion | 61586 Resect nasopharynx skull |
| 58954 Tah rad debulk/lymph remove | 61340 Subtemporal decompression | 61590 Infratemporal approach/skull |
| 58956 Bso omentectomy w/tah | 61343 Incise skull (press relief) | 61591 Infratemporal approach/skull |
| 58957 Resect recurrent gyn mal | 61345 Relieve cranial pressure | 61592 Orbitocranial approach/skull |
| 58958 Resect recur gyn mal w/lym | 61450 Incise skull for surgery | 61595 Transtemporal approach/skull |
| 58960 Exploration of abdomen | 61458 Incise skull for brain wound | 61596 Transcochlear approach/skull |
| 59120 Treat ectopic pregnancy | 61460 Incise skull for surgery | 61597 Transcondylar approach/skull |
| 59121 Treat ectopic pregnancy | 61480 Incise skull for surgery | 61598 Transpetrosal approach/skull |
| 59130 Treat ectopic pregnancy | 61500 Removal of skull lesion | 61600 Resect/excise cranial lesion |
| 59135 Treat ectopic pregnancy | 61501 Remove infected skull bone | 61601 Resect/excise cranial lesion |
| 59136 Treat ectopic pregnancy | 61510 Removal of brain lesion | 61605 Resect/excise cranial lesion |
| 59140 Treat ectopic pregnancy | 61512 Remove brain lining lesion | 61606 Resect/excise cranial lesion |
| 59325 Revision of cervix | 61514 Removal of brain abscess | 61607 Resect/excise cranial lesion |
| 59350 Repair of uterus | 61516 Removal of brain lesion | 61608 Resect/excise cranial lesion |
| 59514 Cesarean delivery only | 61517 Implt brain chemotx add-on | 61610 Transect artery sinus |
| 59525 Remove uterus after cesarean | 61518 Removal of brain lesion | 61611 Transect artery sinus |
| 59620 Attempted vbac delivery only | 61519 Remove brain lining lesion | 61612 Transect artery sinus |
| 59830 Treat uterus infection | 61520 Removal of brain lesion | 61613 Remove aneurysm sinus |

© 2017 Optum360, LLC

CPT © 2017 American Medical Association. All Rights Reserved.

| | | |
|---|---|---|
| 61615 Resect/excise lesion skull | 62192 Establish brain cavity shunt | 63287 Bx/exc idrl imed lesn thrlmb |
| 61616 Resect/excise lesion skull | 62200 Establish brain cavity shunt | 63290 Bx/exc xdrl/idrl lsn any lvl |
| 61618 Repair dura | 62201 Brain cavity shunt w/scope | 63295 Repair laminectomy defect |
| 61619 Repair dura | 62220 Establish brain cavity shunt | 63300 Remove vert xdrl body crvcl |
| 61624 Transcath occlusion cns | 62223 Establish brain cavity shunt | 63301 Remove vert xdrl body thrc |
| 61630 Intracranial angioplasty | 62256 Remove brain cavity shunt | 63302 Remove vert xdrl body thrlmb |
| 61635 Intracran angioplsty w/stent | 62258 Replace brain cavity shunt | 63303 Remov vert xdrl bdy lmbr/sac |
| 61645 Perq art m-thrombect &/nfs | 63050 Cervical laminoplsty 2/> seg | 63304 Remove vert idrl body crvcl |
| 61650 Evasc prlng admn rx agnt 1st | 63051 C-laminoplasty w/graft/plate | 63305 Remove vert idrl body thrc |
| 61651 Evasc prlng admn rx agnt add | 63077 Spine disk surgery thorax | 63306 Remov vert idrl bdy thrclmbr |
| 61680 Intracranial vessel surgery | 63078 Spine disk surgery thorax | 63307 Remov vert idrl bdy lmbr/sac |
| 61682 Intracranial vessel surgery | 63081 Remove vert body dcmprn crvl | 63308 Remove vertebral body add-on |
| 61684 Intracranial vessel surgery | 63082 Remove vertebral body add-on | 63700 Repair of spinal herniation |
| 61686 Intracranial vessel surgery | 63085 Remove vert body dcmprn thrc | 63702 Repair of spinal herniation |
| 61690 Intracranial vessel surgery | 63086 Remove vertebral body add-on | 63704 Repair of spinal herniation |
| 61692 Intracranial vessel surgery | 63087 Remov vertbr dcmprn thrclmbr | 63706 Repair of spinal herniation |
| 61697 Brain aneurysm repr complx | 63088 Remove vertebral body add-on | 63707 Repair spinal fluid leakage |
| 61698 Brain aneurysm repr complx | 63090 Remove vert body dcmprn lmbr | 63709 Repair spinal fluid leakage |
| 61700 Brain aneurysm repr simple | 63091 Remove vertebral body add-on | 63710 Graft repair of spine defect |
| 61702 Inner skull vessel surgery | 63101 Remove vert body dcmprn thrc | 63740 Install spinal shunt |
| 61703 Clamp neck artery | 63102 Remove vert body dcmprn lmbr | 64755 Incision of stomach nerves |
| 61705 Revise circulation to head | 63103 Remove vertebral body add-on | 64760 Incision of vagus nerve |
| 61708 Revise circulation to head | 63170 Incise spinal cord tract(s) | 64809 Remove sympathetic nerves |
| 61710 Revise circulation to head | 63172 Drainage of spinal cyst | 64818 Remove sympathetic nerves |
| 61711 Fusion of skull arteries | 63173 Drainage of spinal cyst | 64866 Fusion of facial/other nerve |
| 61735 Incise skull/brain surgery | 63180 Revise spinal cord ligaments | 64868 Fusion of facial/other nerve |
| 61750 Incise skull/brain biopsy | 63182 Revise spinal cord ligaments | 65273 Repair of eye wound |
| 61751 Brain biopsy w/ct/mr guide | 63185 Incise spine nrv half segmnt | 69155 Extensive ear/neck surgery |
| 61760 Implant brain electrodes | 63190 Incise spine nrv >2 segmnts | 69535 Remove part of temporal bone |
| 61850 Implant neuroelectrodes | 63191 Incise spine accessory nerve | 69554 Remove ear lesion |
| 61860 Implant neuroelectrodes | 63194 Incise spine & cord cervical | 69950 Incise inner ear nerve |
| 61863 Implant neuroelectrode | 63195 Incise spine & cord thoracic | 75952 Endovasc repair abdom aorta |
| 61864 Implant neuroelectrde addl | 63196 Incise spine&cord 2 trx crvl | 75953 Abdom aneurysm endovas rpr |
| 61867 Implant neuroelectrode | 63197 Incise spine&cord 2 trx thrc | 75954 Iliac aneurysm endovas rpr |
| 61868 Implant neuroelectrde addl | 63198 Incise spin&cord 2 stgs crvl | 75956 Xray endovasc thor ao repr |
| 61870 Implant neuroelectrodes | 63199 Incise spin&cord 2 stgs thrc | 75957 Xray endovasc thor ao repr |
| 62005 Treat skull fracture | 63200 Release spinal cord lumbar | 75958 Xray place prox ext thor ao |
| 62010 Treatment of head injury | 63250 Revise spinal cord vsls crvl | 75959 Xray place dist ext thor ao |
| 62100 Repair brain fluid leakage | 63251 Revise spinal cord vsls thrc | 92941 Prq card revasc mi 1 vsl |
| 62115 Reduction of skull defect | 63252 Revise spine cord vsl thrlmb | 92970 Cardioassist internal |
| 62117 Reduction of skull defect | 63265 Excise intraspinl lesion crv | 92971 Cardioassist external |
| 62120 Repair skull cavity lesion | 63266 Excise intrspinl lesion thrc | 92975 Dissolve clot heart vessel |
| 62121 Incise skull repair | 63267 Excise intrspinl lesion lmbr | 92992 Revision of heart chamber |
| 62140 Repair of skull defect | 63268 Excise intrspinl lesion scrl | 92993 Revision of heart chamber |
| 62141 Repair of skull defect | 63270 Excise intrspinl lesion crvl | 93583 Perq transcath septal reduxn |
| 62142 Remove skull plate/flap | 63271 Excise intrspinl lesion thrc | 99184 Hypothermia ill neonate |
| 62143 Replace skull plate/flap | 63272 Excise intrspinl lesion lmbr | 99190 Special pump services |
| 62145 Repair of skull & brain | 63273 Excise intrspinl lesion scrl | 99191 Special pump services |
| 62146 Repair of skull with graft | 63275 Bx/exc xdrl spine lesn crvl | 99192 Special pump services |
| 62147 Repair of skull with graft | 63276 Bx/exc xdrl spine lesn thrc | 99356 Prolonged service inpatient |
| 62148 Retr bone flap to fix skull | 63277 Bx/exc xdrl spine lesn lmbr | 99357 Prolonged service inpatient |
| 62161 Dissect brain w/scope | 63278 Bx/exc xdrl spine lesn scrl | 99462 Sbsq nb em per day hosp |
| 62162 Remove colloid cyst w/scope | 63280 Bx/exc idrl spine lesn crvl | 99468 Neonate crit care initial |
| 62163 Zneuroendoscopy w/fb removal | 63281 Bx/exc idrl spine lesn thrc | 99469 Neonate crit care subsq |
| 62164 Remove brain tumor w/scope | 63282 Bx/exc idrl spine lesn lmbr | 99471 Ped critical care initial |
| 62165 Remove pituit tumor w/scope | 63283 Bx/exc idrl spine lesn scrl | 99472 Ped critical care subsq |
| 62180 Establish brain cavity shunt | 63285 Bx/exc idrl imed lesn cervl | 99475 Ped crit care age 2-5 init |
| 62190 Establish brain cavity shunt | 63286 Bx/exc idrl imed lesn thrc | 99476 Ped crit care age 2-5 subsq |

CPT © 2017 American Medical Association. All Rights Reserved.

© 2017 Optum360, LLC

| | | |
|---|---|---|
| 99477 Init day hosp neonate care | G0341 Percutaneous islet celltrans | G0414 Pelvic ring fx treat int fix |
| 99478 Ic lbw inf < 1500 gm subsq | G0342 Laparoscopy islet cell trans | G0415 Open tx post pelvic fxcture |
| 99479 Ic lbw inf 1500-2500 g subsq | G0343 Laparotomy islet cell transp | |
| 99480 Ic inf pbw 2501-5000 g subsq | G0412 Open tx iliac spine uni/bil | |

# Appendix K — Place of Service and Type of Service

## Place-of-Service Codes for Professional Claims

Listed below are place of service codes and descriptions. These codes should be used on professional claims to specify the entity where service(s) were rendered. Check with individual payers (e.g., Medicare, Medicaid, other private insurance) for reimbursement policies regarding these codes. To comment on a code(s) or description(s), please send your request to posinfo@cms.gov.

| | | |
|---|---|---|
| 01 | Pharmacy | A facility or location where drugs and other medically related items and services are sold, dispensed, or otherwise provided directly to patients. |
| 02 | Telehealth | The location where health services and health related services are provided or received through a telecommunication system. |
| 03 | School | A facility whose primary purpose is education. |
| 04 | Homeless shelter | A facility or location whose primary purpose is to provide temporary housing to homeless individuals (e.g., emergency shelters, individual or family shelters). |
| 05 | Indian Health Service freestanding facility | A facility or location, owned and operated by the Indian Health Service, which provides diagnostic, therapeutic (surgical and non-surgical), and rehabilitation services to American Indians and Alaska natives who do not require hospitalization. |
| 06 | Indian Health Service provider-based facility | A facility or location, owned and operated by the Indian Health Service, which provides diagnostic, therapeutic (surgical and nonsurgical), and rehabilitation services rendered by, or under the supervision of, physicians to American Indians and Alaska natives admitted as inpatients or outpatients. |
| 07 | Tribal 638 freestanding facility | A facility or location owned and operated by a federally recognized American Indian or Alaska native tribe or tribal organization under a 638 agreement, which provides diagnostic, therapeutic (surgical and nonsurgical), and rehabilitation services to tribal members who do not require hospitalization. |
| 08 | Tribal 638 provider-based Facility | A facility or location owned and operated by a federally recognized American Indian or Alaska native tribe or tribal organization under a 638 agreement, which provides diagnostic, therapeutic (surgical and nonsurgical), and rehabilitation services to tribal members admitted as inpatients or outpatients. |
| 09 | Prison/correctional facility | A prison, jail, reformatory, work farm, detention center, or any other similar facility maintained by either federal, state or local authorities for the purpose of confinement or rehabilitation of adult or juvenile criminal offenders. |
| 10 | Unassigned | N/A |
| 11 | Office | Location, other than a hospital, skilled nursing facility (SNF), military treatment facility, community health center, State or local public health clinic, or intermediate care facility (ICF), where the health professional routinely provides health examinations, diagnosis, and treatment of illness or injury on an ambulatory basis. |
| 12 | Home | Location, other than a hospital or other facility, where the patient receives care in a private residence. |
| 13 | Assisted living facility | Congregate residential facility with self-contained living units providing assessment of each resident's needs and on-site support 24 hours a day, 7 days a week, with the capacity to deliver or arrange for services including some health care and other services. |
| 14 | Group home | A residence, with shared living areas, where clients receive supervision and other services such as social and/or behavioral services, custodial service, and minimal services (e.g., medication administration). |
| 15 | Mobile unit | A facility/unit that moves from place-to-place equipped to provide preventive, screening, diagnostic, and/or treatment services. |
| 16 | Temporary lodging | A short-term accommodation such as a hotel, campground, hostel, cruise ship or resort where the patient receives care, and which is not identified by any other POS code. |
| 17 | Walk-in retail health clinic | A walk-in health clinic, other than an office, urgent care facility, pharmacy, or independent clinic and not described by any other place of service code, that is located within a retail operation and provides preventive and primary care services on an ambulatory basis. |
| 18 | Place of employment/ worksite | A location, not described by any other POS code, owned or operated by a public or private entity where the patient is employed, and where a health professional provides on-going or episodic occupational medical, therapeutic or rehabilitative services to the individual. |
| 19 | Off campus-outpatient hospital | A portion of an off-campus hospital provider based department which provides diagnostic, therapeutic (both surgical and nonsurgical), and rehabilitation services to sick or injured persons who do not require hospitalization or institutionalization. |
| 20 | Urgent care facility | Location, distinct from a hospital emergency room, an office, or a clinic, whose purpose is to diagnose and treat illness or injury for unscheduled, ambulatory patients seeking immediate medical attention. |

| 21 | Inpatient hospital | A facility, other than psychiatric, which primarily provides diagnostic, therapeutic (both surgical and nonsurgical), and rehabilitation services by, or under, the supervision of physicians to patients admitted for a variety of medical conditions. |
|---|---|---|
| 22 | On campus-outpatient hospital | A portion of a hospital's main campus which provides diagnostic, therapeutic (both surgical and nonsurgical), and rehabilitation services to sick or injured persons who do not require hospitalization or institutionalization. |
| 23 | Emergency room—hospital | A portion of a hospital where emergency diagnosis and treatment of illness or injury is provided. |
| 24 | Ambulatory surgical center | A freestanding facility, other than a physician's office, where surgical and diagnostic services are provided on an ambulatory basis. |
| 25 | Birthing center | A facility, other than a hospital's maternity facilities or a physician's office, which provides a setting for labor, delivery, and immediate post-partum care as well as immediate care of new born infants. |
| 26 | Military treatment facility | A medical facility operated by one or more of the uniformed services. Military treatment facility (MTF) also refers to certain former U.S. Public Health Service (USPHS) facilities now designated as uniformed service treatment facilities (USTF). |
| 27-30 | Unassigned | N/A |
| 31 | Skilled nursing facility | A facility which primarily provides inpatient skilled nursing care and related services to patients who require medical, nursing, or rehabilitative services but does not provide the level of care or treatment available in a hospital. |
| 32 | Nursing facility | A facility which primarily provides to residents skilled nursing care and related services for the rehabilitation of injured, disabled, or sick persons, or, on a regular basis, health-related care services above the level of custodial care to individuals other than those with intellectual disabilities. |
| 33 | Custodial care facility | A facility which provides room, board, and other personal assistance services, generally on a long-term basis, and which does not include a medical component. |
| 34 | Hospice | A facility, other than a patient's home, in which palliative and supportive care for terminally ill patients and their families is provided. |
| 35-40 | Unassigned | N/A |
| 41 | Ambulance—land | A land vehicle specifically designed, equipped and staffed for lifesaving and transporting the sick or injured. |
| 42 | Ambulance—air or water | An air or water vehicle specifically designed, equipped and staffed for lifesaving and transporting the sick or injured. |
| 43-48 | Unassigned | N/A |
| 49 | Independent clinic | A location, not part of a hospital and not described by any other place-of-service code, that is organized and operated to provide preventive, diagnostic, therapeutic, rehabilitative, or palliative services to outpatients only. |
| 50 | Federally qualified health center | A facility located in a medically underserved area that provides Medicare beneficiaries with preventive primary medical care under the general direction of a physician. |
| 51 | Inpatient psychiatric facility | A facility that provides inpatient psychiatric services for the diagnosis and treatment of mental illness on a 24-hour basis, by or under the supervision of a physician. |
| 52 | Psychiatric facility-partial hospitalization | A facility for the diagnosis and treatment of mental illness that provides a planned therapeutic program for patients who do not require full time hospitalization, but who need broader programs than are possible from outpatient visits to a hospital-based or hospital-affiliated facility. |
| 53 | Community mental health center | A facility that provides the following services: outpatient services, including specialized outpatient services for children, the elderly, individuals who are chronically ill, and residents of the CMHC's mental health services area who have been discharged from inpatient treatment at a mental health facility; 24 hour a day emergency care services; day treatment, other partial hospitalization services, or psychosocial rehabilitation services; screening for patients being considered for admission to state mental health facilities to determine the appropriateness of such admission; and consultation and education services. |
| 54 | Intermediate care facility/individuals with intellectual disabilities | A facility which primarily provides health-related care and services above the level of custodial care to individuals with Intellectual Disabilities but does not provide the level of care or treatment available in a hospital or SNF. |
| 55 | Residential substance abuse treatment facility | A facility which provides treatment for substance (alcohol and drug) abuse to live-in residents who do not require acute medical care. Services include individual and group therapy and counseling, family counseling, laboratory tests, drugs and supplies, psychological testing, and room and board. |
| 56 | Psychiatric residential treatment center | A facility or distinct part of a facility for psychiatric care which provides a total 24-hour therapeutically planned and professionally staffed group living and learning environment. |
| 57 | Non-residential substance abuse treatment facility | A location which provides treatment for substance (alcohol and drug) abuse on an ambulatory basis. Services include individual and group therapy and counseling, family counseling, laboratory tests, drugs and supplies, and psychological testing. |
| 58-59 | Unassigned | N/A |

     CPT © 2017 American Medical Association. All Rights Reserved.     © 2017 Optum360, LLC

| 60 | Mass immunization center | A location where providers administer pneumococcal pneumonia and influenza virus vaccinations and submit these services as electronic media claims, paper claims, or using the roster billing method. This generally takes place in a mass immunization setting, such as, a public health center, pharmacy, or mall but may include a physician office setting. |
|----|----|----|
| 61 | Comprehensive inpatient rehabilitation facility | A facility that provides comprehensive rehabilitation services under the supervision of a physician to inpatients with physical disabilities. Services include physical therapy, occupational therapy, speech pathology, social or psychological services, and orthotics and prosthetics services. |
| 62 | Comprehensive outpatient rehabilitation facility | A facility that provides comprehensive rehabilitation services under the supervision of a physician to outpatients with physical disabilities. Services include physical therapy, occupational therapy, and speech pathology services. |
| 63-64 | Unassigned | N/A |
| 65 | End-stage renal disease treatment facility | A facility other than a hospital, which provides dialysis treatment, maintenance, and/or training to patients or caregivers on an ambulatory or home-care basis. |
| 66-70 | Unassigned | N/A |
| 71 | Public health clinic | A facility maintained by either state or local health departments that provides ambulatory primary medical care under the general direction of a physician. |
| 72 | Rural health clinic | A certified facility which is located in a rural medically underserved area that provides ambulatory primary medical care under the general direction of a physician. |
| 73-80 | Unassigned | N/A |
| 81 | Independent laboratory | A laboratory certified to perform diagnostic and/or clinical tests independent of an institution or a physician's office. |
| 82-98 | Unassigned | N/A |
| 99 | Other place of service | Other place of service not identified above. |

## Type of Service

### Common Working File Type of Service (TOS) Indicators

For submitting a claim to the Common Working File (CWF), use the following table to assign the proper TOS. Some procedures may have more than one applicable TOS. CWF will reject alerts on codes with incorrect TOS designations. CWF will produce alerts on codes with incorrect TOS designations.

The only exceptions to this annual update are:

- Surgical services billed for dates of service through December 31, 2007, containing the ASC facility service modifier SG must be reported as TOS F. Effective for services on or after January 1, 2008, the SG modifier is no longer applicable for Medicare services. ASC providers should discontinue applying the SG modifier on ASC facility claims. The indicator F does not appear in the TOS table because its use depends upon claims submitted with POS 24 (ASC facility) from an ASC (specialty 49). This became effective for dates of service January 1, 2008, or after.

- Surgical services billed with an assistant-at-surgery modifier (80-82, AS) must be reported with TOS 8. The 8 indicator does not appear on the TOS table because its use is dependent upon the use of the appropriate modifier. (See Pub. 100-4 *Medicare Claims Processing*

*Manual,* chapter 12, "Physician/Practitioner Billing," for instructions on when assistant-at-surgery is allowable.)

- Psychiatric treatment services that are subject to the outpatient mental health treatment limitation should be reported with TOS T.

- TOS H appears in the list of descriptors. However, it does not appear in the table. In CWF, "H" is used only as an indicator for hospice. The contractor should not submit TOS H to CWF at this time.

- For outpatient services, when a transfusion medicine code appears on a claim that also contains a blood product, the service is paid under reasonable charge at 80 percent; coinsurance and deductible apply. When transfusion medicine codes are paid under the clinical laboratory fee schedule they are paid at 100 percent; coinsurance and deductible do not apply.

**Note:** For injection codes with more than one possible TOS designation, use the following guidelines when assigning the TOS:

When the choice is L or 1:

- Use TOS L when the drug is used related to ESRD; or

- Use TOS 1 when the drug is not related to ESRD and is administered in the office.

When the choice is G or 1:

- Use TOS G when the drug is an immunosuppressive drug; or

- Use TOS 1 when the drug is used for other than immunosuppression.

When the choice is P or 1:

- Use TOS P if the drug is administered through durable medical equipment (DME); or

- Use TOS 1 if the drug is administered in the office.

The place of service or diagnosis may be considered when determining the appropriate TOS. The descriptors for each of the TOS codes listed in the annual HCPCS update are:

| 0 | Whole blood |
|---|---|
| 1 | Medical care |
| 2 | Surgery |
| 3 | Consultation |
| 4 | Diagnostic radiology |
| 5 | Diagnostic laboratory |
| 6 | Therapeutic radiology |
| 7 | Anesthesia |
| 8 | Assistant at surgery |
| 9 | Other medical items or services |
| A | Used DME |
| D | Ambulance |
| E | Enteral/parenteral nutrients/supplies |
| F | Ambulatory surgical center (facility usage for surgical services) |
| G | Immunosuppressive drugs |
| J | Diabetic shoes |
| K | Hearing items and services |
| L | ESRD supplies |
| M | Monthly capitation payment for dialysis |
| N | Kidney donor |
| P | Lump sum purchase of DME, prosthetics, orthotics |
| Q | Vision items or services |
| R | Rental of DME |
| S | Surgical dressings or other medical supplies |
| U | Occupational therapy |
| V | Pneumococcal/flu vaccine |
| W | Physical therapy |

## Berenson-Eggers Type of Service (BETOS) Codes

The BETOS coding system was developed primarily for analyzing the growth in Medicare expenditures. The coding system covers all HCPCS codes; assigns a HCPCS code to only one BETOS code; consists of readily understood clinical categories (as opposed to statistical or financial categories); consists of categories that permit objective assignment; is stable over time; and is relatively immune to minor changes in technology or practice patterns.

### BETOS Codes and Descriptions:

1. **Evaluation and Management**
   1. M1A   Office visits—new
   2. M1B   Office visits—established
   3. M2A   Hospital visit—initial
   4. M2B   Hospital visit—subsequent
   5. M2C   Hospital visit—critical care
   6. M3   Emergency room visit
   7. M4A   Home visit
   8. M4B   Nursing home visit
   9. M5A   Specialist—pathology
   10. M5B   Specialist—psychiatry
   11. M5C   Specialist—ophthalmology
   12. M5D   Specialist—other
   13. M6   Consultations

2. **Procedures**
   1. P0   Anesthesia
   2. P1A   Major procedure—breast
   3. P1B   Major procedure—colectomy
   4. P1C   Major procedure—cholecystectomy
   5. P1D   Major procedure—TURP
   6. P1E   Major procedure—hysterectomy
   7. P1F   Major procedure—explor/decompr/excis disc
   8. P1G   Major procedure—other
   9. P2A   Major procedure, cardiovascular—CABG
   10. P2B   Major procedure, cardiovascular—aneurysm repair
   11. P2C   Major procedure, cardiovascular—thromboendarterectomy
   12. P2D   Major procedure, cardiovascular—coronary angioplasty (PTCA)
   13. P2E   Major procedure, cardiovascular—pacemaker insertion
   14. P2F   Major procedure, cardiovascular—other
   15. P3A   Major procedure, orthopedic—hip fracture repair
   16. P3B   Major procedure, orthopedic—hip replacement
   17. P3C   Major procedure, orthopedic—knee replacement
   18. P3D   Major procedure, orthopedic—other
   19. P4A   Eye procedure—corneal transplant
   20. P4B   Eye procedure—cataract removal/lens insertion
   21. P4C   Eye procedure—retinal detachment
   22. P4D   Eye procedure—treatment of retinal lesions
   23. P4E   Eye procedure—other
   24. P5A   Ambulatory procedures—skin
   25. P5B   Ambulatory procedures—musculoskeletal
   26. P5C   Ambulatory procedures—inguinal hernia repair
   27. P5D   Ambulatory procedures—lithotripsy
   28. P5E   Ambulatory procedures—other
   29. P6A   Minor procedures—skin
   30. P6B   Minor procedures—musculoskeletal
   31. P6C   Minor procedures—other (Medicare fee schedule)
   32. P6D   Minor procedures—other (non-Medicare fee schedule)
   33. P7A   Oncology—radiation therapy
   34. P7B   Oncology—other
   35. P8A   Endoscopy—arthroscopy
   36. P8B   Endoscopy—upper gastrointestinal
   37. P8C   Endoscopy—sigmoidoscopy
   38. P8D   Endoscopy—colonoscopy
   39. P8E   Endoscopy—cystoscopy
   40. P8F   Endoscopy—bronchoscopy
   41. P8G   Endoscopy—laparoscopic cholecystectomy
   42. P8H   Endoscopy—laryngoscopy
   43. P8I   Endoscopy—other
   44. P9A   Dialysis services (Medicare fee schedule)
   45. P9B   Dialysis services (non-Medicare fee schedule)

3. **Imaging**
   1. I1A   Standard imaging—chest
   2. I1B   Standard imaging—musculoskeletal
   3. I1C   Standard imaging—breast
   4. I1D   Standard imaging—contrast gastrointestinal
   5. I1E   Standard imaging—nuclear medicine
   6. I1F   Standard imaging—other
   7. I2A   Advanced imaging—CAT/CT/CTA; brain/head/neck
   8. I2B   Advanced imaging—CAT/CT/CTA; other
   9. I2C   Advanced imaging—MRI/MRA; brain/head/neck
   10. I2D   Advanced imaging—MRI/MRA; other
   11. I3A   Echography/ultrasonography—eye
   12. I3B   Echography/ultrasonography—abdomen/pelvis
   13. I3C   Echography/ultrasonography—heart
   14. I3D   Echography/ultrasonography—carotid arteries
   15. I3E   Echography/ultrasonography—prostate, transrectal
   16. I3F   Echography/ultrasonography—other
   17. I4A   Imaging/procedure—heart, including cardiac catheterization
   18. I4B   Imaging/procedure—other

4. **Tests**
   1. T1A   Lab tests—routine venipuncture (non-Medicare fee schedule)
   2. T1B   Lab tests—automated general profiles
   3. T1C   Lab tests—urinalysis
   4. T1D   Lab tests—blood counts
   5. T1E   Lab tests—glucose
   6. T1F   Lab tests—bacterial cultures
   7. T1G   Lab tests—other (Medicare fee schedule)
   8. T1H   Lab tests—other (non-Medicare fee schedule)
   9. T2A   Other tests—electrocardiograms
   10. T2B   Other tests—cardiovascular stress tests
   11. T2C   Other tests—EKG monitoring
   12. T2D   Other tests—other

5. **Durable Medical Equipment**
   1. D1A   Medical/surgical supplies
   1. D1B   Hospital beds
   1. D1C   Oxygen and supplies
   1. D1D   Wheelchairs
   1. D1E   Other DME
   1. D1F   Prosthetic/orthotic devices
   1. D1G   Drugs administered through DME

6. **Other**
   1. O1A   Ambulance
   2. O1B   Chiropractic
   3. O1C   Enteral and parenteral
   4. O1D   Chemotherapy
   5. O1E   Other drugs
   6. O1F   Hearing and speech services
   7. O1G   Immunizations/vaccinations

7. **Exceptions/Unclassified**
   1. Y1   Other—Medicare fee schedule
   2. Y2   Other—Non-Medicare fee schedule
   3. Z1   Local codes
   4. Z2   Undefined codes

CPT © 2017 American Medical Association. All Rights Reserved.

© 2017 Optum360, LLC

# Appendix L — Multianalyte Assays with Algorithmic Analyses

The following is a list of administrative codes for multianalyte assays with algorithmic analysis (MAAA) procedures that are usually exclusive to one single clinical laboratory or manufacturer. These tests use the results from several different assays, including molecular pathology assays, fluorescent in situ hybridization assays, and nonnucleic acid-based assays (e.g., proteins, polypeptides, lipids, and carbohydrates) to perform an algorithmic analysis that is reported as a numeric score or probability. Although the laboratory report may list results of individual component tests of the MAAAs, these assays are not separately reportable.

The following list includes the proprietary name and clinical laboratory/manufacturer, an alphanumeric code, and the code descriptor.

The format for the code descriptor usually includes:

- Type of disease (e.g., oncology, autoimmune, tissue rejection)
- Chemical(s) analyzed (e.g., DNA, RNA, protein, antibody)
- Number of markers (e.g., number of genes, number of proteins)

- Methodology(s) (e.g., microarray, real-time [RT]-PCR, in situ hybridization [ISH], enzyme linked immunosorbent assays [ELISA])
- Number of functional domains (when indicated)
- Type of specimen (e.g., blood, fresh tissue, formalin-fixed paraffin embedded)
- Type of algorithm result (e.g., prognostic, diagnostic)
- Report (e.g., probability index, risk score)

MAAA procedures with a Category I code are noted on the following list and can also be found in code range 81500–81599 in the pathology and laboratory chapter. If a specific MAAA test does not have a Category I code, it is denoted with a four-digit number and the letter M. Use code 81599 if an MAAA test is not included on the following list or in the Category I codes. The codes on the list are exclusive to the assays identified by proprietary name. Report code 81599 also when an analysis is performed that may possibly fall within a specific descriptor but the proprietary name is not included in the list. The list does not contain all MAAA procedures.

| Proprietary Name/Clinical Laboratory/Manufacturer | Code | Descriptor |
|---|---|---|
| **Administrative Codes for Multianalyte Assays with Algorithmic Analyses (MAAA)** | | |
| HCV FibroSURE™, LabCorp FibroTest™, Quest Diagnostics/BioPredictive | 0001M | Infectious disease, HCV, six biochemical assays (ALT, A2-macroglobulin, apolipoprotein A-1, total bilirubin, GGT, and haptoglobin) utilizing serum, prognostic algorithm reported as scores for fibrosis and necroinflammatory activity in liver |
| ASH FibroSURE™, LabCorp | 0002M | Liver disease, 10 biochemical assays (ALT, A2-macroglobulin, apolipoprotein A-1, total bilirubin, GGT, haptoglobin, AST, glucose, total cholesterol, and triglycerides) utilizing serum, prognostic algorithm reported as quantitative scores for fibrosis, steatosis, and alcoholic steatohepatitis (ASH) |
| NASH FibroSURE™, LabCorp | 0003M | Liver disease, 10 biochemical assays (ALT, A2-macroglobulin, apolipoprotein A-1, total bilirubin, GGT, haptoglobin, AST, glucose, total cholesterol, and triglycerides) utilizing serum, prognostic algorithm reported as quantitative scores for fibrosis, steatosis, and nonalcoholic steatohepatitis (NASH) |
| ScoliScore™ Transgenomic | 0004M | Scoliosis, DNA analysis of 53 single nucleotide polymorphisms (SNPs), using saliva, prognostic algorithm reported as a risk score |
| HeproDX™, GoPath Laboratories, LLC | 0006M | Oncology (hepatic), mRNA expression levels of 161 genes, utilizing fresh hepatocellular carcinoma tumor tissue, with alpha-fetoprotein level, algorithm reported as a risk classifier |
| NETest (Wren Laboratories, LLC) | 0007M | Oncology (gastrointestinal neuroendocrine tumors), real-time PCR expression analysis of 51 genes, utilizing whole peripheral blood, algorithm reported as a nomogram of tumor disease index |
| | (0008M has been deleted, to report, see 81520) | |
| VisibiliT™ test, Sequenom Center for Molecular Medicine, LLC | 0009M | Fetal aneuploidy (trisomy 21, and 18) DNA sequence analysis of selected regions using maternal plasma, algorithm reported as a risk score for each trisomy |
| **Category I Codes for Multianalyte Assays with Algorithmic Analyses (MAAA)** | | |
| Vectra® DA, Crescendo Bioscience, Inc | 81490 | Autoimmune (rheumatoid arthritis), analysis of 12 biomarkers using immunoassays, utilizing serum, prognostic algorithm reported as a disease activity score (Do not report 81490 with 86140) |
| Corus® CAD, CardioDx, Inc. | 81493 | Coronary artery disease, mRNA, gene expression profiling by real-time RT-PCR of 23 genes, utilizing whole peripheral blood, algorithm reported as a risk score |
| Risk of Ovarian Malignancy Algorithm (ROMA)™, Fujirebio Diagnostics | 81500 | Oncology (ovarian), biochemical assays of two proteins (CA-125 and HE4), utilizing serum, with menopausal status, algorithm reported as a risk score |
| OVA1™, Vermillion, Inc. | 81503 | Oncology (ovarian), biochemical assays of five proteins (CA-125, apolipoprotein A1, beta-2 microglobulin, transferrin, and pre-albumin), utilizing serum, algorithm reported as a risk score |
| Pathwork® Tissue of Origin Test, Pathwork Diagnostics | 81504 | Oncology (tissue of origin), microarray gene expression profiling of >2000 genes, utilizing formalin-fixed paraffin embedded tissue, algorithm reported as tissue similarity scores |

**Appendix L — Multianalyte Assays with Algorithmic Analyses**

| Proprietary Name/Clinical Laboratory/Manufacturer | Code | Descriptor |
|---|---|---|
| PreDx Diabetes Risk Score™, Tethys Clinical Laboratory | 81506 | Endocrinology (type 2 diabetes), biochemical assays of seven analytes (glucose, HbA1c, insulin, hs-CRP, adiponectin, ferritin, interleukin 2-receptor alpha), utilizing serum or plasma, algorithm reporting a risk score |
| Harmony™ Prenatal Test, Ariosa Diagnostics | 81507 | Fetal aneuploidy (trisomy 21, 18, and 13) DNA sequence analysis of selected regions using maternal plasma, algorithm reported as a risk score for each trisomy |
| No proprietary name and clinical laboratory or manufacturer. Maternal serum screening procedures are performed by many labs and are not exclusive to a single facility. | 81508 | Fetal congenital abnormalities, biochemical assays of two proteins (PAPP-A, hCG [any form]), utilizing maternal serum, algorithm reported as a risk score |
| | 81509 | Fetal congenital abnormalities, biochemical assays of three proteins (PAPP-A, hCG [any form], DIA), utilizing maternal serum, algorithm reported as a risk score |
| | 81510 | Fetal congenital abnormalities, biochemical assays of three analytes (AFP, uE3, hCG (any form)), utilizing maternal serum, algorithm reported as a risk score |
| | 81511 | Fetal congenital abnormalities, biochemical assays of four analytes (AFP, uE3, hCG (any form), DIA) utilizing maternal serum, algorithm reported as a risk score (may include additional results from previous biochemical testing) |
| | 81512 | Fetal congenital abnormalities, biochemical assays of five analytes (AFP, uE3, total hCG, hyperglycosylated hCG, DIA) utilizing maternal serum, algorithm reported as a risk score |
| Oncotype DX® (Genomic Health) | 81519 | Oncology (breast), mRNA, gene expression profiling by real-time RT-PCR of 21 genes, utilizing formalin-fixed paraffin embedded tissue, algorithm reported as recurrence score |
| Prosigna® Breast Cancer Assay, NanoString Technologies, Inc. | ● 81520 | Oncology (breast), mRNA gene expression profiling by hybrid capture of 58 genes (50 content and 8 housekeeping), utilizing formalin-fixed paraffin-embedded tissue, algorithm reported as a recurrence risk score |
| MammaPrint®, Agendia, Inc. | ● 81521 | Oncology (breast), mRNA, microarray gene expression profiling of 70 content genes and 465 housekeeping genes, utilizing fresh frozen or formalin-fixed paraffin-embedded tissue, algorithm reported as index related to risk of distant metastasis |
| Oncotype DX® Colon Cancer Assay, Genomic Health | 81525 | Oncology (colon), mRNA, gene expression profiling by real-time RT-PCR of 12 genes (7 content and 5 housekeeping), utilizing formalin-fixed paraffin-embedded tissue, algorithm reported as a recurrence score |
| Cologuard™, Exact Sciences, Inc. | 81528 | Oncology (colorectal) screening, quantitative real-time target and signal amplification of 10 DNA markers (KRAS mutations, promoter methylation of NDRG4 and BMP3) and fecal hemoglobin, utilizing stool, algorithm reported as a positive or negative result (Do not report 81528 with 81275, 82274) |
| ChemoFX®, Helomics, Corp. | 81535 | Oncology (gynecologic), live tumor cell culture and chemotherapeutic response by DAPI stain and morphology, predictive algorithm reported as a drug response score; first single drug or drug combination |
| ChemoFX®, Helomics, Corp. | + 81536 | Oncology (gynecologic), live tumor cell culture and chemotherapeutic response by DAPI stain and morphology, predictive algorithm reported as a drug response score; each additional single drug or drug combination (List separately in addition to code for primary procedure) (Code first 81535) |
| VeriStrat, Biodesix, Inc. | 81538 | Oncology (lung), mass spectrometric 8-protein signature, including amyloid A, utilizing serum, prognostic and predictive algorithm reported as good versus poor overall survival |
| 4Kscore test, OPKO Health Inc. | 81539 | Oncology (high-grade prostate cancer), biochemical assay of four proteins (Total PSA, Free PSA, Intact PSA, and human kallikrein-2 [hK2]), utilizing plasma or serum, prognostic algorithm reported as a probability score |
| CancerTYPE ID, bioTheranostics, Inc. | 81540 | Oncology (tumor of unknown origin), mRNA, gene expression profiling by real-time RT-PCR of 92 genes (87 content and 5 housekeeping) to classify tumor into main cancer type and subtype, utilizing formalin-fixed paraffin-embedded tissue, algorithm reported as a probability of a predicted main cancer type and subtype |
| Prolaris®, Myriad Genetic Laboratories, Inc. | ● 81541 | Oncology (prostate), mRNA gene expression profiling by real-time RT-PCR of 46 genes (31 content and 15 housekeeping), utilizing formalin-fixed paraffin-embedded tissue, algorithm reported as a disease-specific mortality risk score |
| Afirma® Gene Expression Classifier, Veracyte, Inc. | 81545 | Oncology (thyroid), gene expression analysis of 142 genes, utilizing fine needle aspirate, algorithm reported as a categorical result (eg, benign or suspicious) |
| ConfirmMDx® for Prostate Cancer, MDxHealth, Inc. | ● 81551 | Oncology (prostate), promoter methylation profiling by real-time PCR of 3 genes (GSTP1, APC, RASSF1), utilizing formalin-fixed paraffin-embedded tissue, algorithm reported as a likelihood of prostate cancer detection on repeat biopsy |
| AlloMap®, CareDx, Inc | 81595 | Cardiology (heart transplant, mRNA gene expression profiling by real-time qualitative PCR of 20 genes (11 content and 9 housekeeping), utilizing subfraction of peripheral blood, algorithm reported as a rejection risk score |
| | 81599 | Unlisted multianalyte assay with algorithmic analysis |

CPT © 2017 American Medical Association. All Rights Reserved.

© 2017 Optum360, LLC

| Proprietary Name/Clinical Laboratory/Manufacturer | Code | Descriptor |
|---|---|---|
| **Proprietary Laboratory Analyses (PLA)** | | |
| PreciseType® HEA Test, Immucor, Inc. | ● 0001U | Red blood cell antigen typing, DNA, human erythrocyte antigen gene analysis of 35 antigens from 11 blood groups, utilizing whole blood, common RBC alleles reported |
| PolypDX™, Atlantic Diagnostic Laboratories, LLC, Metabolomic Technologies Inc. | ● 0002U | Oncology (colorectal), quantitative assessment of three urine metabolites (ascorbic acid, succinic acid and carnitine) by liquid chromatography with tandem mass spectrometry (LC-MS/MS) using multiple reaction monitoring acquisition, algorithm reported as likelihood of adenomatous polyps |
| Overa (OVA1 Next Generation), Aspira Labs, Inc. Vermillion, Inc. | ● 0003U | Oncology (ovarian) biochemical assays of five proteins (apolipoprotein A-1, CA 125 II, follicle stimulating hormone, human epididymis protein 4, transferrin), utilizing serum, algorithm reported as a likelihood score |
| Gram-Negative Bacterial, Resistance Gene PCR Panel, Mayo Clinic, Check-Points Health BV, Wageningen, Netherlands | ● 0004U | Infectious disease (bacterial), DNA, 27 resistance genes, PCR amplification and probe hybridization in microarray format (molecular detection and identification of AmpC, carbapenemase and ESBL coding genes), bacterial culture colonies, report of genes detected or not detected, per isolate |
| ExosomeDx®, Prostate (IntelliScore), Exosome Diagnostics, Inc. | ● 0005U | Oncology (prostate) gene expression profile by real-time RT-PCR of 3 genes (ERG, PCA3, and SPDEF), urine, algorithm reported as risk score |
| Aegis Drug-Drug Interaction Test, Aegis Sciences Corporation | ● 0006U | Prescription drug monitoring, 120 or more drugs and substances, definitive tandem mass spectrometry with chromatography, urine, qualitative report of presence (including quantitative levels, when detected) or absence of each drug or substance with description and severity of potential interactions, with identified substances, per date of service |
| ToxProtect, Genotox Laboratories LTD | ● 0007U | Drug test(s), presumptive, with definitive confirmation of positive results, any number of drug classes, urine, includes specimen verification including DNA authentication in comparison to buccal DNA, per date of service. See PLA code 0020U for code with the same clinical descriptor; clarify code in this appendix. |
| AmHPR Helicobacter pylori, Antibiotic Resistance Next, Generation Sequencing Panel, American Molecular Laboratories, Inc. | ● 0008U | Helicobacter pylori detection and antibiotic resistance, DNA, 16S and 23S rRNA, gyrA, pbp1,rdxA and rpoB, next generation sequencing, formalin-fixed paraffin-embedded or fresh tissue, predictive, reported as positive or negative for resistance to clarithromycin, fluoroquinolones, metronidazole, amoxicillin, tetracycline and rifabutin |
| DEPArray™HER2, PacificDx | ● 0009U | Oncology (breast cancer), ERBB2 (HER2) copy number by FISH, tumor cells from formalin-fixed paraffin-embedded tissue isolated using image-based dielectrophoresis (DEP) sorting, reported as ERBB2 gene amplified or non-amplified |
| Bacterial Typing by Whole Genome Sequencing, Mayo Clinic | ● 0010U | Infectious disease (bacterial), strain typing by whole genome sequencing, phylogenetic-based report of strain relatedness, per submitted isolate |
| Cordant CORE™, Cordant Health Solutions | ● 0011U | Prescription drug monitoring, evaluation of drugs present by LC-MS/MS, using oral fluid, reported as a comparison to an estimated steady-state range, per date of service including all drug compounds and metabolites |
| MatePair Targeted, Rearrangements, Congenital, Mayo Clinic | ● 0012U | Germline disorders, gene rearrangement detection by whole genome next-generation sequencing, DNA, whole blood, report of specific gene rearrangement(s) |
| MatePair Targeted, Rearrangements, Oncology, Mayo Clinic | ● 0013U | Oncology (solid organ neoplasia), gene rearrangement detection by whole genome next-generation sequencing, DNA, fresh or frozen tissue or cells, report of specific gene rearrangement(s) |
| MatePair Targeted, Rearrangements, Hematologic, Mayo Clinic | ● 0014U | Hematology (hematolymphoid neoplasia), gene rearrangement detection by whole genome next-generation sequencing, DNA, whole blood or bone marrow, report of specific gene |
| OneOme RIghtMed, Pharmacogenomic Test, OneOme, LLC | ● 0015U | Drug metabolism (adverse drug reactions), DNA, 22 drug metabolism and transporter genes, real –time PCR, blood or buccal swab, genotype and metabolizer status for therapeutic decision support |
| BCR-ABL1 major and minor breakpoint fusion transcripts, University of Iowa, Department of Pathology, Asuragen | ● 0016U | Oncology (hematolymphoid neoplasia), RNA, BCR/ABL1 major and minor breakpoint fusion transcripts, quantitative PCR amplification, blood or bone marrow, report of fusion not detected or detected with quantitation |
| JAK2 Mutation, University of Iowa, Department of Pathology, Asuragen | ● 0017U | Oncology (hematolymphoid neoplasia), JAK2 mutation, DNA, PCR amplification of exons 12-14 and sequence analysis, blood or bone marrow, report of JAK2 mutation not detected or detected |
| ThyraMIR, Interpace Diagnostics | ● 0018U | Oncology (thyroid), microRNA profiling by RT-PCR of 10 microRNA sequences, utilizing fine needle aspirate, algorithm reported as a positive or negative result for moderate to high risk of malignancy |
| OncoTarget/, OncoTreat, Columbia University Department of Pathology and Cell Biology, Darwin Health | ● 0019U | Oncology, RNA, gene expression by whole transcriptome sequencing, formalin-fixed paraffin embedded tissue or fresh frozen tissue, predictive algorithm reported as potential targets for therapeutic agents |
| ToxLok, InSource Diagnostics, Agena Bioscience, Inc. | ● 0020U | Drug test(s), presumptive, with definitive confirmation of positive results, any number of drug classes, urine, with specimen verification including DNA authentication in comparison to buccal DNA, per date of service. See PLA code 0007U for code with the same clinical descriptor; clarify code in this appendix. |

| Proprietary Name/Clinical Laboratory/Manufacturer | Code | Descriptor |
|---|---|---|
| Apifiny®, Armune BioScience, Inc. | ● 0021U | Oncology (prostate), detection of 8 autoantibodies (ARF 6, NKX3-1, 5'-UTR-BMI1, CEP 164, 3'-UTR-Ropporin, Desmocollin, AURKAIP-1, CSNK2A2), multiplexed immunoassay and flow cytometry serum, algorithm reported as risk score |
| Oncomine™ Dx Target Test, Thermo Fisher, Scientific | ● 0022U | Targeted genomic sequence analysis panel, non-small cell lung neoplasia, DNA and RNA analysis, 23 genes, interrogation for sequence variants and rearrangements, reported as presence/absence of variants and associated therapy(ies) to consider |
| LeukoStrat® CDx FLT3 Mutation Assay, LabPMM LLC, an Invivoscribe Technologies, Inc. company, Invivoscribe Technologies, Inc. | ● 0023U | Oncology (acute myelogenous leukemia), DNA, genotyping of internal tandem duplication, p.D835, p.I836, using mononuclear cells, reported as detection or non-detection of FLT3 mutation and indication for or against the use of midostaurin |

CPT © 2017 American Medical Association. All Rights Reserved.

© 2017 Optum360, LLC

**-centesis.** Puncture, as with a needle, trocar, or aspirator; often done for withdrawing fluid from a cavity.

**-ectomy.** Excision, removal.

**-orrhaphy.** Suturing.

**-ostomy.** Indicates a surgically created artificial opening.

**-otomy.** Making an incision or opening.

**-plasty.** Indicates surgically formed or molded.

**abdominal lymphadenectomy.** Surgical removal of the abdominal lymph nodes grouping, with or without para-aortic and vena cava nodes.

**ablation.** Removal or destruction of a body part or tissue or its function. Ablation may be performed by surgical means, hormones, drugs, radiofrequency, heat, chemical application, or other methods.

**abnormal alleles.** Form of gene that includes disease-related variations.

**absorbable sutures.** Strands prepared from collagen or a synthetic polymer and capable of being absorbed by tissue over time. Examples include surgical gut and collagen sutures; or synthetics like polydioxanone (PDS), polyglactin 910 (Vicryl), poliglecaprone 25 (Monocryl), polyglyconate (Maxon), and polyglycolic acid (Dexon).

**acetabuloplasty.** Surgical repair or reconstruction of the large cup-shaped socket in the hipbone (acetabulum) with which the head of the femur articulates.

**Achilles tendon.** Tendon attached to the back of the heel bone (calcaneus) that flexes the foot downward.

**acromioclavicular joint.** Junction between the clavicle and the scapula. The acromion is the projection from the back of the scapula that forms the highest point of the shoulder and connects with the clavicle. Trauma or injury to the acromioclavicular joint is often referred to as a dislocation of the shoulder. This is not correct, however, as a dislocation of the shoulder is a disruption of the glenohumeral joint.

**acromionectomy.** Surgical treatment for acromioclavicular arthritis in which the distal portion of the acromion process is removed.

**acromioplasty.** Repair of the part of the shoulder blade that connects to the deltoid muscles and clavicle.

**actigraphy.** Science of monitoring activity levels, particularly during sleep. In most cases, the patient wears a wristband that records motion while sleeping. The data are recorded, analyzed, and interpreted to study sleep/wake patterns and circadian rhythms.

**air conduction.** Transportation of sound from the air, through the external auditory canal, to the tympanic membrane and ossicular chain. Air conduction hearing is tested by presenting an acoustic stimulus through earphones or a loudspeaker to the ear.

**air puff device.** Instrument that measures intraocular pressure by evaluating the force of a reflected amount of air blown against the cornea.

**alleles.** Form of gene usually arising from a mutation responsible for a hereditary variation.

**allogeneic collection.** Collection of blood or blood components from one person for the use of another. Allogeneic collection was formerly termed homologous collection.

**allograft.** Graft from one individual to another of the same species.

**amniocentesis.** Surgical puncture through the abdominal wall, with a specialized needle and under ultrasonic guidance, into the interior of the pregnant uterus and directly into the amniotic sac to collect fluid for diagnostic analysis or therapeutic reduction of fluid levels.

**anastomosis.** Surgically created connection between ducts, blood vessels, or bowel segments to allow flow from one to the other.

**anesthesia time.** Time period factored into anesthesia procedures beginning with the anesthesiologist preparing the patient for surgery and ending when the patient is turned over to the recovery department.

**Angelman syndrome.** Early childhood emergence of a pattern of interrupted development, stiff, jerky gait, absence or impairment of speech, excessive laughter, and seizures.

**angioplasty.** Reconstruction or repair of a diseased or damaged blood vessel.

**annuloplasty.** Surgical plication of weakened tissue of the heart, to improve its muscular function. Annuli are thick, fibrous rings and one is found surrounding each of the cardiac chambers. The atrial and ventricular muscle fibers attach to the annuli. In annuloplasty, weakened annuli may be surgically plicated, or tucked, to improve muscular functions.

**anorectal anometry.** Measurement of pressure generated by anal sphincter to diagnose incontinence.

**anterior chamber lenses.** Lenses inserted into the anterior chamber following intracapsular cataract extraction.

**applanation tonometer.** Instrument that measures intraocular pressure by recording the force required to flatten an area of the cornea.

**appropriateness of care.** Proper setting of medical care that best meets the patient's care or diagnosis, as defined by a health care plan or other legal entity.

**aqueous humor.** Fluid within the anterior and posterior chambers of the eye that is continually replenished as it diffuses out into the blood. When the flow of aqueous is blocked, a build-up of fluid in the eye causes increased intraocular pressure and leads to glaucoma and blindness.

**arteriogram.** Radiograph of arteries.

**arteriovenous fistula.** Connecting passage between an artery and a vein.

**arteriovenous malformation.** Connecting passage between an artery and a vein.

**arthrotomy.** Surgical incision into a joint that may include exploration, drainage, or removal of a foreign body.

**ASA.** 1) Acetylsalicylic acid. Synonym(s): aspirin. 2) American Society of Anesthesiologists. National organization for anesthesiology that maintains and publishes the guidelines and relative values for anesthesia coding.

**aspirate.** To withdraw fluid or air from a body cavity by suction.

**assay.** Chemical analysis of a substance to establish the presence and strength of its components. A therapeutic drug assay is used to determine if a drug is within the expected therapeutic range for a patient.

**atrial septal defect.** Cardiac anomaly consisting of a patent opening in the atrial septum due to a fusion failure, classified as ostium secundum type, ostium primum defect, or endocardial cushion defect.

**attended surveillance.** Ability of a technician at a remote surveillance center or location to respond immediately to patient transmissions regarding rhythm or device alerts as they are produced and received at the remote location. These transmissions may originate from wearable or implanted therapy or monitoring devices.

Appendix M — Glossary

**auricle.** External ear, which is a single elastic cartilage covered in skin and normal adnexal features (hair follicles, sweat glands, and sebaceous glands), shaped to channel sound waves into the acoustic meatus.

**autogenous transplant.** Tissue, such as bone, that is harvested from the patient and used for transplantation back into the same patient.

**autograft.** Any tissue harvested from one anatomical site of a person and grafted to another anatomical site of the same person. Most commonly, blood vessels, skin, tendons, fascia, and bone are used as autografts.

**AVF.** Arteriovenous fistula.

**AVM.** Arteriovenous malformation. Clusters of abnormal blood vessels that grow in the brain comprised of a blood vessel "nidus" or nest through which arteries and veins connect directly without going through the capillaries. As time passes, the nidus may enlarge resulting in the formation of a mass that may bleed. AVMs are more prone to bleeding in patients ages 10 to 55. Once older than age 55, the possibility of bleeding is reduced dramatically.

**backbench preparation.** Procedures performed on a donor organ following procurement to prepare the organ for transplant into the recipient. Excess fat and other tissue may be removed, the organ may be perfused, and vital arteries may be sized, repaired, or modified to fit the patient. These procedures are done on a back table in the operating room before transplantation can begin.

**Bartholin's gland.** Mucous-producing gland found in the vestibular bulbs on either side of the vaginal orifice and connected to the mucosal membrane at the opening by a duct.

**Bartholin's gland abscess.** Pocket of pus and surrounding cellulitis caused by infection of the Bartholin's gland and causing localized swelling and pain in the posterior labia majora that may extend into the lower vagina.

**basic value.** Relative weighted value based upon the usual anesthesia services and the relative work or cost of the specific anesthesia service assigned to each anesthesia-specific procedure code.

**Berman locator.** Small, sensitive tool used to detect the location of a metallic foreign body in the eye.

**bifurcated.** Having two branches or divisions, such as the left pulmonary veins that split off from the left atrium to carry oxygenated blood away from the heart.

**Billroth's operation.** Anastomosis of the stomach to the duodenum or jejunum.

**bioprosthetic heart valve.** Replacement cardiac valve made of biological tissue. Allograft, xenograft or engineered tissue.

**biopsy.** Tissue or fluid removed for diagnostic purposes through analysis of the cells in the biopsy material.

**Blalock-Hanlon procedure.** Atrial septectomy procedure to allow free mixing of the blood from the right and left atria.

**Blalock-Taussig procedure.** Anastomosis of the left subclavian artery to the left pulmonary artery or the right subclavian artery to the right pulmonary artery in order to shunt some of the blood flow from the systemic to the pulmonary circulation.

**blepharochalasis.** Loss of elasticity and relaxation of skin of the eyelid, thickened or indurated skin on the eyelid associated with recurrent episodes of edema, and intracellular atrophy.

**blepharoplasty.** Plastic surgery of the eyelids to remove excess fat and redundant skin weighting down the lid. The eyelid is pulled tight and sutured to support sagging muscles.

**blepharoptosis.** Droop or displacement of the upper eyelid, caused by paralysis, muscle problems, or outside mechanical forces.

**blepharorrhaphy.** Suture of a portion or all of the opposing eyelids to shorten the palpebral fissure or close it entirely.

**bone conduction.** Transportation of sound through the bones of the skull to the inner ear.

**bone mass measurement.** Radiologic or radioisotopic procedure or other procedure approved by the FDA for identifying bone mass, detecting bone loss, or determining bone quality. The procedure includes a physician's interpretation of the results. Qualifying individuals must be an estrogen-deficient woman at clinical risk for osteoporosis with vertebral abnormalities.

**brachytherapy.** Form of radiation therapy in which radioactive pellets or seeds are implanted directly into the tissue being treated to deliver their dose of radiation in a more directed fashion. Brachytherapy provides radiation to the prescribed body area while minimizing exposure to normal tissue.

**breakpoint.** Point at which a chromosome breaks.

**Bristow procedure.** Anterior capsulorrhaphy prevents chronic separation of the shoulder. In this procedure, the bone block is affixed to the anterior glenoid rim with a screw.

**buccal mucosa.** Tissue from the mucous membrane on the inside of the cheek.

**bundle of His.** Bundle of modified cardiac fibers that begins at the atrioventricular node and passes through the right atrioventricular fibrous ring to the interventricular septum, where it divides into two branches. Bundle of His recordings are taken for intracardiac electrograms.

**Caldwell-Luc operation.** Intraoral antrostomy approach into the maxillary sinus for the removal of tooth roots or tissue, or for packing the sinus to reduce zygomatic fractures by creating a window above the teeth in the canine fossa area.

**canthorrhaphy.** Suturing of the palpebral fissure, the juncture between the eyelids, at either end of the eye.

**canthotomy.** Horizontal incision at the canthus (junction of upper and lower eyelids) to divide the outer canthus and enlarge lid margin separation.

**cardio-.** Relating to the heart.

**cardiopulmonary bypass.** Venous blood is diverted to a heart-lung machine, which mechanically pumps and oxygenates the blood temporarily so the heart can be bypassed while an open procedure on the heart or coronary arteries is performed. During bypass, the lungs are deflated and immobile.

**cardioverter-defibrillator.** Device that uses both low energy cardioversion or defibrillating shocks and antitachycardia pacing to treat ventricular tachycardia or ventricular fibrillation.

**care plan oversight services.** Physician's ongoing review and revision of a patient's care plan involving complex or multidisciplinary care modalities.

**case management services.** Physician case management is a process of involving direct patient care as well as coordinating and controlling access to the patient or initiating and/or supervising other necessary health care services.

**cataract extraction.** Surgical removal of the cataract or cloudy lens. Anterior chamber lenses are inserted in conjunction with intracapsular cataract extraction and posterior chamber lenses are inserted in conjunction with extracapsular cataract extraction.

**catheter.** Flexible tube inserted into an area of the body for introducing or withdrawing fluid.

**Centers for Medicare and Medicaid Services.** Federal agency that oversees the administration of the public health programs such as Medicare, Medicaid, and State Children's Insurance Program.

CPT © 2017 American Medical Association. All Rights Reserved.

© 2017 Optum360, LLC

**certified nurse midwife.** Registered nurse who has successfully completed a program of study and clinical experience or has been certified by a recognized organization for the care of pregnant or delivering patients.

**CFR.** Code of Federal Regulations.

**CHAMPUS.** Civilian Health and Medical Program of the Uniformed Services. See Tricare.

**CHAMPVA.** Civilian Health and Medical Program of the Department of Veterans Affairs.

**chemodenervation.** Chemical destruction of nerves. A substance, for example, Botox, is used to temporarily inhibit the transfer of chemicals at the presynaptic membrane, blocking the neuromuscular junctions.

**chemoembolization.** Administration of chemotherapeutic agents directly to a tumor in combination with the percutaneous administration of an occlusive substance into a vessel to deprive the tumor of its blood supply. This ensures a prolonged level of therapy directed at the tumor. Chemoembolization is primarily being used for cancers of the liver and endocrine system.

**chemosurgery.** Application of chemical agents to destroy tissue, originally referring to the in situ chemical fixation of premalignant or malignant lesions to facilitate surgical excision.

**Chiari osteotomy.** Top of the femur is altered to correct a dislocated hip caused by congenital conditions or cerebral palsy. Plate and screws are often used.

**chimera.** Organ or anatomic structure consisting of tissues of diverse genetic constitution.

**choanal atresia.** Congenital, membranous, or bony closure of one or both posterior nostrils due to failure of the embryonic bucconasal membrane to rupture and open up the nasal passageway.

**chondromalacia.** Condition in which the articular cartilage softens, seen in various body sites but most often in the patella, and may be congenital or acquired.

**chorionic villus sampling.** Aspiration of a placental sample through a catheter, under ultrasonic guidance. The specialized needle is placed transvaginally through the cervix or transabdominally into the uterine cavity.

**chronic pain management services.** Distinct services frequently performed by anesthesiologists who have additional training in pain management procedures. Pain management services include initial and subsequent evaluation and management (E/M) services, trigger point injections, spine and spinal cord injections, and nerve blocks.

**cineplastic amputation.** Amputation in which muscles and tendons of the remaining portion of the extremity are arranged so that they may be utilized for motor functions. Following this type of amputation, a specially constructed prosthetic device allows the individual to execute more complex movements because the muscles and tendons are able to communicate independent movements to the device.

**circadian.** Relating to a cyclic, 24-hour period.

**clinical social worker.** Individual who possesses a master's or doctor's degree in social work and, after obtaining the degree, has performed at least two years of supervised clinical social work. A clinical social worker must be licensed by the state or, in the case of states without licensure, must completed at least two years or 3,000 hours of post-master's degree supervised clinical social work practice under the supervision of a master's level social worker.

**clinical staff.** Someone who works for, or under, the direction of a physician or qualified health care professional and does not bill services separately. The person may be licensed or regulated to help the physician perform specific duties.

**clonal.** Originating from one cell.

**CMS.** Centers for Medicare and Medicaid Services. Federal agency that administers the public health programs.

**CO2 laser.** Carbon dioxide laser that emits an invisible beam and vaporizes water-rich tissue. The vapor is suctioned from the site.

**codons.** Series of three adjoining bases in one polynucleotide chain of a DNA or RNA molecule that provides the codes for a specific amino acid.

**cognitive.** Being aware by drawing from knowledge, such as judgment, reason, perception, and memory.

**colostomy.** Artificial surgical opening anywhere along the length of the colon to the skin surface for the diversion of feces.

**commissurotomy.** Surgical division or disruption of any two parts that are joined to form a commissure in order to increase the opening. The procedure most often refers to opening the adherent leaflet bands of fibrous tissue in a stenosed mitral valve.

**common variants.** Nucleotide sequence differences associated with abnormal gene function. Tests are usually performed in a single series of laboratory testing (in a single, typically multiplex, assay arrangement or using more than one assay to include all variants to be examined). Variants are representative of a mutation that mainly causes a single disease, such as cystic fibrosis. Other uncommon variants could provide additional information. Tests may be performed based on society recommendations and guidelines.

**community mental health center.** Facility providing outpatient mental health day treatment, assessments, and education as appropriate to community members.

**computerized corneal topography.** Digital imaging and analysis by computer of the shape of the corneal.

**conjunctiva.** Mucous membrane lining of the eyelids and covering of the exposed, anterior sclera.

**conjunctivodacryocystostomy.** Surgical connection of the lacrimal sac directly to the conjunctival sac.

**conjunctivorhinostomy.** Correction of an obstruction of the lacrimal canal achieved by suturing the posterior flaps and removing any lacrimal obstruction, preserving the conjunctiva.

**constitutional.** Cells containing genetic code that may be passed down to future generations. May also be referred to as germline.

**consultation.** Advice or opinion regarding diagnosis and treatment or determination to accept transfer of care of a patient rendered by a medical professional at the request of the primary care provider.

**continuous positive airway pressure device.** Pressurized device used to maintain the patient's airway for spontaneous or mechanically aided breathing. Often used for patients with mild to moderate sleep apnea.

**core needle biopsy.** Large-bore biopsy needle inserted into a mass and a core of tissue is removed for diagnostic study.

**corpectomy.** Removal of the body of a bone, such as a vertebra.

**costochondral.** Pertaining to the ribs and the scapula.

**CPT.** Current Procedural Terminology. Definitive procedural coding system developed by the American Medical Association that lists descriptive terms and identifying codes to provide a uniform language that describes medical, surgical, and diagnostic services for nationwide communication among physicians, patients, and third parties, used to report professional and outpatient services.

**craniosynostosis.** Congenital condition in which one or more of the cranial sutures fuse prematurely, creating a deformed or aberrant head shape.

**craterization.** Excision of a portion of bone creating a crater-like depression to facilitate drainage from infected areas of bone.

**cricoid.** Circular cartilage around the trachea.

**CRNA.** Certified registered nurse anesthetist. Nurse trained and specializing in the administration of anesthesia.

**cryolathe.** Tool used for reshaping a button of corneal tissue.

**cryosurgery.** Application of intense cold, usually produced using liquid nitrogen, to locally freeze diseased or unwanted tissue and induce tissue necrosis without causing harm to adjacent tissue.

**CT.** Computed tomography.

**cutdown.** Small, incised opening in the skin to expose a blood vessel, especially over a vein (venous cutdown) to allow venipuncture and permit a needle or cannula to be inserted for the withdrawal of blood or administration of fluids.

**cytogenetic studies.** Procedures in CPT that are related to the branch of genetics that studies cellular (cyto) structure and function as it relates to heredity (genetics). White blood cells, specifically T-lymphocytes, are the most commonly used specimen for chromosome analysis.

**cytogenomic.** Chromosomic evaluation using molecular methods.

**dacryocystotome.** Instrument used for incising the lacrimal duct strictures.

**debride.** To remove all foreign objects and devitalized or infected tissue from a burn or wound to prevent infection and promote healing.

**definitive drug testing.** Drug tests used to further analyze or confirm the presence or absence of specific drugs or classes of drugs used by the patient. These tests are able to provide more conclusive information regarding the concentration of the drug and their metabolites. May be used for medical, workplace, or legal purposes.

**definitive identification.** Identification of microorganisms using additional tests to specify the genus or species (e.g., slide cultures or biochemical panels).

**dentoalveolar structure.** Area of alveolar bone surrounding the teeth and adjacent tissue.

**Department of Health and Human Services.** Cabinet department that oversees the operating divisions of the federal government responsible for health and welfare. HHS oversees the Centers for Medicare and Medicaid Services, Food and Drug Administration, Public Health Service, and other such entities.

**Department of Justice.** Attorneys from the DOJ and the United States Attorney's Office have, under the memorandum of understanding, the same direct access to contractor data and records as the OIG and the Federal Bureau of Investigation (FBI). DOJ is responsible for prosecution of fraud and civil or criminal cases presented.

**dermis.** Skin layer found under the epidermis that contains a papillary upper layer and the deep reticular layer of collagen, vascular bed, and nerves.

**dermis graft.** Skin graft that has been separated from the epidermal tissue and the underlying subcutaneous fat, used primarily as a substitute for fascia grafts in plastic surgery.

**desensitization.** 1) Administration of extracts of allergens periodically to build immunity in the patient. 2) Application of medication to decrease the symptoms, usually pain, associated with a dental condition or disease.

**destruction.** Ablation or eradication of a structure or tissue.

**diabetes outpatient self-management training services.** Educational and training services furnished by a certified provider in an outpatient setting. The physician managing the individual's diabetic condition must certify that the services are needed under a comprehensive plan of care and provide the patient with the skills and knowledge necessary for therapeutic program compliance (including skills related to the self-administration of injectable drugs). The provider must meet applicable standards established by the National Diabetes Advisory or be recognized by an organization that represents individuals with diabetes as meeting standards for furnishing the services.

**diagnostic procedures.** Procedure performed on a patient to obtain information to assess the medical condition of the patient or to identify a disease and to determine the nature and severity of an illness or injury.

**dialysis.** Artificial filtering of the blood to remove contaminating waste elements and restore normal balance.

**diaphragm.** 1) Muscular wall separating the thorax and its structures from the abdomen. 2) Flexible disk inserted into the vagina and against the cervix as a method of birth control.

**diaphysectomy.** Surgical removal of a portion of the shaft of a long bone, often done to facilitate drainage from infected bone.

**diathermy.** Applying heat to body tissues by various methods for therapeutic treatment or surgical purposes to coagulate and seal tissue.

**dilation.** Artificial increase in the diameter of an opening or lumen made by medication or by instrumentation.

**dissect.** Cut apart or separate tissue for surgical purposes or for visual or microscopic study.

**DNA.** Deoxyribonucleic acid. Chemical containing the genetic information necessary to produce and propagate living organisms. Molecules are comprised of two twisting paired strands, called a double helix.

**DNA marker.** Specific gene sequence within a chromosome indicating the inheritance of a certain trait.

**dorsal.** Pertaining to the back or posterior aspect.

**drugs and biologicals.** Drugs and biologicals included - or approved for inclusion - in the United States Pharmacopoeia, the National Formulary, the United States Homeopathic Pharmacopoeia, in New Drugs or Accepted Dental Remedies, or approved by the pharmacy and drug therapeutics committee of the medical staff of the hospital. Also included are medically accepted and FDA approved drugs used in an anticancer chemotherapeutic regimen. The carrier determines medical acceptance based on supportive clinical evidence.

**dual-lead device.** Implantable cardiac device (pacemaker or implantable cardioverter-defibrillator [ICD]) in which pacing and sensing components are placed in only two chambers of the heart.

**duplex scan.** Noninvasive vascular diagnostic technique that uses ultrasonic scanning to identify the pattern and direction of blood flow within arteries or veins displayed in real time images. Duplex scanning combines B-mode two-dimensional pictures of the vessel structure with spectra and/or color flow Doppler mapping or imaging of the blood as it moves through the vessels.

**duplication/deletion (DUP/DEL).** Term used in molecular testing which examines genomic regions to determine if there are extra chromosomes (duplication) or missing chromosomes (deletions). Normal gene dosage is two copies per cell except for the sex chromosomes which have one per cell.

**DuToit staple capsulorrhaphy.** Reattachment of the capsule of the shoulder and glenoid labrum to the glenoid lip using staples to anchor the avulsed capsule and glenoid labrum.

**Dx.** Diagnosis.

**DXA.** Dual energy x-ray absorptiometry. Radiological technique for bone density measurement using a two-dimensional projection system in which two x-ray beams with different levels of energy are pulsed alternately and the results are given in two scores, reported as standard deviations from peak bone mass density.

**dynamic mutation.** Unstable or changing polynucleotides resulting in repeats related to genes that can undergo disease-producing increases or decreases in the repeats that differ within tissues or over generations.

**ECMO.** Extracorporeal membrane oxygenation.

**ectropion.** Drooping of the lower eyelid away from the eye or outward turning or eversion of the edge of the eyelid, exposing the palpebral conjunctiva and causing irritation.

**Eden-Hybinette procedure.** Anterior shoulder repair using an anterior bone block to augment the bony anterior glenoid lip.

**EDTA.** Drug used to inhibit damage to the cornea by collagenase. EDTA is especially effective in alkali burns as it neutralizes soluble alkali, including lye.

**effusion.** Escape of fluid from within a body cavity.

**electrocardiographic rhythm derived.** Analysis of data obtained from readings of the heart's electrical activation, including heart rate and rhythm, variability of heart rate, ST analysis, and T-wave alternans. Other data may also be assessed when warranted.

**electrocautery.** Division or cutting of tissue using high-frequency electrical current to produce heat, which destroys cells.

**electrode array.** Electronic device containing more than one contact whose function can be adjusted during programming services. Electrodes are specialized for a particular electrochemical reaction that acts as a medium between a body surface and another instrument.

**electromyography.** Test that measures muscle response to nerve stimulation determining if muscle weakness is present and if it is related to the muscles themselves or a problem with the nerves that supply the muscles.

**electrooculogram (EOG).** Record of electrical activity associated with eye movements.

**electrophysiologic studies.** Electrical stimulation and monitoring to diagnose heart conduction abnormalities that predispose patients to bradyarrhythmias and to determine a patient's chance for developing ventricular and supraventricular tachyarrhythmias.

**embolization.** Placement of a clotting agent, such as a coil, plastic particles, gel, foam, etc., into an area of hemorrhage to stop the bleeding or to block blood flow to a problem area, such as an aneurysm or a tumor.

**emergency.** Serious medical condition or symptom (including severe pain) resulting from injury, sickness, or mental illness that arises suddenly and requires immediate care and treatment, generally received within 24 hours of onset, to avoid jeopardy to the life, limb, or health of a covered person.

**empyema.** Accumulation of pus within the respiratory, or pleural, cavity.

**EMTALA.** Emergency Medical Treatment and Active Labor Act.

**end-stage renal disease.** Chronic, advanced kidney disease requiring renal dialysis or a kidney transplant to prevent imminent death.

**endarterectomy.** Removal of the thickened, endothelial lining of a diseased or damaged artery.

**endomicroscopy.** Diagnostic technology that allows for the examination of tissue at the cellular level during endoscopy. The technology decreases the need for biopsy with histological examination for some types of lesions.

**endovascular embolization.** Procedure whereby vessels are occluded by a variety of therapeutic substances for the treatment of abnormal blood vessels by inhibiting the flow of blood to a tumor, arteriovenous malformations, lymphatic malformation, and to prevent or stop hemorrhage.

**entropion.** Inversion of the eyelid, turning the edge in toward the eyeball and causing irritation from contact of the lashes with the surface of the eye.

**enucleation.** Removal of a growth or organ cleanly so as to extract it in one piece.

**epidermis.** Outermost, nonvascular layer of skin that contains four to five differentiated layers depending on its body location: stratum corneum, lucidum, granulosum, spinosum, and basale.

**epiphysiodesis.** Surgical fusion of an epiphysis performed to prematurely stop further bone growth.

**escharotomy.** Surgical incision into the scab or crust resulting from a severe burn in order to relieve constriction and allow blood flow to the distal unburned tissue.

**established patient.** 1) Patient who has received professional services in a face-to-face setting within the last three years from the same physician/qualified health care professional or another physician/qualified health care professional of the exact same specialty and subspecialty who belongs to the same group practice. 2) For OPPS hospitals, patient who has been registered as an inpatient or outpatient in a hospital's provider-based clinic or emergency department within the past three years.

**evacuation.** Removal or purging of waste material.

**evaluation and management codes.** Assessment and management of a patient's health care.

**evaluation and management service components.** Key components of history, examination, and medical decision making that are key to selecting the correct E/M codes. Other non-key components include counseling, coordination of care, nature of presenting problem, and time.

**event recorder.** Portable, ambulatory heart monitor worn by the patient that makes electrocardiographic recordings of the length and frequency of aberrant cardiac rhythm to help diagnose heart conditions and to assess pacemaker functioning or programming.

**exenteration.** Surgical removal of the entire contents of a body cavity, such as the pelvis or orbit.

**exon.** One of multiple nucleic acid sequences used to encode information for a gene polypeptide or protein. Exons are separated from other exons by non-protein-coding sequences known as introns.

**extended care services.** Items and services provided to an inpatient of a skilled nursing facility, including nursing care, physical or occupational therapy, speech pathology, drugs and supplies, and medical social services.

**external electrical capacitor device.** External electrical stimulation device designed to promote bone healing. This device may also promote neural regeneration, revascularization, epiphyseal growth, and ligament maturation.

**external pulsating electromagnetic field.** External stimulation device designed to promote bone healing. This device may also promote neural regeneration, revascularization, epiphyseal growth, and ligament maturation.

**extracorporeal.** Located or taking place outside the body.

**Eyre-Brook capsulorrhaphy.** Reattachment of the capsule of the shoulder and glenoid labrum to the glenoid lip.

**False Claims Act.** Governs civil actions for filing false claims. Liability under this act pertains to any person who knowingly presents or causes to be presented a false or fraudulent claim to the government for payment or approval.

**fascia.** Fibrous sheet or band of tissue that envelops organs, muscles, and groupings of muscles.

**fasciectomy.** Excision of fascia or strips of fascial tissue.

**fasciotomy.** Incision or transection of fascial tissue.

**fat graft.** Graft composed of fatty tissue completely freed from surrounding tissue that is used primarily to fill in depressions.

**FDA.** Food and Drug Administration. Federal agency responsible for protecting public health by substantiating the safety, efficacy, and security of human and veterinary drugs, biological products, medical devices, national food supply, cosmetics, and items that give off radiation.

**filtered speech test.** Test most commonly used to identify central auditory dysfunction in which the patient is presented monosyllabic words that are low pass filtered, allowing only the parts of each word below a certain pitch to be presented. A score is given on the number of correct responses. This may be a subset of a standard battery of tests provided during a single encounter.

**fissure.** Deep furrow, groove, or cleft in tissue structures.

**fistulization.** Creation of a communication between two structures that were not previously connected.

**flexor digitorum profundus tendon.** Tendon originating in the proximal forearm and extending to the index finger and wrist. A thickened FDP sheath, usually caused by age, illness, or injury, can fill the carpal canal and lead to impingement of the median nerve.

**fluoroscopy.** Radiology technique that allows visual examination of part of the body or a function of an organ using a device that projects an x-ray image on a fluorescent screen.

**focal length.** Distance between the object in focus and the lens.

**focused medical review.** Process of targeting and directing medical review efforts on Medicare claims where the greatest risk of inappropriate program payment exists. The goal is to reduce the number of noncovered claims or unnecessary services. CMS analyzes national data such as internal billing, utilization, and payment data and provides its findings to the FI. Local medical review policies are developed identifying aberrances, abuse, and overutilized services. Providers are responsible for knowing national Medicare coverage and billing guidelines and local medical review policies, and for determining whether the services provided to Medicare beneficiaries are covered by Medicare.

**fragile X syndrome.** Intellectual disabilities, enlarged testes, big jaw, high forehead, and long ears in males. In females, fragile X presents with mild intellectual disabilities and heterozygous sexual structures. In some families, males have shown no symptoms but carry the gene.

**free flap.** Tissue that is completely detached from the donor site and transplanted to the recipient site, receiving its blood supply from capillary ingrowth at the recipient site.

**free microvascular flap.** Tissue that is completely detached from the donor site following careful dissection and preservation of the blood vessels, then attached to the recipient site with the transferred blood vessels anastomosed to the vessels in the recipient bed.

**fulguration.** Destruction of living tissue by using sparks from a high-frequency electric current.

**gas tamponade.** Absorbable gas may be injected to force the retina against the choroid. Common gases include room air, short-acting sulfahexafluoride, intermediate-acting perfluoroethane, or long-acting perfluorooctane.

**Gaucher disease.** Genetic metabolic disorder in which fat deposits may accumulate in the spleen, liver, lungs, bone marrow, and brain.

**gene.** Basic unit of heredity that contains nucleic acid. Genes are arranged in different and unique sequences or strings that determine the gene's function. Human genes usually include multiple protein coding regions such as exons separated by introns which are nonprotein coding sections.

**genome.** Complete set of DNA of an organism. Each cell in the human body is comprised of a complete copy of the approximately three billion DNA base pairs that constitute the human genome.

**habilitative services.** Procedures or services provided to assist a patient in learning, keeping, and improving new skills needed to perform daily living activities. Habilitative services assist patients in acquiring a skill for the first time.

**HCPCS.** Healthcare Common Procedure Coding System.

**HCPCS Level I.** Healthcare Common Procedure Coding System Level I. Numeric coding system used by physicians, facility outpatient departments, and ambulatory surgery centers (ASC) to code ambulatory, laboratory, radiology, and other diagnostic services for Medicare billing. This coding system contains only the American Medical Association's Physicians' Current Procedural Terminology (CPT) codes. The AMA updates codes annually.

**HCPCS Level II.** Healthcare Common Procedure Coding System Level II. National coding system, developed by CMS, that contains alphanumeric codes for physician and nonphysician services not included in the CPT coding system. HCPCS Level II covers such things as ambulance services, durable medical equipment, and orthotic and prosthetic devices.

**HCPCS modifiers.** Two-character code (AA-ZZ) that identifies circumstances that alter or enhance the description of a service or supply. They are recognized by carriers nationally and are updated annually by CMS.

**Hct.** Hematocrit.

**health care provider.** Entity that administers diagnostic and therapeutic services.

**hemilaminectomy.** Excision of a portion of the vertebral lamina.

**hemodialysis.** Cleansing of wastes and contaminating elements from the blood by virtue of different diffusion rates through a semipermeable membrane, which separates blood from a filtration solution that diffuses other elements out of the blood. The blood is slowly filtered extracorporeally through special dialysis equipment and returned to the body. Synonym(s): renal dialysis.

**hemodialysis.** Cleansing of wastes and contaminating elements from the blood by virtue of different diffusion rates through a semipermeable membrane, which separates blood from a filtration solution that diffuses other elements out of the blood.

**hemoperitoneum.** Effusion of blood into the peritoneal cavity, the space between the continuous membrane lining the abdominopelvic walls and encasing the visceral organs.

**heterograft.** Surgical graft of tissue from one animal species to a different animal species. A common type of heterograft is porcine (pig) tissue, used for temporary wound closure.

**heterotopic transplant.** Tissue transplanted from a different anatomical site for usage as is natural for that tissue, for example, buccal mucosa to a conjunctival site.

**HGNC.** HUGO gene nomenclature committee.

**HGVS.** Human genome variation society.

**Hickman catheter.** Central venous catheter used for long-term delivery of medications, such as antibiotics, nutritional substances, or chemotherapeutic agents.

**HLA.** Human leukocyte antigen.

**home health services.** Services furnished to patients in their homes under the care of physicians. These services include part-time or intermittent skilled nursing care, physical therapy, medical social services, medical supplies, and some rehabilitation equipment. Home health supplies and

CPT © 2017 American Medical Association. All Rights Reserved.

© 2017 Optum360, LLC

services must be prescribed by a physician, and the beneficiary must be confined at home in order for Medicare to pay the benefits in full.

**homograft.** Graft from one individual to another of the same species.

**hospice care.** Items and services provided to a terminally ill individual by a hospice program under a written plan established and periodically reviewed by the individual's attending physician and by the medical director: Nursing care provided by or under the supervision of a registered professional nurse; Physical or occupational therapy or speech-language pathology services; Medical social services under the direction of a physician; Services of a home health aide who has successfully completed a training program; Medical supplies (including drugs and biologicals) and the use of medical appliances; Physicians' services; Short-term inpatient care (including both respite care and procedures necessary for pain control and acute and chronic symptom management) in an inpatient facility on an intermittent basis and not consecutively over longer than five days; Counseling (including dietary counseling) with respect to care of the terminally ill individual and adjustment to his death; Any item or service which is specified in the plan and for which payment may be made.

**hospital.** Institution that provides, under the supervision of physicians, diagnostic, therapeutic, and rehabilitation services for medical diagnosis, treatment, and care of patients. Hospitals receiving federal funds must maintain clinical records on all patients, provide 24-hour nursing services, and have a discharge planning process in place. The term "hospital" also includes religious nonmedical health care institutions and facilities of 50 beds or less located in rural areas.

**HUGO.** Human genome organization

**IA.** Intra-arterial.

**ICD.** Implantable cardioverter defibrillator.

**ICD-10-CM.** International Classification of Diseases, 10th Revision, Clinical Modification. Clinical modification of the alphanumeric classification of diseases used by the World Health Organization, already in use in much of the world, and used for mortality reporting in the United States. The implementation date for ICD-10-CM diagnostic coding system to replace ICD-9-CM in the United States was October 1, 2015.

**ICD-10-PCS.** International Classification of Diseases, 10th Revision, Procedure Coding System. Beginning October 1, 2015, inpatient hospital services and surgical procedures must be coded using ICD-10-PCS codes, replacing ICD-9-CM, Volume 3 for procedures.

**ICM.** Implantable cardiovascular monitor.

**ileostomy.** Artificial surgical opening that brings the end of the ileum out through the abdominal wall to the skin surface for the diversion of feces through a stoma.

**iliopsoas tendon.** Fibrous tissue that connects muscle to bone in the pelvic region, common to the iliacus and psoas major.

**ILR.** Implantable loop recorder.

**IM.** 1) Infectious mononucleosis. 2) Internal medicine. 3) Intramuscular.

**immunotherapy.** Therapeutic use of serum or gamma globulin.

**implant.** Material or device inserted or placed within the body for therapeutic, reconstructive, or diagnostic purposes.

**implantable cardiovascular monitor.** Implantable electronic device that stores cardiovascular physiologic data such as intracardiac pressure waveforms collected from internal sensors or data such as weight and blood pressure collected from external sensors. The information stored in these devices is used as an aid in managing patients with heart failure and other cardiac conditions that are non-rhythm related. The data may be transmitted via local telemetry or remotely to a surveillance technician or an internet-based file server.

**implantable cardioverter-defibrillator.** Implantable electronic cardiac device used to control rhythm abnormalities such as tachycardia, fibrillation, or bradycardia by producing high- or low-energy stimulation and pacemaker functions. It may also have the capability to provide the functions of an implantable loop recorder or implantable cardiovascular monitor.

**implantable loop recorder.** Implantable electronic cardiac device that constantly monitors and records electrocardiographic rhythm. It may be triggered by the patient when a symptomatic episode occurs or activated automatically by rapid or slow heart rates. This may be the sole purpose of the device or it may be a component of another cardiac device, such as a pacemaker or implantable cardioverter-defibrillator. The data can be transmitted via local telemetry or remotely to a surveillance technician or an internet-based file server.

**implantable venous access device.** Catheter implanted for continuous access to the venous system for long-term parenteral feeding or for the administration of fluids or medications.

**IMRT.** Intensity modulated radiation therapy. External beam radiation therapy delivery using computer planning to specify the target dose and to modulate the radiation intensity, usually as a treatment for a malignancy. The delivery system approaches the patient from multiple angles, minimizing damage to normal tissue.

**in situ.** Located in the natural position or contained within the origin site, not spread into neighboring tissue.

**incontinence.** Inability to control urination or defecation.

**infundibulectomy.** Excision of the anterosuperior portion of the right ventricle of the heart.

**internal direct current stimulator.** Electrostimulation device placed directly into the surgical site designed to promote bone regeneration by encouraging cellular healing response in bone and ligaments.

**interrogation device evaluation.** Assessment of an implantable cardiac device (pacemaker, cardioverter-defibrillator, cardiovascular monitor, or loop recorder) in which collected data about the patient's heart rate and rhythm, battery and pulse generator function, and any leads or sensors present, are retrieved and evaluated. Determinations regarding device programming and appropriate treatment settings are made based on the findings. CPT provides required components for evaluation of the various types of devices.

**intramedullary implants.** Nail, rod, or pin placed into the intramedullary canal at the fracture site. Intramedullary implants not only provide a method of aligning the fracture, they also act as a splint and may reduce fracture pain. Implants may be rigid or flexible. Rigid implants are preferred for prophylactic treatment of diseased bone, while flexible implants are preferred for traumatic injuries.

**intraocular lens.** Artificial lens implanted into the eye to replace a damaged natural lens or cataract.

**intravenous.** Within a vein or veins.

**introducer.** Instrument, such as a catheter, needle, or tube, through which another instrument or device is introduced into the body.

**intron.** Nonprotein section of a gene that separates exons in human genes. Contains vital sequences that allow splicing of exons to produce a functional protein from a gene. Sometimes referred to as intervening sequences (IVS).

**IP.** 1) Interphalangeal. 2) Intraperitoneal.

**irrigation.** To wash out or cleanse a body cavity, wound, or tissue with water or other fluid.

**Kayser-Fleischer ring.** Condition found in Wilson's disease in which deposits of copper cause a pigmented ring around the cornea's outer border in the deep epithelial layers.

© 2017 Optum360, LLC

CPT © 2017 American Medical Association. All Rights Reserved.

**keratoprosthesis.** Surgical procedure in which the physician creates a new anterior chamber with a plastic optical implant to replace a severely damaged cornea that cannot be repaired.

**keratotomy.** Surgical incision of the cornea.

**krypton laser.** Laser light energy that uses ionized krypton by electric current as the active source, has a radiation beam between the visible yellow-red spectrum, and is effective in photocoagulation of retinal bleeding, macular lesions, and vessel aberrations of the choroid.

**lacrimal.** Tear-producing gland or ducts that provides lubrication and flushing of the eyes and nasal cavities.

**lacrimal punctum.** Opening of the lacrimal papilla of the eyelid through which tears flow to the canaliculi to the lacrimal sac.

**lacrimotome.** Knife for cutting the lacrimal sac or duct.

**lacrimotomy.** Incision of the lacrimal sac or duct.

**laparotomy.** Incision through the flank or abdomen for therapeutic or diagnostic purposes.

**laryngoscopy.** Examination of the hypopharynx, larynx, and tongue base with an endoscope.

**larynx.** Musculocartilaginous structure between the trachea and the pharynx that functions as the valve preventing food and other particles from entering the respiratory tract, as well as the voice mechanism. Also called the voicebox, the larynx is composed of three single cartilages: cricoid, epiglottis, and thyroid; and three paired cartilages: arytenoid, corniculate, and cuneiform.

**laser surgery.** Use of concentrated, sharply defined light beams to cut, cauterize, coagulate, seal, or vaporize tissue.

**LEEP.** Loop electrode excision procedure. Biopsy specimen or cone shaped wedge of cervical tissue is removed using a hot cautery wire loop with an electrical current running through it.

**levonorgestrel.** Drug inhibiting ovulation and preventing sperm from penetrating cervical mucus. It is delivered subcutaneously in polysiloxone capsules. The capsules can be effective for up to five years, and provide a cumulative pregnancy rate of less than 2 percent. The capsules are not biodegradable, and therefore must be removed. Removal is more difficult than insertion of levonorgestrel capsules because fibrosis develops around the capsules. Normal hormonal activity and a return to fertility begins immediately upon removal.

**ligament.** Band or sheet of fibrous tissue that connects the articular surfaces of bones or supports visceral organs.

**ligation.** Tying off a blood vessel or duct with a suture or a soft, thin wire.

**lymphadenectomy.** Dissection of lymph nodes free from the vessels and removal for examination by frozen section in a separate procedure to detect early-stage metastases.

**lysis.** Destruction, breakdown, dissolution, or decomposition of cells or substances by a specific catalyzing agent.

**Magnuson-Stack procedure.** Treatment for recurrent anterior dislocation of the shoulder that involves tightening and realigning the subscapularis tendon.

**maintenance of wakefulness test.** Attended study determining the patient's ability to stay awake.

**Manchester operation.** Preservation of the uterus following prolapse by amputating the vaginal portion of the cervix, shortening the cardinal ligaments, and performing a colpoperineorrhaphy posteriorly.

**mapping.** Multidimensional depiction of a tachycardia that identifies its site of origin and its electrical conduction pathway after tachycardia has been induced. The recording is made from multiple catheter sites within the heart, obtaining electrograms simultaneously or sequentially.

**marsupialization.** Creation of a pouch in surgical treatment of a cyst in which one wall is resected and the remaining cut edges are sutured to adjacent tissue creating an open pouch of the previously enclosed cyst.

**mastectomy.** Surgical removal of one or both breasts.

**McDonald procedure.** Polyester tape is placed around the cervix with a running stitch to assist in the prevention of pre-term delivery. Tape is removed at term for vaginal delivery.

**MCP.** Metacarpophalangeal.

**medial.** Middle or midline.

**mediastinotomy.** Incision into the mediastinum for purposes of exploration, foreign body removal, drainage, or biopsy.

**medical review.** Review by a Medicare administrative contractor, carrier, and/or quality improvement organization (QIO) of services and items provided by physicians, other health care practitioners, and providers of health care services under Medicare. The review determines if the items and services are reasonable and necessary and meet Medicare coverage requirements, whether the quality meets professionally recognized standards of health care, and whether the services are medically appropriate in an inpatient, outpatient, or other setting as supported by documentation.

**Medicare contractor.** Medicare Part A fiscal intermediary, Medicare Part B carrier, Medicare administrative contractor (MAC), or a durable medical equipment Medicare administrative contractor (DME MAC).

**Medicare physician fee schedule.** List of payments Medicare allows by procedure or service. Payments may vary through geographic adjustments. The MPFS is based on the resource-based relative value scale (RBRVS). A national total relative value unit (RVU) is given to each procedure (HCPCS Level I CPT, Level II national codes). Each total RVU has three components: physician work, practice expense, and malpractice insurance.

**metabolite.** Chemical compound resulting from the natural process of metabolism. In drug testing, the metabolite of the drug may endure in a higher concentration or for a longer duration than the initial "parent" drug.

**methylation.** Mechanism used to regulate genes and protect DNA from some types of cleavage.

**microarray.** Small surface onto which multiple specific nucleic acid sequences can be attached to be used for analysis. Microarray may also be known as a gene chip or DNA chip. Tests can be run on the sequences for any variants that may be present.

**mitral valve.** Valve with two cusps that is between the left atrium and left ventricle of the heart.

**moderate sedation.** Medically controlled state of depressed consciousness, with or without analgesia, while maintaining the patient's airway, protective reflexes, and ability to respond to stimulation or verbal commands.

**Mohs micrographic surgery.** Special technique used to treat complex or ill-defined skin cancer and requires a single physician to provide two distinct services. The first service is surgical and involves the destruction of the lesion by a combination of chemosurgery and excision. The second service is that of a pathologist and includes mapping, color coding of specimens, microscopic examination of specimens, and complete histopathologic preparation.

**monitored anesthesia care.** Sedation, with or without analgesia, used to achieve a medically controlled state of depressed consciousness while maintaining the patient's airway, protective reflexes, and ability to respond to stimulation or verbal commands. In dental conscious sedation, the patient is rendered free of fear, apprehension, and anxiety through the use of pharmacological agents.

CPT © 2017 American Medical Association. All Rights Reserved.

© 2017 Optum360, LLC

**monoclonal.** Relating to a single clone of cells.

**multiple sleep latency test (MSLT).** Attended study to determine the tendency of the patient to fall asleep.

**multiple-lead device.** Implantable cardiac device (pacemaker or implantable cardioverter-defibrillator [ICD]) in which pacing and sensing components are placed in at least three chambers of the heart.

**Mustard procedure.** Corrective measure for transposition of great vessels involves an intra-atrial baffle made of pericardial tissue or synthetic material. The baffle is secured between pulmonary veins and mitral valve and between mitral and tricuspid valves. The baffle directs systemic venous flow into the left ventricle and lungs and pulmonary venous flow into the right ventricle and aorta.

**mutation.** Alteration in gene function that results in changes to a gene or chromosome. Can cause deficits or disease that can be inherited, can have beneficial effects, or result in no noticeable change.

**mutation scanning.** Process normally used on multiple polymerase chain reaction (PCR) amplicons to determine DNA sequence variants by differences in characteristics compared to normal. Specific DNA variants can then be studied further.

**myotomy.** Surgical cutting of a muscle to gain access to underlying tissues or for therapeutic reasons.

**myringotomy.** Incision in the eardrum done to prevent spontaneous rupture precipitated by fluid pressure build-up behind the tympanic membrane and to prevent stagnant infection and erosion of the ossicles.

**nasal polyp.** Fleshy outgrowth projecting from the mucous membrane of the nose or nasal sinus cavity that may obstruct ventilation or affect the sense of smell.

**nasal sinus.** Air-filled cavities in the cranial bones lined with mucous membrane and continuous with the nasal cavity, draining fluids through the nose.

**nasogastric tube.** Long, hollow, cylindrical catheter made of soft rubber or plastic that is inserted through the nose down into the stomach, and is used for feeding, instilling medication, or withdrawing gastric contents.

**nasolacrimal punctum.** Opening of the lacrimal duct near the nose.

**nasopharynx.** Membranous passage above the level of the soft palate.

**Nd:YAG laser.** Laser light energy that uses an yttrium, aluminum, and garnet crystal doped with neodymium ions as the active source, has a radiation beam nearing the infrared spectrum, and is effective in photocoagulation, photoablation, cataract extraction, and lysis of vitreous strands.

**nebulizer.** Latin for mist, a device that converts liquid into a fine spray and is commonly used to deliver medicine to the upper respiratory, bronchial, and lung areas.

**nerve conduction study.** Diagnostic test performed to assess muscle or nerve damage. Nerves are stimulated with electric shocks along the course of the muscle. Sensors are utilized to measure and record nerve functions, including conduction and velocity.

**neurectomy.** Excision of all or a portion of a nerve.

**neuromuscular junction.** Nerve synapse at the meeting point between the terminal end of a nerve (motor neuron) and a muscle fiber.

**neuropsychological testing.** Evaluation of a patient's behavioral abilities wherein a physician or other health care professional administers a series of tests in thinking, reasoning, and judgment.

**new patient.** Patient who is receiving face-to-face care from a provider/qualified health care professional or another physician/qualified health care professional of the exact same specialty and subspecialty who belongs to the same group practice for the first time in three years. For OPPS hospitals, a patient who has not been registered as an inpatient or outpatient, including off-campus provider based clinic or emergency department, within the past three years.

**Niemann-Pick syndrome.** Accumulation of phospholipid in histiocytes in the bone marrow, liver, lymph nodes, and spleen, cerebral involvement, and red macular spots similar to Tay-Sachs disease. Most commonly found in Jewish infants.

**Nissen fundoplasty.** Surgical repair technique that involves the fundus of the stomach being wrapped around the lower end of the esophagus to treat reflux esophagitis.

**nonabsorbable sutures.** Strands of natural or synthetic material that resist absorption into living tissue and are removed once healing is under way. Nonabsorbable sutures are commonly used to close skin wounds and repair tendons or collagenous tissue.

**obturator.** Prosthesis used to close an acquired or congenital opening in the palate that aids in speech and chewing.

**obturator nerve.** Lumbar plexus nerve with anterior and posterior divisions that innervate the adductor muscles (e.g., adductor longus, adductor brevis) of the leg and the skin over the medial area of the thigh or a sacral plexus nerve with anterior and posterior divisions that innervate the superior gemellus muscles.

**occult blood test.** Chemical or microscopic test to determine the presence of blood in a specimen.

**ocular implant.** Implant inside muscular cone.

**oophorectomy.** Surgical removal of all or part of one or both ovaries, either as open procedure or laparoscopically. Menstruation and childbearing ability continues when one ovary is removed.

**orthosis.** Derived from a Greek word meaning "to make straight," it is an artificial appliance that supports, aligns, or corrects an anatomical deformity or improves the use of a moveable body part. Unlike a prosthesis, an orthotic device is always functional in nature.

**osteo-.** Having to do with bone.

**osteogenesis stimulator.** Device used to stimulate the growth of bone by electrical impulses or ultrasound.

**osteotomy.** Surgical cutting of a bone.

**ostomy.** Artificial (surgical) opening in the body used for drainage or for delivery of medications or nutrients.

**pacemaker.** Implantable cardiac device that controls the heart's rhythm and maintains regular beats by artificial electric discharges. This device consists of the pulse generator with a battery and the electrodes, or leads, which are placed in single or dual chambers of the heart, usually transvenously.

**palmaris longus tendon.** Tendon located in the hand that flexes the wrist joint.

**paratenon graft.** Graft composed of the fatty tissue found between a tendon and its sheath.

**passive mobilization.** Pressure, movement, or pulling of a limb or body part utilizing an apparatus or device.

**pedicle flap.** Full-thickness skin and subcutaneous tissue for grafting that remains partially attached to the donor site by a pedicle or stem in which the blood vessels supplying the flap remain intact.

**Pemberton osteotomy.** Osteotomy is performed to position triradiate cartilage as a hinge for rotating the acetabular roof in cases of dysplasia of the hip in children.

**penetrance.** Being formed by, or pertaining to, a single clone.

**percutaneous intradiscal electrothermal annuloplasty.** Procedure corrects tears in the vertebral annulus by applying heat to the collagen disc walls percutaneously through a catheter. The heat contracts and thickens the wall, which may contract and close any annular tears.

**percutaneous skeletal fixation.** Treatment that is neither open nor closed and the injury site is not directly visualized. Fixation devices (pins, screws) are placed through the skin to stabilize the dislocation using x-ray guidance.

**pericardium.** Thin and slippery case in which the heart lies that is lined with fluid so that the heart is free to pulse and move as it beats.

**peripheral arterial tonometry (PAT).** Pulsatile volume changes in a digit are measured to determine activity in the sympathetic nervous system for respiratory analysis.

**peritoneal.** Space between the lining of the abdominal wall, or parietal peritoneum, and the surface layer of the abdominal organs, or visceral peritoneum. It contains a thin, watery fluid that keeps the peritoneal surfaces moist.

**peritoneal dialysis.** Dialysis that filters waste from blood inside the body using the peritoneum, the natural lining of the abdomen, as the semipermeable membrane across which ultrafiltration is accomplished. A special catheter is inserted into the abdomen and a dialysis solution is drained into the abdomen. This solution extracts fluids and wastes, which are then discarded when the fluid is drained. Various forms of peritoneal dialysis include CAPD, CCPD, and NIDP.

**peritoneal effusion.** Persistent escape of fluid within the peritoneal cavity.

**pessary.** Device placed in the vagina to support and reposition a prolapsing or retropositioned uterus, rectum, or vagina.

**phenotype.** Physical expression of a trait or characteristic as determined by an individual's genetic makeup or genotype.

**photocoagulation.** Application of an intense laser beam of light to disrupt tissue and condense protein material to a residual mass, used especially for treating ocular conditions.

**physical status modifiers.** Alphanumeric modifier used to identify the patient's health status as it affects the work related to providing the anesthesia service.

**physical therapy modality.** Therapeutic agent or regimen applied or used to provide appropriate treatment of the musculoskeletal system.

**physician.** Legally authorized practitioners including a doctor of medicine or osteopathy, a doctor of dental surgery or of dental medicine, a doctor of podiatric medicine, a doctor of optometry, and a chiropractor only with respect to treatment by means of manual manipulation of the spine (to correct a subluxation).

**PICC.** Peripherally inserted central catheter. PICC is inserted into one of the large veins of the arm and threaded through the vein until the tip sits in a large vein just above the heart.

**PKR.** Photorefractive therapy. Procedure involving the removal of the surface layer of the cornea (epithelium) by gentle scraping and use of a computer-controlled excimer laser to reshape the stroma.

**pleurodesis.** Injection of a sclerosing agent into the pleural space for creating adhesions between the parietal and the visceral pleura to treat a collapsed lung caused by air trapped in the pleural cavity, or severe cases of pleural effusion.

**plication.** Surgical technique involving folding, tucking, or pleating to reduce the size of a hollow structure or organ.

**polyclonal.** Containing one or more cells.

**polymorphism.** Genetic variation in the same species that does not harm the gene function or create disease.

**polypeptide.** Chain of amino acids held together by covalent bonds. Proteins are made up of amino acids.

**polysomnography.** Test involving monitoring of respiratory, cardiac, muscle, brain, and ocular function during sleep.

**Potts-Smith-Gibson procedure.** Side-to-side anastomosis of the aorta and left pulmonary artery creating a shunt that enlarges as the child grows.

**Prader-Willi syndrome.** Rounded face, almond-shaped eyes, strabismus, low forehead, hypogonadism, hypotonia, intellectual disabilities, and an insatiable appetite.

**presumptive drug testing.** Drug screening tests to identify the presence or absence of drugs in a patient's system. Tests are usually able to identify low concentrations of the drug. These tests may be used for medical, workplace, or legal purposes.

**presumptive identification.** Identification of microorganisms using media growth, colony morphology, gram stains, or up to three specific tests (e.g., catalase, indole, oxidase, urease).

**professional component.** Portion of a charge for health care services that represents the physician's (or other practitioner's) work in providing the service, including interpretation and report of the procedure. This component of the service usually is charged for and billed separately from the inpatient hospital charges.

**profunda.** Denotes a part of a structure that is deeper from the surface of the body than the rest of the structure.

**prolonged physician services.** Extended pre- or post-service care provided to a patient whose condition requires services beyond the usual.

**prostate.** Male gland surrounding the bladder neck and urethra that secretes a substance into the seminal fluid.

**prosthetic.** Device that replaces all or part of an internal body organ or body part, or that replaces part of the function of a permanently inoperable or malfunctioning internal body organ or body part.

**provider of services.** Institution, individual, or organization that provides health care.

**proximal.** Located closest to a specified reference point, usually the midline or trunk.

**psychiatric hospital.** Specialized institution that provides, under the supervision of physicians, services for the diagnosis and treatment of mentally ill persons.

**pterygium.** Benign, wedge-shaped, conjunctival thickening that advances from the inner corner of the eye toward the cornea.

**pterygomaxillary fossa.** Wide depression on the external surface of the maxilla above and to the side of the canine tooth socket.

**pulmonary artery banding.** Surgical constriction of the pulmonary artery to prevent irreversible pulmonary vascular obstructive changes and overflow into the left ventricle.

**Putti-Platt procedure.** Realignment of the subscapularis tendon to treat recurrent anterior dislocation, thereby partially eliminating external rotation. The anterior capsule is also tightened and reinforced.

**pyloroplasty.** Enlargement and reconstruction of the lower portion of the stomach opening into the duodenum performed after vagotomy to speed gastric emptying and treat duodenal ulcers.

**qualified health care professional.** Educated, licensed or certified, and regulated professional operating under a specified scope of practice to provide patient services that are separate and distinct from other clinical staff. Services may be billed independently or under the facility's services.

CPT © 2017 American Medical Association. All Rights Reserved.

© 2017 Optum360, LLC

**RAC.** Recovery audit contractor. National program using CMS-affiliated contractors to review claims prior to payment as well as for payments on claims already processed, including overpayments and underpayments.

**radiation therapy simulation.** Radiation therapy simulation. Procedure by which the specific body area to be treated with radiation is defined and marked. A CT scan is performed to define the body contours and these images are used to create a plan customized treatment for the patient, targeting the area to be treated while sparing adjacent tissue. The center of the area to be treated is marked and an immobilization device (e.g., cradle, mold) is created to make sure the patient is in the same position each time for treatment. Complexity of treatment depends on the number of treatment areas and the use of tools to isolate the area of treatment.

**radioactive substances.** Materials used in the diagnosis and treatment of disease that emit high-speed particles and energy-containing rays.

**radiology services.** Services that include diagnostic and therapeutic radiology, nuclear medicine, CT scan procedures, magnetic resonance imaging services, ultrasound, and other imaging procedures.

**radiotherapy afterloading.** Part of the radiation therapy process in which the chemotherapy agent is actually instilled into the tumor area subsequent to surgery and placement of an expandable catheter into the void remaining after tumor excision. The specialized catheter remains in place and the patient may come in for multiple treatments with radioisotope placed to treat the margin of tissue surrounding the excision. After the radiotherapy is completed, the patient returns to have the catheter emptied and removed. This is a new therapy in breast cancer treatment.

**Rashkind procedure.** Transvenous balloon atrial septectomy or septostomy performed by cardiac catheterization. A balloon catheter is inserted into the heart either to create or enlarge an opening in the interatrial septal wall.

**rehabilitation services.** Therapy services provided primarily for assisting in a rehabilitation program of evaluation and service including cardiac rehabilitation, medical social services, occupational therapy, physical therapy, respiratory therapy, skilled nursing, speech therapy, psychiatric rehabilitation, and alcohol and substance abuse rehabilitation.

**respiratory airflow (ventilation).** Assessment of air movement during inhalation and exhalation as measured by nasal pressure sensors and thermistor.

**respiratory analysis.** Assessment of components of respiration obtained by other methods such as airflow or peripheral arterial tone.

**respiratory effort.** Measurement of diaphragm and/or intercostal muscle for airflow using transducers to estimate thoracic and abdominal motion.

**respiratory movement.** Measurement of chest and abdomen movement during respiration.

**ribbons.** In oncology, small plastic tubes containing radioactive sources for interstitial placement that may be cut into specific lengths tailored to the size of the area receiving ionizing radiation treatment.

**Ridell sinusotomy.** Frontal sinus tissue is destroyed to eliminate tumors.

**RNA.** Ribonucleic acid.

**rural health clinic.** Clinic in an area where there is a shortage of health services staffed by a nurse practitioner, physician assistant, or certified nurse midwife under physician direction that provides routine diagnostic services, including clinical laboratory services, drugs, and biologicals and that has prompt access to additional diagnostic services from facilities meeting federal requirements.

**Salter osteotomy.** Innominate bone of the hip is cut, removed, and repositioned to repair a congenital dislocation, subluxation, or deformity.

**saucerization.** Creation of a shallow, saucer-like depression in the bone to facilitate drainage of infected areas.

**Schiotz tonometer.** Instrument that measures intraocular pressure by recording the depth of an indentation on the cornea by a plunger of known weight.

**screening mammography.** Radiologic images taken of the female breast for the early detection of breast cancer.

**screening pap smear.** Diagnostic laboratory test consisting of a routine exfoliative cytology test (Papanicolaou test) provided to a woman for the early detection of cervical or vaginal cancer. The exam includes a clinical breast examination and a physician's interpretation of the results.

**seeds.** Small (1 mm or less) sources of radioactive material that are permanently placed directly into tumors.

**Senning procedure.** Flaps of intra-atrial septum and right atrial wall are used to create two interatrial channels to divert the systemic and pulmonary venous circulation.

**sensitivity tests.** Number of methods of applying selective suspected allergens to the skin or mucous.

**sensorineural conduction.** Transportation of sound from the cochlea to the acoustic nerve and central auditory pathway to the brain.

**sentinel lymph node.** First node to which lymph drainage and metastasis from a cancer can occur.

**separate procedures.** Services commonly carried out as a fundamental part of a total service and, as such, do not usually warrant separate identification. These services are identified in CPT with the parenthetical phrase (separate procedure) at the end of the description and are payable only when performed alone.

**septectomy.** 1) Surgical removal of all or part of the nasal septum. 2) Submucosal resection of the nasal septum.

**Shirodkar procedure.** Treatment of an incompetent cervical os by placing nonabsorbent suture material in purse-string sutures as a cerclage to support the cervix.

**short tandem repeat (STR).** Short sequences of a DNA pattern that are repeated. Can be used as genetic markers for human identity testing.

**sialodochoplasty.** Surgical repair of a salivary gland duct.

**single-lead device.** Implantable cardiac device (pacemaker or implantable cardioverter-defibrillator [ICD]) in which pacing and sensing components are placed in only one chamber of the heart.

**single-nucleotide polymorphism (SNP).** Single nucleotide (A, T, C, or G that is different in a DNA sequence. This difference occurs at a significant frequency in the population.

**sinus of Valsalva.** Any of three sinuses corresponding to the individual cusps of the aortic valve, located in the most proximal part of the aorta just above the cusps. These structures are contained within the pericardium and appear as distinct but subtle outpouchings or dilations of the aortic wall between each of the semilunar cusps of the valve.

**sleep apnea.** Intermittent cessation of breathing during sleep that may cause hypoxemia and pulmonary arterial hypertension.

**sleep latency.** Time period between lying down in bed and the onset of sleep.

**sleep staging.** Determination of the separate levels of sleep according to physiological measurements.

**somatic.** 1) Pertaining to the body or trunk. 2) In genetics acquired or occurring after birth.

**speculoscopy.** Viewing the cervix utilizing a magnifier and a special wavelength of light, allowing detection of abnormalities that may not be discovered on a routine Pap smear.

**speech-language pathology services.** Speech, language, and related function assessment and rehabilitation service furnished by a qualified speech-language pathologist. Audiology services include hearing and balance assessment services furnished by a qualified audiologist. A qualified speech pathologist and audiologist must have a master's or doctoral degree in their respective fields and be licensed to serve in the state. Speech pathologists and audiologists practicing in states without licensure must complete 350 hours of supervised clinical work and perform at least nine months of supervised full-time service after earning their degrees.

**sphincteroplasty.** Surgical repair done to correct, augment, or improve the muscular function of a sphincter, such as the anus or intestines.

**spirometry.** Measurement of the lungs' breathing capacity.

**splint.** Brace or support. 1) dynamic splint: brace that permits movement of an anatomical structure such as a hand, wrist, foot, or other part of the body after surgery or injury. 2) static splint: brace that prevents movement and maintains support and position for an anatomical structure after surgery or injury.

**stent.** Tube to provide support in a body cavity or lumen.

**stereotactic radiosurgery.** Delivery of externally-generated ionizing radiation to specific targets for destruction or inactivation. Most often utilized in the treatment of brain or spinal tumors, high-resolution stereotactic imaging is used to identify the target and then deliver the treatment. Computer-assisted planning may also be employed. Simple and complex cranial lesions and spinal lesions are typically treated in a single planning and treatment session, although a maximum of five sessions may be required. No incision is made for stereotactic radiosurgery procedures.

**stereotaxis.** Three-dimensional method for precisely locating structures.

**Stoffel rhizotomy.** Nerve roots are sectioned to relieve pain or spastic paralysis.

**strabismus.** Misalignment of the eyes due to an imbalance in extraocular muscles.

**surgical package.** Normal, uncomplicated performance of specific surgical services, with the assumption that, on average, all surgical procedures of a given type are similar with respect to skill level, duration, and length of normal follow-up care.

**symblepharopterygium.** Adhesion in which the eyelid is adhered to the eyeball by a band that resembles a pterygium.

**sympathectomy.** Surgical interruption or transection of a sympathetic nervous system pathway.

**tarso-.** 1) Relating to the foot. 2) Relating to the margin of the eyelid.

**tarsocheiloplasty.** Plastic operation upon the edge of the eyelid for the treatment of trichiasis.

**tarsorrhaphy.** Suture of a portion or all of the opposing eyelids together for the purpose of shortening the palpebral fissure or closing it entirely.

**technical component.** Portion of a health care service that identifies the provision of the equipment, supplies, technical personnel, and costs attendant to the performance of the procedure other than the professional services.

**tendon.** Fibrous tissue that connects muscle to bone, consisting primarily of collagen and containing little vasculature.

**tendon allograft.** Allografts are tissues obtained from another individual of the same species. Tendon allografts are usually obtained from cadavers and frozen or freeze dried for later use in soft tissue repairs where the physician elects not to obtain an autogenous graft (a graft obtained from the individual on whom the surgery is being performed).

**tendon suture material.** Tendons are composed of fibrous tissue consisting primarily of collagen and containing few cells or blood vessels. This tissue heals more slowly than tissues with more vascularization. Because of this, tendons are usually repaired with nonabsorbable suture material. Examples include surgical silk, surgical cotton, linen, stainless steel, surgical nylon, polyester fiber, polybutester (Novafil), polyethylene (Dermalene), and polypropylene (Prolene, Surilene).

**tendon transplant.** Replacement of a tendon with another tendon.

**tenon's capsule.** Connective tissue that forms the capsule enclosing the posterior eyeball, extending from the conjunctival fornix and continuous with the muscular fascia of the eye.

**tenonectomy.** Excision of a portion of a tendon to make it shorter.

**tenotomy.** Cutting into a tendon.

**TENS.** Transcutaneous electrical nerve stimulator. TENS is applied by placing electrode pads over the area to be stimulated and connecting the electrodes to a transmitter box, which sends a current through the skin to sensory nerve fibers to help decrease pain in that nerve distribution.

**tensilon.** Edrophonium chloride. Agent used for evaluation and treatment of myasthenia gravis.

**terminally ill.** Individual whose medical prognosis for life expectancy is six months or less.

**tetralogy of Fallot.** Specific combination of congenital cardiac defects: obstruction of the right ventricular outflow tract with pulmonary stenosis, interventricular septal defect, malposition of the aorta, overriding the interventricular septum and receiving blood from both the venous and arterial systems, and enlargement of the right ventricle.

**therapeutic services.** Services performed for treatment of a specific diagnosis. These services include performance of the procedure, various incidental elements, and normal, related follow-up care.

**thoracentesis.** Surgical puncture of the chest cavity with a specialized needle or hollow tubing to aspirate fluid from within the pleural space for diagnostic or therapeutic reasons.

**thoracic lymphadenectomy.** Procedure to cut out the lymph nodes near the lungs, around the heart, and behind the trachea.

**thoracostomy.** Creation of an opening in the chest wall for drainage.

**thyroglossal duct.** Embryonic duct at the front of the neck, which becomes the pyramidal lobe of the thyroid gland with obliteration of the remaining duct, but may form a cyst or sinus in adulthood if it persists.

**total disc arthroplasty with artificial disc.** Removal of an intravertebral disc and its replacement with an implant. The implant is an artificial disc consisting of two metal plates with a weight-bearing surface of polyethylene between the plates. The plates are anchored to the vertebral immediately above and below the affected disc.

**total shoulder replacement.** Prosthetic replacement of the entire shoulder joint, including the humeral head and the glenoid fossa.

**trabeculae carneae cordis.** Bands of muscular tissue that line the walls of the ventricles in the heart.

**trabeculectomy.** Surgical incision between the anterior portion of the eye and the canal of Schlemm to drain the aqueous humor.

**tracheostomy.** Formation of a tracheal opening on the neck surface with tube insertion to allow for respiration in cases of obstruction or decreased patency. A tracheostomy may be planned or performed on an emergency basis for temporary or long-term use.

**tracheotomy.** Formation of a tracheal opening on the neck surface with tube insertion to allow for respiration in cases of obstruction or decreased patency. A tracheotomy may be planned or performed on an emergency basis for temporary or long-term use.

**traction.** Drawing out or holding tension on an area by applying a direct therapeutic pulling force.

**transcranial magnetic stimulation.** Application of electromagnetic energy to the brain through a coil placed on the scalp. The procedure stimulates cortical neurons and is intended to activate and normalize their processes.

**transcription.** Process by which messenger RNA is synthesized from a DNA template resulting in the transfer of genetic information from the DNA molecule to the messenger RNA.

**translocation.** Disconnection of all or part of a chromosome that reattaches to another position in the DNA sequence of the same or another chromosome. Often results in a reciprocal exchange of DNA sequences between two differently numbered chromosomes. May or may not result in a clinically significant loss of DNA.

**trephine.** 1) Specialized round saw for cutting circular holes in bone, especially the skull. 2) Instrument that removes small disc-shaped buttons of corneal tissue for transplanting.

**tricuspid atresia.** Congenital absence of the valve that may occur with other defects, such as atrial septal defect, pulmonary atresia, and transposition of great vessels.

**turbinates.** Scroll or shell-shaped elevations from the wall of the nasal cavity, the inferior turbinate being a separate bone, while the superior and middle turbinates are of the ethmoid bone.

**tympanic membrane.** Thin, sensitive membrane across the entrance to the middle ear that vibrates in response to sound waves, allowing the waves to be transmitted via the ossicular chain to the internal ear.

**tympanoplasty.** Surgical repair of the structures of the middle ear, including the eardrum and the three small bones, or ossicles.

**unlisted procedure.** Procedural descriptions used when the overall procedure and outcome of the procedure are not adequately described by an existing procedure code. Such codes are used as a last resort and only when there is not a more appropriate procedure code.

**ureterorrhaphy.** Surgical repair using sutures to close an open wound or injury of the ureter.

**vagotomy.** Division of the vagus nerves, interrupting impulses resulting in lower gastric acid production and hastening gastric emptying. Used in the treatment of chronic gastric, pyloric, and duodenal ulcers that can cause severe pain and difficulties in eating and sleeping.

**variant.** Nucleotide deviation from the normal sequence of a region. Variations are usually either substitutions or deletions. Substitution variations are the result of one nucleotide taking the place of another. A deletion occurs when one or more nucleotides are left out. In some cases, several in a reasonably close proximity on the same chromosome in a DNA strand. These variations result in amino acid changes in the protein made by the gene. However, the term variant does not itself imply a functional change. Intron variations are usually described in one of two ways: 1) the changed nucleotide is defined by a plus or a minus sign indicating the position relative to the first or last nucleotide to the intron, or 2) the second variant description is indicated relative to the last nucleotide of the preceding exon or first nucleotide of the following exon.

**vascular family.** Group of vessels (family) that branch from the aorta or vena cava. At each branching, the vascular order increases by one. The first order vessel is the primary branch off the aorta or vena cava. The second order vessel branches from the first order, the third order branches from the second order, and any further branching is beyond the third order. For example, for the inferior vena cava, the common iliac artery is a first order vessel. The internal and external iliac arteries are second order vessels, as they each originate from the first order common iliac artery. The external iliac artery extends directly from the common iliac artery and the internal iliac artery bifurcates from the common iliac artery. A third order vessel from the external iliac artery is the inferior epigastric artery and a third

order vessel from the internal iliac artery is the obturator artery. Note orders are not always identical bilaterally (e.g., the left common carotid artery is a first order and the right common carotid is a second order. Synonym(s): vascular origins and distributions.

**vasectomy.** Surgical procedure involving the removal of all or part of the vas deferens, usually performed for sterilization or in conjunction with a prostatectomy.

**vena cava interruption.** Procedure that places a filter device, called an umbrella or sieve, within the large vein returning deoxygenated blood to the heart to prevent pulmonary embolism caused by clots.

**ventricular assist device.** Temporary measure used to support the heart by substituting for left and/or right heart function. The device replaces the work of the left and/or right ventricle when a patient has a damaged or weakened heart. A left ventricular assist device (VAD) helps the heart pump blood through the rest of the body. A right VAD helps the heart pump blood to the lungs to become oxygenated again. Catheters are inserted to circulate the blood through external tubing to a pump machine located outside of the body and back to the correct artery.

**ventricular septal defect.** Congenital cardiac anomaly resulting in a continual opening in the septum between the ventricles that, in severe cases, causes oxygenated blood to flow back into the lungs, resulting in pulmonary hypertension.

**vertebral interspace.** Non-bony space between two adjacent vertebral bodies that contains the cushioning intervertebral disk.

**volar.** Palm of the hand (palmar) or sole of the foot (plantar).

**Waterston procedure.** Type of aortopulmonary shunting done to increase pulmonary blood flow. The ascending aorta is anastomosed to the right pulmonary artery.

**Wharton's ducts.** Salivary ducts below the mandible.

**wick catheter.** Device used to monitor interstitial fluid pressure, and sometimes used intraoperatively during fasciotomy procedures to evaluate the effectiveness of the decompression.

**wound closure.** Closure or repair of a wound created surgically or due to trauma (e.g., laceration). The closure technique depends on the type, site, and depth of the defect. Consideration is also given to cosmetic and functional outcome. A single layer closure involves approximation of the edges of the wound. The second type of closure involves closing the one or more deeper layers of tissue prior to skin closure. The most complex type of closure may include techniques such as debridement or undermining, which involves manipulation of tissue around the wound to allow the skin to cover the wound. The AMA CPT® book defines these as Simple, Intermediate and Complex repair.

**xenograft.** Tissue that is nonhuman and harvested from one species and grafted to another. Pigskin is the most common xenograft for human skin and is applied to a wound as a temporary closure until a permanent option is performed.

**z-plasty.** Plastic surgery technique used primarily to release tension or elongate contracted scar tissue in which a Z-shaped incision is made with the middle line of the Z crossing the area of greatest tension. The triangular flaps are then rotated so that they cross the incision line in the opposite direction, creating a reversed Z.

**ZPIC.** Zone Program Integrity Contractor. CMS contractor that replaced the existing Program Safeguard Contractors (PSC). Contractors are responsible for ensuring the integrity of all Medicare-related claims under Parts A and B (hospital, skilled nursing, home health, provider, and durable medical equipment claims), Part C (Medicare Advantage health plans), Part D (prescription drug plans), and coordination of Medicare-Medicaid data matches (Medi-Medi).

# Appendix N — Listing of Sensory, Motor, and Mixed Nerves

This list contains the sensory, motor, and mixed nerves assigned to each nerve conduction study to improve coding accuracy. Each nerve makes up one single unit of service.

## Motor Nerves Assigned to Codes 95900 and 95907-95913

I. Upper extremity, cervical plexus, and brachial plexus motor nerves

  A. Axillary motor nerve to the deltoid

  B. Long thoracic motor nerve to the serratus anterior

  C. Median nerve

    1. Median motor nerve to the abductor pollicis brevis

    2. Median motor nerve, anterior interosseous branch, to the flexor pollicis longus

    3. Median motor nerve, anterior interosseous branch, to the pronator quadratus

    4. Median motor nerve to the first lumbrical

    5. Median motor nerve to the second lumbrical

  D. Musculocutaneous motor nerve to the biceps brachii

  E. Radial nerve

    1. Radial motor nerve to the extensor carpi ulnaris

    2. Radial motor nerve to the extensor digitorum communis

    3. Radial motor nerve to the extensor indicis proprius

    4. Radial motor nerve to the brachioradialis

  F. Suprascapular nerve

    1. Suprascapular motor nerve to the supraspinatus

    2. Suprascapular motor nerve to the infraspinatus

  G. Thoracodorsal motor nerve to the latissimus dorsi

  H. Ulnar nerve

    1. Ulnar motor nerve to the abductor digiti minimi

    2. Ulnar motor nerve to the palmar interosseous

    3. Ulnar motor nerve to the first dorsal interosseous

    4. Ulnar motor nerve to the flexor carpi ulnaris

  I. Other

II. Lower extremity motor nerves

  A. Femoral motor nerve to the quadriceps

    1. Femoral motor nerve to vastus medialis

    2. Femoral motor nerve to vastus lateralis

    3. Femoral motor nerve to vastus intermedialis

    4. Femoral motor nerve to rectus femoris

  B. Ilioinguinal motor nerve

  C. Peroneal (fibular) nerve

    1. Peroneal motor nerve to the extensor digitorum brevis

    2. Peroneal motor nerve to the peroneus brevis

    3. Peroneal motor nerve to the peroneus longus

    4. Peroneal motor nerve to the tibialis anterior

  D. Plantar motor nerve

  E. Sciatic nerve

  F. Tibial nerve

    1. Tibial motor nerve, inferior calcaneal branch, to the abductor digiti minimi

    2. Tibial motor nerve, medial plantar branch, to the abductor hallucis

    3. Tibial motor nerve, lateral plantar branch, to the flexor digiti minimi brevis

  G. Other

III. Cranial nerves and trunk

  A. Cranial nerve VII (facial motor nerve)

    1. Facial nerve to the frontalis

    2. Facial nerve to the nasalis

    3. Facial nerve to the orbicularis oculi

    4. Facial nerve to the orbicularis oris

  B. Cranial nerve XI (spinal accessory motor nerve)

  C. Cranial nerve XII (hypoglossal motor nerve)

  D. Intercostal motor nerve

  E. Phrenic motor nerve to the diaphragm

  F. Recurrent laryngeal nerve

  G. Other

IV. Nerve Roots

  A. Cervical nerve root stimulation

    1. Cervical level 5 (C5)

    2. Cervical level 6 (C6)

    3. Cervical level 7 (C7)

    4. Cervical level 8 (C8)

  B. Thoracic nerve root stimulation

    1. Thoracic level 1 (T1)

    2. Thoracic level 2 (T2)

    3. Thoracic level 3 (T3)

    4. Thoracic level 4 (T4)

    5. Thoracic level 5 (T5)

    6. Thoracic level 6 (T6)

    7. Thoracic level 7 (T7)

    8. Thoracic level 8 (T8)

    9. Thoracic level 9 (T9)

    10. Thoracic level 10 (T10)

    11. Thoracic level 11 (T11)

    12. Thoracic level 12 (T12)

  C. Lumbar nerve root stimulation

    1. Lumbar level 1 (L1)

    2. Lumbar level 2 (L2)

    3. Lumbar level 3 (L3)

    4. Lumbar level 4 (L4)

    5. Lumbar level 5 (L5)

  D. Sacral nerve root stimulation

    1. Sacral level 1 (S1)

2. Sacral level 2 (S2)
3. Sacral level 3 (S3)
4. Sacral level 4 (S4)

# Sensory and Mixed Nerves Assigned to Codes 95907–95913

I. Upper extremity sensory and mixed nerves
  A. Lateral antebrachial cutaneous sensory nerve
  B. Medial antebrachial cutaneous sensory nerve
  C. Medial brachial cutaneous sensory nerve
  D. Median nerve
    1. Median sensory nerve to the first digit
    2. Median sensory nerve to the second digit
    3. Median sensory nerve to the third digit
    4. Median sensory nerve to the fourth digit
    5. Median palmar cutaneous sensory nerve
    6. Median palmar mixed nerve
  E. Posterior antebrachial cutaneous sensory nerve
  F. Radial sensory nerve
    1. Radial sensory nerve to the base of the thumb
    2. Radial sensory nerve to digit 1
  G. Ulnar nerve
    1. Ulnar dorsal cutaneous sensory nerve
    2. Ulnar sensory nerve to the fourth digit
    3. Ulnar sensory nerve to the fifth digit
    4. Ulnar palmar mixed nerve
  H. Intercostal sensory nerve
  I. Other

II. Lower extremity sensory and mixed nerves
  A. Lateral femoral cutaneous sensory nerve
  B. Medical calcaneal sensory nerve
  C. Medial femoral cutaneous sensory nerve
  D. Peroneal nerve
    1. Deep peroneal sensory nerve
    2. Superficial peroneal sensory nerve, medial dorsal cutaneous branch
    3. Superficial peroneal sensory nerve, intermediate dorsal cutaneous branch
  E. Posterior femoral cutaneous sensory nerve
  F. Saphenous nerve
    1. Saphenous sensory nerve (distal technique)
    2. Saphenous sensory nerve (proximal technique)
  G. Sural nerve
    1. Sural sensory nerve, lateral dorsal cutaneous branch
    2. Sural sensory nerve
  H. Tibial sensory nerve (digital nerve to toe 1)
  I. Tibial sensory nerve (medial plantar nerve)
  J. Tibial sensory nerve (lateral plantar nerve)
  K. Other

III. Head and trunk sensory nerves
  A. Dorsal nerve of the penis
  B. Greater auricular nerve
  C. Ophthalmic branch of the trigeminal nerve
  D. Pudendal sensory nerve
  E. Suprascapular sensory nerves
  F. Other

In the following table, the reasonable maximum number of studies per diagnostic category is listed that allows for a physician or other qualified health care professional to obtain a diagnosis for 90 percent of patients with that same final diagnosis. The numbers denote the suggested number of studies, although the decision is up to the provider.

**Type of Study/Maximum Number of Studies**

| Indication | Limbs Studied by Needle EMG (95860–95864, 95867–95870, 95885–95887) | Nerve Conduction Studies (Total nerves studied, 95907-95913) | Neuromuscular Junction Testing (Repetitive Stimulation 95937) |
|---|---|---|---|
| Carpal Tunnel (Unilateral) | 1 | 7 | — |
| Carpal Tunnel (Bilateral) | 2 | 10 | — |
| Radiculopathy | 2 | 7 | — |
| Mononeuropathy | 1 | 8 | — |
| Polyneuropathy/Mononeuropathy Multiplex | 3 | 10 | — |
| Myopathy | 2 | 4 | 2 |
| Motor Neuronopathy (e.g., ALS) | 4 | 6 | 2 |
| Plexopathy | 2 | 12 | — |
| Neuromuscular Junction | 2 | 4 | 3 |
| Tarsal Tunnel Syndrome (Unilateral) | 1 | 8 | — |
| Tarsal Tunnel Syndrome (Bilateral) | 2 | 11 | — |
| Weakness, Fatigue, Cramps, or Twitching (Focal) | 2 | 7 | 2 |

CPT © 2017 American Medical Association. All Rights Reserved.

© 2017 Optum360, LLC

**Type of Study/Maximum Number of Studies**

| Indication | Limbs Studied by Needle EMG (95860–95864, 95867–95870, 95885–95887) | Nerve Conduction Studies (Total nerves studied, 95907-95913) | Neuromuscular Junction Testing (Repetitive Stimulation 95937) |
|---|---|---|---|
| Weakness, Fatigue, Cramps, or Twitching (General) | 4 | 8 | 2 |
| Pain, Numbness, or Tingling (Unilateral) | 1 | 9 | — |
| Pain, Numbness, or Tingling (Bilateral) | 2 | 12 | — |

# Appendix O — Vascular Families

This table assumes that the starting point is aortic catheterization. This categorization would not be accurate if, for instance, a femoral or carotid artery were catheterized with the blood's flow. The names of the arteries appearing in bold face type in the following table indicate those arteries that are most often the subject of arteriographic procedures.

| First Order | Second Order Branch | Third Order Branch | Beyond Third Order Branches |
|---|---|---|---|
| **Innominate** | **Right Common Carotid** | **Right Internal Carotid** | Right Ophthalmic<br>Right Posterior Communicating<br>Right Middle Cerebral<br>Right Anterior Cerebral |
| | | **Right External Carotid** | Right Superior Thyroid<br>Right Ascending Pharyngeal<br>Right Facial<br>Right Lingual<br>Right Occipital<br>Right Posterior Auricular<br>Right Superficial Temporal<br>Right Internal Maxillary<br>Right Middle Meningeal |
| | **Right Subclavian and Axillary** | **Right Vertebral** | Basilar |
| | | Right Internal Thoracic (Internal Mammary) | |
| | | Right Thyrocervical Trunk | Right Inferior Thyroid<br>Right Suprascapular<br>Right Transverse Cervical |
| | | Right Costocervical Trunk | Right Highest Intercostal<br>Right Deep Cervical |
| | | Right Lateral Thoracic<br>Right Thoracromial<br>Right Humeral Circumflex (A/P) | |
| | | Right Subscapular | Right Circumflex Scapular |
| | | **Right Brachial** | |
| | | Right Deep Brachial | Right Ulnar<br>Right Radial<br>Right Interosseous<br>Right Deep Palmar Arch<br>Right Superficial Palmar Arch<br>Right Metacarpals and Digitals |
| **Left Common Carotid** | **Left Internal Carotid** | Left Ophthalmic<br>Left Posterior Communicating<br>Left Middle Cerebral<br>Left Anterior Cerebral | |
| | **Left External Carotid** | Left Superior Thyroid<br>Left Ascending Pharyngeal<br>Left Facial<br>Left Lingual<br>Left Occipital<br>Left Posterior Auricular<br>Left Superficial Temporal | |
| | | Left Internal Maxillary | Left Middle Meningeal |

**Appendix O — Vascular Families**

| First Order | Second Order Branch | Third Order Branch | Beyond Third Order Branches |
|---|---|---|---|

**Left Subclavian and Axillary**

**Left Vertebral**
Left Internal Thoracic (Internal Mammary)

Left Thyrocervial Trunk
  { Left Inferior Thyroid
  Left Suprascapular
  Left Transverse Cervical

Left Costocervical Trunk
  { Left Hightest Intercostal
  Left Deep Cervical

Left Lateral Thoracic
Left Thoracoacromial
Left Humeral Circumflex (A/P)
Left Subscapular —————————— Left Circumflex Scapular
**Left Brachial**

Left Deep Brachial
  { Left Ulnar
  Left Radial
  Left Interosseous
    { Left Deep Palmar Arch
    Left Superficial Palmar Arch
    Left Metacarpals and Digitals

Intercostals

Bronchials

Recurrent Esophageal

Inferior Phrenic ———————— Superior Suprarenal

**Celiac Trunk**

Left Gastric ———————— Esophageal Branch

Splenic
  { Dorsal Pancreatic ——————— Inferior Transverse Pancreatic
  Great Pancreatic
  Caudal Pancreatic
  Gastroepiploic
  Short Gastrics

Common Hepatic
  Gastroduodenal
    { Posterior Superior Pancreaticoduodenal
    Anterior Superior Pancreaticoduodenal
  Proper Hepatic
    { Left Hepatic
    Right Hepatic
    Cystic
    Gastroepiploic
    Supraduodenal
    Intermediate Hepatic

Middle Suprarenal

**Superior Mesenteric**

Middle Colic

Inferior Pancreaticoduodenal
  { Posterior Inferior Pancreaticoduodenal
  Anterior Inferior Pancreaticoduodenal

Jejunal
Ileocolic
Appendicular
Posterior Cecal
Anterior Cecal
Marginal
Right Colic

| First Order | Second Order Branch | Third Order Branch | Beyond Third Order Branches |
|---|---|---|---|
| **Renal** | Inferior Suprarenal | | |
| Testicular/Ovarian | | | |
| Lumbar | | | |
| Inferior Mesenteric | Left Colic | | |
| | Sigmoid | Rectosigmoid / Superior Rectal | |
| Middle Sacral | | | |
| **Common Iliac** | **Internal Iliac** | Iliolumbar / Lateral Sacral / Superior Gluteal / Umbilical / Superior Vesical / Obturator / Inferior Vesical / Middle Rectal / Inferior Rectal / Internal Pudendal / Inferior Gluteal | |
| | **External Iliac** | Inferior Epigastric | Cremasteric / Pubic |
| | | Deep Circumflex Iliac | Ascending Deep Circumflex Iliac |
| | **Profunda Femoris** | | Medial Descending / Perforating Branches / Lateral Descending / Lateral Circumflex |
| | **Common Femoral** | Deep External Pudendal / Superficial External Pudendal / Ascending Lateral Circumflex Femoral / Descending Lateral Circumflex Femoral / Transverse Lateral Circumflex Femoral | |
| | **Superficial Femoral** | | Geniculate / **Popliteal** / **Anterior Tibial** / **Peroneal** / **Posterior Tibial** |

**Right and Left Main Pulmonary Arteries
(Venous Selective)**

*Reference:* Kadir S. *Atlas of Normal and Variant Angiographic Anatomy.* Philadelphia, Pa: WB Saunders Co; 1991

CPT © 2017 American Medical Association. All Rights Reserved.

# Appendix P — Interventional Radiology Illustrations

## Normal Aortic Arch and Branch Anatomy—Transfemoral Approach

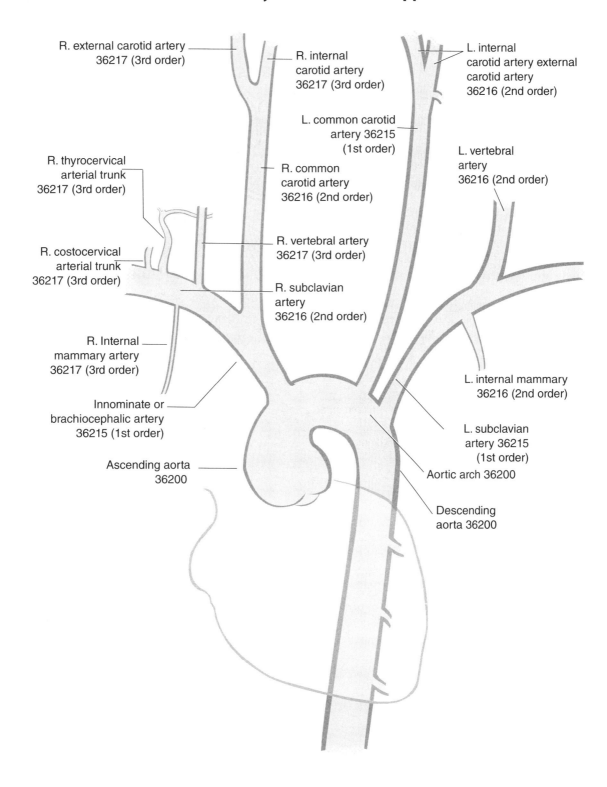

R. external carotid artery
36217 (3rd order)

R. internal
carotid artery
36217 (3rd order)

L. internal
carotid artery external
carotid artery
36216 (2nd order)

L. common carotid
artery 36215
(1st order)

R. thyrocervical
arterial trunk
36217 (3rd order)

R. common
carotid artery
36216 (2nd order)

L. vertebral
artery
36216 (2nd order)

R. costocervical
arterial trunk
36217 (3rd order)

R. vertebral artery
36217 (3rd order)

R. subclavian
artery
36216 (2nd order)

R. Internal
mammary artery
36217 (3rd order)

L. internal mammary
36216 (2nd order)

Innominate or
brachiocephalic artery
36215 (1st order)

L. subclavian
artery 36215
(1st order)

Ascending aorta
36200

Aortic arch 36200

Descending
aorta 36200

## Superior and Inferior Mesenteric Arteries and Branches

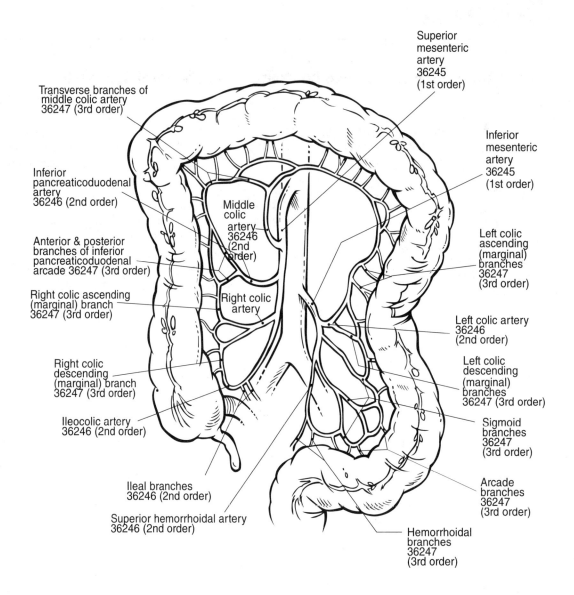

Transverse branches of middle colic artery 36247 (3rd order)

Inferior pancreaticoduodenal artery 36246 (2nd order)

Anterior & posterior branches of inferior pancreaticoduodenal arcade 36247 (3rd order)

Right colic ascending (marginal) branch 36247 (3rd order)

Right colic descending (marginal) branch 36247 (3rd order)

Ileocolic artery 36246 (2nd order)

Ileal branches 36246 (2nd order)

Superior hemorrhoidal artery 36246 (2nd order)

Middle colic artery 36246 (2nd order)

Right colic artery

Superior mesenteric artery 36245 (1st order)

Inferior mesenteric artery 36245 (1st order)

Left colic ascending (marginal) branches 36247 (3rd order)

Left colic artery 36246 (2nd order)

Left colic descending (marginal) branches 36247 (3rd order)

Sigmoid branches 36247 (3rd order)

Arcade branches 36247 (3rd order)

Hemorrhoidal branches 36247 (3rd order)

**Appendix P — Interventional Radiology Illustrations**

## Portal System

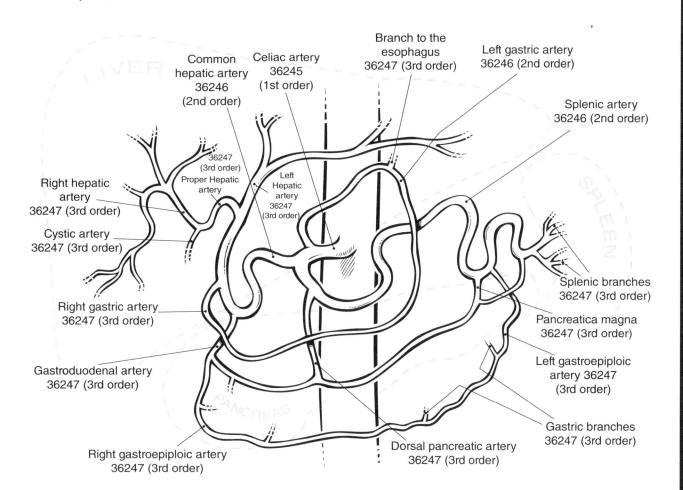

Common hepatic artery
36246
(2nd order)

Celiac artery
36245
(1st order)

Branch to the
esophagus
36247 (3rd order)

Left gastric artery
36246 (2nd order)

Splenic artery
36246 (2nd order)

36247
(3rd order)
Proper Hepatic
artery

Left
Hepatic
artery
36247
(3rd order)

Right hepatic
artery
36247 (3rd order)

Cystic artery
36247 (3rd order)

Splenic branches
36247 (3rd order)

Right gastric artery
36247 (3rd order)

Pancreatica magna
36247 (3rd order)

Left gastroepiploic
artery 36247
(3rd order)

Gastroduodenal artery
36247 (3rd order)

Gastric branches
36247 (3rd order)

Right gastroepiploic artery
36247 (3rd order)

Dorsal pancreatic artery
36247 (3rd order)

LIVER

SPLEEN

PANCREAS

Appendix P — Interventional Radiology Illustrations

## Renal Artery Anatomy—Femoral Approach

Right main renal artery
36245 (1st order)

Left main renal artery
36245 (1st order)

Left anterior
division
36245
(2nd order)

Right anterior
division
36246
(2nd order)

Left segmental
renal arteries
36247
(3rd order)

Right segmental
renal arteries
36247
(3rd order)

Right posterior
division
36246 (2nd order)

Left posterior
divison
36246 (2nd order)

Right accessory lower
pole renal artery
36245 (1st order)

Right accessory lower pole
renal artery arising from
common Iliac artery
36245 (1st order)

CPT © 2017 American Medical Association. All Rights Reserved.

# Upper Extremity Arterial Anatomy—Transfemoral or Contralateral Approach

Subclavian artery R. 36216 (2nd order)
L. 36215 (1st order)

Thoracoacromial artery

Axillary artery
(2nd order) R. 36216
L. 36215 (1st order)

Anterior humeral circumflex artery R. 36217
L. 36216 (2nd order)

Posterior circumflex
humeral artery
(3rd order) R. 36217
(2nd order) L. 36216

Deep brachial artery R. 36217 (3rd order or more)
L. 36217 (3rd order or more)

Brachial artery R. 36217, L. 36217 (3rd order or more)

Superior ulnar collateral artery R. 36217 (3rd order or more)
L. 36217 (3rd order or more)

Radial collateral artery R. 36217, L. 36217 (3rd order or more)

Inferior ulnar collateral artery R. 36217, L. 36217
(3rd order or more)

Recurrent interosseous
artery R. 36217
L. 36217
(3rd order or more)

Radial recurrent artery R. 36217, L. 36217 (3rd order or more)

Common interosseous artery R. 36217, L. 36217
(3rd order or more)

Anterior interosseous artery R. 36217, L. 36217
(3rd order or more)

Ulnar artery
R. 36217
L. 36217
(3rd order or more)

Radial artery R. 36217, L. 36217 (3rd order or more)

Posterior interosseous artery R. 36217, L. 36217
(3rd order or more)

Superficial palmar branch of radial artery
R. 36217, L. 36217 (3rd order or more)

Deep palmar arch R. 36217, L. 36217
(3rd order or more)

Digital
arteries

© 2017 Optum360, LLC          CPT © 2017 American Medical Association. All Rights Reserved.

# Lower Extremity Arterial Anatomy—Contralateral, Axillary or Brachial Approach

External iliac artery 36246 (2nd order)

Aorta 36200

Common iliac artery 36245 (1st order)

Internal iliac artery (aka hypogastric) 36246 (2nd order)

Common femoral artery 36246 (2nd order)

Profunda femoris 36247 artery (3rd order)

Perforating artery branches 36247 (3rd order)

Superficial femoral artery 36247 (3rd order)

Superior lateral genicular artery 36247 (3rd order)

Superior medial genicular artery 36247 (3rd order)

Popliteal artery 36247 (3rd order)

Inferior lateral genicular artery 36247 (3rd order)

Inferior medial genicular artery 36247 (3rd order)

Popliteal artery 36247 (3rd order)

Anterior tibial artery 36247 (3rd order)

Peroneal artery 36247 (3rd order)

Posterior tibial artery 36247 (3rd order)

Posterior tibial artery 36247 (3rd order)

Peroneal artery 36247 (3rd order)

Anterior tibial artery 36247 (3rd order)

Lateral anterior malleolar artery 36247 (3rd order)

Medial anterior malleolar artery 36247 (3rd order)

Posterior view of right leg

Pedis dorsalis artery 36247 (3rd order)

CPT © 2017 American Medical Association. All Rights Reserved.

© 2017 Optum360, LLC

# Portal System

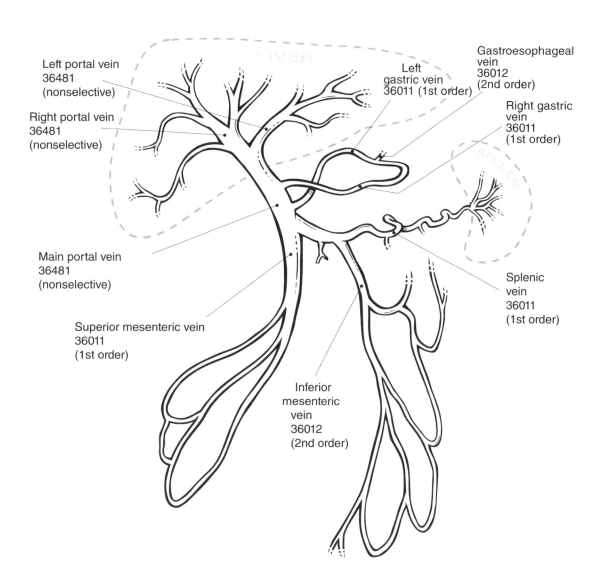

Left portal vein
36481
(nonselective)

Right portal vein
36481
(nonselective)

Main portal vein
36481
(nonselective)

Superior mesenteric vein
36011
(1st order)

Inferior
mesenteric
vein
36012
(2nd order)

Left
gastric vein
36011 (1st order)

Gastroesophageal
vein
36012
(2nd order)

Right gastric
vein
36011
(1st order)

Splenic
vein
36011
(1st order)

CPT © 2017 American Medical Association. All Rights Reserved.

## Coronary Arteries Anterior View

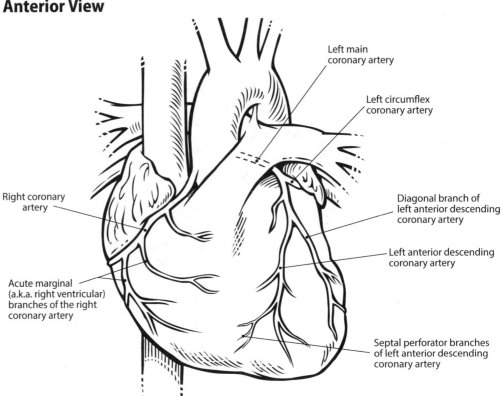

Left main coronary artery

Left circumflex coronary artery

Right coronary artery

Diagonal branch of left anterior descending coronary artery

Left anterior descending coronary artery

Acute marginal (a.k.a. right ventricular) branches of the right coronary artery

Septal perforator branches of left anterior descending coronary artery

## Left Heart Catheterization

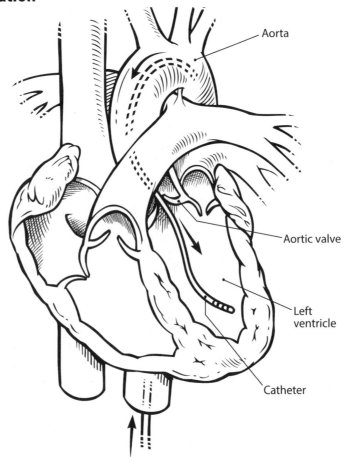

Aorta

Aortic valve

Left ventricle

Catheter

CPT © 2017 American Medical Association. All Rights Reserved.

© 2017 Optum360, LLC

# Heart Conduction System

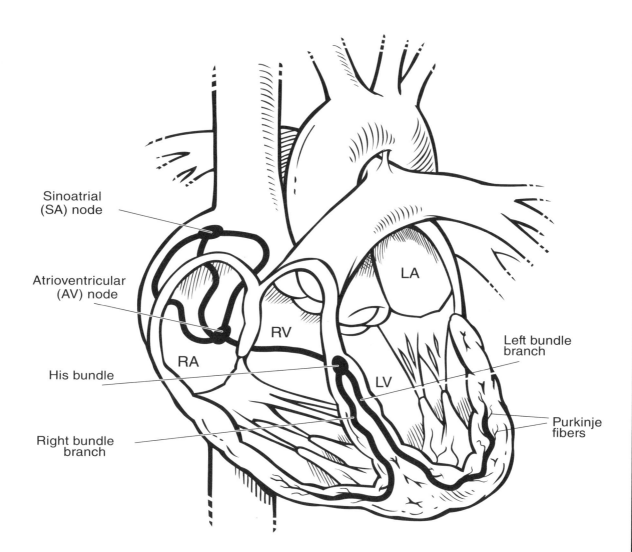

Sinoatrial
(SA) node

Atrioventricular
(AV) node

His bundle

Right bundle
branch

LA

RV

RA

LV

Left bundle
branch

Purkinje
fibers